Tropical Infectious Diseases

Tropical Infectious Diseases
Principles, Pathogens, & Practice

SECOND EDITION

Richard L. Guerrant, MD

Thomas H. Hunter Professor of International Medicine
Director, Center for Global Health
Division of Infectious Diseases and International Health
University of Virginia School of Medicine
Charlottesville, Virginia

David H. Walker, MD

Carmage and Martha Walls Distinguished Chair of Tropical Diseases
Professor and Chairman, Department of Pathology
Director, WHO Collaborating Center for Tropical Diseases
Executive Director
Center for Biodefense and Emerging Infectious Diseases
University of Texas Medical Branch
Galveston, Texas

Peter F. Weller, MD

Professor of Medicine
Harvard Medical School
Co-Chief, Infectious Disease Division
Vice Chair of Research
Department of Medicine
Beth Israel Deaconess Medical Center
Boston, Massachusetts

CHURCHILL LIVINGSTONE
ELSEVIER

ELSEVIER
CHURCHILL
LIVINGSTONE

1600 John F. Kennedy Boulevard
Suite 1800
Philadelphia, PA 19103-2899

TROPICAL INFECTIOUS DISEASES
Principles, Pathogens, & Practice
Second Edition

ISBN 13: 9780443066689
ISBN 10: 0-443-06668-X
Volume 1 Part Number: 9996003310
Volume 2 Part Number: 999600337X

Notice

Knowledge and best practice in this field are constantly changing. As new research and experience broaden our knowledge, changes in practice, treatment and drug therapy may become necessary or appropriate. Readers are advised to check the most current information provided (i) on procedures featured or (ii) by the manufacturer of each product to be administered, to verify the recommended dose or formula, the method and duration of administration, and contraindications. It is the responsibility of the practitioner, relying on his or her own experience and knowledge of the patient, to make diagnoses, to determine dosages and the best treatment for each individual patient, and to take all appropriate safety precautions. To the fullest extent of the law, neither the publisher nor the Editors assume any liability for any injury and/or damage to persons or property arising out or related to any use of the material contained in this book.

Previous edition copyrighted 1999.

ISBN 13: 9780443066689
ISBN 10: 0-443-06668-X

Acquisitions Editor: Tom Hartman
Developmental Editor: Ann Ruzycka Anderson
Project Manager: Cecelia Bayruns
Design Direction: Ellen Zanolle
Cover Designer: Andy Chapman
Marketing Manager: Megan Carr

Printed in the United States of America.

Last digit is the print number: 9 8 7 6 5 4 3 2 1

CONTRIBUTORS

Saad H. Abdalla, Mb,Bs (Khartoum); LRCP, MRCS, FRCPath
Senior Lecturer, Department of Haematology, Imperial College London; Honorary Consultant, Department of Haematology, St. Mary's Hospital, London, United Kingdom
Approach to the Patient in the Tropics with Anemia

Ban Mishu Allos, MD
Assistant Professor of Medicine and Preventive Medicine, Division of Infectious Diseases, Department of Medicine; Assistant Professor, Department of Preventive Medicine, Vanderbilt University School of Medicine, Nashville, TN
Campylobacter *Infections*

Jon Kim Andrus, MD
Chief, Immunization Unit, Family and Community Health, Pan American Health Organization, Washington, DC
Measles

Juanita Angel, MD, PhD
Associate Professor, Instituto de Genética Humana, Pontificia Universidad Javeriana, Bogotá, Columbia
Rotavirus Infections

Gregory M. Anstead, MD, PhD
Assistant Professor, Department of Medicine, University of Texas Health Science Center; Staff Physician, Department of Medicine, University Health System; Staff Physician, Department of Medicine, South Texas Veterans Healthcare System, San Antonio, TX
Histoplasmosis, Blastomycosis, Coccidioidomycosis, and Cryptococcosis; Paracoccidioidomycosis; Penicillioisis Marneffei

Eurico Arruda, MD, PhD
Professor of Microbiology, Department of Cell and Molecular Biology, University of Sao Paulo School of Medicine, Ribeirao Preto, Sao Paulo, Brazil
Respiratory Tract Viral Infections

Ray R. Arthur, PhD
Associate Director for Global Health, National Center for Infectious Diseases, National Centers for Disease Control and Prevention, Atlanta, GA
Surveillance for Emerging Infectious Diseases and Bioterrorism Threats

Paul S. Auerbach, MD, MS, FACEP
Clinical Professor of Surgery, Division of Emergency Medicine, Department of Surgery; Attending Physician, Emergency Medicine, Stanford University Medical Center, Stanford, CA
Animal Poisons in the Tropics; Travel-Related Health Concerns Associated with Extremes of Environment

Ronald C. Ballard, MIBiol, PhD
Chief, Laboratory Reference and Research Branch, Division of STD Prevention, Centers for Disease Control and Prevention, Atlanta, GA
Chlamydia trachomatis *Infections of the Gential Tract (Oculogenital Infections and Lymphogranuloma Venerum)*

Alan G. Barbour, MD
Professor of Medicine and Microbiology and Molecular Genetics, Department of Microbiology and Molecular Genetics and Medicine, University of California at Irvine, Irvine, CA
Relapsing Fever and Other Borrelia *Diseases*

Michele Barry, MD, FACP
Professor of Medicine and Global Health, Department of Medicine and Epidemiology and Public Health, Yale University; Firm Chief, Generalist Firm, Yale–New Haven Hospital, New Haven, CT
Ascariasis

Dan Bausch, MD, MPH&TM
Associate Professor, Department of Tropical Medicine, Tulane School of Public Health and Tropical Medicine; Associate Professor, Department of Medicine, Section of Infectious Diseases, Tulane University Medical Center, New Orleans, LA
Arenavirus Infections

John E. Bennett, MD, MACP
Head, Clinical Mycology Section, Laboratory of Clinical Investigation, National Institute of Allergy and Infectious Diseases; Clinical Center, National Institutes of Health, Bethesda, MD
Entomophthoramycosis, Lobomycosis, Rhinosporidiosis, and Sporotrichosis

Steven L. Berk, MD
Professor of Medicine/Family Medicine and Mirick-Myers Endowed Chair in Geriatric Medicine, Regional Dean, School of Medicine; Internal Medicine and Family Medicine, Texas Tech University Health Sciences Center, Amarillo, TX
Strongyloidiasis

Pascal O. Bessong, BSc (Hons), MSc, PhD
Lecturer, Department of Microbiology, University of Venda for Science and Technology, Thohoyandou, Limpopo Province, South Africa; Research Fellow, Center for Global Health and Myles H. Thaler Center for AIDS and Human Retrovirus Research, University of Virginia, Charlottesville, VA
Human Retroviral Infections in the Tropics

Frank J. Bia, MD, MPH, FACP
Professor of Medicine and Laboratory Medicine, Co-Director, International Health Program, Department of Medicine, Yale School of Medicine, New Haven, CT
Neurologic Disease

Robert E. Black, MD, MPH
Edgar Berman Professor and Chair, Department of International Health, Johns Hopkins University, Baltimore, MD
Nutrition and Miconutrients in Tropical Infectious Diseases

Martin J. Blaser, MD, MACP
Frederick H. King Professor and Chair, Department of Medicine, New York University School of Medicine; Director, Medical Service, Bellevue Hospital Center; Director, Medical Service, Tisch Hospital (NYU Medical Center); Staff Physician, Medical Service, New York Harbor Veterans Affairs Medical Center, New York, NY
Campylobacter *Infections*

Thomas P. Bleck, MD, FACP, FCCM, FCCP, FIDSA, FAAN
The Louise Nerancy Eminent Scholar in Neurology and Professor of Neurology, Neurological Surgery, and Internal Medicine; Director, Neuroscience Intensive Care Unit, Department of Neurology, University of Virginia, Charlottesville, VA
Tetanus; Rabies; Neurologic Disease

David A. Bobak, MD
Associate Professor of Medicine, Division of Infectious Diseases, Department of Medicine, Case Western Reserve University School of Medicine; Staff Physician and Director, Traveler's Healthcare Clinic, Department of Medicine, Case Medical Center/University Hospitals of Cleveland; Staff Physician, Department of Medicine, Louis B. Stokes VA Medical Center, Cleveland, OH
Enteric Clostridium *Infections; Travel-Related Health Concerns Associated with Extremes of Environment*

Luciana L. Borio, MD
Assistant Professor, Department of Medicine, University of Pittsburgh, Pittsburgh, PA; Assistant Professor, Department of Medicine, Johns Hopkins University; Center for Biosecurity of the University of Pittsburgh Medical Center, Baltimore, MD
Smallpox and Monkeypox

Michael D. Bowen, MSc, PhD
Microbiologist, Bioterrorism Rapid Response and Advanced Technology Laboratory, Bioterrorism Preparedness and Response Program, National Center for Infectious Diseases, Centers for Disease Control and Prevention, Atlanta, GA
Arenavirus Infections

Joseph S. Bresee, MD, FAAP
Assistant Professor, Department of Family and Preventive Medicine, Emory University School of Medicine; Lead, Epidemiology Team, Respiratory and Enteric Virus Branch, Division of Viral and Rickettsial Diseases, National Center for Infectious Diseases, Centers for Disease Control and Prevention, Atlanta, GA
Astrovirus, Enteric Adenovirus, and Other Gastroenteritis Viruses

Enrico Brunetti, MD
Assistant Professor, Division of Infectious and Tropical Diseases, Pavia University; Attending Physician, Division of Infectious and Tropical Diseases, IRCCS S. Matteo, Pavia, Italy
Echinococcosis

Fabrizio Bruschi, MD
Professor of Parasitology, Department of Experimental Pathology, MBIE, Università di Pisa, Pisa, Italy
Trichinellosis

Oluma Yoseph Bushen, MD
Fellow, Infectious Disease, Center for Global Health, Division of Infectious Diseases and International Health, University of Virginia, Charlottesville, VA
Cryptosporidiosis

Carlos C. Campbell, MD
Director, Arizona Area Health Education Center, Health Sciences Center, University of Arizona, Tucson, AZ
Malaria

Martin S. Cetron, MD
Director, Department of Global Migration and Quarantine, Centers for Disease Control and Prevention; Adjunct Associate Professor of Medicine, Division of Infectious Diseases, Department of Medicine, Emory University School of Medicine; Adjunct Assistant Professor of Epidemiology, Department of Epidemiology, Rollins School of Public Health, Emory University, Atlanta, GA
Migrant, Immigrant, and Refugee Health

Thomas Cherian, MB, BS, DCH, MD
Scientist, Initiative for Vaccine Research, World Health Organization, Geneva, Switzerland
Haemophilus influenzae *(Including* H. aegyptius*) Infection*

Otavio L. Cintra, MD
Department of Pediatrics, University of Sao Paulo School of Medicine at Ribeirao Preto, Ribeirao Preto, Sao Paulo, Brazil
Respiratory Tract Viral Infections

Richard F. Clark, MD, FACEP, FACMT
Professor, Department of Medicine, University of California at San Diego; Director, Division of Medical Toxicology, UCSD Medical Center; Medical Director, San Diego Division, California Poison Control System, San Diego, CA
Plant Toxins in the Tropics

Myron S. Cohen, MD
J. Herbert Bate Distinguished Professor of Medicine, Microbiology, Immunology and Public Health, Chief, Infectious Diseases, Director, Center for Infectious Diseases, Department of Medicine, University of North Carolina at Chapel Hill; UNC Health Care Systems, Chapel Hill, NC
Sexually Transmitted and Urinary Tract Infections

Robert Colebunders, MD, PhD
Professor of Tropical Diseases, Department of Clinical Sciences, Institute of Tropical Medicine; Professor of Infectious Diseases, Department of Medicine, University of Antwerp, Antwerp, Belgium
Approach to the Patient with HIV and Coinfecting Tropical Infectious Diseases

Ed Cooper, MD, FRCP, FAAP
Clinical Consultant, Partnership for Child Development, Department of Infectious Disease Epidemiology, Imperial College of Science, Technology and Medicine, London, United Kingdom
Trichuriasis

Christina M. Coyle, MD, MS
Associate Professor of Medicine, Department of Medicine, Albert Einstein College of Medicine; Director of Clinical Infectious Disease, Department of Medicine, Jacobi Hospital, Bronx, NY
Cysticercosis

D.W.T. Crompton, OBE, MA, ScD, FRSE
Professor, Institute of Biomedical and Life Sciences, University of Glasgow, Glasgow, Scotland, United Kingdom
Ascariasis

John H. Cross, PhD
Professor, Department of Preventive Medicine and Biometrics, Uniformed Services University of the Health Sciences, Bethesda, MD
Liver, Lung, and Intestinal Fluke Infections

Markus Czub, DVM, PhD
Adjunct Professor, Department of Medical Microbiology, University of Manitoba; Canadian Science Centre for Human and Animal Health, Winnipeg, Manitoba, Canada
Nipah and Hendra Viral Infections

Johanna P. Daily, MD
Harvard School of Public Health, Boston, MA
Hepatobiliary Disease

David Allan Brett Dance, HB, CLB, MSc, FRCPath
Consultant Microbiologist, Derriford Hospital; Regional Microbiologist (Southwest), Health Protection Agency, Plymouth, Devon, United Kingdom
Melioidosis

Mustapha A. Danesi, MB, FRCPI, FMCP, FWACP
Professor, Department of Medicine, College of Medicine, University of Lagos; Consultant Physician and Neurologist, Clinical Department of Medicine, Lagos University Teaching Hospital, Lagos, Lagos State, Nigeria
Neurologic Disease

Chandler R. Dawson, MD
Professor, F.I. Proctor Foundation, Professor, Department of Ophthalmology, University of California, San Francisco, San Francisco, CA
Trachoma

Catherine de Martel, MD, MS
Department of Health Research and Policy, Stanford University School of Medicine, Stanford, CA
Tropical Infectious Diseases and Malignancy

David T. Dennis, MD, MPH, DCMT
Faculty Affiliate, Department of Microbiology, Immunology, and Pathology, Colorado State University; Guest Researcher, Consultant, Division of Vector-Borne Infectious Diseases, Centers for Disease Control and Prevention, Fort Collins, CO
Plague

Ciro A. de Quadros, MD, MPH
Director, International Programs, Albert B. Sabin Vaccine Institute, Washington, DC
Measles

Rebecca Dillingham, MD
Fellow, Center for Global Health, Division of Infectious Disease and International Medicine, University of Virginia Health System, Charlottesville, VA
Social and Cultural Factors in Tropical Medicine: Reframing Our Understanding of Disease; Cyclospora, Isospora, *and* Sarcosystis *Infections*

John E. Donelson, PhD
Professor, Department of Biochemistry, University of Iowa, Iowa City, IA
African Trypanosomiasis (Sleeping Sickness)

J. Stephen Dumler, MD
Professor of Pathology, Division of Medical Microbiology, Department of Pathology, Professor, Cellular and Molecular Medicine Program, The Johns Hopkins University School of Medicine; Associate Director, Division of Medical Microbiology, Department of Pathology, The Johns Hopkins Hospital; Professor, Department of Molecular Microbiology and Immunology, The Johns Hopkins University Bloomberg School of Public Health, Baltimore, MD
Ehrlichioses and Anaplasmosis

Herbert L. DuPont, MD, FACP
Professor of Epidemiology, Department of Epidemiology, University of Texas, School of Public Health; Director, Center for Infectious Disease, University of Texas–Houston,

School of Public Health; Clinical Professor, Department of Medicine, Baylor College of Medicine; Chief, Internal Medicine, Department of Internal Medicine, St. Luke's Episcopal Hospital, Houston, TX
Gastrointestinal Symptoms

Marlene Durand, MD
Assistant Professor, Department of Medicine, Harvard Medical School; Associate Physician, Infectious Disease Unit, Department of Medicine, Massachusetts General Hospital; Director, Infectious Disease Service, Massachusetts Eye and Ear Infirmary, Boston, MA
Ocular Disease

Mark L. Eberhard, PhD
Director, Division of Parasitic Diseases, Centers for Disease Control, Atlanta, GA
Zoonotic Filariasis

Charles Edwards, MB, BS, FRCPC, FACP
Department Head, Department of Medicine, Queen Elizabeth Hospital, St. Michael, Barbados
Leptospirosis

Rachel Barwick Eidex, PhD
Epidemiologist, Division of Global Migration and Quarantine, Centers for Disease Control and Prevention, Atlanta, GA
Yellow Fever

Jerrold J. Ellner, MD, FACP
Professor and Chair, Department of Medicine, University of Medicine and Dentistry of New Jersey/New Jersey Medical School; Professor and Chair, Department of Medicine, University Hospitals, Newark, NJ
Tuberculosis and Atypical Myobacterial Infections

Delia A. Enria, MD, MPH
Director, Instituto Nacional de Enfermedades Virales Humanas, Pergamino, Argentina
Arenavirus Infections

Judith E. Epstein, MD
Assistant Professor, Department of Pediatrics, Uniformed Services University of the Health Sciences; Affiliate Staff, Pediatric Infectious Diseases, National Naval Medical Center, Bethesda, MD; Affiliate Staff, Pediatric Infectious Diseases, Walter Reed Army Medical Center; Director, Malaria Program Clinical Trials, Naval Medical Research Center, Silver Spring, MD
Typhoid Fever

Paul E. Farmer, MD, PhD
Presley Professor of Medical Anthropology, Department of Social Medicine, Harvard Medical School; Chief, Division of Social Medicine and Health Inequalities, Brigham and Women's Hospital; Founding Director, Partners in Health, Boston, MA
Social and Cultural Factors in Tropical Medicine: Reframing Our Understanding of Disease

Heinz Feldmann, MD
Associate Professor, Department of Medical Microbiology, University of Manitoba; Head, Special Pathogens Program, Public Health Agency of Canada, Winnipeg, Manitoba, Canada
Filovirus Infections

Ramon Flick, PhD
Assistant Professor, Center for Biodefense and Emerging Infectious Diseases and WHO Collaborating Center for Tropical Diseases, Department of Pathology, University of Texas Medical Branch, Galveston, TX
Nipah and Hendra Viral Infections; Arenavirus Infections; Bunyaviral Fevers: Rift Valley Fever and Crimean-Congo Hemorrhagic Fever

Kimberley K. Fox, MD, MPH
Adjunct Assistant Professor, Department of Medicine, Emory University, Atlanta, GA; Chief, Asia Regional Activities, Global AIDS Program, US Centers for Disease Control and Prevention, Bangkok, Thailand
Sexually Transmitted and Urinary Tract Infections

Manuel Franco, MD, PhD
Associate Professor, Instituto de Genética Humana, Pontificia Universidad Javeriana, Bogotá, Colombia
Rotavirus Infections

David O. Freedman, MD
Professor of Medicine and Public Health, Division of Geographic Medicine, University of Alabama at Birmingham; Director, UAB Travelers Health Clinic, UAB Health System; Director, Gorgas Course in Clinical Tropical Medicine in Lima, Peru, Gorgas Memorial Institute, Birmingham, AL
Onchocerciasis

Hector H. Garcia, MD, PhD
Associate Professor, Department of Microbiology, Universidad Peruana Cayetano Heredia; Head, Cysticercosis Unit, Instituto de Ciencias Neurologicas, Lima, Peru
Cysticercosis

Robert M. Genta, MD, DTM&H, FACG
Professor and Chair, Department of Pathology, University of Geneva School of Medicine, Geneva, Switzerland
Strongyloidiasis

Robert H. Gilman, MD, DTM&H
Professor, Department of International Health, Johns Hopkins University, Baltimore, MD
Helicobacter pylori *Infections*

Roger I. Glass, MD, PhD
Chief, Viral Gastroenteritis Section, Centers for Disease Control and Prevention, Atlanta, GA
Astrovirus, Enteric Adenovirus, and Other Gastroenteritis Viruses

Jerome Goddard, PhD
Assistant Professor of Medicine, Department of Medicine, The University of Mississippi Medical Center; State Medical Entomologist, General Environmental Services, Mississippi Department of Health, Jackson, MS
Arthropods, Tongue Worms, Leeches, and Arthropod-borne Diseases

Eduardo Gotuzzo, MD, FACP
Director, Instituto de Medicina Tropical "Alexander von Humboldt," Universidad Peruana Cayetano Heredia; Chief, Department of Infectious Diseases, Tropical Medicine and Dermatology, Hospital Nacional Cayetano Heredia, Lima, Peru
Cholera Infections; Brucellosis; Gastrointestinal Symptoms; Tropical Infectious Disease Concerns in Pregnancy

Bruno P. Granwehr, MD
Fellow, Division of Infectious Diseases, Department of Internal Medicine, University of Texas Medical Branch; Masters Student, Clinical Science Graduate Program, Department of Preventive Medicine and Community Health, Graduate School of Biomedical Sciences, University of Texas Medical Branch, Galveston, TX
Japanese Encephalitis and West Nile and Other Flavivirus Infections

John R. Graybill, MD
Professor and Chief, Division of Infectious Diseases, Department of Medicine, University of Texas Health Science Center at San Antonio, San Antonio, TX
Histoplasmosis, Blastomycosis, Coccidioidomycosis, and Cryptococcosis; Paracoccidioidomycosis; Penicillioisis Marneffei

Harry B. Greenberg, MD, FACP
Professor, Departments of Medicine, Microbiology and Immunology, Stanford University School of Medicine, Stanford, CA; Staff Physician, Department of Medicine, Division of Gastroenterology, Veterans Affairs Palo Alto Health Care System, Palo Alto, CA
Rotavirus Infections

Duane J. Gubler, MS, ScD
Director, Asia-Pacific Institute of Tropical Medicine and Infectious Diseases, Chair, Department of Tropical Medicine, Medical Microbiology and Pharmacology, John A. Burns School of Medicine, University of Hawaii, Honolulu, HI
Dengue and Dengue Hemorrhagic Fever

Richard L. Guerrant, MD, FACP
Thomas H. Hunter Professor of International Medicine, Director, Center for Global Health, University of Virginia; Division of Infectious Diseases and International Health, Department of Medicine, University of Virginia Hospital, Charlottesville, VA
Principles of Parasitism: Host–Parasite Interactions; Chemotherapy of Parasitic Diseases; Chemotherapy of Bacterial, Fungal, and Viral Diseases; Enteric Escherichia coli *Infections; Cryptosporidiosis*; Cyclospora, Isospora, *and* Sarcosystis *Infections*

Yezid Gutierrez, MD, MPH&TM, PhD
Adjunct Staff, Department of Laboratory Medicine, The Cleveland Clinic Educational Foundation, Cleveland, OH
Other Tissue Nematode Infections

Frederick G. Hayden, MD
Professor of Internal Medicine and Pathology, Department of Internal Medicine, University of Virginia School of Medicine; Physician, Department of Internal Medicine/Infectious Diseases, University of Virginia Health System, Charlottesville, VA
Respiratory Tract Viral Infections

Donald A. Henderson, MD, MPH
Professor of Medicine and Public Health, Department of Internal Medicine, University of Pittsburgh; Resident Scholar, University of Pittsburgh Medical Center, Center for Biosecurity, Baltimore, MD
Disease Eradication and Control; Smallpox and Monkeypox

Bradley S. Hersh, MD, MPH
Medical Officer, Department of Immunization, Vaccines and Biologicals, World Health Organization, Geneva, Switzerland
Measles

Barbara L. Herwaldt, MD, MPH
Medical Epidemiologist, Division of Parasitic Diseases, Centers for Disease Control and Prevention, Atlanta, GA
Cyclospora, Isospora, *and* Sarcosystis *Infections*

Erik L. Hewlett, MD
Professor, Department of Medicine and Pharmacology, University of Virginia School of Medicine; Attending Physician, Department of Internal Medicine, University of Virginia Hospital, Charlottesville, VA
Pertussis

David R. Hill, MD, DTM&H
Honorary Professor, Department of Infectious and Tropical Diseases, London School of Hygiene and Tropical Medicine; Director, National Travel Health Network and Centre, London, United Kingdom
Intestinal Flagellate and Ciliate Infections

Paul Hoffman, PhD
Associate Professor, Division of Infectious Diseases and International Health, Department of Internal Medicine, University of Virginia Health System, Charlottesville, VA
Legionellosis

Stephen L. Hoffman, MD, DTMH
Chief Executive Officer, Sanaria Inc., Rockville, MD; Adjunct Professor, Department of Preventive Medicine and Biometrics, Uniformed Services University of the Health Sciences, Bethesda, MD
Typhoid Fever; Malaria

Edward W. Hook, III, MD, FACP
Professor of Medicine, Epidemiology, and Microbiology, University of Alabama at Birmingham; Medical Director, STD Control Program, Jefferson County Department of Health, Birmingham, AL
Treponemal Infections

Donald R. Hopkins, MD, MPH
Associate Executive Director, The Carter Center, Atlanta, GA
Dracunculiasis

Duane R. Hospenthal, MD, PhD, FACP, FIDSA, Lt. Col., US Army
Associate Professor of Medicine, Department of Medicine, F. Edward Hébert School of Medicine, Uniformed Services University of the Health Sciences, Bethesda, MD; Chief, Infectious Disease Service, Department of Medicine, Brooke Army Medical Center, Fort Sam Houston, TX; Clinical Associate Professor, Department of Medicine, University of Texas Health Sciences Center at San Antonio, San Antonio, TX
Entomophthoramycosis, Lobomycosis, Rhinosporidiosis, and Sporotrichosis

Peter J. Hotez, MD, PhD
Professor and Chair, Department of Microbiology and Tropical Medicine, The George Washington University, Washington, DC
Hookworm Infections

S. David Hudnall, MD
Professor, Department of Pathology and Laboratory Medicine, The University of Texas Medical Branch, Galveston, TX
Human Herpesvirus Infections

James M. Hughes, MD, FACP
Director, Program in Global Infectious Diseases; Associate Director, Southeastern Center for Emerging Biologic Threats, Emory University School of Medicine; Director, Center for Global Safe Water, Rollins School of Public Health, Atlanta, GA
Surveillance for Emerging Infectious Diseases and Bioterrorism Threats

Raul E. Isturiz, MD, FACP
Chief, Infectious Diseases Section, Centro Medico de Caracas; Chief, Infectious Diseases Section, Centro Medico Docente la Tunidad, Caracas, Venezuela
Tropical Infectious Disease Concerns in Pregnancy

Hamid Jafari, MBBS
Director, Global Immunization Division, National Immunization Program, Centers for Disease Control and Prevention, Atlanta, GA
Enterovirus Infections, Including Poliomyelitis

Maria C. Jaimes, MD
Postdoctoral Fellow, Departments of Medicine, Microbiology and Immunology, Stanford University School of Medicine, Stanford, CA
Rotavirus Infections

Selma M.B. Jeronimo, MD, PhD
Department of Biochemistry, Bioscience Center, Universidade Federal do Rio Grande do Norte, Natal, RN, Brazil
Leishmaniasis

John L. Johnson, MD, FACP
Associate Professor of Medicine and International Health, Division of Infectious Diseases, Department of Medicine, Case Western Reserve University School of Medicine; Staff Physician, Division of Pulmonary and Critical Care Medicine, University Hospitals of Cleveland, Cleveland, OH
Tuberculosis and Atypical Myobacterial Infections

Christopher L. Karp, MD
Boomer Esiason Professor of Pediatrics, Director, Division of Molecular Immunology, Cincinnati Children's Hospital Medical Center, Cincinnati, OH
Approach to the Patient with HIV and Coinfecting Tropical Infectious Diseases

James W. Kazura, MD
Professor, Center for Global Health and Diseases, Case School of Medicine, Case Western Reserve University; Professor, Department of Medicine, University Hospitals of Cleveland, Cleveland, OH
Filariasis

Peter Kern, MD, DTM&H (Hamburg)
Professor of Medicine and Infectious Diseases, Division of Infectious Diseases and Clinical Immunology, University Hospital and Medical Center, Ulm, Germany
Echinococcosis

Gerald T. Keusch, MD
Assistant Provost and Associate Dean for Global Health, Boston University Medical Campus and School of Public Health, Boston, MA
Nutrition and Miconutrients in Tropical Infectious Diseases; Shigellosis

Jay S. Keystone, MD, MSc(CTM), FRCPC
Professor, Department of Medicine, University of Toronto; Staff Physician, Tropical Disease Unit, Toronto General Hospital, Toronto, Ontario, Canada
Health Advice for International Travel; Delusional Parasitosis

Charles H. King, MD, MS, FACP
Associate Professor of International Health, Center for Global Health and Diseases, Case Western Reserve University; Attending Physician, Department of Medicine, University Hospitals of Cleveland, Cleveland, OH
Schistosomiasis

Louis V. Kirchhoff, MD, MPH
Professor, Department of Internal Medicine (Infectious Diseases) and Epidemiology, University of Iowa; Staff Physician, Medical Service, Department of Veterans Affairs Medical Center, Iowa City, IA
American Trypanosomiasis (Chagas' Disease)

Amy D. Klion, MD
Staff Clinician, Laboratory of Parasitic Diseases, National Institute of Allergy and Infectious Disease, National Institutes of Health, Bethesda, MD
Loiasis and Mansonella *Infection*

Keith P. Klugman, MD, PhD
Professor, Department of International Health, Rollins School of Public Health, Professor, Division of Infectious Diseases, School of Medicine, Emory University, Atlanta, GA; Director, Respiratory and Meningeal Pathogens Research Unit, University of the Witwatersrand, Medical Research Council, National Institute for Communicable Diseases, Johannesburg, South Africa
Pneumococcal Infections

Dennis J. Kopecko, PhD
Chief, Laboratory of Enteric and Sexually Transmitted Diseases, Food and Drug Administration, Center for Biologics Evaluation and Research, Bethesda, MD
Shigellosis

Margaret Kosek, MD
Assistant Scientist, Department of International Health, Johns Hopkins Bloomberg School of Public Health, Baltimore, MD
Nutrition and Miconutrients in Tropical Infectious Diseases

Phyllis E. Kozarsky, MD
Professor of Medicine, Department of Medicine/Infectious Diseases; Chief, Geographic Medicine and Travelers' Health Section, Department of Medicine, Emory Unversity School of Medicine, Atlanta, GA
Health Advice for International Travel

Tim Kuberski, MD
Consultant in Infectious Diseases and Tropical Medicine, Private Practice, Glendale, AZ
Angiostrongyliasis

James L. Larson, Jr., MD, FACEP
Assistant Professor, Department of Emergency Medicine, University of North Carolina, Chapel Hill, Chapel Hill, NC
Plant Toxins in the Tropics

James W. Leduc, PhD
Director, Division of Viral and Rickettsial Diseases, National Center for Infectious Diseases, National Centers for Disease Control and Prevention, Atlanta, GA
Surveillance for Emerging Infectious Diseases and Bioterrorism Threats

Stanley M. Lemon, MD
John Sealy Distinguished University Chair and Director, Institute for Human Infections and Immunity, University of Texas Medical Branch at Galveston, Galveston, TX
Viral Hepatitis

Peter Leone, MD
Associate Professor of Medicine, Department of Medicine/Infectious Diseases, University of North Carolina; Medical Director, HIV/STD Prevention and Care Branch, North Carolina Department of Health and Human Services, Chapel Hill, NC
Gonococcal and Other Neisserial Infections

Paul N. Levett, PhD, ABMM, FCCM
Assistant Clinical Director, Provincial Laboratory, Saskatchewan Health, Regina, Saskatchewan, Canada
Leptospirosis

Michael Levin, PhD, FRCP, FRCPCH, F MED SCi
Professor, Department of Paediatrics, Imperial College London; Consultant in Paediatric Infectious Diseases, Department of Paediatrics, St. Mary's Hospital NHS Trust, Paddington, London, United Kingdom
Host Genetics and Susceptibility to Infection

Myron M. Levine, MD, DTPH, FAAP, FACPM
Professor, Departments of Medicine and Pediatrics, Director, Center for Vaccine Development, University of Maryland School of Medicine, Baltimore, MD
Cholera Infections

Aldo A. M. Lima, MD, PhD
Professor, Clinical Research Unit and Institute of Biomedicine/Center for Global Health, Faculty of Medicine; University Hospital, Clinical Research Unit and Institute of Biomedicine, Faculty of Medicine; Pharmacology, Department of Physiology and Pharmacology, Federal University of Ceará, Fortaleza, Ceará, Brasil
Cryptosporidiosis

David L. Longworth, MD
Deputy Chairman, Department of Medicine, Tufts University School of Medicine, Boston, MA; Chairman, Department of Medicine, Baystate Medical Center, Springfield, MA
Cutaneous Lesions

J. Dick MacLean, MD, FRCPC, MRCP(UK), DCMT(Lond)
Professor of Medicine, Director, Department of Medicine, McGill Centre for Tropical Diseases, McGill University; Senior Physician, Department of Medicine, Division of Tropical Diseases, Montreal General Hospital, Montreal, Quebec, Canada
Liver, Lung, and Intestinal Fluke Infections

Alan J. Magill, MD, FACP (COL, MCUSA)
Associate Professor, Department of Preventive Medicine and Biometrics, Uniformed Services University of the Health Sciences, Bethesda, MD; Attending Physician, Infectious Disease Service, Walter Reed Army Medical Center, Washington, DC; Science Director, Walter Reed Army Institute of Research, Silver Spring, MD
Infectious Diseases in Modern Military Forces

Ciro Maguiña, MD
Director, Adjunto del IMT-AVH-UPCH, Departamento de Medicina, Universidad Peruana Cayetano Heredia; Medico Infectologo Tropicalista, Departamento de Medicina Tropical, Hospital Nacional Cayetano Heredia, Lima, Peru
Bartonelloses

James H. Maguire, MD, MPH
Professor and Head, International Health Division, University of Maryland School of Medicine, Baltimore, MD
Babesiosis; Pathogenic and Opportunistic Free-Living Amebas: Acanthamoeba *spp.,* Balamuthia mandrillaris, Naegleria fowleri, *and* Sappina diploidia; *Systemic Coccidia (Toxoplasmosis); Hepatobiliary Disease*

Siddhartha Mahanty, MBBS, MPH
Staff Physician, Malaria Vaccine Development Branch, National Institute of Allergy and Infectious Diseases, National Institutes of Health, Rockville, MD
Liver, Lung, and Intestinal Fluke Infections

El-Sheikh Mahgoub, MD, PhD, FRCPath
Professor of Microbiology, Department of Medical Microbiology and Parasitology, Faculty of Medicine, University of Khartoum; Professor of Medical Education and Research, Sudan Medical Specialisation Board, Khartoum, Sudan
Mycetoma

Susan A. Maloney, MD, MHSc, FAAP
Acting Chief, Immigrant, Refugee, and Migrant Health Branch, Division of Global Migration and Quarantine, Centers for Disease Control and Prevention, Atlanta, GA
Migrant, Immigrant, and Refugee Health

Anthony A. Marfin, MD, MPH, MA
Quarantine Medical Officer, San Francisco Quarantine Station, Division of Global Migration and Quarantine, Centers for Disease Control and Prevention, San Francisco, CA
Yellow Fever

Thomas J. Marrie, MD
Dean of Faculty of Medicine and Dentistry, University of Alberta; University of Alberta Hospital, Edmonton, Alberta, Canada
Legionellosis; Psittacosis; Q Fever

Barry J. Marshall, FRACP, FRS, FAA
NHMRC Senior Principal Research Fellow, Department of Microbiology, University of Western Australia; Consultant Gastroenterologist, Department of Gastroenterology, Sir Charles Gairdner Hospital, Perth, Western Australia, Australia
Helicobacter pylori *Infections*

Gregory J. Martin, MD, FACP, Captain, Medical Corps, US Navy
Associate Professor of Medicine, Department of Internal Medicine, Uniformed Services University, Bethesda, MD; Officer in Charge, US Naval Medical Research Center Detachment, Lima, Lima, Peru
Approach to the Patient in the Tropics with Pulmonary Disease

Tadahiko Matsumoto, MD, DMSc
Clinical Professor, Department of Dermatology, Juntendo University School of Medicine; Clinical Professor, Department of Dermatology, Keio University School of Medicine; Director, Department of Dermatology, Toshiba Hospital, Tokyo, Japan; Clinical Professor, Department of Dermatology, Kurume University School of Medicine, Kurume, Japan; Adjunct Professor, Department of Pathology, Kitasato University School of Medicine, Sagamihara, Japan
Chromoblastomycosis and Phaeohyphomycosis

Steven D. Mawhorter, MD, DTMH
Staff Physician, Department of Infectious Diseases, Cleveland Clinic Foundation, Cleveland, OH; Clinical Assistant Professor, Pennsylvania State University School of Medicine, Hershey, PA
Cutaneous Lesions

James S. McCarthy, MD, FRACP, DH&TM
Associate Professor of Tropical Medicine and Infectious Diseases, School of Population Health, University of Queensland; Staff Specialist, Department of Infectious Diseases, Royal Brisbane and Women's Hospital; Senior Research Fellow, Infectious Diseases and Immunology, Queensland Institute for Medical Research, Herston, Australia
Toxocariasis and Larva Migrans Syndromes; Enterobiasis

Michael R. McGinnis, PhD
Professor, Department of Pathology, University of Texas Medical Branch, Galveston, TX
Dermatophytosis

Paul S. Mead, MD, MPH
Chief, Epidemiology, Molecular Biology and Diagnostic Activity, Bacterial Zoonoses Branch, Division of Vector-Borne Infectious Diseases, National Center for Infectious Diseases, Centers for Disease Control and Prevention, Fort Collins, CO
Plague

Wayne M. Meyers, MD, PhD, DSc (Hon)
Chief, Mycobacteriology, Department of Infectious and Parasitic Disease Pathology, Armed Forces Institute of Pathology, Washington, DC; Research Affiliate, Tulane Regional Primate Research Center, Tulane University, New Orleans, LA
Mycobacterium ulcerans *Infection (Buruli Ulcer); Leprosy*

Samuel I. Miller, MD
Professor, Department of Medicine, Microbiology, and Genome Sciences; Professor, Department of Medicine, University of Washington, Seattle, WA
Nontyphoidal Salmonellosis

James N. Mills, PhD
Chief, Medical Ecology Unit, Division of Viral and Rickettsial Diseases, National Center for Infectious Diseases, Centers for Disease Control and Prevention, Atlanta, GA
Arenavirus Infections; Hantavirus Infections

Michael Minnick, PhD
Professor of Microbiology, Assistant Dean, Division of Biological Sciences, The University of Montana, Missoula, MT
Bartonelloses

Thomas P. Monath, MD, FACP
Chief Scientific Officer, Acambis Inc., Cambridge, MA; Adjunct Professor, Department of Molecular Biology and Immunology, Harvard School of Public Health, Boston, MA
Yellow Fever

Stephan S. Monroe, PhD
Division of Viral and Rickettsial Diseases, National Center for Infectious Diseases, Centers for Disease Control and Prevention, Atlanta, GA
Calicivirus Infections

Thomas A. Moore, MD, FACP
Clinical Associate Professor, Department of Internal Medicine, University of Kansas School of Medicine–Wichita, Wichita, KS
Toxocariasis and Larva Migrans Syndromes; Enterobiasis

Jonathan P. Moorman, MD, PhD
Associate Professor, Department of Internal Medicine, James H. Quillen College of Medicine, East Tennessee State University, Johnson City, TN; Section Chief, Department of Infectious Diseases, James H. Quillen VA Medical Center, Mountain Home, TN
Enteric Clostridium *Infections*

J. Glenn Morris, Jr., MD, MPH&TM
Professor and Chairman, Department of Epidemiology and Preventive Medicine, Professor of Medicine (Infectious Diseases), Professor of Microbiology and Immunology, University of Maryland School of Medicine, Baltimore, MD
"Noncholera" Vibrio *Infections*

Megan Murray, MD, ScD
Assistant Professor, Department of Epidemiology, Harvard School of Public Health; Instructor, Infectious Disease Unit, Massachusetts General Hospital; Instructor, Division of Social Medicine and Health Inequalities, Brigham and Women's Hospital, Boston, MA; Associate Member, Broad Institute, Cambridge, MA
Epidemiology and Biostatistics

K. Darwin Murrell, PhD
Senior Scientist, Centre for Experimental Parasitology, Royal Veterinary and Agricultural University, Copenhagen, Denmark; Adjunct Professor, Department of Preventive Medicine and Biostatistics, Uniformed Services University of the Health Sciences, Bethesda, MD
Trichinellosis

G. Balakrish Nair, PhD, FNA, FNASc
Director, Laboratory Sciences Division, International Centre for Diarrhoeal Diseases Research, Bangladesh, Mohakhali, Dhaka, Bangladesh
"Noncholera" Vibrio *Infections*

Theodore E. Nash, MD
Head, Gastrointestinal Parasites Section, Laboratory of Parasitic Diseases, National Institutes of Allergy and Infectious Diseases, National Institutes of Health, Bethesda, MD
Intestinal Flagellate and Ciliate Infections

Barnett R. Nathan, MD
Assistant Professor, Department of Neurology, University of Virginia, Charlottesville, VA
Tetanus

Anne Nicholson-Weller, MD
Professor of Medicine, Harvard Medical School; Physician in Medicine, Divisions of Infectious Disease and Allergy and Inflammation, Department of Medicine, Beth Israel Deaconess Medical Center, Boston, MA
Immunology, Host Defense, Immunodeficiencies, and Vaccines

Robert L. Norris, MD, FACEP
Associate Professor, Department of Surgery, Stanford University Medical Center; Chief, Department of Emergency Medicine, Stanford Hospital and Clinics, Stanford, CA
Animal Poisons in the Tropics

Thomas B. Nutman, MD
Head, Helminth Immunology Section and Head, Clinical Parasitology Unit, Laboratory of Parasitic Diseases, National Institutes of Health, Bethesda, MD
Filariasis; Loiasis and Mansonella *Infection*

Nigel O'Farrell, MSc, MD, MRCP
Pasteur Suite, Ealing Hospital, London, United Kingdom
Calymmatobacterium granulomatis *Infection (Donovanosis)*

Michael E. Ohl, MD
Research Fellow, Division of Infectious Diseases, Department of Internal Medicine, University of Missouri, Columbia, MO; Research Fellow, Department of Medicine, University of Missouri Medical Center, Seattle, WA
Nontyphoidal Salmonellosis

Juan P. Olano, MD
Associate Professor, Director, Residency Training Program, Department of Pathology, University of Texas Medical Branch, Galveston, TX
Principles of Parasitism: Host–Parasite Interactions; Distinguishing Tropical Infectious Diseases from Bioterrorism

Luis S. Ortega, MD, MPH
Medical Epidemiologist, Division of Global Migration and Quarantine, Centers for Disease Control and Prevention, Atlanta, GA
Migrant, Immigrant, and Refugee Health

Mark A. Pallansch, PhD
Distinguished Consultant, Respiratory and Enteric Viruses Branch, Division of Viral and Rickettsial Diseases, Centers for Disease Control and Prevention, Atlanta, GA
Enterovirus Infections, Including Poliomyelitis

Jean W. Pape, MD
Professor, Department of Medicine, Weill Medical College of Cornell University, New York, NY; Director, GHESKIO Centres, Port-au-Prince, Haiti
Cyclospora, Isospora, *and* Sarcosystis *Infections*

John R. Papp, PhD
Laboratory Reference and Research Branch, Division of STD Prevention, Centers for Disease Control and Prevention, Atlanta, GA
Chlamydia trachomatis *Infections of the Gential Tract (Ocuolgenital Infections and Lymphogranuloma Venerum)*

Julie Parsonnet, MD
Associate Professor, Department of Medicine, and Health Research and Policy, Stanford University School of Medicine, Stanford, CA
Tropical Infectious Diseases and Malignancy

Geoffrey Pasvol, MA, MB ChB, DPhil, FRCP, FRCPE
Professor, Department of Infection and Tropical Medicine, Director, Wellcome Centre for Clinical Tropical Medicine, Imperial College London; Professor, Infection and Tropical Medicine, Northwick Park Hospital, London, United Kingdom
Host Genetics and Susceptibility to Infection; Approach to the Patient in the Tropics with Anemia

Richard D. Pearson, MD, FACP
Professor of Medicine and Pathology, Senior Associate Dean for Medical Education, Departments of Medicine and Pathology, University of Virginia School of Medicine; Professor of Medicine and Pathology, Department of Internal Medicine, University of Virginia Health System, Charlottesville, VA
Chemotherapy of Parasitic Diseases; Chemotherapy of Bacterial, Fungal, and Viral Diseases; Leishmaniasis; Fever and Systemic Symptoms

David A. Pegues, MD
Professor of Clinical Medicine, Division of Infectious Diseases, David Geffen School of Medicine at UCLA; Hospital Epidemiologist, UCLA Healthcare, Los Angeles, CA
Nontyphoidal Salmonellosis

Jacques Pépin, MD, MSc, FRCPC
Professor, Microbiology and Infectious Diseases, Director, Center for International Health, University of Sherbrooke, Sherbrooke, Quebec, Canada
African Trypanosomiasis (Sleeping Sickness)

C. J. Peters, MD
Professor of Pathology and Microbiology, Center for Biodefense and Emerging Infectious Diseases and WHO Collaborating Center for Tropical Diseases, University of Texas Medical Branch, Galveston, TX
Overview of Viral Hemorrhagic Fevers; Arenavirus Infections; Bunyaviral Fevers: Rift Valley Fever and Crimean-Congo Hemorrhagic Fever; Hantavirus Infections; Filovirus Infections; Distinguishing Tropical Infectious Diseases from Bioterrorism

William A. Petri, Jr., MD, PhD, FACP
Wade Hampton Frost Professor of Epidemiology, Professor of Medicine, Microbiology and Pathology, Chief, Division of Infectious Diseases and International Health, Department of Internal Medicine, University of Virginia School of Medicine; Attending Physician, University of Virginia Hospitals, Charlottesville, VA
Enteric Amebiasis

Françoise Portaels, PhD
Professor and Head, Mycobacteriology Unit, Department of Microbiology, Institute of Tropical Medicine, Antwerp, Belgium
Mycobacterium ulcerans *Infection (Buruli Ulcer)*

Thomas C. Quinn, MD, FACP
Professor, Department of Medicine, The Johns Hopkins University, Baltimore, MD; Senior Investigator and Head, International HIV/STD Research Laboratory, Laboratory of Immunoregulation, National Institute of Allergy and Infectious Diseases, National Institutes of Health, Bethesda, MD
Human Retroviral Infections in the Tropics

Didier Raoult, MD, PhD
Professor and Director, Unité des rickettsies, Faculté de Médecine, Marseille, France
Typhus Group Rickettsioses

Steven J. Reynolds, MD, MPH, DTM&H, FRCPC
Assistant Professor, Division of Infectious Diseases, Johns Hopkins School of Medicine; Staff Clinician, National Institute of Allergy and Infectious Diseases, National Institutes of Health, Bethesda, MD;

Scientific Director, NIAID/NIH International Center of Excellence in Research Program, Uganda
Human Retroviral Infections in the Tropics

José M. C. Ribeiro, MD, PhD
Senior Scientist and Section Head, Laboratory of Malaria and Vector Research, National Institute of Allergy and Infectious Diseases, Bethesda, MD
Vector Biology

Pierre E. Rollin, MD
Special Pathogens Branch, Centers for Disease Control and Prevention, Atlanta, GA
Hantavirus Infections; Filovirus Infections

Allan Ronald, MD, MACP
Professor Emeritus, Department of Medicine and Community Health Sciences, University of Manitoba, Winnipeg, Manitoba, Canada
Haemophilus ducreyi *Infections; Sexually Transmitted and Urinary Tract Infections*

Jason Rosé, PhD
Chair, Science Department, Kings Academy High School, Sunnyvale, CA
Rotavirus Infections

Ernesto Ruiz-Tiben, BS, MS, PhD
Technical Director, Dracunculiasis Eradication, The Carter Center, Atlanta, GA
Dracunculiasis

Edward T. Ryan, MD, DTM&H, FACP
Assistant Professor, Department of Medicine, Harvard Medical School; Director, Tropical and Geographic Medicine Center, Division of Infectious Diseases, Massachusetts General Hospital; Assistant Professor, Immunology and Infectious Diseases, Harvard School of Public Health, Boston, MA
Epidemiology and Biostatistics; Ocular Disease

Anthony Sanchez, PhD
Public Health Service Officer, Special Pathogens Branch, Division of Viral and Rickettsial Diseases, Centers for Disease Control and Prevention, Atlanta, GA
Filovirus Infections

Julius Schachter, PhD
Professor of Laboratory Medicine, Department of Laboratory Medicine, University of California, San Francisco, San Francisco, CA
Trachoma

Peter M. Schantz, VMD, PhD
Epidemiologist, Division of Parasitic Diseases, National Center for Infectious Diseases, Centers for Disease Control and Prevention, Atlanta, GA
Echinococcosis

W. Michael Scheld, MD, FACP
Bayer-Gerald L. Mandell Professor of Infectious Diseases, Professor of Internal Medicine, Clinical Professor of Neurosurgery, Director, Pfizer Initiative in International Health, Department of Infectious Diseases and International Health, University of Virginia, Charlottesville, VA
Meningococcal Infections

Eugene R. Schiff, MD, MACP, FRCP, MACG
Professor and Chief, Division of Hepatology, Director, Center for Liver Disease, University of Miami School of Medicine; Jackson Memorial Hospital; Consultant, The Veterans Administration; Cedars Medical Center, Miami, FL
Viral Hepatitis

David A. Schwartz, MD, MS Hyg, FCAP
Visiting Professor, Department of Pathology, Vanderbilt University, Nashville, TN; Guest Scientist, Centers for Disease Control and Prevention, Atlanta, GA
Microsporidiosis

Joseph D. Schwartzman, MD, FAAM
Professor of Pathology, Department of Pathology, Dartmouth Medical School, Hanover, NH; Medical Director of Microbiology and Serology, Department of Pathology, Dartmouth-Hitchcock Medical Center, Lebanon, NH
Systemic Coccidia (Toxoplasmosis)

Elyse G. Seltzer, MD
Senior Director, Clinical Research and Medical Affairs, Vicuron Pharmaceuticals, Inc., King of Prussia, PA
Ascariasis

Arlene C. Seña, MD, MPH
Assistant Professor of Medicine, Department of Medicine, University of North Carolina at Chapel Hill; UNC Health Care Systems, Chapel Hill, NC; Medical Director, Durham County Health Department, Durham, NC
Sexually Transmitted and Urinary Tract Infections

Daniel J. Sexton, MD, FACP
Professor, Department of Medicine, Division of Infectious Diseases, Duke University Medical School; Director, Infection Control Unit, Duke University Medical Center, Durham, NC
Spotted Fever Group Rickettsioses

Trueman W. Sharp, MD, MPH (Capt, MCUSN)
Commanding Officer, US Naval Medical Medical Research Unit No. 3, Cairo, Egypt
Infectious Diseases in Modern Military Forces

Wun-Ju Shieh, MD, MPH, PhD
Medical Officer, Infectious Disease Pathology Activity, Centers for Disease Control and Prevention, Atlanta, GA
Leptospirosis; Arenavirus Infections

Shmuel Shoham, MD
Special Volunteer, Pediatric Oncology Branch of the National Cancer Institute, National Institutes of Health; Assistant Professor, Department of Medicine, Uniformed Services University of the Health Sciences, Bethesda, MD; Attending Physician, Department of Medicine, Washington Hospital Center, Washington, DC
Mucocutaneous and Deeply Invasive Candidiasis

Robert E. Shope, MD (*Deceased*)
Professor of Pathology, Center for Biodefense and Emerging Infectious Diseases and WHO Collaborating Center for Tropical Diseases, Department of Pathology, University of Texas Medical Branch, Galveston, TX
Factors Influencing Geographic Distribution and Incidence of Tropical Infectious Diseases; Bunyaviral Fevers: Rift Valley Fever and Crimean-Congo Hemorrhagic Fever; Japanese Encephalitis and West Nile and Other Flavivirus Infections; Alphavirus Infections

H. H. Shugart, PhD
W.W. Corcoran Professor, Department of Environmental Sciences and Department of Biology, University of Virginia, Charlottesville, VA
Factors Influencing Geographic Distribution and Incidence of Tropical Infectious Diseases

Afzal A. Siddiqui, MPhil, PhD
Associate Professor of Medicine, Department of Internal Medicine, Texas Tech University Health Sciences Center; Health Research Scientist, Thomas E. Creek Veterans Affairs Medical Center, Amarillo, TX
Strongyloidiasis

Upinder Singh, MD
Assistant Professor, Department of Internal Medicine, Stanford University, Stanford, CA
Enteric Amebiasis

Michael B. Smith, MD, MS
Director, Division of Clinical Microbiology, Department of Pathology, University of Texas Medical Branch, Galveston, TX
Dermatophytosis

Bonnie L. Smoak, MD, PhD, MPH (Col, MCUSA)
Associate Professor, Department of Preventive Medicine and Biometrics, Uniformed Services University of the Health Sciences, Bethesda, MD; Director, Division of Preventive Medicine, Walter Reed Army Institute of Research, Silver Spring, MD
Infectious Diseases in Modern Military Forces

Tom Solomon, BA, BM, MRCP, DCH, DTMH, PhD
Senior Lecturer in Neurology, Department of Neurological Science, Senior Lecturer in Medical Microbiology and Tropical Medicine, Department of Medical Microbiology and Genitourinary Medicine, University of Liverpool; Honorary Consultant Neurologist, Walton Centre for Neurology and Neurosurgery; Honorary Consultant Neurologist, Royal Liverpool University Hospital, Liverpool, United Kingdom
Japanese Encephalitis and West Nile and Other Flavivirus Infections; Neurologic Disease

Anastacio de Queiroz Sousa, MD
Associate Professor, Department of Clinical Medicine, Director, Núcleo de Medicina Tropical, Federal University of Ceará; Physician, Hospital São José for Infectious Diseases, Fortaleza, Ceará, Brazil
Meningococcal Infections; Leishmaniasis

Samba O. Sow, MD, MS
Coordinator, Centre pour le Développement des Vaccins–Mali, Centre National d'Appui à la lutte contre la Maladie, Ministry of Health, Bamako, Mali
Cholera Infections

Christina Spiropoulou, PhD
Adjunct Assistant Professor, Department of Microbiology and Immunology, School of Medicine, Emory University; Special Pathogens Branch, Division of Viral and Rickettsial Diseases, Centers for Disease Control and Prevention, Atlanta, GA
Hantavirus Infections

Lawrence R. Stanberry, MD, PhD
John Sealy Distinguished Chair in Pediatrics, Chairman, Department of Pediatrics, Director, Sealy Center for Vaccine Development, Department of Pediatrics, University of Texas Medical Branch, Galveston, TX
Human Herpesvirus Infections

Robert Steffen, MD
Professor of Travel Medicine, Division of Epidemiology and Prevention of Communicable Diseases, Institute of Social and Preventive Medicine, University of Zurich; Director, World Health Organization Collaborating Centre for Travellers' Health, Zurich, Switzerland
Health Advice for International Travel

Theodore S. Steiner, MD, RRCPC
Assistant Professor, Department of Medicine, University of British Columbia, Vancouver, British Columbia, Canada
Enteric Escherichia coli *Infections; Intestinal Coccidia Infection*

Mark C. Steinhoff, MD
Professor, Department of International Health, Johns Hopkins University; Physician, Department of Pediatrics, Johns Hopkins Hospital, Baltimore, MD
Haemophilus influenzae *(Including* H. aegyptius*) Infection*

Dennis L. Stevens, MD, PhD, FACP
Professor, Department of Medicine, University of Washington School of Medicine, Seattle, WA; Chief, Infectious Diseases, Department of Medicine, Veterans Affairs Medical Center, Boise, ID
Streptococcal and Staphylococcal Infections

Kathryn N. Suh, MD, FRCPC
Assistant Professor, Department of Pediatrics, University of Ottawa; Attending Physician, Division of Infectious Diseases, Children's Hospital of Eastern Ontario, Ottawa, Ontario, Canada
Delusional Parasitosis

Martin Tagle, MD
Associate Professor of Medicine, Department of Gastroenterology and Hepatology, Universidad Peruana Cayetano Heredia; Staff Gastroenterologist and Hepatologist, Clinica Anglo-Americana, Lima, Peru
Viral Hepatitis

Herbert B. Tanowitz, MD, FACP
Professor, Department of Pathology and Medicine, Attending Physician, Department of Medicine and Pathology, Albert Einstein College of Medicine; Attending Physician, Department of Medicine, Weiler Hospital, Montefiore Medical Center, Bronx, NY
Introduction to Tapeworm Infections; Cysticercosis; Taenia and Other Tapeworms

Sam R. Telford III, ScD
Associate Professor of Infectious Diseases, Department of Biomedical Sciences, Tufts University School of Veterinary Medicine, North Grafton, MA; Visiting Scientist, Department of Immunology and Infectious Diseases, Harvard School of Public Health, Boston, MA
Babesiosis

Robert B. Tesh, BS, MS, MD
George Dock Distinguished Professor of Pathology, Department of Pathology, University of Texas Medical Branch, Galveston, TX
Sandfly Fever, Oropouche Fever, and Other Bunyavirus Infections; Japanese Encephalitis and West Nile and Other Flavivirus Infections; Alphavirus Infections

Nathan M. Thielman, MD, MPH
Assistant Professor of Medicine, Director of Adult Infectious Diseases Clinic, Department of Medicine, Duke University Medical Center, Durham, NC
Chemotherapy of Bacterial, Fungal, and Viral Diseases; Enteric Escherichia coli *Infections; Gastrointestinal Symptoms*

Elaine Tuomanen, MD, CM
Chair and Full Member, Director of Children's Infection Defense Center, Department of Infectious Diseases, St. Jude Children's Research Hospital, Memphis, TN
Pneumococcal Infections

Luis M. Valdez, MD
Associate Professor, Department of Medicine, Universidad Peruana Cayetano Heredia; Infectious Diseases and Internal Medicine Staff Physician, Associate Director, Department of Medicine, Clinica Anglo Americana (British-American Hospital), Research Associate, Instituto de Medicina Tropical "Alexander Von Humboldt," Lima, Peru
Gastrointestinal Symptoms

Jesus G. Valenzuela, PhD
Vector Molecular Biology Unit, Laboratory of Malaria and Vector Research, National Institute of Allergy and Infectious Diseases, National Institutes of Health, Rockville, MD
Vector Biology

Govinda S. Visvesvara, PhD
Research Microbiologist, Division of Parasitic Diseases, Centers for Disease Control and Prevention, Atlanta, GA
Pathogenic and Opportunistic Free-Living Amebas: Acanthamoeba *spp.,* Balamuthia mandrillaris, Naegleria fowleri, *and* Sappina diploidia

Victoria Wahl-Jensen, MS, PhD
National Research Council Associate, Department of Molecular Virology, United States Army Medical Research Institute of Infectious Diseases, Fort Detrick, MD
Filovirus Infections

David H. Walker, MD
Professor and Chairman, The Carmage and Martha Walls Distinguished Chair in Tropical Diseases, Department of Pathology, Director, World Health Organization Collaborating Center for Tropical Diseases, University of Texas Medical Branch; Chair, Department of Pathology, John Sealy Memorial Hospital, Galveston, TX
Principles of Parasitism: Host–Parasite Interactions; Anthrax; Bartonelloses; Spotted Fever Group Rickettsioses; Typhus Group Rickettsioses; Scrub Typhus; Ehrlichioses and Anaplasmosis; Distinguishing Tropical Infectious Diseases from Bioterrorism

Pramila Walpita, PhD
Research Scientist, Department of Pathology, University of Texas Medical Branch, Galveston, TX; Adjunct Assistant Professor, Department of Pediatric Infectious Diseases, New York University, New York, NY
Nipah and Hendra Viral Infections

Thomas J. Walsh, MD, FACP, FCCP
Senior Investigator, Chief, Immunocompromised Host Section, National Cancer Institute, National Institutes of Health, Bethesda, MD; Adjunct Professor of Pathology, Johns Hopkins University School of Medicine; Adjunct Professor of Medicine, University of Maryland School of Medicine, Baltimore, MD
Mucocutaneous and Deeply Invasive Candidiasis

David A. Walton, MD
Resident Physician, Department of Internal Medicine, Brigham & Women's Hospital, Boston, MA
Social and Cultural Factors in Tropical Medicine: Reframing Our Understanding of Disease

Peter D. Walzer, MD, FACP
ACOS for Research/Professor of Medicine, Research Service, Department of Internal Medicine, VA Medical Center, University of Cincinnati; Attending Physician, Medical Service, Department of Internal Medicine, VA Medical Center, University Hospital, Cincinnati, OH
Pneumocystosis

George Watt, MD, DTM&H
Associate Professor of Tropical Medicine, Department of Clinical Tropical Medicine, Faculty of Tropical Medicine, Mahidol University, Bangkok, Thailand; Associate Professor, Department of Epidemiology, International Health Division, University of Maryland School of Medicine, Baltimore, MD
Scrub Typhus

Douglas M. Watts, MD, PhD
Professor of Pathology, Center for Biodefense and Emerging Infectious Diseases and WHO Collaborating Center for Tropical Diseases, Department of Pathology, University of Texas Medical Branch, Galveston, TX
Bunyaviral Fevers: Rift Valley Fever and Crimean-Congo Hemorrhagic Fever; Japanese Encephalitis and West Nile and Other Flavivirus Infections

Scott C. Weaver, PhD
Director for Tropical and Emerging Infectious Diseases, Professor of Pathology, Microbiology and Immunology, Department of Pathology, University of Texas Medical Branch, Galveston, TX
Alphavirus Infections

Louis M. Weiss, MD, MPH, FACP
Professor, Department of Medicine and Pathology, Albert Einstein College of Medicine; Attending Physician, Department of Medicine (Infectious Diseases), Jack D. Weiler Hospital–Montefiore Medical Center; Attending Physician, Department of Medicine, Bronx Municipal Hospital (Jacobi Medical Center), Bronx, NY
Microsporidiosis

Peter F. Weller, MD, FACP
Professor of Medicine, Department of Medicine, Harvard Medical School; Co-Chief, Infectious Diseases Division, Chief, Allergy and Inflammation Division, Vice Chair for Research, Department of Medicine, Beth Israel Deaconess Medical Center, Boston, MA
Principles of Parasitism: Host–Parasite Interactions; Immunology, Host Defense, Immunodeficiencies, and Vaccines; Chemotherapy of Parasitic Diseases; Chemotherapy of Bacterial, Fungal, and Viral Diseases; Eosinophilia

Jay D. Wenger, MD
Project Manager, National Polio Surveillance Project, New Delhi, India
Meningococcal Infections

Melinda Wharton, MD, MPH, FACP
Acting Deputy Director, National Immunization Program, Centers for Disease Control and Prevention, Atlanta, GA
Diphtheria

A. Clinton White, Jr., MD, FACP
Professor, Infectious Disease Section, Department of Medicine, Department of Immunology, Department of Molecular Virology and Microbiology, Baylor College of Medicine; Chief, Infectious Disease Section, Department of Medicine, Ben Taub General Hospital, Houston, TX
Introduction to Tapeworm Infections; Cysticercosis

Nicholas J. White, OBE, DSc, MD, FRCP, F Med Sci
Professor of Tropical Medicine, Faculty of Tropical Medicine, Mahidol University, Bangkok, Thailand; Professor of Tropical Medicine, Oxford University; Consultant Physician, John Radcliffe Hospital, Oxford, United Kingdom
Malaria

Marc-Alain Widdowson, MA, MSc, VetMB
Medical Epidemiologist, Respiratory and Enteric Virus Branch, Centers for Disease Control and Prevention, Atlanta, GA
Calicivirus Infections

Robert John Wilkinson, MA, PhD, BM, BCh, DTM&H, FRCP
Wellcome Trust Senior Fellow in Clinical Tropical Medicine, Department of Medicine, University of Cape Town; Honorary Physician, Department of HIV/AIDS, GF Jooste Hospital, Manenberg, Cape Town, South Africa; Honorary Consultant Physician, Department of Specialist Medicine, Northwick Park Hospital, Harrow, United Kingdom; Wellcome Trust Senior Fellow in Clinical Tropical Medicine, Department of Medicine, Imperial College London, London, United Kingdom
Host Genetics and Susceptibility to Infection

Mary E. Wilson, MD, FACP
Associate Professor, Department of Medicine, Harvard Medical School; Associate Professor, Department of Population and International Health, Harvard School of Public Health, Boston, MA; Consulting Staff, Department of Medicine, Mount Auburn Hospital, Cambridge, MA
Fever and Systemic Symptoms; Eosinophilia

Murray Wittner, MD, PhD
Professor, Department of Pathology and Parasitology, Attending Physician and Director of Tropical Medicine and Parasitology, Department of Pathology, Albert Einstein College of Medicine; Attending Physician, Department of Pathology, Weiler Hospital, Montefiore Medical Center, Bronx, NY
Introduction to Tapeworm Infections; Cysticercosis; Taenia and Other Tapeworms

Emily J. Wong, MD, FAAP
Assistant Professor, Department of Pediatrics, University of Virginia, Charlottesville, VA
Pertussis

Sherif R. Zaki, MD, PhD
Chief, Infectious Disease Pathology, Centers for Disease Control and Prevention, Atlanta, GA
Leptospirosis; Overview of Viral Hemorrhagic Fevers; Hantavirus Infections; Filovirus Infections

FOREWORD

As the 21st century unfolds, the speciality of tropical medicine is being forced to broaden its scope and skills and to increase its political strength to meet the present challenges to human health in the tropical world. Population expansion continues unabated. As urbanisation intensifies, the public health is compromised and the quality of life is jeopardised. There is an unprecedented level of forced migration. Starvation is rampant in many countries, from the African Sahel, where a current focus is Niger, to North Korea. This has been blamed on climate-related agricultural failure, natural disasters such as locust plagues, and political ineptitude. Climate variation is exposing new areas of the globe to vector-borne tropical diseases. New infectious diseases are emerging, often as a direct result of environmental incursion and ecologic disruption. In tropical developing countries, the increasing prevalence of diabetes mellitus, cardiovascular diseases, bronchial asthma, and other western-style chronic noninfectious diseases adds to human misery and burdens inadequate health services. The global HIV epidemic continues to exact enormous human suffering. Several infections, once programmed for imminent elimination, are resurgent (e.g., poliomyelitis in Indonesia and Yemen) or persistent (e.g., leprosy in Latin America). While impoverished health services struggle to cope, their precious trained medical staff are being recruited to work in western countries.[1,2]

Most of these health disasters in tropical countries have a political background. In 2005, the G8 Summit and some admirable fund-raising events promised to help relieve poverty in Africa, but there is still a lack of real commitment on the part of some of the wealthiest nations and high levels of corruption among the despotic leaders of many of the poorest nations. Reluctance to accept human responsibility for climate change has delayed an appropriately concerted international response. Even the scientific study of tropical infectious diseases is under threat when the research career of such a great authority on plague as Dr. Thomas C. Butler is suspended while he languishes in a federal prison on charges that seem highly inappropriate to those of us who know the man and his work.[3] Inflexible and bigoted dogmas have impeded efforts to constrain the growth of human populations and to control HIV and sexually transmitted infections.

These disturbing and ominous developments make the publication of the magnificent second edition of Guerrant, Walker, and Weller's *Tropical Infectious Diseases: Principles, Pathogens, & Practice* all the more timely, important, and urgent. The new edition builds on the enormous strengths of the first edition, published 6 years ago, by making important innovations and additions. It was surely an editorial master stroke to introduce, early in the book, the absolutely riveting chapter, "Social and Cultural Factors in Tropical Medicine: Reframing Our Understanding of Disease" by Walton, Farmer, and Dillingham. This features a dramatic case history set in Haiti, appropriately styled the "Lazarus effect", which illustrates how much can be achieved in a patient with advanced AIDS and disseminated tuberculosis by using the drugs whose availability is taken for granted in western countries. The authors discuss the scandalous "brain drain" of trained medical staff from the developing world and critically expose some of the naïve economic assumptions underlying the World Health Organisation's unsuccessful rollback malaria campaign. This chapter succeeds in concentrating our attention on "the central irony of 21st century medicine": the persistence of human suffering from infectious diseases, despite our possession of many effective vaccines, treatments, and preventive methods. In my opinion, this new chapter alone justifies the second edition of *Tropical Infectious Diseases* and should help to correct any misapprehension that this book is concerned only with tropical infectious diseases as they affect western, specifically North American, travellers.

As in the first edition, the coverage of the scientific basis of tropical infectious diseases is impressive and extensive. Bioterrorism is now perceived as a threat, resulting in new funding for research on some of the most lethal infections being made available from unusual sources. In the new chapter "Distinguishing Tropical Infectious Diseases from Bioterrorism", Olano, Peters, and Walker help the clinician presented with an index case to distinguish a naturally occurring infection from the first manifestation of a bioterrorist act. This could prove very difficult in those tropical countries where sporadic cases of viral haemorrhagic disease, anthrax, botulism, or plague can occur.

A new chapter on "Tropical Infectious Disease Concerns in Pregnancy" by Isturiz and Gotuzzo will be especially welcomed by those involved in antenatal care in tropical countries. Protection of the physiologically immunosuppressed pregnant woman against life-threatening infections is of paramount importance. The authors discuss the limited role of antimalarial chemoprophylaxis but rightly emphasise the encouraging results of intermittent preventive treatment during pregnancy. However, by far the most impressive results have been achieved by the use of insecticide-treated mosquito nets.[4]

Most of the global health priorities that I have identified are well covered by new or existing chapters: "Migrant, Immigrant, and Refugee Health" by Maloney, Ortega, and Cetron; "Nutrition and Micronutrients in Tropical Infectious Diseases" by Kosek, Black, and Keusch; "Factors Influencing Geographic Distribution and Incidence of Tropical Infectious Diseases" by Shugart and Shope; "Nipah and Hendra Viral Infections" by Flick, Walpita, and Czub; "Respiratory Tract Viral Infections" by Arruda, Cintra, and Hayden; and "Human Retroviral Infections in the Tropics" by Reynolds, Bessong, and Quinn. Despite the specificity of its title, *Tropical Infectious Diseases: Principles, Pathogens, & Practice* provides much that is not strictly tropical infectious diseases. However, if, as I very much hope, there are further editions of this outstandingly valuable reference work, which is fast becoming a classic, the editors should consider whether to expand their horizons to cover the whole of tropical medicine including such important topics as population control, consequences of urbanisation, and western-style noncommunicable diseases. The new edition succeeds, to an even greater extent than the first, in setting new standards of excellence in textbook publishing in the field of tropical infectious diseases.

David A. Warrell
Professor of Tropical Medicine and Infectious Diseases and Founding Director of The Centre for Tropical Medicine (Emeritus), University of Oxford, UK
August 2005

REFERENCES

1. Johnson J: Stopping Africa's medical brain drain. Brit Med J 331:2–3, 2005.
2. Hagopian A, Thompson MJ, Fordyce M, et al: The migration of physicians from sub-saharan Africa to the United States of America: Measures of the African brain drain. http://eprints.ouls.ox.ac.uk/archicve/00000847/01/hagopian_2004.pdf. Accessed August 3, 2005.
3. Murray BE, Anderson KE, Arnold K, et al: Destroying the life and career of a valued physician-scientist who tried to protect us from plague: Was it really necessary? CID 40:1644–1648, 2005.
4. ter Kuile FO, Terlouw DJ, Phillips-Howard PA, et al: Reduction of malaria during pregnancy by permethrin-treated bed nets in an area of intense perennial malaria transmission in western Kenya. Am J Trop Med Hyg 68(Suppl 4):50–60, 2003.

PREFACE

The world of tropical infectious diseases has changed since our first edition of *Tropical Infectious Diseases: Principles, Pathogens, & Practice*. Despite the success and relevance of our first edition to the growing majority of people living in tropical, developing areas, since it was published we have seen the appearance of SARS worldwide, Nipah in southern Asia, and West Nile and monkeypox in the Americas. The continued emergence of AIDS is a global disaster, with the greatest challenges posed in tropical, developing areas. We have also seen the eruption of terrorism, posing unprecedented challenges to distinguish intentional criminal transmission from endemic tropical infectious disease threats, with huge differences in their implications for control.

Hence, we have retained our commitment to combining practical clinical relevance and pragmatic accessibility with algorithms and tables in the "Practice" section for the practicing clinician in the tropics or, increasingly, anywhere that people who have been in the tropics are seen. Our state-of-the-art, well-referenced text also covers the latest developments in immunity, pathogenesis, genetics of virulence, and new molecular approaches to diagnosis and control. It is written by the top experts from around the world, with more than 60 of our 229 authors from outside the United States. Essentially all have extensive, firsthand international experience, representing Asia, Africa, and Latin America, as well as Europe, Australia, and North America.

Responding to popular demand and growing needs, we have added new chapters on "Social and Cultural Factors in Tropical Medicine: Reframing Our Understanding of Disease" by Walton, Farmer and Dillingham; "Distinguishing Tropical Infectious Diseases from Bioterrorism" by Olano, Peters and Walker; "Migrant, Immigrant, and Refugee Health" by Maloney, Ortega, and Cetron; "Delusional Parasitosis" by Suh and Keystone; "Nipah and Hendra Viral Infections" by Flick, Walpita, and Czub; and "Tropical Infectious Disease Concerns in Pregnancy" by Isturiz and Gotuzzo. Other chapters now have major additions addressing environment–disease interactions (Chapter 2 by Shugart and Shope), new color plates especially relevant to animal poisons (Chapter 9 by Norris and Auerbach), surveillance for bioterrorism threats (Chapter 15 by Arthur, LeDuc, and Hughes), Spotted Fever Group Rickettsioses (Chapter 50 by Sexton and Walker), and SARS and metapneumoviruses (Chapter 59 by Arruda, Cintra, and Hayden). Furthermore, entirely new life cycles following our trademark format (with entry of the agent into humans at the 9 o'clock position, bold "boxes" at the top for the resulting acute and chronic human clinical diseases caused, with exit of the agent from the human host at the 3 o'clock position, and spread through vectors/environment outside the human host across the lower half of the cycle) have been added for the spotted fever and typhus rickettsiae, *Borrelia*, *Ehrlichia*, Q fever, *Hymenolepis*, *Dracunculis*, *Diphyllobothrium*, *Babesia*, pertussis, and cholera.

Our authors—the world's authorities on their topics—make this book what it is, the authoritative text in our field. To them we owe a huge debt of gratitude. We also acknowledge our mentors, Maxwell Finland, Charles C. J. Carpenter, Edward W. Hook, Jr., Jerry Mandell, Franz von Lichtenberg, John Edgcomb, Fred Murphy, Joe Grisham, Franklin A. Neva, Thomas H. Weller, and Robert C. Moellering, Jr. who so profoundly shaped our careers. Finally, we thank, once again, our Developmental Editor, Ann Ruzycka Anderson; as well as Mary Ann Winecoff and Sherrill Hebert; and our Production Manager, Cecelia Bayruns, whose labors made this two-volume text possible; and last but most importantly, Nancy, Margie, and Anne, who have again supported us and our sanity amidst deadlines, updates, and reams of galleys to bring this edition to completion.

Richard L. Guerrant, MD

David H. Walker, MD

Peter F. Weller, MD

CONTENTS

VOLUME 1

The Color Plates follow the Contents in Volume 1.

SECTION I

Principles and General Considerations

SECTION II

Pathogens

A. BACTERIAL AND MYCOBACTERIAL INFECTIONS

Color Plates

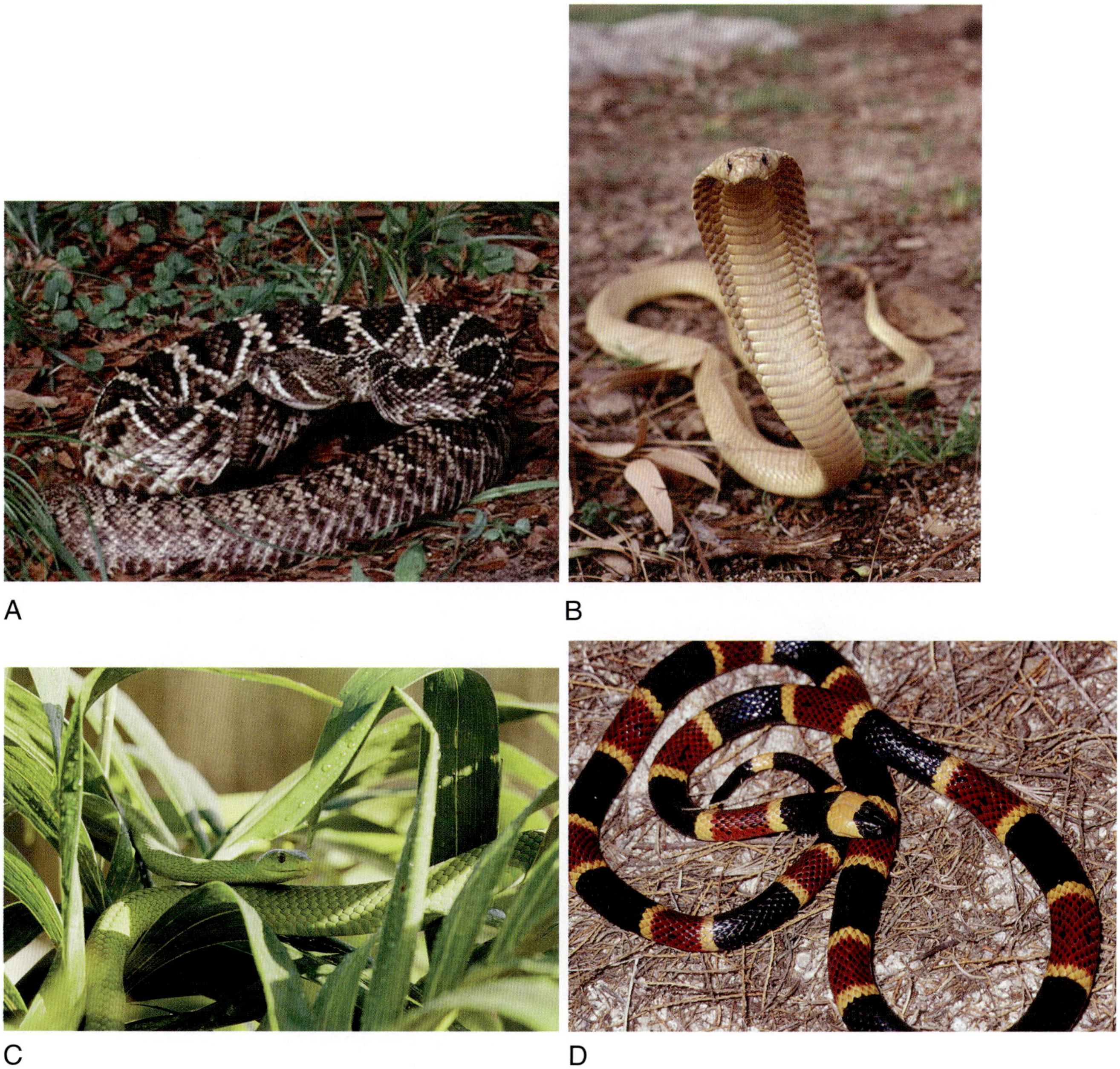

PLATE 9-1 Venomous snakes. *A,* The eastern diamondback rattlesnake (*Crotalus adamanteus*) native to the southeastern United States. This is the largest venomous snake of North America. *B,* The cape cobra (*Naja nivea*) native to South Africa. *C,* The highly venomous green mamba (*Dendroaspis angusticeps*) of Africa. *D,* The eastern coral snake (*Micrurus fulvius*) found in the southeastern United States. While extremely venomous, bites by this shy snake are uncommon. (Photos by Michael Cardwell, Extreme Wildlife Photography.)

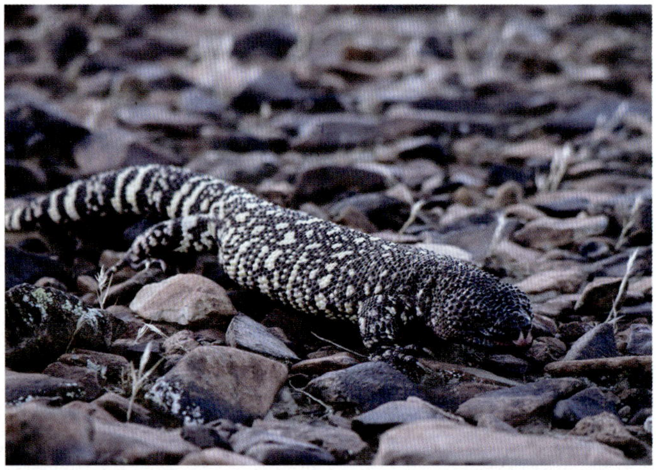

PLATE 9-2 The Mexican beaded lizard (*Heloderma horridum*), native to western Mexico. (Photo by Michael Cardwell, Extreme Wildlife Photography.)

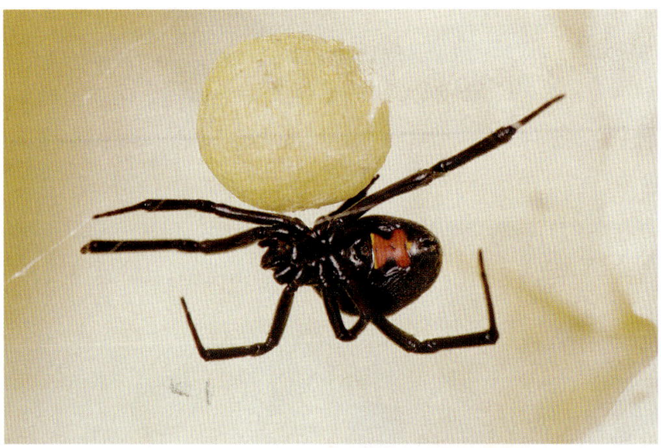

A

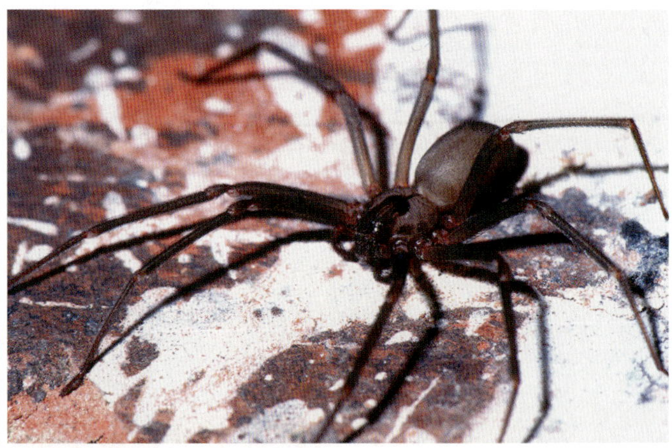

B

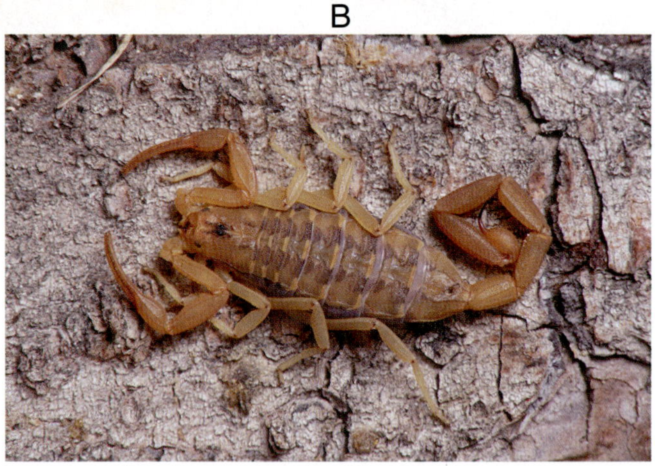

C

PLATE 9-3 Venomous arthropods. *A,* Female western black widow spider (*Latrodectus hesperus*). Note its typical red hour-glass marking on the ventral side of its abdomen. *B,* Brown recluse spider (*Loxosceles reclusa*). Note the violin-shaped marking on the dorsal aspect of the cephalothorax. *C,* Arizona bark scorpion (*Centruroides exilicauda*). (Photos by Michael Cardwell, Extreme Wildlife Photography.)

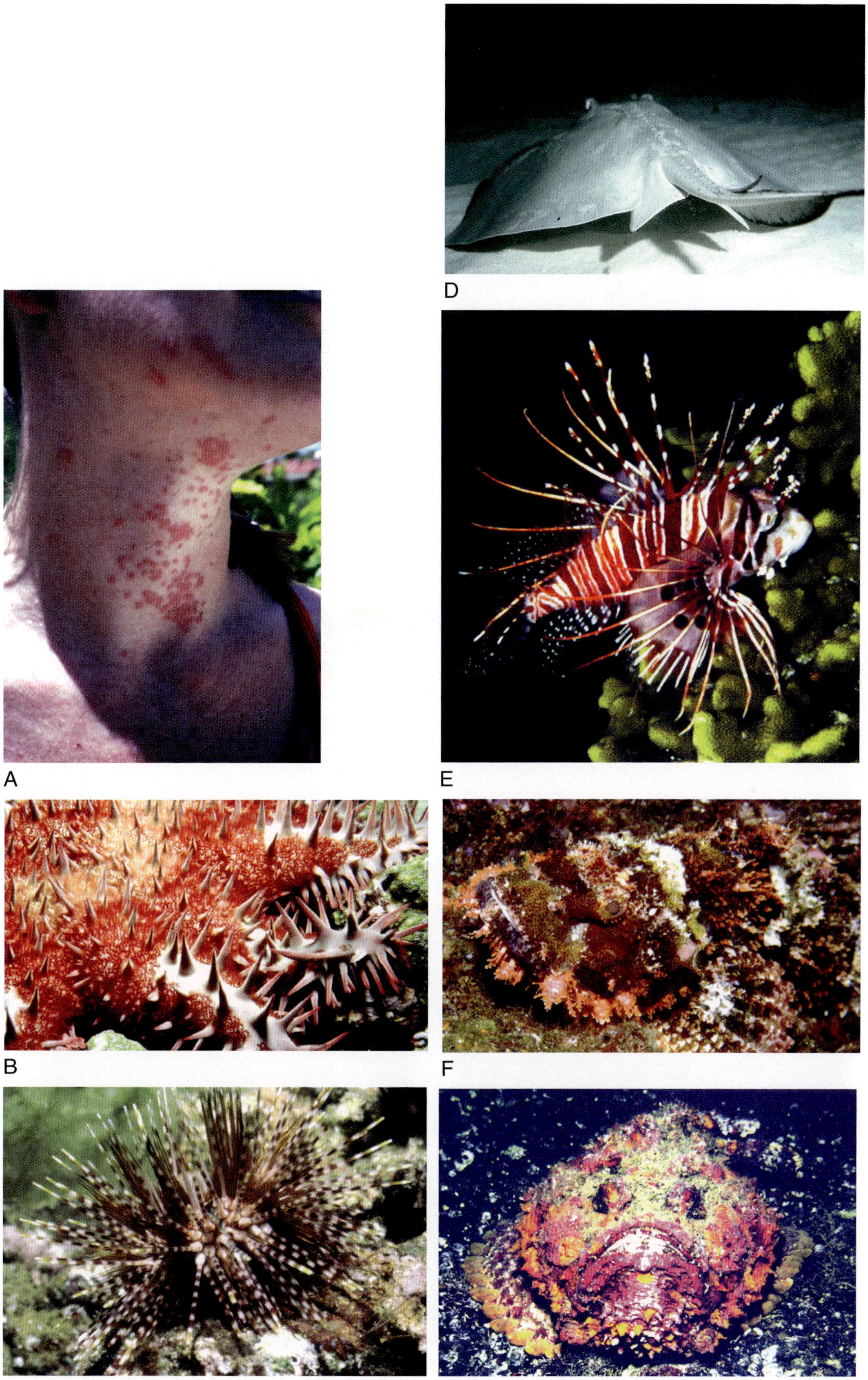

PLATE 9-4 Marine envenomations. *A,* Seabather's eruption on a woman's neck. *B,* Close-up of the spines of a crown of thorns starfish (*Acanthaster planci*). *C,* Striped spiny sea urchin. *D,* Stingray (*Dasyatis americana*) rising from the sandy ocean floor. *E,* Indonesian lionfish (*Pterois* spp.). *F,* Scorpionfish (*Scorpaena* spp.) from the Solomon Islands. *G,* Stonefish (*Synanceja* spp.) in Indonesia. (Photos by Paul Auerbach.)

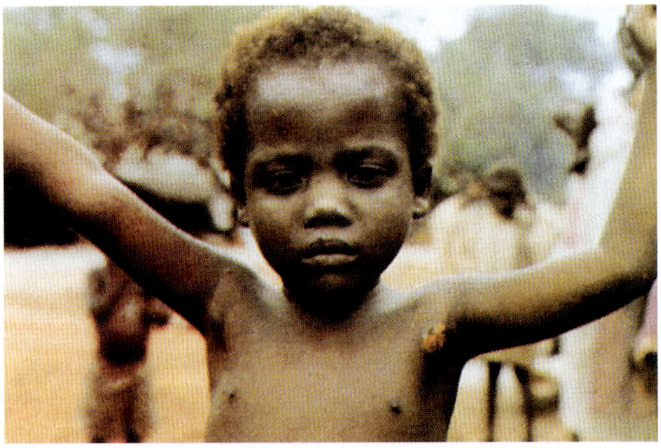

PLATE 44-1 Initial axillary papilloma of yaws. (From Perrine PL, Hopkins DR, Niemel PLA, et al: Handbook of Endemic Treponematoses: Yaws, Endemic Syphilis, and Pinta. Geneva, World Health Organization, 1984.)

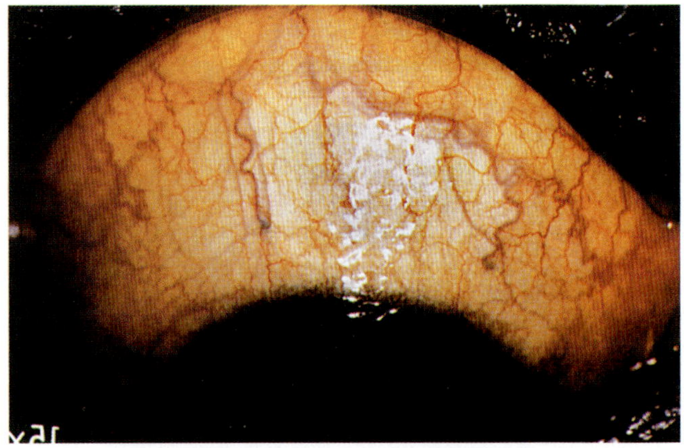

PLATE 46-1 Jaundice and conjuctival suffusion in severe leptospirosis.

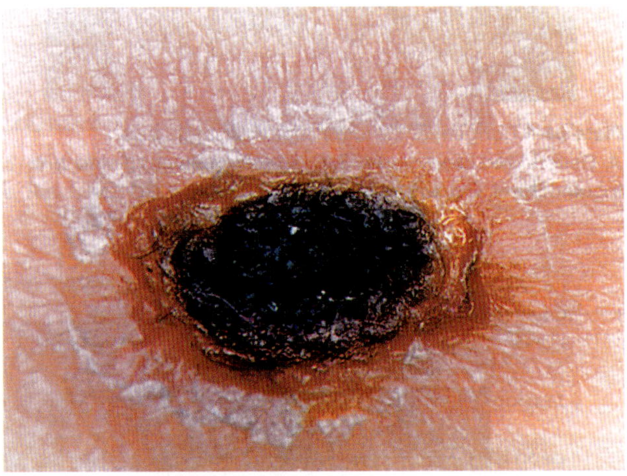

PLATE 52-1 The eschar of scrub typhus represents epidermal and superficial dermal necrosis owing to vascular injury associated with *Orientia tsutsugamushi* at the portal of entry by the bite of a larval chigger.

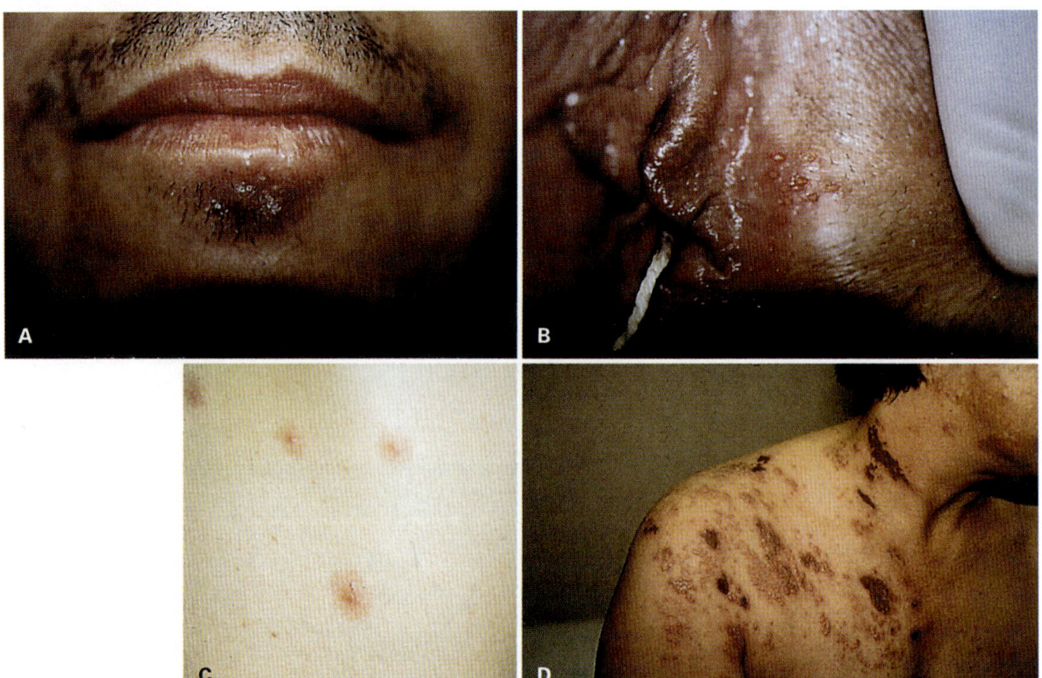

PLATE 57-1 Herpetic skin lesions. *A,* Hepes labialis (primary herpes simplex virus [HSV] type 1). *B,* Herpes genitalis (primary HSV 2). *C,* Varicella (primary varicella-zoster virus [VZV]). *D,* Herpes zoster (secondary VZV).

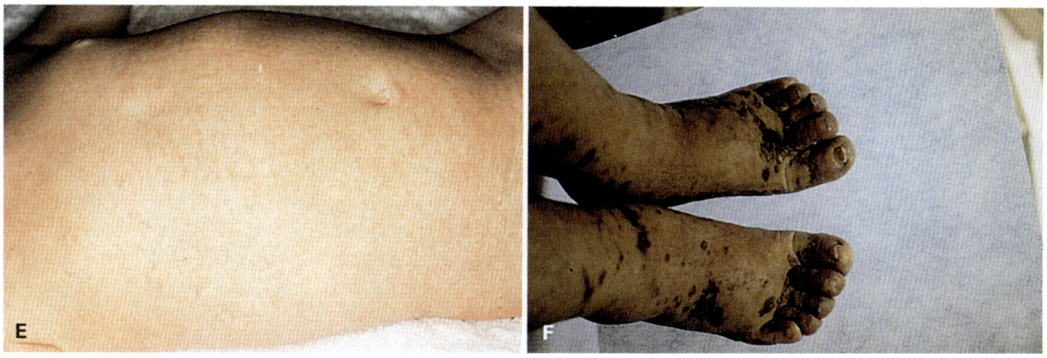

PLATE 57-1 cont'd *E,* Exanthem subitum (primary human herpesvirus [HHV] type 6). *F,* Kaposi's sarcoma (HHV-8). (Courtesy of Stephen Tyring, MD, PhD, University of Texas Medical Branch, Galveston.)

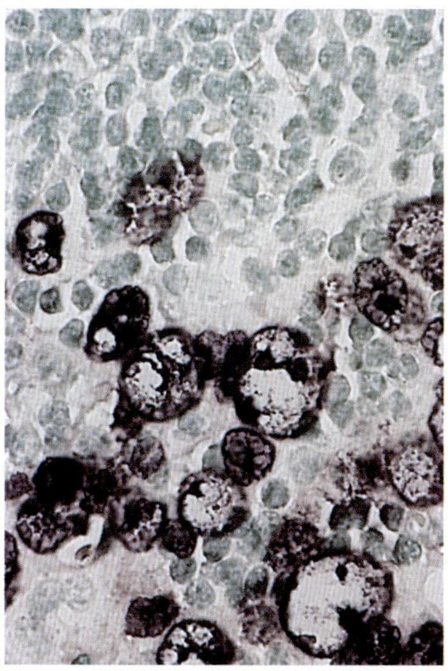

PLATE 57-2 Nasopharyngeal carcinoma. Epstein-Barr virus in situ stain.

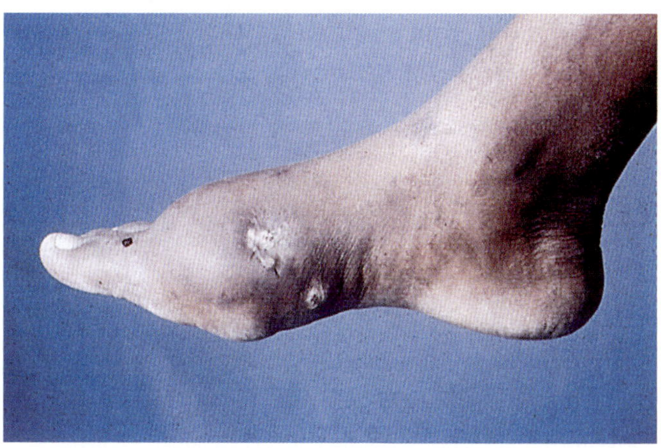

PLATE 78-1 Mycetoma of the foot. Note swelling and sinuses.

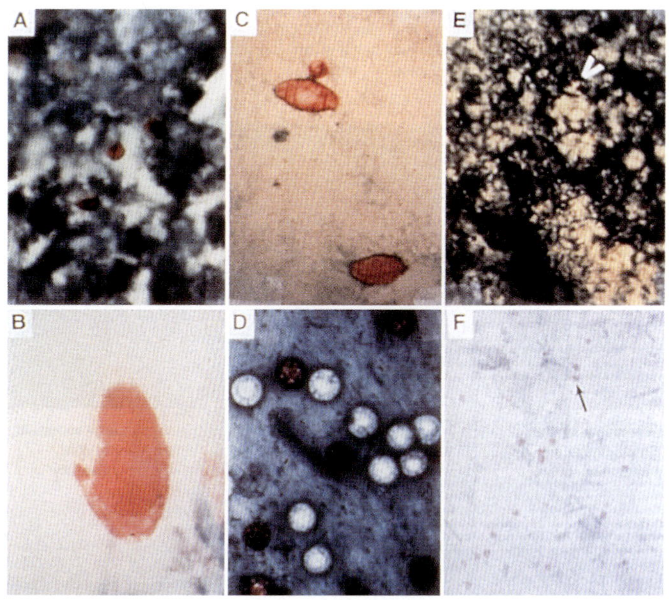

PLATE 88-1 Acid-fast protozoan and other causes of diarrhea in patients with AIDS. (*Cryptosporidium* and *Cyclospora* are important causes of diarrhea in immunologically normal hosts as well.) *A,* Acid-fast *Cryptosporidium* in fecal specimen. B, Acid-fast *Isospora belli* in stool of a Haitian patient with diarrhea. *C, I. belli* and *Cryptosporidium* in a Haitian patient with AIDS and diarrhea. *D,* Acid-fast *Cyclospora cayetanensis* in the stool of a patient with diarrhea. *E,* Acid-fast *Mycobacterium avium-intracellulare* in the stool of a patient with AIDS and diarrhea. *F,* Microsporidia in the stool of a patient with AIDS and diarrhea as seen in modified trichrome stain. (*A,* From Guerrant RL, Bobak DA: Bacterial and protozoal gastroenteritis. N Engl J Med 325:327, 1991. *B* and *C,* Courtesy of Drs. Rosemary Soave and Madeleine Boncy. *D,* Courtesy of Dr. Earl Long. *E,* Courtesy of Dr. Cynthia Sears. *F,* From Weber R, Bryan RT, Owen RL, et al, for the Enteric Opportunistic Infections Working Group: Improved light-microscopical detection of microsporidia spores in stool and duodenal aspirates. N Engl J Med 326:161, 1992.)

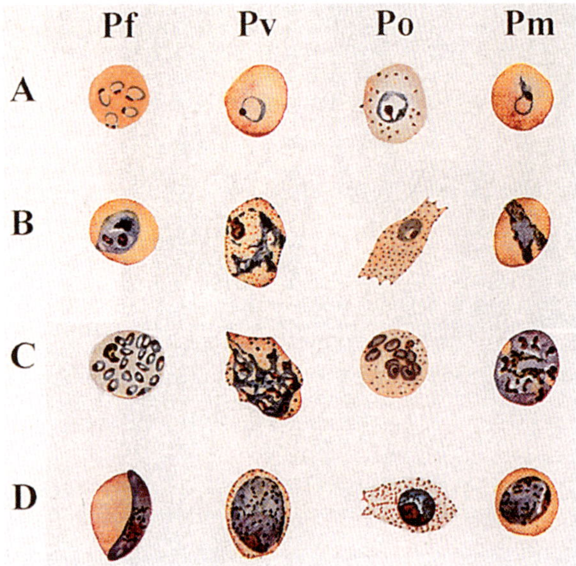

PLATE 90-1 Diagnostic forms of malaria in Giemsa-stained thin blood films. Thick smears (not shown) would show parasite forms after lysis of red blood cells. Columns: Pf, *P. falciparum;* Pv, *P. vivax;* Po, *P. ovale;* Pm, *P. malariae.* Rows: A and B, young and old trophozoites; C, schizonts; D, gameocytes. (Adapted from drawings by Inez Demonet in Brown HW, Neva FA: Basic Clinical Parasitology, 5th ed. Norwalk, CT, Appleton-Century-Crofts, 1983; and World Health Organization: Bench Aids for the Diagnosis of Malaria, 1983.)

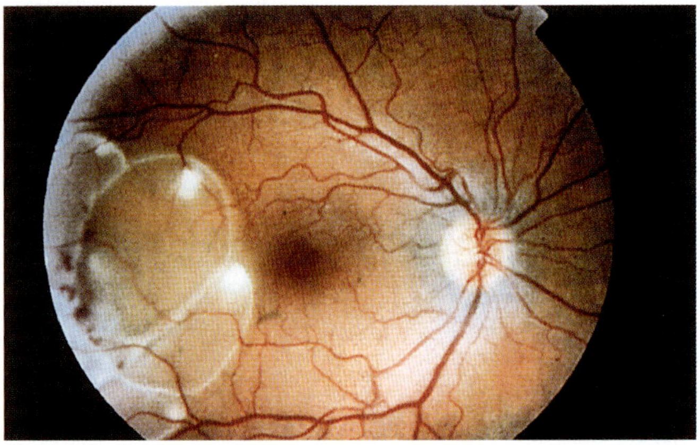

PLATE 115-1 Ocular lesion of *Taenia crassiceps*. Large subretinal mass in the right fundus. (Courtesy of Drs. G. J. Weil, R. S. Chuck, and R. J. Olk, Washington University School of Medicine, St. Louis, MO.)

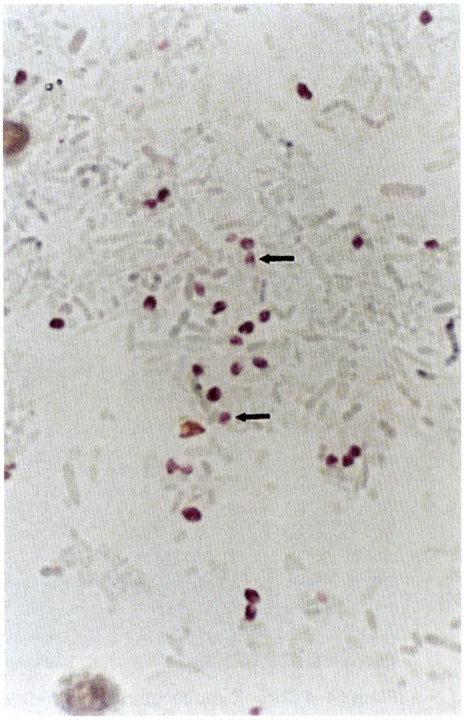

PLATE 96-1 Spores of *Enterocytozoon* in this stool smear stain violet using the Gram-chromotrope technique. Some spores show an equatorial belt *(arrows)* that is helpful for diagnosis (x 1250). (Courtesy of Drs. Hercules Moura and Govinda S. Visvesvara, Centers for Disease Control and Prevention, Atlanta, GA.)

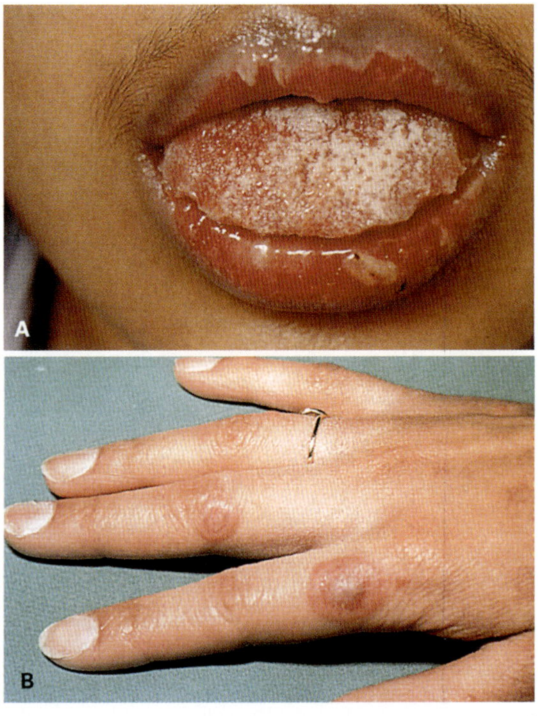

PLATE 126-1 Erythema multiforme of the mouth (*A*) and hand (*B*). (Courtesy of Kenneth J. Tomecki, MD, Cleveland, OH.)

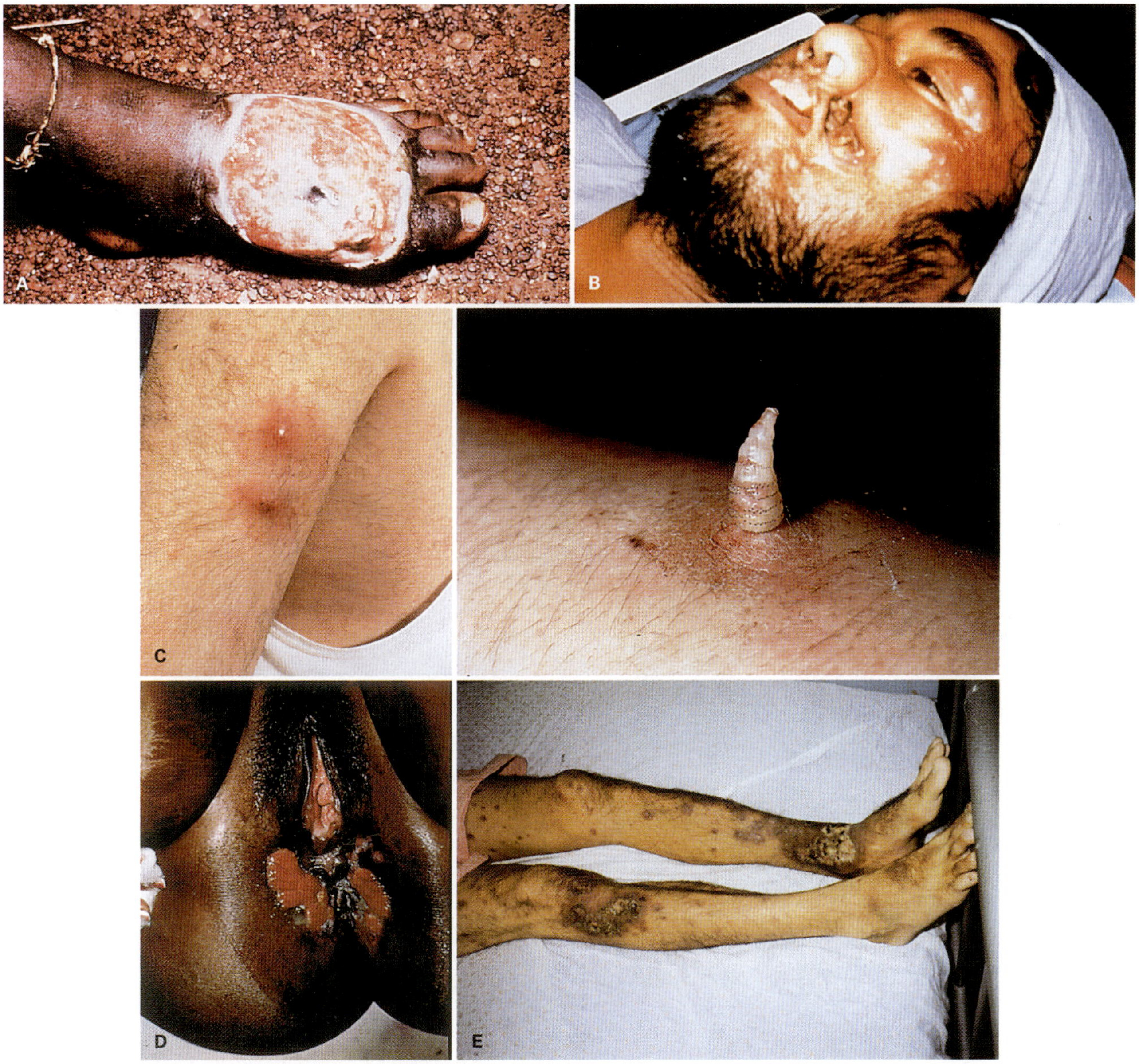

PLATE 126-2 *A,* Tropical phagedenic ulcer. *B,* Buruli ulcer. *C,* Myiasis extruding larva. *D,* Granuloma inguinale. *E,* South American blastomycosis (paracoccidioidomycosis). (*A–C,* Courtesy of Jay S. Keystone, MD. *D* and *E,* Courtesy of R. L. Guerrant, MD, Charlottesville, VA.)

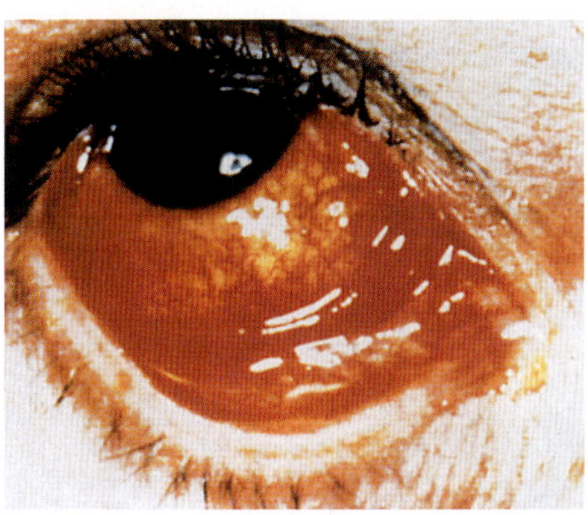

PLATE 129-1 Acute hemorrhagic conjunctivitis due to coxsackievirus A24. (From Yin-Murphy M, Goh KT, Phoon MC, et al: A recent epidemic of acute hemorrhagic conjunctivitis. Am J Ophthalmol 116:213, 1993.)

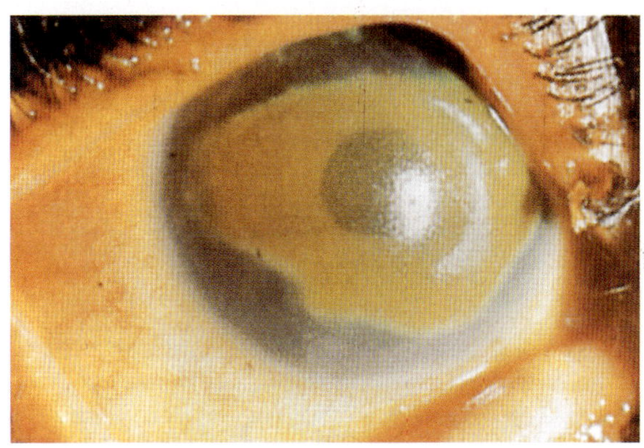

PLATE 129-2 Measles-associated corneal ulceration (superficial) stained with fluorescein. The child was deficient in vitamin A. (From Sandford-Smith J: Eye Diseases in Hot Climates, 2nd ed. Oxford, Butterworth Heinemann, 1990, plate 12c.)

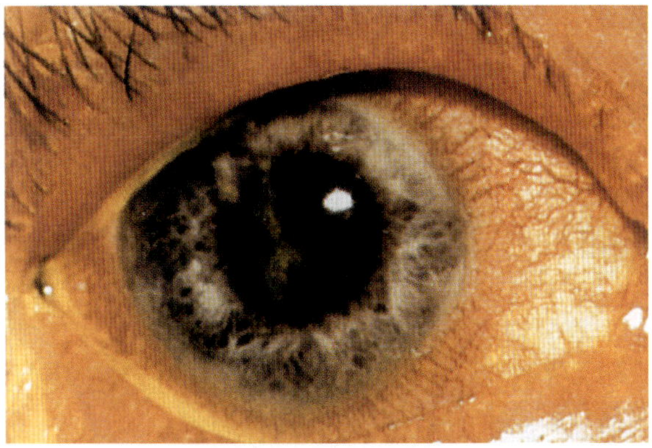

PLATE 129-3 Herpes simplex virus–associated dendritic corneal ulcer stained with fluorescein. Prior to the addition of fluorescein, the cornea appeared normal to the naked eye. (From Sandford-Smith J: Eye Diseases in Hot Climates, 2nd ed. Oxford, Butterworth Heinemann, 1990, plate 7e. Courtesy of Mr. E. Rosen, Manchester, UK.)

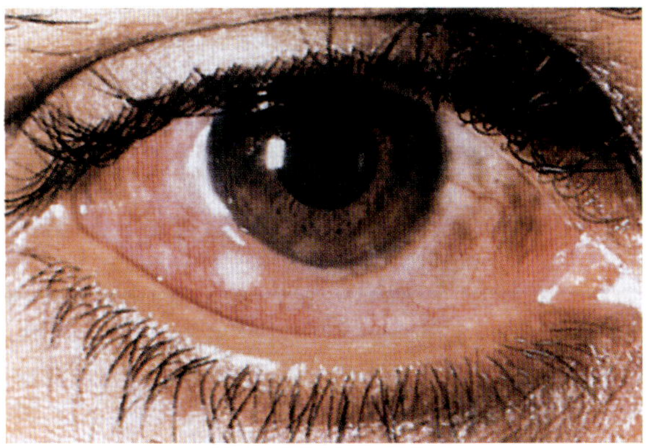

PLATE 129-4 Conjunctival phlyctenule in a patient with pulmonary tuberculosis. (From Helm CJ, Holland GN: Ocular tuberculosis. Surv Ophthalmol 38:229, 1993. Courtesy of Dr. A. M. Mehta, Los Angeles.)

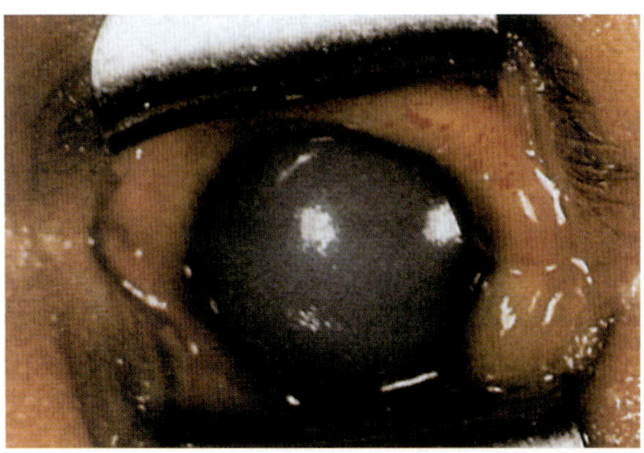

PLATE 129-5 Metastatic bacterial endophthalmitis due to group B β-streptococcus. In this patient, inflammation was predominantly anterior. Note the corneal edema and cloudy and inflamed aqueous. Vitreal inflammation was minimal in the case, but can often be quite pronounced. (From Greenwald MJ, Wohl LG, Sell CH: Metastatic bacterial endophthalmitis: A contemporary reappraisal. Surv Ophthalmol 31:85, 1986.)

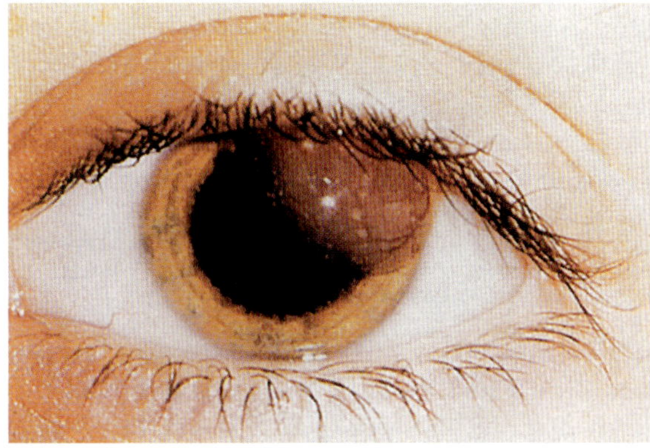

PLATE 129-6 *Rhinosporidium seeberi* conjunctival lesion arising from the superior fornix and extending onto the cornea. Note the fleshy pink appearance and the small white spherules of the lesion. (From Reidy JJ, Sudesh S, Klafter AB, et al: Infection of the conjunctiva by *Rhinosporidium seeberi*. Surv Ophthalmol 41:410, 1997.)

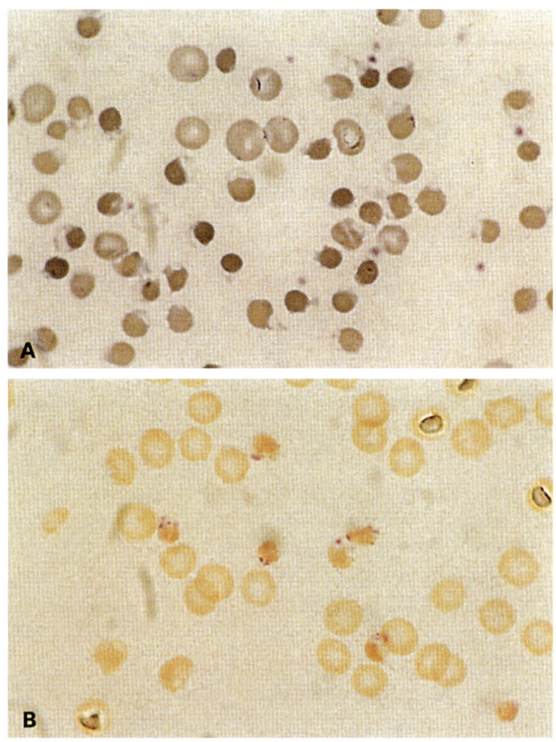

PLATE 131-1 Glucose-6-phosphate dehydrogenase deficiency. *A*, Peripheral blood smear during a hemolytic crisis. Note the irregularly contracted red blood cells with an area of irregular membrane at one end. Where this area is a considerable part of the red blood cell, the term "hemighost" is sometimes used. *B*, Heinz body preparation showing precipitated denatured hemoglobin that is membrane bound. When these Heinz bodies are "pitted" out by the spleen, the appearance is one of irregularly contracted red blood cells and hemighosts.

SECTION I

Principles and General Considerations

1

Principles of Parasitism: Host–Parasite Interactions

JUAN P. OLANO
PETER F. WELLER
RICHARD L. GUERRANT
DAVID H. WALKER

INTRODUCTION

The relationship between two living organisms can be classified as parasitic, symbiotic, or commensal.[1–3] This same classification scheme can be used to describe relationships between microorganisms and more complex living organisms that act as hosts. The term *parasite* is used here in its broad sense to mean a microorganism interacting with another organism (either vertebrate or invertebrate) in the same ecologic niche.

The following definitions are used in this chapter:

Parasitism: Association between two different organisms wherein one benefits at the expense of the other. All infectious agents causing illness belong to this category.

Commensalism: Association between two organisms in which one derives benefit from the other without causing it any harm. This intermediate category is not uniformly accepted. Often, upon detailed analysis, the relationship turns out to be either parasitic or symbiotic.[2]

Symbiosis or *mutualism:* Both organisms benefit from the relationship. The type of relationship also depends on host factors. For example, bacteria normally inhabiting the bowel live in an apparent commensal or (by inhibiting potential pathogens) symbiotic relationship with humans. However, in cases of cirrhosis with consequent hepatic insufficiency, bacteria can become a dangerous source of ammonia that leads to hepatic encephalopathy. A commensal relationship can be transformed into a potentially harmful one. In malnourished people with borderline deficiencies of B-complex vitamins, clinical beriberi can be triggered by administration of broad-spectrum antibiotics. Normally, in this situation bacteria play a symbiotic role by supplying a significant amount of B-complex vitamins.[2]

MICROBIAL FACTORS

Principles of Microbial Evolution and Classification

The earth is approximately 4.5 to 5 billion years old. There is good fossil evidence of microbial life approximately 3.5 billion years ago. Microbial life (stromatolites) was mostly photosynthetic, unicellular, and anaerobic.[1,4] Eukaryotes, bacteria, and archaea evolved from a still hypothetical universal common ancestor.[5–7] Eukaryotes then evolved into protozoans, metazoans, plants, and animals, as we know them today. Moreover, there is strong evidence that primitive eukaryotic cells established relationships with bacterial organisms that later evolved into cytoplasmic organelles, such as chloroplasts in plants and mitochondria in animals.[8]

To put things into perspective, approximately five-sixths of the history of life on Earth has been exclusively microbial. Human beings appeared on the planet only 2 million years ago as very late newcomers to the biosphere. Life was initially anaerobic, but with the appearance of photosynthetic organisms and chloroplasts, oxygen was released into the atmosphere for the first time.[9] Radiation in the upper atmosphere created the ozone layer from molecular oxygen, which then shielded the earth's surface from dangerous radiation. Nucleic acids were therefore protected from harmful mutations. Organisms had to evolve to survive in the presence of oxygen. A few of the ancient anaerobes were able to survive in the highly oxidant atmosphere, and they represent the anaerobes as we know them today.

The phylogeny of living organisms is based on molecular approaches, particularly analysis of ribosomal RNA.[5,6,10] Because of the antiquity of the protein synthesis machinery, these molecules appear to be excellent evolutionary clocks. For prokaryotes, the 16S subunit of ribosomes appears to be the most useful for classification purposes. The number of microbes in the world is tremendous, and relatively few are pathogenic to humans.

Viruses deserve special comment because of their molecular simplicity and at the same time their importance as human pathogens and as possible agents of hereditary changes and cancer.[11,12] A virus is a genetic element with either DNA or

RNA coated by protein of viral origin and sometimes enveloped by lipid material of host origin. Some viruses have enzymes that are necessary for their replication. The only criterion that these organisms fulfill to be considered living organisms is that of reproduction. They are inert particles when outside of the host cell, and once they have access into a cell they become active and the cell is subverted to produce more viral particles. Sometimes the cell dies in the process, and sometimes the relationship is stable. Viral hosts include bacteria, protozoa, animals, and plants.

The classification of viruses is based on different criteria than the ones used for other organisms. There are multiple ways to classify viruses; a simple one is based on the host they infect. Animal viruses have a more refined classification system that goes as high as families. The major criteria are type of nucleic acid, presence or absence of an envelope, manner of replication, and morphologic characteristics.[12,13]

Simpler forms of self-replicating organisms include virusoids and viroids.[14,15] The former are satellite RNAs that are found encapsidated in the proteins encoded by their helper virus (e.g., hepatitis caused by the hepatitis D virus delta agent in conjunction with hepatitis B virus). The viroids are mostly plant pathogens that consist of single-stranded circular RNA molecules.

The concept of "infectious agent" has been revolutionized by the discovery of proteinaceous infectious agents known as prions. These proteins are responsible for neurodegenerative diseases in animals and humans. The protein particles lack nucleic acids but still are able to reproduce and trigger conformational changes in host proteins, leading to cell death.[16,17]

In contrast, protozoa are nucleated, single-cell organisms that, depending on the species, replicate by means as simple as binary fission (e.g., *Trichomonas*) or as complex as involving multiple sexual and asexual stages in both animal and invertebrate hosts (e.g., malaria). Protozoa include amebae (e.g., *Entamoeba histolytica*), flagellates (e.g., *Giardia lamblia*), ciliates (e.g., *Balantidium coli*), and sporozoa (e.g., *Cryptosporidium*). Even more complex are helminths, which are multicellular metazoan organisms with highly developed internal organs, including alimentary and reproductive tracts. The helminths include nematodes (roundworms), cestodes (tapeworms), and trematodes (flukes). Many helminths have complex life cycles with multiple developmental stages both in the animal host and in intermediate invertebrate or vertebrate hosts. Because of their size, helminths, the macroparasites, are solely extracellular pathogens; because of their prolonged life cycles and generation times, their capacity for genetic alteration is diminished compared to smaller, simpler microbes (the microparasites).

Development of Microbial Virulence

Evolution of Virulence

The traditional view assumes that natural selection would favor evolution toward a benign coexistence between host and parasite.[18,19] In other words, virulence was considered an artifact of recent associations between parasites and their hosts. At the logical end, the relationship would become that of commensalism or mutualism. However, this model does not explain epidemiologic observations that in some cases challenge the traditional view. A modern view of evolution of virulence focuses on the trade-off between the benefits that pathogens accrue through increased exploitation of hosts and the costs that result from any effects of disease that reduce transmission to susceptible hosts.[19,20] From this point of view, virulence could be the evolved as well as the primitive stage of the association between host and parasite, depending on the development of enhanced rather than reduced transmission.

According to Levin[19] and Levin and Svanborg-Eden,[20] there are three alternative models to explain evolution of a microparasite's virulence: direct selection, coincidental evolution, and short-sighted within-host selection. The direct selection model states that there is a direct relationship between the parasite's virulence and its rate of infectious transmission. The best documented and often cited example is that of the dramatic changes in virulence that the myxoma virus underwent after being released into the wild in Australia to "control" the population of wild rabbits. In the beginning, rabbit mortality and viral transmission rates were high. As the population of rabbits was decimated, the virulence of the virus decreased and its rate of transmission actually increased. This outcome is explained by the longer survival and duration of the period of shedding of the virus. At the same time, more resistant rabbits increased in number due to the selection process.[21]

According to the coincidental evolution model, the factors responsible for the virulence of a microparasite evolved for some purpose other than to provide the parasite with some advantage within a host or for its transmission to other hosts. Clostridial toxins are good examples in this category. There is no beneficial reason to kill a human host who became infected by *Clostridium tetani* spores from soil in order for the parasite to survive. They are mostly soil bacteria and do not need humans for their survival.[19]

Short-sighted within-host evolution posits that the parasites responsible for the morbidity and mortality of the host are selected for as a consequence of within-host evolution since that produces a local advantage for their survival within the host. The host dies and the rate of transmission would decrease. This is an example of evolutionary myopia in which the long-term consequences of killing a host would not matter to the parasite.[22,23] Natural selection is a local phenomenon that happens at a given time and place and goes perfectly with this model. Bacteria such as *Neisseria meningitidis* that normally live attached to human pharyngeal epithelial cells sometimes invade the central nervous system (CNS) and kill the host. Their replication in the CNS is favored since competition is low and defenses are not as abundant as in the tonsillar areas.[19]

The generation times of mammalian hosts are much longer than those of microorganisms. Therefore, genetic mutations in these hosts, on which natural selection acts, take longer to become part of a large population. Nevertheless, there is evidence that specific microorganisms can exert selective pressure on the gene pool of human hosts. The evidence is strongest for the potentially lethal infections caused by falciparum malaria. In regions of the world where falciparum malaria is endemic, including Africa, there is a high prevalence of genetic mutations that alter hemoglobin structure or synthesis. Falciparum malaria parasites cannot survive in the presence of the mutated forms of hemoglobin, and therefore hosts with specific genetic hemoglobinopathies (the α- and β-thalassemias and hemoglobins S, C, and E) are spared the lethal consequences of falciparum malaria.[24] The selective pressure of malaria on human gene expression is not confined solely to affecting erythrocytes but also likely involves the immune system, cytokines, and other systems.[25]

Other Modes of Altering Virulence and Pathogenicity

Although the selective pressures of evolution generally exert changes over a multitude of centuries, there are other mechanisms that may more rapidly alter microbial pathogenicity, virulence, and drug susceptibility. The expression of mutated genes in microorganisms is heightened when there are greater numbers of organisms and their generation times are brief. Hence, altered gene expression in helminths will be slow to be expressed, whereas in microparasites genetic alterations will be likely to develop. For mycobacterial infections, large numbers of bacilli that persist for a long time facilitate the genetic emergence of drug resistance to a single agent, and this likelihood underlies the principle of using more than a single drug to treat tuberculosis. Even more rapidly dividing microparasites can develop genetic alterations, and this is especially true when the fidelity of genetic replication is poor. This is prominent in human immunodeficiency virus type 1 (HIV-1), whose reverse transcriptase lacks a 3′ exonuclease proofreading activity.[26] Alterations in cell tropism, pathogenicity, and drug sensitivity are frequent in HIV-1 infections. Again, several antiviral agents must be employed concomitantly to circumvent the highly frequent mutations that alter drug susceptibility in HIV-1 strains.

In addition to their own genetic material, many classes of microparasites either contain or are capable of acquiring transferable genetic elements in the form of plasmids, transposons, or bacteriophages. Bacterial virulence factors that are encoded by plasmids include the heat-stable and heat-labile enterotoxins of *Escherichia coli*, the toxins of *Shigella* and enteroinvasive *E. coli*, and the neurotoxin of tetanus. Phage-encoded bacterial virulence determinants include diphtheria toxin, botulinum neurotoxin, and the Shiga-like toxins of enterohemorrhagic *E. coli*. These transferable genetic elements also provide a means for the spread of resistance to antibacterial drugs, an increasing problem in all regions of the world.[27]

Microorganisms and Their Impact on Human Affairs

The overall influence of microorganisms on our daily lives is beneficial. Disease is not the rule with microorganisms, and most of them coexist with the rest of the species in the biosphere without causing any harm to the higher organisms.[1] The beneficial aspects of microbes are innumerable, including innate resistance due to normal flora, antibiotic production, utilization in the dairy and biotechnology industries, enhancement of plant survival due to nitrogen-fixing bacteria, production of natural gas by methanogenic bacteria, and the degradation of crude oil.[1] The impact of infectious diseases on humans includes acute or chronic illness of individuals, widespread effects on infected populations, and comorbid influences on nutrition and development.

Causes of Acute or Chronic Infections in Individuals

One obvious impact of an infectious disease is on the individual infected. Hence, in any region of the world independent of other infectious diseases or malnutrition, the acute infection will cause morbidity and potential mortality in the infected human host. Among otherwise healthy people, the immediate impact of the infection is the symptomatic acute illness. For some infections that have prolonged courses, their impact may also continue over many years. Chronic infections include most of those caused by helminthic parasites, which characteristically live for years; persisting mycobacterial infections; and retroviral infections (HIV-1, HIV-2, and human T-cell lymphotropic virus type 1). Finally, the sequelae of some infections can include the development of neoplasms. Examples include hepatomas associated with chronic hepatitis B and C viral infections, bladder tumors with urinary schistosomiasis, cholangiocarcinomas with biliary fluke infections, and gastric adenocarcinomas and lymphomas associated with *Helicobacter pylori* infections.

Causes of Widespread Infections in Populations

Infectious diseases may affect not only individuals but also large groups of people or entire populations due to epidemic or highly endemic transmission. Throughout human history, a few microorganisms have been responsible for great epidemics and massive numbers of dead or crippled people as a result of infections spreading locally or throughout the world.[28–31] Typhus has had a great impact. Typhus has been associated almost always with situations that involve overcrowding, famine, war, natural disasters, and poverty. The outcomes of several European wars were affected by the morbidity and mortality inflicted by typhus or other diseases on the military. Typhus epidemics were common during the world wars of the 20th century and in the concentration camps where the ecological conditions were ideal for such a disease to spread.[30] Today, typhus and other rickettsioses are still public health problems in some countries, but overall the disease was brought under control after its life cycle was described and antibiotics, insecticides, and public health measures became available.[30]

Bubonic plague, caused by *Yersinia pestis*, is another disease that has shaped history, especially in Europe during the Middle Ages.[31] Millions of people were affected by pandemics that spread throughout the continent. Tuberculosis, smallpox, and measles had a tremendous effect on the native populations of the Americas after Columbus's voyages to the New World. It has been estimated that 90% of the population in Mexico was killed by these pathogens, which were novel to the native residents.

Acquired immunodeficiency syndrome (AIDS) represents the modern pandemic that will continue to affect human history for at least decades. Other examples are cholera and influenza, which are capable of causing pandemics.[32]

In addition to widespread disease caused by epidemic spread of infections, some infectious diseases, because of their highly endemic prevalence in populations, continue to affect large segments of the world's population. These include enteric and respiratory infections, measles, malaria (which still causes 1 to 2 million deaths per year, especially on the African continent), and tuberculosis (which has become the number one killer in the world). Schistosomiasis is an important disease, affecting more than 200 million people worldwide. Furthermore, even the staggering mortality and morbidity of these tropical infectious diseases do not control populations but are associated with population overgrowth. This is true not only across the different countries of the world but also throughout the history of developed countries. Thus, the impact of these infections is not solely on the individual but, because of their highly endemic or epidemic occurrence, on populations. This has consequences on economic, political, and social functioning of entire societies.[33]

Polyparasitism and Effects on Nutrition and Growth

In an otherwise healthy and fully nourished person, a new infection is likely to be the only active infection in that person. In contrast, in regions where enteric and other infections are highly prevalent because of inadequate sanitation and poor socioeconomic conditions, adults and especially children may harbor several infections or be subject to repeated episodes of new enteric pathogens. Thus, the polyparasitism of multiple concurrent or recurrent infections adds a new dimension to the impact of acute infections, not often encountered in developed countries.

Moreover, the subclinical impact of a number of tropical infectious diseases is beginning to become apparent. Increasing data suggest that even "asymptomatic" giardial,[34] cryptosporidial,[35] and enteroaggregative *E. coli*[36] infections may be very important in predisposing to malnutrition, thus reflecting a clinically important impact, even in the absence of overt clinical disease such as diarrhea. Likewise, chronic intestinal helminth infections also have a major impact on nutrition in those with already marginal nutrition. Anthelmintic therapy in these children, who lack symptomatic infections, has led to increases in growth, exercise tolerance, and scholastic performance.[37,38]

Principles of Microbial Metabolism

Microbes are present in every ecosystem of the planet. Therefore, their metabolic pathways are as varied as their ecosystems. Based on the source of energy, they are subdivided into phototrophs (light-derived energy), lithotrophs (inorganic compound-derived energy), and heterotrophs (organic compound-derived energy). Based on the carbon source, microorganisms are either autotrophs (inorganic carbon) or heterotrophs (organic carbon).[1,7] In order to obtain energy from nutrients, organisms need to oxidize food and pass electrons through a chain of electron transporters until they are finally accepted by an oxidizing substance such as oxygen. Some bacteria evolved well before oxygen was present in the earth's atmosphere, and they still use electron acceptors other than oxygen (e.g., H_2S and NO_3). These are anaerobes, and they range from obligate anaerobes to aerotolerant, microaerophilic, and facultative organisms. Most human pathogens are heterotrophs and range from strict anaerobes to obligate aerobes in regard to utilization of oxygen as the final electron acceptor.

MICROBIAL INTERACTIONS WITH HUMAN HOSTS

Just as microorganisms have evolved over centuries or longer, mammalian hosts have evolved to contain and limit the deleterious consequences of infections with diverse microbes. The human immune system is composed of multiple elements, including those of innate immunity and those of adaptive immunity. Many of the elements of innate immunity are more primitive and found in invertebrate organisms, whereas the adaptive immune responses have evolved further in vertebrate hosts. Microorganisms that successfully infect human hosts must, at least in the short term, overcome elements of the host immune system, which then may react further to attempt to control these infections.

Microorganisms that infect humans are exogenous to the host and must colonize or penetrate epithelial barriers to gain access to the host. Except for infections acquired during the intrauterine period, infectious agents must bridge host epithelial surfaces, the keratinized epithelium of the skin, or the mucosal epithelium of the respiratory, gastrointestinal, or genitourinary tracts. Ultimately, there are four types of microbial localization in the host (Fig. 1-1). Some microbes will enter intracellular sites either within the cytoplasm or within vesicular or vacuolar compartments in cells. Other microbes remain extracellular, either at epithelial surfaces or within the host in the blood, lymph, or tissues.

Interactions at Epithelial Barrier Surfaces

The barrier functions occurring at epithelial surfaces are part of the innate host defenses and are important in determining the outcome of interactions of potential pathogens with the host. Interactions at epithelial barriers involved in defense against external microbes include not only the physical properties of the epithelial surfaces but also the overlying mucous phase, the ciliated or other propulsive activities facilitating microbe clearance, and the normal microbial flora.

Normal Flora

Vertebrate warm-blooded organisms, such as humans, are an ideal site for the survival of many microbes and provide

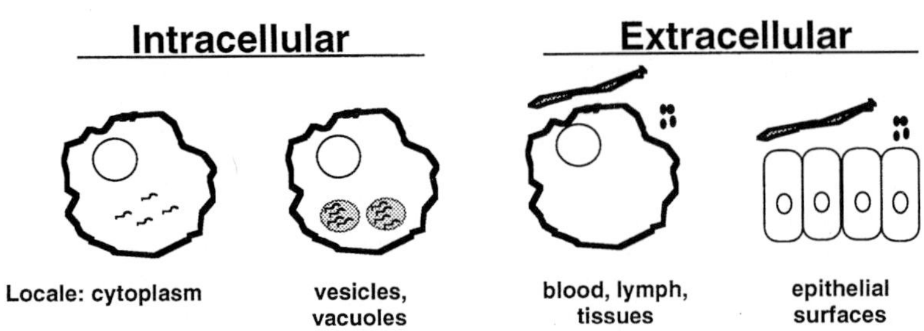

FIGURE 1-1 Microbial localization.

a rich source of organic material and a constant temperature and pH. Microbes coexist with us in and on our bodies, especially on epithelial surfaces where there is contact with the outside world, such as the bowel, upper respiratory tract, mouth, skin, and distal portions of the genitourinary tract.[1,2,39] Most of these microorganisms are highly adapted to live with us and do not cause any harm. The presence of the same type of microorganisms at a particular site in the absence of disease is called colonization. Normal colonizing microbial flora help to limit access by potentially pathogenic microorganisms. One condition predisposing to infection is the alteration of the normal epithelial flora, as occurs with antibiotic therapy, since this may allow for the proliferation of pathogenic organisms normally held in balance by the endogenous normal microbial flora. Examples include *Candida* vaginitis or the development of pseudomembranous colitis due to toxigenic *Clostridium difficile*, which may complicate antibiotic therapy.

Adhesion to the Epithelium

Microorganisms maintain themselves in or on their host by adhesion to cells or the extracellular matrix. Adhesins are encoded by chromosomal genes, plasmids, or phages.[40] They are usually divided into fimbrial and afimbrial adhesins.[41] Fimbrial adhesins are present in organisms such as *Neisseria gonorrhoeae* and are in part responsible for the attachment to genitourinary tract epithelium, preventing the bacteria from being washed out by the urine stream.[42] An example of an afimbrial adhesin is the filamentous hemagglutinin of *Bordetella pertussis*, which is responsible for the attachment of *B. pertussis* to epithelial cells in the respiratory tract.[43] Adhesins attach to receptors in the host. These receptors include proteins, glycolipids, and carbohydrates exposed on the surface of cells or in the extracellular matrix.[40] Integrins are one class of proteins present on eukaryotic cell surfaces that can serve as bacterial receptors.[40] *Helicobacter pylori* binds to Lewis blood group antigen present in the gastric epithelium.[44] *Neisseria* has a ligand that binds to CD66 molecules on epithelial cells.

Some pathogens have even more evolved interactions with the host and activate signal transduction mechanisms in the host cell, which in turn upregulate other molecules that aid in the adhesion process.[2,40] Certain strains of enteropathogenic *E. coli* possess type III secretion or contact-mediated systems.[45] In such cases, the secretion and synthesis of virulence factors is modulated by contact with host surfaces. The systems are complex (more than 20 genes are involved) and have not been elucidated completely at the molecular level.[46,47]

Penetration of the Epithelial Barriers

Some microbes do not have the means to penetrate skin barriers and are only able to gain access through bites produced by arthropods (e.g., rickettsiae, arboviruses, plasmodia, and filariae).[48,49] In such cases, microbes may be introduced by direct inoculation (e.g., rickettsiae, arboviruses, and plasmodia) or may gain access by migrating through the puncture site (filariae). Other microbes (e.g., skin bacteria and fungi) depend on mechanical disruption of the skin (e.g., due to burns, trauma, or intravenous catheters) to invade deeper structures.[50] Still others invade when defenses on mucosal surfaces are lowered due to combined local or generalized immunosuppression and altered mucosal integrity (mucositis) due to chemotherapy or malnutrition (e.g., *Candida* spp. and anaerobic and other enteric bacteria in the bowel). Some microbes do not invade tissues at all and affect the host locally and systemically by liberating toxins at the site of colonization (e.g., diphtheria exotoxin).[40]

For enteric pathogens, some, including poliovirus, *Salmonella typhimurium, Salmonella typhi, Campylobacter jejuni, Yersinia enterocolitica,* and *Yersinia pseudotuberculosis*, gain access to the host across the intestinal epithelium by utilizing uptake in specialized epithelial M cells.[51] Internalization of some microorganisms is also achieved through other mechanisms, such as sequential "zipper-like" encircling of the organisms triggered by bacterial ligands and cellular receptors, as occurs in infections caused by *Listeria monocytogenes.*[40] The trigger mechanism of the bacteria induces massive rearrangements of cytoskeletal proteins such as actin, which results in membrane ruffles, as occurs with shigellosis and salmonellosis.[40]

In the genitourinary tract, invasion of some microbes (e.g., HIV-1) is facilitated by mucosal erosions caused by other infectious agents.[52]

Spread from the Portal of Entry

Once the organisms gain access to the body after overcoming the first lines of defense, they either spread to other sites of the body or reproduce locally and often invade surrounding tissues. Local spread is facilitated by a number of factors, including collagenases, hyaluronidases, fibrinolysis, and other enzymes. They are produced by a wide range of organisms, and the role of these enzymes in invasion is, in some cases, controversial.[2]

Lymphatic spread occurs in most cases once the organisms gain access to subepithelial tissues or serosal surfaces. Lymphatic vessels are distributed in most tissues of the body, with few exceptions such as the brain. Lymph is carried by lymphatic vessels to regional lymph nodes, where it circulates through the node and eventually returns to the systemic circulation through the thoracic duct and the great lymphatic vein. One to three liters of lymph is returned to the systemic circulation every day. Most pathogens are filtered in lymph nodes before reaching the systemic circulation, but some actually reproduce either in the endothelium of lymphatic vessels (e.g., *Mycobacterium leprae*)[2,53] or in tissue macrophages present in the lymph nodes (e.g., *Y. pestis* and *Brucella* spp.) or lymphocytes (HIV and herpesviruses, including Epstein–Barr virus).[54] Some organisms reach the systemic circulation after overwhelming the defenses in the lymph nodes (e.g., *Bacillus anthracis* and *Y. pestis*).

Microorganisms carried in the blood are transported either extracellularly (e.g., most of those causing bacteremia) or intracellularly. Intracellular pathogens are carried by red blood cells (e.g., *Plasmodium*, *Babesia*, Colorado tick fever virus, and *Bartonella*), monocytes (e.g., measles virus, cytomegalovirus, and *Toxoplasma*), or neutrophils (e.g., *Anaplasma phagcytophilum*, *Ehrlichia ewingii*, and some pyogenic bacteria).[2,55]

Once in the blood, by initial lymphatic or hematogenous spread, the microorganisms have access to virtually any site in the body. However, some pathogens exhibit tropism for certain tissues. This tropism depends on multiple factors, including the anatomy of the microcirculation in a given tissue (fenestrated capillaries vs continuous endothelial lining), receptors present on certain endothelial cells, and the presence of mononuclear phagocytic cells in organs such as bone marrow, liver, and spleen.[2] Other less common routes of spread include peripheral nerves (e.g., rabies and varicella-zoster virus), cerebrospinal fluid (after the organisms traverse the blood–brain barrier), and serosal cavities.

Localization in the Host

Microbes that have gained access to the host at or through epithelial barriers then, depending on the properties and size of the pathogens, either have the capacity to seek intracellular sites or remain extracellular (see Fig. 1-1). Mechanisms of host immune responses to the microorganisms vary depending on their sites of localization.

Intracellular Localization

Specific microorganisms use highly developed processes to gain access to and survive within host cells. The microorganisms may be either in the cytoplasm or within vesicular or vacuolar compartments of targeted cells.

Targeting and penetration of cells is governed by the interactions of microbial surface proteins that may engage host cell molecules that function as receptors for the microbial ligands. The entry of malarial parasites into erythrocytes is a good example, and the nature of the erythrocyte receptors used by different malarial parasite species governs which red blood cells are infected. *Plasmodium vivax* binds to the Duffy blood group antigens present on some people's red blood cell membranes. The expression of the Duffy blood group antigen is genetically determined, and this antigen is present mostly in whites and Asians and largely absent in blacks of sub-Saharan African ancestry.[56–59] This genetic absence of a receptor on red blood cells required for vivax malaria's survival explains why vivax malaria is rare in regions of Africa. *Plasmodium vivax* also exhibits a characteristic restriction in the age of erythrocytes it infects. Only young red blood cells and reticulocytes are susceptible to infection, even though the Duffy blood group antigen is present on red blood cells of all ages. The basis for this restriction to younger red blood cells also rests with receptor-mediated limitations. *Plasmodium vivax* parasites contain reticulocyte binding proteins, which recognize and bind to reticulocyte-specific antigens on the red blood cell surface.[60,61] Thus, host cell receptor–microbial ligand interactions have an impact on the geographic range of infections based on host genetic differences in requisite receptor expression and on the specific cells that a microbe may enter.

Another example of the intricacies of microbe-receptor interactions has been recognized with HIV-1. Although CD4 is the primary cellular receptor for HIV entry, binding to CD4 alone is not sufficient for entry of HIV-1 into cells. Cellular coreceptors that are members of the chemokine receptor family of seven-transmembrane G protein–coupled molecules are also important. T-cell tropic strains use the CXCR-4 chemokine receptor and macrophage tropic HIV-1 strains use the CCR-3 and CCR-5 chemokine receptors as coreceptors in concert with CD4. The differences among strains of HIV-1 in their capacities to bind to different chemokine receptor–coreceptors may help explain differences in cell tropism and pathogenicity, the lack of infectability of nonprimate cells, and, for those with genetically altered coreceptors, the apparent resistance to HIV-1 infection of some individuals.[62–65]

Typical of those etiologic agents that have an intracellular localization are viruses. The entry of these agents into cells is increasingly recognized to be dependent on their interactions with specific host cell proteins that act as their "receptors." For instance, host cell molecules that function as viral receptors include multiple isoforms of membrane cofactor protein (CD46), a complement regulatory protein, for measles; the integrin, intracellular adhesion molecule-1 (ICAM-1), for rhinovirus; erythrocyte P antigen for parvovirus B19; and the C3d complement receptor (CR2) for Epstein–Barr virus.[66–69]

Microbes that exist principally within the cytoplasm are sequestered from many immune response mechanisms active on extracellular pathogens, including antibody and phagocytic cells. Viral intracellular proteins will be processed and displayed with class I major histocompatibility complex (MHC) proteins, which enable CD8 cytotoxic T cells to recognize and kill the virally infected cell.

Other microbes are internalized within phagocytic cells, especially macrophages. Once internalized in host cells, organisms such as *Salmonella*, *Mycobacterium*, *Chlamydia*, and *Legionella* use an extraordinary assortment of mechanisms to prevent their phagocytic vacuole from fusing with the host cells' acidifying lysosomes.[70–72] For some parasites, the intracellular environment is an important determinant of parasitism. For example, *Leishmania* and *Coxiella* (unlike other pathogens) benefit from the acidic environment of the macrophage phagolysosome. *Leishmania* use the proton gradient across the lysosome to drive the energy-dependent uptake of two important substrates: glucose and proline.[73] Thus, *Leishmania* amastigotes actually survive in the macrophage phagolysosome because they benefit from its proton gradient and because they avoid activating the processes that normally kill ingested microorganisms. Leishmanial lipophosphoglycan inhibits the action of β-galactosidase, chelates calcium, inhibits protein kinase C and the oxidative burst, and may scavenge toxic oxygen metabolites.[74]

Conversely, other intracellular pathogens such as *Toxoplasma gondii* survive within the macrophage by using an alternative pathway of entry that avoids fusion of the parasitophorous vacuole with lysosomes.[71,75] In contrast, dead or antibody-coated *T. gondii* enter via the Fc receptor and are routed to a different intracellular compartment, which fuses with the lysosome, and are then killed in the phagolysosome.[71,76]

Other organisms, such as *Shigella*, *Listeria*, and *Rickettsia*, breach their vacuolar membrane to multiply freely in the cytoplasm and may also usurp host cellular actin to propel their further spread to neighboring cells, continuing to exploit their intracellular sanctuary.[77–79]

Immune responses against microbes within macrophages rely heavily on class II MHC-mediated presentation of host antigenic peptides to T helper 1 (Th1) types of CD4+ T cells, which then augment the microbicidal activities of the macrophages.

Extracellular Localization

Some types of microbes that remain extracellular typically reside at epithelial surfaces, including bacteria such as *N. gonorrhoeae*, *H. pylori*, *Vibrio cholerae*, and *E. coli*, and helminths such as adult *Ascaris lumbricoides*, hookworms, and *Trichuris trichiura*. Mucosal immune responses, including IgA and leukocytes, participate in host immune reactions to these pathogens.

Other microbes that survive extracellularly are present within the blood, lymph, or tissues of the host, and these organisms include fungi, viruses, bacteria, protozoa, and notably the helminths. Multicellular helminths, due to their large size, remain forever extracellularly and may be found in the blood (e.g., microfilariae), lymph (adult lymphatic filarial worms), tissues (migrating larvae and adult stages of some helminths), and cerebrospinal fluid. Host defense against extracellular pathogens uses antibodies, complement, phagocytic cells, and, for helminths, IgE, eosinophils, and mast cells.[80]

Tissue Damage

There are multiple mechanisms by which microbes inflict damage on host tissues.

Direct Damage or Alteration of Host Cell Function

Host cells can be killed directly by the infectious agent, as in some viral or bacterial infections that are highly cytopathic (e.g., yellow fever virus in hepatocytes and *Salmonella* in macrophages).[81,82] Some microorganisms multiply intracellularly until the cell bursts and dies (e.g., *Rickettsia prowazekii*).[30] Some bacteria, viruses, and other parasites, such as *Shigella*, HIV-1, and *Listeria*, can induce apoptosis of host cells.[54,83,84] Apoptosis is triggered by different mechanisms, such as activation of the interleukin-converting enzyme (ICE) pathway.[85,86] This form of programmed cell death is probably more widespread as a mechanism of cell death in infectious diseases than previously thought.

Damage is sometimes caused by toxins secreted by bacterial cells (exotoxins). In this case, bacteria can either invade host tissues or colonize mucosal sites and then release toxins at the mucosal site that are absorbed systemically and cause distant damage.[87] Exotoxins can act through different pathways that damage the components of the cell membranes such as phospholipids[88] or affect signaling pathways (e.g., *V. cholerae*).[40,89] Other exotoxins, such as streptolysins and listeriolysins, alter membrane permeability. Still others, such as exfoliatin (e.g., *Staphylococcus aureus*) and elastase (e.g., *Pseudomonas* spp.), are capable of degrading extracellular elements.[2] Some toxins are translocated to the intracellular environment, where they affect multiple enzymatic systems. These toxins are classified according to their enzymatic activity, such as adenosine diphosphate (ADP) ribosyl transferase (e.g., diphtheria toxin, *P. aeruginosa* exotoxin A, and pertussis toxin), depurinase (e.g., Shiga toxin), adenylate cyclase (e.g., pertussis hemolysin and anthrax edema factor), and zinc protease (e.g., tetanus).[89] The end result ranges from blockade of protein synthesis and cell death or blockade of exocytosis (especially CNS neurotransmitters at the synaptic cleft)[90,91] to increases of cyclic adenosine monophosphate (AMP) or cyclic guanosine monophosphate (GMP) and changes in cell permeability.[89] Still other organisms, such as *C. difficile*, produce toxins that change basic cell signaling transducers such as Rho to alter cell function or affect their spread. Finally, organisms can interact with host cell or microbial transcriptional regulation of genes (such as iron binding proteins for uropathogenic *E. coli*[87,92]) or cytokine release (such as *H. pylori* or enteroaggregative *E. coli*[36,93–95]) to enhance their survival or elicit pathogenic responses. The evolutionary advantages to a microbe of its remarkable array of traits we call "virulence" hold many of the clues to their control, if we can but truly understand them.

Endotoxins are a subset of lipopolysaccharides present in the outer membrane of gram-negative bacteria that can trigger a wide variety of responses in the host, including massive cytokine release leading to hypotension and shock.[96,97] These deleterious effects occur with high-grade invasion of the blood by gram-negative bacteria, including enteric gram-negative bacteremias and meningococcemia.

Indirect Damage

Damage to the host may also develop as a consequence of immune reactions to the infectious agents. One scheme for classifying immunopathologic responses divides the reactions into four types based on the elements of the immune response involved.[98]

Type I reactions involve elements of strong Th2 responses that lead to increased IgE, eosinophilia, and eosinophil and mast cell activation. Adverse reactions of this type include the development of urticaria (with several helminthic parasites), the occurrence of potentially life-threatening anaphylactic shock in IgE-mediated mast cell degranulation (e.g., triggered by systemic release of antigens from echinococcal cysts[99]), and exuberant eosinophilic infiltration of tissues due to migrating helminth larvae (e.g., Löffler's pneumonia with the pulmonary migration of *Ascaris* larvae).

Type II reactions are also dependent on elements of Th2 cell responses that lead to increased IgM and then IgG antibodies directed toward the infectious agents. These antibodies, if cross-reactive with host antigens, may lead to complement-mediated cytotoxicity or antibody-dependent cell-mediated cytotoxicity by natural killer cells, which have Fc receptors. An example of this type of immunopathologic response is the uncommon hemolytic anemia associated with *Mycoplasma pneumoniae* infection that is mediated by complement-induced hemolysis triggered by IgM (cold agglutinin) antibodies against erythrocyte I antigen.

Type III reactions are caused by the deposition of immune complexes. When neither antibody nor antigen is present in excess of one another, the complexing of antibodies with soluble antigen results in the formation of immune complexes that may cause disease. This may develop acutely as antibody titers rise in the presence of microbial antigens, causing the syndrome of serum sickness. In addition, when soluble antigen is persistently abundant, sustained formation of immune complexes develops, leading to chronic immune complex-mediated tissue damage (especially glomerulonephritis), as found in subacute bacterial endocarditis, chronic hepatitis B antigenemia, and chronic *Plasmodium malariae* infections.[100]

Type IV reactions include adverse reactions mediated by macrophages and cytotoxic T cells. Examples are damage caused by granulomas in leprosy, tuberculosis, tertiary syphilis, and fungal infections. Likewise, granulomas developing around schistosomal eggs, depending on their location, may cause ureteral obstruction or hepatic presinusoidal lesions. Other deleterious inflammatory reactions in this category are mediated by parasite-elicited host cytokines, such as the hepatic fibrosis elicited by schistosomal eggs.

IMMUNE INTERACTIONS

Immune Evasion

The human immune system has evolved in concert with microbes and is very sophisticated, especially with regard to host defenses against microbes, but the system is not perfect. Interactions of the immune system with microbes are an ongoing affair. Microbes have a high mutation rate compared to human beings. Microbes have evolved a diversity of mechanisms that can enable microorganisms to subvert immediate immunologically mediated elimination. Persistence within the host is necessary for the propagation of some parasites.

There are multiple mechanisms by which microbes can persist in the body and evade the immune system. *Tolerance* is defined as specific reduction in the response of the immune system to a given antigen.[101,102] In the case of transplacental infection, the fetus develops a certain degree of tolerance to antigens to which it is exposed. The immune system of fetuses is rather incompletely developed in utero, and microorganisms survive easily. Cytomegalovirus infects the fetus transplacentally and produces extensive damage to multiple tissues. After delivery, infants continue shedding virions for weeks to months because they are unable to destroy the virus. Other mechanisms include the production of superantigens that stimulate a large population of T cells, which then become deleted if the encounter occurs during early development. Exposure to massive amounts of antigen in the circulation can also lead to tolerance.[2,98] Immunosuppression is a well-demonstrated phenomenon that occurs during certain infections caused by viruses, bacteria, protozoa, and helminths. These infections usually involve the lymphoid tissues and macrophages and hamper the immune response.

Intracellular pathogens that are able to spread from cell to cell without exposure to the extracellular compartment can avoid exposure to some elements of the immune system. In other cases, pathogens reside in sites relatively inaccessible to the immune system, such as glandular luminal spaces or kidney tubules. In many infections, antibodies are produced but do not effect microbial killing. Sometimes, antibody avidity is low, the epitopes against which the antibody is directed are not critical to the microorganism's survival, or the mechanism of immune elimination is not antibody dependent.[2]

Other microorganisms have developed means of counteracting specific elements of immune responses, such as production of an IgA-degrading enzyme, IgAase, by certain strains of *N. gonorrhoeae*.[103] Some strains of amebae also produce proteases that destroy complement.[2] Reactivation of infections in old age due to waning immunity has been well demonstrated in cases of tuberculosis and varicella-zoster virus, allowing transmission to new hosts.

One well-studied mechanism of immune evasion is the capability of changing the antigenic structure by genetic mutation or by programmed sequential expression of genes encoding different surface antigens.[104]Antigenic drift and recombination between influenzaviruses affecting humans and animals are well documented. *Borrelia recurrentis* and *Trypanosoma gambiense* are also capable of changing their surface antigens after antibodies control the initial bloodstream infection.[105,106] The new antigens are not recognized by the antibodies, allowing relapse of the infection. Parasites in which sexual reproduction is possible benefit enormously.[107] Genetic variability introduced by crossing over during meiotic divisions is much greater than the variability introduced by asexual reproduction. As many as four crossovers on a single pair of chromosomes have been demonstrated in *P. falciparum*.[108]

Microparasites also have multiple mechanisms by which they can evade the initial line of defense provided by phagocytes. These strategies include killing of the phagocyte (e.g., *Streptococcus pyogenes* and *Entamoeba histolytica*), inhibition of chemotaxis (e.g., *Clostridium perfringens*), decreased internalization of microbes by phagocytic cells (e.g., *T. gondii*), inhibition of opsonins (e.g., *Treponema pallidum*), inhibition of phagolysosome fusion (e.g., *M. leprae* and *Mycobacterium tuberculosis*), and escape from the phagosome into the cytoplasm (e.g., *Rickettsia* spp., *Trypanosoma cruzi*, and *Listeria*).[2,40,70,87] With cell-to-cell spread, microorganisms may be minimally exposed to complement, antibodies, or phagocytes in the extracellular or intravascular spaces.[77,78] Rickettsial infections spread from cell to cell throughout the infected foci in the endothelial layer of the microvasculature.[77,78,89]

Macroparasites, the helminths, have evolved diverse mechanisms that enable them to survive in vivo.[80] Characteristically, helminths live for months to years in infected hosts within the lumen of the bowel, within tissues, or in the blood or lymphatic vessels. Many helminths are in intimate and recurring contact with all elements of the immune system. As a consequence of their size, helminthic worms do not use intracellular mechanisms to evade immune responses but have evolved a number of capabilities that permit their survival. For instance, interference with antigen processing has been well documented in animal models and patients infected with the filarial nematodes *Brugia malayi* and *Onchocerca volvulus*. These helminths produce a family of proteins called the cystatins that are capable of inhibiting proteases responsible for antigen degradation and subsequent presentation through MHC class II pathways in antigen-presenting cells. These proteins are also capable of modulating T cell proliferation and elicit upregulation of IL-10 expression. Other modulators include helminthic derivatives of arachidonic acid such as lipoxin A4, which is capable of blocking production of IL-12 in dendritic cells. Helminthic prostaglandins can also inhibit IL-12 production by dendritic cells. Since helminths have very complex genomes (~21,000 protein encoding genes in some of them), they are capable of producing a large variety of proteins. Some of them are cytokines and related proteins also capable of modulating the host immune response to their advantage. For example, *B. malayi* has been shown to express transforming growth factor (TGF)-β-like proteins capable of binding TGF-β human receptors. Other cytokines include macrophage-migration inhibition factors produced by several nematodes including *B. malayi*. Blockade of effector mechanisms has also been demonstrated in some helminth infections, including proteases that target effector molecules such as eotaxin. Neutrophil proteases can also be inhibited by serpins.

THE EFFECTS OF INFECTIONS ON POPULATIONS

Epidemiology is the study of diseases in populations. Pathogens exist in nature because they reproduce and spread to new hosts. One of the main purposes of epidemiology is the study of how the infectious agent is maintained in nature so that adequate measures can be taken to control the disease.[1,2,109]

Principles of Transmission

The transfer of pathogens in communities involves shedding or excretion of the infectious agent from the host and travel to and entry into a susceptible host. Some organisms are extremely sensitive to environmental conditions such as drying or exposure to sunlight and require close contact between hosts to survive transmission (e.g., *Mycoplasma* spp.). Others are more resistant and can travel to a susceptible host by fomites (e.g., towels, doorknobs, toys, and gloves), vehicles (e.g., food or water), or vectors (e.g., vertebrate animals and arthropods). Transmission of particular diseases can be suspected on the basis of age-specific incidence, geographic and seasonal patterns, and other demographic characteristics. For example, diseases limited to a certain geographic area and season suggest the presence of a vector in the life cycle that determines transmission in that particular region.[1,110]

The way epidemics spread through communities gives some clues to the manner of transmission of an infectious agent.[1,109] Food-borne epidemics are usually explosive, peak in a few days to weeks, and wane abruptly. A large segment of the population is exposed to a common source of infection. In outbreaks involving person-to-person transmission, the number of cases increases slowly, and the disease affects a certain number of susceptible people until it reaches a communicable threshold, after which the number of cases increases slightly faster. If populations are small, the organism dies out before spreading to large segments of the community; that is, a highly communicable stage is never reached.

Other important concepts are those of horizontal and vertical transmission. Horizontal transmission refers to spread of infection from individual to individual in a given population. In contrast, vertical transmission refers to spread of infectious agents from parent to offspring. The latter is important for the maintenance of some arboviruses and rickettsial organisms in their arthropod hosts. They are transmitted transovarially from the female arthropod vector to its offspring. Human pathogens, such as *T. pallidum*, cytomegalovirus, hepatitis B virus, and HIV-1, are also transmitted vertically.

Herd immunity is another important epidemiologic concept. Herd immunity refers to the resistance of a population to a particular disease as a group. For this to occur, a critical proportion of the population must be immune to the pathogen, and once that critical number is reached the rest of the population is protected against the disease. The critical proportion depends on the pathogen and is greater for highly infectious pathogens with long incubation periods and lower for less transmissible pathogens with short incubation periods. For smallpox, the required proportion for herd immunity is approximately 95% and for polio it is 70%. Some diseases have temporal cycles and appear every few years due to variations in herd immunity.[1,28,109,110]

Principles of Nosocomial Infections

These are infections acquired in hospitals and are associated with multiple factors, including immunosuppression (either iatrogenic or due to disease), the presence of infected or colonized patients nearby, transmission by personnel from patient to patient (as fomites or as carriers), invasive procedures that bypass host defense barriers, and the high frequency of antibiotic resistance in the hospital environment. These diseases usually have a more serious outcome than diseases occurring in the community. Some of the etiologic agents are *Pseudomonas aeruginosa*, nearly all Enterobacteriaceae, *C. difficile*, *Enterococcus*, and *S. aureus*.

Principles of Control of Infectious Disease Outbreaks

Control measures can focus on reservoirs (slaughter of infected animals and vaccination). Some pathogens have a human reservoir, and control measures are not as simple and require effective treatment, vaccines, or difficult behavioral changes.[1,110] One safeguard against transmission is keeping water and food supplies free of pathogens. Immunization plays an extremely important role in a relatively few diseases, and herd immunity principles apply. For some diseases, immunity wanes with age, and the adult population becomes susceptible again. Quarantine and isolation are also powerful tools. Quarantine is still used by mutual international agreements for a few diseases (plague, cholera, yellow fever, typhoid fever, and louse-borne relapsing fever). Smallpox was quarantinable before its eradication in the 1970s. Isolation of individual patients is usually applied in hospitals where epidemics of highly resistant and highly transmissible organisms are prone to occur.[111]

Emerging Infectious Diseases

The concept of emerging infectious diseases is not new but has been the focus of attention due to the resurgence of old infectious diseases that were thought to be controlled and the recognition of new pathogens as humans increase their interaction with the biosphere. By definition, an emerging infectious disease is one that has newly appeared in the population or has existed but is rapidly increasing in incidence or geographic range.[112] The list is growing continuously, but the best examples include a wide variety of hemorrhagic fevers and other syndromes caused by viruses such as dengue, arenaviruses, filoviruses, and hantaviruses. Other emerging infections include HIV, cholera with its cyclic pandemics, malaria, yellow fever, cryptosporidiosis, rickettsiosis, ehrlichiosis, and Lyme borreliosis. The factors involved in the emergence or reemergence of infectious diseases are complex and include ecological changes (deforestation, reforestation, flooding, and climatic changes), changes in human demographics and behavior (sexual, cultural, and war), increased international travel, technological advances (organ transplantation and antibiotics), microbial evolution with the appearance of antibiotic-resistant or antigenically distinct strains, and deficiencies in surveillance and public health policy.[108,113–115] The classic triad of microbe, host, and environment is again exemplified.

TROPICAL INFECTIOUS DISEASES

Globally, as assessed in terms of disability-adjusted life years (DALYs), which measures morbidity and mortality,[111] infectious diseases in 1990 accounted for 36.4% of total DALYs. Infectious disease DALYs were considerably in excess of those attributable to cancer (5.9%), heart disease (3.1%), cerebrovascular disease (3.2%), or chronic lung disease (3.5%).[116]

However, these calculations admittedly miss the disproportionate impact of tropical infectious diseases on the still exploding populations living in impoverished, tropical areas, and they grossly underestimate the major developmental impact of common childhood enteric, helminthic, and other infections.[34,117–119] For those caring for individual patients with infectious diseases, appropriate diagnosis and treatment are important considerations for the individual. Even more important is the consideration of approaches that will lead to diminished acquisition of infectious diseases. For some infectious agents, immunization holds promise, as witnessed by the successful global eradication of smallpox and the potential eradication of poliomyelitis. Greater progress in the control of infectious diseases, however, rests with improvements related to socioeconomic conditions of the population at risk. In developed countries, tuberculosis was diminished well before the introduction of the first antimicrobial agents active against *M. tuberculosis* and was attributable to improved socioeconomic conditions. For the major infectious diseases of the tropics, improvements in sanitation, living conditions, and general public health will be critical in helping control the impact of the diverse infectious agents that currently contribute to human morbidity and mortality. The impact of these infections is related not only to their effect on the health of the infected individual but also to their contribution to the morbidity associated with malnutrition and to their larger societal impact as an impediment to the full development of the political, economic, and social potential of entire populations.

REFERENCES

1. Madigan MT, Martinko JM, Parker J: Brock Biology of Microorganisms, 10th ed. Upper Saddle River, NJ, Prentice Hall, 2003.
2. Mims C, Nash A, Stephen J: Mims' Pathogenesis of Infectious Disease, 5th ed. London, Academic Press, 2001.
3. Nelson KE, Masters Williams C, Graham NMH: Infectious Disease Epidemiology: Theory and Practice. Gaithersburg, MD, Aspen, 2001.
4. Schopf JW: Earth's Earliest Biosphere. Its Origin and Evolution. Princeton, NJ, Princeton University Press, 1983.
5. Lepp PW, Brinig MM, Ouverney CC, et al: Methanogenic Archaea and human periodontal disease. Proc Natl Acad Sci 101:6176, 2004.
6. Woese CR: Bacterial evolution. Microbiol Rev 51:221, 1987.
7. Pace NR: A molecular view of microbial diversity and the biosphere. Science 276:734, 1997.
8. Margulis L: Symbiosis in Cell Evolution, 2nd ed. New York, WH Freeman, 1992.
9. Kasting JF: Earth's early atmosphere. Science 259:921, 1993.
10. Olsen GJ, Lane DL, Giovannoni SJ, et al: Microbial ecology and evolution: A ribosomal RNA approach. Annu Rev Microbiol 40:337, 1986.
11. Bishop JM: The molecular genetics of cancer. Science 235:305, 1987.
12. Benjamin T, Vogt PK: Cell transformation by viruses. In Knipe DM, Howley PM, Griffin DE (eds): Field's Virology. New York, Lippincott Williams & Wilkins, 2001.
13. Gelderblom HR: Structure and classification of viruses. In Baron S (ed): Medical Microbiology, 4th ed. Galveston, University of Texas Medical Branch Press, 1996.
14. Francki RB: Encapsidated viroid-like RNA. In Diener TO (ed): The Viroids. New York, Plenum Press, 1987, p 205.
15. Keese P, Synons RH: The structure of viroids and virusoids. In Semanicik JS (ed): Viroids and Viroid-like Pathogens. Boca Raton, Fla, CRC Press, 1986, p 1.
16. Prusiner SB: Shattuck lecture—Neurodegenerative diseases and prions. N Engl J Med 344:1516, 2001.
17. DeArmond SJ, Prusiner SB: Perspectives on prion biology, prion disease pathogenesis, and pharmacologic approaches to treatment. Clin Lab Med 23:1, 2003.
18. Ewald PW: Guarding against the most dangerous emerging pathogens: Insights from evolutionary biology. Emerg Infect Dis 2:245, 1996.
19. Levin BR: The evolution and maintenance of virulence in microparasites. Emerg Infect Dis 2:93, 1996.
20. Levin BR, Svanborg-Eden C: Selection and the evolution of virulence in bacteria: An economical excursion and modest suggestion. Parasitology 100:5103, 1990.
21. Flint SJ, Enquist LW, Racaniello VR, et al: Principles of Virology: Molecular Biology, Pathogenesis, and Control of Animal Viruses. Washington, DC, ASM Press, 2004.
22. Anita R, Levin BR, May RM: Within host population dynamics, and the evolution and maintenance of microparasite virulence. Am Naturalist 144:457, 1994.
23. Bonhoeffer S, Nowak MA: Intrahost versus interhost selection: Viral strategies of immune function impairment. Proc Natl Acad Sci USA 91:8062, 1994.
24. Flint J, Harding RM, Boyce AJ, et al: The population genetics of the haemoglobinopathies. Baillieres Clin Haematol 6:215, 1993.
25. Weatherall DJ, Clegg JB: Genetic variability in response to infection: Malaria and after. Genes Immun 3:331, 2002.
26. Wain-Hobson S: Running the gamut of retroviral variation. Trends Microbiol 4:135, 1996
27. Amyes SG, Gemmell CG: Antibiotic resistance in bacteria. J Med Microbiol 36:4, 1992.
28. Burnet M, White DO: Natural History of Infectious Disease, 4th ed. Cambridge, UK, Cambridge University Press, 1972.
29. McNeill WH: Plagues and Peoples. Garden City, NY, Anchor Press, 1976.
30. Walker DH (ed): Biology of Rickettsial Diseases. Boca Raton, Fla, CRC Press, 1988.
31. Wills C: Yellow Fever and Black Goddess. The Coevolution of Peoples and Plagues. Reading, Mass, Addison-Wesley, 1996.
32. Colwell RR: Global climate and infectious disease: The cholera paradigm. Science 274:2025, 1997.
33. Guerrant RL: Why America must care about tropical medicine: Threats of global health and security from tropical infectious diseases. Am J Trop Med Hyg 59:3, 1998.
34. Simsek Z, Zeyrek FY, Kurcer MA: Effect of *Giardia* infection on growth and psychomotor development of children aged 0–5 years. J Trop Pediatr 50:90, 2004.
35. Checkley W, Gilman RH, Epstein LD, et al: Asymptomatic and symptomatic cryptosporidiosis: Their acute effect on weight gain in Peruvian children. Am J Epidemiol 145:156, 1997.
36. Steiner TS, Lima AA, Nataro JP, et al: Enteroaggregative *Escherichia coli* produce intestinal inflammation and growth impairment and cause interleukin-8 release from intestinal epithelial cells. J Infect Dis 177:88, 1998.
37. Crompton DWT, Montresor A, Nesheim MC, et al (eds): Controlling Disease Due to Helminth Infections. Geneva, World Health Organization, 2003.
38. Stephenson LS: Helminth parasites, a major factor in malnutrition. World Health Forum 15:169, 1994.
39. Isenberg LT, D'Amato RF: Indigenous and pathogenic microorganisms of humans. In Murray PR, Baron EJ, Jorgensen JH, et al (eds): Manual of Clinical Microbiology. Washington, DC, ASM Press; 2003.
40. Finlay B, Falkow S: Common themes in microbial pathogenicity revisited. Microbiol Mol Biol Rev 61:136, 1997.
41. Hultgren SJ, Abraham S, Caparon M, et al: Pilus and nonpilus bacterial adhesins: Assembly and function in cell recognition. Cell 73:887, 1993.
42. Blum G, Falbo V, Caprioli A, et al: Gene clusters encoding the cytotoxic necrotizing factor type 1. Prs-fimbriae and alpha-hemolysin form the pathogenicity island II of the uropathogenic *Escherichia coli* strain J96. FEMS Microbiol Lett 126:189, 1995.
43. Sandros J, Tuomanen E: Attachment factors of *Bordetella pertussis*: Mimicry of eukaryotic cell recognition molecules. Trends Microbiol 96:884, 1993.

44. Boren T, Falk P, Roth KA, et al: Attachment of *Helicobacter pylori* to human gastric epithelium mediated by blood group antigens. Science 262:1892, 1993.
45. Jarvis KG, Giron JA, Jerse AE, et al: Enteropathogenic *Escherichia coli* contains a putative type III secretion system necessary for the export of proteins involved in attaching and effacing lesion formation. Proc Natl Acad Sci USA 92:7996, 1995.
46. von Gijsegem F, Genia S, Boucher C: Conservation of secretion pathways for pathogenicity determinants of plants and animal bacteria. Trends Microbiol 1:175, 1993.
47. Mecsas J, Strauss EJ: Molecular mechanisms of bacterial virulence: Type III secretion and pathogenicity islands. Emerg Infect Dis 2:271, 1996.
48. Garnham PC: Malaria parasites of man: Life cycles and morphology. In Wernsdorfer WH, McGregor I (eds): Malaria. Principles and Practice of Malariology, vol. 1. London, Churchill-Livingstone, 1988, p 61.
49. Manz J, Herbert J: Arboviral encephalitis. In Connor DH, Chandler FW (eds): Pathology of Infectious Diseases. Stamford, Conn, Appleton & Lange, 1997.
50. Schell WA, Salkin IF, McGinnis MR, et al: *Bipolaris*, *Exophiala*, *Scedosporium*, *Sporopthrix* and other dematiaceous fungi. In Murray PR, Baron EJ, Jorgensen JH, et al (eds): Manual of Clinical Microbiology, 8th ed. Washington, DC, ASM Press, 2003.
51. Neutra MR, Pringault E, Kraehenbuhl JP: Antigen sampling across epithelial barriers and induction of mucosal immune responses. Annu Rev Immunol 14:275, 1996.
52. Sewankambo N, Gray RH, Wawer MJ, et al: HIV-1 infection associated with abnormal vaginal flora morphology and bacterial vaginosis. Lancet 350:546, 1997.
53. Cockerell CJ: Leprosy. In Connor DH, Chandler FW (eds): Pathology of Infectious Diseases. Stamford, Conn, Appleton & Lange, 1997.
54. Douek DC: Disrupting T-cell homeostasis: How HIV-1 infection causes disease. AIDS Rev 5:172, 2003.
55. Dumler JS, Walker DH: Ehrlichial infections. In Connor DH, Chandler FW (eds): Pathology of Infectious Diseases. Stamford, Conn, Appleton & Lange, 1997.
56. Chitnis CE, Chaudhuri A, Horuk R, et al: The domain on the Duffy blood group antigen for binding *Plasmodium vivax* and *P. knowlesi* malarial parasites to erythrocytes. J Exp Med 184:1531, 1996.
57. Miller LH, Mason SJ, Clyde DF, et al: The resistance factor to *Plasmodium vivax* in blacks. N Engl J Med 295:302, 1976.
58. Hadley TJ, Peiper SC: From malaria to chemokine receptor: The emerging physiologic role of the Duffy blood group antigen. Blood 87:3077, 1997.
59. Horuk R, Chitnis CE, Darbonne WC, et al: A receptor for the malarial parasite *Plasmodium vivax*: The erythrocyte chemokine receptor. Science 261:1182, 1993.
60. Galinski MR, Barnwell JW: A reticulocyte-binding complex of *Plasmodium vivax* merozoites. Cell 69:1213, 1992.
61. Barnwell JR, Galinski MR: *Plasmodium vivax*: A glimpse into the unique and shared biology of the merozoite. Ann Trop Med Parasitol 89:113, 1995.
62. Choe H, Farzan M, Su NY, et al: The beta-chemokine receptors CCR3 and CCR5 facilitate infection by primary HIV-1 isolates. Cell 85:1135, 1996.
63. Moore JP: Coreceptors: Implications for HIV pathogenesis and therapy. Science 276:51, 1997.
64. Doranz BJ, Berson JF, Rucker J, et al: Chemokine receptors as fusion cofactors for human immunodeficiency virus type 1 (HIV-1). Immunol Res 16:15, 1997.
65. Garred P: Chemokine-receptor polymorphisms: Clarity or confusion for HIV-1 prognosis. Lancet 351:2, 1998.
66. Manchester M, Liszewski MK, Atkinson JP, et al: Multiple isoforms of CD46 (membrane cofactor protein) serve as receptors for measles virus. Proc Natl Acad Sci USA 91:2161, 1994.
67. Greve JM, Davis G, Meyer AM, et al: The major human rhinovirus receptor is ICAM-1. Cell 56:839, 1989.
68. Fingeroth JD, Weis JJ, Tedder TF, et al: Epstein–Barr virus receptor of human B lymphocytes is the C3d receptor CR2. Proc Natl Acad Sci USA 81:4510, 1984.
69. Brown KE, Hibbs JR, Gallinella G, et al: Resistance to parvovirus B19 infection due to lack of virus receptor (erythrocyte P antigen). N Engl J Med 330:1192, 1994.
70. Buchmeier NA, Heffron F: Inhibition of macrophage phagosome-lysosome fusion by *Salmonella typhimurium*. Infect Immun 59:2232, 1991.
71. Walker DH, Valbuena GA, Olano JP: Pathogenic mechanisms of diseases caused by *Rickettsia*. Ann NY Acad Sci 990:1, 2003.
72. Clemens DL, Horwitz MA: Characterization of the *Mycobacterium tuberculosis* phagosome and evidence that phagosomal maturation is inhibited. J Exp Med 181:257, 1995.
73. Zilberstein D, Dwyer DM: Proton motive force-driven active transport of D-glucose and L-proline in the protozoan parasite *Leishmania donovani*. Proc Natl Acad Sci USA 82:1716, 1990.
74. Turco SJ, Descoteaux A: The lipophosphoglycan of *Leishmania* parasites. Annu Rev Microbiol 46:65, 1992.
75. Sibley LD, Weidner E, Krahenbuhl JL: Phagosome acidification blocked by intracellular *Toxoplasma gondii*. Nature 315:416, 1985.
76. Joiner KA, Fuhrman SA, Miettinen HM, et al: *Toxoplasma gondii*: Fusion competence of parasitophorous vacuoles in Fc receptor-transfected fibroblasts. Science 249:641, 1990.
77. Cossart P: Subversion of the mammalian cytoskeleton by invasive bacteria. J Clin Invest 99:2307, 1997.
78. Heinzen RA: Rickettsial actin-based motility: Behavior and involvement of cytoskeletal regulators. Ann NY Acad Sci 990:535, 2003.
79. Portnoy DA, Chakraborty T, Goebel W, et al: Molecular determinants of *Listeria monocytogenes* pathogenesis. Infect Immun 60:1263, 1992.
80. Maizels RM, Yazdanbakhsh M: Immune regulation by helminth parasites: Cellular and molecular mechanisms. Nature Rev Immunol 3:733, 2003.
81. Chen LM, Kaniga K, Galan JE: *Salmonella* spp. are cytotoxic for cultured macrophages. Mol Microbiol 21:1101, 1996.
82. Strano A: Yellow fever. In Connor DH, Chandler FW (eds): Pathology of Infectious Diseases. Stamford, Conn, Appleton & Lange, 1997.
83. Zychlinsky A, Kenny B, Menard R, et al: IpaB mediates macrophage apoptosis induced by *Shigella flexneri*. Mol Microbiol 11:619, 1994.
84. Zychlinsky A, Prevost MC, Sansonetti PJ: *Shigella flexneri* induces apoptosis in infected macrophages. Nature 358:167, 1992.
85. Che NYJ, Smith MR, Thirumalai K, et al: A bacterial invasin induces macrophage apoptosis by binding directly to ICE. EMBO J 15:3853, 1996.
86. Fraser A, Evan G: A license to kill. Cell 85:781, 1996.
87. Bobak DA, Guerrant RL: New developments in enteric bacterial toxins. Adv Pharmacol 23:85, 1992.
88. Walker DH, Firth WT, Ballard JG, et al: Role of phospholipase-associated penetration mechanism in cell injury by *Rickettsia rickettsii*. Infect Immun 40:840, 1983.
89. Finlay BB, Cossart P: Exploitation of mammalian host cell functions by bacterial pathogens. Science 276:718, 1997.
90. Montecucco C, Schiavo G: Mechanism of action of tetanus and botulinum neurotoxins. Mol Microbiol 13:1, 1994.
91. Schiavo G, Benfenati F, Poulain B, et al: Tetanus and botulinum-B neurotoxins block neurotransmitter release by proteolytic cleavage of synaptobrevin. Nature 359:832, 1992.
92. Zhang JP, Normark S: Induction of gene expression in *Escherichia coli* after pilus-mediated adherence. Science 273:1234, 1996.
93. Keates S, Hitti YS, Upton M, et al: *Helicobacter pylori* infection activates NF-kB in gastric epithelial cells. Gastroenterology 113:1099, 1997.
94. Rieder G, Hatz RA, Moran AP, et al: Role of adherence in interleukin-8 induction in *Helicobacter pylori*-associated gastritis. Infect Immun 65:3622, 1997.
95. Guerrant RL, Steiner TS, Lima AA, et al: How intestinal bacteria cause disease. J Infect Dis 179(Suppl 2):S331, 1999.
96. Holst O, Ulmer AJ, Brade H, et al: Biochemistry and cell biology of bacterial endotoxins. FEMS Immunol Med Microbiol 16:83, 1996.
97. Sweet MJ, Hume DA: Endotoxin signal transduction in macrophages. J Leukoc Biol 60:8, 1996.
98. Abbas AK, Lichtman AH: Cellular and Molecular Immunology, 5th ed. Philadelphia, Saunders, 2003.
99. Diaz de Durana MD, Lopez A, Fraj J: Anaphylaxis and cerebral hydatidic disease. Ann Intern Med 126:745, 1997.
100. Abbas AK: Diseases of immunity. In Kumar V, Abbas AK, Fausto N (eds): Robbins and Cotran Pathologic Basis of Disease, 7th ed. Philadelphia, Saunders, 2004.
101. Marrack P, Kappler J: Subversion of the immune system by pathogens. Cell 76:323, 1994.

102. Janeway CA, Travers P, Walport M, et al (eds): Immunobiology, 6th ed. New York, Garland, 2004.
103. Klauser T, Pohlner J, Meyer TF: The secretion pathway of IgA protease-type proteins in gram-negative bacteria. Bioessays 15:799, 1993.
104. Brunham RC, Plummer FA, Stephens RS: Bacterial antigenic variation, host immune response, and pathogen–host coevolution. Infect Immun 61:2273, 1993.
105. Cross GAM, Holder AA, Allen G, et al: An introduction to antigenic variation in trypanosomes. Am J Trop Med Hyg 29:1027, 1980.
106. Saint Girons I, Barbour AG: Antigenic variation in *Borrelia.* Res Microbiol 142:711, 1991.
107. Howard RS, Lively CM: Parasitism, mutation accumulation and the maintenance of sex. Nature 367:554, 1994.
108. Walker-Jonah A, Dolan SA, Gwadz RW, et al: An RFLP map of the *Plasmodium falciparum* genome, recombination rates and favored linkage groups in a genetic cross. Mol Biochem Parasitol 51:313, 1992.
109. Beneson AL: Control of Communicable Diseases in Man, 4th ed. Washington, DC, American Public Health Association, 1985.
110. McGowan JE, Metchock B: Infection control epidemiology and clinical microbiology. In Murray PR, Baron EJ, Pfaller M, et al (eds): Manual of Clinical Microbiology, 8th ed. Washington, DC, ASM Press, 2003.
111. Murray CJL: Quantifying the burden of disease: The technical basis for disability-adjusted life years. In Murray CJL, Lopez AD (eds): Global Comparative Assessments in the Health Sector. Geneva, World Health Organization, 1994.
112. Morse SS: Factors in the emergence of infectious diseases. Emerg Infect Dis 1:7, 1995.
113. Satcher D: Emerging infections: Getting ahead of the curve. Emerg Infect Dis 1:1, 1995.
114. Wilson ME: Travel and the emergence of infectious diseases. Emerg Infect Dis 1:39, 1995.
115. Peiris JS, Yuen KY, Osterhaus AD, et al: The severe acute respiratory syndrome. N Engl J Med 349:2431, 2003.
116. Murray CJL, Lopez AD (eds): The Global Burden of Disease. Cambridge, Mass, Harvard University Press, 1996.
117. Guerrant RL, Kosek M, Lima AAM, et al: Updating the DALYs for diarrhoeal disease. Trends Parasitol 18:191, 2002.
118. Chan M-S: The global burden of intestinal nematode infections—Fifty years on. Parasitol Today 13:438, 1997.
119. Bundy DAP, et al: Health Priorities and Burden of Disease Analysis: Methods and Applications from Global, National and Subnational Studies. Cambridge, Mass, Harvard University Press, 1997.

2

Factors Influencing Geographic Distribution and Incidence of Tropical Infectious Diseases

H. H. SHUGART
ROBERT E. SHOPE

INTRODUCTION

The distribution and incidence of tropical infectious diseases is directly related to geography, evolution, climate, and human factors. The early medical geographers recognized the relationships but were at best only able to document occurrence. Between 1883 and 1886, August Hirsch published in German the second edition of his *Handbook of Geographical and Historical Pathology.*[1] He described in detail the distribution and seasonality of dengue, malaria, smallpox, yellow fever, cholera, plague, typhus, and typhoid fever. He documented the pandemics of cholera, the paradoxical absence of yellow fever from Asia, and the endemicity of dengue and yellow fever in the tropical coastal cities with summer spread to the temperate zone.

A more recent geographer, Jacques May,[2] wrote in the 1950s about the effect of climate and geography on the distribution of malaria, cholera, and other tropical diseases. He traced the origin and travels of cholera, and he related these to the prevailing weather patterns. The reader is referred to at least two other books[3,4] that provide comprehensive maps and discussions of the distribution of tropical infectious diseases.

This chapter builds on the observations and concepts of Hirsch and May. It is not intended to describe the specific distribution of each of the tropical infectious diseases; specific disease chapters of this book do that. Rather, it emphasizes the many natural and human factors, including especially ecology, climate, and human intervention, that influence geographic distribution of agents and diseases and the concepts that govern where and when these diseases appear.

TRACKING AGENTS WITH MOLECULAR EPIDEMIOLOGIC METHODS

In the past, our ability to determine disease distribution and movement was often hindered by inaccurate diagnosis. For instance, clinical signs and symptoms are notoriously insufficient in distinguishing causes of fever, diarrhea, or hemorrhagic disease. The advent of reliable laboratory methods helped to confirm clinical diagnosis. In the past decade, molecular technology has matured so that not only can one map the distribution of the agent and disease but also one can determine the genetic composition of agents by methods employing polymerase chain reaction (PCR) and use this genetic information to map the distribution of geographic variants and track the transport of agents from one geographic site to another.

The newly acquired genetic information also helps us understand how agents evolve focally with their reservoirs. Even agents that are widely distributed, such as those causing rabies, poliomyelitis, dengue, cholera, and acquired immunodeficiency syndrome (AIDS), have regional geographic variation so that the transport and introduction of infection into new areas can be tracked using tools such as monoclonal antibodies and PCR.[5–9] The ability to use PCR to detect the presence of disease organisms in food, flowing water, and groundwater[10–11] coupled with automated sampling and analysis equipment and satellite reporting creates the possibility of monitoring very remote sites for disease presence and potential outbreaks.

ECOLOGY AS A FACTOR IN DISTRIBUTION

Many of the tropical diseases are zoonoses—that is, transmissible in nature from vertebrate animals to humans. The zoonoses are highly sensitive to climatic and other ecological influences. May's classification of infectious diseases[1] has greatly enhanced our conceptual thinking and is fundamental to understanding the basis for the distribution of infectious agents. The term *agent* is used here to mean the infectious entity, including viruses, bacteria, fungi, and parasites. May proposed that agent and number of hosts categorize diseases in the infectious cycle. Two-factor complexes consist of agents transmitted directly from person to person, such as poliovirus. Three-factor complexes involve transmission through a vector or invertebrate intermediate host—that is, a snail, mosquito, or other arthropod. Dengue and malaria, for instance, are transmitted from person to mosquito to person. For the purposes of this chapter, four-factor complexes involve transmission between a nonhuman vertebrate and an arthropod, with humans being usually accidental hosts. Eastern and western encephalitis viruses, for example, are maintained in a reservoir of mosquitoes and birds, with transmission to humans as a spillover from the enzootic cycle.

These cycles have a profound influence on the geographic distribution of the disease agent. An agent transmitted from person to person may persist anywhere that people go and thus have a very wide geographic distribution, affected by human behavior but relatively unaffected by temperature and rainfall. Transmission of a three-factor complex agent is immediately limited geographically by the distribution of the vector or human component of the reservoir. A *reservoir*, as defined by Benenson,[12] is "any person, animal, arthropod, plant, soil, or substance (or combination of these) in which an infectious agent normally lives and multiplies, on which it depends primarily for survival, and where it reproduces itself in such manner that it can be transmitted to a susceptible host." Note that for some tropical infections, such as vector-borne agents, the reservoir is often a combination of the arthropod vector and the vertebrate host because the agent depends on both for survival. Transmission of a four-factor complex agent may be even more restricted because geographic and environmental factors limiting distribution of the reservoir (either the vector or the nonhuman vertebrate), as well as human behavior, will limit the distribution of the infectious disease.

SPECIES DIVERSITY AND FOCALITY IN THE TROPICS

Viruses, parasites, fungi, and bacteria have evolved with their reservoirs from ancestral forms. The evolution of plants and animals in the tropics has generated high species diversity in many taxa. It follows that microorganisms also are diverse in the tropics because each has evolved with specific reservoir hosts. The more diverse the hosts, the more diverse will be the infectious agents. This diversity is also accompanied by focality, an increased degree of spatial localization. Of course, there are exceptions to such focality, namely in birds and bats, which may fly long distances, and human beings, who travel and take along their domestic animals. The microorganisms associated with widely dispersed animals or plants will be less focal.

This focality in the tropics also means that there are probably numerous as yet undescribed agents infecting wild vertebrates and vectors in tropical forests that have the potential to cause disease in people. In 1976, in 1995, and subsequently, Ebola virus emerged from cryptic forest foci in Zaire to cause fatal hemorrhagic human disease. These episodes are a reminder that tropical zoonotic agents may be very focal and hidden in geographically and ecologically limited transmission cycles until people intrude.

Most disease agents are very closely adapted to their vector or vertebrate host. Agents do not easily jump genus and species barriers and thus cannot readily adapt to new environmental conditions when their vector or vertebrate host becomes restricted by a change in environment.

In 1876, Wallace classified and bounded continental and faunal regions.[13] These regions are Nearctic, Neotropical, Palearctic, Oriental, Ethiopian, and Australasian. Theiler and Downs[14] studied the distribution of 280 arboviruses and rodent-associated viruses, and they showed that 247 existed in only one of these regions (Fig. 2-1). Presumably this meant that their vector or vertebrate host was quite specific, and they either were not transported to other regions or there was no available vector or vertebrate in another region to support their cycle of transmission. Thirty were found in two regions and only three in more than two regions. All but one of the viruses that had been discovered in more than one geographic region infected domestic animals, domiciliary mosquitoes (*Aedes aegypti*), or birds and thus had a means of transportation to another region. Viruses that were adapted to rodents were destined to have a very focal distribution because rodents do not fly and, with the exception of the house mouse and the wharf rat, have limited geographic interchange.

The same concepts hold for most bacterial and parasitic tropical agents that have three- or four-factor complexes. Each of the three major species causing human schistosomiasis, for instance, evolved with a different snail. The distribution of each species is limited to that of the snail: *Schistosoma mansoni* with *Biomphalaria* in tropical Africa and Brazil, *Schistosoma haematobium* with *Bulinus* in Africa and the Middle East, and *Schistosoma japonicum* with *Oncomelania* in the Far East. Although the snail is sometimes more widely dispersed than the schistosome, the potential for disease exists wherever the snail resides. Note also that new areas of disease are being created with the construction of dams that provide ecological conditions to support snails. The schistosomes are subsequently introduced to the dam sites by an influx of human populations that bring the parasite with them.

CLIMATE AND DISEASE DISTRIBUTION

Climate is defined as the customary long-term (usually 30 years) pattern of the weather for any given location. *Weather*, on the other hand, is the short-term state of the atmosphere in regard to temperature, rainfall, humidity, and storms. Temperature is the major governing factor for the distribution of many tropical diseases. Reservoir arthropods, snails, and vertebrates have life cycles that are limited by heat and cold. Many of these creatures do not withstand freezing weather and are thus relegated to the tropics because they do not survive winters in the temperate zones. The distribution of the reservoir therefore determines the limits of distribution of the agent and the disease.

TEMPERATURE AND AGENTS

Vector-borne infectious agents have a minimum, optimum, and maximum temperature for their replication in the vector.

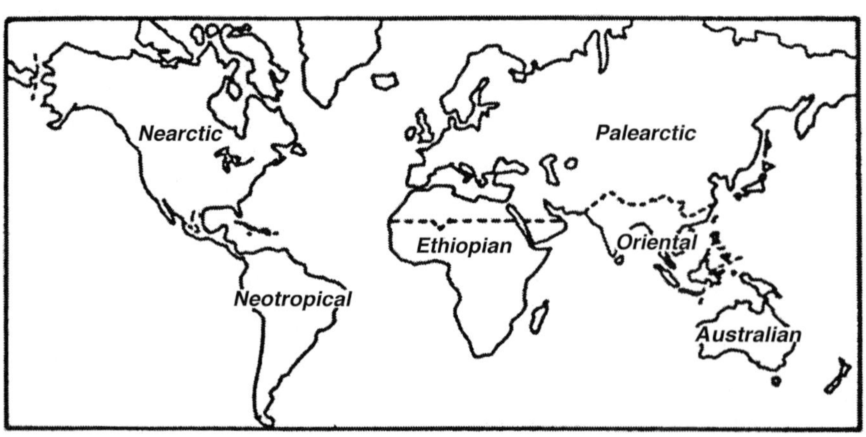

FIGURE 2-1 Wallace's (1876) division of the world into faunal regions, modified by Darlington (1957). (From Darlington PJ Jr: Zoogeography. In: The Geographical Distribution of Animals. New York, Wiley, 1957, p 2.)

The time from imbibing an infectious blood meal until the vector is able to transmit to a vertebrate is the extrinsic incubation period. As a general rule, within limits, tropical agents develop more rapidly and to higher infectious titers at warm temperatures than at cold temperatures. Agents such as *Plasmodium*, arboviruses, vector-borne *Rickettsia*, *Borrelia*, *Trypanosoma*, *Leishmania*, and filariae have an extrinsic incubation at near ambient temperature in an arthropod vector. In these infections, the cycle of transmission can usually proceed more rapidly at higher temperatures. The ambient temperature therefore may limit the distribution of these diseases by restricting the amplification of the agent in areas with a short summer season.

TEMPERATURE AND ARTHROPODS

The temperature also has an effect on the rapidity of development and length of survival of arthropods. Arthropods generally develop more rapidly at warmer temperatures. This means that the eggs hatch earlier, and the passage through life stages is faster, leading in the tropics to early emergence as adults. Warmer temperatures are also usually associated with higher adult arthropod mortality. Immature stages are often less affected by temperature but may not survive extreme cold or heat. The decrease in vector competence attributed to adult mortality may partially compensate for the increase attributed to the more rapid development in the tropics.

The temperature also affects the size of the adult arthropod. Mosquitoes, for instance, are smaller when they develop at warmer temperatures and may therefore require more frequent blood meals. This indirectly makes the smaller mosquito more efficient at transmitting an agent. The aggregate effect of warmer temperatures on arthropods is to increase their efficiency as vectors within broad limits and thus to affect the geographic distribution of the agents they transmit.

TEMPERATURE AND VERTEBRATES

Many vertebrates can adapt to a wide variation in temperature. Some diseases, however, are restricted in distribution to the tropics because the vertebrate reservoirs cannot withstand freezing weather. One such example is rabies in vampire bats.[15]

RAINFALL

Rainfall and other sources of water are essential to the presence of many three- and four-factor complex agents. *Aedes aegypti*, for instance, requires water for development, but this may be in the form of rainfall or as stored drinking water in arid areas. Snails that transmit schistosomiasis require water, and this disease often appears in new geographic sites after dams are constructed and irrigation is instituted.

RAINFALL AND FOOD SUPPLY

The weather may be directly responsible for food or lack of food for the reservoirs of three- and four-factor complex agents. The El Niño or southern oscillation phenomenon has apparently been responsible for periodic increases in wild vertebrate animals such as rodents because of an increase in the food supply following periods of excessive rainfall and warming in the western United States and along the western coast of South America. The El Niño or southern oscillation is a cyclic change in the ocean currents and the atmosphere that occurs approximately every 3 or 4 years. Prior to the 1993 outbreak of hantavirus pulmonary syndrome in the Four Corners area of the western United States, there was a marked increase in food for the rodents, including pine nuts. There was an associated 10-fold increase in the population of *Peromyscus maniculatus*, the rodent reservoir of Sin Nombre virus. These phenomena have been attributed to an El Niño event[16] and illustrate how weather may influence the distribution and incidence of disease.

GEOGRAPHIC BARRIERS TO SPREAD OF AGENTS

Tropical infectious diseases are limited by geographic barriers such as oceans, rivers, mountain ranges, or deserts. Rift Valley fever is an excellent example. This mosquito-borne viral agent is indigenous to sub-Saharan Africa and is believed to have as its reservoir *Aedes* mosquitoes that maintain the virus in mosquito eggs between periods of rain. The eggs are deposited in *dambos* (depressions) in East African pastures. After periods of heavy rain, the eggs hatch and the adult mosquito, transovarially infected, can transmit Rift Valley fever virus to sheep and cattle, which in turn amplify the virus transmission. Rift Valley fever was limited to sub-Saharan Africa until 1977 when it suddenly appeared in the Nile delta, where it infected immunologically virgin populations of sheep, cattle, and an estimated 200,000 people. The barrier of the Sahara Desert was breached. Theories abound to explain the spread of Rift Valley fever, but the most likely are the introduction of (i) an infected domestic animal via Lake Nasser, (ii) infected insects blown on the wind, or (iii) an infected person arriving in Egypt by airplane.[17,18]

LIMITING THE DISTRIBUTION OF TROPICAL INFECTIOUS DISEASES BY PUBLIC HEALTH MEASURES

The distribution of tropical infections can be modified by public health measures. Vaccines, vector control by source reduction and pesticides, treatment, improvement of housing, and drug prophylaxis have been used to limit the distribution of tropical infectious diseases and, at least in the case of smallpox, to eradicate the disease. Several vector-borne diseases, including malaria and yellow fever, were prevalent in the American and Afro-European temperate regions during the 1700s and 1800s. These diseases disappeared outside of the tropics, and some were controlled within the tropics. Sanitation, a raised standard of living, and new technology were primarily responsible. The successes are well-known to most readers. Smallpox was eradicated by 1977 using case finding and vaccination.[19] Major cities were freed of urban yellow fever by control of *A. aegypti* mosquitoes using pesticides and destruction of breeding sites following the methods of General Gorgas.[20] Malaria was eliminated during the 1940s from many temperate zones such as the oases in the Egyptian Western Desert and the islands of Sardinia and Cyprus[21] by mosquito species sanitation. Onchocerciasis in the Americas has been drastically reduced in geographic distribution and incidence by treatment of human carriers with ivermectin.[22] Murine typhus in the southern United States was dramatically controlled with DDT accompanied by diminution of rat populations.[23]

DEMOGRAPHICS AND HUMAN BEHAVIOR AFFECT DISTRIBUTION

Human factors influence the distribution of virtually all tropical infectious diseases. Often, this is because people, in the name of progress, disturb the ecology, thus creating breeding sites for vectors and vertebrate hosts. Examples include the following: First, malaria has become epidemic in the western Amazon region of Brazil, where the population has grown 10-fold since 1970. The immigrants are involved in gold mining and forestry and have settled in areas undergoing rapid deforestation.[24] *Anopheles darlingi* mosquitoes breed in standing water of open-cast mining sites and forest clearings. Initially, people from malaria-endemic regions of Brazil arrived already infected to seed the area. Second, the triatomid bugs that transmit Chagas' disease live in the mud walls of homes in Brazil and Argentina.[25] A change in construction methods to eliminate the bug's hiding places, as well as spraying homes with insecticides with residual activity, in some cases has controlled the insect. Third, in 1995 dengue caused more than 4000 illnesses in the Mexican Rio Grande Valley while at the same time only seven indigenous cases of dengue were reported a few kilometers across the river in the U.S. Rio Grande Valley. This difference has been suggested to be a function of better housing and water supplies on the U.S. side of the Rio Grande.[26] Fourth, construction of dams and irrigation projects create ecological changes often favoring transmission of tropical agents. The Diama Dam in the Senegal River basin was implicated in an outbreak of Rift Valley fever in 1987 in Mauritania.[27] Although the disease was not known to be present in the area before 1987, antibody studies of local inhabitants were positive and led to a warning to local government officials and to the governments sponsoring the dam construction of the risk of an epidemic after the dam was completed. This is an example in which the threat was perceived prior to the epidemic, but the warning was not heeded.

UNKNOWN FACTORS LIMITING DISTRIBUTION: ABSENCE OF YELLOW FEVER FROM ASIA

In some cases, the reason for the distribution of a disease is not intuitively evident. An age-old question is, "Why is there no yellow fever in Asia?" The answer is not known. The yellow fever forest cycle in Africa and South America involves virus, monkey, and mosquito with spillover into humans. Its urban cycle is a three-factor complex involving human beings, *A. aegypti* mosquitoes, and the virus. All of the nonviral factors are present in abundance in Asia, but yellow fever is absent there. Possibly, although unlikely, the virus has never been introduced. Yellow fever is increasingly detected throughout the world in travelers. For instance, in 1996, viremic tourists infected with yellow fever virus near Manaus, Brazil, returned to Switzerland and the United States.[28] One can therefore speculate that the virus must have been introduced by arrival in Asia of viremic persons, in prior times by boat and in recent years by airplane. Possibly, genetically different strains of *A. aegypti* indigenous to Asia are less competent to become infected and transmit yellow fever virus than the mosquitoes of Africa and South America. This hypothesis has been tested in the laboratory. Although many of the strains from Asia had reduced ability to become infected,[29] the differences were relatively small and did not offer a convincing explanation. Possibly, immunity in humans or primates to dengue or other flaviviruses (serologically related to yellow fever) prevented infection. When challenged with yellow fever virus, monkeys immune to dengue had lower viremia levels than did nonimmune monkeys[30]; however, flavivirus immunity in Africa and South America is substantial and does not prevent yellow fever transmission on those continents. Thus, the factor(s) limiting the geographic distribution of yellow fever remains unknown. If, as some believe, it is a numbers game, and the introduction of yellow fever virus has not yet coincided with the presence of *A. aegypti* in sufficient abundance and during the right season to establish an epidemic, then Asia and the rest of the world must maintain careful surveillance and adequate vaccine supplies so that a catastrophic yellow fever epidemic does not occur.

GLOBAL CLIMATE CHANGE AND THE SPREAD OF TROPICAL DISEASES

Gradual warming of the earth's surface by 1°F has been recorded during the past 100 years. This warming trend has been predicted to continue by an international panel of experts constituting the Intergovernmental Panel on Climate Change, with 2000 scientists participating.[31] A few scientists still believe that the warming is a natural cycle that will reverse itself. The strongest arguments that the earth will continue to warm come from computer models of the predicted effects of accumulation of greenhouse gases, including carbon dioxide, that capture outgoing heat radiation, warm the atmosphere, and thus warm the earth's oceans and land. The increasing levels of carbon dioxide are amply documented both by direct atmospheric measurements at Mauna Loa in Hawaii and by sampling of CO_2 trapped in ice cores from glaciers in Greenland and the Antarctic region. It is uncertain that CO_2 emissions from automobiles and industries that burn carbon fuels will be controlled in the near future, and thus there is a risk that the current warming trend will accelerate, and that the earth's warmer climates will expand into higher latitudes and altitudes.

The climate models predict increasing temperatures, especially at night and in the higher latitudes. They also point to drastic changes in rainfall patterns, with some parts of the world having flooding and others drought. More severe and more frequent El Niño events, hurricanes, and typhoons are predicted. Warming will bring melting of the major glaciers and polar ice caps with an increase in the sea level. Conservative models predict that at the current rate of CO_2 accumulation, the temperature will rise approximately 3.5°F and the sea level will elevate approximately 6 in. by 2100. The current concentration of CO_2 is approximately 365 ppm, a level not seen on Earth during the past 160,000 years.

Several studies have projected the effects of warming on the spread and intensity of tropical three-factor and four-factor infectious diseases. According to Jetten and Focks,[32] dengue will increase its transmission intensity by 2 to 10 times in much of its current range with a 2°C rise and will spread to areas not now heavily involved, such as the southern United States, Argentina, the Mediterranean, parts of China, and most of Australia. This prediction takes into account the effects of temperature on adult *A. aegypti* mosquito survival, the parameters of the gonotrophic cycle, the extrinsic incubation period in the mosquito, and the vector size, which affects the frequency of feeding (see Climate and Disease Distribution). According to this model, not only will dengue spread but also the transmission season will be prolonged in much of the mosquito's range, and the risk of secondary infection in younger people, and thus of severe dengue disease, will increase.

Schistosomiasis is a disease caused by trematodes that are obliged to pass part of their life cycle in water and snail hosts. If the climate changes, what are now temperate areas in Europe, Asia, and the Americas are predicted to reach temperatures that will support transmission of human schistosomes in host snails, now limited to the tropics.[33]

According to Killick-Kendrick,[34] leishmaniasis could flourish in southern England by 2025 if the prediction of a 24°C (75°F) summer is correct. He notes that *Phlebotomus perniciosus* has already been found in England; it is an excellent vector of *Leishmania infantum* in southern Europe, could survive the predicted climate, and could maintain the life cycle of *L. infantum* at 24°C. Reservoir hosts such as dogs and immunosuppressed persons are available to support the parasite, and thus the public should be concerned.

Predictions of increased distribution of tropical infectious diseases have also been made for cholera,[35,36] St. Louis and Western equine encephalitis,[37] vampire bat rabies,[38] and malaria.[39,40] The acceptance of these predictions should be qualified, keeping in mind the doubts some scientists harbor about the inevitability of climate change. In addition, the geographic distribution and incidence of diseases are not solely governed by climate. Arguably more important are public health measures, including treatment, drug prophylaxis, immunization, education, and vector control. If the predicted warming is accompanied by technical advances in disease control and an improvement in the standard of living, including housing with screens and air-conditioning, these measures may well dampen the transmission and spread of insect-borne diseases.

THE FUTURE OF GEOGRAPHIC STUDIES

In the past decade, geographic information systems (GIS) have given new tools to the disease ecologist for studying landscape and vegetation. Remote sensing with satellite imagery (Fig. 2-2) has been used to chart surface changes in vegetation and to predict weather patterns such as El Niño or southern oscillation through measurements of ocean surface temperature on a global basis. Predictions of cholera[36] and

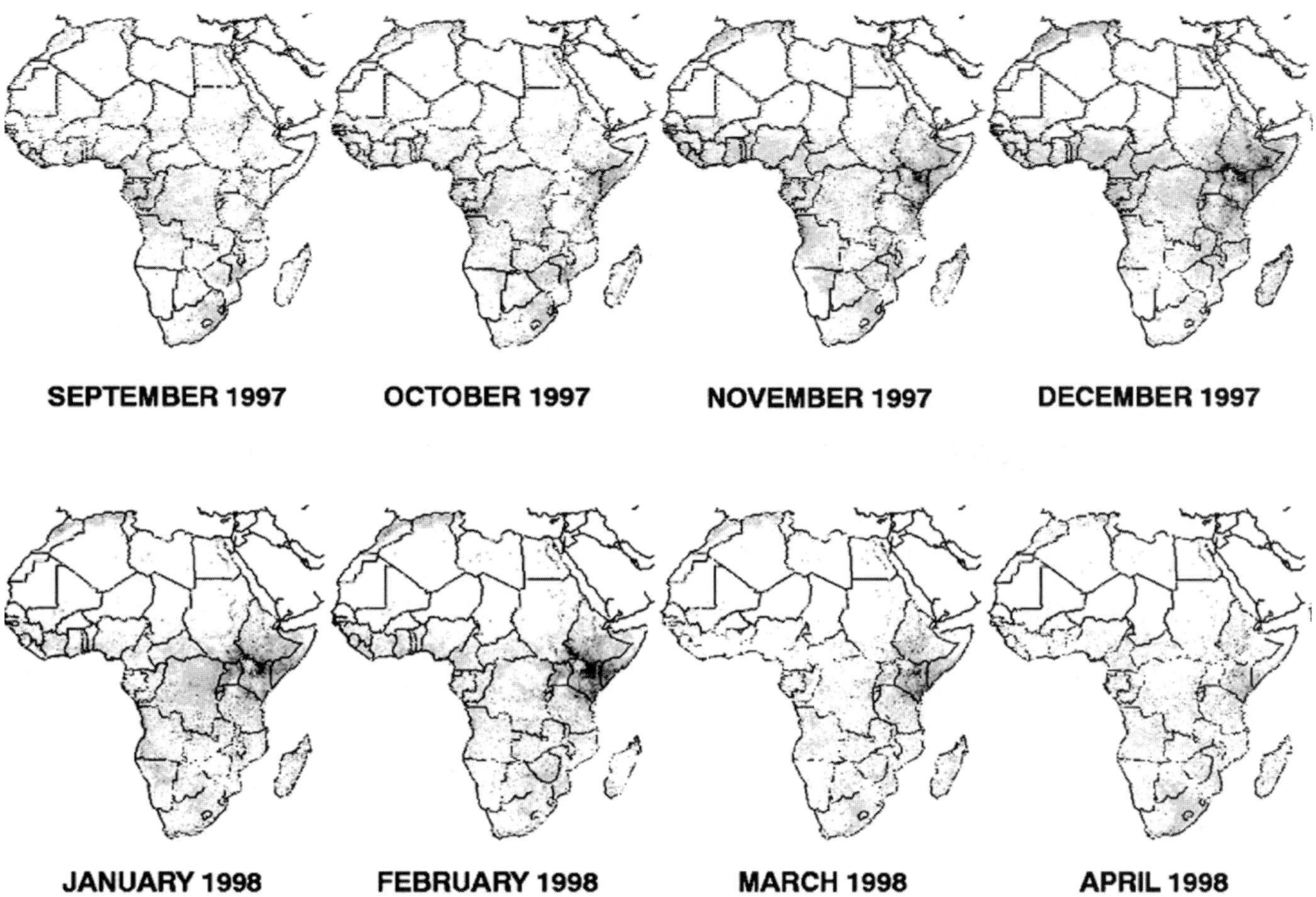

FIGURE 2-2 Monthly Advanced Very High Resolution Radiometer (AVHRR) images of the Normalized Difference Vegetation Index (NDVI) of continental Africa during the 1997–1998 ENSO warm event. Data depicted are the degree of deviation from the long-term mean calculated for the period January 1982 to May 1998 in NDVI units. Darkly shaded areas have received higher than average rainfall and can be used to determine conditions associated with outbreaks of Rift Valley fever. (From Linthicum KJ, Anyamba A, Tucker CJ, et al: Climate and satellite indicators to forecast Rift Valley fever epidemics in Kenya. Science 285:397-400,1999.)

Rift Valley fever[41] outbreaks now appear to be feasible. In the case of Rift Valley fever, analysis of the outbreaks of the disease from 1950 to 1998 indicates the potential to predict the disease as much as 5 months in advance.[42] Can this technology also lead to a better understanding of the distribution and incidence of other three- and four-factor diseases, such as malaria, dengue, and hantavirus pulmonary syndrome?

REFERENCES

1. Hirsch A: Handbook of Geographic and Historical Pathology, ed. 2, 3 vols. Creighton C (trans). London, New Sydenham Society, 1883–1886.
2. May JM: Ecology of Human Disease. New York, MD Publications, 1958.
3. Howe MG (ed): A World Geography of Human Diseases. London, Academic Press, 1977.
4. Learmonth A: Disease Ecology. Oxford, Basil Blackwell, 1988.
5. Smith JS, Orciari LA, Yager PA, et al: Epidemiologic and historical relationships among 87 rabies virus isolates as determined by limited sequence analysis. J Infect Dis 166:296–307, 1992.
6. Rico-Hesse R, Pallansch MA, Nottay BK, et al: Geographic distribution of wild poliovirus type 1 genotypes. Virology 160:311–322, 1987.
7. Rico-Hesse R: Molecular evolution and distribution of dengue viruses type 1 and 2 in nature. Virology 174:479–493, 1990.
8. Karaolis DKR, Lan R, Reeves PR: The sixth and seventh cholera pandemics are due to independent clones separately derived from environmental, nontoxigenic, non-01 *Vibrio cholerae*. J Bacteriol 177:3191–3198, 1995.
9. Louwagie J, Janssens W, Mascola J, et al: Genetic diversity of the envelope glycoprotein from human immunodeficiency virus type 1 isolates of African origin. J Virol 69:263–271, 1995.
10. Waage AS, Vardund T, Lund V, et al: Detection of low numbers of *Salmonella* in environmental water, sewage and food samples by a nested polymerase chain reaction assay. J Appl Microbiol 87:418–428, 1999.
11. Fout GS, Martinson BC, Moyer MWN, et al: A multiplex reverse transcription-PCR method for detection of human enteric viruses in groundwater. Appl Environ Microbiol 69:3158–3164, 2003.
12. Benenson AS: Control of Communicable Diseases Manual, 16th ed. Washington, DC, APHA, 1995.
13. Darlington PJ Jr: Zoogeography: The Geographical Distribution of Animals. New York, Wiley, 1957.
14. Theiler M, Downs WG: Arthropod-Borne Viruses of Vertebrates. New Haven, Conn, Yale University Press, 1973.
15. Acha PN: Epidemiology of paralytic bovine rabies and bat rabies. Bull Off Int Epizool 67:343–382, 1967.
16. Ryan F: Virus X. Boston, Little, Brown, 1997.
17. Sellers RF, Pedgley DW, Tucker MR: Rift Valley fever, Egypt—1977: Disease spread by wind-borne insect vectors? Vet Rec 110:73–77, 1982.
18. Gad AM, Feinsod FM, Allam IH, et al: A possible route for the introduction of Rift Valley fever virus into Egypt during 1977. J Trop Med Hyg 89:233–236, 1986.
19. Fenner R, Henderson DA, Arita I, et al: Smallpox and Its Eradication. Geneva, World Health Organization, 1988.
20. Gorgas WC: Sanitation of tropics with special reference to malaria and yellow fever. JAMA 52:1075–1077, 1909.
21. Soper FL: Species sanitation as applied to the eradication of (A) an invading or (B) an indigenous species. In Proceedings of the Fourth International Congress on Tropical Medicine and Malaria, Washington, DC, May 10–18, 1948, pp 850–857.
22. Cupp EW, Ochoa AO, Collins RC, et al: The effects of multiple ivermectin treatment on infection of *Simulium ochraceum* (Diptera: Simuliidae) with *Onchocerca volvulus* (Filarioidea: Onchocercidae). Am J Trop Med Hyg 40:501–506, 1989.
23. Davis DE: The use of DDT to control murine typhus fever in San Antonio, TX. Public Health Rep 62:449–463, 1947.
24. Camargo LM, Ferreira MU, Krieger H, et al: Unstable hypoendemic malaria in Rondonia (western Amazon region, Brazil): Epidemic outbreaks and work-associated incidence in an agro-industrial rural settlement. Am J Trop Med Hyg 51:16–25, 1994.
25. Nogueira N, Coura JR: American trypanosomiasis (Chagas' disease). In Warren KS, Mahmoud AAF (eds): Tropical and Geographical Medicine, ed. 2. New York, McGraw-Hill, 1990, p 292.
26. Reiter P: Global warming and mosquito-borne disease in USA. Lancet 348:622, 1996.
27. Lederberg J, Shope RE, Oaks SC Jr (eds): Emerging Infections. Washington, DC, National Academy Press, 1992, pp 71–72.
28. Yellow fever in a traveller. Weekly Epidemiol Rec 71:342–343, 1996.
29. Aitken THG, Downs WG, Shope RE: *Aedes aegypti* strain fitness for yellow fever virus transmission. Am J Trop Med Hyg 26:985–989, 1977.
30. Anderson CR, Theiler M: The relative resistance of dengue-immune monkeys to yellow fever virus. Am J Trop Med Hyg 24:115–117, 1975.
31. Houghton JT, Meiro Filho LG, Callander BA, et al: Climate Change, 1995—The Science of Climate Change. Contribution of Working Group I to the Second Assessment Report of the Intergovernmental Panel on Climate Change. Cambridge, UK, Cambridge University Press, 1996.
32. Jetten TH, Focks DA: Potential changes in the distribution of dengue transmission under climate warming. Am J Trop Med Hyg 57:285–297, 1997.
33. Shope RE: Impacts of global climate change on human health: Spread of infectious diseases. In Majumdar SK, Kalkstein LS, Yarnal BM, et al (eds): Global Climate Change: Implications, Challenges and Mitigation Measures. Easton, Pa, Pennsylvania Academy Science, 1992, pp 361–370.
34. Killick-Kendrick R: Leishmaniasis—An English disease of the future? Bull Trop Med Int Health 4:5, 1996.
35. Colwell RR: Global climate and infectious disease: The cholera paradigm. Science 274:2025–2031, 1996.
36. Lipp EK, Huq A, Colwell RR: Effects of global climate change on infectious disease: The cholera model. Clin Microbiol Rev 15:757–770, 2002.
37. Reeves WC, Hardy JL, Reisen WK, et al: Potential effect of global warming on mosquito-borne arboviruses. J Med Entomol 31:323–332, 1994.
38. Shope RE: Infectious diseases and atmospheric change. In White JC (ed): Global Atmospheric Change and Public Health. New York, Elsevier, 1990, pp 47–54.
39. Patz JA, Epstein PR, Burke TA, et al: Global climate change and emerging infectious diseases. JAMA 275:217–223, 1996.
40. Martens WJM, Jetten TH, Rotmans J, et al: Climate change and vector-borne diseases. A global modelling perspective. Global Environ Change 5:195–209, 1995.
41. Linthicum KJ, Bailey CL, Davies FG, et al: Detection of Rift Valley fever viral activity in Kenya by satellite remote sensing imagery. Science 235:1656–1659, 1987.
42. Linthicum KJ, Anyamba A, Tucker CJ, et al: Climate and satellite indicators to forecast Rift Valley fever epidemics in Kenya. Science 285:397–400, 1999.

3

Epidemiology and Biostatistics

EDWARD T. RYAN
MEGAN MURRAY

Epidemiology is the science of investigating the occurrence, causes, and prevention of disease in human populations. Epidemiologic tools may be used to estimate disease frequency, uncover or confirm associations between risk factors and disease occurrence, and define the impact of preventive and curative measures to combat disease. As one of the primary disciplines of the field of public health, epidemiology is of great importance to human health worldwide, especially in the developing world. A fundamental understanding of epidemiologic principles—including basic terminology; study design and hypothesis testing; and data collection, analysis, and interpretation—is, therefore, necessary to the understanding of biomedical sciences.

OVERVIEW AND TERMINOLOGY

Measures of Disease Frequency

Prevalence is a measure of the total number of existing cases of a disease or condition in a specific population at a particular time. Prevalence is usually expressed as a fraction or percentage of a population, but it can also be given as the number of cases per 1000, 10,000, or 100,000 people. In contrast to prevalence, which enumerates *all* cases of a disease, *incidence* is a measure of the number of *new* cases of disease occurring over a specified period. Incidence is, therefore, expressed as the number of cases that occurred in a population of a given size per a unit time. Thus, if a cohort of 1000 individuals is followed for 1 year and 100 of these individuals develop a specific disease, the incidence rate of that disease would be 0.1, or 100 per 1000 per year.

Measures of Effect

In addition to measuring frequency of occurrence of a disease, epidemiologic studies measure the strength of an association between a specific risk factor and the incidence of a disease or medical condition, or between a specific intervention or treatment and the prevention or resolution of a disease. For instance, the effect of a risk factor on disease frequency can be estimated by comparing the incidence of disease in a group that has been exposed to a specific risk factor to the incidence of disease in a group that has not been exposed.

Infectious Disease Terms

There are a number of definitions specific to the epidemiologic study of infectious diseases. A disease that occurs regularly in a population is said to be *endemic*. When a disease occurs at a frequency higher than is expected, it is said to be *epidemic*. A localized epidemic may be referred to as an *outbreak*. Diseases in animals are said to be *enzootic* or *epizootic*. After infection, there often follows a period of *latency*, defined as the duration of time from infection to onset of infectiousness. The period of time immediately following infection may also be an *incubation* period, defined as the time from infection to development of symptomatic disease. If the incubation period is longer than the latent period for a specific disease, individuals may infect others prior to the onset of recognizable illness. An *attack rate* refers to the proportion of a population that develops an infectious disease over a given period. The term *secondary attack rate* refers to the proportion of *exposed* individuals who become ill. The secondary attack rate is often measured among the household members of a known index case, since it is relatively easy to count the number of exposed individuals and follow them over time.

The *basic reproductive number*, often expressed as R_0, is defined as the expected number of secondary infectious cases generated by an average infectious case in a population in which everyone is susceptible. This quantity determines the potential for an infectious agent to start an outbreak, the extent of transmission in the absence of control measures, and the ability of control measures to reduce spread. R_0 can be expressed as a product of the number of contacts each infectious individual has per unit time (k), the probability of transmission per contact between an infectious case and a susceptible person (b), and the mean duration of infectiousness, D:

$$R_0 = bkD$$

Although it is a highly simplified summary of a pathogen's epidemic potential, R_0 may be used to predict outcome following an introduction of an infection into a population. If R_0 is greater than 1, the number of people infected will grow and an epidemic will take place; if R_0 is less than 1, the disease will die out.

In real epidemics, it is useful to replace the *basic reproductive number* with the *effective reproductive number,* denoted R, which is defined as the *actual* average number of secondary cases infected by a primary case. R is usually less than R_0, since it reflects both the impact of control measures instituted over time and the depletion of a susceptible population as previously infected individuals acquire immunity. *Herd immunity* results when a vaccine not only protects a vaccinated individual from contracting an infection but also prevents that individual from spreading the infection to others.

STUDY DESIGN

Understanding scientific–medical studies requires knowledge of a number of fundamental epidemiologic and statistical concepts, the first of which concerns study design. Studies may be designed to measure disease frequency (incidence and prevalence) or to measure an effect (e.g., how effective is drug A compared with drug B in the treatment of individuals with a certain medical condition). A classic type of study that measures disease frequency is a *surveillance study,* which tracks the frequency of a disease in a population over time. It is effectively a reporting system. It may be *active*, in which case people with disease are actively sought, or *passive* where cases are reported that present to medical attention. It may be hospital- or clinic-based or community-based. It may report specific well-defined diseases or, if diagnostic capabilities are limited, it may report syndromes (e.g., the syndrome of ulcerative genital disease as opposed to genital herpes, chancroid, or syphilis, specifically). Surveillance systems are a fundamental tool in public health because they provide critical information on disease burden and changes in disease frequency over time that may alert public health authorities to epidemic disease.

Studies that *measure an effect* may measure the effectiveness of a new drug or vaccine; alternatively, they measure the effect of a possible risk factor on disease frequency (e.g., the effect that smoking has on the risk of developing lung cancer). The optimal study for measuring effect is a *clinical trial*. Randomized clinical trials are prospective studies in which individuals are randomized to one of at least two study arms and followed for the outcome of interest over time. The major advantage of this type of study is that the random nature of group assignment ensures that people in one group will not differ systematically from people in another group in some way that would influence outcome. Another way to say this is that the purpose of randomization is to eliminate potential confounding factors (whether suspected or not suspected) that are associated with both exposure and outcome.

If the random assignment is completely unknown to both the study participants and researchers, it is called a *double-blind randomized trial*. If one of the study arms receives a treatment or intervention and the other receives a placebo, the trial is called a *placebo-controlled trial*. Since it is unethical to offer one group a placebo if there is available a treatment of known benefit, many trials compare the efficacy of a new intervention to that of a standard therapy; these trials are called *equivalence studies*. An example of a randomized double-blind equivalence study would be one that compares the efficacy of two drugs, drug A and drug B, for the treatment of shigellosis. To ensure that both participants and researchers are blinded to the intervention, the drug preparations should look and taste the same, be administered on the same dosing schedule, and given by the same route. Follow-up of the two groups should be identical.

It is often impossible to conduct a clinical trial, especially when the exposure of interest is not an intervention or a treatment but some kind of environmental or genetic factor. In this case, a *cohort study* can be conducted to estimate association between risk factor and outcome. In a cohort study, groups of individuals with different exposure histories are identified and followed over time. As an example, imagine that we want to study the relationship between smoking and lung cancer. We could identify individuals who smoke and those who do not and follow them over time to see if the incidence of lung cancer between the two cohorts is different. This type of study has several possible shortcomings, one of which is that it may take years or decades for an individual to develop a disease or outcome after initial exposure. Another problem inherent in this type of study is the fact that the two cohorts of exposed and unexposed people may differ in ways other than just the basis of the exposure of interest (a *confounding influence*). For example, a confounding influence in our study may be the effect of alcohol consumption on the development of lung cancer (for instance, if individuals who drink heavily were more likely to smoke than those who do not drink heavily).

An alternative study design is a *case-control study*. In this type of study, exposures of people who experience an outcome of interest are compared to exposures of those who have not had such an outcome. This type of study is especially useful for a rare disease or when there is a prolonged period of time between exposure and outcome. Continuing our example of examining the relationship of smoking and lung cancer, in a case-control study, we would identify individuals who have developed lung cancer and a group of "controls" who have not developed lung cancer. We could then ascertain the smoking histories of individuals in the study and try to determine whether they were consistently different between cases and controls. Since case-control studies often involve retrospective collection of exposure data obtained after a subject knows his or her diagnosis, there is a potential for *recall bias*. Another potential problem in case-control studies involves the selection of controls. Ideally, cases should be chosen from the population that gave rise to cases and should be selected without regard to exposure status. Case-control and cohort studies are also referred to as *observational studies,* since there is no intervention.

HYPOTHESIS TESTING

When designing a study, researchers should first *state the hypothesis* that they want to test. For example, "we hypothesize that drug A is effective in treating salmonellosis." The hypothesis should be stated before data are collected. A common pitfall of studies is to first collect data and *then* to analyze data for comparisons that reach statistical significance. Such a fishing expedition may uncover real differences, but may also uncover differences related to chance alone.[1]

A placebo-controlled double-blind randomized trial would be the best way to test our hypothesis that our new drug A is "effective" in treating individuals with salmonella gastroenteritis. When designing this study, researchers should first select relevant and measurable endpoints that will distinguish whether individuals who get the drug "do better." Primary endpoints may be days of diarrhea; days of fever; duration of bacterial shedding of salmonella organisms in stool; and/or the presence or absence of infectious complications, bacteremia, or death. These outcomes should be as clinically relevant and precise as possible; that is, definitions of what constitutes diarrhea and fever should be established before the study is undertaken, the same amount of stool and blood should be collected and processed from all study enrollees to ensure equality of assessment, and data should be recorded and reported as accurately and completely as possible.

After the hypothesis is stated, the researchers should next formulate the *null hypothesis*. In this step, the investigators should assume that no true difference exists between the two study groups (those who get drug A and those who get the placebo). A decision should then be made as to what constitutes a statistically significant result. *Statistical significance* is usually conveyed through a statistic known as the *P value;* results are often considered significant if the *P* value is less than a cut-off value (or "alpha level") of 5%. The *P* value refers to the probability that one would observe a result equal to or more extreme than the study result under the null hypothesis. One way to interpret this is to say that if a difference is shown between the two groups, there is a 95% chance that the difference is true (or a less than 5% chance that the difference is due to chance alone).

The *alpha level* is a cut-off value for a *P* value for a hypothesis test that is often set, somewhat arbitrarily, at 0.05. A *type I error* occurs when the null hypothesis is incorrectly rejected when it is in fact true, that is, when there is no difference between drug A and a placebo. A test with an alpha level of 0.05 should lead to type I errors no more than 5% of the time. Unlike the *P* value that varies with the data, alpha levels are chosen in advance and indicate the specific *P* value that will be considered significant. A *type II (or beta) error* occurs when the null hypothesis is not rejected even when there is truly a difference between the two arms of the study, that is, between drug A and the placebo. Type II errors may occur when a study is not large enough to detect a difference, or when individuals are not followed for an adequate amount of time for differences between groups to become apparent. Most well-designed studies aim for a type II error rate between 10% and 20%. The *power* of a study refers to the probability that the null hypothesis is rejected when it is false, and it is thus given the expression

$$\text{Power} = 1 - \text{Probability of a type II error.}$$

Therefore, most studies aim for 80% to 90% power (i.e., an 80% to 90% chance that if the null hypothesis is not rejected it is correct). It is this power calculation that determines the number of individuals who need to be enrolled in a study.

Only after the hypothesis has been stated and a study appropriately designed and adequately powered should data be collected and stored. Once this is completed, data analysis may begin. In this step, investigators determine the estimated effect of the intervention or exposure, and the probability that the observed difference between the two study groups would occur if no true difference exists in the larger population.

DATA EXPRESSION AND ANALYSIS

Data may be expressed in many ways. When an exposure or outcome is expressed in terms of a continuous variable such as age or weight, the differences between groups may be expressed by comparing *mean* or *median* values for the two groups. Both these statistics are measures of central tendency, meaning that they describe the middle, or average, value of the data. The mean is the *arithmetic* average, which is simply obtained by summing the observations and dividing the sum by the number of observations. For instance, if we measure the days of diarrhea following administration of drug A to patients with salmonellosis, we may find that one patient had diarrhea for 2 days, another for 3 days, another for 4 days, another for 5 days, and another for 20 days. The mean would be a summation divided by the number evaluated (2 + 3 + 4 + 5 + 20 [equals 34] divided by 5 = 6.8). The *median* is the value that divides the data in half; 50% of the observations have values lower than the median, and 50% have values greater than the median. The median is also referred to as the 50th centile. Using the median rather than the mean lessens the impact of outliers, since the actual values of extreme data points do not affect the median. Another way of reducing the effect of extreme outlier observations is to use the *geometric mean,* which is often used with data measured on a logarithmic scale. The geometric mean is calculated by multiplying the observed values and taking the *n*th root, where *n* is the number of observations. For the preceding example, this would be given by

$$\sqrt[5]{(2)(3)(4)(5)(20)} = 4.7.$$

The term *standard deviation* measures the spread of the individual observations around the mean. It is given by the formula

$$s = \sqrt{\Sigma \frac{X - \overline{X}}{n-1}}.$$

where X represents the value of each individual observation, $\overline{X}$ represents the mean, and n represents the number of observations. The *standard error of the mean* indicates the degree of uncertainty in calculating estimate from a sample. A standard error may be calculated from the standard deviation by dividing the standard deviation by a square root of n (with n representing the number of values measured).

Range refers to the interval from the minimum to the maximum value in a set of quantitative measurements. For instance, the arithmetic mean in our example would be 6.8, the geometric mean would be 4.7, the median would be 4, and the range would be 2 through 20.

Data that are *normal* or *normally distributed* are symmetrically distributed around a mean. A classic example of normally distributed data is a bell-shaped curve (e.g., a population-based IQ evaluation; Fig. 3-1).

Characteristics that we might want to study may be measured in a variety of ways. Observed data may be *dichotomous, categorical,* or *continuous.* If data can take only one of two values, they are defined as *dichotomous.* Returning to our smoking and lung cancer example, we could describe smoking in terms of the dichotomous variables "ever" or "never" smoked. *Categorical* observations have values that fit into categories. For example, we might characterize race or ethnicity using a categorical variable. Some data categories describe ascending levels of intensity or severity. For example, we could describe smoking history as "none," "light," "moderate," and "heavy." When categorical data are ordered in this way, they are *ordinal.* Finally, data may be measured on a *continuous* scale. Again, referring to our smoking

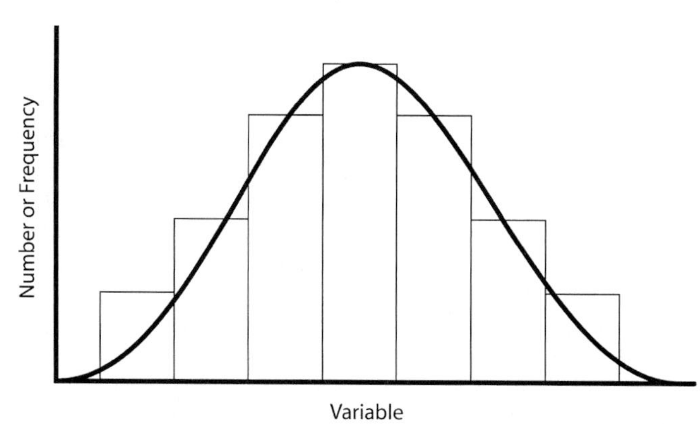

FIGURE 3-1 Normal distribution.

example, we could measure smoking in terms of the number of cigarettes consumed. At analysis, continuous data may be transformed into categorical data (but not vice versa).

Once we have summarized our data into the groups we are comparing, we need to decide whether the data differ between groups. If data are dichotomous, we may compare proportions, for example, the proportion of "ever" smokers who develop lung cancer to "never" smokers who develop lung cancer. For instance, imagine in our study that 5 smokers develop lung cancer out of a cohort of 100, while only 1 of 100 nonsmokers develops lung cancer. These data could be presented in a table of observed frequencies as follows:

	Lung Cancer	No Lung Cancer	Total
Ever smoked	5	95	100
Never smoked	1	99	100
	6	194	200

Under the null hypothesis, we assume that there is no difference in the incidence of lung cancer among smokers and nonsmokers. Given that 6 cases of lung cancer occurred among the 200 people we followed, we can come up with a table of "expected" frequencies under the null hypothesis.

	Lung Cancer	No Lung Cancer	Total
Ever smoked	3	97	100
Never smoked	3	97	100
	6	194	200

We can use the *chi-square test* statistic to ask how likely it would be that we obtained the observed frequencies if the null hypothesis were true. The chi-square statistic is given by the formula

$$X^2 = \sum_{\text{allcells}} \frac{(O-E)^2}{E}$$

where O is observed frequency and E is expected frequency. If the chi-square test is small, this suggests that there is no difference between the groups; if it is large, we assume that a difference exists.

Other statistical tests are available to analyze data. The choice of optimal test depends on a number of variables, including data type and number of groups. For instance, for continuous data that are normally distributed, we could compare the means of two groups using the *t test* for comparing means. When data are not normally distributed, other tests would be required; these usually are based on "order statistics" and include such nonparametric methods as the *Mann-Whitney U Test,* the *Kruskal-Wallis* and the *Wilcoxon matched rank test,* among others. The *ANOVA* (analysis of variance) test may be used to compare more than two groups that are normally distributed. The Mann-Whitney U test is used for evaluating two groups that are not normally distributed, and the Kruskal-Wallis test may be used for evaluating more than two groups that are not normally distributed.

Analysis of data may disclose "associations." For instance, returning to our example of smoking and lung cancer, we may find that smoking and lung cancer are statistically associated. Although variables that are found to be associated with an outcome are often called *risk factors,* a statistical association does not imply a cause and effect relationship between that variable and outcome. The *relative risk* is the probability of an outcome if a risk factor/association is present divided by the probability of the outcome if the risk factor/association is absent. For instance, in our example of the cohort study of smokers and nonsmokers, we imagined a study in which we have followed 100 individuals who smoke and 100 individuals who never smoked. We saw that 5 of the 100 smokers developed cancer (probability 0.05), but that only 1 of 100 nonsmokers developed lung cancer (probability 0.01). The relative risk is, therefore, 0.05 divided by 0.01, or 5. A relative risk of 5 implies that individuals who smoke are five times more likely to develop lung cancer than individuals who do not smoke.

In case-control studies, it is the researcher who determines how many study and control participants are evaluated, and so a true disease frequency in the population as a whole cannot be established. In this case, we cannot estimate the relative risk, since we do not actually know the risk of disease in the unexposed population. An approximation of the relative risk for case control studies is the *odds ratio.* To understand the difference between a risk and an odds ratio, think of the probability (or risk) of throwing a six-sided die in a game of chance and having the die land with six black dots facing up (1 in 6 chance). The odds of throwing a six on the other hand will be the number of times the die will land with six black dots showing divided by the number of times six dots will not be uppermost (1 to 5). An odds ratio is, therefore, the odds of developing an outcome if an association is present, divided by the odds of an outcome if the association is absent. Both the relative risk and the odds ratio are easy to calculate from a 2 × 2 table.

	Lung Cancer	No Lung Cancer	Total
Ever smoked	A	B	A+B
Never smoked	C	D	C+D
	A+C	B+D	A+B+C+D

$$\text{RR} = \frac{A/(A+B)}{C/(C+D)}$$

$$\text{OR} = \frac{[A/(A+C)]/[C/(A+C)]}{[B/(B+D)]/[D/(B+D)]} = \frac{A/C}{B/D} = \frac{AD}{BC}$$

Confidence intervals are a way of combining information about the strength of an association with information about the effects of chance in obtaining the observed results. A 95% confidence interval (CI) is most commonly used. An association is usually reported as an odds ratio (OR) or relative risk (RR) with a 95% CI.

The final stage of analyzing a study is extrapolation. We may extrapolate to an individual or to a group. For instance, based on a relative risk or odds ratio of 5 for smoking and lung cancer, we could conclude that if an individual smoked, he or she may be five times more likely to develop lung cancer than if he or she did not smoke. We may also speak of an *attributable risk percent.* The advantage of this concept is that it allows us to think of a portion of the risk of developing a disease that may be eliminated among those who do not have the risk factor. Attributable risk percentage may be thought of as

$$(\mathrm{RR} - 1/\mathrm{RR}) \times 100\%$$

where RR is relative risk.

For instance, in our study, we found that smoking was associated with a relative risk of 5 of developing lung cancer. This may not seem like an overly large risk of developing lung cancer; however, the attributable risk percent is 5–1/5 = 80%. This suggests that 80% of lung cancer in our study population could have been prevented if our study participants had never smoked.

UNDERSTANDING DIAGNOSTIC LABORATORY TESTS

In many instances, laboratory tests are part of a case definition (e.g., detection of serum antibodies against human immunodeficiency virus [HIV] in a study involving individuals infected with HIV). It should be recalled that a test is often a surrogate marker to distinguish a disease-free group from a diseased group. Assuming a normal distribution in both groups of whatever marker we are measuring (e.g., a serum antibody level), we can imagine that the disease-free and diseased groups do not overlap at all with regard to the specific blood test of interest (Fig. 3-2A). Often, however, the two groups do overlap, and some individuals in the diseased group will have tests with lower values than some of the individuals in the disease-free group (Fig. 3-2B).

In establishing the utility of a test, therefore, we must first establish the reference interval for disease-free individuals. *Sensitivity* and *specificity* of a test are then measured compared with a "gold standard." *Sensitivity* measures the probability that those with a disease will have a positive test when individuals with the disease are identified by the gold standard. *Specificity* measures the probability that those who do not have the disease will test negative by the test being evaluated. There usually is a trade-off between the sensitivity and specificity of a specific test. For example, if we choose *X* as the cutoff value for a positive test on Figure 3-2B of overlapping curves, we will achieve 100% sensitivity—but at the cost of misclassifying many negative cases as positive ones, that is, reducing specificity. Conversely, we could maximize specificity by moving our cutoff value for a positive test rightward to the *Y* position, but in so doing, we would compromise our ability to identify a true case of disease.

For example, imagine that we are evaluating a new test to diagnose schistosomiasis, and imagine that we will compare this test to a gold standard in a village with a population of 1000 individuals of whom 500 actually have schistosomiasis by our gold standard. Imagine that our new test correctly identifies 400 infected individuals but incorrectly identifies 100 truly infected individuals as not having schistosomiasis when in fact they are infected (*false negative*). Also imagine that our new test incorrectly labels 50 individuals as having schistosomiasis who do not (*false positive*).

Test	Gold Standard Disease	Gold Standard Disease-Free
Positive	400 (a)	50 (b)
Negative	100 (c)	450 (d)
	500	500

Sensitivity and specificity are calculated as

$$\text{Sensitivity} = \frac{a}{a+c} = \frac{400}{500} = 0.80 \text{ or } 80\%$$

$$\text{Specificity} = \frac{d}{b+d} = \frac{450}{500} = 0.90 \text{ or } 90\%$$

Our test will, therefore, have a sensitivity of 80% and a specificity of 90%. The actual utility of this test, however, will rest not only on its sensitivity and specificity but also on the prevalence of the disease in question in our population of interest. In our preceding example, there was a 50% prevalence of schistosomiasis (500 infected individuals who lived in a population of 1000). If we assume that the "true" prevalence of schistosomiasis in a different village is 20%, at a population level, the average individual in that village will have a 20% chance of having the disease before the test is performed (in reality, certain individuals will be at higher or lower risk of having schistosomiasis on the basis of age, gender, and other factors).

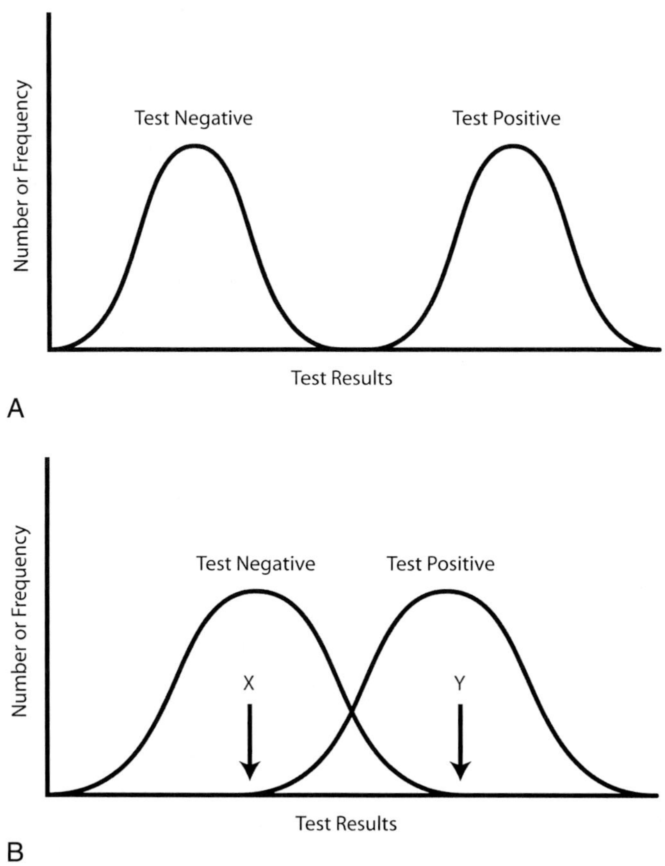

FIGURE 3-2 *A,* Normal distribution in which two groups do not overlap. *B,* Two groups that overlap.

Assuming that we are evaluating 1000 individuals (with 20% of them having the disease), and assuming that we are using our new test with a sensitivity of 80%, we would assume that 160 of the 200 individuals with the disease will be correctly identified by the test:

20% Probability Village X

Test	Gold Standard Disease	Gold Standard Disease-Free
Positive	160	80 false positives
Negative	40 false negatives	720
	200	800

The remaining 20% of these individuals will be incorrectly labeled as negative (n = 40; false negatives). Specificity equals 90%; therefore, 90% of those who are disease-free will be correctly labeled as negative (90% of 800; 720 true negatives). The remaining 10% of individuals who are disease-free will be incorrectly labeled as positive (10% of 800; 80 false positives).

Now let us imagine that we are applying our same test in a different village in which schistosomiasis is much more prevalent and 75% of the population has the disease:

75% Probability Village Y

Test	Gold Standard Disease	Gold Standard Disease-Free
Positive	600	25 false positives
Negative	150 false negatives	225
	750	250

Finally, let us imagine that we use our test in a third village, in which schistosomiasis is much rarer and the true probability of disease is only 2% (only 2% of the population is infected). Then our table would look like this:

2% Probability Village Z

Test	Gold Standard Disease	Gold Standard Disease-Free
Positive	16	98 false positives
Negative	4 false negatives	882
	20	980

Now, let us analyze the predictive value of positive and negative test results in each of these villages. The *positive predictive value* refers to the probability that one who tests positive truly has the disease, while the *negative predictive value* refers to the probability that one who tests negative actually does not have the disease. The crucial point to understand is that the predictive value depends not only on the sensitivity and specificity of the test itself but also on the disease prevalence in the population being evaluated.

Test	Gold Standard Disease	Gold Standard Disease-Free	
Positive	a = Number of individuals diseased and positive	b = Number of individuals disease-free and positive	a + b = total number of test positives
Negative	c = Number of individuals diseased and negative	d = Number of individuals disease-free and negative	c + d = total number of test negatives

The following formulae are used for calculating the predictive value of a positive test and the predictive value of a negative test:

$$\text{Predictive value of a positive test} = \frac{a}{a+b}$$ Proportion of individuals with a positive test who actually have the disease

$$\text{Predictive value of a negative test} = \frac{d}{c+d}$$ Proportion of individuals with a negative test who actually do not have the disease

Using the preceding calculated numbers, and assuming a 2% pretest probability of disease (as in Village Z):

$$\text{Predictive value of a positive test} = \frac{a}{a+b} = \frac{16}{16+98} = 14\%$$

$$\text{Predictive value of a negative test} = \frac{d}{c+d} = \frac{882}{4+882} = 99.5\%$$

Similarly, if we assume a 75% pretest probability as in Village Y,

$$\text{Predictive value of a positive test} = \frac{a}{a+b} = \frac{600}{600+25} = 96\%$$

$$\text{Predictive value of a negative test} = \frac{d}{c+d} = \frac{225}{150+225} = 60\%$$

Therefore, using exactly the same test, with exactly the same sensitivity and specificity, we can generate the following table of positive and negative predictive value of our test in villages with different prevalences of the disease in question:

	Pretest Probability		
	2% (Village Z)	**20% (Village X)**	**75% (Village Y)**
Predictive value of a positive test	14%	66.7%	96%
Predictive value of a negative test	99.5%	94.7%	60%

This means that there is an 86% chance that a positive test obtained in a Village Z with a 2% pretest probability of disease is falsely positive. Similarly, there is a 40% chance that a negative result is in fact falsely negative in Village Y with a pretest probability of disease of 75%. This is despite the fact that we are using the same test with the same sensitivity and specificity in each village. It is, therefore, crucial to understand that the interpretation of laboratory tests (whether in a study or in clinical practice) should be understood in context.

ACKNOWLEDGMENTS

We are grateful to Margaret Bikowski and Sam Riley for assistance with figures. This work was supported in part by a grant from the National Institute of Allergy and Infectious Diseases, Public Health Services U01 AI58935(ETR).

SUGGESTED READINGS

Katz DL: Epidemiology, Biostatistics and Preventive Medicine Review. Philadelphia, WB Saunders, 1997.

Pereira-Maxwell F: A–Z of Medical Statistics: A Comparison of Critical Appraisal. New York, Arnold Publishers/Oxford University Press, 1998.

Riegelman RK: Studying a Study and Testing a Test: How to Read the Medical Evidence, 4th ed. Philadelphia, Lippincott Williams & Wilkins, 2000.

Website for the Centers for Disease Control and Prevention [includes a Data and Statistics section]. www.cdc.gov. Accessed 10/08/04.

Website for the World Health Organization [includes a Research Tools section with statistical information]. www.who.int. Accessed 10/08/04.

4

Social and Cultural Factors in Tropical Medicine: Reframing Our Understanding of Disease

DAVID A. WALTON
PAUL E. FARMER
REBECCA DILLINGHAM

BARRIERS TO CARE AND THE PERSISTENT PATHOGENS: A BIOSOCIAL APPROACH

By the close of the 20th century, the world's ranking infectious pathogens—from well-known malaria and filariasis to the more recently described human immunodeficiency virus (HIV)—could be controlled by the tools of modern medicine and public health. And yet, none of these diseases, or other important "tropical diseases," has been brought to heel. None of them, even those without a nonhuman host, have been eradicated. Some epidemic diseases continue to expand. Still others mutate to become drug-resistant pathogens for which there are no clear therapies. Vaccines, in the event they exist, are not always delivered effectively in the settings in which they are most needed. The cumulative burden of these diseases remains unchanged, and in some cases is growing; this burden weighs most heavily on the world's poorest billion inhabitants.

This chapter examines this central irony of 21st century medicine: the persistence of morbidity and mortality due to infectious diseases years after effective vaccines, cures, suppressive treatments, and preventive strategies have been discovered. The forces inhibiting the successful application of existing scientific knowledge are not primarily biological or cultural; they are, rather, economic and structural barriers to change. Using what may be called a *biosocial model,* this chapter will describe these barriers to health.

Because modern epidemics are almost invariably rooted in social conditions, some long-standing and others changing rapidly, inquiry that does not draw on the social sciences is unlikely to offer a comprehensive or accurate understanding of these plagues. The mechanisms by which social forces shape epidemics are not readily revealed by single methodologies but rather by interdisciplinary research that links qualitative and quantitative methods. A biosocial model calls into question the very term *tropical diseases,* since many of the pathogens discussed in this textbook caused, in the past, significant mortality far from the tropics. The dozen or so diseases grouped under this rubric have little in common in terms of pathogenesis, chronicity of infection, modes of transmission (some are vector-borne, others are not), or efficacy of existing control and treatment strategies. But whether we consider what are often termed the "neglected diseases" (African trypanosomiasis, dengue, leishmaniasis, schistosomiasis, Chagas disease, lymphatic filariasis, and onchocerciasis) or the largest infectious killers (diarrheal and respiratory diseases, HIV, tuberculosis [TB], and malaria), there are important similarities to consider. All of these diseases afflict the poor disproportionately and are linked to social conditions. For each disease, there exist important deliverables: new and improved diagnostics and therapeutics that could affect the distribution and outcomes of these epidemics. In each instance, new discoveries could substantially decrease the morbidity and mortality associated with these persistent pathogens, but social and economic barriers have to date hampered effective control strategies.

The mechanisms by which social forces delay health progress are in large measure those leading to the propagation of new epidemics such as acquired immunodeficiency syndrome (AIDS). We begin this review with a case study of AIDS and TB in rural Haiti, since many of the barriers to care are best seen by closely examining individual illness trajectories and since TB is often the leading cause of death among patients living with HIV disease in resource-poor settings. The case study is followed by a review of structural barriers to effective AIDS prevention and care. Next, a brief description of the economic impact of malaria and the challenges of implementing insecticide-treated bednets (ITNs) illustrates how poverty, the primary social barrier, limits effective implementation of proven prevention strategies. Finally, we will explore the implications of this review for effective control of other leading infectious killers.

AIDS AND TUBERCULOSIS IN HAITI: JOSEPH'S STORY

On the afternoon of March 17, 2003, four men appeared at the public clinic in Lascahobas, Haiti, each carrying a leg of a makeshift stretcher. (The Lascahobas clinic in Central Haiti is a recent partnership between the nonprofit organization Partners in Health/Zanmi Lasante and the Haitian Ministry of Health. It is rural Haiti's second full-service AIDS clinic and also provides a range of other health services.) On the stretcher lay a young man, eyes closed, seemingly unaware of the 5-mile journey he had just taken on the shoulders of his neighbors. When they reached the clinic after the 4-hour trip, they placed the young man, named Joseph, on an exam table. The physician tried to interview him, but Joseph was already stuporous. His brother recounted the dying man's story.

Joseph, 26, had been sick for months. His illness had started with intermittent fevers, followed by coughing, weight loss, weakness, and diarrhea. His family, too poor, they thought, to take him to a hospital, brought Joseph to a traditional healer. Joseph would later explain: "My father sold nearly all that he had—our crops, our land, and our livestock—to pay the healer, but I kept getting worse. My family barely had enough to eat, but they sold everything to try to save me."

Joseph was bed-bound 2 months later. He became increasingly emaciated and soon lost all interest in food. As he later recalled, "My mother, who was caring for me, was taking care of skin and bones."

Faced with what they saw as Joseph's imminent death, his family purchased a coffin. Several days later, a community health worker, employed by the Lascahobas clinic, visited their house. The health worker was trained to recognize the signs and symptoms of TB and HIV and immediately suspected that the barely responsive Joseph might have one or both of these diseases. Hearing that their son might have one last chance for survival, Joseph's parents pleaded with their neighbors to help carry Joseph to the clinic, since he was too sick to travel on a donkey and too poor to afford a ride in a vehicle.

At the clinic, Joseph was diagnosed, as per the community health worker's suspicions, with advanced AIDS and disseminated TB. He was hospitalized and given antiretrovirals and antituberculous medications (Fig. 4-1A). Like his family, however, Joseph, too, had lost faith in the possibility of recovery. He remembers telling his physician, early in the course of his treatment, "I'm dead already, and these medications can't save me."

Despite his doubts, Joseph dutifully took his medications each day, and he slowly began to improve. Several weeks later, he was able to walk. His fevers subsided and his appetite returned. After discharge, he received directly observed therapy (DOT) for both AIDS and TB from a neighbor serving as an *accompagnateur*.[1] After 4 months of therapy, Joseph had gained 30 pounds (Fig. 4-1B).

Now, over a year later, Joseph is employed as an HIV outreach worker, often speaking in front of large audiences about his experience (Fig. 4-1C). "When I was sick ... I couldn't farm the land, I couldn't get up to use the latrine; I couldn't even walk. Now I can do any sort of work. I can walk to the clinic just like anyone else. I care as much about my medications as I do about myself. There may be other illnesses that can break you, but AIDS isn't one of them. If you take these pills, this disease doesn't have to break you."

STRUCTURAL BARRIERS TO EFFECTIVE AIDS AND TUBERCULOSIS CONTROL

Joseph's experience is typical in many ways and instructive in most. He is one of tens of millions worldwide suffering from HIV disease and TB; he lives in great poverty; he sought care unsuccessfully until he simply gave up. His family did what they could to save his life, selling off meager assets and receiving contradictory advice from neighbors and from traditional healers in a country in which trained medical personnel are rare* and most care is fee-for-service. Joseph's experience is exceptional in that he lived in an area of Haiti in which treatment for both AIDS and TB has recently come to be considered a public good and made available to poor patients who cannot pay user fees.[2] Treatment for these two chronic infectious diseases is supervised not by physicians or nurses, who do play a role in the diagnosis of illness, but by community health workers who are also one's neighbors.[3] In the following sections, we review these topics in greater detail by examining an emerging literature that explores socioeconomic barriers to effective care for AIDS and tuberculosis.

The "Brain Drain"

One significant and often-invoked barrier to effective care in resource-poor settings is the lack of medical personnel. In what has been termed the "brain drain," large numbers of physicians and nurses are leaving their home countries in order to pursue opportunities abroad, leaving behind health systems that are understaffed and ill-equipped to deal with the epidemic diseases that ravage local populations.† The World Health Organization (WHO) recommends a minimum of 20 physicians and 100 nurses per 100,000 persons, but recent reports from that body and others have confirmed that many countries, especially in sub-Saharan Africa, fall far short of those targets. Over half of these countries register fewer than 10 physicians per 100,000 population. In contrast, the United States and Cuba boast, respectively, 279 and 596 doctors per 100,000 population. Similarly, the majority of sub-Saharan African countries fail to meet even half of the WHO minimum standard for adequate nursing coverage.‡

These national aggregates, while appalling, do not reveal the further inequalities in health-care staffing within countries. Rural-urban disparities in health-care personnel mirror disparities of both wealth and health. In 1992, the poorest districts in southern Africa reported 5.5 doctors, 188.1 nurses, and 0.5 pharmacists per 100,000 population. The same survey found, in the richest districts, 35.6 doctors, 375.3 nurses, and 5.4 pharmacists per 100,000 population.[4] Nearly 90% of Malawi's population is rural, but over 95% of clinical officers were to be found in urban facilities; 47% of Malawi's nurses were in tertiary care facilities.[5] Even community health workers, trained to provide first-line services to rural populations, often transfer to urban districts. In Kenya, for example, there were only 138 health workers per 100,000 persons in Kenya's rural North Eastern Province in 1989 compared to 688 per 100,000 in Nairobi.[6]

In addition to inter- and intranational transfer of personnel, AIDS itself is contributing to personnel shortages across Africa. Although data on the prevalence of HIV among health professionals is scarce, the available numbers suggest substantial and adverse impacts on an already overburdened health sector. The situation in Malawi is instructive. For example,

---

*The WHO estimates that there are only 27 physicians per 100,000 Haitians. The numbers within the country vary dramatically, with the highest numbers recorded in the area around the capital city. Rural regions, including Joseph's home district (the Central Department), post the lowest coverage: In central Haiti, there are only 2 physicians per 100,000 population (Pan American Health Organization. Health Institutions and Human Resources in Haiti. Updated information as of March 2004. Available at: www.paho.org/English/DD/PED/Health_institutions.ppt.).

†For a complete review of the brain drain phenomenon, see: Physicians for Human Rights: An Action Plan to Prevent Brain Drain: Building Equitable Health Systems in Africa. Boston, Physicians for Human Rights, 2004. See also Joint Learning Initiative: Human Resources for Health: Overcoming the Crisis. Cambridge, MA, Global Equity Initiative, Harvard University, 2004.

‡For health sector statistics, see the WHO's Global Atlas of Infectious Disease (www.who.int/GlobalAtlas) and the United Nations Development Program's Human Development Indicators (hdr.undp.org/statistics/data/).

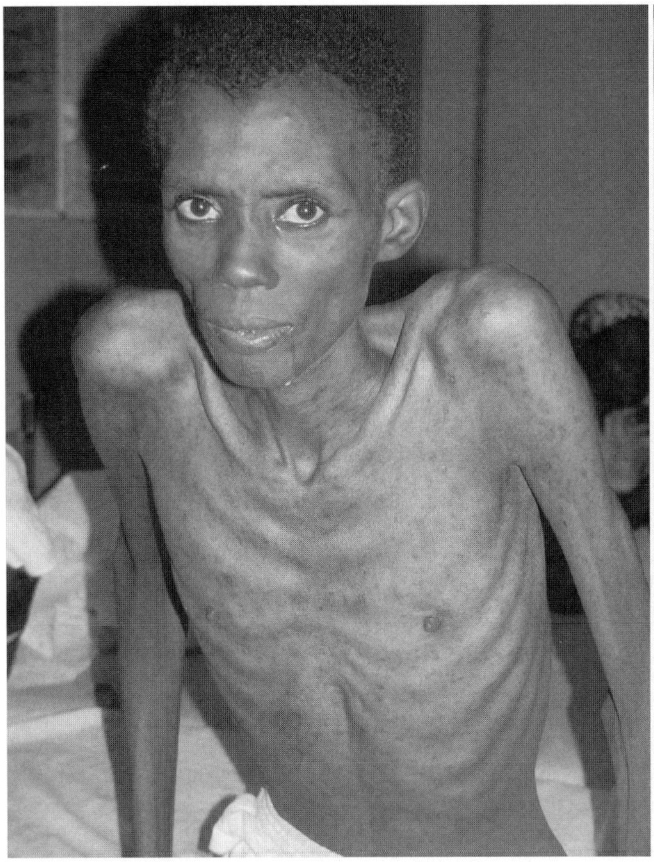

A

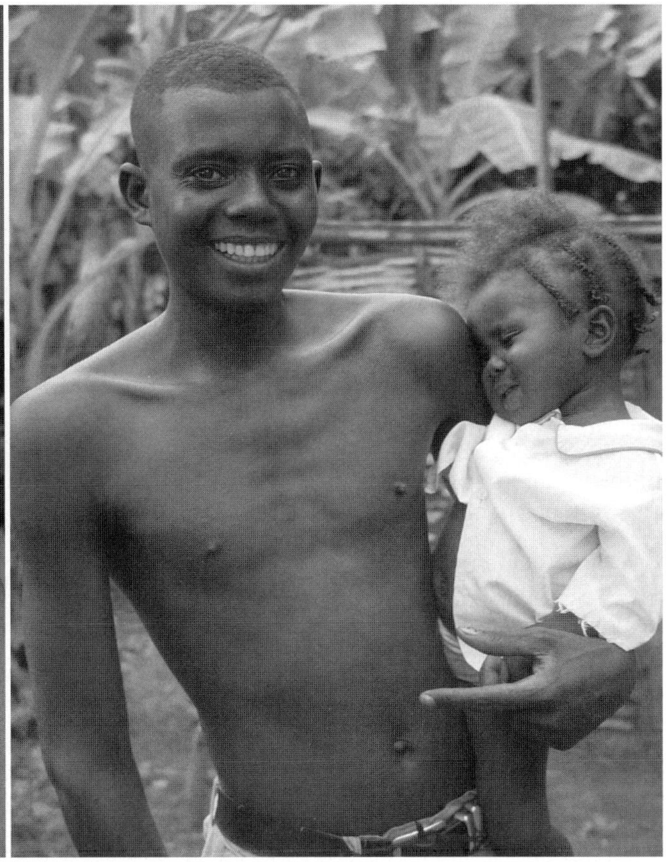

B

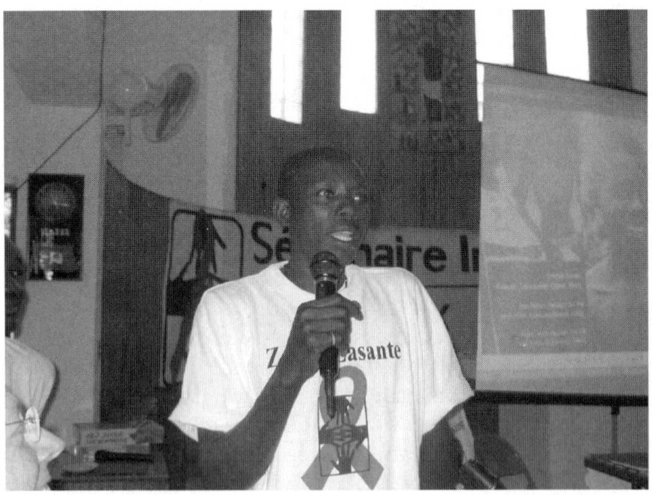

C

FIGURE 4-1 The "Lazarus effect": Effective, accessible treatment for HIV and TB brought Joseph back from the brink of death. His experience, and that of hundreds of thousands of other impoverished patients in rural Haiti now receiving free medical care through a public-private partnership, is renewing his community's faith in the health sector and restoring hope to the destitute sick everywhere. *A,* March 2003: Joseph, before treatment. *B,* September 2003: Joseph after treatment for HIV and TB, with his healthy niece. *C,* August 2004: Joseph speaks at a health and human rights conference. (*A* and *B,* by David Walton; *C,* by Joia Mukherjee. Copyright, Partners in Health. All rights reserved.)

a ranking cause of loss of health-care workers is premature death, often from AIDS.[7] In 1999, it was estimated that 17% to 32% of health-care workers in Botswana had HIV disease, a number expected to increase in the coming years.[8] A recent study that examined the fates of a small cohort of Ugandan physicians found that at least 22 of the 77 doctors who graduated from Makerere Medical School in 1984 had died by 2004, most presumably of AIDS.* Similar numbers have been registered in South Africa, where a small study by the

*Reliable information was obtained for 74 of the 77 graduates, 22 of whom were confirmed dead. "The presumed causes of death (death certificates were not available) were AIDS (11); suicide (six); road traffic injuries, hepatitis, and alcohol related disease (one each); and unknown (two). Five of the suicides were related to knowledge or fear of being HIV positive." Dambisya Y: The fate and career destinations of doctors who qualified at Uganda's Makerere Medical School in 1984: Retrospective cohort study. BMJ 329:600–601, 2004.

South African Human Sciences Research Council found that seroprevalence among health professionals was similar to that among the general population—in this case, 15.7% of all health-care workers surveyed.[9]

The shortage of empowered medical personnel in the areas hardest hit by HIV has profound implications for prevention and treatment efforts in these regions. The cycle of health sector impoverishment, brain drain, and consequent lack of personnel to fill positions, when they are available, conspires against ambitious programs to bring antiretroviral drugs to those living with both AIDS and poverty. The president of Botswana recently declared that one of his country's main obstacles to rapidly expanding HIV/AIDS treatment is "a dearth of doctors, nurses, pharmacists, and other health workers."[10] In South Africa, the departure of nearly 600 pharmacists in 2001, coupled with standing vacancies for 32,000 nurses, has put continued strain on that relatively affluent country's ability to respond to calls for expanded treatment programs.[11,12] In Malawi, only 28% of established nursing posts are filled.[5] Furthermore, the education of medical trainees is also jeopardized as the ranks of the health and academic communities continue to shrink due to migration or disease. The long-term implications are staggering.

A proper biosocial analysis of the brain drain reminds us that health personnel flight—almost always, as this review suggests, from poor to less-poor regions—is not simply a question of desire for more equitable remuneration. Epidemiologic trends and access to the tools of the trade are also relevant, as are working conditions in general. The advent of HIV has led, in many of the settings now losing skilled health personnel, to a sharp rise in tuberculosis incidence; other opportunistic infections have also become, in the eyes of providers, insuperable challenges. Together, these forces have conspired to render the provision of proper care impossible, as the comments of a Kenyan medical resident suggest: "Regarding HIV/AIDS, it is impossible to go home and forget about it. Even the simplest opportunistic infections we have no drugs for. Even if we do, there is only enough for a short course. It is impossible to forget about it....Just because of the numbers, I am afraid of going to the floors. It is a nightmare thinking of going to see the patients. You are afraid of the risk of infection, diarrhea, urine, vomit, blood....It is frightening to think about returning."[13]

Given the impossible situations under which these health-care personnel work, is it any surprise, then, when Randall Tobias, the U.S. government's appointed Global AIDS Coordinator, notes that there are more Ethiopian physicians practicing in Chicago than in all of Ethiopia?[14] In Zambia, only 50 of the 600 doctors trained since the country's independence in 1964 remain in their home country.[12] Nor is it surprising that a 1999 survey of medical students in Ghana in their final year of training revealed that 40 of 43 students planned to leave the country upon graduation.[4]

When providing care for the sick becomes a nightmare for those at the beginning of clinical training, physician "burnout" soon follows among those who carry on in settings of impoverishment. In the public-sector institutions put in place to care for the poorest, the confluence of epidemic disease, lack of resources with which to respond, and user fees have led to widespread burn-out among health workers. Raviola and colleagues offer an important biosocial study linking epidemiology, the experience of providers, and an understanding of the political economy of the Kenyan health-care system. "I don't see a future for the medical profession here," concludes a resident at Kenyatta National Hospital in Nairobi. "Why? It is expensive. You have to invest a lot. There is no government support. People can't afford care here."[13]

In the resource-poor settings upon which this chapter has focused, medical personnel are often precisely those who would conduct research, whether biosocial or conventional, in tropical and infectious diseases. Nurses and other providers are of course similarly affected, but patients and their families are those who pay most dearly for provider burnout, just as they bear the burden of disease and, with the introduction of user fees, much of the cost of responding, however inadequately, to new epidemics and to persistent plagues.

Structural Adjustment and Access to Care

The large-scale socioeconomic forces at work in the differential distribution of sickness and health often stem from decisions made far from hospital wards or even national capitals. Many African countries in fact registered improvements in health systems and indices in the years following independence. Kenya, for example, saw infant mortality decline by more than 58% between 1963 and the early 1990s.[15] However, the economic crises of the 1970s and 1980s left many of these postcolonial nations mired in mounting debts to offshore creditors. African governments needed loans to pay interest on the outstanding debts and to meet basic social spending needs. The World Bank and the International Monetary Fund became the principal creditors in this arena, and these institutions soon found themselves the chief sources of funding for health and development projects in poor countries. Loans came with strict requirements, however: the imposition of sweeping economic "reforms" in favor of a "free market" system designed to stimulate the economy and fix perceived imbalances in trade and government budgets. These economic austerity measures—termed "structural adjustment programs"—had profound and often deleterious effects on the health of many countries, as mandatory reductions of government budgets led to sharp declines in funding for the health sector. In Nigeria, for example, per capita expenditure on health care fell by more than 70% between 1980 and 1987.[16] Some have argued that structural adjustment programs in fact increased risks for HIV infection in Africa.[17]

Cuts in health-care spending led to the closing of public health posts, clinics, and hospitals in many parts of sub-Saharan Africa. Even basic services—from first-aid to prenatal care—were slashed from the operating budgets of many Ministries of Health. Between 1990 and 1992, 14 African countries—all mired in structural adjustment programs—saw at least a 10% decline in the level of polio vaccination. Botswana topped the list with a 24% reduction in polio vaccine coverage during this time.[18]

The collateral damage of economic austerity programs in sub-Saharan Africa also directly affected health-care professionals. Thousands of doctors and nurses across the continent lost their jobs as a result of budget restructuring. Coupled with the brain drain phenomenon, the health sector was further decimated as skilled employees lost their jobs and emigrated overseas. Ghana saw its contingent of doctors more than halved between 1982 and 1992, from 1700 to fewer than 670.[19] In late 2003, an estimated 4000 Kenyan nurses were unemployed secondary to economic policies that restricted recruitment of health workers into the public sector.[20]

User Fees

Another legacy of economic austerity programs is the widespread institution of "user fees" for health services that were formerly free of charge, with the intent of generating revenue for the health sector. Instead of revitalizing the health sector, however, user fees have often sharply reduced the ability of the poor to access medical care. In Ghana, Swaziland, and Congo—three of the first countries to implement user fees—data have shown that making the poor pay for care led to a marked reduction in the utilization of health services.[21]

In an effort to improve access to primary care, specifically maternal and child health, UNICEF and WHO introduced the Bamako Initiative in 1998, with the approval of the Health Ministries of the WHO African Region. The initiative includes the provision of generic essential drugs by donor agencies or national governments to district and village health management committees. These drugs are then sold to the public at a profit, which is then, theoretically, used to buy back the initial stock of drugs and to improve the quality of health centers. But despite widespread support from decision makers and a great deal of positive press, several studies have reported a decline in attendance rates for health services as a result of the user charges stipulated by the Bamako Initiative.[22,23] A longitudinal study conducted in Congo revealed a 40% decrease in health service utilization between 1987 and 1991 after the adoption of the Bamako Initiative.[24]

Similar declines in the utilization of health services after the introduction of cost-sharing were documented elsewhere in the region, including in Tanzania (where utilization of outpatient services in government district hospitals declined by more than 50%), Uganda, Swaziland, and Ghana.[25–28] Despite exemptions for children and the indigent, Mbugua and colleagues found that attendance at rural Kenyan government health facilities plummeted by 41% after user fees were introduced, and rebounded after fees were abolished.[29] In a cross-sectional study of 37 countries in sub-Saharan Africa, even the money-minded World Bank concluded that user fees decreased utilization of health services.[30] Another study revealed that the number of men reporting to sexually transmitted disease (STD) public clinics in Kenya fell by 40% after user charges were introduced in 1989; the authors concluded that the introduction of user fees in STD clinics likely increased the number of untreated STDs in the population.[31] This association has clear implications for HIV treatment and prevention efforts, as HIV is a sexually transmitted disease in much of the world.

Economic Costs and Adherence to HIV Therapy

As HIV treatment programs in resource-poor settings undergo expansion, advocates and pundits alike agree that medication adherence is paramount to the success of these initiatives. But early data have already shown that adherence is significantly reduced in programs in which patients are forced to pay even nominal fees for their medications. Of 137 Ugandan patients being treated with antiretrovirals (ARVs), nearly 33% had dropped out of therapy within 38 weeks; many of them evidenced drug-resistant disease. The cost of therapy was the main reason cited by patients for poor adherence.[32] In Senegal, up until 2000 all patients were required to pay $35 a month for antiretroviral treatment. Indigent patients were exempted from these fees in 2001, and in 2003 the government launched free antiretroviral treatment for all. In a study of adherence during this period, it was noted that over 50% of patients reporting treatment interruption for more than 5 days in 1999–2000 cited financial problems as the chief cause. By 2003, this percentage had dropped to 15%.[33]

Studies from other countries corroborate the negative effects of direct and indirect costs of antiretroviral therapy on adherence. In an analysis of barriers to antiretroviral adherence in Botswana, Weiser and colleagues revealed that nearly 50% of patients who self-reported poor adherence cited financial reasons as the most significant barrier. The authors advised that "patients in Botswana will achieve much higher adherence rates if structural and economic treatment barriers are minimized."[34] These results are similar to those reported by researchers in Uganda, who concluded that "ability to purchase and secure a stable supply of therapy are major barriers to adherence."[35] In Côte d'Ivoire, despite a UNAIDS HIV Drug Access Initiative and public subsidies, the poorest patients were precisely those who did not have access to ARVs.[36]

These studies suggest that charging for ARVs excludes the poor from access to care and also serves to increase the likelihood that acquired resistance will develop through inadequate therapy. In a recent editorial, Mukherjee concludes that "a human rights–based—rather than market-based—approach is the only realistic strategy for an epidemic that is concentrated in the poor and marginalized communities who have neither access to health care nor the ability to pay for treatment."[37]

The economic toll of HIV before the patient is even diagnosed leads to further impoverishment and delays in seeking and receiving effective care. Lessons from the long-entrenched TB epidemic are instructive. In Bangladesh, where all TB services and medications are provided free of charge, the average total loss of income before proper diagnosis and treatment was estimated to be $245, or nearly 4 months of a family's yearly income.[38] Findings were similar in Zambia, where the indirect cost to patients prior to a TB diagnosis was almost 130% of their mean monthly income. These authors found that "most patients required significant financial assistance while seeking care for their disease-related symptoms."[39] In war-torn Sierra Leone, Gibson and colleagues noted that the highest costs to patients were sustained prior to entry into a tuberculosis treatment program, highlighting the economic burden to the patient and family before a diagnosis is even obtained.[40] In Thailand, even after diagnosis at a government hospital, 80% of patients incurred significant costs for travel and food during hospital visits. In the same study, up to 15% of patients were forced to sell household assets and use bank loans to cope with illness-related expenses.[41]

Travel to and from the clinic can exact a significant toll on patients and is an often-significant barrier to care, especially among the poor.[42,43] Data for TB have shown high travel costs to clinic are directly associated with poor compliance, as patients cannot afford regular transportation to pick up their medications every month.[44] These data have obvious implications for HIV treatment programs.

Civil Conflict

The noxious synergy of civil strife and poverty has a well-documented negative impact on the health of the poor. Conflict contributes to the deterioration of existing public health infrastructure in addition to creating conditions that decrease access to clean water and shelter, which can in turn lead to increased incidence of infectious pathogens. Excess morbidity and mortality often result from a near-complete lack of basic health services in and around conflict zones.[45] In an editorial on the violence that engulfed Haiti in 2004, Farmer laments the near-total collapse of the health sector.[46] As easy targets for violence, as well as often being overwhelmed by the consequences of violence, hospitals are increasingly prone to acute staff shortages and stockouts of medications and supplies. The Port-au-Prince hospital—the only university teaching hospital, and the major provider of health care to the poor in the capital city—has been nonfunctional for months at the time of this writing.[47]

The direct impact of conflict on HIV and TB epidemics has also been documented. In Sierra Leone, 23% of tuberculosis clinics closed between 1990 and 1994 secondary to violence and war.[40] The Rwandan genocide in 1994 is believed to have contributed to the expansion of the HIV epidemic to rural areas of that country.[48]

Stigma

The role of stigma as a major barrier to care for HIV patients has been extensively reviewed elsewhere.[49–51] However, recent experiences in resource-poor settings suggest that the introduction of effective HIV treatment and care programs can help destigmatize what was once considered a fatal disease.[52] In communities in rural Haiti, dramatic, visible recoveries after initiation of antiretroviral treatment, dubbed the "Lazarus effect," have led to a sharp decline in HIV-related stigma.[53] While the contours of discrimination vary from country to country, AIDS-related stigma will likely decrease as access to treatment improves and as people come to realize that HIV is a manageable disease.

THE COST OF MALARIA

Malaria's human toll is enormous. An estimated 250 million people suffer from malarial disease each year, and the disease annually kills between 1 million and 2.5 million people, mostly pregnant women and children under 5. The poor disproportionately suffer the consequences of malaria. Fifty-eight percent of malaria mortality occurs in the poorest 20% of the world's population; 90% of malaria mortality is registered in sub-Saharan Africa.[54] The differential magnitude of this burden of mortality is greater than that associated with any other disease.[55] Malaria-associated morbidity is also higher, as documented in a study from Zambia which revealed a 40% greater prevalence of parasitemia in children under 5 in the poorest wealth quintile than in the richest.[56] Despite suffering the greatest consequences of malaria, the poor are precisely those least able to access effective prevention and treatment tools.

Economists describe the complex interactions between malaria and poverty from an opposite but complementary perspective: they delineate ways in which malaria arrests economic development both for individuals and for whole nations. Microeconomic analyses focusing on direct and indirect costs estimate that malaria may consume up to 10% of a household's annual income.[57] A Ghanaian study that categorized the population by income group highlighted the regressive nature of this cost: while the burden of malaria represents only 1% of wealthy families' income, 34% of a poor household's income is consumed by it.[54]

At the national level, macroeconomic analyses estimate that malaria may reduce the per-capita gross national product (GNP) of a disease-endemic country by 50% relative to a non-malarial country. The causes of this drag include high fertility rates, impaired cognitive development of children, decreased schooling, decreased saving, decreased foreign investment, and restriction of worker mobility.[58] Given this enormous cost, it is little wonder that an important review by Sachs and Malaney concludes that "where malaria prospers most, human societies have prospered least."[59]

Rolling Back Malaria

Due in part to differences in vector distribution and climate, resource-rich countries offer few blueprints for malaria control and treatment that are applicable in tropical settings. In 2001, African heads of state endorsed the WHO Roll Back Malaria (RBM) campaign, which prescribes strategies appropriate for sub-Saharan African countries. RBM recommends a three-pronged strategy to reduce malaria-related morbidity and mortality: the use of ITNs, combination antimalarial therapy, and indoor residual spraying.

Some RBM programs have had limited successes, but overall the burden of disease has continued to grow. In fact, annual malaria-attributable mortality increased between 1999 and 2003.[60] While the RBM's own *Africa Malaria Report 2003* is quick to note that morbidity and mortality data collection methods in sub-Saharan Africa are inadequate and indicators may thus lag behind actual outcomes of the ongoing campaigns, they nevertheless acknowledge that "RBM is acting against a background of increasing malaria burden."

Limited success in scaling-up ITN coverage is indicative of the campaign's inadequate acknowledgment of the economic barriers that preclude the destitute sick from accessing critical preventive technologies. Despite proven efficacy and what are considered "reasonable costs,"* the 2003 RBM report reveals disappointing levels of ITN coverage. Of 28 African countries surveyed, only 1.3% (range, 0.2%–4.9%) of households owned at least one ITN, and less than 2% of children sleep under an ITN.[54] Why has the RBM campaign failed to achieve its goals? Do Africans not want to use bednets? Do they not recognize malaria as a health risk? Or have project managers and donors miscalculated most Africans' ability to obtain bednets?

The RBM strategy initially emphasized the importance of commercial markets as sources of ITNs for African populations.[61] A precedent supporting this emphasis is the prior existence in countries such as Madagascar and Mali of local markets for untreated bednets. Presumably, therefore, a demand for bednets existed prior to the RBM campaign, as did a distribution system with points of sale.[62] However, this market approach, even with the application of subsidized social marketing strategies, has not resulted in large increases in coverage in the first years of the RBM campaign.

Several studies have attempted to define willingness to pay (WTP) and actual payment for ITNs in African countries in order to understand why market-based strategies have been unsuccessful. Policy-makers often utilize WTP to determine appropriate pricing for social marketing projects and to project revenue and demand.[63] A cross-sectional study in a rural Nigerian community administered two questionnaires, 1 month apart, to examine community members' WTP for ITNs, actual purchase of ITNs (the second questionnaire was accompanied by the opportunity to buy a subsidized ITN), and factors (such as socioeconomic status and recent history of malarial illness) contributing to hypothetical and actual purchase (n = 453 answering both surveys). The poorest quintile perceived a greater risk of malaria relative to the other quintiles (27.3% vs. 12.9%–21.6%, $p < 0.05$). However, the poorest quintile was least likely to own a net, purchase a net, or express hypothetical WTP. Interestingly, even the most well-off quintile was willing to pay only 51% of the government-set price of the ITN. This finding suggests that even the relatively well-off may not be willing or able to pay for bednets at set prices. The authors of this study concluded that reliance on the sale of nets alone may prove inadequate and that further studies to define the degrees to which costs can be lowered and/or demand increased are needed.[64]

Guyatt and colleagues also offer a critique of the WTP methodology in highland Kenya. Their 2002 study compared the attitudes of people living in homesteads that had been provided with heavily subsidized ITNs (n = 190) to households that had no ITNs and had not been targeted by other health-care initiatives (n = 200). Ninety-seven percent of all households expressed willingness to pay for ITNs. However, only 4% of those willing to pay offered spontaneously to meet the suggested price of 350 KSh (Kenyan shillings). After being prompted that "nets are expensive," 26% of respondents expressed willingness to pay the full price. This study did not actually offer nets for sale; therefore, the number of nets actually purchased cannot be compared. However, this study did contextualize the hypothetical WTP for ITNs by comparing it to other household costs: the price of an ITN equals the cost of sending three children to primary school for a year. In contextualizing the nets' relative cost, the authors call into question the likelihood that families in this district, over half of whom fall below the Kenyan poverty line, would actually be able to purchase ITNs.[65]

Given the documented barriers to purchasing ITNs, especially among the poorest of the poor, many researchers and development professionals involved in malaria programs have called for the free distribution of ITNs, stressing their importance as a public health measure: "the priority for Africa should be to adopt ITNs as a public good—like childhood vaccines."[66]

Adoption of free ITN distribution strategies have been limited, however, by concerns about their feasibility and about clients' misuse of the bednets (for example, as nets for fishing). Evidence from a targeted free distribution program discounts both concerns. In 2001, a Kenyan program sponsored by UNICEF sought to distribute 70,000 ITNs to pregnant women through antenatal clinics. Within 12 weeks, over 50% of the ITNs had reached their intended targets. A 1-year follow-up evaluation of 294 women who had received bednets while pregnant—152 women were from a high-transmission area and 142 from a low-transmission area—revealed that 84% of women in the high-transmission area used the nets throughout their pregnancy. One year later, 77% continued to use the bednets. In the low-transmission area, 57% of women used the bednets during their pregnancy, and 46% continued to use them a year later.[67] These results contradict suppositions that free nets may not be used because recipients do not value them.

Given the scope and magnitude of the challenge posed by malaria, it is unlikely that any one strategy will work for every region or population within a country or across the world. Encouraging results from an employer-based ITN distribution

*ITNs have been proven to be an efficacious and cost-effective public health intervention. A meta-analysis of controlled trials indicates that malaria incidence is reduced by 50% in those who sleep under ITNs compared to those who do not use nets at all (Choi HW, Breman JG, Teutsch SM, et al: The effectiveness of insecticide impregnated bednets in reducing cases of malaria infection: A meta-analysis of published results. Am J Trop Med Hyg 52:377–382, 1995). Even when use of ITNs is compared to use of nontreated nets, the incidence of malaria is reduced by a quarter. On an individual level, the utility of ITNs extends beyond protection from malaria, as several studies suggest that all-cause mortality is reduced in children under 5 to a degree that is greater than the effect attributable to the reduction in malarial disease alone (Nuwaha F: The challenge of chloroquine-resistant malaria in sub-Saharan Africa. Health Policy Plan 16:1–12, 2001). Morbidity, specifically due to anemia, which predisposes children to diarrheal and respiratory illnesses and pregnant women to low-birth-weight infants, is also reduced in populations using ITNs (Bates I, Fenton C, Gruber J, et al: Vulnerability to malaria tuberculosis, an HIV/AIDS infection and disease. Part 1: Determinants operating at individual and household level. Lancet Infect Dis 4:267–277, 2004). In addition, ITNs provide a supplemental benefit in some areas by preventing transmission of lymphatic filariasis, cutaneous leishmaniasis, Chagas disease, and tickborne relapsing fever (Molyneux DH, Nantulya VM: Linking disease control programmes in rural Africa: A pro-poor strategy to reach Abuja targets and millenium development goals. BMJ 328:1129–1132, 2004). At the community level, investigators suggest that the use of an ITN in just one household may reduce the number of mosquito bites in households up to several hundred meters away (Curtis C, Maxwell C, Lemnge M, et al: Scaling-up coverage with insecticide-treated nets against malaria in Africa: Who should pay? Lancet Infect Dis 3:304–307, 2003). The cost of ITNs per disability-adjusted life year (DALY) saved is estimated at $10 to $38, which qualifies it as a "very efficient use of resources and [a] good candidate for public subsidy" (Nuwaha F: The challenge of chloroquine-resistant malaria in sub-Saharan Africa. Health Policy Plan 16:1–12, 2001).

system in Kenya highlight important successes of public-private partnerships, particularly those targeted at working people who have higher and more stable incomes than those in rural subsistence economies.[68] Potential synergies between measles vaccine campaigns and possibly with lymphatic filariasis eradication campaigns have been reported or suggested.[69] Concerns about discomfort associated with sleeping under ITNs or about insecticide toxicities must be addressed through educational campaigns.

The challenge of malaria control will continue to require careful study of appropriate prevention and treatment strategies in the context of our increasingly sophisticated molecular understanding of the pathogen, vector, and host. However, an appreciation for the economic and structural devastation wrought by malaria, like that by diarrhea, AIDS, and tuberculosis, on the most vulnerable populations should heighten our commitment to the critical analysis of how to implement proven strategies to prevent and treat these diseases.

HARNESSING SCIENCE TO CONTROL EPIDEMIC DISEASE: A BIOSOCIAL CHALLENGE

All of what are now often considered tropical diseases—AIDS, African trypanosomiasis, dengue, leishmaniasis, malaria, schistosomiasis, TB, Chagas disease, lymphatic filariasis, and onchocerciasis—are more notable for their differences than for their similarities. Some are caused by viral pathogens; others by parasites or bacteria. Some are vector-borne; others have no known nonhuman hosts. Some of these infections are vaccine-preventable; for others, reliable prevention methods are still under development. While their efficacy varies widely, prevention and/or treatment options are available for each of these diseases. Why, then, do these infections remain ranking causes of death and debility in the 21st century?

In truth, the so-called "tropical" diseases are more linked to social and economic class than to latitude. Although new basic knowledge, especially if generated by "use-inspired basic research,"[70] will lead to improved diagnostic and therapeutic tools, and even as the pace of discovery increases due to our emerging understanding of the genomic structure of the pathogens and vectors in question, it is increasingly clear that social and economic barriers constitute formidable obstacles to the effective and equitable deployment of technologies new and old. As Farmer and Becerra wrote,

> The phenomena that concern us—epidemic and endemic disease—are not solely biological; neither are they purely social. Yet conventional studies typically rely on disciplinary approaches and fail to reveal the full complexity of these epidemics. Only by embracing a transdisciplinary, biosocial approach can we hope to describe fully these "tropical" epidemics, and intervene successfully. For example, when yet another hydroelectric dam alters rates of schistosomiasis or filariasis, we must also study the "behavior" of policymakers at development agencies if we are to understand the distribution and outcome of schistosomiasis and filariasis. When recurrent drug stockouts characterize a tuberculosis control program, the "knowledge, attitudes, beliefs and practices" of patients may have only limited relevance to the emergence of drug resistance, whereas fluctuating drug prices, tariffs, and poor drug quality might prove determinant. When poor bloodscreening practices mean rising rates of American trypanosomiasis, it is an anthropology of blood banking and bloodbankers, rather than scrutiny of patients' notions, that is called for.[71]

In seeking to understand the distribution and outcomes of infectious diseases in a broader social context, it is clear that a rising tide of social inequality is making it increasingly difficult to bring research to the bedside (in fact, many do not sleep in beds, but on mats or worse). This rising outcome gap may well prove the biggest challenge facing epidemic disease control in the coming decades. That is, as we develop new tools—vaccines and other preventives, diagnostics, and drugs—our failure to distribute them equitably means that the poor will do worse than ever. This has been seen starkly as regards TB, malaria, HIV, and other epidemics: although the diseases occur in many settings, virtually all deaths are registered among the poor. From an equity perspective, the situation has gotten worse since new tools were developed.

Not all the news is bad. Structural obstacles can be surmounted, as we saw in considering community-based care for AIDS in rural Haiti, based on previous successful efforts to treat tuberculosis in the same setting.[72] There have also been promising developments in the treatment of visceral leishmaniasis: an estimated 500,000 cases are diagnosed each year in India, Nepal, Bangladesh, East Africa, and parts of Brazil. Each of these settings is beset by socioeconomic barriers to care, and these barriers vary from site to site. In some places, health-care reform has weakened the public delivery systems. In others, such systems are absent or beyond the reach of the majority. But oral miltefosine, the first drug given "orphan" designation in Europe, is a relatively simple treatment and has proven effective in India,[73] where village health workers or mobile teams could administer the drug. It is hoped that miltefosine may also prove effective against post-kala-azar dermal leishmaniasis.

Malaria control, as noted, will require more basic science research. *Anopheles* genome sequencing and genetic manipulation for vector control are already well under way. Bioinformatics and applied genomics will help identify targets for new drugs, vaccines, and diagnostics. In some malaria-endemic areas, novel agents are already available to the fortunate few. The development and evaluation of new therapeutics—single-dose rectal artesunate and the combination pill Lapdap, consisting of two antifolate medications, chlorproguanil and dapsone—are now occurring in tandem with vector elimination campaigns. In KwaZulu Natal in South Africa, DDT reintroduction (indoor residual spraying), combined with the use of artemether-lumefantrine, dropped malaria cases dramatically. Without question, this represents a socially complex intervention that requires an understanding of local conditions and attitudes toward public health, insecticides, and tolerance of drugs with side effects.[74]

We conclude that a great deal more research is required if we are to have better diagnostics; more powerful, less toxic drugs; new control strategies; and effective vaccines for tropical diseases. Without a complementary analysis of social factors like those described in this chapter, however, the long-term deployment of old and new interventions to combat "tropical disease" will risk failure. In some cases, failure will simply maintain the alarmingly unequal topography of health-care outcomes around the globe, even for "easily treatable" diseases. However, as we have learned from the ravages of multidrug-resistant tuberculosis and malaria, failure is an unacceptable option: any efforts that result in failure exacerbate inequalities rather than diminish them, creating infections that are increasingly difficult to treat. Relinquishing our responsibility to treat these diseases in poor people is not an option; rather, we must seek to understand social as well as molecular mechanisms of treatment failure. The social mechanisms may stem from problems with policy-making and implementation, but they will result in the development of resistance to drugs and insecticides, continued unacceptable rates of morbidity and mortality, and the persistence of pathogens that should be controlled thanks to the science of tropical medicine.

ACKNOWLEDGMENT

The authors wish to acknowledge Alice Yang for her invaluable contributions to the conceptualization, research, and revision of this chapter.

REFERENCES

1. For a more detailed discussion of community-based approaches to HIV treatment and care, see Farmer P, Léandre F, Mukherjee JS, et al: Community-based approaches to HIV treatment in resource-poor settings. Lancet 358:404–409, 2001.
2. Walton DA, Farmer PE, Lambert W, et al: Integrated HIV prevention and care strengthens primary health care: Lessons from rural Haiti. J Public Health Policy 25:137–158, 2004.
3. Behforouz HL, Farmer PE, Mukherjee JS: From directly observed therapy to *accompagnateurs:* Enhancing AIDS treatment outcomes in Haiti and in Boston. Clin Infect Dis 38:S429–S436, 2004.
4. Padarath A, Chamberlain C, McCoy D, et al: Health personnel in southern Africa: Confronting misdistribution and brain drain. Regional Network for Equity and Health in Southern Africa (EQUINET), Health Systems Trust, MEDACT (UK), 2003. Available at: www.equinetafrica.org/bibl/docs/healthpersonnel.pdf.
5. Aitken JM, Kemp J: HIV/AIDS, equity, and health sector personnel in southern Africa. Regional Network for Equity in Health in Southern Africa (EQUINET), Oxfam, 2003. Available at: www.equinetafrica.org/bibl/docs/hivpersonnel.pdf.
6. Gupta N, Zurn P, Diallo K, et al: Uses of population census data for monitoring geographical imbalance in the health workforce: Snapshots from three developing countries. Int J Equity Health 2:11, 2003. Available at www.equityhealthj.com/content/2/11.
7. United States Agency for International Development: The Health Sector Human Resource Crisis in Africa: An Issues Paper. Washington, DC, United States Agency for International Development, 2003. Available at: www.dec.org/pdf_docs/PNACS527.pdf.
8. Cohen D: Human Capital and the HIV Epidemic in Sub-Saharan Africa. Geneva, ILO Program on HIV/AIDS and the World of Work, 2002. Available at:www.ilo.org/public/english/protection/trav/aids/publ/wp2_humancapital.pdf.
9. Ncayiyana D: Doctors and nurses with HIV and AIDS in sub-Saharan Africa. BMJ 329:584–585, 2004.
10. Dugger C: Botswana's brain drain cripples war on AIDS. New York Times A10 (November 13, 2003).
11. Katerere K, Matowe L: Effect of pharmacist emigration on pharmaceutical services in southern Africa. Am J Health Syst Pharm 60:1169–1170, 2003.
12. Ogundipe S: Brain drain in Africa stalls anti-HIV campaign. Vanguard (Lagos) (August 10, 2004). Available at: allafrica.com/stories/200408100015.html.
13. Raviola G, Machoki M, Mwaikambo E, et al: HIV, disease plague, demoralization and "burnout": Resident experience of the medical profession in Nairobi, Kenya. Cult Med Psychiatry 26:55–86, 2002.
14. Tobias RL: Global fight against HIV/AIDS: What do we need to do differently. Remarks given at the XV International AIDS Conference, Bangkok, Thailand, July 14, 2004. Available at: www.state.gov/s/gac/rl/rm/2004/34366pf.htm.
15. Kieti Kimalu P: Debt Relief and Health Care in Kenya. Nairobi, Kenya Institute for Public Policy Research and Analysis, 2001. Available at: www.wider.unu.edu/conference/conference-2001-2/poster%20papers/kimalu.pdf.
16. Inter-Church Coalition on Africa. Beyond Adjustment: Responding to the Health Crisis in Africa. Toronto, ICCAF, 1993.
17. Lurie P, Hintzen P, Lowe R: Socioeconomic obstacles to HIV prevention and treatment in developing countries: The roles of the International Monetary Fund and the World Bank. AIDS 9:539–546, 1995.
18. Kamakes J, van der Meer J, Mooren H, et al: Economic adjustment in poor countries is too painful for health care. Bulletin Medicus Mundi 64, 1997. Available at: www.medicusmundi.ch/bulletin/bulletin641.htm.
19. Shoepf BG, Schoepf C, Millen JV: Theoretical therapies, remote remedies: SAPs and the political ecology of poverty and health in Africa. In Kim JY, Millen JV, Irwin A, et al (eds): Dying for Growth: Global Inequality and the Health of the Poor. Monroe, ME, Common Courage Press, 2000, pp 91–125.
20. Lee JW: Speech given in Geneva, Switzerland, at the opening session of the meeting of interested parties, November 3, 2003. Available at: www.who.int/dg/lee/speeches/2003/MIP_Openingsession/en/.
21. Ahrin-Tenkorang D: Mobilizing Resources for Health: The Case for User Fees Revisited. Geneva, Commission on Macroeconomics and Health, World Health Organization, 2000. Available at: www.cmhealth.org/docs/wg3_paper6.pdf.
22. Uzochukwu B, Onwujekwe O: Socio-economic differences and health seeking behaviour for the diagnosis and treatment of malaria: A case study of four local government areas operating the Bamako initiative programme in south-east Nigeria. Int J Equity Health 3:6–12, 2004.
23. Ridde R: Fee-for-services, cost recovery, and equity in a district of Burkina Faso operating the Bamako Iniative. Bull World Health Org 81:532–538, 2003.
24. Haddad S, Fournier P: Quality, cost and utilization of health services in developing countries. A longitudinal study in Zaire. Soc Sci Med 40:743–753, 1995.
25. Hussein AK, Mujinja PG: The effect of the introduction of user charges on previously freely provided health services in government health facilities in Tanzania. East Afr Med J 74:751–757, 1997.
26. Kipp W, Kamugisha J, Jacobs P, et al: User fees, health staff incentives, and service utilization in Kabarole District, Uganda. Bull World Health Org 79:1032–1037, 2001.
27. Yoder R: Are people willing and able to pay for health services? Soc Sci Med 29:35–42, 1989.
28. Waddington C, Enyimayew K: A price to pay: The impact of user charges in Ashanti-Akim District, Ghana. Int J Health Plan Management 4:17–47, 1989.
29. Mbugua J, Bloom G, Segall M: Impact of user charges on vulnerable groups: The case of Kibwezi in rural Kenya. Soc Sci Med 41: 829–835, 1995.
30. Nolan B, Turbat V: Cost Recovery in Public Health Services in Sub-Saharan Africa. Washington, DC, World Bank, 1995.
31. Moses S, Manji F, Bradley JE, et al: Impact of user fees at a referral centre for sexually transmitted diseases in Kenya. Lancet 340: 463–466, 1992.
32. Kamya MR, et al: Treatment outcomes for antiretroviral therapy in a routine clinical setting in Kampala, Uganda. Presented at the 7th International Congress on Drug Therapy in HIV Infection, November 14–19, 2004, Glasgow, Abstract PL4.4.
33. Laniece I, Diop K, Desclaux A, et al: Determinants of long-term adherence to antiretroviral drugs among adults followed for over four years in Dakar, Senegal. Presented at the XV International AIDS Conference, July 11–16, 2004, Bangkok, Abstract We OrB1320. Available at www.iasociety.org/egias/show. asp abstract_id=2175436.
34. Weiser S, Wolfe W, Bangsberg D, et al: Barriers to antiretroviral adherence for patients living with HIV infection and AIDS in Botswana. J Acquir Immune Defic Syndr 34:281–288, 2003.
35. Byakika-Tusiime J, Oyugi JH, Tumwikirize WA, et al: Ability to purchase and secure stable therapy are significant predictors of non-adherence to antiretroviral therapy in Kampala, Uganda. Presented at the 10th Conference on Retroviruses and Opportunistic Infections, February 10–14, 2003, Boston, Abstract 170. Available at: www.aegis.com/conferences/10croi/170.html.
36. Msellati P, Juillet-Amari A, Prudhomme J, et al: Socio-economic and health characteristics of HIV-infected patients seeking care in relation to access to the Drug Access Initiative and to antiretroviral treatment in Côte d'Ivoire. AIDS 17:S63–S68, 2003.
37. Mukherjee J: Basing treatment on rights rather than ability to pay: 3 by 5. Lancet 363:1071–1072, 2004.
38. Croft RA, Croft RP: Expenditure and loss of income incurred by tuberculosis patients before reaching effective treatment in Bangladesh. Int J Tuberc Lung Dis 2:252–254, 1998.

39. Needham DM, Godfrey-Faussett P, Foster SD: Barriers to tuberculosis control in urban Zambia: The economic impact and burden on patients prior to diagnosis. Int J Tuberc Lung Dis 2:811–817, 1998.
40. Gibson N, Boillot F, Jalloh H: The cost of tuberculosis to patients in Sierra Leone's war zone. Int J Tuberc Lung Dis 2:726–731, 1998.
41. Kamolratanakul P, Sawert H, Kongsin S, et al: Economic impact of tuberculosis at the household level. Int J Tuberc Lung Dis 3: 596–602, 1999.
42. Needham DM, Bowman D, Foster SD, et al: Patient care seeking barriers and tuberculosis programme reform: A qualitative study. Health Policy 67:93–106, 2004.
43. Wilkinson D, Floyd K, Gilks CF: Costs and cost-effectiveness of alternative tuberculosis management strategies in South Africa—Implications for policy. S Afr Med J 87:451–455, 1997.
44. Comolet TM, Rakotomalala R, Rajaonarioa H: Factors determining compliance with tuberculosis treatment in an urban environment, Tamatave, Madagascar. Int J Tuberc Lung Dis 2:891–897, 1998.
45. Connolly M, Heymann D: Deadly comrades: War and infectious disease. Lancet 360:S23–S24, 2002.
46. Farmer PE: Political violence and public health in Haiti. New Engl J Med 350:1483–1486, 2004.
47. Kamber M: Haiti's wounds overwhelm a suffering public hospital. New York Times A4 (November 28, 2004).
48. Joint United Nations Programme on HIV/AIDS: 2004 Report on the Global AIDS Epidemic. Geneva, UNAIDS, 2004.
49. Kalichman SC, Simbayi LC: HIV testing attitudes, AIDS stigma, and voluntary HIV counseling and testing in a black township in Cape Town, South Africa. Sex Transm Dis 79:442–447, 2003.
50. Carr RL, Gramling LF: Stigma: A health barrier for women with AIDS. J Assoc Nurses AIDS Care 15:30–39, 2004.
51. de Bruyn T: HIV-related stigma and discrimination—The epidemic continues. Can HIV/AIDS Policy Law Rev 7:8–14, 2002.
52. Médecins sans Frontières South Africa, Department of Public Health at the University of Cape Town, Provincial Administration of the Western Cape, South Africa: Antiretroviral Therapy in Primary Health Care: The Experience of Khayelitsha, Programme in South Africa. Case Study. Geneva, World Health Organization, 2003.
53. Castro A, Farmer P: Understanding and addressing AIDS-related stigma: From anthropological theory to clinical practice in Haiti. Am J Public Health 95:53–59, 2005.
54. World Health Organization. Africa Malaria Report 2003. Geneva, World Health Organization, 2003.
55. Barat LM, Palmer N, Basu S, et al: Do malaria control interventions reach the poor? A view through the equity lens. Am J Trop Med Hyg 71:S174–S178, 2004.
56. Report on the Zambia Roll Back Malaria baseline study undertaken in 10 sentinel districts, July–August 2001. Zambia, RBM National Secretariat, 2001.
57. Russell S: The economic burden of illness for households in developing countries: A review of studies focusing on malaria, tuberculosis, and human immunodeficiency virus/acquired immunodeficiency syndrome. Am J Trop Med Hyg 71:S147–S155, 2004.
58. Malaney P, Spielman A, Sachs J: The malaria gap. Am J Trop Med Hyg 71:S141–S146, 2004.
59. Sachs J, Malaney O: The economic and social burden of malaria. Nature 415:680-685, 2002.
60. Yamey G: Roll Back Malaria: A failing global health campaign. BMJ 328:1086–1087, 2004.
61. World Health Organization: Scaling-up Insecticide-Treated Netting Programmes in Africa. Geneva: World Health Organization, 2002.
62. Lines J, Lengeler C, Cham K, et al: Scaling-up and sustaining insecticide-treated net coverage. Lancet Infect Dis 3:465–466, 2003.
63. Russell S, Fox-Rushby J, Arhin D: Willingness and ability to pay for health care: A selection of methods and issues. Health Policy Plan 10:94–101, 1995.
64. Onwujekwe O, Hanson K, Fox-Rushby J: Inequalities in purchase of mosquito nets and willingness to pay for insecticide-treated nets in Nigeria: Challenges for malaria control interventions. Malar J 3:6, 2004.
65. Guyatt HL, Ochola SA, Snow RW: Too poor to pay: Charging for insecticide-treated bednets in highland Kenya. Trop Med Int Health 7:846–850, 2002.
66. Curtis C, Maxwell C, Lemnge M, et al: Scaling-up coverage with insecticide-treated nets against malaria in Africa: Who should pay? Lancet Infect Dis 3:304–307, 2003.
67. Guyatt H, Ochola S: Use of bednets given free to pregnant women in Kenya. Lancet 362:1549–1550, 2003.
68. Ngugi IK, Chiguzo AN, Guyatt HL: A cost analysis of the employer-based bednet programme in coastal and western Kenya. Health Policy Plan 19:111–119, 2004.
69. Molyneux DH, Nantulya VM: Linking disease control programmes in rural Africa: A pro-poor strategy to reach Abuja targets and millennium development goals. BMJ 328:1129–1132, 2004.
70. Stokes D: Pasteur's Quadrant: Basic Science and Technological Innovation. Washington, DC, Brookings Institution Press, 1997.
71. Farmer PE, Becerra M: Biosocial research and the TDR agenda. TDR News 66:5–7, 2001.
72. Farmer P, Robin S, Ramilus SL, et al: Tuberculosis, poverty, and "compliance": lessons from rural Haiti. Semin Resp Infect 6: 254–260, 1991.
73. Sundar S, Jha TK, Sindermann H, et al: Oral miltefosine for Indian visceral leishmaniasis. N Engl J Med 347:1739–1746, 2002.
74. For more information on the South East African Combination Antimalarial Therapy (SEACAT) Evaluation, a joint project by Mozambique, South Africa, and Swaziland to study the effect of antimalarial therapy on the emergence of resistance, see www.malaria.org.za/Seacat/seacat.html.

5

Nutrition and Micronutrients in Tropical Infectious Diseases

MARGARET KOSEK
ROBERT E. BLACK
GERALD T. KEUSCH

INTRODUCTION

In addition to the toll in morbidity and mortality due to tropical infectious diseases, many infectious diseases common to all regions of the world last longer, are more clinically severe, and are more likely to have a fatal outcome in impoverished regions in the tropics because of the complex interactions between infection, protein-calorie malnutrition, and micronutrient deficiencies. The intent of this chapter is to provide insight into these interactions through a review of the supporting evidence linking the nutritional and micronutrient status of the host, the patency of the immune system, and the course and the outcome of infectious diseases of global importance. Although these interactions generally are accompanied by limited access to education, quality health care, and political instability, the interaction between nutrition and infection has immediate and direct adverse effects on health.

Despite modest improvements in indices during the past 15 years, protein energy malnutrition and micronutrient deficiencies remain highly prevalent in low- and middle-income countries. In 2000, the World Health Organization (WHO) estimated that 26.7% of children younger than the age of 5 years were underweight [weight for age Z (WAZ) <–2], 32.5% were stunted (height for age Z <–2), and 9.4% were wasted [weight for height Z (WHZ) <–2].[1] Of the micronutrients with a demonstrated importance in determining the severity of infectious diseases, it is estimated that clinical vitamin A deficiency (xerophthalmia) affects 4.4 million preschool children and subclinical vitamin A deficiency affects another 127 million.[2] Iron deficiency and consequent anemia is detected in a high proportion of children and adults in developing countries.[3] Zinc deficiency is considered to be common in developing countries and estimates suggest that nearly all low- or middle-income countries have a moderate to high risk of zinc deficiency.[4] It is clear that in developing areas the interaction of malnutrition and infectious disease is a key determinant in health outcomes and an important factor in the transmission and ecology of infectious diseases.

NUTRITION–INFECTION INTERACTIONS: PARADIGMS AND PRINCIPLES

In summarizing the experimental data for the interaction between malnutrition and infection in 1968, Scrimshaw et al. delineated three possible effects that may occur to varying degrees depending on the infectious agent and on the hosts' nutritional status: synergistic, antagonistic, or no effect.[5] The first, synergistic, occurs when the interaction of the infectious agent and nutritional deficiency results in a more adverse clinical outcome than the simple additive combination of the two conditions. This is easy to conceptualize: A malnourished child is more likely to die from a common intercurrent infection, such as pneumonia or dysentery, because of his or her weakened state than a well-nourished child. Alternatively, in more select cases the interaction between the malnutrition and the infection may be antagonistic. In this case, the combined effect of malnutrition and infection is less than expected because the infectious agent replication or pathogenicity is inhibited by the nutritional environment of the host. This may occur when the pathogen has greater requirements for or dependence on a metabolite than the host organism or when the pathology of the infection is dependent on host responses, such as inflammation, that are blunted by malnutrition. Lastly, there may exist circumstances in which the nutritional status of the host and the infectious agent do not interact and outcome is determined independently.

A guiding principle in the relationship between nutrition and infection has been the belief that dietary inadequacy both predisposes to infection and worsens outcome. This long-held principle suggests that nutritional interventions should play a critical role in thwarting the impact of infections. This view is based on observations such as the growth faltering in infants in developing countries that begins between 4 and 6 months of age. At this time, breast milk as an exclusive source of nutrition becomes increasingly inadequate for the growing infant, the available quantity of weaning foods is inadequate, protein content is low and of poor quality, and the availability of other key nutrients such as iron is substandard. Growth faltering in infancy, a good marker of nutritional deprivation,[6] is strongly associated with an increased incidence, duration, and severity of infectious diseases as revealed in numerous prospective studies carried out in areas with a high prevalence of malnutrition.[7–9] Cutaneous anergy was noted to be present in malnourished patients and led to the hypothesis that malnourished individuals suffered disproportionately from infectious diseases because of immune deficits. The relationship between adverse clinical outcomes and protein energy malnutrition is not limited to the developing world. There is a high prevalence of malnutrition in hospitalized adult patients (up to 50% in some studies)[10,11] on medical and surgical wards that is both underrecognized and undertreated by physicians.[12] Studies in these contexts reveal a poorer prognosis for those who are malnourished compared to well-nourished patients and demonstrate that surgical morbidity and mortality can be improved by nutritional rehabilitation prior to surgery.[13–15]

This principle led to attempts to minimize the impact of infectious diseases through food or nutrient supplements during the first year of life. Multiple planned interventions in the 1970s and 1980s sought to demonstrate that the provision of more protein or limiting amino acids to the diet[16,17] and then more energy[18] (when the protein supplements failed to obtain the desired response) would reduce morbidity due to infectious diseases. However, prior to the dramatic success of supplementation with vitamin A in the 1990s interventions to curb the burden of infectious disease through nutritional supplementation were not clear successes.

Concurrent studies also took increasing note that kwashiorkor, the most severe form of protein energy malnutrition, was often preceded by an infection such as acute diarrheal disease,[19] measles,[20] or chicken pox.[21] Prospective birth cohort studies revealed that breast-fed children in impoverished settings grew in parallel to children in industrialized settings. However, when weaning foods were introduced and the incidence of both diarrhea and respiratory illness increased, growth faltering occurred. Even asymptomatic gastrointestinal infections led to growth faltering.[5] Measured observations of children during infectious disease episodes showed that common infections led to anorexia, nutrient malabsorption, micronutrient wasting, and growth deficits.[22–27] Diverse infections often occurred at a rate that continually delayed the ability of a child to achieve adequate catch-up in nutritional status or linear growth, and the child entered a cycle of infections and worsening nutritional status that in the worst cases progressed to kwashiorkor and death.

These observations taken together led to the current thinking of the relationship between nutritional status and infection as bidirectional. Not only could protein energy malnutrition or micronutrient deficiencies worsen infectious disease morbidity but also infections could, through metabolic alterations, lead to deterioration in nutritional and micronutrient status (Fig. 5-1). To maximally diminish the burden of infectious disease in malnourished populations, disease control measures must be instituted in parallel with appropriately targeted nutritional interventions.

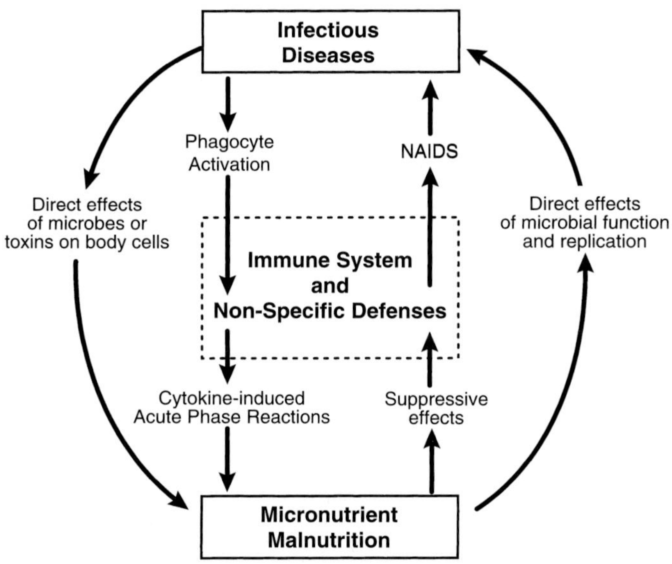

FIGURE 5-1 A schematic representation of the interactions between infectious diseases and malnutrition. These two-way interactions between infectious disease and malnutrition include direct consequences of the infecting microorganisms and indirect (or secondary) effects that involve the immune system and other antigen-nonspecific host defensive organisms. NAIDS, nutritionally acquired immune dysfunction syndromes.

EFFECTS OF MALNUTRITION ON INFECTION

Protein Energy

The degree to which the previous interactions occur and the extent of their actual impact gained clarity when several prospective community-based studies accurately characterized the relationship between anthropometrics and child mortality rates. By analyzing six of the most homogeneous of these studies, Pelletier et al. were able to detect a consistent relationship between the height-for-age index and the relative risk for mortality in under fives.[28,29] Child mortality increased at a compound rate of 5.5 ± 0.8% for each decrement of 0.1 Z score units less than −1. Although a severely malnourished child (with a weight for age of <60% of the reference median or a WAZ of <−3) had 8.4 times the risk of dying as a non-underweight child in the same community, even mild malnutrition (with a weight for age of 70–79% or a WAZ between −1 and −2) had a relative risk of 2.5. This relationship between weight for age and mortality demonstrated consistent accuracy across study sites despite the presence of different pathogens and different rates of stunting and wasting. This relationship was the basis of the population associated risk statistic, a predictive model that inputs the prevalence of weight for age and calculates a percentage of child deaths associated with malnutrition based on the described relationship between WAZ and child mortality.[30] When this model was applied to 53 countries for which reliable anthropometric data were available, it was estimated that 56% of child deaths were attributable to malnutrition's potentiating effects of infectious disease morbidity (Fig. 5-2). Furthermore, because of the high prevalence of mild to moderate malnutrition, 83% of the deaths associated with malnutrition were attributed to mild to moderate, as opposed to severe, malnutrition (Box 5-1).

These findings have been replicated for all-cause child mortality and extended to cause-specific mortality.[31] In these new analyses, 53% of all deaths were attributable to underweight as an underlying cause. Likewise, 61% of diarrhea deaths, 57% of malaria deaths, 52% of pneumonia deaths, and 45% of measles deaths could be attributed to underweight status.

Micronutrients

Micronutrients may have direct effects on the progression of an infection. The availability of key micronutrients in tissues or fluids can influence the growth and replication of infectious agents. For example, iron is required for the propagation of malaria and salmonella, and vitamin B_{12} is required for *Diphyllobothrium latum*. More frequently, micronutrients mediate their effect on morbidity from infectious disease by modulating the immune system. A particular micronutrient deficiency rarely occurs in an isolated manner but often overlaps with other micronutrient deficiencies and protein energy malnutrition. Nevertheless, large prospective field trials have demonstrated the benefits derived from dietary supplements with vitamin A and zinc, which have been shown to reduce the incidence, severity, and duration of various infectious diseases. Data are more limited for iron, vitamin C, and selenium, although in experimental contexts all have shown benefits. Each micronutrient has a specific role in the maintenance of a viable innate and/or adaptive immune response to potential pathogens. Micronutrients with a role in protein synthesis (e.g., thiamine, riboflavin, pantothenic acid, and essential amino acids) are all needed for the production of antibodies. The nonessential amino acids arginine and glutamine appear to provide important benefits for antigen-specific immunity and improved mucosal integrity,[32] and essential polyunsaturated fatty acids are needed to produce prostaglandins, lipoxins,

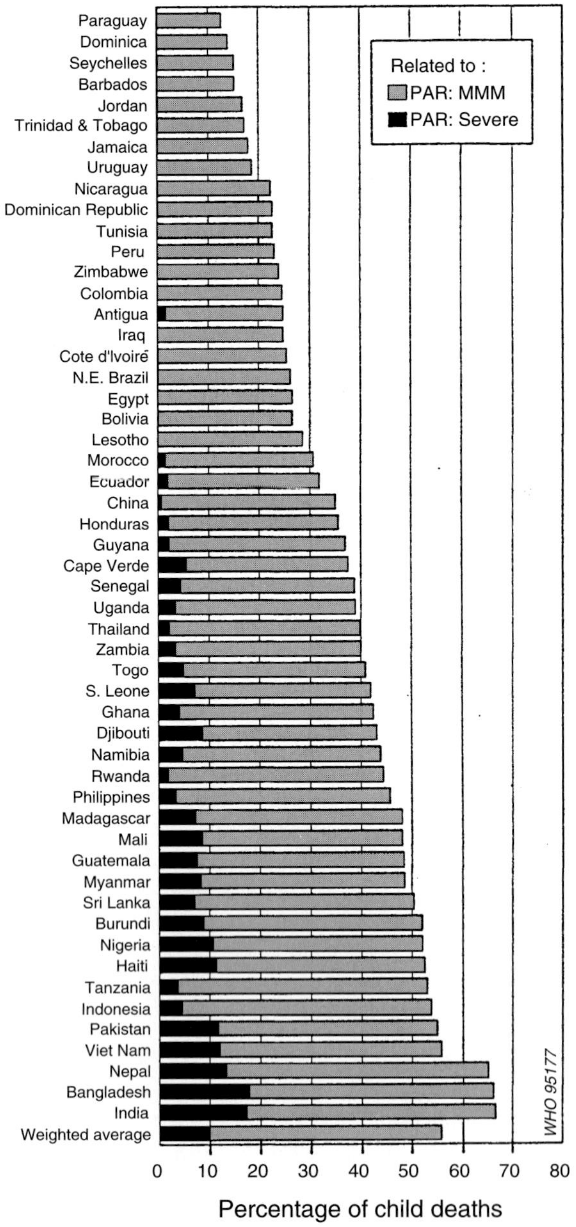

FIGURE 5-2 Population attributable risk (PAR) for child deaths in 52 developing countries due to interactions between mild to moderate malnutrition (PAR: MMM; gray bars) or severe malnutrition (PAR: Severe; black bars) and infection, reported as the percentage of childhood deaths in each country. (From Pelletier DL, Frongillo EA, Schroeder DG, et al: The effects of malnutrition on child mortality in developing countries. Bull WHO 73:443–448, 1995.)

Box 5-1 General Effects of Malnutrition on the Immune System

Protein energy malnutrition
- Decreased mucosal integrity
- Impeded macrophage migration
- Diminished T lymphocyte help in immune responses dependent on mature CD4 cells (cell-mediated immunity)
- Delayed kinetics and deficient antibody responses to certain antigens, particularly polysaccharide
- Depressed amounts of mucosal secretory IgA and specific secretory IgA antibodies in response to mucosal infections
- In vivo consumption of complement, depressed plasma levels of most complement components and activities effecting both alternate and classic pathways of complement activation
- Deficient serum opsonic activity
- ? favors type 2 response

Vitamin A deficiency
- Decreased mucosal integrity
- Altered cytokine expression leads to type 1 immune responses

Zinc deficiency
- Decreased macrophage chemotaxis
- Decreased neutrophil activity
- Decreased T cell response to antigen stimulation
- Favors type 2 responses
- Diminished opsinin activity

Iron deficiency
- Decreased neutrophil chemotaxis and bacteriocidal effects

and thrombaxanes. This review is limited to vitamin A, zinc, iron, vitamin C, and selenium because data in these areas are more complete (Table 5-1).

Vitamin A

Vitamin A modifies the severity of infectious diseases with profound effects on childhood mortality.[33,34] Childhood xerophthalmia, the most reliable indicator of vitamin A deficiency, is linked to a higher risk of morbidity and mortality. Severe untreated xerophthalmia (with corneal involvement) has a high risk of concomitant morbidity, malnutrition, and mortality, with case fatality rates for severe infections ranging from 5% to more than 50%.[35] Milder, noncorneal xerophthalmia, although not blinding, also increases the risk of morbidity and death. Preschool Indonesian children with night blindness (XN), Bitot's spots (X1B), or both conditions (representing "mild xerophthalmia") were three, six, and nine times more likely to die, respectively, within 3 months after diagnosis than their nonxerophthalmic peers.[33] The association was strong and consistent across age, illness, and anthropometric data suggesting a causal role of vitamin A deficiency in exaggerating the risk of early childhood mortality. Excess mortality also extended to siblings of xerophthalmic children. In Nepal, siblings of children with XN or X1B were at 2 or 3 times higher risk of death than children in households with no xerophthalmia.[36] Xerophthalmic "clusters" occur within households, with case siblings being 7 to 13 times more likely to have, or develop, xerophthalmia than children in

Table 5-1 Micronutrient Requirements

	Normal Blood Levels	Treatment (Replacement) Dose	Maintenance Dose or RDA	Symptoms and Signs of Deficiency	Deficiency Effects on Host Defenses	Risk of Toxicity
Vitamin A	25–94 μg/dL	200,000 IU (60,000 RE)* PO qd × 2, at 4 wk, then q 4–6 mo (½ if <12 mo old) or 2440 RE q wk	400–1000 RE/day (1600–5000 IU/day)	Xerophthalmia (night blindness [XN], Bitot's spots [X1B], corneal xerosis, and ulceration necrosis) More severe infections Increased mortality	Lymphoid tissue atrophy with dysfunction of T cells and cell-mediated immunity Impaired antibody production	Skin scaling, headaches, papilledema, lymphadenopathy, hyperostosis, congenital malformations with ≥50,000 IU/day in early pregnancy
Vitamin C	>0.15 mg/dL (>300 mg stores)	100–200 mg/day	10–60 mg/day	Scurvy (perifollicular hemorrhage, weakness)	Impaired phagocyte mobility Impaired phagocytosis Impaired antioxidant activity	Abdominal pain, diarrhea, false-negative stool guaiac, urine glucose
B-complex vitamins						
Thiamine (B_1)	RBC transketolase coefficient <15%	50–100 mg IM or 15–30 mg/day PO	0.3–1.5 mg/day	Beriberi, Wernicke–Korsakoff dementia, nystagmus, ophthalmoplegia	Impaired antibody production	Rare
B_2 (riboflavin)	FAD activity coefficient <1.2	10–15 mg/day PO	0.4–1.7 mg/day	Cheilostomatitis	Impaired antibody production	None known
Niacin (nicotinamide and nicotinic acid)	Low urinary *N*-methyl nicotinamide	50–150 mg nicotinamide (60 mg tryptophan → 1mg niacin)	6–20 mg/day	Pellagra (dermatitis, diarrhea, dementia, death)	Impaired antibody production	Flushing, dry skin, hepatotoxicity with ≥3 g/day
B_6 (pyridoxine)†	>50 ng/mL	5–200 mg/day	0.5–3.0 mg/day	Diarrhea, anemia, seizures	Lymphoid tissue atrophy Impaired humoral and cell-mediated immunity	Sensory neuropathy with >500 mg/day
Folate	4–20 ng/mL	0.4–5.0 mg/day	30–400 μg/day	Macrocytic anemia	Lymphoid tissue atrophy Impaired humoral and cell-mediated immunity	May mask B_{12} deficiency
B_{12}	200–900 pg/mL	100 μg/day cyanocobalamin	0.5–4.0 μg/day	Macrocytic anemia, neuropathy, dementia	Dysfunction of lymphocytes and phagocytes	Rare
Vitamin D_3	Variable (osteomalacia)	2999–4000 IU/day	200–400 IU/day (5–15 mg/day)	Rickets		Hypercalcemia, weakness

Continued

Table 5-1 Micronutrient Requirements—Cont'd

	Normal Blood Levels	Treatment (Replacement) Dose	Maintenance Dose or RDA	Symptoms and Signs of Deficiency	Deficiency Effects on Host Defenses	Risk of Toxicity
Vitamin E	>0.5 mg/dL	30–100 IU (mg) DL-α-tocopherol	6–30 IU mg/day	?Abortion ?Muscular dystrophy	Impaired humoral and cell-mediated immunity Impaired antioxidant activity	Nausea, diarrhea, ↑ bleeding with warfarin sodium with >1 g/day
Vitamin K	Normal clotting	500 μg/day	12–140 μg/day	Bleeding		?Hemolysis
Zinc[‡]	70–130 μg/dL	5 mg tid Zn acetate (15 mg/day × 7 days) = 3.9 mg elemental zinc/day 20 mg elemental zinc/day as zinc gluconate	5–15 mg/day	Dermatitis and enteropathy Increased morbidity (duration) of diarrheal illnesses	Lymphoid tissue atrophy, with dysfunction of T cells and cell-mediated immunity Impaired antibody production Thymic hormone deficiency	Hepatocellular damage and fibrosis Immunologic impairments
Iron	50–170 μg/dL	40–80 mg Fe bid/tid	8–18 mg/day, 30 mg/day in pregnancy	Hypochromic, microcytic anemia	Impaired lymphocyte function Impaired bactericidal function	Hemochromatosis, cirrhosis
Iodine	Urinary 10 μg/dL	150 μg/day	40–150 μg/day	Goiter, hypothyroidism	Delayed antibody production	Iodine-induced hyperthyroidism; *rarely* hypersensitivity
Copper	1.1 μg/mL	2–4 mg/day	1.2–2.0 mg/day	Menkes' disease Anemia, bleeding, depigmentation, kinky hair, brain damage, low plasma ceruloplasmin	Impaired lymphocyte and phagocyte functions	Wison's disease Cirrhosis, impaired metabolism of Fe and Zn
Selenium	100–130 ng/mL	100 μg/day	10–70 μg/day	Keshan's disease Cardiomyopathy, growth retardation, cataracts, impaired sperm production and glutathione peroxidase activity Increased risk of cancer	Impaired lymphocyte and phagocyte functions Impaired antioxidant activity	Damage to liver, brain, heart, and muscle

FAD, flavin adenine dinucleotide; IM, intramuscularly; PO, by mouth; RBC, red blood cell; RDA, recommended daily allowance.
*RE (retinol equivalent) = 1 μg (or 3.33 IU) retinol = 6 μg (or 10 IU) beta-carotene.
[†]Pyridoxal phosphate complexes with the antituberculosis drugs isoniazid and cycloserine.
[‡]Zinc deficiency impairs release of retinol binding protein from liver and impairs retinol conversion to retinal (hence amplifying vitamin A deficiency).

xerophthalmia-free households.[37] This concentration of risk extends to the community: Children living in the vicinity of a xerophthalmic child are more than twice as likely to develop xerophthalmia,[37] and they may also incur a 30% higher risk of mortality than children living in communities virtually free of xerophthalmia.[38]

Intervention trials suggest that vitamin A supplementation modifies the severity, more than the incidence, of certain infectious diseases, as is the general trend with other forms of malnutrition. This effect is most apparent from its impact on all-cause mortality among preschool children. The initial trial conducted in Indonesia found that 1- to 6-year-old children receiving 60,000 μg retinal equivalents (REs) of vitamin A every 6 months died at a 34% lower rate than children in villages not receiving supplements.[39] Seven subsequent trials in Asia and Africa provided vitamin A as a large oral dose (60,000 μg; half dose for children younger than 12 months of age) every 4 to 6 months, a weekly dose of 2440 μg, or half a recommended daily allowance through fortified monosodium glutamate (a popular flavor enhancer). Five trials showed significant reductions in the mortality of children 6 or more months of age, ranging from 19% in Ghana to 54% in southern India,[35] whereas two trials failed to show an impact on mortality. A meta-analysis of these trials revealed a mortality reduction of 23% in all countries and 34% in Asia associated with the use of vitamin A in children older than the age of 6 months.[35] The effect of vitamin A supplementation given earlier than 6 months of age remains controversial.[40–42] However, in 1999, it was estimated that 97 million doses of vitamin A were given, and assuming the all-cause mortality was decreased by 23% in the treated populations, it is estimated that vitamin A supplementation prevented 242,000 deaths in that year alone.[43]

One of the clearest synergistic relationships of a micronutrient and infection is that of vitamin A and measles. Vitamin A treatment can profoundly decrease the morbidity, incidence of secondary complications, and mortality in children with measles. Although the degree of reduction has varied in trials using different doses, a meta-analysis found that the results of randomized controlled trials giving two doses of 200,000 IU vitamin A revealed an overall reduction in all-cause mortality of 67%.[44] The effect of vitamin A on all-cause mortality was greatest in children younger than the age of 2 years, where the decrease in all-cause mortality was 83%.[45] Furthermore, there was a 47% reduction in the incidence of croup and a 77% reduction in pneumonia-specific mortality, and the duration of diarrheal episodes was significantly shortened in the supplemented groups. Vitamin A supplementation is now recommended as standard of care treatment for measles in both developing and developed countries.

The measured impact of the effect of vitamin A for the primary prevention and treatment of diarrhea and respiratory tract infections yields conflicting findings. Several studies have noted a decrease in the duration and severity of diarrheal disease in children receiving vitamin A as primary prophylaxis.[46,47] In children with severe malnutrition and edema, low-dose daily vitamin A supplementation decreased the incidence of diarrhea by 89% (RR = 0.21; 95% CI, 0.07–0.62),[48] and in shigellosis one dose of vitamin A has been shown to increase the percentage of children achieving clinical cure at day 5 following treatment.[49] However, in a meta-analysis of eight double-blind randomized controlled trials of vitamin A prophylaxis no effect on diarrheal disease incidence was found and a mild negative effect (RR = 1.07; 95% CI, 1.02–1.12) was noted on the incidence of respiratory disease.[50] Additionally, vitamin A given as adjunctive therapy in children hospitalized with pneumonia was associated with a decreased oxygen saturation and increased respiratory distress in Peru,[51] and there was a nonsignificant trend toward higher mortality in vitamin A-supplemented children hospitalized with pneumonia in Tanzania.[52]

Children with xerophthalmia or severe malnutrition or any child with measles should be treated according to guidelines from WHO: 200,000 IU of vitamin A orally on presentation, 200,000 IU the following day, and another 200,000 IU dose 2 to 4 weeks following the infection to reestablish liver stores. Children younger than the age of 1 year should receive half doses. The use of vitamin A as routine adjunctive therapy for respiratory infections and diarrhea is not indicated.

Zinc

The classical syndrome of zinc deficiency seen in acrodermatitis enteropathica, a rare genetic disorder, is characterized by dermatitis, linear growth deficits, anorexia, irritability, and chronic diarrhea. Despite the lack of a reliable and widely used indicator of zinc status with which to base estimates of prevalence of this condition, the clinical trials of supplementation showing significant and large impacts on common child diseases in diverse geographic zones and populations indicate that zinc deficiency is a common condition in children in developing regions.[53] Zinc supplementation has been shown to be effective for the primary prevention of diarrhea, respiratory tract infections, and malaria, and trials have indicated a role for zinc in the adjunctive treatment of diarrhea and respiratory tract infections. Trials have demonstrated that zinc-supplemented children have lower mortality and large trials are under way to assess this outcome.

There are 13 studies available that evaluated zinc supplementation as a primary preventive strategy for diarrheal disease in preschool children.[54–67] In 8 of these studies, zinc therapy had a statistically significant protective effect that ranged between 12% and 69%, and in no study was zinc supplementation associated with an increase in the risk of diarrheal illness. A pooled analysis containing the majority of these studies revealed an 18% (95% CI, 7–28) reduction in the incidence of diarrheal disease in supplemented children.[68] Additionally, a study of maternal zinc supplementation during the second and third trimesters of pregnancy noted a 16% decrease in the incidence of diarrhea and a 64% decrease in the incidence of dysentery during the first 6 months of life in children with low birth weights (<2.5 kg).[69] Populations in which plasma zinc concentrations were <9.8 μmol/L, low birth weight or small for gestational age children, and children in the second year of life appear to experience the greatest benefit from zinc supplementation.

A meta-analysis has been performed on 12 studies with data regarding the efficacy of zinc in the treatment of diarrheal disease—5 regarding persistent diarrhea[61,70–73] and 7 regarding acute diarrheal disease.[69–80] For the persistent diarrhea trials, there was a reduction in the duration of illness and a 42% (95% CI, 10–63%) reduction in the composite variable of treatment failure or death in children receiving zinc.[81] WHO recommends the use of zinc along with other vitamins and minerals in cases of persistent diarrhea. Children younger than 12 months of age, males, and children with wasting (WHZ <2) exhibited the greatest treatment benefit. In trials of zinc supplementation in acute diarrhea, the meta-analysis demonstrated that zinc significantly reduced diarrheal duration.[81] There is a WHO UNICEF recommendation that zinc supplements should be used in the treatment of acute diarrhea along with oral rehydration therapy.[82]

There are eight studies that evaluate the role of zinc in the primary prevention of respiratory disease.[54–56,60,61,83] Five of the eight studies reported a decrease in the incidence of acute respiratory tract infections and the protective effect reached significance in three of these studies. No studies reported an increase of respiratory tract infections associated with zinc supplementation. The protective effect ranged from 15% to 88% in the different trials, and a pooled analysis of the majority of these trial estimated a protective effect of 41% (95% CI, 17–59).[68] A trial of zinc as adjunctive therapy in severe acute lower respiratory tract infections in children younger than 2 years of age in Kolkata showed a decreased duration of fever and severity of illness scores in boys but not in girls.[84] This study found no benefit of vitamin A. Another randomized, controlled trial of zinc supplementation as adjunctive therapy of severe pneumonia has shown a significant benefit on recovery.[85]

Findings from three studies on the utility of zinc supplementation for the primary prevention of falciparum malaria are more conflicting. In the Gambia[86] and Papua New Guinea,[59] small studies revealed reductions in health center attendance attributable to falciparum malaria by 30% and 38%, respectively, although only the latter reached statistical significance. In Burkina Faso, a larger study found no difference in the incidence of falciparum malaria diagnosed by active surveillance in zinc-supplemented children. A multicenter trial[87] in Ecuador, Ghana, Tanzania, Uganda, and Zambia revealed no difference in time to reduction of fever or anemia in children receiving zinc as an adjunctive therapy for falciparum malaria.

Zinc given in addition to standard nutritional therapy was associated with lower incidences of morbidity for diarrhea and all-cause mortality in children with severe protein energy malnutrition (PEM).[88] It is clear that zinc, by diminishing the severity of the most prevalent causes of morbidity and mortality of children in developing regions, has an important and as yet unrealized potential to improve global child health. Because supplementation must be at least weekly, the application of this intervention will not be as easy as providing high-dose vitamin A every 6 months. Alternative approaches for primary prevention include supplementing basic foodstuffs or the promotion of the use of animal-based protein, which is a good source of zinc.[89,90] To promote the widespread use of zinc therapy for diarrhea, possible approaches include its incorporation into oral rehydration salts or an active distribution and education campaign of health care providers.

Iron

Iron deficiency, with related anemia, is the most commonly identified micronutrient deficiency globally.[3] Dietary intakes in tropical zones are generally marginal and often confounded by blood loss associated with menstruation or infection with hookworm or schistosomes. Anemia, the most recognizable indicator, may be either a symptom of nutritional deficiency or a response to active infection. Both iron deficiency anemia and the anemia induced by infection lower serum iron levels and therefore may alter the outcome of infections. Many iron intervention studies have been performed since the 1920s and they are well summarized in a review.[91] The analysis of findings is complicated by several factors. The first is the definition of anemia and the failure of many investigators to distinguish between iron deficiency anemia, anemia resulting from infection, and the hereditary hemoglobinopathies (Table 5-2). Furthermore, many studies, especially in the 1970s, were done with parenteral iron dextran as opposed to more physiologic daily oral supplementation. Nevertheless, supplementation with oral iron has been shown to increase hemoglobin and to reduce severe anemia, even in areas with endemic malaria.

Table 5-2 *Iron Deficiency Anemia Versus the Anemia of Infection*

Variable	Iron Deficiency Anemia	Anemia of Infection*
Red blood cell count	Depressed	Depressed
Hemoglobin	Depressed	Depressed
Hematocrit	Depressed	Depressed
Plasma iron	Depressed	*Markedly depressed*
Plasma transferrin	Markedly elevated	*Normal or depressed*
Transferrin saturation	Markedly reduced	Reduced
Plasma ferritin	Markedly reduced	*Normal or increased*
Tissue iron stores	Markedly reduced	*Normal or increased*
Iron therapy	Corrects the anemia	*Fails to correct the anemia*

*Key differences are in *italics*.

Review of trials of iron supplementation indicated that provision of iron results in an increased density of malaria parasites in the blood and possibly clinical malaria.[91] The possible antagonistic relationship for the host between plasmodia and iron is further supported by the efficacy of iron chelators as adjunctive therapy in malaria.[92] A meta-analysis of iron supplementation trials found that iron-supplemented children have more diarrhea.[93] An enteric pathogen that appears to have a complex and possibly antagonistic relation with iron is salmonella. Experimental infection studies in rats have demonstrated both that severe iron deficiency enhanced resistance to infection and that mild deficiency enhanced susceptibility.[94,95] This may explain disparate findings from often cited observational studies that salmonella infections in Guam were often associated with iron-supplemented formula.[96] In general, iron supplementation has not been shown to either increase or decrease the risk of lower respiratory infections.[92]

Vitamin C

Vitamin C decreases the duration but not the incidence of the common cold under normal conditions.[97] However, people undergoing strenuous activity who take vitamin C have been shown to have a decreased incidence of cold symptoms.[98]

Selenium

One of the most novel observations regarding the interaction between a host and an infectious agent came from investigations into the origin and pathogenesis of Keshan's disease, an epidemic cardiomyopathy in China.[99] Epidemiologic investigations revealed that only populations living in areas with selenium-deficient soils developed the disease.[100] Subsequently, blood and tissue samples from cases revealed coxsackie viruses.[101] Laboratory mice fed on selenium-sufficient diets could be infected with a strain of coxsackie virus B4 and developed only mild limited cardiomyopathy, whereas selenium-deficient animals developed a severe cardiomyopathy upon infection with the same coxsackie virus B4 strain.[102] Although this is consistent with Scrimshaw's model of synergistic effects, it was subsequently noted that coxsackie viruses that did not normally exhibit cardiotoxicity in selenium-sufficient animals became cardiotoxic following the passage through selenium-deficient animals. Viral sequencing of the virus after passage through selenium-deficient animals confirmed genotypic changes, whereas strains passed exclusively through selenium-replete animals had no genotypic changes.[103] This appears to an example of a novel type of interaction between host and infectious agent in which the infectious agent increases in virulence because of a specific deficit in the host's nutritional status. Similar findings were reported by the same group in a murine model of influenza A infection.[104] The extent to which the phenomenon of host nutritional status permanently increasing pathogen virulence occurs in nature is unclear, although it is hypothesized to be limited to RNA viruses.

INFECTION-RELATED METABOLIC ALTERATIONS COMPROMISE HOST NUTRITIONAL STATUS

Infectious diseases may produce primary direct losses of body nutrients or secondary losses mediated through the inflammatory cytokine response and catabolic effects (Box 5-2). Loss of iron due to hookworm and schistosomes and loss of macronutrients from geohelminths illustrate the consequences of infectious agents. Direct losses may also result from toxins produced by the pathogen, such as toxigenic strains of enteropathogens that result in sizable losses of electrolytes, water, and bicarbonate. Despite these important examples of direct effects, indirect effects account for the majority of the effects of pathogens on the host's nutritional status. There is an innate link between the immune and endocrine systems, and the metabolic changes associated with even mild infections can have an important effect on the nutritional status of the host. The inflammatory response induces constitutional symptoms, alteration in the metabolism of proteins and carbohydrates, and redistribution of minerals between physiologic compartments.

Box 5-2 Effects of Infection on Host's Nutritional Status

1. Decreased intake (anorexia)
2. Protein catabolism and negative nitrogen balance
3. Depletion of carbohydrate stores
4. Altered fat metabolism
5. Pseudodiabetic state—hyperinsulinemia, increased insulin resistance, raised glucagons and glucocorticoid levels
6. Increased basal metabolic rate
7. Increased gluconeogenesis
8. Decreased absorption (symptomatic and asymptomatic gastrointestinal infections)
9. Micronutrient sequestration (Fe, Zn)
10. Nutrient wasting (Zn loss in diarrhea, protein and vitamin A loss in shigellosis)

Constitutional Symptoms

Constitutional symptoms are a common manifestation of fever, anorexia, malaise, headache, and myalgia: The first two have clear effects on the nutritional status of the host. The hallmark sign of infection, fever, is induced by the release of interleukin-1 (IL-1), IL-6, and tumor necrosis factor-α (TNF-α), which act at the level of the hypothalamus to alter the temperature set point. This host response is believed to be a favorable adaptive response, but it comes at a substantial metabolic cost. For the augmentation of body temperature by 1°C, the basal metabolic rate increases by 12% to 23%.[105] Therefore, with a fever of 40°C, the basal metabolic rate increases approximately 30% to 60% over baseline needs.

Fever is generally accompanied by anorexia. Although the reason for this host response is not clear, its effects can be important. In a well-controlled study in Bangladesh, 41 children with diarrhea between 6 and 35 months of age and an age-matched control group were studied. It was found that children hospitalized with acute watery diarrhea, despite an educational intervention and "coaching," consumed only 47% to 58% of the total calories consumed by the healthy control group. Breast-feeding abrogated the changes to a large extent but not completely. Despite the provision of a nutritionally and culturally appropriate weaning food, the protein intake in normal breast-fed children was 2.5 times that consumed by completely weaned children with diarrhea.[106]

Alterations in Protein Metabolism

Protein catabolism occurs even in subclinical infections.[107,108] Cytokine release triggers skeletal muscle proteolysis via increased levels of corticosteroids by the ubiquitin proteasome pathway,[109,110] and liberated amino acids are taken up in part by the liver, where IL-6-mediated transcriptional regulation leads to the enhancement of transcription and translation of essential acute phase proteins such as C-reactive protein, complement, serum amyloid, and α-antitrypsin while down-regulating synthesis of exported proteins such as albumin and transferrin.[111–113] Despite active proteolysis of muscle, serum amino acids levels are lower than at steady state because of rapid uptake by the liver and immune cells.[114]

Not all amino acids released by proteolysis are recycled; branched amino acids, for example, are used for energy and the released nitrogen is excreted in the urine. Some amino acids, such as phenylalanine, are not recyclable and are also excreted in the urine. The loss of protein, especially during serious infections, is not trivial. It is estimated that in moderate infections, the average daily protein loss is 0.6 g/kg/day, the recommended daily intake for adults. Losses in dysentery are slightly higher (0.9 g/kg/day), and in severe infections, including typhoid fever, daily protein loss approached 1.2 g/kg/day.[115] Although proteolysis may serve in the short-term as a source of amino acids for new protein synthesis, the continuous consumption of proteins must, at a given point, have adverse consequences for the host. Changes are clinically manifest as wasting, and wasting of more than 55% of the lean body mass is incompatible with life, regardless of the cause.[116,117]

Alterations in Carbohydrate Metabolism

The inflammatory response induces a metabolic state characterized by increased gluconeogenesis secondary to cytokine upregulation of the rate-limiting enzyme phosphoenolpyruvate carboxykinase[118] even when exogenous carbohydrate intake is adequate. Serum levels of insulin, glucagon, and corticosteroids are all increased. The metabolic result is a syndrome of hyperinsulinemia, insulin resistance,[119] depressed glycogenesis and fat catabolism,[120] and enhanced peripheral glucose uptake and utilization. Precursor amino acids are deaminated, the nitrogen is converted to urea (which is excreted in urine), and the glucose derived from the carbon backbone is oxidized for energy.

Alterations in Mineral Metabolism

The divalent cations iron and zinc are highly protein bound. During the inflammatory response, significant shifts in the distribution of these minerals occur in physiologic compartments. Iron and zinc are sequestered by the cytokine-induced synthesis of their binding proteins, ferritin and metallothionein. Sequestration of zinc and iron is in direct proportion to the severity of the infection, and zinc levels can fall to half normal levels and iron can become almost undetectable.[121]

GASTROINTESTINAL INFECTIONS

Gastrointestinal infections have a particularly important role in inducing a compromise in host nutritional status. Malabsorption in gastrointestinal illness may result from the epithelial destruction by the pathogen or by the immune response to the pathogen. Even common diarrheal illnesses can have a profound impact on nutrient absorption. In symptomatic rotavirus infection, the most common cause of acute severe diarrheal illness worldwide, there is a 42% decrease in the absorption of nitrogen and fat, a 48% decrement in the absorption of carbohydrates, and a 55% decrease in the total energy absorption.[122] These indices for malabsorption are slightly more severe in both ETEC infections and shigellosis.[25,122] In shigellosis,[123] protein loss is sizable and important, and vitamin A is wasted.[27] Giardiasis and ascariasis lead to the malabsorption of vitamin A.[24] Large losses of zinc also occur in diarrhea.[124]

EFFECTS OF MALNUTRITION ON HOST IMMUNE FUCTION

Innate Immunity: Physical Barriers

The primary physical barrier to infection, the integument, is affected by a wide variety of nutrient deficiencies. Skin lesions are one of the cardinal signs of kwashiorkor. Protein energy malnutrition or even more milder forms of nutritional depletion can be correlated with decreased gastrointestinal mucosal integrity as measured by the lactulose:mannitol ratio.[125] Also, vitamin A deficiency has been found to have a similar effect on gut integrity by the same test.[126] Striking histological changes are noted in the epithelia of vitamin A-deprived animals characterized as metaplastic hyperkeratosis that are rapidly reversible upon vitamin A repletion.[127,128] Although severe zinc deficiency results in characteristic skin lesions,[129] mild to moderate zinc deficiencies also compromise the integrity of the gastrointestinal and respiratory epithelia.[130,131] Indeed, specific nutrient deficiencies are often manifest by epithelial lesions: Dermatosis and mucosal atrophy are noted in pellagra; dermatosis and dermatitis, cheilosis, and angular stomatitis are manifest in pyridoxine deficiency; and subcutaneous atrophy and tissue fragility are seen in scurvy. The nonessential amino acid glutamine also appears to have a role in the maintenance of intestinal epithelial integrity.[32]

Innate Immunity: Phagocytic Cells

Neutrophils and macrophages are the first-line generalized response to invading organisms. There is dispute about diminished neutrophil chemotaxis and adhesion in PEM,[132–134] but there does appear to be a diminished bactericidal killing despite a normal generation of oxidative metabolites.[133,135] Additionally, serum opsininic activity is notably depressed in patients with PEM,[136] and this is likely to further diminish the microbicidal functions of neutrophils. Zinc facilitates neutrophil activity directly[137–139] and indirectly through the stimulation of opsonic activity.[139] Iron deficiency causes a decrease in neutrophil chemotactic activity and bactericidal capacity; the latter is thought to be due in part to diminished myeloperoxidase (an iron-containing enzyme) and in part to hexose monophosphate shunt activities in phagocytic cells.[140] However, there is a balance as high-dose iron infusions depress, at least temporarily, intracellular killing in dialysis patients.[141]

Macrophages play a dual role in host defense. Once activated by lymphokine signals, macrophages may act directly as a microbicidal effector against intracellular pathogens, including viruses, certain bacteria and fungi, as well as protozoa. In addition to these direct functions, macrophages are the key antigen presenting cells for T lymphocyte proliferative responses and cytokine production. Although it is clear that malnourished hosts are at an increased risk of infection due to intracellular pathogens, it is difficult to separate the direct effects on macrophage phagocytosis and microbial function from the indirect effects due to impaired antigen presentation and reduced T cell responses that are necessary to stimulate normal macrophage activation. Despite this, it has been noted in murine models that macrophages from protein-restricted animals are abnormally sensitive to apoptotic stimuli.[142] In children with PEM, a markedly delayed and diminished macrophage migration was noted using the Rebuck window technique.[134] In addition, in murine models diminished adhesion, activation, and delayed phagocytosis were demonstrated.[143,144]

Macrophages appear to have decreased antigen presenting capacity and possibly a diminished capacity for normal coordinated signaling with T cells. A study of activated macrophages from protein-restricted and -sufficient diets revealed that the phagocytosis of *Candida albicans* and the generation of superoxide in response to phorbol myrisate acetate were significantly diminished in the low-protein diet group using cells from both unprimed and BCG-primed animals, suggesting direct effects of malnutrition on the macrophage.[145] The study also evaluated deficits in antigen presentation by using D.10 cells, a standard Th clone derived from AKR mice and incubated with low or normal protein diet macrophages and the soluble antigen conalbumin. This assay measures the resulting incorporation of ^{3}H-thymidine into DNA if antigen presentation is normal. The production of cytokines by the responding T cells, particularly interferon-γ (IFN-γ), then activates the macrophages for intracellular killing and the production of counter-regulatory substances, nitric oxide and prostaglandin E_2 (PGE_2), which dampen the lymphocyte response. No differences in thymidine incorporation were observed using resident or BCG-activated cells, and the expression of Ia, the class II major histocompatibility complex antigen, was only slightly reduced in the low-protein group. The mixed lymphocyte reaction, used to assess the response to particulate allogeneic antigens, was also preserved in the low-protein diet group. However, a marked decrease in macrophage production of NO and PGE_2 was observed, which would be expected to enhance lymphocyte proliferation by diminishing the negative regulatory signals for these cells. Whether this macrophage defect resulted from decreased secretion of IFN-γ by the responding T cells or decreased response of macrophages to IFN-γ signaling is not clear.

There is evidence for both altered intracellular signaling following endotoxin stimulation[146] and altered cytokine responses under multiple experimental conditions in PEM. In one study of cytokine responses, the plasma levels of IL-6 and the p55 and p75 soluble receptors for TNF-α were elevated in children with PEM, especially in the presence of severe PEM with edema, independent of the presence of clinical infection.[147] In contrast, a study on Turkish children without apparent infection found decreased IL-1 levels compared with control subjects, but IL-1 increased during infection in a manner similar to that of the controls.[148] These findings are consistent with prior data in humans showing that in vitro production of IL-1 by lipopolysaccharide (LPS)-stimulated peripheral blood monocytes was depressed in severe PEM compared with controls.[149,150]

In humans with acrodermatitis enteropathica, the monocyte chemotactic response is suppressed and can be normalized by the addition of zinc in vitro.[131,151] In a murine model, zinc deficiency was found to adversely affect monocyte uptake and killing of *Trypanosoma cruzi* in a dose-dependent manner,[152] and zinc-deficient mice exhibited macrophage-mediated depression of T cell proliferation that could be corrected in vitro by the addition of zinc.[153] The extent to which these events occur in common infections in humans is unclear.

Adaptive Immunity

Protein Energy Malnutrition

Protein energy malnutrition profoundly affects the adaptive immune response through diverse mechanisms. Abundant data show that T cells are especially affected, particularly T helper cells, and these deficits are largely mediated through defects in the T cell maturation process. However, important alterations in B cell function, immunoglobulins, and complement are also present. Understanding the effects of PEM is further complicated because study populations almost certainly suffered micronutrient deficiencies at a time when they were not readily identified, and the accurate attribution of immune deficits to one type of undernutrition is not possible.

During the past 150 years, a number of studies have documented a major impact of malnutrition on lymphocytes, long before the concepts of T and B lymphocytes were proposed and methods were developed to identify them. For example, anatomical and histopathologic examination of the thymus, spleen, and lymph nodes in people dying of malnutrition has revealed involution of the thymus and depletion of populations of lymphocytes from the peripheral lymphoid organs, now known to be predominantly populated with T lymphocytes. However, the number of circulating lymphocytes was only mildly diminished or often normal. Later, when it became possible to distinguish T cells from B cells, it was noted that there was a decrease in the number of mature functioning T lymphocytes, an unchanged number of B cells, and an increase in the number of cells that expressed neither T or B cell markers (null cells).[154,155] However, the degree of malnutrition as assessed by anthropometry did not correlate to the percentage of mature and immature T lymphocytes in circulation, and there was considerable individual variation.[155] Studies using monoclonal antibodies to identify lymphocyte subpopulations in Bolivian infants with severe PEM and thymic involution (greater than 90% decrease in thymic size by ultrasonography) have shown a statistically significant decrease in the percentage of mature CD4+ cells, an increase in the percentage of CD1a+ precursor cells and CD8+ Tc and Ts cells, and no change in the percentage of CD21+ B cells in the malnourished compared to normally nourished controls.[156] All these results support a significant deficit affecting the T cell maturation process in individuals with PEM.

The mechanisms that mediate the deficit in T cell maturation are not clear. T cells are so named because stimuli for the maturation of pluripotential lymphocyte precursors along the T lineage are derived from the thymus gland, whereas the maturation signals for B cells are in the bone marrow. The thymus is a compound organ with both epithelial and stromal elements surrounding islands of developing lymphocytes. The thymic epithelium produces a variety of zinc-binding peptides, such as thymosin and thymulin, which have been shown to drive maturation of T lymphocytes in vitro. Lymphocytes from Bolivian children with PEM that are incubated with thymulin in vitro showed an increased percentage of CD4+ cells at the expense of CD1a+ precursors, with no observed change in the percentage of CD21+ B lymphocytes.[156] Studies of lymphocytes of Guatemalan children undergoing incubation with thymosin 5 show consistent findings.[157] These findings taken together strongly suggest that the thymic microenvironment is altered in vivo, and that this alteration causes severe abnormalities in T cell number and function, especially in the maturation of CD4+ cell lines.

Th lymphocytes also differentiate along two functionally polarized lines, Th1 and Th2, under a diverse range of influences, including the cytokine milieu, the nature of the protein ligand, cortisol, norepenephrine, and microbial burden.[158] Th0 cells are stimulated to differentiate into Th1 cells under the influence of IL-12 and produce IL-2, IFN-γ, and TNF-β. IFN-γ stimulates antigen presentation through the upregulation of both major histocompatibility class I and class II molecules on a wide variety of cell types. IL-12, among other things, blocks the differentiation of Th0 cells into Th2 cells. The response mediated by Th1 cells, a type 1 response, is characterized by a strong cell-mediated immune response and phagocytic activity and a relatively weaker humoral response. On the other hand, Th2 cells differentiate under the influence of IL-4 and secrete IL-4, IL-5, IL-10, and IL-13. IL-4, IL-10, and IL-13 stimulate B cell development, antibody production, and immunoglobulin class switching. Furthermore, IL-4 inhibits the differentiation of T0 cells into T1 cells. The response mediated by Th2 cells, type 2 immunity, is characterized by a strong humoral response. The tendency of one response (type 1 or type 2) to limit the other results in polarization of the immune response.

The extent to which PEM alters Th polarization is not well studied. However, in a study of Turkish children with PEM, IL-6 was noted to be significantly elevated, whereas TNF-β levels were not different from those of the control group, leading the authors to conclude that PEM favored a type 2 response.[159] Findings from a murine model support this hypothesis.[160] Delayed-type hypersensitivity skin response is a measure of cell-mediated immunity, which is dependent on Th1 cell activity. Defects in skin test reactivity to recall antigens such as tuberculin and *C. albicans* are prevalent in individuals with PEM. This is not a new observation: During the mid-1960s, prior to the discovery of the T and B lymphocyte lineages and T cell subpopulations, diminished prevalence and size of the tuberculin reaction were observed in African children with PEM compared to better nourished children from the same environment, and the tuberculin response to BCG vaccine was blunted as well.[161,162] Because tuberculosis has long been associated with malnutrition, the adverse effects of PEM on cell-mediated immune responses, the principal host defense against *Mycobacterium tuberculosis*, may be an important determinant of outcome. In fact, one study has shown that peripheral blood monocytes from malnourished tuberculosis patients produced no more IFN-γ when stimulated in vitro than controls, suggesting that defective IFN-γ responses by Th1 cells in malnutrition contribute to the susceptibility of malnourished hosts to tuberculosis.[163]

The percentage of B lymphocytes in the circulation remains in the normal range in PEM patients, consistent with the preservation of the cellularity of B lymphocyte-rich regions of the peripheral lymphoid organs. These cells are functional, and PEM patients usually have elevated serum levels of IgG, IgM, and IgA, especially in the presence of infections. However, normal immunoglobulin levels do not mean that antibody production is normal as well. More important than the total quantity of immunoglobulin are the amount and quality of specific antibody present and the ability of B cells to produce antibodies in response to new antigens.

There are limited data on the production of specific antibodies in PEM patients, mostly from studies using the response to vaccines as the experimental model. The majority of these have involved the use of the T lymphocyte-dependent protein tetanus toxoid and typhoid vaccine, which contains T-dependent protein antigens, the flagellar H antigens of *Salmonella typhi*, and T-independent somatic O antigens. Because of the large body of evidence showing that Th cells are diminished in PEM and the additional information that the immune response seems to be type 2 primed in PEM, the expectation is that PEM will inhibit the response to tetanus toxoid and flagellar H antigens and not significantly effect the response to the O polysaccharide. However, PEM patients appear to respond well to tetanus[164] and to flagellar antigens but not to polysaccharide antigens,[165,166] suggesting that at least some T-dependent responses occur normally but that there is a defect in the response to carbohydrate antigens.[167] Other vaccines have been tested with variable results, sometimes[168–170] but not always[171,172] showing a compromised antibody response. In a study of household contacts of adult cholera patients in Bangladesh, children 1 to 8 years of age were given two oral doses of cholera toxin B subunit, the nontoxic portion of cholera toxin, or placebo within 24 hours of hospitalization of the index adult patient. Although one-third of the children became infected with cholera (half symptomatic with diarrhea), malnourished children (weight for age $<70\%$ of the standard) did not differ from well-nourished children in the concentrations of salivary total IgA, initial serum antitoxin, or vibriocidal antibodies or in their serologic response to colonization, disease, or the toxin B subunit.[173]

Although total IgG levels are normal or elevated in PEM, antipolysaccharide antibodies are commonly of the IgG-2 or IgG-4 subclass. Thus, in response to respiratory infections with encapsulated organisms such as *Streptococcus pneumoniae* or *Haemophilus influenza* type b (Hib), IgG-2 and IgG-4 antibodies are either made locally in the lung or are transported into pulmonary secretions.[174] It is possible that the susceptibility of children with PEM to bacterial encapsulated respiratory pathogens is due to defects in the production of optimal IgG subclass antibodies, but the question has not been fully addressed. On the other hand, trials of the Hib conjugate vaccine in the Gambia effectively eliminated Hib disease, including in children with mild to moderate malnutrition.[175]

Can we make sense of the different vaccine challenges used to elicit antibody responses and the variable results obtained? Unfortunately, clarity and conclusiveness remain illusive. In part, this is because vaccine studies in PEM patients have generally tested the antibody response at the end of 4 weeks or longer following booster doses, and the early response, detectable within days of immunization, has not been examined. However, in real infections (in contrast to immunization), the kinetics of the immune response is crucial to adequate host defenses. Therefore, normal percent seroconversion or even levels of antibody weeks after the original vaccine dose, or even later following a booster dose, do not predict whether the early responses were also normal. In one study of the response to measles vaccine, a delay in specific immune response, measured on days 21 and 42 postimmunization, was noted in children with PEM.[176] The late response may represent a catch-up synthesis of antibody in PEM, sufficient to induce protection against a subsequent infection, but if the early response is delayed or of diminished magnitude in response to the actual infectious agent, then it may not contribute to host defense during infection and may lead to an adverse outcome.

The secretory immune system has also been assessed in individuals with PEM and consistently found to be deficient.[177] For example, a study of the response to measles and oral polio vaccines revealed diminished sIgA levels in saliva and specific IgA antibody responses following immunization of these patients.[178]

When measured in PEM patients, all components of serum complement except C4 have been observed to be significantly reduced, especially C3 and factor B.[179] As a result, both the classical and the alternate pathway are affected, although in vitro assays of complement-dependent hemolysis indicate that the compromise to the antibody-independent and early acting alternate pathway is more severe.[180–182] The high degree of activation of complement and elevated level of circulating complement–antibody complexes and the paradoxical decline in C3 levels in children with PEM and a concurrent infection[178] all suggest that complement activity is at least in part explained by a consumptive process, probably amplified by deficits in synthesis of complement components.[180]

Vitamin A

Despite the large body of data demonstrating a clear benefit of vitamin A on child survival, there is a paucity of data on the mechanisms by which vitamin A deficiency alters immune function. Vitamin A-deficient children have a decreased CD4/CD8 and cell ratio that can normalized with vitamin A.[183] However, the strongest effects of vitamin A deficiency on adaptive immunity are regulated through the induction of a cytokine profile that favors a type 1 over a type 2 response[184–186] that can inhibit antibody responses, especially to polysaccharide antigens.[187] In animal models, high levels of vitamin A augment the type 2 response, even when stimulated by a type 1 antigen such as influenza A.[188] Concern about possible adverse effects of vitamin A on immune responses arose when a defect was noted in the seroconversion rate of 6-month-old children given vitamin A at the time of measles immunization.[183] Because a practical way to give vitamin A was through the delivery structure provided by immunization, this early finding raised concern; however, a group of subsequent studies that measured the immunologic response to measles vaccine at 9 months of age,[189] oral polio vaccine,[190] and DPT[191] vaccine failed to show any adverse event of concurrent vitamin A administration on the antibody response to any of the antigens in these vaccines.

Zinc

Zinc deficiency has diverse effects on adaptive immunity. The most profound deficits induced by zinc deficiency involve T cell-mediated immune responses, especially type 1 responses. Zinc-deficient mice have reduced numbers of T cells, reduced proliferative responses to both mitogens and specific antigens, decreased IL-2 production, and decreased antibody levels to a T-dependent antigen but not a T-independent antigen.[192] All these changes were reversible with zinc supplementation.[151,192,193] These results are consistent with findings in children with PEM in whom nutritional rehabilitation failed to correct thymic gland involution (measured by chest radiographs) until 2 mg/kg/day of zinc was added to their diet. In malnourished children with diminished DTH skin test results, zinc has been demonstrated to augment DTH responsiveness.[194,195] Lymphocyte proliferative responses were greater in children with shigellosis receiving adjunctive zinc therapy than in controls.[196]

Zinc deficiency inhibits thymulin activity and thereby limits both intrathymic and extrathymic T cell differentiation.[197] Zinc deficiency also limits peripheral T cell activation and division through diminished IL-2 production,[198] and by decreasing the activity of NF-κB[199] and downregulating the interaction between IL-2 and IL-2 receptors, the responsiveness of T cells to IL-2 is reduced.[200] In addition to decreased IL-2, production of IFN-γ and TNF-α, cytokines critical for a normal type 1 response, is compromised,[198] whereas the production of the type 2 cytokines IL-4, IL-5, IL-6, and IL-10 remains intact,[198,201] leading to a distinct polarization in T cell response.

Animal studies also support some degree of impairment of B cells due to zinc deficiency, although the effects seem less than those seen in T cells. Pre-B cells and immature B cells, but not mature B cells, are reduced in number during zinc deficiency secondary to glucocorticoid-mediated apoptosis.[202] The patency of the humoral response in zinc deficiency appears to be highly dependent on the antigen. In a murine model, induced zinc deficiency had no detectable effect on the IgM response following immunization with a pneumococcal polysaccharide vaccine,[203] whereas in the same murine model with a T cell-dependent pneumococcal surface protein A vaccine, the IgG response was significantly decreased at both 14 and 28 days. In animals that underwent subsequent pneumococcal challenge, zinc-deficient animals exhibited heavier colonization and were more likely to become septicemic and die than controls.[204] Similar results have been obtained in humans. Two studies of the immunologic response to the oral killed whole cell plus cholera toxin B subunit cholera vaccine demonstrated an increased serum vibriocidal response and a decreased cholera toxin response in zinc-supplemented individuals.[205–207] In one of these studies, fecal anticholera toxin was increased.[205] Vibriocidal antibodies are directed against an LPS antigen and should induce a T-independent response, whereas cholera toxin is a protein and should induce a T-dependent humoral response.

CLINICAL POINTERS

Generally, professionals in public health have accepted the large body of evidence linking malnutrition and infection and act to implement appropriate interventions. Clinicians, however, often fail to recognize malnutrition, particularly milder forms, or to institute and monitor adequate nutritional therapy in patients with concurrent infections. Even mild to moderate malnutrition can be an important determinant in the outcome of an infectious disease. Patient management will be optimized only when clinicians incorporate appropriate nutritional therapy and counseling into clinical practice. Conversely, cytokine-induced losses of muscle mass and body nutrients occur during infections, even in previously well-nourished individuals who receive prompt and effective therapy. These losses can be fully reversed by convalescent feedings and micronutrient supplementation. Despite adequate replacement diets, it generally takes two or three times as long to replete an individual than it took to deplete him or her,[5] and the period of nutritional convalescence will depend on both the chronicity and the severity of the infection. In general, it is recommended that children should receive 30% more calories and 100% more protein to allow for catch-up growth during convalescence. Plentiful early and frequent feedings are especially important for infants and children in order to reinitiate an anabolic state and prevent a cycle of intensified progressive malnutrition often associated with frequent or recurring infections.

Individuals with severe malnourishment (WHZ <–3) greatly benefit from management accorded by structured protocols. Implementation of standardized management protocols in Bangladesh and Brazil has greatly improved outcome measures and decreased case fatality rate following protocol institution.[208,209] Because malnourished patients suffer atrophy of the intestinal mucosa, along with diminished production of hydrochloric acid and digestive enzymes, refeeding may be clinically difficult. Adequate amounts of potassium, phosphate, magnesium, zinc, and other vitamins must be replaced judiciously and energy requirements and intake measured and adjusted carefully during therapy.[210,211] Weight gain must be accurately measured, recorded, and diligently monitored to assess the adequacy of response to therapy. Infections are common and need to be identified and treated early.

Because important forms of malnutrition cause lymphoid atrophy, quick estimation of tonsillar size in a malnourished child provides instantaneous clinical information about the potential functional competence of the immune system. Tonsils virtually disappear during severe malnutrition.

Because vitamin A deficiency is widespread in developing countries, careful eye examinations are a mandatory part of patient evaluation. Both corneal xerophthalmia (xerosis, ulceration, and necrosis) and mild xerophthalmia are authentic clinical indicators that the patient faces an increased risk of morbidity and mortality as well as blindness. Prompt treatment with vitamin A is essential. Because vitamin A deficiency generally occurs in clusters, the presence of xerophthalmia in an index patient should raise the suspicion that family members and possibly the community as a whole share the deficiency. Vitamin A prophylaxis and dietary counseling should extend beyond the index patient. Because vitamin A deficiency increases mortality and the severity of infections before evidence of xerophthalmia, children in most developing countries should receive vitamin A at regular intervals. Although beyond the scope of this chapter, biofortification of the food supply through improvement of the quality of foods rather than supplementation of individuals with vitamin A and other micronutrients is critical if we are to address the nutritional needs of the 9 billion people who will populate Earth by 2050.

Although adequate iron intake is necessary to prevent iron deficiency anemia, caution needs to be exercised in regard to infectious diseases. It is recommended that iron supplements be withheld until initial management of severe malnutrition, which may be accompanied by serious infections. Children who present with infectious diseases and anemia should not be started on iron supplements until the infection is treated. The possible increase in some infections, such as malaria and diarrhea, with routine iron supplementation needs to be considered along with the possible benefits in deciding if this should be done in various settings. High-dose vitamin A administration is a mandatory part of treatment for all children with measles.

Preschool children with diarrhea should receive zinc (20 mg/day for 10–14 days; half this dose for children <6 months old) along with oral rehydration therapy, including increased fluids and continued feeding.

REFERENCES

1. Stephenson LS, Latham MC, Ottesen EA: Global malnutrition. Parasitology 121:S5–S22, 2000.
2. West KP: Extent of vitamin A deficiency among preschool children and women of reproductive age. J Nutr 132:2857S–2866S, 2002.
3. Stoltzfus RJ: Defining iron-deficiency anemia in public health terms: A time for reflection. J Nutr 131:565S–567S, 2001.
4. International Zinc Nutrition Consultative Group (IZiNCG): Technical Document #1. Assessment of the risk of zinc deficiency in populations and options for its control, Hotz C, Brown KH (guest eds). Food Nutr Bull 25(1), 2004.
5. Scrimshaw NS, Taylor CE, Gordon JE: Interactions of nutrition and infection. Monogr Ser World Health Organization 57:3–329, 1968.
6. Habicht JP, Meyers LD, Brownie C: Indicators for identifying and counting the improperly nourished. Am J Clin Nutr 35(5 Suppl): 1241–1254, 1982.
7. Kielmann AA, Taylor CE, DeSweemer C, et al: The Narangwal experiment on interactions of nutrition and infections: II. Morbidity and mortality effects. Indian J Med Res 68(Suppl):21–41, 1978.
8. Mata LJ: The Children of Santa Maria Cauque: A Prospective Field Study of Health and Growth. Cambridge, Mass, MIT Press, 1978.
9. Chen LC, Chowdhury A, Huffman SL: Anthropometric assessment of energy-protein malnutrition and subsequent risk of mortality among preschool aged children. Am J Clin Nutr 33:1836–1845, 1980.
10. Bistrian BR, Blackburn GL, Vitale J, et al: Prevalence of malnutrition in general medical patients. JAMA 235:1567–1570, 1976.
11. Bistrian BR, Blackburn GL, Hallowell E, et al: Protein status of general surgical patients. JAMA 230:858–860, 1974.
12. Correia MI, Campos AC: Prevalence of hospital malnutrition in Latin America: The multicenter ELAN study. Nutrition 19:823–825, 2003.
13. Studley HO: Percentage of weight loss: A basic indicator of surgical risk in patients with chronic peptic ulcer, 1936. Nutr Hosp 16:141–143, 2001.
14. Cannon PR, Wissler RW, Woolridge R: The relationship of protein deficiency to surgical infection. Ann Surg 120:514–525, 1944.
15. Dempsey DT, Mullen JL, Buzby GP: The link between nutritional status and clinical outcome: Can nutritional intervention modify it? Am J Clin Nutr 47(2 Suppl):352–356, 1988.
16. Gordon JE, Scrimshaw NS: Field trial of a newly developed food for prevention of malnutrition. World Rev Nutr Diet 15:256–288, 1972.
17. Gershoff SN, McGandy RB, Suttapreyasri D, et al: Nutrition studied in Thailand. II. Effects of fortification of rice with lysine, threonine, thiamin, riboflavin, vitamin A, and iron on preschool children. Am J Clin Nutr 30:1185–1195, 1977.
18. Rose D, Martorell R: The impact of protein-energy supplementation interventions on child morbidity and mortality. In Hill K (ed): Child Health Priorities for the 1990s. Baltimore, Johns Hopkins University Press, 1990.
19. Gordon JE, Ascoli W, Mata LJ, et al: Nutrition and infection field study in Guatemalan villages, 1959–1964. VI. Acute diarrheal disease and nutritional disorders in general disease incidence. Arch Environ Health 16:424–437, 1968.
20. Netrasiri A, Netrasiri C: Kwashiokor in Bangkok (an analytical study of 54 cases). J Trop Pediatr 1:148–155, 1955.
21. Salomon JB, Gordon JE, Scrimshaw NS: Studies of diarrheal disease in Central America. X. Associated chickenpox, diarrhea and kwashiorkor in a highland Guatemalan village. Am J Trop Med Hyg 15:997–1002, 1966.
22. Martorell R, Yarbrough C, Yarbrough S, et al: The impact of ordinary illnesses on the dietary intakes of malnourished children. Am J Clin Nutr 33:345–350, 1980.
23. Mata LJ, Kromal RA, Urrutia JJ, et al: Effect of infection on food intake and the nutritional state: Perspectives as viewed from the village. Am J Clin Nutr 30:1215–1227, 1977.
24. Mahalanabis D, Simpson TW, Chakraborty ML, et al: Malabsorption of water miscible vitamin A in children with giardiasis and ascariasis. Am J Clin Nutr 32:313–318, 1979.
25. Molla A, Molla AM, Khatun M, et al: Malabsorption of nutrients in children with diarrhoea due to unknown aetiologies. J Pak Med Assoc 43:49–51, 1993.
26. Scrimshaw NS: Effect of infection on nutrient requirements. Am J Clin Nutr 30:1536–1544, 1977.

27. Mitra AK, Alvarez JO, Guay-Woodford L, et al: Urinary retinol excretion and kidney function in children with shigellosis [see comments]. Am J Clin Nutr 68:1095–1103, 1998.
28. Pelletier DL, Frongillo EA Jr, Schroeder DG, et al: The effects of malnutrition on child mortality in developing countries. Bull World Health Organization 73:443–448, 1995.
29. Pelletier DL: The relationship between child anthropometry and mortality in developing countries: Implications for policy, programs and future research. J Nutr 124(10 Suppl):2047S–2081S, 1994.
30. Pelletier DL, Frongillo EA Jr, Schroeder DG, et al: A methodology for estimating the contribution of malnutrition to child mortality in developing countries. J Nutr 124(10 Suppl):2106S–2122S, 1994.
31. Caulfield LE, de Onis M, Blössner M, et al: Undernutrition as an underlying cause of child deaths associate with diarrhea, pneumonia, malaria and measles. Am J Clin Nutr 80:193–198, 2004.
32. van der Hulst RR, van Kreel BK, von Meyenfeldt MF, et al: Glutamine and the preservation of gut integrity. Lancet 341:1363–1365, 1993.
33. Sommer A: Vitamin A, infectious disease, and childhood mortality: A 2 solution? J Infect Dis 167:1003–1007, 1993.
34. Semba RD: Vitamin A, immunity, and infection. Clin Infect Dis 19:489–499, 1994.
35. Sommer A, West KP Jr: Vitamin A Deficiency. New York, Oxford University Press, 1996.
36. Khatry SK, West KP Jr, Katz J, et al: Epidemiology of xerophthalmia in Nepal. A pattern of household poverty, childhood illness, and mortality. The Sarlahi Study Group. Arch Ophthalmol 113:425–429, 1995.
37. Katz J, Zeger SL, West KP Jr, et al: Clustering of xerophthalmia within households and villages. Int J Epidemiol 22:709–715, 1993.
38. Mele L, West KP Jr, Kusdiono PA, et al: Nutritional and household risk factors for xerophthalmia in Aceh, Indonesia: A case–control study. The Aceh Study Group. Am J Clin Nutr 53:1460–1465, 1991.
39. Sommer A, Tarwotjo I, Djunaedi E, et al: Impact of vitamin A supplementation on childhood mortality. A randomised controlled community trial. Lancet 1:1169–1173, 1986.
40. Rahmathullah L, Tielsch JM, Thulasiraj RD, et al: Impact of supplementing newborn infants with vitamin A on early infant mortality: Community based randomised trial in southern India. BMJ 327:254, 2003.
41. West KP Jr, Katz J, Shrestha SR, et al: Mortality of infants <6 mo of age supplemented with vitamin A: A randomized, double-masked trial in Nepal. Am J Clin Nutr 62:143–148, 1995.
42. WHO/CHD Immunisation-Linked Vitamin A Supplementation Study Group: Randomised trial to assess benefits and safety of vitamin A supplementation linked to immunisation in early infancy. Lancet 352:1257–1263, 1998.
43. Ching P, Birmingham M, Goodman T, et al: Childhood mortality impact and costs of integrating vitamin A supplementation into immunization campaigns. Am J Public Health 90:1526–1529, 2000.
44. D'Souza RM, D'Souza R: Vitamin A for treating measles in children. Cochrane Database Syst Rev 1:CD001479, 2002.
45. D'Souza RM, D'Souza R: Vitamin A for the treatment of children with measles—A systematic review. J Trop Pediatr 48:323–327, 2002.
46. Biswas R, Biswas AB, Manna B, et al: Effect of vitamin A supplementation on diarrhoea and acute respiratory tract infection in children. A double blind placebo controlled trial in a Calcutta slum community. Eur J Epidemiol 10:57–61, 1994.
47. Barreto ML, Santos LM, Assis AM, et al: Effect of vitamin A supplementation on diarrhoea and acute lower-respiratory-tract infections in young children in Brazil. Lancet 344:228–231, 1994.
48. Donnen P, Dramaix M, Brasseur D, et al: Randomized placebo-controlled clinical trial of the effect of a single high dose or daily low doses of vitamin A on the morbidity of hospitalized, malnourished children. Am J Clin Nutr 68:1254–1260, 1998.
49. Hossain S, Biswas R, Kabir I, et al: Single dose vitamin A treatment in acute shigellosis in Bangladesh children: Randomised double blind controlled trial [see comments]. BMJ 316:422–426, 1998.
50. Grotto I, Mimouni M, Gdalevich M, et al: Vitamin A supplementation and childhood morbidity from diarrhea and respiratory infections: A meta-analysis. J Pediatr 142:297–304, 2003.
51. Stephensen CB, Franchi LM, Hernandez H, et al: Adverse effects of high-dose vitamin A supplements in children hospitalized with pneumonia. Pediatrics 101:E3, 1998.
52. Fawzi WW, Mbise RL, Fataki MR, et al: Vitamin A supplementation and severity of pneumonia in children admitted to the hospital in Dar es Salaam, Tanzania. Am J Clin Nutr 68:187–192, 1998.
53. Black RE: Zinc deficiency, infectious disease and mortality in the developing world. J Nutr 133:1485S–1489S, 2003.
54. Ninh NX, Thissen JP, Collette L, et al: Zinc supplementation increases growth and circulating insulin-like growth factor I (IGF-I) in growth-retarded Vietnamese children. Am J Clin Nutr 63:514–519, 1996.
55. Sazawal S, Black RE, Bhan MK, et al: Efficacy of zinc supplementation in reducing the incidence and prevalence of acute diarrhea—A community-based, double-blind, controlled trial. Am J Clin Nutr 66:413–418, 1997.
56. Sazawal S, Black RE, Jalla S, et al: Zinc supplementation reduces the incidence of acute lower respiratory infections in infants and preschool children: A double-blind, controlled trial. Pediatrics 102:1–5, 1998.
57. Rosado JL, Lopez P, Munoz E, et al: Zinc supplementation reduced morbidity, but neither zinc nor iron supplementation affected growth or body composition of Mexican preschoolers. Am J Clin Nutr 65:13–19, 1997.
58. Ruel MT, Rivera JA, Santizo MC, et al: Impact of zinc supplementation on morbidity from diarrhea and respiratory infections among rural Guatemalan children. Pediatrics 99:808–813, 1997.
59. Shankar AH, Genton B, Baisor M, et al: The influence of zinc supplementation on morbidity due to *Plasmodium falciparum*: A randomized trial in preschool children in Papua New Guinea. Am J Trop Med Hyg 62:663–669, 2000.
60. Meeks GJ, Witter MM, Ramdath DD: Zinc supplementation: Effects on the growth and morbidity of undernourished Jamaican children. Eur J Clin Nutr 52:34–39, 1998.
61. Penny ME, Peerson JM, Marin M, et al: Randomized, community-based trial of the effect of zinc supplementation, with and without other micronutrients, on the duration of persistent childhood diarrhea Lima, Peru. J Pediatr 135:208–217, 1999.
62. Umeta M, West CE, Haidar J, et al: Zinc supplementation and stunted infants in Ethiopia: A randomised controlled trial. Lancet 355:2021–2026, 2000.
63. Muller O, Becher H, van Zweeden AB, et al: Effect of zinc supplementation on malaria and other causes of morbidity in west African children: Randomised double blind placebo controlled trial. BMJ 322:1567, 2001.
64. Osendarp SJM, Santosham M, Black RE, et al: Effect of zinc supplementation between 1 and 6 mo of life on growth and morbidity of Bangladeshi infants in urban slums. Am J Clin Nutr 76:1401–1408, 2002.
65. Penny ME, Marin RM, Duran A, et al: Randomized controlled trial of the effect of daily supplementation with zinc or multiple micronutrients on the morbidity, growth, and micronutrient status of young Peruvian children. Am J Clin Nutr 79:457–465, 2004.
66. Sur D, Gupta DN, Mondal SK, et al: Impact of zinc supplementation on diarrheal morbidity and growth pattern of low birth weight infants in Kolkata, India: A randomized, double-blind, placebo-controlled, community-based study. Pediatrics 112:1327–1332, 2003.
67. Gupta DN, Mondal SK, Ghosh S, et al: Impact of zinc supplementation on diarrhoeal morbidity in rural children of West Bengal, India. Acta Paediatr 92:531–536, 2003.
68. Zinc Investigators' Collaborative Group (Sazawal S, Black RE, coordinators): Prevention of diarrhea and pneumonia by zinc supplementation in children in developing countries: Pooled analysis of randomized controlled trials. J Pediatr 135:689–697, 1999.
69. Osendarp SJ, van Raaij JM, Arifeen SE, et al: A randomized, placebo-controlled trial of the effect of zinc supplementation during pregnancy on pregnancy outcome in Bangladeshi urban poor. Am J Clin Nutr 71:114–119, 2000.
70. Sachdev HP, Mittal NK, Yadav HS: Oral zinc supplementation in persistent diarrhoea in infants. Ann Trop Paediatr 10:63–69, 1990.
71. Roy SK, Tomkins AM, Mahalanabis D, et al: Impact of zinc supplementation on persistent diarrhoea in malnourished Bangladeshi children. Acta Paediatr 87:1235–1239, 1998.
72. Bhutta ZA, Nizami SQ, Isani Z: Zinc supplementation in malnourished children with persistent diarrhea in Pakistan. Pediatrics 103:e42, 1999.
73. Khatun UHF: Impact of Zinc and Vitamin A supplementation in Malnourished Hospitalized Children Suffering from Persistent Diarrhea. Dhaka, Bangladesh, University of Dhaka, Institute of Nutrition and Food Science, 1998.

74. Sachdev HP, Mittal NK, Mittal SK, et al: A controlled trial on utility of oral zinc supplementation in acute dehydrating diarrhea in infants. J Pediatr Gastroenterol Nutr 7:877–881, 1988.
75. Sazawal S, Black RE, Bhan MK, et al: Zinc supplementation in young children with acute diarrhea in India. N Engl J Med 333:839–844, 1995.
76. Roy SK, Tomkins AM, Akramuzzaman SM, et al: Randomised controlled trial of zinc supplementation in malnourished Bangladeshi children with acute diarrhoea. Arch Dis Child 77:196–200, 1997.
77. Faruque AS, Mahalanabis D, Haque SS, et al: Double-blind, randomized, controlled trial of zinc or vitamin A supplementation in young children with acute diarrhoea. Acta Paediatr 88:154–160, 1999.
78. Dutta P, Mitra U, Datta A, et al: Impact of zinc supplementation in malnourished children with acute watery diarrhoea. J Trop Pediatr 46:259–263, 2000.
79. Strand TA, Chandyo RK, Bahl R, et al: Effectiveness and efficacy of zinc for the treatment of acute diarrhea in young children. Pediatrics 109:898–903, 2002.
80. Hidayat A, Achadi A, Sunoto, et al: The effect of zinc supplementation in children under three years of age with acute diarrhea in Indonesia. Med J Indonesia 7:237–241, 1998.
81. Zinc Investigators' Collaborative Group (Sazawal S, Black RE, coordinators): Therapeutic effects of oral zinc in acute and persistent diarrhea in children in developing countries: Pooled analysis of randomized controlled trials. Am J Clin Nutr 72:1516–1522, 2000.
82. World Health Organization (WHO/FCH/CAH/04.7): WHO–UNICEF Joint Statement on the Clinical Management of Acute Diarrhea, 2004.
83. Bhandari N, Bahl R, Taneja S, et al: Effect of routine zinc supplementation on pneumonia in children aged 6 months to 3 years: Randomised controlled trial in an urban slum. BMJ 324:1358, 2002.
84. Mahalanabis D, Lahiri M, Paul D, et al: Randomized, double-blind, placebo-controlled clinical trial of the efficacy of treatment with zinc or vitamin A in infants and young children with severe acute lower respiratory infection. Am J Clin Nutr 79:430–436, 2004.
85. Brooks WA, Yunus MD, Santosham M, et al: Zinc for severe pneumonia in very young children: Double-blind placebo–controlled trial. Lancet 343:1683–1688, 2004.
86. Bates CJ, Evans PH, Dardenne M, et al: A trial of zinc supplementation in young rural Gambian children. Br J Nutr 69:243–255, 1993.
87. The Zinc Against Plasmodium Study Group: Effect of zinc on the treatment of *Plasmodium falciparum* malaria in children: A randomized controlled trial. Am J Clin Nutr 76:805–812, 2002.
88. Makonnen B, Venter A, Joubert G: A randomized controlled study of the impact of dietary zinc supplementation in the management of children with protein-energy malnutrition in Lesotho. II: Special investigations. J Trop Pediatr 49:353–360, 2003.
89. Neumann CG, Bwibo NO, Murphy SP, et al: Animal source foods improve dietary quality, micronutrient status, growth and cognitive function in Kenyan schoolchildren: Background, study design and baseline findings. J Nutr 133(Suppl 2):3941S–3949S, 2003.
90. Demment MW, Young MM, Sensenig RL: Providing micronutrients through food-based solutions: A key to human and national development. J Nutr 133(Suppl 2):3879S–3885S, 2003.
91. Oppenheimer SJ: Iron and its relation to immunity and infectious disease. J Nutr 131(Suppl 2):616S–633S, 2001.
92. Gera T, Sachdev HPS: Effect of iron supplementation on incidence of infectious illness in children: Systematic review. BMJ 325:2–10, 2002.
93. Müller O, Becher H, van Zweeden AB, et al: Effect of zinc supplementation on malaria and other causes or morbidity in west African children: Randomized double blind placebo controlled trial. BMJ 322:1–6, 2001.
94. Baggs RB, Miller SA: Defect in resistance to *Salmonella typhimurium* in iron-deficient rats. J Infect Dis 130:409–411, 1974.
95. Baggs RB, Miller SA: Nutritional iron deficiency as a determinant of host resistance in the rat. J Nutr 103:1554–1560, 1973.
96. Haddock RL, Cousens SN, Guzman CC: Infant diet and salmonellosis. Am J Public Health 81:997–1000, 1991.
97. Douglas RM, Chalker EB, Treacy B: Vitamin C for preventing and treating the common cold. Cochrane Database Syst Rev 2:CD000980, 2000.
98. Hemila H: Vitamin C and common cold incidence: A review of studies with subjects under heavy physical stress. Int J Sports Med 17:379–383, 1996.
99. Gu BQ: Pathology of Keshan disease. A comprehensive review. Chin Med J (Engl) 96:251–261, 1983.
100. Rayman MP: The importance of selenium to human health. Lancet 356:233–241, 2000.
101. Li Y, Yang Y, Chen H: Detection of enteroviral RNA in paraffin-embedded myocardial tissue from patients with Keshan by nested PCR. Zhonghua Yi Xue Za Zhi 75:344–345, 382, 1995.
102. Bai J: The combined effect of selenium deficiency and viral infection on the myocardium of mice (preliminary study) [author's transl]. Zhongguo Yi Xue Ke Xue Yuan Xue Bao 2:29–31, 1980.
103. Beck MA, Shi Q, Morris VC, et al: Rapid genomic evolution of a non-virulent coxsackievirus B3 in selenium-deficient mice results in selection of identical virulent isolates. Nat Med 1:433–436, 1995.
104. Nelson HK, Shi Q, Van Dael P, et al: Host nutritional selenium status as a driving force for influenza virus mutations. FASEB J 15:1846–1848, 2001.
105. Dubois EF: The Mechanism of Heat Loss and Temperature Regulation. Stanford, Calif, Stanford University Press, 1937.
106. Hoyle B, Yunus M, Chen LC: Breast-feeding and food intake among children with acute diarrheal disease. Am J Clin Nutr 33:2365–2371, 1980.
107. Beisel WR: Interrelated changes in host metabolism during generalized infectious illness. Am J Clin Nutr 25:1254–1260, 1972.
108. Beisel WR: Metabolic response to infection. Annu Rev Med 26:9–20, 1975.
109. Mitch WE, Goldberg AL: Mechanisms of muscle wasting. The role of the ubiquitin–proteasome pathway. N Engl J Med 335:1897–1905, 1996.
110. Tiao G, Fagan J, Roegner V, et al: Energy-ubiquitin-dependent muscle proteolysis during sepsis in rats is regulated by glucocorticoids. J Clin Invest 97:339–348, 1996.
111. Kushner I, Rzewnicki DL: The acute phase response: General aspects. Baillieres Clin Rheumatol 8:513–530, 1994.
112. Healy AM, Gelehrter TD: Induction of plasminogen activator inhibitor-1 in HepG2 human hepatoma cells by mediators of the acute phase response. J Biol Chem 269:19095–19100, 1994.
113. Steel DM, Whitehead AS: The major acute phase reactants: C-reactive protein, serum amyloid P component and serum amyloid A protein. Immunol Today 15:81–88, 1994.
114. Tiao G, Hobler S, Wang JJ, et al: Sepsis is associated with increased mRNAs of the ubiquitin–proteasome proteolytic pathway in human skeletal muscle. J Clin Invest 99:163–168, 1997.
115. Powanda MC: Changes in body balances of nitrogen and other key nutrients: Description and underlying mechanisms. Am J Clin Nutr 30:1254–1268, 1977.
116. Kotler DP, Tierney AR, Wang J, et al: Magnitude of body-cell-mass depletion and the timing of death from wasting in AIDS. Am J Clin Nutr 50:444–447, 1989.
117. Allison DB, Faith MS, Heo M, et al: Hypothesis concerning the U-shaped relation between body mass index and mortality. Am J Epidemiol 146:339–349, 1997.
118. Hill MR, McCallum RE: Identification of tumor necrosis factor as a transcriptional regulator of the phosphoenolpyruvate carboxykinase gene following endotoxin treatment of mice. Infect Immun 60:4040–4050, 1992.
119. Kinney JM: Metabolic responses of the critically ill patient. Crit Care Clin 11:569–585, 1995.
120. Blackburn GL: Lipid metabolism in infection. Am J Clin Nutr 30:1321–1332, 1977.
121. Beisel WR: Zinc metabolism in infection. Prog Clin Biol Res 14:155–179, 1997.
122. Molla A, Molla AM, Sarker SA, et al: Effects of acute diarrhea on absorption of macronutrients during disease and recovery. In Chen LD, Scrimshaw NS (eds): Diarrhea and Malnutrition: Interactions, Mechanisms, and Interventions. New York, Plenum, 1983, pp 143–154.
123. Black RE, Levine M: Intestinal protein loss in shigellosis. Nutr Res 11:1215–1220, 1991.
124. Castillo-Duran C, Vial P, Uauy R: Trace mineral balance during acute diarrhea in infants. J Pediatr 113:452–457, 1988.
125. van der Hulst RR, von Meyenfeldt MF, van Kreel BK, et al: Gut permeability, intestinal morphology, and nutritional depletion. Nutrition 14:1–6, 1998.

126. Thurnham DI, Northrop-Clewes CA, McCullough FS, et al: Innate immunity, gut integrity, and vitamin A in Gambian and Indian infants. J Infect Dis 182(Suppl 1):S23–S28, 2000.
127. McDowell EM, Keenan KP, Huang M: Restoration of mucociliary tracheal epithelium following deprivation of vitamin A. A quantitative morphologic study. Virchows Arch B Cell Pathol Incl Mol Pathol 45:221–240, 1984.
128. McDowell EM, Keenan KP, Huang M: Effects of vitamin A-deprivation on hamster tracheal epithelium. A quantitative morphologic study. Virchows Arch B Cell Pathol Incl Mol Pathol 45:197–219, 1984.
129. Aggett RJ: Severe zinc deficiency. In Mills CR (ed): Zinc in Human Biology. New York, Springer-Verlag, 1989, pp 259–279.
130. Solomons NW: Zinc and copper. In Shils ME, Young VR (eds): Modern Nutrition in Health and Disease. Philadelphia, Lea & Febiger, 1988, pp 238–262.
131. Walsh CT, Sandstead HH, Prasad AS, et al: Zinc: Health effects and research priorities for the 1990s. Environ Health Perspect 102 (Suppl 2):5–46, 1994.
132. Anderson DC, Krishna GS, Hughes BJ, et al: Impaired polymorphonuclear leukocyte motility in malnourished infants: Relationship to functional abnormalities of cell adherence. J Lab Clin Med 101:881–895, 1983.
133. Schopfer K, Douglas SD: Neutrophil function in children with kwashiorkor. J Lab Clin Med 88:450–461, 1976.
134. Kulapongs P, Edelman R, Suskind R, et al: Defective local leukocyte mobilization in children with kwashiorkor. Am J Clin Nutr 30:367–370, 1977.
135. Nayak KC, Sethi AS, Aggarwal TD, et al: Bactericidal power of neutrophils in protein calorie malnutrition. Indian J Pediatr 56:371–377, 1989.
136. Keusch GT, Urrutia JJ, Guerrero O, et al: Serum opsonic activity in acute protein-energy malnutrition. Bull World Health Organization 59:923–929, 1981.
137. Weston WL, Huff JC, Humbert JR, et al: Zinc correction of defective chemotaxis in acrodermatitis enteropathica. Arch Dermatol 113:422–425, 1977.
138. Briggs WA, Pedersen MM, Mahajan SK, et al: Lymphocyte and granulocyte function in zinc-treated and zinc-deficient hemodialysis patients. Kidney Int 21:827–832, 1982.
139. Hasegawa H, Suzuki K, Suzuki K, et al: Effects of zinc on the reactive oxygen species generating capacity of human neutrophils and on the serum opsonic activity in vitro. Luminescence 15:321–327, 2000.
140. Beisel WR: Single nutrients and immunity. Am J Clin Nutr 35(2 Suppl): 417–468, 1982.
141. Deicher R, Ziai F, Cohen G, et al: High-dose parenteral iron sucrose depresses neutrophil intracellular killing capacity. Kidney Int 64: 728–736, 2003.
142. Rivadeneira DE, Grobmyer SR, Naama HA, et al: Malnutrition-induced macrophage apoptosis. Surgery 129:617–625, 2001.
143. Borelli P, Souza IP, Borojevic R, et al: Protein malnutrition: Some aspects of the in vitro adhesion of peritoneal mouse macrophages. Ann Nutr Metab 42:367–373, 1998.
144. Teshima S, Rokutan K, Takahashi M, et al Alteration of the respiratory burst and phagocytosis of macrophages under protein malnutrition. J Nutr Sci Vitaminol (Tokyo) 41:127–137, 1995.
145. Redmond HP, Gallagher HJ, Shou J, et al: Antigen presentation in protein-energy malnutrition. Cell Immunol 163:80–87, 1995.
146. McCarter MD, Naama HA, Shou J, et al: Altered macrophage intracellular signaling induced by protein-calorie malnutrition. Cell Immunol 183:131–136, 1998.
147. Sauerwein RW, Mulder JA, Mulder L, et al: Inflammatory mediators in children with protein-energy malnutrition. Am J Clin Nutr 65:1534–1539, 1997.
148. Aslan Y, Erduran E, Gedik Y, et al: Serum interleukin-1 and granulocyte-macrophage colony-stimulating factor levels in protein malnourished patients during acute infection. Cent Afr J Med 42:179–184, 1996.
149. Bhaskaram P, Sivakumar B: Interleukin-1 in malnutrition. Arch Dis Child 61:182–185, 1986.
150. Kauffman CA, Jones PG, Kluger MJ: Fever and malnutrition: Endogenous pyrogen/interleukin-1 in malnourished patients. Am J Clin Nutr 44:449–452, 1986.
151. Prasad AS: Zinc, infection, and immune function. In Calder PC, Field CJ, Gill HS (eds): Nutrition and Immune Function. New York, CABI, 2002, pp 193–208.
152. Wirth JJ, Fraker PJ, Kierszenbaum F: Zinc requirement for macrophage function: Effect of zinc deficiency on uptake and killing of a protozoan parasite. Immunology 68:114–119, 1989.
153. James SJ, Swendseid M, Makinodan T: Macrophage-mediated depression of T-cell proliferation in zinc-deficient mice. J Nutr 117:1982–1988, 1987.
154. Chandra RK: Rosette-forming T lymphocytes and cell-mediated immunity in malnutrition. Br Med J 3:608–609, 1974.
155. Keusch GT, Cruz JR, Torun B, et al: Immature circulating lymphocytes in severely malnourished Guatemalan children. J Pediatr Gastroenterol Nutr 6:265–270, 1987.
156. Parent G, Chevalier P, Zalles L, et al: In vitro lymphocyte-differentiating effects of thymulin (Zn-FTS) on lymphocyte subpopulations of severely malnourished children. Am J Clin Nutr 60:274–278, 1994.
157. Cruz JR, Chew F, Fernandez RA, et al: Effects of nutritional recuperation on E-rosetting lymphocytes and in vitro response to thymosin in malnourished children. J Pediatr Gastroenterol Nutr 6:387–391, 1987.
158. Spellberg B, Edwards JE Jr: Type 1/type 2 immunity in infectious diseases. Clin Infect Dis 32:76–102, 2001.
159. Dulger H, Arik M, Sekeroglu MR, et al: Pro-inflammatory cytokines in Turkish children with protein-energy malnutrition. Mediators Inflamm 11:363–365, 2002.
160. Yoshino K, Sakai K, Okada H, et al: IgE responses in mice fed moderate protein deficient and high protein diets. J Nutr Sci Vitaminol (Tokyo) 49:172–178, 2003.
161. Harland PS: Tuberculin reactions in malnourished children. Lancet 2:719–721, 1965.
162. Harland PS, Brown RE: Tuberculin sensitivity following b.c.g. vaccination in undernourished children. East Afr Med J 42:233–238, 1965.
163. Bhaskaram P, Sundaramma MN: Peripheral blood monocyte function in malnourished subjects with pulmonary tuberculosis. Eur J Clin Nutr 44:245–248, 1990.
164. Monjour L, Bourdillon F, Korinek AM, et al: Humoral immunity, 5 years after anti-tetanus vaccination, in a group of malaria-infected and malnourished African children. Pathol Biol (Paris) 36:235–239, 1988.
165. Greenwood BM, Bradley-Moore AM, Bradley AK, et al: The immune response to vaccination in undernourished and well-nourished Nigerian children. Ann Trop Med Parasitol 80:537–544, 1986.
166. Mohammed I, Damisah MM: The immunological response to polyvalent meningococcal vaccine in Bauchi State, Nigeria. Trans R Soc Trop Med Hyg 76:351–353, 1982.
167. Keusch GT: Nutritional effects on response of children in developing countries to respiratory tract pathogens: Implications for vaccine development. Rev Infect Dis 13(Suppl 6):S486-S491, 1991.
168. Idris S, El Seed AM: Measles vaccination in severely malnourished Sudanese children. Ann Trop Paediatr 3:63–67, 1983.
169. Powell GM: Response to live attenuated measles vaccine in children with severe kwashiorkor. Ann Trop Paediatr 2:143–145, 1982.
170. Brown RE, Katz M: Failure of antibody production to yellow fever vaccine in children with kwashiorkor. Trop Geogr Med 18:125–128, 1966.
171. Coovadia HM, Parent MA, Loening WE, et al: An evaluation of factors associated with the depression of immunity in malnutrition and in measles. Am J Clin Nutr 27:665–669, 1974.
172. Ifekwunigwe AE, Grasset N, Glass R, et al: Immune responses to measles and smallpox vaccinations in malnourished children. Am J Clin Nutr 33:621–624, 1980.
173. Glass RI, Svennerholm AM, Stoll BJ, et al: Effects of undernutrition on infection with Vibrio cholerae O1 and on response to oral cholera vaccine. Pediatr Infect Dis J 8:105–109, 1989.
174. Reynolds HY: Immunoglobulin G and its function in the human respiratory tract. Mayo Clinic Proc 63:161–174, 1988.
175. Mulholland K, Hilton S, Adegbola R, et al: Randomised trial of Haemophilus influenzae type-b tetanus protein conjugate vaccine [corrected] for prevention of pneumonia and meningitis in Gambian infants. Lancet 349:1191–1197, 1997.

176. Wesley A, Coovadia HM, Watson AR: Immunization against measles in children at risk for severe disease. Trans R Soc Trop Med Hyg 73:710–715, 1979.
177. Chandra RK, Wadhwa M: Nutritional modulation of intestinal mucosal immunity. Immunol Invest 18:119–126, 1989.
178. Chandra RK: Reduced secretory antibody response to live attenuated measles and poliovirus vaccines in malnourished children. BMJ 2:583–585, 1975.
179. Sirisinha S, Edelman R, Suskind R, et al: Complement and C3-proactivator levels in children with protein-calorie malnutrition and effect of dietary treatment. Lancet 1:1016–1020, 1973.
180. Chandra RK: Serum complement and immunoconglutinin in malnutrition. Arch Dis Child 50:225–229, 1975.
181. Suskind R, Edelman R, Kulapongs P, et al: Complement activity in children with protein-calorie malnutrition. Am J Clin Nutr 29:1089–1092, 1976.
182. Keusch GT, Torun B, Johnston RB Jr, et al: Impairment of hemolytic complement activation by both classical and alternative pathways in serum from patients with kwashiorkor. J Pediatr 105:434–436, 1984.
183. Semba RD, Muhilal, Ward BJ, et al: Abnormal T-cell subset proportions in vitamin-A-deficient children. Lancet 341:5–8, 1993.
184. Frankenburg S, Wang X, Milner Y: Vitamin A inhibits cytokines produced by type 1 lymphocytes in vitro. Cell Immunol 185:75–81, 1998.
185. Cantorna MT, Nashold FE, Hayes CE: Vitamin A deficiency results in a priming environment conducive for Th1 cell development. Eur J Immunol 25:1673–1679, 1995.
186. Cantorna MT, Nashold FE, Hayes CE: In vitamin A deficiency multiple mechanisms establish a regulatory T helper cell imbalance with excess Th1 and insufficient Th2 function. J Immunol 152:1515–1522, 1994.
187. Pasatiempo AM, Bowman TA, Taylor CE, et al: Vitamin A depletion and repletion: Effects on antibody response to the capsular polysaccharide of Streptococcus pneumoniae, type III (SSS-III). Am J Clin Nutr 49:501–510, 1989.
188. Cui D, Moldoveanu Z, Stephensen CB: High-level dietary vitamin A enhances T-helper type 2 cytokine production and secretory immunoglobulin A response to influenza A virus infection in BALB/c mice. J Nutr 130:1132–1139, 2000.
189. Benn CS, Aaby P, Bale C, et al: Randomised trial of effect of vitamin A supplementation on antibody response to measles vaccine in Guinea-Bissau, West Africa. Lancet 350:101–105, 1997.
190. Semba RD, Muhilal, Mohgaddam NE, et al: Integration of vitamin A supplementation with the expanded program on immunization does not affect seroconversion to oral poliovirus vaccine in infants. J Nutr 129:2203–2205, 1999.
191. Rahman MM, Mahalanabis D, Hossain S, et al: Simultaneous vitamin A administration at routine immunization contact enhances antibody response to diphtheria vaccine in infants younger than six months. J Nutr 129:2192–2195, 1999.
192. Moulder K, Steward MW: Experimental zinc deficiency: Effects on cellular responses and the affinity of humoral antibody. Clin Exp Immunol 77:269–274, 1989.
193. Cunningham-Rundles C, Cunningham-Rundles S, Iwata T, et al: Zinc deficiency, depressed thymic hormones, and T lymphocyte dysfunction in patients with hypogammaglobulinemia. Clin Immunol Immunopathol 21:387–396, 1981.
194. Golden MH, Harland PS, Golden BE, et al: Zinc and immunocompetence in protein-energy malnutrition. Lancet 1:1226–1228, 1978.
195. Cuevas LE, Almeida LM, Mazunder P, et al: Effect of zinc on the tuberculin response of children exposed to adults with smear-positive tuberculosis. Ann Trop Paediatr 22:313–319, 2002.
196. Raqib R, Roy SK, Rahman MJ, et al: Effect of zinc supplementation on immune and inflammatory responses in pediatric patients with shigellosis. Am J Clin Nutr 79:444–450, 2004.
197. Prasad AS, Meftah S, Abdallah J, et al: Serum thymulin in human zinc deficiency. J Clin Invest 82:1202–1210, 1988.
198. Beck FW, Prasad AS, Kaplan J, et al: Changes in cytokine production and T cell subpopulations in experimentally induced zinc-deficient humans. Am J Physiol 272:E1002–E1007, 1997.
199. Prasad AS, Bao B, Beck FW, et al: Zinc activates NF-kappaB in HUT-78 cells. J Lab Clin Med 138:250–256, 2001.
200. Tanaka Y: A study on the role of zinc on the immune response and body metabolism—A contribution of trace elements. Kobe J Med Sci 35:299–309, 1989.
201. Prasad AS, Beck FW, Grabowski SM, et al: Zinc deficiency: Changes in cytokine production and T-cell subpopulations in patients with head and neck cancer and in noncancer subjects. Proc Assoc Am Physicians 109:68–77, 1997.
202. Fraker PJ, King LE, Laakko T, et al: The dynamic link between the integrity of the immune system and zinc status. J Nutr 130(Suppl 5S): 1399S–1406S, 2000.
203. Strand TA, Aaberge IS, Maage A, et al: The immune response to pneumococcal polysaccharide vaccine in zinc-depleted mice. Scand J Immunol 58:76–80, 2003.
204. Strand TA, Hollingshead SK, Julshamn K, et al: Effects of zinc deficiency and pneumococcal surface protein a immunization on zinc status and the risk of severe infection in mice. Infect Immun 71:2009–2013, 2003.
205. Karlsen TH, Sommerfelt H, Klomstad S, et al: Intestinal and systemic immune responses to an oral cholera toxoid B subunit whole-cell vaccine administered during zinc supplementation. Infect Immun 71:3909–3913, 2003.
206. Qadri F, Ahmed T, Wahed MA, et al: Suppressive effect of zinc on antibody response to cholera toxin in children given the killed, B subunit-whole cell, oral cholera vaccine. Vaccine 22:416–421, 2004.
207. Albert MJ, Qadri F, Wahed MA, et al: Supplementation with zinc, but not vitamin A, improves seroconversion to vibriocidal antibody in children given an oral cholera vaccine. J Infect Dis 187:909–913, 2003.
208. Ahmed T, Ali M, Ullah MM, et al: Mortality in severely malnourished children with diarrhoea and use of a standardised management protocol. Lancet 353:1919–1922, 1999.
209. Cavalcante AA, Pinheiro LM, Monte C, et al: Treatment of malnutrition in Brazil: Simple solutions to common problems. Trop Doct 28: 95–97, 1998.
210. Bhan MK, Bhandari N, Bahl R: Management of the severely malnourished child: Perspective from developing countries. BMJ 326:146–151, 2003.
211. Ahmed T, Ali M, Ullah MM, et al: Mortality in severely malnourished children with diarrhoea and use of a standardised management protocol. Lancet 353:1919–1922, 1999.

6

Host Genetics and Susceptibility to Infection

ROBERT JOHN WILKINSON
MICHAEL LEVIN
GEOFFREY PASVOL

The dawn of the scientific age of medicine in the late 19th century was characterized by the discovery of many of the microorganisms responsible for conditions such as tuberculosis and malaria. At the beginning of the 21st century, the availability of representative whole genome sequences of more than 50 common pathogens heralds a new age of molecular microbiology and parasitology. As a consequence, our consideration of infectious disease tends to be "organism based," with great emphasis on virulence determinants responsible for pathogenicity. In the first half of the 20th century, improvements in living conditions resulted in reduced incidences of many of these infectious diseases, thus emphasizing the importance of the environment as a major influence on the occurrence of infection. Only the rash are trumpeting the death knoll of infectious diseases, however: More people died per day of infection in 2000 than in 1900.

Toward the middle of the 20th century, the concept that the genetic makeup of the host may influence the outcome of infection became apparent, and in this respect malaria served as a prototype. All but a few infectious diseases are characterized clinically by variation in both disease pattern and severity, even in epidemic circumstances, indicating that host response has an important influence on the outcome of disease. A classic study highlighted the importance of host genetic makeup in our susceptibility to infection.[1] The cause-specific risk of dying in adopted children was compared, depending on whether their biologic (genetically related) or adoptive (environmentally related) parent died prematurely before the age of 50 years. The results were striking. The death of a biologic parent resulted in an increased relative risk of dying in the adoptee of 5.8 for infectious diseases, more than for cardiovascular disease (4.5) and much more than for cancers (1.2). The advent of molecular biology embracing the "new genetics" and major advances in our understanding of the structure and function of the immune system have provided tools for the more precise dissection of the role of genetic factors that influence the outcome of infection. One hypothesis is that infection may have been one of the major architects of genes coding for the immune response through generations of natural selection.

GENERAL CONCEPTS

It is rare for a simple Mendelian pattern of inheritance to be apparent when considering the genetic influence on infectious disease. An exception is malaria, in which the parasite's intraerythrocytic lifestyle is influenced by a variety of both red blood cell membrane and hemoglobin variants whose inheritance is relatively simple. As a consequence, malaria has been a very fruitful model for studies of host susceptibility to infectious disease. In most infectious diseases, however, the pattern of inheritance influencing susceptibility is not as clear and is assumed to be complex. Furthermore, the effects of host genes are modified both by environmental factors and by variation in the infecting organism. There are a number of genetic features and general concepts that apply to any consideration of the genetic basis of resistance (or susceptibility) to infection:

1. The traits involved are complex. It is often impossible to find a genetic marker that shows complete cosegregation with a complex trait. The reasons are well stated by Lander and Schork[2]:
    a. Incomplete penetrance and phenocopy: A mutant gene product may have a major influence, but its effect may be compensated for by other mechanisms. Alternatively, a given mutant may give rise to a phenotype that can also arise in the absence of that mutant (phenocopy).
    b. Genetic heterogeneity: Mutations in any one of several genes (e.g., in a biochemical pathway) may give rise to the same phenotype. A good example is given by deficiencies of the interacting complement factors C3, I, or H, which may predispose to infection with encapsulated bacteria.
    c. Polygenic inheritance: Some traits may require the simultaneous presence of variation in multiple genes. This is likely to be the case for most infectious diseases. As more genes influencing susceptibility are discovered, one of the major challenges will be to rank their order of importance.
    d. A high frequency of a disease-associated allele makes the attribution of risk and linkage analysis more difficult. For example, a number of studies have examined the relationship between HLA-DR2 and tuberculosis. The universal problem has been the high general frequency of this allele in the populations under study. Since the HLA-DR2 allele is present in approximately 40% of people in southern India, and in 60% of patients with tuberculosis,[3] a major effect may therefore be missed as a consequence of the difficulty in attributing risk.
2. The protection conferred may only be relative. The possession of red blood cells negative for the Duffy antigen, and the resistance it provides against vivax malaria, is one of the few examples in humans of absolute genetic protection against an infection.[4] In most other circumstances protection is relative. Although people with the sickle cell trait have up to 90% protection against malaria, they can undoubtedly become infected and die of falciparum malaria. Glucose-6-phosphate dehydrogenase (G6PD) deficiency may provide between 50% and 60% protection,

whereas people with α-thalassemia may have as small a margin of protection as 5%.[5] Thus, "protection" is rarely absolute and should only be discussed at the population, rather than the individual, level.

3. The heterozygous rather than homozygous state may confer protection. This is the classic concept of "hybrid vigor." A "double dose" of a protective gene may not be additive in the protection it provides and can even be deleterious. The best example of this phenomenon is in sickle cell carriers (AS), who have a reduced risk of dying of falciparum malaria, whereas the consequences of malaria in a patient with sickle cell disease (SS) may be disastrous.
4. Protection may be highly specific. Protection offered by a genetic trait may be specific on a number of counts. First, protection may exist not only for a disease, for example, malaria, but also for malaria caused by a specific species of parasite. Thus, sickle cell trait carriers are protected against falciparum malaria but not, as far as is known, against the other three *Plasmodium* species in man (i.e., *P. vivax, P. ovale,* and *P. malariae*). Second, protection may be specific for a particular clinical or pathologic form of the disease. An example of this is the class I major histocompatibility complex (MHC) antigen B53, which is associated with protection against both cerebral malaria and severe malarial anemia, whereas the class II haplotype, DRB1*1302, is only protective against anemia.[6] Alternatively, protection may apply to only a particular age group; for example, sickle cell trait carriers living in an endemic area for malaria are mainly protected between the ages of approximately 6 months and 5 years, at the time when passively acquired, antibody-mediated protection from the mother has waned and the individual has not as yet developed actively acquired immunity. Sickle cell trait may hasten the development of acquired immunity.
5. Genetic protection afforded against one disease may result in susceptibility to another. The existence of polymorphism implies that where an apparently deleterious allele persists in a state of balanced polymorphism within a population, there should be selective pressure in favor of that persistence, perhaps mediated by protection against a second disease. For example, homozygosity for a rare polymorphism at position -308 in the tumor necrosis factor-α (TNF-α) promoter region confers a 7.7 times increased risk of dying of cerebral malaria. The persistence of the rare allele in the population at a frequency of 16% implies that it confers protection against another, as yet unidentified infection or disease.[7]

ELEMENTS OF THE IMMUNE SYSTEM

Nonimmune Mechanisms

Molecular genetics has made extraordinary advances in the understanding of the genetic basis and potential treatment of a large number of inherited conditions, some of whose frequency in the tropics is unknown. One such condition is cystic fibrosis caused by a mutation in the chloride transporter cystic fibrosis transmembrane conductance regulator gene (*CFTR*) on chromosome 7.[8] The mutant *CFTR* with phenylalanine at position 508 resists the entry of both *Pseudomonas* and *Salmonella typhi* into epithelial cells.[9,10] Clinically, this gives rise to differing consequences: *Pseudomonas* is not internalized and thereby multiplies to high numbers in abnormally viscid secretions that cannot be cleared. In contrast, there is reason to suspect heterozygosity for the CFTR mutation may confer resistance to typhoid. Another example is the primary ciliary dyskinesias (PCD) including Kartagener's syndrome, in which an abnormality of ciliary action leads to a defect in epithelial clearance with consequent chronic lung infection, which may lead to bronchiectasis, necessitating lung transplantation. Progress in defining the genetic cause of these heterogenous defects has been made as mutations in intermediate-chain dynein (DNAI1; IC78) have been described in some PCD patients.[11]

Innate Immunity

Excepting the unique example of innate protection by red blood cell variants in malaria, the innate system consists of three major elements: serum factors, phagocytic cells, and natural killer (NK) cells. Complement is a proteolytic cascade system consisting of at least 24 serum proteins and 11 membrane-bound proteins. The majority of the complement components are present in the plasma as inactive precursors. Triggering of the complement cascade results in opsonization or lysis of infecting organisms. Chemotactic molecules such as C5a are generated and immune complexes are solubilized. Activation can occur via the binding of antigen-bound IgG or IgM to the first complement C1 (classical pathway). The alternative, antibody-independent pathway involves the activation of C4 and C2 by a plasma serine protease in complex with mannose-binding lectin (MBL), which in turn is bound to suitable carbohydrate ligands present on the surface of bacteria or viruses. The genes for many of the complement components have been identified and the effect of deficiency is listed in Table 6-1. Another line of defense includes lactoferrin, lysozyme, as well as the collectins and defensins. Activation of these molecules can lead directly to lysis of pathogens or to destruction through opsonization or the recruitment of inflammatory cells. The main function of phagocytes is to surround, ingest, and destroy organisms by the process of phagocytosis. Phagocytes, in the form of dendritic cells, also process and present antigens from microorganisms to lymphocytes. A third function of phagocytes is the production of soluble molecules, cytokines and chemokines, which orchestrate the inflammatory process. NK cells belong to a different lineage and can destroy virally infected, embryonic, or tumor cells. Major interest in how phagocytes recognize pathogens has been stimulated by the discovery of the Toll-like receptors (TLRs), whose differential engagement by pathogens can induce overlapping yet distinct patterns of gene expression that contribute to an inflammatory response.[12] In addition, antigen-presenting cells (APCs) employ other pattern recognition receptors, including complement receptor 3 (CR3), scavenger receptors, the mannose receptor, and various other C type lectins such as DC-SIGN.[13] These molecules appear conserved through evolution but the possibility that minor variation within these receptors contributes to susceptibility to infection has attracted attention.[14,15]

Table 6-1 Inherited Conditions Predisposing to Infectious Diseases and Their Genetic Basis

Syndrome	Clinical Features	Defect	Genetic Basis	References
Chronic granulomatous disease	Presents in the first years of life with severe recurrent bacterial and fungal infections	Failure of intracellular O_2^- production	X-linked or autosomal recessive with defects in NADPH oxidase subunits	123–125
X-linked immunodeficiency syndromes	Chronic sinopulmonary infection, chronic diarrhea, and hepatitis			
X-linked agammaglobulinemia	As above	Agammaglobulinemia	Mostly due to mutation in Bruton's tyrosine kinase gene	126
Common variable immunodeficiency	As above		Probable multiple; occasional adult-onset cases homozygous for mutations in ICOS	127, 128
Hyper-IgM syndrome	As above	Lack of IgG, IgA, and IgE	Mutation in CD154 (CD40 ligand)	129
Wiskott–Aldrich syndrome	Eczema, thrombocytopenia, recurrent infections, autoimmune disorders, IgA nephropathy	Mutations in the Wiskott–Aldrich protein, a regulator of platelet and lymphocyte function		130–132
Severe combined immunodeficiency	Severe and persistent infection from early life	Decreased T cells and abnormal thymic differentiation	Mutations in IL-2Rγ, Jak3, IL-7Rα, RAG1, RAG2, Artemis, CD3δ, adenosine deaminase, and CD45	133
C1	SLE-like illness and increased susceptibility to infection	Lack of expression of C1q, C1r, or C1s		134, 135
C3	Increased susceptibility to encapsulated bacteria			136
Factors I and H	As above	Both are cofactors for C3; deficiency therefore gives rise to the same susceptibility		137
C4	Bacterial meningitis	Failure of C4B expression		138
Properdin	Meningococcal disease	X-linked		139
C5–C9	Meningococcal disease			140
Mannose-binding lectins (MBLs)	Unusual and recurrent infection; carriage of hepatitis B	Mutation in codon 52 or 54 of exon 1 of the MBL gene		89, 91, 141

Acquired Immunity

The predominant effector and regulatory cell in the acquired response is the lymphocyte. B lymphocytes produce antibody that attaches to foreign organisms, facilitating their destruction by a number of mechanisms. Their response is regulated by regulatory T cells, mainly CD4+. In addition, cytotoxic T cells, mainly CD8+, can be effector cells that kill infected cells. All T lymphocytes recognize foreign antigen presented by an APC via major histocompatibility complex (MHC) class I and class II molecules. Classical antigen-presentation studies showed that MHC class I molecules present peptides derived from proteins synthesized within the cell, whereas MHC class II molecules present exogenous proteins captured from the environment. Evidence indicates, however, that dendritic cells have a specialized capacity to process exogenous antigens into the MHC class I pathway. This function, known as cross-presentation, provides the immune system with additional flexibility to generate immunity to viruses and tolerance to self.[16]

One of the features of the genes of the MHC region is the high degree of polymorphism. The class I genes encode the antigen-presenting molecules HLA-A, -B, and -C and the class II region genes HLA-DR, -DQ, and -DP. Both regions are located on the short arm of chromosome 6. In between the class I and II regions is the class III region, which encodes a number of genes also involved in the immune response, such as the genes for the complement factors C2 and C4 and factor B and that for the cytokine TNF-α. There is evidence to support the hypothesis that natural selection acts to maintain MHC polymorphism for several reasons. First, unusual allelic frequency distributions occur at MHC loci. Second, the patterns of nucleotide substitution show an enhanced rate of nonsynonymous (amino acid-altering) substitution in the codons encoding the peptide-binding region of the molecules. Third, polymorphisms at certain MHC loci are very long lasting. Fourth, introns at MHC loci are homogenized by recombination and subsequent genetic drift.[17] There is a considerable body of evidence to support the idea that infectious diseases are the main selection force maintaining MHC diversity.[18]

Cytokines

Cytokines, produced by many immune cells, act as soluble effector and regulatory molecules. A very large number of molecules have been described and the literature abounds with studies of association between elevation or depression of a given cytokine and disease. The fact that most cytokine genes are polymorphic has resulted in a large number of studies relating such polymorphism to susceptibility or resistance to various infections (see Table 6-4). In fact, there is considerable redundancy within the cytokine network, with circuits of cytokines acting in tandem to regulate inflammatory processes, and so studies of single cytokines can be poorly informative. Variation with cytokine genes is clearly of most interest when polymorphism is shown to have potential functional correlates, as is the case for the molecules of the MHC.[19]

TECHNIQUES OF GENETIC DISSECTION

It is usual to plan DNA-based dissection of the host response to infection on knowledge of the inheritance of a trait from studies of genetic epidemiology. For example, the association of a particular genotype or phenotype with geographic areas that are, or have been, epidemic for a particular disease strongly suggests a genetic component. A good example is thalassemia, a condition largely found in the tropics but also in Mediterranean countries (e.g., Italy and Cyprus) that have until the mid-20th century been endemic for malaria. One of the earliest such "micromapping" studies carried out was on the island of Sardinia, where a decrease in the frequency of thalassemia and G6PD deficiency coincided with increasing altitude, and malarial transmission was also reduced.[20] Reciprocally, a high frequency of allelic variants conferring susceptibility rather than resistance may be expected to be found in areas that until recently have not been exposed to a specific pathogen.

Association Studies

In case–control studies, people with and without a particular genotype are compared with respect to a number of variables, such as whether they are infected or not, have a higher or lower parasite load, suffer a particular form of the disease, or die or not. An early example of such a study is that of Allison,[21] who determined that normal (AA) controls were more likely to have parasitemia with *Plasmodium falciparum* than people with sickle cell trait (AS). Unfortunately, case–control studies are most susceptible to errors in study design, the most frequent of which is inadequate power (i.e., insufficient numbers). Another pitfall lies in the choice of the control group. For example, regarding malaria, members of a control group of mild asymptomatic cases recruited during the period of a study may, during subsequent infection, develop severe disease. The incidence of some infectious diseases may be related to age and sex and so it is important in these cases to match controls appropriately for age and sex. A third problem is that although association studies can be performed for any DNA polymorphism, they are most meaningful when applied to functionally significant variations in genes that have a clear biologic relation to the trait. Thus, red blood cells containing hemoglobin S reduce parasite growth and multiplication possibly because of leakage of potassium, induction of early sickling, or premature removal of infected red blood cells.[22] Case–control studies are also affected by population admixture. Thus, if a study incorporates a population that is a mix of ancestrally distinct populations that have differing allele frequencies and disease prevalence, false-negative or -positive results may arise. For the previous reasons, findings are often not replicated between studies, and confidence in an association increases if it can be reproduced widely.

A total of 1.42 million single nucleotide polymorphisms (SNPs) exist in the human genome.[23] As high throughput typing techniques develop, there is increased power to detect both spurious and meaningful associations. Statistical handling of large amounts of data will need to be rigorous. Analysis may also better reflect the underlying biological significance of variation. One nascent area is the testing of haplotypes across genes, rather than isolated SNPs within them, for association with infectious disease.[24] Another interesting approach is to relate not the frequency of a single polymorphism within a gene to disease susceptibility but the overall frequency of all polymorphisms within a gene to susceptibility.[14]

Allele-Sharing Methods

A common method compares the observed and expected distributions of the number of alleles between siblings (sib pair analysis). Siblings can share none, one, or two alleles, with an expected proportion of 1:2:1 in the absence of linkage. Increased sharing of an allele would indicate selection. Such an approach has been successfully used in type 1 diabetes. It is a suitable method for microsatellite-based or SNP-based genome mapping and is increasingly applied to a number of common infectious diseases in humans. The results of such studies are then related to the completed human genome and databases of known polymorphisms to identify candidate genes. Further DNA sequencing may be necessary to detect previously undetected polymorphisms.

Linkage Analysis

Gene loci are said to be linked if their alleles do not show independent segregation, implying that the linkage may have some selective advantage. Linkage analysis provides the methodology to quantitate this phenomenon. The application of this method to complex traits is problematic because it necessitates precise modeling. Nevertheless, it has been used in an instance in which simple Mendelian inheritance was suspected. The discovery and cloning of SLC11A1 (formerly referred to as Nramp-1), the product of the *Bcg/Ity/Lsh* locus on chromosome 1 in the mouse and associated with susceptibility to experimental Bacille Calmette–Guérin infection, leishmaniasis, and salmonellosis, created excitement in the field of host genetics and susceptibility to infection.[25–27] The human SLC11A1 is on chromosome 2 but two whole genome-based analyses have not linked SLC11A1 to tuberculosis.[28,29] The fact that some, although not all, association studies have related polymorphism in SLC11A1 to tuberculosis may reflect the greater power of association studies to detect relatively small effects.[30–33] The transmission disequilibrium test (TDT) tests for both linkage and association in families. Although developed to test for linkage in the presence of association, it is increasingly applied to test for association in the presence of linkage. The TDT tests for distortion in transmission of alleles from a heterozygous parent to an affected offspring. A variant that requires a greater study size is the sibTDT, in which unaffected siblings replace the parents. An elegant example of the use of an association study

Table 6-2 Novel Genetic Immunodeficiency Syndromes That Predispose to Intracellular Infection

Molecule	Phenotype	Mutation	References
IFN-γ receptor I	Severe atypical mycobacterial infection	Point mutation at nucleotide 395 that introduces a stop codon	116
IFN-γ receptor II	*M. fortuitum* and *avium* infection	Homozygous dinucleotide deletion at nucleotides 278 and 279, resulting in a premature stop codon	142
IL-12p40	BCG and *Salmonella enteritidis* infection	Large homozygous deletion	143
IL-12β1 receptor subunit	Severe mycobacterial and salmonella infections	A variety of missense and deletion mutations	143, 144
Stat-1	Disseminated BCG or *M. avium* infection	Point mutation at nucleotide position 2116	145

confirmed by an independent TDT analysis relates a SNP at position +874 in the interferon-γ (IFN-γ) gene to susceptibility to tuberculosis in the Cape colored population in South Africa.[34]

INHERITED CONDITIONS PREDISPOSING TO INFECTIOUS DISEASE

A number of well-characterized genetic defects that predispose to infection have been characterized at the molecular level (see Table 6-1). In general, these predispose to severe sepsis and the mutations responsible are so deleterious that they do not persist in populations at other than a minute frequency. The occurrence of such diseases in the tropics is not well documented; thus, their inclusion in a textbook of tropical medicine may be questionable. However, in the past few years major advances in our understanding of immunity to common intracellular pathogens has derived from the analysis of very small numbers of patients (often children) with severe recurrent atypical mycobacterial or *Salmonella* infections. Such individuals have been shown to have mutations in the IL-12- and IFN-γ-driven type 1 cytokine pathway (Table 6-2). This knowledge has prompted the search for less deleterious variants in these genes that may predispose to intracellular infections within populations.[34,35] Thus, a remarkable link exists between the molecular analysis of rare severe childhood infections in developed countries, understanding immunity, and defining genes within which variation may predispose to common infections in the tropics.

STUDIES ON THE GENETIC INFLUENCE OF INFECTIOUS DISEASE IN HUMANS

Table 6-3 shows some HLA associations with infectious disease in humans. Table 6-4 shows non-MHC and class III MHC genes with allelic variants that have been associated with infectious disease. This is intended to be illustrative of

Table 6-3 Summary of Some Reported Associations Between Major Histocompatibility Complex Alleles and Infectious Diseases

Disease	Effect	Allele(s)	Population	References
Protection				
HIV	Reduced progression	DQB1*0302, DRB1*0401	US, hemophiliacs	146
	Diminution in maternally transmitted virus	DRB1*1501 DRB1*1300	Whites, US Black and Hispanic, US	147
	Resistance to infection	A*0205	US, MSM	50
Hepatitis B	Transient infection	DRB1*1302	Multiple	91–93
Dengue shock syndrome	Reduced severity	B13	Thailand	148
Hepatitis C	Reduced severity	DR5	Multiple	71, 94–96
Tuberculosis	Protective	A1 supertype	India	66
Typhoid	Protective	TNFA*2 [308].DRBI*0301 haplotype	Vietnam	149
Falciparum malaria	Reduced severity of cerebral disease and of anemia	B53	Gambia	6
	Reduced anemia	DRB1*1302-DQB1*0501	Gambia	6
Leishmaniasis	Mucosal disease	DR2		150
Filariasis	Reduced elephantiasis	DR3	Indonesia	81
Onchocerciasis	Localized disease	DQB1*0500	West Africa	82
Increased susceptibility				
Dengue shock syndrome	Increased severity	A2	Thailand	148
HIV	More rapid CD4 decline	DQB1*0501–DRB1*0101	US, hemophiliacs	146
	Increased progression to AIDS	DQB1*0603–DRB1*1300, DQB1*0301, DRB1*1400	US, hemophiliacs	146
	More rapid CD4 decline	A1-B8-DR3	US, Scotland	48, 49

Continued

Table 6-3 Summary of Some Reported Associations between Major Histocompatibility Complex Alleles and Infectious Diseases—Cont'd

Disease	Effect	Allele(s)	Population	References
Tuberculosis	Increased severity of pulmonary disease	DR2	Multiple	3, 61–64
	Susceptibility and severity	A3 supertype	India	66
Typhoid	Increased susceptibility	TNFα*1 [-308].DRB1*04 extended haplotype	Vietnam	149
Leprosy	Tuberculoid disease	DRB1*1502	India	84, 85
	Lepromatous disease	DRB1*1501	India	84, 85
Lyme disease	Chronic course	DR2, DR4	US	151, 152
	All forms	A2, C3	Germany	153
Schistosomiasis	Hepatosplenomegaly	B5, B44, DQB1*0201	Multiple	77–80, 154
Filariasis	Elephantiasis	B27, DQ5		81

MSM, men having sex with men.

the types of relationship that have been described rather than being comprehensive. Some of the associations for individual diseases are discussed in more detail in the following sections.

Malaria

Genetic resistance to malarial infection has, of all infections, been best characterized, largely because polymorphisms of the red blood cell membrane and the red blood cell's contents are easily recognized by relatively simple laboratory methods, such as blood group typing, enzyme assays, and hemoglobin electrophoresis (Table 6-5).[4,36] In 1949, J. B. S. Haldane introduced the concept of "balanced polymorphism," whereby carriers of a recessive trait, for example, thalassemia, may be at a selective advantage of surviving severe falciparum malaria compared to both normal people and those with severe thalassemia.[37] This so-called "malaria hypothesis" predicted that the frequency of thalassemia carriers would increase until offset by the resultant increase in the number of severely affected people in the population who would die prematurely, thus achieving a state of balanced polymorphism. α-Thalassemia is usually caused by the deletion of one of the linked pair of α-globin genes. The normal genotype is αα/αα; heterozygotes (αα/α–) are clinically normal, and homozygotes (α–/α–) have a mild anemia. There is good evidence that thalassemia is maintained in Melanesia as a consequence of natural selection by, and protection from, malaria.[5] This may be a result of altered plasmodial surface antigen expression in thalassemic cells.[38] It was thus somewhat surprising that in Espiritu Santo (one of the islands of Vanuatu), the incidence of both the less severe vivax and falciparum

Table 6-4 Non-MHC and Class III MHC Genes with Allele-Specific Associations with Infection

Gene	Allele	Effect	References
Cytokines and Chemokines			
TNF-α	TNFA*2[-308]	Increased severity of falciparum malaria, meningococcal disease, and mucocutaneous leishmaniasis	116, 155, 156
IL-1 complex	IL-1Ra A2-ve/IL-1β+3953) A1 +ve	Increased DTH and pleural tuberculosis	19
IL-8	Haplotype 2	Increased susceptibility to RSV infection	24
IL-10	ATA haplotype	Spontaneous clearance or more rapid fibrosis	99, 100
RANTES	In1.1C allele	Accelerated progression of HIV	57
SDF-1	3′ A/3′ A	Delayed or accelerated progression of HIV	55, 56
Interferon-γ	+874 SNP	Increased susceptibility to tuberculosis	34
Receptors			
CCR2	641 allele	Slower progression of HIV	53
CXP5	32-bp deletion	Slower progression of HIV	52–54
	CCR5P1 haplotype	Rapid progression of HIV	55
IL-12 receptor β1	R214-T365-R378 allele (2)	Increased susceptibility to tuberculosis	35
Vitamin D receptor	VDR tt and ff genotypes	Resistance to tuberculosis and hepatitis B	29, 71
TLR4	Multiple	Increased susceptibility to meningococcal disease	14
TLR5	392 stop codon	Increased susceptibility to Legionnaires' disease	15
Various			
SLC11A1	Various	Susceptibility to tuberculosis	31–33
Haptoglobin	2-2	Increased severity of pulmonary tuberculosis	63, 69, 70
Mannan binding lectin (MBL)	Codon 52, 54, and 57 variants	Increased risk of meningococcal disease and pneumococcal disease; decreased risk of tuberculous meningitis	106, 141

Table 6-5 Red Cell Variants Believed to Provide Protection Against Malaria

Variant	Distribution	Postulated Mechanism	References
Hemoglobinopathies			
Hb S	Sub-Saharan Africa, Indian subcontinent	Premature removal of infected cells, reduced multiplication, induced sickling	22
Hb C	West Africa	Impairment of merozoite release	157
Hb E	Southeast Asia	Increased phagocytosis	158
Hb F	Global	Sensitivity to oxidant stress	159
α-Thalassemia	Global in malaria endemic areas	Increased IgG binding, sensitivity to oxidant stress	5, 38
β-Thalassemia	Mediterranean, Southeast Asia, West Africa	Increased IgG binding, sensitivity to oxidant stress	160
Red cell enzymes			
Glucose-6-phosphate dehydrogenase (G6PD) deficiency	Worldwide	Sensitivity to oxidant stress	40
Pyridoxal kinase	Sporadic	Unknown	161
Red cell membrane			
Melanesian (band III) Ovalocytosis	Melanesia	Reduced invasion	162
Duffy antigen negativity	West Africa mainly; also East Africa	*Plasmodium vivax* only, failure of invasion	163
Blood group O	Worldwide	Poor rosette formation	164
Glycophorin B deficiency	West Africa	Decreased invasion	165

malaria in homozygous thalassemic children aged 0 to 4 years was approximately twice as high as in αα/αα children.[39] The incidence of the rarely severe vivax malaria was particularly high in thalassemia homozygotes younger than 30 months old. The authors postulated that infection by vivax malaria at this age, perhaps because thalassemia is characterized by a mild increase in the number of immature red blood cells (reticulocytes), which are the preferred red blood cell habitat of *P. vivax*, may result in cross-reactive immunity to the lethal effects of *P. falciparum*. Another possibility is that the *P. falciparum* strains present on the island studied may be less virulent, because it is certainly the case that severe falciparum malaria on this island is much less frequent than elsewhere in the world.[39] In another case–control study, the protection of both G6PD-deficient hemizygotes (males) and heterozygote females against falciparum malaria, in both west and east Africa, was demonstrated, resolving an age-old debate on the importance of this genotype in the face of severe falciparum malaria.[40]

Protection against two life-threatening manifestations of malaria, cerebral disease and anemia, is associated in The Gambia with the class I antigen HLA-B53. Protection against anemia only was conferred by the class II extended haplotype DRB1*1302-DQB1*0501.[6] Because HLA-B53 is rare in populations not exposed to malaria, it was proposed that the frequency in The Gambian population studied was due to natural selection. Because red blood cells do not express class I molecules, the site of cytotoxicity is presumably the infected liver cell. Cytotoxic cells do contribute to antimalarial immunity and it was possible to show that a nonamer peptide eluted from the HLA-B53 molecule was able to induce such responses in people exposed to malaria.[41] However, it has been known for more than 30 years that malarial parasites undergo antigenic variation, which can be provoked by the host immune response.[42,43] *Plasmodium falciparum* has no known animal reservoir and thus it is pertinent to bear in mind that the human immune response is conversely almost certainly a powerful selective force on the parasite. Integrated analysis of host and parasite variation is complex but almost certainly will offer powerful future insights.[44] The cytokine TNF-α is encoded by a gene within the MHC class III region on the short arm of chromosome 6 and transcription is under the control of a promoter that lies 5′ to the structural gene. TNF-α, especially when produced in excess, is implicated in the pathogenesis of a number of severe infections, including gram-negative sepsis, tuberculosis, human immunodeficiency virus (HIV) infection, and malaria. Homozygosity for a polymorphism in the promoter region, involving a guanine-for-adenine substitution at position -308 relative to the start codon, is associated with a 7.7 times increased risk of death from cerebral malaria.[7] The functional significance of this polymorphism, however, is controversial. Although it has been shown that people both homozygous and heterozygous for this polymorphism produce significantly more TNF-α in response to lipopolysaccharide (LPS) in vitro,[45] paradoxically two studies of the effect of this polymorphism on transcription showed no effect.[46,47] Recently, a number of non-MHC and class III MHC genes with allele-specific associations with malaria have been described and more examples of these will no doubt follow (Table 6-6). Some of these genetic variants have shown protection against severe disease and others increased susceptibility that may vary, for instance, with the malarial disease phenotype or the population studied, and they would fail to recognize an advantage in the face of some other as yet unidentified selection pressure.

Human Immunodeficiency Virus

There is variability in the natural history of HIV infection. Three categories of infected people have attracted attention: those who progress rapidly, long-term nonprogressers (LTNP),

Table 6-6 Examples of Non-MHC and Class III MHC Genes with Allele-Specific Associations with Malaria

Gene	Variant	Effect	Population	References
Protection				
CR-1	CR1 deficient	Severe disease	Papua New Guinea	166
Fcgamma receptor IIa (CD32)	R131 allele, rather than the RR131 genotype	Severe disease	Children in The Gambia	167
Cd36 gene	Heterozygosity for a non-sense mutation	Severe disease	Kenyan children	168
Intercellular adhesion molecule-1 (ICAM)	ICAM-1Kilifi (change from Lys to Met in the loop that interacts with parasitized red blood cells)	Severe disease	Children in Gabon	169
CD40 ligand (CD40L)	Males hemizygous for the CD40 L-726C (not significant in females)	Severe disease	The Gambia	170
Nitric oxide synthase 2 gene (*NOS2*)	NOS2 (Lambarene) (NOS2-G954C)	Severe and mild disease	Gabon	171
Increased susceptibility				
TNF-α	TNFA*2 [-308].	Increased severity of cerebral malaria	Children in The Gambia	156
TNF-α	TNF-238 A	Increased risk of severe malarial anemia	Children in The Gambia	172
TNF (promoter region)	OCT-1-binding genotype	Increased susceptibility to cerebral malaria	Children in The Gambia	173
Fcgamma receptor IIa (CD32)	HH131 genotype	Severe disease	Children in The Gambia	167
Inducible nitric oxide synthase promoter	Longer forms of CCTTT microsatellite repeat	Severe disease	Adults in Thailand	174
Haptoglobin	Hp1-1	Severe disease	Children in Ghana	175
No effect				
Complement receptor 1 (CD35)	Gene underlying the Knops antithetical antigens S11/S12 and McC(a)/McC(b)	No association	Children in The Gambia	176

and people who are very likely to have been exposed but who do not seroconvert. Initial interest centered on the MHC with reports that rapid progression is associated with the HLA-A1-B8-DR3 extended haplotype.[48,49] It has been reported that the HLA A*0205 is associated with resistance against infection,[50] an observation that fits with a number of reports that ascribe protection against HIV infection to antiviral CD8+ T cells.[51]

The phenomenon of heavily exposed but persistently uninfected people also came to prominence when the coreceptors for HIV infection were described in the mid-1990s. For T-tropic viruses the coreceptor is CXCR-4, and CCR-5 is the coreceptor for M-tropic viral strains. A defective CCR-5 allele, which contains a 32-base pair deletion, prevents expression of CCR-5 at the cell surface. Homozygotes for this mutation are resistant to HIV infection, and infected heterozygotes have slower disease progression, a finding that has been widely reproduced.[52–54] Attendant on the discovery of CXCR-4 and CCR5 as the coreceptors for HIV, a large number of studies have also examined genetic variants in both the chemokine ligands and receptors on susceptibility and the progression of HIV. Thus, a multisite haplotype of the CCR5 regulatory region containing a promoter allele, CCR5P1, that increases CCR5 expression is associated with rapid progression to AIDS, particularly in the early years after infection.[55] HIV-1-infected individuals carrying the CCR2-64I allele progressed to AIDS 2 to 4 years later than individuals homozygous for the common allele.[53] Varying findings, however, have been made with respect to the ligands. For example, a common polymorphism SDF1-3′A exists in the 3′ untranslated region of the stromal-derived factor 1 gene, a ligand of CXCR-4. In the homozygous state, SDF1-3′A/3′A is reported to delay or accelerate the onset of AIDS.[55,56] Similar complexity is revealed by the finding that the downregulating RANTES In1.1C allele, which is in linkage disequilibrium in African Americans with a weaker upregulating RANTES promoter allele (-28G), associates with rapid progression.[57] However, the -28G promoter allele was not associated with rapid progression in a European cohort.[58]

Tuberculosis

Environmental factors are clearly predominant in the development of tuberculosis, so it may be concluded that the role of genetic susceptibility may not be great. However, there are several lines of evidence to suggest that host genes contribute to outcome. There is moderate disease disconcordance between dizygotic and monozygotic twins.[59,60] The relationship between the human SLC11A1 gene and tuberculosis has already been discussed. In addition, an association between pulmonary disease and HLA-DR2 has consistently been reported.[3,61–64] The two largest studies that typed class I alleles failed to detect any association,[62,65] although one study has reported increased frequencies of A3-like supertypes and decreased frequencies of A1-like supertypes in tuberculosis patients.[66]

Two whole genome scans have detected moderate (LOD scores <3) linkage of tuberculosis to different chromosomal regions. In Africa, linkage was found to chromosomes 15q and Xq and in Brazil to chromosome 17q11.2.[28,29] Chromosome 17q11.2 has some interesting candidates, including a number of chemokine genes and the inducible NO synthase gene (*NOS2*). The link to chromosome Xq is also interesting because a male excess of tuberculosis is reported in many populations. Fine mapping has the potential to refine these linkages.[67] However, the lack of a clear major locus for tuberculosis in these studies raises the possibility that most of the genetic component of susceptibility to tuberculosis is dispersed among many loci.[68]

Of the non-MHC genes, there is a substantial body of non-English literature relating haptoglobin 2-2 to the severity of pulmonary tuberculosis, an association that has been reproduced in Africa.[63,69,70] The basis for this is unknown. Homozygotes for a noncoding polymorphism at codon 352 (genotype tt) of the vitamin D receptor gene were significantly underrepresented among Gambians with tuberculosis, an association that was supported by analysis of a separate population of Asians in West London.[29,71] The study from London made a rare attempt to analyze gene–environment interaction by concurrent determination of serum vitamin D levels. Acquired deficiency of vitamin D was far more powerfully associated with tuberculosis than genetic variation in its receptor. Both studies are biologically plausible because 1,25-dihydroxyvitamin D_3 is reported to decrease the intramacrophage growth of *Mycobacterium tuberculosis*.[72]

Research on genetic susceptibility to tuberculosis presents typical, and some exceptional, difficulties with respect to phenotyping. Thus, the determination of susceptibility to develop tuberculosis may best be addressed in children, who are highly susceptible to progression to primary disease. However, culture confirmation of active disease in children is rare and few studies have therefore addressed this with confidence. Because most tuberculosis infection in adults is latent, the phenotyping of control subjects for association studies also presents difficulties. Should controls be tuberculin skin test positive and thus likely to be infected and assumed resistant, or should they be negative? Few, if any, studies have addressed this in detail. The clinical manifestations of reactivation (the most common disease pattern of adults) are quite varied. One possibility is that polymorphic genes affect disease pattern, and some studies have suggested evidence of this.[19,29,73]

Helminthic Infections

An exhaustive and scholarly review of human genetic susceptibility to helminth infection has been published.[74] Two features of helminth infections have attracted genetic study. The first is that, within populations, helminths tend to be overdistributed (i.e., a few people harbor high parasite burdens). Notwithstanding the environmental, behavioral, and parasitic factors that contribute to this feature, there is evidence that the intensity of helminth infection is partially under genetic control. The second feature is that sequelae, particularly of invasive helminth infection, arise because of immunopathology. Thus, fibrosis in schistosomiasis or the dichotomy between microfilaremia or hypersensitivity in filarial infection may have genetic correlates. In particular, a great deal of attention has been paid to the possibility that variants of genes that predispose to atopy protect against helminths. Unfortunately, this exercise has generated as much hot air as hard data.

In contrast, two whole genome-based linkage analyses have productively related the intensity of helminth infection to specific chromosomal regions. In a landmark study of a quantitative trait, microsatellite mapping of 11 informative families in Brazil indicated that the control of intensity of *Schistosoma mansoni* infection mapped to a single region of chromosome 5, most closely to the colony-stimulating factor receptor 1 gene (*CSF1R*) but also to a region containing the genes for the important type 2 cytokines IL-4, -5, and -13.[75] Also, the intensity of *Ascaris* infection was linked to genes on chromosomes 1 and 13, with the most plausible candidate being the B lymphocyte stimulator protein (BlyS).[76]

Hepatosplenic schistosomiasis is believed to be largely due to the immune response to egg antigens, and there have been a number of studies on the role of HLA. Studies from Egypt and a single study from South America have consistently related HLA-B5 to hepatosplenomegaly in *S. mansoni* infection.[77,78] Studies of *Schistosoma japonicum* infection tend to be small, yielding multiple HLA associations, although in the largest of these HLA-B44 was a risk factor for the development of hepatosplenic disease.[79] In a more recent molecular analysis restricted to class II alleles, it was reported that hepatosplenic disease is associated with DQB1*0201.[80]

Lymphatic filariasis caused by *Wuchereria bancrofti* and *Brugia malayi* is characterized by a spectrum of manifestations from asymptomatic microfilaremia to deforming elephantiasis. Tissue damage in elephantiasis is suspected to be immune mediated. In a study of patients with filariasis, the frequency of HLA-B27 and -DQ5 was increased and that of HLA-DR3 decreased in patients with elephantiasis compared to other patients older than age 45.[81] DQB1*0501 has also been associated with patients with localized, as opposed to generalized, onchocerciasis.[82]

Other Diseases

Leprosy

The polar spectrum of clinical leprosy offers an opportunity to investigate the effect of genetic factors on disease expression, but most effort has been directed toward determining susceptibility. An early application of transmission disequilibrium testing suggested linkage of susceptibility to the MHC locus on chromosome 6.[83] At least five studies have indicated an association between leprosy and HLA-DR2, which is strongest for tuberculoid disease. In two studies from India in which molecular typing methods were used, it appears that tuberculoid leprosy associates with DRB1*1502 and lepromatous disease with DRB1*1501.[84,85] However, others concluded that susceptibility to leprosy per se is probably not controlled by HLA-linked genes.[86]

Remarkably, three whole genome scans for leprosy susceptibility in different populations have been reported with entirely different results. The first to be published was a study of the genomes of 224 families from South India containing 245 independent affected sibpairs, mainly with paucibacillary leprosy.

Linkage was found to multiple markers on chromosome 10p13.[87] A later study in Vietnam reported linkage to chromosome 6 but not the MHC, specifically to 17 markers located in a block of approximately 80 kilobases overlapping the 5′ regulatory region shared by the Parkinson's disease gene *PARK2* and the coregulated gene *PACRG*.[88] The same study reproduced the association in a large case–control analysis in Brazil. Also in Brazil, weaker linkage of leprosy to markers on chromosome 17q has been reported.[28] The decaying genome of the leprosy bacillus appears to contain close to the minimum set of genes necessary for mycobacterial survival and thus does not have much scope to vary between populations.[68] How these disparate whole genome scan results will be reconciled remains to be seen.

Hepatitis B and C

A considerable number of studies have been conducted on this subject and on susceptibility to develop hepatocellular carcinoma, which is associated with these infections. In addition, a number of small-scale studies have attempted to associate the response to antiviral therapy with genetic factors. Mutations in codons 52, 54, or 57 in exon 1 of the MBL gene reduces serum MBL levels and may be associated with an opsonic defect. An early analysis showed that a mutation in codon 52 is more common in white, but not Asian, patients with chronic hepatitis B virus (HBV) infection. However, the codon 54 mutation, which in the same study was associated with a greater depression of serum MBL, was not associated with disease.[89] Subsequent studies were not able to associate MBL mutations with hepatitis B.[32,90] An early study associated HLA-DRB1*1302 with transient HBV infection in Gambian adults and children.[91] This association has been replicated in other populations, although a greater protective effect of HLA A*03 was reported for Caucasians.[92,93]

Several studies have reported an association of the HLA DQB1*0301-DRB1*11 extended haplotype with self-limiting HCV infection.[71,94–96] Interestingly, this haplotype is associated with the maintenance of a multispecific CD4+ T helper response to HCV that persists during and after therapy.[97] There is also a trend toward less severe disease with DRB1*11 alleles. Studies of extrahepatic manifestations of chronic HCV have shown an association between DQB1*11 and DRB1*03 with the formation of cryoglobulins.[98] A number of cytokine gene polymorphisms have been studied in the context of HCV infection with variable results. For example, the IL-10 ATA haplotype was reported as more frequent in patients with spontaneous HCV RNA clearance, whereas in another study this haplotype was more frequent among patients with rapid fibrosis.[99,100]

Meningococcal Disease

Most individuals acquiring new strains of meningococci, despite lacking specific antibody for several weeks, do not develop invasive disease following nasopharyngeal acquisition of new strains of meningococci.[101] This suggests that innate immune mechanisms are effective in containing the organism. Host molecules relevant to innate immunity to meningococci include plasma proteins such as complement, mannose-binding lectin, and C-reactive protein, as well as the extensive range of pattern recognition receptors on cell surfaces, such as the TLRs, CD14, and mannose receptors.

Deficiency in terminal components of the complement pathway and properdin with recurrent meningococcal disease are well recognized[102–104] and are shown in Table 6-1. Individuals possessing functional variants in the gene for mannose-binding lectin[105] that lead to reduced plasma concentrations of the protein have increased susceptibility to meningococcal disease.[106]

The host innate immune response to invading microorganisms is triggered following recognition of common structural motifs present on bacteria and viruses through a range of pattern recognition receptors.[107–109] Endotoxin [lipopolysaccharide (LPS)] is able to trigger innate immune responses following recognition by a number of host proteins and surface receptors, including the family of TLRs and the CD14 molecule.[109,110] The importance of TLRs in containing gram-negative organisms was first identified in mice with mutations in the LPS locus.[111] LPS receptor-deficient mice (homologous to TLR-4 deficiency in humans) are unable to respond to bacterial endotoxin and show enhanced susceptibility to infection with *Salmonella*, *Neisseria*, *Escherichia coli*, and other gram-negative organisms.[110–112] An excess of rare TLR-4 coding changes was found in patients with meningococcal disease compared to controls utilizing complete sequencing of the TLR-4 gene ($p = 2 \times 10^{-6}$; odds ratio, 27).[14] This study suggests a critical role for endotoxin sensing in containment of meningococcal disease. TLR-4 is only one of a large number of proteins involved in the detection of endotoxin and other bacterial structures; these include at least nine other proteins in the family of TLRs, CD14, and the accessory proteins including MYD88, MD2, as well as the downstream regulators of cellular activation.[14,109–113] Some or all of these may contribute to the recognition of gram-negative organisms and the activation of defensive host inflammatory responses.

An extensive body of evidence suggests that patients with fulminant and fatal meningococcal disease have an excessive and uncontrolled inflammatory response often under genetic control, with activation involving both cellular and noncellular inflammatory pathways.[114,115] Following the initial report that heterozygosity for the -308 promoter polymorphism in the TNF gene was associated with an increased (2.5 times) risk of death in meningococcal disease,[116] an association between outcome of meningococcal disease and other polymorphisms in the IL-10 and IL-1 pathway has also been reported.[117,118]

Purpura fulminans is the most dramatic complication of meningococcal sepsis, leading to peripheral gangrene and often requiring amputation of limbs and digits. Predisposition to purpura fulminans may also have a genetic basis. A functional polymorphism in the plasminogen activator inhibitor gene is associated with meningococcal outcome.[119] The same applies to the factor V Leiden gene.[120] Patients possessing the 4G allele within the *PAI-1* promoter gene produce higher levels of plasminogen activator inhibitor but are at increased risk of death, confirmed in a much larger subsequent study.[121] These genetic differences in the key regulators of the antithrombotic and thrombolytic pathways likely explain the occurrence of purpura fulminans associated with meningococcal disease.

CLINICAL RELEVANCE

For most practitioners of tropical medicine, the association of disease with genetic polymorphisms may appear attractive intellectually but of very little clinical relevance. We are only on the fringe of discovery of genetic factors influencing host resistance or susceptibility to infection. However, at this relatively early stage, some of the following observations, particularly relating to malaria, have immediate clinical implications and others have more importance for the future:

- Nonimmune carriers of the hemoglobinopathies remain at risk of acquiring malaria. The protection offered by "protective traits" is only relative, and in any case applies only at the population level. Advice to these individuals with regard to antimosquito measures and other precautions to avoid malaria is in no way different from advice to normal people. Patients with sickle cell disease rather than sickle cell trait are at particular risk if they acquire severe malaria.
- People with G6PD deficiency need to avoid a number of potentially harmful oxidant drugs. Primaquine, used in the eradication of the exoerythrocytic forms of vivax and ovale malaria, is one example of a relatively potent oxidant drug that can induce severe hemolysis in a G6PD-deficient person. Chloroquine, on the other hand, is a relatively weak oxidant and only needs to be avoided in severe G6PD deficiency or in people who have had hemolysis in response to the drug in the past. This is one of the best examples of the new area of "pharmacogenetics."
- Errors in determining drug sensitivity of malarial parasites: Parasites cultured in hemoglobin S (Hb S)-containing red blood cells may erroneously appear to be chloroquine resistant. The same parasites, if grown in cells containing Hb A, appear to be sensitive.
- Gene therapy: If a disorder can be shown to be caused, or highly influenced, by a single gene, it may be possible to "replace" the defective gene. An approach to this type of therapy has been described for X-linked severe combined immunodeficiency.[122] This type of approach will not, however, be applicable to diseases such as malaria or tuberculosis, in which susceptibility is likely to be influenced by a large number of genes.
- Vaccination: "Reverse immunogenetics" is the process by which likely T-cell epitopes are either deduced or eluted from MHC molecules shown to be associated with protection. This approach has been used in the identification of peptide epitopes possibly suitable as components for vaccines against malaria. This approach is being applied to a number of other infections. However, it must be borne in mind that adverse effects, as well as protection, can result from inappropriate activation of T cells in many diseases caused by intracellular parasites, emphasizing that caution needs to be taken with this approach.
- Identification of the genetic contribution to complex diseases will lead to an increased understanding of the pathogenesis that will have positive consequences for both diagnosis and treatment.

REFERENCES

1. Sorensen TI, Nielsen GG, Andersen PK, et al: Genetic and environmental influences on premature death in adult adoptees. N Engl J Med 318(12):727–732, 1988.
2. Lander E, Schork N: Genetic dissection of complex traits. Science 265(5181):2037–2048, 1994.
3. Rajalingam R, Mehra NK, Jain RC, et al: Polymerase chain reaction-based sequence-specific oligonuceotide hybridisation analysis of HLA class II antigens in pulmonary tuberculosis: Relevance to disease severity and chemotherapy. J Infect Dis 173(3):669–676, 1996.
4. Livingstone FB: The Duffy blood groups, vivax malaria, and malaria selection in human populations: A review. Hum Biol 56(3):413–425, 1984.
5. Flint J, Hill AV, Bowden DK, et al: High frequencies of alpha-thalassaemia are the result of natural selection by malaria. Nature 321(6072):744–750, 1986.
6. Hill AV, Allsopp CE, Kwiatkowski D, et al: Common West African HLA antigens are associated with protection from severe malaria. Nature 352(6336):595–600, 1991.
7. McGuire W, Hill AV, Allsopp CE, et al: Variation in the TNF-alpha promoter region associated with susceptibility to cerebral malaria. Nature 371(6497):508-510, 1994.
8. Collins FS: Cystic fibrosis: Molecular biology and therapeutic implications. Science 256(5058):774–779, 1992.
9. Pier GB, Grout M, Zaidi T, et al: *Salmonella typhi* uses CFTR to enter intestinal epithelial cells. Nature 393(6680):79–82, 1998.
10. Pier GB: Role of the cystic fibrosis transmembrane conductance regulator in innate immunity to *Pseudomonas aeruginosa* infections. Proc Natl Acad Sci USA 97(16):8822–8828, 2000.
11. Zariwala M, Noone PG, Sannuti A, et al: Germline mutations in an intermediate chain dynein cause primary ciliary dyskinesia. Am J Respir Cell Mol Biol 25(5):577–583, 2001.
12. Janssens S, Beyaert R: Role of Toll-like receptors in pathogen recognition. Clin Microbiol Rev 16(4):637–646, 2003.
13. Gordon S: Pattern recognition receptors: Doubling up for the innate immune response. Cell 111(7):927–930, 2002.
14. Smirnova I, Mann N, Dols A, et al: Assay of locus-specific genetic load implicates rare Toll-like receptor 4 mutations in meningococcal susceptibility. Proc Natl Acad Sci USA 100(10):6075–6080, 2003.
15. Hawn TR, Verbon A, Lettinga KD, et al: A common dominant TLR5 stop codon polymorphism abolishes flagellin signaling and is associated with susceptibility to legionnaires' disease. J Exp Med 198(10):1563–1572, 2003.
16. Heath WR, Carbone FR: Cross-presentation in viral immunity and self-tolerance. Nat Rev Immunol 1(2):126–134, 2001.
17. Hughes AL: Natural selection and the diversification of vertebrate immune effectors. Immunol Rev 190:161–168, 2002.
18. Jeffery KJ, Bangham CR: Do infectious diseases drive MHC diversity? Microbes Infect 2(11):1335–1341, 2000.
19. Wilkinson RJ, Patel P, Llewelyn M, et al: Influence of polymorphism in the genes for the interleukin 1 receptor antagonist and interleukin IL-1b on tuberculosis. J Exp Med 189(12):1863–1874, 1999.
20. Siniscalco M, Bernini L, Filippi G, et al: Population genetics of haemoglobin variants, thalassaemia and glucose-6-phosphate dehydrogenase deficiency, with particular reference to the malaria hypothesis. Bull World Health Organ 34(3):379–393, 1966.
21. Allison A: Protection afforded by sickle cell trait against subtertian malarial infection. BMJ 4857:290–294, 1954.
22. Pasvol G, Weatherall DJ, Wilson RJ: Cellular mechanism for the protective effect of haemoglobin S against *P. falciparum* malaria. Nature 274(5672):701–703, 1978.
23. Sachidanandam R, Weissman D, Schmidt SC, et al: A map of human genome sequence variation containing 1.42 million single nucleotide polymorphisms. Nature 409(6822):928–933, 2001.
24. Hacking D, Knight JC, Rockett K, et al: Increased in vivo transcription of an IL-8 haplotype associated with respiratory syncytial virus disease-susceptibility. Genes Immun 5(4):274–282, 2004.
25. Vidal S, Malo D, Vogan K, et al: Natural resistance to infection with intracellular parasites; Isolation of a candidate gene for *Bcg*. Cell 73(3):469-485, 1993.
26. Plant JE, Blackwell JM, O'Brien AD, et al: Are the Lsh and Ity disease resistance genes at one locus on mouse chromosome 1? Nature 297(5866):510–511, 1982.

27. Bradley DJ: Letter: Genetic control of natural resistance to *Leishmania donovani*. Nature 250(464):353–354, 1974.
28. Jamieson SE, Miller EN, Black GF, et al: Evidence for a cluster of genes on chromosome 17q11–q21 controlling susceptibility to tuberculosis and leprosy in Brazilians. Genes Immun 5(1):46–57, 2004.
29. Bellamy R, Beyers N, McAdam KP, et al: Genetic susceptibility to tuberculosis in Africans: A genome-wide scan. Proc Natl Acad Sci USA 97(14):8005–8009, 2000.
30. El Baghdadi J, Remus N, Benslimane A, et al: Variants of the human NRAMP1 gene and susceptibility to tuberculosis in Morocco. Int J Tuberc Lung Dis 7(6):599–602, 2003.
31. Awomoyi AA, Marchant A, Howson JM, et al: Interleukin-10, polymorphism in SLC11A1 (formerly NRAMP1), and susceptibility to tuberculosis. J Infect Dis 186(12):1808–1814, 2002.
32. Bellamy R, Ruwende C, Corrah T, et al: Variations in the NRAMP1 gene and susceptibility to tuberculosis in West Africans. N Engl J Med 338(10):640–644, 1998.
33. Ryu S, Park YK, Bai GH, et al: 3′ UTR polymorphisms in the NRAMP1 gene are associated with susceptibility to tuberculosis in Koreans. Int J Tuberc Lung Dis 4(6):577–580, 2000.
34. Rossouw M, Nel HJ, Cooke GS, et al: Association between tuberculosis and a polymorphic NFkappaB binding site in the interferon gamma gene. Lancet 361(9372):1871–1872, 2003.
35. Akahoshi M, Nakashima H, Miyake K, et al: Influence of interleukin-12 receptor beta1 polymorphisms on tuberculosis. Hum Genet 112(3):237–243, 2003.
36. Nagel RL: Innate resistance to malaria: The intraerythrocytic cycle. Blood Cells 16(2–3):321–339, 1990.
37. Haldane J: The rate of mutation of human genes. Proc VIIIth Int Congr Genet: 267–272, 1949.
38. Luzzi GA, Merry AH, Newbold CI, et al: Surface antigen expression on *Plasmodium falciparum*-infected erythrocytes is modified in alpha- and beta-thalassemia. J Exp Med 173(4):785–791, 1991.
39. Maitland K, Williams TN, Bennett S, et al: The interaction between *Plasmodium falciparum* and *P. vivax* in children on Espiritu Santo island, Vanuatu. Trans R Soc Trop Med Hyg 90(6):614–620, 1996.
40. Ruwende C, Khoo SC, Snow RW, et al: Natural selection of hemi- and heterozygotes for G6PD deficiency in Africa by resistance to severe malaria. Nature 376(6537):246–249, 1995.
41. Hill AV, Elvin J, Willis AC, et al: Molecular analysis of the association of HLA-B53 and resistance to severe malaria. Nature 360(6403):434–439, 1992.
42. Brown KN, Brown IN: Immunity to malaria: Antigenic variation in chronic infections of *Plasmodium knowlesi*. Nature 208(17):1286–1288, 1965.
43. Brown KN: Antibody induced variation in malaria parasites. Nature 242(5392):49–50, 1973.
44. Bellamy R, Ruwende C, McAdam KP, et al: Mannose binding protein deficiency is not associated with malaria, hepatitis B carriage nor tuberculosis in Africans. Quart J Med 91(1):13–18, 1998.
45. Bouma G, Crusius JB, Oudkerl Pool M, et al: Secretion of tumour necrosis factor α and lymphotoxin α in relation to polymorphisms in the TNF genes and HLA-DR alleles. Relevance for inflammatory bowel disease. Scand J Immunol 43(4):456–463, 1996.
46. Brinkman BM, Zuijdgeest D, Kaijzel EL, et al: Relevance of the tumour necrosis factor alpha (TNF-α) -308 promoter polymorphism in TNF-α gene regulation. J Inflammation 46(1):32–41, 1996.
47. Stuber F, Udalova IA, Book M, et al: -308 tumor necrosis factor (TNF) polymorphism is not associated with survival in severe sepsis and is unrelated to lipopolysaccharide inducibility of the human TNF promoter. J Inflammation 46(1):42–50, 1996.
48. McNeil AJ, Yap PL, Gore SM, et al: Association of HLA types A1-B8-DR3 and B27 with rapid and slow progression of HIV disease. Quart J Med 89(3):177–185, 1996.
49. Kaslow RA, Duquesnoy R, VanRaden M, et al: A1, Cw7, B8, DR3 HLA antigen combination associated with rapid decline of T-helper lymphocytes in HIV-1 infection. A report from the Multicenter AIDS Cohort Study. Lancet 335(8695):927–930, 1990.
50. Liu C, Carrington M, Kaslow RA, et al: Association of polymorphisms in human leukocyte antigen class I and transporter associated with antigen processing genes with resistance to human immunodeficiency virus type 1 infection. J Infect Dis 187(9):1404–1410, 2003.
51. Rowland-Jones SL: Timeline: AIDS pathogenesis: What have two decades of HIV research taught us? Nat Rev Immunol 3(4):343–348, 2003.
52. Marmor M, Sheppard HW, Donnell D, et al: Homozygous and heterozygous CCR5-Delta32 genotypes are associated with resistance to HIV infection. J Acquir Immune Defic Syndr 27(5):472–481, 2001.
53. Smith MW, Dean M, Carrington M, et al: Contrasting genetic influence of CCR2 and CCR5 variants on HIV-1 infection and disease progression. Hemophilia Growth and Development Study (HGDS), Multicenter AIDS Cohort Study (MACS), Multicenter Hemophilia Cohort Study (MHCS), San Francisco City Cohort (SFCC), ALIVE Study. Science 277(5328):959–965, 1997.
54. Barber Y, Rubio C, Fernandez E, et al: Host genetic background at CCR5 chemokine receptor and vitamin D receptor loci and human immunodeficiency virus (HIV) type 1 disease progression among HIV-seropositive injection drug users. J Infect Dis 184(10):1279–1288, 2001.
55. Martin MP, Dean M, Smith MW, et al: Genetic acceleration of AIDS progression by a promoter variant of CCR5. Science 282(5395): 1907–1911, 1998.
56. Brambilla A, Villa C, Rizzardi G, et al: Shorter survival of SDF1-3′A/3′A homozygotes linked to CD4+ T cell decrease in advanced human immunodeficiency virus type 1 infection. J Infect Dis 182(1):311–315, 2000.
57. An P, Nelson GW, Wang L, et al: Modulating influence on HIV/AIDS by interacting RANTES gene variants. Proc Natl Acad Sci USA 99(15): 10002–10007, 2002.
58. Fernandez RM, Borrego S, Marcos I, et al: Fluorescence resonance energy transfer analysis of the RANTES polymorphisms -403G → A and -28G → C: Evaluation of both variants as susceptibility factors to HIV type 1 infection in the Spanish population. AIDS Res Hum Retroviruses 19(5):349–352, 2003.
59. Kallmann F, Reisner D: Twin studies on the significance of genetic factors in tuberculosis. Am Rev Tuberc 47:549–574, 1942.
60. Comstock GW: Tuberculosis in twins: A re-analysis of the Prophit survey. Am Rev Respir Dis 117(4):621–624, 1978.
61. Bothamley GH, Beck JS, Schreuder GMT, et al: Association of tuberculosis and *M. tuberculosis*-specific antibody levels with HLA. J Infect Dis 159(3):549–555, 1989.
62. Singh SP, Mehra NK, Dingley HB, et al: Human leukocyte antigen (HLA)-linked control of susceptibility to pulmonary tuberculosis and association with HLA-DR types. J Infect Dis 148(4):676–681, 1983.
63. Khomenko AG, Litvinov VI, Chukanova VP, et al: Tuberculosis in patients with various HLA phenotypes. Tubercle 71(3):187–192, 1990.
64. Brahmajothi V, Pitchappan RM, Kakkanaiah VN, et al: Association of pulmonary tuberculosis and HLA in south India. Tubercle 72(2):123–132, 1991.
65. Hawkins BR, Higgins DA, Chan SL, et al: HLA typing in the Hong Kong Chest Service/British Medical Research Council study of factors associated with the breakdown to active tuberculosis of inactive pulmonary lesions. Am Rev Respir Dis 138(6):1616–1621, 1988.
66. Balamurugan A, Sharma SK, Mehra NK: Human leukocyte antigen class I supertypes influence susceptibility and severity of tuberculosis. J Infect Dis 189(5):805–811, 2004.
67. Cervino AC, Lakiss S, Sow O, et al: Fine mapping of a putative tuberculosis-susceptibility locus on chromosome 15q11–13 in African families. Hum Mol Genet 11(14):1599–1603, 2002.
68. Cole ST, Eiglmeier K, Parkhill J, et al: Massive gene decay in the leprosy bacillus. Nature 409(6823):1007–1011, 2001.
69. Kharakter ZhZ, Mazhak KD, Pavlenko AV: The role of genetically determined haptoglobin phenotypes in patients with destructive pulmonary tuberculosis. Probl Tuberk 7:50–52, 1990.
70. Kasvosve I, Gomo ZA, Mvundura E, et al: Haptoglobin polymorphism and mortality in patients with tuberculosis. Int J Tuberc Lung Dis 4(8):771–775, 2000.
71. Bellamy R, Ruwende C, Corrah T, et al: Tuberculosis and chronic hepatitis B virus infection in Africans and variation in the vitamin D receptor gene. J Infect Dis 179(3):721–724, 1999.
72. Rockett KA, Brookes R, Udalova I, et al: 1,25-Dihydroxyvitamin D3 induces nitric oxide synthase and suppresses growth of *Mycobacterium tuberculosis* in a human macrophage-like cell line. Infect Immun 66(11):5314–5321, 1998.
73. Hoal-Van Helden EG, Epstein J, Victor TC, et al: Mannose-binding protein B allele confers protection against tuberculous meningitis. Pediatr Res 45(4 Pt 1):459–464, 1999.
74. Quinnell RJ: Genetics of susceptibility to human helminth infection. Int J Parasitol 33(11):1219–1231, 2003.

75. Marquet S, Abel L, Hillaire D, et al: Genetic localisation of a locus controlling their intensity of infection by *Schistosoma mansoni* on chromosome 5q31–q33. Nature Genet 14(2):181–184, 1996.
76. Williams-Blangero S, VandeBerg JL, Subedi J, et al: Genes on chromosomes 1 and 13 have significant effects on Ascaris infection. Proc Natl Acad Sci USA 99(8):5533–5538, 2002.
77. Abdel Salam E, Abdel Khalik A, Abdel Meguid A, et al: Association of HLA class I antigens (A1, B5, B8 and CW2) with disease manifestations and infection in human schistosomiasis mansoni in Egypt. Tissue Antigens 27(3):142–146, 1986.
78. Cabello PH, Krieger H, Lopes JD, et al: On the association between HLA-A1 and B5 and clinical forms of schistosomiasis mansoni. Mem Inst Oswaldo Cruz 86(1):37–40, 1991.
79. Ohta N, Nishimura YK, Iuchi M, et al: Immunogenetic analysis of patients with post-schistosomal liver cirrhosis in man. Clin Exp Immunol 49(3):493–499, 1982.
80. Secor WE, del Corral H, dos Reis MG, et al: Association of hepatosplenic schistosomiasis with HLA-DQB1*0201. J Infect Dis 174(5):1131–1135, 1996.
81. Yazdanbaksh M, Sartono E, Kruize YC, et al: HLA and elephantiasis in lymphatic filariasis. Hum Immunol 44(1):58–61, 1995.
82. Meyer CG, Gallin M, Erttmann KD, et al: HLA-D alleles associated with generalised disease. Localised disease and putative immunity in *Onchocerca volvulus* infection. Proc Natl Acad Sci USA 91(16):7515, 1994.
83. Fine PE, Wolf E, Pritchard J, et al: HLA-linked genes and leprosy: A family study in Karigiri, South India. J Infect Dis 140(2):152–161, 1979.
84. Mehra NK, Rajalingam R, Mitra DK, et al: Variants of HLA-DR2/DR51 group haplotypes and susceptibility to tuberculoid leprosy and pulmonary tuberculosis in Asian Indians. Int J Lepr Other Mycobact Dis 63(2):241–248, 1995.
85. Rani R, Fernandez Vina MA, Zaheer SA, et al: Study of HLA class II alleles by PCR oligotyping in leprosy patients from north India. Tissue Antigens 42(3):133–137, 1993.
86. van Eden W, Gonzalez NM, de Vries RR, et al: HLA-linked control of predisposition to lepromatous leprosy. J Infect Dis 151(1):9–14, 1985.
87. Siddiqui MR, Meisner S, Tosh K, et al: A major susceptibility locus for leprosy in India maps to chromosome 10p13. Nature Genet 27(4):439–441, 2001.
88. Mira MT, Alcais A, Nguyen VT, et al: Susceptibility to leprosy is associated with PARK2 and PACRG. Nature 427(6975):636–640, 2004.
89. Thomas HC, Foster GR, Sumiya M, et al: Mutation in the gene for mannose-binding protein associated with chronic hepatitis B viral infection. Lancet 348(9039):1417–1419, 1996.
90. Hohler T, Wunschel M, Gerken G, et al: No association between mannose-binding lectin alleles and susceptibility to chronic hepatitis B virus infection in German patients. Exp Clin Immunogenet 15(3): 130–133, 1998.
91. Summerfield JA, Ryder S, Sumiya M, et al: Mannose-binding protein gene mutations associated with unusual and severe infections in adults. Lancet 345(8954):886–889, 1995.
92. Hohler T, Gerken G, Notghi A, et al: HLA-DRB1*1301 and *1302 protect against chronic hepatitis B. J Hepatol 26(3):503–507, 1997.
93. Thio CL, Thomas DL, Karacki P, et al: Comprehensive analysis of class I and class II HLA antigens and chronic hepatitis B virus infection. J Virol 77(22):12083–12087, 2003.
94. Peano G, Menardi G, Ponzetto A, et al: HLA-DR5 antigen. A genetic factor influencing the outcome of hepatitis C virus infection? Arch Intern Med 154(23):2733–2736, 1994.
95. Wawrzynowicz-Syczewska M, Underhill JA, Clare MA, et al: HLA class II genotypes associated with chronic hepatitis C virus infection and response to alpha-interferon treatment in Poland. Liver 20(3):234–239, 2000.
96. Yenigun A, Durupinar B: Decreased frequency of the HLA-DRB1*11 allele in patients with chronic hepatitis C virus infection. J Virol 76(4):1787–1789, 2002.
97. Harcourt G, Hellier S, Bunce M, et al: Effect of HLA class II genotype on T helper lymphocyte responses and viral control in hepatitis C virus infection. J Viral Hepatol 8(3):174–179, 2001.
98. Yee LJ: Host genetic determinants in hepatitis C virus infection. Genes Immun 5(4):237–245, 2004.
99. Mangia A, Santoro R, Piattelli M, et al: IL-10 haplotypes as possible predictors of spontaneous clearance of HCV infection. *Cytokine* 25(3):103–109, 2004.
100. Knapp S, Hennig BJ, Frodsham AJ, et al: Interleukin-10 promoter polymorphisms and the outcome of hepatitis C virus infection. Immunogenetics 55(6):362–369, 2003.
101. Cartwright K: Meningococcal carriage and disease. In: Cartwright K (ed) Meningococcal Disease. London, John Wiley and Sons, 1995, pp 115–146.
102. Figueroa J, Andreoni J, Densen P: Complement deficiency states and meningococcal disease. Immunol Res 12(3):295–311, 1993.
103. Linton SM, Morgan BP: Properdin deficiency and meningococcal disease—Identifying those most at risk. Clin Exp Immunol 118(2):189–191, 1999.
104. Fijen CA, Kuijper EJ, Hannema AJ, et al: Complement deficiencies in patients over ten years old with meningococcal disease due to uncommon serogroups. Lancet 2(8663):585–588, 1989.
105. Turner MW: Mannose-binding lectin: The pluripotent molecule of the innate immune system. Immunol Today 17(11):532–540, 1996.
106. Hibberd ML, Sumiya M, Summerfield JA, et al: Association of variants of the gene for mannose-binding lectin with susceptibility to meningococcal disease. Meningococcal Research Group. Lancet 353(9158):1049–1053, 1999.
107. Fearon DT, Locksley RM: The instructive role of innate immunity in the acquired immune response. Science 272(5258):50–53, 1996.
108. Fearon DT: Seeking wisdom in innate immunity. Nature 388(6640):323–324, 1997.
109. Medzhitov R, Janeway CA, Jr: Innate immunity: The virtues of a nonclonal system of recognition. Cell 91(3):295–298, 1997.
110. Beutler B: Toll-like receptors: How they work and what they do. Curr Opin Hematol 9(1):2–10, 2002.
111. Qureshi ST, Gros P, Malo D: The Lps locus: Genetic regulation of host responses to bacterial lipopolysaccharide. Inflamm Res 48(12):613–620, 1999.
112. Beutler B: Tlr4: Central component of the sole mammalian LPS sensor. Curr Opin Immunol 12(1):20–26, 2000.
113. Akira S, Takeda K, Kaisho T: Toll-like receptors: Critical proteins linking innate and acquired immunity. Nat Immunol 2(8):675–680, 2001.
114. Brandtzaeg P, Cartwright K: Pathogenesis of meningococcal infections. In: Cartwright K (ed): Meningococcal Disease. London, John Wiley and Sons, 1995, pp 71–114.
115. van Deuren M, Brandtzaeg P, van der Meer JW: Update on meningococcal disease with emphasis on pathogenesis and clinical management. Clin Microbiol Rev 13(1):144–166, 2000.
116. Nadel S, Newport MJ, Booy R, et al: Variation in the tumor necrosis factor-α gene promoter may be associated with death from meningococcal disease. J Infect Dis 174(4):878–880, 1996.
117. Westendorp RG, Langermans JA, Huizinga TW, et al: Genetic influence on cytokine production in meningococcal disease. Lancet 349(9069):1912–1913, 1997.
118. Read RC, Cannings C, Naylor SC, et al: Variation within genes encoding interleukin-1 and the interleukin-1 receptor antagonist influence the severity of meningococcal disease. Ann Intern Med 138(7):534–541, 2003.
119. Hermans PW, Hibberd ML, Booy R, et al: 4G/5G promoter polymorphism in the plasminogen-activator-inhibitor-1 gene and outcome of meningococcal disease. Meningococcal Research Group. Lancet 354(9178):556–560, 1999.
120. Kondaveeti S, Hibberd ML, Booy R, et al: Effect of the Factor V Leiden mutation on the severity of meningococcal disease. Pediatr Infect Dis J 18(10):893–896, 1999.
121. Haralambous E, Hibberd ML, Hermans PW, et al: Role of functional plasminogen-activator-inhibitor-1 4G/5G promoter polymorphism in susceptibility, severity, and outcome of meningococcal disease in Caucasian children. Crit Care Med 31(12):2788–2793, 2003.
122. Candotti F, Johnston JA, Puck JM, et al: Retroviral-mediated gene correction for X-linked severe combined immunodeficiency. Blood 87(8):3097–3102, 1996.
123. Roesler J, Curnutte JT, Rae J, et al: Recombination events between the p47-phox gene and its highly homologous pseudogenes are the main cause of autosomal recessive chronic granulomatous disease. Blood 95(6):2150–2156, 2000.
124. Porter CD, Kuribayashi F, Parkar MH, et al: Detection of gp91-phox precursor protein in B-cell lines from patients with X-linked chronic granulomatous disease as an indicator for mutations impairing cytochrome b558 biosynthesis. Biochem J 315(Pt 2):571–575, 1996.

125. Liese JG, Jendrossek V, Jansson A, et al: Chronic granulomatous disease in adults. Lancet 347(8996):220–223, 1996.
126. Tsukada S, Saffran DC, Rawlings DJ, et al: Deficient expression of a B cell cytoplasmic tyrosine kinase in human X-linked agammaglobulinemia. Cell 72(2):279–290, 1993.
127. Conley ME, Cooper MD: Genetic basis of abnormal B cell development. Curr Opin Immunol 10(4):399–406, 1998.
128. Grimbacher B, Hutloff A, Schlesier M, et al: Homozygous loss of ICOS is associated with adult-onset common variable immunodeficiency. Nat Immunol 4(3):261–268, 2003.
129. DiSanto JP, Bonnefoy JY, Gauchat JF, et al: CD40 ligand mutations in X-linked immunodeficiency with hyper-IgM. Nature 361(6412):541–543, 1993.
130. Derry JM, Ochs HD, Francke U: Isolation of a novel gene mutated in Wiskott–Aldrich syndrome [published erratum appears in Cell 1994 Dec 2;79(5):following 922]. Cell 78(4):635–644, 1994.
131. Notarangelo LD, Mazza C, Giliani S, et al: Missense mutations of the WASP gene cause intermittent X-linked thrombocytopenia. Blood 99(6):2268–2269, 2002.
132. Zhu Q, Watanabe C, Liu T, et al: Wiskott–Aldrich syndrome/X-linked thrombocytopenia: WASP gene mutations, protein expression, and phenotype. Blood 90(7):2680–2689, 1997.
133. Buckley RH: Molecular defects in human severe combined immunodeficiency and approaches to immune reconstitution. Annu Rev Immunol 22:625–655, 2004.
134. Slingsby JH, Norsworthy P, Pearce G, et al: Homozygous hereditary C1q deficiency and systemic lupus erythematosus. A new family and the molecular basis of C1q deficiency in three families. Arthritis Rheum 39(4):663–670, 1996.
135. Inoue N, Saito T, Masuda R, et al: Selective complement C1s deficiency caused by homozygous four-base deletion in the C1s gene. Hum Genet 103(4):415–418, 1998.
136. Botto M, Fong KY, So AK, et al: Molecular basis of hereditary C3 deficiency. J Clin Invest 86(4):1158–1163, 1990.
137. Colten HR, Rosen FS: Complement deficiencies. Annu Rev Immunol 10:809–834, 1992.
138. Rowe PC, McLean RH, Wood RA, et al: Association of homozygous C4B deficiency with bacterial meningitis. J Infect Dis 160(3):448–451, 1989.
139. Sjoholm AG, Kuijper EG, Tijssen CC, et al: Dysfunctional properdin in a Dutch family with meningococcal disease. N Engl J Med 319(1):33–37, 1988.
140. Fijen CA, Kuijper EJ, Hannema AJ, et al: Complement deficiencies in patients over ten years old with meningococcal disease due to uncommon serogroups. Lancet 2(8663):585–588, 1989.
141. Roy S, Knox K, Segal S, et al: MBL genotype and risk of invasive pneumococcal disease: A case–control study. Lancet 359(9317):1569–1573, 2002.
142. Dorman SE, Holland SM: Mutation in the signal-transducing chain of the Interferon-γ receptor and susceptibility to mycobacterial infection. J Clin Invest 101(11):2364–2369, 1998.
143. Altare F, Durandy A, Lammas D, et al: Impairment of mycobacterial immunity in human interleukin-12 receptor deficiency. Science 280(5368):1432–1435, 1998.
144. Altare F, Ensser A, Breiman A, et al: Interleukin-12 receptor beta1 deficiency in a patient with abdominal tuberculosis. J Infect Dis 184(2):231–236, 2001.
145. Dupuis S, Dargemont C, Fieschi C, et al: Impairment of mycobacterial but not viral immunity by a germline human STAT1 mutation. Science 293(5528):300–303, 2001.
146. Kroner BL, Goedert JJ, Blattner WA, et al: Concordance of human leukocyte antigen haplotype-sharing, CD4 decline and AIDS in hemophilic siblings. Multicenter Hemophilia Cohort and Hemophilia Growth and Development Studies. AIDS 9(3):275–280, 1995.
147. Winchester R, Che NY, Rose S, et al: Major histocompatibility complex class II DR alleles DRB1*1501 and those encoding HLA-DR13 are preferentially associated with a diminution in maternally transmitted human immunodeficiency virus 1 infection in different ethnic groups: Determination by an automated sequence-based typing method. Proc Natl Acad Sci USA 92(26):12374–12378, 1995.
148. Chiewsilp P, Scott RM, Bhamarapravati N: Histocompatibility antigens and dengue hemorrhagic fever. Am J Trop Med Hyg 30(5):1100–1105, 1981.
149. Dunstan SJ, Stephens HA, Blackwell JM, et al: Genes of the class II and class III major histocompatibility complex are associated with typhoid fever in Vietnam. J Infect Dis 183(2):261–268, 2001.
150. Petzl Erler ML, Belich MP, Queiroz Telles F: Association of mucosal leishmaniasis with HLA. Hum Immunol 32(4):254–260, 1991.
151. Kalish RA, Leong JM, Steere AC: Association of treatment-resistant chronic Lyme arthritis with HLA-DR4 and antibody reactivity to OspA and OspB of *Borrelia burgdorferi*. Infect Immun 61(7):2774–2779, 1993.
152. Steere AC, Dwyer E, Winchester R: Association of chronic Lyme arthritis with HLA-DR4 and HLA-DR2 alleles [published erratum appears in N Engl J Med 1991 Jan 10;324(2):129] [see comments]. N Engl J Med 323(4):219–223, 1990.
153. Pfluger KH, Reimers CD, Neubert U, et al: Lyme-borreliosis and possible association with HLA-antigens. Tissue Antigens 33(3):375–381, 1989.
154. Ohta N, Hayashi M, Tormis LC, et al: Immunogenetic factors involved in the pathogenesis of distinct clinical manifestations of schistosomiasis japonica in the Philippine population. Trans R Soc Trop Med Hyg 81(2):292–296, 1987.
155. Cabrera M, Shaw MA, Sharples C, et al: Polymorphism in tumor necrosis factor genes associated with mucocutaneous leishmaniasis. J Exp Med 182(5):1259–1264, 1995.
156. McGuire W, Hill AVS, Allsopp CEM, et al: Severe malarial anaemia and cerebral malaria are associated with separate variants of the TNF promoter region. Paper presented at BSP, London, 1995.
157. Agarwal A, Guindo A, Cissoko Y, et al: Hemoglobin C associated with protection from severe malaria in the Dogon of Mali, a West African population with a low prevalence of hemoglobin S. Blood 96(7):2358–2363, 2000.
158. Chotivanich K, Udomsangpetch R, Pattanapanyasat K, et al: Hemoglobin E: A balanced polymorphism protective against high parasitemias and thus severe *P. falciparum* malaria. Blood 100(4):1172–1176, 2002.
159. Pasvol G, Weatherall DJ, Wilson RJ: Effects of foetal haemoglobin on susceptibility of red cells to *Plasmodium falciparum*. Nature 270(5633):171–173, 1977.
160. Willcox M, Bjorkman A, Brohult J: Falciparum malaria and beta-thalassaemia trait in northern Liberia. Ann Trop Med Parasitol 77(4):335–347, 1983.
161. Martin SK, Miller LH, Kark JA, et al: Low erythrocyte pyridoxal-kinase activity in blacks: Its possible relation to falciparum malaria. Lancet 1(8062):466–468, 1978.
162. Genton B, al-Yaman F, Mgone CS, et al: Ovalocytosis and cerebral malaria. Nature 378(6557):564–565, 1995.
163. Miller LH, Mason SJ, Dvorak JA, et al: Erythrocyte receptors for (*Plasmodium knowlesi*) malaria: Duffy blood group determinants. Science 189(4202):561–563, 1975.
164. Barragan A, Kremsner PG, Wahlgren M, et al: Blood group A antigen is a coreceptor in *Plasmodium falciparum* rosetting. Infect Immun 68(5):2971–2975, 2000.
165. Pasvol G, Wainscoat JS, Weatherall DJ: Erythrocytes deficiency in glycophorin resist invasion by the malarial parasite *Plasmodium falciparum*. Nature 297(5861):64–66, 1982.
166. Cockburn IA, Mackinnon MJ, O'Donnell A, et al: A human complement receptor 1 polymorphism that reduces *Plasmodium falciparum* rosetting confers protection against severe malaria. Proc Natl Acad Sci USA 101(1):272–277, 2004.
167. Cooke GS, Aucan C, Walley AJ, et al: Association of Fcgamma receptor IIa (CD32) polymorphism with severe malaria in West Africa. Am J Trop Med Hyg 69(6):565–568, 2003.
168. Pain A, Urban BC, Kai O, et al: A non-sense mutation in Cd36 gene is associated with protection from severe malaria. Lancet 357(9267):1502–1503, 2001.
169. Kun JF, Klabunde J, Lell B, et al: Association of the ICAM-1Kilifi mutation with protection against severe malaria in Lambarene, Gabon. Am J Trop Med Hyg 61(5):776–779, 1999.
170. Sabeti P, Usen S, Farhadian S, et al: CD40L association with protection from severe malaria. Genes Immun 3(5):286–291, 2002.
171. Kun JF, Mordmuller B, Perkins DJ, et al: Nitric oxide synthase 2(Lambarene) (G-954C), increased nitric oxide production, and protection against malaria. J Infect Dis 184(3):330–336, 2001.

172. McGuire W, Knight JC, Hill AV, et al: Severe malarial anemia and cerebral malaria are associated with different tumor necrosis factor promoter alleles. J Infect Dis 179(1):287–290, 1999.
173. Knight JC, Udalova I, Hill AV, et al: A polymorphism that affects OCT-1 binding to the TNF promoter region is associated with severe malaria. Nature Genet 22(2):145–150, 1999.
174. Ohashi J, Naka I, Patarapotikul J, et al: Significant association of longer forms of CCTTT microsatellite repeat in the inducible nitric oxide synthase promoter with severe malaria in Thailand. J Infect Dis 186(4):578–581, 2002.
175. Quaye IK, Ekuban FA, Goka BQ, et al: Haptoglobin 1-1 is associated with susceptibility to severe *Plasmodium falciparum* malaria. Trans R Soc Trop Med Hyg 94(2):216–219, 2000.
176. Zimmerman PA, Fitness J, Moulds JM, et al: CR1 Knops blood group alleles are not associated with severe malaria in the Gambia. Genes Immun 4(5):368–373, 2003.

7

Disease Eradication and Control

DONALD A. HENDERSON

INTRODUCTION

In 1980, the achievement of smallpox eradication stimulated widespread interest in eradication as public health policy. The smallpox program's success dispelled doubts as to the theoretical feasibility of disease eradication itself and raised hopes that other programs might soon follow. Undertaking intensive, short-term disease control programs with the objective of eliminating a disease has been highly attractive to politicians and health staff alike. The costs of these undertakings are anticipated to be repaid by sharply curtailing preventive measures or stopping them altogether when eradication is achieved.

Smallpox eradication has been succeeded by globally coordinated eradication programs for poliomyelitis[1] and dracunculiasis (Guinea worm infection).[2] Meanwhile, many other diseases have been and continue to be proposed as possible candidates for eradication.

In tropical and industrialized countries alike, there are many who now conceive of disease eradication strategies as a major theme for disease control over the coming decades. The reality of these assumptions must be critically examined because, as history has shown, the price of failed eradication campaigns has been high.

PAST ERADICATION CAMPAIGNS

Many have forgotten that the smallpox eradication campaign was only one in a series of major eradication efforts that date back to early in the 20th century. The possibility of disease eradication was originally suggested by the dramatic successes achieved by early community-wide preventive measures such as vaccination, improved sanitation, nutrition, and vector control. As early as 1888, Charles Chapin, one of America's leading figures in public health, rashly proposed that preventive measures for any disease, if diligently applied, could potentially lead to eradication of that disease.[3] Although Chapin himself did not sustain this argument, others did and most persuasively.[4–6] Thus, throughout the last century, one eradication program after another has been launched, each with lofty expectations and considerable fanfare. These programs, in both their successes and failures, have played important roles in shaping broader public health policies in many countries. None, other than for smallpox, has yet proved successful. In most instances, unfortunately, the failed eradication efforts have left little as a legacy, despite substantial long-term investments in time, energy, and resources. Most of the initiatives have been long forgotten.

The first planned program to eradicate a human disease dates from 1909 when the Rockefeller Foundation launched a hookworm eradication campaign, first in the United States and later extending it to 52 countries on six continents.[7] Its strategy was based on mass screening of children for hookworm infection, their treatment with drugs, and the construction of sanitary facilities. The strategy and the glowing predictions for success were rooted primarily in evangelistic optimism. Nearly 15 years elapsed before the program was critically evaluated. The evaluation showed that the campaign, in fact, had not significantly reduced hookworm infection rates anywhere.[8] The program died a quiet death.

Meanwhile, beginning in 1915, the Rockefeller Foundation launched a yellow fever eradication campaign with the announced expectation of eradicating the disease from the Americas within five years.[9] The foundation anticipated that similar programs in Africa would soon follow. The campaign strategy called for reducing the density in cities and towns of the vector mosquito, *Aedes aegypti*, whose breeding sites were in and near houses. Experience had shown that when mosquito densities were lowered sufficiently, the yellow fever virus ceased to be transmitted.

The campaign proved to be far more difficult and costly than had been anticipated, and so it never extended beyond the Americas. It foundered, finally, when it was discovered in the 1930s that the yellow fever virus had a natural reservoir among jungle mammals, thus making eradication impossible. Abruptly, the strategy shifted to an attempt to eradicate the *A. aegypti* mosquito itself on the premise that even if the yellow fever virus continued to circulate in the jungle, it would be unable to be transmitted in urban settings.[10] However, the task of eradicating a well-established mosquito vector from the whole of the Western Hemisphere proved to be formidable and far beyond the scope of available technology and resources. Efforts gradually waned and finally stopped during the 1970s.[6]

The 1940s brought yet another eradication campaign—against yaws. This was an international effort under the aegis of the World Health Organization (WHO). National yaws programs eventually included 61 countries.[11] The programs sought to eliminate infection by mass screening and treatment with penicillin. After 20 years, however, the yaws program finally had to be abandoned when it was discovered that infected persons who were missed during screening and some with mild or subclinical infection permitted the yaws spirochete to continue to spread despite the best efforts of the field teams.[6]

Finally, in 1955, the most ambitious of all eradication schemes, for malaria, was approved by the World Health Assembly.[12] As with each of the preceding eradication campaigns, the decision to launch the program was more heavily grounded in visionary enthusiasm than in sound science. The malaria eradication strategy relied on the use of a new insecticide, DDT, to be sprayed on the walls of dwellings. Mosquitoes, after biting a patient, customarily settled on adjacent walls, but were killed by DDT and therefore did not further transmit infection. Over a 20-year period, more than $2 billion was expended on national programs extending across all continents.[13] The programs proved to be far more complicated and costly than anyone had anticipated. Insecticide resistance became an increasing problem. From the beginning, it had been known that for most of Africa the basic strategy would not work, in part, because of the presence of mosquito species with quite different behavioral characteristics. However, no answer to this problem was found. By the mid-1970s, yet another large and costly eradication effort had collapsed, leaving as a legacy very little compared to the magnitude of the investment that had been made.

In the 1950s and 1960s, the possibility of smallpox eradication began to be discussed, but politicians and health professionals alike were skeptical of *any* eradication effort.[14] Each of the preceding eradication campaigns had been optimistically launched and had persisted for some 20 to 30 years before it became apparent that the epidemiology and ecology of the respective diseases were different from what had been assumed, that the available technology was inadequate to accomplish the task, and that needed resources were, in any case, far greater than had been budgeted or were available. Not surprisingly, the World Health Assembly, in 1966, did not unanimously welcome the proposal that $2.4 million be designated annually in the regular budget for a greatly strengthened effort to deal with smallpox.[13] Many delegates doubted that the eradication of any disease was possible and others simply did not want to contribute additional funds to a United Nations organization. However, after extended debate, a special smallpox program was approved, albeit by only a two-vote margin. A 10-year goal was suggested. UNICEF (United Nations International Children's Emergency Fund), however, as well as several national assistance agencies, indicated that they would not support any new eradication effort. Indeed, some countries with endemic smallpox initially chose not to participate because of doubts about eradication as a concept.

INTEREST IN ERADICATION IS REVIVED

Over the 11-year period 1967 to 1977, smallpox was eradicated, and this was confirmed officially by the World Health Assembly in 1980. Smallpox vaccination ceased in all countries. Soon a renewed interest in disease eradication arose.

It is notable that there were features about the campaign and about smallpox itself that made eradication more feasible than for any disease previously on the eradication agenda or, for that matter, for any candidate disease.

1. Variola major, the predominant form of smallpox, had a case-fatality rate of 20% to 30% in unvaccinated persons, and being able to spread in any climate was a serious threat to both industrialized and developing countries. Essentially, all countries maintained vaccination programs of some sort whether or not they were endemic. Today, only measles, tuberculosis, and acquired immunodeficiency syndrome (AIDS) pose a threat that begins to approach that of smallpox.
2. There were no animal reservoir and no insect vectors involved in transmission, unlike the situation with malaria and yellow fever, for example.
3. Every infected person developed illness and had a characteristic rash that was readily identifiable by both villagers and health staff. Transmission occurred only during the time the rash was present. On recovery, approximately three-fourths of those who had variola major were left with residual pockmarks on the face, and these lasted for life. Because of these factors, the presence of the virus in any geographic area could be detected readily and outbreaks contained. It was also possible to determine when smallpox infection had been present in an area during previous years, an important determination for remote areas when it became necessary to certify that eradication had been achieved.
4. Outbreaks were reasonably easy to stop. Smallpox spread comparatively slowly in a continuing chain of transmission. Normally, there was an interval of about two weeks between each new generation of cases, and those who were infected usually did not transmit infection to more than two to five additional persons, primarily relatives or close friends. Thus, when a case was detected, it was possible to stop the spread of infection by vaccinating tens to hundreds of potential contacts in an area and to trace the origin of infection to detect other possible outbreaks.
5. An inexpensive, highly thermostable vaccine provided nearly complete protection for periods of 10 to 20 years after a single inoculation. No other vaccine today approaches smallpox vaccine in terms of heat stability, and none provides greater than 95% protection with a single dose of vaccine.

All manner of diseases and conditions have been proposed for eradication since 1980.[15] Some of those mentioned include syphilis, tuberculosis, urban rabies, leprosy, hepatitis B, hunger, traffic accidents, measles, polio, and dracunculiasis.[13,16] Enthusiasm for eradication initiatives stemmed, in part, from the belief that a highly visible, widely publicized eradication target is especially attractive to politicians and the public alike and will garner substantially more funds and support than will programs intended for disease control. Proponents reason that even if programs fail, more money will have been secured for public health and that some good will have been accomplished. Memories of the failed malaria program and the damage this did to the credibility of public health have been little appreciated.

Many of the proposed initiatives for eradication are recognizably meaningless in terms of the accepted definition of eradication: "the purposeful reduction of specific disease prevalence to the point of continued absence of transmission within a specified area by means of a time-limited campaign."[6] Certainly, eradication has no meaning when applied to hunger or traffic accidents, for example. Objections by many to the cavalier use of the term *eradication* resulted in an even more regrettable phrase, "eradication of a disease as a public health problem." Proponents intended the phrase to mean that through control measures, the incidence of a disease would be maintained below some arbitrary level. This was an unfortunate construct, soon discarded as having little meaning. More recently, there has been a growing effort to use the term *elimination* of disease when it is clear that a high degree of control rather than eradication is sought. This term is also misleading as neither reference dictionaries nor scientists are able to distinguish *elimination* from *eradication*. In this chapter, reference is made only to disease eradication as properly defined.

THE FEASIBILITY OF OTHER ERADICATION PROGRAMS

Despite the fact that, for eradication, there were many advantageous attributes intrinsic to both smallpox as a disease and to the program, the eradication effort barely succeeded. Financial support for the program was always precarious despite the fact that every country stood to gain substantially from its eradication. A number of the endemic countries themselves were reluctant participants and some were so torn by civil war that operations could be conducted only during brief intervals in the conflict. Despite the leadership role that WHO played, its internally fragmented leadership made coordinated program operations difficult. To eradicate any disease with less favorable characteristics than those offered by smallpox presents a formidable challenge. Nevertheless there are now two that are in operation—one for polio and one for dracunculiasis.

Polio eradication, as an objective for the Western Hemisphere, was decided on by the Pan American Health Organization in 1985 and a global program by the World Health Assembly in 1988.[1] The basic strategy is similar to that employed for smallpox eradication: (1) special vaccination programs to heighten immunity and (2) surveillance programs to assure that all possible cases of polio are reported, competently investigated, and confirmed. Two special features of the vaccination programs deserve note: (1) national immunization days (NIDs) and (2) "mopping-up campaigns." Countries have scheduled NIDs twice each year during which all children, usually those less than 4 years old, have been vaccinated at collecting points during the cooler months of the year. This is the time of year of the lowest prevalence of enteric viruses that could block growth of the live oral polio vaccine in the intestine. Mopping-up campaigns have been conducted when polio incidence has fallen to very low levels. Such campaigns consist of door-to-door vaccination in the poorest, most densely crowded areas of the country. These are the areas usually found to harbor persistent endemic poliovirus spread.

Five problems have made the eradication of polio far more difficult than was smallpox eradication:

1. In developing countries, polio is nowhere near the problem posed by diseases such as malaria, tuberculosis, and measles. Not surprisingly, few countries were engaged in control programs prior to the advent of the eradication effort. Smallpox, by contrast, was the most feared of all the infectious agents, and all countries had vaccination programs of some sort before global eradication began.
2. In developing countries, polio is far more contagious than smallpox, and thus it is far more difficult to stop its spread. Virtually all children acquire polio infection by 3 to 4 years of age, whereas with smallpox, even in densely populated heavily endemic countries such as India, only 30% of cases were in children younger than 5 years.
3. Polio vaccine is very thermolabile and much less antigenic than smallpox vaccine. Logistically problematic "cold chains" have had to be developed to assure its potency at the point of delivery. In contrast, the smallpox vaccine was stable for 30 days or more even at temperatures of 37°C. Where five or more doses of polio vaccine were normally required to provide protection to 90% or more of recipients, successful vaccination rates for a single smallpox vaccination were consistently more than 95%.
4. Polio surveillance was far more difficult, requiring, as it did, that stool specimens be obtained from all patients within two weeks of illness onset in order to be able to differentiate polio cases from those experiencing paralysis due to other causes. Obtaining, transporting, and identifying specimens posed formidable challenges. In contrast, laboratory confirmation of smallpox cases was seldom needed.
5. A key factor in achieving smallpox eradication was the ability to rapidly stop the spread of disease by vaccinating contacts and neighbors of cases. This was possible because every infected person was readily identifiable and the contacts protected before the disease could spread. For polio, there are perhaps 200 or more infected but asymptomatic individuals for every paralytic case. Thus, a targeted containment program is impossible to execute.

Two impediments to eradication, which were discovered only after the eradication program began, raised questions about its feasibility.[17,18] These impediments relate to the behavior of the attenuated polioviruses, which comprise the live oral polio vaccine (OPV). OPV is the preferred vaccine in most countries, especially in the developing world, because it is considerably less expensive than the inactivated vaccine; it is easier to administer; and it spreads readily in households, serving to protect both the vaccinees and their contacts.[19] Because it quickly provides protection against acquiring and transmitting wild poliovirus, it is everywhere the vaccine of choice for controlling outbreaks. It has been discovered, however, that the vaccine, on rare occasions, can mutate to become paralytogenic and spread from person to person, thus generating an outbreak. Experience to date indicates that such outbreaks may occur after months or even several years of silent spread. A second troubling discovery is the fact that, in certain individuals with a particular genetic defect, the virus may continue to proliferate in the intestinal tract for long periods without symptoms. One individual, who remained asymptomatic, was found to have excreted the virus for upwards of 10 years, excreting a strain which, when tested in monkeys, proved to be paralytogenic. Efforts to treat the infection with a variety of agents proved futile. Nineteen such chronic excretors have been identified but, because few have symptoms, it must be assumed that there are hundreds, perhaps thousands, of such persons who cannot be identified other than by chance isolation of poliovirus from the stool.

Despite these formidable problems, considerable progress has been made in the polio eradication effort. In 2003, the number of cases declined to 773, occurring in 14 countries.[20] However, only three countries appeared to be endemic (India, Pakistan, and Nigeria) by the end of the year. Most cases in the remaining countries represented importations or cases occurring earlier in the year. Both India and Pakistan appeared to be making good progress toward interrupting transmission, but a major setback occurred in Nigeria as a result of uncontrolled polio epidemics in northern Nigeria and subsequent spread of polio throughout Nigeria and to 12 other African countries. Repeated immunization days with mass vaccination are being conducted in all affected areas, and hope is expressed that transmission might be interrupted in 2005. With three additional years being required to confirm that eradication has occurred, this would set the hoped-for year for confirmation of eradication at 2008, fully 8 years beyond the original target date. The cost of the program through 2003 exceeded $3 billion, more than 30 times the cost of the entire smallpox eradication effort.

Dracunculiasis

Prospects are brighter for the eradication of the parasite *Dracunculus medinensis*. An eradication program was agreed on in 1986 by the World Health Assembly with a target for achievement of 1995. Although the program is properly identified as a global eradication program, it involves eradication of the parasite only from generally remote rural areas of a number of tropical African countries as well as isolated areas of India and Pakistan. The strategy is directed toward preventing villagers from ingesting the minute freshwater crustaceans containing the larval parasites. Several methods are used: providing safe water supplies with new wells, destruction of the parasites in water by chemical means, and filtration or boiling of water before ingestion. Through surveys and reports, infected patients are detected, treated, and counseled not to enter the water and so contaminate it.

By 2003, the incidence of dracunculiasis had been reduced from an estimated 3.5 million cases (1986) to only 32,050 cases residing in 4679 villages in 12 countries of tropical Africa.[21] Two-thirds of the cases and infected villages were in Sudan, where continuing civil strife has handicapped operations.

CRITERIA FOR ASSESSING CANDIDATE DISEASES FOR ERADICATION

Before embarking on still more eradication programs, it seems sensible to examine critically the feasibility of such efforts. Five principal determinants are proposed as minimum criteria to be met before an eradication program policy is decided.

1. *There is no natural reservoir for the organism other than humans.* Most infectious agents are *not* candidates for eradication because the responsible organism infects naturally both humans and other mammalian species or may survive naturally in the environment.
2. *The recovered patient ceases to harbor the organism and desirably is immune to later reinfection.* For those diseases in which the organism continues to be present in the body, either in its naturally infectious form or a latent one (e.g., hepatitis B, tuberculosis, varicella), there is little hope for eradication. An eradication effort in such instances would require an effort extending over a generation or more—hardly a feasible proposition given the difficulties in sustaining international commitments to programs for more than 10 to 20 years.
3. *The preventive intervention is affordable, effective, and logistically practicable to apply.* Affordability is critical given the fact that disease candidates for eradication afflict all or most of the poorest countries, where obtaining resources for vaccines that cost as little as $1.00 per dose have so far proved to be difficult. The feasibility of application reflects the realities of the limited transportation, health, and communications infrastructure in so much of the developing world. Vaccines or other treatments that require multiple contacts with the population are beyond local capacities in most developing countries. Thus, long-term treatment regimens, such as are needed in treating tuberculosis, all but preclude the possibility of eradication where such is the only feasible strategy.
4. *The disease is sufficiently important to warrant the effort.* Most countries considered smallpox to be a priority, and virtually all were engaged in control efforts when global eradication began. Thus, contributing resources to a global eradication effort was sound public policy for all countries and all did so. Many developing countries, however, required greater resources than they themselves could provide. International contributions were sought to bridge this gap.

   Poliomyelitis eradication presents another type of challenge because the different countries have much more divergent degrees of interest in such an effort. The industrialized countries have generally accorded high priority to polio control. For the developing countries, however, a disease that produces paralysis in only 1 of 200 infected children, and results in death in only one-tenth of those, inevitably is of less concern than other diseases such as malaria and tuberculosis. Thus, in the polio eradication campaign, the expectation has been that the industrialized countries would provide virtually all funding for the conduct of the program worldwide and that developing countries would cooperate in implementing the program, but at little financial cost to themselves.
5. *Interruption of transmission has been demonstrated to be possible in developed countries and in some developing ones.* An eradication program is a costly investment whose benefits will not be realized unless eradication is achieved. Moreover, as has been apparent in almost every previous eradication program, expectations in terms of strategy, cost, and needed duration of effort have almost always proved to be seriously wrong when finally tested in the field. Accordingly, it would only be prudent to demonstrate empirically, first on a national and then on a regional scale, that the interruption of disease transmission is feasible before embarking on a hemisphere-wide or global effort.

Today, the feasibility of measles eradication is being tested in greatly intensified control programs throughout the Western Hemisphere.[22] Measles poses a special challenge because of the ease and rapidity of its spread and the fact that vaccination of children younger than 9 to 12 months old may be ineffective because of the interference of maternal antibody. Measles transmission has been interrupted for a several-year period in the Caribbean countries and for periods of months in the Americas. However, importations from endemic countries occur repeatedly and are difficult to identify quickly and to control before widespread outbreaks occur. Further experience is clearly needed before the practicability of measles eradication on a wider scale can be assessed.

CONCLUSION

Given history and experience as background, what can be said for the future of eradication as a 21st-century strategy? In considering the prospects, it is necessary to bear in mind that there have been a number of costly eradication campaigns over the past century, but that only smallpox eradication has succeeded, and that by the narrowest of margins. And yet smallpox was by far the easiest of diseases to eradicate. Polio is probably the next most difficult challenge, but the differences in characteristics between the two diseases and the two programs are substantial and many challenges remain. Completing the polio eradication effort requires the continuing execution of vaccination and surveillance programs in the densely crowded Indian subcontinent and in large, all-but-inaccessible areas such as in Congo, Afghanistan, Somalia, and Sudan. Meanwhile, so long as the poliovirus continues to circulate, all other countries have little choice but to maintain their programs of vaccination and surveillance to prevent the virus from being reimported and becoming reestablished.

At this time, one must question the wisdom of even contemplating another eradication effort until the two eradication programs now in progress have been successfully concluded, until the lessons from those programs have been digested, and until the savings from polio eradication have begun to be realized.

Furthermore, there is at this time no candidate disease for which there is a sound scientific basis for eradication, for which the epidemiologic feasibility of doing so is clear, and for which there is a reasonable expectation of political commitment by both afflicted countries and those expected to provide the added resources.

REFERENCES

1. Henderson DA, deQuadros CA: The eradication of poliomyelitis (Albert Sabin Lecture). In Vaccines 95. New York, Cold Spring Harbor Laboratory Press, 1995, p 413.
2. Hopkins DR, Ruiz-Tiben E: Strategies for dracunculiasis eradication. Bull World Health Organ 69:533, 1981.
3. Chapin CV: What changes has the acceptance of the germ theory made in measures for the prevention and treatment in consumption? Fiske Fund Prize Essay. Providence, RI, Providence Press, 1888. Quoted in Soper FL: Rehabilitation of the eradication concept in prevention of communicable diseases. Public Health Rep 80:855, 1965.
4. Cockburn A: The Evolution and Eradication of Infectious Diseases. Baltimore, Johns Hopkins University Press, 1963.
5. Hinman EH: World Eradication of Infectious Diseases. Springfield, IL, Thomas, 1966.
6. Yekutiel P: Eradication of Infectious Diseases: A Critical Study. Basel, S. Karger, 1980.
7. Fosdick RB: The Story of the Rockefeller Foundation. New York, Harper, 1952.
8. Cort WN: Investigations on the control of hookworm disease. I: General introduction. Am J Hyg 1:557, 1921.
9. Strode GK (ed): Yellow Fever. New York, McGraw-Hill, 1951.
10. Duffy J (ed): Ventures in World Health. The Memoirs of Fred Lowe Soper. Washington, DC, Pan American Health Organization, 1977.
11. Guthe T: The treponematoses as a world problem. Brit J Venereal Dis 36:66, 1960.
12. Pampana EJ: A Textbook of Malaria Eradication. London, Oxford University Press, 1963.
13. Fenner F, Henderson DA, Arita I, et al: Smallpox and Its Eradication. Geneva, World Health Organization, 1988.
14. Dubos R: Man Adapting. New Haven, CT, Yale University Press, 1965.
15. Recommendations of the international task force for disease eradication. MMWR 42:1, 1993.
16. Henderson DA: Round table discussion: Lessons from the big eradication campaigns. World Health Forum 2:482, 1981.
17. Fine EM: Gaps in our knowledge about transmission of vaccine-derived polioviruses. Bull World Health Organization 78:358, 2001.
18. Bellmunt A, May G, Zell R, et al: Evolution of poliovirus type I during 5.5 years of prolonged enteral replication in an immunodeficient patient. Virology 265:178, 1999.
19. Sutter RW, Kew OM, Cochi SL: Poliovirus vaccine—live. In Plotkin SA and Orenstein WA (eds): Vaccines. Philadelphia, Saunders, 2004, p 651.
20. World Health Organization: Polio News. Geneva, March 2004.
21. WHO Collaborating Center for Dracunculiasis: Guinea Worm Wrap-Up No.142. Atlanta, GA, Centers for Disease Control and Prevention, April 12, 2004.
22. DeQuadros CA, Olive JM, Hersh BS, et al: Measles elimination in the Americas. JAMA 275:224, 1996.

8

Vector Biology

JOSÉ M.C. RIBEIRO
JESUS G. VALENZUELA

INTRODUCTION

Many parasites, from viruses to nematodes, are transmitted to humans by arthropod vectors, usually by blood-feeding ticks and insects. As noted in several chapters of this book, these invertebrates are important in transmitting some of the most devastating human diseases. Because parts of the life cycle of such parasites are dependent on the life cycle of the vector itself, understanding of the epidemiology and transmission dynamics of these diseases necessarily includes understanding the factors affecting the life cycle of their vectors.

Ticks are specialized mites related to spiders and thus arachnids (having eight legs in the adult stage). Insects are hexapods. Because of the many similarities in their life cycle and transmission of pathogens to humans and other vertebrates, medical entomologists lump ticks and insects as arthropod vectors in medical entomology textbooks.

Although in a few cases pathogens are transmitted mechanically from one host to another by vectors in their attempt to feed, the general rule is for the pathogen to develop an intricate life cycle within the vector host. This life cycle may take from several days to months (as with some tick-borne pathogens). The time taken for the parasite to complete the life cycle within its vector is called the *extrinsic incubation period*. The *intrinsic incubation period* is the time in the vertebrate from infection to the first appearance of symptoms. Some pathogens develop exclusively within the digestive tract of the vector, such as *Trypanosoma cruzi* or *Leishmania* spp., whereas others develop within several compartments of the vector. Thus, *Plasmodium*, *Theileria*, and *Babesia*, as well as most arboviruses, will eventually locate themselves within the salivary glands of the vector, after crossing the gut, disseminating into the hemolymph, and finally invading the salivary glands. Filarial worms, depending on the species, develop in different organs of the vector (muscle, coelomic fat body, or malpighian tubules) and exit the vector by puncturing through its mouthparts while the vector attempts to feed.

VECTOR LIFE CYCLE STRATEGIES

Most blood-sucking arthropods are oviparous, with the exception of some *Diptera* (including the tsetse), which are ovoviviparous (the egg hatches within the uterus and the larva feeds on secretions produced by milk glands). Two basically different growth strategies are observed: those having complete metamorphosis (*holometabolous*; Fig. 8-1) and those having incomplete metamorphosis (*hemimetabolous*; Fig. 8-2). Holometabolous insects follow the model of the butterfly, the caterpillar being very different from the adult animal. Hemimetabolous development follows the cockroach model, the immature animal being similar to the adult. In all cases, the immature animal feeds after coming out of the egg, and molts to a larger stage, shedding its old cuticle in a process called *ecdysis*. The newly emerged insect has a soft cuticle, ingests air or water, and enlarges itself before the cuticle hardens again. This feeding and molting process occurs from two to five times before the arthropod molts to an adult. Before molting to the adult, the general appearance of the insect or tick is similar (only larger) to the newly hatched animal. The last molt in hemimetabolous animals transforms the arthropod into an adult having sexually mature reproductive organs and fully developed wings (in species having wings, they are found only in the adult stage). Also, the adult cuticle is generally different from the immature cuticle. In holometabolous insects (all ticks are hemimetabolous), the last immature molt leads to a pupa, where metamorphosis to the adult stage occurs. All immature stages of holometabolous insects are called *larvae*, whereas all immature stages of hemimetabolous insects are called *nymphs*. In hard ticks (Ixodidae), there are two immature stages: the first is a larva and the second is a nymph.

Nymphs and adults of hemimetabolous insects and ticks thus have the same general appearance (varying in size), usually sharing the same habitat and feeding on the same types of food. However, larvae and adults of holometabolous insects are very different morphologically, have different habitats, and have different feeding habits. Immature and adult ticks, as well as nymphs and adult kissing bugs (triatomids) and bedbugs, all feed solely on blood, while larvae and adults of mosquitoes and sandflies feed on very different things, with only the adult female insect feeding on blood. Thus control of holometabolous insects involves two completely different strategies: those aimed at the immature and those aimed at the adult stages of the vector.

LIFE SPAN, REPRODUCTIVE CAPACITY, AND VECTOR ABUNDANCE

Insects and ticks also vary greatly in their life span and reproductive capacity. Mosquitoes, for example, can complete a life cycle within 1 to 2 weeks, while some ticks may take several years and even more than a decade if food is scarce. Additionally, a single female may produce only a few offspring (such as the tsetse), several hundred (mosquitoes), or thousands (ixodid ticks). Of course, most offspring of such insects never become adults, as only one female needs to achieve maturity to replace the preceding one and keep the vector population size constant. However, changes in the environment that make possible a larger number of larvae and nymphs to become adults can create explosive increases in vector abundance, and thus create epidemic conditions. In the case of mosquitoes, an unusually good rainy season may produce several generations resulting in a large number of adults. Ticks, with their longer life cycles, have populations that can fluctuate on a yearly basis, as can be the case with winter weather fluctuations in New England affecting the density of the deer tick, the vector of Lyme disease. Vector abundance normally exhibits a large variance both temporally and spatially, and this is reflected in the time and spatial dynamics of vector-borne diseases.

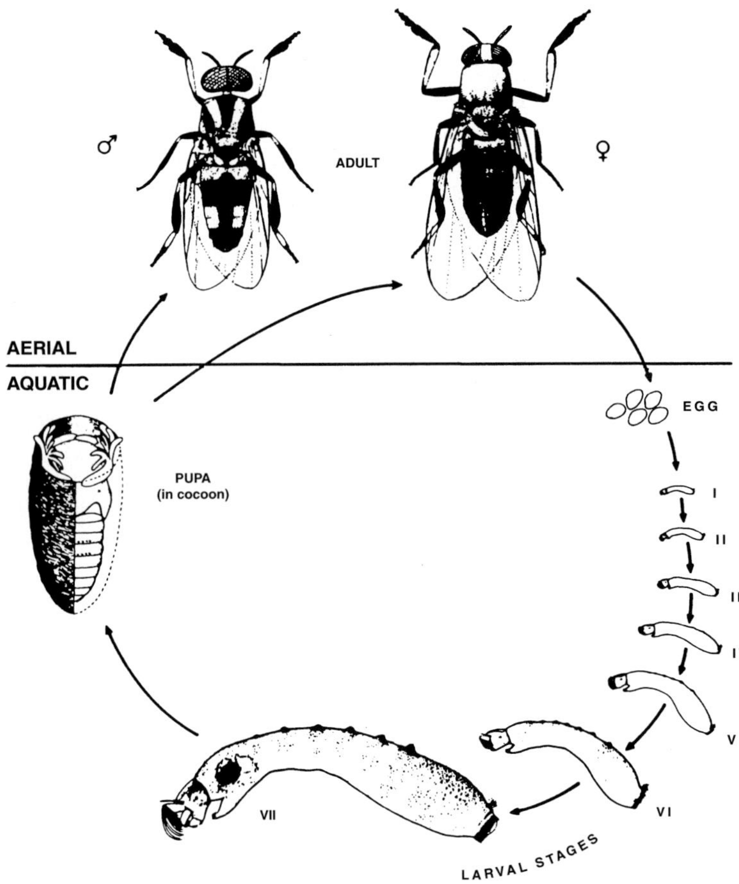

FIGURE 8-1 Life history of a holometabolous insect, represented by the life cycle of a black fly, *Simulium damnosum.* Note the very different aspects of immature and adult insects that share different habitats. (Modified from Beaty BJ, Marquardt WC: The Biology of Disease Vectors. Fort Collins, University Press of Colorado, 1996.)

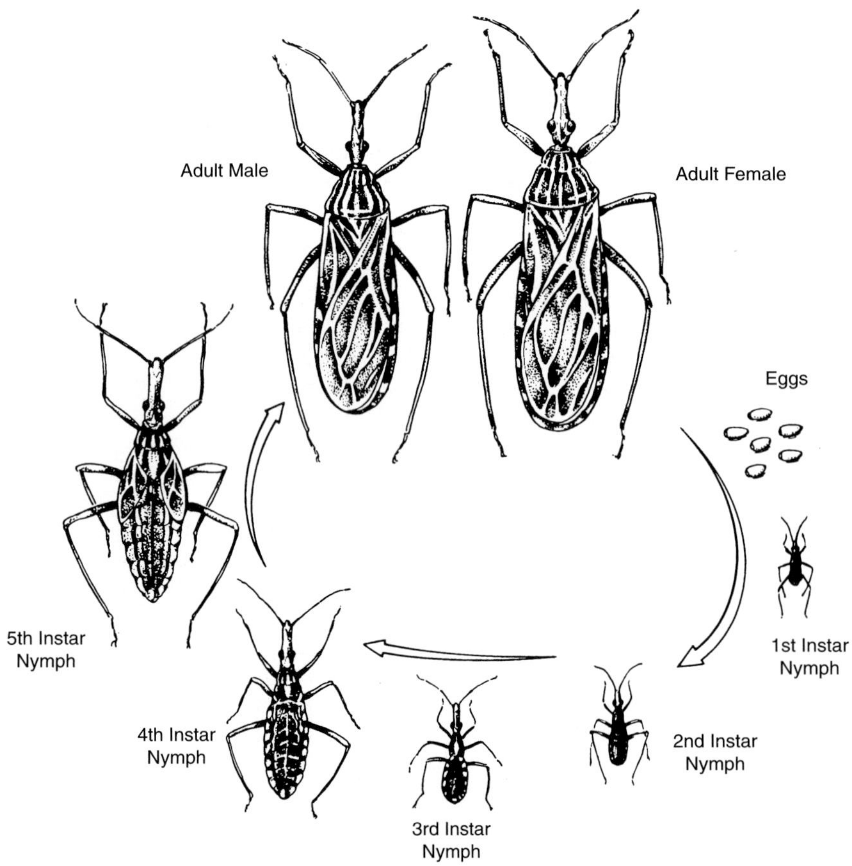

FIGURE 8-2 Life history of a hemimetabolous insect, represented by the life cycle of a triatomine bug, *Rhodnius prolixus.* Note the similar appearance of all instars, which also share the same source of food. (Modified from Beaty BJ, Marquardt WC: The Biology of Disease Vectors. Fort Collins, University Press of Colorado, 1996.)

The life span of a vector relative to the time taken for the parasite to complete its invertebrate life cycle is also very important for understanding the dynamics of vector-borne diseases. For example, most malaria parasites take at least one week to complete their life cycle in the adult female mosquito, but most mosquitoes die of old age before this amount of time. Thus, the longevity of the adult female mosquito is a very important variable determining how many secondary cases a single case of malaria can generate given a certain number of mosquitoes available per person. On the other hand, ticks can outlive most of their rodent hosts, and this can be very important in the perpetuation of viral diseases of short duration (e.g., diseases that either kill the host or to which the host becomes immune) in a small-sized rodent population.

HOST SPECIFICITY

There are two basic strategies followed by those animals that feed on vertebrate blood: a hunting strategy, where the insect actively searches for its prey (most blood-sucking arthropods are micropredators, not parasites), and an ambush strategy, where the insect or tick positions itself to maximize contact with its host or prey. The tsetse, horse fly, and mosquito are good hunters, whereas most ticks and fleas maximize ambush.

The limited size of the brain of invertebrate animals cannot deal with too much information and accordingly they select a group of very distinct variables to make a decision to attack what they think is a host. Visual cues, temperature gradients (including infrared "vision"), and olfaction will mediate host location. For example, some tsetse species are attracted by anything larger than a dog that moves at a certain speed (including a car), are even more attracted if the object smells like cattle urine, and are really excited over a warm surface. Carbon dioxide and water vapor are common attractants to many ticks and hematophagous insects. Recently, the smell of human feet (made possible by the same genus of bacteria that ferments Limburger cheese) was shown to be attractant to *Anopheles gambiae*, a highly anthropophilic (high specificity for feeding on humans) mosquito.

Hematophagous arthropods may become very host-specific or very catholic in their feeding habits depending on the location they choose to start their foraging as well as the cues that each species selects to identify a host. Host specificity is a very important concept for understanding the dynamics of vector-borne diseases, as they have a squared value in the equations of transmission dynamics. For example, a mosquito needs to feed once on a person with malaria to acquire the *Plasmodium* parasite and feed again on another person several days later to deliver the parasite. If only 50% of the population of a particular mosquito species would feed on humans, and only 50% of the mosquitoes feeding on the sick person acquire gametocytes (the parasite stage infectious for the mosquito), then only 50% of this 50%, or only 25% of the entire population, would then transmit the parasite to humans. *An. gambiae* mosquitoes feed almost exclusively on humans (greater than 98%), even when other sources of blood (e.g., cattle) are available, and this is one of the reasons this mosquito is such a good malaria vector. On the other hand, some vectors are relatively nonspecific, and they may become good bridge vectors for transferring zoonotic pathogens, such as *Ixodes scapularis* vectoring *Borrelia burgdorferi* from the white-footed mouse to humans.

VECTOR COMPETENCE

Vector-borne parasites can be very selective in the host species in which they complete development. For example, human malaria can be transmitted only by mosquitoes of the genus *Anopheles*. But there are anopheline mosquito species that serve very poorly or not at all in the invertebrate *Plasmodium* life cycle. This may be due to many biologic reasons varying from the time the mosquito peritrophic matrix is formed (a chitinous dialysis membrane-like structure that forms around the blood meal inside the mosquito gut that may serve as a barrier to the invading parasites), to the mosquito's ability to mount a melanotic reaction to the developing oocyst, and to the sporozoite's ability to find the mosquito salivary gland and survive the mosquito's hemolymph defense system. Other mosquitoes can develop heavy sporozoite infections of the salivary glands, even when feeding on lightly parasitemic hosts. This biologic ability of a vector to serve (or not) in the parasite's life cycle to its infective stage is called *vector competence*. It is actually expressed as the fraction of a particular vector population or species that can transmit the parasite after taking an infectious blood meal. In many cases the term *vector potential* is used synonymously with vector competence, mainly in a context where a potential vector species from a certain geographic area is being investigated for its ability to carry a parasite from another geographic area. For example, a medical entomologist from California may check whether local *Culex* mosquitoes are able to complete the life cycle of a virus found in Japan. The results of such tests of vector competence may indicate the potential for that particular Japanese viral disease to appear in California.

VECTORIAL CAPACITY

Even when determining that a particular arthropod species is competent for the parasite to complete its life cycle, this does not mean that such a vector will be important in maintaining disease transmission in the real world. For example, in the laboratory one may force a mosquito or tick to take a meal from a host it will never find or prefer to feed on in their habitat. Or the life span of the vector may be so short, compared to the extrinsic incubation period, that most of the vectors are dead before transmission occurs. Or the abundance of the vector may be so low that it will not sustain transmission of the pathogen in real-life conditions. To understand the role of a particular vector in the transmission of a particular pathogen, the concept of *vectorial capacity* was developed. Vectorial capacity includes not only the concepts of vector competence but also those of vector abundance, host specificity, vector longevity, and the time taken for the parasite to develop its life cycle within the vector (extrinsic incubation period). Vectorial capacity has a precise numerical meaning that represents the number of infective bites generated by a single case of a particular vector-borne disease, on a per day basis. This concept was developed by workers in the field of malariology and may be adapted to understand several other vector-borne diseases where vector survival is on the same order of magnitude as the extrinsic incubation period (this includes most mosquito–, sandfly–, black fly–, and flea-borne diseases).

In formal numerical terms the vectorial capacity equation can be expressed as:

$$VC = m \cdot a^2 \cdot b \cdot \{p^n/{-\ln p}\}$$

where VC is vectorial capacity (number of mosquito infective bites generated by a single parasitemic patient); m is number of mosquitoes available per person; a is human biting rate; b is vector competence; p is probability of the vector surviving one day; and n is extrinsic incubation period.

This equation can be understood in a very straightforward way by following each term and its relationship to the transmission dynamics of the parasite in the invertebrate host. It is obvious that the number of secondary disease cases of a mosquito-borne disease would be proportional to the number of vectors available per person (Fig. 8-3), that is, the more mosquitoes, the more chance of one case generating another case of malaria. The number of mosquitoes, however, has to be qualified regarding their host specificity, as described previously. If only 10% of the mosquitoes feed on a person, only a maximum of 1% could potentially deliver the parasite back to human hosts, because in order to transmit the disease they would have to feed again on people, assuming that on the second blood feeding the mosquitoes have the same chance of feeding on either a human host or another host (this is a nontested assumption of the MacDonald model!). Vectorial competence would further interfere with the ultimate number of infective bites, as not all vectors may develop the parasite to its infective stage (and that was why "a maximum of 1%" was written in the preceding discussion). The term p^n expresses the number of mosquitoes surviving the length of time associated with the extrinsic incubation period. When collected from the wild, mosquito mortality follows roughly an exponential decay curve,

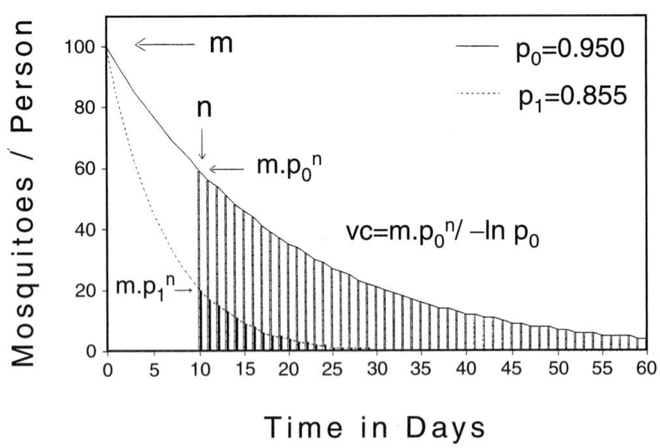

FIGURE 8-3 Graphical representation of two different sets of equal numbers of mosquitoes (100) biting a person infected with malaria at day 0. One set has a daily survival rate of 0.95 whereas the other set has a rate of 0.855. The human biting rate and vector competence are equal to 1 in both mosquito sets. Note that the two sets of mosquitoes die at different rates and continue to bite people without transmitting disease until *n* (extrinsic incubation period) days have elapsed. After this time interval, mosquitoes have infected salivary glands and surviving insects will produce infective bites. The total number of infective bites will be proportional to the number of mosquitoes surviving *n* days multiplied by their life expectancy in days. The result is equal to the vectorial capacity *(VC)* and is numerically equal to the marked areas under the curve. Note that a 10% change in the survival rate leads to a ninefold change in the vectorial capacity.

and thus the number of mosquitoes surviving *n* days would be exactly p^n. For example, if a mosquito has a 90% probability of surviving one day, then the number of mosquitoes that would survive 10 days would be 0.9^{10} or 34.9% of the initial mosquito population (see Fig. 8-3). Thus, at the end of the extrinsic incubation period, only a fraction of the vectors would be delivering the pathogen. However, even considering the number of mosquitoes that survive *n* days, these mosquitoes would not survive forever, and would continue to die. Because most infected mosquitoes do not have their mortality rate changed due to infection with the parasite, we can assume that the daily survival rate of such mosquitoes is still *p*. To calculate the number of infective bites delivered for the remainder of the life of the mosquitoes, one would have to integrate the area under the survival curve for those mosquitoes. We know from calculus that to calculate the area under an exponential with a rate *p*, the solution is $l/{-\ln p}$. Thus the area under the mosquito survivorship curve from day *n* (the extrinsic incubation period) until all mosquitoes are dead represents the vectorial capacity of a particular vector-pathogen association.

The preceding considerations are helpful in understanding the interrelationships of the several variables affecting the transmission dynamics of many vector-borne diseases. For example, it becomes clear that the main parameter affecting vectorial capacity is the term p^n, which has an exponential value. Some of the best mosquito vectors are long-lived when compared with other species. The human biting rate is a quadratic term, whereas mosquito abundance *m* and vector competence *b* are linear terms. Indeed, many poorly anthropophilic vectors such as *Anopheles albimanus* or *Anopheles culicifascies* will only transmit human malaria when they are extremely abundant (and thus the *m* term compensates for the lack of value on a^2). Similarly, *Aedes aegypti* is a poor vector for urban yellow fever in Nigeria (the virus strain was of sylvatic origin), having poor vectorial competence *b*, but when conditions favor extremely abundant mosquito numbers, epidemics have occurred.[1]

The parameters of the previous equation are an extreme simplification of what occurs in real life, but useful insights are obtained even when appreciating its limitations. Many of the terms are considered constants, but in real life they may be functions of other parameters. For example, the extrinsic incubation period changes with temperature; this is an important variable with most malarial and viral pathogens. Increased temperature may reduce incubation time significantly, increasing the vectorial capacity in larger proportion due to the exponential behavior of p^n. Similarly, increased humidity may significantly increase daily survival of mosquitoes (that otherwise may easily die of dehydration), also affecting vectorial capacity in an exponential fashion. The human biting rate of a particular vector species may also change with the repertoire of hosts in a given location. For example, many mosquitoes prefer cattle or horses for a blood meal, but when "progress" arrives and horses and cattle disappear, the same species may start to bite humans preferentially and create a condition for human disease transmission.[2]

BASIC REPRODUCTIVE RATE

To convert the vectorial capacity equation into the basic reproductive rate (R_0) of the particular disease, one has to include the terms that represent the life cycle of the parasite in the human host. These are represented by the number of days that the infection lasts in the vertebrate host, expressed by the disease recovery rate *r* (measured as the probability per day to revert to the nonparasitemic state), and by the probability *c* that the new secondary host will acquire the infection once bitten by the vector. We thus have

$$R_O = VC \cdot c/r$$

It is interesting to note the regulatory effect of vertebrate host immunity on R_O. The more time that a person stays sick (and thus the smaller the recovery rate *r*), the more mosquitoes are infected and the larger the disease R_O. However, in hyperendemic situations people acquire some immunity and the recovery rate is much faster (larger); also, the chance of getting infected by an infective bite (*c*) is smaller due to immunity. Both terms thus conspire to bring down R_O in hyperendemic conditions. Conversely, this is why it is difficult to accomplish sustained control of malaria in hyperendemic conditions: as herd immunity goes down, the disease reproductive rate fights back. In the process of controlling the disease (and thereby reducing immunity), the scenario may change from one of "calm" or "quiet" endemicity to one of severe epidemics.

VECTOR LONGEVITY

The preceding equations are useful for understanding the dynamics of vector-borne diseases when the vector is relatively short-lived with reference to the extrinsic incubation period of the particular pathogen. Other scenarios for transmission can happen where vector longevity, for example, is not an important issue. Ticks are often more long-lived than their vertebrate hosts, as is the case of most rodents. As seen in Chapter 3, population size is an important determinant of the perpetuation of many infectious diseases that leads to lifelong immunity. For example, it is postulated that a human population settlement of at least 200,000 people is necessary to produce enough nonimmune children to sustain measles. One can, however, envision a small population of rodents (fewer than 1000) and their ticks to sustain a virus that produces lifelong immunity by the "ping-pong" effect of the virus being shuttled from the vertebrate to invertebrate hosts on an annual basis. For example, let us imagine a rodent population in sub-Saharan Africa that typically breeds in the annual rainy season, and their ticks, which also feed on an annual cycle. During the rainy season, both larvae and nymphs feed on the rodents simultaneously for a period overlapping two months. Infected nymphs can transmit the virus to nonimmune rodents, and a few days later these rodents transmit the pathogen to larvae, which will feed again only in the next year (after molting to nymphs), when young, nonimmune rodents are available. A disease of short duration, without relapses, conferring lifelong immunity can thus perpetuate itself even within a host population of small size. The same reasoning applies in the absence of vectors if the pathogen can live long enough in the environment to reinfect young mice, as is the case with the North American hantavirus. Because rodents have a relatively short life span, they need a relatively small population size to keep diseases in an enzootic state for a pathogen. On the other hand, rodents can achieve very large population sizes, which makes the situation still worse. This may be one of the explanations for the continuous emergence of pathogens associated with rodent hosts; that is, rapidly generating rodents can maintain cycles of pathogens even when they induce lifelong immunity.

TRANSOVARIAL TRANSMISSION

Some vector-borne pathogens can be transovarially transmitted from the adult female to its offspring. Some mosquitoes can have a small or substantial portion of their eggs containing viruses that will continue their development in the mosquito larvae up to the adult stage. In this case, the first bite of the adult female may inoculate the pathogen into the vertebrate host. Transovarial transmission is often referred to as *vertical* transmission of a pathogen, to differentiate it from *horizontal* transmission, when one vector acquires a pathogen from a vertebrate host. *Sexual* transmission of mosquito-borne viruses was also demonstrated in some rare cases, where male (non–blood feeding) mosquitoes that were infected by the transovarial route could transfer the virus to females via copulation; this also occurs with African swine fever virus in argasid ticks.

In some cases, transovarial transmission of a pathogen is an essential feature of the pathogen life cycle. For example, bovine babesiosis (*Babesia bovis*) is transmitted by the cattle tick (*Boophilus microplus*), which is a single-host tick. *Boophilus* larvae attach to a host, staying with the same animal for life, until the adult female tick takes a large blood meal, drops off, lays thousands of eggs, and dies. There is no way of continuation of the *Babesia* life cycle without transovarial transmission of the protozoa from female to young larvae.

Transovarial transmission may be an important route for the perpetuation of other pathogens that are also transmitted horizontally. For example, a mosquito-borne virus causing epizootics or epidemics might lead to increased herd immunity of the vertebrate hosts that prevents further spread of the virus within the vertebrate population. The virus could perpetuate in nature during the interepidemic period by vertical transmission, until the herd immunity decreases again and a new invasion of the vertebrate population by the pathogen can occur. Even if vertical transmission is relatively inefficient (e.g., if only 10% or less of the offspring become infective), the large number of horizontally infected vectors during epidemic times could lead to a few vertically infected individuals after several mosquito generations, enough to initiate a new epidemic. This is again a case of the ping-pong transmission described previously for tick-borne pathogen scenarios, but due to the much shorter life of mosquitoes, vertical transmission allows for the pathogen to hide within vectors until vertebrate herd immunity goes down.

MODES OF VECTOR-BORNE DISEASE TRANSMISSION

In most cases vectors are not born with parasites they transmit, but rather they get infected while feeding on blood. Once reaching the vector's gut, parasites either continue to live there, such as *Leishmania* and *Trypanosoma*, or they cross the insect midgut epithelium into their vector's hemocoel, an open cavity between the digestive system and the cuticle, filled by hemolymph, the insect's blood, and other insect organs.

Once in the hemolymph, parasites such as *Plasmodium* and several arboviruses will infect their vectors' salivary glands. When vectors salivate into their hosts' skin in their attempt to obtain a blood meal, parasites are thus inoculated. Mosquito-borne parasitic worms can develop in the thoracic muscles, fat body, or Malpighian tubules of their vectors, where they develop to the infectious stage 3 larvae, when they leave the nursing organ back into the hemolymph. These worms are too big to invade the salivary glands, but while the vector is feeding, triggered by the sudden temperature increase, they puncture the vector cuticle actively moving into the vertebrate skin where they attempt to penetrate the tissue through the feeding wound. In many cases the worms just dehydrate before they can achieve their goal, and this is one of the reasons filarial transmissions such as *Wuchereria* are only found in humid places. Gut-dwelling parasites can be transmitted either when they are regurgitated into the vertebrate host, such as *Leishmania* and flea-borne plague, or they can be delivered in the vector feces, such as happens with American trypanosomes. Defecation while feeding is relatively common with vectors because of the relatively huge blood meal, which compresses the insect rectum, and also because of the very rapid water transport from the midgut to the hemolymph and from there to the rectum via the Malpighian tubules, the kidney equivalent in arthropods. Interestingly, desert-dwelling triatomines are not good vectors, because they conserve water so well that they end up not defecating on their hosts. However, rodent reservoirs may acquire the disease while eating the triatomines.

Role of Vector Saliva in Parasite Transmission

Most vector-borne parasites invade their vertebrate hosts in sites were the vector has injected saliva. In the case of salivary-borne pathogens such as malaria, it is important to stress that sporozoites are not delivered into the vertebrate host circulation, as most diagrams show, but rather are released inside the host skin, from where they actively move into the blood circulation. When mosquitoes reach a blood vessel, they suck the blood so fast that all sporozoites end up in the mosquito gut and are lost. *Leishmania* organisms, although not delivered via vector saliva, are delivered in the same wound where salivation occurs, thus the inoculation is coincident with a site exposed to their vector's saliva. Blood feeders' saliva contains an array of pharmacologically active components that assists them to obtain a blood meal. This salivary cocktail includes potent anticoagulants, anti-platelet molecules, vasodilators, and immunomodulators, allowing blood feeders to disarm the vertebrate's hemostatic and inflammatory system to their advantage. This pharmacologically modulated site may become a better location for pathogen establishment; in fact, *Leishmania major* parasites when co-injected into mice with sandfly saliva result in greater infection as compared to inoculation with parasites alone. The same phenomenon has been observed in transmission of viruses by ticks and mosquitoes.

Vertebrate immune responses generated to the bites of arthropod vectors can influence vector feeding and/or the efficiency of pathogen transmission. In the case of ticks, repeated feeding on non-natural hosts results in immune responses that lead to tick rejection. However, immune-mediated tick rejection does not occur, or is milder, when ticks feed on natural hosts. On the other hand, in the case of *Phlebotomus* sandflies, repeated feeding in mice results in delayed type hypersensitivity that causes sandflies to probe and feed faster in these animals. These immune responses, however, have a deleterious effect on some pathogens transmitted by vectors. Immune responses to *Ixodes scapularis* in natural and non-natural hosts result in protection against *Borrelia burgdorferi* infection. Similarly, immune responses to sandflies result in protection against *Leishmania major* infection, and a strong correlation exists between individuals generating immune responses to the sandfly *Lutzomyia longipalpis* and being protected against *Leishmania chagasi* infection. Therefore, in some vector-borne diseases, previous exposure to vector saliva may result in immune responses capable of preventing parasite transmission. It should be emphasized that probably not all immune responses to vector bites are protective against all vector-borne pathogens, as not all individuals respond identically to insect bites. The outcome probably depends on the biology of the pathogen in its vertebrate host. In the case of human malaria, for example, sporozoites tend to leave the bite site within minutes in their journey to the hepatocyte, and thus are not exposed for very long to immune effects of a sensitized skin. However, presentation of circumsporozoite antigen, which remains in the sporozoite trails, will occur in the context of antisaliva immunity. Therefore, the role of saliva in parasite transmission seems to be a two-edged sword phenomenon. In one case, salivary secretions favor the establishment of the pathogen or parasite in vertebrate hosts not previously exposed to salivary components. This enhancement effect may be due to the potent bioactive, anti-inflammatory and immunosuppressive properties of vector's saliva. On the other hand, salivary secretions may decrease transmission of pathogens and parasites in a vertebrate host previously exposed to vector salivary components. This outcome may be due to neutralization of the salivary bioactive components or to indirect killing of the pathogen by cellular immune responses to salivary proteins. Vector salivary secretions are therefore an important component in the transmission of pathogens or parasites and for this reason are being targeted as an alternative approach to control vector-borne diseases.

VECTOR IDIOSYNCRASIES

The following sections are summaries of the life cycle aspects of the most important vectors.

The order Diptera includes all flies, those insects containing only one pair of wings in the adult stage, and a pair of halters, which are atrophied wings. They are all holometabolous, usually having four larval stages or instars, one instar of a nonfeeding pupa, and finally the adult male and female. In some species of mosquitoes and many sandflies, larvae can withstand prolonged periods without food in diapause during the dry or cold season.

Mosquitoes

All larval instar stages of mosquitoes are aquatic. *Aedes* eggs are laid singly at the edge of the water; these embryonate and remain dormant until they are covered by water again.

Culex eggs are laid together in a raft on the surface of the water, while *Anopheles* eggs are laid singly on the water surface or on mud, hatching in both situations after a few days. The female mosquito, depending on the species, may choose either small containers or large bodies of water to lay her eggs. Also, the quality of the water chosen for oviposition will vary with the mosquito species. Usually *Aedes* and *Anopheles* mosquitoes will choose relatively clear water, as the larvae do not withstand much suspended organic matter or scum, whereas *Culex* mosquitoes will thrive in such environments. Thus urban *Culex pipiens* will develop in great numbers in pit latrines, while *Aedes (Stegomyia)* spp. may thrive in small containers containing drinking or rain water. Developmental time from egg to adult may take from 5 days to 3 weeks, depending on the species, temperature, and larval food supply. Only the adult female mosquito feeds on blood, which is used for egg development; usually more than 100 eggs are produced per blood meal. Both male and female mosquitoes take sugar-rich meals, which energize flight. Mosquitoes are vectors of many arboviral diseases such as dengue and yellow fever (transmitted by *Aedes* mosquitoes), malaria (only anopheline mosquitoes transmit human malaria), bancroftian filariasis (mainly by *Culex*, but also *Anopheles* mosquitoes), and brugian filariasis *(Aedes)*.

Sandflies

These insects belong to the family Psychodidae, which also contain the sewer flies. Sandflies are vectors of arboviral, bacterial *(Bartonella)*, and protozoal *(Leishmania)* human diseases. Immature sandflies are terrestrial, the larvae usually inhabiting mature, organically rich soil that has a composition similar to potting soil. Most vectors belong either to the New World genus *Lutzomyia* or to the Old World genus *Phlebotomus*. They may live within human dwellings, but are more commonly associated with peridomestic organic trash, rodent or other vertebrate nests, or forest soil. The immature life cycle of many important vector species is not known precisely. The time from egg to adult can be 45 days or longer depending on temperature. Some species have only one cycle per year, the third instar being the overwintering stage. Only adult female flies feed on blood, and both adults also feed on sugary solutions produced by aphids, fruits, or flower nectar. Adults do not fly well and show a typically "hopping" flight, close to the wall or another surface.

Black Flies

Black fly larvae are all aquatic and need moving water to feed. Most species attach to a substrate within a fast-moving plume of water, where they open their feeding fans to catch nutrients in the form of particulate organic matter. *Simulium neavei* is an important vector of onchocerciasis in central Africa and occurs in lakes where it is attached to the gills of crabs. The flow of water on the gills is sufficient for oxygen exchange in an otherwise calm body of water. Developmental time from egg to adult varies with temperature and species from 2 to nearly 4 months. Adults are good fliers and may disperse with the wind for many miles from their breeding site. Similarly to mosquitoes and sandflies, only the adult female feeds on blood.

Horse Flies and Deer Flies (Tabanids)

These large flies are vectors of *Loa loa* filariasis in West Africa and can also mechanically transmit equine infectious anemia virus between horses. Whether they can also transmit other viruses by mechanical transmission is yet unknown. Carnivorous larvae emerge from eggs deposited in moist grass and soil, where they feed on other insects, such as grubs. Male horse flies feed on vegetable material and do not bite. Females feed by making relatively large and painful cuts in the skin. The flies feed from the hematomas that accumulate in such lesions. They are usually not very efficient feeders, feeding several times per day, often flying directly from one host to another.

Tsetse

The tsetse (the word *tsetse* means fly destructive to cattle; thus the name tsetse fly is redundant) is an ovoviviparous vector of African trypanosomiasis. The female fly has a uterus wherein an individual egg hatches, the resulting larva feeding on secretions provided by milk glands. About every 10 to 15 days, the female fly deposits a large third instar, a larva that burrows into the ground and immediately pupates giving rise later (3 to 4 weeks, or longer) to another adult fly. Both male and female flies feed exclusively on blood. An adult female fly can at most produce six to eight such offspring, half of which are males. Tsetses thus have low reproductive capacity, and their population can be relatively easily controlled by trapping adult flies with ox urine–baited traps. Indeed, capture of 75% of the adult population can reduce the R_0 of the fly population to lower than unity and thus to local extinction. An equivalent effort for mosquitoes would require trapping of more than 95% of the adult population because of their larger reproductive capacity. Different species of tsetse have different host specificities (from crocodiles to wart hogs and humans), as well as different habitat requirements (dry savanna or riverine environments). Accordingly, each particular African trypanosomiasis scenario will be linked to the particularities of the bionomics and life cycle of the particular trypanosome vector.

Fleas (Siphonaptera)

These holometabolous organisms are always associated with the nest of their hosts, and thus a close relationship usually exists between a flea species and its host. This may explain why there are about 200 genera of fleas, while all remaining blood-sucking arthropods make up another 240 genera. Fleas are vectors of rickettsial (murine typhus) and bacterial (plague) pathogens. Also, fleas infected with *Yersinia pestis* develop a "blocked" gut, causing the flea to move from host to host and spread the bacterial pathogen. When the flea's natural zoonotic hosts start to die from disease, the hungry fleas may attack other host species, bridging the pathogen from an epizootic or enzootic to an epidemic cycle. Similarly, fleas that are left in empty burrows may attack anything that looks like food after a period of starvation. Both male and female fleas feed exclusively on blood. Females lay their eggs in the host's nest, the larvae feeding on a mix of organic material comprised of skin keratin mixed with dried host blood that is squirted from the anus of the adult flea while it feeds.

Thus small blood spots found in the bed linen of humans are an indication of flea-feeding activity.

Lice (Anoplura)

These are wingless hemimetabolous insects that live their entire lives associated either with human hair (*Pediculus humanus capitata)* or with the human body, where they stay attached to human clothes *(Pediculus humanus corporis)*. When laid, eggs are attached to hairs or clothes. All instars feed exclusively on blood. The insects are sensitive to a decrease in temperature, so the body variety will survive only in conditions where clothes cannot be washed and changed regularly, as is the case following social turmoil and in homeless populations. Only *P. humanus corporis* is incriminated as a vector of louse-borne typhus and louse-borne relapsing fever. The insecticide DDT was actually discovered in World War II in a program to discover novel pediculicides. The Allies were anticipating huge mortality from louse-borne typhus after the invasion of Italy.

Kissing Bugs (Hemiptera)

Hemiptera is the insect order with the common name of bugs (as flies represent the Diptera). The family Reduviidae has predacious, plant-feeding, and blood-feeding insects. All are hemimetabolous developing through five nymphal instars. The subfamily Triatominae comprises about 125 species in 15 genera, all having exclusively blood-feeding habits. Nymphs and adults live associated with nests, burrows, or habitations of their hosts. Kissing bugs can be very selective for their hosts; some are associated exclusively with birds, others with bats, and so on. Kissing bugs are vectors of *Trypanosoma cruzi*, the causative agent of Chagas' disease. This disease has a zoonotic cycle, as well as an endemic cycle. Thus, vectors maintaining the zoonotic cycle are associated with wildlife or domesticated animals, and vectors associated with human disease are found in the domestic environment. Other species may be found within the peridomestic environment, particularly in chicken pens, stables, woodpiles that harbor rodents, and so forth. Some species of the genera *Triatoma, Panstrongylus*, and *Rhodnius* are highly adapted to the human environment. Nymphs and adults take large meals of blood (5 to 10 times their own weight) in 10 to 30 minutes. They usually attack their victims while the host is sleeping, biting in the face, thus the name kissing bug, or *barbeiros* (barbers) in Portuguese, or *vinchuca* or *chincha* in Spanish. The large meal triggers a diuresis in the bugs, which then defecate while still feeding, depositing *T. cruzi* on its vertebrate host. The life cycle from egg to adult may take from less than 6 months to 2 years depending on the species. Some species (such as most *Rhodnius* spp.) may take only one meal to accumulate all the food they need to molt to the next instar. Others may take two or more meals per instar. *Rhodnius* may go from egg to adult in 6 months, having only 5 meals of blood, each blood meal taking less than 15 minutes. In 6 months of life *Rhodnius* feeds for a total of around 60 minutes before it molts to an adult. During the remaining time the bug is digesting its meal and hiding from predators. Adult females copulate once and are fertilized for life, laying their eggs in the same places in which they hide. Both male and females feed on blood, and may do so several times during adult life. Females lay about 30 eggs per blood meal. With so much time vulnerable to predators, hiding places are very important for kissing bugs. Most domestic species are associated with poor housing construction (mud and stick) that creates small holes and cracks in the walls (most *Triatoma* and *Panstrongylus*), or with dirt floors *(Triatoma dimidiata)*, or with thatched roofs (most *Rhodnius*). Accordingly, endemic Chagas' disease is highly correlated with poverty in rural areas of Central and South America.

Control of kissing bugs is relatively simple compared to that of other vector-borne diseases, and great progress has been made in the last 30 years in reducing domestic Chagas' disease transmission in South America. As zoonotic cycles continue to exist, Chagas' disease may disappear for a time in some areas only to reemerge later as favorable conditions reappear and a bridge from the sylvatic to the human disease cycle takes place. Accordingly, research emphasis on bugs is shifting from domestic species to those that are peridomestic and may serve as bridge vectors.

Ticks (Acari)

For medical entomologic purposes, we can consider ticks as coming in two varieties: hard (family Ixodidae) and soft (family Argasidae). All feed exclusively on blood, but can also produce hygroscopic saliva that captures moisture from the air. Thus these arthropods can survive long periods of time without desiccating. Indeed, some soft ticks can withstand years without a blood meal and without dehydrating. There is, however, a limit to the degree of air humidity at which the saliva can draw water from the atmosphere and this in great part limits the range of different tick species, both on a macro- and a microgeographic area.

Hard Ticks (Ixodidae)

Hard ticks have two immature stages, a six-legged larval stage and an eight-legged nymphal stage; the adults also have eight legs. Ticks are vectors of many arboviral, rickettsial, bacterial, protozoal, and even filarial organisms (the last not of human importance). Ticks can take huge meals compared to their size and stay attached to feed on their hosts for several days to weeks. Adult females take a single blood meal, drop off the host, and produce many hundreds to thousands of eggs before dying. Typically, larval ticks take microliter or submicroliter meals, nymphs will take several microliters, and an adult will take hundreds of microliters to over 1 mL of blood. Thus a mouse can serve well as a host to immature ticks, but a few adult ticks would exsanguinate the animal. Hard ticks can be classified as being one-, two-, or three-host species. For example, the cattle tick *B. microplus* is a one-host tick. Thus larvae coming from eggs deposited in the field ambush a cow and stay with the same animal for life. Two-host ticks will attach to a host as a larva, continue with the host after the nymphal molt, and detach from the vertebrate after the nymphal meal. They molt to adults in the environment and then quest for another host. This strategy allows the tick to use one set of hosts (usually smaller animals) for the immature stages, and another set (usually larger animals) for the adult stages. Many three-host tick species will feed on birds or rodents in their immature stages and on deer or other larger mammals as adults.

There are also three-host species associated with small vertebrates, but in this case the adult female takes smaller meals and lays a smaller number of eggs. Note that transmission of pathogens is potentially greater in three-host tick species, and that transovarial transmission is an important component to be considered.

Depending on the tick species, seasonality of the three life stages is also an important consideration for the transmission dynamics of tick-borne diseases. Seasonality may depend not only on temperature but also on weather cycles in which moisture levels fluctuate. If immature ticks feed on the same hosts at the same time, pathogens might be transmitted from nymphs to larvae. Sometimes larvae and nymphs may feed on the same type of hosts, but several months apart (a good tick strategy to prevent overburdening the food supply). In this case transmission of pathogens from nymphs to larvae would require a chronic infection of the vertebrate host, as is the case with Lyme disease (see the ping-pong effect discussed previously). Tick life cycles take typically less than a year to 2 years and may sustain the parasite in nature while herd immunity of short-lived mammals wanes.

Soft Ticks (Argasidae)

Soft ticks have a variable number of immature stages or instars depending on the species and availability of blood. Unlike hard ticks, which stay attached to their hosts for several days, soft ticks usually take meals lasting from a few minutes to one hour. Some tick species, such as *Ornithodoros coriaceus*, may produce in their hosts large and painful hematomas. Soft ticks are usually associated with nests or burrows of their hosts, or the places where host animals rest. They are vectors of arboviral and bacterial diseases, such as relapsing fever borreliosis.

Trombiculid Mites

These mites are not ticks, but, like ticks, are also acari. They can transmit rickettsial pathogens, such as *Orientia tsutsugamushi* (scrub typhus). Only the six-legged larvae of these mites feed on tissue fluid, nymphs and adults being predacious on other arthropods. Transovarial transmission of the pathogen is thus required for maintenance of disease foci.

VECTOR CONTROL

One can either kill vectors, or avoid their contact by various means, to prevent vector-borne diseases. Note that holometabolous insects have at least two different strategies for their control. One can perform larvicide or adulticide. Insecticides or other control agents will have to be delivered to different sites in the case of most holometabolous insects, depending on whether larvae or adults are being controlled. Malaria control is an example of holometabolous insect control. Malaria is transmitted by several anopheline mosquito species that have different breeding site preferences, different adult resting preferences, and different degrees of anthropophilic behavior. In the case of *An. gambiae*–transmitted malaria in sub-Saharan Africa, the mosquito breeds in small pools of clear, recently collected water, open to the sun for at least part of the day (old water usually contains a myriad of predatory insects, and it may be polluted too, two things that *An. gambiae* larvae dislike). Most of these water pools are associated with human activities, such as tire tracks, irrigation seepages, cattle hoofprints, and so on. Control of larvae in such conditions may be very difficult because of the scattered nature and small size of the sites. On the other hand, the mosquito *An. funestus*, which occurs in the same areas as *An. gambiae*, breeds in permanent bodies of water and avoids predators by hiding in the emerging vegetation. Cleaning of the edges of ponds or introduction of some fish species can provide some control of *An. funestus* breeding. However, both *An. gambiae* and *An. funestus* are very anthropophilic, and rest inside human dwellings, making this behavior amenable to the use of indoor insecticide spraying to kill the adult mosquitoes. Furthermore, one does not need to kill every mosquito as soon as it emerges. Because of the extrinsic incubation period, and because the daily mosquito survival rate is the most crucial parameter for vector capacity, just making life dangerous for the mosquito may reduce its longevity, and have a large impact on malaria transmission. This rationale was actually the basis for exclusive adulticide use of DDT during the malaria eradication attempt of the 1950s. In fact, use of DDT for larvicidal purposes was discouraged, because it would accelerate DDT resistance.

For indoor spraying with an insecticide, one has to make sure that the insect to be controlled is susceptible to the insecticide. The longevity of the insecticidal action on the treated surface varies with the insecticide used, and this factor is important in determining the periodicity and cost of the applications. There are many standardized tests and kits available from the World Health Organization for determining mosquito susceptibility.

Dengue is transmitted by *Ae. aegypti* and *A. albopictus* mosquitoes. These mosquitoes choose small containers with clean water for laying eggs. They lay their eggs singly just above the water line. The eggs embryonate and can sustain further desiccation for many months. When the container is again flooded, the larvae hatch and are the first insects to exploit the new environment. This is a good strategy for avoiding predators, and for being able to molt to the adult before the container dries again. The eggs have also made international trips in exported used tires, the probable mode of introduction of *Ae. albopictus* into the United States. *Ae. aegypti* prefers containers closely associated with humans, whereas *Ae. albopictus* will breed more in the peridomestic environment. In both cases, sanitation around human habitation, as well as changes in habits (such as emptying water in flower pots and other containers) can reduce mosquito breeding. Indoor spraying for *Ae. aegypti* is also effective, but is not so useful for the more exophilic biter *Ae. albopictus*.

Bancroftian filariasis is transmitted by many species of mosquitoes, but the main vector worldwide is *Culex pipiens quinquefasciatus*. Unlike the mosquitoes mentioned previously, *C. pipiens quinquefasciatus* can survive and thrive in highly organic polluted waters that would kill by suffocation any *Aedes* or anopheline larvae. *Culex* larvae have a strong and long siphon tube that allows them to break through the scum of such breeding sites. Indeed, pit latrines and sewers can lead to breeding of enormous numbers of *Culex* mosquitoes, which can make good use of the organic residue. Sanitation measures as well as larvicides can be of use to control such mosquitoes.

Control of river-dwelling black fly larvae involves the introduction of insecticides at regular intervals in rivers and streams, making it important to use appropriate doses of these chemicals to prevent damage to other aquatic life. Great improvement in onchocerciasis control in west Africa was achieved by a coordinated multinational effort in treating most of the Volta River basin.

On the other hand, control of Chagas' disease–transmitting bugs is achieved with indoor residual spraying, which kills all stages of the vector. These bugs also need hiding places such as crevices (common in mud and stick houses) to avoid predators (ants, spiders, birds, rodents—it is a dangerous world for bugs out there). Improvement of economic conditions contributes substantially to Chagas' disease control. Chagas' disease control has been very successful in South America where vector transmission in Brazil was enormously reduced following indoor spraying, together with economic and population changes.

In order to avoid vectors, one can modify human behavior or use chemicals or devices to block vector–human contact. Most vectors have a particular time of day when they search for a meal. Some mosquitoes (such as *Ae. aegypti*) prefer to bite at daybreak or sunset, whereas others (such as *C. pipiens*, *An. gambiae*, and *An. dirus*) prefer to bite in the middle of the night. Planning of human activities around these times may pay off greatly. The British in Southeast Asia during World War II never fought by night and avoided malaria, whereas the Japanese troops became severely malarious by going into the forest at a time when *An. dirus* fed.

Repellents are substances that prevent landing, or probing, and feeding by vectors. Some of these substances possibly act by exciting all chemical receptors in the vectors, so the insect does not know what is occurring, rather than being repelled by a noxious substance. A good repellent has to be volatile, which makes it last a shorter time, and thus frequent applications may be needed for effective control. Some repellents are toxic to children and should be used with care.

Physical means of prevention include house screening and bednets for nighttime-biting vectors. Recently bednets were shown to be more efficient when impregnated with pyrethroid insecticides, and large-scale trials of impregnated bednets for malaria control are being completed. Impregnated bednets are actually an insecticide target device, as the human inside the net acts as bait for the mosquitoes.

It is important to remember that vectors vary considerably in their breeding site choices, as well as in their preferred resting and biting places, and these factors must be taken into consideration for control measures.

REFERENCES

1. Miller BR, Monath TP, Tabachnick WJ, et al: Epidemic of yellow fever caused by an incompetent mosquito vector. Trop Med Parasitol 40:396–399, 1989.
2. Dye C: Approaches to vector control: New and trusted. 5. The epidemiological context of vector control. Trans R Soc Med Hyg 88:147–149, 1994.

ADDITIONAL READING

Beaty BJ, Marquardt WC: The Biology of Disease Vectors. Fort Collins, University of Colorado Press, 1996.

Lane RP, Crosskey RW: Medical Insects and Arachnids. New York, Chapman & Hall, 1993.

Lehane MJ: Biology of Blood Sucking Insects. London, Harper Collins Academic, 1991.

9

Animal Poisons in the Tropics

ROBERT L. NORRIS
PAUL S. AUERBACH

The word *tropical* often conjures up visions of mysterious and deadly creatures creeping or slithering through lush vegetation. What adventure movie or documentary about the jungle is complete without a snake, spider, or scorpion? Hazardous tropical creatures also lurk in the ocean surf and among exotic coral reefs. For most travelers to tropical environments, however, venomous creatures are more of a perceived threat than an actual danger. It is the native human populations in tropical regions of the world on which these creatures take their greatest toll. The purpose of this chapter is to provide a practical overview of the planet's most important terrestrial and marine venomous animals and their poisons. The clinical syndromes that may be anticipated and approaches to management are outlined.

Venomous Snakes

There are approximately 3000 species of snakes, with just over 10% considered dangerously toxic to humans.[1] Venomous snakes are divided into five families, as listed in Table 9-1. All tropical and subtropical and most temperate regions of the world can boast at least one species of venomous snake (Plate 9-1). Notable exceptions include New Zealand, Madagascar, Hawaii, and most of the West Indies.[2]

It is difficult to establish the incidence of venomous snakebite in the world owing to a paucity of reliable data from developing countries. The best estimate to date of worldwide mortality due to venomous snakes comes from a World Health Organization (WHO) report, which suggested 30,000 to 40,000 deaths per year.[3]

SNAKE VENOM AND THE VENOM APPARATUS

Snake venoms, produced in modified salivary glands in the upper jaw and injected through hollow or grooved fangs, are some of the most complex naturally occurring toxins known. Most contain a mixture of proteins (including enzymes), low-molecular-weight (nonenzymatic) polypeptides, metallic ions, and other substances that continue to be researched.[1] To avoid underestimating the potential of any particular snake's venom, one must recognize the complexity of these toxins and anticipate multisystemic manifestations, as in the following discussion.

Viperid venoms (from the family Viperidae) tend to be rich in enzymes such as phospholipase A_2, which adversely affects a variety of cell membranes and metalloproteinases, which directly or indirectly promote coagulopathy, hemorrhage, swelling, and necrosis.[1,4,5] Many of the more lethal fractions of viperid venoms are low-molecular-weight polypeptides that act as neurotoxins, cardiotoxins, myotoxins, and hemotoxins.[1] Although elapid venoms (from the family Elapidae) tend to be simpler in composition than those of the viperids, they are extremely potent, especially in terms of neurotoxicity. Elapid neurotoxins can be divided into those that act presynaptically by inhibiting neurotransmitter release and, more commonly, those that act postsynaptically by blocking acetylcholine effects.[6,7] A number of elapid venoms, especially from several species of spitting cobras, do contain enzymatic components that can cause tissue necrosis.[8] Sea snake venoms all appear to be very similar and contain components with highly potent neurotoxins and myotoxins.[9] The venoms of the burrowing asps (family Atractaspidae) and colubrids (family Colubridae) are more poorly studied at this time. It has become clear, however, that some species of Colubridae, a family of snakes largely thought of as being nonvenomous, are dangerously toxic to humans. These include the boomslang (*Dispholidus typus*), the twig snake (*Thelotornis kirtlandii*), and the Asian keelback snakes (genus *Rhabdophis*).[10]

Clinical Findings

A summary of potential clinical manifestations following venomous snakebite is presented in Box 9-1.[1,11–14] It is important to keep in mind, however, that snake venom poisoning is a complicated disorder that brings into play a number of variables that determine the clinical manifestations and severity of venom poisoning. Such variables include the composition of the snake's venom (which can vary not only by species but also by age, health, and geographic origin of the snake), the factors that led to the bite, and the victim's overall health and body size.[1] It is interesting to note, however, that venomous snakes often bite without injecting any venom. Such "dry bites" occur in approximately 20% to 30% of viperid bites, 50% of elapid bites, and up to 75% of sea snake bites.[15]

Management

First-aid management of venomous snakebite should be aimed at delivering the victim expeditiously to definitive medical care. Beyond that, measures should ideally be judged on their risks vs. benefits. Unfortunately, conclusive studies regarding field management measures for venomous snakebites are sorely lacking. Clearly, however, many techniques recommended in the past are of no proven benefit and may actually worsen the clinical outcome. Examples include incising the bite site, or applying local ice, heat, tourniquets, or electric shocks.[1,16] The victim should be calmed as much as possible, and the bitten extremity can be splinted to limit movement in an effort to reduce pain. While use of mechanical suction has been recommended for many years, evidence suggests that this technique is unable to remove any significant amount of venom from the depot site.[17,18] Furthermore, there is now evidence that mechanical venom extraction devices can cause additional harm to the local tissues.[19]

Table 9-1 Important Venomous Snakes of the World

Family	Subfamily	Genus	Examples and Comments
Viperidae	Viperinae		Old World vipers; Europe; Asia; Africa
		Bitis	
		Vipera	
		Echis	
	Crotalinae		Pit vipers; North, Central, South America; Asia
		Crotalus	Rattlesnake (see Plate 9-1A)
		Agkistrodon	North American cottonmouth, water moccasin, and copperhead
		Bothrops	Central and South American lancehead pit viper
		Trimersurus	Asian pit viper
Elapidae			Old and New World; All Australian terrestrial venomous snakes
		Naja	Cobra (see Plate 9-1B)
		Dendroaspis	Mamba (see Plate 9-1C)
		Bungarus	Krait
		Micrurus	Coral snake (see Plate 9-1D)
		Micruroides	Coral snake
		Oxyuranus	Taipan
		Pseudechis	Australian black snake
		Pseudonaja	Australian brown snake
		Acanthopis	Death adder
Hydrophidae			
	Hydrophinae		Sea snake
	Laticaudinae		Sea krait
Atractaspidae			Burrowing asp
Colubridae			A small percentage of this classically "nonvenomous" family bears rear fangs and modified salivary glands that are, in some cases, capable of causing severe envenomation in humans
		Dyspholidus typus	African boomslang
		Thelotornis kirtlandii	African twig snake, vine snake

Box 9-1 Clinical Findings Following Venomous Snakebite

Viperids (Vipers and Pit Vipers)

Signs and Symptoms

- Pain (often "burning"; may be severe; onset usually very early)
- Soft tissue swelling (may be rapidly progressive; usually confined to subcutaneous tissues)
- Nausea and vomiting
- Diaphoresis
- Ecchymosis/petechiae/purpura
- Hemorrhagic blebs, serous vesicles
- Necrosis
- Bleeding (at essentially any anatomical site)
- Difficulty breathing (due to pulmonary edema or neurotoxicity)
- Bradycardia/tachycardia
- Hypotension/hypertension
- Muscle fasciculations
- Paresthesias
- Muscle paresis/paralysis (uncommon with most viperids)

Laboratory Abnormalities

- Complete blood count: increased hematocrit due to hemoconcentration; decreased hematocrit due to bleeding/hemolysis; decreased platelets (due to consumption); leukocytosis
- Coagulation studies: often abnormal, consistent with consumptive coagulopathy
- Urine: hematuria, myoglobinuria, proteinuria
- Arterial blood gases: in severe cases, hypoxemia, metabolic acidosis
- Others: occasional hyperglycemia and abnormal chemistries consistent with renal dysfunction, liver injury, rhabdomyolysis, cardiac injury

Elapids

Signs and Symptoms

- Pain (may be absent); paresthesias/numbness at bite site
- Soft tissue swelling (usually less than with most viperids)
- Difficulty breathing (due to neurotoxicity)
- Nausea and vomiting
- Diaphoresis
- Muscle fasciculations
- Cranial nerve dysfunction
- Muscle paresis/paralysis (including muscles of respiration)

Laboratory Abnormalities

- Complete blood count: leukocytosis
- Arterial blood gas analysis: in severe cases, hypoxemia, respiratory acidosis

Hydrophids (Sea Snakes)

Signs and Symptoms

- Similar to elapids, plus significant muscle pain

Continued

Box 9-1 Clinical Findings Following Venomous Snakebite—Cont'd

Laboratory Abnormalities
- Chemistries: may demonstrate renal dysfunction (risk of severe hyperkalemia), rhabdomyolysis

Atractaspids (Burrowing Asps)

Signs and Symptoms
- Very similar to viperid venom poisoning, but tend to be less severe

Laboratory Abnormalities
- Coagulation studies: may be prolonged/abnormal
- Serum chemistries: may reveal evidence of liver dysfunction
- Arterial blood gases: hypoxia, hypercarbia
- Electrocardiography: conduction abnormalities

Colubrids

Signs and Symptoms
- Local pain
- Soft tissue swelling
- Ecchymosis
- Lymphadenopathy
- Paresthesias
- Gingival bleeding, epistaxis, hematuria, melena, subcutaneous hemorrhage

Laboratory Abnormalities
- Serum chemistries: may be consistent with renal failure
- Coagulation studies: depletion of fibrinogen and platelets; increased fibrin degradation products
- Urine: hematuria

Another previously recommended first-aid technique was the use of a broad constriction band, applied several inches proximal to the bite to occlude superficial venous and lymphatic return without impeding arterial flow. While there is some evidence that this may limit systemic spread of venom,[20] it may worsen distal swelling and potentially increase local necrosis in viperid bites. If a victim is in a remote area and has been bitten by a potentially lethal snake, the best course of therapy would be application of pressure-immobilization (PI)—a technique pioneered by the Australians and illustrated in Figure 9-1.[21] PI has been demonstrated to reduce venom absorption in animal models of elapid and pit viper snakebite,[22,23] and has been reported anecdotally effective in some human cases.[24–27] It should be realized, however, that strict limitation of venom to the depot site could increase local wound damage. In such a case, the local tissues and perhaps even the extremity may be being sacrificed in an effort to save the victim's life. There is evidence that individuals at risk for snakebite should receive special training on the use of PI to increase the likelihood that it will be applied appropriately if needed.[28]

Hospital management of venomous snakebite begins with sound supportive care. Attention should initially be focused on the victim's airway, breathing, and circulation. Cardiac and pulse oximetry monitoring (if available) should be instituted and intravenous (IV) access should be obtained as soon as possible. Following serious bites by many elapids, respiratory failure due to neuromuscular toxicity can be a problem. If victims show any evidence of respiratory distress or difficulty swallowing or handling secretions, the airway should be protected without delay by endotracheal intubation and their respirations should be supported. Hypotension, often due to venous pooling of blood, should be treated initially with crystalloid infusion. If the blood pressure fails to respond to 20 to 40 mL/kg of crystalloid, then albumin should be added to the resuscitation fluids since it may remain in the leaky vasculature for a longer period of time.[29] Only after an adequate trial of fluid resuscitation should vasopressor agents be added. Blood samples should be drawn for appropriate laboratory studies to include complete blood counts, serum chemistries, renal and liver function studies, coagulation profiles, and typing and screening.

After any immediately life-threatening issues are addressed, a more detailed history can be obtained and an attempt made to identify the offending reptile. If the snake has been brought in with the patient, it should be handled with care, for even a decapitated head can have a bite reflex for up to 1 hour.[30,31] In some regions of the world, such as Australia, aid in identifying the offending species comes in the form of snake venom detection kits, which use a colorimetric, enzyme-linked immunosorbent assay (ELISA) technique to identify the presence of venom in serum, urine, or bite site drainage.[32,33]

The bitten extremity should be marked at two or more sites and the circumferences checked every 15 minutes until it is clear that there is no swelling or that all swelling has stabilized. If any device was used on the extremity in the field in an effort to limit venom spread, caution needs to be used during its removal to prevent the sudden release of venom and lactic acid into the central circulation. If a tourniquet was applied, it should be immediately replaced with a proximal, more loosely fitting constriction band in order to get blood flowing back into the extremity. IV access should be obtained before final removal of any constriction band or pressure-immobilization device. If systemic signs or symptoms of venom poisoning are already present, appropriate antivenom administration should be started before device removal (see later discussion). If systemic signs or symptoms develop after a pressure-immobilization device is removed, the device should be reapplied until antivenom can be started.[34]

Antivenom is the primary therapeutic agent for treatment of snake venom poisoning. The decision to administer antivenom is based on the severity of the victim's symptoms, signs, and laboratory abnormalities. If systemic toxicity is evident, envenomation is at least moderate in severity and the need for antivenom is established. If there are no systemic abnormalities and local findings are minimal (and stable) or absent, then the envenomation is probably mild (or lacking altogether) and antivenom can generally be withheld. Care must be exercised in making these decisions as snake venom poisoning is a dynamic process, and a case that presents as an apparent mild poisoning or even dry bite can progress with time to become severe and life threatening. This is especially true for victims of some sea snake, elapid, and colubrid bites, in whom the onset of symptoms may be delayed for hours.[35,36]

Bites to the lower limb	
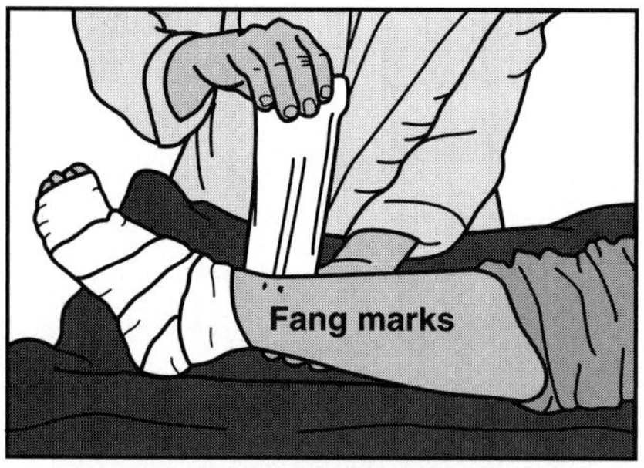	1. Apply a broad pressure bandage over the bite site as soon as possible. Crepe bandages are ideal, but any flexible material may be used. Clothing, towels, etc. may be torn into strips. Pantyhose have been successfully used. Do not take off clothing, as the movement of doing so will promote the movement of venom into the bloodstream. Keep the bitten limb, and the patient, still. Bandage upward from the lower portion of the bitten limb. Even though a little venom may be squeezed upward, the bandage will be more comfortable, and therefore can be left in place for longer if required.
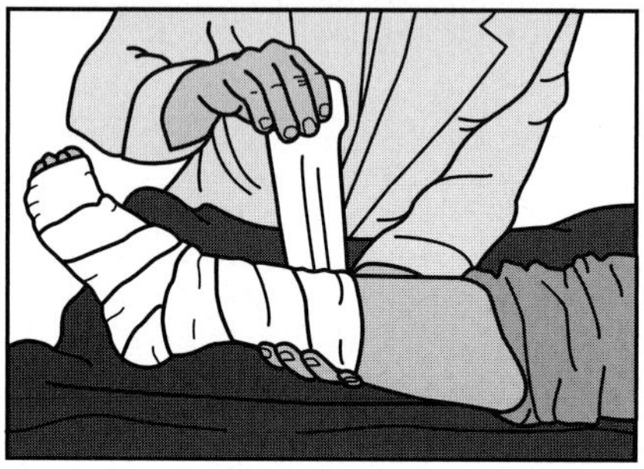	2. The bandage should be as tight as you would apply to a sprained ankle.
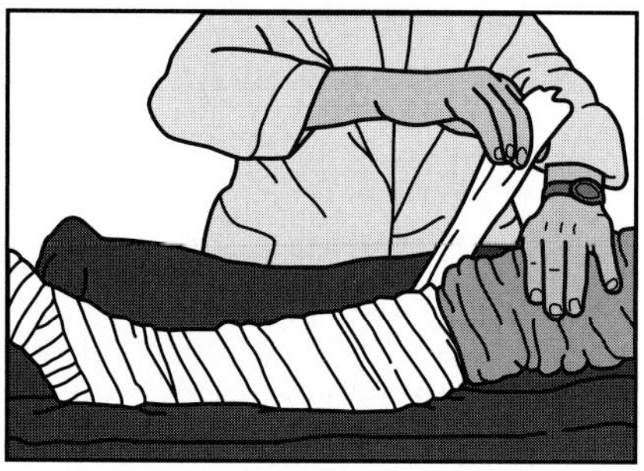	3. Extend the bandage as high as possible up the limb.
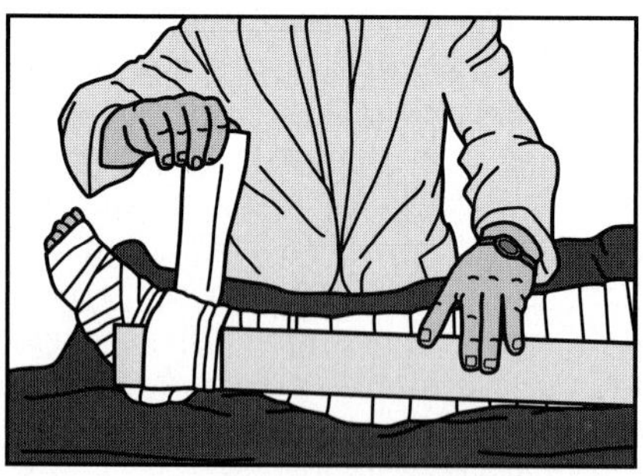	4. Apply a splint to the leg. Any rigid object may be used as a splint: spade, piece of wood or tree branch, rolled up newspapers, etc.
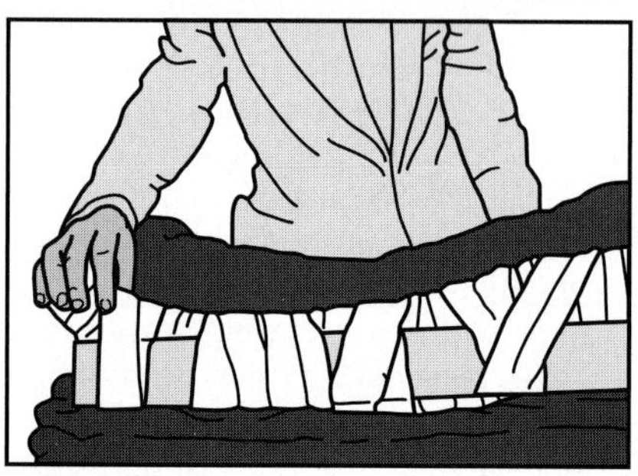	5. Bind it firmly to as much of the leg as possible. Keep the patient still. Lay the patient down to prevent walking or moving around.

FIGURE 9-1 The Australian pressure-immobilization technique for field management of bites and stings by venomous snakes, funnel-web spiders, dangerous scorpions, the box jellyfish, cone snails, and the blue-ringed octopus. (Used with permission from Dr. Ken Winkel, Director, Australian Venom Research Unit, Department of Pharmacology, University of Melbourne [www.avru.org].)

(Continued)

Bites to the hand or forearm	
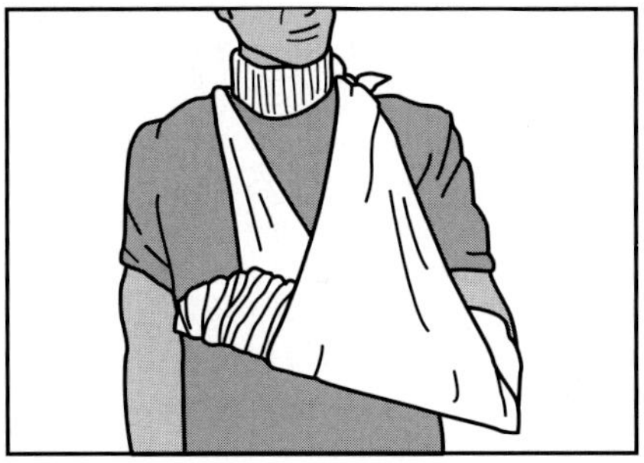	Bandage as much of the arm as possible, starting at the fingers. Use a splint to the elbow. Use a sling to immoblize the arm. Keep the patient still. Lay the patient down to prevent walking or moving around.
Bites to the trunk	If possible apply firm pressure over the bitten area. Do not restrict chest movement. Keep the patient still.
Bites to the head or neck	No first aid for bitten area. Keep the patient still.

FIGURE 9-1 Cont'd.

Antivenoms are either monovalent (covering a single species) or polyvalent (providing coverage for multiple species). An example of a wide-spectrum, polyvalent product is CroFab (Savage Laboratories, Melville, NY), which provides excellent coverage for all North American pit vipers and may be protective in bites by some Central and South America species as well.[37] With few exceptions, there is little to be gained by administering an antivenom that is not designed for use against the offending snake species. A notable exception to this is the efficacy of Australian tiger snake (*Notechis scutatus*) antivenom for sea snake envenomations.[38]

All currently available snake antivenoms are produced from either horse or sheep serum and therefore carry some risk of allergic phenomena (anaphylactic or anaphylactoid reactions or serum sickness; see later discussion). While some (but not all) antivenom manufacturers suggest an intradermal test to predict possible allergy to their products, the sensitivity and specificity of such skin tests are poor.[31,39,40] If a patient has a serious bite and clearly needs antivenom, administration should start without waiting the 20 to 30 minutes it takes to apply and read a skin test.

Before giving antivenom, informed consent should be obtained from the patient when possible and an appropriate dose of epinephrine should be drawn up at the bedside for use in the event of an anaphylactic/anaphylactoid reaction. The patient's intravascular volume should be expanded with crystalloid fluids if his or her cardiovascular status permits.[41] Patients can be premedicated with IV antihistamines (both H_1 and H_2 blockers) if the risk of allergy is felt to be particularly high (as with the use of some less purified products containing more extraneous heterologous proteins, or in a patient with a known allergy to horses or sheep). Premedicating with steroids is of no benefit due to their delayed onset of action.

Snake antivenom should always be given IV, as there is no benefit to local administration,[42] and intramuscular injection results in slower and lower levels of circulating protective antibodies.[43] Guidelines for appropriate starting doses of antivenom can be obtained from product package inserts. The dose to be given should be diluted in approximately 250 to 1000 mL of 5% dextrose in water or saline (approximately 20 mL/kg for young children). The infusion is started very slowly with the physician at the bedside to intervene immediately if an adverse reaction occurs. If the serum is tolerated during the first several minutes of infusion, the rate is increased to complete the infusion in 1 to 2 hours. Further antivenom may be necessary depending on the progression of clinical findings or laboratory abnormalities that might occur following the initial dose. Some manufacturers recommend scheduled redosing of antivenom once initial control of poisoning has been obtained.[44] When adequate antivenom has been administered, the patient generally begins to feel subjectively better and clinical findings stabilize or normalize.

If an anaphylactic/anaphylactoid reaction to the antivenom should occur, the infusion should be immediately halted and the reaction treated in standard fashion with fluids, epinephrine, and further antihistamines as necessary. In this setting, steroids should be given to blunt any delayed second-phase allergic reaction that might occur.[45] Once the reaction is halted, antivenom can often be restarted if necessary based on the severity of venom poisoning.[31] In this scenario, it may help to further dilute the antivenom and run the infusion at a slower rate.

When a victim of severe venom poisoning develops an acute allergic reaction to antivenom, the physician has two choices. Antivenom can be withheld with reliance on supportive care alone. Alternatively, the patient can be placed in an intensive care setting with invasive hemodynamic monitoring and antivenom can be slowly administered while suppressing the reaction with a titrated epinephrine infusion.[46] Consultation with an allergist or toxicologist is helpful. Attempting to desensitize the patient with gradually increasing doses of antivenom is too protracted a process to be beneficial.[31]

Wound care of the bite site includes splinting the extremity with cotton padding between the digits and elevating if soft tissue swelling is present. Tetanus status should be updated as necessary. Prophylactic antibiotics are not necessary.[1,47,48]

Hemorrhagic blebs or serous-filled vesicles should be debrided at 3 to 5 days.[49] Physical therapy is vital to optimal functional recovery and should begin as soon as the patient's condition allows.

Most swelling in snakebites is localized to the subcutaneous tissues. In some cases, however, (especially bites by larger viperids) venom may be deposited deeper into muscle compartments, causing swelling within the confined space.[1] A swollen, ecchymotic, painful extremity may suggest an impending compartment syndrome. In such cases, intracompartmental pressures (ICPs) should be objectively measured (e.g., with a wick catheter). If ICPs exceed capillary perfusion pressure (i.e., greater than approximately 30 mm Hg in a normotensive patient), the extremity should be elevated, antivenom should be given, and a trial of IV mannitol (1 g per kg body weight) can be given (if the patient's blood pressure is adequate). If the victim's ICPs do not return to an acceptable range within one hour of such therapy, a fasciotomy is indicated. Fortunately, this is rarely required.[50]

All patients with evidence of venom poisoning should be admitted to the hospital. Whenever possible, patients who require antivenom or have the potential for sudden cardiovascular or respiratory decompensation should be admitted to an intensive care setting. Owing to the delay in onset of clinical findings with many elapid, sea snake, and some dangerous colubrid species, any victim bitten by one of these should be observed for 24 hours. Following viperid bites, reliable victims who are totally asymptomatic with normal clinical and laboratory findings after 6 hours of observation can be discharged with a responsible adult and instructions to return immediately if symptoms appear. Admitted patients should be closely observed and laboratory values should be rechecked every few hours until stable. Each time the victim voids or defecates, bedside tests to rule out occult blood (as a sign of coagulopathy) should be performed.

At discharge, all victims who received antivenom should be warned of the signs and symptoms of serum sickness. If these occur, they should be treated with steroids until all findings resolve, followed by a weeklong taper. Antihistamines and analgesics may be helpful for symptomatic relief. Any victim who developed a coagulopathy during the acute stage of venom poisoning should be warned that coagulopathy can recur for up to two weeks following envenomation.[51] Such patients should watch for any signs of clinical bleeding and avoid any unnecessary surgery for the next few weeks.

Venomous Lizards

There are only two species of venomous lizards in the world, the Gila monster (*Heloderma suspectum*) and the Mexican beaded lizard (*Heloderma horridum*; Plate 9-2). Gila monsters are found from the southwestern United States into northern Mexico, while beaded lizards are located from central to southern Mexico.[52]

The anatomy, habits, and venoms of these two species are similar, though *H. horridum* reaches substantially larger sizes than does *H. suspectum*. The venom apparatus consists of a pair of multilobar glands in the anterior aspect of the lower jaw with ducts that conduct venom to the bases of teeth on the anterior mandible.[14,53] These loosely attached teeth are grooved to facilitate envenomation. When biting, the lizard may hang on tenaciously and chew, and teeth may be left behind in the wounds. The venom, less complex than most snake venoms, contains hyaluronidase, phospholipase A, proteases, kallikrein, and serotonin.[14,53]

Signs and symptoms of helodermatid venom poisoning may include severe, immediate pain; mild to moderate soft tissue swelling; lymphangitis; local vasospasm; a generalized feeling of weakness; anxiety; nausea and vomiting; tachycardia; tachypnea; and hypotension.[1,53,54] As with snakes, dry bites may occur.[1,54]

The first step in managing the bite of one of these lizards may involve extracting the tenacious creature from the victim's anatomy. This can be accomplished by prying the animal's jaws apart, holding a flame beneath its lower jaw, or submerging the animal in cold water.[55] No first-aid measures are of any proven efficacy, and attention should be directed at delivering the patient as soon as possible to medical care.

Life-supporting measures should be instituted, including endotracheal intubation if necessary (e.g., in the case of profound cardiovascular collapse). Hypotension is treated with IV crystalloid infusion. As with snakebites, albumin may be effective in refractory shock, and pressors are rarely required.[1,53] Laboratory evaluation may reveal a leukocytosis, and coagulation values are usually normal.[1] An electrocardiogram should be obtained, as acute myocardial infarction has been reported following helodermatid bite.[56]

Wounds should be cleansed and irrigated when possible. Punctures can be explored under local anesthesia to rule out retained teeth. While soft tissue radiographs may help in this regard, they are not 100% sensitive.[53] Tetanus status should be updated, but prophylactic antibiotics are unnecessary.[1] Wounds should be dressed and splinted, and adequate analgesics initiated. There is no commercially available antivenom for these bites. Patients with systemic toxicity should be admitted to the hospital, while those with only local findings after several hours of observation can be discharged to a reliable setting with instructions to return if they worsen. Mortality is exceedingly rare and tissue necrosis is not typically seen.[1,55]

Venomous Arthropods

The phylum Arthropoda is truly a cosmopolitan group and comprises approximately 80% of the world's known animal species.[57] Of the venomous arthropods, those of the classes Arachnida (including spiders and scorpions) and Insecta (the stinging insects of the order Hymenoptera) are of major medical importance.

HYMENOPTERA

A significant percentage of the world's population is at risk of life-threatening anaphylactic reactions to Hymenoptera stings. In the United States, for example, somewhere between 0.5% and 5.0% of the population is severely allergic to these venoms.[58] The three superfamilies of major medical importance in this order are the Apoidea (honeybees and bumblebees), the Vespoidea (wasps, yellow jackets, and hornets), and the Formicoidea (ants).

Hymenoptera venoms are complex mixtures of biogenic amines (e.g., acetylcholine, histamine, and serotonin), polypeptides (e.g., melittin and apamin), and enzymes (e.g., phospholipase, hyaluronidase).[59] Fire ant venom is composed primarily of piperidine alkaloids.[59] The venoms of species within a family are very similar and tend to cause more cross-reaction in allergic patients than do venoms from different families.

The types of reactions that can be seen following Hymenoptera stings include a typical, local reaction marked by transient pain, redness, and swelling; a more extensive local reaction with swelling beyond the sting site; a type I (immunoglobulin E–mediated) anaphylactic response with any combination of diffuse urticaria, angioedema, laryngeal edema, bronchospasm, or hypotension; and a delayed, probably immune complex–mediated, reaction.[60] Examples of such delayed reactions include serum sickness and very rare atypical phenomena such as hemolysis, thrombocytopenic purpura, and poorly understood neurologic syndromes such as Guillain-Barré syndrome or transverse myelitis.[59]

Multiple Hymenoptera stings can produce systemic poisoning. Of special interest in this regard are the Africanized honeybees (*Apis mellifera scutellata*), or "killer bees." These bees are located from Argentina northward into the southern United States and differ from domesticated honeybees in that they attack aggressively with less provocation and press an attack to extreme limits, both in terms of the number of bees involved and the distance and time over which they will pursue a victim.[57,61] Their venom, however, appears to be nearly identical to that of the domesticated bee.[57] Systemic poisoning may produce vomiting and diarrhea, headache, abdominal or uterine cramping, diffuse edema, bronchospasm, cardiovascular collapse, and seizures and may initially be difficult to differentiate from an anaphylactic reaction.[60,62,63] The median lethal number of Africanized bee stings has been estimated to be 19 per kilogram body weight.[64]

Fire ant stings are usually multiple owing to this species's habit of swarming onto an intruder and stinging in concert upon release of a pheromone alert signal. Typical local findings following such stings are slightly painful or pruritic papules that become sterile pustules or vesicles over approximately 24 hours. The epidermal covering sloughs in 2 to 3 days, and healing follows.[65]

Management

First-aid measures for routine Hymenoptera stings involve limiting distribution of venom and treating pain and itching. Any retained stinger (common with honeybee stings) should be quickly removed from the wound,[66] and ice should be applied. If a known allergic individual sustains a sting or an anaphylactic reaction occurs in the absence of advanced medical capabilities, a lympho-occlusive constriction band should be applied proximally to the extremity (if possible). If more advanced measures are available in the field, care should proceed per the following discussion. Victims possessing epinephrine self-administration kits should be assisted in their use. All patients with systemic findings following stings should be transported to the hospital as quickly as possible.

Hospital management of a simple local reaction involves continuing cold applications, updating tetanus status as indicated, and the use of antihistamines and mild analgesics as necessary. Secondary infections are rare. Large local reactions can be similarly treated, though oral steroids for a few days are helpful if the symptoms are particularly distressing to the patient.[60]

Anaphylaxis following Hymenoptera stings represents a true emergency, requiring aggressive management of the patient's airway and circulation. Endotracheal intubation is indicated if significant respiratory distress or laryngeal edema or stridor is present. Epinephrine should be administered as soon as available (0.01 mL/kg of a 1:1000 solution intramuscularly, up to a maximum dose of 0.5 mL). If the patient is in profound shock, the epinephrine dose can be diluted to 10 mL and given slowly IV (over 5 to 10 minutes) or an epinephrine infusion can be started and titrated to effect. Hypotensive patients require IV fluid resuscitation and possibly further pressor support. Antihistamines (both H_1 and H_2 receptor blockers) should be started as well. Steroids, orally or intravenously, should be given in an effort to blunt any delayed second phase of anaphylaxis that might occur at 1 to 38 hours following the sting.[45] Patients with significant systemic reactions (e.g., bronchospasm, hypotension, or upper airway swelling) should be hospitalized for further observation. In less severe cases, if the victim is asymptomatic 4 hours after treatment, he or she can be discharged to a reliable environment with instructions to return immediately if symptoms recur.[59] A continued 3-day course of antihistamines and steroids should be prescribed, and the patient should receive an epinephrine self-administration kit (as well as detailed instructions in its use). Patients with systemic reactions should be referred to allergists for potential immunotherapy and should be urged to wear medical alert medallions stating their Hymenoptera allergy. It appears that pediatric patients with systemic reactions limited to dermal manifestations (urticaria) are at no greater risk of developing more severe reactions on re-sting than is the general population, and thus do not need allergy referral[60] (though they should still be prescribed an epinephrine self-administration device). Serum sickness usually presents within 1 week of the sting and may be manifested by urticaria, myalgias, arthralgias, fever, headache, and occasionally renal or neurologic dysfunction. Symptoms can generally be well controlled with oral steroids and antihistamines.[60]

Victims receiving multiple stings and having evidence of systemic toxicity must receive supportive care including oxygen, airway maintenance, and blood pressure support as needed. Hypotension is treated with brisk IV crystalloid infusion and pressor support (epinephrine). These cases often present in similar fashion to anaphylactic shock and can be managed in like fashion.[67]

SPIDERS

While the majority of the many thousands of spider species of the world are venomous, only a few are of major medical importance. Most species lack fangs of sufficient size to penetrate human skin. Two genera of nearly worldwide distribution are of major significance, the widow spiders (*Latrodectus* spp.) and the brown spiders (*Loxosceles* spp.).

Widow Spiders

Widow spiders, with at least 10 species and subspecies, are found from Canada all the way through South America, widely throughout Africa, in the warmer regions of Europe and Asia, and in Australia.[68,69] This is a cosmopolitan spider that is easily transported from one part of the world to another and may be established in areas outside its natural range.[70] It is the female widow spider that poses a threat to humans, as the male is too small to bite through human skin. All female widow spiders have a similar body habitus—a small cephalothorax with a globular abdomen and long, spindly legs (Plate 9-3A). These spiders build sticky, disorganized webs and most victims are bitten when they accidentally contact the web and excite or threaten the spider. The best-known species, and the one on which the majority of research has been done, is the black widow species, *Latrodectus mactans*. In Australia, the indigenous *Latrodectus* species (*L. hasselti*) is known as the redback spider.

The venoms of the different species of widow spiders are all very similar in composition and toxic effects.[71,72] While there are multiple components, the most deleterious is a potent neurotoxin, alpha latrotoxin, which acts at nerve terminals to stimulate the release of neurotransmitters, such as acetylcholine and norepinephrine, resulting in depletion of synaptic vesicles and ultimate blockade of nerve conduction.[72] There is no necrotic or hemolytic component.

The spider's bite is often unnoticed by the patient or may be felt as a slight "pinprick." Local visible tissue changes are minimal. Within an hour, the victim develops local pain that builds in intensity and radiates to regional muscle groups. Bites to the lower extremities may result in significant abdominal muscle pain and spasm, while bites to the upper limbs tend to cause chest pain and tightness (occasionally to the point of dyspnea). Pain peaks after several hours. Vital signs may reveal any combination of tachypnea, tachycardia, hypertension, or fever. Hypertension can be severe enough to precipitate cerebrovascular accidents, congestive heart failure, or myocardial ischemia. Also reported are headache, diaphoresis, nausea, vomiting, restlessness, anxiety, periorbital edema, hyperreflexia, dysrhythmias, and a scarlatiniform or morbilliform skin rash.[73–75] Without treatment, clinical findings (particularly pain) may last up to 72 hours.[41]

Management

There are no first-aid measures of proven benefit for widow spider bites, though local ice may reduce pain. Any victim developing symptoms beyond local mild discomfort should seek prompt medical care.

In the hospital, the victim's airway and cardiorespiratory systems must be evaluated and stabilized as necessary. Attention can then be directed at relieving painful muscle spasms. A number of analgesic approaches have been tried with varying success. While there have been anecdotal successes with the administration of calcium gluconate,[76,77] its overall efficacy appears quite limited.[73,78] A combination of narcotic analgesics and benzodiazepines appears more efficacious.[73] Antivenom (see later discussion) is the fastest, most effective means of relieving significant pain following these bites.[79]

There are no laboratory studies of diagnostic benefit, but the complete blood count often reveals a leukocytosis, and the blood sugar is frequently elevated. Serum creatinine phosphokinase elevations may also be seen, as well as microscopic hematuria and proteinuria. An admission electrocardiogram and chest radiograph are advisable in any victim with evidence of systemic poisoning or with significant underlying medical problems.[41,69,80]

Antivenoms for widow spider bites are produced in several countries, and it appears that these antisera are effective in reversing systemic effects and pain regardless of which *Latrodectus* species is involved.[2,79] All of these agents are heterologous serum products, generally produced in horses, and thus carry some risk of inducing allergic reactions (anaphylactoid responses or serum sickness) in patients. Administration should be done cautiously, according to the manufacturer's recommendations, and with immediate availability of epinephrine.

The indications for administering *Latrodectus* antivenom are somewhat controversial. In the United States, many physicians prefer to withhold antivenom in all but the most serious cases, relying instead on supportive care to see the patient through this rarely fatal disease.[79] In Australia, however, redback spider antivenom is used in the majority of significant bites by these spiders and even in cases where a spider has not been identified, but the patient's presentation is consistent with *Latrodectus* venom poisoning.[81] At the very least, widow spider antivenom should be considered for use in very young or very old patients, patients with obviously severe clinical presentations, patients with severe underlying diseases (cardiac disease, hypertension, obstructive pulmonary disease, etc.), and pregnant women (widow spider venom is a potent abortifacient).[82–84]

Admission to the hospital is advisable for patients with significant symptoms (including pain), particularly very young or very old victims, or those with major underlying medical problems.[85] Adult patients in otherwise good health, with normal vital signs and mild symptoms, can be discharged to a reliable setting. They should follow a course of bed rest and should return if symptoms worsen. All patients should have their tetanus status updated as indicated. The current mortality rate from widow spider venom poisoning is very low,[82,86] though full recovery may take several months.[87]

Brown Spiders

The exact number of brown spider species in the world is unclear, but may exceed 100.[88] They are found in North, Central, and South America; in Europe; in Mediterranean countries; and rarely in Australia.[89,90] The most studied species is the brown recluse (*Loxosceles reclusa*; Plate 9-3B). Most *Loxosceles* are characterized by a violin-shaped marking on the dorsal aspect of the cephalothorax and by the presence of three pairs of eyes (vs. four pairs in most other spiders). Adults are 10 to 15 mm in length and have a leg span of 2 to 3 cm. Unlike widow spiders, both the male and female are dangerous. They are, however, shy and reluctant to bite unless severely antagonized. Most victims are bitten during sleep when they roll over onto a spider in the bed linen or when they put on an article of clothing in which the spider has taken up residence.[91]

Loxosceles venoms, though immunologically distinct, all contain a potent enzyme, sphingomyelinase D, which is probably responsible for cutaneous and subcutaneous tissue necrosis and, in rare cases, hemolysis.[90,92] Dermonecrosis is a result of both venom toxicity and autopharmacologic phenomena within the victim, and appears to involve a cascading pathway of local microvascular damage, complement activation, and stimulation of polymorphonuclear leukocytes (PMNs). Despite the dermonecrotic reputation and potential of this spider's venom, most bites actually result in insignificant lesions that heal spontaneously and completely.[90]

The actual bite is usually painless, and therefore few offending spiders are identified. Within several hours, pruritus, tingling, mild swelling, and redness or blanching at the site may develop.[90,93] During this time, as local tissue ischemia develops, variable pain and tenderness are noted. Within 12 to 18 hours, a small, central blister (clear or hemorrhagic) often forms at the site, surrounded by an irregular zone of erythema or ecchymosis and edema. Within a few days, aseptic necrosis is evident at the bite site with an overlying black eschar. When the eschar sloughs, an open ulcer or crater is left, which may require weeks to months to heal.[90,93] Bites are most severe in fatty regions of the body (buttocks, thighs, etc.).[93] Necrosis rarely involves deeper, more vital structures such as muscles or nerves.[94] Treating physicians faced with a patient with a necrotic wound of unclear etiology should be very careful not to label it as a "brown recluse bite" unless the offending spider has been produced. A better term might be "presumed spider bite" or "presumed arthropod envenomation."[95,96]

Systemic poisoning, termed *viscerocutaneous loxoscelism,* is uncommon, but may be rapidly progressive and severe, especially in children.[71] Onset is generally 24 to 72 hours after the bite and may occur in the absence of any significant cutaneous lesion.[97] Symptoms may resemble a viral illness, with chills, fever, headaches, nausea and vomiting, myalgias, arthralgias, malaise, and weakness. Severe toxicity can lead to hemolysis, thrombocytopenia, disseminated intravascular coagulation (DIC), renal failure, and shock.[90,98]

Management

Prehospital management should focus on local cooling measures to reduce the enzymatic activity of sphingomyelinase D in an attempt to reduce necrosis.[99]

Most victims with a *Loxosceles* bite present with a small- to medium-sized, painful, necrotic-appearing skin lesion of several hours' to a few days' duration. While an in vitro lymphocyte transformation test can confirm a *Loxosceles* bite in patients at approximately 6 weeks after the bite,[100] there is currently no clinically available laboratory method of making the diagnosis on initial presentation. Work continues in an effort to develop a rapid clinical test that can reliably identify when a *Loxosceles* spider is the etiology of a victim's necrotic lesion.

Vital signs should be checked, looking for any evidence of systemic toxicity (tachycardia, tachypnea, hypotension, fever). Laboratory workup should include a complete blood count, platelet count, and urinalysis. If there is evidence of DIC, hemolysis, or hemoglobinuria, further studies should be obtained, including coagulation studies, electrolytes, blood urea nitrogen, serum creatine, blood sugar, liver function tests, and serum haptoglobin, and blood should be typed and screened. The white blood cell count may be elevated and the hemoglobin may drop dramatically in systemic loxoscelism.[71,90]

Controversy abounds over the proper management of brown spider–induced dermonecrosis, and it is important that patients understand that nothing has been definitively proven to limit the degree of tissue damage that may result. Most bites do well with sound conservative wound care measures (cleansing, sterile dressing, splinting, and tetanus prophylaxis as necessary).[49] Local cooling of the bite site should be initiated and continued intermittently for approximately 72 hours.[99] Antibiotic use is controversial, but is certainly indicated if there is any evidence of secondary infection.[49,99] Wound treatment measures that have been recommended in the past include steroids, dapsone, surgery, and hyperbaric oxygen therapy. Steroids, by any route (systemic or intralesional), are of no demonstrated benefit in limiting necrosis.[49,90] Dapsone and colchicine are also unproved but of theoretical benefit owing to their ability to inhibit PMN function.[49,90,101,102] Dapsone can, however, cause dose-dependent hemolytic anemia and methemoglobinemia and is not approved in the United States for use in *Loxosceles* bites.[103,104] It should be reserved for severe lesions in adults.[90] Initial dosage should not exceed 50 mg to 100 mg orally per day (divided every 12 hours), and a glucose-6-phosphate dehydrogenase level should be checked at the time therapy is started.[103] Treatment should continue until the lesion heals or is grafted.[97]

The temptation to surgically excise the bite site in its early stages should be resisted, as it is impossible to predict the extent and ultimate severity of the lesion left to its natural course.[105] Severe-appearing lesions may regress spontaneously with minimal residual scarring.[98] To optimize chances of healing, any required skin grafting should be delayed 6 to 8 weeks until the necrotic process has been completed.[49] Hyperbaric oxygen therapy may be beneficial in severe wounds.[49,106,107] There is, at present, no commercially available *Loxosceles* antivenom in the United States, but a Brazilian antivenom (a polyvalent product that also covers *Phoneutria* spider bites and *Tityus serrulatus* scorpion stings; see later discussion) for *Loxosceles reclusa* and *L. rufescens* does exist,[108] and it is hoped that continued research will yield an effective antivenom for use in any *Loxosceles* bite,[109] particularly if a technique can be developed to identify with certainty the cause of the lesion when patients present without having seen the spider.[110,111]

Management of viscerocutaneous loxoscelism is primarily supportive—ensuring adequate hydration, maintaining electrolyte balance, and giving analgesics as necessary. A short course of systemic steroids (e.g., prednisone, 1 mg/kg/day for 2 to 4 days) may help stabilize erythrocyte membranes and lessen the severity of hemolysis.[71,90,98] Blood products may be needed to treat anemia or thrombocytopenia, and heparin may be added if DIC develops.[90] Hemoglobinuria may necessitate alkalinization of the urine, and dialysis may be required in the face of acute renal insufficiency, though it does not remove venom or hemoglobin from the circulation.[90]

Patients without evidence of systemic toxicity or severe necrosis may be followed as outpatients with daily wound checks, monitoring blood counts, and urinalyses for several days.[90] Patients with systemic toxicity or rapidly expanding lesions should be admitted and have close monitoring for laboratory abnormalities.[105] While there have, to date, been no documented deaths in patients bitten by positively identified brown spiders in the United States, it is clear that *Loxosceles* spiders are capable of severe envenomation, with real potential for mortality, especially in small children.[74]

Miscellaneous Spiders

Other spiders of medical interest include the Australian funnel web spiders (genera *Atrax* and *Hadronyche*), the South American hunting or banana spiders (*Phoneutria* spp.), the aggressive house spider of the U.S. Pacific Northwest (*Tegeneria agrestis*), the wolf spiders (family Lycosidae), and the tarantulas.

The funnel web spiders of Australia and Tasmania are relatively large spiders that can inflict a very painful and potentially fatal bite.[68] The venom is a neurotoxin that stimulates neurotransmitter release from the autonomic nervous system and at neuromuscular junctions.[74] Effects may include salivation, lacrimation, nausea and vomiting, abdominal pain, diarrhea, restlessness, hypertension, muscle twitching, dyspnea, and confusion.[74,89] First-aid therapy involves use of the pressure-immobilization technique (as outlined for snakebites previously), application of ice, and prompt transportation to the hospital.[89] An antivenom is produced in Australia and is effective in severe bites.[89,112]

South American spiders of the genus *Phoneutria* (wandering spiders, huntsman spiders, or banana spiders) can be dangerous.[74] They are large and aggressive, and possess a potent neurotoxic venom that produces severe pain and autonomic overdrive.[74,108] Management may include local anesthetic infiltration, application of local heat, and administration of systemic analgesics or sedatives, or both.[108] There is an antivenom produced in Brazil that is effective for severe bites,[108] which are more likely to occur in very young and very old patients.[113]

While commonly feared because of their large size and "hairy" appearance, most tarantulas (of the suborder Orthognatha) are relatively harmless. While bites can be painful, necrosis and systemic reactions are rare. A problem with many tarantulas is their habit of flicking fine hairs off the dorsum of their abdomens towards a perceived threat. If these "urticating" hairs enter the eyes or mucous membranes, they can cause itching and irritation on both an allergic and a mechanical basis.[105] These barbed, urticating hairs can also penetrate the cornea and cause an acute keratouveitis.[114]

Without doubt, there is still much that needs to be learned about the medical importance of poorly studied spider species. Some species that were previously thought to be medically important have been exonerated of their unjust reputations. Wolf spiders (*Lycosa* spp.) were for some time suspected of causing necrotic lesions in Brazil, but it is now understood that these large hunting spiders are relatively harmless,[115] and it was likely *Loxosceles* spiders causing these clinical findings. Similarly, the white-tail spider in Australia was, for years, erroneously thought to cause necrotic arachnidism, and this has only recently been definitively refuted.[116,117] On the other hand, it has been within the last two decades that the importance of the aggressive house spider or hobo spider (*T. agrestis*) of the U.S. Pacific Northwest has come to light as a cause of necrotic and systemic arachnidism.[118]

Besides the few spider species for which specific therapy exists, such as antivenom for *Latrodectus* bites, the management of spider bites is largely conservative—tetanus prophylaxis, ice, mild analgesics, standard wound care, and antibiotics if secondary infection occurs.

SCORPION VENOM POISONING

There are an estimated 1500 species of scorpions in the world, but only about 25 of these are dangerously toxic to humans.[119] The medically important species in the Old World fall into the genera *Buthus, Androctonus, Leiurus,* and *Buthotus,* and in the New World, *Centruroides* (Plate 9-3C) and *Tityus* are important.[120]

Scorpion venoms have received much research attention in recent years as efforts to isolate the various components proceed. The venoms of scorpions posing a serious threat to human life possess toxins with significant neurologic and cardiovascular effects. These venoms stimulate massive release of neurotransmitters from autonomic nerve terminals, neuromuscular junctions, and the adrenal medulla, resulting in sympathetic, parasympathetic, and paralytic signs and symptoms.[105,120] Pain is a common immediate symptom and may be enhanced by the presence of serotonin in many venoms.[120] Paresthesias may occur as well. Systemic findings are related to venom-induced release of acetylcholine and catecholamines. Such findings may include restlessness, anxiety, roving eye movements, hypersalivation, diaphoresis, nausea, vomiting, hypertension, bradycardia, tachycardia, dysrhythmias, hyperthermia, muscle fasciculations, alternating opisthotonos and emprosthotonos, weakness, paralysis, difficulty speaking or swallowing, dyspnea, wheezing, stridor, pulmonary edema, coma, and death.[120–122] Stings by less toxic scorpions usually result in immediate burning pain and mild local soft tissue swelling or ecchymosis. Allergic reactions to scorpion stings are extremely uncommon.[123] Necrosis is also rare, with the exception of a poorly studied scorpion from Iran and Iraq, *Hemiscorpius lepturus.*[74,124]

Management

First-aid measures for scorpion stings should include local cooling to reduce pain. For neurotoxic scorpions, the Australian pressure-immobilization technique may be beneficial.[89] If the offending scorpion can be safely captured, identification may guide further management.

In the hospital, vital signs should be checked and frequently monitored. Physical examination should assess manifestations of sympathetic, parasympathetic, or neuromuscular excitation. There are no laboratory studies of diagnostic value. Routine tests, if obtained, may demonstrate an increase in white blood cell count, serum glucose, serum amylase, creatinine phosphokinase, renal function values, and mild abnormalities in coagulation values.[122,125] Cerebrospinal fluid pleocytosis has been reported.[122] Victims displaying only local symptoms can be treated on an outpatient basis with ice and appropriate analgesics. Tetanus status should be updated as necessary.

Patients with evidence of systemic envenomation should receive oxygen and cardiac and pulse oximetry monitoring, and should have an IV line established. Endotracheal intubation may be necessary in the face of impending respiratory failure or excessive airway secretions.[122] Central nervous system (CNS) symptoms such as anxiety, restlessness, muscular hyperactivity, and moderate hypertension can usually be treated with bed rest and sedation.[122] Sedative doses of IV benzodiazepines or phenobarbital can be used with close monitoring of respiratory status.[125] Though their efficacy is unproved, adrenergic blocking agents have been recommended for hemodynamically significant supraventricular tachycardia.[120] Antihypertensive agents may be necessary if sedation fails to resolve severe blood pressure elevation.[85] Shock and pulmonary edema may occur in severe cases and may mandate invasive hemodynamic monitoring for adequate resuscitation.[126] Analgesics should be administered as necessary, but narcotics should be given cautiously as there is some evidence of synergistic action with some scorpion venoms.[127]

In many areas of the world, such as South America, Saudi Arabia, India, and Mexico, antivenoms have been prepared against the more dangerous scorpion venoms. Controversy exists, however, regarding the precise indications for and efficacy of these heterologous serum products.[126,128–131] Administration is reasonable in cases of severe envenomation, especially in children not responding promptly to the preceding conservative measures. These antivenoms do carry some risk of anaphylactoid reactions and delayed serum sickness, and their administration should be with similar precautions as outlined previously for snake and spider antivenoms.

Adults stung by potentially dangerous scorpions should be observed for 4 to 6 hours. If significant toxicity appears, they should be admitted to an appropriate hospital unit. If systemic signs and symptoms are absent after several hours of observation, they may be discharged with aftercare instructions to return if they get worse. Owing to the increased severity of envenomations in small children, symptomatic cases and all infants should be admitted to an intensive care setting and monitored closely.[105,125,132]

MISCELLANEOUS VENOMOUS ARTHROPODS

An exhaustive description of all venomous or harmful arthropods is beyond the scope of this chapter. Examples of other arthropods that can cause significant envenomation in humans include centipedes and the larval forms (caterpillars) of the order Lepidoptera (moths and butterflies). The vast majority of bites or stings by these miscellaneous creatures and by unidentified arthropods can be treated satisfactorily with sound supportive care, including local cooling of the wound, elevation and splinting of the involved extremity, updating the tetanus status as necessary, and administering appropriate analgesics. In the rare case of hypotension, IV crystalloid fluids should be initially administered, followed by vasopressor agents if there is a lack of response to volume repletion. If there is concern for an anaphylactic response to the venom, this should be managed as outlined previously under the discussion on Hymenoptera. Wound care should focus on regular cleaning of wounds, removal of any retained foreign bodies (stingers, hairs, spines, etc.), and judicious debridement of clearly necrotic tissue. If secondary infection occurs, appropriate broad-spectrum antibiotics should be administered depending on the clinical scenario. If systemic toxicity is evident, then routine laboratory tests should be obtained (complete blood count, serum electrolytes, renal and liver function studies, blood glucose, coagulation studies, and urinalysis). Depending on the severity of the poisoning and the underlying health of the victim, a chest radiograph and electrocardiogram may be useful.

Marine Envenomations

Ocean-dwelling organisms have developed unique methods of self-defense, and as humans increase their exposure to the marine environment, the possibility of hazardous encounters also increases. It is important that health care providers be familiar with the unique dangers of the aquatic environment, especially the presentation and management of poisonous bites and stings. Most cases of marine venom poisoning occur as acts of self-defense on the part of the creatures and rarely occur without provocation.[133,134]

Stinging invertebrates are among the most common and dangerous marine animals. These organisms envenom by means of dischargeable, stinging, venom-laden barbs contained in organelles known as nematocysts.[135] Millions of microscopic venom-bearing stinging cells (nematocytes) cover the surfaces of the tentacles and are triggered chemically or by tactile stimulation. Venom has direct and indirect effects on the vascular and autonomic nervous systems. Centrally mediated respiratory depression and/or anaphylaxis may occur.[135–137]

Stinging vertebrates typically introduce their venoms to humans via the specialized glands associated with sharp spines, which may be present on their gill covers or dorsal, pectoral, or anal fins. Injuries caused by these animals commonly involve puncture wounds, which may be quite traumatic, in addition to the envenomation. Envenomation syndromes caused by this diverse group of marine animals include sudden cardiogenic death, tissue necrosis, paralysis, anaphylaxis, and a range of enigmatic symptoms and signs specific to the individual animal.[138–150] Venom composition varies among species, but in general has been shown to have a destabilizing effect on cell membranes, in some cases mediated by effects on ion channels.

ENVENOMATIONS BY MARINE INVERTEBRATES

Sponges

Two general syndromes are induced by contact with sponges. The first is a pruritic dermatitis similar to plant-induced allergic dermatitis. A typical offender is the friable Hawaiian or West Indian fire sponge (*Tedania ignis*).[133,151] Within a few hours, but sometimes within 10 to 20 minutes, after skin contact, the victim suffers itching and burning, which may progress to local joint swelling, soft tissue edema, vesiculation, and stiffness, particularly if small pieces of broken sponge are retained in the skin near the interphalangeal or metacarpophalangeal joints. Abraded skin, such as that which has been scraped on stony coral, may allow more rapid or greater absorption of toxin(s).[152] Untreated, mild reactions subside within 3 to 7 days.[153] When large skin areas are involved, the victim may complain of fever, chills, malaise, dizziness, nausea, muscle cramps, and formication. Systemic erythema multiforme or an anaphylactoid reaction may develop a week to 14 days after a severe exposure.[154] The skin may become mottled or purpuric, occasionally after a delay of up to 10 days.[155] The second syndrome is irritant dermatitis that follows penetration of small spicules of silica or calcium carbonate into the skin. In severe cases, surface desquamation of the skin may follow in 10 days to 2 months. No medical intervention can retard this process. Recurrent eczema and persistent arthralgias are rare complications.

To treat, the skin should be gently dried. Spicules should be removed, if possible, using adhesive tape, a thin layer of rubber cement, or a facial peel. As soon as possible, dilute (5%) acetic acid (vinegar) soaks for 10 to 30 minutes three or four times a day should be applied to all affected areas.[133,136,156] Isopropyl alcohol 40% to 70% is a reasonable second choice. Erythema multiforme may require the administration of a systemic glucocorticoid, beginning with a moderately high dose (prednisone 60–100 mg), tapered over 2 to 3 weeks. After the initial decontamination, a mild emollient cream or steroid preparation may be applied to the skin. If the allergic component is severe, particularly if there is weeping, crusting, and vesiculation, a systemic glucocorticoid (prednisone 60–100 mg, tapered over 2 weeks) may be beneficial.

Coelenterates (Cnidaria)

Coelenterates are an enormous group, comprising approximately 10,000 species, at least 100 of which are dangerous to humans. Coelenterates that possess the venom-charged stinging cells are known as cnidaria (nettle). For practical purposes, the cnidaria can be divided into (1) hydrozoans, such as the Portuguese man-of-war; (2) scyphozoans, such as true jellyfish; and (3) anthozoans, such as soft corals, stony corals, and anemones. Fenner divides jellyfishes into three main classes: schyphozoans (true jellyfishes), with tentacles arising at regular intervals around the bell; cubozoans (e.g., "box" jellyfishes), with tentacles arising only from the corners—these may be further divided into carybdeids (e.g., Irukandji), with only one tentacle (except in rare cases) arising from each lower corner of the bell, and chirodropids, which have more than one tentacle in each corner of the bell; and other jellyfishes, such as the hydrozoans (e.g., *Physalia* species).

Clinical Aspects

For clinical purposes, a considerable phylogenetic relationship exists among all stinging species, so that the clinical features of the coelenterate syndrome are fairly constant, with a spectrum of severity. The wise clinician suspects a coelenterate envenomation in all unexplained cases of collapse in the surf, diving accidents, and near drownings. Any victim in distress pulled from marine waters should be carefully examined for one or more cutaneous lesions that may provide the clue to a coelenterate envenomation.

Mild Envenomation. There is usually an immediate pricking or stinging sensation, accompanied by pruritus, paresthesias, burning, throbbing, and radiation of the pain centrally from the extremities to the groin, abdomen, and axillae. The area involved by the nematocysts becomes red-brown-purple, often in a linear whiplike fashion, corresponding to tentacle prints. Other features are blistering, local edema angioedema and wheal formation, as well as violaceous petechial hemorrhages. The papular inflammatory skin rash is strictly confined to the areas of contact and may persist for up to 10 days. If the envenomation is slightly more severe, the aforementioned symptoms, which are evident in the first few hours, can progress over a course of days to local necrosis, skin ulceration, and secondary infection. Untreated, the minor-to-moderate skin disorder resolves over 1 to 2 weeks, with occasional residual hyperpigmentation for 1 to 2 months. Rubbing can cause lichenification. Local hyperhidrosis, fat atrophy, and contracture may occur.[157] Permanent scarring or keloids may result. It has been suggested that sensitization may occur without a definite history of a previous sting, since coelenterates may release antigenic and allergenic venom components into the water.

Moderate and Severe Envenomation. The skin manifestations are similar or intensified and compounded by the onset of systemic symptoms, which may appear immediately or be delayed by several hours:

1. Neurologic: malaise, headache, aphonia, diminished touch and temperature sensation, vertigo, ataxia, spastic or flaccid paralysis, mononeuritis multiplex, Guillain-Barré syndrome, parasympathetic dysautonomia, plexopathy, radial-ulnar-median nerve palsies, brainstem infarction (not a confirmed relationship), delirium, loss of consciousness, convulsions, coma, and death[158–161]
2. Cardiovascular: anaphylaxis, hemolysis, hypotension, small artery spasm, bradyarrhythmias (including electromechanical dissociation and asystole), tachyarrhythmias, vascular spasm, deep venous thrombosis, congestive heart failure, and ventricular fibrillation
3. Respiratory: rhinitis, bronchospasm, laryngeal edema, dyspnea, cyanosis, pulmonary edema, and respiratory failure
4. Musculoskeletal or rheumatologic: abdominal rigidity, diffuse myalgia and muscle cramps, muscle spasm, fat atrophy, arthralgias, reactive arthritis (sero-negative symmetric synovitis with pitting edema),[162] and thoracolumbar pain
5. Gastrointestinal: nausea, vomiting, diarrhea, dysphagia, hypersalivation, and thirst
6. Ocular: conjunctivitis, chemosis, corneal ulcers, corneal epithelial edema, keratitis, iridocyclitis, elevated intraocular pressure, synechiae, iris depigmentation, chronic unilateral glaucoma, and lacrimation[163,164]
7. Other: acute renal failure, lymphadenopathy, chills, fever, and nightmares

Treatment. Therapy is directed at stabilizing major systemic decompensation, opposing the venom's multiple effects, and alleviating pain. Generally, only severe *Physalia* or Cubomedusae stings result in rapid decompensation, unless anaphylaxis is present. Hypotension should be managed with the prompt intravenous administration of crystalloid, such as lactated Ringer's solution. This must be done in concert with detoxification of any nematocysts that are still attached to the victim, to limit the perpetuation of envenomation. Any victim with a systemic component should be observed for a period of at least 6 to 8 hours because rebound phenomena after successful treatment are not uncommon. All elderly victims should undergo electrocardiography and be observed on a cardiac monitor, with frequent checks for arrhythmias. Urinalysis demonstrates the presence or absence of hemoglobinuria, indicating hemolysis.[165] If this is the case, the urine should be alkalinized with bicarbonate to prevent the precipitation of pigment in the renal tubules, while a moderate diuresis (30 to 50 mL/hr) is maintained with a loop diuretic (such as furosemide or bumetanide) or mannitol (0.25 g/kg intravenously every 8 to 12 hours). If there are signs of distal ischemia or an impending compartment syndrome, standard diagnostic and therapeutic measures apply. Vasospasm associated with jellyfish envenomation may be severe, prolonged, and refractory to regional sympathectomy and intra-arterial reserpine or pentoxifylline.[166] *Chironex fleckeri*, the box jellyfish, produces the only coelenterate venom for which specific antivenom exists.

Treatment of Dermatitis. If a person is stung by a coelenterate, the following steps should be taken:

1. Immediately rinse the wound with seawater, not with fresh water. Do not rub the wound with a towel or clothing to remove adherent tentacles. Surf life-savers (lifeguards) in the United States and Hawaii have mentioned that a freshwater hot shower applied with a forceful stream may decrease the pain of an envenomation. If this is successful, one theoretical explanation is that the mechanical effect of the water stream (that dislodges tentacle fragments and/or stinging cells) supercedes the deleterious (sting-stimulating) effect of the hypotonic water. Remove any gross tentacles with forceps or a well-gloved hand. In an emergency, the keratinized palm of the hand is relatively protected, but take care not to become envenomed.
2. Commercial (chemical) cold or ice packs applied over a thin dry cloth or plastic membrane have been shown to be effective when applied to mild or moderate *Physalia utriculus* ("bluebottle") stings.[167] Whether the melt-water from ice applied directly to the skin can stimulate the discharge of nematocysts has not been determined. Applications of hot packs or gentle rinses with hot water are not recommended.
3. Acetic acid 5% (vinegar) is the treatment of choice to inactivate *Chironex fleckeri* toxin. Vinegar will not alleviate the pain from a *Chironex* sting but interrupts the envenomation. The detoxicant should be applied continuously for at least 30 minutes or until the pain is relieved. A sting from the Australian *Physalia physalis*, a relatively recently differentiated species, should not be doused with vinegar, as this may cause discharge of up to 30% of nematocysts.[149]
4. For a sting from *Chironex fleckeri*, the pressure-immobilization technique for venom sequestration is sometimes recommended. If vinegar is immediately available, a liberal dousing should occur and at least 30 seconds should pass before removing the tentacles. After the tentacles are removed, proceed at once with pressure-immobilization. If vinegar is unavailable, remove the tentacles before applying pressure-immobilization.[168] A venolymphatic occlusive tourniquet should be considered only if a topical detoxicant and pressure-immobilization are unavailable, the victim suffers from a severe systemic reaction, and transport to definitive care is delayed. *Chironex* antivenom should be administered intravenously as soon as possible. The intramuscular route is less preferred. The antivenom is supplied in ampoules of 20,000 units by Commonwealth Serum Laboratories, Melbourne, Australia. The initial dose is one ampoule (diluted 1:5 to 1:10 in isotonic crystalloid; dilution with water is not recommended) administered intravenously over 5 minutes, or three ampoules intramuscularly. This has been administered successfully over the years by members of the Queensland Surf Life-Saving Association and the Queensland Ambulance Transport Brigade. Although the antivenom is prepared by hyperimmunizing sheep and adverse reactions reported to date have been rare and mild, the prudent physician is always prepared to treat anaphylaxis or serum sickness.[169] It cannot be overemphasized that the timely administration of antivenom can be lifesaving.[170] In addition to its lifesaving properties, the early administration of antivenom may markedly reduce pain and decrease subsequent skin scarring.[171] Antivenom administration may be repeated once or twice every 2 to 4 hours until there is no further worsening of the skin discoloration, pain, or systemic effects.

For stings from other species, there are substances that may be more specific and, therefore, more effective. Depending on the species, these include isopropyl alcohol (40% to 70%), dilute ammonium hydroxide, sodium bicarbonate (particularly for stings of the sea nettle *Chrysaora quinquecirrha*), olive oil, sugar, urine, and papain (papaya latex [juice] or unseasoned meat tenderizer powdered or in solution). Perfume, aftershave lotion, and high-proof liquor are not particularly efficacious and may be detrimental, as are formalin, ether, and gasoline.

1. Once the wound has been soaked with a decontaminant (e.g., vinegar), remaining (and often "invisible") nematocysts must be removed. The easiest way to do this is to apply shaving cream or a paste of baking soda, flour, or talc and to shave the area with a razor or similar tool. If sophisticated facilities are not available, the nematocysts should be removed by making a sand or mud paste with seawater and using this to help scrape the victim's skin with a sharp-edged shell or piece of wood.
2. A topical anesthetic ointment (lidocaine, 2.5%) or spray (benzocaine, 14%), antihistaminic cream (diphenhydramine or tripelennamine), or mild steroid lotion (hydrocortisone, 1%) may be soothing. These are used after the toxin is inactivated.
3. Victims should receive standard antitetanus prophylaxis. Each wound should be checked at 3 and 7 days after injury for infection. Any ulcerating lesion should be cleaned three times a day and covered with a thin layer of nonsensitizing antiseptic ointment, such as mupirocin.

Prevention. A protocol has been developed to establish the effectiveness of topical agents to block firing of nematocysts.[172] Current research is directed at a combination jellyfish sting inhibitor–sunscreen lotion (Safe Sea: www.nidaria.com) that may prevent discharge of more than 90% of nematocysts that contact protected skin.[173] Failed topical barriers include petrolatum, mineral oil, silicone ointment, cocoa butter, and mechanic's grease.

Seabather's Eruption

Seabather's eruption, commonly termed *sea lice* ("pika-pika" around the Belize barrier reef; "sea poisoning," "sea critters," and "ocean itch" are other names), refers to a dermatitis that results from contact with ocean water.[174] It predominantly involves covered areas of the body and is commonly caused by pinhead-sized (0.5 mm) greenish-brown to black larvae of the thimble jellyfish *Linuche unguiculata*, which breeds in Caribbean waters throughout the summer with a peak in May. A swimmer who encounters the stinging forms usually complains of cutaneous discomfort soon after contact, often while in the water or soon after exiting. The eruption occurs a few minutes to 12 hours after bathing and consists of erythematous and intensely pruritic wheals, vesicles, or papules that persist for 2 to 14 days and then involute spontaneously (Plate 9-4A). When a bathing suit has been worn by a woman, the areas commonly involved include the buttocks, genital region, and breasts. A person at the water's surface (commonly a person who surfaces after a dive) may suffer stings to the exposed neck, particularly if there has been recent motorboat activity in the vicinity, which may disturb and fragment the causative jellyfish. Nematocysts adherent to scalp hair may sting the neck as the hair hangs down. Coalescence indicates a large inoculum. Individual lesions resemble insect bites. Surfers develop lesions on areas that contact the surfboard (chest and anterior abdomen). The rash may also be seen under bathing caps and swim fins or along the edge of the cuffs of wet suits, T-shirts, or "stinger suits."[175] Field management is identical to that for any coelenterate sting (see preceding discussion), with the empirical observation that topical papain may be slightly more effective as an initial decontaminant than vinegar, isopropyl alcohol, or other substances. Substances that are felt to be ineffective include hydrogen peroxide, garlic, antifungal spray, anti–head lice medication, petroleum distillates, fingernail polish, and citrus juice. Further treatment is palliative and consists of calamine lotion with 1% menthol. Because the lesions rarely extend into the dermis, a potent topical corticosteroid may be helpful in mild cases, but benefit is not invariably attained. In a more severe case, an oral or parenteral antihistamine or systemic corticosteroid may be used.

Starfish

Starfish are covered with thorny spines of calcium carbonate crystals held erect by muscle tissue. Glandular tissue interspersed in or underneath the epidermis (integument) produces a slimy venomous substance. The ice pick–like spine of *Acanthaster planci* (Plate 9-4B) can penetrate the hardiest of diving gloves. As the spine enters the skin, it carries venom into the wound, with immediate pain, copious bleeding, and mild edema. The pain is generally moderate and self-limited, with remission over a period of 30 minutes to 3 hours. The wound may become dusky or discolored. Multiple puncture wounds may result in acute systemic reactions, including paresthesias, nausea, vomiting, lymphadenopathy, and muscular paralysis. The wound should immediately be immersed in nonscalding hot water to tolerance (113°F or 45°C) for 30 to 90 minutes or until there is significant pain relief. The pain is rarely severe enough to require local anesthetic infiltration. The puncture wound should be irrigated and explored to remove all foreign material. Because of the stout nature of the spines, it is rare to retain a fragment. However, if any question of a foreign body exists, a soft tissue radiograph often identifies the fractured spine.

Sea Urchins

The venom apparatuses of sea urchins consist of the hollow, venom-filled spines and the triple-jawed globiferous pedicellariae. Venom may also be released from within a thin integumentary sheath on the external surface of the spines of certain urchins (Plate 9-4C).

Urchins may be extremely dangerous to handle; the spines, which are attached to the shell with a modified ball-and-socket joint, are brittle and break off easily in the flesh, lodging deeply and making removal difficult. Pedicellariae are small, delicate seizing organs attached to the stalks scattered among the spines. These are considered to be modified spines with flexible heads.[152] Globiferous pedicellariae are typified by those found in *Toxopneustes pileolus* (flower urchin).

Venomous spines inflict immediate and intensely painful stings. The pain is initially characterized by burning, which rapidly evolves into severe local muscle aching with visible erythema and swelling of the skin surrounding the puncture site or sites. Frequently a spine breaks off and lodges in the victim. Some sea urchin spines contain purplish dye, which may give a false impression of spines left in the skin. Soft tissue density x-ray techniques or magnetic resonance imaging may reveal a radiopaque foreign body. If a spine enters a joint, it may rapidly induce severe synovitis. If multiple spines have penetrated the skin, particularly if they are deeply embedded, systemic symptoms may rapidly develop, including nausea, vomiting, paresthesias, numbness and muscular paralysis, abdominal pain, syncope, hypotension, and respiratory distress. The stings of pedicellariae are often of greater magnitude. Secondary infections and indolent ulceration are common. A delayed hypersensitivity-type reaction ("flare-up") at the site of the puncture(s) has been described, in which the victim demonstrates erythema and pruritus in a delayed fashion (7 to 10 days) post primary resolution from the initial envenomation.[176]

The envenomed body part should immediately be immersed in nonscalding hot water (upper limit 113°F or 45°C) to tolerance for 30 to 90 minutes in an attempt to relieve pain. Any pedicellariae still attached to the skin must be removed or envenomation will continue. This may be accomplished by applying shaving foam and gently scraping with a razor. Embedded spines should be removed with care because they easily fracture. Black or purplish discoloration surrounding the wound after spine removal is often merely spine dye. Although some thin venomous spines may be absorbed within 24 hours to 3 weeks, it is best to remove those that are easily reached. All thick calcium carbonate spines should be removed because of the risk of infection, foreign body encaseation granuloma, or dermoid inclusion cyst. External percussion to achieve fragmentation may prove disastrous if a chronic inflammatory process is initiated in sensitive tissue of the hand or foot. If the spines have acutely entered joints or are closely aligned to neurovascular structures, the surgeon should take advantage of an operating microscope in an appropriate setting to remove all spine fragments. If the spine has entered an interphalangeal joint, the finger should be splinted until the spine is removed to limit fragmentation and further penetration. Infections are common, and deep puncture wounds are an indication for prophylactic antibiotics.

Cone Snails ("Cone Shells")

Most harmful cone snails ("cones") are creatures of shallow Indo-Pacific waters; they are predators that feed by injecting rapid-acting venom by means of a detachable, dartlike radular tooth. Most stings occur on the fingers and hand, as the unknowledgeable fossicker incorrectly handles a hazardous specimen. Mild envenomations resemble bee or wasp stings. The initial pain is followed by localized ischemia, cyanosis, and numbness in the area surrounding the wound. More serious envenomations induce paresthesias at the wound site, which rapidly encompass the limb and then become perioral prior to generalized. Partial paralysis transitions to generalized muscular paralysis causing diaphragmatic dysfunction and respiratory failure. Coma has been observed, and death is attributed to diaphragmatic paralysis or cardiac failure. Other symptoms include dysphagia, syncope, weakness, failing coordination, areflexia, aphonia, dysarthria, diplopia, ptosis, absent gag reflex, blurred vision, and pruritus.

No antivenom is available for cone shell envenomation. The pressure-immobilization technique makes sense and should be applied. Cardiovascular and respiratory support are the usual priorities after a severe envenomation. Edrophonium (10 mg intravenously in an adult) has been suggested as empirical therapy for paralysis. Adverse reactions to edrophonium (anticholinesterase inhibitor) include salivation, nausea, diarrhea, and muscle fasciculations. These can be ameliorated with atropine 0.6 mg IV.

Octopuses

Octopus bites are rare but can result in severe envenomations. Fatalities have been reported from the bites of the Australian blue-ringed (or "spotted") octopuses, *Octopus (Hapalochlaena) maculosus* and *O. (H.) lunulata*. These small creatures, which rarely exceed 20 cm in length with tentacles extended, are found throughout the Indo-Pacific in rock pools, under discarded objects and shells, and in shallow waters.[177]

The venom of *H. maculosa* contains at least one fraction identical to tetrodotoxin, which blocks peripheral nerve conduction by interfering with sodium conductance in excitable membranes.[178] This paralytic agent rapidly produces neuromuscular blockade, notably of the phrenic nerve supply to the diaphragm.

Most victims are bitten on the hand or arm, as they handle the creature.[179] An octopus bite usually consists of two small puncture wounds. The bite goes unnoticed or causes only a small amount of discomfort, described as a minor ache, slight stinging, or a pulsating sensation. Occasionally the site is initially numb, followed in 5 to 10 minutes by discomfort that may spread to involve the entire limb, persisting for up to 6 hours. Within 30 minutes, considerable erythema, swelling, tenderness, heat, and pruritus may develop. By far the most common local tissue reaction is absence of symptoms, a small spot of blood, or a tiny blanched area.[180] More serious symptoms are related predominantly to the neurotoxic properties of the venom. Within 10 to 15 minutes of the bite, the patient notices oral and facial numbness, rapidly followed by systemic progression.[179] Voluntary and involuntary muscles are involved, and the illness may rapidly progress to total flaccid paralysis and respiratory failure. Other symptoms include perioral and intraoral anesthesia (classically, numbness of the lips and tongue), diplopia, blurred vision, aphonia, dysphagia, ataxia, myoclonus, weakness, a sense of detachment, nausea, vomiting, peripheral neuropathy, flaccid muscular paralysis, and respiratory failure, which may lead to death.

First aid at the scene might include the pressure-immobilization technique, although this is as yet unproven for management of octopus bites. Prompt mechanical respiratory assistance has by far the greatest influence on the outcome. Respiratory demise should be anticipated early, and the rescuer should be prepared to provide artificial ventilation, including endotracheal intubation and the application of a mechanical ventilator. The duration of intense clinical venom effect is 4 to 10 hours, after which the victim who has not suffered an episode of significant hypoxia shows rapid signs of improvement. Complete recovery may require 2 to 4 days.

ENVENOMATIONS BY MARINE VERTEBRATES

Stingrays

Stingrays (Plate 9-4D) are usually found in tropical, subtropical, and warm temperate oceans, generally in shallow (intertidal) water areas, such as sheltered bays, shoal lagoons, river mouths, and sandy areas between patch reefs.[181] Rays can enter brackish and fresh waters as well. The venom apparatus of stingrays consists of a bilaterally retroserrate spine or spines and the enveloping integumentary sheath or sheaths. The elongate and tapered vasodentine spine is firmly attached to the dorsum of the tail (whip) by dense collagenous tissue and is edged on either side by a series of sharp retrorse teeth. Along either edge on the underside of the spine are the two ventrolateral glandular grooves, which house the soft venom glands. The entire spine is encased by the integumentary sheath, which also contains some glandular cells. The sting is often covered with a film of venom and mucus.

Stingray "attacks" are purely defensive gestures that occur when an unwary human handles, corners, or steps on a camouflaged creature while wading in shallow waters. The tail of the ray reflexively whips upward and accurately thrusts the caudal spine or spines into the victim, producing a puncture wound or jagged laceration. The integumentary sheath covering the spine is ruptured and venom is released into the wound, along with mucus, pieces of the sheath, and fragments of the spine.

The pain may radiate centrally, peaks at 30 to 60 minutes, and may last for up to 48 hours. The wound is initially dusky or cyanotic and rapidly progresses to erythema and hemorrhagic discoloration, with rapid fat and muscle hemorrhage and necrosis.[182] If discoloration around the wound edge is not immediately apparent, within 2 hours it often extends several centimeters from the wound. Systemic manifestations include weakness, nausea, vomiting, diarrhea, diaphoresis, vertigo, tachycardia, headache, syncope, seizures, inguinal or axillary pain, muscle cramps, fasciculations, generalized edema (with truncal wounds), paralysis, hypotension, arrhythmias, and death.[183,184]

Treatment is directed at combating the effects of the venom, alleviating pain, and preventing infection. If hot water for immersion and irrigation is not immediately available, the wound should be irrigated immediately with nonheated water or saline. If sterile saline or water is not available, tap water may be used. This removes some venom and mucus, and may provide minimal pain relief.

As soon as possible, the wound should be soaked in nonscalding hot water to tolerance (upper limit 113°F or 45°C) for 30 to 90 minutes. During the hot water soak (or at any time, if soaking is not an option), the wound should be explored and debrided of any readily visible pieces of the sting or its integumentary sheath, which would continue to envenom the victim. Cryotherapy can be disastrous. One local remedy, application of half a bulb of onion directly to the wound, has been reported to decrease the pain and perhaps inhibit infection following a sting from the blue-spotted stingray *Dasyatis kuhlii*.[185]

Pain control should be initiated during the first debridement or soaking period. Narcotics may be necessary. Local infiltration of the wound with 1% to 2% lidocaine (Xylocaine) or bupivicaine 0.25% (not to exceed 3–4 mg/kg total dose in adults; not approved in children under the age of 12 years) without epinephrine may be useful. A regional nerve block may be necessary.

After the soaking procedure, the wound should be prepared in a sterile fashion, reexplored, and thoroughly debrided. Wounds should be packed open for delayed primary closure or sutured loosely around adequate drainage in preference to tight closure, which might increase likelihood of wound infection. Another approach that has been mentioned is wound excision followed by packing with an alginate-based wick dressing.[186,187] Prophylactic antibiotics appropriate to cover, among other organisms, the genus *Vibrio* are recommended because of the high incidence of ulceration, necrosis, and infection.

Scorpionfish

Scorpionfish are divided into three groups typified by different genera on the basis of venom organ structure: (1) *Pterois* (zebrafish, lionfish [Plate 9-4E], and butterfly cod), (2) *Scorpaena* (scorpionfish [Plate 9-4F], bullrout, and sculpin), and (3) *Synanceja* (stonefish [Plate 9-4G]). The venom organs are the 12 or 13 (of 18) dorsal, 2 pelvic, and 3 anal spines, with associated venom glands. Although they are frequently large, plumelike, and ornate, the pectoral spines are not associated with venom glands. Each spine is covered with an integumentary sheath, under which venom filters along grooves in the anterolateral region of the spine from the paired glands situated at the base or in the midportion of the spine.

Pterois species carry long, slender spines with small venom glands covered by a thin integumentary sheath. *Scorpaena* species carry longer, heavy spines with moderate-sized venom glands covered by a thicker integumentary sheath. *Synanceja* species carry short, thick spines with large, well-developed venom glands covered by an extremely thick integumentary sheath.

Pain is immediate and intense, with radiation centrally. Untreated, the pain peaks at 60 to 90 minutes and persists for 6 to 12 hours. With a stonefish envenomation, the pain may be severe enough to cause delirium and may persist at high levels for days. The wound and surrounding area are initially ischemic and then cyanotic, with more broadly surrounding areas of erythema, edema, and warmth. Vesicles may form. Rapid tissue sloughing and close surrounding areas of cellulitis, with anesthesia adjacent to peripheral hypesthesia, may be present within 48 hours. Systemic effects include anxiety, headache, tremors, maculopapular skin rash, nausea, vomiting, diarrhea, abdominal pain, diaphoresis, pallor, restlessness, delirium, seizures, limb paralysis, peripheral neuritis or neuropathy, lymphangitis, arthritis, fever, hypertension, respiratory distress, bradycardia, tachycardia, atrioventricular block, ventricular fibrillation, congestive heart failure, pericarditis, hypotension, syncope, and death.[188] The wound is indolent and may require months to heal, only to leave a cutaneous granuloma or marked tissue defect, particularly after a secondary infection or deep abscess. Mild pain may persist for days to weeks.

As soon as possible, the wound or wounds should be immersed in nonscalding hot (upper limit 113°F or 45°C) water to tolerance for up to 90 minutes. Recurrent pain that develops after an interval of 1 to 2 hours may respond to repeat hot water treatment. As soon as is practical, all obvious pieces of spine and sheath fragments should be gently removed from the wound. Vigorous irrigation should be performed with warmed sterile saline to remove any integument or slime. If pain is severe or inadequately controlled (in terms of degree or rapidity of relief) by hot water immersion, local tissue infiltration with 1% to 2% lidocaine without epinephrine, or regional nerve block with an anesthetic such as 0.25% bupivicaine, may be necessary.

Although the spine rarely breaks off in the skin, the wound should be explored to remove any spine fragments, which will otherwise continue to envenom and act as foreign bodies, perpetuating an infection risk and poorly healing wound.

Stonefish antivenom is manufactured by the Commonwealth Serum Laboratories, Melbourne, Australia. In cases of severe systemic reactions from stings of *Synanceja* species, and rarely from other scorpionfish, it is administered intramuscularly. As a rough estimate, one ampoule should neutralize one or two significant stings (punctures).

Sea Snakes

See the previous section on Venomous Snakes.

CONCLUSION

In view of the thousands of species of venomous animals that inhabit this planet, it is testimony to the tolerance of most of these creatures that venom poisoning does not take a greater toll on humanity. While there are specific interventional measures of benefit for some forms of envenomations, such as antivenom for snakebite or hot water immersion for stingray stings, it is often the treating physician's ability to anticipate clinical findings and intervene with sound supportive care that ultimately determines the outcome for the victim.

REFERENCES

1. Russell FE: Snake Venom Poisoning. New York, Scholium International, 1983.
2. Minton SA: Venom Diseases. Springfield, IL, Thomas, 1974.
3. Swaroop S, Grab B: Snakebite mortality in the world. Bull WHO 10:35, 1954.
4. Gutierrez JM, Rucavado A: Snake venom metalloproteinases: Their role in the pathogenesis of local tissue damage. Biochimie 82:841, 2000.
5. Rosenberg P: Pharmacology of phospholipase A2 from snake venoms. In Lee CY (ed): Snake Venoms. Handbook of Experimental Pharmacology, Vol. 52. Berlin, Springer-Verlag, 1979, p 403.
6. Lee CY: Elapid neurotoxins and their mode of action. Clin Toxicol 3:457, 1970.
7. Lee CY: Chemistry and pharmacology of polypeptide toxins in snake venoms. Annu Rev Pharmacol 12:265, 1972.
8. Minton SA, Norris RL: Non–North American venomous reptile bites. In Auerbach PS (ed): Wilderness Medicine: Management of Wilderness and Environmental Emergencies, 3rd ed. St. Louis, Mosby–Year Book, 1995, p 710.
9. Tu AT: Biotoxicology of sea snake venoms. Ann Emerg Med 16:1023, 1987.
10. Weinstein SA, Kardong KV: Properties of Duvernoy's secretions from opisthoglyphous and aglyphous colubrid snakes. Toxicon 32:1161, 1994.
11. Warrell DA, Ormerod LD, Davidson NM: Bites by the night adder (*Causus maculatus*) and burrowing vipers (genus *Atractaspis*) in Nigeria. Am J Trop Med Hyg 25:517, 1976.
12. Gunders AE, Walter HJ, Etzel E: Case of snake-bite by *Atractaspis corpulenta*. Trans R Soc Trop Med Hyg 54:279, 1960.
13. Lee S, Lee CY, Chen YM, et al: Coronary vasospasm as the primary cause of death due to the venom of the burrowing asp, *Atractaspis engaddensis*. Toxicon 24:285, 1986.
14. Minton SA: Venomous bites by nonvenomous snakes: An annotated bibliography of colubrid envenomation. J Wilderness Med 1:119, 1990.
15. Kunkel DB, Curry SC, Vance MV, et al: Reptile envenomations. J Toxicol Clin Toxicol 21:503, 1983–1984.
16. Bucknall NC: Electrical treatment of venomous bites and stings. Toxicon 29:397, 1991.
17. Hardy DL: A review of first aid measures for pitviper bite in North America with an appraisal of Extractor™ suction and stun gun electroshock. In Campbell JA, Brodie ED (eds): Biology of the Pitvipers. Tyler, TX, Selva, 1992, pp 405–414.
18. Alberts MB, Shalit M, LoGalbo F: Suction for venomous snakebite: A study of "mock venom" extraction in a human model. Ann Emerg Med 43:181, 2004.
19. Bush SP, Hegewald KG, Green SM, et al: Effects of a negative pressure venom extraction device (Extractor™) on local tissue injury after artificial rattlesnake envenomation in a porcine model. Wild Environ Med 11:180, 2000.
20. Burgess JL, Dart RC, Egen NB, et al: Effects of constriction bands on rattlesnake venom absorption: A pharmacokinetic study. Ann Emerg Med 21:1086, 1992.
21. Sutherland SK, King K: Management of Snake-Bite Injuries. Huntsville, Australia, Royal Flying Doctor Service of Australia, 1992.
22. Sutherland SK, Harris RD, Coulter AR, et al: First aid for cobra (*Naja naja*) bites. Indian J Med Res 73:266, 1981.
23. Sutherland SK, Coulter AR: Early management of bites by the eastern diamondback rattlesnake (*Crotalus adamanteus*): Studies in monkeys (*Macaca fascicularis*). Am J Trop Med Hyg 30:497, 1981.
24. Murrell G: The effectiveness of the pressure/immobilization first aid technique in the case of a tiger snake bite. Med J Aust 2:295, 1981.
25. Pearn J, Morrison J, Charles N, et al: First-aid for snake-bite: Efficacy of a constrictive bandage with limb immobilization in the management of human envenomation. Med J Aust 2:293, 1981.
26. Balmain R, McClelland KL: Pantyhose compression bandage: First-aid measure for snake bite. Med J Aust 2:240, 1982.
27. Sutherland SK: Pressure immobilization for snakebite in southern Africa remains speculative. South African Med J 85:1039, 1995.
28. Norris RL, Nolan K, Ngo J, et al: Volunteers are unable to properly apply pressure immobilization in a simulated snakebite scenario. Wild Environ Med (accepted for publication, 2005).
29. Schaeffer RC, Carlson RW, Puri VK, et al: The effects of colloidal and crystalloidal fluids on rattlesnake venom shock in the rat. J Pharmacol Exp Ther 206:687, 1978.
30. Kitchens CS, Hunter S, Van Mierop LHS: Severe myonecrosis in a fatal case of envenomation by the canebrake rattlesnake (*Crotalus horridus atricaudatus*). Toxicon 25:455, 1987.
31. Wingert WA, Wainschel J: Diagnosis and management of envenomation by poisonous snakes. South Med J 68:1015, 1975.
32. Reid HA, Theakston RDG: The management of snake bite. Bull WHO 61:885, 1983.
33. Theakston RDG: The application of immunoassay techniques, including enzyme-linked immunosorbent assay (ELISA), to snake venom research. Toxicon 21:341, 1983.
34. Pearn J, Morrison J, Charles N, et al: First-aid for snake-bite: Efficacy of a constrictive bandage with limb immobilization in the management of human envenomation. Med J Aust 2:293, 1981.
35. Tu A, Fulde G: Sea snake bites. Clin Dermatol 5:118, 1987.
36. Christensen PA: The treatment of snakebite. S Afr Med J 43:1253, 1969.
37. Schier JG, Wiener SW, Touger M, et al: Efficacy of Crotalidae polyvalent antivenin for the treatment of hognosed viper (*Porthidium nasutum*) envenomation. Ann Emerg Med 41:391, 2003.
38. Baxter EH, Gallichio HA: Cross-neutralization by tiger snake (*Notechis scutatus*) antivenin and sea snake (*Enhydrina schistosa*) antivenin against several sea snake venoms. Toxicon 12:273, 1974.
39. Corrigan P, Russell FE, Wainschel J: Clinical reactions to antivenin. Toxicon 16:457, 1978.
40. Malasit P, Warrell DA, Chanthavanich P, et al: Prediction, prevention, and mechanism of early (anaphylactic) antivenom reactions in victims of snake bites. BMJ 292:17, 1986.
41. Banner W: Bites and stings in the pediatric patient. Curr Probl Pediatr 18:9, 1988.
42. Chippaux JP: Production and use of snake antivenin. In Tu AT (ed): Reptile Venoms and Toxins, Vol. 5. New York, Marcel Dekker, 1991, p 529.
43. Seifert SA, Boyer LV: Recurrence phenomena after immunoglobulin therapy for snake envenomations: Part 1. Pharmacokinetics and pharmacodynamics of immunoglobulin antivenoms and related antibodies. Ann Emerg Med 37:189, 2001.
44. Package insert CroFab. London, Protherics, Inc. Available at: www.savagelabs.com/images/462531_R1200_CroFab_PI.pdf. (Accessed February 20, 2004.)
45. Ellis AK, Day JH: Diagnosis & management of anaphylaxis. Canadian Med Assoc J 169:307, 2003.
46. Loprinzi CL, Hennessee J, Tamsky L, et al: Snake antivenin administration in a patient allergic to horse serum. South Med J 76:501, 1983.
47. Kerrigan KR, Mertz BL, Nelson SJ, et al: Antibiotic prophylaxis for pit viper envenomation: Prospective, controlled trial. World J Surg 21:369, 1997.
48. Gold BS, Dart RC, Barish RA: Bites of venomous snakes. N Engl J Med 347:347, 2002.
49. Wasserman GS: Wound care of spider and snake envenomations. Ann Emerg Med 17:1331, 1988.
50. Sullivan JB, Wingert WA, Norris RL: North American venomous reptile bites. In Auerbach PS (ed): Wilderness Medicine: Management of Wilderness and Environmental Emergencies. St. Louis, Mosby–Year Book, 1995, p 680.
51. Boyer LV, Seifert SA, Cain JS: Recurrence phenomena after immunoglobulin therapy for snake envenomations: Part 2. Guidelines for clinical management with crotaline Fab antivenom. Ann Emerg Med 37:196, 2001.
52. Kunkel DB: Bites of venomous reptiles. Emerg Med Clin North Am 2:563, 1984.
53. Hooker KR, Caravati EM, Hartsell SC: Gila monster envenomation. Ann Emerg Med 24:731, 1994.
54. Stahnke HL, Heffron WA, Lewis DL: Bite of the gila monster. Rocky Mountain Med J 67:25, 1970.
55. Miller MF: Gila monster envenomation (letter). Ann Emerg Med 25:720, 1995.
56. Bou-Abboud CF, Kardassakis DG: Acute myocardial infarction following a Gila monster (*Heloderma suspectum cinctum*) bite. West J Med 148:577, 1988.

57. Minton SA, Bechtel HB: Arthropod envenomation and parasitism. In Auerbach PS (ed): Wilderness Medicine: Management of Wilderness and Environmental Emergencies. St. Louis, Mosby–Year Book, 1995, p 742.
58. Valentine MD: Anaphylaxis and stinging insect hypersensitivity. JAMA 268:2830, 1992.
59. Iseke R: Hymenoptera envenomation. In Harwood-Nuss AL, Linden CH, Luten RC, et al (eds): The Clinical Practice of Emergency Medicine. Philadelphia, Lippincott-Raven, 1996, p 1456.
60. Reisman RE: Stinging insect allergy. Med Clin North Am 76:883, 1992.
61. Winston ML: The Africanized "killer" bee: Biology and public health. Q J Med 87:263, 1994.
62. Mejia G, Arbelaez M, Henao JE, et al: Acute renal failure due to multiple stings by Africanized bees. Ann Intern Med 104:210, 1986.
63. Weizman Z, Mussafi H, Ishay J, et al: Multiple hornet stings with features of Reye's syndrome. Gastroenterology 89:1407, 1985.
64. Schmidt JO: Allergy to venomous insects. In Graham JM (ed): The Hive and the Honeybee. Hamilton, IL, Dadant & Sons, 1992, p 1209.
65. DeShazo RD, Butcher BT, Banks WA: Reactions to the stings of the imported fire ant. N Engl J Med 323:462, 1990.
66. Visscher PK, Vetter RS, Camazino S: Removing bee stings. Lancet 31:301, 1996.
67. Diaz-Sanchez CL, Lifshitz-Guinzberg A, Ignacio-Ibarra G, et al: Survival after massive (>2000) Africanized honeybee stings. Arch Intern Med 158:925, 1998.
68. Frieberg M, Walls JG: The World of Venomous Animals. Hong Kong, TFH Publications, 1984.
69. Hunt GR: Bites and stings of uncommon arthropods. 1. Spiders. Postgrad Med 70:91, 1981.
70. Horton P: Redback spider is now established in Japan: Bites can be recognised by a unique sign. BMJ 314:1484, 1997.
71. Wong RC, Hughes SE, Voorhees JJ: Spider bites. Arch Dermatol 123:98, 1987.
72. Maretic Z: Latrodectism: Variations in clinical manifestations provoked by *Latrodectus* species of spiders. Toxicon 21:457, 1983.
73. Clark RF, Wethern-Kestner S, Vance MV, et al: Clinical presentation and treatment of black widow spider envenomation: A review of 163 cases. Ann Emerg Med 21:782, 1992.
74. Peters S: A Colour Atlas of Arthropods in Clinical Medicine. London, Wolfe Publishing, 1992.
75. Moss HS, Binder LS: A retrospective review of black widow spider envenomation. Ann Emerg Med 16:188, 1987.
76. Woestman R, Perkin R, Van Stralen D: The black widow: Is she deadly to children? Ped Emerg Care 12:360, 1996.
77. Reeves JA, Allison EJ, Goodman PE: Black widow spider bite in a child. Am J Emerg Med 14:469, 1996.
78. Wingert W: Black widow spider envenomation. Wild Med Letter 12:12, 1995.
79. Graudins A, Padula M, Broady K, et al: Red-back spider (*Latrodectus hasselti*) antivenom prevents the toxicity of widow spider venoms. Ann Emerg Med 37:154, 2001.
80. Edlich RF, Rodeheaver GT, Feldman PS, et al: Management of venomous spider bites. Curr Concepts Trauma Care (Winter):17, 1985.
81. CSL Antivenom Handbook: CSL Red Back Spider Antivenom. Available at: www.toxinology.com/generic_static_files/cslavh_antivenom_redback.html. (Accessed February 16, 2004.)
82. Wingert W: Black widow spider envenomation. Wild Med Lett 12:12, 1995.
83. Russell FE, Marcus P, Streng JA: Black widow spider envenomation during pregnancy: Report of a case. Toxicon 17:188, 1979.
84. Knox I, Cave D: Premature labor precipitated by red-back spider envenomation. Emerg Med (Australia) 5:3, 1993.
85. Russell FE: Venomous bites and stings. In Berkow R (ed): The Merck Manual, 15th ed. Rahway, NJ, Merck Sharp & Dohme, 1987, p 2565.
86. Pneumatikos IA, Galiatsou D, Goe D, et al: Acute fatal toxic myocarditis after black widow spider envenomation. Ann Emerg Med 41:158, 2003.
87. Kobernick M: Black widow spider bite. Am Fam Physician 29:241, 1984.
88. Gertsch WJ, Ennik F: The spider genus *Loxosceles* in North America, Central America, and the West Indes (Araneae, Loxoscelidae). Bull Am Museum Nat History 175:264, 1983.
89. Sutherland SK: Venomous Creatures of Australia. Melbourne, Oxford University Press, 1994.
90. Wasserman GS, Anderson PC: Loxoscelism and necrotic arachnidism. J Toxicol Clin Toxicol 21:451, 1983–1984.
91. Atkins JA, Wingo CW, Sodeman WA, et al: Necrotic arachnidism. Am J Trop Med Hyg 7:165, 1958.
92. Smith CW, Micks DW: A comparative study of the venom and other components of three species of *Loxosceles*. Am J Trop Med Hyg 17:651, 1968.
93. Rees R, Campbell D, Rieger E, et al: The diagnosis and treatment of brown recluse spider bites. Ann Emerg Med 16:945, 1987.
94. Auer Al, Hershey FB: Surgery for necrotic bites of the brown spider. Arch Surg 108:612, 1974.
95. Vetter RS, Cushing PE, Crawford RL, et al: Diagnoses of brown recluse spider bites (loxoscelism) greatly outnumber actual verifications of the spider in four western American states. Toxicon 42:413, 2003.
96. Vetter RS, Bush SP: Reports of presumptive brown recluse spider bites reinforce improbable diagnosis in regions of North America where the spider is not endemic. Clin Infect Dis 35:442, 2002.
97. Wilson DC, King LE: Spiders and spider bites. Dermatol Clin 8:277, 1990.
98. Anderson PC: What's new in loxoscelism—1978. J Mo State Med Assoc 74:549, 1977.
99. King LE: Brown recluse bites: Stay cool. JAMA 254:2895, 1985.
100. Berger RS, Millikan LE, Conway F: An in vitro test for *Loxosceles reclusa* spider bites. Toxicon 11:465, 1973.
101. Hansen RC, Russell FE: Dapsone use for *Loxosceles* envenomation treatment. Vet Hum Toxicol 26:260, 1984.
102. Barrett SM, Romine-Jenkins M, Fisher DE: Dapsone or electric shock therapy for brown recluse spider envenomation? Ann Emerg Med 24:21, 1994.
103. Iserson KV: Methemoglobinemia from dapsone therapy for a suspected brown recluse spider bite. J Emerg Med 3:285, 1985.
104. Bryant SM: Dapsone use in *Loxosceles reclusa* envenomation: Is there an indication? Am J Emerg Med 21:89, 2003.
105. Harves AD, Millikan LE: Current concepts of therapy and pathophysiology in arthropod bites and stings. Part 1. Arthropods. Int J Dermatol 14:543, 1975.
106. Beilman GJ, Winslow CL, Teslow TW: Experimental brown spider bite in the guinea pig: Results of treatment with dapsone or hyperbaric oxygen. J Wild Med 5:287, 1994.
107. Strain GM, Snider TG, Tedford BL, et al: Hyperbaric oxygen effects on brown recluse spider (*Loxosceles*) envenomation in rabbits. Toxicon 29:989, 1991.
108. Lucas S: Spiders in Brazil. Toxicon 26:759, 1988.
109. Araujo SC, Castanheira P, Alvarenga LM, et al: Protection against dermonecrotic and lethal activities of *Loxosceles intermedia* spider venom by immunization with a fused recombinant protein. Toxicon 41:261, 2003.
110. Gomez HF, Krywko DM, Stoecker WV: A new assay for the detection of *Loxosceles* species (brown recluse) spider venom. Ann Emerg Med 39:469, 2002.
111. Krywko DM, Gomez HF: Detection of *Loxosceles* species venom in dermal lesions: A comparison of 4 venom recovery methods. Ann Emerg Med 39:475, 2002.
112. Hartman LJ, Sutherland SK: Funnel-web spider (*Atrax robustus*) antivenom in the treatment of human envenomation. Med J Aust 141:796, 1984.
113. Bucaretchi F, Deus Reinaldo CR, Hyslop S, et al: A clinico-epidemiological study of bites by spiders of the genus Phoneutria. Revista Inst Med Trop Sao Paulo 42:17, 2000.
114. Sandboe FE: Spider keratouveitis. A case report. Acta Ophthalmol Scand 79:531, 2001.
115. Campbell DS, Rees RS, King LE: Wolf spider bites. Cutis 39:113, 1987.
116. White J: Debunking spider bite myths. Med J Aust 179:180, 2003.
117. Isbister GK, Gray MR: White-tail spider bite: A prospective study of 130 definite bites by *Lampona* species. Med J Aust 179:199, 2003.
118. Necrotic arachnidism—Pacific Northwest, 1988–1996. MMWR 45:433, 1996.
119. Polis GA: Introduction. In Polis GA (ed): Biology of Scorpions. Stanford, CA, Stanford University Press, 1990, p 1.
120. Simard JM, Watt DD: Venoms and toxins. In Polis GA (ed): Biology of Scorpions. Stanford, CA, Stanford University Press, 1990, p 414.
121. Bond GR: Antivenin administration for *Centruroides* scorpion sting: Risks and benefits. Ann Emerg Med 21:788, 1992.
122. Berg RA, Tarantino MD: Envenomation by the scorpion *Centruroides exilicauda* (*C. sculpturatus*): Severe and unusual manifestations. Pediatrics 87:930, 1991.

123. King LE, Rees RS: Spider bites and scorpion stings. In Rakel RE (ed): Conn's Current Therapy. Philadelphia, WB Saunders, 1987, p 970.
124. Radmanesh M: Cutaneous manifestations of the *Hemiscorpius lepturus* sting: A clinical study. Intl J Dermatol 37:500, 1998.
125. Rachesky IJ, Banner W, Dansky J, et al: Treatments for *Centruroides exilicauda* envenomation. Am J Dis Child 138:1136, 1984.
126. Gueron M, Sofer S: The role of the intensivist in the treatment of the cardiovascular manifestations of scorpion envenomation. Toxicon 32:1027, 1994.
127. Stahnke HL, Dengler AH: The effect of morphine and related substances on the toxicity of venoms: 1. *Centruroides sculpturatus* Ewing scorpion venom. Am J Trop Med 13:346, 1964.
128. Bawaskar HS, Bawaskar PH: Vasodilators: Scorpion envenoming and the heart (an Indian experience). Toxicon 32:1031, 1994.
129. Ismail M: The treatment of the scorpion envenoming syndrome: The Saudi experience with serotherapy. Toxicon 32:1019, 1994.
130. Freire-Maia L, Campos JA, Amaral CFS: Approaches to the treatment of scorpion envenoming. Toxicon 32:1009, 1994.
131. Gueron M: Is antivenom the most successful therapy in scorpion victims? Toxicon 37:1655, 1999.
132. Rimsza ME, Zimmerman DR, Bergeson PS: Scorpion envenomation. Pediatrics 66:298, 1980.
133. Shattock RM: Injuries caused by wild animals. Lancet 1:412, 1968.
134. Harrison LJ: Dangerous marine life. J Fla Med Assoc 79:633, 1992.
135. Haddad LM, Lee RF, McConnell O, et al: Toxic marine life. In Haddad LM, Winchester JF (eds): Clinical Management of Poisoning and Drug Overdose. Philadelphia, WB Saunders, 1983, p 303.
136. Soppe GG: Marine envenomations and aquatic dermatology. Am Fam Physician 40:97, 1989.
137. Johnson L: A review of bites and stings by venomous animals of southern California: Part II. Arthropods and marine animals. STAT 2:16, 1980.
138. Ronka EKF, Roe WF: Cardiac wound caused by the spine of the stingray (suborder-Masticura). Mil Surg 97:135, 1945.
139. Lester IA: Obituary, Hugo Flecker. Med J Aust 2:809, 1957.
140. Fenner P: Medical frontiers in Australian seas. In Cobcroft M (ed): Fevers and Frontiers. Brisbane, Australia, Amphion, 1990, p 73.
141. Cooper NK: Two cases of near fatal box jellyfish stings sustained in littoral waters of the sultanate of Oman. SPUMS J 2:16, 1985.
142. Bengtson K, Nichols MM, Schnadig V, et al: Sudden death in a child following jellyfish envenomation by *Chiropsalmus quadrumanus*. Case report and autopsy findings [erratum appears in JAMA 266:2834, 1991]. JAMA 266:1404, 1991.
143. Beadnell CE, Rider TA, Williamson JA, et al: Management of a major box jellyfish (*Chironex flecken*) sting. Lessons from the first minutes and hours. Med J Aust 156:655, 1992.
144. Benmeir P, Rosenberg L, Sagi A, et al: Jellyfish envenomation: A summer epidemic. Burns 16:471, 1990.
145. McGoldrick J, Marx JA: Marine envenomations. Part 2: Invertebrates. J Emerg Med 10:71, 1992.
146. Martin JC, Audley I: Cardiac failure following Irukandji envenomation. Med J Aust 153:164, 1990.
147. Roberts J, Kinsey B: Who knew Jack Barnes? A short biography of Dr. John Handyside Barnes—Pioneer medical toxicologist. In Pearn J (ed): Pioneer Medicine in Australia. Brisbane, Australia, Amphion, 1988, p 251.
148. Fenner PJ, Williamson JA, Burnett JW, et al: First aid treatment of jellyfish stings in Australia. Response to a newly differentiated species. Med J Aust 158:498, 1993.
149. Fenner P: Deaths from marine envenomations (with description of the symptoms of ten jellyfish species). In Fenner P (ed): Marine Stinger Guide, 3rd ed. Brisbane, Australia, Surf Life-Saving Association of Australia, 1985, p 1.
150. Williamson J: Classification (with description and medical complications of seven venomous jellyfish). In Williamson J (ed): Some Australian Marine Stings, Envenomations and Poisonings. Brisbane, Australia, Surf Life-Saving Foundation, 1981, p 1.
151. Schwartz S, Meinking T: Venomous marine animals of Florida: Morphology, behavior, health hazards. J Fla Med Assoc 84:433, 1997.
152. Russell FE, Nagabhushanam R: Venomous and Poisonous Marine Invertebrates of the Indian Ocean. New Dehli, India, Oxford and IBH Publishing, 1996.
153. Hadok JC: "Irukandji" syndrome: A risk for divers in tropical waters. Med J Aust 167:649, 1997.
154. Yaffee HS, Stargardtner F: Erythema multiforme from *Tedania ignis*. Arch Dermatol 87:601, 1963.
155. Sims JK, Irei MY: Human Hawaiian marine sponge poisoning. Hawaiian Med J 9:263, 1979.
156. Yaffee HS: Irritation from red sponge. N Engl J Med 282:51, 1970.
157. Burnett JW, Calton GJ: Jellyfish envenomation syndromes updated. Ann Emerg Med 16:1000, 1987.
158. Chand RP, Selliah K: Reversible parasympathetic dysautonomia following stinging attributed to the box-jellyfish (*Chironex fleckeri*). Aust NZ J Med 14:673, 1984.
159. Filling-Katz MR: Mononeuritis multiplex following jellyfish stings. Ann Neurol 15:213, 1984.
160. Meyer PK: Seastroke: A new entity? South Med J 86:777, 1993.
161. Peel N, Kandler R: Localized neuropathy following jellyfish sting. Postgrad Med 66:953, 1990.
162. Weinberg SR: Reactive arthritis following a sting by a Portuguese man-of-war (letter). J Fla Med Assoc 75:280, 1988.
163. Glasser DV, et al: Ocular jellyfish stings. Ophthalmology 92:1414, 1992.
164. Glasser DV, et al: A guinea-pig model of corneal jellyfish envenomation. Toxicon 31:808, 1993.
165. Guess HA, Saviteer PL, Morris RC: Hemolysis and acute renal failure following a Portuguese man-of-war sting. Pediatrics 70:979, 1982.
166. Abu-Nema T, et al: Jellyfish sting resulting in severe hand ischaemia successfully treated with intra-arterial urokinase. Injury: Br J Accident Surg 19:294, 1988.
167. Exton DR, Fenner PJ, Williamson JA: Cold packs: Effective topical analgesia in the treatment of painful stings by Physalia and other jellyfish. Med J Aust 151:625, 1989.
168. Fenner PJ, Williamson JA: Worldwide deaths and severe envenomation from jellyfish stings. Med J Aust 165:658, 1996.
169. Currie B: Clinical implications of research on the box-jellyfish *Chironex fleckeri*. Toxicon 32:1305, 1994.
170. Williamson JA, Callahan VI, Hartwick RF: Serious envenomation by the northern Australian box-jellyfish (*Chironex fleckeri*). Med J Aust 1:13, 1980.
171. Williamson JA, et al: Box-jellyfish venom and humans. Med J Aust 140:444, 1984.
172. Burnett JW, et al: A protocol to investigate the blockade of jellyfish nematocysts by topical agents. Contact Derm 40:56, 1999.
173. Kimball AB, Arambula KZ, Stauffer AR, et al: Efficacy of a jellyfish sting inhibitor in preventing jellyfish stings in normal volunteers. Wild Environ Med 15:102, 2004.
174. Jefferies NJ: Caribbean itch: Eight cases and one who didn't (exercise blue calypso diamond). J R Army Med Corps 143:163, 1997.
175. Tomchik RS, et al: Clinical perspectives on seabather's eruption, also known as sea lice. JAMA 269:1669, 1993.
176. Asada M, et al: A case of delayed hypersensitivity reaction following a sea urchin sting. Dermatologica 180:99, 1990.
177. Sutherland SK, Lane WR: Toxins and mode of envenomation of the common ringed or blue-banded octopus. Med J Aust 1:893, 1969.
178. Sheumack DD, et al: Maculotoxin: A neurotoxin from the venom glands of the octopus *Hapalochlaena maculosa* identified as tetrodotoxin. Science 199:188, 1978.
179. Williamson JA: The blue-ringed octopus bite and envenomation syndrome. Clin Dermatol 5:127, 1987.
180. Williamson JA: The blue ringed octopus. Med J Aust 140:308, 1984.
181. Manowitz NR, Rosenthal RR: Cutaneous-systemic reactions to toxins and venoms of common marine organisms. Cutis 23:450, 1979.
182. Barss P: Wound necrosis caused by the venom of stingrays. Med J Aust 141:854, 1984.
183. Grainger CR: Occupational injuries due to sting rays. Trans R Soc Trop Med Hyg 74:408, 1980.
184. Ikeda T: Supraventricular bigeminy following a stingray envenomation: A case report. Hawaii Med J 48:162, 1989.
185. Whiting SC, Guinea ML: Treating stingray wounds with onions. Med J Aust 168:584, 1998.
186. Fenner PJ: Stingray envenomation: A suggested new treatment. Med J Aust 163:655, 1995.
187. Meyer PK: Stingray injuries. Wild Environ Med 8:24, 1997.
188. Lehmann DF, Hardy JC: Stonefish envenomation (letter). N Engl J Med 329:510, 1993.

10

Plant Toxins in the Tropics

JAMES L. LARSON, Jr.
RICHARD F. CLARK

INTRODUCTION

The study of plant poisoning is termed *phytotoxicology.* This field has not achieved clinical sophistication, in part due to a lack of collaboration between botanists and physicians. Few people possess adequate training in both of these fields. The result has been many poorly documented case reports of plant-related toxicity, often with improper plant identification, using local or common names, and a tendency to combine scientific facts with older fictional accounts.

One of the most significant problems associated with toxic plant exposures is plant identification. Plant toxicity seems to occur consistently on a genus level, although species variation may alter toxicity. Seasonal variations in toxin content, crossbreeding, and changing environmental conditions can all affect toxic potential. Trained botanists often require plant specimens for adequate confirmation of a local species. In addition, the nomenclature of many plant species varies greatly in different regions, making identification more difficult. Common names are often misleading. "Nightshade," for instance, is a name frequently associated with "deadly nightshade" or *Atropa belladonna.* However, the nightshade family, Solanaceae, also includes the edible potato and the poisonous Jerusalem cherry (*Solanum pseudocapsicum*).

Exposures to potentially poisonous plants are common, accounting for an estimated 5% to 10% of all calls to poison control centers. Fortunately, houseplant ingestions result in the majority of these calls, and morbidity and mortality following these incidents are low. Throughout history, the toxic properties of many plants have been described. Information on individual plant toxicity is enormous and constantly expanding. Some plants, such as hemlock, are known to be rapidly fatal when taken in sufficient quantities. Most, however, have not been studied sufficiently. Tropical and subtropical environments harbor numerous species that lack clinical data regarding toxicity.

This chapter covers some of the more common and most toxic species of plants encountered in tropical and subtropical environments (Table 10-1). Identification, pathophysiology, and therapeutic considerations are discussed.

GENERAL MANAGEMENT

History

There is no more important tool in the successful management of plant ingestion than obtaining an accurate history. Timing of the exposure and onset of toxicity, the plant portion and amount ingested, and a description of symptoms are essential to beginning the evaluation. An account of the preparation of the plant or fruit should be obtained. The time of year and seasonal weather conditions should be noted. Potential exposures to other people should be explored.

In order to facilitate identification, portions of the suspected plant should be gathered and brought to the health care facility. Books are often available at emergency departments or through poison control centers and can be used to match common with taxonomic names. If necessary, toxicologists, botanists, or mycologists can often be located through poison centers or local universities.

Physical Examination

Frequently, the health care provider must initiate treatment before reliable identification of the ingested plant can be made. Poisonings by some plant species often present with characteristic physical examination findings (Box 10-1). The most common manifestation of plant toxicity after ingestion is gastroenteritis. Nausea and vomiting can be severe after exposure to numerous plants and can necessitate intravenous fluid repletion. Dehydration with electrolyte imbalance is the main concern following these ingestions. Ricin- and abrin-containing plants (*Ricinus communis* and *Abrus precatoris*) and pokeweed (*Phytolacca americana*) are examples of this type of toxicity. *Philodendron* and other Araecea are also capable of causing gastrointestinal irritation due to the presence of calcium oxalate crystals or other substances within their leaves and stems.

Several classes of plants are known for cardiovascular toxicity. Numerous species of oleander (*Nerium oleander* and *Thevetia peruviana*), foxglove (*Digitalis purpurea*), lily of the valley (*Convallaria majalis*), and red squill (*Urgenia maritima*) all contain cardiac glycosides and can predispose to ventricular dysrhythmias and heart block in severe cases. *Veratrum* and *Rhododendron* species contain toxins that can lead to hypotension and bradycardia. *Aconitum* species, commonly sold as herbal remedies, can impair ion movement through myocyte cell membranes leading to life-threatening dysrhythmias.

Severe neurotoxicity is an uncommon but potentially lethal manifestation of plant poisoning. Water hemlock (*Cicuta* spp.) is responsible for most plant-related fatalities in the United States and can cause refractory status epilepticus after ingestion. Others, such as moonseed (*Menispermum canadense*) and chinaberry (*Melia azedarach*), contain neurotoxic components, but documented cases of neurotoxicity after ingestion are rare. Many plants can produce an altered level of consciousness. *Datura* species such as jimsonweed, deadly nightshade (*Atropa belladonna*), and angels' trumpet (*Brugmansia* spp.) are just a few that contain atropine, scopolamine, and hyoscyamine. Ingestion of the leaves, seeds, or teas made from the seeds of these species produces the classic findings of antimuscarinic toxicity, including dry mouth and skin, hallucinations, tachycardia, urinary retention, and ileus. Others in the tobacco family (*Nicotiana* and *Lobelia* spp.) and poison hemlock (*Conium maculatum*) cause nicotinic receptor stimulation when ingested, resulting in nausea, vomiting, seizures, and paralysis in severe cases.

Table 10-1 Commonly Encountered Toxic Plants

Common Name	Scientific Name	Toxic Parts	Poisonous Principles	Symptoms
Akee	*Blighia sapida*	Fruit	Hypoglycin A	Jamaican vomiting sickness occurs from eating unripe fruit; toxin inhibits gluconeogenesis, leading to profound hypoglycemia; classic symptoms with diaphoresis, nausea, and vomiting, progressing to seizures and coma; much more common in children
Apricot, apple, peach, pear	*Prunus* spp.	Seeds	Amygdalin glycosides	Seeds need to be chewed to release amygdalin that is converted to cyanide by stomach acid; classic symptoms of cyanide poisoning, such as metabolic acidosis, hypotension, coma, and seizures, can occur in large ingestions
Autumn crocus, saffron Glory lily	*Colchicum autumnale* *Gloriosa superba*	All parts	Colchicine	Pain in mouth, throat, and abdomen; severe nausea, vomiting, and diarrhea; symptoms usually appear 2–6 hr after ingestion; bone marrow depression possible, leading to sepsis or other infections after period free of symptoms; peripheral neuropathy and alopecia possible late complications
Beauty of the night, four o'clock	*Mirabilis jalapa*	Root, seed	The alkaloid trigonelline	Irritant to skin, mouth, and throat; causes gastroenteritis
Bird of paradise	*Caesalpinia gilliesii*	Pods, seeds	Unknown	Severe gastroenteritis, dehydration
Bleeding heart Dutchman's breeches	*Dicentra formosa* *Dicentra cucullaria*	Foliage, roots	Isoquinoline alkaloids	Tremors, staggering gait, convulsions, tachypnea, salivation, convulsions; death may be due to respiratory insufficiency and paralysis but is mostly reported from animal exposures
Cassava	*Manihot esculenta*	Fruit or tuber	Linamarin, a cyanogenic glycoside	Tropical ataxic neuropathy can result from eating fruit; neurologic symptoms include optic atrophy, deafness, and peripheral neuropathy; lower extremity weakness is most common sequela; paralysis may occur
Castor bean	*Ricinus communis*	All parts, mainly seeds	Ricin and ricinine (toxalbumins)	Severe nausea, vomiting, and diarrhea; burning sensation in mouth and throat; hemolysis of red blood cells; renal insufficiency; death may be associated with dehydration or systemic poisoning with toxalbumins (rare); 1–3 seeds in a child reported to be lethal
Chinaberry	*Melia azedarach*	Entire plant, especially fruit	Tetranortriterpenoid neurotoxins and other compounds	Has caused serious poisoning in animals (hogs and sheep), including tachypnea, tachycardia, sluggish movements, vomiting; humans develop severe gastroenteritis and weakness; case reports suggest 6–8 fruits may be lethal to a child
Christmas rose Stinking hellabore Lenten rose	*Helleborus niger* *Helleborus foetidus* *Helleborus orientalis*	Rootstocks and leaves	Glycosides ranunculin, hellebrin, others	Inflammation and numbing sensations in mouth; vomiting, diarrhea, and possible convulsions; may have a digitalis-like effect on heart from cardiac glycosides
Daphne	*Daphne mezereum* and other species	Berries, bark, leaves	Daphnin and resin mezerenic acid	Plant intensely irritating, producing vesication when rubbed on skin; ingestion produces burning sensation in mouth, throat, and abdomen; bloody emesis and diarrhea are reported; renal insufficiency, convulsions, and death are possible; case reports are rare
Dieffenbachia, dumbcane	*Dieffenbachia* spp.	All parts	Calcium oxalate and raphide crystals	Irritation of mouth, tongue, lips, and throat; if juice gets in eye, it causes marked burning and inflammation; airway obstruction may occur from swelling

Continued

Table 10-1 Commonly Encountered Toxic Plants—Cont'd

Common Name	Scientific Name	Toxic Parts	Poisonous Principles	Symptoms
Djenkol	*Pithecellobium jiringa*	Seed or bean	Djenkolic acid crystals	Colicky pain in groin and pelvis with nausea, vomiting, and diarrhea; dysuria and hematuria can precede acute renal failure; crystals not always found in urine
Foxglove	*Digitalis purpurea*	Leaves and seeds	Cardiac glycosides, including digitoxin, digitalin, and digitonin	One of the sources of the drug digitalis; in large amounts the active principles cause heart block and ventricular arrhythmias; symptoms begin with severe gastroenteritis and confusion; may cause seizures and death
Golden chain, laburnum	*Laburnum anagyroides*	Flowers, leaves, seeds, bark	The quinolizidine alkaloid cytisine	Dysphagia, mydriasis, agitation, incoordination, vomiting, renal insufficiency; convulsions and coma are possible; action may be similar to nicotine
Poison hemlock, hemlock, spotted hemlock	*Conium maculatum*	All parts	Piperidine alkaloids coniine, γ-coniceine	Resembles nicotine poisoning; gastroenteritis is common along with salivation and urination; weakness may proceed to loss of muscle tone and paralysis; death may occur from respiratory insufficiency
Water hemlock, cowbane, wild carrot, false parsley	*Cicuta maculata* and other species	All parts, mostly the roots	Cicutoxin	Symptoms appear as soon as 15 min after ingestion and include stomach pain, vomiting, salivation, and refractory convulsions; mydriasis and delirium are common; death may occur within 15 min after ingestion of lethal amount
Holly	*Ilix*	Berries	Ilicin or other alkaloids	Nausea, abdominal pain, severe vomiting, and diarrhea
Iris or blue flag	*Iris* sp.	Leaves and root stalks	Irritating resinous substance	Produces severe but not usually serious gastroenteritis; can also cause dermatitis
Jack-in-the-pulpit	*Arisaema triphyllum*	Rhizome	Calcium oxalate crystals	Intense irritation of mouth and throat; burning pain; inflammation of larynx (resembles dumbcane)
Jerusalem cherry, nightshade	*Solanum pseudocapsicum* and other species	Entire plant, especially berries	Solanine and related alkaloids	Headache, abdominal pain, gastroenteritis; convulsions, and coma may occur more commonly in children; respiratory depression rarely reported
Jimson weed, thorn apple	*Datura americana* and other species	All parts, especially seeds	The solanaceous alkaloids atropine, hyoscyamine, and scopolamine	Antimuscarinic symptoms include dry mouth, urinary retention, tachycardia, blurred vision with mydriasis, delirium, hallucinations; temperature may be elevated due to anhydrosis; convulsions and coma are possible; handling leaves or seeds followed by rubbing eyes can cause mydriasis
Lantana	*Lantana camera*	Berries, leaves	Lantadene A, a triterpenoid	Extreme muscular weakness, gastrointestinal irritation, lethargy, cyanosis, and hypotension; animals develop cholestatic jaundice
Larkspur	*Delphinium ajacis* and other species	Entire plant, seeds	Diterpene alkaloids, mainly delphinine	Ingestion in cattle produces gastroenteritis, weakness, respiratory depression, salivation, hypotension, and cardiac arrhythmias; human exposures are rarely reported
Lily of the valley	*Convallaria majalis*	Leaves, flowers, roots	The cardiac glycosides convallarin, convallamarin, and convallatoxin	Cardiac effects similar to other cardiac glycosides; dizziness and vomiting may occur within 1–2 hr after ingestion
Manchineel	*Hippomane mancinella*	Bark, fruit, leaves, and sap	Irritating ester with several triterpene compounds	Severe dermatitis with blistering can occur with contact of the sap or bark; conjuctivitis can result from eye contact; fruit ingestion leads to severe gastroenteritis, and in some cases laryngeal edema from local irritation

Presentation and Treatment

An estimated 5000 people have died in Jamaica since 1886 from ackee poisoning. Children ages 2 to 10 years are most often affected.[5] Symptoms begin with intense vomiting, followed by a quiescent phase that precedes more vomiting, seizures, coma, and death.[6] At the request of the Jamaican Ministry of Health, the U.S. Centers for Disease Control and Prevention investigated a series of patients with Jamaican vomiting sickness between 1989 and 1991. A total of 38 patients were identified. Vomiting was present in 77%, coma in 26%, and seizures in 24%. Eight patients (21%) died.[7] More than 75% of the cases occurred from January to March, and 28 (74%) of the patients were younger than 15 years old. Hypoglycemia with serum glucose levels as low as 3 mg/dL is a hallmark of the disease.[6]

Diagnosis requires recognizing the classic symptoms in association with recent ackee ingestion. Hypoglycemia and acidemia are the main laboratory abnormalities. Excess serum fatty acids can be detected using gas chromatography.[1] Treatment is supportive, focusing on rehydration, electrolyte replacement, and maintenance of normal blood glucose levels.

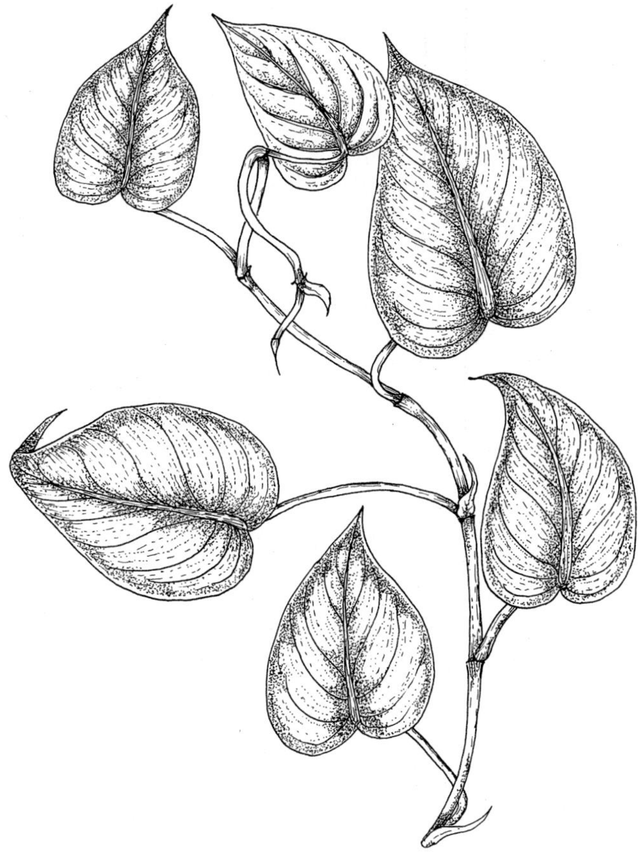

FIGURE 10-2 Philodendron.

Araceae

The Araceae family includes *Philodendron* and *Dieffenbachia* species. Philodendrons are indigenous to areas of Central and South America and can be found as ornamental indoor plants throughout the world[8] (Fig. 10-2). There are more than 275 species in the genus *Philodendron. Dieffenbachia* species are found throughout the tropical Americas and as houseplants. They have large ellipsoid leaves with characteristic pale-yellow central markings (Fig. 10-3).

Toxin

Philodendron and *Dieffenbachia* have cells called idioblasts in their stems and leaves. These idioblasts contain needle-like crystals of calcium oxalate that can be released when a mechanical or chemical stimulus is applied. These cells are cigar-shaped and have a thick, rigid cell wall that forms a "nozzle" shape at either end. Each cell contains a bundle of 100 to 200 projectiles. When firing, the cell membrane covering the nozzle end ruptures and a single projectile is fired two to three cell lengths. Once firing begins, it does not end until all crystals are released.[9] Animal experiments have shown that these calcium oxalate crystals alone do not produce a significant inflammatory response but are released with a proteolytic trypsin-like enzyme.[10] One theory suggests that the toxic substance accompanying the crystals is a bradykinin-like chemical, capable by itself of initiating an inflammatory response in the oral and pharyngeal mucosa.[11,12] Another hypothesis implies that the calcium oxalates or raphide crystals cause initial mechanical tissue damage, allowing the entry of proteolytic enzymes that cause inflammation.[13] The crystals can also penetrate the surface of the cornea and produce a keratoconjunctivitis.[14]

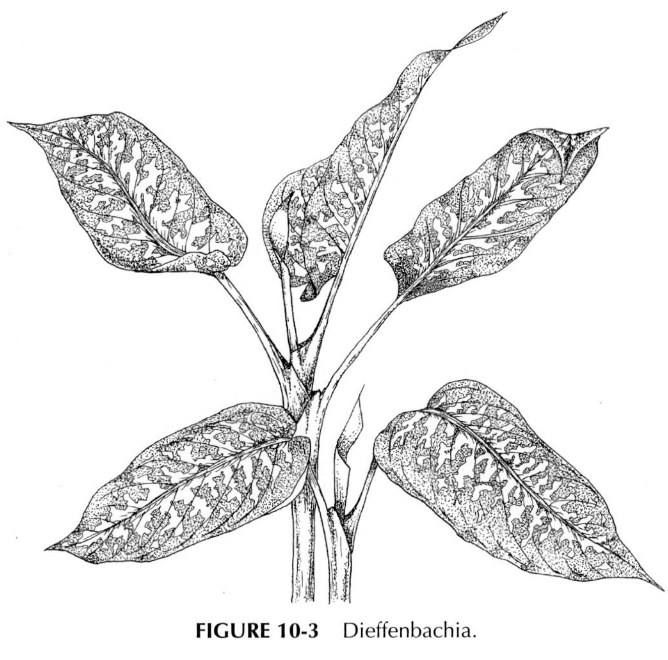

FIGURE 10-3 Dieffenbachia.

Presentation and Treatment

Human toxicity results from mastication of the leaves or stems of the *Philodendron*, *Dieffenbachia*, and other members of the Araceae family. There is an immediate irritation of the mucous membranes, with a burning sensation, salivation, edema, and difficulty speaking. The difficulty in speaking gave *Dieffenbachia* its nickname "dumbcane." A review of 188 exposures to *Dieffenbachia* and *Philodendron* from poison center data in the United States found only four mildly symptomatic cases. The authors concluded that *Dieffenbachia* and *Philodendron* exposures are rarely significant.[15] However, a published case reported severe airway compromise requiring emergency tracheostomy in an elderly man who bit into a *Dieffenbachia* stem thinking it was sugarcane.[12]

Treatment consists of local irrigation to remove the toxin. Observation for pharyngeal and oral swelling and control of the airway should be undertaken if necessary.

Cassava

Cassava (*Manihot esculenta*) provides a major source of calories to approximately 300 million people throughout the tropics, including those in Nigeria, Zaire, Tanzania, Uganda, and Mozambique[16] (Fig. 10-4). The cassava tuber can be processed into several different foods known as garri, fufu, kpokpogari, and cassava flour. The chronic consumption of cassava has been linked to cassavism, the syndrome of tropical ataxic neuropathy (TAN).

Toxin

Cassavism results from the toxin linamarin, a cyanogenic glucoside. Linamarin is hydrolyzed in the intestinal tract by microbial flora releasing cyanide.[17] The cyanide is absorbed at sublethal levels and normally converted to thiocyanate.[18] Several environmental factors, including natural geographic variation in soil composition, influence the cyanogenic potential of cassava. Drought conditions raise the cyanogenic content. The most important factor influencing the development of toxicity seems to be the manner in which the fruit is prepared for consumption. Proper sun drying and thorough cooking of the fruit greatly reduce its toxic potential. Recent studies have also implicated toxins found in some cycads on West Pacific islands and in other tropical countries as causes of TAN.[19]

TAN may be caused by either chronic cyanide or thiocyanate intoxication. During a cassava-related epidemic of TAN in Mozambique that affected more than 1000 people, serum thiocyanate levels in those affected were 30 to 34 μmol/dL (normal, 1 to 4 μmol/dL).[16] A dietary deficiency of sulfur-containing amino acids necessary for cyanide detoxification may also be a factor in the development of TAN.[20] The nutritional requirements of children and pregnant or lactating women make them more likely to show signs of toxicity.

Cyanide inhibits the enzyme cytochrome oxidase, preventing cellular respiration. Thiocyanate inhibits the enzyme fumarase hydratase in the Krebs citric acid cycle. Intact linamarin also inhibits the activity of Na-adenosine triphosphatase (ATPase). Animal studies of TAN have found hypokalemia, swelling, vacuolation of cells, and degeneration of myocardial fibers.[18] It is important to stress that cassavism is a clinical entity distinct from acute cyanide poisoning, and the exact mechanism of toxicity by this fruit is unknown.

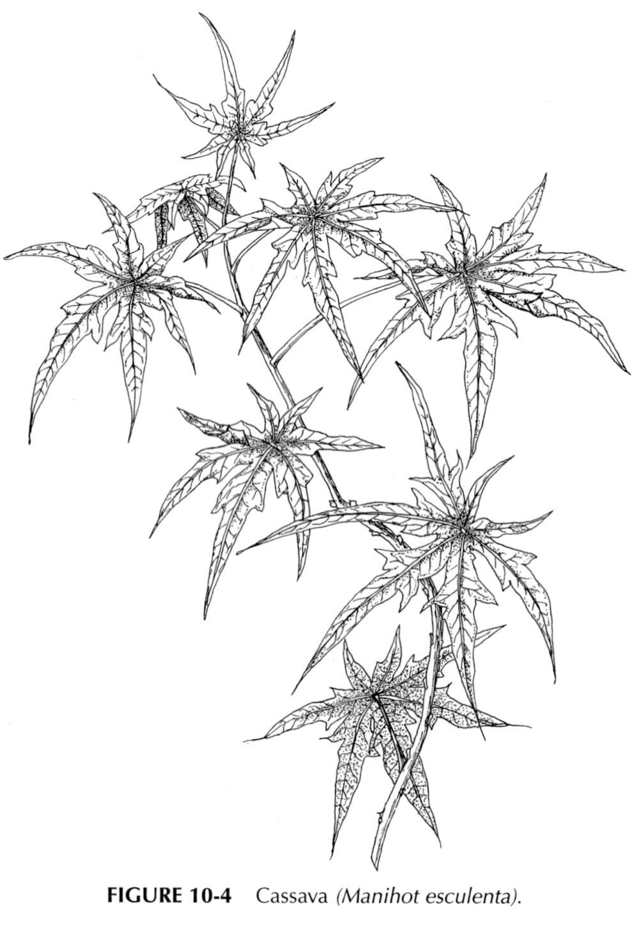

FIGURE 10-4 Cassava *(Manihot esculenta)*.

Presentation and Treatment

Tropical ataxic neuropathy (cassavism) is a syndrome characterized by bilateral primary optic atrophy, bilateral perceptive deafness, myelopathy, and peripheral neuropathy. The diagnosis requires two of these four features to be present.[21] The disease is also known by the local names *konzo* and *mantakassa*. The initial symptom is difficulty walking due to weakened lower extremity musculature. Symmetrical spastic paraparesis with increased muscle tone, hyperreflexia, and bilateral extensor plantar responses usually ensues.[22] Distal sensory loss is rare but the motor deficits are often permanent. One study in Mozambique demonstrated an incidence of ankle clonus in schoolchildren of up to 17%, correlating with high levels of cyanogens concentrations in cassava flour.[23] There is no effective treatment. Prevention of disease through proper food preparation is critical.

Castor Bean and Rosary Pea

The castor bean plant and the rosary pea have similar toxins and are discussed together. *Ricinus communis*, the castor bean plant, is a shrublike herb that grows in the southern United States, Hawaii, and the West Indies. The plant can reach up to 15 ft high with large lobed leaves nearly 3 ft wide. The fruits are oval, covered with spines, and green or red in color. They contain three seeds 1/2 to 3/4 in. in diameter. The seeds are elliptic, smooth, glossy, and mottled with gray, black, brown, and white[24] (Fig. 10-5).

Seeds of *Abrus precator* are known commonly as the rosary pea, precatory bean, prayer bead, and crab's eyes. The rosary

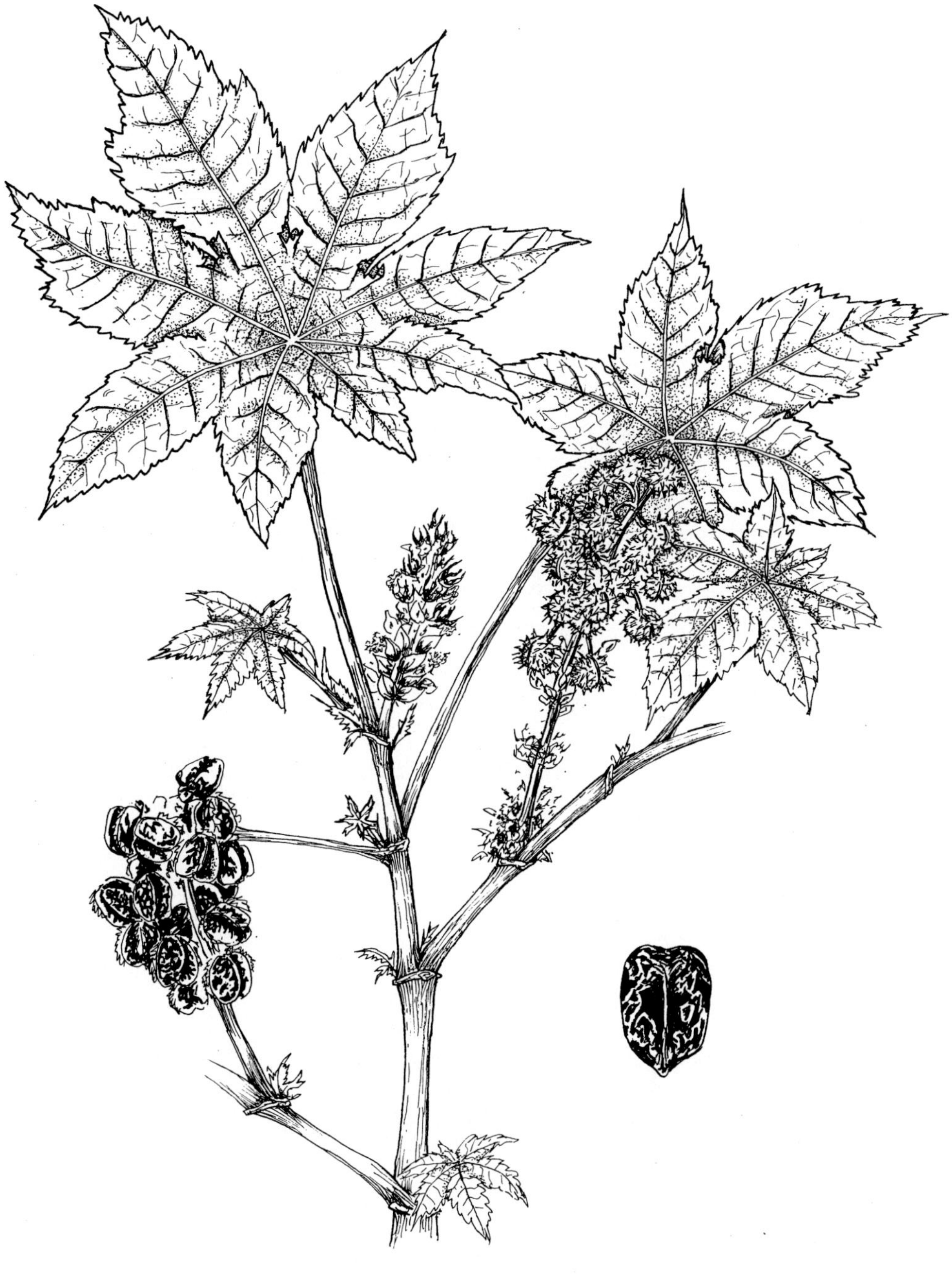

FIGURE 10-5 Castor bean plant *(Ricinus communis)*.

pea is found in Florida, the Caribbean, Hawaii, and Guam.[25] It is a vine with compound leaves and pale red-purple flowers containing toxic scarlet-red and black seeds (Fig. 10-6).

Toxin

Castor beans contain the toxin ricin and the rosary pea contains abrin. Ricin and abrin are considered two of the most potent plant toxins. The estimated lethal dose of ricin in humans is 1.0 mg/kg.[26] They share a similar chemical structure: Each is a glycoprotein composed of peptide subunits named A and B that are linked by a disulfide bridge. The B chain binds to galactose-containing receptors on cell surfaces and facilitates the entry of the A chain.[27] The A chain inactivates the 60S ribosomal subunit of eukaryotic cells and inhibits protein synthesis.[28] It is unclear how bioavailable these toxins are from the gastrointestinal tract.

Presentation and Treatment

Castor beans and rosary peas must have their husks opened (usually by chewing) for severe toxicity to occur.[29] In a review of published castor bean ingestions since 1900, Challoner and McCarron[29] found 424 cases. Eleven deaths were documented. In only 3 cases was the fatal number of beans consumed quantified. Three adults died after eating

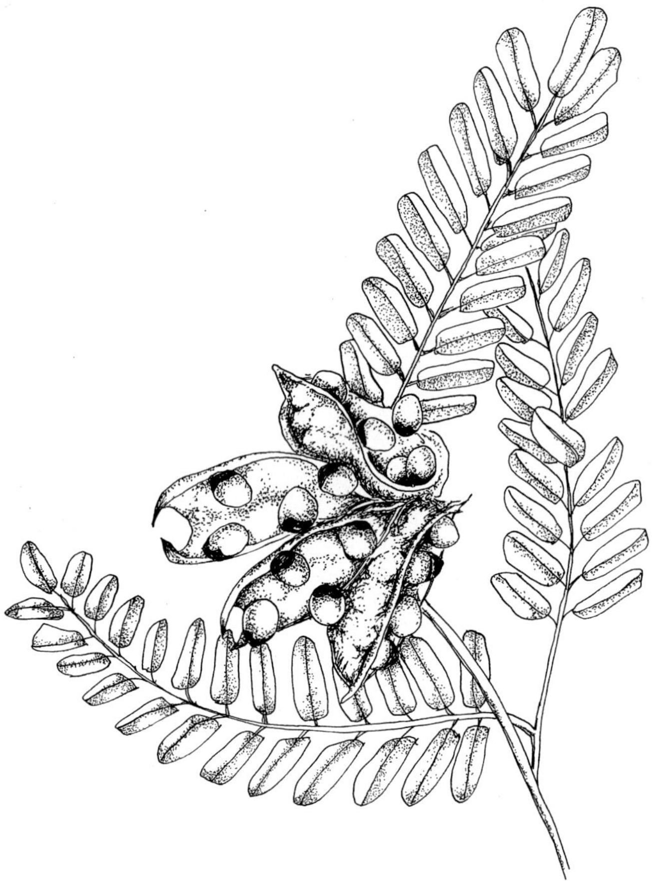

FIGURE 10-6 Rosary pea *(Abrus precatoris)*.

three, five, and six beans. A total of 104 cases in the series were published with a description of clinical findings. Vomiting and diarrhea were the most common symptoms, each occurring more than 80% of the time. The acute gastroenteritis found in the most severe castor bean poisonings can cause dehydration, electrolyte abnormalities, vascular collapse, and death. The multisystem organ damage that can occur from parenteral administration of ricin and abrin has not been well documented in contemporary literature from oral ingestions of these beans, although one case report described self-limited hepatic transaminitis in a child following ingestion of castor beans.[30] Significant quantities of ricin can also be absorbed through inhalation, but this route of exposure is only clinically relevant in biological warfare.

Treatment begins with identifying the bean, determining if the husk was violated, and quantifying the exposure. Symptomatic patients may require admission to the hospital. Supportive care, including aggressive rehydration with intravenous fluids and electrolyte replacement, suffices in most cases. Challoner and McCarron recommend that patients who are asymptomatic but have chewed castor beans should be observed for 6 hours. If no symptoms are evident at that time, they may be discharged home with instructions to return if symptoms develop. Asymptomatic patients who likely did not chew the castor beans can be discharged after a shorter period of observation.[29] Diagnosis and treatment of rosary pea toxicity parallel that of the castor bean.

Djenkol Bean

The djenkol tree (*Pithecellobium jiringa* or *Pithecolobium lobatum*) is found throughout Southeast Asia.[31] Djenkol beans are 3.0 to 3.5 cm in diameter and 1.5 to 2.0 cm thick and have a reddish-brown color. These beans are prepared by frying, boiling, or roasting and are also eaten raw. They are mainly consumed in Thailand, Malaysia, Burma, and Indonesia.[32]

Toxin

Consumption of djenkol beans can cause acute renal failure (djenkolism). Predicting when consumption will cause disease is difficult for several reasons. Djenkolism can occur independent of the method of bean preparation. Cases have also occurred in only one member of a large family that consumed djenkol beans prepared in the same manner. Symptoms may arise in people who have eaten djenkol beans without prior problems, and beans may be safely eaten by former djenkol-poisoned patients without difficulty. Crystals are found in the urine of some patients and in animal models of poisoning, and they are composed of djenkolic acid ($C_7H_{14}O_4N_2S_2$).[31] Despite the isolation of djenkolic acid crystals, the pathophysiology of djenkolism is unclear. Renal biopsies in some patients with djenkolism demonstrate acute tubular necrosis, whereas features of interstitial nephritis are infrequently described. Crystals are not consistently found in the urine of patients with djenkolism, however, arguing against an etiology of mechanical obstruction.[33]

Presentation and Treatment

Males are afflicted by djenkol bean poisoning at a ratio of 9:1 compared to females, and the peak incidence is between September and January when the tree bears fruit.[34] Symptoms include colicky pain in the groin and suprapubic region with vomiting, diarrhea, dysuria, hematuria, and oliguria or anuria.[35] Needle-shaped crystals may be found on urinalysis. Supportive treatment with aggressive rehydration results in resolution of most cases. Djenkolic acid crystals are more soluble in alkaline solutions, and alkalinization of the urine may be of benefit.[32] The prognosis is good in symptomatic cases of djenkolism, as most patients recover with no permanent renal impairment.

Khat

Leaves of the khat bush (*Catha edulis*), found in East Africa and Arabia, are used as a stimulant.[36] Several million people in these areas are habitual khat users, leading to medical and socioeconomic problems. Emigration from Africa and the Middle East has created a market for khat in Europe and the United States.[37,38] *Catha edulis* is a tall evergreen shrub with many centrally located small flowers and podlings. Its leaves are narrow and have serrated borders (Fig. 10-7).

Toxin

The substance responsible for khat intoxication is the alkaloid cathinone (α-aminopropionphenone). Cathinone is very similar in structure and action to amphetamine.[39] Brenneisen and colleagues[36] administered isolated cathinone

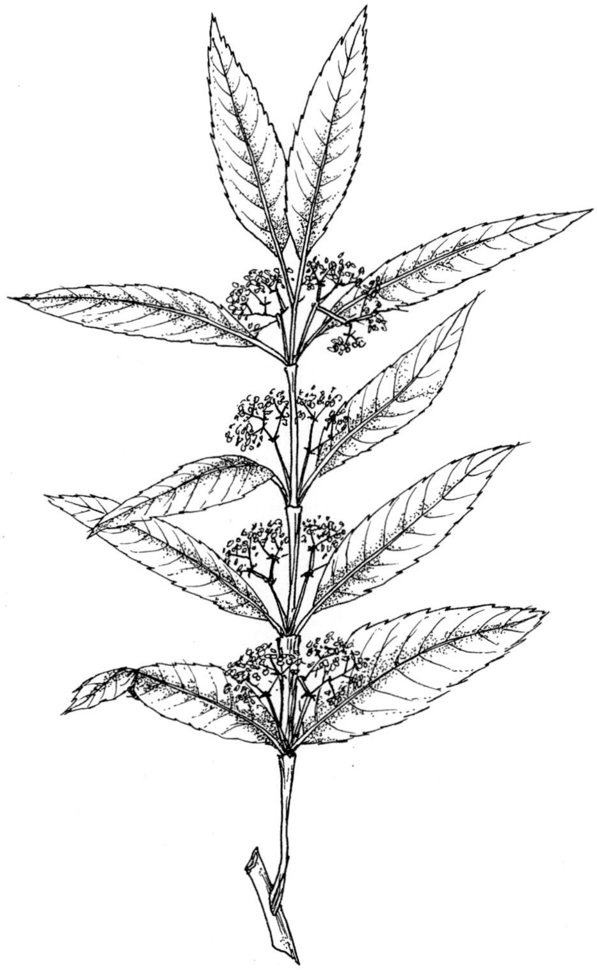

FIGURE 10-7 Khat *(Catha edulis)*.

to volunteers in a double-blind, placebo-controlled crossover study and found increases in blood pressure and heart rate and feelings of euphoria. Khat acts by stimulating the release of norepinephrine and dopamine from presynaptic nerve endings, causing indirect stimulation of the central and sympathetic nervous system.[40]

Presentation and Treatment

Chewing of khat leaves produces a syndrome similar to that of amphetamine intoxication. Khat causes elevated blood pressure, mydriasis, hyperthermia, anorexia, insomnia, increased arousal, and elevated mood. Cerebral hemorrhage, myocardial infarction, and pulmonary edema have been associated with the use of this herb.[41] Khat abuse may cause psychological dependence, aggressive behavior, paranoid ideation, and even psychosis.[39] Fresh leaves are more potent than dried leaves and are preferred by habitual users. Long-term use of khat, especially in conjunction with ethanol and tobacco, may predispose to oral malignancy.[42]

Treatment parallels that of other sympathomimetic poisonings. Benzodiazepines counteract anxiety and agitation. Hyperthermia is an important marker of serious poisoning and may require paralysis, artificial ventilation, and aggressive cooling measures when present. Supportive care measures also include hydration and monitoring for rhabdomyolysis. Patients may require addiction counseling for long-term abstinence.

Lantana

Lantana camara is a flowering ornamental found in the tropical Americas, the West Indies, Southeast Asia, Australia, New Zealand, and South Africa.[43] It is a perennial shrub with square twigs and simple leaves with toothed margins. Small tubular flowers—white, yellow, purple, or pink in color—are found in flat-topped clusters[24] (Fig. 10-8).

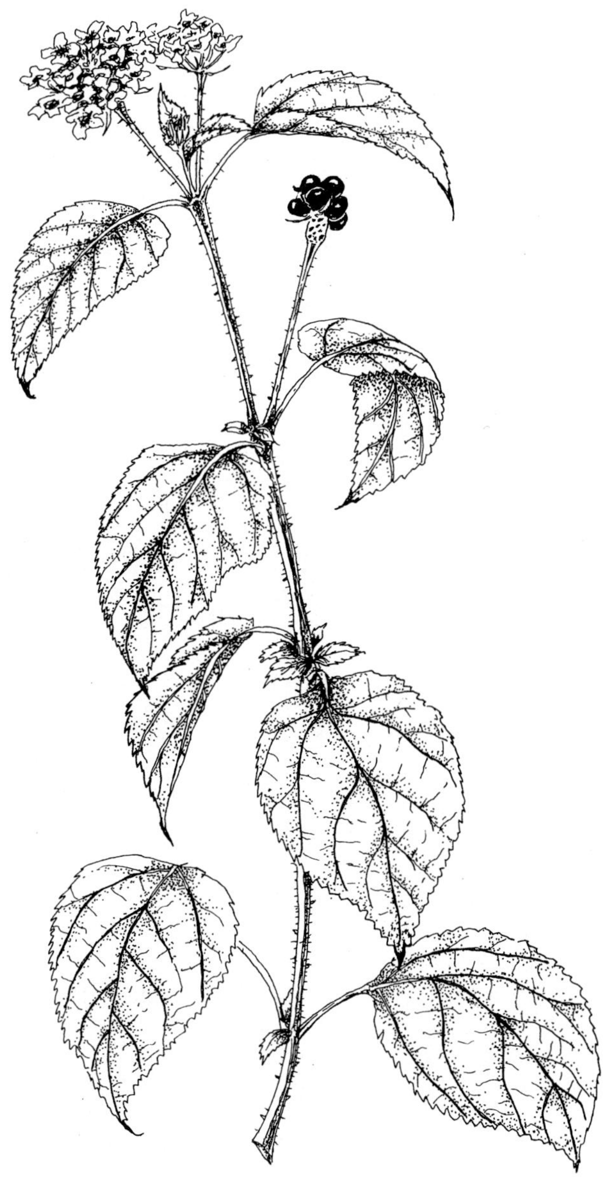

FIGURE 10-8 Lantana *(Lantana camara)*.

Toxin

The toxin responsible for poisoning from lantana has been debated. Most authorities now believe the toxin is a pentacylic triterpenoid chemical known as lantadene A (22-β-angeloxy-3-oxoolean-12-en-28-oic acid) found in lantana leaves and fruit. When administered to animal models, lantadene A can induce cholestasis, hepatotoxcitiy, and photosensitization.[44] However, animal models exposed to purified lantadene A may not demonstrate the same clinical syndrome found in human lantana poisoning.[45] One theory suggests that a separate triterpenoid more recently isolated from these plants, termed lantadene C, may be responsible for some of the heptotoxic activity.[46]

Presentation and Treatment

Human poisoning from *L. camara* is usually the result of children eating the unripe, green fruit. Presenting symptoms include vomiting, diarrhea, weakness, and lethargy. Presenting signs include cyanosis, labored breathing, photophobia, ataxia, decreased deep tendon reflexes, and coma. A 2-year-old child who died after consuming the green fruit of lantana was found to have acute pulmonary edema and circulatory collapse.[47] Consumption of ripe fruit does not cause toxicity.

Treatment is supportive. Gastric lavage may be considered in patients with a history of a large exposure who present within 1 hour of ingestion. Activated charcoal should be administered to all with a history of significant exposure to this plant and those who are symptomatic. All patients should be monitored 4 to 6 hours for signs of toxicity. Liver toxicity may be delayed.

Manchineel

The manchineel tree (*Hippomane mancinella*) is an evergreen found in the West Indies, Central America, the Bahamas, South America, and the west coast of Africa. It is found in coastal regions because of an ability to thrive in a saline environment. The tree grows to 20 to 40 ft in height, has a trunk 1 or 2 ft in diameter, and is covered by smooth gray bark.[48] Manchineel trees produce a round yellow-green fruit known as "guavas."

Manchineels have been described as the most toxic tree on the North American continent.[49] In the United States, it is allowed to grow only in the Florida Everglades and in the Virgin Islands National Park. The aboriginal Carib natives understood the toxic properties of the manchineel tree and used its sap as an arrow poison and as a medicine. The tree is toxic to humans whose skin or mucous membranes contact its irritant sap and those who ingest its fruit or leaves.

Toxin

The leaves, twigs, and bark of the manchineel tree contain a highly irritating latex sap. Adolf and Hecker[48] analyzed manchineel latex to determine the chemical cause of its irritant properties. They found a highly irritating ester of 5β-hydroxy-resiniferonol-6α,7α -oxide with 9-, 11-, and 14-carbon chain fatty acids. The authors also found several triterpenes that proved to be tumor promoting in animal models.

Presentation and Treatment

Skin contact with manchineel sap produces irritation and blisters. Severe dermatitis has occurred even from water falling on those seeking shelter from rain under a manchineel tree. The sap can cause an equally irritating conjunctivitis. In a review of 20 cases of manchineel conjunctivitis, 13 patients showed large corneal epithelial defects that resolved in a mean of 3.75 days.[50] Only 1 patient had a permanent stromal scar 5 years after exposure.

Ingestion of fruit induces lacrimation, salivation, vomiting, diarrhea, and central nervous system depression leading to coma and death.[51] Most non-life-threatening symptoms, such as oral and pharyngeal irritation, seem to subside over several hours.[51] An alkaloid substance resembling physostigmine has been implicated.[52] Ingestion of fruit can also produce life-threatening laryngeal edema through irritant effects on mucosa.

Decontamination is fundamental to the treatment of dermal and ocular exposure. Irrigation with copious amounts of water will limit the exposure. Ocular contact can also be treated with cycloplegics to relieve pain and prophylactic antibiotics while the cornea reepithelializes.

Neurolathyrism

Consumption of the vegetables khesari (*Lathyrus sativus*), found in India, China, Ethiopia, and Nepal, can cause a devastating disease known as neurolathyrism.[53] Khesari is a readily accessible food source in developing countries because it needs no irrigation, fertilizers, or pesticides, and its seeds are high in protein.[54] Consumption of bread or other products produced from this crop can result in toxicity.

Toxin

A neurotoxic amino acid, β-*N*-oxalyamino-L-alanine (BOAA), has been implicated in animal studies as the possible toxin responsible for neurolathyrism. In a primate model, oral consumption of BOAA alone caused a syndrome similar to neurolathyrism. BOAA in vitro inhibits the high-affinity uptake of glutamate transport by isolated synaptosomes, and it may inhibit mitchondrial complex I of the motor cortex and lumbar spinal cord.[55] Intrathecal administration of BOAA to rats demonstrated interference with the transport of aspartic and glutamic acid in spinal nerves.[56] The neuropathologic changes include loss of fibers in the pyramidal tracts of the spinal cord and pallor of the fasciculi gracilis.[16]

Presentation and Treatment

Males are more likely than females to be affected after consuming khesari,[57] and the incidence is highest in the third and fourth decades of life. The syndrome appears after daily consumption of khesari for at least 2 or 3 months. Lathyrism usually occurs during famine conditions when the hearty crop becomes a majority of the diet. Initial symptoms are aching of the waist and rigidity of the calf muscles, known as *lodakas* in India. As symptoms progress, partial or total loss of control over the lower limbs occurs.[53] Some patients have exaggerated knee and ankle reflexes and ankle clonus. Sensory loss is usually absent.[16] The neurologic changes are permanent but nonprogressive, and motor weakness of the upper extremities is rare. No specific therapy has been identified.

Oleander

Naturally occurring cardiac glycosides are found in many plants. The two most common oleanders, *Nerium oleander* and *Thevetia peruviana*, are native to the Mediterranean region and most tropical and subtropical regions around the world, and they are found worldwide as ornamental plants. The flowers of *N. oleander* are white, pink, and dark red, and its fruit is a pair of long narrow pods (Fig. 10-9). *Thevetia peruviana* has yellow flowers and green fruit. Other plants containing cardiac glycosides are shown in Box 10-3.

Toxin

Oleander contains the cardiac glycosides oleandrin, neriine, oleandroside, nerioside, and digitoxigenin.[58,59] Toxicity from oleander has been reported with the consumption of leaves and from the use of oleander twigs as skewers to cook meat.[60] The toxicity of oleander poisoning is indistinguishable from acute digoxin toxicity. Cardiac glycosides inhibit the Na-ATPase pump in cardiac cells. Cardiac intracellular sodium and calcium rise; intracellular potassium falls. The slope of phase 4 in the action potential is increased, resulting in increased automaticity of cardiac cells. Cardiac glycosides also enhance vagal tone and prolong phase 3 of the cardiac action potential in the atrioventricular node and the His–Purkinje conduction system.[61]

Box 10-3 Plants That Contain Cardiac Glycosides

I. Figwort family (Scrophulariaceae)
  A. Foxglove (*Digitalis purpurea*)
II. Lily family (Lillaceae)
  A. Sea onion (*Urginea maritima*)
  B. Lily of the valley (*Convallaria majalis*)
III. Dogbane family (Apocynaceae)
  A. Yellow oleander (*Thevetia peruviana*)
  B. Oleander (*Nerium oleander*)
  C. Wintersweet (*Carissa spectabilis*)
  D. Bushman's poison (*Carissa acokanthera*)
  E. Sea mango (*Cerbera manghas*)
  F. Frangipani (*Plumeria rubra*)
IV. Milkweed family (Asclepiadaceae)
  A. Balloon cotton (*Asclepias fruticosa*)
  B. Redheaded cottonbush (*Asclepias curassavica*)
  C. King's crown (*Calotropis procera*)
  D. Rubber vine (*Cryptostegia grandiflora*)

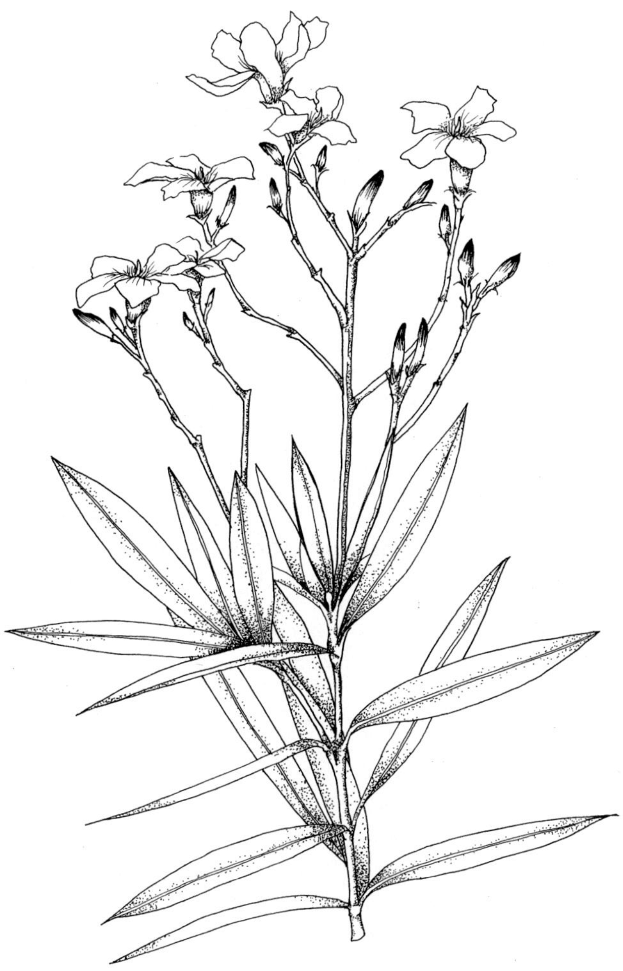

FIGURE 10-9 Oleander *(Nerium oleander)*.

Presentation and Treatment

Accidental poisoning has occurred from chewing oleander flowers or leaves, eating meat cooked over burning oleander branches, and consuming liquids stirred with oleander stems. The ingestion of one oleander leaf is reported to be fatal.[59] The clinical presentation is very similar to acute digoxin poisoning, with nausea and vomiting the initial symptoms. Cardiac toxicity is manifested by many different dysrhythmias. Bradydysrhythmias, including sinus arrest, sinus bradycardia, and atrioventricular nodal blockade, may be seen. Tachydysrhythmias can include atrial tachycardia with block, junctional tachycardia, ventricular tachycardia, and fibrillation. Laboratory abnormalities include profound hyperkalemia.

Treatment of acute oleander ingestion includes gastric decontamination, correction of hyperkalemia, and standard treatment of cardiac dysrhythmias. The advent of specific antibody fragments against digoxin poisoning has revolutionized the care of digoxin-poisoned patients refractory to supportive therapy. The antibody fragments (Fab fragments) bind to and inactivate digoxin, with the resulting complex filtered by the kidney. The use of Fab fragments for the treatment of oleander toxicity in humans is limited to anecdotal case reports;[60] however, a study using high doses of digoxin Fab fragments for the treatment of oleander poisoning in a canine model was successful in reversing both dysrhythmias and hyperkalemia and prevented mortaility.[62] A series from Sri Lanka demonstrated efficacy using multiple doses of activated charcoal in the management of *T. peruviana* poisoning.[63]

Poison Hemlock

Poison hemlock (*Conium maculatum*) is found in North and South America, Europe, and as an ornamental in Asia. It is also known by the common names poison fool's parsley, hemlock, spotted hemlock, and California or Nebraska fern.[64] Poison hemlock grows to a height of 3 to 9 ft (Fig. 10-10). Younger plants have light green leaves that resemble those of a fern and have been mistaken for parsley. The large stems of maturing plants have purple spots. The fleshy white taproot has been mistaken for parsnips. Poison hemlock grows in groups along roadsides, in ditches, and in other uncultivated areas.

Toxin

The toxins in poison hemlock are the piperidine alkaloids coniine and γ-coniceine. The action of coniine is similar to that of nicotine. Animal studies demonstrate that coniine activity on isolated ileum and duodenum is blocked with atropine pretreatment. This implies that coniine stimulates parasympathetic ganglia and explains the observed nicotinic effects following exposure to this plant, which include salivation, mydriasis, and tachycardia, followed by bradycardia. These alkaloids also act as nondepolarizing antagonists at the neuromuscular junction, similar in action to tubocurare.[65] Rhabdomyolysis and acute tubular necrosis have also been reported with poison hemlock ingestion.[66]

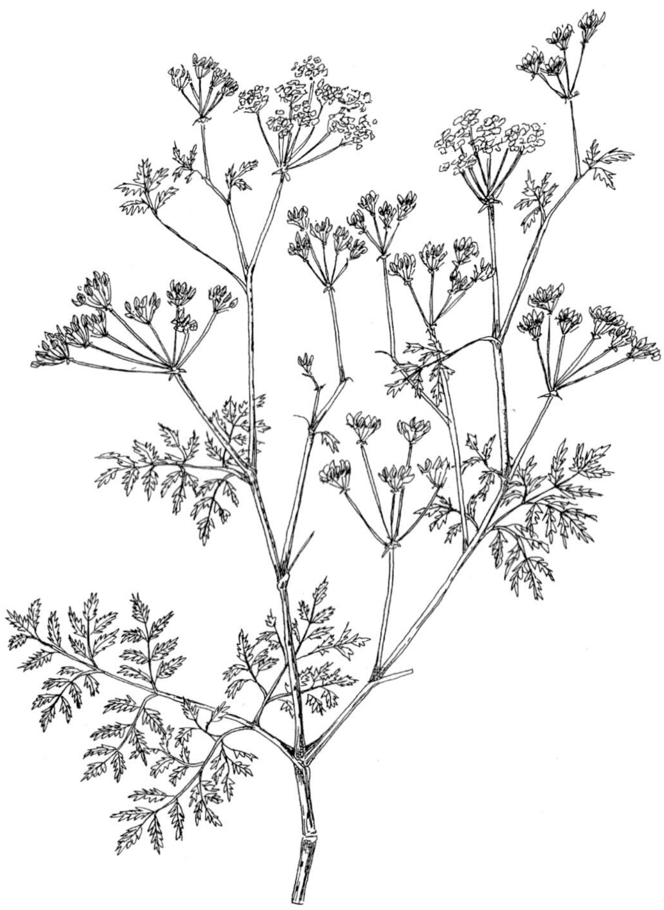

FIGURE 10-10 Poison hemlock *(Conium maculatum)*.

Presentation and Treatment

Symptoms are directly referable to the dual toxicity of the hemlock alkaloids. Salivation, urination, and defecation often precede the loss of tone in skeletal muscle. Death most frequently occurs due to respiratory arrest. There is no antidote; supportive care, including ventilator support and gastric decontamination, should be undertaken when the diagnosis of poison hemlock ingestion is suspected.

Pyrrolizidine Alkaloids

The syndrome of hepatic veno-occlusive disease is found throughout the world associated with consumption of local teas. The disorder has been described in the West Indies, Afghanistan, India, and Israel. The rise in popularity of alternative medicine and the use of herbal teas has led to cases in Europe and the United States.[67,68]

Toxin

The agents responsible for herbal-based hepatic veno-occlusive disease are the pyrrolizidine alkaloids. They are found in Jamaican "bush teas," comfrey (*Symphytum officinale*), grain contaminated with pyrrolizidine-containing weeds,[69] and in many other herbs used to prepare medicinal teas or dietary supplements. Approximately 3% of the world's flowering plants contain toxic pyrrolizidine alkaloids.[70] The dose and duration of exposure required for toxicity are unclear, and no "safe" level of exposure has been established.[71] Pyrrolizidine alkaloids are readily absorbed from the gastrointestinal tract and metabolized by the liver. The alkaloids undergo transformation to inactive or active metabolites by several metabolic pathways; they can be deactivated by *N*-oxidation or by hydrolysis of their ester bonds, or they can be activated by liver microsomal P450 enzymes that convert the alkaloid into a pyrrolic ester. Pyrrolic esters are potent oxidizers that can cause acute hepatotoxicity and cellular necrosis.[72] Chronic hepatotoxicity is also seen with pyrrolizidine alkaloid ingestion, and pathologic findings in animal models of this disease include enlarged hepatocytes.

Veno-occlusive disease results from nonthrombotic occlusion of the small intrahepatic branches of the hepatic vein by loose connective tissue. Damage to the venous endothelium leads to a proliferative fibrotic response resulting in occlusion. Veno-occlusive disease is defined pathologically as a progressive and concentric nonthrombotic occlusion of the lumina of small intrahepatic veins (diameter less than 300 m) by loose connective tissue with necrosis of hepatocytes in centrilobular areas.[71] Since false-negative biopsy results can occur, veno-occlusive disease is primarily a clinical diagnosis.

Presentation and Treatment

The natural history of veno-occlusive disease includes acute and chronic forms. Acute veno-occlusive disease is characterized by ascites, abdominal pain, hepatomegaly, nausea, and vomiting. A cohort of 20 children with suspected pyrrolizidine poisoning in South Africa were examined. The prothrombin time was prolonged in 89% of patients, aspartate aminotransferase was elevated in all patients, and alanine aminotransferase was elevated in 84%. A spectrophotometric test was developed by the investigators that detected pyrrolizidine metabolites in the urine. Mortality in this series was 40%.[73] Chronic veno-occlusive disease presents as cirrhosis with stigmata of liver disease.

Management of hepatic veno-occlusive disease is supportive. Sodium should be restricted and plasma expanders used to maintain oncotic pressure and limit ascites. Spironolactone is recommended for diuresis. Prostaglandin inhibitors are to be avoided to maintain renal blood flow in the presence of decreased intravascular volume.

Water Hemlock

Water hemlock (*Cicuta maculata*) is found throughout North America. Water hemlock belongs to the family Umbelliferae and is related to European water hemlock (*Cicuta virosa*) and English hemlock or water dropwort (*Oenanthe crocata*).[74] Water hemlock is a perennial herb that grows from 3 to 7 ft with clustered, short, and thickened tuberous roots and hairless, purple striped, or mottled stems.[75] They have small, white, heavily scented flowers. Water hemlock roots are chambered (Fig. 10-11). A cut stem reveals yellow oily sap that smells like raw parsnip.[76]

Toxin

The poison isolated from water hemlock is called cicutoxin. Cicutoxin is found in all parts of the plant, with the root containing the highest concentration.[77] Cicutoxin is an unsaturated aliphatic alcohol that acts primarily as a neurotoxin. Virol A is a component of *C. virosa* that has been found to inhibit GABA receptors in an animal model.[78] Poisoning can occur from ingestion or dermal exposure.

Presentation and Treatment

A lethal dose of water hemlock can be contained in one rootstalk (rhizome).[79] Children have died from using the hollow stems as whistles or peashooters.[80] Onset of symptoms can occur within 15 minutes of exposure and initially includes nausea, vomiting, and abdominal pain. Early vomiting may be protective if undigested plant is expelled, but vomiting should not be induced due to the risk of aspiration during convulsions. Severe poisonings result in diaphoresis, salivation, bronchorrhea, and respiratory insufficiency. Death usually follows the development of intractable seizures. Rhabdomyolysis, renal failure, and severe metabolic acidosis may also be seen.[81] An examination of cicuta poisonings reported from 1900 to 1975 revealed 30% mortality.[82]

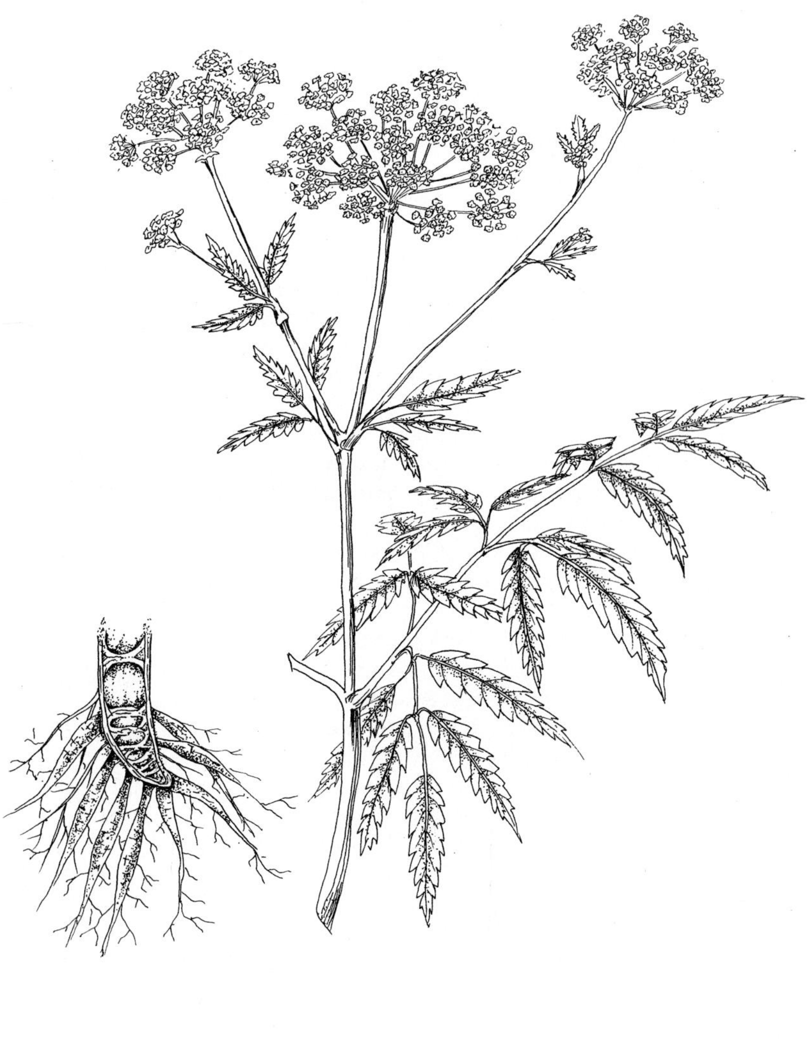

FIGURE 10-11 Water hemlock *(Cicuta maculata)*.

Treatment is supportive; there is no specific antidote. Mechanical ventilation should be used when necessary. Convulsions should be treated with large doses of benzodiazepines or barbiturates. Adequate urine flow should be maintained to reduce the incidence of renal failure in the setting of rhabdomyolysis.

Plant Dermatitis

Plant dermatitis is one of the most common mechanisms by which plants cause human disease. The number of plants that cause dermatitis is legion, and they are found throughout the world. Dermal exposure to some plants can be life threatening.[83] There are four main mechanisms by which plants cause human dermatitis: immediate hypersensitivity, irritant or mechanical dermatitis, phytophotodermatitis, and delayed hypersensitivity.

Urticariogenic plants cause immediate contact dermatitis. Some plants have stinging hairs that introduce irritating plant toxins through mechanical breaks in the skin (e.g., stinging trees of Australia and stinging nettle). Others cause a hypersensitivity response through direct contact alone (e.g., strawberry, castor bean, and chrysanthemum). Contact with these plants causes hives, pruritus, and sometimes anaphylaxis and shock.[84] Treatment of simple urticaria involves use of cold compresses and antihistamines. Systemic reactions may require more intensive therapy.

Many plants cause an irritant contact dermatitis. Simple mechanical irritation through spines or prickly hairs is one method by which plants cause human disease. The thorns of a flowering plant or spines of a cactus can penetrate the skin and cause fungal (*Sporothrix*), bacterial (*Staphylococcus aureus*), and other disease.[84] Chemical irritants are produced by some plants and can cause dermatitis. The manchineel tree, *Dieffenbachia*, and *Philodendron* are examples of plants that exert their toxicity through chemical irritation. Acute clinical findings include erythema, edema, and papular and vesicular reactions. In severe cases, bullae, pustules, and ulcerations may occur. Treatment of mechanical and chemical irritants revolves around removal of the irritating stimulus. This may include manual removal of thorns or copious irrigation of the skin to remove chemical irritants.

Phytophotodermatitis occurs when the skin is exposed to both a plant toxin and ultraviolet radiation. Celery, citrus, Queen Anne's lace, and the common fig can cause a dermatitis characterized by a painful, vesicular, erythematous rash that lasts for 1 or 2 weeks. Healing skin may show hyperpigmentation. Phytophotodermatitis is differentiated from allergic contact dermatitis by its presence only in sun-exposed areas and the finding of hyperpigmentation during healing.[84]

Allergic contact dermatitis results from cell-mediated immunity and is often referred to as a delayed hypersensitivity reaction. Poison ivy, poison oak, mango, and cashew can cause allergic contact dermatitis. The reaction only occurs in those previously exposed and sensitized to the plant. Exposed areas will show erythema, vesiculation, weeping, and pruritus. The lesions heal over several weeks and usually leave no residual scarring or pigmentation. Treatment of phytophotodermatitis and allergic contact dermatitis is similar. In mild cases, antihistamines and topical corticosteroids may provide symptomatic relief. More severe cases warrant the use of oral corticosteroids.[84]

SUMMARY

Tropical plants contain a variety of components that can be toxic to humans and animals. New species and toxins are constantly being discovered and described in all areas of the world. Their effects are still unknown in human exposures. Some varieties, such as water hemlock and ackee, can cause life-threatening toxicity when ingested. More commonly, gastroenteritis is the hallmark of most plant exposures but can lead to weakness and dehydration in severe cases. The more common and better understood toxicities existing among plant species found in tropical and subtropical environments have been presented in this chapter. Most victims of these poisonings survive if administered aggressive support with airway protection and fluid rehydration.

ACKNOWLEDGMENT

We thank Cinnamon Larson for the illustrations used in this chapter.

REFERENCES

1. McTague JA, Forney R: Jamaican vomiting sickness in Toledo, Ohio. Ann Emerg Med 23:1116–1118, 1994.
2. Hardin JW, Arena JM: Human Poisoning from Native and Cultivated Plants. Durham, N.C., Duke University Press, 1974, p 101.
3. Chase GW, Landen WO, Soliman AM: Hypoglycin A content in the aril, seeds and husks of ackee fruit at various stages of ripeness. J Assoc Off Anal Chem 73:318–319, 1990.
4. Feng PC, Patrick SJ: Studies of the action of hypoglycin-A, an hypogycaemic substance. Br J Pharmacol 13:125–130, 1958.
5. Tanaka K, Kean EA, Johnson B: Jamaican vomiting sickness. N Engl J Med 295:461–467, 1976.
6. Hill KR, Bras G, Clearkin KP: Acute toxic hypoglycemia occurring in the vomiting sickness of Jamaica. West Indian Med J 4:91–104, 1955.
7. Figeroa P, Nembhard O, Coleman A: Toxic hypoglycemic syndrome—Jamaica, 1989–1991. MMWR 41:53–55, 1992.
8. Knight TE: Philodendron-induced dermatitis: Report of cases and review of the literature. Cutis 48:375–378, 1991.
9. Rauber A: Observations on the idioblasts of *Dieffenbachia*. Clin Toxicol 23:79–90, 1985.
10. Kuballa B, Lugnier AJ, Anton R: Study of *Dieffenbachia*-induced edema in mouse and rat hindpaw: Respective role of oxalate needles and trypsin-like protease. Toxicol Appl Pharmacol 58:444–451, 1981.
11. Kuballa B, Lugnier A, Anton R: Study of *Dieffenbachia*-induced edema in mouse and rat hindpaw: Respective role of oxalate needles and trypsin-like pritease. Toxicol Appl Pharmacol 58:444–451, 1981.
12. Cumpston KL, Vogel SN, Leiken JB, Erickson TB: Acute airway compromise after brief exposure top a *Dieffenbachia* plant. J Emerg Med 25:391–397, 2003.
13. Walter WG, Khanna PN: Chemistry of the aroids I. *Dieffenbachia seguine*, *amoena*, and *picta*. Econ Bot 26:364–372, 1972.
14. Seet B, Chan WK, Ang CL: Crystalline kerotopathy from *Dieffenbachia* plant sap. Br J Ophthalmol 79:98–99, 1995.
15. Mrvos R, Dean BS, Krenzelok EP: *Philodendron/Dieffenbachia* ingestions: Are they a problem? Clin Toxicol 29:485–491, 1991.
16. Roman GC, Spencer PS, Schoenberg BS: Tropical myeloneuropathies: The hidden Winkler, WO: Report on methods for glucosidal HCN in lima beans. J Assoc Off Agricultural Chem 41:282–287, 1958.
17. Conn, EE: Cyanogenic glycosides. Agric Food Chem 17:519–526, 1973.
18. Kamalu BP: Pathological changes in growing dogs fed on a balanced cassava (*Manihot esculenta* Crantz) diet. Br J Nutr 69:921–934, 1993.
19. Zaninovic V: Possible etiologies for tropical spastic paraparesis and human T lymphotropic virus I-associated myelopathy. Braz J Med Biol Res 37:1–12, 2004.
20. Tor-Agbidye J, Palmer VS, Lasarev MR, et al: Bioactivation of cyanide to cyanate in sulfur amino acid deficiency: Relevance to neurological disease in humans subsisting on cassava. Toxicol Sci 50:228–235, 1999.

21. Njoh J: Tropical ataxic neuropathy in Liberians. Trop Geogr Med 42:92–94, 1990.
22. Spencer PS, Ludolph AC, Kisby GE: Neurologic diseases associated with use of plant components with toxic potential. Environ Res 62:106–113, 1993.
23. Ernesto M, Cardoso AP, Nicala D, et al: Persistent konzo and cyanogen toxicity from cassava in northern Mozambique. Acta Tropica 82:357–362, 2002.
24. Hardin JW, Arena JM: Human Poisoning from Native and Cultivated Plants. Durham, N.C., Duke University Press, 1974, pp 119–121.
25. Lampe KF, McCann MA: AMA Handbook of Poisonous and Injurious Plants. Chicago, American Medical Association, 1985, pp 17–18.
26. Kopferschmitt J, Flesch F, Lugnier A, et al: Acute voluntary intoxication by ricin. Hum Toxicol 2:239–242, 1983.
27. Olsnes S, Refsnes K, Pihl A: Mechanism of action of the toxic lectins abrin and ricin. Nature 249:627–631, 1974.
28. Panter KE, Keeler RF: Piperidine alkaloids of poison hemlock (*Conium maculatum*). In Cheeke P (ed): Toxicants of Plant Origin. Vol. I. Boca Raton, Fla, CRC Press, 1989, pp 109–132.
29. Challoner KR, McCarron M: Castor bean intoxication. Ann Emerg Med 19:1177–1183, 1990.
30. Palatnick W, Tenenbein M: Hepatotoxicity from castor bean ingestion in a child. J Toxicol Clin Toxicol 38:67–69, 2000.
31. Areekul S, Kirdudom P, Chaovanapricha K: Studies on djenkol bean poisoning (djenkolism) in experimental animals. Southeast Asian J Trop Med Pub Health 7:551–558, 1976.
32. Areekul S, Muangman V, Bohkerd C, et al: Djenkol bean as a cause of urolithiasis. Southeast Asian J Trop Med Public Health 9:427–432, 1978.
33. Segasothy M, Swaminathan M, Kong N, et al: Djenkol bean poisoning (djenkolism): An unusual cause of acute renal failure. Am J Kidney Dis 25:63–66, 1995.
34. Suharjono A, Sadatun OE: "Djenkol" intoxication in children. Paediatr Indonesia 8:20–29, 1968.
35. Vachvanichsanong P, Lebel L: Djenkol beans as a cause of hematuria in children. Nephron 76:39–42, 1997.
36. Brenneisen R, Fisch HU, Koelbing U, et al: Amphetamine-like effects in humans of the khat alkaloid cathinone. Br J Clin Pharmacol 30:825–828, 1990.
37. Schechter MD: Dopaminergic nature of acute cathine tolerance. Pharmacol Biochem Behav 36:817–820, 1990.
38. Brown ER, Jarvie DR, Simpson D: Use of drugs at "raves." Scott Med J 40:168–171, 1995.
39. Critchlow S: Khat-induced paranoid psychosis. Br J Psychiatry 150:247–249, 1987.
40. Nencini P, Ahmed AM: Khat consumption: A pharmacologic review. Drug Alcohol Depend 23:19–29, 1989.
41. Halbach H: Medical aspects of the chewing of Khat leaves. Bull World Health Organization 47:21–29, 1972.
42. Kassie F, Darroudi F, Kundi M, et al: Khat (*Catha edulis*) consumption causes genotoxic effects in humans. Int J Cancer 92:329–332, 2001.
43. Sharma OP, Makkar HP, Dawra RK: A review of the noxious plant *Lantana camara*. Toxicon 26:11:975–987, 1988.
44. Sharma OP, Dawra RK, Pattabhi V: Molecular structure, polymorphism and toxicity of lantadene A, the pentacyclic triterpenoid from the hepatotoxic plant *Lantana camara*. J Biochem Toxicol 6:57–63, 1991.
45. Sharma OP, Dawra RK, Makkar HP: Isolation and partial purification of lantana (*Lantana camara* L) toxins. Toxicol Lett 37:165–172, 1987.
46. Sharma OP, Vaid J, Pattabhi V, et al: Biological action of lantadene C, a new hepatotoxicant from Lantana camara var. aculeate. J Biochem Toxicol 7:73–79, 1992.
47. Wolfson SL, Solomons TW: Poisoning by fruit of *Lantana camara*. Am J Dis Child 107:173–176, 1964.
48. Adolf W, Hecker E: On the active principles of the spurge family, X. Skin irritants, cocarcinogens, and cryptic cocarcinogens from the latex of the manchineel tree. J Nat Prod 47:3:482–496, 1984.
49. West E, Arnold LE: The Native Trees of Florida. Gainesville, University of Florida Press, 1946, p 110.
50. Pitts JF, Barker NH, Gibbons DC, et al: Manchineel keratoconjunctivitis. Br J Ophthamol 77:284–288, 1993.
51. Strickland NH, Sanderson NH: Eating a manchineel "beach apple." BMJ 321:428, 2000.
52. Lauter WM, Foote PA: Investigation of the toxic principles of *Hippomane mancinella*. J Am Pharmacol Assoc 44:361–363, 1955.
53. Jahan K, Ahmad K: Studies on neurolathyrism. Environ Res 60:259–266, 1993.
54. Jayaraman KS: Neurolathyrism remains a threat in India. Nature 339:495, 1989.
55. Ravindranath V: Neurolathyrism: Mitchondrial dysfunction in excitotoxicity mediated by L-B-oxalyl aminoalanine. Neurochem Int 40:505–509, 2002.
56. Cheeke PR, Roy DN, Spencer PS: Lathyrogens. In Cheeke P, Pusztai A (eds): Toxicant of Plant Origin. Boca Raton, Fla, CRC Press, 1989, pp 169–201.
57. Xiupyun L: Lathyrus sativus and lathyrism in China. International Network for the Improvement of *Lathyrus savita* and the Eradication of Lathyrism. Lathyrus Lathyrism Newslett Nos. 2.1 and 2.2, 1990.
58. Haynes BE, Bessen HA, Wightman WD: Oleander tea: Herbal draught with death. Ann Emerg Med 14:350–353, 1985.
59. Szabuniewicz M, Schwartz WL, McCrady JD, et al: Experimental oleander poisoning and treatment. Southwestern Vet 25:105–114, 1972.
60. Shumaik GM, Wu AW, Ping AC: Oleander poisoning: Treatment with digoxin-specific Fab antibody fragments. Ann Emerg Med 17:732–735, 1988.
61. Langford SD, Boor PJ: Oleander toxicity: An examination of human and animal toxic exposures. Toxicology 109:1–13, 1996.
62. Clark RF, Selden BS, Curry SC: Digoxin-specific Fab fragments in the treatment of oleander toxicity in a canine model. Ann Emerg Med 20:1073–1077, 1991.
63. De Silva HA, Fonseka MMD, Pathmeswaran A, et al: Multiple-dose activated charcoal for the treatment of yellow oleander poisoning: A single blind, randomized, placebo-controlled trial. Lancet 361:1935–1938, 2003.
64. Cheeke PR, Panter KE, Keeler RF: Piperidine alkaloids of poison hemlock (*Conium maculatum*). In Cheeke P, Rusztai A (eds): Toxicants of Plant Origin. Boca Raton, Fla, CRC Press, 1989, pp 109–132.
65. Bowman WC, Sanghvi IS: Pharmacologic actions of hemlock (*Conium maculatum*) alkaloids. J Pharm Pharmacol 15:1–25, 1963.
66. Scatizzi A, Di Maggio A, Rizzi D, et al: Acute renal failure due to tubular necrosis caused by wildfowl-mediated hemlock poisoning. Renal Failure 15:93–96, 1993.
67. Sperl W, Stuppner H, Gassner I, et al: Reversible hepatic veno-occlusive disease in an infant after consumption of pyrrolizidine-containing herbal tea. Eur J Pediatr 154:112–116, 1995.
68. Ridker PM, Ohkuma S, McDermott WV, et al: Hepatic venocclusive disease associated with the consumption of pyrrolizidine-containing dietary supplements. Gastroenterology 88:1050–1054, 1985.
69. Stewart MJ, Steenkamp V: Pyrrolizidine poisoning: A neglected area in human toxicology. Ther Drug Monit 23:698–708, 2001.
70. Hartmann T, Witte L: Alkaloids: Pyrrolizidine alkaloids: Chemical, biological, and chemoecological aspects. In Pelletier SW (ed): Alkaloids: Chemical and Biological Perspectives. Oxford, Pergamon, 1995, pp 155–233.
71. Abbott PJ: Comfrey: Assessing the low-dose health risk. Med J Aust 149:678–682, 1988.
72. Rollins BJ: Hepatic veno-occlusive disease. Am J Med 81:297–306, 1986.
73. Steenkamp V, Stewart MJ, Zuckerman M: Clinical and analytical aspects of pyrrolizidine poisoning caused by South African traditional medicines. Ther Drug Monit 22:302–306, 2000.
74. Ball MJ, Flather ML, Forfar JC: Hemlock water dropwort poisoning. Postgrad Med J 63:363–365, 1987.
75. Hardin JW, Arena JM: Human Poisoning from Native and Cultivated Plants. Durham, N.C., Duke University Press, 1974, p 107.
76. Lampe KF, McCann MA: AMA Handbook of Poisonous and Injurious Plants. Chicago, American Medical Association, 1985, p 56.
77. Water hemlock poisoning—Maine, 1992. MMWR 43:229–231, 1994.
78. Koji U, Katsuyo O, Takaya Y: Virol A, a toxic trans-polyacetylenic alcohol of *Cicuta virosa*, selectively inhibits the GABA-induced Cl- current in acutely dissociated rat hippocampal CA1 neurons. Brain Res 889:174–180, 2001.
79. Lampe KF, Fagerstrom R: Plant Toxicity and Dermatitis. Baltimore, Williams & Wilkins, 1968, p 130.
80. Miller MM: Water hemlock poisoning. JAMA 101:852–853, 1933.
81. Carlton BE, Tufts E, Girard DE: Water hemlock poisoning complicated by rhabdomyolysis and renal failure. Clin Toxicol 14:87–92, 1979.
82. Starreveld E, Hope MB: Cicutoxin poisoning (water hemlock). Neurology 25:730–734, 1975.
83. Southcott RV, Haegi LA: Plant hair dermatitis. Med J Aust 156:623–632, 1992.
84. Juckett G: Plant dermatitis. Postgrad Med 100:159–171, 1996.

11

Immunology, Host Defense, Immunodeficiencies, and Vaccines

PETER F. WELLER
ANNE NICHOLSON-WELLER

INTRODUCTION

This chapter (1) introduces the basic concepts of the innate and adaptive immune systems and their components; (2) examines how immune responses are regulated and directed to antimicrobial immunity; (3) considers deficiencies of the immune system that predispose to infections; and (4) discusses vaccines and their development. Fuller discussions of these topics are available in major immunology texts[1–3] and in the literature cited in the text.

The field of immunology grew out of early studies of host responses to infectious diseases, and now it is propelled primarily by gene knockouts in inbred strains of mice. The mammalian immune system is complex in both the number of cell types that are involved and the intricate levels of regulation that occur to maintain immunologic homeostasis with the internal and external environments. The scope and physical size of the pathogens that the immune system faces are diverse, ranging from intracellular viruses to very large metazoan parasites (Fig. 11-1). A number of immunologic mechanisms have evolved to handle this broad array of pathogens, and these mechanisms are dependent on the flexible capacity of the human immune system to recognize different foreign antigens. Conceptually, it is convenient to consider the immune system in two parts: innate and adaptive immunity. The innate system is phylogenetically older and the only immune system of simple organisms such as *Drosophila melanogaster* and *Caenorhabditis elegans*. In more complex organisms the innate system is retained, and, beginning at the level of boney vertebrates, an additional adaptive immune system functions. Differences between the innate and adaptive immune systems are summarized in Table 11-1.

INNATE IMMUNITY

Innate immune mechanisms are inherited, invariant, and highly conserved throughout the evolution of nonfungal eukaryotes. These mechanisms have two important attributes: They are always active and they can discriminate what is foreign to the host by recognizing the molecular patterns associated with prokaryotic and fungal pathogens (Tables 11-2 and 11-3). Both the skin and other epithelial surfaces are barriers against pathogens. Further, the mucosal fluid layer found in the respiratory, gastrointestinal, and genitourinary tracts functions as a physical barrier to deter pathogen access to target cells, as well as to supply a medium for washing pathogens away with the motion of peristalsis in the gut or the activity of ciliated epithelium in the airways. Other physical barriers are the various body cavities that are separated from one another by epithelial layers. Importantly, there is nonpathogenic flora, "friendly flora," which normally colonizes surfaces of the host and makes it more difficult for pathogens to colonize. A notable complication of antibiotic therapy is the decimation of antibiotic-sensitive normal flora throughout the host, which gives potential pathogens an advantage. Studies of the normal gut flora have shown that while the host provides unique niches for specific nonpathogenic flora, these organisms have an active role in inducing appropriate differentiation of the host enterocytes, downregulating the inflammatory mediators normally associated with bacterial colonization, and stimulating antibody diversity.[4–6] Thus, normal bacterial flora in the gut exists in a state of mutualism with the host.

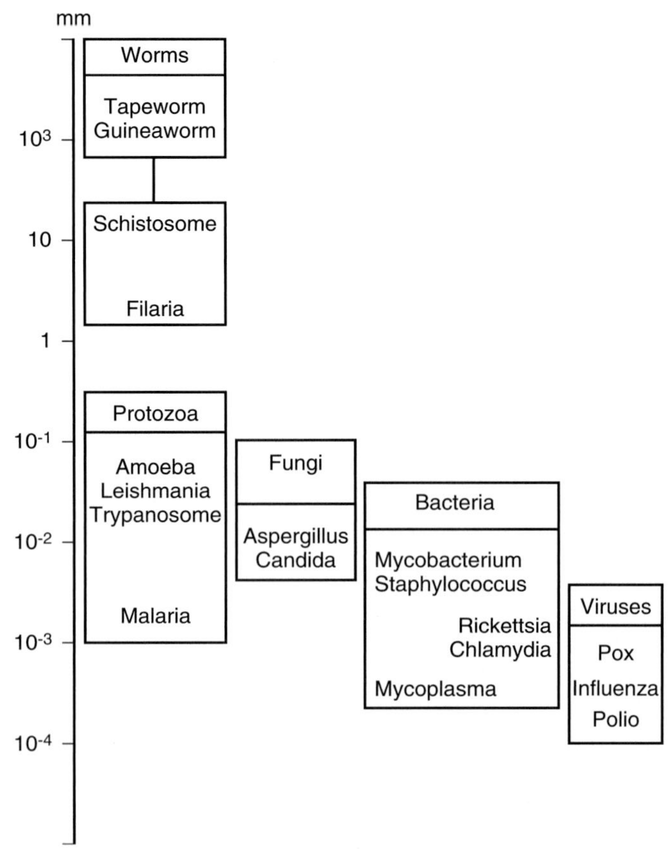

FIGURE 11-1 The infectious agents to which the human immune system must respond are diverse and range in size from large nematode and cestode helminthic parasites to small viral particles.

Table 11-1 Complementary Attributes of the Innate and Adaptive Immune Systems

Attribute	Innate Immunity	Adaptive Immunity
Location of genes	Germline	Germline with significant rearrangements/mutations ocurring in peripheral lymphoid tissues during life
Time of onset	From conception	During life, but only after exposure to specific immunogen
Discrimination of foreignness	Good	Poor
Specificity	Low	High
Capacity to contain invading pathogens	Low	High

Sensors for Pathogens

There are fluid phase molecules as well as cell receptors that can recognize pathogens and trigger an innate immune response. The sensors of innate immunity recognize the vital, conserved molecular patterns that evolved on bacteria and fungi. These molecular motifs, which are not shared by metazoans and higher animals, are called pathogen-associated molecular patterns (PAMPs).[7]

Host Fluid Phase Sensors for PAMPs

Some fluid phase sensors for PAMPs may also be effectors such as the defensins in the mucosal fluids, which bind and kill bacteria. Defensins are a family of cationic proteins in the 3500-kD molecular weight range, which are released by neutrophils and epithelial cells and are abundant in airway and gut secretions.[8] Human cathelicidin, hCAP18, has a distribution similar to defensins. Within the primary granules of neutrophils, hCAP18 is inactive; but once secreted, it is cleaved, yielding two antimicrobial peptides. The antimicrobial activity of both defensins and cathelicidins relies on their capacity to aggregate in microbial cell membranes and disrupt the membrane potential.[8] Located predominantly in the lung, surfactant protein A (SPA) and surfactant protein D (SPD) bind phospholipids and mediate their clearance by phagocytic cells. SPA and SPD can augment the clearance of certain bacteria, and they may be involved in the clearance of apoptotic cells.[9] α and β interferons are stimulated by viral infections and exert antiviral activity by activating NK (natural killer) cells and coordinating an adaptive immune response.[10] Finally, natural antibody, which is almost exclusively IgM, is found in the plasma and body cavity fluids. Since there is no plasma membrane receptor for IgM, the subsequent disposal of the foreign microbe depends entirely on activating the complement cascade, which generates the effectors of host defense. Unlike most antibodies, the specificity of natural antibodies is largely invariant and determined in the germline genes: It is not influenced by T-cell help. Thus, natural antibodies are always present in each host, regardless of the "antigenic experience" of the individual. They are synthesized by the CD5+ or B-1 lymphocytes.

The complement system has three pathways for recognizing PAMPs: (1) the lectin pathway, which uses mannan binding lectin and ficolins as sensors[11]; (2) the classical pathway, which may be activated by direct C1q binding, or indirectly when "natural" IgM antibodies function as a sensor for PAMPs by binding microbial polysaccharides, cardiolipins, and phosphorylcholine and subsequently recruit C1q; and (3) the alternative pathway, which is activated by nonsialyated carbohydrate PAMPs (Fig. 11-2). Serine esterases associated with mannan binding lectin (MASP-1 and MASP-2), and C1q (C1r and C1s) activate C4 and C2 to generate the C3 cleaving enzyme C4b2a shared by both the lectin and classical pathways. C3 activation is significantly amplified compared with other steps in the activation sequence, in part because C3 is present in plasma in higher molar concentrations compared with other complement components. C5 binds to C3b adjacent to C4b2a and once cleaved the resultant C5b condenses with C6, C7, C8, and C9 to form the nonselective C5b-9 channel, while C5a is released in the fluid phase. Although the C5b-9 complex is often referred to as the "membrane attack complex," this is a misnomer. While there is no question that excessive C5b-9 activity is associated with pathology, under normal circumstances C5b-9 has hormone-like activity in that it can stimulate a calcium flux and activate G-coupled protein(s) in host cells, which can lead to a spectrum of cellular responses (reviewed in reference).[12] In terms of host defense, human deficiencies of C5, C6, C7, or C8 and to a lesser extent C9 are associated only with a predisposition to neisserial infections, suggesting that a critical role for C5b-9 is limited to these essential organisms.[13]

Evidence exists that the classical and alternative pathways are slowly turning over C3, and the same is likely for the lectin pathway.[14,15] Both fluid phase and membrane bound inhibitors keep the pathways in check until a PAMP is recognized, then the scale is tipped toward activation, which under most conditions is kept localized and transient.[16] The alternative pathway is activated when C3b is deposited on nonsialylated surfaces, which favors the binding of factor B, the homolog of C2, over the regulator factor H,[17] and can also be recruited when either the lectin or classical pathways have generated bound C3b. After binding to C3b factor B, a proenzyme, is cleaved by factor D to form the C3 cleaving enzyme C3bBb. Adjacent C3b provides a docking site for C5, allowing C3bBb

Table 11-2 Innate Immunity

Barriers	Soluble Mediators	Cellular Mediators
Epithelial surfaces	Natural antibodies	Phagocytes
Mucous layers	Complement	Natural killer (NK) cells
Flushing motions	Cytokines	
Normal microbial flora	Mannan-binding lectin	
	Surfactant proteins A and D	
	Defensins	

Table 11-3 Innate Immunity: Pathways for the Detection of Foreign Particles

Type of Foreign Substance	Fluid Phase Detecting System	Recruits Complement	Cell/Receptor
Viral associated abnormal or deficient MHC class I expression on host cells	—	No	Killer inhibitor receptors (KIRs) of natural killer (NK) cells
LPS	—	No	Toll-like receptor (TLR) 4, CD14
Diacylated bacterial lipoproteins	—	No	TLRs 2, 6
Triacylated bacterial lipoproteins	—	No	TLRs 1, 2
dsRNA	—	No	TLR3
Flagellin	—	No	TLR5
Unmethylated CpG DNA	—	No	TLR9 (intracellular)
Polyglucan carbohydrates	—	No	Glucan receptors dectinol and complement receptor 3 (CR3, CD11b/CD18)
Polymannose carbohydrates	—	No	Mannose-binding receptor (CD206) of macrophages
Polymannose carbohydrates	Mannan-binding lectin (MBL)	Yes	CR1(CD35), CR2(CD21), CR3
Bacterial carbohydrates	Natural Ab (IgM made by CD5+ B cells)	Yes	CR1,CR2,CR3
Nonsialylated carbohydrates	Alternative complement pathway	Yes	CR1,CR2,CR3
Negatively charged surfaces, complexes of anions-cations	Direct C1q binding	Yes	CR1,CR2,CR3
Phospholipids	Surfactant protein A (SPA)	No	Controversial
Phospholipids	Surfactant protein D (SPD)	No	Scavenger receptor

to cleave C5. The remainder of the pathway is shared by all three of the activation pathways.

The complement proteins that potentially remain bound to the PAMP, mannan binding lectin, C1q, C4b, and C3b, are all opsonic and use the same receptor, namely complement receptor 1 or CD35,[18–21] which is expressed on erythrocytes and phagocytes, as well as some other tissues.[22] On erythrocytes, CR1 ligates complement opsonized particles and during passage through the liver and spleen, the particles are removed by resident phagocytes while the erythrocytes return to the circulation, a process known as immune adherence-mediated clearance. C3b, the major complement opsonin, in part because of its molar abundance, facilitates phagocytosis by neutrophils and monocytes. C3b can be further processed by the serine protease factor I to iC3b and then C3dg using as cofactors CR1 or H for the first step, and CR1 for the second step. Regulated processing of C3b generates C3 ligands that engage different receptors, each with distinctive cellular expression. iC3b ligates CR3 (CD11b/CD18), which is expressed on neutrophils and macrophages predominantly; and C3dg ligates CR2 (CD21), which is expressed on B cells and dendritic cells predominantly.

The fluid phase fragments of activation of C4, C3, and C5, namely C4a, C3a, and C5a, are known as anaphylatoxins. They reinforce the inflammatory response, but new appreciation of the widespread expression of receptors for C3a and C5a suggest that these anaphylatoxins are more broadly involved in biology. Indeed, C3a acting in the absence of C3aR potentiates the chemokine CXCL12 for the stimulation of bone marrow B cells, which demonstrates a role for complement in the maturation of the B cells.

Cellular Components

Cellular components of innate immunity include phagocytic cells, NK cells, and the B-1 lymphocytes (those, as mentioned

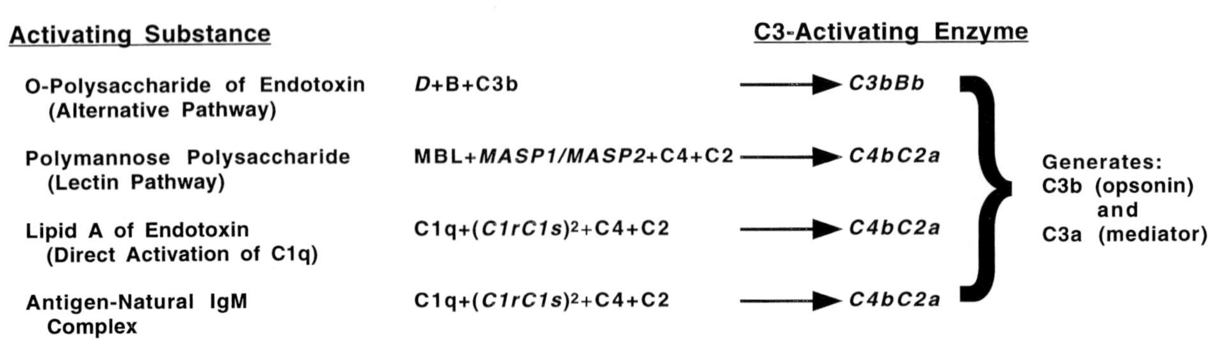

FIGURE 11-2 Complement pathways used in innate immunity. D and B, factors D and B of the alternative complement pathway; MBL, mannan-binding lectin; *MASP1/MASP2*, mannose-binding lectin–activated serine protease 1 and 2, respectively. Enzymes are shown in *italics*. The C5 cleaving enzyme for each of these pathways is the same as the C3 cleaving enzyme, except that it contains another C3b subcomponent that is necessary to bind the C5 substrate.

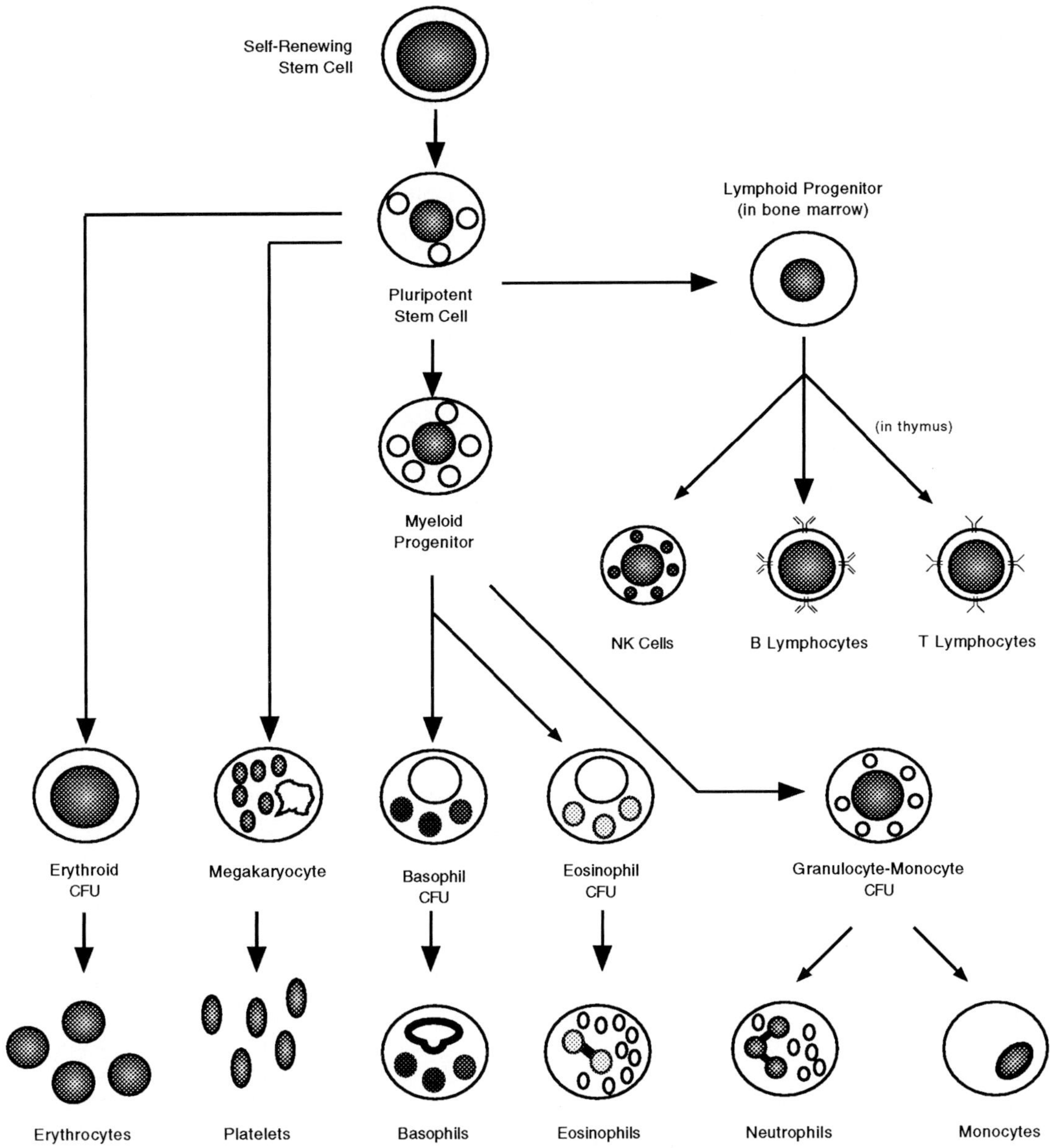

FIGURE 11-3 Cells derived from a common progenitor cell include erythrocytes, platelets, and various types of leukocytes. The leukocytes are lymphocytes (natural killer or NK cells, B cells, and T cells), granulocytes (basophils, eosinophils, and neutrophils), and monocytes, which can further differentiate into macrophages. CFU, colony-forming unit.

previously, responsible for the production of natural antibodies). The phagocytic cells include the neutrophils and monocytes (Fig. 11-3), the latter of which, under the appropriate stimulus, can migrate into the tissues and become macrophages. One well-defined signal for phagocytes to migrate occurs when any of the complement detecting pathways is activated, leading to C5 cleavage and the generation of C5a, which is a potent chemotactic factor for neutrophils and monocytes. A myriad, 43 to date, of polypeptide chemoattractants, termed *chemokines*, also act as chemotactic factors with varying specificities for different classes of leukocytes depending on the expression of their cognate receptor(s).[23] Most often phagocytes depend on the complement system for recognizing the "foreignness" of the particle, and phagocytes then have only to recognize the complement tag, usually C3b or iC3b, using CD35 and CD11a/CD18, respectively, as receptors. However, monocytes and macrophages can recognize polymannose and polyglucan directly by two receptors. The mannose receptor (CD206) (not to be confused with serum MBL) is a C-type lectin,[24,25] and there are two glucan receptors, Dectin-1 and the lectin-binding site of CD11a/CD18.[26,27]

The Toll-like receptors (TLRs) are widely expressed on host cells and are adapted for recognizing a spectrum of PAMPs (see Table 11-3). The intracellular TIR domain of TLRs shares homology with the IL-1 receptor and binds common adaptor proteins that lead to the activation of the transcription factors nuclear factor-κB (NF-κB) and/or interferon-related factor 3 (IRF3).[28] The activation of specific TLRs in different tissue environments is now thought to direct a Th1 or a Th2 pathway of the immune response. The ability of different TLRs to recruit different adaptor proteins and the pairing of different TLRs provides for an appropriate immune response.

NK cells, which are directly cytotoxic to some transformed and bacteria- or virus-infected cells, have novel receptors for detecting these abnormal cells.[29] Some killer Ig-like receptors (KIRs) are stimulated by the normal distribution of MHC class I and have an intracellular immunoreceptor tyrosine-based inhibitory motif (ITIM) domain for inhibition. Thus, these KIRs would deliver a tonic inhibitory signal to the NK cell when it probed a normal cell. However, if the NK cell probed a cell with deficient class 1 expression, such as a virus-infected cell, KIR-mediated inhibition would be interrupted. Other KIRs, whose ligands are unknown, contain an intracellular immunoreceptor tyrosine-based activation motif (ITAM) activation domain. The CD94-NKG2 NK cell receptors are heterodimers with C-type lectin-like activity, and members of this receptor family may signal for either inhibition or activation of the NK cell. The ligands for these NK cell receptors are also host proteins that become induced during cell distress.

B-1 lymphocytes are derived from bone marrow stem cells, but unlike conventional B cells (also known as B-2 lymphocytes), B-1 cells are self-renewing. Mature B-1 lymphocytes do not undergo all the differentiation steps of conventional B cells, and thus have limited opportunity to rearrange and mutate their immunoglobulin genes. This is consistent with the fact that B-1 immunoresponsiveness has been selected over generations of a species to respond to common, invariant immunologic epitopes of pathogens.

Synthesis

The innate immune system has a limited number of responses, all of which are encoded in the germline, meaning the genes originally inherited from the egg and the sperm. In contrast, the adaptive immune system has an almost unlimited array of responses because of ongoing genetic adaptation, which occurs in lymphocytes and is driven by the antigenic exposure of the individual. Why then does the more limited innate immune system persist in higher organisms? There are at least two reasons. First, the adaptive immune system requires time, on the order of days, to generate a useful antibody or cytotoxic T-cell response. In contrast, the innate immune response is operational immediately at the first encounter with a pathogen. Second, the adaptive immune response is not good at recognizing what is foreign, and so it requires the innate system to identify what is foreign and tag the foreign particle.[30] This recognition and tagging process primes adaptive immune responses.[31] On the other hand, the presence of specific antibody also enhances the function of the innate system, for example, antibody enhancement of NK cell function (antibody-dependent cell-mediated cytotoxicity) and the synergistic opsonic activity of specific antibody and complement. Thus, the innate and adaptive immune systems have evolved to function synergistically. Ironically, as vaccines are engineered to be more pure, the vaccine antigen(s) often escape detection by the innate immune system, and thereby become poor immunogens for the adaptive response (see Vaccines). Finally, we have outlined how the innate immune system should work, but all successful pathogens have engineered strategies to avoid some key elements of the innate immune system. These strategies are discussed as the virulence factors in the chapters about specific pathogens.

COMPONENTS OF THE ADAPTIVE IMMUNE SYSTEM

Lymphoid Organs

The lymphoid system can be conceptually divided into a central and a peripheral system. The central system generates the lymphocytes from stem cells in the bone marrow and provides for further differentiation of B cells in the bone marrow and T cells in the thymus. The peripheral lymphoid system, on the other hand, is where the lymphocytes and accessory cells initiate adaptive immune responses. Peripheral lymphoid organs include tonsils, peripheral lymph nodes, spleen, and the mucosal lymphoid systems. In most lymph nodes, as well as in the spleen, lymphocytes are concentrated in the white pulp. T cells are found in the central region and B cells are found in the germinal centers, which are toward the periphery of the organ or node.[1–3]

Cell Types of the Adaptive Immune Response

Many different cell types (see Fig. 11-3) participate in the various types of immune responses. Conventional B-cell development (B-2, not B-1) occurs totally within the bone marrow. As stem cells reproduce themselves, they also give rise to cells that will pass through the pro- and pre-B-cell lineages, eventually giving rise to mature B cells, which leave the bone marrow. The B cell receptor is comprised of membrane bound monomeric IgM, which conveys the antigenic specificity for the cell, and two associated invariant signalling molecules, Igα and Igβ. During B-cell maturation in the marrow, the heavy and light chain immunoglobulin genes are rearranged, allowing for a large repertoire of specificities. Most of the mature but naive B cells released from the marrow do not survive because they do not have access to the follicles of the peripheral lymphoid system. Activated B cells localize in the germinal centers of lymph nodes, and in that site further mutations of the immunoglobulin heavy and light chain genes occur, and selection leads to B cells capable of secreting high-affinity antibodies.[1–3] The immunoglobulin product of a B cell always has the same specificity as the Ig of the receptor. The properties of the five classes of human immunoglobulins are presented in Table 11-4.

T-cell precursors are generated in the bone marrow and migrate to the thymus where T-cell receptor (TCR) gene rearrangement takes place. The V, J, D, and C region genes come together to form the αβ and γδ TCRs. There is one specificity associated with each TCR, and after gene rearrangement to form the αβ TCR and γδ TCR, the TCR is expressed on the cell surface. TCR diversity is even greater than that for immunoglobulin owing to the large number of J and D region genes. Close to the time when TCR gene rearrangement occurs, the cells begin expressing several important accessory molecules (CD4, CD8, CD2, and CD3). During the process of T-cell maturation in the thymus, two other important maturation steps occur: positive and negative selection. During positive selection only

Table 11-4 Physical, Chemical, and Biologic Properties of Human Immunoglobulins

Property	IgM	IgG	IgA	IgD	IgE
Molecular weight (kD)	970	160	170–340	184	188
Serum concentration (mg/dL)	45–150	800–1500	90–325	0–8	<0.025
Light chains	κ or λ	κ or λ	κ or λ	κ or λ	κ or λ
Heavy chains (subgroups)	μ	γ1, γ2, γ3, or γ4	α1 or α2	δ	ε
J chain	Yes	No	In dimeric form	No	No
Time of synthesis*	First	Later			
Half-life in serum (days)	5	23	6	3	2.5
Localization	Serum	Serum, amniotic fluid, tissues	Serum, secretions, tears, colostrum, saliva, gastrointestinal and genitourinary tracts	Serum	Serum, tissues
Complement activation					
Classical pathway	++++	++	0	0	0
Alternative pathway	+	+	+	+	+
Opsonic activity	++	++++	0		
Lytic activity†	++++	++	0		
Inhibition of bacterial adherence	+	+	+++		
Viral neutralization	++	++	++		
Reaginic activity	0	Only IgG4	0	0	++++

*Because IgM antibody is produced early in infection and usually does not persist after months, IgM antibody can be a indicator of recent infection. Further, IgM antibody does not cross the placenta (in contrast to IgG), so IgM antibodies against a pathogen in a neonate are indicative of intrauterine or postnatal infection of the child and are independent of maternal antibodies.
†Only through activation of complement.

those T cells which react with self-MHC can mature. During negative selection most T cells that recognize "self-peptides" are eliminated.[1–3]

T and B lymphocytes are the only cells that recognize specific antigens. B cells not only produce antibody, they also function as antigen-presenting cells. In contrast to B cells, T cells are also major regulators of the immune response and are involved in cell-mediated immunity.[1–3] While lymphocytes are the cell populations most identified with immune responses, the functioning of these cells is dependent on other types of cells arriving in sufficient numbers at the site where foreign antigen is found.

Leukocyte Trafficking to Sites of Pathogen Invasion

A critical step in the immune system's response to pathogens is to recruit cells to enter an area of pathogen invasion or inflammation. Specific cell populations within the bloodstream are recruited to sites of pathogen invasion by interacting with molecules on the surface of the endothelium lining blood vessels or cavities. Innate immune sensors direct the release of IL-1β and TNF-α by cells at the site of pathogen invasion, which leads to the upregulation of E- and P-selectins on the surface of adjacent endothelial cells. Leukocytes, in contrast, express L-selectin constitutively. Initially, cells in the circulation are slowed down by weak binding orchestrated by the E- and P-selectins binding their counterreceptors, which are specific carbohydrates on the leukocytes.[32] While rolling adjacent to the site of inflammation, the cells receive a second signal through a chemokine or chemotactic receptor that activates the leukocyte's integrins for attachment to integrin ligands on enothelial cells. As a result of integrin ligation and signaling,[33] the leukocyte flattens and arrests on the endothelium, prior to migrating between or through endothelial cells and across the extracellular matrix to the focus of infection. The process of leukocyte migration from the intravascular space to the extravascular space is known as diapedesis. A remarkable feature of diapedesis is that different integrin signals lead to the emigration of specific subpopulations of leukocytes.[34]

MAJOR HISTOCOMPATIBILITY COMPLEX

The major histocompatibility complex (MHC), also designated HLA for "human leukocyte antigen," is expressed on the surfaces of a large variety of cells and is translated from a region of highly polymorphic genes.[1–3] A number of very elegant studies in mice led to the MHC's being recognized as responsible for immune responses, and the region to which these genes mapped was called the Ir region for immune response genes.[35] These genes were subsequently shown to be necessary for activation of helper T lymphocytes, which are necessary for the production of T-dependent antibody. Later it was recognized that T cells do not recognize free or soluble antigens, but rather peptides of antigens that are bound to MHC. The MHC has two types of gene products: class I and class II. Class I consists of a transmembrane heavy chain, which is complexed to soluble β_2-microglobulin. All cells, with the sole exception of erythrocytes, express class I. Class II is composed of an α and β transmembrane chain and is predominantly expressed on antigen-presenting cells. Both classes of MHC contain a "groove" in which processed peptide binds.[36]

MHC and Antigen Presentation

The manner in which MHC class I and II molecules are synthesized and assembled determines which types of pathogenic peptides can be bound by them (Fig. 11-4). Some of the

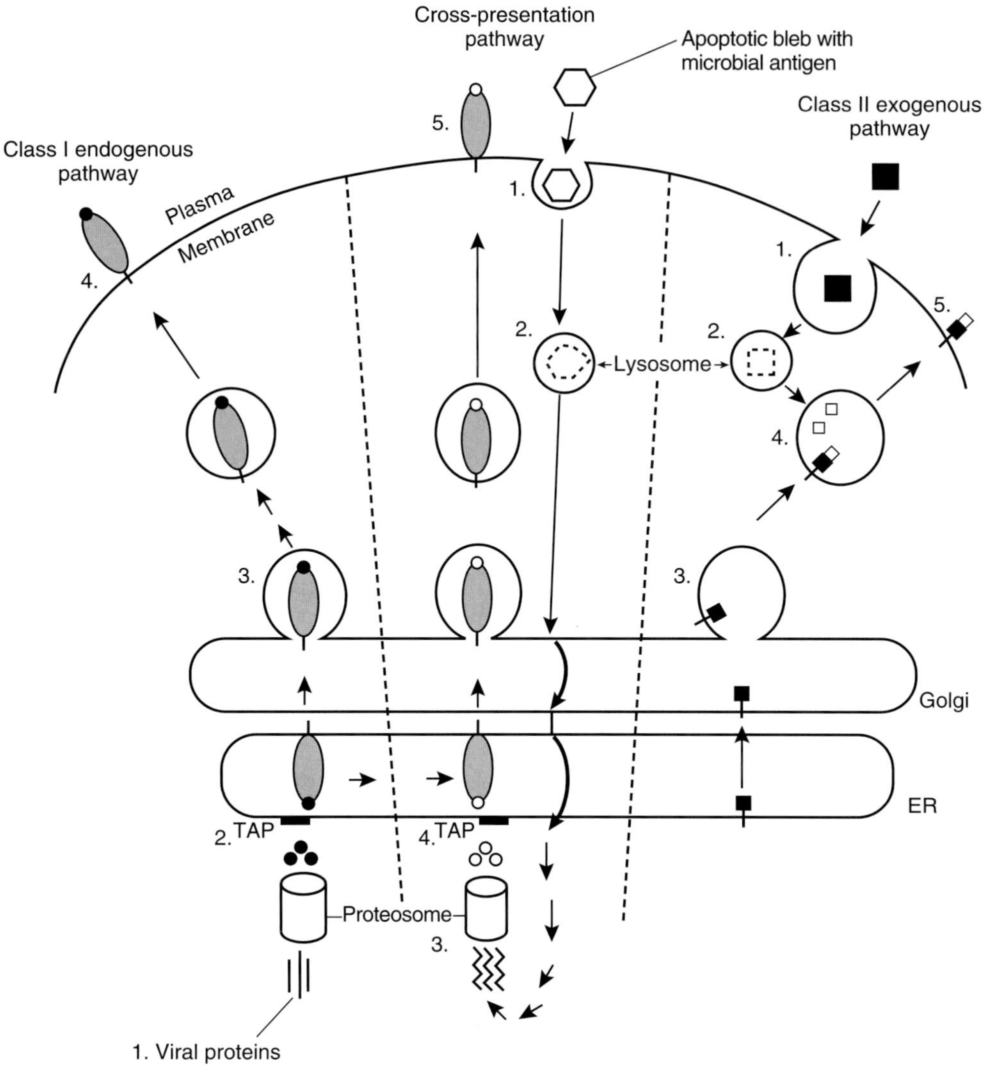

FIGURE 11-4 The pathways for processing antigens for presentation with major histocompatibility complex (MHC) molecules. Intracellular antigens (*left*), such as those derived from viruses, are degraded in the proteosome (1); complexed with TAP (transporter associated with antigen processing) (2); exported from the Golgi as an MHC class I antigen peptide complex (3), which are then expressed on the outer plasma membrane (4). Extracellular antigens (*right*) are phagocytosed or endocytosed (1), and degraded in lysosomes (2). Class II MHC molecules are synthesized and leave the Golgi in vesicles (3) that fuse with late endosomes containing antigenic peptides allowing the peptides to complex with MHC class II proteins (4); and the peptide–MHC class II complexes move to the plasma membrane (5). Cross-presentation (*center*) occurs when exogenous antigens, usually in a complex with apoptotic debris, are internalized by phagocytosis or endocytosis (1); move through a lysosomal compartment (2) to the proteosome (3). Thereafter, the degraded peptides are bound to TAP (4) for movement into the endoplasmic reticulum (ER) and Golgi for complexing with MHC class I proteins for transport and expression at the plasma membrane (5).

proteins synthesized endogenously by the host cell's ribosomes, as is the case for viral proteins, are normally degraded in the constitutive proteosome, an organelle designed to break down denatured or nonessential proteins to peptides. In the case of an intracellular infection, "immunoproteosomes" are induced by IFNγ and replace some of the constitutive proteosomes. The two types of proteosomes have distinctive proteolytic specificities and thereby enhance the repertoire of available peptides being presented to T cells.[37] Some of these peptides are transported into the endoplasmic reticulum (ER) by the TAPs (transporters of antigen presentation), where peptides usually of 8 to 9 amino acids in length are loaded into the groove of nascently synthesized class I molecules. Finally, the MHC class I–peptide complex is transported through the Golgi complex and exocytosed to the cell surface.[38] Nonself peptides (foreign, e.g., viral, peptides) complexed with the MHC will be recognized. The T cells that recognize foreign peptides complexed to class I MHC activate cytotoxic CD8+ T cells, which specifically lyse the virus-infected cell (Fig. 11-5). Because, potentially, any nucleated cell could be infected with a virus, all cells in the body, except erythrocytes, express class I MHC and are thereby scrutinized by T cells for evidence of a foreign peptide. Host peptides are also presented by class I MHC, but are generally not recognized, since self-recognizing T cells are eliminated in the thymus and never circulate. Those T cells reacting with host peptides with low affinity can be removed in the periphery.

A different pathway of antigen presentation is followed for molecules synthesized outside the cell, such as those from the extracellular pathogen *Streptococcus pneumoniae*. In this case, antigen-presenting cells, which are primarily monocytes, macrophages, dendritic cells, and B lymphocytes, sample the extracellular milieu. This sampling might take the form of phagocytosis of particles, such as bacteria, by monocytes or macrophages, or endocytosis and pinocytosis of soluble samples by any of the antigen-presenting cells. The larger antigens are proteolytically degraded, and eventually the derived peptides end up in an endocytic vesicle, which contains class II MHC. The class II MHC was previously synthesized in the ER and then packaged in an endosomal compartment by the Golgi complex of the antigen-presenting cell. In an elegant process, antigenic peptides bind to the class II MHC and then are expressed on the surface of the antigen-presenting cell.[39]

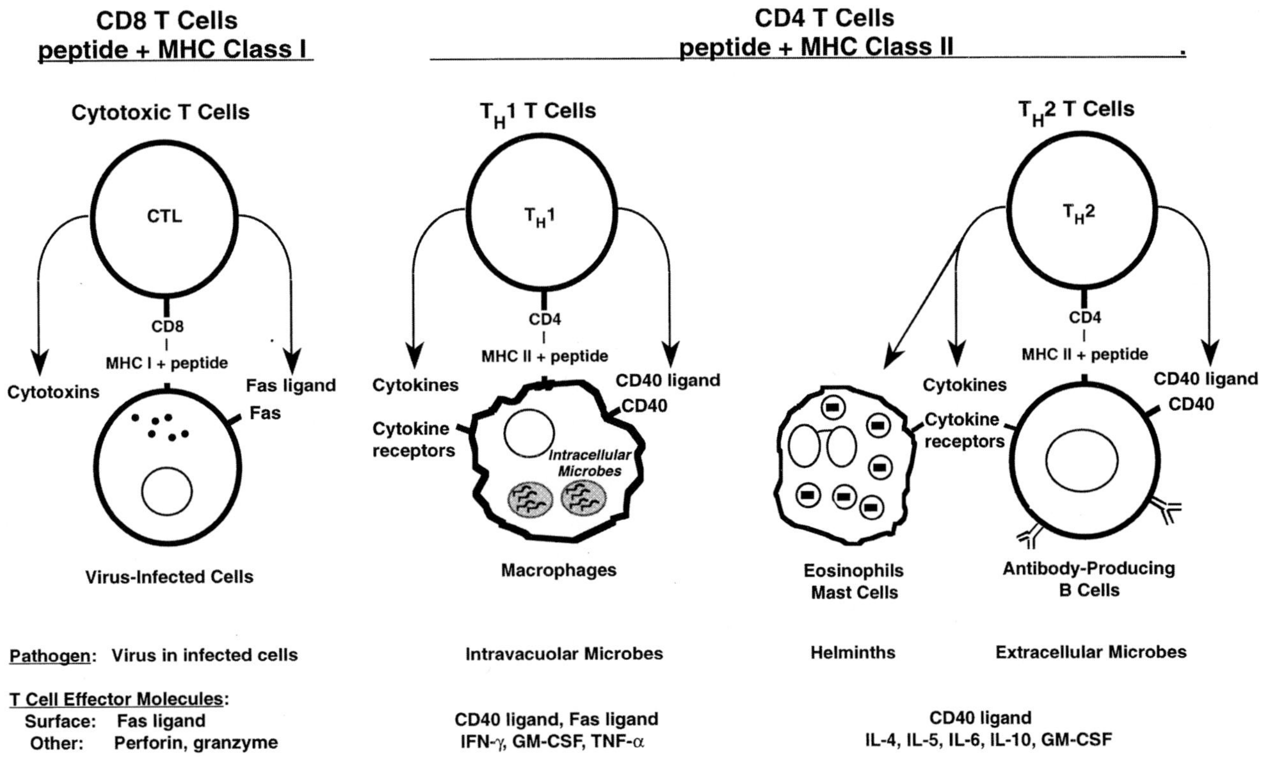

FIGURE 11-5 Responses of T-lymphocyte subsets to infectious agents. CD8+ T cells respond to antigens from intracellular pathogens, such as viruses, presented with class I major histocompatibility complex (MHC) molecules. These cytolytic CD8+ T cells lyse infected target cells by release of toxic proteins (perforin, granzyme) and by induction of apoptosis (programmed cell death) by engagement of Fas. CD4+ T cells can be directed to develop into T helper 1 (Th1) cells that stimulate macrophage killing of intracellular pathogens (cell-mediated immunity) or T helper 2 (Th2) cells that produce antibody or enhance eosinophil- and mast cell–mediated responses to helminthic parasites. GM-CSF, granulocyte-macrophage colony–stimulating factor; IFN-γ, interferon-γ; IL-4, etc., interleukins; TNF-α, tumor necrosis factor-α.

It is the CD4+ helper T cells that recognize antigens bound to class II MHC. Again, as in the case of peptides expressed with class I MHC, the majority of peptides bound to class II MHC will be host-derived, but there will no T cells to react with the host peptides because those T cells will have been previously eliminated in the thymus by negative selection.

Two addenda to the classic distinction of class I and class II pathways of antigen presentation are necessary. First, although class I and class II MHC are efficient at presenting peptide antigens, lipid and glycolipid antigens, such as those derived from *Mycobacterium* species, are presented by CD1 proteins. Distinguishing features of the CD1 proteins are that they have limited diversity and their cytoplasmic tails target them to distinct endosomal compartments for the potential loading of lipids from different intracellular pathogens.[40] The second addendum to the class I/class II paradigm is the concept of "cross presentation." Cross presentation occurs when an antigen made outside the antigen-presenting cell is internalized by endocytosis or phagocytosis and instead of complexing with class II MHC, it is routed to a compartment containing class I MHC (see Fig. 11-4).[41,42] At least one pathway involves digestion in the proteosome and complexing of the peptide with class I in the ER in the usual manner. Antigenic material that is from apoptotic infected cells or complexed with heat shock proteins from stressed or necrotic cells is favored for cross presentation.[43,44]

Reason for MHC Diversity

In humans, the MHC, or HLA, genes are located on chromosome 6. There are three major polymorphic genes for class I (A, B, and C).[1–3] Because these genes are codominant, a cell will commonly express six different MHC class I molecules (three from each parent). The class II polymorphic genes are DR, DP, and DQ, all composed of α and β chains. Many individuals also have a gene for an extra DR β chain, either of which can combine with the DR α chain. Thus, class II MHC heterozygous individuals can express eight different polymorphic alleles (four from each parent). The reason an individual needs so many possible MHC proteins is to be able to generate a diverse array of grooves in the MHC molecules, such that there would be a groove to fit at least some antigens from each potential pathogen. Although this strategy works most of the time, there are some MHC types that have been linked to susceptibility to certain pathogens (see Tables 8-2 and 8-3), or to an increased frequency of certain immunologic diseases. The reason the human species maintains such a large and diverse MHC repertoire likely relates to the capacity to respond to numerous and diverse pathogens. Although an evolving pathogen might find a susceptible MHC-"deficient" type in a few individuals, others in the population will have different and functional MHC types and therefore will not be susceptible to the altered pathogen.

Costimulation

Activation of T cells is not accomplished solely by the TCR complex binding to antigen in the cleft of the MHC. If this were so, then self-reacting T cells that escape negative selection in the thymus could induce autoimmune responses. Control of T-cell activation is in part regulated by a number of accessory molecules that must be engaged in order for the T cell to respond. These regulatory molecules are called "costimulatory" molecules.[45] While the presence of CD28 on T cells is constitutive, its ligands on the antigen-presenting cell, CD80 and CD86 (previously known as B7.1 and B7.2), are induced when innate immunity recognizes the PAMPs.[46] Ligation of lymphocyte CD40 ligand (CD154) by CD40 on the antigen-presenting cell stimulates the production of cytokines and allows for activation of integrins, which provide stable adhesion between the two cells and thereby enhances the possibility of stimulating an immune response.[47]

Complement C3 fragment C3dg can effect another type of costimulation. Antigens can directly interact with a B cell's immunoglobulin receptor and trigger a proliferative response. If, however, the antigen is first recognized as foreign by the complement system and tagged with C3b, which is processed to C3dg, the threshold amount of antigen needed to evoke a B-cell response is lowered by a factor of 10,000.[31] One reason C3dg-tagged antigen is efficient is that the CD21/CD19 signaling complex is costimulated with the antigen receptor. CD21 is the receptor for C3dg, while CD19 gives positive signaling to B cells.

The ability of the innate immune system to appropriately recognize pathogens and upregulate costimulatory molecules on antigen-presenting cells provides an important control over the immune system: Interaction between a peripheral lymphocyte that binds a self-antigen on an antigen-presenting cell that lacks costimulatory molecules leads to functional paralysis of the lymphocyte, or tolerance (*vide infra*).[48]

Anergy and Tolerance

Anergy is a state of global immunologic unresponsiveness, which can be remedied by removal or addition of one or more factors.[1–3] For instance, an abundance of IL-10 leads to downregulation of molecules on antigen-presenting cells such that they are unable to activate T cells to respond in the presence of specific antigen. Removal of IL-10 from the system leads to restoration of responsiveness.

Tolerance is different from a state of anergy and occurs when the immune system is unable to respond to specific antigens.[1–3] Therefore, all other immune responses would occur normally except for the response to the specific antigen to which the organism has been made tolerant. There are multiple steps in the immune response that are susceptible to tolerance, and these steps are used as a safeguard to prevent the immune system from reacting against itself, so-called autoimmunity. During development, most T cells in the periphery are tolerant to self-antigens because those cells avidly reacting with self-antigens are eliminated in the thymus during "negative selection." Immature B cells that react with multivalent self-antigens are destroyed by programmed cell death, or apoptosis, a process referred to as "clonal deletion." Immature B cells that react with soluble self-antigens are rendered inactive by the downregulation of their surface IgM and their signaling potential. Finally, when CD4+ T cells bind an antigen-presenting cell expressing antigen-MHC but no costimulatory molecules, these T cells will be rendered tolerant. Tolerance can be induced experimentally in animals and has been shown to be partially dependent on the form and the route of administration of the antigen. High doses of antigen, orally administered antigen, or repetitive doses of low concentrations of antigen may all lead to tolerance. Successful vaccine strategies must avoid inducing tolerance.

MATURATION OF IMMUNE RESPONSES AND ANTIMICROBIAL IMMUNITY

Immune responses, initiated as outlined earlier, are subject to regulation that for antimicrobial immunity selects elements of the immune system adapted to contain specific pathogens and also regulates immune responses to minimize damage to surrounding cells and tissues due to uncontrolled inflammatory reactions.[1–3]

Cytotoxic CD8+ T Cells

The presentation of cytosolic antigens, notably those of viral pathogens, will utilize class I MHC proteins and elicit responses of CD8+ T cells (see Fig. 11-4). Cytotoxic T cells are recruited by two mechanisms: (1) cross presentation by dendritic cells of host cellular debris containing microbial antigens, which leads to IL-2-dependent recruitment; and (2) in the case of antigen presentation by a nondendritic APC, the simultaneous binding of a CD4 helper T cell and a naive antigen-specific CD8 to the APC (see Fig. 11-5). CD8+ T cells are capable of eliminating infected cells by several mechanisms, including the release of granule-derived cytotoxins (granzyme, perforin) and the Fas ligand engagement of target cell Fas to elicit apoptosis (programmed cell death). Cytotoxic T cells also release cytokines that contribute to host defense. For instance, these cells release IFN-γ, which inhibits viral replication and activates macrophage for intracellular killing and antigen presentation.

CD4+ T Cells and Class II Presentation

Presentation of peptide antigens via class II MHC proteins is capable of stimulating CD4+ T cells. These cells differentiate from a common Th0 progenitor into cells with distinct phenotypes referred to as Th1 or Th2 cells. These two subsets of T helper cells were first defined in murine systems and have been further refined based on studies of murine strains infected with protozoal parasites, such as *Leishmania*, and helminthic parasites, such as schistosomes.[49,50] The T helper cell subsets are defined by the cytokines they produce. Th1 cells are characterized by IL-2, IFN-γ, and IL-12 production. In contrast, Th2 responses are associated with IL-4, IL-5, IL-10, and IL-13 production. The two T helper subsets and the dominant cytokines of each are cross-regulatory: IFN-γ from Th1 cells inhibits development of Th2 cells, and IL-10 and transforming growth factor-β (TGF-β) made by Th2 cells inhibit Th1 development. In humans, unlike mice, there is more variability in T helper cells, especially among the cytokines they produce.

The processes whereby T helper cells differentiate into Th1 or Th2 subsets are currently thought to be influenced by the type of immature dendritic cell and its enviroment when it first presents the microbial antigen.[51] Because the type of the immature dendritic cell defines its repertoire of PAMP receptors, a given microbial antigen may preferentially be presented by a phenotypically distinct dendritic cell. In addition, the tissue microenvironment, with its distinctive exposure to foreign antigens and array of innate immune cells, influences the ability of resident immature dendritic cells to polarize T helper cells. Surrounding macrophages and NK cells that are stimulated by foreign antigens provide signals that bias the immature dendritic cell toward Th1, whereas stimulated mast cells and eosinophils bias the immature dendritic cell toward Th2.

Th1 Responses: Cell-Mediated Immunity and Delayed Type Hypersensitivity

For intracellular pathogens that live within vesicles or vacuoles, such as mycobacteria, neither antibody nor cytotoxic T cells have access to the pathogens. Rather, macrophages harboring these pathogens must be activated by antigen-specific Th1 lymphocytes to kill the pathogens, a process called cell-mediated immunity.[52] The antigen-committed Th1 cells first recognize their cognate microbial peptide complexed with MHC class II on the surface of an infected macrophage, and then this lymphocyte secretes macrophage-activating cytokines, including IFN-γ, TNF-α, and granulocyte-monocyte colony-stimulating factor (GM-CSF). CD40 ligand on the Th1 lymphocyte engages CD40 on macrophages and also contributes to macrophage activation. The "classically" activated macrophage uses upregulated nitric oxide and oxygen radicals to aid in killing of pathogens in phagolysosomes.[53] A less productive form of Th1 immunity is known as delayed type hypersensitivity. Contact dermatitis, such as sensitivity to poison ivy, is a common form of delayed type hypersensitivity.

Th2 Responses: Antibody Production and Immediate Hypersensitivity

Th2 responses are important for host defense against extracellular pathogens, and Th2 cells participate in this in two different ways. First, Th2 cells are critical in activating B cells to produce antibodies. Activated Th2 cells express the CD40 ligand that must interact with CD40 on the surface of the B cell, and produce specific cytokines, such as IL-4 and IL-6, which stimulate B cells and promote isotype switching, whereby immunoglobulin synthesis matures from IgM to include other classes of immunoglobulins (see Table 11-4). Antibodies can function to directly neutralize some pathogens and toxins, to opsonize pathogens facilitating their phagocytosis by cells such as macrophages and neutrophils, and to activate complement for enhanced opsonization or lysis of some bacteria. Antibody may also enhance NK cell functions by means of antibody-dependent cellular cytotoxicity. A second role of Th2 cells is to "alternatively" activate macrophages to produce Th2 cytokines instead of Th1 cytokines. The end result is that the macrophage becomes more efficient at presenting peptides from extracellular microbes. Epithelioid cells and granulomatous fibrosis are the histologic hallmarks of alternatively activated macrophages.[53]

Activation of the Th2 pathway can lead to immediate hypersensitivity, an IgE-dependent form of allergy. The reaction is initiated when IgE antibodies that are bound via their Fc region to the IgE receptors, principally on mast cells, bind their specific antigens ("allergens"). Crosslinking of the IgE receptors on these cells stimulates the activation and release of mediators from these cells. IL-4 from Th2 lymphocytes strongly promotes the synthesis of IgE; the Th2 cytokines IL-5 and GM-CSF stimulate eosinophil differentiation and activation; and IL-4 acts on mast cells. IgE, eosinophils, and mast cells are involved in host defense against the extracellular helminthic parasites. On the other hand, a dysregulated Th2 response leads to chronic inflammation, asthma being a prime example.[54]

Regulatory T Cells

Although it was speculated for some time that there might be a subset of regulatory T cells (T_R), it was not until these cells could be identified by cell surface markers that definitive studies could be performed. In both mice and humans, the major population of T_R is CD25+, CD4+. CD25 is the α-chain of the high affinity IL-2 receptor. T_R have rearranged T cell receptors and are antigen specific; many of them react with host antigens. Once activated, the T_R secretes IL-10 and TGF-β and suppresses the immune response nonspecifically. The importance of T_R has been shown in mice and humans. Mice that are depleted of CD25+, CD4+ lymphocytes rapidly develop autoimmune disease; and in humans genetic deficiency of Foxp3 transcription factor, which is downstream of CD25 signaling, is associated with IPEX (immune dysregulation, polyendocrinopathy, enteropathy, and X-linked syndrome).[55] In normal subjects, lymphocytes reacting with self-antigens with high affinity are eliminated in the thymus. T_R are favored to bind lymphocytes that react with self- or nonself-antigens with low affinity, and thus are favored to remove self-reacting lymphocytes in the periphery. T_R proliferate in the periphery and are very radiosensitive. Loss of T_R may have a significant role in the development of autoimmune complications commonly seen after chemotherapy and/or radiation therapy.

IMMUNOPATHOLOGY

Autoimmunity

Tolerance to self is essential to maintain normal body functions. As discussed earlier (see Anergy and Tolerance), this is accomplished at multiple steps beginning early in development and continuing for the life of the organism. Autoimmune disease occurs when there is a breaking of tolerance to self-antigens. The autoimmune response may result from the incomplete elimination of autoreactive clones by the thymus. Alternatively, autoimmune responses may be elicited when normally hidden, sequestered self-antigens are released into the lymphoid environment and activate T cells. Lastly, autoimmune responses may be the result of the activation of formerly anergic T-cell self-reactive clones. Several genetic factors have been clearly associated with a risk of acquiring autoimmune disease. First, certain MHC alleles predispose to autoimmune disease, such as the association of the class I MHC B27 allele with ankylosing spondylitis. One possible explanation for why a specific MHC type is associated with a particular autoimmune syndrome is that the MHC protein is more likely to bind a target host autoantigen. The converse, lack of peptide binding to MHC, is the explanation for the association of some host MHC types with susceptibility to specific pathogens (see Chapter 8, Table 8-1).

A second genetically determined risk factor for the development of autoimmune disease is the genetic deficiency of an early complement component. The relative risks for the deficiencies are C1q greater than C4 greater than C2.[56] A mild form of systemic lupus erythematosus (SLE) is associated with C2 deficiency, moderated SLE disease is associated with C4 deficiency, while a pernicious SLE-like syndrome is almost invariably associated with C1q deficiency.[57] There are at least two potential reasons why the absence of an early complement component predisposes to autoimmunity: (1) it is more difficult to clear potential autoantigens; and (2) it is more difficult to clear antigen-antibody immune complexes once they are formed.[58] Additional risk factors for autoimmune disease include the genetically determined upregulation of costimulatory molecules and a functional deficiency of T_R.

Other Forms of Immunopathology

Immune responses to infections may contribute to pathologic changes in other ways. When neither antibody nor antigen is singularly present in excess of the other, the complexing of antibodies with soluble antigen results in the formation of immune complexes that may cause disease. This may develop acutely as antibody titers rise, causing the syndrome of serum sickness. In addition, when soluble antigen is persistently abundant, there is sustained formation of immune complexes, leading to chronic immune complex–mediated tissue damage, as found in subacute bacterial endocarditis and chronic *Plasmodium malariae* infections.

The recruitment and activation of phagocytes in response to infections also may contribute to tissue damage owing to the exuberant local release of leukocyte granule enzymes and other proteins and generation of oxidants. Thus, the pyogenic response of neutrophils to bacterial infections can be partially deleterious, as with the chronic neurologic sequelae following bacterial meningitis in children. Likewise, eosinophil activation in response to helminthic infections and allergic diseases, such as asthma, can damage host cells.[54]

A serious condition known variously as hematophagocytic syndrome (HPS), hematophagocytic lymphohistiocytosis, and reactive macrophage activation syndrome is associated with macrophages in the bone marrow and spleen ingesting erythrocytes and sometimes nucleated blood cells.[59] The Th1 cytokines INF-γ and TNF-α are largely responsible for the abnormally activated macrophages. A subgroup of those with a familial form of HPS have mutations in their perforin gene. More commonly, the condition is nonfamilial and associated with certain infections, including Epstein-Barr virus, herpes 6, malaria, and *Salmonella* infections; and HPS may also be associated with autoimmune conditions and leukemia.

IMMUNODEFICIENCIES

Genetic deficiencies (see Chapter 8, Table 8-1), as well as acquired defects in the immune system may be associated with susceptibility to infections, and the pattern of infection—affected tissue and specific pathogen(s)—gives insight as to the defect (Table 11-5).[60,61] Many of the classic neonatal phenotypes of severe immunodeficiency states have now been recognized with a more moderate phenotype in adults. Thus, an appreciation of immunodeficient states is relevant for any age. The new onset of infection in a previously healthy host

Table 11-5 Genetic Deficiencies Affecting Lymphocyte Functions

Disease	Defective Gene Product	Resulting Defects
T cells		
Severe combined immunodeficiency (SCID)		
X-linked SCID	IL-2/IL-4 receptor γ chain	T-cell proliferation, lymphopenia, antibody production, hypogammaglobulinemia
Non-X-linked SCID	JAK-3 kinase	T-cell proliferation, lymphopenia, antibody production, hypogammaglobulinemia
Adenosine deaminase deficiency	Adenosine deaminase	T-cell proliferation, lymphopenia, antibody production, hypogammaglobulinemia
Purine nucleoside phosphorylase deficiency	Purine nucleoside phosphorylase	T-cell function, decreased CD3+ cells
T-cell immunodeficiencies	IL-2, CD3ε, CD3γ, or ZAP 70 tyrosine kinase	Infections, autoimmunity, allergies
HLA class II deficiency	C II TA; RFX 5	Impaired cell-mediated immunity
HLA class I deficiency	TAP2	Impaired cell-mediated immunity
DiGeorge syndrome		Thymic aplasia, cardiac abnormalities
Wiskott-Aldrich syndrome	WASP	Thrombocytopenia, low IgM, high IgA
Ataxia-telangiectasia	ATM	Low IgA, CD3 and CD4 cells
Immune dysfunction, polyendocrinopathy, enteropathy, and X-linked syndrome (IPEX)	FOX3p	Severe autoimmunity
B cells		
X-linked hypogammaglobulinemia		Low antibodies
X-linked immunodeficiency with hyper IgM	CD 40 ligand	High IgM, low IgG and IgA
Common variable immunodeficiency		Low IgG and poor antibody response
IgA deficiency		Decreased IgA

Table 11-6 Patterns of Infections Associated with Specific Immune Defects

Site/Organism	Typical Onset	Disease-Associated Defect
Recurrent meningitis		
Neisseria meningitidis	>12 years	Complement deficiency in properdin, C5, C6, C7, C8 or C9
S. pneumoniae, and other species	After trauma or surgery	
Severe aphthous ulcers	Anytime	Neutropenia, HIV
Sinopulmonary infections		
S. pneumoniae, S. pyogenes	Neonatal	IgG deficiency, C3 deficiency, congenital neutropenia, dysfunctional PMN
H. influenza, N. meningitides	Anytime	Common variable IgG deficiency
Pulmonary infections	Childhood–adult	Deficiencies of IFNγ, IFNγR, IL-12 or IL-12R
Atypical mycobacteria		
Nocardia spp.	Adult	Alveolar proteinosis
Herpes virus I or II	Infancy	NK cell deficiency
Severe EBV infection	Infancy–adult	X-linked lymphoproliferative disease
Bacteremia		
S. pneumoniae, S. pyogenes, H. influenza, N. meningitidis	Anytime	HIV, hypo- or asplenia
Salmonella (nontyphoidal)	—	HIV, hemoglobinopathies, Bartonellosis, deficiencies of IFNγ, IFNγR, IL-12 or IL-12R
Neisseria gonorrhoeae	Sexually active	Complement deficiency in properdin, C5, C6, C7, C8, or C9
Skin infections		
S. aureus	Childhood	Leukocyte adhesion deficiency (deficiency or dysfunction of β2 integrins)
	—	Job's syndrome
Chronic granulomatous disease (genetic defects in neutrophil NADPH oxidase, impaired respiratory burst, and H_2O_2	Infancy–adult	*S. aureus, Salmonella* spp., *Burkholderia cepacia, Serratia marcescens, Nocardia asteroides, Aspergillus* spp., and *Chromobacterium violaceum*
Strongyloides stercoralis	Anytime	HTLV-1, glucocorticoid use, lymphoma
M. tuberculosis relapse	Anytime	HIV, glucocorticoid use

can herald the presence of an underlying acquired disease such as a hematologic malignancy and HIV infection, which are important to rule out first. The issue as to when it is relevant to consider a genetically determined immunodeficient state depends on the family history, age of the patient, and chronicity and pattern of infections; there are no easy rules. However, there are some recurrent themes such as the similar susceptibility of patients deficient in either IgG, neutrophils, or complement C3; and some "signature" organisms, such as the association of *Aspergillius* spp. and *Burkholderia cepacia* (Table 11-6).

VACCINES

The capacity to elicit protective immunity against infectious agents was first achieved 200 years ago with the utilization of *vaccinia* (cowpox) by Jenner to protect against smallpox. The word *vaccination* derives from this first success. Immunization was critical in eradicating smallpox from the world and underlies the approach to the global eradication of other infections, including poliomyelitis. With the vaccines currently recommended by the World Health Organization (WHO) Expanded Programme on Immunization, significant mortality or morbidity from several infections can be prevented in children and adults. Among early childhood diseases, measles accounts for more deaths during childhood than any other vaccine-preventable disease. In 2002, WHO estimated that there were 30 to 40 million cases of measles with more than 700,000 deaths, mostly occurring in developing countries. Thus, at present, delivering available vaccines to at-risk populations is as great a problem as the development of new vaccines. WHO maintains a web site giving the immunization status of any given country or region for the previous year: www.who.int/vaccines-surveillance/DataDown.htm.

Immune Responses

Early vaccines were based on the administration of either killed or live attenuated organisms in the hope that they would stimulate protective immune responses. Organisms treated with formalin are nonviable but still immunogenic. Attenuated human viruses are derived by passaging virus in culture on nonhuman cells during which the virus mutates and loses its pathogenicity but retains its immunogenicity for humans. Based on experience and the evolving understanding of immune responses, both the limitations of existing approaches and newer strategies to elicit the development of protective immunity are being appreciated. Rational approaches to vaccine development will take account of: (1) the need to engage the innate immune system so that co-stimulatory molecules on the antigen-presenting cell are upregulated, (2) the immunization site most likely to engage effective dendritic cells, and (3) the means to avoid T_R cell blunting of the immune response. In addition, the immune condition of the subject must be considered. The efficacy of immunizing infants with live attenuated viral vaccines is compromised by maternally acquired antibody, so that immunizations with measles, mumps, and rubella must be delayed until about one year of age. The immune system of children under age 2 is incapable of responding to immunization with bacterial polysaccharides, such as those needed for pneumococcal and *Haemophilus influenzae* type b (Hib) vaccinations. The conjugation of the bacterial polysaccharide with a carrier protein, as now employed in conjugate *H. influenzae* and *S. pneumoniae* vaccines, facilitates Th2 cell interactions. This occurs because the B cell specific for the microbial polysaccharide will internalize the carbohydrate-carrier complex via its B cell Ig receptor and process and then present in a MHC class II complex the carbohydrate as well as peptides from the carrier protein on its surface. This allows the B cell, which can only make Ig against the carbohydrate, to receive additional T-cell help from T cells that recognize the carrier protein peptides. With this additional T-cell help, a B cell is more efficiently stimulated to produce protective antibodies directed to the bacterial polysaccharides. This strategy circumvents the age limitation in the development of immune responses, enabling such conjugate vaccines to be administered effectively to infants, those most at risk of serious infections.

In addition to the chemical form of the immunogen, immune responses are governed by the site of immunization and by the presence of agents that can bolster immune responses. While intravenous administration of antigen can lead to tolerance of B and T cells, intradermal or subcutaneous administration facilitates uptake of antigen by antigen-presenting dendritic cells, thereby enhancing immune responses.[62] Administration of antigens at mucosal surfaces (e.g., intranasally or orally) may be less effective in terms of stimulating systemic immunity because dendritic cells in these areas are programmed to dampen immune responses. Nevertheless mucosal immunity can be important in preventing the spread of pathogens. Coadministration of an immunogen with adjuvants, substances that stimulate innate immunity, can enhance and influence the nature of the immune response. In diphtheria-pertussis-tetanus (DPT) immunizations, *Bordetella pertussis* functions as both an adjuvant and an immunogen. Aluminum hydroxide gel, alum, an adjuvant currently approved for use in humans, elicits a predominantly Th2-type T-cell response, leading to enhanced antibody formation. In contrast to some infections, Th1-type CD4+ T-cell responses with enhanced intracellular killing or cytotoxic CD8+ T-cell responses will be needed to ensure effective immune responses after immunization. Ongoing research is actively evaluating different strategies to develop newer adjuvants to enhance the efficacy of immunizations.

Cytokines are potential biologic agents that might have utility in directing specific types of immune responses. In experimental animal systems, the coadministration of the cytokine IL-12 with a vaccine can promote strong Th1 responses. Problems associated with cytokine use are toxicity and cost. Further, it is not known how administration of cytokines might influence responses to other organisms that person might harbor.

Vaccine Formulations and Delivery

The ideal attributes for a vaccine are: (1) safe for all ages; (2) effective, long-lasting immunity; (3) requires only a single, or two closely spaced, immunizations; (4) provides protection within 2 weeks; (5) can be delivered without need of a needle and syringe; (6) may be administered in a formulation with other vaccines; (7) is stable at high and low temperatures; and (8) is inexpensive to produce.[63]

The initial era of vaccine development was based on the use of killed or attenuated whole organisms as immunogens. Usually these produced reasonable immune responses because of their recruitment of innate immunity, but in some cases they are associated with adverse reactions. Examples of adverse reactions would include the encephalopathic responses to the older formulations of killed *Bordetella pertussis* vaccine and the allergy to contaminating egg protein of influenza vaccine, which is produced by growing the virus in chicken eggs. To avoid such issues, many newer vaccines use purified molecules as immunogens.

Subunit Approach to Vaccines

Subunit vaccines are composed of purified recombinant proteins or synthetic peptides encoding defined epitopes of potential pathogens. Four reasons have led to the recent emphasis on using subunits of organisms as vaccines: (1) avoidance of the potential toxicities of whole organisms, such as those associated with killed pertussis vaccine; (2) provision of more stable vaccines, especially as compared with the care needed to keep live, attenuated strain vaccines active; (3) obviation of the high cost of growing fastidious organisms or organisms with complicated life cycles, such as malarial parasites; and (4) the feasibility of the subunit approach using molecular biologic recombinant technology.

Although there are benefits to recombinant subunit vaccines, one limitation is they are not very immunogenic when administered by themselves. Highly purified immunogens may not stimulate the innate immune system and fail to upregulate the costimulatory molecules on antigen-presenting cells, and thus fail to induce an immune response. The advantage of using whole organisms is that the innate immune system can recognize the organism as foreign, and thereby use complement and the upregulation of costimulatory molecules to induce an immune response.

One way to compensate for their lack of immunogenicity is to combine the purified subunits with more immunogenic adducts or administer them with newer adjuvants. A complex of the recombinant immunogen and recombinant complement C3dg is an appealing adduct because of its potential to recruit not only the B cell receptor, but also the CD21/CD19 complex, which potentiates the B cell response. Newer and more potent adjuvants include MF59, which is a lipid-detergent mixture containing squalene; F127, a copolymer that can be mixed with the immunogen and other immunomodulators at a cool temperature and, when injected, the mixture gels at body temperature providing a solid phase depot of immunoreactants; and the use of unmethylated CpG DNA, which is able to directly Toll-like receptor 9, which in humans is primarily expressed on B cells and plasmacytoid dendritic cells.[64,65] Although the development of new adjuvants is a burgeoning field, acceptance of this technology for human use has lagged because of concerns of inducing autoimmunity.[66]

DNA Vaccines

A major innovation in vaccine delivery systems developed in the 1990s has been the transfection of mammalian cells with "naked DNA." This method of vaccination simply requires that the coding DNA for the candidate vaccine antigen be placed into a plasmid, usually containing a strong eukaryotic promoter such as cytomegalovirus. Purified plasmid in saline is then injected intradermally or intramuscularly and transfection of cells occurs. The transfected cells produce the candidate antigen, which, being intracellular, is processed and then expressed on the cell surface via class I MHC. If the cell is lysed, additional candidate antigen is released, which can then be processed via the extracellular class II pathway, or the cross-presentation pathway (see Fig. 11-4). Thus, via this methodology it is possible to generate MHC class I– and MHC class II–dependent responses to the candidate antigen.

Advantages of this method are that no adjuvants are required, the vaccine does not require special storage because DNA is stable, and the purification of plasmid DNA is relatively simple compared with purification of recombinant proteins. It is possible to enhance DNA vaccine efficacy by the coinjection of other plasmid DNA, which either contains the coding regions for molecules that will function as adjuvants or includes noncoding regions of DNA that themselves elicit adjuvant activity. Notably, the costimulatory molecules CD80 and CD86 have been incorporated into plasmid DNA, as well as the coding region for IL-12. Thus, one can attempt to direct the nature of the ensuing immune response via the local production of these molecules. For cytokines, this approach is particularly attractive, as the plasmid DNA stays local when injected intramuscularly.

There are potential drawbacks to the use of DNA vaccines. The most serious concern would be that the plasmid DNA becomes integrated into the genome, where any number of integration-related problems may later appear, such as the activation of oncogenes. Other concerns are that the long-term production of candidate vaccine antigen might induce tolerance to the antigen rather than a protective immune response. Additionally, there is the worry that the use of DNA vaccines may lead to autoimmune diseases, owing to lysis of the cells and release of cellular components including DNA.

Vaccine Delivery Systems

Molecular biologic approaches also enable novel methods of introducing immunogens into hosts that are not dependent on adjuvants. One promising approach is to incorporate the DNA coding sequence for the relevant antigen into a microbial vector that can be made innocuous and suitable for administration to humans. Several vectors, including genetically altered, avirulent *Salmonella* bacteria, vaccinia virus, bacille Calmette-Guérin (BCG) mycobacteria, as well as edible plants are being studied. In addition, formulations of vaccines that allow transdermal or transmucosal immunization would greatly facilitate large scale, or emergency immunization programs.

CONCLUSION

Vaccines already exist that protect against life-threatening infections (e.g., rabies, diphtheria), and that can eradicate major diseases (e.g., smallpox, and maybe polio), prevent diseases in susceptible populations by the immunization of surrogates (e.g., rubella immunization to prevent congenital rubella syndrome, tetanus immunization to prevent neonatal tetanus), limit morbidity (e.g., hepatitis A), and prevent late sequelae of infections (e.g., prevention of hepatitis B–associated neoplasms). Further, new insights from a fuller understanding of immunology coupled with recombinant technology offer the possibility of making current vaccines more effective and developing new vaccines for important infectious diseases, such as HIV, TB, and malaria. Yet the fact that over 1 million children die each year of diseases for which we already have vaccines (vaccine-preventable disease) underscores the social and economic factors that limit access to this highly effective means of disease prevention.

REFERENCES

1. Janeway CA, Jr, Travers P, Walport M, et al: Immunobiology: The Immune System in Health and Disease, 6th ed. London, Garland Publishing, 2004.
2. Abbas AK, Lichtman AH: Cellular and Molecular Immunology. Philadelphia, W.B. Saunders, 2003.
3. Paul WE: Fundamental Immunology. Philadelphia, Lippincott, Williams and Wilkins, 2003.
4. Hooper LV, Wong MH, Thelin A, et al: Molecular analysis of commensal host-microbial relationships in the intestine. Science 291:881–884, 2001.
5. Kelly D, Campbell JI, King TP, et al: Commensal anaerobic gut bacteria attenuate inflammation by regulating nuclear-cytoplasmic shuttling of PPAR-gamma and RelA. Nat Immunol 5:104–112, 2004.
6. Rhee KJ, Sethupathi P, Driks A, et al: Role of commensal bacteria in development of gut-associated lymphoid tissues and preimmune antibody repertoire. J Immunol 172:1118–1124, 2004.
7. Medzhitov R, Janeway CA, Jr: Innate immunity: The virtues of a nonclonal system of recognition. Cell 91:295–298, 1997.
8. Yang D, Biragyn A, Hoover DM, et al: Multiple roles of antimicrobial defensins, cathelicidins, and eosinophil-derived neurotoxin in host defense. Annu Rev Immunol 22:181–215, 2004.
9. Hickling TP, Clark H, Malhotra R, et al: Collectins and their role in lung immunity. J Leukoc Biol 75:27–33, 2004.
10. Nguyen KB, Salazar-Mather TP, Dalod MY, et al: Coordinated and distinct roles for IFN-alpha beta, IL-12, and IL-15 regulation of NK cell responses to viral infection. J Immunol 169:4279–4287, 2002.
11. Holmskov U, Thiel S, Jensenius JC: Collections and ficolins: Humoral lectins of the innate immune defense. Annu Rev Immunol 21:547–578, 2003.
12. Nicholson-Weller A, Halperin JA: Membrane signaling by complement C5b-9, the membrane attack complex. Immunol Res 12:244–257, 1993.
13. Figueroa J, Andreoni J, Densen P: Complement deficiency states and meningococcal disease. Immunol Res 12:295–311, 1993.
14. Manderson AP, Pickering MC, Botto M, et al: Continual low-level activation of the classical complement pathway. J Exp Med 194:747–756, 2001.
15. Pangburn MK, Muller-Eberhard HJ: Relation of putative thioester bond in C3 to activation of the alternative pathway and the binding of C3b to biological targets of complement. J Exp Med 152:1102–1114, 1980.
16. Morgan BP, Harris CL: Regulation in the Activation Pathways. San Diego, Academic Press, 1999, Chapter 3.
17. Meri S, Pangburn MK: Discrimination between activators and nonactivators of the alternative pathway of complement: Regulation via a sialic acid/polyanion binding site on factor H. Proc Natl Acad Sci USA 87:3982–3986, 1990.
18. Klickstein LB, Bartow TJ, Miletic B, et al: Identification of distinct C3b and C4b recognition sites in the human C3b/C4b receptor (CR1, CD35) by deletion mutagenesis. J Exp Med 168:1699–1717, 1988.
19. Krych M, Hourcade D, Atkinson JP: Sites within the complement C3b/C4b receptor important for the specificity of ligand binding. Proc Natl Acad Sci USA 88:4353–4357, 1991.
20. Klickstein LB, Barbashov S, Liu T, et al: Complement receptor type 1 (CR1, CD35) is a receptor for C1q. Immunity 7:345–355, 1997.
21. Ghiran I, Barbashov SF, Klickstein LB, et al: Complement receptor 1/CD35 is a receptor for mannan-binding lectin. J Exp Med 192:1797–1808, 2000.
22. Klickstein LB, Moulds JM: CR1. In Morley BJ, Walport MJ (eds): The Complement Facts Book. New York, Academic Press, 2000, pp 136–145.

23. Rot A, von Andrian UH: Chemokines in innate and adaptive host defense: Basic chemokinese grammar for immune cells. Annu Rev Immunol 22:891–928, 2004.
24. Ezekowitz RA, Sastry K, Bailly P, et al: Molecular characterization of the human macrophage mannose receptor: Demonstration of multiple carbohydrate recognition-like domains and phagocytosis of yeasts in Cos-1 cells. J Exp Med 172:1785–94, 1990.
25. Taylor ME, Conary JT, Lennartz MR, et al: Primary structure of the mannose receptor contains multiple motifs resembling carbohydrate-recognition domains. J Biol Chem 265:12156–12162, 1990.
26. Willment JA, Gordon S, Brown GD: Characterization of the human beta-glucan receptor and its alternatively spliced isoforms. J Biol Chem 276:43818–43823, 2001.
27. Thornton BP, Vetvicka V, Pitman M, et al: Analysis of the sugar specificity and molecular location of the beta-glucan-binding lectin site of complement receptor type 3 (CD11b/CD18). J Immunol 156:1235–1246, 1996.
28. McGettrick AF, O'Neill LA: The expanding family of MyD88-like adaptors in Toll-like receptor signal transduction. Mol Immunol 41:577–582, 2004.
29. McQueen KL, Parham P: Variable receptors controlling activation and inhibition of NK cells. Curr Opin Immunol 14:615–621, 2002.
30. Medzhitov R, Janeway CA, Jr: Decoding the patterns of self and nonself by the innate immune system. Science 296:298–300, 2002.
31. Dempsey PW, Allison ME, Akkaraju S, et al: C3d of complement as a molecular adjuvant: Bridging innate and acquired immunity. Science 271:348–350, 1996.
32. Lowe JB: Glycan-dependent leukocyte adhesion and recruitment in inflammation. Curr Opin Cell Biol 15:531–538, 2003.
33. Kim M, Carman CV, Springer TA: Bidirectional transmembrane signaling by cytoplasmic domain separation in integrins. Science 301:1720–1725, 2003.
34. Laudanna C, Kim JY, Constantin G, et al: Rapid leukocyte integrin activation by chemokines. Immunol Rev 186:37–46, 2002.
35. Benacerraf B: A hypothesis to relate the specificity of T lymphocytes and the activity of I region-specific Ir genes in macrophages and B lymphocytes. J Immunol 120:1809–1812, 1978.
36. Madden D: The three-dimensional structure of peptide-MHC complexes. Annu Rev Immunol 13:587–622, 1995.
37. Yang Y: Generation of major histocompatibility complex class I antigens. Microbes Infect 5:39–47, 2003.
38. Paulsson KM, Wang P: Quality control of MHC class I maturation. FASEB J 18:31–38, 2004.
39. Bryant PW, Lennon-Dumenil AM, Fiebiger E, et al: Proteolysis and antigen presentation by MHC class II molecules. Adv Immunol 80:71–114, 2002.
40. Moody DB, Porcelli SA: Intracellular pathways of CD1 antigen presentation. Nat Rev Immunol 3:11–22, 2003.
41. Sigal LJ, Crotty S, Andino R, et al: Cytotoxic T-cell immunity to virus-infected non-haematopoietic cells requires presentation of exogenous antigen. Nature 398:77–80, 1999.
42. Castellino F, Boucher PE, Eichelberg K, et al: Receptor-mediated uptake of antigen/heat shock protein complexes results in major histocompatibility complex class I antigen presentation via two distinct processing pathways. J Exp Med 191:1957–1964, 2000.
43. Li Z, Menoret A, Srivastava P: Roles of heat-shock proteins in antigen presentation and cross-presentation. Curr Opin Immunol 14:45–51, 2002.
44. Winau F, Kaufmann SH, Schaible UE: Apoptosis paves the detour path for CD8 T cell activation against intracellular bacteria. Cell Microbiol 6:599–607, 2004.
45. Sharpe AH, Freeman GJ: The B7-CD28 superfamily. Nat Rev Immunol 2:116–126, 2002.
46. Fearon DT, Locksley RM: The instructive role of innate immunity in the acquired immune response. Science 272:50–53, 1996.
47. Sims TN, Dustin ML: The immunological synapse: Integrins take the stage. Immunol Rev 186:100–117, 2002.
48. Appleman LJ, Boussiotis VA: T cell anergy and costimulation. Immunol Rev 192:161–180, 2003.
49. Reiner SL, Locksley RM: The regulation of immunity to *Leishmania major*. Annu Rev Immunol 13:151–177, 1995.
50. Sher A, Coffman RL: Regulation of immunity to parasites by T cells and T cell-derived cytokines. Annu Rev Immunol 10:385–409, 1992.
51. Mazzoni A, Segal DM: Controlling the Toll road to dendritic cell polarization. J Leukoc Biol 75:721–730, 2004.
52. Mackaness GB: The influence of immunologically committed lymphoid cells on macrophage activity in vivo. J Exp Med 129:973–992, 1969.
53. Ma J, Chen T, Mandelin J, et al: Regulation of macrophage activation. Cell Mol Life Sci (60):2334–2346, 2003.
54. Cohn L, Elias JA, Chupp GL: Asthma: Mechanisms of disease persistence and progression. Annu Rev Immunol 22:789–815, 2004.
55. Sakaguchi S: Naturally arising CD4+ regulatory T cells for immunologic self-tolerance and negative control of immune responses. Annu Rev Immunol 22:531–562, 2004.
56. Walport MJ: Complement. Second of two parts. N Engl J Med 344:1140–1144, 2001.
57. Bowness P, Davies KA, Norsworthy PJ, et al: Hereditary C1q deficiency and systemic lupus erythematosus. QJM 87:455–464, 1994.
58. Manderson AP, Botto M, Walport MJ: The role of complement in the development of systemic lupus erythematosus. Annu Rev Immunol 22:431–456, 2004.
59. Henter JI, Elinder G, Ost A: Diagnostic guidelines for hemophagocytic lymphohistiocytosis. The FHL Study Group of the Histiocyte Society. Semin Oncol 18:29–33, 1991.
60. Fischer A, Cavazzana-Calvo M, De Saint Basile G, et al: Naturally occurring primary deficiencies of the immune system. Annu Rev Immunol 15:93–124, 1997.
61. Rosenzweig SD, Holland SM: Phagocyte immunodeficiencies and their infections. J Allergy Clin Immunol 113:620–626, 2004.
62. Belyakov IM, Hammond SA, Ahlers JD, et al: Transcutaneous immunization induces mucosal CTLs and protective immunity by migration of primed skin dendritic cells. J Clin Invest 113:998–1007, 2004.
63. Levine MM, Sztein, MB: Vaccine development strategies for improving immunization: the role of modern immunology. Nat Immunol 5:460–464, 2004.
64. Coeshott CM, Smithson SL, Verderber E, et al: Pluronic® F127-based systemic vaccine delivery systems. Vaccine 22:2396–2405, 2004.
65. Klinman DM, Currie D, Gursel I, et al: Use of CpG oligodeoxynucleotides as immune adjuvants. Immunol Rev 199:201–216, 2004.
66. Sesardic D, Dobbelaer R: European union regulatory developments for new vaccine adjuvants and delivery systems. Vaccine 22:2452–2456, 2004.

12

Tropical Infectious Diseases and Malignancy

CATHERINE DE MARTEL
JULIE PARSONNET

INTRODUCTION

Cancer is commonly considered a disease of the industrialized world. Many maintain that the modern lifestyle—with its cigarettes, poor diet, and exposure to environmental pollutants—is the pre-eminent cause of cancer, and that malignancy is a price paid for development. Epidemiologic data largely support this viewpoint. Annual age-standardized cancer mortality rates per 100,000 population regularly range above 100 for females and 150 for males in industrialized nations, extending as high as 400 for certain urban minority populations in the United States. Cancer incidence and mortality rates are typically far lower in developing countries.[1,2] For example, Sri Lanka reports mortality rates of 65.3 for males and 62.9 for females.[3] Without question, the proportion of all deaths due to cancer in industrialized nations far exceeds that in the developing tropical nations.

It is incorrect, however, to conclude that cancer is not an important concern in developing countries. One must keep in mind that cancer remains a disease of the elderly. In poorer tropical countries, where acute infectious diseases, maternal and infant mortality, and trauma afflict all to many children and young adults, crude cancer rates—unadjusted for the age structure of the population—appear disproportionately low. Among the elderly of developing countries, however, as in industrialized nations, cancer is a leading cause of death. In fact, developing countries already bear the brunt of the world's cancer. Of the estimated 10.06 million new cases of cancer worldwide in 2000, 5.38 million (53.46%) occurred in the developing world, and this is almost certainly an underestimate.[3,4] In most developing countries, cancer registries are incomplete or nonexistent.[5] Moreover, cancer diagnosis, when registered, is often based on incomplete information, as diagnostic capabilities are limited and postmortem examinations are rare. Thus, the number, types, and distribution of cancer cases are not known with any reasonable degree of certainty.[4]

Despite these limitations, certain trends are apparent. The demographic and epidemiologic transitions that accompany economic development have led to a gradually increasing median age and a growing proportion of older persons throughout the world. At present, approximately 8% of the population of developing countries is over age 60; this figure is expected to rise to 20% by 2050.[6] This trend, together with growing tobacco use, urbanization, industrialization, and disposable income, foretell a rapid increase in chronic disease, including cancers, in all but the very poorest countries.[7] Indeed, cancer is already a major public health challenge in some developing areas. Reported age-standardized mortality rates for both sexes and all sites are considerably higher today in tropical South America than they are in North America.[3] Nevertheless, it should not be assumed that populations of developing countries are homogeneous. Bassett and colleagues[8,9] have pointed out the extreme differences in cancer patterns of European and African residents of Harare, Zimbabwe. In a study of bladder cancers in Durban, South Africa, 95% of the tumors in whites and 30% in Africans were transitional cell carcinoma, while 53% of the African patients, but only 2% of the whites, had squamous cell carcinoma. Ova of *Schistosoma haematobium* were seen in microscopic sections of the bladder tumors in 85% of the patients with squamous cell carcinoma, but in only 10% of the patients with transitional cell carcinoma.[10] Such studies can be extremely useful in unraveling the etiology and epidemiology of cancer among populations by pinpointing differences in risk factors.

As an increasing proportion of the world's cancer burden falls on the developing countries, the demand will grow for costly and sophisticated resources for diagnosis and treatment of malignancies. All developing countries combined, with 84% of the world's population, account for only 11% of global health spending.[11] Therefore the inevitable increase in cancer incidence in tropical countries in future decades will provide a powerful economic incentive to focus on prevention to any extent possible. The questions are: what should we prevent and how do we prevent it?

INFECTION AS A PREVENTABLE CAUSE OF CANCER

Acute infectious diseases are universally recognized as the major cause of premature mortality in developing countries, particularly among infants and children. Ironically, it is now evident that, among adults, many cancers are also caused by infectious diseases. Such an idea is not new. Early in the last century, Johannes Andreas Grib Fibiger received the Nobel Prize for reporting (incorrectly, as it turned out) that a nematode could cause malignant tumors in the stomachs of rats. Before they were discredited, Fibiger's ideas inspired others to explore similar avenues of research.[12] Thus began a field of research in infection-related malignancy. In this regard, Fibiger's work remains important to this day. He initiated a field of research but also illustrated its pitfalls. Determining true causal associations can be difficult. Moreover, even distinguishing true cancers from infection-induced proliferative lesions can be challenging.

That infection might lead to malignancy is often greeted with surprise and skepticism by individuals in developed countries, and belies ignorance about cancers that afflict developing countries. A popular book about cancer published in 1995 claimed that, "Viral infection appears to play a role in only a tiny minority of cancer.... Granting even that viruses may play a heretofore undiscovered role in other cancer, it is probably fair to say that undue attention has been given to this particular collection of agents. The same could be said for infectious agents more generally."[13] Until recently, infectious agents that cause cancer were termed "rare and inconsequential." This view, though widely held 10 years ago, is now known to be erroneous. Worldwide, infection remains among the most important causes of cancer. The International Agency of Research on Cancer (IARC) estimates conservatively that 15.6% of all malignancies, and 21% in developing countries, are attributable to infectious agents.[14] In some countries, the proportion is substantially higher. For example, in The Gambia in the late 1990s, 62.5% of malignancies in men affected either the liver (of which 84% were considered attributable to hepatitis B or C) or stomach (at least 55% estimated to result from *Helicobacter pylori* infection). In Gambian women, 57% of cancers affect the liver, stomach, or uterine cervix (95% attributable to human papillomavirus, HPV).[5,15] In terms of overall mortality age-adjusted numbers, cancers of the stomach for men and cervix uteri for women both rank second worldwide, while liver cancer ranks third and sixth for men and women, respectively.[3] Thus, while cancer may be widely perceived as a consequence of industrial and environmental pollutants, in actuality, infection with certain cosmopolitan pathogens is second only to smoking as a cause of death from malignancy (Fig. 12-1). In addition, certain agents such as *Opisthorchis viverrini* and human T-cell leukemia virus type 1 (HTLV-1) are significant causes of certain cancers in restricted geographic areas. While the number of cases is not extensive, these viruses are of interest in elucidating mechanisms of oncogenesis.

The impact of pathogen-induced malignancy is particularly pronounced in countries in the transition from third world to first world economies. Adults in these populations who were infected with carcinogenic microbes such as hepatitis B virus (HBV) or *H. pylori* in childhood are experiencing a rapid increase in life expectancy. Since each year of chronic

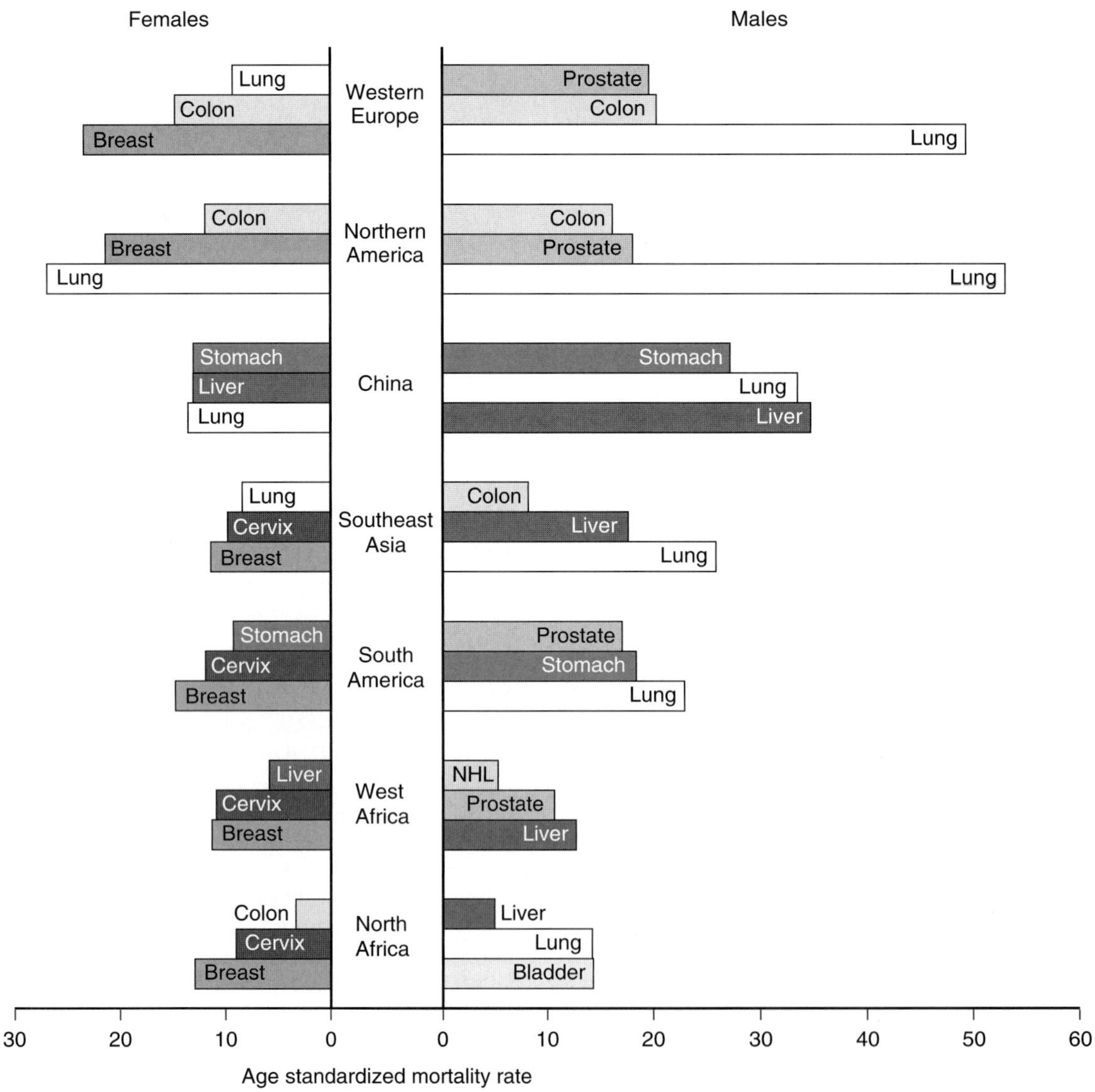

FIGURE 12-1 Estimates of the three leading causes of cancer death, by region. (Adapted from Ferlay J, Bray F, Pisani P, et al: GLOBOCAN 2000: Cancer Incidence, Mortality and Prevalence Worldwide, Version 1.0. IARC CancerBase No. 5. Lyon, IARC Press, 2001. Limited version available from: www-dep.iarc.fr/globocan/globocan.htm. Last updated on 03/02/2001.)

infection adds to the cumulative cancer risk, the number of cancer cases related to infection in early life would be expected to parallel the overall increase in longevity.

Yet, in many respects, the predominance of infection-related cancer can be looked upon as good news. Infectious diseases are often preventable or treatable; therefore, knowledge of specific infectious causes and the epidemiology of the pathogens involved provide a blueprint for control of those particular malignancies. The feasibility of control is demonstrated by the dramatic decline in infection-related malignancy in industrialized nations. Gastric and cervical cancers, for example, were among the leading causes of cancer death in the United States as recently as 1945, but are now far less prominent. The decline of cancer at these sites occurred without the benefit of vaccines or specific interventions. Rather, general improvements in socioeconomic status, sanitation, and hygiene appear to be responsible for the substantial reductions in infection-related malignancy, as they have for many other kinds of infectious diseases in industrialized nations.

While chronic infections are significant causes of cancer in developing countries, they are not the only important class of carcinogenic exposure. In developing countries, as throughout the world, the primacy of cigarette smoking cannot be overstressed. Lung cancer alone accounts for 12.8% of all new malignancies diagnosed worldwide.[3] Where cigarettes remain too expensive for the average person, they currently play a small role in causing malignancy. In many countries, as socioeconomic conditions improve, the prevalence of cigarette smoking rises accordingly, auguring poorly for the future. Also important is the relative absence of fresh fruits and vegetables from the diets of poorer countries. Exposure to dietary carcinogens such as mycotoxins and nitrates also magnify the cancer risk. Thus, although cancers related to infection may be quite common in developing countries, attention must be paid to other factors that can also be addressed by public health interventions.

INFECTIONS THAT CAUSE CANCER

Many infectious agents have been posited to cause cancer. The IARC biannually reviews epidemiologic and basic science information on putative cancer-causing agents. It then classifies these agents as definite, probable, possible, or unlikely causes of cancer. To date, they have carried out extensive evaluations of liver flukes, schistosomes, *H. pylori,* hepatitis viruses, human herpesvirus 8 (HHV-8), HPV, HTLV, human immunodeficiency virus (HIV), and Epstein-Barr virus (EBV; Table 12-1).

Table 12-1 *Infectious Agents Purported to Cause Malignancy*

Organism	Tumor	IARC Classification*	Attributable Fraction†
Viruses			
Hepatitis B	Hepatocellular carcinoma	Group 1	60%
Hepatitis C	Hepatocellular carcinoma and MALT lymphoma	Group 1	24%
Papillomaviruses 16 and 18	Cervical, anogenital cancers	Group 1	90%–98% for all viruses
Papillomaviruses 31 and 33	Cervical, anogenital cancers	Group 2A	
Papillomaviruses 2 and other papillomaviruses	Cervical, anogenital cancers	Group 2B	
HTLV-1	Adult T-cell leukemia	Group 1	1%
Epstein-Barr virus	Burkitt's lymphoma	Group 1	81%
	Non-Hodgkin's lymphoma	Group 1	
	Hodgkin's disease	Group 1	49%
	Nasopharyngeal carcinoma	Group 1	
	Gastric adenocarcinoma	NS	
HHV-8	Kaposi's sarcoma	Group 2A	
HIV-1	ID related cancers	Group 1	
HIV-2	ID related cancers	Group 2A	
Bacteria			
Helicobacter pylori	Gastric adenocarcinoma	Group 1	55%
	Gastric lymphoma		75%
Campylobacter jejuni	Immunoproliferative small intestinal disease (IPSID)	NS	
Mycobacterium ulcerans	Squamous cell carcinoma (skin)	NS	
Salmonella typhi	Cholangiocarcinoma	NS	
Chronic or recurrent UTIs	Bladder cancer	NS	
Chronic osteomyelitis or wound infections	Squamous cell carcinoma	NS	
Parasites			
Opisthorchis viverrini	Cholangiocarcinoma	Group 1	
Clonorchis sinensis	Cholangiocarcinoma	Group 2A	
Schistosoma haematobium	Bladder cancer	Group 1	4%
Schistosoma japonicum	Hepatocellular and rectal cancers	Group 2B	

*From "Overall Evaluations of Carcinogenicity to Humans" as evaluated in IARC Monographs Volumes 1–82. Web site: 193.51.164.11/monoeval/crthall.html. Last updated January 9, 2004, consulted April 7, 2004.
†From references 14 and 15.

Other infectious agents that have not yet been evaluated by the IARC, but are suspected of causing cancer, are also listed in Table 12-1. Because the great majority of these pathogens are reviewed elsewhere in this book, we will not discuss their life cycles, epidemiology, or clinical manifestations. Instead, we focus here on the general features and control of the principal infection-induced malignancies.

A simplified scheme of infection-related oncogenesis can be used to categorize the malignancies into one of two types: either tumors caused by the integration of oncogenic DNA into the host cell or those induced by chronic inflammation. Basically, all types of oncogenic agents enhance cell growth. The mechanisms by which this occurs can be quite variable, however, ranging from expression of viral oncogenes for cell growth factors to stimulation of growth by inflammatory intermediaries. Agents with oncogenes, however, directly immortalize cells, while inflammatory carcinogenic agents do not. Moreover, it is thought that immunosuppression may be important for development of malignancies related to oncogene integration. This is not thought to be the case for inflammation-related malignancy; in fact, immunosuppression, by lessening the inflammatory response, could potentially protect against inflammation-related cancers. This was highlighted in a recent review by Smukler and Ratner who state "the observed lack of a significant increase in the incidence of hepatocellular carcinoma [in HIV infected patients] may be caused, in part, by a possible reduction in HBV-induced hepatic damage in HIV coinfected people. Immune impairment in HIV-positive patients leads to higher HBV replication levels with less severe liver damage because of a blunted HBV-specific immune response and less consequent cirrhosis."[16] A disproportionate lack of necrotizing inflammation in HIV-HBV coinfected subjects supports this possibility.[17] Finally, cancers related to inflammation appear to occur only after a long incubation period. There is no such temporal relationship between oncogenic viruses and cancer. This latter point is most readily demonstrated by the short incubation period between EBV infection and the development of Burkitt's lymphoma in young children in sub-Saharan Africa.

The importance of inflammation in inducing cancer was first exemplified by two diseases not uncommon to the tropics: chronic, draining osteomyelitis and Buruli ulcers (caused by *Mycobacterium ulcerans*). These chronic, inflammatory conditions, if left untreated, cause aggressive squamous-cell carcinomas.[18] In each instance, carcinogenesis appears to depend not on specific oncogenic genes or gene products produced by the infectious agent, but rather on the organism's ability to persist despite the host's efforts to combat its presence. Inflammation is thought to induce cancer by stimulating production of reactive oxygen and nitrogen species that damage DNA, proteins, and membranes. Inflammation may also increase the proliferative rate of infected tissues, promoting development of tumors. Proliferation is a promutagenic effect, permitting more cells to be susceptible to DNA damage and mutation. It also fosters selective growth of mutant clones.[19–23] We now recognize that many infections, including *H. pylori*, *S. haematobium*, *O. viverrini*, and HBV, are at least in part linked to cancer by their ability to foster an inflammatory response. In support of this, phenotypes of *H. pylori* that cause more inflammation are more closely related to malignancy.[24] Treatment of *S. haematobium* and *O. viverrini* leads to marked decreases in inflammatory cells within the bladder and liver, respectively, and associated declines in chromosomal damage.

As stated previously, the risk of developing inflammation-related cancer also appears to be intimately tied to the duration of the inflammatory process. This has been particularly well established for HBV infection but appears also to be the case for *H. pylori* and probably other agents as well.[25,26] The chronicity of infection implies that the carcinogenic effects of infection are likely to be promotional rather than resulting from a single initiating event.

Oncogenic viruses—such as EBV, HTLV-1, HHV-8, and human papillomaviruses—may lead more directly to cancer by integration of viral oncogenes or oncogene promoters into nuclear DNA. Resultant viral oncoproteins may for instance interact with and inactivate host tumor suppressor proteins such as p53, uncoupling normal growth control processes and leading to cellular transformation.[27,28] Oncogenic viruses may also induce production of cell growth factors, stimulating the host cell's reproduction, and accordingly their own. Other viruses, such as HIV, are not direct carcinogens but, by limiting the host's immune response, foster carcinogenic effects of normally more innocuous agents. For example, HIV-related cellular immunodeficiency fosters carcinogenesis by chronic colonizers such as EBV and permits infection with HHV-8, an unusual agent in immunocompetent hosts, with resultant Kaposi's sarcoma (KS). KS in persons with HIV infection occurs at a rate thousands of times higher than in the non-HIV population.[29] In HIV-infected patients, lymphomas also occur at much higher rates than in the general population. Although the specific cause remains to be determined, much evidence points to the activity of lymphotropic viruses, particularly EBV. Whereas both EBV and HTLV-1 have long been implicated in the development of lymphoid malignancies, additional viral and bacterial agents are now thought to have lymphoproliferative activity. These include HHV-8, hepatitis C virus (HCV), *H. pylori*, *Borrelia burgdorferi*, and possibly *Campylobacter jejuni*.[30–33]

The etiology of infection-induced cancer is made more complex by multifactorial causality of certain tumors on the one hand, and multiple outcomes following certain infections on the other. The importance of a specific agent in causing malignancy (its "attributable risk") depends on its prevalence. For example, in high-incidence areas of hepatitis, primary hepatocellular carcinoma (HCC) is commonly associated with chronic infection with HBV or HCV. Shin and associates[34] found strong evidence that HBV and HCV were independent risk factors for HCC in Korea, where liver cancer mortality is reported to be the highest in the world. In areas where hepatitis viruses are less prevalent, they will be a less common factor in HCC. In Sweden, for example, Kaczynski and coworkers tested 113 HCC patients for serologic or immunocytochemical evidence of such infection. They found no signs of chronic HBV infection, and HCV reactivity occurred in only 7 of 64 patients.[35] Thus, chronic viral hepatitis appeared to play a minor role in induction of HCC in Sweden, where alcohol-related cirrhosis is a much more common risk factor.

Certain infections may be important, but not sufficient, for the induction of cancer. Just as most smokers do not get lung cancer, most infections with potentially carcinogenic pathogens do not proceed to a malignancy. For example, the large and diverse group of HPVs is implicated in causation of a variety of proliferative conditions, some of which (warts, epithelial cysts, intraepithelial neoplasias, anogenital, orolaryngeal and oropharyngeal papillomas, keratoacanthomas, and other types of hyperkeratoses) are relatively benign. At least 90% of cancers of the cervix and more than 50% of other anogenital cancers are attributed to certain high-risk HPV types that may act as solitary carcinogens or in concert with cofactors. The progression of HPV-associated squamous epithelial lesions to cervical cancer may be enhanced by certain concurrent sexually transmitted agents, such as herpes simplex virus or chlamydia, and is clearly associated with HIV-induced immunosuppression.[15] Aflatoxin B1 is widely considered to be a cocarcinogen with HBV; although either is capable of inducing HCC, the combination appears to behave synergistically in regions where both agents are endemic.[36] Although 90% of the world's population is thought to be infected with EBV, the two tumors classically linked to EBV occur in limited geographic areas. Burkitt's lymphoma is found in hyperendemic malarial areas of Africa and New Guinea, and nasopharyngeal carcinoma in parts of Asia, suggesting the presence of specific, geographically limited, cofactors.[37,38]

PREVENTION OF INFECTION-RELATED MALIGNANCIES

Each carcinogenic pathogen has unique features that may facilitate or frustrate efforts to control or prevent the associated cancers. Prevention at the primary level—that is, by blocking an initial infection—may be accomplished in the case of hepatitis B by immunization of infants with a recombinant DNA or plasma-derived vaccine. Such vaccine has already proved effective in protecting inoculated children against chronic carriage and hepatocellular carcinoma.[38,40] In Taiwan, an intensive vaccination program in newborns began in 1984. The incidence of hepatocellular carcinoma in children 6 to 9 years of age declined from 0.52 per 100,000 children for those born before the program to 0.13 for those born after, a reduction by a factor of four. Since 1991, HBV vaccine is recommended as part of the WHO's Expanded Programme on Immunizations (EPI). It is currently given as part of routine childhood immunizations in 141 countries with a global coverage rising from 15% in 1996 to around 45% in 2002. Unfortunately, it is the only vaccine currently available that is specifically targeted at an infection-induced malignancy in humans. Promising evaluation of a vaccine against HPV types 16 and 18, responsible for up to 70% of cervical cancers worldwide, has recently been reported, suggesting a need to consider vaccine delivery strategy targeting young women before the onset of sexual activity.[41–43] Other efforts are underway to develop vaccines against viral, bacterial, and parasitic agents, including EBV, HTLV-1, *H. pylori*, and *Schistosoma* species. Unfortunately, vaccine development often constitutes high-risk research for pharmaceutical companies. In helminthology in particular, the diminishing focus of research on vaccine development, the diminution of grant funding, the difficulty to publish papers in prestigious journals, and the ensuing decline in the number of trainees in helminthes laboratories render the prospect of successful vaccines still far away.[44,45]

In the absence of vaccines, primary prevention depends largely on global public health measures and education. Prevention programs for schistosomiasis include education of the public in proper disposal of excreta to avoid contact with contaminated water. Infection with the oriental liver flukes *Opisthorchis* and *Clonorchis* can be prevented by refraining from eating raw or partially fermented freshwater fish. Educational campaigns in endemic areas of northeastern Thailand and elsewhere have had only limited success in dislodging long-ingrained traditional dietary practices. *H. pylori* infection appears to diminish in conjunction with improved household sanitation and hygiene. For HPV and HIV infection, "safe sex" practices may limit transmission (although this has been poorly studied for HPV), while for HCV, global testing of blood supplies and drug rehabilitation programs can control its spread. Only for EBV infection is primary prevention of infection unlikely to be attained by public health measures.

Secondary prevention, intended to impede the development of an existing infection to an advanced stage, is the rationale behind the Papanicolaou smear for signs of premalignant changes that may lead to cervical cancer. This cancer prevention strategy has proved an extraordinarily cost-effective method of health promotion. Where the Papanicolaou smear is widely employed, cervical cancer rates have plummeted. Some authors have also suggested that therapeutic vaccines may have a role to play in regression of cervical lesions related to HPV in humans.[28] Other secondary prevention strategies include case finding and chemotherapy of trematode and *H. pylori* infections. To date, however, very few prevention programs have been studied in terms of long-term efficacy or cost-effectiveness. Fendrick and colleagues evaluated how effective *Helicobacter pylori* treatment would need to be for it to be a cost-effective strategy for gastric cancer prevention (Fig. 12-2). In the United States, $50,000 is considered a reasonable amount to pay for 1 year of life. Despite the low incidence of gastric cancer in the United States, screening 40-year-olds for *H. pylori* and treating all infected persons would only need to be 20% effective for it to be cost-effective. The screening and treatment strategy would be even more cost-effective in high-risk populations such as Japanese Americans.[46] Despite these promising numbers, results of the first randomized trial of *H. pylori* eradication to prevent gastric cancer have been discouraging, showing little difference between treatment and placebo groups.[47] However, methodological issues in this study left open to question whether *H. pylori* eradication may yet be a cost-effective strategy to prevent stomach cancer.

As mentioned previously, the epidemiology of carcinogenic pathogens is closely related to the social and economic characteristics of the human population that harbors them, and disease prevalence may change without biomedical intervention. Improvements in the storage, transportation, and processing of foods, and particularly the dissemination of refrigeration, appear to be responsible for the dramatic decline in gastric cancer in industrialized countries in recent decades. Knowledge of the transmission and ecology of *H. pylori* had nothing to do with this decrease. However,

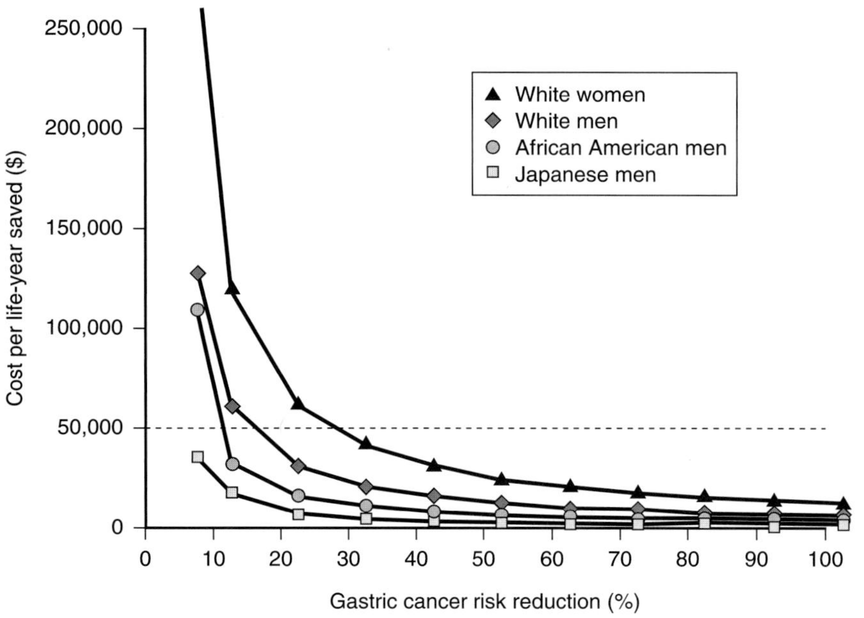

FIGURE 12-2 Example of sensitivity analysis. Risk reduction of cancer attributable to *H. pylori* eradication in a simulated cohort of men and women 40-years old serologically screened for *H. pylori* and treated when positive (no follow-up testing). Studies such as this one are the basis for ongoing secondary prevention studies to see if treatment of infection can prevent malignancy. (Adapted from Fendrick AM, Chernew ME, Hirth RA, et al: Clinical and economic effects of population-based *Helicobacter pylori* screening to prevent gastric cancer. Arch Intern Med 159[2]:142–148, 1999.)

known risk factors cannot always be easily altered. For example, early age at first intercourse and number of sexual partners are strongly associated with risk of cervical cancer, but are related to broad secular sociocultural trends. As technologies become more widespread, human behavior and activities evolve, and other emerging pathogens such as HIV appear, we can anticipate further changes in the epidemiology of infection-induced cancers.

REFERENCES

1. Pisani P, Parkin DM, Bray F, et al: Estimates of the worldwide mortality from 25 cancers in 1990. Int J Cancer 83(1):18–29, 1999.
2. Parkin DM, Pisani P, Ferlay J: Estimates of the worldwide incidence of 25 major cancers in 1990. Int J Cancer 80(6):827–841, 1999.
3. Ferlay J, Bray F, Pisani P, et al: GLOBOCAN 2000: Cancer Incidence, Mortality and Prevalence Worldwide, Version 1.0. IARC CancerBase No. 5. Lyon, France, IARC Press, 2001. Limited version available from: www.dep-iarc.fr/globocan/globocan.htm. Last updated on 03/02/2001.
4. Parkin DM, Bray F, Ferlay J, et al: Estimating the world cancer burden: Globocan 2000. Int J Cancer 94(2):153–156, 2001.
5. Bah E, Parkin DM, Hall AJ, et al: Cancer in The Gambia: 1988–97. Br J Cancer 84(9):1207–1214, 2001.
6. World Population Prospects: The 2002 Revision Highlights. New York, Population Division of the Department of Economic and Social Affairs of the United Nations Secretariat, United Nations, 2003, pp 47–50.
7. Jones SB. Cancer in the developing world: A call to action. BMJ 319(7208):505–508, 1999.
8. Bassett MT, Chokunonga E, Mauchaza B, et al: Cancer in the African population of Harare, Zimbabwe, 1990–1992. Int J Cancer 63(1):29–36, 1995.
9. Bassett MT, Levy L, Chokunonga E, et al: Cancer in the European population of Harare, Zimbabwe, 1990–1992. Int J Cancer 63(1):24–28, 1995.
10. Groeneveld AE, Marszalek WW, Heyns CF: Bladder cancer in various population groups in the greater Durban area of KwaZulu-Natal, South Africa. Br J Urol 78(2):205–208, 1996.
11. Schieber G, Maeda A: Health care financing and delivery in developing countries. Health Aff (Millwood) 18(3):193–205, 1999.
12. Weisse AB: Barry Marshall and the resurrection of Johannes Fibiger. Hosp Pract (Off Ed) 31(9):105–112, 116, 1996.
13. Proctor R: Cancer Wars. New York, Basic Books, 1995.
14. Pisani P, Parkin DM, Munoz N, et al: Cancer and infection: Estimates of the attributable fraction in 1990. Cancer Epidemiol Biomarkers Prev 6(6):387–400, 1997.
15. Bosch FX, de Sanjose S: Chapter 1: Human papillomavirus and cervical cancer—Burden and assessment of causality. J Natl Cancer Inst Monogr (31):3–13, 2003.
16. Smukler AJ, Ratner L: Hepatitis viruses and hepatocellular carcinoma in HIV-infected patients. Curr Opin Oncol 14(5):538–542, 2002.
17. Colin JF, Cazals-Hatem D, Loriot MA, et al: Influence of human immunodeficiency virus infection on chronic hepatitis B in homosexual men. Hepatology 29(4):1306–1310, 1999.
18. Evans MR, Etuaful SN, Amofah G, et al: Squamous cell carcinoma secondary to Buruli ulcer. Trans R Soc Trop Med Hyg 93(1):63–64, 1999.
19. Rosin MP, Saad el Din Zaki S, Ward AJ, et al: Involvement of inflammatory reactions and elevated cell proliferation in the development of bladder cancer in schistosomiasis patients. Mutat Res 305(2):283–292, 1994.
20. Lynch D, Mapstone N, Clarke A: Cell proliferation in *Helicobacter pylori* associated gastritis and the effect of eradication therapy. Gut 36(3):346–350, 1995.
21. Tarao K, Ohkawa S, Shimizu A, et al: Significance of hepatocellular proliferation in the development of hepatocellular carcinoma from anti-hepatitis C virus-positive cirrhotic patients. Cancer 73(4):1149–1154, 1994.
22. Noffsinger AE, Hui YZ, Suzuk L, et al: The relationship of human papillomavirus to proliferation and ploidy in carcinoma of the anus. Cancer 75(4):958–967, 1995.
23. Mann DL, Martin P, Hamlin-Green G, et al: Virus production and spontaneous cell proliferation in HTLV-I-infected lymphocytes. Clin Immunol Immunopathol 72(3):312–320, 1994.
24. Huang J, Zheng G, Sumanac K, et al: Meta-analysis of the relationship between cagA seropositivity and gastric cancer. Gastroenterology 125(6):1636–1644, 2003.
25. Payne RJ, Nowak MA, Blumberg BS: Analysis of a cellular model to account for the natural history of infection by the hepatitis B virus and

its role in the development of primary hepatocellular carcinoma. J Theor Biol 159(2):215–240, 1992.
26. Blaser MJ, Chyou PH, Nomura A: Age at establishment of *Helicobacter pylori* infection and gastric carcinoma, gastric ulcer, and duodenal ulcer risk. Cancer Res 55(3):562–565, 1995.
27. Werness BA, Levine AJ, Howley PM: Association of human papillomavirus types 16 and 18 E6 proteins with p53. Science 248(4951):76–79, 1990.
28. Mauser A, Saito S, Appella E, et al: The Epstein-Barr virus immediate-early protein BZLF1 regulates p53 function through multiple mechanisms. J Virol 76(24):12503–12512, 2002.
29. Emmanoulides C, Miles SA, Mitsuyasu RT: Pathogenesis of AIDS-related Kaposi's sarcoma. Oncology (Huntingt) 10(3):335–341; discussion: 342–350, 1996.
30. Cathomas G: Human herpes virus 8: A new virus discloses its face. Virchows Arch 436(3):195–206, 2000.
31. Luppi M, Barozzi P, Maiorana A, et al: Human herpesvirus-8 DNA sequences in human immunodeficiency virus-negative angioimmunoblastic lymphadenopathy and benign lymphadenopathy with giant germinal center hyperplasia and increased vascularity. Blood 87(9):3903–3909, 1996.
32. Parsonnet J, Isaacson PG: Bacterial infection and MALT lymphoma. N Engl J Med 350(3):213–215, 2004.
33. Lecuit M, Abachin E, Martin A, et al: Immunoproliferative small intestinal disease associated with *Campylobacter jejuni*. N Engl J Med 350(3):239–248, 2004.
34. Shin HR, Lee CU, Park HJ, et al: Hepatitis B and C virus, *Clonorchis sinensis* for the risk of liver cancer: A case-control study in Pusan, Korea. Int J Epidemiol 25(5):933–940, 1996.
35. Kaczynski J, Hansson G, Hermodsson S, et al: Minor role of hepatitis B and C virus infection in the etiology of hepatocellular carcinoma in a low-endemic area. Scand J Gastroenterol 31(8):809–813, 1996.
36. Lunn RM, Zhang YJ, Wang LY, et al: p53 mutations, chronic hepatitis B virus infection, and aflatoxin exposure in hepatocellular carcinoma in Taiwan. Cancer Res 57(16):3471–3477, 1997.
37. Morrow RH, Jr: Epidemiological evidence for the role of falciparum malaria in the pathogenesis of Burkitt's lymphoma. IARC Sci Publ (60):177–186, 1985.
38. Lo KW, Huang DP: Genetic and epigenetic changes in nasopharyngeal carcinoma. Semin Cancer Biol 12(6):451–462, 2002.
39. Whittle H, Jaffar S, Wansbrough M, et al: Observational study of vaccine efficacy 14 years after trial of hepatitis B vaccination in Gambian children. BMJ 325(7364):569–573, 2002.
40. Chang MH, Chen CJ, Lai MS, et al: Universal Hepatitis B vaccination in Taiwan and the incidence of hepatocellular carcinoma in children. N Engl J Med 336(26):1855–1859, 1997.
41. Koutsky LA, Ault KA, Wheeler CM, et al: A controlled trial of a human papillomavirus type 16 vaccine. N Engl J Med 347(21):1645–1651, 2002.
42. Lowy DR, Frazer IH: Chapter 16: Prophylactic human papillomavirus vaccines. J Natl Cancer Inst Monogr (31):111–116, 2003.
43. Harper DM, Franco EL, Wheeler C, et al: Efficacy of a bivalent virus-like particle vaccine in prevention of infection with human papilloma virus types 16 and 18 in young women: A randomised controlled trial. Lancet 364(9447):1757–1765, 2004.
44. Pearce EJ: Progress towards a vaccine for schistosomiasis. Acta Trop 86(2–3):309–313, 2003.
45. Colley DG, LoVerde PT, Savioli L: Infectious disease. Medical helminthology in the 21st century. Science 293(5534):1437–1438, 2001.
46. Fendrick AM, Chernew ME, Hirth RA, et al: Clinical and economic effects of population-based *Helicobacter pylori* screening to prevent gastric cancer. Arch Intern Med 159(2):142–148, 1999.
47. Wong BC, Lam SK, Wong WM, et al: *Helicobacter pylori* eradication to prevent gastric cancer in a high-risk region of China: A randomized controlled trial. JAMA 291(2):187–194, 2004.

13

Chemotherapy of Parasitic Diseases

RICHARD D. PEARSON
PETER F. WELLER
RICHARD L. GUERRANT

INTRODUCTION

A large number of drugs are used in the treatment of parasitic diseases, which is not surprising given the genetic diversity and varying life cycles of parasites. This chapter provides an overview of therapy based on phylogenetic and clinical factors. The treatment of helminth infections is summarized in sections on intestinal and systemic nematodes, trematodes, and cestodes. The therapy of protozoal infections follows and is divided into the treatment of malaria, luminal parasites, the kinetoplastida, and other systemic protozoal infections. A number of generalizations emerge from this approach that help in organizing an otherwise vast amount of information. In addition, the treatment of specific parasitic infections is addressed in detail. More complete discussions of the pharmacology and mechanisms of action of the antiparasitic drugs are found elsewhere.[1,2] Substantial additional information about indications, dosing, and toxicity is available in the Medical Letter on Drugs and Therapeutics, Drugs for parasitic infections (www.medicalletter.org),[3] as summarized in the tables in this chapter.

TREATMENT OF INTESTINAL NEMATODES

The benzimidazoles, albendazole and mebendazole, have broad spectra of activities against intestinal nematodes, including *Ascaris lumbricoides*, *Trichuris trichiura*, *Ancylostoma duodenale*, *Necator americanus*, *Enterobius vermicularis*, and others (Table 13-1). Albendazole is particularly attractive because of its pharmacokinetics. It is effective in the treatment of most intestinal helminth infections when administered as a single dose, and it has been used successfully in mass treatment programs in developing countries. Pyrantel pamoate is active against the hookworms, *A. lumbricoides*, *E. vermicularis*, and some other intestinal nematodes, but it is not effective against *T. trichiura*. The benzimidazoles and pyrantel pamoate have replaced a number of older anthelminthics such as piperazine, which are more toxic or less effective but are still used in some developing areas. Ivermectin is recommended for the treatment of *Strongyloides stercoralis*. Thiabendazole, which is no longer manufactured in the United States, was previously the drug of choice, but it has substantial untoward effects. Some still use it in people with disseminated hyperinfection. Albendazole has some activity against *S. stercoralis*, but even with high-dose prolonged therapy, failures may occur.

Albendazole, because of its broad spectrum of activity and favorable pharmacokinetics, has emerged as the drug of choice for the treatment of common intestinal nematode infections.[4] Mass treatment programs employing a single dose of albendazole to treat intestinal helminth infections have improved the nutritional status and fitness of malnourished children in Africa.[5,6] Albendazole is also effective in treating cutaneous larva migrans.[7] It is the drug of choice for echinococcal infections[8,9] and used for neurocysticercosis.[10] It is also used for the treatment of intestinal, ocular, and disseminated microsporidiosis due to *Encephalitozoon (Septata) intestinalis* and other microsporidia in patients with acquired immunodeficiency syndrome (AIDS), but not all microsporidia are susceptible.[11] Albendazole binds to tubulin in susceptible parasites, inhibits microtubule assembly, and decreases glucose absorption. It can also inhibit fumarate reductase in helminths.

Albendazole is poorly water soluble, but it is well absorbed when administered with a fatty meal. There is rapid first-pass metabolism in the liver to albendazole sulfoxide, which has excellent anthelminthic activity. The serum half-life of albendazole sulfoxide is 8 or 9 hours, and the concentration in cerebrospinal fluid (CSF) is 40% of that in serum. Concurrent administration of dexamethasone, which is frequently administered to patients being treated for neurocysticercosis to prevent cerebral edema, increases the serum levels by approximately 50%.[12] The concentration of albendazole sulfoxide in echinococcal cysts is approximately 25% of that in serum. Elimination of albendazole sulfoxide and other metabolites of albendazole is primarily through the kidney.

Albendazole is usually well tolerated when given as a single dose for the treatment of intestinal nematode infections, although some patients develop gastrointestinal discomfort or experience migration of adult *A. lumbricoides* from the nose or mouth or in the stool. Albendazole is embryotoxic in animals and contraindicated during pregnancy. High-dose, prolonged therapy for echinococcal disease is occasionally complicated by alopecia, reversible bone marrow suppression, or hepatocellular injury.

Mebendazole was widely used for the treatment of the common intestinal helminths prior to the introduction of albendazole.[13] It also kills the adults and has some activity against invasive larvae of *Trichinella spiralis*.[14] Mebendazole selectively binds to helminthic tubulin, blocks its assembly into microtubules, and inhibits glucose uptake, leading to depletion of glycogen stores and ultimately parasite death. Glucose metabolism is not affected in humans.

Mebendazole is only slightly soluble in water and is relatively poorly absorbed from the gastrointestinal tract,[13] which limits its effectiveness against tissue-dwelling helminths. The serum half-life of absorbed drug is 2.5 to 5.5 hours. It is metabolized in the liver and excreted in the urine. Mebendazole is relatively well tolerated in the doses used to treat intestinal helminths. Transient abdominal pain and diarrhea occur in a small number of recipients. Prolonged, high-dose therapy used in the treatment of echinococcal liver cysts has been associated with alopecia, hepatocellular injury, and transient bone marrow suppression with severe, but reversible, neutropenia. Mebendazole is contraindicated during pregnancy.

Thiabendazole has a broad spectrum of activity, but because of its toxicity, its systemic use has been limited to the treatment

Table 13-1 Treatment of Nematode (Roundworm) Infections

Infection	Drug	Adult Dosage	Pediatric Dosage
Ancylostoma caninum (*Eosinophilic enterocolitis*)			
Drug of choice:	Albendazole[a]	400 mg once	400 mg once
	or Mebendazole	100 mg bid × 3 days	100 mg bid × 3 days
	or Pyrantel pamoate[a]	11 mg/kg (max. 1 g) × 3 days	11 mg/kg (max. 1 g) × 3 days
	or Endoscopic removal		
Ancylostoma duodenale, see Hookworm			
Angiostrongyliasis (*Angiostrongylus cantonensis*, *Angiostrongylus costaricensis*)			
Angiostrongylus cantonensis	see footnote[b]		
Angiostrongylus costaricensis	see footnote[c]		
Anisakiasis (*Anisakis* spp.)			
Treatment of choice:	Surgical or endoscopic removal[d]		
Ascariasis (*Ascaris lumbricoides, roundworm*)			
Drug of choice:[e]	Albendazole[a]	400 mg once	400 mg once
	or Mebendazole	100 mg bid × 3 days or 500 mg once	100 mg bid × 3 days or 500 mg once
	or Ivermectin[a]	150–200 μg/kg once	150–200 μg/kg once
Baylisascariasis (*Baylisascaris procyonis*)			
Drug of choice:	See footnote[f]		
Capillariasis (*Capillaria philippinensis*)			
Drug of choice:	Mebendazole[a]	200 mg bid × 20 days	200 mg bid × 20 days
Alternatives:	Albendazole[a]	400 mg daily × 10 days	400 mg daily × 10 days
Cutaneous larva migrans (*creeping eruption, dog and cat hookworm*)			
Drug of choice:	Albendazole[a]	400 mg daily × 3 days	400 mg daily × 3 days
	or Ivermectin[a]	200 μg/kg daily × 1–2 days	200 μg/kg daily × 1–2 days
	or Thiabendazole	Topically	Topically
Dracunculus medinensis (guinea worm) infection			
Drug of choice:	See footnote[g]		
Enterobius vermicularis (pinworm) infection			
Drug of choice:[h]	Pyrantel pamoate	11 mg/kg base once (max. 1 g); repeat in 2 wk	11 mg/kg base once (max. 1 g); repeat in 2 wk
	or Mebendazole	100 mg once; repeat in 2 wk	100 mg once; repeat in 2 wk
	or Albendazole[a]	400 mg once; repeat in 2 wk	400 mg once; repeat in 2 wk
Filariasis			
Wuchereria bancrofti, Brugia malayi, Brugia timori			
Drug of choice:[i,j]	Diethylcarbamazine[k]	Day 1: 50 mg po Day 2: 50 mg tid Day 3: 100 mg tid Days 4 through 14: 6 mg/kg/day in 3 doses	Day 1: 1 mg/kg po Day 2: 1 mg/kg tid Day 3: 1–2 mg/kg tid Days 4 through 14: 6 mg/kg/day in 3 doses
Loa loa			
Drug of choice:[j,l]	Diethylcarbamazine[k,*]	Day 1: 50 mg, p.o. Day 2: 50 mg tid Day 3: 100 mg tid Days 4 through 21: 9 mg/kg/day in 3 doses	Day 1: 1 mg/kg p.o. Day 2: 1 mg/kg tid Day 3: 1–2 mg/kg tid Days 4 through 21: 9 mg/kg/day in 3 doses
Mansonella ozzardi			
Drug of choice:[j]	See footnote[m]		

Continued

Table 13-1 Treatment of Nematode (Roundworm) Infections—Cont'd

Infection	Drug	Adult Dosage	Pediatric Dosage
Mansonella perstans			
Drug of choice:[j]	Albendazole[a]	400 mg bid × 10 days	400 mg bid × 10 days
	or Mebendazole[a]	100 mg bid × 30 days	100 mg bid × 30 days
Mansonella streptocerca			
Drug of choice:[j,n]	Diethylcarbamazine	6 mg/kg/d × 14 days	6 mg/kg/day × 14 days
	Ivermectin[a]	150 μg/kg once	150 μg/kg once
Tropical pulmonary eosinophilia (TPE)[o]			
Drug of choice:	Diethylcarbamazine	6 mg/kg/day in 3 doses × 12–21 days	6 mg/kg/day in 3 doses × 12–21 days
Onchocerca volvulus (river blindness)			
Drug of choice:	Ivermectin[p]	150 μg/kg once, repeated every 6–12 mo until asymptomatic	150 μg/kg once, repeated every 6–12 mo until asymptomatic
Gnathostomiasis (*Gnathostoma spinigerum*)			
Treatment of choice:[q]	Albendazole[a]	400 mg bid × 21 days	400 mg bid × 21 days
	or Ivermectin[a]	200 μg/kg/day × 2 days	200 μg/kg/day × 2 days
	± Surgical removal		
Gongylonemiasis (*Gongylonema* sp.)[r]			
Treatment of choice:	Surgical removal		
	or Albendazole[a]	10 mg/kg/day × 3 days	10 mg/kg/day × 3 days
Hookworm infection (*Ancylostoma duodenale, Necator americanus*)			
Drug of choice:	Albendazole[a]	400 mg once	400 mg once
	or Mebendazole	100 mg bid × 3 days or 500 mg once	100 mg bid × 3 days or 500 mg once
	or Pyrantel pamoate[a]	11 mg/kg (max. 1 g) × 3 days	11 mg/kg (max. 1 g) × 3 days
Moniliformis *moniliformis* infection			
Drug of choice:	Pyrantel pamoate[a]	11 mg/kg once, repeat twice, 2 wk apart	11 mg/kg once, repeat twice, 2 wk apart
Oesophagostomum *bifurcum*			
Drug of choice:	See footnote[s]		
Strongyloidiasis (*Strongyloides stercoralis*)			
Drug of choice:[t]	Ivermectin	200 μg/kg/day × 2 days	200 μg/kg/day × 2 days
Alternative:	Albendazole[a]	400 mg bid × 7 days	400 mg bid × 7 days
	or Thiabendazole	50 mg/kg/day in 2 doses × 2 days (max 3 g/day)	50 mg/kg/day in 2 doses × 2 days (max 3 g/day)
Trichinellosis (*Trichinella spiralis*)			
Drugs of choice:	Steroids for severe symptoms		
	plus		
	mebendazole[a]	200–400 mg tid × 3 days, then 400–500 mg tid × 10 days	200–400 mg tid × 3 days, then 400–500 mg tid × 10 days
Alternative:	Albendazole[a]	400 mg bid × 8–14 days	400 mg bid × 8–14 days
Trichostrongylus infection			
Drug of choice:	Pyrantel pamoate[a]	11 mg/kg base once (max. 1 g)	11 mg/kg once (max. 1 g)
Alternative:	Mebendazole[a]	100 mg bid × 3 days	100 mg bid × 3 days
	or Albendazole[a]	400 mg once	400 mg once

Infection	Drug	Adult dosage	Pediatric dosage
Trichuriasis (*Trichuris trichiura*, whipworm)			
Drug of choice:	Mebendazole	100 mg bid × 3 days or 500 mg once	100 mg bid × 3 days or 500 mg once
Alternative:	Albendazole[a]	400 mg × 3 days	400 mg × 3 days
	Ivermectin[a]	200 µg/kg/day × 3 days	200 µg/kg/day × 3 days
Visceral larva migrans (*Toxocariasis*)[u]			
Drug of choice:	Albendazole[a]	400 mg bid × 5 days	400 mg bid × 5 days
	Mebendazole[a]	100–200 mg bid × 5 days	100–200 mg bid × 5 days

[a]An approved drug but considered investigational for this condition by the FDA.

[b]Most patients have a self-limited course and recover completely. Analgesics, corticosteroids, and careful removal of CSF at frequent intervals can relieve symptoms from increased intracranial pressure (Lo Re III V, Gluckman SJ: Am J Med 114:217, 2003). No anthelminthic drug is proven to be effective and some patients have worsened with therapy (Slom TJ, et al: N Engl J Med 346:668, 2002). In one report, however, mebendazole and a corticosteroid appeared to shorten the course of infection (Tsai, H-C, et al: Am J Med 111:109, 2001).

[c]The efficacy of anthelmintic therapy in humans has not been documented.

[d]Repiso Ortega A, et al: Gastroenterol Hepatol 26:341, 2003. Successful treatment of a patient with anisakiasis with albendazole has been reported (Moore DA, et al: Lancet 360:54, 2002).

[e]Nitazoxanide has activity against *Ascaris* and some other nematodes. It is FDA approved as a pediatric oral suspension for treatment of *Cryptosporidium* in immunocompetent children younger than 12 years old and for *Giardia* (Medical Letter 45:29, 2003). It may also be effective for mild to moderate amebiasis (Diaz E, et al: Am J Trop Med Hyg 68:384, 2003). Nitazoxanide is available in 500-mg tablets and an oral suspension; it should be taken with food.

[f]No drugs have been demonstrated to be effective. Albendazole 25 mg/kg/day × 20 days started as soon as possible (up to 3 days after possible infection) might prevent clinical disease and is recommended for children with known exposure (ingestion of racoon stool or contaminated soil) (MMWR 50:1153, 2002; Gavin PJ, Shulman, ST: Pediatr Infect Dis 22:651, 2003), Mebendazole, thiabendazole, levamisole, or ivermectin could be tried if albendazole were not available. Steroid therapy may be helpful, especially in eye and CNS infections. Ocular baylisascariasis has been treated successfully using laser photocoagulation therapy to destroy the intraretinal larvae.

[g]Treatment of choice is slow extraction of worm combined with wound care (Greenaway C: CMAJ 170:495, 2004). Ten days' treatment with metronidazole 250 mg tid in adults and 25 mg/kg/day in three doses in children is not curative but decreases inflammation and facilitates removal of the worm. Mebendazole 400–800 mg/day × 6 days has been reported to kill the worm directly.

[h]Since all family members are usually infected, treatment of the entire household is recommended by some experts.

[i]Most symptoms caused by adult worm. Single dose combination of albendazole (400 mg) with either ivermectin (200 mcg/kg) or diethylcarbamazine (6 mg/kg) is effective for reduction or suppression of *W. bancrofti* microfilaria but does not kill the adult forms (D Addiss et al, Cochrane Database Syst Rev 2004; CD003753).

[j]Antihistamines or corticosteroids may be required to decrease allergic reactions due to disintegration of microfilariae from treatment of filarial infections, especially those caused by *Loa loa*. Endosymbiotic *Wolbachia* bacteria may have a role in filarial development and host response, and may represent a new target for therapy. Treatment with doxycycline 100 or 200 mg/d × 4-6 wks in lymphatic filariasis and onchocerciasis has resulted in substantial loss of *Wolbachia* with subsequent block of microfilariae production and absence of microfilaria when followed for 24 months after treatment (A Hoerauf et al, Med Microbiol Immunol 2003; 192:211; A Hoerauf et al, BMJ 2003; 326:207).

[k]For patients with microfilaria in the blood, Medical Letter consultants would start with a lower dosage and scale up as indicated. Multi-dose regimens have been shown to provide more rapid reduction in microfilaria than single-dose diethylcarbamazine, but microfilaria levels are similar 6-12 mos after treatment (LD Andrade et al, Trans R Soc Trop Med Hyg 1995; 89:319; PE Simonsen et al, Am J Trop Med Hyg 1995; 53:267). A single dose of 6 mg/kg is used in endemic areas for mass treatment (J Figueredo-Silva et al, Trans R Soc Trop Med Hyg 1996; 90:192; J Noroes et al, Trans R Soc Trop Med Hyg 1997; 91:78).

[l]In heavy infections with *Loa loa*, rapid killing of microfilariae can provoke an encephalopathy. Apheresis has been reported to be effective in lowering microfilarial counts in patients heavily infected with *L. loa* (Ottesen EA: Infect Dis Clin North Am 7:619, 1993). Albendazole has also been used to reduce microfilaremia (Klion AD, et al: J Infect Dis 168:202, 1993; Kombila M et al: Am J Trop Med Hyg 58:458, 1998). Albendazole may be useful for treatment of loiasis when diethylcarbamazine is ineffective or cannot be used, but repeated courses may be necessary (Klion AD, et al: Clin Infect Dis 29:680, 1999). The use of ivermectin in loiasis has been associated with life-threatening encephalopathy. Diethylcarbamazine, 300 mg once/week, has been recommended for prevention of loiasis (Nutman TB, et al: N Engl J Med 319:752, 1988).

[m]Diethylcarbamazine has no effect. Ivermectin 200 µg/kg once, has been effective.

[n]Diethylcarbamazine is potentially curative due to activity against both adult worms and microfilariae. Ivermectin is only active against microfilariae.

[o]Relapse occurs and can be treated with diethylcarbamazine.

[p]Annual treatment with ivermectin, 150 µg/kg, can prevent blindness due to ocular onchocerciasis (Mabey D, et al: Ophthalmology 103:1001, 1996). Diethylcarbamazine should not be used for treatment of this disease.

[q]de Gorgolas M, et al: J Travel Med 10:358, 2003. All patients should be treated with a medication regardless of whether surgery is attempted.

[r]Eberhard ML, Busillo C: Am J Trop Med Hyg 61:51, 1999; Wilson ME, et al: Clin Infect Dis 32:1378, 2001.

[s]Albendazole or pyrantel pamoate may be effective (Ziem JB, et al: Ann Trop Med Parasitol 98:385, 2004).

[t]In immunocompromised patients or disseminated disease, it may be necessary to prolong or repeat therapy or to use other agents. Veterinary parenteral and enema formulations of ivermectin have been used in severely ill patients unable to take oral medications (Chiodini PL, et al: Lancet 355:43, 2000; Orem J, et al: Clin Infect Dis 37:152, 2003; Tarr PE: Am J Trop Med Hyg 68:453, 2003). The dose of thiabendazole recommended is likely to be toxic and may have to be decreased.

[u]Optimum duration of therapy is not known. Some Medical Letter consultants would treat for 20 days. For severe symptoms or eye involvement, corticosteroids can be used in addition.

Derived from the *Medical Letter on Drugs and Therapeutics*, Drugs for parasitic infections, www.medicalletter.org, August 2004. Recommendations that differ from those of the medical letter are marked with an asterisk.

of strongyloidiasis. It is also used topically for the treatment of cutaneous larva migrans.[15] Ivermectin is recommended for uncomplicated strongyloidiasis, although some experts consider thiabendazole the treatment of choice for those with disseminated hyperinfection. The mechanism of action of thiabendazole is thought to be similar to that of mebendazole and albendazole. Gastrointestinal side effects, including nausea, vomiting, and diarrhea, are common. Other side effects include dizziness, tinnitus, and other neurological effects as well as elevated liver enzymes. It is contraindicated during pregnancy. Topically applied thiabendazole used in the treatment of cutaneous larva migrans is well tolerated.[15]

Pyrantel pamoate[16] is a depolarizing neuromuscular blocking agent that is active against *E. vermicularis*, the hookworms, and *A. lumbricoides*. It is poorly absorbed after oral administration. It is usually well tolerated. Some recipients experience transient gastrointestinal side effects or, less commonly, headache, drowsiness, insomnia, dizziness, or hypersensitivity reactions. It is not recommended for use during pregnancy. The muscles of susceptible nematodes undergo depolarization and an increase in spike discharge frequency that leads to a short period of calcium-dependent stimulation resulting in irreversible paralysis of the worms. They are subsequently expelled in the feces. Pyrantel also inhibits helminthic acetylcholinesterases. Piperazine, which paralyzes worms by causing hyperpolarization, and pyrantel are mutually antagonistic and should not be administered together.

Ivermectin, a macrocyclic lactone produced by *Streptomyces avermitilis*, has a broad spectrum of activity against helminths and arthropods. It is the drug of choice for the treatment of strongyloidiasis[17,18] and for onchocerciasis. Ivermectin is well absorbed after oral administration. It is highly protein bound, has a serum half-life of 12 hours, and accumulates in adipose tissue and in the liver. It is subject to enterohepatic recirculation and eliminated in the stool. Ivermectin activates the opening of gated-chloride channels that are found only in susceptible helminths and arthropods. The result is an influx of chloride ions and paralysis of the pharyngeal pumping mechanism of helminths. It is well tolerated when used for the treatment of strongyloidiasis. However, failures with ivermectin have been noted, leading to the use of multiple doses at weekly intervals in immunocompromised patients with disseminated disease or the use of other drugs. Ivermectin is widely used in veterinary practice for the treatment of nematodes such as the dog heart worm, *Dirofilaria immitis*.

TREATMENT OF SYSTEMIC NEMATODES

Diethylcarbamazine is the drug of choice for several systemic filarial nematode infections, including those caused by *Wuchereria bancrofti*, *Brugia malayi*, *Brugia timori*, and *Loa loa,* and for people with tropical pulmonary eosinophilia[19,20] (see Table 13-1). Diethylcarbamazine is not directly toxic to microfilariae but promotes the host's killing of microfilariae of these species and also promotes damage or killing of adult worms. It can be used prophylactically to prevent *L. loa* infections in endemic areas. Diethylcarbamazine kills microfilariae of *Onchocerca volvulus*, but it is not used for the treatment of onchocerciasis because the rapid release of parasite antigens as well as lipopolysaccharide derived from filarial harbored *Wolbachia* endiosymbionts often elicits severe systemic and ocular inflammatory reactions. Ivermectin, which is associated with much less severe reactions, is the drug of choice.

Diethylcarbamazine, a piperazine derivative, is well absorbed orally and has a half-life of 8 hours. The parent drug and its metabolites are excreted through the kidney. Side effects include those attributable directly to the drug and those that result from the release of parasite antigens and *Wolbachia* lipopolysaccharide. Side effects include nausea, vomiting, anorexia, headache, malaise, weakness, arthralgias, and, rarely, acute psychotic reactions. In patients with *W. bancrofti* or *B. malayi* infection, localized swelling or nodules may develop along lymphatics during treatment, or there may be transient lymphedema or hydrocele formation. Diethylcarbamazine is no longer used in patients with onchocerciasis because it can elicit the Mazzotti reaction, which is characterized by hypotension, pruritus, fever, tachycardia, wheezing, chorioretinitis, and uveitis secondary to the release of microfilarial antigens and *Wolbachia* lipopolysaccharide. Life-threatening encephalopathy has been reported in patients with heavy *L. loa* infections who received the drug.[21] Although the mechanism of diethylcarbamazine is uncertain, diethylcarbamazine enhances in vivo killing of filariae, resulting in their destruction by the host's immune system.

Ivermectin is the drug of choice for the treatment of onchocerciasis,[22,23] killing microfilariae in the skin and eye. It does not kill adult *O. volvulus*, but it decreases production of microfilariae. Retreatment is usually necessary at 6- to 12-month intervals. Ivermectin has activity against microfilaria of *W. bancrofti*, *B. malayi*, and *L. loa*, but it does not kill the adult worms. Profits from the use of ivermectin for the treatment of the dog heart worm, *D. immitis*, have permitted the manufacturer to provide the drug free to people with onchocerciasis in developing areas.

TREATMENT OF CESTODES AND TREMATODES

Among the platyhelminths, praziquantel is active against adult cestodes (tapeworms) in the human intestinal tract (Table 13-2) and most trematodes that infect humans (Table 13-3).[24,25] The principal exception is *Fasciola hepatica*, which responds to the veterinary fasciolide, triclabendazole, and to bithionol.[26,27] Both albendazole and praziquantel kill cysticerci of *Taenia solium* in the central nervous system (CNS) and can be used in the treatment of neurocysticercosis.[28,29] Corticosteroids are often administered concomitantly to reduce the inflammatory response elicited by released cysticercal antigens and the increase in intracranial pressure that can result. The concurrent use of corticosteroids increases the CSF level of albendazole and decreases that of praziquantel. Albendazole is preferred by many for the treatment of neurocysticercosis. Prolonged albendazole therapy cures more than one-third of patients with *Echinococcus granulosus* cysts, and it is given to people with echinococcal cysts prior to and during percutaneous drainage procedures or surgery to prevent seeding of the peritoneum. It is also used for the suppression of inoperable *Echinococcus multilocularis* infections. The adverse effects of these anthelminthic drugs are summarized in Box 13-1.

Praziquantel is rapidly taken up by susceptible platyhelminths. Studies of the tapeworm *Hymenolepis diminuta* indicate that praziquantel causes blebs in the neck of the tapeworm and the release of calcium from endogenous stores, which results in paralysis and expulsion of the worm from the gastrointestinal tract.[30] In the case of schistosomes, praziquantel

Table 13-2 Treatment of Cestode (Tapeworm) Infections

Infection	Drug	Adult Dosage	Pediatric Dosage
Adult (intestinal stage)			
Diphyllobothrium latum **(fish),** ***Taenia saginata*** **(beef),** ***Taenia solium*** **(pork),** ***Dipylidium caninum*** **(dog)**			
Drug of choice:	Praziquantel[a]	5–10 mg/kg once	5–10 mg/kg once
Alternative:	Niclosamide	2 g once	50 mg/kg once
Hymenolepsis nana **(dwarf tapeworm)**			
Drug of choice:	Praziquantel[a]	25 mg/kg once	25 mg/kg once
Alternative:	Nitazoxanide[a,b]	500 mg × 3 days[c]	1–3 yr: 100 mg bid × 3 days[c] 4–11 yr: 200 mg bid × 3 days[c]
Larval (tissue stage)			
Echinococcus granulosus (hydatid cyst)			
Drug of choice:[d]	Albendazole	400 mg bid × 1–6 mo	15 mg/kg/day (max. 800 mg) × 1–6 mo
Echinococcus multilocularis			
Treatment of choice:	See footnote[e]		
Taenia solium (*Cysticercosis*)			
Treatment of choice:	See footnote[f]		
Alternative:	Albendazole	400 mg bid × 8–30 days; can be repeated as necessary	15 mg/kg/day (max. 800 mg) in 2 doses × 8–30 days; can be repeated as necessary
	or Praziquantel[a]	50–100 mg/kg/day in 3 doses × 30 days	50–100 mg/kg/day in 3 doses × 30 days

[a]An approved drug but considered investigational for this condition by the FDA.
[b]Nitazoxanide is FDA approved as a pediatric oral suspension for treatment of *Cryptosporidium* in immunocompetent children younger than 12 years old and for *Giardia* (Medical Letter 45:29, 2003). It may also be effective for mild to moderate amebiasis (Diaz E, et al: Am J Trop Med Hyg 68:384, 2003). Nitazoxanide is available in 500-mg tablets and an oral suspension; it should be taken with food.
[c]Juan JO, et al: Trans R Soc Trop Med Hyg 96:193, 2002.
[d]Patients may benefit from surgical resection or percutaneous drainage of cysts. Praziquantel is useful preoperatively or in case of spillage of cyst contents during surgery. Percutaneous aspiration–injection–reaspiration (PAIR) with ultrasound guidance plus albendazole therapy has been effective for management of hepatic hydatid cyst disease (Smego, RA, Jr et al: Clin Infect Dis 37:1073, 2003).
[e]Surgical excision is the only reliable means of cure. Reports have suggested that in nonresectable cases use of albendazole or mebendazole can stabilize and sometimes cure infection (Craig P: Curr Opin Infect Dis 16:437, 2003).
[f]Initial therapy for patients with inflammed parenchymal cysticerosis should focus on symptomatic treatment with antiseizure medication. Treatment of parenchymal cysticerci with albendazole or praziquantel is controversial. (Maguire, JM: N Engl J Med 350:215, 2004). Patients with live parenchymal cysts who have seizures should be treated with albendazole together with steroids (6 mg dexamethsone or 40–60 mg prednisone daily) and an antiseizure medication (Garcia HH, et al: N Engl J Med 350:249, 2004). Patients with subarachnoid cysts or giant cysts in the fissures should be treated for at least 30 days (Proaño JV, et al: N Engl J Med 345:879, 2001). Surgical intervention or CSF diversion are indicated for obstructive hydocephalus; prednisone 40 mg/day may be given with surgery. Arachnoiditis, vasculitis, or cerebral edema are treated with prednisone 60 mg/day or dexamethasone 4–6 mg/day together with albendazole or praziquantel (White, AC Jr.: Annu Rev Med 51:187, 2000). Any cysticercoidal drug may cause irreparable damage when used to treat ocular or spinal cysts, even when corticosteroids are used. An ophthamalic exam should always precede treatment to rule out intraocular cysts.
Derived from *Medical Letter on Drugs and Therapeutics*, Drugs for parasitic infections, www.medicalletter.org, August 2004.

Table 13-3 Treatment of Trematode (Fluke) Infections

Infection	Drug	Adult Dosage	Pediatric Dosage
Fluke, hermaphroditic, infection			
Clonorchis sinensis (Chinese liver fluke)			
Drug of choice:	Praziquantel	75 mg/kg/day in 3 doses × 1 day	75 mg/kg/day in 3 doses × 1 day
	or Albendazole[a]	10 mg/kg × 7 days	10 mg/kg × 7 days
Fasciola hepatica (sheep liver fluke)			
Drug of choice:[b]	Triclabendazole	10 mg/kg once or twice[c]	10 mg/kg once or twice[c]
Alternative:[d]	Bithionol	30–50 mg/kg on alternative days × 10–15 doses	30–50 mg/kg on alternative days × 10–15 doses
Fasciolopsis buski, Heterophyes heterophyes, Metagonimus yokogawai (intestinal flukes)			
Drug of choice:	Praziquantel[a]	75 mg/kg/day in 3 doses × 1 day	75 mg/kg/day in 3 doses × 1 day
Metorchis conjunctus (North American liver fluke)[e]			
Drug of choice:	Praziquantel[a]	75 mg/kg/day in 3 doses × 1 day	75 mg/kg/day in 3 doses × 1 day
Nanophyetus salmincola			
Drug of choice:	Praziquantel[a]	60 mg/kg/day in 3 doses × 1 day	60 mg/kg/day in 3 doses × 1 day
Opisthorchis viverrini (Southeast Asian liver fluke)			
Drug of choice:	Praziquantel[a]	75 mg/kg/day in 3 doses × 1 day	75 mg/kg/day in 3 doses × 1 day
Paragonimus westeramani (lung fluke)			
Drug of choice:	Praziquantel[a]	75 mg/kg/day in 3 doses × 2 days	75 mg/kg/day in 3 doses × 2 days
Alternative:[f]	Bithionol	30–50 mg/kg on alternative days × 10–15 doses	30–50 mg/kg on alternative days × 10–15 doses

Continued

Table 13-3 Treatment of Trematode (Fluke) Infections—Cont'd

Infection	Drug	Adult Dosage	Pediatric Dosage
Schistosomiasis (*Bilharziasis*)			
S. haematobium			
Drug of choice:	Praziquantel	40 mg/kg/day in 2 doses × 1 day	40 mg/kg/day in 2 doses × 1 day
S. japonicum			
Drug of choice:	Praziquantel	60 mg/kg/day in 3 doses × 1 day	60 mg/kg/day in 3 doses × 1 day
S. mansoni			
Drug of choice:	Praziquantel	40 mg/kg/day in 2 doses × 1 day	40 mg/kg/day in 2 doses × 1 day
Alternative:	Oxamniquine[g]	15 mg/kg once[h]	20 mg/kg/day in 2 doses × 1 day[h]
S. mekongi			
Drug of choice:	Praziquantel	60 mg/kg/day in 3 doses × 1 day	60 mg/kg/day in 3 doses × 1 day

[a]An approved drug but considered investigational for this condition by the FDA.

[b]Unlike infections with other flukes, *Fasciola hepatica* infections may not respond to praziquantel. Triclabendzole (Egaten, Novartis) may be safe and effective but data are limited (Graham CS, et al: Clin Infect Dis 33:1, 2001). It is available from Victoria Pharmacy, Zurich, Switzerland (www.pharmaworld.com; 41-1-211-24-32) and should be given with food for better absorption. A single study has found that nitazoxanide has limited efficacy for treating fascioliasis in adults and children (Favennec L, et al: Aliment Pharmocol Ther 17:265, 2003).

[c]Richter J, et al: Curr Treat Option Infect Dis 4:313, 2002.

[d]Nitazoxanide is FDA approved as a pediatric oral suspension for treatment of *Cryptosporidium* in immunocompetent children younger than 12 years old and for *Giardia* (Medical Letter, 45:29, 2003). It may also be effective for mild to moderate amebiasis (Diaz E, et al: Am J Trop Med Hyg 68:384, 2003). Nitazoxanide is available in 500-mg tablets and an oral suspension; it should be taken with food.

[e]MacLean JD, et al: Lancet 347:154, 1996.

[f]Triclabendazole may be effective in a dosage of 5 mg/kg once/day × 3 days or 10 mg/kg bid × 1 day (Calvopiña M, et al: Trans R Soc Trop Med Hyg 92:566, 1998).

[g]Oxamniquine has been effective in some areas in which praziquantel is less effective (Stelma FF, et al: J Infect Dis 176:304, 1997). Oxamniquine is contraindicated in pregnancy.

[h]In East Africa, the dose should be increased to 30 mg/kg, and in Egypt and South Africa to 30 mg/kg/day × 2 days. Some experts recommend 40–60 mg/kg over 2–3 days in all of Africa (Shekhar KC: Drugs 42:379, 1991).

Derived from *Medical Letter on Drugs and Therapeutics*, Drugs for parasitic infections, www.medicalletter.org, August 2004.

Box 13-1 Adverse Effects of Anthelminthic Drugs

Drugs Used for Nematode Infections

Albendazole (Albenza [GlaxoSmithKline])
- **Occasional:** abdominal pain; migration of *Ascaris* through mouth and nose; reversible alopecia; increased serum transaminase activity
- **Rare:** leukopenia; rash; renal toxicity

Diethylcarbamazine citrate USP* (Hetrazan)
- **Frequent:** severe allergic or febrile reactions in patients with microfilariae in the blood or skin; gastrointestinal disturbances
- **Rare:** encephalopathy (with treatment of heavy *Loa loa* infection)

Ivermectin (Stromectol [Merck])
- **Occasional:** Mazzotti-type reaction seen in onchocerciasis, including fever, pruritus, tender lymph nodes, headache, joint and bone pain
- **Rare:** hypotension

Mebendazole (Vermox [McNeil])
- **Occasional:** diarrhea, abdominal pain, migration of *Ascaris* through mouth and nose
- **Rare:** leukopenia, agranulocytosis, hypospermia

Pyrantel pamoate (Antiminth [Pfizer])†
- **Occasional:** gastrointestinal disturbances, headache, dizziness, rash, fever

Drugs Used for Cestode and Trematode Infections

Albendazole (Albenza [GlaxoSmithKline])—see above

Bithionol* (Bitin [Tanabe, Japan])
- **Frequent:** photosensitivity reactions, vomiting, diarrhea, abdominal pain, urticaria
- **Rare:** leukoplakia, toxic hepatitis

Oxamniquine (Vansil [Pfizer])†
- **Occasional:** headache, fever, dizziness, somnolence, nausea, diarrhea, rash, insomnia, hepatic enzyme changes, ECG changes, EEG changes, orange-red discoloration of urine
- **Rare:** seizures, neuropsychiatric disturbances

Praziquantel (Biltricide [Bayer])
- **Frequent:** abdominal pain, diarrhea, malaise, headache, dizziness
- **Occasional:** sedation, fever, sweating, nausea, eosinophilia, fatigue
- **Rare:** pruritus, rash, edema, hiccups

*Available from the CDC Drug Service, Centers for Disease Control and Prevention, Atlanta, GA 30333; telephone (404) 639-3670; evenings, weekends, and holidays (404) 639-2888.

†Not available in the United States.

damages the tegument, resulting in intense vacuolation and increased permeability to calcium.[31] Adult schistosomes are paralyzed and translocated to the liver through the portal circulation. Sequestered antigens are exposed on the parasite's surface allowing for the binding of antibodies and phagocytes and immune destruction of the parasite.

Praziquantel is well absorbed after oral administration. There is extensive first-pass metabolism, and the metabolites, which are inactive, are excreted in the urine. Praziquantel is approximately 80% protein bound; the serum half-life is 4 to 6 hours. The concentration in the CSF is approximately 15% to 20% of that in plasma.[32] The concurrent administration of corticosteroids, which is often done in patients undergoing treatment for neurocysticercosis to decrease inflammation in the brain, reduces the CSF concentrations of praziquantel and may decrease its efficacy.

Praziquantel is frequently associated with mild, transient side effects, including headaches, lassitude, dizziness, nausea, vomiting, and abdominal discomfort, but these are seldom severe enough to interrupt therapy. Apparent untoward reactions due to the release of parasite antigens have been reported in patients treated for schistosomiasis and pulmonary paragonimiasis. Increased intracranial pressure resulting from the release of cysticercal antigens is a potentially life-threatening event in patients receiving praziquantel for neurocysticercosis, and corticosteroids are usually administered concurrently.[33,34] Praziquantel is contraindicated in people with cysticerci in the eye or spinal cord because of the deleterious consequences of local inflammatory reactions. The concurrent administration of cimetidine, ketoconazole, or miconazole can inhibit the metabolism of praziquantel and increase serum levels.

Niclosamide is active against adult tapeworms in the gastrointestinal tract.[35] It is very poorly absorbed, which limits its spectrum of activity to intestinal organisms. It is thought to uncouple oxidative phosphorylation in the mitochondria of adult cestodes, and it may also interfere with anaerobic metabolism. As the adult tapeworm dies, there is destruction of the scolex and proximal portion with expulsion of the remainder of the worm in the feces.

Niclosamide is usually well tolerated, but it can cause mild gastrointestinal or systemic symptoms and, rarely, a rash. It kills adult *T. solium*, but the disintegration of the worm and the release of viable ova into the intestinal lumen raise the theoretical possibility of autoinfection. For this reason, many physicians prefer praziquantel for intestinal *T. solium* infection. When niclosamide is used, it is often followed by a purge to expedite removal of the worm. In the case of *Hymenolepis nana*, 5 to 7 days of niclosamide are needed to cure infection, whereas a single dose of praziquantel is effective, and it is consequently preferred.

Oxamniquine is an alternative to praziquantel for the treatment of *Schistosoma mansoni* infections.[36] Although the precise mechanism of its action is uncertain, it produces marked alterations in the tegument of adult schistosomes, but it does so over a period of days, in contrast to praziquantel, which acts in hours. Higher doses of oxamniquine are recommended for treatment in some areas of Egypt and equatorial Africa. Oxamniquine is well absorbed orally and has a half-life of 1.0 to 2.5 hours. The parent drug and its metabolites are cleared through the kidney and can produce an orange or red discoloration of the urine. Potential side effects include dizziness, drowsiness, skin rash, and gastrointestinal disturbances, including abdominal pain, diarrhea, nausea, vomiting, and loss of appetite. Seizures occur rarely. Oxamniquine is contraindicated in people with epilepsy and during pregnancy.

TREATMENT OF SYSTEMIC PROTOZOAL INFECTIONS: MALARIA, BABESIOSIS, AND TOXOPLASMOSIS

Malaria

The prophylaxis (Table 13-4; Box 13-2) and treatment of malaria (Table 13-5; see Box 13-2) are of great importance in

Table 13-4 *Drugs Used for Prevention of Malaria*

Infection	Drug	Adult Dosage	Pediatric Dosage
Malaria, prevention of[a]			
Chloroquine-sensitive areas[b]			
Drug of choice:	Chloroquine phosphate[c,d]	500 mg (300 mg base), once/wk[e]	5 mg/kg base once/wk, up to adult dose of 300 mg base[e]
Chloroquine-resistant areas[b]			
Drug of choice:	Atovaquone/proguanil[d,f]	1 adult tab/day[g]	11–20 kg: 1 peds tab/day[f,g] 21–30 kg: 2 peds tabs/day[f,g] 31–40 kg: 3 peds tabs/day[f,g] >40 kg: 1 adult tab/day[f,g]
	or Mefloquine[d,h,i]	1 adult tablet (250 mg) once/wk[e]	5–10 kg: 1/8 tab once/wk[e] 11–20 kg: 1/4 tab once/wk[e] 21–30 kg: 1/2 tab once/wk[e] 31–45 kg: 3/4 tab once/wk[e] >45 kg: 1 tab once/wk[e]
	or Doxycycline[d,j]	100 mg daily[k]	2 mg/kg/day, up to 100 mg/day[k]
Alternatives:	Primaquine[j,l]	30 mg base daily[m]	0.6 mg/kg base daily
	or Chloroquine phosphate plus	500 mg (300 mg base) once/wk[e]	5 mg/kg base once/wk, up to 300 mg base[e]
	proguanil[n]	200 mg once/day	<2 yr: 50 mg once/day 2–6 yr: 100 mg once/day

Continued

Table 13-4 Drugs Used for Prevention of Malaria—Cont'd

Infection	Drug	Adult Dosage	Pediatric Dosage
			7–10 yr: 150 mg once/day >10 yr: 200 mg once/day
Malaria, self-presumptive treatment[o]			
Drug of choice	Atovaquone/proguanil[j,f]	4 adult tabs daily × 3 days	<5 kg: not indicated 5–8 kg: 2 peds tabs once/day × 3 days 9–10 kg: 3 peds tabs once/day × 3 days 11–20 kg: 1 adult tab once/day × 3 days 21–30 kg: 2 adult tabs once/day × 3 days 31–40 kg: 3 adult tabs once/day × 3 days >40 kg: 4 adult tabs once/day × 3 days
	or Quinine sulfate	650 mg q8h × 3–7 day[p]	30 mg/kg/d in 3 doses × 3–7 day[p]
	plus		
	doxycycline[j,k]	100 mg bid × 7 day	4 mg/kg/d in 2 doses × 7 day
	or Mefloquine[h]	750 mg followed 12 hrs later by 500 mg	15 mg/kg followed 12 hrs later by 10 mg/kg

[a]No drug regimen guarantees protection against malaria. If fever develops within 1 year (particularly within the first 2 months) after travel to malarious areas, travelers should be advised to seek medical attention. Insect repellents, insecticide-impregnated bed nets, and proper clothing are important adjuncts for malaria prophylaxis (Medical Letter 45:41, 2003). Malaria in pregnancy if particularly serious for both mother and fetus; therefore, prophylaxis is indicated if exposure cannot be avoided.

[b]Chloroquine-resistant *P. falciparum* occurs in all malarious areas except Central America west of the Panama Canal Zone, Mexico, Haiti, the Dominican Republic, and most of the Middle East (choloroquine resistant has been reported in Yemen, Oman, Saudi Arabia, and Iran). For treatment of multiple drug-resistant *P. falciparum* in Southeast Asia, especially Thailand, where resistance to mefloquine is frequent, atovaquone/proguanil, artesunate plus mefloquine, or artemether plus mefloquine may be used (Luxemburger JC, et al: Trans R Soc Trop Med Hyg 88:213, 1994; Karbwang J, et al: Trans R Soc Trop Med Hyg 89:296, 1995).

[c]In pregnancy, chloroquine prophylaxis has been used extensively and safely.

[d]For prevention of attack after departure from areas where *P. vivax* and *P. ovale* are endemic, which includes almost all areas where malaria is found (except Haiti), some experts prescribe in addition primaquine phosphate 30 mg base/day or, for children, 0.6 mg base/kg/day during the last 2 weeks of prophylaxis. Others prefer to avoid the toxicity of primaquine and rely on surveillance to detect cases when they occur, particularly when exposure was limited or doubtful. See below.

[e]Beginning 1 or 2 weeks before travel and continuing weekly for the duration of stay and for 4 weeks after leaving.

[f]Atovaquone plus proguanil is available as a fixed-dose combination tablet: adult tablets (Malarone; 250 mg atovaquone/100 mg proguanil) and pediatric tablets (Malarone Pediatric; 62.5 mg atovaquone/25 mg proguanil). To enhance absorption, it should be taken with food or a milky drink. Atovaquone/proguanil should not be given to pregnant women or patients with severe renal impairment (creatinine clearance <30 mL/min). There have been several isolated reports of resistance in *P. falciparum* in Africa (Schwartz E, et al: Clin Infect Dis 37:450, 2003; Farnert A, et al: BMJ 326:628, 2003).

[g]Beginning 1 or 2 days before travel and continuing for the duration of stay and for 1 week after leaving. In one study of malaria prophylaxis, atovaquone/proguanil was better tolerated than mefloquine in nonimmune travelers (Overbosch D, et al: Clin Infect Dis 33:1015, 2001).

[h]Adverse effects including nausea, vomiting, diarrhea, dizziness, disturbed sense of balance, toxic psychosis, and seizures can occur. Mefloquine should not be used for treatment of malaria in pregnancy unless there is no other treatment option because of increased risk for stillbirth Nosten F, et al: Clin Infect Dis 28:808, 1999). It should be avoided for treatment of malaria in people with active depression or with a history of psychosis or seizures and should be used with caution in people with psychiatric illness. Mefloquine can be given to patients taking α-blockers if they do not have an underlying arrhythmia; it should not be used in patients with conduction abnormalities. Mefloquine should not be given together with quinine, quinidine, or halofantrine, and caution is required in using quinine, quinidine, or halofantrine to treat patients with malaria who have taken mefloquine for prophylaxis. Resistance to mefloquine has been reported in some areas, such as the Thailand–Myanmar and Thailand–Cambodia borders and in the Amazon basin, where 25 mg/kg should be used. In the United States, a 250-mg tablet of mefloquine contains 228 mg mefloquine base. Outside the United States, each 275-mg tablet contains 250 mg base.

[i]Mefloquine has not been approved for use during pregnancy. However, it has been reported to be safe for prophylactic use during the second or third trimester of pregnancy and possibly during early pregnancy as well (CDC Health Information for International Travel, 2003–2004, p 111; Smoak BL, et al: J Infect Dis 176:831, 1997). For pediatric doses less than half a tablet, it is advisable to have a pharmacist crush the tablet, estimate doses by weighing, and packing them in gelatin capsules. There are no data for use in children <5 kg, but based on dosages in other weight groups, a dose of 5 mg/kg can be used. Mefloquine is not recommended for patients with cardiac conduction abnormalities, and patients with a history of depression, seizures, psychosis, or psychiatric disorders should avoid mefloquine prophylaxis. Resistance to mefloquine has been reported in some areas, such as the Thailand–Myanmar and Thailand–Cambodia borders; in these areas, atovaquone/proguanil or doxycycline should be used for prophylaxis.

[j]An approved drug but considered investigational for this condition by the FDA.

[k]Beginning 1 or 2 days before travel and continuing for the duration of stay and for 4 weeks after leaving. Use of tetracyclines is contraindicated in pregnancy and in children younger than 8 years old. Doxycycline can cause gastrointestinal disturbances, vaginal moniliasis, and photosensitivity reactions.

[l]Primaquine phosphate can cause hemolytic anemia, especially in patients whose red cells are deficient in glucose-6-phosphate dehydrogenase. This deficiency is most common in African, Asian, and Mediterranean peoples. Patients should be screened for G-6-PD deficiency before treatment. Primaquine should not be used during pregnancy.

[m]Studies have shown that daily primaquine beginning 1 day before departure and continued until 3–7 days after leaving the malaria area provides effective prophylaxis against chloroquine-resistant *P. falciparum* (Baird JK, et al: Clin Infect Dis 37:1659, 2003). Some studies have shown less efficacy against *P. vivax*. Nausea and abdominal pain can be diminished by taking with food.

[n]Proguanil (Paludrine–Wyeth Ayerst, Canada; AstraZeneca, United Kingdom), which is not available alone in the United States but is widely available in Canada and Europe, is recommended mainly for use in Africa south of Sahara. Prophylaxis is recommended during exposure and for 4 weeks afterwards. Proguanil has been used in pregnancy without evidence of toxicity (Phillips-Howard PA, Wood D: Drug Saf 14:131, 1996).

[o]A traveler can be given a treatment course of atovaquone/proguanil or pyrimethamine/sulfadoxine for presumptive self-treatment of febrile illness. This approach should be used only in very rare circumstances when a traveler cannot promptly receive medical care.

[p]In Southeast Asia, relative resistance to quinine has increased and treatment should be continued for 7 days.

Derived from *Medical Letter on Drugs and Therapeutics*, Drugs for parasitic infections, www.medicalletter.org, August 2004.

Table 13-5 Drugs Used for the Treatment of Malaria

Infection	Drug	Adult Dosage	Pediatric Dosage
***P. falciparum*[a] acquired in areas of chloroquine resistance**			
Oral[b]			
Drugs of choice:	Atovaquone/proguanil[c]	4 adult tabs daily × 3 days	<5 kg: not indicated 5–8 kg: 2 peds tabs once/day × 3 days 9–10 kg: 3 peds tabs once/day × 3 days 11–20 kg: 1 adult tab once/day × 3 days 21–30 kg: 2 adult tabs once/day × 3 days 31–40 kg: 3 adult tabs once/day × 3 days >40 kg: 4 adult tabs once/day × 3 days
	or Quinine sulfate	650 mg q8h × 3–7 days[d]	30 mg/kg/day in 3 doses × 3–7 days
	plus		
	doxycycline[e,f]	100 mg bid × 7 days	4 mg/kg/day in 2 doses × 7 days
	or plus		
	tetracycline[e,f]	250 mg qid × 7 days	6.25 mg/kg qid × 7 days
	or plus[g]		
	clindamycin[e,h]	20 mg/kg/day in 3 doses × 7 days[i]	20 mg/kg/day in 3 doses × 7 days
Alternatives:	Mefloquine[j]	750 mg followed 12 hr later by 500 mg	15 mg/kg followed 12 hr later by 10 mg/kg
	or Artesunate[k]	4 mg/kg/day × 3 days	4 mg/kg/day × 3 days
	plus		
	mefloquine[j]	750 mg followed 12 hr later by 500 mg	15 mg/kg followed 12 hr later by 10 mg/kg
***P. vivax*[l] acquired in areas of chloroquine resistance**			
Oral[l]			
Drug of choice:	Quinine sulfate	650 mg q8h × 3–7 days[d]	30 mg/kg/day in 3 doses × 3–7 days[d]
	plus		
	doxycycline[e,f]	100 mg bid × 7 days	4 mg/kg/day in 2 doses × 7 days
	or Mefloquine[j]	750 mg followed 12 hr later by 500 mg	15 mg/kg followed 12 hr later by 10 mg/kg
Alternatives:	Chloroquine	25 mg base/kg in 3 doses over 48 hr	
	plus		
	primaquine[m]	30 mg base daily × 14 days	0.6 mg/kg/day × 14 days
All *Plasmodium* except **chloroquine-resistant *P. falciparum*[a]** and **chloroquine-resistant *P. vivax*[l]**			
Oral[b]			
Drug of choice:	Chloroquine phosphate[n]	1 g (600 mg base), then 500 mg (300 mg base) 6 hr later, then 500 mg (300 mg base) at 24 and 48 hr	10 mg base/kg (max. 600 mg base), then 5 mg base/kg 6 hr later, then 5 mg base/kg at 24 and 48 hr
All *Plasmodium*			
Parenteral			
Drug of choice:[o]	Quinidine gluconate[p]	10 mg/kg loading dose (max. 600 mg) in normal saline over 1–2 hr followed by continuous infusion of 0.02 mg/kg/min until PO therapy can be started	10 mg/kg loading dose (max. 600 mg) in normal saline over 1–2 hr followed by continuous infusion of 0.02 mg/kg/min until PO therapy can be started
	OR Quinine dihydrochloride[p]	20 mg/kg loading dose in 5% dextrose over 4 hr, followed by 10 mg/kg over 2–4 hr q8h (max. 1800 mg/day) until PO therapy can be started	20 mg/kg loading dose in 5% dextrose over 4 hr, followed by 10 mg/kg over 2–4 hr q8h (max. 1800 mg/day) until PO therapy can be started
Alternative:	Artemether[q]	3.2 mg/kg IM, then 1.6 mg/kg daily × 5–7 days	3.2 mg/kg IM, then 1.6 mg/kg daily × 5–7 days

Continued

Table 13-5 Drugs Used for the Treatment of Malaria—cont'd

Infection	Drug	Adult Dosage	Pediatric Dosage
Prevention of relapses: ***P. vivax and P. ovale*** **only**			
Drug of choice:	Primaquine phosphate[m]	30 mg base/day × 14 days	0.6 mg base/kg/day × 14 days

[a]Chloroquine-resistant *P. falciparum* occurs in all malarious areas except Central America west of the Panama Canal Zone, Mexico, Haiti, the Dominican Republic, and most of the Middle East (chloroquine resistance has been reported in Yemen, Oman, Saudi Arabia, and Iran). For treatment of multiple drug-resistant *P. falciparum* in Southeast Asia, especially Thailand, where resistance to mefloquine is frequent, atovaquone/proguanil, artesunate plus mefloquine, or artemether plus mefloquine may be used (Luxemburger JC, et al: Trans R Soc Trop Med Hyg 88:213, 1994; Karbwang J, et al: Trans R Soc Trop Med Hyg 89:296, 1995).

[b]Uncomplicated or mild malaria may be treated with oral drugs.

[c]Atovaquone plus proguanil is avaliable as a fixed-dose combination tablet: adult tablets (Malarone; 250 mg atovaquone/100 mg proguanil) and pediatric tablets (Malarone Pediatric; 62.5 mg atovaquone/25 mg proguanil). To enhance absorption, it should be taken with food or a milky drink.* Some experts recommend dividing the daily dose and giving it bid to decrease the gastrointestinal side effects. Atovaquone/proguanil should not be given to pregnant women or patients with severe renal impairment (creatinine clearance <30mL/min). There have been several isolated reports of resistance in *P. falciparum* in Africa (Schwartz E, et al: Clin Infect Dis 37:450, 2003; Farnert A, et al: BMJ 326:628, 2003).

[d]In Southeast Asia, relative resistance to quinine has increased and treatment should be continued for 7 days.

[e]An approved drug but considered investigational for this condition by the FDA.

[f]Use of tetracyclines in contraindicated in pregnancy and in children younger than 8 years old.

[g]Fansidar is no longer recommended by the CDC nor used by most experts in North America because of widespread resistance and the potential for severe hypersensitivity reactions to sulfadoxine. Fansidar tablets contain 25 mg of pyrimethamine and 500 mg of sulfadoxine. The treatment dose is 3 tablets once for adults. For children it is $\frac{1}{4}$ tablet once for those <5 kg, $\frac{1}{2}$ tablet once for 5–10 kg, 1 tablet once for 11–20 kg, $1\frac{1}{2}$ tablet once for 21–30 kg, 2 tablets once for 31–40 kg, and 3 tablets once for >40 kg. Resistance to pyrimethamine-sulfadoxine has been reported from Southeast Asia, the Amazon basin, sub-Saharan Africa, Bangladesh, and Oceania.

[h]For use in pregnancy.

[i]Lell B, Kremsner PG: Antimicrob Agents Chemother 46:2315, 2002.

[j]At this dosage, adverse effects including nausea, vomiting, diarrhea, dizziness, disturbed sense of balance. toxic psychosis, and seizures can occur. Mefloquine should not be used for treatment of malaria in pregnancy unless there is no other treatment option because of increased risk for stillbirth (Nosten F, et al: Clin Infect Dis 28:808, 1999). It should be avoided for treatment of malaria in people with active depression or with a history of psychosis or seizures and should be used with caution in people with psychiatric illness. Mefloquine can be given to patients taking α-blockers if they do not have an underlying arrhythmia; it should not be used in patients with conduction abnormalities. Mefloquine should not be given together with quinine, quinidine, or halofantrine, and caution is required in using quinine, quinidine, or halofantrine to treat patients with malaria who have taken mefloquine for prophylaxis. Resistance to mefloquine has been reported in some areas, such as the Thailand–Myanmar and Thailand–Cambodia borders and in the Amazon basin, where 25 mg/kg should be used. In the United States, a 250-mg tablet of mefloquine contains 228 mg mefloquine base. Outside the United States each 275-mg tablet contains 250 mg base.

[k]Nosten F, et al: Lancet 356:297, 2000; van Vugt, M: Clin Infect Dis 35:1498, 2002.

[l]*P. vivax* with decreased susceptibility to chloroquine is a significant problem in Papua New Guinea and Indonesia. There are also a few reports of resistance from Myanmar, India, the Solomon Islands, Vanuatu, Guyana, Brazil, Colombia, and Peru.

[m]Primaquine phosphate can cause hemolytic anemia, especially in patients whose red cells are deficient in glucose-6-phosphate dehydrogenase. This deficiency is most common in African, Asian, and Mediterranean peoples. Patients should be screened for G6PD deficiency before treatment. Primaquine should not be used during pregnancy.

[n]If chloroquine phosphate is not available, hydroxychloroquine sulfate is as effective; 400 mg of hydroxychloroquine sulfate is equivalent to 500 mg of chloroquine phosphate.

[o]Exchange transfusion has been helpful for some patients with high-density (>10%) parasitemia, altered mental status, pulmonary edema, or renal complications (Miller KD, et al: N Engl J Med 321:65, 1989).

[p]Continuous ECG, blood pressure, and glucose monitoring is recommended, especially in pregnant women and young children. For problems with quinidine availability, call the manufacturers (Eli Lilly, 800-545-5979) or the CDC Malaria Hotline (770-488-7788). Quinidine may have greater antimalarial activity than quinine. The loading dose should be decreased or omitted in patients who have received quinine or mefloquine. If more than 48 hours of parenteral treatment is required, the quinine or quinidine dose should be reduced by 30% to 50%.

[q]Limited studies on efficacy except with *P. falciparum*; not FDA approved or available in the United States (Artemether-Quinine Meta-Analysis Study Group: Trans R Soc Trop Med Hyg 95:637, 2001; Marsh K: East Afr Med J 79:619, 2002).

Derived from *Medical Letter on Drugs and Therapeutics*, Drugs for parasitic infections, www.medicalletter.org, August 2004.

Box 13-2 Adverse Effects of Antimalarial Drugs

Artemether* (Artenam [Arenco, Belgium])
Occasional: neurologic toxicity, possible increase in length of coma, increased convulsions, prolongation of Q–Tc interval
Artesunate* (Guilin No. 1 Factory, People's Republic of China)
Occasional: ataxia, slurred speech, neurologic toxicity, possible increase in length of coma, increased convulsions, prolongation of Q–Tc interval
Atovaquone (Mepron [GlaxoSmithKline]; Malarone [with proguanil [GlaxoSmithKline])
Occasional: abdominal pain, nausea, vomiting, diarrhea, headache
Chloroquine HCl and chloroquine phosphate (Aralen [Sanofi], and others)
Occasional: pruritus; vomiting; headache; confusion; depigmentation of hair; skin eruptions; corneal opacity; weight loss; partial alopecia; extraocular muscle palsies; exacerbation of psoriasis, eczema, and other exfoliative dermatoses; myalgias; photophobia
Rare: irreversible retinal injury (especially when total dosage exceeds 100 g, discoloration of nails and mucous membranes, nerve-type deafness, peripheral neuropathy and myopathy, heart block, blood dyscrasias, hematemesis
Mefloquine (Lariam [Roche])
Frequent: vertigo, lightheadedness, nausea, other gastrointestinal disturbances, nightmares, visual disturbances, headache, insomnia
Occasional: confusion, psychological disturbance
Rare: psychosis, hypotension, convulsions, coma, paresthesias
Primaquine phosphate USP
Frequent: hemolytic anemia in glucose-6-phosphate dehydrogenase deficiency
Occasional: neutropenia, gastrointestinal disturbances, methemoglobinemia
Rare: CNS symptoms, hypertension, arrhythmias
Proguanil* (Paludrine [Wyeth–Ayerst, Canada; AstraZeneca, United Kingdom], or with atovaquone, Malarone [GlaxoSmithKline])
Occasional: oral ulceration, hair loss, scaling of palms and soles, urticaria
Rare: hematuria (with large doses), vomiting, abdominal pain, diarrhea (with large doses), thrombocytopenia
Quinine dihydrochloride* and sulfate (many manufacturers)
Frequent: cinchonism (tinnitus, headache, nausea, abdominal pain, visual disturbance)
Occasional: deafness, hemolytic anemia, other blood dyscrasias, photosensitivity reactions, hypoglycemia, arrhythmias, hypotension, drug fever
Rare: blindness, sudden death if injected too rapidly

*Not available in the United States.

the tropics. The use of long-sleeved clothing, screens, and bed nets, the application of insect repellants with diethylmetatolumide to exposed skin, and the use of permethrin or related residual insecticides on clothing and bed nets reduce the risk of Anopheline mosquito bites and transmission of malaria, but chemoprophylaxis is still necessary.[37–39]

Chloroquine is the drug of choice for the prophylaxis and treatment of malaria caused by chloroquine-sensitive *Plasmodium vivax*, *Plasmodium ovale*, *Plasmodium malariae*, and *Plasmodium falciparum*.[3,37–39] Primaquine is used to prevent later relapses of *P. vivax* and *P. ovale*. It is the only currently available drug that is active against hypnozoites of those species.

Plasmodium falciparum and, to a lesser extent, *P. vivax* are notable among protozoa for their propensity to develop resistance to chemotherapeutic agents. Chloroquine resistance is widespread among *P. falciparum*. Only in Central America west of the Panama Canal, Haiti, adjacent areas of the Dominican Republic, and some areas of the Middle East can *P. falciparum* isolates be considered sensitive. Chloroquine-resistant *P. vivax* is well documented in Indonesia and some other areas,[40] but they are still focal and limited in number. Doxycycline, the fixed combination of atovaquone–proguanil (Malarone), or mefloquine can be used for chemoprophylaxis in areas where chloroquine-resistant *P. falciparum* or *P. vivax* are endemic.[3,37–39] The untoward effects of mefloquine, particularly its neuropsychiatric side effects, have been a source of increasing concern and limit its use.[41] Daily primaquine is another option in special circumstances. Quinine sulfate with tetracycline, treatment doses of mefloquine, or treatment doses of atovaquone–progunail (in uncomplicated cases) are used for the therapy of acute chloroquine-resistant *P. falciparum* malaria. Halofantrine has been used for chloroquine-resistant malaria in Africa, but it is associated with prolonged QT interval and sudden death. It should be avoided unless no alternatives are available.

Resistance to mefloquine and quinine has emerged in rural areas of Thailand, elsewhere in Southeast Asia, and some other regions. Artesunate and other artemisinin derivatives, which have not been approved by the U.S. Food and Drug Administration (FDA), are used in Southeast Asia and some other areas of the world for the treatment of resistant *P. falciparum* infections. Specific recommendations for malaria prophylaxis and treatment depend on the infecting species and site of acquisition. The Centers for Disease Control and Prevention (CDC) provides recommendations for specific countries.[37] Drugs used for the treatment and prevention of malaria are summarized in Tables 13-4 and 13-5.

Chloroquine, a 4-aminoquinoline, remains the drug of choice for the prophylaxis and treatment of chloroquine-sensitive *P. vivax*, *P. ovale*, *P. malariae*, and *P. falciparum* malaria. Its mechanism of action has been extensively studied. It is concentrated in the hemoglobin-containing digestive vesicles of asexual intraerythrocytic parasites. Chloroquinine inhibits the parasite's heme polymerase that incorporates ferriprotoporphyrin IX, which is potentially toxic to the parasite, into insoluble, nontoxic, crystalline hemozoin.[42] Chloroquine-resistant strains of *P. falciparum* actively transport chloroquine out of the intraparasitic compartment. Although this can be blocked by calcium channel inhibitors in vitro, chloroquine resistance has not been effectively reversed in humans. Hydroxychloroquine (Plaquenil) is also effective for prophylaxis against chloroquine-sensitive *Plasmodium* species.

Chloroquine has a bitter taste, but it is well absorbed from the gastrointestinal tract. The half-life, which varies, averages 4 days, permitting once-weekly administration for prophylaxis. Approximately half of the parent drug is excreted unchanged in the urine and the remainder is metabolized in the liver. Chloroquine is generally well tolerated when used at the doses recommended for the prophylaxis and treatment of malaria. Side effects include headache, nausea, vomiting, blurred vision, dizziness, and fatigue. Some Africans and African Americans experience pruritus, which responds to antihistamines. Rare side effects include depigmentation of hair, exacerbation of psoriasis, blood dyscrasias, seizures, neuropsychiatric effects, and reactions in people with porphyria. Retinal damage has occurred in people receiving chloroquine at high doses for the treatment of rheumatologic disorders, but it has not been documented as a problem in people taking it weekly over many years for malaria prophylaxis.[43] Chloroquine has been used for chemoprophylaxis during pregnancy.

Children are more sensitive to the toxic effects of chloroquine than adults, and cardiopulmonary collapse and death have occurred following accidental overdoses and in adults attempting suicide. As little as 1 g of chloroquine can be fatal in children unless treatment is initiated with mechanical respiration, diazepam to control seizures, and blood pressure support.[44] An intravenous preparation of chloroquine is available outside the United States, but it must be given slowly and with great caution because of its propensity to produce respiratory depression, heart block, hypotension, cardiovascular collapse, and seizures.

Primaquine, an 8-aminoquinoline, is the only drug currently available that can eradicate hypnozoites of *P. vivax* and *P. ovale* in the liver. It is administered to people with *P. vivax* and *P. ovale* infections to prevent relapses. Relatively resistant strains of *P. vivax* have been reported from the Southwest Pacific, Southeast Asia, South America, and East Africa.[45–47] People infected with such strains often respond to higher doses of primaquine. Primaquine can also be used in special circumstances for prophylaxis against chloroquine-resistant *P. falciparum* and other forms of malaria, but recipients must be tested to ensure that they do not have glucose-6-phosphate dehydrogenase (G6PD) deficiency.[48] Primaquine plus clindamycin is an alternative to trimethoprim-sulfamethoxazole for the treatment of *Pneumocystis jiroveci* pneumonia in people who cannot tolerate sulfonamides.

Primaquine is well absorbed orally and rapidly converted to carboxyprimaquine, which has a half-life of approximately 7 days. The precise mechanism of action is unknown, but it is thought to interfere with mitochondrial function and possibly the transport of vesicles in the parasite. Primaquine is generally well tolerated, although some recipients experience abdominal cramps, epigastic distress, and nausea. The major concern is hemolysis in people with G6PD deficiency.[49] The G6PD status of the recipient should be determined before it is administered. Altered dosage schedules can be used in Africans with G6PD deficiency. Rarely, primaquine causes neutropenia, methemoglobinemia, hypertension, or arrhythmias. Primaquine is contraindicated during pregnancy and in breast-feeding mothers because life-threatening hemolysis may occur in the fetus or baby if they are G6PD deficient. Travelers should be warned not to give the drug to fellow travelers who have not been screened for G6PD deficiency.

Quinine sulfate, a cinchona alkaloid, is the oldest of the antimalarials.[50] With the exception of quinine-resistant *P. falciparum* strains in Thailand and adjacent areas of Southeast Asia, quinine is effective against all four *Plasmodium* species, including chloroquine-resistant *P. falciparum*. The mechanism of its action is unknown, but quinine is thought to act at the level of the parasites' hemoglobin-containing digestive vesicle and may interfere with ferriprotoporphyrin IX metabolism.

Quinine has a very bitter taste. It is rapidly absorbed after oral administration and has a half-life of 16 to 18 hours in people with malaria. It is metabolized in the liver, and the native drug and its metabolites are excreted in the urine. Quinine has the poorest therapeutic-to-toxicity ratio of any antimalarial drug. The side effects, known collectively as cinchonism, include tinnitus, decreased hearing, headache, nausea, vomiting, dysphoria, and visual disturbances. They are dose related and reversible.

Quinine has also been associated with severe hypoglycemia in people with heavy *P. falciparum* infections due to the utilization of glucose by the parasites and release of insulin from the pancreas.[51] Hypoglycemia can be prevented or treated by the administration of intravenous glucose. Rare complications with quinine include massive hemolysis in patients with heavy *P. falciparum* infections resulting in hemoglobinuria and renal failure (blackwater fever), cutaneous hypersensitivity reactions, agranulocytosis, and hepatitis. Quinine can cause respiratory paralysis in people with myasthenia gravis. It stimulates uterine contractions and can produce abortions, but it has saved the lives of many pregnant women with *P. falciparum* malaria.

Quinidine gluconate, the stereoisomer of quinine, is recommended for the intravenous treatment of patients with acute malaria who cannot take quinine by mouth.[52,53] Quinidine gluconate is well-known for its role in the treatment of ventricular ectopy. Its side effects include prolongation of the Q-T interval, arrhythmias, and hypotension, particularly if it is infused too rapidly. People receiving intravenous quinidine should be monitored in an intensive care setting and changed to the oral quinine as soon as they can take medications by mouth. Where it is available, intravenous quinine dihydrochloride can be used if quinidine is not available. It, too, can produce myocardial depression, peripheral vascular collapse, respiratory depression, and death. Patients must be monitored closely during its infusion. Intravenous therapy with either drug should be terminated as soon as the patient is able to take oral drugs.

Mefloquine, a quinoline methanol compound derived from quinine, has been widely used for the prophylaxis and treatment of chloroquine-resistant *P. falciparum* malaria.[54] It is active against all four *Plasmodium* species, including those that are resistant to chloroquine. Mefloquine-resistant strains of *P. falciparum* are common in rural areas of Thailand and adjacent countries, and they have been reported from some other areas.

Mefloquine is available for oral administration only, and it is slowly and incompletely absorbed. It is 99% protein bound and has a variable half-life ranging from 6 to 23 days, with a mean of approximately 14 days. It is metabolized and excreted slowly through the bile and feces. Mefloquine appears to interfere with the food vacuoles of the intraerythrocytic asexual stage of the parasite.

Considerable attention has been paid to the untoward effects of mefloquine.[41] It is reasonably well tolerated in most recipients, although it can cause transient nausea, dizziness, vivid dreams, fatigue, and lassitude. Less common, but of substantial concern, are neuropsychiatric reactions that include anxiety, depression, acute psychosis, and seizures. Mefloquine is therefore contraindicated in people with a history of epilepsy or psychiatric problems. It can depress atrial–ventricular conduction and should not be used by patients with cardiac conduction defects. Mefloquine may be used in people taking β-blockers if they have no underlying arrhythmias. Mefloquine also has antibacterial activity, and it can inactivate the live oral typhoid vaccine (*Salmonella typhi* Ty21a) if administered concurrently. Rare side effects include exfoliative erythroderma, agranulocytosis, and paresthesias. Mefloquine is not approved by the FDA for use during pregnancy or in children who weigh less than 15 kg, but it is used in situations in which the potential benefits are judged to outweigh the risks.[55]

Halofantrine, a 9-phenanthrenemethanol, has activity against the asexual, intraerythrocytic stages of chloroquine-sensitive and chloroquine-resistant strains of *P. falciparum*, *P. vivax*, *P. ovale*, and *P. malariae*. It is not approved for use in the United States, but it is used in Africa. Halofantrine is variably absorbed after oral administration; higher levels are obtained if the drug is taken with a fatty meal. The half-life of the native drug is 1 or 2 days and that of its active metabolite is 3 to 5 days. It is excreted primarily in the feces. Halofantrine produces prolongation of the Q-T interval and has been associated with sudden death, presumably due to cardiac arrhythmias.[56]

Doxycycline taken daily provides effective prophylaxis against all *Plasmodium* species. Either tetracycline or doxycycline can be administered with quinine to treat acute chloroquine-resistant malaria. They do not act quickly enough to be used alone. The tetracyclines are well absorbed after oral administration, and they are generally well tolerated. They can produce gastrointestinal symptoms. Doxycycline can also cause severe esophagitis if it does not pass through to the stomach. Consequently, it should be taken with a full glass of water and the recipient should remain upright for 1 hour after ingestion. Other potential untoward effects include photosensitivity dermatitis, *Candida albicans* vaginitis, and antibiotic-associated colitis. Finally, tetracyclines should not be used in children younger than 8 years of age because of the potential for dental staining or in pregnant women.

Pyrimethamine alone or with sulfonamides has been used in the prevention and treatment of malaria, but resistance is now widespread. The two inhibit sequential steps in the folic acid metabolic pathway. Sulfonamides reduce the activity of dihydropteroate synthetase and reduce the binding of *p*-aminobenzoic acid to it. Pyrimethamine preferentially inhibits dihydrofolate reductase in susceptible parasites. Fansidar[57] is a fixed combination of pyrimethamine (25 mg) and sulfadoxine (500 mg), a long-acting sulfonamide with a half-life of 5 to 9 days. It has been associated with life-threatening cutaneous hypersensitivity reactions in people allergic to sulfonamides and is no longer marketed in the United States.

The most recent advance in the prevention and treatment of malaria is the fixed combination of atovaquone and proguanil (Malarone, adult tablets contain atovaquone 250 mg and proguanil 100 mg). It can be used for prophylaxis in areas with chloroquine-resistant *P. falciparum* and for the treatment of uncomplicated *P. falciparum* infections.[58,59] Malarone is better tolerated than mefloquine or doxycycline. Atovaquone used as a single drug also has activity against *Pneumocystis jiroveci*.[60]

Atovaquone is a highly lipophilic compound with low aqueous solubility. Administration with food enhances its absorption twofold. Plasma concentrations do not increase proportionately with dose. Atovaquone is highly protein bound, with a half-life exceeding 60 hours. There is extensive enterohepatic cycling, and it is eventually excreted unchanged in the feces. Atovaquone selectively inhibits electron transport at the level of the cytochrome bc_1 complex, which results in collapse of the parasite's mitochondrial membrane potential. It also affects pyrimidine biosynthesis, which is obligatorily coupled to electron transport in *Plasmodium* through ubiquinone/ubiquinol. Resistance develops rapidly when atovaquone is used alone to treat malaria. It is generally well tolerated but can cause gastrointestinal side effects, including nausea, vomiting, and diarrhea, as well as skin rash and pruritus.

Proguanil is slowly absorbed after oral administration. The serum level falls to zero within 24 hours, so it must be taken daily for prophylaxis. Its triazine metabolite, cycloguanil, inhibits dihydrofolate reductase in susceptible *Plasmodium*. Resistance is well documented among *Plasmodium* species when the drug is used alone. Proguanil also acts synergistically with atovaquone to collapse mitochondrial membrane potential in *Plasmodium*. It is generally well tolerated. At higher doses it can cause nausea, vomiting, abdominal pain, and diarrhea. Hematological effects occur rarely.

The combination of atovaquone–proguanil (Malarone) is administered daily, starting 1 or 2 days before exposure, during travel, and for 7 days after the last potential exposure. It is generally well tolerated, but abdominal pain, nausea, vomiting, diarrhea, headache, pruritus, and rash may occur. Asymptomatic, transient elevations of liver enzymes have been observed with treatment doses of Malarone.

Artemisinin and its derivatives, which include artesunate, artemether, and arteether, are sesquiterpene lactones derived from the Chinese herbal medication for malaria, quinghaosu, which comes from the wormwood plant, *Artemisin annua*.[61,62] They are endoperoxide-containing compounds. In the presence of intraparasitic iron, they are thought to be converted into free radicals and other intermediates that alkylate specific malarial proteins and act rapidly to kill intraerythrocytic parasites. They are usually administered with a second antimalarial drug to prevent relapses. Although not licensed for use in the United States, artesunate and other artemisinin derivatives are widely used in Thailand and elsewhere to treat patients with mefloquine-resistant and/or quinine-resistant *P. falciparum* malaria.[61,62] The route of administration varies; some are administered orally, whereas others are given intravenously, intramuscularly, or by suppository. They are rapidly cleared from the circulation. Adverse effects are infrequent and mild. They include abdominal pain, diarrhea, and drug fever. Decreased reticulocytes and neutrophils and cerebellar dysfunction have been observed. Contact dermatitis has also been associated with sesquiterpene lactones. Neuropathic effects have been reported in dogs given chronic, high-dose therapy. The short half-life of the artemisinin derivatives and concern about potential neurotoxicity have precluded their use for malaria prophylaxis.

Toxoplasmosis, Babesiosis, and Pneumocystis Pneumonia

Like *Plasmodium* species, *Toxoplasma gondii* and *Babesia* species are important pathogens of the phylum Apicomplexa. The medications used to treat them and their untoward effects are summarized in Box 13-3 and Table 13-6. They include

Box 13-3 Adverse Effects of Drugs Used to Treat Other Protozoa

Atovaquone (Mepron [GlaxoSmithKline])
Frequent: rash, nausea
Occasional: nausea, vomiting, diarrhea, rash
Dapsone (Jacobus)
Frequent: rash, transient headache, gastrointestinal irritation, anorexia, infectious mononucleosis–like syndrome
Occasional: cyanosis due to methemoglobinemia and sulfhemoglobinemia; other blood dyscrasias, including hemolytic anemia; nephrotic syndrome; liver damage; peripheral neuropathy; hypersensitivity reactions; increased risk of lepra reactions; insomnia; irritability; uncoordinated speech; agitation; acute psychosis
Rare: renal papillary necrosis, severe hypoalbuminemia, epidermal necrolysis, optic atrophy, agranulocytosis, neonatal hyperbilirubinemia after use in pregnancy
Pyrimethamine USP (Daraprim [GlaxoSmithKline])
Occasional: blood dyscrasias, folic acid deficiency
Rare: rash, vomiting, convulsions, shock, possibly pulmonary eosinophilia, fatal cutaneous reactions with pyrimethamine-sulfadoxine (Fansidar)
Spiramycin (Rovamycine [Aventis])
Occasional: gastrointestinal disturbances
Rare: allergic reactions

several of the antimalarial drugs discussed previously and the antibiotics clindamycin, azithromycin and spiramycin that act at the ribosomal level. Pyrimethamine and sulfadiazine are recommended for the treatment of toxoplasmosis. Clindamycin is an alternative to sulfadiazine for people with sulfonamide allergies. The macrolide, spiramycin, is recommended for the treatment of toxoplasmosis during pregnancy. Atovaquone plus azithromycin are now the first choice for babesiosis. Clindamycin and quinine are effective but more toxic. Trimethoprim-sulfamethoxazole, dapsone (a sulfone widely used in the treatment of leprosy), and several other drugs used for protozoal diseases are used in the treatment of *Pneumocystis jiroveci* as summarized in Table 13-6.

TREATMENT OF INTESTINAL AND VAGINAL PROTOZOA

Several major luminal pathogens, *Entamoeba histolytica*, *Giardia lamblia*, and *Trichomonas vaginalis*, which live in anaerobic conditions in the intestine or vagina, are susceptible to metronidazole or tinidazole.[63,64] The latter recently gained FDA approval (Table 13-7). The recommended treatment of these and other intestinal protozoal infections and the associated untoward effects are summarized in Tables 13-7 and Box 13-4, respectively. *Cryptosporidium*, which has been responsible for major water-borne epidemics in North America and elsewhere and is an important pathogen in people with AIDS, is resistant to most antimicrobial agents. Nitazoxanide has proven to be effective for cryptosporidiosis in immunocompetent children. Unfortunately, failures have been common in those with AIDS.[65] Nitazoxanide, which is available in oral formulation, is also approved for the treatment of giardiasis in children. Trimethoprim-sulfamethoxazole, which inhibits successive steps in the folic acid pathway, is effective for the treatment of *Isospora belli* and *Cyclospora cayetanensis*. Ciprofloxacin, a fluoroquinolone antibiotic that acts on topoisomerase II, is an alternative. Albendazole is used to treat intestinal microsporidiosis due to *Encephalitozoon [Septata] intestinalis* and ocular and disseminated disease caused by some other microsporidia species.

Metronidazole, a nitroimidazole that is active only under anaerobic conditions, is used in the treatment of *E. histolytica*, *G. lamblia*, and *T. vaginalis* as well as for anaerobic bacterial diseases. It is activated by reduction of its 5-nitro group through a sequence of intermediate steps involving microbial electron transport proteins of low redox potential. It is concentrated in anaerobic organisms and serves as an electron sink.

Metronidazole is rapidly absorbed after oral administration and has a half-life of 8 hours. More than half of each dose is

Box 13-4 Adverse Effects of Drugs Used in the Treatment of Luminal Protozoal Infections

Diloxanide furoate* (Furamide [Boots, United Kingdom])
Frequent: flatulence
Occasional: nausea, vomiting, diarrhea
Rare: diplopia, dizziness, utricaria, pruritus
Furazolidone* (Furoxone [Roberts])
Frequent: nausea, vomiting
Occasional: allergic reactions, including pulmonary infiltration, hypotension, utricaria, fever, vesicular rash; hypoglycemia; headache
Rare: hemolytic anemia in glucose-6-phosphate dehydrogenase deficiency and neonates, disulfiram-like reaction with alcohol, monoamine oxidase inhibitor interactions, polyneuritis
Iodoquinol (Yodoxin [Glenwood], others)
Occasional: rash, acne, slight enlargement of the thyroid gland, nausea, diarrhea, cramps, and pruritus
Rare: optic neuritis, optic atrophy, loss of vision, peripheral neuropathy after prolonged use in high dosage (for months); iodine sensitivity
Metronidazole (Flagyl [Searle], others)
Frequent: nausea, headache, metallic taste, anorexia
Occasional: vomiting, diarrhea, insomnia, weakness, stomatitis, vertigo, tinnitus, paresthesias, rash, dry mouth, dark urine, urethral burning, disulfiram-like reaction with alcohol, candidiasis
Rare: seizures, encephalopathy, pseudomembranous colitis, ataxia, leukopenia, peripheral neuropathy, pancreatitis
Nitazoxanide (Alinia [Romark])
Occasional: gastrointestinal side effects
Ornidazole* (Tiberal [Roche, France])
Occasional: dizziness, headache, gastrointestinal disturbances
Rare: reversible peripheral neuropathy
Paromomycin (aminosidine; Humatin [Monarch]; Leshcutan* [Teva, Israel])
Frequent: gastrointestinal disturbances with oral use
Occasional: vestibular nerve damage (mainly auditory) and renal damage when aminosidine is given IV; vertigo; pancreatitis
Tinidazole (Tindamax [Presutti])
Occasional: metallic taste, nausea, vomiting, rash
Albendazole (see Box 13-1)

*Not available in the United States.

Table 13-6 Treatment of Other Protozoal Diseases

Infection	Drug	Adult Dosage	Pediatric Dosage
Acanthamoeba keratitis			
Drug of choice:	See footnote[a]		
Amebic Meningoencephalitis, primary and granulomatous			
Naegleria			
Drug of choice:	Amphotericin B[b,c]	1.5 mg/kg/day in 2 doses × 3 days, then 1 mg/kg/day × 6 days	1.5 mg/kg/day in 2 doses × 3 days, then 1 mg/kg/day × 6 days
Acanthamoeba			
Drug of choice:	See footnote[d]		
Balamuthia mandrillaris			
Drug of choice:	See footnote[e]		
Sappinia diploidea			
Drug of choice:	See footnote[f]		
Babesiosis (*Babesia microti*)			
Drugs of choice:[g]	Clindamycin[h]	1.2 g bid IV or 600 mg tid PO × 7–10 days	20–40 mg/kg/day PO in 3 doses × 7–10 days
	plus quinine[h]	650 mg tid PO × 7–10 days	25 mg/kg/day PO in 3 doses × 7–10 days
	or Atovaquone[h]	750 mg bid × 7–10 days	20 mg/kg bid × 7–10 days
	plus azithromycin[h]	600 mg daily × 7–10 days	12 mg/kg daily × 7–10 days
Microsporidiosis			
Ocular (*Encephalitozoon hellem, Encephalitozoon cuniculi, Vittaforma corneae [Nosema corneum]*)			
Drug of choice:	Albendazole:[h]	400 mg bid	
	plus fumagillin[i]		
Disseminated (*E. hellem, E.cuniculi, E. intestinalis, Pleistophora* sp., *Trachipleistophora* sp., *Brachiola vesicularum*)			
Drug of choice:[j]	Albendazole[h]	400 mg bid	
Pneumocystis jiroveci (formerly *carinii*) pneumonia (PCP)[k]			
Drug of choice:	Trimethoprim/sulfamethoxazole (TMP)	TMP 15 mg/kg/day, SMX 75 mg/kg/day, PO or IV in 3 or 4 doses × 14–21 days	TMP 15 mg/kg/day, SMX 75 mg/kg/day, PO or IV in 3 or 4 doses × 14–21 days
Alternatives:	Primaquine[h,l]	30 mg base PO daily × 21 days	
	plus clindamycin[h]	600 mg IV q6h × 21 days, or 300–450 mg PO q6h × 21 days	
	or Trimethoprim[h]	5 mg/kg tid × 21 days	
	plus dapsone	100 mg daily × 21 days	
	or Pentamidine	3–4 mg/kg IV daily × 14–21 days	3–4 mg/kg IV daily x 14–21 days
	or Atovaquone	750 mg bid × 21 days	1–3 mo: 30 mg/kg/day 4–24 mo: 45 mg/kg/day >24 mo: 30 mg/day
Primary and secondary prophylaxis[m]			
Drug of choice:	Trimethoprim/sulfamethoxazole (TMP)	1 tab (single or double strength) daily	TMP 150 mg/m², SMX 750 mg/m² in 2 doses on 3 consecutive days/wk
Alternatives:[n]	Dapsone[h]	50 mg bid, or 100 mg daily	2 mg/kg/day (max. 100 mg) or 4 mg/kg (max. 200 mg) each wk
	or Dapsone[h]	50 mg daily or 200 mg each wk	
	plus pyrimethamine[o]	50 mg or 75 mg each wk	
	or Pentamidine aerosol	300 mg inhaled monthly via *Respirgard II* nebulizer	≥5 yr: 300 mg inhaled monthly via *Respirgard II* nebulizer
	or Atovaquone[h]	1500 mg daily	1–3 mo: 30 mg/kg/day 4–24 mo: 45 mg/kg/day >24 mo: 30 mg/kg/day

Continued

Table 13-6 *Treatment of Other Protozoal Diseases—Cont'd*

Infection	Drug	Adult Dosage	Pediatric Dosage
Toxoplasmosis (*Toxoplasma gondii*)[p]			
Drugs of choice:[q,r]	Pyrimethamine[s]	25–100 mg/day × 3–4 wk	2 mg/kg/day × 3 days, then 1 mg/kg/day (max. 25 mg/day) × 4 wk[t]
	plus		
	sulfadiazine	1–1.5 g qid 3–4 wk	100–200 mg/kg/day × 3–4 wk

[a]For treatment of keratitis caused by Acanthamoeba, concurrent topical use of 0.1% propamidine isethionate (Brolene) plus neomycin-polymyxin B-gramicidin ophthalmic solution has been successful (Hargrave SL, et al: Ophthalmology 106:952, 1999). In some European countries, propamidine is not available and hexamidine (Desmodine) has been used (Seal DV: Eye 17:893, 2003). In addition, 0.02% topical polyhexamethylene biguanide (PHMB) and/or chlorhexadine has been used successfully in a large number of patients (Tabin G, et al: Cornea 20:757, 2001; Wysenbeek YS, et al: Cornea 19:464, 2000). PHMB is available from Leiter's Park Avenue Pharmacy, San Jose, CA (800-292-6773; www.leiterrx.com). The combination of chlorhexadine, natamycin (pimaricin), and debridement has also been successful (Kitagawa K, et al: Jpn J Ophthalmol 47:616, 2003).

[b]*Naegleria* infection has been treated successfully with intravenous and intrathecal use of both amphotericin B and miconazole plus rifampin and with amphotericin B, rifampin, and ornidazole (Seidel J, et al: N Engl J Med 306:346, 1982; Jain R, et al: Neurol India 50:470, 2002). Other reports of successful therapy are less well documented.

[c]An approved drug but considered investigational for this condition by the FDA.

[d]Strains of *Acanthamoeba* isolated from fatal granulomatous amebic encephalitis are usually susceptible in vitro to pentamidine, ketoconazole, flucytosine, and (less so) to amphotericin B. Chronic *Acanthamoeba* meningitis has been successfully treated in two children with a combination of oral trimethoprim/sulfamethoxazole, rifampin, and ketoconazole (Singhal T, et al: Pediatr Infect Dis J 20:623, 2001) and in an AIDS patient with fluconazole, sulfadiazine, and pyrimethamine combined with surgical resection of the CNS lesion (Seijo Martinez M, et al: J Clin Microbiol 38:3892, 2000). Disseminated cutaneous infection in an immunocompromised patient has been treated successfully with IV pentamidine isethionate, topical chlorhexidine, and 2% ketoconazole cream, followed by oral itraconazole (Slater CA, et al: N Engl J Med 331:85, 1994).

[e]A free-living leptomyxid ameba that causes subacute to fatal granulomatous CNS disease. Several cases of *Balamuthia* encephalitis have been successfully treated with flucytosine, pentamidine, fluconazole, and sulfadiazine plus either azithromycin or clarithromycin (phenothiazines were also used) combined with surgical resection of the CNS lesion (Deetz TR, et al: Clin Infect Dis 37:1304, 2003; Jung S, et al: Arch Pathol Lab Med 128:466, 2004).

[f]A free-living ameba not previously known to be pathogenic to humans. It has been successfully treated with azithromycin, IV pentamidine, itraconazole, and flucytosine combined with surgical resection of the CNS lesion (Gelman BB, et al: J Neuropathol Exp Neurol 62:990, 2003).

[g]Exchange transfusion has been used in severely ill patients and those with high (>10%) parasitemia (Hatcher JC, et al: Clin Infect Dis 32:1117, 2001). In patients who were not severely ill, combination therapy with atovaquone and azithromycin was as effective as clindamycin and quinine and may have been better tolerated (Krause PJ, et al: N Engl J Med 343:1454, 2000).

[h]An approved drug but considered investigational for this condition by the FDA.

[i]Ocular lesions due to *E. hellem* in HIV-infected patients have responded to fumagillin eyedrops prepared from Fumidil-B (bicyclohexyl ammonium fumagillin) used to control a microsporidial disease of honey bees (Diesenhouse MG: Am J Ophthalmol 115:293, 1993), available from Leiter's Park Avenue Pharmacy. For lesions due to *V. corneae*, topical therapy is generally not effective and keratoplasty may be required (Davis RM, et al: Ophthalmology 97:953, 1990).

[j]Molina J-M, et al: J Infect Dis 171:245, 1995. There is no established treatment for *Pleistophora*. For disseminated disease due to *Trachipleistophora* or *Brachiola*, itraconazole 400 mg PO once/day plus albendazole may also be tried (Coyle CM, et al: N Engl J Med 351:42, 2004).

[k]Pneumocystis has been reclassified as a fungus. In severe disease with room air $PO_2 \le 70$ mmHg or Aa gradient ≥35 mmHg, prednisone should also be used (Gagnon S, et al: N Engl J Med 323:1444, 1990; Caumes E, et al: Clin Infect Dis 18:319, 1994).

[l]Primaquine phosphate can cause hemolytic anemia, especially in patients whose red cells are deficient in glucose-6-phosphate dehydrogenase. This deficiency is most common in African, Asian, and Mediterranean peoples. Patients should be screened for G6PD deficiency before treatment. Primaquine should not be used during pregnancy.

[m]Primary/secondary prophylaxis in patients with HIV can be discontinued after CD4 count increases to $>200 \times 10^6$/L for >3 months.

[n]An alternative trimethoprim/sulfamethoxazole regimen is one DS tab 3x/week. Weekly therapy with sulfadoxine 500 mg/pyrimethamine 25 mg/leucovorin 25 mg was effective PCP prophylaxis in liver transplant patients (Torre-Cisneros J, et al: Clin Infect Dis 29:771, 1999).

[o]Plus leucovorin 25 mg with each dose of pyrimethamine.

[p]In ocular toxoplasmosis with macular involvement, corticosteroids are recommended in addition to antiparasitic therapy for an anti-inflammatory effect.

[q]To treat CNS toxoplasmosis in HIV-infected patients, some clinicians have used pyrimethamine 50–100 mg/day (after a loading dose of 200 mg) with sulfadiazine and, when sulfonamide sensitivity developed, have given clindamycin 1.8–2.4 g/day in divided doses instead of the sulfonamide. Atovaquone plus pyrimethamine appears to be an effective alternative in sulfa-intolerant patients (Chirgwin K, et al: Clin Infect Dis 34:1243, 2002). Treatment is followed by chronic suppression with lower dosage regimens of the same drugs. For primary prophylaxis in HIV patients with $<100 \times 10^6$/L CD4 cells, trimethoprim-sulfamethoxazole, pyrimethamine with dapsone, or atovaquone with or without pyrimethamine can be used. Primary or secondary prophylaxis may be discontinued when the CD4 count increases to $>200 \times 10^6$/L for more than 3 months (USPHS/IDSA Guidelines for the Treatment of Opportunistic Infections in Adults and Adolescents with HIV, 2004).

[r]Women who develop toxoplasmosis during the first trimester of pregnancy can be treated with spiramycin (3–4 g/day). After the first trimester, if there is no documented transmission to the fetus, spiramycin can be continued until term. If transmission has occurred in utero, therapy with pyrimethamine and sulfadiazine should be started (Montoya JG, Liesenfeld O: Lancet 363:1965, 2004). Pyrimethamine is a potential teratogen and should be used only after the first trimester.

[s]Plus leucovorin 10–25 mg with each dose of pyrimethamine.

[t]Congenitally infected newborns should be treated with pyrimethamine every 2 or 3 days and a sulfonamide daily for about 1 year (Remington JS, Desmonts G: In Remington JS, Klein JO (eds), Infectious Disease of the Fetus and Newborn Infant, 5th ed. Philadelphia: Saunders, 2001, p. 290).

Derived from the *Medical Letter on Drugs and Therapeutics*, Drugs for parasitic infections, www.medicalletter.org, August 2004.

Table 13-7 Treatment of Luminal Protozoa

Infection	Drug	Adult Dosage	Pediatric Dosage
Amebiasis (*Entamoeba histolytica*)			
Asymptomatic			
Drug of choice:	Iodoquinol	650 mg tid × 20 days	30–40 mg/kg/day (max. 2 g) in 3 doses × 20 days
	or Paromomycin	25–35 mg/kg/day in 3 doses × 7 days	25–35 mg/kg/day in 3 doses × 7 days
Alternative:	Diloxanide furoate[a]	500 mg tid × 10 days	20 mg/kg/day in 3 doses × 10 days
Mild to moderate intestinal disease[b]			
Drug of choice:[c]	Metronidazole	500–750 mg tid × 7–10 days	35–50 mg/kg/day in 3 doses × 7–10 days
	or Tinidazole[d]	2 g once daily × 3 days	50 mg/kg/day (max. 2 g) in 1 dose × 3 days
Severe intestinal and extraintestinal disease[b]			
Drug of choice:	Metronidazole	750 mg tid × 7–10 days	35–50 mg/kg/day in 3 doses × 7–10 days
	or Tinidazole[d]	2 g once daily × 5 days	50 mg/kg/day (max. 2 g) × 5 days
Balantidiasis (*Balantidium coli*)			
Drug of choice:	Tetracycline[e,f]	500 mg qid × 10 days	40 mg/kg/day (max. 2 g) in 4 doses × 10 days
Alternatives:	Metronidazole[e]	750 mg tid × 5 days	35–50 mg/kg/day in 3 doses × 5 days
	Iodoquinol[e]	650 mg tid × 20 days	40 mg/kg/day in 3 doses × 20 days
Blastocystis hominis **infection**			
Drug of choice:	See footnote[g]		
Cryptosporidiosis (*Cryptosporidium*)			
Non-HIV infected			
Drug of choice:	Nitazoxanide[c]	500 mg bid × 3 days[e]	1–3 yr: 100 mg bid × 3 days 4–11 yr: 200 mg bid × 3 days
HIV infected			
Drug of choice:	See footnote[h]		
Cyclosporiasis (*Cyclospora cayetanensis*)			
Drug of choice:[i]	Trimethoprim/sulfamethoxazole[e] (TMP)	TMP 160 mg/SMX 800 mg (1 DS tab) bid × 7–10 days	TMP 5 mg/kg, SMX 25 mg/kg bid × 7–10 days
Dientamoeba fragilis **infection**[j]			
Drug of choice:	Iodoquinol	650 mg tid × 20 days	30–40 mg/kg/day (max. 2 g) in 3 doses × 20 days
	or Paromomycin[e]	25–35 mg/kg/day in 3 doses × 7 days	25–35 mg/kg/day in 3 doses × 7 days
	or Tetracycline[e,f]	500 mg qid × 10 days	40 mg/kg/day (max. 2 g) in 4 doses × 10 days
	or Metronidazole	500–750 mg tid × 10 days	20–40 mg/kg/day in 3 doses × 10 days
Giardiasis (*Giardia duodenalis*)			
Drug of choice:	Metronidazole[e]	250 mg tid × 5 days	15 mg/kg/day in 3 doses × 5 days
	Nitazoxanide[c]	500 mg bid × 3 days	1–3 yr: 100 mg q12h × 3 days 4–11 yr: 200 mg q12h × 3 days
	Tinidazole[d]	2 g once	50 mg/kg once (max. 2 g)
Alternatives:[k]	Paromomycin[e,l]	25–35 mg/kg/day in 3 doses × 7 days	25–35 mg/kg/day in 3 doses × 7 days
	Furazolidone	100 mg qid × 7–10 days	6 mg/kg/day in 4 doses × 7–10 days
	Quinacrine[a]	100 mg tid × 5 days	2 mg/kg tid × 5 days (max. 300 mg/day)
Isosporiasis (*Isospora belli*)			
Drug of choice:[m]	Trimethoprim/sulfamethoxazole[e] (TMP)	TMP 160 mg/SMX 800 mg (1 DS tab) bid × 10 days	TMP 5 mg/kg, SMX 25 mg/kg bid × 10 days

Continued

Table 13-7 Treatment of Luminal Protozoa—Cont'd

Infection	Drug	Adult Dosage	Pediatric Dosage
Microsporidiosis			
Intestinal (*Enterocytozoon bieneusi, Encephalitozoon [Septata] intestinalis*)			
E. bieneusi[n]			
Drug of choice:	Fumagillin	60 mg/day PO × 14 days	
E. intestinalis			
Drug of choice:	Albendazole[e]	400 mg bid × 21 days	
Trichomoniasis (*Trichomonas vaginalis*)			
Drug of choice:[o]	Metronidazole	2 g once or 500 mg bid × 7 days	15 mg/kg/day orally in 3 doses × 7 days
	or Tinidazole[d]	2 g once	50 mg/kg once (max. 2 g)

[a]The drug is not available commercially, but as a service can be compounded by Panorama Compounding Pharmacy, 6744 Balboa Blvd, Van Nuys, CA 91406 (800-247-9767) or Medical Center Pharmacy, New Haven, CT (203-688-6816).

[b]Treatment should be followed by a course of iodoquinol or paromomycin in the dosage used to treat asymptomatic amebiasis.

[c]Nitazoxanide is FDA approved as a pediatric oral suspension for treatment of *Cryptosporidium* in immunocompetent children younger than 12 years old and for *Giardia* (Medical Letter 45:29, 2003). It may also be effective for mild to moderate amebiasis (Diaz E, et al: Am J Trop Med Hyg 68:384, 2003). Nitazoxanide is available in 500-mg tablets and an oral suspension; it should be taken with food.

[d]A nitro-imidazole similar to metronidazole, tinidazole was recently approved by the FDA and appears to be as effective and better tolerated than metronidazole. It should be taken with food to minimize GI adverse effects. For children and patients unable to take tablets, a pharmacist may crush the tablets and mix them with cherry syrup (Humco and others). The syrup suspension is good for 7 days at room temperature and must be shaken before use. Ornidazole, a similar drug, is also used outside the United States.

[e]An approved drug but considered investigational for this condition by the FDA.

[f]Use of tetracyclines is contraindicated in pregnancy and in children younger than 8 years old.

[g]Clinical significance of these organisms is controversial; metronidazole 750 mg tid × 10 days, iodoquinol 650 mg tid × 20 days, or trimethoprim-sulfamethoxazole 1 DS tab bid × 7 days have been reported to be effective (Stenzel DJ, Borenam, PFL: Clin Microbiol Rev 9:563, 1996; Ok UZ, et al: Am J Gastroenterol 94:3245, 1999). Metronidazole resistance may be common (Haresh K, et al: Trop Med Int Health 4:274, 1999) Nitazoxanide has been effective in children (Diaz E, et al: Am J Trop Med Hyg 68:384, 2003).

[h]Nitazoxanide has not consistently been shown to be superior to placebo in HIV-infected patients (Amadi B, et al: Lancet 360:1375, 2002). A small randomized, double-blind trial in symptomatic HIV-infected patients who were not receiving HAART found paromomycin similar to placebo (Hewitt RG, et al: Clin Infect Dis 31:1084, 2000).

[i]HIV-infected patients may need higher dosage and long-term maintenance (A Kansouzidou et al: J Trav Med 11:61, 2004).

[j]Norberg A, et al: Clin Microbiol Infect 9:65, 2003.

[k]Albendazole 400 mg daily × 5 days alone or in combination with metronidazole may also be effective (Hall A, Nahar Q: Trans R Soc Trop Med Hyg 87:84, 1993; Dutta AK, et al: Indian J Pediatr 61:689, 1994; Cacopardo B, et al: Clin Ter 146:761, 1995). Combination treatment with standard doses of metronidazole and quinacrine given for 3 weeks has been effective for a small number of refractory infections (Nash TE, et al: Clin Infect Dis, 33:22, 2001). In one study, nitazoxanide was used successfully in high doses to treat a case of Giardia resistant to metronidazole and albendazole (Abboud P, et al: Clin Infect Dis 32:1792, 2001).

[l]Not absorbed; may be useful for treatment of giardiasis in pregnancy.

[m]In immunocompetent patients usually a self-limited illness. Immunosuppressed patients may need higher doses, longer duration (TMP/SMX qid × 10 days, followed by bid × 3 weeks), and long-term maintenance. In sulfonamide-sensitive patients, pyrimethamine 50–75 mg daily in divided doses (plus leucovorin 10–25 mg/day) has been effective.

[n]Oral fumagillin (Sanofi Recherche, Gentilly, France) has been effective in treating *E. bieneusi* (Molina J-M, et al: N Engl J Med 346:1963, 2002) but has been associated with thrombocytopenia. Highly active antiretroviral therapy (HAART) may lead to microbiologic and clinical response in HIV-infected patients with microsporidial diarrhea (USPHS/IDSA Guidelines for the Treatment of Opportunistic Infections in Adults and Adolescents with HIV, 2004). Octreotide (Sandostatin) has provided symptomatic relief in some patients with large-volume diarrhea.

[o]Sexual partners should be treated simultaneously. Metronidazole-resistant strains have been reported and can be treated with higher doses of metronidazole (2–4 g/day × 7–14 days) or with tinidazole (Hager WD: Sex Transm Dis 31:343, 2004).

Derived from the *Medical Letter on Drugs and Therapeutics*, Drugs for parasitic infections, www.medicalletter.org, August 2004.

It is administered intravenously over a prolonged period of time. Amphotericin B binds to sterols, such as ergosterol, and is thought to damage the cytoplasmic membrane of leishmania much as it does the membranes of susceptible fungi. Untoward effects including fever, chills, malaise, nausea, anorexia, and vomiting accompany administration. Both acute and chronic nephrotoxicity and resulting electrolyte abnormalities are common.

Liposomal amphotericin B (AmBisome) is the only drug approved for the treatment of visceral leishmaniasis in the United States.[97,98] Direct delivery of drug to the reticuloendothelial system by liposomes is theoretically attractive since leishmanias reside in mononuclear phagocytes. Liposomal amphotericin B is relatively well tolerated in comparison to amphotericin B deoxycholate. Other lipid-associated amphotericin B preparations also appear to be effective but have been less extensively studied. Although liposomal amphotericin B is considered the drug of choice for the treatment of visceral leishmaniasis in the United States and other industrialized countries, the high cost has limited its use in the rest of the world. Therapeutic failures have been reported in people with cutaneous leishmaniasis treated with liposomal amphotericin B.

Miltefosine (hexadecylphosphocholine) is the only orally administered drug with activity against *Leishmania* species. It is currently used in India, where resistance to pentavalent antimony is common, for the treatment of visceral leishmaniasis.[99–101] Preliminary studies suggest that miltefosine may also be useful in the treatment of cutaneous leishmaniasis but at higher doses than those used for visceral leishmaniasis.[102] Further studies are needed to define the role of miltefosine in the treatment of visceral leishmaniasis in areas of the world other than India and in the treatment of cutaneous and mucosal leishmaniasis.

Miltefosine was developed initially as an antineoplastic agent. Although the precise mechanism of action is uncertain, it is known to interact with membrane constituents. It affects cell signaling pathways by inhibiting phosphokinase C and protein kinase C. It also interferes with the synthesis of glycosylphosphatidylinositol membrane anchors, which are important in leishmania and related kinetoplastids. Miltefosine is relatively well tolerated, but nausea, vomiting, and motion sickness may occur. Elevations of transaminases, BUN, and creatinine have been noted but usually resolve with continuation of the drug. The side effects seldom result in premature termination of therapy in patients treated for visceral leishmaniasis.

A number of other drugs have been used in the treatment of leishmaniasis. They include the imidazole antifungals, ketoconazole,[103] itraconazole,[104] and fluconazole,[105] which inhibit ergosterol biosynthesis. The imidazoles vary in their activity against different *Leishmania* species. They have most often been used for the treatment of cutaneous leishmaniasis, but failures occur. Pentamidine isethionate is an alternative for the treatment of visceral and cutaneous leishmaniasis, but it is associated with serious side effects. Preliminary data indicate that paromomysin administered intravenously has activity against pentavalent antimony-resistant *L. donovani*. Paromomycin has also been used topically with methylbenzethonium chloride in soft white paraffin for the treatment of cutaneous leishmaniasis caused by *L. major* and some other *Leishmania* species.[106] A number of other drugs and approaches have been studied, but the data are insufficient to recommend their general use.

TREATMENT OF ECTOPARASITIC DISEASES

The major ectoparasites of humans, lice and scabies, are treated with malathion, permethrin, or alternative drugs (Table 13-9; Box 13-6).

Table 13-9 Treatment of Ectoparasites

Infection	Drug	Adult Dosage	Pediatric Dosage
Lice infestation (*Pediculus humanus, P. capitis, Phthirus pubis*)[a]			
Drug of choice:	0.5% Malathion[b]	Topically	Topically
	or 1% Permethrin[c]	Topically	Topically
Alternative:	Pyrethrins with piperonyl butoxide[c]	Topically	Topically
	or Ivermectin[d,e]	200 µg/kg × 3, days 1, 2, and 10	200 µg/kg × 3 days 1, 2, and 10
Scabies (*Sarcoptes scabiei*)			
Drug of choice:	5% Permethrin	Topically[f]	Topically[f]
Alternatives:[g]	Ivermectin[d,h]	200 µg/kg once[f]	200 µg/kg once[f]
	or 10% Crotamiton	Topically once/daily × 2 days	Topically once/daily × 2 days

[a]For infestation of eyelashes with *P. pubis* lice, use petrolatum; TMP/SMX has also been used (Meinking TL; Curr Probl Dermatol 24:157, 1996). For pubic lice, treat with 5% permethrin or ivermectin as for scabies. TMP/SMX has also been effective together with permethrin for head lice. (Hipolito RB, et al: Pediatrics 107:E30, 2001).

[b]Yoon KS, et al: Arch Dermatol 139:994, 2003.

[c]A second application is recommended 1 week later to kill hatching progeny. Some lice are resistant to pyrethrins and permethrin (Meinking TL, et al: Arch Dermatol 138:220, 2002).

[d]An approved drug but considered investigational for this condition by the FDA.

[e]Ivermectin is effective against adult lice but has no effect on nits (Jones KN, English JC III: Clin Infect Dis 36:1355, 2003).

[f]In some cases, treatment may need to be repeated in 10–14 days.

[g]Lindane (gamma-benzene hexachloride; Kwell) should be reserved as a second-line agent. The FDA has recommended it should not be used for immunocompromised patients, young children, the elderly, and patients <50 kg.

[h]Ivermectin, either alone or in combination with a topical scabicide, is the drug of choice for crusted scabies in immunocompromised patients (del Giudice P: Curr Opin Infect Dis 15:123, 2004). The safety of oral ivermectin in pregnancy and young children has not been established.

Derived from the *Medical Letter on Drugs and Therapeutics*, Drugs for parasitic infections, www.medicalletter.org, August 2004.

Box 13-6 Adverse Effects of Drugs Used in the Treatment of Ectoparasites

Crotamiton (Eurax [Westwood–Squibb])
  Occasional: rash, conjunctivitis
Malathion (Ovide [Medicis])
  Occasional: local irritation
Permethrin (Nix [GlaxoSmithKline], Elimite [Allergan]),
Pyrethrins and piperonyl butoxide (RID [Pfizer], others)
  Occasional: allergic reactions

REFERENCES

1. Pearson RD: Agents active against parasites and *Pneumocystis*. In Mandell GL, Bennett JE, Dolin R (eds): Principles and Practice of Infectious Diseases, 6th ed. Philadelphia, Elsevier Science, 2005, pp 568–603.
2. Liu LX, Weller PF: Antiparasitic drugs. N Engl J Med 334:1178–1184, 1996.
3. Anonymous: Drugs for parasitic infections. Med Lett Drugs Ther (www.medicalletter.com), August 2004.
4. Jagota SC: Albendazole, a broad-spectrum anthelmintic, in the treatment of intestinal nematode and cestode infections: A multicenter study in 480 patients. Clin Ther 8:226–231, 1986.
5. Stephenson LS, Latham MC, Adams EJ, et al: Weight gain of Kenyan school children infected with hookworm, *Trichuris trichiura*, and *Ascaris lumbricoides* is improved following once- or twice-yearly treatment with albendazole. J Nutr 123:656–665, 1993.
6. Adams EJ, Stephenson LS, Latham MC: Physical activity and growth in Kenyan school children with hookworm, *Trichuris trichiura* and *Ascaris lumbricoides* infections are improved after therapy with albendazole. J Nutr 124:1199–1206, 1994.
7. Albanese G, Venturi C, Galbiati G: Treatment of larva migrans cutanea (creeping eruption): A comparison between albendazole and traditional therapy. Intern J Dermatol 40:67–71, 2001.
8. Keshmiri M, Baharvahdat H, Fattahi SH, et al: Albendazole versus placebo in treatment of echinococcosis. Trans R Soc Trop Med Hyg 95:190–194, 2001.
9. Wilson JF, Rausch RL, McMahon BJ, et al: Parasiticidal effect of chemotherapy in alveolar hydatid disease: Review of experience with mebendazole and albendazole in Alaskan Eskimos. Clin Infect Dis 15:234–249, 1992.
10. Cruz I, Cruz ME, Carrasco F, et al: Neurocysticercosis: Optimal dose treatment with albendazole. J Neurol Sci 133:152–154, 1995.
11. Dore GJ, Marriott DJ, Hing MC, et al: Disseminated microsporidiosis due to *Septata intestinalis* in nine patients infected with the human immunodeficiency virus: Response to therapy with albendazole. Clin Infect Dis 211:70–76, 1995.
12. Jung H, Hurtado M, Medina MT, et al: Dexamethasone increases plasma levels of albendazole. J Neurol 237:279–280, 1990.
13. Keystone JS, Murdoch JK: Mebendazole. Ann Intern Med 91:582–586, 1979.
14. Levin ML: Treatment of trichinosis with mebendazole. Am J Trop Med Hyg 32:980–983, 1983.
15. Blackwell V, Vega-Lopez F: Cutaneous larva migrans: Clinical features and management of 44 cases presenting in the returning traveller. Br J Dermatol 145:434–437, 2001.
16. Rayes D, De Rosa MJ, Spitzmaul G, et al: The anthelmintic pyrantel acts as a low efficacious agonist and an open-channel blocker of mammalian acetylcholine receptors. Neuropharmacology 41:238–245, 2001.
17. Naquira C, Jimenez G, Guerra JG, et al: Ivermectin for human strongyloidiasis and other intestinal helminths. Am J Trop Med Hyg 40:304–309, 1989.
18. Datry A, Hilmarsdottir I, Mayorga-Sagastume R, et al: Treatment of *Strongyloides stercoralis* infection with ivermectin compared with albendazole: Results of an open study of 60 cases. Trans R Soc Trop Med Hyg 88:344–345, 1994.
19. Ottesen EA: Efficacy of diethylcarbamazine in eradicating infection with lymphatic-dwelling filariae in humans. Rev Infect Dis 7:341–356, 1985.
20. Eberhard ML, Dickerson JW, Hightower AW, et al: Bancroftian filariasis: Long-term effects of treatment with diethylcarbamazine in a Haitian population. Am J Trop Med Hyg 45:728–733, 1991.
21. Carme B, Boulesteix J, Boutes H, et al: Five cases of encephalitis during treatment of loiasis with diethylcarbamazine. Am J Trop Med Hyg 44:684–690, 1991.
22. Taylor HR, Pacque M, Munoz B, et al: Impact of mass treatment of onchocerciasis with ivermectin on the transmission of infection. Science 250:116–118, 1990.
23. Pacque M, Munoz B, Greene BM, et al: Community-based treatment of onchocerciasis with ivermectin: Safety, efficacy, and acceptability of yearly treatment. J Infect Dis 163:381–385, 1991.
24. Pearson RD, Guerrant RL: Praziquantel: A major advance in anthelminthic therapy. Ann Intern Med 99:195–198, 1983.
25. King CH, Mahmoud AA: Drugs five years later: Praziquantel. Ann Intern Med 110:290–296, 1989.
26. Farid Z, Trabolsi B, Boctor F, et al: Unsuccessful use of praziquantel to treat acute fascioliasis in children. J Infect Dis 154:920–921, 1986.
27. Farid Z, Mansour N, Kamal M, et al: The treatment of *Fasciola hepatica* infection in children. Trop Geogr Med 42:95–96, 1990.
28. Sotelo J, Torres B, Rubio-Donnadieu F, et al: Praziquantel in the treatment of neurocysticercosis: Long-term follow-up. Neurology 35:752–755, 1985.
29. Norman RM, Kapadia C: Cerebral cysticercosis: Treatment with praziquantel. Pediatrics 78:291–294, 1986.
30. Prichard RK, Bachmann R, Hutchinson GW, et al: The effect of praziquantel on calcium in *Hymenolepis diminuta*. Mol Biochem Parasitol 5:297–308, 1982.
31. Xiao S-H, Friedman PA, Catto BA, et al: Praziquantel-induced vesicle formation in the tegument of male *Schistosoma mansoni* is calcium dependent. J Parasitol 70:177–179, 1984.
32. Thomas H, Andrews P, Mehlhorn H: New results on the effect of praziquantel in experimental cysticercosis. Am J Trop Med Hyg 31:803–810, 1982.
33. Markwalder K, Hess K, Valavanis A, et al: Cerebral cysticercosis: Treatment with praziquantel. Report of two cases. Am J Trop Med Hyg 33:273–280, 1984.
34. Sotelo J, Escobedo F, Rodriguez-Carbajal J, et al: Therapy of parenchymal brain cysticercosis with praziquantel. N Engl J Med 310:1001–1007, 1984.
35. Pearson RD, Hewlett EL: Niclosamide therapy for tapeworm infections. Ann Intern Med 102:550–551, 1985.
36. Butterworth AE, Sturrock RF, Ouma JH, et al: Comparison of different chemotherapy strategies against *Schistosoma mansoni* in Machakos District, Kenya: Effects on human infection and morbidity. Parasitology 103:339–355, 1991.
37. Health Information for International Travel 2003–2004. U.S. Department of Health and Human Services, Public Health Service, Centers for Disease Control and Prevention, Atlanta, GA (www.cdc.gov).
38. Wellems TE, Miller LH: Two worlds of malaria. N Engl J Med 349:1496–1498, 2003.
39. Jong EC, Nothdurft HD: Current drugs for antimalarial chemoprophylaxis: A review of efficacy and safety. J Travel Med 8(suppl 3):S48–S56, 2001.
40. Schwartz IK, Lackritz EM, Patchen LC: Chloroquine-resistant *Plasmodium vivax* in Indonesia. N Engl J Med 324:927, 1991.
41. Rendi-Wagner P, Noedl H, Wernsdorfer WH, et al: Unexpected frequency, duration and spectrum of adverse events after therapeutic dose of mefloquine in healthy adults. Acta Tropica 81:167–173, 2002.
42. Slater AFG, Cerami A: Inhibition by chloroquine of a novel haem polymerase enzyme activity in malaria trophozoites. Nature 355:167–169, 1992.
43. Lange WR, Frankenfield DL, Moriarty-Sheehan M, et al: No evidence for chloroquine-associated retinopathy among missionaries on long-term malaria prophylaxis. Am J Trop Med Hyg 51:389–392, 1994.
44. Riou B, Barriot P, Rimailho A, et al: Treatment of severe chloroquine poisoning. N Engl J Med 318:1–6, 1988.
45. Arias AE, Corredor A: Low response rate of Colombian strains of *Plasmodium vivax* to classical antimalarial therapy. Trop Med Parasitol 40:21–23, 1989.

46. Luzzi GA, Warrell DA, Barnes AJ, et al: Treatment of primaquine resistant *Plasmodium vivax* malaria. Lancet 340:310, 1992.
47. Smoak BL, DeFraites RF, Magill AJ, et al: *Plasmodium vivax* infections in U.S. Army troops: Failure of primaquine to prevent relapse in studies from Somalia. Am J Trop Med Hyg 56:231–234, 1997.
48. Baird JK, Lacy MD, Basri H, et al: United States Naval Medical Research Unit 2 Clinical Trials Team. Randomized, parallel placebo-controlled trial of primaquine for malaria prophylaxis in Papua, Indonesia. Clin Infect Dis 33:1990–1997, 2001.
49. Clyde DF: Clinical problems associated with the use of primaquine as a tissue schizontocidal and gametocytocidal drug. Bull World Health Organ 59:391–395, 1981.
50. Krogstad DJ, Herwaldt BL, Schlesinger PH: Antimalarial agents: Specific treatment regimens. Antimicrob Agents Chemother 32:957–961, 1988.
51. White JN, Warrell DA, Chanthavanich P, et al: Severe hypoglycemia and hyperinsulinemia in falciparum malaria. N Engl J Med 309:61–66, 1983.
52. Phillips RE, Warrell DA, White NJ, et al: Intravenous quinidine for the treatment of severe falciparum malaria. N Engl J Med 312:1273–1278, 1985.
53. Miller KD, Greenberg AE, Campbell CC: Treatment of severe malaria in the United States with a continuous infusion of quinidine gluconate and exchange transfusion. N Engl J Med 321:65–70, 1989.
54. Anonymous: Development of mefloquine as an antimalarial drug. Bull World Health Organ 61:169–178, 1983.
55. Steketee RW, Wirima JJ, Hightower AW, et al: The effect of malaria and malaria prevention in pregnancy on offspring birthweight, prematurity, and intrauterine growth retardation in rural Malawi. Am J Trop Med Hyg 55(suppl 1):31–41, 1996.
56. Bradley DJ: Antimalarial prophylaxis. Manufacturers recommend more stringent guidelines for halofantrine. BMJ 308:721, 1994.
57. Pearson RD, Hewlett EL: Use of pyrimethamine-sulfadoxine (Fansidar) in prophylaxis against chloroquine-resistant *Plasmodium falciparum* and *Pneumocystis carinii*. Ann Intern Med 106:714–718, 1987.
58. Marra F, Salzman JR, Ensom MH: Atovaquone-proguanil for prophylaxis and treatment of malaria. Ann Pharmacother 37:1266–1275, 2003.
59. Overbosch D, Schilthuis H, Bienzle U, et al: Malarone International Study Team. Atovaquone-proguanil versus mefloquine for malaria prophylaxis in nonimmune travelers: Results from a randomized, double-blind study. Clin Infect Dis 33:1015–1021, 2001.
60. Anonymous. Atovaquone for *Pneumocystis* pneumonia. Med Lett Drugs Ther 35:28–29, 1993.
61. Meshnick SR, Taylor TE, Kamchonwongpaisan S: Artemisinin and the antimalarial endoperoxides: From herbal remedy to targeted chemotherapy. Microbiol Rev 60:301–315, 1996.
62. Newton PN, Angus BJ, Chierakul W, et al: Randomized comparison of artesunate and quinine in the treatment of severe falciparum malaria. Clin Infect Dis 37:7–16, 2003.
63. Powell SJ, Wilmot AJ, Wisdon-Dew R: Further trials of metronidazole in amoebic dysentery and amoebic liver abscess. Ann Trop Med Parasitol 61:511–514, 1967.
64. Welsh JS, Rowsell BJ, Freeman C: Treatment of intestinal amoebiasis and giardiasis: Efficacy of metronidazole and tinidazole compared. Med J Aust 1:469–471, 1978.
65. Scaglia M, Atzori C, Marchetti G, et al: Effectiveness of aminosidine (paromomycin) sulfate in chronic *Cryptosporidium* diarrhea in AIDS patients: An open, uncontrolled, prospective clinical trial. J Infect Dis 170:1349–1350, 1994.
66. Soderman WA Jr: Amebiasis (clinical seminar). Am J Dig Dis 16:51–60, 1971.
67. Simon M, Shookhoff HB, Terner H, et al: Paromomycin in the treatment of intestinal amebiasis. A short course of therapy. Am J Gastroenterol 48:504–511, 1967.
68. Wolfe MS: Nondysenteric intestinal amebiasis: Treatment with diloxanide furoate. JAMA 224:1601–1604, 1973.
69. Fisher AK, Walter FG, Szabo S: Iodoquinol associated seizures and radiopacity. J Toxicol Clin Toxicol 31:113–120, 1993.
70. Oakley GP Jr: The neurotoxicity of the halogenated hydroxyquinolines. JAMA 225:395–397, 1973.
71. Anonymous. Nitazoxanide (Alinia)—A new anti-protozoal agent. Med Lett Drugs Ther 45:29–31, 2003.
72. Amadi B, Mwiya M, Musuku J, et al: Effect of nitazoxanide on morbidity and mortality in Zambian children with cryptosporidiosis: A randomized controlled trial. Lancet 360:1375–1380, 2002.
73. White AC Jr: Nitazoxanide: An important advance in anti-parasitic therapy. Am J Trop Med Hyg 68:382–383, 2003.
74. Pearson RD: Treatment of intestinal parasites in children with nitazoxanide. Curr Infect Dis Rep 6:25–26, 2004.
75. Gordin FM, Simon GL, Wofsy CB, et al: Adverse reactions to trimethoprim-sulfamethoxazole in patients with acquired immunodeficiency syndrome. Ann Intern Med 100:495–499, 1984.
76. Milord F, Pepin J, Loko L, et al: Efficacy and toxicity of eflornithine for treatment of *Trypanosoma brucei gambiense* sleeping sickness. Lancet 340:652–655, 1992.
77. Milord F, Loko L, Ethier L, et al: Eflornithine concentrations in serum and cerebrospinal fluid of 63 patients treated for *Trypanosoma brucei gambiense* sleeping sickness. Trans R Soc Trop Med Hyg 87:473–477, 1993.
78. Paulos C, Paredes J, Vasquez I, et al: Pharmacokinetics of a nitrofuran compound, nifurtimox, in healthy volunteers. Int J Clin Pharmacol Ther Toxicol 27:454–457, 1989.
79. Andrade SG, Magalhaes JB, Pontes AL: Evaluation of chemotherapy with benznidazole and nifurtimox in mice infected with *Trypanosoma cruzi* strains of different types. Bull World Health Organ 63:721–726, 1985.
80. de Andrade AL, Zicker F, de Oliveira RM, et al: Randomised trial of efficacy of benznidazole in treatment of early *Trypanosoma cruzi* infection. Lancet 348:1407–1413, 1996.
81. Coura JR, de Abreu LL, Willcox HP, et al: Comparative controlled study on the use of benznidazole, nifurtimox and placebo, in the chronic form of Chagas' disease, in a field area with interrupted transmission. I. Preliminary evaluation. Rev Soc Bras Med Trop 30:139–144, 1997.
82. Docampo R, Moreno SN: Current chemotherapy of human African trypanosomiasis. Parasitol Res 90(suppl 1):S10–S103, 2003.
83. Nok A: Arsenicals (melarsoprol), pentamidine and suramin in the treatment of human African trypanosomiasis. Parasitol Res 90:71–79, 2003.
84. Doua F, Miezan TW, Sanon Singaro JR, et al: The efficacy of pentamidine in the treatment of early-late stage *Trypanosoma brucei gambiense* trypanosomiasis. Am J Trop Med Hyg 55:586–588, 1996.
85. Pepin J, Khonde N: Relapses following treatment of early-stage *Trypanosoma brucei gambiense* sleeping sickness with a combination of pentamidine and suramin. Trans R Soc Trop Med Hyg 90:183–186, 1996.
86. Pearson RD, Hewlett EL: Pentamidine for the treatment of *Pneumocytis carinii* pneumonia and other parasitic diseases. Ann Intern Med 103:782–786, 1985.
87. Pepin J, Milord F, Khonde A, et al: Gambiense trypanosomiasis: Frequency of, and risk factors for, failure of melarsoprol therapy. Trans R Soc Trop Med Hyg 88:447–452, 1994.
88. Pepin J, Milord F, Khond AN, et al: Risk factors for encephalopathy and mortality during melarsoprol treatment of *Trypanosoma brucei gambiense* sleeping sickness. Trans R Soc Trop Med Hyg 89:92–97, 1995.
89. Milord F, Pepin J, Loko L, et al: Efficacy and toxicity of eflornithine for treatment of *Trypanosoma brucei gambiense* sleeping sickness. Lancet 340:652–655, 1992.
90. Politi C, Carrin G, Evans D, et al: Cost-effectiveness analysis of alternative treatments of African gambiense trypanosomiasis in Uganda. Health Econ 4:273–287, 1995.
91. Bacchi CJ, Nathan HC, Livingston T, et al: Differential susceptibility to DL-α-difluoromethylornithine in clinical isolates of *Trypanosoma brucei rhodesiense*. Antimicrob Agents Chemother 34:1183–1188, 1990.
92. Herwaldt BL, Berman JD: Recommendations for treating leishmaniasis with sodium stibogluconate (Pentostam) and review of pertinent clinical studies. Am J Trop Med Hyg 46:296–306, 1992.
93. Grogl M, Thomason FN, Franke ED: Drug resistance in leishmaniasis: Its implications in systemic chemotherapy of cutaneous and mucocutaneous disease. Am J Trop Med Hyg 47:117–126, 1992.
94. Berman JD: Chemotherapy for leishmaniasis: Biochemical mechanisms, clinical efficacy, and future strategies. Rev Infect Dis 10:560–586, 1988.
95. Mishra M, Biswas UK, Jha DN, et al: Amphotericin versus pentamidine in antimony-unresponsive kala-azar. Lancet 340:1256–1257, 1992.
96. Thakur CP, Sinha GP, Pandey AK, et al: Daily versus alternate-day regimen of amphotericin B in the treatment of kala-azar: A randomized comparison. Bull World Health Organ 72:931–936, 1994.

97. Berman JD: U.S. Food and Drug Administration approval of AmBisome (liposomal amphotericin B) for treatment of visceral leishmaniasis. Clin Infect Dis 28:49–51, 1999.
98. Meyerhoff A: U.S. Food and Drug Administration approval of AmBisome (liposomal amphotericin B) for treatment of visceral leishmaniasis. Clin Infect Dis 28:42–48; discussion 49–51, 1999.
99. Sundar S, Jha TK, Thakur CP, et al: Oral miltefosine for Indian visceral leishmaniasis. N Engl J Med 347:1739–1746, 2002.
100. Jha TK, Sundar S, Thakur CP, et al: Miltefosine, an oral agent, for the treatment of Indian visceral leishmaniasis. N Engl J Med 341:1795–1800, 1999.
101. Sundar S, Makharia A, More DK, et al: Short-course oral miltefosine for treatment of visceral leishmaniasis. Clin Infect Dis 31:1110–1113, 2000.
102. Soto J, Toledo J, Gutierrez P, et al: Treatment of American cutaneous leishmaniasis with miltefosine, an oral agent. Clin Infect Dis 33:E57–E61, 2001.
103. Navin TR, Arana BA, Arana FA, et al: Placebo-controlled clinical trial of sodium stibogluconate (Pentostam) versus ketoconazole for treating cutaneous leishmaniasis in Guatemala. J Infect Dis 165:528–534, 1992.
104. Dogra J, Aneja N, Behari Lal B, et al: Cutaneous leishmaniasis in India: Clinical experience with itraconazole (R51 211 Janssen). Int J Dermatol 29:661–662, 1990.
105. Alrajhi AA, Ibrahim EA, De Vol EB, et al: Fluconazole for the treatment of cutaneous leishmaniasis caused by *Leishmania major*. N Engl J Med 346:891–895, 2002.
106. el-On J, Halevy S, Grunwald MH, Weinrauch L: Topical treatment of Old World cutaneous leishmaniasis caused by *Leishmania major*: A double-blind control study. J Am Acad Dermatol 27:227–231, 1992.

14

Chemotherapy of Bacterial, Fungal, and Viral Diseases

NATHAN M. THIELMAN
RICHARD L. GUERRANT
PETER F. WELLER
RICHARD D. PEARSON

INTRODUCTION

This chapter provides an overview of major antibacterial, antimycobacterial, antifungal, and antiviral agents but does not include comprehensive information about the pharmacology, indications, dosing, or toxicities of all the chemotherapeutic agents used in the treatment of tropical infectious diseases. The treatment of specific infections is more thoroughly addressed in Section II, Pathogens. Additionally, drugs used against opportunistic infections and potentially serious drug interactions in human immunodeficiency syndrome (HIV)-infected patients are summarized. More complete discussions are found in pharmacology textbooks, and substantial additional information about indications, dosing, and toxicities may be found in *Medical Letters on Drugs and Therapeutics.*

ANTIBACTERIAL DRUGS

Antibiotics, their pharmacology and indications, form the topic of entire textbooks. The increasingly worrisome emergence of resistance among bacteria has nearly outstripped even the impressive burgeoning of new antibiotics, and effective therapy often requires isolation of the pathogen and sensitivity testing to specific antimicrobial agents. Furthermore, infections in immunocompromised hosts or in "privileged sites," such as cerebrospinal fluid (CSF) or endocarditic vegetations, often require bactericidal agents or synergistic antibiotic combinations. Treatment of common infections such as pneumonia, meningitis, and sepsis is fraught with increasing difficulty because of resistant organisms. For example, *Streptococcus pneumoniae* is increasingly resistant to penicillin and sometimes to cephalosporins and macrolides. *Listeria monocytogenes,* an important cause of meningitis, is resistant to even third-generation cephalosporins. Ampicillin is recommended for its treatment. Macrolides are indicated for "atypical" pneumonia caused by *Mycoplasma pneumoniae, Chlamydia pneumoniae,* or *Legionella pneumoniae.* In addition to gram-negative bacilli, staphylococci, particularly methicillin-resistant *Staphylococcus aureus* and *Candida*, have emerged as important causes of nosocomial infection. Adverse effects of antibiotics are also common, ranging from hypersensitivity reactions, including rash, fever, and anaphylaxis, most often seen with sulfonamides and β-lactam antibiotics, to nephrotoxicity, especially with aminoglycosides. Antibiotic-associated colitis or superinfections can occur with most antibiotics but are especially common with those whose broad spectrum alters the normal oropharyngeal, bowel, and other flora. This section focuses on selective principles of antibiotic therapy within the major classes of antibacterial drugs and lists the infections for which these agents are generally the drug of choice or a primary alternative. These are summarized in Table 14-1.

Shown in Figure 14-1 are the various mechanisms by which antibacterial agents exert either bactericidal or bacteriostatic activity against different microorganisms. The major

Table 14-1 Selected Antibacterial Drugs

Drug	Infections for Which Drug Is a Top Choice or a Primary Alternative	Some Important Infections *Not* Treated by Drug
Bacterial Cell Wall Inhibitors		
β-Lactams	*Streptococcus**	Gram-negatives
• Penicillins	*Enterococcus** (with aminoglycoside)	β-Lactamase-producing *Staphylococcus aureus*
	*Staphylococcus** (if sensitive)	*Legionella*
	Neisseria meningitidis	
	Bacillus anthracis	
	Clostridium perfringens, Clostridium tetani	
	Anaerobes (oropharyngeal)	
	Pasteurella multocida	
	Spirillum minus	
	Streptobacillus moniliformis	
	Actinomyces	
	Leptospira	
	Treponema pallidum, Treponema pertenue	
	Capnocytophaga canimorsus (DF-2) (+ aminoglycoside)	

Continued

Table 14-1 Selected Antibacterial Drugs—Cont'd

Drug	Infections for Which Drug Is a Top Choice or a Primary Alternative	Some Important Infections *Not* Treated by Drug
Bacterial Cell Wall Inhibitors		
• Aminopenicillins: Ampicillin, amoxicillin	*Enterococcus* (with aminoglycoside) *Listeria monocytogens* (± gentamicin) *Proteus mirabilis** *Eikenella corrodens**	*Legionella* β-Lactamase-producing Gram-negatives *Staphylococcus aureus* *Haemophilus influenzae*
+β-Lactamase inhibitor Amoxicillin + clavulanate Ampicillin + sulbactam	β-Lactamase-producing *H. influenzae* *S. aureus* *Escherichia coli* *Klebsiella pneumoniae* *Moraxella (Branhamella) catarrhalis* Anaerobes	*Legionella* *Acinetobacter* *Pseudomonas* *Citrobacter* *Enterobacter* *Serratia*
• Penicillinase-resistant penicillins: Cloxacillin, dicloxacillin, nafcillin, oxacillin, flucloxacillin	*Staphylococcus** (penicillinase +)	MRSA *Enterococcus*
• Carboxy- and ureidopenicillins +β-Lactamase inhibitor: Ticarcillin + clavulanate Piperacillin + tazobactam	*Pseudomonas aeruginosa** (+ aminoglycoside) *Enterobacter* *Escherichia coli* *Klebsiella pneumoniae* *Proteus* spp. *Providencia stuartii* *Acinetobacter* *Bacteroides* Some polymicrobial infections (e.g., diabetic foot ulcer)	Some enterococci *Legionella* *Campylobacter jejuni* *Listeria*
• Cephalosporins:		*All cephalosporins:*
1st generation (cephalothin et al)	Methicillin-susceptible *Staphylococcus aureus,* streptococci (penicillin-susceptible), *E. coli, Klebsiella,* Proteus* (indole +),	Enterococci MRSA *Listeria* *Legionella*
2nd generation (cefuroxime et al)	*Providencia*, Moraxella (Branhamella) catarrhalis*	
3rd generation: cefotaxime, ceftriaxone	*Neisseria gonorrhoeae** (or cefixime or cefpodoxime) *Haemophilus ducreyi; Salmonella,* Borrelia burgdorferi* meningitis, *Campylobacter fetus*	
ceftazidime	*Pseudomonas aeruginosa** *Pseudomonas pseudomallei** (melioidosis)	
4th generation: cefepime	*Pseudomonas aeruginosa, Enterobacter, Klebsiella pneumoniae*	
• Monobactam: Aztreonam	Gram-negatives	All gram-positives
• Carbapenems: Imipenem, meropenem	*Campylobacter fetus* *Enterobacter** (with aminoglycoside) *Acinetobacter** *Citrobacter freundii* *Serratia*	MRSA *Pseudomonas capacia* *Xanthomonas (Stenotrophomonas) maltophilia* *Enterococcus faecium* *Corynebacterium* JK group *Legionella*
Vancomycin	MRSA Penicillin-resistant pneumococci (with ceftriaxone or cefotaxime) *Bacillus cereus, Bacillus subtilis* *Corynebacterium* JK group	All gram-negatives
Plasma Membrane Active Agent		
Daptomycin†	*Enterococcus* *Staphylococcus aureus* MRSA	All gram-negatives Anaerobes

Table 14-1 Selected Antibacterial Drugs—Cont'd

Drug	Infections for Which Drug Is a Top Choice or a Primary Alternative	Some Important Infections *Not* Treated by Drug
Inhibitors of Bacterial Ribosomal Actions		
Macrolides		
Erythromycin	*Corynebacterium diphtheriae* (with antitoxin) Streptococci (in penicillin- and cephalosporin-allergic patients) *Campylobacter jejuni,* Bartonella* *Bartonella henselae, quintana* (or ciprofloxacin for *B. henselae*) *Bordetella pertussis* *Haemophilus ducreyi* (or ceftriaxone or azithromycin) *Legionella* *Chlamydia trachomatis* (inclusion conjunctivitis, pneumonia) *Mycoplasma pneumoniae* (alt. tetracycline) *Ureaplasma urealyticum*	Most gram-negatives
Clarithromycin[‡]	*Helicobacter pylori** (or tetracycline + metronidazole + bismuth)	
Azithromycin	*C. trachomatis* (trachoma, urethritis, cervicitis)	
Aminoglycosides		
Streptomycin Gentamicin	*Yersinia pestis* (plague); *Francisella tularensis* (in combination with ampicillin for *Enterococcus, Listeria* or with tetracycline for *Brucella, Pseudomonas mallei*)	Monotherapy for any organism[‖]
Tobramycin, amikacin	(in combination with ureidopenicillins for *P. aeruginosa*)	
Tetracyclines[§]	*Brucella** (+ aminoglycoside) *Calymmatobacterium granulomatis Vibrio** (alt. cefotaxime for *Vibrio vulnificus*), *Chlamydia psittaci, Chlamydia pneumoniae* (TWAR), *Chlamydia trachomatis* (urethritis, cervicitis, LGV) *Rickettsia, Ehrlichia, Borrelia recurrentis, Borrelia burgdorferi*	Most hospital-acquired bacteria
Clindamycin	Anaerobes, toxic streptococci, staphylococci (preferred by some)	All gram-negatives
Chloramphenicol	*Bacteroides** (oropharyngeal strains; or penicillin)	Enterococci MRSA
Linezolid	*Enterococcus* MRSA Highly penicillin-resistant *Streptococcus pneumoniae*	Gram-negatives Anaerobes
Quinupristin/dalfopristin (Synercid)	Vancomycin-resistant *Enterococcus faecium*	*Enterococcus faecalis* Gram-negatives Anaerobes
DNA Gyrase Inhibitors		
Fluoroquinolones[¶]		
All →	Most enteric gram-negative bacilli,* including *Salmonella** (typhi and others), *Shigella,* Vibrio cholerae, Campylobacter jejuni*	
Ciprofloxacin	*Plus: Bartonella henselae* (cat-scratch bacillus), *Neisseria gonorrhoeae, Haemophilus ducreyi, Pseudomonas aeruginosa**	Anaerobes, streptococci
Ofloxacin	*Plus: Neisseria gonorrhoeae, Chlamydia trachomatis*	Anaerobes, streptococci
Levofloxacin, gatifloxacin, moxifloxacin	*Plus:* β-lactam-resistant *S. pneumoniae* *Plus:* β-lactam-resistant *S. pneumoniae* *Pseudomonas aeruginosa (ciprofloxacin, levofloxacin)**	Some anaerobes

Continued

Table 14-1 Selected Antibacterial Drugs—Cont'd

Drug	Infections for Which Drug Is a Top Choice or a Primary Alternative	Some Important Infections *Not* Treated by Drug
Bacterial Folate Antagonists		
Sulfonamides		
Trimethoprim-sulfamethoxazole	*Moraxella (Branhamella) catarrhalis* *Yersinia enterocolitica** *Aeromonas* *Burkholderia cepacia** *Stenotrophomonas maltophilia** *Nocardia*	*Campylobacter jejuni* Enterococci Anaerobes Most *Pseudomonas* species
Other		
Metronidazole	*Clostridium difficile* *Bacteroides** (gastrointestinal strains) Bacterial vaginosis	Aerobic bacteria

MRSA, methicillin-resistant *S. aureus*; LGV, lymphogranuloma venereum; VRE, vancomycin-resistant enterococci.
*Confirm sensitivity as resistance is increasing (e.g., *Streptococcus pneumoniae* requiring cefotaxime, ceftriaxone, or, for high-level resistance, vancomycin plus rifampin or levofloxacin, gatifloxacin, or moxifloxacin).
†FDA-approved for complicated skin and skin structure infections.
‡Clarithromycin is not recommended for use in pregnancy or in patients receiving terfenadine therapy who have pre-existing cardiac abnormalities.
§Tetracyclines are generally not recommended for pregnant women or for children less than 8 years of age.
||Aminoglycosides are useful only in combination therapy.
¶Fluoroquinolones are generally not recommended for children or pregnant women.
See Choice of antibacterial agents. Treatment Guidelines from The Medical Letter 2:13–24, 2004, for doses, toxicities, and alternatives.

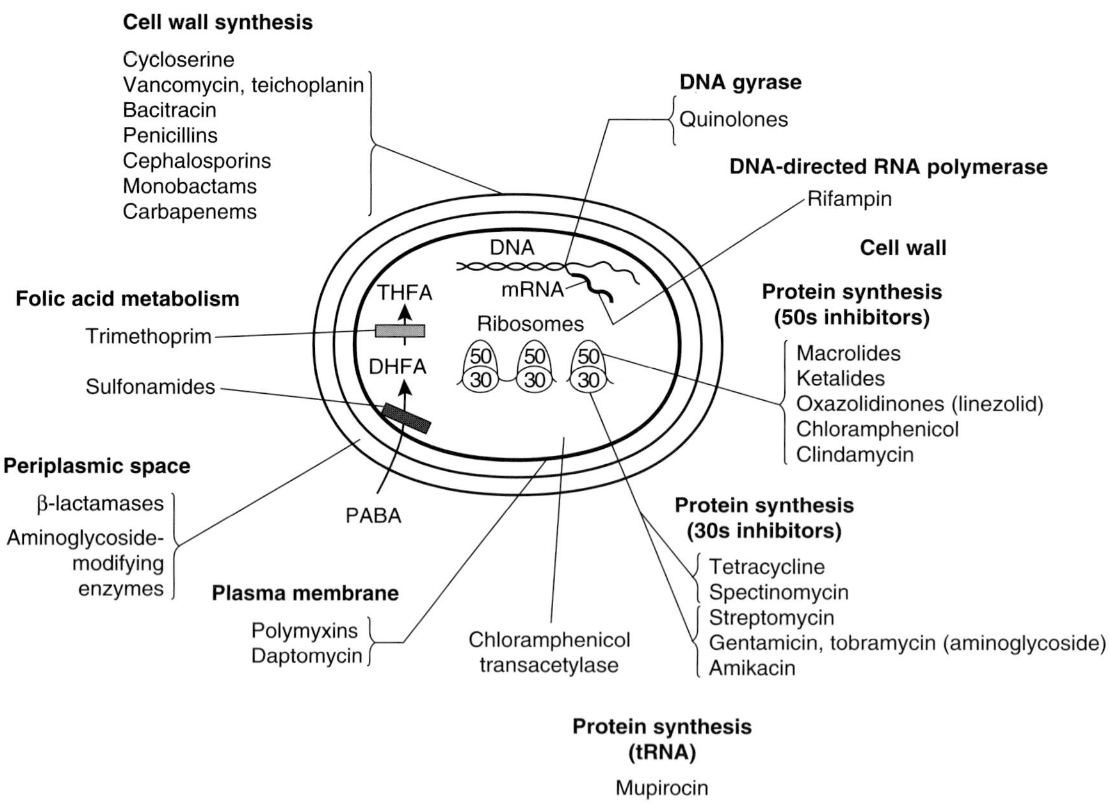

FIGURE 14-1 Antimicrobial sites of bactericidal or bacteriostatic action on microorganisms. The five general mechanisms are (1) inhibition of synthesis of the cell wall, (2) damage to the outer membrane, (3) modification of nucleic acid and DNA synthesis, (4) modification of protein synthesis (at ribosomes), and (5) modification of energy metabolism within the cytoplasm (at folate cycle). DHFA, dihydrofolate; PABA, para-aminobenzoic acid; THFA, tetrahydrofolate. (Adapted from Brody TE, Larner J, Minneman K, et al: Human Pharmacology: Molecular to Clinical, 3rd ed. St. Louis, Mosby–Year Book, 1998.)

bacterial cell wall inhibitors are β-lactam agents (such as penicillins, cephalosporins, and carbapenems) and vancomycin. Penicillins differ in their absorption, protein-binding characteristics, metabolism, and renal excretion, but in general all are well distributed throughout the body. In the presence of inflammation, CSF concentrations rise to around 5% of those in plasma. Adjustments in dosages of penicillin are generally not necessary until renal clearance decreases below 30 mL per minute. Penicillin G and penicillin V are active against most non-β-lactamase–producing gram-positive and gram-negative cocci. Ampicillin and amoxicillin exhibit broader gram-negative coverage than penicillin does, but increasing resistance among *Haemophilus influenzae, Shigella,* and *Salmonella* has been seen in recent years. Penicillinase-resistant penicillins (e.g., methicillin, nafcillin, dicloxacillin) inhibit staphylococci and streptococci. The carboxypenicillins (carbenicillin and ticarcillin) have extended activity against *Pseudomonas aeruginosa* and other gram-negative bacilli. Because they are readily destroyed by β-lactamases, these agents are useful primarily when combined with a β-lactamase inhibitor. Ureidopenicillins (e.g., piperacillin, mezlocillin, and azlocillin) also exhibit extended activity against gram-negative organisms (including *Pseudomonas*), while retaining activity against streptococci. The combination of piperacillin with the β-lactamase inhibitor tazobactam renders this ureidopenicillin more effective against β-lactamase producing bacteria.

Cephalosporins are classified into generations based on their spectrum of antimicrobial activity. In general, first-generation cephalosporins have good activity against gram-positive organisms and moderate activity against gram-negative bacilli such as *Escherichia coli.* Some second-generation cephalosporins, such as cefotaxime, have enhanced activity against *Haemophilus* and gram-negative bacilli, but less activity than first-generation cephalosporins against staphylococci. Third-generation cephalosporins, in general, have less activity against staphylococci and more activity against streptococci, Enterobacteriaceae, *Neisseria,* and *Haemophilus* spp. Notably, ceftazidime and cefoperazone have less activity against streptococci but improved activity against *P. aeruginosa.* Third-generation cephalosporins, like penicillins, are widely distributed into body compartments. Cefotaxime and ceftriaxone enter the CSF and are widely used to treat meningitis. Ceftizoxime (and cefepime) also can be used to treat meningitis. Most cephalosporins are eliminated by renal mechanisms. Cefoperazone and ceftriaxone are primarily excreted by the biliary route. A relatively new category, fourth-generation cephalosporins, includes cefepime, which is approved for use in the United States. Fourth-generation cephalosporins have activity against both gram-positive cocci (comparable to that of cefotaxime or ceftriaxone) and excellent activity against *P. aeruginosa* (comparable to that of ceftazidime).

Penicillins are generally well tolerated. The most important life-threatening side effect is a type I hypersensitivity reaction, which occurs in up to 0.05% of treatment courses. A morbilliform skin eruption occurs in 3% to 5% of patients. Occasionally, penicillin can cause seizures when given in high doses, particularly in patients with concomitant renal failure. The incidence of anaphylaxis with cephalosporins is even less than that seen with penicillins. It is estimated that fewer than 5% of those who have anaphylactic reactions to penicillin are at risk for such a reaction with a cephalosporin.

The carbapenems—imipenem, meropenem, and ertapenem—all administered intravenously, are β-lactam antibiotics that are relatively resistant to β-lactamases. Because imipenem is hydrolyzed by a renal dihydropeptidase, it is combined with a renal dehydropeptidase inhibitor, cilastatin. Imipenem and meropenem reach therapeutic concentrations in CSF in patients with meningitis; however, imipenem may cause seizures in patients with underlying brain injury or impaired renal clearance. Clinical experience suggests that carefully adjusting imipenem dosing according to renal function or the use of meropenem may help decrease the risk of seizures. Imipenem and meropenem have excellent activity against gram-positive and gram-negative aerobes and anaerobes. Unlike imipenem and meropenem, ertapenem has minimal activity against *P. aeruginosa* or *Acinetobacter.* It offers the advantage of once daily dosing for infections caused by susceptible organisms.

Vancomycin, a glycopeptide cell wall inhibitor unrelated to β-lactams, is not absorbed orally and is primarily used intravenously. It is eliminated by glomerular filtration and is not removed by hemodialysis or peritoneal dialysis. Dosage should be adjusted in patients with impaired creatinine clearance. Vancomycin is useful for gram-positive (but not for gram-negative) bacteria, particularly methicillin-resistant *S. aureus* and methicillin-resistant coagulase-negative staphylococci. Oral vancomycin effectively treats *Clostridium difficile*–associated diarrhea; however, metronidazole is equally effective, less expensive, and perhaps less likely to foster the emergence of vancomycin-resistant enterococci. Vancomycin occasionally causes "red-man syndrome," a histamine-mediated phenomenon characterized by erythema, especially around the head and neck, sometimes with hypotension. Vancomycin also can be ototoxic, particularly at higher plasma concentrations or when given in combination with aminoglycosides.

Some new agents with activity targeting gram-positive bacteria have become available in recent years. Daptomycin, a cyclic lipopeptide that binds to and depolarizes bacterial plasma membranes, resulting in cell death, was recently approved by the U.S. Food and Drug Administration (FDA) for the treatment of complicated skin and skin structure infections and appears to be similar in efficacy to vancomycin for this indication. It offers the advantage of once daily dosing and is a reasonable alternative to vancomycin. Linezolid, an oxazolidinone that inhibits protein synthesis at the bacterial ribosome has clinically useful activity against both *Enterococcus faecium* and *faecalis,* including many vancomycin-resistant enterococci and methicillin-resistant staphylococci. It has the advantage of being dosed orally, but its long-term use has been limited primarily by concerns for treatment-associated thrombocytopenia. Quinupristin/dalfopristin, a combination of streptogramins, also inhibits bacterial protein synthesis. It is active against methicillin-resistant *S. aureus* and *E. faecium,* including vancomycin-resistant strains, but not against *E. faecalis.* Disadvantages of quinupristin/dalfopristin include the requirement for infusion via a central venous catheter and frequent dose-limiting myalgias.

The macrolide antibiotics include erythromycin, clarithromycin, azithromycin, and dirithromycin. Erythromycin has broad gram-positive activity (including *S. pneumoniae, Streptococcus pyogenes,* and *Corynebacterium diphtheriae*) and inhibits *Bordetella pertussis,* legionellae, mycoplasmas, and chlamydiae. Erythromycin is distributed throughout the body but does not achieve adequate concentrations to treat meningitis. The most common adverse effects of erythromycin are gastrointestinal. Transient hearing loss can be seen, especially at high doses. Clarithromycin is associated with fewer gastrointestinal side effects. Its spectrum of activity includes that of erythromycin plus activity against atypical mycobacteria and some *H. influenzae* spp. It is two to four times more active than erythromycin against staphylococci and streptococci. Azithromycin is better absorbed and better tolerated than erythromycin; it has an extremely long half-life and can be given once daily for 5 days. It is two to four times less active than erythromycin against staphylococci and streptococci but it is more active against *H. influenzae.* A single 1-g dose is effective for genital chlamydial infections. Erythromycin and clarithromycin should never be coadministered with terfenadine or astemizole because of potential cardiac toxicity (such as torsades de pointes). Recently approved by the FDA, telithromycin is the first of a new class of antibiotics, ketalides, which are structurally similar to macrolides but demonstrate enhanced activity against multidrug-resistant *S. pneumoniae.* Telithromycin is approved for acute bacterial exacerbation of chronic bronchitis, acute bacterial sinusitis, and mild to moderately severe community-acquired pneumonia.

Aminoglycosides are not absorbed orally but are given primarily by either intravenous or intramuscular injection. The antimicrobial spectrum of activity of aminoglycosides is limited to aerobic and facultative gram-negative bacilli. Nephrotoxicity occurs in 5% to 25% of patients and ototoxicity (vestibular or auditory) in 0.5% to 3.0% of patients. Renal toxicity is usually reversible, whereas ototoxicity often is not. Toxicity can typically be avoided by careful monitoring of blood levels and serial measurements of serum creatinine.

Tetracyclines are broad-spectrum agents that may be administered either orally or intravenously. They are typically well absorbed (best absorbed in the fasting state because tetracyclines chelate with divalent metals), widely distributed in body fluids, and renally excreted. Tetracyclines are the drug of choice for Rocky Mountain spotted fever, ehrlichiosis, and chlamydial infections; *Borrelia burgdorferi,* mycoplasmas, *Vibrio cholerae, Brucella* spp., and *Pseudomonas pseudomallei* are usually susceptible. Increasing resistance renders them less useful against many other bacterial strains. Tetracyclines may cause discoloration of teeth and bones in children less than 8 years of age and may cause photosensitivity in any patient.

Chloramphenicol (another inhibitor of bacterial ribosomal activity) is active against a broad range of aerobic and anaerobic gram-positive and gram-negative bacteria, chlamydiae, rickettsiae, and *Mycoplasma* spp. It is well absorbed from the gastrointestinal tract and can be given intravenously. Chloramphenicol is widely distributed throughout the body and, because of its lipid solubility, achieves high concentrations in brain tissue and CSF. The dose should be reduced in patients with hyperbilirubinemia. Chloramphenicol may cause reversible bone marrow suppression in adults receiving 4 g or more per day and causes aplastic anemia in 1 in 24,000 to 40,000 recipients. It has also been associated with optic neuritis and with gray baby syndrome in premature infants.

Clindamycin is well absorbed orally and can be given by intramuscular or intravenous dosing as well. Clindamycin penetrates most body compartments except brain tissue and CSF. Concentrations are inadequate to treat meningitis or other brain infections except toxoplasmosis. The half-life of clindamycin is prolonged in severe liver disease. It is active against most gram-positive cocci (except enterococci) and many anaerobes. Clindamycin causes diarrhea in up to 20% of patients and pseudomembranous colitis in 3% to 5% of patients. It is rarely associated with hepatotoxicity and allergic reactions such as rash.

The quinolones constitute another class of antibacterials, DNA gyrase inhibitors, which inhibit DNA synthesis in bacterial but not mammalian cells. They are well absorbed orally and distributed widely. Absorption of several quinolones is impaired in the presence of magnesium, aluminum, calcium, zinc, and iron. Because the newer fluoroquinolones such as levofloxacin, gatifloxacin, and moxifloxacin have good activity against increasingly penicillin-resistant pneumococci, they are often considered for treatment of community-acquired pneumonia. Quinolones are effective against most Enterobacteriaceae, *Haemophilus* spp., gram-negative cocci, legionellae, mycoplasmas, and chlamydiae. Moxifloxacin also has activity against anaerobes. These agents are not the therapy of choice for infections with staphylococci and penicillin-susceptible streptococci. Although generally well tolerated, all quinolones can cause gastrointestinal upset and central nervous system (CNS) side effects, the latter occurring more commonly in the elderly. Because quinolones cause arthropathy in immature animals, they are not recommended for use in children or pregnant women. Quinolones decrease the clearance of theophylline.

Folic acid synthesis is inhibited by both trimethoprim and sulfonamides. The combination trimethoprim-sulfamethoxazole provides a potent sequential inhibition of folic acid synthesis and is useful in treating *S. aureus, S. pyogenes, S. pneumoniae, E. coli, Proteus mirabilis, Shigella* spp., *Salmonella* spp., *Pseudomonas cepacia, Pseudomonas pseudomallei, Yersinia enterocolitica,* and *Neisseria gonorrhoeae.* It is also useful in treating several protozoal infections, including *Pneumocystis carinii, Isospora belli,* and *Cyclospora cayetanensis.* Hypersensitivity reactions, Stevens-Johnson syndrome, and hematologic toxicities are some of the more common or serious complications of therapy with sulfamethoxazole.

ANTIMYCOBACTERIAL DRUGS

The agents used for mycobacterial infections and their toxicities are summarized in Table 14-2. Susceptible strains of *Mycobacterium tuberculosis* are treated with isoniazid and rifampin with or without pyrazinamide, for 6 to 9 months. Where significant resistance (i.e., >4% to isoniazid) is possible, a four-drug regimen with isoniazid, rifampin, pyrazinamide, and either ethambutol or streptomycin is used until the sensitivities are known. In cases of multiple drug resistance, additional agents are required to achieve a minimum of three or more drugs to which the organism is susceptible. In addition, clarithromycin or azithromycin, ethambutol, and rifabutin are used in treatment of *Mycobacterium avium–intracellulare* complex infections in persons with acquired immunodeficiency syndrome (AIDS).

ANTIFUNGAL DRUGS

The therapeutic armamentarium against fungi is expanding (Table 14-3). For many years, amphotericin B was the only

Table 14-2 Antimycobacterial Drugs

Drugs	Main Adverse Effects
Primary Agents Against *Mycobacterium tuberculosis**	
Isoniazid (PO or IM, 5 mg/kg/day; 10–20 mg/kg/day for children; max. 300 mg/day for adults and children)	Hepatic toxicity, peripheral neuropathy
Rifampin (PO or IV, 10–20 mg/kg/day to 600 mg/day)	Hepatic toxicity, flulike syndrome
Pyrazinamide (PO 15–30 mg/kg/day to 1.5–2.5 g/day)	Hepatic toxicity, arthralgias, hyperuricemia
Ethambutol (Myambutol PO, 15–25 mg/kg/day)	Optic neuritis
Streptomycin (IM 15 mg/kg/day; 20–30 mg/kg/day for children)	Vestibular toxicity, renal damage
Alternative Antimycobacterial Drugs	
Capreomycin (Capastar IM 15 mg/kg/day; 15–30 mg/kg/day for children; max. 1 g)	Auditory and vestibular toxicity, renal damage
Kanamycin (Kantrex et al IM or IV 15 mg/kg/day; 15–30 mg/kg/day for children; max. 1 g)	Auditory and renal toxicity
Amikacin (Amikin IM or IV 15 mg/kg/day; 15–30 mg/kg/day for children)	
Cycloserine (Seromycin et al PO 250–500 mg bid; 10–20 mg/kg/day; max. 1 g)	Psychiatric symptoms, seizures
Ethionamide (Trecator-SC PO 250–500 mg bid; 15–20 mg/kg/day; max. 1 g)	Gastrointestinal disturbances, hepatic toxicity
Ciprofloxacin (Cipro PO 250–750 mg bid for adults only)	
Ofloxacin (Floxin PO 600–800 mg/day for adults only)	
Para-aminosalicyclic acid (PAS; Teebacin PO 4–6 g bid; 75 mg/kg bid for children; max. 12 g)	Gastrointestinal disturbances
Clofazimine (Lamprene PO 100–200 mg; 1 mg/kg in children)	Gastrointestinal disturbances; ichthyosis; pigmentation of cornea, retina, skin
Additional Agents Particularly Useful for MAC[†]	
Clarithromycin PO 500 mg bid	↑ Rifabutin and AZT levels
Azithromycin PO 500 mg qd (500 mg 3 × wk when used as a component of MAC treatment regimen)	
Clarithromycin 500 mg bid or azithromycin 1200 mg qwk or 300 mg qd (for MAC prophylaxis)	
Rifabutin PO 300–450 mg qd	

AZT, zidovudine; MAC, *Mycobacterium avium–intracellulare* complex.
*See Drugs for tuberculosis. Med Lett Drugs Ther 37:67–70, 1995, and Med Lett Drugs Ther 37:87–94, 1995, for details regarding indications, doses, and toxicities.
[†]See Table 14-11 for additional details.

Table 14-3 Systemic Antifungal Drugs

Antifungal Agent	Diseases for Which This Is the Drug of Choice or a Primary Alternative	Antifungal Agent	Diseases for Which This Is the Drug of Choice or a Primary Alternative
Amphotericin* (0.5–1.5 mg/kg IV)	Aspergillosis Blastomycosis Candidiasis (deep) (± flucytosine) Coccidioidomycosis (± flucytosine) Cryptococcosis Histoplasmosis Mucormycosis Paracoccidioidomycosis Sporotrichosis (systemic)	Oral azoles[†] Fluconazole (100–200 mg/day PO)	Candidiasis[‡] (oropharyngeal, esophageal, vaginal) Coccidioidomycosis (requires 400–800 mg/day PO) Cryptococcosis (200 mg/day PO, for suppression)
		Ketoconazole (400–800 mg/day PO)	Pseudallescheriasis (ketoconazole or miconazole) *Madurella mycetomatis*[§] Blastomycosis

Continued

Table 14-3 Systemic Antifungal Drugs—Cont'd

Antifungal Agent	Diseases for Which This Is the Drug of Choice or a Primary Alternative	Antifungal Agent	Diseases for Which This Is the Drug of Choice or a Primary Alternative
Itraconazole (200 mg qd or bid PO)	Blastomycosis Histoplasmosis Pseudallescheriasis Paracoccidioidomycosis Sporotrichosis (cutaneous, itraconazole or saturated solution of potassium iodide) Chromomycosis (*Fonsecaea pedrosi* et al)		Alternative for Candidiasis (oropharyngeal, esophageal) Coccidioidomycosis Histoplasmosis Paracoccidioidomycosis
		Voriconazole (6 mg/kg IV q12h × 1 day, then 4 mg/kg IV q12h, then 200 mg bid PO)	Invasive aspergillosis Refractory infection with *Scedosporium apiospermum* or *Fusarium* spp.
		Echinocandin Caspofungin (70 mg IV × 1 day, then 50 mg IV once/day)	Invasive aspergillosis Deep *Candida* infections

*Amphotericin B is given IV over about a 2- to 4-hour interval once a day or in double doses every other day. The duration of therapy with the drug usually ranges from 4 to 12 weeks. To decrease the severity of the initial reaction to the drug, if the patient is not dangerously ill, some clinicians begin with a 1-mg test dose, followed in 2 to 4 hours, if no severe reaction occurs, by a full therapeutic dose. Pretreatment with acetaminophen (Tylenol and others), aspirin, or hydrocortisone 25 mg IV can decrease the severity of the reactions. Treatment with meperidine (Demerol and others) 25 mg IV can shorten the duration of fever and chills.

†The optimal duration of treatment with the oral azole drugs is unclear. Depending on the disease, these drugs are continued for weeks or months or, particularly in AIDS patients, indefinitely. With ketoconazole and itraconazole, AIDS patients may have lower serum concentrations.

‡For patients with oropharyngeal disease, clotrimazole troches five times daily or nystatin solution (100,000 units/mL) 5 mL qid may be effective and are relatively inexpensive. For patients with fluconazole-resistant esophageal disease, amphotericin B 0.3 mg/kg IV can be used. *Candida krusei* infections are usually resistant to fluconazole. *Candida glabrata* infections are often resistant. Bladder irrigation with 50 mg/L of amphotericin B in sterile water has been used to treat *Candida cystitis*.

§Actinomycetoma (with *Actinomadura madurae, Nocardia,* et al) requires streptomycin + sulfamethoxazole-trimethoprim or dapsone.

Modified from Systemic antifungal drugs. Med Lett Drugs Ther 38:12, 1996; see also Antifungal drugs. Treatment guidelines. Medical Letter 3:7–14, 2005.

drug available for the treatment of most systemic fungal infections. Its untoward effects and requirement for parenteral administration are problematic (Table 14-4). Lipid-associated and liposomal amphotericin preparations, which may be less toxic, have recently become available. In the United States, these agents are approved only for treatment of aspergillosis in patients who are refractory to, or intolerant of, conventional amphotericin B therapy. The introduction of the azoles—ketoconazole, fluconazole, itraconazole, and voriconazole—which are less toxic than amphotericin B and can be administered orally, constituted major advances. The echinocandin caspofungin has excellent clinical activity against *Aspergillus* spp. and *Candida* spp. and a favorable safety profile.

Table 14-4 Toxicities of the Antifungal Drugs

Drug	Toxicity
Amphotericin B	Systemic: fever, chills, headache, hypotension, tachycardia Gastrointestinal: nausea and vomiting Nephrotoxicity (may be decreased by sodium loading): hypomagnesemia, hypokalelmia, renal tubular acidosis Hematologic: anemia, thrombocytopenia, mild leukopenia
Flucytosine	Bone marrow depression (increased with renal impairment if dosage adjustments are not made)
Itraconazole	Gastrointestinal: nausea, abdominal pain Drug interactions: increases levels of terfenadine and cisapride, which can be fatal; rhabdomyolysis if used concurrently with cyclosporine, lovastatin, simvastatin; absorption dependent on gastric acidity, decreased by H_2 blockers and antacids; others
Ketoconazole	Gastrointestinal intolerance, mild hepatotoxicity Others: rash, itching, dizziness, gynecomastia Endocrine: gynecomastia, altered libido, decreased potency, menstrual irregularity Drug interactions: increases levels of terfenadine and cisapride, which can be fatal; others
Fluconazole	Allergic: rash, Stevens-Johnson syndrome (rare), anaphylaxis (rare) Others: serious hepatotoxicity (rare) Drug interactions: increases levels of terfenadine and cisapride, which can be fatal; others
Voriconazole	Similar to other azoles except that approximately 30% have transient visual disturbances following dosing
Caspofungin	Generally well tolerated; pruritus and headache are most common

ANTIVIRAL DRUGS AND THE TREATMENT OF OPPORTUNISTIC INFECTIONS IN PATIENTS WITH AIDS

The major antiviral agents and their indications and major toxicities are shown in Tables 14-5 and 14-6. The treatment of HIV infection is changing rapidly, and favored regimens combine nucleosides and protease inhibitors (PIs) or non-nucleoside reverse transcriptase inhibitors (NNRTIs) (see Table 14-6). Potentially serious drug interactions can occur, especially when protease inhibitors, which can affect the cytochrome P-450 enzyme system in the liver, are used concurrently with antimycobacterial, antifungal, or other agents. Drugs that induce or inhibit the cytochrome P-450 system and their effects on substrate drugs are noted in Table 14-7, and other important drug interactions and cumulative toxicities are summarized in Tables 14-8 through 14-10. The approaches to treatment of opportunistic infections in patients with HIV infection are summarized in Table 14-11. Updated treatment recommendations from the U.S. Department of Health and Human Services are frequently posted at http://www.aidsinfo.nih.gov.

Table 14-5 *Antiviral Drugs (Other Than Antiretroviral Agents)**

Antiviral (with Representative Adult Dose)	Virus or Disease for Which This is a First-Line Drug	Toxicity
Acyclovir (Zovirax and others) (IV or PO to 800 mg 5 ×/day × 5–10 days)	HSV, VZV	Gastrointestinal disturbances, crystalline nephropathy, headache, rash
Valacyclovir (Valtrex) (prodrug of acyclovir) (up to PO 1 g tid)	HSV, VZV	Similar to acyclovir; prolonged high doses may cause TTP/HUS
Famciclovir (Famvir) (prodrug of penciclovir) (PO 500 mg bid/tid)	HSV, localized VZV	Headache, nausea, diarrhea
Amantadine (Symmetrel) or rimantadine (Flumadine) (PO 200 mg/day × 5 days)	Influenza A	CNS anxiety, insomnia, confusion (usually minor, less with rimantadine)
Ganciclovir (Cytovene) (IV 5 mg/kg 1–2 ×/day)	CMV retinitis, pneumonia, others	Neutropenia, thrombocytopenia
Foscarnet (Foscavir) (IV 40–60 mg/kg q8h)	For resistant CMV, HSV, VZV	Renal dysfunction, hypocalcemia
Cidofovir (Vistide) (IV 5 mg/kg q2wk)	CMV retinitis (chronic suppression)	Nephrotoxicity, neutropenia, metabolic acidosis, uveitis, ocular hypotony
Interferon-alfa (Roferon-A, Intron-A, Alferon N) (SC or IM 3–10 million units 3 ×/wk × 4–6 mo) or Pegylated interferon-alfa 2b (PEG-Intron) (1 μg/kg once/wk SC × 48 wk)	Chronic hepatitis B, C[†], D	Flulike symptoms, marrow suppression, et al
Ribavirin (Virazole) (aerosol 12–18 hr/day × 3–7 days, or IV)	RSV, Lassa fever, Sabia virus, CCHF, some hantavirus infections	Teratogenic, embryotoxic, hemolytic anemia
Ribavirin (Rebetrol, Rebetron) (1000–1200 mg/d PO)	Hepatitis C[†]	
Trifluridine (Viroptic) (topical, 1 drop 1% q2h × 10 days)	Ocular and mucocutaneous HSV	—
Vidarabine (Vira-A)	(HSV, VZV before acyclovir)	
Lamivudine (Epivir HBV) (100 mg PO 1 × /day × 1–3 yr)	Hepatitis B	Generally well tolerated; rare headache, nausea, dizziness
Fomiversen (Vitravene) (330 μg intravitreally q2wk × 2, then 2 ×/mo)	CMV retinitis	Iritis, vitritis, increased intraocular pressure and vision changes
Valgancyclovir (Valcyte) (prodrug of gancyclovir) (900 mg PO bid × 21 days followed by 900 mg once daily)	CMV retinitis, others	Similar to gancyclovir
Gancyclovir intraocular implant (Vitrasert) (4.5 mg intraocularly q5–8mo)	CMV retinitis	Late retinal detachment
Oseltamivir (Tamiflu) (75 mg PO bid × 5 days for treatment; 75 mg PO once daily for prevention)	Influenza A or B treatment (within 36 hr) and prevention	Nausea and vomiting
Zanamivir (Relenza) (10 mg bid × 5 days by inhaler)	Influenza A or B treatment (within 2 days)	Nasal and throat discomfort, bronchospasm
Pencyclovir (Denavir) (1% cream applied q2h while awake × 4 days)	Orolabial HSV	

HSV, herpes simplex virus; VZV, varicella-zoster virus; TTP, thrombotic thrombocytopenic purpura; HUS, hemolytic-uremic syndrome; CMV, cytomegalovirus; RSV, respiratory syncytial virus; CCHF, Crimean-Congo hemorrhagic fever; CNS, central nervous system.

*See Drugs for non-HIV viral infections. Med Lett Drugs Ther 44(W1123A), 2002, for full information about dosing, indications, and toxicities.

†For Hepatitis C infections, inferon and ribavirin are coadministered.

Table 14-6 Antiretroviral Drugs (with Usual Doses and Main Adverse Effects)

Antiretroviral	Main Adverse Effects	Antiretroviral	Main Adverse Effects
Reverse Transcriptase (RT) Inhibitors		***Protease Inhibitors***	
Nucleoside and Nucleotide Analogs			
Zidovudine (AZT, Retrovir) PO 200 mg tid or 300 mg bid	Anemia, neutropenia, nausea and vomiting, hemolytic anemia, malaise, myopathy, confusion, hepatitis	Saquinavir (Invirase PO 600 mg tid; Fortovase PO 1200 mg tid)	Diarrhea; nausea; abdominal pain; poor bioavailability, especially with Invirase. ↓ levels with rifampin, rifabutin; antihistamine toxicity
Didanosine (dideoxyinosine, ddI, Videx) PO 125–200 mg bid; Videx EC, PO 400 mg qd	Neuropathy, pancreatitis, gastrointestinal upset, ↓ absorption with itraconazole, ketaconazole, and possibly dapsone	Ritonavir (Norvir) PO 600 mg q12h	Diarrhea; nausea and vomiting; paresthesias; transaminitis; asthenia; levels reduced by rifampin, rifabutin, dexamethasone; other drug toxicities
Zalcitabine (dideoxycytidine, ddC, Hivid) PO 0.75 mg tid	Neuropathy, rash, stomatitis, esophageal ulceration, pancreatitis, fever	Indinavir (Crixivan) PO 800 mg q8h	Renal stones, hyperbilirubinemia, gastric hypoacidity (↓ ddI absorption), other drug toxicities
Stavudine (d4T, Zerit) PO 40 mg bid (30 mg bid if <60 kg)	Neuropathy, transaminitis, rarely pancreatitis, lipoatrophy		
Lamivudine (3TC, Epivir) PO 150 mg bid or PO 300 mg qd	Gastrointestinal upset, rare pancreatitis	Nelfinavir (Viracept) PO 750 mg tid with food or PO 1250 mg bid with food	Diarrhea, asthenia, nausea, abdominal pain, headache, rash
Zidovudine + lamivudine (Combivir) 1 tablet PO bid	See above		
Tenofovir disoproxil Fumarate (Viread) 300 mg PO bid	Asthenia, headache, renal insufficiency		
Abacavir (Ziagen) 300 mg PO qd	Hypersensitivity reaction (can be fatal)		
Emtricitabine (FTC, Emtriva) 200 mg PO qd	Headache, nausea, skin hyperpigmentation	Atazanavir (Regataz) 400 mg once daily	Indirect hyperbilirubinemia, prolonged PR interval, hyperglycemia, fat maldistribution.
Abacavir + lamivudine + Zidovudine (Trizivir) 1 tablet PO bid	See above		
Abacavir + lamivudine (Epzicom) 1 tablet qd	See above		
Tenofovir + emtricitabine (Truvada) 1 tablet qd	See above		
Non-nucleoside RT Inhibitors			
Efavirenz (Sustiva) 600 mg PO qd	Rash, vivid dreams, dizziness, insomnia, impaired concentration	Lopinavir/ritonavir (Kaletra) 400 mg lopinavir + 100 mg ritonavir PO bid, with food	Diarrhea, nausea, vomiting, asthenia, liver function test abnormalities, glucose abnormalities, hyperlipidemia, fat maldistribution
Nevirapine (Viramune) PO 200 mg bid	Rash		
Delavirdine (Rescriptor) PO 400 mg tid	Rash	Fosamprenavir (Lexiva) 1400 mg PO bid	Diarrhea, nausea, vomiting, fat maldistribution, skin rash, hyperglycemia, lipid abnormalities
		Fusion Inhibitors	
		Enfuvirtide (T-20, Fuzeon)	Local injection site reactions, increased rate of bacteria pneumonia, hypersensitivity reaction

See Drugs for HIV Infection. Med Lett Drugs Ther 43(W1119A), 2001, and U.S. Department of Health & Human Services: Guidelines for the Use of Antiretroviral Agents in HIV-1 Infected Adults & Adolescent. Available at www.aidsinfo.nih.gov.

Table 14-7 Drugs That Should Not Be Used with PI or NNRTI Antiretrovirals

Drug Category*	Calcium Channel Blocker	Cardiac Drugs	Lipid-lowering Agents	Antimycobacterial Drugs[†]	Antihistamine Drugs[‡]	Gastrointestinal Drugs[‡§]	Neuroleptic Drugs	Psychotropic Drugs	Ergot Alkaloids (Vasoconstrictor)	Herbs	Other
Protease Inhibitors (PIs)											
Indinavir	(none)	(none)	Simvastatin Lovastatin	Rifampin Rifapentine	Astemizole Terfenadine	Cisapride	Pimozide	Midazolam[#] Triazolam	Dihydroergotamine (DHE 45) ergotamine[¶] (various forms) ergonovine methylergonovine	St. John's wort	Atazanavir
Ritonavir[‖]	Bepridil	Amiodarone Flecainide Propafenone Quinidine	Simvastatin Lovastatin	Rifapentine	Astemizole Terfenadine	Cisapride	Pimozide	Midazolam[#] Triazolam	Dihydroergotamine (DHE 45) ergotamine[¶] (various forms) ergonovine methylergonovine	St. John's wort	
Saquinavir	(none)	(none)	Simvastatin Lovastatin	Rifampin Rifabutin, Rifapentine	Astemizole Terfenadine	Cisapride	Pimozide	Midazolam[#] Triazolam	Dihydroergotamine (DHE 45) ergotamine[¶] (various forms) ergonovine methylergonovine	St. John's wort Garlic supplements	
Nelfinavir	(none)	(none)	Simvastatin Lovastatin	Rifampin Rifapentine	Astemizole Terfenadine	Cisapride	Pimozide	Midazolam[#] Triazolam	Dihydroergotamine (DHE 45) ergotamine[¶] (various forms) ergonovine methylergonovine	St. John's wort	
Amprenavir Fosamprenavir[‖]	Bepridil	(none)	Simvastatin Lovastatin	Rifampin Rifapentine	Astemizole Terfenadine	Cisapride	Pimozide	Midazolam[#] Triazolam	Dihydroergotamine (DHE 45) ergotamine[¶] (various forms) ergonovine methylergonovine	St. John's wort	Delavirdine
Lopinavir (LPV) + Ritonavir (RTV)	(none)	Flecainide Propafenone	Simvastatin Lovastatin	Rifampin** Rifapentine	Astemizole Terfenadine	Cisapride	Pimozide	Midazolam[#] Triazolam	Dihydroergotamine (DHE 45) ergotamine[¶] (various forms) ergonovine methylergonovine	St. John's wort	
Atazanavir	Bepridil	(none)	Simvastatin Lovastatin	Rifampin Rifapentine	Astemizole Terfenadine	Cisapride Proton pump inhibitors	Pimozide	Midazolam[#] Triazolam	Dihydroergotamine (DHE 45) ergotamine[¶] (various forms) ergonovine methylergonovine	St. John's wort	Indinavir Irinotecan

Continued

Table 14-7 *Drugs That Should Not Be Used with PI or NNRTI Antiretrovirals—Cont'd*

Drug Category*	Calcium Channel Blocker	Cardiac Drugs	Lipid-lowering Agents	Antimycobacterial Drugs[†]	Antihistamine Drugs[‡]	Gastro–intestinal Drugs[‡§]	Neuroleptic Drugs	Psychotropic Drugs	Ergot Alkaloids (Vasoconstrictor)	Herbs	Other
Non-nucleoside Reverse Transcriptase Inhibitors (NNRTIs)											
Nevirapine	(none)	(none)	(none)	Rifampin Rifapentine[†]	(none)	(none)	(none)	(none)	(none)	St. John's wort	
Delavirdine	(none)	(none)	Simvastatin Lovastatin	Rifampin Rifapentine[†] Rifabutin	Astemizole Terfenadine	Cisapride H_2 blockers Proton pump inhibitors	(none)	Alprazolam Midazolam[#] Triazolam	Dihydroergotamine (DHE 45) ergotamine[¶] (various forms) ergonovine methylergonovine	St. John's wort	Amprenavir Fosamprenavir
Efavirenz	(none)	(none)	(none)	Rifapentine[†]	Astemizole Terfenadine	Cisapride	(none)	Midazolam[#] Triazolam	Dihydroergotamine (DHE 45) ergotamine[¶] (various forms) ergonovine methylergonovine	St. John's wort	

*Certain listed drugs are contraindicated based on theoretical considerations. Thus, drugs with narrow therapeutic indices and suspected metabolic involvement with cytochrome P-450–3A, –2D6, or unknown pathways are included in this table. Actual interactions may or may not occur among patients.

[†]HIV patients being treated with rifapentine have a higher rate of TB relapse than those treated with other rifamycin-based regimens; an alternative agent is recommended for this population.

[‡]Astemizole and terfenadine are not marketed in the United States.

[§]The manufacturer of cisapride has a limited-access protocol in place for patients meeting specific clinical eligibility criteria.

[#]Midazolam can be used with caution as a single dose and given in a monitored situation for procedural sedation.

[¶]This is likely a class effect.

[||]Each 150-mg amprenavir Agenerase capsule has 109 IU (International Units) of vitamin E, and 1 mL of amprenavir oral solution has 46 IU of vitamin E. At FDA-approved doses, the daily amount of vitamin E in Agenerase is 58-fold increase over the federal government reference daily intake for adults. Patients should be cautioned to avoid supplemental doses of vitamin E. Multivitamin products containing minimal amounts of vitamin E are likely acceptable.

**In one small study, higher doses of RTV or LPV/RTV offset rifampin-inducing activity of LPV. Of note, 28% of subjects discontinued due to increases in LFTs. The safety of this combination is still under evaluation.

Suggested Alternatives

Cerivastatin (no longer marketed in the United States), simvastatin, lovastatin: pravastatin and fluvastatin have the least potential for drug-drug interactions; atorvastatin should be used with caution, using the lowest possible starting dose and monitoring closely; no pharmacokinetic data or safety data are available for coadministration of rosuvastatin with the antiretroviral agents.

Rifabutin: clarithromycin, azithromycin (MAI prophylaxis); clarithromycin, azithromycin, ethambutol (MAI treatment)

Astemizole, terfenadine (no longer marketed in the United States): desloratadine, loratadine, fexofenadine, cetirizine

Midazolam, triazolam: temazepam, lorazepam

From U.S. Department of Health and Human Services: Guidelines for the Use of Antiretroviral Agents in HIV-1 Infected Adults and Adolescents. Available at www.aidsinfo.nih.gov.

Table 14-8 *Drug Interactions Between Antiretrovirals and Other Drugs: PIs, NNRTIs, and NRTIs*

Drugs Affected	Drug Interactions Requiring Dose Modifications or Cautious Use		
	Indinavir (IDV)	**Ritonavir* (RTV)**	**Saquinavir† (SQV)**
Antifungals			
Ketoconazole	Levels: IDV ↑ 68% Dose: IDV 600 mg tid	Levels: ketoconazole ↑ 3 × Dose: use with caution; do not exceed 200 mg ketoconazole daily	Levels: SQV ↑ 3 × Dose: if ketoconazole dose is >200 mg/d, monitor for excessive diarrhea, nausea, abdominal discomfort, and adjust doses accordingly
Voriconazole	Levels: no significant changes in AUC of azole or IDV (healthy subjects) Dose: standard	No data, but potential for bidirectional inhibition between voriconazole and PIs; monitor for toxicities	No data, but potential for bidirectional inhibition between voriconazole and PIs; monitor for toxicities
Antimycobacterials			
Rifampin	Levels: IDV (unboosted) ↓ 89%; IDV (boosted) ↓ 87% Contraindicated	Levels: RTV ↓ 35% Dose: no change Increased liver toxicity possible Coadministration may lead to loss of virologic response if RTV sole PI Alternative antimycobacterial agents, such as rifabutin, should be considered	Levels: SQV ↓ 84% Contraindicated unless using RTV+SQV Dose: SQV/RTV 400/400 mg bid, rifampin 600 mg qd or 3 ×/week
Rifabutin	Levels: IDV ↓ 32%; rifabutin ↑ 2 × Dose: ↓ rifabutin to 150 mg qd or 300 mg 3 ×/wk. IDV 1000 mg tid If RTV boosted, use rifabutin dosing recommendations for coadministration with RTV; continue current dose of boosted IDV	Levels: rifabutin ↑ 4 × Dose: ↓ rifabutin to 150 mg qd or 3 ×/week† RTV: Maintain current dose if sole PI or part of a boosted regimen	Levels: SQV ↓ 40% Contraindicated unless using SQV/RTV Dose: rifabutin 150 mg qd or 3 ×/week†
Clarithromycin	Levels: Clarithromycin ↑ 53% No dose adjustment	Levels: Clarithromycin ↑ 77% Dose: adjust clarithromycin dose for moderate and severe renal impairment	Levels: Clarithromycin ↑ 45% SQV ↑ 177% No dose adjustment
Oral contraceptives	Levels: norethindrone ↑ 26% Ethinylestradiol ↑ 24% No dose adjustment	Levels: ethinyl estradiol ↓ 40% Use alternative or additional method	No data
Lipid-Lowering Agents			
Simvastatin Lovastatin Atorvastatin	Levels: potential for large increase in statin levels; avoid concomitant use Levels: potential for increase in AUC; use lowest possible starting dose of atorvastatin with careful monitoring	Levels: potential for large increase in statin levels; avoid concomitant use Levels: 450% ↑ when administered with SQV/RTV combination Use lowest possible starting dose of atorvastatin with careful monitoring	Levels: potential for large increase in statin levels; avoid concomitant use Levels: 450% ↑ when administered with SQV/RTV combination Use lowest possible starting dose of atorvastatin with careful monitoring
Pravastatin	No data	Levels: 50% ↓ when administered with SQV/RTV combination; no dose adjustment needed	Levels: 50% ↓ when administered with SQV/RTV combination No dose adjustment needed

Continued

Table 14-8 Drug Interactions Between Antiretrovirals and Other Drugs: PIs, NNRTIs, and NRTIs—Cont'd

	Drug Interactions Requiring Dose Modifications or Cautious Use		
Drugs Affected	**Indinavir (IDV)**	**Ritonavir* (RTV)**	**Saquinavir[†] (SQV)**
Anticonvulsants			
Carbamazepine Phenobarbitol Phenytoin	Carbamazepine markedly ↓ IDV AUC Consider alternative agent	Carbamazepine: ↑ serum levels when coadministered with RTV Use with caution Monitor anticonvulsant levels	Unknown but may markedly ↓ SQV levels Monitor anticonvulsant levels
Methadone	No change in methadone levels	Methadone ↓ 37% Monitor and titrate dose if needed May require ↑ methadone dose	Methadone AUC ↓ 20%; when coadministered with SQV/RTV 400/400 mg BID Dose: no adjustment for this PI regimen, but monitor and titrate to methadone response if necessary
Erectile Dysfunction Agents			
Sildenafil	Sildenafil AUC ↑ threefold; use cautiously Start with reduced dose of 25 mg every 48 hours, and monitor for adverse effects	Sildenafil AUC ↑ 11-fold Use cautiously Start with reduced dose of 25 mg every 48 hours, and monitor for adverse effects	Sildenafil AUC ↑ twofold Use a 25-mg starting dose of sildenafil
Vardenafil	Vardenafil AUC ↑ 16-fold IDV (unboosted) AUC ↓ 30% Dose: consider sildenafil instead of verdenafil if IDV unboosted Do not exceed vardenafil 2.5 mg in 72 hours if administered with RTV	Vardenafil AUC ↑ 49-fold RTV AUC ↓ 20% Dose: Vardenafil: start with a 2.5-mg dose, and do not exceed a single 2.5-mg dose in 72 hours RTV: maintain current dose	No data but vardenafil AUC may be substantially increased Start with a 2.5-mg dose, and do not exceed a single 2.5-mg dose in 24 hours Do not exceed a single 2.5-mg dose in 72 hours if administered with RTV
Tadalafil	Concomitant administration will result in substantial increase in tadalafil AUC and half-life (normal = 17.5 hr) Start with a 5-mg dose, and do not exceed a single dose of 10 mg every 72 hours	Tadalafil AUC ↑ 124% Start with a 5-mg dose, and do not exceed a single dose of 10 mg every 72 hours	Concomitant administration will result in substantial increase in tadalafil AUC and half-life (normal = 17.5 hr) Start with a 5-mg dose, and do not exceed a single dose of 10 mg every 72 hours
Miscellaneous	Grapefruit juice ↓ IDV levels by 26% Vitamin C ≥ 1 g/d ↓ IDV AUC by 14% and Cmin by 32% Itraconazole: reduce IDV (unboosted) dose to 600 mg TID; do not exceed 200 mg itraconazole twice daily RTV boosted regimen: see RTV	Many possible interactions Desipramine ↑ 145%; reduce dose Trazadone AUC ↑ 60%; use lowest dose, and monitor for CNS and CV adverse effects Theophylline ↓ 47%; monitor theophylline levels	Grapefruit juice ↑ SQV levels Dexamethasone ↓ SQV levels RTV boosted regimen: see RTV

Drugs Affected	Drug Interactions Requiring Dose Modifications or Cautious Use		
	Nelfinavir (NFV)	Amprenavir (APV)	Fosamprenavir (fos-APV)
Antifungals			
Ketoconazole	No dose adjustment necessary	Levels: APV ↑ 31% Ketoconazole ↑ 44% Dose: standard	Presumably similar interactions (an increase in both APV and ketoconazole levels) and recommendation as APV Consider ketoconazole dose reduction if dose is > 400 mg/d If fos-APV/r: use with caution; do not exceed 200 mg ketoconazole daily
Voriconazole	No data, but potential for bidirectional inhibition between voriconazole and PIs exists; monitor for toxicities	No data, but potential for bidirectional inhibition between voriconazole and PIs exists; monitor for toxicities	Presumably similar interaction and recommendation as APV
Antimycobacterials			
Rifampin[§]	Levels: NFV ↓ 82% Should not be coadministered	Levels: APV AUC ↓ 82% No change in rifampin AUC Should not be coadministered	Presumably similar interaction and recommendation as APV
Rifabutin	Levels: NFV ↓ 32% Rifabutin ↑ 2 × Dose: ↓ rifabutin to 150 mg qd or 300 mg 3 ×/week ↑ NFV dose to 1000 mg tid	Levels: APV AUC ↓ 15% rifabutin ↑ 193% Dose: No change in APV dose; decrease rifabutin to 150 mg qd or 300 mg 3 ×/week[†] If RTV boosted, use rifabutin dosing recommendations for coadministration with RTV; continue current dose of boosted APV	Similar interaction and recommendation as APV if fos-APV unboosted If RTV boosted fos-APV, dose reduce rifabutin to 150 mg QOD or 3 ×/wk[†]
Clarithromycin	No data	Levels: APV AUC ↑ 18% No change in clarithromycin AUC No dose adjustment	Presumably similar interaction and recommendation as APV
Oral contraceptives	Levels: norethindrone ↓ 18% ethinyl estradiol ↓ 47% Use alternative or additional method	Levels: ↑ ethinyl estradiol and norethindrone levels; APV levels ↓ 20% Do not coadminister; alternative methods of contraception are recommended	Presumably similar interaction as APV Do not coadminister; alternative methods of contraception are recommended
Lipid-lowering Agents			
Simvastatin	Avoid concomitant use Simvastatin AUC ↑ 505%—not recommended	Levels: potential for large increase in statin levels Avoid concomitant use	Presumably similar interaction and recommendation as APV
Lovastatin	Potential for large increase in Lovastatin AUC—not recommended		
Atorvastatin (ATO)	ATO AUC ↑ 74%—use lowest possible starting dose or atorvastatin with careful monitoring	ATO levels have potential for large increase Use lowest possible starting dose of atorvastatin with careful monitoring	ATO AUC ↑ 150% Maximum ATO dose of 20 mg/d; use with careful monitoring and consider alternative agent
Pravastatin	No data	No data	No data

Continued

Table 14-8 Drug Interactions Between Antiretrovirals and Other Drugs: PIs, NNRTIs, and NRTIs—Cont'd

	Drug Interactions Requiring Dose Modifications or Cautious Use		
Drugs Affected	**Nelfinavir (NFV)**	**Amprenavir (APV)**	**Fosamprenavir (fos-APV)**
Anticonvulsants			
Carbamazepine Phenobarbitol Phenytoin	Unknown but may decrease NFV levels substantially Monitor anticonvulsant levels and virologic response Consider obtaining NFV levels	Unknown, but may decrease APV levels substantially Monitor anticonvulsant levels and virologic response Consider obtaining APV levels	Presumably similar interaction and recommendation as APV
Methadone	NFV may decrease methadone levels but minimal effect on maintenance dose Monitor and titrate dose if needed May require ↑ methadone dose	Methadone levels ↓ 13% APV Cmin ↓ 25% Monitor and titrate methadone if needed	Presumably similar interaction and recommendation as APV
Erectile Dysfunction Agents			
Sildenafil	Sildenafil AUC ↑ 2–11-fold; use cautiously Start with reduced dose of 25 mg every 48 hours, and monitor for adverse effects	Sildenafil AUC ↑ 2–11-fold; use cautiously Start with reduced dose of 25 mg every 48 hours, and monitor for adverse effects	Similar interaction and recommendations as APV
Vardenafil	No data but vardenafil AUC may be substantially increased Start with a 2.5-mg dose, and do not exceed a single 2.5-mg dose in 24 hours Do not exceed 2.5 mg in 72 hours if administered with RTV	No data, but vardenafil AUC may be substantially increased Start with a 2.5-mg dose, and do not exceed a single 2.5 mg dose in 24 hours Do not exceed 2.5 mg in 72 hours if administered with RTV	Similar interaction and recommendations as APV
Tadalafil	Concomitant administration will result in substantial increase in tadalafil AUC and half-life (normal = 17.5 hr) Start with a 5-mg dose, and do not exceed a single dose of 10 mg every 72 hours	Tadalafil half-life = 17.5 hours Concomitant administration will result in substantial increase in tadalafil AUC and half-life (normal = 17.5) Start with a 5-mg dose, and do not exceed a single dose of 10 mg every 72 hours	Similar interaction and recommendations as APV

Drugs Affected	Drug Interactions Requiring Dose Modifications or Cautious Use: Atazanavir (ATV)	Lopinavir (LPV)
Antifungals		
Ketoconazole	No dosage adjustment necessary	Levels: LPV AUC ↓ 13%; ketoconazole ↑ threefold Dose: use with caution; do not exceed 200 mg ketoconazole daily
Voriconazole	No data, but potential for bidirectional inhibition between voriconazole and PIs exists; monitor for toxicities	No data, but potential for bidirectional inhibition between voriconazole and PIs exists; monitor for toxicities
Antimycobacterials		
Rifampin[§]	Should not be coadministered	Levels: LPV AUC ↓ 75%; should not be coadministered A safe and effective dose of LPV/r that can be given with rifampin has not been established[§]
Rifabutin	Levels: rifabutin AUC ↑ 2.5-fold Dose: ↓ rifabutin dose to 150 mg qod or 3 ×/wk[†] ATV dose standard	Levels: rifabutin AUC ↑ threefold; 25-O-desacetyl metabolite ↑ 47.5-fold Dose: decrease rifabutin dose to 150 mg qod or 3 ×/week; LPV/r: standard
Clarithromycin	Levels: clarithromycin AUC ↑ 94% and may cause QTc prolongation Clarithromycin active metabolic concentrations are significantly reduced Dose: ↓ clarithromycin dose by 50%; consider alternative therapy	Levels: ↑ clarithromycin AUC 77% Dose: adjust clarithromycin dose for moderate and severe renal impairment
Oral contraceptives	Levels: ethinyl estradiol AUC ↑ 48%, norethindrone AUC ↑ 110% Dose: use lowest effective dose or alternative methods	Levels: ethinyl estradiol ↓ 42% Use alternative or additional method
Lipid-lowering Agents		
Simvastatin Lovastatin Atorvastatin (ATO)	Levels: potential for large increase in statin levels; avoid concomitant use Atorvastatin levels have potential for large increase Use lowest possible starting dose of atorvastatin with careful monitoring	Levels: potential for large increase in statin levels Avoid concomitant use Atorvastatin AUC ↑ 5.88-fold Use lowest possible starting dose of atorvastatin with careful monitoring
Pravastatin	No data	Paravastatin AUC ↑ 33%; no dosage adjustment necessary
Anticonvulsants		
Carbamazepine Phenobarbitol Phenytoin	Unknown but may decrease ATV levels substantially Monitor anticonvulsant levels	Many possible interactions: carbamazepine: ↑ levels when coadministered with RTV Use with caution; monitor anticonvulsant levels Phenytoin: ↓ levels of LPV, RTV, and ↓ levels of phenytoin when administered together; avoid concomitant use
Methadone	No data	Methadone AUC ↓ 53% Monitor and titrate dose if needed May require ↑ methadone dose

Continued

Table 14-8 Drug Interactions Between Antiretrovirals and Other Drugs: PIs, NNRTIs, and NRTIs—Cont'd

	Drug Interactions Requiring Dose Modifications or Cautious Use	
Drugs Affected	**Atazanavir (ATV)**	**Lopinavir (LPV)**
Erectile Dysfunction Agents		
Sildenafil	Sildenafil levels have potential for increase Start with reduced dose of 25 mg every 48 hours, and monitor for adverse effects	Sildenafil AUC ↑ 11-fold in combination with RTV; use cautiously Start with reduced dose of 25 mg every 48 hours, and monitor for adverse effects
Vardenafil	No data, but vardenafil AUC may be substantially increased Start with a 2.5-mg dose, and do not exceed a single 2.5-mg dose in 24 hours Do not exceed 2.5 mg in 72 hours if administered with RTV	No data, but vardenafil AUC may be substantially increased Start with a 2.5-mg dose, and do not exceed a single 2.5-mg dose in 72 hours
Tadalafil	Concomitant administration will result in substantial increase in tadalafil AUC and half-life (normal = 17.5 hr); start with a 5-mg dose, and do not exceed a single dose of 10 mg every 72 hours	Tadalafil AUC ↑ 124% when coadministered with RTV Start with a 5-mg dose, and do not exceed a single dose of 10 mg every 72 hours
Miscellaneous	Diltiazem AUC ↑ 125%, ↓ diltiazem dose by 50%; ECG monitoring is recommended Calcium channel blockers: caution is warranted; dose titration should be considered; ECG monitoring is recommended ATV inhibits UGT and may interfere with irinotecan metabolism; avoid concomitant use H_2-receptor antagonists: reduced ATV concentrations are expected with simultaneous administration; separate dosing by 12 hours Antacids and buffered medications: reduced ATV concentrations are expected with simultaneous administration; give ATV 2 hr before or 1 hr after these medications RTV boosted regimen: see RTV	See Miscellaneous RTV recommendations, below

Drugs Affected	Drug Interactions Requiring Dose Modifications or Cautious Use: Nevirapine (NVP)	Delavirdine (DLV)	Efavirenz (EFV)
Antifungals			
Ketoconazole	Levels: ketoconazole ↓ 63% NVP ↑ 15% to 30% Dose: not recommended	No data	No data
Voriconazole	No data, but potential for bidirectional interaction between voriconazole and NNRTIs exists; monitor for toxicities and voriconazole effectiveness	No data, but potential for bidirectional inhibition between voriconazole and delaviridine exists; monitor for toxicities	No data, but potential for bidirectional interaction between voriconazole and NNRTIs exists; monitor for toxicities and voriconazole effectiveness
Antimycobacterials			
Rifampin	Levels: NVP ↓ 20% to 58% Virologic consequences are uncertain; the potential for additive hepatotoxicity exists Use of this combination is not recommended; however, if used, coadministration should be done with careful monitoring	Levels: DLV ↓ 96% Contraindicated	Levels: EFV ↓ 25% Dose: consider ↑ EFV to 800 mg qd
Rifabutin	Levels: NVP ↓ 16% No dose adjustment[‖]	Levels: DLV ↓ 80% Rifabutin ↑ 100% Not recommended	Levels: EFV unchanged Rifabutin ↓ 35% Dose: ↑ rifabutin dose to 450–600 mg qd or 600 mg 3 ×/wk[‖] EFV: standard
Clarithromycin	Levels: NVP ↑ 26% Clarithromycin ↓ 30% Monitor for efficacy or use alternative agent	Levels: clarithromycin ↑ 100%, DLV ↑ 44% Dose-adjust for renal failure	Levels: clarithromycin ↓ 39% Monitor for efficacy, or use alternative agent
Oral contraceptives	Levels: ethinyl estradiol ↓ approx 20%; use alternative or additional methods	No data	Levels: ethinyl estradiol ↑ 37% No data on other component Use alternative or additional methods

Continued

Table 14-8 Drug Interactions Between Antiretrovirals and Other Drugs: PIs, NNRTIs, and NRTIs—Cont'd

Drugs Affected	Drug Interactions Requiring Dose Modifications or Cautious Use		
	Nevirapine (NVP)	**Delavirdine (DLV)**	**Efavirenz (EFV)**
Lipid-lowering Agents			
Simvastatin Lovastatin	No data	Levels: potential for large increase in statin levels; avoid concomitant use	No data
Pravastatin	No data	No data	No data
Anticonvulsants			
Carbamazepine Phenobarbitol Phenytoin	Unknown Use with caution Monitor anticonvulsant levels	Unknown but may decrease DLV levels substantially Monitor anticonvulsant levels	Use with caution Monitor anticonvulsant levels
Methadone	Levels: NVP unchanged Methadone ↓ significantly Titrate methadone dose to effect	No data	Levels: methadone ↓ significantly Titrate methadone dose to effect
Miscellaneous	No data	May increase levels of dapsone, warfarin, and quinidine Sildenafil: potential for increased concentrations and adverse effects; use cautiously Start with reduced dose of 25 mg every 48 hours and monitor for adverse effects Vardenafil: no data, but vardenafil AUC may be substantially increased Start with a 2.5-mg dose, and do not exceed a single 2.5-mg dose in 24 hours Tadalafil: no data, but concomitant administration will likely result in substantial increase in tadalafil AUC and half-life (normal = 17.5 hr) Start with a 5-mg dose, and do not exceed a single dose of 10 mg every 72 hours Atorvastatin levels have potential for large increase; use lowest possible starting dose of atorvastatin with careful monitoring	Monitor warfarin when used concomitantly

Drugs Affected	Zidovudine (ZDV)	Stavudine (d4T)	Didanosine (ddI)	Tenofovir (TDF)
	Drug Interactions Requiring Dose Modifications or Cautious Use			
Methadone	No data	Levels: d4T ↓ 27%; methadone unchanged No dose adjustment	Levels: EC ddI unchanged Buffered ddI AUC ↓ 63%; methadone unchanged Dose: no change in EC ddI. May consider buffered ddI dose to increase or maintain standard	No data
Miscellaneous				
Ribavirin	Ribavirin inhibits phosphorylation of ZDV; this combination should be avoided if possible, or closely monitor virologic response	No data	Coadministration not recommended; ribavirin increases the intracellular levels of the active metabolite of ddI and may cause serious toxicities	No data
Didanosine	No data	Peripheral neuropathy, lactic acidosis, and pancreatitis seen with this combination; use with caution and only if potential benefit outweighs potential risks	No data	Levels: ddI AUC ↑ by 44%; Cmax ↑ by 28% Monitor for ddI-associated toxicities For patients > 60 kg, 250 mg/day of ddI EC is recommended
Atazanavir (ATV)	No data	No data	Buffered ddI + ATV simultaneously: Levels: ↓ AUC of ATV 87%; take ATV (with food) 2 hr before or 1 hr after buffered ddI No interaction is expected with ddI-EC; however, dosing should be at different times, as ATV should be taken with food and ddI-EC on an empty stomach	ATV 400 + TDF 300 Levels: ATV AUC ↓ 25% and Cmin ↓ by 40%; TDF AUC ↑ by 24%; avoid concomitant use ATV + RTV 300/100 mg qd + TDF 300 mg qd Levels: ATV AUC ↓ by 25% and Cmin by 23%; ATV Cmin was higher with RTV than ATV without RTV Consider ATV + RTV (300/100 mg qd) for coadministration with TDF (300 mg qd); however, pharmacokinetic, safety, and virologic data are limited

Continued

Table 14-8 Drug Interactions Between Antiretrovirals and Other Drugs: PIs, NNRTIs, and NRTIs—Cont'd

	Drug Interactions Requiring Dose Modifications or Cautious Use			
Drugs Affected	**Zidovudine (ZDV)**	**Stavudine (d4T)**	**Didanosine (ddI)**	**Tenofovir (TDF)**
Indinavir (IDV)	No data	No data	Buffered ddI and IDV simultaneously: Levels: ↓ AUC of IDV; take IDV 1 hr before or after buffered ddI	No data
Lopinavir/ritonavir	No data	No data	No data	LPV/r 400/100 AUC ↓ 15%; TDF AUC ↑ 34%; clinical significance of interaction is unknown
Lamivudine plus (Abacavir or Didanosine)	No data	No data	No data	High rate of early virologic nonresponse with 3TC and ABC plus TDF; combination should be avoided
Cidofovir Ganciclovir Valganciclovir	No data	No data	ddI + oral ganciclovir (GCV): ddI AUC ↑ 111%; GCV AUC ↓ 21%; Appropriate doses for the combination of ddI and oral GCV have not been established	Possibly competes for active tubular secretion with tenofovir; may increase serum concentration of these drugs and/or tenofovir Monitor for dose-related toxicities

*Drugs for which plasma concentrations may be decreased by coadministration with ritonavir: anticoagulants (warfarin), anticonvulsants (phenytoin, divaproex, lamotrigine), antiparasitics (atovaquone).

†Rifabutin 3 ×/wk is recommended if CD4 cell count is <100/mm³.

‡Some drug interaction studies were conducted with Invirase. May not necessarily apply to use with Fortovase.

§Limited data on RTV-SQV and LPV-RTV demonstrate that RTV compensates, to a degree, for rifampin induction. In one small study, higher doses of ritonavir (up to 400 mg per dose) or an increased dose of LPV/RTV 800/200 mg were needed to offset rifampin-inducing activity of LPV; the standard dose of rifampin was used in these studies. Of note, 28% of subjects discontinued due to increases in LFTs. The safety of this combination is not established. If coadministered, close monitoring is recommended, as is measuring LPV concentrations.

‖These recommendations apply to regimens that do not include PIs, which can substantially increase rifabutin levels.

From U.S. Department of Health and Human Services: Guidelines for the Use of Antiretroviral Agents in HIV-1 Infected Adults and Adolescents. Available at www.aidsinfo.nih.gov.

Table 14-9 Drug Effects on Concentration of Protease Inhibitors (PIs)

Drug Affected	Ritonavir	Saquinavir*	Nelfinavir	Amprenavir	Lopinavir/Ritonavir	Atazanavir
Protease Inhibitors						
Indinavir (IDV)	Levels: IDV ↑ 2–5 × Dose: 400/400 mg or 800/100 mg or 800/200 mg IDV/RTV bid Caution: renal events may be increased with higher IDV concentrations	Levels: IDV no effect SQV ↑ 4–7 ×[†] Dose: insufficient data	Levels: IDV ↑ 50%; NFV ↑ 80% Dose: limited data for IDV 1200 mg bid + NFV 1250 mg bid	Levels APV AUC ↑ 33% Dose: not established	Levels: IDV AUC and Cmin ↑ Dose: IDV 600 mg bid	Coadministration of these agents is not recommended because of potential for additive hyperbilirubinemia
Ritonavir (RTV)	No data	Levels: RTV no effect SQV ↑ 20 ×[†‡] Dose: 1000/100 mg SQV (sgc or hgc)/ RTV bid or 400/ 400 mg bid	Levels: RTV no effect; NFV ↑ 1.5 × Dose: RTV 400 mg bid + NFV 500–750 mg bid	Levels: APV AUC ↑ 2.5–3.5-fold Dose: 600/100 mg APV/RTV bid, or 1200/200 mg APV/RTV qd	Lopinavir is co-formulated with ritonavir as Kaletra	ATV/r 300/100 ↑ ATV AUC by 238%
Saquinavir (SQV)	No data	No data	Levels: SQV ↑ 3–5 ×; NFV ↑ 20%[†] Dose: standard NFV; Fortovase 800 mg tid or 1200 mg bid	Levels: APV AUC ↓ 32% Dose: insufficient data	Levels: SQV[†] AUC and Cmin ↑ Dose: SQV 1000 mg bid, LPV/r standard	SQV 1200 mg qd + ATV 400 qd ↑ SQV AUC by 449%; no formal recommendation
Nelfinavir (NFV)	No data	No data	No data	Levels: APV AUC ↑ 1.5-fold Dose: insufficient data	Levels: LPV ↓ 27%; NFV ↑ 25% Dose: insufficient data	
Amprenavir (APV)	No data	No data	No data	No data	APV: AUC and Cmin increased relative to APV without RTV; APV AUC and Cmin reduced relative to APV + RTV; LPV Cmin may be decreased relative to LPV/r Dose: APV 600–750 mg bid; LPV/r standard, or consider dose increase to 533/133 mg bid Consider monitoring PI concentrations	No data
Fosamprenavir (fos-APV)	Fos-APV: AUC and Cmin ↑ 100% and 400%, respectively, with 200 mg RTV ARV-experienced should receive boosted regimen	Levels: APV AUC ↓ 32% Dose: insufficient data	No data	No data	Fos-APV: Cmin ↓ 64% (at dose of 700 mg bid with 100 mg bid of RTV) LPV: Cmin ↓ 53% (at LPV/r dose of 400/100) Should not be coadministered; doses are not established	No data
Lopinavir/ Ritonavir (LPV/RTV)	No data	No data	No data	No data	No data	No information with LPV/ ATV; RTV 100 mg ↑ ATV AUC by 238%

*Several drug interaction studies have been completed with saquinavir given as Invirase or Fortovase. Results from studies conducted with Invirase may not be applicable to Fortovase.
[†]Study conducted with Fortovase.
[‡]Study conducted with Invirase.
From U.S. Department of Health and Human Services: Guidelines for the Use of Antiretroviral Agents in HIV-1 Infected Adults and Adolescents. Available at www.aidsinfo.nih.gov.

Table 14-10 Drug Effects on Concentration of NNRTIs

Drug Affected	Nevirapine	Delavirdine	Efavirenz
PIS and NNRTIs			
Indinavir (IDV)	Levels: IDV ↓ 28% NVP no effect Dose: IDV 1000 mg q8h, or consider IDV/RTV NVP standard	Levels: IDV ↑ >40% DLV no effect Dose: IDV 600 mg q8h DLV standard	Levels: IDV ↓ 31% Dose: IDV 1000 mg q8h, or consider IDV/RTV EFV standard
Ritonavir (RTV)	Levels: RTV ↓ 11% NVP no effect Dose: standard	Levels: RTV ↑ 70% DLV no effect Dose: DLV standard RTV: no data	Levels: RTV ↑ 18% EFV ↑ 21% Dose: standard
Saquinavir* (SQV)	Levels: SQV ↓ 25% NVP no effect Dose: consider SQV-sgc/RTV 400/400 or 1000/100 bid or SQV-hgc/RTV 1000/100 bid	Levels: SQV[†] ↑ 5 × DLV no effect Dose: Fortovase 800 mg tid, DLV standard (monitor transaminase levels)	Levels: SQV[†] ↓ 62% EFV ↓ 12% SQV is not recommended to be used as sole PI when EFV is used Dose: Consider SQV-sgc/RTV 400/400
Nelfinavir (NFV)	Levels: NFV ↑ 10% NVP no effect Dose: standard	Levels: NFV ↑ 2 × DLV ↓ 50% Dose: no data (monitor for neutropenic complications)	Levels: NFV ↑ 20% Dose: standard
Amprenavir (APV)	No data	Levels: APV AUC ↑ 130% DLV AUC ↓ 61% Dose: coadministration not recommended	Levels: APV AUC ↓ 36% Dose: Add RTV 200 mg to standard APV dose, or consider APV/RTV 450/200 mg EFV dose standard
Fosamprenavir (fos-APV)	No data	Presumably similar PK affects as APV Dose: coadministration not recommended	Levels: fos-APV Cmin ↓ 36% (when dosed at 1400 mg qd with 200 mg of RTV) Dose: 1400 mg qd with 300 mg qd of RTV or 700 mg bid with 100 mg bid of RTV
Lopinavir/Ritonavir (LPV/RTV)	Levels: LPV Cmin ↓ 55% Dose: consider LPV/r 533/133 mg bid NVP dose standard	Levels: LPV levels expected to increase Dose: insufficient data	Levels: LPV AUC ↓ 40% EFV no change Dose: consider LPV/r 533/133 mg bid EFV dose standard
Atazanavir (ATV)	No data A decrease in ATV levels is expected	No data	Levels: ATV AUC ↓ 74% EFV no change Dose: Recommend ATV/r 300/100 mg each given once daily with food EFV standard
Nevirapine (NVP)	No data	No data	Levels: NVP no effect EFV: AUC ↓ 22%
Delavirdine (DLV)	No data	No data	No data

*Several drug interaction studies have been completed with saquinavir given as Invirase or Fortovase. Results from studies conducted with Invirase may not be applicable to Fortovase.
[†]Study conducted with Invirase.
From U.S. Department of Health and Human Services: Guidelines for the Use of Antiretroviral Agents in HIV-1 Infected Adults and Adolescents. Available at www.aidsinfo.nih.gov.

Table 14-11 Drugs Used Against Selected Opportunistic Infections

Infection/Drug	Usual Prophylactic or Suppressive Doses
Pneumocystis pneumonia (PCP)	
Trimethoprim (TMP)-sulfamethoxazole (SMX)/day PO or IV TMP 15 mg/kg/day × 3 wk	PO 1 double-strength (DS) tab qd or 3 ×/wk (e.g., 800 mg SMX + 160 mg TMP)
Pentamidine isethionate IV 3–4 mg/kg/day × 3 wk	300 mg inhaled monthly
Trimetrexate (+ folinic acid 20 mg/m² q6h × 3 wk) IV 45 mg/m² × 3 wk	—
Dapsone (+ trimethoprim 5 mg/kg tid PO × 3 wk) PO 100 mg/day × 3 wk	PO 100 mg 2 ×/wk or PO 100 mg/day + 50 mg pyrimethamine 2 ×/wk
Atovaquone PO 750 mg bid × 3 wk	—
Clindamycin (300 mg PO—600 mg IV qid × 3 wk) and primaquine (15 mg base PO qd × 3 wk)	—
Prednisone, in addition to TMP/SMX, if patient acutely ill, pO_2 <70 mm Hg (40 mg bid × 5 days, then 40 mg qd × 5 days, then 20 mg qd × 11 days)	—
Toxoplasmosis	
Pyrimethamine PO 50–100 mg qd and sulfadiazine PO 1.0–1.5 g q6h, or pyrimethamine + clindamycin	Pyrimethamine PO 25–50 mg qd and sulfadiazine 0.5–1.0 g q6h for suppression
Cryptosporidiosis	
Aminosidine (paromomycin) PO 500–750 mg qid	—
Nitazoxanide PO 0.5–1.0 g bid × 14 days	—
Mucosal candidiasis	
Nystatin PO 0.5–1.0 mU 3–5 ×/day or clotrimazole 10 mg 5 ×/day	—
Fluconazole PO 100–200 mg qd	—
Ketoconazole PO 200–400 mg qd	—
Cryptococcosis	
Amphotericin B 0.7–1.0 mg/kg/day + 5 FC 25 mg/kg PO qid, then fluconazole 400 mg PO × 8 wk	Fluconazole 200 mg PO qd for suppression
Herpes simplex virus (HSV) or varicella-zoster virus (VZV) infections	
Acyclovir 200–800 mg PO 5 ×/day or 10 mg/kg IV q8h × 1–2 wk for VZV	For suppression: 400 mg PO bid
Foscarnet 40 mg/kg IV q8h	40 mg/kg IV qd
Cytomegalovirus (CMV) infections	
Ganciclovir IV 5 mg/kg q12h	For suppression: IV 5–6 mg/kg qd or 5 ×/wk or PO 1 g tid po 1 g tid
Intraocular gancyclovir implant + valgancyclovir 900 mg PO bid with food × 14–21 days, then valgancyclovir 900 mg/day	
Foscarnet	
IV 60–90 mg/kg q8–12h	IV 90–120 mg/kg qd
Cidofovir (beware of nephrotoxicity)	
Mycobacterium-avium complex (MAC)	
Clarithromycin PO 500 mg bid *or* Azithromycin PO (500 mg/day or some use 500 mg 3 ×/wk) + Ethambutol 15–25 mg/kg/day + Rifabutin 300 mg PO qd	For primary prophylaxis: Azithromycin 1200 mg/PO/week or Clarithromycin 500 mg PO bid
Syphilis	
Penicillin	
IM 2.4 million units benzathine weekly × 1–3 wk or doxycycline 100 mg PO bid × 2–4 wk or IV 12–24 million units/day × 2 wk or IM 2.4 million units procaine qd × 10 days with 500 mg probenecid PO bid (one of the latter 2 regimens needed for neurosyphilis)	

From Bartlett JG, Gallant JE: The 2004 Abbreviated Guide to Medical Management of HIV Infection. Available from Johns Hopkins AIDS Service at http://www.hopkins-aids.edu/publications/publications.html.

SUGGESTED READINGS

Antifungal drugs. Treatment guidelines. Medical Letter 3:7–14, 2005.
Bartlett JG: Community-acquired pneumonia in adults: guidelines for management. The Infectious Disease Society of America. Clin Infect Dis 26:811–838, 1998.
Bartlett JG, Gallant JE: The 2004 Abbreviated Guide to Medical Management of HIV Infection. Available from Johns Hopkins AIDS Service at http://www.hopkins-aids.edu/publications/publications.html. Accessed 12/8/04.
Bartlett JG, Mundy LM: Community-acquired pneumonia. N Engl J Med 333:1618–1624, 1995.
Choice of antibacterial drugs. Treatment Guidelines from the Medical Letter 2:13–26, 2004.
Drugs for AIDS and associated infections. Med Lett Drugs Ther 37:87–94, 1995.
Drugs for HIV infection. Med Lett Drugs Ther 43(W1119A), 2001.
Drugs for non HIV-viral infections. Med Lett Drugs Ther 44(W1123A), 2002.
Drugs for tuberculosis. Med Lett Drugs Ther 37:67–70, 1995.
Musher DM, Spindel SJ: Community-acquired pneumonia. Curr Clin Top Infect Dis 16:102–124, 1996.
Piscitelli SC, Flexner C, Minor JR, et al: Drug interactions in patients infected with human immunodeficiency virus. Clin Infect Dis 23:685–693, 1996.
Systemic antifungal drugs. Med Lett Drugs Ther 38:10–12, 1996.
U. S. Department of Health and Human Services: Guidelines for the Use of Antiretroviral Agents in HIV-1 Infected Adults and Adolescents. Available at www.aidsinfo.nih.gov. Accessed 12/8/04.

15

Surveillance for Emerging Infectious Diseases and Bioterrorism Threats

RAY R. ARTHUR
JAMES W. LEDUC
JAMES M. HUGHES

INTRODUCTION

Despite advances in science, technology, and medicine that have improved disease prevention and management, endemic and emerging infectious diseases continue to pose threats to domestic and global health. Established diseases such as malaria, tuberculosis (TB), and human immunodeficiency virus (HIV) infection still proliferate, fueled in part by antimicrobial resistance.[1,2] The increasing speed and volume of international travel, migration, and trade create new opportunities for microbial spread, and the prospect of a deliberate release of pathogenic microbes underscores the importance of preparedness to address the unexpected.[3] The example of severe acute respiratory syndrome (SARS), a previously unknown disease that spread rapidly across countries and continents in 2003, illustrates the vulnerability of the global community to new microbial threats and highlights the need for increased vigilance and strengthened response capacity.[4,5]

The current state of readiness to address new disease agents is outlined in the 2003 Institute of Medicine report, *Microbial Threats to Health: Emergence, Detection, and Response*.[6] Building on the Institute's 1992 report,[7] which sought to dispel complacency about the risk of infectious diseases, the new report calls for raised awareness and aggressive global action to address the developments of the intervening decade. These developments include the continued evolution of antimicrobial resistance, the ongoing threat of an influenza pandemic, the increased transborder spread of contagious diseases, the upsurge in infections arising from animal reservoirs, and the threat of intentional biological attacks, as well as the availability of new technologies for diagnosing and preventing disease and for linking public health practitioners around the world.

Recent domestic challenges have included the introduction of West Nile encephalitis[8,9] and monkeypox[10] into the United States, the anthrax episodes of fall 2001,[11] and multistate outbreaks involving contaminated food products.[12–14] Internationally, public health officials have faced the emergence of Nipah virus[15] and SARS,[4] the intensified global spread of dengue,[16,17] Ebola outbreaks of unprecedented magnitude,[18] and the direct avian-to-human transmission of influenza.[19,20] Each of these examples illustrates the global implications of local problems, the role of strong health intelligence networks in addressing emerging infections, and the importance of data on the incidence of natural background diseases in recognizing unusual disease events.[21]

PUBLIC HEALTH SURVEILLANCE

Public health surveillance is the continuous and systemic collection, analysis, interpretation, and feedback of systematically collected information used to inform public health decision making.[22] Timely community health information in the hands of trained experts is the foundation for recognition of threats to health. To intervene successfully to treat existing infections and prevent the onset of new ones, disease surveillance systems need to provide a continuous, accurate, and near real-time overview of a population's health. Surveillance systems must be sensitive in terms of their ability to detect outbreaks and other significant changes in community health status over time, and they must be flexible in adapting to changing health intelligence needs. Given the increasing pace of international travel and globalization and the threat of intentional outbreaks, surveillance activities need to extend beyond the monitoring of disease burden to include the capacity to quickly recognize unusual, unexpected, or unexplained disease patterns. Because many emerging infectious agents are zoonotic, it is also important to integrate veterinary disease reporting networks into systems that monitor diseases of humans.

Astute clinicians and microbiologists are essential for early detection of threats at the clinical front lines. In the United States, surveillance for notifiable diseases is conducted by state and local health departments, which receive reports from physicians, nurses, and laboratorians who are often the first to observe and report unusual illnesses or syndromes. States voluntarily report nationally notifiable diseases to the Centers for Disease Control and Prevention (CDC) through the National Electronic Telecommunications System for Surveillance (NETSS). To expedite national disease reporting, CDC, in collaboration with the Council of State and Territorial Epidemiologists (CSTE), has developed a standards-based system for collecting and distributing electronic disease reports from local health departments to state and federal public health authorities. The infectious disease surveillance component of this developing Public Health Information Network (PHIN) is the National Electronic Disease Surveillance System (NEDSS). NEDSS is designed to standardize and facilitate the collection of electronic disease information on nationally notifiable diseases within local health jurisdictions directly from healthcare providers to local health authorities.[23] Limited resources have, however, precluded the establishment of a fully integrated health surveillance system that connects health departments and care providers.

Starting in 1994, CDC launched a two-phase initiative to strengthen domestic capacity to respond to the dual threats of endemic and emerging infections. The publication of

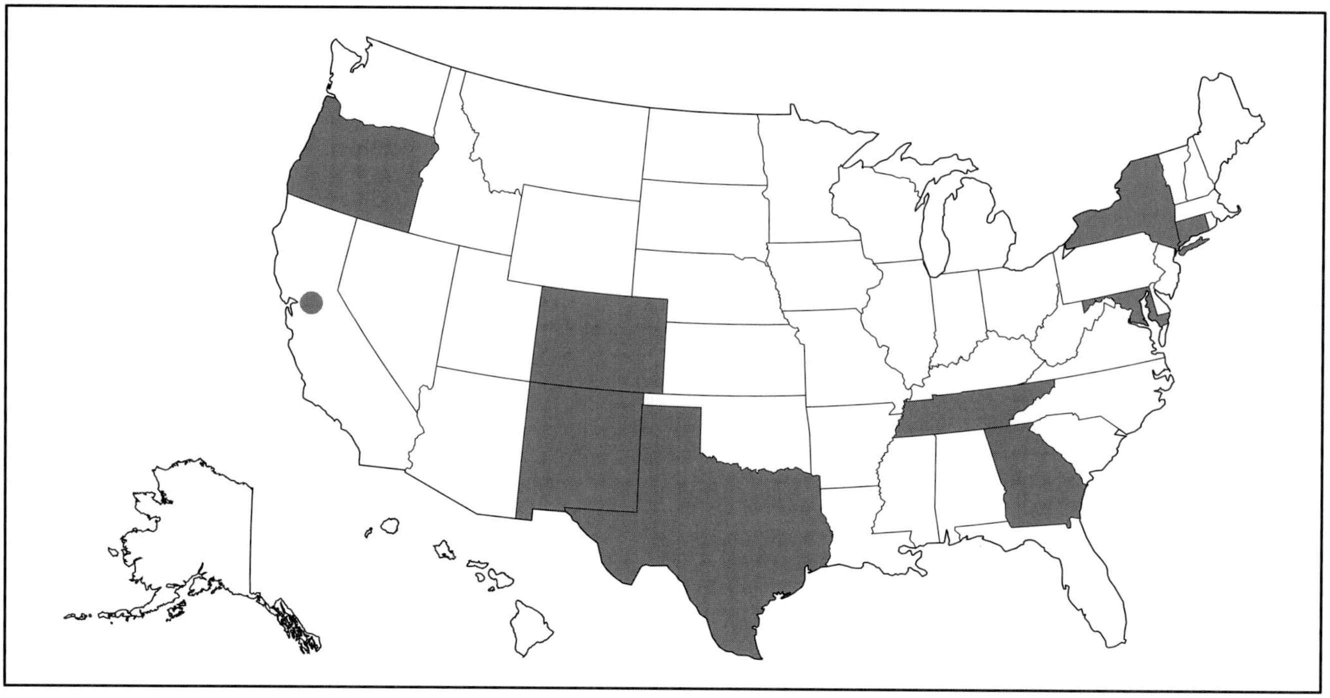

FIGURE 15-1 Distribution of Emerging Infections Programs (EIPs), a network of state health departments and their collaborators in local health departments, academic institutions, and clinical settings, coordinated by the Centers for Disease Control and Prevention, 2004. Surveillance population: approximately 44 million.

two strategy documents[24,25] led to the launching of new surveillance initiatives, including the Emerging Infections Program (EIP), a national network for population-based surveillance and research[26] (Fig. 15-1). Several provider-based sentinel surveillance networks were established in collaboration with emergency room physicians, infectious disease specialists, and travel medicine specialists to provide early warning of events that might be missed by public health surveillance. Additional enhancements to the surveillance effort include development of the National Molecular Subtyping Network for Foodborne Disease Surveillance (PulseNet) as an early warning system for foodborne diseases, support for the Gonococcal Isolate Surveillance Project (GISP) to monitor antimicrobial resistance in *Neisseria gonorrhoeae*, strengthened surveillance for diseases of current concern (e.g., West Nile encephalitis), and surveillance for outbreaks that might be due to acts of bioterrorism.

The CDC also works in partnership with the World Health Organization (WHO), ministries of health, foundations, development agencies, and other federal agencies to promote national, regional, and international disease surveillance. Recognition of the global nature of the emergence and spread of infectious diseases stimulated the development of a third strategy document focused on CDC's efforts to enhance global capacity for disease surveillance and outbreak response.[27] The document presents six priority areas for protecting domestic and global health, among which are global initiatives for disease control, international outbreak assistance, and a global approach to disease surveillance. CDC's international activities include creation of the United States–Mexico Border Infectious Disease Surveillance (BIDS) system, development of the Global Emerging Infections Sentinel Network (GeoSentinel), and provision of technical assistance to regional disease surveillance networks in Africa, Asia, Latin America, and the circumpolar regions of Canada and Europe, as well as to WHO's disease-specific global networks.

WHO manages global disease surveillance and response through a composite of partnerships and networks for gathering, verifying, and analyzing international disease intelligence, mainly to support global and regional efforts to eradicate certain diseases, such as polio, and to protect the global community against diseases with pandemic potential. The oldest of these networks is the global influenza surveillance network, which was established more than 50 years ago and has served as the prototype for the design and implementation of subsequent systems (see later discussion).[28] A recent addition to the disease-specific surveillance approach is DengueNet, a web-based network for gathering and sharing information on dengue and dengue hemorrhagic fever.

To respond to the increasing number of emerging and rapidly spreading infectious diseases, WHO has developed a global "network of networks" that links local, regional, national, and international networks of laboratories and medical centers into a mega-surveillance network for early warning and response.[29] Formal partners include ministries of health, WHO Collaborating Centers, WHO country and regional offices, and international military groups such as the Global Emerging Infections System of the U.S. Department of Defense (DoD-GEIS). Outbreak reports are also received from nongovernmental organizations, relief workers, private clinics, individual scientists, and public health practitioners. Additional information is provided by Health Canada's Global Public Health Intelligence Network (GPHIN), an electronic tool used by WHO since 1997, which scans Internet news sites for reports of outbreaks and unusual disease events.

Global surveillance networks all operate within the framework of the International Health Regulations, which outline WHO's authority and member states' obligations in reporting and preventing the spread of infectious disease. The International Health Regulations require official reporting of only three diseases: plague, cholera, and yellow fever.[30] Outbreaks of these diseases are reported in WHO's *Weekly Epidemiological Record* and electronically through postings on the Internet. Recognizing the limitations of the regulations in the era of emerging and reemerging diseases and spurred by the SARS experiences of 2003, WHO and its member states have undertaken a revision of the document. During the 56th World Health Assembly (WHA), two resolutions were passed, one specific to SARS (WHA56.29) and the other adding impetus to the revision efforts (WHA56.28). The resolutions seek to secure enhanced collaboration with WHO in responding to infectious disease outbreaks. In recognition of the role of animals in the spread of human disease and the potential for infectious disease dissemination due to international travel and trade, the resolution prompted by the SARS experience also urges member states to "ensure collaboration, when appropriate, with veterinary, agricultural and other relevant agencies involved in animal care and research on, and planning and implementation of, preventive and control measures."[31]

Whereas the International Health Regulations provide the legal framework for global control of infectious diseases, WHO's Global Outbreak Alert and Response Network (GOARN) is the operational arm, that is, the mechanism by which WHO's partners respond to outbreaks of international importance.[29] GOARN activities are described in the following section.

EXAMPLES OF SPECIALIZED SURVEILLANCE AND RESPONSE NETWORKS

Global Influenza Surveillance Network

Established in 1952, this global network of more than 100 virus laboratories in 83 countries monitors influenza activity and collects the viral isolates that determine the composition of the following year's influenza vaccines[32] (Fig. 15-2). The isolates are characterized by WHO Collaborating Centers in the United Kingdom, Japan, Australia, and the United States. In addition to guiding the annual composition of recommended vaccines, the network operates as an early warning system for the appearance of influenza variants and novel strains that could signal the emergence of an influenza pandemic.

Global Laboratory Network for Poliomyelitis Eradication

International disease eradication strategies include a strong surveillance component. To support the Global Polio Eradication Initiative, WHO established the Global Laboratory Network for Poliomyelitis Eradication,[33] which uses molecular techniques to determine whether wild-type polio is circulating in areas undergoing eradication efforts. Genomic sequencing capabilities and collaboration among network laboratories have allowed the tracking of virus

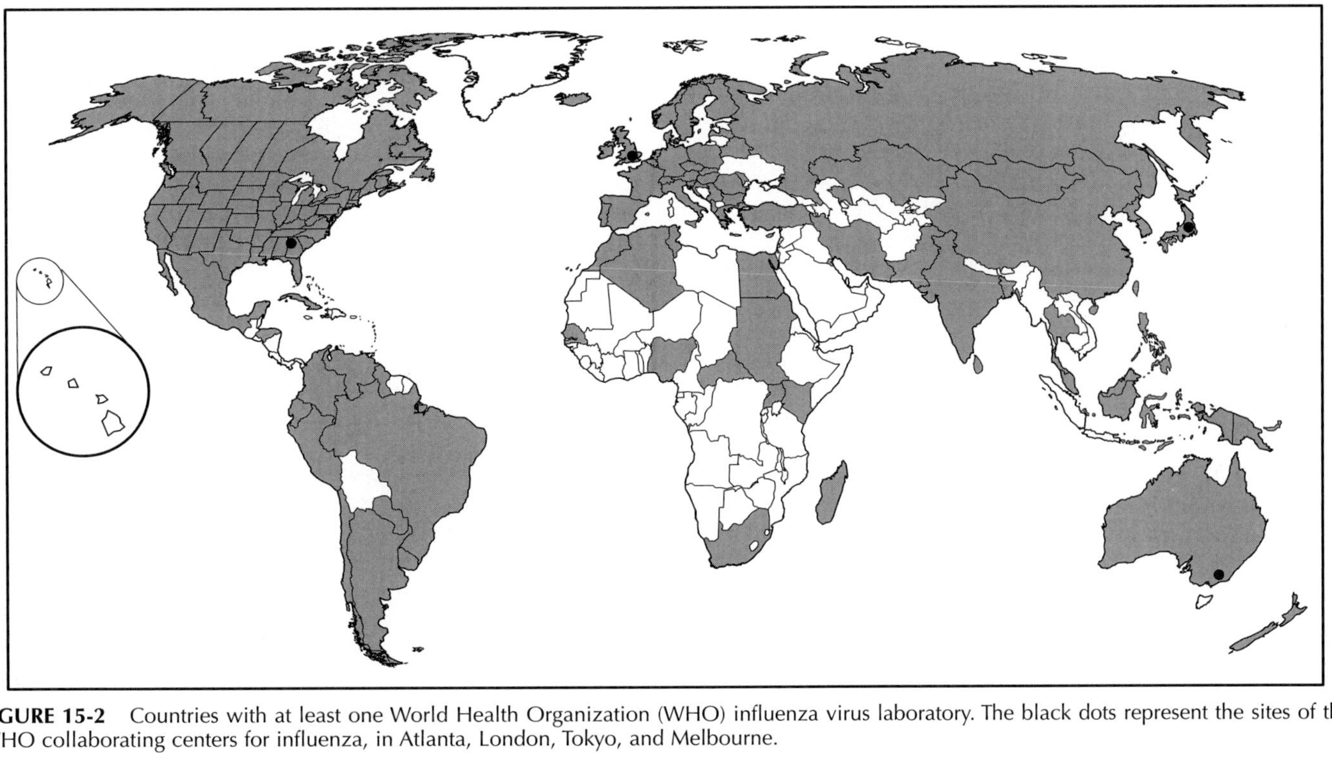

FIGURE 15-2 Countries with at least one World Health Organization (WHO) influenza virus laboratory. The black dots represent the sites of the WHO collaborating centers for influenza, in Atlanta, London, Tokyo, and Melbourne.

strains within and among countries and the identification of the origin of viruses imported into polio-free countries.[34]

Global *Salmonella* Surveillance System (Global Salm-Surv)

Started in 2000, WHO's Global Salm-Surv is a global network of laboratories and individuals involved in isolation, identification, and antimicrobial resistance testing of *Salmonella* and surveillance of salmonellosis. The goal is to enhance the capacity and quality of *Salmonella* surveillance, serotyping, and antimicrobial resistance testing throughout the world. Global Salm-Surv conducts an electronic discussion group, international training courses for microbiologists and epidemiologists, external quality assurance testing, and focused research projects on topics such as surveillance enhancement and burden of illness. Member institutions enter their top 15 *Salmonella* serotypes yearly in a web-based country databank that can be searched for serotype frequency nationally, regionally, or globally.

Global Project on Antituberculosis Drug Resistance Surveillance

Surveillance of antimicrobial resistance is fundamental for understanding trends, developing treatment guidelines, and assessing the effectiveness of interventions. In 1994, WHO, the International Union against Tuberculosis and Lung Disease (IUATLD), and other partners launched the Global Project on Antituberculosis Drug Resistance Surveillance in response to growing concern about drug resistance and its impact on TB control. The purpose of this network of reference laboratories is to measure the prevalence of anti-TB drug resistance in several countries using standard methods and to study the correlation between the level of drug resistance and treatment policies in those countries.

Global Outbreak Alert and Response Network

GOARN was launched in 2000 as a mechanism for combating international disease outbreaks, ensuring the rapid deployment of appropriate technical assistance to affected areas, and contributing to long-term epidemic preparedness and capacity building. GOARN electronically links more than 120 partner institutions and surveillance networks, which together possess the expertise, skills, and resources for rapid outbreak detection, verification, and response.[29] The coordinated response to the large Ebola hemorrhagic fever outbreak in Uganda in 2000 demonstrated the merit of the principles on which the network is based and functions.[18,35] The importance of GOARN was also evident in 2003, when WHO coordinated the unprecedented global response to SARS. Through GOARN, WHO mobilized the international public health, clinical, and research communities to rapidly identify and characterize the causative agent and to contain the spread of this new infectious agent, providing a new standard for future responses to global microbial threats.[36]

Laboratory Response Network

The Laboratory Response Network (LRN) was established by CDC in 1999 to respond quickly to acts of chemical and biological terrorism, emerging infectious diseases, and other public health threats and emergencies. The more than 120 federal, state, and local public health, veterinary, military, environmental, and international laboratories in the network have progressively stringent levels of safety, containment, and technical proficiency that enable them to recognize, rule out, confirm, or definitively characterize highly infectious agents using standardized protocols and reagents and to maintain communication through a secure web site.

The value of the LRN was demonstrated during the SARS epidemic, when validated reagents and protocols were rapidly distributed within weeks of the discovery of the etiologic agent (SARS-associated coronavirus [SARS-CoV7]) thereby providing diagnostic testing capability to each state.

CRITICAL ROLE OF THE LABORATORY

Microbiology laboratories play a critical role in surveillance for emerging infectious diseases and bioterrorism threats by identifying the microbial cause of syndromes, detecting and reporting new or unusual pathogens, and assessing antimicrobial resistance.[6,37] To carry out this role, laboratories require well-equipped and safe facilities, adequate human and financial resources, access to needed reagents, and robust quality control.

Accurate etiologic diagnosis is dependent on standardization of and scrupulous attention to a series of essential procedures. These include the collection of appropriate clinical specimens, careful handling of specimens, accurate and complete labeling, and access to relevant clinical information to guide the testing process. Laboratorians also benefit from knowledge of the local epidemiologic situation. The chain of events is completed when the laboratory provides results to the attending medical staff to guide clinical management of the patient and to the epidemiologist for trend analysis, monitoring, and response. Specimen collection requires an understanding of the samples needed (e.g., whole blood, serum, cerebrospinal fluid); proper containers for safe transport outside the clinical facility; complete labeling with information on the source and the time of collection relative to clinical status; proper packaging for shipping; and compliance with regulations for transport. The laboratory to which the specimens are being sent should be notified in advance about the shipment to facilitate assistance with customs clearance and transport.

The critical needs of the laboratory center around three basic resources: equipment and supplies to conduct the required tests, reagents to test for the pathogens of interest, and trained staff to perform the testing. Although each of these requirements may be a limiting factor in the recognition of emerging infections, the availability of high-quality diagnostic reagents may be the most critical, especially for viral diseases. Laboratories often have adequate reagents for diseases known to occur locally but not for viral illnesses that occur in other parts of the world. Ensuring the quality of serologic tests also requires inclusion of positive and negative control sera that might be difficult to obtain, especially for diseases of low incidence. If reagents are not commercially available, the laboratory must rely on its own locally produced reagents or on reagents supplied by others that may not have benefited from appropriate quality control during production.

For some agents, such as influenza, dengue, and hantaviruses, commercially available diagnostic kits that can be used in settings with minimal laboratory facilities have overcome this obstacle. Nonetheless, the user, who may not be a trained laboratorian, still needs to collect the specimen appropriately and interpret the results correctly.

One of the most important aspects of a global strategy for monitoring of emerging diseases, especially those caused by viruses, is ensuring the proper level of biosafety containment and strict adherence to biosafety procedures to allow safe handling of pathogenic organisms. The importance of biosafety precautions was demonstrated by the recurrence of SARS-CoV in Singapore, Taiwan, and China in late 2003 to early 2004 due to laboratory acquired infections.[38–40] Most organisms are classified in one of four distinct biosafety levels, depending on the seriousness of the disease they produce, their transmissibility, and the availability of effective treatment or vaccines.[41] Biosafety levels 3 and 4 are required for handling the most dangerous pathogens and require highly specialized facilities. The physical plant required to support a biosafety level 4 laboratory is considerable, and maintenance expenses are high. Consequently, only a few exist in the world, and all serve as major referral laboratories.

Laboratory diagnosis is not confined, however, to state-of-the-art facilities. The use of field laboratories can be a factor in the rapid containment of outbreaks of emerging infectious diseases. During the 2000–2001 outbreak of Ebola hemorrhagic fever in Uganda, laboratory testing was performed at a field laboratory established by CDC and supplemented by additional testing at CDC and other reference centers.[18] The availability of the field lab was determined to be a key logistic element in containing the outbreak rapidly.[42]

Pathology laboratories also make critical contributions to the identification of new and emerging infectious diseases.[43] Pathologists have had a frontline role in identifying the causal agents, describing the pathogenetic processes, and guiding the early phases of the epidemiologic investigations of several recently described diseases, including hantavirus pulmonary syndrome,[44] new variant Creutzfeldt-Jakob disease,[45] and SARS.[46] Clinicopathologic studies have also been useful in delineating the pathogenesis of emerging infectious diseases such as West Nile virus encephalomyelitis.[47] Immunologic and molecular methods, including immunohistochemistry (IHC), in situ hybridization, and polymerase chain reaction (PCR), have revolutionized the ability of pathologists to diagnose and study infectious diseases and are likely to ensure an increasing role of pathology as an active partner in surveillance activities.[43]

COMMUNICATIONS

A final component of surveillance is the ability to rapidly and reliably exchange information on disease incidence and distribution, preferably in real time. Disease intelligence relies on formal and informal networks for dissemination and sharing of timely, accurate information on occurrences and outbreaks of infectious diseases and diffusion of prevention recommendations. One of the key lessons that emerged from the 2003 global SARS epidemic was the importance of networks of laboratory scientists, clinicians, and public health experts, aided by electronic communications, in rapidly generating the scientific basis for public health action. It was the "virtual" international network of laboratories, linked by a secure web site and daily teleconferences, that identified the causative agent and developed early diagnostic tests. The laboratory network served as a model for groups of clinical and epidemiologic experts who shared and compiled the data needed to track the outbreak and assess the effectiveness of containment measures.

In the current electronic era, countries are increasingly aware of the value of network-facilitated early warning systems, rapid information exchange, and technology transfer for the control of infectious agents. Technologies developed and enhanced over the last several years have stimulated the creation of web-based public health tools for improving national and international disease reporting and facilitating emergency communications. In the United States, CDC communicates breaking surveillance information to public health officials through two electronic networks: the Epidemic Information Exchange (Epi-X), a secure mechanism for sharing health surveillance information on outbreaks and other unusual events, and the Health Alert Network (HAN), which links local, state, and federal health agencies and provides an electronic platform for emergency alerts and long distance training. In similar fashion, the Eurosurveillance Project, funded by the European Commission, promotes the diffusion and exchange of information on communicable diseases in Europe. Globally, WHO shares information through the Outbreak Verification List distributed weekly by electronic mail, the WHO Disease Outbreak News on the WHO web site, and the *Weekly Epidemiological Record*. Supplementing these mechanisms are less formal networks of individuals and organizations, such as GPHIN, the web-based application that scans global electronic news media for information on health risks and the Program for Monitoring Emerging Diseases (ProMED), a web-based reporting system.

Another essential component of information exchange during infectious disease outbreaks is risk communication. Any outbreak of a novel or reemerging infectious disease is likely to be characterized by scientific uncertainties and high levels of concern that public health officials will be challenged to harness and guide. Since the 2001 anthrax attacks and the 2003 global SARS outbreaks, CDC and WHO have been actively involved in efforts to incorporate risk communication into public health practice.

SUMMARY

Future challenges posed by infectious agents are difficult to predict but certainly include the continuing threat of an influenza pandemic, a recurrence of SARS, the emergence of other zoonotic agents that cross the species barrier to humans, the emergence of new bacterial strains that are more virulent or resistant to antibiotics, the possible deliberate release of pathogenic microbes by terrorists, and the likelihood of increased spread of dengue, cholera, West Nile virus, yellow fever, and foodborne diseases. The best defense against these mobile and resilient pathogens is timely and reliable infectious disease information obtained through global public health surveillance.[29] The international community has made important strides in developing networks for detecting and reporting infectious disease events and enhancing capacity for clinical and laboratory surveillance. Continued commitment and support are needed to optimize the use of these systems to improve the detection of unusual disease events, strengthen the ability to share disease intelligence, and inform prevention and containment efforts.

REFERENCES

1. Bloland PB: Drug resistance in malaria. Geneva, World Health Organization, 2001.
2. WHO: WHO global strategy for containment of antimicrobial resistance. Geneva, World Health Organization, 2001.
3. Insitute of Medicine: Biological threats and terrorism: Assessing the science and response capabilities. Workshop summary. Washington, DC, National Academy Press, 2002.
4. Berger A, Drosten C, Doerr HW, et al: Severe acute respiratory syndrome (SARS)—paradigm of an emerging viral infection. J Clin Virol 29:13–22, 2004.
5. IOM: Learning from SARS: Preparing for the next disease outbreak. Washington, DC, National Academies Press, 2004.
6. IOM: Microbial threats to health: Emergence, detection, and response. Washington, DC, National Academies Press, 2003.
7. IOM: Emerging infections: Microbial threats to health in the United States. Washington, DC, National Academy Press, 1992.
8. Petersen LR, Roehrig JT: West Nile virus: A reemerging global pathogen. Emerg Infect Dis 7:611–614, 2001.
9. Petersen LR, Marfin AA, Gubler DJ: West Nile virus. JAMA 290:524–528, 2003.
10. Reed KD, Melski JW, Graham MB, et al: The detection of monkeypox in humans in the Western Hemisphere. N Engl J Med 350:342–350, 2004.
11. Jernigan DB, Raghunathan PL, Bell BP, et al: Investigation of bioterrorism-related anthrax, United States, 2001: Epidemiologic findings. Emerg Infect Dis 8:1019–1028, 2002.
12. CDC: Multistate outbreak of *Salmonella* serotype Typhimurium infections associated with drinking unpasteurized milk—Illinois, Indiana, Ohio, and Tennessee, 2002–2003. MMWR 52:613–615, 2003.
13. CDC: Public health dispatch: Multistate outbreak of hepatitis A among young concert attendees—United States, 2003. MMWR 52:844–845, 2003.
14. Jay MT, Garrett V, Mohle-Boetani JC, et al: A multistate outbreak of *Escherichia coli* O157:H7 linked to consumption of beef tacos at a fast-food restaurant chain. Clin Infect Dis 39:1–7, 2004.
15. Chua K, Bellini W, Rota P, et al: Nipah virus: A recently emergent deadly paramyxovirus. Science 288:1432–1435, 2000.
16. Messer WB, Gubler DJ, Harris E, et al: Emergence and global spread of a dengue serotype 3, subtype III virus. Emerg Infect Dis 9:800–809, 2003.
17. WHO: Dengue/dengue haemorrhagic fever: Situation in 2000. Wkly Epidemiol Rec 75:193–196, 2000.
18. CDC: Outbreak of Ebola hemorrhagic fever—Uganda, August 2000–January 2001. MMWR 50:73–77, 2001.
19. CDC: Isolation of avian influenza A (H5N1) viruses from humans—Hong Kong, May–December 1997. MMWR 46:205–207, 1997.
20. Hien TT, Liem NT, Dung NT, et al: Avian influenza A (H5N1) in 10 patients in Vietnam. N Engl J Med 350:1179–1188, 2004.
21. Heymann DL: The microbial threat in fragile times: Balancing known and unknown risks. Bull World Health Organ 80:179, 2002.
22. CDC: Updated guidelines for evaluating public health surveillance systems: Recommendations from the guidelines working group. MMWR 50(RR-13), 2001.
23. NEDSS Working Group: National Electronic Disease Surveillance System (NEDSS): A standards-based approach to connect public health and clinical medicine. J Public Health Manag Pract 7:43–50, 2001.
24. CDC: Addressing emerging infectious disease threats: A prevention strategy for the United States. Atlanta, Centers for Disease Control and Prevention, 1994.
25. CDC: Preventing emerging infectious diseases: A strategy for the 21st century. Atlanta, Centers for Disease Control and Prevention, 1998.
26. Pinner RW, Rebmann CA, Schuchat A, et al: Disease surveillance and the academic, clinical, and public health communities. Emerg Infect Dis 9:781–787, 2003.
27. CDC: Protecting the nation's health in an era of globalization: CDC's global infectious disease strategy. Atlanta, Centers for Disease Control and Prevention, 2002.
28. Heymann DL, Rodier GR: Global surveillance of communicable diseases. Emerg Infect Dis 4:362–365, 1998.
29. Heymann DL, Rodier GR: Hot spots in a wired world: WHO surveillance of emerging and re-emerging infectious diseases. Lancet Infect Dis 1:345–353, 2001.
30. WHO: International Health Regulations, 3rd annotated ed. Geneva, World Health Organization, 1983.
31. WHO: Revision of the International Health Regulations. World Health Assembly resolution WHA 56.28. Geneva, World Health Organization, 2003.
32. WHO: WHO global influenza surveillance network, 2004. http://www.who.int/csr/disease/influenza/surveillance/en/. Accessed 1/28/05.
33. CDC: Laboratory surveillance for wild poliovirus and vaccine-derived poliovirus, 2000–2001. MMWR 51:369–371, 2002.
34. CDC: Progress toward global eradication of poliomyelitis, 2001. MMWR 51:253–256, 2002.
35. WHO: Global outbreak alert and response network, 2005. http://www. who.int/csr/outbreaknetwork/en/. Accessed 3/24/05.
36. Heymann DL: The international response to the outbreak of SARS in 2003. Philos Trans R Soc Lond B Biol Sci 359:1127–1129, 2004.
37. McGowan JE Jr, Tenover FC: Confronting bacterial resistance in healthcare settings: A crucial role for the microbiologist. Nat Rev Microbiol 2:251–258, 2004.
38. Lim PL, Kurup A, Gopalakrishna G, et al: Laboratory-acquired severe acute respiratory syndrome. N Engl J Med 350:1740–1745, 2004.
39. WHO: Severe acute respiratory syndrome in Taiwan, China, 2003. http://www.who.int/csr/don/2003_12_17/en/. Accessed 1/28/05.
40. WHO: Investigation into China's recent SARS outbreak yields important lessons for global public health, 2004. http://www.wpro.who.int/sars/docs/update/update_07022004.asp. Accessed 1/28/05.
41. CDC/NIH: Biosafety in microbiological and biomedical laboratories. 4th ed. Washington, DC, Government Printing Office, 1999.
42. Maurice J: The Uganda Ebola outbreak—not all negative. Bull World Health Organ 78:1476–1477, 2000.
43. Zaki SR, Paddock CD: The emerging role of pathology in infectious diseases. In Scheld WM, Craig WA, Hughes JM (eds): Emerging Infections 3. Washington, DC, ASM Press, 1999.
44. Goldsmith CS, Elliott LH, Peters CJ, et al: Ultrastructural characteristics of Sin Nombre virus, causative agent of hantavirus pulmonary syndrome. Arch Virol 140:2107–2122, 1995.
45. Will RG, Ironside JW, Zeidler M, et al: A new variant of Creutzfeldt-Jakob disease in the UK. Lancet 347:921–925, 1996.
46. Goldsmith CS, Tatti KM, Ksiazek TG, et al: Ultrastructural characterization of SARS coronavirus. Emerg Infect Dis 10:320–326, 2004.
47. Guarner J, Shieh WJ, Hunter S, et al: Clinicopathologic study and laboratory diagnosis of 23 cases with West Nile virus encephalomyelitis. Hum Pathol 35:983–990, 2004.

SECTION II

Pathogens

A. BACTERIAL AND MYCOBACTERIAL INFECTIONS

16

Enteric Escherichia coli *Infections*

THEODORE S. STEINER
NATHAN M. THIELMAN
RICHARD L. GUERRANT

INTRODUCTION

Diarrheal illnesses constitute one of the leading infectious causes of death and disability worldwide. It is estimated that approximately 2.5 million children die annually from diarrheal illnesses, the vast majority in Africa, Asia, and Latin America.[1] In a World Bank index of overall disease burden, disability-adjusted life years (DALYs) lost, diarrheal illnesses accounted for 7.3% of the total DALYs lost worldwide in 1990, nearly twice that due to sexually transmitted diseases, including acquired immunodeficiency syndrome (AIDS), and three times that due to malaria.[2] Furthermore, the World Bank DALY calculation for diarrhea counts predominantly its mortality, largely ignoring its even more staggering impact on morbidity and malnutrition.[3] Of the varied bacterial pathogens known to cause diarrhea worldwide, enterovirulent *Escherichia coli* collectively constitutes one of the most common, if not the most common, causes of diarrheal illness in tropical regions, particularly where sanitation facilities are limited.[4–6]

E. coli is the major aerobic organism of the normal intestinal flora, with around 10^{6-8} colony-forming units per gram of stool. Although the majority of isolates remain nonpathogenic gut commensals, diverse sets of virulence determinants confer this versatile species with virtually the entire range of pathogenic mechanisms by which bacteria cause diarrhea. Depending on how one deconstructs the complex range of diarrheagenic virulence traits in *E. coli,* anywhere between 5 and 10 different categories can easily be defined. This chapter emphasizes the five major types for which pathogenicity in outbreaks or volunteer studies has been established: enterotoxigenic *E. coli* (ETEC), enteropathogenic *E. coli* (EPEC), enteroaggregative *E. coli* (EAEC), enterohemorrhagic *E. coli* (EHEC), and enteroinvasive *E. coli* (EIEC). Also reviewed is diffusely adherent *E. coli* (DAEC), which has been variably associated with diarrhea in epidemiologic studies.

AGENT

E. coli is a short, non-spore-forming, often fimbriate gram-negative bacillus that grows readily on simple culture media or synthetic media with as little as glycerol or glucose as its only nutrient. With the exception of many enteroinvasive strains, most *E. coli* organisms are first identified as lactose-fermenting gram-negative rods on routine culture medium. Other biochemical characteristics include indole production, lack of citrate fermentation, positive methyl red test, and negative urease and Voges-Proskauer reactions. *E. coli* is further characterized by a relatively complex serotyping scheme involving 173 O (lipopolysaccharide), 80 K (capsular), and 56 H (flagellar) antigens, all of which can be subdivided into partial antigens. Although the final number of *E. coli* serotypes is enormously high, 50,000 to 100,000 or more, the number of pathogenic serotypes in gastrointestinal infections is fairly limited (Table 16-1). The current serotyping scheme

***Table 16-1** Serogroups Associated with Enterovirulent* Escherichia coli

Category	Predominant O Serogroups
Enterotoxigenic (ETEC)	*LT:* 1, 6, 7, 8, 9, 128 *LT + ST:* 11, 15, 20, 25, 27, 60, 63, 75, 78, 80, 85, 88, 89, 99, 101, 109, 114, 139, 153 *ST:* 12, 78, 115, 148, 149, 153, 159, 166, 167
Enterohemorrhagic (EHEC)	157, 26, 103, 111, 113, + some 50 others
Enteroinvasive (EIEC)	11, 28, 29, 112, 115, 124, 136, 143, 144, 147, 152, 164, 167, 173
Enteropathogenic (EPEC)	18, 26, 44, 55, 86, 111, 114, 119, 125, 126, 127, 128, 142, 145, 157, 158
Enteroaggregative (EAggEC)	3, 15, 44, 51, 77, 78, 86, 91, 92, 111, 113, 126, 141, 146
Diffusely adherent (DAEC)	75, 15, 126

establishes O and H antigens based on bacterial agglutination; the K antigen is determined by gel immunoprecipitation or phage typing.[7] Each of the major categories of diarrheagenic *E. coli* falls into a relatively, but not absolutely, restricted set of these O:H serotypes, which has proved useful in understanding both the pathogenesis and epidemiology of enteric *E. coli* infections.

EPIDEMIOLOGY

Despite the worldwide ubiquity of *E. coli,* most enteric *E. coli* infections are seen in the developing world where sanitation facilities are limited. In community-based studies in Bangladesh and Brazil, ETEC alone accounted for up to 15% to 20% of cases of diarrhea[4,8] and, overall, ETEC is regarded as the leading identified cause of traveler's diarrhea,[9,10] having been isolated in over half of the cases investigated in some studies.[11,12] Young children in the tropics are particularly prone to ETEC infections. In one prospective longitudinal study, ETEC was identified as the cause of diarrhea as many as two to three times per year per infant.[13] Like most enteropathogens, ETEC infection is acquired by ingesting contaminated food or water, and infants are at particular risk at weaning. The infective dose of ETEC is relatively high in the normal host, ranging from 10^6 to 10^{10} colony-forming units.[14,15]

EPEC was the first group of *E. coli* shown to cause diarrhea. In the 1940s, epidemiologic investigations implicated EPEC isolates in outbreaks of community-acquired and nosocomial infantile diarrhea in Great Britain.[16] In these initial reports, mortality rates exceeded 50% in some cases.[16] Although EPEC is no longer considered a common cause of diarrhea in most developed nations, sporadic cases and outbreaks have been reported in Great Britain, Finland, and the United States.[17–21] Numerous studies in tropical or developing areas have demonstrated a convincing association of EPEC in infants with diarrhea,[21–26] and in some studies EPEC was identified as the most common bacterial cause of diarrhea in the youngest children.[26–28] Recent hospitalization has been identified as an important risk factor for EPEC diarrhea in children in São Paulo, Brazil.[21] Older studies have suggested bottle feeding as a risk factor for EPEC diarrhea,[16,29] and more recent series have demonstrated that breastfeeding is protective.[21,28]

EAEC, classically identified by its ability to adhere to HEp-2 cells and glass slides in a "stacked-brick" pattern, is implicated as a significant cause of persistent diarrhea (greater than 14 days) in developing regions (identified on the map with an asterisk [*]).[22,30–33] This endemic pediatric diarrhea was initially felt to be the predominant disease caused by EAEC, but more recent studies have demonstrated that EAEC is nearly as common as ETEC as a potential cause of adult travelers' diarrhea and also causes outbreak and episodic infections in developed countries.[34–38] EAEC has also been identified as a cause of chronic diarrhea in patients with AIDS.[39–42]

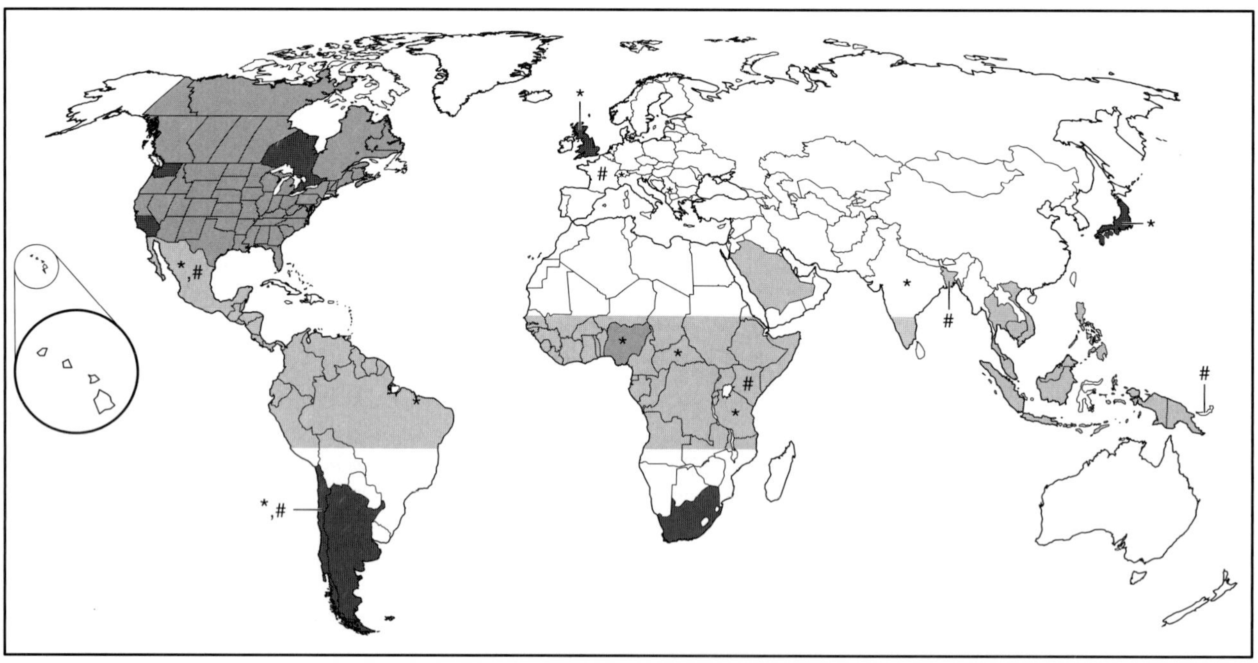

Enteric *Escherichia coli*

- Enterohemorrhagic *E. coli* (EHEC), more prevalent in industrialized regions, but outbreaks also have been recognized in South Africa and Swaziland.
- Major outbreaks of EHEC.
- Enterotoxigenic *E. coli* and enteropathogenic *E. coli*, more prevalent in developing, tropical regions.

Note: A number of epidemiologic studies have linked enteroaggregative *E. coli* (*) or diffusely adherent *E. coli* (#) with either acute or persistent diarrhea.

Diffusely adhering *E. coli,* so named because of its HEp-2 pattern of adherence, has been variably associated with diarrhea in a number of epidemiologic studies (identified on the map by the number mark [#]).[25,43–47] In the largest of these, Levine and colleagues[46] examined 1081 samples from children with diarrhea and matched controls in Chile. An association between DAEC and diarrhea increased with age, plateauing at a relative risk of 2.1 at 48 to 60 months of age. The increasing list of epidemiologic studies that examine the importance of EAEC and DAEC in pediatric diarrhea is exhaustive; the reader is referred to several excellent reviews for a comprehensive summary.[48–50]

Although infection with *E. coli* O157:H7 and other EHEC is primarily recognized in developed countries, this pathogen also occasionally plagues the developing world. The majority of outbreaks worldwide are reported in the United States, Canada, the United Kingdom, and Japan, where foods originating from or contaminated by bovine sources are typically implicated.[51–54] EHEC has also been isolated in a number of tropical or developing areas, including Chile, Argentina, India, South Africa, and Swaziland.[55–58] Like most of the other enterovirulent *E. coli,* sporadic cases of *E. coli* O157:H7 peak during the warm weather months.[59]

EIEC, which taxonomically is more closely related to *Shigella* than to other *E. coli,* probably accounts for only 1% to 2% of endemic diarrheal episodes.[60] EIEC infections can be readily transmitted via contaminated food, and the largest outbreak (226 persons affected) in the United States was attributed to contamination of imported Camembert cheese with EIEC serogroup O124.[61]

CLINICAL MANIFESTATIONS

Dictated by diverse sets of virulence determinants, the clinical manifestations of the different types of enterovirulent *E. coli* vary from cholera-like watery secretion with ETEC to dysentery indistinguishable from shigellosis with EIEC. The clinical characteristics of various enteric *E. coli* infections are summarized in Table 16-2. ETEC characteristically causes an acute watery diarrhea within 8 to 72 hours after ingestion, which ranges from a mild self-limited illness to dehydrating cholera-like purging.[14,15] Typically, stools are watery and without evidence of inflammation. Fever is usually low-grade or absent. Beyond the diarrhea, ETEC infections in infants and children interrupt normal feeding patterns and lead to diminished long-term linear growth.[4,13]

EPEC infections can be devastating to the neonate. Classically, mortality rates of 25% to 70% have been reported in outbreaks where clinical illness is typically characterized by vomiting, low-grade fever, and profuse watery diarrhea. In subjects with experimental EPEC infection, fecal lactoferrin levels are significantly elevated, demonstrating the inflammatory nature of this disease.[62] EPEC may persist, as evidenced in a U.S. day-care center outbreak in which infants' symptoms lasted for a mean of 18 days.[17]

EAEC is prominently linked with persistent diarrhea in children. Fever and grossly bloody stools are rarely associated with clinical infection,[22,31] but fecal lactoferrin levels are often elevated in children with EAEC infections whether they have diarrhea or not, the latter having significant growth shortfalls, suggesting that EAEC causes malnutrition and intestinal inflammation, with or without diarrhea.[63] It is notable that in some epidemiologic studies EAEC has not been associated with diarrhea[43,47,64] and that different strains have variably caused diarrhea in human volunteer studies.[65,66,66A] This observation is partly explained by heterogeneous expression of virulence determinants, but host factors may also be relevant. It was recently shown that travelers with a particular genotype in the interleukin (IL)-8 promoter are more likely to develop symptomatic diarrhea with EAEC infection. The importance of this and other naturally occurring polymorphisms in EAEC infection in other settings remains to be known.

Little is known about the clinical characteristics of DAEC enteric infections, which have been inconsistently associated with diarrhea (except in older children 18 to 60 months of age). One study found a particular association of DAEC with vomiting.[67] However, its pathogenicity is clouded by two studies involving 51 volunteers challenged with three different DAEC strains.[65,68] Only one individual developed diarrhea. As with EAEC, not all DAEC isolates (as defined by HEp-2 adherence) possess the necessary virulence traits to cause disease. For example, in one case-control study, only DAEC isolates that expressed the *afa* locus were statistically associated with diarrhea.[69]

E. coli O157:H7 and other EHEC cause diarrhea, hemorrhagic colitis, hemolytic-uremic syndrome (HUS), thrombotic thrombocytopenic purpura (TTP), and sometimes death. Although infection with *E. coli* O157:H7 typically begins as nonbloody diarrhea, in most cases that come to medical attention the diarrhea becomes bloody by the second or third day of illness. Fevers are seen in fewer than one-third of patients and vomiting in about half. Fecal leukocytes or lactoferrin are typically seen in less than 40% of patients with symptomatic EHEC infection. Uncomplicated infections typically resolve in about 1 week. Infection with *E. coli* O157:H7 has been confused with a number of other gastrointestinal disorders such as appendicitis, inflammatory bowel disease, and ischemic colitis.[51,70] Local complications may include bowel perforation, toxic megacolon, and stricture.[59,70,71] The most devastating sequela, HUS (a constellation of microangiopathic hemolytic anemia, thrombocytopenia, and acute renal failure), occurs most frequently in children between 1 and 4 years of age and in the elderly.[72] The overall rate of HUS in sporadic cases of bloody diarrhea with *E. coli* O157:H7 is between 5% and 10%.[59] A number of studies point to preexisting EHEC infection in 75% to 95% of children presenting with HUS.[73–76] It is often difficult to document microbiologic evidence of EHEC infection at the onset of HUS symptoms, as persons with HUS typically seek medical attention around 6 to 12 days after the onset of diarrhea, when the EHEC stool counts are decreasing.[77] Reported risk factors for the development of HUS in patients with EHEC diarrhea include the extremes of age,[78] leukocytosis,[79] diminished P1 antigen expression on red blood cells,[80] the use of antimotility agents, and possibly prior antimicrobial therapy (see later discussion).[51,81]

As with shigellosis, EIEC infection typically causes watery diarrhea, followed by dysenteric stools with mucus, fecal leukocytes, and scant blood. Fever, severe abdominal cramps, and malaise are common.

Table 16-2 *Clinical Features of Enteric* Escherichia coli *Infections*

Type of *E. coli*	Epidemiology/Setting	Incubation Period	Diarrhea	Additional Features	Sequelae
ETEC	Young children to adults in developing world Travelers to tropics	10–72 hr	Acute watery	Nausea, abdominal cramping; with or without low grade fevers	Interrupted feeding patterns leading to diminished linear growth
EPEC	Infants in developing world	As short as 9–12 hr	Acute persistent Watery	Positive fecal lactoferrin, vomiting, fever, dehydration	Mortality rates up to 25%–70% reported
EAEC	Children in developing world	20–48 hr	Persistent	Fever in 12%; grossly bloody stools in up to one third of patients	May interfere with normal growth patterns
	Travelers to tropics	Unknown	Acute; occasionally persistent	More likely than ETEC to have positive fecal lactoferrin	Occasional persistence
EHEC	All ages Primarily in United States, Canada, Europe, cone of South America	12–60 hr	Acute bloody diarrhea (progressing to hemorrhagic colitis in 38%–61%); occasionally nonbloody diarrhea	Fecal leukocytes or lactoferrin in 30%–40%; Fevers in 0%–32%; abdominal pain; moderate leukocytosis	Progression to HUS/TTP in 2%–8%; rarely death; complications greatest at extremes of age; Long-term renal damage may occur following HUS
EIEC	All ages Primarily in developing regions; occasional outbreaks in industrialized countries	As short as 10–18 hr	Acute watery diarrhea followed by dysentery	Fecal leukocytes or lactoferrin elevated; gross purulence, blood, mucus may be seen in stool; severe abdominal cramps	Hypoglycemia, especially if malnourished
DAEC	Pathogenicity most established in children ages 24–60 months	Unknown	Acute in 3 studies; persistent in 1; not associated with diarrhea in multiple studies	Nausea/vomiting prominent in one study	Unknown

HUS, hemolytic-uremic syndrome; TTP, thrombotic thrombocytopenic purpura.

PATHOGENESIS AND IMMUNITY

Summarized in Table 16-3 are the major known virulence determinants for enterovirulent *E. coli*, including their genetic traits, mechanisms of action, and relevant experimental models. Also noted are other enteric bacteria expressing similar virulence determinants, illustrating that the diverse range of virulence traits demonstrated in *E. coli* infections are representative of those present in the majority of bacterial enteropathogens. While not dealt with elsewhere in this book, such organisms as *Aeromonas, Plesiomonas, Klebsiella, Citrobacter, Enterobacter,* and *Yersinia* may produce enterotoxins, as noted in Table 16-3, and may be important enteric pathogens, more often in cooler, temperate climates.

Enterotoxigenic *E. coli*

In order for ETEC to be fully pathogenic, the organism must both colonize the small intestine and elaborate one or more enterotoxins. After ingestion in contaminated food or water, ETEC with fimbrial colonization factor antigens (CFAs) attach and multiply in situ, thereby overcoming the peristaltic defense mechanism in the proximal small intestine. CFA-I, CFA-II, CFA-IV, and others are distinguished from the type 1 pili, common to almost all *E. coli*, by their ability to agglutinate erythrocytes in the presence of D-mannose. Although most ETEC isolates are associated with at least one of the classic CFA types, other additional attachment factors (such as PCFO159, PCFO166, E8775, CS 7, and CS 17), yet to be fully characterized, may also participate in small intestine colonization.[82–85]

ETEC is defined primarily by the heat-labile (LT) and heat-stable (ST) toxins it elaborates. Of the four known enterotoxins (LT-I, LT-II, STa, and STb) produced by ETEC, LT-I and STa are best established as important secretagogues in humans, and pathogenic strains typically elaborate one or both of these toxins. The LT-I family of toxins are high-molecular-weight proteins (84,000 to 86,000 daltons) remarkably similar to cholera toxin in structure and function. The deduced amino acid sequences of the single enzymatically active (A) subunit and the five binding (B) subunits of LT-I demonstrate approximately 80% homology with that of cholera toxin, and its secretory effect is blocked by antisera to cholera toxin.[86] Given this degree of structural similarity with cholera toxin, it is not surprising that the mechanism of action of LT enterotoxin is nearly identical to that of cholera toxin (Fig. 16-1). After binding to a GM_1 ganglioside receptor (or to a 130- to 140-kDa glycoprotein receptor 20 to 30 times more prevalent in intestinal brush border than the binding site for cholera toxin[87]) like cholera toxin, LT activates adenylate cyclase via NAD-dependent adenosine diphosphate (ADP) ribosylation of Gs_{α}. The resultant increase in intracellular cyclic adenosine monophosphate (cAMP) ultimately stimulates chloride secretion and inhibits sodium absorption, leading to the voluminous watery stools characteristic of this infection. The ST toxin family, which bears significant homology with

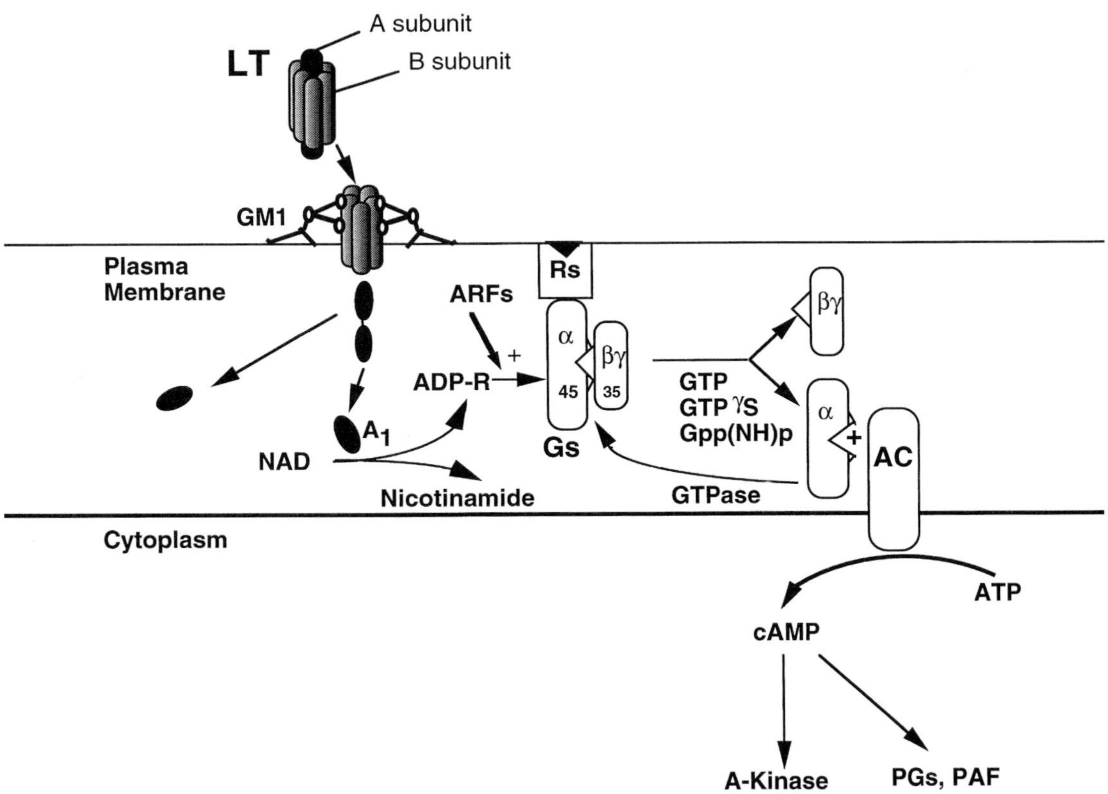

FIGURE 16-1 Heat-labile toxin (LT), a homologue of cholera toxin, binds to a monosialoganglioside receptor (GM1) via its B subunits, and the A_1 subunit is released from B_5 and A_2 by cleavage of a disulfide bond. This enzymatically active peptide catalyzes the dissolution of NAD to nicotinamide and, in the presence of adenosine diphosphate (ADP) ribosylation factors (ARFs), ADP ribosylates Gs_{α}, which then dissociates from the βγ subunit to activate adenylate cyclase. Cyclic adenosine monophosphate (cAMP) formation, catalyzed by adenylate cyclase, stimulates water and electrolyte secretion by intestinal epithelial cells via protein kinase A, prostaglandin (PG) synthesis, and possibly platelet-activating factor (PAF). ATP, adenosine triphosphate; GTP, guanosine triphosphate.

Table 16-3 Pathogenic Mechanisms of Enterovirulent Escherichia coli

Category*	Virulence Determinant	Genetic Locus	Mechanism	Experimental Model	Enteric Bacteria Expressing Similar Virulence Determinants
ETEC[†]	CFA-I-IV	Plasmid	Colonization	MRHA	
	LT I and II	LT-I (plasmid) LT-II (chromosome)	Adenylate cyclase → secretion	18-hr rabbit ileal loops and CHO/Y1 cells	LT-like toxins: *Vibrio cholerae, Klebsiella, Enterobacter, Aeromonas hydrophila, Plesiomonas shigelloides, Campylobacter, Salmonella*
	ST-I (ST_a)	Plasmid	Guanylate cyclase → secretion	4–6 hr rabbit ileal loops and suckling mice	ST-like toxins: *Yersinia enterocolitica, Citrobacter freundii*, non-O1 vibrios, EAEC
	ST-II (ST_b)	Plasmid	Cyclic nucleotide–independent HCO_3 secretion	Piglet loop	
EHEC[†]	SLT-I and II SLT-IIvh and IIvp	Phage	Toxins bind to Gb3 receptor, Glycosidase cleaves adenosine-4324 in 28S rRNA of 60S ribosomal subunits to halt protein synthesis	HeLa cell cytotoxicity	Shiga toxin: *Shigella dysenteriae* type 1
	Intimin	Locus of enterocyte effacement (LEE) (chromosomal pathogenicity island)	Intimate adherence to Tir (see below), leading to pedestal formation	Fluorescent actin staining (FAS), pedestal formation	EPEC, *Citrobacter rodentium*, REPEC
	Type III secretion system (TTSS)	LEE	Intimate attachment via Tir injected into cell membrane; actin rearrangement, pedestal formation		EPEC shares many similar genes, although pedestals are qualitatively different; TTSS found in many plant and animal pathogens (e.g., REPEC, *Citrobacter rodentium, Salmonella, Yersinia)*
	TTSS effectors: Tir	LEE	Binding to intimin, recruitment of actin condensation		
	EspA	LEE	Part of needle complex		
	EspB,D	LEE	Form pores in host cell membrane for effector delivery		
	EspF	LEE	Causes host cell apoptosis		
	EspG, H	LEE	Possibly mediates invasion		
	Map	LEE	Mitochondrial damage		
	NleA	Non-LEE PAI	Target unknown; localizes to Golgi apparatus		
	Accessory toxins: ToxB EspP Ehx (RTX toxin) StcE	pO157 plasmid	Implicated in adhesion, cytotoxicity, tissue edema	Various	Homologues in many pathogenic bacteria

EIEC[†]	IpaA, B, C IpgD (invasion and adhesin proteins)	Plasmid	Cell invasion and spread	Séreny test	Invasion plasmid: *Shigella* spp.
	IscA	Plasmid	Actin nucleation, leading to intracellular spread	Actin microfilament formation and cytoplasmic motility	*Shigella* spp.
	SepA	Plasmid	Serine protease autotransporter (SPATE)		Various
EPEC[†]	Bundle-forming pilus	60-MDa EAF plasmid (bfpA)	Localized adherence (LA)	LA to HEp-2 cells	
	Intimin/Tir	Chromosomal LEE	Tir injected into host cell gets tyrosine phosphorylated and binds intimin on bacterial surface	FAS, pedestal formation	EHEC, *Citrobacter rodentium*, REPEC
	TTSS	LEE, additional PAIs	Similar effectors as in EHEC, above		
	flagellin	*fliC* (chromosome)	Motility; IL-8 release via TLR5 activation	Motility and cytokine release	*Salmonella*, EAEC, EHEC
EAEC[†]	Aggregative adherence fimbriae (AAF)	*aggA* (60-MDa AA plasmid)	Aggregative adherence (AA), biofilm formation	HEp-2 or HeLa cell AA	
	EAST1	*astA* (AA plasmid)	Guanylate cyclase → secretion	Rabbit ileal loops and Ussing chambers	Found in many EHEC, other *E. coli*
	Dispersin	*aap* (AA plasmid)	Regulated deaggregation during colonization		
	Pet	Plasmid	Cleavage of fodrin, leading to cytoskeletal damage	Ussing chamber; cytotoxicity	Other SPATE family members
	Pic	*pic/set* locus on chromosome	Mucinase		
	ShET-1	*pic/set* locus on chromosome	Possible enterotoxin	Ussing chamber	*Shigella*
	flagellin	*fliC* (chromosomal)	IL-8 release via TLR5 activation	Motility, cytokine release	*Salmonella*, EPEC, EHEC
DAEC	Fimbrial adhesin (F1845)	Chromosome	Binding to CD55 (decay accelerating factor) leading to unique cytopathology	Diffuse adherence (DA) to HEp-2 cells	Uropathogenic *E. coli*
	Afimbrial adhesin (AIDA-I)	Plasmid	DA	DA to HEp-2 cells	

CFA, colonization factor antigen; LEE, locus of enterocyte effacement; LT, heat-labile toxin; MRHA, mannose-resistant hemagglutination; PAI, pathogenicity island, REPEC, rabbit enteropathogenic *E. coli*; SLT, Shiga-like toxin; ST, heat-stable toxin.

*See Table 16-1.

[†]Pathogenicity in humans established in outbreaks or volunteer studies.

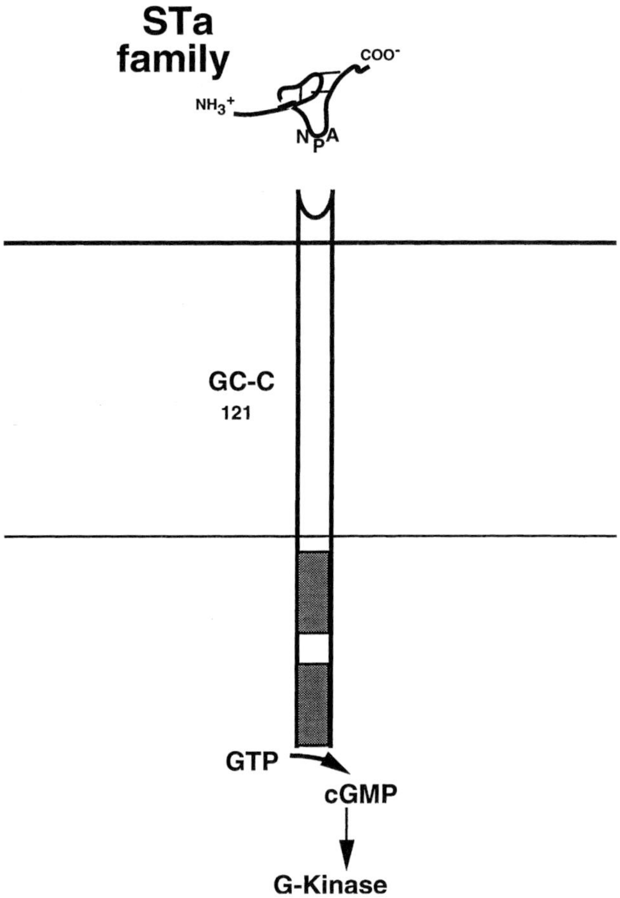

FIGURE 16-2 Heat-stable enterotoxin (ST), an 18– to 19–amino acid peptide, binds to an extracellular domain of guanylate cyclase (GC-C) to increase cyclic guanosine monophosphate (cGMP), which activates G kinase, ultimately leading to altered sodium and chloride transport via phosphorylation of membrane proteins. GTP, guanosine triphosphate.

the endogenous intestinal peptide guanylin, also causes fluid and electrolyte secretion.[88] The major ST toxin responsible for diarrhea in humans, STa, is an 18– to 19– amino -acid enterotoxin with no subunit structure, which contains three disulfide bonds important for biologic activity. As shown in Figure 16-2, STa binds to an extracellular domain of guanylate cyclase, resulting in increased intracellular levels of cyclic guanosine monophosphate (cGMP), which ultimately leads to decreased absorption of sodium and increased chloride secretion.

In addition to *Vibrio cholerae*, occasional other bacteria, including *Klebsiella, Enterobacter, Morganella, Aeromonas, Plesiomonas, Campylobacter,* and *Salmonella* species, have been shown to elaborate LT-like toxins.[5,89–94] An STa-like peptide toxin, EAST-1, is produced by many EAEC and EHEC isolates and causes fluid secretion in a cGMP-dependent manner.[95,96]

Enteropathogenic *E. coli*

Unlike in ETEC, secretory exotoxin elaboration does not play a role in the pathogenesis of EPEC. The basic pathogenic feature of these organisms is the attaching-and-effacing lesion, which is characterized by degeneration of the microvillus brush border, with cupping and pedestal formation of the plasma membrane at sites of bacterial attachment, noted histologically[97] (Fig. 16-3). Figure 16-4 depicts the four-stage model of EPEC pathogenesis, proposed by Donnenberg and Kaper,[98] as well as the mechanism of its invasive capacity. Localized adherence is mediated by the bundle-forming pilus, which is primarily encoded by the *bfpA* gene. A chromosomal *dsbA* gene that encodes a periplasmic enzyme capable of disulfide bond catalysis also appears to be necessary at this step. Adherent bacteria then express a type III secretion system (TTSS) "needle complex," which penetrates the host cell membrane and injects bacterial proteins, most notably Tir. After injection, Tir is tyrosine phosphorylated, leading to recruitment of cytoskeletal elements that form a tall pedestal upon which the bacterium sits. The *eae* gene product, intimin, sits in the bacterial cell wall and binds directly to Tir, helping to anchor the bacterium to the pedestal. A number of additional proteins secreted by the TTSS have been identified, some of which reside in the chromosomal pathogenicity island known as the LEE (locus of enterocyte effacement), which was clearly identified as a virulence trait in EPEC strains in human volunteer studies.[99] Additional non-LEE TTSS effectors have been recently described, adding additional complexity to the question of how EPEC causes diarrhea.[100,101] Several of these effectors appear to modulate host signaling and are required for full pathogenicity in closely

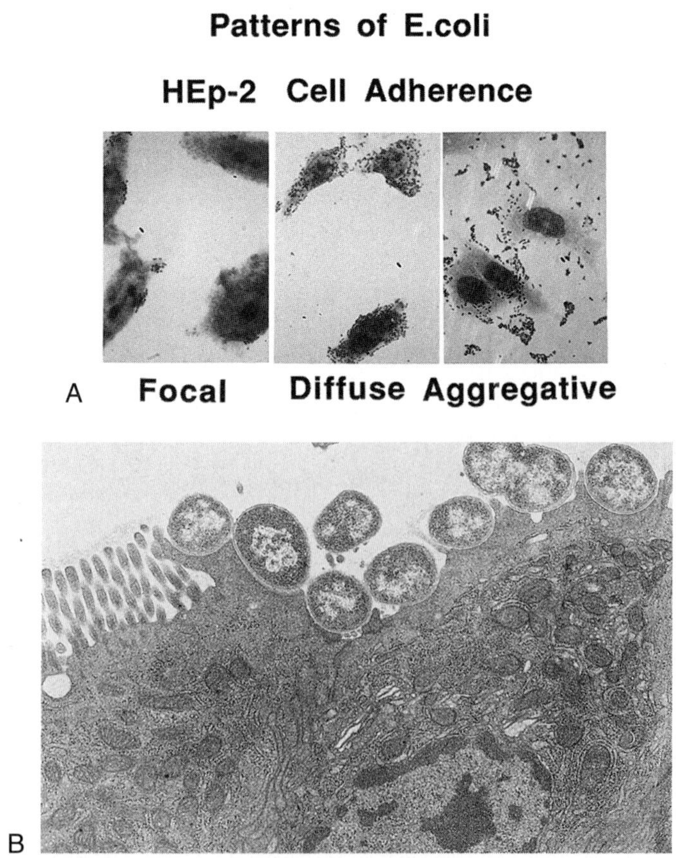

FIGURE 16-3 *A,* Three types of HEp-2 cell attachment: locally adherent enteropathogenic *E. coli* (EPEC, *left*), diffusely adherent *E. coli* (DAEC, *center*), and enteroaggregative *E. coli* (*right*). *B,* EPEC attachment and effacement on human enterocytes in a patient with diarrhea. (From Rothbaum R, McAdams AJ, Giannella R, et al: A clinicopathologic study of enterocyte-adherent *Escherichia coli:* A cause of protracted diarrhea in infants. Gastroenterology 83:441, 1982.)

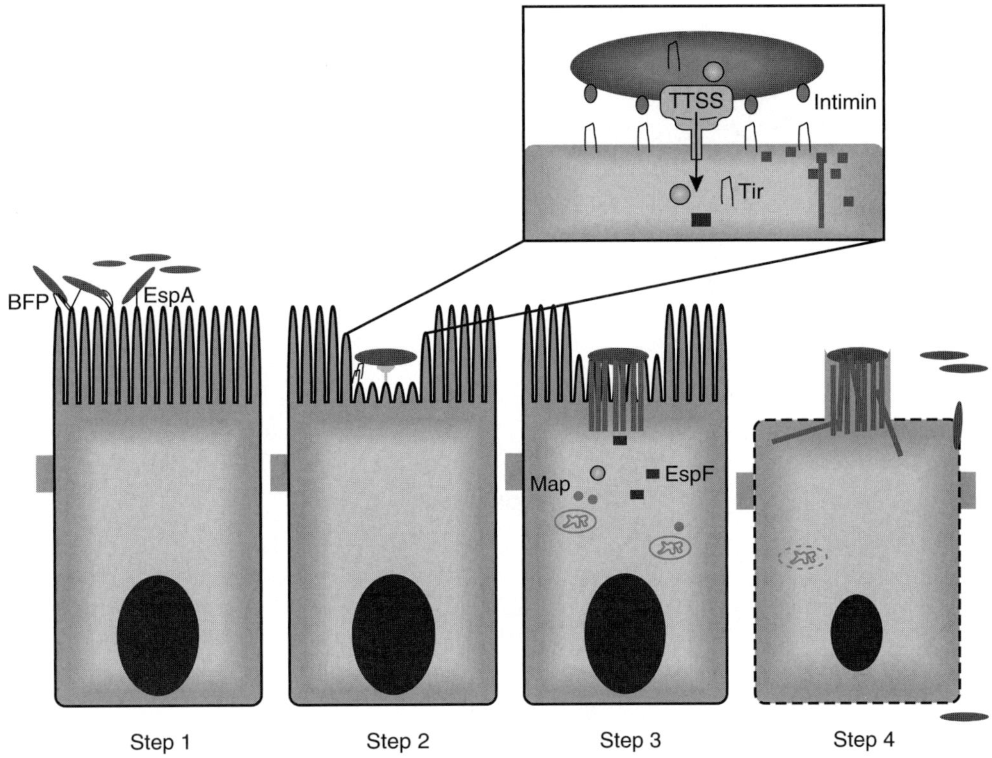

FIGURE 16-4 Four-stage model of EPEC (and EHEC) pathogenesis. Step 1: Bacteria contact the epithelial surface and adhere loosely via bundle-forming pili (BFP) and EspA projections. Step 2: Intimate attachment begins as bacteria inject Tir and other effectors via the type three secretion system (TTSS). Tir inserts into the host cell membrane and binds intimin on the bacterial surface. Meanwhile, host proteins are recruited to the cytoplasmic tail of Tir and begin cytoskeletal rearrangements. Step 3: Actin recruited to the contact point with the bacteria forms an elongated pedestal. TTSS effectors alter host cell physiology. Shown are Map, which damages mitochondria, and EspF, which causes apoptosis. Step 4: Pedestal formation and cell damage continue, leading to loss of membrane and mucosal barrier integrity. In addition, invasion of bacteria can occur at this stage. (Modified from Donnenberg MS, Kaper JB: Enteropathogenic *Escherichia coli*. Infect Immun 60:3953, 1992; and Tesh VL, O'Brien AD: Adherence and colonization mechanisms of enteropathogenic and enterohemorrhagic *Escherichia coli*. Microb Pathol 12:245, 1992.)

associated animal pathogens (*Citrobacter rodentium*, rabbit enteropathogenic *E. coli*). A list of known TTSS effectors of EPEC and other pathogenic proteins is given in Table 16-3. Although EPEC organisms do not cause keratoconjunctivitis in guinea pigs, a property classically associated with invasive *Shigella* and EIEC, invasion has been observed in clinical specimens, in vivo experimental models, and a variety of epithelial cell types in vitro.[102–107] Exactly how any of these epithelial cell changes lead to diarrhea has not been fully worked out. Incubation of EPEC with polarized epithelial monolayers results in decreased transepithelial resistance, possibly reflecting an increase in permeability that could contribute to diarrhea.[108] In addition, the loss of microvilli likely leads to malabsorption.[109]

The role of immune responses in EPEC infection is uncertain. The distinctively different age-specific attack rates may be explained by the development of immunity following colonization or infection with EPEC. Certain TTSS effector proteins, especially intimin and Tir, are highly immunogenic in mice.[110] Alternatively, the loss of age-specific receptors may account for the dramatic drop in EPEC infection in patients older than 6 months of age.[111] Several lines of evidence suggest that breast milk may provide passive immunity against EPEC infection. In addition to the association of EPEC infection with bottle feeding, secretory IgA to the EPEC adherence factor (EAF) and oligosaccharide fractions of human colostrum and breast milk have been shown to inhibit localized adhesion of EPEC to HEp-2 cells.[112,113]

Enterohemorrhagic *E. coli*

At least two virulence traits, attaching-and-effacing ability and Shiga-like toxin elaboration, confer pathogenicity to EHEC organisms. Like EPEC, EHEC cause filamentous actin accumulation at the site of attachment in association with "cup and pedestal" formation.[114] As in EPEC, this is achieved through the actions of genes on a chromosomal pathogenicity island analogous to the LEE. However, there are some differences between EPEC and EHEC pedestals; notably, EHEC Tir does not require tyrosine phosphorylation in order to initiate pedestal formation.[115]

What distinguishes EPEC from EHEC more obviously are the Shiga-like toxins (SLTs) of EHEC. These toxins, which are structurally and functionally similar to the Shiga toxin from *Shigella dysenteriae I*, are also referred to as verotoxins, reflecting their cytotoxicity for Vero cells. Thus, EHEC has been variably referred to in the literature as STEC and VTEC. Current convention is to label as EHEC only those organisms that have both attaching-and-effacing ability and express one or both SLTs.[48] At least two immunologically distinct SLTs, both with one A and five B subunits, have been described. The 70-kDa SLT-I is virtually identical to Shiga toxin and is neutralizable by antiserum against Shiga toxin. The smaller 60-kDa SLT-II is neutralized by antibodies to neither Shiga toxin nor SLT-I.[116,117]

Although SLTs alone are capable of stimulating bloody fluid accumulation and mucosal injury in multiple animal models,[118,119] SLT production does not appear to be requisite for developing diarrhea in EHEC infections.[120] In severe disease, particularly when bloody diarrhea is present, it is thought that SLTs gain systemic access and that they, particularly SLT-II, play a central role in the development of HUS. It is proposed that SLTs, which inhibit protein synthesis in a number of cell lines in vitro, do so in endothelial cells (Fig. 16-5), ultimately causing them to detach and expose platelets to the subendothelium, thus initiating coagulation.[121,122] The receptor for the SLT B subunit, globotriosyl ceramide or Gb3, is highly expressed in several of

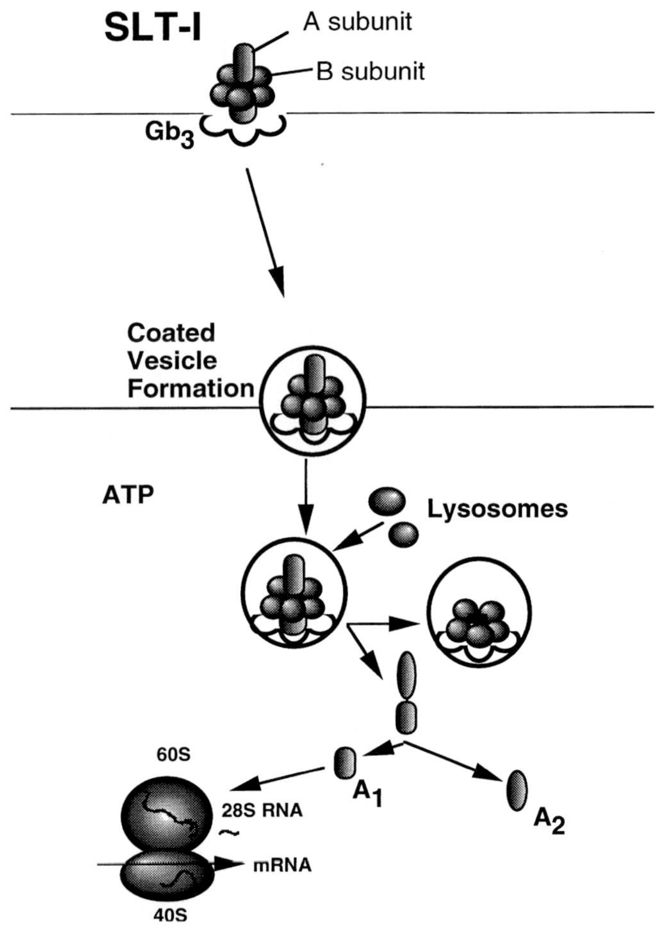

FIGURE 16-5 Shiga-like toxins (SLTs) I and II produced by enterohemorrhagic *E. coli* bind to globotriosyl ceramide (Gb_3) via B subunits and undergo receptor-mediated endocytosis. The A subunit, after release into the cytoplasm, is proteolytically degraded to A_1 and A_2 fragments. The former binds to the 60S ribosome and cleaves an adenine residue at position 4324 in 28S ribosomal RNA, thereby halting protein synthesis and causing cell death. ATP, adenosine triphosphate.

the target organs of EHEC/HUS, including the colon, kidneys, and brain.[123–126] In addition, in rabbits SLT-I has been shown to induce a thrombotic microvascular angiopathy similar to that seen in humans with HUS.[118] Epidemiologic data suggest that SLT-II may be more important than SLT-I for progression of *E. coli* O157:H7 infection to HUS.[53,127,128]

The role of antibodies in protecting against EHEC infection or its complications remains unknown. Although the epidemiologic observation of increased rates of infection and complications in young children and the elderly may suggest a role for immunity in preventing infection, reports of recurrent hemorrhagic colitis and HUS associated with recurrent *E. coli* O157:H7 infections argue against a key role for protective immunity.[59,129,130] However, there is hope that a bovine vaccine raised to adherence factors of EHEC may prevent colonization with these organisms and thereby eliminate spread to humans.

Enteroaggregative *E. coli*

Data from several volunteer studies demonstrate marked variability in EAEC pathogenicity in adults.[65,66,131] It is possible that this category of *E. coli*, defined primarily by a phenotypic assay (stacked-brick HEp-2 cell adherence), includes subsets of *E. coli* with varied (or no) virulence traits. However, phylogenetic analysis suggests that there are three distinct subfamilies of EAEC with common traits, indicating that EAEC is not as heterogeneous a class of bacteria as was once thought. Moreover, there is clinical evidence that strains with a "typical" adherence pattern and strains that express the transcriptional regulator *aggR* and genes in its regulon are more likely to be pathogenic than atypical strains.[38,132]

There are a number of identified virulence traits in EAEC. The characteristic HEp-2 adherence is mediated by flexible bundle-forming fimbrial structures, aggregative adherence fimbriae (AAF), of which at least three distinct types exist. The AAF are encoded by two separate gene clusters on the 60-MDa AA plasmid.[133] Also encoded on the plasmid is Pet, a member of the serine protease autotransporter toxin family. Pet cleaves host cytoskeletal proteins and may be responsible for many of the cytotoxic effects of EAEC in vitro. An additional plasmid protein, dispersin, is expressed during EAEC infection, and serves to release AAF attachments to allow for bacterial dispersion.[134] Many EAEC isolates also encode a plasmid-borne enterotoxin, designated EAST-1, which bears significant homology with the enterotoxin domains of ST and guanylin.[96]

In addition to the plasmid virulence traits noted previously, EAEC strain 042 (the prototype pathogenic in volunteers) expresses several chromosomal virulence traits. One of these proteins, Pic, is a mucinase that likely contributes to the distinctive intestinal adherence of EAEC.[135,136] The opposite strand from Pic in the same location encodes a protein, ShET-1, that was first identified as an enterotoxin in *Shigella flexneri*.[137] Finally, EAEC 042 expresses a highly inflammatory flagellin, which causes IL-8 release from epithelial cells in vitro and appears to be responsible for most if not all of the inflammatory response to EAEC.[138]

Diffusely Adherent *E.coli*

Less is known about DAEC pathogenesis than about other *E. coli* pathotypes. The diffusely adherent phenotype can be mediated by either fimbrial (F1845) or afimbrial (AIDA-1) adhesins.[139,140] These adhesins are homologous to Afa/Dr adhesins found on many uropathogenic *E. coli*, and bind to decay accelerating factor (CD55), leading to clustering of this protein in the cell membrane and unique ultrastructural changes.[141–144] Toxic effects include loss of tight junction integrity[145] and basolateral cytokine release.[146]

Enteroinvasive *E. coli*

Like *Shigella*, EIEC penetrates and multiplies within colonic epithelial cells, eventually causing cell death and the exuberant host inflammation responsible for much of the dysenteric clinical syndrome. A large 140-MDa plasmid that has extensive homology with the invasion plasmid of *Shigella* species mediates these virulence properties.[147] The invasion plasmid encodes a TTSS that injects effectors IpaA, B, and C and IpgD, which recruit epithelial cell signaling to create cytoskeletal rearrangements that permit entry of the bacterium (reviewed in Kaper and colleagues[48]). An additional plasmid-encoded protein, IcsA, localizes to one pole of the bacterial outer membrane where it binds neural Wiskott–Aldrich syndrome protein (N-WASP), leading to actin condensation. This polar actin condensation pushes the bacterium through the cytoplasm and ultimately into adjacent cells, leading to horizontal spread through the epithelium.[148,149] Other virulence traits expressed by some EIEC isolates include plasmid-encoded enterotoxins, which may explain the watery diarrhea often seen in early stages of EIEC infection.[150,151] It was also recently shown that EIEC can trigger inflammation in intestinal epithelial cells by activating the host protein Nod1.[152]

DIAGNOSIS

Because of the ubiquity of *E. coli* in fecal material, definitive diagnosis of enteric infections with enterovirulent *E. coli* often involves sophisticated techniques to detect the virulence traits themselves, many of which are beyond the scope of most clinical diagnostic laboratories. Of the enterovirulent *E. coli,* EHEC is most easily identified because of the dominant prevalence of serotype O157:H7. Because *E. coli* O157:H7, unlike most *E. coli,* does not ferment sorbitol, sorbitol-MacConkey agar is used as a screening medium. Presumptive diagnosis of *E. coli* O157:H7 infection can be made when sorbitol-negative (clear) *E. coli* isolates are shown to agglutinate in the presence of *E. coli* O157 antiserum.[153] However, non-O157 EHEC isolates, which can cause human disease, will be missed by this method. Newer immunologic techniques that detect SLT-I and SLT-II in stool are therefore in widespread use.[154] Screening for EHEC by one of these methods is recommended for all bloody stool samples received in diagnostic laboratories.[155]

The enteroadherent *E. coli* types (EPEC, EAEC, and DAEC) are classically identified by the HEp-2 cell adherence assay in which HEp-2 cells are incubated with *E. coli* isolates, washed, stained, and then examined microscopically for adherence patterns. EPEC attaches in focal aggregates (local adherence), EAEC adheres to both HEp-2 cells and glass in a stacked-brick pattern, and as suggested by the name, DAEC adheres in a diffuse pattern to cells (but not glass). Although a number of technical variations in the HEp-2 cell adherence assay have been described, it appears that the so-called CVD (Center for Vaccine Development, University of Maryland) method or a modification of the UTH (University of Texas, Houston) method to include a 2- to 4-hour postwash incubation is best able to distinguish all three patterns.[156,157] A simpler version using prefixed HEp-2 cells was shown to be 92% sensitive for detection of EAEC.[158] EAEC may also be sensitively identified by biofilm formation when grown in rich media in the absence of cells, although the specificity appears lower than with HEp-2 cells.[159]

ETEC is distinguished by establishing the presence of characteristic enterotoxins or the genes which encode them. LT or ST can be identified using tissue culture techniques (such as the Chinese hamster ovary cell elongation assay for LT)[160] or cyclic GMP elevations in T84 cells for ST.[88] Less cumbersome techniques include several commercially available immunoassays.[161,162] Genetic techniques using DNA probes or PCR have also been used.[163–167]

DNA tests for EPEC, EAEC, and DAEC have also been used with varying degrees of success. The most useful of these for EPEC are the EAF and *eaeA* probes, which detect the adherence plasmid and LEE pathogenicity island, respectively. The AA probe for EAEC (which recognizes a portion of the AA plasmid)[168] has been shown to be highly sensitive and specific in some studies, but it is clear that probe-negative strains predominate in clinical disease in some areas of the world. Newer probes targeting *aggR*, *pic/set*, and *aap* appear promising, but larger studies are pending.[169,170] Probes for the Afa/Dr adhesins of DAEC are also being studied.

Classically, EIEC was identified using the animal model of invasion, such as the Séreny test in which invasion is demonstrated in the conjunctiva of guinea pigs.[171] More recently, molecular techniques using DNA probes and PCR have shown promise as highly sensitive and specific alternatives to the more classic diagnostic methods.[172,173]

TREATMENT

Rehydration

As with all diarrheal diseases, replacement of lost fluid and electrolytes is the cornerstone of therapy. This is best accomplished with the oral rehydration formulation recommended by the World Health Organization (Table 16-4). The formulation is based on the physiologic observation that intestinal absorption of sodium is coupled to that of glucose, and that addition of glucose to sodium-containing solutions drives sodium absorption even in the face of ongoing intestinal secretion. Simple and inexpensive, oral rehydration therapy has been credited with saving up to 1 million lives per year.[174] Oral rehydration is preferred over intravenous therapy for several reasons: It is more physiologic (with an intact thirst mechanism, overhydration is avoided), less expensive, less painful, safer (no risk of intravenous catheter infections), and much easier to administer in developing countries.

Successful use of oral rehydration therapy begins with a careful assessment of the patient's hydration status. Guidelines for assessing dehydration in children are listed in Table 16-5. In addition, assessment of capillary refill time,[175] urine output, and urine specific gravity may be useful measures of dehydration and response to rehydration therapy.[176] Oral rehydration is recommended for those with mild to moderate dehydration. When severe dehydration (10% or

Table 16-4 Oral Rehydration Formulas

WHO Formula		Home Recipe	
Ingredient	**Amount***	**Ingredient**	**Amount***
NaCl	3.5 g	Table salt	½–¾ tsp
$NaHCO_3$	2.5 g	Baking soda	½ tsp
KCl	1.5 g	Orange juice	1 cup
Glucose	20 g	Table sugar†	4 level tsp

WHO, World Health Organization.
*Per liter (1.05 qt) of clean water.
†Food-based oral rehydration formulations, prepared by replacing table sugar with 50 to 60 g of cereal flour or 200 g of mashed boiled potato, may help to reduce fluid output.

Table 16-5 Evaluation of Dehydration in Patients with Diarrhea

Variable	Mild (3%–5% Body Weight)	Moderate (6%–9% Body Weight)	Severe (≥10% Body Weight)
Blood pressure	Normal	Normal	Normal to reduced
Heart rate	Normal	Increased	Increased*
Quality of pulses	Normal	Normal or slightly decreased	Moderately decreased
Skin turgor†	Normal	Decreased	Decreased
Mucous membranes	Slightly dry	Dry	Dry
Eyes	Normal	Sunken orbits	Deeply sunken orbits
Tears	Present	Absent	Absent
Extremities	Warm, normal capillary refill	Delayed capillary refill	Cool, mottled
Mental status	Normal	Normal to listless	Normal to lethargic or comatose
Urine output	Slightly decreased	Moderately decreased	Severely decreased to anuric

*Bradycardia may develop in severe cases.
†May not be reliable in the presence of severe malnutrition.
Adapted from Bern C, Martines J, deZoysa I, et al: The magnitude of the global problem of diarrheal disease: A ten-year update. Bull World Health Organ 70:705, 1992.

more of body weight) is present, intravenous therapy with normal saline or Ringer's lactate is recommended, and serum electrolytes should be measured and corrected if oral therapy cannot be given first. As soon as dehydration has been corrected, age-appropriate refeeding can further reduce stool output, decrease the duration of diarrhea, and improve nutritional values.[176–178]

Antimicrobial Therapy

In placebo-controlled trials published in the early 1980s, tetracycline, trimethoprim-sulfamethoxazole, and trimethoprim alone were all shown to decrease the duration of diarrhea in either naturally acquired ETEC infection or in volunteers experimentally infected with the organism.[179,180] Since then, a number of studies of *E. coli* isolates in developing countries have reported increased resistance to multiple antimicrobials, including ampicillin and trimethoprim-sulfamethoxazole.[181–186] Fortunately, the vast majority of *E. coli* isolates remain sensitive to fluoroquinolones,[183–185,187] and multiple studies have demonstrated the efficacy of these agents in the treatment of traveler's diarrhea, including the subgroups infected with ETEC and EAEC.[37,187–190] Abbreviated courses of quinolone therapy for 3 days[187,191] or even single dose[188] have documented efficacy in patients with traveler's diarrhea. Rarely, ciprofloxacin resistance has emerged in multidrug-resistant *E. coli* isolates from travelers treated with ciprofloxacin.[191] Effective therapy for EAEC-associated traveler's diarrhea using the nonabsorbable antibiotic rifamixin has also been demonstrated in a small clinical trial.[192] Ciprofloxacin was also effective in curing EAEC diarrhea in a small group of HIV-infected patients.[40] Specific therapy for DAEC has not been studied. Several reports suggest the efficacy of antibiotics in managing EPEC infections,[97,193,194] although the only controlled trial specifically addressing EPEC infections was with 49 Ethiopian children in whom serotype O111:B4 predominated.[194] In this series, complete resolution of diarrhea was seen within 3 days in 73% of cases receiving trimethoprim-sulfamethoxazole (and in 76% in those receiving mecillinam) vs. 7% in controls, and bacteriologic cure was confirmed in 53% of those receiving antibiotics vs. none in the control group. In addition to rehydration therapy and antibiotics, parenteral nutrition supplementation may be helpful in the severely malnourished patient with EPEC infection.[97] In multiple regions worldwide, antimicrobial resistance among EPEC isolates is emerging[195–197]; if feasible, antimicrobial selection should be guided by susceptibility testing.

The role of antimicrobial treatment in EHEC disease remains uncertain. Although most *E. coli* O157:H7 is susceptible in vitro to antibiotics such as ampicillin, carbenicillin, gentamicin, cephalothin, chloramphenicol, quinolones, trimethoprim, and trimethoprim-sulfamethoxazole,[78,198–200] exposure of the organism to sublethal concentrations of trimethoprim-sulfamethoxazole, ciprofloxacin, and tetracycline has been reported to increase SLT release.[201] Of note, ciprofloxacin also stimulates increased release of endotoxin from *E. coli*,[202,203] which can result in significant cytokine release from whole blood and human peripheral blood monocytes.[204,205] There is limited clinical evidence that antibiotics may be harmful in EHEC infection, including a prospective but nonrandomized study,[206] suggesting an association between antibiotic use and progression to HUS. Among retrospective studies from several outbreaks, antibiotics did not appear to influence the duration of symptoms.[78,207] In one retrospective case series of 20 patients with *E. coli* O157:H7 infection, treatment with trimethoprim-sufamethoxazole was significantly associated with the development of HUS.[79] However, other studies report an association of appropriate antimicrobial therapy for more than 24 hours with lack of progression to HUS.[81] In the only prospective randomized therapeutic trial in EHEC diarrhea, the duration of symptoms was not significantly reduced by trimethoprim-sulfamethoxazole, although treatment was begun relatively late in the illness.[208] In addition, the preceding prospective study found a trend toward the development of HUS in the group not receiving antibiotics, although this did not reach statistical significance.[208] A recent meta-analysis of nine studies (six retrospective and three prospective) did not show a higher risk of HUS following antibiotic administration.[209]

Bacillary dysentery associated with EIEC typically responds to appropriate antimicrobials targeting shigellosis. As with *Shigella* species, antibiotic susceptibility patterns vary geographically, and antimicrobials such as ampicillin and trimethoprim-sulfamethoxazole may not be effective against EIEC. Resistance to third-generation cephalosporins and quinolones, including nalidixic acid, is less common.[210,211]

Other Therapies

Bismuth Subsalicylate

In addition to oral rehydration therapy and specific antimicrobial therapy, a number of other agents may help to treat enteric *E. coli* infections. Bismuth subsalicylate has been used ever since the early 1900s as an antidiarrheal agent, and several studies have validated its efficacy in treating diarrhea caused chiefly by enterovirulent *E. coli*.[212] Its efficacy in preventing and treating ETEC infections has been shown in volunteers fed ETEC, as well as in field trials.[213,214] In addition, in a recent randomized placebo-controlled trial in which the most commonly isolated potential pathogen was *E. coli* with EPEC serotypes, bismuth subsalicylate effected a significant reduction in duration of diarrhea, duration of hospitalization, and stool output in infants and young children with acute watery diarrhea.[215] Nonetheless, antidiarrheal drugs including bismuth subsalicylate are generally not recommended in treating infants with acute diarrhea caused by any pathogen.[176]

Antimotility Agents

Loperamide shortens the time to the last unformed stool in traveler's diarrhea and may offer some modest benefit in patients infected with ETEC during the first 24 hours of combination therapy with ciprofloxacin; however, antimotility agents may mask fluid losses and should not be used in children.[216–218] The safety of antimotility agents in EIEC infections is uncertain. Murphy and associates[219] reported no adverse effects in 42 adult patients with dysentery who received loperamide in combination with ciprofloxacin and, compared with 46 receiving ciprofloxacin alone, this regimen resulted in fewer unformed stools and a shorter duration of diarrhea.[219] Nonetheless, the modest symptomatic improvement seen with antimotility agents in this disease must be weighed against reports of adverse outcomes associated with their use in inflammatory diarrheal illnesses.[220,221] Given reports associating antimotility agents with the development of HUS,[81,222,223] and increased risk of central nervous system manifestations in HUS[224] in EHEC infections, they should clearly be avoided in patients suspected of having hemorrhagic colitis.

Probiotics

There has been significant enthusiasm for the use of live bacterial preparations as "natural" remedies for gastrointestinal illness. While live-culture yogurt has antibacterial activity in vitro,[225] it had no significant clinical effect in rabbit EPEC infection in one study.[226] Yogurt was shown to be no more effective than milk in treating acute diarrhea in malnourished children.[227] Newer probiotic preparations containing defined organisms have shown more promise. One such organism, *Lactobacillus* GG, shortens the duration of acute diarrhea in children with rotavirus infection but not bacterial diarrhea.[228–230] In one trial, prophylactic administration of *Lactobacillus* GG to undernourished children in Peru did decrease the incidence of diarrheal episodes (5.21 episodes/child/year vs. 6.02 for placebo; $p < 0.05$).[231] *Lactobacillus* GG was also shown to prevent traveler's diarrhea in two randomized, blinded, placebo-controlled studies, although the effect was limited to travelers to particular areas (Turkey, North Africa).[232,233] In summary, there is currently no evidence to support the routine use of any probiotic preparation in the prevention or treatment of *E. coli* enteric infection, although this remains an area of active investigation.

PREVENTION AND CONTROL

As with the vast majority of pathogens causing diarrheal illness, proper sanitation and hygiene aimed at diminishing the risk of fecal-oral transmission is important for the prevention of enteric *E. coli* infections. Culturally sensitive education on the use of soap and handwashing after defecation and before eating or preparing foods and improvements in the disposal of human waste are the simplest and, perhaps overall, the most effective means of preventing disease caused by most enteric *E. coli*.[234–238] Numerous studies have demonstrated the protective benefits of breastfeeding in preventing diarrheal diseases, including those associated with ETEC and EPEC.[21,239,240] Not only does breastfeeding diminish the risk of fecal-oral exposure from exposure to weaning foods, but breast milk likely affords immunologic protection[241] and may contribute oligosaccharides and other substances which interfere with attachment of *E. coli* to intestinal epithelium.[112,113] Programs which address deficiencies in micronutrients such as vitamin A and zinc have also been shown to improve the severity of diarrhea in developing regions.[242–245]

Those traveling to the tropics should be advised to eat only those foods that are thoroughly cooked and served piping hot, or fresh fruits that can be peeled. In general, chemoprophylaxis for traveler's diarrhea is not recommended. People who are at high risk of complications from traveler's diarrhea, such as those with diabetes, inflammatory bowel disease, advanced AIDS, or those on immunosuppressive drugs, should be warned that agents such as *Cryptosporidium* are not prevented by antibiotics and may cause far worse disease than ETEC or EAEC. Moreover, the increasing antibiotic resistance of certain pathogens (e.g., *Campylobacter* in Thailand) makes chemoprophylaxis less attractive.

Given the striking association of EHEC infection with bovine sources in developed countries, preventive efforts have focused primarily on inspection of food products and new microbiologic quality standards.[246] Increased industrialization of food supplies in developing countries and greater sharing of food sources globally multiply the potential for outbreaks with enteric *E. coli* such as EHEC and other gastrointestinal pathogens. Stricter governmental and industrial standards may help prevent widespread point-source outbreaks.

Vaccine development targeting *E. coli* enteric infections is an active field of study. Several trials of a combined oral inactivated cholera/CT-B subunit vaccine to prevent traveler's diarrhea due to ETEC have had promising results.[247–251] This vaccine is available in Europe and Australia and was recently marketed in Canada (Dukoral, Aventis Pasteur) but is not available in the United States. Additional human vaccines against ETEC and EHEC are under development. In addition, a vaccine to prevent EHEC colonization of beef cattle is undergoing trials.

REFERENCES

1. Kosek M, Bern C, Guerrant RL: The global burden of diarrhoeal disease, as estimated from studies published between 1992 and 2000. Bull World Health Organ 81:197, 2003.
2. World Bank: World Development Report 1993. Washington, DC, World Bank, 1993.
3. Guerrant RL, Kosek M, Lima AA, et al: Updating the DALYs for diarrhoeal disease. [Erratum appears in Trends Parasitol 18:281, 2002.] Trends Parasitol 18:191, 2002.
4. Black RE, Merson MH, Huq I, et al: Incidence and severity of rotavirus and *Escherichia coli* diarrhoea in rural Bangladesh. Implications for vaccine development. Lancet 1:141, 1981.
5. Guerrant RL, Moore RA, Kirschenfeld PM, et al: Role of toxigenic and invasive bacteria in acute diarrhea of childhood. N Engl J Med 293:567, 1975.
6. Moyenuddin M, Rahman KM, Sack DA: The aetiology of diarrhoea in children at an urban hospital in Bangladesh. Trans R Soc Trop Med Hyg 81:299, 1987.
7. Orskov F, Orskov I: *Escherichia coli* serotyping and disease in man and animals [review]. Can J Microbiol 38:699, 1992.
8. Guerrant RL, Kirchhoff LV, Shields DS, et al: Prospective study of diarrheal illnesses in northeastern Brazil: Patterns of disease, nutritional impact, etiologies, and risk factors. J Infect Dis 148:986, 1983.
9. Levine MM: *Escherichia coli* that cause diarrhea: Enterotoxigenic, enteropathogenic, enteroinvasive, enterohemorrhagic, and enteroadherent. J Infect Dis 155:377, 1987.
10. DuPont HL: Traveler's diarrhea. In Blaser MJ, Smith PD, Ravdin JI, et al (eds): Infections of the Gastrointestinal Tract. New York, Raven Press, 1995, p 299.
11. Merson MH, Morris GK, Sack DA, et al: Travelers' diarrhea in Mexico. A prospective study of physicians and family members attending a congress. N Engl J Med 294:1299, 1976.
12. Sack DA, Kaminsky DC, Sack RB, et al: Enterotoxigenic *Escherichia coli* diarrhea of travelers: A prospective study of American Peace Corps volunteers. Johns Hopkins Med J 141:63, 1977.
13. Black RE, Brown KH, Becker S, et al: Longitudinal studies of infectious diseases and physical growth of children in rural Bangladesh. II. Incidence of diarrhea and association with known pathogens. Am J Epidemiol 115:315, 1982.
14. DuPont HL, Formal SB, Hornick RB, et al: Pathogenesis of *Escherichia coli* diarrhea. N Engl J Med 285:1, 1971.
15. Levine MM, Caplan ES, Waterman D, et al: Diarrhea caused by *Escherichia coli* that produce only heat-stable enterotoxin. Infect Immun 17:78, 1977.
16. Taylor J, Powell BW, Wright J: Infantile diarrhea and vomiting: A clinical and bacteriological investigation. BMJ 2:117, 1949.
17. Bower JR, Congeni BL, Cleary TG, et al: *Escherichia coli* O114: Nonmotile as a pathogen in an outbreak of severe diarrhea associated with a day care center. J Infect Dis 160:243, 1989.
18. Viljanen MK, Peltola T, Junnila SY, et al: Outbreak of diarrhoea due to *Escherichia coli* O111:B4 in schoolchildren and adults: Association of Vi antigen-like reactivity. Lancet 336:831, 1990.
19. Hill SM, Phillips AD, Walker-Smith JA: Enteropathogenic *Escherichia coli* and life threatening chronic diarrhoea. Gut 32:154, 1991.
20. Kotler DP, Orenstein JM: Chronic diarrhea and malabsorption associated with enteropathogenic bacterial infection in a patient with AIDS. Ann Intern Med 119:127, 1993.
21. Blake PA, Ramos S, MacDonald KL, et al: Pathogen-specific risk factors and protective factors for acute diarrheal disease in urban Brazilian infants. J Infect Dis 167:627, 1993.
22. Cravioto A, Tello A, Navarro A, et al: Association of *Escherichia coli* HEp-2 adherence patterns with type and duration of diarrhoea. Lancet 337:262, 1991.
23. Echeverria P, Taylor DN, Bettelheim KA, et al: HeLa cell-adherent enteropathogenic *Escherichia coli* in children under 1 year of age in Thailand. J Clin Microbiol 25:1472, 1987.
24. Echeverria P, Orskov F, Orskov I, et al: Attaching and effacing enteropathogenic *Escherichia coli* as a cause of infantile diarrhea in Bangkok. J Infect Dis 164:550, 1991.
25. Echeverria P, Serichantalerg O, Changchawalit S, et al: Tissue culture–adherent *Escherichia coli* in infantile diarrhea. J Infect Dis 165:141, 1992.
26. Gomes TA, Blake PA, Trabulsi LR: Prevalence of *Escherichia coli* strains with localized, diffuse, and aggregative adherence to HeLa cells in infants with diarrhea and matched controls. J Clin Microbiol 27:266, 1989.
27. Cravioto A, Reyes RE, Ortega R, et al: Prospective study of diarrhoeal disease in a cohort of rural Mexican children: Incidence and isolated pathogens during the first two years of life. Epidemiol Infect 101:123, 1988.
28. Robins-Browne RM, Still CS, Miliotis MD, et al: Summer diarrhoea in African infants and children. Arch Dis Child 55:923, 1980.
29. Giles C, Sangster G, Smith J: Epidemic gastroenteritis of infants in Aberdeen during 1947. Arch Dis Child 24:45, 1949.
30. Bhan MK, Khoshoo V, Sommerfelt H, et al: Enteroaggregative *Escherichia coli* and *Salmonella* associated with nondysenteric persistent diarrhea. Pediatr Infect Dis J 8:499, 1989.
31. Bhan MK, Raj P, Levine MM, et al: Enteroaggregative *Escherichia coli* associated with persistent diarrhea in a cohort of rural children in India. J Infect Dis 159:1061, 1989.
32. Wanke CA, Schorling JB, Barrett LJ, et al: Potential role of adherence traits of *Escherichia coli* in persistent diarrhea in an urban Brazilian slum. Pediatr Infect Dis J 10:746, 1991.
33. Fang GD, Lima AA, Martins CV, et al: Etiology and epidemiology of persistent diarrhea in northeastern Brazil: A hospital-based, prospective, case-control study. J Pediatr Gastroenterol Nutr 21:137, 1995.
34. Cohen MB, Hawkins JA, Weckbach LS, et al: Colonization by enteroaggregative *Escherichia coli* in travelers with and without diarrhea. J Clin Microbiol 31:351, 1993.
35. Adachi JA, Jiang ZD, Mathewson JJ, et al: Enteroaggregative *Escherichia coli* as a major etiologic agent in traveler's diarrhea in 3 regions of the world. Clin Infect Dis 32:1706, 2001.
36. Gascon J, Vargas M, Quinto L, et al: Enteroaggregative *Escherichia coli* strains as a cause of traveler's diarrhea: A case-control study. J Infect Dis 177:1409, 1998.
37. Glandt M, Adachi JA, Mathewson JJ, et al: Enteroaggregative *Escherichia coli* as a cause of traveler's diarrhea: Clinical response to ciprofloxacin. Clin Infect Dis 29:335, 1999.
38. Jiang ZD, Greenberg D, Nataro JP, et al: Rate of occurrence and pathogenic effect of enteroaggregative *Escherichia coli* virulence factors in international travelers. J Clin Microbiol 40:4185, 2002.
39. Gassama A, Sow PS, Fall F, et al: Ordinary and opportunistic enteropathogens associated with diarrhea in Senegalese adults in relation to human immunodeficiency virus serostatus. Int J Infect Dis 5:192, 2001.
40. Wanke CA, Gerrior J, Blais V, et al: Successful treatment of diarrheal disease associated with enteroaggregative *Escherichia coli* in adults infected with human immunodeficiency virus. J Infect Dis 178:1369, 1998.
41. Mayer HB, Wanke CA: Enteroaggregative *Escherichia coli* as a possible cause of diarrhea in an HIV-infected patient. N Engl J Med 332:273, 1995.
42. Wanke CA, Mayer H, Weber R, et al.: Enteroaggregative *Escherichia coli* as a potential cause of diarrheal disease in adults infected with human immunodeficiency virus. J Infect Dis 178:185, 1998.
43. Giron JA, Jones T, Millan-Velasco F, et al: Diffuse-adhering *Escherichia coli* (DAEC) as a putative cause of diarrhea in Mayan children in Mexico. J Infect Dis 163:507, 1991.
44. Begaud E, Jourand P, Morillon M, et al: Detection of diarrheogenic *Escherichia coli* in children less than ten years old with and without diarrhea in New Caledonia using seven acetylaminofluorene-labeled DNA probes. Am J Trop Med Hyg 48:26, 1993.
45. Jallat C, Livrelli V, Darfeuille-Michaud A, et al: *Escherichia coli* strains involved in diarrhea in France: High prevalence and heterogeneity of diffusely adhering strains. J Clin Microbiol 31:2031, 1993.
46. Levine MM, Ferreccio C, Prado V, et al: Epidemiologic studies of *Escherichia coli* diarrheal infections in a low socioeconomic level peri-urban community in Santiago, Chile. Am J Epidemiol 138:849, 1993.

47. Baqui AH, Sack RB, Black RE, et al: Enteropathogens associated with acute and persistent diarrhea in Bangladeshi children less than 5 years of age. J Infect Dis 166:792, 1992.
48. Kaper JB, Nataro JP, Mobley HL: Pathogenic *Escherichia coli*. Nat Rev Microbiol 2:123, 2004.
49. Okeke IN, Nataro JP: Enteroaggregative *Escherichia coli*. Lancet Infect Dis 1:304, 2001.
50. Nataro JP, Steiner TS: Enteroaggregative and Diffusely Adherent *Escherichia coli*. San Diego, CA, Elsevier Science (USA), 2002, p 189.
51. Griffin PM, Tauxe RV: The epidemiology of infections caused by *Escherichia coli* O157: H7, other enterohemorrhagic *E. coli*, and the associated hemolytic uremic syndrome. Epidemiol Rev 13:60, 1991.
52. Karmali MA: Infection by verocytotoxin-producing *Escherichia coli*. Clin Microbiol Rev 2:15, 1989.
53. Thomas A, Chart H, Cheasty T, et al: Vero cytotoxin–producing *Escherichia coli*, particularly serogroup O 157, associated with human infections in the United Kingdom: 1989–91. Epidemiol Infect 110:591, 1993.
54. World Health Organization: Food safety—Enterohemorrhagic *Escherichia coli* infection, Japan. Weekly Epidemiol Rec 71:267, 1996.
55. Cordovez A, Prado V, Maggi L, et al: Enterohemorrhagic *Escherichia coli* associated with hemolytic-uremic syndrome in Chilean children. J Clin Microbiol 30:2153, 1992.
56. Ghosh AR, Nair GB, Naik TN, et al: Entero-adherent *Escherichia coli* is an important diarrhoeagenic agent in infants aged below 6 months in Calcutta, India. J Med Microbiol 36:264, 1992.
57. Lopez EL, Contrini MM, Devoto S, et al: Incomplete hemolytic-uremic syndrome in Argentinean children with bloody diarrhea. J Pediatr 127:364, 1995.
58. Isaacson M, Canter PH, Effler P, et al: Haemorrhagic colitis epidemic in Africa (letter) [see comments]. Lancet 341:961, 1993.
59. Griffin PM: *Escherichia coli* O157:H7 and other enterohemorrhagic *Escherichia coli*. In Blaser MJ, Smith PD, Ravdin JI, et al (eds): Infections of the Gastrointestinal Tract. New York, Raven Press, 1995, p 739.
60. Acheson DWK, Keusch GT: *Shigella* and enteroinvasive *Escherichia coli*. In Blaser MJ, Smith PD, Ravdin JI, et al (eds): Infections of the Gastroinstestinal Tract. New York, Raven Press, 1995, p 763.
61. Marier R, Wells JG, Swanson RC, et al: An outbreak of enteropathogenic *Escherichia coli* foodborne disease traced to imported French cheese. Lancet 2:1376, 1973.
62. Miller JR, Barrett LJ, Kotloff K, et al: A rapid test for infectious and inflammatory enteritis. Arch Intern Med 154:2660, 1994.
63. Steiner TS, Lima AAM, Nataro JP, et al: Enteroaggregative *Escherichia coli* produce intestinal inflammation and growth impairment and cause interleukin-8 release from intestinal epithelial cells. J Infect Dis 177:88, 1998.
64. Lanata CF, Black RE, Maurtua D, et al: Etiologic agents in acute vs persistent diarrhea in children under three years of age in peri-urban Lima. Peruvian Acta Paediatr Suppl 381:32, 1992.
65. Mathewson JJ, Johnson PC, DuPont HL, et al: Pathogenicity of enteroadherent *Escherichia coli* in adult volunteers. J Infect Dis 154:524, 1986.
66. Nataro JP, Levine MM, Savarino S, et al: Volunteer studies of enteroaggregative *Escherichia coli*. Abstract B-315; 82. Presented at the General Meeting of the American Society of Microbiology, Atlanta, GA, May 16–20, 1993.
66A. Jiang ZD, Okhuysen PC, Guo DC, et al: Genetic susceptibility to enteroaggregative *E. Coli* diarrhea: Polymorphism in the interleukin-8 promoter region. J Infect Dis 188:506, 2003.
67. Poitrineau P, Forestier C, Meyer M, et al: Retrospective case-control study of diffusely adhering *Escherichia coli* and clinical features in children with diarrhea. J Clin Microbiol 33:1961, 1995.
68. Tacket CO, Moseley SL, Kay B, et al: Challenge studies in volunteers using *Escherichia coli* strains with diffuse adherence to HEp-2 cells. J Infect Dis 162:550, 1990.
69. Germani Y, Begaud E, Duval P, et al: Prevalence of enteropathogenic, enteroaggregative, and diffusely adherent *Escherichia coli* among isolates from children with diarrhea in new Caledonia. J Infect Dis 174:1124, 1996.
70. Hunt CM, Harvey JA, Youngs ER, et al: Clinical and pathological variability of infection by enterohaemorrhagic (Vero cytotoxin producing) *Escherichia coli* [see comments]. J Clin Pathol 42:847, 1989.
71. de la Hunt MN, Morris KP, Coulthard MG, et al: Oesophageal and severe gut involvement in the haemolytic uraemic syndrome. Br J Surg 78:1469, 1991.
72. Cohen MB, Giannella RA: Hemorrhagic colitis associated with *Escherichia coli* O157:H7. Adv Intern Med 37:173, 1992.
73. Karmali MA, Petric M, Lim C, et al: Sensitive method for detecting low numbers of verotoxin-producing *Escherichia coli* in mixed cultures by use of colony sweeps and polymyxin extraction of verotoxin. J Clin Microbiol 22:614, 1985.
74. Neill MA, Tarr PI, Clausen CR, et al: *Escherichia coli* O157:H7 as the predominant pathogen associated with the hemolytic uremic syndrome: A prospective study in the Pacific Northwest. Pediatrics 80:37, 1987.
75. Cleary TG: Cytotoxin-producing *Escherichia coli* and the hemolytic uremic syndrome. Pediatr Clin North Am 35:485, 1988.
76. Lopez EL, Diaz M, Grinstein S, et al: Hemolytic uremic syndrome and diarrhea in Argentine children: The role of Shiga-like toxins. J Infect Dis 160:469, 1989.
77. Tarr PI, Neill MA, Clausen CR, et al: *Escherichia coli* O157:H7 and the hemolytic uremic syndrome: Importance of early cultures in establishing the etiology. J Infect Dis 162:553, 1990.
78. Griffin PM, Ostroff SM, Tauxe RV, et al: Illnesses associated with *Escherichia coli* O157:H7 infections: A broad clinical spectrum. Ann Intern Med 109:705, 1988.
79. Pavia AT, Nichols CR, Green DP, et al: Hemolytic-uremic syndrome during an outbreak of *Escherichia coli* O157:H7 infections in institutions for mentally retarded persons: Clinical and epidemiologic observations. J Pediatr 116:544, 1990.
80. Taylor CM, Milford DV, Rose PE, et al: The expression of blood group P1 in post-enteropathic haemolytic uraemic syndrome. Pediatr Nephrol 4:59, 1990.
81. Cimolai N, Carter JE, Morrison BJ, et al: Risk factors for the progression of *Escherichia coli* O157:H7 enteritis to hemolytic-uremic syndrome [see comments]. [Published erratum appears in J Pediatr 116:1008, 1990.] J Pediatr 116:589, 1990.
82. Binsztein N, Jouve MJ, Viboud GI, et al: Colonization factors of enterotoxigenic *Escherichia coli* isolated from children with diarrhea in Argentina. J Clin Microbiol 29:1893, 1991.
83. Svennerholm AM, McConnell MM, Wiklund G: Roles of different putative colonization factor antigens in colonization of human enterotoxigenic *Escherichia coli* in rabbits. Microb Pathog 13:381, 1992.
84. Oyofo BA, el-Etr SH, Wasfy MO, et al: Colonization factors of enterotoxigenic *E. coli* (ETEC) from residents of northern Egypt. Microbiol Res 150:429, 1995.
85. Knutton S, Lloyd DR, McNeish AS: Identification of a new fimbrial structure in enterotoxigenic *Escherichia coli* (ETEC) serotype O148:H28 which adheres to human intestinal mucosa: A potentially new human ETEC colonization factor. Infect Immun 55:86, 1987.
86. Lockman H, Kaper JB: Nucleotide sequence analysis of the A2 and B subunits of *Vibrio cholerae* enterotoxin. J Biol Chem 258:13722, 1983.
87. Griffiths SL, Critchley DR: Characterisation of the binding sites for *Escherichia coli* heat-labile toxin type I in intestinal brush borders. Biochim Biophys Acta 1075:154, 1991.
88. Forte LR, Eber SL, Turner JT, et al: Guanylin stimulation of Cl- secretion in human intestinal T84 cells via cyclic guanosine monophosphate. J Clin Invest 91:2423, 1993.
89. Gardner SE, Fowlston SE, George WL: In vitro production of cholera toxin–like activity by *Plesiomonas shigelloides*. J Infect Dis 156:720, 1987.
90. Jertborn M, Svennerholm AM: Enterotoxin-producing bacteria isolated from Swedish travellers with diarrhoea. Scand J Infect Dis 23:473, 1991.
91. Klipstein FA, Engert RF: Immunological relationship of the B subunits of *Campylobacter jejuni* and *Escherichia coli* heat-labile enterotoxins. Infect Immun 48:629, 1985.
92. Molina NC, Peterson JW: Cholera toxin-like toxin released by *Salmonella* species in the presence of mitomycin C. Infect Immun 30:224, 1980.
93. Sandefur PD, Peterson JW: Neutralization of *Salmonella* toxin–induced elongation of Chinese hamster ovary cells by cholera antitoxin. Infect Immun 15:988, 1977.
94. Schultz AJ, McCardell BA: DNA homology and immunological cross-reactivity between *Aeromonas hydrophila* cytotonic toxin and cholera toxin. J Clin Microbiol 26:57, 1988.
95. Savarino S, McVeigh A, Watson J, et al: Enteroaggregative *Escherichia coli* heat-stable enterotoxin is not restricted to enteroaggregative *E. coli*. J Infect Dis 173:1019, 1996.

96. Savarino S, Fasano A, Watson J, et al: Enteroaggregative *Escherichia coli* heat-stable enterotoxin 1 represents another subfamily of *E. coli* heat-stable toxin. PNAS 90:3093, 1993.
97. Rothbaum R, McAdams AJ, Giannella R, et al: A clinicopathologic study of enterocyte-adherent *Escherichia coli:* A cause of protracted diarrhea in infants. Gastroenterology 83:441, 1982.
98. Donnenberg MS, Kaper JB: Enteropathogenic *Escherichia coli* [review]. Infect Immun 60:3953, 1992.
99. Donnenberg MS, Tacket CO, James SP, et al: Role of the eaeA gene in experimental enteropathogenic *Escherichia coli* infection [see comments]. J Clin Invest 92:1412, 1993.
100. Deng W, Puente JL, Gruenheid S, et al: Dissecting virulence: Systematic and functional analyses of a pathogenicity island. Proc Natl Acad Sci USA 101:3597, 2004.
101. Gruenheid S, Sekirov I, Thomas NA, et al: Identification and characterization of NleA, a non-LEE-encoded type III translocated virulence factor of enterohaemorrhagic *Escherichia coli* O157:H7. Mol Microbiol 51:1233, 2004.
102. Donnenberg MS, Donohue-Rolfe A, Keusch GT: Epithelial cell invasion: An overlooked property of enteropathogenic *Escherichia coli* (EPEC) associated with the EPEC adherence factor. J Infect Dis 160:452, 1989.
103. Francis CL, Jerse AE, Kaper JB, et al: Characterization of interactions of enteropathogenic *Escherichia coli* O127:H6 with mammalian cells in vitro. J Infect Dis 164:693, 1991.
104. Miliotis MD, Koornhof HJ, Phillips JI: Invasive potential of noncytotoxic enteropathogenic *Escherichia coli* in an in vitro Henle 407 cell model. Infect Immun 57:1928, 1989.
105. Moon HW, Whipp SC, Argenzio RA, et al: Attaching and effacing activities of rabbit and human enteropathogenic *Escherichia coli* in pig and rabbit intestines. Infect Immun 41:1340, 1983.
106. Tzipori S, Robins-Browne RM, Gonis G, et al: Enteropathogenic *Escherichia coli* enteritis: Evaluation of the gnotobiotic piglet as a model of human infection. Gut 26:570, 1985.
107. Ulshen MH, Rollo JL: Pathogenesis of *Escherichia coli* gastroenteritis in man—Another mechanism. N Engl J Med 302:99, 1980.
108. Canil C, Rosenshine I, Ruschkowski S, et al: Enteropathogenic *Escherichia coli* decreases the transepithelial electrical resistance of polarized epithelial monolayers. Infect Immun 61:2755, 1993.
109. Rothbaum RJ, Partin JC, Saalfield K, et al: An ultrastructural study of enteropathogenic *Escherichia coli* infection in human infants. Ultrastruct Pathol 4:291, 1983.
110. Ghaem-Maghami M, Simmons CP, Daniell S, et al: Intimin-specific immune responses prevent bacterial colonization by the attaching-effacing pathogen *Citrobacter rodentium*. Infect Immun 69:5597, 2001.
111. Donnenberg MS: Enteropathogenic *E. coli*. In Blaser MJ, Smith PD, Ravdin JI, et al (eds): Infections of the Gastrointestinal Tract. New York, Raven Press, 1995, p 709.
112. Cravioto A, Tello A, Villafan H, et al: Inhibition of localized adhesion of enteropathogenic *Escherichia coli* to HEp-2 cells by immunoglobulin and oligosaccharide fractions of human colostrum and breast milk. J Infect Dis 163:1247, 1991.
113. Silva ML, Giampaglia CM: Colostrum and human milk inhibit localized adherence of enteropathogenic *Escherichia coli* to HeLa cells. Acta Paediatr 81:266, 1992.
114. Knutton S, Baldwin T, Williams PH, et al: Actin accumulation at sites of bacterial adhesion to tissue culture cells: Basis of a new diagnostic test for enteropathogenic and enterohemorrhagic *Escherichia coli.* Infect Immun 57:1290, 1989.
115. DeVinney R, Stein M, Reinscheid D, et al: Enterohemorrhagic *Escherichia coli* O157:H7 produces Tir, which is translocated to the host cell membrane but is not tyrosine phosphorylated. Infect Immun 67:2389, 1999.
116. Padhye VV, Zhao T, Doyle MP: Production and characterisation of monoclonal antibodies to Verotoxins 1 and 2 from *Escherichia coli* of serotype O157:H7. J Med Microbiol 30:219, 1989.
117. Strockbine NA, Marques LR, Newland JW, et al: Two toxin-converting phages from *Escherichia coli* O157:H7 strain 933 encode antigenically distinct toxins with similar biologic activities. Infect Immun 53:135, 1986.
118. Richardson SE, Rotman TA, Jay V, et al: Experimental verocytotoxemia in rabbits. Infect Immun 60:4154, 1992.
119. Padhye VV, Beery JT, Kittell FB, et al: Colonic hemorrhage produced in mice by a unique vero cell cytotoxin from an *Escherichia coli* strain that causes hemorrhagic colitis. J Infect Dis 155:1249, 1987.
120. Tzipori S, Karch H, Wachsmuth KI, et al: Role of a 60-megadalton plasmid and Shiga-like toxins in the pathogenesis of infection caused by enterohemorrhagic *Escherichia coli* O157:H7 in gnotobiotic piglets. Infect Immun 55:3117, 1987.
121. O'Brien AD, Holmes RK: Shiga and Shiga-like toxins [review]. Microbiol Rev 51:206, 1987.
122. Su C, Brandt LJ: *Escherichia coli* O157:H7 infection in humans [review]. Ann Intern Med 123:698, 1995.
123. Hughes AK, Ergonul Z, Stricklett PK, et al: Molecular basis for high renal cell sensitivity to the cytotoxic effects of shigatoxin-1: Upregulation of globotriaosylceramide expression. [Erratum appears in J Am Soc Nephrol 14(5):following table of contents "Note: Ergonal Z [corrected to Ergonul Z]", 2003.] J Am Soc Nephrol 13:2239, 2002.
124. Eisenhauer PB, Chaturvedi P, Fine RE, et al: Tumor necrosis factor alpha increases human cerebral endothelial cell Gb3 and sensitivity to Shiga toxin. Infect Immun 69:1889, 2001.
125. Utsunomiya I, Ren J, Taguchi K, et al: Immunohistochemical detection of verotoxin receptors in nervous system. Brain Res Brain Res Protoc 8:99, 2001.
126. Ren J, Utsunomiya I, Taguchi K, et al: Localization of verotoxin receptors in nervous system. Brain Res 825:183, 1999.
127. Scotland SM, Willshaw GA, Smith HR, et al: Properties of strains of *Escherichia coli* belonging to serogroup O157 with special reference to production of Vero cytotoxins VT1 and VT2. Epidemiol Infect 99:613, 1987.
128. Ostroff SM, Tarr PI, Neill MA, et al: Toxin genotypes and plasmid profiles as determinants of systemic sequelae in *Escherichia coli* O157:H7 infections. J Infect Dis 160:994, 1989.
129. Siegler RL, Griffin PM, Barrett TJ, et al: Recurrent hemolytic uremic syndrome secondary to *Escherichia coli* O157:H7 infection. Pediatrics 91:666, 1993.
130. Robson WL, Leung AK, Miller-Hughes DJ: Recurrent hemorrhagic colitis caused by *Escherichia coli* O157:H7. Pediatr Infect Dis J 12:699, 1993.
131. Nataro JP: Enteroaggregative and diffusely adherent *Escherichia coli.* In Blaser MJ, Smith PD, Ravdin JI, et al (eds): Infections of the Gastrointestinal Tract. New York, Raven Press, 1995, p 727.
132. Sarantuya J, Nishi J, Wakimoto N, et al: Typical enteroaggregative *Escherichia coli* is the most prevalent pathotype among *E. coli* strains causing diarrhea in Mongolian children. J Clin Microbiol 42:133, 2004.
133. Nataro JP, Deng Y, Maneval DR, et al: Aggregative adherence fimbriae I of enteroaggregative *Escherichia coli* mediate adherence to HEp-2 cells and hemagglutination of human erythrocytes. Infect Immun 60:2297, 1992.
134. Sheikh J, Czeczulin JR, Harrington S, et al: A novel dispersin protein in enteroaggregative *Escherichia coli*. J Clin Invest 110:1329, 2002.
135. Henderson IR, Czeczulin J, Eslava C, et al: Characterization of pic, a secreted protease of *Shigella flexneri* and enteroaggregative *Escherichia coli*. Infect Immun 67:5587, 1999.
136. Behrens M, Sheikh J, Nataro JP: Regulation of the overlapping pic/set locus in *Shigella flexneri* and enteroaggregative *Escherichia coli*. Infect Immun 70:2915, 2002.
137. Vargas M, Gascon J, Jimenez De Anta MT, et al: Prevalence of *Shigella* enterotoxins 1 and 2 among *Shigella* strains isolated from patients with traveler's diarrhea. J Clin Microbiol 37:3608, 1999.
138. Steiner TS, Nataro JP, Poteet-Smith CE, et al: Enteroaggregative *Escherichia coli* expresses a novel flagellin that causes IL-8 release from intestinal epithelial cells. J Clin Invest 105:1769, 2000.
139. Bilge SS, Clausen CR, Lau W, et al: Molecular characterization of a fimbrial adhesin, F1845, mediating diffuse adherence of diarrhea-associated *Escherichia coli* to HEp-2 cells. J Bacteriol 171:4281, 1989.
140. Benz I, Schmidt MA: Cloning and expression of an adhesin (AIDA-I) involved in diffuse adherence of enteropathogenic *Escherichia coli.* Infect Immun 57:1506, 1989.
141. Peiffer I, Servin AL, Bernet-Camard MF: Piracy of decay-accelerating factor (CD55) signal transduction by the diffusely adhering strain *Escherichia coli* C1845 promotes cytoskeletal F-actin rearrangements in cultured human intestinal INT407 cells. Infect Immun 66:4036, 1998.

142. Guignot J, Breard J, Bernet-Camard MF, et al: Pyelonephritogenic diffusely adhering *Escherichia coli* EC7372 harboring Dr-II adhesin carries classical uropathogenic virulence genes and promotes cell lysis and apoptosis in polarized epithelial caco-2/TC7 cells. Infect Immun 68:7018, 2000.
143. Peiffer I, Guignot J, Barbat A, et al: Structural and functional lesions in brush border of human polarized intestinal Caco-2/TC7 cells infected by members of the Afa/Dr diffusely adhering family of *Escherichia coli*. Infect Immun 68:5979, 2000.
144. Guignot J, Peiffer I, Bernet-Camard MF, et al: Recruitment of CD55 and CD66e brush border-associated glycosylphosphatidylinositol-anchored proteins by members of the Afa/Dr diffusely adhering family of *Escherichia coli* that infect the human polarized intestinal Caco-2/TC7 cells. Infect Immun 68:3554, 2000.
145. Peiffer I, Blanc-Potard AB, Bernet-Camard MF, et al: Afa/Dr diffusely adhering *Escherichia coli* C1845 infection promotes selective injuries in the junctional domain of polarized human intestinal Caco-2/TC7 cells. Infect Immun 68:3431, 2000.
146. Betis F, Brest P, Hofman V, et al: Afa/Dr diffusely adhering *Escherichia coli* infection in T84 cell monolayers induces increased neutrophil transepithelial migration, which in turn promotes cytokine-dependent upregulation of decay-accelerating factor (CD55), the receptor for Afa/Dr adhesins. Infect Immun 71:1774, 2003.
147. Sansonetti PJ, d'Hauteville H, Ecobichon C, et al: Molecular comparison of virulence plasmids in *Shigella* and enteroinvasive *Escherichia coli*. Ann Microbiol (Paris) 134A:295, 1983.
148. Kocks C, Marchand JB, Gouin E, et al: The unrelated surface proteins ActA of Listeria monocytogenes and IcsA of *Shigella flexneri* are sufficient to confer actin-based motility on *Listeria innocua* and *Escherichia coli* respectively. Mol Microbiol 18:413, 1995.
149. Suzuki T, Mimuro H, Suetsugu S, et al: Neural Wiskott-Aldrich syndrome protein (N-WASP) is the specific ligand for *Shigella* VirG among the WASP family and determines the host cell type allowing actin-based spreading. Cell Microbiol 4:223, 2002.
150. Fasano A, Kay BA, Russell RG, et al: Enterotoxin and cytotoxin production by enteroinvasive *Escherichia coli*. Infect Immun 58:3717, 1990.
151. Nataro JP, Seriwatana J, Fasano A, et al: Identification and cloning of a novel plasmid-encoded enterotoxin of enteroinvasive *Escherichia coli* and *Shigella* strains. Infect Immun 63:4721, 1995.
152. Kim JG, Lee SJ, Kagnoff MF: Nod1 is an essential signal transducer in intestinal epithelial cells infected with bacteria that avoid recognition by toll-like receptors. Infect Immun 72:1487, 2004.
153. Chapman PA, Daly CM: Comparison of Y1 mouse adrenal cell and coagglutination assays for detection of *Escherichia coli* heat labile enterotoxin. J Clin Pathol 42:755, 1989.
154. Kehl KS, Havens P, Behnke CE, et al: Evaluation of the Premier EHEC assay for detection of Shiga toxin producing *Escherichia coli*. J Clin Microbiol 35:2051, 1997.
155. Guerrant RL, Van Gilder T, Steiner TS, et al: Practice guidelines for the management of infectious diarrhea. Clin Infect Dis 32:331, 2001.
156. Haider K, Faruque SM, Albert MJ, et al: Comparison of a modified adherence assay with existing assay methods for identification of enteroaggregative *Escherichia coli*. J Clin Microbiol 30:1614, 1992.
157. Vial PA, Mathewson JJ, Dupont HL, et al: Comparison of two assay methods for patterns of adherence to HEp-2 cells of *Escherichia coli* from patients with diarrhea. J Clin Microbiol 28:882, 1990.
158. Miqdady MS, Jiang ZD, Nataro JP, et al: Detection of enteroaggregative *Escherichia coli* with Formalin-preserved HEp-2 cells. J Clin Microbiol 40:3066, 2002.
159. Wakimoto N, Nishi J, Sheikh J, et al: Quantitative biofilm assay using microtiter plate to screen for enteroaggregative *Escherichia coli*. Am J Trop Med Hyg 71:687, 2004.
160. Guerrant RL, Brunton LL, Schnaitman RC, et al: Cyclic adenosine monophosphate and alteration of Chinese hamster ovary cell morphology: A rapid, sensitive in vitro assay for the enterotoxins of *Vibrio cholerae* and *Escherichia coli*. Infect Immun 10:320, 1974.
161. Scotland SM, Willshaw GA, Said B, et al: Identification of *Escherichia coli* that produces heat-stable enterotoxin STA by a commercially available enzyme-linked immunoassay and comparison of the assay with infant mouse and DNA probe tests. J Clin Microbiol 27:1697, 1989.
162. Speirs J, Stavric S, Buchanan B: Assessment of two commercial agglutination kits for detecting *Escherichia coli* heat-labile enterotoxin. Can J Microbiol 37:877, 1991.
163. Baldini MA, Kaper JB, Levine MM, et al: Plasmid-mediated adhesin in enteropathogenic *Escherichia coli*. J Pediatr Gastroenterol Nutr 2:534, 1983.
164. Echeverria P, Taylor DN, Seriwatana J, et al: A comparative study of enterotoxin gene probes and tests for toxin production to detect enterotoxigenic *Escherichia coli*. J Infect Dis 153:255, 1986.
165. Gicquelais KG, Baldini MM, Martinez J, et al: Practical and economical method for using biotinylated DNA probes with bacterial colony blots to identify diarrhea-causing *Escherichia coli*. J Clin Microbiol 28:2485, 1990.
166. Saez-Llorens X, Guzman-Verduzco LM, Shelton S, et al: Simultaneous detection of *Escherichia coli* heat-stable and heat-labile enterotoxin genes with a single RNA probe. J Clin Microbiol 27:1684, 1989.
167. Wernars K, Delfgou E, Soentoro PS, et al: Successful approach for detection of low numbers of enterotoxigenic *Escherichia coli* in minced meat by using the polymerase chain reaction. Appl Environ Microbiol 57:1914, 1991.
168. Baudry B, Savarino SJ, Vial P, et al: A sensitive and specific DNA probe to identify enteroaggregative *Escherichia coli*, a recently discovered diarrheal pathogen. J Infect Dis 161:1249, 1990.
169. Okeke IN, Lamikanra A, Czeczulin J, et al: Heterogeneous virulence of enteroaggregative *Escherichia coli* strains isolated from children in southwest Nigeria. J Infect Dis 181:252, 2000.
170. Zamboni A, Fabbricotti SH, Fagundes-Neto U, et al: Enteroaggregative *Escherichia coli* virulence factors are found to be associated with infantile diarrhea in Brazil. J Clin Microbiol 42:1058, 2004.
171. Sereny B: Experimental shigella keratoconjunctivitis: A preliminary report. Acta Microbiol Acad Sci Hung 2:293, 1955.
172. Oberhelman RA, Kopecko DJ, Venkatesan MM, et al: Evaluation of alkaline phosphatase-labelled ipaH probe for diagnosis of *Shigella* infections. J Clin Microbiol 31:2101, 1993.
173. Ye LY, Lan FH, Zhu ZY, et al: Detection of *Shigella* and enteroinvasive *Escherichia coli* using polymerase chain reaction. J Diarrhoeal Dis Res 11:38, 1993.
174. Hirschhorn N, Greenough WB: Progress in oral rehydration therapy. Sci Am 264:50, 1991.
175. Saavedra JM, Harris GD, Li S, et al: Capillary refilling (skin turgor) in the assessment of dehydration. Am J Dis Child 145:296, 1991.
176. American Academy of Pediatrics, Provisional Committee on Quality Improvement, Subcommittee on Acute Gastroenteritis: Practice parameter: The management of acute gastroenteritis in young children. Pediatrics 97:424, 1996.
177. Santosham M, Fayad IM, Hashem M, et al: A comparison of rice-based oral rehydration solution and "early feeding" for the treatment of acute diarrhea in infants. J Pediatr 116:868, 1990.
178. Brown KH, Gastanaduy AS, Saavedra JM, et al: Effect of continued oral feeding on clinical and nutritional outcomes of acute diarrhea in children. J Pediatr 112:191, 1988.
179. Merson MH, Sack RB, Islam S, et al: Disease due to enterotoxigenic *Escherichia coli* in Bangladeshi adults: Clinical aspects and a controlled trial of tetracycline. J Infect Dis 141:702, 1980.
180. DuPont HL, Reves RR, Galindo E, et al: Treatment of travelers' diarrhea with trimethoprim/sulfamethoxazole and with trimethoprim alone. N Engl J Med 307:841, 1982.
181. Lester SC, del Pilar Pla M, Wang F, et al: The carriage of *Escherichia coli* resistant to antimicrobial agents by healthy children in Boston, in Caracas, Venezuela, and in Qin Pu, China. N Engl J Med 323:285, 1990.
182. Murray BE, Mathewson JJ, DuPont HL, et al: Emergence of resistant fecal *Escherichia coli* in travelers not taking prophylactic antimicrobial agents. Antimicrob Agents Chemother 34:515, 1990.
183. Bourgeois AL, Gardiner CH, Thornton SA, et al: Etiology of acute diarrhea among United States military personnel deployed to South America and west Africa. Am J Trop Med Hyg 48:243, 1993.
184. Oyofo BA, el-Gendy A, Wasfy MO, et al: A survey of enteropathogens among United States military personnel during Operation Bright Star '94, in Cairo, Egypt. Mil Med 160:331, 1995.
185. Sharp TW, Thornton SA, Wallace MR, et al: Diarrheal disease among military personnel during Operation Restore Hope, Somalia, 1992–1993. Am J Trop Med Hyg 52:188, 1995.
186. Hyams KC, Bourgeois AL, Merrell BR, et al: Diarrheal disease during Operation Desert Shield [see comments]. N Engl J Med 325:1423, 1991.
187. Mattila L, Peltola H, Siitonen A, et al: Short-term treatment of traveler's diarrhea with norfloxacin: A double-blind, placebo-controlled study during two seasons. Clin Infect Dis 17:779, 1993.

188. Salam I, Katelaris P, Leigh-Smith S, et al: Randomised trial of single-dose ciprofloxacin for travellers' diarrhoea. Lancet 344:1537, 1994.
189. Ericsson CD, Johnson PC, Dupont HL, et al: Ciprofloxacin or trimethoprim-sulfamethoxazole as initial therapy for travelers' diarrhea. A placebo-controlled, randomized trial. Ann Intern Med 106:216, 1987.
190. Thornton SA, Wignall SF, Kilpatrick ME, et al: Norfloxacin compared to trimethoprim/sulfamethoxazole for the treatment of travelers' diarrhea among U.S. military personnel deployed to South America and west Africa. Mil Med 157:55, 1992.
191. Wistrom J, Gentry LO, Palmgren AC, et al: Ecological effects of short-term ciprofloxacin treatment of travellers' diarrhoea. J Antimicrob Chemother 30:693, 1992.
192. Infante RM, Ericsson CD, Jiang ZD, et al: Enteroaggregative *Escherichia coli* diarrhea in travelers: Response to rifaximin therapy. Clin Gastroenterol Hepatol 2:135, 2004.
193. Clausen CR, Christie DL: Chronic diarrhea in infants caused by adherent enteropathogenic *Escherichia coli*. J Pediatr 100:358, 1982.
194. Thoren A, Wolde-Mariam T, Stintzing G, et al: Antibiotics in the treatment of gastroenteritis caused by enteropathogenic *Escherichia coli*. J Infect Dis 141:27, 1980.
195. Gross RJ, Rowe B, Threlfall EJ: *Escherichia coli* O142.H6: A drug-resistant enteropathogenic clone? J Hyg (Lond) 94:181, 1985.
196. Moyenuddin M, Wachsmuth IK, Moseley SL, et al: Serotype, antimicrobial resistance, and adherence properties of *Escherichia coli* strains associated with outbreaks of diarrheal illness in children in the United States. J Clin Microbiol 27:2234, 1989.
197. Olukoya DK, Daini O, Alabi SA, et al: Antimicrobial resistance patterns and plasmids of enteropathogenic *Escherichia coli* isolated in Nigeria. Eur J Epidemiol 4:306, 1988.
198. Pai CH, Gordon R, Sims HV, et al: Sporadic cases of hemorrhagic colitis associated with *Escherichia coli* O157:H7. Clinical, epidemiologic, and bacteriologic features. Ann Intern Med 101:738, 1984.
199. Tarr PI, Neill MA, Christie DL, et al: *Escherichia coli* O157:H7 hemorrhagic colitis (letter). N Engl J Med 318:1697, 1988.
200. Ratnam S, March SB, Ahmed R, et al: Characterization of *Escherichia coli* serotype O157:H7. J Clin Microbiol 26:2006, 1988.
201. Walterspiel JN, Ashkenazi S, Morrow AL, et al: Effect of subinhibitory concentrations of antibiotics on extracellular Shiga-like toxin I. Infection 20:25, 1992.
202. Cohen J, McConnell JS: Release of endotoxin from bacteria exposed to ciprofloxacin and its prevention with polymyxin B. Eur J Clin Microbiol 5:13, 1986.
203. Crosby HA, Bion JF, Penn CW, et al: Antibiotic-induced release of endotoxin from bacteria in vitro. J Med Microbiol 40:23, 1994.
204. Bailly S, Fay M, Ferrua B, et al: Ciprofloxacin treatment in vivo increases the ex vivo capacity of lipopolysaccharide-stimulated human monocytes to produce IL-1, IL-6 and tumour necrosis factor-alpha. Clin Exp Immunol 85:331, 1991.
205. Prins JM, Kuijper EJ, Mevissen ML, et al: Release of tumor necrosis factor alpha and interleukin 6 during antibiotic killing of *Escherichia coli* in whole blood: Influence of antibiotic class, antibiotic concentration, and presence of septic serum. Infect Immun 63:2236, 1995.
206. Wong CS, Jelacic S, Habeeb RL, et al: The risk of the hemolytic-uremic syndrome after antibiotic treatment of *Escherichia coli* O157:H7 infections [see comment]. N Engl J Med 342:1930, 2000.
207. Ostroff SM, Kobayashi JM, Lewis JH: Infections with *Escherichia coli* O157:H7 in Washington State. The first year of statewide disease surveillance. JAMA 262:355, 1989.
208. Proulx F, Turgeon JP, Delage G, et al: Randomized, controlled trial of antibiotic therapy for *Escherichia coli* O157:H7 enteritis. J Pediatr 121:299, 1992.
209. Safdar N, Said A, Gangnon RE, et al: Risk of hemolytic uremic syndrome after antibiotic treatment of Escherichia coli O157:H7 enteritis: a meta-analysis [see comment]. JAMA 288:996, 2002.
210. Matsushita S, Yamada S, Kudoh Y, et al: Biochemical characteristics, growth on selective media, antimicrobial susceptibility, and diarrheagenic toxin production of enteroinvasive *Escherichia coli*. Kansenshogaku Zasshi 64:734, 1990.
211. Prado D, Lopez E, Liu H, et al: Ceftibuten and trimethoprim-sulfamethoxazole for treatment of *Shigella* and enteroinvasive *Escherichia coli* disease. Pediatr Infect Dis J 11:644, 1992.
212. Bierer DW: Bismuth subsalicylate: History, chemistry, and safety [review]. Rev Infect Dis 12(Suppl 1):S3, 1990.
213. DuPont HL, Sullivan P, Pickering LK, et al: Symptomatic treatment of diarrhea with bismuth subsalicylate among students attending a Mexican university. Gastroenterology 73:715, 1977.
214. DuPont HL, Ericsson CD, Johnson PC, et al: Prevention of travelers' diarrhea by the tablet formulation of bismuth subsalicylate. JAMA 257:1347, 1987.
215. Figueroa-Quintanilla D, Salazar-Lindo E, Sack RB, et al: A controlled trial of bismuth subsalicylate in infants with acute watery diarrheal disease. N Engl J Med 328:1653, 1993.
216. DuPont HL, FloresSanchez J, Ericsson CD, et al: Comparative efficacy of loperamide hydrochloride and bismuth subsalicylate in the management of acute diarrhea. Am J Med 88:15S, 1990.
217. Johnson PC, Ericsson CD, DuPont HL, et al: Comparison of loperamide with bismuth subsalicylate for the treatment of acute travelers' diarrhea. JAMA 255:757, 1986.
218. Taylor DN, Sanchez JL, Candler W, et al: Treatment of travelers' diarrhea: Ciprofloxacin plus loperamide compared with ciprofloxacin alone. A placebo-controlled, randomized trial. Ann Intern Med 114:731, 1991.
219. Murphy GS, Bodhidatta L, Echeverria P, et al: Ciprofloxacin and loperamide in the treatment of bacillary dysentery. Ann Intern Med 118:582, 1993.
220. DuPont HL, Hornick RB: Adverse effect of Lomotil therapy in shigellosis. JAMA 226:1525, 1973.
221. Walley T, Milson D: Loperamide related toxic megacolon in *Clostridium difficile* colitis (letter). Postgrad Med J 66:582, 1990.
222. Tapper D, Tarr P, Avner E, et al: Lessons learned in the management of hemolytic uremic syndrome in children. J Pediatr Surg 30:158, 1995.
223. Cimolai N, Basalyga S, Mah DG, et al: A continuing assessment of risk factors for the development of *Escherichia coli* O157:H7–associated hemolytic uremic syndrome. Clin Nephrol 42:85, 1994.
224. Cimolai N, Morrison BJ, Carter JE: Risk factors for the central nervous system manifestations of gastroenteritis-associated hemolytic-uremic syndrome. Pediatrics 90:616, 1992.
225. Kotz CM, Peterson LR, Moody JA, et al: In vitro antibacterial effect of yogurt on *Escherichia coli*. Digest Dis Sci 35:630, 1990.
226. Gotteland M, Pochart P, Dabbech M, et al: In vivo effect of yogurt on excretion of enteropathogen *Escherichia coli* RDEC-1 during acute diarrhea in the just-weaned rabbit. J Pediatr Gastroenterol Nutr 14:264, 1992.
227. Bhatnagar S, Singh KD, Sazawal S, et al: Efficacy of milk versus yogurt offered as part of a mixed diet in acute noncholera diarrhea among malnourished children. J Pediatr 132:999, 1998.
228. Isolauri E, Juntunen M, Rautanen T, et al: A human *Lactobacillus* strain (*Lactobacillus casei* sp strain GG) promotes recovery from acute diarrhea in children. Pediatrics 88:90, 1991.
229. Guandalini S, Pensabene L, Zikri MA, et al: *Lactobacillus* GG administered in oral rehydration solution to children with acute diarrhea: a multicenter European trial [see comment]. J Pediatr Gastroenterol Nutr 30:54, 2000.
230. Shornikova AV, Isolauri E, Burkanova L, et al: A trial in the Karelian Republic of oral rehydration and *Lactobacillus* GG for treatment of acute diarrhoea. Acta Paediatr 86:460, 1997.
231. Oberhelman RA, Gilman RH, Sheen P, et al: A placebo-controlled trial of *Lactobacillus* GG to prevent diarrhea in undernourished Peruvian children [see comment]. J Pediatr 134:15, 1999.
232. Oksanen PJ, Salminen S, Saxelin M, et al: Prevention of travellers' diarrhoea by *Lactobacillus* GG. Ann Med 22:53, 1990.
233. Kollaritsch H, Holst H, Grobara P, et al: Prophylaxe der reisediarrhoe mit *Saccharomyces boulardii*. Ergebnisse einer plazebokontrollierten doppelblindstudie. Fortschr Med 111:152, 1993.
234. Black RE, Dykes AC, Anderson KE, et al: Handwashing to prevent diarrhea in day-care centers. Am J Epidemiol 113:445, 1981.
235. Esrey SA, Habicht JP: Epidemiologic evidence for health benefits from improved water and sanitation in developing countries [review]. Epidemiol Rev 8:117, 1986.
236. Feachem RG: Interventions for the control of diarrhoeal diseases among young children: Promotion of personal and domestic hygiene. Bull World Health Organ 62:467, 1984.
237. Henry FJ, Rahim Z: Transmission of diarrhoea in two crowded areas with different sanitary facilities in Dhaka, Bangladesh. J Trop Med Hyg 93:121, 1990.
238. Stanton BF, Clemens JD: An educational intervention for altering water-sanitation behaviors to reduce childhood diarrhea in urban Bangladesh. II. A randomized trial to assess the impact of the

intervention on hygienic behaviors and rates of diarrhea. Am J Epidemiol 125:292, 1987.

239. Cruz JR, Gil L, Cano F, et al: Breast milk anti–*Escherichia coli* heat-labile toxin IgA antibodies protect against toxin-induced infantile diarrhea. Acta Paediatr Scand 77:658, 1988.
240. Long KZ, Wood JW, VasquezGariby E, et al: Proportional hazards analysis of diarrhea due to enterotoxigenic *Escherichia coli* and breast feeding in a cohort of urban Mexican children. Am J Epidemiol 139:193, 1994.
241. Tacket CO, Losonsky G, Link H, et al: Protection by milk immunoglobulin concentrate against oral challenge with enterotoxigenic *Escherichia coli*. N Engl J Med 318:1240, 1988.
242. Stansfield SK, Pierre-Louis M, Lerebours G, et al: Vitamin A supplementation and increased prevalence of childhood diarrhoea and acute respiratory infections. Lancet 342:578, 1993.
243. Barreto ML, Santos LM, Assis AM, et al: Effect of vitamin A supplementation on diarrhoea and acute lower-respiratory-tract infections in young children in Brazil. Lancet 344:228, 1994.
244. Sazawal S, Black RE, Bhan MK, et al: Zinc supplementation in young children with acute diarrhea in India [see comments]. N Engl J Med 333:839, 1995.
245. Walser BL, Lima AAM, Guerrant RL: Effects of high-dose oral vitamin A on diarrheal episodes among children with persistent diarrhea in a northeast Brazilian community. Am J Trop Med Hyg 54:582, 1996.
246. Guerrant RL, Theno DM: *Escherichia coli* O157:H7. N Engl J Med 333:1711, 1995.
247. Qadri F, Ahmed T, Ahmed F, et al: Safety and immunogenicity of an oral, inactivated enterotoxigenic *Escherichia coli* plus cholera toxin B subunit vaccine in Bangladeshi children 18–36 months of age. Vaccine 21:2394, 2003.
248. Qadri F, Wenneras C, Ahmed F, et al: Safety and immunogenicity of an oral, inactivated enterotoxigenic *Escherichia coli* plus cholera toxin B subunit vaccine in Bangladeshi adults and children. Vaccine 18:2704, 2000.
249. Cohen D, Orr N, Haim M, et al: Safety and immunogenicity of two different lots of the oral, killed enterotoxigenic *Escherichia coli*-cholera toxin B subunit vaccine in Israeli young adults. Infect Immun 68:4492, 2000.
250. Wiedermann G, Kollaritsch H, Kundi M, et al: Double-blind, randomized, placebo controlled pilot study evaluating efficacy and reactogenicity of an oral ETEC B-subunit-inactivated whole cell vaccine against travelers' diarrhea (preliminary report). J Travel Med 7:27, 2000.
251. Savarino SJ, Hall ER, Bassily S, et al: Oral, inactivated, whole cell enterotoxigenic *Escherichia coli* plus cholera toxin B subunit vaccine: Results of the initial evaluation in children. PRIDE Study Group. J Infect Dis 179:107, 1999.

17

Typhoid Fever*

JUDITH E. EPSTEIN
STEPHEN L. HOFFMAN

INTRODUCTION

Typhoid fever is an acute systemic illness caused by infection with *Salmonella enterica* subspecies *enterica* serotype Typhi. It is characterized by (1) prolonged fever, (2) sustained bacteremia without endothelial or endocardial involvement, and (3) bacterial invasion of and multiplication within the mononuclear phagocytic cells of the liver, spleen, lymph nodes, and Peyer's patches. Paratyphoid fever is a pathologically and clinically similar, but generally milder, illness that is caused by many serotypes of the genus *Salmonella* but most commonly by *Salmonella* serotypes Paratyphi A, Schottmuelleri, and Hirschfeldii. Enteric fever refers to either typhoid or paratyphoid fever.

Although Hippocrates may have written about typhoid fever, it was not until the early 19th century that French workers described the clinical and pathologic features of *dothiénentérite* (boil of the intestine), which was endemic in Paris. In 1829, Pierre Louis first called it *typhöide* meaning "typhus-like," but he did not distinguish between the typhoid of Paris and the typhus that was then common in Great Britain. Thus both typhoid and typhus take their names from the Greek *typhos,* which means "smoke" and refers to the apathy and confusion associated with fever that are such prominent features of the fully developed clinical syndromes and also refers to the belief that the diseases had their origin in miasmic vapors. In 1837, William Wood Gerhard, a former student of Louis working in Philadelphia, clearly differentiated typhoid from typhus fever, both clinically and pathologically. He wrote: "The anatomical characters of these varieties of fevers are peculiar to themselves and it is [as] impossible to substitute the lesion of the follicles of the small intestine observed in typhoid fever from [for] the pathological phenomena of typhus as it is by other treatment or means to transform the eruption of measles into the pustules of smallpox."

In 1880, Eberth described *Bacillus typhosus* in histologic sections of mesenteric lymph nodes and the spleen. Four years later, Gaffky successfully cultured *Salmonella* Typhi and stressed that the infection was waterborne and not airborne. In 1896, Achard and Bensaude isolated *S.* Paratyphi B and first used the term *paratyphoid fever.* In the same year, Widal described the eponymous reaction, and Wright from England and Pfeiffer from Germany introduced the first vaccination against typhoid.

Until 1948, there were no other major advances in the prevention, diagnosis, or treatment of typhoid fever. Modifications of the first inactivated whole-cell vaccines were used for prevention, Widal's test and culture were used for diagnosis, and patient management was supportive, the outcome being highly dependent on the quality of nursing care. In 1948, Woodward and colleagues,[1] who were working in Malaysia to determine if chloramphenicol was effective in treating scrub typhus, found that one of their suspected scrub typhus patients had typhoid fever and that chloramphenicol rapidly cleared the bacteremia and markedly shortened the duration of the illness. Until the emergence of resistance, chloramphenicol was the antimicrobial agent of choice for treating both typhoid and paratyphoid fever. In the 1970s and 1980s, live oral attenuated[2–4] and Vi capsular polysaccharide[5,6] *S.* Typhi vaccines were developed and shown to be effective in large field trials. By the mid 1990s, these vaccines had replaced whole-cell vaccines in adults and children older than 2 years of age. More recently, a Vi capsular polysaccharide-conjugate vaccine has been shown to be even more effective than the previous vaccines[7,8] and it is expected that it will replace the other vaccines in the coming years. Fortunately, as drug resistance has emerged to existing antibiotics, new drugs such as fluoroquinolones and third-generation cephalosporins have proven successful in the treatment of typhoid fever. Nevertheless, there is concern that drug resistance may outpace the effectiveness of available drugs. It is hoped the availability of the genomic sequence of *S.* Typhi[9] will provide the foundation for new methods of prevention, diagnosis, and treatment of typhoid fever.

AGENT

Salmonella is the most complex genus in the family Enterobacteriaceae, with more than 2400 serotypes currently listed in the Kauffman-White scheme. Because multiple nomenclature systems are used, classification of the organism can be confusing. Previously, salmonellae were classified as having three distinct "species": *S. choleraesuis, S. typhi,* and *S. enteritidis.* Most of the described serotypes belonged to the species *S. enteritidis.* Salmonellae were further grouped (A, B, C, etc.) based on somatic O antigen and further divided into serotypes (1, 2, 3, etc.) based on flagellar H antigens.[10]

All *Salmonella* and *Arizona* isolates are now considered to be a single species (*Salmonella enterica*), separated into seven distinct subgroups: I, II, IIIa, IIIb, and IV through VI. Subgroup I contains most of the *Salmonella* serotypes responsible for human disease. Based on this new schema, the complete name for all isolates is designated as, for example, *Salmonella enterica* subspecies *enterica* serotype Typhi. However, due to wide clinical use and familiarity, it is still appropriate to address them as, for example, *Salmonella* Typhi, as long as it is understood that these organisms are a serotype of the species *Salmonella enterica* and not a distinct species. In this chapter, the name *S.* Typhi will be used throughout. All salmonellae grow on simple media; however, specimens are usually cultured on a selective medium, such as *Salmonella-Shigella*

*All material in this chapter is in the public domain, with the exception of any borrowed figures or tables. The opinions or assertions herein are those of the authors and are not to be construed as official or as reflecting the views of the U.S. Navy or the naval service at large.

the liver, spleen, lymph nodes, and Peyer's patches of the ileum. Our knowledge of the sequence of events following ingestion of an infective dose of S. Typhi is derived from studies of human volunteers and chimpanzees experimentally infected with S. Typhi and of mice infected with *Salmonella enteritidis* and *Salmonella* Typhimurium. However, this information is incomplete, and the theories of pathogenesis are not well substantiated.[14,56] For example, there is still no well-documented explanation of the pathogenesis of the mental confusion and other central nervous system manifestations that led to the disease being called typhoid.

Proposed Sequence of Events

Mucosal Penetration

After ingestion, the organisms pass through the upper gastrointestinal tract to the small intestine, where they either invade directly or multiply for several days before invading. Since fewer than 5% of the villi have organisms attached, it is hypothesized that there are specific receptor sites on the villi, but these receptors have not been identified. Stool cultures are positive for several days after S. Typhi ingestion and then become negative until after the onset of clinical illness. Human volunteer studies have shown that invasion can take place in the jejunum, and animal studies suggest that it occurs in the ileum. The M cells, epithelial cells that overlie the Peyer's patches, are the potential sites where S. Typhi is internalized and transported to the underlying lymphoid tissues.[62] After penetration, the organisms pass to the intestinal lymphoid follicles and the draining mesenteric lymph nodes; some also pass into the systemic circulation where they are filtered out by the reticuloendothelial cells of the liver and spleen. The salmonellae are able to prevent acidification of the phagosomes, survive, and multiply within the mononuclear phagocytic cells of the lymphoid follicles, lymph nodes, liver, and spleen. At this stage, there are subtle degenerative, proliferative, and granulomatous changes in the villi, crypt glands, and lamina propria of the small bowel and in the mesenteric lymph glands. These changes are reversible and unassociated with clinical symptoms.

Dissemination and Organ Invasion

At a critical point (which is probably a function of number of bacteria, bacterial virulence, and the host's immune response), a sufficient number of organisms and possibly other mediators that induce clinical symptoms are released from this sequestered intracellular habitat in the intestinal and mesenteric lymph system and pass through the thoracic duct and into the general circulation. This marks the end of the incubation period, which may last from 3 to 60 days, but is usually 7 to 14 days.

During this bacteremic phase, the organisms may invade any organ but are most commonly found in the liver, spleen, bone marrow, gallbladder, and Peyer's patches in the terminal ileum.[56,63] They invade the gallbladder either directly from the bloodstream or from the bile and then reappear in the intestine, where they are excreted in the stool and reinvade through the intestinal wall. At most tissue sites the organisms are again taken up by, and multiply within, the mononuclear phagocytic cells.

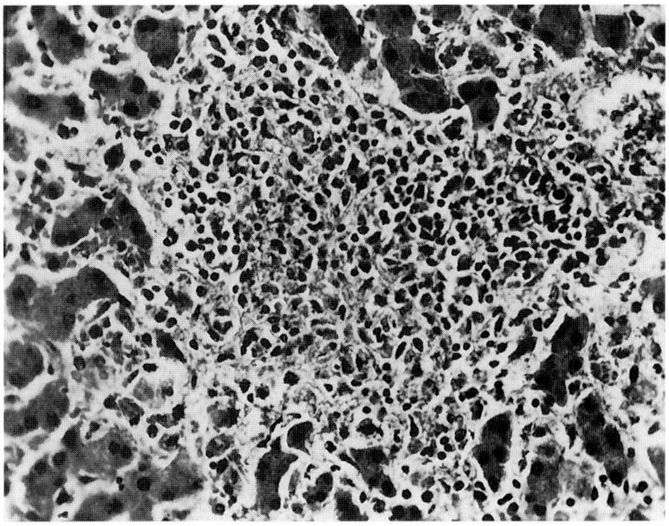

FIGURE 17-2 A typhoid nodule in the liver during the stage of active invasion. This lesion is principally composed of macrophages (*center*) with variable numbers of lymphocytes and plasma cells (*periphery*). (×305.) (Courtesy of the Armed Forces Institute of Pathology, Neg. No. 72-4603.)

Pathology

The basic histologic finding in typhoid fever is infiltration of tissues by macrophages (typhoid cells) containing bacteria, erythrocytes, and degenerated lymphocytes. Aggregates of these macrophages are called typhoid nodules (Fig. 17-2). They are most commonly found in the intestine, mesenteric lymph nodes, spleen, liver, and bone marrow, but may be found in the kidneys, testes, and parotid glands.

Intestine

In the intestine, there are four classic pathologic stages. *Hyperplastic* changes begin during the first week of illness and primarily involve Peyer's patches of the ileum and solitary lymphoid follicles of the cecum, but may involve any lymphoid tissue in the intestine. Almost all infiltrative cells are mononuclear; typhoid nodules are common. If the hyperplasia does not resolve, *necrosis* of the intestinal mucosa develops, usually after 7 to 10 days of clinical illness (Fig. 17-3). *Sloughing* of the mucosa follows and results in the development of an *ulcer*, which may bleed (see Fig. 17-3). The ulcers conform in shape and distribution to the location of the lymphoid follicles are largest in the ileum, and are almost always found on the antimesenteric border of the intestines. These ulcers may perforate into the peritoneal cavity.[64] Perforations are single and measure less than 1 cm in 80% of cases, and 90% are found within 60 cm of the ileocecal valve. When healing takes place, it is usually complete, without scarring.

Mesenteric Lymph Nodes, Spleen, and Liver

In the mesenteric lymph nodes, the sinusoids are enlarged and distended by large collections of macrophages and reticuloendothelial cells. The nodes become soft and swollen and often contain areas of focal necrosis. The spleen is enlarged, red, soft, and congested. Its serosal surface may have

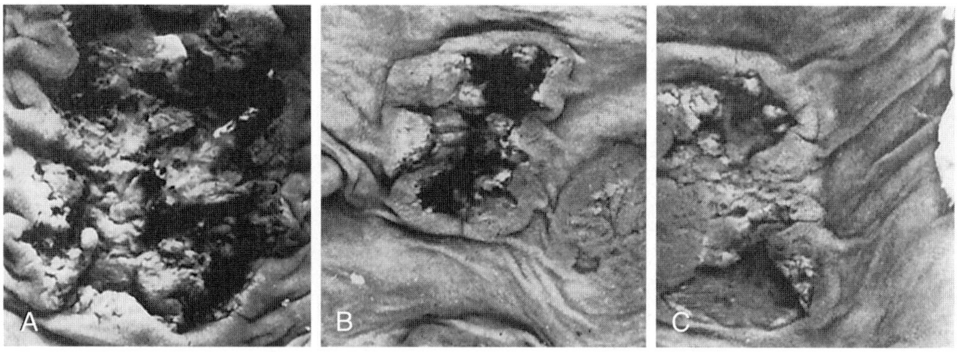

FIGURE 17-3 Peyer's patches in the ileum showing several stages in a single specimen. *A,* Active ulceration. *B,* Necrosis. *C,* The sloughing of necrotic tissue has left the muscularis bare. (Courtesy of the Armed Forces Institute of Pathology, Neg. No. 64-3208-2.)

a fibrinous exudate. Microscopically, the red pulp is congested and contains typhoid nodules. The liver is usually enlarged. Hypertrophy and hyperplasia of the Kupffer cells produce the typhoid nodules. There is frequently focal hepatic necrosis and cloudy swelling of hepatocytes. The gallbladder is usually slightly hyperemic and may, in rare instances, show evidence of cholecystitis.

Other Organs

These are less frequently involved during typhoid fever and usually have lesions attributed to toxic factors. The heart may be flabby with dilated ventricles, and microscopically there is often a nonspecific pattern of necrosis with degeneration and fatty infiltration of the myocardial cells. The lungs may develop an interstitial pneumonitis and bronchitis, and skeletal muscles may show Zenker's degeneration. The most common lesion found in the kidneys is swelling and albuminous degeneration of the proximal tubular epithelium, but interstitial nephritis, glomerulonephritis, and pyelonephritis have been noted. Central nervous system changes have been poorly described, but ring hemorrhages, capillary thrombi, perivenous demyelinating leukoencephalitis, and meningitis have been reported. Occasionally, focal lesions such as osteomyelitis, brain abscess, and spleen and liver abscesses have been reported. These lesions are almost always characterized by a polymorphonuclear instead of a mononuclear response. Salmonellae stimulate phagocytosis of neutrophils, red blood cells, and platelets by histiocytes within the bone marrow stroma.[65] This may be one of the mechanisms behind the pancytopenia commonly seen in typhoid fever.

Pathogenesis of Organ Dysfunction and Toxemia

A hypothesis for the pathogenesis of typhoid fever must explain (1) the inflammatory and necrotic changes at the sites of multiplication of the organism in the intestine, liver, spleen, and lymph nodes; (2) the prolonged pyrexia and toxemia; and (3) the pathologic changes and functional derangements in organs such as the heart, lungs, brain, and kidneys, where typhoid nodules and *S.* Typhi are generally not found.

Until the 1970s, most authorities thought that the necrotic changes in the intestine, liver, spleen, and lymph nodes were the result of tissue hypoxia secondary to small vessel occlusion by typhoid nodules, and that the systemic manifestations and dysfunction of other organs were caused by circulating endotoxin.[66] There is evidence that neither small vessel occlusion nor circulating endotoxin play a major role in the pathogenesis of typhoid fever.[67,68]

Endotoxin

The role of endotoxin in the pathogenesis of typhoid fever is unclear.[69] Investigators at the University of Maryland showed that when *S.* Typhi endotoxin was initially injected into human volunteers, it produced chills, fever, headaches, myalgias, anorexia, nausea, thrombocytopenia, and leukopenia, as in typhoid fever.[66] After these volunteers had received repeated injections of endotoxin, they became unresponsive (tolerant) to it, but when the tolerant subjects were challenged with *S.* Typhi, they developed classic typhoid fever. Since typhoid fever is an unrelenting, sustained illness when not treated with antibiotics, the fact that the volunteers developed tolerance to endotoxin suggests that circulating endotoxin does not cause the symptoms and signs of naturally acquired typhoid fever. Furthermore, the facts that endotoxin-tolerant volunteers developed typhoid fever after rechallenge, and that circulating endotoxin as detected by limulus assay is not present in many patients with typhoid fever, make it even less likely that circulating endotoxin plays a major role in the pathogenesis of the disease.[68]

Immune Complexes and Other Immunologic Reactions

Several investigators have found circulating immune complexes in patients with typhoid fever, and others have noted immune complexes in renal biopsy specimens taken from typhoid patients with glomerulonephritis and nephrotic syndrome. The significance of these complexes is unknown. Other investigators have hypothesized that some of the less common central nervous manifestations of typhoid fever, such as Guillain-Barré syndrome, perivenous leukoencephalitis, and transverse myelitis, are due to an immune reaction, but there is no good evidence to support these hypotheses.

Disseminated Intravascular Coagulation

Although there have been several reports of clinically classic disseminated intravascular coagulation (DIC) in typhoid patients, this is a rare complication. On the other hand, many patients with *S.* Typhi infections have laboratory evidence of DIC without bleeding and may have localized DIC within organs.[68]

Metabolic and Nutritional Factors

Various authors have suggested that anemia, vitamin deficiencies, zinc and other trace metal deficiencies, thyroid dysfunction, tryptophan metabolites, other amino acids, and the time of day that infection occurs or treatment is initiated are all important in the pathogenesis of the disease and the host's ability to mobilize adequate defenses. Although it is likely that many of these factors may be important in determining the ultimate expression of the disease, it is unlikely that any of them are the major determinants of how the disease is expressed or how the host defends against the infection.

Proposed Pathogenesis

The unique feature of typhoid fever is the relationship between *S.* Typhi and macrophages in the liver, spleen, intestinal lymphoid follicles, and mesenteric lymph nodes. Macrophages can produce an array of functionally active cytokines. These include tumor necrosis factor-α (TNF-α), interleukin-1 (IL-1), and interferon-α and -β (IFN-α, IFN-β). Macrophages are also an important source of arachidonate metabolites and reactive oxygen intermediates. These macrophage products can cause cellular necrosis, recruitment of other inflammatory cells, stimulation of the immune system, vascular instability, initiation of the clotting mechanism, bone marrow depression, fever, and other abnormalities associated with typhoid fever. It is likely that *S.* Typhi endotoxin stimulates the macrophages to release these substances, which locally mediate the intestinal and hepatocellular necrosis found in the disease, and which, when released systemically, cause most of the other manifestations of the disease.[69]

Although immune complexes, other immune reactions, and metabolic disturbances probably cause some of the less common manifestations of the disease, it is doubtful that they play a significant role in the pathogenesis of the major features.

IMMUNOLOGIC RESPONSE

Typhoid fever induces both systemic and local humoral and cellular immune responses. Although there have been many descriptive studies of the immune responses associated with infection with *S.* Typhi, and with immunization with typhoid vaccines, the roles of specific immune mechanisms in the development of resistance to reinfection with *S.* Typhi, the pathogenesis of typhoid, and complete elimination of bacteria from infected persons have not been clearly established.[70,71] Some have suggested that infection with typhoid confers long-lasting immunity to reinfection, but the high incidence of typhoid fever in young adults in endemic areas and the results of volunteer studies indicate that this is not the case. Fifteen volunteers who had ingested 10^5 organisms and developed acute typhoid fever were rechallenged with 10^5 organisms (expected to cause infection in 25% of nonimmune persons) a mean of 20 months after the first infection. Five (33%) developed acute typhoid fever again (T.F. Woodward, personal communication). The fact that hospital-based studies indicate that the incidence of severe typhoid fever is higher in older adolescents and young adults than in young children suggests that an acquired immune response may play a role in the pathogenesis of severe disease. Relapse may reflect the inadequate development of an appropriate anti–*S.* Typhi immune response.

Antibodies

S. Typhi–specific secretory immunoglobulin A (IgA) in the small intestine may be important in determining whether mucosal penetration takes place. A study from India has reported that patients with typhoid fever have lower levels of IgA in intestinal secretions than do controls.[72] *S.* Typhi–specific IgA has been demonstrated in the feces and intestinal fluid of volunteers immunized with the oral typhoid vaccine, Ty21a.

Development of specific antibodies during typhoid fever has been well documented.[72,73] Circulating IgG, IgM, and in some cases IgA antibodies to *S.* Typhi O, H, Vi, and porin antigens have been identified. Not all persons with typhoid fever develop antibodies to these antigens. Fourfold titer rises to O, H, and Vi antigens were documented in 75%, 75%, and 40%, respectively, of volunteers experimentally infected with *S.* Typhi. Immunization with the Vi antigen vaccine and the oral vaccine, Ty21a (see following Vaccines section), respectively, induces antibodies to Vi antigen and O antigen (IgG and IgA), and immunization with the killed typhoid vaccines can induce antibodies to O, H, and Vi antigens. It has not been proven that these antibodies are responsible for the protective immunity found after administration of these vaccines. However, the developers of the Vi vaccine attribute the vaccine-induced protection entirely to antibodies against Vi antigen. Work has only recently begun to determine the fine specificity of antigen-specific antibody responses.

Cellular Immune Responses

A major characteristic of typhoid fever is the activation of macrophages.[73–75] Phagocytosis is a major host defense mechanism, and substances released from macrophages, including cytokines, reactive oxygen intermediates, and arachidonic acid metabolites, probably play a significant role in the pathogenesis of the disease. Several small studies in India have suggested that patients who do not develop cell-mediated immunity as measured by the leukocyte migration inhibition test have an increased incidence of complications and relapse, but investigators in Sri Lanka using similar techniques did not find this relationship. Immune cells may also play an important role in the protective immunity induced by immunization, but this response has not been adequately characterized.[76] It has been proposed that the protective immunity induced by immunization with the oral typhoid vaccine Ty21a may be mediated by antibody-dependent cellular cytotoxicity involving IgA antibodies against *S.* Typhi and CD4+ T cells, since volunteers immunized with Ty21a have been shown to develop this immune response.

CLINICAL MANIFESTATIONS

The clinical presentation of typhoid fever is variable, but nearly all patients have fever and most have a headache.[77,78] The range of clinical manifestations and severity of the illness varies, depending on the patient population. Clinicians who see outpatients in an endemic area of the developing world will find that their typhoid patients are moderately ill, that fewer than 10% will require hospitalization, that complications are rare, and that the case-fatality rate will be less than 1%. Hospital-based physicians in the same area will see typhoid patients who are much sicker; have a greater range of symptoms, signs, and complications; and have a case-fatality rate that may range from 1% to 30%. If one sees typhoid patients in the developed world, nearly all patients will be hospitalized, but the clinical severity, complications, and case-fatality rates will be comparable to those in outpatients in the developing world. In many cases, the most severely ill patients will have been sicker for longer periods than those who are moderately ill, but this is not always so. The strain of S. Typhi, the number of organisms ingested, the general and nutritional condition and immunologic status of the patient, and, possibly, the genetic makeup of the host may influence the clinical presentation.

Untreated Typhoid Fever

After ingestion of the organisms, 10% to 20% of patients will have transient diarrhea. These patients, as well as all others, remain asymptomatic during the incubation period, which usually lasts 7 to 14 days but can be as short as 3 days and as long as 60 days, depending on the number of organisms ingested. As the stage of sustained bacteremia develops, the incubation period ends and the patient notices the onset of fever, which classically increases daily in a stepwise fashion but may be remittent or sustained. At this point, the patient will usually have a flulike syndrome with headache and malaise and will frequently have a sore throat, anorexia, nausea, abdominal pain, and myalgias, but may have any of the symptoms listed in Table 17-3. By the end of the first week after the onset of symptoms, the fever is sustained, and the patient is often toxic and may have any of the symptoms and signs listed in Tables 17-3 and 17-4.

Table 17-3 Symptoms Expected on Admission in Hospitalized Typhoid Patients in Endemic Areas of the Developing World

Symptom	Percent
Fever	99
Weakness	99
Anorexia	85
Headache	85
Dizziness	80
Abdominal pain	50
Nausea	50
Chills	50
Diarrhea	45
Constipation	40
Cough or chest discomfort	35
Vomiting	35
Myalgia/arthralgia	35
Confusion	25
Sore throat	20
Decreased hearing	15
Blood in stool or melena	12
Epistaxis	10
Dysuria	2
Seizures	2

Table 17-4 Physical Signs Expected on Admission in Hospitalized Typhoid Patients in Endemic Areas of the Developing World

Common		Less Common	
Sign	Percent	Sign	Percent
Fever	98	Disorientation	25
Coated tongue	95	Relative bradycardia	15
Apathy	70	Rales or rhonchi	15
Hepatomegaly	50	Delerium	15
Abdominal pain	45	Severe toxicity	10
Rose spots	0–50	Decreased hearing	10
Moderate illness	45	Stiff neck	10
Toxicity	45	Stupor	2
Splenomegaly	35	Focal neurologic findings	1

The fever remains sustained during the second week and by the third week begins to come down spontaneously by lysis. Intestinal perforation or hemorrhage, or both, can occur at any stage of the illness, but these findings classically occur during the third week. The illness can go on for several months, although by the end of the fourth week the temperature usually returns to normal, and except for patients with metastatic foci in whom cholecystitis, osteomyelitis, and soft tissue abscesses may develop, most patients have recovered. It is at this stage that most relapses occur.

Clinical Course and Manifestations in Patients Who Receive Antimicrobials

Antimicrobials shorten the course, reduce the rate of complications if begun early, reduce the case-fatality rate, and some may increase the relapse rate.[78] During volunteer studies in Maryland, more than 400 patients with typhoid fever were treated within 3 days of the onset of fever and the complication and case-fatality rates were zero.

Symptoms

The approximate frequencies of symptoms and signs expected to be found in hospitalized patients in endemic areas of the developing world are summarized in Tables 17-3 and 17-4. Before hospitalization, most of these patients will have been ill for 6 to 12 days, most will have seen a healthcare provider at some point, and most will have received short courses of antibiotics. Fever is universal and, although present daily, is usually higher in the late afternoon and evening. Chills and dull frontal or diffuse headaches are common. The headaches often prevent patients from sleeping comfortably. Most patients are anorectic. They complain of abdominal pain, but cannot localize it well. Both diarrhea and constipation are common; normal bowel function is unusual.[50,77] Children frequently have diarrhea. Bloody dysentery is occasionally encountered. The incidence of cough and chest discomfort varies considerably. Sore throats are common during the first week of illness, but less common later. Dysuria is more commonly encountered in parts of the world where *S. haematobium* is endemic. Epistaxis, which was a common finding in the preantibiotic era, is much less common now. Seizures are occasionally reported, being more common in children less than 5 years of age. If the patient's family is interviewed, a history of intermittent confusion during peak illness is frequently reported.

Signs

On physical examination, the patient is generally moderately ill to toxic; however, 10% to 15% of patients will be severely toxic and may be hyperpyretic. The patient will be apathetic, lying immobile in bed, often staring blankly, but will be arousable. About 10% of patients are severely agitated and 5% obtunded. Disorientation is common, as is frank delirium.[50,77] Stupor and coma are infrequent. If the patient is hypovolemic from blood loss or dehydration, hypotension or shock may be present. Characteristic gram-negative septic shock is uncommon on admission, but may occur after intestinal perforation, in patients with severe typhoid fever without obvious perforation, and as a preterminal event. Relative bradycardia, once considered to be a classic finding in typhoid fever, in actuality is encountered in fewer than 25% of patients.[23,77] Rose spots, which are blanching, red, maculopapular lesions measuring 2 to 4 mm, are most frequently found on the abdomen and chest, but can be found on the extremities and back.[23] Rose spots are less frequently found in dark-skinned patients. The tongue may be covered with a thick, "furry" white-to-brown coating that spares the bright red tips and edges. The incidence of respiratory findings varies, but signs consistent with bronchitis (15%) are more common than those of lobar consolidation (1% to 8%).

The abdominal examination is frequently difficult to interpret. In classic descriptions, the abdomen is said to be "doughy," and the examiner easily palpates loops of bowel filled with air and fluid and finds diffuse lower quandrant tenderness. In some reports, diffuse abdominal pain with moderate guarding has often been described.[77] Frequently, it is difficult for the examiner to be certain that perforation has not occurred. The spleen or liver is enlarged in 30% to 50% of patients, and although both organs can become quite large, more commonly they are moderately enlarged, with the liver palpable 2 or 3 cm below the right costal margin and the spleen palpable on deep inspiration or 1 or 2 cm below the left costal margin. They are both usually soft and moderately tender. Occult blood is found in the stool of 20% to 30% of patients.

Complications and Unusual Manifestations

Intestinal Perforation

Intestinal perforation occurs in about 3% of hospitalized patients. It usually occurs during the third week of illness, but can happen during the first week.[64,79] The patient with perforation has the usual symptoms of typhoid fever and complains of severe abdominal pain that is often localized to the right lower quandrant, but may be diffuse. Bowel sounds are absent in 50% of cases. About 75% of patients will have guarding, rebound tenderness, and rigidity, particularly in the right lower quadrant.[50,64,80,81] Some patients will have an absence of hepatic dullness because of free air in the abdomen, but a pneumoperitoneum is present on radiography in only 50% to 70% of patients. Perforation causes a marked sudden rise in pulse, fall in blood pressure, and onset of severe pain. In most patients, the diagnosis is not difficult. However, as noted previously, approximately 25% of patients will not have classic findings of peritonitis and perforation, and in these patients the diagnosis is difficult. It is sometimes difficult to decide whether a patient has perforation, impending perforation, or just severe typhoid abdominal pain. In the appropriate clinical setting, a rising white blood cell count with a shift to the left is suggestive of perforation, but this probably occurs in fewer than half of the patients with perforation.

Intestinal Hemorrhage

Intestinal hemorrhage occurs in up to 15% of cases. Patients may or may not be toxic. The bowel usually does not perforate, and bleeding is sometimes heavy enough to cause shock.[50] If blood replacement can keep up with losses, the hemorrhaging is usually a self-limiting process, not requiring surgery. About 25% of patients with typhoid fever have minor bleeding that does not require transfusion.

Neuropsychiatric Manifestations

In the past 25 years, reports from India,[82] Papua New Guinea,[21] Indonesia,[83,84] and Africa (particularly Nigeria)[85] have documented a wide spectrum of neuropsychiatric manifestations of typhoid fever. In some series, half the patients have had disorders of mental status. The most common findings are disturbances of the level of consciousness that range from disorientation to delirium, obtundation, stupor, and coma. Delirium, stupor, and coma are grave prognostic signs associated with case-fatality rates that have exceeded 40%. Delirium often persists after the temperature and metabolic abnormalities have returned to normal, and there is no good explanation for its pathogenesis.

Other less commonly encountered central nervous system findings are seizures, typhoid meningitis, encephalomyelitis, transverse myelitis with spastic paraplegia, peripheral or cranial neuritis, and Guillain-Barré syndrome. Psychotic syndromes, including schizophrenia-like illnesses, mania, depression, and catatonia, have all been described, especially in Africa.

Cardiovascular Manifestations

Myocarditis occurs in 1% to 5% of typhoid patients,[86,87] whereas nonspecific electrocardiographic changes occur in 10% to 15% of patients. Patients with myocarditis may have no cardiovascular symptoms or may have chest pains, congestive heart failure, arrhythmias, or cardiogenic shock. When myocarditis occurs in young children, it is frequently a serious complication. Electrocardiographic findings are the same as in any myocarditis. Pericarditis rarely occurs, but "peripheral vascular collapse" without other cardiac findings is increasingly being described. Deep venous and arterial thromboses are uncommon.

Hepatobiliary Manifestations

Mild asymptomatic elevations of transaminases are common in typhoid fever.[86,87] Jaundice with or without major elevations of hepatic enzymes occurs in 1% to 2% of patients, as does acute cholecystitis. Acute or chronic cholecystitis may occur months to years after an episode of typhoid fever. Culture of stones or bile yields *S.* Typhi in these cases.

Genitourinary Manifestations

About 25% of patients excrete *S.* Typhi in the urine at some point during their illness.[86,87] Transient proteinuria is the most common urinary abnormality and in some cases is due to an immune complex–mediated glomerulonephritis. On occasion the glomerulonephritis may present as renal failure or nephrotic syndrome, and in these cases the prognosis is poor. In severely ill patients, acute tubular necrosis may develop, and in patients with severe intravascular hemolysis, which may or may not be associated with glucose-6-phosphate dehydrogenase (G6PD) deficiency, renal failure can occur. Both pyelonephritis and cystitis also occur in typhoid patients.

Other Complications

DIC is rarely of clinical importance, but thrombocytopenia, hypofibrinogenemia, elevated prothrombin (PT) and partial thromboplastin times (PTT), and elevated levels of fibrin degradation products are found in most patients.[68] The hemolytic-uremic syndrome and severe intravascular hemolysis have been reported. Because of the sustained bacteremia, focal infections can develop at any site of the body, but these occur rarely. The most common sites of infection are in the bones (extremities, spine, ribs), but infections have been reported in the brain, liver, spleen, muscles, breast, thyroid, salivary glands, and cervical lymph nodes. In the past, thrombophlebitis, parotitis, and decubitus ulcers were common complications but they now occur rarely.

Relapse

Relapse occurred in 5% to 10% of patients in the preantibiotic era, and although initial reports in the 1950s and 1960s suggested that relapse increased to 10% to 20% in antibiotic-treated patients, most series have not reported increased relapse rates in appropriately treated patients.[88] Fever generally returns about 2 weeks after the cessation of antibiotic therapy or, in untreated patients, about 2 weeks after defervescence. However, relapse can occur during convalescence when the patient is afebrile but is still symptomatic and on antibiotics, and it has been reported several months after the initial illness. The relapse syndrome is usually, but not always, milder than the initial syndrome.

Typhoid in Children under 5 Years of Age

S. Typhi infections have been acquired congenitally, and there have been many case reports in neonates. The clinical presentation in children less than 5 years of age, and especially those less than 1 year of age, is less predictable than in adults.[50] It ranges from an extremely mild illness, often diagnosed as a viral infection, but treated with antimicrobials, to severe typhoid fever with hospital mortality rates reaching 30%. Children with typhoid fever frequently have diarrhea and vomiting, and up to 20% may have convulsions. Typhoid meningitis, although reported in adults and older children, is found almost exclusively in children less than 5 years old. Paratyphoid fever, particularly in infants, may also cause severe disease with high case-fatality and complication rates. In Indonesia, paratyphoid in children is often caused by the multiple antimicrobial–resistant *S.* Oranienburg.

Geographic Variations

Reports from India,[82] Papua New Guinea,[21] Indonesia,[83,84] and some areas of Africa[85] have described patients with abnormal levels of consciousness or shock who have a much higher case-fatality rate than those with normal mental status. These cases of severe typhoid fever with high mortality have rarely been reported from the Americas. It is not clear if the difference in severity is a function of the host, the bacteria, or epidemiologic factors. In areas of endemic schistosomiasis, a syndrome of prolonged, intermittent fever and *Salmonella* bacteremia associated with mild active chronic schistosomiasis has been documented. The pathogenesis of this syndrome is unknown; however, it may be linked to the abnormal immune response seen in chronic schistosomiasis or the tegmental attachment of bacteria to the adult schistosome worm. Chronic *Salmonella* urinary carriage is common in areas with endemic *S. haematobium* and is undoubtedly related to the obstructive uropathy of urinary schistosomiasis. These patients may experience intermittent fever and bacteremia secondary to the resultant pyelonephritis. Patients with opisthorchiasis (liver fluke infection) may have intrahepatic as opposed to gallbladder carriage, and these persons may have asymptomatic carriage or recurrent cholangitis.

Chronic Carriers

A person who excretes the organism in the stool 1 year after the initial illness is considered to be a carrier. Although 20% of typhoid patients will excrete the organism for 2 months after the onset of illness and 10% for 3 months, only about 3% of patients go on to become carriers.[23] The prevalence is higher in females and in the elderly and is probably correlated with the prevalence of cholelithiasis. Most carriers are asymptomatic, and in some series up to 25% could not give a history compatible with acute typhoid fever. Persons with abnormalities of the genitourinary system, including schistosomiasis, have a much higher prevalence of urinary carriage than those with a normal system.

Laboratory Findings

At the time of hospital admission, most patients will be moderately anemic, have an elevated erythrocyte sedimentation rate, and a platelet count reduced to about 150,000. The white blood cell count will often be about 5000/μL to 6000/μL, but may range from 1200/μL to over 20,000/μL. The differential count is usually normal or shifted slightly to the left, but there may be a relative lymphocytosis, especially later in the disease. The cerebrospinal fluid is usually normal in typhoid fever. Most patients will have a slightly elevated PT and PTT, decreased fibrinogen levels, and circulating fibrin degradation products. Serum enzymes, for example, aspartate transaminase (AST) and alanine transaminase (ALT), are usually elevated to twice normal, as is the serum bilirubin. Hyponatremia and hypokalemia are commonly encountered but are usually not severe. Renal function is usually normal. The urine often has low levels of protein and a few white blood cells.

DIAGNOSIS

The diagnosis of typhoid fever is suspected by the clinician, suggested by assays that identify *Salmonella* antibodies, antigens, or DNA, and confirmed by isolation of the organism. Widal's reaction is indicative of typhoid fever in only 40% to 60% of patients at the time of admission,[89] and although the organism can be isolated from 95% of patients, identification takes at least 18 hours and often 3 to 4 days.[90,91] Thus, investigations are under way to develop more sensitive laboratory methods for making the rapid, presumptive diagnosis of typhoid fever.

Isolation of the Organism

Culturing bone marrow aspirates (BMAs) is the single most sensitive method of isolating S. Typhi from patients with typhoid fever.[90,92,93] The diagnosis of typhoid cannot be excluded, and the sensitivity of other diagnostic techniques cannot be established without a BMA culture. If a BMA culture cannot be obtained, culturing 8 to 15 mL of whole blood, intestinal secretions, and stool will identify 85% to 90% of patients with typhoid fever.[92] A major limitation of conventional culture techniques is that it takes a minimum of 48 hours, and often 72 hours, from specimen acquisition until identification of the organism in culture. Work carried out in Indonesia indicates that when the mononuclear cell fraction of blood is cultured, a procedure that concentrates organisms and presumably removes inhibitory serum factors, or when organisms are concentrated by lysis centrifugation, 100% of cultured organisms can be identified within 18 hours of specimen acquisition.[94]

BMA cultures are positive in 80% to 95% of patients, even if patients have been taking antibiotics for several days, and regardless of how long they have been ill.[90,92,93] The blood culture is positive in 40% to 80% of patients. When experimentally infected human volunteers had daily cultures prior to antibiotic therapy (the mean number of cultures was 5.8), only 75% had positive blood cultures. In the Dade County, Florida, epidemic (see previous Epidemiology discussion), only 55% of hospitalized patients with typhoid fever had positive blood cultures.[23] The sensitivity of blood cultures is greatest during the first week of illness, is reduced by prior ingestion of antibiotics, and is directly related to the quantity of blood cultured and the ratio of culture broth to blood. Repeating blood cultures may improve the yield. Reports from South Africa indicated that culturing blood clots in the presence of streptokinase was 50% more sensitive than culturing whole blood.[95] This finding was not confirmed in studies in Indonesia.[93] Culturing intestinal secretions using a duodenal string capsule has been shown to have a sensitivity of 60% to 80%.[92,96] The sensitivity can be improved by culturing two specimens and leaving the string capsule in overnight, and may increase during the third week of illness.[96] In a single study, culturing skin snips of Rose spots had a sensitivity of 63%.[90] A 1-g stool culture is reportedly more sensitive than a rectal swab culture, but is more difficult to obtain. A single-admission rectal swab culture can be expected to detect S. Typhi in 30% to 40% of patients[90,92]; the sensitivity increases with the length of illness. Because of irregular shedding, several stool cultures may be necessary to identify carriers. Urine cultures are reported to be positive in 5% to 10% of patients, except in areas endemic for *S. haematobium,* where the positivity rate increases markedly. S. Typhi has also been isolated from the cerebrospinal fluid, peritoneal fluid, mesenteric lymph nodes, resected intestine, pharynx, tonsils, abscesses, bone, and other sites.

Bone marrow aspirates and blood are cultured directly into bottles containing liquid broth media. A subculture from the blood culture bottles may be isolated into Taurocholate Infusion Broth (0.5% bile salt broth with 5 g Na Taurocholate in 1 L nutrient broth). Cultures are then further subcultured to selective media such as XLD, MacConkey, or *Salmonella-Shigella* agar, from which suspect colonies are picked for identification. When colonies appear, they are identified by PCR using nested fliC and Vi-associated primers or, most commonly, by using standard biochemical reactions and incubation with specific antisera. A staphylococcal protein A coagglutination technique can be used to identify colonies as soon as they appear on culture plates.[95]

After isolation, the organism should be tested for antimicrobial sensitivity. If it is resistant to chloramphenicol, it should be checked for the presence of R plasmids encoding for multiple antibiotic resistance. So-called "quinolone-resistant" strains, which generally have minimum inhibitory concentrations of the fluoroquinolones within the susceptible range of the interpretive criteria of the NCCLS, are characterized by resistance to nalidixic acid.

Serologic and Other Tests

Widal's Test

The standard serologic test in use for the diagnosis of typhoid fever has been Widal's reaction, which measures agglutinating antibodies to the O and H antigens of S. Typhi. Numerous studies have shown that the sensitivity, specificity, and predictive values of this test vary dramatically among laboratories. This wide variation is caused by differences in patient populations, antigens, and techniques. Thus, if physicians do not know the sensitivity, specificity, and predictive values for the test in their laboratory and in their patient population, the results are almost uninterpretable. On the other hand, if these values are known, Widal's test can be of some use.

Widal's test is inherently nonspecific because (1) S. Typhi shares O and H antigens with other *Salmonella* serotypes[15,23] (see Table 17-2); (2) S. Typhi shares cross-reacting epitopes with other Enterobacteriaceae; and (3) H antibody titers remain elevated for long periods after infection or immunization. Widal's test has a low sensitivity because (1) a significant number of culture-positive patients never develop detectable antibody as measured by this test; and (2) in those who do develop an antibody titer, the titer frequently begins to rise before the onset of clinical disease, making it difficult to demonstrate a fourfold rise in titer.

Studies in endemic areas have shown the sensitivity of a single elevated O antibody titer (≥1:40 in Mexico and Indonesia, ≥1:480 in Zimbabwe) to vary from 50% to 90% and the specificity of the same titer to vary from 70% to 99%. In Indonesia, an O antibody titer of 1:40 or greater measured by the rapid, Widal's slide agglutination test (results available to the physician within 45 minutes of specimen acquisition) was shown to have a positive predictive value of 96%.[89] Although not useful when negative, when the test was positive the health-care provider could be 96% certain that the patient had typhoid fever. A rapid tube test for *Salmonella* O9 antibody using magnetic particles has been reported.[97] The sensitivity of a single H titer is similar, but the specificity is much lower. In endemic areas, a fourfold rise in O or H antibody titer is generally found in fewer than 40% of culture-positive patients. In nonendemic areas, the sensitivity is usually the same as in endemic areas, whereas the specificity is generally higher. A Vi agglutination reaction has been used for screening for *S.* Typhi carriers. The reported sensitivity and specificity are 70% to 80% and 80% to 95%, respectively.

Rapid tests, which include the enzyme-linked immunosorbent assay (ELISA), dipstick assays, latex agglutination, and monoclonal antibodies, have been developed.[98–100] Although these tests are in use in some laboratories, they are not yet readily available for general use.

DNA Probes and Polymerase Chain Reaction

DNA probes have been developed for identifying *S.* Typhi from bacterial culture isolates and directly from blood.[101,102] However, these tests are not yet commercially available. PCR assays have been utilized by a number of groups for rapid diagnosis of *S.* Typhi infection in blood specimens from patients with typhoid fever, but these also are not yet in routine clinical use.[103–105] Such assays, utilizing primers based on the flagellin gene and the Vi antigen, can be used to detect genomic *S.* Typhi DNA in 12 hours or less,[106] with a high degree of sensitivity and specificity.

Differential Diagnosis

Endemic Areas

During the first week of illness, it is difficult to clinically distinguish typhoid fever from many other febrile illnesses. Thus, the physician must suspect typhoid fever, order appropriate cultures, and consider treatment prior to obtaining bacteriologic confirmation. During the second week of febrile illness, the range of possibilities is narrowed, particularly if the other locally prevalent diseases that can cause prolonged fever are known. These include other bacterial diseases such as endocarditis, brucellosis, tularemia, tuberculosis, and abscesses; rickettsial infections such as typhus; protozoan infections such as malaria, visceral leishmaniasis, amebic liver abscess, and toxoplasmosis; viral infections such as influenza or dengue fever; and noninfectious diseases such as connective tissue diseases and lymphoproliferative disorders.

Physicians practicing in the tropics frequently see patients with fevers lasting for 7 to 10 days who have nonspecific clinical findings compatible with typhoid and negative bacteriologic tests and who recover either without antimicrobial treatment or after empirical treatment with a broad-spectrum antibiotic. It is likely that many of these patients do have viral infections. It should be noted that the spleen in typhoid fever is generally considerably smaller and softer than the spleen in malaria.

Developed Countries

Unless there is an epidemic, most cases will be imported. The physician must remember to take a travel history, suspect typhoid fever in febrile patients returning from endemic areas, and order appropriate cultures. The differential diagnosis will include those diseases prevalent in the areas visited, as outlined previously, and all other causes of prolonged fever. Typhoid should also be suspected in patients who have not traveled and who have prolonged fever.

If the diagnosis of typhoid fever is considered, and particularly if the patient is toxic or has had previous antibiotics, a bone marrow aspirate culture should be used as a primary diagnostic tool.

TREATMENT

In most cases of typhoid fever, successful treatment requires prompt diagnosis, use of an appropriate antibiotic, and bed rest at home. In many endemic areas, more than 90% of patients are managed in this way, and case-fatality rates for such patients are less than 1%.[86,107] In some areas of Indonesia, India, Nepal, and a number of countries in Africa, 20% to 30% of patients with typhoid who are admitted to the hospital are severely ill, and unless they receive intensive care, appropriate doses of corticosteroids, and surgery, when indicated, may have case-fatality rates of 10% to 50%.[21,83–85,108] Management of hospitalized patients requires (1) proper use of antibiotics; (2) good nursing care; (3) adequate nutrition; (4) careful attention to fluid and electrolyte balance; (5) prompt diagnosis and treatment of intestinal perforation, intestinal bleeding, and other complications; and (6) the use of high-dose corticosteroids in severely ill patients.

Antibiotic Selection

Medications that are appropriate for the treatment of typhoid fever include ampicillin, amoxicillin, cefotaxime, ceftriaxone, chloramphenicol, trimethoprim-sulfamethoxazole, or a fluoroquinolone.[109] Of these, fluoroquinolones have been found to result in the shortest fever-clearance times. Azithromycin has also recently been shown to be effective. Oral therapy is indicated for uncomplicated disease and parenteral therapy is required for severe illness. Choice of a specific antibiotic is based on the expected or known susceptibility of the organism. Caution must be applied when interpreting results of susceptibility testing. Although *S.* Typhi is often susceptible in vitro to drugs including cephalexin, aminoglycosides, furazolidone, and second-generation cephalosporins, use of these drugs has often resulted in treatment failure.

Multidrug-Resistant Typhoid Fever

Infection acquired in India, Pakistan, and Egypt is routinely resistant to multiple antibiotics (ampicillin, chloramphenicol, trimethoprim-sulfamethoxazole). For typhoid fever attributable to such strains, appropriate treatment includes a 10- to 14-day course of ceftriaxone or a 5- to 7-day course of ofloxacin or ciprofloxacin, although more prolonged courses of treatment may be necessary. The widely available fluoroquinolones (ofloxacin, ciprofloxacin, and perfloxacin) are all of equivalent efficacy; however, norfloxacin should not be used to treat typhoid fever because of suboptimal bioavailability. See the discussion under "Fluoroquinolones" regarding the use of fluoroquinolones in the pediatric population. Azithromycin may also be considered for the treatment of multidrug resistant strains.

Quinolone-Resistant Strains

Treatment failures with fluoroquinolones have been reported in infections caused by nalidixic acid–resistant strains. Such relatively quinolone-resistant strains have emerged as an increasingly important clinical problem in the last decade, becoming endemic in a number of areas including southern Vietnam and northern India.[110,111] Although optimal treatment for quinolone-resistant uncomplicated typhoid fever has not been established, options include azithromycin (8–10 mg/kg/dose) for 7 days, a third-generation cephalosporin given for 10 to 14 days, or a fluoroquinolone (20 mg/kg/day) given for 10 to 14 days (given that one can generally achieve levels of the drug that surpass the MIC). Shorter courses of fluoroquinolones have been less satisfactory in the treatment of quinolone-resistant strains.[110] A randomized controlled study found that azithromycin 20 mg/kg/day for 5 days was more effective than ofloxacin 8 mg/kg/day for 5 days for nalidixic acid–resistant enteric fever.[112] For severe disease with quinolone-resistant strains, ceftriaxone or cefotaxime are recommended; fluoroquinolones may be used as a second-line alternative. In the case of *S.* Typhi strains with MIC values of ciprofloxacin of ≥ 2 μg/mL, a third generation cephalosporin or azithromycin should be used.

Specific Antibiotics

Chloramphenicol

Prior to the emergence of drug-resistant strains of *S.* Typhi, chloramphenicol was the most effective and widely used antibiotic for treating typhoid fever patients and the standard against which all other antibiotics were judged. It produces defervescence and relief of symptoms in most patients within 3 to 4 days, reduced the pre–antibiotic era case-fatality rates of 10% to 15% to 1% to 4%, and cures approximately 90% of patients with chloramphenicol-sensitive strains.[87,107] Most studies have shown that in acute chloramphenicol-sensitive *S.* Typhi infections, chloramphenicol produces more rapid defervescence than do ampicillin, amoxicillin, and trimethoprim-sulfamethoxazole, and a higher rate of clinical cure than ampicillin. However, the emergence of multidrug-resistant typhoid fever (MDRTF) has lessened its usefulness. In addition, it does not reduce the relapse rate, has no effect on the convalescent excretor or chronic carrier, and causes aplastic anemia in 1 in every 10,000 to 50,000 patients. In the treatment of susceptible strains, chloramphenicol has the advantage of being inexpensive and rarely associated with any short-term side effects noticeable to the patient.

Fluoroquinolones

In the late 1980s and 1990s, with the emergence of MDRTF, fluoroquinolones, including ciprofloxacin, norfloxacin, and oflaxacin, were shown to be effective agents for the treatment of typhoid fever.[113–117] For typhoid fever caused by susceptible strains, evidence suggests that the fluoroquinolones provide the most effective therapy for typhoid fever even when given as short courses of 3 to 7 days. Pooling data from 17 clinical trials conducted with ciprofloxacin, oflaxacin, fleroxacin, and perfloxacin, the mean fever clearance time was less than 4 days and cure rates were greater than 96%.[116] Most recent studies suggest that, as compared to chloramphenicol, trimethoprim-sulfamethoxazole, and even the third-generation cephalosporins, the fluoroquinolones act more rapidly and have lower rates of stool carriage.[117–119] Relapse after treatment with fluoroquinolones has generally been reported to be less than that with chloramphenicol or the cephalosporins.

Use of fluoroquinolones in animal models has resulted in cartilage damage and, thus, according to Food and Drug Administration (FDA) product labeling, use has generally been contraindicated in patients less than 18 years of age. Perfloxacin, a fluoroquinolone once widely used in France, has been associated with several cases of presumed arthropathy in the pediatric population.[120] However, overall, the data acquired on the short-term use of fluoroquinolones to treat infections such as typhoid fever and dysentery in the pediatric population has been reassuring with regard to safety and tolerability.[121] Thus, in specific situations, such as in the treatment of typhoid fever caused by multidrug resistant strains, their use is considered to be justified by many infectious disease experts.[121]

Third-Generation Cephalosporins

Studies in animals indicate that the third-generation cephalosporins are quite effective in the acid environment of reticuloendothelial cells and that particularly cefoperazone, but also ceftriaxone, is excreted in high concentration into the biliary tract. The in vivo activity of these compounds against *S.* Typhi has been attributed to these characteristics. Ceftriaxone, cefixime, cefotaxime, and cefoperazone (all third-generation cephalosporins) have acceptable efficacy in the treatment of typhoid fever. In the past 2 decades, these compounds, particularly ceftriaxone and cefoperazone, have been shown in a number of studies to be at least as effective in treating typhoid fever as chloramphenicol.[122] The third-generation oral cephalosporin cefixime has been shown to be effective in the treatment of uncomplicated typhoid fever due to MDRTF *S.* Typhi, although short-course treatment with cefixime appears less effective than short-course treatment with ofloxacin.[123]

Ampicillin, Amoxicillin, and Trimethoprim-Sulfamethoxazole

These drugs are all effective against *S.* Typhi with R plasmid–mediated resistance to chloramphenicol, but R plasmid–mediated resistance to ampicillin and to trimethoprim is increasingly recognized. The dosage regimens listed in Table 17-5 will provide the best available cure rates and the lowest relapse rates. Treatment with these antibiotics does not prevent gallbladder carriage.

Table 17-5 Antimicrobial Therapy of Typhoid and Paratyphoid Fever

Antibiotic	Route of Administration*	Daily Dosage (mg/kg/day)	Doses per Day	Duration (Days)
Chloramphenicol	PO/IV	PO:50–75, IV:100 (Usual adult dose: 2 g/day)	4	14–21
Trimethoprim-sulfamethoxazole	PO/IV	8† (Adults 320† mg/day)	2	14
Amoxicillin	PO	75–100	3	14
Ampicillin	IV/IM	100	4	10–14
Ceftriaxone	IV	50–75 (Adults: 2–4 g/day)	1	10–14
Cefotaxime	IV	40–80 (Adults: 2–4 g/day)	3	10–14
Cefixime	PO	15–20 (Adults: 200–400 mg/day)	2	10–14
Ciprofloxacin or Ofloxacin§	PO/IV	15–20‡	2	5–14§
Azithromycin	PO	8–10 (Adults: 500 mg/day)	1	7

*For severe typhoid, parenteral therapy is indicated.
†The dosage refers to the trimethoprim component.
‡The generally recommended dosage is 15 mg/kg/day except for treatment of quinolone-resistant strains, for which 20 mg/kg/day is recommended.
§For uncomplicated typhoid fever, the generally recommended duration is 5–7 days for fully susceptible strains (3-day courses also shown to be effective, particularly for epidemics); 5–7 days for multidrug–resistant strains; 10–14 days for quinolone-resistant strains. For severe typhoid fever, 10–14 days is recommended.

Azithromycin

Although not yet approved by the FDA for treating typhoid, there are considerable data indicating that the macrolide azithromycin provides an alternative therapeutic option for the treatment of uncomplicated typhoid fever. It possesses in vitro activity against *S.* Typhi.[124,125] It has been studied in a number of randomized comparative clinical trials. In India, a randomized comparative study in 77 adults demonstrated that 7 days of azithromycin was at least as effective as 14 days of chloramphenicol in treating typhoid fever with susceptible strains (100% vs. 94% cure at 14 days post start of treatment with no prolonged fecal carriage in either group). In Egyptian children aged 4 to 17 years, 31 of 34 children (91%) were cured after 7 days of azithromycin and none had relapses as compared to 29 of 30 (97%) cured with ceftriaxone with 4 (14%) relapses.[126] In a randomized controlled comparison of 5 days of azithromycin or 5 days of ofloxacin in 88 adult patients with multidrug-resistant or nalidixic acid–resistant typhoid fever, those treated with azithromycin had a shorter fever clearance (135 vs. 174 hours) and had no positive fecal cultures at the end of treatment, as compared to 41% of those treated with ofloxacin.[112] A comparative study in Egypt of azithromycin and ciprofloxacin, each given for 7 days, demonstrated that the drugs were similarly effective clinically and against the infectious agent.[115]

Other

Although effective in vitro against *S.* Typhi, sulfonamides, tetracyclines, and aminoglycosides are ineffective in vivo, probably because they are ineffective at the low pH of the phagolysomes that contain intracellular *S.* Typhi in reticuloendothelial cells. Aztreonam has had a variable success rate and thus is not considered first-line therapy.

Supportive, Nutritional, and Nursing Care

Toxic patients with typhoid fever are frequently immobile or agitated, anorectic or incapable of eating, and highly febrile. They must be turned and bathed frequently, fed intravenously or carefully by mouth, and cooled with a cooling blanket or by using tepid sponge baths supplemented by a fan to enhance evaporation. They must be protected against aspiration and observed for signs of intestinal perforation or hemorrhage and shock. Many authorities recommend avoidance of antipyretics, since they are reported to cause precipitous drops in temperature and hypotension; however, they may be used if the temperature remains over 39.5°C after other measures have been tried. Patients who do not have a paralytic ileus, suspected perforation, or severe abdominal pain should be encouraged to eat whatever they like, since maintenance of good nutritional status is more important than an unsubstantiated concern about some foods precipitating intestinal perforation or hemorrhage. Vitamin supplementation is recommended. Some patients may require total parenteral nutrition, but this is infrequent.

Fluid and Electrolyte Balance

Most patients can be managed without intravenous therapy. Patients with severe typhoid fever have poor oral intake, high insensible water losses, and tend to become dehydrated with hyponatremia and hypokalemia. Vomiting or diarrhea exacerbates the situation. Initial fluid replacement therapy should provide for maintenance needs, insensible losses, and replacement for dehydration. A typical 50-kg patient who is not in shock will require 3 to 4 L of fluid the first day. Thereafter, records of input and output should be kept and used in managing the patient. If possible, electrolyte determinations should be performed frequently. If not possible, the patient should receive liberal quantities of sodium chloride and potassium unless renal failure is suspected.

Corticosteroids

Since the observations of Woodward and colleagues in 1951,[108] the use of corticosteroids in severe typhoid fever has been controversial. Corticosteroids dramatically shorten the toxic febrile stage in typhoid fever, but until 1982 there was no proof that they reduced mortality. Studies in Indonesia by Hoffman, Punjabi, and colleagues have shown that prompt administration of high-dose dexamethasone reduces mortality in patients with severe typhoid fever without increasing the incidence of complications, carriers, or relapse among survivors.[83,84] The results of these studies have led to the recommendation by the Antimicrobial Agents Committee of the Infectious Diseases Society of America that patients with suspected typhoid fever who are delirious, obtunded, stuporous, comatose, or in shock (severe typhoid fever) should immediately receive dexamethasone or an equivalent corticosteroid.[127] After starting antimicrobial therapy, an initial dose of 3 mg/kg of dexamethasone should be administered by slow intravenous infusion over 30 minutes. This is followed by 1 mg/kg of dexamethasone given at the same rate every 6 hours for eight additional doses, the total duration of corticosteroid therapy being 48 hours. Patients with normal mental and circulatory status do not require corticosteroids, but those with borderline mental or circulatory status should be monitored every 15 minutes in an intensive care unit. If their condition deteriorates, they should receive dexamethasone or an equivalent corticosteroid immediately because a delay in institution of this therapy has been shown to significantly increase mortality.

Treatment of Complications

Intestinal Perforation

Generalized peritonitis and large quantities of pus are often found in patients with intestinal perforation, while walling off of the perforation is infrequent. If a well-trained surgeon, anesthesiologist, and operating room staff and the necessary equipment are available, operative management of typhoid perforation is indicated.[79–81] If these are not available, the choice between operative and nonoperative management is controversial and must be individualized.

In all cases the patient should be started on appropriate antibiotics for *S.* Typhi depending on the local resistance pattern; placed on nasogastric suction; resuscitated with fluids, blood, and oxygen as needed; and given corticosteroids, if severely toxic. In addition, further antibiotics need to be added to provide coverage for the gram-negative rods and anaerobes that constitute the intestinal flora.

It is preferable to stabilize the patient before surgery, but the operation should not be delayed for more than several hours after diagnosis. At operation, the ileum, as well as the cecum and proximal large bowel, should be examined for perforations, and one of several procedures should be performed; for example, intestinal resection and primary anastomosis, or wedge excision, or debridement of the ulcer with primary closure of the perforation. Most surgeons will suture sites of impending perforation with serosa-to-serosa approximation. The peritoneal cavity is then lavaged and the abdomen is closed, with or without drainage. Standard postoperative care is practiced. As the interval between perforation and surgery increases and the preoperative status of the patient worsens, the case-fatality rate increases. Mortality rates of 10% to 32% have been reported.

Intestinal Hemorrhage

In most cases, intestinal hemorrhage, even when massive, can be managed with general supportive care and vigorous replacement of blood. Occasionally the use of platelets, fresh-frozen plasma to replace clotting factors, or intestinal resection will be necessary, but this is uncommon. If the patient does not have an abnormal level of consciousness or shock, the case-fatality rate will be less than 1%.

Other Complications

Renal failure, pneumonia, respiratory failure, myocarditis, arrhythmias, cardiac failure, shock, meningitis, localized abcesses, arthritis, osteomyelitis, hemolytic anemia, and cholecystitis are all occasionally encountered and should be managed with antimicrobials and standard medical or surgical practices.[86] DIC may sometimes be clinically significant, in which case platelet, blood, and clotting factor transfusions may be necessary. There is no evidence that heparin therapy is useful in typhoid.

Relapse

Relapse should be treated in the same way as the first attack.

Management of Carriers

In the absence of cholelithiasis, the majority of carriers can be cured by a prolonged course of antibiotics targeted to the susceptibility of the organism. Cure rates of approximately 80% have been reported with oral ampicillin or amoxicillin 100 mg/kg/day, plus probenecid 30 mg/kg/day taken for 3 months; trimethoprim-sulfamethoxazole, one double-strength tablet twice daily, for 3 months; or 750 mg of ciprofloxacin twice daily for 4 weeks.[128–130] In the presence of cholelithiasis, the preceding regimen should be tried before surgical intervention is considered, but in most cases antimicrobial treatment alone will not be successful and cholecystectomy, as well as the same antimicrobial regimen, is required. A cure rate of 80% to 90% can be obtained with combined surgical and antimicrobial treatment. In some patients with cholelithiasis, *Salmonella* carriage can be eliminated with ciprofloxacin alone.[129,130] Some chronic urinary carriers of *S.* Typhi are infected with *Schistosoma haematobium.* The schistosomiasis should be treated first, and then the patient should receive an antibiotic.

Prognosis

The prognosis is dependent on the patient population and the geographic area of the world. In an epidemic in developed countries, patients will generally be seen and treated promptly, have a case-fatality rate of less than 1%, and have a low incidence of complications. The majority of patients in endemic areas will be treated as outpatients and have case-fatality and complication rates comparable to those expected in an epidemic in developed countries.

In Central and South America, hospitalized patients are reported to have mortality rates of less than 1%. In some endemic areas, including Indonesia, Nigeria, India, and Nepal, severe typhoid fever (abnormal level of consciousness or shock) is common among hospitalized patients. These patients with severe typhoid fever may have a mortality rate as high as 50% if they are not treated with high-dose dexamethasone therapy.[21,82–85,108]

Nearly all studies report much lower complication, case-fatality, relapse, and carrier rates with paratyphoid fever. There have been a number of reports of particularly severe paratyphoid fever in young children and infants, in whom complication and case-fatality rates have been similar to those in patients with typhoid fever.

PREVENTION AND CONTROL

Nonendemic Areas

In developed countries, prevention is now the responsibility of sanitation, water supply, and public health officials. Individuals need not take any special precautions. Chronic carriers should be identified and treated. In the past, considerable time and money were devoted to screening food handlers, but in many countries this is no longer considered necessary. In the event of an epidemic, the source of the infection must be identified and eliminated, and any breakdown in the water delivery and sewage systems must be repaired. The general populace must be informed of the need to adhere to standard hygiene practices.

Endemic Areas

People can minimize their chances of developing enteric fever by paying careful attention to the quality of the food and water that they ingest and by receiving immunizations. *S.* Typhi in water is killed by heating to 57°C, iodination, or chlorination. *S.* Typhi in food is killed at the same temperature, but the food must be heated uniformly for several minutes. Travelers to or residents of endemic areas should drink only boiled or bottled water; avoid eating fresh, uncooked vegetables or unpeeled fruit that has not been thoroughly washed in iodinated or chlorinated water; and use discretion when eating in restaurants or at food stalls. Reduction of endemicity will depend on improvements in water supply and sewage systems and education of the populace as to proper hygiene and food and water preparation practices. Mass immunization can be extremely useful.

Vaccines

In the United States, there are two vaccines currently available for immunization against typhoid: (1) the oral Ty21a vaccine, an oral, live, attenuated vaccine (Vivotif Berna vaccine, manufactured from the Ty21a strain of *S.* Typhi by the Swiss Serum and Vaccine Institute); and (2) the intramuscular ViCPS vaccine, a Vi capsular polysaccharide vaccine (Typhim Vi, manufactured by Aventis Pasteur). The efficacy of these vaccines is expected to be between 50% and 75%. See Table 17-6 for recommendations on usage. The intramuscular heat-phenol-inactivated vaccine (manufactured by Wyeth-Ayerst) has been discontinued and is no longer available for use. A Vi capsular polysaccharide-protein conjugate vaccine has recently been shown to be more effective than all other vaccines[7,8] and it is hoped that it will be introduced for general use soon. Vivaxim is a combined hepatitis A/typhoid fever vaccine (HA/Vi), which has been licensed for vaccination of travelers in Europe, but is not available in the United States.[131]

Oral Ty21a Vaccine

The Ty21a vaccine, agalactose epimerase (gal E) mutant of *S.* Typhi, was developed by Germanier as an oral vaccine.[2–4] In contrast to the whole-cell vaccine, it has minimal to no side effects. In volunteers in Maryland, five to eight doses conferred 87% protection against an ID_{50}. Field studies suggest an inverse relation between the level of transmission of typhoid in an area and protective efficacy. In 6- to 7-year-old Egyptians (incidence in controls, 46/100,000/year), the protective efficacy was 96% after 3 years.[3] In 6- to 21-year-old Chileans (incidence in controls, 103/100,000/year), the efficacy was 67% after 3 years,[2] and in 3- to 19-year-old Indonesians (incidence in controls, 1206/100,000/year), the efficacy of the liquid and enteric-coated formulations was 53% and 42% after 2.5 years, respectively.[4] The vaccine does not contain Vi antigen and is thought to induce a protective cellular immune response. However, the vaccine has not been

*Table 17-6 Dosage and Schedule for Typhoid Fever Vaccination**

Vaccination	Age	Dose/Mode of Administration	No. of Doses	Dosing Interval	Boosting Interval
Oral, Live, Attenuated TY21a Vaccine					
Primary series	6 years or older	1 capsule†/oral	4	48 hours	Not applicable
Booster	6 years or older	1 capsule†/oral	4	48 hours	Every 5 years
Vi Capsular Polysaccharide Vaccine					
Primary series	2 years or older	0.50 mL/intramuscular	1	Not applicable	Not applicable
Booster	2 years or older	0.50 mL/intramuscular	1	Not applicable	Every 2 years

*Per *2004 Centers for Disease Control and Prevention Recommendations.*
†Administer with cool liquid no warmer than 37°C (98.6°F).

shown to induce either cellular or humoral immunity in children less than 2 years of age.[132,133] It is not recommended for use in children less than 6 years of age.

Parenteral ViCPS Vaccine

This vaccine was developed and studied by Robbins and coworkers.[5,6] In 5- to 44-year-old Nepalese (incidence in controls, 654/100,000/year), a single injection of the vaccine was not associated with significant side effects and conferred a protective efficacy of 72% after 17 months.[5] In South African schoolchildren (approximate incidence in controls, 470/100,000/year), the Vi vaccine had a protective efficacy of approximately 64% during 21 months of surveillance.[6] The Vi vaccine was associated with an efficacy of 73% (95% confidence interval [CI], 32%–89%) in protecting against infection among 1260 students immunized before an outbreak of typhoid fever occurring in a middle school in the People's Republic of China and an efficacy of 71% (95% CI, −9% to 92%) in protecting 441 students immunized during the outbreak, results which support its use as a public health tool.[134] It is thought that antibodies to Vi antigen are responsible for the protective immunity. However, the Vi vaccine does not induce protective antibody levels in young children nor does it produce a booster reponse.[135,136] It is not recommended for use in children less than 2 years of age.

Whole-Cell Typhoid Vaccines

These vaccines have now been discontinued from use. The first parenteral killed typhoid vaccine was introduced in 1896. By 1912, all U.S. military personnel were required to receive it, but it was not until the 1960s that the vaccine's efficacy was established in field trials.[137] The WHO sponsored trials in typhoid-endemic areas of Poland, Yugoslavia, Guyana, and the then Soviet Union, and demonstrated that both phenol- and acetone-inactivated vaccines offered 51% to 88% protection to children and young adults. The acetone-inactivated vaccine, which preserves Vi antigen, was moderately more effective than the phenol-inactivated vaccine. Studies at the University of Maryland showed that the same vaccines used in the WHO studies gave 67% protection to volunteers who ingested an ID_{25} (10^5 organisms) of *S.* Typhi, but did not offer any protection to those who ingested an ID_{50} (10^7 organisms).[137] The heat- and phenol-inactivated typhoid vaccines had been the only available vaccine for children younger than 2 years of age. However, the vaccines have been associated with a relatively high rate of adverse events, with local and systemic side effects reported in 25% to 50% of recipients[138] and their use has been discontinued in the United States.

S. Typhi Vi Conjugate Vaccine

Given that the two licensed vaccines confer only a maximum of 75% protective immunity and do not protect or are not recommended for young children, this conjugate vaccine was developed and has shown promising results. *S. typhi* Vi conjugate vaccine (Vi-rEPA) is composed of Vi bound to a nontoxic recombinant protein which is antigenically identical to *Pseudomonas aeruginosa* exotoxin A (rePA).[139] Based on initial demonstrations of safety and immunogenicity,[140] a double-blind, placebo-controlled, randomized trial was conducted in 11,091 children 2 to 5 years of age in 16 communes in Dong Thap Province, Vietnam (incidence in controls, 358/100,000/year).[7] The vaccine was safe, immunogenic, with a protective efficacy of 91.5% (95% CI, 77.1% to 96.6%; $p < 0.001$) over 27 months of active surveillance. In all of the 36 children evaluated 1 month after the second immunization, there was a 10-fold increase in serum IgG Vi antibodies. During a subsequent 19-month period of passive surveillance, protective efficacy was 82.4% (95% CI, 22.3% to 99.1%).[8]

Vaccine Recommendations

Routine typhoid vaccination should be given to laboratory workers likely to work with *S.* Typhi, household contacts of known *S.* Typhi carriers, and those traveling to or living in areas where typhoid is endemic. This includes most countries of the developing world. Routine vaccination is not recommended in those countries where the incidence is low, as in the United States and Europe, not even during disasters or for family contacts. During disasters or in refugee camps in endemic areas, mass immunization should be considered, recognizing that provision of safe food and water is of primary importance.

Immunization

See Table 17-6 for schedule and dosage of vaccines, as recommended by the Centers for Disease Control and Prevention.

Ty21a

Children who are 6 years of age and older and adults should take one capsule every 2 days for a total of four capsules.[109] The capsule should be taken with cool liquid approximately 1 hour prior to intake of a meal. Capsules should be kept refrigerated.[4] The liquid formulation of Ty21a, which may be useful in administering the vaccine to children, is not available in the United States, but is used in many locations throughout the world. The vaccine manufacturer recommends reimmunization with the entire four-dose series every 5 years in the case of continued or renewed exposure to *S.* Typhi.

Since Ty21a is a live attenuated vaccine, it should not be given to immunocompromised persons, including those infected with HIV. Antimicrobial medications should be avoided during the week prior to administration of the first dose and for the week after the fourth dose of Ty21a. Administration of proguanil hydrochloride should be delayed until 10 or more days after the fourth dose of Ty21a.

Vi Capsular Polysaccharide Vaccine

Immunization may be given to people 2 years of age and older and consists of a single 0.5-mL (25-μg) dose administered intramuscularly. The vaccine manufacturer recommends that a booster dose be given every 2 years for continued or renewed expsosure to *S.* Typhi.

Adverse Reactions

Adverse reactions to Ty21a are minimal. These may include abdominal discomfort, nausea, vomiting, fever, headache, rash, or urticaria. Adverse reactions to the ViCPS vaccine are also minimal: fever (0%–1%), headache (1.5%–3%), and local reactions of erythema of induration of 1 cm or greater (7%) have been reported.

Recommendations for Children under 2 Years of Age and for Pregnant Women

There are no available data concerning the efficacy of either of the licensed vaccines for use in children under 2 years of age. Evidence exists to suggest that breastfeeding and careful preparation of formula may reduce the risk of infection in endemic regions.[109] No safety data are available for the use of typhoid vaccines in pregnant women.

REFERENCES

1. Woodward TE, Smadel JE, Ley HL, et al: Preliminary report on the beneficial effect of chloromycetin in the treatment of typhoid fever. Ann Intern Med 2:131–134, 1948.
2. Levine MM, Black RE, Ferreccio C, et al: Large-scale field trial of Ty21a live oral typhoid vaccine in enteric-coated capsule formulation. Lancet 1049–1052, 1987.
3. Wahdan MH, Serie C, Cerisier Y, et al: A controlled field trial of live *Salmonella typhi* strain Ty21a oral vaccine against typhoid: Three-year results. J Infect Dis 145:292–295, 1985.
4. Simanjuntak CH, Paleologo FP, Punjabi NH, et al: Oral immunisation against typhoid fever in Indonesia with Ty21a vaccine. Lancet 338:1055–1059, 1991.
5. Acharya IL, Lowe CU, Thapa R, et al: Prevention of typhoid fever in Nepal with the Vi capsular polysaccharide of *Salmonella typhi.* N Engl J Med 317:1101–1104, 1987.
6. Klugman KP, Koornhof HJ, Schneerson R, et al: Protective activity of Vi capsular polysaccharide vaccine against typhoid fever. Lancet 2:1165–1169, 1987.
7. Lin FY, Ho VA, Khiem HB, et al: The efficacy of a *Salmonella typhi* Vi conjugate vaccine in two-to-five-year-old children. N Engl J Med 334:1263–1269, 2001.
8. Mai NL, Phan VB, Vo AH, et al: Persistent efficacy of Vi conjugate vaccine against typhoid fever in young children. N Engl J Med 349:1390–1391, 2003.
9. Parkhill J, Dougan G, James KD, et al: Complete genomic sequence of multiple drug resistant *Salmonella enterica* serovar Typhi CT18. Nature 413:848–852, 2001.
10. Koneman EW, Allen SD, Janda WM, et al: The Enterobacteriaceae. Color Atlas and Textbook of Diagnostic Microbiology, 4th ed. Philadelphia, J.B. Lippincott, 1992, pp 105–184.
11. McClelland M, Sanderson KE, Spieth J, et al: The complete genome sequence of *Salmonella enterica* serovar Typhimurium LT2. Nature 413:852–856, 2001.
12. Blattner FR, Plunkett G III, Bloch CA, et al: The complete genome sequence of *Escherichia coli* K-12. Science 277:1453–1474, 1997.
13. Wain J, House D, Parkhill J, et al: Unlocking the genome of the human typhoid bacillus. Lancet Infect Dis 2:163–170, 2002.
14. Edelman R, Levine MM: Summary of an international workshop on typhoid fever. Rev Infect Dis 8:329–349, 1986
15. Osler W: Principles and Practices of Medicine, 7th ed. New York, Appleton, 1909, pp 57–105.
16. Centers for Disease Control and Prevention. Summary of notifiable diseases—United States, 2002. MMWR 51:70–76, 2002.
17. Sinha A, Sazawal S, Kumar R, et al: Typhoid fever in children aged less than 5 years. Lancet 354:734–737, 1999.
18. Lin FY, Vo AH, Phan VB, et al: The epidemiology of typhoid fever in the Dong Thap Province, Mekong Delta region of Vietnam. Am J Trop Med Hyg 62:644–648, 2000.
19. Typhoid vaccines. Wkly Epidemiol Rec 75:257–264, 2000.
20. Crump JA, Luby SP, Mintz ED: The global burden of typhoid fever. Bull World Health Org 82:346–353, 2004.
21. Rogerson SJ, Spooner VJ, Smith TA, et al: Hydrocortisone in chloramphenicol-treated severe typhoid fever in Papua New Guinea. Trans R Soc Trop Med Hyg 85:113–116, 1991.
22. Mermin JH, Townes JM, Gerber M, et al: Typhoid fever in the United States, 1985–1994: Changing risks of international travel and increasing antimicrobial resistance. Arch Intern Med 158:633–638, 1998.
23. Hoffman TA, Ruiz CJ, Counts GW, et al: Waterborne typhoid fever in Dade County, Florida: Clinical and therapeutic evaluations of 105 bacteremic patients. Am J Med 59:481–487, 1975.
24. Typhoid fever—San Antonio, Texas. MMWR 30:540, 545–546, 1981.
25. Taylor JP, Shandera WX, Betz TG, et al: Typhoid fever in San Antonio, Texas: An outbreak traced to a continuing source. J Infect Dis 149:553–557, 1984.
26. Lin FYC, Becke JM, Groves C: Restaurant-associated outbreak of typhoid fever in Maryland: Identification of carrier facilitated by measurement of serum Vi antibodies. J Clin Microbiol 26:1194–1197, 1988.
27. Birkhead GS, Morse DL, Levine WC, et al: Typhoid fever at a resort hotel in New York: A large outbreak with an unusual vehicle. J Infect Dis 167:1228–1232, 1993.
28. Typhoid fever—Skagit County, Washington. MMWR 39:749–751, 1990.
29. Pradier C, Keita-Perse O, Bernard E, et al: Outbreak of typhoid fever on the French Riviera. Eur J Clin Microbiol Infect Dis 19:464–467, 2000.
30. Olsen SJ, Bleasdale SC, Magnano AR, et al: Outbreaks of typhoid fever in the United States, 1960–99. Epidemiol Infect 130:13–21, 2003.
31. Colquhoun J, Weetech RS: Resistance to chloramphenicol developing during treatment of typhoid fever. Lancet 2:621–623, 1950.
32. Gupta A: Multidrug-resistant typhoid fever in children: Epidemiology and therapeutic approach. Pediatr Infect Dis J 13:134–140, 1994.
33. Mirza SH, Beeching NJ, Hart CA: Multi-drug resistant typhoid: A global problem. J Med Microbiol 44:317–319, 1996.
34. Rowe B, Ward LR, Threlfall EJ: Multidrug-resistant *Salmonella* typhi: A worldwide epidemic. Clin Infect Dis 24(Suppl 1):S106–S109, 1997.
35. Alsoub H, Uwaydah AK, Matar I, et al: A clinical comparison of typhoid fever caused by susceptible and multidrug-resistant strains of *Salmonella typhi*. Br J Clin Pract 51:8–10, 1997.
36. Wain J, Diep TS, Ho VA, et al: Quantitation of bacteria in blood of typhoid fever patients and relationship between counts and clinical features, transmissibility, and antibiotic resistance. J Clin Microbiol 36:1683–1687, 1998.
37. Hoa NT, Diep TS, Wain J, et al: Community-acquired septicaemia in southern Viet Nam: The importance of multidrug-resistant *Salmonella typhi*. Trans R Soc Trop Med Hyg 92:503–508, 1998.
38. Threlfall EJ, Ward LR, Skinner JA, et al: Ciprofloxacin-resistant *Salmonella typhi* and treatment failure. Lancet 353:1590–1591, 1999.
39. Threlfall EJ, Ward LR: Decreased susceptibility to ciprofloxacin in *Salmonella enterica* serotype typhi, United Kingdom. Emerg Infect Dis 7:448–450, 2001.
40. Mermin JH, Vilar R, Carpenter J, et al: A massive epidemic of multidrug-resistant typhoid fever in Tajikistan associated with consumption of municipal water. J Infect Dis 179:1416–1422, 1999.
41. Parry C, Wain J, Chinh NT, et al: Quinolone-resistant *Salmonella typhi* in Vietnam. Lancet 351:1289, 1998.
42. Wain J, Hoa NT, Chinh NT, et al: Quinolone-resistant *Salmonella typhi* in Viet Nam: Molecular basis and clinical response to treatment. Clin Infect Dis 25:1404–1410, 1997.
43. Mehta G, Randhawa VS, Mohapatra NP: Intermediate susceptibility to ciprofloxacin in *Salmonella typhi* strains in India. Eur J Clin Microbiol Infect Dis 20:760–761, 2001.
44. Saha Sk, Talukder SY, Islam M, et al: A highly ceftriaxone-resistant *Salmonella typhi* in Bangladesh. Pediatr Infect Dis J 18:387, 1999.
45. Ackers ML, Puhr ND, Tauxe RV, et al: Laboratory-based surveillance of *Salmonella* serotype typhi infections in the United States: Antimicrobial resistance on the rise. JAMA 283:2668–2673, 2000.
46. Wasfy Mo, French R, Ismail TF, et al: Trends of multiple-drug resistance among *Salmonella* serotype typhi isolates during a 14-year period in Egypt. Clin Infect Dis 35:1265–1268, 2002.
47. Gautam V, Gupta NK, Chaudhary U, et al: Sensitivity pattern of *Salmonella* serotypes in Northern India. Braz J Infect Dis 6:281–287, 2002.
48. Saha SK, Saha S, Ruhulamin M, et al: Decreasing trends of multiresistant *Salmonella typhi* in Bangladesh. J Antimicrob Chemother 39:554–556, 1997.

49. Tjaniadi P, Lesmana M, Subekti D, et al: Antimicrobial resistance of bacterial pathogens associated with diarrheal patients in Indonesia. Am J Trop Med Hyg 68:666–670, 2003.
50. Butler T, Islam A, Kabir I, et al: Patterns of morbidity and mortality in typhoid fever dependent on age and gender: Review of 552 hospitalized patients with diarrhea. Rev Infect Dis 13:85–90, 1991.
51. Duggan MB, Beyer L: Enteric fever in young Yoruba children. Arch Dis Child 50:67–71, 1975.
52. Vollaard AM, Ali S, van Asten HA, et al: Risk factors for typhoid and paratyphoid fever in Jakarta, Indonesia. JAMA 291:2607–2615, 2004.
53. Saha SK, Baqui AH, Hanif M, et al: Typhoid fever in Bangladesh: Implications for vaccination policy. Pediatr Infect Dis J 20(5):521–524, 2001.
54. Le Page P, Bogaerts J, Van Goethem C, et al: Community acquired bacteremia in African children. Lancet 1:1458–1461, 1987.
55. Reller ME, Olsen SJ, Kressel AB, et al: Sexual transmission of typhoid fever: A multistate outbreak among men who have sex with men. Clin Infect Dis 37:141–144, 2003.
56. Hornick RB, Greisman SE, Woodward TE, et al: Typhoid fever: Pathogenesis and immunologic control. Part 1. N Engl J Med 283:686–691, 1970.
57. Blaser MJ, Newman LS: A review of human salmonellosis: I. Infective dose. Rev Infect Dis 4:1096–1106, 1982.
58. Gorden J, Small PLC: Acid resistance in enteric bacteria. Infect Immun 61:364–367, 1993.
59. Dunstan SJ, Stephens HA, Blackwell JM, et al: Genes of the class II and class III major histocompatibility complex are associated with typhoid fever in Vietnam. J Infect Dis 183:261–268, 2001.
60. Gotuzzo E, Frisancho O, Sanchez J, et al: Association between the acquired immunodeficiency syndrome and infection with *Salmonella typhi* or *Salmonella paratyphi* in an endemic typhoid area. Arch Intern Med 151:381–382, 1991.
61. Crewe-Brown HH, et al: Invasive *Salmonella* species and HIV infection. In Proceedings of the 12th World AIDS Conference, Geneva, Switzerland, June 28–July 3, 1998, 284 (abstract).
62. Kohtaba S, Yokobata H, Yabuuchi E: Cytopathogenic effect of *Salmonella typhi* GIFU 10007 on M cells of murine ileal Peyer's patches in ligated ileal loops: An ultrastructural study. Microbiol Immunol 30:1225–1237, 1986.
63. Rubin RH, Weinstein L: Salmonellosis: Microbiologic, Pathologic, and Clinical Features. New York, Stratton Intercontinental, 1977.
64. Bitar R, Tarpley J: Intestinal perforation in typhoid fever: A historical and state-of-the-art review. Rev Infect Dis 7:257–271, 1985.
65. Fame TM, Englehard D, Riley HD Jr: Hemophagocytosis accompanying typhoid fever. Pediatr Infect Dis 5:367–369, 1986.
66. Hornick RB, Greisman SE, Woodward TE, et al: Typhoid fever: Pathogenesis and immunologic control. Part 2. N Engl J Med 283:739–746, 1970.
67. Greisman SE, Hornick RB, Wagner HN, et al: The role of endotoxin during typhoid fever and tularemia in man: IV. The integrity of the endotoxin tolerance mechanisms during infection. J Clin Invest 48:613–629, 1969.
68. Butler T, Bell WR, Levin J, et al: Typhoid fever: Studies of blood coagulation, bacteremia, and endotoxemia. Arch Intern Med 138:407–410, 1978.
69. Hornick RB, Greisman S: On the pathogenesis of typhoid fever. Arch Intern Med 138:357–359, 1978.
70. Forrest BD, LaBrooy LT, Breyer L, et al: The human humoral immune response to *Salmonella typhi* Ty21a. J Infect Dis 163:336–345, 1991.
71. Levine MM, Ferreccio C, Black RE, et al: Progress in vaccines against typhoid fever. Prev Inf Dis 11(Suppl 3):S552–S557, 1989.
72. Rajagopalan P, Kumar R, Malaviya AN: Immunological studies in typhoid fever. I. Immunoglobulins, C3, antibodies, rheumatoid factor and circulation immune complexes in patients with typhoid fever. Clin Exp Immunol 44:68–73, 1981.
73. Thevanesam V, Arseculeraine SC, Weliange LV, et al: Cell mediated and humoral immune responses in human typhoid fever. Trop Geogr Med 34:13–17, 1982.
74. Murphy JR, Wasserman SS, Baqar S, et al: Immunity to *Salmonella typhi:* Considerations relevant to measurement of cellular immunity in typhoid-endemic regions. Clin Exp Immunol 75:228–233, 1989.
75. Mabel TJ, Paniker CKJ: The role of cell-mediated immunity in typhoid. Asian J Infect Dis 3:69–75, 1979.
76. Tagliabue A, Villa L, De Magistris MT, et al: IgA-driven T cell–mediated anti-bacterial immunity in man after live oral Ty 21a vaccine. J Immunol 137:1504–1510, 1986.
77. Stuart BM, Pullen RL: Typhoid: Clinical analysis of three hundred and sixty cases. Arch Intern Med 78:629–661, 1946.
78. Klotz SA, Jorgensen JH, Buckwold FJ, et al: Typhoid fever. An epidemic with remarkably few clinical signs and symptoms. Arch Intern Med 144:533–537, 1984.
79. Eustache J-M, Kreis DJ: Typhoid perforation of the intestine. Arch Surg 118:1269–1271, 1983.
80. Meier DE, Imediegwu OO, Tarpley JL: Perforated typhoid enteritis: Operative experience with 108 cases. Am J Surg 157:423–427, 1989.
81. Kim J-P, Oh S-K, Jarrett F: Management of ileal perforation due to typhoid fever. Ann Surg 181:88–91, 1975.
82. Khosla SN: Changing patterns of typhoid (a reappraisal). Asian Med J 25:185–198, 1982.
83. Hoffman SL, Punjabi NH, Kumala S: Reduction of mortality in chloramphenicol-treated severe typhoid fever by high-dose dexamethasone. N Engl J Med 310:82–88, 1984.
84. Punjabi NH, Hoffman SL, Edman DC, et al: Treatment of severe typhoid fever in children with high dose dexamethasone. Pediatr Infect Dis J 7:598–600, 1988.
85. Osuntokun BO, Bademosi O, Ogunremi K, et al: Neuropsychiatric manifestations of typhoid fever in 959 patients. Arch Neurol 27:7–13, 1972.
86. Woodward TE, Smadel JE: Management of typhoid fever and its complications. Ann Intern Med 60:144–157, 1964.
87. Rowland HAK: The complications of typhoid fever. Am J Trop Med Hyg 64:143–148, 1961.
88. Butler T, Rumans L, Arnold K: Response of typhoid fever caused by chloramphenicol-susceptible and chloramphenicol-resistant strains of *Salmonella typhi* to treatment with trimethoprim-sulfamethoxazole. Rev Infect Dis 4:551–561, 1982.
89. Hoffman SL, Flanigan TP, Klaucke D, et al: The Widal slide agglutination test, a valuable rapid diagnostic test in typhoid fever patients at the Infectious Diseases Hospital of Jakarta. Am J Epidemiol 123:869–875, 1986.
90. Gilman RH, Terminel M, Levine MM, et al: Relative efficacy of blood, urine, rectal swab, bone-marrow and rose-spot cultures for recovery of *Salmonella typhi* in typhoid fever. Lancet 1:1211–1213, 1975.
91. Wicks ACB, Holmes GS, Davidson L: Endemic typhoid fever: A diagnostic pitfall. QJM 40:341–354, 1971.
92. Hoffman SL, Punjabi NH, Rockhill RC, et al: Duodenal string-capsule culture compared with bone-marrow, blood, and rectal-swab cultures for diagnosing typhoid and paratyphoid fever. J Infect Dis 149:157–161, 1984.
93. Hoffman SL, Edman DC, Punjabi NH, et al: Bone marrow aspirate culture superior to streptokinase clot culture and 8 ml 1:10 blood-to-broth ratio blood culture for diagnosis of typhoid fever. Am J Trop Med Hyg 35:836–869, 1986.
94. Rubin FA, McWhirter PD, Burr D, et al: Rapid diagnosis of typhoid fever: Identification of *Salmonella typhi* within 18 hours of specimen acquisition by culture of the mononuclear cell/platelet fraction of blood. J Clin Microbiol 28:825–827, 1990.
95. Rockhill RC, Lesmana M, Moechtar MA, et al: Detection of *Salmonella* C1, D and V1 antigens, by coagglutination, in blood cultures from patients with *Salmonella* infection. Southeast Asian J Trop Med Public Health 11:441–445, 1980.
96. Benavente L, Gotuzzo E, Guerra J, et al: Diagnosis of typhoid fever using a string capsule device. Trans R Soc Trop Med Hyg 78:564–565, 1984.
97. Lim PL, Tam FCH, Cheong YM, et al: One-step 2-minute test to detect typhoid-specific antibodies based on particle separation in tubes. J Clin Microbiol 36:2271–2278, 1998.
98. House D, Bishop A, Parry C, et al: Serology of typhoid fever in an area of endemnicity and its relevance to diagnosis. J Clin Microbiol 39:1002–1007, 2001.
99. Hatta M, Goris MG, Heerkens E, et al: Simple dipstick assay for the detection of *Salmonella typhi*–specific IgM antibodies and the evolution of the immune response in patients with typhoid fever. Am J Trop Med Hyg 66:416–421, 2002.

100. Gasem MH, Smits HL, Goris MG, et al: Evaluation of a simple and rapid dipstick assay for the diagnosis of typhoid fever. J Med Microbiol 51:173–177, 2002.
101. Rubin FA, Kopecko DJ, Sack RB, et al: Evaluation of a DNA probe for identifying *Salmonella typhi* in Peruvian and Indonesian bacterial isolates. J Infect Dis 157:1051–1053, 1988.
102. Rubin FA, McWhirter PD, Punjabi NH, et al: Use of a DNA probe to detect *Salmonella typhi* in the blood of patients with typhoid fever. J Clin Microbiol 27:1112–1114, 1989.
103. Chaudhry R, Laxmi BV, Nisar N, et al: Standardisation of polymerase chain reaction for the detection of *Salmonella typhi* in typhoid fever. J Clin Pathol 50:437–439, 1997.
104. Haque A, Ahmed N, Peerzada A, et al: Utility of PCR in diagnosis of problematic cases of typhoid. Jpn J Infect Dis 54:237–239, 2001.
105. Kumar A, Arora V, Bashamboo A, et al: Detection of *Salmonella typhi* by polymerase chain reaction: Implications in diagnosis of typhoid fever. Infect Genet Evol 2:107–110, 2002.
106. Massi MN, Shirakawa T, Gotoh A, et al: Rapid diagnosis of typhoid fever by PCR assay using one pair of primers from flagellin gene of *Salmonella typhi*. J Infect Chemother 9:233–237, 2003.
107. Rowland HAK: The treatment of typhoid fever. J Trop Med Hyg 64:101–111, 1961.
108. Woodward TE, Hall HE, Dias-Rivera R, et al: Treatment of typhoid fever. II. Control of clinical manifestations with cortisone. Ann Intern Med 34:10–19, 1951.
109. American Academy of Pediatrics Red Book: 2003 Report of the Committee on Infectious Diseases, 26th ed. Elk Grove Village, IL, American Academy of Pediatrics, 2003, pp 541–547, 693–694.
110. Parry CM: The treatment of multidrug-resistant and nalidixic acid-resistant typhoid fever in Viet Nam. Trans R Soc Trop Med Hyg 98:413–422, 2004.
111. Renuka K, Kapil A, Kabra SK, et al: Reduced susceptibility to ciprofloxacin and gyra gene mutation in North Indian strains of *Salmonella enterica* serotype Typhi and serotype Paratyphi A. Microb Drug Resist 10:146–153, 2004.
112. Chinh NT, Parry CM, Ly NT, et al: A randomized comparison of azithromycin and ofloxacin for treatment of multidrug-resistant or nalidixic acid-resistant enteric fever. Antimicrob Agents Chemother 44:1855–1859, 2000.
113. Soe GB, Overturf GD: Treatment of typhoid fever and other systemic salmonelloses with cefotaxime, ceftriaxone, cefoperazone, and other newer cephalosporins. Rev Infect Dis 9:719–736, 1987.
114. Tran TH, Bethell DB, Nguyen TT, et al: Short course of ofloxacin for treatment of multidrug-resistant typhoid. Clin Infect Dis 20:917–923, 1995.
115. Girgis NJ, Butler T, Frenck RW, et al: Azithromycin versus ciprofloxacin for treatment of uncomplicated typhoid fever in a randomized trial in Egypt that included patients with multidrug resistance. Antimicrob Agents Chemother 43:1441–1444, 1999.
116. Parry CM, Hien TT, Dougan G, et al: Typhoid fever. N Engl J Med 347:1770–1782, 2002.
117. ThanhPhuong CX, Kneen R, ThanhMai TT, et al: Comparative study of cefixime and ofloxacin for treatment of uncomplicated typhoid fever in Vietnamese children. Third Asia-Pacific Symposium on Typhoid Fever and Other Salmonellosis, Bali, Indonesia, December 8–10, 1997, Abstract T-6, p 79.
118. Muhdoch DA, Banatvaia NA, Bone A, et al: Epidemic ciprofloxacin resistant *Salmonella typhi* in Tasjikistan. Lancet 351:339, 1998.
119. White NJ, Parry CM: The treatment of typhoid fever. Curr Opin Infect Dis 9:298–302, 1996.
120. Alghasham AA, Nahata MC: Clinical use of fluoroquinolones in children. Ann Pharmacother 34:347–359, 2000.
121. Pegues DA, Ohl ME, Miller SI: *Salmonella* species including *Salmonella* Typhi. In Mandell GL, Bennet JE, Dolin R (eds): Principles and Practices of Infectious Diseases. New York, Churchill Livingstone, 2005, pp 2636–2654.
122. Herzog CH: New trends in the chemotherapy of typhoid fever. Acta Trop 37:275–280, 1980.
123. Cao XT, Kneen R, Nguyen TA, et al: A comparative study of ofloxacin and cefixime for treatment of typhoid fever in children. The Dong Nai Pediatric Center Typhoid Study Group. Pediatr Infect Dis J 18:245–248, 1999.
124. Jones K, Felmingham D, Ridgeway G: In vitro activity of azithromycin (CP-62,993), a novel macrolide, against enteric pathogens. Drugs Exp Clin Res 14:613–615, 1988.
125. Metchok B: In vitro activity of azithromycin compared with other macrolides and oral antibiotics against *Salmonella typhi*. J Antimicrob Chemother 25(Suppl A):29–31, 1990.
126. Frenck WF, Nakhla I, Sultan Y, et al: Azithromycin versus ceftriaxone for the treatment of uncomplicated typhoid fever in children. Clin Infect Dis 31:1134–1138, 2000.
127. McGowan JE, Chesney PJ, Crossley KB, et al: Guidelines for the use of systemic glucocorticosteroids in the management of selected infections. J Infect Dis 165:1–13, 1992.
128. Gotuzzo E, Carillo C: Quinolones in typhoid fever. Infect Dis Clin Pract 3:345–351, 1994.
129. Freerksen E, Rosenfeld M, Freerksen R, et al: Treatment of chronic *Salmonella* carriers. Chemotherapy 23:192–210, 1977.
130. Rodriguez-Noriega E, Andrade-Villanueva J, Amaya-Tapia G: Quinolones in the treatment of *Salmonella* carriers. Rev Infect Dis 11:S1179–S1187, 1989.
131. Beran J, Chlibek R, Weber F: A combined dual-chamber typhoid/hepatitis A vaccine as a booster dose in hepatitis A primed adults. Vaccine 21:4650–4654, 2003.
132. Levine MM, Taylor DN, Fenereccio C: Typhoid vaccines come of age. Pediatr Infect Dis J 8:374–381, 1989.
133. Murphy JR, Grez L, Schlesinger L, et al: Immunogenicity of S. typhi Ty21a vaccine for young children. Infect Immun 59:4291–4293, 1991.
134. Yang HH, Kilgore PE, Yang LH, et al: An outbreak of typhoid fever, Xing-An County, People's Republic of China, 1999: Estimation of the field effectiveness of Vi polysaccharide typhoid vaccine. J Infect Dis 183:1775–1780, 2001.
135. Robbins JD, Robbins JB: Re-examination of the protective role of the capsular polysaccharide (Vi antigen) of *Salmonella typhi*. J Infect Dis 150:436–449, 1984.
136. Keitel WA, Bond NL, Zahradnik JM, et al: Clinical and serological responses following primary and booster immunization with *Salmonella typhi* Vi polysaccharide vaccines. Vaccine 12:195–199, 1994.
137. Ivanoff B, Levine MM, Lambert PH: Vaccination against typhoid fever: Present status. Bull World Health Org 72:957–971, 1994.
138. Engels EA, Falagas ME, Lau J, et al: Typhoid fever vaccines: A meta-analysis of studies on efficacy and toxicity. BMJ 316:110–116, 1998.
139. Szu SC, Stone AL, Robbins JD et al: Vi capsular polysaccharide-protein conjugates for prevention of typhoid fever: Preparation, characterization, and immunogenicity in laboratory animals. J Exp Med 166:1510–1524, 1987.
140. Kossaczka Z, Lin FY, Ho VA, et al: Safety and immunogenicity of Vi conjugate vaccines for typhoid fever in adults, teenagers, and 2- to 4-year-old children in Vietnam. Infect Immun 67:5806–5810, 1999.

18

Nontyphoidal Salmonellosis

DAVID A. PEGUES
MICHAEL E. OHL
SAMUEL I. MILLER

INTRODUCTION

Nontyphoidal *Salmonella* species have been isolated from most animals, including domestic and wild mammals, reptiles, and birds, and are a major source of foodborne disease throughout the developed and developing world.[1] *Salmonella* is readily transmitted to humans by contaminated food or poor sanitation. Infection most often results in self-limited acute gastroenteritis; less frequently, bacteremia with or without focal infection occurs. The widespread distribution of *Salmonella* in the environment; its increasing prevalence in the global food chain; and its virulence and adaptability have an enormous medical, public health, and economic impact worldwide.

AGENT

Salmonella is a genus of the family of Enterobacteriaceae. Like other members of the family, the organisms are gram-negative non-spore-forming facultatively anaerobic bacilli that measure 2 to 3 by 0.4 to 0.6 microns in size.[2] The genome sequences of *Salmonella typhimurium* strain LT2 consists of 4,857,432 base pairs and 5599 coding sequences, including 204 pseudogenes.[3] Although the genome is remarkably similar to that of other Enterobacteriaceae, the 8% of genes unique to subtype 1 *Salmonella* may be involved in adaptation to warm-blooded hosts.

The genus *Salmonella* has two species: *Salmonella choleraesuis*, with six subspecies (I, II, IIIa, IIIb, IV, and VI), and *Salmonella bongor*, which formerly was subspecies V.[4] *S. choleraesuis* subspecies I contains almost all the serotypes pathogenic for humans. Because *S. choleraesuis* refers to both a species and a serotype, the species designation *Salmonella enterica* has been recommended and widely adopted. According to the current *Salmonella* nomenclature system, the full taxonomic designation *Salmonella enterica* subspecies *enterica* serotype *typhimurium* can be shortened to *Salmonella* serotype *typhimurium* or *Salmonella typhimurium*.

Members of the seven *Salmonella* subspecies can be grouped into one of more than 2400 serotypes (serovars) according to somatic O, surface Vi, and flagellar H antigens and habitats (Table 18-1).[5] For simplicity, most *Salmonella* serotypes are named for the city in which they were defined,

Table 18-1 Salmonella *Species, Subspecies, Serotypes, and Their Usual Habitats*

Salmonella Species and Subspecies	Serotypes Within Subspecies (No.)	Usual Habitat
S. enterica subsp. *enterica* (I)	1454	Warm-blooded animals
S. enterica subsp. *salmae* (II)	489	Cold-blooded animals and the environment*
S. enterica subsp. *arizonae* (IIIa)	84	Cold-blooded animals and the environment*
S. enterica subsp. *diarizonae* (IIIb)	324	Cold-blooded animals and the environment*
S. enterica subsp. *houtenae* (IV)	70	Cold-blooded animals and the environment*
S. enterica subsp. *indica* (VI)	12	Cold-blooded animals and the environment*
S. bongori (V)	20	Cold-blooded animals and the environment*
Total	2463	

*Isolates of all species and subspecies have occurred in humans.
Adapted from Brenner FW, Villar RG, Angulo FJ, et al: Salmonella nomenclature. J Clin Microbiol 38:2465–2467, 2000.

and the serotype is often used as the species designation.[4] Although serotyping of all surface antigens can be used for formal identification, most laboratories perform a few simple agglutination reactions that define specific O-antigen serogroups, designated as groups A, B, C_1, C_2, D, and E *Salmonella*.[6]

EPIDEMIOLOGY

Incidence

In many countries the incidence of human *Salmonella* infections has increased markedly, although good population-based surveillance data are mostly lacking. In the United States, the incidence rate of nontyphoidal *Salmonella* infection has doubled in the last two decades, with an estimated 1.4 million cases occurring annually.[7,8] In 2002, the incidence rate of salmonellosis (17.7 per 100,000 population) was highest among 10 potentially foodborne diseases under active surveillance and varied little by geographic region (Fig. 18-1).[9] In 2001, *S. typhimurium, S. enteritidis,* and *S. newport* were the three most common serotypes, together accounting for half of all laboratory-confirmed cases of human salmonellosis.[10] Nontyphoidal *Salmonella* causes a small but significant proportion of diarrhea among travelers[11] and among young children in developing countries.[12] The incidence of salmonellosis is highest during the rainy season in tropical climates and during May to October in temperate climates in the Northern hemisphere, coinciding with the peak in foodborne outbreaks.

Reservoirs and Transmission to Humans

In humans, nontyphoidal *Salmonella* infections are most often associated with food products and are the most frequently identified agent of foodborne disease outbreaks (Fig. 18-2).[13]

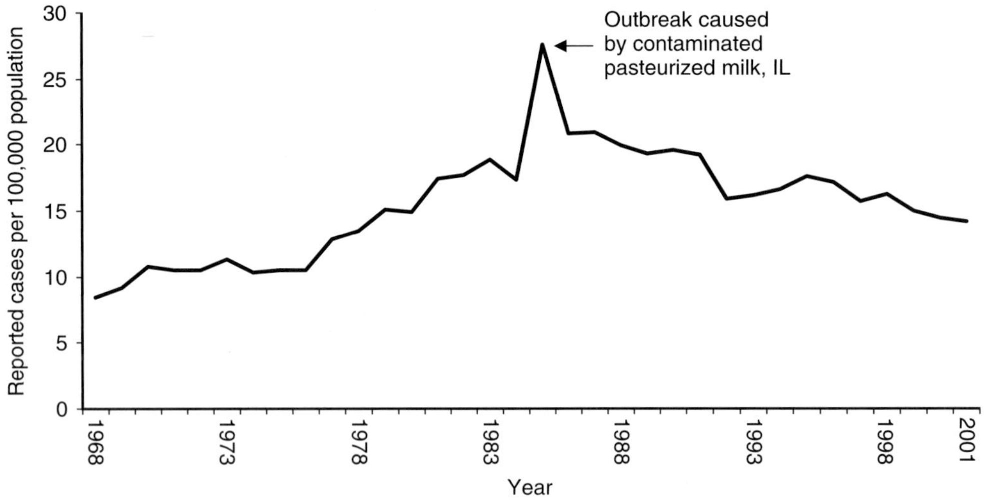

FIGURE 18-1 Incidence rate per 100,000 population of laboratory-confirmed *Salmonella, Campylobacter, Shigella,* and *E. coli* O157:H7 infections by selected sites in the United States, Foodborne Diseases Active Surveillance Network, 2002. (From Centers for Disease Control and Prevention. Preliminary FoodNet Data on the Incidence of Foodborne Illnesses—Selected Sites, United States, 2002. MMWR 52:340–343, 2003.)

Food of animal origin, including meat, poultry, eggs, and dairy products, can become contaminated with *Salmonella.*[13] Eating uncooked or inadequately cooked foods cross-contaminated with these products may lead to human infection. In the developed world, acquisition of nontyphoidal salmonellosis most often is associated with consumption of poultry and eggs,[13,14] but a wide range of food vehicles have been implicated in transmission to humans.[13,15] Although foodborne outbreaks predominate, waterborne outbreaks of salmonellosis also have been reported.[16] Salmonellosis associated with exotic pets is a resurgent public health problem, with an estimated 3% to 5% of all cases of salmonellosis in humans associated with exposure to exotic pets, especially reptiles.[15]

Antimicrobial Resistance

Antimicrobial resistance among human nontyphoidal *Salmonella* isolates is increasing worldwide and is likely due, in part, to the widespread use of antimicrobial agents for the empirical treatment of febrile syndromes and as growth promoters in animal production.[17,18] High rates of resistance (>50% to 100%) to chloramphenicol, trimethoprim-sulfamethoxazole, and ampicillin have been reported from Africa, Asia, and South America. Multidrug-resistant nontyphoidal *Salmonella* has now emerged in developed countries, including the United States (Table 18-2 and Fig. 18-3).[19] Individuals with resistant *Salmonella* isolates are more likely than those with susceptible ones to have been treated with an antimicrobial agent recently, to have systemic infections, to be hospitalized, and to die of their infection.[19,20]

Of particular concern is the worldwide emergence of a distinct strain of multidrug-resistant *S. typhimurium,* characterized as definitive phage type 104 (DT104), that is resistant to at least five antimicrobials—ampicillin, chloramphenicol, streptomycin, sulfonamides, and tetracyclines.[21] The DT104 strain has broad host reservoirs and is difficult to control in domestic livestock, leading to its widespread clonal dissemination among food animals, especially cattle, and humans in Europe,

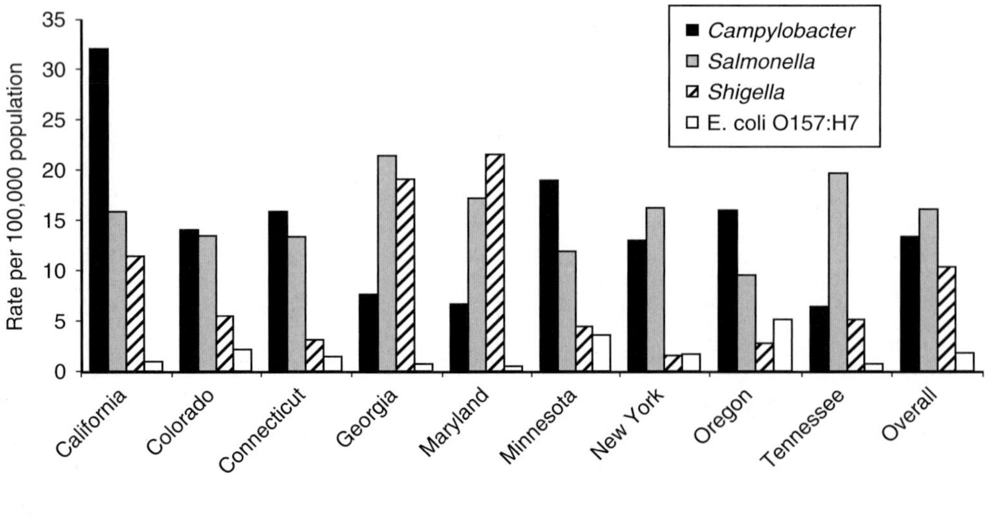

FIGURE 18-2 Incidence rate per 100,000 population of nontyphoidal salmonellosis by year, United States, 1968–2001. (From Centers for Disease Control and Prevention. Summary of Notifiable Diseases, United States, 2001. MMWR 50:96, 2003.)

Table 18-2 Antimicrobial Resistance of Salmonella *Isolates, United States, 2000*

	***Salmonella* Typhi (N=177)**	***Salmonella* Non-Typhi (N=1378)**
	N (% Resistant)	**N (% Resistant)**
Amikacin	2 (1.1)	0 (0)
Amoxicillin–clavulanic acid	0 (0)	54 (4)
Ampicillin	16 (9)	219 (16)
Cefoxitin	3 (1.7)	43 (3)
Ceftriaxone	0 (0)	18 (1.3)
Cephalothin	2 (1.1)	54 (4)
Chloramphenicol	19 (11)	138 (10)
Ciprofloxacin	0 (0)	5 (0.4)
Gentamicin	1 (0.6)	37 (3)
Nalidixic acid	41 (23)	34 (2)
Streptomycin	18 (11)	223 (16)
Sulfamethoxazole	21 (12)	235 (17)
Tetracycline	19 (11)	256 (19)
Trimethoprim-sulfamethoxazole	16 (9)	29 (2)

Adapted from Centers for Disease Control and Prevention. NARMS 2000 Annual Report. Available at http://www.cdc.gov/narms/annuals.htm.

the United States, Canada, and the Middle and Far East.[21–24] Although no more virulent than susceptible *S. typhimurium* strains, infection with DT104 may be associated with greater morbidity and mortality, likely reflecting inadequate empirical antimicrobial therapy.[25]

Outbreaks and sporadic cases of nontyphoidal *Salmonella* resistant to third-generation cephalosporins have been reported in both developed and developing countries.[26] Resistance to third-generation cephalosporins is conferred by conjugative plasmid-encoded β-lactamases from functional groups 1 (AmpC) and 2 (TEM).[26,27] Recent surveys in the United States found that 5.1% of *Salmonella* isolates from cattle and pigs and 1.6% of isolates from humans were ceftriaxone resistant (MIC ≧16 μg/mL).[28] Quinolone-resistant *Salmonella* strains have emerged among human and animals, and resistance is due to mutations of the intracellular targets DNA gyrase (*gyrA* or *gyrB*) or topoisomerase IV, or to overproduction of efflux pumps.[29–31] Emergence of quinolone resistance among human *Salmonella* isolates clearly is linked with the use of fluoroquinolones as growth promoters in food animals.[18,32]

Salmonella enteritidis

S. enteritidis associated with shell eggs emerged in the 1980s as the predominant *Salmonella* serotype and source of foodborne disease in the United States and some other countries.[14,33] Infection of egg-laying and broiler poultry flocks with *S. enteritidis* is widespread, although the mechanism of transmission from farm to farm is not known. Infection localizes to the ovaries and upper oviduct tissue and is transmitted to the forming egg before shell deposition.[34] An estimated 2.3 million of 69 billion shell eggs produced annually in the United States contain *S. enteritidis*.[35] Outbreaks of *S. enteritidis* infection have been associated with ingestion of uncooked or lightly cooked eggs (e.g., sunny side up), egg-containing food products, and inadequately cooked poultry.[14,36] Although cooking of eggs until all liquid yolk is solidified kills *S. enteritidis*, the use of pasteurized egg products remains the safest alternative for institutions and the general public.

International Spread of Salmonellosis

Changes in food consumption and the rapid growth of international trade in agricultural food products have facilitated the dissemination of new *Salmonella* serotypes associated with fresh fruits and vegetables.[37] Human or animal feces may contaminate the surface of fruits and vegetables and may not be removed by washing. Recent foodborne outbreaks of salmonellosis associated with fresh produce include cantaloupe, tomatoes, unpasteurized orange juice, cilantro, and raw seed sprouts. Soaking seeds in sodium hypochlorite can reduce, but does not eliminate, the risk of sprout-associated illness, and thus immunocompromised persons should not eat sprouts.[38] Manufactured food items also pose an enormous potential hazard of foodborne salmonellosis in developed countries because of their centralized production and wide-scale distribution. Recent outbreaks associated with manufactured food products include ice cream (United States, *S. enteritidis*), pasteurized milk (United States, *S. typhimurium*), powdered milk products and infant formula (Canada and United States, *S. tennessee*), unpasteurized goat milk cheese (France, *S. paratyphi*), and ready-to-eat snacks.

Transmission in Hospitals and Other Care Facilities

Although health care–associated salmonellosis is infrequent, such infections have been associated with substantial morbidity and mortality.[39] Although nosocomial transmission of *Salmonella* from patients to health-care workers has been associated with handling soiled linen, noncompliance with barrier precautions, and fecally incontinent residents,[40] the risk of transmission from health-care workers to patients appears to be low if infection control measures are observed carefully.[41] In contrast, the risk of nosocomial fecal-oral transmission to neonates and infants from acutely or chronically infected family members is high, because of relative gastric achlorhydria and the buffering capacity of ingested breast milk and formula.[42] High-iron infant formulas may further increase the risk of infant salmonellosis compared with breast feeding.[43] Contaminated enteral feeding and crowding also have been associated with nosocomial transmission among pediatric patients.[44] Control of outbreaks in day care centers may be difficult because of the need for frequent diaper changing and the higher rate and longer duration of convalescent carriage in the preschool age group.[45]

The elderly are at increased risk for *Salmonella* bacteremia and extraintestinal infection due to debility, underlying illnesses, and waning immunity. Residents of long-term care facilities may be at particular risk of salmonellosis because many of these institutions have only limited infection control programs.[46] From 1975 through 1987, nontyphoidal *Salmonella* was the most common cause of foodborne outbreaks reported from long-term care facilities in the United States, accounting for 52% of outbreaks and 81% of outbreak-associated deaths.[46]

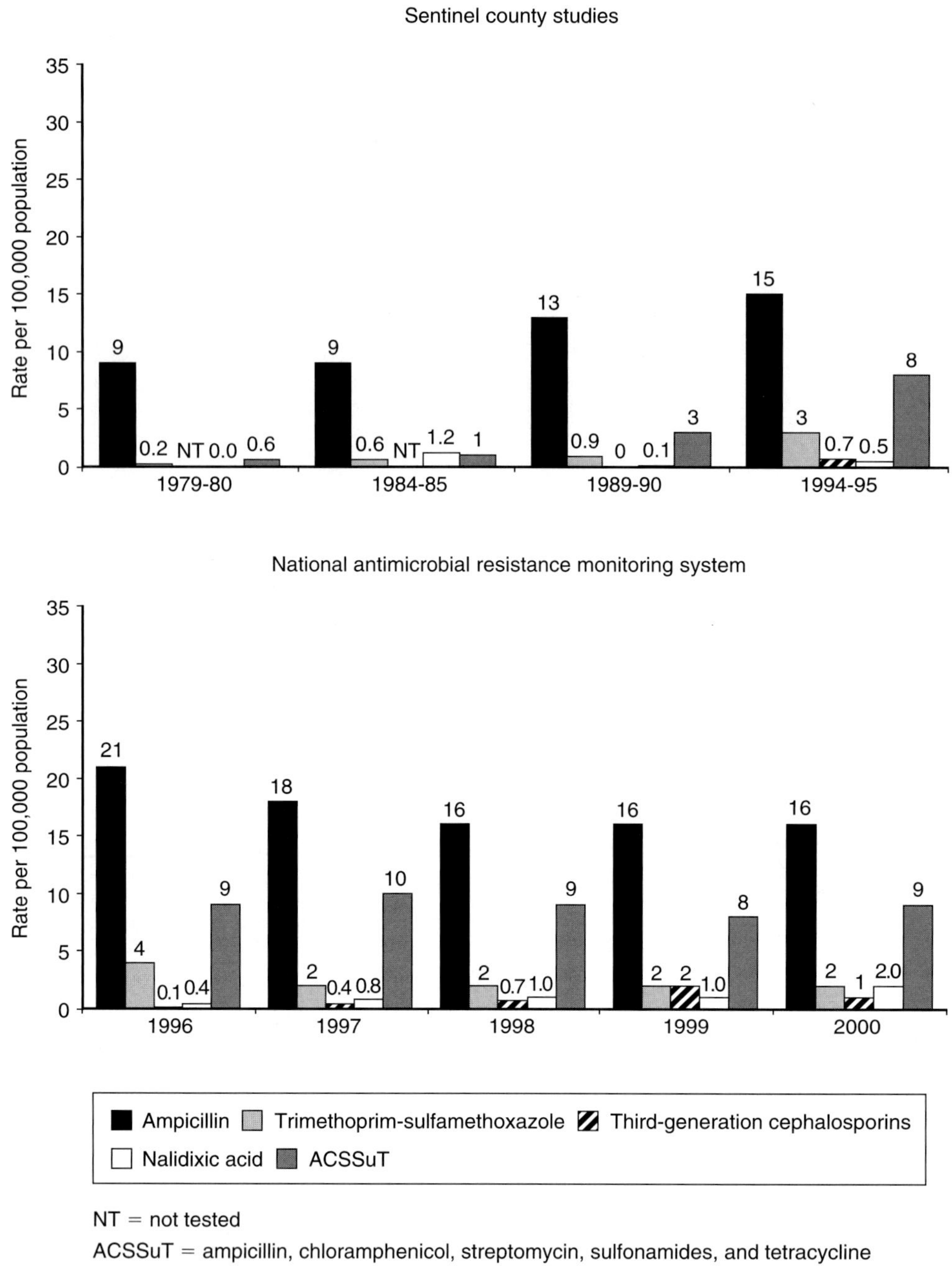

FIGURE 18-3 Summary of long-term trends in antimicrobial resistance in non-typhi *Salmonella* isolates, United States, 1979–2000. (From Centers for Disease Control and Prevention. NARMS 2000 Annual Report. Available at http://www.cdc.gov/narms/annuals.htm.)

DISEASE

Clinical Manifestations

Gastroenteritis

Infection with nontyphoidal *Salmonella* most often results in self-limited acute gastroenteritis that is indistinguishable from that due to many other enteric bacterial pathogens. Within 6 to 48 hours after ingestion of contaminated food or water, nausea, vomiting, and diarrhea occur.[47] In most cases, stools are loose, of moderate volume, and without blood. In rare cases, stool may be watery and of large volume ("cholera-like") or of small volume associated with tenesmus ("dysentery-like"). Fevers (38°C to 39°C), abdominal cramping, nausea, vomiting, and chills frequently are reported. Headache, myalgias, and other systemic symptoms also can occur. Microscopic examination of stools shows neutrophils and, less frequently, red blood cells. Infrequently, *Salmonella* can cause a syndrome of pseudoappendicitis or can mimic the intestinal changes of inflammatory bowel disease.[47] Toxic megacolon is a rare but potentially life-threatening complication.[48]

Diarrhea is usually self-limited, typically lasting for 3 to 7 days.[47] Diarrhea that persists for more than 10 days should suggest another diagnosis. If fever is present, it usually resolves within 48 to 72 hours. Occasionally, patients require hospitalization for dehydration, and death occurs infrequently. In the United States, nontyphoidal *Salmonella* infections result in an estimated rate of hospitalization of 2.2 per 1 million population and 582 deaths per year.[8] A disproportionate number of these deaths occur among the elderly, especially those residing in long-term care facilities, and among immunocompromised patients.[14,46,49,50]

After resolution of gastroenteritis, the mean duration of carriage of nontyphoidal *Salmonella* in the stool is 4 to 5 weeks and varies by *Salmonella* serotype.[45] Antimicrobial therapy may increase the duration of carriage.[45] In addition, a higher proportion of neonates have prolonged carriage; in one study, 50% of neonates were still excreting *Salmonella* at 6 months.[51] However, the delayed clearance of infection in neonates does not result in permanent carriage, as almost all chronic carriers are adults.[45,51]

Bacteremia

Classically, *S. choleraesuis* and *S. dublin* produce a syndrome of sustained bacteremia with fever, but any *Salmonella* serotype can cause bacteremia.[47] From 1% to 4% of immunocompetent individuals with *Salmonella* gastroenteritis have positive blood cultures.[45] The proportion is greater for infants, the elderly, and the immunocompromised, including those with acquired immunodeficiency syndrome (AIDS).[50,52–56] *Salmonella* has a propensity for infection of vascular sites, and high-grade or persistent bacteremia suggests an endovascular infection.[57] The risk of endovascular infection complicating *Salmonella* bacteremia is estimated to be 10% to 25% in persons over 50 years of age, usually involves the aorta, and most commonly results from seeding atherosclerotic plaques or aneurysms.[58,59] Mortality rates range from 14% to 60% and are lower with prompt diagnosis and combined medical and surgical therapy.[60,61]

Salmonellosis and HIV Infection

HIV-infected individuals have up to a 20- to 100-fold increased risk of salmonellosis compared with the general population.[50] *Salmonella* is more likely to cause severe invasive disease in persons with AIDS compared with infection in immunocompetent persons and those with AIDS-related complex or asymptomatic HIV infection, including fulminant diarrhea, acute enterocolitis, rectal ulceration, recurrent bacteremia, meningitis, and death despite antimicrobial therapy.[62,63] In studies among HIV-infected persons in Africa, *Salmonella* species were one of the most frequent cause of bacteremia, were often multidrug resistant, and were associated with high mortality (24% to 80%) and recurrence rates (43%).[64,65] Focal infections due to nontyphoidal *Salmonella* are infrequent among HIV-infected individuals, most often occurring among those with CD4 counts below 100/mm^3.[63]

Recurrent nontyphoidal *Salmonella* bacteremia is an AIDS-defining illness that apparently results from incomplete clearance of the primary infection owing to impaired cell-mediated immunity. Without maintenance antimicrobial therapy, up to 45% of individuals with HIV infection will have recurrent bacteremia.[62] Among those with HIV, the incidence of recurrent nontyphoidal *Salmonella* bacteremia has declined, likely owing to the direct bactericidal activity of antiretrovirals on *Salmonella* species, the impact of HAART on immune reconstitution, and the use of trimethoprim-sulfamethoxazole for the prevention of *Pneumocystis* pneumonia.[62,66,67]

Localized Infections

Localized infections develop in approximately 5% to 10% of persons with *Salmonella* bacteremia, and the presentation may be delayed.[68] Extraintestinal complications of salmonellosis and their management are summarized in Table 18-3.

Chronic Carrier State

The chronic carrier state is defined as the persistence of *Salmonella* in stool or urine for periods longer than 1 year. From 0.2% to 0.6% of patients with nontyphoidal salmonellosis develop chronic carriage,[69] a lower frequency than that observed in *S. typhi* infection.[58,70,71] The frequency of chronic carriage is higher in women, in persons with biliary abnormalities or concurrent bladder infection with *Schistosoma haematobium*, and in infants.[55,72]

PATHOGENESIS AND IMMUNITY

Interactions with Gastrointestinal Tract and Induction of Enteritis

Salmonella infections begin with the ingestion of bacteria in contaminated food or water. Investigations of point source outbreaks suggest that as few as 10^3 bacteria may produce nontyphoidal gastroenteritis in many of those exposed and that the ingested dose is an important determinant of incubation period and disease severity.[73] Gastric acidity represents the initial barrier to *Salmonella* colonization, and conditions that increase gastric pH significantly increase susceptibility to infection.[74]

After passage to the small intestine, salmonellae must evade host antimicrobial factors secreted into the intestinal lumen, including antimicrobial peptides, bile salts, and secretory IgA, and traverse a protective mucous barrier before encountering intestinal epithelial cells.[75,76] Salmonellae express multiple fimbriae that contribute to tight adherence to intestinal epithelial cells in culture and are required for colonization in animal models.[77]

Microscopy reveals that salmonellae invade intestinal epithelial cells by a morphologically distinct process termed bacteria-mediated endocytosis (Fig. 18-4).[78,79] Shortly after bacteria adhere to the apical epithelial surface, profound cytoskeletal rearrangements occur in the host cell, disrupting the normal epithelial brush border and inducing formation of membrane ruffles that reach out and enclose adherent bacterial in large vesicles. This process resembles the membrane ruffling induced in many cell types by growth factors and is functionally distinct from receptor-mediated endocytosis, the mechanism by which many other pathogens enter nonphagocytic cells.[80] Following bacterial internalization, a fraction of *Salmonella*-containing vesicles transcytose to the basolateral membrane, and the apical epithelial brush border reconstitutes. The epithelial cell type that serves as the principal portal for *Salmonella* invasion is uncertain. In the mouse enteric fever model, salmonellae preferentially adhere to and enter the specialized microfold cells (M cells) that overlie lymphoid tissue within Peyer's patches.[81] In bovine and rabbit models of enteritis, however, salmonellae do not appear to interact preferentially with M cells but instead adhere to and invade intestinal enterocytes diffusely.[82] It is possible that M cells are the

Table 18-3 Extraintestinal Infectious Complications of Salmonellosis

Site	Incidence	Risk Factors	Manifestations	Complications	Mortality	Diagnosis	Treatment
Endocarditis[58,149]	0.2% to 0.4%	Preexisting valvular heart disease	Valvular vegetation, infected mural thrombus	Valve perforation, relapse (20% to 25%), pericarditis	~70%	Blood culture, echocardiography	Early valve surgery + 6 wk P ceph 3,* P amp,† P/PO quinolone‡
Arteritis[60,150,151]	Rare	Atherosclerosis, aortic aneurysm, endocarditis, prosthetic graft, myelodysplasia	Prolonged fever, pain in back, chest, or abdomen	Mycotic aneursym, aneurysm rupture, aortoenteric fistula, vertebral osteomyelitis	14% to 60%	Blood culture, CT or nuclear scan	Early surgical bypass + 6 wk P ceph 3, P amp,† P/PO quinolone
Central nervous system[152–154]	0.1% to 0.9%	Infants (especially neonates)	Meningitis, ventriculitis, brain abscess, subdural empyema, encephalopathy	Seizures, mental retardation, hydrocephalus, brain infarction, relapse	~20% to 60%	CSF culture, CT or MRI scan	≥3 wk P ceph 3, P amp,† carbapenem
Pulmonary[58,68]	Rare	Lung malignancy, structural lung disease, sickle cell anemia	Pneumonia	Lung abscess, empyema, bronchopleural fistula	~25% to 60%	Respiratory culture, chest radiograph	≥2 wk P/PO abx§
Bone[155,156]	<1%	Sickle cell anemia, male gender, connective tissue disease, immunosuppression	Femur, tibia, humerus, lumbar vertebrae	Relapse, chronic osteomyelitis	Very low	Bone radiograph	≥4 wk P ceph 3,* P amp,† P/PO quinolone‡ + surgery for sequestra
Joint—reactive[157,158]	0.6%	HLA-B27, antibiotic therapy	≥3 Joints involved (especially knee, ankle, wrist, and sacroiliac)	Prolonged symptoms (mean duration, 5.5 mo)	Negligible	Joint fluid examination and culture	Nonsteroidal anti-inflammatory agent
Joint—septic[159]	0.1% to 0.2%	Osteoarthritis, connective tissue disease, sickle cell disease, prosthetic joint	Knee, hip, shoulder	Joint destruction osteomyelitis	Very low	Joint fluid examination and culture	Repeated needle aspiration + ≥4 wk P/PO abx

Muscle/soft tissue[160]	Rare	Local trauma, male gender, diabetes, HIV infection	Abscess, pyomyositis	Osteomyelitis, endovascular infection, frequent relapse	~33%	Ultrasonography, aspiration	Drainage + ≥2 wk P abx
Hepatobiliary[161]	Rare	Cholelithiasis, cirrhosis, amebic abscess, echinococcal cyst, hepatocellular carcinoma	Hepatomegaly, cholecystitis, hepatic abscess	Rupture with secondary peritonitis, subphrenic abscess, spontaneous bacterial peritonitis	~10%	Ultrasonography, aspiration	Drainage + ≥2 wk P abx
Splenic	Rare	Sickle cell anemia, splenic cyst, splenic hematoma	Splenomegaly	Left-sided empyema, subphrenic abscess, rupture with secondary peritonitis	<10%	Ultrasonography, aspiration	≥2 wk P abx, ± percutaneous drainage or splenectomy
Urinary[53,162]	0.6%	Urolithiasis, malignancy, renal transplantation	Cystitis, pyelonephritis	Renal abscess, interstitial nephritis, relapse	~20%	Urine culture, ultrasonography	Removal of structural abnormality + 1 to 2 wk P abx + ≥6 wk PO quinolone or TMP-SMX
Genital[58]	Rare	Pregnancy, renal transplantation	Ovarian abscess, testicular abscess, prostatitis, epididymitis	Abscess	Very low	Ultrasonography, aspiration	Drainage of collection + 1 to 2 wk P abx + ≥6 wk PO quinolone or TMP-SMX
Soft tissue[163]	<1%	Local trauma immunosuppression	Pustular dermatitis, subcutaneous abscess, wound infection	Septic thrombophlebitis, endophthalmitis	~15%	Drainage culture	≥2 wk P abx + drainage of collection

CSF, cerebrospinal fluid; CT, computerized tomography; MRI, magnetic resonance imaging; TMP-SMX, trimethoprim-sulfamethoxazole.
*Pceph 3, parenteral third generation cephalosporin.
†Pamp, parenteral ampicillin.
‡P/PO FQ, parenteral or oral fluoroquinolone.
§P/PO, parenteral or oral antimicrobial (e.g., quinolone, ampicillin, TMP-SMX, chloramphenicol or third-generation cephalosporin).

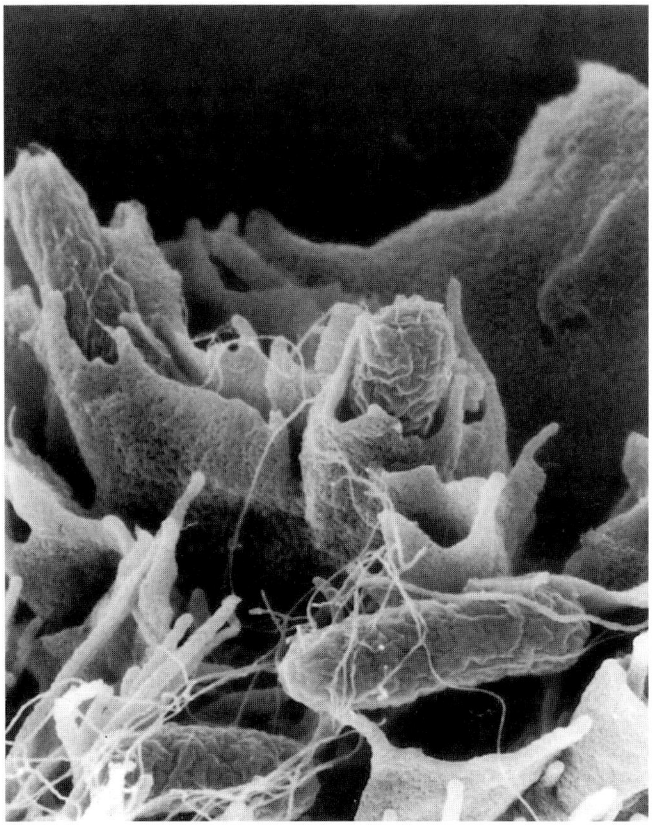

FIGURE 18-4 Scanning electron micrograph showing *Salmonella typhimurium* entering a Hep-2 cell through bacteria-mediated endocytosis. Membrane ruffles extend from the cell surface, enclosing and internalizing adherent bacteria. (Reprinted with permission from Ohl ME, Miller SI: Salmonella: A model for bacterial pathogenesis. Annu Rev Med 52:259–274, 2001. ©2001 by Annual Reviews. www.annualreviews.org.)

principal portal of entry in the enteric fever syndrome and that generalized invasion of enterocytes plays a greater role in the enteritis induced by nontyphoidal *Salmonella* serotypes.

Salmonellae encode a type III secretion system (TTSS) within pathogenicity island 1 (the SPI-1 TTSS) that is required for bacteria-mediated endocytosis and intestinal epithelial invasion. Type III secretion systems are complex macromolecular machines that have evolved to subvert host cell function through the translocation of virulence proteins directly from the bacterial cytoplasm into the host cell. Two SPI-1 translocated proteins, SipC and SipA, promote membrane ruffling and *Salmonella* invasion through direct interactions with the actin cytoskeleton. The SipC protein inserts into the host cell plasma membrane and directly nucleates actin polymerization at the site of *Salmonella* attachment.[83] The SipA protein further enhances actin polymerization through stabilization of actin filaments and reduction of the critical concentration for polymerization.[84] Additional SPI-1 translocated proteins contribute to *Salmonella* invasion by targeting members of the Rho family of monomeric GTP-binding proteins (G proteins). Rho family members, including cdc42, rac, and rho, regulate the structure and dynamics of the actin cytoskeleton and are required for formation of the membrane ruffles that mediate *Salmonella* internalization. The SPI-1 translocated proteins SopE and SopE2 directly activate rac1 and cdc42 in vitro by acting as GDP/GTP exchange factors (GEFs) and induce membrane ruffling following microinjection into epithelial cells.[85,86] SopB is an additional SPI-1 translocated protein that acts as an inositol polyphosphatase within the host cell.[87] Among other effects, this activity indirectly stimulates Rho GTPases and promotes membrane ruffling.[88] Overall, available data indicate that SipA and SipC act in concert with downstream cellular effectors of activated Rho GTPases to initiate and spatially direct the actin rearrangements that lead to *Salmonella* internalization.

In addition to invasion of intestinal epithelial cells, *Salmonella* serotypes clinically associated with gastroenteritis induce a secretory response in intestinal epithelium and initiate recruitment and transmigration of neutrophils into the intestinal lumen.[89] The SPI-1 TTSS is also required for these responses in tissue culture and animal models of enteritis. Stimulation of Rho GTPase signaling by SopE and SopE2 also leads to activation of MAP kinase pathways and synthesis of proinflammatory cytokines, including the neutrophil chemoattractant IL-8.[86,90] In addition to its role in invasion, the inositol polyphosphatase activity of SopB leads to accumulation of D-*myo*-inositol-1,4,5,6 tetrakisphosphate in epithelial cells.[91] The increased concentration of this compound ultimately leads to an increase in cellular basal chloride secretion, with associated fluid flux. The SPI-1 translocated proteins SopA and SopD also contribute to intestinal secretory and inflammatory responses in ligated ileal loops, but the molecular basis of these effects remains unclear.[89,92]

Following *Salmonella* invasion, intestinal inflammation may result from activation of the innate immune system through stimulation of proinflammatory receptors present on phagocytes and the basolateral surface of intestinal epithelia. This includes activation of Toll-like receptor 4 (Tlr4) by LPS and Tlr5 by bacterial flagellin.[93,94] Intestinal inflammation probably contributes to fluid secretion and diarrhea through disruption of the epithelial barrier and increased water flux by an exudative mechanism.

Salmonellae also utilize the SPI-1 TTSS to deliver proteins that down-regulate the host inflammatory response associated with *Salmonella* invasion. The SptP protein inactivates Rho GTPase signaling by acting as a GTPase-activating protein (Rho GAP).[95] This directly opposes the activity of SopE and SopE2 and reduces membrane ruffling and proinflammatory signaling following bacterial invasion. In addition, the SspH1 and AvrA proteins inhibit NF-kB activation and related host cell cytokine synthesis.[96,97] These SPI-1 translocated proteins may promote bacterial persistence in the host by maintaining host cell integrity and allowing evasion of the host immune response. The presence of SPI-1 translocated proteins with opposing molecular actions (e.g., SopE and SptP) suggests temporal ordering of protein function, with initial activity of SPI-1 proteins associated with invasion and proinflammatory signaling and subsequent activity of anti-inflammatory proteins.

Interactions with Macrophages and Systemic Infection

Salmonellae are facultative intracellular pathogens, and available data from both animal models of infection and humans with enteric fever suggest that bacterial replication within macrophages is essential for production of systemic disease.

The role of intracellular bacterial replication in human gastroenteritis due to nontyphoidal serotypes is less clear, but it is likely that the ability of salmonellae to resist killing by macrophages contributes to the cases of bacteremia and systemic infection occasionally associated with nontyphoidal *Salmonella* infection in humans.

Multiple *Salmonella* regulatory proteins are required for bacterial adaptation to the intracellular environment and replication within macrophages. The PhoP/PhoQ two-component regulatory system senses the intracellular environment and induces transcription of more than 40 *Salmonella* genes required for survival within macrophages.[98] Activation of the PhoP/PhoQ regulon leads to widespread modifications in the protein and lipopolysaccharide components of the bacterial inner and outer membranes.[99,100] These surface modifications confer resistance to antimicrobial factors within the phagosome, including antimicrobial peptides. PhoP/PhoQ regulated lipopolysaccharide modifications include addition of aminoarabinose, ethanolamine, palmitate, and 2-hydroxymryistate to lipid A, thus altering the charge density and fluidity of the outer membrane and discouraging antimicrobial peptide insertion in the membrane.[100,101] In addition, PhoP/PhoQ-regulated modifications in lipid A structure produce a lipopolysaccharide molecule with significantly less proinflammatory signaling activity, which may facilitate bacterial survival within host tissues.[100]

Salmonellae express several enzymes that inactivate microbicidal reactive oxygen and nitrogen species produced within the macrophage. Resistance to nitric oxide (NO) and related reactive nitrogen compounds results in part from bacterial synthesis of homocysteine, an NO antagonist.[102] *Salmonella* mutants unable to synthesize homocysteine due to inactivation of the *metL* gene are hypersensitive to NO and are less virulent. In addition, salmonellae produce at least one superoxide dismutase that inactivates reactive oxygen species.[103]

Recently three laboratories have described a second *Salmonella* type III secretion system that is necessary for survival in the macrophage and establishment of systemic infection.[104–106] Encoded in *Salmonella* pathogenicity island 2 (SPI-2), this system is expressed by intracellular bacteria and translocates proteins across the membrane of the *Salmonella*-containing vacuole (SCV) into the macrophage cytosol.[107] SPI-2 translocated proteins appear to prevent the maturation of the SCV into a mature phagolysosome, thus creating an intracellular compartment favorable for bacterial replication. Several SPI-2 translocated proteins, including SifA, SifB, SseJ, SopD2, PipB, and PipB2 localize to the surface of the SCV and may alter its fusion with other membranous compartments within the macrophage.[108–112] Two additional SPI-2 translocated proteins, SspH2 and SseI, interact with the actin cytoskeleton surrounding the SCV and probably contribute to remodeling of vacuole-associated actin networks.[107] Recent studies indicate that SPI-2 mediated modifications in the SCV lead to exclusion of the NADPH oxidase and inducible nitric oxide synthase from the vacuolar membrane, allowing the bacterium to evade the reactive oxygen and nitrogen species produced by these enzymes.[113,114]

SpvB is a *Salmonella* virulence protein that is secreted into the macrophage cytoplasm, possibly by the SPI-2 TTSS, and ADP-ribosylates monomeric actin (G-actin), thus promoting disassembly of actin networks around the vacuole.[107,115] SpvB promotes bacterial dissemination beyond the intestine in animals and bacteremia in humans.[116] Other bacterial factors, including incompletely characterized cytotoxin genes and genes required for synthesis of essential nutrients and iron acquisition, also are important in systemic pathogenesis.[117–119]

Host Response and Immunity

The innate immune system senses invasive *Salmonella* infections using Toll-like receptors that recognize conserved elements of bacterial structure, including recognition of LPS by Tlr4, bacterial lipoproteins by Toll-like receptor 2 (Tlr2), and flagellin by Tlr5.[94] Activation of these receptors on phagocytes and epithelia leads to synthesis of cytokines that orchestrate the acute inflammatory response and instruct the subsequent antigen-specific immune response. Mice lacking a functional Tlr4 response are highly susceptible to *Salmonella* infection, confirming the importance of this initial response to infection.[120] Studies in mice demonstrate that the initial control of *S. typhimurium* replication in host tissue requires recruitment and activation of macrophages.[121] In both mice and humans, macrophage activation and efficient killing of *Salmonella* is associated with production of IFN-γ, Il-12, and TNF-1.[122–124] Mice with targeted disruptions in these genes are highly susceptible to infection. In addition, humans with mutations in the IFN-γ and Il-12 receptor genes develop severe infections with nontyphoidal *Salmonella* serotypes.[125,126]

Although the innate immune system is able to suppress initial *Salmonella* replication, final clearance of infection and immunity to rechallenge requires a Th1-type CD4 T-cell response and production of specific antibodies by B cells.[124] This is supported by the observation that mice lacking mature CD4 cells (H2I;AB-/- mice) or B cells (lgh-6-/- mice) are unable to control *Salmonella* infection.[124,127,128] The importance of cellular immunity in controlling *Salmonella* infection in humans is demonstrated by the extreme susceptibility of individuals with HIV infection, lymphoproliferative diseases, or immune suppression following transplantation.[50,52,53,62,129]

DIAGNOSIS

Isolation and Identification

Freshly passed stool is preferred for the isolation of *Salmonella.* Stool is plated directly onto agar plates. Low-selective media, such as MacConkey agar and deoxycholate agar, and intermediate-selective media, such as *Salmonella-Shigella*, xylose-lysine-deoxycholate, or Hektoen agar, are widely used to screen for both *Salmonella* and *Shigella* species. New selective chromogenic media, such as CHROMagar and COMPASS agar, are more specific than other selective media, reduce the need for confirmatory testing and time to identification, and increasingly are used for the primary isolation and presumptive identification of *Salmonella* from clinical stool specimens.[130]

In addition to plating stool onto primary media, tetrathionate- and selenite-based enrichment broths are often used to facilitate the recovery of low numbers of organisms.[130] Highly *Salmonella*-selective media, such as selenite with brilliant green, should be reserved for use in stool cultures of suspected carriers and for outbreaks. Bismuth sulfite agar, which contains an indicator of hydrogen sulfite production and does not contain lactose, can be used for the detection of the 1% of Salmonella strains (including most *Salmonella* serogroup C strains) that ferment lactose.[131]

After primary isolation, possible *Salmonella* isolates can be tested in commercial identification systems or inoculated into screening media such as triple sugar iron and lysine iron agar. Rapid, IgM antibody-based serologic tests have been developed and may supplement stool culture for the diagnosis of acute *Salmonella* infection.[132] Isolates with typical biochemical profiles for *Salmonella* should be serogrouped with commercially available polyvalent antisera or sent to a reference or public health laboratory for complete serogrouping.

Molecular Typing

Subtyping methods frequently are used for epidemiologic purposes to differentiate strains of common *Salmonella* serotypes. Phenotyping methods may be useful for characterizing outbreak-associated strains and sporadic multidrug-resistant isolates, and include bacteriophage typing, plasmid profile analysis, antimicrobial susceptibility, and biotyping. More discriminative genotyping techniques, including ribotyping, pulsed-field gel electrophoresis, insertion sequences analysis, PCR-based fingerprinting, and multilocus sequence typing, have been used in epidemiologic studies to differentiate strains within a given serotype. Genomic DNA analysis using microarrays may complement the other genotyping methods.[133] However, lack of standardization and time requirement limit the widespread use of these genotyping techniques.

TREATMENT

Gastroenteritis

Salmonella gastroenteritis is usually a self-limited disease, and therapy primarily should be directed to the replacement of fluid and electrolyte losses. In a large meta-analysis, antimicrobial therapy for uncomplicated nontyphoidal *Salmonella* gastroenteritis, including short-course or single-dose regimens with oral fluoroquinolones, amoxicillin, or trimethoprim-sulfamethoxazole, did not significantly decrease the length of illness, including duration of fever or diarrhea, and was associated with an increased risk of relapse, positive culture after 3 weeks, and adverse drug reactions.[134] Therefore, antimicrobials should not be used routinely to treat uncomplicated nontyphoidal *Salmonella* gastroenteritis or to reduce convalescent stool excretion.

Although less than 5% of all patients with *Salmonella* gastroenteritis develop bacteremia, certain individuals are at increased risk for invasive infection and may benefit from preemptive antimicrobial therapy. Antimicrobial therapy should be considered for neonates, persons older than 50 years, and those with immunosuppression or cardiac valvular or endovascular abnormalities, including prosthetic vascular grafts. Treatment consists of an oral or intravenous antimicrobial administered for 48 to 72 hours or until the patient becomes afebrile. Longer treatment may result in a higher rate of chronic carriage and relapse. For susceptible organisms, treatment with an oral fluoroquinolone, trimethoprim-sulfamethoxazole, or amoxicillin is adequate. Occasionally, antimicrobial prophylaxis has been required to control institutional outbreaks, particularly in long-term care facilities and pediatrics wards, where compliance with infection control measures may be difficult.[135]

Although fluoroquinolones are not recommended for administration to children less than 10 years of age, they may have a role in treating severe nontyphoidal salmonellosis in this age group. In a small study, seven children with severe typhoidal or nontyphoidal salmonellosis who did not improve on conventional therapy improved rapidly when treated with oral perfloxacin (12 mg/kg daily for 7 days).[136] In addition, a double-blind placebo-controlled trial in Turkey demonstrated that intravenous immunoglobulin (500 mg/kg on days 1, 2, 3, and 8) in combination with cefoperazone when administered to preterm neonates with *S. typhimurium* infection reduced the rate of mortality, complications, and duration of antimicrobial therapy compared with treatment with cefoperazone alone, a finding that merits further study.[137]

Bacteremia

Because of the increasing prevalence of antimicrobial resistance, empirical therapy for life-threatening bacteremia or focal infection suspected to be caused by nontyphoidal *Salmonella* should include a third-generation cephalosporin and a fluoroquinolone until susceptibilities are known. It is also important to document whether the bacteremia is high grade (i.e., >50% of three or more blood cultures are positive) and, if so, to search for endovascular abnormalities by echocardiogram or other imaging techniques, such as CT or indium-labeled WBC scan. Low-grade bacteremia not involving vascular structures should be treated with intravenous antimicrobial therapy for 7 to 14 days. Six weeks of intravenous therapy with a β-lactam antibiotic, such as ampicillin or ceftriaxone, is recommended to treat documented or suspected endovascular infection. Intravenous ciprofloxacin followed by prolonged oral therapy may be an option, but published clinical experience is limited.[61] Chloramphenicol should not be used to treat endovascular infection because of high failure rates.[57,138] In addition, early surgical resection of infected aneurysms or other infected endovascular sites is recommended.[60,61] Patients with infected prosthetic vascular grafts that could not be resected have been maintained successfully on chronic suppressive oral therapy.[139]

Recurrent *Salmonella* Bacteremia in Individuals with AIDS

In persons with AIDS and a first episode of *Salmonella* bacteremia, 1 to 2 weeks of intravenous antimicrobial therapy followed by 4 weeks of oral fluoroquinolone therapy (e.g., ciprofloxacin 500 to 750 mg twice daily) should be administered to attempt eradication of the organism and to decrease the risk of recurrent bacteremia.[140] Persons who relapse following 6 weeks of antimicrobial therapy should receive long-term suppressive therapy with an oral fluoroquinolone or trimethoprim-sulfamethoxazole. Fluoroquinolones and zidovudine have a synergistic antibacterial effect against *Salmonella*; administration of both drugs may dramatically decrease the risk of recurrent infection.[141] Although data are lacking, trimethoprim-sulfamethoxazole may be a good choice for long-term suppressive therapy of salmonellosis if the organism is susceptible because of its efficacy in prevention of other opportunistic infections, including *Pneumocystis* pneumonia.

Chronic Carrier State

Chronic carriage of nontyphoidal *Salmonella* is managed similarly to typhoid carriage. Amoxicillin (3 g for adults or 100 mg/kg for children divided three times a day for 3 months), trimethoprim-sulfamethoxazole (one double-strength tablet twice a day for 3 months), and ciprofloxacin (750 mg twice daily for 4 weeks) are effective in eradication of chronic carriage associated with susceptible strains, with cure rates of more than 80%.[142,143] The high concentration of amoxicillin and fluoroquinolones in bile and the superior intracellular penetration of fluoroquinolones are theoretical advantages over trimethoprim-sulfamethoxazole. Cost considerations favor the use of amoxicillin for treating carriage of susceptible organisms. However, antimicrobial agents are infrequently effective in eradicating the carrier state if anatomic abnormalities, such as biliary or kidney stones, are present. In such cases, surgery combined with antimicrobial therapy often is required for eradication.[69] Chronic suppressive antimicrobial therapy should be considered for those patients with persistent carriage in whom no anatomic abnormality can be identified or who relapse after cholecystectomy.

PREVENTION AND CONTROL

The prevention and control of salmonellosis require both an understanding of the complex cycles of transmission and ongoing surveillance to characterize trends in *Salmonella* occurrence and to identify outbreaks. Control of foodborne salmonellosis requires barriers to the introduction and multiplication of *Salmonella* from the farm to the table.[144] Recognition of foodborne outbreaks requires that clinicians have a high index of suspicion, order the appropriate laboratory test, and promptly report positive culture results to local public health departments. Vaccination of feed animals, limiting the use of antimicrobials as growth promoters, and improved food safety practices should further reduce the burden of foodborne salmonellosis. The use of algorithms and rapid molecular subtyping have improved the ability to detect clusters and outbreaks of salmonellosis.[145] Establishment of cooperative international surveillance systems has facilitated rapid data exchange for the prevention of human salmonellosis associated with the widely distributed agricultural and manufactured foods.[146,147]

Although most cases of *Salmonella* infection occur sporadically, large numbers of persons potentially may become infected when commercial kitchens serve *Salmonella*-contaminated foods that have been insufficiently cooked or mishandled. Commercial food service establishments can reduce the risk of foodborne *Salmonella* illness by not serving food containing raw or undercooked eggs, by using pasteurized eggs whenever possible, and by avoiding cross-contamination of food items. Use of pasteurized eggs for all recipes calling for bulk pooled eggs is recommended for all long-term care facilities and hospitals.[46]

The most cost-effective approach to the control of salmonellosis in food handlers is attention to good personal hygiene and maintenance of time-temperature standards for food handling. Routine screening of food handlers for carriage after gastroenteritis is common before allowing individuals to return to work. However, there seems to be little justification for this approach, since few outbreaks are related to specific food handlers, prolonged carriage in food handlers after gastroenteritis is rare, and the number of organisms present is small. Therefore, it is reasonable to allow individuals to return to work after diarrhea is resolved. Two consecutive negative stool samples should be required only for food handlers whose work involves touching unwrapped foods that are consumed raw or served without further cooking. Routine surveillance of food handlers for asymptomatic stool carriage of *Salmonella* is not recommended.

To limit the risk of nosocomial transmission to patients and health-care workers, patients excreting *Salmonella* should be managed with Standard Precautions, including the use of barrier precautions, such as gloves, when performing direct patient care or handling soiled articles. Control of *Salmonella* outbreaks in long-term care facilities or neonatal care areas may be difficult because of poor compliance with isolation precautions and the increased susceptibility of these patients.[148] Although *Salmonella* infection in newborns, the elderly, or immunocompromised can be severe, the risk of transmission of *Salmonella* from health-care workers to patients appears to be very small.[41] Once health-care workers are asymptomatic and passing formed stool, they should be allowed to return to work if Standard Precautions are observed. However, local and state regulations should be followed, since some require work exclusion for health-care workers with salmonellosis until two or more stool cultures obtained at least 24 hours apart are negative.

REFERENCES

1. Committee on *Salmonella*: An Evaluation of the *Salmonella* Problem. Washington DC, National Academy of Science, 1969.
2. Farmer JJ: Enterobacteriaceae: Introduction and identification. In Murray PR, Baron EJ, Pfaller M, et al (eds): Manual of Clinical Microbiology, 7th ed. Washington, DC, American Society for Microbiology, 1999, pp. 442–458.
3. McClelland M, Sanderson KE, Spieth J, et al: Complete genome sequence of *Salmonella enterica* serovar *typhimurium* LT2. Nature 413:852–856, 2001.
4. Popoff MY, Bockemühl J, Brenner FW: Supplement 1998 (No. 42) to the Kauffmann-White scheme. Res Microbiol 151:63–65, 2000.
5. Brenner FW, Villar RG, Angulo FJ, et al: *Salmonella* nomenclature. J Clin Microbiol 38:2465–2467, 2000.
6. Boop CA, Brenner FW, Wells JG, et al: *Escherichia*, *Shigella*, and *Salmonella*. In: Murray PR, Baron EJ, Pfaller M, Tenover FC, Yolken RH (eds): Manual of Clinical Microbiology, 7th ed. Washington, DC, American Society for Microbiology, 1999, pp. 467–471.
7. Ackers ML, Puhr ND, Tauxe RV, et al: Laboratory-based surveillance of *Salmonella* serotype *typhi* infections in the United States: antimicrobial resistance on the rise. JAMA 283:2668–2673, 2000.
8. Mead PS, Slutsker L, Dietz V, et al: Food-related illness and death in the United States. Emerg Infect Dis 5:607–625, 1999.
9. Centers for Disease Control and Prevention: Preliminary FoodNet data on the incidence of foodborne illnesses—selected sites, United States, 2002. MMWR 52:340–343, 2003.
10. Centers for Disease Control and Prevention: Summary of Notifiable Diseases, United States, 2001. MMWR 50:96, 2003.
11. Gorbach SL, Kean BH, Evans DG, et al: Travelers' diarrhea and toxigenic *Escherichia coli*. N Engl J Med 292:933–936, 1975.
12. Saidi SM, Iijima Y, Sang WK, et al: Epidemiological study on infectious diarrheal diseases in children in a coastal rural area of Kenya. Microbiol Immunol 41:773–778, 1997.

13. Todd EC: Epidemiology of foodborne diseases: a worldwide review. World Health Stat Q 50:30–50, 1997.
14. Mishu B, Koehler J, Lee LA, et al: Outbreaks of *Salmonella enteritidis* infections in the United States, 1985–1991. J Infect Dis 169:547–552 1994.
15. Woodward DL, Khakhria R, Johnson WM: Human salmonellosis associated with exotic pets. J Clin Microbiol 35:2786–2790, 1997.
16. Angulo FJ, Tippen S, Sharp DJ, et al: A community waterborne outbreak of salmonellosis and the effectiveness of a boil water order. Am J Public Health 87:580–584, 1997.
17. Spika JS, Waterman SH, Hoo GW, et al: Chloramphenicol-resistant *Salmonella newport* traced through hamburger to dairy farms: a major persisting source of human salmonellosis in California. N Engl J Med 316:565–570, 1987.
18. Chiu CH, Wu TL, Su LH, et al: The emergence in Taiwan of fluoroquinolone resistance in Salmonella enterica serotype choleraesuis. N Engl J Med 346:413–419, 2002.
19. Lee LA, Puhr ND, Maloney EK, et al: Increase in antimicrobial-resistant *Salmonella* infections in the United States, 1989–1990. J Infect Dis 170:128–134, 1994.
20. Helms M, Vastrup P, Gerner-Smidt P, et al: Excess mortality associated with antimicrobial drug-resistant *Salmonella typhimurium*. Emerg Infect Dis 8:490–495, 2002.
21. Humphrey T: *Salmonella typhimurium* definitive type 104: a multiresistant *Salmonella*. Int J Food Microbiol 67:173–186, 2001.
22. Casin I, Breuil J, Brisabois A, et al: Multidrug-resistant human and animal *Salmonella typhimurium* isolates in France belong predominantly to a DT104 clone with the chromosome- and integron-encoded beta-lactamase PSE-1. J Infect Dis 179:1173–1182, 1999.
23. Glynn MK, Bopp C, Dewitt W, et al: Emergence of multidrug-resistant *Salmonella enterica* serotype *typhimurium* DT104 infections in the United States. N Engl J Med 338:1333–1338, 1998.
24. Beaudin BA, Brosnikoff CA, Grimsrud KM, et al: Susceptibility of human isolates of *Salmonella typhimurium* DT104 to antimicrobial agents used in human and veterinary medicine. Diagn Microbiol Infect Dis 42:17–20, 2002.
25. Allen CA, Fedorka-Cray PJ, Vazquez-Torres A, et al: In vitro and in vivo assessment of *Salmonella enterica* serovar *typhimurium* DT104 virulence. Infect Immun 69:4673–4677, 2001.
26. Barguellil F, Burucoa C, Amor A, et al: In vivo acquisition of extended-spectrum beta-lactamase in *Salmonella enteritidis* during antimicrobial therapy. Eur J Clin Microbiol Infect Dis 14:703–706, 1995.
27. Winokur PL, Vonstein DL, Hoffman LJ, et al: Evidence for transfer of CMY-2 AmpC beta-lactamase plasmids between *Escherichia coli* and *Salmonella* isolates from food animals and humans. Antimicrob Agents Chemother 45:2716–2722, 2001.
28. Centers for Disease Control and Prevention: NARMS 2000 Annual Report. Available at http://www.cdc.gov/narms/annuals.htm. Accessed 8/26/04.
29. Giraud E, Cloeckaert A, Kerboeuf D, et al: Evidence for active efflux as the primary mechanism of resistance to ciprofloxacin in *Salmonella enterica* serovar *typhimurium*. Antimicrob Agents Chemother 44:1223–1228, 2000.
30. Heisig P: High-level fluoroquinolone resistance in a *Salmonella typhimurium* isolate due to alterations in both gyrA and gyrB genes. J Antimicrob Chemother 32:367–377, 1993.
31. Randall LP, Cooles SW, Sayers AR, et al: Association between cyclohexane resistance in *Salmonella* of different serovars and increased resistance to multiple antibiotics, disinfectants and dyes. J Med Microbiol 50:919–924, 2001.
32. Threlfall EJ, Frost JA, Ward LR, et al: Increasing spectrum of resistance in multiresistant *Salmonella typhimurium*. Lancet 347:1053–1054, 1996.
33. Rodrigue DC, Tauxe RV, Rowe B: International increase in *Salmonella enteritidis*: a new pandemic? Epidemiol Infect 105:21–27, 1990.
34. Keller LH, Benson CE, Krotec K, et al: *Salmonella enteritidis* colonization of the reproductive tract and forming and freshly laid eggs of chickens. Infect Immun 63:2443–2449, 1995.
35. Hope BK, Baker R, Edel ED, et al: An overview of the *Salmonella enteritidis* risk assessment for shell eggs and egg products. Risk Anal 22:203–218, 2002.
36. Centers for Disease Control and Prevention: Outbreaks of *Salmonella* serotype enteritidis infection associated with eating raw or undercooked shell eggs—United States, 1996–1998. MMWR 49:73–79, 2000.
37. Altekruse SF, Cohen ML, Swerdlow DL: Emerging foodborne diseases. Emerg Infect Dis 3:285–293, 1997.
38. Brooks JT, Rowe SY, Shillam P, et al: *Salmonella typhimurium* infections transmitted by chlorine-pretreated clover sprout seeds. Am J Epidemiol 154:1020–1028, 2001.
39. Weikel CS, Guerrant RL: Nosocomial salmonellosis [editorial]. Infect Control 6:218–220, 1985.
40. Wall PG, Ryan MJ: Faecal incontinence in hospitals and residential and nursing homes for elderly people. BMJ 312:378, 1996.
41. Tauxe RV, Hassan LF, Findeisen KO, et al: Salmonellosis in nurses: lack of transmission to patients. J Infect Dis 157:370–373, 1988.
42. Wilson R, Feldman RA, Davis J, et al: Salmonellosis in infants: the importance of intrafamilial transmission. Pediatrics 69:436–438, 1982.
43. Haddock RL, Cousens SN, Guzman CC: Infant diet and salmonellosis. Am J Public Health 81:997–1000, 1991.
44. Bornemann R, Zerr DM, Heath J, et al: An outbreak of *Salmonella* serotype *saintpaul* in a children's hospital. Infect Control Hosp Epidemiol 23:671–676, 2002.
45. Buchwald DS, Blaser MJ: A review of human salmonellosis. 2. Duration of excretion following infection with nontyphi *Salmonella*. Rev Infect Dis 6:345–356, 1984.
46. Levine WC, Smart JF, Archer DL, et al: Foodborne disease outbreaks in nursing homes, 1975 through 1987. JAMA 266:2105–2109, 1991.
47. Saphra I, Winter JW: Clinical manifestations of salmonellosis in man: an evaluation of 7779 human infections identified at the New York Salmonella Center. N Engl J Med 256:1128, 1957.
48. Chaudhuri A, Bekdash BA: Toxic megacolon due to *Salmonella*: a case report and review of the literature. Int J Colorectal Dis 17:275–279, 2002.
49. Lim E, Koh WH, Loh SF, et al: Non-typhoidal salmonellosis in patients with systemic lupus erythematosus: a study of fifty patients and a review of the literature. Lupus 10:87–92, 2001.
50. Celum CL, Chaisson RE, Rutherford GW, et al: Incidence of salmonellosis in patients with AIDS. J Infect Dis 156:998–1002, 1987.
51. Szanton VL: Epidemic salmonellosis. Pediatrics 20:794–808, 1957.
52. Han T, Sokal JE, Neter E: Salmonellosis in disseminated malignant diseases: a seven-year review (1959–1965). N Engl J Med 276: 1045–1052, 1967.
53. Mussche MM, Lameire NH, Ringoir SM: *Salmonella typhimurium* infections in renal transplant patients: report of five cases. Nephron 15:143–150, 1975.
54. Barrett-Connor E: Bacterial infection and sickle cell anemia: an analysis of 250 infections in 166 patients and a review of the literature. Medicine 50:97–112, 1971.
55. Neves J, Raso P, Marinko PP: Prolonged septicemic salmonellosis intercurrent with *Schistosomiasis mansoni* infection. J Trop Med Hyg 74:79, 1971.
56. Sperber SJ, Schleupner CJ: Salmonellosis during infection with human immunodeficiency virus. Rev Infect Dis 9:925–934, 1987.
57. Parsons R, Gregory J, Palmer DL: *Salmonella* infections of the abdominal aorta. Rev Infect Dis 5:227–231, 1983.
58. Cohen JI, Bartlett JA, Corey GR: Extra-intestinal manifestations of *Salmonella* infections. Medicine 66:349–388, 1987.
59. Benenson S, Raveh D, Schlesinger Y, et al: The risk of vascular infection in adult patients with nontyphi *Salmonella* bacteremia. Am J Med 110:60–63, 2001.
60. Shimoni Z, Pitlik S, Leibovici L, et al: Nontyphoid *Salmonella* bacteremia: age-related differences in clinical presentation, bacteriology, and outcome. Clin Infect Dis 28:822–827, 1999.
61. Hsu RB, Tsay YG, Chen RJ, et al: Risk factors for primary bacteremia and endovascular infection in patients without acquired immunodeficiency syndrome who have nontyphoid salmonellosis. Clin Infect Dis 36:829–834, 2003.
62. Angulo FJ, Swerdlow DL: Bacterial enteric infections in persons infected with human immunodeficiency virus. Clin Infect Dis 21(Suppl 1): S84–S89, 1995.
63. Fernández Guerrero ML, Ramos JM, Núñez A, et al: Focal infections due to non-typhi *Salmonella* in patients with AIDS: report of 10 cases and review. Clin Infect Dis 25:690–697, 1997.
64. Wolday D, Erge W: Antimicrobial sensitivity pattern of *Salmonella*: comparison of isolates from HIV-infected and HIV-uninfected patients. Trop Doct 28:139–141, 1998.
65. Gordon MA, Banda HT, Gondwe M, et al: Non-typhoidal salmonella bacteraemia among HIV-infected Malawian adults: high mortality and frequent recrudescence. Aids 16:1633–1641, 2002.

66. Casado JL, Valdezate S, Calderon C, et al: Zidovudine therapy protects against *Salmonella* bacteremia recurrence in human immunodeficiency virus-infected patients. J Infect Dis 179:1553–1556, 1999.
67. Hung CC, Hsieh SM, Hsiao CF, et al: Risk of recurrent non-typhoid *Salmonella* bacteraemia after early discontinuation of ciprofloxacin as secondary prophylaxis in AIDS patients in the era of highly active antiretroviral therapy. Aids 15:645–647, 2001.
68. Aguado JM, Ramos JM, Garcia-Corbeira P, et al: The clinical spectrum of focal infection due to nontyphoid *Salmonella*: 32 years' experience. Med Clin (Barc) 103:293–298, 1994.
69. Musher DM, Rubenstein AD: Permanent carriers of nontyphosal *Salmonellae*. Public Health Rep 132:869–872, 1973.
70. Stuart BM, Pullen RL: Typhoid: clinical analysis of three hundred and sixty cases. Arch Intern Med 78:629–661, 1946.
71. Roland HA: The complications of typhoid fever. J Trop Med Hyg 64:143–152, 1961.
72. Balfour AE, Lewis R, Ahmed S: Convalescent excretion of *Salmonella enteritidis* in infants. J Infect 38:24–25, 1999.
73. Mintz ED, Cartter ML, Hadler JL, et al: Dose-response effects in an outbreak of *Salmonella enteritidis*. Epidemiol Infect 112:13–23, 1994.
74. Gianella RA, Broitman SA, Zamcheck N: Gastric acid barrier to ingested microorganisms in man: studies in vivo and in vitro. Gut 13:251–256, 1972.
75. Michetti P, Mahan MJ, Slauch JM, et al: Monoclonal secretory immunoglobulin A protects mice against oral challenge with the invasive pathogen *Salmonella typhimurium*. Infect Immun 60:1786–1792, 1992.
76. Selsted ME, Miller SI, Henschen AH, et al: Enteric defensins: antibiotic peptide components of intestinal host defense. J Cell Biol 118:929–936, 1992.
77. van der Velden AW, Baumler AJ, Tsolis RM, et al: Multiple fimbrial adhesins are required for full virulence of *Salmonella typhimurium* in mice. Infect Immun 66:2803–2808, 1998.
78. Takeuchi A: Electron microscopic studies of experimental *Salmonella* infection. 1. Penetration into the intestinal epithelium by *Salmonella typhimurium*. Am J Pathol 50:109–136, 1967.
79. Francis CL, Starnbach MN, Falkow S: Morphological and cytoskeletal changes in epithelial cells occur immediately upon interaction with *Salmonella typhimurium* grown under low-oxygen conditions. Mol Microbiol 6:3077–3087, 1992.
80. Pace J, Hayman MJ, Galán JE: Signal transduction and invasion of epithelial cells by *S. typhimurium*. Cell 72:505–514, 1993.
81. Jones BD, Ghori N, Falkow S: *Salmonella typhimurium* initiates murine infection by penetrating and destroying the specialized epithelial M cells of the Peyer's patches. J Exp Med 180:15–23, 1994.
82. Watson PR, Paulin SM, Bland AP, et al: Characterization of intestinal invasion by *Salmonella typhimurium* and *Salmonella dublin* and effect of a mutation in the invH gene. Infect Immun 63:2743–2754, 1995.
83. Hayward RD, Koronakis V: Direct nucleation and bundling of actin by the SipC protein of invasive *Salmonella*. Embo J 18:4926–4934, 1999.
84. Zhou D, Mooseker MS, Galan JE: Role of the *S. typhimurium* actin-binding protein SipA in bacterial internalization. Science 283: 2092–2095, 1999.
85. Friebel A, Ilchmann H, Aepfelbacher M, et al: SopE and SopE2 from *Salmonella typhimurium* activate different sets of RhoGTPases of the host cell. J Biol Chem 276:34035–34040, 2001.
86. Hardt W-D, Chen L-M, Schuebel KE, et al: *S. typhimurium* encodes an activator of Rho GTPases that induces membrane ruffling and nuclear responses in host cells. Cell 93:815–826, 1998.
87. Norris FA, Wilson MP, Wallis TS, et al: SopB, a protein required for virulence of *Salmonella dublin*, is an inositol phosphate phosphatase. Proc Natl Acad Sci USA 95:14057–14059, 1998.
88. Zhou D, Chen LM, Hernandez L, et al: A *Salmonella* inositol polyphosphatase acts in conjunction with other bacterial effectors to promote host cell actin cytoskeleton rearrangements and bacterial internalization. Mol Microbiol 39:248–259, 2001.
89. Zhang S, Kingsley RA, Santos RL, et al: Molecular pathogenesis of *Salmonella* enterica serotype typhimurium-induced diarrhea. Infect Immun 71:1–12, 2003.
90. Hobbie S, Chen LM, Davis RJ, et al: Involvement of mitogen-activated protein kinase pathways in the nuclear responses and cytokine production induced by *Salmonella typhimurium* in cultured intestinal epithelial cells. J Immunol 159:5550–5559, 1997.
91. Eckmann L, Rudolf MT, Ptasznik A, et al: D-myo-Inositol 1,4,5, 6-tetrakisphosphate produced in human intestinal epithelial cells in response to *Salmonella* invasion inhibits phosphoinositide 3-kinase signaling pathways. Proc Natl Acad Sci USA 94:14456–14460, 1997.
92. Wood MW, Rosqvist R, Mullan PB, et al: SopE, a secreted protein of *Salmonella dublin*, is translocated into the target eukaryotic cell via a sip-dependent mechanism and promotes bacterial entry. Mol Microbiol 22:327–338, 1996.
93. Gewirtz AT, Navas TA, Lyons S, et al: Cutting edge: bacterial flagellin activates basolaterally expressed TLR5 to induce epithelial proinflammatory gene expression. J Immunol 167:1882–1885, 2001.
94. Akira S: Mammalian Toll-like receptors. Curr Opin Immunol 15:5–11, 2003.
95. Fu Y, Galan JE: A salmonella protein antagonizes Rac-1 and Cdc42 to mediate host-cell recovery after bacterial invasion. Nature 401:293–297, 1999.
96. Collier-Hyams LS, Zeng H, Sun J, et al: Cutting edge: *Salmonella* AvrA effector inhibits the key proinflammatory, anti-apoptotic NF-kappa B pathway. J Immunol 169:2846–2850, 2002.
97. Haraga A, Miller SI: A *Salmonella enterica* serovar *typhimurium* translocated leucine-rich repeat effector protein inhibits NF-kappa B-dependent gene expression. Infect Immun 71:4052–4058, 2003.
98. Miller SI, Kukral AM, Mekalanos JJ: A two-component regulatory system (*phoP phoQ*) controls *Salmonella typhimurium* virulence. Proc Natl Acad Sci USA 86:5054–5058, 1989.
99. Guina T, Yi EC, Wang H, et al: A PhoP-regulated outer membrane protease of *Salmonella enterica* serovar *typhimurium* promotes resistance to alpha-helical antimicrobial peptides. J Bacteriol 182:4077–4086, 2000.
100. Guo L, Lim K, Gunn JS, et al: Regulation of lipid A modifications by *Salmonella typhimurium* virulence genes *phoP-phoQ*. Science 276: 250–253, 1997.
101. Guo L, Lim KB, Poduje CM, et al: Lipid A acylation and bacterial resistance against vertebrate antimicrobial peptides. Cell 95:189–198, 1998.
102. Groote MA, Testerman T, Xu Y, et al: Homocysteine antagonism of nitric oxide-related cytostasis in *Salmonella typhimurium*. Science 272: 414–417, 1996.
103. Vazquez-Torres A, Jones-Carson J, Baumler AJ, et al: Extraintestinal dissemination of *Salmonella* by CD18-expressing phagocytes. Nature 401:804–808, 1999.
104. Shea JE, Hensel M, Gleeson C, et al: Identification of a virulence locus encoding a second type III secretion system in *Salmonella typhimurium*. Proc Natl Acad Sci USA 93:2593–2597, 1996.
105. Valdivia RH, Falkow S: Fluorescence-based isolation of bacterial genes expressed within host cells. Science 277:2007–2011, 1997.
106. Ochman H, Soncini FC, Solomon F, et al: Identification of a pathogenicity island required for *Salmonella* survival in host cells. Proc Natl Acad Sci USA 93:7800–7804, 1996.
107. Miao EA, Brittnacher M, Haraga A, et al: *Salmonella* effectors translocated across the vacuolar membrane interact with the actin cytoskeleton. Mol Microbiol 48:401–415, 2003.
108. Freeman JA, Ohl ME, Miller SI: The *Salmonella enterica* serovar *typhimurium* translocated effectors SseJ and SifB are targeted to the Salmonella-containing vacuole. Infect Immun 71:418–427, 2003.
109. Brumell JH, Goosney DL, Finlay BB: SifA, a type III secreted effector of *Salmonella typhimurium,* directs *Salmonella*-induced filament (Sif) formation along microtubules. Traffic 3:407–415, 2002.
110. Brumell JH, Tang P, Zaharik ML, et al: Disruption of the *Salmonella*-containing vacuole leads to increased replication of *Salmonella enterica* serovar *typhimurium* in the cytosol of epithelial cells. Infect Immun 70:3264–3270, 2002.
111. Knodler LA, Celli J, Hardt WD, et al: *Salmonella* effectors within a single pathogenicity island are differentially expressed and translocated by separate type III secretion systems. Mol Microbiol 43:1089–1103, 2002.
112. Knodler LA, Vallance BA, Hensel M, et al: *Salmonella* type III effectors PipB and PipB2 are targeted to detergent-resistant microdomains on internal host cell membranes. Mol Microbiol 49:685–704, 2003.
113. Chakravortty D, Hansen-Wester I, Hensel M: *Salmonella* pathogenicity island 2 mediates protection of intracellular *Salmonella* from reactive nitrogen intermediates. J Exp Med 195:1155–1166, 2002.
114. Vazquez-Torres A, Xu Y, Jones-Carson J, et al: *Salmonella* pathogenicity island 2-dependent evasion of the phagocyte NADPH oxidase. Science 287:1655–1658, 2000.

115. Lesnick ML, Reiner NE, Fierer J, et al: The *Salmonella* spvB virulence gene encodes an enzyme that ADP-ribosylates actin and destabilizes the cytoskeleton of eukaryotic cells. Mol Microbiol 39:1464–1470, 2001.
116. Fierer J, Krause M, Tauxe R, et al: *Salmonella typhimurium* bacteremia: association with the virulence plasmid. J Infect Dis 166:639–642, 1992.
117. Reitmeyer JC, Peterson JW, Wilson KJ: *Salmonella* cytotoxin: a component of the bacterial outer membrane. Microb Pathog 1:503–510, 1986.
118. Hoiseth SK, Stocker BA: Aromatic-dependent *Salmonella typhimurium* are non-virulent and effective as live vaccines. Nature 291:238–239, 1981.
119. Kingsley R, Rabsch W, Stephens P, et al: Iron supplying systems of *Salmonella* in diagnostics, epidemiology and infection. FEMS Immunol Med Microbiol 11:257–264, 1995.
120. Bernheiden M, Heinrich JM, Minigo G, et al: LBP, CD14, TLR4 and the murine innate immune response to a peritoneal *Salmonella* infection. J Endotoxin Res 7:447–450, 2001.
121. Mastroeni P: Immunity to systemic *Salmonella* infections. Curr Mol Med 2:393–406, 2002.
122. Mastroeni P, Harrison JA, Robinson JH, et al: Interleukin-12 is required for control of the growth of attenuated aromatic-compound-dependent salmonellae in BALB/c mice: role of gamma interferon and macrophage activation. Infect Immun 66:4767–4776, 1998.
123. Everest P, Roberts M, Dougan G: Susceptibility to *Salmonella typhimurium* infection and effectiveness of vaccination in mice deficient in the tumor necrosis factor alpha p55 receptor. Infect Immun 66:3355–3364, 1998.
124. Hess J, Ladel C, Miko D, et al: *Salmonella typhimurium* aroA infection in gene-targeted immunodeficient mice: major role of CD4+ TCR-alpha beta cells and IFN-gamma in bacterial clearance independent of intracellular location. J Immunol 156:3321–3326, 1996.
125. de Jong R, Altare F, Haagen IA, et al: Severe mycobacterial and *Salmonella* infections in interleukin-12 receptor-deficient patients. Science 280:1435–1438, 1998.
126. Jouanguy E, Doffinger R, Dupuis S, et al: IL-12 and IFN-gamma in host defense against mycobacteria and salmonella in mice and men. Curr Opin Immunol 11:346–351, 1999.
127. Mastroeni P, Simmons C, Fowler R, et al: Igh-6(-/-) (B-cell-deficient) mice fail to mount solid acquired resistance to oral challenge with virulent *Salmonella enterica* serovar *typhimurium* and show impaired Th1 T-cell responses to Salmonella antigens. Infect Immun 68:46–53, 2000.
128. Nauciel C: Role of CD4+ T cells and T-independent mechanisms in acquired resistance to *Salmonella typhimurium* infection. J Immunol 145:1265–1269, 1990.
129. Wolfe MS, Louria DB, Armstrong D, et al: Salmonellosis in patients with neoplastic disease: a review of 100 episodes at Memorial Cancer Center over a 13-year period. Arch Intern Med 128:546–554, 1971.
130. Perez JM, Cavalli P, Roure C, et al: Comparison of four chromogenic media and Hektoen agar for detection and presumptive identification of *Salmonella* strains in human stools. J Clin Microbiol 41:1130–1134, 2003.
131. Ruiz J, Nunez ML, Diaz J, et al: Comparison of five plating media for isolation of *Salmonella* species from human stools. J Clin Microbiol 34:686–688, 1996.
132. Oracz G, Feleszko W, Golicka D, et al: Rapid diagnosis of acute *Salmonella* gastrointestinal infection. Clin Infect Dis 36:112–115, 2003.
133. Garaizar J, Porwollik S, Echeita A, et al: DNA microarray-based typing of an atypical monophasic *Salmonella enterica* serovar. J Clin Microbiol 40:2074–2078, 2002.
134. Sirinavin S, Garner P: Antibiotics for treating salmonella gut infections. Cochrane Database Syst Rev 93:CD001167, 2000.
135. Lightfoot NF, Ahmad F, Cowden J: Management of institutional outbreaks of *Salmonella* gastroenteritis. J Antimicrob Chemoth 26:37–46, 1990.
136. Gendrel D, Raymond J, Legall MA, et al: Use of pefloxacin after failure of initial antibiotic treatment in children with severe salmonellosis. Eur J Clin Microbiol Infect Dis 12:209–211, 1993.
137. Gokalp AS, Toksoy HB, Turkay S, et al: Intravenous immunoglobulin in the treatment of *Salmonella typhimurium* infections in preterm neonates. Clin Pediatr (Phila) 33:349–352, 1994.
138. Cohen PS, O'Brien TF, Schoenbaum SC, et al: The risk of endothelial infection in adults with *Salmonella* bacteremia. Ann Intern Med 89:931–932, 1978.
139. Donabedian H: Long-term suppression of *Salmonella* aortitis with an oral antibiotic. Arch Inter Med 149:1452–1453, 1989.
140. Jacobson MA, Hahn SM, Gerberding JL, et al: Ciprofloxacin for *Salmonella* bacteremia in the acquired immunodeficiency syndrome (AIDS). Ann Intern Med 110:1027–1029, 1989.
141. Lewin CS, Allen RA, Amyes SG: Antibacterial activity of fluoroquinolones in combination with zidovudine. J Med Microbiol 33:127–131, 1990.
142. Freerksen E, Rosenfield M, Freerksen R: Treatment of chronic *Salmonella* carriers. Chemotherapy 23:192, 1977.
143. Ferreccio C, Morris JG, Jr, Valdivieso C, et al: Efficacy of ciprofloxacin in the treatment of chronic typhoid carriers. J Infect Dis 157:1235–1239, 1988.
144. Hogue A, White P, Guard-Petter J, et al: Epidemiology and control of egg-associated *Salmonella enteritidis* in the United States of America. Rev Sci Tech 16:542–553, 1997.
145. Bender JB, Hedberg CW, Boxrud DJ, et al: Use of molecular subtyping in surveillance for *Salmonella enterica* serotype *typhimurium*. N Engl J Med 344:189–195, 2001.
146. Fisher IST, Rowe B, Bartlett CLR, et al: 'Salm-Net'-laboratory-based surveillance of human salmonella infections in Europe. PHLS Microbiol Dig 11:181, 1994.
147. Hastings L, Burnens A, de Jong B, et al: Salm-Net facilitates collaborative investigation of an outbreak of *Salmonella tosamanga* infection in Europe. Commun Dis Rep Rev 6:R100–R102, 1996.
148. Standaert SM, Hutcheson RH, Schaffner W: Nosocomial transmission of *Salmonella* gastroenteritis to laundry workers in a nursing home. Infect Control Hosp Epidemiol 15:22–26, 1994.
149. Pace F, Fanfarillo F, Giorgino F, et al: *Salmonella enteritidis* pericarditis: case report and review of the literature. Ann Ital Med Int 17:189–192, 2002.
150. Soravia-Dunand VA, Loo VG, Salit IE: Aortitis due to *Salmonella*: report of 10 cases and comprehensive review of the literature. Clin Infect Dis 29:862–868, 1999.
151. Chiu CH, Ou JT: Risk factors for endovascular infection due to nontyphoid salmonellae. Clin Infect Dis 36:835–836, 2003.
152. Huang LT, Ko SF, Lui CC: Salmonella meningitis: clinical experience of third-generation cephalosporins. Acta Paediatr 86:1056–1058, 1997.
153. Lee WS, Puthucheary SD, Omar A: Salmonella meningitis and its complications in infants. J Paediatr Child Health 35:379–382, 1999.
154. Karim M, Islam N: Salmonella meningitis: report of three cases in adults and literature review. Infection 30:104–108, 2002.
155. Banky JP, Ostergaard L, Spelman D: Chronic relapsing salmonella osteomyelitis in an immunocompetent patient: case report and literature review. J Infect 44:44–47, 2002.
156. Santos EM, Sapico FL: Vertebral osteomyelitis due to salmonellae: report of two cases and review. Clin Infect Dis 27:287–295, 1998.
157. Ekman P, Kirveskari J, Granfors K: Modification of disease outcome in *Salmonella*-infected patients by HLA-B27. Arthritis Rheum 43: 1527–1534, 2000.
158. Buxton JA, Fyfe M, Berger S, et al: Reactive arthritis and other sequelae following sporadic *Salmonella typhimurium* infection in British Columbia, Canada: a case control study. J Rheumatol 29:2154–2158, 2002.
159. Chen JY, Luo SF, Wu YJ, et al: Salmonella septic arthritis in systemic lupus erythematosus and other systemic diseases. Clin Rheumatol 17:282–287, 1998.
160. Collazos J, Mayo J, Martínez E, et al: Muscle infections caused by *Salmonella* species: case report and review. Clin Infect Dis 29:673–677, 1999.
161. Lee CC, Poon SK, Chen GH: Spontaneous gas-forming liver abscess caused by *Salmonella* within hepatocellular carcinoma: a case report and review of the literature. Dig Dis Sci 47:586–589, 2002.
162. Ramos JM, Aguado JM, García-Corbeira P, et al: Clinical spectrum of urinary tract infections due on nontyphoidal *Salmonella* species Clin Infect Dis 23:388–390, 1996.
163. Behr MA, McDonald J: Salmonella neck abscess in a patient with beta-thalassemia major: case report and review. Clin Infect Dis 23:404–405, 1996.

19

Shigellosis

GERALD T. KEUSCH
DENNIS J. KOPECKO

INTRODUCTION

Shigellosis, a disease typically associated with poverty, poor hygiene, and crowded living conditions, remains a common cause of diarrhea, dysentery, and death in developing countries as well as an important contributor to childhood malnutrition.[1] In 1999, the estimated global mortality due to shigellosis was 1.1 million, with 99% of the deaths occurring in the developing world.[2] In such settings, *Shigella* spp. cause 5% to 15% of all diarrhea cases and the majority of bloody diarrhea or dysentery episodes in infants and children seeking care in clinics or hospitals. In contrast, in the United States, *Shigella* accounts for less than 1% of documented intestinal infections. Moreover, most patients have mild-to-moderate watery diarrhea indistinguishable from that due to other causes such as rotavirus; therefore, the diarrhea is not investigated microbiologically and thus goes unreported. The Centers for Disease Control and Prevention (CDC) recently estimated that there are more than 440,000 cases of shigellosis annually in the United States,[3] although the number of documented cases is in the range of 10,000 to 20,000 per year. For reasons that are not well understood, transmission of the most virulent serotype, *Shigella dysenteriae* type 1, occurs almost exclusively in developing countries.[4] This organism is responsible for large-scale, often devastating epidemics, now often in settings of humanitarian emergencies with large numbers of refugees, such as the 1994 outbreak among Rwandan refugees, killing an estimated 30,000 people in just a few weeks.[5] In wealthier countries, *Shigella sonnei*, the least virulent *Shigella* species, is the most prevalent, with significant outbreaks occurring among the increasing number of young children in day-care centers, where inadequate hygienic conditions facilitate person-to-person spread of infection.[3]

AGENT

Dysentery has been a well-characterized syndrome since antiquity. However, it was just over a century ago, during a severe outbreak in Japan, that the first complete description of the prototypic *Shigella* species was accomplished by Kiyoshi Shiga,[6] for whom the organism was ultimately named. Dysentery, the prototypic classic presentation of shigellosis, consists of a triad of findings, including the frequent passage of small-volume bloody stools, abdominal cramps, and tenesmus (the painful straining to pass stool), and is often referred to as bacillary dysentery to distinguish it from amebic dysentery, the other major cause of the syndrome in the tropics, caused by the protozoan *Entamoeba histolytica*.

Shigella, a gram-negative rod-shaped organism that grows aerobically and anaerobically, is a highly host-adapted member of the family Enterobacteriaceae that naturally infects humans and nonhuman primates such as gibbons, gorillas, and rhesus monkeys.[7] It cannot be differentiated from *Escherichia coli* by contemporary criteria of DNA relatedness, and were it discovered today it would be classified within the genus *Escherichia*.[8] While genetic analysis indicates that the different shigella serotypes evolved from various *E. coli* serotypes, *Shigella* has remained a separate genus because of its historic separation and distinctive clinical illnesses. Unlike most *E. coli* and *Salmonella* strains, *Shigella* does not possess flagella and is nonmotile. There are a number of biochemical differences between *Shigella* and other Enterobacteriaceae, but these are of no particular importance for diagnosis or, apparently, for virulence.

The original isolate described by Shiga is now known as *S. dysenteriae* serotype 1. At least 11 additional serotypes of this species have been described, and new putative strains continue to be reported. Over the 4 decades following the original description of the prototype organism, three additional *Shigella* species, most containing a number of serotypes, subtypes, or phage (or colicin) types, were described.[1] These include, in decreasing order of the severity of illness they cause, *S. flexneri*, *S. boydii*, and *S. sonnei*. Although *S. dysenteriae* can be readily distinguished from the other three species by its inability to ferment mannitol, in practice the four species are identified primarily by their inability to utilize lactose or produce H_2S, and then distinguished by serologic characteristics.

EPIDEMIOLOGY

Shigella are present wherever humans exist. Direct spread from one person to another is a major route of transmission, facilitated by the very low inoculum of organisms required for infection. For example, experimental human studies have shown that just 10 to 100 *S. dysenteriae* 1 will cause infection in many and clinical disease in 10% to 20% of nonimmune subjects.[9] Transmission is fecal-oral, generally secondary to initial contamination of the hands with infected feces. Failure to hand wash results in the transfer of organisms directly to the mouth or to an inanimate object subsequently handled by another susceptible person. *Shigella* may also be transferred from feces or via contaminated hands to food or water, allowing the organisms to multiply and cause common-source outbreaks. Fly species attracted to human feces can also serve this transfer role to food or water, especially where sanitary facilities are poor. In such settings, the use of traps to reduce the fly population is reported to diminish the incidence of shigellosis.[10] The organisms have also been transmitted sexually, via anal-oral contact. These multiple routes promote the efficient transmission of *Shigella* infection, even though the genus is not hardy outside the human intestinal tract. Because environmental and major animal reservoirs do not exist, it is theoretically possible to control the incidence of infection by effective environmental sanitation of fecal waste.

The incidence of shigellosis is highest in children 1 to 5 years of age, presumably because good personal hygiene is more difficult to achieve in the young and because they have not yet acquired specific immunity. In many disease-endemic countries *Shigella* infections peak during the hot

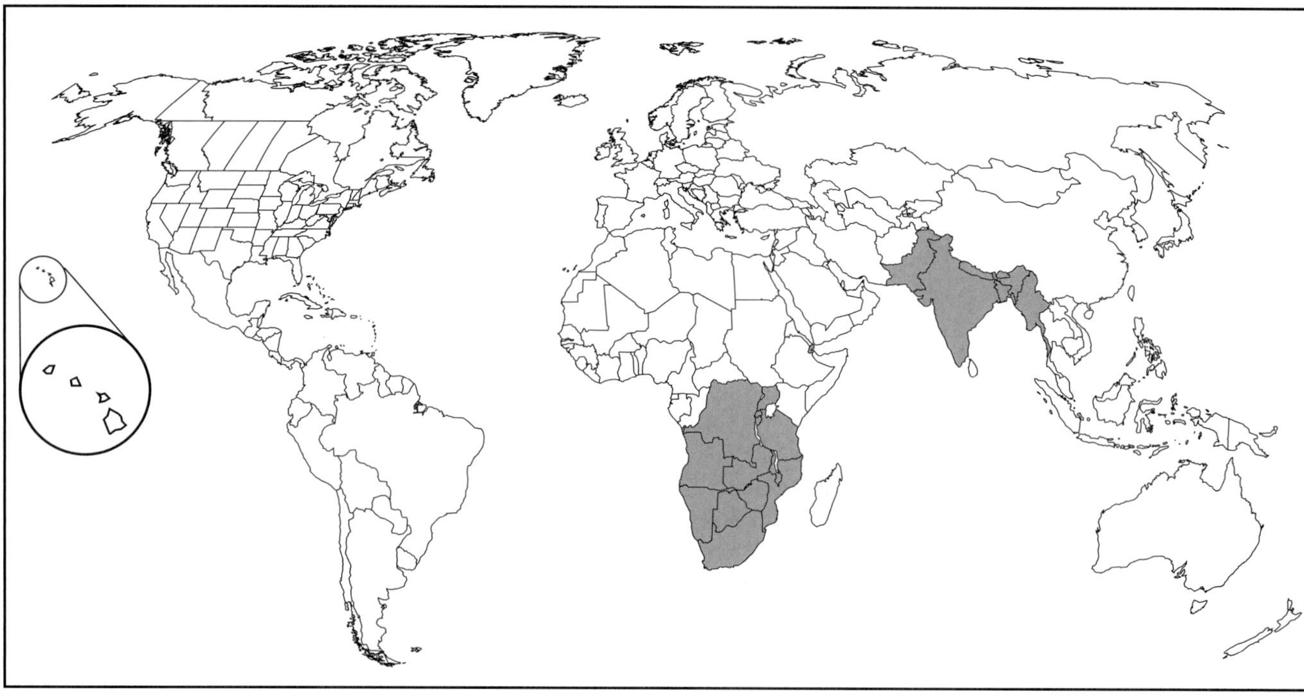

■ *Shigella dysenteriae* type 1, major areas of endemicity

dry season, when water for hand washing and washing food and cooking utensils can be in short supply. In some countries, however, peaks occur in the rainy season, as the rains wash contaminated feces from the environment into drinking water sources. In the United States, shigellosis is common in infant day-care centers, where nonimmune young children cluster and good hygiene is difficult to maintain. Similar conditions on reservations for native Americans also place them at high risk for shigellosis.

Even though the organisms are present worldwide, the distribution of the four *Shigella* species is closely related to social and economic development. Although the explanation is uncertain, *S. dysenteriae* type 1 diminished in prevalence and then virtually disappeared as a cause of clinical disease following World War I, and was replaced by *S. flexneri* spp. Following World War II, however, *S. flexneri* was progressively replaced in industrialized countries by *S. sonnei* while remaining the predominant isolate in developing countries. Again the reason is unclear; however, it has been hypothesized that contamination of water in developing countries with *Plesiomonas shigelloides,* which can express the same O antigen as *S. sonnei*, induces a common O-antigen-specific immunity.[11] Perhaps signaling its evolutionary origins, the fourth species, *S. boydii,* is present primarily in the Indian subcontinent and has always been an uncommon isolate elsewhere.

S. dysenteriae type 1, the only epidemic member of the genus, re-emerged in 1969 in a major outbreak in Mexico and Central America, resulting in several hundred thousand deaths. Subsequent epidemics in South Asia and Africa signaled the return of this organism to prominence throughout the developing world.[1]

DISEASE

Symptoms of shigellosis typically begin 24 to 72 hours after ingestion of the organism, with malaise and fever, followed shortly by diarrhea, usually watery at the outset. This may evolve into bloody diarrhea or the prototypical manifestation of *Shigella* infection, dysentery, which is characterized by the frequent passage of small volume, grossly bloody and mucoid stools (Fig. 19-1), accompanied by tenesmus, which

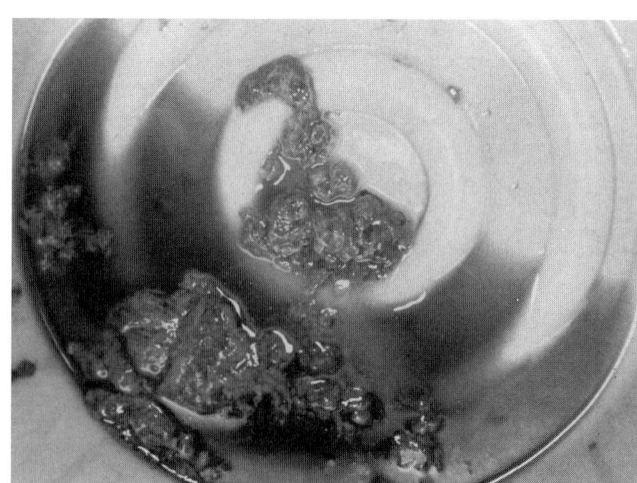

FIGURE 19-1 Typical dysenteric stool, a small-volume 5- to 10-mL stool containing bloody fluid and mucus. Such stools may be passed 30 or more times per day.

is painful straining at defecation. These manifestations result from inflammation and ulceration of the colonic mucosa and an intense proctitis. Dysentery is not an invariable consequence of *Shigella* infection, and is in large part determined by the identity and virulence of the infecting strain. Thus, most patients with *S. sonnei* infections never develop dysentery, whereas the reverse is true for *S. dysenteriae* type 1 infection.

Shigella dysentery is associated with profound anorexia.[12] Because the stomach and small bowel are not involved in shigellosis, neither vomiting nor severe dehydration are prominent manifestations, although mild-to-moderate dehydration may occur as a result of stool water losses, increased insensible water loss from fever, and reduced food and fluid intake. In contrast, the intensity of the proctitis can be so severe that rectal prolapse occurs, especially in small children with *S. dysenteriae* type 1 or *S. flexneri* infection.[13] Functional intestinal obstruction and toxic megacolon is another complication due to severe inflammation (Fig. 19-2), most commonly with *S. dysenteriae* type 1 infection.[14] Although infection with *Shigella* usually does not progress beyond the lamina propria, colonic or distal ileal perforation is a rare complication, occurring most typically in neonates or malnourished children.[15] Bacteremia due to the infecting *Shigella* organism itself or other Enterobacteriaceae may be present, usually in malnourished or immunocompromised patients.[16]

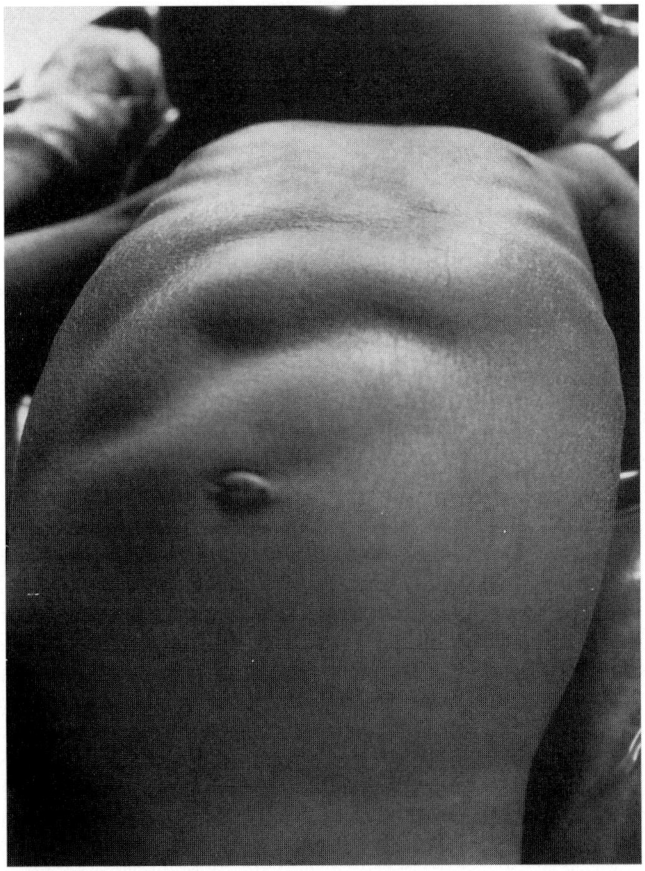

FIGURE 19-2 Bangladeshi child with toxic megacolon caused by *Shigella dysenteriae* type 1 infection. The dilated loops of bowel are clearly outlined on the abdominal wall.

Shigellosis is associated with a number of systemic complications. Generalized motor seizures can be the presenting feature of disease in some patients, especially young children with high fever.[17] The seizures appear to be more common with *S. sonnei* and are rarely recurrent. Patients with shigellosis may become profoundly obtunded or even comatose, usually in association with metabolic aberrations such as severe hypoglycemia and hyponatremia.[18] Hypoglycemia occurs in the face of starvation and an inadequate gluconeogenic response and may be profound (< 1 mmol/L). Hyponatremia is associated with dysenteric forms of shigellosis, and in Bangladesh serum sodium concentrations less than 125 mmol/L are present in approximately 50% of all patients with severe *S. dysenteriae* type 1 and 25% of those with *S. flexneri* infection. This is due to sodium loss in the stool plus secretion of antidiuretic hormone in amounts inappropriate for the serum sodium concentration, possibly triggered by the profound hypoalbuminemia and decreased intravascular oncotic pressure found in many patients with severe dysentery.[19]

The most dramatic systemic complication of shigellosis is hemolytic-uremic syndrome (HUS), a thrombotic microangiopathy characterized by hemolytic anemia, thrombocytopenia, and oliguric renal failure. It occurs in *S. dysenteriae* type 1 infection, usually first noted 1 to 5 days after the appearance of the dysentery, often as the intestinal disease is subsiding.[19] Both the renal failure and the hemolytic anemia can be severe, whereas the thrombocytopenia is usually less so, with platelet counts in the range of 25,000 to 100,000/mm^3 and without bleeding manifestations except in the gut. HUS is often incomplete; each of the three findings can occur in isolation.[20] Shigellosis can also have a profound effect on nutrition in children, and wherever shigellosis is hyperendemic, as in Bangladesh, it is a major contributor to the high prevalence of malnutrition for two main reasons:

1. Patients with shigellosis have increased energy requirements owing to the effects of fever (see Chapter 5).[21]
2. The metabolic consequences of the inflammatory cytokines released in the host response result in muscle protein catabolism, altered priorities for protein synthesis, and decreased nutrient intake because of anorexia.

In addition, these patients lose considerable amounts of protein in the gut owing to epithelial cell death, ulceration, and the transudation of serum into the colonic lumen,[22] which exacerbates the negative nitrogen balance induced by the infection. In developing countries, the more severe *Shigella* infections due to *S. dysenteriae* type 1 and *S. flexneri* almost double the subsequent rate of persistent (> 14 days) diarrhea and increase mortality by 10-fold.[23]

PATHOGENESIS AND IMMUNITY

As they exit the infected host in stool, shigellae are acid resistant. This is the consequence of growth phase–regulated activation of a glutamate-dependent acid-resistance system,[24] transcriptionally regulated by the alternative sigma factor RpoS of RNA polymerase, which is induced only during the stationary phase of the growth cycle.[1,25] This property allows the organisms to tolerate exposure to pH below 2.5 for several hours. This facilitates their survival during passage through the acidic environment of the stomach and accounts in large part for the low oral infectious dose of *Shigella*. Stationary-phase growth occurs when shigellae are present in the distal colon, endowing them with a property as they are about to be excreted in feces that increases the likelihood that they will successfully colonize the next susceptible host they encounter. Once past the stomach shigellae invade host cells of the terminal ileum and colon and multiply within the cytoplasm, sequestered from extracellular host defenses. This efficient host cell invasion ability also contributes to the low inoculum required for infection by these organisms. Interestingly, organisms in the acid-resistant state do not efficiently invade mammalian cells, and once past the stomach, shigellae downregulate acid-resistance genes and transcriptionally upregulate invasion genes. Invasion of the intestinal epithelium proceeds by means of a complex mechanism mediated by both microbial and host proteins.[2,26,27] Intimate biochemical "cross-talk" signals between *Shigella* and various host cell types activate specific bacterial genes necessary for virulence. These include the type 3 secretion system and invasion mediators and leads to essential host cell responses, such as cytoskeletal actin rearrangements and inflammation.[3]

Our understanding of the invasion process and the ensuing host-mediated pathogenesis of disease has undergone dramatic extensions in the past decade as a result of both new cell biology studies and revolutionary findings of pathogen-recognition receptors for innate immunostimulation.[28] On the basis of the results of early molecular genetic studies of *Shigella*, combined with tissue culture invasion assays, *Shigella* was thought simply to employ a set of genes encoded on a large 180- to 220-kb plasmid, termed ipaB, ipaC, and ipaD (for *i*nvasion *p*lasmid *a*ntigens) to induce bacterial uptake by a phagocytosis-like process at the luminal surface of intestinal mucosal cells. Following ingestion, the organisms reached the cytoplasm within a host cell membrane-bound endosome (Fig. 19-3).[29] Subsequent lysis of the endosome membrane released bacteria into the cell cytoplasm, where they multiplied, leading ultimately to death of the host cell. It seemed reasonable to presume that pathogen-induced host mucosal cell death was responsible for the colitis that characterizes dysentery. New information dramatically changed the paradigm of *Shigella* pathogenesis, and the pathologic consequences of shigellosis are now thought to be due largely to an imbalanced inflammatory over-response to the pathogen that results in formidable local intestinal tissue damage.

The mucus-covered epithelium constitutes a major line of defense against most enteric microbes because they cannot cross this tight epithelial cell monolayer barrier. In addition, it is endowed with both intracellular and extracellular receptors to recognize microbial invasion and activate the innate immune system.[15] Because *Shigella* requires mucosal invasion to cause disease, it has developed unique molecular strategies to breach the mucosal barrier. Convincing evidence now exists that shigellae initially traverse the mucosa, not through epithelial cells as originally believed, but rather through M cells, specialized for antigen processing.[30] Organisms thus reach the underlying lymphoid follicles, apparently without disrupting the M cells, and encounter and are phagocytosed by resident macrophages. Following lysis of the phagosomal vacuole, shigellae are released into the cytoplasm, where they multiply, leading to apoptosis, or programmed cell death, of infected macrophages.[31] This process is triggered by caspase 1, activated by the *ipaB* gene product,[32] a critical bacterial virulence factor involved in invasion as well. With macrophage death, intracellular stores of the mature inflammatory cytokines interleukin-1β (IL-1β) and IL-18 are released.[33] In addition, as demonstrated by infection of differentiated intestinal epithelial cell monolayers in culture, invasive organisms such as *Shigella*, but not noninvasive organisms such as normal flora *E. coli*, result in the toll-like receptor (TLR)-4-mediated upregulation of proinflammatory cytokine genes[16] and an increase in epithelial cell secretion of cytokines such as IL-8 and tumor necrosis factor-α (TNF-α).[34] Studies of rectal samples from acutely ill or convalescing shigellosis patients show a pattern of IL-1, IL-4, IL-6, IL-8, TNF-α, and gamma interferon (IFN-γ) production; severe illness is associated with markedly increased IL-1β, IL-6, TNF-α, and IFN-γ expression.[14] IL-1β and IL-8 both induce the migration and activation of polymorphonuclear neutrophils (PMNs), resulting in the local recruitment of PMNs to the lamina propria, in preparation for their transmigration between the epithelial cells to the gut lumen.[35]

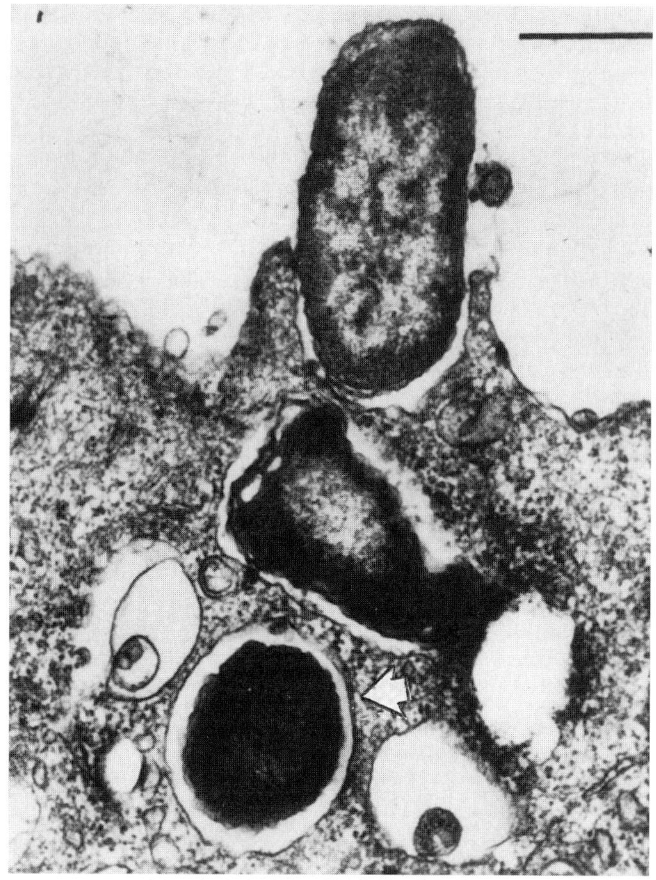

FIGURE 19-3 Invasion of cultured HeLa cell monolayers by *Shigella flexneri*. The bacterial cell at the top of the figure has initiated the reorganization of the epithelial cell cytoskeleton, and the actin-based movement of the host cell membranes to form a phagocytic vacuole is evident. The two pseudopods of host cell origin will fuse at the top, engulfing the bacterium within a membrane-bounded endosome. An organism within an endosome is present at the lower portion of the photomicrograph (*arrowhead*).

Shigella lipopolysaccharide (LPS) is a critical signal for PMN adherence and migration. The LPS is translocated in an active form from the luminal (apical) to the mucosal (basal) side of intestinal epithelial cells, where it interacts with circulating host LPS-binding protein and is then recognized by the PMN ligand, CD14. This sequence of events leads to upregulation and activation of the PMN adherence ligand CD11b/CD18, which is required for transepithelial migration.[36] Other yet uncharacterized *Shigella* factors apparently mediate the migration of PMNs between the epithelial cells (paracellular pathway), which disrupts the integrity of the tight junctions and allows *Shigella* and other luminal bacteria to breach the mucosal epithelium in large numbers. Their access to the basolateral epithelial surface triggers the pathogen recognition TLRs, leading to further upregulation of proinflammatory cytokines.[16]

Thus, invasion of the epithelial mucosa actually involves three processes: a primary translocation across the mucosa via M cells, a secondary invasion process in which the bacteria released from dead macrophages or translocated across the mucosa invade the basolateral surface of the mucosa, and a tertiary amplification of epithelial cell invasion when the tight junction is disrupted and organisms invade through the damaged barrier. All three are essential to disease pathogenesis. In the rabbit model, for example, if the action of IL-1 is blocked by pretreatment with IL-1 receptor antagonist,[37] or if neutrophil chemotaxis and migration are prevented by antibody to PMN surface determinants essential to this process, for example, anti-CD18,[23] the progression of the infection is halted and no clinical disease ensues. *Shigella*, long believed to be directly responsible for tissue destruction and the ensuing immune response, which was thought to clear the infection, clearly activates innate immune responses that are both defensive (PMN-mediated killing of shigellae) and offensive (destabilization of epithelial cohesion and mucosal damage). Specifically, *Shigella* infection activates PMNs and triggers degranulation, damaging surrounding tissue,[38] while the organisms are efficiently trapped within and killed by the PMNs via a mechanism that does not require oxygen.[39] The inflammatory response in shigellosis is in reality a double-edged sword,[40] and the resulting innate immune response imbalance to some degree mimics the immunologic overresponse seen in inflammatory bowel diseases.[15]

The invasion of intestinal epithelial cells itself is dependent on a microbial needle-like secretion apparatus (termed type III) that injects the effector *ipa* invasins through the host cell membrane into the periplasm to initiate the invasion process into M cells, macrophages, and absorptive epithelial cells.[14] These effectors modulate the activities of Cdc42, Rac, and Rho, which are small GTPases that control actin polymerization and the cellular extensions involved in the macropinocytic uptake of *Shigella*. Lysis of the endosomal membrane proceeds via the actions of IpaB and IpaC, releasing organisms into the cytoplasm. *Shigella* mutants that cannot lyse the endosomal vacuole also cannot multiply and are essentially avirulent. As the bacteria in the cytoplasm multiply, actin filaments are polymerized at one pole of the bacterium and are bundled to form an actin tail.[41] Other host cell proteins also are deposited in the actin tail, including plastin (an actin-binding isoform of fimbrin), vinculin (involved in linking actin bundles to the plasma membrane), and filamin (an actin gelation protein).[14,42,43] This process is energized by the microbial protein IcsA, an adenosine triphosphatase (ATPase) necessary for actin polymerization.[44] IcsA mutant strains, which fail to generate an actin tail, do not move within the cell and are of reduced virulence. Actin polymerization at the tail end pushes the organism forward, and for this reason it is often referred to as the "actin motor." The unipolar localization of IcsA, the nucleator of the actin tail, is dependent on normal LPS, inasmuch as LPS mutants show aberrant surface localization of IcsA.[45] The actin motor can drive shigellae to the plasma membrane, where they push out from the surface in long, membrane-bound protrusions (dubbed "fireworks" as studied in nonconfluent cultured cells)[46] (Fig. 19-4). In confluent cells, these protrusions are found in the intermediate junction regions, below the tight junctions, where epithelial cells contact one another, and constitute a unique mechanism for intercellular spread of shigellae.[47] The protrusions indent the membrane of the adjacent cell so that the organism within becomes surrounded by both the cell membrane of the protrusion and the cell membrane of the second cell. When this double-membraned endosome is lysed, the organisms are released into the cytoplasm of the latter. Further evidence that such protrusions are involved in cell-to-cell invasion is the requirement for host cell E-cadherin, a calcium-dependent cell adhesion molecule localized to the intermediate junctions.[48] In cells that lack the ability to produce E-cadherin, abortive protrusions develop in which the bacteria fail to intimately interact with the inner face of the host membrane and lose contact with actin inside the protrusions. The final stage of intercellular invasion, lysis of the double cell membrane itself, is mediated via IpaB, IpaC, and IpgC.[49] In vivo, secondary epithelial cell invasion by *Shigella* is followed by cell-to-cell invasion and bacterial multiplication. This results in necrosis and sloughing of infected epithelial cells, creating focal microulcerations of the mucosa, primarily in the terminal ileum and colon, with the intensity of infection greatest in

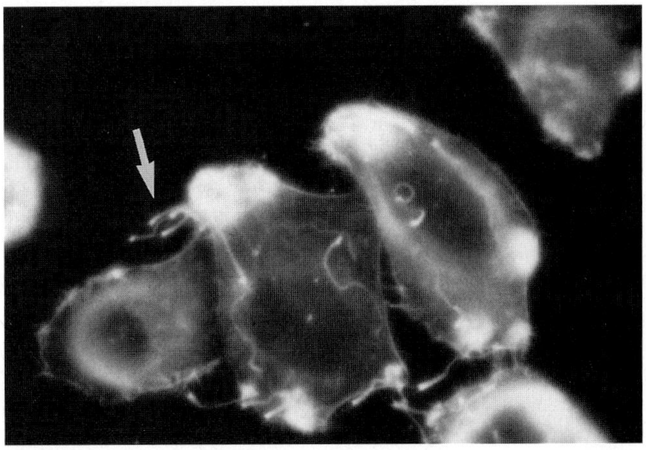

FIGURE 19-4 Intracellular movement of *Shigella flexneri* within HeLa cells, stained with fluorescein-labeled phalloidin, which specifically binds to polymerized actin. The actin tails are labeled and may be seen as bright streaks within the cytoplasm as the organism is pushed forward by the "actin motor" created by actin polymerization. Organisms that have moved out to the plasma membrane and are protruding from the plane of the membrane, the so-called fireworks, are indicated by the arrow.

the rectum and distal colon. The basis for this preferential localization in the colon is not presently understood.

These inflammatory processes persist longer in children than in adults, perhaps reflecting the immunologic immaturity in young children. Clearance of disease symptoms likely involves a combination of normal intestinal cell turnover, killing of *Shigella* by the innate defenses (e.g., PMNs), down-modulation of inflammation, and the development of specific immunity for final pathogen clearance. Epidemiologic evidence indicates that immunity to *Shigella* is serotype-specific, based on LPS; however, the precise nature of protective immunity, for example, mucosal immunoglobulin A (IgA) versus serum IgG, is not known.

S. dysenteriae type 1, but no other species of *Shigella,* makes a cytolethal protein toxin called Shiga toxin. This toxin binds to glycolipid receptors on the surface of cells, which leads to its uptake via a process of receptor-mediated endocytosis.[50] The active enzymatic portion of the toxin is transported to the Golgi region and then in retrograde fashion to the endoplasmic reticulum, where it catalytically and irreversibly inhibits host ribosomal protein synthesis. Although the role of Shiga toxin in human disease has not been fully clarified, experiments in monkeys comparing infection with isogenic wild-type virulent *S. dysenteriae* type 1 and a Shiga toxin$^-$ mutant differing only in toxin production demonstrate that toxin$^-$ *S. dysenteriae* 1 causes uncomplicated shigellosis and toxin-producing strains cause more severe gut inflammation, ulceration, and capillary damage.[51] Shiga toxin–producing *Shigella,* but not nontoxigenic species, are epidemiologically linked to the development of HUS. This association is strengthened by the finding that serotypes of *E. coli* that produce the structurally and biochemically similar Shiga toxins 1 and 2 are also strongly associated with HUS.[52]

DIAGNOSIS

Specific diagnosis of *Shigella* infection depends primarily on isolation of the organism from microbiologic cultures of a stool or rectal swab sample, preferably the former because of the better yield. Samples that cannot be cultured rapidly (best at the bedside) should be inoculated onto transport media such as buffered glycerol-saline, the preferred transport medium for isolation of *Shigella,* or Cary-Blair medium. It is best to use both a moderately selective medium for gram-negative organisms, such as MacConkey[46] or deoxycholate citrate agar (DCA), and a more highly selective medium such as xylose-lysine-deoxycholate (XLD),[47] Hektoen enteric (HE), or *Salmonella-Shigella* (SS) agar.[48] *Shigella,* as well as *Salmonella,* fails to change the color of the pH indicator in the agar because of its inability to ferment lactose, allowing the technician to pick putatively pathogenic lactose-negative colonies for further identification, for example, subculture to triple sugar iron (TSI) agar or Kligler iron agar (KIA). On these media, *Shigella* are nonmotile, produce an alkaline slant and acid butt owing to their inability to ferment lactose aerobically in the slope and the anaerobic fermentation of glucose in the butt, and do not produce hydrogen sulfide or gas. Isolates that fulfill these criteria can be confirmed and speciated by serologic methods, using specific grouping antisera.

In many areas of the tropics, microbiological tests are not readily available, and the diagnosis must be based on clinical and simple laboratory features. Many practitioners in endemic areas still believe that dysentery is more commonly amebic in etiology, but there is ample evidence that patients with the dysentery syndrome, including both children and adults, are far more likely to be infected with *Shigella.*[53] The clinical and laboratory features and stool examination in amebic and bacillary dysentery differ. A very short prehospitalization illness, high fever, and abundant fecal leukocytes (> 50 neutrophils per high-power field) are highly suggestive of shigellosis.[54] In the absence of microscopy or culture capability to make the specific diagnosis, patients with frank dysentery should be presumed to have shigellosis and treated empirically for this infection. In the field setting, the diagnosis of clinical dysentery can be established by community health workers who either observe the characteristic dysenteric stool or obtain a history of bloody stools from the mothers, who have been shown to be reliable historians of stool character.[55]

Modern rapid methods for diagnosis of *Shigella* infection have been developed. These include fluorescent antibody staining for *S. dysenteriae* type 1, which appears to have high sensitivity (92%) and specificity (93%),[56] immunomagnetic isolation followed by polymerase chain reaction[57] or monoclonal antibodies[58] for identification, and isotope- or enzyme-labeled DNA probes for virulence markers specific for *Shigella*, some of which are also present in the much rarer *Shigella*-like enteroinvasive *E. coli.*[59,60] To date, with one exception, no reliable rapid method is commercially available or in routine use anywhere. The exception is an enzyme immunoassay for Shiga toxin that can be done directly on stool and is indicative of the presence of a Shiga toxin–producing *S. dysenteriae* type 1 or *E. coli* serotype, such as O157. This test is in use in some developed countries for rapid diagnosis of *E. coli* O157 and other Shiga toxin-producing *E. coli* infections.[61] Serologic antibody testing is useful for epidemiologic studies but not for diagnosis of acute disease, especially in endemic areas where the majority of the population is seropositive from prior exposure.[62]

TREATMENT AND PROGNOSIS

Antimicrobial therapy is the cornerstone of treatment for shigellosis. In the absence of effective antimicrobial therapy, mortality due to *Shigella* infection is appreciable, especially from infection with *S. dysenteriae* type 1, which has been associated with a mortality rate in excess of 10%, particularly in the young and the elderly.[63] Although *S. sonnei* is generally a mild, self-limited infection in developed countries, infection with any *Shigella* species can be lethal in the malnourished or immunocompromised patient in developing countries. However, antimicrobial therapy given within 72 hours of symptoms not only brings prompt resolution of the dysenteric symptoms but also prevents the more serious complications of the infection.[64] All persons who have dysentery and presumed *Shigella* infection should therefore be treated with an appropriate antimicrobial agent when first seen; the results of culture and susceptibility testing, if available, can then be used to modify the initial therapy if necessary.

To be useful in the treatment of shigellosis in the tropics, an antimicrobial agent should be active in vitro against the infecting strain of *Shigella;* should be safe for use in children under 5 years of age, who are the target for the majority of *Shigella* infections; preferably can be administered orally; should be demonstrated to be efficacious in controlled trials; and is inexpensive.[65] Because of the increasing prevalence of multiple drug–resistant strains, selection of an appropriate agent has become increasingly difficult. The older oral agents chloramphenicol and tetracycline are no longer effective because of the high prevalence of resistance. For the same reason, trimethoprim-sulfamethoxazole and ampicillin, until recently the drugs of choice for the treatment of shigellosis, are no longer useful in most developing countries.[66] Some drugs that are effective in vitro, such as oral extended-spectrum cephalosporins (e.g., cefixime), are ineffective in vivo,[67] as are nonabsorbable agents, such as furazolidone, despite advertising claims to the contrary.

Thus, current options for treating *Shigella* infections in the tropics are limited (Table 19-1). Oral agents shown to be effective in clinical trials against multiply resistant strains are nalidixic acid (to which most strains of *S. dysenteriae* type 1 but not *S. flexneri* are now resistant), the fluoroquinolones such as ciprofloxacin and others, the β-lactam agent pivamdinocillin,[68] and azithromycin.[69] The parenteral agent ceftriaxone has also shown efficacy, even when given for just 2 days.[70] The major concern with the recommendation of ceftriaxone for severe disease due to resistant strains is that the drug may not be available in the community, will be more expensive than established oral drugs, and requires parenteral administration. The overall guiding principles in the choice of an agent for shigellosis in developing countries include availability, cost, and the pattern of resistance in the community. Short-course (3-day) ciprofloxacin, shown to be effective, can therefore reduce the costs of treatment.[71] The danger is the selection of resistance if the drug is overly and indiscriminately used.[72] If shigellosis is suspected on the basis of clinical findings, empiric antimicrobial treatment is recommended. If the patient does not improve within 48 hours, then infection with a *Shigella* strain resistant to the drug being used or infection with another organism should be suspected, and therapy changed to an appropriate alternative agent. It is essential to know the resistance pattern in each geographic area to devise an empirical strategy of first- and second-line drugs, and this requires a surveillance system with an adequate testing laboratory, neither of which may be available in developing countries.

Because patients with shigellosis are rarely severely dehydrated, intravenous rehydration is not necessary. Oral rehydration therapy is generally sufficient to reverse the mild-to-moderate dehydration that may occur. Severe hyponatremia can be treated IV with either normal saline, or if close monitoring is available, a 3% NaCl solution. Administration of 12 mL/kg body weight of the latter will raise the serum sodium concentration by 10 mmol/L. The danger is that rapid correction of hyponatremia can be accompanied by central nervous system complications.

Patients with shigellosis should be fed to the extent they are willing to eat (breast milk or solid foods, depending on age) to prevent acute hypoglycemia as well to militate against the development or aggravation of malnutrition. Feeding may be limited because of diminished appetite, at least until the infection is controlled with antimicrobial therapy.[73]

Table 19-1 *Antimicrobial Agents for Treatment of Shigellosis in Tropical Countries*

Agent	Adult Dose	Pediatric Dose*	Frequency†	Duration	Comment
Nalidixic acid	500 mg	15 mg/kg	4 times daily	5 days	Most strains of *Shigella dysenteriae* type 1 now resistant.
Pivamdinocillin	400 mg	25 mg/kg	4 times daily	5 days	Not widely available, generic name is pivmecillinam outside the United States.
Fluoroquinolones	‡	10 mg/kg	Twice daily	3 days	Not approved for use in children in some countries; risk of toxicity in children is small when used in standard dose and duration.
Azithromycin	500 mg on day 1; 250 mg thereafter	10 mg/kg on day 1; 5 mg/kg thereafter	Once daily	5 days	Clinical trials have not been conducted in children.
Trimethoprim-sulfamethoxazole	160 mg trimethoprim–800 mg sulfamethoxazole	4 mg/kg trimethoprim – 20 mg/kg sulfamethoxazole	Twice daily	5 days	Most *Shigella flexneri* and *S. dysenteriae* type 1 strains are resistant.
Ampicillin	500 mg	25 mg/kg	4 times daily	5 days	Most *S. flexneri* and *S. dysenteriae* type 1 strains in tropical countries are resistant.

*Maximum pediatric dose is adult dose.
†Single-dose therapy with ciprofloxacin 1 g, or norfloxacin 800 mg, is effective for non–*S. dysenteriae* type 1 infections.
‡Ciprofloxacin (500 mg), norfloxacin (400 mg), and enoxacin (200 mg) have all been found to be effective in clinical trials.

Restoration of nutritional status is most rapidly achieved if a high-calorie, preferably high-quality protein-rich diet can be provided during convalescence. But, because it takes considerably longer to replenish nutrient stores than it does to create the deficit during infection, the parents of a child recovering from shigellosis must be encouraged to feed their child more than normal during the prolonged convalescent period, until satisfactory weight gain has occurred.

Treatment of complications of disease is largely supportive. Patients with seizures do not need anticonvulsant therapy, since more than one seizure is uncommon.[46] Where readily available, anticonvulsants are often given before the cause of the seizure becomes apparent. Patients with HUS may require both transfusions and peritoneal dialysis. Even with these interventions, mortality from *S. dysenteriae*–associated HUS remains higher than in HUS associated with other infections.[74,75] Whether this is because the underlying infection is more severe or because facilities for managing these complications in areas where *S. dysenteriae* type 1 outbreaks occur are often poor, or both, is uncertain. Toxic megacolon can be associated with a mortality rate as high as 50%.[47] Colectomy, which may be necessary in treating megacolon due to ulcerative colitis in developed countries, is rarely an option in developing countries because long-term care for a child with a colectomy usually is unavailable. If perforation occurs in this setting, simple surgical repair and primary closure in two layers plus aggressive fluid therapy are recommended. Rectal prolapse will resolve on its own as the infection wanes; in the interim, the prolapsed tissues should be kept moist and protected against injury. Suspected bacteremia or sepsis should be treated with parenteral, broad-spectrum antibiotics.

PREVENTION AND CONTROL

Because of the importance of person-to-person transmission and the low inoculum requirement, the primary method of preventing *Shigella* infections is good personal hygiene. Caretakers of children should wash their hands after defecating and after caring for infants who have defecated, and always before preparing food.[70] Hand washing with soap is preferred, but if soap is not available in a village setting then traditional practice of washing with an abrasive substance (e.g., sand or ash) or even with water alone is better than not washing. In addition to the difficulties encountered in changing established behaviors such as inadequate hand washing, a further limitation of this approach in developing countries is that water is often not available. Although flies are not a major means of dissemination of *Shigella,* in settings with poor hygiene practices and an inadequate environmental sanitation infrastructure, fly control reduces the prevalence of infection.[76]

The other approach to prevent *Shigella* infection is immunization. However, it has proved difficult to develop safe and effective vaccines for shigellosis, in part because the key protective antigens and the mechanism of protective immunity remain unclear. Pioneering early vaccine studies demonstrated that protective immunity against shigellosis is serotype-specific. For example, when two groups of children of over 10,000 each were immunized with different streptomycin-dependent multivalent live oral vaccines, protection was documented against the serotypes and species included in the vaccine they received.[77] Clinical data in experimental human shigellosis models support this concept, as previous infection protects against reinfection with the same *Shigella* species and serotype.[78,79] However, the specific and relative roles of humoral versus cell-mediated responses and mucosal versus systemic immunity in recovery from infection remain uncertain, hampering the development of effective vaccines. Because traditional parenteral killed vaccines have been ineffective,[80] attention has shifted to alternative approaches, including the use of oral immunization with live attenuated *Salmonella typhi* expressing *Shigella* LPS genes[78] or with live attenuated *Shigella* strains,[81] immunization with cloned virulence factors,[82] and the use of parenteral LPS-protein conjugates.[83] To date, no acceptable safe and sufficiently effective vaccine has been developed, although multiple approaches have been tried. On the basis of its role in severe disease in the rhesus monkey model,[39] a simple approach to protect against HUS due to *S. dysenteriae* type 1 or Shiga toxin–producing *E. coli* infections would be to immunize against the toxins involved, using simple toxoids or more complex, genetically inactivated toxin molecules or subunits.[84] Such a vaccine should also decrease the incidence of HUS due to *S. dysenteriae* type 1, as well as Shiga toxin–producing *E. coli*, but this remains to be demonstrated.

REFERENCES

1. Keusch GT, Bennish ML: Shigellosis. In Evans AS, Brachman PS (eds): Bacterial Infections of Humans, 3rd ed. New York, Plenum Press, 1998.
2. Kotloff KL, Winickoff JP, Clemens JD, et al: Global burden of *Shigella* infections: Implications for vaccine development and implementation of control strategies. Bull WHO 77:651–666, 1999.
3. Mead P, Slutsker L, Griffin PM, et al: Food-related illness and death in the United States. Emerg Infect Dis 5:607–625, 1999.
4. Guerrant RL, Kosek M, Moore S, et al: Magnitude and impact of diarrheal diseases. Arch Med Res 33:351–355, 2002.
5. Goma Epidemiology Group: Public health impact of Rwandan refugee crisis: What happened in Goma, Zaire, in July 1994? Lancet 345:339–344, 1995.
6. Shiga K: Ueber den Dysenterie-Bacillus (*Bacillus dysenteriae*). Zentralbl Bakteriol Orig 24:913–918, 1898.
7. Banish LD, Sims R, Sack D, et al: Prevalence of shigellosis and other enteric pathogens in a zoolgic collection of primates. J Am Vet Med Assoc 203:126–132, 1993.
8. Lan R, Reeves PR: *Escherichia coli* in disguise: Molecular origins of *Shigella*. Microbes Infect 4:1125–1132, 2002.
9. DuPont HL, Levine MM, Hornick RB, et al: Inoculum size in shigellosis and implications for expected mode of transmission. J Infect Dis 159:1226–1228, 1989.
10. Levine OS, Levine MM: Houseflies (*Musca domestica*) as mechanical vectors of shigellosis. Rev Infect Dis 13:688–696, 1991.
11. Sack DA, Hoque AT, Huq A, et al: Is protection against shigellosis induced by natural infection with *Pleisiomonas shigelloides?* Lancet 343:1413–1415, 1994.
12. Rahman MM, Kabir I, Mahalanabis D, et al: Decreased food intake in children with severe dysentery due to *Shigella dysenteriae* 1 infection. Eur J Clin Nutr 46:833–838, 1992.
13. Huskins WC, Griffiths JK, Faruque AS, et al: Shigellosis in neonates and young infants. J Pediatr 125:14–22, 1994.
14. Christianson KA: Toxic megacolon complicating shigellosis. J R Coll Surg Edinb 32:109–110, 1987.
15. Hamadani JD, Azad MT, Chowdhury JJ, et al: Intestinal perforation in a child with *Shigella dysenteriae* type 1 infection: A rare complication. J Diarrhoeal Dis Res 12:225–226, 1994.
16. Struelens MJ, Pate D, Kabir I, et al: *Shigella* septicemia: Prevalence, presentation, risk factors, and outcome. J Infect Dis 152:784–790, 1985.
17. Khan WA, Dhar U, Salam MA, et al: Central nervous system manifestations of childhood shigellosis: Prevalence, risk factors, and outcome. Pediatrics 103:E18, 1999.

18. Bennish ML: Potentially lethal complications of shigellosis. Rev Infect Dis 13(suppl 4):S319–S324, 1991.
19. Koster F, Levin J, Walker L, et al: Hemolytic-uremic syndrome after shigellosis: Relation to endotoxemia and circulating immune complexes. N Engl J Med 298:927–933, 1978.
20. Lopez EL, Contrini MM, Devoto S, et al: Incomplete hemolytic-uremic syndrome in Argentinean children with bloody diarrhea. J Pediatr 127:364–367, 1995.
21. Kosek M, Black RE, Keusch GT: Nutrition and micronutrients in tropical infectious diseases. In Guerrant RL, Walker DH, Weller PF (eds): Tropical Infectious Diseases, 2nd ed. Philadelphia, Churchill Livingstone, 2005, Chapter 5.
22. Bennish ML, Salam MA, Wahed MA: Enteric protein loss during shigellosis. Am J Gastroenterol 88:53–57, 1993.
23. Ahmed F, Ansaruzzaman M, Haque E, et al: Epidemiology of postshigellosis persistent diarrhea in young children. Pediatr Infect Dis J 20:525–530, 2001.
24. Bhagwat AA, Bhagwat M: Comparative analysis of transcriptional regulatory elements of glutamate-dependent acid-resistance systems of *Shigella flexneri* and *Escherichia coli* 0157:H7. FEMS Microbiol Lett 234:139–147, 2004.
25. Small P, Blankenhorn D, Welty D, et al: Acid and base resistance in *Escherichia coli* and *Shigella flexneri:* Role of rpoS and growth pH. J Bacteriol 176:1729–1737, 1994.
26. Fernandez MI, Sansonetti PJ: Effector molecules of *Shigella* pathogenesis and host responses. In Hecht GA (ed): Microbial Pathogenesis and the Intestinal Epithelial Cell. Washington, DC, ASM Press, 2003, Chapter 25.
27. Fleckenstein JM, Kopecko DJ: Breaching the mucosal barrier by stealth: An emerging pathogenic mechanism for enteroadherent bacterial pathogens. J Clin Invest 107:27–30, 2001.
28. Girardin SE, Sansonetti PJ, Philpott DJ: Intracellular vs extracellular recognition of pathogens—common concepts in mammals and flies. Trends Microbiol 10:193–199, 2002.
29. Maurelli AT: *Shigella* inside and out: Lifestyles of the invasive and dysenteric. ASM News 58:603–608, 1992.
30. Perdomo JJ, Cavaillon JM, Huerre M, et al: Acute inflammation causes epithelial invasion and mucosal destruction in experimental shigellosis. J Exp Med 180:1307–1319, 1994.
31. Zychlinsky A, Prevost MC, Sansonetti PJ: *Shigella flexneri* induces apoptosis in infected macrophages. Nature 358:167–169, 1992.
32. Zychlinsky A, Kenny B, Menard R, et al: IpaB mediates macrophage apoptosis induced by *Shigella flexneri.* Mol Microbiol 11:619–627, 1994.
33. Zychlinsky A, Fitting C, Cavaillon JM, et al: Interleukin-1 is released by murine macrophages during apoptosis induced by *Shigella flexneri.* J Clin Invest 94:1328–1332, 1994.
34. Jung HC, Eckmann L, Yang SK, et al: A distinct array of proinflammatory cytokines is expressed in human colon epithelial cells in response to bacterial invasion. J Clin Invest 95:55–65, 1995.
35. Perdomo JJ, Guonon P, Sansonetti PJ: Polymorphonuclear leukocyte transmigration promotes invasion of colonic epithelial monolayer by *Shigella flexneri.* J Clin Invest 93:633–643, 1994.
36. Wright SD, Ramos RA, Hermanowski-Vosatka A, et al: Activation of the adhesive capacity of CR3 on neutrophils by endotoxin: Dependence on lipopolysaccharide binding protein and CD14. J Exp Med 173:1281–1286, 1991.
37. Sansonetti PH, Arondel J, Cavaillon J-M, et al: Role of interleukin-1 in the pathogenesis of experimental shigellosis. J Clin Invest 96:884–892, 1995.
38. Renesto P, Mounier J, Sansonetti PJ: Induction of adherence and degranulation of polymorphonuclear leukocytes: A new expression of the invasive phenotype of *Shigella flexneri.* Infect Immun 64:719–723, 1996.
39. Mandi-Mulec I, Weiss J, Zychlinsky A: *Shigella flexneri* is trapped in polymorphonuclear leukocyte vacuoles and efficiently killed. Infect Immun 65:110–115, 1997.
40. Smith JA: Neutrophils, host defense, and inflammation: A double edged sword. J Leukocyte Biol 56:672–686, 1994.
41. Bernardini ML, Mounier J, d'Hautville H, et al: Identification of *icsA,* a plasmid locus of *Shigella flexneri* that governs bacterial intra- and intercellular spread through interaction with F-actin. Proc Natl Acad Sci USA 86:3867–3871, 1989.
42. Kadurugamuwa JL, Rohde M, Wehland J, et al: Intercellular spread of *Shigella flexneri* through a monolayer mediated by membranous protrusions and associated with reorganization of the cytoskeletal protein vinculin. Infect Immun 59:3463–3471, 1991.
43. Prevost MC, Lesourd M, Arpin M, et al: Unipolar reorganization of F-actin layer at bacterial cell division and bundling of actin filaments by plastin correlate with movement of *Shigella flexneri* within HeLa cells. Infect Immun 60:4088–4099, 1992.
44. Goldberg MB, Parsot C, Barzu O, et al: Unipolar localization and ATPase activity of IcsA, a *Shigella flexneri* protein involved in intracellular movement. J Bacteriol 175:2189–2196, 1993.
45. Sandlin RC, Lampel KA, Keasler SP, et al: Avirulence of mutants of *Shigella flexneri:* Requirement of O antigen for correct unipolar localization of IcsA in the bacterial outer membrane. Infect Immun 63:229–237, 1995.
46. Sandlin RC, Goldberg MB, Maurelli AT: Effect of O side-chain length and composition on the virulence of *Shigella flexneri* 2a. Mol Microbiol 22:63–73, 1996.
47. Vasselon T, Mounier J, Hellio R, et al: Movement along actin filaments of the perijunctional area and de novo polymerization of cellular actin are required for *Shigella flexneri* colonization of epithelial Caco-2 cell monolayers. Infect Immun 60:1031–1040, 1992.
48. Sansonetti PJ, Mounier J, Prevost MC, et al: Cadherin expression is required for the spread of *Shigella flexneri* between epithelial cells. Cell 76:829–839, 1994.
49. Allaoui A, Mounier J, Prevost MC, et al: *IcsB:* An *S. flexneri* gene necessary for the lysis of protrusions during intracellular spread. Mol Microbiol 6:1605–1616, 1992.
50. Acheson DW, Kane AV, Keusch GT: Shiga toxins. Methods Mol Biol 145:41–63, 2000.
51. Fontaine A, Arondel J, Sansonetti PJ: Role of Shiga toxin in the pathogenesis of bacillary dysentery studied using a tox^- mutant of *Shigella dysenteriae* I. Infect Immun 56:3099–3109, 1988.
52. Karmali MA, Petric M, Lim C, et al: The association between idiopathic hemolytic uremic syndrome and infection by Verocytotoxin-producing *Escherichia coli.* J Infect Dis 151:775–782, 1985.
53. Townes JM, Quick R, Gonzales OY, et al: Etiology of bloody diarrhea in Bolivian children: Implications for empiric therapy. J Infect Dis 175:1527–1530, 1997.
54. Speelman P, McGlaughlin R, Kabir I, et al: Differential clinical features and stool findings in shigellosis and amoebic dysentery. Trans R Soc Trop Med Hyg 81:549–551, 1987.
55. Ronsmans C, Bennish ML, Wierzba T: Diagnosis and management of dysentery by community health workers. Lancet 2:552–555, 1988.
56. Albert MJ, Ansaruzzaman M, Alim AR, et al: Fluorescent antibody test for rapid diagnosis of *Shigella dysenteriae* type 1 infection. Diagn Microbiol Infect Dis 15:359–361, 1992.
57. Islam D, Linberg AA: Detection of *Shigella dysenteriae* type 1 and *Shigella flexneri* in feces by immunomagnetic isolation and polymerase chain reaction. J Clin Microbiol 30:2801–2806, 1992.
58. Islam D, Tzipori S, Islam M, et al: Rapid detection of *Shigella dysenteriae* and *Shigella flexneri* in faeces by an immunomagnetic assay with monoclonal antibodies. Eur J Clin Microbiol Infect Dis 12:25–32, 1993.
59. Oberhelman RA, Kopecko DJ, Venkatesan MM, et al: Evaluation of alkaline phosphatase–labeled ipaH probe for diagnosis of *Shigella* infections. J Clin Microbiol 31:2101–2104, 1993.
60. Echeverria P, Sethabutr O, Pitarangsi C: Microbiology and diagnosis of infections with *Shigella* and enteroinvasive *E. coli.* Rev Infect Dis 13(suppl 4):S220–S225, 1991.
61. Kehl KS, Havens P, Behnke CE, et al: Evaluation of the premier EHEC assay for detection of Shiga toxin–producing *Escherichia coli.* J Clin Microbiol 35:2051–2054, 1997.
62. Cam PD, Pal T, Lindberg AA: Immune response against lipopolysaccharide and invasion plasmid encoded antigens of shigellae in Vietnamese and Swedish dysentery patients. J Clin Microbiol 31:454–457, 1993.
63. Bennish ML, Wojtyniak BJ: Mortality due to shigellosis: community and hospital data. Rev Infect Dis 13(suppl 4):S245–S251, 1991.
64. Bennish ML, Levy S: Antimicrobial resistance of enteric pathogens. In Blaser MJ, Smith PD, Ravdin JI, et al (eds): Infections of the Gastrointestinal Tract. New York, Raven Press, 1995, pp 1499–1523.
65. Bennish ML, Salam MA: Rethinking options for the treatment of shigellosis. J Antimicrob Chemother 30:243–247, 1992.
66. Sack RB, Rahman M, Yunus M, et al: Antimicrobial resistance in organisms causing diarrheal disease. Clin Infect Dis 24 (suppl 1): S102–S105, 1997.
67. Salam MA, Seas C, Khan WA, et al: Treatment of shigellosis. 4. Cefixime is ineffective in shigellosis in adults. Ann Intern Med 123:505–508, 1995.

68. Ekwall M, Jonsson M: A comparison of the combination pivmecillinam/pivampicillin and cotrimoxazole in the treatment of convalescent carriers of *Salmonella* and *Shigella*. Scand J Infect Dis 16:99–102, 1984.
69. Khan WA, Seas C, Dhar U, et al: Treatment of shigellosis: 5. Comparison of azithromycin and ciprofloxacin: A double-blind, placebo-controlled, randomized clinical trial. Ann Intern Med 126:697–703, 1997.
70. Eidlitz-Marcus T, Cohen YH, Nussinovitch M, et al: Comparative efficacy of two- and five-day courses of ceftriaxone for treatment of severe shigellosis in children. J Pediatr 123:822–824, 1993.
71. The Zimbabwe, Bangladesh, South Africa (Zimbasa) Dysentery Study Group: Multicenter, randomized, double blind clinical trial of short course versus standard course oral ciprofloxacin for *Shigella dysenteriae* type 1 dysentery in children. Pediatr Infect Dis J 21:1136–1141, 2002.
72. Ashkenazi S, Levy I, Kazaronovski V, et al: Growing antimicrobial resistance of Shigella isolates. J Antimicrob Chemother 51427–429, 2003.
73. Molla AM, Molla AM: Effect of antibiotics on food intake and absorption of nutrients for children with diarrhea due to *Shigella*. Rev Infect Dis 13(suppl 4):S347–S350, 1991.
74. Nathoo KJ, Sanders JA, Siziya S, et al: Haemolytic uraemic syndrome following *Shigella dysenteriae* type 1 outbreak in Zimbabwe: A clinical experience. Cent Afr J Med 41:267–274, 1995.
75. Chopra M, Wilkinson D, Stirling S: Epidemic shigella dysentery in children in northern Kwazulu-Natal. S Afr Med J 87:48–51, 1997.
76. Cohen D, Green M, Block C, et al: Reduction of transmission of shigellosis by control of houseflies (*Musca domestica*). Lancet 337:993–997, 1991.
77. Mel D, Gangarosa EJ, Radovanovic ML, et al: Studies on vaccination against bacillary dysentery. 6. Protection of children by oral immunization with streptomycin-dependent *Shigella* strains. Bull World Health Organ 45:457–464, 1971.
78. DuPont HL, Hornick RB, Snyder MJ, et al: Immunity in shigellosis. 2. Protection induced by oral live vaccine or primary infection. J Infect Dis 125:12–16, 1972.
79. Herrington DA, Van de Verg L, Formal SB, et al: Studies in volunteers to evaluate candidate *Shigella* vaccines: Further experience with a bivalent *Salmonella typhi–Shigella sonnei* vaccine and protection conferred by previous *Shigella sonnei* disease. Vaccine 8:353–357, 1990.
80. Formal SB, Hale TL, Kapfer C: *Shigella* vaccines. Rev Infect Dis 11(suppl 3):S547–S551, 1989.
81. Phalipon A, Sansonetti P: Live attenuated *Shigella flexneri* mutants as vaccine candidates against shigellosis and vectors for antigen delivery. Biologicals 23:125–134, 1995.
82. Turbyfill KR, Hartman AB, Oaks EV: Isolation and characterization of a Shigella flexneri invasin complex subunit vaccine. Infect Immun 68:6624–6632, 2000.
83. Cohen D, Ashkenazi S, Green MS, et al: Double-blind vaccine-controlled randomised efficacy trial of an investigational *Shigella sonnei* conjugate vaccine in young adults. Lancet 349:155–159, 1997.
84. Acheson DW, Levine MM, Kaper JB, et al: Protective immunity to Shiga-like toxin I following oral immunization with Shiga-like toxin I B-subunit-producing *Vibrio cholerae* CVD 103-HgR. Infect Immun 64:355–357, 1996.

20

Campylobacter *Infections*

BAN MISHU ALLOS
MARTIN J. BLASER

INTRODUCTION

Campylobacters are bacteria that often produce an acute gastrointestinal illness. Infections with these organisms occur in every part of the world, including arctic, temperate, and tropical climates.[1] In developing countries, especially those in tropical areas, they are hyperendemic and important causes of morbidity and possibly mortality in young children. *Campylobacter* infections also are an important cause of diarrhea in persons residing in developed countries who travel to developing countries in the tropics.[2,3]

AGENT

Campylobacter species are microaerophilic, comma-shaped, gram-negative rods that were first recognized as causes of infectious abortion in animals in the early twentieth century[4] and later were determined also to cause infectious abortion in women.[5] Over the next decades, the organisms were reported to cause bacteremia, meningitis, endocarditis, and abscesses in immunocompromised patients.[6,7] A group of related organisms also were isolated from the blood of patients with diarrhea.[8] During the last three decades of the twentieth century, campylobacters were recognized as one of the most common bacterial causes of diarrhea worldwide.

Although the organisms were first called *Vibrio*, they were assigned to a new genus, *Campylobacter,* in 1973[9]; this scheme was later modified so that the opportunistic organism was called *Campylobacter fetus*, and the related vibrios were called *Campylobacter jejuni* and *Campylobacter coli*.[10] In 2000, the complete genome of *Campylobacter jejuni* was sequenced.[11]

The use of filtration with antibiotic-free culture systems[12] and other newer techniques[13,14] have led to the recognition that many other "atypical" species of *Campylobacter* and closely related genera also may produce human disease[15] (Table 20-1). Such species include *C. fetus*, *Campylobacter upsaliensis*, *Campylobacter hyointestinalis*, *Campylobacter lari*, *Helicobacter cinaedi*, *Helicobacter fennelliae*, *Arcobacter cryaerophila*, *Arcobacter butzleri*, *Campylobacter jejuni* subspecies *doyleii*, *Campylobacter concisus*, *Campylobacter mucosalis*, *Campylobacter rectus*, and *Campylobacter sputorum*. New pathogenic species of *Campylobacter* are being identified with some regularity.

In tropical countries such as South Africa, such "atypical" campylobacters comprise more than 50% of the *Campylobacter* species isolated.[16–18] In contrast, in the United States and other developed nations, *C. jejuni* accounts for greater than 95% of *Campylobacter* species isolated.[19] Other studies of *Campylobacter*, in Thailand,[20] Hong Kong,[21] and the Central African Republic,[22] show a higher incidence of *C. coli* relative to that seen in industrialized nations. However, since methods designed to optimize detection of *C. jejuni* might not support growth of other species, the contribution of these organisms to the burden of human disease may be underestimated.

Campylobacters grow best at the body temperatures of warm-blooded animals. Optimal growth for *C. jejuni* is at 42°C at which campylobacters will survive only a few days, but at 4°C they can persist for weeks in substances such as water, feces, urine, or milk.[23] Similarly, the organism may flourish and grow in an alkaline environment but will not last 5 minutes at pH less than 2.3.[23]

EPIDEMIOLOGY

The epidemiology of *Campylobacter* infections is markedly different in tropical developing countries than in the developed world (Table 20-2). Infections are hyperendemic among young children. In tropical countries such as Bangladesh, South Africa, The Gambia, Zaire, India, Australia, Indonesia, and China, the rate of isolation of *Campylobacter* is greatest in infants and declines with age.[24] Although national surveillance programs for campylobacteriosis do not exist in developing countries, estimates from laboratory-based surveillance suggest that the incidence of this infection among children less than 5 years of age may be more than 100 times higher than the rate among children in developed nations.[25] Campylobacters frequently can be isolated from asymptomatic children and adults in developing countries.[26] In contrast, in developed countries, infection is almost always recognized in association with illness, recognized asymptomatic infections are uncommon, and young children are not at greatest risk.

In the developing nations mentioned previously, breastfed children are usually protected, but a high rate of infection with concomitant watery diarrhea is observed after they are weaned.[27] In addition to early weaning, close proximity to animals and lack of toilets are important risk factors for the development of early-childhood diarrheal illnesses in general, and those caused by *Campylobacter* in particular.[25,28] The apparent absence of multiple infections within a household[29] suggests that person-to-person transmission is not an important mode of spread, even in developing countries. Infections in adults and older children usually are asymptomatic and durations of excretion are short, suggesting that acquired immunity is protective. The importance of acquired protective immunity is further supported by studies in developing countries showing that rising serum antibodies to *Campylobacter* are associated with a lower rate of infection.[30,31]

Outbreaks of *Campylobacter* infection, which occur regularly in developed countries, do not occur in developing countries because of this high level of immunity. Campylobacters are ubiquitous in the environment in tropical climates and infections occur year-round. The late summer and early fall peak in the incidence of *Campylobacter* infections observed in temperate climates is not seen in tropical countries.[24,26,32]

Table 20-1 *Clinical and Epidemiologic Features Associated with "Atypical" Campylobacters and Related Organisms*

Species	Clinical Presentation	Epidemiologic Data
C. coli	Fever, diarrhea, abdominal pain	Clinically and epidemiologically similar to *C. jejuni*
C. fetus	Bacteremia, sepsis, meningitis, vascular infection, abortion	Found in healthy sheep and cattle; may cause spontaneous abortion and infertility
C. upsaliensis	Watery diarrhea, low-grade fever, abdominal pain	Found in dogs, cats; may have autumn seasonality in tropical countries
C. lari	Abdominal pain, diarrhea	Seagulls colonized; transmitted to human via contaminated water
C. hyointestinalis	Watery or bloody diarrhea, vomiting, abdominal pain	Causes proliferative enteritis in swine
H. fennelliae, H. cinaedi	Chronic mild diarrhea, proctitis, abdominal cramps	Increased in homosexual men and in children in developing countries; may cause bacteremia in HIV+ hosts
C. jejuni subspecies *doylei*	Diarrhea	Role as a human pathogen not established
A. cryaerophila	Diarrhea, rarely bacteremia	Isolated from mussels in brackish water
A. butzleri	Fever, diarrhea, abdominal pain, nausea; rarely bacteremia	Enzootic in nonhuman primates
C. sputorum	Pulmonary, axillary, groin, and perianal abscesses	Has been isolated from dairy cows
H_2-requiring campylobacters*	Periodontitis; less commonly, diarrhea	Role as a human pathogen not established
H. pullorum	Uncommon human pathogen; occasionally associated with diarrhea, rarely bacteremia	Isolated from asymptomatic hens and from hens with hepatitis
H. rappini	Gastroenteritis; few case reports document bacteremia	Animal reservoir not known

*Includes *C. rectus*, *C. curvus*, and *C. concisus*.

Although rotavirus, enterotoxigenic *Escherichia coli*, and *Shigella* infections are more common than *Campylobacter* as causes of diarrhea in tropical countries,[28,33,34] campylobacters are the most common bacterial cause of community-acquired diarrhea in developed countries.[35,36] However, even in developing countries, *Campylobacter* infections are increasing and in some areas surpassing *Shigella* and *E. coli* as causes of diarrhea.[37] Furthermore, the prevalence of *Campylobacter* infections is higher in tropical climates than in cooler ones. Even among healthy, asymptomatic children in countries such as Bangladesh, South Africa, The Gambia, and Central African Republic, *Campylobacter* may be isolated from 10% to 40% of children

Table 20-2 *Clinical and Epidemiologic Characteristics of* Campylobacter *Infections in Developed versus Tropical Developing Countries*

Characteristic	Developed Countries	Developing Countries
Peak age group affected	15–29 yr	<2 yr
Endemicity of infection	Endemic	Hyperendemic
Occurrence of outbreaks	Common	Rare
Seasonality	Summer and fall peaks	Year-round
Predominant mode of transmission	Food-borne	Uncertain
Clinical expression	Inflammatory	Noninflammatory
Asymptomatic infection	Uncommon	Usual
Nature of diarrhea	Inflammatory*	Watery
Abdominal cramps	Common	Rare
Bacterial load in stools of infected persons	High	Low
Presence of immunity in typical adult	No	Yes

*Stools frequently contain gross or occult blood, and leukocytes.

from a single culture.[26,29,38–40] *Campylobacter* infection is one of the most common causes of diarrhea among travelers to developing countries[41] and in Thailand is the most common cause.[31,42]

Most human infections with *Campylobacter* in developing countries occur because of consumption of or exposure to animals or their products. Campylobacters live as commensals in the gastrointestinal tract of a variety of animals, especially avian species. Not surprisingly, campylobacters are frequently isolated from poultry and other animals in developing countries,[43–48] but the extent of the contribution of this source to human illness has not been determined.[49] In Africa, campylobacters also have been isolated from surface domestic water sources used for human consumption[50] and from diary products.[51] The main vehicles of human infection in developed countries are water, milk, raw meat, and most importantly, poultry. Person-to-person transmission of *Campylobacter* is infrequent in both developed and developing countries.

DISEASE

In developing countries, the clinical consequences of infection with *Campylobacter* differ from those seen in the developed world. When children in tropical settings develop diarrhea as a result of *Campylobacter* infection, it frequently is watery and there usually is little or no evidence of an inflammatory process.[52] Although symptomatic infection is most likely to occur during the first few months and years of life, asymptomatic infections outnumber symptomatic ones by 2 to 1, even among children less than 5 years of age.[53] Infection among children in tropical countries is quite common; more than two infections per year are likely during the first 5 years of life.[29,53] Among young children in Bangladesh, the estimated rate is eight *Campylobacter* infections per year.[26]

In developed areas, *Campylobacter* infections usually produce an acute gastrointestinal illness that is indistinguishable from illness caused by other "inflammatory" enteric bacteria such as *Salmonella* and *Shigella*. Illness usually begins abruptly with abdominal cramps and diarrhea. Children in developing countries who develop symptomatic *Campylobacter* infection also typically experience loose stools with mucus, along with fever and vomiting.[54] However, although half of *Campylobacter*-infected patients presenting for medical attention in developed countries have bloody diarrhea,[35] in tropical climates the diarrhea usually does not contain blood. Less than one third of *Campylobacter*-infected children in Thailand have bloody stools; most have mucoid stools that are neither watery nor bloody; about one third have watery diarrhea.[20,54] *Campylobacter* infection among persons living in tropical areas also are less likely to produce abdominal cramps.[26] The illness usually resolves within 1 to 2 weeks; about 20% of patients will have relapsing symptoms lasting several weeks. Although *Campylobacter* infections occur frequently in HIV-infected persons residing in developed countries,[55] a similar phenomenon is not always observed in developing nations.[56–58]

Complications of *Campylobacter* infections are rare and usually the result of local invasion. Massive gastrointestinal hemorrhage may occur. Other complications include cholecystitis, pancreatitis, obstructive hepatitis, and splenic rupture.[59–62] Neonatal sepsis and death can occur if the mother is infected during the third trimester.[63] Extraintestinal complications of *Campylobacter* infections are rare[64] but are more common in malnourished children. Such complications include bacteremia, meningitis, and purulent arthritis. Infection may lead to fulminant sepsis and death. The postinfection complication, Guillain-Barré syndrome (GBS), occurs at an estimated rate of 1 per 2000 infections.[65] A particularly severe form of GBS, acute motor axonal neuropathy, occurs in seasonal epidemics among children in rural China and also may be associated with preceding *C. jejuni* infection.[66] Reactive arthritis also may occur after *Campylobacter* infection and is most common in persons who carry the HLA-B27 phenotype.[67–69] *C. jejuni* was recently implicated as a cause of immunoproliferative small intestine disease (a form of lymphoma) in a 45-year-old woman in Cameroon.[70]

In patients in developed countries, the pathologic lesion of *Campylobacter* enteritis is infiltration of the lamina propria with acute and chronic inflammatory cells and destruction of epithelial glands with crypt abscess formation.[71] The site of tissue injury is usually the jejunum, ileum, and colon.[71,72] This nonspecific colitis may be indistinguishable from ulcerative colitis or Crohn's disease; hence the importance of diagnosing this treatable infection before immunosuppressive therapy is given for inflammatory bowel disease. The pathology of *Campylobacter* enteritis among patients in tropical and developing countries has not been well described but, based on the clinical presentation, is presumably milder.

PATHOGENESIS AND IMMUNITY

Three factors important in the ability of *Campylobacter* to produce illness include the dose of organisms reaching the small intestine, the host's immunity to the organism, and the virulence of the particular strain. Infection leads to multiplication of the organism in the intestine. The number of bacterial cells required to cause illness is unknown, but a high dose is likely needed to infect 50% of subjects.[73] In general, the higher the inoculum, the shorter the incubation period (usually 1 day to 1 week) and the higher the attack rate.

In developed countries, *Campylobacter*-infected persons shed between 10^6 and 10^9 colony-forming units (CFU) per gram of stool.[23] However, the intestinal bacterial load is lower among similarly infected persons in developing nations.[30] Furthermore, in developing areas, the duration and number of organisms excreted are highest in infants and decline with age, also consistent with increasing acquisition of immunity.[54]

Characteristics of campylobacters that enable them to adhere to and invade intestinal cells include the presence of flagella, high-molecular-weight plasmids, superficial adhesins, fimbriae, and chemotactic factors.[73–80,81] Campylobacters must be flagellated to colonize, invade, and cause disease.[82] Although the bacteria do not possess fimbriae per se, fimbriae-like filaments enable the organisms to attach to epithelial cells.[83] Additionally, several *C. jejuni* surface proteins (e.g., PEB1, CadF) appear to function in attachment and subsequent colonization and invasion.[83] Invasion of epithelial cells by *C. jejuni* results in cellular injury and, ultimately, in diarrhea. The mechanism of invasion is complex and not completely understood.[84]

Despite early reports to the contrary,[85] the low level of enterotoxin production that occasionally has been observed

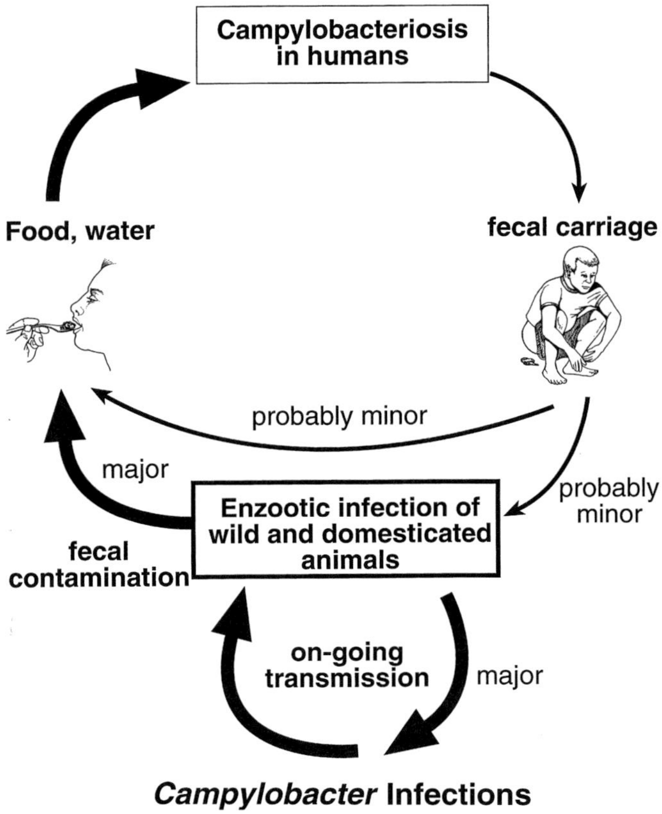

in vitro does not appear to be important in the pathogenesis of *Campylobacter* infections.[81,86] Enterotoxin production cannot be demonstrated in vivo, and infected patients do not form antibodies against enterotoxin.[87] All *C. jejuni* isolates possess a gene that codes for cytolethal distending toxin; however, not all isolates produce this toxin, and its role in causing disease is not established.[88]

Specific immunity to *Campylobacter* may be acquired. In developing countries where these infections are hyperendemic, infection and illness rates decline with age, again suggesting the acquisition of immunity. Volunteer studies also have shown that short-term specific immunity to *Campylobacter* occurs.[73,89] Humoral immunity appears to play an important role in containing *Campylobacter* infection. After infection, serum antibodies (IgA, IgG, and IgM) peak in 2 to 4 weeks, then rapidly decline.[90] The importance of humoral immunity is further supported by studies showing that in hypogammaglobulinemic patients, *Campylobacter* infections are severe, prolonged, and difficult to eradicate.[91] Children in tropical settings develop steadily rising serum IgA antibodies to *Campylobacter*. Once these high levels are achieved, IgG levels, which also rise through early childhood, begin to decline.[54,92,93] These data suggest that frequent exposure to *Campylobacter* leads to the development of solid "gut immunity," which precludes sensitization of IgG-producing cells. Such gut immunity correlates well with the declining incidence of infection with age, the lower proportion of infections that are symptomatic, and the reduced bacterial level and duration of excretion.[54]

Persons with human immunodeficiency virus (HIV) infection have more frequent, persistent, severe, and extraintestinal *Campylobacter* infections than the general population in developed nations.[94,95] Although these observations could suggest that cellular immunity also plays an important role in protection against *Campylobacter*, many such patients have defects in humoral responses as well.

Serum killing of *Campylobacter* species occurs via complement-mediated bactericidal activity.[96] This could explain why bacteremia due to *Campylobacter* species is uncommon except in immunodeficient persons, or is due to the serum-resistant *C. fetus*.[96] Serum-resistant campylobacters have been isolated from the cerebrospinal fluid of patients with meningitis.[97]

DIAGNOSIS

In developing countries, the simplest and most inexpensive method for diagnosis of *Campylobacter* infection is direct examination of stools after Gram or Wright staining. Stools also can be directly examined for the presence of white blood cells or lactoferrin and erythrocytes, which are nonspecific findings associated with inflammatory agents but that also suggest the presence of a bacterial enteric pathogen, such as *Campylobacter*.

The gold standard for detection of *Campylobacter* infection is culture of the organism from stool, blood, or other site of infection. Because *Campylobacter* infection cannot be differentiated from infections due to other bacterial enteric pathogens on clinical grounds, isolation of the organism using a selective technique is the only way to make the diagnosis with certainty. Cephalothin-containing selective media will suppress most fecal flora while permitting the growth of most *C. jejuni* strains. However, some *Campylobacter* species (and even a few *C. jejuni* strains) are cephalothin-susceptible, and must be isolated on less selective media or on antibiotic-free media after filtration of the stool sample. In tropical countries, many patients may have mixed infections with *Campylobacter* and other enteric pathogens.[20,54] Therefore, the precise contribution of *Campylobacter* infection to these children's illnesses may be difficult to assess.

Campylobacter infection also may be mistaken for inflammatory bowel disease. *Campylobacter* enterocolitis may produce crypt abscesses (which are frequent in ulcerative colitis) and granulomas (which are common in Crohn's disease).[71,72,98] Persons suspected of having inflammatory bowel disease should have cultures for several different *Campylobacter* species performed as part of their diagnostic workup.

Serologic testing occasionally may be useful for detecting recent *Campylobacter* infection.[96,99] However, this technique is unlikely to be helpful in tropical developing countries where infection is hyperendemic and background infection rates are high. Polymerase chain reaction (PCR) to detect *Campylobacter* in stools is beginning to be used in some clinical laboratories in developed nations.[100,101] However, the clinical significance of a positive PCR assay in a patient in a developing country might be difficult to interpret and the costs associated with such testing preclude wide usage.

TREATMENT AND PROGNOSIS

Antimicrobial treatment of *Campylobacter* infections, if initiated early in the illness, reduces the duration of bacterial excretion in stools.[102,103] However, most patients with *Campylobacter* enteritis, and certainly those with asymptomatic or mild infection, do not need antimicrobial therapy. Even patients whose symptoms lead them to seek medical care may not require measures other than encouragement to keep well hydrated. Occasionally, intravenous fluids are needed, especially in the very young and very old. In developing countries, oral hydration solutions are the best method of maintaining fluid and electrolyte balance, unless volume depletion is severe. The prognosis for most patients with *Campylobacter* infection is favorable; symptoms usually resolve within 1 week without antimicrobial therapy.

Antibiotics should be given to *Campylobacter*-infected patients in certain high-risk groups or clinical circumstances. Because *Campylobacter* infection may have deleterious effects on the fetus, pregnant women should receive prompt therapy.[63] Similarly, HIV-infected or other immunocompromised patients should receive antibiotics. With the expanding HIV epidemic in developing countries, extraintestinal infection will be increasingly common. Immunocompetent persons with fever greater than 38.3°C (101°F), bloody stools, symptoms lasting more than 1 week, or worsening symptoms also may benefit from antimicrobial therapy.

Campylobacters are susceptible to a wide variety of antimicrobial agents, including macrolides, quinolones, nitrofurans, and aminoglycosides. Care should be taken before prescribing tetracycline because more than 20% of campylobacters are resistant.[104,105] Susceptibility to ampicillin, metronidazole, and trimethoprim-sulfamethoxazole is variable. There is almost universal resistance of *Campylobacter* to cephalosporins, penicillin, vancomycin, and rifampin.

Erythromycin remains the treatment of choice for most patients with infections due to *Campylobacter*. Erythromycin has low toxicity, has a relatively narrow spectrum of activity, and is inexpensive. Because erythromycin stearate is incompletely absorbed, it can exert a local effect throughout the bowel, in addition to its systemic effects. In most developed countries, the rate of erythromycin resistance among *Campylobacter* species has remained under 10%.[106–108] Higher rates of resistance have been reported from developing countries, such as Thailand,[33] but resistance remains low in other countries, such as India and Kenya.[109–110] The rate of erythromycin resistance is substantially higher among *C. coli* strains.[105,111–113] The newer macrolides, azithromycin and clarithromycin, have excellent activity against *Campylobacter*.[114–117] Although they achieve higher concentrations in tissue, they provide little clinical advantage over erythromycin and are considerably more expensive. Strains resistant to erythromycin also will be resistant to these newer macrolides. The activity of clindamycin against *C. jejuni* is equivalent to that of erythromycin.

At one time, it appeared that quinolones, such as ciprofloxacin, had emerged as the treatment of choice for bacterial diarrhea in general and for *Campylobacter* enteritis in particular.[118] Unfortunately, rapidly emerging resistance of campylobacters to quinolones in tropical regions and in other parts of the world has limited their effectiveness.[103,119,120] Widespread use of fluoroquinolones in poultry has led to the transfer of antibiotic-resistant strains to humans.[121–122] Nalidixic acid resistance commonly but not invariably crosses with resistance to ciprofloxacin.[105] Resistance to this agent has paralleled the increasing resistance to fluoroquinolones.

In special circumstances when therapy is required, and when a patient is intolerant of many agents or when a strain has an unusual antibiotic resistance pattern, alternative agents such as chloramphenicol may be used; nearly all campylobacters are susceptible to chloramphenicol.[105,123] This agent is especially useful in tropical developing countries because of its low cost. For persons with bacteremia and other extraintestinal suppurative infections, gentamicin and imipenem are active against campylobacters and the rate of resistance to these agents is less than 1%. Gentamicin is ineffective against *Campylobacter* in the gut; therefore, oral therapy with an effective, absorbable drug also must be given.

PREVENTION AND CONTROL

Campylobacters are so ubiquitous in the environment of most tropical developing nations that there is no possibility of reducing the reservoirs of infection. Rather, prevention must focus on interrupting the path of transmission to humans from animals, animal products, or environmental sources contaminated by animals or humans. Poultry, livestock, pets, and wild animals are the major reservoirs. Therefore, as for many bacterial enteric pathogens, a basic tenet of prevention is adequate hand washing; this is especially important in tropical areas for people who handle animals and food within a household. Especially important is the awareness of the necessity for proper cooking and storage of foods of animal origin.

The safe disposal of sewage and the protection and purification of water supplies also are fundamental to control of most diseases due to enteric pathogens, including *Campylobacter*. Programs to improve water safety in developing countries may impact the number of infections.[124] Excreta from sheep, cattle, and wild and domestic birds should not be allowed to contaminate a community's water supplies. Chlorination reliably inactivates *Campylobacter*.[125]

Control of *Campylobacter* infections in developing countries will likely be difficult unless an effective vaccine is developed. Because of the diversity of serotypes of *C. jejuni*, the possibility of vaccination for prevention of infection must be based on group antigens. Since *Campylobacter* infection of humans is "accidental" given that humans are not required for completion of their life cycle, the natural acquisition of immunity in developing countries and the identification of group antigens suggest that vaccination will be feasible. There is no proven benefit of antibiotic prophylaxis to prevent *Campylobacter* infection in travelers to tropical and subtropical environments.

REFERENCES

1. Nachamkin I: Campylobacter and Arcobacter. In Murray PR, Baron EJ, Pfaller MA, et al (eds): Manual of Clinical Microbiology. Washington, DC, American Society for Microbiology 1995, pp. 483–491.
2. Gallardo F, Gascon J, Ruiz J, et al: *Campylobacter jejuni* as a cause of traveler's diarrhea: clinical features and antimicrobial susceptibility. J Travel Med 5:23–26, 1998.
3. Shlim DR, Hoge CW, Rajah R, et al: Persistent high risk of diarrhea among foreigners in Nepal during the first 2 years of residence. Clin Infect Dis 29:613–616, 1999.
4. MacFadyean F, Stockman S: Report of the Department Committee Appointed by the Board of Agriculture and Fisheries to Inquire into Epizootic Abortion. Vol. 3. London, HMSO, 1909 (abstract).
5. Vinzent R, Dumas J, Picard N: Septicemie grave au cours de la grossesse due a un vibrion: avortement consecutive. Bull Acad Natl Med 131:90–93, 1947.
6. Bokkenheuser V: *Vibrio fetus* infection in man. 1. Ten new cases and some epidemiologic observations. Am J Epidemiol 91:400–409, 1970.

7. Franklin B, Ulmer DD: Human infection with *Vibrio fetus*. West J Med 120:200–204, 1974.
8. King EO: Human infections with *Vibrio fetus* and a closely related *vibrio*. J Infect Dis 101:119–129, 1957.
9. Vernon M, Chatlain R: Taxonomic study of the genus Campylobacter (Sebald and Vernon) and designation of the neotype strain for the type species. *Campylobacter fetus* (Smith and Taylor) Sebald and Vernon. Int J Syst Bacteriol 23:122–134, 1973.
10. Smibert RM: The genus Campylobacter. Ann Rev Microbiol 32:700–773, 1978.
11. Parkhill J, Wren BW, Mungall K, et al: The genome sequence of the food-borne pathogen *Campylobacter jejuni* reveals hypervariable sequences. Nature 403:665–668, 2000.
12. Megraud F, Elharrif Z: Isolation of Campylobacter species by filtration. Eur J Clin Microbiol 4:437–438, 1985.
13. Lastovica AJ, LeRoux E: Efficient isolation of *Campylobacter upsaliensis* from stools. J Clin Microbiol 39:4222–4223, 2001.
14. Burnens AP, Nicoleg J: Three supplementary diagnostic tests for Campylobacter species and related organisms. J Clin Microbiol 31:708–710, 1994.
15. Lastovica AJ, Skirrow MB: Clinical significance of Campylobacter and related species other than *Campylobacter jejuni* and *C. coli*. In Nachamkin I, Blaser MJ (eds): Campylobacter, 2nd ed. Washington DC, ASM Press, 2000, pp. 89–120.
16. Lastovica A, Engel ME, Blaser MJ: Atypical campylobacters and related organisms. In Blaser MJ, Smith PD, Ravdin JI, et al (eds): Infections of the Gastrointestinal Tract. Philadelphia, Lippincott, Williams and Wilkins, 2002, pp. 741–762.
17. Lastovica AJ, Le Roux E: Prevalence and distribution of Campylobacter spp. in the diarrhoeic stools and blood cultures of pediatric patients. Acta Gastroenterol Belg 56:34, 1993.
18. Le Roux E, Lastovica AJ: The Cape Town Protocol: how to isolate the most campylobacters for your dollar, pound, franc, yen, etc. In Lastovica AJ, Newell DG, Lastovica EE (eds): Proceedings of the 9th International Workshop on Campylobacter, Helicobacter and Related Organisms. Cape Town, South Africa, September 15–19, 1997. Cape Town, Institute of Child Health, 1998, pp. 30–33.
19. Tauxe RV: Epidemiology of *Campylobacter jejuni* infections in the United States and other industrialized nations. In Nachamkin I, Blaser MJ, Tompkins LS (eds): *Campylobacter jejuni*—Current Strategy and Future Trends. Washington DC, American Society of Microbiology, 1992, pp. 9–19.
20. Taylor DN, Echeverria P, Pitarangsi C, et al: The influence of strain characteristics and immunity on the epidemiology of Campylobacter infections in Thailand. J Clin Microbiol 26:863–868, 1988.
21. Ho BSW, Wong WT: A one-year survey of Campylobacter enteritis and other forms of bacterial diarrhea in Hong Kong. J Hyg 94:55–60, 1985.
22. Georges-Courbot MC, Baya C, Beraud AM, et al: Distribution and serotypes of *Campylobacter jejuni* and *Campylobacter coli* in enteric Campylobacter strains isolated from children in the Central African Republic. J Clin Microbiol 23:592–594, 1986.
23. Blaser MJ, Hardesty HL, Powers B, et al: Survival of *Campylobacter fetus* subsp. *jejuni* in biological milieus. J Clin Microbiol 11:309–313, 1980.
24. Oberhelman RA, Taylor DN: Campylobacter infections in developing countries. In Nachamkin I, Blaser MJ (eds): Campylobacter, 2nd ed. Washington DC, ASM Press, 2000, pp. 139–153.
25. Coker AO, Isokpehi RD, Thomas BN, et al: Human Campylobacteriosis in developing countries. Emerg Infect Dis 8:237–243, 2002.
26. Glass RI, Stoll BJ, Huq MI, et al: Epidemiology and clinical features of endemic *Campylobacter jejuni* infection in Bangladesh. J Infect Dis 148:292–296, 1983.
27. Megraud F, Boudraa G, Bessaoud K, et al: Incidence of Campylobacter infection in infants in western Algeria and the possible protective role of breast feeding. Epidemiol Infect 105:73–78, 1990.
28. Guerrant RL, Kirchhoff LV, Shields DS, et al: Prospective study of diarrheal illnesses in northeastern Brazil: patterns of disease, nutritional impact etiologies, and risk factors. J Infect Dis 148:986–997, 1983.
29. Blaser MJ, Glass RI, Imdadul Hugh M, et al: Isolation of *Campylobacter fetus* subsp. *jejuni* from Bangladeshi children. J Clin Microbiol 12:744–747, 1980.
30. Taylor DN, Perlman DM, Echeverria PD, et al: Campylobacter immunity and quantitative excretion rates in Thai children. J Infect Dis 168:754–758, 1993.
31. Walz SE, Baqar S, Beecham HJ, et al: Pre-exposure anti-*Campylobacter jejuni* immunoglobulin A levels associated with reduced risk of Campylobacter diarrhea in adults traveling to Thailand. Am J Trop Med Hyg 65:652–656, 2001.
32. Georges MC, Wachsmuth IK, Meunier DM, et al: Parasitic, bacterial and viral enteric pathogens associated with diarrhea in the Central African Republic. J Clin Microbiol 19:571–575, 1984.
33. Oyofo BA, Subekti D, Tjaniadi P, et al: Enteropathogens associated with acute diarrhea in community and hospital patients in Jakarta, Indonesia. FEMS Immunol Med Microbiol 34:139–146, 2002.
34. Brooks JT, Shapiro RL, Kumar L, et al: Epidemiology of sporadic bloody diarrhea in rural Western Kenya. Am J Trop Med Hyg 68:671–677, 2003.
35. Blaser MJ, Wells JG, Feldman RA, et al: The Collaborative Diarrhea Disease Study Group: *Campylobacter* enteritis in the United States: a multicenter study. Ann Intern Med 98:360–365, 1983.
36. MacDonald KL, O'Leary MJ, Cohen ML, et al: *Escherichia coli* O157: H7, an emerging gastrointestinal pathogen. JAMA 259:3567–3570, 1988.
37. Bodhidatta L, Vithayasai N, Eimpokalarp B, et al: Bacterial enteric pathogens in children with acute dysentery in Thailand: increasing importance of quinolone-resistant Campylobacter. Southeast Asian J Trop Med Pub Health 33:752–757, 2002.
38. Bokkenheuser VD, Richardson NJ, Bryner JH, et al: Detection of enteric campylobacteriosis in children. J Clin Microbiol 9:227–232, 1979.
39. Georges-Courbot MC, Beraud-Cassel AM, Gouandjim I, et al: Prospective study of enteric Campylobacter infections in children from birth to 6 months in the Central African Republic. J Clin Microbiol 23:592–594, 1987.
40. Billingham JD: Campylobacter enteritis in The Gambia. Trans R Soc Trop Med Hyg 75:641–644, 1981.
41. DuPont HL, Ericsson CD: Drug therapy: prevention and treatment of traveler's diarrhea. N Engl J Med 328:1821–1827, 1993.
42. Sanders JW, Isenbarger DW, Walz SE, et al: An observational clinic-based study of diarrheal illness in deployed United States military personnel in Thailand: presentation and outcome of *Campylobacter* infection. Am J Trop Med Hyg 67:533–538, 2002.
43. Coker AO, Isokpehi RD, Thomas BN, et al: Zoonotic infections in Nigeria: overview from a medical perspective. Acta Trop 76:59–63, 2000.
44. Raji MA, Adekeye JO, Kwaga JK, et al: Bioserogroups of Campylobacter species isolated from sheep in Kaduna State, Nigeria. Small Rumin Res 37:215–221, 2000.
45. Osano O, Arimi SM: Retail poultry and beef as sources of *Campylobacter jejuni*. East Afr Med J 76:141–143, 1999.
46. Quinones-Ramirez EI, Vazquez-Salinas C, Rodas-Suarez OR, et al: Frequency of isolation of *Campylobacter* from roasted chicken samples from Mexico City. J Food Prot 63:117–119, 2000.
47. Aquino MHC, Pacheco APG, Ferreira MCS, et al: Frequency of isolation and identification of thermophilic campylobacters from animals in Brazil. Vet J 164:159–161, 2002.
48. Harvey SA, Winch PJ, Leontsini E, et al: Domestic poultry-raising practices in a Peruvian shantytown: implications for control of *Campylobacter jejuni*-associated diarrhea. Acta Tropica 86:41–54, 2003.
49. Oberhelman RA, Gilman RH, Sheen P, et al: *Campylobacter* transmission in a Peruvian shantytown: a longitudinal study using strain typing of Campylobacter isolates from chickens and humans in household clusters. J Infect Dis 187:260–269, 2003.
50. Obi CL, Potgieter N, Bessong PO, et al: Scope of potential bacterial agents of diarrhea and microbial assessment of quality of river water sources in rural Venda communities in South Africa. Water Sci Tech 47:59–64, 2003.
51. Vaishnavi C, Singh S, Singh K: Bacterial profile of dairy products in Chandigarh. Trop Gastroenterol 23:72–75, 2002.
52. Taylor DN: Campylobacter infections in developing countries. In Nachamkin I, Blaser MJ, Tompkins LS (eds): *Campylobacter jejuni*—Current Strategy and Future Trends. Washington DC, American Society of Microbiology, 1992, pp. 20–30.
53. Calva JJ, Ruiz-Palacioz GM, Lopez-Vidal AB, et al: Cohort study of intestinal infection with campylobacter in Mexican children. Lancet 1:503–506, 1988.
54. Blaser MJ, Black RE, Duncan DJ, et al: *Campylobacter-jejuni*-specific serum antibodies are elevated in Bangladeshi children. J Clin Microbiol 21:146–147, 1985.

55. Snijders F, Kuijper EJ, de Wever B, et al: Prevalence of Campylobacter-associated diarrhea among patients infected with Human Immunodeficiency Virus. Clin Infect Dis 24:1107–1113, 1997.
56. Awole M, Gebre-Selassie S, Kassa T, et al: Isolation of potential bacterial pathogens from the stool of HIV-infected and HIV-non-infected patients and their antimicrobial susceptibility patterns in Jimma Hospital, south west Ethiopia. Ethiopian Med J 40:353–364, 2002.
57. Gwavava C, Chihota VN, Gangaidzo IT, et al: Dysentery in patients infected with human immunodeficiency virus in Zimbabwe: an emerging role for *Schistosoma mansoni* and *Escherichia coli* O157? Ann Trop Med Parasitol 95:509–513, 2001.
58. Germani Y, Minssart P, Vohito M, et al: Etiologies of acute, persistent, and dysenteric diarrheas in adults in Bangui, Central African Republic, in relation to Human Immunodeficiency Virus serostatus. Am J Trop Med Hyg 59:1008–1014, 1998.
59. Pitkanen T, Ponka A, Petersson T, et al: Campylobacter enteritis in 188 hospitalized patients. Arch Intern Med 143:215–219, 1983.
60. Gerritsen van der Hoop A, Veringa EM: Cholecystitis caused by *Campylobacter jejuni*. Clin Infect Dis 17:133, 1993.
61. Ezpeleta C, de Ursua PR, Obregon F, et al: Acute pancreatitis associated with *Campylobacter jejuni* bacteremia. Clin Infect Dis 15:1050, 1992.
62. Wood CJ, Fleming V, Turridge J, et al: *Campylobacter* peritonitis in continuous ambulatory peritoneal dialysis: report of eight cases and a review of the literature. Am J Kidney Dis 19:257–263, 1992.
63. Simor AE, Ferro S: *Campylobacter jejuni* infection occurring during pregnancy. Eur J Clin Microbiol Infect Dis 9:142–144, 1990.
64. Skirrow MB, Jones DM, Sutcliffe E, et al: *Campylobacter* bacteremia in England and Wales, 1981–91. Epidemiol Infect 110:567-573, 1993.
65. Mishu B, Blaser MJ: Role of infection due to *Campylobacter jejuni* in the initiation of Guillain-Barré syndrome. Clin Infect Dis 17:104–108, 1993.
66. Ho TW, Mishu B, Li CY, et al: Guillain-Barré syndrome in northern China. Relationship to *Campylobacter jejuni* infection and anti-glycolipid antibodies. Brain 118:597–605, 1995.
67. Gumpel JM, Martin C, Sanderson PJ: Reactive arthritis associated with *Campylobacter* enteritis. Ann Rheum Dis 40:64–65, 1981.
68. Bremell T, Bjelle A, Svedhem A: Rheumatic symptoms following an outbreak of *Campylobacter* enteritis: a five year follow-up. Ann Rheum Dis 50:934–938, 1991.
69. Rautelin H, Koota K, von Essen R, et al: Waterborne *Campylobacter jejuni* epidemic in a Finnish hospital for rheumatic diseases. Scand J Infect Dis 22:321–326, 1990.
70. Lecuit M, Abachin E, Martin A, et al: Immunoproliferative small intestine disease associated with *Campylobacter jejuni*. N Engl J Med 350:239–248, 2004.
71. Blaser MJ, Parsons RB, Wang WLL: Acute colitis caused by *Campylobacter fetus* ss. *jejuni*. Gastroenterol 78:448–453, 1980.
72. Price AB, Jewkes J, Sanderson PJ: Acute diarrhea: *Campylobacter* colitis and the role of rectal biopsy. J Clin Pathol 32:990–997, 1979.
73. Black RE, Levine MM, Clements ML, et al: Experimental *Campylobacter jejuni* infection in humans. J Infect Dis 157:474–479, 1988.
74. Caldwell MB, Guerry P, Lee EC, et al: Reversible expression of flagella in *Campylobacter jejuni*. Infect Immun 50:941–943, 1985.
75. Grant CCR, Konkel ME, Cleplak W, et al: Role of flagella in adherence, internalization, and translocation of *Campylobacter jejuni* in nonpolarized and polarized epithelial cell cultures. Infect Immun 61:1764–1771, 1993.
76. Yao R, Burr DH, Doig P, et al: Isolation of motile and non-motile insertional mutants of *Campylobacter jejuni*: the role of motility in adherence and invasion of eukaryotic cells. Mol Microbiol 14:883–893, 1994.
77. Bacon DJ, Alm RA, Burr DH, et al: Involvement of a plasmid in virulence of *Campylobacter jejuni*. Infect Immun 68:4384–4390, 2000.
78. Pei Z, Burucoa C, Grignon B, et al: Mutation in the *peb1A* locus of *Campylobacter jejuni* reduces interactions with epithelial cells and intestinal colonization of mice. Infect Immun 66:938–943, 1998.
79. Yao R, Burr DH, Guerry P: CheY-mediated modulation of *Campylobacter jejuni* virulence. Mol Microbiol 23:1021–1031, 1997.
80. Doig P, Yao R, Burr DH, et al: An environmentally regulated pilus-like appendage involved in *Campylobacter* pathogenesis. Mol Microbiol 20:885–894, 1996.
81. Wassenaar TM, Blaser MJ: Pathophysiology of *Campylobacter jejuni* infections in humans. Microbes Infect:1:1023–1033, 1999.
82. Wassenaar TM, Bleumink-Pluym NMC, Van DerZeijst BAM: Inactivation of *Campylobacter jejuni* flagellin genes by homologous recombination demonstrates that *flaA* but not *flaB* is required for invasion. EMBO J 10:2055–2061, 1991.
83. Doig P, Yao R, Burr DH, et al: An environmentally regulated pilus-like appendage involved in *Campylobacter* pathogenesis. Mol Microbiol 20:885–894, 1996.
84. Hu L, Kopecko DJ: Interactions of Campylobacter with eukaryotic cells: gut luminal colonization and mucosal invasion mechanisms. In Nachamkin I, Blaser MJ (eds): Campylobacter, 2nd ed. Washington DC, ASM Press, 2000, pp. 191–215.
85. Lindblom GB, Johny M, Khalil K, et al: Enterotoxigenicity and frequency of *Campylobacter jejuni*, *C. coli*, and *C. laridis* in human and animal stool isolates from different countries. FEMS Microbiol Lett 54:163–168, 1990.
86. Wassenaar TM: Toxin production by *Campylobacter* spp. Rev Clin Microbiol 10:466–476, 1997.
87. Perez-Perez GI, Taylor DN, Echeverria PD, et al: Lack of evidence of enterotoxin involvement in pathogenesis of *Campylobacter* diarrhea. In Nachamkin I, Blaser MJ, Tompkins LS (eds): *Campylobacter jejuni*—Current Strategy and Future Trends. Washington DC, American Society of Microbiology, pp. 184–192, 1992.
88. Pickett CL, Pesci EC, Cottle DL, et al: Prevalence of cytolethal distending toxin production in *Campylobacter jejuni* and relatedness of *Campylobacter* sp *cdtB* genes. Infect Immun 64:2070–2078, 1996.
89. Black RE, Perlman D, Clements ML, et al: Human volunteer studies with *Campylobacter jejuni*. In Nachamkin E, Blaser MJ, Tompkins LS (eds): *Campylobacter jejuni*—Current Strategy and Future Trends. Washington DC, American Society of Microbiology, pp. 207–215, 1992.
90. Blaser MJ, Duncan D: Human serum antibody response to *Campylobacter jejuni* infection as measured in an enzyme-linked immunosorbent assay. Infect Immun 44:292–298, 1984.
91. Melamed I, Bujanover Y, Igra YS, et al: *Campylobacter* enteritis in normal and immunodeficient children. Am J Dis Child 137:752–753, 1983.
92. Blaser MJ, Taylor DN, Echeverria P: Immune response to *Campylobacter jejuni* in a rural community in Thailand. J Infect Dis 153:249–254, 1986.
93. Blaser MJ, Black RE, Duncan DJ, et al: *Campylobacter jejuni*–specific antibodies are elevated in healthy Bangladeshi children. J Infect Dis 151:227–235, 1985.
94. Sorvillo FJ, Lieb LE, Waterman SH: Incidence of campylobacteriosis among patients with AIDS in Los Angeles County. J Acquir Immune Defic Syndr Hum Retrovirol 4:598–602, 1991.
95. Tee W, Mijch A: *Campylobacter jejuni* bacteremia in Human Immunodeficiency Virus (HIV)-infected and non-HIV-infected patients: comparison of clinical features and review. Clin Infect Dis 26:91–96, 1998.
96. Blaser MJ, Smith PF, Kohler PA: Susceptibility of *Campylobacter* isolates to the bactericidal activity in human serum. J Infect Dis 151:227–235, 1985.
97. Blaser MJ, Perez GP, Smith PF, et al: Extraintestinal *Campylobacter jejuni* and *Campylobacter coli* infections: host factors and strain characteristics. J Infect Dis 153:552–559, 1986.
98. Surawicz CM, Belic L: Rectal biopsy helps to distinguish acute self-limited colitis from idiopathic inflammatory bowel disease. Gastroenterol 86:104–113, 1984.
99. Mishu B, Patton CM, Blaser MJ: Microbiologic characteristics of *Campylobacter jejuni* strains isolated from patients with Guillain-Barré syndrome (abstract). Clin Infect Dis 17:538, 1993.
100. Maher M, Finnegan C, Collins E, et al: Evaluation of culture methods and a DNA probe-based PCR assay for detection of *Campylobacter* species in clinical specimens of feces. J Clin Microbiol 41:2980–2986, 2003.
101. Kulkarni SP, Lever S, Logan JM, et al: Detection of campylobacter species: a comparison of culture and polymerase chain reaction based methods. J Clin Pathol 55: 749–753, 2002.
102. Goodman LJ, Trenholme GM, Kaplan RL, et al: Empiric antimicrobial therapy of domestically acquired acute diarrhea in urban adults. Arch Intern Med 150:541–546, 1990.
103. Petruccelli BP, Murphy GS, Sanchez JL, et al: Treatment of traveler's diarrhea with ciprofloxacin and loperamide. J Infect Dis 165:557–560, 1992.

104. Vanhoof R, Vanderlinden MP, Dierickx R, et al: Susceptibility of *Campylobacter fetus* subsp. *jejuni* to twenty-nine antimicrobial agents. Antimicrob Agents Chemother 14:553–556, 1978.
105. Reina J, Ros MJ, Serra A: Susceptibilities to 10 antimicrobial agents of 1,220 *Campylobacter* strains isolated from 1987 to 1993 from feces of pediatric patients. Antimicrob Agents Chemother 38:2917–2920, 1994.
106. Brunton WA, Wilson A, Macrae RM: Erythromycin-resistant campylobacters. Lancet 2:1385, 1978.
107. Taylor DE, Chang N, Garner RS, et al: Incidence of antibiotic resistance and characterization of plasmids in *Campylobacter jejuni* strains isolated from clinical sources in Alberta, Canada. Can J Microbiol 32:28–32, 1986.
108. Walder M, Forsgren A: Erythromycin-resistant campylobacters. Lancet 2:1201, 1978.
109. Prasad KN, Mathur SK, Dhole TN, et al: Antimicrobial susceptibility and plasmid analysis of *Campylobacter jejuni* isolated from diarrhoeal patients and healthy chickens in northern India. J Diarrhoeal Dis Res 12:270–273, 1994.
110. Shapiro RL, Kumar L, Phillips-Howard P, et al: Antimicrobial-resistant bacterial diarrhea in rural Western Kenya. J Infect Dis 183:1701–1704, 2001.
111. Taylor DN, Blaser MJ, Echeverria P, et al: Erythromycin-resistant *Campylobacter* infections in Thailand. Antimicrob Agents Chemother 31:438–442, 1987.
112. Speelman P, Struelens MJ, Sanyal SC, et al: Detection of *Campylobacter jejuni* and other potential pathogens in traveler's diarrhea in Bangladesh. Scand J Gastroenterol 18:19–23, 1983.
113. Hirschl AM, Wolf D, Berger J, et al: In vitro susceptibility of *Campylobacter jejuni* and *Campylobacter coli* isolated in Austria to erythromycin and ciprofloxacin. Int J Med Microbiol 272:443–447, 1990.
114. Endtz HP, Broeren M, Mouton RP: In vitro susceptibility of quinolone-resistant *Campylobacter jejuni* to new macrolide antibiotics. Eur J Clin Microbiol Infect Dis 12:48–50, 1993.
115. Kirst HA, Sides GD: New directions for macrolide antibiotics: pharmacokinetics and clinical efficacy. Antimicrob Agents Chemother 33:1419–1422, 1989.
116. Taylor DE, Chang N: In vitro susceptibilities of *Campylobacter* and *Campylobacter coli* to azithromycin and erythromycin. Antimicrob Agents Chemother 35:1917–1918, 1991.
117. Kitzis MD, Goldstein FW, Miegi M, et al: In vitro activity of azithromycin against various gram-negative bacilli and anaerobic bacteria. Antimicrob Agents Chemother 25:15–18, 1990.
118. Ruiz-Palacios GM: Norfloxacin in the treatment of bacterial enteric infections. Scand J Infect Dis 48:S55–S63, 1986.
119. Kuschner RA, Trofa AF, Thomas RJ, et al: Use of azithromycin for the treatment of *Campylobacter* enteritis in travelers to Thailand, an area where ciprofloxacin resistance is prevalent. Clin Infect Dis 21: 536–541, 1995.
120. Cardinale E, Dromigny J-A, Tall F, et al: Fluoroquinolone susceptibility of *Campylobacter* strains, Senegal. Emerg Infect Dis 9:1479–1481, 2003.
121. Smith KE, Besser JM, Hedberg CW, et al: Quinolone-resistant *Campylobacter jejuni* infections in Minnesota, 1992–1998. N Engl J Med 340:1525–1532, 1999.
122. Allos BM, Blaser MJ: *Campylobacter* species. In Yu VL, Weber, Raoult (eds): Antimicrobial Therapy and Vaccines, 2nd ed. New York, Apple Trees Productions, 2002, pp. 169–171.
123. Sagara H, Mochizuki A, Okamura N, et al: Antimicrobial resistance of *Campylobacter jejuni* and *Campylobacter coli* with special reference to plasmid profiles of Japanese clinical isolates. Antimicrob Agents Chemother 31:713–719, 1987.
124. Quick RE, Venczel LV, Mintz ED, et al: Diarhoea prevention in Bolivia through point-of-use water treatment and safe storage: a promising new strategy. Epidemiol Infect 122:83–90, 1999.
125. Blaser MJ, Smith PF, Wang WLL, et al: Inactivation of *Campylobacter jejuni* by chlorine and monochloramine. Appl Environ Microbiol 51:307–311, 1986.

21

Cholera Infections

MYRON M. LEVINE
EDUARDO GOTUZZO
SAMBA O. SOW

INTRODUCTION

Cholera is a diarrheal illness caused by *Vibrio cholerae* O1 (and less often by serogroup O139), which in its severe form, cholera gravis, can rapidly and fatally dehydrate adults as well as children. Besides its clinical severity in the individual patient, cholera is one of the few bacterial diseases that is capable of true pandemic spread. Since 1961, when the seventh pandemic caused by *V. cholerae* O1 biotype El Tor began on the island of Sulawesi, El Tor cholera has progressively extended to involve all the inhabited continents. Since cholera is spread by contaminated water and food vehicles, its transmission is facilitated wherever populations are not served by treated water supplies and sanitation.

Several events in the last decade of the 20th century exemplify the epidemiologic and clinical importance of cholera and demonstrate why it commands special attention among practitioners of clinical and preventive tropical medicine. These events included

1. The return of cholera to Latin America in 1991, after a century of absence, and its rapid dissemination leading to more than 1 million cases by 1994[1];
2. The explosive outbreak of El Tor cholera in Rwandan refugees in Goma, Zaire, resulting in approximately 70,000 cases and 12,000 deaths in July 1994[2,3];
3. The appearance in 1992–1993 of epidemic cholera in the Indian subcontinent, caused for the first time by a *Vibrio cholerae* serogroup other than O1, so-called O139 Bengal.[4,5]

AGENT

Medical historians debate whether cholera existed in ancient populations in the Indian subcontinent and the Middle East or only emerged in the early 19th century as a new infectious disease of humans. What is incontestable is that at least seven distinct pandemics of cholera have occurred since the first was recorded in 1817. The first six pandemics originated in the Ganges delta from which they spread progressively to involve other countries and continents. During the third and fourth pandemics, John Snow made hallmark descriptions of the epidemiology of cholera, suggesting that it was a contagion and incriminating its spread via sewage-contaminated municipal water.[6] Incredibly, these insights were made several decades before Robert Koch isolated the causative bacterium in Egypt in 1883, during the fifth pandemic.[7]

In the 1950s, investigators in India demonstrated that cell-free supernatants of *V. cholerae* caused fluid accumulation in isolated loops of rabbit intestine, thereby implying the existence of an enterotoxin.[8] In the late 1960s, cholera enterotoxin was purified to homogeneity and shown to be composed of two different types of subunits noncovalently linked.[9] Also in the late 1960s, oral glucose/electrolyte solutions were shown to be effective in rehydrating patients with mild and moderate cholera, a clinical breakthrough that eventually revolutionized the therapy of diarrheal dehydration of all etiologies.[10]

V. cholerae, a motile gram-negative facultative anaerobe with a unipolar flagellum, prefers alkaline (pH 6–10), brackish (elevated sodium) environments. This chitinase-producing species comprises part of the autochthonous flora of brackish water environments where it is closely associated with zooplankton and other fauna having chitinous exoskeletons.[11] *V. cholerae* is a well-defined species based on biochemical tests and DNA homology studies,[12] but one that is not homogeneous with regard to the potential to cause epidemic human disease. Taxonomists currently recognize more than 200 serogroups of *V. cholerae*. Within the species, an important discrimination exists among strains with respect to the production of cholera enterotoxin (CT), O serogroup, and the potential for epidemic spread. Prior to 1992, only enterotoxigenic *V. cholerae* within the O1 serogroup were recognized as the etiologic agents of endemic and epidemic cholera. Within the O1 serogroup, there exist two main serotypes, Inaba and Ogawa, and two biotypes, classical and El Tor.[12] Whereas either biotype can cause the spectrum of clinical manifestations from asymptomatic infection to cholera gravis, the ratio of mild to severe cases is higher for the El Tor biotype. Characteristics that differentiate the El Tor biotype include a resistance to polymyxin B, ability to agglutinate chicken erythrocytes, and a susceptibility to specific typing phages. El Tor tend to be much hardier than classical biotype vibrios and survive better in the environment and in the intestine of humans. Even as *V. cholerae* El Tor has spread worldwide for almost 4 decades in the form of the seventh cholera pandemic, classical biotype *V. cholerae* persisted in the Ganges delta, along with El Tor, throughout much of this time.

V. cholerae O1 strains can shift between Inaba and Ogawa, with the change more often going from Ogawa to Inaba.[12] DNA sequence analysis of genes (*rfb*) encoding the O1 antigen reveals that the sequences for Inaba and Ogawa antigens are almost identical and that some serotype shifts are the consequence of minor alterations in the sequence of *rfbT*.[13,14]

Beginning in late 1992, large-scale epidemics of typical clinical cholera caused by a serogroup other than O1 were reported in India and Bangladesh,[4,5] marking the first time that epidemic disease was attributed to another serogroup. Molecular analysis of the causative agent, so-called O139 Bengal, reveals that it possesses the identical virulence attributes and other characteristics as *V. cholerae* El Tor (e.g., sequences encoding cholera toxin and toxin coregulated pili, resistance to polymyxin).[12] It appears that the epidemic O139 strain was derived by a deletion event in the genes that encode O1 of an El Tor strain followed by the acquisition of a large fragment of new DNA encoding O139. During 1993, O139 spread to multiple other Asian countries (e.g., Thailand,

Burma, Pakistan, China) and importations were also reported in the United States and United Kingdom. At this time, it was feared that these epidemiologic events might be the harbingers of an eighth cholera pandemic with O139 as the etiologic agent. However, in 1995 and 1996 the incidence of O139 diminished in the Indian subcontinent and this serogroup disappeared from several countries that it had invaded in the previous 2 years. Since O139 disease has become endemic in Bengal, health authorities for the past decade have maintained surveillance to see whether O139 disease resurges and spreads to other continents in pandemic form.

There also exist O1 and O139 strains that do not produce CT, do not cause cholera, and are not involved in epidemics. By contrast, there are sporadic *V. cholerae* strains of serogroups other than O1 or O139 that are associated with diarrhea or other clinical syndromes such as bacteremia; however, these other serogroups do not cause explosive epidemics or have pandemic potential.

EPIDEMIOLOGY

Incidence and Geographic Distribution

A defining feature of the epidemiology of cholera viewed from a global perspective is that, because of its pandemic nature, the disease ebbs and flows across vast geographic distances over time. The Ganges delta is the ancestral home of cholera, where it has persisted in the past in interpandemic periods as "Asiatic cholera." As the seventh pandemic of El Tor cholera has progressively disseminated since the early 1960s from its origin on the island of Sulawesi in Indonesia, it has become endemic in many areas where it first appeared in epidemic form. Thus, cholera is now endemic in the Philippines; in several countries in Southeast Asia; in multiple countries in sub-Sahara Africa; and (during the 1990s) in Peru, Ecuador, and a number of other Latin American countries.

Typically, when cholera newly invades an immunologically naive population, the highest incidence is observed in young adult males. However, as the disease becomes increasingly endemic, the incidence increases in women and children; eventually, the peak incidence is found in young children.

Seasonality

In most endemic areas, cholera exhibits a seasonal pattern with months of high and low incidence.[15] When a new cholera season begins, the disease typically appears simultaneously in multiple geographically separate foci. This pattern has also been seen as cholera invades new territory. For example, in 1991 when the cholera invasion of South America began with an explosive and extensive epidemic in Peru, large outbreaks appeared almost simultaneously in three distinct cities spanning a 900-kilometer stretch along the Pacific Coast.[15]

Reservoirs of Infection

Since humans are the only known host of cholera and chronic carriers are extremely rare, it was previously assumed

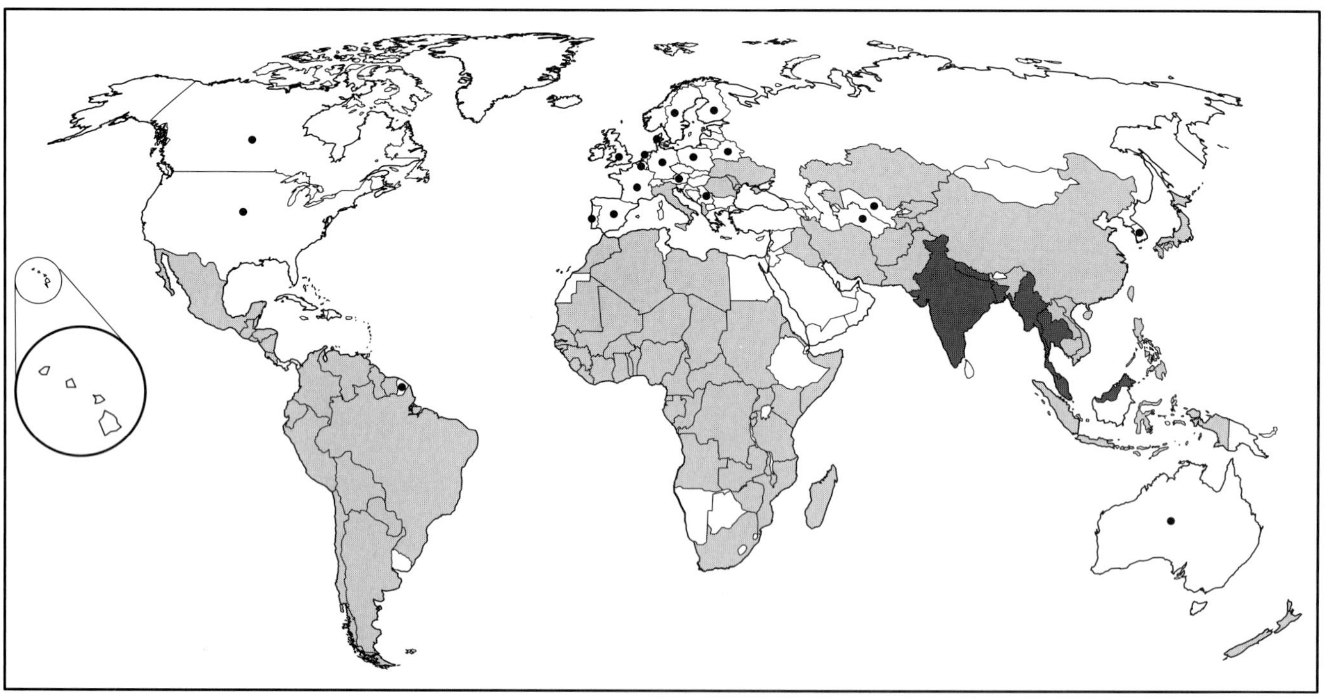

Cases of cholera since 1990

- *Vibrio cholerae* O1
- *Vibrio cholerae* O1 and/or O139
- • Imported cases only

Note: Cholera likely occurs in some unshaded areas; shaded areas show those reported to the World Health Organization between 1990 and 2003.

that in endemic areas mild and asymptomatic infections serve as the reservoir to maintain the disease until the next cholera season when conditions would once again favor enhanced transmission. However, this explanation was unable to account for a number of the epidemiologic observations. Epidemiologists' views on what might comprise the reservoirs of cholera infection underwent radical change because of a series of events in the 1980s that occurred along the Gulf of Mexico Coast of the United States. The appearance of a single case of cholera in Texas in 1973 in a fisherman caused by an unusual highly hemolytic El Tor Inaba strain[16] followed 5 years later by an outbreak of approximately two dozen cases of the identical strain in which poorly cooked seafood was incriminated as the vehicle,[17] led to the identification of an environmental focus of infection in the Gulf of Mexico. This El Tor Inaba strain was found to constitute autochthonous flora of the brackish waters of Gulf estuaries, where it was associated with shrimp and other crustacea eaten as local seafood.

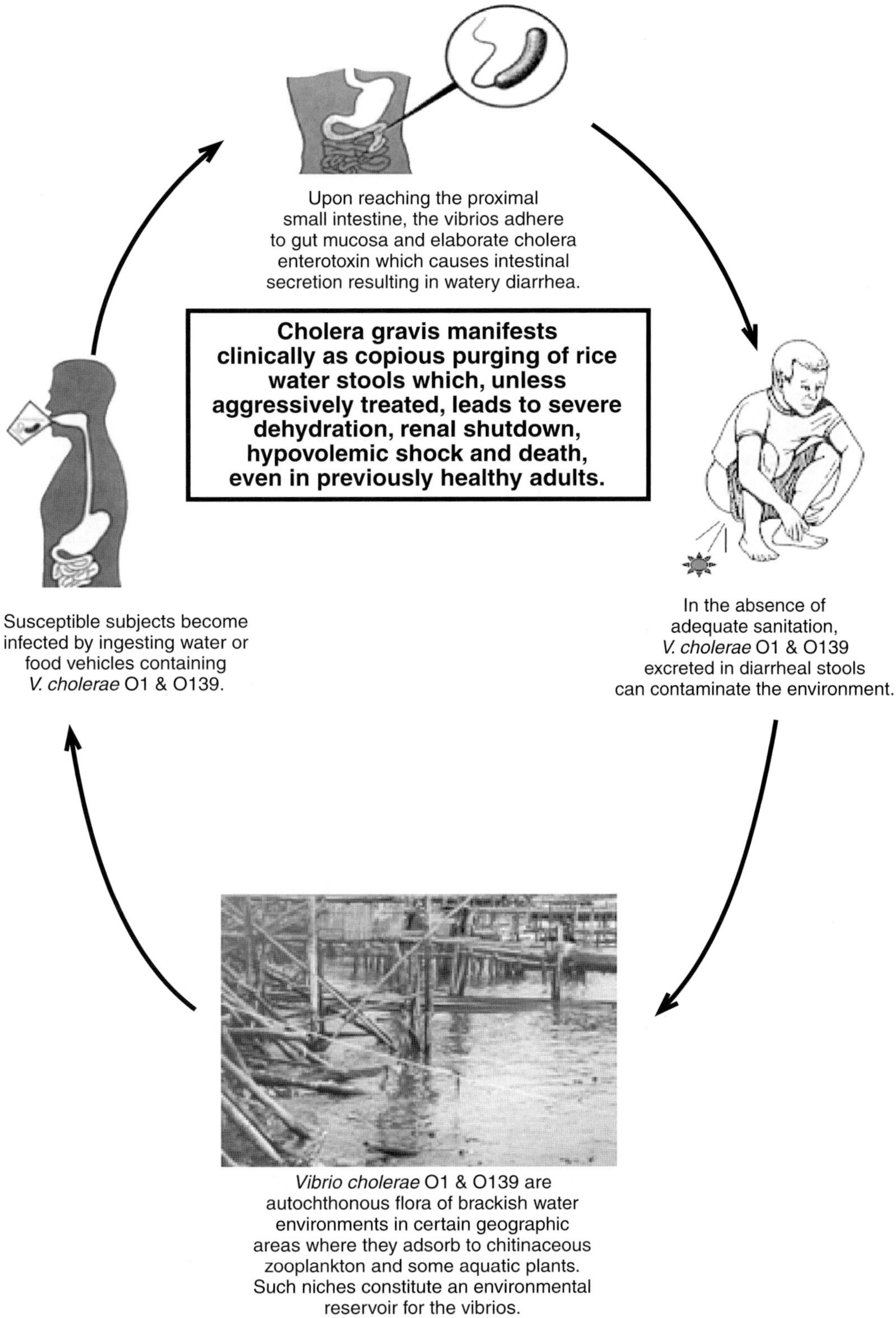

Identification of a similar environmental focus of free-living enterotoxigenic *V. cholerae* O1 El Tor in Queensland, Australia, further supported the contention that, at least in some instances, brackish water environmental niches serve as the reservoir of *V. cholerae* O1.[18]

Colwell[11] reports that *V. cholerae* can enter a "viable but nonculturable" state that allows them to survive harsh environmental conditions by means of a kind of bacterial hibernation. When the toxigenic *V. cholerae* eventually encounter favorable conditions of temperature, salinity, pH, and so on, they can rejuvenate, regaining the potential to actively metabolize and grow.[11] These may also be the conditions under which zooplankton blooms occur.

Modes of Transmission

Most of our knowledge about the vehicles of transmission of cholera stems from case-control investigations, which have demonstrated a number of distinct routes for waterborne transmission and an array of food vehicles.[19,20] Contaminated water remains an important vehicle of transmission in many parts of the world.[20] When El Tor cholera struck Latin America in explosive fashion in 1991, faulty municipal water and sewage systems, contaminated surface waters, and unsafe domestic water storage methods resulted in extensive waterborne cholera transmission.[21,22] Beverages prepared with contaminated water and sold by street vendors, ice, and even commercial bottled water have been incriminated.[23]

V. cholerae O1 may gain access to food in a primary manner, as by the natural association of vibrios with the chitinous exoskeletons of shrimp, crabs, and oysters in certain estuarine environments,[11,17,24] or food may be secondarily contaminated during preparation or handling.[25] The most commonly implicated food vehicle worldwide has been raw or undercooked seafood, including mussels, shrimps, oysters, cockles, clams, fish, salt fish, and ceviche (uncooked fish or shellfish marinated in lemon or lime juice).

Cooked grains, beans, and rice with sauces have also been repeatedly incriminated in cholera transmission. A small inoculum of enterotoxigenic *V. cholerae* introduced by an infected food handler into one of these types of food and stored without refrigeration can increase by several logs within 8 to 12 hours. In several instances, cholera has been transmitted by vegetables or fruit irrigated with raw sewage or doused with sewage to freshen them.[26]

During outbreaks or seasonal epidemics, cholera may be spread via multiple modes of transmission. Depending on local culture and customs, climate, and other factors, certain modes and vehicles of transmission predominate.[27] Finally, if pathogenic *V. cholerae* O1 and O139 persist in environmental reservoirs, then transmission across long distances can occur via the ballast water of large ships, as they intake ballast water in one port and discharge it prior to entering another port thousands of miles away.[28]

Epidemiologists, with few exceptions, recognize that person-to-person contact spread of cholera virtually never occurs. Transmission is essentially always via food or water vehicles.

International Surveillance and Disease Notification

Since cholera was the disease for which modern public health surveillance and reporting was first organized, it bears the code 001 in the international classification of diseases. Moreover, along with plague and yellow fever, by international convention, cholera is a notifiable disease. In 1994, 94 countries, the largest number ever, reported cholera to the World Health Organization (WHO), signifying the cumulative effect of epidemics in Africa, Asia, and Latin America. Nevertheless, for reasons involving trade, fear of food embargoes, and effects on tourism, many countries delay reporting cholera cases to the WHO or do not report at all. For example, from international health statistics in the late 1980s, Bangladesh would appear to have had little or no cholera. Yet at the same time as those "official" statistics were generated, large-scale field trials were carried out to evaluate cholera vaccines in which hundreds of confirmed cases were documented.[29]

Host Risk Factors

Known host factors that greatly increase the risk of developing cholera gravis include blood group O,[30] hypochlorhydria,[31,32] and a lack of background immunity.[33] In both endemic and epidemic situations, persons of blood group O are clearly at much greater risk of developing cholera gravis than persons of other blood groups.[30,34] When cholera invades a new, immunologically naive population, persons with hypochlorhydria (e.g., with partial gastrectomy) have often been the index case.[35] In endemic areas, the highest incidence of cholera usually is seen in children 1 to 4 years of age. The age-specific incidence falls thereafter and the prevalence and geometric mean titer of serum vibriocidal antibody rise, as increasing immunity is acquired.[36] However, there is one interesting exception to this pattern: Women of childbearing age exhibit a high incidence.[15]

Molecular Epidemiology

Molecular biologic techniques have been applied to analyze *V. cholerae* O1 and O139 strains in order to determine relationships and to deduce the origin or derivation of strains. The techniques include Southern blotting of restricted chromosomal DNA with specific probes, examination of restriction fragment length polymorphism (RFLP, ribotyping), pulsed-field gel electrophoresis (PFGE), multilocus enzyme electrophoresis (MEE, electropherotyping), comparison of DNA sequences, polymerase chain reaction methods, and full or partial genome sequencing.[37–41] Application of these molecular subtyping methods has revealed that there are four major clonal groups of *V. cholerae* O1 El Tor strains worldwide called: (1) seventh pandemic; (2) U.S. Gulf Coast; (3) Australia; (4) Latin America. The U.S. Gulf Coast and Australian strains, each representing an environmental reservoir, are closely related. The seventh pandemic and Latin American strains are also similar. It has also been shown that the O139 epidemic strains of 1992–1994 are closely related (indeed, virtually identical) to strains of the El Tor seventh pandemic clone.

DISEASE

The incubation period is usually 18 to 40 hours but can be as short as 12 hours or as long as 72 hours, depending on the inoculum ingested and the susceptibility of the host.

11. Colwell RR: Global climate and infectious disease: The cholera paradigm. Science 274:2025, 1996.
12. Kaper JB, Morris JG Jr, Levine MM: Cholera. Clin Microbiol Rev 8:48, 1995.
13. Stroeher UH, Karageorgos LE, Morona R, et al: Serotype conversion in *Vibrio cholerae* O1. Proc Natl Acad Sci USA 89:2566, 1992.
14. Ito T, Hiramatsu K, Ohshita Y, et al: Mutations in the rfbT gene are responsible for the Ogawa to inaba serotype conversion in *Vibrio cholerae* O1. Microbiol Immunol 37:281, 1993.
15. Glass RI, Becker S, Huq I, et al: Endemic cholera in rural Bangladesh, 1966–1980. Am J Epidemiol 116:959, 1982.
16. Weissman JB, DeWitt WE, Thompson J, et al: A case of cholera in Texas, 1973. Am J Epidemiol 100:487, 1974.
17. Blake PA, Allegra DT, Snyder JD, et al: Cholera—A possible endemic focus in the United States. N Engl J Med 302:305, 1980.
18. Rogers RC, Cuffe RG, Cossins YM, et al: The Queensland cholera incident of 1977. 2. The epidemiological investigation. Bull World Health Org 58:665, 1980.
19. Blake PA: Epidemiology of cholera in the Americas. Gastroenterol Clin North Am 22:639, 1993.
20. Sack DA, Sack RB, Nair GB, et al: Cholera. Lancet 363:223, 2004.
21. Swerdlow DL, Mintz ED, Rodriguez M, et al: Waterborne transmission of epidemic cholera in Trujillo, Peru: Lessons for a continent at risk. Lancet 340:28, 1992.
22. Ries AA, Vugia DJ, Beingolea L, et al: Cholera in Piura, Peru: A modern urban epidemic. J Infect Dis 166:1429, 1992.
23. Blake PA, Rosenberg ML, Florencia J, et al: Cholera in Portugal, 1974. II. Transmission by bottled mineral water. Am J Epidemiol 105:344, 1977.
24. Lowry PW, Pavia AT, McFarland LM, et al: Cholera in Louisiana. Widening spectrum of seafood vehicles. Arch Intern Med 149:2079, 1989.
25. St. Louis ME, Porter JD, Helal A, et al: Epidemic cholera in West Africa: The role of food handling and high-risk foods. Am J Epidemiol 131:719, 1990.
26. Cohen J, Schwartz T, Klasmer R, et al: Epidemiological aspects of cholera El Tor outbreak in a non-endemic area. Lancet 2:86, 1971.
27. Gunnlaugsson G, Einarsdottir J, Angulo FJ, et al: Funerals during the 1994 cholera epidemic in Guinea-Bissau, West Africa: The need for disinfection of bodies of persons dying of cholera. Epidemiol Infect 120:7, 1998.
28. McCarthy SA, Khambaty FM: International dissemination of epidemic *Vibrio cholerae* by cargo ship ballast and other nonpotable waters. Appl Environ Microbiol 60:2597, 1994.
29. Clemens JD, Sack DA, Harris JR, et al: Field trial of cholera vaccines in Bangladesh: Results from three year follow-up. Lancet 335:270, 1990.
30. Glass RI, Holmgren J, Haley CE, et al: Predisposition for cholera of individuals with O blood group. Possible evolutionary significance. Am J Epidemiol 121:791, 1985.
31. Nalin DR, Levine MM, Rhead J, et al: Cannabis, hypochlorhydria, and cholera. Lancet 2:859, 1978.
32. Nalin DR, Levine RJ, Levine MM, et al: Cholera, non-*Vibrio cholera,* and stomach acid. Lancet 2:856, 1978.
33. Mosley WH, Ahmad S, Benenson AS, et al: The relationship of vibriocidal antibody titre to susceptibility to cholera in family contacts of cholera patients. Bull World Health Org 38:777, 1968.
34. Tacket CO, Losonsky G, Nataro JP, et al: Extension of the volunteer challenge model to study South American cholera in a population of volunteers predominantly with blood group antigen O. Trans R Soc Trop Med Hyg 89:75, 1995.
35. Gitelson S: Gastrectomy, achlorhydria and cholera. Isr J Med Sci 7:663, 1971.
36. Mosley WH, McCormack WM, Ahmed A: Report of the 1966–67 cholera field trial in rural East Pakistan. 2. Results of the serological surveys in the study population—The relationship of case rate to antibody titre and an estimate of the inapparent infection rate with *Vibrio cholerae*. Bull World Health Org 40:187, 1969.
37. Evins GM, Cameron DN, Wells JG, et al: The emerging diversity of the electrophoretic types of *Vibrio cholerae* in the Western Hemisphere. J Infect Dis 172:173, 1995.
38. Cameron DN, Khambaty FM, Wachsmuth IK, et al: Molecular characterization of *Vibrio cholerae* O1 strains by pulsed-field gel electrophoresis. J Clin Microbiol 32:1685, 1994.
39. Faruque SM, Roy SK, Alim AR, et al: Molecular epidemiology of toxigenic *Vibrio cholerae* in Bangladesh studied by numerical analysis of rRNA gene restriction patterns. J Clin Microbiol 33:2833, 1995.
40. Faruque SM, Ahmed KM, Alim AR, et al: Emergence of a new clone of toxigenic *Vibrio cholerae* O1 biotype El Tor displacing *V. cholerae* O139 Bengal in Bangladesh. J Clin Microbiol 35:624, 1997.
41. Faruque SM, Chowdhury N, Kamruzzaman M, et al: Genetic diversity and virulence potential of environmental *Vibrio cholerae* population in a cholera-endemic area. Proc Natl Acad Sci USA 101:2123, 2004.
42. Nalin DR, Levine MM, Hornick RB, et al: The problem of emesis during oral glucose-electrolytes therapy given from the onset of severe cholera. Trans R Soc Trop Med Hyg 73:10, 1979.
43. Bennish ML, Azad AK, Rahman O, et al: Hypoglycemia during diarrhea in childhood. Prevalence, pathophysiology, and outcome. N Engl J Med 322:1357, 1990.
44. Levine M, Kaper J, Black RE, et al: New knowledge on pathogenesis of bacterial enteric infections as applied to vaccine development. Microbiol Rev 47:510, 1983.
45. Tacket CO, Losonsky G, Nataro JP, et al: Safety and immunogenicity of live oral cholera vaccine candidate CVD 110, a delta ctxA delta zot delta ace derivative of El Tor Ogawa *Vibrio cholerae*. J Infect Dis 168:1536, 1993.
46. Silva TM, Schleupner MA, Tacket CO, et al: New evidence for an inflammatory component in diarrhea caused by selected new, live attenuated cholera vaccines and by El Tor and O139 *Vibrio cholerae*. Infect Immun 64:2362, 1996.
47. Stokes NR, Zhou X, Meltzer SJ, et al: Transcriptional responses of intestinal epithelial cells to infection with *Vibrio cholerae*. Infect Immun 72:4240, 2004.
48. Levine MM, Black RE, Clements ML, et al: Volunteer studies in development of vaccines against cholera and enterotoxigenic *Escherichia coli*: A review. In Holme T, Holmgren J, Merson MH, et al (eds): Acute Enteric Infections in Children: New Prospects for Treatment and Prevention. Amsterdam, Elsevier/North-Holland Biomedical, 1981, p 443.
49. DiRita VJ: Co-ordinate expression of virulence genes by ToxR in *Vibrio cholerae*. Mol Microbiol 6:451, 1992.
50. Taylor RK, Miller VL, Furlong DB, et al: Use of phoA gene fusions to identify a pilus colonization factor coordinately regulated with cholera toxin. Proc Natl Acad Sci USA 84:2833, 1987.
51. Thelin KH, Taylor RK: Toxin-coregulated pilus, but not mannose-sensitive hemagglutinin, is required for colonization by *Vibrio cholerae* O1 El Tor biotype and O139 strains. Infect Immun 64:2853, 1996.
52. Herrington DA, Hall RH, Losonsky G, et al: Toxin, toxin-coregulated pili, and the toxR regulon are essential for *Vibrio cholerae* pathogenesis in humans. J Exp Med 168:1487, 1988.
53. Hall RH, Losonsky G, Silveira AP, et al: Immunogenicity of *Vibrio cholerae* O1 toxin-coregulated pili in experimental and clinical cholera. Infect Immun 59:2508, 1991.
54. Levine MM, Kaper JB, Herrington D, et al: Volunteer studies of deletion mutants of *Vibrio cholerae* O1 prepared by recombinant techniques. Infect Immun 56:161, 1988.
55. Fasano A, Baudry B, Pumplin DW, et al: *Vibrio cholerae* produces a second enterotoxin, which affects intestinal tight junctions. Proc Natl Acad Sci USA 88:5242, 1991.
56. Trucksis M, Galen JE, Michalski J, et al: Accessory cholera enterotoxin (Ace), the third member of a *Vibrio cholerae* virulence cassette. Proc Natl Acad Sci USA 90:5267, 1993.
57. Waldor MK, Mekalanos JJ: Lysogenic conversion by a filamentous phage encoding cholera toxin. Science 272:1910, 1996.
58. Davis BM, Waldor MK: Filamentous phages linked to virulence of *Vibrio cholerae*. Curr Opin Microbiol 6:35, 2003.
59. Waldor MK, Rubin EJ, Pearson GD, et al: Regulation, replication, and integration functions of the *Vibrio cholerae* CTXphi are encoded by region RS2. Mol Microbiol 24:917, 1997.
60. Clements ML, Levine MM, Young CR, et al: Magnitude, kinetics, and duration of vibriocidal antibody responses in North Americans after ingestion of *Vibrio cholerae*. J Infect Dis 145:465, 1982.
61. Levine MM, Young CR, Hughes TP, et al: Duration of serum antitoxin response following *Vibrio cholerae* infection in North Americans: Relevance for seroepidemiology. Am J Epidemiol 114:348, 1981.
62. Losonsky GA, Tacket CO, Wasserman SS, et al: Secondary *Vibrio cholerae*–specific cellular antibody responses following wild-type homologous challenge in people vaccinated with CVD 103-HgR live

oral cholera vaccine: Changes with time and lack of correlation with protection. Infect Immun 61:729, 1993.
63. Glass RI, Svennerholm AM, Khan MR, et al: Seroepidemiological studies of El Tor cholera in Bangladesh: Association of serum antibody levels with protection. J Infect Dis 151:236, 1985.
64. Losonsky GA, Lim Y, Motamedi P, et al: Vibriocidal antibody responses in North American volunteers exposed to wild-type or vaccine *Vibrio cholerae* O139: Specificity and relevance to immunity. Clin Diagn Lab Immunol 4:264, 1997.
65. Hasan JA, Huq A, Tamplin ML, et al: A novel kit for rapid detection of *Vibrio cholerae* O1. J Clin Microbiol 32:249, 1994.
66. Qadri F, Hasan JA, Hossain J, et al: Evaluation of the monoclonal antibody-based kit Bengal SMART for rapid detection of *Vibrio cholerae* O139 synonym Bengal in stool samples. J Clin Microbiol 33:732, 1995.
67. Nato F, Boutonnier A, Rajerison M, et al: One-step immunochromatographic dipstick tests for rapid detection of *Vibrio cholerae* O1 and O139 in stool samples. Clin Diagn Lab Immunol 10:476, 2003.
68. Seas C, DuPont HL, Valdez LM, et al: Practical guidelines for the treatment of cholera. Drugs 51:966, 1996.
69. Mahalanabis D, Choudhuri AB, Bagchi NG, et al: Oral fluid therapy of cholera among Bangladesh refugees. Johns Hopkins Med J 132:197, 1973.
70. Carpenter CCJ: The treatment of cholera: Clinical science at the bedside. J Infect Dis 166:2, 1992.
71. Patra FC, Mahalanabis D, Jalan KN, et al: Is oral rice electrolyte solution superior to glucose electrolyte solution in infantile diarrhoea? Arch Dis Child 57:910, 1982.
72. Molla AM, Sarker SA, Hossain M, et al: Rice-powder electrolyte solution as oral-therapy in diarrhoea due to *Vibrio cholerae* and *Escherichia coli*. Lancet 1:1317, 1982.
73. Hossain MS, Salam MA, Rabbani GH, et al: Rice-ORS versus glucose-ORS in management of severe cholera due to *Vibrio cholerae* O139 Bengal: A randomized, controlled clinical trial. J Health Popul Nutr 21:325, 2003.
74. Gotuzzo E, Seas C, Echevarria J, et al: Ciprofloxacin for the treatment of cholera: A randomized, double- blind, controlled clinical trial of a single daily dose in Peruvian adults. Clin Infect Dis 20:1485, 1995.
75. Khan WA, Saha D, Rahman A, et al: Comparison of single-dose azithromycin and 12-dose, 3-day erythromycin for childhood cholera: A randomised, double-blind trial. Lancet 360:1722, 2002.
76. Nair GB, Shimada T, Kurazono H, et al: Characterization of phenotypic, serological, and toxigenic traits of *Vibrio cholerae* O139 bengal. J Clin Microbiol 32:2775, 1994.
77. Khan WA, Bennish ML, Seas C, et al: Randomised controlled comparison of single-dose ciprofloxacin and doxycycline for cholera caused by *Vibrio cholerae* 01 or 0139. Lancet 348:296, 1996.
78. Alam AN, Alam NH, Ahmed T, et al: Randomised double blind trial of single dose doxycycline for treating cholera in adults. BMJ 300: 1619, 1990.
79. Quick RE, Venczel LV, Gonzalez O, et al: Narrow-mouthed water storage vessels and in situ chlorination in a Bolivian community: A simple method to improve drinking water quality. Am J Trop Med Hyg 54:511, 1996.
80. D'Aquino M, Teves SA: Lemon juice as a natural biocide for disinfecting drinking water. Bull Pan Am Health Org 28:324, 1994.
81. McCormack WM, Chowdhury AM, Jahangir N, et al: Tetracycline prophylaxis in families of cholera patients. Bull World Health Org 38:787, 1968.
82. Weber JT, Mintz ED, Canizares R, et al: Epidemic cholera in Ecuador: Multidrug-resistance and transmission by water and seafood. Epidemiol Infect 112:1, 1994.
83. Sanchez JL, Vasquez B, Begue RE, et al: Protective efficacy of oral whole-cell/recombinant-B-subunit cholera vaccine in Peruvian military recruits. Lancet 344:1273, 1994.
84. Taylor DN, Cardenas V, Sanchez JL, et al: Two year study of the protective efficacy of the oral whole cell plus recombinant B subunit (WC/rBS) cholera vaccine in Peru. J Infect Dis 181: 1667, 2000.
85. Levine MM, Kaper JB: Live oral cholera vaccine: From principle to product. Bull Inst Pasteur 93:243, 1995.
86. Tacket CO, Cohen MB, Wasserman SS, et al: Randomized, double-blind, placebo-controlled, multicentered trial of the efficacy of a single dose of live oral cholera vaccine CVD 103-HgR in preventing cholera following challenge with *Vibrio cholerae* O1 El tor Inaba three months after vaccination. Infect Immun 67:6341, 1999.
87. Legros D, Paquet C, Perea W, et al: Mass vaccination with a two-dose oral cholera vaccine in a refugee camp. Bull World Health Org 77:837, 1999.
88. Kotloff KL, Wasserman SS, O'Donnell S, et al: Safety and immunogenicity in North Americans of a single dose of live oral cholera vaccine CVD 103-HgR: Results of a randomized, placebo-controlled, double-blind crossover trial. Infect Immun 60:4430, 1992.
89. Suharyono, Simanjuntak C, Witham N, et al: Safety and immunogenicity of single-dose live oral cholera vaccine CVD 103-HgR in 5-9-year-old Indonesian children. Lancet 340:689, 1992.
90. Simanjuntak CH, O'Hanley P, Punjabi NH, et al: The safety, immunogenicity, and transmissibility of single-dose live oral cholera vaccine CVD 103-HgR in 24 to 59 month old Indonesian children. J Infect Dis 168:1169, 1993.
91. Lagos R, Avendano A, Prado V, et al: Attenuated live oral cholera vaccine strain CVD 103-HgR elicits significantly higher serum vibriocidal antibody titers in persons of blood group O. Infect Immun 63:707, 1995.
92. Gotuzzo E, Butron B, Seas C, et al: Safety, immunogenicity, and excretion pattern of single-dose live oral cholera vaccine CVD 103-HgR in Peruvian adults of high and low socioeconomic levels. Infect Immun 61:3994, 1993.
93. Lagos R, San Martin O, Wasserman SS, et al: Palatability, reactogenicity and immunogenicity of engineered live oral cholera vaccine CVD 103-HgR in Chilean infants and toddlers. Pediatr Infect Dis J 18:624, 1999.
94. Tacket CO, Losonsky G, Nataro JP, et al: Onset and duration of protective immunity in challenged volunteers after vaccination with live oral cholera vaccine CVD 103-HgR. J Infect Dis 166:837, 1992.
95. Richie E, Punjabi NH, Sidharta Y, et al: Efficacy trial of single-dose live oral cholera vaccine CVD 103-HgR in North Jakarta, Indonesia, a cholera-endemic area. Vaccine 18:2399, 2000.
96. Calain P, Chaine JP, Johnson E, et al: Can oral cholera vaccination play a role in controlling a cholera outbreak? Vaccine 22:2444, 2004.
97. Mahon BE, Mintz ED, Greene KD, et al: Reported cholera in the United States, 1992–1994: A reflection of global changes in cholera epidemiology. JAMA 276:307, 1996.
98. Taylor DN, Rizzo J, Meza R, et al: Cholera among Americans living in Peru. Clin Infect Dis 22:1108, 1996.

22

"Noncholera" Vibrio Infections

J. GLENN MORRIS, Jr.
G. BALAKRISH NAIR

AGENT

Cholera is a well-recognized (and highly feared) disease in tropical areas. As investigators in the early part of this century began to acquire an understanding of the "cholera bacillus" (*Vibrio cholerae*), it became apparent that these bacteria could be divided into two groups: those that agglutinated with serum from cholera patients (designated as O group 1 strains) and those that failed to agglutinate (designated as "nonagglutinating" or "noncholera" vibrios).[1,2] This latter group consisted primarily of environmental isolates that were thought to be nonpathogenic, although there was early speculation that they might be responsible for "paracholera" syndromes. Firm evidence of the pathogenicity of these strains did not emerge until the 1950s when the first outbreaks due to noncholera strains were identified and investigated. As data accumulated, it became increasingly clear that many of the strains were so distinct from *V. cholerae* as to constitute separate species.[3,4]

It is now recognized that within the species *V. cholerae* there are well over 200 O groups. Strains in serogroup O1 were regarded as the sole cause of epidemic cholera until 1992, when *V. cholerae* strains subsequently classified as O139 (syn. Bengal) first appeared and spread in epidemic form across the Indian subcontinent.[5,6] *V. cholerae* in serogroups other than O1 and O139 are generally defined as "noncholera" or "nonepidemic" vibrios. However, it should be recognized that serogroup is not a consistent marker for pathogenicity, as there are environmental *V. cholerae* O1 and O139 strains that do not carry the genes for standard virulence factors such as cholera toxin,[7] while strains in other serogroups (such as O37) have been found to be closely related genetically to epidemic O1 strains and have caused outbreaks of cholera-like illness.[8,9] Toxigenic strains of *V. cholerae* serogroup O141 have been associated with sporadic cholera-like diarrhea and bloodstream infections in the United States[10]; localized outbreaks of diarrheal illness have been caused by O10 and O12 strains in 1994 in Peru,[11] O6 and O14 strains in Khmer refugee camps in Thailand,[12] and O10 strains in India.[13] In general, however, non-O1/O139 *V. cholerae* strains have been associated with mild, sporadic illness, or with asymptomatic colonization.[14]

Fujino and coworkers first isolated what we now know as *V. parahaemolyticus* from clinical samples and from shirasu (dried sardines) associated with an outbreak of gastroenteritis that occurred in Osaka in 1950. Over the subsequent decade, many other outbreaks in Japan incriminated a halophilic, hemolytic gram-negative organism similar to that described by Fujino. The vehicles in these outbreaks were usually raw fish, shellfish, and cucumbers in brine. The names *Pasteurella parahaemolytica, Pseudomonas enteritis,* and *Oceanomonas parahaemolytica* were all suggested before taxonomic studies firmly placed the organism within the genus *Vibrio.*[15,16] The current serotyping scheme recognizes 75 combinations of O and K serotypes of *V. parahaemolyticus*. While early studies did not show a linkage between specific serogroups and virulence, a new *V. parahaemolyticus* clonal group that appears to have increased virulence has emerged during the past decade: these strains are found in a limited number of serogroups (O3:K6, O4:K68, O1:K25, O1:KUT) and appear to be responsible for a pandemic of *V. parahaemolyticus* gastroenteritis that has affected nine countries including the United States.[17,18]

In addition to *V. cholerae* and *V. parahaemolyticus,* nine other *Vibrio* species that can infect humans (or that have been isolated from humans) are now recognized. *V. fluvialis,*[19,20] *V. furnissi,*[21] *V. hollisae,*[22] and *V. mimicus*[23,24] have been associated primarily with diarrheal disease. *V. alginolyticus* and *V. damsela*[22] generally cause wound infections. *V. vulnificus,* initially described in 1979 as a "lactose-positive marine *Vibrio,*" is recognized as an important cause of septicemia in alcoholics and immunosuppressed hosts; cases have been reported primarily from Korea, Taiwan, and the Gulf Coast region of the United States.[25–27] A newly described biogroup of *V. vulnificus*, biogroup 3, has been implicated in serious wound infections associated with exposure to live tilapia in Israel.[28] Descriptions of infections with *V. cincinnatiensis,*[29] *V. carchariae,*[30] and *V. metschnikovii*[31,32] have been restricted to case reports, and the significance of their isolation from humans remains to be determined. Table 22-1 lists the *Vibrio* species associated with human illness, together with data on numbers of reported cases and deaths in the United States for 1999.[33] Numerous other *Vibrio* species (currently totaling at least 50) inhabit the marine environment, but are not known to be pathogenic to humans.

EPIDEMIOLOGY

Incidence

V. parahaemolyticus is the most commonly isolated noncholera vibrio. In Japan, it has traditionally been implicated as the cause of at least one-fourth of food-borne disease cases.[16] After having shown a decreasing trend in recent years, *V. parahaemolyticus* cases started to increase again around 1994 in Japan. Between 1996 and 1998, the number of cases more than doubled, with 12,346 cases in 850 incidents reported in 1998; this increase appears to be linked with the appearance of the new clonal group of pandemic *V. parahaemolyticus* strains in serogroups O3:K6, O4:K68, O1:K25, and O1:KUT.[34] Diarrheal cases attributed to strains in these groups have also been rapidly increasing in Bangladesh, India, Taiwan, and other southeast Asian countries since 1996, as well as in the United States.[34–38]

Table 22-1 Vibrio *Species Implicated as Causes of Human Disease and Number of Deaths Associated with Infection with These Species*

Vibrio Species	Clinical Presentation			No. of Cases (No. of Deaths)*
	Gastroenteritis	Wound or Ear Infection	Septicemia	
V. cholerae				
Epidemic (O1, O139)	++	(+)	—	5 (0)[†]
Nonepidemic	++	+	+	45 (0)
V. mimicus	++	+	—	10 (0)
V. parahaemolyticus	++	+	(+)	116 (1)
V. fluvialis	++	+	+	19 (0)
V. furnissii	++	—	—	1 (0)
V. hollisae	++	+	(+)	13 (0)
V. vulnificus	+	++	++	83 (31)[‡]
V. alginolyticus	—	++	—	28 (0)
V. damsela	—	++	—	2 (0)
V. cincinnatiensis	—	—	(+)	0 (0)
V. carchariae	—	(+)	—	0 (0)
V. metschnikovii	(+)	—	(+)	1 (0)

++, Most common clinical presentation; +, neither rare nor most common clinical presentation; (+), rare clinical presentation.

*Data reflect *Vibrio* infections reported to the Centers for Disease Control and Prevention during 1999. Data are from the 24 states that reported cases; for many of these states, reporting of *Vibrio* infections is not routine, and consequently numbers may not reflect the true number of cases. Data were kindly provided by R. Tauxe, U.S. Centers for Disease Control and Prevention, Atlanta.

[†]Data include 4 cases associated with foreign travel.

[‡]The 31 reported deaths are from a group of 75 cases for which data on death were available.

From Morris JG Jr: Cholera and other types of vibrioses: A story of human pandemics and oysters on the half shell. Clin Infect Dis 37:272–280, 2003.

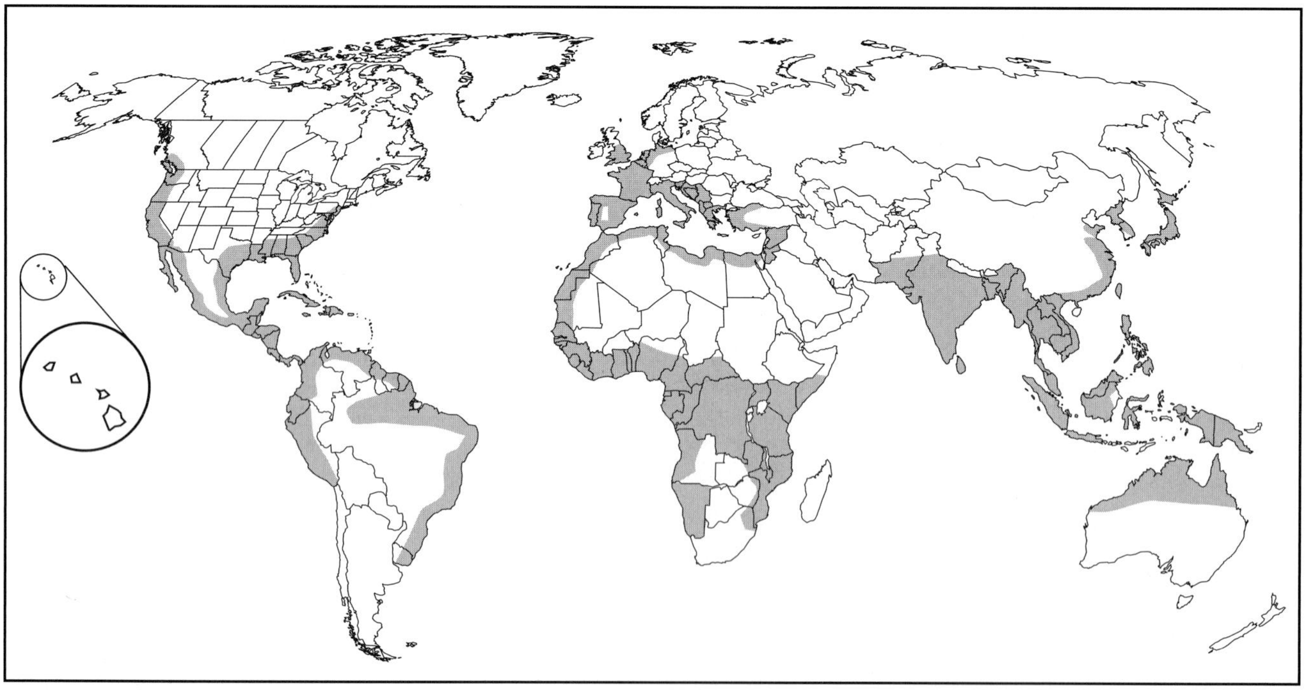

V. cholerae in O groups other than O1 or O139 Bengal has been isolated from 2% to 3% of patients with diarrheal illness in tropical areas (including travelers).[14] As seen with other *Vibrio* species, isolation rates appear to be higher in coastal areas: an isolation rate of 16.4% was reported from Cancún, Mexico,[39] as compared with no isolations in a study in Mexico City.[40] In Calcutta, a cholera-endemic area, the isolation rate for nonepidemic strains of *V. cholerae* among patients hospitalized with diarrhea has been reported to vary between 2.7% and 4.9%, with no temporal clustering of any particular serogroup and no pronounced seasonality.[41]

In a 13-year study in Florida,[41] *V. hollisae* was the third most common *Vibrio* species (after *V. parahaemolyticus* and *V. cholerae*) isolated from patients with diarrhea. Population-based data on rates of isolation of this and other *Vibrio* species from patients with diarrhea in tropical areas are limited; however, it is likely that they are responsible for substantively fewer cases of illness than are *V. cholerae* and *V. parahaemolyticus*. *V. vulnificus* is the most common cause of vibrio-associated sepsis in the United States; incidence in coastal areas has been estimated to be in the range of 0.5 cases/100,000 population per year.[42,43] While population-based data are lacking, incidence rates appear to be higher in Korea and Taiwan.[26,44]

Carriage

Long-term human carriage of *Vibrio* species is unusual; chronic carriers do not appear to play a role in the epidemiology of the disease. However, short-term carriage or asymptomatic infections may be relatively common. From a cohort of 479 physicians attending a meeting in New Orleans who agreed to submit stool samples, 51 stool samples were positive for noncholera vibrios (*V. parahaemolyticus*, nonepidemic *V. cholerae*, *V. vulnificus*, *V. fluvialis*, and *V. mimicus*), of which 36 had been collected from individuals reporting no recent diarrheal illness.[45] In a large study conducted in Iran in 1971, 1.6% of pilgrims returning from Mecca were estimated to be carriers of noncholera *V. cholerae* (compared with 0.015% of persons leaving for Mecca). Isolations of this organism from stool cultures obtained from the contacts of these pilgrims increased over the following 6 months and decreased thereafter. Of these contacts, 60% reported diarrheal illness.[46] In a study in Calcutta, 15.3% of family contacts of *V. parahaemolyticus* diarrhea cases were found to be carrying the organism, with excretion continuing for up to 5 days.[47] Carriage of *Vibrio* species by wild and domestic animals is also well described: nonepidemic *V. cholerae* has been isolated from dogs in Calcutta[48]; from cows, goats, dogs, and chickens in India[49]; from ducks in Denmark[50]; from seagulls in England; and from horses, lambs, and bison in Colorado.[51]

Transmission

Transmission pathways are shown in the following "life cycle." The marine or estuarine environment serves as the primary reservoir for these organisms. However, there is also the possibility of secondary contamination of food and water sources by feces from infected humans and animals.

Noncholera *Vibrio* Infections

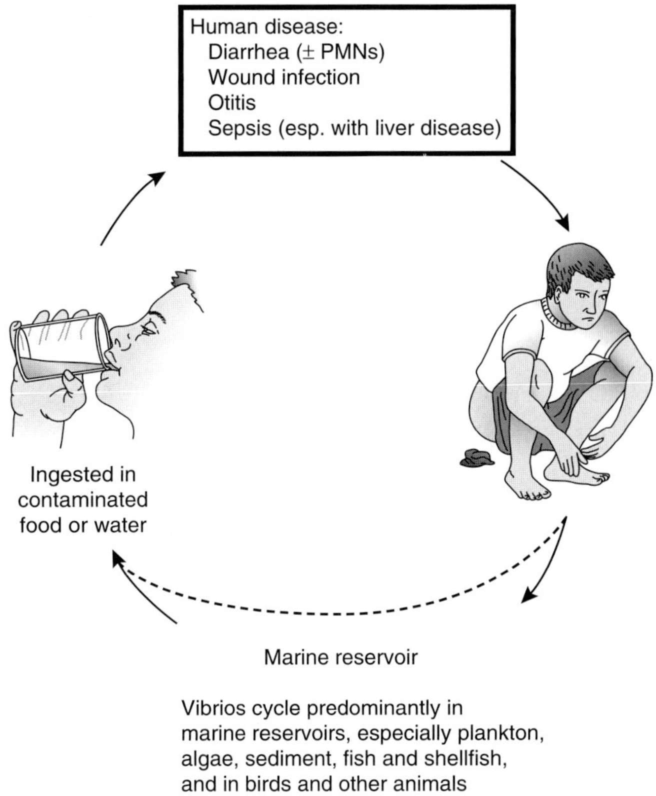

In temperate regions, virtually all cases can be linked back to seafood, particularly raw or undercooked seafood.[42] Raw oysters are commonly implicated in transmission; while U.S. *V. cholerae* and *V. vulnificus* cases have always been significantly associated with raw oyster consumption,[52,53] there were major U.S. *V. parahaemolyticus* outbreaks linked with oysters in 1997 (Washington State) and 1998 (Texas, New York, Connecticut, and Washington State).[54] The pattern is less clear in tropical areas, possibly because of the increased risk of fecal contamination of food and water sources, or cross-contamination of foods by seafood vehicles. For example, in the previously noted study in Cancún,[39] home-prepared gelatin was the only statistically significant risk factor identified in a case-control study; however, the organism was isolated from 86% of untreated well water samples, 92% of sewage samples, and 21% of seafood samples. Similarly, a waterborne outbreak of noncholera *V. cholerae* occurred in the Sudan in 1968 due to contamination of surface water next to a well.[55]

Ecology/Distribution/Seasonality

Vibrios are ubiquitous in the marine environment. While most are halophilic (i.e., require salt for growth), *V. cholerae* can grow in freshwater, and has been isolated from freshwater lakes.[56,57] In temperate climates, counts of vibrio bacteria vary seasonally: in the summer (when water temperatures exceed 20°C), vibrios can easily be isolated from water, suspended particulate matter, plankton, algae, sediment, fish, and shellfish; during the winter months, they decline markedly in number and are found primarily in sediments.[15,58] Among other possible natural reservoirs, egg masses of the nonbiting midge *Chironomous* spp (Diptera) have recently been shown to harbor *V. cholerae*.[59] Vibrio counts are independent of the level of fecal coliforms; that is, these are naturally occurring, free-living organisms that can be present in "pristine" waters that are free of fecal contamination.

Vibrio counts in oysters tend to be particularly high, with numbers of *V. parahaemolyticus* and *V. vulnificus* that may be 100 times higher than the surrounding water.[58] In a survey conducted by the Food and Drug Administration (FDA), non-O1 *V. cholerae* could be isolated from 14% of randomly selected oyster shell stock.[60] Studies along the Gulf Coast and in Chesapeake Bay indicate that virtually all summer-harvested oysters carry *V. vulnificus* and/or *V. parahaemolyticus*, with counts that can exceed 10^4/g of oyster meat.[54,58,61] *V. cholerae* and *V. vulnificus* can shift to a "viable but nonculturable" form, which may permit them to survive for extended periods in the environment under adverse conditions.[62–64] *V. cholerae* (and possibly other species) also have the ability to acquire a "rugose" morphology, associated with the production of a surface polysaccharide that promotes cell aggregation and provides protection to the organism by formation of biofilm-like masses of cells.[65]

As noted previously, vibrios are ubiquitous: they can be found in marine environments, estuaries, and freshwater throughout the world. Human illness due to vibrios shares a similar distribution, although patterns of illness vary from region to region, depending, in part, on cultural factors. In Japan, where consumption of seafood (including raw and undercooked seafood) is relatively common, *V. parahaemolyticus* accounts for a large proportion of food-borne illness. *V. vulnificus* has emerged as a significant health problem in Korea and Taiwan, linked again with consumption of raw or undercooked seafood.[26,44] In the United States, where vibrio infections appear to be less common, outbreaks and sporadic cases are concentrated along the Atlantic, Gulf, and Pacific coastlines.

In temperate areas illness tends to follow a seasonal pattern,[42] which can be correlated with levels of the causative organism in the environment. There have been suggestions that increasing water temperatures in coastal areas in the United States (possibly related to global warming) have served as a co-factor in the increasing incidence of *V. parahaemolyticus* in this country.[66] Seasonality is less apparent in tropical areas.

Host Factors

In cases of vibrio gastroenteritis, factors such as sex, race, or blood group have not shown any consistent correlation with disease. The median age of persons with vibrio gastroenteritis varies with geographic location. In Cancún, Mexico, for example, children less than 1 year of age were at highest risk of infection with nonepidemic *V. cholerae*,[39] whereas in Bangladesh and Thailand cases tended to occur in older children and adults. In a survey of 14 sporadic nonepidemic *V. cholerae* infections in the United States,[52] the median patient age was 45, which may reflect the older age of the population that consumes raw oysters. Factors that decrease gastric acidity may increase the risk of infection.

Host factors play a much more important role in the epidemiology of sepsis due to *Vibrio* species. Virtually all patients with sepsis due to *V. vulnificus* and nonepidemic *V. cholerae* have an underlying chronic medical illness.[25–27,42,53,67,68] Those with liver disease, such as alcoholic cirrhosis or hemochromatosis, are especially at risk. Based on the number of cases reported to the Florida Health Department between 1981 and 1992, the annual rate of illness from *V. vulnificus* infection in adults with self-reported liver disease in Florida who ate raw oysters was 7.2 per 100,000 adults, 80 times the rate for adults without known liver disease who ate raw oysters (0.09 cases per 100,000 population).[53] The risk of sepsis due to *V. parahaemolyticus* also appears to be increased by the presence of underlying chronic illness, although the association does not appear to be as strong as that seen with *V. cholerae* and *V. vulnificus*. Again, there are suggestions that risk is increased in patients with decreased gastric acidity.

DISEASE

Primary clinical presentations vary by species and may include gastroenteritis, wound and ear infections, and septicemia.

Vibrio-associated gastroenteritis is similar to that seen with other enteric pathogens, with patients reporting diarrhea, abdominal pain, and, to a lesser degree, nausea and vomiting. In studies of sporadic noncholera *V. cholerae* cases identified retrospectively on the basis of stool cultures, illness has been relatively severe. Among 14 sporadic cases identified in a study in the United States,[52] the median duration of illness was 6.4 days. All of these patients had diarrhea, 71% had fever, but only 21% had nausea and vomiting. One-fourth of these patients had bloody diarrhea. Experimental infections in normal, healthy volunteers[69] and cases identified through outbreak investigations[70,71] have been associated with less severe disease, with median durations of illness ranging from 12 to 24 hours. The incubation period in outbreaks ranged from 12 to 24 hours; the median incubation period in volunteers[69] was 10 hours (range, 5.5 to 96 hours).

V. parahaemolyticus produces a similar spectrum of gastrointestinal illness. In a summary of clinical data from 202 patients with *V. parahaemolyticus* gastroenteritis that were reported to the Centers for Disease Control and Prevention (CDC) between 1973 and 1998, manifestations included diarrhea (98%), abdominal cramps (89%), nausea (76%), vomiting (55%), and fever (52%).[35] In both the United States and Japan, illness tends to be mild, with a median duration (in U.S. foodborne outbreaks) of 2.4 days.[35] Bloody stools were noted in 29% of *V. parahaemolyticus* cases reported to the CDC.[35] There are also rare reports of more severe illness: a dysentery-like syndrome may occur in association with infection,[72,73] hypotension and shock occurred in three of five *V. parahaemolyticus* cases in one outbreak in Great Britain, and there were 20 deaths among the 272 patients involved in the Japanese outbreak where *V. parahaemolyticus* was first identified.[15] The incubation period for *V. parahaemolyticus* generally ranges from 4 to 48 hours, with most illness occurring 12 to 24 hours after exposure. *Vibrio* species have been isolated from seawater-exposed wounds[14,42] and have been implicated as a cause of otitis and, rarely, pneumonia associated with near-drowning episodes.[14] While infection can occur in normal hosts, complications, including sepsis, are more likely in persons who are immunocompromised or have chronic underlying illnesses.[42]

Septicemia, due primarily to encapsulated strains of *V. vulnificus* and *V. cholerae*, occurs almost exclusively in persons who have underlying liver disease, are alcoholic, diabetic, or in some way immunocompromised.[25–27,67,68] One-third of patients with *V. vulnificus* septicemia present in shock.[25–27] Thrombocytopenia is common, and there is often evidence of disseminated intravascular coagulation; gastrointestinal bleeding is not infrequent. The mortality rate is greater than 50%, with mortality exceeding 90% among patients who become hypotensive within the first 24 hours of hospitalization. Three-fourths of patients with *V. vulnificus* septicemia have characteristic bullous skin lesions[3,25–27]; identification of these skin lesions in the appropriate epidemiologic setting should prompt aggressive, specific therapy for this pathogen. While there are fewer data on patients with *V. cholerae* septicemia, the clinical presentation is comparable to that seen with *V. vulnificus* (although skin lesions do not appear to be as prominent); the mortality rate in a recent case series from Taiwan was 47%, with a rate in excess of 60% noted in an older U.S. series.[67,68]

PATHOGENESIS

It is likely that nonepidemic *V. cholerae* strains cause gastroenteritis through a number of different mechanisms, analogous to the multiplicity of mechanisms described for diarrheagenic *Escherichia coli*. Some *V. cholerae* strains outside of O groups 1 and 139 Bengal carry the genes for and produce cholera toxin (CT).[8,63] In one study in Bangladesh, CT-producing strains were isolated from 29% of cases of sporadic non-O1 *V. cholerae* gastroenteritis; patients infected with these strains had more severe illness, with greater weight loss, a significantly higher specific gravity on admission, and more prolonged and profuse diarrhea.[74] Most other studies, however, show that the production of CT is relatively uncommon among clinical isolates of nonepidemic serotypes of *V. cholerae*.[14,75]

A subgroup of *V. cholerae* strains produces a heat-stable enterotoxin (designated NAG-ST[76]) that closely resembles the heat-stable enterotoxin of enterotoxigenic *E. coli*. Volunteer studies, as well as epidemiologic studies of outbreak and sporadic cases of nonepidemic *V. cholerae* disease, suggest that these strains, tentatively designated enterotoxigenic *V. cholerae*, are a cause of diarrheal disease in humans.[12,68] Recently, the presence of a toxin gene cluster related to the family of RTX toxins was shown in several environmental isolates of *V. cholerae*, including non-O1 and O1, CT-negative strains. The RTX toxins genes encode a product that is responsible for a cytotoxic activity observed when mammalian cells are exposed to *V. cholerae* cells, suggesting that this toxin could be responsible for some of the pathogenic properties of the nonepidemic strains of *V. cholerae*.[77] While this and a number of other virulence factors have been proposed for nonepidemic *V. cholerae* strains,[78] the role of these factors in disease causation is not completely clear. In studies in volunteers,[68] two out of three nonepidemic *V. cholerae* strains tested did not cause human disease, suggesting that many, if not most, of the strains outside of known pathogenic subgroups are nonpathogenic commensals.

The pathogenicity of *V. parahaemolyticus* isolates has traditionally been correlated with the production of the thermostable direct hemolysin (Vp-TDH), which is responsible for the beta hemolysis seen when these isolates are plated on Wagatsuma agar.[15,79,80] Original studies in Japan showed that this phenomenon, named the Kanagawa phenomenon after the prefecture in Japan where it was discovered, was present in 96% of clinical isolates but in only 1% of environmental isolates. Volunteer studies also demonstrated the importance of Vp-TDH: Kanagawa-positive strains produced diarrhea whereas doses of up to 10^9 Kanagawa-negative strains failed to do so in 15 volunteers.[81] Furthermore, studies with isogenic mutants have shown that deletion of the Vp-TDH gene results in loss of enterotoxic activity in laboratory models (Ussing chamber and rabbit ileal loop assays).[82]

A second group of hemolysins, known as Vp-TDH-related hemolysins, or Vp-TRH, can be found in certain clinical isolates, especially those that are Kanagawa-negative.[83–85] These hemolysins are genetically related to Vp-TDH (they share around 70% sequence homology) but are more diverse (less than 2.8% divergence among most Vp-TDH vs. 16% between two subgroups of Vp-TRH). Studies of *V. parahaemolyticus* from the west coast of the United States and from Thailand have linked clinical illness with isolation of urease-positive, Kanagawa-negative strains from stool cultures.[86,87] These strains, in turn, have been shown almost always to carry the *tdh* gene.[88,89] Screening for urease production may permit identification of a subset of *V. parahaemolyticus* isolates that are Kanagawa-negative but are nonetheless virulent in humans. Whole genome sequence comparisons between *V. cholerae* and *V. parahaemolyticus* show that the two organisms use distinct mechanisms to establish infection with the genes of a type III secretion system (TTSS) being identified in the genome of *V. parahaemolyticus* but not *V. cholerae*.[90] The TTSS is a central virulence factor of diarrhea-causing bacteria such as shigella, salmonella, and enteropathogenic *E. coli*, which cause gastroenteritis by invading or intimately interacting with intestinal epithelial cells. Infection with *V. parahaemolyticus* results in B-cell responses and an acute inflammatory response that is self-limiting and less severe than that observed in patients with shigellosis but more severe than that seen in patients with cholera.[91]

Encapsulation appears to be a key virulence factor for strains which cause septicemia.[92,93] All *V. vulnificus* strains can produce a polysaccharide capsule. A majority of nonepidemic strains of *V. cholerae* also produce a capsule, with the degree of encapsulation correlating significantly with the risk of sepsis.[94] *V. cholerae* O1 strains (i.e., epidemic cholera strains) are not encapsulated and have not been associated with septicemia. Interestingly, *V. cholerae* O139 Bengal strains are encapsulated[95] and do appear to be able to cause septicemia in susceptible hosts. Encapsulation provides vibrios with protection against serum bactericidal activity and allows bacteria to resist opsonization and phagocytosis. Antibodies directed against the capsular polysaccharide are protective in animal models.[96]

DIAGNOSIS

Although some *Vibrio* species will grow on media routinely used for isolating stool pathogens, identification is often difficult. A selective medium made with thiosulfate, citrate, bile salts, and sucrose (TCBS agar) has become the standard medium used in microbiology laboratories for the isolation of these organisms. With the exception of a few strains of *V. hollisae*, all pathogenic vibrios will grow on this medium, producing colonies that are yellow (sucrose fermenters such as *V. cholerae*) or blue-green (nonsucrose fermenters such as *V. parahaemolyticus*). Isolates from wounds and blood will grow on any standard culture medium, including blood agar.

Table 22-2 Tests for Differentiation of Selected Vibrio *Species*

Test	*V. cholerae* O1 and Non-O1	*V. mimicus*	*V. parahaemolyticus*	*V. fluvialis*	*V. furnissi*	*V. hollisae*	*V. vulnificus*
Oxidase	+	+	+	+	+	+	+
NO_3-NO_2 + 1% NaCl	+	+	+	+	+	+	+
Indole + 1% NaCl	+	+	+	–	–	+/–	+
Voges-Proskauer + 1% NaCl	+/–	–	–	–	–	–	–
Urease	–	–	–/+	–	–	–	–
Lysine decarboxylase + 1% NaCl	+	+	+	–	–	–	+
Ornithine decarboxylase + 1% NaCl	+	+	+	–	–	–	+/–
Arginine dihydrolase + 1% NaCl	–	–	–	+	+	–	–
Fermentation of							
Sucrose	+	–	–	+	+	–	–/+
Lactose	(+)/–	+/–	–	–	–	–	+
L-Arabinose	–	–	+	+	+	+	–
Gas from glucose	–	–	–	–	+	–	–
Growth in nutrient broth							
0% NaCl	+	+	–	–	–	–	–
3% NaCl	+	+	+	+	+	+	+
6% NaCl	+/–	+/–	+	+/–	+/–	+/–	+/–
8% NaCl	–	–	+	–	–	–	–
10% NaCl	–	–	–	–	–	–	–
Susceptibility to O/129							
10 μg	S*	S	R	R	R	R	S
150 μg	S*	S	S	S	S	S	S
Growth on TCBS	Y	G	G	Y	Y	G/–	G/Y

+, most strains positive; –, most strains negative; +/– or –/+, variable reaction (predominant reaction shown as the numerator); ( ), delayed reaction; G, green colonies; R, resistant; S, susceptible; Y, yellow colonies; TCBS, thiosulfate citrate bile salts sucrose agar.
*Recent cotrimoxazole-resistant isolates in Calcutta also show resistance to pteridine.
From Janda JM, Powers C, Bryant AG, et al: Current perspectives on the epidemiology and pathogenesis of clinically significant *Vibrio* species. Clin Microbiol Rev 1:245–267, 1988.

Confirmation of the genus and identification of the species can be accomplished using standard biochemical panels (Table 22-2). It is important to remember that many vibrios are halophilic: the addition of 1% NaCl to growth media is often necessary to prevent false-negative reactions. When examining environmental samples, especially water samples, concentration procedures or selective enrichment broths may be needed.

Serotyping[97] is available for *V. cholerae* through the National Institute of Health, Tokyo, and may prove useful in analysis of outbreak-related strains. PCR and probe-based methods for identification of critical genes in many of these species are increasingly available on an experimental basis.[98–100] Similarly, there are increasing data on typing of strains by pulsed-field gel electrophoresis (PFGE) and multilocus sequence typing (MLST).[101]

TREATMENT AND PROGNOSIS

Treatment

As in any diarrheal disease, volume repletion is the most important element of therapy in patients with vibrio gastroenteritis. Antimicrobial therapy in cholera has been shown to reduce the duration of diarrhea and the excretion of vibrios. While there are no controlled trials of therapy in vibrio gastroenteritis, the use of antimicrobial therapy in more severe cases would appear to be reasonable. Based on in vitro susceptibility data (and data from clinical trials in cholera) tetracycline or ciprofloxacin appear to be the drugs of choice for therapy.

Wound infections require appropriate débridement and antimicrobial therapy; again, tetracycline or ciprofloxacin appear to be reasonable choices. For patients with septicemia, rapid initiation of antimicrobial therapy is critical, with studies suggesting that prognosis is worsened when therapy is delayed.[25] As with any patient with septicemia and shock, supportive care (ideally in an intensive care unit setting) is essential. Although no controlled trials are available, a combination of minocycline (100 mg q12h po) and cefotaxime (2.0 g q8h iv) or use of a "newer" fluoroquinolone has been recommended for treatment of sepsis caused by *V. vulnificus*,[102,103] and would appear to be reasonable in management of sepsis caused by other *Vibrio* species.

It has been shown in animal models that hyperimmune serum directed against the *V. vulnificus* capsular polysaccharide

however, the organism has been isolated with a prevalence of 10% to 25%, a finding that implicates nosocomial transmission as the primary form of acquisition for this organism.[27] McFarland and colleagues[28] studied 428 hospitalized patients and found that only 7% were culture positive for *C. difficile* on admission. An additional 21% of these patients acquired *C. difficile* during hospitalization, and 37% of this subset eventually developed a diarrheal illness.

Clostridium difficile can be isolated in 15% to 25% of patients with antibiotic-associated diarrhea and in 95% to 100% of patients with PMC.[5] In a prospective study, Gerding and associates[29] found that 30% of hospitalized adult patients with diarrhea had stools that were culture positive for *C. difficile* and determined that 87% of the cases of *C. difficile* colitis were nosocomially acquired. The results of several other studies indicate that as many as 1 in 100 hospitalized patients who receive antibiotics may develop *C. difficile* colitis, although the actual risk varies among institutions studied.[30]

Transmission and Prevalence

Whereas most types of anaerobic infections are generally believed to arise from endogenous sources, *C. difficile* infection is usually acquired nosocomially.[4] Evidence for the method of transmission of the organism is found in institutional outbreaks, in animal models of disease, and in multiple epidemiologic studies of *C. difficile*-induced colitis.[4,25,27,29] The major disease-related reservoirs of *C. difficile* include human carriers and environmental surfaces. Clabots and colleagues[31] noted a direct correlation between the likelihood of *C. difficile* acquisition and the length of hospital admission. In another study, McFarland and coworkers[28] found that 21% of patients became newly colonized with *C. difficile* during their hospital stay, and that the organism was cultured at a higher frequency from patients who were exposed to *C. difficile*-positive roommates. These investigators also found that the organism was frequently isolated from hospital environmental surfaces. *Clostridium difficile* spores are generally resistant to commonly used disinfectants, a finding that may help explain the high isolation rate of the organism from nosocomial surfaces.In this same study, up to 59% of health care workers caring for *C. difficile*-positive patients were found to be culture positive as well. This result helps to explain the high rate of nosocomial transmission of the organism. Notably, the use of vinyl gloves by hospital workers markedly reduces transmission of *C. difficile*.[32]

Risk Factors

Clostridium difficile colitis was initially described in association with clindamycin use. *Clostridium difficile* infections are still most frequently observed in patients receiving antibiotics, particularly in conjunction with hospitalization. Antimicrobials with activity against obligate anaerobic bacteria alter the normal microbial ecosystem and appear to put the patient at greatest risk of *C. difficile* infection.[5,33] In contrast, antimicrobials with little or no anaerobic activity appear to pose somewhat less of a risk. Classically, ampicillin, clindamycin, and cephalosporins are the agents believed to be most commonly associated with the development of *C. difficile* colitis[34–36] (Box 23-1). Clindamycin appears to have the highest relative risk. In one study, 10% to 20% of patients receiving this antibiotic developed diarrhea, and approximately 2% developed PMC.[37] The β-lactams, however, have probably been responsible for a greater number of cases of *C. difficile*-related disease, likely owing to the common use of this class of antibiotic.[25,34] The risk of *C. difficile* colitis appears to increase with the use of multiple antimicrobial agents, as well as with more prolonged courses of antibiotic treatment.[29,38–40] Brown and colleagues[39] found that greater than 10 days of antibiotic administration was a significant risk factor for the development of diarrhea due to *C. difficile*.

Box 23-1 Agents Implicated in *Clostridium difficile*-Associated Infections

Antimicrobials	***Antineoplastics***
Ampicillin/amoxicillin*	Doxorubicin
Cephalosporins*	Cisplatin
Clindamycin*	Cyclophosphamide
Other penicillins	Fluorouracil
Erythromycin	Methotrexate
Chloramphenicol	
Sulfonamides	
Imipenem-cilastatin	
Tetracyclines	
Trimethoprim	
Quinolones	
Rifampin	
Aminoglycosides†	
Metronidazole†	
Vancomycin†	

*Commonly associated.
†Rarely associated.

Although certain antibiotics carry a higher relative risk for the development of *C. difficile*-related disease, essentially all antibiotics have been reported to cause *C. difficile* colitis. Antimicrobials that are less commonly associated with *C. difficile* infections include the macrolides, chloramphenicol, the sulfonamides, the quinolones, tetracycline, and penicillins other than ampicillin and amoxicillin.[41] One report suggested that newer fluoroquinolones with broader antimicrobial activity, such as gatifloxacin, may be associated with increased incidence of *C. difficile* disease compared to those with more narrow spectrum.[42] Rare reports have described *C. difficile* with vancomycin, rifampin, and even metronidazole.[25,39] Therefore, disease due to *C. difficile* must be considered in any patient with diarrhea who has recently received any type of antibacterial agent. Notably, several case reports have also implicated antineoplastic drugs as occasional causes of *C. difficile* colitis (e.g., fluorouracil, methotrexate, cisplatin, doxorubicin, and cyclophosphamide).[43] These agents may act by altering the microecology of the gastrointestinal tract, either by intrinsic antimicrobial properties or by disruption of mucosal integrity.

Other, nonpharmacologic risk factors for the development of *C. difficile* infections have been reported in several studies and include advanced age, severe underlying illnesses, prolonged hospitalization, nasogastric intubation, fecal or urinary incontinence, intensive care unit stays, and recent surgery, especially involving the gastrointestinal tract.[38–40] In addition, recent studies support the concept that immune responses may protect against infection.[44] In one study, the presence of an initial antibody response to toxin A was associated with protection against recurrence of *C. difficile* diarrhea.[45]

DISEASE

Clostridium difficile infections represent a broad range of clinical disease, including asymptomatic carriage; mild, self-limited diarrhea; severe diarrhea; PMC; and toxic megacolon. A history of 5 to 10 days of antimicrobial exposure is typical. In some cases, however, there may be shorter incubation periods, and in others there may be delays of up to 10 weeks before the onset of symptoms is noted. Most commonly, patients present with mild diarrhea and lower abdominal cramping but with few systemic symptoms. In mild cases, symptoms may resolve simply with withdrawal of the offending antibiotic. Mucus may be present in the stools, but frankly bloody diarrhea occurs in only 5% to 10% of cases.[14,25] In patients with true colitis, fever, nausea, anorexia, dehydration, significant abdominal cramping or pain, and leukocytosis are usually present.[5,26,46,47] In certain cases, patients may have up to 20 loose stools per day. Patients with severe or fulminant colitis, however, may actually develop ileus, a complication that occurs most frequently in the elderly.[26,27]

Pseudomembranous plaques are present in up to 10% of cases of antimicrobial-induced colitis and usually indicate severe *C. difficile* disease.[46,48] In these cases, colonoscopy reveals the pathognomonic yellow-white plaques adherent to an erythematous mucosa. The lesions are generally found in the rectosigmoid and descending colon but, occasionally, can also be present throughout the intestinal tract. The plaques range in size from 2 to 10 mm and are composed of fibrin, mucus, necrotic epithelial cells, and leukocytes. In certain cases, the lesions can coalesce to form extensive areas of involvement. PMC due to *C. difficile* can lead to significant protein loss and result in hypoalbuminemia.[49]

Paralytic ileus, colonic dilation, and toxic megacolon represent a spectrum of rare but serious complications of PMC. With these complications, diarrhea often subsides and the patient may eventually develop abdominal distention and extreme pain. Also, the physical examination reveals features of an acute abdomen. In these situations, the risk of intestinal perforation is significant and precludes sigmoidoscopy. Surgery, when required, is difficult and is generally associated with a marked increase in mortality.[49]

PATHOGENESIS

Unlike many bacterial causes of inflammatory colitis, *C. difficile* is noninvasive. The pathogenesis of *C. difficile*-induced colitis is a result of one or both of two heat-labile exotoxins (toxin A and toxin B) produced by the organism in the setting of an altered colonic flora.[24,50,51] Approximately 25% of colonizing strains do not produce toxins and are not pathogenic. In general, toxigenic strains produce both toxins A and B. The relative amounts of each toxin produced by any one strain are variable and do not necessarily correlate with severity of disease. Toxin A is a 308-kDa enterotoxin and cytotoxin that leads to disruption of intestinal intercellular junctions, hemorrhagic fluid secretion, mucosal damage, and inflammation in animal models.[24] Toxin A likely binds to mucosal cells via a glycoprotein receptor on human intestinal epithelial cell surfaces, and the cellular uptake of toxin A has several characteristics of a receptor-mediated endocytic process.[52] The major intracellular target of toxin is the monoglucosylation of the Rho family of small G proteins. Rho proteins regulate a variety of cellular functions, most notably actin microfilament organization.[53,54] In addition, toxin A may exert some of its effects via a Rho-independent pathway, signals likely triggered directly by cell binding.[55] A key factor in the pathophysiology of PMC is the generation of an intense inflammatory response, a reaction that is likely elicited by toxin A-induced cytokine release (interleukins-1, -6, and -8 and tumor necrosis factor) from chemotactic neutrophils, monocytes, mast cells, and epithelial cells found in the tissues of the intestinal mucosa.[51,56,57]

Toxin B is an approximately 270-kDa protein that exerts cytotoxic effects toward certain tissue culture cell lines that can be up to 1000 times greater than that observed for toxin A.[51,52] Toxin B, however, does not exert enterotoxic activity in most animal models. Although it is clear that toxin A is critical to the development of clinical disease, roles for toxin B are less clear.[24] Intriguingly, toxin B also appears to inactivate the Rho proteins in certain cell types. Thus, differences in the biologic actions of toxins A and B must be related to differences in cell binding, mechanisms of cellular uptake, Rho-independent effects of the toxins, or a combination of these. Toxin A-negative, toxin B-positive strains of *C. difficile* have been shown to clearly induce serious disease.[58,59]

DIAGNOSIS

The diagnosis of *C. difficile* infection relies heavily on clinical acumen as well as appropriate laboratory evaluation.[20] A patient producing three or more unformed stools per day for at least 2 days in the setting of exposure to antimicrobial or antineoplastic agents can be considered to have the syndrome of antibiotic-associated diarrhea.[60,61] Endoscopy can be used to visualize pseudomembranes, which, if present, are highly suggestive of *C. difficile*-induced colitis.[4,29] This technique, however, is expensive, not always readily available, and runs the risk of serious complications, including colonic perforation. Therefore, endoscopy is not generally recommended except for the unusual and critically ill patient who would benefit from an immediate diagnosis of PMC so as to avoid exploratory laparotomy. In the vast majority of cases, laboratory evaluation is the preferred diagnostic approach, and several techniques are currently in use.

The cytotoxin (or tissue culture) assay detects primarily toxin B in stool filtrates by observing the characteristic cytotoxic changes that this toxin produces in standardized tissue culture cell lines. Because the vast majority of toxigenic *C. difficile* strains produce both toxins A and B, this assay is considered diagnostic of toxigenic *C. difficile*-induced colitis. The assay is time-consuming and requires trained technologists to examine the cell lines for cytotoxic effect. The diagnosis can be confirmed by neutralization of the cytotoxic effect using antitoxin specific for *C. difficile*. The sensitivity of the cytotoxic assay ranges from 70% to 100%, with a specificity of 95% to 99%.[20,60,62]

A correctly performed stool culture is extremely sensitive in detecting the presence of *C. difficile*. The specificity of culture is low, however, because culture techniques do not distinguish between nontoxigenic (and therefore nonpathogenic) and toxigenic strains of the organism. In addition, culture requires several days to achieve isolation and identification of the organism.[20,60]

The enzyme immunoassay (EIA) detects the presence of toxins A or B in stool filtrates and is a faster technique for diagnosing *C. difficile* infection. The specificity of this technique approaches that of the cytotoxin assay (75% to 100%), but the sensitivity of various commercial kits varies from 63% to 94%. Because of this wide variation in sensitivity, the performance history of any particular kit must be known to ascertain its clinical usefulness for any specific patient.[20,63] These assays are widely used and can be performed on two or three specimens to increase diagnostic yield.[64]

The latex agglutination (LA) test, although initially thought to detect the presence of toxins A or B, in fact detects the unrelated but *C. difficile*-specific enzyme, glutamate dehydrogenase.[65] LA tests are relatively insensitive compared to other assays (48% to 68%).[20,60] Furthermore, this antigen-based test, like stool culture, cannot distinguish nontoxigenic from toxigenic strains.

Fecal lactoferrin testing by latex agglutination provides a sensitive measure of inflammatory enteritis and correlates well with EIA and cytotoxin assays in patients with *C. difficile* infections.[66,67] As with a fecal leukocyte test, a positive fecal lactoferrin test in a patient with antibiotic-associated diarrhea should alert the clinician to the possibility of *C. difficile* colitis but is not diagnostic of the syndrome and should be followed by one of the specific tests listed previously.

Polymerase chain reaction (PCR) can detect toxigenic *C. difficile* by amplification of the toxin A or B gene or both genes. This research-based assay is under development and appears to be extremely sensitive.[68,69] If specificity issues and turnaround time can be improved, the test may prove valuable in the future.

TREATMENT AND PROGNOSIS

Initial Therapy

In patients with mild *C. difficile*-associated diarrhea, cessation of the offending antimicrobial, if possible, may be all that is required. Specific therapy is indicated for patients with more severe or persistent symptoms and also for those patients who require continuation of their original antimicrobial agents (Table 23-1). Initial therapy with oral metronidazole 250 mg four times daily, or oral vancomycin 125-mg capsules four times daily or a 500-mg intravenous preparation given orally, appears to be equally efficacious, with cure rates greater than 95% when administered for 10 days.[5,70,71] Some symptomatic improvement is usually seen within 24 to 72 hours of initiating therapy, although diarrhea and colitis may persist for several additional days. Metronidazole has generally been proposed as the therapy of choice because this agent is inexpensive and may reduce an important potential problem of vancomycin—selection for the emergence of other vancomycin-resistant organisms.[5] Vancomycin is preferred during pregnancy or lactation and is employed when patients fail to respond to metronidazole within the first 3 to 5 days.

Table 23-1 *Treatment of* Clostridium difficile-*Associated Disease*

Antibiotic	Cure Rate (%)	Relapse Rate (%)	References
Metronidazole* 250 mg PO qid × 10 days	>95	~5	5, 25, 71
Vancomycin 125 mg PO qid × 10 days	>95	~15	5, 71, 72, 75
Teicoplanin 100 mg bid × 10 days	>95	~8	72
Bacitracin 25,000 units PO qid × 10 days	~80	~30	74, 75

bid, twice a day; PO, by mouth; qid, four times a day.
*Relapses should be re-treated with the initial regimen because greater than 90% will achieve cures; relapse rates were not significantly different from those of vancomycin in trials using both antimicrobial therapies.

The relapse rates for metronidazole and vancomycin are similar (4% to 20%). The experience with oral teicoplanin 100 mg twice daily for 10 days is very limited, but in initial reports, this agent appears to have a similar response rate to that of oral vancomycin.[72] Agents such as bacitracin and cholestyramine have inferior cure or relapse profiles and should not be used as initial therapy.[73–75]

Although oral metronidazole is well absorbed from the upper gastrointestinal tract, bactericidal concentrations of the drug in feces can be measured in patients with inflammatory diarrhea.[76] Major side effects of metronidazole include nausea, the development of a metallic taste, and a disulfiram-like reaction that occurs with ingestion of alcohol. Oral vancomycin is not appreciably absorbed and is excreted unchanged in the stool. For patients who cannot take oral therapy or in whom oral therapy may be unreliable (notably patients with abdominal surgery, or those with ileus or toxic megacolon), intravenous metronidazole appears to be effective and bacteriocidal fecal concentrations can be achieved.[76,77] If ileus is present, oral metronidazole or oral vancomycin (500 mg four times daily) can be instilled via nasogastric tubes with documented efficacy.[5,70,78] Intravenous vancomycin, in contrast, does not undergo appreciable gastrointestinal excretion and should not be used for the treatment of *C. difficile*-associated disease.

Relapses

Up to 20% of patients treated for *C. difficile*-associated disease will have relapse after cessation of therapy. These relapses usually occur within 2 weeks after initial therapy is discontinued. Relapse is probably due to the persistence of antibiotic-resistant *C. difficile* spores rather than the development of antibiotic resistance of the vegetative organism. In patients with relapse, re-treatment with the initial agent will result in a greater than 90% cure rate.[5,70] Multiple empirical regimens have been evaluated in patients who suffer two or more recurrences. Most of these regimens focus on efforts to repopulate the normal colonic flora. Perhaps most encouraging is the use of *Saccharomyces boulardii* in combination with standard antimicrobial therapy in patients with recurrent infection. A blinded, controlled study demonstrated a reduced rate of relapse with this particular combination therapy when compared with standard antimicrobial therapy alone.[79] There are anecdotal reports of successful therapy using metronidazole followed by oral *Lactobacillus*,[80] vancomycin in combination with rifampin or cholestyramine,[81–83] tapering or pulse doses of vancomycin,[84] rectal instillation of stool or mixed broth cultures,[85] and intravenous immune globulin.[86,87] None of these therapies appear to be uniformly effective, and their use is empirical for any particular patient. With increasingly worrisome antibiotic-resistant enteric organisms (e.g., vancomycin-resistant enterococci), clearly the need is increasing for chemotherapeutic or immunologic agents (other than antimicrobials) that block the dramatic effects of the toxin(s),[88] such as antitoxic antibody, pharmacologic blockers such as phospholipase A_2 or cyclooxygenase inhibitors, or platelet-activating factor antagonists.[89]

PREVENTION AND CONTROL

Clostridium difficile-associated disease is in general acquired nosocomially in the context of concurrent antimicrobial therapy. Prevention and control efforts, therefore, are targeted at interrupting the horizontal transmission of the organism and restricting the use of antimicrobials. Although no specific barrier methods have been completely effective, it appears likely that the use of gloves, hand washing, and the enteric isolation of symptomatic infected patients reduce transmission of the organism.[28,32,39,90–92] It is less clear whether isolation of asymptomatic carriers is helpful.[31]

Environmental surfaces in rooms of patients with *C. difficile*-associated disease have a high rate of *C. difficile* contamination, with resistant spores presenting a challenge in terms of disinfection.[28] Disinfection of the contaminated hospital environment with hypochlorite, formaldehyde, or glutaraldehyde solutions reduces the amount of *C. difficile* cultured from these surfaces. Therefore, although no well-controlled trials of environmental disinfection have been published, this may be an important adjunctive measure to reduce nosocomial transmission of the organism.[92,93]

Given that there is a strong association of *C. difficile* colitis with antibiotic use, restricting the use of the more common offending agents would likely be helpful in controlling the incidence of *C. difficile*-related disease. Restriction of clindamycin use has been reported to reduce the incidence of *C. difficile*-associated diarrhea, but few additional studies have addressed this issue.[39,94,95] Furthermore, the majority of studies that have examined prophylactic measures in the setting of outbreaks instituted multiple control measures simultaneously, thus making it difficult to distinguish the relative merits of any individual intervention.

Prophylactic therapy for patients already receiving antimicrobials is not well studied. One trial using *S. boulardii* during antimicrobial administration and for 2 weeks thereafter did demonstrate a reduction of antibiotic-associated diarrhea.[79] In this study, the incidence of *C. difficile*-associated diarrhea was reduced when compared with placebo but did not reach statistical significance. Other agents reported to be useful for prophylaxis include bovine *C. difficile* antibodies and *Lactobacillus* in the form of yogurt or acidophilus milk.[80,96] Initial results appear promising, but further clinical testing is required to determine the true utility of these regimens.

OTHER ENTERIC *CLOSTRIDIUM* INFECTIONS

Clostridium perfringens

Clostridium perfringens type C has been the cause of both sporadic and epidemic cases of necrotizing enteritis. Clinical entities such as *Darmbrand* ("bowel gangrene") in postwar Germany during the 1940s and pigbel[97] in the Papua New Guinea highlands have been attributed to this organism, which elicits alpha and beta toxins capable of causing the enteritis. Poor nutrition and episodic dietary indulgence have been associated with these entities, with investigators suggesting that a low level of digestive enzymes in people with low protein dietary intake may prevent normal inactivation of bacterial toxins.[98] Clinically, previously healthy patients present with a necrotizing enteritis syndrome that may include anorexia, nausea, vomiting, abdominal pain, and hematochezia and may progress to sepsis. Complications are common and include peritonitis secondary to bowel perforation, ileus, and chronic scarring leading to malabsorption, obstruction, or fistulas.

Multiple lines of evidence in animal and human models suggest that it is the beta toxin of *C. perfringens* type C that is responsible for clinical disease.[98–100] Serum beta antitoxin titers were significantly increased after illness with pigbel in 12 of 21 cases in Papua New Guinea, and administration of type C antiserum resulted in a 30% decrease in the need for surgery, reducing mortality from 43% to 19%.[97,101] Finally, active immunization against the beta toxin has proved to be effective in preventing pigbel.[99,100]

Therapy for these enteritides includes bowel decompression, supportive care, and surgical resection of involved bowel in patients who have perforation, sepsis, or a palpable mass lesion. Antiserum to *C. perfringens* type C containing beta antitoxin can be administered. The active beta toxin vaccine can be used prophylactically in areas where disease is likely to occur.

Clostridium botulinum

Clostridium botulinum is the cause of botulism and is due to intoxication with a group of similar clostridial neurotoxins (types A to G) that predominantly affect the peripheral neuromuscular junction and autonomic synapses.[102] Although classically associated with food-borne, wound, and infantile presentations, an inhalational form in the setting of bioterrorism has been discussed.[102] All forms lead to similar neurologic presentations.

Food-borne botulism is most frequently recognized during outbreaks and appears to be due to ingestion of toxins found in home-canned vegetables, fruits, and fish products.[103] The toxin is absorbed in the duodenum and jejunum, passes into the bloodstream, and acts at peripheral cholinergic synapses much like tetanus toxin to proteolytically cleave synaptobrevin II to prevent the vesicular docking and extracellular release of acetylcholine; this induces paralysis in the motor system and autonomic dysfunction in autonomic ganglia and parasympathetic nerve terminals.[102,104]

Food-borne botulism develops 24 to 36 hours after ingestion of the toxin and may initially cause diarrhea, dry mouth, and nausea.[102] Evidence of cranial nerve dysfunction soon follows—notably blurred vision, diplopia, dysphagia, and dysarthria—eventually spreading to the upper and lower extremities and the respiratory musculature.[104,105] Autonomic dysfunction may lead to constipation, alterations in heart rate and blood pressure, and urinary retention.[106] Treatment of botulism is primarily supportive, with particular attention given to ventilatory support.[102,104] Antitoxin therapy with equine serum is available, although no controlled trials have been performed. Purgatives may be given initially for contaminated food still present in the gastrointestinal tract, but they should be avoided in the presence of ileus.

Clostridium tetani is reviewed in Chapter 43. Other clostridial infections causing myonecrosis or gangrene (often in combination with other anaerobes or staphylococci or streptococci) are beyond the scope of this chapter and are reviewed in standard textbooks of infectious diseases.[97]

SUMMARY

Clostridium difficile infection is a common cause of nosocomial diarrhea that generally occurs in the setting of antimicrobial exposure. Infections require the presence of both the *C. difficile* organism and its unique enterotoxin, toxin A. *Clostridium difficile* infections comprise a spectrum of disease ranging from mild diarrhea to toxic megacolon and death. Treatment with oral metronidazole or vancomycin is effective, and prevention of nosocomial horizontal transmission by barrier techniques, antimicrobial restriction, and enteric isolation may deter future outbreaks.

REFERENCES

1. Guerrant RL, Hughes JM, Lima NL, et al: Diarrhea in developed and developing countries: Magnitude, special settings, and etiologies. Rev Infect Dis 12(Suppl 1):S41–S50, 1990.
2. Johnson S, Gerding DN: *Clostridium difficile*-associated diarrhea. Clin Infect Dis 26:1027–1034; quiz 1035–1036, 1998.
3. Wilcox MH: *Clostridium difficile*—Setting the scene. J Antimicrob Chemother 41(Suppl C):1–3, 1998.
4. Gerding DN, Johnson S, Peterson LR, et al: *Clostridium difficile*-associated diarrhea and colitis. Infect Control Hosp Epidemiol 16:459–477, 1995.
5. Bartlett JG: Clinical practice. Antibiotic-associated diarrhea. N Engl J Med 346:334–339, 2002.
6. Riley TV, Cooper M, Bell B, et al: Community-acquired *Clostridium difficile*-associated diarrhea. Clin Infect Dis 20(Suppl 2):S263–S265, 1995.
7. Forward LJ, Tompkins DS, Brett MM: Detection of *Clostridium difficile* cytotoxin and *Clostridium perfringens* enterotoxin in cases of diarrhoea in the community. J Med Microbiol 52:753–757, 2003.
8. Riley TV, O'Neill GL, Bowman RA, et al: *Clostridium difficile*-associated diarrhoea: Epidemiological data from Western Australia. Epidemiol Infect 113:13–20, 1994.
9. Ayyagari A, Sharma P, Venkateswarlu K, et al: Prevalence of *Clostridium difficile* in pseudomembranous and antibiotic-associated colitis in north India. J Diarrhoeal Dis Res 4:157–160, 1986.
10. Akhtar SQ: Isolation of *Clostridium difficile* from diarrhoea patients in Bangladesh. J Trop Med Hyg 90:189–192, 1987.
11. Oyofo BA, Subekti D, Tjaniadi P, et al: Enteropathogens associated with acute diarrhea in community and hospital patients in Jakarta, Indonesia. FEMS Immunol Med Microbiol 34:139–146, 2002.
12. Pinto LJ, Alcides AP, Ferreira EO, et al: Incidence and importance of *Clostridium difficile* in paediatric diarrhoea in Brazil. J Med Microbiol 52:1095–1099, 2003.
13. Maraki S, Georgiladakis A, Tselentis Y, et al: A 5-year study of the bacterial pathogens associated with acute diarrhoea on the island of Crete, Greece, and their resistance to antibiotics. Eur J Epidemiol 18:85–90, 2003.
14. Tedesco FJ, Barton RW, Alpers DH: Clindamycin-associated colitis. A prospective study. Ann Intern Med 81:429–433, 1974.
15. Bartlett JG, Onderdonk AB, Cisneros RL, et al: Clindamycin-associated colitis due to a toxin-producing species of Clostridium in hamsters. J Infect Dis 136:701–705, 1977.
16. Hall I, O'Toole E: Intestinal flora in new-born infants: With a description of a new pathogenic anaerobe, *Bacillus difficilis*. Am J Dis Child 49: 390–402, 1935.
17. Bartlett JG, Onderdonk AB, Cisneros RL: Clindamycin-associated colitis in hamsters: Protection with vancomycin. Gastroenterology 73:772–776, 1977.
18. Wilson KH: The microecology of *Clostridium difficile*. Clin Infect Dis 16(Suppl 4):S214–S218, 1993.
19. Delmee M: Laboratory diagnosis of *Clostridium difficile* disease. Clin Microbiol Infect 7:411–416, 2001.
20. Wilkins TD, Lyerly DM: *Clostridium difficile* testing: After 20 years, still challenging. J Clin Microbiol 41:531–534, 2003.
21. Viscidi R, Willey S, Bartlett JG: Isolation rates and toxigenic potential of *Clostridium difficile* isolates from various patient populations. Gastroenterology 81:5–9, 1981.
22. Eglow R, Pothoulakis C, Itzkowitz S, et al: Diminished *Clostridium difficile* toxin A sensitivity in newborn rabbit ileum is associated with decreased toxin A receptor. J Clin Invest 90:822–829, 1992.
23. Wada N, Nishida N, Iwaki S, et al: Neutralizing activity against *Clostridium difficile* toxin in the supernatants of cultured colostral cells. Infect Immun 29:545–550, 1980.
24. Borriello SP: Pathogenesis of *Clostridium difficile* infection. J Antimicrob Chemother 41(Suppl C):13–19, 1998.
25. Kelly CP, Pothoulakis C, LaMont JT: *Clostridium difficile* colitis. N Engl J Med 330:257–262, 1994.
26. Fekety R, Shah AB: Diagnosis and treatment of *Clostridium difficile* colitis. JAMA 269:71–75, 1993.
27. Bartlett JG: *Clostridium difficile*: History of its role as an enteric pathogen and the current state of knowledge about the organism. Clin Infect Dis 18(Suppl 4):S265–S272, 1994.
28. McFarland LV, Mulligan ME, Kwok RY, et al: Nosocomial acquisition of *Clostridium difficile* infection. N Engl J Med 320:204–210, 1989.
29. Gerding DN, Olson MM, Peterson LR, et al: *Clostridium difficile*-associated diarrhea and colitis in adults. A prospective case-controlled epidemiologic study. Arch Intern Med 146:95–100, 1986.
30. Silva J Jr: Update on pseudomembranous colitis. West J Med 151: 644–648, 1989.
31. Clabots CR, Johnson S, Olson MM, et al: Acquisition of *Clostridium difficile* by hospitalized patients: Evidence for colonized new admissions as a source of infection. J Infect Dis 166:561–567, 1992.
32. Johnson S, Gerding DN, Olson MM, et al: Prospective, controlled study of vinyl glove use to interrupt *Clostridium difficile* nosocomial transmission. Am J Med 88:137–140, 1990.
33. Vollaard EJ, Clasener HA, van Saene HK, et al: Effect on colonization resistance: An important criterion in selecting antibiotics. DICP 24: 60–66, 1990.
34. Golledge CL, McKenzie T, Riley TV: Extended spectrum cephalosporins and *Clostridium difficile*. J Antimicrob Chemother 23:929–931, 1989.
35. Silva J, Fekety R, Werk C, et al: Inciting and etiologic agents of colitis. Rev Infect Dis 6(Suppl 1):S214–S221, 1984.
36. Bartlett JG: *Clostridium difficile*: Clinical considerations. Rev Infect Dis 12(Suppl 2):S243–S251, 1990.
37. Gurwith MJ, Rabin HR, Love K: Diarrhea associated with clindamycin and ampicillin therapy: Preliminary results of a cooperative study. J Infect Dis 135(Suppl):S104–S110, 1977.
38. McFarland LV, Surawicz CM, Stamm WE: Risk factors for *Clostridium difficile* carriage and *C. difficile*-associated diarrhea in a cohort of hospitalized patients. J Infect Dis 162:678–684, 1990.
39. Brown E, Talbot GH, Axelrod P, et al: Risk factors for *Clostridium difficile* toxin-associated diarrhea. Infect Control Hosp Epidemiol 11:283–290, 1990.
40. Thibault A, Miller MA, Gaese C: Risk factors for the development of *Clostridium difficile*-associated diarrhea during a hospital outbreak. Infect Control Hosp Epidemiol 12:345–348, 1991.
41. Bartlett JG: Antimicrobial agents implicated in *Clostridium difficile* toxin-associated diarrhea of colitis. Johns Hopkins Med J 149:6–9, 1981.
42. Gaynes R, Rimland D, Killum E, et al: Outbreak of *Clostridium difficile* infection in a long-term care facility: Association with gatifloxacin use. Clin Infect Dis 38:640–645, 2004.
43. Anand A, Glatt AE: *Clostridium difficile* infection associated with antineoplastic chemotherapy: A review. Clin Infect Dis 17:109–113, 1993.

44. Kyne L, Warny M, Qamar A, et al: Asymptomatic carriage of *Clostridium difficile* and serum levels of IgG antibody against toxin A. N Engl J Med 342:390–397, 2000.
45. Kyne L, Warny M, Qamar A, et al: Association between antibody response to toxin A and protection against recurrent *Clostridium difficile* diarrhoea. Lancet 357:189–193, 2001.
46. Knoop FC, Owens M, Crocker IC: *Clostridium difficile*: Clinical disease and diagnosis. Clin Microbiol Rev 6:251–265, 1993.
47. Bartlett JG: Leukocytosis and *Clostridium difficile*-associated diarrhea. Am J Gastroenterol 95:3023–3024, 2000.
48. Counihan TC, Roberts PL: Pseudomembranous colitis. Surg Clin North Am 73:1063–1074, 1993.
49. Rybolt AH, Bennett RG, Laughon BE, et al: Protein-losing enteropathy associated with *Clostridium difficile* infection. Lancet 1:1353–1355, 1989.
50. Borriello SP, Davies HA, Kamiya S, et al: Virulence factors of *Clostridium difficile*. Rev Infect Dis 12(Suppl 2):S185–S191, 1990.
51. Bongaerts GP, Lyerly DM: Role of toxins A and B in the pathogenesis of *Clostridium difficile* disease. Microb Pathog 17:1–12, 1994.
52. Lyerly DM, Krivan HC, Wilkins TD: *Clostridium difficile*: Its disease and toxins. Clin Microbiol Rev 1:1–18, 1988.
53. Just I, Wilm M, Selzer J, et al: The enterotoxin from *Clostridium difficile* (ToxA) monoglucosylates the Rho proteins. J Biol Chem 270: 13932–13936, 1995.
54. Dillon ST, Rubin EJ, Yakubovich M, et al: Involvement of Ras-related Rho proteins in the mechanisms of action of *Clostridium difficile* toxin A and toxin B. Infect Immun 63:1421–1426, 1995.
55. Pothoulakis C, Sullivan R, Melnick DA, et al: *Clostridium difficile* toxin A stimulates intracellular calcium release and chemotactic response in human granulocytes. J Clin Invest 81:1741–1745, 1988.
56. Steiner TS, Flores CA, Pizarro TT, et al: Fecal lactoferrin, interleukin-1beta, and interleukin-8 are elevated in patients with severe *Clostridium difficile* colitis. Clin Diagn Lab Immunol 4:719–722, 1997.
57. Flegel WA, Muller F, Daubener W, et al: Cytokine response by human monocytes to *Clostridium difficile* toxin A and toxin B. Infect Immun 59:3659–3666, 1991.
58. Alfa MJ, Kabani A, Lyerly D, et al: Characterization of a toxin A-negative, toxin B-positive strain of *Clostridium difficile* responsible for a nosocomial outbreak of *Clostridium difficile*-associated diarrhea. J Clin Microbiol 38:2706–2714, 2000.
59. Johnson S, Kent SA, O'Leary KJ, et al: Fatal pseudomembranous colitis associated with a variant *Clostridium difficile* strain not detected by toxin A immunoassay. Ann Intern Med 135:434–438, 2001.
60. Gerding DN, Brazier JS: Optimal methods for identifying *Clostridium difficile* infections. Clin Infect Dis 16(Suppl 4):S439–S442, 1993.
61. Fekety R: Guidelines for the diagnosis and management of *Clostridium difficile*-associated diarrhea and colitis. American College of Gastroenterology, Practice Parameters Committee. Am J Gastroenterol 92:739–750, 1997.
62. Peterson LR, Kelly PJ: The role of the clinical microbiology laboratory in the management of *Clostridium difficile*-associated diarrhea. Infect Dis Clin North Am 7:277–293, 1993.
63. Whittier S, Shapiro DS, Kelly WF, et al: Evaluation of four commercially available enzyme immunoassays for laboratory diagnosis of *Clostridium difficile*-associated diseases. J Clin Microbiol 31:2861–2865, 1993.
64. Manabe YC, Vinetz JM, Moore RD, et al: *Clostridium difficile* colitis: An efficient clinical approach to diagnosis. Ann Intern Med 123:835–840, 1995.
65. Willis DH, Kraft JA: Confirmation that the latex-reactive protein of *Clostridium difficile* is a glutamate dehydrogenase. J Clin Microbiol 30:1363–1364, 1992.
66. Guerrant RL, Araujo V, Soares E, et al: Measurement of fecal lactoferrin as a marker of fecal leukocytes. J Clin Microbiol 30:1238–1242, 1992.
67. Schleupner MA, Garner DC, Sosnowski KM, et al: Concurrence of *Clostridium difficile* toxin A enzyme-linked immunosorbent assay, fecal lactoferrin assay, and clinical criteria with *C. difficile* cytotoxin titer in two patient cohorts. J Clin Microbiol 33:1755–1759, 1995.
68. Kato N, Ou CY, Kato H, et al: Identification of toxigenic *Clostridium difficile* by the polymerase chain reaction. J Clin Microbiol 29:33–37, 1991.
69. Kuhl SJ, Tang YJ, Navarro L, et al: Diagnosis and monitoring of *Clostridium difficile* infections with the polymerase chain reaction. Clin Infect Dis 16(Suppl 4):S234–S238, 1993.
70. Olson MM, Shanholtzer CJ, Lee JT Jr, et al: Ten years of prospective *Clostridium difficile*-associated disease surveillance and treatment at the Minneapolis VA Medical Center, 1982–1991. Infect Control Hosp Epidemiol 15:371–381, 1994.
71. Teasley DG, Gerding DN, Olson MM, et al: Prospective randomised trial of metronidazole versus vancomycin for *Clostridium-difficile*-associated diarrhoea and colitis. Lancet 2:1043–1046, 1983.
72. de Lalla F, Nicolin R, Rinaldi E, et al: Prospective study of oral teicoplanin versus oral vancomycin for therapy of pseudomembranous colitis and *Clostridium difficile*-associated diarrhea. Antimicrob Agents Chemother 36:2192–2196, 1992.
73. Mogg GA, Arabi Y, Youngs D, et al: Therapeutic trials of antibiotic associated colitis. Scand J Infect Dis Suppl:41–45, 1980.
74. Young GP, Ward PB, Bayley N, et al: Antibiotic-associated colitis due to *Clostridium difficile*: Double-blind comparison of vancomycin with bacitracin. Gastroenterology 89:1038–1045, 1985.
75. Dudley MN, McLaughlin JC, Carrington G, et al: Oral bacitracin vs vancomycin therapy for *Clostridium difficile*-induced diarrhea. A randomized double-blind trial. Arch Intern Med 146:1101–1104, 1986.
76. Bolton RP, Culshaw MA: Faecal metronidazole concentrations during oral and intravenous therapy for antibiotic associated colitis due to *Clostridium difficile*. Gut 27:1169–1172, 1986.
77. Kleinfeld DI, Sharpe RJ, Donta ST: Parenteral therapy for antibiotic-associated pseudomembranous colitis. J Infect Dis 157:389, 1988.
78. Apisarnthanarak A, Razavi B, Mundy LM: Adjunctive intracolonic vancomycin for severe *Clostridium difficile* colitis: Case series and review of the literature. Clin Infect Dis 35:690–696, 2002.
79. Surawicz CM, Elmer GW, Speelman P, et al: Prevention of antibiotic-associated diarrhea by *Saccharomyces boulardii*: A prospective study. Gastroenterology 96:981–988, 1989.
80. Gorbach SL: Lactic acid bacteria and human health. Ann Med 22: 37–41, 1990.
81. Pruksananonda P, Powell KR: Multiple relapses of *Clostridium difficile*-associated diarrhea responding to an extended course of cholestyramine. Pediatr Infect Dis J 8:175–178, 1989.
82. Moncino MD, Falletta JM: Multiple relapses of *Clostridium difficile*-associated diarrhea in a cancer patient. Successful control with long-term cholestyramine therapy. Am J Pediatr Hematol Oncol 14:361–364, 1992.
83. Buggy BP, Fekety R, Silva J Jr: Therapy of relapsing *Clostridium difficile*-associated diarrhea and colitis with the combination of vancomycin and rifampin. J Clin Gastroenterol 9:155–159, 1987.
84. Tedesco FJ, Gordon D, Fortson WC: Approach to patients with multiple relapses of antibiotic-associated pseudomembranous colitis. Am J Gastroenterol 80:867–868, 1985.
85. Tvede M, Rask-Madsen J: Bacteriotherapy for chronic relapsing *Clostridium difficile* diarrhoea in six patients. Lancet 1:1156–1160, 1989.
86. Salcedo J, Keates S, Pothoulakis C, et al: Intravenous immunoglobulin therapy for severe *Clostridium difficile* colitis. Gut 41:366–370, 1997.
87. Leung DY, Kelly CP, Boguniewicz M, et al: Treatment with intravenously administered gamma globulin of chronic relapsing colitis induced by *Clostridium difficile* toxin. J Pediatr 118:633–637, 1991.
88. Lima AA, Lyerly DM, Wilkins TD, et al: Effects of *Clostridium difficile* toxins A and B in rabbit small and large intestine in vivo and on cultured cells in vitro. Infect Immun 56:582–588, 1988.
89. Fonteles M, Fang G, Thielman NM, et al: Role of platelet activating factor in the inflammatory and secretory effects of *Clostridium difficile* toxin A. J Lipid Mediat Cell Signal 11:133–143, 1995.
90. Nolan NP, Kelly CP, Humphreys JF, et al: An epidemic of pseudo-membranous colitis: Importance of person to person spread. Gut 28:1467–1473, 1987.
91. Bettin K, Clabots C, Mathie P, et al: Effectiveness of liquid soap vs. chlorhexidine gluconate for the removal of *Clostridium difficile* from bare hands and gloved hands. Infect Control Hosp Epidemiol 15:697–702, 1994.
92. Struelens MJ, Maas A, Nonhoff C, et al: Control of nosocomial transmission of *Clostridium difficile* based on sporadic case surveillance. Am J Med 91:138S–144S, 1991.
93. Kaatz GW, Gitlin SD, Schaberg DR, et al: Acquisition of *Clostridium difficile* from the hospital environment. Am J Epidemiol 127:1289–1294, 1988.
94. Pear SM, Williamson TH, Bettin KM, et al: Decrease in nosocomial *Clostridium difficile*-associated diarrhea by restricting clindamycin use. Ann Intern Med 120:272–277, 1994.

95. Climo MW, Israel DS, Wong ES, et al: Hospital-wide restriction of clindamycin: Effect on the incidence of *Clostridium difficile*-associated diarrhea and cost. Ann Intern Med 128:989–995, 1998.
96. Lyerly DM, Bostwick EF, Binion SB, et al: Passive immunization of hamsters against disease caused by *Clostridium difficile* by use of bovine immunoglobulin G concentrate. Infect Immun 59:2215–2218, 1991.
97. Murrell TG, Roth L, Egerton J, et al: Pig-bel: Enteritis necroticans. A study in diagnosis and management. Lancet 1:217–222, 1966.
98. Lawrence G, Walker PD: Pathogenesis of enteritis necroticans in Papula New Guinea. Lancet 1:125–126, 1976.
99. Lawrence G, Shann F, Freestone DS, et al: Prevention of necrotising enteritis in Papua New Guinea by active immunisation. Lancet 1:227–230, 1979.
100. Lawrence GW, Lehmann D, Anian G, et al: Impact of active immunisation against enteritis necroticans in Papua New Guinea. Lancet 336:1165–1167, 1990.
101. Murrell TG: Pig-bel—Epidemic and sporadic necrotizing enteritis in the highlands of New Guinea. Australas Ann Med 16:4–10, 1967.
102. Arnon SS, Schechter R, Inglesby TV, et al: Botulinum toxin as a biological weapon: Medical and public health management. JAMA 285:1059–1070, 2001.
103. MacDonald KL, Cohen ML, Blake PA: The changing epidemiology of adult botulism in the United States. Am J Epidemiol 124:794–799, 1986.
104. Hughes JM, Blumenthal JR, Merson MH, et al: Clinical features of types A and B food-borne botulism. Ann Intern Med 95:442–445, 1981.
105. Weber JT, Hibbs RG Jr, Darwish A, et al: A massive outbreak of type E botulism associated with traditional salted fish in Cairo. J Infect Dis 167:451–454, 1993.
106. Vita G, Girlanda P, Puglisi RM, et al: Cardiovascular-reflex testing and single-fiber electromyography in botulism. A longitudinal study. Arch Neurol 44:202–206, 1987.

24

Helicobacter pylori *Infections*

BARRY J. MARSHALL
ROBERT H. GILMAN

INTRODUCTION

Helicobacter pylori colonizes the mucus layer of the human stomach and causes inflammation termed *active chronic gastritis.*[1] *H. pylori* can easily be identified using simple techniques available in all microbiology laboratories. The bacterium infects more than half of the population of the world, is more common in tropical countries, and in some people it causes peptic ulceration or gastric cancer. In the tropics it may be associated with reduced gastric acid,[2] increased diarrhea, and malnutrition.[3] *H. pylori* can be diagnosed by direct examination of gastric mucosal biopsy tissue obtained at endoscopy, or noninvasively using serology, a urea breath test, or a fecal antigen test. Cure of the infection is possible in most patients with a two-week treatment using combinations of antimicrobial agents and acid-lowering drugs.[4] In the tropics, due to poor sanitation, reinfection is common.[5–7] For this reason there is currently much interest in the development of an oral vaccine to prevent new infections.

AGENT

H. pylori is the type strain of a new genus of spiral-shaped bacteria named *Helicobacter*. Their morphology and sheathed flagella may facilitate motility in the mucus layer of the gastrointestinal tract. *H. pylori* is microaerophilic, which means that it prefers a reduced amount of oxygen for growth, but is not anaerobic. This is probably the environment found in the mucus layer of the gut, a transitional zone between the anaerobic lumen and the oxygenated mucosa. The characteristics and growth requirements of *H. pylori* are listed next.

Morphologically, *H. pylori* is a gram-negative spiral, 3.5 μm long × 0.6 μm thick, with 1.5 wavelengths and four to seven sheathed flagella at one end of the organism, as shown in Figure 24-1. In tissues *H. pylori* appears spiral and lies close to the gastric epithelial cells and in the mucus glands. Squashed or smeared fresh gastric biopsy specimens may be stained by Gram stain or examined by phase contrast microscopy.[8,9] In histologic sections *H. pylori* stains well with Giemsa, toluidine blue, or silver stains. Hematoxylin and eosin (H&E) stain does not adequately demonstrate *H. pylori*.

In culture, *H. pylori* appears longer and spiral forms are not as obvious. Usually comma shapes and U-shapes (unseparated dividing organisms) are seen.[10]

Culture

H. pylori is microaerophilic, growing in reduced O_2 at 37°C in 4 to 6 days on fresh (preferably) chocolate or blood agar. The "*Campylobacter* atmosphere" generated by a commercial *Campylobacter* kit in a gas jar provides atmosphere for *H. pylori* culture. If available, a 10% CO_2 incubator also provides excellent growth conditions. "*Campylobacter*" atmospheres are also available as premixed cylinders that can be used to fill a sealable plastic bag with a moist paper towel inside. If nothing else is available, a candle jar with moist paper towels in the bottom will provide an adequate atmosphere, and even gas-generating methods such as the "steel wool and Alka Seltzer" idea of Pennie and colleagues[11] can be used.

Selective Media

Although *H. pylori* can be isolated easily from gastric biopsy samples onto nonselective media, 20% of patients have bacterial contamination of the biopsy, and overgrowth of commensal flora will make isolation of *H. pylori* difficult. To maximize the isolation rate, a selective medium can be made by adding vancomycin, trimethoprim, and amphotericin to the culture medium.[12] Ready-made selective media for *H. pylori* culture are available,[13] or *Campylobacter* isolation media such as Skirrow's medium may also be used.[14]

Identification

On blood or chocolate agar, transparent or pale-yellow 1- to 2-mm "water spray" colonies appear after 3 to 6 days. They are strongly positive for catalase, oxidase, and rapid urease. In the last-named test, a pink color is observed within 5 minutes of applying a colony to Christensen's urea agar. The organism may also be grown in broth such as shaking tubes of *Brucella* broth[15] or in gas-permeable shaking bags[16] in a CO_2 incubator, or in fermenters.[17]

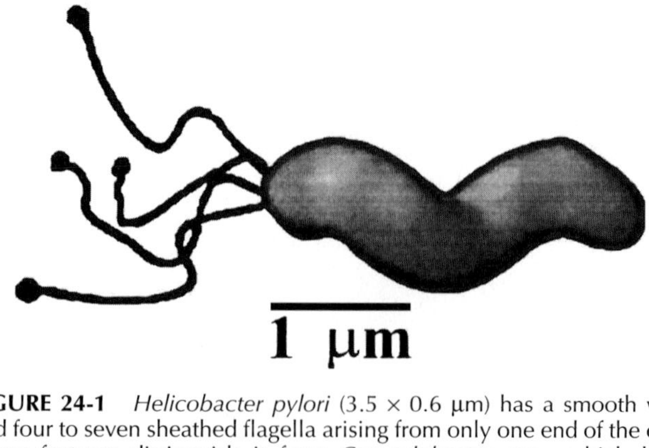

FIGURE 24-1 *Helicobacter pylori* (3.5 × 0.6 μm) has a smooth wall and four to seven sheathed flagella arising from only one end of the cell. These features distinguish it from *Campylobacter* spp., which have rough cell walls and a single, thinner, unsheathed flagellum at each end of the cell. Other *Helicobacter* spp. have distinguishing features such as many flagella and axial filaments (*H. felis* from cats) or flagella sprouting from the sides of the organism (*H. mustelae* from ferrets). Mature organisms appear as spiral forms with 1.5 wavelengths.

Pitfalls

When subculturing *H. pylori*, one should always examine the Gram's stain morphology of *H. pylori* as well as perform the biochemical identification tests described earlier. Contaminating organisms may appear similar to the naked eye and are often urease, oxidase, or catalase positive.

EPIDEMIOLOGY AND TRANSMISSION

H. pylori infects more than 70% of persons in most developing countries and about 30% of persons in developed countries. In societies that have recently emerged to affluence (such as Japan), *H. pylori* is still quite common and infects most persons over the age of 40 years.

H. pylori is acquired in childhood, probably by the fecal-oral route. The bacterium has been isolated from the feces of children in The Gambia[18] and polymerase chain reaction (PCR) techniques have demonstrated the genome of the organism in water from Peru.[5] In developing countries, children may be infected at the rate of 15% per annum so that most of the population is infected by adulthood. The initial infection with *H. pylori* may be somewhat precarious in that some children lose the infection spontaneously for a time but then reacquire it from the environment. This may occur several times before the child maintains a stable permanent gastric infection.[19] Initially the infection may spread from one parent to one of the children in the family, then spread to other family members, siblings, or the uninfected parent by fecal contamination, and even aerosols of vomitus.[20,21] Thus the infection is transmitted from one generation to the next, but young children appear to amplify the infection rate.[22]

The exact mechanism of spread is still somewhat controversial. *H. pylori* DNA is sometimes present in the dental plaque of some infected persons,[23] but actual live organisms are only very rarely culturable from the oral cavity. Thus the organisms might occasionally be carried to the mouth in gastric reflux, but probably do not live in the mouth. Oral-oral spread of *H. pylori* seems possible but has been hard to demonstrate. For example, in Belgium, investigators studied infants born to 67 infected mothers but could detect only one new *H. pylori* infection by breath test during a 12-month period.[24] This may mean that most new infections in developing countries are fecal-oral, that is, from other children, relatives, or from environmental sources. The prevalence rate in developing countries, as compared with Western countries, is shown in Figure 24-2.

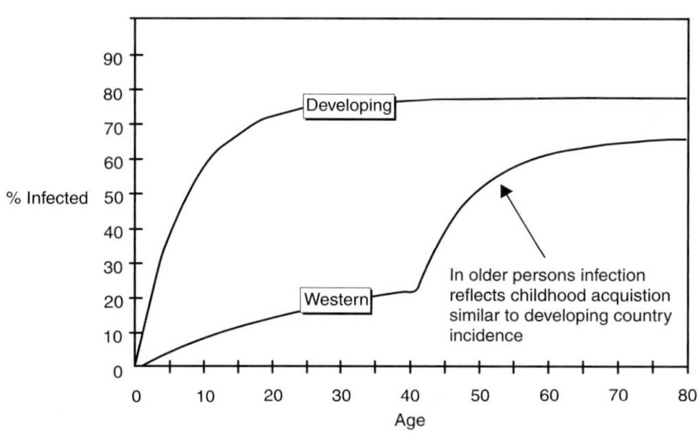

FIGURE 24-2 The prevalence of *Helicobacter pylori* in developing and Western countries. In developed countries, *H. pylori* is decreasing in prevalence so that most of the infections are in those over the age of 50 years who likely acquired the infection during childhood. The infection in young persons is only seen in immigrants from high-risk countries.

PATHOGENESIS

Acute Infection

Immediately after ingestion by a healthy person, it is thought that the urease enzyme of *H. pylori* enables the bacterium to survive in acid by generating ammonia and bicarbonate from urea present in the gastric juice:[25] Vague symptoms of epigastric discomfort then commence 72 hours after ingestion of the organism. Gastric acid secretion may initially increase, associated with varying degrees of epigastric discomfort[26] followed by vomiting episodes.[20,27] Symptoms usually settle after several days as the bacterium induces achlorhydria. The cause of the achlorhydria is unknown; however, it might involve the action of a bacterial toxin,[28] ammonia, or the presence of cytokines, especially interleukin-1β.[29]

In the tropics, achlorhydria has long been associated with malnutrition and susceptibility to enteric infections such as *V. cholerae* and enterotoxigenic *E. coli* infections.[30,31] So far, *H. pylori* infection is the only known environmental agent proven to cause achlorhydria. Since the acute infection is associated with long periods when the gastric acid barrier is impaired, *H. pylori* may increase susceptibility to the other enteric pathogens and thus be an important pathogen in the pediatric age group.[32] Perhaps related to the achlorhydria, acute *H. pylori* infection is associated with a mild growth arrest,[33] and in a few studies infected children grow up shorter than controls.[34,35]

The achlorhydria of acute *H. pylori* is "chemically induced" and is reversible, unlike that seen after many years of the chronic *H. pylori* infection, where atrophy of gastric mucosa causes acid secretion to be irreversibly diminished (see following discussion).[32]

Attachment

H. pylori has several attachment mechanisms that enable it to selectively colonize gastric mucosa but not intestinal mucosa. To various degrees, *H. pylori* is adherent to Lewis B antigen,[36] phosphatidylethanolamine,[37] and ganglioside GM_3,[38] all of which are present on the gastric mucus epithelial cells. In addition, *H. pylori* synthesizes Lewis X antigen which may be a mechanism of "molecular mimicry" to make the organism similar to the host tissue, thus attenuating the immune response.[39] Once attached, *H. pylori* induces the production of interleukin-8 (IL-8) which in turn attracts neutrophils.[40] If deep colonization occurs in the acid secreting mucosa, secretion of IL-1 by inflammatory cells may inhibit acid secretion

Cytotoxins

The effect of *H. pylori* on the gastric mucosa is more severe when the bacterium produces cytotoxins. The most notable of these is CagA, which is one component of about 30 genes in the cagA pathogenicity island. This structure, present in most

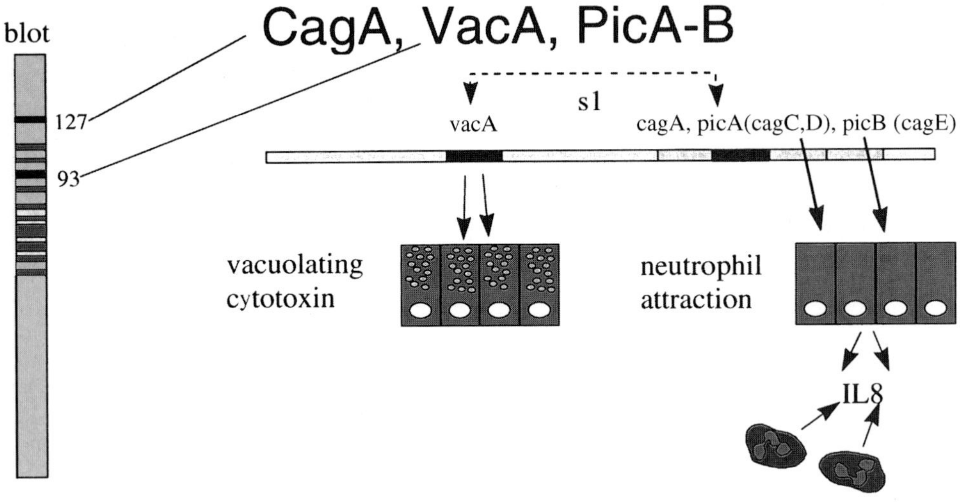

FIGURE 24-3 Relationships of cytotoxin genes and proteins. The left side diagrams a representative immunoblot pattern of a patient with a duodenal ulcer and *Helicobacter pylori* infection. The 127-kDa band is the cytotoxin-associated gene A (*cagA*) product. The cagA pathogenicity island has a higher guanine + cytosine content than the rest of the *H. pylori* genome. This suggests that the *cagA* gene group has long ago been imported from a different genus. The *vacA* (vacuolating toxin A) gene has two main subunits (s and m), and these can each be in two subtypes (s1, s2, and m1, m2). When s2 is present, the cytotoxic potential of the organism is very weak and is not usually associated with peptic ulcer, and the CagA island is usually absent.

strains, codes for a "Type IV" secretion system. This causes a hollow pilus-like structure to form which then injects the CagA toxin protein into the epithelial cell. CagA toxin emulates at least two growth-factors causing the epithelial cell to adopt a less structured, more mobile, primitive form. Thus the integrity of the gastroduodenal epithelium is compromised and nutrients are able to leak up from between the cells and towards the *H. pylori*. In developed countries, CagA is present in only 60% of strains, whereas in most tropical or developing countries (Peru is a good example) more than 90% of strains are CagA-positive.

Linked to the cagA island is a propensity for such isolates to produce VacA toxin of a more virulent subtype. VacA is a membrane pore which leads to leaky intracellular organelles and the appearance of "vacuoles" in the cells. The two *vacA* subunits "s" and "m" can each exist in two forms, s1 or s2, and m1 or m2; only s1 (m1 or m2) are associated with active cytotoxin (Fig. 24-3).[41] Other toxins are BabA (Blood-Group Antigen Binding Toxin A)[42] and iceA (Induced with Contact to Epithelium). Toxin-producing strains (cagA, vacA, BabA) are more likely to be present in persons with duodenal ulcer or with gastric cancer because they upregulate the degree of mucosal inflammation. This effect is also modulated by various interleukin polymorphisms in the patient, such as IL-1β and its receptor so that some individuals with a virulent strain could experience a 5–50 fold increased risk of cancer from a *H. pylori* infection.[43,44]

DISEASE ASSOCIATIONS AND CLINICAL MANIFESTATIONS

Active Chronic Gastritis

Chronic gastritis refers to the histological presence of mononuclear cells (lymphocytes and plasma cells) in the gastric mucosa. Histologic chronic gastritis is associated very closely with *H. pylori* and there are few patients with this finding who do not have the organism.[45] There is also a variable amount of neutrophilic infiltration of the mucosa, typically invading the necks of mucous glands. This latter appearance gives the name "active" or "acute" to the typical histologic appearance of "active chronic gastritis."[46] Because the cause of chronic gastritis was unknown before the discovery of *H. pylori*, the terminology was confusing and nonstandardized. In most of the literature, terms such as "atrophic gastritis," "superficial gastritis," "simple gastritis," "antral gastritis," and "type 1 gastritis" all refer to the histology of *H. pylori* infection. The various classifying and descriptive terms for the lesion have been well described in several papers.[47–49]

In the antrum of the stomach, *H. pylori* is most numerous on the surface of the epithelium (beneath the mucus layer) but it also lives in the mucus-secreting glands. In the body of the stomach (corpus), almost all of the organisms are found on the surface. The inflammation tends to collect near the bacteria. Thus in the corpus, the appearance is that of a "superficial gastritis," whereas in the antrum, the inflammation is deeper. In either place the lesion can be associated with lymphoid follicles.[50]

In the long-standing case of chronic active superficial gastritis, the superficial inflammation includes a predominance of PMNs. In contrast, in the deep portion of the glands below the necks the inflammation is predominantly chronic with lymphocytes surrounding destroyed remnants of gastric deep glands; an appearance that has been called the glandular lymphocytic adherence lesion. As this deep inflammation becomes more extensive, the deep glands become islands separated by chronic inflammation, they are less tightly packed, and their depth decreases. This decrease is called chronic atrophic gastritis. Another way deep glands are replaced is through intestinal metaplasia. The degree of deep glands lost through either inflammation or intestinal metaplasia determines how extensive is the chronic atrophic gastritis.[51] Chronic atrophic gastritis is a precancerous lesion probably due to the effects of long-term hypochlorhydria and the resultant presence of abnormal gastric flora. In general, inflammation, both superficial and deep, is more severe in the antrum, less in the corpus, and least in the cardia.[52] In both the antrum and the corpus, the preceding lesions may be associated with lymphoid follicles. Lymphoid follicles are rarely seen in the gastric mucosa except after *H. pylori* infection.[53]

Attachment of the bacterium causes damage to the cytoskeleton of the epithelial cells so that they bulge out rather than maintain a flat luminal surface. Under periodic acid–Schiff staining, the apical mucus content of infected gastric mucosa is less than normal and cells are shorter. These changes have been termed the destructive mucin lesion of the covering gastric epithelium.[49,54]

Over the lifetime of the infected person, inflammation may destroy the glandular elements (atrophy) and intestinal cells often replace gastric mucus-secreting epithelium (intestinal metaplasia). The resulting atrophic gastritis is the final "burned out" phase of *H. pylori* infection, usually seen in older persons. In tropical countries, however, where *H. pylori* may have been present from a very early age, atrophic gastritis may be seen in young adults and is believed to be a major risk factor for gastric cancer.[55]

Duodenal and Gastric Ulcer

The most obvious disease associated with *H. pylori* is peptic ulceration (Fig. 24-4). More than 90% of duodenal ulcers are associated with toxin-producing *H. pylori.*[56] When a patient with a duodenal ulcer does not have *H. pylori* infection, etiologic factors such as Zollinger-Ellison syndrome or nonsteroidal anti-inflammatory drug (NSAID) use are likely.[57]

In gastric ulcer, two causes prevail, and many patients will exhibit both. Most gastric ulcers have *H. pylori* and these can be identified by presence of the bacterium or chronic gastritis. The stomach is also directly exposed to ingested agents such as an NSAID and is more likely than the duodenum to ulcerate in response to these agents. Therefore, in the United States, about 50% of gastric ulcers are not associated with histologic chronic gastritis or *H. pylori* but are caused by NSAIDs.[48]

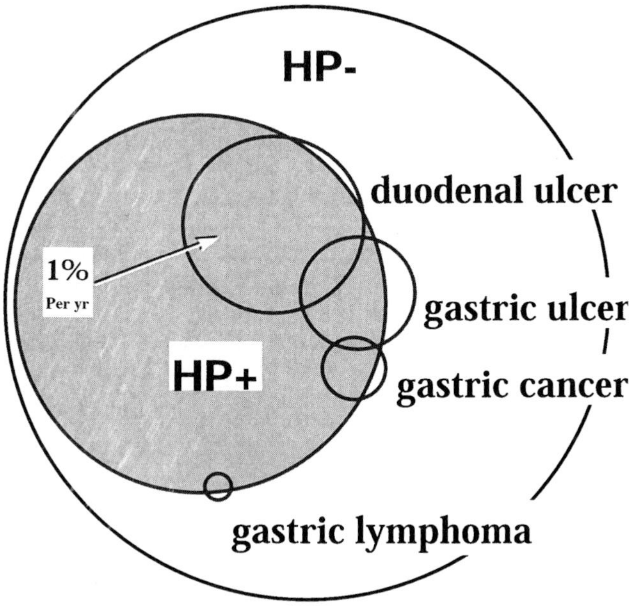

FIGURE 24-4 Disease associations with *Helicobacter pylori* (HP). The large circle represents a typical population in a developed country where 60% of persons are *not* infected with *H. pylori.* The darker circle represents the 40% of persons who *are* infected with *H. pylori.* Even so, nearly all the duodenal ulcers and gastric ulcers occur in the *H. pylori*–positive group. Each year, 1% of infected patients undergo transition from asymptomatic gastritis to symptomatic peptic ulcer. Note that most gastric adenocarcinomas and gastric mucosa–associated lymphoid tissue (B-cell) lymphomas also occur in the *H. pylori*–positive persons. Controversy reigns as to the role of *H. pylori* in persons with dyspepsia but in whom ulcers are not found: Should *H. pylori* be treated in these persons, or ignored?

In tropical countries where NSAIDs are less widely used and *H. pylori* is very common, most gastric ulcers are caused by *H. pylori.*[58] Perhaps because of this, gastric ulcers are more likely to be malignant and require endoscopy and biopsy for histologic examination.

The proposed causation of duodenal ulcer is as follows. Persons with *H. pylori,* but with colonization mainly in the antrum, have high acid secretion but a defective mucosal barrier. Inflammation in the antrum impairs the growth of D cells (which make somatostatin) and thus decreases their inhibitory effects on the gastrin-producing G cells. This results in higher gastrin production, which may in turn, over the lifetime of the patient, cause a hyperplasia of the acid-secreting mucosa. Gastric mucus cells normally present in the duodenal bulb become colonized with *H. pylori,* seeded from the infection present in the antrum. Neutrophil invasion of the duodenal epithelium (duodenitis) increases susceptibility to ulceration. Inflammation is more severe when the *H. pylori* secretes CagA, thus associating the cytotoxin with duodenal ulcer.[59,60]

All persons with peptic ulcer should be tested for *H. pylori* and treated with antimicrobial agents when evidence of the infection exists.[4,61] Ulcer recurrence is less than 10% when *H. pylori* is eradicated, whereas more than 90% of ulcers recur when the bacterium persists.[62] Thus, most patients are cured of their ulcer disease with effective antibiotic treatment.[63]

Gastric Cancer

Adenocarcinoma

Worldwide, gastric cancer is the second most common cancer, the high prevalence areas being Brazil, Colombia, Korea, China, and Japan. *H. pylori* infection affects more than half the population in these countries.[63] The incidence of gastric cancer has declined in the United States since 1930. It was the most common cancer, but now it ranks about ninth.[64]

H. pylori confers an approximately sixfold risk of gastric cancer, accounting for about half of all gastric cancers.[63] Thus, in most tropical countries where *H. pylori* is prevalent, gastric cancer is also common. In India, Bangladesh, the Middle East, southern China, and some African countries, however, *H. pylori* is prevalent but gastric cancer is not. This paradox suggests that genetic, dietary, and other unknown environmental factors are also important in the etiology of adenocarcinoma.[64,65]

The proposed chain of events in gastric carcinoma starts with a very early (age 1 to 5 years) infection with *H. pylori* so that the corpus mucosa is damaged during childhood. In this setting, ulcers are unlikely but a large area of the stomach is involved in the process. Damaged areas coalesce into chronic atrophic gastritis and acid secretion diminishes, eventually allowing other organisms to colonize the stomach.[66–68] In this setting, nitrates can be changed to nitrites and then to nitrosamines, which are carcinogenic. In the presence of ammonia, inflammation itself can cause nitrosamines to form in the mucosa. Inflammation is more severe when the *H. pylori* secretes toxin, thus associating several cytotoxins with gastric cancer.

The Ulcer-Cancer Controversy

It has been well demonstrated that CagA toxin–positive strains of *H. pylori* are associated with both duodenal ulcer (a high-acid state) and stomach cancer (a low-acid state). Paradoxically, patients who have duodenal ulcer are protected from developing stomach cancer. This implies that acid protects from the carcinogenic effects of *H. pylori*. Even in Japan, where stomach cancer is common, it is quite rare for a person with duodenal ulcer to develop the malignancy.[69]

One proposed explanation for this is the age of acquisition of the infection. In a tropical country where *H. pylori* is acquired in early childhood and nutrition may be poor, the infection causes severe damage to the acid-secreting area of the stomach.[55] Poor nutrition probably also assists this tendency to develop an asymptomatic low-acid state.[70]

Various factors are associated with the development of gastric cancer associated with *H. pylori* infection. These include the presence of hypochlorhydria due to infection, virulence of the infecting strain, genetic factors of the host, micronutrients in the diet, and geographical location of the patient. Thus, even if CagA toxin is present, the patient may never develop a duodenal ulcer but may be susceptible to gastric cancer in later life.[3]

If *H. pylori* is acquired in late childhood or in the adult years, then the infection tends to affect mainly the antrum of the stomach, leaving the acid-secreting part of the stomach (the corpus) intact. High acid secretion allows the development of duodenal ulcer disease.

Lymphoma

H. pylori eradication therapy should be the initial step in the treatment of proven or suspected gastric lymphoma. Up to 90% of mucosa-associated lymphoid tissue (MALT) lymphomas are associated with *H. pylori*.[71] These indolent B-cell lymphomas are sometimes driven by continuing *H. pylori* antigenic stimulus and regress when *H. pylori* infection is treated.[72,73] Apparent cure of MALT lymphoma occurs in 70% of patients in whom *H. pylori* is eradicated.[74]

DIAGNOSIS

The diagnosis of *H. pylori* may be by invasive or noninvasive methods, or both, as shown in Table 24-1. Endoscopic biopsy of gastric mucosa is the usual invasive method, although invasive methods can include blind biopsy, nasogastric aspiration, or the gastric string test.[75] Noninvasive tests are primarily serologic tests that detect IgG antibody to *H. pylori*, urea breath tests (UBT) to detect gastric urease, and fecal antigen tests.

Invasive Tests

Histology

For histologic study from intact mucosa, mucosal biopsy specimens are taken away from any visible lesion. This allows the pathologist to separate true inflammation (active chronic gastritis) from changes due to acute ulcer healing. Biopsies for

Table 24-1 Accuracy of Diagnostic Tests for Helicobacter pylori *Infection in 268 Patients Undergoing Esophagogastroduodenoscopy*

Tests	Sensitivity (%)	Specificity (%)	Positive Predictive Value (%)	Negative Predictive Value (%)
Invasive				
Biopsy: Chronic inflammation*	100	66.3	84.4	100
Biopsy: Acute inflammation†	86.7	93.7	96.2	79.5
Biopsy: Warthin-Starry silver stain‡	93.1	99.0	99.4	88.7
CLOtest rapid urease test§	89.6	100	100	84.1
Noninvasive				
^{13}C-urea breath test‖	90.2	95.8	97.5	84.3
Fecal Antigen Test**	94.1	91.8	93.4	92.6
Serum IgG¶	91.3	91.6	95.2	85.3
Serum IgA	71.1	85.3	89.8	61.8

*Chronic inflammation present in gastric antral biopsies.
†Acute inflammation present in gastric antral biopsies.
‡Warthin-Starry stain of gastric antral biopsy.
§Urease test conducted on gastric antral biopsy with results ascertained at 24 hours.
‖^{13}C-urea breath test 60 minutes after administration of 150 mg ^{13}C-labeled urea.
**Data from Vaira D, Malfertheiner P, Megraud F, et al: Diagnosis of *Helicobacter pylori* infection with a new non-invasive antigen-based assay. HpSA European study group. Lancet 354(9172):30–33, 1999.
¶Serum antibodies to *H. pylori*.
Data from Cutler AF, Havstad S, Ma CK, et al: Accuracy of invasive and noninvasive tests to diagnose *Helicobacter pylori* infection. Gastroenterology 109:136, 1995.

H. pylori should be in addition to biopsies taken to exclude malignancy. At least two or, preferably, three biopsies need to be taken to detect *H. pylori* histologically. One biopsy can be taken from the greater curve of the antrum, one from the mid-corpus, and a third from the lesser curve angular notch.[75] In addition to routine H&E sections, the specimens should be stained with Giemsa or a silver stain such as Warthin-Starry or Genta stain.[76]

Culture

Culture methods have been described earlier. Cultures may be moistened with a single drop of saline and transported to the laboratory in a sterile tube the same day. In some studies, organisms have remained viable in snap frozen biopsies.[77]

Culture has also been performed from blind gastric mucosal biopsies, from gastric aspirates, and from gastric string tests. These methods are less sensitive than culture of biopsies and are not widely used. Biopsy material, gastric mucus, and gastric juice can, of course, also be examined with polymerase chain reaction (PCR) or immunologic methods to detect *H. pylori,* but at present these are not reproducible in different laboratories and have no particular advantage over culture or histology.

Urease Test

The ability of *H. pylori* to produce urease allows one to rapidly detect the organism in gastric biopsy material. Typically, the mucosal biopsy specimen is placed in a medium containing urea and a pH indicator. If urease (or *H. pylori*) is present, urea is converted to ammonia and the pH rises with a subsequent color change.[78] *H. pylori* is a prolific urease producer so that the reaction occurs in a few minutes in biopsies from infected patients. Since the test is so specific for *H. pylori,* once a positive urease test has been noted, other diagnostic material is often unnecessary and may be discarded to save expense.[79]

Noninvasive Tests

Infection is almost always accompanied by a rise in specific IgG antibody to *H. pylori.* IgM is present in some persons during the acute infection but has not been well studied because acute infections are rarely documented. IgA is present in 80% of persons with *H. pylori* so it can be used to diagnose the infection when present, but the absence of IgA does not exclude infection. Thus, in most cases, IgG is the best predictor of *H. pylori* infection (Fig. 24-5).

Tests to detect IgG come as a laboratory-based multi-well enzyme-linked immunosorbent assay (ELISA) kit, which is the most accurate serologic test. In properly selected patients, sensitivity and specificity reach 95%. In patients who have been treated for *H. pylori* infection in the preceding two years, IgG may remain positive and give an incorrect positive result even in persons who no longer have *H. pylori* infection.[80] For this reason the urea breath test is a better choice for follow-up. However, if carefully validated methods are used, serology can be used as a somewhat less accurate predictor of bacterial eradication. In Mexican patients, a 10% drop in ELISA absorbance at one year predicated *H. pylori* eradication in 84% of treated patients.[81]

A fecal antigen test for *H. pylori* is less sensitive than the urea breath test at detecting *H. pylori* after treatment, but fecal tests are ideal when the UBT is unavailable, and in very young children.

As well as being present in blood, small amounts of IgG may be detected in urine and gingival secretions. The latter two sources allow initial diagnosis from urine specimens and saliva.

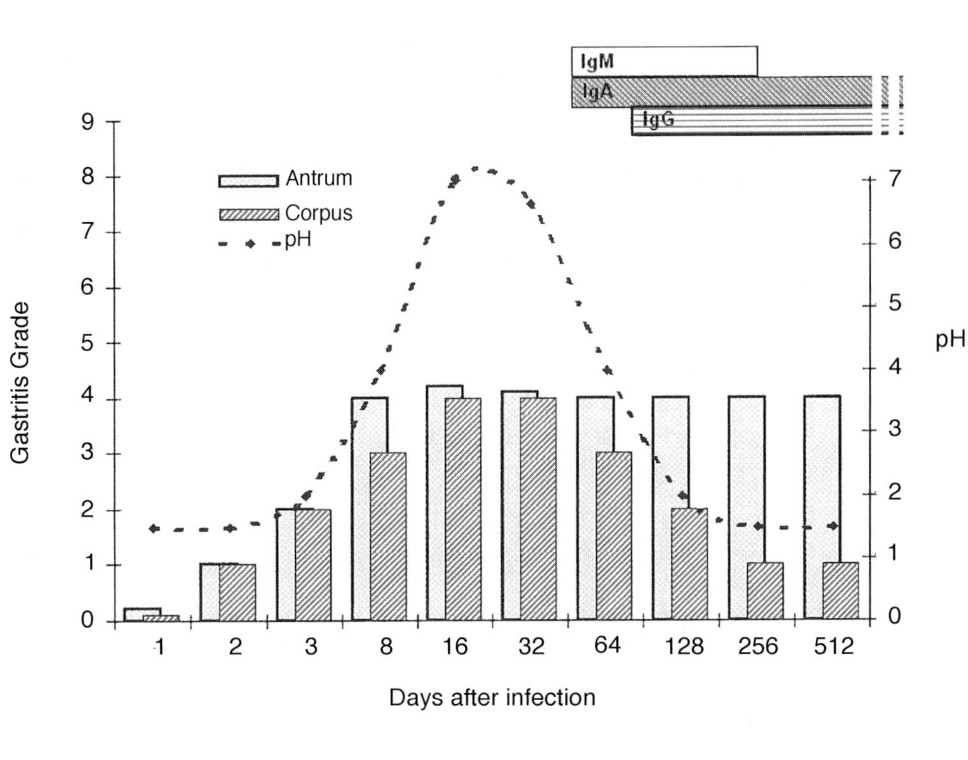

FIGURE 24-5 The natural history of *Helicobacter pylori* infection. The horizontal axis shows the time scale in days over 18 months. The left vertical axis is gastritis grade as represented in the columns showing antral and corpus mucosa inflammation graded 0 to 4. The right vertical axis shows the pH of gastric juice on a scale of 0 to 7. Note that corpus mucosa inflammation (*hatched vertical bars*) subsides after 3 months, whereas antral inflammation remains. As the corpus mucosa returns to near normal, acid secretion revives and gastric pH (*dotted line*) falls to normal acidic levels. Variable early responses are seen in IgA and IgM. IgG is present after the fourth week and remains as the most stable antibody response in nearly all infected persons.

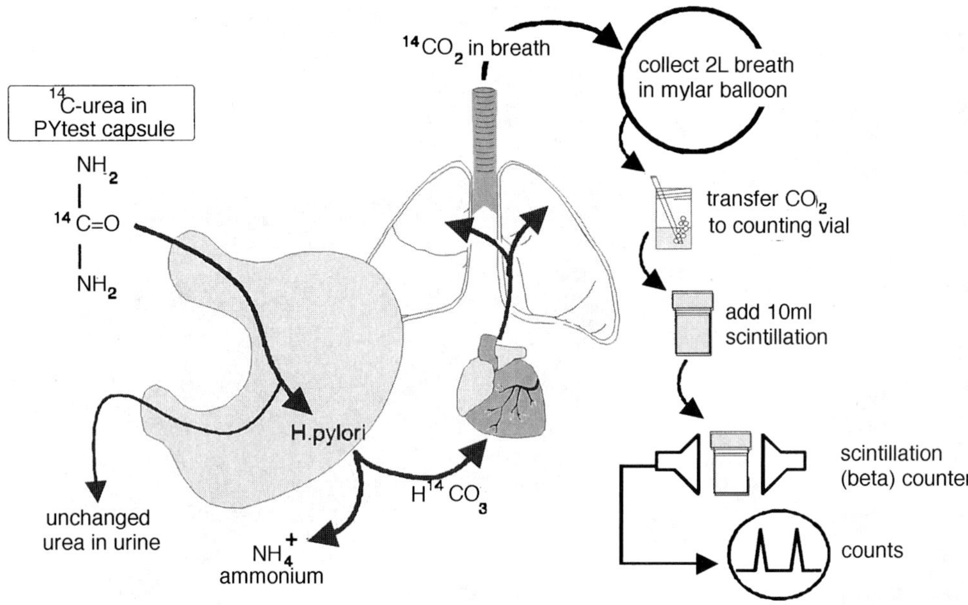

FIGURE 24-6 The urea breath test. Urea labeled with an isotope of carbon (a capsule of ^{14}C-urea in this illustration) is swallowed by the fasted patient. Ten to 15 minutes later, a breath sample is collected into a balloon, processed as shown, and then counted in a scintillation counter. $^{14}CO_2$ can be detected in the breath of a patient infected with *Helicobacter pylori*. When *H. pylori* is not present, the urea remains intact and there is no $^{14}CO_2$ in the breath. Unchanged ^{14}C-urea is excreted in the urine. Since more than 90% of the isotope is excreted within 3 days, radiation exposure is exceedingly small, about the same as natural background in 24 hours (0.3 mrem). In the ^{13}C-urea breath test, the patient first swallows a high-fat meal or drink, which serves to delay gastric emptying. Ten minutes later, a baseline breath sample is collected and a solution of isotope is swallowed. Diagnostic breath samples are collected 20 to 40 minutes later. Breath samples are analyzed in an isotope ratio mass spectrometer.

Breath Tests

Urea breath tests rely on the breakdown of isotope-labeled urea by urease (from *H. pylori*) in the stomach (Fig. 24-6). The C^{14} UBT only takes 10 minutes and requires a single breath sample. The C^{13} test takes 40 minutes and requires a baseline plus a 20–30 minute test sample. Both tests are highly accurate and the choice of which to use depends on availability and cost. Although the C^{14} UBT uses a trace of radioactive carbon, the dose is very small—equal to less than 24 hours of background exposure, so it is not excluded from use in women or children.[82]

Diagnostic Criteria for Research Studies

Table 24-1 gives comparative data on the accuracy of various diagnostic tests as observed by Cutler and associates and Vaira and coworkers.[83,84] Although histology is accurate, these data reflect the results obtained by an expert pathologist with considerable experience in *H. pylori* diagnosis. Accuracy is quite variable among community pathologists, depending on their experience and the technical excellence of the staining methods used.

For clinical research, concordance between two different methods is necessary to prove the presence or absence of *H. pylori*. Good combinations for initial diagnosis would be histology and culture, urease test and culture, histology and serology, or urease test and serology.

In developing countries, noninvasive "indirect" methods of diagnosis are less helpful in demonstrating cure after therapy, probably due to frequent exposure and reinfection with *H. pylori*. Positive serology in a highly endemic site frequently does not reverse. In addition, even "direct" tests such as UBT and stool antigen tests are more difficult to interpret due to false-positive results.

Proof of cure requires demonstration of sterile gastric mucosa, by two tests, 4 weeks after completion of therapy. Alternatively, two negative tests (UBT or fecal antigen) will suffice, the first at 4 weeks post therapy and the second at 6 to 8 weeks post therapy.

TREATMENT OF *H. PYLORI* IN THE TROPICS

What is the role of treatment of *H. pylori* infection in the tropics? In many ways, treatment is similar to that in the United States, where eradication is prescribed for patients with peptic ulcer disease and the rare patient with gastric lymphoma.

In the tropics, regimens containing metronidazole are much less effective. Furazolidone is an alternative to metronidazole in a 10-day regimen that includes bismuth and amoxicillin. In some countries (i.e., Peru, Bangladesh, and Turkey), there is rapid recurrence even after successful eradication of *H. pylori* from the stomach. *Eradication* is defined as the absence of *H. pylori* at least 4 weeks after the last dose of antimicrobial therapy was given.[6] Reinfection is most likely caused by fecal contamination of water or food.

By sheer experience, several rules can be stated about eradication of *H. pylori*:

- In vitro sensitivity to an antibiotic does not predict in vivo efficacy. Therefore, use tested antibiotic combinations that are proven to work.

- Acid appears to protect *H. pylori* from antibiotics; therefore, the most successful treatments include strong acid suppression with proton pump inhibitors.
- Eradication rates peak between seven and 14 days of treatment. Do not use treatments shorter than seven days (cure rate is lower) or longer than 14 days (cure rate does not increase, but side effects increase).
- *H. pylori* does not develop resistance to the following drugs: amoxycillin, bismuth, tetracycline, and furazolidone. Therefore they may be reused, and sensitivity testing for them is not required.
- *H. pylori* quickly becomes resistant to the following drugs: metronidazole (and other "idazoles"), clarithromycin (and other "thromycins"), and rifabutin. Box 24-1 outlines doses used in therapy, while Table 24-2 gives treatment options.

PREVENTION AND CONTROL

In developing countries, *H. pylori* recurrence after successful treatment occurs at rates 10 to 20 times higher than in developed countries. In addition, bacterial counts of *H. pylori* in gastric biopsies taken in recurrence are similar to those in biopsies taken prior to treatment. The high reinfection rate and lack of change in the *H. pylori* bacterial counts suggest there is little natural immunity after infection.

The rapid recurrence of *H. pylori* infection in some areas means that its treatment in impoverished tropical areas needs to be based on objectives that have a likelihood of some success. Goals for control of infection will have to be tempered with the additional need for improved sanitation. Thus, for example, antimicrobial treatment of the majority of the world's population living in tropical, developing areas to eradicate *H. pylori* for the purpose of preventing cancer would be unrealistic at present. On the other hand, prevention of gastric ulcer and duodenal ulcer recurrence for periods of a year or two might have some utility even where recurrence is high. Ethnic and cultural factors are also worth considering. For example, in Malaysia, prevalence rates among the Malays ranged from 12% to 29%, while the Chinese ranged from 27% to 58%, and Indians were between 49% and 52%.[85]

The role that treatment will have in reversing the progress of precancerous lesions to cancer is not known. Evidence suggests that treatment may reverse dysplasia but not intestinal metaplasia. In patients with severe intestinal metaplasia associated with atypical changes or dysplasia, it is probably worthwhile at present to attempt to eradicate *H. pylori* from the mucosa. In patients with gastric lymphoma, a condition seen more commonly in developed countries, eradication is mandatory because tumor regression occurs when *H. pylori* infection is treated. There is no evidence to date, however, that eradicating *H. pylori* in patients with gastric cancer will affect the course except to prevent further new cancers.

Reinfection with *H. pylori* makes vaccine use highly attractive in some countries yet the high reinfection rates suggest that finding an effective vaccine may be quite difficult. Vaccines need to work in children to prevent early infection in order to protect against ulcer disease and gastric cancer. As noted previously, natural immunity to reinfection is weak, thus another possible use for the vaccine will be to prevent recurrence of *H. pylori* infection after effective antimicrobial therapy.

Box 24-1 Treatments in Common Usage

- Omeprazole 20 mg BID, clarithromycin 500 mg BID, and amoxycillin 1g BID (7–10 days)
- Omeprazole 20 mg BID, clarithromycin 250 mg BID, and metronidazole 400 mg BID (7 days)
- Bismuth (subsalicylate or citrate) 1 tablet QID*, tetracycline 500 mg QID, metronidazole 250 mg QID (1 g to 1.5 g daily) (10–14 days)
- Rabeprazole 20 mg BID, amoxicillin 1 g BID, levofloxacin 250 mg BID (10 days)
- Omeprazole 20 mg BID, amoxicillin 1 g BID, furazolidone 200 mg BID, and bismuth subsalicylate (De-Nol) 240 mg (2 tabs) BID (14 days)

*Addition of a proton pump inhibitor probably enhances the cure rate.

Table 24-2 Treatment Options for Helicobacter pylori*

Group	Description	Duration
A†	**Bismuth**	
	Ranitidine bismuth citrate (RBC) 400 mg BID	14 days
	Bismuth subsalicylate (Pepto Bismol) 525 mg (2 tabs) QID	14 days
	Bismuth subcitrate (DeNol) 120 mg (1 tab) QID	14 days
B	**Penicillin**	
	Amoxicillin IG BID	7 or 10 or 14 days
C	**Macrolide**	
	Clarithromycin 500 mg BID‡	7 or 10 or 14 days
	Josamycin 1000 mg BID	7 days
D	**Nitroimidazole**	
	Metronidazole 500 mg BID or TID‡	7 or 10 or 14 days
	Tinidazole 1000 mg daily	7 or 10 or 14 days
E	**Tetracycline**	
	Tetracycline 500 mg QID	14 days
F	**Quinolone**	7 or 10 or 14 days
	Ofloxacin 500 mg BID	7–14 days
	Levofloxacin 250 mg BID	7–14 days
	Ciprofloxacin 500 mg BID	14 days
G	**Nitrofurans**	
	Furazolidone 200 mg BID‡	7 or 10 or 14 days
H	**Ansamycin**	
	Rifabutin 150 mg BID	14 days
I	**Proton Pump Inhibitors (use double a normal dose)**	
	Omeprazole 20 mg BID	
	Esomeprazole 40 mg BID	
	Lansoprazole 30 mg BID	
	Pantoprazole 40 mg BID	
	Rabeprazole 20 mg BID	

*Treatment priorities are normally: IBC→IBD→IBEG. For penicillin allergy choose ICD or IAED→IFH.

†When Pepto Bismol is not available, substitute DeNol 1 tablet QID. RBC is not available in all countries.

‡Side effects are likely as doses of clarithromycin, metronidazole and furazolidone increase.

H. pylori infection is one of the most common infections in the tropics, significantly associated with peptic ulcer disease, gastric cancer, and possibly with other enteric infections. New diagnostic, therapeutic, and preventive measures will undoubtedly determine the evolving approaches to better controlling the consequences of *H. pylori* infections worldwide.

REFERENCES

1. Marshall BJ, Warren JR: Unidentified curved bacilli in the stomach of patients with gastritis and peptic ulceration. Lancet 1:1311, 1984.
2. Braga LL, Marshall BJ, Moreno H, et al: *Helicobacter pylori*: Gastritis, peptic ulcer and gastric cancer in developing countries. In Guerrant RL, de Souza MA, Nations MK (eds): At the Edge of Development: Health Crises in a Transitional Society. Durham, NC, Carolina Academic Press, 1996.
3. Sullivan PB, Thomas JE, Wight DG, et al: *H. pylori* infection in Gambian children with chronic diarrhea and malnutrition. Arch Dis Child 65:189, 1990.
4. Soll AH: Medical treatment of peptic ulcer disease. JAMA 275:622, 1996.
5. Hulten K, Han SW, Enroth H, et al: *Helicobacter pylori* in the drinking water in Peru. Gastroenterology 110:1031, 1996.
6. Ramirez-Ramos A, Gilman RH, Leon-Barua R, et al: Rapid recurrence of *Helicobacter pylori* infection in Peruvian patients after successful eradication. Clin Infect Dis 25:1027, 1997.
7. Soto G, Bautista CT, Roth DE, et al: *Helicobacter pylori* reinfection is common in Peruvian adults after antibiotic eradication therapy. J Infect Dis 188:1263, 2003.
8. Marshall BJ, McGechie DB, Rogers PAR, et al: Pyloric campylobacter infection and gastroduodenal disease. Med J Aust 149:439, 1985.
9. Pinkard KJ, Harrison B, Capstick JA, et al: Detection of *Campylobacter pyloridis* in gastric mucosa by phase contrast microscopy. J Clin Pathol 39:112, 1986.
10. Buck GE, Smith JS: Medium supplementation for growth of *Campylobacter pyloridis*. J Clin Microbiol 25:597, 1987.
11. Pennie RA, Zunino JN, Rose E, et al: Economical, simple method for the production of the gaseous environment required for the cultivation of *Campylobacter jejuni*. J Clin Microbiol 20:320, 1984.
12. Krajden S, Bohnen J, Anderson J, et al: Comparison of selective and nonselective media for recovery of *Campylobacter pylori* from antral biopsies. J Clin Microbiol 25:1117, 1987.
13. Hachem CY, Clarridge JE, Evans DG, et al: Which is the best medium for isolation of *Helicobacter pylori* from gastric mucosal biopsies? (abstract). Am J Gastroenterol 89:1287, 1994.
14. Tee W, Fairley S, Smallwood R, et al: Comparative evaluation of three selective media and a nonselective medium for the culture of *Helicobacter pylori* from gastric biopsies. J Clin Microbiol 29:2587, 1991.
15. Shadowen RD, Sciortino CV: Improved growth of *Campylobacter pylori* in a biphasic system. J Clin Microbiol 27:1744, 1989.
16. Secker DA, Tompkins DS, Alderson G: Gas-permeable lifecell tissue culture flasks give improved growth of *Helicobacter pylori* in a liquid medium. J Clin Microbiol 29:1060, 1991.
17. Mendz GL, Hazell SL: Amino acid utilization by *Helicobacter pylori*. Int J Biochem Cell Biol 27:1085, 1995.
18. Thomas JE, Gibson GR, Darboe MK, et al: Isolation of *Helicobacter pylori* from human faeces. Lancet 340:1194, 1992.
19. Klein PD, Gilman RH, Leon-Barua R, et al: The epidemiology of *Helicobacter pylori* in Peruvian children between 6 and 30 months of age (abstract). Am J Gastroenterol 89:1306, 1994.
20. Mitchell JD, Mitchell HM, Tobias V: Acute *Helicobacter pylori* infection in an infant, associated with gastric ulceration and serological evidence of intra-familial transmission. Am J Gastroenterol 87:382, 1992.
21. Fecal and oral shedding of *Helicobacter pylori* from healthy infected adults. JAMA 282:2240, 1999.
22. Mitchell JD, Mitchell HM, Tobias V: Acute *Helicobacter pylori* infection in an infant, associated with gastric ulceration and serological evidence of intra-familial transmission. Am J Gastroenterol 87:382, 1992.
23. Nguyen AM, Engstrand L, Genta RM, et al: Detection of *Helicobacter pylori* in dental plaque by reverse transcription–polymerase chain reaction. J Clin Microbiol 31:783, 1993.
24. Blecker U, Lanciers S, Keppens E, et al: Evolution of *Helicobacter pylori* positivity in infants born from positive mothers (abstract). Am J Gastroenterol 89:1334, 1994.
25. Marshall BJ, Barrett LJ, Prakash C, et al: Urea protects *Helicobacter (Campylobacter) pylori* from the bactericidal effect of acid. Gastroenterology 99:697, 1990.
26. Morris A, Nicholson G: Ingestion of *Campylobacter pyloridis* causes gastritis and raised fasting gastric pH. Am J Gastroenterol 82:192, 1987.
27. Graham DY, Alpert LC, Smith JL, et al: Iatrogenic *Campylobacter pylori* infection is a cause of epidemic achlorhydria. Am J Gastroenterol 83:974, 1988.
28. Hoffman JS, King WW, Fox JG, et al: Rabbit and ferret parietal cell inhibition by Helicobacter species. Dig Dis Sci 40:147, 1995.
29. McGowan CC, Cover TL, Blaser MJ: *Helicobacter pylori* and gastric acid: Biological and therapeutic implications. Gastroenterology 110:926, 1996.
30. Shahinian ML, Passaro DJ, Swerdlow DL, et al: *Helicobacter pylori* and epidemic *Vibrio cholerae* O1 infection in Peru. Lancet 355:377, 2000.
31. Evans C, Gilman RH, Rabbani GH, et al. Gastric acid secretion and enteric infection in Bangladesh. Trans R Soc Trop Med Hyg 91:681, 1997.
32. Gilman RH, Partanen R, Brown K, et al: Decreased gastric acid secretion and bacterial colonization of the stomach in severely malnourished Bangladeshi children. Gastroenterology 94:1308, 1988.
33. Passaro DJ, Taylor DN, Gilman RH, et al. Growth slowing after acute *Helicobacter pylori* infection is age-dependent. J Pediatr Gastroenterol Nutr 35:522, 2002.
34. Takahashi M, Kimura H, Watanabe K: *Helicobacter pylori* infection in patients with idiopathic short stature. Pediatr Int 44:277, 2002.
35. Bravo LE, Mera R, Reina JC, et al: Impact of *Helicobacter pylori* infection on growth of children: A prospective cohort study. J Pediatr Gastroenterol Nutr 37:614, 2003.
36. Borén T, Falk P, Roth KA, et al: Attachment of *Helicobacter pylori* to human gastric epithelium mediated by blood group antigens. Science 262:1892, 1993.
37. Lingwood CA, Huesca M, Kuksis A: The glycerolipid receptor for *Helicobacter pylori* (and exoenzyme S) is phosphatidylethanolamine. Infect Immun 60:2470, 1992.
38. Kamisago S, Iwamori M, Tai T, et al: Role of sulfatides in adhesion of *Helicobacter pylori* to gastric cancer cells. Infect Immun 64:624, 1996.
39. Chan NW, Stangier K, Sherburne R, et al: The biosynthesis of Lewis X in *Helicobacter pylori*. Glycobiology 5:683, 1995.
40. Crabtree JE, Xiang Z, Lindley IJ, et al: Induction of interleukin-8 secretion from gastric epithelial cells by a cagA negative isogenic mutant of *Helicobacter pylori*. J Clin Pathol 48:967, 1995.
41. Atherton JC, Cao P, Peek RM Jr, et al: Mosaicism in vacuolating cytotoxin alleles of Helicobacter pylori. Association of specific *vacA* types with cytotoxin production and peptic ulceration. J Biol Chem 270:17771, 1995.
42. Pride DT, Meinersmann RJ, Blaser MJ: Allelic variation within *Helicobacter pylori* babA and babB. Infect Immun 69:1160, 2001.
43. El Omar EM, Carrington M, Chow WH, et al: Interleukin-1 polymorphisms associated with increased risk of gastric cancer. Nature 404:398, 2000.
44. Figueiredo C, Machado JC, Pharoah P: *Helicobacter pylori* and interleukin 1 genotyping: an opportunity to identify high-risk individuals for gastric carcinoma. J Natl Cancer Inst 94:1680, 2002.
45. Drumm B, Sherman P, Cutz E, et al: Association of *Campylobacter pylori* on the gastric mucosa with antral gastritis in children. N Engl J Med 316:1557, 1987.
46. Warren JR, Marshall B: Unidentified curved bacilli on gastric epithelium in active chronic gastritis (letter). Lancet 1:1273, 1983.
47. el-Zimaity HM, Graham DY, al-Assi MT, et al: Interobserver variation in the histopathological assessment of *Helicobacter pylori* gastritis. Hum Pathol 27:35, 1996.
48. Maaroos HI, Kekki M, Villako K, et al: The occurrence and extent of *Helicobacter pylori* colonization and antral and body gastritis profiles in an Estonian population sample. Scand J Gastroenterol 25:1010, 1990.
49. Recavarren-Arce S, Gilman RH, León-Baruá R, et al: Chronic atrophic gastritis: Early diagnosis in a population where *Helicobacter pylori* infection is frequent. Clin Infect Dis 25:1006, 1997.
50. Genta RM, Hammer HW, Graham DY: Gastric lymphoid follicles in *Helicobacter pylori* infection: Frequency, distribution and response to triple therapy. Hum Pathol 24:577, 1993.

51. Kuipers EJ, Uyterlinde AM, Pena AS, et al: Long-term sequelae of *Helicobacter pylori* gastritis. Lancet 345:1525, 1995.
52. Logan RP, Walker MM, Misiewicz JJ, et al: Changes in the intragastric distribution of *Helicobacter pylori* during treatment with omeprazole. Gut 36:12, 1995.
53. Warren JR: Gastric pathology associated with *Helicobacter pylori*. Gastroenterol Clin North Am 29:705, 2000.
54. Recavarren-Arce S, Leon Barua R, Cok J, et al: *Helicobacter pylori* and progressive gastric pathology that predisposes to gastric cancer. Scand J Gastroenterol 181(Suppl):51, 1991.
55. Recavarren S, León Baruá R, Rodriguez C, et al: *Helicobacter pylori*–associated chronic gastritis in Peruvian adolescents is very common and severe. J Clin Gastroenterol 20:335, 1995.
56. Rauws EA, Langenberg W, Houthoff HJ, et al: *Campylobacter pyloridis*–associated chronic active antral gastritis: A prospective study of its prevalence and the effects of antibacterial and antiulcer treatment. Gastroenterology 94:33, 1988.
57. Sonnenberg A, Townsend WF: Testing for *Helicobacter pylori* in the diagnosis of Zollinger-Ellison syndrome. Am J Gastroenterol 86:606, 1991.
58. Weir WR, Goodgame R, Kiire CF, et al: Campylobacter-like organisms and gastritis in Africa. Trans R Soc Trop Med Hyg 82:172, 1988.
59. Eaton KA, Krakowka S: *H. pylori* strain differences and their role in early, transient neutrophilic inflammation in gnotobiotic piglets (abstract). Gastroenterology 100(Suppl 4):A100, 1996.
60. Wyatt JI, Rathbone B, Dixon MF, et al: *C. pyloridis* and acid induced gastric metaplasia in the pathogenesis of duodenitis. J Clin Pathol 40:841, 1987.
61. Cotton P: NIH consensus panel urges antimicrobials for ulcer patients, skeptics concur with caveats (news). JAMA 271:808, 1994.
62. Hopkins RJ, Girardi LS, Turney EA: Relationship between *Helicobacter pylori* eradication and reduced duodenal and gastric ulcer recurrence: A review. Gastroenterology 110:1244, 1996.
63. Rauws EA, Tytgat GN: Cure of duodenal ulcer associated with eradication of *Helicobacter pylori*. Lancet 335:1233, 1990.
64. Munoz N, Franceshi S: Epidemiology of gastric cancer and perspectives for prevention. Salud Publica Mex 39:318, 1997.
65. León-Baruá R, Berendson-Seminario R, Recavarren-Arce S, et al: Geographic factors probably modulating alternative pathways in *Helicobacter pylori*–associated gastroduodenal pathology: A hypothesis. Clin Infect Dis 25:1013, 1997.
66. Siurala M, Isokoski M, Varis K, et al: Prevalence of gastritis in a rural population. Biopsy study of subjects selected at random. Scand J Gastroenterol 3:211, 1968.
67. Correa P, Cuello C, Duque E, et al: Gastric cancer in Colombia. III. The natural history of precursor lesions. J Natl Cancer Inst 57:1027, 1976.
68. Kuipers EJ, Uyterlinde AM, Pena AS, et al: Long term sequelae of *H. pylori* gastritis. Lancet 345:1525, 1995.
69. Uemura N, Okamoto S, Yamamoto S: *Helicobacter pylori* infection and the development of gastric cancer. N Engl J Med 345:784, 2001.
70. El-Omar EM, Oien K, El-Nujumi A, et al: *Helicobacter pylori* infection and chronic gastric acid hyposecretion. Gastroenterology 113:15, 1997.
71. Wotherspoon AC, Ortiz Hidalgo C, Falzon MR, et al: *Helicobacter pylori*–associated gastritis and primary B-cell gastric lymphoma. Lancet 338:1175, 1991.
72. Hussell T, Isaacson PG, Crabtree JE, et al: The response of cells from low-grade B-cell gastric lymphomas of mucosa-associated lymphoid tissue to *Helicobacter pylori*. Lancet 342:571, 1993.
73. Stolte M, Eidt S: Healing gastric MALT lymphomas by eradicating *H. pylori*? Lancet 342:568, 1993.
74. Bayerdorffer E, Neubauer A, Eidt S, et al, for the Malt-Lymphoma Study Group, Germany: Double-blind treatment of early gastric malt-lymphoma patients by *Helicobacter pylori* eradication. Gastroenterology 106(Suppl 2):370, 1994.
75. El-Zimaity HMT, Al Assi MT, Genta RM: Confirmation of successful therapy of *Helicobacter pylori* infection: Number and site of biopsies or a rapid urease test. Am J Gastroenterol 90:1962, 1995.
76. Genta RM, Robason GO, Graham DY: Simultaneous visualization of *Helicobacter pylori* and gastric morphology: A new stain. Hum Pathol 25:221, 1994.
77. Peterson WL, Graham DY, Marshall B, et al: Clarithromycin as monotherapy for eradication of *Helicobacter pylori*: A randomized, double-blind trial. Am J Gastroenterol 88:1860, 1993.
78. Marshall BJ, Warren JR, Francis GJ, et al: Rapid urease test in the management of *Campylobacter pyloridis*–associated gastritis. Am J Gastroenterol 82:200, 1987.
79. Szeto ML, Pounder RE, Hamilton Dutoit SJ, et al: Rapid urease test provides specific identification of *Campylobacter pylori* in antral mucosal biopsies. Postgrad Med J 64:935, 1988.
80. Cutler AF, Prasad VM: Long-term follow-up of *Helicobacter pylori* serology after successful eradication. Am J Gastroenterol 91:85, 1996.
81. Mohar A, Ley C, Guarner J: Eradication rate of *Helicobacter pylori* in a Mexican population at high risk for gastric cancer and use of serology to assess cure. Am J Gastroenterol 97:2530, 2002.
82. Leide-Svegborn S, Stenstrom K, Olofsson M: Biokinetics and radiation doses for carbon-14 urea in adults and children undergoing the *Helicobacter pylori* breath test. Eur J Nucl Med 26:573, 1999.
83. Cutler AF, Havstad S, Ma CK, et al: Accuracy of invasive and noninvasive tests to diagnose *Helicobacter pylori* infection. Gastroenterology 109:136, 1995.
84. Vaira D, Malfertheiner P, Megraud F, et al: Diagnosis of *Helicobacter pylori* infection with a new non-invasive antigen-based assay. HpSA European study group. Lancet 354:30, 1999.
85. Goh KL, Parasakthi N: The racial cohort phenomenon: Seroepidemiology of *Helicobacter pylori* infection in a multiracial South-East Asian country. Eur J Gastroenterol Hepatol 13:177, 2001.

25

Meningococcal Infections

W. MICHAEL SCHELD
JAY D. WENGER
ANASTACIO DE QUEIROZ SOUSA

INTRODUCTION

Meningococcal infections continue to pose serious problems worldwide and are influenced by multiple factors, including geography, season, climate, serogroup, and population demographics.[1,2] Although focal outbreaks and epidemics occur in more developed areas, the incidence of epidemic meningococcal meningitis and meningococcemia exhibits high geographic variability. The classic example is the so-called meningitis belt of sub-Saharan Africa (Fig. 25-1), where hyperendemic and epidemic meningococcal serogroup A disease occurs regularly (see later discussion).[1,2] Indeed, nearly 250,000 cases were recorded in this area in 1996, one of the worst outbreaks on record.[3] Meningococcal infections continue to pose an important public health threat in the tropics because mortality is unacceptably high and serious neurologic and other sequelae are not infrequent.

History

The syndrome of epidemic meningitis with a purpuric rash was identified by Viesseux in 1805, who described an epidemic of "malignant purpuric fever" surrounding Geneva, Switzerland.[4] Danielson and Mann recorded the first observations of meningococcemia and resultant meningitis in the United States in 1806 and many of the early descriptions were collated in a treatise by Elisha North of Connecticut in 1811.[5,6] Then, as now, the fulminant nature of some cases was frightening to physicians and laypersons alike; for example, the following was written by the Reverend Festus Foster of Petersham, Massachusetts, in a letter to the editor of *The Worchester Spy* dated March 6, 1811[4]:

> I hasten to give you a sketch of the spotted fever in this place. It made its first appearance about the beginning of January last; but the instances were few and distant from each other, until last week. Although it had proved fatal in most instances, seven only had died belonging to this town previous to the 25th of February. Since that time the disorder has come upon us like a flood of mighty waters. We have buried eight persons within the last eight days. About twelve or fifteen new cases appeared on Thursday last; many of them very sudden and violent. This was the most melancholy and alarming day ever witnessed in this place. Seven or eight physicians were continually engaged in the neighborhood north of the meeting house, and I believe not one half hour passed in the forenoon without presenting a new case. Pale fear and extreme anxiety were visible in every countenance....

Anton Weichselbaum of Vienna first isolated meningococci in 1887. The organisms were obtained from the cerebrospinal fluid (CSF) of six patients with meningitis and were initially named *Diplococcus intracellularis meningitidis*. The lumbar puncture was introduced by Quincke in 1891 and the major CSF alterations associated with meningitis were well recognized by the turn of the century.[4] The first truly significant therapeutic modality for any form of meningitis was developed by Simon Flexner in 1913 and consisted of systemic and intrathecal administration of antimeningococcal antisera raised in horses. Although toxic, antisera therapy reduced the mortality of meningococcal meningitis from approximately 80% to 30% during World War I and for decades thereafter. The first successful account of therapy of meningococcal meningitis with an antimicrobial agent was published in 1937[7,8]; nine patients survived after receiving subcutaneous and intraspinal injections of sulfanilamide and the sole death occurred despite eradication of the organism from CSF. Although sulfonamide resistance among meningococci was common by the mid 1960s and led to the abandonment of this class of agents for the treatment and prophylaxis of meningococcal disease, this event spurred interest in the development of immunoprophylaxis, leading to several safe and effective meningococcal vaccines. Despite these achievements, serious meningococcal epidemics continue and the mortality associated with meningococcemia remains significant despite the introduction of newer antimicrobial agents.

AGENT

Neisseria species are non-spore-forming, oxidase-positive, nonmotile, gram-negative cocci (measuring approximately 0.8 μm by 0.6 μm) that usually appear as biscuit- or kidney-shaped diplococci on smears of infected fluids. Since other organisms may appear similar morphologically, identification rests on biochemical and immunologic techniques. Sugar fermentation reactions are usually sufficient for speciation within the genus *Neisseria*.[9] Meningococci characteristically ferment glucose and maltose to acid. The organisms grow rapidly on blood, chocolate, gonococcal, or enriched Mueller-Hinton agar in a moist 3% to 10% CO_2 environment at 35°C to 37°C. A modified Thayer-Martin medium is employed for meningococcal isolation from contaminated sites, as in detection of the carrier state. The organism is rather fastidious, susceptible to drying and chilling, so all specimens should be inoculated promptly.

The ultrastructural characteristics of meningococci are complex. Surface components include capsular polysaccharide, fimbriae or pili, lipopolysaccharide (LPS), and outer membrane proteins (OMPs); several of these structures are important virulence determinants (see later discussion).[4,9] Major classification schemes of meningococci divide organisms into serogroups based on structural differences among capsular polysaccharides and agglutination reactions with specific antisera. Invasive isolates are uniformly encapsulated, whereas carrier strains are often unencapsulated (nongroupable). The serogroups have very

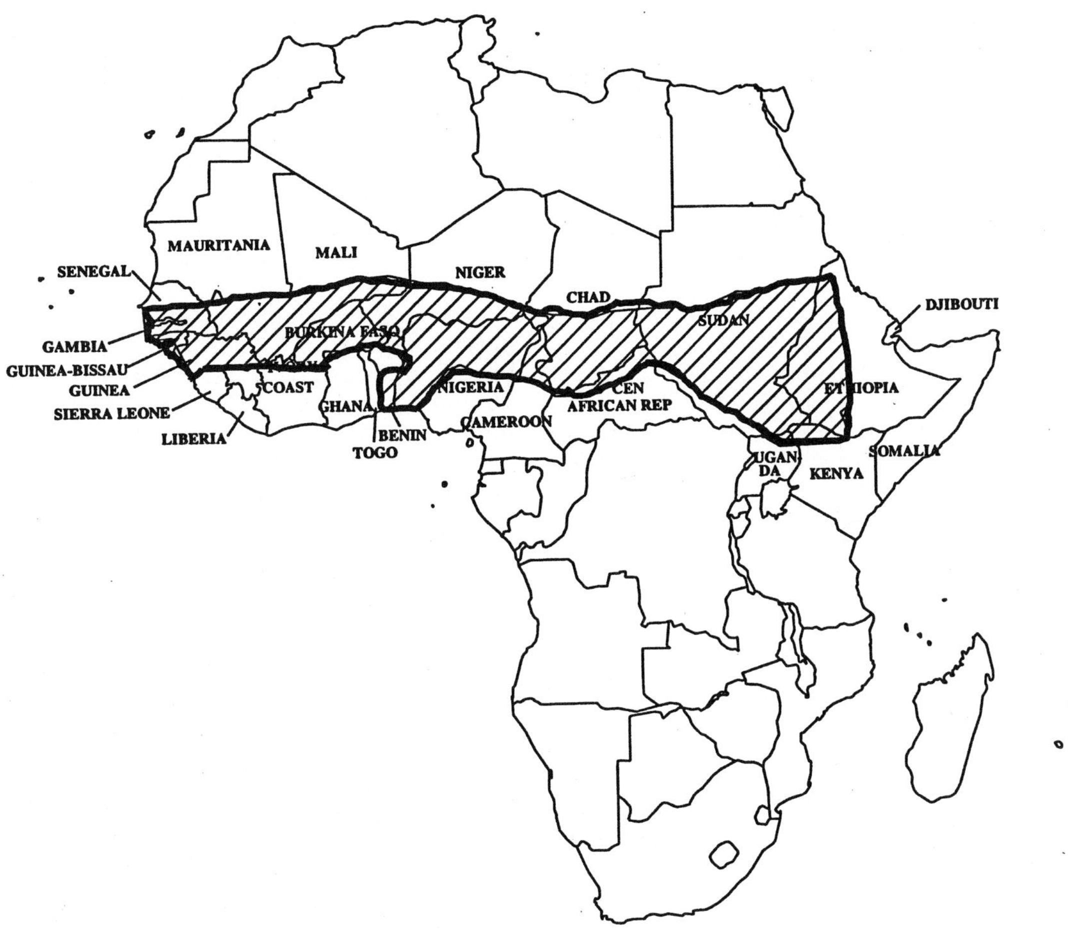

FIGURE 25-1 The sub-Saharan Africa "meningitis belt."

important epidemiologic and prevention-related implications. Thirteen serogroups are currently recognized[4,9–11] and designated A, B, C, D, E, H, I, K, L, X, Y, Z, and W-135. Most meningococcal disease is caused by organisms in serogroups A, B, C, and Y, although the proportion of cases caused by serogroup W-135 is increasing in some areas.[4] Recent epidemiologic trends for the three major serogroups are discussed in the following section.

Further classification of meningococci within serogroups into serotypes is based largely on the analysis of OMP profiles in the cell envelope.[4,12] Variations in protein porB are currently classified into serotypes 1 through 21. This classification scheme is useful in epidemiologic studies and as a basis for the preparation of subtype vaccines. Further classification into subserotypes is based on variations in protein porA.[13] Subserotypes P1.1 through P1.16 are currently recognized. Variations in LPS are utilized for subdivision into immunotypes (L1 through L12).[1,10,14–17] Techniques for subclassification of meningococci are generally available only in research or reference laboratories but are extremely useful in epidemiologic studies. In addition to classification by serogroup, serotype, subserotype, and LPS immunotype, many reports have focused on multilocus enzyme electrophoresis.[18–21] This latter technique led to the realization that epidemics caused on a worldwide basis by a strain of serogroup A meningococci are derived from a single clone. The availability of the sequence of the meningococcal genome, coupled with the lack of serogroup B vaccine, has fostered the use of this database for the development of a noncapsular vaccine approach designated "reverse vaccinology."[22]

EPIDEMIOLOGY

Transmission and Carriage

Neisseria meningitidis disease is exclusive to humans. No intermediate host, animal transmission, or reservoir has been proved. The human nasopharynx is the natural reservoir for meningococci; transmission is facilitated by airborne droplets or close personal contact. Meningococcal colonization may result in an asymptomatic carrier state (which is most common) or endemic, hyperendemic (i.e., in the meningitis belt between epidemics at approximately 10–50 cases per 100,000 per year), or epidemic disease.[2,4,10] Meningococci persist asymptomatically in the nasopharynx for periods ranging from several weeks to months to as long as 1 to 2 years.[23] During this colonization phase, protective antibodies to the strain are usually induced.[24,25] Carriage rates in most civilian populations range from 5% to 15%, but may be much higher in certain populations in which conditions conducive to outbreaks of meningococcal disease exist, such as extreme crowding and mixing of populations in military recruit training camps. The implications of transmission and carriage on the pathogenesis and immunology of meningococcal disease are described later.

Although, as noted previously, at least 13 capsular serogroups of meningococci have been described, most human disease is caused by serogroups A, B, C, Y, and W-135, and these strains cause nearly all outbreaks of disease. This section describes recent epidemiologic trends for the major serogroups.

Serogroup A

Serogroup A organisms are the most common cause of large epidemics.[26] These outbreaks may lead to incidence rates as high as 300 to 1000 cases per 10^5 population.[2] For example, the annual incidence reached 370 cases per 100,000 population in the greater São Paulo area in 1974, with 31,000 cases reported per year.[1,2,4] Attack rates are highest in children and young adults and some investigators have reported that, compared with the age distribution of disease in endemic cases, higher proportions of the disease occur in older children during epidemics.[27,28] Even with optimal treatment the mortality rate is still approximately 5% to 10% in patients with meningococcal meningitis[29] and approximately 20% of survivors have neurologic sequelae, including mental retardation and hearing loss.[30]

In some areas of the world, serogroup A meningococcal epidemics recur in a vaguely periodic pattern.[26] The African meningitis belt (see Fig. 25-1) is the best studied and the classic representative of this phenomenon. Although meningococcal infections were not recorded in the area until the 1880s, large outbreaks still occur regularly. The region, stretching from Ethiopia in the east to The Gambia in the west, frequently experiences epidemic disease and in some countries epidemics occur every 8 to 12 years. Figure 25-2 shows the incidence of disease and outbreak history in a typical meningitis belt country, Niger, for a 70-year period. This area of sub-Saharan Africa is dry with an average yearly rainfall of 300 mm and with winter seasons that feature warm, dry, and dusty winds (the harmattan).[26,31] Outbreaks typically begin with the onset of the dry season in January and end abruptly with the coming of the rains in May or June.[2,4] Although conjectural, the distinct seasonality is striking and may be related to the drying effect on mucous membranes, seasonal transmission of respiratory viruses, or other factors.[32]

Olyhoek and colleagues[18] studied strains from epidemic waves from the 1950s through the early 1980s in an effort to assess the role of specific serogroup A meningococcal strains in these outbreaks. Individual epidemics and most waves of epidemics occurring over a number of years were invariably due to single strains. Although multiple strains could be identified during interepidemic periods, nearly all disease during outbreaks was caused by a single strain. No specific microbiologic characteristics were identified among the outbreak strains, which could account for the apparently increased virulence in epidemic potential, but this work suggests that strain characteristics are linked with epidemic disease.[2]

Major epidemics in the meningitis belt are heralded by a "shift to the right" toward older age groups (i.e., adolescents instead of 5- to 9-year-old children), a predictive feature of explosive epidemics in this area.[4,10] It is possible that introduction of new strains into populations that have not previously (or at least recently) been exposed to them leads to higher attack rates in older children compared to endemic or hyperendemic disease.[2,20] This could occur without assuming the new organisms have any inherent increased invasiveness or transmission potential. Introduction of newer strains with different antigenic determinants into the population places older children and young adults at risk since they have never "seen" this strain and may not be immunologically protected as they were from previously circulating strains.[2,33]

In 1996, the biggest wave of meningococcal meningitis outbreaks ever recorded hit West Africa.[3] An estimated 250,000 cases and 25,000 deaths occurred in Niger, Nigeria, Burkina Faso, Chad, and other countries and paralyzed medical care systems locally. The outbreak stopped with the spring rains as usual but continued into the next winter season.[2] The strain isolated was from the III-1 clone, which has

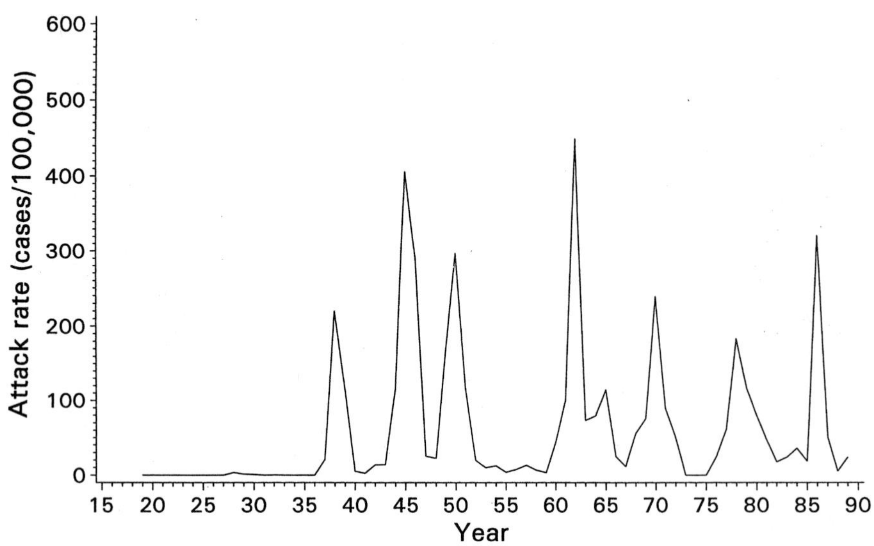

FIGURE 25-2 The epidemiology of meningitis in Niger (a country located in the "meningitis belt") from 1919 through 1989. (From Riedo FX, Plikaytis BD, Broome CV: Epidemiology and prevention of meningococcal disease. Pediatr Infect Dis J 14:643, 1995.)

caused a series of outbreaks in Africa since 1988, according to the Centers for Disease Control and Prevention (CDC).

Serogroup C

Large-scale outbreaks due to serogroup C have occurred frequently in the tropics in recent years. For example, the attack rate was 517 cases per 100,000 inhabitants during a serogroup C epidemic in Upper Volta (now Burkina Faso) in 1979 and recent studies documented an attack rate of 400 to 450 per 100,000 children up to 8 years of age in the Faroe Islands.[4,10]

Large serogroup A outbreaks such as those seen in Africa have not occurred in the developed world for over 2 decades.[1] In fact, in most developed countries, meningococcal disease in general, usually caused by serogroup B, C, or Y meningococci, has slowly decreased in incidence (Fig. 25-3). However, in the late 1980s and early 1990s, disturbing small outbreaks and an increased incidence of serogroup C disease were identified in a number of countries, particularly Canada.[34,35] The outbreaks usually involved between 5 and 20 children or young adults in small geographic areas and the fatality rate (10% to 15%) and burden of serious sequelae caused increasing alarm. Most of the recent Canadian outbreaks and cases were caused by one specific serogroup C strain, designated enzyme type ET-15.[36] This ET type increased in Canadian strain collections from 5% of all invasive isolates in 1985 to over 65% by 1990 and resulted in a large-scale immunization program (see later discussion). The ET-15 strain and four other closely related clonal strains were also implicated in a marked increase in outbreaks of serogroup C meningococcal disease in the United States, and this serogroup is among the most prevalent causes of meningococcal meningitis in that country (Table 25-1). Multiple outbreaks of serogroup C meningococcal disease have occurred recently and mass immunization campaigns were conducted in more than 10 separate sites between 1990 and 1993.[34] A clear increase in both recognized outbreaks and vaccine use for outbreak control occurred in the early 1990s. The U.S. outbreaks usually involved 5 to 15 persons in small communities or institutions, occurred with the same seasonal pattern as endemic disease (peak disease rates in the winter and early spring), were distributed widely over the country, and had a case-fatality rate that did not differ from the U.S. endemic disease rate observed previously.[2,34] Institutional outbreaks

Table 25-1 Neisseria meningitidis *Serogroups Responsible for Invasive Disease: United States, 1995*

Serogroup	Percentage of Isolates
C	32
B	24
Y	31
W-135	6
A	<1

Adapted from Broome CV, Wenger JD, Schuchat A, et al: Changing epidemiology of bacterial meningitis in the United States. Presented at the 36th Interscience Conference on Antimicrobial Agents and Chemotherapy, New Orleans, LA, September 1996, abstract S64.

tended to be of short duration, often with all cases occurring within 1 or 2 weeks, which differed from community-wide outbreaks, which tended to occur over a period of several months. Among community-wide outbreaks, affected persons tend to be older than those with endemic disease, again reflecting the possible introduction of strains of serogroup C meningococci that were "new" to the local populations. Indeed, this was confirmed by ET studies, which showed that 8 of the 13 most recent U.S. outbreaks were caused by closely related strains very similar to the Canadian ET-15.[2,34] These recent outbreaks have led to an increased understanding of the efficacy of the serogroup C meningococcal vaccine.[37]

Serogroup B

Group B organisms, especially B:15:P1.16, have recently emerged as important pathogens in northern Europe, causing serious local outbreaks peaking in the 10- to 20-year-old age group. The continued high prevalence of serogroup B meningococcal disease has important implications because of the current lack of a widely available vaccine effective against this serogroup.

In the early 1990s, increasing rates of meningococcal disease in the general population and focal outbreaks were documented in Oregon.[34,38] The overall rate of disease, which had been in the range of 1 to 2 cases per 100,000 population, similar to that in the United States in general, rose steadily to

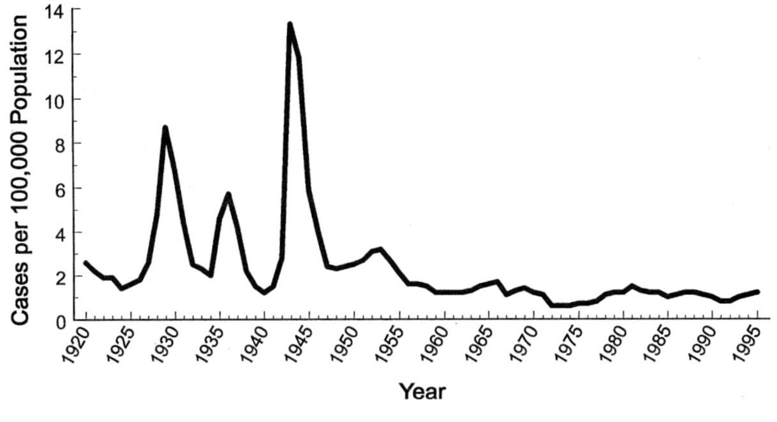

FIGURE 25-3 The incidence of reported meningococcal disease in the United States by year, 1920–1995.

approximately 5 cases per 100,000. The age distribution in the cases also rose, consistent with epidemic disease caused by the other serogroups, but data soon showed that most of the cases were caused by serogroup B. Further subtyping data identified an enzyme type strain previously seen only very rarely in the United States, designated ET-301. This strain caused 80% of all serogroup B disease in Oregon (Fig. 25-4) and was closely related to other strains identified by Caugant and colleagues as the ET-5 complex.[39,40] Strains from this group have caused increased rates of disease, usually with overall incidence rates between 5 and 15 cases per 100,000 population per year in Norway, the Netherlands, Cuba, and throughout much of Latin America in the 1980s and early 1990s. In contrast to serogroup A and C outbreaks, which even in the absence of large-scale immunization programs usually run their course over a period of 2 to 3 years in a given area, serogroup B ET-5 outbreaks tend to cause prolonged elevations of disease rates in the same areas, persisting for up to a decade.[41] Although its precise origin is unknown, the ET-5 clone had marched through much of Europe, then through Latin America prior to its arrival in Oregon. The appearance of the ET-5 clone was gradual over many years as suggested by the disease rates, but the general epidemiologic pattern of disease was similar to endemic patterns in most respects, including seasonality, sex distribution (favoring males), and mortality rates. The shift in age distribution was again consistent with introduction of a new strain into an antigenically virgin population, as noted previously with serogroup A and C outbreaks. In the absence of an effective vaccine and in order to evaluate the potential for other preventive measures, a study of risk factors for meningococcal disease was performed by the CDC and the Oregon and Washington state health departments.[42] Cases (120) and controls (250) were stratified by age above or below 18 years. Among those less than 18 years of age, the presence of a mother who smoked in the house was the overwhelming risk factor for disease, even when controlling for other socioeconomically related factors, including household crowding and educational status. Among those over 18 years of age, smoking or exposure to smoke was the only other significant risk factor in addition to underlying disease. A modifiable risk factor, smoking contributed strongly to disease acquisition in all age groups and suggests that 30% of all meningococcal disease in the outbreaks was attributable to smoking. Antismoking measures should be a useful public health measure during meningococcal outbreaks.[2,42]

Finally, as in the preceding discussion, meningococcal meningitis is primarily a disease of children and young adults. Fewer than 10% of cases occur in patients over 45 years old. Although meningococcal meningitis is unusual in this age group, 33% of sporadic meningococcal disease occurred in adults in a recent 5-year, population-based study from Atlanta.[43] Underlying conditions such as multiple myeloma, congestive heart failure, asplenia, and infection with human immunodeficiency virus (HIV) were prevalent in adults over 25 years of age with meningococcal infection but were unusual in

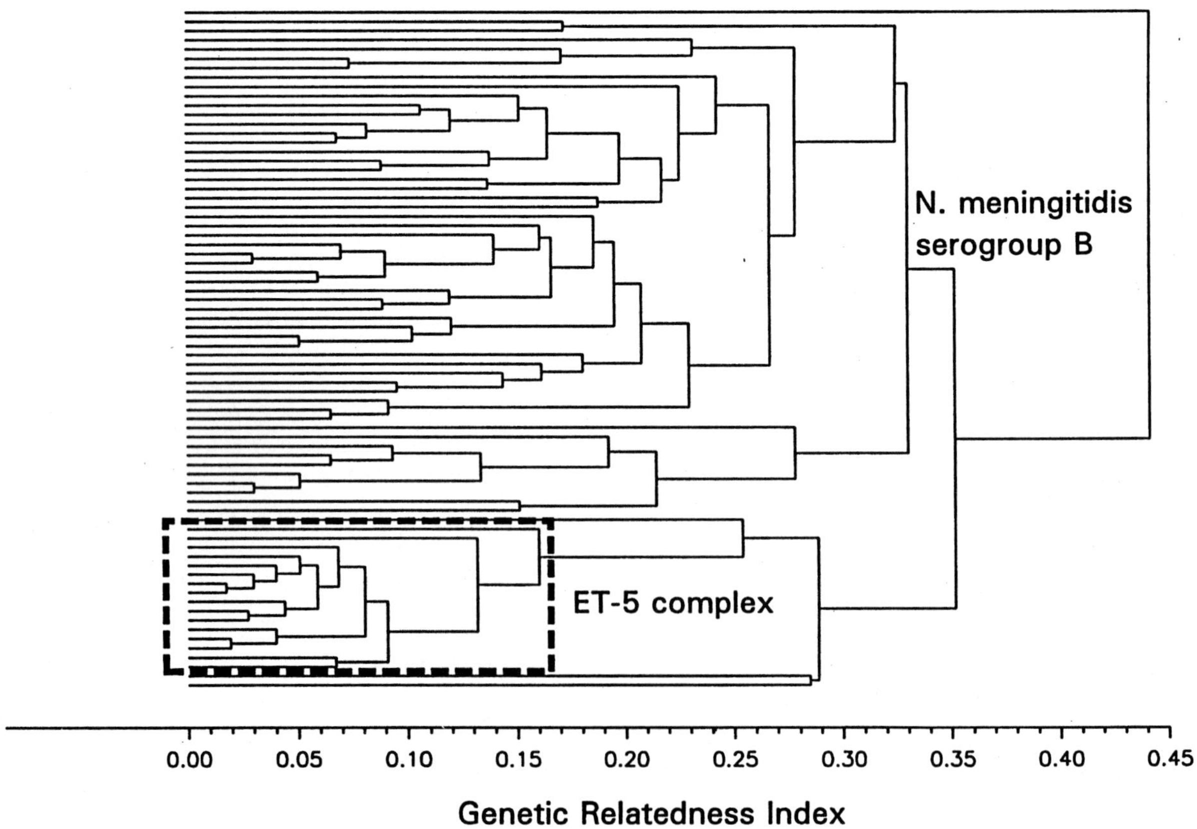

FIGURE 25-4 Multilocus enzyme electrophoresis dendrogram of serogroup B meningococci showing the location of the enzyme type 5 (ET-5) complex.

the 18- to 24-year-old group (i.e., normal, nonimmunosuppressed persons).

CLINICAL MANIFESTATIONS

The clinical manifestations of meningococcal disease can vary considerably, ranging from transient fever and bacteremia to fulminant disease with death ensuing within hours of the onset of symptoms. Wolfe and Birbara[44] described four major clinical syndromes:

1. *Bacteremia without sepsis.* In the setting of an upper respiratory illness or viral exanthem, blood cultures are drawn which are reported as positive for *N. meningitidis,* often after discharge. Occult bacteremia with recovery in the absence of antimicrobial therapy is rare, but serum concentrations of bacteria in children are often low, from 22 to 325 organisms per milliliter of blood in one report.[45]
2. *Meningococcemia without meningitis.* The patient is clinically septic with signs of malaise, weakness, headache, and hypotension developing shortly after admission or before in the presence or absence of skin rash and leukocytosis.
3. *Meningitis with or without meningococcemia.* Headache, fever, and meningeal signs predominate with a cloudy CSF. The state of the sensorium varies from fully alert to deeply obtunded. The deep tendon and superficial reflexes are unaltered and there are no pathologic reflexes.
4. *Meningoencephalitis.* Profound obtundation with meningeal signs and a cloudy CSF are characteristic. Furthermore, the deep tendon reflexes and superficial reflexes are either absent or, rarely, hyperactive and pathologic reflexes are frequently present.

Variations of these scenarios have been reported and the patient may progress from one to another during the course of disease.[4,9]

It is worth noting that the wide range of clinical expressions requires a high index of suspicion for meningococcal disease, especially in an endemic situation with sporadic cases. Meningococcal meningitis appears to differ somewhat from other forms of bacterial meningitis. For example, in a review of 53 cases of meningococcal meningitis by Carpenter and Petersdorf,[46] headache, confusion, and stiff neck occurred as symptoms in less than half of the patients. In infants and small children, fever and vomiting are often the only early clue to central nervous system (CNS) involvement, and these patients are frequently brought to the hospital only after an insidious impairment in consciousness or convulsions occur.[9] Evidence of meningeal irritation is common, except in the very young and very old. In classic early studies, Feigin and Dodge[47] observed that focal neurologic signs and seizures were less common in meningococcal meningitis when compared to pneumococcal meningitis or disease due to *Haemophilus influenzae.* Levels of consciousness across the spectrum were very similar with all three meningeal pathogens. Focal cerebral involvement in meningococcal meningitis is rare. The symptoms and signs of bacterial meningitis are listed in Table 25-2. With the preceding exception, meningococcal meningitis is similar to other forms of bacterial meningitis in presentation. Myalgias are particularly

Table 25-2 Symptoms and Signs of Bacterial Meningitis

Symptom or Sign	Percentage
Headache	≥90
Fever	≥90
Meningismus	≥85
Alteration in consciousness	≥80
Petechiae/purpura	≈50
Vomiting	≈30
Seizures	≈30
Focal neurologic findings	≈25
Myalgias	≈20
Ocular palsies	≈10
Hemiparesis	<5
Papilledema	<1

frequent in meningococcal disease and suggest this diagnosis over other bacterial pathogens. Focal findings, including cranial nerve deficits, are less frequent with meningococcal meningitis when compared with pneumococcal disease.[4,9,47] Finally, papilledema is rare in all forms of bacterial meningitis and suggests an alternative diagnosis.

Although petechiae progressing to purpuric lesions are a classic harbinger of meningococcemia with or without meningitis, some patients display a nonpetechial, nonpurpuric maculopapular eruption. These rashes, seen early in the syndrome, were described extensively by military physicians in the 1940s and 1950s.[44,48] The maculopapular rash resembles a viral exanthem, particularly rubella, and is evanescent, lasting hours to at most 2 days. Intense myalgias are often present during this rash. The petechial eruption is characterized by discrete lesions 1 mm to 2 mm in diameter, most frequently on the trunk and lower extremities, rapidly progressing to more extensive ecchymotic lesions (Figs. 25-5 and 25-6). Petechiae are common in pressure areas from clothing and rarely are vesicular or characterized by desquamation. Petechiae correlate with thrombocytopenia and coagulopathy, particularly disseminated intravascular coagulation (DIC). Response of petechiae early in the disease to therapeutic modalities is an important prognostic variable that can be assessed at the

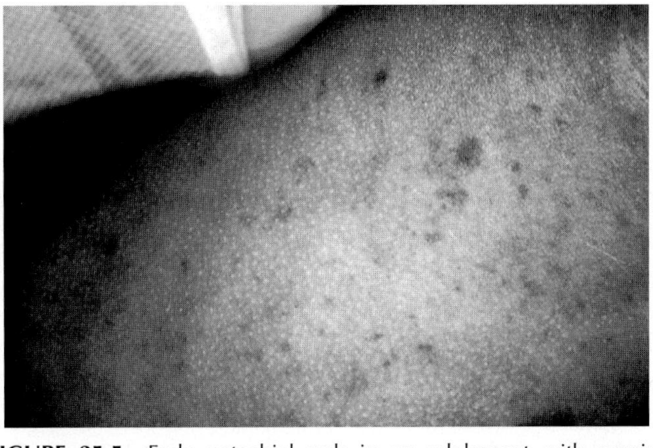

FIGURE 25-5 Early petechial rash in an adolescent with meningococcemia.

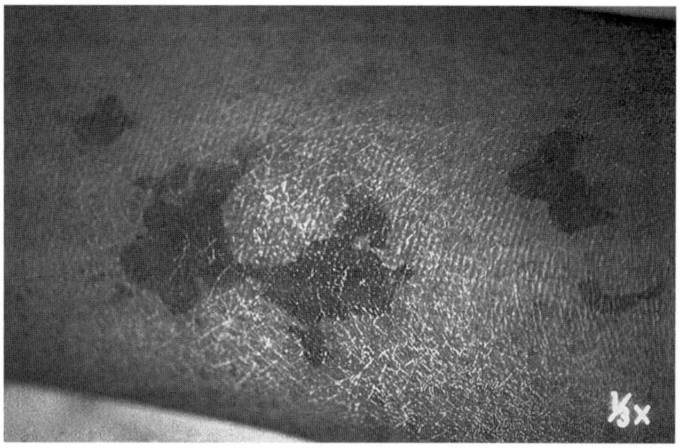

FIGURE 25-6 Diffuse ecchymotic eruption in a case of meningococcemia.

bedside by proper attention to the number of lesions and progression within a defined area of the skin.[4,9]

Although the differential diagnosis is wide (Box 25-1), the presence of petechiae and fever with an altered sensorium is a medical emergency. Shock or the syndrome of purpura fulminans may dominate the clinical picture. Usually, the manifestations are of "cold shock" with peripheral vasoconstriction and cyanotic poorly perfused extremities in the presence of a diffuse purpuric eruption with systemic acidosis. The outlook is poor, especially when other complications, including the acute respiratory distress syndrome, DIC, renal failure, and myopericarditis, are present. The classic Waterhouse-Friderichsen syndrome is characterized by the following: (1) sudden onset of febrile illness, (2) petechial hemorrhages in the skin and mucous membranes, (3) cardiovascular collapse, and (4) DIC. Approximately 10% to 20% of meningococcal infections are dominated by this fulminant septicemia.[4,9,49]

Complications of meningococcemia and meningitis are related to shock and raised intracranial pressure, respectively. Other complications may be quite prominent and are somewhat unusual when compared with other forms of bacterial meningitis, including arthritis, pericarditis, myocarditis, conus medullaris syndrome, and cranial nerve palsies of the sixth, seventh, and eighth cranial nerves.[9,47,50–54] Pericarditis may be an immunologic reaction or secondary to toxins since many cases occur following bacteriologic eradication of the organism.[55]

Box 25-1 Differential Diagnosis of Fever, Altered Sensorium, and Petechial Rash

- Meningococcal disease
- Rickettsial infections (e.g., Rocky Mountain spotted fever)
- *Staphylococcus aureus* endocarditis
- *Streptococcus pneumoniae, Haemophilus influenzae* (especially with splenectomy)
- Septic shock
- Viral meningitis
- Viral hemorrhagic fevers
- "Noninfectious": thrombotic thrombocytopenic purpura (TTP), hemolytic-uremic syndrome (HUS), vasculitis, etc.

Pericardial involvement appears to be more frequent in the convalescent phase of the disease and in cases due to serogroup C meningococci.[52] Serious complications are often evident after eradication of the microorganism from blood and other body fluids. Myocarditis associated with meningococcal infection is manifested by a gallop rhythm, heart failure, pulmonary edema, and high central venous pressures in the face of poor peripheral perfusion. Cardiac glycosides are often prescribed, but evidence of therapeutic value is lacking. Although myocarditis is present in more than 50% of patients who die of meningococcal disease, clinically symptomatic heart failure is unusual. It does appear, however, that acute meningococcemia with myocarditis has a higher mortality rate than when this complication is absent.[4,9,55]

Respiratory Tract Infections

Although nasopharyngeal colonization with meningococci renders sputum cultures hazardous in the interpretation of suspected meningococcal pneumonia, this syndrome has been recognized for more than 80 years.[56,57] Bacteremic meningococcal pneumonia is rare, and therefore blood cultures are often of no value. Serogroup Y organisms are often responsible for meningococcal pneumonia, although the recent emergence of serogroup Y strains in the Chicago area documented a variety of presentations out of proportion to pneumonia.[58] In a classic 1977 study utilizing transtracheal cultures to establish the diagnosis in U.S. Air Force recruits,[59] serogroup Y meningococcal pneumonia was characterized by a history of cough, chest pain, fever, chills, and a previous upper respiratory infection in more than 50% of patients. Rales and fever were nearly uniform and evidence of pharyngitis was present in over 80% of patients. Multiple lobar involvement was common (40%), but the right-lower and right-middle lobes were involved most frequently. No deaths occurred in this series of 68 patients.[59]

The association of meningococcal invasive disease with a preceding upper respiratory tract infection has been noted by many authors. Although common, the role of viral upper respiratory tract disease as a causal factor in systemic meningococcal disease remains problematic. Meningococcal clearance is clearly hindered in the presence of an upper respiratory tract infection, particularly influenza, but efforts at control of upper respiratory tract infections have only infrequently had an impact on the incidence of invasive meningococcal disease. Meningococcal pneumonia is unusual; for example, in a study of the cause of community-acquired pneumonia in Finland, this organism was isolated from only 6 of 162 cases.[60] In addition, the association of contact of cases with a prior symptom of upper respiratory tract infection has been implicated as a cause of serious meningococcal disease by several authors. The implication that inflammation in the nasopharynx is the predecessor to bacteremic disseminated meningococcal disease remains conjectural, but meningococcal disease incidence and severity both rise during influenza epidemics.[61]

A review[62] of 58 patients with meningococcal pneumonia over a 25-year period documented a shift in antimicrobial therapy from predominantly penicillin to cephalosporins; overall fatality was 8.6%. The serogroups responsible were as follows: Y, 44%; B, 18%; W-135, 16%; and C, 14%.

Fulminant meningococcal supraglottitis was first reported in 1995, with five more reports subsequently, and is characterized by fever, sore throat, muffled voice, and dysphagia with swollen supraglottic tissues seen on fiberoptic laryngoscopy, plain films, or cervical CT scans.[63]

Meningococcal Urethritis

Meningococci have been isolated from the urethra and can be the etiologic agent in cases of urethritis.[9,64] Association with oral-genital sex and acquisition of the organism has been suggested. In homosexual males, the organism was isolated from the oral pharynx in 93% versus 6% from the rectum and only 1% from the urethra.[65] Nevertheless, β-lactamase-producing meningococci (although very rare overall) have been most often isolated from urogenital sources.

Chronic Meningococcemia

This unusual syndrome, characterized by persistent meningococcal bacteremia associated with low-grade fever, rash, and arthritis, has been increasingly reported in recent years. The syndrome is very similar to that observed with chronic gonococcemia for which it is often mistaken.[66] Rompalo and associates[67] compared the isolation of gonococci with that of meningococci from blood or synovial fluid cultures from 1970 to 1972 with similar studies from 1980 through 1983. The ratio of gonococcal to meningococcal isolates changed from 15:1 in the earlier period to 9:5 for the period 1980 to 1983. Systemic meningococcal infection should be considered in the patient with the acute arthritis-dermatitis syndrome, commonly ascribed to *Neisseria gonorrhoeae* (see Chapter 26).

Meningococcemia in the Setting of Complement Deficiency

As discussed in the following secitons, complement or properdin deficiency predisposes persons to the occurrence of systemic meningococcal disease.[4,9,68,69] Interestingly, the degree of severity of the meningococcal infection is often less and case-fatality rates are low when terminal complement components are affected. In all other respects, the clinical course is similar to that outlined previously. The specific complement and properdin deficiencies associated with systemic meningococcal infection are outlined in the following discussion.

PATHOGENESIS AND IMMUNITY

As stated previously, meningococcal disease is exclusive to humans. The meningococcal carrier state is fundamental to the development of invasive disease.[2,4,9,10] Approximately 6% of the population develops nasopharyngeal colonization with *N. meningitidis* yearly. Nasopharyngeal carriage rates vary markedly with age and the population under study but are approximately 5% to 15%, rising from 0.5% in children 3 to 48 months old to approximately 20% to 40% in young adults. Carriage persists for weeks to months and occasionally years and largely accounts for the increased risk of disease in household contacts of an index case. Although uncharacterized host and environmental factors, including prior viral upper respiratory tract infection, contribute to containment of infection or invasion, host immunity also plays an important role. Those persons recently colonized with meningococci appear to be at greatest risk of invasive disease.[23]

The age-specific incidence of meningococcal infection is inversely proportional to the presence of serum bactericidal antibodies against serogroups A, B, and C. More than 50% of infants possess bactericidal antibody at the time of birth as a result of transplacental transfer. Immunoglobulin G (IgG) antibody to serogroup B polysaccharide, however, is lacking in neonates. This contributes to the occurrence of serogroup B meningococcal disease in this age group, and since serogroup B meningococcal capsular antigen is identical to the capsular polysaccharides of *Escherichia coli* K1 and certain types of serogroup B streptococci, these organisms are also major causes of neonatal sepsis and meningitis.[70] The inverse link between occurrence of invasive disease and bactericidal antibody was first documented during an outbreak of serogroup C meningococcal meningitis among U.S. Army recruits in 1968.[24]

Although recovery from invasive meningococcal disease generally confers lifelong immunity against the homologous serogroup, this is not the major immunizing process. Nasopharyngeal colonization, particularly with serogroup B, C, or Y, may elicit the development of bactericidal activity, primarily directed against the colonizing strain but also active against heterologous organisms within 5 to 12 days of acquisition.[4] Nasopharyngeal colonization with nongroupable meningococci or *Neisseria lactamica,* virtually nonpathogenic organisms, may confer protective immunity against other meningococci with invasive potential. The carriage rates of pathogenic meningococci are far too low in children to account for antibody formation and the importance of other cross-reacting organisms, outside the genus *Neisseria,* has also been proposed. Paradoxically, an exuberant IgA response to meningococci may actually enhance the development of systemic disease.

In addition to bactericidal antibody, an intact complement system is also a component of the host's defenses against invasive meningococcal disease. Recurrent or chronic neisserial infections have been associated with rare isolated deficiencies of late complement components (C5, C6, C7, or C8, and perhaps C9).[68,69] Screening for complement defects is useful in families with recurrent or chronic neisserial infections and perhaps for individuals after only one episode of invasive meningococcal disease.[71] Complement deficiency also appears to predispose to meningitis caused by nongroupable meningococci and *Neisseria*-related bacteria (i.e., *Moraxella* or *Acinetobacter* species).[72] Depletion of early complement components (C1, C3, or C4) because of an underlying disorder such as nephrotic syndrome, hepatic failure, the presence of C3 nephritic factor, or multiple myeloma may predispose to the first episode of invasive meningococcal disease.[4] Properdin deficiency or dysfunction, with normal concentrations, also predisposes to invasive meningococcal disease; this defect is reversible with vaccination.[68,73] Asplenic states also increase the risk of serious infections by encapsulated organisms, especially *H. influenzae* or *Streptococcus pneumoniae,* but also meningococci. Although all of the preceding factors (particularly recent colonization with a pathogenic strain in a nonimmune host) undoubtedly contribute to the pathogenesis of overt meningococcal disease, the precise determinants

Box 25-2 Putative Meningococcal Virulence Factors

Capsular polysaccharide
Pili
IgA protease
Lipopolysaccharide (endotoxin)
Outer membrane proteins
Outer membrane vesicles or blebs
Metabolic pathways (e.g., iron)

contributing to the clinical illness (as opposed to the usual outcome of asymptomatic carriage) are poorly defined. Even during epidemics, only 1 in 1000 to 5000 colonized patients develops disease.[4,10,23] Various predisposing factors have been proposed to explain this discrepancy, including crowding, low socioeconomic status, poor general health, a preceding upper viral respiratory tract infection, and alcoholism.[1] Simultaneous outbreaks of meningococcal and influenza infections have been described in institutional and community settings.[61] The role of viral infections in the enhancement of meningococcal dissemination is unproved[32,61,74] and the precise factors that contribute to the development of overt clinical illness are at present poorly understood.

The time from nasopharyngeal acquisition to bloodstream invasion is short, usually 10 days or less. The incubation period may also be quite short, since "secondary" cases commonly occur within 1 to 4 days of the index case.[4,9] Once the organism is blood-borne, more than 90% of meningococcal disease is manifested as meningitis or meningococcemia. As noted previously, the clonal nature, even among clones of closely related organisms, suggests the complex interplay among virulence characteristics.[4]

The putative meningococcal virulence characteristics are listed in Box 25-2. As noted previously, all isolates from invasive infections are encapsulated (i.e., serogroup-positive), but 20% to more than 50% of isolates from carriers are unencapsulated (nontypable). The capsular polysaccharide appears to be essential to virulence, probably because of its antiphagocytic properties which allow the organism to escape host-phagocytic clearance mechanisms within the CSF or bloodstream. Pili are protein surface appendages composed of identical pilin repeated subunits and are very similar within the genus *Neisseria*. Cross-reacting antibodies bind to a short peptide sequence (residue 69–94) of gonococcal pili that is essential to receptor binding function, with perhaps a similar adhesion-promoting function among meningococci. Fresh meningococcal isolates from carriers and patients with clinical infection contain 7 to 40 pili per diplococcus.[75] Pili are important mediators of meningococcal adhesion to human nonciliated columnar nasopharyngeal epithelial cells,[76] an important early step in the development of the carrier state. Extracellular proteases that cleave the IgA1 heavy chain in the hinge region are elaborated by pathogenic *Neisseria* species (i.e., meningococci and gonococci). Although the role of IgA proteases in the pathogenesis of disease is controversial, these enzymes may promote invasion at the pharyngeal portal of entry. Meningococcal LPS resembles *H. influenzae* LPS by a lack of the O-antigenic polysaccharide side chain found in enteric bacteria despite a smooth phenotype and proven virulence and is more properly referred to as a lipooligosaccharide (LOS). LPS is clearly important in the genesis of an array of the clinical manifestations of meningococcemia and meningitis.[4,14,15] Although the specific role for OMPs in meningococcal virulence is unclear, these organisms release substantial amounts of cell surface material in the form of outer membrane vesicles or blebs containing OMPs and LPS during growth in vitro and in vivo in the absence of cell lysis, a process exacerbated by antimicrobial agents. These outer membrane vesicles or blebs represent relevant vehicles for CNS tissue damage during meningococcal infection.[77] Finally, tissue invasion may also be facilitated by the ability of meningococci to obtain iron from transferrin, hemoglobin, and lactoferrin. Animals subjected to iron overload are more susceptible to fatal meningococcal infection.

DIAGNOSIS

Patients with a petechial or purpuric eruption, fever, and altered sensorium represent a medical emergency; the differential diagnosis is listed in Box 25-1. Between 50% and 75% of children with meningococcemia have a purpuric or petechial rash, principally on the trunk and lower extremities. Petechiae are found in the skin, mucous membranes, and conjunctivae but not in the nail beds.[78] A similar rash is sometimes seen on the trunk and extremities in echovirus type 9 meningitis, acute staphylococcal endocarditis, and rarely pneumococcal or *H. influenzae* meningitis, except in asplenic patients.[79,80] In the tropics, various viral hemorrhagic fevers (e.g., dengue, Crimean-Congo, Ebola) may present with fulminant ecchymotic lesions, fever, and altered consciousness. Rickettsial infections may also present with a similar picture. Petechial rashes should be promptly examined microscopically in the initial evaluation of a patient with suspected meningococcemia after aspiration or making a "touch preparation" on a glass slide; approximately 70% of these preparations will reveal the organisms usually within vacuolated neutrophils if meningococcemia is present (Fig. 25-7). In approximately 20% to 25% of patients with meningococcemia, the organisms

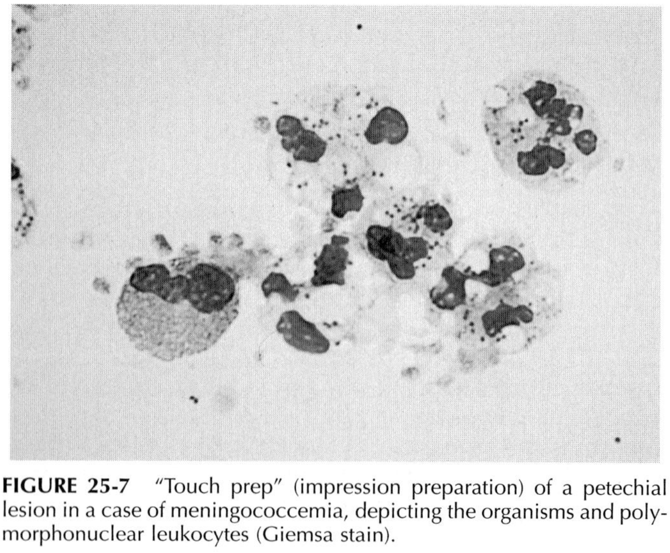

FIGURE 25-7 "Touch prep" (impression preparation) of a petechial lesion in a case of meningococcemia, depicting the organisms and polymorphonuclear leukocytes (Giemsa stain).

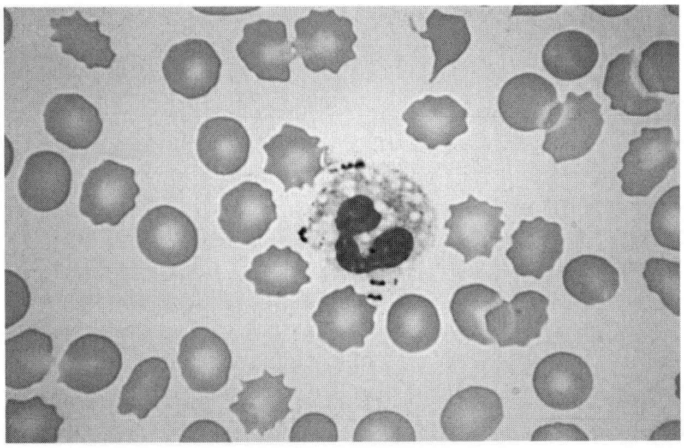

FIGURE 25-8 Buffy coat preparation of a peripheral blood smear in meningococcemia, displaying leukocyte-associated meningococci (Wright's stain).

may be visualized on the peripheral blood smear, especially in a buffy coat preparation (Fig. 25-8). Although the sensitivity is low, this simple test can be quite valuable in the initial approach.

The gold standard for the definitive diagnosis of invasive meningococcal disease remains culture of the organism from a normally sterile body fluid; the CSF and blood are the most common sites of positive cultures by the preceding techniques.[4,9] It is worth noting that CSF cultures are often positive in the presence of suspected meningococcemia, even in the absence of clinical signs of overt meningitis.[81] Meningococci are often cultured from CSF specimens that appear virtually normal by cytologic and chemical analyses in the early phases of illness. The mean concentration of meningococci in CSF specimens is approximately 10^5 colony-forming units (CFU) per milliliter with a wide range from approximately 10^2 CFU/mL to greater than 10^7 CFU/mL.[82,83]

The diagnosis of meningococcal meningitis requires examination of the CSF. As discussed previously, culture remains the gold standard and CSF Gram's stains in the presence of meningococcal meningitis have an overall sensitivity of approximately 70% in untreated patients. Other CSF values are highly variable. In an analysis of 58 patients with meningococcal meningitis,[46] the median leukocyte count was approximately 1200/mm^3, with a range of less than 10/mm^3 to more than 65,000/mm^3. Polymorphonuclear leukocytes predominate overwhelmingly in untreated patients. CSF protein concentrations range from 25 mg/100 mL to more than 800 mg/100 mL, with a median value of approximately 150 mg/100 mL, while 75% of CSF specimens reveal glucose concentrations below 40 mg/100 mL. All of these values may be altered significantly by prior antimicrobial treatment.[4,9,46]

Detection of meningococcal antigen in CSF by various techniques, including counterimmunoelectrophoresis, latex agglutination, and cold agglutination, have demonstrated variable sensitivity and specificity despite the capability of detecting 0.5 μg or less of meningococcal antigen under standardized test conditions.[9,82] False negative results are common.[84] Meningococcal antigen may be detected in urine by these techniques despite negative CSF specimens. These tests should only be considered in Gram's stain–negative cases. CSF concentrations of lactic dehydrogenase or neuraminidase are elevated in meningococcal meningitis.[85,86] Although the concentrations of these enzymes appear to be higher in meningococcal disease than in the other two major forms of bacterial meningitis, the utility of these tests in individual patient management is unclear.

Recently, the polymerase chain reaction (PCR) has been applied to the diagnosis of invasive meningococcal disease. For example, Ni and colleagues[87] examined 54 CSF samples with appropriate controls by PCR in a blinded fashion. The sensitivity and specificity of PCR for the diagnosis of meningococcal meningitis were both 91%. PCR may be most appropriate in Gram stain-negative cases, especially in patients receiving prior antimicrobial therapy, but requires special techniques and is expensive. Multiplex PCR has proven effective in the diagnosis of meningococcal disease, especially in the setting of prior antimicrobial administration.[88,89] The technique can be used to rapidly type strains of critical value in an evolving epidemic.[40] A more broad-based PCR technique utilizing 16sRNA may differentiate bacterial from viral meningitis, even in partially treated or Gram stain-negative cases,[90] but is not specific for meningococcal disease and not widely available. Nevertheless, in selected cases, PCR is a valuable adjunct for the diagnosis of meningococcal infections where resources are available. In most tropical regions during an epidemic, meningococcal meningitis is treated empirically without attempt at specific microbiologic or cytologic confirmation. Neuroimaging is virtually never indicated in suspected meningococcal meningitis or meningococcemia.

TREATMENT AND PROGNOSIS

Antimicrobial Therapy

Penicillin G 300,000 units/kg/day intravenously (IV), in divided doses every 2 to 4 hours, or ampicillin 300 to 400 mg/kg/day, in divided doses every 4 hours, are the preferred antibiotics for the treatment of invasive meningococcal disease.[4,9,91] A 5-day course of therapy is adequate for most cases of uncomplicated meningococcal meningitis (although some authorities recommend treatment durations of 3 days). Meningococcal resistance to penicillin has been reported.[92] β-lactamase-producing isolates are still very rare,[93] but penicillin-resistant strains that do not produce β-lactamase appear to have a reduced affinity for penicillin-binding proteins (e.g., PBP-2 and PBP-3) and have been reported from Spain, the United Kingdom, and other countries.[94,95] In Spain, the number of relatively penicillin-resistant meningococcal isolates reached 20% in 1989.[94] However, in the United States in 1991, only 3 of 100 isolates submitted to the CDC had minimum inhibitory concentrations (MICs) of penicillin of 0.125 μg/mL.[96] Because of the low frequency of resistance in some areas, routine sensitivity testing of meningococcal isolates is not indicated; nevertheless, surveillance for resistance should continue. Meningitis due to relatively penicillin-resistant meningococci (MICs in the range of 0.1 μg/mL to 0.8 μg/mL) has been managed successfully with currently recommended doses of penicillin or a third-generation cephalosporin (e.g., cefotaxime, ceftriaxone). These latter agents are preferred alternatives to penicillin; first- and second-generation cephalosporins and sulfonamides are unreliable.[4,9,97–100] Chloramphenicol is an effective substitute in the penicillin-allergic patient at a dosage of 100 mg/kg/day up to a maximum of 4 g/day total dose,[4,9,10] as chloramphenicol-resistant meningococci, although reported, remain rare.[101] Chloramphenicol is often the preferred agent in resource-limited settings and is often administered in an oily vehicle by the intramuscular (IM) route to sustain chloramphenicol concentrations in blood over prolonged periods of time.[4,10] Recent studies in the United Kingdom have suggested that immediate administration by general practitioners of penicillin in the office setting as soon as the diagnosis is suspected may lead to improvement in the mortality rate.[102,103] Urgent administration of antimicrobial agents is indicated on suspicion of invasive meningococcal disease; prehospitilization administration may reduce mortality.[104]

Supportive Care

Meningococcemia is often complicated by vascular collapse and shock. Multisystem organ failure is not infrequent. Meningococcal LPS is a potent toxin and initiates a cascade of events characterized by the release of multiple proinflammatory cytokines.[105] Girardin and coworkers[106] have demonstrated that serum concentrations of tumor necrosis factor-α (TNF-α), interleukin-1 (IL-1), and interferon-γ (INF-γ) correlate with the severity of meningococcemia in children. Waage and associates[105,107–109] studied this problem extensively during the recent epidemics in Norway. It is clear that high serum concentrations of IL-6 and IL-1 are associated with a fatal outcome in children. IL-1 was exclusively detected in patients with high concentrations of IL-6, TNF-α, and LPS and a rapidly fatal outcome. Extensive complement activation also occurs in fulminant cases of meningococcemia. Complement activation products in concert with other mediators may contribute to multisystem organ failure and death in severe cases. Despite this newfound knowledge, adjunctive therapy with specific polyclonal or monoclonal antibodies to proinflammatory cytokines remains investigational at the time of this writing and is of unproven benefit in fulminant meningococcemia.[110] Despite the suggestion that the Waterhouse-Friderichsen syndrome is mediated in part by adrenal hemorrhage, the use of corticosteroids remains controversial. Although corticosteroids may be of benefit in some forms of bacterial meningitis, high doses are associated with a worse outcome in sepsis and septic shock. In suspected invasive meningococcal disease, corticosteroids are best avoided.[111] In addition, the routine use of heparin in the therapy of DIC is not recommended. Some authorities recommend heparin if the patient is actively bleeding; the benefit of this approach remains unproved and may be harmful.[9,112,113] The administration of heparin did, however, appear to reduce the complications of digit and extremity necrosis, a dreaded complication, in a small noncontrolled series of patients with purpura fulminans[114] and deserves further evaluation. Other major life-threatening processes such as renal failure; systemic acidosis; the acute respiratory distress syndrome; meningococcal pneumonia; nosocomial pneumonia due to aspiration; and neurologic sequelae, including coma, diabetes insipidus, and raised intracranial pressure, may need to be addressed during the acute phase. Obviously, these problems are best approached in the intensive care unit environment.[4,9,98–100] During epidemics, such complications may easily overwhelm public health resources in resource-limited settings. Pericarditis may occur insidiously in the convalescent phase of the illness. Meningococci are not usually found in the pericardial fluid, and cardiac tamponade is unusual.[52]

Despite aggressive supportive care and the administration of appropriate antimicrobial agents, the outcome for patients with fulminant meningococcemia is often poor. A modality that deserves further study is plasmapheresis. This technique has been attempted, although on an extremely limited scale, in desperately ill patients and may lead to a rapid decrease in serum TNF-α concentrations and improved mortality and morbidity rates.[115] Although controlled clinical trials have not been performed, the outcome in the severely ill patients studied in these trials is much better than expected when compared with historical controls. Venovenous diafiltration or extracorporeal membrane oxygenation has also been utilized, apparently with some success, in meningococcemia,[116,117] but these techniques also remain experimental at this time. However, administration of the N-terminal fragment of recombinant bactericidal permeability increasing (rBPI21) protein improves functional outcome of children with meningococcemia, but the study was not large enough to detect a mortality benefit.[118]

Meningococcemia results in profound depletion of serum protein C concentrations. Administration of recombinant protein C may limit the extent of tissue necrosis (and reduce mortality),[119] but further data is needed. This modality is expensive, precluding use in many areas.

Prognostic indicators for the outcome from meningococcemia have been evaluated. One system developed by Kornelisse and colleagues, based on serum potassium, platelet, and C-reactive protein concentrations, and base excess, predicts survival or death in 86% of patients.[120]

Finally, meningococcemia is associated with supranormal plasma concentrations of plasminogen activator inhibitor (PAI-1). Children with a functional deletion/insertion (46–56) polymorphism in the promoter region of PAI-1 produce higher concentrations and are at increased risk of coagulopathy and death from meningococcemia.[121]

PREVENTION AND CONTROL

Chemoprophylaxis

Following the documented efficacy of sulfonamides for therapy of meningococcal meningitis, it became apparent that these agents could eliminate the carrier state for prolonged periods.[9,100] Eradication of the carrier state during epidemics led to a decline in the number of cases.[48] Chemoprophylaxis to prevent "secondary" cases is now well established. Unfortunately, following a serogroup B meningococcal epidemic at Fort Ord, California, in 1963 and the widespread recognition of sulfonamide resistance, this group of agents is no longer reliable. Similarly, other agents active against meningococci in vitro have been tested and have failed to eradicate the carrier state, including erythromycin, trimethoprim, cephalexin, nalidixic acid, and oxytetracycline. Many authorities have hypothesized that eradication of the carrier state is dependent on achieving bactericidal concentrations in tears and saliva.[122]

Several agents reliably eradicate the carrier state, although for a varying duration of time. Minocycline eradicates the carrier state rapidly and eradication persists for up to 6 to 10 weeks after treatment.[9,123] Unfortunately, vertiginous reactions limit the usefulness of this agent. Rifampin is also highly effective but can result in the emergence of rifampin-resistant meningococci in approximately 10% to 27% of the patients receiving this agent.[124] Ciprofloxacin, ofloxacin, and azithromycin[125] have been shown in controlled studies to eradicate nasopharyngeal carriage following a single dose for up to 1 month in a high proportion (95% or more of subjects).[126,127] Similarly, a single dose of ceftriaxone (250 mg IM in adults and 125 mg for children under 15 years of age) is also highly effective.[128] Currently, rifampin is the recommended therapy for meningococcal prophylaxis at a dosage of 600 mg every 12 hours in adults and 10 mg/kg every 12 hours in children (both for 2 days).[9] This recommendation also concludes that quinolones and ceftriaxone in a single dose are highly effective and compliance is assured.[129]

The group at greatest risk of secondary cases of meningococcal disease includes household contacts of the index case and these persons should certainly receive chemoprophylaxis. Similar high-risk situations occur in closed populations, including college dormitories, military barracks, nursery schools, day-care centers, and chronic care hospitals.[130] The use of chemoprophylactic agents in these groups should be individualized based on the intensity of exposure. Health-care personnel rarely require chemoprophylaxis except when intimate contact (such as mouth-to-mouth resuscitation)[48] with the index patient is performed.[131] Exposure to cases of meningococcal pneumonia is usually recognized too late to afford protection to health-care workers through chemoprophylaxis. The index case should also receive chemoprophylaxis prior to leaving the hospital if treated with penicillin or ampicillin, as these agents do not predictably eliminate the carrier state.

Immunoprophylaxis

Shortly after the recognition of sulfonamide-resistant meningococci, and the obvious implications for prevention of secondary cases through chemoprophylaxis, efforts to develop immunogenic vaccines against the major meningococcal serogroups intensified.[132] While immunity is variable following vaccination, no current commercially available meningococcal polysaccharide vaccine is immunogenic in children under 24 months of age and therefore chemoprophylaxis is a primary strategy in day-care centers. Conjugate vaccines are urgently needed (see later discussion). Large-scale studies have clearly documented the immunogenicity and protective efficacy of vaccines against serogroups A and C meningococci. The use of these vaccines in developing countries has markedly increased in recent years, as discussed in the following sections.

Serogroup A

Gotschlich and coworkers[133] conclusively demonstrated the protective activity of bactericidal antibody against capsular polysaccharide. Serogroup A polysaccharide vaccines seem to be immunogenic in older children and adults, but are unreliable in children less than 2 years of age. In addition, protection from a single dose is limited to less than 3 years in children who receive the vaccine between the ages of 1 and 4 years.[27,134] In older children, efficacy declines slowly over 3 years but long-term duration has not been studied. Thus, routine infant immunization has never been recommended with these vaccines[135–138] and their primary use has been in emergency campaigns.[139]

For maximum efficacy, emergency mass immunization of populations at risk requires early recognition of the outbreak and rapid mobilization of immunization. Thus, markers of outbreaks are critically needed at the local level quickly. Moore and colleagues[140] evaluated the pattern of meningococcal epidemics in Burkina Faso and found that 2 consecutive weeks of 15 cases per 100,000 population was a good early predictor of a major outbreak and could be used to trigger immunization. As shown in Figure 25-9, mass immunization of a population in Nairobi, Kenya, prevented a large number of cases, but many more cases could have been prevented if immunization had been started earlier. This concept has now been integrated into an emergency response plan by the World Health Organization (WHO), which outlines necessary steps to accurately identify and respond to outbreaks.[139] Even with accurate detection and rapid response, however, it is estimated that only about 60% of outbreak-related cases can be prevented by this strategy. Prevention of additional cases, and ultimate prevention of outbreaks altogether, require more effective vaccines.

Following the example provided by the *H. influenzae* type b conjugate vaccines, preparations of serogroup A, C, or W-135 polysaccharide chemically conjugated to proteins have been evaluated in clinical trials.[141–144] Conceptually, the conjugated product will perform as a T cell dependent antigen, which induces larger immune responses in infants, primes immunologic memory, and can lead to booster responses with subsequent doses. The introduction of similar conjugated vaccines into routine immunization programs in Africa appears to be the only effective way to prevent future epidemics. Indeed, this approach has already proven feasible. Chemoprophylaxis is impractical in resource-limited settings (e.g., the sub-Saharan meningitis belt) to control meningococcal disease. The first major worldwide epidemic of serogroup W-135 disease followed the hajj (the annual pilgrimage of Muslims to Mecca) in 2000 and spread throughout areas of Africa (e.g., Burkina Faso) and Europe through 2002. A conjugate vaccine, developed and deployed rapidly against serogroups A, W-135, and C produced a dramatic decline in cases during 2003 to 2004.

The meningococcal vaccine project, a collaboration of the WHO, CHI/Path, and the Gates Foundation, with a new manufacturer (the Serum Institute of India) is on target to produce a cheap (approximately 40¢/dose) serogroup A meningococcal conjugate vaccine by 2009. The goal is to target high-risk groups, ages 1 to 29 years, in 18 countries, a total population of approximately 270 million.

Serogroup C

The serogroup C polysaccharide vaccine shares many of the characteristics of the serogroup A polysaccharide vaccine (in the United States, the only licensed meningococcal vaccine is a combination of serogroups A, C, Y, and W-135 antigens, but monovalent A, monovalent C, and bivalent A–C are available in other areas). Again, the serogroup C vaccine is not effective in children less than 2 years of age.[129] In addition, 7 to 10 days is required following immunization to reach appreciable antibody levels, so rapid immunization is essential to maximize

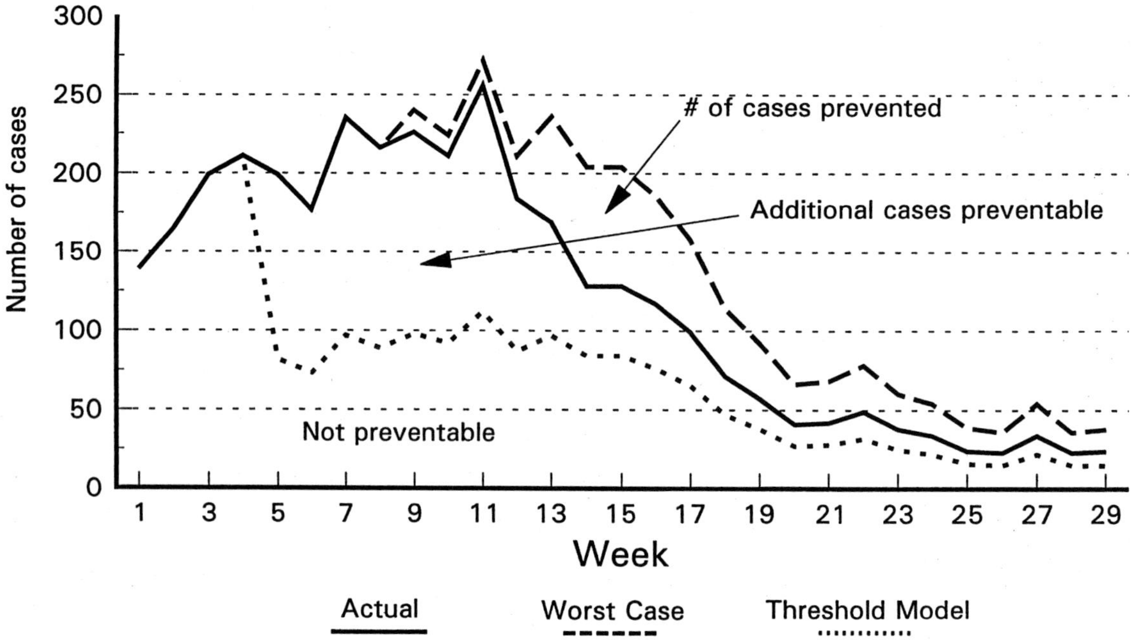

FIGURE 25-9 The epidemic curve from a serogroup A meningococcal disease epidemic in Nairobi, Kenya, in 1989. The solid line shows the actual number of cases that occurred by week, including those that occurred after mass immunization campaigns. The hatched line shows modeled data with the estimated number of cases that would have occurred without any vaccination program. The space between these two lines represents the number of cases actually prevented. However, the dotted line shows modeled data of the number of cases that would have been prevented if immunization had been carried out according to the time line set forth in the current WHO guidelines and clearly shows that a much larger number of cases were preventable by mass vaccination. (From Pinner RW, Onyango F, Perkins BA, et al: Epidemic meningococcal disease in Nairobi, Kenya—1989. J Infect Dis 166:359, 1992; and unpublished data from the Centers for Disease Control and Prevention, Atlanta, GA.)

impact in an epidemic. Serogroup C outbreaks, such as those described earlier in Canada, usually involve a small number of individual cases, so that recognition of the outbreak and accurate characterization of a population at risk are difficult. The advisory committee for immunization practices has recently addressed many of these issues in guidelines for the control of serogroup C outbreaks.[129]

Although the efficacy of serogroup C vaccines has been clearly established in studies of U.S. Army recruits by Artenstein and associates,[145] the efficacy and impact of large-scale immunization campaigns for serogroup C meningococcal disease following local focal outbreaks in the United States and Canada have been difficult to evaluate. However, in several instances, additional cases occurred in the same population during the next meningococcal disease season, which raises questions about the utility of immunization campaigns and the assessment of the efficacy of the vaccine delivered in this fashion.[2] For example, in Gregg County, Texas, high rates of disease occurred for three consecutive years in spite of large immunization programs. A case-control study revealed that the vaccine was 85% protective, but additional studies demonstrated only a relatively small proportion of the population at risk had received vaccine in the early mass campaigns, leaving a large segment of the population unvaccinated.[146] This illustrates the lack of herd immunity following meningococcal vaccination; current preparations protect only those who receive the vaccine. Complete immunization coverage with a polysaccharide vaccine approach is critical to halting epidemic disease. As with serogroup A disease, conjugate serogroup C meningococcal vaccines promise to provide a means to prevent not only epidemic but also endemic infections.[142] The experience with serogroup C conjugate vaccine in the United Kingdom is illuminating. Although rates vary widely in Europe, the annual incidence of meningococcal disease in the United Kingdom is higher than in the United States (e.g., approximately 3–5 cases/100,000 population/year vs. 1.0–1.5 cases/100,000 population/year). In 1997, the serotype distribution in the United Kingdom was as follows: B, 54%; C, 38%; other, 8%; and most deaths due to serogroup C occurred in children less than 2 years of age and in adolescents 15 to 20 years old. Licensed serogroup C vaccines have conjugated the polysaccharide to CRM-197 mutant diphtheria toxin or tetanus toxoid.[147] The former was launched in the United Kingdom in 1999 (approximately 18 million doses in children less than 18 years of age from November 1999 through October 2000). Routine vaccination was offered at 2, 3, and 4 months of age with varying schedules in older children. High serum bactericidal titers (e.g., greater than 1:8) correlating with efficacy were induced by 4 months of age with a brisk memory response evoked upon booster administration after 1 year. The vaccine efficacy was an approximately 90% reduction in serogroup C disease in the vaccinated group,[148] while no change in serogroup B disease occurred in the United Kingdom overall. In addition, carriage was reduced (although low)[149] and invasive disease declined approximately 67% in the unvaccinated older population.[150] Although this approach is extremely promising, vaccine efficacy was lost greater than 1 year after vaccination in the 2, 3, and 4 month target group when examined 4 years afterward.[151] It is hoped that changes to this "accelerated" schedule and/or uniform boosters will reverse this trend.

Serogroup B

Since the polysaccharide antigen of serogroup B meningococci displays cross-reactivity with human neural tissue, development of vaccines based on the polysaccharide antigen has proved exceedingly difficult and, indeed, there is currently no vaccine available for the prevention of serogroup B disease. There is likely a strong immunologic tolerance to the presentation of this antigen.[152] Thus, efforts to create a serogroup B vaccine have been recently directed at the OMPs of the organism. Although several candidate vaccines have been prepared which display moderate efficacy in older children, efficacy in children less than 4 years of age has not been shown, and this is a major problem for widespread use of the vaccine.[153–156] In addition to OMP vaccines and polysaccharide-protein conjugates, other approaches to the development of new vaccines against meningococci are currently under study, including vaccines developed to detoxify lipooligosaccharide, an anti-idiotype antibody approach, novel surface proteins, peptide mimics, or a mucosal vaccine approach.[9,132,157,158]

Many other meningococcal polysaccharide-conjugate vaccine are under development. Aventis has produced a quadrivalent (A, C, Y, W-135) meningococcal polysaccharide vaccine conjugated to 48 μg of diphtheria toxid (Menactra) and have submitted a New Drug Application to the Food and Drug Administration targeting persons ages 11 to 55 years in the United States. The vaccine is expensive (estimates $70–$80/dose exclusive of administration costs) and does not protect the youngest, most vulnerable group (e.g., less than 1 year of age). The advisory committee on immunization practices is evaluating further data on efficacy, pharmacoeconomics, target populations, implementation, and so forth. Other approaches have complexed meningococcal conjugates to established antigens for potential routine childhood immunizations (e.g., DTPw-hepatitis B-HiB-meningococcal serogroups A and C or Hib-meningococcal serogroup C). These have been developed by major multinational pharmaceutical firms and expense may prelude widespread uptake in resource-limited settings.

REFERENCES

1. Reido FX, Plikaytis BD, Broome CV: Epidemiology and prevention of meningococcal disease. Rev Infect Dis 4:71, 1983.
2. Wenger JD, Perkins BA: Patterns in the emergence of epidemic meningococcal disease. In Scheld WM, Armstrong DA, Hughes JM (eds): Emerging Infections 1. Washington, DC, American Society for Microbiology, 1998, p 125.
3. Anonymous: Cerebrospinal meningitis in Africa. Wkly Epidemiol Rep 42:318, 1996.
4. Roos KL, Tunkel AR, Scheld WM: Acute bacterial meningitis in children and adults. In Scheld WM, Whitley RJ, Durack DT (eds): Infections of the Central Nervous System, 2nd ed. Philadelphia, Lippincott-Raven, 1997, p 335.
5. Danielson L, Mann E: The first American account of cerebrospinal meningitis. Rev Infect Dis 5:969, 1983.
6. North E: Concerning the epidemic of spotted fever in New England. Rev Infect Dis 2:811, 1980.
7. Schwentker FF, Gelman S, Long PH: The treatment of meningococcic meningitis with sulfanilamide. Landmark article April 24, 1937; JAMA 251:788, 1984.
8. Scheld WM, Mandell GL: Sulfonamides and meningitis. JAMA 251:791, 1984.
9. Apicella MA: *Neisseria meningitidis*. In Mandell GL, Bennett JE, Dolin R (eds): Principles and Practice of Infectious Diseases, 4th ed. New York, Churchill Livingstone, 1995, p 1896.
10. Scheld WM: Meningococcal diseases. In Warren KS, Mahmoud AAF (eds): Tropical and Geographical Medicine, 2nd ed. New York, McGraw-Hill, 1990, p 798.
11. Ashton FE, Ryan A, Diena B, et al: A new serogroup (L) of *Neisseria meningitidis*. J Clin Microbiol 17:722, 1983.
12. Frasch CE, Zollinger WE, Poolman JT: Serotype antigens of *Neisseria meningitidis* and a proposed scheme for designation of serotypes. Rev Infect Dis 7:504, 1985.
13. Frasch CE, Zollinger WD, Poolman JT: Proposed schema for identification of serotypes of *Neisseria meningitidis*. In Schoolnik GK (ed): The Pathogenic *Neisseria*. Washington, DC, American Society for Microbiology, 1985, p 519.
14. Gamian A, Beurret M, Michon F, et al: Structure of the L2 lipopolysaccharide core oligosaccharides of *Neisseria meningitidis*. J Biol Chem 267:922, 1992.
15. Jones DM, Borrow R, Fox AJ, et al: The lipooligosaccharide immunotype as a virulence determinant in *Neisseria meningitidis*. Microbiol Pathol 13:219, 1992.
16. Verheul AFM, Snippe H, Poolman JT: Meningococcal lipopolysaccharides: Virulence factor and potential vaccine component. Microbiol Rev 57:34, 1993.
17. Estabrook MM, Baker CJ, Griffiss JM: The immune response of children to meningococcal lipooligosaccharides during disseminated disease is directed primarily against two monoclonal antibody-defined epitopes. J Infect Dis 167:966, 1993.
18. Olyhoek T, Crowe BA, Achtman M: Clonal population structure of *Neisseria meningitidis* serogroup A isolated from epidemics and pandemics between 1915 and 1983. Rev Infect Dis 9:665, 1987.
19. Crowe BA, Wall RA, Kusecek B, et al: Clonal and variable properties of *Neisseria meningitidis* isolated from cases and carriers during and after an epidemic in the Gambia, West Africa. J Infect Dis 159:686, 1989.
20. Moore PS, Reeves MW, Schwartz B, et al: Intercontinental spread of an epidemic group A *Neisseria meningitidis* strain. Lancet 2:260, 1989.
21. Caugant DA, Mocca IF, Frasch CE, et al: Genetic structure of *Neisseria meningitidis* populations in relation to serogroup, serotype, and outer membrane protein pattern. J Bacteriol 169:2781, 1987.
22. Rappuoli R: Reverse vaccinology, a genome-based approach to vaccine development. Vaccine 19:2688, 2001 .
23. Broome CV: The carrier state: *Neisseria meningitidis*. J Antimicrob Chemother 18(Suppl A):25, 1986.
24. Goldschneider I, Gotschlich EC, Artenstein MS: Human immunity to the meningococcus. I. The role of humoral antibodies. J Exp Med 129:1307, 1969.
25. Griffiss JM, Brandt BL, Jarvis GA: Natural immunity to *Neisseria meningitidis*. In Vedros NA (ed): Evolution of Meningococcal Disease, Vol. 2. Boca Raton, FL, CRC Press, 1987, p 99.
26. Riedo FX, Plikaytis BD, Broome CV: Epidemiology and prevention of meningococcal disease. Pediatr Infect Dis J 14:643, 1995.
27. Pinner RW, Onyango F, Perkins BA, et al: Epidemic meningococcal disease in Nairobi, Kenya—1989. J Infect Dis 166:359, 1992.
28. Peltola H, Kataja JM, Makela PH: Shift in age distribution of meningococcal disease as predictor of an epidemic? Lancet 2:595, 1982.
29. Jackson LA, Wenger JD: Laboratory-based surveillance for meningococcal disease in selected areas, United States, 1989–1991. MMWR 42:21, 1993.
30. Baraff LJ, Lee SI, Schriger DL: Outcomes of bacterial meningitis in children: A meta-analysis. Pediatr Infect Dis J 12:389, 1993.
31. Greenwood BM: Epidemiology of meningitis in tropical Africa. In Williams DW (ed): Bacterial Meningitis. London, Academic Press, 1987, p 61.
32. Moore PS, Hierholzer J, De Witt W, et al: Respiratory viruses and mycoplasma as cofactors for epidemic group A meningococcal meningitis. JAMA 264:1271, 1990.
33. Greenwood BM, Blakebrough IS, Bradley AK, et al: Meningococcal disease and season in sub-Saharan Africa. Lancet 1:1339, 1984.
34. Jackson LA, Schuchat A, Reeves MW, et al: Serogroup C meningococcal outbreaks in the United States. An emerging threat. JAMA 273:383, 1995.
35. Whalen CM, Hockin JC, Ryan A, et al: The changing epidemiology of invasive meningococcal disease in Canada, 1985 through 1995. Emergence of a virulent clone of *Neisseria meningitidis*. JAMA 273:390, 1995.

36. Ashton FE, Ryan JA, Borczyk A, et al: Emergence of a virulent clone of *Neisseria meningitidis* serotype 2a that is associated with meningococcal group C disease in Canada. J Clin Microbiol 29:2489, 1991.
37. Hume SE: Mass voluntary immunization campaigns for meningococcal disease in Canada: Media hysteria. JAMA 267:1833, 1992.
38. Serogroup B meningococcal disease—Oregon, 1994. MMWR 44:121, 1995.
39. Reeves MW, Perkins BA, Diermeyer M, et al: Epidemic-associated *Neisseria meningitidis* detected by multilocus enzyme electrophoresis. Emerg Infect Dis 1:53, 1995.
40. Caugant DA, Froholm LO, Bovre K, et al: Intercontinental spread of a genetically distinctive complex of clones of *Neisseria meningitidis* causing epidemic disease. Proc Natl Acad Sci USA 83:4927, 1986.
41. Fischer M, Perkins BA: *Neisseria meningitidis* serogroup B: Emergence of the ET-5 complex. Semin Pediatr Infect Dis 8:50, 1997.
42. Fischer M, Hedberg K, Cardosi P, et al: Epidemic meningococcal disease and tobacco smoke: A risk factor study in the Pacific Northwest (abstract). Presented at 10th International Pathogenic *Neisseria* Conference, Baltimore, MD, September 8–13, 1996.
43. Stephens DS, Hajjeh RA, Baughman WS, et al: Sporadic meningococcal disease in adults: Results of a 5-year population-based study. Ann Intern Med 123:937, 1995.
44. Wolfe RE, Birbara C: Meningococcal infections at an army training center. Am J Med 44:243, 1968.
45. Sullivan TD, LaScolea LJ: *Neisseria meningitidis* bacteremia in children: Quantitation of bacteremia and spontaneous clinical recovery without antibiotic therapy. Pediatrics 80:63, 1987.
46. Carpenter RR, Petersdorf RG: The clinical spectrum of bacterial meningitis. Am J Med 33:262, 1987.
47. Feigin RD, Dodge PR: Bacterial meningitis: Newer concepts of pathophysiology and neurologic sequelae. Pediatr Clin North Am 23:541, 1976.
48. Feldman HA: Meningococcal infections. Adv Intern Med 18:117, 1972.
49. Frederiks JAM: Meningococcal meningitis. In Vinken RJ, Bruyn GW, Klawans HL, et al (eds): Handbook of Clinical Neurology. Amsterdam, Elsevier, 1988, p 21.
50. Gotschall RA: Conus medullaris syndrome after meningococcal meningitis. N Engl J Med 286:882, 1972.
51. Herman RA, Rubin HA: Meningococcal pericarditis without meningitis presenting as tamponade. N Engl J Med 290:143, 1974.
52. Morse JR, Oretsky MI, Hudson JA: Pericarditis as a complication of meningococcal meningitis. Ann Intern Med 74:212, 1971.
53. Pierce I, Cooper E: Meningococcal pericarditis, clinical features and therapy in five patients. Arch Intern Med 129:918, 1972.
54. Maron BJ, Macoul KL, Benaron P: Unusual complications of meningococcal meningitidis. Johns Hopkins Med J 131:64, 1972.
55. Brasier AR, Macklis JD, Vaughn D, et al: Myopericarditis as an initial presentation of meningococcemia. Unusual manifestations of infection with serotype W135. Am J Med 82:641, 1987.
56. Putsch RW, Hamilton JD, Wolinsky E: *Neisseria meningitidis,* a respiratory pathogen. J Infect Dis 121:48, 1970.
57. Irwin RS, Woelk WK, Coudon WL: Primary meningococcal pneumonia. Ann Intern Med 82:493, 1975.
58. Racoosin JA, Whitney CG, Conover C, et al: Emergence of *Neisseria meningitidis* serogroup Y disease. Presented at 36th Interscience Conference on Antimicrobial Agents and Chemotherapy, New Orleans, LA, September 15–18, 1996, abstract LB28.
59. Koppes GM, Ellenbogen C, Gebhart RJ: Group Y meningococcal disease in United States Air Force recruits. Am J Med 62:661, 1977.
60. Kerttula Y, Leinonen M, Koskela M, et al: The etiology of pneumonia, application of bacterial serology and basic laboratory methods. J Infect 14:21, 1987.
61. Hubert B, Watier L, Garnerin P, et al: Meningococcal disease and influenza-like syndrome: A new approach to an old question. J Infect Dis 166:542, 1992.
62. Winstead JM, McKinsey DS, Tasker S, et al: Meningococcal pneumonia: Characterization and review of cases seen over the past 25 years. Clin Infect Dis 30:87, 2000.
63. Schwam E, Cox J: Fulminant meningococcal supraglottitis: An emerging infectious syndrome? Emerg Infect Dis 5:464, 1999.
64. Faur YC, Weisburd MH, Wilson ME: Isolation of *Neisseria meningitidis* from the genitourinary tract and anal canal. J Clin Microbiol 2:178, 1975.
65. Salet IE, Frasch CE: Seroepidemiologic aspects of *Neisseria meningitidis* in homosexual men. Can Med Assoc J 126:38, 1982.
66. Frank ST, Gomez RM: Chronic meningococcemia. Mil Med 133:918, 1968.
67. Rompalo AM, Hood EW, Roberts PL, et al: The acute arthritis dermatitis syndrome. The changing importance of *Neiserria gonorrhoeae* and *Neisseria meningitidis.* Arch Intern Med 147:281, 1987.
68. Densen P, Weiler JM, Griffiss JM, et al: Familial properdin deficiency and fatal bacteremia. Correction of the bactericidal defect by vaccination. N Engl J Med 316:922, 1987.
69. Ross SC, Rosenthal PJ, Berberich HM, et al: Killing of *Neisseria meningitidis* by human neutrophils: Implications for normal and complement deficient individuals. J Infect Dis 155:1266, 1987.
70. Smith AL: Neonatal bacterial meningitis. In Scheld WM, Whitley RJ, Durack DT (eds): Infections of the Central Nervous System, 2nd ed. Philadelphia, Lippincott-Raven, 1997, p 313.
71. Ross SC, Densen P: Complement deficiency states and infection: Epidemiology, pathogenesis and consequences of neisserial and other infections in an immune deficiency. Medicine (Baltimore) 63:243, 1984.
72. Figen CAP, Kuijper EJ, Tjia HG, et al: Complement deficiency predisposes for meningitis due to nongroupable meningococci and *Neisseria*-related bacteria. Clin Infect Dis 18:780, 1994.
73. Sjoholm AG, Kuijper EJ, Tijsen CC, et al: Dysfunctional properdin in a Dutch family with meningococcal disease. N Engl J Med 319:33, 1988.
74. Krasinski K, Nelson JO, Butler S: Possible association of mycoplasma and viral respiratory infections with bacterial meningitis. Am J Epidemiol 125:499, 1987.
75. Pinner R, Spellman P, Stephens DS: Evidence for functionally distinct pili expressed by *Neisseria meningitidis.* Infect Immun 59:3169, 1991.
76. Rayner CFJ, Dewar A, Moxon ER, et al: The effect of variations in the expression of pili on the interaction of *Neisseria meningitidis* with human nasopharyngeal epithelium. J Infect Dis 171:113, 1995.
77. Wispelwey B, Hansen EJ, Scheld WM: *Haemophilus influenzae* outer membrane vesicle induced blood-brain barrier permeability during experimental meningitis in the rat. J Clin Invest 82:1339, 1988.
78. Harter DH, Jubelt B: Bacterial infections. In Rowland LP (ed): Merritt's Textbook of Neurology. Philadelphia, Lea & Febiger, 1984, p 53.
79. Dodge PR, Swartz MN: Bacterial meningitis—A review of selected aspects II: Special neurologic problems, postmeningitic complications and clinicopathological correlations. N Engl J Med 272:954, 1965.
80. Tunkel AR, Scheld WM: Acute meningitis. In Mandell GL, Bennett JE, Dolin R (eds): Principles and Practice of Infectious Diseases, 4th ed. New York, Churchill Livingstone, 1995, p 831.
81. Levin S, Painter MB: The treatment of acute meningococcal infection in adults. Ann Intern Med 64:1049, 1966.
82. Feldman WE: Relation of concentrations of bacteria and bacterial antigen in cerebrospinal fluid to prognosis in patients with bacterial meningitis. N Engl J Med 296:433, 1977.
83. Feldman WE: Concentrations of bacteria in cerebrospinal fluid of patients with bacterial meningitis. J Pediatr 88:549, 1976.
84. McCracken GH: Rapid identification of specific etiology in meningitis. J Pediatr 88:706, 1976.
85. O'Toole RD, Goode L, Howe C: Neuraminidase activity in bacterial meningitis. J Clin Invest 50:979, 1971.
86. Beaty HN: Cerebrospinal fluid lactic dehydrogenase and its isoenzymes in infection of the central nervous system. N Engl J Med 279:1197, 1968.
87. Ni H, Knight AI, Cartwright K, et al: Polymerase chain reaction for diagnosis of meningococcal meningitis. Lancet 340:1432, 1993.
88. Seward RJ, Towner KJ: Evaluation of a PCR-immunoassay technique for detection of *Neisseria meningitidis* in cerebrospinal fluid and peripheral blood. J Med Microbiol 49:451, 2000.
89. Diggle MA, Clarke SC: Detection and genotyping of meningococci using a nested PCR approach. J Med Microbiol 52:51, 2003.
90. Saravolatz LD, Manzor O, VanderVelde N, et al: Broad-range bacterial polymerase chain reaction for early detection of bacterial meningitis. Clin Infect Dis 36:40, 2003.
91. McCracken GH, Nelson JD, Kaplan SL, et al: Consensus report: Antimicrobial therapy for bacterial meningitis in infants and children. Pediatr Infect Dis J 6:501, 1987.
92. Van Esso D, Fontanals D, Uriz S, et al: *Neisseria meningitidis* strains with decreased susceptibility to penicillin. Pediatr Infect Dis 6:438, 1987.

93. Dillon JR, Pauze M, Yeung KH: Spread of penicillinase-producing and transfer plasmids from the gonococcus to *Neisseria meningitidis.* Lancet 1:779, 1983.
94. Saez-Nieto JA, Lujan R, Berron S, et al: Epidemiology and molecular basis of penicillin-resistant *Neisseria meningitidis* in Spain: A 5-year history (1985–1989). Clin Infect Dis 14:394, 1992.
95. Woods CR, Smith AL, Wasilauskas BL, et al: Invasive disease caused by *Neisseria meningitidis* relatively resistant to penicillin in North Carolina. J Infect Dis 170:453, 1994.
96. Jackson LA, Tenover FC, Baker C, et al: Prevalence of *Neisseria meningitidis* relatively resistant to penicillin in the United States, 1991. J Infect Dis 169:438, 1994.
97. Trallero EP, Garcia Arenzana JM, Ayestaran I, et al: Comparative activity in vitro of 16 antimicrobial agents against penicillin-susceptible meningococci and meningococci with diminished susceptibility to penicillin. Antimicrob Agents Chemother 33:1622, 1989.
98. Scheld WM: Bacterial meningitis, brain abscess, and other suppurative intracranial infections. In Fauci AS, Braunwald E, Isselbacher KJ, et al (eds): Harrison's Principles of Internal Medicine, 14th ed. New York, McGraw-Hill, 1998, p 2419.
99. Tunkel AR, Scheld WM: Acute meningitis. In Stein JH, Daly WJ, Easton JK, et al (eds): Internal Medicine, 5th ed. St. Louis, Mosby–Year Book, 1998, p 1402.
100. Scheld WM: Bacterial meningitis. In Rakel RE (ed): Conn's Current Therapy—1999. Philadelphia, WB Saunders, 1999, p 105.
101. Galimand M, Gerbaud G, Guibourdenche M, et al: High-level chloramphenicol resistance in *Neisseria meningitidis.* N Engl J Med 339:868, 1998.
102. Cartwright K, Reilly S, White D, et al: Early treatment with parenteral penicillin in meningococcal disease. BMJ 305:143, 1992.
103. Strang JR, Pugh EJ: Meningococcal infections: Reducing the case fatality rate by giving penicillin before admission to hospital. BMJ 305:141, 1992.
104. Barquet N, Domingo P, Cayla JA, et al: Prognostic factors in meningococcal disease. Development of a bedside predictive model and scoring system. JAMA 278:491, 1997.
105. Waage A, Brandtzaeg P, Halstensen A, et al: The complex pattern of cytokines in serum from patients with meningococcal septic shock. J Exp Med 169:333, 1989.
106. Girardin E, Grau GE, Dayr JM, et al: Tumor necrosis factor and interleukin-1 in the serum of children with severe infectious purpura. N Engl J Med 319:397, 1988.
107. Brandtzaeg P, Bryn K, Kierulf P, et al: Meningococcal endotoxin in lethal septic shock plasma studies by gas chromatography, mass spectroscopy, ultracentrifugation and electron microscropy. J Clin Invest 89:816, 1992.
108. Brandtzaeg P, Ovstebo R, Kierulf P: Compartmentalization of lipopolysaccharide production correlates with clinical presentation in meningococcal disease. J Infect Dis 166:650, 1992.
109. Monsalve F, Rucabado L, Salvador A, et al: Myocardial depression in septic shock caused by meningococcal infection. Crit Care Med 12:1021, 1984.
110. Westendorp RGJ, Langermans JAM, de Bel CE, et al: Release of tumor necrosis factor: An innate host characteristic that may contribute to the outcome of meningococcal disease. J Infect Dis 171:1057, 1995.
111. Belsey MA, Hoffpauir CW, Smith MHD: Dexamethasone in the treatment of acute bacterial meningitis: The effect of study design on the interpretation of results. Pediatrics 44:503, 1969.
112. Corrigan JJ Jr, Jordan CM: Heparin therapy in septicemia with disseminated intravascular coagulation. Effect on mortality and on correction of hemostatic defects. N Engl J Med 283:778, 1970.
113. Denmark TC, Knight EL: Cardiovascular and coagulation complications of group C meningococcal disease. Arch Intern Med 127:238, 1971.
114. Kuppermann N, Inkelis SH, Saladino R: The role of heparin in the prevention of extremity and digit necrosis in meningococcal purpura fulminans. Pediatr Infect Dis J 13:867, 1994.
115. Drapkin MS, Wisch JS, Gelfand JA, et al: Plasmapheresis for fulminant meningococcemia. Pediatr Infect Dis J 8:399, 1989.
116. Best C, Walsh J, Sinclair J, et al: Early haemo-diafiltration in meningococcal septicaemia. Lancet 347:202, 1995.
117. Champion MP, Murdoch IA, Sajjanhar T, et al: Extracorporeal membrane oxygenation for refractory shock in fulminant meningococcal sepsis. Lancet 347:201, 1996.
118. Giroir BP, Scannon PJ, Levin M: Bactericidal/permeability-increasing protein—Lessons learned from the phase III, randomized, clinical trial of rBPI21 for adjunctive treatment of children with severe meningococcemia. Crit Care Med 29(Suppl 7):S130, 2001.
119. Rintala E, Kauppila M, Seppala OP, et al: Protein C substitution in sepsis-associated purpura fulminans. Crit Care Med 28:2373, 2000.
120. Kornelisse RF, Hazelzet JA, Hop WCJ, et al: Meningococcal septic shock in children: Clinical and laboratory features, outcome, and development of a prognostic score. Clin Infect Dis 25:640, 1997.
121. Hermans PW, Hibberd ML, Booy R, et al: 4G/5G promoter polymorphism in the plasminogen-activator-inhibitor-1 gene and outcome of meningococcal disease. Lancet 354:556, 1999.
122. Hoeprich PD: Prediction of antimeningococcic chemoprophylactic efficacy. J Infect Dis 123:125, 1971.
123. Guttler RB, Counts GW, Avent CK, et al: Effect of rifampin and minocycline on meningococcal carrier rates. J Infect Dis 124:199, 1971.
124. Weidner CE, Dunkel TB, Pettyjohn FS, et al: Effectiveness of rifampin in eradicating the meningococcal carrier state in a relatively closed population: Emergence of resistant strains. J Infect Dis 124:172, 1971.
125. Girgis N, Sultan Y, Frenck RW Jr, et al: Azithromycin compared with rifampin for eradication of nasopharyngeal colonization by *Neisseria meningitidis.* Pediatr Infect Dis J 17:816, 1998.
126. Gilja HO, Halstensen A, Digranes A, et al: Single-dose ofloxacin to eradicate tonsillopharyngeal carriage of *Neisseria meningitidis.* Antimicrob Agents Chemother 37:2024, 1993.
127. Pugsley MP, Dworzack DI, Horowitz EA, et al: Efficacy of ciprofloxacin in treatment of nasopharyngeal carriers of *Neisseria meningitidis.* J Infect Dis 156:211, 1987.
128. Schwartz B: Chemoprophylaxis for bacterial infections: Principles of and application to meningococcal infection. Rev Infect Dis 13(Suppl 2):S170, 1991.
129. Control and prevention of meningococcal disease and control and prevention of serogroup C meningococcal disease: Evaluation and management of suspected outbreaks: Recommendations of the Advisory Committee on Immunization Practices (ACIP). MMWR 46:1, 1997.
130. The Meningococcal Disease Surveillance Group: Analysis of endemic meningococcal disease by serogroup and evaluation of chemoprophylaxis. J Infect Dis 134:201, 1976.
131. Artenstein MS, Ellis RE: The risk of exposure to a patient with meningococcal meningitis. Mil Med 133:474, 1968.
132. Peltola H: Vaccines against bacterial meningitis. In Scheld WM, Whitley RJ, Durack DT (eds): Infections of the Central Nervous System, 2nd ed. Philadelphia, Lippincott-Raven, 1997, p 1041.
133. Gotschlich EC, Goldschneider I, Artenstein MS: Human immunity to the meningococcus IV. Immunogenicity of the group A and group C polysaccharides in human volunteers. J Exp Med 129:1367, 1969.
134. Reingold AL, Broome CV, Hightower AW, et al: Age-specific differences in duration of clinical protection after vaccination with meningococcal polysaccharide A vaccine. Lancet 2:114, 1985.
135. Kayhty H, Karanko V, Peltola H, et al: Serum antibodies to capsular polysaccharide vaccine of group A *Neisseria meningitidis* followed for three years in infants and children. J Infect Dis 142:861, 1980.
136. Peltola H, Makela PH, Kayhty H, et al: Clinical efficacy of meningococcus group A capsular polysaccharide vaccine in children three months to five years of age. N Engl J Med 297:686, 1977.
137. Gold R, Lepow ML, Goldschneider I, et al: Kinetics of antibody production to group A and to group C meningococcal polysaccharide vaccines administered during the first six years of life: Prospects for routine immunization of infants and children. J Infect Dis 140:690, 1979.
138. Lennon D, Gellin B, Hood D, et al: Successful intervention in a group A meningococcal outbreak in Auckland, New Zealand. Pediatr Infect Dis J 11:617, 1992.
139. World Health Organization Working Group: Control of epidemic meningococcal disease. World Health Organization Practical Guidelines. Geneva, Foundation Marcel Merieux, 1995.
140. Moore PS, Plikaytis BD, Bolan GA, et al: Detection of meningitis epidemics in Africa: A population-based analysis. Int J Epidemiol 21:155, 1992.
141. Twumasi PAJ, Kumah S, Leach A, et al: A trial of a group A plus group C meningococcal polysaccharide-protein conjugate vaccine in African infants. J Infect Dis 171:632, 1995.

142. Lieberman JM, Chiu SS, Wong VK, et al: Safety and immunogenicity of a serogroups A/C *Neisseria meningitidis* oligosaccharide-protein conjugate vaccine in young children. JAMA 275:1499, 1996.
143. Fairley CK, Begg N, Borrow R, et al: Conjugate meningococcal serogroup A and C vaccine: Reactogenicity and immunogenicity in United Kingdom infants. J Infect Dis 174:1360, 1996.
144. Leach A, Twumasi PA, Kumah S, et al: Induction of immunologic memory of Gambian children by vaccination in infancy with a group A plus group C meningococcal polysaccharide-protein conjugate vaccine. J Infect Dis 175:200, 1997.
145. Artenstein MS, Gold R, Zimmerly JG, et al: Prevention of meningococcal disease by group C polysaccharide vaccine. N Engl J Med 282:417, 1970.
146. Rosenstein N, Levine O, Taylor J, et al: Persistant serogroup C meningococcal disease outbreak in a vaccinated population, Gregg County, Texas (abstract). Presented at 36th Interscience Conference on Antimicrobial Agents and Chemotherapy, New Orleans, LA, September 15–18, 1996.
147. Soriano-Gabarro M, Stuart JM, Rosenstein NE: Vaccines for the prevention of meningococcal disease in children. Sem Pediatr Infect Dis 13:182, 2002.
148. Ramsay ME, Andrews N, Kaczmarski EB, et al: Efficacy of meningococcal serogroup C conjugate vaccine in teenagers and toddlers in England. Lancet 357:195, 2001.
149. Maiden MC, Stuart JM, The UK meningococcal carriage group: Carriage of serogroup C meningococci 1 year after meningococcal C conjugate polysaccharide vaccination. Lancet 359:1829, 2002.
150. Ramsay ME, Andrews NJ, Trotter CL, et al: Herd immunity from meningococcal serogroup C conjugate vaccination in England: Database analysis. BMJ 326:365, 2003.
151. Trotter CL, Andrews NJ, Kaczmarski EB, et al: Effectiveness of meningococcal serogroup C conjugate vaccine 4 years after introduction. Lancet 364:365, 2004.
152. Frasch CE: Vaccines for prevention of meningococcal disease. Clin Microbiol Rev 42:318, 1996.
153. Sierra GV, Campa HC, Varcacel NM, et al: Vaccine against group B *Neisseria meningitidis:* Protection trials and mass vaccination results in Cuba. NIPH Ann 14:195, 1991.
154. Bjune G, Hoiby EA, Gronnesby JK, et al: Effect of an outer membrane vesicle vaccine against group B meningococcal disease in Norway. Lancet 338:1093, 1991.
155. Boslego J, Garcia J, Cruz C, et al: Efficacy, safety, and immunogenicity of a meningococcal vaccine group B (15:P1.3) outer membrane protein vaccine in Iquique, Chile. Chilean National Committee for Meningococcal Disease. Vaccine 13:821, 1995.
156. Moraes JC, Perkins BA, Camargo MCC, et al: Protective efficacy of a serogroup B meningococcal vaccine in São Paulo, Brazil. Lancet 340:1074, 1992.
157. Westerink MAJ, Campagnari AA, Wirth MA, et al: Development and characterization of an anti-idiotype antibody to the capsular polysaccharide of *Neisseria meningitidis* serogroup C. Infect Immun 56:1120, 1988.
158. Bowe F, Lavelle EC, McNeela EA, et al: Mucosal vaccination against serogroup B meningococci: Induction of bactericidal antibodies and cellular immunity following intranasal immunization with NadA of *Neisseria meningitidis* and mutants of *Escherichia coli* heat-labile enterotoxin. Infect Immun 72:4052, 2004.

26

Gonococcal and Other Neisserial Infections

PETER LEONE

INTRODUCTION AND THE AGENT

The sexually transmitted disease commonly known as gonorrhea is caused by the bacterium *Neisseria gonorrhoeae*. *N. gonorrhoeae* is a gram-negative diplococcus that is aerobic, nonmotile, and non-spore-forming. It belongs to the family Neisseriaceae, which contains the genera *Neisseria, Moraxella, Eikenella, Simonsiella, Alysiella, Kingella*, and *Acinetobacter*.[1] The genus *Neisseria* is composed of 10 species, all of human origin. Despite their human origin, two of these species are pathogenic to humans: *N. gonorrhoeae* and *N. meningitidis*.[2] The latter is an etiologic agent of a common form of bacterial meningitis (see Chapter 25). *N. gonorrhoeae* is the cause of urethritis, cervicitis, pelvic inflammatory disease (PID), and associated infections and is distantly related to *Neisseria lactamica*, which can occasionally be a human pathogen. All *Neisseria* species are oxidase-positive, but only *N. gonorrhoeae* typically invades the upper reproductive tract; 20% of women with gonococcal cervicitis develop PID.[3] Gonorrhea is occasionally invasive, and 0.3% to 3.0% of mucosal infections progress to disseminated gonococcal infection (DGI).[4] Perhaps the most important impact of gonorrhea is facilitation of acquisition of human immunodeficiency virus (HIV)[5,6] and shedding of HIV in semen.[7]

EPIDEMIOLOGY

Although the overall incidence of gonorrhea has declined since 1975, it remains the second most commonly reported communicable disease in the United States. The case rate of U.S. gonococcal infection decreased from 371.5 per 100,000 population in 1986 to 116.2 per 100,000 in 2003.[8] The 2003 rate is the lowest ever reported for the United States. Even with the continued decline in the gonorrhea rate, the rates remain high regionally—in the Southeast; among some ethnic groups—African Americans and Hispanics; and among certain behavioral risk groups—men who have sex with men (MSM), as well as adolescents.[8] The highest incidence of gonorrhea occurs in adolescents and young adults.[9] In 2003, 15- to 19-year-olds showed the highest rate among females while 20- to 24-year-olds had the highest rates among males.[8] These elevated rates may reflect their greater number of partners, the higher likelihood of unprotected intercourse, and choice of partners, who themselves have a higher incidence of disease. A recent population-based survey of adolescents in the United States found relatively low overall prevalence of gonorrhea, 0.43%, with little variation in prevalence by sex or age but substantial differences by ethnicity. The prevalence rate for African Americans was approximately 2%, which was 36 and 14 times greater for white men and women, respectively.[10]

The global incidence of gonorrhea remains high with an estimated 62 million new cases each year.[11,12] Rates for the disease remain low in most of Europe and are relatively higher in developing countries. Importation of gonorrhea from other countries accounts for 14% to 25% of cases of gonorrhea diagnosed in Europe.[13] Accurate information on the incidence and prevalence of gonorrhea is lacking for most of these countries. Gonococcal infection is often underdiagnosed and underreported. Infection distribution is uneven with the highest rates in sub-Saharan Africa, South and Southeast Asia, the Caribbean, and Latin America. This is also true in developed countries where prevalence is highest in the most marginalized individuals socially and economically. Prevalence studies suggest that lower socioeconomic factors, ethnic minority status, and younger age are major determinants of disease acquisition.

Poverty is a risk factor for gonorrhea, as indicated by the higher rates of disease in the rural southern United States, large inner cities, and within minority groups.[9] Impoverished groups often have limited access to health care, are reluctant to seek prompt treatment for disease, may engage in drug or substance abuse, and often populate concentrated areas with high disease rates. In the United States, poverty is often reflected by minority status, which helps explain higher disease rates within various ethnic groups. In 2003, African Americans accounted for 70.7% of total reported cases of gonorrhea in the United States.[8] The rate of gonorrhea for African Americans was 20 times higher than among whites in 2003 (655.8 cases per 100,000 vs. 32.7). The infection rate of gonorrhea among American Indian/Alaskan natives (103.5) and among Hispanics (71.7) was 3 and 2 times higher, respectively, than the rate among non-Hispanic white Americans.[8] These disparities in reported rates of infection further illustrate the greater impact of gonorrhea on minority groups.[9,14] Ethnicity itself is not a risk factor but rather a surrogate marker for social and behavioral factors. If these factors were more easily quantifiable, they could be more clearly separated from the larger category of ethnic background.

Transmission

Gonorrhea may be the sexually transmitted disease (STD) most efficiently spread from person to person. Transmission following a single episode of vaginal intercourse is approximately 70% to 80% from male to female and 20% to 30% from female to male.[15,16] Transmission through either receptive or insertive rectal intercourse may be less efficient than by vaginal intercourse. Oral-genital transmission is probably the least common and least efficient means of transmission. Although specific rates are not available, it has been reported that transmission is greater through fellatio than cunnilingus.[17] In MSM, oral-genital contact may account for up to 50% of all urethral infections. Consequently, oral-genital contact can be viewed as a risk factor for acquisition of urethral gonorrhea.[18]

As with other STDs, gonorrhea prevalence and transmission can be partially explained by applying the concept of "core group" transmitters. By definition, members of the core group are individuals who are more likely to become infected and more likely to transmit the disease to others. As a result of their high level of sexual activity and frequency of partner change, these individuals have the greatest influence in sustaining the epidemic of gonorrhea.[19]

CLINICAL MANIFESTATIONS

The clinical manifestations of gonorrhea are numerous and vary from local asymptomatic disease to dissemination. The initial site of infection, the infecting strain of gonorrhea, host immunity, and other coinfections all influence the spectrum of clinical disease experienced by the patient.

Gonococcal Infection in Men

In men, gonococcal urethritis is the most common manifestation of infection. Following inoculation of the anterior male urethra, *N. gonorrhoeae* attaches to and infects columnar epithelial cells. The incubation period may range from 24 hours to 14 days, but 75% of men develop symptoms (dysuria and discharge) within 4 days of infection.[20,21] Dysuria usually precedes the development of purulent discharge by approximately 24 hours. Although 90% of newly acquired infections are symptomatic, about 50% of all infections in the community have few to no symptoms.[22] If left untreated, gonococcal urethritis usually resolves over the course of several weeks, with the majority of cases becoming asymptomatic within 6 months.[23]

Since the widespread availability of effective antimicrobial therapy in the 1940s, local complications in men have become rare. Local complications do occur, however, as evident from the gonococcal cause of about 10% of acute epididymitis. Other complications include acute or chronic prostatitis, orchitis, seminal vesiculitis, posterior urethritis, and infection of Tyson's and Cowper's glands.[24]

The patient's sexual practice may be a major indication of the potential site of infection. In homosexual males, the rectum is the only site of gonococcal infection in 40% of reported cases. Rectal infection occurs through direct inoculation by receptive anal intercourse and often results in symptomatic disease.[25,26] Symptoms can be quite mild with only pruritus and painless rectal discharge. Conversely, patients can experience severe rectal pain and bloody, mucopurulent discharge. Diagnosis is best made by anoscopy and culture, since external inspection may reveal few signs of infection. Without treatment the patient can become a chronic, asymptomatic carrier. Pharyngeal infection occurs in up to 25% of homosexual men and 7% of heterosexual men who engage in oral-genital contact with an infected partner. Over 90% of pharyngeal infections are asymptomatic but can produce an exudative pharyngitis or tonsillitis. The pharynx is the only site of infection in 5% of patients with gonococcal infection. Pharyngeal infection clears spontaneously in nearly all cases within 12 weeks of infection.[27–30]

Gonococcal Infection in Women

The clinical presentation of gonorrhea in women is varied, and about 50% of women with endocervical infection are asymptomatic. Although the columnar epithelial cells of the endocervix are the initial site of infection, up to 30% of women with untreated infection develop upper reproductive tract infection or PID.[31,32] In the presence of endocervical infection, infection usually also involves the urethra.

The incubation period for gonorrhea is longer in women than in men but is usually less than 10 days. The clinical presentation is highly variable and includes vaginal discharge secondary to mucopurulent cervicitis (MPC), abnormal menstrual bleeding, and anorectal discomfort.[25,32] Dysuria is also a common symptom of gonococcal infection in women. It is often mistaken for acute bacterial cystitis and should be suspected in young, sexually active women with pyuria in the absence of bacteria. Women who present with dysuria should have a pelvic examination as well as examination of the urethra for inflammatory exudate, and visualization of the cervix for signs of endocervical involvement and specimen collection.

PATHOGENESIS AND IMMUNITY

Infection with *N. gonorrhoeae* encompasses several specific stages. These include (1) attachment, (2) local proliferation with subsequent colonization of the mucosal cell surface, (3) penetration or invasion, and (4) local inflammatory response or dissemination.[4] Most, if not all, of these stages involve cell surface components that may be subject to phase or antigenic variations. Phase variation refers to the ability of the organism to turn the expression of a gene on or off. In the case of one such gene, gonococcal pilin, the gonococcus has a pilin expression locus, *pilE*, and multiple, silent pilin incomplete variant copies, *pilS*.[33] Gene conversion occurs with the movement of a sequence from a *pilS* locus into the *pilE* expression locus. Incorporation of a *pilS* sequence that alters the structure of the pili results in antigenic variation, but if incorporation of the sequence blocks transcription of or expression of functional pili, phase variation occurs.

We use pilin as an example of this process. Several other outer membrane structures also undergo phase variation, antigenic variation, or both. These include Opa (opacity-related protein), LOS (lipo-oligosaccharide), and PilC (a pilus-associated attachment protein).[34–38]

Attachment

Following introduction of gonococci onto a mucosal site, gonococci attach to the surface of columnar epithelial cells. Initial attachment is mediated by pili—filamentous, outer membrane appendages composed of multiple subunits.[39] Human challenge studies suggest pili are important for infection, since Pil-negative variants are noninfectious.[40] In addition, these studies demonstrated that multiple pilin variants can be present in a single infection.[41,42] Little is known about the precise mechanism of pilin-associated adherence to epithelial cells, although a putative host cell receptor was identified as CD46, or membrane cofactor protein.[43] Antibodies raised against pili have been shown to block attachment of gonococci to epithelial cells.[33] Subsequent studies have demonstrated that protective pilin antibodies have been directed at the highly variable pilin epitopes. This may explain why there is such a high degree of pilin antigenic variation by gonococci in vivo, since it allows evasion of the first line of host immunity.

Attachment by pili may be further influenced by the PilC proteins: PilC1 and PilC2 are proteins that copurify with pilin and also undergo phase variation.[44] They play a key role in epithelial cell adherence, but there is uncertainty about how they interact with pilin, or how they assist with cell attachment.[45] Gonococcal attachment and invasion are associated with actin rearrangements, membrane ruffling, pedestal formation, and recruitment of phosphorylated host cell proteins and receptors.[46]

Two other outer membrane structures, Opa and gonococcal LOS, are also involved in attachment and invasion of the host cell. The interaction of gonococcal LOS to the human asialoglycoprotein receptor (ASGP-R) allows entry into primary human urethral epithelial cells.[47] Opa proteins are a family of 11 or 12 related proteins that increase the colonial opacity of gonorrhea when viewed under a dissecting microscope.[42] Opa proteins undergo frequent phase and antigenic variation, with up to four or five different Opa genes being simultaneously expressed with a change in frequency of about 0.001 per cell per generation.[48]

Opa antigenic variation is regulated by translational frame shifting, which is due to a high-frequency, spontaneous variation in the number of CTCTT oligonucleotide repeats in the signal encoding sequence of the Opa region.[38] Each Opa contains two hypervariable regions (HV-1 and HV-2), which are surface-exposed and promote the intimate attachment of gonococci to the host cell.[49,50] Experimental infection in the urethra of male volunteers suggests the need for Opa phenotypic expression for infection to occur.[51,52] In addition, Opa is necessary for endocytosis by eukaryotic cells.[53] Antibodies directed against these regions decrease cell adherence, but no cross-reacting Opa antibodies have been found to block adherence. Several studies suggest that only a few Opa types may be able to mediate cellular attachment or induce endocytosis.[53] Opa binding sites that have been identified include heparin sulfate proteoglycans and carcinoembryonic antigen–like cell adhesion molecules (CEACAMs, formerly referred to as CD66 antigens).[54,55] Expression of different members of the CEACAMs family may explain preferential binding of gonococci to particular cells, since various Opa variants exhibit different binding specificities for various CEACAMs family members.[56]

CEACAM engagement on professional phagocytic cells results in the activation of the host cell Src tyrosine kinases, Hck and Fgr, which is then followed by Rac activation. Rac activation, in turn, triggers cytoskeletal rearrangement and internalization of the gonococcus.[57]

Although Opa is important in the pathogenesis of gonococcal infection, gonococcal isolates from the upper genital tract of women are less likely to express Opa than isolates from the lower genital tract.[58] It is possible that the initial lower tract infection involves Opa but the subsequent production of antibodies directed against Opa exerts pressure for the selection of gonococcal strains that do not express Opa. These Opa-negative strains then ascend the genital tract (by means other than transcellular migration) to cause upper tract infection. Antibodies directed against Opa may have protective benefits in women with gonococcal infection, since the presence of antibodies to increasing number of Opa variants was correlated with a lower risk of developing salpingitis after an episode of cervical infection.[59] This antibody response does not result in protection from acquisition of gonococcal infection. The role of Opa in the pathogenesis of infection is the subject of study in several laboratories.

Gonococci express a heterogeneous mixture of LOS in their outer membrane. The LOS of *N. gonorrhoeae* differs from that of other gram-negative bacteria by the absence of the O-antigenic side chains but possesses similar core oligosaccharide and lipid A.[60] LOS mediates bacterium-bacterium adherence and plays a role in epithelial cell invasion. LOS is known to produce a marked inflammatory response, which is responsible for many of the signs and symptoms associated with gonococcal infection. It causes inflammation by inducing complement activation, lysis of host cells, and the local production of tumor necrosis factor (TNF). These mechanisms cause much of the tissue damage associated with upper tract disease. The exuberant host immune response to gonococcal infection, while leading to control of infection, can account for many of the signs and symptoms of disease. Gonococci are able to escape host defense mechanisms directed against LOS by at least three different means: (1) mimicking the host glycolipids, (2) phase and antigenic variation, and (3) sialylation of the terminal core sugar, which results in masking of LOS.[60] This inhibits antibody recognition of LOS and prevents effective formation and deposition of the terminal complement complex on the gonococcal outer membrane. The presence of sialic acid on gonococcal LOS confers serum resistance but also inhibits Opa-mediated entry into some cells.[61,62] In summary, Por, Opa, and LOS each have individual profound effects on bacterial trafficking across the human genital tract epithelial barrier and influence the effects of one another when they are expressed in combination.[63]

Proliferation

In vivo, free iron is a limiting nutrient for gonococcal proliferation. The ability of gonococci to acquire iron, either in the form of lactoferrin or transferrin, is required for successful colonization of human genital epithelium.[64]

Free iron is scarce in host mucosal sites primarily because high-affinity iron-binding proteins, human transferrin and lactoferrin, act to bind free iron and reduce its availability.[4] In response to iron deprivation, gonococci produce receptors (Tbp1 and Tbp2) for binding human transferrin and human lactoferrin (LBP-1).[33] On binding of transferrin and lactoferrin to the receptors, iron is released and transported across the periplasmic space to the cytoplasmic membrane via a ferric iron–binding protein and hence into the cytoplasm.

Gonococci are able to undergo intracellular replication, both within phagocytic vacuoles and within columnar epithelial cells. Gonococci grow in both aerobic and anaerobic environments.[65] This adaptive response helps gonococci evade phagocytic attack. By utilizing oxygen, gonococci compete with the oxidative metabolism of phagocytic cells and contribute to the development of an anaerobic environment. Unique proteins expressed under these anaerobic conditions may allow survival and replication within leukocyte phagolysosomes. Survival of gonococci in the vaginal tract appears to be enhanced by one of two multidrug-resistance efflux systems (MtrCDE). The MtrCDE system appears to undergo hormonal regulation, suggesting that the secretory stage of the mammalian reproductive cycle, through the effect of progesterone, may inhibit gonococcal survival in vivo.[66]

Local Invasion

Following attachment to mucosal cells, gonococci become engulfed in a process known as parasite-directed endocytosis. This process appears to be enhanced by the outer membrane protein Por (Proteins IA and IB).[67] Porins are trimeric protein structures that form anion-selective transmembrane channels. There are two structurally related forms: PorA and PorB. Por is expressed constitutively and does not undergo high-frequency phase or antigenic variation. Antigenic variation probably occurs by low-frequency mutations of Por.[68] Purified Por exhibits several functions believed to be important in cellular invasion. One is the ability to insert itself into the host cell membrane and collapse the membrane potential.[66,69] The second is its ability to bind calmodulin. As such, it may be able to induce the endocytosis of gonococci into epithelial cells, blunt the polymorphonuclear (PMN) leukocyte oxidative burst, and block phagolysosomal fusion. Por selectively inhibits PMN granule fusion with plasma membrane to downregulate oxidative metabolism.[70] Por is also a basis for strain serotyping.[71] Normal human serum can kill circulating gonococci through the activation of complement and the deposition of terminal complement complex on the cell surface.[60] Disseminated gonococcal isolates are typically serum-resistant and can induce defective deposition of the terminal complement complex on the outer membrane.[60] PorA appears to be crucial to the development of serum resistance, since most invasive strains express PorA. Both PorA and PorB strains cause local infection, although PorB strains are more common.[72]

Gonococcal Adaptation to Avoid Host Immunity

In order for *N. gonorrhoeae* to survive, it has developed strategies to avoid host defense mechanisms. Examples of these strategies include antigenic and phase variation of Opa, Pil, and LOS.[33,35,37] Four other mechanisms also play an important role in protection from host attack: (1) masking of gonococcal antigen (sialylation of LOS); (2) mimicry (the similarity of terminal LOS sugars to host glycolipids); (3) release of immunoglobulin A (IgA) 1 protease, which cleaves and thus inactivates mucosal IgA; and (4) blocking antigen.[73] This last strategy involves the blocking of mucosal defenses by the binding of antibodies to a reduction modifiable protein (Rmp). Unlike the antigenic variability associated with Por, Opa, and Pil, Rmp has relative antigenic stability within the species and the genus *Neisseria*.[74–77] Rmp is physically associated with Por on the outer membrane of gonococci and is highly immunogenic for non-complement-fixing antibodies. The antibodies directed against Rmp bind to the Por-Rmp complex and block the effective deposition of complement-fixing anti-Por antibodies.[78] Once bound, antibodies to Rmp increase the deposition of C3 and C9 and redirect terminal complement complex to nonlytic sites.[79–81] The presence of anti-Rmp antibodies also correlates with an increased risk of gonococcal mucosal infection.[82] Rmp is closely related to the outer membrane protein 3 (OmpA) of *Escherichia coli* and the class 4 protein of meningococcus.[80] It is possible that Rmp antibodies are acquired in the absence of gonococcal infection by colonization of the intestinal tract by *E. coli* or by nasopharyngeal colonization with meningococcus. In essence, gonococci can use the host immune response against other organisms as its way of preventing an effective response to itself.

Sialylation of LOS on gonococci also prevents the binding of bactericidal antibodies and interferes with the deposition of complement by forming a pseudocapsule on gonococci. This provides a partial immunogenic cover to neighboring Por.[73]

DIAGNOSIS

Cervical or urethral exudate should be examined by Gram's stain and by culture. Mucopurulent cervicitis is defined by the presence of a yellow-green discoloration on a swab after insertion into the endocervix. In the absence of infection, the swab would remain white or be coated by a clear mucoid discharge. Culture or other diagnostic tests should be used to differentiate gonococcal cervicitis from other causes of cervical inflammation such as chlamydia and herpes simplex. The endocervical Gram's stain sensitivity is only 50% and must demonstrate intracellular gram-negative diplococci to discriminate between *N. gonorrhoeae* and other *Neisseria* and gram-negative species that normally inhabit the vagina and cervix.[24] Whenever possible, it is essential to confirm the diagnosis of gonococcal infection through either culture or through direct or amplified genetic probes.

Other local sites of infection in women include gonococcal proctitis, which is found in 35% to 50% of women with cervicitis and is usually asymptomatic. It can be the only site of infection in 5% of women.[32,83] If symptoms are present, they are similar to those shown by men. Although sore throat and pharyngitis in the STD clinic are often associated with a history of fellatio, gonorrhea or other sexually transmitted infections are not usually isolated.[83,84] Most pharyngeal infections are asymptomatic and clear spontaneously. Pharyngeal gonorrhea is found in 10% to 20% of women with endocervical infection,[84] is associated with an apparent increased risk of dissemination, and has been associated with sexual transmission.[27,84]

Local infection of the endocervix extends to the uterus, fallopian tubes, or adjacent structures in about 15% of women.[31,85,86] Factors contributing to upper tract infections include menstruation, use of an intrauterine device (IUD), a history of douching, adolescent age, or previous history of PID. Clinical signs and symptoms of upper tract infection involve some or all of a constellation including lower abdominal pain, dyspareunia, abnormal menstrual bleeding, adnexal and cervical motion tenderness, fever, and other complaints consistent with an intra-abdominal infection. Endocervical Gram's stain may be helpful and yield a presumptive diagnosis by the presence of intracellular gram-negative diplococci, but it is negative in 40% to 60% of women with PID.[24] Therefore, the diagnosis of PID is usually made on clinical grounds and cannot be distinguished from nongonococcal PID. None of the clinical signs and symptoms have both high sensitivity or specificity for PID. Use of three clinical variables—a high erythrocyte sedimentation rate, fever, and adnexal tenderness—correctly classified only 65% of laparoscopically diagnosed PID.[87] Because of the lack of a diagnostic clinical sign or symptom, the differential diagnosis remains broad and includes ectopic pregnancy, urinary tract infection, pyelonephritis, appendicitis, proctocolitis, and endometriosis.

Early diagnosis and treatment are essential to preventing the complications of PID. Infertility is strongly associated with a history of PID and occurs with increasing frequency: in 11% of women who have had one episode, in 23% with two episodes, and in 75% with three or more episodes of PID. Other sequelae include chronic pelvic pain and ectopic pregnancy.[24,88]

Other urogenital complications from gonorrhea in women include perihepatitis (Fitz-Hugh–Curtis syndrome), which presents as acute right or bilateral upper quadrant tenderness, frequently with signs and symptoms of PID.[89] Infection of Bartholin's gland duct presents with local erythema and pus at the posterior third of the labia majora.

Infection with gonorrhea during pregnancy is similar in clinical presentation to that in nonpregnant women. However, in women with gonococcal infection, there are higher rates of spontaneous abortion, premature rupture of membranes, acute chorioamnionitis, postpartum endometriosis, and premature delivery.[90,91] Asymptomatic women may transmit infection throughout the pregnancy and postpartum periods. In particular peripartum transmission to the newborn may result in infection of the conjunctiva, rectum, or respiratory tract.[92] Gonococcal ophthalmia can be prevented by routine screening for endocervical infection during pregnancy and by the prophylactic use of 1% silver nitrate, erythromycin, or tetracycline ophthalmic solution.[93] These agents may not be available in developing countries. A single application of povidone-iodine 2.5% is an inexpensive alternative with a broad spectrum of activity against chlamydia, gonococcus, HIV, and herpes simplex.[94,95] Given the high rates of tetracycline-resistant *N. gonorrhoeae* (TRNG), tetracycline may no longer be adequate as prophylactic therapy.[4]

Disseminated Disease

DGI is relatively rare, occurring in 0.5% to 3.0% of untreated mucosal infections.[4] The majority of DGI occurs in persons with asymptomatic mucosal infection. This may be partially due to infection by a distinct clone that typically causes minimally symptomatic mucosal infection but is prone to systemic dissemination. This clone exhibits the AHU auxotype, PorIA serovar, and serum-resistant phenotype. Host factors are also important with women, accounting for about 70% of disseminated disease and bacteremia, often beginning during menses. Patients with terminal complement component deficiency are particularly susceptible to systemic infection with the gonococcus and meningococcus.[96]

The clinical manifestations of DGI are a result of gonococcal bacteremia, although patients typically lack the classic signs of bacteremia, that is, high fever, leukocytosis, or systemic toxicity.[4] The most common presentation of DGI is polyarthritis. Gonococcal arthritis can, however, present as monarticular arthritis, the most common cause of acute arthritis in young adults. An important clinical finding that helps differentiate gonococcal arthritis from other infectious causes is tenosynovitis, which often occurs over the involved joint and is sometimes accompanied by erythema.[97] Skin lesions, which typically occur throughout this period, appear as sparse, pustular lesions with surrounding erythema on the distal extremities. Lesions are present in 50% to 75% of patients but number fewer than 30 in most cases.[98,99]

Purulent arthritis is a later manifestation of the arthritis-dermatitis syndrome associated with DGI and occurs in approximately 30% to 40% of patients with DGI. Synovial fluid cultures are usually sterile but are more frequently positive in patients with synovial fluid leukocyte counts greater than 40,000/μL.[100] Blood and skin lesion cultures are usually also sterile, with the overall yield of blood cultures being less than 30% but decreasing with the duration of clinical illness.[101] This may be due to the intermittent, low level of bacteremia, the extraordinary nutritional requirements of the gonorrhea strains most likely to disseminate, and the role of immunocomplex deposition as a cause of local inflammation.

Other manifestations of DGI include mild pericarditis, endocarditis, and meningitis (each of which is seen in fewer than 3% of patients with DGI).[100–102]

To confirm the diagnosis of DGI, cultures should be obtained from all mucosal sites. In more than 80% of patients, gonococci can be isolated from genital, rectal, or pharyngeal cultures. In cases in which cultures are negative from all mucosal sites, isolation of *N. gonorrhoeae* from the sexual partners may be the only means of confirming the diagnosis.

Culture

The gold standard for detection of *N. gonorrhoeae* has been the culture. The widespread use of nucleic acid amplification tests (NAATs) may signify a change in this long-standing standard. The main benefits of culture are high specificity and the ability to do additional studies, such as antimicrobial susceptibility testing on culture isolates. The disadvantages of culture can be substantial in developing countries because of the stringent storage and transport requirements of culture media, the fastidious growth requirements of *N. gonorrhoeae*, and the delay in obtaining results. Test performance, available technology, cost, and prevalence of gonorrhea must be taken into account when selecting diagnostic tests to be used for identifying gonococcal infection. Ideally, the test should be highly sensitive, specific, rapid, and inexpensive.[103]

The yield of gonococcal culture largely depends on the anatomic site of the culture and the use of selective or nonselective media. Selective media contain several antibodies to prevent the overgrowth of genitourinary, enteric, and oral flora. Modified Thayer-Martin (MTM) is probably the most widely used selective medium, with an overall sensitivity of 80% to 95% for isolation of *N. gonorrhoeae*. Other selective media include NYC (New York City), Martin-Lewis (ML), and GC-Lect. There are significant differences among these media. MTM lacks serum and inhibits the growth of 3% to 10% of *N. gonorrhoeae* strains because of its high concentration of vancomycin (3 μg/mL) relative to other media. Additionally, it is difficult to predict when vancomycin-sensitive strains may be present, because of geographic variation in prevalence. Vancomycin-sensitive strains are more likely to be found in heterosexuals, whites, and asymptomatic carriers. Moreover, growth of vancomycin-sensitive strains largely depends on the size of the inoculum; smaller inocula are more likely to be inhibited. GC-Lect medium has some advantage over MTM for the isolation of vancomycin-sensitive strains owing to its lower concentration of vancomycin (2 μg/mL) and the presence of supplemental nutrients. NYC medium is serum-enriched and also has a vancomycin concentration of 2 μg/mL. NYC medium is translucent and therefore facilitates both the selection of oxidase-positive colonies and viewing under a stereomicroscope. Production variability and increased cost render NYC less useful than MTM.

To prevent the overgrowth of gonococcal colonies with normal flora, it is best to use selective media in sites with a higher concentration of easily cultured bacteria, such as the rectum, pharynx, and endocervix. Nonselective media can be used for urethral specimens from men with symptomatic urethritis because of the high concentration of gonococci relative to that of other genital flora.

In women, a single culture of the endocervix is usually sufficient for isolation of gonococci because infection usually involves the cervix. It is rare to detect infection in other sites without first finding it in the cervix. For women who have undergone a hysterectomy, urethral cultures are indicated. Consideration of culturing the accessory gland ducts, pharynx, and rectum is based on clinical presentation, site of sexual contact, and cost.

Gram's Stain

Low cost and rapidity of diagnosis make Gram's stain of clinical specimens an important test for the evaluation of gonorrhea in the clinical setting. Gram's stain is considered positive if neutrophils with intracellular gram-negative diplococci are observed. It is considered negative in the absence of gram-negative diplococci, and equivocal following observation of extracellular gram-negative or morphologically atypical-appearing organisms.[103,104] Because it is not possible to distinguish *N. meningitidis* from *N. gonorrhoeae* by Gram's stain, it is sometimes necessary to confirm the diagnosis through culture. Other nonpathogenic *Neisseria* species are usually not present as intracellular organisms.

The sensitivity and specificity of the Gram's stain smear varies, depending on the site of infection and the presence or absence of symptoms. For symptomatic urethritis in men, the high sensitivity and specificity, 95% and 98%, respectively, suffices for diagnosis.[104–107] In asymptomatic males, the sensitivity is significantly lower and requires a culture to rule out gonococcal infection. Lower sensitivity (40% to 60%) is also seen in Gram's stains of endocervical samples from symptomatic women, although it retains a high specificity in these cases. Owing to high specificity, it is possible to make a presumptive diagnosis on the basis of a positive smear. The high intraobserver variability in preparing and reading endocervical Gram's stains renders unreliable the reading of a negative Gram's stain.[103,106] Although sometimes useful, the Gram's-stained smear of the rectum, pharynx, and other sites should be used only in conjunction with cultures or other diagnostic tests to confirm diagnosis.

Nucleic Acid Amplification Tests

NAAT methodology involves amplification of specific *N. gonorrhoeae* DNA or RNA sequences by polymerase chain reaction (PCR), strand displacement assay (SDA), or transcription-mediated assay (TMA). Commercially available ligase chain reaction (LCR) is no longer available. NAATs have reported sensitivities and specificities from urethral and endocervical specimens that are comparable to culture.[108,109] The advantages of these tests over culture are the rapidity of results and the high sensitivity compared with culture. The latter has allowed testing for *N. gonorrhoeae* by NAATs to be applied to urine specimens and vaginal swabs.[110] Urine-based testing permits screening of populations outside the traditional clinic setting and identification of the asymptomatic carrier of *N. gonorrhoeae* without invasive testing. First-generation NAATs had difficulties with cross-reactivity with nongonococcal *Neisseria* species. Second-generation NAATs approach zero cross-reactivity with nongonococcal species and have the added advantage of being able to simultaneously identify *N. gonorrhoeae* and *Chlamydia trachomatis*. Studies with TMA have demonstrated excellent performance diagnosing anorectal or pharyngeal infection.[111]

The high sensitivity of NAATs has a trade-off in that specificity is not 100%. There can be false-positive results when screening is performed in low-prevalence populations.[112] Caution must be given to use of NAATs in screening asymptomatic populations. Even with reported high specificity, there is reason to be concerned that a poor positive predictive value with vaginal swabs may occur with PCR and could still be an issue for TMA and SDA.[113]

Other Diagnostic Tests

Specimen collection, transportation, and storage issues all contribute to failure in culture identification of gonococcal infection.[114] With the development of nonculture diagnostic tests, it is increasingly possible to confirm the diagnosis through other methods: enzyme immunoassays, DNA probes, and DNA amplification assays.[108,115,116] These diagnostic methods potentially offer more rapid results and higher sensitivity than culture. DNA probe assays for gonorrhea have a reported sensitivity of 93% to 99% and specificity of 98% to 99.5%.[117] One DNA probe, PACE 2, combines probes against *N. gonorrhoeae* and *C. trachomatis* into a single test with sensitivity and specificity comparable to the single probe for *N. gonorrhoeae*.[118] In addition, not all nonculture tests produce gonococcal isolates that may be used for antimicrobial susceptibility testing. For this reason, it is best that they not replace the use of ongoing surveillance systems. In the future, commercially available NAATs may identify resistance genes. Correlation of genetic markers of resistance to clinical isolates will still need to be made prior to widespread use of this technology as part of resistance monitoring.

TREATMENT

Antimicrobial Resistance

Control of gonococcal disease has depended heavily on the use of highly effective and preferably single-dose antibiotic therapy.[118] As early as the 1950s, however, reduced susceptibility to penicillin was reported.[119] Unfortunately, antimicrobial resistance has continued to evolve and spread since that time. Antibiotic resistance remains disproportionately represented in less developed nations and in socially marginalized groups. The reasons for the development of resistance are complex but can be attributed to four major factors: (1) poor compliance with prescribed therapy, (2) inadequate dosing of antibiotics, (3) circumstances causing low or inadequate antibiotic serum levels, and (4) conditions favoring the selection of resistance mutations (such as the widespread use of antimicrobial agents in the general population).

Antibiotic resistance occurs through two main mechanisms: chromosomal and plasmid-mediated resistance. Chromosomal resistance is encoded at several different loci and usually occurs as a stepwise, incremental resistance pattern. The single exception to stepwise chromosomal resistance is spectinomycin, to which high-level resistance occurs after a single alteration to the ribosomal target.[120,121] Plasmid resistance usually occurs as a one-step change to high-level resistance and rapidly spreads through a population.

Therapeutic regimens should be based on the knowledge of the in vitro sensitivity of prevalent gonococci in the immediate region. A strong argument can be made that regional susceptibility patterns are more important than strain susceptibility in a given individual.[122] This is especially important because most treatment occurs prior to obtaining the antimicrobial susceptibilities on a particular gonococcal isolate. Increasing minimum inhibitory concentrations (MICs) to antimicrobial therapy partially explains the rise in treatment failure, which further highlights the importance of monitoring resistance patterns in order to accurately select treatment regimens. In turn, this can further the discovery of new resistance patterns as they develop. Ideally, this monitoring should be a continuous surveillance program. Owing to financial constraints, point prevalence studies at repeated intervals can be performed to follow temporal changes in susceptibility patterns.

The specific incidence of antibiotic resistance is geographically variable, but effective treatment is a common challenge in several countries. In the United States, the Far East, and western and central Africa,[123] treatment with penicillin and tetracycline is unreliable owing to the appearance in gonococci of plasmids that produce β-lactamase, resulting in penicillinase-producing *N. gonorrhoeae* (PPNG); of plasmids that mediate high-level TRNG; and emergence over many decades of chromosomally mediated penicillin- and tetracycline-resistant *N. gonorrhoeae* (CMRNG).[123–125] PPNG strains are characterized by the production of β-lactamase and have MICs for penicillin greater than or equal to 16 μg/mL. CMRNG strains are characterized by the lack of β-lactamase production and have penicillin MICs less than 8 μg/mL. A strain can have plasmid-mediated resistance to both penicillin and tetracycline (PPNG-TRNG). Chromosomal-resistant strains usually have MICs less than or equal to 2 μg/mL for tetracycline, penicillin, or cefoxitin. In general, chromosomal resistance occurs through alterations in antimicrobial-binding proteins or through decreased net permeability of the gonococcal outer membrane.[119,126]

In reaction to widespread penicillin and tetracycline resistance, the Centers for Disease Control and Prevention (CDC) in 1987 ceased to recommend the first-line use of these agents for treatment of gonorrhea. It then began advocating the use of third-generation cephalosporins and selected fluoroquinolones.[127,128] Fortunately, ceftriaxone continues to be effective with no reported resistance. Cefixime had been the only oral cephalosporin recommended by the CDC for the treatment of uncomplicated gonococcal infection. The sole company manufacturing cefixime ceased manufacturing it in the United States in July 2002, and the drug is no longer available in the United States.[129]

Cefpodoxime has recently been advocated as a replacement for cefixime.[130] There is some concern, however, regarding the potential emergence of strains resistant to the use of a 200-mg dose of cefpodoxime and a similar concern of emerging resistance to cefixime should it again become widely available. The clinical data for cefpodoxime are sparse, at best, with only one clinical trial reported in the literature. Although it appears cefpodoxime therapy at 200 mg and 400 mg is equivalent, only two patients were treated with the 200-mg dose.[131] Monitoring for the emergence of resistance or evidence of clinical treatment failure is recommended for areas where cefpodoxime is used as first-line treatment for uncomplicated gonococcal infection.

The concern over potential cefixime resistance stems from application of a therapeutic index, defined by the ratio of peak serum concentration to MIC. The recommended therapeutic index is a ratio greater than 3 to 4:1, as determined by the use of penicillin G for the treatment of gonococcal urethritis.[132] Antimicrobial agents with a therapeutic index greater than 4 are highly effective in curing gonorrhea. Relative to other therapies, cefixime demonstrates a low peak serum level. The recommended dose of cefixime, 400 mg PO, produces a peak serum level of 4 μg/mL, while 500 mg of ceftriaxone IM produces peak serum concentrations of 42 to 45 μg/mL. This concentration is more than 1000 times greater than the MIC for *N. gonorrhoeae*.[133,134]

Of greater concern is the emergence of fluoroquinolone resistance (QNRG), which has been noted in the Far East, Australia, Africa, Europe, and (most recently) the United States.[135] Fluoroquinolone resistance is chromosomally mediated and affects all members of this class of drug. Ciprofloxacin is decreasing in effectiveness in most areas of the United States and Africa. QNRG is endemic in Hawaii and California with increases in QNRG seen in Washington state and Massachusetts. Widespread increases in QNRG have been noted in MSM throughout the United States. This prompted the CDC to issue behavior-specific recommendations on treatment of gonorrhea. Because prevalence does not appear to be high among heterosexuals, broad-based changes have not been made for heterosexuals. Concern does arise for the willingness of men to identify MSM activity in areas where the stigma of homosexuality remains high. As a result, it may be prudent to have gender-specific recommendations for treatment where the prevalence for QNRG remains high for MSM. The trend in increasing prevalence of QNRG warrants close surveillance and adherence to several recommendations regarding the use of fluoroquinolones for gonorrhea:

1. Avoiding use of fluoroquinolones to treat gonorrhea in natives of, or travelers from, Asia or the western Pacific countries, Hawaii, or California (owing to prevalence of high-level resistance)
2. Avoiding use of fluoroquinolones to treat gonorrhea in MSM. Consideration should be given to avoid use of fluoroquinolones in all men and women with gonorrhea where QNRG in MSM is a concern, since men may not disclose MSM activity and women have a high rate of asymptomatic infection with *N. gonorrhoeae*
3. Using only the recommended doses of fluoroquinolones (500 mg of ciprofloxacin or 400 mg of ofloxacin when they are used for treatment of gonorrhea)
4. Prescribing single-dose therapy with the additional use of azithromycin or doxycycline, which may retard the selection of resistance

Antimicrobial Therapy

Ideally, antimicrobial therapy for gonorrhea should be safe, be inexpensive, and achieve rapid serum and tissue levels at least three to four times greater than the MIC of the infecting gonococcal strain. Treatment regimens for uncomplicated gonorrhea should cure at least 95% of infections by a single dose of therapy. In 2002, the CDC recommended two fluoroquinolones—oral ciprofloxacin 500 mg and oral ofloxacin 400 mg—or two broad-spectrum cephalosporins—oral cefixime 400 mg or IM ceftriaxone 125 mg—for the treatment of uncomplicated gonorrhea.[136] The continued evolution of gonococcal resistance has led to significant changes to the 2002 recommendations. The ideal therapeutic index (ratio of peak serum concentration to MIC of 3 to 4:1) is achieved with the recommended regimens of cefixime or ceftriaxone. Ciprofloxacin achieves peak serum concentrations of 2.5 μg/mL following a single 500-mg oral dose and should be adequate for treating gonococcal strains with decreased susceptibilities (MIC of 0.125 to 0.5 μg/mL). Ciprofloxacin-resistant strains are defined as having an MIC greater than 1.0 μg/mL and nonresponsive to the recommended dose.[124] Ceftriaxone, cefixime, and ciprofloxacin all clear *N. gonorrhoeae* in less than 24 hours from the urethral mucosa and semen of men.[137] Because of the rapid clearance of infection and the high potency of the recommended treatment regimens, test of cure is not indicated following treatment for uncomplicated gonorrhea with current cephalosporin regimens. The high rate of coinfection with chlamydia in most geographic areas—15% to 20% among men and 30% to 50% among women—necessitates empirical treatment of chlamydia infection with all gonorrhea treatment regimens.[138,139] Current recommendations in the United States call for either ceftriaxone 125 mg IM or cefixime 400 mg PO (not currently available in the United States) or spectinomycin 2.0 g IM plus treatment for possible coinfection with *C. trachomatis* with either single-dose azithromycin 1.0 g PO, or with doxycycline 100 mg PO two times per day for 7 days.[139,140] Ciprofloxacin and ofloxacin are contraindicated in pregnant and nursing women, and relatively contraindicated in children less than 18 years of age. Persons who may have acquired gonorrhea in Asia, the Pacific Rim (including Hawaii), California, and other areas such as England and Wales with high rates of QNRG should not be treated with fluoroquinolones.[141] The CDC has now added MSM as a group for whom for whom alternatives to fluoroquinolones should be used for the treatment of gonorrhea. An additional consideration for choice of therapy given the recent increase in syphilis in MSM is that ciprofloxacin and ofloxacin are not active against *Treponema pallidum* and are therefore not effective against incubating syphilis. Consideration should be given to using a regimen containing ceftriaxone or azithromycin where syphilis prevalence remains high.[142]

Alternative regimens for those unable to take cephalosporins or quinolones include spectinomycin 2 g IM, kanamycin 2 g IM, or gentamicin 240 mg IM.[136,143,144] Because of the low risk of cross-reactions between penicillin and cephalosporins with single-dose therapy, cephalosporins may be used in patients with penicillin allergies, unless there is a history of an immediate IgE-mediated hypersensitivity reaction.

Pharyngeal gonococcal infection may be treated with ceftriaxone 125 mg IM. An alternative regimen for those unable to be treated with cephalosporins is ciprofloxacin 500 mg or ofloxacin 400 mg PO.[136] When considering alternative regimens, it is important to note that spectinomycin is ineffective against pharyngeal infection.[143] Its use in the United States has been limited to pregnant women who are unable to take cephalosporins.

Gonorrhea in pregnancy is best treated with ceftriaxone 250 mg IM, plus a regimen active against *C. trachomatis* with erythromycin base 500 mg PO, four times a day for 7 days, or amoxicillin 500 mg PO three times a day for 7 days, or azithromycin 1.0 g PO.[136,143] Pregnant women for whom cephalosporins are contraindicated may be treated with spectinomycin 2 g IM once. Pregnant women should have rectal and endocervical cultures for *N. gonorrhoeae* obtained 3 to 7 days following therapy as a test of cure.

DGI requires hospitalization for observation of response to therapy and to assure compliance. The recommended initial regimen for DGI is ceftriaxone 1 g IM or IV every 24 hours.[136,143] If patients are allergic to cephalosporins, therapy should include spectinomycin 2 g IM every 12 hours.[136] Resolution of symptoms usually occurs within 24 to 48 hours of initiation of therapy. In patients with a prompt clinical response to therapy and whose compliance is likely, therapy can be completed on an outpatient basis, with an oral regimen of cefixime 400 mg twice per day or cefpodoxime 400 mg twice per day, or (if QRNG is not a consideration) ciprofloxacin 500 mg twice per day or ofloxacin 400 mg twice per day to complete 7 to 10 days of total antibiotic therapy.[136]

Meningitis and endocarditis require high-dose intravenous therapy with a highly active agent that achieves adequate tissue levels in the site of infection, such as ceftriaxone 1 to 2 g IV every 12 hours. The duration of therapy should be a minimum of 10 to 14 days for gonococcal meningitis and a minimum of 4 weeks for gonococcal endocarditis.[136]

PID requires prompt treatment to reduce the incidence of chronic infection, chronic pelvic pain, and infertility. Women must be evaluated to distinguish PID from appendicitis and ectopic pregnancy. Severely ill women—those with high fever, severe pain, or inability to tolerate oral fluids—should be treated in the hospital until they are afebrile and have clinically improved. Outpatient therapy is best limited to nonpregnant, compliant women with mild-to-moderate disease. Follow-up examination is performed within 48 to 72 hours to monitor for clinical improvement in signs and symptoms. The two main therapeutic options appear in Table 26-1.

PREVENTION AND CONTROL

Despite widely available effective therapy, the persistence of gonorrhea at epidemic levels demonstrates the failure of current control programs. Persistence of STDs in a community can be described by the equation[145]

$$Ro = BcD$$

Where Ro (the reproductive rate) is greater than 1, the disease will increase in prevalence in the community. The reproductive rate is dependent on the efficiency of transmission (B), the rate of sexual partner change (c), and the duration of infectiveness (D). Attempts to reduce the reproductive rate can be directed at interventions that may alter these factors.

Barrier methods remain one of the most effective means of reducing the transmission of gonorrhea.[146] For men, this

Table 26-1 Therapy for Pelvic Inflammatory Disease in Women

Outpatient Therapy	Inpatient Therapy*
Option A Ceftriaxone 250 mg IM *or* Cefoxitin 2.0 g IM with probenecid 1.0 g PO *plus* Doxycycline 100 mg PO, twice per day for 14 days Option B Ofloxacin 400 mg PO, twice per day for 14 days *plus* Metronidazole 500 mg PO, twice per day for 14 days	Option A Cefoxitin 2.0 g IV every 6 hours *or* Cefotetan 2.0 g IV every 12 hours *plus* Doxycycline 100 mg IV every 12 hours Option B Clindamycin 900 mg IV every 8 hours *plus* Gentamicin loading dose IV or IM (2 mg/kg of body weight), followed by a maintenance dose (1.5 mg/kg) every 8 hours

*IV therapy should be continued for a minimum of 48 hours after clinical improvement and, once the patient is switched to oral therapy, completed with doxycycline 100 mg PO twice per day for a total of 14 days of antimicrobial therapy.[9]

includes the use of latex or polyurethane condoms. The current version of the female polyurethane condom has been demonstrated to reduce the transmission of trichomoniasis, but studies evaluating its effectiveness in reducing the transmission of gonorrhea have not been published.[147] The major drawbacks to all barrier methods are noncompliance and unacceptability. The female condom presents identical problems. These issues are further complicated by male resistance to the use of the female condom.

Methods which allow more autonomy in initiation by females include the use of vaginal microbicidal agents. When used intravaginally, the currently available agent, nonoxynol-9, reduces the risk of gonorrhea by 10% to 70%.[148] Since nonoxynol-9 is a detergent that can disrupt the lipid bilayers of cell membranes, it can cause mucosal irritation and ulcers and thus increase the risk of HIV transmission. As a result, nonoxynol-9 as means of gonorrhea prevention is no longer recommended.

Vaccines offer the hope of reducing the efficiency of transmission. Crude killed, whole-cell vaccines have been tried in humans and primates, but they are likely to be more toxic than subunit vaccines and offered no protection in human trials.[149] To date, subunit vaccines directed against Pil and Por have not prevented infection in human volunteers.[150,151] Future vaccines may target PilC, TbpB (an immunogenic component of the transferrin receptor), or FrpB (a partially conserved outer membrane iron-repressed protein).[60] DNA vaccines offer a highly promising approach to effective immunogenic response but have yet to be studied for a gonococcal vaccine. A recent study using a DNA vaccine for priming an antibody response to PorB resulted in a high titer and long-lasting antibody response in an animal model.[152]

Until the availability of an effective vaccine, behavioral intervention remains a crucial strategy for reducing the spread of gonorrhea. Behavioral intervention aims to increase condom use/acceptability and to both delay sexual debut and reduce the rate of partner change. Transmission of gonorrhea is further influenced by factors that affect health-care utilization. The essential components of an effective control program are providing increased access to health care, providing the opportunity for treatment at the earliest presentation of symptoms, identifying high-risk groups for targeted interventions, screening high-risk asymptomatic patients for infection, identifying and treating sexual partners of patients with gonorrhea, and rescreening those identified with infection 3 to 4 months after treatment.[136]

REFERENCES

1. Bovre K: Neisseriaceae. In Kreig RR, Holt JG (eds): Bergey's Manual of Systemic Bacteriology. Baltimore, Williams & Wilkins, 1984, p 228.
2. Vedros NA: Neisseria. In Kreig RR, Holt JG (eds): Bergey's Manual of Systemic Bacteriology. Baltimore, Williams & Wilkins, 1984, p 290.
3. Hook EW III, Holmes KK: Gonococcal infections. Ann Intern Med 102:229–243, 1985.
4. Handsfield HH, Sparling PF: *Neisseria gonorrhoeae*. In Mandell GL, Bennett JE, Dolin R (eds): Principles and Practice of Infectious Diseases. New York, Churchill Livingstone, 1995, p 190.
5. Mertens TE, Hayes RJ, Smith PG: Epidemiologic methods to study the interactions between HIV infection and other sexually transmitted diseases. AIDS 4:57–65, 1990.
6. Laga M, Manoka T, Kivuvu M, et al: Non-ulcerative sexually transmitted diseases are risk factors for HIV-1 transmission in women: Results from a cohort study. AIDS 7:95–102, 1993.
7. Cohen MS, Hoffman IF, Royce RA, et al: Reduction of concentration of HIV-1 in semen after treatment of urethritis: implications for prevention of sexual transmission of HIV-1. Lancet 349:1868–1873, 1997.
8. Centers for Disease Control and Prevention: Sexually Transmitted Disease Surveillance, 2003. Atlanta, GA, U.S. Department of Health and Human Services, September 2004.
9. Barnes RC, Holmes KK: Epidemiology of gonorrhea: Current perspectives. Epidemiol Rev 6:1–30, 1984.
10. Miller WC, Ford CA, Morris M, et al: Prevalence of chlamydial and gonococcal infections among adolescents in the United States. JAMA 291:2229–2236, 2004.
11. Gerbase AC, Rowley JT, Heymann DHL, et al: Global prevalence and incidence estimates of selected curable STDs. Sex Transm Infect 74:S12–S16, 1998.
12. World Health Organization: Gonorrhoea estimates. In Global prevalence and incidence of selected curable sexually transmitted infections. Available at WHO/HIV_AIDS/(2001).02;WHO/CDS/EDC/(2001). Overview and Estimates, Geneva, WHO, 2001.
13. De Schryver A, Meheus A: International travel and sexually transmitted diseases. World Health Statist Q 42:90–99, 1989.
14. Centers for Disease Control and Prevention: Unpublished data, 1998.
15. Holmes KK, Johnson DW, Trostle HJ: An estimate of the risk of men acquiring gonorrhea by sexual contact with infected females. Am J Epidemiol 91:170–174, 1970.

16. Hooper RR, Reynolds GH, Jones OG, et al: Cohort study of venereal disease. 1. The risk of gonorrhea transmission from infected women to men. Am J Epidemiol 108:136–144, 1978.
17. Sackel SG, Alpert S, Fiumara NJ, et al: Orogenital contact and the isolation of *Neisseria gonorrhoeae, Mycoplasma hominis*, and *Ureaplasma urealyticum* from the pharynx. Sex Transm Dis 6:64–68, 1979.
18. Lafferty WE, Hughes JP, Hansfield HH: Sexually transmitted diseases in men who have sex with men. Sex Transm Dis 24:272–278, 1997.
19. Hethcote HW, Yorke JA: Gonorrhoea transmission dynamics and control. In Levin S (ed): Lecture Notes in Biomathematics, 56. New York, Springer-Verlag, 1984, p 99.
20. Jacobs NF, Kraus SJ: Gonococcal and nongonococcal urethritis in men. Ann Intern Med 82:7–12, 1975.
21. Harrison WO, Hooper RR, Wiesner PJ, et al: A trial of minocycline given after exposure to prevent gonorrhea. N Engl J Med 300:1074–1078, 1979.
22. Handsfield HH, Lipman TO, Hamisch JP, et al: Asymptomatic gonorrhea in men: Diagnosis, natural course, prevalence, and significance. N Engl J Med 290:117–123, 1974.
22. Pelouze PS: Gonorrhea in the Male and Female. Philadelphia, WB Saunders, 1941.
24. Hook EW, Handsfield HH: Gonococcal infection in the adult. In Holmes KK, Mardh PA, Sparling PF, et al (eds): Sexually Transmitted Diseases. New York, McGraw-Hill, 1990.
25. Klein EJ, Fisher LS, Chow AW, et al: Anorectal gonococcal infection. Ann Intern Med 86:340–346, 1977.
26. Lebedeff DA, Hochman EB: Rectal gonorrhea in men: Diagnosis and treatment. Ann Intern Med 92:463–466, 1980.
27. Tice AW, Rodriguez VL: Pharyngeal gonorrhea. JAMA 246:2717–2719, 1981.
28. Bro-Jørgenson A, Jensen T: Gonococcal pharyngeal infection: Report of 110 cases. Br J Vener Dis 49:491–499, 1973.
29. Janda WM, Bonhoff M, Morello JA, et al: Prevalence and site-pathogen studies of *Neisseria meningitidis* and *N. gonorrhoeae* in homosexual men. JAMA 244:2060–2064, 1980.
30. Wallin J, Siegel MS: Pharyngeal *Neisseria gonorrhoeae*: Colonizer or pathogen? BMJ 1:1462–1463, 1979.
31. McCormack WM, Stumuchar RJ, Johnson K, et al: Clinical spectrum of gonococcal infection in women. Lancet 1:1182–1185, 1977.
32. Barlow D, Phillips I: Gonorrhea in women: Diagnostic, clinical, and laboratory aspects. Lancet 1:761–764, 1978.
33. Alcorn TM, Cohen MS: Gonococcal pathogenesis: Adaptation and immune evasion in the human host. Curr Opin Infect Dis 7:310, 1994.
34. Elkins CE, Sparling PF: Immunobiology of *Neisseria gonorrhoeae*. In Quinn TC, Gallin J, Fauci AS (eds): Sexually Transmitted Diseases, Vol. 8. Advances in Host Defense Mechanisms. New York, Raven Press, 1992, p 113.
35. Seifert HS: Questions about gonococcal pilus phase and antigenic variation. Mol Microbiol 21:433–440, 1996.
36. Bergstrom S, Robbins K, Koomey JM, et al: Piliation control mechanisms in *Neisseria gonorrhoeae*. Proc Natl Acad Sci USA 83:3890–3894, 1986.
37. Apicella MA, Shero M, Jarvis GA, et al: Phenotypic variation in epitope expression of the *Neisseria gonorrhoeae* lipooligosaccharide. Infect Immun 55:1755–1761, 1987.
38. Stern A, Brown M, Nickel P, et al: Opacity genes in *Neisseria gonorrhoeae*: Control of phase and antigenic variation. Cell 47:61–71, 1986.
39. Cohen MS, Sparling PF: Mucosal infection with *Neisseria gonorrhoeae*. J Clin Invest 89:1699–1705, 1992.
40. Kellogg DS, Peacock WL, Deacon WE, et al: Clonal variation and virulence in *N. gonorrhoeae*. J Bacteriol 85:1274–1279, 1963.
41. Seifert HS, Wright CJ, Jerse AE, et al: Multiple gonococcal pilin antigenic variants are produced during experimental human infections. J Clin Invest 93:2744–2749, 1994.
42. Swanson J, Barrera O, Sola J, et al: Expression of outer membrane protein II by gonococci in experimental gonorrhea. J Exp Med 168:2121–2129, 1988.
43. Kallstrom H, Liszewski MK, Atkinson JP, et al: Membrane cofactor protein (MCP or CD46) is a cellular pilus receptor for pathogenic *Neisseria*. Mol Microbiol 25:639–647, 1997.
44. Rudel T, Scheurerpflug F, Meyer TF: *Neisseria* PilC protein identified as type-4 pilus tip-located adhesion. Nature 373:357–359, 1995.
45. Virji M, Heckels JE: The role of common and type-specific pilus antigenic domains in adhesion and virulence of gonococci for human epithelial cells. J Gen Microbiol 130:1089–1095, 1984.
46. Merz AJ, So M: Interactions of pathogenic neisseriae with epithelial cell membranes. Annu Rev Cell Dev Biol 16:423–457, 2000.
47. Harvey HA, Jennings MP, Campbell CA, et al: Receptor-mediated endocytosis of *Neisseria gonorrhoeae* into primary human urethral epithelial cells: The role of the asialoglycoprotein receptor. Mol Microbiol 42:659–672, 2004.
48. Meyer LW: Rates of in vitro changes in gonococcal colony opacity phenotypes. Infect Immun 37:481–485, 1982.
49. Bhat KS, Gibbs CP, Barrera O, et al: The opacity proteins of *Neisseria gonorrhoeae* strain MS 11 are encoded by a family of 11 complete genes. Mol Microbiol 5:1889–1901, 1991.
50. Connell TD, Shaffer P, Cannon JG: Characterization of the repertoire of the hypervariable regions in the protein II (opa) gene family of *Neisseria gonorrhoeae*. Mol Microbiol 4:439–449, 1990.
51. Swanson J, Barrera O, Sola J, et al: Expression of outer membrane protein II by gonococci in experimental gonorrhea. J Exp Med 168:2121–2129, 1988.
52. Jerse AE, Cohen MS, Drown PM, et al: Multiple gonococcal opacity proteins are expressed during experimental urethral infection in the male. J Exp Med 179:911–920, 1994.
53. Weel JF, Hopman CT, Van Putten JP: In situ expression and localization of *Neisseria gonorrhoeae* opacity proteins in infected epithelial cells: Apparent role of opa proteins in cellular invasion. J Exp Med 6:1395–1405, 1991.
54. Virji M, Watt, SM, Barker, S, et al: The N-domain of the human CD66a adhesion molecule is a target for Opa proteins of *Neisseria meningitidis* and *Neisseria gonorrhoeae*. Mol Microbiol 22:929–939, 1996.
55. Chen T, Belland RJ, Wilson J, Swanson J: Adherence of pilus-Opa-gonococci to epithelial cells in vitro involves heparan sulfate. J Exp Med 182:511–517, 1995.
56. Bos MP, Gruner F, Belland RJ: Differential recognition of members of the carcinoembryonic antigen family by Opa variants of *Neisseria gonorrhoeae*. Infect Immun 65:2353–2361, 1997.
57. Hauck CR, Meyer TF, Lang F, Gulbins E: CD66-mediated phagocytosis of Opa52 *Neisseria gonorrhoeae* requires a Src-like tyrosine kinase- and Rac1-dependent signaling pathway. EMBO J 17:443–454, 1998.
58. Draper DL, James JF, Brooks GF, et al: Comparison of virulence markers of peritoneal and fallopian tube isolates with endocervical *Neisseria gonorrhoeae* isolates from women with salpingitis. Infect Immun 27:882–888, 1980.
59. Plummer FA, Chubb H, Simonsen JN, et al: Antibodies to opacity proteins (opa) correlate with a reduced risk of gonococcal salpingitis. J Clin Invest 93:1748–1755, 1994.
60. Sparling PF, Elkins C, Wyrick PB, et al: Vaccines for bacterial sexually transmitted infections: A realistic goal? Proc Natl Acad Sci USA 91:2456–2463, 1994.
61. Parsons NJ, Curry A, Fox AJ, et al:. The serum resistance of gonococci in the majority of urethral exudates is due to sialylated lipopolysaccharide seen as a surface coat. FEMS Microbiol Lett 69:295–299, 1992.
62. Van Putten JP: Phase variation of lipopolysaccharide directs interconversion of invasive and immuno-resistant phenotypes of *Neisseria gonorrhoeae*. EMBO J 12:4043–4051, 1993.
63. Gorby GL, Ehrhardt AF, Apicella MA, Elkins C: Invasion of human fallopian tube epithelium by *Escherichia coli* expressing combinations of a gonococcal porin, opacity-associated protein, and chimeric lipo-oligosaccharide. J Infect Dis 184:460–472, 2001.
64. Anderson JE, Hobbs MM, Biswas GD, Sparling PF: Opposing selective forces for expression of the gonococcal lactoferrin receptor. Mol Microbiol 48:1325–1337, 2003.
65. Knapp JS, Clark VL: Anaerobic growth of *Neisseria gonorrhoeae* coupled to nitrite reduction. Infect Immun 76:176–181, 1984.
66. Jerse AE, Sharma ND, Simms AN, et al: A gonococcal efflux pump system enhances bacterial survival in a female mouse model of genital tract infection. Infect Immun 71:5576–5582, 2003.
67. Layh-Schmitt SG, Schmitts S, Buchanan TM: Interaction of non-piliated *Neisseria gonorrhoeae* strain 7122 and protein IA with an epithelial cell monolayer. Int J Med Microbiol Viral Parasitol Infect Dis 271:158–170, 1989.
68. Lynch EC, Blake MS, Gotschlich EC, et al: Studies of porins spontaneously transferred from whole cells and reconstituted from purified proteins of *Neisseria gonorrhoeae* and *Neisseria meningitidis*. Biophys J 45:104–107, 1984.

69. Young JDE, Blake MS, Mauro A, et al: Properties of the major outer membrane protein from *Neisseria gonorrhoeae* incorporated into model lipid membranes. Proc Natl Acad Sci USA 80:3831–3835, 1983.
70. Lorenzen DR, Gunther D, Pandit JF, et al: Neisseria gonorrhoeae porin modifies the oxidative burst of human professional phagocytes. Infect Immun 68:6215–6222, 2000.
71. Knapp JS, Tam MR, Nowinski RC, et al: Serological classification of *Neisseria gonorrhoeae* with use of monoclonal antibodies to gonococcal outer membrane protein I. J Infect Dis 150:44–48, 1984.
72. Brunham RC, Plummer F, Slaney L, et al: Correlation of auxotype and protein 1 type with expression of disease due to *Neisseria gonorrhoeae*. J Infect Dis 152:339–343, 1985.
73. Jarvis GA: Recognition and control of neisserial infection by antibody and complement. Trends Microbiol 3:198–201, 1995.
74. Britigan BE, Cohen MS, Sparling PF: Gonococcal infections: A model of molecular pathogenesis. N Engl J Med 312:1683–1694, 1985.
75. Heckels JE, Virji M: Antigenic variation of gonococcal pili: Immunochemical and biological studies. In Schoolnik GK, Brooks GF, Falkow S (eds): Pathogenic Neisseriae: Proceedings of the Fourth International Symposium on the Pathogenic Neisseriae. Washington, DC, American Society for Microbiology, 1985, p 288.
76. Fischer SH, Rest RF: Gonococci possessing only certain PII outer membrane proteins stimulate and adhere to human neutrophils. Infect Immun 56:1574–1579, 1988.
77. Hagblom P, Segal E, Billyard E, et al: Intragenic recombination leads to pilus antigenic variation in *Neisseria gonorrhoeae*. Nature 315:156–158, 1985.
78. Rice PA: Molecular basis for serum resistance in *Neisseria gonorrhoeae*. Clin Microbiol Rev 2:S112–S117, 1989.
79. Rice PA, Vayo HE, Tam MR, et al: Immunoglobulin G antibodies directed against protein III block killing of serum-resistant *Neisseria gonorrhoeae* by immune serum. J Exp Med 164:1735–1748, 1986.
80. Gotschlich EC, Blake MS, Seiff M: The DNA sequence of the structural gene of gonococcal protein III and the flanking region containing a repetitive sequence: Homology of protein III with enterobacterial OmpA proteins. J Exp Med 165:471–482, 1987.
81. Joiner KA, Scales R, Warren KA, et al: Mechanism of action of blocking immunoglobulin G for *Neisseria gonorrhoeae*. J Clin Invest 76:1765–1772, 1985.
82. Plummer FA, Chubb H, Simonsen JN, et al: Antibody to Rmp (outer membrane protein 3) increases susceptibility to gonococcal infection. J Clin Invest 91:339–343, 1993.
83. Kinghorn GR, Rashid S: Prevalence of rectal and pharyngeal infection in women with gonorrhea in Sheffield. Br J Vener Dis 55:408–410, 1979.
84. Wiesner PJ, Tronca E, Bonin P, et al: Clinical spectrum of pharyngeal gonococcal infections. N Engl J Med 288:181–185, 1973.
85. Holmes KK, Eschenbach DA, Knapp JS: Salpingitis: Overview of etiology and epidemiology. Am J Obstet Gynecol 138:893–900, 1980.
86. Westrom L: Incidence, prevalence and trends of acute pelvic inflammatory disease and its consequence in industrialized countries. Am J Obstet Gynecol 138:880–892, 1980.
87. Simms I, Warburton F, Westrom L: Diagnosis of pelvic inflammatory disease: Time for a rethink. Sex Trams Infect 79:491–494, 2003.
88. Sweet RL: Pelvic inflammatory disease. Hosp Pract 28(suppl):25–30, 1993.
89. Lopez-Zeno JA, Keith LG, Berger GS: The Fitz-Hugh–Curtis syndrome revisited: Changing perspectives after half a century. J Reprod Med 30:567–582, 1985.
90. Edwards LE, Barrada MI, Harmann AA, et al: Gonorrhea in pregnancy. Am J Obstet Gynecol 132:637–641, 1978.
91. Schulz KF, Cates W Jr, O'Mara RR: Pregnancy loss, infant death, and suffering: Legacy of syphilis and gonorrhea in Africa. Genitourin Med 63:320–325, 1987.
92. Alexander ER: Gonorrhea in the newborn. Ann N Y Acad Sci 549:180–186, 1988.
93. Hammerchlag MR, Cummings C, Roblin PM, et al: Efficacy of neonatal ocular prophylaxis for the prevention of chlamydial and gonococcal conjunctivitis. N Engl J Med 320:369–372, 1989.
94. Isenberg SJ, Apt L, Wood M: A controlled trial of povidone-iodine as prophylaxis against ophthalmia neonatorum. N Engl J Med 332:562–566, 1995.
95. Isenberg SJ, Apt L, Del Signore M, et al: A double application approach to ophthalmia neonatorum prophylaxis. Br J Ophthalmol 87:1449–1452, 2003.
96. Ellison RT III, Cord JG, Kohler PF, et al: Underlying complement deficiency in patients with disseminated gonococcal infection. Sex Transm Dis 14:20–204, 1987.
97. Zenilman JA: Gonorrhea. In Rein MF, Mandell GC (eds): Atlas of Infectious Diseases, Vol 5. Sexually Transmitted Disease. New York, Churchill Livingstone, 1996, pp 1.2–1.19.
98. Handsfield HH, Wiesner PJ, Holmes KK: Treatment of the gonococcal arthritis-dermatitis syndrome. Ann Intern Med 84:661–667, 1976.
99. O'Brien JP, Goldenberg DL, Rice PA, et al: Disseminated gonococcal infection: A prospective analysis of 49 patients and a review of the pathophysiology and immune mechanisms. Medicine (Baltimore) 2:395–406, 1983.
100. Holmes KK, Counts GW, Beaty HN: Disseminated gonococcal infection. Ann Intern Med 74:979–993, 1971.
101. Masi AT, Eisenstein BI: Disseminated gonococcal infection (DGI) and gonococcal arthritis (GCA). 2. Clinical manifestations, diagnosis, complications, treatment and prevention. Semin Arthritis Rheum 10:173–197, 1981.
102. Sayeed ZA, Bhaduri U, Howell E, et al: Gonococcal meningitis: A review. JAMA 219:1730–1731, 1972.
103. Rothenberg RB, Simon R, Chipperfield E, et al: Efficacy of selected diagnostic tests for sexually transmitted diseases. JAMA 235:49–51, 1976.
104. McCutchan JA: Epidemiology of venereal urethritis: Comparison of gonorrhea and nongonococcal urethritis. Rev Infect Dis 6:669–688, 1984.
105. Morello JM, Janda WM, Doern GU: Neisseria and Branhamella. In Belows A, Hausler WJ, Hermann KL, et al (eds): Manual of Clinical Microbiology, 5th ed. Washington, DC, American Society for Microbiology, 1991, p 258.
106. Ison CA: Laboratory methods in genitourinary medicine: Methods of diagnosing gonorrhea. Genitourin Med 66:453–459, 1990.
107. Jacobs NF, Kraus SJ: Gonococcal and nongonococcal urethritis in men: Clinical and laboratory differentiation. Ann Intern Med 82:7–12, 1975.
108. Ching S, Lee H, Hook EW, et al: Ligase chain reaction for detection of *Neisseria gonorrhoeae* in urogenital swabs. J Clin Microbiol 33:3111–3114, 1995.
109. Moncada J, Schachter J, Hook EW, et al: The effect of urine testing in evaluations of the sensitivity of the Gen-probe APTIMA Combo 2 Assay on endocervical swabs for *Chlamydia trachomatis* and *Neisseria gonorrhoeae*. Sex Transm Dis 31:273–277, 2004.
110. Mahony JB, Luinstra KE, Tyndall M, et al: Multiplex PCR for detection of *Chlamydia trachomatis* and *Neisseria gonorrhoeae* in genitourinary specimens. J Clin Microbiol 33:3049–3053, 1995.
111. Lachica ML, Fujikawa BK, Fahlk LD, et al: Use of the Aptima Combo2 nucleic acid amplification test for *Chlamydia trachomatis* and *Neisseria gonorrhoeae* in pharyngeal and rectal specimens. 103rd American Society of Microbiology meeting, Washington, DC, 2003.
112. Katz AR, Effler PV, Ohye RG, et al: False-positive gonorrhea test results with a nucleic acid amplification test: The impact of low prevalence on positive predictive value. Clin Infect Dis 38:814–819, 2004.
113. Klausner JD: The NAAT is out of the bag. Clin Infect Dis 38:820–821, 2004.
114. Ehret JM, Judson RN, Biddle JW: Gonorrhea. In Wentworth J, Judson FN (eds): Laboratory Methods for the Diagnosis of Sexually Transmitted Diseases. Washington, DC, American Public Health Association, 1984, p 43.
115. Thomason JL, Gelbart SM, Sobeiski VJ, et al: Effectiveness of Gonozyme for detection of gonorrhea in low-risk pregnant and gynecologic populations. Sex Transm Dis 16:28–31, 1989.
116. Hale YM, Melton ME, Lewis JS, et al: Evaluation of the PACE 2 *Neisseria gonorrhoeae* assay by three public health laboratories. J Clin Microbiol 31:451–453, 1993.
117. Iwen PC, Walker RA, Warren KL, et al: Evaluation of the nucleic acid-based test (PACE 2C) for simultaneous detection of *Chlamydia trachomatis* and *Neisseria gonorrhoeae* in endocervical specimens. J Clin Microbiol 33:2587–2591, 1995.
118. Franks AG: Successful combined treatment of penicillin-resistant gonorrhea. Am J Med 5c:211:553, 1946.
119. Sparling PF: Antibiotic resistance in the gonococcus. In Roberts RB (ed): The Gonococcus, Vol 1. New York, Wiley, 1977, p 111.
120. Cannon JG, Sparling PF: The genetics of the gonococcus. Annu Rev Microbiol 38:111–133, 1984.

121. Maness MJ, Foster GC, Sparling PF: Ribosomal resistance to streptomycin and spectramycin in *Neisseria gonorrhoeae*. J Bacteriol 120:1293–1299, 1974.
122. Philpot CR, Tapsall JW: Single-dose antibiotic therapy for the treatment of uncomplicated anogenital gonorrhea. Med J Aust 146:254–256, 1987.
123. Van Dyck E, Crabbe F, Nzila N, et al: Increasing resistance of *Neisseria gonorrhoeae* in West and Central Africa. Sex Transm Dis 24:32–37, 1997.
124. Fox K, Knapp JS, Holmes KK, et al: Antimicrobial resistance in *Neisseria gonorrhoeae* in the United States, 1988–1994: The emergence of decreased susceptibility to the fluoroquinolones. J Infect Dis 175S:1396–1403, 1997.
125. Knapp JS, Mesola VP, Neal SW, et al: Molecular epidemiology, in 1994, of *Neisseria gonorrhoeae* in Manila and Cebu City, Republic of the Philippines. Sex Transm Dis 24:2–7, 1997.
126. Chopra I, Hawkey PM, Hinton M: Tetracyclines, molecular and clinical aspects. J Antimicrob Chemother 29:245–277, 1992.
127. Antibiotic-resistant strains of *Neisseria gonorrhoeae*: Policy guidelines for detection, management, and control. MMWR 36(suppl 5):15, 1987.
128. 1993 Sexually transmitted diseases guidelines. MMWR 42(RR-14):1, 1993.
129. Centers for Disease Control and Prevention: Notice to readers: discontinuation of cefixime tablets—U.S. MMWR 51:1052, 2002.
130. California Department of Health Services, Sexually Transmitted Diseases (STD) Control Branch: California gonorrhea treatment guidelines. June 25, 2003.
131. Novak E, Paxton LM, Tubbs HJ, et al: Orally administered cefpodoxime proxetil for treatment of uncomplicated gonococcal urethritis in males: A dose-response study. Antimicrob Agents Chemother 36:1764–1765, 1992.
132. Jaffe HW, Schroeter AL, Reynolds GH, et al: Pharmacokinetic determinants of penicillin cure of gonococcal urethritis. Antimicrob Agents Chemother 15:587–591, 1979.
133. Neu HC, Chin NX, Labthavikul P: Comparative in vitro activity and beta-lactamase stability of PR 17027, a new orally active cephalosporin. Antimicrob Agents Chemother 26:174–180, 1984
134. Patel IH, Kaplan SA: Pharmacokinetic profile of ceftriaxone in man. Am J Med 77(suppl 4C):17–25, 1984.
135. Fluoroquinolone-resistant *Neisseria gonorrhoeae*, San Diego, 1997. MMWR 47:405–408, 1998.
136. Centers for Disease Control and Prevention: Sexually Transmitted Diseases Treatment Guidelines 2002. MMWR 51:1–80, 2002.
137. Haizlip J, Isbey SF, Hamilton HA, et al: Time required for elimination of *Neisseria gonorrhoeae* from the urogenital tract in men with symptomatic urethritis: Comparison of oral and intramuscular single-dose therapy. Sex Transm Dis 22:145–148, 1995.
138. Jaschek G, Gaydos CA, Welsh LE, et al: Direct detection of *Chlamydia trachomatis* in urine specimens from symptomatic and asymptomatic men by using a rapid polymerase chain reaction assay. J Clin Microbiol 31:1209–1212, 1993.
139. Batteiger BE, Jones RB: Chlamydial infections. Infect Dis Clin North Am 1:55–81, 1987.
140. Centers for Disease Control and Prevention: Increases in fluoroquinolone-resistant *Neisseria gonorrhoeae* among men who have sex with men—United States, 2003, and revised recommendations for gonorrhea treatment, 2004. MMWR 53:335–338, 2004.
141. Tanaka M, Matsumoto T, Kobayashi I, et al: Emergence of in vitro resistance to fluoroquinolones in *Neisseria gonorrhoeae* isolated in Japan. Antimicrob Agents Chemother 39:2367–2370, 1995.
142. Hook EW III, Roddy RE, Handsfield HH, et al. Ceftriaxone therapy for incubating and early syphilis. J Infect Dis 158:881–884, 1988.
143. Moran JS, Zenilman JM: Therapy for gonococcal infections: Options in 1989. Rev Infect Dis 12(suppl 6):S633–S644, 1990.
144. Lule G, Behets FM, Hoffman IF, et al: STD/HIV control in Malawi and the search for affordable and effective urethritis therapy: A first field evaluation. Genitourin Med 70:384–388, 1994.
145. May, R, Anderson R: Transmission dynamics of HIV infection. Nature 326:137–142, 1987.
146. Centers for Disease Control and Prevention: Update: Barrier protection against HIV infection and other sexually transmitted diseases. MMWR 30:589, 1993.
147. Soper DE, Shoupe D, Shangold GA, et al: Prevention of vaginal trachomoniasis by compliant use of the female condom. Sex Transm Dis 20:137–139, 1993.
148. Louv WC, Austin H, Alexander WJ, et al: A clinical trial of nonoxynol-9 for preventing gonococcal and chlamydial infections. J Infect Dis 158:518–523, 1988.
149. Greenberg L, Diena B, Ashton F, et al: Gonococcal vaccine studies in Inuvik. Can J Public Health 65:29–33, 1974.
150. Barbosa-Cesnik CT, Gerbase A, Heymann D: STD vaccines—an overview. Genitourin Med 73:336–342, 1997.
151. Adimora AA, Sparling PF, Cohen MS: Vaccines for classic sexually transmitted diseases (review). Infect Dis Clin North Am 8:859–876, 1994.
152. Zhu W, Thomas CE, Sparling PF: Immunization of mice with a plasmid encoding *Neisseria gonorrhoeae* PorB protein by intramuscular injection and epidermal particle bombardment. Vaccine 22:660–669, 2004.

27

Haemophilus ducreyi *Infections*

ALLAN RONALD

Haemophilus ducreyi (really an *Actinobacillus*) is a leading cause (along with syphilis and herpes simplex virus) of genital ulcers. Most prevalent in tropical developing areas, it likely predisposes to increased HIV acquisition and is an important target of sexually transmitted disease (STD) control programs.

AGENT

The organism *H. ducreyi* no longer is classified taxonomically by 16S rRNA within the *Haemophilus* genus but rather is more properly cited within the *Actinobacillus* cluster.[1] The organisms stain faintly with Gram's stain and are arranged in "school of fish" or "railway tracks" patterns. *H. ducreyi* is fastidious and grows best on media supplemented with vitamins, vancomycin to inhibit growth of gram-positive organisms, and charcoal to absorb toxic substances.[2] *H. ducreyi* has a capsule, pili, and several virulence factors.[3]

EPIDEMIOLOGY

H. ducreyi is spread only through sexual transmission. The organism has no known reservoir other than persons with ulcers that may not be clinically obvious and does not preclude individuals, particularly female sex workers, from transmitting it. The annual global incidence of chancroid has been reduced dramatically in the past decade and is now probably below 2 million. More than 99% of cases occur in developing countries, particularly southern Africa and India. Following exposure, uncircumcised men are three times more susceptible to infection. Among female sex workers in developing countries in the 1980s, as many as 10% had ulcers and were transmitting *H. ducreyi*.[4] *H. ducreyi* is readily transmitted between heterosexual partners during unprotected intercourse, with a risk of infection that exceeds 50%.[4] Chancroid also enhances the probability of HIV transmission. *H. ducreyi* ulceration recruits lymphocytes and macrophages to the mucosal surface and provides an easy target of entry for HIV from the genital secretions of the sexual partner.[5] HIV-infected

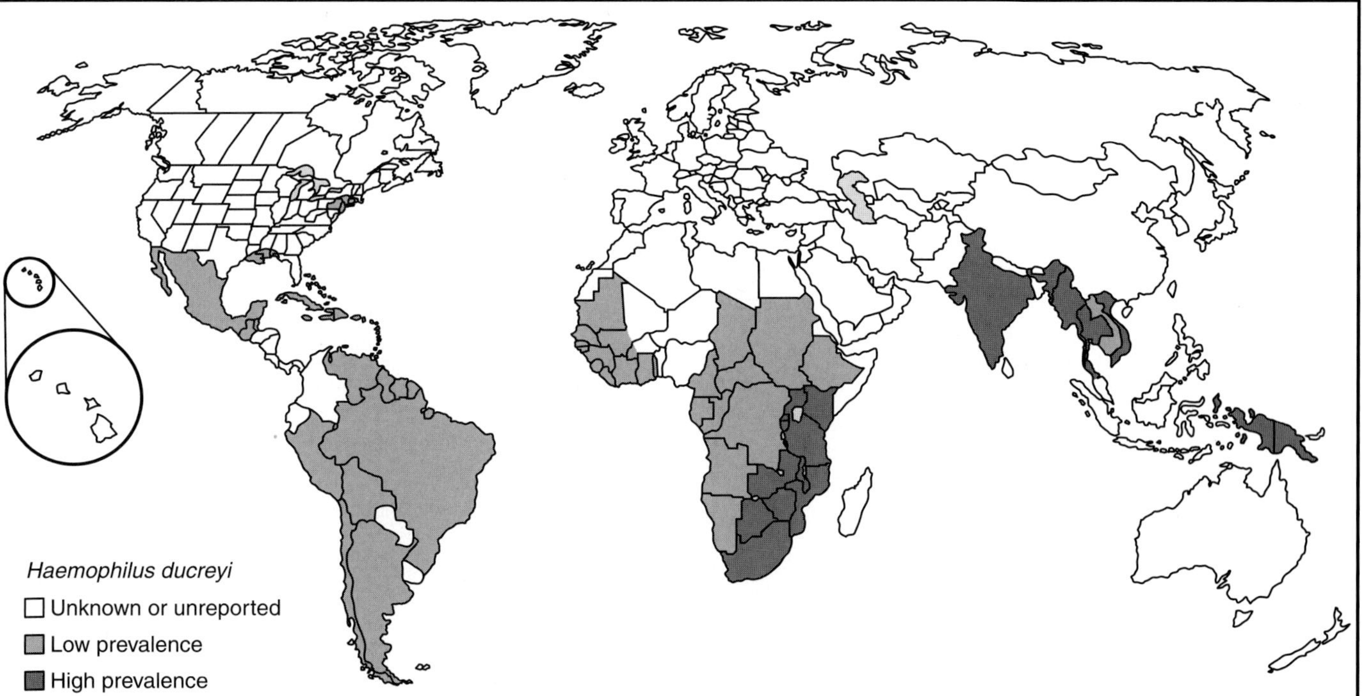

Note: Low prevalence of chancroid in southern United States, New York City area, the Caribbean, Latin America, and most of Africa. High prevalence in eastern and southern Africa, India, Thailand, and Indochina.
No recent global studies have ascertained the current prevalence of chancroid around the world so 1999 estimates are being used. However, *H. ducreyi* appears to have been controlled, reduced dramatically in incidence, and even eradicated from certain areas of the world during the past 5 years. For instance, there have been very few cases reported in East Africa, an area where chancroid was occurring in 10,000s annually during the 1980s and early 1990s.

persons who acquire chancroid excrete the virus in the ulcer and expose subsequent sexual partners to a substantive risk of infection. In some societies, the contribution of chancroid to the HIV epidemic may be as much as one-quarter of the total incidence of HIV infection.[6]

DISEASE

Chancroid is an ulcerating disease characterized by multiple shaggy undermining lesions on the genitalia. *H. ducreyi* does not cause systemic, invasive infection. The ulcers are usually painful, often quite superficial, and in about 40% of patients, associated with inguinal lymphadenitis. If untreated, the adenitis proceeds to bubo formation and may drain spontaneously, creating an inguinal abscess. In men, about half the ulcers occur on the prepuce and the rest on the glans, in the urethra, on the penile shaft, and on the scrotum and adjacent skin. Kissing lesions are common. In women the lesions occur commonly at the vestibular entrance, particularly on the posterior fourchette. However, numerous lesions are frequently widely present on the inner aspects of the labia majora and on the labia minora. Women with chancroid have a median of four ulcers.

Despite the apparent classic features of chancroid, numerous studies have shown that clinical etiologic identification and differentiation from syphilis, genital herpes, and granuloma inguinale is not possible.[7] As a result, syndromic management to include chancroid is essential for all patients with genital ulcer disease (GUD) if chancroid is endemic in the region.

PATHOGENESIS

H. ducreyi has cytotoxic and hemolytic proteins that are important determinants of virulence in both animal models and in human volunteer studies.[3] Attachment and invasion of epithelial cells are also necessary for virulence. The host response is predominantly mononuclear with a preponderance of activated T lymphocytes and macrophages.

DIAGNOSIS

H. ducreyi can be transported in supplemented thioglycollate transport media and kept for up to 24 hours at 4°C. However, ideally the culture should be plated immediately onto specially prepared chocolate media.[2] Growth is optimal at 32°C in a CO_2 environment with 100% humidity. A candle jar with a moistened paper towel provides a satisfactory environment. Growth often is not apparent before 48 hours. The opaque yellow-gray colony can usually be moved intact across the agar surface. Biochemical studies have limited use. Polymerase chain reaction (PCR) technology has been adapted to identify *H. ducreyi* from genital ulcer specimens and, when combined with PCR primers and probes for *Treponema pallidum* and herpes simplex virus, can identify the cause of GUD in most patients. Serologic tests for chancroid are neither specific nor sensitive.

TREATMENT

Chancroid can be effectively treated with erythromycin and with the fluoroquinolones. Most strains are resistant to ampicillin, tetracycline, and sulfonamides. Erythromycin is prescribed for 7 days in a dose of 500 mg three times a day.[8] Ciprofloxacin can be prescribed as a single daily dose of 500 mg.[8] Both regimens have cure rates in excess of 90%. Inguinal buboes should be incised or aspirated if they become fluctuant.

PREVENTION

Chancroid prevention requires implementation of conventional STD control initiatives. Primary prevention strategies include promotion of safer sex, widespread use of condoms, and partner referral with empiric treatment of contacts. Efforts to encourage early diagnosis through self-referral and appropriate syndromic treatment at the first point of contact with the health system are also important strategies. Routine examination of sex workers with empirical treatment of genital ulceration with regimens effective against chancroid and syphilis reduces the reservoir of this pathogen and rapidly reduces the incidence of chancroid. No vaccine is currently available. However, STD control measures are effective, even in resource-limited societies, and should be a high priority within the health-care system.

REFERENCES

1. Dewhirst FE, Paster BI, Olsen I, Fraser GJ: Phylogeny of 54 representative strains of species in the family Pasteurellaceae as determined by comparison of 16S rRNA sequences. J Bacteriol 174:2002–2013, 1992.
2. Trees DL, Morse SA: Chancroid and *Hemophilus ducreyi*: an update. Clin Microbiol Rev 8:357–375, 1995.
3. Spinola SM, Bauer ME, Munson JS II: Immunopathogenesis of *Hemophilus ducreyi* infection (chancroid). Infect Immun 70:1667–1676, 2002.
4. Plummer FA, D'Costa LJ, Nsanze H, et al: Epidemiology of chancroid and *Hemophilus ducreyi* in Nairobi. Lancet 2:1293–1295, 1983.
5. King R, Gough J, Ronald A, et al: An immunohistochemical analysis of naturally occurring chancroid. J Infect Dis 174:427–430, 1996.
6. Steen R: On eradicating chancroid. Bull World Health Org 79:818–826, 2001.
7. Ndinya-Achola JO, Kihara AN, Fisher LD, et al: Presumptive specific clinical diagnosis of genital ulcer disease (GUD) in a primary health care setting in Nairobi. Int J STD AIDS 7:201–205, 1996.
8. Malonza IM, Tyndall MW, Ndinya-Achola JO, et al: A randomized double-blind placebo-controlled trial of single dose ciprofloxacin versus azithromycin for the treatment of chancroid in Nairobi, Kenya. J Infect Dis 180:1886–1893, 1999.

28

Haemophilus influenzae (*Including* H. aegyptius) *Infection*

MARK C. STEINHOFF
THOMAS CHERIAN

INTRODUCTION

Haemophilus influenzae is among the most common causes of bacterial meningitis and other invasive infections in infants and young children throughout the world. Historically in the developing world, it has not been recognized as a vaccine-preventable cause of serious morbidity, long-term disability, and death. The availability of an effective vaccine against *H. influenzae* type b (Hib), which can virtually eliminate Hib disease, underscores the importance of determining the burden of vaccine-preventable illness caused by Hib. It also deserves recognition as a tropical illness in view of its global swath of illness and death.[1]

The related *Haemophilus aegyptius* is responsible for epidemic acute purulent conjunctivitis. This infection is more common in the developing world, for reasons that are not well understood. The epidemics of purpuric fever in Brazil caused by a strain of *H. aegyptius* are not a recent problem, and similar epidemics have not occurred elsewhere.

AGENTS

F. Pfeiffer in 1889 first described the "influenza bacillus" in Germany during an influenza epidemic, mistakenly reporting it as the cause of influenza. The genus *Haemophilus* ("blood-loving" in Greek) was formally named in 1920, to mark its requirement for blood substances in artificial media.

H. influenzae is a small, fastidious gram-negative bacterium that requires hemin (X factor) and nicotinamide adenine dinucleotide (NAD, or V factor) for growth on artificial media. NAD is not available in routine blood agar, which accounts for its apparent absence in laboratories that do not use chocolate agar (made by heating blood so that red blood cells lyse and release V factor), or supplemented media such as Fildes or Leventhal agar. The organism elaborates a polysaccharide capsule that permits classification into six distinct capsular serotypes (a through f). The capsular subtype b (Hib) has caused over 90% of all invasive infections. In addition, *H. influenzae* can be biochemically typed into six biotypes (I through VI). The biotypes and the capsular serotypes are distinct typing methods, not correlated with each other. The entire Hib chromosome was sequenced in 1995, the first free-living organism to be DNA sequenced.

The older *H. aegyptius* is found within *H. influenzae* biotype III and is closely related to serotype c. It was initially described by Robert Koch in Egypt in 1883 during an epidemic of conjunctivitis and subsequently isolated by Weeks. It is still referred to as the Koch-Weeks bacillus. Genomic analyses suggest that *H. aegyptius* is identical to *H. influenzae* with DNA homology of 80% to 100%. In 1984, a new clonal epidemic strain of *H. aegyptius* with unique pathogenic properties appeared in Brazil,[1] causing Brazilian purpuric fever (BPF). The specific clone has caused all cases of BPF and has some unique features that differentiate it from other *H. aegyptius* strains, though its growth requirements appear to be identical to those of *H. influenzae*. BPF has declined in importance since the 1990s.

EPIDEMIOLOGY

H. influenzae is part of the normal human nasopharyngeal flora and spreads by the airborne or direct contact routes from person to person. Nonencapsulated strains are frequently found in the upper respiratory tract. Among encapsulated strains, invasive type b is carried by 2% to 4% of children in North America. Carriage of type b organisms can occur in up to 30% of children in developing countries and in children in day-care centers in North America.[2] The Hib serotype causes most invasive disease, including bacteremia, meningitis, epiglottitis, pneumonia and empyema, septic arthritis, and cellulitis. In North America and Europe, the peak incidence of invasive Hib disease is from 6 to 12 months of age; in West Africa and India, the peak incidence is from 6 to 8 months.[3,4] Figure 28-1 and the map summarize data on incidence of Hib disease.[5,6] Among Eskimo and Native American children under 5 years of age, rates of Hib meningitis of up to 254 per 100,000 have occurred.[6] Data from developing countries are limited, but studies from Asia show lower incidences compared with Africa.[6–8]

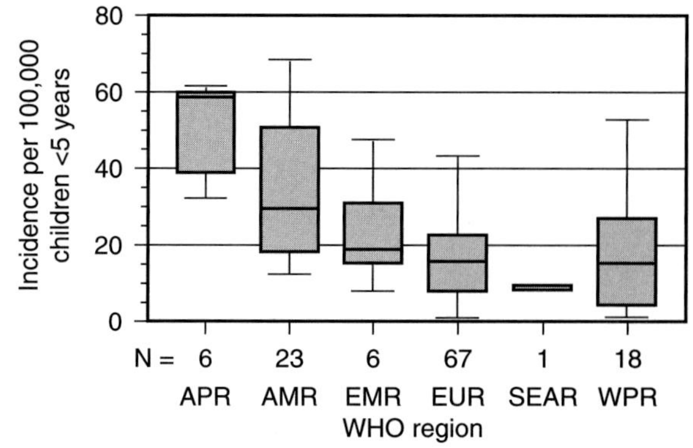

FIGURE 28-1 Incidence (mean, quartiles, range) of Hib meningitis in children under 5 years of age, by WHO region (excludes studies in special-risk groups). AMR, Americas; APR, Asia and Pacific Rim; EMR, Eastern Mediterranean region; EUR, Europe; SEAR, Southeast Asia region; WPR, Western Pacific region. (Adapted from *Haemophilus influenzae* type b [Hib] meningitis in the pre-vaccine era: A global review of incidence, age distributions, and case-fatality rates. WHO/V&B/02.18. Geneva, Switzerland, WHO, 2002.)

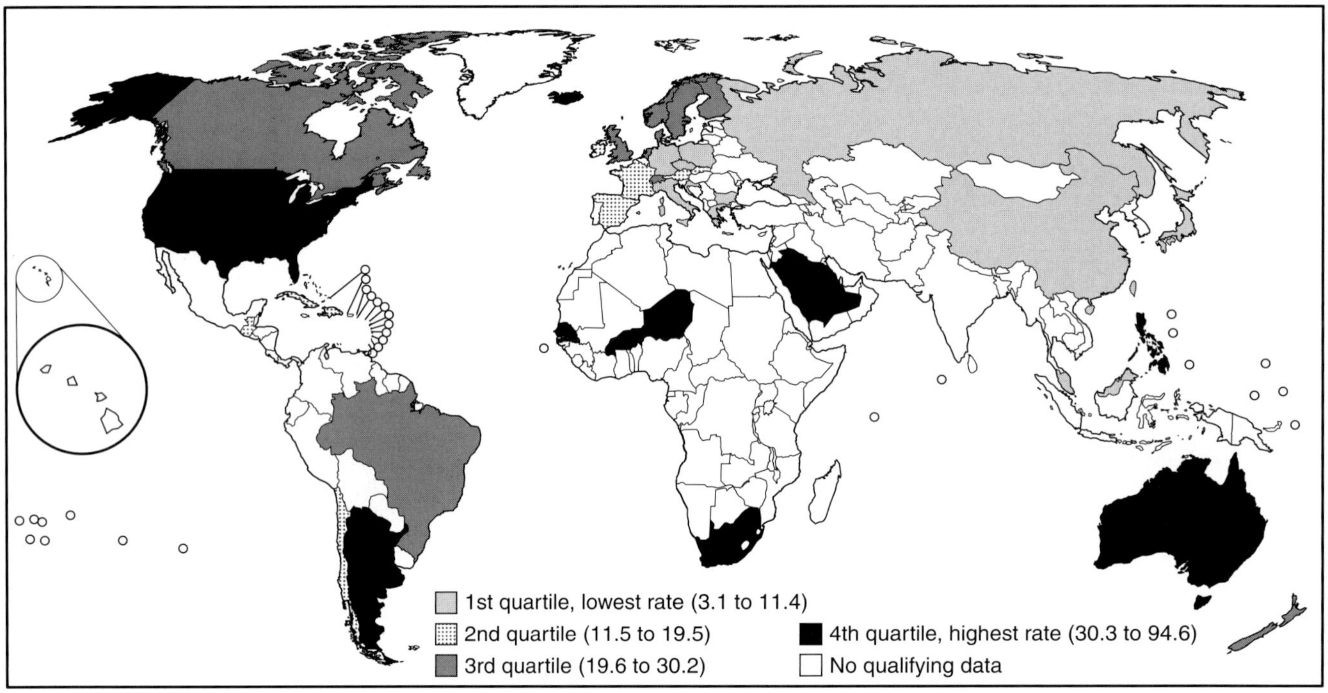

Country specific incidence, by quartile, of Hib meningitis per 100,000 children <5 years of age in the pre-vaccine era, 46 countries. (Adapted from *Haemophilus influenzae* type b (Hib) meningitis in the pre-vaccine era: a global review of incidence, age distributions, and case-fatality rates. WHO/V&B/02.18. Geneva, Switzerland: WHO 2002).

The epidemiology of *H. aegyptius* is not well described. It causes epidemics of purulent conjunctivitis, and outbreaks have occurred in both developed and developing countries. Preexisting trachoma is a major risk factor for epidemic conjunctivitis. In 1984, an outbreak of purpuric fever caused by *H. aegyptius* occurred in São Paulo, Brazil.[9] Although this organism is a common cause of conjunctivitis throughout the world, bacteremia was not reported prior to the epidemic of BPF in 1984. The majority of persons with conjunctivitis and with BPF have been children. The principal route of transmission seems to be direct inoculation from fingers to conjunctiva, but airborne spread may also occur.

DISEASE

Unencapsulated *H. influenzae* strains may cause sinusitis, otitis media, and bronchitis and may also cause pneumonia in children in developing regions or in adults with immune defects. Hib strains cause meningitis, bacteremia, pneumonia, epiglottitis, septic arthritis, pericarditis, and occult febrile bacteremia, as well as placentitis and peripartum septicemia in mothers. A small proportion of invasive disease is caused by other capsular types, notably, a and f.

About half of all reported invasive infections caused by Hib are meningitis, and before the introduction of Hib vaccine, Hib accounted for the majority of childhood bacterial meningitis cases worldwide, outside the meningococcal belt of Africa.[5,6] The clinical characteristics of Hib meningitis are similar among children of developing or developed countries, although the case-fatality rates may reach 40% in the former. Complications include subdural effusions, and central nervous system (CNS) sequelae occur in 11% to 40% of survivors of Hib meningitis, with deafness being a common finding. Hib epiglottitis was common in older children in North America and Europe but is rarely reported in developing countries.[4] Hib pneumonia is said to be infrequent in developed countries. However, in developing countries data on Hib pneumonia are mixed; lung tap and Hib vaccine studies indicate that Hib may cause from 4% to 30% of severe pneumonias in hospitalized patients.[10–13]

H. aegyptius produces a purulent vascular conjunctivitis, which often is bilateral and otherwise not pathognomonic. However, BPF is a unique syndrome.[9] It is a rapidly progressing illness with onset usually within a week of purulent conjunctivitis. Widespread petechiae followed by purpura, vascular collapse, and death usually occur within 1 to 2 days of the onset of the febrile illness. Although milder cases have been described, BPF appears to have a fulminant course with a high mortality rate.

PATHOGENESIS

Carriage of Hib in the nasopharynx is mediated by pili, which facilitate attachment to epithelial cells, and an immunoglobulin (Ig) A1 protease protects the organism from mucosal antibodies. Carriage increases following infection with influenza or other viruses. Most carried strains are nonencapsulated. Following carriage, encapsulated strains may invade the bloodstream and infect secondary sites, whereas nonencapsulated strains mainly cause disease by contiguous spread.

Type b strains have a pentose polysaccharide capsule composed of repeating units of phosphoribosyl phosphate (PRP), which is a critical virulence factor. The other serotypes have hexose polysaccharide capsules and are far less frequent in invasive disease. It has been known since the 1930s era of serotherapy that IgG antibody directed against the capsular polysaccharide can be used for therapy and is protective in an animal model. Specific anti-PRP antibody mediates opsonophagocytosis and is correlated with protection. The age-specific incidence of disease in human infants is inversely correlated with levels of serum anti-PRP antibody.[14]

H. aegyptius does not have a polysaccharide capsule, and the pathogenesis of conjunctivitis or BPF is not understood. The BPF clone has a lipooligosaccharide that varies significantly from non-BPF strains, and this clone possesses a unique pilin protein.[15] However, neither characteristic has been proved to have a specific role in its virulence. The role of host defenses is unknown.

DIAGNOSIS

H. influenzae is diagnosed by microbiologic isolation of the organism from a sterile site such as cerebrospinal fluid (CSF), blood, lung puncture, joint, or bone. The characteristic small, flat, colorless colonies are seen on subculture on chocolate agar. Hib excretes capsular polysaccharide, which can be seen by antigen detection techniques with latex agglutination in the blood, CSF, and urine. The sensitivity of urine antigen tests is variable, and false positives may occur in colonized children or those who have recently received Hib vaccine.

H. aegyptius is diagnosed by culture, usually from the conjunctiva. The BPF clone is present in blood cultures from patients with the syndrome, as well as in conjunctival cultures.

TREATMENT

Ampicillin or chloramphenicol has been the treatment of choice for all forms of invasive *H. influenzae* disease, but resistance to ampicillin emerged during the 1970s and to chloramphenicol in the 1990s and has reduced their usefulness in many regions.[4,16] Third-generation cephalosporins should be used for initial treatment depending on local susceptibility patterns. Cefotaxime 200 mg/kg/day in four doses or ceftriaxone 100 mg/kg once daily are regimens of first choice. Treatment for meningitis and sepsis syndromes should be continued for 7 to 10 days. Osteomyelitis requires a longer course of therapy, usually 2 weeks of parenteral therapy followed by 2 to 4 weeks of an oral regimen.

Controlled trials in children with Hib meningitis have shown that dexamethasone 0.15 mg/kg every 6 hours, given for 2 to 4 days with a third-generation cephalosporin reduces the occurrence of hearing loss, probably by modifying the inflammatory response. This may be less effective in the more advanced cases typically admitted to hospitals in developing regions.[17] *H. aegyptius* conjunctivitis has been treated both topically and systemically. Systemic treatment is preferred and, in particular, whenever outbreaks of BPF occur, systemic treatment is mandatory to forestall invasive disease. *H. aegyptius* has become resistant to ampicillin and chloramphenicol. Third-generation cephalosporins are effective alternatives. Trimethoprim-sulfamethoxazole can also been used for the treatment of conjunctivitis. Therapeutic efficacy studies in BPF are limited. Supportive measures are critical, however, to ensure survival when the clinical syndrome has fully developed.

PREVENTION

The virtual elimination of invasive Hib disease in many regions by vaccine is an outstanding success story of modern public health.[14] Polysaccharide PRP vaccines were effective in older children but were immunologically ineffective in infants at greatest risk. Conjugation of the polysaccharide to proteins stimulates a T cell–dependent antibody response in infants, with immunologic priming. Four different Hib PRP-protein conjugate vaccines effective in infants are now available. The vaccines have similar efficacy but differ in immunologic details. Hib meningitis virtually disappeared a few years after the introduction of protein-conjugated Hib PRP vaccines for infants in 1991 in the United States. This status was achieved even though the level of immunization among infants was lower than 80% in many urban regions, suggesting that reduction of carriage in vaccinees had a herd effect that resulted in protection of unvaccinated infants.[18] The experience of rapid disappearance of Hib meningitis within 1 to 2 years of introduction of routine immunization was replicated in Europe,[19] South America,[20] and West Africa.[21,22]

Current U.S. practice is to administer three doses of oligosaccharide-CRM_{197} conjugate Hib vaccine (HbOC) or PRP-T vaccine at 2, 4, and 6 months of age or two doses of PRP-OMP at 2 and 4 months, with a booster at 5 to 18 months. Because of the success of universal infant immunization in developed countries, and the reports of high efficacy of Hib conjugate vaccine in the prevention of invasive disease,[20,21,23] the World Health Organization (WHO) recommends the use of this vaccine wherever Hib disease is present.[24] Hib vaccines combined with diphtheria-tetanus-pertussis (DTP) vaccine are in use in the United States, and combination vaccines with Hib, DTP, and IPV are available elsewhere.

Passive immunization with monthly injections of human IgG can prevent Hib disease although this is not feasible in developing regions. Preventive treatment of unvaccinated household infant contacts with rifampicin is recommended in North America to reduce the 1% to 4% secondary attack rate in household and day-care contacts.

H. aegyptius is spread by hands and fomites. Eye-to-eye transmission can be reduced by hand washing and early effective treatment.

REFERENCES

1. Peltola H: Worldwide *Haemophilus influenzae* type b disease at the beginning of the 21st century: Global analysis of the disease burden 25 years after the use of the polysaccharide vaccine and a decade after the advent of conjugates. Clin Microbiol Rev 13:302–317, 2000.
2. Gessner BD, Sutanto A, Steinhoff M, et al: A population survey of *Haemophilus influenzae* type b nasopharyngeal carriage prevalence in Lombok Island, Indonesia. Pediatr Infect Dis J 17:S200–S204, 1998.
3. Bijlmer HA: World-wide epidemiology of *Haemophilus influenzae* meningitis: Industrialized versus non-industrialized countries. Vaccine 9 (suppl):S5–S9, 1991.
4. INCLEN Invasive Bacterial Infections Surveillance (IBIS) Group: Are *Haemophilus influenzae* infections a significant problem in India? A prospective study and review. Clin Infect Dis 34:949–957, 2002.

5. Funkhouser A, Steinhoff MC, Ward J: *Haemophilus influenzae* disease and immunization in developing countries. Rev Infect Dis 13:S542–S554, 1991.
6. *Haemophilus influenzae* type b (Hib) meningitis in the pre-vaccine era: A global review of incidence, age distributions, and case-fatality rates. WHO/V&B/02.18. Geneva, Switzerland, WHO, 2002.
7. Supachai R-N, Treleaven SC, Chunsuttiwat S, et al: Prospective population-based incidence of *Haemophilus influenzae* type b meningitis in Thailand. Vaccine 22:975–983, 2004.
8. Kim JS, Jang YT, Kim JD, et al: Incidence of Haemophilus *influenzae* type b and other invasive diseases in South Korean children. Vaccine 22:3952–3962, 2004.
9. Brazilian Purpuric Fever Study Group: *Haemophilus aeqypticus* bacteraemia in Brazilian purpuric fever. Lancet 2:761–763, 1987.
10. Hughes JR, Sinha DP, Cooper MR, et al: Lung tap in childhood: Bacteria, viruses, and mycoplasmas in acute lower respiratory tract infections. Pediatrics 44:477–485, 1969.
11. Mulholland K, Hilton S, Adegbola R, et al: Randomized trial of *Haemophilus influenzae* type b–tetanus protein conjugate for prevention of pneumonia and meningitis in Gambian infants. Lancet 349:1191–1197, 1997.
12. Gessner BD, Sutanto A, Linehan M, et al: Incidences of vaccine-preventable *Haemophilus influenzae* type b pneumonia and meningitis in Indonesian children: Hamlet-randomized vaccine probe design. Lancet 365:43–52, 2005.
13. De Andrade ALSS, de Andrade JG, Martelli CMT, et al: Effectiveness of *Haemophilus influenzae* b conjugate vaccine on childhood pneumonia: A case-control study in Brazil. Int J Epidemiol 33:173–181, 2004.
14. Robbins JB, Schneerson R, Anderson P, et al: The 1996 Albert Lasker Medical Research Awards. Prevention of systemic infections, especially meningitis, caused by *Haemophilus influenzae* type b: Impact on public health and implications for other polysaccharide-based vaccines. JAMA 276:1181–1185, 1996.
15. Rubin LG: Phase-variable expression of the 145-kDa surface protein of Brazilian purpuric fever case-clone strains of *Haemophilus influenzae* biogroup *aegyptius*. J Infect Dis 171:713–717, 1995.
16. Weinberg GA, Spizer ED, Murray PR, BOSTID Haemophilus Susceptibility Study Group: Antimicrobial susceptibility patterns of *Haemophilus* isolates from children in eleven developing nations. Bull World Health Organ 68:179–184, 1990.
17. Qazi SA, Khan MA, Mughal N, et al: Dexamethasone and bacterial meningitis in Pakistan. Arch Dis Child 75:482–488, 1996.
18. Adams WG, Deaver KA, Cochi SL, et al: Decline of childhood *Haemophilus influenzae* type b (Hib) disease in the Hib vaccine era. JAMA 269:221–226, 1993.
19. Peltola H, Kilpi T, Anttila M: Rapid disappearance of *Haemophilus influenzae* type b meningitis after routine childhood immunization with conjugate vaccines. Lancet 340:592–594, 1992.
20. Lagos R, Horwitz I, Toro J, et al: Large scale, postlicensure, selective vaccination of Chilean infants with PRP-T conjugate vaccine: Practicality and effectiveness in preventing invasive *Haemophilus influenzae* type b infections. Pediatr Infect Dis J 15:216–222, 1996.
21. Adegbola RA, Usen SO, Weber M, et al: Haemophilus influenzae type b meningitis in The Gambia after introduction of a conjugate vaccine. Lancet 354:1091–1092, 1999.
22. Steinhoff MC: *Haemophilus influenzae* type b infections are preventable everywhere. Lancet 349:1186–1187, 1997.
23. Wenger JD, DiFabio J-L, Landaverde JM, et al: Introduction of Hib conjugate vaccines in the non-industrialized world: Experience in four "newly adopting" countries. Vaccine 18:736–742, 2000.
24. Global Programme for Vaccines and Immunization (GPV): The WHO Position Paper on *Haemophilus influenzae* type b conjugate vaccines. Wkly Epidemiol Rec 73:64–68, 1998.

29

Calymmatobacterium granulomatis *Infection* (*Donovanosis*)

NIGEL O'FARRELL

INTRODUCTION

Donovanosis is a cause of genital ulceration found in a few diverse tropical countries. The condition has been known under many names, including serpiginous ulceration of the groin, ulcerating granuloma of the pudenda, granuloma genito-inguinale, infective granuloma, granuloma inguinale tropicum, chronic venereal sores, granuloma venereum, and, more commonly, granuloma inguinale. This variation in terminology has led to many cases of donovanosis being mistaken for lymphogranuloma venereum (see Chapter 48), a condition caused by *Chlamydia trachomatis serovars* L1–L3.

Donovanosis was first described by Macleod, Professor of Surgery in Calcutta in 1882[1] and the causative organism was recognised by Donovan in Madras in 1905.[2] Until recently, the organism has been classified as *Calymmatobacterium granulomatis*, a gram-negative bacillus. However, based on evidence of a phylogenetic similarity of 99% with *Klebsiella pneumoniae* and *K. rhinoscleromatis*, a proposal has been put forward that the organism be reclassified as *K. granulomatis comb nov*.[3] Lesser phylogenetic similarities with *Klebsiella* spp. have also been reported and further confirmatory studies are needed to determine whether *C. granulomatis* is indeed a unique species.[4]

AGENT

Classical Donovan bodies measure 1.5 × 0.7 μm and are usually found in macrophages and epithelial cells of the stratum malphigii. Characteristically there is a large mononuclear cell 25 to 90 μm in diameter with intra-cytoplasmic cysts filled with deeply stained Donovan bodies.[5] Initial attempts to culture the causative organism were unconvincing until 1943 when Anderson reported its isolation on the yolk sac of chick embryos and proposed a new genus, *Donovania*, and species, *granulomatis*.[6,7] Electron microscopy studies typically show organisms with gram-negative morphology and a large capsule but no flagella. Filiform vesicular protrusions may be seen on a corrugated cell wall.[8]

EPIDEMIOLOGY

Donovanosis has an unusual geographic distribution. Currently, it is found in Papua, New Guinea, South Africa—KwaZulu-Natal and Eastern Transvaal, parts of India and Brazil, and in aboriginal communities in Australia. Sporadic cases are occasionally reported elsewhere in Southern Africa, the West Indies, and South America. The largest epidemic recorded was in Papua, New Guinea, where 10,000 cases were reported in a population of 15,000 between 1922–1952.[9]

Following the recent move to syndromic reporting of sexually transmitted infections (STIs) in many developing countries, routine reporting of donovanosis has diminished considerably even in endemic areas. Prior to this change, a significant epidemic emerged in Durban, South Africa, where 3153 cases were reported from the main STI clinic in 1997.[10] Donovanosis also accounted for 11% and 16% of genital ulcers in men and women, respectively, in an earlier Durban study.[11,12] In Papua, New Guinea, the incidence of donovanosis is now decreasing but the condition was the second most common cause of genital ulceration in five health centers in 1989–1990.[13] In Pondicherry, south India, donovanosis accounted for 14% of genital ulcer cases in an STI clinic between 1993–1997.[14] In the Northern Territory region of Australia, reported cases decreased to less than 10 per year by 2002 from an estimated 300 cases in 1998, following the introduction of an eradication program.[15,16]

Donovanosis is generally regarded as an STI, albeit one with low infectivity. The case for sexual transmission is supported by the following: a history of sexual exposure before the appearance of lesions, increased incidence in most sexually active age groups, anal lesions in homosexual men practicing receptive anal intercourse, genital infection predominant, frequent concomitant STIs, and outbreaks linked to sex work. Although infection with donovanosis in sexual partners of index cases is not invariable, epidemiological treatment is advised, as lesions may not always be immediately obvious.

DISEASE

The incubation period is uncertain. Experimental lesions have been induced in humans 50 days after inoculation and this duration is probably a reasonable estimate.[17] The condition usually starts as a firm papule or subcutaneous nodule that subsequently ulcerates. Four types of lesions are reported: (1) Ulcerogranulomatous—the most common type—beefy-red, nontender, fleshy ulcers that bleed readily to the touch; (2) Hypertrophic or verrucous type—usually with a raised irregular edge, sometimes dry; (3) Necrotic—offensive-smelling ulcer causing tissue destruction; (4) Sclerotic or cicatricial lesion with fibrous and scar tissue.

The genital area is affected in 90% of cases and the inguinal region in 10% (Fig. 29-1). The usual sites of infection are, in men, coronal sulcus (Fig. 29-2), prepuce, and frenum, and in women, the labia minora and fourchette. Cervical lesions are uncommon but may mimic carcinoma. Extragenital lesions occur in 6% of cases and are usually associated with genital disease. Sites of infection include lip, gums, cheek, palate, pharynx, neck, nose, larynx, and chest.[18] Lymph gland enlargement is uncommon. Disseminated donovanosis is rare

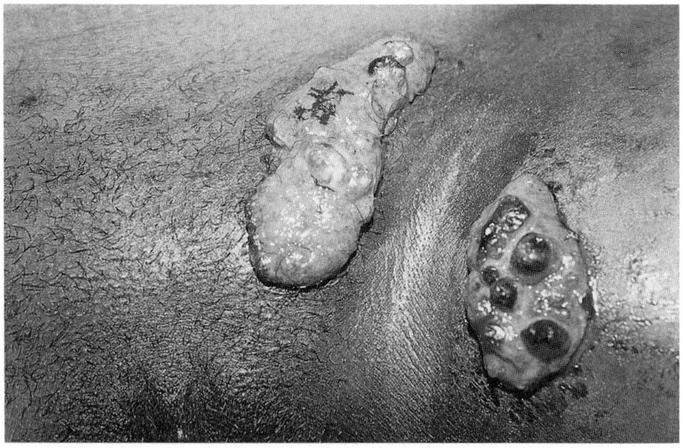

FIGURE 29-1 Inguinal lesions of donovanosis.

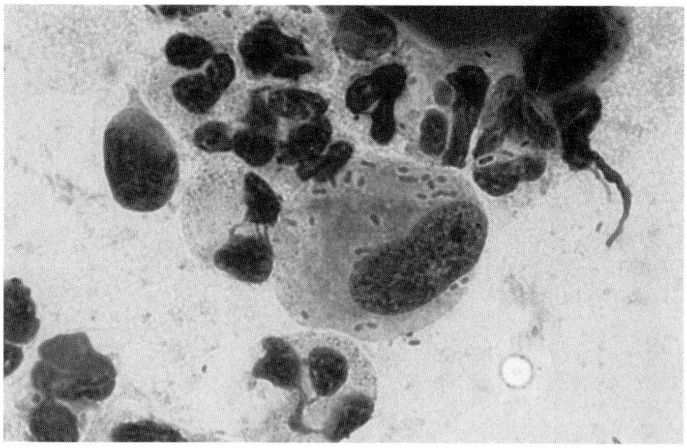

FIGURE 29-3 Tissue smear stained by rapid Giemsa (RapiDiff) technique showing numerous Donovan bodies in a monocyte.

but secondary spread to liver and bone may occur and is often associated with pregnancy and cervical lesions. Extragenital lesions may be difficult to differentiate from rhinoscleroma caused by *Klebsiella rhinoscleromatis.* Carcinoma is a serious but rare complication.

As a cause of genital ulceration that bleeds readily, it is not surprising that donovanosis is a risk factor for HIV infection. In Durban, the proportion of men diagnosed with donovanosis and HIV increased significantly as the duration of lesions increased suggesting that HIV was acquired through sexual intercourse despite ulceration.[19]

DIAGNOSIS

In endemic areas, a clinical diagnosis of genital donovanosis by experienced observers has a reasonably high positive predictive value.[20] If possible, confirmation of the diagnosis should be made before antibiotics are given so that definitive treatment can be given. The diagnosis is made by identifying intracellular Donovan bodies, sometimes capsulated, within large mononuclear cells in smears obtained either from tissue smears or biopsy samples (Fig. 29-3).

Tissue smears can be performed cheaply and quickly in busy clinics. However, to achieve the maximum positive yield, specimens must be prepared carefully. Debris should be removed from the ulcer by gently rolling a cotton-tipped swab across the lesion to minimize bleeding. Another swab should then be both rolled firmly across the ulcer to collect material and then across a glass slide so that material is spread evenly. The slide is air dried and stained by a rapid Giemsa method using eosin and thiazine solutions.[21] If multiple swabs are taken to detect other pathogens and donovanosis is suspected clinically, the tissue smear should be taken first so that an adequate amount of material can be collected.

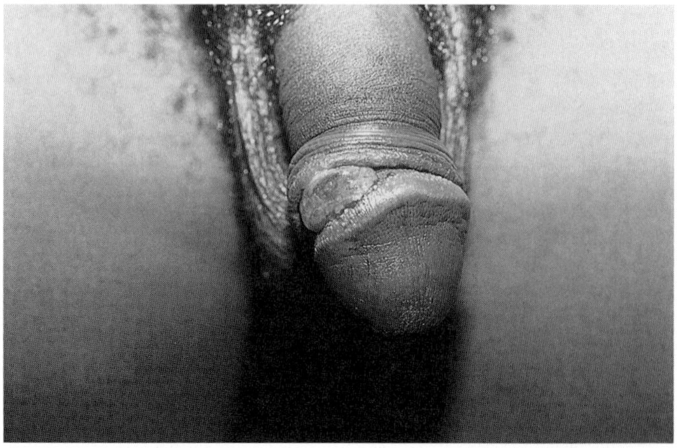

FIGURE 29-2 Typical penile donovanosis lesion.

In clinics where patients are likely to return, a crushed tissue smear using a slow overnight Giemsa method is preferable.[22] Pieces of tissue obtained by using a forceps and scalpel from the advancing surface of the ulcer are crushed between two slides and then stained.[23] If time and resources allow, biopsy specimens may offer a greater chance of confirming the diagnosis. The best stains to use are either Giemsa or silver. Histologic changes of donovanosis show epithelial proliferation with a heavy inflammatory infiltrate of plasma cells, neutrophils, and few lymphocytes. Biopsy is invariably required to confirm the diagnosis for necrotic and sclerotic ulcers and sometimes for hypertrophic lesions.

Culture of the causative organism has recently been the subject of a resurgence of interest. After a gap of 35 years, culture was reported from two centers in 1997—in Durban using a monocyte coculture system[24] and in Darwin, Australia, with a modified chlamydia culture system using human epithelial cell lines.[25]

Polymerase chain reaction (PCR) methods have also been developed for donovanosis.[4,26] In Darwin, amplification of *Klebsiella*-like sequences was achieved using primers targeting the phoE gene. A diagnostic PCR was developed using the observation that two unique base changes in the phoE gene eliminate Hae111 restriction sites enabling clear differentiation from closely related species of *Klebsiella*.[26,27] A colorimetric PCR test has since been developed for use in diagnostic laboratories.[28]

Serologic testing with an indirect immunofluorescence method using tissue sections from known donovanosis cases has been undertaken but the sensitivity of this method is low for early lesions.[29] Other diagnostic methods, now superseded, include antigen detection, complement fixation, and skin tests.

In communities where donovanosis is prevalent, practitioners should have a high index of suspicion and be able to make a reasonably accurate clinical diagnosis in most cases. However, other causes of genital ulceration—primary syphilis, condylomata lata of secondary syphilis (see Chapter 44), chancroid (see Chapter 27) and large HIV-associated herpes ulcers (see Chapter 76)—should also be considered. Amebiasis (see Chapter 86) and carcinoma may mimic necrotic donovanosis. Dual infection with one or more of the classical causes of genital ulcers should always be considered, particularly if there is a delay in seeking medical attention. In developed countries, a history of travel to and sex in an endemic country (see Chapter 132) may point to a diagnosis of donovanosis.[30]

TREATMENT AND PROGNOSIS

WHO guidelines recommend azithromycin 1 g followed by 500 mg daily until all lesions have healed.[31] In Australia, either azithromycin 1 g weekly for 4 to 6 weeks or 500 mg once daily for 1 week were both effective.[32] The CDC recommends azithromycin 1 g weekly for at least 3 weeks or until all lesions have healed.[33] Other antibiotics should probably be given for 3 weeks or until all lesions are healed and include: co-trimoxazole 160–800 mg twice daily, ciprofloxacin 750 mg twice daily, doxycycline 100 mg twice daily. Gentamicin 1 mg/kg 3 times daily intramuscularly or intravenously can be given if there is no response in the first few days with other regimens. Ceftriaxone, norfloxacin, and trovofloxacin have also proved effective. Surgery may have to be undertaken for intractable lesions that cause gross tissue destruction.

The introduction of syndromic STI management has significant implications for the management of donovanosis. Traditional syndromic algorithms for genital ulcers have advised treating for syphilis and chancroid although, more recently, herpes management has also been included. Optimal treatment for donovanosis differs from chancroid and areas with significant prevalences of donovanosis should therefore have their own local algorithms that will ensure adequate treatment for possible cases. A good example of this local approach is in Australia where azithromycin is the drug of choice when donovanosis is suspected amongst aboriginals.[16] In the past, azithromycin has often been excluded from treatment protocols because of cost but its price has decreased considerably and it should now be the universal first choice treatment for donovanosis.

A neglected aspect in the management of donovanosis is the psychologic distress to which some patients, particularly those with long-standing disease, are subjected to. The importance of case management for donovanosis is therefore still very important. Many patients present with long-standing disease and previously have sought health care elsewhere. In these cases confirmation of the diagnosis should be sought so that specific treatment can be given for donovanosis. Patients should be seen in a confidential setting and informed that they have an unusual condition that will respond to antibiotics over time. Poor genital hygiene may be a predisposing factor[18] and the need to wash behind the foreskin in men with subpreputial lesions should be mentioned. The report that azithromycin for 1 week is effective is particularly important for the management of patients who have to travel long distances.

It is unclear whether HIV alters the response of donovanosis ulcers to treatment. In Durban, the clinical response to treatment was unaltered in HIV-positive pregnant women[34] but in India, ulcers in HIV-positive subjects took slightly longer to heal than in HIV-negative subjects.[35] Although there is no data about azithromycin for donovanosis in HIV-positive subjects, it would be surprising if it were not shown to be effective.

PREVENTION AND CONTROL

The fact that significant numbers of donovanosis cases are found in only a few geographic locations makes the condition particularly suitable for targeted initiatives for disease control. In Papua, New Guinea, the large epidemic was controlled by annual examination, registration of the population, compulsory treatment, and assistance from the police in detaining patients reluctant to cooperate with the authorities.[9] Also in Papua, in the Goilala District, where 3.4% of the local population were infected with donovanosis, successful control measures included house-to-house visits with on-site medical examinations.[36] When antibiotics first became available in the United States, donovanosis elimination programs were initiated by some states. More recently a donovanosis eradication program targeting aboriginal and Torres Strait Islander populations in Australia commenced in 1996.[16] This intervention has reduced the number of cases significantly and owes much to strong political commitment supported with resources to heighten awareness of donovanosis at the primary health-care level.

Female sex workers have been implicated as source contacts of index cases in the United States[37] and Papua, New Guinea,[38] and usually have detectable lesions if infected. Clearly health-care providers working with sex workers in donovanosis endemic areas should be targeted to increase awareness of donovanosis.

Control of genital ulcers is one strategy that could be important in limiting the spread of HIV.[39] It is therefore noteworthy that the numbers of cases of HIV attributable to heterosexual sex is still very low in the Northern Territory, Australia, where a sustained program to eliminate donovanosis has now been in place for some years.[15] Global eradication of donovanosis remains a distinct possibility but will require significant inputs from those in endemic areas if it is to be accepted onto the WHO disease eradication agenda.[40]

REFERENCES

1. McLeod K: Precis of operations performed in the wards of the first surgeon, Medical College Hospital, during the year 1881. Indian Med Gaz 17:113, 1882.
2. Donovan C: Medical cases from Madras General Hospital. Indian Med Gaz 40:411, 1905.
3. Carter J, Bowden FJ, Bastian I, et al: Phylogenetic evidence for reclassification of *Calymmatobacterium granulomatis* as *Klebsiella granulomatis comb nov*. Int J Syst Bacteriol 49:1695, 1999.
4. Kharsany AB, Hoosen AA, Kiepala P, et al: Phylogenetic analysis of *Calymmatobacterium granulomatis* based on 16S sequences. J Med Microbiol 48:841, 1999.
5. Pund ER, Greenblatt RB: Specific histology of granuloma inguinale. Arch Path 23:224, 1937.

6. Anderson K: The cultivation from granuloma inguinale of a micro-organism having the characteristics of Donovan bodies in the yolk sacs of chick embryos. Science 97:560, 1943.
7. Anderson K: An etiologic consideration of *Donovania granulomatis* cultivated from three cases in embryonic yolk. J Exp Med 81:25, 1945.
8. Kharsany AB, Hoosen AA, Naicker T, et al: Ultrastructure of *Calymmatobacterium granulomatis*: Comparison of culture with tissue biopsy specimens. J Med Microbiol 47:1069, 1998.
9. Vogel LC, Richens J: Donovanosis in Dutch South New Guinea: History, evolution of the epidemic and control. PNG Med J 32:203, 1989.
10. Annual report of the Medical Officer of Health for Durban 1997.
11. O'Farrell N, Hoosen AA, Coetzee K, et al: Genital ulcer disease in men in Durban, South Africa. Genitourin Med 67:327, 1991.
12. O'Farrell N, Hoosen AA, Coetzee K, et al: Genital ulcer disease in women in Durban, South Africa. Genitourin Med 67:322, 1991.
13. Hudson BJ, van der Meidjen W, Lupiwa T, et al: A survey of sexually transmitted diseases in five STD clinics in Papua, New Guinea. PNG Med J 37:152, 1994.
14. Thappa DM, Singh S, Singh A: HIV infection and sexually transmitted diseases in a referral STD centre in South India. Sex Transm Inf 75:191, 1999.
15. Department of Heath and Community Services. Northern Territory AIDS/ STD Program Surveillance Update: Vol. 3(No. 2), 2002.
16. Miller P: Donovanosis control or eradication? A situation review of donovanosis in Aboriginal and Torres Strait Islander populations in Australia. Commonwealth Department of Health and Aged Care, 2001.
17. Greenblatt RB, Diernst RB, Pund ER, et al: Experimental and clinical granuloma inguinale. JAMA 113:1109, 1939.
18. Rajam RV, Rangiah PN: Donovanosis. WHO Monograph Series No. 24, Geneva, 1954.
19. O'Farrell N, Windsor I, Becker P: Risk factors for HIV-1 in heterosexual attenders at a sexually transmitted diseases clinic in Durban. S Afr Med J 80:17, 1991.
20. O'Farrell N, Hoosen AA, Coetzee KD, et al: Genital ulcer disease: Accuracy of clinical diagnosis and strategies to improve control in Durban, South Africa. Genitourin Med 70:7, 1994.
21. O'Farrell N: A rapid staining technique for the diagnosis of granuloma inguinale (donovanosis). Genitourin Med 66:200, 1990.
22. Sehgal VN, Jain MK: Tissue section Donovan Bodies—Identification through slow-Giemsa (overnight) technique. Dermatologica 174:228, 1987.
23. Cannefax GR: The technique of the tissue spread method for demonstrating Donovan Bodies. J Vener Dis Inf 201:201, 1948.
24. Kharsany AB, Hoosen AA, Kiepala P, et al: Growth and cultural characteristics of *Calymmatobacterium granulomatis*: The aetiological agent of granuloma inguinale (donovanosis). J Med Microbiol 46:579, 1997.
25. Carter J, Hutton S, Sriprakash KS, et al: Culture of the causative organism for donovanosis (*Calymmatobacterium granulomatis*). J Clin Micro 35:487, 1997.
26. Bastian I, Bowden FJ: Amplification of *Klebsiella*-like sequences from biopsy samples from patients with donovanosis. Clin Infect Dis 23:1328, 1996.
27. Carter JS, Bowden FJ, Sriprakash KS, et al: Diagnostic polymerase chain reaction for donovanosis. Clin Infect Dis 28:1168, 1999.
28. Carter JS, Kemp DJ: A colorimetric detection system for *Calymmatobacterium granulomatis*. Sex Transm Inf 76:134, 2000.
29. Freinkel AL, Dangor Y, Koornhoff HJ, et al: A serological test for Granuloma inguinale. Genitourin Med 68:269, 1992.
30. Morrone A, Toma L, Franco G, et al: Donovanosis in developed countries: Neglected or misdiagnosed disease? Int J STD & AIDS 14:288, 2003.
31. WHO Guidelines for the Management of Sexually Transmitted Infections. 2003.
32. Bowden FJ, Mein J, Plunkett C, et al: Pilot study of azithromycin in the treatment of genital donovanosis. Genitourin Med 72:17, 1994.
33. CDC. Sexually transmitted diseases treatment guidelines. MMWR 51:RR6, 2002.
34. Hoosen AA, Mphatsoe M, Kharsany AB, et al: Granuloma inguinale in association with pregnancy and HIV infection. Int J Gynecol Obstet 53:133, 1996.
35. Jamkhedkar PP, Hira SK, Shroff HJ, et al: Clinico-epidemiologic features of granuloma inguinale in the era of acquired immune deficiency syndrome. Sex Transm Dis 25:196, 1998.
36. Zigas V: A donovanosis project in Goilala 1951–1954. PNG Med J 14:148, 1951.
37. Rosen T, Tschen JA, Ramsdell W, et al: Granuloma inguinale. J Am Acad Dermatol 11:433, 1984.
38. Maddocks I: Donovanosis in Papua. PNG Med J 10:49, 1967.
39. O'Farrell N: Genital ulcers, stigma, HIV and STI control in sub-Saharan Africa. Sex Trans Inf 78:143, 2002.
40. O'Farrell N: Global eradication of donovanosis: An opportunity for limiting the spread of HIV-1 infection. Genitourin Med 71:27, 1995.

30

Pneumococcal Infections

ELAINE TUOMANEN
KEITH P. KLUGMAN

INTRODUCTION

Acute respiratory infections are the leading cause of infectious disease mortality[1] and morbidity among children in developing countries[2] (Fig. 30-1). Until 1965, acute respiratory infections caused 25% of all deaths in children younger than 5 years old in European countries with adult life expectancy greater than 45 years compared to 4% of childhood deaths in countries with adult life expectancy greater than 70 years. During the 1980s, acute respiratory infections caused a mean of 18.8% of mortality in children younger than 5 years old in developing countries.[2] An analysis has shown that the percentage of infant mortality attributable to pneumonia is increased as the infant mortality rate increases.[3] Most fatal pneumonia in children is caused by *Haemophilus influenzae* or *Streptococcus pneumoniae*,[4] and the pneumococcus is also the most important cause of pneumonia in adults.[5,6] The pneumococcus is also a leading bacterial pathogen in the cause of meningitis throughout the world, including tropical countries.[7] It is estimated that approximately three of every four children on Earth will have had at least one episode of acute otitis media by the age of 3 years and the pneumococcus is the leading bacterial pathogen responsible for between 25% and 50% of cases of acute otitis media.[8] The pneumococcus is an important cause of sinusitis[9] and can also rarely cause other infections, such as peritonitis (associated with infections of the reproductive organs[10] or with the nephrotic syndrome),[11] endocarditis, septic arthritis, osteomyelitis, epidural and brain abscesses, as well as soft tissue infections.[12]

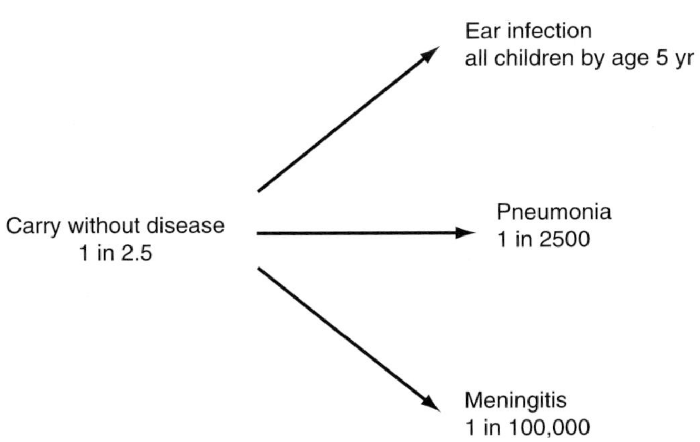

FIGURE 30-1 Prevalence of pneumococcal infection in children.

AGENT

The pneumococcus is a Gram-positive coccus that is usually identified on the basis of optochin susceptibility and bile solubility. It can also be identified by its reaction with specific antisera. There are 90 pneumococcal serotypes described.[13]

Although the first observation of the organism now known as *S. pneumoniae* was made by Klebs in 1875,[14] the significance of this observation eluded him[15] and the discovery of the organism is often credited to Pasteur[16] and Sternberg,[17] who in 1881 passaged the organism from human saliva in rabbits and noticed that it caused a fatal septicemia in the animals. After much debate, it was recognized in 1883 to be a cause of lobar pneumonia by Friedländer.[18]

Fifty years later, driven by a desire to understand the lethal events in pneumococcal pneumonia, Griffith[19] and Alloway[20] demonstrated that the capsular polysaccharide was the essence of virulence of pneumococci, and capsular production could be naturally transferred as a heritable trait by an exogenous chemical substance, the transforming principle. In 1944, Avery and colleagues[21] showed that the transforming principle was DNA. During the next 50 years, the study of pneumococcal infection produced the first nonprotein vaccine,[22] suggested mechanisms for the action of penicillin and antibiotic tolerance,[23] and uncovered the complex structure and inflammatory properties of gram-positive peptidoglycan.[24,25] Historically, the pneumococcus has thus provided a rich resource for the discovery of important tenets in medicine.[26]

EPIDEMIOLOGY

Although primary immunodeficiencies, including immunoglobulin subclass deficiencies, predispose to pneumococcal infection, by far the most important risk factors in adults in developed countries are smoking and chronic obstructive pulmonary disease, as well as underlying systemic diseases such as liver failure, renal failure, alcoholism, sickle cell disease, lymphoma, and leukemia. Invasive pneumococcal disease is common, however, in crowded communities as disparate as the crowded huts of rural villages in Papua New Guinea[27] and the jails of modern urban America.[28] The disease is more common in winter, probably due to increased carriage[29] and increased antecedent viral infections at that time of the year.

The emergence of human immunodeficiency virus (HIV) infection as a specific risk factor for invasive pneumococcal disease was first described when an excess of pneumococcal pneumonias was found among patients with acquired immunodeficiency syndrome (AIDS) in 1984.[30] The incidence of pneumococcal bacteremia in AIDS patients was subsequently shown to be approximately 100 times greater than that in patients without AIDS.[31] In some African countries, HIV is now the dominant risk factor for invasive pneumococcal disease in adults[32,33] and children.[34] Risk factors for invasive pneumococcal disease in HIV-infected people include a CD4 count of less than 200 cells per microliter, a previous history of pneumonia, and a serum albumin value less than 3 g/dL.[35] HIV-infected patients with pneumonia have an increased incidence of bacteremia and, in particular, recurrent bacteremias.[9,36] In a study on invasive pneumococcal disease in a cohort of sex workers in Nairobi, there was a pneumococcal bacteremia rate of 2.38% per annum with a recurrence rate of 19.1% in those who previously had had pneumococcal bacteremia. The distribution of disease associated with bacteremia was somewhat unusual in that although the majority of cases had pneumonia, 30% had sinusitis and 11% had occult bacteremia.[9] These workers also noted a large decline in the CD4 count (mean of 105/μL) during the acute infection. HIV-infected patients usually respond well to standard antibiotic therapy.[9,36] Molecular analysis of repeat episodes of pneumococcal bacteremia in Kenya have documented reinfection with a serotype different from that previously isolated, coinfection with more than one serotype at the same time, and relapse with recurrent disease caused by a serotype identical to that previously isolated from the patient.[37] Data suggest that pediatric serotypes are more common in HIV-infected people,[32,38] particularly women.[32]

Antibiotic Resistance

Penicillin resistance of the pneumococcus was first described by Hansman and Bullen in Australia in 1967.[39] Until the 1980s, the focus of resistance was Papua New Guinea, South Africa, and Spain[40]; although the incidence of resistance in most developed countries remained low, very few data were available from developing countries. The 1990s witnessed a dramatic increase in resistance worldwide, including Southeast Asia.[41] Studies in Pakistan,[42] South Africa,[43,44] and elsewhere have documented a similar rate of resistance in isolates obtained from nasopharyngeal swabs from children attending outpatient clinics, or on admission to hospital, compared with isolates from blood and cerebrospinal fluid (CSF). This allows the possibility of determining the incidence of resistance in small field trials that focus on nasopharyngeal carriage. Such studies have been reported from many countries, including the Central African Republic,[45] Zambia,[46] and Malawi.[47] Although a direct association between the total use of antibiotics in a given country and antibiotic resistance has not been documented in developing countries, this association has been documented for the pneumococcus in Europe.[48] Antimicrobial agents are freely available in most developing countries, but there are some poor countries with populations not exposed to antibiotics and these populations may harbor pneumococci with very low levels of resistance. Such a situation has been documented in Lesotho[49] and in Nepal.[50] Macrolide resistance is increasingly common in pneumococci but may be expected to be more common in developed countries where these more expensive drugs are widely used. In developing communities, mass treatment with azithromycin for trachoma may increase the isolation of macrolides-resistant pneumococci, particularly if these strains are preexistent in the community.[50,51] Among the oral agents, resistance to trimethoprim-sulfamethoxazole is of particular concern because of its widespread use in the treatment of pneumonia, as prophylaxis in HIV-infected patients in developing countries, and its ability to select multiresistant strains.[47] Fansidar therapy for malaria

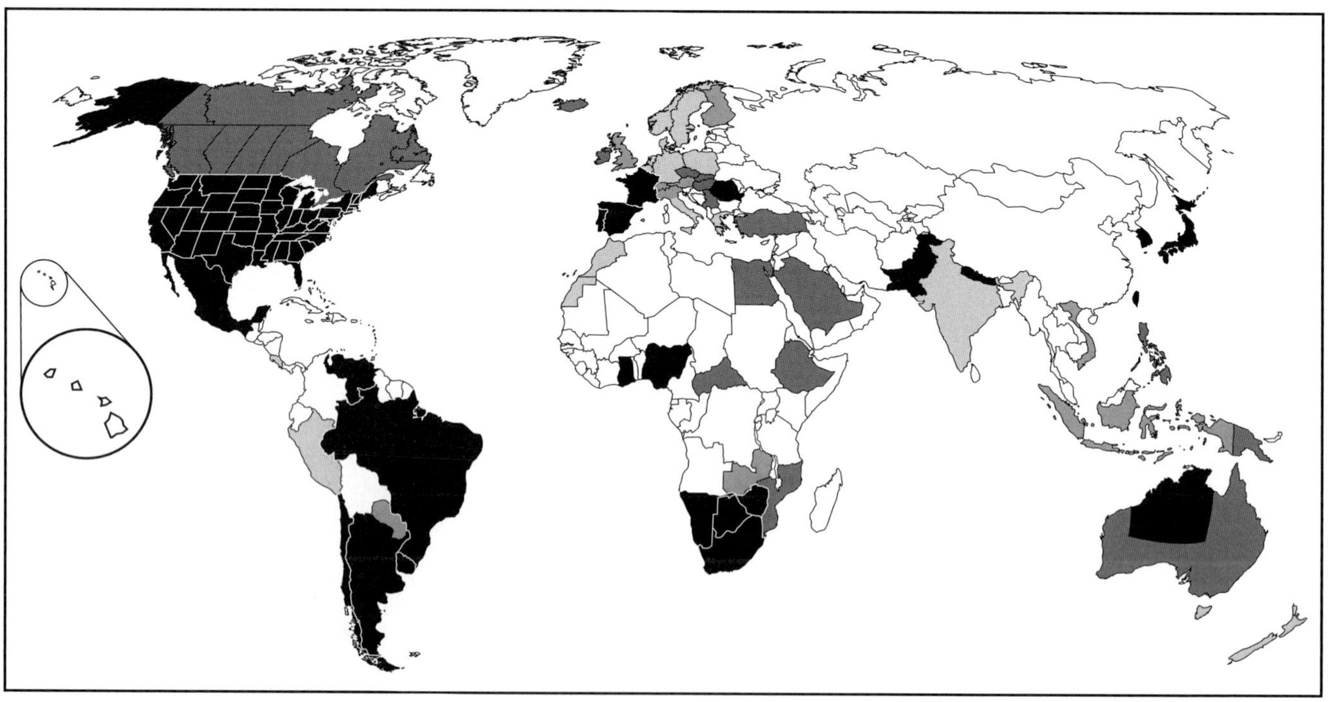

Global prevalence of penicillin resistance in the pneumococcus

□ Unknown
■ <5%
■ 5–10%
■ 10–25%
■ >25%

has been shown to select trimethoprim sulfamethoxazole resistance in pneumococci isolated from the nasopharynx of exposed children in Malawi.[52]

PATHOGENESIS AND IMMUNITY

Only with the very recent advent of genome sequencing and new genetic strategies amenable to mutation of gram-positive bacteria have the actual components of the pneumococcus that orchestrate disease become approachable. Sequences of several pneumococcal genomes have been published[53,54] and functional genomic screening, such as by signature tagged mutagenesis or microarray analysis, has identified many new virulence determinants and their regulatory mechanisms (Fig. 30-2).[55–60]

Targeting Pneumococci to Several Niches in the Host

Pneumococci are harbored asymptomatically in the nasopharynx by approximately 50% of the population at any given time.[61] Pneumococci bind to nasopharyngeal cells by several protein "adhesins," the most dominant of which is choline-binding protein A (CbpA). CbpA binds secretory component of IgA on the surface of the epithelium, allowing the bacteria to enter and translocate across the cell.[62,63]

Progression to overt disease is more frequent upon acquisition of a new serotype[64] or following a viral respiratory tract infection, particularly influenza.[65] On gaining access to the lung, pneumococci adhere to and invade cytokine-activated lung and endothelial cells by binding to the platelet-activating factor (PAF) receptor on activated cells. Pneumococci bound to the PAF receptor are internalized and migrate across eukaryotic cells in a vacuole, suggesting this as a route of entry for invasive disease.[66] The ability of PAF receptor antagonists to block internalization and transmigration in vitro and to interrupt progression from pneumonia to bacteremia in animal models is consistent with this pathogenetic mechanism.

Invasion is the result of the coordinate activity of several virulence determinants. The activities of individual adhesive ligands appear to be controlled by several global regulatory pathways that adjust the bacterial surface composition in response to environmental cues.[56] High-frequency phase variation in colonial morphology is a marker for a reversible transition between virulent (transparent colonies) and avirulent (opaque colonies) phenotypes.[67] Modulation of virulence is also seen in mutants in two component signal transduction systems.[68] Invasion and host tissue damage are potentiated by the production of pneumolysin, a 53-kDa, thiol-activated, pore-forming cytolysin, and by the production of hydrogen peroxide.[69,70] Once in the bloodstream, progression to pneumococcal meningitis usually occurs in conjunction with a high-grade septicemia. Invasion of the subarachnoid space may relate to the ability of the pneumococci to bind to and traverse cerebral vascular endothelial cells by binding to the PAF receptor using cell wall choline and CbpA.[71]

Inflammation in Response to Pneumococcal Cell Wall

Whereas surface proteins are the key players in the recognition and invasion of host cells by pneumococci, it is the cell wall that is responsible for initiating inflammation. Like classic Gram-positive bacteria, the cell wall is composed of interlinked disaccharide peptides that form a network.[24] This backbone is decorated with a polyribitol teichoic acid, which

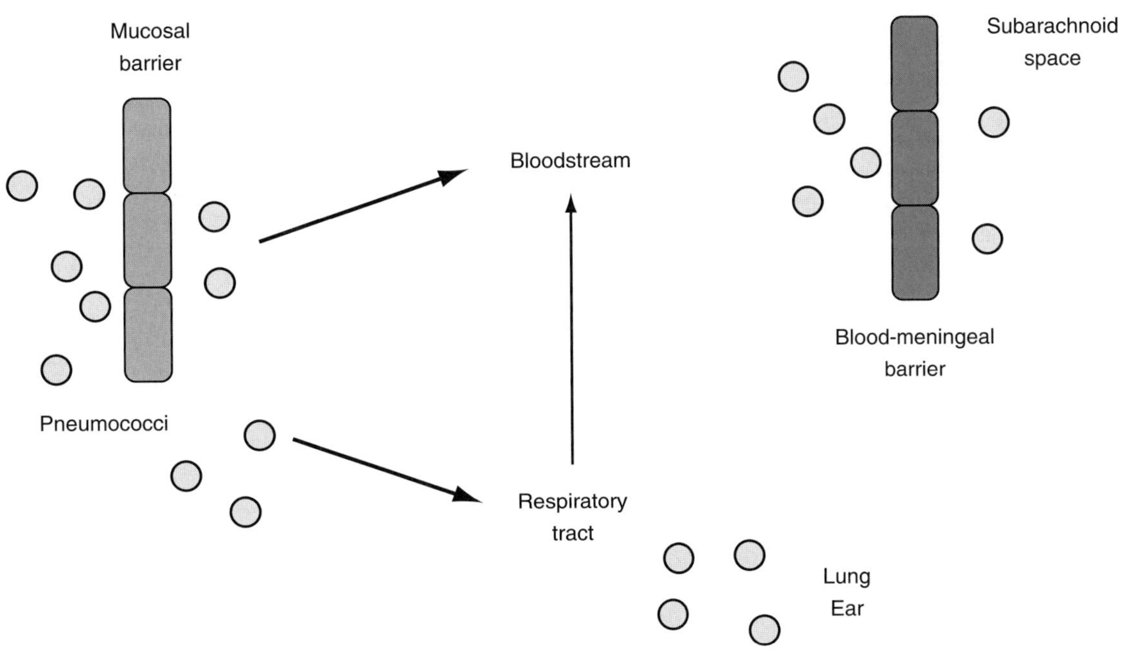

FIGURE 30-2 Pathogenesis of pneumococcal infection.

is unusual in that it contains phosphorylcholine.[72] The phosphorylcholine and the chemical composition of the cell wall building blocks are critical to the inflammatory activity of the cell wall.[25] The choline is also the docking station for the family of secreted choline-binding proteins. It has recently been realized that virtually all respiratory pathogens decorate a surface determinant with choline, presumably to avoid detection by the innate immune system's C-reactive protein.[73,74]

All the signs and symptoms of pneumococcal pneumonia, otitis media, and meningitis can be produced by instilling purified, protein-free pneumococcal cell wall into the appropriate organ.[25,75] The greater the release of cell wall during infection, the greater the inflammatory response and the more acute the course of disease.[76] This broad, potent inflammatory activity resembles Gram-negative bacterial endotoxin. The cell wall interacts with all elements of the acute inflammatory response. Components of the cell wall bind to CD14,[77] lipopolysaccharide (LPS)-binding protein,[78] and other soluble carrier proteins that then present the cell wall to Toll-like receptor 2.[79] Intracellular cell wall is recognized by NOD2.[80–82] These interactions activate transcription of acute phase response genes through NF-κB.[80] This results in the production of cytokines (particularly interleukin-1 and tumor necrosis factor), chemokines (such as PAF), and procoagulant activity.

Some secreted proteins and cell wall components are directly cytotoxic in that they kill eukaryotic cells. This toxicity can arise either by necrosis or by apoptosis. Pneumolysin and hydrogen peroxide and probably the cell wall have been shown to induce apoptosis of epithelial, endothelial, neuronal, and immune cells.[83–85]

Clearance

Clearance of pneumococci involves recruitment of leukocytes in a $ß_2$ integrin-dependent fashion and subsequent phagocytosis. Depending on the chemistry of the capsule, phagocytosis can be avid or fail completely. The most virulent serotypes are 3, 4, and 6.[86] Type-specific anti-capsular antibody is the critical element in protective immunity. Phagocytosis is also promoted by the strong ability of the cell wall to fix complement and the ability of the acute phase reactant, C-reactive protein, to bind to the phosphorylcholine of the pneumococcal teichoic acid.[87,88] Furthermore, the teichoic acid serves as a ligand for the defense collagens (mannose-binding protein, macrophage scavenger receptor, and surfactant protein D), which accelerate clearance.[89,90]

DIAGNOSIS

Pneumococcal infections are diagnosed primarily by culture of the organism from appropriate clinical samples, such as CSF, blood, pleural fluid, or purulent sputum. Confirmation of a pneumococcal cause of otitis media requires tympanocentesis. Although not routinely used diagnostically, lung puncture is required to establish the true cause of pneumonia. Other approaches to diagnosis include the detection of pneumococcal antigen, especially in CSF, and interest has recently focused on the molecular diagnosis of pneumococcal infection using the polymerase chain reaction (PCR). In this regard, a number of genes have been used as targets, including the autolysin and pneumolysin genes,[37] the penicillin-binding protein 2B gene,[38] *lytA*,[91] *psaA*,[92] DNA polymerase 1,[93] and the 16S recombinant RNA gene.[94] Detection of urinary antigen may be useful in adults.[95]

DISEASES: TREATMENT AND PROGNOSIS

Meningitis

The mainstay of treatment of pneumococcal meningitis in developing countries has been intravenous penicillin or ampicillin, usually given in combination with chloramphenicol. The emergence of penicillin resistance led to a prospective comparative study of the outcome of the combination of penicillin and chloramphenicol in the treatment of penicillin-resistant versus penicillin-susceptible pneumococcal meningitis. This study showed that patients with penicillin-resistant strains responded poorly to the combination of penicillin and chloramphenicol, with 80% of patients having a poor outcome without change of therapy.[96] The bactericidal activity of chloramphenicol appears to be diminished against penicillin-resistant strains.[96,97] This has led to the situation that the third-generation cephalosporins, cefotaxime, or ceftriaxone are preferred in the management of pneumococcal meningitis where resistant strains are common. The decision as to which drugs can be used for empirical therapy will depend on the resources of the country and the knowledge of the prevalence of resistant strains in that country. The emergence of cephalosporin resistance in pneumococci in the United States,[98] together with evidence of increased CSF bactericidal activity against these strains after the addition of vancomycin,[99] suggests that vancomycin should be added empirically to cephalosporin for management of pneumococcal meningitis. The decision to use combination therapy will depend on the prevalence of strains with minimum inhibitory concentration of cefotaxime or ceftriaxone greater than 2 μg/mL. Dexamethasone is widely given as adjunctive therapy for the management of pneumococcal meningitis, and a meta-analysis supports the use of the drug for 2 days in the treatment of childhood pneumococcal meningitis,[100] as does a more recent study in adults.[101]

Pneumonia

The clinical spectrum of pneumococcal pneumonia is wide, including a rapid onset of high fever with rigors in young adults and an insidious disease with few physical signs in the elderly. Splenectomized patients are at risk of particularly rapid-onset disease. Signs associated with greater severity of disease include age older than 65 years, underlying illness, a respiratory rate greater than 30 breaths per minute in adults, shock, multiple organ involvement, multilobar disease, and a poor white blood cell response (less than 4×10^9 cells per liter).[102]

Empirical treatment for moderate pneumonia in many developing countries has been trimethoprim-sulfamethoxazole. Although data are lacking on the impact of resistance to this drug combination on the outcome of pneumonia therapy, the drug fails to eradicate resistant pneumococci from children with otitis.[103] Also, because pneumococcal resistance to ß-lactams does not influence the outcome of pneumonia treated with these agents,[104] oral amoxicillin appears to be the drug of choice and indeed has been shown to be superior[105] for management of pneumococcal pneumonia in the outpatient setting.

Intravenous management with penicillin or ampicillin is appropriate treatment for severe infections. In penicillin-allergic patients, new fluoroquinolones that are highly active against pneumococci are probably the drugs of choice,[102] although their cost may be prohibitive in developing countries. Very severe pneumonias may be treated with combination therapy using a ß-lactam and macrolides based on observational studies,[106,107] but prospective randomized trials of combination therapy have not been performed.

Otitis Media

In terms of the penetration of drugs into the middle ear, the spectrum of activity of different agents against pneumococci, and retained activity against resistant strains, high-dose amoxicillin is the most appropriate oral agent for the management of otitis media.[108]

PREVENTION AND CONTROL

Pneumococcal disease was the first infection to be prevented by a nonprotein vaccine. Due to the work of Griffith, Tillet, Finland, Heidelberger, MacLeod, and Austrian, the capsular polysaccharide has come to be recognized as a critical component of vaccine efficacy (reviewed in Musher and associates[109] and Broome and Breiman[110]). The geographic distribution of serotypes differs by region, making a universal vaccine based on a reasonable number of capsular types complicated and costly to compose.[111] The currently approved vaccines consist of the capsular polysaccharides from 23 of the most common serotypes.[110] After many comprehensive studies, there is now overwhelming evidence that this vaccine is approximately 60% efficacious for protection against invasive disease in the general population, but it fails to protect the segments of the population most susceptible to disease: children younger than the age of 2 years or the elderly who are medically compromised.[110,112–114] The vaccine also does not protect against pneumonia,[115] and it may enhance disease in HIV-infected people who are not on antiretroviral therapy.[116] The basis for the ineffectiveness is the inability to elicit a T cell–dependent immune response. This can be overcome by conjugating a protein to the polysaccharide, a process successfully used to introduce a seven-valent pneumococcal vaccine in the United States in 2000.[117] Seven- and nine-valent pneumococcal conjugate vaccines are highly effective in preventing sepsis and meningitis in children due to vaccine serotypes,[118,119] even in HIV-infected children.[119] The vaccine reduces radiographically proven pneumonia by 25% in fully immunized children[119] and induces herd immunity in the population.[117] Although the vaccine reduces pneumococcal otitis, its overall efficacy against otitis is reduced by serotype replacement.[120] A major pneumococcal virulence determinant optimal for vaccine formulation remains to be identified. The advantage of choosing a pneumococcal protein determinant is that protection may be extended to capsular types not in the vaccine formulation.

Antibiotic prophylaxis has been attempted in communities such as Papua New Guinea with high rates of disease,[27,121] but because of the emergence of resistance it is reserved for patients at particularly high risk, for example, children with sickle cell disease.[122] These patients require pneumococcal vaccine after 2 years of age[120] and are a priority group to receive conjugate pneumococcal vaccine. Conjugate vaccines have also been shown to interrupt the transmission of antibiotic-resistant strains[123–125]; however, cost remains a major barrier to their introduction in developing countries. A recent study has shown that conjugate vaccine reduces hospitalization of children with viral-associated pneumonia, presumably by preventing pneumococcal superinfection.[126]

REFERENCES

1. World Health Report. Geneva, Switzerland, World Health Organization, 1999.
2. Garenne M, Ronsmans C, Campbell H: The magnitude of mortality from acute respiratory infections in children under 5 years in developing countries. World Health Stat Q 45:180, 1992.
3. Williams BG, Gouws E, Boschi-Pinto C, et al: Estimates of world-wide distribution of child deaths from acute respiratory infections. Lancet Infect Dis 2:25, 2002.
4. Shann F: The management of pneumonia in children in developing countries. Clin Infect Dis 21(Suppl 3):S218, 1995.
5. Sullivan RJ Jr, Dowdle WR, Marine WM, et al: Adult pneumonia in a general hospital. Etiology and host risk factors. Arch Intern Med 129:935, 1972.
6. Musher DM: Pneumococcal pneumonia including diagnosis and therapy of infection caused by penicillin-resistant strains. Infect Dis Clin North Am 5:509, 1991.
7. Pecoul B, Varaine F, Keita M, et al: Long-acting chloramphenicol versus intravenous ampicillin for treatment of bacterial meningitis. Lancet 338:862, 1991.
8. Klein JO: Otitis media. Clin Infect Dis 19:823, 1994.
9. Gilks CF, Ojoo SA, Ojoo JC, et al: Invasive pneumococcal disease in a cohort of predominantly HIV-1 infected female sex-workers in Nairobi, Kenya. Lancet 347:718, 1996.
10. Sirotnak AP, Eppes SC, Klein JD: Tuboovarian abscess and peritonitis caused by *Streptococcus pneumoniae* serotype 1 in young girls. Clin Infect Dis 22:993, 1996.
11. Gorensek MJ, Lebel MH, Nelson JD: Peritonitis in children with nephrotic syndrome. Pediatrics 81:849, 1988.
12. Musher DM: *Steptococcus pneumoniae*. In Mandell GL, Bennet JE, Dolin R (eds): Principles and Practice of Infectious Diseases. New York, Churchill Livingstone, 1995, pp 1811
13. Henrichsen J: Six newly recognized types of *Streptococcus pneumoniae*. J Clin Microbiol 33:2759, 1995.
14. Klebs E: Beitrage zur kenntnis der schistomyceten. 4.Die monadinen. Arch Exp Pathol Pharmakol 4:409, 1875.
15. White B: The Biology of Pneumococcus. Cambridge, Mass., Harvard University Press, 1979.
16. Pasteur L: Sur une maladie nouvelle, provoquee par la salive d'un enfant mort de la rage. C Acad Sci 10:159, 1881.
17. Sternberg G: A fatal form of septicaemia in the rabbit produced by subcutaneous injection of human saliva. Natl Board Health Bull 2:781, 1881.
18. Friedländer C: Die mikrokokken der pneumonie. Fortschr Med 1, 1883.
19. Griffith F: The significance of pneumococcal types. J Hyg 27:113, 1928.
20. Alloway J: Further observatons on the use of pneumococcus extracts in effecting transformation of type in vitro. J Exp Med 57:265, 1933.
21. Avery OT, MacLeod CM, McCarty M: Studies on the chemical nature of the substance inducing transformation of pneumococcal types. J Exp Med 79:137, 1944.
22. Austrian R, Douglas RM, Schiffman G, et al: Prevention of pneumococcal pneumonia by vaccination. Trans Assoc Am Phys 89:184, 1976.
23. Tomasz A, Albino A, Zanati E: Multiple antibiotic resistance in a bacterium with suppressed autolytic system. Nature 227:138, 1970.
24. Garcia-Bustos J, Tomasz A: A biological price of antibiotic resistance: Major changes in the peptidoglycan structure of penicillin-resistant pneumococci. Proc Natl Acad Sci USA 87:5415, 1990.
25. Tuomanen E, Liu H, Hengstler B, et al: The induction of meningeal inflammation by components of the pneumococcal cell wall. J Infect Dis 151:859, 1985.
26. Watson DA, Musher DM, Jacobson JW, et al: A brief history of the pneumococcus in biomedical research: A panoply of scientific discovery. Clin Infect Dis 17:913, 1993.
27. Hansman D, Glasgow H, Sturt J, et al: Increased resistance to penicillin of pneumococci isolated from man. N Engl J Med 284:175, 1971.

28. Hoge CW, Reichler MR, Dominguez EA, et al: An epidemic of pneumococcal disease in an overcrowded, inadequately ventilated jail. N Engl J Med 331:643, 1994.
29. Gray BM, Turner ME, Dillon HC Jr: Epidemiologic studies of *Streptococcus pneumoniae* in infants. The effects of season and age on pneumococcal acquisition and carriage in the first 24 months of life. Am J Epidemiol 116:692, 1982.
30. Simberkoff MS, El Sadr W, Schiffman G, et al: *Streptococcus pneumoniae* infections and bacteremia in patients with acquired immune deficiency syndrome, with report of a pneumococcal vaccine failure. Am Rev Respir Dis 130:1174, 1984.
31. Redd SC, Rutherford GW 3rd, Sande MA, et al: The role of human immunodeficiency virus infection in pneumococcal bacteremia in San Francisco residents. J Infect Dis 162:1012, 1990.
32. Buie KA, Klugman KP, von Gottberg A, et al: Gender as a risk factor for both antibiotic resistance and infection with pediatric serogroups/serotypes in HIV-infected and uninfected adults with pneumococcal bacteremia. J Infect Dis 189:1996, 2004.
33. Gordon SB, Chaponda M, Walsh AL, et al: Pneumococcal disease in HIV-infected Malawian adults: Acute mortality and long-term survival. AIDS 16:1409, 2002.
34. Madhi SA, Petersen K, Madhi A, et al: Increased disease burden and antibiotic resistance of bacteria causing severe community-acquired lower respiratory tract infections in human immunodeficiency virus type 1-infected children. Clin Infect Dis 31:170, 2000.
35. Gebo KA, Moore RD, Keruly JC, et al: Risk factors for pneumococcal disease in human immunodeficiency virus-infected patients. J Infect Dis 173:857, 1996.
36. Janoff EN, Breiman RF, Daley CL, et al: Pneumococcal disease during HIV infection. Epidemiologic, clinical, and immunologic perspectives. Ann Intern Med 117:314, 1992.
37. Jordens JZ, Paul J, Bates J, et al: Characterization of *Streptococcus pneumoniae* from human immunodeficiency virus-seropositive patients with acute and recurrent pneumonia. J Infect Dis 172:983, 1995.
38. Fry AM, Facklam RR, Whitney CG, et al: Multistate evaluation of invasive pneumococcal diseases in adults with human immunodeficiency virus infection: Serotype and antimicrobial resistance patterns in the United States. J Infect Dis 188:643, 2003.
39. Hansman D, Bullen MM: A resistant pneumococcus. Lancet 2:264, 1967.
40. Klugman KP: Pneumococcal resistance to antibiotics. Clin Microbiol Rev 3:171, 1990.
41. Song JH, Lee NY, Ichiyama S, et al: Spread of drug-resistant *Streptococcus pneumoniae* in Asian countries: Asian Network for Surveillance of Resistant Pathogens (ANSORP) Study. Clin Infect Dis 28:1206, 1999.
42. Mastro TD, Nomani NK, Ishaq Z, et al: Use of nasopharyngeal isolates of *Streptococcus pneumoniae* and *Haemophilus influenzae* from children in Pakistan for surveillance for antimicrobial resistance. Pediatr Infect Dis J 12:824, 1993.
43. Koornhof HJ, Wasas A, Klugman K: Antimicrobial resistance in *Streptococcus pneumoniae*: A South African perspective. Clin Infect Dis 15:84, 1992.
44. Friedland IR, Klugman KP: Antibiotic-resistant pneumococcal disease in South African children. Am J Dis Child 146:920, 1992.
45. Rowe AK, Deming MS, Schwartz B, et al: Antimicrobial resistance of nasopharyngeal isolates of *Streptococcus pneumoniae* and *Haemophilus influenzae* from children in the Central African Republic. Pediatr Infect Dis J 19:438, 2000.
46. Woolfson A, Huebner R, Wasas A, et al: Nasopharyngeal carriage of community-acquired, antibiotic-resistant *Streptococcus pneumoniae* in a Zambian paediatric population. Bull World Health Organization 75:453, 1997.
47. Feikin DR, Davis M, Nwanyanwu OC, et al: Antibiotic resistance and serotype distribution of *Streptococcus pneumoniae* colonizing rural Malawian children. Pediatr Infect Dis J 22:564, 2003.
48. Bronzwaer S, Cars O, Buchholz U, et al: A European study on the relationship between antimicrobial use and antimicrobial resistance. Emerging Infect Dis 8:278, 2002.
49. Mthwalo M, Wasas A, Huebner R, et al: Antibiotic resistance of nasopharyngeal isolates of *Streptococcus pneumoniae* from children in Lesotho. Bull World Health Organization 76:641, 1998.
50. Fry AM, Jha HC, Lietman TM, et al: Adverse and beneficial secondary effects of mass treatment with azithromycin to eliminate blindness due to trachoma in Nepal. Clin Infect Dis 35:395, 2002.
51. Leach AJ, Shelby-James TM, Mayo M, et al: A prospective study of the impact of community-based azithromycin treatment of trachoma on carriage and resistance of *Streptococcus pneumoniae*. Clin Infect Dis 24:356, 1997.
52. Feikin DR, Dowell SF, Nwanyanwu OC, et al: Increased carriage of trimethoprim/sulfamethoxazole-resistant *Streptococcus pneumoniae* in Malawian children after treatment for malaria with sulfadoxine/pyrimethamine. J Infect Dis 181:1501, 2000.
53. Tettelin H, Nelson KE, Paulsen IT, et al: Complete genome sequence of a virulent isolate of *Streptococcus pneumoniae*. Science 293:498, 2001.
54. Hoskins J, Alborn WE Jr, Arnold J, et al: Genome of the bacterium *Streptococcus pneumoniae* strain R6. J Bacteriol 183:5709, 2001.
55. Hava DL, Camilli A: Large-scale identification of serotype 4 *Streptococcus pneumoniae* virulence factors. Mol Microbiol 45:1389, 2002.
56. Hava DL, LeMieux J, Camilli A: From nose to lung: The regulation behind *Streptococcus pneumoniae* virulence factors. Mol Microbiol 50:1103, 2003.
57. Lau GW, Haataja S, Lonetto M, et al: A functional genomic analysis of type 3 *Streptococcus pneumoniae* virulence. Mol Microbiol 40:555, 2001.
58. Polissi A, Pontiggia A, Feger G, et al: Large-scale identification of virulence genes from *Streptococcus pneumoniae*. Infect Immun 66:5620, 1998.
59. Sebert ME, Palmer LM, Rosenberg M, et al: Microarray-based identification of htrA, a *Streptococcus pneumoniae* gene that is regulated by the CiaRH two-component system and contributes to nasopharyngeal colonization. Infect Immun 70:4059, 2002.
60. Mei JM, Nourbakhsh F, Ford CW, et al: Identification of *Staphylococcus aureus* virulence genes in a murine model of bacteraemia using signature-tagged mutagenesis. Mol Microbiol 26:399, 1997.
61. Austrian R: Some aspects of the pneumococcal carrier state. J Antimicrob Chemother 18(Suppl A):35, 1986.
62. Hammerschmidt S, Talay SR, Brandtzaeg P, et al: SpsA, a novel pneumococcal surface protein with specific binding to secretory immunoglobulin A and secretory component. Mol Microbiol 25:1113, 1997.
63. Zhang JR, Mostov KE, Lamm ME, et al: The polymeric immunoglobulin receptor translocates pneumococci across human nasopharyngeal epithelial cells. Cell 102:827, 2000.
64. Gray BM, Converse GM 3rd, Dillon HC Jr: Epidemiologic studies of *Streptococcus pneumoniae* in infants: Acquisition, carriage, and infection during the first 24 months of life. J Infect Dis 142:923, 1980.
65. McCullers JA, Rehg JE: Lethal synergism between influenza virus and *Streptococcus pneumoniae*: Characterization of a mouse model and the role of platelet-activating factor receptor. J Infect Dis 186:341, 2002.
66. Cundell DR, Gerard NP, Gerard C, et al: *Streptococcus pneumoniae* anchor to activated human cells by the receptor for platelet-activating factor. Nature 377:435, 1995.
67. Weiser JN, Austrian R, Sreenivasan PK, et al: Phase variation in pneumococcal opacity: Relationship between colonial morphology and nasopharyngeal colonization. Infect Immun 62:2582, 1994.
68. Throup JP, Koretke KK, Bryant AP, et al: A genomic analysis of two-component signal transduction in *Streptococcus pneumoniae*. Mol Microbiol 35:566, 2000.
69. Spellerberg B, Cundell DR, Sandros J, et al: Pyruvate oxidase as a determinant of virulence in *Streptococcus pneumoniae*. Mol Microbiol 19:803, 1996.
70. Paton JC, Lock RA, Lee CJ, et al: Purification and immunogenicity of genetically obtained pneumolysin toxoids and their conjugation to *Streptococcus pneumoniae* type 19F polysaccharide. Infect Immun 59:2297, 1991.
71. Ring A, Weiser JN, Tuomanen EI: Pneumococcal trafficking across the blood–brain barrier. Molecular analysis of a novel bidirectional pathway. J Clin Invest 102:347, 1998.
72. Tomasz A: Choline in the cell wall of a bacterium: Novel type of polymer-linked choline in Pneumococcus. Science 157:694, 1967.
73. Weiser JN, Pan N, McGowan KL, et al: Phosphorylcholine on the lipopolysaccharide of *Haemophilus influenzae* contributes to persistence in the respiratory tract and sensitivity to serum killing mediated by C-reactive protein. J Exp Med 187:631, 1998.
74. Gould JM, Weiser JN: The inhibitory effect of C-reactive protein on bacterial phosphorylcholine platelet-activating factor receptor-mediated adherence is blocked by surfactant. J Infect Dis 186:361, 2002.

75. Ripley-Petzoldt ML, Giebink GS, Juhn SK, et al: The contribution of pneumococcal cell wall to the pathogenesis of experimental otitis media. J Infect Dis 157:245, 1988.
76. Tuomanen E, Pollack H, Parkinson A, et al: Microbiological and clinical significance of a new property of defective lysis in clinical strains of pneumococci. J Infect Dis 158:36, 1988.
77. Pugin J, Heumann ID, Tomasz A, et al: CD14 is a pattern recognition receptor. Immunity 1:509, 1994.
78. Weber JR, Freyer D, Alexander C, et al: Recognition of pneumococcal peptidoglycan: An expanded, pivotal role for LPS binding protein. Immunity 19:269, 2003.
79. Yoshimura A, Lien E, Ingalls RR, et al: Cutting edge: Recognition of gram-positive bacterial cell wall components by the innate immune system occurs via Toll-like receptor 2. J Immunol 163:1, 1999.
80. Spellerberg B, Rosenow C, Sha W, et al: Pneumococcal cell wall activates NF-kappa B in human monocytes: Aspects distinct from endotoxin. Microb Pathog 20:309, 1996.
81. Pauleau AL, Murray PJ: Role of nod2 in the response of macrophages to toll-like receptor agonists. Mol Cell Biol 23:7531, 2003.
82. Girardin SE, Travassos LH, Herve M, et al: Peptidoglycan molecular requirements allowing detection by Nod1 and Nod2. J Biol Chem 278:41702, 2003.
83. Braun JS, Sublett JE, Freyer D, et al: Pneumococcal pneumolysin and H(2)O(2) mediate brain cell apoptosis during meningitis. J Clin Invest 109:19, 2002.
84. Braun JS, Novak R, Herzog KH, et al: Neuroprotection by a caspase inhibitor in acute bacterial meningitis. Nat Med 5:298, 1999.
85. Colino J, Snapper CM: Two distinct mechanisms for induction of dendritic cell apoptosis in response to intact *Streptococcus pneumoniae*. J Immunol 171:2354, 2003.
86. Briles DE, Crain MJ, Gray BM, et al: Strong association between capsular type and virulence for mice among human isolates of *Streptococcus pneumoniae*. Infect Immun 60:111, 1992.
87. Mold C, Rodgers CP, Kaplan RL, et al: Binding of human C-reactive protein to bacteria. Infect Immun 38:392, 1982.
88. Winkelstein JA, Tomasz A: Activation of the alternative complement pathway by pneumococcal cell wall teichoic acid. J Immunol 120:174, 1978.
89. Polotsky VY, Fischer W, Ezekowitz RA, et al: Interactions of human mannose-binding protein with lipoteichoic acids. Infect Immun 64:380, 1996.
90. Dunne DW, Resnick D, Greenberg J, et al: The type I macrophage scavenger receptor binds to gram-positive bacteria and recognizes lipoteichoic acid. Proc Natl Acad Sci USA 91:1863, 1994.
91. McAvin JC, Reilly PA, Roudabush RM, et al: Sensitive and specific method for rapid identification of *Streptococcus pneumoniae* using real-time fluorescence PCR. J Clin Microbiol 39:3446, 2001.
92. Morrison KE, Lake D, Crook J, et al: Confirmation of psaA in all 90 serotypes of *Streptococcus pneumoniae* by PCR and potential of this assay for identification and diagnosis. J Clin Microbiol 38:434, 2000.
93. Friedland LR, Menon AG, Reising SF, et al: Development of a polymerase chain reaction assay to detect the presence of *Streptococcus pneumoniae* DNA. Diagn Microbiol Infect Dis 20:187, 1994.
94. Radstrom P, Backman A, Qian N, et al: Detection of bacterial DNA in cerebrospinal fluid by an assay for simultaneous detection of *Neisseria meningitidis*, *Haemophilus influenzae*, and streptococci using a seminested PCR strategy. J Clin Microbiol 32:2738, 1994.
95. Roson B, Fernandez-Sabe N, Carratala J, et al: Contribution of a urinary antigen assay (Binax NOW) to the early diagnosis of pneumococcal pneumonia. Clin Infect Dis 38:222, 2004.
96. Friedland IR, Klugman KP: Failure of chloramphenicol therapy in penicillin-resistant pneumococcal meningitis. Lancet 339:405, 1992.
97. Friedland IR, Shelton S, McCracken GH Jr: Chloramphenicol in penicillin-resistant pneumococcal meningitis. Lancet 342:240, 1993.
98. Bradley JS, Connor JD: Ceftriaxone failure in meningitis caused by *Streptococcus pneumoniae* with reduced susceptibility to beta-lactam antibiotics. Pediatr Infect Dis J 10:871, 1991.
99. Klugman KP, Friedland IR, Bradley JS: Bactericidal activity against cephalosporin-resistant *Streptococcus pneumoniae* in cerebrospinal fluid of children with acute bacterial meningitis. Antimicrobial Agents Chemother 39:1988, 1995.
100. McIntyre PB, Berkey CS, King SM, et al: Dexamethasone as adjunctive therapy in bacterial meningitis. A meta-analysis of randomized clinical trials since 1988. JAMA 278:925, 1997.
101. De Gans J, van de Beek D for the European Dexamethasone in Adulthood Bacterial Meningitis Study Investigators: Dexamethasone in adults with bacterial meningitis. N Engl J Med 347:1549, 2002.
102. Mandell LA, Bartlett JG, Dowell SF, et al: Update of practice guidelines for the management of community-acquired pneumonia in immunocompetent adults. Clin Infect Dis 37:1405, 2003.
103. Leiberman A, Leibovitz E, Piglansky L, et al: Bacteriologic and clinical efficacy of trimethoprim-sulfamethoxazole for treatment of acute otitis media. Pediatr Infect Dis J 20:260, 2001.
104. Klugman KP: Bacteriological evidence of antibiotic failure in pneumococcal lower respiratory tract infections. Eur Respir J Suppl 36:3S, 2002.
105. Straus WL, Qazi SA, Kundi Z, et al: Antimicrobial resistance and clinical effectiveness of co-trimoxazole versus amoxicillin for pneumonia among children in Pakistan: Randomised controlled trial. Pakistan Co-trimoxazole Study Group. Lancet 352:270, 1998.
106. Waterer GW, Somes GW, Wunderink RG: Monotherapy may be suboptimal for severe bacteremic pneumococcal pneumonia. Arch Intern Med 161:1837, 2001.
107. Baddour LM, Yu VL, Klugman KP, et al: Combination therapy lowers mortality among severely ill patients with pneumococcal bacteremia. Am J Respir Crit Care Med 170:440, 2004.
108. Dagan R: Achieving bacterial eradication using pharmacokinetic/pharmacodynamic principles. Int J Infect Dis 7(Suppl 1):S21, 2003.
109. Musher DM, Watson DA, Dominguez EA: Pneumococcal vaccination: Work to date and future prospects. Am J Med Sci 300:45, 1990.
110. Broome CV, Breiman RF: Pneumococcal vaccine—Past, present, and future. N Engl J Med 325:1506, 1991.
111. Lee CJ, Banks SD, Li JP: Virulence, immunity, and vaccine related to *Streptococcus pneumoniae*. Crit Rev Microbiol 18:89, 1991.
112. Fedson DS, Shapiro ED, LaForce FM, et al: Pneumococcal vaccine after 15 years of use. Another view. Arch Intern Med 154:2531, 1994.
113. Shapiro ED, Berg AT, Austrian R, et al: The protective efficacy of polyvalent pneumococcal polysaccharide vaccine. N Engl J Med 325:1453, 1991.
114. Hirschmann JV, Lipsky BA: The pneumococcal vaccine after 15 years of use. Arch Intern Med 154:373, 1994.
115. Mangtani P, Cutts F, Hall AJ: Efficacy of polysaccharide pneumococcal vaccine in adults in more developed countries: The state of the evidence. Lancet Infect Dis 3:71, 2003.
116. French N, Nakiyingi J, Carpenter LM, et al: 23-valent pneumococcal polysaccharide vaccine in HIV-1-infected Ugandan adults: Double-blind, randomised and placebo controlled trial. Lancet 355:2106, 2000.
117. Whitney CG, Farley MM, Hadler J, et al: Decline in invasive pneumococcal disease after the introduction of protein–polysaccharide conjugate vaccine. N Engl J Med 348:1737, 2003.
118. Black SB, Shinefield HR, Ling S, et al: Effectiveness of heptavalent pneumococcal conjugate vaccine in children younger than five years of age for prevention of pneumonia. Pediatr Infect Dis J 21:810, 2002.
119. Klugman KP, Madhi SA, Huebner RE, et al: A trial of a 9-valent pneumococcal conjugate vaccine in children with and those without HIV infection. N Engl J Med 349:1341, 2003.
120. Eskola J, Kilpi T, Palmu A, et al: Efficacy of a pneumococcal conjugate vaccine against acute otitis media. N Engl J Med 344:403, 2001.
121. Douglas RM, Sturt J: Letter: Penicillin-resistant pneumococci and pneumonia. Med J Aust 1:82, 1975.
122. Wong WY, Overturf GD, Powars DR: Infection caused by *Streptococcus pneumoniae* in children with sickle cell disease: Epidemiology, immunologic mechanisms, prophylaxis, and vaccination. Clin Infect Dis 14:1124, 1992.
123. Mbelle N, Huebner RE, Wasas AD, et al: Immunogenicity and impact on nasopharyngeal carriage of a nonavalent pneumococcal conjugate vaccine. J Infect Dis 180:1171, 1999.
124. Dagan R, Givon-Lavi N, Zamir O, et al: Effect of a nonavalent conjugate vaccine in carriage of antibiotic-resistant *streptococcus pneumoniae* in daycare centers. Pediatr Infect Dis J 22:532, 2003.
125. Talbot TR, Poehling KA, Hartert TV, et al: Reduction in high rates of antibiotic-nonsusceptable invasive pneumococcal disease in Tennessee after introduction of the pneumococcal conjugate vaccine. Clin Infect Dis 39:641, 2004.
126. Madhi SA, Klugman KP: Vaccine Trials Group: A role for *streptococcus pneumoniae* in virus-associated pneumonia. Nat Med 10:811, 2004.

31

Streptococcal and Staphylococcal Infections

DENNIS L. STEVENS

Streptococcus pyogenes Infections

Group A streptococcus (GAS) causes disease in every continent on Earth and is unique among human pathogens in its ability to cause a wide variety of clinical infections and postinfectious sequelae.[1] Further, in its coevolution with humans, *Streptococcus pyogenes* has developed a myriad of molecular strategies to neutralize or bind directly to most of the important host defense molecules produced by the human host.[2] Thus, in pathogenesis of both acute GAS infections and the well-known postinfectious sequelae, it is the specific host response or altered host response to this unique pathogen that accounts for the morbidity and mortality. This chapter emphasizes these host–microbe relationships to explain the unique epidemiologic and pathogenic features of *S. pyogenes* and, in the next section, *Staphylococcus aureus*.

AGENT

S. pyogenes is a gram-positive, catalase-negative coccus that divides in a single plane, thus forming chains of bacteria, particularly in liquid cultures. Lancefield[3] developed a classification scheme based on acid-extractable polysaccharide of streptococci and, to date, groups of streptococci from A to O have been defined by such typing. Typing of strains has been simplified through the development of commercially available rapid latex agglutination schemes. Although the bacitracin susceptibility test has proved very reliable as a presumptive marker for group A, both false negative and false positive results are problematic. GAS may be grown aerobically or anaerobically and, in general, growth is enhanced in the presence of 10% carbon dioxide.

EPIDEMIOLOGY

The epidemiology of GAS infections is a dynamic process geographically and temporally. The declining prevalence and severity of both rheumatic fever (RF) and scarlet fever caused by GAS throughout the 20th century in much of the Western world may have been related to improved socioeconomic conditions, timely antibiotic treatment of streptococcal pharyngitis, and secondary prophylaxis for RF.[4] However, these declines are more likely due to cyclic variation in the virulence of the organism. The recent outbreaks of pharyngitis, acute RF, and the newly recognized streptococcal toxic shock syndrome (strep TSS) support this concept.

The reservoirs of *S. pyogenes* in nature are the skin and mucous membranes of humans, and nearly 5% of all people, regardless of age, carry the organism in their throats. In the recent past, RF was much more common in the United States, particularly in the northern states. Currently, RF is very uncommon in the United States but is prevalent in developing countries, many of which are in tropical environments.[4] Impetigo is also more common in tropical areas, though elevation above sea level is also a factor that increases the prevalence of disease.[1] It is likely, though unproven, that skin carriage is higher in tropical areas than temperate climates, though the inverse is true for carriage of GAS in the throat. Recently, invasive GAS infections, such as strep TSS and necrotizing fasciitis, have been described with increased frequency in North America and Europe[5–15] and subsequently throughout tropical areas as well. The diversity of infectious diseases caused by group A streptococcus is illustrated in Box 31-1.

DISEASES

GAS, perhaps more than any other pathogen, has the ability to cause diverse infections. The clinical characteristics of each of these are described in the following sections.

Pharyngitis and the Asymptomatic Carrier

The baseline streptococcal pharyngeal carriage rate is roughly 5%, but reaches rates of 15% to 50% in school-age children in temperate climates during epidemics of GAS pharyngitis. Transmission occurs via aerosolized droplets from the upper airway of one host to another. GAS pharyngitis is most common in children 5 to 15 years of age who live in temperate climates. The cardinal manifestations of GAS pharyngitis include sore throat, submandibular and anterior cervical adenopathy, fever of greater than 38°C, and pharyngeal erythema with exudates. Acute pharyngitis is sufficient

Box 31-1 Streptococcal Infections and Sequelae

Cellulitis
Erysipelas
Impetigo
Mastoiditis
Myonecrosis
Necrotizing fasciitis
Otitis media
Peritonsillar abscess
Pharyngitis
Pneumonia
Poststreptococcal glomerulonephritis
Rheumatic fever
Sinusitis
Streptococcal toxic shock syndrome

to induce antibody against M protein, SLO, Dnase, and hyaluronidase, and, if present, pyrogenic exotoxins. GAS pharyngitis may proceed to scarlet fever, bacteremia, suppurative head and neck infections, Strep TSS, carrier state, RF, or poststreptococcal glomerulonephritis. Thus, the outcomes depend on the interaction between specific streptococcal virulence factors with immunologic defense molecules of the human host.

During GAS epidemics, particularly where RF or a poststreptococcal glomerulonephritis is prevalent, treatment of asymptomatic carriers may be necessary, and programs that use monthly injection of benzathine penicillin effectively reduce the incidence of GAS pharyngitis as well as RF.

Scarlet Fever

In recent years, outbreaks of scarlet fever in the United States and Great Britain have often been associated with strains of GAS-producing pyrogenic exotoxin C.[16] The cases have been notably mild and the illness has been referred to as "pharyngitis with rash." Historically, this form was known as benign scarlet fever, though scarlet fever has not always been a mild disease: Around 1900 mortality rates of 25% were common in temperate climates on both sides of the Atlantic.

Scarlet fever has been divided into the following types: mild, moderate, toxic, and septic. Thus, benign scarlet fever may be either mild or moderate, and the fatal or malignant form may be either septic or toxic. Historically, the toxic cases invariably began with a severe sore throat, marked fever, delirium, skin rash, and painful cervical lymph nodes. In severe toxic cases, fulminating fevers of 107°F, pulse rates of 130 to 160 beats per minute, severe headache, delirium, convulsions, little if any skin rash, and death within 24 hours were the usual findings. These cases occurred before the advent of antibiotics, antipyretics, and anticonvulsants, and deaths were the result of uncontrolled seizures and hyperpyrexia. The term *septic scarlet fever* refers to the form characterized by local invasion of the soft tissues of the neck and complications such as upper airway obstruction, otitis media with perforation, profuse mucopurulent drainage from the nose, bronchopneumonia, and death. Note that necrotizing fasciitis and myositis were not previously observed in association with scarlet fever.

Soft Tissue Infections

Erysipelas

Erysipelas is caused exclusively by *S. pyogenes* and is characterized by the abrupt onset of fiery-red swelling of the face or extremities.[17] Distinctive features are well-defined margins, particularly along the nasolabial fold; a scarlet or salmon-red color; rapid progression; and intense pain. Flaccid bullae filled with clear fluid may develop during the second to third day of illness, yet extension to deeper soft tissues, bacteremia, and shock occur only rarely. Surgical débridement is rarely required and treatment with penicillin is very effective. Swelling may progress despite treatment, though fever, pain, and intense redness diminish usually within 24 to 48 hours. Desquamation of the involved skin occurs 5 to 10 days into the illness and scarring of the skin does not occur. Infants and elderly adults are most commonly afflicted. Erysipelas has become less severe since the early 1900s even before antibiotic treatment became available.

Streptococcal Pyoderma (Impetigo Contagiosa)

The thick, crusted skin lesions of streptococcal pyoderma frequently have a golden-brown color resembling dried serum.[17] Children between 2 and 5 years of age are most commonly infected. Epidemics occur throughout the year in tropical areas or during the summer months in more temperate climates and are usually associated with poor hygiene. Initially, colonization of the unbroken skin occurs either exogenously from patients with impetiginous lesions or endogenously by contamination of the skin with oropharyngeal organisms. Development of impetiginous lesions requires 10 to 14 days and is initiated by minor trauma such as an abrasion or insect bite, which facilitates intradermal inoculation. Patients with impetigo should receive penicillin, particularly when numerous sites of the skin are involved, though treatment does not prevent poststreptococcal glomerulonephritis. Topical treatment with an agent effective against gram-positive bacteria, such as bacitracin or mupirocin, is also effective. About 50% of cases of impetigo currently are caused by *S. aureus.*

Cellulitis

GAS may invade the epidermis and subcutaneous tissues, resulting in local swelling, erythema, and pain.[17] The skin becomes indurated and, in contrast to erysipelas, is a pinkish color. Patients with lymphedema secondary to lymphoma, filariasis, or surgical node dissection (mastectomy, carcinoma of the prostate, etc.) are predisposed to development of GAS cellulitis, as are those with chronic venous stasis and superficial dermatophyte infection of the toes. Saphenous vein donor site cellulitis may be due to group A, C, or G streptococci. Cellulitis associated with a primary focus (e.g., an abscess or boil) is more likely caused by *S. aureus.* Aspiration of the leading-edge and punch biopsy yield a causative organism in 15% and 40% of cases, respectively. Patients respond quickly to penicillin, though in some cases where staphylococcus is of concern, nafcillin or oxacillin may be a better choice, or one may need cover for methicillin-resistant *S. aureus* (MRSA) infection (discussed later in this chapter). If bluish or violet discoloration develops or if bullae become apparent, a deeper infection such as necrotizing fasciitis or myositis should be considered (see Necrotizing Fasciitis). Particularly when such patients demonstrate systemic toxicity, a serum creatine phosphokinase level should be obtained and, if elevated, prompt surgical inspection and debridement should be performed.

Lymphangitis

Cutaneous infection with bright red streaks ascending proximally is most commonly associated with GAS, though groups C and G have also been implicated. Prompt antibiotic treatment is mandatory because bacteremia and systemic toxicity develop rapidly once infected lymphatic fluid reaches the thoracic ducts.

Necrotizing Fasciitis

Necrotizing fasciitis, originally called streptococcal gangrene, is a deep-seated infection of the subcutaneous tissue that results in progressive destruction of fascia and fat but may spare the skin itself.[17] Within the first 24 hours, swelling, heat, erythema, and tenderness develop and rapidly spread proximally and distally from the original focus. During the next 24 hours, the erythema darkens, changing from red to purple to blue, forming blisters and bullae that contain clear, yellow fluid.[18] The purple areas become frankly gangrenous and extensive necrosis of the subcutaneous tissue ensues. Patients become increasingly toxic and develop shock and multiorgan failure. In the past, aggressive fasciotomy and débridement and application of Dakin's solution topically achieved mortality rates as low as 20%, even before antibiotics were available. The increased severity of necrotizing fasciitis that has occurred among recent cases of Strep TSS relative to shock, multiorgan failure, and mortality could be due to the increased virulence of GAS itself.

Myositis and Myonecrosis

Historically, streptococcal myositis has been an extremely uncommon GAS infection, and only 21 cases were documented from 1900 to 1985.[19] Recently, an increased prevalence of GAS myositis has been reported in the United States, Norway, and Sweden.[5,6,20] Translocation of GAS from an asymptomatic infection of the pharynx to the muscle site must occur hematogenously because penetrating trauma is not usually a major factor. Further, most patients have not reported symptomatic pharyngitis or tonsillitis. Severe pain at the site of infection may be the only presenting symptom; swelling and erythema may be the only signs of infection. Muscle compartmental syndromes may develop rapidly. In most cases a single muscle group is involved; however, because patients frequently have bacteremia, there may be other sites of myositis or abscess. Distinguishing streptococcal myositis from spontaneous gas gangrene caused by *C. perfringens* or *C. septicum* may be difficult, although the presence of crepitus or gas in the tissue would favor a diagnosis of clostridial infection. Myositis is easily distinguished from necrotizing fasciitis anatomically by means of surgical exploration or incisional biopsy, though clinical features of both conditions overlap and 30% to 40% of patients may have both. Though soft tissue radiography, computed tomography (CT), and magnetic resonance imaging (MRI) may be useful in localizing the site of infection, these generally show only edema or soft tissue swelling and do not distinguish myonecrosis or myositis from soft tissue damage due to blunt trauma. Increasing quantities of muscle enzymes in the serum may provide a useful clinical clue of deep infection. In published reports, the case-fatality rate of necrotizing fasciitis is between 20% and 50%, whereas that of GAS myositis is between 80% and 100%. Aggressive surgical débridement is of extreme importance because of the poor efficacy of penicillin described in human cases as well as in experimental streptococcal models of myositis (see Treatment).

Streptococcal Toxic Shock Syndrome

In the mid-1980s, reports of invasive GAS infections associated with bacteremia, deep soft-tissue infection, shock, and multiorgan failure began to appear in the medical literature from North America and Europe.[5,20] Though all ages may be affected, the greatest increases have occurred among previously healthy persons from 15 to 50 years of age. Mortality rates of 30% to 70% have been described in patients with Strep TSS, in spite of aggressive modern treatment measures. The Strep TSS is defined as any GAS infection associated with the sudden onset of shock and organ dysfunction.

Acquisition of Group A Streptococcus and Predisposing Factors

The most common sites of infection resulting in Strep TSS are soft tissue infections (necrotizing fasciitis, myonecrosis), pneumonia, postpartum sepsis, septic joint, peritonitis, and empyema. For soft tissue infection, the portals of entry are surgical site, chickenpox, insect bites, slivers, burns, and minor abrasions. The portal of entry of streptococci could not be ascertained in 45% of cases. Many of these occurred at the exact site of minor local nonpenetrating traumas (muscle strain, ankle sprain, subcutaneous hematoma, etc.). Early on, the only symptoms may be fever and severe pain. In adults, a virus-like prodrome suggestive of influenza precedes the onset of Strep TSS by several days. The use of nonsteroidal anti-inflammatory drugs (NSAIDs) to treat pain or suppress fever may mask the presenting symptoms or predispose the patient to more severe complications such as shock.

Symptoms

Pain is a common initial symptom of Strep TSS, is abrupt in onset and severe, and may not be associated with tenderness or physical findings. The pain most commonly involves an extremity, but may also mimic peritonitis, pelvic inflammatory disease, acute myocardial infarction, or pericarditis.

Physical Findings

Fever is the most common presenting sign, although on admission to the hospital 10% of patients in one report had profound hypothermia secondary to shock. Confusion may be present in over half of the patients and, in some, it progresses to coma or combativeness. In our report,[5] 80% of patients had tachycardia and 55% had systolic blood pressure of less than 110 mmHg on admission. Although 45% of patients had normal blood pressure (systolic pressure > 110 mm Hg) on admission, in all of these patients hypotension developed within the subsequent 4 hours. Soft tissue infection evolved to necrotizing fasciitis or myositis in 70% of patients, and in these cases surgical débridement, fasciotomy, or amputation was required. An ominous sign was the progression of soft tissue swelling to formation of vesicles and then bullae, which took on a violaceous or bluish coloration. Among patients with no soft tissue infection on admission, a variety of clinical presentations were observed; these included endophthalmitis, myositis, perihepatitis, peritonitis, myocarditis, and overwhelming sepsis. Patients who experience shock and multiorgan failure without clinical evidence of local infection have a worse prognosis because definitive diagnosis and surgical débridement may be delayed.

Laboratory Test Results

Evidence of renal involvement was apparent at the time of admission by the presence of hemoglobinuria and elevated serum creatinine level. The serum albumin level was moderately low (3.3 g/dL) on admission and dropped further (2.3 g/dL) by 48 hours. Hypocalcemia, including ionized hypocalcemia, was detectable early in the hospital course. The serum creatine phosphokinase (CPK) level is a useful test to detect deeper soft tissue infections, such as necrotizing fasciitis or myositis.

The initial laboratory studies demonstrated only mild leukocytosis, but a dramatic left shift (43% of white blood cells were band forms, metamyelocytes, and myelocytes). The mean platelet count was normal on admission but dropped to approximately 120,000 cells/mm^3 within 48 hours, frequently in the absence of criteria for disseminated intravascular coagulopathy (DIC).

Bacteriologic Cultures

GAS was isolated from blood in 60% of cases, and from deep tissue specimens in 95%.

Clinical Course

Shock was apparent early in the course and management was complicated by profound capillary leak.[5] Adult respiratory distress syndrome (ARDS) occurred frequently (55%) and complicated fluid resuscitation. Renal dysfunction preceded hypotension in many patients and progressed or persisted for 48 to 72 hours despite treatment. In all patients who survived, serum creatinine levels returned to normal within 4 to 6 weeks. Overall 30% to 70% of patients have died despite aggressive treatment, including administration of intravenous fluids, colloid, pressors, and mechanical ventilation; and surgical intervention, including fasciotomy and débridement, exploratory laparotomy, intraocular aspiration, amputation, and hysterectomy.

Characteristics of Clinical Isolates of Group A Streptococci

M protein types 1, 3, 12, and 28 of GAS have been the most common isolates from patients with shock and multiorgan failure in studies made worldwide. These same strains have also been found in increased numbers from patients with pharyngitis, erysipelas, and asymptomatic carriers. Pyrogenic exotoxin A or B, or both, have been found in isolates from the majority of patients with severe infection. Infections in Norway, Sweden, and Great Britain have been primarily due to M protein type 1 strains of GAS that produce pyrogenic exotoxin B.

POSTINFECTIOUS SEQUELAE

Rheumatic Fever

The prevalence of acute RF (ARF) in the Western world decreased dramatically after World War II (0.5 to 1.88 cases per 100,000 school-age children per year).[21] In contrast, in India and Sri Lanka the prevalence of ARF has remained 140 per 100,000 for children between 5 and 19 years of age. Socioeconomic factors seem to be important because the highest rates in all countries have been among the impoverished in large cities. Although improved living conditions and the development of penicillin have had important roles in reducing the prevalence of ARF in the United States, the decreases had actually begun before antibiotics were available. In recent years there has been a resurgence of ARF among U.S. military recruits and in the civilian population among predominantly white middle-class children.[22] A particularly frightening aspect of these recent civilian cases has been the low incidence of symptomatic pharyngitis (24% to 78%). Thus, our modern primary prevention strategy (diagnosis of acute GAS pharyngitis with penicillin treatment within 10 days) would not have prevented ARF in these cases.[23]

Variations in the expression of virulence factors of "rheumatogenic strains" of *S. pyogenes* may best explain these fluctuations in ARF. M protein types isolated from RF patients (i.e., types 1, 3, 5, 6, 14, 18, 19, and 24)[4] have a common antigenic domain that is immunologically cross-reactive with human heart tissue. Understanding this molecular mimicry holds great promise for the elucidation of the immune mechanisms resulting in clinical ARF. One other marker for rheumatogenicity is the mucoid appearance of fresh pharyngeal isolates from patients with ARF. In recent times in the United States, such strains have been of type 18.

Although certain M protein types are strongly associated with ARF, such strains may cause other GAS infections as well. For example, types 1 and 3 have also been associated with poststreptococcal glomerulonephritis and Strep TSS. Further, epidemics of pharyngitis caused by type 1 are not invariably associated with epidemics of RF. That host factors determine the clinical outcome of GAS infection is suggested by the observation that persons with certain human leukocyte antigen (HLA) class II antigens are predisposed to development of ARF. Further, Stollerman[21] suggests that a gradual acquisition of susceptibility to ARF by schoolchildren occurs after repeated infections. This is supported by the observations of Ayoub and associates, which state that ARF is uncommon in children less than 2 years old and that antibody response to streptococcal antigens is exaggerated in children with ARF compared with those with GAS pharyngitis alone.[24] In addition, Zabriskie and colleagues[25] have shown that patients with ARF demonstrate increased expression of the B-cell alloantigen D8/17 in comparison with unaffected family members, including identical twins. That some strains of GAS can cause ARF in any person is suggested by the observation that the attack rate of ARF can vary from 388 cases per 100,000, as seen in soldiers in World War II, to 1 per 100,000 today. Such fluctuations among relatively homogeneous populations separated in time suggest changes in the relative rheumatogenicity of GAS and not unique host factors.

The clinical manifestations of ARF are multiple and, because each is not specific for ARF, several criteria must be met to establish a definitive diagnosis.[4] Simply put, two major manifestations or one major and two minor manifestations plus, in either case, evidence of an antecedent GAS infection are required for definitive diagnosis. The major manifestations and the frequency with which they occur during first attacks of ARF are as follows: arthritis (75%), carditis (40% to 50%), chorea (15%), and subcutaneous nodules (< 10%). The minor manifestations are fever, arthralgia, heart block, the presence of acute phase reactants in the blood (C-reactive protein, leukocytosis, and elevated erythrocyte sedimentation rate), and prior history of ARF or rheumatic heart disease. Carditis, when present, occurs during the first 3 weeks of illness and may involve the pericardium, myocardium, and endocardium. Patients with pericarditis may have chest pain or pericardial effusion, whereas those with myocarditis may have intractable heart failure. Manifestations of acute endocarditis include the development of new murmurs of mitral regurgitation or aortic regurgitation, the latter being sometimes associated with a low-pitched apical mid-diastolic flow murmur (Carey-Coombs murmur). Murmurs of mitral stenosis and aortic stenosis are not detected acutely during first attacks of ARF but are chronic manifestations of rheumatic heart disease. Migratory arthritis involves several joints, most frequently the knees, ankles, elbows, and wrists, in more than 50% of patients.

Each involved joint has evidence of inflammation that characteristically resolves within 2 to 3 weeks with no progression to chronic arthritis or articular damage. Subcutaneous nodules occur several weeks into the course of ARF and are found over bony surfaces or tendons. They last only 1 to 2 weeks and have, in some cases, been associated with severe carditis. Erythema marginatum is an evanescent, nonpainful, erythematous eruption occurring on the trunk or proximal extremities. Individual lesions can develop and disappear within minutes, but the process may wax and wane over several weeks or months. Sydenham's chorea often occurs later in the course than other manifestations of ARF and is characterized by rapid nonpurposeful choreiform movements of the face, hands, and feet. Attacks usually disappear during sleep but may persist for 2 to 4 months.

Poststreptococcal Glomerulonephritis

Acute glomerulonephritis (AGN) can follow either pharyngeal or skin infection and is associated with GAS strains possessing M protein types 12 and 49, respectively.[1] During epidemics of skin or pharyngeal infection produced by a nephritogenic strain, attack rates of 10% to 15% have been documented with latent periods of 10 days after pharyngitis and 3 weeks after pyoderma. Nonspecific symptoms include lethargy, malaise, headache, anorexia, and dull back pain. The classic signs of AGN are all related to fluid overload and are manifested initially by edema, both dependent and periorbital. Hypertension develops in most patients and is usually mild. Severe cases may be characterized by ascites, pleural effusion, encephalopathy, and pulmonary edema, though evidence of heart failure per se is lacking. Evidence of glomerular damage by renal biopsy has been documented in nearly 50% of contacts of siblings with AGN, suggesting that, as in ARF, subclinical disease is not uncommon after infection with certain strains of GAS. Unlike RF, but similar to scarlet fever, glomerulonephritis occurs most commonly in children between 2 and 6 years of age. Like ARF and scarlet fever, AGN may affect several members of the same family. Recurrences or secondary attacks occur only rarely and there is little to suggest that AGN progresses to chronic renal failure.

The differential diagnosis of poststreptococcal AGN must include Henoch-Schönlein disease, polyarteritis nodosa, idiopathic nephrotic syndrome, leptospirosis, hemolytic-uremic syndrome (*Escherichia coli* O157:H7), and malignant hypertension. The diagnosis is simpler if there has been a recent history of symptomatic GAS pharyngitis, impetigo, or scarlet fever. Elevated or rising antibody titers to streptococcal antigens such as ASO, anti-DNase A or B, or antihyaluronidase are helpful, though ASO concentration may be low in patients with pyoderma. A careful urinalysis to document proteinuria and hematuria should be performed, but it is mandatory to demonstrate red blood cell casts because the latter is the hallmark of glomerular injury. The blood urea nitrogen and creatinine values are elevated and, if nephrotic syndrome is present, the serum cholesterol level may be elevated and serum albumin concentration low. Twenty-four-hour excretion of protein is usually less than 3 g and total hemolytic complement and C3 levels are markedly reduced. The potential role of streptococcal infections in predisposing to other syndromes such as pediatric autoimmune neuropsychiatric disorder associated with streptococcal infection (PANDAS) remains unclear.[26]

PATHOGENESIS AND IMMUNITY

S. pyogenes is a unique human pathogen because it causes multiple and distinct clinical syndromes and has developed unique ways to interact with and neutralize host defense mechanisms. Some of these virulence factors facilitate invasion, inhibit phagocytosis, and contribute to pathogenesis.

Adherence of cocci to the mucosal epithelium is a crucial step in the pathogenesis of pharyngitis and RF and it occurs via the complex interaction of fibronectin-binding protein, lipoteichoic acid, peptidoglycan, and M protein with cell surface structures including fibronectin. It is unclear if penetration of epithelial cells is important in the pathogenesis of pharyngitis but it is important in invasive diseases such as bacteremia. How GAS penetrates cells or migrates between cell junctions to reach the deeper tissue is not understood. Studies by Hanski and Caparon[27] suggest that carbon dioxide and oxygen may alter expression of M protein and fibronectin-binding protein. Once within the tissues, the organism evades the host's inflammatory defenses by destroying or inactivating complement-derived chemoattractants (C5a peptidase),[28] dysregulating endogenous complement inhibitory factors (factor H),[29] and binding or inactivating immunoglobulin (M protein and M protein–like proteins). Expression of M protein, in the absence of type-specific antibody, protects the GAS from phagocytosis by polymorphonuclear leukocytes (PMNs) and monocytes, and secretion of streptolysin O (SLO) in high concentration destroys approaching phagocytes. Distal to the focus of infection, lower concentrations of SLO stimulate PMN adhesion to endothelial cells, effectively preventing continued granulocyte migration.

Cytokines, in particular tumor necrosis factor (TNF), are produced by monocytes and lymphocytes in response to many different GAS factors, including peptidoglycan, SLO, and SPEB. These cytokines play important roles in the development of fever, shock, and multiorgan failure associated with Strep TSS, but are also responsible for the fever and rash associated with scarlet fever. A unique feature of the pyrogenic exotoxins and some M protein fragments is their ability to interact with certain V_{β}jb regions of the T-cell receptor in the absence of classic antigen processing by antigen-presenting cells (APCs). In the nonimmune host, SLO, SPEA, and other streptococcal components stimulate host cells to produce TNF and interleukin-1 (IL-1). In addition, the superantigens associated with GAS induce not only IL-1 and TNF-α from monocytes but induce clonal proliferation of T lymphocytes with massive production of the lymphokines, interferon-γ (INF-γ), IL-2, and TNF-β. These monokines and lymphokines together then mediate hypotension and stimulate leukostasis, resulting in shock, microvascular injury, multiorgan failure, and, if excessive, death.

Bacterial Cell Structure and Extracellular Products

Capsule

Some strains of GAS possess luxuriant capsules of hyaluronic acid, resulting in large mucoid colonies on blood agar. In recent times this mucoid phenotype has been associated with M protein types 1, 3, and 18 strains isolated from patients during epidemics of streptococcal pharyngitis and secondary RF.[4]

M Proteins

Over150 different M types of GAS are recognized, based either on antibody recognition typing of the M protein expressed or by sequencing of the *emm* gene itself. M protein is a coiled α helix consisting of four regions of repeating amino acids (A–D): A proline-glycine–rich region serves to intercalate the protein into the bacterial cell wall, and a hydrophobic region acts as a membrane anchor. Region A near the N-terminal is highly variable, and antibodies to this region confer type-specific protection, likely due to enhanced opsonization of the M protein.[29] Within the more conserved B–D regions lies an area that binds one of the complement regulatory proteins (factor H). The net effect is to stearically inhibit antibody binding and complement-derived opsonin deposition, thus effectively camouflaging the organism against immune surveillance. M protein also inhibits the phagocytosis of *S. pyogenes* by PMNs, though this property can be overcome by type-specific antisera. Kotb and associates have shown that fragments of M protein can also act as superantigens.[30] The regulation of M-protein synthesis is not firmly established but may be controlled by genetic elements of a *vir* gene composed of an upstream control sequence coupled to gene segments coding for M protein, immunoglobulin-binding proteins, and C5a peptidase.[28] Observations by Lancefield[3] suggest that the quantity of M protein produced decreases with passage on artificial media and conversely increases rapidly with passage through mice. During untreated pharyngitis, the quantity of M protein produced by an infecting strain progressively decreases during convalescence.

Cell Wall

The cell wall, which is composed of a peptidoglycan backbone with integral lipoteichoic acid (LTA) components, provides a rigid exoskeleton containing the delicate cytoplasmic and genomic elements of the bacteria. Besides their structural functions, both peptidoglycan and LTA have important interactions with the host immune system (see later discussion).

Hyaluronic Acid Capsule

This structure confers a mucoid appearance to colonies of GAS. Its role in pathogenesis has yet to be defined. Strains that are highly mucoid likely adhere to and invade epithelial cells less well than nonmucoid strains. However, a keratinocyte receptor (CD44) has been shown to bind to hyaluronic acid capsule. Once a barrier has been breached, the capsule may provide protection from phagocytosis and in general these mucoid strains are more virulent if injected subcutaneously.[31]

Cytoplasmic Membrane

Little is known about the function and composition of the cytoplasmic membrane, though it is clear that it does serve as an effective barrier to the external milieu and also is the site of cell wall synthesis, which is in turn orchestrated by five different penicillin-binding proteins (PBPs) found within membrane fragments. The regulation of cell-wall degradation and synthesis during chain elongation is a dynamic process whose control is a reflection of the metabolic activity of the cell. Interestingly, this process becomes dysregulated in the presence of cell wall–active antibiotics. All PBPs are expressed during log-phase growth of GAS, and it is at this stage that penicillin's effects are greatest.[32]

Streptolysin O

SLO belongs to a family of oxygen-labile, thiol-activated cytolysins (TACs) and causes the broad zone of beta hemolysis surrounding colonies of GAS on blood agar plates. TAC toxins bind to cholesterol moieties on eukaryotic cell membranes, creating toxin-cholesterol aggregates that contribute to cell lysis via a colloid-osmotic mechanism. Exogenous cholesterol inhibits hemolysis both in vitro and in situations where serum cholesterol is high (e.g., nephrotic syndrome); thus, elevated antistreptolysin (ASO) titers occur because either cholesterol or anti-ASO antibody "neutralizes" SLO. Several TAC toxins, including SLO, have been cloned and sequenced and there exists striking homology among SLO, perfringolysin O, and pneumolysin in a 13– to 15–amino acid sequence upstream from the cysteine residue.[33] The significance of SLO in pathogenesis is discussed later in this chapter.

Deoxyribonucleases A, B, C, and D

Expression of deoxyribonucleases (DNases) in vivo elicits production of anti-DNase antibody during and after infection. Antibodies to DNase A and DNase B have proved useful in the serologic diagnosis of pharyngeal and skin infections.[1,17] The importance of these enzymes in the pathogenesis of GAS infections has not been proved.

Hyaluronidase

The extracellular enzyme hyaluronidase hydrolyzes the hyaluronic acid in deeper tissues and may facilitate the spread of GAS infections along fascial planes. Its clinical importance is unknown; however, a rise in antihyaluronidase titers follows GAS infections in general, especially those involving the skin.

Pyrogenic Exotoxins A, B, C, MF, and SSA

The pyrogenic exotoxins A, B, C, MF, and SSA, also called scarlatina toxins and erythrogenic toxins, function to induce lymphocyte blastogenesis, potentiate endotoxin-induced shock,[34] induce fever, suppress antibody synthesis, and act as superantigens.[35,36]

The gene for pyrogenic exotoxin A (*speA*) is transmitted by bacteriophage,[37] and stable toxin production depends on lysogenic conversion in a manner analogous to that for diphtheria toxin production by *Corynebacterium diphtheriae.* Factors that control SPEA production are not yet understood, though the quantity of SPEA produced can vary dramatically from decade to decade.[38] Historically, SPEA-producing strains have been associated with severe cases of scarlet fever and, more recently, with Strep TSS.[5]

Although all strains of GAS are endowed with genes for SPEB (*speB*), as with SPEA, the quantity of toxin produced varies greatly. SPEB is related to the proteinase precursor and the role of each in pathogenesis has only recently been investigated.[39,40]

Pyrogenic exotoxin C (SPEC), like SPEA, is bacteriophage-mediated and its expression is likewise highly variable. Hallas[16] demonstrated that mild cases of scarlet fever in England have been associated with strains of GAS-producing SPEC.

Streptococcal superantigen (SSA) has recently been described in an M protein type 3 GAS strain isolated from a patient with Strep TSS.[41] This toxin has similar characteristics to those of other pyrogenic toxins and also functions as a superantigen. Its distribution among strains of GAS and its role in pathogenesis has not been defined.

Mitogenic factor (MF) has all the features of other pyrogenic exotoxins and is a potent inducer of cytokines and lymphokines and has been found in most strains of GAS examined.[42,43]

Many other superantigens have been described from GAS, though the role that they play in pathogenesis remains to be determined.[44]

Protein F

Protein F is a fibronectin-binding protein, which, in conjunction with peptidoglycan, lipoteichoic acid and M protein, plays an important role in adherence of GAS to epithelial surfaces.[44] Production of protein F is inversely related to carbon dioxide concentrations in the milieu.[27]

C5A Peptidase

C5A peptidase, an enzyme produced by most strains of GAS and some strains of group B streptococcus, cleaves the complement activation factor C5A and may thus impede the migration of phagocytes to the site of infection.[28]

TREATMENT

Emergence of Erythromycin Resistance

The first erythromycin-resistant strain of *S. pyogenes* (GAS) was isolated in Great Britain in 1959 and, by 1975, resistant strains had also been isolated in the United States, Canada, and Japan. Although the prevalence of erythromycin resistance among GAS strains has remained low (3.6% to 4.0%) in most western countries, in Japan resistance increased from 8.5% to 72% between 1971 and 1974. Similarly, erythromycin resistance had been a rare finding in Sweden; however, in 1984, an epidemic of pharyngitis (294 cases) caused by erythromycin-resistant GAS was reported. Marked increases in erythromycin resistance have also been documented in Finland, Australia, and Spain, and recently, Pittsburgh.

Sulfonamide Resistance

Sulfonamide resistance currently is reported in fewer than 1% of GAS isolates.

Therapeutic Failure of Penicillin

The major problem in the treatment of GAS infections with penicillin is a lack of in vivo efficacy, despite in vitro susceptibility to penicillin. Penicillin failure in pharyngitis, tonsillitis, or mixed infections has been attributed to inactivation of penicillin in situ by β-lactamases produced by co-colonizing organisms such as *Bacteroides fragilis* or *S. aureus.* For example, this factor contributes to the 10% to 25% bacteriologic failure rate of penicillin treatment of GAS pharyngitis. Further, active selection of such β-lactamase-producing organisms following treatment with penicillin is well documented and leads to bacteriologic failure in 40% to 80% of patients. In support of the role of β-lactamase in bacteriologic failures, Smith and Kaplan described cure rates of 90% in such failures if the second treatment consisted of amoxacillin plus clavulanate compared with only a 29% cure with a second regimen of penicillin.[45] In addition, antibiotics that are unaffected by β-lactamase activity (e.g., amoxicillin with clavulanate, erythromycin, or clindamycin) have a greater efficacy than penicillin in patients with recurrent GAS tonsillitis. In penicillin-allergic patients with acute GAS pharyngitis, erythromycin, cephalosporins, and clindamycin are reasonable alternatives, and all have had greater bacterologic efficacy than penicillin in clinical trials.

Genotypic penicillin tolerance could also explain penicillin's lack of efficacy in tonsillitis or pharyngitis. Tolerant strains demonstrate a slower rate of growth, a slower rate of bacterial killing by penicillin, and an absence of β-lactam-induced cell lysis. Penicillin-tolerant GAS strains have been isolated from 11 of 18 cases of penicillin treatment failures of acute tonsillitis compared with 0 of 15 from successfully treated patients. Penicillin-tolerant strains have also caused epidemics of pharyngitis.

Recently, reports that describe penicillin's reduced efficacy in the treatment of severe streptococcal infections in humans (i.e., streptococcal bacteremia, pneumonia, myositis, and Strep TSS) have surfaced. Studies in animals demonstrated that penicillin was effective if given early or if small numbers of GAS were used to initiate infection. With larger inocula, or if treatment was delayed, penicillin was no more effective than placebo. Thus, penicillin's efficacy declined as the infection became more severe. In comparative trials in animal models of GAS myonecrosis and necrotizing fasciitis, clindamycin had excellent efficacy even if treatment was delayed up to 16 hours. Recently it was demonstrated that GAS organisms in log-phase cultures produce five PBPs, whereas in the stationary phase they do not.[32] Thus, in fulminant infections, GAS organisms have reached a stationary phase of growth and subsequent treatment with penicillin fails due to an absence of its high-affinity targets, the PBPs. Clindamycin's greater efficacy could be due to its ability to suppress virulence factor production (M protein and pyrogenic exotoxin), its longer postantibiotic effect, its indifference to in vivo inoculum or stage of growth, and its ability to attenuate TNF synthesis by human monocytes.

Staphyloccus aureus Infections

In tropical climates, the most common *S. aureus* infection is pyomyositis, though impetigo, cellulitis, carbuncles, and furuncles are also very common. In cities where intravenous drug abuse is prevalent, endocarditis and bacteremia have also been described. *Staphylococcus epidermidis* is also an important cause of intravascular, central nervous system shunt, and prosthetic joint infections. Similarly, *Staphylococcus saprophyticus* and *Staphylococcus intermedius* cause urinary tract infection and infected dog bites, respectively, in western cultures and likely cause similar problems in tropical countries as well.

AGENT

Staphylococci are gram-positive cocci that divide in two planes, thus yielding the classic clusters of cocci. *S. aureus* colonies cause beta hemolysis on sheep blood agar plates and appear as large moist colonies that may develop a golden hue with prolonged growth or when incubated at room temperature for a few hours.

EPIDEMIOLOGY

The normal reservoir of *S. aureus* and *S. epidermidis* is human skin. In addition, the nasal passage may harbor *S. aureus* and may provide an inoculum for those with recurrent furunculosis. *S. aureus* causes infection in healthy persons as well as compromised patients and is distributed among all peoples of the world. Clinical settings with specific staphylococcal infections are listed in Box 31-2.

Box 31-2 Staphylococcal Infections

- Bacteremia
- Cavernous sinus thrombosis
- Cellulitis
- Endocarditis
- Furunculosis
- Impetigo
- Myositis
- Necrotizing fasciitis
- Osteomyelitis
- Pneumonia
- Septic arthritis
- Staphylococcal scalded skin syndrome
- Staphylococcal toxic shock syndrome
- Suppurative thrombophlebitis
- Surgical incision site infection

DISEASES

Folliculitis, Carbuncles, and Abscesses

Abscesses can develop from skin organisms introduced into the deeper tissue, from seeding of the skin from hematogenous sources such as bacteremia associated with endocarditis, or contiguously from infectious foci in the lung or gastrointestinal tract. In the former case, hair follicles serve as a portal of entry for a number of bacterial species, though *S. aureus* is the most common cause of localized folliculitis. Recurrent folliculitis is most common in black males in association with shaving (folliculitis barbae). Folliculitis can progress to small subcutaneous abscesses (furuncles), which either resolve with antibiotic treatment alone or progress to form very large, exquisitely painful carbuncles that require surgical drainage as well as antibiotics. Certain individuals seem predisposed to develop recurrent *S. aureus* infections (recurrent furunculosis) and most have underlying factors such as poor hygiene, nasal carriage of staphylococcus, or neurodermatitis. Though it is suggested that diabetic patients are prone to such infections, there are few data to support this concept. In contrast, patients with Job's syndrome classically have recurrent *S. aureus* infections. In addition, these patients have eosinophilia and high levels of immunoglobulin E (IgE) antibody in serum.

Treatment of recurrent furunculosis may require surgical incision and drainage as well as antistaphylococcal antibiotics such as nafcillin parenterally or dicloxacillin orally. Prevention is difficult, but some success has been realized with intranasal bacitracin or mupirocin ointment and hexachlorophene (pHisoHex) baths (in adults). Prophylactic antibiotics should be used only in severe cases.

Sebaceous glands empty into hair follicles and the ducts, if blocked (sebaceous cyst), may resemble a staphylococcal abscess or may become secondarily infected. Chronic folliculitis is uncommon except in acne vulgaris where normal flora, for example, *Propionibacterium acnes,* may play a role. Hidradenitis suppurativa occurs in either acute or chronic forms and can lead to recurrent axillary or pudendal abscesses.

Impetigo

Impetigo contagiosa is caused by *S. pyogenes,* and bullous impetigo by *S. aureus.* Both skin lesions may have an early bullous stage but then appear as thick crusts with a golden-brown color. Streptococcal lesions are most common in children 2 to 5 years of age, and epidemics may occur in settings of poor hygiene and particularly in children from lower socioeconomic conditions in tropical climates. It is important to recognize impetigo because of its potential relationship to poststreptococcal glomerulonephritis.

Pyomyositis

Pyomyositis is usually due to *S. aureus,* is common in tropical areas but rare in temperate climates, and commonly there is no known portal of entry. The most common presenting features are muscle pain (100%) and fever (81%).[46] Blood cultures are positive in 14.3% of cases and common complications are bronchopneumonia (23.1%) and empyema (19.2%) and mortality is low (7.7%). In one series there was an association with tuberculosis of the dorsal-lumbar spine.[46] Infection remains localized and shock does not occur, unless strains produce toxic shock syndrome toxin-1 (TSST-1) or certain enterotoxins. In contrast, *S. pyogenes* may induce a primary myositis referred to as streptococcal necrotizing myositis, which is associated with severe systemic toxicity. Such infections have been described recently as part of the Strep TSS.

Empyema

S. aureus is the most common cause of empyema in the pediatric age group in tropical areas and has the highest prevalence in the hottest most humid months.[47] Predisposing conditions were prior pustular skin lesions, measles, chickenpox, and blunt trauma to the chest. Only 4% of strains have been methicillin-resistant *S. aureus* (MRSA), but this could increase dramatically in the future. Chest tube drainage was effective in 78% of cases; however, the remaining patients required decortication.[47]

Endocarditis

S. aureus is an important cause of acute endocarditis worldwide. Intravenous drug abuse is the most common risk factor and in 50% of cases involves the right side of the heart. Still, fulminant staphylococcal bacteremia with endocarditis can occur in patients with no risk factors. The major complications regardless of cause are acute destruction of the aortic valve with sudden-onset pulmonary edema. In such cases, it may be necessary to replace the aortic valve immediately to prevent the development of left ventricular dilatation and subsequent myocardopathy. Patients with right-sided endocarditis are less prone to cardiovascular collapse but may develop multiple staphylococcal abscesses of the lung. Regardless of the location of the vegetations, some patients develop metastatic abscesses of the liver, spleen, bones, and kidney. (See also later discussion of MRSA.)

Staphylococcal Toxic Shock Syndrome

Epidemiology

Toxic shock syndrome associated with *S. aureus* infections was originally referred to as TSS,[48] though in this chapter this syndrome is designated Staph TSS to distinguish it from Strep TSS. Between 77% and 93% of cases of Staph TSS have occurred in females and the vast majority (> 90%) of these women were white and 15 to 19 years of age.[49–54] The incidence of Staph TSS was highest in 1980 and ranged from 2.4 to 16 per 100,000 population.[52,53,55–58] Because most of these studies were performed using similar techniques and case definitions, the differences in incidence of disease likely represented bona fide epidemiologic variations—with northern California having the lowest[58] and Colorado[57] having the highest infection rates. Following the peak of reported cases of Staph TSS in 1980, a marked and persistent decline ensued. Numerous epidemiologic studies established that the illness was associated with females during their menstrual cycles and that *S. aureus* colonization and infection within the vagina played a significant role.[49–57] The toxin, TSST-1, was isolated from *S. aureus*[59,60] and found to be produced by over 90% of *S. aureus* strains isolated from menstrual cases of Staph TSS.[61]

The marked decline in the incidence of Staph TSS that began in 1981 has many possible explanations. First, there may have been enhanced reporting of cases in 1980 owing to extensive media coverage. Second, this decline could be related to education of the patients at risk, loss of virulence of the microbe, or acquisition of immunity to the putative toxins by a significant segment of the population. Lastly, some suggest that the reduced prevalence was due to removal of Rely tampons. Clearly, the last does not explain this epidemiologic phenomenon fully because menstrual cases of Staph TSS continue to occur. For further discussions about the epidemiologic studies implicating tampons, and Rely in particular, the reader is referred to the literature.[49–52,62,63]

Also in the early 1980s it was established that nonmenstrual cases of Staph TSS occurred among both sexes, regardless of age, and were associated with surgical procedures such as rhinoplasty with Teflon stents or nasal packing.[64] Nonmenstrual cases have also been described in association with a variety of primary *S. aureus* infections, including cutaneous infection, postsurgical or postpartum infection, focal tissue infection, and pneumonia with or without antecedent influenza infection.[65] In contrast to menstrual cases of Staph TSS, TSST-1 has been detected in only half of strains isolated from patients with nonmenstrual Staph TSS.[61,64] Finally, staphylococcal enterotoxin B (SEB) and, to a lesser extent, enterotoxins A (SEA) and C (SEC) have been found in the remaining strains.[66–69] In addition, case reports suggest that strains that produce TSST-1 together with SEC may be more likely to cause fatalities,[67,68] but luckily both toxins are rarely found together in the same strain.[69]

Clinical Presentation

A prodromal period of 2 to 3 days precedes the physical manifestations of Staph TSS and consists of malaise, myalgia, and chills.[70] Fever begins soon thereafter, followed by symptoms of lightheadedness, modest confusion, and lethargy. The majority of patients develop diarrhea early in the course. Symptoms of hypovolemia, due in part to capillary leak and diarrhea, then predominate and include hyperventilation, palpitations, and dizziness on standing. Confusion, a prominent feature of Staph TSS, may affect some patients' ability to recognize the seriousness of their illness, resulting in delayed treatment.

When patients are first examined, fever, tachycardia, tachypnea, and hypotension are usually present. A transient, erythematous rash has been observed in over 50% of patients and may be either diffuse or patchy in distribution.[70] Many patients have marked peripheral vasodilation associated with high cardiac output and thus erythematous skin may represent maximal capillary dilation due to toxins or endogenous mediators. The capillary leak mentioned previously may not be apparent until fluid resuscitation has been undertaken. Desquamation of skin, particularly at sites of a previous erythematous rash, occurs between 7 and 14 days.[70]

Pathogenesis and Immunity

There is little doubt that TSST-1 and staphylococcal enterotoxins are the major virulence factors associated with cases of Staph TSS. There is substantial evidence that the genetic determinants for TSST-1 and SEB are neither plasmid- nor bacteriophage-mediated and that the gene is a variably expressed, mobile element, likely a transposon.[71] There has been intense research to elucidate the environmental and genetic control mechanisms responsible for enhanced toxin production. Clearly, neutral pH, iron, trace elements such as magnesium and calcium, as well as oxygen enhance TSST-1 production.[63] Toxin is produced mainly during the late log phase and early stationary phases of growth.

Extrapolation of these findings to the apparent increased risk of menstrual Staph TSS with tampon use in 1980 has been more difficult if not controversial. Some suggest that tampons could (1) increase vaginal partial oxygen pressure, at least during placement, thereby stimulating toxin synthesis by colonizing strains of *S. aureus,* (2) supply surfactants that could increase toxin production, and (3) bind magnesium and shift the growth kinetics of staphylococci toward enhanced toxin production.[65] Thus, modest quantities of these toxins, locally produced, interact with the immune system, first at the site of infection and then systemically.

Monocytes, as well as a mononuclear cell line, have the ability to bind TSST-1 and staphylococcal enterotoxins. In addition, these toxins bind to specific sites on the V_{β}jb region of the T-lymphocyte receptor (TCR). Simultaneous binding to both monocyte and T lymphocyte results in T-cell proliferation (blastogenesis) and activation of both cell types via the superantigen mechanism.[72] Recent studies have shown that activation of the T cell via this mechanism requires the appropriate toxin, viable T lymphocytes bearing a specific V repertoire, and either a viable APC, a nonviable APC, or a fragment of the major histocompatibility complex (MHC) class II receptor.[73] Other accessory molecules may also participate in the docking between MHC class II and TCR. One of the T-lymphocyte binding sites for enterotoxin appears to be CD4.[74] CD4 site binding could serve to stabilize the complex between the TCR and MHC class II. Further, blocking of other surface molecules such as ICAM-1, CD11a, CD28, or CD2 with monoclonal antibodies effectively prevented T-cell proliferation in the presence of SEB.[75]

The consequences of superantigen stimulation of the immune system are T-lymphocyte proliferation and generation of vast quantities of the lymphokines IL-2, INF-γ, and TNF-β[72,76,77] as well as the monokines TNF-α, IL-1, and IL-6,[35,76] yet the dynamics of production are quite different for each. Specifically, during the first 24 hours, production of TNF by peripheral blood mononuclear cells (PBMCs) predominates. By 48 hours, TNF-β is detectable, and at 72 hours, equal quantities of TNF-α and TNF-β can be measured.[76]

The control mechanism of cytokine production via the superantigen mechanism is poorly understood, but both counterregulatory cytokines and accelerated programmed cell death are likely involved. For example, the conventional wisdom regarding T-cell proliferation describes the initial proliferation of T cells in response to superantigens followed by the rapid depletion of T-cell subsets bearing the specific V repertoire through accelerated programmed cell death or apoptosis.[67] T-lymphocyte dynamics have been studied in a mouse model of SEB-induced shock.[78,79] There was clear evidence of V-selective clonal expansion 24 to 48 hours after administration of SEB.[78,79] On day 3, clonally expanding cells became depleted through accelerated programmed cell death (apoptosis) resulting in anergy.[78,79] McCormack and colleagues[80] demonstrated that this expansion-deletion sequence occurs predictably in vivo when high concentrations of a superantigen are used. However, deletions also occur using low dosages. In fact, concentrations that were insufficient to cause T-cell blastogenesis in vivo were still capable of depleting specific V subsets of T lymphocytes.[80] Using sublethal concentrations of a superantigen, Miethke and coworkers[81] demonstrated that 4 to 6 hours after in vivo challenge with SEB, BALB/c mice became resistant to an otherwise lethal dose of SEB plus D-galactosamine.[81] These authors demonstrated that PBMCs harvested from such animals during this time lost the ability to release lymphokines such as TNF-β and IL-2.[81] They hypothesized that endogenous corticosteroids released in response to the first wave of lymphokines induced by SEB may have suppressed T-cell responsiveness. Though this might be an adequate explanation, counterregulatory cytokines likely play a more important role. For example, 10 ng/mL of IL-10, a regulatory cytokine produced by the Th2 subset of CD4+ helper T lymphocytes, inhibited synthesis of TNF-β and INF-γ production by TSST-1-stimulated PBMCs by 68% and 86%, respectively.[82] The relevance of this endogenous control mechanism in vivo is uncertain since only 72 pg/mL of IL-10 was produced in vitro by PBMCs stimulated with TSST-1,[82] a concentration well below that used in the in vitro studies. Krakauer[82] points out that exogenous administration of recombinant IL-10 might be a rational treatment for superantigen-induced disease. Recent studies showing that IL-10 protected animals from lethal challenge support this hypothesis[83] (see also discussion under Treatment). Interestingly, IL-10 did not inhibit T-lymphocyte blastogenesis,[82] suggesting that IL-10 works largely by inhibiting transcriptional events.

Though the previously described animal models of superantigen injection demonstrate lethality, what is the evidence that *S. aureus* toxins such as TSST-1 or the enterotoxins cause an illness resembling Staph TSS? The animal model that has been best studied in this regard is the rabbit whiffle ball model. Briefly, sterile plastic chambers are implanted beneath the skin of rabbits and allowed to mature over the course of 3 to 4 weeks. Strains of *S. aureus* are then inoculated into these chambers and physiologic measurements of blood chemistries, blood pressure, pulse, temperature, and mortality are recorded. Scott and coworkers[84] and Rasheed and colleagues,[85] using this model, and De Azevedo and associates,[86] using an implanted uterine diffusion chamber model, demonstrated that strains producing TSST-1 were more likely to induce a toxic shock–like syndrome than strains that did not produce TSST-1. Strains of *S. aureus* that produced altered TSST-1 toxins lacking the ability to induce mitogenicity were nontoxic in the rabbit whiffle ball chamber model,[87] though the reason for the loss of mitogenicity was unexplained. Subsequently, using both genetically altered SEC mutants and peptide fragments of SEC to stimulate lymphocyte proliferation in vitro, it was determined that toxin binding to the α helix of the MHC class II portion of the APC was critically important in the induction of lymphocyte blastogenesis.[88]

The role of TSST-1 in inducing a TSS-like illness is also supported by the demonstration that a neutralizing monoclonal antibody prevented illness in rabbits challenged with a TSST-1-producing strain of *S. aureus.*[89] Parsonnet and colleagues[90] have also developed a slow infusion model that allows the investigation of purified, recombinant, and genetically altered toxins.

Treatment and Prognosis

Patients diagnosed as having Staph TSS will be profoundly hypotensive, tachycardic, and febrile, and may have evidence of coagulopathy. The general supportive measures described in the previous section apply to Staph TSS as well. Clearly, in menstrual cases, early removal of the tampon and irrigation of the vaginal vault are important. Similarly, in nonmenstrual cases, surgical débridement, drainage, and removal of stents and packing are vital.[91]

Antibiotic treatment based on in vitro susceptibility would suggest that nafcillin, first- or second-generation cephalosporins, vancomycin, clindamycin, erythromycin, and fluoroquinolones would be reasonable choices. A variety of these antibiotics have been used in the last 15 years, and the mortality rate for Staph TSS remains at about 3% for menstrual cases and is two- to threefold higher for nonmenstrual cases.[63]

As with Strep TSS, shock and organ failure in patients with Staph TSS is clearly the consequence of the deleterious effects of extracellular proteinaceous toxins on the immune system. Thus, antibiotics that suppress protein (toxin) synthesis might be more efficacious than cell wall–active antibiotics, as has been described in the previous section. Clindamycin in concentrations that are either above the minimal inhibitory concentration (MIC)[92] or below it[93] suppress TSST-1 synthesis by strains of *S. aureus*. Parsonnet and coworkers[94] demonstrated that clindamycin, erythromycin, rifampin, and fluoroquinolones all suppressed TSST-1 synthesis by greater than 90%. In contrast, five different β-lactam antibiotics, including nafcillin and cephalosporins, increased measurable TSST-1 in culture supernatants, probably by releasing intracellular stores of toxin in part by causing direct lysis or by increasing the permeability of the cell wall.[94] Unfortunately, there has been no controlled clinical trial comparing different antibiotics; however, these results suggest that antibiotic susceptibility alone may not necessarily predict success.

The potential use of immunoglobulin to treat Staph TSS has a sound basis (see also the section on Strep TSS Treatment). First, many investigators have demonstrated that patients who develop Staph TSS have low to absent antibody titers against TSST-1 or enterotoxins or both.[63] Second, the general population in both the United States and Europe has significant antibody titers against these toxins and titers increase with age.[63] This latter finding is supported by the observation that pooled immunoglobulin preparations have high titer antibody against TSST-1.[63] Finally, there are recent data in experimental animals that antibody which neutralizes TSST-1 is therapeutic.[95,96] There have been no prospective studies done in humans.

The usefulness of corticosteroids in shock has been studied for many years. Corticosteroid therapy is not currently considered to be an effective treatment in the United States, though some centers in Europe currently use this treatment. Todd[91] advocates corticosteroids for patients with "severe Staph TSS unresponsive to initial antibiotic therapy."

TREATMENT

Cellulitis

Because of the diverse causes of cellulitis, empirical choices of antibiotic therapy depend greatly on the clinical factors described previously. Once cultures and sensitivities are available, choices are much easier and more specific. The physician must first decide if the patient's illness is severe enough to require parenteral treatment either in the hospital or on an outpatient basis. For presumed streptococcal or staphylococcal cellulitis, nafcillin, cephalothin, cefuroxime, vancomycin, or erythromycin are good choices. Cefazolin and ceftriaxone have less activity against *S. aureus* than cephalothin, though clinical trials have shown a high degree of efficacy. Ceftriaxone may be a useful choice for outpatient treatment because of once-per-day dosing. Similarly, teicoplanin, like vancomycin, has excellent activity against *S. pyogenes* and both *S. aureus* and *S. epidermidis* and may be given once per day by intravenous or intramuscular injection. For patients being treated with oral drugs, dicloxacillin, cefuroxime axetil, cefpodoxime, or erythromycin (or clarithromycin or azithromycin) are effective treatments. For known group A, B, C, or G streptococcal infections, penicillin or erythromycin should be used orally or parenterally. In serious group A streptococcal infections, clindamycin is superior to penicillin. This is probably because in this type of infection, wherein large numbers of bacteria are present, streptococci are in a stationary phase of growth and do not express a full complement of PBPs. In contrast, clindamycin is not affected by inoculum size or stage of growth. In addition, clindamycin suppresses production of extracellular toxins by both *S. aureus* and *S. pyogenes*.

Methicillin-Resistant *S. aureus* Infections

During the last 15 years, there has been a slow but steady increase in the prevalence of MRSA in all communities of the world, including Indonesia, Japan, India, North and South America, and Europe. Until 2002, these strains were all associated with hospital-associated (HA) MRSA infections and the greatest risk factors were prior hospitalization, surgical procedures, and recent antibiotic exposure, particularly fluoroquinolones, β-lactam antibiotics, and vancomycin. Currently, a dramatic increase in community-associated (CA) MRSA infections has been reported. These are most commonly associated with soft tissue infections, though pneumonia, toxic shock syndrome, and necrotizing soft tissue infections have been described.[97,98] Vancomycin has been the drug of choice, though it is slowly bactericidal and does not penetrate tissues, particularly the lung, very well. Linezolid has been shown to be an effective agent for skin and soft-tissue infections, bacteremia, and pneumonia caused by MRSA. Recently, daptomycin, which is rapidly bactericidal, has also been approved for MRSA skin and skin structure infections. Clinical trials are under way for an indication in MRSA endocarditis, though it is not yet approved for this purpose. Unfortunately, HA MRSA strains are also resistant to many other antibiotics. CA MRSA strains are less likely to be resistant to trimethoprim-sulfamethoxazole and tetracyclines, but inducible clindamycin resistance has emerged as a potential problem in 20% to 30% of strains. These dynamic changes in the susceptibility of *S. aureus* cause great difficulty in recommending specific treatments for both HA and CA MRSA. The clinician must factor in the prevalence of MRSA in his or her environment and the seriousness of the infection in selecting empiric antibiotics. It is more important than ever to obtain cultures and rely on sensitivities to guide subsequent treatment.

PREVENTION AND CONTROL

Prevention and control of streptococcal and staphylococcal infections and their sequelae are best accomplished by careful personal hygiene and prompt treatment of early infections. Extensive regimens to eradicate carriage may have a role in selected cases of recurring infections.

REFERENCES

1. Stevens DL: Streptococcal infections. In Goldman L, Bennett JC (eds): Cecil Textbook of Medicine, 20th ed. Philadelphia, WB Saunders, 1996, pp 1585–1590.
2. Stevens DL, Bryant AE, Yan S, et al: Factors controlling host range and pathogenesis of group A streptococcal infections. In Verduin CM, Watson DA, van Dijk H, et al (eds): Constitutional Resistance to Infection. Austin, TX, RG Landes, 1995, pp 15–24.
3. Lancefield RC: Current knowledge of type specific M antigens of group A steptococci. J Immunol 89:307–313, 1962.
4. Bisno AL: Group A Streptococcal infections and acute rheumatic fever. N Engl J Med 325:783–793, 1991.
5. Stevens DL, Tanner MH, Winship J, et al: Reappearance of scarlet fever toxin A among streptococci in the Rocky Mountain West: Severe group A streptococcal infections associated with a toxic shock-like syndrome. N Engl J Med 32:1–7, 1989.
6. Martin PR, Hoiby EA: Streptococcal serogroup A epidemic in Norway 1987–1988. Scand J Infect Dis 22:421–429, 1990.
7. Holm S: Fatal group A streptococcal infections. Presented at the 89th Meeting of the American Society of Microbiology, New Orleans, May 15–19, 1989.
8. Wheeler MC, Roe MH, Kaplan EL, et al: Outbreak of group A streptococcus septicemia in children. Clinical, epidemiologic, and microbiological correlates. JAMA 266:533–537, 1991.
9. Gaworzewska ET, Coleman G: Correspondence: Group A streptococcal infections and a toxic shock–like syndrome. N Engl J Med 321:1546, 1989.
10. Schwartz B, Facklam RR, Breiman RF: changing epidemiology of group A streptococcal infection in the USA. Lancet 336:1167–1171, 1990.
11. Bartter T, Dascal A, Carroll K, et al: "Toxic strep syndrome": Manifestation of group A streptococcal infection. Arch Intern Med 148:1421–1424, 1988.
12. Hribalova V: *Streptococcus pyogenes* and the toxic shock syndrome. Ann Intern Med 108:772, 1988.
13. Greenberg RN, Willoughby BG, Kennedy DJ, et al: Hypocalcemia and "toxic" syndrome associated with streptococcal fasciitis. South Med J 76:916–918, 1983.
14. Jackson MA, Olson LC, Burry VF: Pediatric group A streptococcal (GAS) disease with multi-organ dysfunction. In Program and Abstracts of the Interscience Conference on Antimicrobial Agents and Chemotherapy, 1990.
15. Thomas JC, Carr SJ, Fujioka K, et al: Community-acquired group A streptococcal deaths in Los Angeles Country. J Infect Dis 160:1086–1087, 1989.
16. Hallas G: The production of pyrogenic exotoxins by group A streptococci. J Hyg (Camb) 95:47–57, 1985.
17. Bisno Al, Stevens DL: Streptococcal infections in skin and soft tissues. N Engl J Med 334:240–245, 1996.
18. Maleney FL: Hemolytic streptococcus gangrene. Arch Surg 9:317–364, 1924.
19. Adams EM, Gudmundsson S, Yocum DE, et al: Streptococcal myositis. Arch Intern Med 145:1020–1023, 1985.
20. Holm SE, Norrby A, Bergholm AM, et al: Aspects of pathogenesis of serious group A streptococcal infections in sweden, 1988–1989. J Infect Dis 166:31–37, 1992.
21. Stollerman GH: Rheumatic Fever and Streptococcal Infection. New York, Grune & Stratton, 1975.
22. Veasy LG, Wiedmeier SE, Orsmond GS: Resurgence of acute rheumatic fever in the intermountain area of the United States. N Engl J Med 316:421–427, 1986.
23. Wannamaker LW, Rammelkamp CH Jr, Deeny FW, et al: Prophylaxis of acute rheumatic fever by treatment of the preceding streptococcal infection with various amounts of depot penicillin. Am J Med 10:673–695, 1951.
24. Ayoub EM, Barrett DJ, Maclaren NK, et al: Association of class II human histocompatibility leukocyte antigens with rheumatic fever. J Clin Invest 77:2019–2026, 1986
25. Zabriskie JB, Lavenchy D, Williams RC Jr, et al: Rheumatic-fever associated B-cell alloantigens as identified by monoclonal antibodies. Arthritis Rheum 28:1047–1051, 1985.
26. Stinger HS, Loiselle CR, Lee O, et al: Anti-basal ganglia iantibodies in PANDA. Mov Disord 19:406–415, 2004.
27. Hanski E, Caparon M: Protein F, a fibronectin-binding protein, is an adhesin of the group A streptococcus *Streptococcus pyogenes*. Proc Natl Acad Sci USA 89:6172–6176, 1992.
28. Cleary PP, Peterson J, Chen C, et al: Virulent human strains of group G streptococci express as C5a peptidase enzyme similar to that produced by group A streptococci. Infect Immun 59:2305–2310, 1991.
29. Fischetti VA: Streptococcal M protein. Sci Am 264:58–65, 1991.
30. Kotb M, Ohnishi H, Majumdar G, et al: Temporal relationship of cytokine release by peripheral blood mononuclear cells stimulated by the streptococcal superantigen pep M5. Infect Immun 61:1194–1201, 1993.
31. Moses AE, Zalcman K, Yaron S, et al: M Protein any hyaluronic acid capsule both contribute to the capacity of mucoid goup A streptococci to resist phagocytic killing in human blood. In Program and Abstracts of the 33rd Meeting of the Infectious Disease Society of America, 1995.
32. Stevens DL, Yan S, Bryant AE: Penicillin Binding protein expression at different growth stages determines penicillin efficacy in vitro and in vivo: An explanation for the inoculum effect. J Infect Dis 167:1401–1405, 1993.
33. Tweten RK: Nucleotide sequence of the gene for perfringolysin O (theta-toxin) from *Clostridium perfringens:* Significant homology with the genes for streptolysin O and pneumolysin. Infect Immum 56:3235–3240, 1998.
34. Stevens DL: Invasive group A streptococcus infections. Clin Infect Dis 14:2–13, 1992.
35. Fast DJ, Schlievert PM, Nelson RD: Toxic shock syndrome–associated staphylococcal and streptococcal pyrogenic toxins are potent inducers of tumor necrosis factor production. Infect Immum 57:291–294, 1989.
36. Hackett SP, Stevens DL: Streptococcal toxic shock syndrome: Synthesis of tumor necrosis factor and interleukin-1 by monocytes stimulated with pyrogenic exotoxin A and streptolysin O. J Infect Dis 165:879–885, 1992.
37. Yu CE, Ferretti JJ: Molecular epidemiologic analysis of the type A streptococcal exotoxin (erythrogenic toxin) gene (speA) in clinical *Streptococcus pyogenes* strains. Infect Immun 57:3715–3719, 1989.
38. Kohler W, Gerlach D, Knoll H: Streptococcal outbreaks and erythrogenic toxin type A. Zentralbl Bakt Hyg 266:104–115, 1987.
39. Kappur V, Majesky MW, Li LL, et al: Cleavage of interleukin 1 (IL-1) precursor to produce active IL-1 by a conserved extracellular cysteine protease from *Streptococcus pyogenes.* Proc Natl Acad Sci USA 90:7676–7680, 1993.
40. Herwald H, Collin M, Muller-Esterl W, et al: Streptococcal cysteine proteinase releases kinnis: A novel virulence mechanism. J Exp Med 184:1–9, 1996.
41. Mollick JA, Miller GG, Musser JM, et al: A novel superantigen isolated from pathogenic strains of *Streptococcus pyogenes* with aminoterminal homology to staphylococcal enterotoxins B and C. J Clin Invest 92:710–719, 1993.
42. Iwasaki M, Igarashi H, Hinuma Y, et al: Cloning, characterization and overexpression of a *Streptococcus pyogenes* gene encoding a new type of mitogenic factor. FEBS Lett 331:187–192, 1993.
43. Norrby-Teglund A, Newton D, Kotb M, et al: Superantigenic properties of the group A streptococcal exotoxin SpeF (MF). Infect Immun 62:5227–5233, 1994.
44. Proft T, Moffat SL, Berkahn CJ, et al: Identification and characterization of novel superantigens from *Streptococcus pyogenes*. J Exp Med 189:89–101, 1999.
45. Smith TD, Huskins WC, Kim KS, et al: Efficacy of beta-lactamase-resistant penicillin and influence of penicillin tolerance in eradicating streptococci from pharynx after failure of penicillin therapy for group A streptococcal pharyngitis. J Pediatr 6:601–607, 1987.
46. Malhotra P, Singh S, Sud A, et al: Tropical pyomyositis: Experience of a tertiary care hospital in northwest India. J Assoc Physicians India 48:1057–1059, 2000.
47. Baranwal AK, Singh M, Marwaha RK, et al: Empyema thoracis: A 10-year comparative review of hospitalised children from shouth Asia. Arch Dis Child 88:1009–1014, 2003.

48. Todd J, Fishaut M: Toxic-shock syndrome associated with phase-group-1 staphylococci. Lancet 2:1116–1118, 1978.
49. Broome CV: Epidemiology of toxic shock syndrome in the United States: Overview. Rev Infect Dis 11:S14–21, 1989.
50. Davis JP, Chesney PJ, Wand PJ, et al: The Investigation and Laboratory Team: Toxic shock syndrome: Epidemiologic features, recurrence, risk factors, and prevention. N Engl J Med 303:1429–1435, 1980.
51. Shands KN, Schmidt GP, Dan BB, et al: Toxic shock syndrome in menstruating women. N Engl J Med 303:1436–1442, 1980.
52. Schlech WF, Shands KN, Reingold AL, et al: Risk factors for the development of toxic shock syndrome: Association with a tampon brand. JAMA 248:835–839, 1982.
53. Osterholm MT, Davis JP, Gibson RW, et al: Tri-state toxic-shock syndrome study. I. Epidemiologic findings. J Infect Dis 145:431–440, 1982.
54. Latham RH, Kehrberg MW, Jacobson JA, et al: Toxic shock syndrome in Utah: A case-control and surveillance study. Ann Intern Med 96:906–908, 1982.
55. Helgerson SD, Foster LR: Toxic shock syndrome in Oregon. Ann Intern Med 96:909–911, 1982.
56. Osterholm MT, Forfang JC: Toxic shock syndrome in Minnesota: Result of an active-passive surveillance system. J Infect Dis 145:458–464, 1982.
57. Todd JK, Wiesenthal AM, Ressman M, et al: Toxic shock syndrome. II. Estimated occurrence in Colorado as influenced by case ascertainment methods. Am J Epidemiol 122:857–867, 1985.
58. Petitti DB, Reingold AL, Chin J: The incidence of toxic shock syndrome in northern California: 1972–1983. JAMA 255:368–372, 1986.
59. Schlievert PM, Shands KN, Dan BB, et al: Identification and characterization of an exotoxin from *Staphylococcus aureus* associated with toxic-shock syndrome. J Infect Dis 143:509–516, 1981.
60. Bergdoll MS, Crass BA, Reiser RF, et al: A new staphylococcal entertoxin, entertoxin F, associated with toxic-shock-syndrome *Staphylococcus aureus* isolates. Lancet 1:1017–1021, 1981.
61. Bonventre PF, Weckbach L, Harth G, et al: Distribution and expression of toxic shock syndrome toxin 1 gene among *Staphylococcus aureus* isolates of toxic shock syndrome and non-toxic shock syndrome origin. Rev Infect Dis 11:S90–S95, 1989.
62. Mittag H-C: Toxic Shock Syndrome and the Other Staphylococcal Toxicoses. Stuttgart, Schattauer, 1988.
63. Bergdoll MS, Chesney PJ: Toxic Shock Syndrome. Boca Raton, FL, CRC Press, 1991.
64. Jacobson JA, Kasworm E, Daly JA: Risk of developing toxic shock syndrome associated with toxic shock syndrome toxin 1 following nongenital staphylococcal infection. Rev Infect Dis 11:S8–S13, 1989.
65. Murray DL, Ohlendorf DH, Schlievert PM: Staphylococcal and streptococcal superantigens: Their role in human diseases. ASM News 61:229–235, 1995.
66. Crass BA, Bergdoll MS: Involvement of staphylococcal entertoxins in nonmenstrual toxic shock shyndrome. J Cin Microbiol 23:1138–1139, 1986.
67. Schlievert PM: Staphylococcal enterotoxin B and toxic shock syndrome toxin 1 are significantly associated with non-menstrual TSS. Lancet 1:1149–1150, 1986.
68. Crass BA, Bergdoll MS: Toxin involvement in toxic shock syndrome. J Infect Dis 153:918–926, 1986.
69. Bohach GA, Kreiswirth BN, Novick RP, et al: Analysis of toxic shock syndrome isolates producing staphylococcal enterotoxins B and C1 with use of Southern hybridization and immunologic assays. Rev Infect Dis 11:S75–S81, 1989.
70. Chesney PJ: Clinical aspects and spectrum of illness of toxic shock syndrome: Overview. Rev Infect Dis 11:S1–S13, 1989.
71. Kreiswirth BN, Projain SJ, Schlievert PM, et al: Toxic shock syndrome toxin 1 is encoded by a variable genetic element. Rev Infect Dis 11:S83–S88, 1989.
72. Marrack P, Kappler JW: The staphylococcal enterotoxins and their relatives. Science 248:705–711, 1990.
73. See RH, Kum WWS, Chang AH, et al: Induction of tumor necrosis factor and interleukin-1 by purified staphylococcal toxic shock syndrome toxin 1 requires the presence of both monocytes and T lymphocytes. Infect Immun 60:2612–2618, 1992.
74. Bavari S, Ulrich RG: Staphylococcal enterotoxin A and toxic shock syndrome toxin compete with CD4 for human major histocompatibility complex class II binding. Infect Immum 63:423–429, 1995.
75. Krakauer T: Costimulatory receptors for the superantigen staphylococcal enterotoxin B on human vascular endothelial cells and T cells. J Leukos Biol 56:458–463, 1994.
76. Hackett SP, Stevens DL: Superantigens associated with staphylococcal and streptococcal toxic shock syndromes are potent inducers of tumor necrosis factor beta synthesis. J Infect Dis 168:232–235, 1993.
77. Norrby-Teglund A, Norgren M, Holm SE, et al: Similar cytokine induction profiles of a novel streptococcal exotoxin, MF, and pyrogenic exotoxins A and B. Infect Immum 62:3731–3738, 1994.
78. MacDonald HR, Baschieri S, Lees RK: Clonal expansion precedes anergy and death of Vbeta8+ peripheral T cells responding to staphylococcal enterotoxin B in vivo. Eur J Immunol 21:1963–1996, 1991.
79. Kawabe Y, Ochi A: programmed cell death and extrathymic reduction of Vbeta8 + CD4 T cells in mice tolerant to *Staphylococcus aureus* enterotoxin B. Nature 349:245–248, 1991.
80. McCormack JE, Callahan JE, Kappler J, et al: Profound deletion of mature T cells in vivo by chronic exposure to exogenous superantigen. J Immunol 150:3785–3792, 1993.
81. Miethke T, Wahl C, Heeg K, et al: Acquired resistance to superantigen-induced T cell shock. V selective T cell unresponsiveness unfolds directly from a transient state of hyperreactivity. J Immunol 150:3776–3784, 1993.
82. Krakauer T: Inhibition of toxic shock syndrome toxin-1-induced cytokine production and T cell activation by interleukin-10, interleukin-4, and dexamethasone. J Infect Dis 172:988–992, 1995.
83. Bean AGD, Freiberg RA, Andrade S, et al: Interleukin 10 protects mice against staphylococcal enterotoxin B-induced lethal shock. Infect Immun 61:4937–4939, 1993.
84. Scott DF, Kling JM, Kirkland JJ, et al: Characterization of *Staphylococcus aureus* isolates from patients with toxic shock syndrome, using polyethylene infection chambers in rabbits. Infect Immun 39:383–387, 1983.
85. Rasheed JK, Arko RJ, Freely JC, et al: Acquired ability of *Staphylococcus aureus* to produce toxic shock associated protein and resulting illness in a rabbit model. Infect Immun 47:598–604, 1985.
86. De Azavedo JCS, Foster TJ, Hartigan PJ, et al: Expression of the cloned toxic shock syndrome toxin 1 gene (tst) in vivo with a rabbit uterine model. Infect Immun 50:304–309, 1985.
87. Bonventre PF, Heeg H, Cullen C, et al: Toxicity of recombinant toxic shock syndrome toxin 1 and mutant toxins produced by *Staphyloccus aureus* in a rabbit infection model of toxic shock syndrome. Infect Immun 61:793–799, 1993.
88. Hoffmann ML, Jablonski LM, Crum KK, et al: Predictions of T-cell receptor- and major histocompatibility complex-binding sites on staphylococcal enterotoxin C1. Infect Immun 62:3396–3407, 1994.
89. Best GK, Scott DF, Kling JM, et al: Protection of rabbits in an infection model of toxic shock syndrome (TSS) by a TSS toxin-1-specific monoclonal antibody. Infect Immun 56:998–999, 1988.
90. Parsonnet J, Gillis ZA, Richter AG, et al: A rabbit model of toxic shock syndrome that uses a constant, subcutaneous infusion of toxic shock syndrome toxin 1. Infect Immun 55:1070–1076, 1987.
91. Todd JK: Therapy of toxic shock syndrome. Drugs 39:856–861, 1990.
92. Wexler DE, Nelson RD, Cleary PP: Human neutrophil chemotactic response to group A streptococci: Bacteria-mediated interference with complement-derived factors. Infect Immun 39:239–246, 1983.
93. Dickgiesser N, Wallach U: Toxic shock syndrome toxin-1 (TSST-1): Influence of its production by subinhibitory antibiotic concentrations. Infect Immun 15:351–353, 1996
94. Parsonnet J, Modern PA, Giacobbe K: Effect of subinhibitory concentrations of antibiotics on production of toxic shock syndrome toxin-1 (TSST-1). Presented at the 32nd Meeting of Infectious Disease Society of America, Orlando, FL, Oct 7–9, 1994.
95. Bonventre PF, Thompson MR, Adinolfi LE, et al: Neutralization of toxic shock sydrome toxin 1 by monoclonal antibodies in vitro and in vivo. Infect Immun 56:135–141, 1988.
96. Melish ME, Frogner KS, Hirata SA, et al: Human gamma globulin therapy in experimental toxic shock syndrome (TSS). In Program and abstracts of the American Society for Microbiology, Atlanta, 1987, p 57.
97. Stevens DL: Community-acquired Staphylococcus aureus infections: Increasing virulence and emerging methicillin resistance in the new millennium. Curr Opin Infect Dis 16:189–191, 2003.
98. Miller LG, Perdreau-Remington F, Rieg G, et al: Necrotizing fasciitis caused by community-associated methicillin-resistant *Staphylococcus aureus* in Los Angeles. N Engl J Med 352:1445–1453, 2005.

32

Pertussis

EMILY J. WONG
ERIK L. HEWLETT

INTRODUCTION

Pertussis, or whooping cough, remains a significant cause of morbidity and mortality worldwide. Despite the availability of vaccines effective in preventing infection by *Bordetella pertussis*, an estimated 50 million cases occur each year, resulting in 300,000 deaths. The majority of these cases occur in developing countries, where malnutrition and limited supportive care contribute to the case fatality rate in infants, which can reach 4%.[1,2] Even in countries where pertussis vaccination is widely available, there is still a significant burden of pertussis disease, particularly in adolescents and adults.[3–9]

AGENT

Pertussis is caused by coccobacillary organisms from the genus *Bordetella*. *B. pertussis* and *B. parapertussis* are responsible for whooping cough illness in humans; there are additional *Bordetella* species, including *B. bronchiseptica*, *B. avium*, *B. hinzii*, *B. holmesii*, and *B. trematum*.[10–14] Although *B. bronchiseptica* is primarily an animal pathogen, it can cause respiratory illness in humans, often via transmission from animals.[15,16]

Both *B. pertussis* and *B. parapertussis* have been isolated from patients with clinical pertussis, and there are cases in which dual infection has been documented.[17] However, *B. parapertussis* does not produce pertussis toxin, one of the major virulence factors of *B. pertussis* contributing to severity of disease,[18,19] and infection with *B. parapertussis* is rare in infants less than 6 months old. Therefore, *B. pertussis* is believed to be the predominant cause of severe pertussis disease and mortality and is the focus of the World Health Organization (WHO) pertussis surveillance.[2]

EPIDEMIOLOGY

Pertussis has a worldwide distribution, but the lack of active surveillance in many countries has resulted in a paucity of reliable data from some regions of the world, particularly Africa. Historically, pertussis has persisted in communities as an endemic disease with 3- to 5-year periodic cycles of epidemics. Recent outbreaks have occurred in settings associated with crowded living conditions (e.g., military units, the Hajj pilgrimage, oil refinery workers)[20–22] and communities with low vaccination rates (e.g., Afghanistan).[23]

Reported incidences of disease in unimmunized populations are as high as 6000 per 100,000 child-years <15 years of age and 18,000 per 100,000 child-years <5 years of age.[2,24] Following pertussis vaccine introduction, incidence drops to <20 per 100,000 person-years,[2,9,25] but can rise to rates of 300 to 500 cases per 100,000 person-years owing to disease in adolescents and adults.[4,7,26]

Prior to the introduction of whole-cell pertussis vaccine, many infants had passive immunity from maternally transmitted antibodies. Pertussis was primarily an illness of young children (aged 2 to 10 years), who thereby acquired natural immunity that was subsequently boosted through repetitive exposures in the community. As a result of widespread use of pertussis vaccine, there has been a shift in the age distribution of pertussis cases. Infants are born unprotected owing to the lack of maternal pertussis antibodies. Following immunization, young children acquire immunity that wanes as they approach adolescence. This susceptible older population is now capable of transmitting pertussis to each other and to the next generation of infants. In a number of countries, an initial decrease in pertussis disease was followed by a rise in incidence years later, with a higher proportion of cases occurring in adolescents, adults, and infants, and a lower proportion occurring in young children.[5,6,8,9] Although pertussis immunization remains effective, its duration of protection is limited, resulting in a growing number of susceptible older individuals and infants without passively acquired antibodies.

DISEASE

Pertussis infection is acquired by the transmission of *B. pertussis* via aerosol droplet during close exposure to a person with active infection. An asymptomatic incubation period ranging from 1 to 3 weeks is followed by the catarrhal phase, with symptoms including rhinorrhea, watery eyes, dry cough, mild conjunctival injection, malaise, and low-grade fever.[27] This phase can be clinically indistinguishable from many other upper respiratory tract infections and lasts approximately 1 week. As the illness progresses to the paroxysmal phase, infected individuals may develop the characteristic paroxysmal cough—a series of short expiratory bursts—followed by an inspiratory gasp that produces the typical whoop. Paroxysms and whoop are relatively uncommon in infants, who may have episodes of apnea as the sole manifestation of disease. Associated with the paroxysmal cough are the symptoms of post-tussive emesis, cyanosis, facial flushing, and syncope.[3,28,29] Patients, especially those who are unimmunized, may exhibit leukocytosis with lymphocyte predominance.

During the paroxysmal phase, which can last for weeks to months, there can be significant morbidity and mortality, especially in developing countries where malnutrition and dehydration lead to greater severity of disease.[30] The principal complications include pneumonia (caused by *B. pertussis* or other pathogens), conjunctival hemorrhages, ulceration of the lingual frenulum, rectal prolapse, and central nervous system (CNS) dysfunction. CNS abnormalities can present as encephalopathy or seizures and are seen more frequently in infants and young children.[8,31]

Following the paroxysmal phase, the convalescent phase is a time when paroxysms decrease in frequency and intensity. The duration of this phase can be several months, and exposure to other respiratory pathogens or even simple stimuli such as cold air, can precipitate recurrence of the paroxysmal cough.

Bordetella pertussis: Transmission and immunity

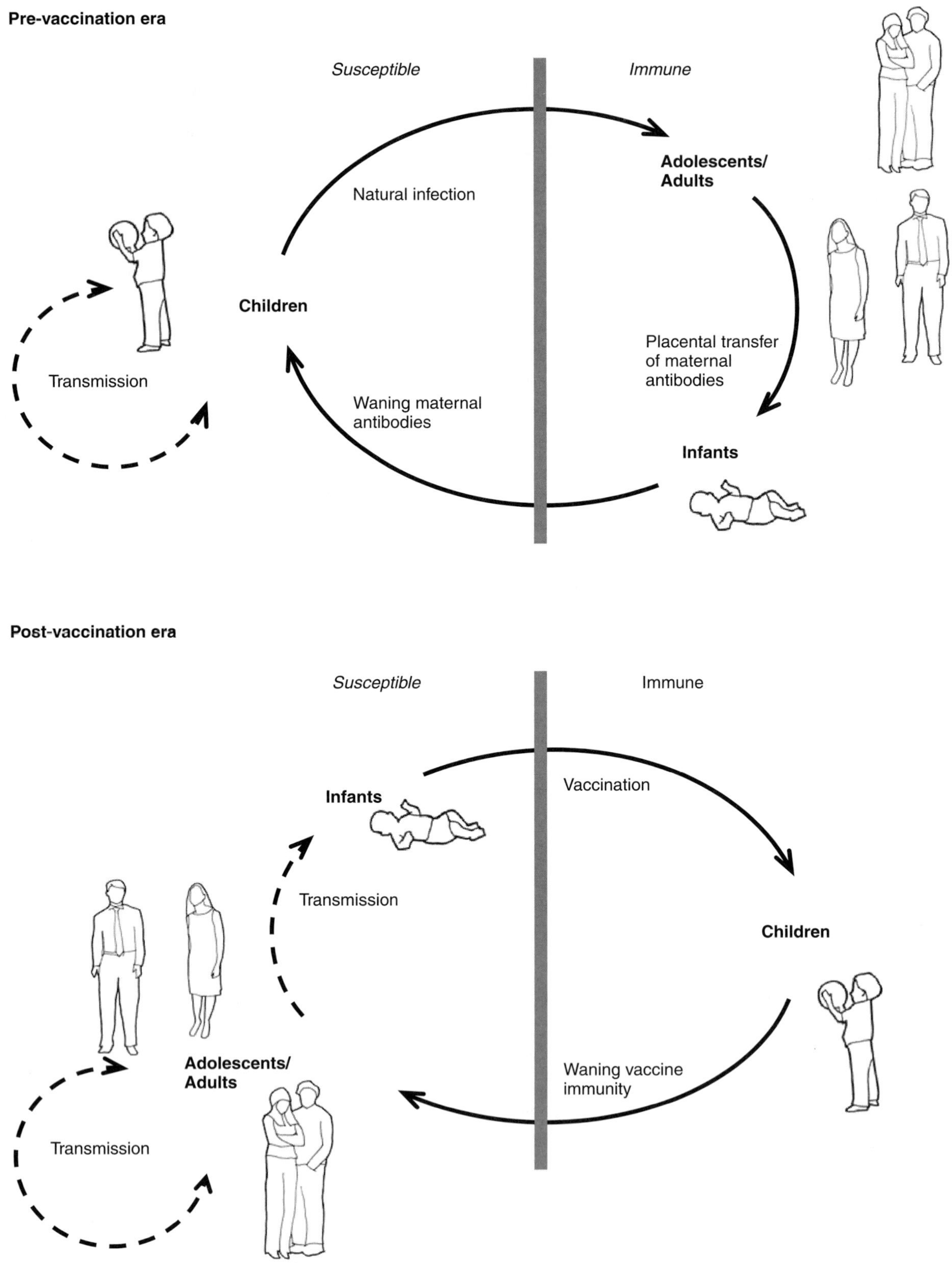

PATHOGENESIS

B. pertussis produces a number of virulence factors that interact in an orchestrated sequence of events required for development of the clinical disease of pertussis. Despite knowledge of the mechanisms of action of several of these factors at the cellular and molecular level, their exact target tissues and pathophysiology remain a matter of speculation. A current working model for the pathogenesis of pertussis involves adhesins, toxins, and other virulence factors.[32–34] The adherence factors—filamentous hemagglutinin (FHA), pertactin (PRN), and fimbriae (FIM)—appear to be involved in the attachment of *B. pertussis* to ciliated respiratory epithelia, but no single factor is absolutely essential to establishment of infection. The release of tracheal cytotoxin (TCT), a breakdown product of the bacterial peptidoglycan, causes ciliostasis and death of the tracheal ciliated epithelial cells. Adenylate cyclase toxin (ACT) produces an accumulation of cyclic adenosine monophosphate (cAMP) intracellularly, which impairs the function of leukocytes and may affect other cell types. Other pathogenic factors produced by *B. pertussis* (dermonecrotic toxin, tracheal colonization factor, and an autotransporter/serum resistance factor, BrkA) have also been described.

The best-known product of *B. pertussis* is pertussis toxin (PT),[35] which induces lymphocytosis, enhances insulin secretion, inhibits intracellular signal transduction, and impairs the function of phagocytes. As the only component that seems to disseminate systemically, PT appears to be the main contributor to the more severe manifestations of disease and the resulting sequelae. However, the target tissues of PT that are responsible for specific symptoms remain to be elucidated.[36]

DIAGNOSIS

Historically, the diagnosis of pertussis infection has been limited by a lack of a sensitive and specific diagnostic method that is also practical for widespread use. Isolation of the *B. pertussis* organism by culture by use of Bordet-Gengou agar or newer media is very specific but has low sensitivity, even in experienced laboratories. Epidemiologic studies and vaccine efficacy trials have used serology to diagnose pertussis infection by detecting antibodies against pertussis or pertussis components in the serum. However, there is not yet a fully standardized methodology for pertussis serology, and published studies have used a variety of serologic case definitions.[4,5,29,37] Serology has limited clinical utility when an acute diagnosis is needed, especially if paired acute and convalescent sera are required for diagnosis.

Polymerase chain reaction (PCR) assays for *B. pertussis* are highly sensitive and specific and are increasingly available for routine diagnosis in clinical settings.[3,38] Because PCR does not require a viable organism, the diagnosis of pertussis infection can sometimes be made in patients who have already received treatment with antibiotics or who present for care later in the course of illness.[39] Recent advancements in PCR allow discrimination between *B. pertussis* and *B. parapertussis*.[40–42] Despite its advantages, PCR cannot identify phenotypic variations among pertussis strains or potential antibiotic resistance that can be detected using culture isolates; it is also more costly and is less widely available in developing countries.

Diagnosis of a clinical case of pertussis can be made on the basis of clinical presentation when specimens are not available or in areas where laboratory diagnosis is not possible. WHO recommends that a clinical case of pertussis be diagnosed by a physician or be defined as a cough lasting at least 2 weeks with at least one of the following symptoms: paroxysms of coughing, inspiratory whooping, or post-tussive vomiting without other apparent cause. A case that meets the clinical case definition and is supported by a laboratory test is considered a laboratory-confirmed case.[2]

TREATMENT

Supportive therapy is critical for infants with pertussis disease, who are at the greatest risk for complications and neurologic sequelae. They often require hospitalization for close monitoring, frequent nasotracheal suctioning, supplemental oxygen, and parenteral hydration and nutrition. There has been little advancement in specific antimicrobial therapy for pertussis in the past 25 years. Although some antibiotics have been shown to eliminate *B. pertussis* from the respiratory tract, thereby reducing transmission of the organism, their efficacy in reducing the severity and duration of disease appears dependent on early initiation of therapy. Erythromycin (particularly the estolate ester) is recommended at a dose of 40 to 50 mg/kg/d (maximum 2g/d) divided into 4 doses, for a full 14-day course to prevent bacteriologic relapse.[43–46] The newer macrolides—clarithromycin and azithromycin—have good in vitro activity against pertussis and supportive clinical experience. Although there are no standard doses for pertussis, studies suggest clarithromycin 7.5 mg/kg (maximum 500 mg) twice a day for 7 days, or azithromycin 10 mg/kg/d (maximum 500 mg) on day 1 then 5 mg/kg/d (maximum 250 mg) for 4 subsequent days.[47–49] When a macrolide is not available or cannot be tolerated, trimethoprim-sulfamethoxazole can be used, but there are few published reports of its use in pertussis treatment.[50–52] Adjunctive therapy with corticosteroids[53] or β_2-adrenergic agonists[54,55] may be of some symptomatic benefit in severely affected individuals, but their efficacies are uncertain and require further study.

PREVENTION

In the prevaccine era, immunity to pertussis infection was acquired and maintained through clinical disease followed by repetitive exposure to *B. pertussis* as it circulated in the community. It was soon recognized that acquisition of antibodies to the organism correlated with resistance to infection.[56] In the 1950s, a killed, whole-cell pertussis vaccine, combined with diphtheria and tetanus toxoids and aluminum-containing adjuvants (DTwP vaccine), was developed and widely used throughout the world. This vaccine has been shown in trials to have an efficacy of greater than 80% if properly prepared. Unfortunately, there has been significant variability in the vaccine product made by different manufacturers, resulting in lower efficacy with some products.[57]

In some countries, the use of the whole-cell vaccine has been limited by its associated reactogenicity, including pain, swelling, fever, anorexia, and vomiting.[58,59] In younger children and infants, there were reports of encephalopathy and neurologic sequelae temporally associated with DTwP but no conclusive evidence that DTwP causes CNS damage.[58,60]

Because of the concern over the safety of DTwP, several acellular pertussis (aP) vaccines were developed using PT and one or more of the following components: PRN, FHA, or FIM.[61] These vaccines have similar efficacy and decreased reactogenicity compared with whole-cell vaccines. Currently they are licensed and available in combination with diphtheria and tetanus toxoids (DTaP) in most developed countries. However, the complexity of producing purified vaccine components entails a production cost that is unreasonable for most developing countries.

WHO continues to recommend use of whole-cell pertussis vaccine in developing countries because of its lower cost of production and its greater availability, especially in countries that manufacture their own vaccine. In countries where the reactogenicity of the whole-cell vaccine is an issue and may cause decreased acceptance of pertussis immunization, WHO recommends use of the acellular vaccine.[62]

The duration of protection from whole-cell vaccines is 10 to 12 years[3] but is yet to be determined for aP vaccines. It has been observed that some *B. pertussis* strains isolated from previously vaccinated individuals have genetic variations in the components, suggesting possible postvaccinal adaptation of the organism.[2] Although the relevance of these observations to vaccine efficacy is not established, it is clear that the immunity induced by vaccines received in childhood wanes with time. Countries that instituted routine pertussis immunization in the 1950s observed a drop in pertussis incidence and then a resurgence in cases with a greater proportion in adolescents and adults.[2–7,9] Countries with recent pertussis programs are reporting similar changes. For example, following the initiation of infant pertussis immunization in Senegal, there was a decline in incidence in every age group and up to 79% reduction in children 6 to 23 months old. During an 8-year period, the median age of individuals experiencing pertussis rose from 4.1 to 6.2 years of age, and cases in children less than 5 years old dropped from 60% to 38% percent.[63]

Clinical trials of the newer aP vaccines have been conducted in adolescents and adults, demonstrating safety and immunogenicity.[3,64,65] In the one adult efficacy trial in the United States, the aP vaccine appeared to provide protection against infection, but there were too few cases to demonstrate efficacy definitively.[26] Acellular pertussis vaccines are now licensed and available for use in older individuals in Europe, Canada, and Australia. New recommendations to vaccinate adolescents have been made in Germany, France, and Canada; the vaccination of health-care and child care workers is recommended in the European Union and required in Germany.[3,9,66] It is anticipated that the U.S. Centers for Disease Control (CDC) will make recommendations for the immunization of health-care and child care workers against pertussis if the aP vaccine is approved for use in adults.[67,68]

WHO has not yet issued recommendations for the immunization of adults against pertussis. As childhood vaccination programs are implemented in developing countries, the age distribution of pertussis is shifting toward older individuals. A greater proportion of infants will be born to mothers with waning immunity and exposed to adults with greatest risk for infection. However, in these countries, the acellular pertussis vaccines may be unavailable or prohibitive because of cost, an important consideration in the development of future recommendations for adult immunization.

REFERENCES

1. Crowcroft NS, Stein C, Duclos P, Birmingham M: How best to estimate the global burden of pertussis? Lancet Infect Dis 3:413–418, 2003.
2. Pertussis surveillance: a global meeting, Geneva, 16–18 October 2000. Geneva, World Health Organization, 2001. http://www.who.int/vaccines-documents/DocsPDF01/www605.pdf. Accessed 11/13/04.
3. von Konig CH, Halperin S, Riffelmann M, Guiso N: Pertussis of adults and infants. Lancet Infect Dis 2:744–750, 2002.
4. Strebel P, Nordin J, Edwards K, et al: Population-based incidence of pertussis among adolescents and adults, Minnesota, 1995–1996. J Infect Dis 183:1353–1359, 2001.
5. Baron S, Njamkepo E, Grimprel E, et al: Epidemiology of pertussis in French hospitals in 1993 and 1994: thirty years after a routine use of vaccination. Pediatr Infect Dis J 17:412–418, 1998.
6. Campins-Marti M, Cheng HK, Forsyth K, et al: Recommendations are needed for adolescent and adult pertussis immunisation: rationale and strategies for consideration. Vaccination 20:641–646, 2001.
7. Zielinski A, Rosinska M, Czarkowski M, Rudowska J: The effectiveness of vaccination with whole-cell pertussis vaccine by age group in Poland 1996–2001. Scand J Infect Dis 36:114–118, 2004.
8. Pertussis—United States, 1997–2000. MMWR 51:73–76, 2002.
9. National Advisory Committee on Immunization: Prevention of pertussis in adolescents and adults. CCDR Canada Communicable Disease Report 29:1–9, 9/1/2003. http://www.hc-sc.gc.ca/pphb-dgspsp/publicat/ccdr-rmtc/03pdf/acs-dcc-29-5-6.pdf. Accessed 11/13/04.
10. von Wintzingerode F, Gerlach G, Schneider B, Gross R: Phylogenetic relationships and virulence evolution in the genus *Bordetella*. In Hacker J, Kaper JB (eds): Pathogenicity islands and the evolution of pathogenic microbes. Berlin-Heidelberg, 2002, pp 177–199.
11. Parton R: New perspectives on *Bordetella* pathogenicity. J Med Microbiol 44:233–235, 1996.
12. Funke G, Hess T, Vandamme P: Characteristics of *Bordetella hinzii* strains isolated from a cystic fibrosis patient over a 3-year period. J Clin Microbiol 34:966–969, 1996.
13. Njamkepo E, Delisle F, Hagege I, et al: *Bordetella holmesii* isolated from a patient with sickle cell anemia: analysis and comparison with other *Bordetella holmesii* isolates. Clin Microbiol Infect Dis 6:131–136, 2000.
14. Vandamme P, Heyndrickx M, Vancanneyt M, et al: *Bordetella trematum* sp. nov., isolated from wounds and ear infections in humans, and reassessment of Alcaligenes denitrificans Ruger and Tan 1983. Int J Syst Bacteriol 46:849–858, 1996.
15. Bauwens JE, Spach DH, Schacker TW, et al: *Bordetella bronchiseptica* pneumonia and bacteremia following bone marrow transplantation. J Clin Microbiol 30:2474–2475, 1992.
16. Gueirard P, Weber C, Coustumier AL, Guiso N: Human *Bordetella bronchiseptica* infection related to contact with infected animals: persistence of bacteria in host. J Clin Microbiol 33:2002–2006, 1995.
17. Iwata S, Aoyama T, Goto A, et al: Mixed outbreak of *Bordetella pertussis* and *Bordetella parapertussis* in an apartment house. Dev Biol Stand 73:333–341, 1991.
18. Wirsing von Konig CH, Finger H: Role of pertussis toxin in causing symptoms of *Bordetella parapertussis* infection. Eur J Clin Microbiol Infect Dis 13:455–458, 1994.
19. Liese JG, Renner C, Stojanov S, Belohradsky BH: Clinical and epidemiological picture of *B. pertussis* and *B. parapertussis* infections after introduction of acellular pertussis vaccines. Arch Dis Child 88:684–687, 2003.
20. Klement E, Uliel L, Engel I, et al: An outbreak of pertussis among young Israeli soldiers. Epidemiol Infect 131:1049–1054, 2003.
21. Wilder-Smith A, Earnest A, Ravindran S, Paton NI: High Incidence of pertussis among Hajj pilgrims. Clin Infect Dis 37:1270–1272, 2003.
22. Pertussis outbreak among adults at an oil refinery—Illinois, Aug–Oct 2002. MMWR 52:1–4, 2003.
23. Afghanistan health update. World Health Organization, 2003. http://www.who.int/csr/don/en/pertussisoutbreak.pdf. Accessed 11/13/04.
24. Preziosi MP, Yam A, Wassilak SG, et al: Epidemiology of pertussis in a West African community before and after introduction of a widespread vaccination program. Am J Epidemiol 155:891–896, 2002.
25. Fung KS, Yeung WL, Wong TW, So KW, Cheng AF: Pertussis—a re-emerging infection? J Infect 48:145–148, 2004.

26. Ward J, Partridge S, Chang S, et al: Acellular pertussis vaccine efficacy and epidemiology of pertussis in adolescents and adults: NIH multicenter adult pertussis trial (APERT). Acellular Pertussis Vaccine Conference (NIAID, FDA, CDC, AAP, NVP). 11/12/00.
27. Lapin JH: Whooping Cough. Springfield, IL, Thomas, 1943.
28. Tozzi AE, Rava L, Ciofi degli Atti ML, and Progetto Pertosse Working Group: Clinical presentation of pertussis in unvaccinated and vaccinated children in the first six years of life. Pediatrics 112:1069–1075, 2003.
29. Senzilet LD, Halperin SA, Spika JS, et al and Sentinel Health Unit Surveillance System Pertussis Working Group: Pertussis is a frequent cause of prolonged cough illness in adults and adolescents. Clin Infect Dis 32:1691–1697, 2001.
30. Wright PE: Pertussis in developing countries: definition of the problem and prospects for control. Rev Infect Dis 13:S528–S534, 1991.
31. Halperin SA, Marrie TJ: Pertussis encephalopathy in an adult: case report and review. Rev Infect Dis 13:1043–1047, 1991.
32. Hewlett EL: Pertussis: current concepts of pathogenesis and prevention. Pediatr Infect Dis J 16:S78–S84, 1997.
33. Locht C, Antoine R, Jacob-Dubuisson F: *Bordetella pertussis*, molecular pathogenesis under multiple aspects. Curr Opin Microbiol 4:82–89, 2001.
34. Mattoo S, Foreman-Wykert AK, Cotter PA, Miller JF: Mechanisms of Bordetella pathogenesis. Front Biosci 6:E168–E186, 2001.
35. Locht C, Antoine R: *Bordetella pertussis* protein toxins. In Alouf JE, Freer JH (eds): The Comprehensive Sourcebook of Bacterial Protein Toxins, 2nd ed. London, Academic Press, 1999, pp 130–146.
36. Schaeffer LM, Weiss AA: Pertussis toxin and lipopolysaccharide influence phagocytosis of *Bordetella pertussis* by human monocytes. Infect Immun 69:7635–7641, 2001.
37. Gilberg S, Njamkepo E, Du C, et al: Evidence of *Bordetella pertussis* infection in adults presenting with persistent cough in a French area with very high whole-cell vaccine coverage. J Infect Dis 186:415–418, 2002.
38. Lingappa JR, Lawrence W, West-Keefe S, et al: Diagnosis of community-acquired pertussis infection: comparison of both culture and fluorescent-antibody assays with PCR detection using electrophoresis or dot blot hybridization. J Clin Microbiol 40:2908–2912, 2002.
39. Edelman K, Nikkari S, Ruuskanen O, et al: Detection of *Bordetella pertussis* by polymerase chain reaction and culture in the nasopharynx of erythromycin-treated infants with pertussis. Pediatr Infect Dis J 15:54–57, 1996.
40. Reizenstein E, Johansson B, Mardin L, et al: Diagnostic evaluation of polymerase chain reaction discriminative for *Bordetella pertussis*, *B. parapertussis*, and *B. bronchiseptica*. Diagn Microbiol Infect Dis 17:185–191, 1993.
41. Qin X, Turgeon DK, Ingersoll BP, et al: *Bordetella pertussis*. PCR: simultaneous targeting of signature sequences. Diagn Microbiol Infect Dis 43:269–275, 2002.
42. Cloud JL, Hymas WC, Turlak A, et al: Description of a multiplex *Bordetella pertussis* and *Bordetella parapertussis* LightCycler PCR assay with inhibition control. Diagn Microbiol Infect Dis 46:189–195, 2003.
43. Steketee RW, Wassilak SGF, Adkins WN II, et al: Evidence for a high attack rate and efficacy of erythromycin prophylaxis in a pertussis outbreak in a facility for the developmentally disabled. J Infect Dis 157:434–440, 1988.
44. Hoppe JE and Erythromycin Study Group: Comparison of erythromycin estolate and erythromycin ethylsuccinate for treatment of pertussis. Pediatr Infect Dis J 11:189–193, 1992.
45. Dodhia H, Crowcroft NS, Bramley JC, Miller E: UK guidelines for use of erythromycin chemoprophylaxis in persons exposed to pertussis. J Public Health Med 24:200–206, 2002.
46. Guris D: Treatment and chemoprophylaxis. In: Guidelines for the Control of Pertussis Outbreaks. Atlanta, Centers for Disease Control and Prevention, 2003, Chapter 3.
47. Langley JM, Halperin SA, Boucher FD, et al: Azithromycin is as effective as and better tolerated than erythromycin estolate for the treatment of pertussis. Pediatrics 114:e96–e101, 2004. http://www.pediatrics.org/cgi/content/full/114/1/e96.
48. Aoyama T, Sunakawa K, Iwata S, et al: Efficacy of short-term treatment of pertussis with clarithromycin and azithromycin. J Pediatr 129:761–764, 1996.
49. Pichichero ME, Hoeger WJ, Casey JR: Azithromycin for the treatment of pertussis. Pediatr Infect Dis J 22:847–849, 2003.
50. Heininger U, Cherry JD, Stehr K, et al, and Pertussis Vaccine Study Group: Comparative efficacy of the Lederle/Takeda acellular pertussis component DTP (DTaP) vaccine and Lederle whole-cell component DTP vaccine in German children after household exposure. Pediatrics 102:546–553, 1998.
51. Christie CD, Glover AM, Willke MJ, et al: Containment of pertussis in the regional pediatric hospital during the Greater Cincinnati epidemic of 1993. [see comment]. Infect Control Hosp Epidemiol 16:556–563, 1995.
52. Hoppe JE, Halm U, Hagedorn HJ, Kraminer-Hagedorn A: Comparison of erythromycin ethylsuccinate and co-trimoxazole for treatment of pertussis. [Erratum in Infection 17:330, 1989.] Infection 17:227–231, 1989.
53. Roberts I, Gavin R, Lennon D: Randomized controlled trial of steroids in pertussis. Pediatr Infect Dis J 11:982–983, 1992.
54. Krantz I, Norrby SR, Trollfors B: Salbutamol vs. placebo for treatment of pertussis. Pediatr Infect Dis 4:638–640, 1985.
55. Mertsola J, Viljanen MK, Ruuskanen O: Salbutamol in the treatment of whooping cough. Scand J Infect Dis 18:593–594, 1986.
56. Vaccination against whooping-cough: final report to the Whooping-Cough Immunization Committee of the Medical Research Council and to the Medical Officers of Health for Battersea and Wandsworth, Bradford, Liverpool, and Newcastle. Br Med J 1:994–1000, 1959.
57. Fine PEM, Clarkson JA: Reflections on the efficacy of pertussis vaccines. Rev Infect Dis 9:866–883, 1987.
58. Adverse effects of pertussis and rubella vaccines. Washington, DC, National Academy Press, 1991, pp 1–367.
59. Hodder SL, Mortimer EA II: Epidemiology of pertussis and reactions to pertussis vaccine. Epidemiol Rev 14:243–267, 1992.
60. Peter G, Easton JG, Halsey NA, and Committee on Infectious Diseases: The relationship between pertussis vaccine and brain damage: Reassessment. Pediatrics 88:397–400, 1991.
61. Hewlett EL, Cherry JD: New and improved vaccines against pertussis. In Cobon GS, Kaper JB, Woodrow GC, et al (eds): New Generation Vaccines, Chapter 30. New York, 1997, pp 387–416.
62. Pertussis vaccine. Geneva, World Health Organization, 2004. http://www.who.int/vaccines/en/pertussis.shtml. Accessed 11/13/04.
63. Preziosi MP, Yam A, Wassilak SG, et al: Epidemiology of pertussis in a West African community before and after introduction of a widespread vaccination program.[see comment]. Am J Epidemiol 155:891–896, 2002.
64. Keitel WA, Muenz LR, Decker MD, et al: A randomized clinical trial of acellular pertussis vaccines in healthy adults: dose-response comparisons of 5 vaccines and implications for booster immunization. J Infect Dis 180:397–403, 1999.
65. Halperin SA, Smith B, Russell M, et al: Adult formulation of a five component acellular pertussis vaccine combined with diphtheria and tetanus toxoids and inactivated poliovirus vaccine is safe and immunogenic in adolescents and adults. Pediatr Infect Dis J 19:276–283, 2000.
66. Calendrier vaccinal 2004: Avis du conseil supérieur d'hygiène publique de France, 19 mars 2004. BEH 28–29, 121–132, 2004. http://www.invs.sante.fr/beh/2004/28_29/beh_28_29_2004.pdf. Accessed 12/20/04.
67. Immunization of Health-Care Workers: Recommendations of the Advisory Committee on Immunization Practices (ACIP) and the Hospital Infection Control Practices Advisory Committee (HICPAC). MMWR 46:1–42, 12/26/97. http://www.cdc.gov/mmwr/preview/mmwrhtml/00050577.htm. Accessed 11/13/04.
68. Guidelines for Preventing Health-Care–Associated Pneumonia, 2003. MMWR 53:1–36, 3/26/04. http://www.cdc.gov/mmwr/preview/mmwrhtml/rr5303a1.htm. Accessed 11/13/04.

33

Legionellosis

THOMAS J. MARRIE
PAUL HOFFMAN

INTRODUCTION

From July 21 to 24, 1976, the 58th Annual Convention of the American Legion was held at a hotel in Philadelphia. One hundred eighty-two of the attendees at the convention developed pneumonia.[1] One hundred forty-seven (81%) were hospitalized and 29 (16%) died. This outbreak of pneumonia, of apparent unknown cause, triggered an exhaustive epidemiologic and microbiologic investigation by the Centers for Disease Control and Prevention (CDC) culminating in the isolation of a new microorganism, *Legionella pneumophila*, approximately 6 months later.[2]

It soon became apparent from analysis of stored serum samples that this organism had caused disease prior to 1976, and prospective studies showed that the spectrum of illness ranged from a nonpneumonic, mild, self-limited febrile illness (Pontiac fever)[3] to a pneumonic illness that varied from mild to severe. The latter was often accompanied by multisystem disease.[1,4] The pneumonic form of the illness following infection with *Legionella* is referred to as Legionnaires' disease.

AGENT

There are more than 30 species in the family Legionellaceae.[5] *Legionella pneumophila* serogroup 1 accounts for most of the cases of Legionnaires' disease. Legionellaceae are gram-negative, aerobic, non-spore-forming bacilli that measure 0.3 to 0.9 μm wide by 2 to 20 μm long. These organisms require special media for growth. Charcoal yeast extract agar buffered to pH 6.9 and containing α-ketoglutarate along with cefamandole, polymyxin B, and anisomycin to prevent growth of other microorganisms is the primary medium used for isolation of these organisms. Addition of α-ketoglutaric acid to the medium promotes growth of *Legionella* likely by stimulation of oxygen-scavenging enzymes.

These organisms are visualized poorly, if at all, by Gram stain. In tissue, silver impregnation stains such as the Dieterle or Warthin–Starry method allow visualization of the organism.

EPIDEMIOLOGY

Once the microorganism had been isolated, it was characterized and diagnostic reagents became available. In 1981, 5 years after the initial outbreak, England and colleagues[6] reported on the first 1000 cases of sporadic Legionnaires' disease in the United States. The authors noted that most cases occurred during June to October—71% of patients were male, and 88% were white. During the 2 weeks before onset of this illness, 37% had traveled overnight, 29% had visited a hospital, and 5% had been hospitalized 2 days before onset of illness. Twenty-three percent lived within sight of a construction or excavation site, and 32% had been exposed to a construction or excavation.

As we have learned more about the epidemiology of this disease, these were all seminal observations. With these original observations in mind, it is instructive to examine the report of Marston and associates,[7] which analyzed *Legionella* surveillance data on 3254 patients reported to the CDC from 1980 through 1989. Disease rates did not vary by year but were higher in the northern states and during the summer. The mean age of patients with Legionnaires' disease was 52.7 years compared with 34.7 years for the U.S. population. In contrast to earlier reports, people with Legionnaires' disease were now more likely to be black. They were also more likely to be smokers and have diabetes, cancer, acquired immunodeficiency syndrome (AIDS), or end-stage renal disease. Indeed, the observed number of cases among patients with AIDS was 42-fold higher than expected. Risk factors for mortality in the study of Marston and coworkers were older age, male sex, nosocomial acquisition of disease, immunosuppression, end-stage renal disease, and cancer. Twenty-three percent of the cases were nosocomially acquired.

Soon after the description of Legionnaires' disease, it was evident that cases could occur sporadically or in clusters. Furthermore, these cases could be community or nosocomially acquired. As with most infectious diseases, outbreaks provided an opportunity to learn about the mechanisms of transmission of Legionnaires' disease. In most instances, *Legionella* is transmitted to humans by inhalation of aerosols containing the bacteria. Outbreaks have been associated with exposure to a variety of aerosol-producing devices, including showers,[8,9] a grocery store mist machine,[10] cooling towers,[11–16] whirlpool spas,[17,18] decorative fountains, and evaporative condensers.[19,20] It is also likely that aspiration of contaminated potable water by immunosuppressed patients is a mechanism whereby *Legionella* is acquired.[21,22]

Legionellae thrive in natural and complex water distribution systems. In Nova Scotia, 6 of 7 Halifax hospitals studied had *Legionella* spp. in the potable water supply, whereas only 3 of 32 other hospitals in Nova Scotia had this microorganism in the potable water.[23] *Legionella pneumophila* multiplies in potable water that contains amebae but not in filtered amebae-free water.[24] Amebae are natural hosts for legionellae.[25]

Legionellosis is believed to occur worldwide, but data are limited or nonexistent for many countries. It is likely that legionellosis is very uncommon in areas without water heaters and complex water distribution systems. However, even in these areas, aspiration of contaminated natural water, such as following boating accidents, can result in Legionnaires' disease. Legionnaires' disease has been found throughout North America, Europe, the United Kingdom, Argentina and Brazil in South America, Singapore, Thailand, and Australia. A few cases of Legionnaires' disease have been reported in India. The major problem is that serologic tests and culture for legionellae are not available in most tropical countries. Indeed, Harris and Beeching[26] state that the Western approach to the management of pneumonia "with hospitalization and administration of antibiotics to cover typical and 'atypical'

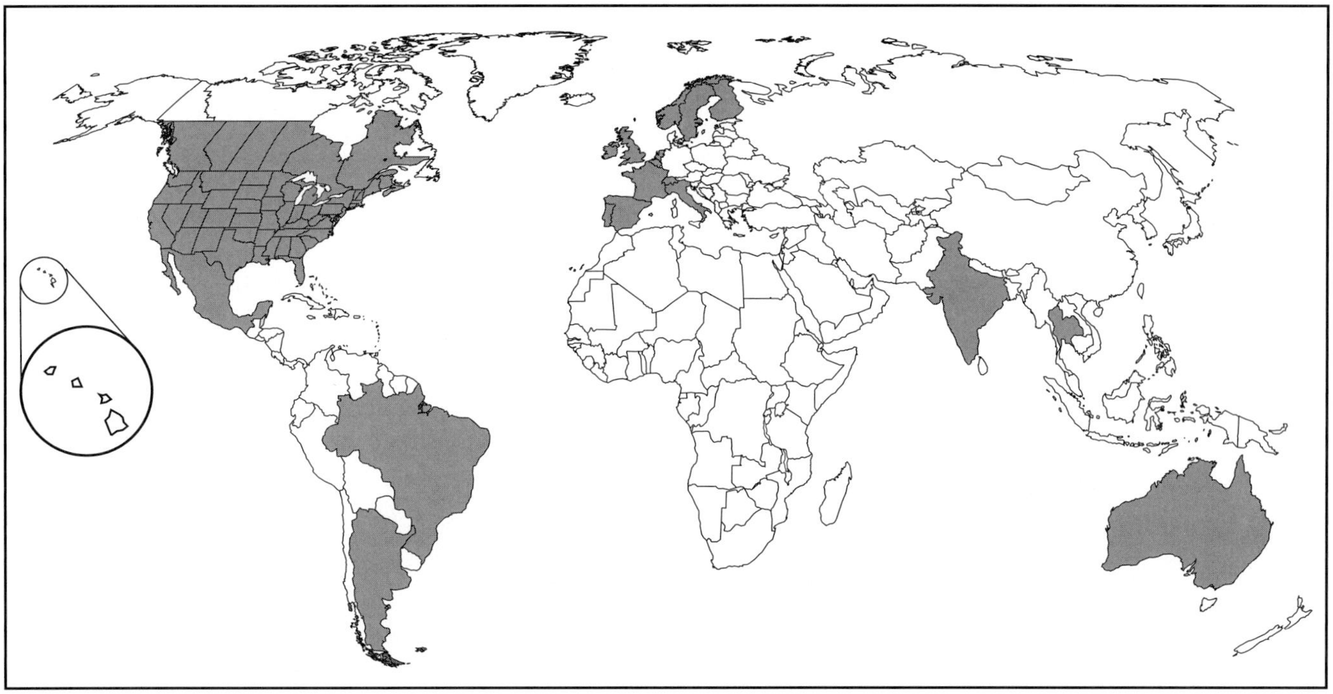

Human cases of *Legionella pneumophila* infection

■ Known distribution

[e.g., *Legionella*] organisms is not appropriate for much of the tropics." However, in areas where studies have been carried out, *Legionella* and Legionnaires' disease have been found. This situation is exemplified by data from Singapore. There were 144 cases of Legionnaires' disease from 1991 to 1995, and there was widespread contamination of water (33% of 2774 cooling towers and 18.8% of 16 outdoor fountains) by *Legionella* in that country.[27]

DISEASE

Legionellosis consists of two diseases: Pontiac fever and Legionnaires' disease. The former is a self-limited febrile illness. The incubation period is 24 to 48 hours. There is a 90% or greater attack rate among those exposed, and recovery occurs in approximately 1 week. Malaise, myalgia, fever, chills, headache, and nonproductive cough are common symptoms. There is no pneumonia.[28]

Legionnaires' disease is a pneumonic illness with a wide spectrum of severity and frequency of extrapulmonary manifestations. The following is a typical case history for this disease:

> A 32-year-old man, a nonsmoker and nondrinker, was admitted in July 1979 with a 1-week history of chills, rigors, and sweats, followed by anorexia, nausea, vomiting, and diarrhea. Subsequently, he developed a nonproductive cough with progressive dyspnea, wheezing, right pleuritic chest pain, and headache. His temperature was 39.5°C with evidence of pneumonic changes in the right upper lobe. The leukocyte count was 17.2×10^9/L, and the serum sodium was 123 mEq/L. Despite penicillin and later tetracycline therapy, there was progressive respiratory distress with spread of the pneumonic infiltrate over a 4-day period to involve the entire right lung and the left lingula. On the sixth hospital day, further progression of the pneumonia resulted in respiratory failure, and assisted ventilation was required. Erythromycin gluceptate (500 mg intravenously every 6 hours) was started with reduction in temperature after 8 days and improvement in the pneumonic process allowing extubation. A normochromic normocytic anemia and elevated liver enzymes developed. He was discharged after 22 days in the hospital. Antibody titers against *L. pneumophila* were 1:64 (acute) and 1:64,000 (convalescent).

*Table 33-1 Comparison of Selected Features of Nosocomial Legionnaires' Disease from Three Reports**

Feature	Korvick and Yu[29]	Kirby et al.[4]	Marrie et al.[30]
No. studied	65	20	55
Male:female ratio	62:3	14:6	33:22
Mean age (yrs)	59.2	52.3	58.6
No. died	16 (24.6)	14 (70)	35 (63.3)
Immunosuppressed	27 (41.5)	18 (90)	40 (73)
Malignancy	19 (29)	7 (35)	16 (29)
Assisted ventilation	NS	NS	33 (60)
Cough	60 (92)	14 (70)	37 (67)
Chills	50 (77)	6 (30)	37 (67)
Diarrhea	30 (47)	3 (15)	12 (22)
Dyspnea	23 (36)	7 (35)	35 (64)
Chest pain	21 (33)	11 (55)	8 (15)
Hemoptysis	22 (34)	6 (30)	1 (2)
Legionella isolated	5 (8)	NS	40 (70)

NS, not stated.
*Numbers in parentheses refer to percentage.

Initially, patients with Legionnaires' disease have a non-productive cough, but later in the course of the illness it can be productive. Occasionally, hemoptysis occurs and the clinical picture may mimic pulmonary embolus.

Rales and signs of consolidation are evident on examination. There may be relative bradycardia. Some patients have watery diarrhea and headache; confusion and lethargy dominate the clinical picture in others. The pneumonia may continue to progress despite appropriate treatment, and respiratory failure may ensue. In severe Legionnaires' disease, clinical improvement is not seen for 4 or 5 days after appropriate antibiotic therapy has been instituted.

Disseminated intravascular coagulation, thrombocytopenia, rhabdomyolysis, glomerulonephritis, pyelonephritis, pericarditis, and pancreatitis may complicate the clinical course. Hyponatremia and hypophosphatemia are common.

Table 33-1 summarizes selected features of nosocomial Legionnaires' disease as reported from three different institutions.[29,30]

The radiographic manifestations of Legionnaires' disease consist of alveolar opacities that may be segmental or lobar and unilateral or bilateral. Pleural effusions occur. Progression of the opacities is common (Fig. 33-1). Indeed, in severe Legionnaires' disease, progression of the pneumonia continues for 4 or 5 days after institution of appropriate antibiotic therapy. Examination of pulmonary tissue infected by *Legionella* reveals a fibrinopurulent lobar pneumonia or bronchopneumonia.[31] Polymorphonuclear leukocytes, predominantly neutrophils, and

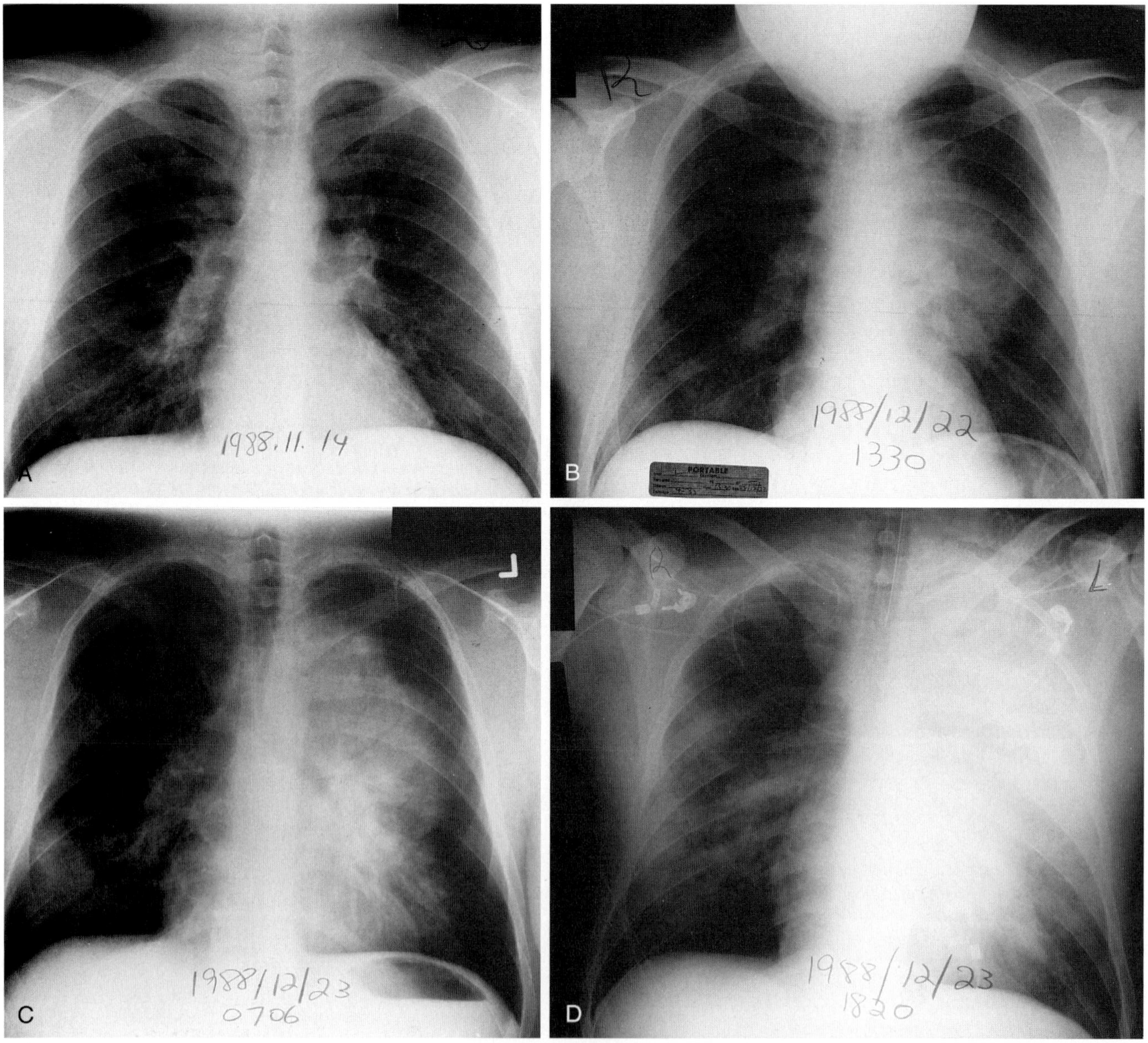

FIGURE 33-1 *A–D,* Serial chest radiographs of a 42-year-old man with chronic lymphocytic leukemia who was admitted December 22, 1988, with Legionnaires' disease. The rapid progression of the pneumonia is evident. The radiograph dated November 14, 1988 (*A*) was taken when he was well.

macrophages are found within the alveoli. Leukocytoclasis is a common feature. A mixed interstitial inflammatory pattern may accompany the airspace inflammation. Thrombosis of small vessels, septic vasculitis, and alveolar wall necrosis can occur.

PATHOGENESIS AND IMMUNITY

The legionellae are intracellular parasites of protozoa in natural environments, and humans become infected by inhalation of aerosols containing bacteria or amoeba laden with the organisms.[32] In the lung, *Legionellae* are actively phagocytized by alveolar macrophages, in which they abrogate phagosome–lysosome fusion and replicate in an endosome surrounded by the endoplasmic reticulum.[33] It is generally believed that *Legionella* plies a common infection strategy in both natural hosts and human macrophages[34] as depicted in Figure 33-2. The legionellae are naturally invasive but can enter alveolar macrophages by coiling phagocytosis or following opsonization with complement or antibodies. Once intracellular, the bacteria-laden endosome recruits small vesicles, mitochondria, and ribosomes and within 4 to 6 hours becomes enveloped by the endoplasmic reticulum, establishing the replicative endosome.[33] Bacterial growth initiates between 4 and 6 hours postinfection and continues in macrophages for 24 hours, at which time the macrophage disintegrates and the bacteria are released. Macrophage death is due to apoptosis that is activated early in infection.[35] The released bacteria are often phagocytized by other macrophages, and the cycle is repeated.

A new developmental form of *L. pneumophila* has been identified and characterized in natural hosts and in nonphagocytic HeLa cell cultures that resembles a cyst or spore.[36,37] Mature intracellular forms (MIFs) stain red with Gimenez stain, whereas vegetative replicating bacteria do not retain the red stain and are counterstained green.[37] The cystlike MIF is highly infectious, metabolically dormant, and can persist in potable water for long periods of time. In natural hosts, MIFs appear between 48 and 72 hours postinfection and are not

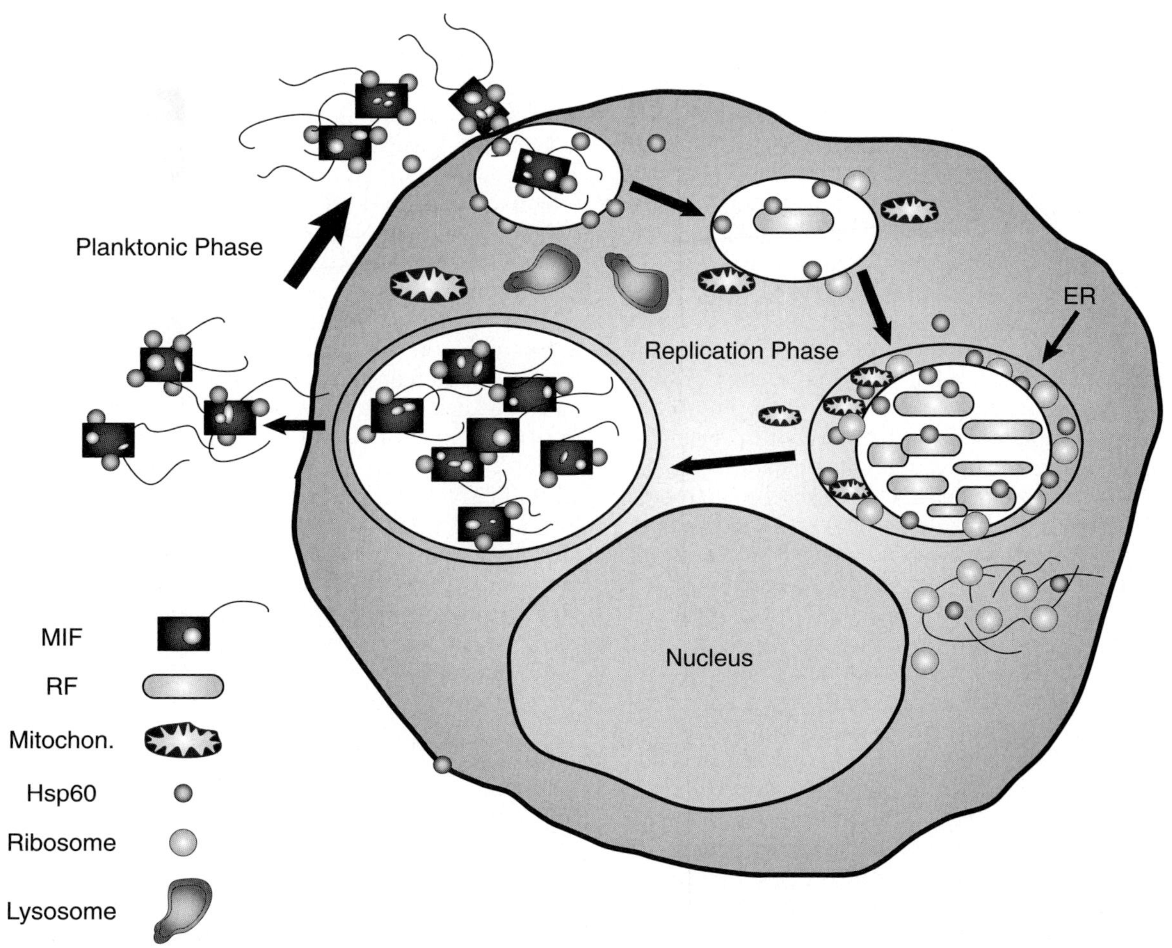

FIGURE 33-2 *Legionella pneumophila* developmental cycle. *Legionella pneumophila* enters natural hosts and macrophages by phagocytosis. The bacteria are invasive of nonphagocytic cell lines. Depicted are the mature intracellular forms (MIFs) entering a host cell and contained within an endosomal membrane. Displayed on the surface of MIFs that stain red by the Gimenez stain is Hsp60, a surface-associated protein that promotes attachment and invasion. The endosome does not fuse with lysosomes and recruits vesicles, mitochondria, and ribosomes. The *Legionella*-laden endosome becomes surrounded by the endoplasmic reticulum (ER), producing a replication-proficient environment. During this period, MIFs germinate into vegetative replicative forms (RF) and no longer stain red with Gimenez stain. The bacteria initiate rounds of replication, and late in infection the RFs differentiate into the nonreplicating MIFs. Following destruction of the host cell, MIFs are released into the environment. MIFs are initially motile, but they lose motility after 24 hours and further differentiate into a planktonic cyst that can remain infectious for extended periods while between hosts.

appreciably observed in macrophages due to early apoptotic death. It has been suggested that MIFs likely represent the transmissible form of the disease and offer an explanation for why Legionnaires' disease is not a communicable disease in humans.[37]

It is noteworthy that in a murine model of Legionnaires' disease, inoculation of *L. pneumophila*–infected *Hartmannella vermiformis* resulted in an eight-fold increase in intrapulmonary *L. pneumophila*.[38] These observations are consistent with reports that *L. pneumophila* harvested from amoeba are more infectious upon reinfection than are in vitro–grown bacteria. MIFs are also approximately 100-fold more infectious than in vitro–grown bacteria. Since airborne amebae are found in water aerosols,[8] they may serve as a reservoir or transmission vehicle for delivery of highly infectious MIFs to humans.

Virulence of *Legionella* is considered multifactoral and complex since the bacteria must not only establish the replicative endosome but also acquire all nutrients from the host cell, including amino acids, organic acids, iron, and other micronutrients.[39,40] Avirulent mutants do not replicate in macrophages and are defective in expression of transmission traits that include sensitivity to sodium chloride, osmotic resistance, motility, and surface location of heat shock protein 60 (Hsp60).[41,42] Genetic analysis reveals that most mutations associated with avirulence map to two chromosomal locations that encode components of a type IV secretion system. The system named Dot/Icm (defect in organelle trafficking/intracellular multiplication) delivers both DNA and proteins into host cells, but little is known about how effector proteins alter host cellular functions.[43,44] One of the delivered proteins, Hsp60, has been shown to block organelle trafficking when attached to latex beads, suggesting an unusual role for heat shock proteins in bacterial pathogenesis.[45] A functional type IV secretion system and the effectors it delivers are required early in invasion of host cells, but once the replicative phagosome is produced, the functions of the Dot/Icm proteins are dispensable.[46] Interestingly, if these proteins are not present in the progeny of spent cells, they are noninfectious upon reinoculation. Within the context of a developmental cycle, *Legionella* alternates between a vegetative replicative form (RF) and a planktonic MIF survival form that upon entry into a new host must germinate back into the RF.[36,37] The genes associated with regulation of each developmental form are in the early stages, but MIF formation does require regulators of stationary phase, such as sigma factor RpoS, RelA (produces alarmone ppGpp).[47]

Early studies established that immunity against *L. pneumophila* required development of a cellular immune response.[48] Antibodies are not effective against *L. pneumophila* because opsonized bacteria are more efficiently phagocytized. Interactions of *Legionella* with murine macrophages also induce an array of cytokines and chemokines. An interleukin-1β (IL-1β) response is produced upon binding of the bacteria to macrophages.[49] Interestingly, IL-12 and interferon-γ (IFN-γ) are commonly detected in serum of infected patients or in animal models, but in macrophage culture, *Legionella* specifically represses IL-12 production.[50] It is now believed that most of the IL-12 is produced by dendritic cells.[51] Among the cytokines detected in murine models or in human infection are IL-1α, IL-1β, IL-4, IL-6, IL-12, and IL-18. The lack of viable markets for vaccines against *Legionella* has limited research initiatives in this area. In one study, vaccination of guinea pigs with the purified major outer membrane protein OmpS protected guinea pigs against an LD_{100} lethal challenge, whereas immunization with purified Hsp60 provided little protection.[52] Production of IFN-γ has a protective effect by promoting activation of macrophages. Activated macrophages limit the intracellular replication of *Legionella* by decreasing the expression of transferrin receptors and limiting the availability of iron to the bacteria.[53]

Legionella pneumophila serves as a model system for the study of innate immunity because as an aquatic pathogen of protozoa, it has not evolved mechanisms to evade the human immune system. In this regard, human infection represents a dead end or failure in the life cycle of *Legionella* and provides an explanation for why immunocompromised people are so susceptible to infection.[34] Thus, whatever *Legionella* can do to interfere with the host immune system occurs by chance and not by the design of evolution.

DIAGNOSIS

A high index of suspicion is necessary in diagnosing sporadic cases of Legionnaires' disease. Outbreaks of pneumonia usually trigger a workup for *Legionella*, so these are easier to diagnose.

Isolation of the organism from respiratory secretions is the definitive diagnostic method. Detection of *Legionella* antigen in urine by enzyme-linked immunosorbent assay (ELISA) is approximately 80% sensitive and more than 95% specific.[54,55] This test is readily available for *L. pneumophila* serogroup 1. Diagnostic kits are also available for detection of antigens of *L. pneumophila* 1 to 6. *Legionella* antigen is excreted in the urine for days to weeks (rarely up to 1 year) after the onset of pneumonia.

Demonstration of a fourfold rise in antibody titer between acute and convalescent serum samples using an indirect immunofluorescence whole-cell assay can also be used to diagnose Legionnaires' disease. Up to 12 weeks may be required to demonstrate a fourfold rise in antibody, so serology is not useful for the acute management of this disease. A single or static titer of 1:256 or greater is no longer considered satisfactory for the diagnosis of Legionnaires' disease.[56] Polymerase chain reaction (PCR) applied to respiratory secretions, pulmonary tissue, or pleural fluid is currently undergoing evaluation as a diagnostic method.[57,58] In particular, PCR of material obtained by throat swab is an attractive approach, but the sensitivity and specificity of such a strategy have yet to be defined.

TREATMENT AND PROGNOSIS

Erythromycin has been considered to be the drug of choice. It should be given in a dose of 1 g intravenously every 6 hours. At this dosage, reversible ototoxicity may occur.[59] Rifampin (300 mg twice daily) orally should be given until clinical improvement occurs, at which time it can be discontinued. Relapses occur with treatment of less than 21 days' duration.

Azithromycin is also effective in the treatment of Legionnaires' disease.[60] Quinolones and doxycycline are also active against *L. pneumophila*, and they have been used to treat Legionnaires' disease.

Early administration of antibiotics (within 8 hours of admission to hospital) to patients with severe Legionnaires' disease has been associated with better outcomes.[61]

PREVENTION AND CONTROL

When cases of nosocomial Legionnaires' disease are diagnosed, the potable water distribution system of the hospital should be cultured for *Legionella*. If legionella is found, heating the water to 160°F (70°C) for several days and then flushing hot water throughout all the outlets can result in temporary reduction of the concentration of *Legionella* in the water. Hyperchlorination or the addition of copper and silver ions to the water supply can also control contamination of the potable water and result in cessation of outbreaks of nosocomial Legionnaires' disease. If legionellaceae cannot be eradicated from the water supply, all organ transplant recipients and all those who are receiving corticosteroids should not drink the water and should not shower in the water. In addition, on-site or nearby cooling towers should have the coolant water cultured for *Legionella*.

Outbreaks of Legionnaires' disease onboard cruise ships and at flower shows emphasize the importance of surveillance for this infection and control of *Legionella* in a variety of water distribution systems.[62]

REFERENCES

1. Fraser DW, Tsai TR, Orenstein W, et al, and the Field Investigation Team: Legionnaires' disease—Description of an epidemic of pneumonia. N Engl J Med 297:1189, 1977.
2. McDade JE, Shepard CC, Fraser DW, et al: Legionnaires' disease. Isolation of a bacterium and demonstration of its role in other respiratory diseases. N Engl J Med 297:1197, 1977.
3. Glick TH, Gregg MB, Berman B, et al: Pontiac fever. An epidemic of unknown aetiology in a health department. I. Clinical and epidemiological aspects. Am J Epidemiol 107:149, 1978.
4. Kirby BD, Snyder KM, Meyer RD, et al: Legionnaires' disease: Clinical features of 24 cases. Ann Intern Med 89:297, 1978.
5. Brenner DJ: Classification of the legionellae. Semin Respir Infect 2:190, 1987.
6. England AC, Fraser DW, Plikaytis RD, et al: Sporadic legionellosis in the United States: The first thousand cases. Ann Intern Med 94:164, 1981.
7. Marston BJ, Lipman HB, Breiman RF: Surveillance for Legionnaires' disease. Risk factors for morbidity and mortality. Arch Intern Med 154:2417, 1994.
8. Breiman RF, Fields BS, Sanden GN, et al: Association of shower use with Legionnaires' disease: Possible role of amoebae. JAMA 263:2924, 1990.
9. Hanrahan JP, Morse DL, Scharf VB, et al: A community hospital outbreak of legionellosis: Transmission by potable hot water. Am J Epidemiol 125:639, 1987.
10. Mahoney FJ, Hoge CW, Farley TA, et al: Community-wide outbreak of Legionnaires' disease associated with a grocery store mist machine. J Infect Dis 165:736, 1992.
11. Dondero TJ Jr, Rendtorff RC, Mallison GF, et al: An outbreak of Legionnaires' disease associated with a contaminated air-conditioning cooling tower. N Engl J Med 302:365, 1980.
12. Klaucke DN, Vogt RL, LaRue D, et al: Legionnaires' disease: The epidemiology of two outbreaks in Burlington, Vermont, 1980. Am J Epidemiol 119:382, 1984.
13. Addiss DG, Davis JP, LaVenture M, et al: Community-acquired Legionnaires' disease associated with a cooling tower: Evidence of longer-distance transport of *Legionella pneumophila*. Am J Epidemiol 130:557, 1989.
14. Mitchell E, O'Mahoney M, Watson JM, et al: Two outbreaks of Legionnaires' disease in Bolton Health District. Epidemiol Infect 104:159, 1990.
15. O'Mahoney MC, Stanwell-Smith RE, Tillett HE, et al: The Stafford outbreak of Legionnaires' disease. Epidemiol Infect 104:361, 1990.
16. Garbe PL, Davis BJ, Weisfeld JS, et al: Nosocomial Legionnaires' disease: Epidemiologic demonstration of cooling towers as a source. JAMA 254:521, 1985.
17. Outbreak of pneumonia associated with a cruise ship. MMWR 43:521, 1994.
18. Vogt RL, Hudson PJ, Orciari L, et al: Legionnaires' disease and a whirlpool spa [Letter]. Ann Intern Med 107:596, 1987.
19. Cordes LG, Fraser DW, Skaliy P, et al: Legionnaires' disease outbreak at an Atlanta, Georgia country club: Evidence for spread from an evaporative condenser. Am J Epidemiol 111:425, 1980.
20. Breiman RF, Cozen W, Fields BS, et al: Role of air-sampling in investigation of an outbreak of Legionnaires' disease associated with exposure to aerosols from an evaporative condenser. J Infect Dis 161:1257, 1990.
21. Marrie TJ, Haldane D, MacDonald S, et al: Control of nosocomial Legionnaires' disease by using sterile potable water for high risk patients. Epidemiol Infect 107:591, 1991.
22. Venezia RA, Agresta MD, Hanley EM, et al: Nosocomial legionellosis associated with aspiration of nasogastric feeding diluted in tap water. Infect Control Hosp Epidemiol 15:529, 1994.
23. Marrie TJ, Green P, Burbridge S, et al: *Legionellaceae* in the potable water of Nova Scotia hospitals and Halifax residences. Epidemiol Infect 112:143, 1994.
24. Wadowsky RM, Butler LJ, Cook MK, et al: Growth-supporting activity for *Legionella pneumophila* in tap water cultures and implication of hartmannellid amoebae as growth factors. Appl Environ Microbiol 54:2677, 1988.
25. Rowbotham TJ: Current views on the relationship between amoebae, *Legionellae*, and men. Isr J Med Sci 22:678, 1986.
26. Harris AD, Beeching NJ: Pneumonia in adults: A guide to diagnosis and management in the district hospital. Tropical Doct 21:9, 1991.
27. Committee on Epidemic Diseases: Legionellosis surveillance in Singapore, 1991–1995. Epidemiol News Bull 22:13, 1996.
28. Kaufman A, McDade J, Patton C, et al: Pontiac fever: Isolation of the etiologic agent (*Legionella pneumophila*) and demonstration of its mode of transmission. Am J Epidemiol 114:337, 1981.
29. Korvick JA, Yu VL: Legionnaires' disease: An emerging surgical problem. Ann Thorac Surg 43:341, 1987.
30. Marrie TJ, Haldane D, Bezanson G: Nosocomial Legionnaires' disease: Clinical and radiographic patterns. Can J Infect Dis 3:253, 1992.
31. Winn WC, Myerowitz RL: The pathology of the *Legionella* pneumonias. Hum Pathol 12:401, 1981.
32. Edelstein PH, Meyer RD: Legionnaires' disease. A review. Chest 85:114–120, 1984.
33. Swanson MS, Isberg RR: Identification of *Legionella pneumophila* mutants that have aberrant intracellular fates. Infect Immun 64:2585, 1996.
34. Hoffman PS: Invasion of eukaryotic cells by *Legionella pneumophila*: A common strategy for all hosts? Can J Infect Dis 8:139, 1997.
35. Zink SD, Pedersen L, Cianciotto NP, et al: The Dot/Icm type IV secretion system of *Legionella pneumophila* is essential for the induction of apoptosis in human macrophages. Infect Immun 70:1657, 2002.
36. Faulkner G, Garduno RA: Ultrastructural analysis of differentiation in *Legionella pneumophila*. J Bacteriol 184:7025, 2002.
37. Garduno RA, Garduno E, Hiltz M, et al: Intracellular growth of *Legionella pneumophila* gives rise to a differentiated form dissimilar to stationary-phase forms. Infect Immun 70:6273, 2002.
38. Brieland J, McClain M, Health L, et al: Coinoculation with *Hartmannella vermiformis* enhances replicative *Legionella pneumophila* lung infection in a murine model of Legionnaires' disease. Infect Immun 64:2449, 1996.
39. Cianciotto NP: Pathogenicity of *Legionella pneumophila*. Int J Med Microbiol 291:331, 2001.
40. James BW, Mauchline WS, Fitzgeorge RB, et al: Influence of iron-limited continuous culture on physiology and virulence of *Legionella pneumophila*. Infect Immun 63:4224, 1995.
41. Catrenich CE, Johnson W: Characterization of the selective inhibition of growth of virulent *Legionella pneumophila* by supplemented Mueller–Hinton medium. Infect Immun 57:1862, 1989.
42. Byrne B, Swanson MS: Expression of *Legionella pneumophila* virulence traits in response to growth conditions. Infect Immun 66:3029, 1998.
43. Sadosky AB, Wiater LA, Shuman HA: Identification of *Legionella pneumophila* genes required for growth within and killing of human macrophages. Infect Immun 61:5361, 1993.
44. Berger KH, Isberg RR: Two distinct defects in intracellular growth complemented by a single genetic locus in *Legionella pneumophila*. Mol Microbiol 7:7, 1993.

45. Garduño RA, Garduño E, Hoffman PS: Surface-associated Hsp60 chaperonin of *Legionella pneumophila* mediates invasion in a HeLa cell model. Infect Immun 66:4602, 1998.
46. Roy CR, Berger KH, Isberg RR: *Legionella pneumophila* DotA protein is required for early phagosome trafficking decisions that occur within minutes of bacterial uptake. Mol Microbiol 28:663, 1998.
47. Bachman MA, Swanson MS: Genetic evidence that *Legionella pneumophila* RpoS modulates expression of the transmission phenotype in both the exponential phase and the stationary phase. Infect Immun 72:2468, 2004.
48. Horwitz MA: Cell-mediated immunity in Legionnaires' disease. J Clin Invest 71:1686, 1983.
49. Retzlaff C, Yamamoto Y, Okubo S, et al: *Legionella pneumophila*–heat shock protein induced increase of interleukin-1β mRNA involves protein kinase C signaling in macrophages. Immunology 89:281, 1996.
50. Matsunaga K, Yamaguchi H, Klein TW, et al: *Legionella pneumophila* suppresses macrophage interleukin-12 production by activating the p42/44 mitogen-activated protein kinase cascade. Infect Immun 71:6672, 2003.
51. Kikuchi T, Kobayashi T, Gomi K, et al: Dendritic cells pulsed with live and dead *Legionella pneumophila* elicit distinct immune responses. J Immunol 172:1727, 2004.
52. Weeratna R, Stamler DA, Edelstein PH, et al: Human and guinea pig immune responses to *Legionella pneumophila* protein antigens: Vaccination of guinea pigs with OmpS, but not Hsp60, induces cell-mediated and protective immunity. Infect Immun 62:3454, 1994.
53. Nash TW, Libby DM, Horwitz MA: IFN-gamma-activated human alveolar macrophages inhibit the intracellular multiplication of *Legionella pneumophila*. J Immunol 140:3978, 1988.
54. Kohler RB: Legionella antigenuria: Testing and interpretation. Clin Microbiol Newslett 12:185, 1990.
55. Ruf B, Schurman D, Horbach I, et al: Prevalence and diagnosis of *Legionella pneumophila:* A 3-year prospective study with emphasis on application of urinary antigen detection. J Infect Dis 162:1341, 1990.
56. Plouffe JF, File TM Jr, Breiman RF, et al: Reevaluation of the definition of Legionnaires' disease: Use of urinary antigen. Clin Infect Dis 20: 1286, 1995.
57. Matsiota-Bernard P, Pitsouni E, Legakis N, et al: Evaluation of commercial amplification kit for detection of *Legionella pneumophila* in clinical specimens. J Clin Microbiol 32:1503, 1994.
58. Ramirez JA, Ahkee S, Tolentino A, et al: Diagnosis of *Legionella pneumophila*, *Mycoplasma pneumoniae*, or *Chlamydia pneumoniae* lower respiratory tract infections using the polymerase chain reaction on a throat swab. Diagn Microbiol Infect Dis 24:7, 1996.
59. Swanson DJ, Sung RJ, Fine MJ, et al: Erythromycin ototoxicity: Prospective assessment with serum concentrations and audiograms in a study of patients with pneumonia. Am J Med 92:61, 1992.
60. Plouffe J, Breiman R, Fields B, et al: Azithromycin in the treatment of *Legionella pneumonia* requiring hospitalization. Clin Infect Dis 37:1475, 2003.
61. Gacouin A, Le Tulzo Y, Lavoue S, et al: Severe pneumonia due to *Legionella pneumophila*: Prognostic factors, impact of delayed appropriate antimicrobial therapy. Intensive Care Med 28:686, 2002.
62. Regan CM, McCann B, Syed Q, et al: Outbreak of Legionnaires' disease on a cruise ship: Lessons for international surveillance and control. Commun Dis Public Health Jun 6:152, 2003.

34

Melioidosis

DAVID ALLAN BRETT DANCE

INTRODUCTION

Melioidosis is the name given to any infection caused by the gram-negative bacillus *Burkholderia pseudomallei*. Previously considered an esoteric and rare disease, melioidosis has emerged over the past 20 years as an important cause of morbidity and mortality in Southeast Asia and northern Australia, and is also endemic in other tropical regions. More recently still, it has attracted attention as a potential bioweapon, and *B. pseudomallei* has been classified as a "Category B" agent by the US Centers for Disease Control.[1]

ORGANISM

Melioidosis was first recognized as a fatal "glanders-like" illness in Burma in 1911 by Alfred Whitmore.[2] The genetic similarity of the causative organism to that of glanders, *Burkholderia mallei*, has been confirmed by modern taxonomists, supporting Whitmore's proposal of the specific epithet *pseudomallei*. Animal and human infections with Whitmore's bacillus were later recognized by Stanton and Fletcher in the Federated Malay States.[3] They considered the disease to be a zoonosis and coined the term *melioidosis*, derived from the Greek μηλίσ (glanders or distemper of asses). Workers in French Indochina subsequently showed that the organism was really an environmental saprophyte.[4] Over 400 French and American soldiers contracted the disease during the wars in Southeast Asia.[5] Since the mid-1970s, melioidosis has emerged as an important infection in parts of Thailand, and it is being increasingly recognized elsewhere.[6,7]

B. pseudomallei was previously classified in various genera (e.g., *Malleomyces, Pfeifferella, Actinobacillus, Bacillus, Pseudomonas*), but along with other members of ribosomal RNA (rRNA) homology group II of the genus *Pseudomonas* (e.g., *Pseudomonas cepacia*), it was assigned to the new genus, *Burkholderia*, by Yabuuchi in 1992.[8]

EPIDEMIOLOGY

Geographic Distribution

The main area of melioidosis endemicity is Southeast Asia. The disease has also been recognized as endemic to tropical Australia since 1949, possibly introduced by troops returning from endemic areas at the end of the World War II.[9] It is estimated that 2000 to 5000 cases occur each year in Thailand,[10] while up to 50 cases are diagnosed annually in both Singapore and Australia. In recent years it has become clear that the disease is also prevalent in China[11] and the Indian subcontinent,[12] which has been the source of infection of several recent cases diagnosed in Britain.

It is likely that the true distribution of melioidosis extends beyond Southeast Asia and northern Australia. Sporadic cases have been reported from the Pacific islands, central Africa, Central and South America, and the Caribbean.[6,7] The disease is probably underdiagnosed in many of these regions, because relatively sophisticated laboratory facilities are necessary to confirm the diagnosis. Furthermore, reports of cases in Iran and an epizootic that occurred in France during the 1970s[13] suggest that infection may be transmitted in nontropical regions.

Reservoirs and Transmission

B. pseudomallei is readily isolated from soil and surface water in endemic areas, particularly from rice paddies.[14] Using selective media it may be recovered from 68% to 78% of rice fields in Thailand.[15,16] Some arabinose-assimilating environmental isolates originally thought to be *B. pseudomallei* have now been assigned to a new, avirulent species, *Burkholderia thailandensis*.[17] *B. pseudomallei* is thought to persist in clay layers during the dry season, from which it recolonizes the surface mud and water during the rainy season.[18] The physical, chemical, and biologic factors that influence environmental colonization with *B. pseudomallei* are poorly understood.[19]

Humans and a wide range of animals are thought usually to become infected by inoculation or contamination of wounds or mucosae with soil or surface water, although a specific exposural incident is only identified in 6% to 25% of cases.[20,21] Infections occurred in a disproportionate number of helicopter crewmen during the Vietnam War, possibly through inhalation of aerosols generated by the rotors.[22] Two recent outbreaks in Australia have been traced to potable water supplies, although the mode of transmission was uncertain.[23,24] There is no evidence that ingestion or insect vectors play a role in transmission. Although melioidosis has been observed in a wide range of animal species (including rodents, primates, sheep and goats, pigs, cattle, horses, deer, dogs and cats, dolphins, koalas, kangaroos, camels, crocodiles, and birds), transmission from animals to humans has rarely been reported,[25] and person-to-person spread is also extremely uncommon.[26] Iatrogenic infection from contaminated injections and laboratory-acquired infections have also been reported occasionally, resulting in the classification of *B. pseudomallei* as a containment level 3 pathogen.

Descriptive Epidemiology

Melioidosis predominantly affects people in regular contact with soil and water (e.g., rice farmers in Southeast Asia and aboriginals in Australia). In northeastern Thailand, melioidosis accounts for 18% of community-acquired septicemia,[27] and in the Northern Territory of Australia it is the commonest cause of fatal community-acquired sepsis.[21] In a review of the epidemiology of culture-positive melioidosis seen over a 5-year period in Ubon Ratchathani in northeastern Thailand, the average annual incidence was estimated as 4.4 per 100,000 population, with evidence of space-time clustering.[20]

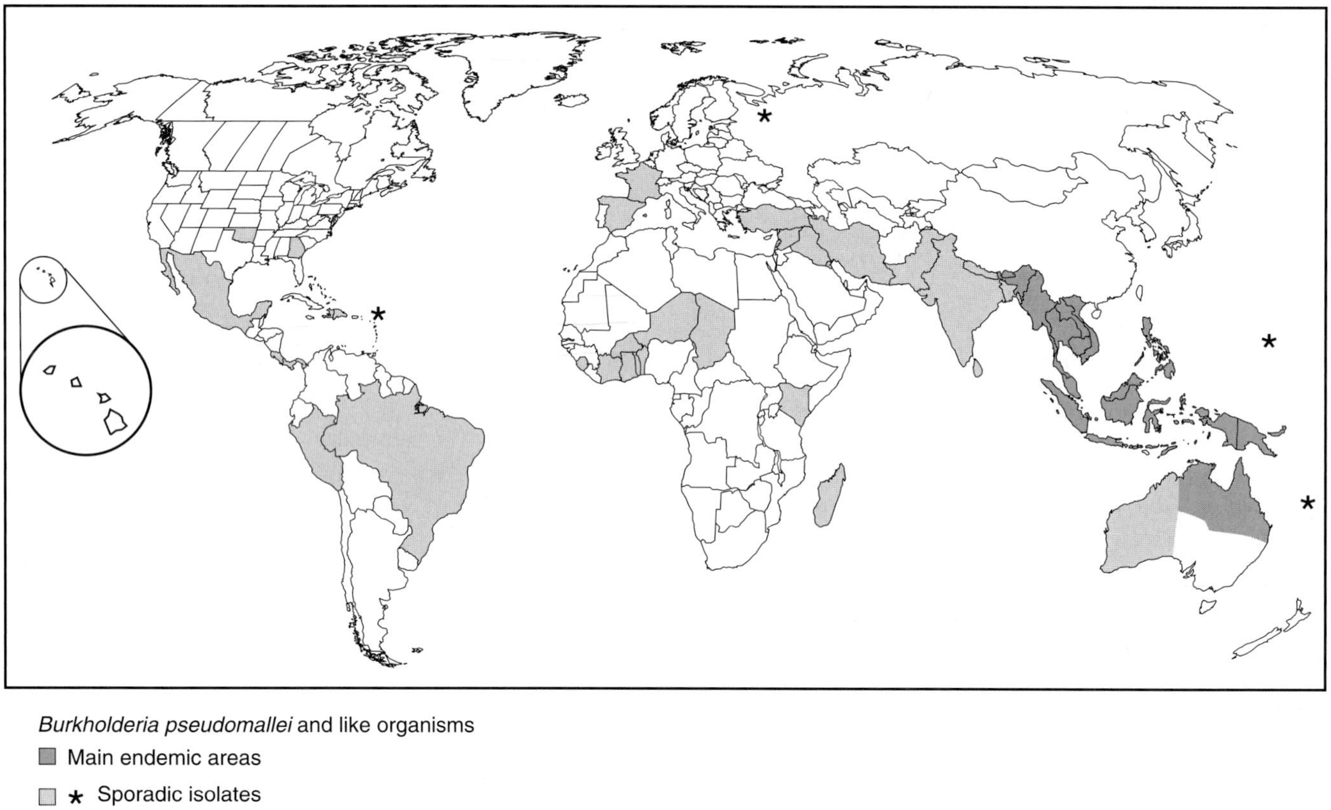

All age groups were affected, with the peak incidence occurring from age 40 to 60 years. The male-female ratio is only 3:2 in Thailand, but is much higher in Australia and Singapore, probably because of differences in exposure to soil during rice farming. The reported incidence is up to tenfold higher in parts of Australia, probably reflecting better ascertainment. Wherever the disease occurs, it is markedly seasonal, approximately 75% of cases presenting during the rainy season, with the highest incidence occurring during especially heavy monsoons.[21] Most cases appear to be recently acquired,[28] but the disease may remain latent for as long as 29 years.[29] The presence of underlying diseases, such as diabetes mellitus, chronic renal failure, immunosuppressive treatments including steroids, thalassemia, chronic liver disease, chronic lung disease (including cystic fibrosis), and kava consumption, which are found in 60% to 80% of cases,[20,21,30,31] is an important risk factor for melioidosis. The association with diabetes mellitus is particularly strong and may increase the relative risk of infection by up to 100-fold.[20] Perhaps surprisingly, there is no evidence that human immunodeficiency virus infection predisposes to melioidosis.

DISEASE

The clinical spectrum of *B. pseudomallei* infection is extremely broad, and melioidosis has been referred to as "the remarkable imitator."[32] The majority of infections are subclinical, although melioidosis may run a fulminant, rapidly fatal course, particularly in the immunocompromised. None of the clinical classifications of melioidosis is entirely satisfactory. Infections may be acute or chronic and localized or disseminated, but one form of the disease may progress to another and individual patients are often difficult to categorize. Several reviews have summarized the clinical manifestations of melioidosis.[2,3,5,21,22,27,33–35]

Mild and Subclinical Infections

In endemic areas such as northeastern Thailand, 80% of children have antibodies to *B. pseudomallei* by the time they are 4 years old,[36] yet melioidosis is uncommon, so the majority of infections are presumably mild or asymptomatic. A flulike illness associated with seroconversion has been reported from Australia.[37]

Latent Infections

Melioidosis is unusual for a bacterial infection in that long periods of latency have been observed before the disease has become clinically apparent.[29] Recrudescent infections in veterans of the Vietnam War have given rise to the nickname "Vietnamese time bomb."[38] Relapses usually occur at times of intercurrent stress (e.g., other acute infections, burns or trauma, malignancies, diabetes mellitus), when cellular immunity is likely to be suppressed. The sites and mechanisms of persistence are unknown, although clinically silent, chronic, localized foci of melioidosis in the lung, liver, or spleen have been reported in animals. The proportion of seropositive patients who harbor latent infection, and are therefore at risk of relapse, is also uncertain.

Septicemic Melioidosis

Approximately 50% to 60% of cases of culture-positive melioidosis have positive blood cultures.[20,21] Most of these present clinically as community-acquired sepsis syndrome, with a short history (median, 6 days; range, 1 day to 2 months) of high fever and rigors, although some have a less acute, typhoidal illness with a swinging fever, often associated with profound weight loss.[27] Patients with multiple, noncontiguous foci of infection, which probably reflect bacteremia at some stage, behave similarly. Only half have evidence of a primary focus of infection, usually in the lung or skin and subcutaneous tissues. Confusion, stupor, jaundice, and diarrhea may also be prominent features. Initial investigations usually reveal anemia, a neutrophil leukocytosis, coagulopathy, and evidence of renal and hepatic impairment. Such patients often deteriorate rapidly, developing widespread metastatic abscesses, particularly in the lungs, liver, and spleen, and metabolic acidosis with Kussmaul's breathing. Once septic shock has supervened, the untreated mortality approaches 95%, with many patients dying within 48 hours of hospital admission. Other poor prognostic features include absence of fever, leukopenia, azotemia, and abnormal liver function tests.[27]

If the patient survives this acute phase, the manifestations of the multiple septic foci which result from bacteremic dissemination become prominent. Any site or tissue may be involved, but the most common foci are the lungs, liver, spleen, prostate, and skin and soft tissues. An abnormal chest radiograph is found in 60% to 80% of patients, the most common pattern being widespread, nodular shadowing[39] (Fig. 34-1). Multiple liver and splenic abscesses are also common[40] (Fig. 34-2). Cutaneous pustules or subcutaneous abscesses occur in 10% to 20% of cases[27] (Fig. 34-3). Secondary lesions may occur in any other tissue or organ (e.g., kidneys, bones and joints, brain). "Neurological melioidosis," characterized by peripheral motor weakness, brain stem encephalitis, aseptic meningitis, and respiratory failure, is now thought to reflect direct invasion of the central nervous system rather than being toxin-mediated.[21,41]

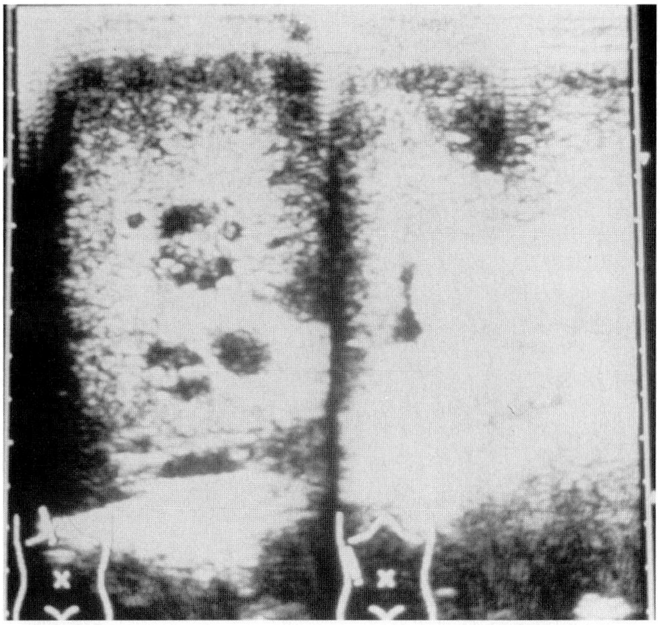

FIGURE 34-2 Abdominal ultrasound showing multiple liver abscesses in a patient with septicemic melioidosis ("Swiss cheese liver"). A similar picture may be seen in the spleen. (From Dance DAB: Melioidosis, glanders, and tularaemia. Med Int 107:4508–4511, 1992.)

Localized Melioidosis

The most common site of localized melioidosis is the lung, usually in the form of a subacute cavitating pneumonia accompanied by profound weight loss, which is often confused with tuberculosis[42] (Fig. 34-4). Relative sparing of the apices and the infrequency of hilar adenopathy may help to distinguish the two.[39] There is a predilection for the upper lobes, although any lung zone may be affected. Complications include pneumothorax, empyema, and purulent pericarditis, and ultimately progression to septicemia.

Acute suppurative parotitis (Fig. 34-5) is a characteristic manifestation of melioidosis in Thai children, accounting for

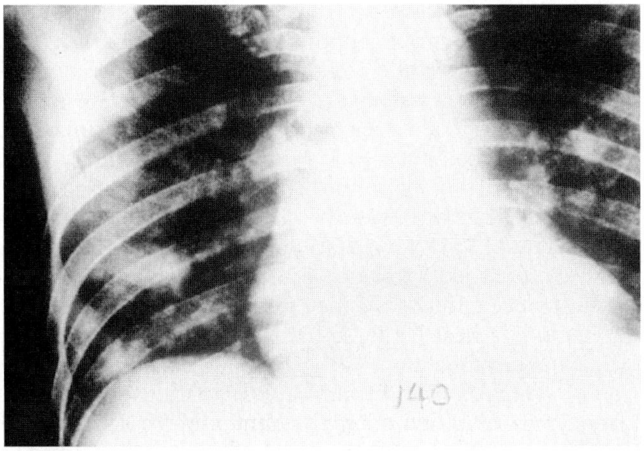

FIGURE 34-1 Chest radiograph of a patient with septicemic melioidosis showing multiple foci of consolidation ("blood-borne pneumonia"). (From Dance DAB: Melioidosis. In Cook G [ed]: Manson's Tropical Diseases, 20th ed. London, WB Saunders, 1996, pp 925–930.)

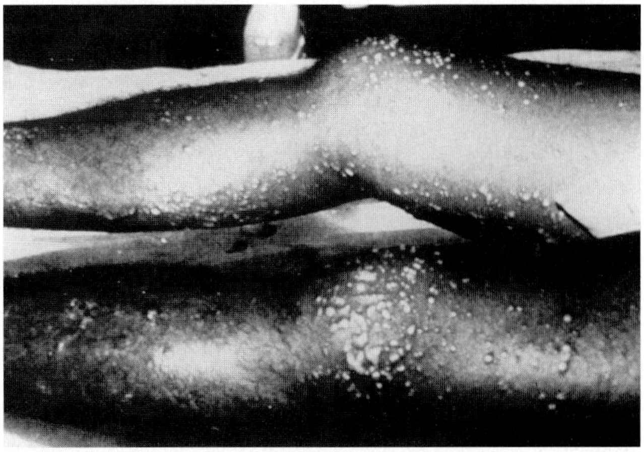

FIGURE 34-3 Multiple pustules on the legs of a rice farmer with nephrotic syndrome, treated with steroids. Gram stain of pus revealed numerous *Burkholderia pseudomallei* organisms. (From Dance DAB: Melioidosis, glanders, and tularaemia. Med Int 107:4508–4511, 1992.)

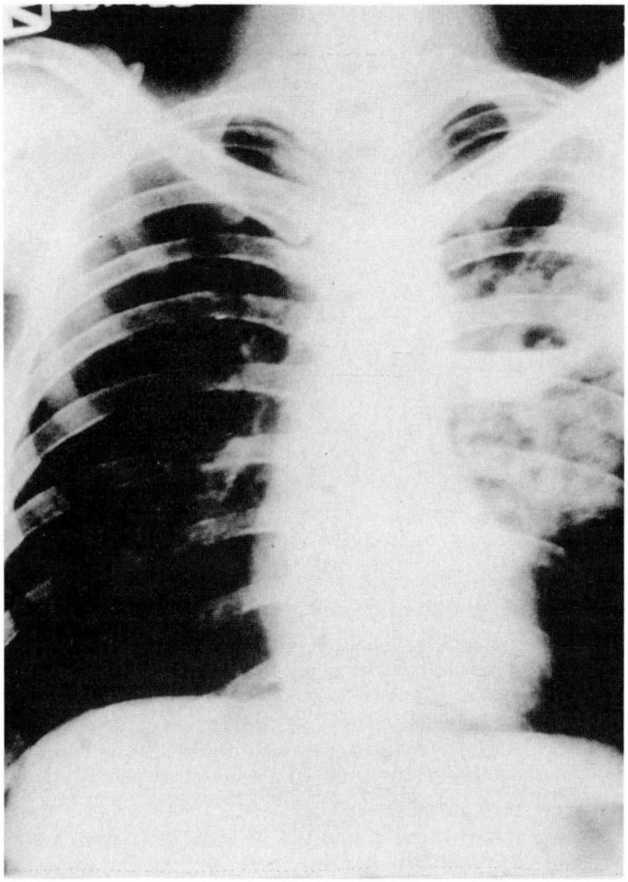

FIGURE 34-4 Chest radiograph of a patient with localized pulmonary melioidosis showing extensive consolidation and cavitation. (From Pitt TL, Dance DAB: Melioidosis and *Pseudomonas pseudomallei.* Public Health Lab Serv Microbiol Digest 8:127–130, 1991.)

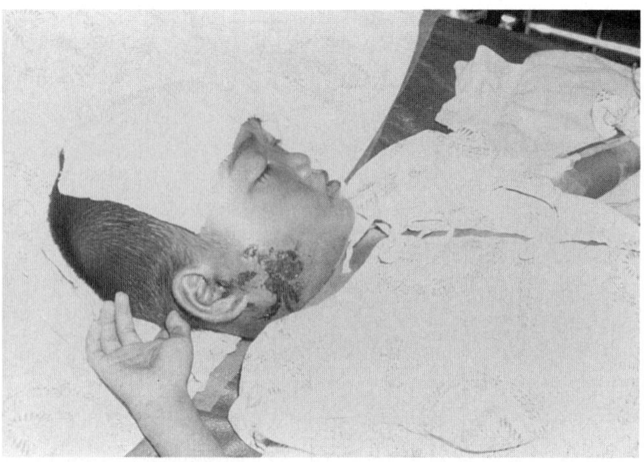

FIGURE 34-5 Child with acute suppurative parotitis. In this case the overlying skin is involved, an abscess has ruptured into the auditory canal, and there is facial nerve palsy. The child was also septicemic. (From Dance DAB: Melioidosis, glanders, and tularaemia. Med Int 107:4508–4511, 1992.)

approximately one-third of pediatric cases,[43,44] but has rarely been reported elsewhere. This strong age-site association probably reflects ascending infection after oral contamination with muddy water. Most cases are unilateral and result in parotid abscesses that require surgical drainage, although they may rupture spontaneously into the auditory canal. Facial nerve palsy and septicemia are rare complications.

Although the lung and parotid are the most common foci for localized *B. pseudomallei* infection, any other organ or tissue may be affected. Well-described examples include cutaneous and subcutaneous abscesses, lymphadenitis, osteomyelitis and septic arthritis, liver or splenic abscesses, cystitis, pyelonephritis, prostatic abscesses, epididymo-orchitis, keratitis, and brain abscesses.

Pathology

B. pseudomallei is essentially a pyogenic organism, but lesions of melioidosis may vary from an acute, necrotizing inflammation with abscess formation to a chronic granulomatous inflammation, depending on the duration of the infection, and sometimes a mixed picture is seen.[45] It is difficult to make a specific histopathologic diagnosis, but features which may be helpful include the presence of intracellular "globi" of gram-negative bacilli combined with giant cells against a background of acute necrotizing inflammation.[46]

PATHOGENESIS

The pathogenesis of melioidosis is poorly understood and until recently had been relatively little studied. The outcome of infection with *B. pseudomallei* depends on the balance between the host's immune system, the virulence of the infecting strain, and the size and route of the initial inoculum. Abscesses or granulomas occur at the site of primary infection, from which invasion of the bloodstream may ensue leading to septicemia and metastatic seeding of other tissues. A high level of bacteremia (> 50 CFU/mL) is associated with a fatal outcome.[47]

Bacterial Virulence Factors

The advent of molecular techniques, including the sequencing of the *B. pseudomallei* genome, as well as comparison with the closely related, avirulent *B. thailandensis*, have greatly facilitated studies of *B. pseudomallei* virulence. The organism possesses several potential virulence determinants and strains of the organism undoubtedly vary in virulence.[48] Lipopolysaccharide (LPS) is presumably important during septicemia, although the biologic effects of *B. pseudomallei* LPS differ from those of enterobacterial LPS.[49] An extracellular polysaccharide capsule is undoubtedly a key virulence factor, although its precise role remains to be defined.[50] Other possible virulence determinants include a heat-labile, lethal exotoxin with a molecular weight of approximately 31 kD, which appears to act by inhibition of synthesis of macromolecules[51]; various other toxins and enzymes (e.g., hemolysin, lecithinase, lipase, and proteases[52]); a siderophore (malleobactin)[53]; flagella[54]; acid phosphatase[55]; and type III secretion systems.[56]

There is increasing evidence that *B. pseudomallei* is able to survive intracellularly,[57] which probably contributes to the recalcitrant nature of melioidosis, its potential for long periods of latency, and its tendency to relapse.[58] Spread between cells appears to occur in a manner similar to, but different from, that which occurs with *Listeria monocytogenes*, involving actin rearrangement into a comet tail appearance within membrane protrusions, and leading to cell death through apoptosis.[59]

Host Defense

As already mentioned, clinically apparent melioidosis is an opportunistic infection. There is some evidence that innate, humoral, and cell-mediated immunity all contribute to defense against the disease. Evidence from studies in experimental animals suggests that antibodies to the exotoxin, LPS, flagellin, flagellin-LPS conjugates, and capsular polysaccharides may all have some protective effect. In human infections, the level of antibody to O-PSII, but not O-PSI, was significantly higher in patients who survived melioidosis than in those who died.[60] Production of interferon-gamma appears to be particularly important in protection in some mouse models.[61] The fact that C57BL/6 mice are considerably more resistant to infection by *B. pseudomallei* than BALB/c mice also suggests a role for cellular immunity in host defense.[62] On the other hand, an overaggressive host response may actually contribute to pathogenesis, and raised levels of several pro-inflammatory cytokines have been found to be associated with a poor outcome in human melioidosis.[63–65]

DIAGNOSIS

Melioidosis is difficult to diagnose on clinical grounds alone, so, where possible, laboratory confirmation by detection of *B. pseudomallei* or of corresponding antibodies should be sought. This requires relatively sophisticated facilities, which are not available in many endemic areas. Because of the potential for latency, the diagnosis should be considered in any patient who has ever visited an endemic area who presents with septicemia or abscesses, particularly if there is evidence of an underlying disease such as diabetes mellitus.

Microscopy and Culture

The organism should be sought in blood, pus, sputum, urine, or any other specimen appropriate to the clinical presentation. Microscopy of a gram-stained smear may reveal bipolar or unevenly staining gram-negative rods, but this has a low specificity and sensitivity. Direct immunofluorescent microscopy may be helpful in endemic areas, but is not widely available.[66] Isolation and identification of *B. pseudomallei* is diagnostic, since asymptomatic carriage has never been reported. The organism grows readily on most laboratory media, although it may take 48 hours or more to develop characteristic colonial morphology. The sensitivity of culture may be increased by the use of selective media.[67] Culture of a throat swab alone using these selective techniques has an overall sensitivity of 36% for the diagnosis of melioidosis (79% in sputum-positive patients), which is particularly useful in children or others who cannot produce sputum.[68] Identification of cultures may be conducted using conventional biochemical tests, commercial kits, or agglutination, but may be delayed or incorrect because many microbiologists are not familiar with the characteristics of the organism. Consequently, if melioidosis is suspected, the laboratory should always be warned to ensure that appropriate techniques and containment measures are employed.

Detection of Antigens and Nucleic Acids

Several rapid diagnostic techniques for the detection of *B. pseudomallei* antigens and nucleic acids have been developed, but most of these currently have suboptimal sensitivity when used directly on clinical samples and are not widely available.[69,70] Techniques like latex agglutination are, however, useful for rapid identification of the organism in plate or broth cultures.[71,72]

Detection of Antibodies

The serodiagnostic test most widely used in endemic areas is an indirect hemagglutination (IHA) test, which detects IgM antibodies to crude heat-stable antigens (probably predominantly LPS).[73] The test is poorly standardized, and there is considerable interlaboratory variation between the titers regarded as positive. Both false negatives and false positives are seen, the latter being a particular problem in endemic areas as a result of high background seropositivity. Nonetheless, a single high titer (>1:40) in someone from a nonendemic area, or a rising titer, may be diagnostically useful. Enzyme-linked immunosorbent assays (ELISAs), which detect IgG antibodies, appear to give similar results. Assays which detect specific IgM (indirect immunofluorescence, ELISA) correlate better with disease activity,[74–77] and are thus more useful in endemic areas and, along with measurement of C-reactive protein,[78] in follow-up of patients on treatment. A number of assays employing more purified antigens have been reported to have better sensitivity and specificity than the IHA test,[79,80] but none of these tests have been subjected to a large scale, multicenter analysis.

TREATMENT AND PROGNOSIS

Supportive Treatment

Patients with septicemic melioidosis usually require aggressive supportive treatment and should ideally be managed in an intensive care unit. Particular attention should be paid to correction of volume depletion and septic shock, respiratory and renal failure, and hyperglycemia or ketoacidosis. Abscesses should be drained whenever possible.

Specific Treatment

B. pseudomallei is intrinsically resistant to many antibiotics, including aminoglycosides and early β-lactams. A complete lack of response to penicillin and gentamicin, a combination often used in the empirical treatment of septicemia in the tropics, is characteristic of melioidosis.[27]

Until the mid-1980s, various empirical combination regimens were used to treat melioidosis, usually including a tetracycline, chloramphenicol, and co-trimoxazole. Several recent studies, which have been well summarized elsewhere,[35,81] have provided a sound evidence base for the treatment of severe melioidosis. Treatment comprises two phases, an acute phase, the aim of which is to reduce mortality, and an eradication phase, the aim of which is to reduce the risk of relapse. The acute mortality of acute severe melioidosis can be substantially reduced by newer β-lactam agents such as ceftazidime, imipenem, and cefoperazone-sulbactam, with or without co-trimoxazole.[82–86] Very recently, dramatic success has been achieved in Darwin, northern Australia, using meropenem plus co-trimoxazole with adjunctive G-CSF, the mortality from melioidosis septic shock falling from 95% to 10%.[87] This work needs repeating in a randomized, prospective study. Ceftazidime (120 mg/kg/day), imipenem, or meropenem (50 mg/kg/day) is currently the treatment of choice and should be given for 2 to 4 weeks according to the clinical response. Amoxicillin-clavulanate therapy is associated with a higher failure rate,[88] and ceftriaxone and cefotaxime should not be used.[89] Unfortunately, all these new antibiotics are extremely expensive, and so practitioners in many endemic areas will have to continue using chloramphenicol succinate (100 mg/kg/day), doxycycline (4 mg/kg/day), and co-trimoxazole (trimethoprim 10 mg/kg/day and sulfamethoxazole 50 mg/kg/day), either individually or in combination, which are known to give inferior outcomes.

Following parenteral treatment, prolonged oral antibiotics are needed to prevent relapse, which occurs in up to 23% of patients,[28,58] and is more common in patients with more severe disease. This can be reduced to less than 10% if antibiotics are given for a total of 20 weeks.[90] The combination of chloramphenicol (40 mg/kg/day), doxycycline (4 mg/kg/day), and co-trimoxazole (10 mg plus sulfamethoxazole 50 mg/kg/day) has been associated with a lower relapse rate than amoxicillin and clavulanate (60 mg amoxicillin plus clavulanic acid 15 mg/kg/day), although this may have been accounted for by differences in compliance, so either regimen is probably adequate.[90] Amoxicillin and clavulanate is preferable in children and in pregnant or lactating women because of lower toxicity. The fluoroquinolones, with or without azithromycin, and doxycycline alone are all associated with unacceptable relapse rates.[91–93] It is possible that the chloramphenicol component of the regimen is not necessary,[93] and further prospective studies are needed to determine whether co-trimoxazole alone is adequate for eradication.[21,87] In patients with mild localized disease, the preceding oral regimens may be used, although the optimal agents and duration of treatment remain to be defined.

Outcome and Follow-up

Even with optimal treatment, the mortality from acute severe melioidosis is high (30% to 47%). In patients who survive, there is often chronic morbidity resulting both from the disease itself and the underlying conditions. Patients require long-term follow-up to detect relapse. Susceptibility tests should be carried out on isolates obtained during or after treatment, since resistance may emerge in 5% to 10% of cases.[94]

PREVENTION AND CONTROL

B. pseudomallei is ubiquitous in the environment in endemic areas, so it is difficult for those whose occupations involve soil and water contact to avoid exposure. It might be worthwhile for those particularly at risk (e.g., diabetic patients) to avoid rice farming, or use hand and foot protection, although the effectiveness of this has not been evaluated. Elimination of the organism from soil using disinfectants was attempted in the French outbreak,[13] but is probably futile. There is no *B. pseudomallei* vaccine licensed for human use, although experimental vaccines are under development and have been used in animals.[95] The organism should be handled in containment level 3 facilities in the laboratory. Patients should ideally be nursed in standard isolation, although person-to-person spread is very rare.

REFERENCES

1. Rotz LD, Khan AS, Lillibridge SR, et al: Public health assessment of potential biological terrorism agents. Emerg Infect Dis 8:225, 2002.
2. Whitmore A: An account of a glanders-like disease occurring in Rangoon. J Hyg 13:1, 1913.
3. Stanton AT, Fletcher W: Melioidosis. Studies from the Institute of Medical Research, Federated Malay States, 21. London, John Bale & Son and Danielson, 1932.
4. Chambon L: Isolement du bacille de Whitmore à partir du milieu extérieur. Ann Inst Pasteur 89:229, 1955.
5. Sanford JP: *Pseudomonas* species (including melioidosis and glanders). In Mandell GL, Bennett JE, Dolin R (eds): Principles and Practice of Infectious Diseases, 4th ed. New York, Churchill Livingstone, 1995, p 2003.
6. Dance DAB: Melioidosis: The tip of the iceberg? Clin Microbiol Rev 4:52, 1991.
7. Dance DAB: Melioidosis as an emerging global problem. Acta Trop 74:115, 2001.
8. Yabuuchi E, Kosako Y, Oyaizu H, et al: Proposal of *Burkholderia* gen. nov and transfer of seven species of the genus *Pseudomonas* homology group II to the new genus, with the type species *Burkholderia cepacia* (Palleroni and Holmes 1981) comb. nov. Microbiol Immunol 36:1251, 1992.
9. Fournier J: La mélioïdose et le B. de Whitmore. Controverses épidémiologiques et taxonomiques. Bull Soc Pathol Exot 58:753, 1965.
10. Dharakul T, Songsivilai S: Recent developments in the laboratory diagnosis of melioidosis. J Infect Dis Antimicrob Agents 13:77, 1995.
11. Li L, He YW: *Pseudomonas pseudomallei* and melioidosis in China. Chin Med J (Engl) 105:775, 1992.
12. John TJ, Jesudason MV, Lalitha MK, et al: Melioidosis in India: The tip of the iceberg? Indian J Med Res 103:62, 1996.
13. Mollaret HH: L'affaire du jardin des plantes ou comment la mélioïdose fit son apparition en France. Med Mal Infect 18:643, 1988.
14. Strauss JM, Groves MG, Mariappan M, et al: Melioidosis in Malaysia. II. Distribution of *Pseudomonas pseudomallei* in soil and surface water. Am J Trop Med Hyg 18:698, 1969.
15. Nachiangmai N, Patamasucon P, Tipayamonthein B, et al: *Pseudomonas pseudomallei* in southern Thailand. Southeast Asian J Trop Med Public Health 16:83, 1985.
16. Wuthiekanun V, Smith MD, Dance DAB, et al: Isolation of *Pseudomonas pseudomallei* from soil in north-eastern Thailand. Trans R Soc Trop Med Hyg 89:41, 1995.
17. Brett PJ, DeShazer D, Woods DE: *Burkholderia thailandensis* sp. nov., a *Burkholderia pseudomallei*–like species. Int J Systemat Bacteriol 48:317, 1998.
18. Thomas AD, Forbes-Faulkner J, Parker M: Isolation of *Pseudomonas pseudomallei* from clay layers at defined depths. Am J Epidemiol 110:515, 1979.
19. Inglis TJJ, Mee BJ, Chang BJ. The environmental microbiology of melioidosis. Rev Med Microbiol 12:13, 2001.
20. Suputtamongkol Y, Hall AJ, Dance DAB, et al: The epidemiology of melioidosis in Ubon Ratchatani, northeast Thailand. Int J Epidemiol 23:1082, 1994.
21. Currie BJ, Fisher DA, Howard DM, et al: Endemic melioidosis in tropical northern Australia: a 10-year prospective study and review of the literature. Clin Infect Dis 31:981, 2000.
22. Howe C, Sampath A, Spotnitz M: The *pseudomallei* group: A review. J Infect Dis 124:598, 1971.

23. Currie BJ, Mayo M, Anstey NM, et al: A cluster of melioidosis cases from an endemic region is clonal and linked to the water supply using molecular typing of *Burkholderia pseudomallei* isolates. Am J Trop Med Hygiene 65:177, 2001.
24. Inglis TJJ, Garrow SC, Henderson M, et al: *Burkholderia pseudomallei* traced to water treatment plant in Australia. Emerg Infect Dis 6:56, 2000.
25. Low Choy J, Mayo M, Janmaat A, et al: Animal melioidosis in Australia. Acta Trop 74:153, 2000.
26. Kunakorn M, Jayanetra P, Tanphaichitra D: Man-to-man transmission of melioidosis. Lancet 337:1290, 1991.
27. Chaowagul W, White NJ, Dance DAB, et al: Melioidosis: A major cause of community-acquired septicemia in northeastern Thailand. J Infect Dis 159:890, 1989.
28. Currie BJ, Fisher DA, Anstey NM, et al: Melioidosis: Acute and chronic disease, relapse and re-activation. Trans R Soc Trop Med Hyg 94:301, 2000.
29. Chodimella U, Hoppes WL, Whalen S, et al: Septicemia and suppuration in a Vietnam veteran. Hosp Pract 32:219, 1997.
30. Suputtamongkol Y, Chaowagul W, Chetchotisakd P, et al: Risk factors for melioidosis and bacteremic melioidosis. Clin Infect Dis 29:408, 1999.
31. O'Carroll MR, Kidd TJ, Coulter C, et al: *Burkholderia pseudomallei*: Another emerging pathogen in cystic fibrosis. Thorax 58:1087, 2003.
32. Poe RH, Vassallo CL, Domm BM: Melioidosis: The remarkable imitator. Am Rev Respir Dis 104:427, 1971.
33. Leelarasamee A, Bovornkitti, S: Melioidosis: Review and update. Rev Infect Dis 11:413, 1989.
34. Punyagupta S: Melioidosis: Review of 686 cases and presentation of a new clinical classification. In Punyagupta S, Sirisanthana T, Stapatayavong B (eds): Melioidosis. Bangkok, Bangkok Medical Publisher, 1989, p 217.
35. White NJ. Melioidosis. Lancet 361:1715, 2003.
36. Kanaphun P, Thirawattanasuk N, Suputtamongkol Y, et al: Serology and carriage of *Pseudomonas pseudomallei:* A prospective study in 1000 hospitalized children in Northeast Thailand. J Infect Dis 167:230, 1993.
37. Ashdown LR, Johnson RW, Koehler JM, et al: Enzyme-linked immunosorbent assay for the diagnosis of clinical and subclinical melioidosis. J Infect Dis 160:253, 1989.
38. Goshorn RK: Recrudescent pulmonary melioidosis. A case report involving the so-called "Vietnamese Time Bomb." Indiana Med 80:247, 1987.
39. Dhiensiri T, Puapairoj S, Susaengrat W: Pulmonary melioidosis: Clinical-radiologic correlation in 183 cases from northeastern Thailand. Radiology 166:711, 1988.
40. Vatcharapreechasakul T, Suputtamongkol Y, Dance DAB, et al: *Pseudomonas pseudomallei* liver abscesses: A clinical, laboratory, and ultrasonographic study. Clin Infect Dis 14:412, 1992.
41. Woods ML, Currie BJ, Howard DM, et al: Neurological melioidosis: Seven cases from the Northern Territory of Australia. Clin Infect Dis 15:163, 1992.
42. Everett ED, Nelson RA: Pulmonary melioidosis. Observations in thirty-nine cases. Am Rev Respir Dis 112:331, 1975.
43. Dance DAB, Davis TME, Wattanagoon Y, et al: Acute suppurative parotitis caused by *Pseudomonas pseudomallei* in children. J Infect Dis 159:654, 1989.
44. Lumbiganon P, Viengnonda S: Clinical manifestations of melioidosis in children. Pediatr Infect Dis J 14:136, 1995.
45. Piggott JA, Hockholzer L: Human melioidosis. A histopathologic study of acute and chronic melioidosis. Arch Pathol 90:101, 1970.
46. Wong KT, Putucheary SD, Vadivelu J: The histopathology of human melioidosis. Histopathology 26:51, 1995.
47. Walsh AL, Smith MD, Wuthiekanun V, et al: Prognostic significance of quantitaive bacteremia in septicemic melioidosis. Clin Infect Dis 21:1498, 1995.
48. Miller WR, Pannell L, Cravitz L, et al: Studies on certain biological characteristics of *Malleomyces mallei* and *Malleomyces pseudomallei*. II. Virulence and infectivity for animals. J Bacteriol 55:127, 1948.
49. Matsuura M, Kawahara K, Ezaki T, et al: Biological activities of lipopolysaccharide of *Burkholderia (Pseudomonas) pseudomallei*. FEMS Microbiol Lett 137:79, 1996.
50. Reckseidler SL, DeShazer D, Sokol PA, et al: Detection of bacterial virulence genes by subtractive hybridization: identification of capsular polysaccharide of *Burkholderia pseudomallei* as a major virulence determinant. Infect Immun 69:34, 2001.
51. Mohamed R, Nathan S, Embi N, et al: Inhibition of macromolecular synthesis in cultured macrophages by *Pseudomonas pseudomallei* exotoxin. Microbiol Immunol 33:811, 1989.
52. Ashdown LR, Koehler JM: Production of hemolysin and other extracellular enzymes by clinical isolates of *Pseudomonas pseudomallei*. J Clin Microbiol 28:2331, 1990.
53. Yang H, Kooi CD, Sokol PA: Ability of *Pseudomonas pseudomallei* malleobactin to acquire transferrin-bound, lactoferrin-bound, and cell-derived iron. Infect Immun 61:656, 1993.
54. Chua KL, Chan YY, Gan YH. Flagella are virulence determinants of *Burkholderia pseudomallei*. Infect Immun 71:1622, 2003.
55. Dejsirilert S, Butraporn R, Chiewsilp D, et al: High activity of acid phosphatase of *Pseudomonas pseudomallei* as a possible attribute relating to its pathogenicity. Jap J Med Sci Biol 42:39, 1989.
56. Stevens MP, Friebel A, Taylor LA, et al: A *Burkholderia pseudomallei* type III secreted protein, BopE, facilitates bacterial invasion of epithelial cells and exhibits guanine nucleotide exchange factor activity. J Bacteriol 185:4992, 2003.
57. Jones AL, Beveridge TJ, Woods DE: Intracellular survival of *Burkholderia pseudomallei*. Infect Immun 64:782, 1996.
58. Chaowagul W, Suputtamongkol Y, Dance DAB, et al: Relapse in melioidosis: incidence and risk factors. J Infect Dis 168:1181, 1993.
59. Breitbach K, Rottner K, Klocke S, et al: Actin-based motility of *Burkholderia pseudomallei* involves the Arp 2/3 complex, but not N-WASP and Ena/VASP proteins. Cell Microbiol 5:385, 2003.
60. Charuchaimontri C, Suputtamongkol Y, Nilakul C, et al: Antilipopolysaccharide II: An antibody protective against fatal melioidosis. Clin Infect Dis 29:813, 1999.
61. Santanirand P, Harley VS, Dance DAB, et al: Obligatory role of gamma interferon for host survival in a murine model of infection with *Burkholderia pseudomallei*. Infect Immun 67:3593, 1999.
62. Leakey AK, Ulett GC, Hirst RG: BALB/c and C57BL/6 mice infected with virulent *Burkholderia pseudomallei* provide contrasting animal models for the acute and chronic forms of melioidosis. Microb Pathogenesis 24:269, 1998.
63. Suputtamongkol Y, Kwiatkowski D, Dance DAB, et al: Tumor necrosis factor in septicemic melioidosis. J Infect Dis 165:561, 1992.
64. Friedland JS, Suputtamongkol Y, Remick DG, et al: Prolonged elevations of interleukin-8 and interleukin-6 concentrations in plasma and of leukocyte interleukin-8 mRNA levels during septicemic and localized *Pseudomonas pseudomallei* infection. Infect Immun 60:2402, 1992.
65. Simpson AJH, Smith MD, Weverling GJ, et al: Prognostic value of cytokine concentrations (tumour necrosis factor, interleukin 6 and interleukin 10) and clinical parameters in severe melioidosis. J Infect Dis 181:621, 2000.
66. Walsh AL, Smith MD, Wuthiekanun V, et al: Immunofluorescence microscopy for the rapid diagnosis of melioidosis. J Clin Pathol 47:377, 1994.
67. Wuthiekanun V, Dance DAB, Wattanagoon Y, et al: The use of selective media for the isolation of *Pseudomonas pseudomallei* in clinical practice. J Med Microbiol 33:121, 1990.
68. Wuthiekanun V, Suputtamongkol Y, Simpson AJH, et al: Value of throat swab in the diagnosis of melioidosis. J Clin Microbiol 39:3801, 2001.
69. Desakorn V, Smith MD, Wuthiekanun V, et al: Detection of *Pseudomonas pseudomallei* antigen in urine for the rapid diagnosis of melioidosis. Am J Trop Med Hyg 51:627, 1994.
70. Haase A, Brennan M, Barrett S, et al: Evaluation of PCR for diagnosis of melioidosis. J Clin Microbiol 36:1039, 1998.
71. Anuntagool N, Naigowit P, Petkanchanapong V, et al: Monoclonal antibody-based rapid identification of *Burkholderia pseudomallei* in blood culture fluid from patients with community-acquired septicaemia. J Med Microbiol 49:1075, 2000.
72. Wuthiekanun V, Anuntagool N, White NJ, et al: Short report: A rapid method for the differentiation of *Burkholderia pseudomallei* and *Burkholderia thailandensis*. Am J Trop Med Hygiene 66:759, 2002.
73. Ashdown LR: Indirect haemagglutination test for melioidosis. Med J Aust 147:364, 1987.
74. Ashdown LR: Relationship and significance of specific immunoglobulin M antibody response in clinical and subclinical melioidosis. J Clin Microbiol 14:361, 1981.
75. Khupulsup K, Petchclai B: Application of indirect hemagglutination test and indirect fluorescent antibody test for IgM antibody for diagnosis of melioidosis in Thailand. Am J Trop Med Hyg 35:366, 1986.

76. Kunakorn M, Boonma P, Khupulsup K, et al: Enzyme-linked immunosorbent assay for immunoglobulin M specific antibody for the diagnosis of melioidosis. J Clin Microbiol 28:1249, 1990.
77. Kunakorn M, Petchclai B, Khupulsup K, et al: Gold blot for detection of immunoglobulin M (IgM)- and IgG-specific antibodies for rapid serodiagnosis of melioidosis. J Clin Microbiol 29:2065, 1991.
78. Ashdown LR: Serial C-reactive protein levels as an aid to the management of melioidosis. Am J Trop Med Hyg 46:151, 1992.
79. Sermswan RW, Wongratanacheewin S, Anuntagool N, et al: Comparison of the polymerase chain reaction and serological tests for diagnosis of septicemic melioidosis. Am J Trop Med Hyg 63:146, 2000.
80. Wongratanacheewin S, Sermswan RW, Anuntagool N, et al: Retrospective study on the diagnostic value of IgG ELISA, dot immunoassay and indirect haemagglutination in septicemic melioidosis. Asian Pacific J Allerg Immunol 19:129, 2001.
81. Samuel M, Ti Y: Interventions for treating melioidosis (Cochrane Methodology Review). In The Cochrane Library, Issue 4, 2003, Chichester, UK: John Wiley & Sons, Ltd.
82. White NJ, Dance DAB, Chaowagul W, et al: Halving the mortality of severe melioidosis by ceftazidime. Lancet 2:697, 1989.
83. Sookpranee M, Boonma P, Susaengrat W, et al: Multicenter prospective randomized trial comparing ceftazidime plus co-trimoxazole with chloramphenicol plus doxycycline and co-trimoxazole for treatment of severe melioidosis. Antimicrob Agents Chemother 36:158, 1992.
84. Suputtamongkol Y, Rajchanuwong A, Chaowagul W, et al: Ceftazidime vs. amoxicillin/clavulanate in the treatment of severe melioidosis. Clin Infect Dis 19:846, 1994.
85. Simpson AJH, Suputtamongkol Y, Smith MD, et al: Comparison of imipenem and ceftazidime as therapy for severe melioidosis. Clin Infect Dis 29:381, 1999.
86. Chetchotisakd P, Porramitikul S, Mootsikapun P, et al: Randomized, double-blind, controlled study of cefoperazone-sulbactam plus cotrimoxazole versus ceftazidime plus cotrimoxazole for the treatment of severe melioidosis. Clin Infect Dis 33:29, 2001.
87. Cheng AC, Stephens DP, Anstey NM, et al: Adjunctive granulocyte colony-stimulating factor for treatment of septic shock due to melioidosis. Clin Infect Dis 38:32, 2004
88. Suputtamongkol Y, Rajchanuwong A, Chaowagul W, et al: Ceftazidime vs. amoxicillin/clavulanate in the treatment of severe melioidosis. Clin Infect Dis 19:846, 1994.
89. Chaowagul W, Simpson AJH, Suputtamongkol Y, et al: Empirical cephalosporin treatment of melioidosis. Clin Infect Dis 28:1328, 1999.
90. Rajchanuvong A, Chaowagul W, Suputtamongkol Y, et al: A prospective comparison of co-amoxiclav and the combination of chloramphenicol, doxycycline, and co-trimoxazole for the oral maintenance treatment of melioidosis. Trans R Soc Trop Med Hyg 89:546, 1995.
91. Chaowagul W, Suputtamongkol Y, Smith MD, et al: Oral fluoroquinolones for maintenance treatment of melioidosis. Trans R Soc Trop Med Hyg 91:599, 1997.
92. Chaowagul W, Simpson AJH, Suputtamongkol Y, et al: A comparison of chloramphenicol, trimethoprim-sulfamethoxazole, and doxycycline with doxycycline alone as maintenance therapy for melioidosis. Clin Infect Dis 29:375, 1999.
93. Chetchotisakd P, Chaowagul W, Mootsikapun P, et al: Maintenance therapy of melioidosis with ciprofloxacin plus azithromycin compared with cotrimoxazole plus doxycycline. Am J Trop Med Hyg 64:24, 2001.
94. Dance DAB, Wuthiekanun V, Chaowagul W, et al: The antimicrobial susceptibility of *Pseudomonas pseudomallei*. Emergence of resistance in vitro and during treatment. J Antimicrob Chemother 24:295, 1989.
95. Warawa J, Woods DE: Melioidosis vaccines. Expert Rev Vaccines 1:477, 2002.

35

Diphtheria

MELINDA WHARTON

INTRODUCTION

Diphtheria is caused by infection with *Corynebacterium diphtheriae,* a gram-positive bacillus. Toxigenic strains of *C. diphtheriae* produce a powerful exotoxin that is responsible for the most severe manifestations of the disease.

Prior to the introduction of effective childhood vaccination programs, diphtheria was a major cause of childhood mortality. In 1884, Löffler reported isolation of the organism from patients with diphtheria and demonstration of its pathogenicity in animals. He hypothesized that a potent poison was formed at the site of the local lesion because the organism was usually found only in the site of inoculation in the respiratory tract. In 1888, Roux and Yersin reported that sterile filtrates from cultures of the diphtheria bacillus were lethal to guinea pigs, with development of lesions identical to those found in animals infected with the organism. This was followed by the demonstration of immunity in animals that had received iodine-treated toxin, and the passive transfer of this immunity to other animals by Behring in 1890. In 1894, Roux and Martin used equine antitoxin for treatment of children, with dramatic reduction in mortality. The first vaccines were mixtures of toxin and antitoxin; these were replaced by diphtheria toxoid in the 1920s.

The organism is usually transmitted by direct person-to-person contact. Both symptomatic persons with diphtheria and asymptomatic carriers can transmit the organism, although symptomatic persons are thought to be more highly infectious than carriers. Transmission by fomites may occur, and milk-borne outbreaks have been reported.

In temperate climates, epidemics of respiratory diphtheria are seen in susceptible populations, with a seasonal increase in the fall and winter. Mortality rates of 5% to 10% are typically reported. In tropical climates, cutaneous infection is thought to typically occur repeatedly in childhood, conferring immunity. Because toxin is poorly absorbed from cutaneous sites, systemic manifestations of diphtheria toxin are less commonly seen in the cutaneous form.

AGENT

Corynebacteria are taxonomically related to the mycobacteria and *Nocardia. C. diphtheriae* is a pleomorphic, nonmotile, gram-positive bacillus. A selective medium containing tellurite is essential for primary isolation. Four biotypes—gravis, mitis, intermedius, and belfanti—can be distinguished based on colonial morphology on tellurite blood agar and biochemically.[1]

Although other virulence factors exist, the most significant virulence factor is diphtheria toxin, a 58-kD protein produced by strains carrying β-corynebacteriophage. The phage encodes the toxin, and nontoxigenic strains can be converted to toxin production by this phage. Toxin production is controlled by a regulatory protein, diphtheria toxin regulatory protein (DtxR), which is encoded by the bacterial chromosome. Toxin production is inhibited by iron, which binds to DtxR. The DtxR-iron complex then binds to the diphtheria toxin gene operator, repressing synthesis of toxin.[2]

Rarely, other *Corynebacterium* species (*C. pseudotuberculosis* and *C. ulcerans*) can produce toxin. Sequence analysis of 16S ribosomal RNA has demonstrated that these species are closely related to *C. diphtheriae.*[3]

EPIDEMIOLOGY

Diphtheria occurs worldwide, but where effective childhood immunization programs have been implemented, dramatic reductions in diphtheria morbidity and mortality have resulted. In industrialized countries, routine immunization of infants and young children in the 1940s and 1950s led to dramatic reductions in diphtheria incidence. Although clinical diphtheria is now rare in most developed countries, circulation of *C. diphtheriae* may persist in selected populations within those countries. Circulation of toxigenic *C. diphtheriae* has been documented in Canada and in the United States.[4,5]

In developing countries, diphtheria toxoid was included in the Expanded Programme on Immunization beginning in the 1970s. Vaccination coverage of infants with three doses of diphtheria toxoid in developing countries rose from 5% in 1974 to 46% by 1985 and 79% by 1992.[6] From 70,000 to 90,000 cases of diphtheria were reported each year during the 1970s to the World Health Organization (WHO); by the 1990s, this had decreased to 22,000 to 27,000 cases each year, representing a decrease worldwide of about 70% over a 20-year period. The reduction in reported cases of diphtheria globally during this period was largely due to reductions in reported cases of diphtheria in developing countries.[7]

A major diphtheria epidemic began in the Russian Federation in 1990 and subsequently spread throughout the former Soviet Union. By early 1996, approximately 125,000 cases and 4000 deaths had been reported in the new independent states of the former Soviet Union.[8] Although the factors that led to this epidemic are not completely understood, delayed immunization of young children and lack of routine booster immunization of adults contributed to susceptibility of the population. Population movements following the dissolution of the Soviet Union facilitated spread within the new independent states. Molecular typing has demonstrated that the outbreak was associated with the emergence of an epidemic clone of *C. diphtheriae* biotype gravis in Russia, although other strains circulated concurrently.[9] Russian-manufactured diphtheria toxoid was used throughout the Soviet Union prior to the country's dissolution; in several case-control studies, the vaccine was demonstrated to be highly effective in prevention of diphtheria.[10,11] In response to the epidemic, vaccine coverage of both children and adults has increased in most countries of the former Soviet Union, and the incidence of disease has been dramatically reduced.

Diphtheria epidemics among adolescents and young adults have also been reported in a number of developing countries. Prior to the introduction of routine immunization programs, diphtheria was predominantly a disease of young children in developing countries, with little disease among those 15 years of age and older.[6] As vaccination programs are introduced, the incidence of disease decreases among the children targeted by those programs and the average age of patients with diphtheria increases.[12] Outbreaks in Jordan, Lesotho, Algeria, China, and Ecuador have been reported.[6,13–15] The common features of these epidemics were that they occurred following a period of high immunization coverage among young children and that cases of diphtheria were predominately reported among adolescents and young adults, populations not covered by the immunization program.

In tropical and subtropical climates, *C. diphtheriae* was a common cause of cutaneous infection prior to the introduction of vaccination programs. In these areas, repeated exposure early in life was thought to result in immunity, and severe manifestations of diphtheria were infrequent.[16,17] Cutaneous diphtheria is thought to serve as the primary reservoir of *C. diphtheriae* in endemic areas where poverty, crowding, and poor hygiene are prevalent. In temperate climates, respiratory diphtheria exhibits a marked seasonality, with seasonal increases in the autumn and winter.

Group A *Streptococcus* is frequently isolated from cases of both respiratory and cutaneous diphtheria. It is unknown if one infection predisposes to the other, or if they are frequently co-isolated, because both infections may be associated with similar risk factors.

DISEASE

Following an incubation period of 2 to 5 days, the illness begins with malaise, sore throat, anorexia, and low-grade fever. The hallmark of respiratory diphtheria is the pseudomembrane (Fig. 35-1), which may be seen in the posterior oropharynx, and may extend into the larynx or trachea or upward into the nose. The pseudomembrane is composed of fibrin, cellular debris, and bacteria and may be white, gray, or black, and is typically firmly adherent, resulting in bleeding if forcibly removed. The membrane usually begins on the tonsils or posterior pharynx, but can spread upward into the nasopharynx or in severe cases into the trachea and bronchi. Soft-tissue swelling of the neck results in the so-called bull-necked appearance. In vaccinated persons, the membrane may be follicular and nonconfluent.

The most serious complications of diphtheria are respiratory obstruction, if the membrane is extensive, and complications due to distant effects of the toxin, most commonly myocarditis or neuropathy. Myocarditis typically occurs 7 to 14 days after onset of disease, but may occur as early as the first week or as late as 6 weeks after onset of illness. Electrocardiographic abnormalities may be detected in the absence of clinical signs or symptoms of myocardial involvement. The most common electrocardiographic abnormalities are flattening and inversion of T waves, ST-segment changes,

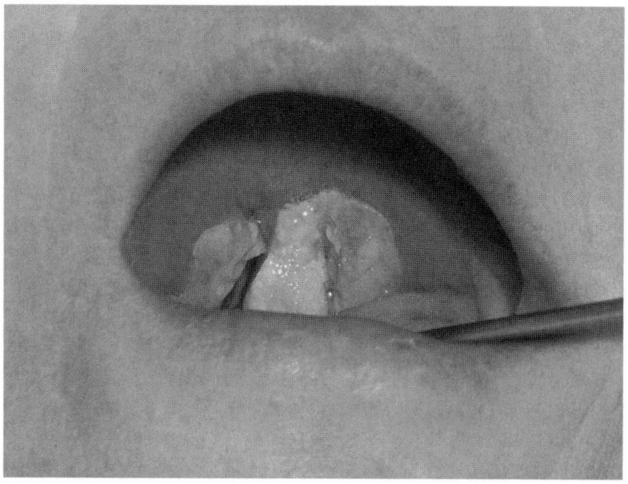

FIGURE 35-1 Pseudomembrane in a patient with respiratory diphtheria. (Courtesy of Dr. Peter Strebel, Centers for Disease Control and Prevention, Atlanta, GA.)

and conduction abnormalities, including complete heart block. The prognosis appears to be worse in cases of diphtheria myocarditis with conduction disturbances or ventricular ectopy.[18,19] Use of artificial pacemakers may be required, but even with ventricular pacing, a high mortality has been reported among patients with severe conduction abnormalities.[20,21] Permanent cardiac damage due to diphtheria myocarditis is rare, but recovery may be prolonged. Pathologically, scattered foci of hyaline and granular degeneration are seen early in the course, followed by fibrosis.

Neuropathy may be seen either early or late in the course of illness. Palatal neuropathy and other cranial nerve palsies are often seen early in the course—as early as the first week of illness—while ocular palsies, diaphragmatic paralysis, and paralysis of limbs are generally seen later in the course of illness. Electrophysiologic studies demonstrate slowing of conduction, prolongation of distal motor latency, and, in severe cases, conduction block. Diaphragmatic paralysis may necessitate ventilatory support. If the patient survives, complete recovery is expected. Pathologic changes include segmental demyelination of nerve fibers within sensory ganglia and demyelination of adjacent peripheral nerves and anterior and posterior roots.

Other complications include renal failure, thrombocytopenia, and coagulation abnormalities. Disseminated intravascular coagulation may occur in severe cases.

Cutaneous diphtheria may occur as a secondary infection following impetigo, other skin infections, or injury (Fig. 35-2). Primary diphtheria typically begins as a vesicle or pustule that progresses to a punched-out ulcer, most commonly seen on the extremities. Lesions may be single or multiple. The ulcer initially is painful and covered with a dark pseudomembrane, but later becomes anesthetic. Healing usually occurs spontaneously over 6 to 12 weeks, but the course may be more prolonged.[22] Complications due to systemic absorption of diphtheria toxin may be seen, but are uncommon. Cutaneous diphtheria is more common in tropical and subtropical areas than in temperate areas.

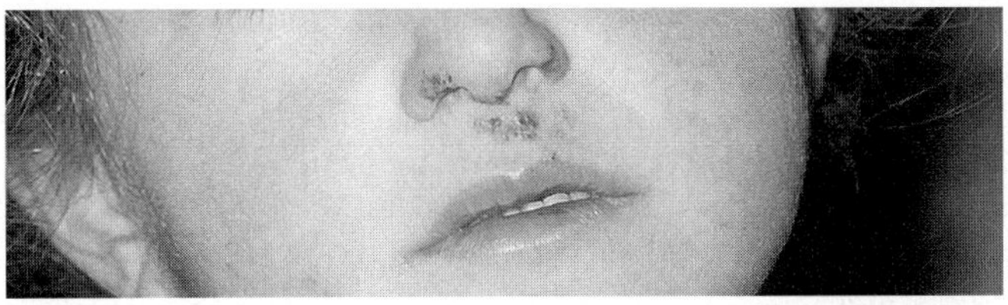

FIGURE 35-2 Cutaneous diphtheria in a child with nasal diphtheria. (Courtesy of Dr. Linda Quick, Centers for Disease Control and Prevention, Atlanta, GA.)

PATHOGENESIS

Diphtheria toxin is a 58-kD protein comprising 535 amino acid residues. It is synthesized as a single polypeptide but in its active form is proteolyzed to two polypeptide chains linked by a disulfide bond. The C-terminal B fragment (345 residues) contains the transmembrane and receptor-binding domains, and the N-terminal A fragment (190 residues) contains the catalytic domain. On the cell surface, diphtheria toxin binds to heparin-binding epidermal growth factor precursor, and the toxin-receptor complex undergoes receptor-mediated endocytosis. The A fragment is then translocated across the endocytic membrane into the cytosol. In the acidic environment of the endosome, protonation of specific residues within the transmembrane domain facilitates penetration of the endoplasmic membrane.[23] Once in the cytosol, the catalytic domain catalyzes the transfer of adenosine diphosphate (ADP)–ribose from nicotinamide adenine dinucleotide (NAD) to elongation factor-2, halting protein synthesis and resulting in cell death.[24] Although diphtheria toxin is the major virulence factor in *C. diphtheriae,* other virulence factors exist. Nontoxigenic *C. diphtheriae* strains can cause typical respiratory diphtheria with pseudomembrane, although toxin-related complications such as myocarditis and neuropathy are not seen. Invasive disease due to nontoxigenic strains of *C. diphtheriae* is well documented.[25]

DIAGNOSIS

The diagnosis of diphtheria is often made initially on clinical grounds. Because of the importance of early treatment with diphtheria antitoxin, clinicians should not wait for laboratory confirmation to initiate treatment.

The diagnosis is confirmed by isolation of *C. diphtheriae* from the site of infection. Use of a selective culture medium containing tellurite is essential to primary isolation; therefore, the clinical laboratory must be alerted that diphtheria is suspected.

For evaluation of patients with suspected respiratory diphtheria, both nasopharyngeal and throat swabs should be obtained. Nasopharyngeal swabs are obtained by inserting the swab through one nostril beyond the anterior nares. The swab is gently advanced along the floor of the nasal cavity under the middle turbinate until the pharyngeal wall is reached. Force must not be used to overcome any obstruction. For throat swabs, the pharynx should be clearly visible and well illuminated and the tongue depressed with an applicator. The throat is swabbed without touching the tongue or the buccal mucosa. The membrane should be rubbed vigorously, with slight pressure and a rotating movement applied to the swab. The edge of the membrane should be lifted and the area beneath it swabbed. For suspected cases of diphtheria infection of nonrespiratory sites, the lesions should be cleansed with sterile normal saline and any crusted material removed, and the swab pressed firmly into the lesion.[1]

Once isolated, the organism should be characterized by biotype and evaluated for production of toxin. The standard method of toxigenicity testing is the Elek immunoprecipitation test. A polymerase chain reaction (PCR) assay for the *tox* and *dtxR* genes has been developed. PCR may be performed directly on clinical specimens, providing a rapid confirmatory test.[26]

The differential diagnosis of respiratory diphtheria includes bacterial and viral pharyngitis, infectious mononucleosis, Vincent's angina, acute epiglottitis, and peritonsillar abscess.

TREATMENT AND PROGNOSIS

The mainstay of treatment of diphtheria is diphtheria antitoxin. Because diphtheria antitoxin does not neutralize intracellular diphtheria toxin, it is essential that it be given as early in the course of illness as possible; prognosis clearly worsens the later in the course of illness that antitoxin is administered. Often it is necessary to make the decision to administer antitoxin on clinical grounds, before laboratory confirmation is available.

Available preparations of diphtheria antitoxin are of equine origin and, as with any heterologous serum, may produce immediate or delayed reactions. A history of prior horse serum exposure or allergy should be obtained and the patient tested for hypersensitivity by skin or eye testing prior to administration of the product. During hypersensitivity testing or infusion of diphtheria antitoxin, a 1:1000 solution of epinephrine should be available and ready for emergency use if needed.

For skin testing, 0.1 mL of a 1:100 dilution of diphtheria antitoxin in physiologic saline is injected intracutaneously. A wheal 1 cm or more in diameter at 20 minutes indicates sensitivity. In persons with a history of allergy to equine serum, 0.05 mL of a 1:1000 dilution should be administered. A negative test does not preclude the occurrence of serum reactions.

For eye testing, one drop of a 1:10 dilution of diphtheria antitoxin in physiologic saline is instilled in the lower lid of one eye and one drop of physiologic saline is instilled in the other eye for comparison. At 20 minutes, conjunctivitis and lacrimation indicate sensitivity, and the eye should be treated with one drop of a 1:100 solution of epinephrine.

If there is no history of hypersensitivity to equine serum and the sensitivity test is negative, the total recommended dose of antitoxin should be given without delay. The dose is determined by the site and extent of local disease and the severity and duration of illness. For anterior nasal diphtheria, 10,000 to 20,000 units of diphtheria antitoxin is recommended, with increasing doses for the tonsillar form (15,000–25,000 units), pharyngeal or laryngeal diphtheria of 48 hours or less duration (20,000–40,000 units), nasopharyngeal disease (40,000–60,000 units), and extensive disease of greater than 3 days' duration or with brawny swelling of the neck (80,000–120,000 units). The preferred route of administration is intravenous because peak antitoxin levels may not be reached for several days following intramuscular administration. The patient should be carefully monitored during administration of antitoxin and the infusion stopped if there are signs of shock.

If the patient is sensitive to horse serum, the indications for use of diphtheria antitoxin should be re-evaluated. If antitoxin is indicated, the patient should be desensitized; standard protocols for desensitization are published.[27]

Toxin-mediated complications are uncommon in cutaneous diphtheria, but have occurred. Use of antitoxin may be indicated in patients with extended, multiple pseudomembranous lesions.[22]

Although antimicrobial agents are of secondary importance in the treatment of diphtheria, they will hasten clearing of the organism and may result in less risk of transmission of diphtheria to others. Agents of choice are penicillin or erythromycin, which are highly active against *C. diphtheriae*. Until the patient can swallow easily, parenteral administration is recommended, with dosages of intramuscular procaine penicillin G (25,000–50,000 units/kg/day for children and 1.2 million units/day for adults in two divided doses) or parenteral erythromycin (40–50 mg/kg/day with a maximum dosage of 2 g/day). Once the patient can swallow easily, oral erythromycin in four divided doses or oral penicillin 125 to 250 mg four times a day can be substituted to complete the 14-day course of therapy.[28] In mild cases, oral therapy may be used for the complete course of treatment. Erythromycin resistance has been reported in areas where erythromycin has been used widely for treatment of cutaneous diphtheria; likewise, tetracycline and rifampin resistance have also been reported.[29,30]

Without antitoxin treatment, respiratory diphtheria is frequently fatal, with case-fatality rates of 30% to 50% reported. With introduction of diphtheria antitoxin for treatment of diphtheria, mortality has decreased to 5% to 10% in most series. In diphtheria, receipt of antitoxin within the first 2 to 3 days of illness is clearly associated with reduced mortality. Disease in vaccinated persons is usually mild.

PREVENTION AND CONTROL

Vaccination of infants with diphtheria toxoid in combination with tetanus toxoid and whole-cell pertussis vaccines (DTP) in many countries of the world has resulted in dramatic reductions in diphtheria incidence globally. In developing countries, the highest priority for diphtheria prevention and control is to reach a high coverage rate for the primary series of three doses of DTP in infants. In endemic areas, infant immunization will protect young children from diphtheria, although it will not prevent continued circulation of the organism, and immunity of older children and adults will be maintained by re-exposure. Frequent skin infections due to *C. diphtheriae* are thought to contribute to maintenance of population immunity in countries where diphtheria is endemic.[6]

Effective childhood immunization programs do not result in eradication of the organism, but do result in reduced circulation; at that point, disease may be seen among adolescents and young adults—especially those who did not receive a primary series when the immunization program was just beginning. Additional immunization strategies must be considered in the context of overall national health priorities, but additional doses of diphtheria toxoid at school entry are indicated if outbreaks occur among schoolchildren, and a dose at school leaving may be operationally the easiest to implement if disease is occurring among adolescents and young adults.[6]

Once a case is recognized, the following measures are recommended to limit further spread. Strict isolation should be maintained until elimination of the organism is demonstrated by negative cultures of two samples obtained at least 24 hours apart after completion of antimicrobial therapy. Close contacts (household members and other persons with a history of direct contact with the case-patient) should be identified and evaluated for signs and symptoms of diphtheria. As soon as nasopharyngeal and pharyngeal swabs are obtained for culture, antimicrobial prophylaxis should be administered regardless of prior vaccination status. Recommended regimens include a single dose of intramuscular benzathine penicillin G (600,000 units for children less than 6 years of age and 1.2 million units for persons older than 6 years of age) or a 7- to 10-day course of oral erythromycin (40 mg/kg/day for children and 1 g/day for adults). Although there is some evidence that erythromycin may be more effective at eradication of the carrier state than penicillin, a single dose of benzathine penicillin administered intramuscularly may be preferred if compliance is in doubt. Persons who continue to harbor the organism after treatment with either agent should receive an additional 10-day course of erythromycin and follow-up cultures should be obtained. Vaccination status of contacts should be assessed and, if indicated, vaccine administered. Surveillance of close contacts should be maintained for at least 7 days, but hospitalization in the absence of clinical illness is not indicated.[28] Reporting of cases of diphtheria to public health authorities is required by law in many countries.

For control of epidemic diphtheria in the former Soviet Union, the European Region of WHO recommended early diagnosis and proper management of diphtheria cases, rapid investigation and standard treatment of contacts, and rapidly increasing population immunity by attaining high coverage among children through routine vaccination—95% coverage with four doses of DTP in all districts—and administration of a single dose of age-appropriate formulation of diphtheria toxoid to the entire population. Additional doses were also recommended for certain adult age groups and a booster should be given every 10 years to adults, especially travelers to endemic areas. Although optimal control has not yet been achieved in all countries of the former Soviet Union, the effectiveness of this strategy for outbreak control is now well established.[31,32]

In the United States and many other developed countries, diphtheria toxoid is administered to children less than 7 years of age with tetanus toxoid and acellular pertussis vaccine (DTaP); DTaP may also be combined with other vaccines in combination vaccines that decrease the number of injections that need to be administered simultaneously. U.S. immunization authorities recommend that children receive DTaP at 2, 4, and 6 months of age, with booster doses at 15 to 18 months and 4 to 6 years. Adult formulation tetanus and diphtheria toxoids (Td) are recommended every 10 years, beginning at age 11 to 12 years. Travelers to diphtheria-endemic areas are at risk of contracting diphtheria and should be age-appropriately immunized prior to travel.[33]

REFERENCES

1. Efstratiou A, Maple PAC: Laboratory Diagnosis of Diphtheria. The Expanded Programme on Immunization in the European Region of WHO. Copenhagen, World Health Organization, 1994.
2. Tao X, Schiering N, Zeng H, et al: Iron, DtxR, and the regulation of diphtheria toxin expression. Mol Microbiol 14:191, 1994.
3. Pascual C, Lawson PA, Farrow JA, et al: Phylogenetic analysis of the genus *Corynebacterium* based on 16S rRNA gene sequences. Int J Syst Bacteriol 45:724, 1995.
4. Wilson CR, Casson RI, Wherrett B, et al: Toxigenic diphtheria in two isolated northern communities. Arctic Med Res Suppl:346, 1991.
5. Toxigenic *Corynebacterium diphtheriae*—Northern Plains Indian community, August–October 1996. MMWR 46:506, 1997.
6. Galazka AM, Robertson SE: Diphtheria: Changing patterns in the developing world and the industrialized world. Eur J Epidemiol 11:107, 1995.
7. Galazka AM, Robertson SE, Oblapenko GP: Resurgence of diphtheria. Eur J Epidemiol 11:95, 1995.
8. Update: Diphtheria epidemic—New independent states of the former Soviet Union, January 1995–March 1996. MMWR 45:693, 1996.
9. Popovic T, Kombarova SY, Reeves MW, et al: Molecular epidemiology of diphtheria in Russia, 1985–1994. J Infect Dis 174:1064, 1996.
10. Hardy IR, Dittman S, Sutter RW: Current situation and control strategies for resurgence of diphtheria in the newly independent states of the former Soviet Union. Lancet 347:1739, 1996.
11. Vitek C, Brennan M, Gotway C, et al: Risk for diphtheria among children associated with increasing time since last booster vaccination. In Abstracts of the 37th Interscience Conference on Antimicrobial Agents and Chemotherapy, Toronto, Canada, September 28–October 1, 1997, Abstract G-9.
12. Loevinsohn BP: The changing age structure of diphtheria patients: Evidence for the effectiveness of EPI in the Sudan. Bull World Health Org 68:353, 1990.
13. Khuri-Bulos N, Hamzah Y, Sammerrai SM, et al: The changing epidemiology of diphtheria in Jordan. Bull World Health Org 66:65, 1988.
14. Van Geldermalsen AA, Wenning U: A diphtheria epidemic in Lesotho, 1989: Did vaccination increase the population susceptibility? Ann Trop Paediatr 13:13, 1993.
15. Youwang Y, Jianming D, Young X, et al: Epidemiological features of an outbreak of diphtheria and its control with diphtheria toxoid immunization. Int J Epidemiol 21:807, 1992.
16. Bray JP, Burt EB, Potter EV, et al: Epidemic diphtheria and skin infections in Trinidad. J Infect Dis 126:34, 1972.
17. Montgomery J: Carriage of *Corynebacterium diphtheriae* in children of the Eastern Highlands Province. Papua New Guinea Med J 27:20, 1984.
18. Naiditch MJ, Bower AG: Diphtheria: A study of 1433 cases observed during a ten-year period at the Los Angeles Country Hospital. Am J Med 17:229, 1954.
19. Bethell DB, Dung NM, Loan HT, et al: Prognostic value of electrocardiographic monitoring of patients with severe diphtheria. Clin Infect Dis 20:1259, 1995.
20. Stockins BA, Lanas FT, Saavedra JG, et al: Prognosis in patients with diphtheria myocarditis and bradyarrhythmias: Assessment of results of ventricular pacing. Br Heart J 72:190, 1994.
21. Dung NM, Kneen R, Kiem N, et al: Treatment of severe diphtheritic myocarditis by temporary insertion of a cardiac pacemaker. Clin Infect Dis 35:1425, 2002.
22. Höfler W: Cutaneous diphtheria. Int J Dermatol 30:845, 1991.
23. Choe S, Bennett MJ, Fujii G, et al: The crystal structure of diphtheria toxin. Nature 357:216, 1992.
24. Collier RJ: Diphtheria toxin: Mode of action and structure. Bacteriol Rev 39:54, 1975.
25. Patey O, Bimet F, Riegel P, et al: Clinical and molecular study of *Corynebacterium diphtheriae* systemic infections in France. J Clin Microbiol 35:441, 1997.
26. Nakao H, Popovic T: Development of a direct polymerase chain reaction for detection of diphtheria toxin gene. J Clin Microbiol 35:1651, 1997.
27. American Academy of Pediatrics: Passive immunization. In Pickering LK (ed): Red Book: 2003 Report of the Committee on Infectious Diseases, 26th ed. Elk Grove Village, IL, American Academy of Pediatrics, 2003, pp 60–63.
28. Farizo KM, Strebel PM, Chen RT, et al: Fatal respiratory disease due to *Corynebacterium diphtheriae:* Case report and review of guidelines for management, investigation, and control. Clin Infect Dis 16:59, 1993.
29. Maple PA, Efstratiou A, Tseneva G, et al: The in-vitro susceptibilities of toxigenic strains of *Corynebacterium diphtheriae* isolated in northwestern Russia and surrounding areas to ten antibiotics. J Antimicrob Chemother 34:1037, 1994.
30. Wilson AP: Treatment of infection caused by toxigenic and non-toxigenic strains of *Corynebacterium diphtheriae.* J Antimicrob Chemother 35:717, 1995.
31. De Zoysa A, Efstratiou A: Eighth International Meeting of the European Laboratory Working Group on Diphtheria and the Diphtheria Surveillance Network—June 2004: Progress is needed to sustain control of diphtheria in European Region. Eurosurveillance 9:13, 2004.
32. Dittman S: Epidemic diphtheria in the newly independent states of the former USSR—Situation and lessons learned. Biologicals 25:179, 1997.
33. CDC: Fatal respiratory diphtheria in a U.S. traveler to Haiti—Pennsylvania, 2003. MMWR 52:1285, 2004.

36

Tuberculosis and Atypical Mycobacterial Infections

JOHN L. JOHNSON
JERROLD J. ELLNER

INTRODUCTION

Tuberculosis (TB) is a chronic necrotizing granulomatous disease caused by the acid-fast bacillus *Mycobacterium tuberculosis* or the closely related species *M. bovis* and *M. africanum*. It is spread primarily by inhalation of aerosolized infectious droplet nuclei from patients with active pulmonary TB. The lungs are the main portal of entry. The most common manifestation of TB in humans is pulmonary disease, but nearly all organ systems can be involved. The most frequent sites of extrapulmonary disease are the lymph nodes, pleura, and bones and joints.

TB occurs worldwide, but more than 95% of cases and 98% of deaths occur in developing countries. Miliary and meningeal TB in children and TB occurring in human immunodeficiency virus (HIV)-coinfected people are important causes of death in areas of high prevalence. *Mycobacterium bovis* is still a significant cause of human disease in developing countries unless infected and diseased cattle are identified and destroyed in skin test programs and milk is pasteurized.

AGENT

Mycobacterium tuberculosis is a slender nonmotile bacillus approximately 2 to 4 μm in length. It is an obligate aerobic organism and grows best in tissues with high ambient oxygen tensions, such as the apices of the lung or the renal cortex. The cell wall consists of a waxy coat containing mycolic acid and other complex lipopolysaccharides. This unique cell wall gives members of the genus *Mycobacterium* their characteristic acid-fast staining property. After staining with carbol fuchsin, mycobacteria are not decolorized by washing with acid alcohol. Mycobacteria take up other stains, such as Gram stain, poorly. *Mycobacterium tuberculosis* typically appears as a slender solid or beaded organism, and virulent strains are often aggregated in clumps in culture. The complete genome of a virulent laboratory strain of *M. tuberculosis* H37Rv was the first to be sequenced,[1] leading to new knowledge about the pathogenesis and virulence of tuberculosis and promising to accelerate the identification of new targets for diagnostic testing, treatment, and vaccine development.

Mycobacterium africanum can be reliably distinguished from *M. tuberculosis* only by biochemical testing. The clinical features, drug susceptibility, and outcomes of *M. africanum* disease are similar to those of *M. tuberculosis*. The bovine tubercle bacillus, *M. bovis*, shares greater than 95% DNA homology with *M. tuberculosis* and causes disease in humans, cattle, deer, badgers, and other animals. Speciation can be performed only by specialized laboratories. Most strains are niacin positive, do not reduce nitrate, and are resistant to pyrazinamide.

Tuberculosis is predominantly spread by droplet nuclei that are generated during coughing and sneezing by people with active pulmonary TB. Direct transmission by heavily infected body secretions from fistulas and skin lesions occurs infrequently. Cutaneous TB from direct inoculation occurs rarely in pathologists ("prosector's wart") and laboratory workers. Fomites (eating utensils, clothing, and bedding) play no role in TB transmission among humans. Large droplet nuclei rapidly settle out of air currents or are removed by the mucociliary ladder in the upper airway and present little danger. Bacteria in small droplets are rapidly killed by drying and exposure to ultraviolet (UV) light. Tubercle bacilli in droplet nuclei measuring 1 to 5 μm in diameter remain suspended in air for long periods, where they can be inhaled and reach the distal airspaces to establish a primary focus of infection. The number of bacilli needed to produce infection is low; infection in humans may occur when as few as one to five bacilli impact in a terminal alveolus.

The risk of infection is related to the duration and severity of exposure to infectious droplet nuclei. The length of exposure must generally be prolonged; brief casual exposures usually do not result in infection.[2] The density of infectious droplet nuclei in the air in proximity to an active TB case is related to the smear status of the index case (bacillary density), cough frequency, and the number of air exchanges (ventilation) in the area. Because up to 1000 to 10,000 acid-fast bacilli (AFB) per milliliter of sputum must be present for a positive AFB smear,[3] smear-positive people are the most important sources of transmission of TB in the community. Approximately 30% to 60% of people heavily exposed to smear-positive individuals with pulmonary TB become infected. For programmatic purposes, AFB smear-negative patients usually are considered to be noninfectious. In fact, they may account for up to 17% of new cases.[4] Crowded housing also leads to increased transmission of TB due to repeated and prolonged exposure and decreased air exchanges. Most transmission of TB occurs in household contacts—that is, people living in the same residence with an infectious smear-positive case. Intimate contact such as sharing a bed with a patient with TB poses the greatest risk.

EPIDEMIOLOGY

TB is a major global health problem. Up to one-third of the world's population is infected with *M. tuberculosis*. The World Health Organization (WHO) estimates that 8 million new TB cases and 1.9 million deaths occurred in 2000 due to TB, making it the second leading cause of death due to an identified infectious pathogen worldwide, exceeded only by HIV/AIDS.[5,6] Most of the burden of TB falls on developing countries: More than 95% of all TB cases and 98% of all deaths due to TB occur in developing countries, especially those in sub-Saharan Africa and Asia. Up to 7% of all deaths and 26% of preventable deaths in developing countries are due to TB.[7,8] TB predominantly affects young adults in their most productive years of life and has substantial impact on economic development.

Tuberculosis also is increasingly an urban problem. Two-thirds of the world's population will live in cities by 2025; many will live in crowded, substandard housing with poor ventilation in large cities in developing countries in Asia and Africa.

Tuberculosis and Human Immunodeficiency Virus Interactions

HIV infection currently is the greatest risk factor known for the progression of latent *M. tuberculosis* infection to active TB and for the rapid progression of new infection to TB. Thirty to 40% of all new TB cases in many African countries occur in HIV-coinfected people, with rates as high as 60% to 70% in some eastern and southern African nations.[5] Increasing rates of HIV coinfection in countries such as Botswana have led to rapid increases in the incidence of TB despite the introduction of more effective TB treatment strategies using the Directly Observed Therapy, Short Course (DOTS) strategy.[9] In 2000, at least 11.4 million people were infected by HIV and *M. tuberculosis*; the majority live in Asia and sub-Saharan Africa. Globally, approximately 11% of all new TB cases—double the percentage in 1990—occur in HIV-infected people.[5,10]

The cumulative risk of developing active TB in HIV-infected people is markedly higher than the 5% to 10% lifetime risk in tuberculin skin test (TST)-positive HIV-noninfected people.[11,12] The reported risk of developing active TB in HIV-infected people is approximately 8% per year among TST-positive people.[13–16] Increasing TB cases among HIV-infected people also pose a threat to public health because TB can be spread to both HIV-infected and HIV-noninfected people in the community.

The clinical manifestations of TB in HIV-coinfected people are highly dependent on which infection (HIV or TB) occurs first and the degree of immunosuppression. In developing countries with a high prevalence of TB, many people become infected with *M. tuberculosis* during childhood and early adolescence. Most will not develop active TB after primary infection. People with latent TB infection who later become coinfected with HIV have a subsequent 5% to 8% annual risk of developing reactivation TB. The risk depends on the severity of HIV-related immunosuppression. TB developing early after HIV infection when CD4 counts are high presents predominantly as pulmonary disease with typical clinical and radiographic manifestations. With advanced HIV-related immunosuppression, the presentation becomes more atypical (lower lobe noncavitating infiltrates and intrathoracic adenopathy) with an increase in extrapulmonary disease.

People who are infected with HIV and who then later become infected with *M. tuberculosis* frequently develop rapidly progressive primary TB. Active sputum smear–positive TB developed within 4 months in 37% of HIV-infected people exposed to two TB patients in a group home for HIV-infected people in San Francisco.[17] In a nosocomial TB outbreak in Italy, 8 of 18 HIV-infected patients exposed to a single sputum smear–negative TB patient developed active TB, 7 within 60 days of diagnosis of the index case.[18] In areas with a high prevalence of TB, HIV-infected people successfully treated for TB also are at increased risk to develop recurrent TB due to reinfection. In a prospective study of South African mine workers, 62% of relapses in HIV-infected adults were due to reinfection compared to 6% in HIV-noninfected individuals.[19]

Despite good clinical and microbiologic responses to TB chemotherapy,[20–24] the development of active TB in HIV-infected people appears to be associated with shortened survival[24,25] due to enhanced cytokine expression and increased HIV replication.[26] TB is now the leading cause of death in HIV-infected people globally, especially in sub-Saharan Africa, where it has been found at postmortem examination in 40% to 54% of HIV-infected adults.[27,28] Globally, 13% of all deaths due to TB occur in HIV-infected people[5]; this proportion will likely continue to increase due to the increasing occurrence of HIV infection in populations already infected with *M. tuberculosis*.

Tuberculin Skin Test

Tuberculin skin testing is widely used in epidemiologic surveys to assess the prevalence and estimate the annual rate of TB infection and in clinical practice to assess whether a person has been infected with *M. tuberculosis*. Many commercial purified protein derivative (PPD) antigens are available and are standardized by comparison with an international standard PPD-S in human subjects. Five tuberculin units (equivalent to 0.0001 mg of the international standard) is the dose widely used for tuberculin skin testing. Skin testing should be performed by intradermal injection (Mantoux method) of 5 tuberculin units of antigen in 0.1 mL, usually into the skin of the volar surface of the forearm. Correctly placed injections produce an immediate raised wheal. The test should be read as the number of millimeters of palpable induration present after 48 to 72 hours.

The operating characteristics of the test are dependent on the population tested, the amount of nonspecific cross-reactions (generally small reactions) due to exposure and infection with environmental mycobacteria, and the cut point used. Most people with reactions greater than 10 mm are infected with *M. tuberculosis*. A cut point of 5 mm is recommended when testing HIV-infected people. The presence of a positive tuberculin test indicates only prior infection with *M. tuberculosis* and not active disease. In fact, up to one-fourth of newly diagnosed patients with active pulmonary TB have negative tuberculin reactions.

False-negative PPD tests can be caused by protein-calorie malnutrition, other diseases such as sarcoidosis and HIV infection, intercurrent viral infections, and immunosuppressive drugs such as corticosteroids. False-positive reactions are often due to cross-reactions with environmental mycobacteria. The size of a previously positive tuberculin reaction may wane over time. Repeated testing of such a patient may result in the perception of new TST conversion suggesting recent infection. Two-step tuberculin tests in which PPD testing is repeated on people with a negative initial PPD skin test 1 week later can be used to identify this booster phenomenon. If the second PPD test is reactive, the positive test should be ascribed to boosting rather than to recent infection.

It is not possible to definitively distinguish between positive PPD skin reactions due to *M. tuberculosis* infection and reactions due to previous bacille Calmette–Guérin (BCG) vaccination. Reactions due to BCG vaccination wane with time. The larger the reaction, the more likely it is due to *M. tuberculosis* infection. Routine BCG vaccination in infancy has little impact on the size of the TST reaction in adults; however, it may be a confounding factor in people revaccinated at school age or adolescence.[29]

Recent knowledge about the important role of T lymphocytes and interferon-γ (IFN-γ) in tuberculosis has led to the development of in vitro diagnostic assays to detect tuberculous infection. QuantiFERON-TB is a new test based on antigen-specific stimulation of IFN-γ release from mononuclear cells in a peripheral blood sample from a person being evaluated for latent TB infection.[30,31] Mycobacterial and control antigens are incubated with the blood sample overnight and the amount of IFN-γ in the supernatant is measured. The use of mycobacterial antigens including early secreted antigen-6 (ESAT-6) and culture filtrate protein-10 that are found in MTB, but not in BCG or most other nontuberculous mycobacteria, enhances the specificity of this new test. This assay offers the advantages that it can be done in a single visit, there is little interobserver variability, and there are no boosted responses.

DISEASE

Risk Factors for Progression from Infection to Active Tuberculosis

Most people infected by *M. tuberculosis* do not develop active TB. In such people, infection is typically marked only by the development of a positive PPD skin test. Five percent to 10% of HIV-noninfected people develop active TB during their lifetime.[11] The risk is greatest in the first 2 years following infection and then declines. The risk of developing TB is associated with more intense exposure and is higher for people infected through contact with an index sputum smear-positive TB case.[2] The age at the time of TB infection is also important. People who become infected in infancy, adolescence, or old age are more likely to develop active TB.

The risk of developing progressive primary or reactivation TB is increased in immunocompromised people; the degree of risk varies with the underlying disease-impairing host defenses. The risk of developing TB among HIV-infected people was 79-fold greater than in HIV-noninfected people in one study[13] and may be up to 170-fold higher in patients with acquired immunodeficiency syndrome (AIDS).[32] People with silicosis, end-stage renal disease, certain malignancies such as head and neck cancers and lymphomas, poorly controlled diabetes mellitus, chronic malnutrition, rapid weight loss, chronic treatment with corticosteroids and other immunosuppressive drugs, and those who smoke tobacco are also at increased risk of developing TB, although the relative risk is much less than that of HIV-infected people. The duration and dose of corticosteroid use associated with an increased risk of TB are unknown; however, treatment for less than 3 or 4 weeks with doses of 15 mg of prednisone or less daily probably causes little increased risk.

Primary Tuberculosis

TB infection is usually acquired by the inhalation of droplet nuclei containing viable tubercle bacilli that are phagocytosed by alveolar macrophages to establish a primary nidus of infection. In the nonimmune host, the bacilli multiply intracellularly, kill the cell, and then spread to the draining hilar lymph nodes or to the bloodstream via the thoracic duct. Most primary infections are asymptomatic, but some people develop fever, nonproductive cough, dyspnea, and, occasionally, erythema nodosum. Symptoms are more common in children than adults. Crepitations from alveolar consolidation and focal wheezes due to bronchial compression by enlarged intrathoracic lymph nodes may be present. Lesions demonstrable on chest film include small patchy alveolar infiltrates in the middle and lower lung fields, often with unilateral hilar adenopathy. Bronchial compression by enlarged nodes may produce upper or middle lobe collapse. Small transient pleural effusions occur in 10% of patients.

The vast majority of immunocompetent people develop an effective immune response against TB and contain their primary infection, leaving only small calcified parenchymal scars (Ghon complex), usually in the middle and lower lung fields. If the corresponding draining hilar lymph node is visible, the radiographic lesion is termed a Ranke complex (Fig. 36-1A). Small scars due to arrested lesions from seeding of tubercle bacilli to the apical regions of the lung at the time of primary infection are known as Simon's foci (Fig. 36-1B). In many people, however, residua of the primary focus are undetectable on subsequent chest x-ray films.

Following primary infection, immunocompetent people develop specific acquired resistance to reinfection. Although incompletely understood, the protective immune mechanisms appear to include T lymphocyte–dependent activation of macrophages to destroy tubercle bacilli. Specific acquired resistance is long-lasting, possibly due to repeated primary but clinically latent foci of infection. Conditions such as HIV infection associated with immunosuppression may lead to lowered resistance to exogenous reinfection.[19] Reinfection is most likely to contribute substantially to new cases of TB in areas of high prevalence and transmission.

Progressive Primary Tuberculosis

People who fail to develop specific acquired immune responses following primary TB infection may develop progressive primary TB. This form of disease is most common in young children, the immunocompromised, and the elderly. Miliary or meningeal disease may result after widespread hematogenous dissemination of tubercle bacilli. The clinical presentation is frequently cryptic with nonspecific symptoms such as malaise and fatigue or fever of unknown origin.[33] Progressive primary disease in young adults presents with fever, productive cough, night sweats, weight loss, and upper lobe cavitary lesions, which can be reliably distinguished from reactivation TB only when recent PPD skin test conversion has been documented.[34]

Reactivation (Postprimary Tuberculosis)

Although acquired immune responses are crucial to mycobacterial killing and the prevention of progressive pulmonary or disseminated disease after primary infection, they do not totally eradicate all viable tubercle bacilli. Low numbers of dormant, slowly metabolizing organisms persist in small,

pleural fluid cultures are significantly more likely to be positive in HIV-positive patients.[91] Inoculation of liquid as well as solid culture media enhances diagnosis.

In HIV-noninfected persons, tuberculous pleurisy is generally a self-limited condition with spontaneous resolution of the effusion even without specific anti-TB treatment. Unfortunately, 41% to 65% of these patients will later develop active TB, the majority within the first 3 years after the episode of pleurisy.[92,93] Tuberculous pleurisy responds extremely well to modern chemotherapy regimens. Isoniazid (INH) and rifampicin given daily for 9 months, or daily for 1 month followed by twice-weekly treatment for 5 or 8 months, cures more than 98% of patients.[94,95] Six-month short-course regimens including pyrazinamide are also highly effective. If the clinical suspicion for TB is high and pleural biopsy is unavailable or the biopsy histology and special stains are negative, another reasonable option is empirical treatment with specific anti-TB chemotherapy with repeat PPD skin testing and reevaluation in 4 to 6 weeks. Repeated thoracocenteses are unnecessary. Intrapleural corticosteroids are of little value. A tapering course of adjunctive oral corticosteroids (prednisolone, 0.75 mg/kg/day) given during the first 2 or 3 months of anti-TB treatment was shown in one placebo-controlled study to increase the rate of resolution of symptoms and pleural fluid resorption but did not alter the extent of residual pleural thickening.[96] Corticosteroids probably are of marginal benefit in patients with small effusions and mild symptoms.

Large necrotic tuberculous foci or cavities occasionally rupture into the pleural space to produce a true tuberculous empyema. The pleural fluid is thick and cloudy with a high density of bacilli. An etiologic diagnosis usually can be established quickly by simple microscopy and culture of the pleural fluid. Tuberculous empyemas are usually associated with far-advanced cavitary disease. Treatment is difficult, may need to be prolonged, and should be given in conjunction with a chest consultant.[97] Drainage or decortication is often required. Secondary complications include extension through the chest wall producing chest wall abscesses and draining fistulas.

Tuberculous Lymphadenitis

Lymphadenitis is the most common extrapulmonary manifestation of TB seen in developing countries. Although less frequent in developed nations, it is a significant problem in immigrants from high-prevalence countries in Asia and Africa. *Mycobacterium tuberculosis* is the most common cause of mycobacterial lymphadenitis worldwide. In developed nations with a low prevalence of TB, atypical mycobacteria, including *Mycobacterium avium–intracellulare* complex (MAC) and *Mycobacterium scrofulaceum*, are frequent isolates in pediatric cases.[98] Lymphadenitis may be a complication of primary infection, reactivation disease, or contiguous spread. It is more common in young children and women and may be more frequent among Asians and Pacific islanders.[99] Stigmas of active or remote pulmonary disease were present on chest radiographs in 39% of cases in one large series from Hong Kong.[100]

The cervical lymph nodes are most commonly involved; this form of disease is known as scrofula. The affected nodes characteristically are nontender and cause little pain. Tuberculous lymphadenitis is more likely to involve nodes in the supraclavicular and posterior fossae. Lymphadenitis due to atypical mycobacteria is more likely to be present with disease in the submandibular and high anterior cervical lymph node groups.[101] The nodes are firm on palpation initially but may become matted and fluctuant as they become necrotic. Draining sinuses form frequently. Systemic symptoms such as fever, weight loss, and failure to thrive are common. Definitive diagnosis requires recovery of the organism on smears and cultures of aspirated material, draining pus, or lymph node biopsy material. The diagnostic yields, from AFB smears and culture of lymph node biopsies, were 56% and 69%, respectively, in one large study from Finland.[102] In hospitals where cytopathology is available, fine- or wide-needle aspiration cytology with AFB and hematoxylin and eosin (H&E) staining and mycobacterial culture is another useful diagnostic option.[103,104] AFB or caseation was seen in 75% of simple lymph node aspirates done for suspected tuberculous lymphadenitis at a teaching hospital in Zambia; 85% of these patients were HIV seropositive.[104]

Six- to 12-month short-course chemotherapy regimens including isoniazid and rifampicin (plus pyrazinamide for the first 2 months) are the mainstays of therapy. New enlarged nodes may appear and previously swollen lymph nodes may persist or enlarge slightly during or after chemotherapy; this is not a sign of treatment failure and such patients may be carefully followed.[105]

Routine surgical excision or aspiration confers no benefit or disadvantage and should be avoided.[105] Surgical management (total excision of involved nodes) should be reserved for diagnostic biopsy when necessary and for complications such as persistent draining sinuses and compromise of vital contiguous structures.

Bone and Joint Tuberculosis

Skeletal TB affects mainly large weight-bearing joints (Table 36-1). Most cases involving synovial joints present with monarticular arthritis; however, spinal disease may occur at multiple levels. In cases of spondylitis, the most common sites are the lower thoracic and lumbar spine (48%–67% of cases).[106] Tuberculous osteomyelitis usually involves the metaphyseal regions of bones where the blood supply is greatest.

Most skeletal TB in infants and children is associated with progressive primary TB, whereas in older children and adults it usually results from reactivation of a previous hematogenously seeded focus[107] or by hematogenous seeding after breakdown of a long-latent focus in the kidney, lymph nodes, or other organs.[106] Spread from contiguous lymphatic structures (e.g., from the kidney or parietal pleura to para-aortic lymph nodes and then to the lumbar spine) may be important in the pathogenesis of some cases of tuberculous spondylitis.

***Table 36-1** Joints Involved with Skeletal Tuberculosis*

Affected Joint	Percentage of Cases
Spine	50
Hip	15
Knee	15
Wrist, ankle, others	20

TB affecting synovial joints produces a combination of arthritis and osteomyelitis. The main complaint is usually the insidious onset of pain and swelling in the affected joint. A history of trauma to the affected joint preceded the onset of tuberculous arthritis in one-fourth of patients in one study.[107]

In tuberculous spondylitis, the principal symptom is local or radicular pain (10%–30% of cases). Symptoms of spinal cord compression are more common with cervical spondylitis because the spinal canal is narrower at this level. Neurologic deficits tend to be symmetrical and slowly progressive over weeks to months, in contrast to the asymmetrical and rapidly evolving symptoms of neoplastic spinal cord compression. Spinal cord compression can occur due to extrinsic compression by caseous material, necrotic bone, vertebral subluxation, or direct tuberculous inflammation of the dura mater and meninges.[108] Lower extremity weakness, easy fatigability, loss of bowel and bladder control, and fever may occur.

Tuberculous spondylitis usually affects the vertebral body more than the posterior spinal elements (Fig. 36-4). Multiple vertebral levels may be involved. The initial site of disease is usually the subchondral region of the anterior portion of the vertebral body with preservation of the joint space. Proliferation of granulation tissue, pannus formation, and caseous necrosis then occur. Local disease may progress to involve the disk space and adjacent vertebrae. Collapse of the vertebral body may result in kyphosis or severe gibbus deformities. Necrotic debris tracks outward, limited by ligamentous and fascial planes. In the spine, the caseous material is limited anteriorly by the thick anterior spinous ligament and thus tends to bulge laterally, producing the typical fusiform appearance of the paraspinous (Pott's) abscess. Pus may dissect along other planes resulting in extrapleural, posterior cervical, retropharyngeal, and psoas abscesses.

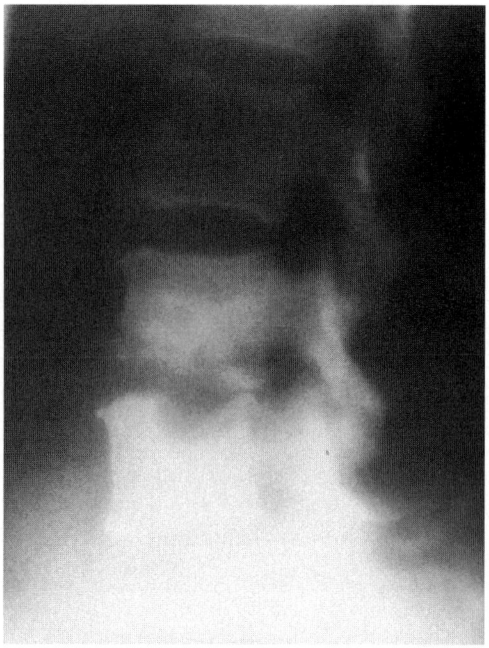

FIGURE 36-4 Tuberculous spondylitis. Lytic lesion involving the anterior and inferior aspect of the L3 vertebra and the posterior and superior aspects of the L4 vertebra with early sparing of the disk space.

Box 36-1 Radiographic Features of Tuberculous Spondylitis

- Multiple levels of involvement
- Narrowing and destruction of the intervertebral space
- Destruction of both adjacent vertebral bodies
- Collapse (anterior wedging) of the vertebral bodies
- Paraspinous "cold" abscess formation–fusiform mass
- Kyphosis/gibbus deformity

The differential diagnosis includes other infectious and neoplastic spondylitides. Radiographic findings may be helpful (Box 36-1) but are nonspecific. Sparing of the disk space and destruction of the vertebral pedicles suggest spinal metastatic disease rather than tuberculous spondylitis.

The absence of pulmonary disease does not exclude the diagnosis of osseous TB. Fifty percent of patients with skeletal TB had normal chest films in one large series.[109] Positive TSTs occur in 77% to 100%. In the absence of concomitant pulmonary disease to obtain clinical specimens for diagnosis, biopsy of the affected bone with culture and histologic examination are usually necessary for definitive diagnosis. Aspirate or biopsy material is positive for tuberculosis in 50% to 71% of cases.[109,110] In cases with joint involvement, simple aspiration with AFB smear and culture should be the initial diagnostic procedure. AFB smears and cultures of joint fluid are positive in 25% and 60% to 94% of cases, respectively.[107–111] Synovial biopsy has a higher yield and is valuable when simple aspiration is nondiagnostic and the diagnosis remains obscure.

Several well-done controlled clinical trials by the British Medical Research Council demonstrated that most patients do well with prolonged (12–24 months) chemotherapy with isoniazid- and rifampicin-containing regimens. Prolonged bed rest, plaster casts, and routine surgical debridement added little or no additional benefit.[112–115] Spinal surgery is not indicated for the majority of patients. Severe neurologic deficits at the time of presentation, severe spinal instability, deterioration in neurologic status, and failure of neurologic signs to improve after several months of chemotherapy are indications for surgical treatment. Progression of disease should be assessed on clinical and neurologic as well as radiographic grounds. Modern short-course regimens including isoniazid, rifampicin, ethambutol, and pyrazinamide may be utilized. The duration of treatment required is controversial and should be individualized based on the patient's response to therapy. Many authorities recommend at least 12 months of therapy.

Miliary Tuberculosis

The term *miliary tuberculosis* is used to describe disseminated TB resulting from hematogenous spread associated with characteristic lesions on chest radiography. Miliary lesions are diffuse 1- or 2-mm rounded opacities scattered throughout all lung fields and are named for their resemblance to millet seeds. Early lesions may be indistinct and easily missed (Fig. 36-5A). Advanced lesions may coalesce and appear as larger rounded lesions that occasionally cavitate (Fig. 36-5B). In developing countries with a high prevalence of TB, most

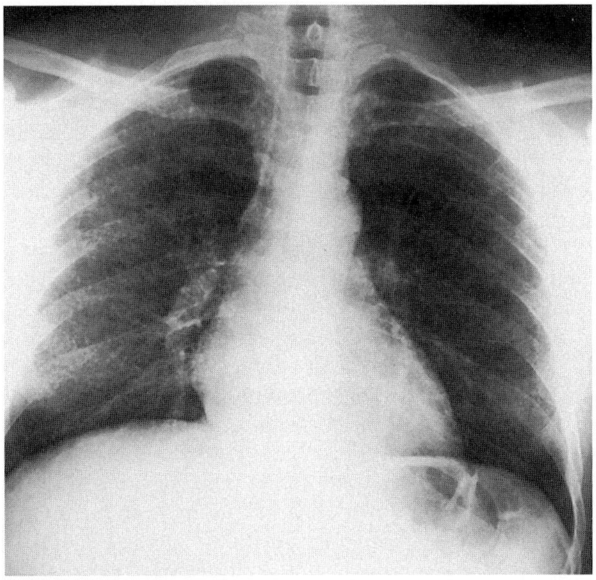

A

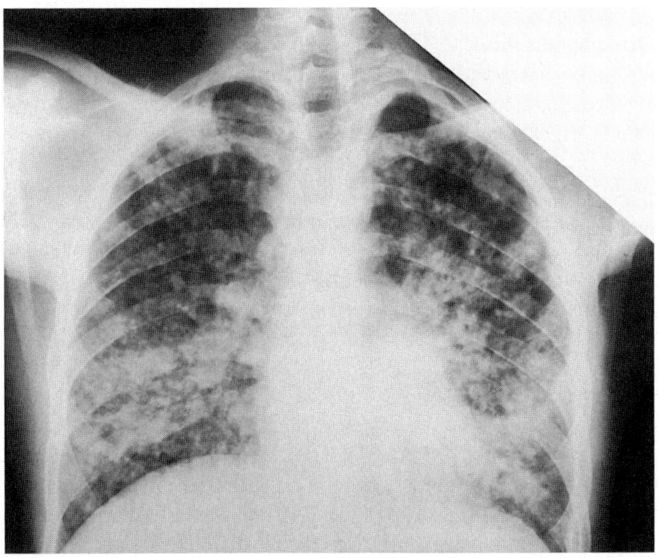

B

FIGURE 36-5 *A*, Early miliary tuberculosis. Diffuse 1- or 2-mm rounded opacities involve all lung fields. *B*, Coalescence of smaller lesions in advanced miliary disease.

cases occur following primary infection. In industrialized countries, the majority of cases arise from breakdown and hematogenous seeding from old latent foci in the lung or other organs. Pathologically, the pulmonary lesions consist of aggregates of macrophages and lymphocytes in granulomas with or without caseous necrosis. In severely immunocompromised patients, such as patients with advanced AIDS, little tissue inflammation may be present and many bacilli may be visible.

Systemic symptoms predominate in patients with miliary TB despite the numerous pulmonary lesions. The chest is generally clear to auscultation. A minority have lymphadenopathy or hepatosplenomegaly. Choroidal tubercles, which are raised white-yellow plaques visible in the choroid on fundoscopic examination, are pathognomonic but occur in fewer than 15% of cases. Fever, weight loss, and failure to thrive are frequent, and miliary TB may be a cause of fever of unknown origin in the elderly.[33] Hematologic abnormalities ranging from leukopenia to leukemoid reactions occur in 10% of cases.[116] Patients may present with headache, confusion, personality change, and focal neurologic deficits due to concomitant central nervous system (CNS) involvement with tuberculous meningitis.

The diagnosis of miliary TB is usually straightforward when typical radiographic lesions are present. The PPD skin test is positive in only 52% to 72% of cases.[117–120] Patients with neurologic symptoms and signs should undergo lumbar puncture and cerebrospinal fluid (CSF) examination. Hyponatremia may be a clue to the syndrome of inappropriate secretion of antidiuretic hormone due to CNS disease. The diagnostic yields of sputum AFB smears and culture, urine and gastric aspirate culture, and tissue biopsies in patients with miliary TB are listed in Table 36-2.

Routine mycobacterial cultures may take 3 or more weeks to become positive. In urgent situations, when available, fiberoptic bronchoscopy with transbronchial lung biopsy has a diagnostic yield of 75% to 100%.[118,124,125] When classic necrotizing granulomas are present, a presumptive diagnosis can be reached quickly. When sputum examination is unrevealing, other tissue sites may be biopsied. Bone marrow aspiration and biopsy with smear and culture should be strongly considered in patients with hematologic abnormalities. Liver and lymph node biopsies also have high diagnostic yields. Treatment with the standard short-course regimens described later is recommended for cases of miliary TB.

Table 36-2 Yield of Diagnostic Studies in Miliary Tuberculosis (Percentage with Positive Histology or Culture)

	Sputum						
Series	**AFB Smears**	**Culture**	**Gastric Aspirate Culture**	**Urine Culture**	**Bone Marrow Biopsy and Culture**	**Liver Biopsy**	**Lymph Node Biopsy**
Berger and Samortin[121]	—	50	—	—	80	100	100
Munt[119]	33	63	—	14	33	67	62
Gelb et al.[120]	—	55	—	23	100	82	60
Grieco and Chmel[122]	—	—	—	—	—	60	80
Bobrowitz[123]	18	66	—	—	—	—	—
Maartens et al.[118]	33	62	75	33	86	100	100
Kim et al.[124]	33	76	100	59	45	59	—

Tuberculous Meningitis

TB involves the CNS in three ways. Tuberculomas are parenchymal mass lesions that produce focal symptoms by acting as space-occupying lesions. Tuberculous spondylitis can result in spinal cord compression or radiculopathy. The most frequent form of CNS TB is tuberculous meningitis. Tuberculous meningitis is the most life-threatening form of extrapulmonary TB and was uniformly fatal before the advent of antituberculous chemotherapy. It is still a leading cause of death and chronic disability in infants and children with TB.[126]

Unlike areas of the developing world with a high prevalence of TB where the infant or child develops tuberculous meningitis in the setting of progressive primary infection or miliary disease, in more developed nations tuberculous meningitis is more frequently seen in adults and the elderly in association with reactivation TB. The HIV pandemic has also been associated with increased case rates of CNS TB. Tuberculous meningitis occurs five times more frequently in HIV-infected people than those who are HIV seronegative.[127] Five percent to 10% of HIV-infected patients with TB have CNS involvement, predominantly as meningitis.[21,127–129] Tuberculous meningitis resembles many other forms of chronic meningitis. It occurs without other evidence of extracranial TB in a significant minority of cases, further increasing difficulties in diagnosis.

Tuberculous meningitis usually results from the rupture of a subependymal tuberculous focus into the CSF provoking a brisk local inflammatory and immunologic response.[130,131] The severe inflammatory responses in the subarachnoid space cause most of the symptoms and ultimate morbidity of tuberculous meningitis. Pathologic lesions include (1) a thick gelatinous basilar exudate capable of entrapping cranial nerves and blood vessels and blocking normal CSF resorptive pathways; (2) a severe arteriolitis and perivasculitis with subsequent endarteritis and thrombosis of nutrient vessels to the brain parenchyma, resulting in ischemia and infarction; and (3) severe comorbidity due to debility and secondary infection.

Adults may develop tuberculous meningitis in the setting of progressive primary disease or miliary TB similar to children. However, they may also develop it due to late meningeal seeding and subependymal tubercle formation from bacilli spread systemically from the breakdown of small cryptic smoldering or previously dormant renal and osseous foci.[130] Most cases have other clinical or radiographic stigmas of TB in other extracranial sites, but a few have no other apparent evidence of TB outside of the CNS.

Common clinical manifestations at the time of presentation for medical attention include headache, fever, irritability, and, in children, episodes of protracted vomiting. Fever is present in 47% to 100% of cases,[132,133] and meningismus is present in 57% to 90% of cases[134,135]; decreased level of consciousness, papilledema, and cranial nerve palsies (most commonly of the sixth cranial nerve, followed by palsies of the third, fourth, and seventh cranial nerves) are seen less frequently. The clinical presentation of tuberculous meningitis is similar in HIV-positive and -negative people.[127,136]

In adults, the presentation of tuberculous meningitis is similar to many other forms of chronic meningitis, with fever, meningismus, headache, and an abnormal level of consciousness.[123] The combination of leptomeningeal signs, especially new or evolving cranial nerve palsies, a chest film picture consistent with TB, and a CSF profile of hypoglycorrhachia with lymphocytic pleocytosis should suggest the diagnosis.

The duration of symptoms prior to hospital admission varies from a few days to 6 months. Initial TSTs were positive in 31% to 61% of adult[137,138] and 50% to 96% of pediatric cases.[126,139] Sputum smears and cultures or gastric aspirate cultures were positive in 14% to 51% of cases.[134,140] The chest radiograph is helpful diagnostically: 44% to 88% of all adult and pediatric patients have radiographic abnormalities compatible with pulmonary TB.[135,141] Approximately 20% will have a miliary pattern. Bone marrow biopsy and liver biopsy are other good sites for diagnostic sampling in miliary disease. Computed tomography (CT) and nuclear magnetic resonance imaging of the head, where available, are useful in detecting concomitant tuberculomas and complications such as hydrocephalus. Hyponatremia is present in 37% to 73% of patients[142,143] due to the syndrome of inappropriate antidiuretic hormone secretion.[144] Due to the increased incidence of tuberculous meningitis in HIV-infected people, patients should be offered HIV testing.

The usual CSF findings consist of hypoglycorrhachia (CSF glucose <40 mg/dL) in 32% to 88% of patients,[142,145] elevated protein levels, and a lymphocytic pleocytosis with 100 to 500 cells per milliliter.[146] This pattern of abnormalities is generally the same across all age groups. The fluid is usually clear or ground glass in appearance. Markedly elevated protein levels (>500 mg/dL) and xanthochromic fluid may occasionally be seen in severe cases complicated by hydrocephalus with spinal subarachnoid block. An early predominance of polymorphonuclear leukocytes occurs in 6% to 45% of cases.[133,134]

The CSF glucose characteristically declines as the disease progresses. A rising CSF protein may signal the development of obstruction to CSF recirculation due to worsening basilar or spinal arachnoiditis. With appropriate treatment, the CSF findings normalize in the following order: glucose, CSF protein, and CSF cell counts.[140] CSF abnormalities may take up to 3 to 6 months to resolve completely.[147]

The yield from direct AFB smears of CSF ranges from 0% to 87%.[135,143] CSF mycobacterial cultures are positive in 40% to 83%.[135,148] Examination of fluid from the last tube collected at lumbar puncture, larger volumes of CSF (5–20 mL), or staining the clot (pellicle), if one forms, may increase the yield of direct AFB smears. Newer techniques, including measurement of CSF adenosine deaminase, antibodies against mycobacterial proteins, polymerase chain reaction (PCR) analysis, and assays to detect mycobacterial antigens, have been developed but have not entered widespread use due to limited sensitivity and specificity.[149–151]

A high level of clinical suspicion, however, is necessary to diagnose many cases of tuberculous meningitis. Only one-fourth to one-third of patients will have a history of exposure to a known case of TB, although such information should be sought. The chest x-ray, if consistent with TB, provides an important diagnostic clue. Acid-fast smears and cultures of secretions and tissues from other organs may provide important supportive evidence. Sputum examination should be performed in patients with pulmonary involvement. Cultures of gastric aspirates may be useful alternatives in children. The yields of sputum and gastric aspirate smears and cultures range from 14% to 51%.[134,140]

Lumbar puncture and examination of the CSF form the cornerstones of diagnosis in tuberculous meningitis. The differential diagnosis of subacute or chronic lymphocytic meningitis, with or without hypoglycorrhachia, is broad and includes fungal meningitis, "aseptic" viral meningitis, parasitic infestations of the CNS, acute syphilitic meningitis, brain abscesses, subdural hematomas, carcinomatous meningitis, and other rarer diseases.[152] The most important differential diagnostic concern in immunocompromised patients is cryptococcal meningitis. The immediate diagnostic value of the lumbar puncture lies in the rapid exclusion of bacterial meningitis and subarachnoid hemorrhage and the demonstration of cell counts and chemistries consistent with tuberculous meningitis. Multiple lumbar punctures (up to three to four taps of 10–20 mL of CSF) are indicated if the diagnosis remains in doubt as the yield from cultures and smears increases with serial taps[135] and the evolution of CSF chemistries and cell counts (development of lymphocytic pleocytosis and progressive fall in glucose) can be followed.

Most of the first-line anti-TB drugs achieve good levels in the CSF. In the presence of meningeal inflammation, isoniazid achieves levels in the CSF comparable to those in the blood.[153] Rifampicin levels are 20% to 50% of those in the peripheral blood.[154] Ethambutol, pyrazinamide, and ethionamide all penetrate into the CNS relatively well. The notable exceptions are the aminoglycosides that penetrate even inflamed meninges poorly.

Modern short-course chemotherapy regimens (described later) including isoniazid, rifampicin, pyrazinamide, and ethambutol achieve good cure rates.[155] Most authorities treat tuberculous meningitis for at least 1 year. Evidence suggests that the adjunctive administration of corticosteroids (given as prednisone 1 mg/kg/day up to a maximum of 60 mg/day or its equivalent for the first 4–6 weeks of treatment) is beneficial in cases of tuberculous meningitis with depressed levels of consciousness, hydrocephalus, stroke, and cranial nerve palsies or other focal neurologic abnormalities.[135,156–158] Corticosteroids may achieve these salutary effects by blunting severe local inflammation with vasculitis and entrapment of small cerebral blood vessels and cranial nerves. The corticosteroid dosage is tapered after 4 to 6 weeks depending on the clinical response of the patient. Antituberculous chemotherapy alone may be adequate in less severe cases.

Elevated intracranial pressure (ICP) and hydrocephalus are common in tuberculous meningitis, especially in children. Ventriculoatrial or -peritoneal shunting procedures may be required for neurologic deterioration despite appropriate antituberculous chemotherapy and ICP-reducing measures, progressively increasing ICP, and the presence of severe hydrocephalus on imaging studies. The overall prognosis is determined by the severity of neurologic involvement at the time of presentation and the duration of illness.[126,132,135,145,159,160] Comatose patients have the highest mortality and the greatest risk of permanent neurologic sequelae.

Renal and Genital Tuberculosis

Renal TB is typically a disease of young and middle-aged adults. Most cases of renal TB arise by secondary hematogenous spread of bacilli to the renal cortex from pulmonary lesions either at the time of initial TB infection or due to late breakdown of an old caseous focus. Because of the high renal blood flow, some renal seeding probably occurs in nearly all people at the time of primary infection. These small renal lesions become arrested after the development of effective cell-mediated immunity but may reactivate to produce disease years or decades later.

Renal TB is characterized by caseous lesions that may necrose and destroy functioning renal parenchyma. Lesions heal by scarring, contraction, and fibrosis. Ureteral fibrosis may lead to strictures or hydronephrosis and obstructive uropathy. Renal TB also may present as interstitial nephritis.

Any portion of the lower genitourinary tract can be involved secondarily by antegrade infection from the infected urine.[161] Bilateral disease is frequently present. Acute or chronic renal failure is an uncommon manifestation but can occur when there has been advanced destruction of both kidneys or bilateral ureteral obstruction. The most frequent presenting symptoms are dysuria (34%), hematuria (27%), and abdominal or flank pain (10%).[162] Fever, weight loss, and night sweats and other systemic symptoms are uncommon. Bladder involvement presents with dysuria, nocturia, or sterile cystitis. Renal TB may also be asymptomatic and discovered incidentally during the evaluation of an abnormal routine urinalysis showing sterile pyuria or microscopic hematuria.

The urinalysis was abnormal in 93% of patients in one large series, with hematuria occurring in 12% and hematuria and pyuria in 34%.[163] Urine AFB smears are positive in 50% to 70% of cases, and cultures for *M. tuberculosis* are positive in 25% to 95% of patients.[164] Nearly all patients have reactive PPD skin tests. Approximately three-fourths of patients with renal TB have abnormal chest films consistent with active or remote TB. Intravenous pyelography (IVP) is the standard mode of imaging and allows good visualization of the upper and lower genitourinary tract. The IVP is abnormal in more than 90% of patients, with classic findings suggestive of renal TB present in approximately one-half.[146] Characteristic abnormalities include cortical scarring, papillary necrosis, calcifications, caliceal dilation, and strictures of the collecting system. The ureters may be shortened and dilated ("pipe stem") or show single or multiple ("beaded") strictures. Strictures may develop while patients are on anti-TB treatment.

The mainstay of treatment of renal TB is short-course chemotherapy. Concomitant corticosteroid treatment has been advocated by some to prevent ureteral strictures but no controlled clinical trials have been performed. Surgical treatment was once widely used for extirpation of infected necrotic tissue but is now reserved for treatment of complications. Whenever possible, surgical treatment should be delayed to allow completion of 4 to 6 weeks of anti-TB chemotherapy before surgery. Partial or complete nephrectomy may be necessary to remove destroyed kidneys or treat cases of recurrent cystitis. Ureteral dilation and reconstructive procedures may be required to treat ureteral strictures.

The most common sites of involvement of the female genital tract are the fallopian tubes, endometrium, and ovaries.[165] TB of the female genital tract is usually due to hematogenous spread to the affected organs and differs from genitourinary TB in men in this respect. The urinary tract is often not affected. Women with genitourinary TB usually present with menorrhagia, pelvic pain, vaginal discharge, or infertility. The mean age at onset is in the fifth decade of life. Most patients are nulliparous. The general physical examination is often unremarkable. Female genitourinary tract TB can be diagnosed by endometrial biopsy, curettage, or culture of menstrual blood during the first 2 days of flow.

Nearly all males with genital TB present with a mass lesion (usually painless) in the epididymis, prostate, and, less frequently, the testis[166]; 90% have concomitant active renal TB. The diagnosis can be established by biopsy of the lesion.

Tuberculous Pericarditis

Tuberculous pericarditis arises most frequently by direct spread from involved mediastinal lymph nodes or adjacent pulmonary lesions and from hematogenous seeding. Pericardial effusion is the most common clinical manifestation. Pericardial effusions usually form slowly. In chronic cases, up to several liters of fluid can accumulate with massive pericardial enlargement. The fluid is initially thin and watery but becomes cloudy and more exudative with progressive disease. Healing by fibrosis can result in pericardial calcification and constrictive pericarditis, the most serious complication.

The onset is insidious in three-fourths of cases. Cough, chest pain, dyspnea, orthopnea, pedal edema, and night sweats are the most frequent symptoms. Fever is present in 73% to 97% of patients[167,168] and signs of pericardial disease with cardiomegaly, tachycardia, pulsus paradoxus, muffled heart sounds, hepatomegaly, jugular venous distention, ascites, and peripheral edema occur in 34% to 84% of cases.[167–169] Ten percent of 240 patients in one large series from South Africa presented with acute pericardial tamponade.[170] Concomitant pleural effusions are present in approximately one-half of patients.

The diagnosis may be difficult to confirm. Sputum samples can be examined when pulmonary lesions are present; however, these are absent in many cases. Pericardiocentesis usually reveals an exudative fluid. Direct AFB smears of pericardial fluid are rarely positive and the yield on culture is 50% to 59%.[168,170] Pericardial biopsy with histologic examination and culture of the affected tissue has a higher diagnostic yield of 70% to 83%.[168,170] In high TB prevalence areas, tuberculous pericarditis is usually the most common cause of pericardial disease in adults, and empirical anti-TB treatment may be considered. It is important to note that 5% to 17% of patients in large older case series had negative tuberculin reactions. Tuberculin anergy is even more frequent in immunosuppressed people such as AIDS patients with tuberculous pericarditis. Therefore, the absence of a positive tuberculin skin test does not exclude the diagnosis.

Treatment with standard short-course chemotherapy is effective in most cases. A minority of patients develops congestive heart failure and elevated venous pressure due to constrictive pericarditis; these patients may require pericardiectomy. Early surgical drainage does not alter late progression to constrictive pericarditis or mortality,[170] but does decrease the need for repeat pericardiocentesis and the need for later drainage procedures.[171] Pericardiectomy is indicated for life-threatening or recurrent tamponade or persistently elevated venous pressure.[171] Adjunctive corticosteroid treatment can reduce granulomatous inflammation and decrease later complications. In a placebo-controlled trial of prednisolone (60 mg three times a day for 1 month, 30 mg three times a day for 1 month, 15 mg three times a day for 2 weeks, and 5 mg/day for 1 week) added to short-course chemotherapy in patients with constrictive pericarditis, prednisolone therapy was associated with more rapid improvement in symptoms, decreased need for pericardiectomy, and decreased mortality.[171,172] Adjunctive corticosteroid therapy also has been shown to decrease mortality in HIV-infected people with tuberculous pericarditis.[173]

Abdominal Tuberculosis

Although rare in industrialized countries, abdominal involvement by TB is still a common cause of abdominal disease and ascites in developing nations. Gastrointestinal TB usually arises from swallowing infected sputum or drinking unpasteurized milk. *Mycobacterium bovis* may be the etiologic agent in cases acquired by the latter mechanism. *Mycobacterium tuberculosis* and atypical mycobacteria frequently involve the abdominal lymph nodes and viscera in patients with advanced AIDS.

TB can involve the gastrointestinal tract at all levels. Ulcerating masses can occur in esophagus and stomach and present with gastrointestinal bleeding or perforation. The terminal ileum, with its rich submucosal lymphoid tissue, is the area of the bowel most frequently involved by TB. Disease in the distal ileum may mimic Crohn's disease or patients may present with "tuberculous typhlitis" with fever, obstruction, gastrointestinal bleeding, or perforation and an acute abdomen.

Widespread disease with lymph node and serosal involvement presents as tuberculous peritonitis and ascites. Clinical manifestations are described in several excellent reviews.[174,175] Abdominal pain, swelling, weight loss, and anorexia are the most frequent presenting complaints. Sixty-two percent are febrile (often low-grade fever) and 80% have ascites on physical examination.[174] Most cases have an insidious onset, although ascites may accumulate rapidly and a few patients present with peritonitis and an acute abdomen. This indolent presentation must be distinguished from mesenteric spread of primary abdominal cancers with diffuse abdominal carcinomatosis. When symptoms are acute, the diagnosis of TB is often unsuspected and made at the time of laparotomy for suspected cholecystitis, appendicitis, or pelvic inflammatory disease. Findings on physical examination are nonspecific and the classic finding of a "doughy" abdomen with a palpable mass is infrequent. Pathologically, widespread mesenteric thickening, ascites, and tubercles studding the peritoneum, omentum, and other viscera are present.

The diagnosis is difficult in patients without findings of other pulmonary or extrapulmonary disease. PPD skin tests are often negative and do not exclude the diagnosis. The ascitic fluid is usually a clear, straw-colored exudate with a lymphocytic pleocytosis. The fluid may be transudative with little or no elevation of the total protein when TB peritonitis complicates preexisting cirrhosis. The bacillary burden in ascitic fluid is low and AFB smears are usually negative. Culture of small volumes of ascitic fluid has a diagnostic yield of only 40% to 50%[175,176] but increased to 85% when 1 L of fluid was examined.[177] Plain films of the abdomen may show signs of ascites, dilated loops of small bowel, or calcifications. A chest x-ray should always be obtained to search for concomitant pulmonary TB or pleural effusion, which was present in 58% of patients in one large study.[174] Barium studies may show areas of bowel narrowing. Ultrasonography and CT scanning of the abdomen, when available, are useful in demonstrating the presence of ascites and lymphadenopathy and involvement of other viscera. Biopsy is often necessary to confirm the diagnosis. Blind needle biopsy of the peritoneum has a diagnostic yield of 64% but carries the potential risk of bowel injury and hemorrhage. Open laparotomy avoids these risks, is well tolerated, and is nearly 100% diagnostic. When available, directed laparoscopic biopsy is the diagnostic test of choice. It is safe and allows biopsies to be taken from directly visualized lesions with a diagnostic yield of 84% to 100%.[177,178] Short-course anti-TB chemotherapy regimens are highly effective for the treatment of abdominal TB.

Other Rare Forms of Tuberculosis

Direct inoculation of the tubercle bacillus into the skin following trauma can produce chancre-like lesions (firm, ulcerating, nontender nodules) in people without prior TB infection or large warty lesions in sensitized people usually involving the hands in adults or the feet in children.[179,180] Lupus vulgaris is another form of cutaneous TB believed to arise by seeding of the skin from another endogenous tuberculous focus. The lesions most commonly involve the neck and face and begin as reddish-brown papules. Large plaques with peripheral "apple jelly" nodules may develop as the lesions grow. The lesions are not painful. The diagnosis is made by biopsy with special stains and mycobacterial culture. High clinical suspicion is essential because tuberculin skin tests are negative in many of these patients and more than half of patients do not have other evidence of active TB.[181]

Ocular forms of TB include ulcerative or nodular conjunctivitis, scleritis, uveitis, and choroidal tubercles. Phlyctenular keratoconjunctivitis, characterized by elevated pink or white nodules at the limbus, is a particular form of conjunctivitis in children that is believed to be a hypersensitivity reaction to mycobacterial proteins and is rarely associated with active TB. Choroidal tubercles are small, round, white or gray lesions in the choroid of the posterior eye pathognomonic of miliary TB.

TB can also involve the larynx, paranasal sinuses, salivary glands, and oral cavity. Laryngeal disease is most frequently, but not always, seen in conjunction with extensive pulmonary TB. Sinus lesions appear as masses or ulcers. The middle ear may be infected by direct spread of bacilli via the eustachian tube or hematogenously. Painless chronic drainage from otitis media is highly suspicious of TB.

Globally, TB is the leading cause of primary adrenal insufficiency. Adrenal gland involvement was present in more than 50% of patients with disseminated TB.[182] Chronic and, rarely, acute adrenal insufficiency may be the presenting signs of tuberculosis.

PATHOGENESIS AND IMMUNITY

The interaction between *M. tuberculosis* and the host is influenced by the genetics of both. It is assumed that certain humans express enhanced levels of innate resistance, although the immunogenetic basis for this is not understood. Strains of *M. tuberculosis* also differ in their virulence and their induction of host cytokines that may modify the granulomatous tissue reaction as well as the TST. After inhalation, droplet nuclei containing small numbers of viable tubercle bacilli are deposited in the terminal airspaces. The initial site of exposure/infection is most often in the lower or middle lobes due to the higher ventilation of these lung regions. The potential interaction of ingested bacilli with antibody is an important area of current investigation. In the lung, tubercle bacilli are phagocytosed by alveolar macrophages and dendritic cells. Tubercle bacilli have the capacity to invade alveolar type 2 epithelial cells as well. The initial interactions also involve Toll-like receptors (TLRs) on the phagocyte surface that are ligated by the lipoglycan lipoarabinomannan. Phagocytosis, invasion, and ligation of TLRs result in the production of chemokines that attract blood monocytes and lymphocytes to form an inflammatory focus.

More than half of intensely exposed household contacts fail to manifest *M. tuberculosis* infection presumably due to innate resistance. Bronchoalveolar lavage cells from exposed household contacts demonstrate an increased frequency of *M. tuberculosis*–reactive IFN-γ-producing cells that may contribute to local protection. The innate local host defenses that prevent establishment of infection manifest by tuberculin skin test conversion in exposed people are not understood. The current understanding of events associated with the establishment of a latent focus of infection is as follows: In the immunologically naive host lacking sufficient innate resistance, the bacilli have the capacity to multiply intracellularly, ultimately leading to necrotic cell death with release of more bacilli into the alveolar space. T cells drawn to the inflammatory focus do not have immunologic memory. Nonetheless, certain T cell populations (e.g., γδ T cells and natural killer cells) may activate alveolar macrophage and monocyte killing of the bacteria to provide some local control of the infection. Bacilli released by lysed cells spread from the alveolar spaces to the regional lymph nodes, however, and then hematogenously throughout the body.

Subsequent events are determined by the development of specific acquired resistance. In the absence of a competent immune response, tissue inflammation and damage are minimal. The clinical presentation is atypical with predominance of lower lobe disease, noncavitary opacities, and extrapulmonary manifestations. Immunodeficient hosts, infants, and children may develop miliary disease and TB meningitis.

However, more than 95% of infected humans control the infection and have no clinical symptoms. In them, the initial interactions between the bacillus and host cells lead to induction of specific acquired immunity against *M. tuberculosis*. This immunity controls the primary infection and maintains foci of persistent organisms as clinically latent. Macrophages infected with tubercle bacilli and dendritic cells present mycobacterial antigens to T cells with appropriate antigen-specific receptors triggering expansion of memory immune cells. After initial infection with *M. tuberculosis*, alveolar macrophages release multiple cytokines, including IL-1, IL-6, IL-12, TNF-α, and granulocyte macrophage-colony stimulating factor (GM-CSF), as well as the chemokines IL-8 and RANTES (*r*egulated upon *a*ctivation, *n*ormal *T* cell *e*xpressed and *s*ecreted), which facilitate recruitment of lymphocytes and monocytes into the lung.[183,184] Pulmonary macrophages also release the deactivating factors IL-10 and transforming growth factor-β (TGF-β). The balance of cytokines and receptors expressed by antigen presenting cells determines whether T cell differentiation occurs along the Th1 pathway generally associated with protective immunity or the Th2 pathway in which antibody formation dominates. This nomenclature derives from murine systems, in which CD4 cells comprise two functionally distinct populations that differ in requirements for costimulatory factors and antigen presenting cells. Th1 cells produce IFN-γ and IL-2, enhance macrophage microbicidal activity, and augment DTH. Th2 cells produce predominantly deactivating cytokines, including IL-4, IL-5, IL-6, and IL-10, and favor B cell growth and antibody production. Th1 and Th2 lymphocyte populations have important cross-regulatory functions. For example, IFN-γ produced by Th1 cells inhibits proliferation of Th2 cells, whereas IL-10 and IL-4 inhibit Th1 cell function.[185] Humans show similar patterns of cytokine production.

CD4 T lymphocytes play an important role in immune defenses against TB. Depletion of CD4 cells in mice results in uncontrolled BCG infection,[186] whereas adoptive transfer of CD4 cells from sensitized animals confers protection against TB.[187] The risk of developing pulmonary TB and severe forms of extrapulmonary disease correlates with declining CD4 lymphocyte counts in HIV-infected people.[188,189] The tremendously increased risk of reactivation of a clinically latent TB infection in HIV-infected people redefines the concept of latency. Clearly, active immune surveillance involving CD4 lymphocytes is essential for controlling bacterial replication at these sites. In addition to CD4 cells, CD8 cells contribute to protective immunity.[190,191] The role of γδ T cells, $CD4^-CD8^-$, and natural killer cells to acquired immunity is unclear. Evidence has emerged supporting a role for antibody in protection, requiring a rethinking of basic concepts of immunity and pathogenesis.[192,193]

As noted previously, *M. tuberculosis* antigen-specific T cells (CD4 and CD8) produce critical macrophage-activating factors, including GM-CSF and IFN-γ. Activated macrophages are capable of intracellular killing of mycobacteria and forming granulomas, further limiting dissemination of the organism. A second function of specific T cells is to serve as cytotoxic effector cells to lyse macrophages that are overladen with bacilli. The organisms thus released are killed either directly or after ingestion by newly recruited activated macrophages. The cytokine TNF-α is produced by cells that are infected with *M. tuberculosis* or exposed to mycobacterial antigens and has diverse roles in TB. It is critical to the formation of granulomas but also contributes to morbidity as a cause of fever, wasting, and hypotension. The development of effective specific acquired immunity responses occurs concomitantly with the development of specific DTH responses demonstrated by a reactive tuberculin skin test, which can usually be detected 4 to 6 weeks after initial TB infection.

In people who develop protective immune responses, the initial focus of infection usually heals by fibrosis or after undergoing caseation and calcification. Regional lymph nodes also heal over several months. Small numbers of viable tubercle bacilli may survive in these foci for decades in a dormant state. Breakdown of these foci in the setting of waning immunity due to aging, immunosuppressive medications, HIV infection, or other medical illnesses as discussed previously can result in reactivation of the previously well-contained infection, leading to clinically apparent disease.

Protective immune responses against TB developed after primary infection usually protect against subsequent exogenous reinfection with other strains of *M. tuberculosis*. Studies using restriction fragment length polymorphism DNA fingerprinting, however, indicate that recent infection and exogenous reinfection and progressive TB disease may contribute substantially to TB morbidity in densely crowded slums in high-burden countries[194] and in immunocompromised groups such as alcoholics residing in public shelters[195] and HIV-infected patients in large urban areas.[196,197] Reinfection TB has also been documented to occur in HIV-infected people in Africa[19] and may be most important in crowded urban areas of developing countries and in closed environments, principally mines, where high rates of TB disease and transmission occur.

During the period of clinical latency, effective host defenses against the development of active TB are characterized by strong Th1-like patterns presumably reprimed at local sites of bacterial replication. IL-12 appears to be the critical cytokine in the development of protective immunity and IFN-γ in its expression. Genetic defects in the expression of these cytokines or their receptors lead to predisposition to disseminated mycobacterial infections.

When the immune host is exposed to mycobacterial antigens as occurs in postprimary and reactivation TB, a brisk in situ DTH response occurs and may contribute to tissue damage. This is the case in pleural TB and TB peritonitis, pericarditis, and meningitis. When the balance between mycobacterial replication and host immunity shifts, usually because of immunosuppression, reactivation TB ensues. At the pulmonary focus there is a vigorous inflammatory response with unregulated expression of cytokines. The immune response no longer controls bacterial replication, contributing instead to tissue damage. The sputum contains high levels of IFN-γ, TNF-α, and other cytokines.[198] Patients with progressive TB show a Th2 pattern with depression of DTH, in vitro blastogenesis, and production of IL-2 and IFN-γ. Their circulating T cells express IL-4, and serum immunoglobulin G levels to *M. tuberculosis* proteins are increased. The inflammatory response leads to programmed cell death or apoptosis and development of cavities. Systemically, there is overproduction of the immunosuppressive cytokines TGF-β and IL-10, which depress IFN-γ expression.[199] As patients are treated, the suppression by these cytokines diminishes, unmasking a protracted primary defect in T cell function. This acquired immunosuppression may be a factor in bacterial persistence and the requirement for lengthy courses of chemotherapy as well as the increased risk of reinfection seen in treated TB patients.

With the sequencing of the genome of *M. tuberculosis* it is possible to explore the role of differences in virulence of the organism in pathogenesis. For example, certain strains, such as CDC1551, appear to induce more cytokine production, larger granulomas, and more DTH.[200] The relative role of host and bacterial genetics as opposed to acquired comorbidities in influencing the progression of infection and disease is an area of active research.

Drug Resistance

Soon after the introduction of streptomycin for the treatment of TB, treatment failures due to drug resistance were noted when patients were treated with single agents. Drug resistance develops from random chromosomal mutations, which occur spontaneously at low rates in wild-type strains of *M. tuberculosis*. The rate of natural resistance varies for specific agents: 1 in 0.5×10^4 bacilli for ethambutol, 1 in 3.5×10^6 for isoniazid, 1 in 3.8×10^6 for streptomycin, and 1 in 3.1×10^8

for rifampicin. Combination chemotherapy was introduced in the 1950s to overcome acquired drug resistance by ensuring that sufficient numbers of drugs were given such that all organisms present in a patient were susceptible to one or more of the drugs used. Solid caseous foci contain approximately 10^2 to 10^4, whereas cavitary lesions contain approximately 10^7 to 10^9 bacilli.[201] The probability of a single tubercle bacillus being resistant to more than one drug is the product of the probabilities of resistance to each drug. A cavitary lesion before treatment may already contain 10 to 1000 organisms resistant to a single drug, but it is unlikely that such a lesion contains bacilli resistant to two or more drugs; for example, 1 in $10^6 \times 1$ in 10^6 = only 1 in 10^{12} bacilli would be expected to be resistant to both drugs.

Monotherapy, inappropriate treatment regimens, or the addition of a single drug to the regimen of patients failing treatment select for the outgrowth (clinical resistance) of populations of mutant resistant organisms and the development of multiple drug-resistant TB. The presence of multiple drug resistance limits options for successful treatment and cure of the patient and may lead to the spread of drug-resistant TB to others in the community.

The term *primary drug resistance* refers to the presence of resistance to one or more antituberculous medications in a patient who has never been treated for TB. Primary drug resistance rates are a reflection of natural drug resistance and the successful application of TB treatment by the TB control program in the community. *Acquired drug resistance* refers to drug resistance in patients with a prior history of TB treatment. Acquired drug resistance is often due to poor compliance, poor absorption or bioavailability of drugs, and the addition of single agents to the regimens of patients who are already failing treatment (Box 36-2). Poorly organized TB treatment programs can lead to the rapid development of drug resistance in both developing and industrialized countries.

The term *multidrug resistant* (MDR) TB refers to *M. tuberculosis* isolates resistant to at least isoniazid and rifampicin. The development of rifampicin resistance is a crucial event because overall success rates with four-drug short-course initial and retreatment regimens in patients with isoniazid or streptomycin resistance are only slightly less than those with fully drug-susceptible organisms,[202] whereas treatment outcomes in the presence of both isoniazid and rifampicin resistance are poor. Multiple drug resistance necessitates the use of more toxic, more expensive, and less effective second- and third-line agents for TB treatment. Many developing countries cannot afford these second- and third-line agents.

Box 36-2 Factors Associated with Acquired Drug Resistance

- Incomplete or intermittent therapy
- Physician error
- Inadequate initial treatment regimen
- Patient noncompliance
- Inappropriate isoniazid preventive therapy (failure to exclude active tuberculosis)

Rates of drug resistance vary widely nationally and regionally and reflect differing methods used in drug-resistance surveys. During the past decade, WHO and the International Union Against Tuberculosis have conducted surveys of resistance rates against first-line anti-TB drugs from 58 countries or regions.[203] Areas of high single and multiple drug resistance have been reported from both industrialized and developing countries. For newly diagnosed patients the median prevalence of resistance to at least one first-line drug in the most recent WHO/International Union Against Tuberculosis and Lung Disease (IUATLD) survey was 11% and ranged from 2% in Uruguay to 37% in Estonia.[203] The median prevalence of MDR TB was 1.0% in new TB cases, with the highest rates of up to 14% in areas of China and the former Soviet Union. The prevalence of drug-resistant and MDR TB is higher in previously treated individuals.[204] Taking a careful history regarding prior TB treatment and exposure to individuals with known drug-resistant TB is the most important way to identify patients at risk for having drug-resistant TB.

DIAGNOSIS

Routine methods for the diagnosis of TB are based on demonstration of the organism on smears and cultures obtained from infected secretions or tissues from affected organs. Newer methods involve the detection of specific *M. tuberculosis* antigens or antibodies to mycobacterial proteins and the identification of specific *M. tuberculosis* DNA in clinical specimens.

Standard procedures begin with microscopic examination of smears made from potentially infected secretions and tissues and culture of these materials on a variety of media. Hot and cold carbol fuchsin (Ziehl–Neelsen and Kinyoun) methods are the most widely used. The number of bacilli that must be present in a sample for a positive AFB smear has been estimated to be 10^3 to 10^4/mL,[3,205] but good laboratories with experienced microscopists who spend adequate time examining slides likely have a lower threshold for detection. The use of fluorochrome stains such as auramine–rhodamine allows more rapid screening of sputum smears with a sensitivity comparable to those of the Ziehl–Neelsen or Kinyoun methods. The rate of sputum smear positivity is dependent on the bacillary load, which is in turn dependent on the extent of disease and the presence of cavitary lesions. Pretreatment smears are negative in 22% to 61% of new pulmonary TB cases and are more common in patients with minimal and noncavitary disease.[206–209]

Clinical specimens can be cultured on a variety of media. The most popular are opaque egg-based Löwenstein–Jensen and clear oleic acid–albumin agar-based Middlebrook media. Löwenstein–Jensen medium is inexpensive but small early colonies can be detected earlier on transparent agar-based media. Cultures should be examined weekly until positive or for 8 weeks. Organisms from positive cultures are then speciated using morphologic and biochemical techniques to identify them as *M. tuberculosis* or atypical mycobacteria. Using conventional egg- or agar-based media, 4 to 8 weeks are required for cultures to become positive, especially for paucibacillary and smear-negative samples. The long culture period is due to the long dividing times of mycobacteria (12–18 hours), which means that 3 or more weeks are required for growth from a single cell to a visible colony on solid media. Drug susceptibility testing by conventional techniques requires an additional 2 to 4 weeks.

Sputum specimens can be collected at the time of examination, in the early morning, and as overnight pooled collections. Early morning specimens are preferred because these sample the tracheobronchial secretions that have collected in the airways overnight and have a higher yield and a lower contamination rate. Multiple specimens should be examined. The diagnostic yield increases with up to five specimens but most of the enhanced yield is achieved with the first three samples.[210] Sputum can also be induced by the inhalation of normal or hypertonic (3%) saline aerosols in adults unable to spontaneously produce sputum. The resulting secretions are thinner than spontaneously expectorated sputum and the laboratory must be made aware that the sample is an induced specimen to prevent it from being discarded as unsatisfactory. In children and young adults unable to produce sputum, gastric aspiration can be performed, preferably in the early morning before the patient rises, to sample respiratory secretions that have been swallowed and pooled in the stomach. Mycobacteria die quickly in acidic stomach contents, and gastric aspirates should be processed promptly or neutralized with buffer. The sensitivity of AFB smears of gastric aspirates is only 23% to 30%; however, positive smears are highly reliable for the diagnosis of TB.[211,212]

Where available, bronchoscopy is useful for diagnosis in cases in which sputum specimens are repeatedly negative and other samples are unavailable and an empirical trial of treatment is inadvisable. Samples can be obtained by washing, brushing, bronchoalveolar lavage, and transbronchial lung biopsy. Specimens obtained at bronchoscopy are rarely the only positive specimens in patients with TB when final culture results are available.[213–215] The principal value of bronchoscopy, therefore, is in allowing the diagnosis to be established quickly in seriously ill or immunocompromised patients (including patients with AIDS) by demonstrating necrotizing granulomas or AFB in histologic sections of tissue.[118,214–216] Transbronchial biopsy with the fiberoptic bronchoscope may be particularly valuable for the rapid evaluation of suspected cases of miliary disease.[118,125,217]

Newer methods have been developed to shorten the time needed to diagnose TB and perform drug susceptibility testing.[218,219] Systems based on automated or semiautomated detection of growth in enriched liquid media can detect growth more rapidly than detection of visible colonies on solid media. Radiometric culture methods such as the BACTEC 460 system rely on the detection of radioactive ^{14}C released from a labeled palmitic acid substrate in liquid media by metabolically active mycobacteria and significantly shorten the time until detection of a positive culture. Nonradiometric systems such as the mycobacterial growth indicator tube based on oxygen quenching in the presence of replicating mycobacteria are also entering clinical use. Using appropriate decontamination methods and culture media, it is possible to directly inoculate susceptibility testing media from clinical specimens, eliminating the lengthy primary culture step.

Traditional systems for speciating mycobacteria have relied on biochemical parameters, colonial morphology and rate of growth, and gas or liquid chromatography. Rapid methods using DNA probes have been developed that bind specifically to mycobacterial RNA from a single species; binding is detected photometrically. Probes are commercially available for *M. tuberculosis* complex (includes *M. tuberculosis* and *M. bovis*), *M. avium* complex, *M. avium*, *M. intracellulare*, *M. kansasii*, and *M. gordonae*. These tests require only a few hours to perform.

Ideal diagnostic techniques would allow direct detection of mycobacteria in clinical specimens. The numbers of bacilli in most clinical specimens are small, necessitating the use of concentration methods, very sensitive assays, or procedures that amplify mycobacterial components to detectable levels. Several nucleic acid amplification assays have been developed for mycobacterial diagnosis based on PCR, strand displacement or transcription-mediated amplification, reporter phage, and ligase chain reaction methods. In general, these tests have performed well on smear-positive respiratory specimens (sensitivity, 82%–100%; specificity, 93%–100%) but less so on smear-negative specimens (sensitivity, 51%–88%; specificity, 97%–100%).[218] Molecular amplification tests are expensive and require significant infrastructure and staff training for reliable performance.

Conventional drug susceptibility testing against first-line anti-TB drugs can be performed using the critical concentration or indirect proportion methods on solid media but requires 2 or 3 weeks to perform after a positive culture is obtained.[220,221] The time to obtain results is reduced using enriched liquid culture systems such as the BACTEC 460 system. Resistance to rifampicin is due in the great majority of cases to mutations in a short sequence of the *rpo b* gene of the bacterial RNA polymerase, and rapid PCR-based methods have been developed to assess whether resistance to rifampicin is present. Resistance to other drugs is due to a variety of mechanisms and mutations, and rapid genotypic testing for resistance is not currently feasible. Rapid phenotypic tests for resistance using luciferase reporter phage[222,223] and amplified bacteriophage techniques[224] are also in late development or commercially available. Because they are simpler and use existing laboratory equipment and skills, they may be more affordable and widely applicable.

TREATMENT

Modern TB treatment is based on the use of potent short-course, multiple-drug regimens that sterilize the sputum rapidly. TB treatment is divided into two phases—the initial intensive phase lasting 1 or 2 months that kills the rapidly dividing, rapidly metabolizing organisms, followed by a 4- to 6-month continuation phase that kills the remaining slowly metabolizing organisms.

The most useful first-line drugs for TB treatment include isoniazid, rifampicin, ethambutol, pyrazinamide, and streptomycin. Adult and pediatric dosages are summarized in Table 36-3. Combination therapy with these agents forms the foundation of current TB chemotherapy.

First-Line Drugs

Streptomycin

Streptomycin was introduced for the treatment of tuberculosis in 1948 soon after its discovery. It must be given parenterally and penetrates most body spaces and tissues, including inflamed meninges. The initial use of streptomycin

*Table 36-3 Dosages of First-Line Antituberculosis Drugs Used in Adults and Children**

Drug	Daily Dose	Twice Weekly Dose	Thrice Weekly Dose
Isoniazid	5 mg/kg PO (10–15 mg/kg in children); maximum 300 mg/day	15 mg/kg PO (20–30 mg/kg in children); maximum 900 mg/dose	15 mg/kg PO (20–30 mg/kg in children); maximum 900 mg/dose
Rifampicin	10 mg/kg PO (10–20 mg/kg in children); maximum 600 mg/day	10 mg/kg PO (10–20 mg/kg in children); maximum 600 mg/day	10 mg/kg PO (10–20 mg/kg in children); maximum 600 mg/day
Pyrazinamide	Weight 40–55 kg = 1000 mg; 56–75 kg = 1500 mg; above 76 kg = 2000 mg PO (15–30 mg/kg in children); maximum 2 g/day	Weight 40–55 kg = 2000 mg; 56–75 kg = 3000 mg; above 76 kg = 4000 mg PO (50–70 mg/kg in children); maximum 4 g/dose	Weight 40–55 kg = 1500 mg; 56–75 kg = 2500 mg; above 76 kg = 3000 mg PO (50–70 mg/kg in children); maximum 3 g/dose
Ethambutol†	Weight 40–55 kg = 800 mg; 56–75 kg = 1200 mg; above 76 kg = 1600 mg PO (15–25 mg/kg in children);	Weight 40–55 kg = 2000 mg; 56–75 kg = 2800 mg; above 76 kg = 4000 mg PO (50 mg/kg in children);	Weight 40–55 kg = 1200 mg; 56–75 kg = 2000 mg; above 76 kg = 2400 mg PO (25–30 mg/kg in children)
Streptomycin	15 mg/kg IM (20–40 mg/kg in children); maximum 1 g/day	25–30 mg/kg IM (adults and children); maximum 1.5 g/dose	25–30 mg/kg IM (adults and children); maximum 1.5 g/dose

IM, intramuscularly; PO, orally.
*Children younger than 12 years old.
†Ethambutol is not recommended for treatment in children younger than 12 years old who cannot be reliably monitored for ophthalmologic toxicity but should be considered in cases of drug-resistant tuberculosis.

monotherapy for cavitary TB in the 1940s was quickly followed by the observation that following initial remarkable improvement, after 3 months of treatment up to 80% of patients treated with streptomycin had streptomycin-resistant bacilli.[225] When combined in various regimens with subsequent agents, such as isoniazid, para-aminosalicylic acid, and ethambutol, streptomycin proved highly useful in TB treatment. Streptomycin is a first-line bactericidal agent with a minimum inhibitory concentration (MIC) against *M. tuberculosis* of 8 μg/mL. Streptomycin is usually given by intramuscular (IM) injection at a dose of 15 mg/kg/day (up to 1 g/day) for the first 1 or 2 months of treatment. The drug is renally excreted and the dose should be decreased in patients with underlying renal insufficiency. Major side effects include ototoxicity (vestibular more than hearing loss) and nephrotoxicity and are related to the cumulative dose.

Isoniazid

Isoniazid (isonicotinic acid hydrazide) was introduced for the treatment of tuberculosis in 1952. Isoniazid is a mycobactericidal drug with an MIC against *M. tuberculosis* of 0.05 to 0.2 μg/mL. It is well absorbed when administered orally (PO) with good tissue and CNS penetration. It can also be administered parenterally by IM injection. Usual doses are 5 mg/kg/day up to 300 mg/day in adults. Higher doses can be given when intermittent dosing is used (twice- or three-times-weekly administration); however, these should not exceed 900 mg/dose because of the increased risk of neurotoxicity, specifically seizures.

The frequency of adverse reactions to isoniazid in HIV-noninfected patients is approximately 5%.[226] The most common adverse reactions are rash, fever, peripheral neuropathy, and jaundice. Rarer adverse events include neutropenia, thrombocytopenia, seizures, encephalopathy, antinuclear antibody–positive small-vessel vasculitis, dyspepsia, red blood cell aplasia, optic neuritis, methemoglobinemia, urinary retention, and pellagra. Severe and rarely fatal hepatitis may occur during isoniazid preventive therapy. Elevations of serum aminotransferases occur in 10% to 20% of all subjects receiving isoniazid preventive therapy.[227] These increases, developing during the initial weeks of therapy, are generally asymptomatic and frequently resolve despite continuation of the drug. People who consume ethanol (especially on a daily basis), those with preexisting liver disease, and pregnant and postpartum black and Hispanic women are at increased risk of hepatotoxicity.[228,229] Hepatotoxicity is usually reversible if the medication is stopped when initial symptoms of hepatotoxicity, including nausea, anorexia, malaise, and dull upper abdominal discomfort, occur. Health care workers and patients need to be aware of these symptoms and the importance of stopping INH treatment and seeking medical attention if they occur.

Isoniazid therapy is also associated with the development of a dose-dependent peripheral sensorimotor neuropathy via interactions with pyridoxine and pyridoxal-5-phosphate metabolism. Peripheral neuropathy develops in only 1% to 2% of well-nourished patients receiving 3 to 5 mg/kg/day of isoniazid, but it is also more frequent in malnourished people, pregnant women, and patients with diabetes mellitus, chronic renal failure, and alcoholism. Isoniazid peripheral neuropathy can be prevented or reversed in nearly all cases by supplemental oral pyridoxine 25 to 50 mg/day. Where available, pyridoxine supplementation should be given to all patients receiving INH.

Rifampicin

Rifampicin is a first-line bactericidal agent that inhibits DNA-dependent RNA polymerase, leading to the death of the bacilli. Rifampicin is well absorbed with good penetration of inflamed meninges. The MIC against *M. tuberculosis* is approximately 0.5 μg/mL. The usual dose is 10 mg/kg/day (up to 600 mg/day). Rifampicin is a potent hepatic enzyme inducer and has many clinically significant drug interactions affecting the dosing of other medications, such as warfarin sodium (Coumadin), theophylline, and HIV protease inhibitors. Rifampicin increases the metabolism of estrogens and can result in decreased efficacy of hormonal contraceptive and breakthrough bleeding. The principal side effects are gastrointestinal intolerance, skin rashes, cholestatic jaundice, and hepatitis. A flulike syndrome characterized by malaise, fever, chills, headache, and myalgias can occur and is more frequent with intermittent dosing. Hemolytic anemia and thrombocytopenia are rare complications but require permanent discontinuation of the drug. Body secretions, including urine, sweat, and tears, appear orange or orange-red during rifampicin treatment.

Ethambutol

Ethambutol is primarily a mycobacteriostatic agent given to prevent the emergence of drug resistance to other first-line drugs. It has low CSF penetration. The MIC is 1 to 5 μg/mL. Usual dosages are 15 to 25 mg/kg/day. The drug is renally excreted and the dosage should be reduced in patients with renal insufficiency. The most important side effect of ethambutol is retrobulbar neuritis, which presents as blurred vision or decreased peripheral and color vision. The frequency of ocular toxicity is lower at the 15 mg/kg/day dose that is recommended when ethambutol is continued after the intensive phase of therapy. Patients receiving ethambutol should be instructed about symptoms of ocular toxicity. Simple visual acuity and color vision screening at follow-up clinic visits may help detect this complication early. Ethambutol should not be prescribed for young children who cannot report visual symptoms reliably. Ocular toxicity is reversible in most cases after discontinuation of the drug.

Pyrazinamide

Pyrazinamide is an important first-line bactericidal agent first used in TB treatment in the 1950s. Early concerns about hepatotoxicity relegated it to a minor role until the 1970s, when a series of important clinical trials conducted by the British Medical Research Council clearly established its important role in rapid sterilization of tuberculous lesions with resultant shortening of the duration of chemotherapy from 9 to 12 months to 6 months. Pyrazinamide is highly active in the acidic intracellular environment against organisms in macrophages. It has good tissue penetration, including the CSF. Usual doses are 15 to 30 mg/kg/day, up to 2 g/day. The most frequent side effects are gastrointestinal intolerance, hepatotoxicity, arthralgias, asymptomatic hyperuricemia due to blockade of urate excretion, and, rarely, acute gouty arthritis. Pyrazinamide does not appear to further increase the risk of hepatotoxicity when used in combination with isoniazid and rifampicin.[230] Minor arthralgias occur frequently and can usually be treated with salicylates or nonsteroidal inflammatory agents such as indomethacin while continuing the drug. The major value of pyrazinamide is its early sterilizing activity against intracellular organisms during the initial intensive phase of treatment.[231]

Thiacetazone

Thiacetazone is an inexpensive mycobacteriostatic drug that is widely used in developing countries in Africa, usually at a dose of 150 mg/day in combination with isoniazid and streptomycin in a 12-month daily treatment regimen consisting of 1 or 2 months of isoniazid, thiacetazone, and streptomycin followed by 10 months of isoniazid and thiacetazone. It is available in a combination formulation with isoniazid for convenient dosing. Thiacetazone has been associated with an increased incidence of cutaneous drug reactions, including severe Stevens–Johnson syndrome, in HIV-infected children and adults.[232–235] It should be considered a second-line agent when adequate supplies of rifampicin and pyrazinamide are available.

Second-Line Antituberculosis Drugs

Several other agents are available for retreatment of TB and the treatment of known or suspected drug-resistant TB cases. As a whole, these drugs are more toxic, less well tolerated, and less effective for TB treatment. Their use is indicated only for drug-resistant TB and as substitute agents when first-line drugs cannot be tolerated by the patient. Treatment involving second-line drugs also must be given for long durations of 12 to 24 months. Several of these agents must be given parenterally. Many are not readily available in developing countries due to their expense. Table 36-4 summarizes some important points about these agents.

Initial Tuberculosis Treatment Regimens

Many national and international organizations have published excellent comprehensive guidelines for TB treatment that are very valuable for clinicians.[236–239] This section discusses general principles of treatment (Box 36-3) and some suggested highly effective short-course regimens. The use of such regimens is feasible and highly cost-effective under program conditions.[240,241] Although the availability of regular supplies of high-quality drugs and the prescribing of adequate regimens in adequate doses for adequate durations are essential, it is important to stress the critical roles of the health care team, patient adherence to treatment, social factors, and political commitment in achieving good outcomes in TB control.

Four drugs should be prescribed initially unless local drug-resistance rates to first-line anti-TB drugs are known to be low (<2%).[236] Treatment with rifampicin, isoniazid, and pyrazinamide is critical to the success of 6-month short-course regimens. Rifampicin and isoniazid should be given for the entire duration of 6-month regimens for optimal efficacy. Pyrazinamide is necessary only during the first 2 months of treatment of drug-susceptible TB. Where available, the use of fixed-dose combination tablets decreases the number of pills to be taken, lessens the risk that patients may take only some of their drugs, and is strongly recommended by WHO.[238]

Table 36-4 Second-Line Antituberculosis Drugs

Drug	Pharmacokinetics/Mechanism of Action	Daily Dose for Children and Adults (Maximum Dose)	Common Side Effects
Para-aminosalicylic acid (PAS)	Inhibits mycobacterial dihydropteroate synthetase; well absorbed after oral dosing	150 mg/kg/day (12 g) PO	Gastric upset, sodium load, nausea, vomiting, diarrhea
Ethionamide	Structurally similar to isoniazid; well absorbed PO; good CSF penetration; renally excreted	15–20 mg/kg/day (1 g) PO	Gastrointestinal upset, hepatotoxicity, rash
Kanamycin	Binds to 30S subunit of bacterial ribosome; inhibits protein synthesis; given IM; renally excreted	15–30 mg/kg/day (1 g) IM	Ototoxicity, nephrotoxicity
Capreomycin	Similar to other aminoglycosides; given IM; poor CSF penetration; renally excreted	15–30 mg/kg/day (1 g) IM	Nephrotoxicity, ototoxicity
Cycloserine	Analogue of D-alanine; inhibits cell wall synthesis; well absorbed PO	15–20 mg/kg/day (1 g) PO	Psychosis, seizures, depression, headache, personality change, rash, vertigo
Fluroquinolones (ofloxacin, levofloxacin)	Inhibits topoisomerase II (DNA-gyrase); well absorbed PO; parenteral preparations of some drugs available; renal excretion	PO	Gastrointestinal upset, dizziness, tremor, confusion, seizures, photosensitivity

CSF, cerebrospinal fluid; IM, intramuscularly; PO, orally.

Patient compliance is a crucial factor in treatment failure and the development of acquired drug resistance. Whenever possible, TB treatment should be administered as directly observed therapy (DOT), where a health care worker or lay supervisor observes the patient swallow each dose of medications. DOT has been shown to be a highly effective (and cost-effective) strategy for TB treatment in both industrialized and developing countries.[240,242]

The following 6-month regimens have been shown to be highly effective in initial TB treatment[231,243,244]:

1. Two months of daily isoniazid, rifampicin, ethambutol, and pyrazinamide followed by 4 months of isoniazid and rifampicin administered two or three times weekly
2. Two weeks of daily isoniazid, rifampicin, ethambutol, and pyrazinamide followed by 6 weeks of twice weekly isoniazid, rifampicin, ethambutol, and pyrazinamide followed by 4 months of twice weekly isoniazid and rifampicin
3. Six months of three times weekly isoniazid, rifampicin, and pyrazinamide

Box 36-3 Important Principles in Treatment of Tuberculosis

- Use combination chemotherapy with at least two drugs to which the patient's organism can reasonably be expected to be susceptible.
- Never add a single drug to a failing regimen.
- The principal role of bacteriostatic drugs is to prevent emergence of resistant organisms during combination chemotherapy.
- Adequate doses of bioavailable drugs must be given consistently for an adequate duration of time for cure to be achieved.
- Both the patient and the physician share responsibility for successful treatment.

If drug susceptibility testing is performed and the isolate is fully drug susceptible, ethambutol may be discontinued. If the patient cannot tolerate pyrazinamide, excellent results may be achieved in patients with fully susceptible TB with 9 months of isoniazid and rifampicin. Six months of treatment with the previous regimens is generally adequate for patients with pulmonary tuberculosis who have satisfactory clinical and bacteriologic responses to treatment. Based on data suggesting that patients with initial cavitary disease who do not convert their sputum cultures to negative after 2 months of treatment are at high risk for relapse, some authorities now recommend extending treatment for an additional 3 months with INH and rifampicin for such patients.[236]

In developing countries with limited supplies of rifampicin, 2 months of daily ethambutol, isoniazid, rifampicin, and pyrazinamide followed by 6 months of daily isoniazid and ethambutol[238] or 6 months of isoniazid and thiacetazone[239] are widely used, although relapse rates are higher than with regimens containing rifampicin during the entire course of treatment.[246] Longer treatment regimens without a potent rifampicin and pyrazinamide-containing intensive phase, such as 2 months of daily isoniazid, thiacetazone, and streptomycin followed by 10 months of isoniazid and thiacetazone, can also be utilized but are associated with lower cure rates and high rates of cutaneous drug reactions in areas with a high prevalence of HIV coinfection.[233–235,245]

Patients should be instructed to cover their mouth and nose with a handkerchief or tissue when coughing. Masks and an initial period of respiratory isolation are desirable for hospitalized patients with smear-positive disease, where available. These measures can be discontinued when the number of bacilli visible on sputum smears and cough frequency decrease. Short-course chemotherapy regimens rapidly sterilize the sputum. Sputum smears may take longer to clear than sputum cultures, especially when rifampicin-containing regimens are used. Sputum smear-positive, culture-negative status was observed during the first 4 to 20 weeks of treatment in 20% of patients in one large series.[208] This phenomenon presumably is due to the visualization of nonviable organisms on sputum smears. Adequate respiratory isolation facilities are not available in many hospitals, however, and the primary emphasis in infection control should be on maintaining a high clinical suspicion for TB and the rapid diagnosis and treatment of infectious sputum smear-positive individuals.

Routine monitoring of hepatic function tests is not recommended. Proper patient education about TB, the need for full completion of treatment, and common side effects is important. In addition to DOT visits, patients should routinely be seen in the clinic on a monthly basis to review progress. At a minimum, the sputum should be examined monthly until conversion, at the end of treatment, and whenever clinical symptoms warrant. Seventy-seven percent to 90% of patients treated with rifampicin-containing short-course regimens should be culture negative (more than 75% smear negative) after completing 2 months of treatment, and essentially all should be culture negative after 3 months.[240,247–250] Reduction in cough frequency, resolution of fever and chest pain, and weight gain are the most important clinical signs of response to treatment. Defervescence occurred within 2 weeks in 64% to 93% of patients with pulmonary TB treated with rifampicin-containing regimens.[251,252] Serial chest radiography should not routinely be used to monitor response to treatment. One-fourth to one-third of patients with good clinical and microbiologic responses to treatment have worsening of radiographic lesions during the initial months of treatment. Chest films should be taken when the clinical course is complicated by new hemoptysis, poor response to treatment, or other significant changes in the patient's condition. In cases of poor response to treatment, if the chest film has not improved after 3 months of treatment, noncompliance, malabsorption of anti-TB drugs, drug-resistant TB, an incorrect initial diagnosis, or other concomitant chest disease should be considered. An end-of-treatment film may be helpful as a future baseline for comparison.

Patients should be instructed to return to the clinic promptly for medical attention when symptoms of drug toxicity occur. Early signs of hepatotoxicity (nausea, malaise, anorexia, and upper abdominal discomfort) should be emphasized. Minor drug reactions may be managed symptomatically with continuation of anti-TB treatment. Moderate or severe suspected drug reactions should be treated by discontinuation of TB treatment, appropriate medical management, and serial observation of the patient until the reaction subsides. At the discretion of the treating clinician, stepwise reinstitution of the anti-TB drugs at full dosage beginning with the least likely offending drug may be considered on a case-by-case basis, or alternative drugs may be substituted. The use of desensitization schedules with escalating doses of drugs such as isoniazid is not recommended. The reintroduction process should not be prolonged to avoid long periods of monotherapy. The implicated drug should be discontinued if the reaction occurs during rechallenge and the regimen modified appropriately by the addition of new replacement drugs. Most adverse drug reactions to anti-TB drugs are reversible upon discontinuation of the offending medication.

There are several promising developments in the treatment of TB. Rifapentine, a long-acting rifamycin, has been shown to be effective when administered once weekly during the continuation phase of treatment in HIV-noninfected patients.[253] New compounds including PA-824, a nitroimidazopyran active against slowly dividing organisms, are in early testing.[254] Newer fluoroquinolones, including levofloxacin, gatifloxacin, and moxifloxacin, are highly active against *M. tuberculosis* and may allow shortening of treatment to less than 6 months. In a trial from India, 4- and 5-month regimens including an initial intensive phase containing ofloxacin, INH, rifampicin, and pyrazinamide were highly successful in patients with smear-positive tuberculosis, resulting in relapse rates of less than 4%.[255]

Special Situations

Pediatric Tuberculosis

Microbiologic confirmation of the diagnosis of TB is difficult in young children and the decision to treat is often based on known close contact with an infectious smear-positive case, compatible clinical symptoms and radiographic findings, and lack of response to empirical treatment with broad-spectrum antibiotics targeted against common bacterial pathogens. Regimens used in children are comparable to those in adults with appropriate dose modifications[236] (see Table 36-3). Local formularies should be consulted about available preparations of anti-TB drugs for children. Ethambutol should be avoided in infants and young children who cannot report symptoms of ophthalmologic toxicity. Radiographic and clinical response should be monitored, with improvement expected over 2 or 3 months. Intrathoracic lymphadenopathy may take up to 2 years to fully resolve in children, and the persistence of lymphadenopathy is not, in itself, an indication for prolonged therapy.

Pregnancy and Lactation

TB treatment regimens used in pregnant and lactating women are similar to regimens used in nonpregnant women.[236,256,257] Few data are available on the potential teratogenicity of pyrazinamide and some programs avoid its use in pregnancy. Isoniazid and rifampicin have good long-term safety records in pregnant and lactating women, and daily treatment with isoniazid and rifampicin for 9 months is highly effective in drug-susceptible TB. Treatment of drug-resistant TB during pregnancy is complex, and such patients should be evaluated by a specialist. Successful treatment of MDR TB during pregnancy has been reported.[258]

The risk of isoniazid hepatotoxicity may be increased during pregnancy and the early postpartum period. Aminoglycosides should be avoided during pregnancy due to the risk of irreversible ototoxicity in the fetus. Pregnant women are more susceptible to development of isoniazid-associated peripheral neuropathy and should receive pyridoxine 25 to

50 mg/day while on TB treatment. Breast-feeding is safe while on TB chemotherapy.[259]

Extrapulmonary TB

Extrapulmonary TB is associated with lower bacillary burdens than pulmonary disease; therefore, extrapulmonary disease can generally be treated with standard short-course regimens that are effective for pulmonary disease.[243,260] Owing to the serious implications of relapsed disease at sites of potentially limited drug penetration, most clinicians treat miliary, meningeal, and skeletal TB for 12 or more months. Adjunctive surgical debridement and stabilization of bone and joint tuberculosis should be considered in addition to chemotherapy on a case-by-case basis. There is evidence from controlled clinical trials that short courses of corticosteroids (1 mg/kg/day prednisone or the equivalent rapidly tapered over 4 to 6 weeks) may be useful in cases of tuberculous meningitis, pericarditis, and severe serofibrinous pleurisy. Corticosteroids have also been used in cases of extensive pulmonary TB with severe clinical toxicity or acute respiratory failure. Corticosteroids can be given safely in conjunction with anti-TB chemotherapy.

Tuberculosis Treatment in Human Immunodeficiency Virus–Coinfected Patients

The treatment of choice for pulmonary TB in HIV-infected patients is short-course combination chemotherapy with regimens including isoniazid, rifampicin, ethambutol, and pyrazinamide that are effective in more than 95% of patients with drug-susceptible TB when administered for a full course of treatment.[20,21,23,24,64] Due to increased relapse rates (in some instances with acquired rifampicin resistance) in HIV-infected patients treated with twice-weekly therapy, daily treatment during the intensive phase and at least thrice-weekly treatment during the continuation phase are highly recommended.[261,262] In contrast, regimens that do not include rifampicin as a principal component are associated with an increased incidence of severe cutaneous hypersensitivity reactions, lower rates of sputum conversion, higher treatment failure and relapse rates, and increased mortality compared with rifampicin-containing regimens in HIV-infected patients.[233,245,263]

Compliance is critical to good outcomes in the treatment of TB in HIV-infected people. DOT may be especially valuable in this setting.[264] Ambulatory treatment is fully satisfactory for the majority of patients with uncomplicated disease.

When treated with appropriate regimens, clinical and microbiologic responses to treatment are comparable to responses in HIV-noninfected patients. An extended duration of anti-TB chemotherapy is not routinely indicated in HIV-infected patients[23]; however, the microbiologic response to therapy should be closely monitored with serial sputum examinations. Treatment should be prolonged if the response to treatment is slow or otherwise unsatisfactory.[236]

Rarely, patients being started on anti-TB chemotherapy develop transient worsening of fever, lymphadenitis, cerebral tuberculomas, pulmonary infiltrates, pleural effusions, or other signs and symptoms of TB—so-called paradoxical reactions. Paradoxical reactions occur in HIV-uninfected people but appear to be more frequent in HIV-infected patients and in some studies have occurred more frequently in patients being started on antiretroviral therapy and anti-TB treatment at the same time.[265] Paradoxical reactions usually occur within the first 2 months of antiretroviral therapy, often during the initial 2 to 3 weeks of treatment, and may be more frequent in patients with low CD4 counts. The cause of paradoxical reactions is unclear; however, they may be due to reconstitution of host immune responses and heightened inflammatory responses after beginning anti-TB and possibly antiretroviral therapy.[266] Clinical deterioration should be ascribed to paradoxical reactions only after careful evaluation for treatment failure, malabsorption, noncompliance, drug toxicity, or another concomitant opportunistic infection. Mild paradoxical reactions are usually self-limited and may be treated symptomatically. Some authorities recommend a short course of several weeks of prednisone or methylprednisolone beginning at 1 mg/kg/day for patients with severe paradoxical reactions.[236]

Two studies of HIV-infected South African and Haitian adults assessing whether secondary prophylaxis with INH after initial treatment could prevent recurrent TB showed a 55% to 82% decrease in recurrent disease in patients receiving INH.[267,268] Patients with advanced HIV infection benefited the most, leading some authorities to recommend expansion of preventive therapy guidelines to include secondary INH prophylaxis in patients with advanced HIV/AIDS living in areas with a high prevalence of TB.

The timing of initiating antiretroviral therapy and the antiretroviral drugs and regimens used in treating HIV-infected patients with TB who are not currently on antiretroviral therapy is an evolving area of clinical practice. Rifampicin is a potent hepatic microsomal enzyme inducer and alters the metabolism of many drugs. Antiretroviral therapy with protease inhibitors and nonnucleoside reverse transcriptase inhibitors has significant drug interaction during rifampicin therapy, resulting in low serum concentrations of the antiretroviral drugs and high rifampicin levels. In severely immunosuppressed patients (CD4 count $< 200\ \mu L^{-1}$) deaths due to HIV-related complications may occur early during TB treatment. Therefore, many authorities recommend beginning concomitant antiretroviral therapy early. Rifabutin has fewer drug interactions and, where available, can be used as an alternative to rifampicin. Other options include using antiretroviral therapy regimens including efavirenz and avoiding protease inhibitors initially. For patients with a lesser degree of HIV-related immunosuppression, it may be best to optimally treat TB before beginning antiretroviral therapy. Recommendations and guidelines are rapidly changing and the clinician should consult with a specialist skilled in the treatment of both TB and HIV/AIDS for assistance.

Drug-Resistant Tuberculosis

From a tuberculosis control program standpoint, drug-resistant *M. tuberculosis* isolates are as infectious and virulent as drug-susceptible strains.[269,270] The clinical presentation of drug-resistant TB is similar to that of drug-susceptible TB; however, drug-resistant TB is difficult to treat and associated with worse outcomes.

Whereas initial isoniazid or streptomycin monoresistance has only minimal impact on the outcome of 6 months of treatment with rifampicin-containing short-course regimens,[202] the presence of rifampicin resistance or resistance to both isoniazid and rifampicin (MDR TB) are serious. Prolonged treatment with more toxic and expensive agents is required. Although initial studies reporting clinical outcomes among MDR TB patients were discouraging, recent work shows improving trends, with as many as 80% of patients responding to treatment.[271] With appropriate consultation and supervision, community-based therapy for MDR TB has been successful in some settings.[272] Patients have improved outcomes when their treatment regimen contains a minimum of three drugs to which their isolate is susceptible.[273] A single agent should never be added to a failing regimen.

Cases of drug-resistant TB should be managed by specialized units and consultants whenever possible because treatment requires a good laboratory and access to more expensive and toxic drugs. Retreatment of treatment failures, relapses, and cases of suspected drug-resistant TB should be carefully monitored and administered as DOT. Under program conditions, failures and relapses of TB after an initial course of short-course chemotherapy are rarely multiple drug resistant. Routine drug susceptibility testing of initial pretreatment isolates, although optimal, is not absolutely necessary. Patients with acquired drug resistance to isoniazid or isoniazid and streptomycin can still be cured by retreatment regimens such as the standard 8-month IUATLD retreatment regimens consisting of 2 months of streptomycin, ethambutol, isoniazid, rifampicin, and pyrazinamide, followed by 1 month of ethambutol, isoniazid, rifampicin, and pyrazinamide, and concluding with 5 months of daily or three-times-weekly isoniazid, ethambutol, and rifampicin.[239] Drug susceptibility testing should be performed in patients with treatment failure or relapse, especially after unsuccessful retreatment.

The most important management principle in treating patients with resistance to one or more drugs is the administration of at least two new drugs to which the patient's isolate is susceptible. Initial isoniazid monoresistance can be treated with the retreatment regimens described previously; with a 9-month regimen of rifampicin, ethambutol, and pyrazinamide for 2 months followed by rifampicin and ethambutol for 7 months[274]; or with 6 months of rifampicin, ethambutol, and pyrazinamide.[236] Patients whose isolates are resistant to rifampicin alone may be treated with INH and ethambutol for 18 months or INH, pyrazinamide, and streptomycin for 9 months.[275]

Treatment for MDR TB (resistant to at least INH and rifampicin) involves prolonged therapy and the use of drugs with substantial side effects. Patients with suspected MDR TB should be managed in consultation with a specialist experienced in the management of MDR TB. General principles of management include the initial use of five drugs that are likely to be active, including an injectable, until sputum cultures are negative, then continuing with three drugs. The most efficacious (bactericidal) drugs available should be used in adequate and tolerable doses for an adequate duration. If the patient is failing standard short-course treatment with INH, rifampicin, pyrazinamide, and ethambutol and MDR TB is suspected, one approach is to add a fluoroquinolone such as ofloxacin or levofloxacin, an injectable drug such as kanamycin or amikacin, and possibly ethionamide. Authorities recommend continuing treatment for at least 12 to 15 months after sputum culture conversion. In the setting of localized disease, continued sputum positivity, massive hemoptysis, or inability to tolerate medical treatment, surgical resection of diseased lung tissue may play an adjunctive role in the treatment of MDR TB.[276,277] Detailed information about the treatment of drug-resistant TB can be obtained from several excellent sources.[239,278–281]

PREVENTION AND CONTROL

Tuberculosis Control

There are three principal strategies for the prevention and control of TB. Primary preventive measures include BCG vaccination and interruption of transmission, case finding, and treatment. Preventive therapy—the administration of drugs given after a person has become infected by *M. tuberculosis* to prevent the development of active TB—is an approach targeted at secondary prevention of new cases.

Due to their higher bacillary burden, sputum smear–positive people with active TB (50% of all TB cases) are the principal source of TB transmission in the community. The highest priority in TB control programs and the fundamental approach advocated by IUATLD and WHO is the rapid identification and treatment of new cases of sputum smear–positive pulmonary TB detected through passive case finding. Because these infectious cases transmit TB to others, treatment of smear-positive cases benefits the affected individual and the community. When fully implemented, efficient case finding and effective treatment of smear-positive TB cases can quickly reduce mortality due to TB and the incidence of the disease in high-prevalence areas.

Bacille Calmette–Guérin Vaccination

Bacille Calmette-Guérin is a living attenuated strain of *M. bovis* derived by serial passage in culture by Calmette and Guérin between 1908 and 1918. It is the basis of several inexpensive, safe vaccines widely used for the prevention of TB. BCG is a component of the United Nations Expanded Programme on Immunizations and is the world's most widely used vaccine. It is usually given as a single intradermal injection soon after birth.

Results of 21 large clinical trials of various BCG vaccines have yielded conflicting data about the efficacy of BCG in the prevention of TB. Protective efficacy ranged from −10% to 81% in these studies.[282] Meta-analyses of these studies suggest that BCG vaccines are approximately 50% protective against the development of TB.[283] In some tropical countries, such as Malawi, BCG vaccine protects against leprosy but not TB. The protective efficacy of BCG vaccines against TB was decreased or absent in trials done in countries closer to the equator, possibly due to the higher frequency of naturally occurring infection with nontuberculous mycobacteria in these areas, which may be cross-protective against TB. Several different strains of BCG are used in making BCG vaccines. Genomic studies comparing various BCG strains have identified deletions, duplications, and single nucleotide polymorphisms that may also account for some of the difference in protection among various BCG vaccines.[284] In contrast to data showing variable prevention of pulmonary TB, there is more solid evidence that BCG is approximately 85% effective in preventing miliary and meningeal TB, the two most life-threatening forms of TB, in childhood.[285] The protective efficacy and duration of protection of BCG vaccination in immunocompromised people, such as those infected with HIV, are unclear.

Complications of BCG vaccination are infrequent and consist mainly of local lymphadenopathy or lymphadenitis; disseminated disease is rare. The rate of complications may be slightly higher in HIV-infected people but is still very low,[286] and WHO recommends that BCG vaccination be administered to infants early in life, even when the mother is known or suspected of being HIV infected. BCG vaccination should be withheld only from people with symptomatic HIV infection.[287]

Vaccines against TB that are under development include DNA vaccines, protein and peptide vaccines with new adjuvants, recombinant BCG and other live vectors expressing immunodominant mycobacterial antigens, naturally or rationally attenuated strains of mycobacteria, and nonpeptide vaccines.[288] Several candidate vaccines are entering human testing.

Treatment of Latent TB Infection

Treatment of latent TB infection, formerly termed TB preventive therapy, has two principal benefits—an individual health benefit through prevention of TB and an important benefit to the community wherein decreased transmission and new *M. tuberculosis* infections will lead to an eventual lowering of case rates in the entire population. Interest in the use of isoniazid to prevent TB disease in people with previous *M. tuberculosis* infection began in the late 1950s. In HIV-noninfected people, 6 to 12 months of isoniazid preventive therapy was clearly shown to provide long-term health benefits. Isoniazid decreases the occurrence of TB by approximately 65% (range, 25%–92%)[289]; protection lasts up to 19 years and may be lifelong.[290]

Effectiveness is strongly correlated with the duration of preventive therapy and patient compliance. Maximal benefit in HIV-noninfected people was observed with 6 to 12 months of isoniazid preventive therapy, with no further advantage resulting from treatment exceeding 1 year.[291] In a large study from Eastern Europe, the protective efficacy of isoniazid preventive therapy in patients with fibrotic residual lesions on chest radiography was only slightly reduced with 6 months of treatment, from 75% to 65%, compared with 12 months of therapy, whereas side effects were more frequent with the longer regimen.[292] Efficacy increases with compliance and was as high as 90% in highly compliant patients in some clinical trials; however, even patients with intermittent compliance over a sustained course of therapy benefit substantially from isoniazid preventive therapy.[12] Based on the previous data, 9 months of treatment with isoniazid is now the recommended regimen for treatment of latent TB infection for children and most adults. Three months of treatment with isoniazid and rifampicin has also been shown to be effective for the prevention of tuberculosis.[293–295]

The principal safety consideration regarding isoniazid preventive therapy is isoniazid-related hepatotoxicity. In a placebo-controlled trial of 6 to 12 months of isoniazid preventive therapy, the overall incidence of hepatotoxicity was 0.5%.[296] The incidence of hepatotoxicity increased with age, from 0.3% in people 20 to 34 years old to 1.2% in patients 35 to 49 years old, and with increased length of therapy. Ethanol consumption (especially on a daily basis), preexisting liver disease, possibly pregnancy, and the postpartum period[228,229] are also associated with hepatotoxicity.

Data from seven controlled clinical trials have shown that preventive therapy is also effective in PPD-positive (PPD ≥5 mm) HIV-infected people.[297] Six to 12 months of isoniazid, 3 months of INH plus rifampicin, and 2 or 3 months of rifampicin and pyrazinamide provide approximately 56% to 60% short-term protection against TB. The combination of rifampicin and pyrazinamide is no longer recommended for treatment of latent TB infection because of an increased rate of severe hepatotoxicity and fulminant hepatic failure.[298] PPD-negative and anergic individuals have not been shown to benefit from preventive therapy against TB.[293,299,300]

The duration of the protective effect of TB preventive therapy in HIV-infected people is unknown.[301] Data from Zambia and Uganda suggest that benefits extend for 1 to 3 years[302,303] and may be longer after treatment with rifampicin-containing regimens.[302]

Decisions to prescribe isoniazid preventive therapy should balance the risks of developing active TB and the risk of isoniazid toxicity. HIV-infected people, close household contacts of smear-positive TB patients, and recent PPD skin test converters are among those at highest risk of developing active TB. Other groups of people with positive PPD skin tests for whom TB preventive therapy should be considered are listed in Box 36-4. Active TB must be excluded prior to beginning preventive therapy.

The daily dosage of isoniazid for preventive therapy is 5 mg/kg (10 mg/kg in children) up to a maximum dose of 300 mg. Isoniazid can also be given twice weekly at a dose of 15 mg/kg up to a maximum dose of 900 mg when supervised preventive therapy is warranted, although the protective efficacy of intermittent regimens has not been studied. Pyridoxine 25 to 50 mg/day should be administered to prevent INH-associated peripheral neuropathy. Routine biochemical monitoring of serum transaminases in patients receiving isoniazid preventive therapy is of limited value in people younger than 35 years of age but should be considered in older people, drinkers, and those with underlying liver disease. When serum liver function tests are monitored, discontinuation of isoniazid should be considered if the levels exceed three to five times the upper limit of normal. All people receiving isoniazid preventive therapy should be instructed to seek medical attention if symptoms of hepatotoxicity, such as malaise, dark urine, nausea,

Box 36-4 Tuberculin Skin Test–Positive Patients for Whom Tuberculosis Preventive Therapy Should Be Considered

- HIV-infected patients and people at high risk for HIV such as intravenous drug users
- Close contacts of new infectious TB cases (especially sputum smear–positive cases)
- Recent purified protein derivative skin test converters
- People with underlying medical conditions placing them at high risk of developing TB (poorly controlled diabetes mellitus, prolonged corticosteroid therapy, leukemia, Hodgkin's disease, head and neck cancer, end-stage renal disease, conditions associated with rapid weight loss, and chronic protein-calorie malnutrition)
- Recent immigrants from countries with a high prevalence of TB
- Institutionalized people (prisons, nursing homes, etc.)

and abdominal pain, develop and should be seen at the clinic at least monthly.

Only limited experience is available with drugs other than isoniazid for preventive therapy in patients who have been exposed to known or suspected cases of drug-resistant TB or where INH was not tolerated. Treatment with 4 months of daily rifampicin[295] has been used in instances in which the index TB case is resistant to INH or in which the patient could not tolerate INH. Six months of ethambutol plus pyrazinamide or pyrazinamide plus ofloxacin have been used as preventive therapy in high-risk patients who were infected after exposure to cases of MDR TB, although side effects, mainly gastrointestinal intolerance, have been frequent with the latter regimen.

ATYPICAL MYCOBACTERIA

Several species of mycobacteria other than *M. tuberculosis* have been implicated as important human pathogens in the past three decades. Although the number of cases of disease due to these organisms is much less than those due to *M. tuberculosis* in developing countries, atypical mycobacteria are responsible for many serious infections in immunocompromised people in the United States and Europe, including disseminated *M. avium* complex (MAC) disease in patients with advanced AIDS. Several species cause chronic pulmonary disease and lymphadenitis, the most common clinical manifestations of disease in HIV-noninfected people (Table 36-5).

Disease due to representative species will be discussed. The reader is referred to the excellent comprehensive reviews by Wolinsky,[304] Pitchenik and Fertel,[305] and Wallace[306] for further information.

There are several important distinctions between human disease due to nontuberculous mycobacteria and TB. Atypical mycobacteria are less virulent human pathogens and tend to produce disease in immunocompromised people or people with underlying structural lung disease. Pulmonary disease, lymphadenitis, and disseminated disease are the most common clinical manifestations of disease due to atypical mycobacteria. Nontuberculous mycobacteria are environmental organisms and many species can be isolated from soil, water, dust, milk, and birds or animals in temperate climates. There is little evidence of human-to-human transmission of these organisms, and patients with atypical mycobacterial disease are generally not considered infectious to others. Lastly, many of these organisms can colonize humans without producing invasive disease.

Nontuberculous mycobacteria are usually classified based on the rapidity of growth on solid media and the production of pigment when incubated in light (photochromogens) or darkness (scotochromogens; Runyon classification). Photochromogens (group I) include *M. kansasii, M. marinum,* and *M. simiae*; scotochromogens (group II) include *M. scrofulaceum, M. szulgai, M. xenopi, M. gordonae,* and *M. flavescens*; nonchromogens (group III) include *M. avium–intracellulare, M. ulcerans, M. gastri, M. terrae, M. triviale,* and *M. malmoense*; and rapid growers (group IV) include *M. fortuitum, M. abscessus, M. chelonae,* and *M. smegmatis*. Nontuberculous mycobacteria cannot be reliably distinguished from M. tuberculosis by AFB smear microscopy and positive smears should be presumed to indicate active TB until proven otherwise. Speciation is difficult and time-consuming and was previously done only by reference laboratories using colonial morphology, pigment production, and biochemical testing methods. Recently, several species- or species group-specific DNA probes have become available (GenProbe) that allow rapid differentiation of *M. tuberculosis, M. kansasii,* MAC, and the common laboratory water-borne contaminant *M. gordonae*.

Table 36-5 *Common Disease Syndromes Associated with Atypical Mycobacterial Species in Humans*

Syndrome	Species
Chronic pulmonary disease	*M. avium–intracellulare* (MAC) complex *M. kansasii* *M. abscessus* *M. xenopi* *M. fortuitum* complex *M. simiae* *M. malmoense* *M. szulgai*
Skin and soft tissue infections	*M. marinum* (swimming pool or fish tank granulomas) *M. fortuitum* complex *M. chelonae* *M. abscessus* *M. ulcerans* (Buruli ulcer) *M. haemophilum*
Skeletal infections	*M. fortuitum* complex MAC complex *M. kansasii* *M. marinum* *M. terrae*
Lymphadenitis	MAC complex *M. scofulaceum* *M. fortuitum* complex *M. malmoense* *M. kansasii* *M. haemophilum* *M. genavense*
Disseminated disease	MAC complex *M. kansasii* *M. scofulaceum* *M. fortuitum* complex *M. chelonae* *M. haemophilum*

Lymphadenitis

Nontuberculous mycobacteria are a common cause of pediatric cervical lymphadenitis. Most children present with unilateral submandibular and high anterior cervical lymph node enlargement.[98] Most are afebrile, appear healthy, and no immunologic abnormalities can be detected. The pathogenesis is unclear but may be related to oropharyngeal trauma from teething and the fact that young children commonly put objects in their mouths. MAC is now the most frequently recovered species, replacing *M. scrofulaceum* and *M. fortuitum*.[98] Many children with nontuberculous lymphadenitis have positive PPD skin tests. Tuberculin skin tests may be useful in suggesting an underlying mycobacterial cause of the enlarged nodes but are not helpful in distinguishing cases due to *M. tuberculosis* and other nontuberculous mycobacteria. The chest x-ray is usually normal in children with lymphadenitis due to nontuberculous mycobacteria. A tuberculous cause is more likely when associated pulmonary stigmas are present and the supraclavicular and posterior cervical nodes are affected.

The treatment of choice is surgical—total excision of the affected nodes. Incision and drainage and simple biopsy are not recommended because they frequently result in the formation of chronically draining fistulas and sinus tracts requiring difficult cleanup surgery. Antibiotic treatment has not previously been shown to be useful; however, experience with regimens that contain newer agents, such as clarithromycin and fluoroquinolones, has been limited and these drugs may play a role in the future treatment of this condition.

Skin and Soft Tissue Infections

Mycobacterium marinum causes chronic papular lesions and cellulitis when inoculated into the skin traumatized in association with exposure to fresh or saltwater marine environments, including fish tanks. Tenosynovitis can occur if deeper structures are injured, and rarely a sporotrichoid picture with nodules developing proximal to the site of the initial lesion may occur. The diagnosis is made by history, a consistent appearance of the lesion, and biopsy and culture. *Mycobacterium marinum* grows best at low temperatures, and culture at 28 to 30°C (rather than 37°C) is required for optimal isolation. *Mycobacterium haemophilum* and *M. fortuitum* also produce nodular skin lesions, usually in severely immunocompromised people. Deep chronic lower extremity skin ulcers are produced by *M. ulcerans* in tropical Africa (Buruli ulcer) and Australia. *Mycobacterium ulcerans* produces a potent family of toxins, the mycolactones, which are responsible for the severe, protracted local tissue destruction.[307] *Mycobacterium kansasii, M. fortuitum, M. chelonae,* and MAC can also produce skeletal disease, frequently involving the hand, which resembles TB but usually requires surgical treatment.

Chronic Pulmonary Disease

MAC, *M. kansasii, M. malmoense, M. fortuitum, M. xenopi,* and *M. chelonae* are the most common nontuberculous mycobacteria causing chronic respiratory disease. Concomitant chronic obstructive pulmonary disease (COPD), pneumoconioses (especially silicosis), chronic bronchiectasis, head and neck and lung cancers, and alcoholism are recognized risk factors for disease due to nontuberculous mycobacteria. Fast-growing species such as *M. fortuitum* and *M. chelonae* sometimes produce chronic pneumonia in patients with rheumatoid lung disease, achalasia, cystic fibrosis, and underlying lipoid pneumonia. Nontuberculous mycobacteria may also colonize the lower airway without producing invasive disease, especially in the presence of other chronic structural lung diseases. Therefore, care must be taken to distinguish between colonization and invasive disease. Bronchoscopes and respiratory therapy equipment can become contaminated with water-borne nontuberculous mycobacteria if not properly decontaminated between uses. Diagnostic criteria established by the American Thoracic Society for the diagnosis of nontuberculous mycobacteria as etiologic pathogens in patients with compatible clinical and radiographic findings require persistently positive AFB smears and isolation of the organism by moderately heavy growth in culture from two or more sputum or bronchoscopic specimens and the exclusion of other possible causes such as TB or other endemic mycoses such as histoplasmosis or cryptococcosis.[308] Despite retrospective series claiming subtle differences between the chest radiographic findings in pulmonary diseases due to nontuberculous mycobacteria and *M. tuberculosis*, in day-to-day clinical practice the radiographic findings in these two conditions are indistinguishable. Apical fibrocavitary disease with scarring, contraction, and volume loss are the most common findings.

Disease Due to *M. avium–intracellulare* Complex

The MAC is a group of slowly growing mycobacteria that cause cervical lymphadenitis and chronic, slowly progressive necrotizing pneumonia in HIV-noninfected children and adults, respectively, and disseminated disease in patients with AIDS.

Chronic Pulmonary Disease

Clinical series from the pre-HIV era emphasized the role of MAC as a cause of chronic necrotizing apical pneumonia similar to TB in elderly men with COPD, bronchiectasis, remote TB, or lung cancer.[309] The underlying lung disease was believed to predispose to colonization with MAC, which then resulted in a chronic, slowly progressive, necrotizing pneumonia in a small number of individuals. Patients presented with chronic productive cough, weight loss, fever, and night sweats with fibrocavitary infiltrates on chest film.

In industrialized countries such as the United States, the prevalence of chronic pulmonary disease due to MAC appears to be increasing[310] for unclear reasons, and the spectrum of disease has widened recently. MAC disease has been described as presenting as slowly progressive middle lung field noncavitating nodular infiltrates and persistent cough without fever or weight loss in middle-aged, nonsmoking women with no prior history of respiratory disease.[311,312] Fibrocavitary lesions are much less common in these patients. Chest CT scans demonstrated nodular interstitial disease and bronchiectasis in these patients, which was believed to be due to the nontuberculous mycobacterial disease. Many of these patients succumbed to slowly progressive respiratory failure.

Treatment of pulmonary MAC disease requires prolonged multiple-drug chemotherapy. The organism is highly resistant to many drugs used to treat TB. Recurrence after treatment is frequent. The course of the disease and long-term outcome vary significantly among patients; however, substantial morbidity is common and some patients die of slowly progressive respiratory failure and cor pulmonale. In HIV-noninfected people, cavitary lung disease due to MAC is often indolent, and in some patients noncavitary disease improves or resolves without treatment. In people with concomitant lung diseases such as bronchiectasis or COPD, treatment of the underlying condition with smoking cessation, bronchodilators, and antibiotics should be optimized. MAC is resistant in vitro to many antibiotics. When treatment is necessary, multiple drugs should be used and, when possible, isolates should be submitted to a reference laboratory for susceptibility testing. The new azalide and macrolide antibiotics, azithromycin and clarithromycin, are highly active against MAC. One suggested initial regimen is clarithromycin or azithromycin, rifampicin, ethambutol, and amikacin or streptomycin for 2 or 3 months followed by clarithromycin or azithromycin, rifampicin, and ethambutol for a total of 24 months.[313] Treatment of pulmonary MAC disease must be prolonged. Side effects are frequent, and early consultation with a unit experienced with the management of these patients is advised whenever possible.

Disseminated Disease in Human Immunodeficiency Virus–Infected Patients

Although TB is the most common serious mycobacterial disease affecting HIV-infected people worldwide, disseminated MAC infection is a common late opportunistic infection among HIV-infected people in the United States and Europe. The incidence of disseminated MAC disease has decreased greatly due to the advent of highly active antiretroviral therapy and effective chemoprophylaxis. Disseminated MAC disease has been infrequently reported in HIV-infected patients from developing countries in Africa,[314,315] despite the fact that the organism is present in great numbers in the soil and water.[316] Disseminated MAC infection in patients with AIDS usually presents with fever, chronic diarrhea, night sweats, anorexia, hepatosplenomegaly, abdominal lymphadenopathy, fatigue, and weight loss.[317] Severe anemia and elevated serum alkaline phosphatase are often present. In contrast to HIV-noninfected patients, significant pulmonary disease due to MAC is uncommon in patients with AIDS.

Disseminated MAC infection occurs late in the course of HIV infection and contributes significantly to morbidity and mortality.[318,319] The median peripheral blood CD4 lymphocyte count at the time of diagnosis in several studies was less than 50/μL, and disseminated MAC infection has been reported only rarely in patients with CD4 counts greater than 100/μL. The pathogenesis of disseminated MAC infection in AIDS is unclear. The frequent isolation of MAC from the sputum or stool of patients with AIDS before the diagnosis of disseminated MAC disease suggests that primary infection via inhalation or ingestion of the organism usually precedes disseminated disease.

The diagnosis of disseminated MAC infection in AIDS is usually straightforward. Blood cultures are positive in more than 90% of cases; bone marrow, liver, and lymph node biopsies also have very high diagnostic yields. Although MAC has significant in vitro resistance to many antimycobacterial drugs, treatment with newer drug regimens has led to improvement in symptoms, clearing of mycobacteremia, and increased survival. The new macrolides and azalides, clarithromycin and azithromycin, are highly active against MAC. Combination therapy with clarithromycin 500 mg twice daily or azithromycin 600 mg once daily plus ethambutol 15 mg/kg/day is highly effective. The addition of an aminoglycoside[320] or rifabutin[321] adds little to the effectiveness of treatment with a macrolide plus ethambutol. Rifabutin has significant interactions with many antiretroviral drugs. Chemoprophylaxis against disseminated MAC infection is now recommended by many authorities for HIV-infected people whose CD4 lymphocyte counts are less than 50/μL.[322] Azithromycin 1200 mg once weekly and clarithromycin 500 mg twice daily are the most widely used regimens and decrease the incidence of disseminated MAC infection by approximately 60%.[323,324] Rifabutin can be used alternatively for preventive therapy in people who are intolerant of macrolides but is less effective. Data from several clinical trials have shown that chemoprophylaxis against MAC can be safely discontinued in patients who have a sustained increase in their CD4 count to greater than 100/μL for more than 3 months after beginning antiretroviral therapy.

Disease Due to *M. kansasii*

Mycobacterium kansasii causes chronic pulmonary disease similar to reactivation TB and disseminated disease in patients with advanced AIDS. Disease due to this pathogen occurs sporadically throughout the world but is most common in the central and southwestern United States and in England and Wales. In HIV-noninfected patients with pulmonary disease, treatment with isoniazid, rifampicin, and ethambutol for 18 to 24 months or until sputum cultures have been negative for 12 months is recommended.[308] *Mycobacterium kansasii* usually responds well to treatment. The duration of therapy required in patients with AIDS is unknown.

Treatment

Treatment of disease due to nontuberculous mycobacteria is long and difficult. Few clinical trials have been done to guide therapy. Atypical mycobacteria are usually resistant to most anti-TB drugs, although several other classes of chemotherapeutic drugs have activity against some species. The value of drug susceptibility testing in guiding treatment is controversial, and reliable testing is available only through a few specialized laboratories. Susceptibility testing is best established in the treatment of *M. kansasii* disease and for assessing susceptibility to macrolides and azalides for MAC infection.

The effectiveness of drug therapy is highly variable, even with combination therapy. Thorough surgical debridement is important in localized disease. *Mycobacterium marinum* infections limited to superficial tissue can be treated with doxycycline, trimethoprim-sulfamethoxazole, or ciprofloxacin. Deeper or extensive infections require treatment with combination therapy with rifampicin, ethambutol, and possibly streptomycin. Sulfonamides, cefoxitin, amikacin, ciprofloxacin, and imipenem are active against *M. fortuitum*. Infections due to *M. scrofulaceum* should be treated with the same regimens used for MAC infections.[325] Treatment of MAC and *M. kansasii* infections was described earlier. The reader is encouraged to consult the published guidelines of the American and British Thoracic Societies for detailed information about the treatment of specific mycobacterial infections.[308,326]

REFERENCES

1. Cole ST, Brosch R, Parkhill J, et al: Deciphering the biology of *Mycobacterium tuberculosis* from the complete genome sequence. Nature 393:537, 1998.
2. Grzybowski S, Barnett GD, Styblo K: Contacts of cases of active pulmonary tuberculosis. Bull Int Union Tuberc 50:90, 1975.
3. Yeager H, Lacy J, Smith LR, et al: Quantitative studies of mycobacterial populations in sputum and saliva. Am Rev Respir Dis 95:998, 1967.
4. Behr MA, Warren SA, Salamon H, et al: Transmission of *Mycobacterium tuberculosis* from patients smear-negative for acid-fast bacilli. Lancet 353:444, 1999.
5. Corbett EL, Watt CJ, Walker N, et al: The growing burden of tuberculosis: Global trends and interactions with the HIV epidemic. Arch Intern Med 163:1009, 2003.

6. Frieden TR, Sterling TR, Munsiff SS, et al: Tuberculosis. Lancet 362:887, 2003.
7. Murray CJ, Styblo K, Rouillon A: Tuberculosis in developing countries: Burden, intervention and cost. Bull Int Union Tuberc Lung Dis 65:6, 1990.
8. Kochi A: The global tuberculosis situation and the new control strategy of the World Health Organization. Tubercle 72:1, 1991.
9. De Cock KM, Chaisson RE: Will DOTS do it? A reappraisal of tuberculosis control in countries with high rates of HIV infection. Int J Tuberc Lung Dis 3:457, 1999.
10. Dolin PJ, Raviglione MC, Kochi A: Global tuberculosis incidence and mortality during 1990–2000. Bull WHO 72:213, 1994.
11. Comstock GW, Livesay VT, Woolpert SF: The prognosis of a positive tuberculin reaction in childhood and adolescence. Am J Epidemiol 99:131, 1974.
12. O'Brien RJ, Perriens JH: Preventive therapy for tuberculosis in HIV infection: The promise and the reality. AIDS 9:665, 1995.
13. Selwyn PA, Hartel D, Lewis VA, et al: A prospective study of the risk of tuberculosis among intravenous drug users with human immunodeficiency virus infection. N Engl J Med 320:545, 1989.
14. Guelar A, Gatell JM, Verdejo J, et al: A prospective study of the risk of tuberculosis among HIV-infected patients. AIDS 7:1345, 1993.
15. Moreno S, Baraia-Etxaburu J, Bouza E, et al: Risk for developing tuberculosis among anergic patients infected with HIV. Ann Intern Med 119:194, 1993.
16. Antonucci G, Girardi E, Raviglione MC, et al: Risk factors for tuberculosis in HIV-infected persons. A prospective cohort study. The Gruppo Italiano di Studio Tubercolosi e AIDS (GISTA). JAMA 274:143, 1995.
17. Daley CL, Small PM, Schecter GF, et al: An outbreak of tuberculosis with accelerated progression among persons infected with the human immunodeficiency virus. An analysis using restriction-fragment-length polymorphisms. N Engl J Med 326:231, 1992.
18. Di Perri G, Cruciani M, Danzi MC, et al: Nosocomial epidemic of active tuberculosis among HIV-infected patients. Lancet 2:1502, 1989.
19. Sonnenberg P, Murray J, Glynn JR, et al: HIV-1 and recurrence, relapse, and reinfection of tuberculosis after cure: A cohort study in South African mineworkers. Lancet 358:1687, 2001.
20. Chaisson RE, Schecter GF, Theuer CP, et al: Tuberculosis in patients with the acquired immunodeficiency syndrome. Clinical features, response to therapy, and survival. Am Rev Respir Dis 136:570, 1987.
21. Small PM, Schecter GF, Goodman PC, et al: Treatment of tuberculosis in patients with advanced human immunodeficiency virus infection. N Engl J Med 324:289, 1991.
22. Jones BE, Otaya M, Antoniskis D, et al: A prospective evaluation of antituberculosis therapy in patients with human immunodeficiency virus infection. Am J Respir Crit Care Med 150:1499, 1994.
23. Perriens JH, St. Louis ME, Mukadi YB, et al: Pulmonary tuberculosis in HIV-infected patients in Zaire. A controlled trial of treatment for either 6 or 12 months. N Engl J Med 332:779, 1995.
24. Ackah AN, Coulibaly D, Digbeu H, et al: Response to treatment, mortality, and CD4 lymphocyte counts in HIV-infected persons with tuberculosis in Abidjan, Cote d'Ivoire. Lancet 345:607, 1995.
25. Whalen C, Horsburgh CR, Hom D, et al: Accelerated course of human immunodeficiency virus infection after tuberculosis. Am J Respir Crit Care Med 151:129, 1995.
26. Wallis RS, Vjecha M, Amir-Tahmasseb M, et al: Influence of tuberculosis on human immunodeficiency virus (HIV-1): Enhanced cytokine expression and elevated beta 2-microglobulin in HIV-1-associated tuberculosis. J Infect Dis 167:43, 1993.
27. Ansari NA, Kombe AH, Kenyon TA, et al: Pathology and causes of death in a group of 128 predominantly HIV-positive patients in Botswana, 1997–1998. Int J Tuberc Lung Dis 6:55, 2002.
28. Lucas SB, Hounnou A, Peacock C, et al: The mortality and pathology of HIV infection in a west African city. AIDS 7:1569, 1993.
29. Karalliedde S, Katugaha LP, Uragoda CG: Tuberculin response of Sri Lankan children after BCG vaccination at birth. Tubercle 68:33, 1987.
30. Streeton JA, Desem N, Jones SL: Sensitivity and specificity of a gamma interferon blood test for tuberculosis infection. Int J Tuberc Lung Dis 2:443, 1998.
31. Mazurek GH, LoBue PA, Daley CL, et al: Comparison of a whole-blood interferon gamma assay with tuberculin skin testing for detecting latent *Mycobacterium tuberculosis* infection. JAMA 286:1740, 2001.
32. Anonymous: Tuberculosis and AIDS—Connecticut. MMWR 36:133, 1987.
33. Proudfoot AT, Akhtar AJ, Douglas AC, et al: Miliary tuberculosis in adults. Br Med J 2:273, 1969.
34. Stead WW, Kerby GR, Schlueter DP, et al: The clinical spectrum of primary tuberculosis in adults. Confusion with reinfection in the pathogenesis of chronic tuberculosis. Ann Intern Med 68:731, 1968.
35. Khan MA, Kovnat DM, Bachus B, et al: Clinical and roentgenographic spectrum of pulmonary tuberculosis in the adult. Am J Med 62:31, 1977.
36. Palmer PE: Pulmonary tuberculosis—Usual and unusual radiographic presentations. Semin Roentgenol 14:204, 1979.
37. Segarra R, Sherman DJ, Rodriguez-Aguero J: Lower lung field tuberculosis. Am Rev Respir Dis 87:37, 1963.
38. Barza M, Weinstein L: Uncommon presentations of pulmonary tuberculosis in adults. Postgrad Med 51:143, 1972.
39. Davis SD, Yankelevitz DF, Williams T, et al: Pulmonary tuberculosis in immunocompromised hosts: Epidemiological, clinical, and radiological assessment. Semin Roentgenol 28:119, 1993.
40. Goodman PC: Pulmonary tuberculosis in patients with acquired immunodeficiency syndrome. J Thorac Imaging 5:38, 1990.
41. McAdams HP, Erasmus J, Winter JA: Radiologic manifestations of pulmonary tuberculosis. Radiol Clin North Am 33:655, 1995.
42. Schaaf HS, Beyers N, Gie RP, et al: Respiratory tuberculosis in childhood: The diagnostic value of clinical features and special investigations. Pediatr Infect Dis J 14:189, 1995.
43. Houwert KA, Borggreven PA, Schaaf HS, et al: Prospective evaluation of World Health Organization criteria to assist diagnosis of tuberculosis in children. Eur Respir J 11:1116, 1998.
44. Donald PR, Fourie PB, Grange JM: Tuberculosis in Childhood. Pretoria, South Africa, J.L. Van Shaik, 1999.
45. Greenberg SD, Frager D, Suster B, et al: Active pulmonary tuberculosis in patients with AIDS: Spectrum of radiographic findings (including a normal appearance). Radiology 193:115, 1994.
46. Keiper MD, Beumont M, Elshami A, et al: CD4 T lymphocyte count and the radiographic presentation of pulmonary tuberculosis. A study of the relationship between these factors in patients with human immunodeficiency virus infection. Chest 107:74, 1995.
47. Lucas SB, Peacock CS, Hounnou A, et al: Disease in children infected with HIV in Abidjan, Cote d'Ivoire. BMJ 312:335, 1996.
48. Pitchenik AE, Burr J, Suarez M, et al: Human T-cell lymphotropic virus-III (HTLV-III) seropositivity and related disease among 71 consecutive patients in whom tuberculosis was diagnosed. A prospective study. Am Rev Respir Dis 135:875, 1987.
49. Pitchenik AE, Cole C, Russell BW, et al: Tuberculosis, atypical mycobacteriosis, and the acquired immunodeficiency syndrome among Haitian and non-Haitian patients in south Florida. Ann Intern Med 101:641, 1984.
50. Handwerger S, Mildvan D, Senie R, et al: Tuberculosis and the acquired immunodeficiency syndrome at a New York City hospital: 1978–1985. Chest 91:176, 1987.
51. Louie E, Rice LB, Holzman RS: Tuberculosis in non-Haitian patients with acquired immunodeficiency syndrome. Chest 90:542, 1986.
52. Reider HL, Cauthen GM, Comstock GW, et al: Epidemiology of tuberculosis in the United States. Epidemiol Rev 11:29, 1989.
53. Rieder HL, Cauthen GM, Bloch AB, et al: Tuberculosis and acquired immunodeficiency syndrome—Florida. Arch Intern Med 149:1268, 1989.
54. Tuberculosis and acquired immunodeficiency syndrome—New York City. MMWR 36:785, 1987.
55. Perlman DC, el-Sadr WM, Nelson ET, et al: Variation of chest radiographic patterns in pulmonary tuberculosis by degree of human immunodeficiency virus-related immunosuppression. Clin Infect Dis 25:242, 1997.
56. Shafer RW, Goldberg R, Sierra M, et al: Frequency of *Mycobacterium tuberculosis* bacteremia in patients with tuberculosis in an area endemic for AIDS. Am Rev Respir Dis 140:1611, 1989.
57. Kramer F, Modilevsky T, Waliany AR, et al: Delayed diagnosis of tuberculosis in patients with human immunodeficiency virus infection. Am J Med 89:451, 1990.
58. Modilevsky T, Sattler FR, Barnes PF: Mycobacterial disease in patients with human immunodeficiency virus infection. Arch Intern Med 149:2201, 1989.
59. Long R, Maycher B, Scalcini M, et al: The chest roentgenogram in pulmonary TB patients seropositive for human immunodeficiency virus type 1. Chest 99:123, 1991.

60. Brindle RJ, Nunn PP, Githui W, et al: Quantitative bacillary response to treatment in HIV-associated pulmonary tuberculosis. Am Rev Respir Dis 147:958, 1993.
61. Elliott AM, Namaambo K, Allen BW, et al: Negative sputum smear results in HIV-positive patients with pulmonary tuberculosis in Lusaka, Zambia. Tuberc Lung Dis 74:191, 1993.
62. Klein NC, Duncanson FP, Lenox TH 3rd, et al: Use of mycobacterial smears in the diagnosis of pulmonary tuberculosis in AIDS/ARC patients. Chest 95:1190, 1989.
63. Perronne C, Ghoubontni A, Leport C, et al: Should pulmonary tuberculosis be an AIDS-defining diagnosis in patients infected with HIV? Tuberc Lung Dis 73:39, 1992.
64. Theuer CP, Hopewell PC, Elias D, et al: Human immunodeficiency virus infection in tuberculosis patients. J Infect Dis 162:8, 1990.
65. Di Perri G, Cazzadori A, Vento S, et al: Comparative histopathological study of pulmonary tuberculosis in human immunodeficiency virus-infected and non-infected patients. Tuberc Lung Dis 77:244, 1996.
66. Cauthen GM, Dooley SW, Onorato IM, et al: Transmission of *Mycobacterium tuberculosis* from tuberculosis patients with HIV infection or AIDS. Am J Epidemiol 144:69, 1996.
67. Cruciani M, Malena M, Bosco O, et al: The impact of human immunodeficiency virus type 1 on infectiousness of tuberculosis: A meta-analysis. Clin Infect Dis 33:1922, 2001.
68. Carvalho AC, DeRiemer K, Nunes ZB, et al: Transmission of *Mycobacterium tuberculosis* to contacts of HIV-infected tuberculosis patients. Am J Respir Crit Care Med 164:2166, 2001.
69. Klausner JD, Ryder RW, Baende E, et al: *Mycobacterium tuberculosis* in household contacts of human immunodeficiency virus type 1-seropositive patients with active pulmonary tuberculosis in Kinshasa, Zaire. J Infect Dis 168:106, 1993.
70. Nunn P, Mungai M, Nyamwaya J, et al: The effect of human immunodeficiency virus type-1 on the infectiousness of tuberculosis. Tuberc Lung Dis 75:25, 1994.
71. Espinal MA, Perez EN, Baez J, et al: Infectiousness of *Mycobacterium tuberculosis* in HIV-1-infected patients with tuberculosis: A prospective study. Lancet 355:275, 2000.
72. Wallgren A: The time-table of tuberculosis. Tubercle 29:245, 1948.
73. Saks AM, Posner R: Tuberculosis in HIV positive patients in South Africa: A comparative radiological study with HIV negative patients. Clin Radiol 46:387, 1992.
74. Frye MD, Pozsik CJ, Sahn SA: Tuberculous pleurisy is more common in AIDS than in non-AIDS patients with tuberculosis. Chest 112:393, 1997.
75. Allen JC, Apicella MA: Experimental pleural effusion as a manifestation of delayed hypersensitivity to tuberculin PPD. J Immunol 101:481, 1968.
76. Fujiwara H, Tsuyuguchi I: Frequency of tuberculin-reactive T-lymphocytes in pleural fluid and blood from patients with tuberculous pleurisy. Chest 89:530, 1986.
77. Shimokata K, Kawachi H, Kishimoto H, et al: Local cellular immunity in tuberculous pleurisy. Am Rev Respir Dis 126:822, 1982.
78. Ribera E, Ocana I, Martinez-Vazquez JM, et al: High level of interferon gamma in tuberculous pleural effusion. Chest 93:308, 1988.
79. Ribera E, Espanol T, Martinez-Vazquez JM, et al: Lymphocyte proliferation and gamma-interferon production after "in vitro" stimulation with PPD. Differences between tuberculous and nontuberculous pleurisy in patients with positive tuberculin skin test. Chest 97:1381, 1990.
80. Barnes PF, Fong SJ, Brennan PJ, et al: Local production of tumor necrosis factor and IFN-gamma in tuberculous pleuritis. J Immunol 145:149, 1990.
81. Hodsdon WS, Luzze H, Hurst TJ, et al: HIV-1-related pleural tuberculosis: Elevated production of IFN-gamma, but failure of immunity to *Mycobacterium tuberculosis*. AIDS 15:467, 2001.
82. Levine H, Szanto PB, Cugell DW: Tuberculous pleurisy. An acute illness. Arch Intern Med 122:329, 1968.
83. Berger HW, Mejia E: Tuberculous pleurisy. Chest 63:88, 1973.
84. Sibley JC: A study of 200 cases of tuberculous pleurisy with effusion. Am Rev Tuberc 62:314, 1950.
85. Ellner JJ: Pleural fluid and peripheral blood lymphocyte function in tuberculosis. Ann Intern Med 89:932, 1978.
86. Ellner JJ: Suppressor adherent cells in human tuberculosis. J Immunol 121:2573, 1978.
87. Hurwitz S, Leiman G, Shapiro C: Mesothelial cells in pleural fluid: TB or not TB? S Afr Med J 57:937, 1980.
88. Valdes L, Pose A, San Jose E, et al: Tuberculous pleural effusions. Eur J Intern Med 14:77, 2003.
89. Scharer L, McClement JH: Isolation of tubercle bacilli from needle biopsy specimens of parietal pleura. Am Rev Respir Dis 97:466, 1968.
90. Levine H, Metzger W, Lacera D, et al: Diagnosis of tuberculous pleurisy by culture of pleural biopsy specimen. Arch Intern Med 126:269, 1970.
91. Luzze H, Elliott AM, Joloba ML, et al: Evaluation of suspected tuberculous pleurisy: Clinical and diagnostic findings in HIV-1-positive and HIV-negative adults in Uganda. Int J Tuberc Lung Dis 5:746, 2001.
92. Patiala J: Initial tuberculous pleuritis in the Finnish armed forces in 1939–1945 with special reference to eventual post-pleuritic tuberculosis. Acta Tuberc Scand Suppl 15:1, 1954.
93. Roper WH, Waring JJ: Primary serofibrinous pleurisy with effusion in military personnel. Am Rev Tuberc 71:616, 1955.
94. Dutt AK, Moers D, Stead WW: Short-course chemotherapy for pleural tuberculosis. Nine years' experience in routine treatment service. Chest 90:112, 1986.
95. Dutt AK, Moers D, Stead WW: Tuberculous pleural effusion: 6-month therapy with isoniazid and rifampin. Am Rev Respir Dis 145:1429, 1992.
96. Lee CH, Wang WJ, Lan RS, et al: Corticosteroids in the treatment of tuberculous pleurisy. A double-blind, placebo-controlled, randomized study. Chest 94:1256, 1988.
97. Sahn SA, Iseman MD: Tuberculous empyema. Semin Respir Infect 14:82, 1999.
98. Wolinsky E: Mycobacterial lymphadenitis in children: A prospective study of 105 nontuberculous cases with long-term follow-up. Clin Infect Dis 20:954, 1995.
99. Gonzalez OY, Teeter LD, Thanh BT, et al: Extrathoracic tuberculosis lymphadenitis in adult HIV seronegative patients: A population-based analysis in Houston, Texas, USA. Int J Tuberc Lung Dis 7:987, 2003.
100. Lau SK, Kwan S, Lee J, et al: Source of tubercle bacilli in cervical lymph nodes: A prospective study. J Laryngol Otol 105:558, 1991.
101. Appling D, Miller RH: Mycobacterium cervical lymphadenopathy: 1981 update. Laryngoscope 91:1259, 1981.
102. Huhti E, Brander E, Paloheimo S, et al: Tuberculosis of the cervical lymph nodes: A clinical, pathological and bacteriological study. Tubercle 56:27, 1975.
103. Lau SK, Wei WI, Hsu C, et al: Efficacy of fine needle aspiration cytology in the diagnosis of tuberculous cervical lymphadenopathy. J Laryngol Otol 104:24, 1990.
104. Bem C, Patil PS, Elliott AM, et al: The value of wide-needle aspiration in the diagnosis of tuberculous lymphadenitis in Africa. AIDS 7:1221, 1993.
105. British Thoracic Society Research Committee: Short course chemotherapy for lymph node tuberculosis: Final report at 5 years. Br J Dis Chest 82:282, 1988.
106. Gorse GJ, Pais MJ, Kusske JA, et al: Tuberculous spondylitis. A report of six cases and a review of the literature. Medicine (Baltimore) 62:178, 1983.
107. Berney S, Goldstein M, Bishko F: Clinical and diagnostic features of tuberculous arthritis. Am J Med 53:36, 1972.
108. Hodgman JR, Skinsnes DH, Leong CY: The pathogenesis of Pott's paraplegia. J Bone Joint Surg Am 49:1167, 1967.
109. Newton P, Sharp J, Barnes KL: Bone and joint tuberculosis in greater Manchester 1969–79. Ann Rheum Dis 41:1, 1982.
110. Davies PD, Humphries MJ, Byfield SP, et al: Bone and joint tuberculosis. A survey of notifications in England and Wales. J Bone Joint Surg Br 66:326, 1984.
111. Hold J: The value of histological and bacteriological examination in the tuberculosis of bones and joints. Acta Orthop Scand 35:91, 1964.
112. Medical Research Council Working Party on Tuberculosis of the Spine: First report: A controlled trial of ambulant outpatient treatment and in-patient rest in bed in the management of tuberculosis of the spine in young Korean patients on standard chemotherapy. J Bone Joint Surg Br 55:678, 1973.
113. Medical Research Council Working Party on Tuberculosis of the Spine: Fifth report: A five-year assessment of controlled trials of in-patient and out-patient treatment and of plaster-of-Paris jackets for tuberculosis of the spine in children on standard chemotherapy. Studies in Masan and Pusan, Korea. J Bone Joint Surg Br 58B:399, 1976.

114. Medical Research Council Working Party on Tuberculosis of the Spine: Sixth report: Five-year assessments of controlled trials of ambulatory treatment, debridement and anterior spinal fusion in the management of tuberculosis of the spine. Studies in Bulawayo (Rhodesia) and in Hong Kong. J Bone Joint Surg Br 60B:163, 1978.
115. Medical Research Council Working Party on Tuberculosis of the Spine: Eighth report: A 10-year assessment of a controlled trial comparing debridement and anterior spinal fusion in the management of tuberculosis of the spine in patients on standard chemotherapy in Hong Kong. J Bone Joint Surg Br 64:393, 1982.
116. Glasser RM, Walker RI, Herion JC: The significance of hematologic abnormalities in patients with tuberculosis. Arch Intern Med 125:691, 1970.
117. Sahn SA, Neff TA: Miliary tuberculosis. Am J Med 56:494, 1974.
118. Maartens G, Willcox PA, Benatar SR: Miliary tuberculosis: Rapid diagnosis, hematologic abnormalities, and outcome in 109 treated adults. Am J Med 89:291, 1990.
119. Munt PW: Miliary tuberculosis in the chemotherapy era: With a clinical review in 69 American adults. Medicine (Baltimore) 51:139, 1972.
120. Gelb AF, Leffler C, Brewin A, et al: Miliary tuberculosis. Am Rev Respir Dis 108:1327, 1973.
121. Berger HW, Samortin TG: Miliary tuberculosis: Diagnostic methods with emphasis on the chest roentgenogram. Chest 58:586, 1970.
122. Grieco MH, Chmel H: Acute disseminated tuberculosis as a diagnostic problem. A clinical study based on twenty-eight cases. Am Rev Respir Dis 109:554, 1974.
123. Bobrowitz ID: Active tuberculosis undiagnosed until autopsy. Am J Med 72:650, 1982.
124. Kim JH, Langston AA, Gallis HA: Miliary tuberculosis: Epidemiology, clinical manifestations, diagnosis, and outcome. Rev Infect Dis 12:583, 1990.
125. Burk JR, Viroslav J, Bynum LJ: Miliary tuberculosis diagnosed by fibreoptic bronchoscopy and transbronchial biopsy. Tubercle 59:107, 1978.
126. Ramachandran P, Duraipandian M, Nagarajan M, et al: Three chemotherapy studies of tuberculous meningitis in children. Tubercle 67:17, 1986.
127. Berenguer J, Moreno S, Laguna F, et al: Tuberculous meningitis in patients infected with the human immunodeficiency virus. N Engl J Med 326:668, 1992.
128. Shafer RW, Kim DS, Weiss JP, et al: Extrapulmonary tuberculosis in patients with human immunodeficiency virus infection. Medicine (Baltimore) 70:384, 1991.
129. Bouza E, Martin-Scapa C, Bernaldo de Quiros JC, et al: High prevalence of tuberculosis in AIDS patients in Spain. Eur J Clin Microbiol Infect Dis 7:785, 1988.
130. Auerbach O: Tuberculous meningitis: Correlation of therapeutic results with the pathogenesis and pathologic changes. I. General considerations and pathogenesis. Am Rev Tuberc 64:408, 1951.
131. Rich AR, McCordock HA: The pathogenesis of tuberculous meningitis. Johns Hopkins Hosp Bull 52:5, 1933.
132. Idriss ZH, Sinno AA, Kronfol NM: Tuberculous meningitis in childhood. Forty-three cases. Am J Dis Child 130:364, 1976.
133. Barrett-Connor E: Tuberculous meningitis in adults. South Med J 60:1061, 1967.
134. Klein NC, Damsker B, Hirschman SZ: Mycobacterial meningitis. Retrospective analysis from 1970 to 1983. Am J Med 79:29, 1985.
135. Kennedy DH, Fallon RJ: Tuberculous meningitis. JAMA 241:264, 1979.
136. Dube MP, Holtom PD, Larsen RA: Tuberculous meningitis in patients with and without human immunodeficiency virus infection. Am J Med 93:520, 1992.
137. Crocco JA, Blecker MJ, Rooney JJ Jr, et al: Tuberculous meningitis in adults: Clinical analysis. NY State J Med 80:1231, 1980.
138. Stockstill MT, Kauffman CA: Comparison of cryptococcal and tuberculous meningitis. Arch Neurol 40:81, 1983.
139. Zarabi M, Sane S, Girdany BR: The chest roentgenogram in the early diagnosis of tuberculous meningitis in children. Am J Dis Child 121:389, 1971.
140. Hinman AR: Tuberculous meningitis at Cleveland Metropolitan General Hospital 1959 to 1963. Am Rev Respir Dis 95:670, 1967.
141. Sumaya CV, Simek M, Smith MH, et al: Tuberculous meningitis in children during the isoniazid era. J Pediatr 87:43, 1975.
142. Haas EJ, Madhavan T, Quinn EL, et al: Tuberculous meningitis in an urban general hospital. Arch Intern Med 137:1518, 1977.
143. Karandanis D, Shulman JA: Recent survey of infectious meningitis in adults: Review of laboratory findings in bacterial, tuberculous, and aseptic meningitis. South Med J 69:449, 1976.
144. Smith J, Godwin-Austen R: Hypersecretion of anti-diuretic hormone due to tuberculous meningitis. Postgrad Med J 56:41, 1980.
145. Lincoln EM, Sordillo SVR, Davies PA: Tuberculous meningitis in children. A review of 167 untreated and 74 treated patients with special reference to early diagnosis. J Pediatr 57:807, 1960.
146. Fishman RA: The Cerebrospinal Fluid in Diseases of the Nervous System. Philadelphia, WB Saunders, 1980, p 265.
147. Lepper MH, Spies HW: The present status of the treatment of tuberculosis of the central nervous system. Ann NY Acad Sci 106:106, 1963.
148. Ogawa SK, Smith MA, Brennessel DJ, et al: Tuberculous meningitis in an urban medical center. Medicine (Baltimore) 66:317, 1987.
149. Miorner H, Sjobring U, Nayak P, et al: Diagnosis of tuberculous meningitis: A comparative analysis of 3 immunoassays, an immune complex assay and the polymerase chain reaction. Tuberc Lung Dis 76:381, 1995.
150. Kaur A, Basha A, Ranjan M, et al: Poor diagnostic value of adenosine deaminase in pleural, peritoneal & cerebrospinal fluids in tuberculosis. Indian J Med Res 95:270, 1992.
151. Seth P, Ahuja GK, Bhanu NV, et al: Evaluation of polymerase chain reaction for rapid diagnosis of clinically suspected tuberculous meningitis. Tuberc Lung Dis 77:353, 1996.
152. Ellner JJ, Bennett JE: Chronic meningitis. Medicine (Baltimore) 55:341, 1976.
153. DesPrez RM, Boone IU: Metabolism of O^{14}-isoniazid in humans. Am Rev Respir Dis 84:42, 1961.
154. Tuchman AJ, Berger S, Daras M: Cerebrospinal fluid penetration of anti-infective agents. South Med J 77:1443, 1984.
155. Donald PR, Schoeman JF, Van Zyl LE, et al: Intensive short course chemotherapy in the management of tuberculous meningitis. Int J Tuberc Lung Dis 2:704, 1998.
156. Girgis NI, Farid Z, Kilpatrick ME, et al: Dexamethasone adjunctive treatment for tuberculous meningitis. Pediatr Infect Dis J 10:179, 1991.
157. Escobar JA, Belsey MA, Duenas A, et al: Mortality from tuberculous meningitis reduced by steroid therapy. Pediatrics 56:1050, 1975.
158. Schoeman JF, Van Zyl LE, Laubscher JA, et al: Effect of corticosteroids on intracranial pressure, computed tomographic findings, and clinical outcome in young children with tuberculous meningitis. Pediatrics 99:226, 1997.
159. Kilpatrick ME, Girgis NI, Yassin MW, et al: Tuberculous meningitis—Clinical and laboratory review of 100 patients. J Hyg (London) 96:231, 1986.
160. Smith AL: Tuberculous meningitis in childhood. Med J Aust 1:57, 1975.
161. Wise GJ, Marella VK: Genitourinary manifestations of tuberculosis. Urol Clin North Am 30:111, 2003.
162. Simon HB, Weinstein AJ, Pasternak MS, et al: Genitourinary tuberculosis. Clinical features in a general hospital population. Am J Med 63:410, 1977.
163. Christensen WI: Genitourinary tuberculosis: Review of 102 cases. Medicine (Baltimore) 53:377, 1974.
164. Lattimer JK: Renal tuberculosis. N Engl J Med 273:208, 1965.
165. Sutherland AM: Gynaecological tuberculosis: Analysis of a personal series of 710 cases. Aust N Z J Obstet Gynaecol 25:203, 1985.
166. Gorse GJ, Belshe RB: Male genital tuberculosis: A review of the literature with instructive case reports. Rev Infect Dis 7:511, 1985.
167. Hageman JH, D'Esopo ND, Glenn WW: Tuberculosis of the pericardium. A long-term analysis of forty-four proved cases. N Engl J Med 270:327, 1964.
168. Rooney JJ, Crocco JA, Lyons HA: Tuberculous pericarditis. Ann Intern Med 72:73, 1970.
169. Fowler NO, Manitsas GT: Infectious pericarditis. Prog Cardiovasc Dis 16:323, 1973.
170. Strang JI, Kakaza HH, Gibson DG, et al: Controlled clinical trial of complete open surgical drainage and of prednisolone in treatment of tuberculous pericardial effusion in Transkei. Lancet 2:759, 1988.
171. Strang JIG, Nunn AJ, Johnson DA, et al: Management of tuberculous constrictive pericarditis and tuberculous pericardial effusion in Transkei: Results at 10 years follow-up. Q J Med 97:525, 2004.

172. Strang JI, Kakaza HH, Gibson DG, et al: Controlled trial of prednisolone as adjuvant in treatment of tuberculous constrictive pericarditis in Transkei. Lancet 2:1418, 1987.
173. Hakim JG, Ternouth I, Mushangi E, et al: Double blind randomised placebo controlled trial of adjunctive prednisolone in the treatment of effusive tuberculous pericarditis in HIV seropositive patients. Heart 84:183, 2000.
174. Bastani B, Shariatzadeh MR, Dehdashti F: Tuberculous peritonitis—Report of 30 cases and review of the literature. Q J Med 56:549, 1985.
175. Burack WR, Hollister RM: Tuberculous peritonitis. A study of forty-seven proved cases encountered by a general medical unit in twenty-five years. Am J Med 28:510, 1960.
176. Karney WW, O'Donoghue JM, Ostrow JH, et al: The spectrum of tuberculous peritonitis. Chest 72:310, 1977.
177. Singh MM, Bhargava AN, Jain KP: Tuberculous peritonitis. An evaluation of pathogenetic mechanisms, diagnostic procedures and therapeutic measures. N Engl J Med 281:1091, 1969.
178. Jorge AD: Peritoneal tuberculosis. Endoscopy 16:10, 1984.
179. Kakakhel KU, Fritsch P: Cutaneous tuberculosis. Int J Dermatol 28:355, 1989.
180. Wortman PD: Pulmonary and cutaneous tuberculosis. J Am Acad Dermatol 27:459, 1992.
181. Marcoval J, Servitje O, Moreno A, et al: Lupus vulgaris. Clinical, histopathologic, and bacteriologic study of 10 cases. J Am Acad Dermatol 26:404, 1992.
182. Slavin RE, Walsh TJ, Pollack AD: Late generalized tuberculosis: A clinical pathologic analysis and comparison of 100 cases in the preantibiotic and antibiotic eras. Medicine (Baltimore) 59:352, 1980.
183. Sadek MI, Sada E, Toossi Z, et al: Chemokines induced by infection of mononuclear phagocytes with mycobacteria and present in lung alveoli during active pulmonary tuberculosis. Am J Respir Cell Mol Biol 19:513, 1998.
184. Wallis RS, Ellner JJ: Cytokines and tuberculosis. J Leukoc Biol 55:676, 1994.
185. Maggi E, Parronchi P, Manetti R, et al: Reciprocal regulatory effects of IFN-gamma and IL-4 on the in vitro development of human Th1 and Th2 clones. J Immunol 148:2142, 1992.
186. Muller I, Cobbold SP, Waldmann H, et al: Impaired resistance to *Mycobacterium tuberculosis* infection after selective in vivo depletion of L3T4+ and Lyt-2+ T cells. Infect Immun 55:2037, 1987.
187. Orme IM: Characteristics and specificity of acquired immunologic memory to *Mycobacterium tuberculosis* infection. J Immunol 140:3589, 1988.
188. Jones BE, Young SM, Antoniskis D, et al: Relationship of the manifestations of tuberculosis to CD4 cell counts in patients with human immunodeficiency virus infection. Am Rev Respir Dis 148:1292, 1993.
189. Barnes PF, Bloch AB, Davidson PT, et al: Tuberculosis in patients with human immunodeficiency virus infection. N Engl J Med 324:1644, 1991.
190. Cho S, Mehra V, Thoma-Uszynski S, et al: Antimicrobial activity of MHC class I-restricted CD8+ T cells in human tuberculosis. Proc Natl Acad Sci USA 97:12210, 2000.
191. Lewinsohn DA, Heinzel AS, Gardner JM, et al: *Mycobacterium tuberculosis*-specific CD8+ T cells preferentially recognize heavily infected cells. Am J Respir Crit Care Med 168:1346, 2003.
192. Teitelbaum R, Glatman-Freedman A, Chen B, et al: A mAb recognizing a surface antigen of *Mycobacterium tuberculosis* enhances host survival. Proc Natl Acad Sci USA 95:15688, 1998.
193. Glatman-Freedman A: Advances in antibody-mediated immunity against *Mycobacterium tuberculosis*: Implications for a novel vaccine strategy. FEMS Immunol Med Microbiol 39:9, 2003.
194. van Rie A, Warren R, Richardson M, et al: Exogenous reinfection as a cause of recurrent tuberculosis after curative treatment. N Engl J Med 341:1174, 1999.
195. Nardell E, McInnis B, Thomas B, et al: Exogenous reinfection with tuberculosis in a shelter for the homeless. N Engl J Med 315:1570, 1986.
196. Alland D, Kalkut GE, Moss AR, et al: Transmission of tuberculosis in New York City. An analysis by DNA fingerprinting and conventional epidemiologic methods. N Engl J Med 330:1710, 1994.
197. Small PM, Hopewell PC, Singh SP, et al: The epidemiology of tuberculosis in San Francisco. A population-based study using conventional and molecular methods. N Engl J Med 330:1703, 1994.
198. Ribeiro-Rodrigues R, Resende Co T, Johnson JL, et al: Sputum cytokine levels in patients with pulmonary tuberculosis as early markers of mycobacterial clearance. Clin Diagn Lab Immunol 9:818, 2002.
199. Hirsch CS, Toossi Z, Othieno C, et al: Depressed T-cell interferon-gamma responses in pulmonary tuberculosis: Analysis of underlying mechanisms and modulation with therapy. J Infect Dis 180:2069, 1999.
200. Manca C, Tsenova L, Barry CE 3rd, et al: *Mycobacterium tuberculosis* CDC1551 induces a more vigorous host response in vivo and in vitro, but is not more virulent than other clinical isolates. J Immunol 162:6740, 1999.
201. Canetti G: Present aspects of bacterial resistance in tuberculosis. Am Rev Respir Dis 92:687, 1965.
202. Mitchison DA, Nunn AJ: Influence of initial drug resistance on the response to short-course chemotherapy of pulmonary tuberculosis. Am Rev Respir Dis 133:423, 1986.
203. Espinal MA, Laszlo A, Simonsen L, et al: Global trends in resistance to antituberculosis drugs. N Engl J Med 344:1294, 2001.
204. Espinal MA, Laserson K, Camacho M, et al: Determinants of drug-resistant tuberculosis: Analysis of 11 countries. Int J Tuberc Lung Dis 5:887, 2001.
205. Hobby GL, Holman AP, Iseman MD, et al: Enumeration of tubercle bacilli in sputum of patients with pulmonary tuberculosis. Antimicrob Agents Chemother 4:94, 1973.
206. Dutt AK, Stead WW: Short-course chemotherapy. The Arkansas experience. Chest 80:724, 1981.
207. Gunnels JJ, Bates JH, Swindoll H: Infectivity of sputum-positive tuberculous patients on chemotherapy. Am Rev Respir Dis 109:323, 1974.
208. Kim TC, Blackman RS, Heatwole KM, et al: Acid-fast bacilli in sputum smears of patients with pulmonary tuberculosis. Prevalence and significance of negative smears pretreatment and positive smears post-treatment. Am Rev Respir Dis 129:264, 1984.
209. Narain R, Rao MS, Chandrasekhar P, et al: Microscopy positive and microscopy negative cases of pulmonary tuberculosis. Am Rev Respir Dis 103:761, 1971.
210. Kubica GP, Gross WM, Hawkins JE, et al: Laboratory services for mycobacterial diseases. Am Rev Respir Dis 112:773, 1975.
211. Berean K, Roberts FJ: The reliability of acid fast stained smears of gastric aspirate specimens. Tubercle 69:205, 1988.
212. Klotz SA, Penn RL: Acid-fast staining of urine and gastric contents is an excellent indicator of mycobacterial disease. Am Rev Respir Dis 136:1197, 1987.
213. Danek SJ, Bower JS: Diagnosis of pulmonary tuberculosis by flexible fiberoptic bronchoscopy. Am Rev Respir Dis 119:677, 1979.
214. So SY, Lam WK, Yu DY: Rapid diagnosis of suspected pulmonary tuberculosis by fiberoptic bronchoscopy. Tubercle 63:195, 1982.
215. Wallace JM, Deutsch AL, Harrell JH, et al: Bronchoscopy and transbronchial biopsy in evaluation of patients with suspected active tuberculosis. Am J Med 70:1189, 1981.
216. Kennedy DJ, Lewis WP, Barnes PF: Yield of bronchoscopy for the diagnosis of tuberculosis in patients with human immunodeficiency virus infection. Chest 102:1040, 1992.
217. Willcox PA, Benatar SR, Potgieter PD: Use of the flexible fibreoptic bronchoscope in diagnosis of sputum-negative pulmonary tuberculosis. Thorax 37:598, 1982.
218. Watterson SA, Drobniewski FA: Modern laboratory diagnosis of mycobacterial infections. J Clin Pathol 53:727, 2000.
219. Dunlap NE, Bass J, Fujiwara P, et al: Diagnostic standards and classification of tuberculosis in adults and children. Am J Respir Crit Care Med 161:1376, 2000.
220. Kent PT, Kubica GP: Public Health Mycobacteriology: A Guide for the Level III Laboratory. Atlanta, Centers for Disease Control, 1985.
221. Canetti G, Fox W, Khomenko A, et al: Advances in techniques of testing mycobacterial drug sensitivity, and the use of sensitivity tests in tuberculosis control programmes. Bull WHO 41:21, 1969.
222. Banaiee N, Bobadilla-del-Valle M, Riska PF, et al: Rapid identification and susceptibility testing of *Mycobacterium tuberculosis* from MGIT cultures with luciferase reporter mycobacteriophages. J Med Microbiol 52:557, 2003.
223. Riska PF, Su Y, Bardarov S, et al: Rapid film-based determination of antibiotic susceptibilities of *Mycobacterium tuberculosis* strains by using a luciferase reporter phage and the Bronx Box. J Clin Microbiol 37:1144, 1999.

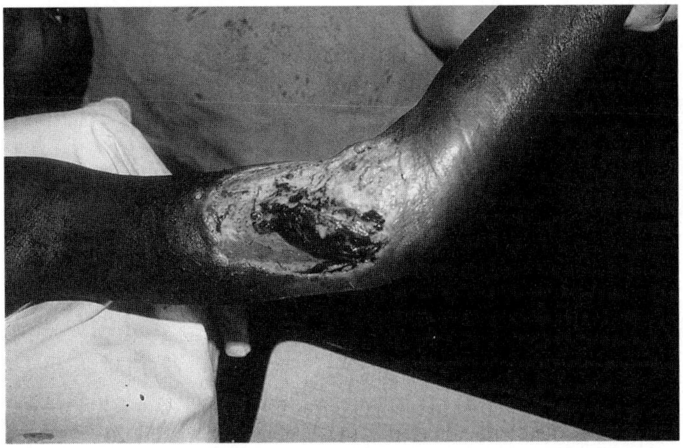

FIGURE 37-7 Plaque/edematous lesion extending from wrist to axilla with a large ragged ulcer at the elbow of a 10-year-old boy in Benin.

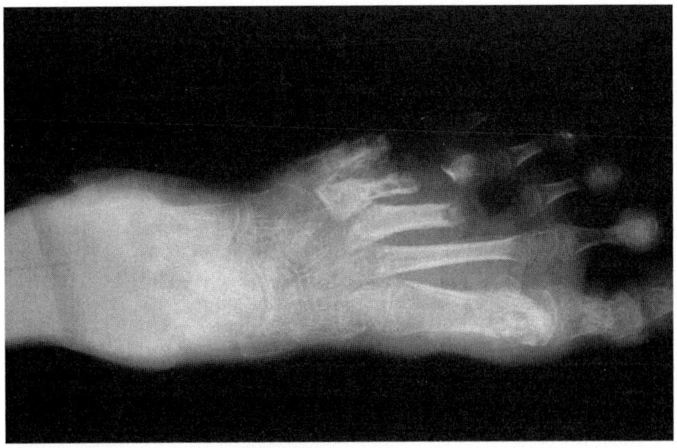

FIGURE 37-8 Radiograph shows contiguous osteomyelitis of the phalanges and metatarsal bones directly under a major ulcer of *M. ulcerans* disease on the dorsum of the foot.

Edematous Form

The edematous lesion is characterized by diffuse, firm, nonpitting thickening of the skin, with margins that frequently are clinically imperceptible. Lesions are not painful. Often there are color changes of the skin. Size of lesions ranges from small (5 cm in diameter) to massive, sometimes involving an entire extremity or even most of the trunk. There usually is no history or microscopic evidence of a nodule.[43]

Microscopically, there is massive contiguous coagulation necrosis similar to that of the other forms already mentioned. AFB are most plentiful in the deepest layers of the panniculus and fascia. Many lesions suggest that the AFB tend to proliferate along and just above the fascial plane. Necrosis extends far beyond the limits of spread of AFB.

Metastatic Disease

Potentially, *M. ulcerans* may enter the lymphatic system or bloodstream from any form of BU; however, it probably occurs more frequently with disseminated forms. Although clinical lymphadenopathy is not a feature of BU, local and regional lymph nodes reveal invasion of the afferent lymphatic vessels and cortical sinuses, often with extension into the medullary areas with necrosis. Targets for metastatic spread seem to be limited to skin and bone. Osteomyelitis, either contiguous (osteitis; Fig. 37-8) or metastatic, is seen in 10% to 15% of BU patients (Fig. 37-9).[44–46] Hematogenous spread appears to involve the epiphyseal/metaphyseal level initially in the long bones of the limbs, but the bones of the hands and feet are likewise affected.[38] Sometimes the soft tissue surrounding a bone is damaged to the extent that the bone becomes infarcted. Severe deformity and amputations are common sequelae of bone involvement. Microscopically, there is coagulation necrosis of the bone marrow and destruction of the trabeculae of the cancellous area of bones.

PATHOGENESIS AND IMMUNITY

The pathogenesis of early *M. ulcerans* infection is related closely to at least two known properties of the etiologic agent: optimal growth at 30° to 33°C and elaboration of a potent toxin.[22] Temperature requirement favors onset of lesions in skin. Toxin destroys tissue, providing a nutrient medium for bacillary proliferation and separating the organism from contact with immunocompetent cells. In vitro, the toxin is also directly immunosuppressive to both B and T cells.[11] Variations in clinical and histopathologic presentations of BU suggest that some individuals have innate resistance, some develop resistance early and others late, and a few seem to be totally anergic.

The skin test reagent "burulin" is a purified sonicate of cultured *M. ulcerans*. Intracutaneous inoculation of this reagent reveals that most BU patients do not show a delayed-type hypersensitivity response to *M. ulcerans* components early in the infection but do mount a cell-mediated response as healing begins.[47] This correlates well with the histopathologic appearance of delayed-type hypersensitivity granulomas in older lesions as they begin to heal. Presumably, the immunosuppressive effect on T cells, previously noted, and the immunologically isolated status of BU lesions resulting from the local necrosis limit the sensitization of immunocompetent cells in

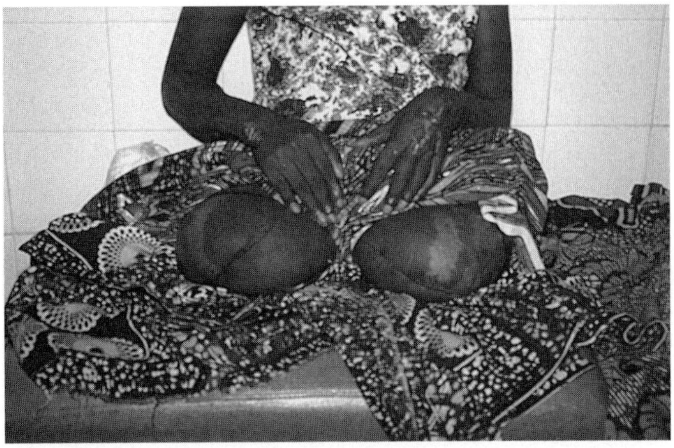

FIGURE 37-9 Amputations resulting from metastatic spread to bone of lower extremities. There is also spread to both wrists in this 13-year-old girl in Benin.

early and advancing stages of the disease.[11] The ultimate effect is T cell anergy, which prevents the development of the Th1 cellular response. Eventually there is sufficient immunostimulation by antigens of *M. ulcerans* to promote proliferation of peripheral blood mononuclear cells and production of γ-interferon to facilitate a Th1-type granulomatous response.[12,46,48,49] Sera from patients show humoral antibodies to soluble *M. ulcerans* antigens; however, their importance in pathogenesis and usefulness for diagnosis have not been defined.[50] Following the granulomatous stage, lesions heal by scarring.

Data on coinfection of BU and HIV are insufficient to establish increased susceptibility of patients with HIV/AIDS to BU. However, anecdotal observations suggest that BU disease is more aggressive in HIV-infected patients.[51]

DIAGNOSIS

The experienced observer in endemic areas usually can make an accurate clinical diagnosis.[52,53] In ulcerated lesions, Ziehl-Neelsen stains of smears of exudates from the undermined edge often reveal clusters of extracellular AFB (Fig. 37-10). The same material, after decontamination, may be used for culture on Löwenstein-Jensen or other suitable mycobacterial media. Incubation temperature must be 30° to 32°C. Transport media may be employed if stains and cultures cannot be performed locally. Molecular biologic analysis of exudates or biopsy specimens using PCR techniques are available for the identification of *M. ulcerans*.[16,54,55]

Specimens for histopathologic analysis should come from the edge of the ulcer and include all levels down to and including the fascia. In nonulcerative disease (plaque or edematous), specimens should be taken from the presumed center of the lesion. Ellipses of tissue are diagnostically more productive than punch biopsy specimens. The differential diagnosis is extensive. In specimens studied at the Armed Forces Institute of Pathology (AFIP), where the primary clinical diagnosis was BU, the authors noted the following histopathologic diagnoses:

- Infections: staphylococcal abscess, tropical phagedenic ulcer, tuberculosis, atypical mycobacterioses (other than *M. ulcerans*), Majocchi's granuloma, epididymitis, phycomycosis, phaeohyphomycosis, African histoplasmosis, filariasis, and leishmaniasis.
- Neoplasias: squamous and basal cell carcinomas, Kaposi's sarcoma, lymphoma, osteosarcoma, and a large variety of benign tumors of the skin such as fibromas and lipomas.
- Miscellaneous lesions: stasis ulcer, calcinosis cutis, epidermal cyst, gouty tophus, and foreign body granuloma.

TREATMENT AND PROGNOSIS

A number of therapeutic drug trials are under study and some are promising, but none has had sufficient evaluation to permit recommendation. Excisional surgery remains the recommended therapy (Figs. 37-11 and 37-12). To inhibit metastatic spread, surgeons should prescribe antibiotic therapy before surgery and continue this therapy postoperatively for 2 to 3 weeks. Rifampin and clarithromycin combined is the most frequently used regimen.

Papules and nonulcerated nodules are widely excised and usually closed primarily.[56] This procedure is usually curative.[57]

Plaques and edematous disease are excised widely down to or through the fascia if necrotic. Any involved muscle should be excised. Determining the limits of lateral extension of disease is often difficult. Experienced surgeons may be able to determine these limits by palpation, but exploratory incisions and blunt dissections are useful to establish the lines of excision.[44] Marginal recurrences are frequent and must be further excised. Sometimes the involvement of skin is so extensive (e.g., loss of 75% of the skin of the trunk) that the very insult of the surgery is life-threatening. Split-skin autografting is usually performed after sufficient granulation tissue has developed. Small ulcers may be excised and closed primarily.

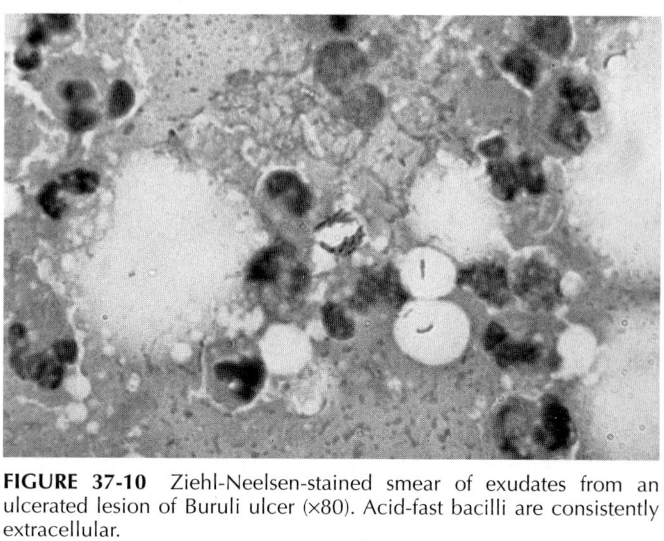

FIGURE 37-10 Ziehl-Neelsen-stained smear of exudates from an ulcerated lesion of Buruli ulcer (×80). Acid-fast bacilli are consistently extracellular.

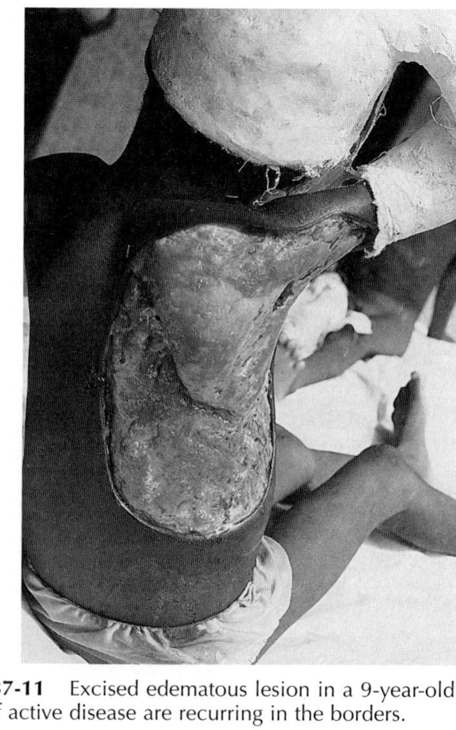

FIGURE 37-11 Excised edematous lesion in a 9-year-old girl in Togo. Pockets of active disease are recurring in the borders.

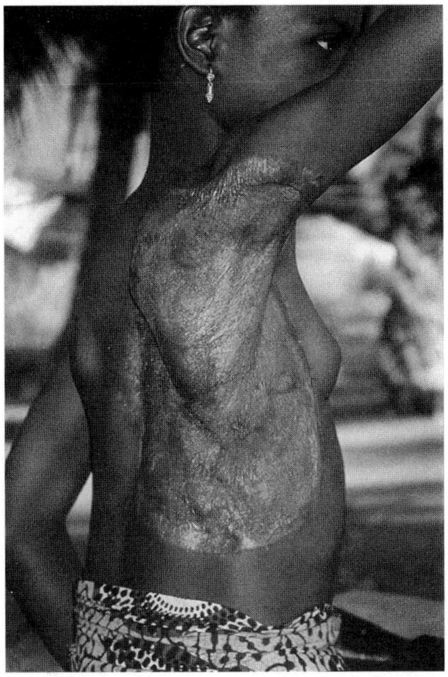

FIGURE 37-12 Patient in Figure 37-11 seen 5 years after complete excision and autologous split-skin grafting.

Large ulcers are excised using the principles described previously to determine the extent of excision. Postoperative care, especially physiotherapy, is essential for the prevention of contractures (Fig. 37-13). It is most important that the skin graft eventually covers the lesion completely because actinic radiation is strong in most endemic areas, resulting in cancers in nonpigmented surfaces. Bone lesions should be managed by specialists; however, management of bone lesions is outlined in a WHO manual.[52] Heat therapy without surgical excision is successful for appropriate lesions but must be applied assiduously, keeping the base of ulcers at 40°C by fully controlled heating jackets.[58] Open heat-cradles seldom meet the requirement.

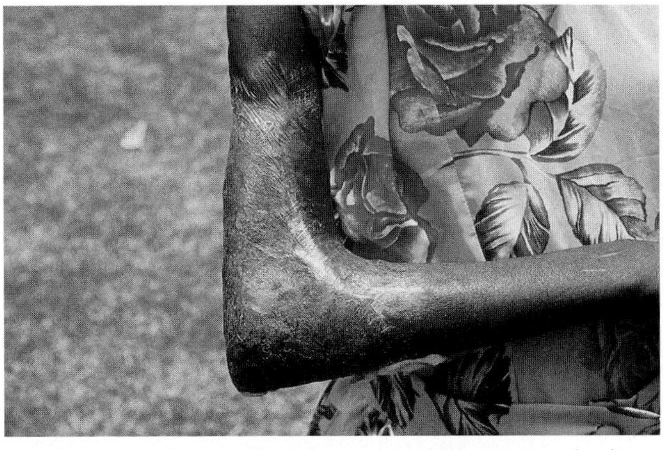

FIGURE 37-13 Frozen elbow from contracture scarring of a large, healed Buruli ulcer in a Ghanian girl.

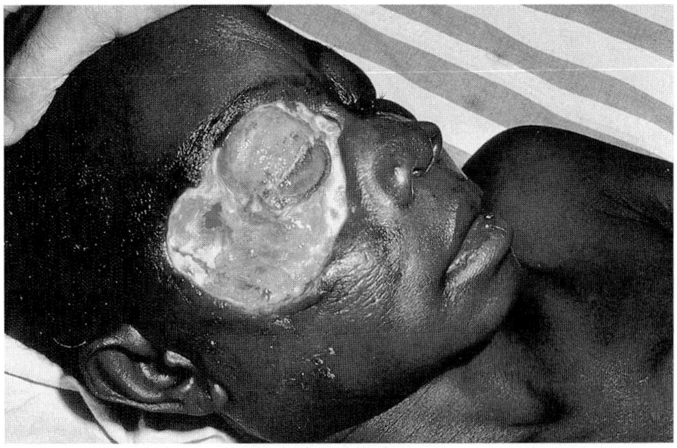

FIGURE 37-14 Patient in Congo who lost an eye from a major ulcerative lesion of Buruli ulcer.

Prognosis is unpredictable. Surgically managed early small lesions have an excellent prognosis. However, any lesion may recur locally or spread metastatically after initial therapy, threatening the loss of significant tissue, and increasing the danger of cosmetic and disabling deformities and amputations.[59] Secondary septicemia, tetanus, and gas gangrene sometimes are fatal. Without initial appropriate treatment, patients are likely to become severely disabled, increasing the stigma of the disease (Fig. 37-14). These patients are prone to developing psychosocial problems and become a socioeconomic burden to the community and the health-care delivery system.[4,60]

PREVENTION

In tropical rural settings where BU is endemic and scantily dressed children work and play, protection against contamination of the skin is virtually impossible. Although wearing long trousers reduces rates of infection, achieving this measure is not feasible.[24] Protected water supplies in villages reduces exposure to *M. ulcerans*–contaminated sources, but in most endemic countries, providing wells is not a priority. Thus, environmentally oriented plans for the control of BU are not likely to succeed, leaving vaccination programs the only viable alternative.

Vaccination with a single BCG inoculation protects against BU, but the effect against infection wanes after 6 to 12 months.[61,62] Nevertheless, the longstanding policy of neonatal vaccination with BCG, intended to prevent disseminated tuberculosis, does reduce the rate of osteomyelitis in BU-infected patients.[46] Because repeated BCG vaccination provides long-lasting protection against leprosy, plans are under way to test this approach for the control of BU.[63] Subunit vaccines based on virulence factors or antigens of *M. ulcerans* are being studied.[64]

REFERENCES

1. Clancey JK, Dodge OG, Lunn HF, et al: Mycobacterial skin ulcers in Uganda. Lancet 2:951, 1961.
2. Cook A: Mengo hospital notes. Makerere Medical School Library, Kampala, Uganda, 1897. (Cited in BMJ 2:37, 1970.)
3. Asiedu K, Scherpbier R, Raviglione M (eds), for WHO: Buruli ulcer: *Mycobacterium ulcerans* infection. WHO/CDS/CPE/GBUI/2000.1, 2000.

4. Aujoulat I, Johnson C, Zinsou C, et al: Psychosocial aspects of health seeking behaviours of patients with Buruli ulcer in southern Benin. Trop Med Int Health 8:750, 2003.
5. MacCallum P, Tolhurst JC, Buckle G, et al: A new mycobacterial infection in man. J Pathol Bacteriol 60:93, 1948.
6. Portaels F, Chemlal K, Elsen P, et al: *Mycobacterium ulcerans* in wild animals. Rev Sci Tech 20:252, 2001.
7. Daffe M, Vernerot A, Levy Frebault VV: The phenolic mycoside of *Mycobacterium ulcerans*: structure and taxonomic implications. J Gen Microbiol 138:131, 1992.
8. Rogall T, Flohr T, Böttger, EC: Differentiation of *Mycobacterium* species by direct sequencing of amplified DNA. J Gen Microbiol 136:1915, 1990.
9. Chemlal K, Huys G, Fonteyne PA, et al: Evaluation of PCR-restriction profile analysis, IS*2404* restriction fragment length polymorphism and amplified fragment length polymorphism fingerprinting for identification and typing of *Mycobacterium ulcerans* and *M. marinum*. J Clin Microbiol 39:3272, 2001.
10. Read RG, Heggie CM, Meyers WM, et al: Cytotoxic activity of *Mycobacterium ulcerans*. Infect Immun 9:1114, 1974.
11. Pimsler M, Sponsler TA, Meyers WM: Immunosuppressive properties of the soluble toxin from *Mycobacterium ulcerans*. J Infect Dis 157:577, 1988.
12. George KM, Chatterjee D, Gunawardana G, et al: Mycolactone: a polyketide toxin from *Mycobacterium ulcerans* required for virulence. Science 283:854, 1999.
13. Mve-Obiang A, Lee RE, Portaels F, et al: Heterogeneity of mycolactone toxins produced by *Mycobacterium ulcerans*: Implications on virulence. Infect Immun 71:774, 2003.
14. Stinear TP, Mve-Obiang A, Small PLC, et al: Giant plasmid-encoded polyketide synthases produce the macrolide toxin of *Mycobacterium ulcerans*. Proc Natl Acad Sci USA 101:1345, 2004.
15. Portaels F, Fonteyne PA, De Beenhouwer H, et al: Variability of 3′ end of 16S rRNA sequence of *Mycobacterium ulcerans* is related to geographic origin of isolates. J Clin Microbiol 34:962, 1996.
16. Stinear TP, Ross BC, Davies JK, et al: Identification and characterization of IS2404 and IS2606: two distinct repeated sequences for detection of *Mycobacterium ulcerans* by PCR. J Clin Microbiol 37:1018, 1999.
17. Faber WR, Pereira Arias-Bouda LM, Zeegelaar JE, et al: First reported case of *Mycobacterium ulcerans* infection in a patient from China. Trans R Soc Trop Med Hyg 94:277, 2000.
18. Tsukamura M, Kaneda K, Imaeda T, et al: A taxonomic study on a *Mycobacterium* which caused skin ulcer in a Japanese girl and resembled *Mycobacterium ulcerans*. Kekkaku 64:1, 1989.
19. Veitch MGK, Johnson PDR, Flood PE, et al: A large localized outbreak of *Mycobacterium ulcerans* infection on a temperate southern Australian island. Epidemiol Infect 119:313, 1997.
20. Portaels F: Contribution a l'étude des mycobactéries de l'environment au Bas-Zaire. Ann Soc Belge Med Trop 53:373, 1973.
21. Horsburgh CR Jr, Meyers WM: Buruli ulcer. In Horsburgh CR Jr, Nelson AM (eds): Pathology of Emerging Infections. Washington, DC, American Society for Microbiology, 1997, Chap 7, p. 119.
22. Meyers WM: Mycobacterial infections of the skin. In Doerr W, Seifert G (eds): Tropical Pathology, 2nd ed. Berlin, Springer Verlag, 1995, p. 291.
23. Meyers WM, Tignokpa N, Priuli GB, et al: *Mycobacterium ulcerans* infection (Buruli ulcer): first reported patients from Togo. Br J Dermatol 134:1116, 1996.
24. Marston BJ, Diallo MO, Horsburgh CR Jr, et al: Emergence of Buruli ulcer disease in the Daloa region of Côte d'Ivoire. Am J Trop Med Hyg 52:219, 1995.
25. Debacker M, Aguiar J, Steunou C, et al: *Mycobacterium ulcerans* disease (Buruli ulcer) in a rural hospital, south Benin, 1997–2001. Emerg Infect Dis 10:1391, 2004.
26. Ross BC, Johnson PDR, Oppedisano F, et al: Detection of *Mycobacterium ulcerans* in environmental samples during an outbreak of ulcerative disease. Appl Environ Microbiol 63:4135, 1997.
27. Ross BC, Marino L, Oppedisano F, et al: Development of a PCR assay for rapid diagnosis of *Mycobacterium ulcerans* infection. J Clin Microbiol 35:1696, 1997.
28. Mitchell PJ, Jerrett IV, Slee KJ: Skin ulcers caused by *Mycobacterium ulcerans* in koalas near Bairnsdale, Australia. Pathology 16:256, 1984.
29. Trott KA, Stacy BA, Lifland BD, et al: Characterization of a *Mycobacterium ulcerans*–like infection in a colony of African tropical clawed frogs (*Xenopus tropicalis*). Comp Med 54:309, 2004.
30. Walsh DS, Meyers WM, Krieg RE, et al: Transmission of *Mycobacterium ulcerans* to the nine-banded armadillo. Am J Trop Med Hyg 61:694, 1999.
31. Marsollier L, Aubry J, Saint-André JP, et al: Ecologie et mode de transmission de *Mycobacterium ulcerans*. Pathol Biol 51:490, 2003.
32. Meyers WM, Shelly WM, Connor DH, et al: *Mycobacterium ulcerans* infections developing at the sites of trauma to skin. Am J Trop Med Hyg 23:919, 1974.
33. Debacker M, Zinsou C, Aguiar J, et al: First case of *Mycobacterium ulcerans* disease (Buruli ulcer) following a human bite. Clin Infect Dis 36:e67, 2003.
34. Hofer M, Hirschel B, Kirschner P, et al: Disseminated osteomyelitis from *Mycobacterium ulcerans* after a snakebite. N Engl J Med 328:1007, 1993.
35. Evans MR, Mawdsley J, Bull R, et al: Buruli ulcer in a visitor to London. Br J Dermatol 149:907, 2003.
36. Bär W, Rüsch-Gerdes S, Richter E, et al: *Mycobacterium ulcerans* infection in a child from Angola: diagnosis by direct detection and culture. Trop Med Int Health 3:189, 1998.
37. Journeau P, Fitoussi F, Jehanno P, et al: Buruli's ulcer: three cases diagnosed and treated in France. J Pediatr Orthop B 12:229, 2003.
38. Pszolla N, Sarkar MR, Strecker W, et al: Buruli ulcer: a systemic disease. Clin Infect Dis 37:e78, 2003.
39. Semret M, Koromihis G, MacLean JD, et al: *Mycobacterium ulcerans* infection (Buruli ulcer): first reported case in a traveler. Am J Trop Med Hyg 61:689, 1999.
40. Connor DH, Lunn F: Buruli ulceration: a clinicopathologic study of 38 Ugandans with *Mycobacterium ulcerans* infection. Arch Pathol 81:183, 1966.
41. Guédénon A, Zinsou C, Josse R, et al: Traditional treatment of Buruli ulcer in Benin. Arch Dermatol 131:741, 1995.
42. Hayman J: Clinical features of *Mycobacterium ulcerans* infection. Aust J Dermatol 26:67, 1985.
43. Abalos FMV, Aguiar J, Guédénon A, et al: *Mycobacterium ulcerans* infection (Buruli ulcer): a case report of the disseminated nonulcerative form. Ann Diagn Pathol 4:376, 2000.
44. Portaels F, Zinsou C, Aguiar J, et al: Les atteintes osseuses dans l'ulcère de Buruli: à propos de 73 cas. Bull Séanc Acad R Sci Outre-Mer 49:161, 2003.
45. Lagarrigue V, Portaels F, Meyers WM, et al: L'ulcère de Buruli: attention aux atteintes osseuses! A propos de 33 cas observés au Bénin. Med Trop 60:262, 2000.
46. Portaels F, Aguiar J, Debacker M, et al: *Mycobacterium bovis* BCG vaccination as prophylaxis against *Mycobacterium ulcerans* osteomyelitis in Buruli ulcer disease. Infect Immun 72:62, 2004.
47. Stanford JL: Immunologically important constituents of mycobacteria: antigens. In Ratledge C, Stanford JL (eds): Biology of the Mycobacteria. New York, Academic Press, 1983, p. 113.
48. Gooding TM, Johnson PDR, Campbell DE: Immune response to infection with *Mycobacterium ulcerans*. Infect Immun 69:1704, 2001.
49. Pahlaven A, Wright DJM, Andrews C, et al: The inhibitory action of *Mycobacterium ulcerans* soluble factor on monocyte/T cell cytokine production and NFkB function. J Immunol 163:3928, 1999.
50. Dobos KM, Spotts EA, Marston BJ, et al: Serologic response to culture filtrate antigens of *Mycobacterium ulcerans* during Buruli ulcer disease. Emerg Infect Dis 6:158, 2000.
51. Johnson RC, Ifebe D, Hans-Moevi A, et al: Disseminated *Mycobacterium ulcerans* disease in an HIV-positive patient: a case study. AIDS 16:1704, 2002.
52. Buntine J, Croft K (eds), for WHO: The management of *Mycobacterium ulcerans* disease (Buruli ulcer). WHO/CDS/CPE/GBUI/2001.2, 2001.
53. Portaels F, Johnson PDR, Meyers WM (eds), for WHO: Diagnosis of *Mycobacterium ulcerans* disease (Buruli ulcer). WHO/CDS/CPE/GBUI/2001.3, 2001.
54. Stinear TP, Jenkin GS, Davies JK, et al: *Mycobacterium ulcerans* in the environment from an endemic region in South Eastern Australia with sequence-capture PCR. Appl Environ Microbiol 66:3206, 2000.
55. Rondini S, Mensah-Quainoo E, Troll H, et al: Development and application of real-time PCR assay for quantification of *Mycobacterium ulcerans* DNA. J Clin Microbiol 41:4231, 2003.
56. Uganda Buruli Group: Clinical features and treatment of pre-ulcerative Buruli lesions (*Mycobacterium ulcerans* infection). BMJ 2:390, 1970.
57. Evans MR, Phillips R, Etuaful SN, et al: An outreach education and treatment project in Ghana for the early stage of *Mycobacterium ulcerans* disease. Trans R Soc Trop Med Hyg 97:159, 2003.

58. Meyers WM, Shelly WM, Connor DH: Heat treatment of *Mycobacterium ulcerans* infections without surgical excision. Am J Trop Med Hyg 23:924, 1974.
59. Aguiar J, Steunou C: Les ulcères de Buruli en zone rurale au Bénin: prise en charge de 635 cas. Méd Trop 57:83, 1997.
60. Asiedu K, Etuaful S: Socioeconomic implications of Buruli ulcer in Ghana: a three-year review. Am J Trop Med Hyg 59:1015, 1998.
61. Uganda Buruli Group: BCG vaccination against *Mycobacterium ulcerans* infection (Buruli ulcer). Lancet 1:111, 1969.
62. Smith PG, Revill WDL, Lukwago E, et al: The protective effect of BCG against *Mycobacterium ulcerans* disease: a controlled trial in an endemic area of Uganda. Trans R Soc Trop Med Hyg 70:449, 1976.
63. Karonga Prevention Trial Group: Randomised controlled trial of single BCG, repeated BCG, or combined BCG and killed *Mycobacterium leprae* vaccine for prevention of leprosy and tuberculosis in Malawi. Lancet 348:17, 1996.
64. Tanghe A, Content J, Van Vooren JP, et al: Protective efficacy of a DNA vaccine encoding antigen 85A from *Mycobacterium bovis* BCG against Buruli ulcer. Infect Immun 69:5403, 2001.

38

Leprosy

WAYNE M. MEYERS

INTRODUCTION

Leprosy is a chronic infection by *Mycobacterium leprae,* affecting mainly the cooler body areas: skin, upper respiratory passages, anterior segments of eyes, superficial segments of peripheral nerves, and testes. The traditional, pervasive, social stigma attached to leprosy may be traced to the disfigurement, deformity, mutilations, and blindness related to damage to these tissues. In cultures influenced by Judeo-Christian orthodoxy, the ostracism leprosy patients suffer is frequently severe and, in part, attributable to what is called leprosy in the Old Testament.[1] The Hebrew word *tsara'ath* was translated *lepra* in the Septuagint, the first Greek version of the Old Testament (third century BC). Subsequent Latin and English translations of the Bible used *lepra* and *leprosy*, respectively. The original Hebrew word denoted a group of diseases, none of which had recognizable clinical features of leprosy, and referred generally to ceremonial uncleanness.[2] Cultures never influenced by Judaic laws, however, frequently had or have similar attitudes toward leprosy—for example, the Chinese as early as the eighth century BC.[3] To ameliorate the stigma of the disease, the International Leprosy Association in 1948 abandoned the word "leper" for "leprosy patient."[4] Today, the term "Hansen's disease" is a frequent synonym for leprosy.[5] Prevention of disability and conservation of cosmetic integrity are of utmost importance to preserve productivity and social acceptance.

AGENT

M. leprae, measuring 0.5 μm × 4.0 to 7.0 μm, is an acid-fast bacillus (AFB) in the order Actinomycetales and family Mycobacteriaceae. The Ziehl–Neelsen method stains *M. leprae* in smears, but in tissue sections the Fite-Faraco method is optimal. Acid-fastness is related to mycolic acid in the cell wall.[6] Staining properties of *M. leprae* in skin smears or biopsy specimens are important in the rapid assessment of the therapeutic efficacy of antileprotics. Viable organisms stain solidly, and as they degenerate, stain irregularly, then become granular, and eventually non-acid-fast. Persistence of bacillary carcasses in tissues or in smears can be established by silver staining techniques.[7] In multibacillary patients such carcasses may remain in macrophages for several years after the leprosy bacilli have lost acid-fastness.

In 1873, in Norway, Hansen proposed that the bacillary bodies he saw in unstained tissue fluids from lepromatous nodules were the cause of leprosy. This was the first mycobacterium and the first etiologic agent of a chronic disease identified in humans. The leprosy bacillus is apparently an obligate intracellular parasite; however, investigators occasionally report in vitro cultivation in cell-free media. All such claims remain unsubstantiated.[8] Because *M. leprae* is, as yet, noncultivable, identification of candidate organisms as *M. leprae* depends on ancillary criteria, as follows: (1) fails to grow on routine mycobacteriologic media; (2) infects the foot pads of mice in a manner consistent with that of *M. leprae*[9]; (3) acid-fastness is abolished by exposure to pyridine[10]; (4) invades nerves in humans or experimental hosts; (5) suspensions of killed bacilli produce a characteristic pattern ("lepromin reaction") when injected into the skin of leprosy patients with each of the various clinical forms[11]; (6) produces phenolic glycolipid–1 (PGL-1), a presumed species-specific antigen[12]; and (7) contains species-specific DNA sequences.[13] Cell walls of *M. leprae* contain arabinogalactan, mycolates, peptidoglycan, and protein.[14] Constituents of the cell wall appear to play a significant role in the *M. leprae*–host cell interaction, both in protecting the parasite and in stimulating immune responses.[15–18] The *M. leprae* genome contains 3,268,203 base pairs with a G + C % of 57.79. Only 1604, or 49.5%, of the genes encode proteins, compared with 3959, or 90.8%, for *Mycobacterium tuberculosis*. This represents a massive deficit of metabolic capabilities for *M. leprae* that probably explains why it has not been cultivated in vitro.[19] The assumed gene decay may be related to the long multiplication time of 13 days for *M. leprae,* as observed in the foot pads of immunologically intact mice, and to the normally long incubation periods of leprosy. In less resistant hosts such as nude mice, generation times may be as short as 26 hours,[20] approaching that of 18 hours for *M. tuberculosis*. This may help explain the short incubation periods in some highly susceptible infants under 1 year of age.[21] Preferential localization of lesions of leprosy to cooler body locations,[22] selective growth in foot pads of normal mice, and the marked susceptibility of armadillos (body temperature 32 to 35°C) suggest that the optimal growth temperature for *M. leprae* is lower than 37°C.[23]

EPIDEMIOLOGY

Leprosy and its transmission do not require a tropical environment. Historically, the disease has afflicted people in nearly every part of the world, including countries traversed by the Arctic Circle. Today the higher prevalences in the tropics are best attributable to socioeconomic factors. In 1995 the World Health Organization (WHO) estimated that there were 1.83 million people in the world with active leprosy.[24] This represents a marked reduction in the global prevalence of leprosy in the several previous decades (12 to 15 million); however, the annual reported incidence of new patients (approximately 700,000) remains unchanged. A considerable portion of the reduction in total numbers of patients may be artificial and attributable to the redefinition of a case of leprosy. Today only individuals who receive chemotherapy for leprosy are counted as cases. Prevalence rates vary: Of all patients, southern Asia has 75% (India alone, 65%); Africa, 12%; and the Americas, 8%. In the United States there are an estimated 6000 people with a history of leprosy, with 133 new patients reported in 2003, 26 of whom were born in the United States.[25]

Infected humans are the most common source of leprosy; however, nonhuman reservoirs are well known. Naturally acquired leprosy was first detected in armadillos in Louisiana in 1974 and infects up to one-half of the armadillos in some foci.[26,27] Similarly, indigenous leprosy has been detected in chimpanzees and monkeys in West Africa and elsewhere.[28–30] Humans may acquire leprosy from wild infected armadillos,[31,32] and possibly from other zoonotic sources in other geographic areas. There is no evidence for transmission of leprosy by insects or any other vector.

Prevalence of disease seldom exceeds 5% in most large populations. In adults, the male-to-female ratio is 2 to 3:1, but in children, it is 1 to 1. Specific immunologic parameters in subjects in Ethiopia suggest that occupational contacts, for example, health care workers, have the highest sensitization rates to *M. leprae* (58%), followed by household contacts (47%), and noncontacts in endemic areas (29%).[33] In most populations living in endemic areas, 5% to 10% of infected persons develop progressive clinical disease.[34] Children usually constitute 20% to 30% of all cases detected.[35] The role of genetic factors is unclear: In some ethnic groups, certain HLA-DR types are associated with the particular type of leprosy, but not necessarily with susceptibility.[36,37]

Lower prevalences of leprosy correlate directly with the availability of adequate housing and level of living standards. This is perhaps the best explanation for the disappearance of leprosy from northern Europe beginning just after the Middle Ages, and explains the tendency for leprosy to prevail today in the underprivileged areas of the world, primarily the tropics. Other public health factors common to the tropics may influence the prevalence of leprosy. For example, there is a markedly increased frequency of intestinal nematode infections in lepromatous leprosy in Brazil and probably in most tropical climates. Diniz and colleagues attribute this to a modulation of the host immune response by these parasites: down-regulation of the Th1 and up-regulation of the Th2 responses.[38]

DISEASE

Leprosy is a paradigm for the understanding of the range of clinical and pathologic interactions between variable host responses and a bacterium with relatively stable virulence. The immune response determines the position of a patient in the classic spectrum of disease forms described in Table 38-1, which reflects the popular Ridley–Jopling classification.[39] The WHO classification of leprosy for field workers is assumed to be based on the bacterial burden in tissues: *paucibacillary* (PB), patients with skin smears negative for AFB, or five or fewer cutaneous lesions; and *multibacillary* (MB), those with skin smears positive for AFB, or more than five lesions.[40] Some versions of the WHO classification suggest that skin smears be excluded. Observations by the author indicate that a system based only on number of lesions is prone to errors in classification that can be moderated by the use of skin smears for AFB, or by histopathologic analysis.

The immunologic capability of an individual, including patients, in relation to *M. leprae*, is assessed by the intradermal inoculation of 0.1 mL of *lepromin*, a suspension of heat-killed *M. leprae* (1.6×10^8 organisms per milliliter), obtained today from experimentally infected armadillos.[11] The response is evaluated by measuring the diameter of induration at the injection site 3 to 4 weeks postinoculation (Mitsuda reaction).[41] Because high percentages of all normal populations react,[42] this skin test is never diagnostic but is useful in the classification of disease: Tuberculoid leprosy and borderline tuberculoid leprosy patients are strongly positive (>5 mm); lepromatous leprosy, weakly or nonreactive (0 to 2 mm); and borderline lepromatous and midborderline have intermediate reactions (3 to 5 mm; see Table 38-1).

Table 38-1 Clinical and Histopathologic Classification of Leprosy

Clinical Features	Histopathologic Features
Tuberculoid (TT)	
Few well-defined anesthetic macules or plaques; neural involvement common	Granulomas with or without giant cells; rare bacilli; nerves damaged; no subepidermal freezone
Borderline Forms	
Borderline tuberculoid (BT)	
More lesions, borders less distinct; neural involvement common	Similar to TT but with occasional bacilli, usually in nerves; subepidermal freezone
Midborderline (BB)	
More lesions than BT, borders vague; neural involvement common	Epithelioid cells and histiocytes; focal lymphocytes; increased cellularity of nerves; bacilli readily found, mostly in nerves; subepidermal freezone
Borderline lepromatous (BL)	
Numerous lesions, borders vague; less neural damage than in BB	Histiocytes, few epithelioid cells, some foamy cells; bacilli plentiful in nerves and histiocytes; subepidermal freezone
Lepromatous (LL)	
Multiple macules, nodules, or diffuse infiltrations; symmetrically distributed neural lesions develop late	Foamy histiocytes with large numbers of bacilli; few lymphocytes; numerous bacilli in nerves; minimal intraneural cellular infiltration; subepidermal freezone
Indeterminate (I)	
Vaguely defined, hypopigmented, or erythematous macules	Small lymphocytic infiltrates around nerves and appendages; rare bacilli, usually in nerves

Based on Ridley DS, Jopling WH: Classification of leprosy according to immunity: a five-group system. Int J Lepr 34:255, 1966.

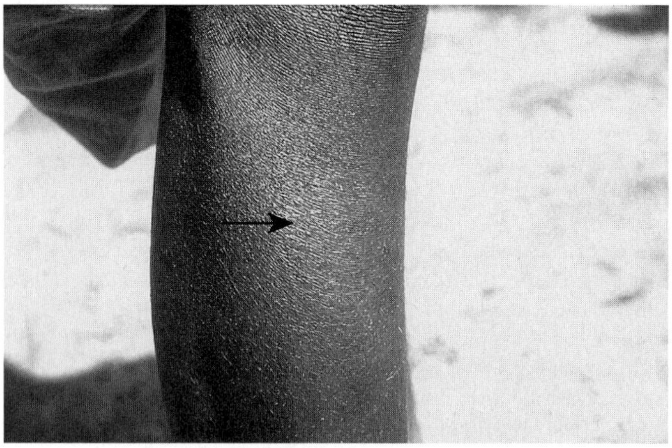

FIGURE 38-1 Indeterminate leprosy *(arrow)* on the leg of an Indian patient. The lesion is hypopigmented with vague borders.

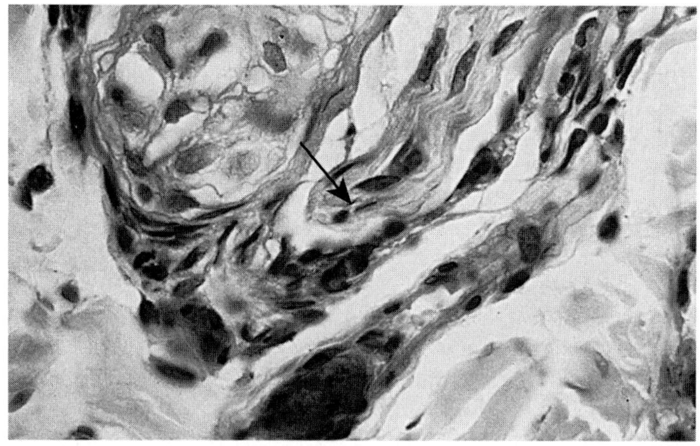

FIGURE 38-3 Indeterminate leprosy. Note the single acid-fast bacillus *(arrow)* in a nerve twig of a parallel Fite–Faraco-stained section of lesion shown in Figure 38-2.

Modifications of this test using a high concentration of leprosy bacilli show that lepromatous patients cannot clear *M. leprae* from the reaction site, whereas tuberculoid patients destroy the bacilli efficiently.[43] Thus, survival and multiplication of the etiologic agents in macrophages determine the form of leprosy: If macrophages destroy *M. leprae* rapidly, minimal or no lesions develop, but if macrophages do not control multiplication of *M. leprae,* severe disseminated disease follows. While there is considerable evidence that the level of cell-mediated immunity to *M. leprae* determines the progress of disease, the precise mechanisms are poorly defined. In lepromatous patients there may be anergy to a variety of antigens, but most strikingly and most consistently to those of *M. leprae.*[44]

Indeterminate Leprosy

Indeterminate leprosy (I) is usually the earliest lesion and presents as poorly defined macules, mildly hypopigmented in dark skin and slightly erythematous in lighter skin (Fig. 38-1). Texture, the amount of hair, sensation, and sweating in the lesion are, at most, only slightly changed. Histopathologically, there are a few lymphocytes around neurovascular bundles (Fig. 38-2). These changes are nonspecific unless AFB are found in nerves, arrectores pilorum muscles, or in the subepidermal area (Fig. 38-3).[45] Diagnosis of indeterminate lesions often requires close cooperation between the histopathologist and clinician. Lesions may self-heal, remain unchanged for long periods, or progress to other forms of leprosy.

Tuberculoid Leprosy

Tuberculoid leprosy (TT) patients have a single or few lesions, which may be macular or infiltrated. Borders are well defined and often finely papulated (Figs. 38-4 and 38-5). Sensation and sweating are impaired in lesions, and hair is frequently absent. Cutaneous nerves and peripheral nerve trunks are often enlarged in the region of lesions (Fig. 38-6). Sections of skin show epithelioid cell granulomas that invade nerves and often the epidermis (Fig. 38-7). AFB are rare and are found most consistently in nerves, papillary dermis, or arrectores pilorum muscles (Fig. 38-8).

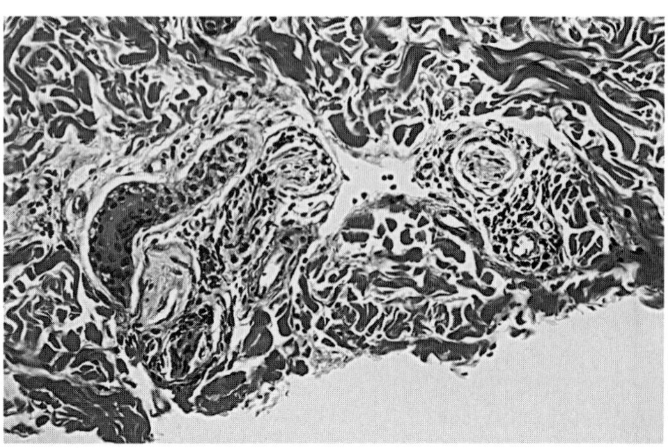

FIGURE 38-2 Indeterminate leprosy showing infiltration of a few lymphocytes around nerves and vessels in the lower dermis. Nerves are intact.

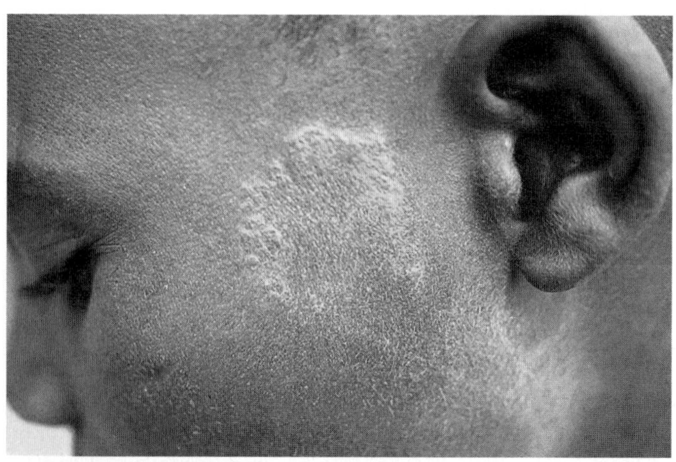

FIGURE 38-4 Early tuberculoid leprosy on the cheek of an Angolan boy. The lesion is hypopigmented with well-defined papular borders and is mildly hypoesthetic. Early lesions on the face often have only slight or no sensory changes.

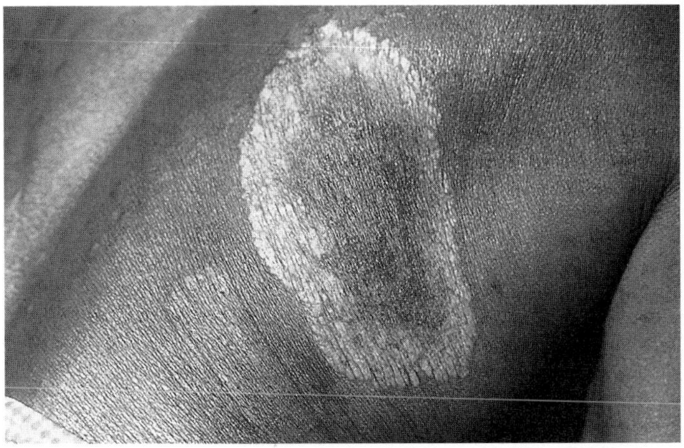

FIGURE 38-5 Tuberculoid leprosy. A Congolese patient with a single anesthetic lesion that developed over 13 years. Note healed atrophic repigmented center and active hypopigmented and infiltrated edge.

Borderline Leprosy

Borderline leprosy has three major subgroups: borderline tuberculoid (BT; Fig. 38-9), midborderline (BB), and borderline lepromatous (BL). This area of the spectrum is unstable, especially BB. BT lesions resemble those of TT but often are more numerous, and definition of their margins is less distinct. In BL there are widespread plaques and nodules. Histopathologically, the quality of the granulomas ranges from hyperergic with few AFB in BT, to nearly anergic with many AFB in histiocytes and nerves in BL. Damage to cutaneous and peripheral nerves develops early and is often severe and widespread (Fig. 38-10). Reversal reactions (type 1) are common, with resulting neuropathic changes, especially in the hands, feet, and face.

Lepromatous Leprosy

Lepromatous leprosy (LL) infiltrates nearly the entire skin, but the cellular exudates are heaviest in the cooler areas, such as the ears, the central portion of the face, and the extensor surfaces of the thighs and forearms (Fig. 38-11). Physical examination may easily miss the subtle macules of early LL.

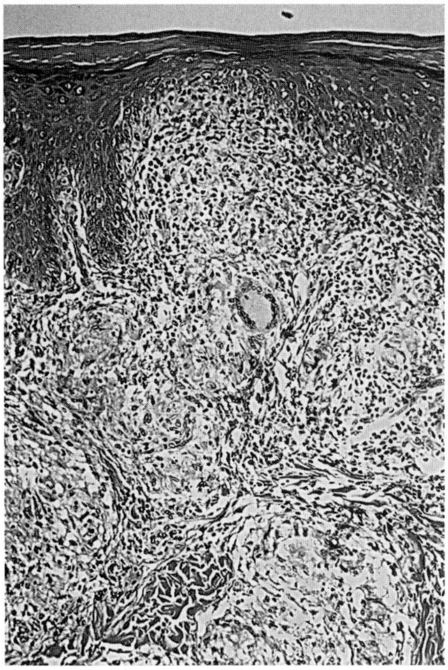

FIGURE 38-7 Tuberculoid leprosy. Granulomas composed of epithelioid cells, giant cells, and lymphocytes replace the dermis and invade the epidermis.

Damage to nerves develops slowly but relentlessly. There is insensitivity of hands and feet and loss of some body hair (e.g., eyebrows) at later stages. Other areas involved are the upper respiratory tract from the nasal mucosa to the larynx, the eye, lymph nodes, and testes. Sterility and gynecomastia may follow leprous orchitis. Histopathologically, macrophages densely infiltrate the dermis but leave a subepidermal clear zone (Fig. 38-12). Nerves are rather well preserved until late. AFB abound in nerves, macrophages, blood vessel walls, and arrectores pilorum muscles, with many AFB in clumps and globi (Fig. 38-13).

Other Manifestations of Leprosy

Occasionally in LL, especially in relapsing patients, elevated firm nodules appear in the skin. Histologically, the

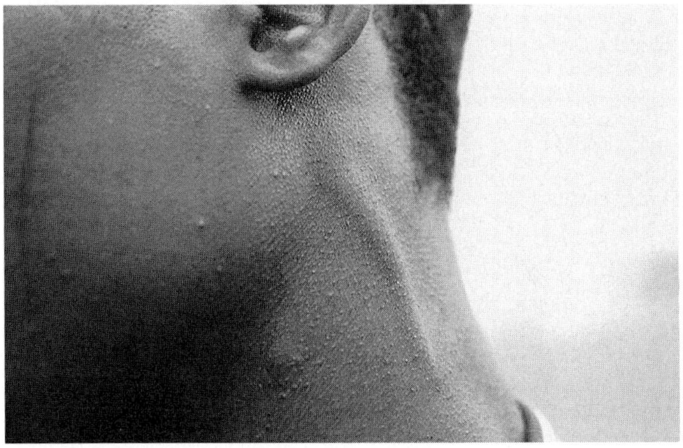

FIGURE 38-6 Thickened great auricular nerve in tuberculoid leprosy. The healing lesion of leprosy is barely visible anterior to the ear.

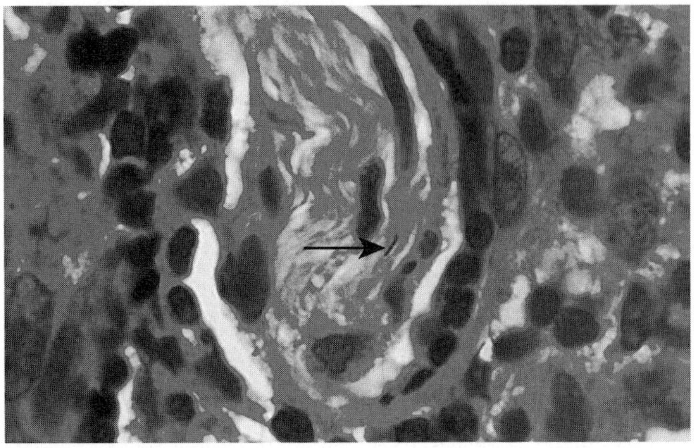

FIGURE 38-8 Damaged dermal nerve in lesion of tuberculoid leprosy. The nerve contains two acid-fast bacilli *(arrow)*.

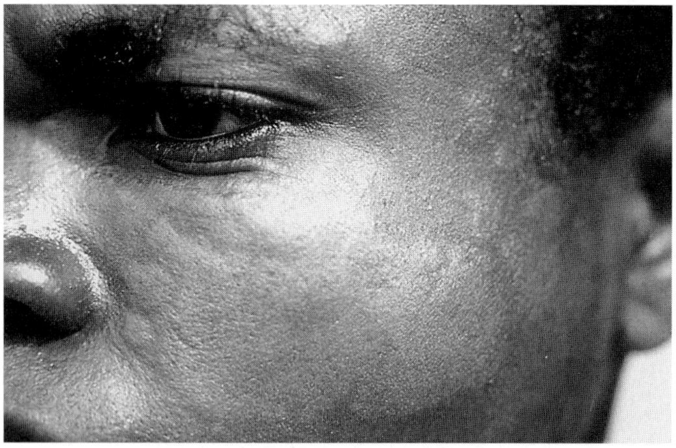

FIGURE 38-9 Borderline tuberculoid leprosy in a Congolese patient undergoing a mild reversal reaction. The multiple lesions are sharply delineated, infiltrated, and erythematous. Peripheral nerve trunks were painful, enlarged, and tender.

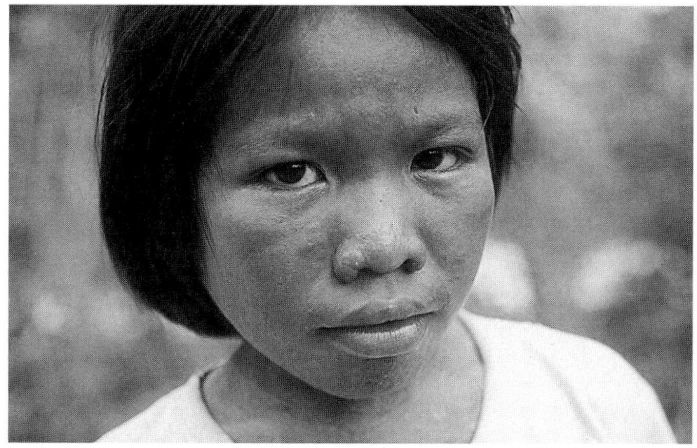

FIGURE 38-11 Lepromatous leprosy showing heaviest infiltrations of skin over the central portion of the face. The eyebrows are thinned.

macrophages resemble fibrocytes arranged in whorls, as in dermatofibromas, and contain numerous AFB. These lesions are called *histoid* leprosy.[46]

In patients of Latin American ancestry, particularly Mexicans, there is a highly anergic form of LL called *Lucio's leprosy.* Infiltration of skin is so diffuse that the diagnosis is often missed. In advanced stages, *Lucio's phenomenon* may develop, characterized by obstructive vasculitis causing dermal infarcts and ulcers (Fig. 38-14), often involving massive areas of the skin.

Occasionally *pure neural leprosy* affects peripheral nerves in the absence of cutaneous lesions. Biopsy specimens of nerves may show any form of leprosy, but most are borderline disease. On presentation patients have one or more painful enlarged peripheral nerves accompanied by sensory loss, paresis, or muscular wasting.

Reactions

The course of leprosy is often punctuated by acute reactional episodes. Reactions are classified into two categories: type 1, or reversal reactions (Fig. 38-15), and type 2, or *erythema nodosum leprosum* (ENL; Fig. 38-16).

Reversal reactions are most frequent in borderline leprosy and represent an episodic upgrading of cell-mediated immunity. Existing cutaneous lesions become swollen and erythematous. Neuritis is common and is responsible for much of the sensory loss and deformities of borderline leprosy. By repeated reversal reactions, borderline lesions may gradually upgrade toward tuberculoid disease. Today, with defined short-term therapeutic regimens for treatment, both the clinician and the pathologist are confronted with the problem of differentiating relapsing leprosy from upgrading reversal reactions. The following criteria have been formulated[47,48]: *relapse*—increased number of lesions, skin smear positive for AFB (BB and BL patients), tissue reaction inconsistent with reversal reaction, and favorable response to antileprosy therapy; *reversal reaction*—exacerbation of sites of previous lesions, skin smear negative, tissue reaction suggesting reversal reaction, and rapid response to anti-inflammatory therapy (e.g., corticosteroids).

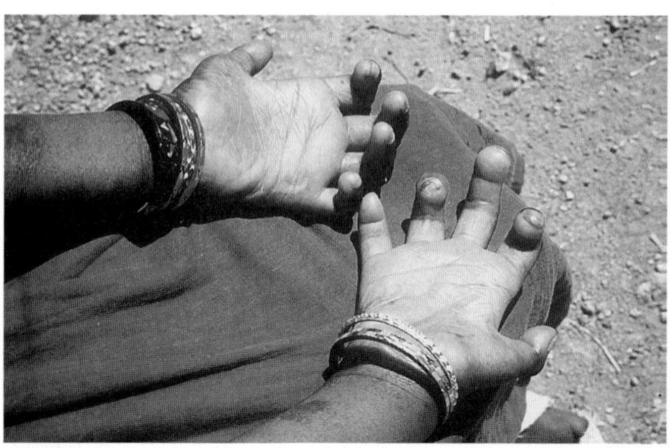

FIGURE 38-10 Mutilated and deformed insensitive hands of a Pakistani woman due to multiple peripheral neuropathies of borderline leprosy. Note flattening of palms from loss of thenar and hypothenar eminences.

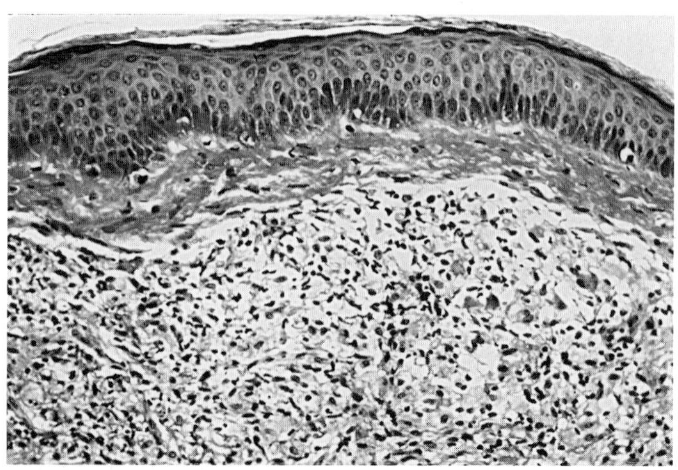

FIGURE 38-12 Lepromatous leprosy showing subepidermal clear zone and replacement of the dermis by vacuolated macrophages.

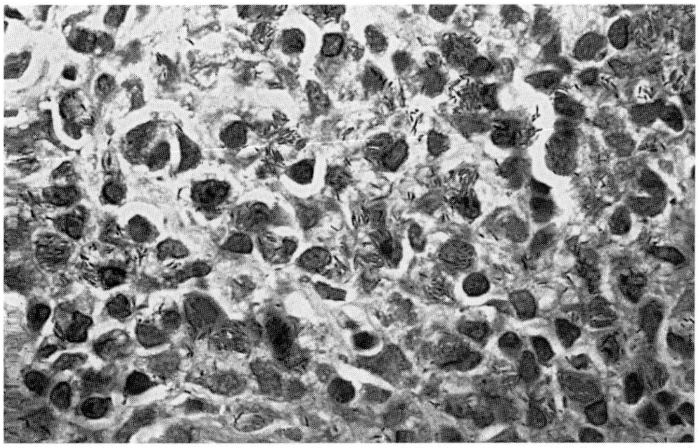

FIGURE 38-13 High-power magnification of a Fite–Faraco-stained section of Figure 38-12 showing massive numbers of acid-fast bacilli in macrophages.

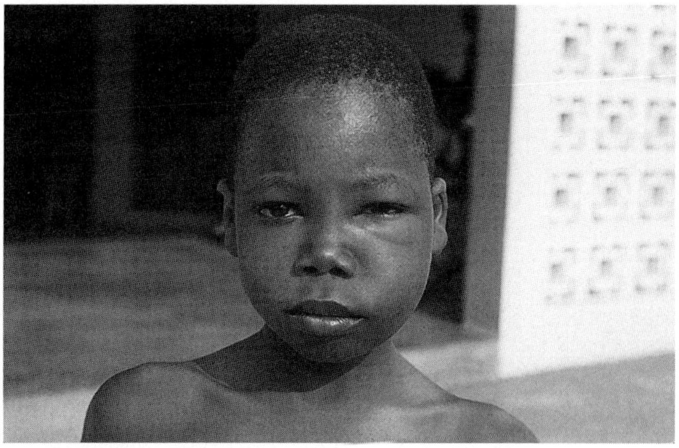

FIGURE 38-15 Early reversal reaction in a Congolese boy with a borderline tuberculoid lesion on the face. Note the swollen left side of the face with slight ipsilateral facial palsy. Corticosteroid therapy rapidly reduced the swelling and restored full facial nerve function.

Lepromin-positive patients with IgM antibodies to PGL-1 are at greatest risk of reversal reactions, suggesting participation of both humoral and cell-mediated components.[49] Sensitized T lymphocytes proliferate in reversal reactions, releasing cytokines that call in and activate macrophages.[50] Tissue reaction shows edema, increased numbers of lymphocytes, epithelioid cells, and giant cells. This is the only instance where hyperergic lesions of leprosy may show necrosis in granulomas and dermal nerves. Increased TNF-α may provoke this necrosis.[51]

Erythema nodosum leprosum (ENL) develops in approximately half of all lepromatous patients. Clinically, there is rapid onset of tender subcutaneous nodules, often accompanied by fever, synovitis, and iridocyclitis. ENL lesions resemble the Arthus phenomenon and probably are related to immunocomplexes that form locally by the release of antigens of *M. leprae* that combine with circulating antibody and probably modulate the T-lymphocyte populations in situ. There are, for example, increased numbers of T helper cells within lesions,[52] and TNF-α is increased.[53] Histopathologically, neutrophils usually infiltrate the lesion, often accompanied by vasculitis and ulceration. Elevation of serum amyloid A and C-reactive protein may help establish the diagnosis in atypical lesions.[54] Secondary amyloidosis in LL is seen most frequently in patients with chronic ENL.

PATHOGENESIS AND IMMUNITY

In humans, direct skin-to-skin contact or fomites may transmit leprosy,[55] but the nasorespiratory route is believed to be most common.[56] Secretions from the nasal mucosa of untreated lepromatous patients contain large numbers of viable leprosy bacilli.[57] *M. leprae* bacilli, after drying in the shade, in India, remain viable for up to 5 months, and in wet soil for 46 days.[58] Thus, the leprosy bacilli could be carried in aerosols and contaminate the nasal mucosa, perhaps first binding to fibronectin and then to fibronectin receptors on mucosal cells.[59] Transmission through mother's milk or transplacental infection is plausible. Breast tissue and mother's milk of multibacillary patients may contain large numbers of *M. leprae,* putting their nursing infants at risk.[60] There is increasing evidence for placental transmission of leprosy. Cord blood contains *M. leprae*–specific IgA and IgM antibodies,

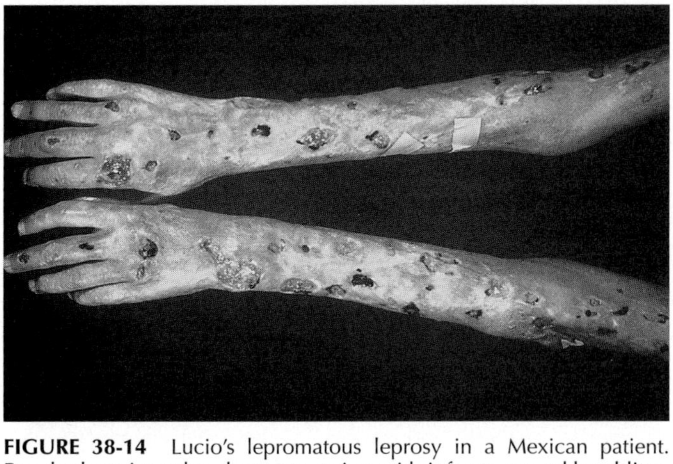

FIGURE 38-14 Lucio's lepromatous leprosy in a Mexican patient. Punched-out irregular ulcers are at sites with infarcts caused by obliterative vasculitis of dermal and subcutaneous vessels.

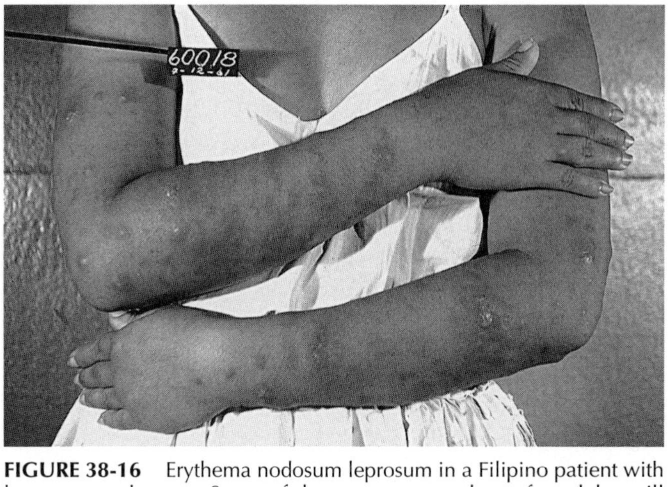

FIGURE 38-16 Erythema nodosum leprosum in a Filipino patient with lepromatous leprosy. Some of the numerous tender, soft nodules will rupture and discharge pus.

and titers of these antibodies rise in some infants of lepromatous mothers over 3 to 24 months after birth.[61,62] Leprosy in infants under 1 year of age is well known. In one series of 49 such infants, the youngest patient was 2 months old at diagnosis,[21] and the mother had clinical leprosy in only about half of these infants. This implies that during gestation the mother had a transient subclinical *M. leprae* bacteremia.

Bacteremia is common in multibacillary leprosy and in up to 15% of paucibacillary patients.[63,64] Invasion and multiplication of *M. leprae* in dermal lymphatic and vascular endothelial cells probably plays a major role in the hematogenous spread of the bacillus.[65,66] Scollard and associates have demonstrated that *M. leprae* invades peripheral nerves via the blood (and possibly lymphatic) vessels of the perineurium, gaining access to the endoneurial compartment.[67] Infection of endothelial cells by *M. leprae* may lead to ischemia of nerve, contributing to peripheral neuritis. The Schwann cell of peripheral nerves is the classic target for *M. leprae*. Rambukkana and coworkers have shown that laminin-2 in the basal lamina of the Schwann cell–axon unit binds to *M. leprae*, and ultimately that the α-dystroglycan receptor of the Schwann cells binds with laminin-2.[68] This may be one mechanism by which Schwann cells become infected.

Disturbances in the modulation of T lymphocyte–macrophage function in the different forms of leprosy are well known. Total numbers of circulating T lymphocytes may be decreased in advanced lepromatous disease, but T-cell subset ratio variations are not consistent.[69] In lesions, however, T helper (CD4+) cells predominate in tuberculoid leprosy, and T suppressor (CD8+) lymphocytes predominate in lepromatous disease.[70,71] Increased suppressor cell activity in lepromatous leprosy may be induced by lepromin[72] or PGL-1,[73] and may in part be related to infiltration of paracortical areas of lymph nodes by *M. leprae*–laden macrophages.[74]

Much is known about the immunologic perturbations in leprosy, which have been extensively reviewed.[75] Protective mechanisms against leprosy, the contribution of the T-cell subsets, cytokine networks, and macrophage bactericidal mechanisms, for example, remain unresolved.[76]

Classically, CD4+ T lymphocytes recognize specific antigens when associated with HLA and produce interferon-γ (IFN-γ), which activates macrophages. Macrophages from lepromatous patients, once activated by cytokines, have the capacity to kill and clear *M. leprae*.[77] Production of interleukin-2 (IL-2) and IFN-γ, however, is deficient in lepromatous patients. This suppression may represent an effect of CD8+ T suppressor cells by reducing proliferation of sensitized T cells and inhibiting activation of macrophages. IL-2 restores proliferation of lymphocytes and IFN-γ production in response to specific stimulation.[75,78,79] Injection of IL-2 and IFN-γ into lepromatous lesions increases the influx of CD4+ T cells, activating macrophages and reducing bacillary load.[80,81] These cytokines may have therapeutic value but do provoke tumor necrosis factor–α (TNF-α), which may be associated with reversal reactions in skin and peripheral nerves.[82]

The immune response, as it may relate to the spectrum of disease forms in leprosy, may be summarized as follows: In tuberculoid leprosy the response is that of Th1-like T cells, and in lepromatous leprosy there is a Th2 response producing cytokines IL-4 and IL-10.[83] These different immunologic responses of the host determine, in large measure, the different clinical and histopathologic forms in the spectrum of leprosy (see Table 38-1).

DIAGNOSIS

The cardinal signs of leprosy are hypoesthetic lesions of the skin, enlarged peripheral nerves, and AFB in skin smears. In the absence of another clear diagnosis, any one of these observations suggests leprosy. Delay in diagnosis is often prolonged following the first visit to a physician for leprosy-related symptoms; in the United States, this period averages 1 to 1.5 years. Such delay may result in irreversible sequelae.

Physical Examination

History of contact or residence in endemic areas raises suspicion of leprosy in a patient with chronic lesions of the skin. Experienced observers can often make the diagnosis clinically. Histopathologic evaluation is, however, strongly recommended for confirmation of the diagnosis and classification.

The entire skin surface should be examined. Vague changes are best seen in direct sunlight. Peripheral nerves are palpated for enlargement and tenderness. Cutaneous nerves in or near lesions may be enlarged. Unexplained damage to hands or feet, or any muscle weakness (e.g., clawhand or footdrop) or sensory deficit strongly suggests peripheral neuropathy. Lepromatous patients may have a chronic stuffy nose.

Sensory changes in lesions are tested for light touch with a few fibers of cotton or calibrated nylon bristles, and for heat–cold discrimination by warm and cool water in test tubes. Sensory changes are the most important criterion for clinical diagnosis; thus, repeated testing is recommended in doubtful situations.

Skin Smears

Skin smears are obtained from multiple sites (usually six to eight) and should include the edge of macules or plaques, nodules, both earlobes, and the nasal mucosa. Skin smears are made by squeezing a fold of skin between thumb and forefinger, and making a short shallow slit in the skin with a razor blade or scalpel. The instrument is then turned at a right angle to the slit, and the sides of the slit are scraped. The fluid thus obtained is spread on a slide over a circle approximately 1 cm in diameter, heat-fixed, and stained by the Ziehl–Neelsen method. Evaluation of the smears must be performed by experienced personnel to avoid misinterpretation (e.g., reagents may be contaminated with AFB).[84]

Serologic tests for the *M. leprae*–specific PGL-1 antigen and antibodies to PGL-1 are available.[85–87] Specificity is high, and most lepromatous patients are positive. Paucibacillary patients, however, are frequently nonreactive. Other serologic tests based on proteins of *M. leprae* are under study.[88] Multibacillary patients have PGL-1 antigen in serum and urine.[89,90] DNA technology is able to detect small numbers of *M. leprae* in tissue sections, skin, and nasal smears. Because of potential contamination in laboratories in endemic areas, all data from DNA findings must be interpreted carefully and correlated clinicopathologically.[13,34,91] Sera from lepromatous patients may give false-positive reactions for syphilis in cardiolipin-based assays.

Histopathologic Studies

Biopsy specimens should be taken from the edges of lesions and should include the entire thickness of the skin and subcutaneous tissue. Occasionally, damaged nerves may appear only in the subcutaneous tissue. Punch biopsy specimens are most convenient, but should be as large as is cosmetically acceptable for the site chosen. The specimen should be fixed in 10% buffered formalin for routine evaluation. If DNA studies are anticipated, the specimen must be preserved in 70% ethyl alcohol.[92] To demonstrate *M. leprae* optimally in tissue sections, the Fite–Faraco method is essential.[93] A diagnosis of leprosy is made only when the evidence is convincing; "consistent with leprosy" must be avoided in histopathologic evaluations.

Differential Diagnosis

Only a few of the extensive list of differential diagnoses can be given here; they are listed in three categories:

1. *Changes in pigmentation.* Superficial mycoses, scars, birthmarks, postinflammatory changes, and cutaneous filariasis (onchocerciasis and streptocerciasis)[94]
2. *Infiltrated lesions.* Leishmaniasis, lymphoma, granuloma annulare, granuloma multiforme (Mkar disease),[95] lupus erythematosus, psoriasis, pityriasis rosea, sarcoidosis, and neurofibromatosis
3. *Peripheral neuropathies.* Syringomyelia, lead toxicity, diabetes mellitus, primary amyloidosis, and familial hypertrophic neuropathy

TREATMENT AND PROGNOSIS

Because of known drug-resistant strains of *M. leprae*, especially to dapsone and rifampin, monotherapy with any antileprotic is proscribed.[96,97] The type of antibacterial multidrug therapeutic (MDT) regimen employed is usually based on the WHO simplified classification of the disease, that is, PB or MB, and utilizes the WHO recommended combination of drugs,[98–100] as follows:

Single lesion regimen: Some clinicians treat patients who have only a single skin lesion with a single dose combination of rifampin 600 mg, ofloxacin 400 mg, and minocycline 100 mg. In the author's view, there are insufficient long-term follow-up data on efficacy to recommend the general use of this therapeutic approach. Such patients should be treated at least by the PB regimen.

Paucibacillary regimen: Rifampin 600 mg given once monthly under supervision, plus dapsone 100 mg/day for 6 months. Treatment is then discontinued.

Multibacillary regimen: Rifampin 600 mg and clofazimine 300 mg are given once monthly under supervision, plus dapsone 100 mg/day and clofazimine 50 mg/day for at least 12 months; however, some authorities recommend continuation of treatment for 24 months.[83] If hyperpigmentation of skin by clofazimine is not acceptable, prothionamide, ethionamide, or minocycline may be substituted.

Doses of the WHO regimens for children are given in Table 38-2.[101]

In the United States, the National Hansen's Disease Programs (NHDP) recommends the following regimens[102]:

For PB disease: dapsone 100 mg daily plus rifampin 600 mg daily, for 12 months

For MB disease: dapsone 100 mg daily plus rifampin 600 mg daily and clofazimine 50 mg daily, for 24 months

Note: The NHDP recommends that rifampin be given monthly (600 mg) if the patient is currently taking corticosteroids.

Apart from the increasing prevalence of drug resistance of strains of *M. leprae*, multidrug regimens are recommended for their potential for elimination of "persisting" organisms. Persisting *M. leprae* organisms are those leprosy bacilli that are susceptible to the drugs used in therapy, but which can still be identified in small numbers from patients who respond satisfactorily clinically. Such organisms may be responsible for relapses following therapy. Relapse rates following MDT are low but acceptable by most authorities—less than 1% in one large series of patients.[103] A follow-up, however, of 5368 patients for a mean of 10.8 years by Cellona and colleagues showed an absolute relapse rate of 3%; but of particular concern were rates as high as 13% in some subsets of patients.[104] In most populations of patients, relapses are highest in PB patients, suggesting that some patients are wrongly classified. In the experience of histopathologists, clinicians using the WHO system often misclassify MB patients and place them in the PB category. Thus, such patients are apt to be undertreated. There are anecdotal reports of highly bacilliferous patients with relapse rates of up to 20%.[105] Although results of the WHO MDT appear excellent, long-term follow-up is essential.[106] Resistance to all of the drugs in the WHO MDT regimen has been occasionally reported.[107] In view of these various reports of relapse rates, recommendations for MDT regimens should be given regular reappraisal, especially regarding kinds and dosage of drugs and duration of therapy, with special emphasis on long-term follow-up.

Several other potent antileprosy drugs and combinations are under clinical trial and may eventually be included in multidrug regimens. Among these are the fluoroquinolones pefloxicin and ofloxacin, the macrolide clarithromycin, and the tetracycline minocycline.[108–112]

Efficacy of chemotherapy in lepromatous patients can be assessed by clinical progress and the staining property of *M. leprae* in skin smears or biopsy specimens. The response of tuberculoid and borderline patients is best measured by the clinical response and histopathologic evaluation. Viability of *M. leprae* in patients can be determined by mouse foot pad inoculation or by a variety of other, more rapid metabolic assays.[113]

Table 38-2 *World Health Organization Regimens for Multidrug Therapy Regimen for Leprosy in Children*

Weight (kg)	Percentage of Adult Dose
15–30	50
30–45	75
>45	100

From Jopling WH: Handbook of Leprosy. London, Heinemann, 1984.

Care of insensitive hands and feet and correction of physical deformities are essential to the comprehensive treatment of the affected patient. This is an extensive topic, and the reader is directed to appropriate texts on the subject.[114–116]

Therapy for Reactions

Reactions in leprosy are considered a medical emergency. Appropriate treatment should be instituted immediately and the patient followed closely.

Reversal Reaction

If the reaction is accompanied by peripheral neuritis, the affected part is immobilized by a splint, and analgesics and corticosteroids given orally. Up to 80 mg of prednisone daily is given initially and tapered off over 2 to 3 months to a minimally effective level as long as neuritis persists. If long-term prednisone therapy is required, an alternate-day regimen may be attempted. Although suggested by some, the usefulness of clofazimine as an adjunct to corticosteroids in reversal reactions has not been established.[117] Antileprosy therapy is continued during treatment for reactions.

Erythema Nodosum Leprosum

Because all MDT regimens for MB leprosy contain clofazimine, which has significant anti-inflammatory activity, severe ENL is encountered less frequently today. In milder forms of ENL, therapy may require only mild analgesics. Severe ENL requires more aggressive therapy, especially when there is iritis, neuritis, cutaneous ulceration, or orchitis. Thalidomide is the most active drug for ENL, and the initial dose is 100 mg three to four times daily.[118] This dosage is then tapered to the minimum effective level. Clofazimine may also be increased to up to 300 mg/day, but an effect is not usually observed until after use for 4 to 6 weeks. Thalidomide is prescribed only for males and nonfertile females, and some clinicians will administer the drug only to inpatients under direct supervision. Efficacy of thalidomide may depend in part on inhibition of TNF-α production, but other cytokines are probably also affected.[75] If thalidomide cannot be used, prednisone is given as for reversal reactions. Iridocyclitis is a serious complication; local corticosteroids must be added to systemic anti-inflammatory treatment and ophthalmologic consultation obtained.

PREVENTION AND CONTROL

There are no recommendations for prevention of infection in endemic areas. Chemoprophylaxis of close contacts may be useful but is probably not appropriate for large populations.[119,120]

Current control programs are based on the principles that (1) the number of contagious patients is reduced by chemotherapy, and (2) the surveillance of contacts will detect early leprosy. Execution of these principles requires intensive programs in education of the public and training of medical personnel to diagnose leprosy and deliver treatment. A rapid low-cost test for PGL-1 detection offers promise for the identification of contacts of leprosy patients at risk and could be incorporated into control programs.[121] Skin tests specific for leprosy would represent a marked advance in early diagnosis and are under study.[122,123] If such a skin test is considered successful, in view of the fact that many exposed individuals do not go on to develop disease, the ethical management of positive skin reactors without clinical findings must be resolved.

Effective vaccination offers the best approach to the elimination of leprosy infection in humans.[124] Initial evaluation in Venezuela of the WHO vaccine composed of heat-killed *M. leprae* plus bacille Calmette–Guérin (BCG) did not show protection against leprosy.[125] A single BCG vaccination gives varying levels of protection in different geographic areas. A study in Malawi, however, employing repeated BCG vaccinations gave an overall protection rate of 50% against leprosy, with 95% protection in children under 15 years of age.[126] Other trials of vaccines based on cultivable mycobacteria (*Mycobacterium w* and the ICRC bacillus) are in progress in India.[127,128] The development of potential vaccines based on subunit mycobacterial antigens are in the early planning stages.[83]

In contrast to the association of tuberculosis with human immunodeficiency virus (HIV), HIV infection may not be a significant risk factor for leprosy in most populations.[129,130] In some populations in Africa, HIV infection has an overall 2.2 relative risk for leprosy, and up to 23% of the multibacillary infections were HIV-infected.[131] Thus, the eventual effect of HIV infection on control of leprosy remains undetermined.

There is cautious optimism that rigorous application of the WHO MDT regimens will interrupt transmission of leprosy and diminish the incidence. The goal of WHO is to eliminate leprosy as a public health problem, that is, to achieve a prevalence of active leprosy of one patient or less per 10,000 population in all countries. Initially, the year 2000 was set as the time goal for achieving this level of elimination; however, this goal was not reached and has been extended to 2005, and programs that give special attention to the higher endemic foci have been established. To maintain patient confidence and provide more complete care, it should be mandatory that all such programs include resources for follow-up and management of the physical disabilities and social stigma of patients who have completed fixed-duration therapeutic regimens.[83,132] The integration of leprosy control operations into the general health care programs of most countries today makes this goal a formidable task.

REFERENCES

1. Brody SJ: The Disease of the Soul: Leprosy in Medieval Literature. Ithaca, NY, Cornell University Press, 1974.
2. Lieber E: Skin diseases: contagion and sin in the Old Testament. Int J Dermatol 33:593, 1994.
3. Skinsnes OK: Leprosy in society. 2. The pattern of concept and reaction to leprosy in Oriental antiquity. Lepr Rev 35:106, 1964.
4. Leprosy News and Notes. Fifth International Leprosy Congress—1948. The words "leper" and "leprosy." Int J Lepr 16:243, 1948.
5. Frist T: Don't Treat Me Like I Have Leprosy. London, International Federation of Antileprosy Associations (ILEP), 1996.
6. Barksdale L, Kim KS: Mycobacterium. Bacteriol Rev 41:217, 1977.
7. Wabitsch KR, Meyers WM: Histopathologic observations on the persistence of *Mycobacterium leprae* in the skin of multibacillary leprosy patients under chemotherapy. Lepr Rev 59:341, 1988.
8. Kato L: Leprosy associated mycobacteria: implications. Acta Leprol 7:1, 1989.
9. Shepard CC: The experimental disease that follows the injection of human leprosy bacilli into foot pads of mice. J Exp Med 112:445, 1960.

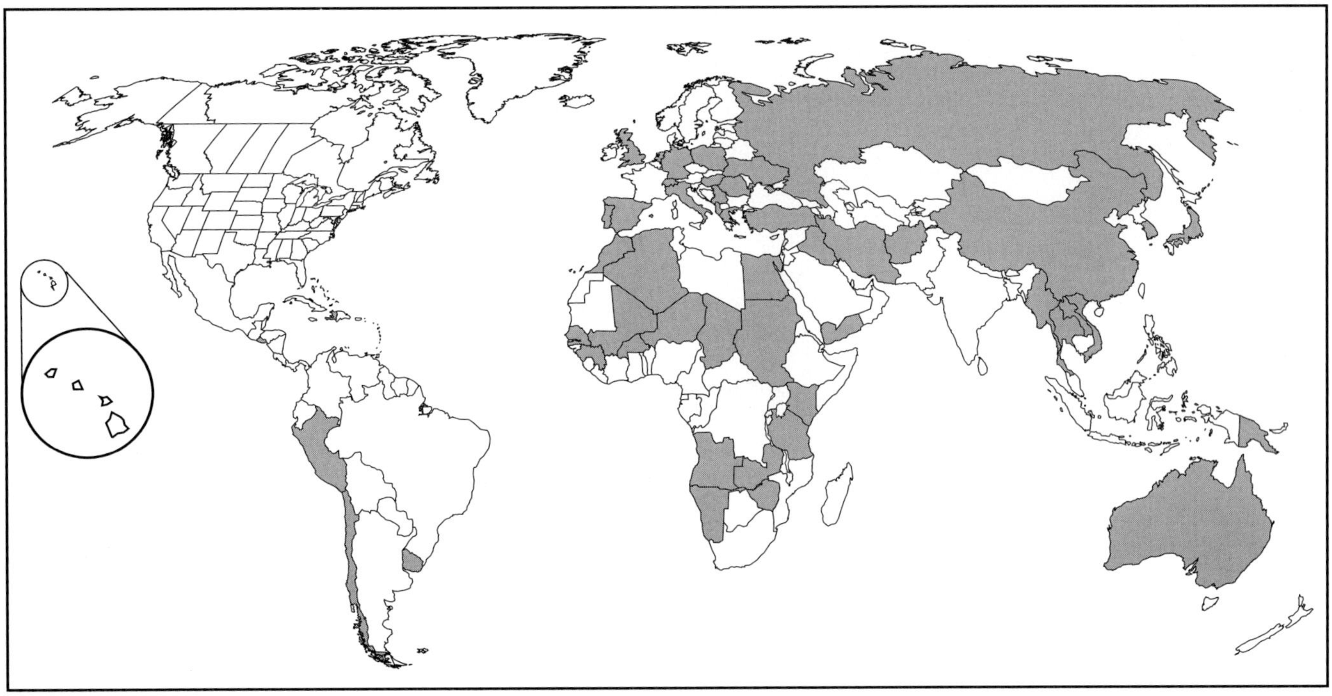

Countries with cases of human infection with *Bacillus anthracis*

■ Global distribution

not only this result but also can transport anthrax organisms in contaminated parts of the carcass and in their own feces over substantial distances. Thus, the cycle of deposition of spores in the soil and their consumption by herbivores continues. The best example of the ability of spores to survive in the soil is the biological warfare experiments on Gruinard Island off the western coast of Scotland.[3] Explosive release of spores in 1942 and 1943 resulted in soil contamination that persisted until 1986 when extensive formaldehyde decontamination was successfully accomplished. Where anthrax in domestic animals has been a problem in the past, it may remain so unless effective preventive vaccination is implemented and maintained.

Humans become incidentally infected when contacting spores on dead animals or their meat, hides, hair, or wool. The most common form of the disease, cutaneous anthrax, occurs when spores enter skin damaged by a cut or abrasion in persons involved in butchering or skinning an infected animal or working with the wool, hair, or hide in an industry that may be thousands of miles away.[1,2,6,7,16–21] There is circumstantial evidence that biting flies transmit anthrax not only to humans but also among animals.[21,22] Ingestion of raw or undercooked meat may cause a severe enteric disease that has been described mainly in tropical Africa and Asia. Inhalation of spores causes illness mainly in manufacturing settings, including the domestic weaving of contaminated wool.[1,2,23–26]

DISEASE

The four clinical forms of human anthrax—cutaneous, oral-oropharyngeal, gastrointestinal, and inhalational—are determined by the portal of entry of the etiologic bacterium. More than 90% of cases are cutaneous, and even if untreated 80% or more of these infections remain localized. A high proportion of patients with inhalational, oropharyngeal, gastrointestinal, and oral-oropharyngeal forms and approximately 20% of patients with the cutaneous form develop systemic bacteremia and succumb to the fatal effects of the anthrax toxins.

Cutaneous Anthrax

Cutaneous anthrax occurs mainly on the exposed parts of the body, usually the hands, fingers, arms, face, or neck.[1–3,17–22,27] In greater than 90% of cases, there is a single lesion. After an incubation period of 1 to 7 days (usually 2 or 3 days), local pruritus is the initial symptom, followed within a day by a papule a few millimeters in diameter. Usually, on the second day one or more vesicles appear on the papule or in a ring around it. After enlargement or coalescence of the vesicles during the subsequent 1 to 3 days, the papule ruptures, forming a round 0.5- to 3-cm ulcer that dries to become a depressed, brown eschar that turns black, thick, and adherent to the underlying tissue during the next few days (Fig. 39-2). A characteristic feature of the eschar is that it is painless, and unless it is superinfected there is no pus. Many patients are afebrile, having no systemic signs or symptoms; others have headache, anorexia, nausea, malaise, and fever. Other significant clinical manifestations are regional lymphadenopathy and nonpitting edema around the eschar. The severity and extent of the edema are related to the overall severity of the infection and to the location of the lesion in an area with loose connective tissue. The edema itself can be fatal, particularly in the head and neck; tracheotomy may be required to

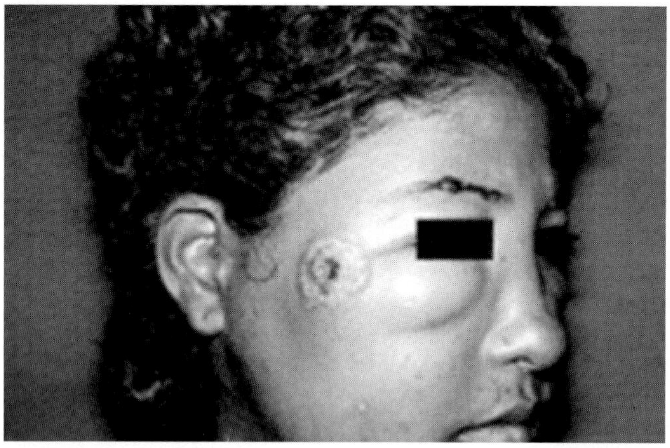

FIGURE 39-2 Eschar of cutaneous anthrax that developed over a 5-day period from a small painless pruritic papule to a hemorrhagic bulla. The 20-year-old woman had been tending grazing goats. (Sethuraman G, Thappa DM, Karthikeyan K: Cutaneous anthrax. Postgrad Med J 76:472, 2000.)

avoid asphyxiation. Septicemic anthrax, whether occurring in association with cutaneous, gastrointestinal, or inhalational anthrax, is characterized by hematogenous lesions in the meninges and gastrointestinal tract in a substantial proportion of cases, as well as by the systemic effects of the toxin.[28,29] The local cutaneous lesion resolves slowly over 2 to 6 weeks, apparently without any effect of treatment and frequently with little trace after healing of the already established pathologic processes. In rare cases, complicating gangrene may require skin grafting and surgical reconstruction, particularly of the eyelid.

The skin lesion usually manifests edema involving, most prominently, the upper dermis (Fig. 39-3), with formation of a subepidermal bulla that is sloughed, leaving an ulcer. The fully formed eschar comprises coagulation necrosis of the skin with anthrax bacilli, vasculitis, edema, hemorrhage, and leukocytic exudate extending deep into the subcutaneous fat but not the skeletal muscle.[29,30] Experimental subcutaneous inoculation of spores into chimpanzees demonstrated dose-dependent development of septicemic anthrax, with death occurring between days 3 and 7 after inoculation of 5×10^3 to 5×10^4 spores.[31] There was gelatinous edema of the surrounding skin and hemorrhagic necrosis of the draining lymph nodes.

Oral-Oropharyngeal and Gastrointestinal Anthrax

Infection following the ingestion of meat of infected animals has been described frequently in Africa and Asia.[5–8,32,33] In oral-oropharyngeal anthrax, the pathologic lesions are visible, a history of eating raw or slightly cooked meat an average of 2 days beforehand is usually obtained, and epidemiologic association with cases of cutaneous anthrax is evident.[32] Presenting symptoms include swelling of the neck, fever, sore throat, and dysphagia.[32–34] Examination reveals soft tissue edema, regional lymphadenopathy, and mucosal lesions of the tonsils, posterior pharynx, base of the tongue, or hard palate. The lesion is initially congested and edematous and undergoes necrosis and ulceration by the end of the first week; early in the second week a pseudomembrane forms over the ulcer. A substantial portion of these patients recover following antibiotic treatment, but severely ill patients develop respiratory distress and may die of septicemic toxemia. The pathologic findings include mucosal ulceration, necrosis of underlying tissue, the presence of an overlying pseudomembrane, and hemorrhagic regional lymph nodes.

Gastrointestinal anthrax incidence is erratic, which presumably explains why infected animals are so regularly eaten. An outbreak of gastrointestinal anthrax occurred affecting 143 of 155 persons 15 to 72 hours after eating the meat of a dead zebra (91% gastrointestinal, 9% oropharyngeal).[34] Nine children died within 48 hours. Abdominal radiographs revealed gaseous distention, air-fluid levels, and ascites. Illness begins with low-grade fever, headache, and congestion of the face and conjunctivae followed 24 hours later by abdominal pain, nausea, vomiting, an ill-defined right lower

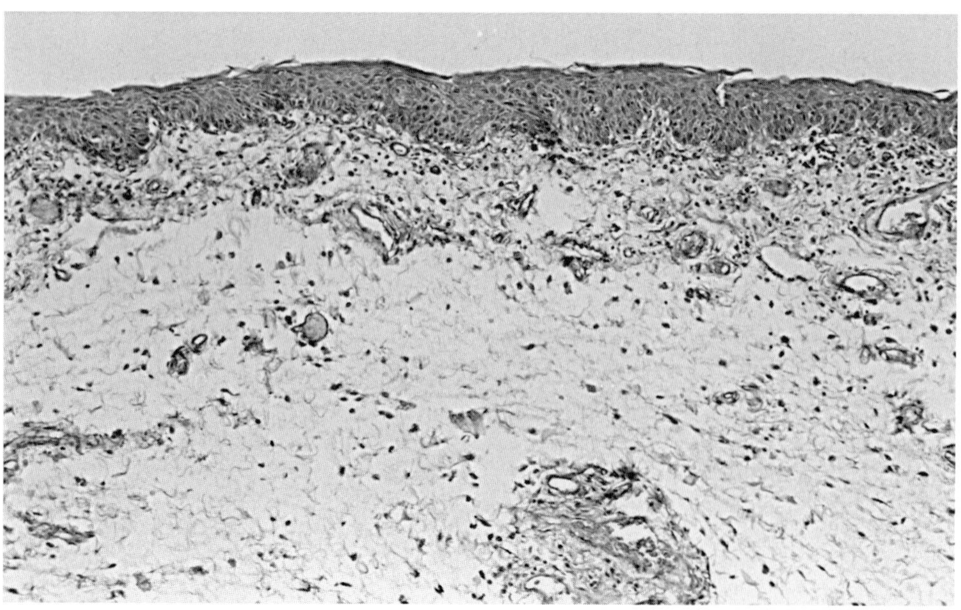

FIGURE 39-3 Photomicrograph of skin in a case of cutaneous anthrax showing typical, marked dermal edema resulting in separation of collagen fibers together with vascular ectasia and a patchy mixed inflammatory cell infiltrate. (H&E stain; ×160.) (Courtesy of Dr MJ Hale, The South African Institute for Medical Research.)

quadrant or periumbilical mass, abdominal distention, ascites, and hypovolemia.[35] Subsequent rapid increase in abdominal girth, paroxysmal abdominal pain, and occasionally gastrointestinal bleeding lead to shock. Exploratory laparotomy reveals abundant ascites and large, soft mesenteric lymph nodes, especially in the ileocecal region, and edema of the cecum, ascending colon, or a segment of small intestine. Infection presumably results from penetration of the mucosa by spores and subsequent germination to the vegetative form. In his experimental studies of anthrax in sheep, Pasteur had to mix the bacterial spores with feed containing thistle, probably to provide a mechanical lesion through which the spores entered the mucosa. The portal of entry is considered to be the cecum, ascending colon, or terminal ileum, where the pathologic findings are a solitary hemorrhagic, necrotic, edematous mucosal lesion and hemorrhagic mesenteric lymphadenitis, analogous to the lymphatic spread of fatal cutaneous or oral-oropharyngeal anthrax.[36] Cases in which the gastric mucosa contained the apparent primary lesions have also been described.[29] Patients with gastrointestinal anthrax present with fever, anorexia, nausea, and vomiting and later develop severe abdominal pain.[5–8] At least half the cases are fatal owing to septicemic toxemia and in some cases hemorrhagic, bacillus-laden ascites or gastrointestinal hemorrhage.

Inhalational and Meningeal Anthrax

Inhalational anthrax occurs as an industrial disease associated with contaminated wool, hair, or other animal products, or as bioterrorism (see Chapter 15).[23–26,37] *B. anthracis* spores inhaled in particles smaller than 5 μm in diameter are transported to the mediastinal lymph nodes, where they germinate, replicate, and secrete toxins that cause massive hemorrhage, edema, and necrosis in these nodes. The organisms and their toxins disseminate hematogenously with a nearly uniformly fatal outcome unless an effective antibiotic is used early in the illness.

Although anthrax meningoencephalitis is considered to result from hematogenous spread after entry in the skin, gastrointestinal tract, or lungs and from lymphogenous spread to the regional lymph nodes, patients have been described in whom no primary lesion was identified.[38] The case-fatality rate is around 34% even with treatment.

PATHOGENESIS AND IMMUNITY

After germination, *B. anthracis* secretes three plasmid-encoded proteins: protective antigen, lethal factor, and edema factor, which act in combination as toxins.[3] Protective antigen, an 83-kD protein, binds by its C-terminal to a cell surface receptor, is cleaved by a host protease (furin) to yield a 63-kD polypeptide, and assembles into a heptameric β-barrel that is capable of binding lethal factor or edema factor. After endocytosis of the protective antigen-lethal factor/edema factor complex, acid-mediated conformational change, and insertion of the heptamer pore into the endocytic membrane, the lethal toxin and/or edema toxin are transported into the host cell cytoplasm.[39–41] Edema factor, an 89-kD protein, is a calmodulin-dependent adenylate cyclase that increases the intracellular cyclic adenosine monophosphate (AMP), resulting in the interstitial edema occurring around the eschar.[42] Lethal factor is a zinc metalloprotease[43] with activity that digests mitogen-activated protein kinases 1, 2, 3, 4, 6, and 7.[44] Pathogenicity of *B. anthracis* requires the presence of the plasmid-encoded, antiphagocytic, poly-D-glutamic acid capsule.[45] A key pathologic lesion apparently explaining the lethal hemorrhagic meningitis and hematogenous hemorrhagic pneumonia of disseminated anthrax is vasculitis.[46] The induction of apoptosis in endothelial cells by lethal toxin may play a role in the vascular lesions.[47]

Immunity to anthrax requires immunization in which protective antigen is the most important stimulus of toxin-neutralizing antibodies although antigens of lethal factor, the spore, and cell wall also contribute to protection.

DIAGNOSIS

The diagnosis of anthrax depends on recognition of the cutaneous or oropharyngeal lesion, typical signs and symptoms, history of exposure or potential exposure to an infected animal or its products, and laboratory confirmation by examination of a gram-stained smear of vesicle fluid, skin or oropharyngeal ulcer base, ascites, or pleural or cerebrospinal fluid; culture; immunohistochemical identification of *B. anthracis;* or serologic studies. The preceding pruritus, ring of vesicles, black eschar, absence of pain and pus, and presence of edema surrounding the cutaneous lesion are diagnostically suggestive. The differential diagnosis of cutaneous anthrax includes staphylococcal boil, syphilitic chancre, ulceroglandular tularemia or plague, rickettsial eschar, brown recluse spider bite, burn wound, ecthyma gangrenosa, milker's nodule, and orf. The differential diagnosis of oral-oropharyngeal anthrax includes diphtheria and peritonsillar abscess. Gastrointestinal anthrax and anthrax meningitis could present with similar signs and symptoms to gastroenteritis or meningitis caused by many agents. In its early stages, inhalational anthrax resembles influenza or other viral upper respiratory infections. An important diagnostic clue is radiographic widening of the mediastinum owing to edema, hemorrhage, and necrosis. Diagnosis, especially in samples of animal blood, is confirmed by the M'Fadyean stain, which demonstrates a pink capsule surrounding dark-blue, often square-ended bacilli.[3,48] Nonhemolytic tenacious colonies of nonmotile, penicillin-sensitive, gram-positive bacilli are recovered from vesicle fluid, eschar, tonsillar ulcer, blood, ascites, or cerebrospinal fluid on 5% sheep blood agar. Specific identification is achieved by lysis with a specific γ-bacteriophage or by staining with monoclonal antibodies to the capsule and cell wall antigens.

A specific inhibition enzyme immunoassay for antibodies directed against purified protective antigen has been used to establish a diagnosis in cases of cutaneous anthrax.[9,30]

TREATMENT

Cutaneous anthrax had a case-fatality rate of 16% in the preantibiotic era during the period 1933–1938. One physician cared for 116 cases of cutaneous anthrax between 1933 and 1955, using antianthrax serum in the first 21 cases, sulfonamides in the 56 patients between 1939 and 1947, and penicillin, a tetracycline (27 patients), chloramphenicol (7 patients), or erythromycin (2 patients), thereafter.[17] After 1933, no deaths occurred as all the treatment regimens proved to be of increasing effectiveness. Early in its use penicillin was administered in doses as low as 50,000 to 100,000 units daily.[49] After doses of 100,000 to 200,000 units/d for 3 days, no bacteria could be recovered from 90% of the cutaneous lesions. Two million units of intravenous penicillin sterilizes blister fluid in 5 hours.

For cutaneous anthrax, oral potassium penicillin V (30 mg/kg body weight per day in four divided doses every 6 hours for 5 to 7 days) is recommended. In more severely ill patients, intramuscular procaine penicillin G aqueous (34,000 units/kg body weight per day divided into two equal doses given every 12 hours) is often given. For penicillin-allergic patients, tetracycline, ciprofloxacin, erythromycin, or chloramphenicol can be used.

For systemic anthrax (septicemic, inhalational, gastrointestinal, or oropharyngeal) high-dose intravenous penicillin G is the treatment of choice. Ciprofloxacin (400 mg intravenously every 12 hours or 100 mg doxycycline intravenously every 12 hours) has been used to treat systemic anthrax sepsis.[34] Streptomycin, erythromycin, and tetracycline have also been used. Intensive supportive care is often necessary.

Surgical excision of the cutaneous lesion or incision of a subcutaneous or tonsillar lesion does not improve the outcome nor does it yield any drainage of pus because there is none. Indeed, exacerbation of the local injury may ensue.

PREVENTION AND CONTROL

Prevention of human anthrax depends on prevention of animal anthrax as has largely been achieved in Europe and the United States. In Zimbabwe during the period October 1979–1980 when civil and military conditions stopped effective animal vaccination programs, there were more than 6000 cases of human anthrax compared with fewer than 500 cases during the entire period 1923–1977.[20–22] In South Africa, animal vaccinations provided free, beginning in 1923, reduced the annual outbreaks of anthrax in cattle from approximately 1000 to fewer than three.[48] The effective veterinary vaccine consists of viable *B. anthracis* spores that contain the plasmid for production of protective antigen, lethal factor, and edema factor but lack the plasmid with genes for synthesis of the capsule.[48] Control measures include quarantine of animals on farms where cases have been confirmed, vaccination of all livestock on the farm and adjacent areas, treatment of animals with antibiotics (antibiotics must not be given 10 days before or after vaccination to avoid killing the live attenuated bacterial vaccine), isolation and destruction of infected animals, incineration or burial of infected carcasses with slaked lime, and disinfection of the premises with 5% formaldehyde.

Humans are protected by public awareness programs regarding the dangers of contact with the infected animals or their meat and products. Vaccines have been developed for human use; a live spore vaccine similar to the Sterne veterinary vaccine has been used effectively in the former USSR.[50] Dynaport produces a nonliving vaccine that contains protective antigen and requires a primary series of inoculations as well as booster vaccinations.

Prophylactic antibiotics are ineffective in preventing inhalational anthrax unless given for 6 days, preferably in conjunction with vaccination on days 1 and 15.[51] Oral penicillin prophylaxis has been used following ingestion of known contaminated meat and after cutaneous injection of virulent organisms.

REFERENCES

1. Christie AB: Anthrax. In Infectious Diseases: Epidemiology and Clinical Practice, Vol 23. Edinburgh, Churchill Livingstone, 1974, p 787.
2. Brachman PS: Anthrax. In Wehrle PF, Top FH (eds): Communicable and Infectious Diseases, 9th ed. St Louis, Mosby-Year Book, 1981, p 119.
3. LaForce FM: Anthrax. Clin Infect Dis 19:1009, 1994.
4. Fox MD, Boyce JM, Kaufmann AF, et al: An epizootiologic study of anthrax in Falls County, Texas. J Am Vet Med Assoc 170:327, 1977.
5. Bhat P, Mohan DN, Srinivasa H: Intestinal anthrax with bacteriological investigations. J Infect Dis 152:1357, 1985.
6. Kunanusont C, Limpakarnjanarat K, Foy HM: Outbreak of anthrax in Thailand. Ann Trop Med Parasitol 84:507, 1990.
7. Sekhar PC, Singh RS, Sridhar MS, et al: Outbreak of human anthrax in Ramabhadrapuram village of Chittoor district in Andhra Pradesh. Indian J Med Res 91:448, 1990.
8. Alizad A, Ayoub EM, Makki N: Intestinal anthrax in a two-year-old child. Pediatr Infect Dis J 14:394, 1995.
9. Read TD, Peterson SN, Tourasse N, et al: The genome sequence of *Bacillus anthracis* Ames and comparison to closely related bacteria. Nature 423:81, 2003.
10. Liu H, Bergman NH, Thomason B, et al: Formation and composition of the *Bacillus anthracis* endospore. J Bacteriol 186:164, 2004.
11. Bourgogne A, Drysdale M, Hilsenbeck SG, et al: Global effects of virulence gene regulators in a *Bacillus anthracis* strain with both virulence plasmids. Infect Immun 71:2736, 2003.
12. Turnbull PC, Doganay M, Lindeque PM, et al: Serology and anthrax in humans, livestock and Etosha National Park wildlife. Epidemiol Infect 108:299, 1992.
13. Lindeque PM, Turnbull PC: Ecology and epidemiology of anthrax in the Etosha National Park, Namibia. Onderstepoort J Vet Res 61:71, 1994.
14. Tuchili LM, Pandey GS, Sinyangwe PG, et al: Anthrax in cattle, wildlife and humans in Zambia. Vet Rec 132:487, 1993.
15. Dragon DC, Rennie RP: The ecology of anthrax spores: tough but not invincible. Can Vet J 36:295, 1995.
16. MacDonald WD: Anthrax: report of a fatal case involving the cutaneous and gastrointestinal systems. N Engl J Med 226:949, 1942.
17. Gold H: Anthrax: a report of one hundred seventeen cases. Arch Intern Med 96:387, 1955.
18. Parvizpour D: Human anthrax in Iran: an epidemiological study of 468 cases. Int J Zoonoses 5:69, 1978.
19. Taylor JP, Dimmitt DC, Ezzell JW, et al: Indigenous human cutaneous anthrax in Texas. South Med J 86:1, 1993.
20. Davies JCA: A major epidemic of anthrax in Zimbabwe: I. Cent Afr J Med 28:291, 1982.
21. Davies JCA: A major epidemic of anthrax in Zimbabwe: II. Cent Afr J Med 29:8, 1983.
22. Davies JCA: A major epidemic of anthrax in Zimbabwe: the experience at the Beatrice Road Infectious Diseases Hospital, Harare. Cent Afr J Med 31:176, 1985.
23. Brachman PS: Inhalation anthrax. Ann NY Acad Sci 353:83, 1980.
24. Eurich FW: The history of anthrax in the wool industry of Bradford, and of its control. Lancet 1:57, 1926.
25. LaForce FM: Woolsorters' disease in England. Bull NY Acad Med 54:956, 1978.
26. Elkina AV: The epidemiology of a pulmonary form of anthrax. Zh Mikrobiol Epidemiol Immunobiol 48:112, 1971.
27. Aksaray N, Cinaz P, Coskun U, et al: Cutaneous anthrax. Trop Geogr Med 42:168, 1990.
28. Abramova FA, Grinberg LM, Yampolskaya OV, et al: Pathology in inhalational anthrax in 42 cases from the Sverdlovsk outbreak of 1979. Proc Natl Acad Sci USA 90:2291, 1993.
29. Dutz W, Kohout E: Anthrax. Pathol Annu 6:209, 1971.
30. Shieh WJ, Guarner J, Paddock C, et al: The critical role of pathology in the investigation of bioterrorism-related cutaneous anthrax. Am J Pathol 163:1901–1910, 2003.
31. Berdjis CC, Gleiser CA: Experimental subcutaneous anthrax in chimpanzees. Exp Mol Pathol 3:63, 1964.

32. Sirisanthana T, Navachareon N, Tharavichitkul P, et al: Outbreak of oral-oropharyngeal anthrax: an unusual manifestation of human infection with *Bacillus anthracis*. Am J Trop Med Hyg 33:144, 1984.
33. Doganay M, Almac A, Hanagasi R: Primary throat anthrax. Scand J Infect Dis 18:415, 1986.
34. Beatty ME, Ashford DA, Griffin PM, et al: Gastrointestinal anthrax. Arch Intern Med 164:2527, 2003.
35. Kanafani ZA, Ghossain A, Sharara AI, et al: Endemic gastrointestinal anthrax in 1960s Lebanon: clinical manifestations and surgical findings. Emerg Infect Dis 9:520, 2003.
36. Derizhanov SM: Pathologic Anatomy and Pathogenesis of the Intestinal Form of Anthrax. Smolensk, Russia, Smolensk Institute of Pathology Anatomy, Western Oblast Government Printing House, 1935.
37. Walker DH, Yampolska O, Grinberg LM: Death at Sverdlovsk: what have we learned? Am J Pathol 144:1135, 1994.
38. George S, Mathai D, Balraj V, et al: An outbreak of anthrax meningoencephalitis. Trans R Soc Trop Med Hyg 88:206, 1994.
39. Klimpel KR, Molloy SS, Thomas G, et al: Anthrax toxin protective antigen is activated by a cell surface protease with the sequence specificity and catalytic properties of furin. Proc Natl Acad Sci USA 89:10277, 1992.
40. Novak JM, Stein M-P, Little SF, et al: Functional characterization of protease-treated *Bacillus anthracis* protective antigen. J Biol Chem 267:17186, 1992.
41. Singh Y, Klimpel KR, Arora N, et al: The chymotrypsin-sensitive site, FFD^{315}, in anthrax toxin protective antigen is required for translocation of lethal factor. J Biol Chem 269:29039, 1994.
42. Little SF, Leppla SH, Burnett JW, et al: Structure-function analysis of *Bacillus anthracis* edema factor by using monoclonal antibodies. Biochem Biophys Res Commun 199:676, 1994.
43. Klimpel KR, Arora N, Leppla SH: Anthrax toxin lethal factor contains a zinc metalloprotease consensus sequence which is required for lethal toxin activity. Mol Microbiol 13:1093, 1994.
44. Chopra AP, Boone SA, Liang X, et al: Anthrax lethal factor proteolysis and inactivation of MAPK kinase. J Biol Chem 278: 9402, 2003.
45. Uchida I, Sekizaki T, Hashimoto K, et al: Association of the encapsulation of *Bacillus anthracis* with a 60 megadalton plasmid. J Gen Microbiol 131:363, 1985.
46. Grinberg LM, Abramova FA, Yampolskaya OV, et al: Quantitative pathology of inhalational anthrax. I. Quantitative microscopic findings. Mod Pathol 14:482, 2001.
47. Kirby JE: Anthrax lethal toxin induces human endothelial cell apoptosis. Infect Immun 72:430, 2004.
48. Anthrax control and research, with special reference to national programme development in Africa: memorandum from a WHO meeting. Bull World Health Organ 72:13, 1994.
49. LaBoccetta AC: Anthrax: 36 human cases of the external type treated successfully with penicillin. Am J Med Sci 216:407, 1948.
50. Shlyakhov EN, Rubinstein E: Human live anthrax vaccine in the former USSR. Vaccine 12:727, 1994.
51. Friedlander AM, Welkos SL, Pitt MLM, et al: Postexposure prophylaxis against experimental inhalation anthrax. J Infect Dis 167:1239, 1993.

40

Bartonelloses

DAVID H. WALKER
CIRO MAGUIÑA
MICHAEL MINNICK

INTRODUCTION

The genus *Bartonella* includes *B. bacilliformis,* the etiologic agent of a sandfly-transmitted febrile hemolytic anemia (Oroya fever) and chronic cutaneous angiomatosis (verruga peruana) endemic to Andean tropical Peru, Ecuador, and Colombia; *B.* (formerly *Rochalimaea*) *quintana,* the causative agent of trench fever during World Wars I and II and currently among the louse-infested poor; *B. henselae,* the major cause of cat-scratch disease (Table 40-1); *B.* (formerly *Rochalimaea*) *vinsonii,* until recently not considered to be a pathogen; *B. elizabethae,* an etiologic agent of infective endocarditis (as are *B. henselae, B. quintana,* and *B. vinsonii*); and several newly discovered species and others formerly assigned to the genus *Grahamella,* that cause persistent asymptomatic infections of wild rodents in both tropical and temperate regions.[1–5] In immunocompromised persons, particularly those infected with human immunodeficiency virus (HIV), *B. henselae* and *B. quintana* cause opportunistic infections, frequently manifested as cutaneous bacillary angiomatosis resembling verruga peruana.[6] Bartonellae are members of the α-Proteobacteria group, which also contains the genera *Rickettsia, Ehrlichia,* and *Brucella,* and *Agrobacterium tumefaciens,* a plant pathogen, all of which have evolved from a common ancestor.

Pre-Columbian evidence of South American bartonellosis includes artistic representations in pottery and stone as well as lesions in a mummy.[7–9] The Spanish conquistadors in Ecuador and soldiers dispatched to quell the rebellion of Diego de Almagro developed illnesses characterized by systemic symptoms and numerous cutaneous lesions that persisted for months, which were documented by chronicles contemporary with the events. The verruga peruana form of the illness was described in colonial times and was illustrated by a medical photograph in the 1856 medical thesis of Dr. Tomás Salazar. The acute hemolytic form of *B. bacilliformis* infection occurred catastrophically during the construction of Peru's Central Railway, which includes 61 bridges from Lima to Oroya, from which the designation Oroya fever is derived.[7,8,10] At least 7000 workers died between 1869 and 1873 as the railroad construction passed from 1000 to 3000 m above sea level, roughly along the Rimac River valley, where the sandfly vector abounds. The city of Oroya, at 3800 m elevation, has always been free of the disease. The connection between

Table 40-1 Etiology and Transmission of Human Bartonelloses

Agent	Disease	Vector
B. bacilliformis	Oroya fever (acute) Verruga peruana (chronic)	*Lutzomyia verrucarum* (sandfly)
B. quintana	Trench fever	*Pediculus humanus corporis* (louse)
	Bacillary angiomatosis Endocarditis	
B. henselae	Cat-scratch disease	Cats and *Ctenocephalides felis* (flea)
	Bacillary angiomatosis Endocarditis	
B. elizabethae and *B. vinsonii*	Endocarditis	Presumably fleas and ticks

Oroya fever and verruga peruana was vividly and dramatically demonstrated by a Peruvian medical student, Daniel Carrión, who, seeking to prove that the cutaneous disease was infectious, had himself inoculated experimentally with material from a patient's skin lesion.[7–11] Only as death from severe febrile disease and anemia approached did he realize that the verruga had contained the etiologic agent of Oroya fever. Both manifestations of the infection are now known as Carrión's disease. The Peruvian physician Alberto Barton is credited with the first visualization of the causative bacteria within circulating erythrocytes of patients with Oroya fever in 1905. Battistini, a Peruvian physician working in collaboration with Noguchi's laboratory at the Rockefeller Institute, was apparently the first to regularly cultivate *B. bacilliformis,* and in 1926 Noguchi purportedly cultivated the organism from verruga lesions obtained from Peru.

During the severe trench fever epidemic involving a million persons during World War I, *B. quintana* was considered to be related to rickettsiae because it was found in lice and could not be cultivated.[12] In 1961 Vinson and Fuller[13] reported the isolation of the etiologic agent after prolonged cultivation on blood agar; subsequent infection of human volunteers with this isolate fulfilled Koch's postulates.[14]

Visualization of bacteria in silver-stained lesions of cat-scratch disease in 1983 and the discovery in 1990 that the sequence of a polymerase chain reaction (PCR) product of the 16S ribosomal DNA (rDNA) from bacillary angiomatosis lesions was the same as that from a novel species, *B. henselae,* isolated from the blood of immunocompromised patients, were important milestones in the elucidation of the medical importance of this organism.[15–19] Subsequently, cat-scratch disease patients were shown to develop antibodies to *B. henselae* and to be infected with this bacterium.[20]

AGENTS

B. bacilliformis is an aerobic, facultative intracellular 1- to 3-μm pleomorphic bacillus with a poorly staining gram-negative cell wall and 2 to 16 unipolar flagella conferring a high degree of motility.[21] *B. henselae* exhibits a characteristic twitching movement and has been demonstrated to have type IV pili.[22] *B. henselae* and *B. quintana* are metabolically rather inert in that they test negative for glucose oxidation, indole production, nitrate reduction, and catalase, oxidase, and urease activity.

Bartonellae require hemin, with *B. quintana* having the highest hemin requirement for growth among bacteria.[23] *B. quintana* has five heme receptors that are all expressed and are predicted to be β-barrel outer membrane proteins with eight transmembrane domains and four extracellular loops. The *ialA* invasion gene of *B. bacilliformis* is a dinucleoside polyphosphate hydrolase more similar to eukaryotic plant diadenosine tetraphosphate hydrolases than to the bacterial enzymes.[24] It is considered likely that it removes the toxic substrate that accumulates during invasion and oxidative stress generated by host defenses with useful ATP as a byproduct of its catabolism.

Growth of bartonellae is slow, requires 5% CO_2, hemin, and an optimal temperature of 35°C for *B. quintana* and *B. henselae* and 28°C for *B. bacilliformis*.

EPIDEMIOLOGY

The reservoir host of *B. bacilliformis* is the human, who may remain persistently bacteremic for months after recovery from the clinical illness.[25–28] A wildlife reservoir was postulated, since isolated cases have occurred in persons exposed to vectors for a single night in deserted areas.[29] However, no confirmed isolations of *B. bacilliformis* have been obtained from fauna in the endemic areas. The classically accepted vector in Peru is the female hematophagous sandfly, *Lutzomyia verrucarum*, which is found in narrow river valleys between 500 and 3200 m above sea level. More recently, cases have occurred in high rainforest regions.[30] South American bartonellosis also occurs in Colombia and Ecuador, where *L. verrucarum* is absent.[31] The most likely vector in Colombia is the highly anthropophilic *L. columbiana,* but at present the disease is apparently seldom documented in Colombia.[12,27] The probable vectors in Ecuador, where cases occur in low-lying coastal areas as well as the Andes, are unknown. Although sandflies are incompletely studied in South America, more than 500 different species have been described with two thirds of them in the Americas, more than 60 in Ecuador, and approximately 120 in Peru.[32,33] Serologic studies suggest that in endemic areas more than 60% of the population has been infected.[34] In such populations 0.5% to 10% are bacteremic at any given time.[25,27,35] A prospective population-based study in an endemic site identified a high incidence (12.7 infections/100 person-years) that was greatest in children less than 5 years of age and declined with age.[35] The affected pediatric population commonly belongs to a low income population. Higher incidence was associated with the increased humidity, temperature, and sandfly population during El Niño–influenced weather. As expected with a human reservoir and transmission by indoor sandfly bites in the evening and night, 70% of cases clustered in 18% of households. Mothers in endemic areas expect the verruga to occur in their children and are concerned if, after a certain febrile illness that they consider to be bartonellosis, the children do not develop the skin lesions, fearing more severe complications and death. Epidemics occur when immunologically naive persons are exposed to the infection because of population migration or introduction of infected sandflies.[7,28]

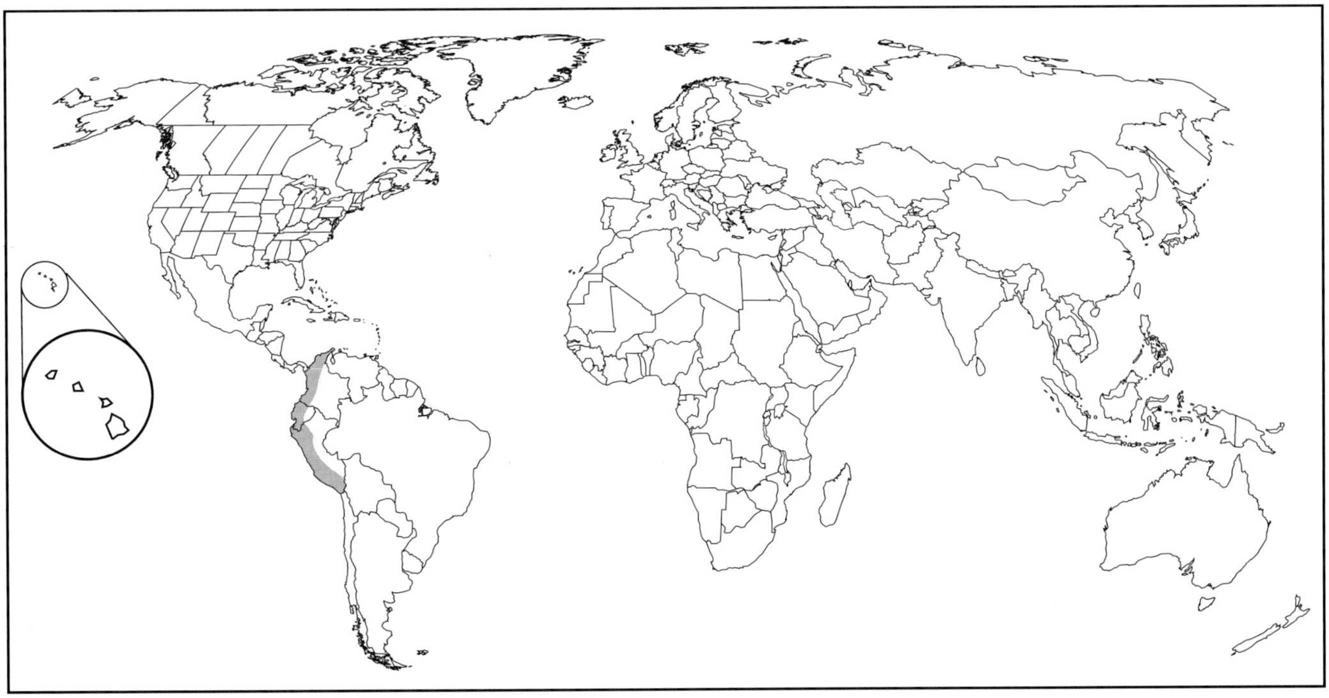

Bartonella bacilliformis

Global distribution

The human louse, *Pediculus humanus corporis,* was recognized as the human-to-human vector of epidemic trench fever in the European theaters of World Wars I and II. *B. quintana* infections have also occurred in the past in North Africa, Ethiopia, Japan, China, Mexico, and Bolivia and more recently in the United States and France among immunocompromised patients, particularly those with HIV infection, as well as among homeless persons who abuse alcohol.[12,13,36–40] After immunocompetent persons recover from untreated *B. quintana* infection, asymptomatic bacteremia may continue for months. It is likely that *B. quintana* is a prevalent but as yet poorly recognized agent of human infections in the tropics.[41]

The reservoir of *B. henselae* is the domestic cat throughout the world, particularly in warm, humid climates where *Ctenocephalides felis* cat fleas thrive.[42,43] A substantial proportion of domestic cats are infected, and bacteremia is prolonged, lasting months to more than a year.[42,44] Cat fleas transmit *B. henselae* between cats and possibly by contaminating cat scratch or bite wounds with flea feces.[45,46] The bacteria remain infectious in flea feces for prolonged periods. There are two genotypes of *B. henselae* that have variable prevalences in different geographic regions with imperfect concordance between the distributions of human and cat genotypes.[47,48] Cat-scratch disease and other manifestations of *B. henselae* infection occur throughout the tropics, although their particular manifestations in some of these areas are yet to be described.

Bartonella endocarditis, most frequently caused by *B. quintana* or *B. henselae*, is not related to the immune status of the host but rather to the risk factors for infection.[49] Case reports of endocarditis caused by *B. elizabethae* or *B. vinsonii* subsp. *berkhoffii,* of myocarditis caused by *B. washoensis*, of neuroretinitis caused by *B. grahamii,* and of bacteremia caused by *B. vinsonii* subsp. *arupensis* are difficult to link with the natural reservoir-vector cycles.[50,51] Conversely high seroprevalence of antibodies to rat-associated *B. elizabethae* among urban intravenous drug abusers has not been correlated with clinical manifestations.[52]

DISEASES

The incubation period of South American bartonellosis is considered to be 21 days (from Carrión's experimental case) with a range of 1 to 30 weeks and a mean of 2 months. The two clinical forms of the disease—Oroya fever and verruga peruana—may occur sequentially, sometimes with an intervening clinically silent period, or either form may occur alone.[7,10,26–28,53,54] The usual gradual onset of systemic symptoms of malaise, somnolence, anorexia, myalgia, headache, pain in the back and extremities, chills, and fever accompany erythrocyte parasitization levels as high as 100%. The mononuclear phagocytic system removes and destroys a major portion of the infected red blood cells after 2 to 4 weeks, resulting in severe anemia with erythrocyte counts in some cases below $10^6/\mu L$, accompanied by hepatosplenomegaly, generalized lymphadenopathy, jaundice, dyspnea, and mental status changes.[27,55,56] The facultative intracellular bartonellae invade endothelial cells, particularly in skin and lymph nodes. Patients with severe infection develop pericardial effusion, myocarditis, coma, convulsions, delirium, acute respiratory distress, anasarca, acute renal failure, and multiple organ failure.[57,58] Infection during pregnancy may result in transplacental infection, abortion, fetal death, and maternal death. The duration of Oroya fever is between 1 and 6 weeks with variation from mild to fatal in approximately 40% of patients during the pre-antibiotic era, 8% currently in hospital settings, 88% in a recent outbreak in a remote rural area, and 0.7% in a contemporary population-based study.[28,56] Death frequently occurs owing to infection-induced immunodeficiency and consequent opportunistic infections that intervene in 30% of cases caused by bacteria (e.g., salmonellae, staphylococci, or *Mycobacterium tuberculosis*), protozoa (e.g., *Toxoplasma* or amoebae), fungi (e.g., *Histoplasma* or *Pneumocystis*), and viruses (e.g., herpesvirus or hepatitis B virus).[11] Salmonellosis was formerly the most frequent fatal complication in hospitalized patients.[59] Inversion of the T lymphocyte helper and suppressor subset ratio and development of skin test anergy reflect transient immunosuppression underlying the appearance of opportunistic infections.[60] Persistent bacteremia by *Bartonella bacilliformis* has been described in a splenectomized patient.[61]

Two to 20 weeks after recovery from Oroya fever or without any preceding illness, arthralgia, fever, and a series of crops of verrucae appear as painless erythematous 0.2- to 4-cm papules, sessile or subdermal nodules, or large angioma-like cutaneous lesions (Fig. 40-1). The lesions are prone to bleed and occur particularly on the head and extremities; sometimes they also occur on the nasal, conjunctival, and oral mucosa, but they

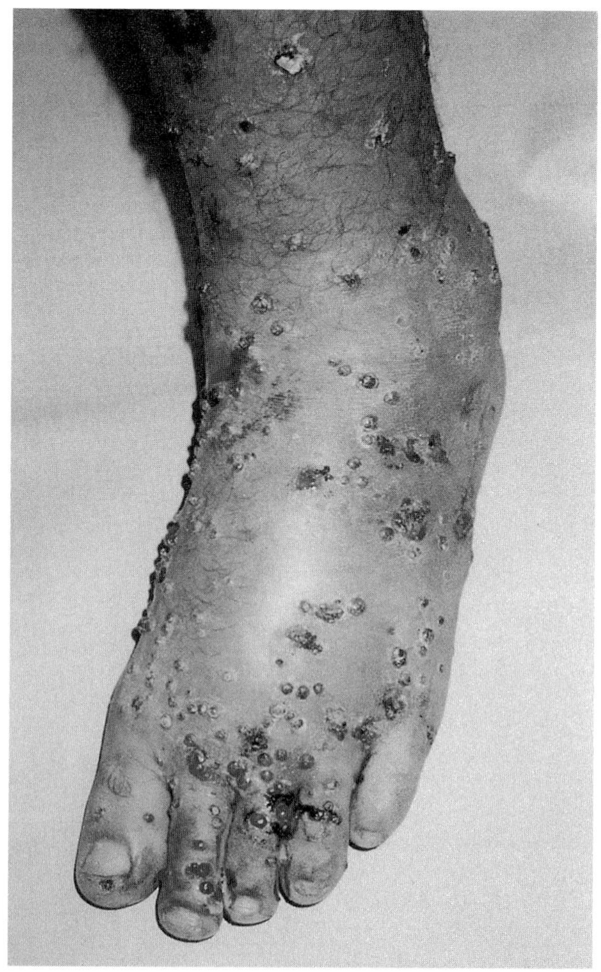

FIGURE 40-1 Verruga peruana skin lesions on the foot and leg of a patient from Peru infected with *B. bacilliformis.*

have never been described in internal organs. Histologically, these lesions consist of proliferations of vascular endothelial cells and dermal dendrocytes with interspersed macrophages, lymphocytes, and plasma cells.[62–64] In verrucae, bartonellae are observed extracellularly.[62,63] Individual verrucae dry up and slough in a few weeks, leaving no scars. Crops of verrucae can occur for months or exceptionally for years.[65,66] In an endemic area, 11% of infections were acute hematic Oroya fever; 37% of the infected population had verruga peruana preceded by symptoms of Oroya fever, 31.5% developed verruga peruana without preceding acute hematic illness, and 20.5% were asymptomatic. Overall only 7% of this medically underserved population were hospitalized, and none died.[35] In an outbreak in a nonendemic area where the disease had not previously occurred, 77.5% of the population developed antibodies against *B. bacilliformis*, 13.8% had symptoms (fever, headache, and bone and joint pain) of Oroya fever, and verruga peruana occurred in 17.6% with only 4.8% of the population manifesting the biphasic course.[67]

Trench fever or acute *B. quintana* infection has a variable incubation period that averages 8 days.[12,14,36] The clinical course varies from mild and afebrile to moderately severe with a long clinical course and numerous relapses. Some patients suffer a single febrile episode of 4 to 5 days often accompanied by malaise, headache, pain that is particularly severe in the shins, and an evanescent rash that is visible mainly in lightly pigmented skin. Other patients have continuous fever for up to 6 weeks or a course with three to eight periodic febrile episodes of about 5 days' duration from which the name *B. quintana* is derived. Contemporary *B. quintana* infection of homeless alcoholic persons is typically manifested only as fever unless associated with *Bartonella* endocarditis.[37–39] Yet among homeless French persons, 14% are bacteremic, 80% of whom are afebrile. Prolonged *B. quintana* bacteremia can persist for 300 to 443 days after onset. In Europe, chronic lymphadenopathy has been associated with granulomatous *B. quintana* infection of the lymph nodes.[68] Immunocompromised patients, especially those with the acquired immunodeficiency syndrome (AIDS), develop disseminated angioma-like lesions of the skin and viscera, bacillary angiomatosis, and bacillary peliosis that are indistinguishable from those produced by *B. henselae*.[6,16]

The clinical manifestations of *B. henselae* infection include cat-scratch disease, unilateral follicular conjunctivitis, neuroretinitis, retinochoroiditis, encephalitis, meningitis, encephalopathy, persistent or relapsing febrile bacteremia, hepatosplenic lesions, infective endocarditis, osteomyelitis, atypical pneumonia, erythema nodosum, bacillary angiomatosis, bacillary peliosis, and inflammatory or vasoproliferative lesions in virtually any organ.[6,16–19,42,47,69–79] Cat-scratch disease is manifest as a papule at the site of inoculation of organisms by cat scratch or bite and regional lymphadenopathy with or without fever in 25% to 60% of patients 3 to 12 days after injury and 1 to 2 weeks before onset of constitutional symptoms. *B. henselae* stimulates an inflammatory reaction in immunocompetent hosts manifest most often as regional (epitrochlear, axillary, and/or cervical) lymphadenopathy that resolves in a median of 7 weeks and undergoes suppuration in 15%. Peruvian studies have detected antibodies to *B. henselae* and *B. clarridgeiae*.[80,81] The formation of mature granulomas leads to the elimination of the organisms. In immunocompromised patients, *B. henselae* and *B. quintana* infections stimulate the proliferation and migration of endothelial cells, resulting in cutaneous bacillary angiomatosis and in some patients similar vascular proliferations in the spleen and liver (bacillary peliosis), lymph node, lung, bone, gastrointestinal tract, brain, mouth, nose, and anus.[82] The lesions resemble verruga peruana with lobular proliferations of endothelial cells.[83] They also contain neutrophils, leukocytoclastic debris, and extracellular amorphous granular material that is revealed by Warthin-Starry silver staining to be microcolonies of bartonellae. Although *B. henselae* and *B. quintana* are facultative intracellular bacteria, intracellular bartonellae (Rocha-Lima bodies) are not characteristic of *B. henselae* and *B. quintana* bacillary angiomatosis.[22] In some patients, the disseminated lesions are neither angioma-like nor granulomatous but rather a mixture of nonspecific inflammation and fibrosis.

Bartonella endocarditis affects mainly middle aged patients who present with fever (83%), often develop emboli (43%) from the large vegetations that involve the aortic valve more often than the mitral valve, and occasionally suffer renal failure owing to mesangioproliferative glomerulonephritis.[49] *Bartonella henselae* most often affects previously damaged valves, and *B. quintana*, previously normal valves. Chronic myocarditis has been reported in association with evidence for *Bartonella* infections.[84,85]

PATHOGENESIS AND IMMUNITY

In Oroya fever, the facultatively intracellular *B. bacilliformis* is introduced into the vasculature by the bite of a sandfly and is taken up by endothelial cells of capillaries, sinusoidal lining cells, and red blood cells.[86–88] Bartonellae induce invaginations in the erythrocyte cell membrane by a small uncharacterized molecule—deformin—and enter the red blood cell using proteins encoded in a two-gene locus together with motive force from flagella.[21,89–93] Entry of *B. bacilliformis* into endothelial cells is dependent on Rho-GTPase, which is activated by the bacteria.[94] *Bartonella quintana* circulate inside 0.001% to 0.005% of human erythrocytes, sequestered from immune attack.[95] Although in vitro cultivation of *B. quintana* in human red blood cells shortens the cells' lifespan, anemia does not occur in marked contrast with extravascular hemolysis in Oroya fever.[95,96] Experimental infection of rats with *B. tribocorum* having deletions in the type IV secretion components *virB4* or *virD4* demonstrated the requirement of these genes for establishment of intraerythrocytic infections.[97]

The pathogenesis of enhanced angiogenesis in *Bartonella*-associated verruga peruana, bacillary angiomatosis, and peliosis may involve endothelial mitogenic factors (e.g., GroEL) secreted by the bacteria, paracrine and autocrine angiogenic effects of vascular endothelial growth factor from macrophages and overlying epidermis, interleukin (IL)–1β from macrophages and IL-8 and angiopoetin 2 from endothelial cells, inhibition of endothelial apoptosis by an unidentified bacterial component, and possibly decreased levels of antiangiogenic IL-12 and IFN-γ in immunocompromised persons.[98–100]

Host defenses against bartonellae involve strong cell-mediated immunity associated with delayed-type sensitivity and Th1-type cytokines (IFN-γ and IL-12). Homeless persons with chronic *B. quintana* bacteremia lack specific antibodies and have lower production of TNF-α, IL-1β, and IL-6 by peripheral blood mononuclear cells and greater production of immunosuppressive IL-10 after *B. quintana* stimulation, which may

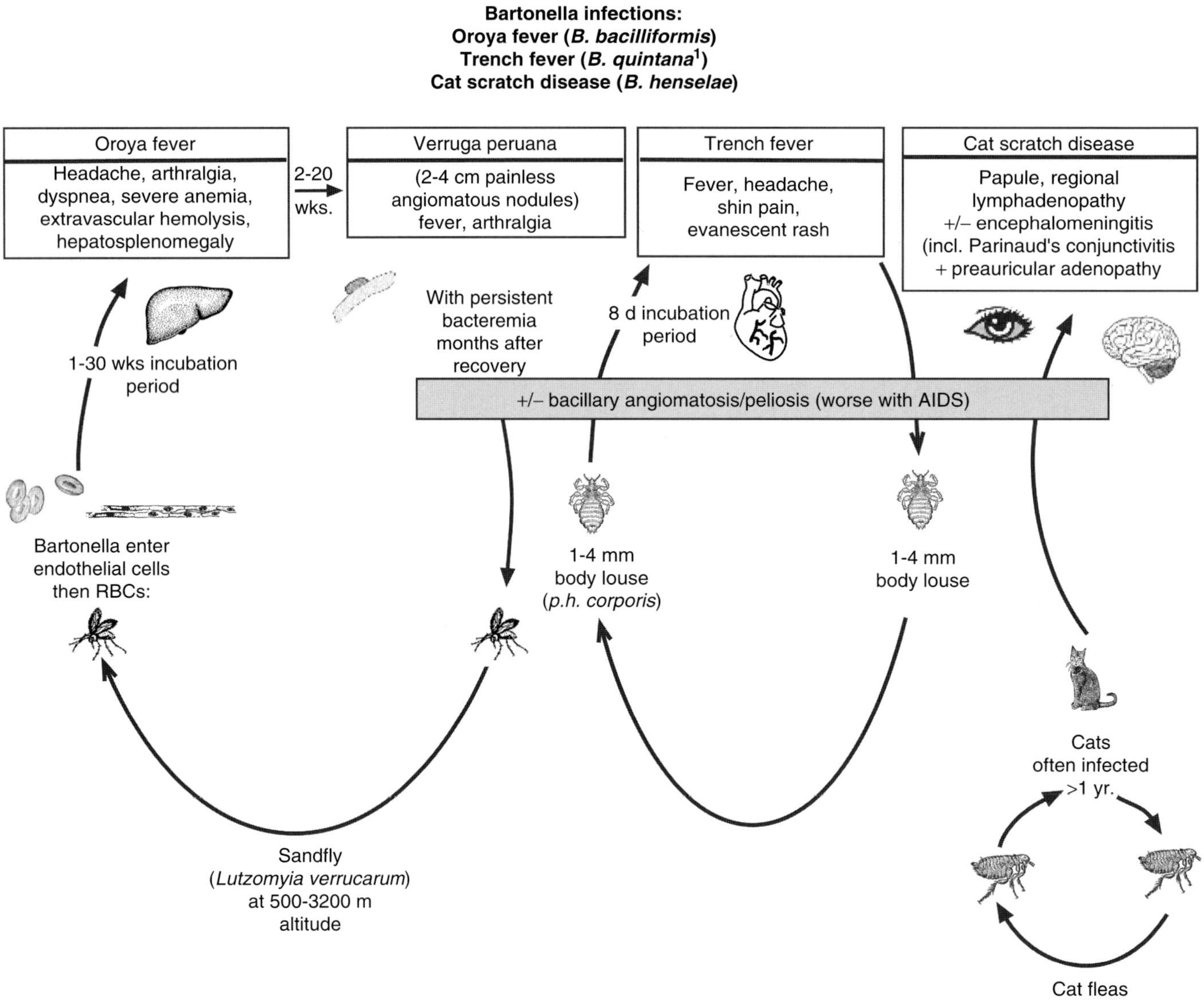

underlie the failure of the immune system to clear the infection.[101] Antibodies clear bartonellae when they are released from infected erythrocytes.[102]

DIAGNOSIS

Oroya fever, with an early clinical differential diagnosis including typhoid fever, malaria, brucellosis, hepatitis, tuberculosis, leptospirosis, sepsis, sylvatic yellow fever, typhus, paracoccidioidomycosis, histoplasmosis, hematologic malignancy, and hemolytic or aplastic anemia, can be diagnosed by detection of *B. bacilliformis* within erythrocytes in stained blood smears (Fig. 40-2). Caution is recommended, however, because of the frequency of artifacts.[27,53] Epidemiologic data are essential. The bacteria can be cultivated from blood in 71% to 83% of cases by incubating for up to 6 weeks at 28°C on Columbia agar supplemented with 5% defibrinated blood or other blood- or hemin-supplemented media, with detection of colonies after a average of 18 days. Diagnosis can also be achieved by PCR even on blood spotted onto a card and can be differentiated from other bartonellae.[35,103–105] Serologic diagnosis of *B. bacilliformis* infection can be established by enzyme immunoassay, IgM or IgG indirect immunofluorescence, indirect hemagglutination and immunoblot detection of a 17- or 18-kDa antigen.[34,67] The diagnosis of verruga peruana, for which the clinical differential diagnosis includes hemangiomas, pyogenic granuloma, bacillary angiomatosis, Kaposi's sarcoma, chickenpox, molluscum contagiosum, and malignant melanoma can be confirmed by histopathology.[62,66,106] Culture of *B. bacilliformis* from the skin lesions is difficult because of frequent contamination and its slow growth rate.

The diagnosis of cat-scratch disease, which formerly relied upon clinical criteria, delayed-type hypersensitivity to a crude skin test material derived from human infected tissues containing antigens of *B. henselae,* and histopathology, now can be established by immunofluorescence antibody (IFA) test, enzyme immunoassay serology, culture, or PCR of lymph node aspirate or biopsy.[20,70] IFA serology provides best results with low passage bacterial antigen cocultivated with cells.

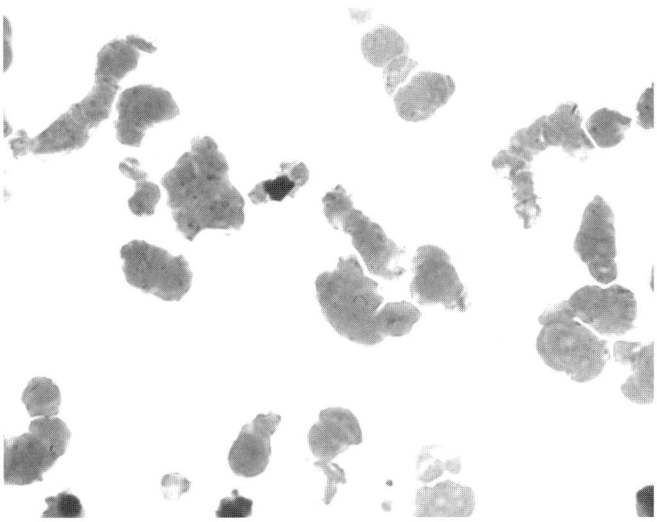

FIGURE 40-2 Peripheral blood smear of a Peruvian patient with Oroya fever. A high portion of erythrocytes contain *Bartonella bacilliformis*.

Agar-grown antigens yield lower titers, and end point titers vary with different commercial products. Thus, a fourfold rise in titer or seroconversion is more convincing than a single high titer. Enzyme immunoassay serology for cat-scratch disease detects IgM antibodies in 53% of sera during the first 3 months, reverting to negative thereafter. IgG antibodies are detected in 92% although initially negative in 28% followed by seroconversion. IgG antibodies are still detectable in only 25% of patients after 1 year.[80] There is considerable serologic cross-reactivity between *B. quintana* and *B. henselae*. Bacteremia with *B. quintana* or *B. henselae* can be diagnosed by saponin or EDTA freeze-thaw lysis of erythrocytes to release intracellular bartonellae, followed by centrifugation and incubation at 35°C in a humid 5% CO_2 atmosphere on chocolate or Columbia blood agar for more than a month, for colonial growth to be visible.[48,107] Organisms are identified by twitching motility in wet mounts, immunofluorescent staining with specific antibodies, and molecular methods. In a recent large series of cases of cat-scratch disease, *B. henselae* DNA was detected by PCR in 31% of lymph node biopsies and 55% of lymph node aspirates, and *B. henselae* was isolated from 27% of lymph node biopsies and 11% of lymph node aspirates after a median of 21 days.[48] The most cost-effective diagnosis of cat-scratch disease relies on the combination of clinical manifestations and serology. The etiologic diagnosis of bacillary angiomatosis and *Bartonella* endocarditis can be established on resected tissues by a combination of histopathology and immunohistology, PCR, or culture.[37,83,108] Bartonella antibodies are usually absent in immunocompromised patients with bacillary angiomatosis. Bartonella endocarditis is diagnosed more effectively by real-time PCR than by culture, and an IFA titer of at least 800 is strongly supportive of the diagnosis.[48,109] The species of bartonella endocarditis can be determined by cross-absorption immunoblotting.[110]

TREATMENT

Oroya fever was treated traditionally with chloramphenicol (50 mg/kg/d up to 3 g/d) and after defervescence with half the dose for 10 days because of chloramphenicol's activity against salmonellosis, a classically described life-threatening secondary infection.[56,111] In recent years, therapeutic failure with chloramphenicol due to overwhelming infections (e.g., *Pseudomonas* sp, *Enterobacter* sp, *Acinetobacter* sp) has changed the drug of choice to ciprofloxacin in children and adults. The dosage of ciprofloxacin for the acute phase is 500 mg bid orally for 10 days. The dosage for children younger than 15 years is 250 mg bid orally for 10 days.[112] Mutations of *gyrA* in organisms grown in the presence of ciprofloxacin suggest the potential development of resistance.[113] Transfusions of packed red blood cells may be needed to treat the severe anemia in approximately 10% of patients. It must be remembered that throughout the disease the bone marrow is hyperactive, liberating immature erythrocyte precursors. Once the infection is under control, recovery from anemia is surprisingly prompt. For severe cerebral complications (coma, convulsions due to cerebral hypoxia, and edema), short courses of dexamethasone have been employed.[111] The verrucae can be treated with oral rifampin (10 mg/kg/d for 14 to 21 days), which is more effective and convenient than the formerly used streptomycin. Alternative drugs are oral erythromycin, ciprofloxacin, and azithromycin.[66,112,114,115]

The signs of uncomplicated cat-scratch disease are mainly the manifestations of an effective immune response, and antibiotic treatment has little or no effect on the course of disease although azithromycin may hasten the resolution of lymphadenopathy.[116] In vitro susceptibility tests for *B. quintana* and *B. henselae* correlate poorly with clinical experience. Many antimicrobial agents are bacteriostatic, but aminoglycosides such as gentamicin are bactericidal against *B. henselae*.[114,117] Ocular bartonellosis is treated with doxycycline (100 mg every 12 hours) because of superior ocular penetration with a 2- to 4-week course in immunocompetent patients and 4 months or longer in immunocompromised patients.[78] In practice, bacillary angiomatosis is treated with oral doxycycline (100 mg twice a day) or oral erythromycin (0.5 to 1.0 g four times a day) for 2 to 3 months and longer if resolution is incomplete or relapse occurs. Oral tetracycline, minocycline, chloramphenicol, clarithromycin, and azithromycin have also been used successfully. In a series of 101 patients with bartonella endocarditis, among whom 12 died and two suffered relapses, full recovery was more likely if the patient was treated with an aminoglycoside, and survival was more likely if the patient was treated for a minimum of 14 days with an aminoglycoside.[49] Endocarditis and, in many cases, bacteremia and visceral bacillary angiomatosis or peliosis are treated intravenously. *Bartonella* endocarditis requires cardiac valve replacement in 76% of cases usually for hemodynamic reasons. The intraerythrocytic niche of *B. quintana* presents a therapeutic challenge. Testing of antimicrobial agents against intraerythrocytic *B. quintana* revealed that doxycycline, fluoroquinolones, and β-lactams are not bactericidal, gentamicin and rifampin are bactericidal at 4 μg/mL, but the peak intraerythrocytic concentration of gentamicin (0.26 μg/mL) occurs after 24 hours and is not bactericidal.[96] Most likely gentamicin kills *B. quintana* only after its release from red blood cells. Chronic *B. quintana* bacteremia in homeless persons was effectively cleared by treatment with gentamicin (3 mg/kg in one IV dose daily) for 14 days followed by oral doxycycline (200 mg/d) for 28 days.[118]

PREVENTION AND CONTROL

Control efforts for *B. bacilliformis* infections are directed mainly against adult sandflies. Peridomestic exposure to *Lutzomyia* is reduced by spraying houses, nearby animal shelters, and other structures with residual insecticides and by the use of fine-mesh screens. Area control of sylvan sandflies is not currently achievable, and resistance to insecticides is at least a potential concern. Individual protection using insect repellants and fine-mesh bednets is feasible and in endemic areas should focus on infants and children. An effective measure for workers in endemic areas is to leave the dangerous areas before dusk and set up camp elsewhere; in the Andes, a relatively short distance may mean a difference of several hundred meters in elevation.

Reduction in *B. henselae* transmission can be achieved via elimination of cat fleas and avoidance of traumatic injury by cats. Prophylaxis for *Mycobacterium avium* complex infections or other reasons with macrolides seems to protect also against *Bartonella* infections in HIV-infected persons.[119]

Control of trench fever depends on destroying human body lice with insecticides and improved socioeconomic conditions that make it possible to kill lice as clothes are washed routinely in hot, soapy water. Intensive treatment of human infections would reduce the reservoir of *B. quintana*.

Reduction of infection in the known reservoirs of bartonelloses, for example, humans (*B. bacilliformis* and *B. quintana*) and cats (*B. henselae*), could be theoretically be accomplished by vaccination. It is also conceivable that an agent for which there is no nonhuman reservoir, such as *B. bacilliformis* and *B. quintana*, might eventually be eradicated.

REFERENCES

1. Brenner DJ, O'Connor SP, Winkler HH, et al: Proposals to unify the genera *Bartonella* and *Rochalimaea,* with descriptions of *Bartonella quintana* comb. nov., *Bartonella henselae* comb. nov., *Bartonella vinsonii* comb. nov., and *Bartonella elizabethae* comb. nov., and to remove the family *Bartonellaceae* from the order *Rickettsiales.* Int J Syst Bacteriol 43:777, 1993.
2. Castle KT, Kosoy M, Lerdthusnee K, et al: Prevalence and diversity of *Bartonella* in rodents of northern Thailand: a comparison with *Bartonella* in rodents from southern China. Am J Trop Med Hyg 70:429, 2004.
3. Birtles RJ, Harrison TG, Saunders NA, et al: Proposal to unify the genera *Grahamella* and *Bartonella* with descriptions of *Bartonella talpae* comb. nov., *Bartonella peroymsci* comb. nov., and three species, *Bartonella grahamii* sp. nov., *Bartonella taylorii* sp. nov., and *Bartonella doshiae* sp. nov. Int J Syst Bacteriol 45:1, 1995.
4. Birtles RJ, Harrison TG, Molyneux DH: *Grahamella* in small woodland mammals in the U.K.: isolation, prevalence and host specificity. Ann Trop Med Parasitol 88:317, 1994.
5. Daly JS, Worthington MG, Brenner DJ, et al: *Rochalima elizabethae* sp. nov. isolated from a patient with endocarditis. J Clin Microbiol 31:872, 1993.
6. Relman DA: Bacillary angiomatosis and *Rochalimaea* species. Curr Clin Top Infect Dis 14:205, 1994.
7. Schultz MG: A history of bartonellosis (Carrión's disease). Am J Trop Med Hyg 17:503, 1983.
8. Alexander B: A review of bartonellosis in Ecuador and Colombia. Am J Trop Med Hyg 52:354, 1995.
9. Allison MJ, Pezzia A, Gerszten E, et al: A case of Carrión's disease associated with human sacrifice from the Huari culture of southern Peru. Am J Phys Anthropol 41:295, 1974.
10. Leonard J: Daniel Carrión and Carrión's disease. Bull Pan Am Health Organ 25:258, 1991.
11. Garcia-Caceres U, Garcia FU: Bartonellosis: an immunodepressive disease and the life of Daniel Alcides Carrión. Am J Clin Pathol 95:S58, 1991.
12. Byam W, Carrol JH, Churchill JH, et al: Trench fever: a louse-borne disease. In Frowde H (ed): Lice and Their Menace to Man. London, Hodder & Stoughton, Oxford University Press, 1919.
13. Vinson JW, Fuller HS: Studies on trench fever. I. Propagation of rickettsia-like microorganisms from a patient's blood. Pathol Microbiol 24:152, 1961.
14. Vinson JW, Varela G, Molina-Pasquel C: Trench fever. III. Induction of clinical disease in volunteers inoculated with *Rickettsia quintana* propagated on blood agar. Am J Trop Med Hyg 18:713, 1969.
15. Wear DJ, Margileth AM, Hadfield TL, et al: Cat scratch disease: a bacterial infection. Science 221:1403, 1983.
16. Relman DA, Loutit JS, Schmidt TM, et al: An approach to the identification of uncultured pathogens: the agent of bacillary angiomatosis. N Engl J Med 323:1573, 1990.
17. Slater LN, Welch DF, Hensel D, et al: A newly recognized fastidious gram-negative pathogen as a cause of fever and bacteremia. N Engl J Med 323:1587, 1990.
18. Regnery RL, Anderson BE, Clarridge JE III, et al: Characterization of a novel *Rochalimaea* species, *R. henselae* sp. nov., isolated from blood of a febrile, human immunodeficiency virus–positive patient. J Clin Microbiol 30:265, 1992.
19. Welch DF, Pickett DA, Slater LN, et al: *Rochalimaea henselae* sp. nov., a cause of septicemia, bacillary angiomatosis, and parenchymal bacillary peliosis. J Clin Microbiol 30:275, 1992.
20. Regnery RL, Olson JG, Perkins BA, et al: Serologic response to *"Rochalimaea henselae"* antigen in suspected cat-scratch disease. Lancet 339:1443, 1992.
21. Scherer DC, DeBuron-Connors I, Minnick MF: Characterization of *Bartonella bacilliformis* flagella and effect of antiflagellin antibodies on invasion of human erythrocytes. Infect Immun 61:4962, 1993.
22. Batterman HJ, Peek JA, Loutit JS, et al: *Bartonella henselae* and *Bartonella quintana* adherence to and entry into cultured human epithelial cells. Infect Immun 63:4553, 1995.
23. Minnick M, Sappington K, Smitherman L, et al: Five-member gene family of *Bartonella quintana*. Infect Immun 71:814, 2003.
24. Cartwright J, Britton P, Minnick M, et al: The *ialA* invasion gene of *Bartonella bacilliformis* encodes a (di)nucleoside polyphosphate hydrolase of the MutT motif family and has homologs in other invasive bacteria. Biochem Biophys Res Comm 256:474, 1999.
25. Weinman D, Pinkerton H: Carrión's disease. IV. Natural sources of bartonella in the endemic zone. Proc Soc Exp Biol Med 37:596, 1937.
26. Herrer A: Carrión's disease. II. Presence of *Bartonella bacilliformis* in the peripheral blood of patients with the benign form. Am J Trop Med Hyg 2:645, 1953.
27. Groot H: Human bartonellosis or Carrión's disease. In Gradwohl RBH, Soto LB, Felsenfeld O (eds): Clinical Tropical Medicine. St Louis, Mosby-Year Book, 1951, p 615.
28. Gray GC, Johnson AA, Thornton SA, et al: An epidemic of Oroya fever in the Peruvian Andes. Am J Trop Med Hyg 42:215, 1990.
29. Birtles RJ, Canalez JJ, Ventosilla P, et al: Prevalence and genotype analysis of *Bartonella* species isolated from intra-domicillary animals in bartonellosis-endemic regions of Peru. In Kazar J, Toman R (eds): Rickettsiae and Rickettsial Diseases. Bratislava, Slovakia, Slovak Academy of Sciences, 1996, p 611.
30. Maco V, Maguiña C, Tirado A, et al: *Bartonella bacilliformis* confirmed by histopathology in the high forest of Peru. Rev Inst Med Trop S Paulo 46:171, 2004.
31. Hertig M: Phlebotomus and Carrión's disease. Am J Trop Med 22:1, 1942.
32. Tesh RB, Guzman H: Sand flies and the agents they transmit. In Beaty JB, Marquardt WC (eds): The Biology of Disease Vectors. Vol 9. Niwot, University Press of Colorado, 1996, p 117.
33. Pérez JE: Studies on *Lutzomyia* spp. vectors of leishmaniasis in Peru. PhD thesis, University of Liverpool, UK, 1995.
34. Knobloch J, Solano ML, Alvarez GO, et al: Antibodies to *Bartonella bacilliformis* as determined by fluorescence antibody test, indirect haemagglutination and ELISA. Trop Med Parasitol 36:183, 1985.
35. Chamberlin J, Laughlin L, Romero S, et al: Epidemiology of endemic *Bartonella bacilliformis*: a prospective cohort study in a Peruvian mountain valley community. J Infect Dis 186:983, 2002.
36. Vinson JW: Louse-borne diseases worldwide. Trench fever. In Proceedings of the International Symposium on the Control of Lice and Louse-borne Diseases, Washington, DC, Dec 4–6, 1972, p 76.
37. Drancourt M, Mainardi JL, Brouqui P, et al: *Bartonella (Rochalimaea) quintana* endocarditis in three homeless men. N Engl J Med 332:419, 1995.

38. Spach DH, Kanter AS, Dougherty MJ, et al: *Bartonella (Rochalimaea) quintana* bacteremia in inner-city patients with chronic alcoholism. N Engl J Med 332:424, 1995.
39. Spach DH, Callis KP, Paauw DS, et al: Endocarditis caused by *Rochalimaea quintana* in a patient infected with human immunodeficiency virus. J Clin Microbiol 31:692, 1993.
40. Jackson LA, Spach DH, Kippen DA, et al: Seroprevalence to *Bartonella quintana* among patients at a community clinic in downtown Seattle. J Infect Dis 173:1023, 1996.
41. Raoult D, Birtles RJ, Montoya M, et al: Survey of three bacterial louse-associated diseases among rural Andean communities in Peru: prevalence of epidemic typhus, trench fever, and relapsing fever. Clin Infect Dis 29:434, 1999.
42. Koehler JE, Glaser CA, Tappero JW: *Rochalimaea henselae* infection: a new zoonosis with the domestic cat as reservoir. JAMA 271:531, 1994.
43. Ueno H, Muramatsu Y, Chomel BB, et al: Seroepidemiological survey of *Bartonella (Rochalimaea) henselae* in domestic cats in Japan. Microbiol Immunol 39:339, 1995.
44. Kordick DL, Wilson KH, Sexton DJ, et al: Prolonged *Bartonella* bacteremia in cats associated with cat-scratch disease patients. J Clin Microbiol 33:3245, 1995.
45. Chomel BB, Kasten RW, Floyd-Hawkins KA, et al: Experimental transmission of *Bartonella henselae* by the cat flea. J Clin Microbiol 34:1952, 1996.
46. Higgins JA, Radulovic S, Jaworski DC, et al: Acquisition of the cat scratch disease agent *Bartonella henselae* by cat fleas (Siphonaptera: Pulicidae). J Med Entomol 33:490, 1996.
47. Bergmans AMC, Schellekens JFP, VanEmbden JDA, et al: Predominance of two *Bartonella henselae* variants among cat-scratch disease patients in the Netherlands. J Clin Microbiol 34:254, 1996.
48. Fournier P, Mainardi J, Raoult D: Value of microimmunofluorescence for diagnosis and follow-up of *Bartonella* endocarditis. Clin Diag Lab Immunol 9:795, 2002.
49. Raoult D, Fournier P, Vandenesch F, et al: Outcome and treatment of *Bartonella* endocarditis. Arch Intern Med 163:226, 2003.
50. Kosoy M, Murray M, Gilmore R, et al: *Bartonella* strains from ground squirrels are identical to *Bartonella washoensis* isolated from a human patient. J Clin Microbiol 41:645, 2003.
51. Roux V, Eykrn S, Wyllie S, Raoult D: *Bartonella vinsonii* subsp. *Berkhoffii* as an agent of afebrile blood culture-negative endocarditis in a human. J Clin Microbiol 38:1698, 2000.
52. Comer JA, Diaz T, Vlahov D, et al: Evidence of rodent-associated *Bartonella* and *Rickettsia* infections among intravenous drug users from central and east Harlem, New York City. Am J Trop Med Hyg 65:855, 2001.
53. Weinman D: The bartonella group. In Dubos RJ, Hirsch JG (eds): Bacterial and Mycotic Infections of Man. Vol. 43. Philadelphia, Lippincott, 1965, p 775.
54. Maguiña C: Bartonellosis o Enfermedad de Carrión. Nuevos Aspectos de una Vieja Enfermedad. Lima, A.F.A. Editores Importadores, 1998.
55. Reynafarje C, Ramos J: The hemolytic anemia of human bartonellosis. Blood 17:562, 1961.
56. Maguiña C, Gotuzzo E: Bartonellosis: new and old. Infect Dis Clin North Am 14:1, 2000.
57. Strong RP, Tyzzer EE, Brues CT, et al: Report of First Expedition to South America, 1913. Cambridge, Mass, Harvard University Press, 1915.
58. Maguiña C: Estudio de 145 casos de bartonelosis humana. Doctoral thesis, Universidad Peruana Cayetano Heredia, Lima, Peru, 1993.
59. Cuadra M: Salmonellosis complication in human bartonellosis. Tex Rep Biol Med 14:97, 1956.
60. Patrucco R: Estudio de los parametros immunologicos en pacientes portadores de la enfermedad de Carrión. Diagnostico 12:138, 1983.
61. Henriquez C, Hinojosa JC, Ventosilla P, et al: Report of an unusual case of persistent bacteremia by *Bartonella bacilliformis* in a splenectomized patient. Am J Trop Med Hyg 71:53, 2004.
62. Arias-Stella J, Lieberman PH, Erlandson RA, et al: Histology, immunohistochemistry, and ultrastructure of the verruga in Carrión's disease. Am J Surg Pathol 10:595, 1986.
63. Recavarren S, Lumbreras H: Pathogenesis of the verruga of Carrión's disease. Am J Pathol 66:461, 1972.
64. Cáceres-Ríos H, Rodríguez-Tafur J, Bravo-Puccio F, et al: Verruga peruana: an infectious endemic angiomatosis. Crit Rev Oncog 6:47, 1995.
65. Maguiña C, Romero I, Soto N, et al: Natural history of Peruvian wart and the use of western blot, preliminary report. Folia Dermatologica 13:36, 2004.
66. Maguiña-Vargas C, Cok J, Gilman R, et al: Prospective study of new episodes of Peruvian wart. Dermatol Per 13:189, 2003.
67. Kosek M, Lavarello R, Gilman R, et al: Natural history of infection with *Bartonella bacilliformis* in a nonendemic population. J Infect Dis 182:865, 2000.
68. Raoult D, Drancourt M, Carta A, et al: *Bartonella (Rochalimaea) quintana* isolation in patient with chronic adenopathy, lymphopenia, and a cat. Lancet 343:977, 1994.
69. Caniza MA, Granger DL, Wilson KH, et al: *Bartonella henselae*: etiology of pulmonary nodules in a patient with depressed cell-mediated immunity. Clin Infect Dis 20:1505, 1995.
70. Dolan MJ, Wong MT, Regnery RL, et al: Syndrome of *Rochalimaea henselae* adenitis suggesting cat scratch disease. Ann Intern Med 118:331, 1993.
71. Hadfield TL, Warren R, Kass M, et al: Endocarditis caused by *Rochalimaea henselae*. Hum Pathol 24:1140, 1993.
72. Koehler JE, Quinn FD, Berger TG, et al: Isolation of *Rochalimaea* species from cutaneous and osseous lesions of bacillary angiomatosis. N Engl J Med 327:1625, 1992.
73. Lucey D, Dolan MJ, Moss CW, et al: Relapsing illness due to *Rochalimaea henselae* in immunocompetent hosts: implication for therapy and new epidemiological associations. Clin Infect Dis 14:683, 1992.
74. Mohle-Boetani J, Koehler JE, Berger TG, et al: Bacillary angiomatosis and bacillary peliosis in patients infected with human immunodeficiency virus: clinical characteristics in a case-control study. Clin Infect Dis 22:794, 1996.
75. Slater LN, Pitha JV, Herrera L, et al: *Rochalimaea henselae* infection in acquired immunodeficiency syndrome causing inflammatory disease without angiomatosis or peliosis. Arch Pathol Lab Med 118:33, 1994.
76. Stone JE, Gorensek MJ, Del Toro J, et al: Encephalitis associated with cat scratch disease—Broward and Palm Beach counties, Florida, 1994. Arch Dermatol 131:254, 1995.
77. Wade N, Levi L, Jones M, et al: Optic disk edema associated with peripapillary serous retinal detachment: an early sign of systemic *Bartonella henselae* infection. Am J Ophthalmol 130:327, 2000.
78. Cunningham E, Koehler J: Ocular bartonellosis. Am J Ophthalmol 130:340, 2000.
79. Verdon R, Geffray L, Collet T, et al: Vertebral osteomyelitis due to *Bartonella henselae* in adults: a report of 2 cases. Clin Infect Dis 35: e141, 2002.
80. Metzkor-Cotter E, Kletter Y, Avidor B, et al : Long-term serological analysis and clinical follow-up of patients with cat scratch disease. Clin Infect Dis 37:1149, 2003.
81. Huarcaya E, Maguiña C, Merello J, et al: A prospective study of cat-scratch disease in Lima, Peru. Rev Inst Med Trop S Paulo 44:325, 2002.
82. Conley T, Slater L, Hamilton K: *Rochalimaea* species stimulate human endothelial cell proliferation and migration *in vitro*. J Lab Clin Med 124:521, 1994.
83. LeBoit PE, Berger TG, Egbert BM, et al: Bacillary angiomatosis: the histopathology and differential diagnosis of a pseudoneoplastic infection in patients with human immunodeficiency virus disease. Am J Surg Pathol 13:909, 1989.
84. Meininger G, Nadasdy T, Hruban R, et al: Chronic acute myocarditis following acute *Bartonella henselae* infection. Am J Surg Pathol 25:1211, 2001.
85. Wesslen L, Ehrenborg C, Holmberg M, et al: Subacute bartonella infection in Swedish orienteers succumbing to sudden unexpected cardiac death or having malignant arrhythmias. Scand J Infect Dis 33:429, 2001.
86. Pinkerton H, Weinman D: Carrión's disease. I. Behavior of the etiological agent within cells growing or surviving in vitro. Proc Soc Exp Biol Med 37:587, 1937.
87. Pinkerton H, Weinman D: Carrión's disease. II. Comparative morphology of the etiological agent in Oroya fever and verruga peruana. Proc Soc Exp Biol Med 37:591, 1937.
88. Cuadra M, Takano J: The relationship of *Bartonella bacilliformis* to the red blood cell as revealed by electron microscopy. Blood 33:708, 1969.

89. Benson LA, Kar S, McLaughlin G, et al: Entry of *Bartonella bacilliformis* into erythrocytes. Infect Immun 54:347, 1986.
90. Garcia FU, Wojta J, Hoover RL: Interactions between live *Bartonella bacilliformis* and endothelial cells. J Infect Dis 165:1138, 1992.
91. Mernaugh G, Ihler GM: Deformation factor: An extracellular protein synthesized by *Bartonella bacilliformis* that deforms erythrocyte membranes. Infect Immun 60:937, 1992.
92. Xu Y, Lu Z, Ihler GM: Purification of deformin, an extracellular protein synthesized by *Bartonella bacilliformis* which causes deformation of erythrocyte membranes. Biochem Biophys Acta 1234:173, 1995.
93. Mitchell SJ, Minnick MF: Characterization of a two-gene locus from *Bartonella bacilliformis* associated with the ability to invade human erythrocytes. Infect Immun 63:1552, 1995.
94. Verma A, Davis G, Ihler G: Infection of human endothelial cells with *Bartonella bacilliformis* is dependent on Rho and results in activation of Rho. Infect Immun 68:5960, 2000.
95. Rolain J, Foucault C, Guieu R, et al: *Bartonella quintana* in human erythrocytes. Lancet 360:226, 2002.
96. Rolain J, Maurin M, Mallet M, et al: Culture and antibiotic susceptibility of *Bartonella quintana* in human erythrocytes. Antimicrob Agent Chemother 47:614, 2003.
97. Schulein R, Dehio C: The VirB/VirD4 type IV secretion of *Bartonella* is essential for establishing intraerythrocytic infection. Mol Microbiol 46:1053, 2002.
98. Garcia FU, Wojta J, Broadley KN, et al: *Bartonella bacilliformis* stimulates endothelial cells *in vitro* and is angiogenic *in vivo*. Am J Pathol 136:1125, 1990.
99. Minnick M, Smitherman L, Samuels D: Mitogenic effect of *Bartonella bacilliformis* on human vascular endothelial cells and involvement of GroEL. Infect Immun 71:6933, 2003.
100. Dehio C: Recent progress in understanding *Bartonella*-induced vascular proliferation. Curr Opin Microbiol 6:61, 2003.
101. Capo C, Amirayan-Chevillard N, Brouqui P, et al: *Bartonella quintana* bacteremia and overproduction of interleukin-10: model of bacterial persistence in homeless people. J Infect Dis 187:837, 2003.
102. Seubert A, Schulein R, Dehio C: Bacterial persistence within erythrocytes: a unique pathogenic strategy of *Bartonella* spp. Int J Med Microbiol 291:555, 2002.
103. Birtles RJ. Differentiation of *Bartonella* species using restriction endonuclease analysis of PCR-amplified 16S rRNA genes. FEMS Microbiol Lett 129:261, 1995.
104. Roux V, Raoult D. The 16S-23S or rRNA intergenic spacer region of *Bartonella (Rochalimaea)* species is longer than usually described in other bacteria. Gene 156:107, 1995.
105. Henriquez C, Infante B, Merello J, et al: Identification de *Bartonella bacilliformis* por metodos moleculares. Rev Med Hered 13:58, 2002.
106. Gonzales C, Maguiña C, Munoz S, et al: Bartonelosis (fiebre de la Oroya o verruga peruana). Reporte de un caso: revision de la literatura. Rev Chilena Dermatol 18:298, 2004.
107. Tierno PM Jr, Inglima K, Parisi MT: Detection of *Bartonella (Rochalimaea) henselae* bacteremia using BacT/alert blood culture system. Am J Clin Pathol 104:530, 1995.
108. Min K, Reed JA, Welch DF, et al: Morphologically variable bacilli of cat scratch disease are identified by immunocytochemical labeling with antibodies to *Rochalimaea henselae*. Am J Clin Pathol 101:607, 1994.
109. Zeaiter Z, Fournier P, Greub G, et al: Diagnosis of *Bartonella* endocarditis by a real-time nested PCR assay using serum. J Clin Microbiol 41:919, 2003.
110. Houpikian P, Raoult D: Western immunoblotting for *Bartonella* endocarditis. Clin Diag Lab Immunol 10:95, 2003.
111. Llanos-Cuentas A, Maguiña-Vargas C, Warrell DA: Bartonellosis. In Weatherall DJ, Ledingham JGG, Warrell DA (eds): Oxford Textbook of Medicine. Vol. 1. Oxford, Oxford University Press, 1996, p 773.
112. Rolain JM, Brouqui P, Koehler JE, et al: Recommendations for treatment of human infections caused by *Bartonella* species. Antimicrob Agents Chemother 48:1921, 2004.
113. Minnick MF, Wilson ZR, Smitherman LS, Samuels DS. *gyrA* mutations in ciprofloxacin-resistant *Bartonella bacilliformis* strains obtained in vitro. Antimicrob Agents Chemother 47:383, 2003.
114. Maurin M, Gasquet S, Ducco C, et al: MICs of 28 antibiotic compounds for 14 *Bartonella* (formerly *Rochalimaea*) isolates. Antimicrob Agents Chemother 39:2387, 1995.
115. Gotuzzo E, Maguiña C: Treatment of bartonellosis (letter). J Travel Med 2:278, 1995.
116. Bass J, Freitas B, Freitas A: Prospective randomized double blind placebo-controlled evaluation of azithromycin for treatment of cat scratch disease. Pediatric Infect Dis J 17:447, 1999.
117. Maurin M, Raoult D: Antimicrobial susceptibility of *Rochalimaea quintana, Rochalimaea vinsonii,* and the newly recognized *Rochalimaea henselae*. J Antimicrob Chem 332:587, 1993.
118. Foucault C, Raoult D, Brouqui P: Randomized open trial of gentamicin and doxycycline for eradication of *Bartonella quintana* from blood in patients with chronic bacteremia. Antimicrob Agent Chemother 47:2204, 2003.
119. Koehler J, Sanchez M, Tye S, et al: Prevalence of *Bartonella* infection among human immunodeficiency virus–infected patients with fever. Clin Infect Dis 37:559, 2003.

41

Brucellosis

EDUARDO GOTUZZO

INTRODUCTION

In 1885, Sir David Bruce described "a disease of long duration with fever, profuse perspiration, splenomegaly, frequent relapses, rheumatoid or neuralgic pain, swelling of the joints and orchitis" seen in his patients in Malta, and he isolated the pathogen from the spleen of his autopsy studies.[1] Brucellosis still poses important problems in animals and humans in some regions of the world.[2–4]

AGENT

Brucella is a slow-growing, aerobic, catalase-positive, nonmotile gram-negative coccobacillus in the α-proteobacteria (α-2 group) with *Bartonella (Rochalimaea) henselae* and *Agrobacterium tumefaciens*.[5,6] The *Brucella* species that infect humans are all now considered to be biovars of *B. melitensis* (the cause of Malta fever with the goat reservoir), but traditionally have also included *B. abortus* (the cause of Bang's diseases and abortions in cattle), *B. suis* (from aborting swine), *B. canis* (from aborting beagle dogs), and two other organisms that are considered nonpathogenic to humans that have been isolated from sheep and wood rats, respectively (*B. ovis* and *B. neotomae*).[7,8]

EPIDEMIOLOGY

Brucellosis presents two epidemiologically different profiles (Table 41-1):

1. In developed countries, brucellosis is typically an occupational disease in abbatoir workers,[9] butchers, veterinarians, and farmers, usually affecting adult men (and occasionally family members), who become infected through the skin and conjunctiva. It is usually caused by *B. abortus*.[10,11]
2. In endemic countries, principally three important regions, infections are associated with *B. melitensis*. These regions include Mediterranean countries (Spain, Portugal, Italy, and Greece), Middle Eastern countries (Iran, Iraq, Kuwait, Saudi Arabia, Israel, and Jordan),[12,13] and Latin American countries (Peru, Argentina, and Mexico).[12,14–18] In these regions, males and females are equally infected and 20% to 25% of cases are children. Infections are typically acquired through the consumption of dairy products, especially nonpasteurized goat cheese and untreated milk.[19,20] Recently, two cases of *B. melitensis* were reported in Bangkok, which signifies the re-appearance of brucellosis in Thailand after 36 years.[21]

Some outbreaks, including those in family groups, have been reported from common sources, often from contaminated edible products.[22–28] *B. melitensis* may symptomatically infect up to 50% of family members.[20,29] A Saudi Arabian study evaluated household members of patients with acute brucellosis through serological screening; two members or more tested positive in 42% of the families. The risk factor in these families was raw milk ingestion.[30] The lowest attack rates are in young children, probably related to food habits rather than to immunity. Evidence does not support human-to-human transmission, except in rare cases of infection via bone marrow transplantation,[31] blood transfusion, and a possible case of transmission to a sexual partner via the organism in semen.[32] Women develop more severe brucellosis[20,32,33] with more articular involvement[29] and more severe thrombocytopenia[34] with *B. melitensis* infections. The other two *Brucella* organisms of human importance are *B. abortus*, whose reservoir is cattle, and *B. suis,* which is an enzootic disease in swine. *B. canis* has infected only a few dog breeders.[35,36]

As in other developed areas, in the United States, *B. abortus* has been the most frequent cause of brucellosis, as noted in reports from Iowa and Texas.[9,37,38] Since 1986, the Centers for Disease Control and Prevention (CDC) has listed brucellosis as a notifiable disease of low frequency, with fewer than 50 human cases per year, most likely because of the bovine brucellosis eradication program. More than 60% of U.S. cases

Table 41-1 Brucellosis: Epidemiologic and Clinical Differences

	Brucella abortus	*Brucella melitensis*
Prinicipal reservoir	Cattle	Goats
Transmission	Worker's disease: veterinarians, farmers, butchers	Consumption of nonpasteurized goat cheese
Age	Adults 20–45 yr	All ages, 25% children
Sex	>95% male	50% female
Geographic location	United States	Arabian countries; Latin America: Peru, Mexico, Argentina; Mediterranean countries: Spain, Italy, France, Greece, Portugal
Pathogenicity	Low	High
Subclinical-clinical case ratio	8:1	<1:1
Clinical pattern	Mild disease; no chronic form; mortality <0.1%	More severe form, frequent relapses: chronic form 1%–5%; motality 1%
Outbreaks	Rare	Frequent in the United States with imported dairy products
Family cases	Rare	Occasional

occur in Texas and California, and only 5% to 10% are recognized and/or reported.[39] *B. melitensis* has also been reported in travelers to endemic areas where the use of antacids and H_2-receptor inhibitors has been considered as a risk factor, in addition to the consumption of "typical" local food prepared with unpasteurized cheese or milk.[40]

Brucellosis is an emerging disease in travellers to Latin America, the Middle East, and the Mediterranean coast, especially among people who receive antacids or eat unpastuerized cheese.[41] *Brucella* is one of the most infectious bacteria to laboratory personnel through aerosols.[41,42] However, with the new biohazard precautions and the use of biologic safety hoods, laboratory infections have become infrequent.[43,44]

CLINICAL MANIFESTATIONS

It is useful to stratify the different clinical presentations of brucellosis due to *B. melitensis*.[45] However, it is less helpful in the evaluation of patients with *B. abortus* or *B. suis* infections, because chronic or recurring forms are infrequent.

Acute Form (Classical Febrile Brucellosis)

In acute *B. melitensis* infections, patients typically present with evening fever (100°F or greater), with profuse or patchy sweating, malaise, headache, and weight loss (3 to 10 kg in 1 to 2 weeks). Half of these patients have arthralgias and one-third have arthritis, often with myalgias and back pain.

Mild anemia, leukopenia, and hepatic involvement are frequent,[46–50] but psychiatric and urologic complications are rare. Constipation is common in endemic brucellosis; however, patients may present with diarrhea and fever, especially travelers from developed countries.

Relapsing or Undulant Form (Malta Fever)

This is the "classical pattern" described by Bruce[1] and is observed after 2 months with the disease. In the preantibiotic era, 75% of patients developed this form, with rare cases persisting beyond 1 year. This form represents 25% to 30% of cases in endemic areas and usually reflects incomplete treatment, failure of standard treatment, or lack of a proper initial diagnosis and therapy.

Hepatic involvement and arthritis are common, as is a mild depressive mood, and occasionally uveitis and orchiepididymitis in young males.[51] This form may also present as a fever of unknown origin (FUO).[52]

Chronic Brucellosis

Two patterns of chronic brucellosis (lasting more than 1 year) may be seen. The first is a cyclic course with back pain, arthralgias, sweating, and depressive mood. This pattern is very similar to the chronic fatigue syndrome and occurs more frequently in women, especially women older than 40 years of age.

The second chronic form is localized brucellosis: spondylitis or uveitis (or episcleritis) without fever or systemic symptoms. This form is frequent in adults (representing 5% to 10% of cases in endemic areas), affects both sexes equally, but is rare in children.

In addition to the preceding clinical forms, the following sections detail complications (often localized) that may be seen (listed in order of decreasing frequency).

Arthritis

The frequency of arthritis depends on the criteria used and whether the series is prospective or not; some have counted arthralgias as arthritis. Several forms of arthritis are listed in Table 41-2.

Peripheral arthritis is the most common presentation, affecting young adults and children; most cases involve monarticular arthritis in the knee or hip.[45,53] However, some patients have polyarthritis and other rheumatoid-like syndromes. Peripheral arthritis likely involves two pathogenic mechanisms: (1) *Reactive arthritis* is associated with poly- or pauciarticular involvement, where *Brucella* is not isolated from the joint. This form is associated with high circulating immune complex levels,[54] has a good prognosis, and often remits spontaneously.[13,55–57] (2) Alternatively, *infectious monarticular arthritis* can occur in which the organism is able to be isolated from synovial fluid when the proper culture medium is used. The prognosis depends on appropriate antibiotic treatment. Low levels of lactate in synovial fluids have been reported to be associated with the isolation of *Brucella* from the joint.[58] Even biopsy of the synovial fluid does not distinguish between reactive and infectious arthritis (both are exudative and inflammatory); only the clinical pattern and the appropriate culture can define which process is involved. More unusual forms include sternoclavicular arthritis[59,60] and extra-articular rheumatism (tendinitis, bursitis, and fibrositis) seen in approximately 10% of adult women.

Sacroileitis is the second most frequent articular lesion.[44,61] It is usually unilateral, more frequent in young adults, seen in both sexes, and often associated with pain on movement (Lasègue's sign). The bone scan is helpful in diagnosis.

Spondylitis occurs in 5% to 10% of patients with brucellar arthritis.[45,53,62] A Hungarian study noted the association of human leukocyte antigen (HLA)-B27 with brucellar spondyloarthritis[63]; however, this association is less impressive in our Peruvian familial studies of brucellar arthritis.[64–66] Narrowing of the disk space (diskitis) is the earliest sign; however, the presence of lytic and blastic lesions and the erosion of the anterosuperior

***Table 41-2** Arthritis in Brucellosis Related to Age and Clinical Form*

Brucellosis Clinical Form	Brucellar Arthritis	Peripheral Arthritis	Sacroileitis	Spondylitis	Age
Acute	20%–35%	Frequent	Frequent	Rare	Children, young adults
Subacute	25%–40%	Common	Frequent	Common	Young adults, children
Chronic	40%–60%	Rare	Rare	Frequent	Mainly >40 yr

Table 41-3 Differential Diagnosis of Tuberculous versus Brucellar Spondylitis

	Tuberculous Spondylitis	Brucellar Spondylitis
Age	Young adults (20–40 yr)	>40 yr old
Sex	More common in males	Slightly more frequent in females
Main localization	Dorsal	Lumbar
Two or more vertebrae	<10%	20%–30%
Paravertebral abscess	Very common	10%–20%
Radiography	Lytic lesion (rare, blastic)	Lytic and blastic lesion
Sequelae (gibbus or humpback deformity)	Common	Rare

part of the vertebral body ("parrot peak") is the most characteristic presentation.[67–69] This form is rare in children; most patients are older than 40 years of age. Important differential diagnostic considerations are other infectious spondylitis such as tuberculous (Table 41-3) and *Staphylococcus aureus* spondylitis. *S. aureus* spondylitis is painful and presents with fever, a symptom less commonly seen with tuberculous spondylitis and occasionally in brucellar spondylitis, given that it is a late complication. A recent report describes an Italian couple whose only symptom was spondylitis-generated pain.[70] Their pain was exacerbated by lying down, which differs it from ostearthropathic pain, which improves with rest. In addition, brucellar spondylitis, with its diskitis and reduction of the intervertebral space, must be distinguished from neoplastic metastasis that affect vertebral bodies.

Hepatitis

Although the presence of hepatomegaly is frequent (50% to 70%) and increased alkaline phosphatase is common, clinical hepatitis is less frequent and is detected in approximately 3% to 6% of adults. In the case of *B. melitensis,* the finding of granulomas is infrequent in the United States,[71] but we have noted that granulomatous hepatitis confirmed by electron microscopy is common in Latin America and may occur in association with the development of a cell-mediated immune response.[49,50] Sometimes more severe forms of hepatitis with bone and hematologic changes are seen.[11,43,72,73] In the 1940s, severe hepatitis was a common cause of death, as reported in an autopsy study.[74]

Hematologic Involvement

Mild anemia and leukopenia with lymphocytosis are common in uncomplicated brucellosis.[75–77] We have found that the degree of lymphopenia is correlated with the severity of brucellosis.[77] Bone marrow aspiration frequently shows iron deficiency (up to 35%, even in males); the absence of iron has been associated with more aggressive courses in animals,[48] a finding that could explain the greater severity of brucellosis in women than in men.[29,33,34] While three of four males studied had normal values of iron deposits in bone marrow, only 6 of 18 females had normal iron stores ($P<0.02$). We also have found severe thrombocytopenia to be associated with brucellosis in 6 of 485 males and 21 of 605 females ($P<0.05$).[34] Severe thrombocytopenia may require steroid therapy, and in some patients with persistent thrombocytopenia after 2 months of treatment and proven bacteriologic cure, splenectomy may be necessary.[34,78]

Rare complications of brucellosis include Evans's syndrome,[76,77] with pancytopenia and cytophagocytosis,[79–82] which can be confused with malignant histiocytosis. Pancytopenia is caused by granulomas in bone marrow.[47] Severe thrombocytopenia may cause fatal central nervous system (CNS) hemorrhage.

Neurologic Involvement

Neurobrucellosis is reported in 1% to 5% of adults, but is a rare complication in children.[83–86] It usually involves meningitis or encephalitis. The cerebrospinal fluid (CSF) is similar to that in other chronic meningitides with increased lymphocytes and protein; CSF cultures are positive in 10% to 20% of cases.[87] The clinical pattern is characterized by fever, headache, neck rigidity, and altered consciousness. In contrast to tuberculous meningitis, the cranial nerves are usually not involved in neurobrucellosis. Guillain-Barré syndrome can be seen in young adults with acute brucellosis; brain abscesses are rare.[88–92] The CNS may also be involved in *Brucella* endocarditis or from bleeding in severe thrombocytopenia; both are associated with a poor prognosis.

Other Complications

One of the risk factors for travelers from developed countries to endemic areas is the use of antacids or H_2-receptor antagonists. In these patients, gastrointestinal symptoms are frequent, mainly subacute diarrhea (although among residents of endemic areas, constipation is more common).[40,93]

Brucella endocarditis can occur in a previously normal aortic valve (50% to 70% of *Brucella* endocarditis), and it remains the leading cause of death in brucellosis.[83,84] When the patient recovers, the valve becomes calcified. Despite some reported success with medical treatment alone, most experts recommend valve replacement and 2 to 3 months of antibiotic therapy.[94–96]

In chronic brucellosis (with *B. melitensis*), psychiatric disorders are common: These include "brucellar neurasthenia," chronic fatigue, amnesia, and depression.[97,98] In the preantibiotic era, suicide was one of the causes of death.[99,100] Symptoms often persist after the infection is cured; antidepressant or other symptomatic therapy may be required for 3 to 6 months.

Eye Involvement

Eye involvement is an unusual complication that may occur in subacute or chronic forms of brucellosis. Anterior or posterior uveitis is the most common ocular manifestation of *Brucella* infection.[101,102] Panuveitis often results in loss of vision.[103–106] Other ocular lesions include papilledema, optic neuritis, and episcleritis.[105–109] In patients without proper treatment, secondary glaucoma, cataracts, retinal detachment, and phthisis bulbi have been reported.[101–104]

Pulmonary Involvement

Pulmonary involvement constitutes an important complication in the bioterrorism era. In an extensive review of 450 brucellosis patients in Greece, 31 had a respiratory pathologic findings at the time of diagnosis. Patients mainly had lobar pneumonia and presented with an interstitial pattern in chest x-rays.[110]

Brucellosis in Children and Pregnancy

Brucellosis produces mild to moderate disease in children, but the chronic form is rare. Relapses in children are usually due to incomplete treatment. Hepatitis and arthritis are often seen in children. The arthritis is usually peripheral, but hip or knee arthritis may be seen.[12,15,111–113]

Brucellosis during pregnancy is associated with poor fetal prognosis with a high rate of abortion, miscarriage, prematurity, and fetal death.[17,83,114] In a recently extensive case series from Saudi Arabia that included pregnant women with brucellosis, the incidence of spontaneous abortion in the first and second trimesters was 43%, whereas the incidence of intrauterine fetal death in the third trimester was 2%.[115] The study also reported the beneficial effect of prompt treatment with cotrimoxazole or cotrimoxazole/rifampin over fetal prognosis.[115] In another Peruvian series of pregnant women with brucellosis, early treatment with rifampin for 6 weeks plus an aminoglycoside greatly improved the fetal prognosis.[116] A few cases of congenital brucellosis have been reported, but early diagnosis and proper treatment should prevent most congenital infection.

HIV and Brucellosis

Regarding brucellosis among HIV patients, a Spanish series reported 12 cases properly diagnosed (8 with culture positive to *Brucella* spp. and 4 with high anti-Brucella antibody titers, with a median CD4 count of 544 (136–1006). In this series, the clinical pattern and response to therapy was similar to what is expected in non-HIV patients: 2 of 12 had initial relapses, although no additional microbiologic relapses were seen in 18 months of followup.[117] It should be noted that there are other reports that have described more frequent relapse in HIV patients.[118,119]

PATHOGENESIS AND IMMUNITY

Brucella infections are likely acquired via small or subclinical skin abrasions, conjunctival inoculation, or perhaps less commonly via the respiratory route. *B. melitensis* is more

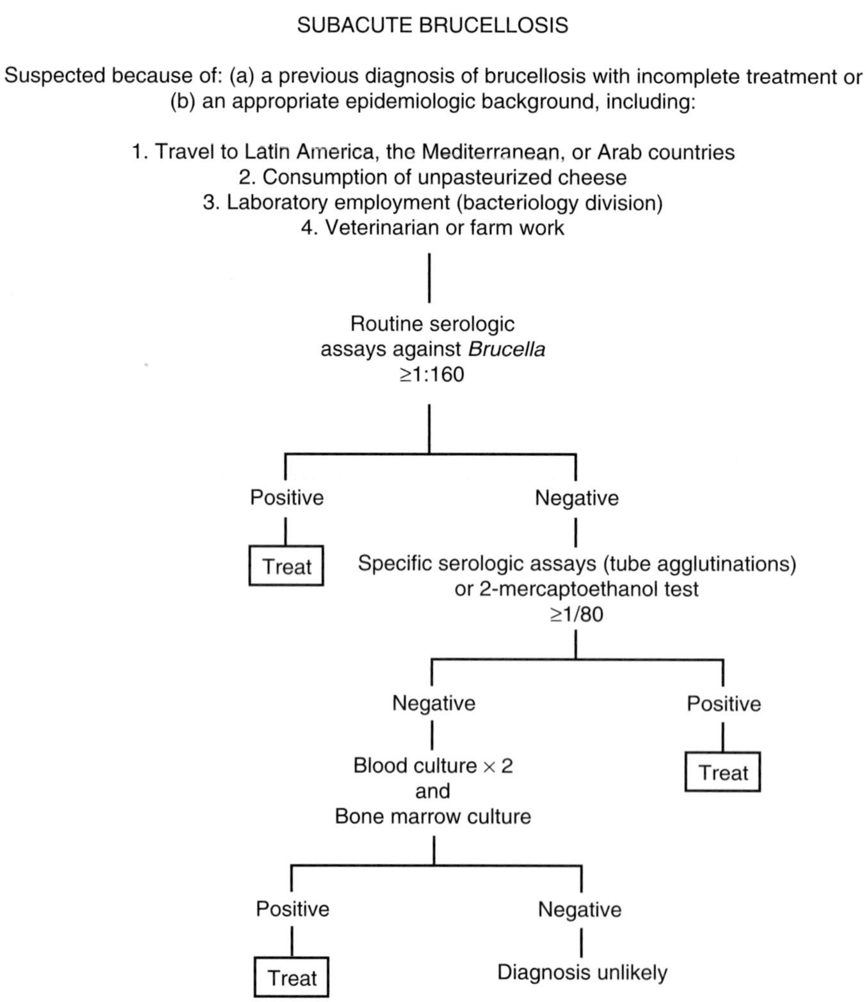

FIGURE 41-1 Algorithm for the diagnosis and treatment of subacute brucellosis.

acid- and serum-resistant and is likely acquired frequently via oral ingestion. The 2- to 3-week incubation period likely involves invasion, perhaps analogous to typhoid fever, with multiplication in macrophages since the organism is able to survive intracellularly. Its smooth lipopolysacchride (LPS) appears to be responsible for the resistance of *Brucella* to serum.

The tendency of *B. abortus* to localize in placental tissue in cattle may well relate to the enrichment of placental tissue with erythritol, which may stimulate the growth of this organism.[120] Furthermore, unlike *B. melitensis* and *B. suis,* which tend to cause abscesses in experimental animals, *B. abortus* tends to cause granuloma formation in mice.[121] Immune responses, initially immunoglobulin M (IgM) then proceeding to IgG, clearly do not provide full protective immunity, since relapsing disease can occur. The role of cell-mediated immunity is suggested by the formation of granulomas and likely determines the characteristic recovery from and partial resistance to subsequent reinfection.

DIAGNOSIS

Since the protean clinical and routine laboratory manifestations are not specific to brucellosis, a thorough history of occupation, travel, and consumption of unpasteurized milk or milk products is key to making the diagnosis (Figs. 41-1 and 41-2). Although it requires biosafety level 3 precautions, the isolation of *Brucella* provides a definitive diagnosis. The best procedure is bone marrow culture,[122,123] with a yield of 92% (vs. 70% with two blood cultures; $P<0.001$) and with faster growth (4.32 days vs. 6.65 days; $P<0.01$) in our prospective study. The best medium, Ruiz-Castañeda,[122,124] was modified by Carrillo through the addition of sodium polyethylene sulfonate (SPS) and cysteine. With the new DuPont Isolator and Bactec techniques, the isolation is improved.[125,126] Bone marrow culture is especially important in difficult clinical cases with epidemiologic suspicion of brucellosis, and when serologic tests are negative (as seen in relapsing uveitis,[104] unexplained fever, or with hematologic abnormalities).[3] However, in routine evaluations, the diagnosis of brucellosis is usually made by serology[124,127]; in a large series in the United States, only 17% of cases had bacteriologic isolation.[37]

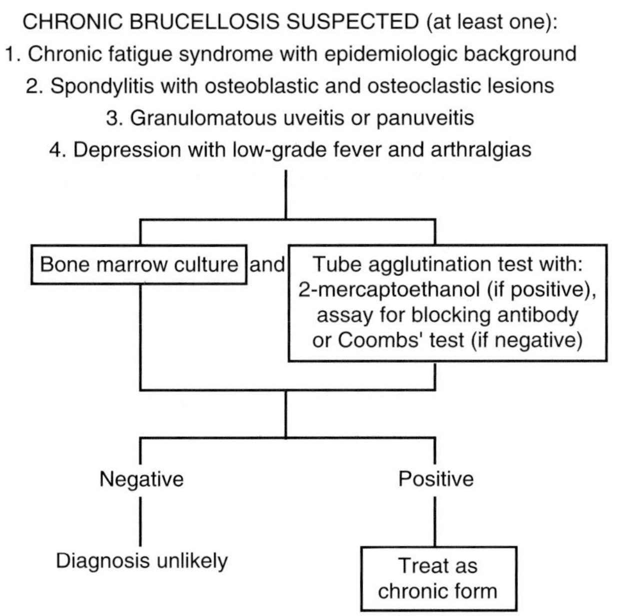

FIGURE 41-2 Algorithm for the diagnosis and treatment of chronic brucellosis.

In Spain and Peru, the rose bengal test remains an inexpensive, sensitive, and specific test; however, it is not useful in follow-up of patients or in diagnosing relapses.[14,120,128,129] In these cases, 2-mercaptoethanol (2-ME) is used to detect IgG antibody.[129,130] However, well-standardized *Brucella* antigen (usually from the smooth, cross-reacting *B. abortus* strain, which may miss rough *B. canis* infections) and dilution to exclude false-negative prozone effects are key to the diagnosis. Antigens often used in "febrile agglutinins" are frequently nonspecific with cross-reactions from cholera, tularemia, or *Yersinia* infections. Polymerase chain reaction (PCR) methods using ribosomal RNA are under development.[131] In Germany, they have lately been using PCR enzyme-linked immunosorbent assay (ELISA) and real-time PCR assays with promising results.[132]

BRUCELLA AS A BIOTERRORISM AGENT

Brucella is listed as a potential agent for a biologic attack by the CDC. *Brucella* spp. carries risk mainly because its aerosols are easy to prepare and disseminate. Even 10 to 100 bacteria can produce human disease, and it poses substantial risk for laboratory acquired infection.[133–135] In the laboratory, attack rates can be as high as 30% to 100% depending on the inoculum size and the worker's position. *Brucella* needs to be handled with the biosafety guidelines of a level 3 organism.[136–138] The strategy chosen for combination antibiotic prophylaxis and serologic follow-up of exposed workers is provided in a recent report from Quebec after a large exposure of workers to *B. melitensis*.[139] A model to evaluate the economic impact and potential medical care in a brucellosis postattack intervention was reviewed with emphasis on pulmonary aerosol use.[140]

TREATMENT AND PROGNOSIS

Although several antibiotics have in vitro activity against *Brucella,* effective agents must be active intracellularly, produce a rapid decrease in fever, reduce or treat complications, and have a low rate of relapse. Because of the high rate of relapse with monotherapy, two antibiotics are usually recommended.[88,141–144]

The drug of choice is tetracycline because of its intracellular bactericidal activity against *Brucella*[145] and because it has a low rate of relapse and a large international experience showing its efficacy.[146–149] The gastrointestinal tolerance of tetracyclines is poor and there is interaction with milk, antacids, or meals. Doxycycline has fewer side effects and its twice-daily use after meals is well tolerated. However, patients should avoid sun exposure because it occasionally causes photosensitivity.

Doxycycline should be used in combination with another antibiotic (Box 41-1). The World Health Organization (WHO) recommends 6 weeks of the combination of doxycycline with rifampicin 600 to 900 mg/day.[43] Doxycycline for 6 weeks can also be combined with streptomycin (or netilmicin), one dose daily for 2 weeks, with good results.[146,150,151] However, rifampicin may increase the clearance of doxycycline and reduce the doxycycline half-life in serum (mainly in rapid acetylators)[152];

Box 41-1 Treatment of Brucellosis

Adults: Doxycycline* PO 100 mg bid × 6 weeks plus rifampicin PO 600 to 900/day × 6 weeks or streptomycin or netilmicin IM once a day × 14 days
Children ≥ 7 years old: Same treatment as adults (only 4 weeks)
Children < 7 years old: Rifampicin 10 mg/kg/day × 4 weeks plus streptomycin or netilmicin once a day × 14 days or co-trimoxazole × 4 weeks
Pregnancy: Rifampicin 600 mg/day × 6 weeks plus streptomycin or netilmicin once a day × 14 days

*In the chronic form, a prolonged course of doxycycline 100 mg/day × 6 weeks more may be indicated along with antidepressant drugs as needed.

frequent relapses have been seen with this combination. A meta-analysis from five Spanish trials shows a significant rate of relapse with rifampicin plus doxycycline in comparison with streptomycin and doxycycline.[35] In a study in Spain, azithromycin and gentamicin were used to treat 10 brucellosis patients; the cure rate was 7 out of 10 but the relapse rate was high. These results do not favor the use of azithromycin in brucellosis.[153] In children, the relapse rate is low when receiving 4 weeks of treatment.[12,15]

In pregnant women and children younger than 7 years of age, tetracyclines are contraindicated. Some studies have described the use of rifampicin in combination with aminoglycoside (or co-trimoxazole).[12,15,17,83,145]

PREVENTION AND CONTROL

Because brucellosis is a zoonosis, the best control measure is prevention, with pasteurization of dairy products and use of gloves and masks by veterinarians and farmers. In the laboratory, careful adherence to safety guidelines and precautions is imperative.[145]

As a zoonosis in domestic animals, brucellosis is prevented by serologic testing and elimination of infected cattle and by routine pasteurization of milk. In addition, immunization of calves with a *B. abortus* strain 19 vaccine and of goats with a *B. melitensis* strain rev-1 vaccine is helpful. Some have used a live attenuated *Brucella* vaccine in persons at high risk, but this is not widely available. Improved animal husbandry and use of animal control measures and milk pasteurization have substantially reduced brucellosis in many areas.

REFERENCES

1. Bruce D: Note on discovery of a micrococcus in Malta Fever. Practitioner 39:161–170, 1887.
2. Roux J: Épidémiologie et prévention de la brucellose. Bull World Health Org 57:179–194, 1979.
3. Thimm BM: Brucellosis: Distribution in Man, Domestic and Wild Animals. Berlin, Springer-Verlag, 1982.
4. Lulu AR, Araj GF, Kahteeb MI, et al: Human brucellosis in Kuwait: A prospective study of 400 cases. Q J Med 66:39–54, 1988.
5. Moreno E, Stackebrandt E, Dorsch M, et al: *Brucella abortus* 16S rRNA and lipid A reveal a phylogenetic relationship with members of the alpha-2 subdivision of the class *Proteobacteria.* J Bacteriol 172:3569–3576, 1990.
6. DeLay J, Mannheim W, Segers P, et al: Ribosomal ribonucleic acid cistron similarities and taxonomic neighborhood of *Brucella* and CDC group Vd. Int J Syst Bacteriol 37:35–42, 1987.
7. Verger JM, Grimont F, Grimont PAD, et al: *Brucella,* a monospecific genus as shown by desoxyribonucleic acid hybridizaion. Int J Syst Bacteriol 35:292–295, 1985.
8. Corbel MJ: International Committee on Systemic Bacteriology Subcommittee on the Taxonomy of *Brucella.* Int J Syst Bacteriol 38:450–452,1988.
9. Buchanan TM, Hendricks SI, Patton DM, et al: Brucellosis in the United States 1960–1972, an abbatoir-associated disease. Part III. Epidemiology and evidence for acquired immunity. Medicine (Baltimore) 53:427–439, 1974.
10. Annual Summary 1983. Reported morbidity and mortality in the United States. MMWR 32:18, 1984.
11. Spink WW: Family studies on brucellosis. Am J Med Sci 227:128–133, 1954.
12. Abo-Shehada MN, Odeh JS, Abu-Essud M, et al: Seroprevalence of brucellosis among high risk people in northern Jordan. Int J Epidemiol 25:450–454, 1996.
13. Gottesman G, Vanunu D, Maayan MC, et al: Childhood brucellosis in Israel. Pediatr Infect Dis J 15:610–615, 1996.
14. Ariza J: Brucelosis 1984. Med Interna (Barcelona) 2:113–164, 1984.
15. Lubani MM, Dudin KI, Sharda DC, et al: A multicenter therapeutic study of 1100 children with brucellosis. Pediatr Infect Dis 8:75–78, 1989.
16. Norton WL: Brucellosis and rheumatic syndromes in Saudi Arabia. J Rheumatol 43:810–813, 1984.
17. Zavala-Trujillo I, Nava-Zavala A, Guerra-Cáceres J, et al: Brucellosis. Infect Dis Clin North Am 8:225–241, 1994.
18. Corbel MJ: Brucellosis: An overview. Emerg Infect Dis 3:213–221, 1997.
19. Castell-Monsalve J, Rullan JV, Peiro Callizo EF, et al: Epidemic outbreak of 81 cases of brucellosis following the consumption of fresh cheese without pasteurization. Rev Esp Salud Publica 70:303–311, 1996.
20. Gotuzzo E, Carrillo C, Seas C, et al: Caracteristicas epidemiológicas y clínicas de la Brucelosis en 39 grupos familiares. Rev Esp Intern Infect Microbiol Clin 7:519–523, 1989.
21. Manosuthi W, Thummakul T, Vighagool A, et al: A case report—Brucellosis: Re-emerging disease in Thailand. Southeast Asian J Trop Med Public Health 35:109–112, 2004.
22. Young EJK, Suvanno-Parent V: Brucellosis outbreak attributed to ingestion of unpasteurized goat cheese. Arch Intern Med 135:240–243, 1975.
23. Rivero-Puente A, Maravi-Pomo E, Burusco MJ, et al: Monograph of Brucellosis. Pamplona, Spain, Universidad de Navarra, 1978.
24. Spink WW: The Nature of Brucellosis. Minneapolis, MN, University of Minnesota Press, 1956, pp 207–208.
25. Monit Mad Kour M: Brucellosis. Cambridge, UK, Butterworths, 1989.
26. Mousa ARM, Elhag KM, Hkogall M, et al: The nature of human brucellosis in Kuwait, study of 379 cases. J Infect Dis 10:211–220, 1988.
27. Damdhere M, Bhagwat R, Sainini G: Outbreak of brucellosis in family. Indian J Med Sci 18:145–149, 1964.
28. Eckman MR: Brucellosis linked to Mexican cheese. JAMA 232:636–637, 1975.
29. Gotuzzo E, Seas C, Guerra J, et al: Brucellar arthritis—Study of 39 Peruvian families. Ann Rheum Dis 46:506–509, 1987.
30. Almuncef MA, Memish ZA, Balbky HH, et al: Importance of screening household members. Epidemiol Infect 132:533–540, 2004.
31. Naparsteck E, Block CS, Slavin S: Transmission of brucellosis in bone marrow transplantation. Lancet 1:574–575, 1982.
32. Goossens H, Marcelis L, Dekeyser P, et al: *Brucella melitensis*: Person-to-person transmission? Lancet 1:773, 1983.
33. Gotuzzo E, Carrillo C, Seas C, et al: Caracteristicas epidemiólogicas y clinicas de la brucelosis en 50 grupos familiares. Rev Med Hered 1:8–13, 1990.
34. Ulloa V, Rojas J, Gotuzzo E: Púrpura trombocitopénica asociada a Brucelosis. Rev Med Hered 3:87–93, 1992.
35. Carmichael LE: Canine brucellosis: Isolation, diagnosis, transmission. Proc US Livestock Sanit Assoc 71:517–527, 1967.
36. Carmichael LE: Contagious abortion in beagles. Hounds Hunting 64:14, 1967.

37. Buchanan TM, Sulzeir CR, Frix MK, et al: Brucellosis in the United States, 1960–1972, an abbatoir-associated disease. Part II. Diagnostic aspects. Medicine (Baltimore) 53:415–425, 1974.
38. Brucellosis surveillance—Annual summary 1978. MMWR 1979.
39. Wise RI: Brucellosis in the United Status: Past, present, and future. JAMA 244:2318–2322, 1980.
40. Arnow PM, Smaron M, Ormiste V: Brucellosis in a group of travelers to Spain. JAMA 251:505–507, 1984.
41. Memish ZA, Balkhy HH: Brucellosis and international travel. J Travel Med 11:49–55.
42. Pike RM: Laboratory-associated infections. Summary and analysis of 3921 cases. Health Lab Sci 13:105–114, 1976.
43. Elberg SS: A guide to the diagnosis, treatment and prevention of brucellosis. Bull World Health Org 81:31, 1981.
44. Sanford JP: Brucella pneumonia. Semin Respir Infect 12:24–27, 1997.
45. Gotuzzo E, Carrillo C: Brucella arthritis. In Espinoza L, Goldberg D, Arnett F, et al (eds): Infections in the Rheumatic Disease. Orlando, FL, Grune & Stratton, 1988, pp 31–41.
46. Martin-Moreno S, Soto-Guzmán O, Bernardo-de-Quiros J, et al: Pancytopenia due to hemophagocytosis in patients with brucellosis: A report of four cases. J Infect Dis 147:445–449, 1983.
47. Lynch EC, McKechnie JC, Alfrey CP Jr: Brucellosis with pancytopenia. Ann Intern Med 69:319–322, 1968.
48. Garcia P, Yrivarren JL, Argumans C, et al: Evaluación de la mèdula ósea en pacientes con brucelosis. Correlación clinicopatholǒgica. Rev Enferm Infect y Microbiol Clin 8:37–42, 1990.
49. Fernández-Guerrero ML, Diás-Curiel M, Cortez-Cansino JM: Hepatic granulomas in brucellosis (letter). Ann Intern Med 92:572, 1980.
50. Recavarren S, Gotuzzo E: Patogenesis de la hepatitis granulomatosa por Brucella; Estudios ultraestucturales. Acta Med Peru 4:39–50, 1975.
51. Colmenero JD, Reguera JM, Martos F, et al: Complications associated with *Brucella melitensis* infection: A study of 530 cases. Medicine 75:195–211, 1996.
52. Farid Z, Trabolsi B, Yassin W, et al: Acute brucellosis presenting as fever of unknown origin (FUO). Trans R Soc Trop Med Hyg 74:402–404, 1980.
53. Gotuzzo E, Alarcón G, Bocanagra T, et al: Articular involvement in human brucellosis. A retrospective analysis of 304 cases. Semin Arthritis Rheum 12:245–255, 1982.
54. Bocanagra T, Gotuzzo E, Alarcón G, et al: Circulating immune complexes in acute fever and brucellosis. Clin Res 29:381, 1981.
55. Alarcón GS, Bocanagra T, Gotuzzo E, et al: Reactive arthritis associated with brucellosis: HLA studies. J Rheumatol 8:621–625, 1981.
56. Bocanagra T, Gotuzzo E, Castañeda O, et al: Rheumatic manifestations of brucellosis. Ann Rheum Dis 45:526–528, 1986.
57. Brito M, Gonzales-Dias J, Marques J, et al: Brucelosis osteoarticular. Rev Esp Reumatol Enferm Osteoarthritis (Barcelona) 15:219–236, 1972.
58. Mavridis AK, Drosos AA, Tsolas O, et al: Lactate levels in brucella arthritis. Rheumatol Int 4:169–171, 1984.
59. Ibáñez R, Ruiz P, Garciá-Chillón AG, et al: Sternoclavicular brucellosis. J Rheumatol 14:183–185, 1987.
60. Berrocal A, Gotuzzo E, Calvo A, et al: Sternoclavicular brucellar arthritis: A report of seven cases and a review of the literature. J Rheumatol 20:1184–1186, 1993.
61. Feldman JL, Menkes GJ, Weil B, et al: Les sacro-iléites infectieuses. Édude multicentrique sue 214 observations. Rev Rheumatol Med Osteartic 48:83–91, 1981.
62. Ariza J, Gudiol F, Valverde J, et al: Brucellar spondylitis: A detailed analysis based on current findings. Rev Infect Dis 7:656–664, 1985.
63. Hodinka L, Gomor B, Meretey K, et al: HLA-B27 associated spondyloarthritis in chronic brucellosis. Lancet 1:499, 1978.
64. Alarcón G, Gotuzzo E, Hinostroza S, et al: Brucella-induced reactive arthritis HLA studies (abstract). Clin Res 28:820A, 1980.
65. Alarcón G, Gotuzzo E, Hinostroza S, et al: HLA studies in brucellar spondylitis. Clin Rheumatol 4:312–314, 1985.
66. Alarcón G, Gotuzzo E, Hinostroza S, et al: Familial studies in human brucellosis. Tissue Antigens 26:77–79, 1985.
67. Ibero I, Vela P, Pascual E: Arthritis of shoulder and spinal cord compression due to *Brucella* disc infection. Br J Rheumatol 36:377–381, 1997.
68. Pons P: Spondylitis melitoccocita. Ann Med 5:227, 1929.
69. Roux H, Peloux Y, Gaborit P, et al: Les manifestations ostéoarticulaires de la brucellose. Encycl Med Chir Paris 14:1–10, 1983.
70. Taliani G, Bartoloni A, Tosí A, et al: Lumbar pain in a married couple who likes cheese—Brucella strikes again! Clin Exp Rheumatol 22:477–480, 2004.
71. Young EJ: Brucella melitensis hepatitis: The absence of granulomas. Ann Intern Med 91:414–417, 1979.
72. Bruguera M, Cervantes F: Hepatic granulomas in brucellosis. Ann Intern Med 92:571–572, 1980.
73. Spink WW, Hoffbauer FW, Walker WW, et al: Histopathology of the liver in human brucellosis. J Lab Clin 34:40, 1949.
74. Arias Stella J: Brucellosis. Contribución al conocimiento patológico. Ann Fac Med (Peru) 34:429–517, 1951.
75. Calder RM, Steen C, Baker L: Blood studies in brucellosis. JAMA 112:1893–1898, 1939.
76. Carcelén A, Gutiérrez LD, Rojas O: Sindromes hematológicos. Rev Sanid Nav Peru 4:117–130, 1968.
77. Crosby E, Llosa L, Miro Quesada M, et al: Hematologic changes in brucellosis. J Infect Dis 150:419–424, 1984.
78. McGaraty WC, Serafin D: Indications for splenectomy. Am J Surg 115:355–363, 1968.
79. Dorantes S: Cuadros hematológicos severos en brucelosis. Bol Med Hosp Infant Mexico 24:235–247, 1967.
80. Stoll DB, Blum S, Pasuale D, et al: Thrombocytopenia with decreased megakaryocytes. Ann Intern Med 94:170–175, 1981.
81. Young EJ, Corbel MJ (eds): Brucellosis. Clinical and Laboratory Aspects. Boca Raton, FL, CRC Press, 1989.
82. Zuazu J, Duran J, Julia A: Hemofagocitosis en brucelosis aguda. Rev Clin Esp 152:213–233, 1981.
83. Young EJ: Human brucellosis. Rev Infect Dis 5:821–842, 1983.
84. al Deeb SM, Yaqub BS, Sharif HS, et al: Neurobrucellosis: Clinical characteristics, diagnosis and outcome. Neurology 39:498–501, 1989.
85. Bashir R, Al-Kawl Z, Harder EJ, et al: Nervous system brucellosis: Diagnosis and treatment. Neurology 35:1576–1581, 1985.
86. Bouza E, Garcia de la Torre M, Parras F, et al: Brucellar meningitis. Rev Infect Dis 9:810–822, 1987.
87. Corbel MJ: Microbiology of the genus Brucella. In Young EJ, Corbel MJ (eds): Brucellosis: Clinical and Laboratory Aspects. Boca Raton, FL, CRC Press, 1989, pp 53–72.
88. Dalrymple-Champneys W: Undulant fever, a neglected problem. Lancet 1:429–477, 1950.
89. Oliveri RI, Matera G, Foca A, et al: Polyradiculoneuropathy with cerebrospinal fluid albuminocytological dissociation due to neurobrucellosis. Clin Infect Dis 23:833–834, 1996.
90. Riestra-Castañeda R, González-Garrido A, González-Cornejo S: Brucellosis and polyneuroradiculomyeloencephalitis. A case report. Arch Med Res 27:331–333, 1996.
91. Lubani MM, Dudin KI, Araj GF, et al: Neurobrucellosis in children. Pediatr Infect Dis 8:79–82, 1989.
92. Mousa AR, Koshy TS, Araj GF, et al: *Brucella* meningitis: Presentation, diagnosis and treatment: A prospective study of ten cases. Q J Med 60:873–875, 1986.
93. Ablin J, Mevorach D, Eliakim R: Brucellosis and the gastrointestinal tract. The odd couple. J Clin Gastroenterol 24:25–29, 1997.
94. Cohen N, Golik A, Alon I, et al: Conservative treatment for *Brucella* endocarditis. Clin Cardiol 20:291–294, 1997.
95. Saadeh AM, Abu-Farsakh NA, Omari HZ: Infective endocarditis and occult splenic abscess caused by *Brucella melitensis* infection: A case report and review of the literature. Acta Cardiol 51:279–285, 1995.
96. Quiroga J, Miralles A, Farinola T, et al: Surgical treatment of *Brucella* endocarditis. Cardiovasc Surg 4:227–230, 1996.
97. Martin WJ, Nichols DR, Beahrs OH: Chronic localized brucellosis. Arch Intern Med 107:75–80, 1961.
98. Spink WW: What is chronic brucellosis? Ann Intern Med 35:358–374, 1951.
99. Rodríguez-Torres A, Fermosa J, Landinez R: Causas de muerte en brucelosis. Rev Med Hosp Obrero Lima 12:315–327, 1965.
100. Pacheco G, Thiago de Mello M: Brucellose. Monografias do Instituto Oswaldo Cruz. Rio de Janeiró, Serviço Gráfico do Instituto Brasileiro de Geografia e Estadística, 1956, pp 402–441
101. Woods A: Endogenous Uveitis. Baltimore, Williams & Wilkins, 1960.

102. Tobaru L: Uveitis: Aspectos Clinicos y Etiologicos. Estudio Prospectivo de 28 Casos, Lima, Peru, (specialty thesis, oftalmologìa). Lima, Peru, Universidad Pervana Cayetano Heredia, 1983.
103. Carbone A, Rolando I, Gotuzzo E, et al: La brucelosis lesiones oftalmológicas. Diagnostico 12:196–202, 1983.
104. Rolando I, Carbone A, Gotuzzo E, et al: Circulating immune complexes in the pathogenesis of human brucellar uveitis. Chibret Int J Ophthalmol 3:30–38, 1985.
105. Rolando I, Carbone A, Haro D, et al: Retinal detachment in chronic brucellosis. Am J Ophthalmol 99:733–734, 1985.
106. Rolando I, Tobaru L, Hinostroza S, et al: Clinical manifestations of 25 *Brucella* uveitis. Ophthalmic Pract 5:12–17, 1987.
107. Dolgatova EL: Ocular status of patients with brucellosis. Vestn Oftalmol 113:37–38, 1997.
108. Lyall M: Ocular brucellosis. Trans Ophthalmol Soc UK 93:689–697, 1973.
109. Oppermann A, Royer I, Joubert L, et al: La brucellose oculaire. Ann Anat Pathol 3:499–502, 1969.
110. Pappas G, Bosilkovski M, Akritidis N, et al: Brucellosis and the respiratory system. Clin Infec Dis 37:95–99, 2003.
111. Chattas A, Ramaccio HF, Zamar R, et al: Brucelosis en el niño. Gaceta Sanitaria (Argentina) 6:69–77, 1963.
112. Shan PM, Joshi VG: Brucellosis in children. Indian Pediatr 4:226–231, 1967.
113. Vallejo JG, Stevens AM, Dutton RV, et al: Hepatosplenic abscesses due to *Brucella melitensis*: Report of a case involving a child and review of the literature. Clin Infect Dis 22:485–489, 1996.
114. Criscuolo E, DiCarlo FB: El aborto y otras manifestaciones ginecobstétricas en el curso de la brucelosis humana. Rev Fac Cienc Min Educ Univ Cordoba 12:321–330, 1954.
115. Khan MY, Mah MW, Memish ZA: Brucellosis in pregnant women. Clin Infect Dis 32:1172–1177, 2001.
116. D'Onadío G: Brucelosis y gestación: cuadro clínico y pronóstico materno-fetal (Thesis Bachelor's degree in Medicine). Lima, Peru, Universidad Peruana Cayetano Heredia, 2003.
117. Moreno S, Ariza J, Espinosa FJ, et al: Brucellosis in patients infected with the human immunodeficiency virus. Eur J Clin Microbiol Infect Dis 17:319–26, 1998.
118. Ibarra V, Blanco JR, Metola L, et al: Relapsing brucellosis in a patient infected with the human immunodeficiency virus (HIV). Clin Microbiol Infect 9:1259–1260, 2003.
119. Fernandez Reyes JL, Rosa Jimenez F, Banez Sanchez F, et al: Acute brucellosis and human immunodeficiency virus infection. Current status (letter). Ann Med Interna 17:275.
120. Keppie J, Williams AE, Witt K, et al: The role of erythritol in the tissue localisation of the brucellae. Br J Exp Pathol 46:104–110, 1965.
121. Young EJ, Gomez CI, Yawn DH, et al: Comparison of *Brucella abortus* and *Brucella melitensis* infections of mice and their effect on acquired cellular resistance. Infect Immun 26:680–685, 1997.
122. Gotuzzo E, Carrillo C, Guerra J, et al: Evaluation of diagnostic methods for brucellosis. Value of bone marrow culture. J Infect Dis 153:122–125, 1986.
123. Diaz R, Moriyon I: Laboratory techniques in the diagnosis of human brucellosis. In Young EJ, Corbel MK (eds): Brucellosis: Clinical and Laboratory Aspects. Boca Raton, FL, CRC Press, 1989, pp 73–84.
124. Ruiz-Castañeda M, Tovar R, Velez R: Studies on brucellosis in Mexico. Comparative study of various diagnostic tests and classification of the isolate bacteria. J Infect Dis 70:97–102, 1942.
125. Yagupsky P, Peled N, Press J, et al: Comparison of BACTEC 9240 Peds Plus medium and isolator 1.5 microbial tube for detection of *Brucella melitensis* from blood cultures. J Clin Microbiol 35:1382–1384, 1997.
126. Gedikoglu S, Helvaci S, Ozakin C, et al: Detection of *Brucella melitensis* by BACTEC NR 730 and BACTEC 9120 systems. Eur J Epidemiol 12:649–650, 1996.
127. Williams E: Brucellosis. Practitioner 226:1507–1514, 1982.
128. Rodríguez-Torres A, Fermosa J, Landinez R: Brucelosis. Medicina (B Aires) 48:3126, 1983.
129. Garrillo C, Sanchez-Grinan E, Gotuzzo E, et al: Evaluación de las metodologiás diagnósticas en brucellosis, según las diferentes formas clinicas. Presented at Congreso Pervano de Medicina Interna, Lima, Peru, October 29–31, 1984, abstract 102.
130. Baldi PC, Miguel SE, Fossati CA, et al: Serological follow-up of human brucellosis by measuring IgG antibodies to lipopolysaccharide and cytoplasmic proteins of *Brucella* species. Clin Infect Dis 22:446–455, 1996.
131. Herman L, DeRidder G: Identification of *Brucella* spp. by using the polymerase chain reaction. Appl Environ Microbiol 58:2099–2101, 1992.
132. Al Dahouk S, Tomaso H, Nockler K, et al: The detection of *Brucella* spp. using PCR-ELISA and real-time PCR assays. Clin Lab 50:387–394, 2004.
133. Leggiadro RJ: The threat of biological terrorism—A public health and infection control reality. Infect Control Hosp Epidemiol 9:5–14, 2000.
134. Rosenbloom M, Leikin JB, Vogel SN, et al: Biological and chemical agents: A brief synopsis. Am J Ther 9:5–14, 2002.
135. Noah DL, Huebner KD, Darling RG, et al: The history and threat of biological warfare and terrorism. Emerg Med Clin North Am 20:255–271, 2002.
136. Sewell DL: Laboratory-associated infections and biosafety. Clin Microbiol Rev 8:389–405, 1995.
137. Yagupsky P, Peled N, Riesenberg K, et al: Exposure of hospital personnel of *Brucella melitensis* and occurrence of laboratory-acquired disease in endemic area. Scand J Infect Dis 32:31–35, 2000.
138. Staszkiewicz J, Lewis CM, Colville J, et al: Outbreak of *Brucella melitensis* among microbiology laboratory workers in a community hospital. J Clin Microbiol 29:531–543, 1991.
139. Robichaud S, Libman M, Behr M, et al: Prevention of laboratory-acquired brucellosis. Clin Infect Dis 38:119–122, 2004.
140. Kaufmann A, Meltzer M, Schmid G: The economic impact of bioterrorism attack: Are prevention and postattack intervention programs justifiable? Emerg Infect Dis 3:83–94, 1997.
141. Al-Majed SA, Al-alka AD, Al-Mitwalli A, et al: Use of antibiotics in the treatment of human brucellosis. Curr Ther Res 57:175, 1986.
142. Carrillo C, Gotuzzo E, Adachi J, et al: Sensibilidad antimicrobiana in vitro de cepas de *Brucella melitensis* aisladas en un area endémica (Lima, Perú). Rev Esp Quimioter 6:309–313, 1993.
143. Conti R, Parenti F: Rifampicin therapy for brucellosis, flavobacterium meningitis and cutaneous leishmaniasis. Rev Infect Dis 5(Suppl 3). S600–S605, 1994.
144. Daikos GK, Pappaolyzos N, Marketos N, et al: Trimethoprim-sulfamethoxazole in brucellosis. J Infect Dis 128(Suppl):S731–S733, 1973.
145. Solera J, Martinez-Alfaro E, Espinosa A: Recognition and optimum treatment of brucellosis. Drugs 53:245–256, 1997.
146. Akova M, Uzun O, Akalin HE, et al: Quinolones in treatment of human brucellosis: Comparative trial of ofloxacin-rifampicin versus doxycycline-rifampicin. Antimicrob Agents Chemother 37:1831–1834, 1993.
147. Ariza J, Gudiol F, Pallares R, et al: Treatment of human brucellosis with doxycycline plus rifampin or doxycycline plus streptomycin: A randomized double-blind study. Ann Intern Med 117:25–30, 1992.
148. Bosch J, Linares J, López de Goicochea MJ, et al: In vitro activity of ciprofloxacin, ceftriaxone and five other antimicrobial agents against 95 strains of *Br. melitensis*. J Antimicrob Chemother 17:459–461, 1986.
149. Farid Z, Miale A, Omar S, et al: Antibiotic treatment of acute brucellosis caused by *Br. melitensis*. J Trop Med Hyg 64:157–163, 1961.
150. Solera J, Espinosa A, Martinez-Alfaro E, et al: Treatment of human brucellosis with doxycycline and gentamicin. Antimicrob Agents Chemother 41:80–84, 1997.
151. Solera J, Espinosa A, Geijo P, et al: Treatment of human brucellosis with netilmicin and doxycycline. Clin Infect Dis 22:441–445, 1996.
152. Colmenero JD, Fernández-Gallardo LC, et al: Possible implication of doxycycline-rifampin interaction for treatment of brucellosis. Antimicrob Agent Chemother 38:2798–2802, 1994.
153. Solera J, Beato JL, Martinez-Alfaro E, et al: Azitromycin and gentamicin therapy for the treatment of humans with brucellosis. Clin Infect Dis 32:506–509, 2001.

42

Plague

DAVID T. DENNIS
PAUL S. MEAD

INTRODUCTION

Definition

Plague in humans is a severe febrile illness caused by the gram-negative bacillus, *Yersinia pestis*. Historically, it is synonymous with catastrophic epidemics. *Y. pestis* is maintained in nature as a zoonotic infection of rodents and their fleas in scattered foci in large areas of Asia, Africa, and the Americas. It is an incidental infection of humans and mammals other than rodents. Humans acquire infection most often by the bite of rodent fleas, occasionally by handling or ingesting infected animal tissues, or by inhaling contagious airborne particles. The vast majority of cases of human plague now occur in underserved Third World populations where sanitation is poor and persons live in close association with rodent reservoirs of infection. The principal clinical forms of plague are bubonic, septicemic, and pneumonic. Bubonic (lymphadenitic) plague accounts for 85% or more of primary plague cases. Septicemic and pneumonic plagues occur most often as secondary complications of bubonic plague, but may arise directly from primary infections. All forms of plague are curable if they are diagnosed and treated early. However, delays in treatment can rapidly lead to potentially fatal overwhelming infection and endotoxemia. Although plague has a high epidemic potential, preventive steps can be taken to reduce risks of exposure, and outbreaks can be readily halted using standard public health measures. Cases should be reported to health authorities immediately so that appropriate investigative and control measures can be implemented without delay. Reporting and control of the disease is mandated by national and international health regulations. Recently, concern has been raised over plague as a potential weapon of terrorism; *Y. pestis* has been classified as a Category A select agent subject to federal laws governing its management and transport. Medical and public health preparedness and response plans have been developed to counter the threat of its potential misuse.[1,2]

History

Three pandemics of plague have been recorded. In the Justinian pandemic (circa 542–767 AD), it is thought that plague moved from upper Egypt to the Mediterranean and spread from there to Europe and Asia Minor, ultimately causing an estimated 40 million deaths. The second plague pandemic began in Central Asia early in the 14th century, caused epidemics in China and India, and moved along caravan routes to the Near and Middle East. Entering Messina by ship in 1347, plague swept swiftly through Europe and the British Isles, receiving the epithet "Black Death." Medieval plague killed a quarter or more of the affected populations at its height and was followed by successive epidemics in the European region over the next several centuries. The last global surge of plague, the third (modern) pandemic, arose in the latter half of the 19th century in Yunnan Province, China, struck Hong Kong in 1894, and spread from there by rat-infested steamships to port cities throughout the world, including several in the United States.[3–5] Within 30 years of its appearance in Hong Kong, the third plague pandemic had resulted in 26 million human cases and more than 12 million deaths, most of them in India.[3]

The plague bacillus was first identified in Hong Kong in 1894 by Alexandre Yersin, who isolated the organism from enlarged lymph nodes (buboes) of plague victims.[6] In 1898, Paul-Louis Simond, a French scientist sent to investigate epidemic plague in Bombay, identified the plague bacillus in the tissues of dead rats and subsequently proposed that the organism was transmitted from rat to rat, and from rats to humans by rat fleas.

After 1900, the global spread of plague was limited by regulations that controlled rats in ports and imposed inspection and rat-proofing of ships. *Y. pestis* did, however, become newly established among urban and rural rodent populations in many previously unaffected areas of the Americas, Europe, Africa, and Asia, resulting in scattered zoonotic foci that still exist throughout the world today.[7,8] In San Francisco, between 1900 and 1908, major outbreaks of rat-borne plague killed more than 200 persons. By 1908, plague was epizootic in ground squirrels in counties surrounding the city,[5] and in subsequent years spread to wild rodent populations throughout California and other states in the western third of the country. The last outbreak of urban plague and of person-to-person pneumonic transmission in the United States occurred in a slum area of Los Angeles in 1924–1925.

By the middle of the 20th century, cities in the United States and elsewhere had enforced higher sanitary standards and building codes, effective insecticides and rodenticides had become widely available, and several classes of antibiotics had been shown to be efficacious in treating plague. Most human plague since then has been sporadic and rural in distribution. Outbreaks have been relatively slow to develop and readily controlled by a combination of surveillance, early diagnosis and treatment, and flea and rat suppression.[9] The major exceptions to this generalization were the large rat-borne plague epidemics that occurred from 1962 to 1975 in war-torn Vietnam and in the 1990s in Madagascar.[6,10]

Plague is one of the three diseases (plague, cholera, yellow fever) subject to quarantine under World Health Organization (WHO) international health regulations.[11] In 1994, articles of these regulations were used to prevent potential spread of plague from India after a reported outbreak of pneumonic plague there evoked local panic and an exaggerated international response to the perceived health emergency.[12,13]

AGENT

General Microbiology

Y. pestis is a nonmotile, nonsporulating, gram-negative coccobacillus in the family Enterobacteriaceae.[4,14] It is microaerophilic, oxidase- and urease-negative, non–lactose-fermenting, and biochemically unreactive. The organism is nonfastidious and is highly infective to laboratory rodents. *Y. pestis* grows slowly but well on a wide variety of common media (e.g., brain-heart infusion broth, sheep blood agar, chocolate agar, and MacConkey agar). Routine specimens can be safely handled under BSL-2 procedures, but manipulation of isolates requires BSL-3 measures to adequately protect laboratory workers.[14] Growth occurs across a wide range of temperature (4°C to 40°C) and pH (5.0 to 9.6), but is optimal at 28°C and pH 7.4. Incubation at 37°C for 24 hours on agar yields pinpoint, transparent colonies that are easily overlooked, especially if there is contamination of the culture by other bacteria. At 48 hours, colonies are typically gray, 1 mm to 2 mm in diameter, and have an irregular "hammered metal" appearance when viewed under magnification. In broth, *Y. pestis* grows in flocculent clumps, typically attached to the sides of the tube in downwardly projecting stalactite forms that leave a clear broth. With polychromatic stains such as Wayson, Wright, or Giemsa, plague bacilli from clinical specimens demonstrate a characteristic bipolar appearance resembling closed safety pins (Fig. 42-1). Although *Y. pestis* is not truly encapsulated, it produces an envelope that contains the unique fraction 1 (F1) glycoprotein surface antigen.

Decoding of the entire genome of the plague bacillus shows that it only recently evolved from *Y. pseudotuberculosis*.[15,16] It is highly adapted to rodents and their fleas and does not long persist outside them. In the environment, it is rapidly killed by temperatures above 40°C and by desiccation.

Y. pestis Virulence Factors

Y. pestis expresses several virulence factors that are important for its survival in rodents, humans, and fleas.[4,17–19] Most genes encoding these virulence factors reside on three plasmids, *Pst* (9.5 kb), *Lcr* (approximately 70 kb), and *pFra* (approximately 110 kb). The *Pst* plasmid encodes a temperature-dependent plasminogen activator (Pla) and a bacteriocin (pesticin). The plasminogen activator, a bacterial surface protease, is important for survival of *Y. pestis* in fleas. This protease facilitates the formation of a bolus of blood and aggregated bacteria in the flea midgut, which blocks the flea's proventriculus and leads to regurgitation of infective material when the "blocked" flea attempts to feed (see Epizootic Plague). Pesticin promotes iron uptake by *Y. pestis*.

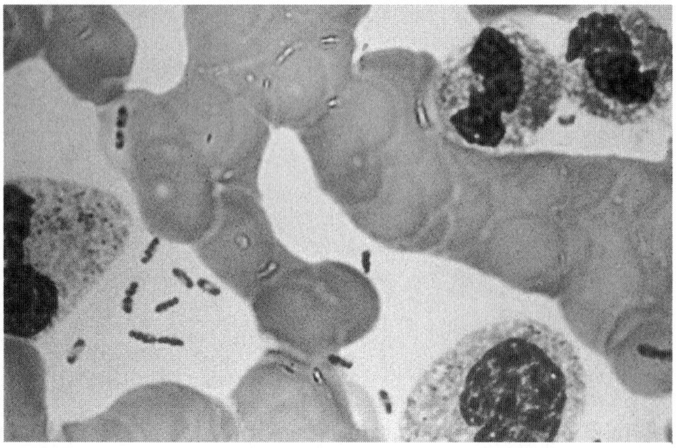

FIGURE 42-1 Peripheral blood smear from a patient with plague septicemia, showing characteristic bipolar-staining *Yersinia pestis* (Wright's stain, oil immersion).

The low calcium response plasmid (*Lcr*) encodes gene products active in low calcium environments. The products include various outer surface proteins (Yops) and a soluble V antigen, thought to be essential to *Y. pestis* survival in macrophages. Factors associated with the approximately 70-kb plasmid inhibit the production by macrophages of interferon-gamma (IFN-γ) and tumor necrosis factor–alpha (TNF-α).

The *pFra* plasmid contains genes for the fraction 1 (F1) envelope glycoprotein antigen and a murine exotoxin. F1 antigen is produced only by organisms growing at 30°C or greater. *Y. pestis* strains expressing F1 antigen are able to resist phagocytosis in the absence of opsonizing antibodies. The murine toxin (Ymt) is highly toxic to mice and rats, but is not known to be toxic in humans. In the flea midgut, Ymt (recently recognized to be phospholipidase D) plays a critical role in protecting *Y. pestis* from a cytotoxic digestion product of blood plasma. The emergence in *Y. pestis* of the single responsible gene (*ymt*) did, by adapting the bacillus to fleas, radically separate the natural history of the plague bacillus from that of the enteropathogenic *Yersinia* spp.[20]

Chromosomally encoded virulence factors include a lipopolysaccharide endotoxin and a factor controlling the absorption of exogenous iron. Endotoxin is responsible for complement activation and release of cytokines. When *Y. pestis* is grown on media with Congo red, a heme-analogue dye, iron absorption is indicated by pigment production. Strains that do not produce pigment have diminished virulence in mammals and are unable to induce blocking in the flea gut. Hemin storage locus (*hms*) products expressed in the low temperature (28°C or less) environment of the flea assist in forming blockages of the flea gut necessary for efficient transmission.[18–20] A chromosomally encoded product, the pH 6 antigen (Psa), inhibits phagocytosis of *Y. pestis* in mammals.

Y. pestis Biotypes

Y. pestis isolates can be classified into biotypes based on their ability to ferment glycerol and reduce nitrate. Three biotypes have been associated with respective plague pandemics.[21] Relict populations of the Antiqua biotype are found in Africa, southeastern Russia, and Central Asia; the Mediaevalis biotype is found around the Caspian Sea; and the Orientalis biotype in Asia and the Western Hemisphere. Typing based on ribosomal gene characteristics supports these distinctions. Considering their adaptation to diverse ecologies worldwide, wild *Y. pestis* strains are quite uniform, although finer genomic analyses have recently demonstrated subtle and evolving differences.[22,23]

Y. pestis Life Cycle

Y. pestis is a zoonotic infection that principally involves wild and domestic rodents, and their various flea species (Fig. 42-2).

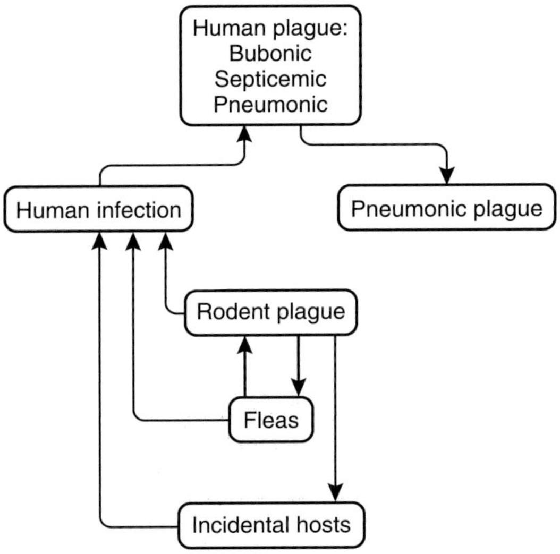

FIGURE 42-2 *Yersinia pestis* cycles, demonstrating the interrelationships of its rodent reservoir, flea vector, and incidental mammalian hosts, including humans. In the usual situation, *Y. pestis* is transmitted from rodent to rodent, and occasionally from rodent to human or other incidental mammalian host, by an infective rodent flea. Pet dogs and cats can bring infective rodent fleas into the home environment. Infection may be transmitted directly from rodent to rodent by cannibalism, and from infected animal to predator or to human by ingestion. Humans may also acquire infection by accidental percutaneous inoculation while handling contaminated tissues or fluids. Plague pneumonia can be transmitted from one person to another and, rarely, from cats to persons, by infective respiratory droplets.

Plague spreads from rodents to humans when humans intrude into the natural (wild) cycle, or when commensal rodents become infected and transmission is established in homes and other communal settings. Human-to-human transmission may result from close and unprotected exposure to persons with respiratory plague. Transmission from person to person by the human flea, *Pulex irritans*, is controversial. Studies of plague transmission in the 20th century suggest that spread by the human flea, if it occurs, is inefficient and uncommon; however, human fleas have been proposed as an important factor in the rapid spread of plague in Europe during the Black Death.

EPIDEMIOLOGY

Ecology

More than 200 species of mammals and 150 species of fleas have been found to be naturally infected with *Y. pestis*. However, few of these hosts are important for maintaining enzootic or epizootic life cycles, and fewer still pose a significant risk to humans. The natural history of *Y. pestis* is complex, and an understanding of the organism's ecology and life cycle is helpful in defining its epidemiology and designing control and prevention strategies (Box 42-1).[7–9,24–26]

Enzootic Plague

In its natural reservoir hosts, infection with the plague bacillus is often unnoticed. This is characteristic of enzootic

Box 42-1 Plague Foci

North American Plague Foci

Wild rodent plague has been reported west of the 100th meridian in 17 contiguous western states and in some areas of adjacent Canada and Mexico.[7,8,25] The major plague sites are the southwestern focus, comprising mainly semi-arid grassland plateaus, foothills, and forested uplands of northeastern Arizona, most of New Mexico, southern Utah, and southern Colorado; the Pacific Coast focus, comprising mostly valley grassland, foothills, and the montane habitat of California and southern Oregon; the Great Basin focus, encompassing parts of Utah, Nevada, and southern Idaho; and the Rocky Mountain and northern focus, comprising mostly northern Colorado, Wyoming, and Montana.

The principal rodent hosts in the southwestern focus are various burrowing ground squirrels (*Spermophilus* spp.), prairie dogs (primarily *Cynomys gunnisoni*), wood rats (*Neotoma* spp.), antelope ground squirrels (*Ammospermophilus* spp.), deer mice (*Peromyscus maniculatis*), and related species. The major rodent hosts in the various niches of the Pacific Coast focus include *Spermophilus* spp., especially the California ground squirrel (*S. beecheyi*), the golden-mantled ground squirrel (*S. lateralis*), chipmunks (various *Tamias* spp.), deer mice and other *Peromyscus* spp., and voles (*Microtus* spp.). Other important hosts in the United States include various small ground squirrels (*S. elegans, S. beldingi,* and *S. townsendi*) in the Rocky Mountain and Great Basin regions, and the black-tailed prairie dog (*Cynomys ludovicianus*) in the Great Plains region. Epizootics of plague have recently occurred in urban tree squirrel (*Sciurus niger*) populations in cities along the eastern foothills of the Colorado Rocky Mountains, but pose a small risk to humans because these squirrels are parasitized by nonanthropophagic fleas.

Since 1950, a few cities in the United States have rarely been found to have *Y. pestis*–infected rats (e.g., Tacoma, San Francisco, Los Angeles, Dallas). However, no widespread epizootics or human plague cases have resulted, possibly because the rats have been infested with only small numbers of fleas or with flea species that are inefficient vectors of *Y. pestis*.

The principal fleas transmitting plague among wild rodent epizootic hosts in the United States include various ground squirrel fleas (*Oropsylla montana* [*Diamanus montanus*], *Hoplopsyllus anomalus, Thrassis* spp., *Opisocrostis* spp., *Oropsylla idahoensis*), prairie dog fleas (*Opisocrostis* spp.), wood rat fleas (*Orchopeas* spp.), and chipmunk fleas (*Eumolpianus eumolpi*).[7,8,25] *Or. montana* is the most important vector of *Y. pestis* to persons in the United States because it is a competent host that readily feeds on a wide range of rodents, and on other mammals, including humans.

Continued

Box 42-1 Plague Foci—Cont'd

South American Plague Foci

In South America, active enzootic plague foci exist in Brazil, Bolivia, Peru, and Ecuador, and have been described previously in Paraguay, Argentina, and Venezuela. *Y. pestis* infection in these foci has been variously found in commensal rats (*Rattus* spp.), cotton rats (*Sigmodon* spp.), rice rats (*Oryzomys* spp.), field mice (*Akodon* spp.), cane mice (*Zygodontomys* spp.), wild cavies, and domesticated guinea pigs (*Cavia* and *Galea* spp.).[3,26] Domestic guinea pigs are reared in homes for food in the Andean region and are considered a potential commensal risk of infection to humans; human plague outbreaks in the Andean region, including a recent extensive bubonic plague epidemic in northern Peru and a mixed bubonic/pneumonic plague outbreak in Ecuador, have been suspected to be associated in the domestic environment with infected guinea pigs as well as *R. rattus*. A previously active plague area in northeastern Brazil has been quiescent over the past 20 years. The various fleas that serve as principal vectors in South American foci are *X. cheopis* on *Rattus* spp. and *Polygenis* and *Pleochaetis* spp. on wild rodents. *Pulex irritans,* the human flea (which also parasitizes domesticated guinea pigs), has been implicated as a potential transmitter of plague to humans in some Andean outbreaks.

African Plague Foci

Widely scattered active plague foci exist in East and South Africa, including Democratic Republic of the Congo (previously Zaire), Uganda, Kenya, Tanzania, Zambia, Zimbabwe, Mozambique, Botswana, South Africa, Namibia, and Angola, and on the Indian Ocean island of Madagascar.[3,7,26] Less active foci exist in some northern Africa states (e.g., Libya, Algiers). The principal wild rodent hosts in Africa include gerbils (*Tatera* and *Desmodillus* spp.), swamp rats (*Otomys* spp.), various grass mice (*Arvicanthis* spp.), multimammate mice (*Mastomys* spp.), and commensal rats (*Rattus* spp.). One scenario describes plague in grassland gerbil populations spreading to multimammate mice in agricultural fields, and then to commensal rats in villages, resulting in human plague outbreaks. The principal flea vectors of wild rodent hosts are *Xenopsylla* and *Dinopsyllus* spp., while *X. cheopis* and *X. braziliensis* are the principal flea species involved in transmission among commensal rats and to man.

Asian Plague Foci

The most important Eurasian plague hosts are gerbils (various *Meriones* spp.) in Iran, Kurdistan, Transcaucasia, other areas around the Caspian Sea, and the plains of southeastern Russia and Khazakstan; marmots (*Marmota* spp.) in Central Asia, including mountainous Khazakstan, northeastern China, Mongolia, Manchuria, and in Transbaikalia; and ground squirrels (*Spermophilus* spp.) in Mongolia, northern-central China, the central Asian plains and steppes, and some areas around the Caspian Sea.[3,7,26] The primary flea vectors on gerbils are *Xenopsylla* and *Nosopsyllus* spp.; on marmots, various *Oropsylla, Rhadinopsylla,* and *Citellophilus* spp.; and on ground squirrels, *Citellophilus* and *Neopsylla* spp.

In India, the gerbil, *Tatera indica*, has been described as the principal wild rodent maintenance host.[3,7,26] Although it lives principally in open grassland sites in its natural state, it does invade agricultural fields and village peripheries. Other maintenance hosts include *Mellardia meltada,* various field mice, and palm squirrels (*Funambulus* spp.). The important commensal rat species are *Bandicota bengalensis, Bandicota indica, R. rattus,* and *R. norvegicus*. The primary vectors of plague in India are *X. cheopis* and *Xenopsylla astia*.

The principal rodent hosts in Myanmar, Vietnam, and Indonesia are *R. rattus* subsp. *diardii* and the Polynesian rat (*Rattus exulans*).[3,7,26] *R. rattus* subsp. *flavipectus* is an important host in southern China. *R. norvegicus* and the bandicoot, *B. indicus,* have been described as important hosts in Vietnam. The shrew, *Suncus murinus,* has been described as a possibly important host of plague in Vietnam and Indonesia. *X. cheopis* is the principal vector of plague in southern China, Myanmar, Vietnam, and Indonesia; *X. astia* (a less efficient vector) is also found on rats in Myanmar and Vietnam. *Stivalius cognatus,* a rat flea, is considered to be an important secondary vector of plague in Indonesia.

infections among rodents in remote, sparsely populated areas, such as the semiarid or arid grassland steppes of Central Asia and the savannahs of eastern Africa.[7–9,25,26] Fleas become infected by feeding on bacteremic rodents; although infection sickens or kills some enzootic hosts, most tolerate the infection and noticeable population die-offs do not usually occur. Although nonrodent mammals, such as predatory carnivores, do not serve as reservoirs of infection, they may contribute to the maintenance of zoonotic cycles by transporting infective fleas from one rodent population to another. Enzootic transmission generally places humans at a small risk of incidental infection, and associated cases are typically infrequent and sporadic.

Epizootic Plague

In epizootic plague, infection spreads rapidly among susceptible rodent populations transmitted by efficient flea vectors (both rodents and fleas serve as amplifying hosts of *Y. pestis*).[7,8,24–26] Epizootics often result in die-offs of affected rodent populations and accelerated dispersal of their fleas. Spread of infective fleas to rodents living in close association with humans can pose a serious threat in residential areas. Prairie dogs are highly susceptible and sensitive epizootic hosts in the southwestern United States, and epizootics can quickly kill off colonies over wide areas, sometimes in close proximity to suburban developments.

Historically, urban epidemics and pandemic spread of plague have been linked to epizootics involving the commensal rodents *Rattus rattus* and *R. norvegicus.* The smaller, domestic, roof or black rat (*R. rattus*) is considered the most dangerous plague host. Since ancient times, this adaptable and clever rodent has lived in intimate domestic association with humans in Asia, the Middle East, and Africa. Its migration to Europe allowed the rapid spread of plague there during the medieval period.

15. Achtman M, Zurth K, Morelli G, et al: *Yersinia pestis*, the cause of plague, is a recently emerged clone of *Yersinia pseudotuberculosis*. Proc Natl Acad Sci USA 24:14043, 1999.
16. Parkhill J, Wren BW, Thompson NR, et al: Genome sequence of *Yersinia pestis*, the causative agent of plague. Nature 413:523, 2001.
17. Brubaker RR: Factors promoting acute and chronic diseases caused by yersiniae. Clin Microbiol Rev 4:309, 1991.
18. Carniel E: Evolution of pathogenic *Yersinia*, some lights in the dark. Adv Exp Med Biol 529:3, 2003.
19. Hinnebusch BJ: Bubonic plague: A molecular genetic case history of the emergence of an infectious disease. J Mol Med 75:645, 1997.
20. Hinnebusch BJ, Rudolph AE, Cherepenov P, et al: Role of murine toxin in survival of *Yersinia pestis* in the midgut of the vector flea. Science 296:733, 2002.
21. Guiyoule A, Grimont F, Iteman I, et al: Plague pandemics investigated by ribotyping of *Yersinia pestis* strains. J Clin Microbiol 32:634, 1994.
22. Guiyoule A, Rasoamanana B, Buchrieser C, et al: Recent emergence of new variants of *Yersinia pestis* is Madagascar. J Clin Microbiol 35:2826, 1997.
23. Radnedge L, Agron PG, Worsham PL, et al: Genome plasticity in *Yersinia pestis*. Microbiology 148:1687, 2002.
24. Pollitzer R, Meyer KF: The ecology of plague. In May JH (ed): Studies in Disease Ecology. New York, Hefner, 1961, p 433.
25. Barnes AM: Surveillance and control of bubonic plague in the United States. Symp Zool Soc London 50:237–270, 1982.
26. Gratz NG: Rodent reservoirs and flea vectors of natural foci of plague. In Plague Manual: Epidemiology, Distribution, Surveillance and Control. Geneva, World Health Organization, 1999, p 63.
27. Dennis DT, Orloski K: Plague! In Bernstein E, Tomchuck L, Brant J, et al (eds): 1996 Medical and Health Annual. Chicago, Encyclopaedia Brittanica, 1996, p 160.
28. Saxena VK, Vergese T: Ecology of flea-transmitted zoonotic infection in village Mamla, District Beed. Curr Sci 71:800, 1996.
29. Craven RB, Maupin GO, Beard ML, et al: Reported cases of human plague infections in the United States, 1970–1991. J Med Entomol 30:758, 1993.
30. Gage KL, Dennis DT, Orloski KA, et al: Cases of cat-associated plague in the western U.S., 1977–1998. Clin Infect Dis 30:893, 2000.
31. Mann JM, Martone WJ, Boyce JM, et al: Endemic human plague in New Mexico: Risk factors associated with infection. J Infect Dis 140:397, 1979.
32. Christie AB, Chen TH, Elberg SS: Plague in camels and goats: Their role in human epidemics. J Infect Dis 141:724, 1980.
33. World Health Organization: Human plague in 2000 and 2001. Wkly Epidemiol Rec 78:130, 2003.
34. Chanteau S, Ratsifasoamanana L, Rasoamanana B, et al: Plague, a reemerging disease in Madagascar. Emerg Infect Dis 4:101, 1998.
35. Dennis DT: Plague as an emerging disease. In Scheld WM, Craig WA, Hughes JM (eds): Emerging Infections 2. Washington, DC, ASM Press, 1998, p 169.
36. Butler T, Bell WR, Nguyen NL, et al: *Yersinia pestis* infection in Vietnam. I. Clinical and hematological aspects. J Infect Dis 129(Suppl):S78, 1974.
37. Butler T: A clinical study of bubonic plague: Observations on the 1970 Vietnam epidemic with emphasis on coagulation studies, skin histology and electrocardiograms. Am J Med 53:268, 1972.
38. Hull HF, Montes JM, Mann JM: Septicemic plague in New Mexico. J Infect Dis 155:113, 1987.
39. Butler T, Levin J, Nguyen NL, et al: *Yersinia pestis* infection in Vietnam. II. Quantitative blood cultures and detection of endotoxin in the cerebrospinal fluid of patients with meningitis. J Infect Dis 133:493, 1976.
40. Crook LD, Tempest B: Plague—A clinical review of 27 cases. Arch Intern Med 152:1253, 1992.
41. Hull HF, Montes JM, Mann JM: Plague masquerading as gastrointestinal illness. West J Med 145:485, 1986.
42. Wu Lien-Teh: A Treatise on Pneumonic Plague. Geneva, League of Nations Health Organization, 1926.
43. Becker TM, Poland JD, Quan TJ, et al: Plague meningitis—A retrospective analysis of reported cases in the United States, 1970–1979. West Med J 147:554, 1987.
44. Dennis D, Meier F: Plague. In Horsburgh CR, Nelson AM (eds): Pathology of Emerging Infections. Washington, DC, ASM Press, 1997, p 21.
45. Finegold MJ: Pathogenesis of plague: A review of plague deaths in the United States during the last decade. Am J Med 45:549, 1968.
46. Burmeister RW, Tigertt WD, Overholt EL: Laboratory-acquired pneumonic plague: Report of a case and review of previous cases. Ann Intern Med 56:789, 1962.
47. Cornelis GR: *Yersinia* type III secretion: Send in the effectors. J Cell Biol 158:401, 2002.
48. Sing A, Rost D, Tvardovskaia N, et al: *Yersinia* V-antigen exploits toll-like receptor 2 and CD14 for interleukin 10–mediated immunosuppression. J Exp Med 196:1017, 2002.
49. Kopp E, Medzhitov R: A plague on host defense. J Exp Med 196:1009, 2002.
50. Sodhi A, Sharma RK, Batra HV, et al: Mechanism of rLcrV and rYopB mediated immunosuppression in murine peritoneal macrophages. Mol Immunol 41:767, 2004.
51. Kerschen EJ, Cohen DA, Kaplan AM, et al: The plague virulence protein YopM targets the innate immune response by causing a global depletion of NK cells. Infect Immun 72:4589, 2004.
52. Mann JM, Schmid GP, Stoetz PA, et al: Peripatetic plague. JAMA 247:46, 1982.
53. Centers for Disease Control and Prevention: Imported plague—New York City, 2002. MMWR 52:725, 2003.
54. Morse SA, Kellogg RB, Perry S: Detecting biothreat agents: The laboratory response network. ASM News 69:433, 2003.
55. Butler T, Hudson BW: The serological response to *Yersinia pestis* infection. Bull WHO 55:39, 1977.
56. Chanteau S, Rahalison L, Ralafiarisoa L, et al: Development and testing of a rapid diagnostic test for bubonic and pneumonic plague. Lancet 361:211, 2003.
57. Centers for Disease Control and Prevention. Fatal human plague—Arizona and Colorado, 1996. MMWR 46:617, 1997.
58. Boulanger L, Ettestad P, Fogarty J, et al: Gentamicin and tetracyclines for the treatment of human plague: Review of 75 cases in New Mexico, 1985–1999. Clin Infect Dis 38:663, 2004.
59. Frean JA, Arntzen L, Capper T, et al: In vitro activities of 14 antibiotics against 100 human isolates of *Yersinia pestis* from a southern African plague focus. Antimicrob Agents Chemother 40:2646, 1996.
60. Russell P, Eley SM, Bell DL, et al: Doxycycline or ciprofloxacin prophylaxis and therapy against experimental *Yersinia pestis* infection in mice. J Antimicrob Chemother 37:769, 1996.
61. Galimand M, Guiyoule A, Gerbaud G, et al: Multidrug resistance in *Yersinia pestis* mediated by a transferable plasmid. N Engl J Med 337:677, 1997.
62. Centers for Disease Control and Prevention. Prevention of plague. Recommendations of the Advisory Committee on Immunization Practices (ACIP). MMWR 45:1, 1996.
63. World Health Organization: Technical guide for a system of plague surveillance. Wkly Epidemiol Rec 14:149, 1973.
64. Fritz CL, Dennis DT, Tipple MA, et al: Surveillance for pneumonic plague in the United States during an international emergency: A model for control of imported emerging diseases. Emerg Infect Dis 2:30, 1996.
65. Titball RW, Williamson ED, Dennis DT: Plague. In Plotkin SA, Orenstein WA (eds): Vaccines, 4th ed. Philadelphia, WB Saunders, 2004, p 999.

43

Tetanus

BARNETT R. NATHAN
THOMAS P. BLECK

INTRODUCTION

Tetanus remains a significant health concern throughout the world. In 1975 Edsal estimated that about 1 million cases of the disease occurred annually in the world.[1] In the United States and other developed countries the number of cases and deaths from tetanus has fallen significantly over the last 40 years.[2,3] However, in the tropics and particularly the developing countries in these regions, tetanus, particularly neonatal tetanus, continues to be a significant cause of morbidity and mortality, with neonatal tetanus having an up to 90% mortality rate.[4,5] Technological advances such as pharmacologic muscle relaxants and ventilatory support have made the treatment of acute tetanus possible. Unfortunately, many of these techniques are not readily available in the developing world. Fortunately, an effective vaccine *is* available, and immunization programs are clearly effective in reducing mortality, particularly from neonatal tetanus.[6]

Tetanus was described very early in the history of medicine, with both the Egyptians and the Greeks recording the muscle rigidity and trismus that characterize the disease.[7,8] In the 18th century, tetanus was thought to be a result of nerve injury,[9] and the muscle spasms were also at times confused with the convulsions of epilepsy. In the 19th century, Sir William Gowers described quite accurately the typical appearance of a patient with tetanus: "Tetanus is a disease of the nervous system characterized by persistent tonic spasm, with violent brief exacerbations. The spasm almost always commences in the muscles of the neck and jaw, causing closure of the jaws (trismus, lockjaw), and involves muscles of the trunk more than those of the limbs. It is always acute in onset, and a very large proportion of those who are attacked die."[10] Nicolaier reported a strychnine-like toxin from anaerobic soil bacteria in 1884,[11] and 6 years later Behring and Kitasato demonstrated that immunization with an inactivated extract of this bacterium prevented tetanus.[12]

In the 18th century neonatal tetanus was known as the "7-day disease" in the Americas[13] and as the "9-day fits in Dublin"[14] because it usually presents about 1 to 2 weeks postpartum. In 1846, Sims conjectured that neonatal tetanus resulted from placing infants on their backs, thereby compressing the occiput and occluding the blood supply to the medulla.[15] In 1887, 3 years after Nicolaier's report, Beumer determined that the umbilicus was the portal of entry for neonatal tetanus.[16]

AGENT

Clostridium tetani is a slender, obligate anaerobic bacillus measuring 0.5 to 1.7 μm × 2.1 to 18.1 μm.[17] Although classified as a gram-positive organism, it may stain variably, especially in tissue or older cultures.[18] Most strains are slightly motile, and have abundant peritrichous flagella during growth.[19] The mature organism loses its flagella and forms a spherical terminal spore,[20] producing a profile like that of a squash racket (Fig. 43-1).[21] The spores resist extremes of temperature and moisture and they are stable at atmospheric oxygen tension. The spores can survive indefinitely and are viable after exposure to ethanol, phenol, or formalin. Death of the spores can be ensured by exposure to 100°C for 4 hours, autoclaving at 121°C and 103 kPa (15 psi) for 15 minutes, or with iodine, glutaraldehyde, or hydrogen peroxide.

Spores can be isolated from animal feces and therefore are ubiquitous in the environment. In small numbers they can be found in the soil and even on carpets, and hence any breach in skin defenses such as wounds, burns, animal bites, human bites,[22] and even insect bites may result in inoculation of the spores.[23] Close to 80% of tetanus cases in the United States between 1972 and 1989 were the result of acute injuries (with equal contributions from punctures and lacerations as the acute wound type likely to cause tetanus), while only 20% were the result of more chronic wounds.[24] There was only a slight preponderance of patients acquiring tetanus while indoors as compared with outdoors (29% vs. 21%).[24] In many series, however, between 7% and 21% of tetanus cases are cryptogenic.[25]

In culture, the bacterium grows best at 37°C and will grow on a variety of media (including blood agar) as long as oxygen is excluded. Standard anaerobic isolation techniques, such as placing the sample in an anaerobic transport system, are important in the culture of the organism. However, diagnostic and therapeutic decisions should not be made based on the culture, since cultures are frequently negative in patients with clinical tetanus, and routine bacteriologic studies do not

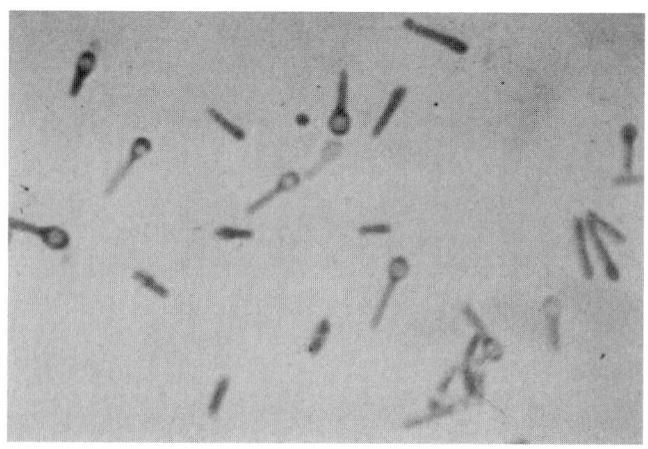

FIGURE 43-1 Gram's stain of a culture of *Clostridium tetani*. (Original magnification ×1000.) (From Bleck T, Brauner JS: Tetanus. In Scheld WM, Whitley RJ, Durack DT [eds]: Infections of the Central Nervous System, 2nd ed. New York, Raven Press, 1996; courtesy of P. C. Schrechenberger and A. Kuritza.)

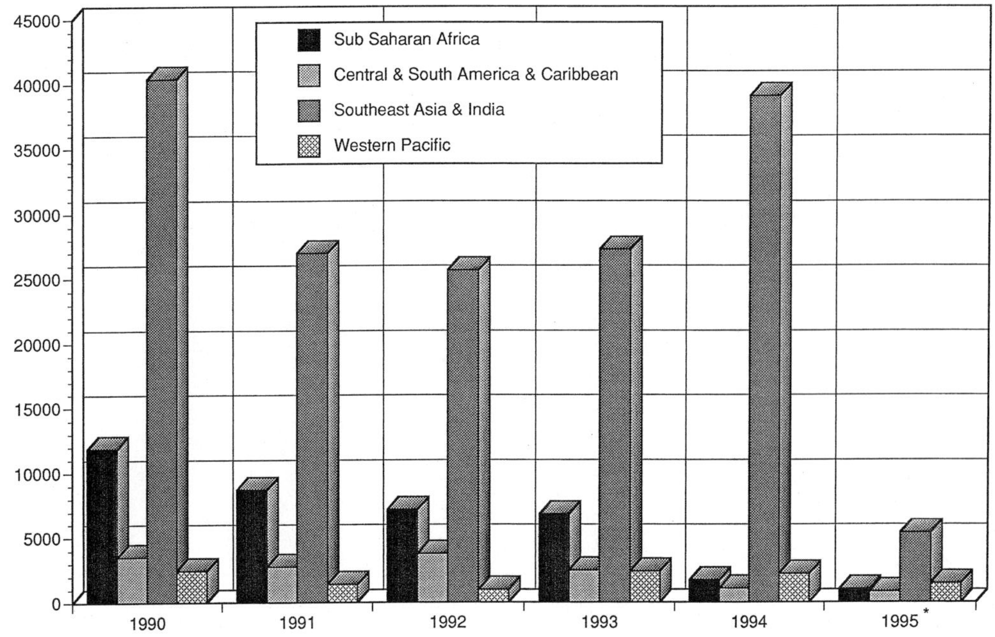

FIGURE 43-2 Reported annual incidence of all tetanus cases (including neonatal) by tropical region for years 1990 to 1995. Values along the abscissa represent the total number of cases reported to WHO. *No report from India in 1995. (Adapted from World Health Organization: Global programme on vaccines: Total tetanus incidence data. 1996. Available at: gopher://gopher.who.ch:70/11/.whosis/.gpvis/.incidence/.total-tetanus.)

indicate whether a strain of *C. tetani* carries the plasmid required for toxin production.

EPIDEMIOLOGY

About 1 million cases of tetanus occur annually worldwide, suggesting an incidence of approximately 18 per 100,000 population per year,[1] but this number has a high degree of uncertainty because reported cases of tetanus are significantly lower than this estimate. In tropical and developing countries tetanus continues to be a significant problem, with more than 45,000 cases reported in 1994. Figure 43-2 demonstrates the total number of reported tetanus cases throughout the tropical world. In the tropics and developing countries the number of neonatal cases has also dropped more than 50% while the total number of cases of tetanus has remained relatively stable. Figure 43-3 demonstrates the number of reported neonatal tetanus cases throughout the tropics. Neonatal tetanus

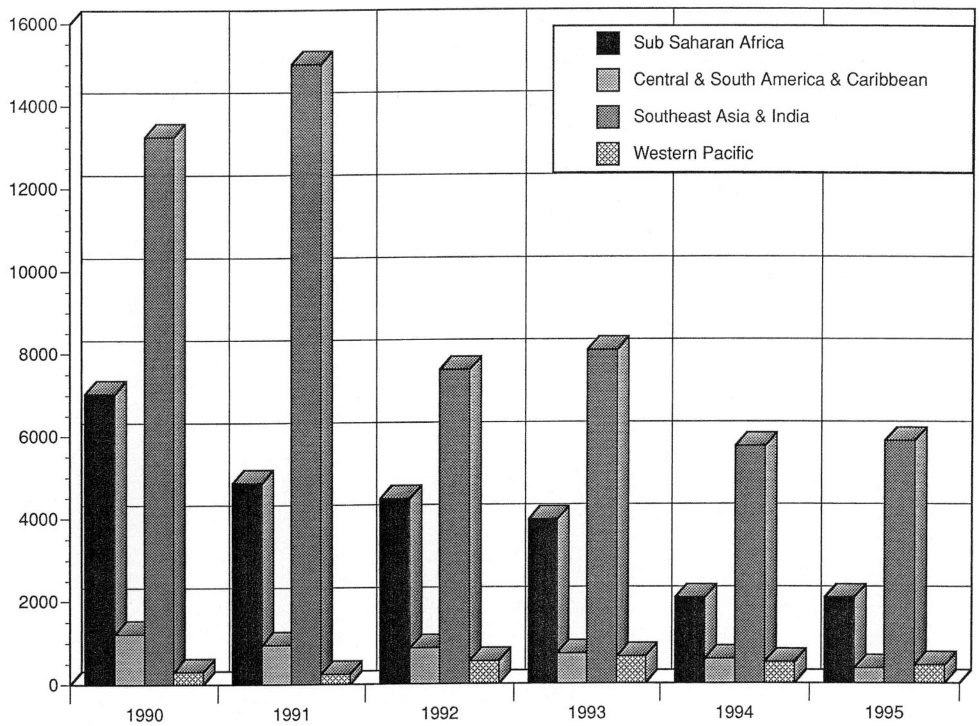

FIGURE 43-3 Reported annual incidence of neonatal tetanus by tropical region for years 1990 to 1995. Values along the abscissa represent total number of cases reported to WHO. (Adapted from World Health Organization: Global programme on vaccines: Neonatal tetanus incidence data. 1996. Available at: gopher://gopher.who.ch:70/11/.whosis/.gpvis/.incidence/.neonatal-tetanus.)

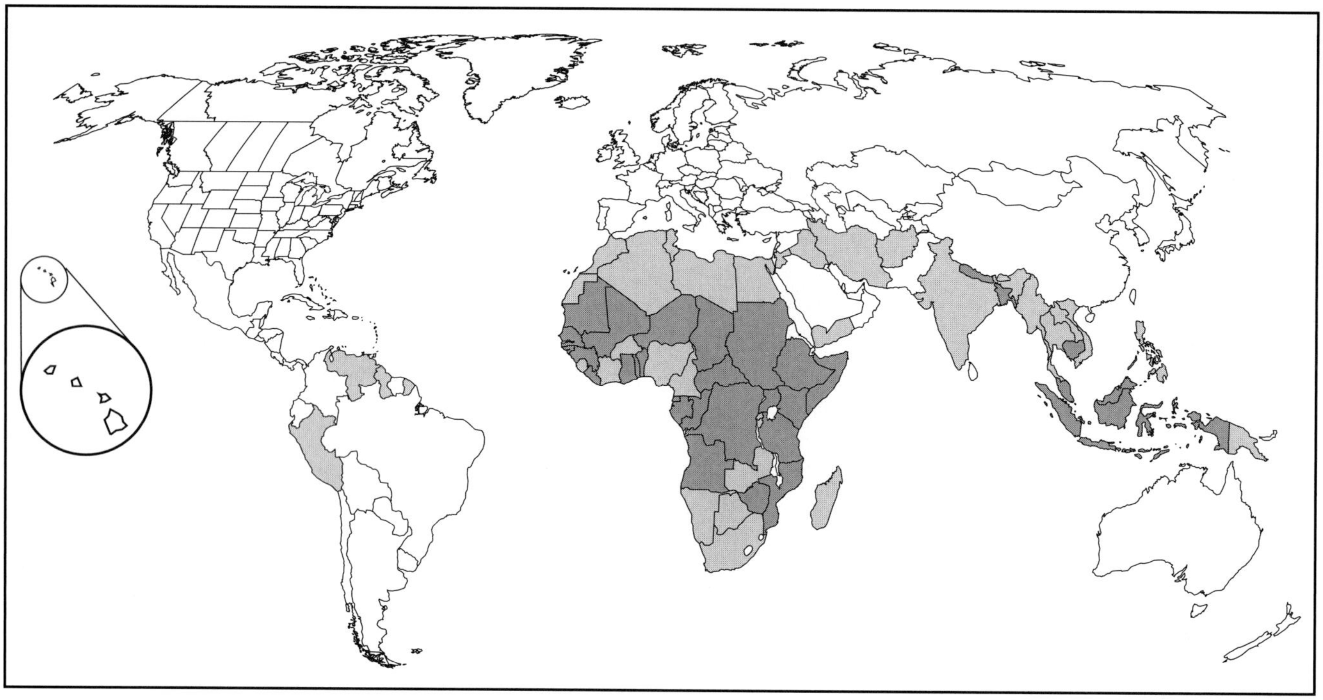

Estimated neonatal tetanus mortality rates, 1991 (per 1000 live births).

□ Fewer than 1

▨ 1–5

■ more than 5

accounts for approximately half of the total number of cases worldwide and has up to a 90% mortality rate.[4,5] Eighty percent of worldwide neonatal tetanus cases occur in Bangladesh, China, Ethiopia, India, Indonesia, Kenya, Nepal, Nigeria, Pakistan, Somalia, Sudan, Uganda, Vietnam, and Zaire.[26] There is an estimated total of 120,000 deaths annually in the African region due to neonatal tetanus, which accounts for 10% to 30% of infant deaths in many countries.[27] In 1994 an estimated 500,000 deaths from neonatal tetanus occurred worldwide, but since the 1980s it is estimated that the number of deaths from neonatal tetanus has been cut in half through vaccination before or during pregnancy and with clean delivery and cord care practices.[26] Vaccinating the mother at this stage gives her long-term protection but, also importantly, protects the newborn during the first few weeks of life. Figure 43-4 demonstrates a decrease in the number of all tetanus cases, but particularly neonatal tetanus, since 1990. The World Health Organization has established the goal of eliminating maternal and neonatal tetanus by 2005,[28] but reality in the forms of war and inadequate resources has delayed this achievement.

DISEASE

Tetanus is classified into four clinical subtypes: generalized, localized, cephalic, and neonatal. These four clinical subtypes represent the site of toxin action, either predominantly at the neuromuscular junction or at more central inhibitory systems. Incubation time (the time from spore inoculation to first symptoms) for all clinical types seems to vary depending on the ultimate severity of the disease, with more severe disease developing more quickly (8.3 ± 4.7 days) and mild disease taking longer (11 ± 6.7 days).[29] The length of the incubation period also varies with the distance of the inoculation site from the central nervous system (CNS), so that injuries to the lower extremities have longer incubation periods than those occurring at more proximal sites.

Generalized tetanus is the most commonly recognized form of the disease. Trismus, or lockjaw, is the most common presenting sign. It is caused by rigidity of the masseter muscles, which in turn prevents the opening of the mouth, and its severity can be gauged by measuring the distance between the upper and lower teeth with the mouth maximally opened. Trismus results in the classic and characteristic risus sardonicus (Fig. 43-5), a facial expression which consists of lateral extension of the corners of the mouth, raised eyelids, and wrinkling of the forehead. These facial features may at times be subtle and may require comparisons with old photographs or confirmation of a change by the patient's family or friends.

Involvement of other muscle groups can then follow the onset of trismus: first the neck, then the thorax and abdomen, and finally the extremities. Tetanic spasms or generalized spasms resemble opisthotonus, decerebrate posturing, or even seizures, and are elicited by both external (noises, drafts of air, touching the patient) or internal (full bladder, coughing) stimuli. The tetanic spasms last for a few seconds to minutes and occur at irregular intervals. These spasms are extremely painful, and full consciousness is retained; this helps differentiate them from seizures or decerebrate posturing. Tetanospasmin is epileptogenic in experimental models, but true epileptic seizures in tetanus are rare. Respiratory compromise is the

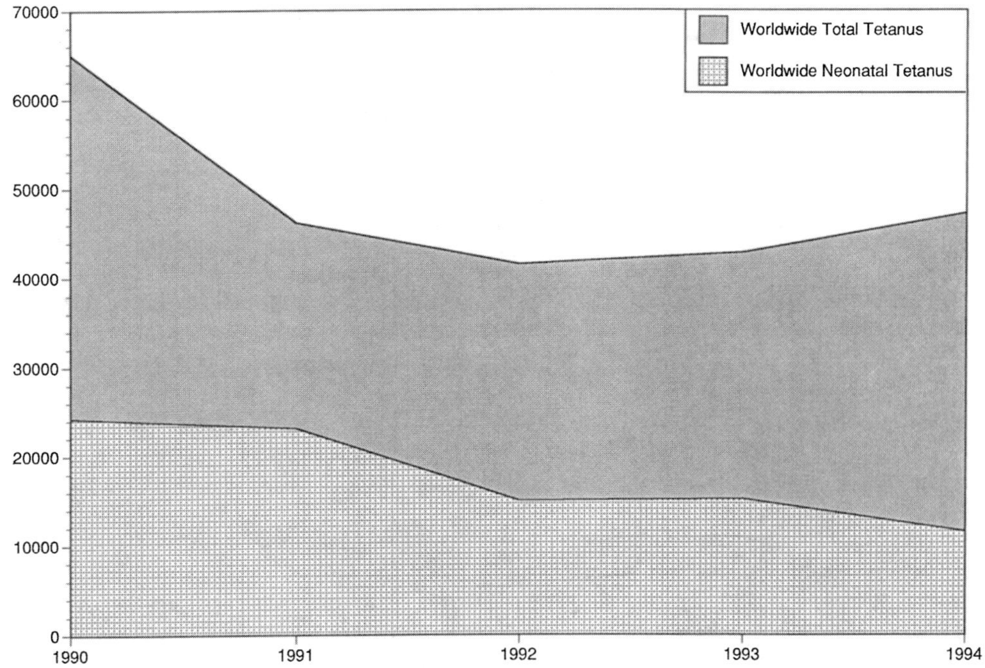

FIGURE 43-4 Total number of all tetanus cases and total neonatal tetanus cases reported worldwide from 1990 to 1994. The total number of cases is represented along the abscissa. Note the trend in the decreasing number of cases in this 5-year period, particularly in neonatal tetanus, likely due to increases in immunization worldwide. (Adapted from World Health Organization: Global programme on vaccines: Total tetanus incidence data. 1996. Available at: gopher://gopher.who.ch:70/11/.whosis/.gpvis/.incidence/.total-tetanus; and World Health Organization: Global programme on vaccines: Neonatal tetanus incidence data. 1996. Available at: gopher://gopher.who.ch:70/11/.whosis/.gpvis/.incidence/.neonatal-tetanus.)

most serious early problem in generalized tetanus. Spasm of the glottis may occur and results in death via asphyxiation. The diaphragm and abdominal musculature are also frequently affected and this can result in apnea. This effect may be either central or directly at the neuromuscular junction (NMJ),[30] causing paralysis of these muscles. Deep tendon reflexes are usually hyperactive. After several days of illness, autonomic dysfunction, usually a hypersympathetic state, is noted in patients with severe tetanus. Autonomic dysfunction is now the leading cause of death in tetanus patients.[31] It is characterized by labile hypertension and tachycardia, arrhythmias, peripheral vascular constriction, diaphoresis, pyrexia, increased carbon dioxide output, increased urinary catecholamine excretion, and sometimes hypotension. The disease may continue to progress for 10 to 14 days, reflecting the time it takes for the toxin to be transported to the CNS. Recovery then begins, usually taking about 4 weeks. Without antitoxin, the disease persists for as long as the toxin is produced. Because toxin is produced in insufficient quantities to stimulate an immune response, patients who survive tetanus have little in the way of natural immunity and recurrent tetanus is well documented.[32,33]

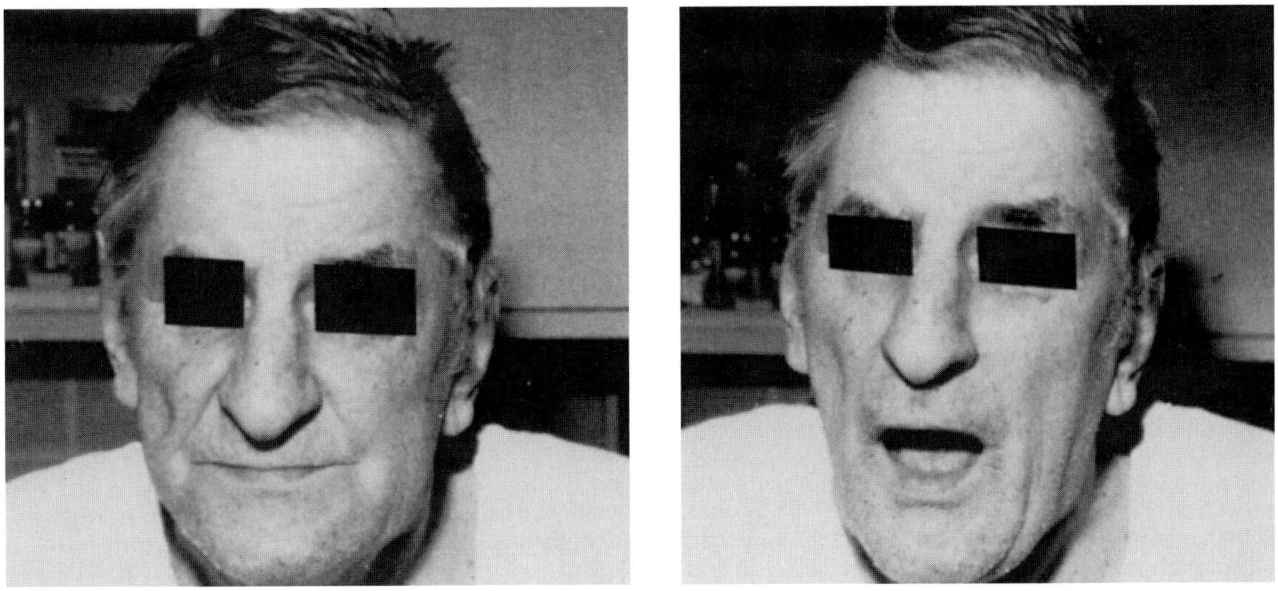

FIGURE 43-5 The photograph on the left demonstrates risus sardonicus. Note the straightened upper lip at rest. The photograph on the right demonstrates trismus. The patient was instructed to open his mouth as fully as possible. (From Bleck T, Brauner JS: Tetanus. In Scheld WM, Whitley RJ, Durack DT [eds]: Infections of the Central Nervous System, 2nd ed. New York, Raven Press, 1996.)

Localized tetanus is characterized by fixed rigidity of the muscles at or near the site of injury. This may be mild, may persist for months, and usually resolves spontaneously. The muscle may be painful, and deep tendon reflexes may be brisk. The toxin may affect the NMJ, causing weakness, as well as rigidity. Partial immunity to the toxin may be responsible for preventing further hematogenous spread and generalized tetanus,[34] but unless treated, localized tetanus frequently evolves to the generalized form.

Cephalic tetanus occurs with injuries to the head or at times is associated with *C. tetani* infections of the middle ear.[35] Patients have weakness of the facial musculature, and facial paresis is common.[36] Dysphagia[37] and extraocular muscle[38] involvement also have been reported. The incubation period is usually 1 to 2 days. This is an unusual form of tetanus, and it too can evolve to the generalized form if left untreated.

Neonatal tetanus is a generalized form of the disease and is far more common in developing countries than in the developed world. It is the leading cause of neonatal mortality in many parts of the world, and of the diseases that can be vaccinated against it is second only to measles as a cause of childhood death.[39] It usually follows an infection of the umbilical stump, often because of improper wound care. In addition, a lack of maternal immunity to tetanus, which, if present, would be passively transferred to the neonate, is necessary for the development of this disease. Four factors seem to play a role in developing neonatal tetanus: (1) the length of the stump (a shorter stump appears to increase the risk), (2) the care with which the cord is ligated, (3) the cleanliness of the instruments and dressings, and (4) the cleanliness of the environment.[40] The incubation period is from 1 to 10 days postpartum, and the mortality rate is up to 90%, with the largest numbers of deaths in the first week of the disease. The infants usually are weak, irritable, and unable to suck. Tetanic spasms occur later, and the opisthotonic posturing must be differentiated from neonatal seizures or other metabolic or congenital abnormalities that cause posturing in this age group. The hypersympathetic state described previously also is common and is frequently the cause of death. Developmental retardation is common in those who survive.[41]

PATHOGENESIS AND IMMUNITY

The spores of *C. tetani* germinate and the bacteria proliferate when the redox potential of the tissue is low. Once the bacteria are growing, two exotoxins are produced: tetanospasmin and tetanolysin. The clinical significance of tetanolysin is unclear. It may aid in the damage of viable tissue near the wound site, lowering the redox potential and allowing for continued growth of anaerobes, perhaps by disrupting membrane channels.[42,43] There also is evidence that tetanolysin can cause electrocardiographic abnormalities and disseminated intravascular coagulation when given systemically in experimental animals.[44]

Tetanospasmin, or "tetanus toxin," is believed to cause all the typical clinical manifestations of tetanus. It is synthesized as a single 151-kD (1315–amino acid) chain.[45–46] This molecule is then cleaved by a bacterial protease into a heavy chain and a light chain, connected by a disulfide bridge.[47] The disulfide bridge is necessary for the activity of the toxin.[48] The more commonly accepted fragments are those derived from papain treatment, which cleaves the heavy chain at lysine 865, about 50 kD from the C-terminal end.[49] This is termed the *C fragment*, whereas the light chain and the N-terminal end, still linked by the disulfide bridge, are variously called the *B fragment* or the *A-B fragment*. These chains are thought to affect different phases of toxin binding, cell entry, and toxicity. The DNA for this polypeptide resides on a single plasmid[50]; strains of *C. tetani* that do not have this plasmid have no toxigenic properties. Tetanospasmin inhibits neurotransmitter release at the presynaptic terminal,[51] and this accounts for the clinical presentation of tetanus. The toxin first binds to the presynaptic membrane and then must pass through it[52]; how this occurs is not entirely clear. Some studies suggest it does so through uncoated vesicles.[53,54] Other studies have demonstrated that it can produce pores in phospholipid and ganglioside vesicles,[55] suggesting perhaps another method of toxin entry. The toxin enters the cytoplasm via an acidic vacuole (similarly to diphtheria toxin). Other toxins, such as cholera, must enter via the Golgi apparatus before membrane translocation.[56] Once in the cytoplasm of the presynaptic terminal, tetanospasmin cleaves the protein (synaptobrevin) that "docks" the neurotransmitter-filled vesicle to the membrane, ultimately for fusion and then release.[57] Thus, because synaptobrevin is cleaved, the vesicle is unable to fuse with the membrane and the neurotransmitter cannot be released.

Tetanospasmin travels via retrograde transport back to the cell body and can then cross several orders of synaptically connected neurons. This process allows the toxin to move from the NMJ of alpha motor neurons to the spinal cord and ultimately to the brain, and helps explain its effects on the NMJ, autonomic function, and the CNS. The heavy chain of the toxin is necessary for the retrograde transport of the toxin to the cell body.[58] Tetanospasmin is also spread hematogenously but must still enter the CNS via neurons and retrograde transport. Any toxin that has not entered a neuron is potentially accessible to antitoxin antibody, but toxin that is intraneuronal or intraaxonal is not, and this helps explain the delay in improvement for several days after initiation of treatment.

Once transported to the spinal cord, tetanospasmin affects the inhibitory neurons. These neurons use either glycine or γ-aminobutyric acid (GABA) and normally inhibit the alpha motor neurons. Without this inhibition, the motor neuron increases its firing rate, ultimately causing rigidity of the muscle innervated by this neuron. More clinically relevant is the fact that without this inhibition, the normal relaxation of antagonist muscles is impaired, and the characteristic tetanic spasm occurs, in response to movement or stimulation. The toxin is transported into the brainstem,[59] but the clinical relevance of this is unclear.

Tetanospasmin disinhibits sympathetic reflexes at the spinal cord level, implying that hyperadrenergic findings do not depend on the hypothalamus or brain stem[60]; however, the development of the syndrome of inappropriate antidiuretic hormone (SIADH) secretion may support hypothalamic involvement.[61] Patients with tetanus occasionally develop bradycardia and hypotension,[62] as well as disruption of gastric motility,[63] indicating that parasympathetic function is also disrupted.

The effects of tetanospasmin at the NMJ have been established for more than 40 years.[64] More recent studies show a presynaptic defect in the release of acetylcholine (similar to botulism) demonstrated by single-fiber electromyography (EMG).[65]

NMJ recovery presumably depends on sprouting new synapses, but the original junctions eventually recover, after which the new ones are pruned. Although frequently overlooked, there may be significant weakness in tetanus, and the tetanospasmin effect on the NMJ is likely the reason.

DIAGNOSIS AND DIFFERENTIAL DIAGNOSIS

The diagnosis of tetanus is primarily clinical. A clinical picture of trismus, muscle rigidity, stimulus-induced tetany, and a history of a wound or injury within the last 3 weeks is highly suggestive of generalized tetanus. Likewise, a newborn with a poor suck and increased muscle rigidity and spasms, in the setting of poor umbilical hygiene and a mother with no immunization history, likely has neonatal tetanus. EMG may demonstrate findings consistent with increased excitability of the motor neurons as well as NMJ blockade, although this is not specific for tetanus. *C. tetani* is rarely cultured from the wound, and in any case a positive culture does not prove the presence of the disease. Blood and serum studies are usually normal or nonspecific, and cerebrospinal fluid (CSF) is usually normal. For the most part, laboratory studies help evaluate for other entities in the differential diagnosis.

Symptoms caused by strychnine, a direct antagonist at the glycine receptor, mimic tetanus. Abdominal muscle rigidity between spasms is more common in tetanus than strychnine toxicity, and trismus frequently occurs later with strychnine. A history of strychnine intoxication may be elicited, and the toxin may be found in the serum, urine, or gastric contents. Dystonic reactions to dopamine antagonists may be confused with tetanus; however, torticollis and oculogyric crisis can be seen in the former but never with tetanus. A brief trial of an anticholinergic agent, such as benztropine or diphenhydramine, which usually relieves dystonic reactions, can further differentiate dystonia from tetanus. Tetany produced by hypocalcemia or alkalosis is usually accompanied by Chvostek's sign (spasm of the facial muscles elicited by tapping on the facial nerve in the region of the parotid gland) and Trousseau's phenomenon (tapping the palm and eliciting palmar spasm). Tetany from these metabolic causes usually involves the extremities rather than the axial musculature, and trismus is much less common. Associated serologic studies confirm the diagnosis. Generalized seizures may be confused with tetanus, but the former, by definition, involves a loss of consciousness. Both, however, respond to benzodiazepines. Conversion reaction or "pseudotetanus" is a disorder in which the patient's movements resemble tetanus. Patients with psychiatric disease can at times be distracted, their movements or postures inconsistent, and there may be a history suggestive of secondary gain. Finally, while the nuchal rigidity of meningitis may resemble the neck stiffness of tetanus, the CSF in tetanus is invariably normal.

TREATMENT

A patient with generalized tetanus or neonatal tetanus requires the facilities and the expertise of an intensive care unit (ICU) to survive. A review of 335 consecutive tetanus patients revealed that survival drastically improved after the development of ICUs (44% mortality vs. 15%) and that the major improvement came from prevention of death due to respiratory failure.[66] The mainstays of treatment include (1) neutralizing existing toxin before it enters the nervous system, (2) inhibiting further production of tetanus toxin, (3) muscle relaxation and sedation, (4) management of autonomic instability, and (5) ventilatory, nutritional, and general ICU support. A time-based protocol that the authors have found effective in generalized tetanus is shown in Box 43-1.

Treatment of generalized tetanus should begin with administration of human tetanus immunoglobulin (HTIG). Blake and colleagues[67] demonstrated that a single dose of 500 IU is as effective as the standard dose of 3000 to 5000 IU. The smaller amount can be given as a single dose; this is important as each intramuscular (IM) injection is a potential stimulus for a tetanic spasm. Equine antitetanic serum may be more readily available, particularly in developing regions, but it has a much higher incidence of adverse reactions. It is dosed at 10,000 to 1 million units IM. Once the tetanus toxin has entered the motor neuron, it is no longer possible to neutralize it with the antibody. Intrathecal administration of HTIG is possible (although not approved by the U.S. Food and Drug Administration [FDA]) and some authors report that it may be advantageous[68]; however, other studies have failed to demonstrate a benefit.[69] Debriding the portal of entry does not change the course of the disease, although it may help prevent secondary infection. Antibiotic treatment should be initiated at the outset. In the only study comparing metronidazole and penicillin, the former was superior with significantly less progression of the disease, shorter hospitalization, and improved survival.[70] This may not represent a beneficial effect of metronidazole as much as a negative effect of penicillin, which is a GABA antagonist.[71] The dose of metronidazole is 500 mg intravenously (IV) every 6 hours for 7 to 10 days.

Muscle relaxation is best accomplished with benzodiazepines or baclofen. Diazepam, lorazepam, and midazolam are all effective. With all three agents, very large doses are required to control tetanic spasms; doses in excess of 500 mg/24 hr of diazepam, 200 mg/24 hr of lorazepam, and 0.1 to 0.3 mg/kg/hr of midazolam may be required. Intrathecal administration of baclofen also is effective.[72,73] If GABA receptor agonists, such as benzodiazepines or baclofen, are unsuccessful in controlling the muscle spasms, then neuromuscular blockade is necessary. Vecuronium (6 to 8 mg/hr) or pancuronium bromide as a bolus of 0.1 mg/kg, then infusion of 0.3 to 0.6 mg/kg/min, can be used. Vecuronium is preferred, since it is less likely to cause autonomic instability. A recent case report demonstrated the *in*effectiveness of rocuronium in controlling tetany and spasms.[74] Of course, when paralytic agents are used, the patient must be intubated and ventilated with positive pressure. More likely, the patient will need to be intubated on presentation; this is done so as to protect the airway, which may occlude during tetanic spasms. Control of autonomic instability can be achieved with a variety of agents. Intravenous labetalol, a combined α- and β-blocker, is the treatment of choice. Esmolol, clonidine, and morphine sulfate are also effective. Magnesium sulfate infusions can help with many aspects of the disease.[75] For bradycardia and hypotension, a temporary pacemaker may be necessary for the former, while fluid boluses and sympathomimetics (e.g., norepinephrine) may be required for the latter. The nutritional requirements of tetanus patients may be extraordinary, but once they are sedated and their spasms and autonomic activity suppressed, their nutritional requirements are similar to those of other critically

Box 43-1 Management Protocol for Generalized Tetanus

I. Diagnosis and stabilization: first hour after presentation
  A. Assess airway and ventilation. If necessary, prepare for endotracheal intubation and neuromuscular junction blockade (e.g., vecuronium 0.1 mg/kg).
  B. Obtain samples for antitoxin level, strychnine and dopamine antagonist assays, electrolytes, blood urea nitrogen, creatinine, creatine kinase, and urinary myoglobin determination. If meningitis is part of the patient's differential diagnosis, perform a lumbar puncture.
  C. Determine the portal of entry, incubation period, period of onset, and immunization history.
  D. Administer benztropine 1 to 2 mg intravenously (IV) or diphenhydramine 50 mg IV to aid in excluding a dystonic reaction (see text for caveat).
  E. Administer a benzodiazepine IV (diazepam in 5-mg increments, or lorazepam in 2-mg increments) to control spasms and decrease rigidity. Initially, employ a dose adequate to produce sedation and minimize reflex spasms. If this dose compromises the airway or ventilation, intubate using a short-acting neuromuscular blocking agent prior to transferring the patient to a quiet, darkened area of the intensive care unit.

II. Early management phase: first 24 hours
  A. Administer human tetanus immunoglobulin (HTIG), 500 units intramuscularly (IM).
  B. At a different site, administer IM an absorbed tetanus toxoid such as tetanus-diphtheria vaccine 0.5 mL or diphtheria-tetanus-pertussis vaccine 0.5 mL, as appropriate for age. Adsorbed tetanus toxoid without diphtheria toxoid is available for patients with a history of reaction to diphtheria toxoid; otherwise, the correct combination for the patient's age should be employed.
  C. If intrathecal administration of antitoxin is being considered, it should be administered at this point.
  D. Begin metronidazole 500 mg IV every 6 hours for 7 to 10 days.
  E. Perform a tracheostomy after placement of an endrotracheal tube and under neuromuscular junction blockade if spasms produce any degree of airway compromise, or if dysphagia or difficulty managing secretions occurs.
  F. Debride the wound if this is indicated for its own management (this has no apparent effect on the course of tetanus).
  G. Place a soft, small-bore nasal feeding tube or a central venous hyperalimentation catheter.
  H. Administer benzodiazepines as needed to control spasms and produce sedation. If adequate control is not achieved, institute long-term neuromuscular junction blockade (e.g., with a vecuronium infusion or intermittent pancuronium injections). Continue benzodiazepines for sedation with electroencephalographic monitoring to ensure somnolence.
  I. Initiate physical therapy for pulmonary toilet and passive range-of-motion exercises as soon as the patient has been stabilized pharmacologically. Additional sedation should be given before each treatment, and again during the treatment if the therapy provokes spasms.

III. Intermediate management phase: next 2 to 3 weeks
  A. Treat sympathetic hyperactivity with IV labetalol 0.25 to 1.0 mg/min or morphine 0.5 to 1.0 mg/kg/hour. Consider epidural blockade with local anesthetics. Avoid diuretics for blood pressure control, because volume depletion will worsen autonomic instability.
  B. If hypotension is present, place a pulmonary artery catheter and an arterial line, and administer fluids, dopamine, or norepinephrine.
  C. Sustained bradycardia usually requires a pacemaker. Atropine or isoproterenol may be useful during pacemaker placement. External pacing should be avoided unless the patient is under neuromuscular junction blockade.
  D. Begin prophylactic heparin to prevent pulmonary embolism.
  E. Use a flotation bed, if possible, to prevent skin breakdown and peroneal nerve palsies. Otherwise, ensure frequent turning and employ antirotation boots.
  F. Maintain benzodiazepines until neuromuscular junction blockade, if employed, is no longer necessary, and the severity of spasms has diminished substantially. Taper the dose over 14 to 21 days.
  G. Begin rehabilitation planning.

IV. Convalescent stage: 2 to 6 weeks
  A. When spasms are no longer present, begin physical therapy. Many patients require supportive psychotherapy.
  B. Before discharge, administer another dose of the appropriate tetanus toxoid combination.
  C. Schedule a third dose of toxoid to be given 4 weeks after the second.

Adapted from Bleck T, Brauner JS: Tetanus. In Scheld WM, Whitley RJ, Durack DT (eds): Infections of the Central Nervous System, 2nd ed. New York, Raven Press, 1996.

ill patients. Gastric emptying may be impaired, and therefore, central venous nutrition may be necessary.

There is no standard regimen for the treatment of neonatal tetanus; however, it is treated much like generalized tetanus. Tetanus antitoxin should be administered to neutralize the tetanospasmin that has not yet entered neurons. Human antitetanic immunoglobulin is preferred with a single dose of 3000 to 5000 units IM, but as noted previously a smaller dose may also be effective (although not specifically tested in children). Equine antitoxin is more widely used because of its availability, but serum sickness or allergic reactions are, of course, a significant concern. A single dose of 5000 units of equine antiserum is appropriate. A recent study in neonatal tetanus failed to show any advantage for intrathecal antitoxin.[70] Although debridement of the wound or infected umbilical stump may be surgically indicated, there is no evidence that debridement itself helps prevent progression of the disease. Eradication of the organism can be accomplished with penicillin 100,000 units/kg/day, although penicillin, being a GABA antagonist, can theoretically act synergistically with tetanospasmin and worsen spasms. Metronidazole may be a better choice. Sedation and muscle relaxation of the neonate can be accomplished with a variety of agents including, for acute control of spasms, paraldehyde 0.3 mL/kg IM or diazepam 1 to 2 mg/kg IM or IV; and for chronic sedation, phenobarbital 5 mg/kg every 6 hours, or diazepam 1 to 2 mg/kg every 6 hours. Chronic ICU support must also be maintained as described previously for generalized tetanus.

PREVENTION AND CONTROL

Active immunization with tetanus toxoid is one of the most effective preventive measures in medicine. Preventing one case of tetanus saves enough health-care expense to immunize several thousand people.[76] Active immunization with three IM injections of alum-adsorbed tetanus toxoid (10 lyophilized units, 0.5 mL) provides almost complete immunity for 5 years. Routine immunization in the infant begins at 6 weeks to 2 months of age with two other immunizations at 1- to 2-month intervals. A fourth vaccination should be given 1 year after the third, and a fifth at 4 to 6 years of age. Children under 7 years of age should receive the combined diphtheria-tetanus-pertussis (DTP) vaccine, while the tetanus-diphtheria (Td) vaccine is recommended for those older than seven. Several studies demonstrate that the pertussis component of the vaccine can be given in acellular rather than cellular form with fewer side effects and better efficacy in preventing pertussis.[77] This DTP vaccine has been approved by the FDA.[78] The complete series must be given to ensure adequate antibody titers. Routine boosters should be administered every 10 years.

In the developing world, neonatal tetanus remains a significant problem owing to large numbers of unimmunized women of childbearing age. Recently, a single dose of tetanus toxoid was administered to unimmunized pregnant women in their third trimester; both the mothers and their babies developed protective antibody titers.[79] Studies have also demonstrated that both human immunodeficiency virus–infected adults and infants have the ability to develop protective tetanus antibody titers.[80,81]

Immunization after an injury that might cause tetanus (contaminated wound, puncture, burn, frostbite, avulsion, and crush injury) should be performed if no tetanus booster has been given within the last 5 years. An injured patient should be boosted with the adsorbed Td vaccine if none has been administered within the last 10 years. If a prior immunization history is unavailable, then a series of three monthly Td injections should be performed. HTIG should also be administered (250 to 500 IU) to a patient with no clear previous vaccination history, particularly if the wound is likely to cause tetanus. Most authors agree that both HTIG and tetanus toxoid can be given simultaneously, as long as different sites are used. Tables 43-1 and 43-2 represent the current recommendations of the American College of Emergency Physicians for immunization after injury in children less than 7 years of age and older children and adults.[82]

On the horizon are other methods of immunization. Sustained-release tetanus toxoid may be available in the future, allowing for a vaccination schedule with fewer doses.[83] Oral immunization has been demonstrated in mice by genetically engineering a mutant live *Salmonella typhi* strain to carry a fragment of the tetanospasmin gene (fragment C),[84] and oral or nasal administration of liposome-incorporated tetanus toxoid may be possible.[85]

Table 43-1 Guide to Tetanus Prophylaxis in Wound Management in Children under 7 Years Old

Patient's History of Adsorbed Tetanus Toxoid	Clean Minor Wounds		All Other Wounds	
	DPT (or Td)	HTIG	DPT (or Td)	HTIG
Less than three doses or unknown	Yes*	No	Yes*	Yes
Three or more doses	No†	No	No‡	No

DPT, diphtheria-pertussis-tetanus vaccine; HTIG, human tetanus immunoglobulin; Td, tetanus-diphtheria vaccine.
*The primary immunization series should be completed.
†Yes, if the routine immunization schedule has lapsed (to make up for missed doses).
‡Yes, if the routine immunization schedule has lapsed, or if more than 5 years since the last dose of tetanus toxoid.
Adapted from Tetanus immunization for adults and children in the ED. Information paper. ACEP Online August 1996; available at: http//www.acep.org/policy/PM000604.htm.

Table 43-2 Guide to Tetanus Prophylaxis in Wound Management in Children Older Than 7 Years of Age and Adults

Patient's History of Adsorbed Tetanus Toxoid	Clean Minor Wounds		All Other Wounds	
	Td	HTIG	Td	HTIG
Less than three doses or unknown	Yes	No	Yes	Yes
Three or more doses	No*	No	No†	No

HTIG, human tetanus immunoglobulin; Td, tetanus-diphtheria toxoids adsorbed (for use in adults and children over 7 years of age).
*Yes, if more than 10 years since last dose.
†Yes, if more than 5 years since last dose.
Adapted from Tetanus immunization for adults and children in the ED. Information paper. ACEP Online August 1996; available at: http://www.acep.org/policy/PM000604.htm.

REFERENCES

1. Edsall G: Introduction. In Edsall G (ed): Proceedings of the Fourth International Conference on Tetanus Dakar, Senegal. Lyon, France, Fondation Merieux, 1975, pp 19–20.
2. Summary of notifiable disease, 1988. MMWR 38:39, 1989.
3. Tetanus—United States, 1982–1984. MMWR 34:601–611, 1985.
4. Schofield F: Selective primary health care: Strategies for control of disease in the developing world. 22. Tetanus: A preventable problem. Rev Infect Dis 8:144–156, 1986.
5. Cvjetanovic B, Grab B, Uemura K, et al: Epidemiological model of tetanus and its use in the planning of immunization programmes. Int J Epidemiol 1:125–137, 1972.

6. Bjerregaard P, Steinglass R, Mutie DM, et al: Neonatal tetanus mortality in coastal Kenya: A community survey. Int J Epidemiol 22:163–169, 1993.
7. Ghalioungui P: Magic and Medical Science in Ancient Egypt. London, Hodder & Stoughton, 1963.
8. Adams F: The Extant Works of Aretaeus, the Cappadocian. London, Sydenham Society, 1856.
9. Cullen W: First Lines of the Practice of Physic. Dublin, 1791. Cited in Mettler CA, Mettler FA: History of Medicine. Philadelphia, Blakiston, 1947, pp 157–175.
10. Gowers WR: A Manual of Diseases of the Nervous System. Philadelphia, Blackiston, 1888.
11. Nicolaier A: Üeber Infectiösen Tetanus. Dtsch Med Wochenschr 10:842–844, 1884.
12. Behring E, Kitasato S: Üeber das Zustandekommen der Diphtherie-Immunität und der Tetanus-Immunität bei Thieren. Dtsch Med Wochenschr 16:1113–1114, 1890.
13. de Ulloa A: Noticias Americanas: Entretenimientos Physicohistorios. Madrid, 1772. Cited in Mettler CA, Mettler FA: History of Medicine. Philadelphia, Blakiston, 1947, pp 745–746.
14. Clarke J: An account of a disease which until lately proven fatal to a great number of infants in the Lying-In Hospital of Dublin. Med Facts Observ 3:78–104, 1792. Cited in Mettler CA, Mettler FA: History of Medicine. Philadelphia, Blakiston, 1947, p 746.
15. Sims JM: Trismus nascentium: Its pathology and treatment. Am J Med Sci 11:363–379, 1846.
16. Beumer O: Zur aetologischen Bedeutung der Tetanus-Bacillen. Berl Klin Wochenschr 541–543, 575–577, 1887. Cited in Mettler CA, Mettler FA: History of Medicine. Philadelphia, Blakiston, 1947.
17. Cato EP, George WL, Finegold SM: Genus *Clostridium prazemozski* 1880, 23AL. In Smeath PHA, Mair NS, Sharpe ME, et al (eds): Bergey's Manual of Systematic Bacteriology, Vol 2. Baltimore, Williams & Wilkins, 1986, pp 1141–1200.
18. Hatheway CL: Bacterial sources of clostridial neurotoxins. In Simpson LL (ed): Botulinum neurotoxin and tetanus toxin. San Diego, Academic Press, 1989, pp 4–24.
19. Willis AT: Clostridium: The spore-bearing anaerobes. In Parker MT (ed): Topley and Wilson's Principles of Bacteriology, Virology and Immunity, Vol 2. Baltimore, Williams & Wilkins, 1983, pp 442–475.
20. Hoeniger JFM, Tauschel HD: Sequence of structural changes in cultures of *Clostridium tetani* grown on a solid medium. J Med Microbiol 7:425–432, 1974.
21. Bleck TP, Brauner JS: Tetanus. In Scheld WM, Whitley RJ, Marra CM (eds): Infections of the Central Nervous System, 3rd ed. New York, Lippincott Williams & Wilkins, 2004, pp 625–648.
22. Mugati GI, Dixon MS: Tetanus following human bite. Br J Plast Surg 45:614–615, 1992.
23. Tonge BL: Tetanus from chigger flea sores. J Trop Pediatr 35:94, 1989.
24. Sutter RW, Orenstein WA, Wassilak SG: Tetanus. In Hoeprich PD, Jordan MC, Ronald AR (eds): Infectious Diseases, 5th ed. Philadelphia, JB Lippincott, 1994, pp 1175–1185.
25. Adams EB: The prognosis and prevention of tetanus. S Afr Med J 42:739–743, 1968.
26. Available at http://www.who.int/vaccines/en/neotetanus.shtml. Accessed 1/30/05.
27. Health Communications and Public Relations: Childhood diseases in Africa: Neonatal tetanus. World Health Organization Fact Sheet No. 109. March 1996.
28. Available at http://www.who.int/vaccines-documents/DocsPDF02/www692.pdf. Accessed 1/30/05.
29. Brauner JS, Rios Vieira SR, Bleck TP: Changes in severe accidental tetanus mortality in ICU during two decades in Brazil. Intensive Care Med 28:930–935, 2002.
30. Veronesi R, Focaccia R: The clinical picture. In Veronesi R (ed): Tetanus: Important new concepts. Amsterdam, Excerpta Medica, 1981, pp 183–206.
31. Luisto M, Iivanainen M: Tetanus of immunized children. Dev Med Child Neurol 35:351–355, 1993.
32. Spenney JG, Lamb RN, Cobbs CG: Recurrent tetanus. South Med J 64:859, 1971.
33. Brust JCM, Richter RW: Tetanus in the inner city. NY State Med J 74:1735–1742, 1974.
34. Risk WS, Bosch EP, Kimura J, et al: Chronic tetanus: Clinical report and histochemistry of muscle. Muscle Nerve 4:363–366, 1981.
35. Patel JC, Kale PA, Mehta BC: Otogenic tetanus: Study of 922 cases. In Patel JC (ed): Proceedings of the First International Conference on Tetanus, Bombay, November 8–10, 1963. The Study Group of Tetanus, King Edward Memorial Hospital, 1965, pp 640–644.
36. Dastur FD, Shahani MT, Dastoor DH, et al: Cephalic tetanus: Demonstration of a dual lesion. J Neurol Neurosurg Psychiatry 40:782–786, 1977.
37. Lathrop DL, Griebel M, Horner J: Dysphagia in tetanus: Evaluation and outcome. Dysphagia 4:173–175, 1989.
38. Saltissi S, Hakin RN, Pearce J: Ophthalmoplegic tetanus. BMJ 1:437, 1976.
39. Progress toward the global elimination of neonatal tetanus 1989–1993. MMWR 43:885–887, 893–894, 1994.
40. Schofield FD, Tucker VM, Westbrook GR: Neonatal tetanus in New Guinea: Effect of active immunization in pregnancy. BMJ 2:785–789, 1961.
41. Anlar B, Yalaz K, Dizmen R: Long-term prognosis after neonatal tetanus. Dev Med Child Neurol 31:76–80, 1989.
42. Rottem S, Groover K, Habig WH, et al: Transmembrane diffusion channels in *Mycoplasma gallisepticum* induced by tetanolysin. Infect Immun 58:598–602, 1990.
43. Blumenthal R, Habig WH: Mechanisms of tetanolysin-induced membrane damage: Studies with black lipid membranes. J Bacteriol 157:321–323, 1984.
44. Hardegree MC, Palmer AE, Duffin N: Tetanolysin: In vivo effects in animals. J Infect Dis 123:51–60, 1971.
45. Craven CJ, Dawson DJ: The chain composition of tetanus toxin. Biochim Biophys Acta 317:277–285, 1973.
46. Matsuda M: The structure of tetanus toxin. In Simpson LL (ed): Botulinum Neurotoxin and Tetanus Toxin. San Diego, Academic Press, 1989, pp 69–92.
47. Bergey GK, Habig WH, Bennett JI, et al: Proteolytic cleavage of tetanus toxin increases activity. J Neurochem 53:155–161, 1989.
48. Krieglstein K, Henschen A, Weller U, et al: Arrangement of disulfide bridges and positions of sulfhydryl groups in tetanus toxin. Eur J Biochem 188:39–45, 1990.
49. Helting TB, Zwisler O: Structure of tetanus toxin. 1. Breakdown of the toxin molecule and discrimination between polypeptide fragments. J Biol Chem 12:1147–1153, 1977.
50. Fisel U, Jarausch W, Goretzki K, et al: Tetanus toxin: Primary structure, expression in *E. coli*, and homology with botulinum toxins. EMBO J 5:2495–2502, 1986.
51. Bleck TP: Pharmacology of tetanus. Clin Neuropharmacol 9:103–120, 1986.
52. Middlebrook JL: Cell surface receptors for protein toxins. In Simpson LL (ed): Botulinum Neurotoxin and Tetanus Toxin. San Diego, Academic Press, 1989, pp 95–119.
53. Schwab ME, Thoenen H: Selective binding, uptake, and retrograde transport of tetanus toxin by nerve terminals in the rat iris. J Cell Biol 77:1–13, 1978.
54. Montesano R, Roth J, Robert A, et al: Non-coated membrane invaginations are involved in binding and internalization of cholera and tetanus toxins. Nature 296:651–653, 1982.
55. Schmid MF, Robinson JP, DasGupta BR: Direct visualization of botulinum neurotoxin–induced channels in phospholipid vesicles. Nature 364:827–830, 1993.
56. Orlandi PA, Curran PK, Fishman PH: Brefeldin A blocks the response of cultured cells to cholera toxin. J Biol Chem 268:12010–12016, 1993.
57. Schiavo G, Benfenati F, Poulain B, et al: Tetanus and botulinum-B neurotoxins block neurotransmitter release by proteolytic cleavage of synaptobrevin. Nature 359:832–835, 1992.
58. Evinger C, Erichsen JT: Transsynaptic retrograde transport of fragment C of tetanus toxin demonstrated by immunohistochemical localization. Brain Res 380:383–388, 1986.
59. Dumas M, Schwab ME, Thoenen H: Retrograde axonal transport of specific macromolecules as a tool for characterizing nerve terminal membranes. J Neurobiol 10:179–197, 1979.
60. Parr GH, Wellhoner HH: The action of tetanus toxin in preganglionic sympathetic reflex discharges. Naunyn Schmiedebergs Arch Pharmacol 276:437–445, 1973.
61. Potgieter PD: Inappropriate ADH secretion in tetanus. Crit Care Med 11:417–418, 1983.
62. Ambache N, Lippold OCH: Bradycardia of central origin produced by injections of tetanus toxin into the vagus nerve. J Physiol (Lond) 108:186–196, 1949.

63. Habermann E: Tetanus. In Vinken PJ, Bruyn GW (eds): Handbook of Clinical Neurology, Vol 33. Amsterdam, North-Holland, 1978, pp 491–547.
64. Harvey AM: The peripheral action of tetanus toxin. J Physiol (Lond) 96:348–365, 1939.
65. Fernandez JM, Ferrandiz M, Larrea L, et al: Cephalic tetanus studied with single fibre EMG. J Neurol Neurosurg Psychiatry 46:862–866, 1983.
66. Trujillo MH, Castillo A, España J, et al: Impact of intensive care management on the prognosis of tetanus. Chest 92:63–65, 1987.
67. Blake PA, Feldman RA, Buchanan TM, et al: Serologic therapy of tetanus in the United States. JAMA 236:42–44, 1976.
68. Gupta PS, Kapoor R, Goyal S, et al: Intrathecal human tetanus immune globulin in early tetanus. Lancet 2:439–440, 1980.
69. Begue RE, Lindo-Soriano I: Failure of intrathecal antitoxin in the treatment of neonatal tetanus. J Infect Dis 164:619–620, 1991.
70. Ahmadsyah I, Salim A: Treatment of tetanus: An open study to compare the efficacy of procaine penicillin and metronidazole. BMJ 291:648–650, 1985.
71. Goonetilleke A, Harris JB: Clostridial neurotoxins. J Neurol Neurosurg Psychiatry 2004;75(Suppl 3):35–39.
72. Müller H, Börner U, Zierski J, et al: Intrathecal baclofen for treatment of tetanus-induced spasticity. Anesthesiology 66:76–79, 1987.
73. Saissy JM, Demazière J, Vitris M, et al: Treatment of severe tetanus by intrathecal injections of baclofen without artificial ventilation. Intensive Care Med 18:241–244, 1992.
74. Anandaciva S, Koay CW: Tetanus and rocuronium in the intensive care unit. Anaesthesia 51:505–506, 1996.
75. Attygalle D, Rodrigo N: New trends in the management of tetanus. Expert Rev Anti Infect Ther 2:73–84, 2004.
76. Bleck TP: Tetanus. Dis Mon 37:547–603, 1991.
77. Gustafsson L, Hallander HO, Olin P, et al: A controlled trial of a two component accellular, a five component acellular and a whole cell pertussis vaccine. N Engl J Med 334:349–355, 1996.
78. Food and Drug Administration approval of an acellular pertussis vaccine for the initial four doses of the diphtheria, tetanus, and pertussis vaccination series. MMWR 45:676–677, 1996.
79. Dastur FD, Awatramani VP, Chitre SK, et al: A single dose vaccine to prevent neonatal tetanus. J Assoc Physicians India 41:97–99, 1993.
80. Kurtzhals JAL, Kjeldsen K, Heron I, et al: Immunity against diphtheria and tetanus in human immunodeficiency virus–infected Danish men born 1950–1959. APMIS 100:803–808, 1992.
81. Barbi M, Biffi MR, Binda S, et al: Immunization in children with HIV seropositivity at birth: Antibody response to polio vaccine and tetanus toxoid. AIDS 6:1465–1469, 1992.
82. American College of Emergency Physicians: Tetanus Immunization for Adults and Children in the Emergency Department. 2000. Available at http://www.acep.org/library/pdf/tetanusipfinal.pdf. Accessed 1/30/05.
83. Chang AC, Gupta RK: Stabilization of the tetanus toxoid in poly (DL-lactic-co-glycolic acid) microspheres for controlled release of the antigen. J Pharm Sci 85:129–132, 1996.
84. Stevenson A, Roberts M: Intranasal immunisation against tetanus with an attenuated *Bordetella bronchiseptica* vector expressing FrgC: improved immunogenicity using a Bvg-regulated promoter to express FrgC. Vaccine 22:4300–4305, 2004.
85. Alpar HO, Bowen JC, Brown MRW: Effectiveness of liposomes as adjuvants of orally and nasally administered tetanus toxoid. Int J Pharm 88:335–344, 1992.

B. SPIROCHETAL INFECTIONS

44 Treponemal Infections

EDWARD W. HOOK, III

INTRODUCTION

Treponemal infections of humans have a worldwide distribution and include both venereal syphilis, caused by *Treponema pallidum* subsp. *pallidum* and the endemic treponematoses, which include yaws (*T. pallidum* subsp. *pertenue*), pinta (*Treponema carateum*), and endemic syphilis (*T. pallidum* subsp. *endemicum*). Although venereal syphilis is a worldwide problem associated with sexual transmission by persons with multiple sexual partners, endemic treponematoses are primarily childhood diseases that are most common in tropical regions and are usually spread from person to person by direct, nonsexual contact. Nonetheless, there are numerous important similarities in the causative agents, the natural history of infection, diagnostic tests, and therapy that translate into similar approaches to management. In this chapter, before discussing the individual diseases, we address the common microbiologic, clinical, and therapeutic elements of these infections.

AGENTS

The pathogenic treponemes are thin, motile, organisms that are approximately 0.15 μm in diameter and 6 to 50 μm in length. The treponemes pathogenic for humans (*T. pallidum* subsp. *pallidum*, *pertenue*, and *endemicum* and *T. carateum*) are indistinguishable from one another microscopically and serologically.[1,2] Pathogenic treponemes cannot be cultivated for prolonged periods in vitro, although *T. pallidum* has been successfully cultivated for periods of days. Unlike the *T. pallidum* subspecies, which can also be propagated in small animals such as rabbits and hamsters, *T. carateum* can only be grown in primates. Despite these similarities, studies utilizing polymerase chain reaction amplification and restriction endonuclease cleavage of the genetic sequences flanking the region coding for a 15-kDa lipoprotein have been used for the first time to successfully and reliably differentiate *T. pallidum* subsp. *pallidum* from *T. pallidum* subsp. *pertenue* and *endemicum* (the authors were unable to evaluate *T. carateum* because, inasmuch as it cannot be propagated in nonprimates, there are no examples of this organism in existing treponemal strain banks).[3] Using dark field microscopy for visualization, pathogenic treponemes typically have 6 to 14 regularly coiled spirals, and viable organisms move with a spinning, corkscrew motility, often flexing at the midpoint. The organism is tapered at either end and has an outer membrane that, unlike the typical protein-rich membranes of most bacteria, is largely made up of phospholipids with relatively few surface-exposed proteins.[4,5] Some investigators have suggested that the relatively protein-deficient surface structure of treponemes may be related to the tendency for these infections to progress despite their capacity to elicit high-titer, diagnostic antibody responses to what are most often non-surface-exposed internal antigens. Between the organisms' outer membrane and the cell wall are six axial fibrils (three at either end), which contribute to the typical motility of the organism.

EPIDEMIOLOGY

Syphilis and the endemic treponematoses originate following inoculation of pathogenic organisms at mucosal or cutaneous surfaces. Infection is facilitated by breaks (microscopic or otherwise) in epithelial surfaces. Infectivity of treponemal infections may vary somewhat according to the histopathologic location of the organisms within lesions.[6] In yaws, the treponemes are predominantly present in the epidermis, unlike syphilis, in which organisms tend to be deeper and are found in the dermis or at the dermal–epidermal junction. Subsequent to inoculation and following an incubation period that not uncommonly may be a matter of weeks, the organisms cause primary cutaneous lesions at the site of inoculation. Primary lesions are most often solitary, but the lesion serves as a focus for subsequent spread of the organism, both locally through scratching and systemically via hematogeneous routes to cause a more generalized rash and other lesions typical of the specific diseases. Following the early stages of clinical disease, which tend to be somewhat self-limited and resolve without treatment, infections enter latent stages. People with latent infections may experience periodic relapse for periods of as long as 5 years, at which time they are again infectious to others. During intervals when infected people are lesion-free, with the exception of congenital transmission of syphilis, they are not infectious to others. Untreated people with latent infections are also at risk of long-term sequelae of chronic infection. Unlike syphilis, central nervous system disease and perinatal transmission are believed to be rare, if not undescribed, in people with the endemic treponematoses. Because the treponemes are too thin to be readily visualized by light microscopy, diagnosis of infection may be made using dark-field microscopy of material from clinical lesions. Dark-field microscopy, however, is not readily available in the majority of settings where patients with syphilis or endemic treponematoses are encountered, and thus the diagnosis is often made on the basis of the clinical presentation or serologic diagnosis.

DIAGNOSIS

The diagnosis of treponemal infections is most often accomplished using serologic tests. No serologic assays have been created specifically for the diagnosis of endemic treponematoses.[1,2] However, since no currently available commercial tests can serologically distinguish between antibody responses to syphilis and the endemic treponematoses, tests designed for syphilis[7] diagnosis have been and continue to be routinely utilized for diagnosis of yaws, pinta, and endemic syphilis. Two basic types of serologic tests are utilized to detect antibodies to the treponemes that cause syphilis and endemic treponematoses[1,7,8]: nontreponemal tests, which detect antibodies reactive with cardiolipin (diphosphatidylglycerol), which is also a normal component of many tissues, and, for evaluation of sera from patients found to be positive in nontreponemal tests, a "confirmatory" serologic test using specific treponemal antigens. The two-stage testing procedure is recommended in most instances because of the tendency for a small proportion (1% to 3%) of many populations to have false-positive nontreponemal serologic tests for syphilis.

The two most widely used nontreponemal tests are the VDRL (Venereal Disease Research Laboratory) test and the rapid plasma reagin (RPR) test.[1,8] Each test is based on flocculation reactions occurring when antibodies to treponemes react with a cardiolipincholesterol–lecithin antigen. Whereas the VDRL test can only use sera for testing and is slightly cheaper to perform, the RPR assay, which can be performed using either serum or plasma, is somewhat easier to perform and read. Both tests are usually performed using doubling dilutions of sera, allowing quantification of results, which can then be utilized to evaluate changes in antibody titers over time in response to therapy. People with treponemal infections typically develop serologic test reactivity within a few days after the appearance of primary infectious lesions at the site of inoculation.[1] Antibody titers then rise rapidly in the early stages of disease, falling either in response to therapy or more slowly after the manifestations of early infection resolve and the infection enters the latent stage. Following successful therapy, in many but not all patients, antibody titers will decline to low levels or even become nonreactive when tested using nontreponemal serologic tests.

False-positive serologic test results for syphilis (and other pathogenic treponemal infections) occur in 1 to 3% of most populations.[1,8] Biologic false-positive (BFP) test results may be transient or chronic, most often result in relatively low-titer serologic assay results (reactive in dilutions of 1:4 or less), and are identified by the fact that sera from patients with BFP nontreponemal test results rarely react in the treponemal serologic tests used to confirm the presence of pathogenic treponemal infection. Transient BFP results may occur in people with viral infections, following vaccinations, may be due to drug or other allergic reactions, or may occur in pregnancy. An increased prevalence of chronic BFP syphilis test reactivity is seen in people with chronic infections (endocarditis, leprosy, tuberculosis, human immunodeficiency virus [HIV] infection, etc.), with chronic inflammatory disorders (lupus erythematosus, rheumatoid arthritis, and antiphospholipid antibody syndrome), in parenteral drug users, and so on. Malarial infections are often cited as a cause of BFP syphilis tests in the tropics. BFP treponemal antibody test results may also be seen in people who do not have any of the processes sometimes associated with increased test reactivity. BFP serologic tests for syphilis are usually reactive at low (1:4 dilution or less) titers, although a small proportion of people with BFP have higher titers. In many developing nations, where BFP may be common, endemic treponematoses are present, syphilis as well as other genital ulcer diseases (chancroid and genital herpes) are present, and it may be difficult to obtain treponemal test results, clinicians use titers above 1:8 to define "active syphilis" to guide therapeutic decision making. Although this approach probably has numerous exceptions, it is a useful generalization for resource-limited settings.

As mentioned previously, reactivity in treponemal serologic assays designed for syphilis diagnosis is utilized to distinguish people with treponemal infections from those with BFPs. Prototypal treponemal assays include the fluorescent treponemal antibody absorption (FTA-ABS) and microhemagglutination assay–*Treponema pallidum* (MHA-TP) assays, which, like all treponemal tests, are based on the reactivity of antitreponemal antibodies from people with syphilis or endemic treponematoses with prepared antigens from *T. pallidum*. In the FTA-ABS test, the antigens of rabbit-propagated *T. pallidum* are detected using indirect immunofluorescence microscopy, whereas in the MHA-TP, prepared *T. pallidum* antigens are bound to turkey red blood cells and used to detect antitreponemal antibodies in a hemagglutination assay. Although the MHA-TP test may be used quantitatively, in most instances treponemal serologic tests are used only as confirmatory tests to help distinguish people infected with one of the pathogenic treponemes from those with BFPs. Although less thoroughly studied than nontreponemal tests, false-positive assays do occur with treponemal tests as well. Thus, there is little benefit to the use of these more complex, more expensive tests for screening purposes. In addition, although in some patients with syphilis (and, by extension, the endemic treponematoses) treponemal test reactivity may return to a nonreactive state following therapy, in the majority of patients it does not. These tests are not routinely recommended to follow the response to therapy.

TREATMENT AND PROGNOSIS

All treponemal infections appear to continue to be uniquely sensitive to relatively low doses of penicillin G.[1,8,9] The susceptibility of *T. pallidum* to the activity of long-acting benzathine penicillin, combined with the relatively long incubation period during which recently infected people are not infectious to others and the fact that these organisms only infect humans, makes pathogenic treponemal infections theoretically eradicable. For early infections, the recommended therapy usually consists of benzathine penicillin G, which provides low levels of penicillinemia for 2 or 3 weeks following a single injection. Using such therapy, cure rates for patients with early, active infections are 95% to 97%. In adults, the recommended therapy for syphilis is 2.4 million units of benzathine penicillin G given intramuscularly, whereas for endemic treponematoses 1.2 million units is recommended.[7,9] Although many other antimicrobial agents, including other penicillins, cephalosporins, tetracyclines, and macrolide antibiotics, are also active against *T. pallidum* subsp. *pallidum* (and probably other pathogenic treponemes as well), the low cost and efficacy of single-dose therapy have made benzathine penicillin G the therapeutic agent of choice worldwide. Quinolone antibiotics, aminoglycosides, and sulfa drugs are not effective for treponemal infections. In some instances, it is possible that intercurrent therapy for other infections may also be beneficial for unappreciated treponemal infections, modifying the natural history of infection and reducing or eliminating infectivity.

Capitalizing on the ready availability of a diagnostic serologic test and the high efficacy of therapy using long-acting penicillins in the late 1940s and early 1950s, the World Health Organization outlined a strategy for eradication of endemic treponematoses using mass treatment with long-acting penicillin for large numbers of people or even entire populations.[7,10,11] In this plan, based on the results of serologic surveys that provided reliable estimates of the seroprevalence of infection, for populations with a prevalence of active yaws in excess of 10%, treatment of entire populations was recommended, whereas for populations with medium (5% to 10%) prevalence, treatment was to be administered to all children younger than 15 years of age and all contacts of infectious cases.[7] For populations with a lower (less than 5%) prevalence, rather than mass treatment, aggressive therapy of active cases and all household and other contacts was recommended. Other critical components of proposed programs for eradication of endemic treponematoses included careful follow-up to detect the anticipated small numbers of treatment failures, aggressive retreatment of those treatment failures and their contacts, and follow-up surveillance to prevent resurgence of disease. The yaws eradication campaigns resulted in a dramatic reduction in the prevalence of these infections. However, possibly as a result of the failure of intensive follow-up and the persistence of small foci of infection, since the late 1980s yaws has again become more common in Africa, areas of the South Pacific, and Southeast Asia.

CLINICAL PRESENTATION

The endemic treponematoses (and syphilis) cannot be distinguished from each other microbiologically or serologically. For people with early disease in endemic areas the clinical features and epidemiologic settings in which patients are encountered usually permit accurate presumptive diagnosis. In contrast, it may be quite difficult to accurately distinguish sporadically occurring treponemal infections from one another or to ascertain which infection has caused reactive treponemal serologic test results in a patient with latent or previously treated disease. The following sections describe the typical presentations and course of human treponemal infections.

Yaws

Yaws is a disease of children (peak incidence at age 2 to 10 years) that is most common in warm, humid regions, including South and Central America, the Caribbean, equatorial Africa, and the equatorial islands of Southeast Asia.[7,10,11] The prevalence and incidence of yaws declined markedly during the yaws eradication campaigns of the 1950s, but in recent years the disease has again become more common. The infection is spread mainly by direct exposure to infectious lesions containing treponemes, possibly facilitated when compared with secondary

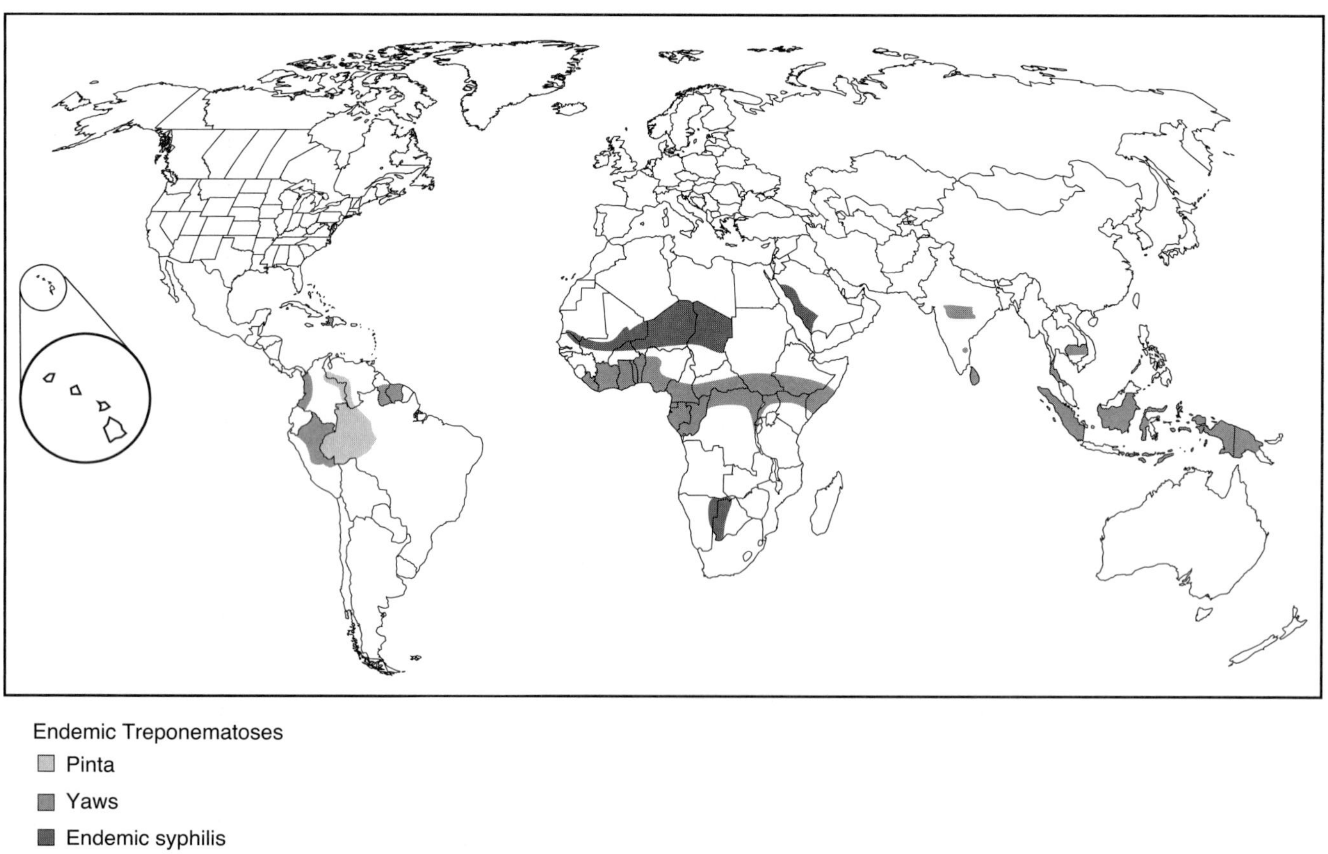

syphilis by the epidermal location of organisms within cutaneous lesions.[6] The transmission of yaws is said to be enhanced by the presence of lesions (scrapes, abrasions, etc.), which may increase the infectiousness of inoculated treponemes, as well as social conditions that may increase the likelihood of direct contact between infected and uninfected people, such as crowding and deficiencies in community sanitation (e.g., lack of water for bathing and washing clothes).

The clinical manifestations of yaws vary over the course of the infection. An initial (primary) lesion appears at the site of inoculation after an incubation period of approximately 3 weeks (range, 9 to 90 days). The primary lesion is initially papular and typically enlarges to become a papilloma several centimeters in diameter (Fig. 44-1 and Plate 44-1). The primary papilloma (also referred to as a frambesioma or mother yaw) is a highly infectious lesion that may reveal numerous spirochetes upon examination of lesion exudate by dark-field microscopy and may persist untreated for as long as 3 to 6 months, after which time it resolves spontaneously. Prior to actual development of the primary papule, and while it is present in the primary stage, *T. pallidum* subsp. *pertenue* disseminates hematogenously, lymphatogenously, and through autoinoculation to give rise to secondary yaws. Local spread is facilitated by the pruritic nature of cutaneous lesions. Unlike syphilis, dissemination of *T. pallidum* subsp. *pertenue* is not known to cause neurologic disease or to be passed transplacentally to cause congenital infection.

The presentations of secondary yaws are quite varied and include a spectrum of cutaneous lesions as well as involvement of lymph nodes, bone (periostitis), and cartilage. Most cutaneous lesions are infectious to others and may appear anywhere on the body, presenting as macules, papules, nodules, or hyperkeratotic lesions, any of which may ulcerate. Unless suprainfection occurs, cutaneous lesions tend to heal (either spontaneously after periods of as long as 6 months or following therapy) without scarring. Interestingly, climate may influence the number and morphology of yaws lesions. Lesions tend to be fewer in number and are more likely to be macular during arid periods (or in arid regions) when papillomas are found mainly in moist parts of the body, such as the axillae, skin folds, and mucosal surfaces.

In patients with secondary yaws, nonsuppurative lymphadenitis presenting as swelling and tenderness of nodes draining cutaneous lesions is not uncommon. Periosteal and

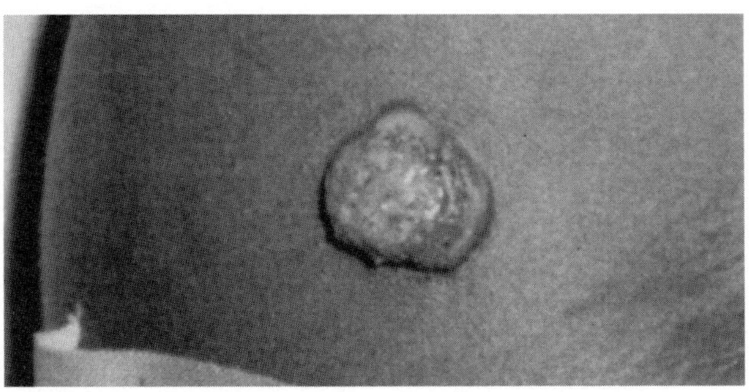

FIGURE 44-1 Initial, solitary yaws papilloma (frambesioma) on the upper thigh. (From Perine PL, Hopkins DR, Niemel PLA, et al: Handbook of Endemic Treponematoses: Yaws, Endemic Syphilis, and Pinta. Geneva, World Health Organization, 1984.)

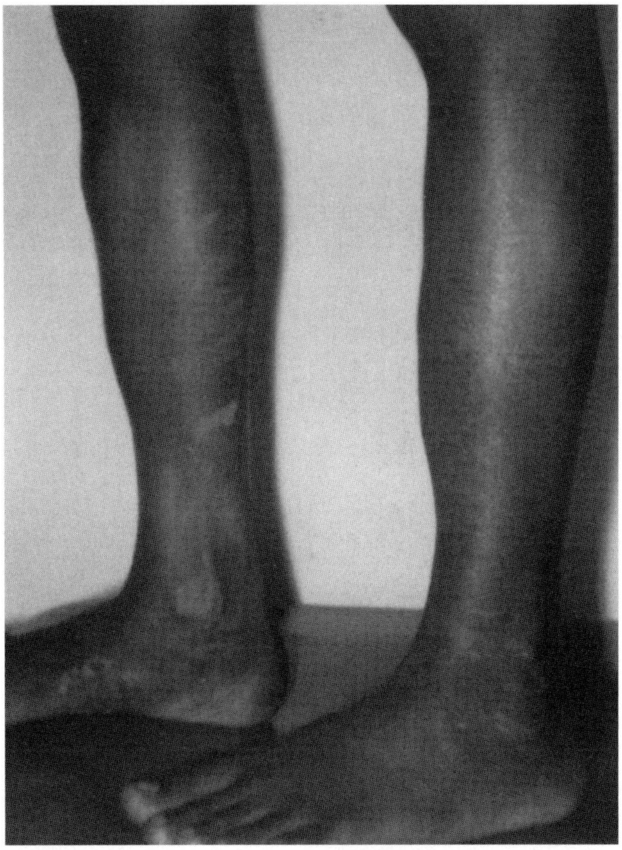

FIGURE 44-2 Bony deformity of the tibiae due to yaws osteoperiostitis. (From Perine PL, Hopkins DR, Niemol PLA, et al: Handbook of Endemic Treponematoses: Yaws, Endemic Syphilis, and Pinta. Geneva, World Health Organization, 1984.)

cartilaginous involvement may lead to pain, swelling, and local tenderness in patients with secondary yaws. Also characteristic of secondary yaws is the time course of untreated infection in which lesions resolve and then recur after a latent period when no lesions are present, most often in warm, moist body areas (the axillae, anus, and around the mouth). After 5 years, secondary recurrences are rarely seen, if at all. Over the natural history of untreated disease, the total duration of infectiousness to others is estimated to be 12 to 18 months.

Similar to syphilis, approximately 10% of patients with yaws may develop lesions of late infection that, although not infectious to others, may be disfiguring. Chronic periosteal involvement and resultant scarring may lead to disfiguring lesions, including the so-called saber shins, a bony deformity of the tibiae (Fig. 44-2). In addition, nodular lesions of late yaws may destroy cartilaginous structures such as the nose, an irreversible process known as gangosa.

Endemic Syphilis

Like yaws, endemic syphilis, previously also referred to as *bejel* (Arabic), is a readily transmissible disease of children.[7] Although previously widespread among nomadic and seminomadic populations of North Africa, southwest Asia, and the eastern Mediterranean basin, endemic syphilis is now most common among nomads living in the Arabian peninsula and along the southern border of the African Sahara desert. As might be inferred by its distribution, unlike yaws, which is more common in humid regions, endemic syphilis is more common in dry, arid regions.

Endemic syphilis is highly transmissible by contact with inanimate objects, such as shared drinking vessels, as well as by direct lesion contact contributing to spread.[7] Endemic syphilis is most common among children aged 2 to 15 years, who participate in the spread of infection to family members and others as well as provide a reservoir of infection.

Although often not clinically apparent, the primary lesions of endemic syphilis are nonetheless an important source of infection to others. The initial lesions, resulting from either direct or indirect inoculation, are painless mucous patches occurring on oral mucosal surfaces. The mucous patches of endemic syphilis are pale or white shallow ulcerations that may occur anywhere within the mouth. These lesions in turn may give rise to secondary lesions that may present as angular stomatitis (split papules) or more widely disseminated papular cutaneous lesions similar to those seen in yaws. Also similar to yaws, patients with endemic syphilis may experience a wide variety of secondary cutaneous lesions (papillomas, macules, and rashes of all types and locations) as well as periostitis, which may cause permanent bony deformity. Patients with late stages of endemic syphilis may also experience destruction of nasopharyngeal cartilage, causing gangosa.

Pinta

Of all the human treponematoses, the least is known about pinta and its causative agent.[7] Pinta was only recognized as a treponemal disease in 1938 after demonstration of spirochetes in a lesion exudate from a patient with pinta. Unlike other *T. pallidum* subspecies, *T. pallidum* subsp. *carateum* causes infection only in man and higher primates and cannot be propagated in smaller, relatively inexpensive laboratory animals such as rabbits. As a result, there are no examples of the organism in treponemal strain banks for study.

The distribution of pinta is limited to the New World, having been described in semiarid regions of the Caribbean and South and Central America. Further distinguishing it from other endemic treponematoses, pinta is most common in young adults (peak incidence, age 15 to 30 years) and has a long duration of skin lesions and chronic cutaneous changes that result from untreated infection.

The primary lesion of pinta, most commonly occurring on exposed surfaces such as the legs, foot, forearm, or back of the hand, begins as a papule that gradually enlarges through local extension. These lesions may become hyperkeratotic and, over a period of 3 to 9 months, may change from a copper to a slate-blue color. Regional lymphadenopathy may be seen in patients with pinta. The later stage of pinta is also characterized by its cutaneous manifestations, which may be hyper- or hypopigmented. Unlike other treponematoses, the findings of late pinta are limited to the skin. Deep tissue or organ involvement has not been described.

Syphilis

Syphilis and its causative agent, *T. pallidum* subsp. *pallidum*, are the best studied of all pathogenic human treponemal diseases. The disease has been recognized by clinicians and medical scientists for approximately 500 years, and currently utilized diagnostic tests for human treponemal infections (dark-field microscopy and both treponemal and nontreponemal serologic testing) were developed to assist in the diagnosis and management of this disease and are applicable to diagnosis and management of endemic treponematoses on the basis of cross-reactivity with other *T. pallidum* subspecies. Similarly, most current treatments of nonsyphilitic treponemal infections are based on extrapolation of data from studies of syphilitic patients. Thus, despite the fact that syphilis is transmitted from sexual contact and follows a somewhat different natural history (particularly in its later stages), this infection provides the basis for most current understanding of all pathogenic treponemal infections in humans.

Syphilis has a worldwide distribution, but there is substantial regional variation in its prevalence.[8] Infection tends to be more common in developing countries, and among developed countries the prevalence of syphilis in the United States is 5 to 10 times higher than in any other nation. The infection is primarily transmitted through direct contact with infectious lesions, although parenteral transmission through needle sharing in the context of drug use and transmission through transfusion of unscreened whole blood account for a small number of cases.

The peak incidence of syphilis occurs among sexually active people aged 18 to 40 years, particularly in the context of having multiple sexual partners. Unlike the endemic treponematoses, syphilis may be transmitted to children born to infected mothers, giving rise to congenital infection as well.

The primary lesion of syphilis or the chancre typically occurs at sites of sexual exposure after an incubation period of approximately 3 weeks.[8] Although genital locations are most common, chancres are occasionally seen at other sites of inoculation, including the anus, cutaneous surfaces, and the oral cavity. A classic syphilitic chancre typically begins as a papule that quickly ulcerates to form a solitary, painless, clean-based ulcer approximately 8 to 15 mm in diameter. Untreated, such lesions may persist for 3 to 6 weeks prior to resolving without scarring. Soon after or at approximately the time when primary lesions resolve, the secondary manifestations of infection occur (primary lesions may persist in 10% to 15% of patients with secondary manifestations). Secondary lesions are highly varied in appearance and location. Cutaneous manifestations are most common. The so-called classic rash of secondary syphilis is composed of palmar or plantar, or palmar and plantar macular, lesions that may be 0.5 to 2.0 cm in diameter and are painless. The spectrum of cutaneous manifestations of secondary syphilis, however, is vast, giving rise to reference to this infection as the "great imitator." Secondary syphilitic skin rashes may be generalized or focal; macular, papular, pustular, or a combination thereof; and resemble a wide variety of other cutaneous dermatoses. In addition to skin rashes, patients with secondary syphilis may develop highly infectious, heaped-up, papillomatous masses referred to as condylomata lata, mucous patches, and systemic lymphadenopathy. Although fever and other severe systemic manifestations are not common in patients with secondary syphilis, the disease is systemic and it is not unusual for patients to complain of generalized malaise. A small proportion of secondary syphilis patients may develop

of the pathogen by the *Ixodes* spp. ticks is rare or nonexistent. Ticks usually acquire the infection when they feed as larvae or nymphs on small mammals or birds. After the molt, the nymphs or adults feed on other mammals and birds, thus perpetuating the *Borrelia* spp. in nature. The usual hosts for the adult ticks are large mammals, such as deer. Humans most commonly become infected through the bite of nymphs, which are small enough to go unnoticed. Unlike argasid ticks, which feed for only short periods of time and transmit the spirochetes from the start of feeding, ixodid ticks feed for several days before dropping off. *Borrelia burgdorferi* and other Lyme borreliosis species must migrate from the midgut to the salivary glands over 1 or 2 days before they begin to enter the host.

Lyme borreliosis is the most common vector-borne disease in the United States, primarily in the northeastern and north central regions, and throughout much of Europe.[2,26] The risk of infection is highly focal, though, and it depends on the characteristics of the environment and the degree of exposure to infected nymphs. A canopied forest with an undergrowth of grass and low shrubs is a typical landscape. Humans come in contact with ticks through recreational and work activities in these environments and also around their homes, which may abut forests and wood stands. Unlike some *Ornithodoros* species, the *Ixodes* ticks that transmit Lyme borreliosis do not reside in dwellings.

DISEASE

The clinical hallmark of relapsing fever is the sudden onset of two or more episodes of fever spaced by afebrile periods of greater well-being (Table 45-4).[24,27–29] The temperature may reach 43°C and is usually above 39°C. In the louse-borne form, the first episode of unremittent fever lasts 3 to 6 days and is typically followed by a single milder episode. During tick-borne relapsing fever, there are multiple febrile periods of 1 to 3 days each, as observed in the temperature pattern of two cases (Fig. 45-2). In both forms of relapsing fever, the intervals between fevers are generally from 4 to 14 days. The first fever episode ends by crisis, which is characterized by rigors, hyperpyrexia, and elevations of pulse and blood pressure over approximately 15 to 30 minutes. This phase is followed by a few to several hours of profuse diaphoresis, falling temperature, and hypotension. Deaths from untreated

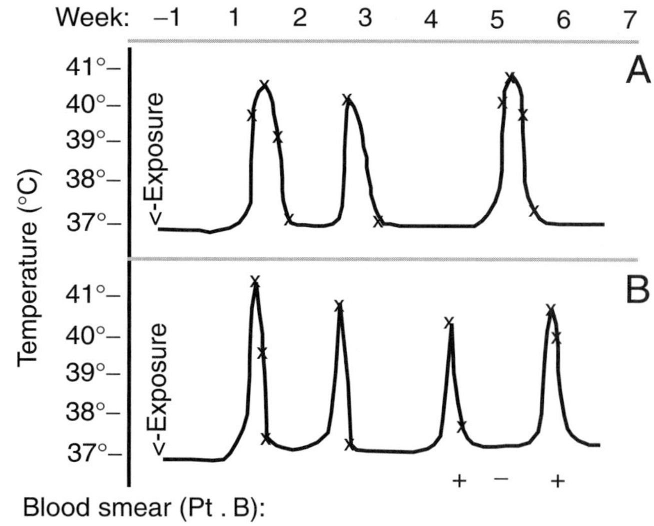

FIGURE 45-2 *A* and *B,* Temperature curves in two cases of tick-borne relapsing fever. The exposure to ticks occurred 1 week before onset of first fever. The *X*s on the curves indicate when temperatures were taken. Wright-stained blood smears of the patient in (*B*) were examined and were assessed as positive (+) or negative (–) with respect to the presence of spirochetes (see Fig. 45-4).

relapsing fever are most common during the crisis and its immediate aftermath.

Accompanying the first and subsequent fevers are headache, neck stiffness, arthralgia, myalgia, and nausea. The person with relapsing fever may complain of dizziness and have an unsteady gait. On examination, the patient may be delirious or apathetic. Sometimes, the initial presentation is stupor or coma. A nonproductive cough is common during louse-borne relapsing fever and may, in combination with high fever and myalgias, suggest influenza.

Most patients with relapsing fever have splenomegaly, which may present as abdominal or left shoulder pain. A frequent feature in early descriptions of relapsing fever was jaundice. More than half of patients with louse-borne relapsing fever and approximately 10% of patients with tick-borne relapsing fever have enlarged livers and clinical or laboratory evidence of hepatitis. There are elevated levels of hepatic transaminases and unconjugated bilirubin and also moderately prolonged prothrombin and partial thromboplastin times.

Table 45-4 Clinical and Laboratory Features of Tick-Borne RF, Louse-Borne RF, and Lyme Borreliosis

Characteristic	Tick-Borne RF	Louse-Borne RF	Lyme Borreliosis
Fever ≥39°C	Common	Common	Rare
Duration without treatment	Days–weeks	Days	Weeks–years
Fever relapses	Multiple	Few	None
Local skin rash	No	No	Common
Neurologic involvement	Common	Rare	Common
Joint involvement	No	No	Common
Spirochetes on blood smear	Yes	Yes	No
Antibiotic therapy	Several doses	Single or few doses	Several doses
Jarisch–Herxheimer reaction	Moderate	Moderate–severe	Mild

RF, relapsing fever.

Cholestasis is not prominent. If the albumin concentration is low, it is more likely the consequence of preexisting malnutrition or ongoing leakage of fluids into tissues than the hepatic dysfunction.

In louse-borne relapsing fever, epistaxis and skin petechiae and ecchymoses are common. They probably are attributable to thrombocytopenia, impaired production of clotting factors by the liver, and/or blockage of small vessels by aggregates of spirochetes. Epistaxis and petechiae are less common in tick-borne relapsing fever than in louse-borne relapsing fever. Platelet counts may fall below 50,000/μL. Leukocyte counts are usually in the normal range or only slightly elevated; there may be leukopenia during the crisis. A mild-to-moderate normocytic anemia is common.

Although louse-borne relapsing fever patients often present with delirium, apathy, or stiff neck, these are more likely the effect of the bacteremia than specific invasion of the central nervous system.[30] Direct neurologic involvement is more common in tick-borne relapsing fever. Meningitis and meningoencephalitis are serious consequences of this invasion. There may be residual hemiplegia or aphasia. Cranial neuritis, most commonly of the seventh or eighth cranial nerves, typically first appears during the second or third febrile period of tick-borne relapsing fever. The presentation is unilateral or bilateral Bell's palsy or deafness. Other neurologic manifestations during tick-borne relapsing fever are radiculopathy and myelitis. Unilateral or bilateral iridocyclitis or panophthalmitis may leave the patient with permanent visual impairment.

Myocarditis appears to be common in louse-borne and tick-borne relapsing fever and may be the proximate cause of death in many cases.[31,32] The most common evidence of myocarditis is gallops on cardiac auscultation and a prolonged QTc interval by electrocardiogram. Some patients have cardiomegaly and pulmonary edema on chest radiographs.

Relapsing fever during pregnancy frequently leads to abortion or stillbirth. There may be transplacental transmission of the infection, or a newborn may be infected at birth.[33,34] Congenital malformations as a consequence of relapsing fever have not been reported.

During early infection with *B. burgdorferi*, *B. afzelii*, or *B. garinii*, the frequent skin manifestation is erythema migrans, a erythematous patch or target-like skin lesion at the site of the tick bite.[35] During dissemination of the infection, erythema migrans lesions may appear in numerous locations. Temperatures of 39°C or higher are uncommon during Lyme borreliosis. The greatest morbidity with Lyme borreliosis occurs in patients with late or chronic infections (i.e., those lasting several weeks to years).[2] In these patients, there is chronic oligoarthritis, debilitating dysfunction of the central and/or peripheral nervous system, or a persistent inflammatory skin disorder.

In fatal cases of relapsing fever, the usual gross findings are widespread petechiae, enlarged spleen and liver, and an edematous, congested brain.[24,27,30] The most common general findings on histologic examination of autopsy cases are swelling of endothelial cells, microvascular leakage, perivascular mononuclear cell infiltrates, microabscesses, and hemorrhages. Fatal cases of louse-borne relapsing fever frequently have myocarditis with histiocytic infiltrates and microhemorrhages. The spleen and liver, but not the kidneys or adrenals, often have focal areas of necrosis. Although bleeding is a common complication of louse-borne relapsing fever, evidence of intravascular coagulation is not prominent.

The spirochetes can be detected in tissue sections with Warthin–Starry or modified Dieterle silver stains or by immunofluorescence.[36] Borrelias are primarily extracellular organisms. They move through or between endothelial cells as they leave the blood for tissues, but they do not appear to proliferate in these or phagocytic cells. The spirochetes are usually found in perivascular locations, sometimes as tangles of bacteria. In autopsy cases and experimentally infected animals, spirochetes are commonly found in the spleen, liver, brain, eye, and kidney. In the brain, the spirochetes are around the meninges.[30,37] In general, the severity of relapsing fever directly correlates with the number of spirochetes in the blood.[38]

Fatalities from Lyme borreliosis only are extremely rare.[2] The usual pathologic specimen is a skin biopsy, which if taken from the leading edge of the expanding skin rash can reveal spirochetes by silver stain or immunofluroescence.[36] Biopsies of synovial tissue of patients with frank arthritis reveal acute and chronic inflammation with proliferative synovium.[39] The presence of spirochetes in joint tissue can be demonstrated by polymerase chain reaction but almost never by microscopy.

PATHOGENESIS AND IMMUNITY

A *Borrelia* infection of humans almost always begins with contact with a tick or louse bearing the spirochetes. Less commonly, the disease is acquired through accidental inoculation of infected blood; by contact of blood with abraded or lacerated skin, mucous membranes, or the conjunctiva; or, rarely, by transplacental transmission from mother to fetus.[33,34] Transmission to humans by aerosol, fomites, human saliva, urine, feces, or sexual contact has not been documented.

A single spirochete is sufficient to initiate relapsing fever.[40] Having gained access to the blood, the organisms multiply there at a rate of one cell division every 6 to 12 hours until they number 10^5 to 10^8 per milliliter of blood. The incubation period between the exposure and the onset of fever is 3 to 12 days. From the blood, the spirochetes may invade the central nervous system, eye, liver, and other organs. Persistence of the spirochetes in the blood for up to several weeks is achieved by the population staying one step ahead of the host's immune response through the strategy of multiphasic antigenic variation.[41,42]

Recurrence of fever after the initial and subsequent immune responses is the result of regrowth of the spirochete population in the blood. Early microbiologists and immunologists recognized that the new crop of borrelias were antigenically distinct from the original infecting organism.[43] The populations that predominated during each relapse were assigned different serotype names. For example, a rat infected with serotype A had serotypes B and C in the blood during the first and second relapse, respectively. However, the order of serotype appearance is not absolutely fixed: Sometimes, serotype C may follow serotype A instead of serotype B in the relapse sequence. Characteristically, antiserum to serotype A could passively protect mice from infection with serotype A but not serotypes B or C. Similarly, antisera against serotypes C or B were effective against the homologous serotype but not against others.

The varying antigens that determine serotype identity are a set of outer membrane lipoproteins called variable membrane proteins as a group. These proteins are of two sizes: variable small proteins (Vsps) of approximately 20 kilodaltons and variable large proteins (Vlps) of approximately 40 kilodaltons. A single strain of *B. hermsii* may be capable of producing 30 to 40 different variable major proteins, about equally divided in number between Vsps and Vlps. There can be as little as 30% identity in amino acid sequences between two different variable major proteins of the same strain of a relapsing fever *Borrelia* sp., a feature that accounts for the lack of cross-reactivity between antisera.[44]

There is a complete or near-complete variable membrane protein gene (*vmp*) for each Vsp or Vlp protein. In any single cell at any given time, only one *vmp* gene is expressed, usually at a site near the end of a linear plasmid. The other 30 or 40 *vmp* genes in the genome are silent in their storage locations on other linear plasmids. The expression site, in distinction from the silent sites, has a promoter in front of the *vmp* gene. A different *vmp* gene spontaneously replaces the one at the expression site at an estimated frequency of 10^{-4} to 10^{-3} per cell generation.[45] The newly appearing serotype is still in low numbers at the time the immune system responds to the first serotype with an outpouring of antibodies and, thus, escapes as the original infecting serotype is cleared from the blood.

There are two ways in which a *vmp* gene at the expression site is replaced by another. The most common mechanism is a nonreciprocal, unidirectional recombination between two linear plasmids.[41,42] A simplified representation of such a switch in these genes is shown in Figure 45-3. The recombination has the features of a gene conversion: The unchanged donor sequence is a silent *vmp* and the target sequence is the *vmp* gene at the expression site. The boundaries for the recombination are regions of sequence identity between silent and expression sites around and flanking the 5′ and 3′ ends of the expressed and silent genes.

The second mechanism by which a new *vmp* gene is expressed is an intramolecular rather than the intermolecular recombination between two plasmids. For the second mechanism to occur, there must be an untranscribed *vmp* gene downstream from the expressed gene and in the same orientation.[46] A deletion between short direct repeats at the 5′ ends of each of the two genes effectively excises the sitting gene.

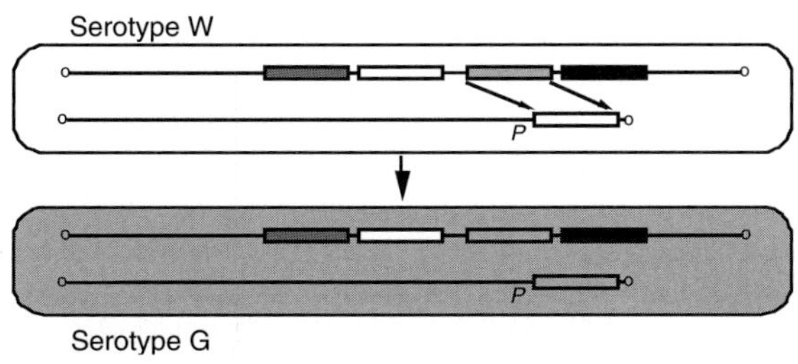

FIGURE 45-3 Schematic representation of molecular events in an antigenic switch from serotype W (*white*) or serotype G (*gray*) in relapsing fever *Borrelia* spp. In this switch, there is an intermolecular gene conversion in which the donor sequence is a silent *vmp* gene in a tandem array of silent genes, which are denoted by white, black, or dark or light gray boxes, on a linear plasmid. The target sequence is an extra copy of the white *vmp* gene that is next to the telomere (o) of another linear plasmid and downstream from a promoter. The light gray *vmp* gene at the silent location is unchanged in the recombination.

The one behind moves up with deletion to take its place next to the promoter. After this deletion, the newly expressed gene is susceptible to additional small gene conversions that provide further diversity of the *vmp* genes.

Variable membrane proteins also have a role in tissue localization during infection. Within a given species, certain serotypes can invade the brain, whereas other serotypes, identical but for the variable membrane protein, cannot.[47] Some species of *Borrelia*, such as *B. duttoni* in Africa and *B. turicatae* in North America, are particularly neurotropic.[30]

Lyme borreliosis begins as a local infection, which manifests as a skin rash approximately 1 or 2 weeks after a tick has attached for at least 24 hours.[2,48] In the skin, the spirochetes move centrifugally, thus enlarging the diameter of the lesion over several days to weeks. In many patients, the borrelias also circulate in the blood during acute infection but at a density that is undetectable by light microscopy of unconcentrated blood. If fever occurs during Lyme borreliosis, it is mild. During the bacteremia, the infection disseminates to other organs and tissues, commonly the joints, heart, and nerves and brain. Late manifestations of Lyme borreliosis are the result of persistence of spirochetes and the provocation of inflammation in the tissues and organs, mainly the brain and nerves, skin, heart, and large joints, rather than the reappearance of spirochetes in the blood. The pathogen's persistence, albeit in low numbers, in tissues occurs in the face of a continued antibody response and appears to be the consequence of antigenic variation in a set of surface lipoproteins—the Vls proteins—that are homologous to the Vlp proteins of relapsing fever species.[41]

In animals infected with relapsing fever *Borrelia* spp., immunoglobulin M (IgM) antibodies alone are sufficient to limit or eliminate infection from the blood.[49,50] Experimental animals with deficient T cell function, such as nude mice, clear spirochetes from the blood as effectively as their immunocompetent counterparts.[51] Whether T cells play a more important role in long-term protection from infection or in control of the infection in the central nervous system is not known. Because specific antibodies, even Fab monomers, to outer membrane proteins can kill borrelias in the absence of complement or phagocytes,[52] deficiencies in the latter immune effectors may not hinder clearance of borrelias from the blood. Immune deficiencies that do increase severity of relapsing fever in experimental animals are the absence of the spleen and impaired B-cell function.

During infection, animals and human patients have antibodies to a number of different components of spirochetes, but only those directed against the Vsps and Vlps appear to be effective in controlling infection.[45] Antibodies to flagella as well as other components of the *Borrelia* sp. are found in patients convalescent from relapsing fever, but these antibodies do not provide protection by passive immunization. The immune response is often not successful in clearing borrelias from the brain, cerebrospinal fluid, or eye.[30] In these locations, relapsing fever spirochetes, much like *Treponema pallidum*, can persist for years.

Infection with *B. burgdorferi* or another Lyme borreliosis agent is more severe, in terms of tissue inflammation, in mice with profound immune deficiencies, but the infection is not fatal.[2] Among immunocompetent mice, the degree of tissue pathology and spirochete burden is determined by genetic factors of both the host and the pathogen.[48] Experimental animals can be passively protected by immune sera alone.

In some cases, depending on the specificities of the antisera, administration of immune sera can clear infection. Although cell-mediated immunity to *B. burgdorferi* appears not to play a necessary or even sufficient role in an effective immune response to infection or vaccination, T cell responses to a pathogen or host antigen may be responsible for a form of reactive arthritis of one or a few large joints that a minority of untreated patients in North America experience.[39]

DIAGNOSIS

Recurrent fevers at intervals of a few to several days suggest the diagnosis of relapsing fever. If these are accompanied by the crisis phenomenon—hepatomegaly or splenomegaly, thrombocytopenia with normal white count, cranial neuritis in the case of tick-borne relapsing fever, or jaundice and petechiae in the case of louse-borne relapsing fever—and an epidemiologic history of exposure to lice or soft-bodied ticks, then relapsing fever is highly likely. In the absence of a full constellation of typical features, relapsing fever may be confused with rickettsioses, malaria, typhoid fever, brucellosis, Colorado tick fever, dengue, leptospirosis, rat-bite fever, or meningococcemia, depending on the epidemiologic circumstances. Patients with louse-borne relapsing fever may have epidemic typhus as well. In early Lyme borreliosis, there is usually, but not always, a prominent localized erythematous rash and mild fever. Late Lyme borreliosis may mimic a number of other infectious and noninfectious disorders.[2] The few geographic areas where both Lyme borreliosis and relapsing fever occur are far western North America and some areas bordering the Mediterranean.

If the diagnosis of relapsing fever is suspected, a smear or wet mount of the blood should be prepared during a febrile period. Once the temperature is declining or has returned to the normal range without the aid of antipyretics, visual detection of spirochetes in blood is very unlikely. Giemsa or Wright stains of a methanol-fixed thin smear usually reveal the spirochetes if the concentration of microorganisms in the blood is greater than 10^5 per milliliter (Fig. 45-4).

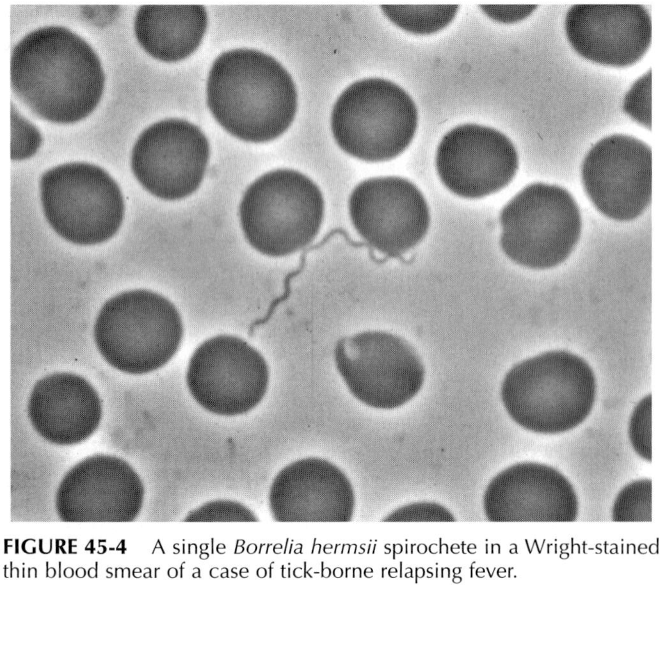

FIGURE 45-4 A single *Borrelia hermsii* spirochete in a Wright-stained thin blood smear of a case of tick-borne relapsing fever.

In hospitals and clinics with automated procedures for blood smear analysis, a manual examination of the blood smear should be requested. As many as 200 oil immersion fields should be viewed before judging the smear negative.

With a thick smear, concentrations of 10^4 or more organisms per milliliter of blood can be detected. If Giemsa or Wright stain is used, the slide should first be dehemoglobinized, such as with 0.5% acetic acid. This step can be omitted if the smear is treated with acridine orange[53] or fluorescein-labeled anti-*Borrelia* antibody[45] and then examined under ultraviolet light.

Phase contrast or dark-field microscopy reveals motile spirochetes in blood diluted in phosphate-buffered saline under a cover slip and examined at approximately 400× magnification. Coiling, uncoiling, and bending movements of the spirochetes as they swim among the erythrocytes are telltale signs. Centrifugation of the anticoagulated blood in a capillary tube and examination of the buffy coat by microscopy improve the limit of detection of microscopy to 10^3 spirochetes per milliliter of blood.[54,55]

When relapsing fever is suspected but spirochetes are not directly visualized, inoculation of blood or cerebrospinal fluid into young mice or rats may reveal a *Borrelia* sp.[56] Most inbred or outbred strains are suitable for this purpose. Infection of the mouse can be enhanced by sublethal gamma irradiation, treatment with cyclophosphamide, the severe combined immunodeficiency phenotype, or splenectomy.[45,47,57,58] The tail vein, saphenous vein, or orbital sinus blood of the inoculated mice should be examined daily for the presence of the spirochetes for 7 days.

In vitro cultivation is an alternative to animal inoculation for recovery of the organism from blood, cerebrospinal fluid, or tissues, but this is not a widely available procedure. Kelly's medium and its most commonly used derivative, BSK medium, support the growth of most *Borrelia* spp.[59–61] Selection from contaminants is achieved by supplementation of the medium with rifampin, phosphomycin, aminoglycosides, and/or amphotericin B. Tubes of medium are inoculated with several drops of blood or other specimen and incubated at 34° to 36°C in tightly capped tubes for up to 2 weeks. Samples of the cultures are examined every day or other day by dark-field or phase contrast microscopy. More rapid than culture for direct detection is the polymerase chain reaction, which has been used to study *B. hermsii* and *B. turicatae* in blood, brain, cerebrospinal fluid, and joint tissues of mice[38] and to confirm *B. duttonii* infection of humans.[19]

Serologic assays have seldom been of value for the confirmation of relapsing fever because of lack of standardization, limited availability, and generally low specificity of whole cell assays. Elevated titers of antibodies that bind to the *Proteus* OX-K antigen in the Weil–Felix agglutination assay occur in relapsing fever,[62] but this assay is less commonly offered than in the past. Enzyme-linked immunosorbent assay (ELISA) and immunofluorescence assay (IFA), which are based on whole cells, are available at some reference laboratories. They are of greatest diagnostic value when paired (i.e., acute and convalescent sera) and changes in titer are assessed. Without access to these resources, the more widely available ELISA assay for antibodies to *B. burgdorferi* may provide enough cross-reactivity that convalescent sera from some relapsing fever patients will give positive reactions. For these ELISA results to be considered supportive of the diagnosis of relapsing fever, the Western blot assay for Lyme borreliosis and reagin-based and treponeme-specific assays for syphilis should be negative. An immunoassay using a recombinant form of GlpQ protein, which is found in relapsing fever *Borrelia* spp. but not in the LB *Borrelia* spp., demonstrated higher specificity than whole cell assays in studies of both tick-borne and louse-borne relapsing fever.[63,64]

In contrast to relapsing fever, laboratory confirmation of the diagnosis of Lyme borreliosis usually rests on measurement of antibodies to a Lyme borreliosis *Borrelia* spp. and not on direct recovery or detection of the agent.[65] Even during early infection, when the organisms are disseminating, organisms cannot be detected by microscopy of the blood. There are two options for serologic testing: (1) a whole cell-based ELISA followed by confirmatory immunoblot for those samples with positive or borderline reaction and (2) a subunit ELISA based on a conserved region of Vls proteins of *B. burgdorferi*. The sensitivity and specificity of the so-called "two-tiered" approach and the subunit assay are approximately the same. The serologic assays do not have a place as screening tests for Lyme borreliosis because of their low predictive value in situations in which the a priori likelihood of the Lyme borreliosis is low. Unlike syphilis, for which screening tests may be justified for disease control and prevention, there is no evidence of person-to-person transmission of *B. burgdorferi*.

Analysis of the cerebrospinal fluid is indicated in cases of suspected relapsing fever or Lyme borreliosis when there are signs of meningitis or meningoencephalitis.[30] Documentation of a mononuclear pleocytosis and/or mildly to moderately elevated protein levels in the cerebrospinal fluid provides justification for use of intravenous antibiotic therapy of tick-borne relapsing fever and Lyme borreliosis. Lumbar puncture analysis under these conditions also rules out most other non-viral infectious causes of meningitis. Standard bacterial, mycobacterial, and fungal cultures of the cerebrospinal fluid are negative if the cause of the disease is relapsing fever or Lyme borreliosis.

TREATMENT AND PROGNOSIS

Relapsing fever was one of the first infections to be treated with an antimicrobial agent; Paul Ehrlich and colleagues administered organic arsenicals to patients with relapsing fever, and these medications were used for this purpose until the discovery of penicillin and tetracycline. Since that time, these antibiotics have been the drugs of choice for this and other *Borrelia* infections. The minimum inhibitory concentrations of penicillin and tetracycline for *Borrelia* spp. in broth medium are less than 0.1 μg/mL.[9,66,67] *Borrelia* spp. are also susceptible to cephalosporins, macrolides, chloramphenicol, coumermycins, and vancomycin,[68] but there is less laboratory and clinical experience with these antibiotics. Borrelias are not susceptible to rifampin, metronidazole, and sulfa drugs and are relatively resistant to most quinolones and aminoglycosides. However, there is no evidence that *Borrelia* spp. have acquired resistance to any antibiotics. In the case of relapsing fever, the effectiveness of the antibiotic therapy can be assessed by observing the clearance of spirochetes from the blood. Within 4 to 8 hours of the first dose of an effective antibiotic, most patients will no longer have detectable spirochetes in the blood.

Single doses of 100 mg of doxcycline, 500 mg of tetracycline, or 500 mg of erythromycin stearate or ethyl succinate are effective oral antibiotic treatment for adults with louse-borne relapsing fever.[69–71] For all children, the oral dose of erythromycin is 12.5 mg kg^{-1} up to 500 mg. For children older than 8 years of age, the oral dose of doxycycline is 2 mg kg^{-1} up to 100 mg, and the oral dose of tetracycline is 12.5 mg kg^{-1} up to 500 mg. An alternative single-dose oral treatment is chloramphenicol at 500 mg for adults and 12.5 to 25 mg kg^{-1} up to 500 mg for children.[72] The overall recurrence rate after antibiotic treatment is less than 5%. Tetracyclines appear to have better efficacy and are preferred over erythromycin, except for pregnant and nursing women and for children younger than 9 years old. When the patient cannot take tetracycline by mouth, the intravenous dose is 250 or 500 mg for adults. Parenteral treatment with intramuscular penicillin G. procaine is 600,000 to 800,000 units for adults and 400,000 units for children. If louse-borne typhus is suspected, the recommended antibiotics are doxycycline or chloramphenicol, but single doses will not be sufficient.

Tick-borne relapsing fever cases occur either sporadically or in limited outbreaks. Although the evidence on management is mostly anecdotal, accumulated clinical experience indicates that there is a recurrence rate of 20% or higher after single-dose treatment of tick-borne relapsing fever.[27,73,74] From their residence in the brain, protected by the blood–brain barrier, tick-borne relapsing fever spirochetes can reinvade the blood once antibiotic levels have declined below minimum inhibitory concentrations.[68,75] The preferred treatment for adults, therefore, is tetracycline 500 mg or 12.5 mg kg^{-1} orally every 6 hours for 10 days, or doxycycline 100 mg twice daily for 10 days. When tetracyclines are contraindicated, the alternative is erythromycin 500 mg or 12.5 mg kg^{-1} orally every 6 hours for 10 days. If a β-lactam antibiotic is given, it should be administered intravenously rather than orally, especially if central nervous system involvement is suspected or confirmed by examination. Three million units of penicillin G every 4 hours or 2 g ceftriaxone once a day or in two divided doses for 10 to 14 days for adults is effective intravenous treatment for Lyme borreliosis and from animal studies would likely also be effective for relapsing fever with neurologic involvement.

In general, the treatment of Lyme borreliosis is similar to that of tick-borne relapsing fever.[2,76] Two recommended oral therapies for adults with uncomplicated, early disease are doxycycline, 100 mg twice daily, or amoxicillin, 500 mg three times daily, for 14 to 21 days. When central nervous system involvement is documented or suspected, parenteral antibiotics as described in the preceding paragraph are recommended. In some cases of Lyme borreliosis, either oral or parenteral antibiotics are continued for up to 1 month.

Jarisch–Herxheimer Reaction

Relapsing fever is one of the few infections for which antibiotic therapy poses a significant risk of death or further morbidity, for reasons other than anaphylaxis or overdosage. Within a few hours of the first dose of an antibiotic of most any type, 80% to 90% of patients with louse-borne relapsing fever and 30% to 40% of patients with tick-borne relapsing fever experience a worsening of symptoms.[77,78] In a minority of patients, the reaction is life-threatening or fatal. A mild Jarisch–Herxheimer reaction (J-HR) occurs during the first day after start of antibiotics for some patients with early localized or disseminated Lyme borreliosis.

J-HR is essentially the same as the "crisis" that soon follows the appearance of neutralizing antibodies in the blood. In both situations, the borrelial cells are lysed, and their contents are released into the circulation. Within 1 or 2 hours, the patient experiences intense rigors and becomes restless and apprehensive. The temperature elevates 1°C or 2°C, and the pulse rate and blood pressure rise. This is followed during the next few hours by profuse sweating, exhaustion, a decline in temperature, a fall in blood pressure, and leukopenia.

In an animal model of the J-HR, the same changes in temperature and white cell count occur after treatment of infected mice with ampicillin or infusion of ruptured spirochetes. The abundant lipoproteins of the spirochetes likely act on the Toll-like receptor 2 of macrophages and other cells.[11,79] This ligand-receptor binding induces the release of inflammatory cytokines.[80] Levels of tumor necrosis factor (TNF), interleukin (IL)-6, and IL-8 increase severalfold over pretreatment levels during the J-HR in patients treated for louse-borne relapsing fever.[81]

Therapy with penicillin in comparison to tetracyclines has a somewhat lower risk of producing a severe J-HR,[71] but this may be at the cost of a delay in illness resolution and possibly a higher disease recurrence risk.[71,82] Administration of corticosteroids, pentoxifylline, antipyretics, or naloxone has been of limited or no benefit in reducing morbidity or mortality from J-HR. Infusion of antibodies to human TNF prior to administration of the penicillin reduced the severity of J-HR in a clinical trial,[83] but this treatment is very expensive.

Anticipation of the reaction and provision of monitoring or constant nursing attention will permit resuscitative measures, such as volume expansion and digoxin, to be started promptly. Placement of an intravenous line with an infusion of saline before administering the antibiotic is recommended. The pathophysiology of J-HR includes low systemic resistance and dilatation of the vasculature, increased tissue demands for oxygen from fever and inflammation, and myocardial dysfunction. If all of these aspects are addressed, for example, by increasing the blood volume, providing an inotropic agent, and reduction of core body temperature by tepid water sponge baths or acetaminophen, the chances of recovery from a severe J-HR or from a severe crisis are improved.

Untreated louse-borne relapsing fever and tick-borne relapsing fever historically have had mortality rates of 10% to 70% and 4% to 10%, respectively. With timely treatment with appropriate antibiotics, the death rates are reduced to 2% to 5% for the louse-borne form and to less than 2% for tick-borne relapsing fever. Malnourished individuals, infants, and pregnant women are at a higher risk of more severe disease. Prognosis is poorer if the patient is stuporous or comatose on admission or if there is diffuse bleeding, myocarditis, poor hepatic function, bronchopneumonia, or coinfection with typhus, typhoid,[84] or malaria. The mortality rate from J-HR in louse-borne relapsing fever is approximately 5%. Some patients have survived the crisis or J-HR only to die suddenly later the same day or the next, perhaps from an arrhythmia.

Mortality from Lyme borreliosis is rare and is probably attributable to cardiac conduction abnormalities during myocarditis. There have been no recorded fatalities from J-HR with Lyme borreliosis. Some patients with chronic arthritis do not substantially benefit in the short term from one or two courses of antibiotic therapy, but many eventually show improvement.

PREVENTION AND CONTROL

Louse-borne relapsing fever can be prevented by avoiding infestation or contact with human body and possibly head lice. Although humans are reservoirs of the infection, there is no direct human-to-human transmission, with the exception of transplacental or perinatal transmission or contact with blood. The body louse lives in clothing and only attaches to the skin when feeding. Reduction of crowding, improved personal hygiene, and better access to washing facilities greatly decreases the potential for louse-borne diseases. More specific and immediate measures for delousing patients and household or shelter contacts are bathing, shaving of the scalp, and application of one of the following: 1% lindane shampoo (Kwell) or powder; 0.5% permethrin powder; 1% permethrin soap, lotion, or shampoo; 10% DDT powder; 5% carbaryl powder; or 1% malathione powder.[27,85] The insecticides can be mixed with talcum powder. Infested clothes and bedding materials should washed in water that is at least 60°C and with either soap or 7% (w/v) DDT. If possible, the clothing and bedding should then be ironed.

Log cabins and similar wood structures in forested areas are a particular risk for tick-borne relapsing fever when rodents nest in roofs, walls, and woodpiles, under eaves and porches, and in burrows under the house. In other natural environments, ticks may be in caves or natural shelters where animals sleep and nest. In inhabited areas, ticks may be in thatched roofs, mud walls, and crawl spaces under houses. In more agrarian environments, domestic animals, such as pigs, goats, and sheep, may be reservoirs for infection of humans, if the livestock are adjacent to the living quarters and the ticks have access to the human household. Sleeping on floors of buildings with suspected infestation should be avoided. Beds are preferably metal and at a distance from walls. Insecticide-impregnated mosquito nets around the bed may be useful. For entry into infested caves, DEET can be applied to the exposed skin, and permethrin can be sprayed on clothing. Efforts should be made to make structures rodent-proof.[62,86] Interiors of buildings infested with *Ornithodoros* ticks can be sprayed or fumigated with 0.5% diazinon, 0.5% malathion, or 0.5% lindane.

Empirical evidence suggests that when *Ornithodoros* tick bites do occur on an occasional basis, such as during exploration of a cave or vacation in a cabin located in an area endemic for tick-borne relapsing fever, prophylactic tetracycline (500 mg orally four times daily for 2 or 3 days) will reduce the risk of infection if taken within 2 days of the exposure. This regimen may also prevent illness after accidental inoculation with infected blood or culture medium in the laboratory, hospital, or clinic.

Currently, there is no vaccine for either louse-borne relapsing fever or tick-borne relapsing fever. A would-be developer of such a vaccine faces the challenge of the several serotypes that a single strain presents to the host. Until a conserved antigen is identified, the prospects for a successful vaccine are poor. A vaccine against Lyme borreliosis was approved for commercial use in the United States, but it is no longer on the market or available.[26]

REFERENCES

1. Felsenfeld O: *Borrelia*. Strains, Vectors, Human and Animal Borreliosis. St. Louis, MO, Warren H. Greene, 1971.
2. Steere AC: Lyme disease. N Engl J Med 345:115–125, 2001.
3. Barbour AG: *Borrelia*: A diverse and ubiquitous genus of tick-borne pathogens. In Scheld WM, Craig WA, Hughes JM (eds): Emerging Infections 5. Washington, DC, ASM Press, 2001, pp 153–174.
4. Bunikis J, Garpmo U, Tsao J, et al: Typing of relapsing fever group strains, including newly discovered species in hard ticks. Emerg Infect Dis 10:1661–1664, 2004.
5. James AM, Liveris D, Wormser GP, et al: *Borrelia lonestari* infection after a bite by an *Amblyomma americanum* tick. J Infect Dis 183:1810–1814, 2001.
6. Paster BJ, Dewhirst FE: Phylogenetic foundation of spirochetes. J Mol Microbiol Biotechnol 2:341–344, 2000.
7. Holt SC: Anatomy and chemistry of spirochetes. Microbiol Rev 38:114–160, 1978.
8. Barbour AG: Cultivation of *Borrelia*: A historical overview. Int Med J Microbiol 263:11–14, 1986.
9. Barbour AG, Hayes SF: Biology of *Borrelia* species. Microbiol Rev 50:381–400, 1986.
10. Takayama K, Rothenberg RJ, Barbour AG: Absence of lipopolysaccharide in the Lyme disease spirochete, *Borrelia burgdorferi*. Infect Immun 55:2311–2313, 1987.
11. Vidal V, Scragg IG, Cutler SJ, et al: Variable major lipoprotein is a principal TNF-inducing factor of louse-borne relapsing fever. Nat Med 4:1416–1420, 1998.
12. Ferdows MS, Serwer P, Griess GA, et al: Conversion of a linear to a circular plasmid in the relapsing fever agent *Borrelia hermsii*. J Bacteriol 178:793–800, 1996.
13. Barbour AG: Specificity of *Borrelia*–tick vector relationships. In Gillespie S, Smith G, Osbourn A (eds): SGM Symposium 63: Microbe–Vector Interactions in Vector-Borne Disease. Cambridge, UK, Cambridge University Press, 2004.
14. Hoogstraal H: Ticks and spirochetes. Acta Trop 36:133–136, 1979.
15. Dworkin MS, Anderson DE Jr, Schwan TG, et al: Tick-borne relapsing fever in the northwestern United States and southwestern Canada. Clin Infect Dis 26:122–131, 1998.
16. Davis H, Vincent JM, Lynch J: Tick-borne relapsing fever caused by *Borrelia turicatae*. Pediatr Infect Dis J 21:703–705, 2002.
17. Dworkin MS, Shoemaker PC, Fritz CL, et al: The epidemiology of tick-borne relapsing fever in the United States. Am J Trop Med Hyg 66:753–758, 2002.
18. Trape JF, Godeluck B, Diatta G, et al: The spread of tick-borne borreliosis in West Africa and its relationship to sub-Saharan drought. Am J Trop Med Hyg 54:289–293, 1996.
19. Dupont HT, La Scola B, Williams R, et al: A focus of tick-borne relapsing fever in southern Zaire. Clin Infect Dis 25:139–144, 1997.
20. Korenberg EI: Borrelioses. In Pokrovsky VI (ed): Epidemiology of Infectious Diseases: A Manual. Moscow, Meditsina, 1993, pp 382–391.
21. Anda P, Sanchez-Yebra W, del Mar Vitutia M, et al: A new *Borrelia* species isolated from patients with relapsing fever in Spain. Lancet 348:162–165, 1996.
22. Felsenfeld O, Goldstein HB, Wolf RH, et al: The relationship of ribosomal activity to lymphoid tissue histology in *Borrelia* infection. Exp Mol Pathol 12:225–234, 1970.
23. Mitiku K, Mengistu G: Relapsing fever in Gondar, Ethiopia. East Afr Med J 79:85–87, 2002.
24. Bryceson A, Parry E, Perine P, et al: Louse-borne relapsing fever: A clinical and laboratory study of 62 cases in Ethiopia and a reconsideration of the literature. Q J Med 153:129–170, 1970.
25. Barbour AG, Fish D: The biological and social phenomenon of Lyme disease. Science 260:1610–1616, 1993.
26. Steere AC, Coburn J, Glickstein L: The emergence of Lyme disease. J Clin Invest 113:1093–1101, 2004.
27. Southern P, Sanford J: Relapsing fever. A clinical and microbiological review. Medicine 48:129–149, 1969.
28. Chung H, Chang F: Relapsing fever: Clinical and statistical study of 337 cases. Chin Med J 55:6–33, 1939.
29. Rijkels D: Louse-borne relapsing fever in Ethiopia. Trop Geographr Med 23:335–340, 1971.
30. Cadavid D, Barbour AG: Neuroborreliosis during relapsing fever: Review of the clinical manifestations, pathology, and treatment of infections in humans and experimental animals. Clin Infect Dis 26:151–164, 1998.
31. Wengrower D, Knobler H, Gillis S, et al: Myocarditis in tick-borne relapsing fever. J Infect Dis 149:1033, 1984.
32. Judge D, Samuel I, Perine P, et al: Louse-borne relapsing fever in man. Arch Pathol 97:136–140, 1974.
33. Fuchs PC, Oyama AA: Neonatal relapsing fever due to transplacental transmission of *Borrelia*. J Am Med Assoc 208:690–692, 1969.
34. Brasseur D: Tick-borne relapsing fever in a premature infant. Ann Trop Paediatr 5:161–162, 1985.
35. Berger BW: Current aspects of Lyme disease and other *Borrelia burgdorferi* infections. Dermatol Clin 15:247–255, 1997.
36. Duray PH: The surgical pathology of human Lyme disease: An enlarging picture. Am J Surg Pathol 11:47–60, 1987.
37. Cadavid D, Pachner AR, Estanislao L, et al: Isogenic serotypes of *Borrelia turicatae* show different localization in the brain and skin of mice. Infect Immun 69:3389–3397, 2001.
38. Pennington PM, Allred CD, West CS, et al: Arthritis severity and spirochete burden are determined by serotype in the *Borrelia turicatae*–mouse model of Lyme disease. Infect Immun 65:285–292, 1997.
39. Steere AC, Glickstein L: Elucidation of Lyme arthritis. Nat Rev Immunol 4:143–152, 2004.
40. Schuhardt VT, Wilkerson M: Relapse phenomena in rats infected with single spirochetes (*Borrelia recurrenis* var. turicatae). J Bacteriol 62:215–219, 1951.
41. Barbour AG: Antigenic variation of relapsing fever *Borrelia* spp. and other bacterial pathogens. In Craig NL, Craigie R, Gellert M, et al (eds): Mobile DNA II. Washington, DC, American Society for Microbiology, 2002.
42. Barbour AG: Antigenic variation in *Borrelia*: Relapsing fever and Lyme borreliosis. In Craig A, Scherf A (eds): Antigenic Variation. London, Academic Press, 2003, pp 319–356.
43. Barbour AG: Immunobiology of relapsing fever. Contrib Microbiol Immunol 8:125–137, 1987.
44. Rich SM, Sawyer SA, Barbour AG: Antigen polymorphism in *Borrelia hermsii*, a clonal pathogenic bacterium. Proc Natl Acad Sci USA 98:15038–15043, 2001.
45. Stoenner HG, Dodd T, Larsen C: Antigenic variation of *Borrelia hermsii*. J Exp Med 156:1297–1311, 1982.
46. Restrepo BI, Barbour AG: Antigen diversity in the bacterium *B. hermsii* through "somatic" mutations in rearranged *vmp* genes. Cell 78:867–876, 1994.
47. Cadavid D, Thomas DD, Crawley R, et al: Variability of a bacterial surface protein and disease expression in a possible mouse model of systemic Lyme borreliosis. J Exp Med 179:631–642, 1994.
48. Barbour AG: *Borrelia* infections: Relapsing fever and Lyme disease. In Cunningham MW, Fujinami RS (eds): Effects of Microbes on the Immune System. Philadelphia, Lippincott, Williams & Wilkins, 2000, pp 57–70.
49. Alugupalli KR, Gerstein RM, Chen J, et al: The resolution of relapsing fever borreliosis requires IgM and is concurrent with expansion of B1b lymphocytes. J Immunol 170:3819–3827, 2003.
50. Barbour AG, Bundoc V: *In vitro* and *in vivo* neutralization of the relapsing fever agent *Borrelia hermsii* with serotype-specific immunoglobulin M antibodies. Infect Immun 69:1009–1015, 2000.
51. Newman K Jr, Johnson RC: T-cell-independent elimination of *Borrelia turicatae*. Infect Immun 45:572–576, 1984.
52. Sadziene A, Jonsson M, Bergstrom S, et al: A bactericidal antibody to *Borrelia burgdorferi* is directed against a variable region of the OspB protein. Infect Immun 62:2037–2045, 1994.
53. Sciotto CG, Lauer BA, White WL, et al: Detection of *Borrelia* in acridine orange-stained blood smears by fluorescence microscopy. Arch Pathol Lab Med 107:384–386, 1983.
54. Cobey FC, Goldbarg SH, Levine RA, et al: Short report: Detection of borrelia (relapsing fever) in rural Ethiopia by means of the quantitative buffy coat technique. Am J Trop Med Hyg 65:164–165, 2001.
55. Matton P, Van Melckebeke H: Bovine borreliosis: Comparison of simple methods for detection of the spirochaete in the blood. Trop Anim Health Prod 22:147–152, 1990.
56. Chohan IS: Tick-borne relapsing fever in Kashmir: Mice inoculation—A diagnostic method of choice. Indian J Pathol Bacteriol 10:289–294, 1967.
57. Barbour AG, Barrera O, Judd RC: Structural analysis of the variable major proteins of *Borrelia hermsii*. J Exp Med 158:2127–2140, 1983.

58. Meleney HE: Relapse phenomena of *Spironema recurrentis*. J Exp Med 48:65–82, 1928.
59. Barbour AG: Isolation and cultivation of Lyme disease spirochetes. Yale J Biol Med 57:521–525, 1984.
60. Kelly R: Cultivation of *Borrelia hermsi*. Science 173:443–444, 1971.
61. Cutler SJ, Fekade D, Hussein K, et al: Successful in-vitro cultivation of *Borrelia recurrentis*. Lancet 343:242, 1994.
62. Boyer KM, Munford RS, Maupin GO, et al: Tick-borne relapsing fever: An interstate outbreak originating at Grand Canyon National Park. Am J Epidemiol 105:469–479, 1977.
63. Schwan TG, Schrumpf ME, Hinnebusch BJ, et al: GlpQ: An antigen for serological discrimination between relapsing fever and Lyme borreliosis. J Clin Microbiol 34:2483–2492, 1996.
64. Porcella SF, Raffel SJ, Schrumpf ME, et al: Serodiagnosis of louse-borne relapsing fever with glycerophosphodiester phosphodiesterase (GlpQ) from *Borrelia recurrentis*. J Clin Microbiol 38:3561–3571, 2000.
65. Bunikis J, Barbour AG: Laboratory testing for suspected Lyme disease. Med Clin North Am 86:311–340, 2002.
66. Barbour AG: Laboratory aspects of Lyme borreliosis. Clin Microbiol Rev 1:399–414, 1988.
67. Barbour AG, Todd WJ, Stoenner HG: Action of penicillin on *Borrelia hermsii*. Antimicrob Agents Chemother 21:823–829, 1982.
68. Kazragis RJ, Dever LL, Jorgensen JH, et al: In vivo activities of ceftriaxone and vancomycin against *Borrelia* spp. in the mouse brain and other sites. Antimicrob Agents Chemother 40:2632–2636, 1996.
69. Butler T, Jones PK, Wallace CK: *Borrelia recurrentis* infection: Single-dose antibiotic regimens and management of the Jarisch–Herxheimer reaction. J Infect Dis 137:573–577, 1978.
70. Perine PL, Teklu B: Antibiotic treatment of louse-borne relapsing fever in Ethiopia: A report of 377 cases. Am J Trop Med Hyg 32:1096–1100, 1983.
71. Seboxa T, Rahlenbeck SI: Treatment of louse-borne relapsing fever with low dose penicillin or tetracycline: A clinical trial. Scand J Infect Dis 27:29–31, 1995.
72. World Health Organization: WHO Model Prescribing Information. Drugs Used in Bacterial Infections. Geneva, World Health Organization, 2001.
73. Horton J, Blaser M: The spectrum of relapsing fever in the Rocky Mountains. Arch Intern Med 145:871–873, 1985.
74. Cherry J: The prevention and treatment of tick-borne relapsing fever with special reference to aureomycin and terramycin. Trans R Soc Trop Med Hyg 49:563–573, 1955.
75. Schuhardt V, Hemphill E: Brain involvement as a possible cause of relapse after treatment in spirochaetal relapsing fever. Science 103:422–423, 1946.
76. Steere AC: Duration of antibiotic therapy for Lyme disease. Ann Intern Med 138:761–762, 2003.
77. Bryceson AD, Cooper KE, Warrell DA, et al: Studies of the mechanism of the Jarisch–Herxheimer reaction in louse-borne relapsing fever: Evidence for the presence of circulating *Borrelia* endotoxin. Clin Sci 43:343–354, 1972.
78. Bryceson A: Clinical pathology of the Jarisch–Herxheimer reaction. J Infect Dis 133:696–704, 1976.
79. Scragg IG, Kwiatkowski D, Vidal V, et al: Structural characterization of the inflammatory moiety of a variable major lipoprotein of *Borrelia recurrentis*. J Biol Chem 275:937–941, 2000.
80. Hirschfeld M, Kirschning CJ, Schwandner R, et al: Cutting edge: Inflammatory signaling by *Borrelia burgdorferi* lipoproteins is mediated by toll-like receptor 2. J Immunol 163:2382–2386, 1999.
81. Negussie Y, Remick DG, DeForge LE, et al: Detection of plasma tumor necrosis factor, interleukins 6, and 8 during the Jarisch–Herxheimer reaction of relapsing fever. J Exp Med 175:1207–1212, 1992.
82. Warrell DA, Perine PL, Krause DW, et al: Pathophysiology and immunology of the Jarisch–Herxheimer-like reaction in louse-borne relapsing fever: Comparison of tetracycline and slow-release penicillin. J Infect Dis 147:898–909, 1983.
83. Fekade D, Knox K, Hussein K, et al: Prevention of Jarisch–Herxheimer reactions by treatment with antibodies against tumor necrosis factor alpha. N Engl J Med 335:311–315, 1996.
84. Anderson TR, Zimmerman LE: Relapsing fever in Korea. A clinicopathologic study of eleven fatal cases with special attention to association with salmonella infections. Am J Pathol 31:1083–1109, 1955.
85. Garnham P, Davis C, Heisch R, et al: An epidemic of louse-borne relapsing fever in Kenya. Trans R Soc Trop Med Hyg 41:141–170, 1947.
86. Paul WS, Maupin G, Scott-Wright AO, et al: Outbreak of tick-borne relapsing fever at the north rim of the Grand Canyon: Evidence for effectiveness of preventive measures. Am J Trop Med Hyg 66:71–75, 2002.

46

Leptospirosis

WUN-JU SHIEH
CHARLES EDWARDS
PAUL N. LEVETT
SHERIF R. ZAKI

INTRODUCTION

Leptospirosis is a zoonotic disease caused by pathogenic spirochetes of the genus *Leptospira.* In 1907, Stimson described the microorganism in renal tubules of a patient who died of so-called yellow fever.[1] The spirochete was first isolated in Japan by Inada and coworkers in 1915,[2] nearly 30 years after Weil described the clinical disease in 1886.[3] Its relatively recent discovery belies the long history of leptospirosis, which was probably known much earlier in China and Japan by names such as "rice harvest jaundice" and "autumn fever."[4,5]

AGENTS

Leptospires (from the Greek *leptos*, "fine," and *speira*, "a coil") are thin, finely coiled, filamentous spirochetes measuring 6 to 20 μm in length and 0.1 μm in width, with characteristic curved or hooked ends. The genus *Leptospira* contains both pathogenic and nonpathogenic strains. Traditionally, pathogenic leptospires have been included in the species *L. interrogans*, which contains at least 250 antigenically distinct variants known as serovars.[6,7] The genus *Leptospira* was reclassified, based on DNA relatedness,[8–10] into 16 species including at least 7 pathogenic species: *L. interrogans*, *L. borgpetersenі*, *L. inadai*, *L. noguchii*, *L. santarosai*, *L. weillii*, and *L. kirschneri.* Identification of *Leptospira* isolates is important because different serovars cause different clinical diseases and have different host specificities.

EPIDEMIOLOGY

Leptospirosis is an infectious disease of worldwide distribution. Because it is most prevalent in areas where diagnostic capabilities are limited, and because its clinical presentation varies, few reliable data on its global incidence are available. Nevertheless, this disease has been described as the most common zoonosis affecting many species of wild and domestic animals, such as rodents, livestock, wild mammals, dogs, and cats.[6] Human infection can occur either through direct contact with infected animals or, much more commonly, through indirect contact with water or soil contaminated by the urine of infected animals.[11] Person-to-person transmission is extremely rare since man is a dead-end host for leptospiral dissemination.[5] In contrast, leptospires can survive for long periods in the renal tubules of infected animals without causing illness. Most human infections occur in young adult men and children and result from occupational or environmental exposure.[11] Epidemiologic studies indicate that infection is commonly associated with certain occupations, such as farmer,

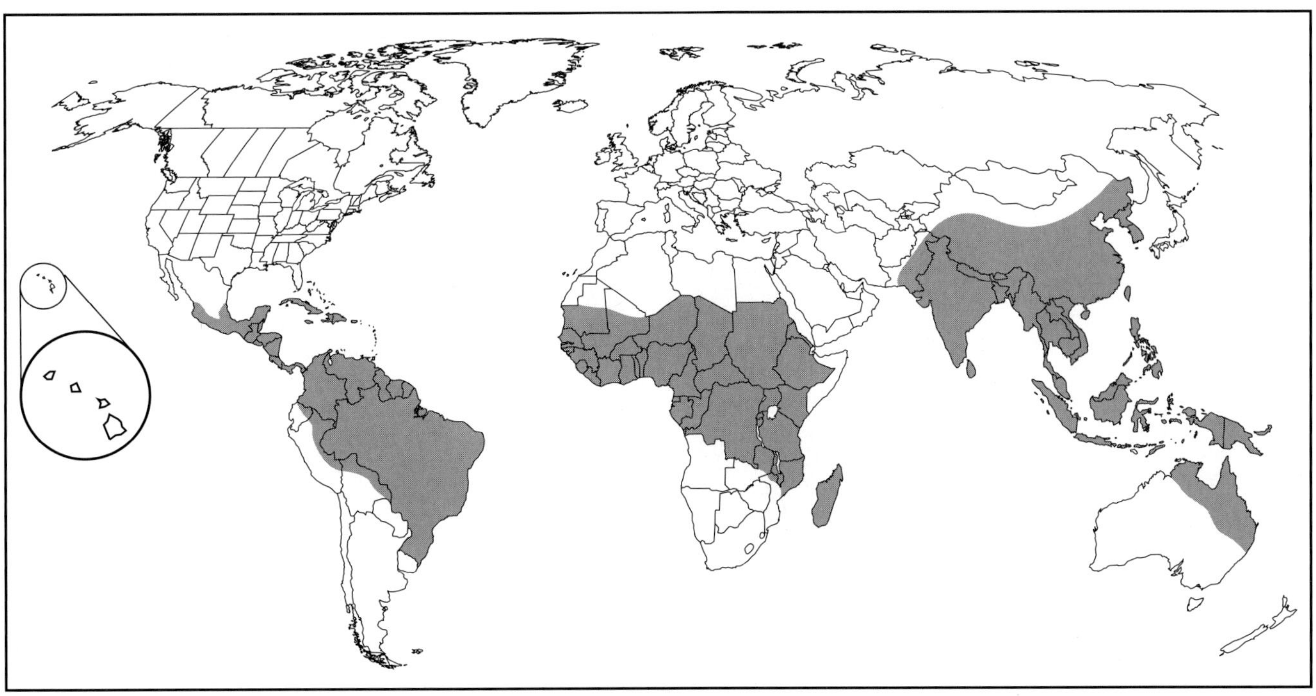

Leptospira spp.

sewage worker, veterinarian, and animal handler. Leptospirosis can also be transmitted during recreational activities, such as hiking, picnicking, swimming, and canoeing.[12–15]

Leptospires can survive in untreated water for months or years, but it cannot survive desiccation or salt water.[11] Only sporadic cases of leptospirosis are seen in arid climates and deserts. In comparison, the disease is endemic in tropical and temperate areas, areas with heavy precipitation, and areas with high levels of subsurface water. Hence, China, Southeast Asia, Africa, and South and Central America have immense areas where the disease is endemic. Leptospirosis occurs sporadically in these areas, with a peak seasonal incidence in summer; large epidemics have been reported after periods of unusually heavy rainfall and monsoons.

DISEASE

The incubation period of leptospirosis ranges from 2 to 26 days (usually 7 to 12). In general, it can be divided into two distinct clinical syndromes: 90% of patients present with a mild anicteric febrile illness, and 10% are severely ill with jaundice and other manifestations (Weil's syndrome). Both anicteric and icteric leptospirosis may follow a biphasic course. In the first or septicemic phase, patients usually present with an abrupt onset of fever, chills, headache, myalgias, skin rashes, nausea, vomiting, conjunctival suffusion, and prostration. The fever may be high and remittent, reaching a peak of 40°C before defervescence. Conjunctival suffusion is characteristic and usually appears on the third or fourth day (Plate 46-1). Myalgias usually involve the muscles in the calf, abdomen, and paraspinal region and can be severe. When present in the neck, myalgias may cause nuchal rigidity reminiscent of meningitis. In the abdomen, myalgia may mimic acute abdomen, leading to confusion with surgical intraabdominal emergencies.[15–17] The cutaneous manifestations in mild leptospirosis include transient urticarial, macular or maculopapular, erythematous, or purpuric rash.[18] The first phase lasts 3 to 9 days, followed by 2 or 3 days of defervescence, after which the second or "immune" phase develops.

The second phase is characterized by leptospiruria and correlates with the appearance of IgM antibodies in the serum. Fever and earlier constitutional symptoms recur in some patients, and signs of meningitis, such as headaches, photophobia, and nuchal rigidity, may develop. Central nervous system (CNS) involvement in leptospirosis most commonly occurs as aseptic meningitis.[19–21] Complications such as optic neuritis, uveitis,[22,23] iridocyclitis,[24] chorioretinitis,[25] and peripheral neuropathy occur more frequently in the immune phase[26] (Fig. 46-1). Prolonged or recurrent uveitis was demonstrated in 2% of patients with onset several months after symptoms of clinical leptospirosis.[27]

In icteric leptospirosis, persistent high fever and jaundice may obscure the two phases.[26] The severe form of leptospirosis is usually associated with hepatic dysfunction, renal insufficiency, hemorrhage, myocarditis,[28,29] and a high mortality. Hemorrhage can occur as petechiae, purpura, conjunctival hemorrhage, gastrointestinal hemorrhage, and pulmonary hemorrhage. Severe pulmonary hemorrhage has been described in China,[30] Korea,[31] and since 1996 in Nicaragua,[32,33] where patients died of pulmonary hemorrhage with no significant renal dysfunction or jaundice (Fig. 46-2). Other, less common manifestations of leptospirosis are generalized lymphadenopathy,[32,34] pharyngitis, acalculous cholecystitis,[17,35] and adult respiratory distress syndrome.[36]

Most of the routine laboratory tests show nonspecific findings. The white blood cell count can be low, normal, or elevated, but it is usually associated with a left shift. Mild anemia and thrombocytopenia are common; hemolytic anemia and disseminated intravascular coagulation have been described in severe cases.[37]

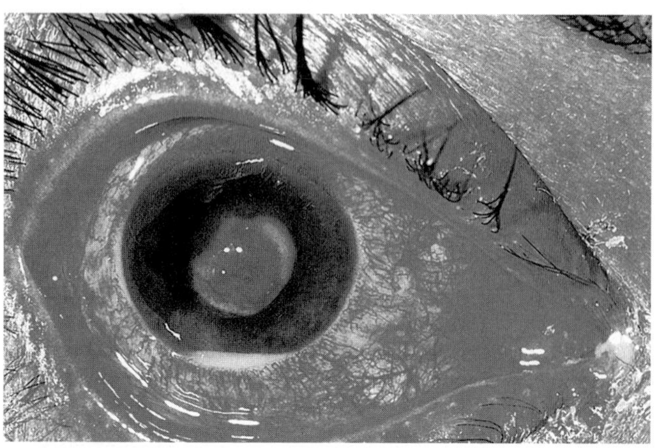

FIGURE 46-1 Hypopyon uveitis with posterior synechiae. (Courtesy of Dr. S. R. Rathinam, Aravind Eye Hospital, Madurai, India.)

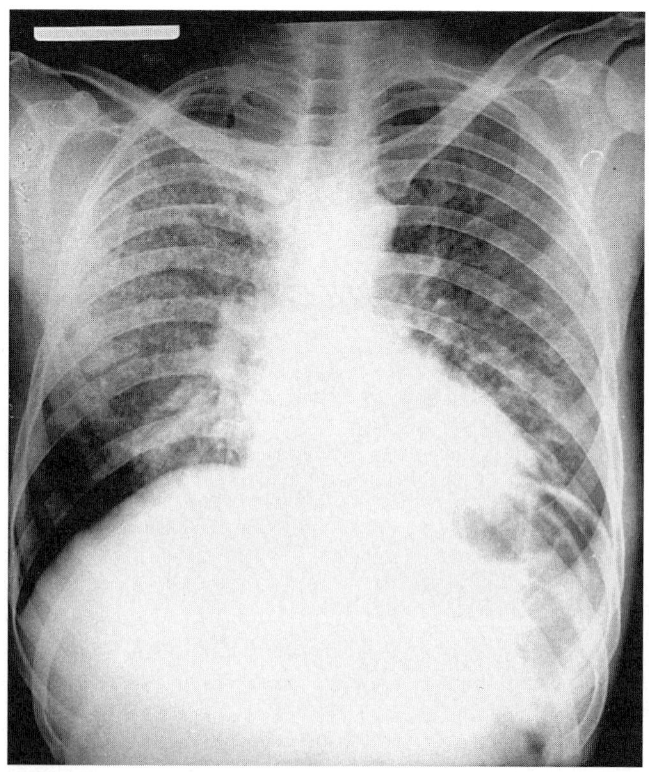

FIGURE 46-2 Bilateral pulmonary infiltrates as seen in chest radiograph of a patient who died of massive pulmonary hemorrhage.

Thrombocytopenia is found in more than 50% of patients and is significantly associated with renal failure.[38,39] Liver, renal, and CNS involvement may be present in any combination. Liver involvement may be mild or severe, with bilirubin levels reaching 60 to 80 mg/dL in extreme cases.[40] Hepatomegaly occurs more often in icteric disease but is observed in as many as 15% of anicteric cases. Serum alkaline phosphatase, lactate dehydrogenase, aspartate aminotransferase, and alanine aminotransferase may all be elevated.[41] Usually, the levels are two or three times greater than the upper limits of normal and infrequently reach the higher ranges typical of acute viral hepatitis. Hyperamylasemia occurs frequently in severe disease, but pancreatitis is rare. Proteinuria, pyuria, hematuria, and hyaline or granular casts are common findings on urinalysis, even in the absence of renal dysfunction.[42] Renal function impairment is primarily a result of tubular damage; however, hypovolemia may play a critical role in the subsequent development of renal insufficiency.[43,44] In the cerebrospinal fluid (CSF), neutrophils usually predominate in the early course of meningitis but are surpassed by lymphocytes after the seventh day. The CSF protein level may be normal or elevated up to 300 mg/dL, while the glucose concentration is normal. Although abnormal CSF findings are reported in as many as 80% of leptospirosis cases, only half of the patients are symptomatic.

Various electrocardiographic and chest radiographic abnormalities are common in patients with leptospirosis.[45,46] Arrhythmias or significant cardiac irritability was documented in 35% of patients who were subjected to continuous cardiac monitoring for 24 hours.[26] The significant arrhythmias were atrial fibrillation, flutter, and tachycardia. Premature ventricular contractions are common and can progress to ventricular fibrillation. Echocardiograms on 88 patients in one study revealed pericarditis and small pericardial effusions in 6% of patients.[26] The chest radiographic abnormalities can include pulmonary edema, diffuse pneumonitis, nonsegmental or basal linear opacities, and pleural effusions.[47,48]

The prognosis of leptospirosis depends on the severity of the disease and associated complications. Anicteric leptospirosis usually has a good prognosis, but fatal pulmonary hemorrhage and myocarditis have been reported in anicteric cases.[32,33]

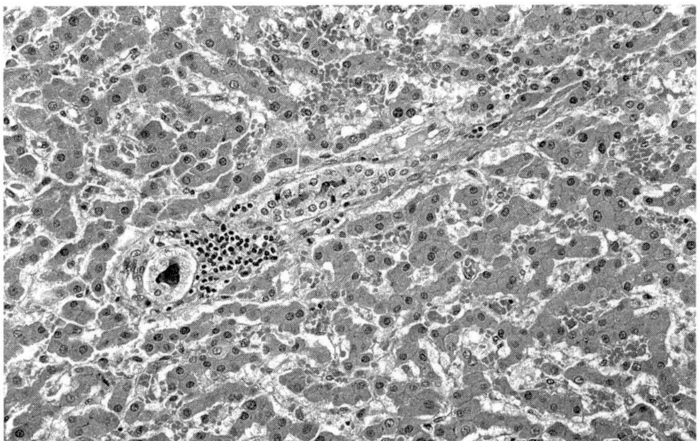

FIGURE 46-3 Low-power magnification of liver that shows a portal area infiltrated with a moderate number of lymphocytes. Note prominent portal ductal and canalicular bile plugs, sinusoidal dilation, and hypertrophic Kupffer cells containing phagocytosed erythrocytes. (H&E; original magnification ×50.)

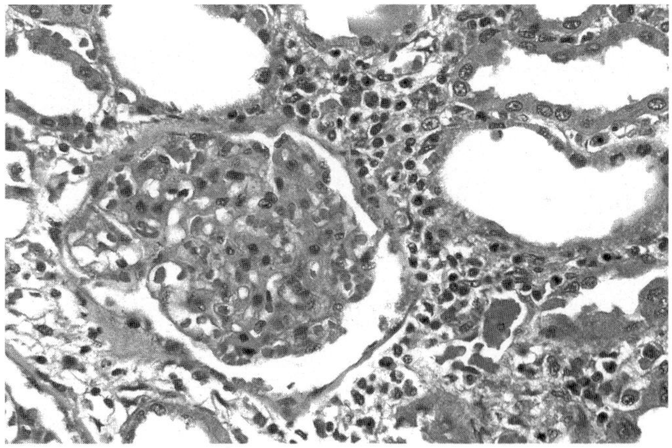

FIGURE 46-4 Photomicrograph of kidney showing tubular dilation and an interstitial mononuclear infiltrate. Note swelling and focal denudation of tubular epithelial lining cells. (H&E; original magnification ×100.)

The case fatality rate for Weil's syndrome is 15% to 40% and is higher for patients older than age 60 years.[49]

In fatal cases, various degrees of jaundice are usually present.[41] Generalized petechiae or ecchymosis in the skin and most internal organs also occur commonly. Microscopically, systemic vasculitis with endothelial injury is seen. The damaged endothelial cells usually show different degrees of swelling, necrosis, and denudation. The main histopathologic changes are usually found in the liver, kidney, heart, and lungs.[32,41,50–52] Hepatic lesions include mild degenerative changes in hepatocytes, prominent hypertrophy and hyperplasia of Kupffer cells, erythrophagocytosis, and cholestasis[53] (Fig. 46-3). Focal necrosis with occasional acidophilic bodies may occur, but there is no particular zonal distribution of the necrosis. Mild to moderate mononuclear cell infiltrates are present in portal tracts. In the kidney, the main histopathologic feature is diffuse tubulointerstitial inflammation characterized by a cellular infiltrate including lymphocytes, plasma cells, macrophages, and polymorphonuclear leukocytes (Fig. 46-4). Tubular necrosis is also a common finding. Glomeruli show mild hyperplasia of mesangial cells and occasional infiltration with inflammatory cells.[54] Grossly, the lungs are heavy and severely congested, with focal areas of hemorrhage. Microscopically, the lungs show congestion with foci of intraalveolar hemorrhage[32] (Fig. 46-5). In some cases, pulmonary lesions include diffuse alveolar damage and variable degrees of airspace disorganization.

PATHOGENESIS

The leptospires can penetrate abraded skin or intact mucous membranes, after which they enter the circulation and rapidly disseminate to various tissues.[7] Penetration and invasion of tissues are presumably accomplished through a burrowing motion produced by a pair of axial filaments and release of hyaluronidase.[55] The dissemination and proliferation of the spirochetes in various tissues results in a systemic illness with a broad spectrum of clinical manifestations, including fever, headache, chills, myalgia, abdominal pain, and conjunctival suffusion; more severe manifestations include renal failure, jaundice, meningitis, hypotension, hemorrhage, and hemorrhagic pneumonitis (Fig. 46-6).

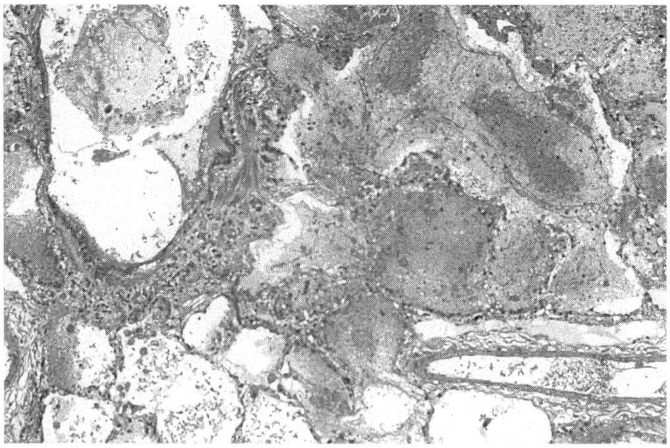

FIGURE 46-5 Lung in a fatal case with massive pulmonary hemorrhage. Extensive hemorrhage and fibrin are seen within the alveoli. Note mild interstitial inflammatory response and sloughing of bronchial epithelium. (H&E; original magnification ×25.)

The pathogenesis of leptospirosis is not fully understood (see Fig. 46-6); there is a marked disparity between the profound clinical illness and the paucity of histologic lesions. In the septicemic (first) phase of human infections and experimental animal models, vascular injury is seen in various organs.[43,56–60] Spirochetes can be found in the walls of capillaries and medium- and large-sized vessels[32] (Fig. 46-7). The exact mechanism of vascular damage is not clear. A direct toxic effect of the leptospires has been proposed to cause the vascular injury, but no bacterial endotoxin has been demonstrated. In the immune (second) phase of illness, the host immune response, including immune complex deposition, may play a role in endothelial injury.[28,38]

DIAGNOSIS

The differential diagnosis of leptospirosis depends on the epidemiology of acute febrile illnesses in the particular area.

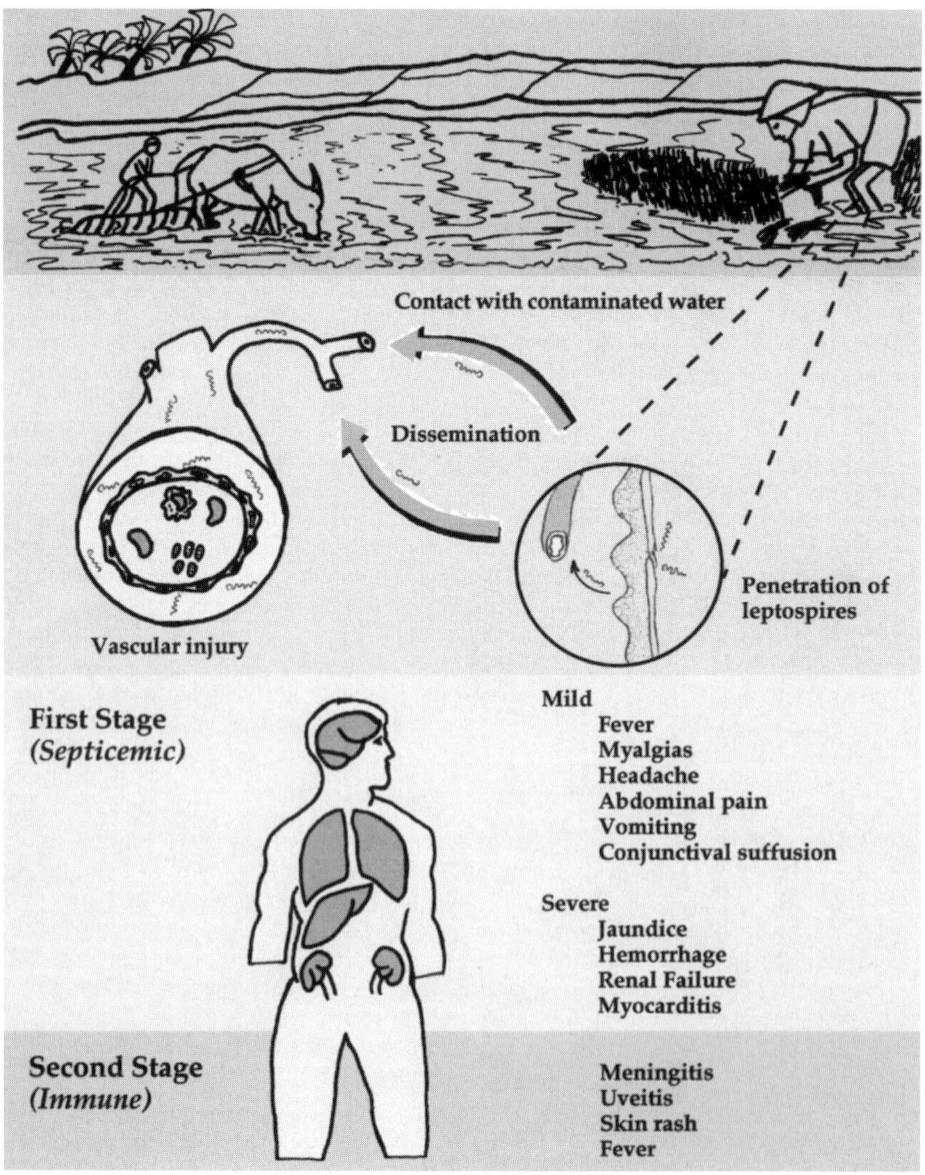

FIGURE 46-6 Pathogenesis and clinical characteristics of leptospirosis. (Courtesy of Nadia Zaki.)

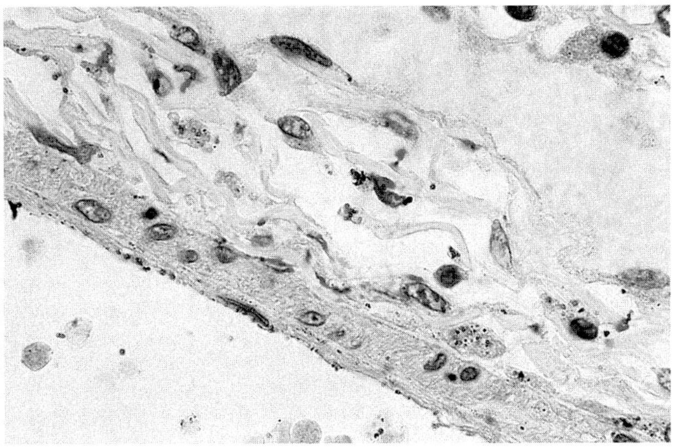

FIGURE 46-7 High-power magnification of a medium-size pulmonary vessel showing intact and granular forms of leptospires. Note mononuclear cells within the vessel wall and focal denudation of endothelial cells. (Immunoalkaline phosphatase staining; original magnification ×25.)

A high index of suspicion is needed in endemic areas, and leptospirosis must be considered when a patient presents with acute onset of fever, headache, and myalgia. However, in locations where dengue fever or malaria is also present, the differentiation may be very difficult because of the similar clinical manifestations. Laboratory confirmation is crucial, especially when these diseases are occurring simultaneously during the rainy season. Other conditions to be considered in the differential diagnosis include influenza, meningitis or encephalitis, viral hepatitis, rickettsioses, typhoid fever, Kawasaki syndrome, septicemia, toxoplasmosis, brucellosis, yellow fever, hantavirus infection, and Legionnaires' disease. When the patient presents with jaundice during or after an acute febrile illness, leptospirosis must be differentiated from other causes of jaundice. The high level of bilirubin seen in Weil's disease with mild to modest elevation of transaminases assists in the differentiation from viral hepatitis, which usually has a much higher level of transaminases for any given level of bilirubin. A high serum creatine phosphokinase concentration or thrombocytopenia would also favor a diagnosis of leptospirosis. A good history should help to differentiate patients with alcoholic hepatitis.

The definitive diagnosis of leptospirosis depends on laboratory findings. The presence of leptospires may be confirmed by direct detection of the organisms or indirectly by serologic methods. Direct methods include microscopy, antigen detection, DNA detection, and culture. Microscopic methods include examination of tissue samples by dark field, histological staining, and immunohistochemical (IHC) staining methods. Visualization of leptospires by dark field microscopic examination of body fluids such as blood, urine, CSF, or dialysate fluid is insensitive and lacks specificity.[61] Approximately 10^4 leptospires/ml are necessary for one cell per field to be visible by dark field microscopy.[62]

The Dieterle, Steiner, and Warthin–Starry silver impregnation stains can demonstrate leptospires in tissues and body fluids; these silver stains also need special expertise in interpretation since confusion with nerve fibers, cell membrane fragments, and fibrin filaments can occur. IHC staining techniques using immunoalkaline phosphatase[17,32,63] or immunoperoxidase[64] staining methods can readily demonstrate leptospiral antigens and intact leptospira in various tissues (Fig. 46-8). Examination of postmortem human tissues, such as kidney, liver, lymph node, and lung, by the immunoalkaline phosphatase method has proved to be a valuable tool in the investigation of leptospirosis outbreaks.[32]

An antigen detection assay was described,[65] but this assay has not been applied widely. Isolation of leptospires in culture from clinical material is a definitive diagnostic test. However, isolation of leptospires requires special media,[66,67] and unless there is a high index of suspicion cultures are rarely performed while the patient is bacteremic during the acute phase of the illness. Leptospires grow slowly, and cultures may not be positive until several weeks after collection. These factors combine to lower the recovery rate of leptospires and render culture almost invariably unhelpful for individual patient management.

Several polymerase chain reaction (PCR) primer pairs have been described for amplification of leptospires, but few have been shown to amplify leptospiral DNA from human or veterinary clinical material, and only two methods have been subjected to extensive clinical evaluation.[68,69] Both approaches have limitations: The primers described by Merien and colleagues[70] amplify a 331-base pair (bp) fragment of the *rrs* (16S rRNA) gene of both pathogenic and nonpathogenic leptospires, whereas the G1/G2 primers described by Gravekamp and associates[71] do not amplify *L. kirschneri* serovars, necessitating the use of two primer pairs for detection of all pathogenic serovars.[72] Using these two primer pairs, leptospiral DNA has been amplified from serum,[68,69,71] urine,[68,69,73] aqueous humor,[74] CSF,[69,75,76] and a number of tissues obtained at autopsy.[77] Sensitive real-time PCR assays have been developed, one targeting an 87-bp section of the 16S rRNA gene using TaqMan probe chemistry[78] and another targeting the LipL32 virulence factor gene using SYBR green chemistry.[79]

Because of the difficulties associated with culturing leptospires and the generally low index of clinical suspicion at the time of presentation, the majority of cases of leptospirosis are diagnosed by serology. The reference standard assay is the microscopic agglutination test (MAT), in which live antigens representing different serogroups of leptospires are reacted with serum samples and then examined for agglutination by

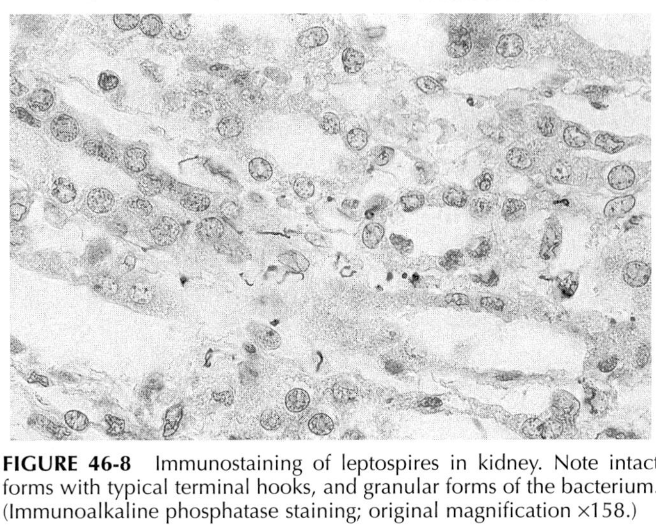

FIGURE 46-8 Immunostaining of leptospires in kidney. Note intact forms with typical terminal hooks, and granular forms of the bacterium. (Immunoalkaline phosphatase staining; original magnification ×158.)

dark field microscopy.[80] This test requires significant expertise and resources to perform and interpret, and its use is restricted to a few reference laboratories.

A serologically confirmed case of leptospirosis is defined by a fourfold rise in MAT titer to one or more serovars between acute phase and convalescent serum specimens run in parallel. A titer of at least 1:800 in the presence of compatible symptoms is strong evidence of recent or current infection.[11] Suggestive evidence for recent or current infection includes a single titer of at least 1:200 obtained after the onset of symptoms.[81]

Cross-reactions occur between different serogroups, especially in acute phase samples.[82] Cross-reactivity in acute samples is due to IgM antibodies, which may persist for several years.[83] The MAT is a serogroup-specific assay and cannot be used to interpret reliably the identity of the infecting serovar.[84] Knowledge of the presumptive serogroup may be of epidemiological value in determining potential exposures to animal reservoirs.

Diagnostic application of the MAT is limited by low sensitivity when acute serum samples are tested.[85] Other agglutination assays that detect total immunoglobulins, such as the indirect hemagglutination assay, suffer from similarly low sensitivities on acute specimens but have high sensitivities when acute and convalescent specimens are tested.[82] IgM antibodies are detectable from the fifth day of illness, and commercial IgM detection assays are available in different formats.[82,86–89] Use of these assays as screening tests offers the potential to enhance the diagnostic capacity of many laboratories, especially those in developing countries, where most cases of leptospirosis occur.

TREATMENT AND PROGNOSIS

Death seldom ensues in anicteric leptospirosis, and treatment with antibiotics within the first 4 days of illness will reduce the duration of illness and alleviate the symptoms. Either oral doxycycline 100 mg twice daily for 7 days or penicillin 2.4 to 3.6 million units/day in divided doses for 7 days is effective in shortening the clinical course.[90,91] An in vitro study has suggested that cefotaxime has better minimum inhibitory concentration levels than penicillin and may serve as an alternative choice. Jarisch–Herxheimer-type reactions can be seen after initiation of antibiotic treatment.[92] Unless there is a high index of suspicion, most cases are not confirmed at an early stage. Treatment therefore has to be early and empirical when the diagnosis is considered in the appropriate setting.

Patients presenting with severe disease are usually jaundiced or have renal insufficiency as part of Weil's disease. They should be treated with meticulous attention to electrolyte balance and rehydration to prevent anuric renal failure. If early signs of renal failure or prerenal azotemia are present, aggressive rehydration over 48 to 72 hours with intensive monitoring of the outcome may be beneficial.[93] If acute renal failure occurs, peritoneal dialysis, hemodialysis, or continuous venovenous hemofiltration are all effective therapies. The jaundice requires no treatment. Patients should have serial electrocardiograms performed, and if any abnormality is detected, they should be placed under continuous electrocardiographic monitoring. The treatment of arrhythmias in patients with myocarditis should be evaluated and appropriate treatment instituted. Aggressive specific therapy for presenting signs, such as hemorrhage, hypotension, respiratory failure, or change in level of consciousness, is warranted. Controversy still exists as to whether antibiotics are of any value in the treatment of Weil's disease. From several clinical studies, it was concluded that penicillin has little effect on the clinical outcome of severe leptospirosis, except for leptospiruria.[92,94,95] In any controversy, patients should be given the benefit of the doubt. Intravenous penicillin or cefotaxime should therefore be given in this group of patients. It was also suggested that all patients with anicteric leptospirosis be treated irrespective of the time in the course of illness. Further studies need to be done with more clearly defined criteria for severe disease and patient exclusion to answer the question as to the efficacy of antibiotics in Weil's disease.

PREVENTION AND CONTROL

Strategies to prevent and control leptospirosis focus mainly on reducing direct contact with infected animals and contaminated water or soil.[11] The risk of contact with infected animals may be reduced by the institution of appropriate sanitation measures among veterinarians, farmers, and others who handle animals. Since rodents are important natural reservoirs for leptospires, reduction of rodent populations can reduce the incidence of human leptospirosis in endemic areas. However, in places with poverty and poor sanitation, reduction of exposure to rodents may be difficult. Prevention of indirect exposure, or exposure to contaminated water or soil, is more difficult, but a common recommendation is to wear rubber boots and protective clothing and, where possible, to avoid exposure to contaminated rivers, streams, still water, and mud.

Prevention programs for domestic animals have long included leptospira vaccines.[96–99] Effective vaccines are available for cattle, swine, and dogs. The vaccine for cattle generally includes *L. interrogans* serovar *hardjo*; the vaccine for swine usually includes serovars *pomona*, *grippotyphosa*, *canicola*, and *icterohaemorrhagiae*; and the vaccine for dogs includes *L. interrogans* serovars *canicola* and *icterohaemorrhagiae*. Vaccinated dogs are protected against clinical leptospirosis but continue to shed live leptospires. Immunization of humans is not a common practice, but trials of human vaccines to specific serovars have been attempted successfully in mines in Japan and rice fields in Italy and Spain. Vaccine trials are under way in China, Korea, and Cuba. The major problem with vaccination of humans is that immunity is serovar specific, and it is very difficult to select all the potentially important serovars for the vaccines.[100–102]

To be effective, the vaccine must include the serovar(s) responsible for the majority of infections in the community. In addition, the incidence of disease should be high enough to justify immunization of people considered to be at high risk for leptospirosis.

REFERENCES

1. Stimson AM: Note on an organism found in yellow fever tissue. Public Health Rep 22:541, 1907.
2. Inada R, Ido Y, Hoki R, et al: The etiology, mode of infection and specific therapy of Weil's disease. J Exp Med 23:377, 1916.

3. Weil A: Ueber eine eigentumliche, mit Milztumor, Icterus, und Nephritis einhergehende akute Infektionskrankheit. Dtsch Arch Klin Med 39:209, 1886.
4. Everard JD: Leptospirosis. In Cox FEG (ed): Illustrated History of Tropical Diseases. London, The Wellcome Trust, 1996, p 110.
5. Faine S: Brief history of leptospirosis. Leptospira Leptospirosis:1, 1993.
6. Torten M, Marshall RB: Leptospirosis. In Beran GW (ed): Handbook of Zoonoses. Boca Raton, CRC Press, 1994, p 245.
7. Farrar WE: *Leptospira* species (leptospirosis). In Mandell GL (ed): Principles and Practice of Infectious Diseases, 4th ed. New York, Churchill Livingstone, 1995, p 2137.
8. Yasuda PH, Steigerwalt AG, Sulzer KR, et al: Deoxyribonucleic acid relatedness between serogroups and serovars in the family Leptospiraceae with proposals for seven new *Leptospira* species. Int J Syst Bacteriol 37:407, 1987.
9. Perolat P, Chappel RJ, Adler B, et al: *Leptospira fainei* sp. nov., isolated from pigs in Australia. Int J Syst Bacteriol 48:851, 1998.
10. Brenner DJ, Kaufmann AF, Sulzer KR, et al: Further determination of DNA relatedness between serogroups and serovars in the family Leptospiraceae with a proposal for *Leptospira alexanderi* sp. nov. and four new *Leptospira* genomospecies. Int J Syst Bacteriol, 49:839, 1999.
11. Faine S: Guidelines for the Control of Leptospirosis. Geneva, World Health Organization, 1982, p 1.
12. Anderson DC, Folland DS, Fox MD, et al: Leptospirosis: A common-source outbreak due to leptospires of the grippotyphosa serogroup. Am J Epidemiol 107:538, 1978.
13. Feigin RD, Anderson DC: Human leptospirosis. CRC Crit Rev Clin Lab Sci 5:413, 1975.
14. Anonymous: Outbreak of leptospirosis among white-water rafters—Costa Rica, 1996. MMWR 46:577, 1997.
15. Morgan J, Bornstein SL, Karpati AM, et al: Outbreak of leptospirosis among triathlon participants and community residents in Springfield, Illinois, 1998. Clin Infect Dis 34:1593, 2002.
16. Berman SJ, Tsai CC, Holmes K, et al: Sporadic anicteric leptospirosis in South Vietnam. A study in 150 patients. Ann Intern Med 79:167, 1973.
17. Guarner J, Shieh WJ, Morgan J, et al: Leptospirosis mimicking acute cholecystitis among athletes participating in a triathlon. Hum Pathol 32:750, 2001.
18. Fraser DW, Glosser JW, Francis DP, et al: Leptospirosis caused by serotype Fort-Bragg. A suburban outbreak. Ann Intern Med 79:786, 1973.
19. Sperber SJ, Schleupner CJ: Leptospirosis: A forgotten cause of aseptic meningitis and multisystem febrile illness. South Med J 82:1285, 1989.
20. Heath CW Jr, Alexander AD, Galton MM: Leptospirosis in the United States. Analysis of 483 cases in man, 1949–1961. N Engl J Med 273:915, 1965.
21. Edwards GA, Domm BM: Human leptospirosis. Medicine (Baltimore) 39:117, 1960.
22. Watt G: Leptospirosis as a cause of uveitis. Arch Intern Med 150:1130, 1990.
23. Rathinam SR, Rathnam S, Selvaraj S, et al: Uveitis associated with an epidemic outbreak of leptospirosis. Am J Ophthalmol 124:71, 1997.
24. Beeson PB, Hankey DD, Cooper CF Jr: Leptospiral iridocyclitis; Evidence of human infection with *Leptospira pomona* in the United States. J Am Med Assoc 145:229, 1951.
25. Hines MT: Immunologically mediated ocular disease in the horse. Vet Clin North Am Large Anim Pract 6:501, 1984.
26. Edwards CN, Nicholson GD, Hassell TA, et al: Leptospirosis in Barbados. A clinical study. West Indian Med J 39:27, 1990.
27. Alexander A, Baer A, Fair JR, et al: Leptospiral uveitis; Report of a bacteriologically verified case. AMA Arch Opthalmol 48:292, 1952.
28. de Brito T, Morais CF, Yasuda PH, et al: Cardiovascular involvement in human and experimental leptospirosis: Pathologic findings and immunohistochemical detection of leptospiral antigen. Ann Trop Med Parasitol 81:207, 1987.
29. Lee MG, Char G, Dianzumba S, et al: Cardiac involvement in severe leptospirosis. West Indian Med J 35:295, 1986.
30. Dai B: Advances in research on leptospira and human leptospirosis in China. Chin Med Sci J 7:239, 1992.
31. Park SK, Lee SH, Rhee YK, et al: Leptospirosis in Chonbuk Province of Korea in 1987: A study of 93 patients. Am J Trop Med Hyg 41:345, 1989.
32. Zaki SR, Shieh WJ: Leptospirosis associated with outbreak of acute febrile illness and pulmonary haemorrhage, Nicaragua, 1995. The Epidemic Working Group at Ministry of Health in Nicaragua. Lancet 347:535, 1996.
33. Trevejo RT, Rigau-Perez JG, Ashford DA, et al: Epidemic leptospirosis associated with pulmonary hemorrhage—Nicaragua, 1995. J Infect Dis 178:1457, 1998.
34. van Crevel R, Speelman P, Gravekamp C, et al: Leptospirosis in travelers. Clin Infect Dis 19:132, 1994.
35. Monno S, Mizushima Y: Leptospirosis with acute acalculous cholecystitis and pancreatitis. J Clin Gastroenterol 16:52, 1993.
36. de Koning J, van der Hoeven JG, Meinders AE: Respiratory failure in leptospirosis (Weil's disease). Neth J Med 47:224, 1995.
37. Trowbridge AA, Green JB 3rd, Bonnett JD, et al: Hemolytic anemia associated with leptospirosis. Morphologic and lipid studies. Am J Clin Pathol 76:493, 1981.
38. Edwards CN, Nicholson GD, Hassell TA, et al: Thrombocytopenia in leptospirosis: The absence of evidence for disseminated intravascular coagulation. Am J Trop Med Hyg 35:352, 1986.
39. Edwards CN, Nicholson GD, Everard CO: Thrombocytopenia in leptospirosis. Am J Trop Med Hyg 31:827, 1982.
40. Ramos-Morales F, Diaz-Rivera RS, Cintron-Rivera AA, et al: The pathogenesis of leptospiral jaundice. Ann Intern Med 51:861, 1959.
41. Arean VM: The pathologic anatomy and pathogenesis of fatal human leptospirosis (Weil's disease). Am J Pathol 40:393, 1962.
42. Gendro NY, Prieur J, Gaufroy X, et al: Leptospirosis in French Polynesia: 120 case reports. Med Trop (Mars) 52:21, 1992.
43. Arean VM: Studies on the pathogenesis of leptospirosis. II. A clinicopathologic evaluation of hepatic and renal function in experimental leptospiral infections. Lab Invest 11:273, 1962.
44. Magaldi AJ, Yasuda PN, Kudo LH, et al: Renal involvement in leptospirosis: A pathophysiologic study. Nephron 62:332, 1992.
45. Ragnaud JM, Dupon M, Echinard E, et al: Pulmonary manifestations in severe ictero-hemorrhagic leptospirosis. Ann Med Interne (Paris) 138:282, 1987.
46. Ramachandran S: Electrocardiographic abnormalities in leptospirosis. J Trop Med Hyg 78:210, 1975.
47. Im JG, Yeon KM, Han MC, et al: Leptospirosis of the lung: Radiographic findings in 58 patients. Am J Roentgenol 152:955, 1989.
48. Wang CP, Chu CW, Lu FL: Studies on anicteric leptospirosis. 3. Roentgenologic observations of pulmonary changes. Chin Med J (Engl) 84:298, 1965.
49. Centers for Disease Control: Annual summary—1984. MMWR 33:1986.
50. Sinniah R, Boonpucknovig V, Sinniah B: Spirochaetal and leptospiral diseases. In Doerr D (ed): Tropical Pathology. Berlin, Springer-Verlag, 1995, p 223.
51. Dooley JR, Ishak KG: Leptospirosis. In Binford CH (ed): Pathology of Tropical and Extraordinary Diseases. Washington, DC, Armed Forces Institute of Pathology, 1976.
52. Pierce PF, Utz JP, Lack EE: Leptospirosis. In Connor DH (ed): Pathology of Infectious Diseases. Stamford, Conn, Appleton & Lange, 1997, p 615.
53. De Brito T, Machado MM, Montans SD, et al: Liver biopsy in human leptospirosis: A light and electron microscopy study. Virchows Arch Pathol Anat Physiol Klin Med 342:61, 1967.
54. Penna D, De Brito T, Pupo AA, et al: Kidney biopsy in human leptospirosis. Am J Trop Med Hyg 12:896, 1963.
55. Miller NG, Froehling RC, White RJ: Activity of leptospires and their products on L cell monolayers. Am J Vet Res 31:371, 1970.
56. Alves VA, Gayotto LC, De Brito T, et al: Leptospiral antigens in the liver of experimentally infected guinea pig and their relation to the morphogenesis of liver damage. Exp Toxicol Pathol 44:425, 1992.
57. Alves VA, Gayotto LC, Yasuda PH, et al: Leptospiral antigens (*L. interrogans* serogroup *ictero-haemorrhagiae*) in the kidney of experimentally infected guinea pigs and their relation to the pathogenesis of the renal injury. Exp Pathol 42:81, 1991.
58. De Brito T, Prado MJ, Negreiros VA, et al: Detection of leptospiral antigen (*L. interrogans* serovar *copenhageni* serogroup Icterohaemorrhagiae) by immunoelectron microscopy in the liver and kidney of experimentally infected guinea-pigs. Int J Exp Pathol 73:633, 1992.
59. Arean VM, Henry JB: Studies on the pathogenesis of leptospirosis. IV. The behavior of transaminases and oxidative enzymes in experimental leptospirosis: A histochemical and biochemical assay. Am J Trop Med Hyg 13:430, 1964.

60. De Brito T, Bohm GM, Yasuda PH: Vascular damage in acute experimental leptospirosis of the guinea-pig. J Pathol 128:177, 1979.
61. Vijayachari P, Sugunan AP, Umapathi T, et al: Evaluation of darkground microscopy as a rapid diagnostic procedure in leptospirosis. Indian J Med Res 114:54, 2001.
62. Turner LH: Leptospirosis. 3. Maintenance, isolation and demonstration of leptospires. Trans R Soc Trop Med Hyg 64:623, 1970.
63. Meites E, Jay MT, Deresinski S, et al: Reemerging leptospirosis, California. Emerg Infect Dis 10:406, 2004.
64. Alves VA, Yasuda PH, Yamashiro EH, et al: An immunohistochemic assay to localize leptospires in tissue specimens. Rev Inst Med Trop Sao Paulo 28:170, 1986.
65. Saengjaruk P, Chaicumpa W, Watt G, et al: Diagnosis of human leptospirosis by monoclonal antibody-based antigen detection in urine. J Clin Microbiol 40:480, 2002.
66. Faine S: Acid-treated, heated serum derivative for culture media for *Leptospira*. Appl Microbiol 17:185, 1969.
67. Levett PN: Leptospirosis. Clin Microbiol Rev 14:296, 2001.
68. Brown PD, Gravekamp C, Carrington DG, et al: Evaluation of the polymerase chain reaction for early diagnosis of leptospirosis. J Med Microbiol 43:110, 1995.
69. Merien F, Baranton G, Perolat P: Comparison of polymerase chain reaction with microagglutination test and culture for diagnosis of leptospirosis. J Infect Dis 172:281, 1995.
70. Merien F, Amouriaux P, Perolat P, et al: Polymerase chain reaction for detection of *Leptospira* spp. in clinical samples. J Clin Microbiol 30:2219, 1992.
71. Gravekamp CH, van de Kemp EA: Detection of leptospiral DNA by PCR in serum from patients with copenhageni infections. In Kobayashi Y (ed): Leptospirosis. Proceedings of the Leptospirosis Research Conference 1990. Tokyo, University of Tokyo Press, 1991, p 151.
72. Gravekamp C, Van de Kemp H, Franzen M, et al: Detection of seven species of pathogenic leptospires by PCR using two sets of primers. J Gen Microbiol 139:1691, 1993.
73. Bal AE, Gravekamp C, Hartskeerl RA, et al: Detection of leptospires in urine by PCR for early diagnosis of leptospirosis. J Clin Microbiol 32:1894, 1994.
74. Merien F, Perolat P, Mancel E, et al: Detection of *Leptospira* DNA by polymerase chain reaction in aqueous humor of a patient with unilateral uveitis. J Infect Dis 168:1335, 1993.
75. Vinetz JM, Glass GE, Flexner CE, et al: Sporadic urban leptospirosis. Ann Intern Med 125:794, 1996.
76. Romero EC, Billerbeck AE, Lando VS, et al: Detection of *Leptospira* DNA in patients with aseptic meningitis by PCR. J Clin Microbiol 36:1453, 1998.
77. Brown PD, Carrington DG, Gravekamp C, et al: Direct detection of leptospiral material in human postmortem samples. Res Microbiol 154:581, 2003.
78. Smythe LD, Smith IL, Smith GA, et al: A quantitative PCR (TaqMan) assay for pathogenic *Leptospira* spp. BMC Infect Dis 2:13, 2002.
79. Levett PN, Morey RE, Galloway RL, et al: Detection of pathogenic leptospires by real-time quantitative PCR. J Med Microbiol 54:45, 2005.
80. Levett PN: Leptospira and Leptonema. In Murray PR (ed): Manual of Clinical Microbiology. Washington, DC, ASM Press, 2003, p 929.
81. Centers for Disease Control and Prevention: Case definitions for infectious conditions under public health surveillance. MMWR Recomm Rep 46:1, 1997.
82. Levett PN, Branch SL, Whittington CU, et al: Two methods for rapid serological diagnosis of acute leptospirosis. Clin Diagn Lab Immunol 8:349, 2001.
83. Cumberland P, Everard CO, Wheeler JG, et al: Persistence of anti-leptospiral IgM, IgG and agglutinating antibodies in patients presenting with acute febrile illness in Barbados 1979–1989. Eur J Epidemiol 17:601, 2001.
84. Levett PN: Usefulness of serologic analysis as a predictor of the infecting serovar in patients with severe leptospirosis. Clin Infect Dis 36:447, 2003.
85. Cumberland P, Everard CO, Levett PN: Assessment of the efficacy of an IgM-ELISA and microscopic agglutination test (MAT) in the diagnosis of acute leptospirosis. Am J Trop Med Hyg 61:731, 1999.
86. Winslow WE, Merry DJ, Pirc ML, et al: Evaluation of a commercial enzyme-linked immunosorbent assay for detection of immunoglobulin M antibody in diagnosis of human leptospiral infection. J Clin Microbiol 35:1938, 1997.
87. Smits HL, Ananyina YV, Chereshsky A, et al: International multicenter evaluation of the clinical utility of a dipstick assay for detection of *Leptospira*-specific immunoglobulin M antibodies in human serum specimens. J Clin Microbiol 37:2904, 1999.
88. Smits HL, van der Hoorn MA, Goris MG, et al: Simple latex agglutination assay for rapid serodiagnosis of human leptospirosis. J Clin Microbiol 38:1272, 2000.
89. Bajani MD, Ashford DA, Bragg SL, et al: Evaluation of four commercially available rapid serologic tests for diagnosis of leptospirosis. J Clin Microbiol 41:803, 2003.
90. McClain JB, Ballou WR, Harrison SM, et al: Doxycycline therapy for leptospirosis. Ann Intern Med 100:696, 1984.
91. Kocen RS: Leptospirosis. A comparison of symptomatic and penicillin therapy. Br Med J 5286:1181, 1962.
92. Oie S, Hironaga K, Koshiro A, et al: In vitro susceptibilities of five *Leptospira* strains to 16 antimicrobial agents. Antimicrob Agents Chemother 24:905, 1983.
93. Nicholson GD, Edwards CN, Hassell TA, et al: Urinary diagnostic indices in the management of leptospirosis. Selection of patients for dialysis therapy. West Indian Med J 38:33, 1989.
94. Watt G, Padre LP, Tuazon ML, et al: Placebo-controlled trial of intravenous penicillin for severe and late leptospirosis. Lancet 1:433, 1988.
95. Edwards CN, Nicholson GD, Hassell TA, et al: Penicillin therapy in icteric leptospirosis. Am J Trop Med Hyg 39:388, 1988.
96. Banker DD: Modern practice in immunization. 11. Other bacterial and miscellaneous vaccines. Indian J Med Sci 22:743, 1968.
97. Bey RF, Johnson RC: Leptospiral vaccines in dogs: Immunogenicity of whole cell and outer envelope vaccines prepared in protein-free medium. Am J Vet Res 43:831, 1982.
98. Bolin CA, Cassells JA, Zuerner RL, et al: Effect of vaccination with a monovalent *Leptospira interrogans* serovar *hardjo* type hardjo-bovis vaccine on type hardjo-bovis infection of cattle. Am J Vet Res 52:1639, 1991.
99. Kerr DD, Marshall V: Protection against the renal carrier state by a canine leptospirosis vaccine. Vet Med Small Anim Clin 69:1157, 1974.
100. Philip NA, Tennent RB: Leptospirosis: A report from one practice on the use of a leptospiral vaccine for a period of three years. N Z Med J 65(Suppl 15):13, 1966.
101. Shenberg E, Torten M: A new leptospiral vaccine for use in man. I. Development of a vaccine from *Leptospira* grown on a chemically defined medium. J Infect Dis 128:642, 1973.
102. Torten M, Shenberg E, Gerichter CB, et al: A new leptospiral vaccine for use in man. II. Clinical and serologic evaluation of a field trial with volunteers. J Infect Dis 128:647, 1973.

47

Trachoma

CHANDLER R. DAWSON
JULIUS SCHACHTER

INTRODUCTION

Trachoma is a chronic conjunctivitis that progresses to scarring of the conjunctiva, painful inturned eyelashes, and corneal scarring with blindness. Blinding trachoma is still highly endemic in many developing countries, where 84 million people have active, infectious trachoma, 7.6 million have trachomatous inturned eyelids needing corrective surgery, and 6 million are blind from the disease.[1,2]

The disease was once found throughout the world but has disappeared from temperate climates with industrialization and improving socioeconomic and hygienic conditions. Today, most trachoma is found in tropical and subtropical areas. It is endemic in many countries in Africa, was common in the southern Mediterranean and Middle East, and can be found in countries of South Asia, some parts of China, Australasia, and South and Central America.[2]

Blinding endemic trachoma of developing countries is caused by infections with *Chlamydia trachomatis* serovars A, B, Ba, or C. Eye infection caused by the sexually transmitted *C. trachomatis* serovars D through K can produce conjunctivitis resembling the early inflammatory phases of endemic trachoma, but without conjunctival scarring and blindness.

A major effort to control blinding trachoma was established by the World Health Organization (WHO) in 1997 as the "Global Elimination of Blinding Trachoma by 2020 (GET 2020)."

AGENT

Biologic Characteristics

C. trachomatis, the causative agent of trachoma, is one of three species within the genus *Chlamydia* that are human pathogens.[3] *C. trachomatis* causes trachoma. It also contains serovars that cause genital tract disease and is now identified as the most common sexually transmitted bacterial pathogen (see Chapter 48). *C. psittaci* is almost ubiquitous among avian species and causes the human disease psittacosis, but it also includes other strains of mammalian origin (see Chapter 49). *C. pneumoniae* is a human pathogen with a worldwide distribution.[4] It is a major cause of respiratory disease and is an etiologic candidate in cardiovascular disease.

Chlamydiae have a complex cell wall (similar to gram-negative bacteria in composition), both DNA and RNA, prokaryotic ribosomes, and metabolic enzymes that would permit independent existence, except that they lack energy-production mechanisms. Moulder[5] thus termed the chlamydiae to be "energy parasites" and credited their obligate intracellular parasitism to this trait.

An unusual characteristic of the obligately intracellular chlamydiae is their developmental growth cycle. The extracellular form of the organism is the elementary body, and it alone is infectious and is responsible for cell-to-cell spread and person-to-person transmission. Following attachment, the elementary body enters the host cell, apparently by a receptor-mediated endocytosis process. If the particles are viable, or do not have antibody attached, they prevent lysosomal fusion and undergo replication in the phagosome. Within 6 to 8 hours of ingestion, the elementary body is reorganized into a reticulate body (the only form that replicates). This larger, thin-walled form diverts the host cell's synthetic functions for its own metabolic purpose and proceeds to divide by binary fission. The reticulate bodies are not infectious. After 18 to 24 hours, the reticulate bodies become reorganized into elementary bodies and thus become infectious again. Subsequently, elementary bodies may disrupt and exit the host cell to infect new cells. The full cycle takes about 72 to 96 hours for the trachoma biovar. These intracytoplasmic collections of elementary bodies constitute the inclusions that may be seen in cytologic smears stained by Giemsa or immunofluorescence methods.

Although all chlamydiae share a genus-specific antigen, there is little DNA homology among *C. trachomatis, C. psittaci,* and *C. pneumoniae* strains.[3] These three species of chlamydiae are distinguished by several features. The elementary body of *C. pneumoniae* is pear-shaped with a large periplasmic space, whereas the elementary bodies of the other two species are round with little or no periplasmic space. The inclusions of *C. trachomatis* accumulate glycogen and thus stain with iodine, whereas the inclusions of *C. psittaci* and *C. pneumoniae* do not. The inclusions of *C. trachomatis* are more compact than those of *C. psittaci* and *C. pneumoniae*. A fourth difference is their response to sulfonamides: *C. trachomatis* is sensitive, but *C. psittaci* and *C. pneumoniae* are not.

C. trachomatis can be further subdivided into strains that cause lymphogranuloma venereum (LGV) and strains that cause oculogenital infections. They differ significantly in their biologic activity. LGV strains are more invasive and can infect many tissues in addition to epithelial cells (e.g., lymph node invasion, forming the characteristic bubo). This property permits more active cell-to-cell transmission in cell culture and the use of animal inoculation (e.g., mouse) for diagnostic purposes. The oculogenital strains, constituting the trachoma biovar, consist of at least 12 serotypes.[6] They are not readily invasive in tissue culture and in vivo grow only in columnar and squamocolumnar epithelial cells (conjunctivae, respiratory tract, urethra, cervix, rectal mucosa).

Previously, it has not been possible to identify biologic properties that differentiate the serovars associated with blinding trachoma from those of the trachoma biovar associated with genital tract disease. Recently, however, two sets of genes have been identified that suggest such a differentiation. The polymorphic membrane protein gene designated *pmpH* has been shown to differ in ways that are consistent with each of these three disease-causing groups of *Chlamydia trachomatis*.[7] This observation suggests distinct evolutionarily divergent patterns for this gene.

More exciting, because of the functional implication, have been the findings relevant to the presence of a tryptophan synthase.[8] This enzyme converts indole into tryptophan. The isolates from trachoma do not have the enzyme, whereas isolates of genital tract origin do (whether they are LGV or trachoma biovars). Gamma-interferon is an important host response to chlamydial infection and is known to interfere with the completion of the chlamydial developmental cycle. Its action is thought to be due to tryptophan depletion. In vitro interferon's inhibitory effect in cell culture can be reversed by adding indole, if the chlamydiae possess a functional tryptophan synthase. This "indole rescue" was only observed with isolates of genital tract origin. This likely represents selection for a survival characteristic of the organism. The authors posit that presence of the enzyme allows for productive infection in the genital tract where normal flora may produce indole, thus allowing the chlamydiae to escape the interferon effect.

Antigenic Composition and Diversity

Human strains of *C. trachomatis* have been classified into more than 18 serovariants (serovars) and 2 biovariants (biovars): the trachoma biovar (serovars A through K and type variants) and the LGV biovar (serovars L1 to L3).[8] Infections with the trachoma biovar strains are limited to columnar mucous epithelium resulting in ocular infections, inclusion conjunctivitis, and trachoma, as well as genital tract infections. Serovars A, B, Ba, and C are typically associated with endemic trachoma, whereas all the serovars have been found in the genital tract (although generally with a preponderance of serovars D and E). Virulence differences have yet to be identified that could account for this distribution of serovars. Even between the biovariants, the molecular basis of virulence differences is unknown.

All chlamydiae share a common lipopolysaccharide (LPS), which is similar in structure but less complex than LPS from gram-negative bacteria.[9] Significantly, the chlamydial LPS is antigenically distinct from that of most other bacteria and represents an important target for culture-independent diagnostic assays. Another essential antigenic component is the surface-exposed major outer membrane protein (MOMP).[10] The MOMP is antigenically complex and displays both serovar-specific antigens and antigens shared by *C. trachomatis* strains that cause human infection.[11] The latter antigen is also used for culture-independent detection of *C. trachomatis*. Consequently, diagnostic assays that detect LPS will identify all chlamydial species, whereas assays that detect MOMP will not identify *C. psittaci* or *C. pneumoniae*. Unlike the LPS antigens, the MOMP antigens are targets of host immunity. This conclusion has been supported by an association of immune protection with serovar specificity and by in vitro neutralization of infectivity using anti-MOMP monoclonal antibodies.[12]

EPIDEMIOLOGY

Trachoma has a worldwide distribution, and blinding trachoma is still a major public health problem in sub-Saharan Africa; in the Middle Eastern crescent; in Central, South, and East Asia; and in limited areas of the Americas, Australasia, and the Pacific islands.[1,2] Nonblinding trachoma is present in a much larger region of these same areas, which includes most of the drier subtropical and tropical countries. Trachoma was once prevalent and severe in many countries of Europe, North America, and Asia, but it regressed and disappeared with the rising living standards that accompanied industrialization and economic development.

Trachoma rarely occurs with the living conditions in developed countries and in many urban communities of developing countries. In persons with clinically healed trachoma, however, there may be recurrences of active disease, following treatment with topical corticosteroids, with recurrent atopic conjunctivitis, and in old age. This recurrent adult disease usually does not present a significant public health risk, however.

In communities with blinding trachoma, most children are infected by the age of 1 or 2 years, and active inflammatory trachoma is most prevalent in 2- to 5-year-olds. The prevalence of active disease then declines steadily, although some adults continue to have signs of active disease.[13] Thus children are the chief reservoir of ocular chlamydial infection in communities with endemic trachoma. Blinding lesions (inturned eyelids and corneal scarring) are the outcome of earlier severe or moderate-intensity inflammatory disease. These blinding sequelae are generally observed in adults but may occur in childhood as the result of very severe inflammatory disease.

Risk Factors

Trachoma is associated with poverty. Economic development appears to eliminate or reduce the severity of the disease. Transmission of the disease is by direct or indirect contact with infected material (e.g., hands, clothing, towels) and by flies. Among the environmental features of greatest importance are the presence of young children in the household, crowding, and the unavailability of safe water and household latrines.[14,15] The behavioral risk factors associated with the severity of trachoma are primarily the lack of facewashing of young children and the lack of latrines in households.

In many endemic areas, the open disposal of human and animal wastes contributes to an increase in the fly population. The flies that cluster on children's eyes to feed on ocular discharges can transfer these discharges to the eyes of other children in the same family within 15 to 30 minutes.[16–18] Children with endemic trachoma also harbor *C. trachomatis* in the upper respiratory and gastrointestinal tracts.[19] Thus, transmission may also occur by aerosol droplet spread and fecal contamination of fomites, as well as by flies.

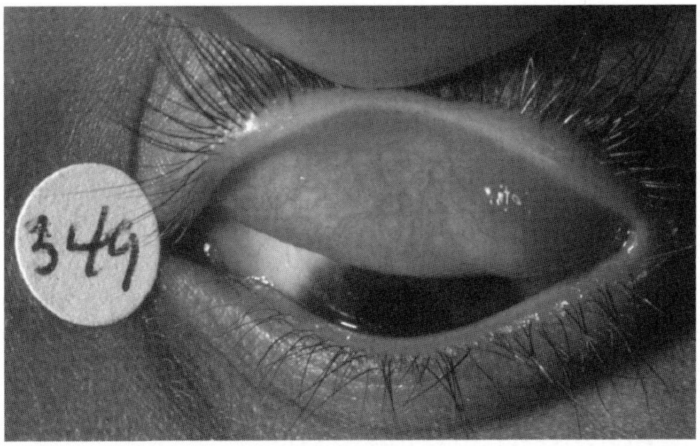

FIGURE 47-1 Active infectious trachoma. The presence of lymphoid follicles (white, avascular spots) in a bed of punctate dilated capillaries and diffuse infiltration (papillary infiltration) on the conjunctiva of the upper eyelid indicates active, presumably infectious, trachoma in this Tunisian child. (The numbered label was used to identify the child in a therapy trial.)

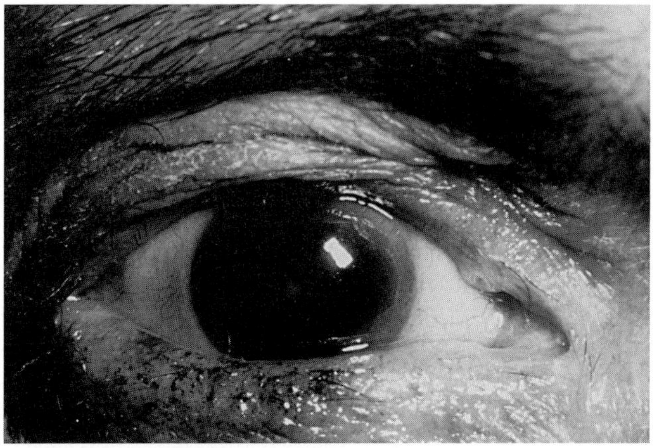

FIGURE 47-3 Trachomatous trichiasis. Conjunctival scarring acquired in childhood has caused gradual contraction of the lid margins producing inturned lashes (trichiasis and entropion) from the lower lid, which abrade the cornea.

DISEASE

In communities with endemic trachoma, the disease often has inapparent or gradual onset. Initially, trachoma presents as conjunctivitis characterized by the formation of lymphoid follicles in the subconjunctival tissue and inflammatory infiltration (papillary hypertrophy) of the conjunctiva (Fig. 47-1). In children under 2 years of age, the papillary reaction with inflammatory thickening of the conjunctiva may be the predominant sign, and follicles may not be a prominent sign. The disease involves the entire conjunctiva, but its effects are most noticeable on the upper tarsus, which has been selected as a diagnostically critical area for examination to represent the degree of trachomatous inflammation and scarring.[20]

As chronic trachoma progresses, it causes scarring of the conjunctiva (Fig. 47-2), with fine linear and small stellate scars in milder cases, or broad confluent or synechial scars in severe cases. With severe scarring, there is distortion of the lids, particularly of the upper tarsus, to produce inturned eyelashes (Fig. 47-3). The disease also can destroy the mucus-secreting conjunctival goblet cells and injure the lacrimal glands and tear ducts. Thus, constant corneal abrasion by the inturned eyelashes and deficient tear secretion can lead to corneal ulceration followed by opacification and visual loss. The deep trachomatous scarring in the upper tarsus and fornix may also produce defects in lid closure with exposure of the cornea, which also predisposes to traumatic and infectious damage to the cornea (Fig. 47-4).

During its inflammatory infectious phases, trachoma produces lesions of the cornea ranging from fine punctate defects in the epithelium (epithelial keratitis) to infiltrates of the superficial stromal connective tissue and superficial neovascularization (vascular pannus). A unique characteristic of trachoma is the formation of lymphoid follicles at the conjunctival-corneal junction (limbus), which on resolution

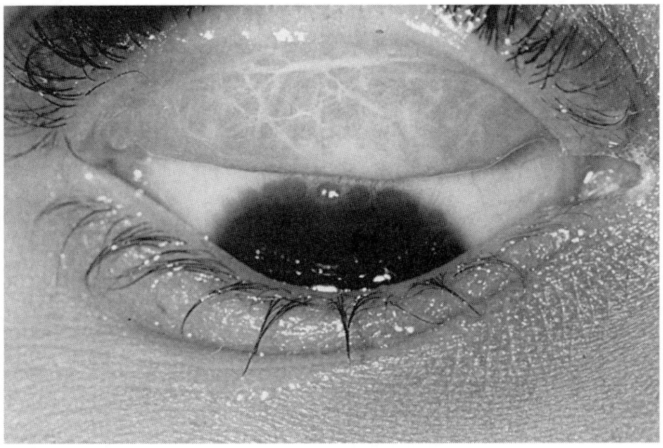

FIGURE 47-2 Trachoma scarring and Herbert's pits in a 6-year-old Tunisian child. The scars are a network of white lines on the conjunctiva of the upper eyelid. Between the scars there are still a few follicles and a diffuse inflammatory infiltrate. The lid margin has been pulled inward so the orifices of the meibomian glands appear to open on the conjunctival surface. Herbert's pits are seen here as circular round depressions at the conjunctival-corneal border. They are found only with trachoma.

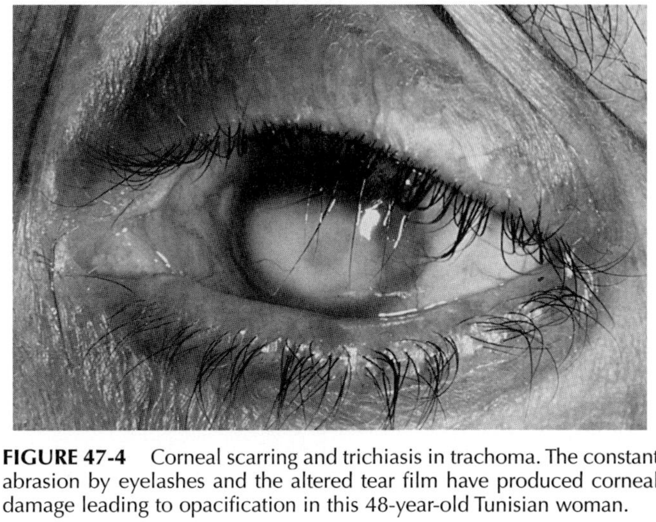

FIGURE 47-4 Corneal scarring and trichiasis in trachoma. The constant abrasion by eyelashes and the altered tear film have produced corneal damage leading to opacification in this 48-year-old Tunisian woman.

leave characteristic depressions at the limbus called Herbert's peripheral pits (see Fig. 47-2).

The degree of conjunctival scarring is directly proportional to the intensity and duration of inflammation.[21] Very severe scarring occurs in children as young as 4 or 5 years of age. Inturned eyelids are uncommon at this age, however, and tend to occur in late adolescence and early adult life, long after the active inflammatory disease has subsided. This late onset of inturned lids in adults may be due to repeated episodes of infection with the development of more scarring and the gradual contraction of the lid margin.

The older MacCallan classification is rarely used now, and there are two related systems recommended by the World Health Organization (WHO) to describe the clinical findings.[20,22] For this clinical evaluation, signs involving the upper tarsal conjunctiva are used as a convenient index of the disease process. These conjunctival signs include lymphoid follicles, diffuse infiltration and papillary hypertrophy, conjunctival scarring, inturned eyelashes, and corneal opacity.

The detailed WHO descriptive system emphasizes the grading of the intensity of inflammatory disease on the basis of tarsal follicles and of diffuse inflammation and papillary hypertrophy. Cicatricial signs include conjunctival scarring, inturned eyelashes, and corneal opacity.[20] This detailed description has been useful for clinical research in field studies.

A simplified description was introduced in 1987 by the WHO for use by primary health-care workers (Box 47-1).[22] This simplified system was developed for use by nonspecialist health workers in developing countries, using a handlight and loupe for examination. A specific series of interventions is linked to the clinical findings.

To identify the presence or absence of trachoma in a community, individual cases must have at least two of the following signs: (1) follicles in the upper tarsal conjunctiva, (2) limbal follicles or their sequelae, Herbert's pits (see Fig. 47-2), (3) typical conjunctival scarring, and (4) vascular pannus more extensive at the superior limbus.[20] Communities with blinding trachoma have a high prevalence of older persons with severe visual loss caused by corneal opacity and a substantial prevalence of potentially disabling trachomatous lesions, specifically inturned eyelashes.[13] These irreversible changes are the long-term outcome of prolonged or recurrent inflammatory disease of moderate or severe intensity. Communities with nonblinding trachoma may have a low incidence of potentially blinding lesions and little if any visual loss from trachoma.

In communities with blinding trachoma, chlamydial infection is always present, but other ocular microbial pathogens appear to contribute significantly to the intensity of trachoma and to the lesions that impair vision.

Box 47-1 Simplified Description of Trachoma for Primary Eye Care

Trachoma follicles	Five or more lymphoid follicles on the central area of the upper tarsal conjunctiva
Trachomatous inflammation	Diffuse inflammation of the tarsal conjunctiva that obscures more inflammation than half of the normal deep tarsal vessels
Trachomatous scarring	Any characteristic scarring of the tarsal conjunctiva
Trichiasis or entropin	At least one or more deviated lashes touching the eyeball
Corneal opacity	Easily visible corneal opacity or scarring over the pupil

From Thylefors B, Dawson CR, Jones BR, et al: A simple system for the assessment of trachoma and its complications. Bull World Health Org 65:477, 1987.

PATHOGENESIS AND IMMUNITY

The host response of the human conjunctiva in trachoma is characterized both clinically and histologically by the presence of lymphoid follicles with germinal centers.[23–25] In the early stages of trachoma, the epithelial and subepithelial tissues are infiltrated with lymphocytes and polymorphonuclear leukocytes. Where the conjunctiva is bound down over the tarsal plate, the epithelium is elevated by infiltrating inflammatory cells to form papillae with vascular tufts and folds of epithelium between the elevations.

Early in the disease, collections of lymphocytes appear in the submucosa just beneath the epithelium or deeper within the connective tissue. These early follicles do not have germinal centers and appear to consist mostly of small lymphocytes. As the disease progresses, the collections of lymphocytes develop into lymphoid germinal centers, with an outside layer of small, dense lymphocytes and an inner center of lighter-staining cells with more cytoplasm. Unlike central lymph nodes, these lymphoid follicles are displaced toward the surface. The lymphocytes of the subepithelial follicles appear to be infiltrating the overlying conjunctival epithelium, which is flattened and loosened over the follicle itself, allowing ready access of foreign material into the follicle. Lymphoid follicles in the conjunctiva can also occur deeper in the connective tissue and are not necessarily adjacent to the conjunctival epithelium. Between follicles, the epithelium and submucosal layers are diffusely infiltrated with lymphocytes and some polymorphonuclear cells.

In more advanced stages of trachoma, the follicle itself becomes necrotic, and connective tissue forms in and around the follicles, producing scarring. The formation of Herbert's pits by follicles at the corneoscleral junction (limbus) is evidence that the follicle (during its formation in this confined space) can erode the connective tissue without causing any overt ulceration or connective tissue reaction with scarring.

Macrophages are frequently found in the epithelium and in the follicles themselves. Plasma cells appear to be distributed throughout the conjunctiva. Between the follicles, there is marked lymphocytic infiltration. In addition, the capillaries are dilated, and the whole conjunctival layer is thickened by the cellular infiltration with the formation of papillary villi. As scarring takes place, islands of epithelium between the elevated papillae may become trapped and form epithelial-lined cysts, which fill with desquamated debris to form yellow structures, clinically identified as "post-trachomatous degeneration." Progressive scarring produces inward deformation of the lid margins with inturned eyelashes (trichiasis and entropion), which constantly abrade the cornea to produce corneal scarring and blindness.[23]

DIAGNOSIS

The laboratory methods for diagnosis of *C. trachomatis* in patients with trachoma are essentially the same procedures that have been used to diagnose chlamydial genital tract infections (see Chapter 48). There have been many evaluations of the sensitivity and specificity of these tests for diagnosis of sexually transmitted diseases. It is far more difficult to perform rigorous evaluations in trachoma-endemic areas because of the difficulties in maintaining cold chains and establishing appropriate "gold standards" for comparison. In developing countries, the time-honored Giemsa stain may still be of use in detecting chlamydial inclusions in conjunctival scrapings from some cases of severe active trachoma.[26] Antigen detection methods, such as direct fluorescent antibody (DFA) and enzyme immunoassay (EIA) are also of some use, but they are less sensitive than the newer amplified DNA tests.[27] These are probably the tests of choice for field studies because they do not require maintenance of a cold chain and the specimens can be sent back to reference laboratories or be tested locally.

C. trachomatis can be identified in cytologic scrapings or in tissue specimens by recognition of characteristic intracytoplasmic inclusions.[26] Such identification in conjunctival epithelial cells, and less frequently in cervical epithelial cells, constituted the only technique available at the time when trachoma and oculogenital diseases were first recognized, at the turn of the 20th century, until the organism was isolated in embryonated eggs in 1957 by T'ang and associates in Beijing.[28]

This diagnostic approach has been supplanted by the use of cell culture isolation methods and by the use of modern nonculture diagnostic tests that detect chlamydial antigens or genes. For many years, the most sensitive method for identification of *C. trachomatis* infection of the genital tract was isolation in cell culture. Direct methods of detection of chlamydial DNA (DNA probes) have not been more sensitive than EIA procedures. However, the introduction of amplified DNA technology, such as the polymerase chain reaction (PCR) or ligase chain reaction (LCR), in the mid-1990s revolutionized chlamydial diagnostics.[29,30] These tests are highly specific and are more sensitive than any other diagnostic tests, including culture. The broad-based use of LCR or PCR has greatly improved the management of genital infections by *C. trachomatis*, but has not yet been applied in trachoma control.

Isolation

The method of choice for recovery of *C. trachomatis* is by cell culture using McCoy, HeLa-229, BHK-21, or L-929 cells. A necessary step in cell cultivation of *C. trachomatis* strains other than LGV is centrifugation of the inoculum onto the cells. In addition, the cells are treated to enhance infection; Gordon and colleagues, who developed the modern cell culture technique, used irradiation of McCoy cells.[31] Cycloheximide has been substituted for irradiation, and cycloheximide-treated McCoy cells are the most widely used cultivation method at present.[32] Specimen material is inoculated into individual vials with cell sheets on coverslips within them or into wells of microtiter plates that have been implanted with cells. They can be examined at 48 to 96 hours after inoculation. Intracytoplasmic inclusions can be recognized by iodine, Giemsa, or more commonly by fluorescent antibody (FA) staining. Iodine stain only identifies *C. trachomatis* strains. FA stains are more sensitive and can be species-specific (to MOMP) or genus-specific (to LPS).

Antigen and Nucleic Acid Probes

In recent years, other nonculture diagnostic methods have been evaluated and widely used, including DFA, EIA, and DNA probe methods. There are a number of DFA kits commercially available. Although they differ primarily in their specificity and in their ease of laboratory use, the general principle is the same. A cytologic smear is fixed (at which stage it can be stored), stained with a fluorescein-conjugated monoclonal antibody, and examined by ultraviolet microscopy. Elementary bodies are recognized as small apple-green dots. When the test is performed by experienced persons, the sensitivity can be as high as 90%, but is more often 70% to 80%. The specificity is usually 98% or greater. Thus, it is an excellent screening test for high-risk populations, but less useful in low-prevalence populations.[27,33]

The EIA class of tests is designed for immunochemical detection of dissolved antigenic components. The tests have been designed with the use of plastic to absorb chlamydial LPS or with antigen capture in a sandwich format.[34]

Both DFA and EIA are technologically easier and are less difficult to transport than cell culture. However, they have lower sensitivity and specificity. The DFA has the advantage of a verifiable sample quality, rapidity (as little as 30 minutes), and no restriction as to specimen site. EIA requires less training and experience because its indicator is more objective; it is more suitable for batch processing, and it can be automated.

Direct nucleic acid probes are commercially available. They are less sensitive than culture, although they are highly specific.[34] In contrast, the amplified DNA technology, exemplified by LCR and PCR, is far more sensitive than cell culture and is extremely specific.[29,30,35] The chlamydial genes can be detected in epithelial cell specimens and in male and female urine samples.[36,37] Although noninvasive sampling (urine) is important for diagnosing sexually transmitted diseases, conjunctival swabs are still needed to collect specimens for trachoma.

Except for the DFA smears, specimens for trachoma should be kept at 5°C (i.e., on ice) for transport from the field. As with antigen detection methods, there is the drawback that no propagated organism is available for further identification (e.g., serologic markers, or testing for antibiotic sensitivity). Also, direct detection methods may be more expensive than culture.

Serologic and Immunologic Diagnostic Methods

Although a variety of serologic methods have been used in the past to detect antibodies, the indirect immunofluorescence method, first developed by Bernkopf and then by McComb and Nichols, has been simplified and standardized in an indirect microimmunofluorescence (MIF) test by Wang and associates.[38] At present, this is the most commonly used test for evaluation of host response to trachoma or to oculogenital *C. trachomatis* agents. For LGV, the complement fixation (CF) test can be used, although the MIF test remains more sensitive and specific. The MIF test employs yolk sac–grown or cell culture–grown *C. trachomatis* of all known immunotypes as antigen. Antigen dots are placed on a slide in a specific pattern. They are attached to the slide in a diluted yolk sac suspension. Serial dilutions of serum, tears, or local secretions are applied, followed by fluorescein-conjugated antihuman globulin. An obvious advantage of the test is that the conjugate may be prepared against any immunoglobulin class, thus permitting titration of IgG-, IgM-, or IgA-specific antibody. A counterstain is added to the conjugate to permit clearer identification of specific fluorescence in the dots to which antibody-containing serum has been applied. If differentiation among antibodies to specific immunotypes is sought, the antigens can be evaluated separately. For many purposes, antigen pools can be used.

A CF test is available to measure host response to any chlamydial infection.[39] It is still the most commonly used test for psittacosis and LGV, but it is too insensitive for trachoma or oculogenital infections. Usually, the antigen for the CF is obtained from a yolk sac–grown LGV strain and is prepared by boiling and treatment with phenol.

TREATMENT AND CONTROL

WHO initiated a major effort to control blinding trachoma in 1997 as the "Global Elimination of Blinding Trachoma by 2020 (GET 2020)."[2] A nongovernmental organization, the International Trachoma Initiative (ITI) was established in 2001 to distribute azithromycin donated by Pfizer Inc. for trachoma control. The ITI assists Ministries of Health in affected countries to develop systematic national trachoma control programs.

In trachoma-endemic regions, the goal of trachoma intervention programs is the elimination of trachoma as a blinding disease. The new programs are based on four components, the SAFE strategy: surgery to correct inturned eyelids; antibiotics to eliminate the reservoir of chlamydial infection in the community and to reduce inflammation in individuals; promotion of personal hygiene, with emphasis on facial cleanliness in young children; and environmental changes to reduce transmission of trachoma through the elimination of human fecal material and provision of pure water supplies.[40]

Surgery

The surgical correction of inturned eyelids (trichiasis) from trachoma is carried out with tarsal rotation procedures.[41] In many programs, these procedures are done by trained nurses or general physicians, less frequently by ophthalmologists. Recurrent trichiasis after surgery has been observed regularly, for example, 11% after 1 year in Vietnam.[42] A comparison of surgical cases done by ophthalmologists or by trained eye care workers in Ethiopa showed no difference in the rates of recurrence at 6 months (14.6%) in the two groups.[43]

For patients blind from trachomatous corneal scarring, corneal transplant surgery has a poor outcome. The reduced flow of tears, loss of mucus from goblet cell destruction, exposure by distorted lids, and inadequate follow-up care all contribute to graft failure in such patients.

Antibiotics

The objectives of antibiotic treatment are to reduce the pool of chlamydial infection in the community and the severity of active trachoma, and thus of the risk of blindness, in individual cases. Sulfonamides, tetracyclines, erythromycin, other macrolides and azalides, and rifampin are effective against trachoma. Most control programs utilized topical tetracycline ointment from the 1950s to the mid-1990s. Antibiotic treatment in endemic communities (active trachoma in more than 20% of children) has been based on the supervised application of antibiotic to all persons in a community ("mass therapy").[20]

The advent of oral azithromycin has led to a renewed interest in trachoma control because it is effective with one to three doses and can be taken by children as young as 6 months old.[44] The compliance is very high with a single dose, and the drug is well tolerated. The new recommendation for this community treatment is azithromycin, given as a single dose (20 mg/kg body weight for children, or 1 g for adults; height can be used as a surrogate for weight in children).[40] Because Pfizer Inc. has donated oral azithromycin for trachoma control (135 million doses committed), there is no cost of this antibiotic to programs involved in trachoma control, but there are still substantial costs for distributing it to large populations.

Initial case control studies showed that oral azithromycin was as effective or better than topical oxytetracycline ointment.[44–46] A subsequent trial of village-wide oral azithromycin (1 dose weekly for 3 weeks) compared to oxytetracyline ointment (1 dose daily for 42 days) in Egypt, Tanzania, and Gambia showed a substantial reduction of chlamydial infection by both treatments, but only a modest effect on clinically active trachoma.[47] The new goal of antimicrobial treatment is the elimination of chlamydial eye infection and thus of infectious trachoma. Elimination of trachoma in one village in Tanzania was achieved by an initial azithromycin dose (94% compliance) and topical tetracycline to active cases for 18 months.[48] In practice, mass treatment is carried out in communities or regions with 10% or more active trachoma in children. It is apparent that in most of these areas about 5% of the children have trachoma-like follicular conjunctivitis that is not caused by chlamydial infection.

The evaluation of antibiotic treatment has been based on the clinical diagnosis of active trachoma. After treatment, however, clinical trachoma activity is no longer an adequate surrogate for chlamydial eye infection, because the clinical signs of disease persist after the infection has resolved.[49] To determine the need for further rounds of mass treatment, it will be necessary to test for chlamydial eye infection, preferably by one of the nucleic acid amplification tests.

Face Washing and Hygiene

Personal hygiene intervention is based on studies indicating that failure to wash the faces of young children is a significant risk factor for trachoma.[15] Face washing has been incorporated into studies of antibiotic treatment.[50]

Environment

Environmental controls include the provision of latrines to reduce fly density and provision of adequate water supplies by building wells or distribution systems.[14–16] These activities are important for community development; they are capital intensive and do not have an immediate effect on infectious trachoma.[51]

REFERENCES

1. Thylefors B, Negrel AD, Pararajasegaram R, et al: Global data on blindness. Bull World Health Org 73:115, 1995.
2. Mariotti S: New steps toward eliminating blinding trachoma. N Engl J Med 351:2004, 2004.
3. Moulder JW: Order Chlamydiales and family Chlamydiaceae. In Krieg NR (ed): Manual of Systematic Bacteriology, Vol. 1. Baltimore, Williams & Wilkins, 1984, p 729.
4. Grayston JT, Campbell LA, Kuo CC, et al: A new respiratory tract pathogen: *Chlamydia pneumoniae* strain TWAR. J Infect Dis 161:618, 1990.
5. Moulder JW: Intracellular parasitism: Life in an extreme environment. J Infect Dis 130:300, 1974.
6. Wang SP, Grayston JT: Three new serovars of *Chlamydia trachomatis*: Da, Ia, and L2a. J Infect Dis 163:403, 1991.
7. Stothard DR, Toth GA, Batteiger BE: Polymorphic membrane protein H has evolved in parallel with the three disease-causing groups of *Chlamydia trachomatis*. Infect Immun 71:1200, 2003.
8. Caldwell HD, Wood H, Crane D, et al: Polymorphisms in *Chlamydia trachomatis* tryptophan synthase genes differentiate between genital and ocular isolates. J Clin Invest 111:1757, 2003.
9. Nurminen M, Leinonen M, Saikku P, et al: The genus-specific antigen of *Chlamydia*: Resemblance to the lipopolysaccharide of enteric bacteria. Science 220:1279, 1983.
10. Caldwell HD, Kromhout J, Schachter J: Purification and partial characterization of the major outer membrane protein of *Chlamydia trachomatis*. Infect Immun 31:1161, 1981.
11. Stephens RS, Wagar EA, Schoolnik GK: High-resolution mapping of serovar-specific and common antigenic determinants of the major outer membrane protein of *Chlamydia trachomatis*. J Exp Med 167:817, 1988.
12. Zhang YX, Stewart SJ, Caldwell HD: Protective monoclonal antibodies to *Chlamydia trachomatis* serovar- and serogroup-specific major outer membrane protein determinants. Infect Immun 57:636, 1989.
13. Courtright P, Sheppard J, Schachter J, et al: Trachoma and blindness in the Nile Delta: Current patterns and projections for the future in the rural Egyptian population. Br J Ophthalmol 73:536, 1989.
14. Courtright P, Sheppard J, Lane S, et al: Latrine ownership as a protective factor in inflammatory trachoma in Egypt. Br J Ophthalmol 75:322, 1991.
15. West SK, Congdon N, Katala S, et al: Facial cleanliness and risk of trachoma in families. Arch Ophthalmol 109:855, 1991.
16. Jones BR: The prevention of blindness from trachoma. Trans Ophthalmol Soc UK 95:16, 1975.
17. Emerson PM, Lindsay SW, Alexander N, et al: Role of flies and provision of latrines in trachoma control: Cluster-randomized controlled trial. Lancet 363:1093, 2004.
18. Miller K, Pakpour N, Yi E, et al: Pesky trachoma suspect finally caught. Brit J Ophthalmol 88:750, 2004.
19. Malaty R, Zaki S, Said ME, et al: Extraocular infections in children in areas with endemic trachoma. J Infect Dis 143:853, 1981.
20. Dawson CR, Jones BR, Tarizzo ML: A Guide to Trachoma Control. Geneva, World Health Organization, 1981.
21. Dawson CR, Juster R, Marx R, et al: Limbal disease in trachoma and other ocular chlamydial infections: Risk factors for corneal vascularisation. Eye 3(Pt 2):204, 1989.
22. Thylefors B, Dawson CR, Jones BR, et al: A simple system for the assessment of trachoma and its complications. Bull World Health Org 65:477, 1987.
23. al-Rajhi AA, Hidayat A, Nasr A, et al: The histopathology and the mechanism of entropion in patients with trachoma. Ophthalmology 100:1293, 1993.
24. Taylor HR, Prendergast RA, Dawson CR, et al: An animal model for cicatrizing trachoma. Invest Ophthalmol Vis Sci 21:422, 1981.
25. Duke-Elder S: System of Ophthalmology, Vol. 8. London, Henry Kingston, 1963.
26. Yoneda C, Dawson CR, Daghfous T, et al: Cytology as a guide to the presence of chlamydial inclusions in Giemsa-stained conjunctival smears in severe endemic trachoma. Br J Ophthalmol 59:116, 1975.
27. Schachter J, Moncada J, Dawson CR, et al: Nonculture methods for diagnosing chlamydial infection in patients with trachoma: A clue to the pathogenesis of the disease? J Infect Dis 158:1347, 1988.
28. T'ang F-F, Chang H-L, Huang Y-T, et al: Studies on the etiology of trachoma with special reference to isolation of the virus in chick embryo. Chin Med J 75:429, 1957.
29. Bobo L, Munoz B, Viscidi R, et al: Diagnosis of *Chlamydia trachomatis* eye infection in Tanzania by polymerase chain reaction/enzyme immunoassay. Lancet 338:847, 1991.
30. Schachter J, Stamm WE, Quinn TC, et al: Ligase chain reaction to detect *Chlamydia trachomatis* infection of the cervix. J Clin Microbiol 32:2540, 1994.
31. Gordon FB, Harper IA, Quan AL, et al: Detection of *Chlamydia (Bedsonia)* in certain infections of man. I. Laboratory procedures: Comparison of yolk sac and cell culture for detection and isolation. J Infect Dis 120:451, 1969.
32. Ripa KT, Mardh PA: Cultivation of *Chlamydia trachomatis* in cycloheximide-treated McCoy cells. J Clin Microbiol 6:328, 1977.
33. Stamm WE: Diagnosis of *Chlamydia trachomatis* genitourinary infections. Ann Intern Med 108:710, 1988.
34. Clarke LM, Sierra MF, Daidone BJ, et al: Comparison of the Syva Micro Trak enzyme immunoassay and Gen-Probe PACE 2 with cell culture for diagnosis of cervical *Chlamydia trachomatis* infection in a high-prevalence female population. J Clin Microbiol 31:968, 1993.
35. Bobo L, Coutlee F, Yolken RH, et al: Diagnosis of *Chlamydia trachomatis* cervical infection by amplified DNA with an enzyme immunoassay. J Clin Microbiol 28:1968, 1990.
36. Jaschek G, Gaydos CA, Welsh LE, et al: Direct detection of *Chlamydia trachomatis* in urine specimens from symptomatic and asymptomatic men by using a rapid polymerase chain reaction assay. J Clin Microbiol 31:1209, 1993.
37. Chernesky MA, Lee H, Schachter J, et al: Diagnosis of *Chlamydia trachomatis* urethral infection in symptomatic and asymptomatic men by testing first-void urine in a ligase chain reaction assay. J Infect Dis 170:1308, 1994.
38. Wang S-P, Kuo CC, Grayston JT: A simplified method for immunological typing of trachoma-inclusion conjunctivitis-lymphogranuloma venereum organisms. Infect Immun 7:356, 1973.
39. Schachter J: Chlamydiae. In Noel R, Conway de Marcario E, Fahey JL, et al (eds): Manual of Clinical Laboratory Immunology, 4th ed. Washington, DC, American Society for Microbiology, 1992, p 661.
40. Mecaskey JW, Knirsch, CA, Kumaresan JA, et al: The possibility of eliminating blinding trachoma. Lancet Infect Dis 3:728, 2003.
41. Reacher MH, Munoz B, Alghassany A, et al: A controlled trial of surgery for trachomatous trichiasis of the upper lid. Arch Ophthalmol 110:667, 1992.
42. Thanh TT, Khandekar R, Luong VQ, et al: One year recurrence of trachomatous trichiasis in routinely operated Cuenod Nataf procedure cases in Vietman. Brit J Ophthalmol 88:1114, 2004.
43. Alemayehu W, Melese M, Bejiga A, et al: Surgery for trichiasis by ophthalmologists versus integrated eye care workers: A randomized trial. Ophthalmology 111:578, 2004.
44. Bailey RL, Arullendran P, Whittle HC, et al: Randomised controlled trial of single-dose azithromycin in treatment of trachoma. Lancet 342:453, 1993.
45. Tabbara KF, Abu-el-Asrar A, al-Omar O, et al: Single-dose azithromycin in the treatment of trachoma. A randomized, controlled study. Ophthalmology 103:842, 1996.
46. Dawson CR, Schachter J, Sallam S, et al: A comparison of oral azithromycin with topical oxytetracycline/polymycin for the treatment of trachoma in children. Clin Infect Dis 24:363, 1997.
47. Schachter J, West SK, Mabey D, et al: Azithromycin in control of trachoma. Lancet 354:630, 1999.
48. Solomon AW, Holland MJ, Alexander ND, et al: Mass treatment with a single-dose of azithromycin for trachoma. N Engl J Med 351:1962, 2004.
49. Bird M, Dawson CR, Schachter J, et al: Does the diagnosis of trachoma adequately identify ocular chlamydial infection in trachoma-endemic areas? J Infect Dis 187:1669, 2003.
50. West S, Munoz B, Lynch M, et al: Impact of face-washing on trachoma in Kongwa, Tanzania. Lancet 345:155, 1995.
51. Kuper H, Solomon AW, Buchan J, et al: A critical review of the SAFE strategy for the prevention of blinding trachoma. Lancet Infect Dis 3:372, 2003.

48

Chlamydia trachomatis *Infections of the Genital Tract (Oculogenital Infections and Lymphogranuloma Venereum)*

RONALD C. BALLARD
JOHN R. PAPP

INTRODUCTION

Chlamydia trachomatis is primarily a human pathogen associated with medically important oculogenital infections. They are classified under the order Chlamydiales and family Chlamydiaceae. A proposal to separate members of the family Chlamydiaceae into two genera, *Chlamydia* and *Chlamydophila,*[1] has not been widely accepted by many workers in the field.[2] This reclassification would largely affect *C. pneumoniae,* which causes respiratory infections in man, and *C. psittaci,* which causes a variety of infections relevant to veterinary medicine, some of which are known zoonotic agents. There have been no proposed changes to the taxonomic classification of *C. trachomatis* associated with human infections. This chapter deals exclusively with those infections of the genital tract caused by *C. trachomatis*.

Diseases caused by *C. trachomatis* have been recognized since ancient times. Trachoma, the blinding eye disease, which is spread from eye to eye, was known in China in the 27th century BC, while its complications were described in Egypt in the Ebers papyrus as early as the 19th century BC (see Chapter 47).[3] Although the communicable nature of the disease was obvious to early workers, the etiologic agent was not demonstrated until 1907 when Halberstaedter and Prowazek[4] succeeded in infecting orangutans with material obtained from the eyes of trachoma patients. They described intracytoplasmic inclusion bodies in conjunctival epithelial cells from infected animals and maintained that the small granules they saw within the inclusions represented the etiologic agent.[4] They later demonstrated similar inclusion bodies in epithelial cells obtained from trachoma patients. Similar inclusion bodies were subsequently found in cases of nongonococcal ophthalmia neonatorum and in the cervix of the mother and the urethra of the father of a baby who presented with an eye infection, and in urethral scrapings from a number of men with nongonococcal urethritis (NGU).[5,6]

Meanwhile, an infection of the inguinal lymph nodes (climatic bubo), frequently seen in the tropics, was first recognized as a sexually transmitted disease (STD) by Rost in 1912,[7] while a similar disease, lymphogranuloma inguinale, had been well documented in more temperate climates.[8] Subsequently, these two diseases were found to be identical, a situation that had long been suspected on both clinical and pathologic grounds.

In many respects, investigations to determine the cause of the disease now called lymphogranuloma venereum (LGV) mirror those previously described for trachoma and other chlamydial infections of the genital tract. Thus, in the early 1920s, both Gamna[9] and Favre[10] described intracytoplasmic inclusion bodies in material obtained from patients with LGV, and Gamna also found them in guinea pigs previously inoculated with pus obtained from human cases.[11] In 1930, Hellerstrom and Wassen[12] succeeded in transmitting the infection to monkeys by intracerebral inoculation, which resulted in the development of meningoencephalitis. Soon afterward, mice were infected by the same route, and lesions similar to those seen in humans were produced in monkeys and marmosets.[13]

A close relationship between these organisms and the causative agent of psittacosis was suggested in 1942 when sera from patients with trachoma or inclusion conjunctivitis were found to fix complement in the presence of LGV and psittacosis antigen.[14] These organisms were initially grouped together as the PLT (psittacosis-lymphogranuloma-trachoma) group of atypical "viruses" and later as chlamydial organisms.

AGENT

Developmental Cycle

Chlamydiae are obligate intracellular bacteria with a unique biphasic life cycle (Fig. 48-1). The cycle is initiated by the attachment of an infectious elementary body to the surface of a susceptible cell. The mechanism by which chlamydiae attach to the host cell has not been fully elucidated, though electrostatic and receptor interactions have been postulated.[15,16] Once attached, the metabolically inactive elementary body (approximate size: 350 nm in diameter) enters the cell by phagocytosis, but the resulting phagocytic vacuole does not fuse with primary lysosomes. The prevention of lysosomal fusion is thought to be mediated by chlamydial surface antigens and dependent on the presence of living elementary bodies, since heat-killed or antibody-treated organisms are rapidly sequestered into phagolysosomes.[17] While in the phagocytic vacuole, the elementary body remains intact and undergoes reorganization to form, within 8 hours, what is known as the initial or reticulate body. This is a much larger (800–1000 nm in diameter) metabolically active particle that is unable to survive outside the host cell, but can replicate by binary fission to produce

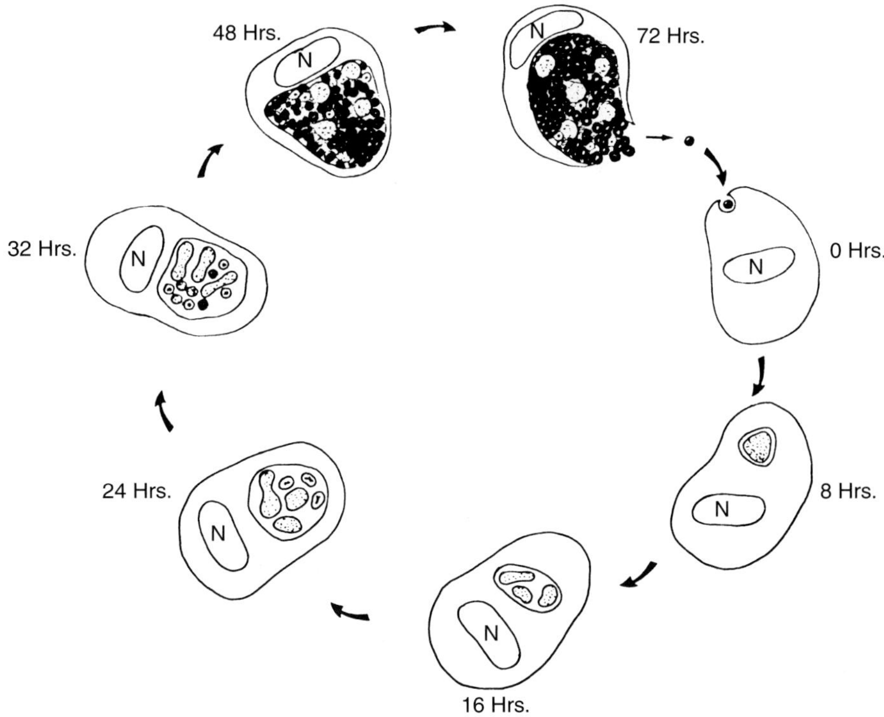

FIGURE 48-1 Schematic representation of the chlamydial developmental cycle. 0 hour: ingestion; 8 hours: reorganization into reticulate body; 16 to 24 hours: multiplication of reticulate bodies; 32 to 48 hours: multiplication and reorganization into elementary bodies; 72 hours: release of elementary bodies. N, cell nucleus.

further reticulate bodies. After approximately 20 hours, the inclusion, which has formed in the cytoplasm of the host cell, contains numerous reticulate bodies. Thereafter, reorganization of these particles to form elementary bodies occurs on a 1:1 basis. By 40 hours post infection, the inclusion contains large numbers of mature elementary bodies and a smaller number of reticulate bodies that are continuing to undergo division and reorganization. An increase in chlamydial infectivity associated with further production of elementary bodies continues until 48 to 72 hours post infection, when lysis of the host cell takes place and liberation of the contents of the mature inclusion occurs. The chlamydial development cycle thus takes approximately 2 to 3 days to complete. However, there is some variation as LGV strains generally have shorter development cycles than *C. trachomatis* strains associated with ocular and genital infections.

Subtypes of *Chlamydia trachomatis*

Chlamydiae are antigenically complex, possessing antigens that demonstrate specificity at the genus, species, and subspecies levels. Antigenic cross-reactivity, as measured by the indirect microimmunofluorescence test,[18] has been used to classify isolates of *C. trachomatis* into 15 serovars (Table 48-1). The serovars are usually, but not exclusively, associated with distinct chlamydial infections; thus serovars A through C have generally been associated with hyperendemic trachoma, serovars D through K with oculogenital infections, while the L serovars have been associated with LGV.[19] These serovar-specific epitopes reside largely within two domains in the major outer membrane protein (MOMP) of the organism,[20] whereas the immunodominant genus-specific epitope is associated with the heat-stable lipopolysaccharide.

Table 48-1 Human Diseases Caused by Chlamydiae

Species	Biovars	Disease
C. trachomatis	A, B, Ba, C	Hyperendemic blinding trachoma
	D-K	Acute urethritis, cervicitis
		Adult and neonatal conjunctivitis
		Salpingitis, proctitis, epididymitis, Reiter's disease
		Neonatal pneumonia
	L_1, L_2, + L_3	Lymphogranuloma venereum
		Proctocolitis
C. psittaci	Many, uncharacterized	Pneumonia, endocarditis, abortion
C. pneumoniae	? Only one	Community-acquired pneumonia
		Bronchitis
		? Circulatory disease

As expected, polymorphisms within the gene that encodes the MOMP, *ompA*, parallel the designations assigned by seovar analysis.[21] Genotype determination has proven to be useful in epidemiologic studies since it can be accomplished directly from clinical specimens without the need to isolate the organism.[22] The *ompA* polymorphisms provide a higher level of discrimination by identifying variants within the parent genotype. These variants may be useful in determining sexual networks and assessing the impact on immune selection.

DISEASE

Oculogenital Infections

In terms of their clinical manifestations, genital infections caused by serovars D through K of *C. trachomatis* closely parallel those caused by *Neisseria gonorrhoeae*, since they share the same cell target, namely, columnar epithelial cells. However, generally, infections caused by *C. trachomatis* tend to produce milder symptoms than those caused by *N. gonorrhoeae*, probably because *C. trachomatis* infection elicits a less severe acute inflammatory reaction.

Infections of the Genital Tract in Men

Chlamydial infection of the urethra results in the development of NGU. *C. trachomatis* is the causative agent in approximately 50% of cases of NGU, while other possible causes include *Mycoplasma genitalium* and *Ureaplasma urealyticum*. Clinically, chlamydia-positive and chlamydia-negative NGU cannot be differentiated on the basis of signs or symptoms. The incubation period of NGU (including chlamydial urethritis) is longer than that of gonorrhoea, varying from 1 to 3 weeks in the majority of cases, and the onset of symptoms of NGU is more insidious. These symptoms include dysuria, appearance of a clear or white urethral discharge, and occasionally frequency of micturition. Many patients may be asymptomatic or minimally symptomatic, which results in prolonged periods when they may be infectious to their sexual partner. Despite these mild manifestations, it is often difficult to differentiate between gonococcal and chlamydial infections on clinical grounds alone and, indeed, the two infections may coexist in up to 30% of cases of acute gonococcal urethritis.[23] *C. trachomatis* is also a frequent cause of postgonococcal urethritis (PGU), which follows treatment (normally single dose) of mixed gonococcal-chlamydial infections with an antibiotic that is active against *N. gonorrhoeae* but not against *C. trachomatis*. In industrialized societies, PGU is usually symptomatic, but in the developing world, the majority of cases are apparently either asymptomatic or minimally symptomatic.[24]

C. trachomatis, along with *N. gonorrhoeae*, has emerged as a major cause of acute epididymitis in sexually active young men. Chlamydiae were initially isolated from epididymal aspirates obtained from patients in the United States who were all under 35 years of age and who presented with concomitant urethritis. This contrasted with the findings in older men who did not present with urethritis and from whom only gram-negative bacilli could be isolated.[25] Studies of the role of *C. trachomatis* in the etiology of acute epididymitis in mineworkers in South Africa have also indicated that chlamydial infection is probably more important than gonococcal infection as a cause of this complication in developing societies.[24] In contrast, a role for *C. trachomatis* in the etiology of chronic abacterial prostatitis remains speculative despite the proven link between *N. gonorrhoeae* and acute bacterial prostatitis.[26]

Infections of the Genital Tract in Women

The endocervix is the most common site of infection with *C. trachomatis* in women. In many cases, the infection may be completely asymptomatic. However, those with symptoms may complain of vaginal discharge, dysuria, or lower abdominal pain. On examination, the cervix may appear normal or may be severely eroded with follicular hypertrophy and an associated mucopurulent endocervical discharge. Likewise, chlamydial infection of the urethra in women may either be asymptomatic or associated with urethral symptoms such as dysuria and frequency. *C. trachomatis* has been implicated in over 60% of cases of the so-called acute urethral syndrome in women. The infection is characterized by the presence of urethral symptoms together with a sterile pyuria.[27]

Ascending spread of *C. trachomatis* from the endocervical canal to the endometrium, fallopian tubes, and peritoneal cavity is the most serious complication of both asymptomatic and symptomatic chlamydial infection in women. The organism is capable of inducing a plasma cell endometritis, acute and chronic salpingitis, and full-blown peritonitis with associated perihepatitis (Fitz-Hugh–Curtis syndrome) and periappendicitis. Infected pregnant women are at risk of developing late postpartum endometritis. Resolution of these upper genital tract infections may result in chronic pelvic pain, tubal infertility, or ectopic pregnancy. However, a body of evidence has accumulated that the majority of cases of chlamydial salpingitis are symptom-free and that these cases of so-called "silent PID" may contribute significantly to tubal infertility.[28]

Other Infections in Adults

C. trachomatis may cause a proctitis and pharyngitis in both men and women, and accidental inoculation of the eye may result in the development of adult inclusion conjunctivitis. *C. trachomatis* may be associated with 50% of cases of sexually acquired reactive arthritis (SARA) by acting as a trigger to precipitate the disease in genetically predisposed (HLA-B27-positive) persons.[29] In a few cases, the urethritis and arthritis may be accompanied by both the conjunctivitis and the mucocutaneous lesions classically associated with Reiter's disease.

Neonatal Chlamydial Infections

Neonatal inclusion conjunctivitis has long been recognized as the result of an infection transmitted from mothers to their babies during passage through the birth canal. With the advent of sensitive tissue culture techniques, it became apparent that some babies delivered vaginally through an infected cervix developed a mucopurulent conjunctivitis. The onset of the disease is generally insidious, following an incubation period of 1 to 3 weeks. Hyperemia, chemosis, and a discharge that becomes progressively purulent are the most prominent features of the infection. However, lymphoid follicles, which are characteristically found in adult chlamydial infections of the eye, are notably absent unless the infection persists for more

tuberculosis, since an adenosine deaminase level of greater than 43 IU/L in pleural fluid is believed to be sensitive and specific for tuberculosis.

PATHOGENESIS AND IMMUNITY

Human infection with *Chlamydia psittaci* follows inhalation of contaminated aerosols shed by infected birds. The mechanism whereby *C. psittaci* is introduced into a flock of birds is poorly understood. Many investigators think that wild birds, which can be infected by the same strains as domestic flocks, play a major role in this process.[25] It is likely that vertical transmission occurs in flocks.[25]

In turkeys *C. psittaci* infects epithelial cells and macrophages in the respiratory tract.[26] This is followed by septicemia and localization of the organisms in epithelial cells and macrophages in various organs.[26] It is still unclear whether humoral or cell-mediated immunity is the most important host defense against *C. psittaci*. The major outer membrane protein (MOMP) has been identified as a protective antigen.[27,28] Plasmid DNA expressing *C. psittaci* serovar A MOMP was used to vaccinate turkeys and was shown to be effective.[29]

DIAGNOSIS

A high index of suspicion is necessary to make the diagnosis of psittacosis. Confirmation is by serologic test—the microimmunofluorescence test is more sensitive and species-specific than the complement fixation test (CF). *C. psittaci* may also be isolated in tissue culture, but most laboratories do not have the capability of cultivating chlamydiae. An antibody titer of 1:64 by the CF test is considered diagnostic. A fourfold rise in titer is also diagnostic. The CF test is genus-specific and does not distinguish *C. trachomatis* from *C. pneumoniae* or *C. psittaci* infection. *C. psittaci* DNA can be detected in respiratory secretions using polymerase chain reaction. Wong and associates[30] studied 78 patients in whom a diagnosis of psittacosis was made on the basis of appropriate clinical symptoms following exposure to sick birds. The CF test identified 36 of 78 (46%) as positive, while the microimmunofluorescence (MIF) test identified 48 of 78 (61%). The investigators used eight strains of *C. psittaci* in the MIF test. Others have noted that the MIF test can be falsely negative.[20] Thus, more than one strain of *C. psittaci* should be used in the MIF test. Wong and coworkers[30] noted four serologic reaction patterns among their 78 patients: (1) positive CF and MIF tests (46%), (2) anticomplementary or negative CF test and positive MIF test (15%), (3) positive serologic response to *C. pneumoniae* (9%), and (4) negative antibody titer using both CF and MIF tests (29%).

TREATMENT AND PROGNOSIS

Treatment is with tetracycline or doxycycline for 10 to 21 days.[2] Response to treatment is usually prompt. Some patients have severe fatigue that persists for 2 to 3 months following resolution of the acute illness. A longer course of treatment has been recommended to prevent relapse. Erythromycin is an alternative to treatment with a tetracycline but may be less efficacious in severe cases. There is less than a 1% mortality rate in treated cases.

PREVENTION AND CONTROL

Infected birds should be treated with tetracycline, chlortetracycline, or doxycycline for at least 45 days. Ideally, all imported birds should be treated prophylactically for *C. psittaci*. The Centers for Disease Control and Prevention has issued recommendations for the control of *C. psittaci* among humans and birds, and these should be used when ever a case of psittacosis is encountered. All cases of psittacosis should be reported to a medical officer of public health for appropriate follow-up and tracing of infected birds.[31]

REFERENCES

1. Harris RL, Williams TW: Contribution to the question of pneumotyphus: a discussion of the original article by J. Ritter in 1880. Rev Infect Dis 7:119, 1985.
2. Macfarlane JT, Macrae AD: Psittacosis. Br Med Bull 39:163, 1983.
3. Kaltenboeck B, Kousoulas KG, Storz J: Structures of and allelic diversity and relationships among the major outer membrane protein (*ompA*) genes of the four chlamydial species. J Bacteriol 175:487, 1993.
4. Buttery RB, Wreighitt TG: Outbreak of psittacosis associated with a cockatiel. Lancet 2:742, 1987.
5. Maffei C, Ditanislao F, Pausi P, et al: Psittacosis of non-avian origin. Lancet 2:806, 1984.
6. Beer RJ, Bradford WP, Hart RJ: Pregnancy complicated by psittacosis acquired from sheep. BMJ 284:1156, 1982.
7. Regan RJ, Datnan JRE, Treharne JD: Infective endocarditis with glomerulonephritis associated with cat chlamydia (*C. psittaci*) infection. Br Heart J 42:349, 1979.
8. van Buuren CE, Dorrestein GM, van Dijk JE: *Chlamydia psittaci* infections in birds: a review in the pathogenesis and histopathological features. Vet Q 16:38, 1994.
9. Esposito AL: Pulmonary infections acquired in the workplace: a review of occupation associated pneumonia. Clin Chest Med 13:355, 1992.
10. Lardner AJ, Lett S, Harvey E, et al: Human psittacosis linked to a bird distributor in Mississippi—Massachusetts and Tennessee 1992. MMWR 41:794, 1992.
11. Helm CW, Smart GE, Cumming AD, et al: Sheep-associated severe *Chlamydia psittaci* infection in pregnancy. Int J Gynaecol Obstet 28:369, 1989.
12. Yung AP, Grayson ML: Psittacosis: a review of 135 cases. Med J Aust 148:228, 1988.
13. Semel JD: Cutaneous findings in a case of psittacosis. Arch Dermatol 120:1227, 1984.
14. Shee CD: Cerebellar disturbance in psittacosis. Postgrad Med J 64:382, 1988.
15. Mason AB, Jenkins P: Acute renal failure in fulminant psittacosis. Respir Med 88:239, 1994.
16. Day CJ, Fawcett IW: Psittacosis and acute thrombocytopenic purpura. J R Soc Med 85:360, 1992.
17. Tsapas G, Klonizakis I, Casakos K, et al: Psittacosis and arthritis. Chemotherapy 37:143, 1991.
18. Wong KF, Chan JKC, Chan CH, et al: Psittacosis-associated hemophagocytic syndrome. Am J Med 91:204, 1991.
19. Murray HW, Twazon CU: Atypical pneumonias. Med Clin North Am 64:507, 1980.
20. Gherman RB, Leventis LL, Miller RC: Chlamydial psittacosis during pregnancy: a case report. Obstet Gynecol 86:648, 1995.
21. Verweij PE, Meis JFGM, Eijk R, et al: Severe human psittacosis requiring artificial ventilation: case report and review. Clin Infect Dis 20:440, 1995.
22. Macfarlane JT, Miller AC, Roderick Smith WH, et al: Comparative radiographic features of community-acquired legionnaires' disease, pneumococcal pneumonia, mycoplasma pneumonia and psittacosis. Thorax 39:28, 1984.
23. Coutts H, MacKenzie S, White RJ: Clinical and radiographic features of psittacosis infection. Thorax 40:530, 1985.
24. Orriols R, Munoz X, Drobnic Z, et al: High adenosine deaminase activity in pleural effusion due to psittacosis. Chest 101:881, 1992.

25. Andersen AA, Vanrompay D: Avian chlamydiosis. Rev Sci Tech 19:396, 2000.
26. Vanrompay D, Mast J, Ducatelle R, et al: *Chlamydia psittaci* infections in turkeys: pathogenesis of infection in avian serovar A, B and D. Vet Microbiol 47:245, 1995.
27. Hatch TP, Vance DW, Al-Hossainey E: Identification of a major envelope protein in *Chlamydia* species. J Bacteriol 146:426, 1981.
28. Caldwell HD, Kromhout J, Schachter J: Purification and characterization of the major outer membrane protein of *Chlamydia trachomatis*. Infect Immun 31:1161, 1981.
29. Vanrompay D, Cox E, Volckaert G, et al: Turkeys are protected from infection with *Chlamydia psittaci* by plasmid DNA vaccination against the major outer membrane protein. Clin Exp Immunol 118:49, 1999.
30. Wong KH, Skelton SK, Daugharty H: Utility of complement fixation and microimmunofluorescence assays for detecting serologic responses in persons with clinically diagnosed psittacosis. J Clin Microbiol 32:2417, 1994.
31. Centers for Disease Control: Compendium of measures to control *Chlamydia psittaci* infection among humans (psittacosis) and birds (avian chlamydiosis). MMWR 49:1, 2000.

50

Spotted Fever Group Rickettsioses

DANIEL J. SEXTON
DAVID H. WALKER

INTRODUCTION

Rickettsia species of the spotted fever group (SFG) cause human diseases in tropical Africa, Asia, Australia, South America, Central America, and Mexico. During the past decade, several new rickettsial diseases have been discovered (e.g., tick-associated lymphadenopathy and flea-borne spotted fever), and the recognized geographic range of known rickettsial diseases such as rickettsialpox has expanded from urban to suburban and rural areas, and African tick bite fever and Japanese spotted fever to new countries. Rickettsial infections are often neglected and are poorly recognized by physicians in many tropical and subtropical locations. Indeed, despite a number of recent reports describing rickettsial diseases in new locations or the discovery of new rickettsiae, medical science has focused insufficient efforts in the diagnosis and antimicrobial treatment of rickettsial infections in subtropical and tropical areas, and thus it is likely that much remains to be discovered.

ORGANISMS

Rickettsiae are small (0.3 × 1.0 μm) obligately intracellular bacteria with a gram-negative cell wall that reside free in the cytosol of human endothelial cells and various cells of their arthropod hosts. The family Rickettsiaceae contains the genera *Rickettsia* and *Orientia*. The genus *Rickettsia* is divided into the typhus and spotted fever groups on the basis of antigenic differences in the immunodominant lipopolysaccharides (LPS) the presence of outer membrane protein A (OmpA) in SFG rickettsiae, and evolutionary genetic relationships.[1] OmpA serves as an adhesin and contains a series of hydrophilic tandem repeat units that vary in number and order, and OmpB, also an adhesin, is a 135-kD S-layer protein, which is the processed form of a 168-kD precursor.[2–6] Species- and strain-specific epitopes are located on these proteins.[7–10] Molecular approaches to the taxonomy of *Rickettsia* species reveal very close genetic relationships that in other genera such as *Orientia* would lump many of these organisms into a smaller number of named species.[11,12] For example, *R. africae* and *R. parkeri* show minimal differences as do *R. japonica* and the proposed new species "*R. heilongjiangiensis*."[13,14] The genetic conservatism of these bacteria may be explained by their intracellular location and prolonged survival in arthropod hosts mitigating immune selective pressure. Rickettsiae have gone through remarkable gene reduction with a genome as small as 1.1 Mb and rely upon the cytosolic environment and their effective transport systems for amino acids, phosphorylated sugars, and ATP as well as utilizing their own metabolic enzymes. Approximately one-half of the known species of SFG rickettsiae cause disease in humans; the remainder have been isolated only from arthropods. Species of SFG rickettsiae known to cause human disease include *R. rickettsii, R. conorii, R. africae, R. australis, R. sibirica, R. japonica, R. honei, R. parkeri, R. slovaca, R. felis, R. aeschlimannii*, and *R. akari*.

During the first decade of the 20th century, a young American investigator, Howard Ricketts, discovered that ticks were vectors of a then mysterious illness known as Rocky Mountain spotted fever (RMSF), that the causative organism (which he isolated in guinea pigs) circulated in nature between ticks and mammals, and that infected ticks transmitted the causative organism to their progeny.[15] Ricketts's discoveries paved the way for later investigators, who discovered other rickettsial diseases occurring between the tropics of Capricorn and Cancer, which are the focus of this chapter.

EPIDEMIOLOGY

Although SFG rickettsioses were identified in some tropical countries in the first half of the 20th century—*R. conorii* (Tunisia, Kenya, South Africa, India), *R. rickettsii* (Mexico, Colombia, Brazil), and *R. australis* (Australia)—in general, rickettsiology had scarcely investigated these parts of the world.[16–20] Recently, investigations using powerful and sensitive molecular tools have identified a myriad of varieties of SFG rickettsiae in patients and arthropods associated with disease in many parts of the world, including *R. africae, R. parkeri, R. honei, R. japonica, R. felis, R. sibirica* (mongolotimoniae strain), *R. slovaca*, and *R. aeschlimannii*.[21–23] The geographic distribution of the rickettsiae is not as narrowly focal as was believed; for example, *R. sibirica* strains cause disease in Asia, Europe, and Africa; *R. africae*/*R. parkeri* strains in Africa, Eurasia, North and South America; and *R. honei* in southern Australia and Thailand.[24,25] In some instances, such as *R. felis*, which is maintained transovarially in cat fleas that have been distributed throughout the world in felines, or *R. akari* that is maintained transovarially in mites carried by domestic mice, a worldwide distribution can be explained. Others rely upon unproven hypotheses such as transportation of infected ticks on migratory birds.

SFG rickettsiae are associated mainly with ticks, with the exceptions of *R. akari* (*Liponyssoides sanguineus*, mites) and *R. felis* (*Ctenocephalides felis*, cat fleas; Table 50-1). The geographic distribution of the *Rickettsia* is determined largely by

Table 50-1 Epidemiology of Spotted Fever Group Rickettsioses Listed in Order of Decreasing Clinical Severity

Agent	Disease	Geographic Distribution	Maintenance in Nature	Human Transmission
R. rickettsii	Rocky Mountain spotted fever, Brazilian spotted fever	North and South America	Transovarial maintenance in *Dermacentor, Rhipicephalus*, and *Amblyomma* ticks; less extensive horizontal transmission from tick to mammal to tick	Tick bite
R. conorii	Boutonneuse fever, Mediterranean spotted fever, Kenya tick typhus, Israeli spotted fever, Indian tick typhus, Astrakhan spotted fever	Mediterranean basin, Africa, Asia	Transovarial maintenance in *Rhipicephalus* ticks	Tick bite
R. sibirica	North Asian tick typhus	Russia, China, Mongolia, Pakistan, Kazakhstan, Kirgiziya, Tadzhikistan, France, Niger, Mali, South Africa	Transovarial maintenance in *Dermacentor*, *Haemaphysalis*, and *Hyalomma* ticks; horizontal transmission from tick to mammal to tick	Tick bite
R. japonica	Japanese spotted fever	Japan, China	Presumably a transovarial tick host	Tick bite
R. australis	Queensland tick typhus	Eastern Australia	Transovarial transmission in *Ixodes* ticks	Tick bite
R. akari	Rickettsialpox	United States, Ukraine, Croatia, possibly worldwide	Transovarial transmission in *Liponyssoides sanguineus* mites; horizontal transmission from mite to mouse to mite	Mite bite
R. honei	Flinders Island spotted fever	Southern Australia, Thailand	Transovarial transmission in *Aponomma* ticks	Tick bite
R. africae/R. parkeri	African tick bite fever	Sub-Saharan Africa, Caribbean, North and South America	Transovarial maintenance in *Amblyomma* ticks	Tick bite
R. felis	Flea-borne spotted fever	North and South America, Africa, Europe, presumably worldwide	Transovarial transmission in *Ctenocephalides felis* fleas	Unknown
R. slovaca	Tick-borne lymphadenopathy; *Dermacentor*-borne necrosis, eschar, lymphadenopathy	Europe	Transovarian transmission in *Dermacentor* ticks	Tick bite
R. aeschlimannii	Not named	Southern Europe, Africa	Presumably transovarian transmission in *Hyalomma* ticks	Tick bite

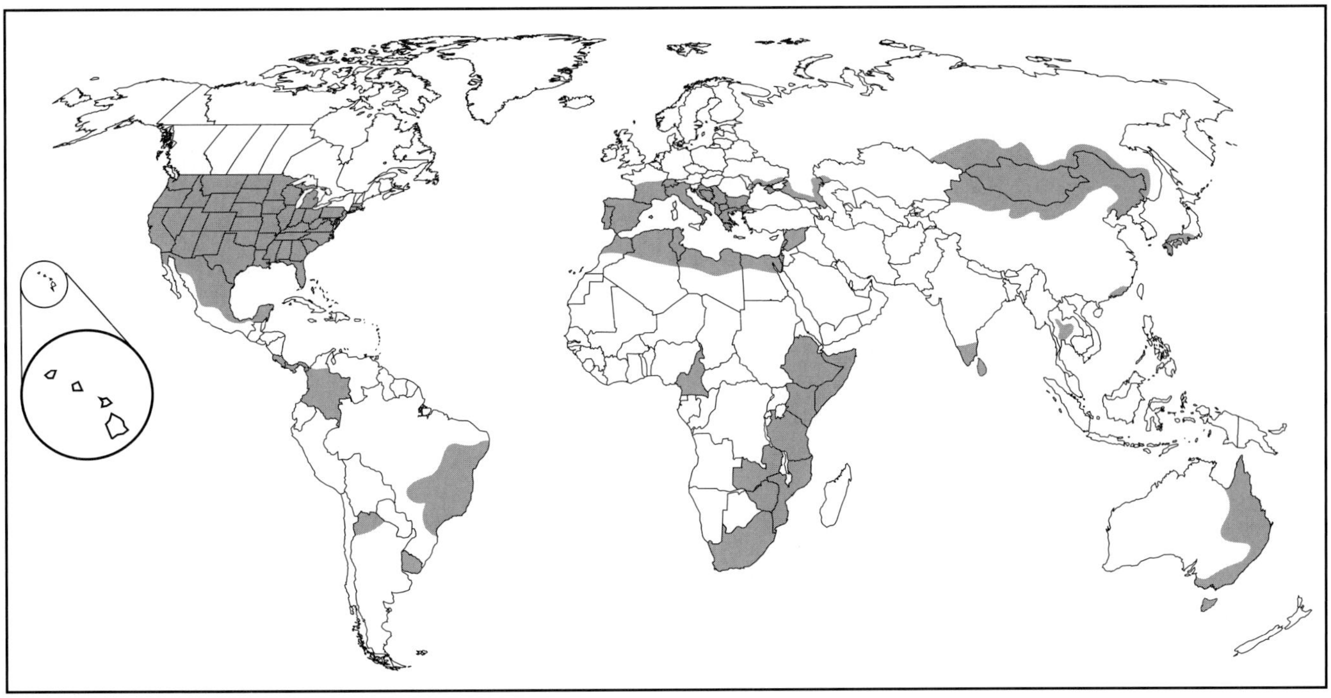

Rickettsiae of the Spotted Fever Group

that of its arthropod host in which vertical transovarian transmission from one generation to the next is the major mechanism of maintenance in nature.[26] Highly pathogenic bacteria such as *R. rickettsii* have a deleterious effect on their tick host resulting in death of the infected tick lineage after several generations of transovarian passage.[27] This harmful interaction correlates with a low prevalence (less than one *R. rickettsii*-infected *Dermacentor* tick per 1000 ticks) even in endemic regions.[28] These highly virulent rickettsiae rely upon their virulence for horizontal transmission to establish new infected tick lines by growth in a vertebrate host and generation of high titers of rickettsiae in the blood to be acquired by feeding ticks. In contrast, some less pathogenic organisms such as *R. africae* are present in up to 80% of their host ticks with which they appear to have a successful relationship. Some SFG species such as *R. peacockii*, *R. montanensis*, *R. massiliae*, *R. amblyommii*, and *R. rhipicephali* have never been associated with human disease.

SFG rickettsiae are transmitted during feeding of the tick or mite when rickettsiae are inoculated in arthropod saliva into the person's skin. The epidemiology thus is determined by climatological factors that affect tick activity and human activities that bring persons in contact with infected ticks. Tick prevalence and questing behavior seeking a host for a blood meal are affected by temperature and humidity, which vary dramatically from one region to another. Indeed, in most endemic locations there is a demarcated seasonal occurrence of rickettsial infections.

Rickettsia conorii is highly associated with *Rhipicephalus sanguineus* brown dog ticks, particularly in the Mediterranean basin including southern Europe, North Africa, and the Middle East. The rarity of recognized tick bite suggests transmission by larval and nymphal ticks. Likely the most prevalent SFG rickettsiosis in the world, African tick bite fever was recognized as a distinct illness by the 1930s although subsequently confused with *R. conorii* infections. Nearly 60 years later, the agent was identified as *R. africae*, which is transmitted by highly aggressive *Amblyomma hebraeum* ticks in southern Africa and by *A. variegatum* in this tick's geographic distribution in sub-Saharan Africa and the West Indies. Outbreaks involving clusters of travelers in rural areas and soldiers in southern Africa and many cases among febrile patients in Cameroon suggest that *R. africae* may cause a very high incidence of infections among indigenous persons as well as travelers returning from endemic regions.[29]

The extremely close genetic and antigenic relationship between *R. africae* and *R. parkeri* and the recent description of an African tick bite fever–like disease in a patient infected with *R. parkeri* in Virginia suggests that the same or similar disease occurs in North America where *Amblyomma maculatum* and *A. americanum* are the tick hosts. A similar SFG rickettsial disease in Uruguay associated with *A. triste* tick bite and the presence of *R. parkeri* in *Amblyomma* ticks in Brazil and Uruguay may indicate the distribution of this infection throughout the Americas where infected *Amblyomma* vectors occur.

RMSF has been documented in the United States, Mexico, Costa Rica, Panama, Colombia, Brazil, and Argentina.[30–32] The principal vectors of *R. rickettsii* in the tropics are *R. sanguineus* and *A. cajennense*. However, *A. cajennense* has also been described as a host of an unidentified SFG rickettsia in Veracruz, Mexico, and *R. rickettsii* has also been isolated from rabbit ticks (*Haemaphysalis leporispalustris*) collected in Costa Rica.[33,34] *R. australis* infection has been found along the entire eastern coastal region of Australia from Cairns, Queensland, to Gippsland in eastern Victoria.[35]

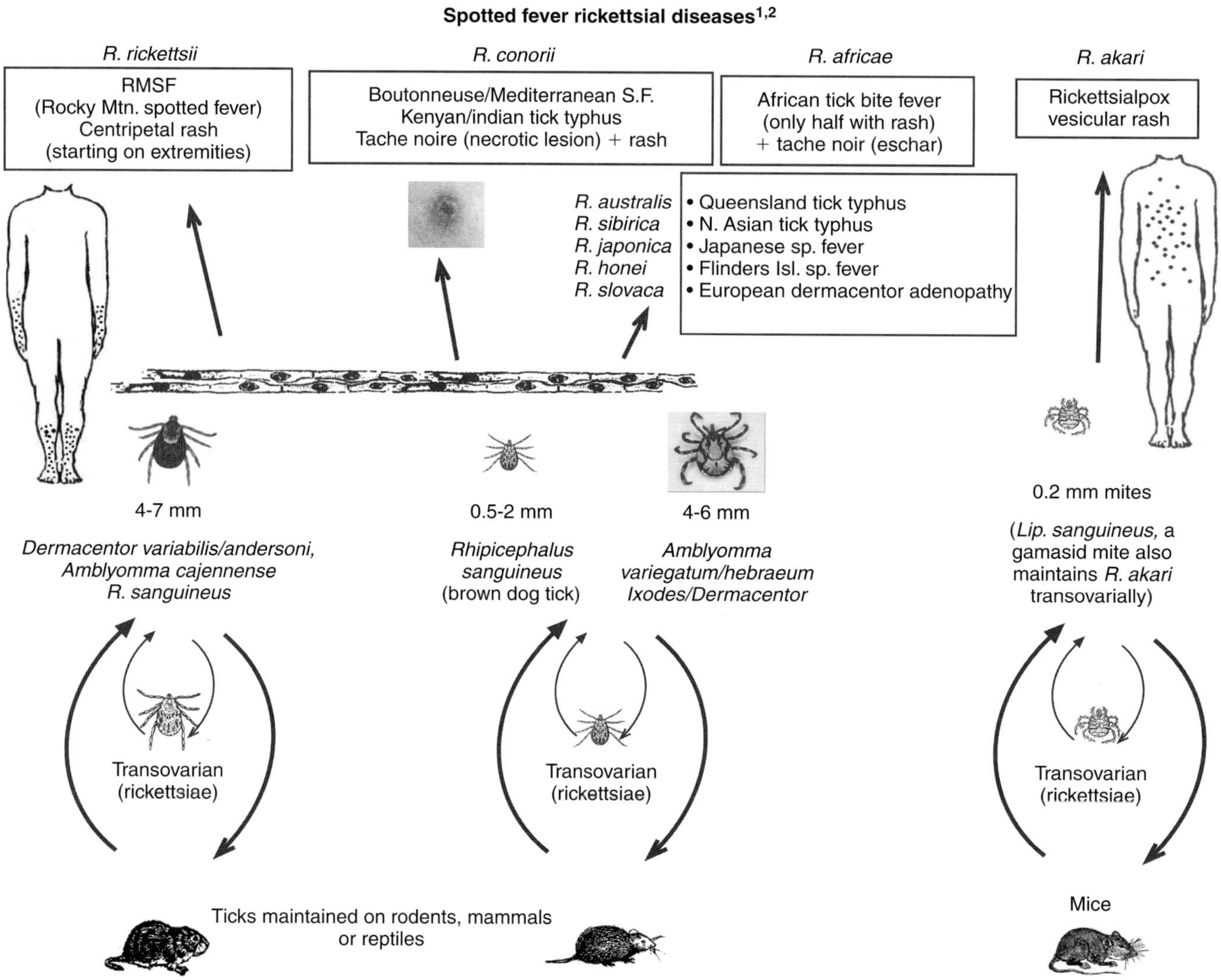

The primary vector of *R. australis* is *Ixodes holocyclus* (the scrub tick), although there is also a single report of isolation of *R. australis* from *Ixodes tasmani*.[36] *I. holocyclus* is the principal man-biting tick in Australia, but it also feeds on a wide array of domestic and wild animals, many of which have been shown to have antibodies against SFG rickettsiae.[35,37]

The mite-borne SFG rickettsial species, *R. akari,* the cause of the human disease rickettsialpox, has been isolated only in temperate areas of the Northern Hemisphere such as the United States, Ukraine, Croatia, and Korea.[38,39] However, recent reports describing a case of rickettsialpox in a man from North Carolina and another in a patient from Turkey suggest that rickettsialpox may occur much more widely and in nonurban areas.[40]

Investigations in the tropics using contemporary tools are beginning to yield important information about rickettsial diseases in these locations. The most definitive studies, cultivation of rickettsiae from samples of human patients, have been accomplished recently for *R. africae* and *R. sibirica* (mongolotimoniae strain). Clinical studies of patients with acute febrile illness suspected to be dengue, typhoid, or malaria in whom these diagnoses have been excluded have shown by IgM serology and immunoblotting that SFG rickettsioses are prevalent in study sites in Latin America and Africa.[41–43] Investigation of clinical samples by polymerase chain reaction (PCR) have identified candidate agents such as *R. felis* and *R. aeschlimannii*.[44,45] PCR studies of vectors in the endemic and outbreak areas have yielded similar candidate agents, but with weaker association as human pathogens.

Frequently, serosurveys of healthy subjects are undertaken with the aim of assessing the incidence of undiagnosed infections. For SFG rickettsiae, these studies are usually difficult to interpret owing to crossreactivity among SFG rickettsiae because of shared antigens such as the LPS. Conclusions that highly virulent organisms such as *R. rickettsii* are causing a high prevalence of asymptomatic infections are unlikely to be valid. Indeed the vast majority of *Rickettsia* identified in the tick populations to which the subjects are exposed (e.g., *R. montanensis*) have no evidence of pathogenicity.

SFG rickettsioses have been diagnosed serologically by neither rickettsial isolation nor PCR identification of the etiologic species of *Rickettsia* in Thailand, Hong Kong, and Sri Lanka.[46–49] Serosurveys have revealed significant presence of antibodies to SFG rickettsiae among persons in Taiwan, the Philippines, Hainan Island, Indonesia, Mexico, Brazil, and many sub-Saharan African countries.[50–53]

DISEASES

SFG rickettsioses vary in severity from a case-fatality rate of 23% in untreated RMSF to illness that is in some patients afebrile and never reported to be fatal (*R. slovaca, R. aeschlimannii*; see Table 50-1). Because of their severity and occurrence in tropical countries (RMSF and boutonneuse fever), high prevalence (African tick bite fever), and unique clinical presentation (*R. slovaca*–associated tick-borne lymphadenopathy), these entities will be described individually.

Rocky Mountain Spotted Fever

After an incubation period of 2 to 14 (average 7) days, RMSF usually begins with fever, muscle aches, and headache.[54,55] Early in the course, nausea, vomiting, and abdominal pain occur frequently. Occasionally patients manifest these symptoms and abdominal tenderness leading to consideration of acute surgical abdomen and exploratory laparotomy. Rash usually appears on day 3 to 5 after onset of fever. Rocky Mountain spotless fever occurs in 10% to 15% patients. Such cases may end fatally. Rash may be absent or difficult to recognize in African-American patients. The rash classically begins on the wrists and ankles, spreads centripetally, and in 36% to 82% involves the palms and soles often late in the course; however, there is wide variability in the evolution, distribution, and appearance of skin rash in patients with RMSF. Some patients with RMSF have localized rashes on one body region or rashes that appear late in onset of illness manifesting only as small number of petechial lesions.[56] Skin necrosis or gangrene occurs in a small but important minority of patients—particularly those in whom diagnosis and treatment are delayed.[57]

Neurological complications such as meningoencephalitis, coma, and seizures may be life-threatening. CSF pleocytosis and/or elevated protein concentration may be seen in up to half of patients who undergo lumbar puncture. Focal neurologic deficits, meningismus, ataxia, photophobia, or transient deafness may also occur and lead to diagnostic confusion with other infectious diseases. Pulmonary manifestations including cough, radiographic alveolar infiltrates, interstitial pneumonia, and pleural effusions may be present in some cases. Adult respiratory distress syndrome (ARDS) may require mechanical ventilation and supplemental oxygen. In such cases, there is minimal myocardial dysfunction with noncardiogenic pulmonary edema caused by increased vascular permeability associated with intense rickettsial infection of the pulmonary microcirculation. However, the same vasculitic process may involve the heart, resulting in histologic and electrocardiographic changes typical of myocarditis or produce heart block in other patients. Thus, careful assessment of cardiac function is needed to distinguish patients with RMSF complicated by ARDS from those with heart failure due to *Rickettsia*-induced myocarditis. In severe cases, increased vascular permeability results in edema, hypovolemia, decreased glomerular filtration, and prerenal azotemia. In patients with severe hypotensive shock, oliguric acute renal failure may be associated with acute tubular necrosis. Aside from a petechial rash, severe hemorrhagic phenomena seldom occur. Similarly, despite frequent thrombocytopenia, true disseminated intravascular coagulation is rare.[58,59]

Boutonneuse Fever (Mediterranean Spotted Fever)

Boutonneuse fever differs from RMSF in a lower untreated case fatality rate (4% vs. 23%); the presence of a *tache noire* (eschar); a 1-cm focus of vascular rickettsial infection and injury leading to epidermal and dermal necrosis at the site of tick bite inoculation of rickettsiae in 72% of cases; and lower incidence of myalgia, petechiae, stupor, and cough.[60] Illness can be severe in patients with underlying disease such as cardiac failure or diabetes, old age, alcoholism, and glucose-6-phosphate dehydrogenase deficiency.[61]

African Tick Bite Fever

African tick bite fever (ATBF) is a milder illness than RMSF, and fatalities are rare. After an incubation period of 5 to 7 days, patients with ATBF suffer abrupt onset of fever (59%–100%), nausea, fatigue, headache (62%–83%), myalgia (63%–87%), nuchal myalgia (81%), eschars (53%–100%), which are typically multiple (21%–54%), regional painful lymphadenopathy (40%–100%), rash (15%–46%) that is either maculopapular (14%–26%) or vesicular (0%–21%), and aphthous stomatitis (0%–11%).[62,63]

Patients from Uruguay suspected to have infection with closely related *R. parkeri* also had eschars and painful lymphadenopathy more often than rash.[64] The North American patient infected with *R. parkeri* suffered multiple eschars, regional lymphadenopathy, fever, headache, myalgia, and maculopapular rash.[23]

Other SFG Rickettsioses

Rickettsia slovaca infection occurs in Europe during the cold months when *Dermacentor* ticks attach, usually to the occipital scalp, followed 7 to 9 days later by the presence of an eschar and painful regional (often cervical) lymphadenopathy, seldom accompanied by fever or rash.[65] The complication of prolonged alopecia at the site of the eschar (24%) and aesthenia persisting even after doxycycline treatment suggests the possibility of co-involvement of other factors or agents.

Although other SFG rickettsioses are clinically similar, it should be noted that there is growing recognition of severe cases of Japanese spotted fever, including a fatal case and patients with meningoencephalitis, multiorgan failure, and coagulopathy.[66] The recognized incidence of rickettsialpox has risen owing to more attention to evaluation of eschars in the wake of bioterrorist-associated cases of cutaneous anthrax. *Rickettsia sibirica* infections were diagnosed among a group of paleontologists doing field investigations in Mongolia, and human infections with a novel strain have been documented in France and Africa.[67]

PATHOGENESIS AND IMMUNITY

SFG rickettsiae grow and undergo reactivation of virulence in the salivary glands of ticks and mites from which they are inoculated into the dermis of the skin during tick feeding. Presumably rickettsiae spread via lymphatic vessels to the regional lymph nodes and subsequently hematogenously throughout the body. These obligately intracellular bacteria grow mainly in endothelial cells and to a lesser extent in macrophages. They enter the endothelium by attachment to a cell membrane protein by rickettsial OmpA and OmpB, induce cytoskeletal rearrangements resulting in phagocytosis, and rapidly lyse the phagosomal membrane, escaping into the cytosol where they replicate by binary fission.[7,68–70] SFG rickettsiae stimulate actin-based mobility via their protein RickA, which activates the host's Arp 2/3 complex that triggers nucleation of actin polymerization.[71,72] The actin tail that forms at one pole of the SFG *Rickettsia* propels it through the cytosol and via filopodia to the extracellular space or for cell-to-cell spread.

SFG rickettsiae injure endothelial cells by stimulation of their production of reactive oxygen species that damage cell membranes by lipid peroxidation.[73] The most important pathophysiologic effect of endothelial injury is increased vascular permeability leading to edema (see the Diseases section).[74,75] SFG rickettsiae manipulate the endothelial cells to serve as an efficient host for their growth by inhibiting apoptosis via activation of NF-κB, leading to inhibition of caspases 3, 8, and 9 and inhibition of release of cytochrome C from mitochondria.[76]

Immunity to SFG rickettsiae is mediated principally by T lymphocytes. Both CD4 and CD8 T lymphocytes secrete proinflammatory cytokines, especially IFN-γ, which along with TNF-α, IL-1β, and RANTES activate endothelial cells, macrophages, and hepatocytes to kill intracellular rickettsiae via synthesis of nitric oxide and hydrogen peroxide and/or limitation of available tryptophan via its degradation by indoleamine-2,3-dioxygenase.[77] It is particularly noteworthy that following human infection by *R. africae,* serum levels of the immune mediators IFN-γ, TNF-α, and RANTES are elevated.[78] CD8 lymphocytes provide a critical host defense with perforin-dependent elimination of infected cells by MHC class I–dependent cytotoxic T lymphocyte activity.[79] Dampening of the infection early in the course by innate immunity includes NK cell activation with secretion of IFN-γ.[80] Antibodies to OmpA and OmpB, but not lipopolysaccharide, contribute to control of infection and are effective in preventing reinfection.[81]

DIAGNOSIS

The clinical diagnosis of SFG rickettsiosis is often difficult. This difficulty is underscored by the fact that cases are sometimes only first suspected at autopsy even in areas where sophisticated medical care and diagnostic testing are available.[82] Fever, headache, and myalgias are nearly universal features of SFG rickettsial infections, but such symptoms are present in many other infectious diseases. Skin rash occurs in most but not all patients with *R. conorii, R. australis,* and *R. rickettsii* infection, but occurs in only half of patients with *R. africae* infection. A localized necrotic skin lesion (an eschar or *tache noire*) commonly occurs at the site of rickettsial inoculation by tick bite in patients with infection caused by *R. conorii* (except in Israel), *R. australis, R. japonica, R. africae, R. slovaca, R. aeschlimannii,* and *R. honei,* and by mite bite for *R. akari.* Rarely, such eschars may occur in patients with *R. rickettsii* infection as well.[83] It is important to note that skin rash, eschar, and a history of tick bite may be absent or easily overlooked in some patients with SFG rickettsial infections; thus the absence of a rash or history of tick bite should not eliminate the possibility of a rickettsial disease in a febrile patient with other compatible symptoms, signs, and laboratory abnormalities such as thrombocytopenia, mental status changes, or renal insufficiency. On the other hand, a history of a recent tick bite or tick contact can be of enormous help in diagnosing SFG rickettsioses in a patient with fever and nonspecific symptoms such as myalgias, headache, and gastrointestinal complaints. Similarly when present, an eschar is often a critical clinical diagnostic sign of SFG rickettsioses, but the presence or absence of an eschar is not in itself diagnostic of SFG rickettsiosis as similar lesions occur in scrub typhus, cutaneous anthrax, tularemia, primary syphilis, and chancroid.

The diagnosis of a SFG rickettsial infection can be established by isolation or molecular detection of the causative organism from blood or tissue and by immunohistochemical methods that visualize SFG rickettsiae in skin biopsy specimens.[84–89] *R. conorii* and *R. africae* have also been detected in circulating endothelial cells using immunomagnetic beads to capture the detached endothelial cells and immunocytologic techniques to demonstrate the rickettsiae.[90] SFG rickettsial infection can be confirmed using a variety of serologic methods.[91–93] Most of the standard serologic techniques, such as the microimmunofluorescent antibody test, cannot distinguish among infections with the different SFG rickettsial species. In addition, PCR technology has been used to diagnose SFG rickettsial infections, but its diagnostic sensitivity remains to be proven to be adequate, particularly early in the course of disease.[94–97]

Because SFG rickettsial infections often begin with nonspecific symptoms and because subsequent physical and laboratory findings such as a skin rash and thrombocytopenia are easily confused with an array of other diseases prevalent in the tropics, the clinical diagnosis of SFG rickettsial infections must rest on a synthesis of epidemiologic factors such as season of the year, possible exposure to ticks or tick-infested environments, and the clinical findings. It is difficult (and sometimes impossible) to initially distinguish SFG rickettsial infections from dengue; typhoid fever; malaria; drug reaction; and exanthematous viral infections such as measles, rubella, and arboviral and enteroviral disease. Occasionally, severe infection due to *R. rickettsii* or *R. conorii* can mimic meningococcemia, staphylococcal bacteremia, toxic shock syndrome, leptospirosis, viral hemorrhagic fever, or thrombotic thrombocytopenic purpura.

TREATMENT AND PROGNOSIS

Two drugs are the mainstays of treatment of all SFG rickettsial diseases: tetracycline and chloramphenicol. Tetracyclines such as doxycycline are generally the preferred agents, even for young children.[98] Despite the fact that doxycycline is safe and appropriate as initial therapy of children with suspected RMSF (and other SFG rickettsioses), there is evidence that unfounded fears of toxicity may result in a hesitancy to use this drug as empiric therapy for RMSF. For example, fewer than 5% of children presenting to a Texas children's hospital with a suspected rickettsiosis actually received doxycycline or chloramphenicol as initial theapy.[99] An analysis of the outcome of 6338 patients with RMSF reported to the Centers for Disease Control and Prevention from 1981 to 1990 suggested that older patients, those treated with chloramphenicol only, patients not receiving a tetracycline as primary therapy, and those with delay in institution of therapy greater than 5 days had higher mortality rates.[100] Chloramphenicol is the preferred agent for pregnant women and for persons with severe illness in whom it is difficult or impossible to distinguish between a rickettsial infection and meningococcal infection. Quinolones have been shown to have activity against SFG rickettsiae *in vitro*, and in boutonneuse fever quinolones have been shown to be as effective as doxycycline in reduction in the duration of fever and are apparently superior in the rapidity of amelioration of other symptoms.[101,102] Although azithromycin and clarithromycin have been shown to provide equivalent successful outcome as chloramphenicol in children with mild Mediterranean spotted fever, neither they nor fluoroquinolones can be recommended at the present time for patients with moderate or severe SFG rickettsiosis. Duration of treatment of SFG rickettsial infections has not been studied systematically in a large cohort of humans. Although treatment regimens using doxycycline to treat *R. conorii* infection for time periods as short as 1 to 2 days have been reported to be as efficacious as 10-day regimens, similar studies have not been undertaken for treatment of other SFG rickettsiae such as *R. rickettsii* and *R. australis*.[103] Additionally, relapse of *R. conorii* infection in children treated with short courses of doxycycline has been reported.[104] In light of these data, most authorities recommend that tetracycline, chloramphenicol, or ciprofloxacin be continued for 7 days or until the patient has been afebrile for at least 48 hours and is improving clinically.

PREVENTION AND CONTROL

The tick vectors of SFG rickettsiae are widespread, and control of tick populations is generally not feasible. A vaccine is not available for any SFG rickettsia. Thus, avoidance of tick bite is the only preventive method available. Tick repellants and protective clothing reduce the risk of tick exposure, but are less acceptable to persons in a warm, humid environment. Regular inspection and removal of ticks from the body prior to inoculation of rickettsiae-infected saliva also reduces the likelihood of infection.

REFERENCES

1. Vishwanath S: Antigenic relationships among the rickettsiae of the spotted fever and typhus groups. FEMS Microbiol Lett 81:341, 1991.
2. Anderson BE, McDonald GA, Jones DC, et al: A protective protein antigen of *Rickettsia rickettsii* has tandemly repeated, near-identical sequences. Infect Immun 58:2760, 1990.
3. Hackstadt T, Messer R, Cieplak W, et al: Evidence for proteolytic cleavage of the 120-kilodalton outer membrane protein of rickettsiae: Identification of an avirulent mutant deficient in processing. Infect Immun 60:159, 1992.
4. Gilmore RD Jr: Comparison of the *rompA* gene repeat regions of rickettsiae reveals species-specific arrangements of individual repeating units. Gene 125:97, 1993.
5. Crocquet-Valdes PA, Weiss K, Walker DH: Sequence analysis of the 190-kDa antigen-encoding gene of *Rickettsia conorii* (Malish 7 strain). Gene 140:115, 1994.
6. Bouyer DH, Stenos J, Crocquet-Valdes P, et al: *Rickettsia felis*: Molecular characterization of a new member of the spotted fever group. Int J Syst Evol Microbiol 51:339, 2001.
7. Li H, Lenz B, Walker DH: Protective monoclonal antibodies recognize heat-labile epitopes on surface proteins of spotted fever group rickettsiae. Infect Immun 56:2587, 1988.
8. Anacker RL, Mann RE, Gonzales C: Reactivity of monoclonal antibodies to *Rickettsia rickettsii* with spotted fever and typhus group rickettsiae. J Clin Microbiol 25:167, 1987.
9. Walker DH, Feng H, Saada JI, et al: Comparative antigenic analysis of spotted fever group rickettsiae from Israel and other closely related organisms. Am J Trop Med Hyg 52:569, 1995.
10. Walker DH, Liu Q, Yu X, et al: Antigenic diversity of *Rickettsia conorii*. Am J Trop Med Hyg 47:78, 1992.
11. Stothard DR, Fuerst PA: Evolutionary analysis of the spotted fever and typhus groups of *Rickettsia* using 16S rRNA gene sequences. Syst Appl Microbiol 18:52, 1995.
12. Lee JH, Park HS, Jung KD, et al: Identification of the spotted fever group rickettsiae detected from *Haemaphysalis longicornis* in Korea. Microbiol Immunol 47:301, 2003.
13. Xu W, Raoult D: Distribution of immunogenic epitopes on the two major immunodominant proteins (rOmpA and rOmpB) of *Rickettsia conorii* among the other rickettsiae of the spotted fever group. Clin Diagn Lab Immunol 4:753, 1997.
14. Fournier PE, Dumler JS, Greub G, et al: Gene sequence-based criteria for identification of new *Rickettsia* isolates and description of *Rickettsia heilongjiangensis* sp. nov. J Clin Microbiol 41:5456, 2003.
15. Walker DH: Rocky Mountain spotted fever: A disease in need of microbiological concern. Clin Microbiol Rev 2:227, 1989.
16. Conor AL, Bruch A: Une fièvre éruptive observée en Tunisie. Bull Soc Pathol Exot 3:492, 1910.
17. Andrew R, Bonnin JM, Williams S: Tick typhus in north Queensland. Med J Aust 2:253, 1946.
18. Patino L, Afanador A, Paul JH: A spotted fever in Tobia, Colombia: Preliminary report. Am J Trop Med Hyg 17:639, 1937.
19. Dias E, Martins AV: Spotted fever in Brazil. Am J Trop Med 19:103, 1939.
20. Bustamante ME: Una nueva rickettsioisis en Mexico. Existencia de la fiebre manchada Americana en los estados de Sinaloa y Sonora. Rev Inst Salub Enferm Trop 4:189, 1943.
21. Kelly PJ, Beati L, Mason PR, et al: *Rickettsia africae* sp. nov., the etiological agent of African tick bite fever. Int J Syst Bacteriol 46:611, 1996.
22. Uchida T, Uchiyama T, Kumano K, et al: *Rickettsia japonica* sp. nov., the etiological agent of spotted fever group rickettsiosis in Japan. Int J Syst Bacteriol 42:303, 1992.
23. Paddock CD, Summer JW, Comer JA, et al: *Rickettsia parkeri*: A newly recognized cause of spotted fever rickettsiosis in the United States. Clin Infect Dis 38:805, 2004.
24. Stewart RS: Flinders Island spotted fever: A newly recognized endemic focus of tick typhus in Bass Strait. Part 1. Clinical and epidemiological features. Med J Aust 154:94, 1991.
25. Graves SR, Dwyer BW, McColl D, et al: Flinders Island spotted fever: A newly recognized endemic focus of tick typhus in Bass Strait. Part 2. Serological investigations. Med J Aust 154:99, 1991.
26. Kelly PJ, Mason PR: Transmission of a spotted fever group rickettsia by *Amblyomma hebraeum* (Acari:Ixodidae). Med Entomol 28:598, 1991.
27. Niebylski ML, Schrumpf ME, Burgdorfer W, et al: *Rickettsia peacocki* sp. nov., a new species infecting wood ticks, *Dermacentor andersoni*, in Western Montana. Int J Syst Bacteriol 47:446, 1997.
28. Walker DH, Fishbein DB: Epidemiology of rickettsial diseases. Eur J Epidemiol 7:237, 1991.
29. Smoak BL, McClain JB, Brundage JF, et al: An outbreak of spotted fever rickettsiosis in U.S. Army troops deployed to Botswana. Emerg Infect Dis 2:217, 1996.
30. Sexton DJ, Corey GR, Dietze R, et al: Brazilian spotted fever in Espirito Santo, Brazil: Description of a focus of infection in a new endemic region. Am J Trop Med Hyg 49:222, 1993.
31. Calero MC, Nunez JM, Silva Gotyia R: Rocky Mountain spotted fever in Panama. Report of two cases. Am J Trop Med Hyg 1:631, 1952.
32. Fuentes LG: Primer caso de fiebre de las Montanas Rocosas en Costa Rica, America Central. Rev Latinoam Microbiol 21:167, 1979.
33. Bustamante ME, Varela G: III. Estudios de fiebre manchada en Mexico: Hallazgo del *Amblyomma cajennense* naturalmente infectado, en Veracruz. Rev Inst Salub Enferm Trop 7:75, 1946.
34. Fuentes L, Calderon A, Hun L: Isolation and identification of *Rickettsia rickettsii* from the rabbit tick (*Haemaphysalis leporispalustris*) in the Atlantic zone of Costa Rica. Am J Trop Med Hyg 34:564, 1985.

35. Sexton DJ, Dwyer B, Kemp R, et al: Spotted fever group rickettsial infections in Australia: A review. Rev Infect Dis 13:876, 1991.
36. Pickens EG, Bell EJ, Lackman DB, et al: Use of mouse serum in identification and serologic classification of *Rickettsia akari* and *Rickettsia australis*. J Immunol 94:883, 1965.
37. Sexton DJ, Banks J, Graves S, et al: Prevalence of antibodies to spotted fever group rickettsiae in dogs from southeastern Australia. Am J Trop Med Hyg 45:243, 1991.
38. Huebner RJ, Stamps P, Armstrong C: Rickettsialpox—A newly recognized rickettsial disease. I. Isolation of the etiological agent. Public Health Rep 61:1605, 1946.
39. Radulovic S, Feng H-M, Morovic M, et al: Isolation of *Rickettsia akari* from a patient in a region where Mediterranean spotted fever is endemic. Clin Infect Dis 22:216, 1996.
40. Krusell A, Comer JA, Sexton DJ: Rickettsialpox in North Carolina: A case report. Emerg Infect Dis 8:727, 2002.
41. Zavala-Velazquez JE, Yu X-J, Walker DH: Unrecognized spotted fever group rickettsiosis masquerading as dengue fever in Mexico. Am J Trop Med Hyg 55:157, 1996.
42. Ndip LM, Bouyer DH, DaRosa APAT, et al: Acute spotted fever rickettsiosis among febrile patients, Cameroon. Emerg Infect Dis 10:432, 2004.
43. Ndip LM, Fokam EB, Bouyer EH, et al: Detection of *Rickettsia africae* in patients and ticks along the coastal region of Cameroon. Am J Trop Med Hyg 71:363, 2004.
44. Zavala-Velazquez JE, Zavala-Castro JE, Vado-Solis I, et al: Identification of *Ctenocephalides felis* fleas as a host of *Rickettsia felis*, the agent of a spotted fever rickettsiosis in Yucatan, Mexico. Vector Borne Zoonotic Dis 2:69, 2002.
45. Pretorius A-M, Birtles RJ: *Rickettsia aeschlimannii:* A new pathogenic spotted fever group rickettsia, South Africa. Emerg Infect Dis 8:874, 2002.
46. Kularatne SAM, Edirisingha JS, Gawarammana IB, et al: Emerging rickettsial infections in Sri Lanka: The pattern in the hilly central province. Trop Med Int Health 8:803, 2003.
47. Sirisanthana T, Pinyopornpanit V, Sirisanthana V, et al: First cases of spotted fever group rickettsiosis in Thailand. Am J Trop Med Hyg 50:682, 1994.
48. Cohen MAH, Cheng AFB, Leung NWY: A fatal case of rickettsial spotted fever in Hong Kong—Lion Rock fever. J Hong Kong Med Assoc 41:185, 1989.
49. Tseng RYM, Ho AKC, Li CK, et al: Spotted fever in Hong Kong. Ann Trop Paediatr 12:255, 1992.
50. Feng HM, Chen TS, Lin BH, et al: Serologic survey of spotted fever group rickettsiosis on Hainan Island of China. Microbiol Immunol 35:687, 1991.
51. Kelly PJ, Mason PR, Matthewman LA, et al: Seroepidemiology of spotted fever group rickettsial infections in humans in Zimbabwe. J Trop Med Hyg 94:304, 1991.
52. Dupont HT, Brouqui P, Faugere B, et al: Prevalence of antibodies to *Coxiella burnetii, Rickettsia conorii,* and *Rickettsia typhi* in seven African countries. Clin Infect Dis 21:1126, 1995.
53. Takada N, Fujita H, Yano Y, et al: Serosurveys of spotted fever and murine typhus in local residents of Taiwan and Thailand compared with Japan. Southeast Asian J Trop Med Public Health 24:354, 1993.
54. Kaplowitz LG, Fischer JJ, Sparling PF: Rocky Mountain spotted fever: A clinical dilemma. Curr Clin Top Infect Dis 2:89, 1981.
55. Helmick CG, Bernard KW, D'Angelo LJ: Rocky Mountain spotted fever: Clinical, laboratory, and epidemiological features of 262 cases. J Infect Dis 150:480, 1984.
56. Sexton DJ, Corey GR: Rocky Mountain "spotless" and "almost spotless" fever: A wolf in sheep's clothing. Clin Infect Dis 15:439, 1992.
57. Kirkland KB, Marcom PK, Sexton DJ, et al: Rocky Mountain spotted fever complicated by gangrene: Report of six cases and review. Clin Infect Dis 16:629, 1993.
58. Rao AK, Schapira M, Clements ML, et al: A prospective study of platelets and plasma proteolytic systems during the early stages of Rocky Mountain spotted fever. N Engl J Med 318:1021, 1988.
59. Elghetany MT, Walker DH: Hemostatic changes in Rocky Mountain spotted fever and Mediterranean spotted fever. Am J Clin Pathol 112:159, 1999.
60. Raoult D, Weiller PJ, Chagnon A, et al: Mediterranean spotted fever: Clinical, laboratory and epidemiological features of 199 cases. Am J Trop Med Hyg 35:845, 1986.
61. Raoult D, Zuchelli P, Weiller PJ, et al: Incidence, clinical observations and risk factors in the severe form of Mediterranean spotted fever among patients admitted to hospital in Marseilles 1983–1984. J Infect 12:111, 1986.
62. Raoult D, Birtles RJ, Montoya M, et al: Survey of three bacterial louse-associated diseases among rural Andean communities in Peru: Prevalence of epidemic typhus, trench fever, and relapsing fever. Clin Infect Dis 29:434, 1999.
63. Jensenius M, Ueland T, Fournier PE, et al: Systemic inflammatory responses in African tick-bite fever. J Infect Dis 187:1332, 2003.
64. Raoult D, Lakos A, Fenollar F, et al: Spotless rickettsiosis caused by *Rickettsia slovaca* and associated with *Dermacentor* ticks. Clin Infect Dis 34:1331, 2002.
65. Kodama K, Senba T, Yamauchi H, et al: Japanese spotted fever associated with multiorgan failure. J Infect Chemother 7:247, 2001.
66. Conti-Diaz IA . Rickettsiosis por *Rickettsia conorii* (fiebre botonosa del Mediterráneo o fiebre de Marsella). Estado actual en Uruguay. Rev Med Uruguay 17:119, 2001.
67. Lewin MR, Bouyer DH, Walker DH, et al: *Rickettsia sibirica* infection in members of scientific expeditions to northern Asia. Lancet 362: 1201, 2003.
68. Li H, Walker DH: Characterization of rickettsial attachment to host cells by flow cytometry. Infect Immun 60:2030, 1992.
69. Walker TS: Rickettsial interactions with human endothelial cells *in vitro*: Adherence and entry. Infect Immun 44:205, 1984.
70. Uchida T, Yu XJ, Uchiyama T, et al: Identification of a unique spotted fever group rickettsia from humans in Japan. J Infect Dis 159:1122, 1989.
71. Teysseire N, Chiche-Portiche C, Raoult D: Intracellular movements of *Rickettsia conorii* and *R. typhi* based on actin polymerization. Res Microbiol 143:821, 1992.
72. Gouin E, Egile C, Dehoux P, et al: The RickA protein of *Rickettsia conorii* activates the Arp2/3 complex. Nature 427:457, 2004.
73. Santucci LA, Gutierrez PL, Silverman DJ: *Rickettsia rickettsii* induces superoxide radical and superoxide dismutase in human endothelial cells. Infect Immun 60:5113, 1992.
74. Harrell GT, Aikawa JK: Pathogenesis of circulatory failure in Rocky Mountain spotted fever. Alteration in the blood volume and the thiocyanate space at various stages of the disease. Arch Intern Med 83:331, 1949.
75. Davidson MG, Breitschwerdt EB, Walker DH, et al: Vascular permeability and coagulation during *Rickettsia rickettsii* infection in dogs. Am J Vet Res 51:165, 1990.
76. Feng HM, Walker DH: Mechanisms of intracellular killing of *Rickettsia conorii* in infected human endothelial cells, hepatocytes, and macrophages. Infec Immun 68:6729, 2000.
77. Joshi SG, Francis CW, Silverman DJ, et al: Nuclear factor κB protects against host cell apoptosis during *Rickettsia rickettsii* infection by inhibiting activation of apical and effector caspases and maintaining mitochondrial integrity. Infec Immun 71:4127, 2003.
78. Walker DH, Olano JP, Feng HM: Critical role of cytotoxic T lymphocytes in immune clearance of rickettsial infection. Infec Immun 69:1841, 2001.
79. Billings AN, Feng HM, Olano JP, et al: Rickettsial infection in murine models activates an early anti-rickettsial effect mediated by NK cells and associated with production of gamma interferon. Am J Trop Med Hyg 65:52, 2001.
80. Feng HM, Whitworth T, Olano JP, et al: Fc-dependent polyclonal antibodies and antibodies to outer membrane proteins A and B, but not to lipopolysaccharides, protect SCID mice against fatal *Rickettsia conorii* infection. Infec Immun 72:2222, 2004.
81. Paddock CD, Greer PW, Freebee, et al: Hidden mortality attributable to Rocky Mountain spotted fever: Immunohistochemical detection of fatal, serologically unconfirmed disease. J Infect Dis 179:1469, 1999.
82. Jensenius M, Fournier PE, Vene S, et al: African tick bite fever in travelers to rural Sub-equatorial Africa. Clin Infect Dis 36:1411, 2003.
83. Walker DH, Gay RM, Valdes-Dapena M: The occurrence of eschars in Rocky Mountain spotted fever. J Am Acad Dermatol 4:571, 1981.
84. Kaplowitz LG, Lange JV, Fischer JJ, et al: Correlation of rickettsial titers, circulating endotoxin, and clinical features in Rocky Mountain spotted fever. Arch Intern Med 143:1149, 1983.

85. Marrero M, Raoult D: Centrifugation-shell vial technique for rapid detection of Mediterranean spotted fever rickettsia in blood culture. Am J Trop Med Hyg 40:197, 1989.
86. Walker DH, Cain BG, Olmstead PM: Laboratory diagnosis of Rocky Mountain spotted fever by immunofluorescent demonstration of *Rickettsia rickettsii* in cutaneous lesions. Am J Clin Pathol 69:619, 1978.
87. Walker DH, Occhino C, Tringali GR, et al: Pathogenesis of rickettsial eschars: The tache noire of boutonneuse fever. Hum Pathol 19:1449, 1988.
88. Montenegro MR, Mansueto S, Hegarty BC, et al: The histology of "taches noires" of boutonneuse fever and demonstration of *Rickettsia conorii* in them by immunofluorescence. Virchows Arch 400:309, 1983.
89. Raoult D, De Micco C, Gallais H, et al: Laboratory diagnosis of Mediterranean spotted fever by immunofluorescent demonstration of *Rickettsia conorii* in cutaneous lesions. J Infect Dis 150:145, 1984.
90. Drancourt M, George F, Brouqui P, et al: Diagnosis of Mediterranean spotted fever by indirect immunofluorescence of *Rickettsia conorii* in circulating endothelial cells isolated with monoclonal antibody-coated immunomagnetic beads. J Infect Dis 166:660, 1992.
91. Teysseire N, Raoult D: Comparison of western immunoblotting and microimmunofluorescence for diagnosis of Mediterranean spotted fever. J Clin Microbiol 30:455, 1992.
92. Raoult D, Dasch GA: Line blot and western blot immunoassays for diagnosis of Mediterranean spotted fever. J Clin Microbiol 27:2073, 1989.
93. Kleeman KT, Hicks JL, Anacker RL, et al: Early detection of antibody to *Rickettsia rickettsii*: A comparison of four serological methods: indirect hemagglutination, indirect fluorescent antibody, latex agglutination, and complement fixation. In Burgdorfer W, Anacker RL (eds): Rickettsiae and Rickettsial Diseases. New York, Academic Press, 1981, p 171.
94. Tzianabos T, Anderson B, McDade J: Detection of *Rickettsia rickettsii* in clinical specimens by using polymerase chain reaction technology. J Clin Microbiol 27:2866, 1989.
95. Sexton DH, Kanj SS, Wilson K, et al: The use of polymerase chain reaction as a diagnostic test for Rocky Mountain spotted fever. Am J Trop Med Hyg 50:59, 1994.
96. Williams WJ, Radulovic S, Dasch GA, et al: Identification of *Rickettsia conorii* infection by polymerase chain reaction in a soldier returning from Somalia. Clin Infect Dis 19:93, 1994.
97. Tange Y, Matsumoto M, Okada T, et al: Detection of DNA of causative agent of spotted fever group rickettsiosis in Japan from the patient's blood sample by polymerase chain reaction. Microbiol Immunol 38:665, 1994.
98. Peter G, Halsey NA, Marcuse EK, et al (eds): 1997 Red Book: Report of the Committee on Infectious Diseases, 24th ed. Elk Grove Village, IL, American Academy of Pediatrics, 1997.
99. Purvis JJ, Edwardes MS: Doxycyline use for rickettsial disease in pediatric patients. Pediatr Infect Dis J 19:871, 2000.
100. Holman RC, Paddock CD, Curns AT, et al: Analysis of risk factors for fatal Rocky Mountain spotted fever: Evidence for superiority of tetracyclines for therapy. J Infect Dis 184:1437, 2001.
101. Ruiz-Beltrán R, Herrero-Herrero JI: Evaluation of ciprofloxacin and doxycycline in the treatment of Mediterranean spotted fever. Eur J Clin Microbiol Infect Dis 11:427, 1992.
102. Jabarit-Aldighieri N, Torres H, Raoult D: Susceptibility of *Rickettsia conorii, R. rickettsii,* and *Coxiella burnetii* to PD 127,391, PD 131,628, ofloxacin, and ciprofloxacin. Antimicrob Agents Chemother 36:2529, 1992.
103. Bella F, Espejo E, Uriz S, et al: Randomized trial of 5-day rifampin versus 1-day doxycycline therapy for Mediterranean spotted fever. J Infect Dis 164:433, 1991.
104. Yugupsky P, Gross EM: Relapse of Israeli spotted fever treated with doxycycline. Trans R Soc Trop Med Hyg 79:139, 1981.

51

Typhus Group Rickettsioses

DAVID H. WALKER
DIDIER RAOULT

INTRODUCTION

Murine typhus, usually misdiagnosed as another ailment, is among the most prevalent febrile illnesses occurring in the tropics.[1–5] Louse-borne typhus is not only one of the most devastating infections in world history but also a continuing cause of morbidity and mortality among isolated, impoverished populations in tropical locations.[6] Like spotted fever group rickettsiae (see Chapter 50), typhus group rickettsiae are small, obligately intracellular, gram-negative bacteria that have an arthropod host as at least a portion of their ecologic niche.

Two pathogenic *Rickettsia* species are classified in the typhus group: *R. prowazekii* (epidemic louse-borne typhus, recrudescent typhus, and flying squirrel–associated typhus) and *R. typhi* (murine typhus). Typhus infections were first described by Fracastorius in 1546 based on his observations during an epidemic in Italy in 1528. Luis de Toro described an epidemic of a previously unknown, frequently fatal, acute febrile illness among soldiers in Spain in 1557.[7] The disease was undoubtedly epidemic louse-borne typhus based on the appearance of a macular rash on days 4 to 7 of disease, neurologic and other characteristic signs and symptoms, winter seasonality, and even association of illness with contact with clothing of the ill. As many as half of the deaths among Napoleon's 700,000 soldiers during the Russian campaign of 1812 were caused by typhus, just one example of the tremendous effect of typhus on history. Boissier de Sauvage named the disease exanthematic typhus to distinguish it from typhoid.[8] Not until 1836 was the differentiation of typhus fever and typhoid fever determined by Gerhard on the basis of the intestinal lesions of typhoid fever. Typhus was proved to be transmitted by human body lice by Nicolle in 1909, for which he was awarded the Nobel Prize in 1928. That the cause was an intracellular infectious agent with bacterial morphology was demonstrated by a series of investigations building one upon another performed by Ricketts, Anderson, Goldberger, von Prowazek, da Rocha-Lima, and Wolbach between 1910 and 1922. Milder forms of typhus described by Brill in 1898 in New York among emigrees from Russia and other European typhus zones and by Paullin in 1913 in Atlanta were proved during the 1930s to be recrudescence of louse-borne *R. prowazekii* infection and rat flea–transmitted *R. typhi* infection, respectively.[9–14]

Antibiotic-resistant *R. prowazekii* strains have been developed, and both *R. prowazekii* and *R. typhi* are aerosol-transmitted biothreats.[15–17]

AGENTS

Typhus group rickettsiae have a small (1.1×10^6 bp) genome; a 135-kD major, immunodominant S-layer protein arranged tetragonally on the cell wall surface, peptidoglycan, and abundant lipopolysaccharide.[18–22] Typhus group rickettsiae are highly adapted to the intracellular environment with its high potassium content and availability of compounds such as adenosine triphosphate (ATP), amino acids, and phosphorylated sugars such as uridine diphosphoglucose for which the rickettsiae possess specific transport mechanisms to their advantage in obtaining these molecules from the host cell cytoplasm.[23]

The bioenergetics of typhus group rickettsiae includes the production of ATP via the tricarboxylic acid cycle, one or more electron transport systems, and five ADP/ATP translocases. Early in the infection cycle when host cytoplasmic ATP concentration is high, the ADP/ATP translocases exchange ATP of the host for ADP from the rickettsiae. Later when host cell ATP is depleted, the ADP/ATP translocases are down-regulated so as not to reverse the exchange mechanism, and citrate synthase, which is a component of the tricarboxylic acid cycle, is highly expressed.[24,25] Interestingly, *Rickettsia* and mitochondria diverged from a common ancestor 1.5–2 billion years ago.[26] The rickettsial obligately intracellular lifestyle has resulted in marked genome reduction, reflecting the loss of genes required for extracellular competition. The single circular genome contains fewer than 900 genes, numerous split genes with internal stop codons, and relics of obsolete genes. Among the 41 pseudogenes of *R. typhi* are all six cytochrome oxidase genes, which are active in *R. prowazekii*. Conversely the *metK* enzyme for synthesis of S-adenosylmethionine is inactivated by mutation in *R. prowazekii* but not in *R. typhi*. Both have S-adenosylmethionine transporters.[27] A unique feature of *Rickettsia* is the presence of many in-frame palindromic sequence insertions with locations compatible with normal conformation and function of the proteins.[28]

The rickettsial ecologic cycle involves adaptation to two very different hosts: an arthropod and a warm-blooded mammal. The availability of nutrients and oxygen and other conditions vary tremendously between them. Rickettsiae contain unusual split *spoT* genes, each component of which may be functional in the stringent response—an increase in diguanosine pentaphosphate in response to starvation in the unfed arthropod or other stress—by catabolism of the toxic molecules to the energy resource ATP.[29] Rickettsiae also contain a family of autotransporters and some of the type IV secretion components but lack others that are not useful in the intracellular environment.[25,26]

EPIDEMIOLOGY

Typhus group rickettsiae that are pathogenic for humans have an insect vector (louse or flea) and are transmitted mainly in the insect's feces. *R. prowazekii* infects a high proportion of southern flying squirrels (*Glaucomys volans*) in the eastern United States and is transmitted among flying squirrels by

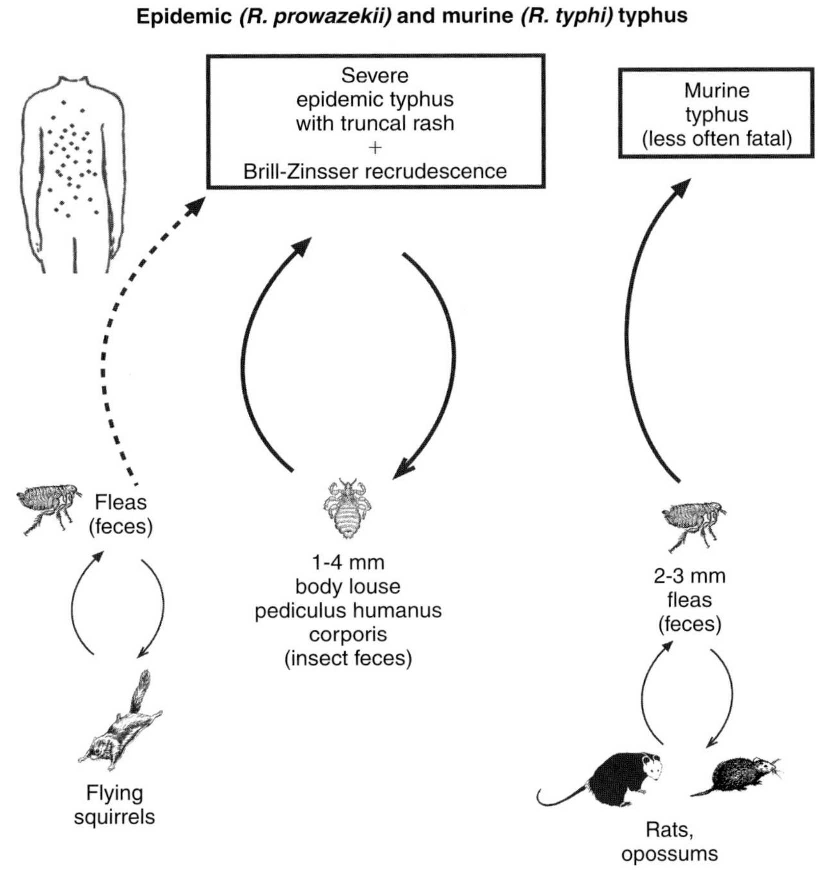

their own species of louse and flea without deleterious effects to the reservoir or arthropod hosts.[30] Human infection is likely the result of the deposition of flea feces upon humans whom the fleas will bite when the opportunity arises. The appearance of typhus fever in southern Europe during the 1500s suggests that it could have been introduced as a latent infection in a returning conquistador. Typhus was also described in Mexico nearly contemporaneously in 1545. Native Americans might have established the louse-human cycle after having become infected by contact with flying squirrels in eastern North America or Mexico. Transmission of *R. prowazekii* by human body lice (*Pediculus humanus corporis*) does not involve a high degree of adaptation of the rickettsia and the louse. Growth of rickettsiae to great quantities in the louse gut epithelium results not only in highly infectious louse feces but also in rupture of the intestine of the louse; extravasation of blood into the hemocoel, turning the louse's body red; and death of the louse.[31] Lice do not maintain *R. prowazekii* transovarially.

After recovery from the acute infection, *R. prowazekii* persists in many persons as an asymptomatic, latent infection. Years or decades later, presumably owing to waning immunity, the rickettsial infection reactivates as a milder, rarely fatal, bout of typhus fever with sufficient rickettsemia to infect a portion of body lice feeding on the patient. Lice do not tolerate febrile body temperatures and leave patients to seek a new host. These infected lice may transmit rickettsiae to nonimmune subjects and ignite an epidemic under conditions of general lousiness. Recrudescent typhus usually occurs less than 10 years after acute typhus fever but may occur more than 30 years afterward. Most descriptions of louse-borne typhus are of epidemics such as occurred in Europe during and after World War I involving 30 million cases and 3 million deaths in Russia alone.[32] In impoverished, cold, mountainous areas such as the tropical Andes of Peru, Guatemala, Mexico, and Ethiopia and other countries in Africa and Asia, louse-borne typhus is an endemic disease.[6,33–39] Since the civil war in central Africa, typhus that had disappeared for 25 years reemerged in Rwanda, Burundi, and Congo and is apparently becoming endemic.[34,35] It has also reappeared after 30 years in Algeria and Russia, and an autochthonous case was diagnosed in a homeless person in France in 2003.[36–39] *Pediculus humanus corporis* lice are strictly adapted to humans and live in the clothing rather than on the body, to which they go five times a day to feed. In the endemic *R. prowazekii* situation, there are localized outbreaks of infection mainly among the young, since older persons are mostly immune and serve as the reservoir for these outbreaks when they suffer sporadic cases of recrudescent typhus. Travel and lousiness are capable of introducing *R. prowazekii* into other areas, including warm locations in the tropics where the highly susceptible nonimmune population could suffer an epidemic. Lessons learned from the epidemic of louse-borne typhus that affected between 45,000 and 100,000 patients during the civil war in Burundi are that epidemic

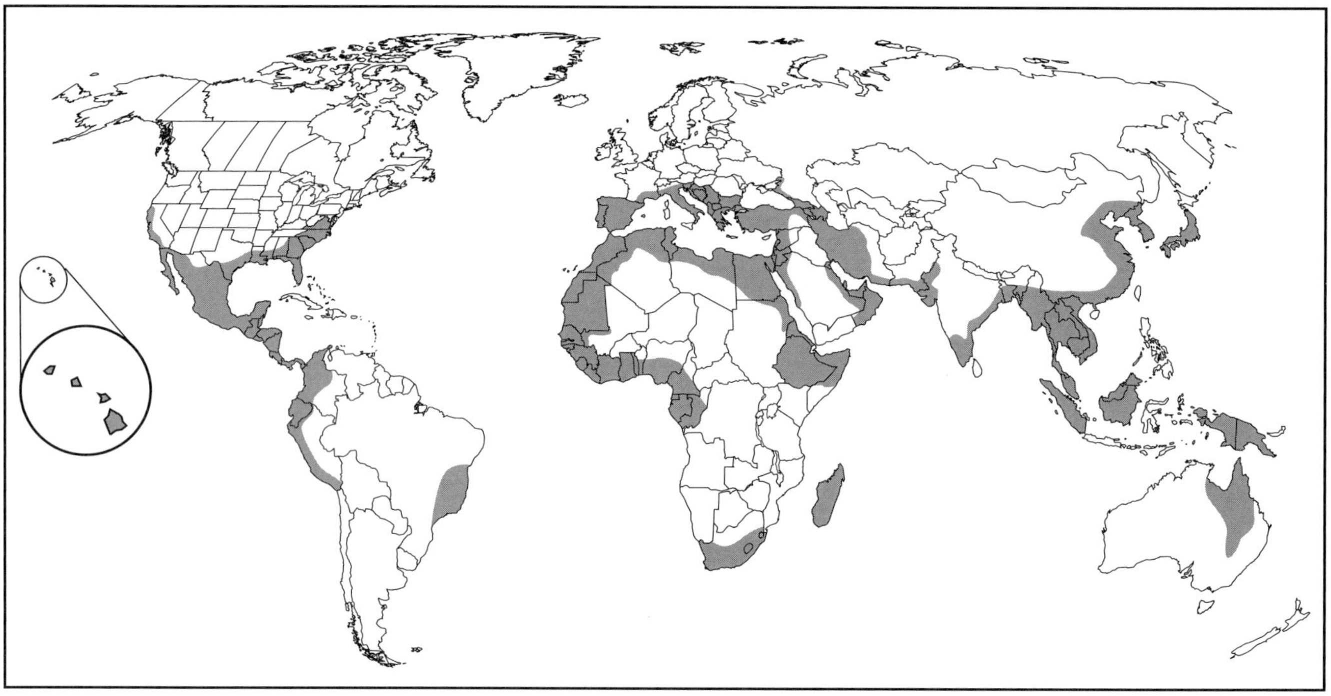

Rickettsia typhi

typhus with many fatalities can smolder in louse-infested populations of prisons and refugee camps for years without an accurate diagnosis and the disorder of war severely impedes effective epidemic control.[34,40,41] The occurrence of patients with evidence of latent *R. prowazekii* infection in populations where body lice are present emphasizes the need for vigilance.[42]

R. typhi occurs worldwide, particularly in warm, humid, coastal environments of the tropics and subtropics.[1,3–5,43–53] Prevalent in many areas although seldom investigated, murine typhus turns up frequently as recent studies in southern India, Indonesia, and Philippines have shown.[54–56] Among displaced Khmers at the Thai-Cambodian border, 70% of patients with

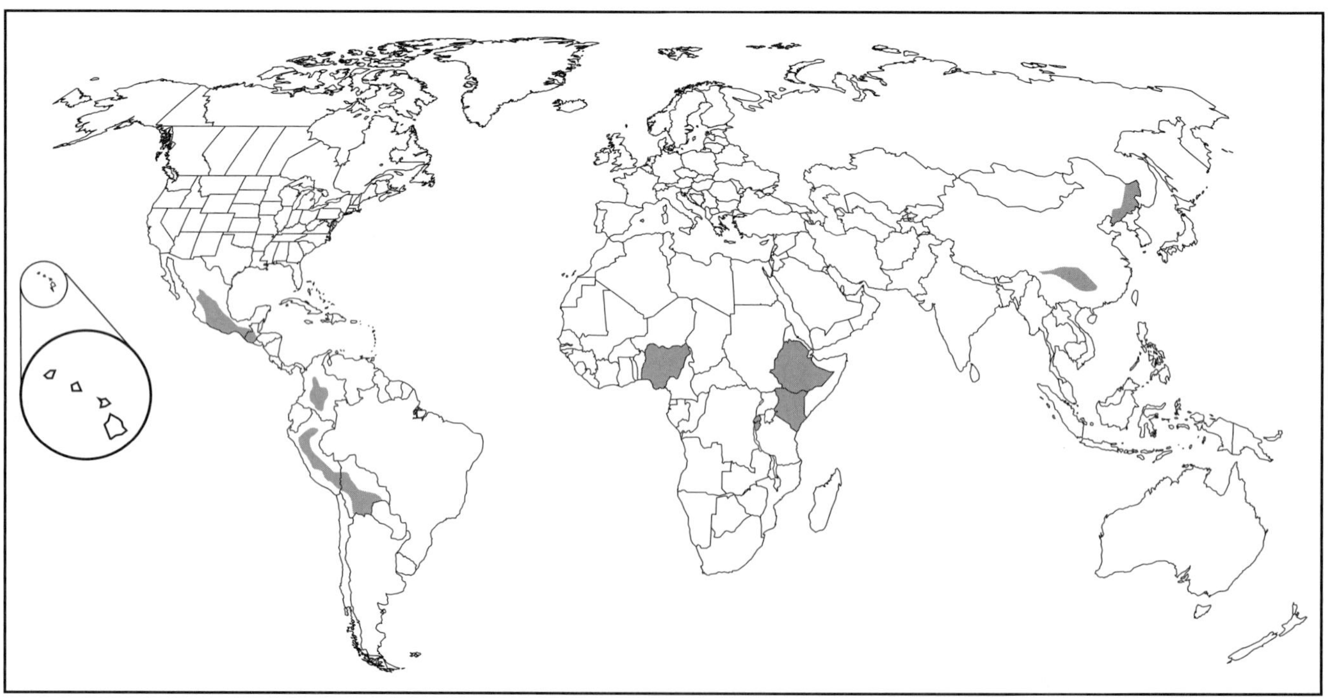

Rickettsia prowazekii

unexplained fever had murine typhus.[4] In Thailand and Laos, murine typhus is one of the most common cause of acute febrile illnesses. Although there are field and laboratory data for seven genera and 11 species of fleas, three species of lice, and three species of mites serving as vectors of *R. typhi,* the epidemiologic and ecologic evidence in most parts of the world points to the Oriental rat flea, *Xenopsylla cheopis,* as the major vector and peridomestic *Rattus* species as the critical vertebrate host. Generally rickettsiae-laden flea feces are scratched into the pruritic fleabite wound. However, a smaller fraction of infections is probably caused by fleabite. *R. typhi* might also be transmitted by rubbing infected flea feces into the conjunctival mucous membrane or by inhalation of rickettsiae from dried flea feces, in which rickettsiae have been demonstrated to survive by an unknown mechanism for years. *R. typhi* is maintained mainly by horizontal transmission from infected flea to rat to uninfected flea. Fleas remain infected for the rest of a normal life span and pass the infection transovarially to a small fraction of their offspring. Rats are highly susceptible to infection with *R. typhi,* develop sufficient rickettsemia to infect fleas imbibing their blood, and do not usually show any signs of illness. Murine typhus can spread inland along lines of transportation wherever *Rattus, X. cheopis,* and *R. typhi* are carried. Spread of inland foci occurred in the United States in the 1930s and 1940s.[57,58] Subsequent to the severe diminution in the incidence of murine typhus associated with DDT dusting and rat control, murine typhus has persisted in southern Texas and southern California, apparently in the absence of rat fleas. Cat fleas, *Ctenocephalides felis,* are the vector, and opossums are a vertebrate host of the rickettsiae and possibly serve as a reservoir.[59–61] Cycles involving other fleas and mammals such as in *Monopsyllus sciurorum sciurorum* fleas and the European fat dormouse might be present but as yet undetected elsewhere, including the tropics.[62]

Although in some instances history of exposure to rat- and rat flea–infested environments can be obtained from the patient, usually the murine typhus patient is not aware of exposure.[52,63,64] Fleabite is seldom recalled. A substantial proportion of patients are food handlers or are exposed to a focus with infected rats and rat fleas at work or home, usually unknowingly.[57]

DISEASES

The typhus fevers have clinical similarities with differences in severity according to host factors and the greater virulence of *R. prowazekii.*[65,66] Contemporary series describe the diseases when ameliorated by antirickettsial treatment.[46,52,63] Recrudescent typhus is milder, presumably because of the stimulation of anamnestic immunity. It is not clear whether flying squirrel–associated typhus is apparently milder because of the general prior good health, nutrition, living conditions, and medical care of the patients as compared with poor, malnourished, neglected cases of louse-borne typhus or whether the eastern United States flying squirrel strains are less virulent.[67–70] Murine typhus is substantially less severe than louse-borne typhus, even though among hospitalized patients 10% are admitted to the intensive care unit and 1% to 4% die.[63,64,71]

A contemporary series of 60 patients with epidemic typhus in Ethiopia was characterized clinically by fever and headache (100%), chills (82%), rash (recognized only in 38% of these patients with pigmented skin), conjunctivitis (53%), muscle tenderness (70%), nausea (32%), vomiting (10%), abdominal pain (30%), jaundice (17%), cough (38%), photophobia (33%), and no fatalities.[6] Laboratory evaluation demonstrated mild, normocytic, normochromic anemia (48%); thrombocytopenia (43%); mildly elevated serum aspartate transaminase (63%), alanine transaminase (35%), serum bilirubin (20%), lactate dehydrogenase (82%), creatine kinase (31%), blood urea nitrogen (31%), and creatinine (2%); and mild hypoproteinemia (38%). In the preantibiotic era, the fatality rate of epidemic typhus was usually at least 10% and as high as 60% under some circumstances. In the Polish series studied by Wolbach following World War I, there was a prodrome of 1 day or longer in 88%; onset characterized by fever (100%), headache (89%), chills (74%), and myalgias (54%); and admission physical examination revealing rash (100%), conjunctival injection (87%), and rales (74%).[72] Rash appeared on day 5 as pink 2- to 6-mm macules, usually on the trunk, followed by appearance on the extremities with usual sparing of face, palms, and soles. During the course, marked delirium (48%), coma (6%), hemorrhagic rash (34%), gangrene (4%), and opportunistic bronchopneumonia (10%) occurred, and 13.3% of patients died. The patients of the Burundi epidemic suffered from prominent myalgia as well as fever, delirium, stupor, confusion, dry cough, conjunctivitis, and the frequently prominent feature of constipation. Even in the darkly pigmented patients, a rash was often visible in the axilla (Fig. 51-1).[34,40] Chest roentgenograms frequently reveal interstitial pneumonia. Flying squirrel–associated typhus has been characterized by fever (100%),

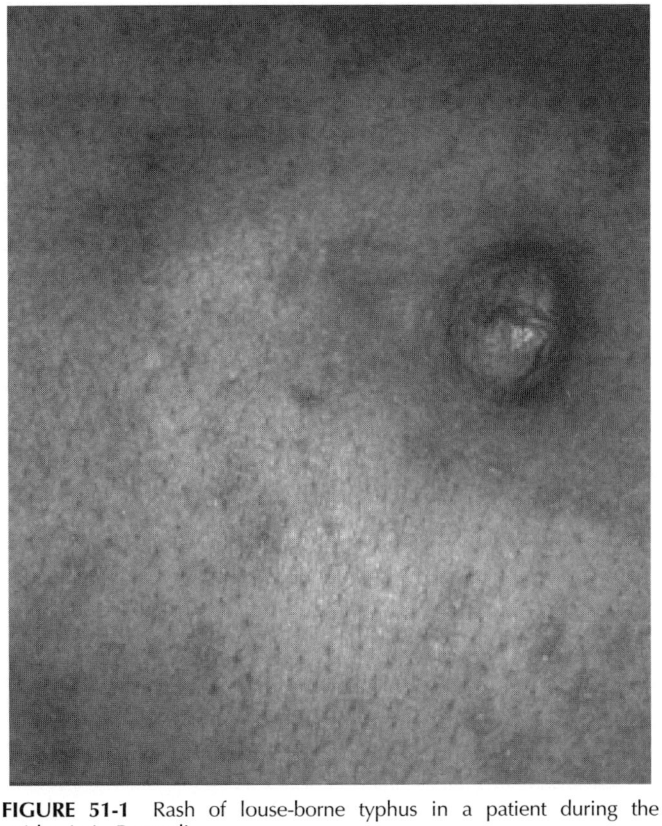

FIGURE 51-1 Rash of louse-borne typhus in a patient during the epidemic in Burundi.

headache (81%), maculopapular rash (66%), confusion (44%), and myalgia (42%).[69] Patients with Brill-Zinsser recrudescent typhus suffer fever, intense headache, myalgia, nausea, dulled sensorium, congested conjunctiva, constipation, and maculopapular rash appearing on the back and abdomen on days 5–7 and spreading rapidly.

In contemporary murine typhus series from Thailand, southern Texas, and Greece, after an incubation period of 1–2 weeks the clinical manifestations have been fever (98% to 100%), headache (42% to 100%, occurring less frequently in children), chills (64% to 92%), rash (2% to 71% with recognition dependent largely on darkness of skin pigmentation), myalgia (45% to 71%), nausea (31% to 59%), vomiting (23% to 40%), diarrhea (5% to 26%), abdominal pain (11% to 31%), jaundice (3% to 11%), confusion (2% to 8%), and seizures (2% to 4%).[4,5,46,52,63] The rash is macular or maculopapular (78%) and is petechial in less than 10%.[46] Murine typhus in pediatric patients is frequently mild, with half of the Thai patients suffering only nocturnal fever with normal daytime activities.[73] Experiments in human volunteers in the preantibiotic era documented an incubation period of 8 to 16 days (mean, 11.1 days), a prodrome usually of 2 days' duration, rash appearing in 79% of patients usually after 4 days of illness, and an average duration of fever of 12 days.[74] A series of 30 hospitalized pediatric cases of murine typhus had more clinical and laboratory manifestations: fever (100%), rash (80%), headache (77%), abdominal pain (60%), vomiting (43%), cough (40%), thrombocytopenia (60%), hyponatremia (66%), and hypoalbuminemia (46%).[75] In some patients, the signs, symptoms, and cerebrospinal fluid (CSF) mononuclear cell–predominant pleocytosis and increased protein concentration are similar to the findings in viral and leptospiral meningoencephalitis.[76] On the other hand, central nervous system (CNS) abnormalities may occur in patients with normal CSF. Chest radiographs are abnormal in 20% or more of patients, who have pulmonary infiltrates, atelectasis, pulmonary edema, or pleural effusions.[63] Laboratory evaluation of the pathophysiology reveals thrombocytopenia (48%); hyponatremia (60%); hypocalcemia (79%); elevated serum urea (27%) and creatinine (21%); hypoalbuminemia (89%); and elevated serum aspartate transaminase (90%), alanine transaminase (73%), alkaline phosphatase (60%), lactate dehydrogenase (87%), and creatine kinase (21%).[63] Complications may include acute renal failure (usually prerenal azotemia), respiratory failure requiring intubation, severe CNS disease, hematemesis, intracerebral hemorrhage, cardiac conduction abnormalities, intravascular hemolysis due in some cases to glucose-6-phosphate dehydrogenase deficiency or hemoglobinopathy, and exploratory laparotomy for suspected acute surgical abdomen.[46,52,63,76,77]

PATHOGENESIS AND IMMUNITY

Typhus group rickettsiae attach to the surface of endothelial cells, rapidly stimulate their entry by induced phagocytosis, and quickly escape from the phagosome into the cytosol, where they divide rather slowly (every 8 to 10 hours) by binary fission.[78] Only after the endothelial cell is greatly distended with rickettsiae does it burst, resulting in its death and release of the organisms for another cycle of infection. The macrophage is a target cell for a smaller fraction of the rickettsiae. Injury to the infected endothelium results in vascular lesions in the skin, brain, and other organs manifested as rash, encephalitis, myositis, and increased vascular permeability.[72,79] The last results in edema, hypovolemia, hypotension, hypoalbuminemia, azotemia, and hyponatremia. Only a very small portion of infected, injured blood vessels thrombose, and ischemic necrosis occurs only rarely.[72] Typhus rickettsiae have phospholipase activity that is hypothesized to play a role in entry, escape from the phagosome, and cell injury.[80] Analysis of the genomes of *R. prowazekii* and *R. typhi* has revealed several candidates for membranolytic function including *tlyA*, *tlyC*, *pldA*, and a gene with similarity to the patatin protein family, the main storage protein of potatoes, which also has phospholipase A activity.[25,26] Current evidence is strongest for expression and activity of phospholipase D (*pldA*) and typhus hemolysin C (*tlyC*).[81,82] Another potential virulence factor is *sodB*, an ortholog of an iron-associated superoxide dismutase, which is predicted to remove reactive oxygen species and favor rickettsial intracellular survival.[25] In vitro data suggest that rickettsial infection of endothelium and macrophages stimulates secretion of prostaglandin E_2, prostaglandin I_2, leukotriene B_4, and platelet-activating factor, which along with interleukin-1 (IL-1), tumor necrosis factor–α (TNF-α), and other cytokines has been hypothesized to account for some of the pathophysiologic effects of typhus.[83–85] It is unclear whether the concentrations and locations of secretion of these mediators are likely to account in part for aspects of the disease not caused directly by rickettsial killing of endothelial cells.

Typhus lesions are composed of small blood vessels with swollen endothelium and perivascular accumulation of lymphocytes and macrophages.[72] Intradermal rickettsial inoculation is accompanied by prompt recruitment of perivascular infiltration of CD8 and CD4 T lymphocytes in immune humans.[86] Typhus rickettsiae are killed intracellularly and extracellularly by nitric oxide synthesized by murine macrophages, and potentially and more importantly by endothelial cells, activated by IFN-γ and TNF-α.[87,88] IFN-γ and CD8 T lymphocytes are critical effectors of immune clearance of *R. typhi* in vivo in mice.[89] Cytotoxic T lymphocytes recognize typhus rickettsial antigens on infected major histocompatibility antigen-matched cells.[90] Protective immunity appears to be mediated mainly by cellular mechanisms of adaptive immunity, but natural immunity and antibodies are likely to contribute as well.[91] *R. prowazekii* resides in a latent state in the lymph nodes of healthy persons long after recovery from acute typhus fever, but the mechanism of reactivation of *R. prowazekii* is poorly understood.[92]

DIAGNOSIS

The nonspecific flulike symptoms of typhus fevers prior to the appearance of the exanthem, which never occurs in many patients, particularly the dark-skinned populations of the tropics, are nearly impossible to recognize as louse-borne typhus or murine typhus.[4,6,63] Typhus was confounded historically with malaria and typhoid and is frequently misdiagnosed as these two diseases currently.[34,39,40,110]

Prominent cough and pulmonary signs may suggest pneumonia or bronchitis; neurologic signs with or without CSF abnormalities raise the diagnostic consideration of viral or bacterial meningoencephalitis; gastrointestinal symptoms and abdominal tenderness may suggest viral and bacterial enterocolitis or acute surgical abdomen; elevated hepatic enzymes or jaundice suggests the possibility of viral hepatitis. In addition, the differential diagnosis includes typhoid fever; malaria; leptospirosis; arboviral, enteroviral, filoviral, and arenaviral infections; meningococcemia; measles; secondary syphilis; and toxic shock syndrome. The clinical response of typhus group rickettsioses to treatment with chloramphenicol is often interpreted erroneously as support for a diagnosis of typhoid fever. Even in areas where typhus infections are well known to the medical community, the initial correct clinical diagnosis of typhus is made in only 5% to 10% of cases.[63] The Burundi epidemic of typhus, after years of smoldering activity, was recognized only by the investigation of the death of an emergently repatriated Swiss nurse. Murine typhus is among the most prevalent febrile illnesses in the tropics but usually remains misdiagnosed in those seeking medical attention and undiagnosed in those who have no access to health care. Typhus group infections also occur in travelers returning from endemic areas including southern Europe and southeast Asia.[93–96]

Often the first clue to the occurrence of a typhus group infection is a serologic result, even the least sensitive and least specific of which are not necessarily available in many tropical locations. Although the serologic diagnosis of rickettsial diseases is generally retrospective, the relatively long incubation period and lateness in the course when typhus infection is usually considered allows time for the generation of the detectable antibody response in the first serum sample of some patients.[97] The extensive cross-reactivity among typhus group rickettsiae permits use of any one of them as a test antigen, but does not allow easy demonstration of which agent stimulated the antibody response, since fewer than half of patients with epidemic typhus have a fourfold higher titer against *R. prowazekii* than against *R. typhi*. Cross-absorption, although capable of specific diagnosis, is laborious, expensive, and seldom undertaken.[98] The accepted standard is the indirect immunofluorescent antibody assay (IFA), which requires an ultraviolet microscope that seldom is available in the tropical setting.[99] An IgG titer of 128 or an IgM titer of 32 is considered to be diagnostic. Serodiagnosis can be achieved from blood spotted onto filter paper and mailed to a reference laboratory.[100] The indirect immunoperoxidase antibody assay requires only a light microscope and performs with equivalent sensitivity and specificity to the IFA.[4,5,52] In Thailand, the diagnostic criterion for this test in murine typhus is a fourfold or greater rise in titer to at least 200 or a single titer of either 400 or 800, depending on the serologic titers in the healthy local population. Comparison of a rapid, simple dot ELISA with IFA and the historic, but now archaic, Weil-Felix *Proteus* agglutination test demonstrated that the sensitivity and specificity of the dot ELISA were 89% and 98%, respectively, and of the *Proteus* OX-19 agglutination, 72% and 98%, respectively, at a cut-off titer of 320.[97,101] In certain settings, even *Proteus* OX-19 agglutination is a useful tool in recognizing the occurrence of typhus fevers. Whether or not patients with recrudescent typhus produce IgM antibodies to *R. prowazekii*, among which are those that cross-react with and agglutinate *Proteus* OX-19, is controversial.[102]

Immunohistologic demonstration of typhus group rickettsiae in a cutaneous biopsy or necropsy tissues also establishes the diagnosis of a typhus group infection.[79,103,104] An etiologic diagnosis of a specific *Rickettsia* species infection requires isolation and identification of the obligate intracellular organisms in living cells of cell culture (most effectively the shell vial centrifugation-enhanced system), inoculated animals, or embryonated eggs, or polymerase chain reaction (PCR) amplification of DNA of a rickettsial gene and species identification by restriction fragment length polymorphism analysis or sequencing.[105–108] While these methods are not routinely available owing to cost and the paucity of scientists with expertise in rickettsiology, their application on a selective basis to establish the presence of the various typhus fevers in a particular region would stimulate awareness of the presence of these infections. *Rickettsia prowazekii* can be detected by PCR on lice removed from patients even after sent via mail to a reference laboratory.[109] Ultimately, timely presumptive diagnosis of the individual patient relies on knowledgeable clinical suspicion, and implementation of public health measures to control epidemic typhus or rats and rat fleas depends on a precise diagnosis. A bioterrorism attack of aerosol-transmitted typhus would be very unlikely to be considered diagnostically before the onset of rash, possibly not even then.[17]

TREATMENT

Patients with typhus infections treated before severe hypotension, acute renal or respiratory failure, severe CNS disease, or other complications occur usually respond dramatically to antirickettsial therapy, particularly doxycycline, with defervescence within 48 to 72 hours.[46,52,63] Louse-borne typhus fever has been treated successfully in some settings with a single 200-mg oral dose of doxycycline.[34] Single-dose doxycycline treatment has greater than 80% efficacy in murine typhus but is not recommended because relapses may occur.[52] The current recommendations are to treat with oral doxycycline (100 mg twice daily), oral tetracycline (25 to 50 mg/kg/d in four divided doses), or chloramphenicol (60 to 75 mg/kg/d in four divided doses). Patients who are comatose or vomiting can be treated intravenously, and doxycycline or chloramphenicol is recommended for patients with renal failure. Pregnant patients should be evaluated individually and treated with either chloramphenicol (early trimester) or doxycycline (late trimester) if necessary. Treatment should, if possible, be continued for 2 to 3 days after defervescence to avoid relapse. The fluoroquinolone ciprofloxacin has been associated with treatment failure and should not be used.[39,107,110,111] Clinical experience, the intracellular niche, and the presence of β-lactamase and several multidrug transport analogs in the genomes emphasize the natural resistance of *R. prowazekii* and *R. typhi* to most classes of antibiotics.[25,26] The lack of therapeutic response of the 63% of pediatric patients with murine typhus to treatment with a third-generation cephalosporin is a typical situation;[75] in louse-borne typhus, the outcome can be fatal.[110] It is advisable to avoid giving sulfa-containing antimicrobials to patients suspected of having a typhus infection because these drugs actually exacerbate the disease. Strains of *R. prowazekii* resistant to chloramphenicol[15] or tetracycline have been selected in the laboratory, and transformation to antimicrobial resistance has been performed by molecular methods.[112] Thus, the specter of a bioterrorism attack with *R. prowazekii* or *R. typhi* resistant to all antibiotics is a threat that has not been addressed. Supportive care, including intensive care nursing, avoidance of pressure sores, dialysis, mechanical ventilation with supplemental oxygen, transfusions, amputation of gangrenous extremities, and antimicrobial treatment of opportunistic pneumonia may be required in some severely ill patients.

PREVENTION AND CONTROL

Control of epidemic and highly prevalent endemic typhus fevers depends on marked reduction in the vector and, in some cases, the reservoir populations. Murine typhus decreased from more than 5000 cases reported annually in the southern United States during the 1940s to fewer than 100 annual cases currently following repeated dusting of rat passageways with DDT, killing rats, and modifying buildings to prevent entry of rats. Epidemics of human louse-borne typhus have been curtailed by use of insecticides such as lindane power for delousing, and washing clothes in hot water to kill the lice. Dusting powder containing 1% permethrin applied in doses of 30 to 50 mg per adult on both inside and outside of clothing and on bedding can be repeated at 6-week intervals to kill lice. Some louse populations are resistant to some of insecticides.[113] The large Burundi epidemic was controlled by immediate treatment of patients with 200 mg of doxycycline.[34] Vaccination has been used with some apparent success to prevent louse-borne typhus.[113] Killed *R. prowazekii* vaccines required boosters and seemed to reduce the severity of illness in persons whose protection was only partial. A live attenuated strain was used as an effective vaccine under epidemiologic conditions where dose-dependent local and systemic reactions during the 2- to 3-day period after immunization, mild to moderate symptomatic infection 9 to 14 days after inoculation in approximately 14% of recipients, and the possibility of reversion to virulence were acceptable. Use of such vaccines may be no more than a theoretical possibility at present because none are licensed or produced. Development of a highly effective, safe vaccine that would provide protection against all rickettsial infections is a feasible goal.[114] However, the lack of awareness of the true disease burden of these infections by public health agencies and the unlikeliness of commercial profit to be gained from the perceived target populations of the neglected poor in the tropics mitigate against vaccine development.

REFERENCES

1. Traub R, Wisseman CL, Farhang-Azad A: The ecology of murine typhus—a critical review. Trop Dis Bull 75:237, 1978.
2. Al-Awadi AR, Al-Kazemi N, Ezzat G, et al: Murine typhus in Kuwait in 1978. Bull World Health Organ 60:283, 1982.
3. Brown AE, Meek SR, Maneechai N, et al: Murine typhus among Khmers living at an evacuation site on the Thai-Kampuchean border. Am J Trop Med Hyg 38:168, 1988.
4. Duffy PE, Le Guillouzic H, Gass RF, et al: Murine typhus identified as a major cause of febrile illness in a camp for displaced Khmers in Thailand. Am J Trop Med Hyg 43:520, 1990.
5. Wilde H, Pornsilapatip J, Sokly T, et al: Murine and scrub typhus at Thai-Kampuchean border displaced persons camps. Trop Geogr Med 43:363, 1991.
6. Perine PL, Chandler BP, Krause DK, et al: A clinico-epidemiological study of epidemic typhus in Africa. Clin Infect Dis 14:1149, 1992.
7. De Toro L: De la fiebre epidemica y nueva, en latin punticular, vulgarmente tabardillo y pintas. Burgos, Spain, Felipe Junta, 1574. Reprint Madrid, Imprenta de J Cosano, 1941.
8. Raoult D, Woodward T, Dumler J: The history of epidemic typhus. Infect Dis Clin North Am 18:127, 2004.
9. Brill NE: An acute infectious disease of unknown origin. Am J Med Sci 139:484, 1910.
10. Paullin JE: Typhus fever with a report of cases. South Med J 6:36, 1913.
11. Zinsser H, Castaneda MR: On the isolation from a case of Brill's disease of a typhus strain resembling the European type. N Engl J Med 209:815, 1933.
12. Zinsser H: Varieties of typhus virus and the epidemiology of the American form of European typhus fever (Brill's disease). Am J Hyg 20:513, 1934.
13. Maxcy KF: An epidemiological study of endemic typhus (Brill's disease) in the southeastern United States with special reference to its mode of transmission. Public Health Rep 41:2967, 1926.
14. Dyer RE, Rumreich A, Badger LF: Typhus fever. A virus of the typhus type derived from fleas collected from wild rats. Public Health Rep 46:334, 1931.
15. Weiss E, Dressler HR: Increased resistance to chloramphenicol in *Rickettsia prowazekii* with a note on failure to demonstrate genetic interaction among strains. J Bacterial 83:409, 1962.
16. Azad A, Radulovic S: Pathogenic rickettsiae as bioterrorism agents. Ann NY Acad Sci 990:734, 2003.
17. Walker DH: Principles of the malicious use of infectious agents to create terror: reasons for concern for organisms of the genus *Rickettsia*. Ann NY Acad Sci 990:1, 2003.
18. Vishwanath S: Antigenic relationships among the rickettsiae of the spotted fever and typhus groups. FEMS Microbiol Lett 81:341, 1991.
19. Carl M, Dobson ME, Ching W-M, et al: Characterization of the gene encoding the protective paracrystalline-surface-layer protein of *Rickettsia prowazekii*: presence of a truncated identical homolog in *Rickettsia typhi*. Proc Natl Acad Sci USA 87:8237, 1990.
20. Hahn M, Kim K, Kim I, et al: Cloning and sequence analysis of the gene encoding the crystalline surface layer protein of *Rickettsia typhi*. Gene 133:129, 1993.
21. Hahn M, Chang W: Expression and purification of the crystalline surface layer protein of *Rickettsia typhi*. Microbiol Immunol 40:233, 1996.
22. Roux V, Raoult D: Phylogenetic analysis of the genus *Rickettsia* by 16S rDNA sequencing. Res Microbiol 146:385, 1995.
23. Winkler HH: *Rickettsia* species (as organisms). Annu Rev Microbiol 44:131, 1990.
24. Andersson SGE: Bioenergenetics of the obligate intracellular parasite *Rickettsia prowazekii*. Biochem Biophys Acta 1365:105, 1998.
25. McLeod MP, Qin X, Karpathy SE, et al: The complete genome sequence of *Rickettsia typhi* and comparison with other rickettsiae. J Bacteriol 186:5842, 2004.
26. Andersson SGE, Zomorodipour A, Andersson JO, et al: The genome sequence of *Rickettsia prowazekii* and the origin of mitochondria. Nature 396:113, 1998.
27. Tucker AM, Winkler HH, Driskell LO, et al: *S*-Adenosylmethionine transport in *Rickettsia prowazekii*. J Bacteriol 185:3031, 2003.
28. Ogata H, Aduc S, Abergel C, et al: Protein coding palindromes are a unique but recurrent feature in *Rickettsia*. Genome Res 12:808, 2002.
29. Gaywee J, Xu WL, Radulovic S, et al: The *Rickettsia prowazekii* invasion gene homolog (*invA*) encodes a nudix hydrolase active on adenosine (5′)-pentaphospho-(5′)-adenosine. Mol Cell Proteomics 1:179, 2002.
30. Sonenshine DE, Bozeman FM, Williams MS, et al: Epizootiology of epidemic typhus (*Rickettsia prowazekii*) in flying squirrels. Am J Trop Med Hyg 27:339, 1978.
31. Houhamdi L, Fournier P, Fang R, et al: An experimental model of human body louse infection with *Rickettsia prowazekii*. J Infect Dis 186:1639, 2002.
32. Patterson KD: Typhus and its control in Russia, 1870–1940. Med Hist 37:361, 1993.
33. Raoult D, Birtles RJ, Montoya M, et al: Survey of louse-associated diseases among rural Andean communities in Peru: prevalence of epidemic typhus, trench fever, and relapsing fever. Clin Infect Dis 29:434, 1999.
34. Raoult D, Ndihokubwayo JB, Tissot-Dupont H, et al: Outbreak of epidemic typhus associated with trench fever in Burundi. Lancet 352:353, 1998.
35. Fournier PE, Ndihokubwayo JB, Guidran J, et al: Human pathogens in body and head lice. Emerg Infect Dis 8:1515, 2001.
36. Mokrani K, Fournier PE, Dalichaouche M, et al: Reemerging threat of epidemic typhus in Algeria. J Clin Microbiol 42:3898, 2004.

37. Tarasevich I, Rydkina E, Raoult D: Epidemic typhus in Russia. Lancet 352:1151, 1998.
38. Badiaga S, Brouqui P, Raoult D: Autochthonous epidemic typhus associated with *Bartonella quintana* bacteremia in a homeless person. Am J Trop Med Hyg, 2005, in press.
39. Niang M, Brouqui P, Raoult D: Epidemic typhus imported from Algeria. Emerg Infect Dis 5:716, 1999.
40. Ndihokubwayo J-B, Raoult D: Le typhus epidemique en Afrique. Medecine Tropicale 59:181, 1999.
41. Raoult D, Roux V, Ndihokubwaho JB, et al: Jail fever (epidemic typhus) outbreak in Burundi. Emerg Infect Dis 3:357, 1997.
42. Alcantara VE, Gallardo EG, Hong C, et al: Typhus group rickettsiae antibodies in rural Mexico. Emerg Infect Dis 10:549, 2004.
43. Azad AF: Epidemiology of murine typhus. Annu Rev Entomol 35:553, 1990.
44. Gross EM, Arbeli Y, Bearman JE, et al: Spotted fever and murine typhus in the Negev Desert region of Israel, 1981. Bull World Health Organ 62:301, 1984.
45. Graves SR, Banks J, Dwyer B, et al: A case of murine typhus in Queensland. Med J Aust 156:650, 1992.
46. Tselentis Y, Babalis T, Chrysanthis D, et al: Clinicoepidemiological study of murine typhus on the Greek Island of Evia. Eur J Epidemiol 8:268, 1992.
47. Corwin A, Habib M, Watts D, et al: Community-based prevalence profile of arboviral, rickettsial, and hantaan-like viral antibody in the Nile River Delta of Egypt. Am J Trop Med Hyg 48:776, 1993.
48. Takada N, Fujita H, Yano Y, et al: Serosurveys of spotted fever and murine typhus in local residents of Taiwan and Thailand compared with Japan. Southeast Asian J Trop Med Public Health 24:354, 1993.
49. Strickman D, Tanskul P, Eamsila C, et al: Prevalence of antibodies to rickettsiae in the human population of surburban Bangkok. Am J Trop Med Hyg 51:149, 1994.
50. Gray GC, Rodier GR, Matras-Maslin VC, et al: Serologic evidence of respiratory and rickettsial infections among Somali refugees. Am J Trop Med Hyg 52:349, 1995.
51. Letjaief AO, Yacoub S, Dupont HT, et al: Seroepidemiological survey of rickettsial infections among blood donors in central Tunisia. Trans R Soc Trop Med Hyg 89:266, 1995.
52. Silpapojakul K, Chayakul P, Krisanapan S: Murine typhus in Thailand: clinical features, diagnosis and treatment. Q J Med 86:43, 1993.
53. Dupont HT, Brouqui P, Faugere B, et al: Prevalence of antibodies to *Coxiella burnetii, Rickettsia conorii,* and *Rickettsia typhi* in seven African countries. Clin Infect Dis 21:1126, 1995.
54. Mathai E, Lloyd G, Cherian T, et al: Serological evidence for the continued presence of human rickettsioses in southern India. Ann Trop Med Parasitol 95:395, 2001.
55. Richards AL, Faisal Rusjdi EA, Kelly DJ, et al: Evidence of *Rickettsia typhi* and the potential for murine typhus in Jayapura, Irian Jaya, Indonesia. Am J Trop Med Hyg 66:431, 2002.
56. Camer GA, Alejandria M, Amor M, et al: Detection of antibodies against spotted fever group *Rickettsia* (SFGR), typhus group *Rickettsia* (TGR), and *Coxiella burnetii* in human febrile patients in the Philippines. Jpn J Infect Dis 56:26, 2003.
57. Tucker CB, Woodring TV, Essick HC: An outbreak of endemic typhus fever in Nashville, Tennessee. Am J Public Health 31:917, 1941.
58. Topping NH: Apparent recent extension of typhus in the United States. Am J Trop Med Hyg 23:37, 1943.
59. Farhang-Azad A, Traub R, Sofi M, et al: Experimental murine typhus infection in the cat flea, *Ctenocephalides felis* (Siphonaptera: Pulicidae). J Med Entomol 21:675, 1984.
60. Williams SG, Sacci JB, Jr., Schriefer ME, et al: Typhus and typhuslike rickettsiae associated with opossums and their fleas in Los Angeles County, California. J Clin Microbiol 30:1758, 1992.
61. Sorvillo FJ, Gondo B, Emmons R, et al: A suburban focus of endemic typhus in Los Angeles County: Association with seropositive domestic cats and opossums. Am J Trop Med Hyg 48:269, 1993.
62. Trilar T, Radulovic S, Walker DH: Identification of a natural cycle involving *Rickettsia typhi* infection of *Monopsyllus sciurorum sciurorum* fleas from the nests of the fat dormouse. Eur J Epidemiol 10:757, 1994.
63. Dumler JS, Taylor JP, Walker DH: Clinical and laboratory features of murine typhus in South Texas, 1980 through 1987. JAMA 266:1365, 1991.
64. Miller ES, Beeson PB: Murine typhus fever. Medicine (Baltimore) 25:1, 1946.
65. Walker DH: The role of host factors in the severity of spotted fever and typhus rickettsioses. Ann NY Acad Sci 590:10, 1990.
66. McDade JE: Evidence supporting the hypothesis that rickettsial virulence factors determine the severity of spotted fever and typhus group infections. Ann NY Acad Sci 590:20, 1990.
67. McDade JE, Shepard CC, Redus MA, et al: Evidence of *Rickettsia prowazekii* infections in the United States. Am J Trop Med Hyg 29:277, 1980.
68. Duma RJ, Sonenshine DE, Bozeman FM, et al: Epidemic typhus in the United States associated with flying squirrels. JAMA 245:2318, 1981.
69. CDC: Epidemic typhus associated with flying squirrels—United States. MMWR 31:555, 1982.
70. Ackley AM, Peter WJ: Indigenous acquisition of epidemic typhus in the eastern United States. South Med J 74:245, 1981.
71. Stuart BM, Pullen RL: Endemic (murine) typhus fever: clinical observations of 180 cases. Ann Intern Med 23:520, 1945.
72. Wolbach SB, Todd JL, Palfrey FW: The Etiology and Pathology of Typhus. Cambridge, Mass, League of Red Cross Societies at the Harvard University Press, 1922.
73. Silpapojakul K, Chupuppakarn S, Yuthasompob S, et al: Scrub and murine typhus in children with obscure fever in the tropics. Pediatr Infect Dis J 10:200, 1991.
74. Woodward TE: Murine typhus fever: its clinical and biologic similarity to epidemic typhus. In Walker DH (ed): Biology of Rickettsial Diseases. Boca Raton, Fla, CRC Press, 1988, p 79.
75. Fergie JE, Purcell K, Wanat D: Murine typhus in South Texas children. Pediatr Infect Dis J 19:535, 2000.
76. Silpapojakul K, Ukkachoke C, Krisanapan S: Rickettsial meningitis and encephalitis. Arch Intern Med 151:1753, 1991.
77. Shaked Y, Shpilberg O, Samra Y: Involvement of the kidneys in Mediterranean spotted fever and murine typhus. Q J Med 87:103, 1994.
78. Walker TS: Rickettsial interactions with human endothelial cells in vitro: adherence and entry. Infect Immun 44:205, 1984.
79. Walker DH, Parks FM, Betz TG, et al: Histopathology and immunohistologic demonstration of the distribution of *Rickettsia typhi* in fatal murine typhus. Am J Clin Pathol 91:720, 1989.
80. Ojcius DM, Thibon M, Mounier C, et al: pH and calcium dependence of hemolysis due to *Rickettsia prowazekii*: comparison with phospholipase activity. Infect Immun 63:3069, 1995.
81. Renesto P, Dehoux P, Gouin E, et al: Identification and characterization of a phospholipase D-superfamily gene in rickettsiae. J Infect Dis 188:1276, 2003.
82. Whitworth T, Bouyer D: Personal communication, 2004.
83. Walker TS, Brown JS, Hoover CS, et al: Endothelial prostaglandin secretion: effects of typhus rickettsiae. J Infect Dis 162:1136, 1990.
84. Walker TS, Dersch MW, White WE: Effects of typhus rickettsiae on peritoneal and alveolar macrophages: Rickettsiae stimulate leukotriene and prostaglandin secretion. J Infect Dis 163:568, 1991.
85. Walker TS, Mellott GE: Rickettsial stimulation of endothelial platelet-activating factor synthesis. Infect Immun 61:2024, 1993.
86. Dumler JS, Wisseman CL Jr: Preliminary characterization of inflammatory infiltrates in response to *Rickettsia prowazekii* reinfection in man: Immunohistology. Acta Virol 36:45, 1992.
87. Turco J, Winkler HH: Role of nitric oxide synthase pathway in inhibition of growth of interferon-sensitive and interferon-resistant *Rickettsia prowazekii* strains in L929 cells treated with tumor necrosis factor alpha and gamma interferon. Infect Immun 61:4317, 1993.
88. Turco J, Liu H, Gottlieb SF, et al: Nitric oxide-mediated inhibition of the ability of *Rickettsia prowazekii* to infect mouse fibroblasts and mouse macrophagelike cells. Infect Immun 66:558, 1998.
89. Walker DH, Popov V, Feng H-G: Establishment of a novel endothelial target mouse model of a typhus group rickettsiosis: evidence for critical roles for gamma interferon and CD8 T-lymphocytes. Lab Invest 80:1361, 2000.
90. Rollwagen F, Dasch G, Jerrells T: Mechanisms of immunity to rickettsial infection: characterization of a cytotoxic effector cell. J Immunol 136: 1418, 1986.
91. Rollwagen F: Role of natural killer cells in the early clearance of *Rickettsia typhi* in mice. In Eisensten T, Bullock W, Hanna N (eds): Host Defenses and Immunomodulation to Intracellular Pathogens. New York, Plenum Press, 1998.

92. Price WH, Emerson H, Nagel H, et al: Ecologic studies on the interepidemic survival of louse-borne epidemic typhus fever. Am J Hyg 67:154, 1958.
93. Hassan IS, Ong EL: Fever in the returned traveller: remember murine typhus! J Infect 31:173, 1995.
94. Wilson ME, Brush AD, Meany MC: Murine typhus acquired during short-term urban travel. Am J Med 87:233, 1989.
95. Parola P, Vogelaers D, Roure C, et al: Murine typhus in travelers returning from Indonesia. Emerg Infect Dis 4:677, 1998.
96. Gikas A, Doukakis S, Pediaditis J, et al: Murine typhus in Greece: epidemiological, clinical, and therapeutic data from 83 cases. Trans R Soc Trop Med Hyg 96:250, 2002.
97. Silpapojakul K, Pradutkanchana J, Pradutkanchana S, et al: Rapid, simple serodiagnosis of murine typhus. Trans R Soc Trop Med Hyg 89:625, 1995.
98. La Scola B, Rydkina L, Ndihokubwayo, et al: Serological differentiation of murine typhus and epidemic typhus using cross-absorption and Western blotting. Clin Diagn Lab Immunol 7:612, 2000.
99. Ormsbee R, Peacock M, Philip R, et al: Serologic diagnosis of epidemic typhus fever. Am J Epidemiol 105:261, 1977.
100. Fenollar F, Raoult D: Diagnosis of rickettsial diseases using samples dried on blotting paper. Clin Diagn Lab Immunol 6:483, 1999.
101. Kelly DJ, Chan CT, Paxton H, et al: Comparative evaluation of a commercial enzyme immunoassay for the detection of human antibody to *Rickettsia typhi*. Clin Diagn Lab Immunol 2:356, 1995.
102. Eremeeva ME, Balayeva NM, Raoult D: Serological response of patients suffering from primary and recrudescent typhus: comparison of complement fixation reaction, Weil-Felix test, microimmunofluorescence and immunoblotting. Clin Diagn Lab Immunol 1:318, 1994.
103. Stasko T, De Villez RL: Murine typhus: a case report and review. J Am Acad Dermatol 7:377, 1982.
104. Walker DH, Feng HM, Ladner S, et al: Immunohistochemical diagnosis of typhus rickettsioses using an anti-lipopolysaccharide monoclonal antibody. Mod Pathol 10:1038, 1997.
105. Carl M, Tibbs CW, Dobson ME, et al: Diagnosis of acute typhus infection using the polymerase chain reaction. J Infect Dis 161:791, 1990.
106. Walker D, Bouyer D: Rickettsia. In Baron E, Pealler M, Yolken R (eds): Manual for Clinical Microbiology. Washington, DC, ASM Press, 2003, p 1005.
107. Birg ML, La Scola B, Roux V, et al: Isolation of *Rickettsia prowazekii* from blood by shell vial cell culture. J Clin Microbiol 37:3722, 1999.
108. Schriefer ME, Sacci JB Jr, Dumler JS, et al: Identification of a novel rickettsial infection in a patient diagnosed with murine typhus. J Clin Microbiol 32:949, 1994.
109. Roux V, Raoult D: Body lice as tools for diagnosis and surveillance of reemerging diseases. J Clin Microbiol 37:596, 1999.
110. Zanetti G, Francioli P, Tagan D, et al: Imported epidemic typhus. Lancet 352:1709, 1998.
111. Laferl H, Fournier PE, Seiberl G, et al: Murine typhus poorly responsive to ciprofloxacin: a case report. J Travel Med 9:103, 2002.
112. Rachek LI, Hines A, Tucker AM, et al: Transformation of *Rickettsia prowazekii* to erythromycin resistance encoded by the *Escherichia coli ereB* gene. J Bacteriol 182:3289, 2000.
113. Wisseman CL Jr: Concepts of louse-borne typhus control in developing countries: the use of the living attenuated E strain typhus vaccine in epidemic and endemic situations. In Kohn A, Klingberg MA (eds): Immunity in Viral and Rickettsial Diseases. New York, Plenum Press, 1972, p 97.
114. Valbuena GV, Jordan JM, Walker DH: T cells mediate cross-protective immunity between typhus group rickettsiae and spotted fever group rickettsiae. J Infect Dis 190:1221, 2004.

52

Scrub Typhus

GEORGE WATT
DAVID H. WALKER

INTRODUCTION

Scrub typhus is a chigger-borne zoonosis which is of greatest public health importance in tropical Asia and the islands of the western Pacific Ocean. The clinical disease and vector mite were described in China in AD 313; the epidemiology and clinical course were recounted in a Chinese poem of AD 610.[1] The causative organism was discovered in Japan by studies of Nagayo and Ogata and their coworkers in the 1920s and early 1930s. By 1935, scrub typhus had been recognized in India, Sumatra (Indonesia), Formosa (Taiwan), the Philippines, northern Australia, the former Indochina (Vietnam), Malaya (Malaysia), Burma (now Myanmar), and New Guinea.[2] Scrub typhus became known to the West during World War II when an estimated 18,000 cases occurred in Allied soldiers; there were 30,000 cases in Japanese troops.

AGENT

In 1924, Nagayo and colleagues[3] observed stained intracellular organisms in macrophages from tissue smears of humans and animals, but were unable to cultivate the microbes that did not pass through bacterial filters. In 1930, Nagayo and coworkers isolated and passaged the microorganisms in Descemet's membrane by inoculation of the anterior chamber of the rabbit eye.[4] One year earlier, in 1929, Ogata and Unro[5] propagated the organism through 80 passages in rabbit testis and observed them stained in macrophages, and in 1932 Ogata and associates[6] developed intraperitoneal infection of mice as a valuable method of rickettsial isolation.

Although the organisms meet the general definition of rickettsiae (small [0.5×1.2 to 3.0 μm], obligate intracellular, arthropod-borne bacteria), they have been reclassified into a separate genus, *Orientia*.[7] By 16S ribosomal RNA (rRNA) phylogeny, they are closely related (98.5% to 99.9%) to one another and substantially less closely related (90.2% to 90.6% homology) to organisms of the genus *Rickettsia*. Their cell wall differs strikingly from that of *Rickettsia* ultrastructurally, in its unique component proteins, and in the lack of lipopolysaccharide and peptidoglycan.[7–11] The 56-kD outer envelope protein comprises 20% of the cellular protein and has alternating hydrophobic and hydrophilic regions consistent with a transmembrane protein containing four hydrophilic variable domains of 16 to 40 amino acids of varying sequences with epitopes that are strain-specific and others that are shared with some or all strains. There is 59% to 82% overall amino acid homology among the various strains.[9] The antigenic and genetic diversity of this major outer membrane protein is vastly different than in the classic Kato, Karp, and Gilliam strains. Other major surface-exposed proteins are 110, 47, and 25 kD in molecular mass and also manifest antigenic diversity.[12,13]

Heat shock proteins of 58 to 60 kD and 11 kD, analogues of GroEL and GroES, have species-specific DNA sequences.[14] Genetic analysis of 111 strains of *O. tsutsugamushi* from Thailand based on restriction patterns of the products of polymerase chain reaction (PCR) amplification of the 58- to 60-kD heat shock protein showed 35 *groE* genotypes.[15] Each geographic area had its own particular genotypes that were highly restricted to specific localities with little spread. Isolates from other countries also showed considerable variability that was unique to each country. Despite the enormous genetic and antigenic variability, the organism seems genetically stable; the 22- and 56-kD protein genes of rickettsiae from isolates from a chigger colony obtained 26 years apart were identical. These data suggest a large number of isolated, independent chigger lineages of *O. tsutsugamushi* with a long history of divergent evolution.

EPIDEMIOLOGY

The disease or its etiologic agent has been documented within a triangle with apices in the Primorje region of the Russian Far East, northern Australia, and Afghanistan.

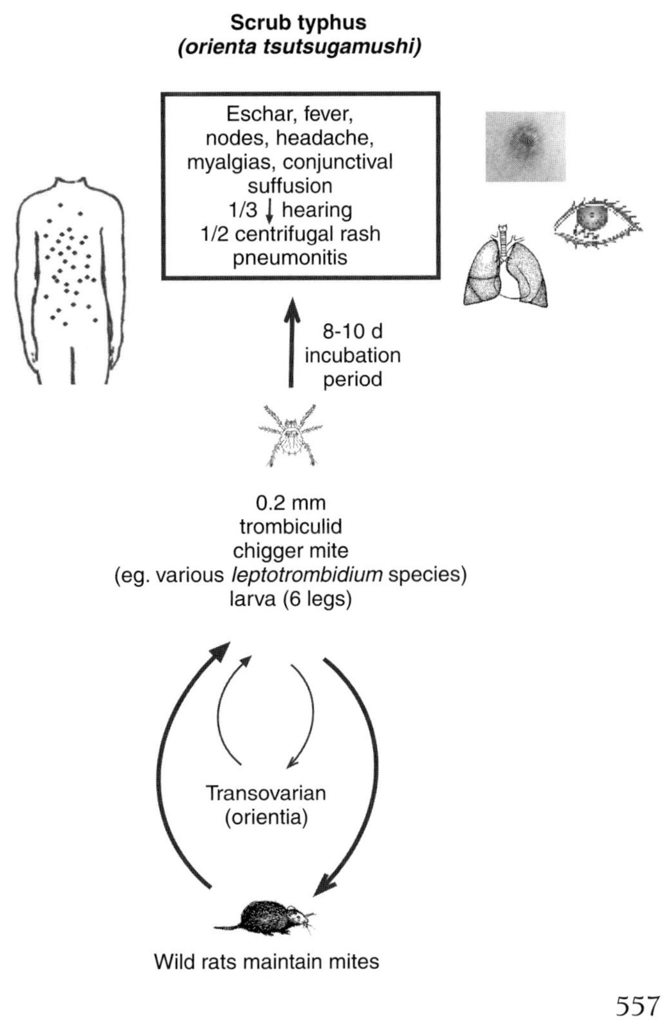

Endemic areas range from typical tropical secondary growth (scrub) vegetation to temperate zones (e.g., Kashmir, Korea, and Mount Fuji) and even the Himalayas above 3000 m elevation.[2,16,17] The ecologic factors underlying the reemergence of scrub typhus that has been documented recently in southern India, Sri Lanka, and the Maldives are not known.[18,19] Active rice fields appear to be an important underappreciated ecological niche of transmission, and agricultural exposure including on oil palm and rubber plantations and forestry poses a major risk. The etiologic agent, *O. tsutsugamushi,* is maintained by efficient transovarial transmission in trombiculid mites and is transmitted to humans by the larval mite (chigger) during feeding.[20,21] Only the six-legged larva is parasitic, feeding for 2 to 10 days on the tissue juices of the skin. The eight-legged nymphs and adults are predators that live in the forest floor. The chiggers are not host-specific, and wild rats are susceptible to long-lasting infections. The rats are key to the population density of the chiggers but are not a reservoir of *O. tsutsugamushi*; only a low proportion of chiggers acquire *O. tsutsugamushi* from infected rats, and chiggers infected by feeding neither develop a generalized infection nor transmit the organisms transovarially to their offspring.[16]

Transmission to humans occurs during the seasonal activity of the chigger, which is determined by temperature and humidity: *Leptotrombidium akamushi* transmission occurred in Japan during July to September when the temperature is above 25°C but seems to have disappeared; *Leptotrombidium pallidum* transmission occurs in Japan, Korea, and the Primorje region of Russia in two peaks, autumn to winter and late spring to early summer at 18°C to 20°C; *Leptotrombidium scutellare* transmission occurs in Japan, China, and Malaysia only in autumn and winter at 18°C to 20°C; and transmission by *Leptotrombidium deliense, Leptotrombidium fletcheri,* and *Leptotrombidium arenicola* occurs in warm, humid tropical areas year-round.[2] The efficiency of transovarian transmission varies from mite to mite and temporally in individual mites.[22,23] Infection of female mites results not only in transovarial maintenance of *Orientia* but also in sex ratio distortion in favor of females, further enhancing transovarian transmission.[24]

Disease transmission occurs in rural and suburban areas as well as in villages, but inhabitants of city centers are not at risk. Most cases go undiagnosed because symptoms and signs are often nonspecific and commercial diagnostic tests are generally not available. Where prospective, longitudinal studies have been performed, as in peninsular Malaysia, a high incidence has been observed. Scrub typhus was the cause of 18.3% and 23.3% of febrile admissions at two hospitals.[25] In two communities the incidence of *O. tsutsugamushi* was 3.9% and 3.2% per month; the seroprevalence was 48% and 53% with an age-dependent increase to greater than 80% above age 44 years.[26] Exposure to remote scrub and forested areas of Laos, Vietnam, and Cambodia resulted in seroconversion at a rate of 484 per 1000 person-years.[27] It appears that pathogenicity is age-dependent and varies geographically. In the preantibiotic era, the case-fatality rate in Japan was 30% (15% in 11- to 20-year-olds, 20% in 21- to 30-year-olds, and 59% in those above age 60 years).[28] In Taiwan the case-fatality rate was 11% (5% in children and 45% in the elderly). In the Pescadores Islands, the case-fatality rate was only 3%. Among Allied troops during World War II, outbreaks were usually associated with the early stage of development of a camp when chiggers were plentiful, with case-fatality rates ranging from less than 1% to more than 30%.[29]

DISEASE

The chigger bite can occur on any part of the body, is painless, and is not usually remembered by the patient.[30] An eschar forms at the bite site in about half of primary infections and a third of secondary infections. The eschar begins as a small, painless papule and develops during the 6- to 20-day (average 10-day) incubation period. It enlarges, undergoes central necrosis, and acquires a blackened scab (Plate 52-1). The eschar is usually well developed by the time fever appears. Regional lymph nodes are enlarged and sometimes tender. Fever and headache begin abruptly and are frequently accompanied by myalgias and malaise. Hearing loss concurrent with fever occurs in about one-third of cases and is a very useful diagnostic clue.[31] Conjunctival hyperemia and generalized lymphadenopathy are frequently occurring, diagnostically helpful physical signs.[32] A transient macular rash may appear at the end of the first week of illness. The rash appears on the trunk, becomes maculopapular, and spreads peripherally. However, it is often difficult to detect on dark-skinned persons. The systemic involvement was demonstrated by gastric endoscopic observations that paralleled the cutaneous manifestations in the 23% of scrub typhus patients who had gastrointestinal symptoms.[33] The vascular pathology and pathophysiology are emphasized in the report of a scrub typhus patient with retinal hemorrhages and increased vascular permeability observed by fluorescein retinal angiography.[34]

Cough, tachypnea, and infiltrates on chest radiography are among the most frequent presentations of scrub typhus.[35] Tachypnea sometimes progresses to dyspnea, the patient becomes cyanotic, and full-blown adult respiratory distress syndrome (ARDS) may ensue. ARDS is associated with older age and preceding infiltrates on chest radiographs in patients with scrub typhus who have a higher risk of dying, but if they recover, have no serious sequelae.[36] Relative bradycardia is the main cardiac manifestation.[37,38] Confusion, apathy, and other mild personality changes are common. Convulsions and coma occur only rarely.[39] In a patient with severe encephalomyelitis, MRI lesions were observed in locations corresponding to the neurologic deficits and the usual distribution of pathologic lesions.[40] Severe disease associated with delayed diagnosis may be associated with ARDS, acute renal failure, hypotensive shock, and occasionally disseminated intravascular coagulation.

PATHOGENESIS AND IMMUNITY

Human volunteers fed upon by infected chiggers developed a febrile illness with an eschar and regional lymphadenopathy after an 8- to 10-day incubation period during which organisms were apparently inoculated from the salivary glands of the chiggers into the dermis and subsequently spread to the regional lymph nodes and bloodstream.[21] Bacteremia was detected 1 to 3 days before onset of fever.

The target cells of *O. tsutsugamushi* in humans are endothelial cells throughout the body, macrophages, and cardiac myocytes.[41,42] Organisms have been identified in pleural, pericardial, and peritoneal cells in spleen and liver, and mononuclear cells circulating in the blood.

Evaluation of the results of both experimental animal infections and studies in cell culture is confounded by the unclear relevance of the target cells in these models. In mice, the route of inoculation determines the distribution of rickettsiae: peritoneal serosa, exudate, and adjacent organ capsules after intraperitoneal inoculation; macrophages, including Kupffer cells, splenic sinusoid–lining cells, lymph node sinus–lining cells, and interstitial cells of the lung, kidney, and adrenal with subcutaneous or intramuscular inoculation; and meningeal cells following intracerebral inoculation.[43] The apparent lack of significant endothelial cell infection in these models renders interpretation of their relevance problematic.

The basic histopathologic lesions, disseminated perivasculitis, and focal interstitial mononuclear infiltrations associated with edema appear to reflect the host response to endothelial infection.[44] Thrombotic lesions are rare.[42] The most important lesions are interstitial pneumonia with alveolar edema, hemorrhage, occasionally hyaline membranes, interlobular septal edema, and meningoencephalitis.[41,42,44,45] Correspondingly, the causes of death are respiratory failure, central nervous system (CNS) involvement with coma, and peripheral vascular collapse.[41] Other lesions include pleural effusions, splenomegaly, erythrophagocytosis, and leukophagocytosis in the spleen, liver, and lymph nodes; bone marrow hyperplasia; multifocal interstitial nephritis; and interstitial and perivascular myocarditis, which is pathophysiologically insignificant.[41,42,44,45]

O. tsutsugamushi attaches to its host cell via a surface protein, enters by stimulating phagocytosis, escapes from the phagosome, and replicates by binary fission in the cytosol. Spread to infect other cells occurs via budding projections from the infected cell contacting a neighboring cell, which engulfs the host membrane–bound or free bacterium.[2,46] Within the new cell, the organism enters the cytosol by lysing the intervening host cell membranes.

Studies of the interaction of *O. tsutsugamushi* with endothelial cells or macrophages in cell culture have elucidated some of the fundamental pathogenesis of scrub typhus. Neutralization of *O. tsutsugamushi* infectivity by antibodies directed against epitopes of the 56-kDa major cell wall protein suggests that it plays a role in adhesion and/or entry into the host cell on which heparan sulfate glucosaminoglycan is a receptor.[47] *O. tsutsugamushi* are moved intracellularly to the microtubule organizing center where replication occurs.[48] Antibody-opsonized organisms escape from the phagosomes of polymophonuclear leukocytes, but their intracellular movement is altered. Although orientiae can inhibit apoptosis of human macrophages by reducing intracellular release of calcium ions from endoplasmic reticulum, cells heavily infected with orientiae undergo apopotic cell death in association with decreased expression of anti-apoptotic bcl-2, decreased actin stress fiber polymerization, and decreased cellular focal adhesion kinase and paxillin.[49]

Immunity to *O. tsutsugamushi* is incomplete, with frequent reinfections. Immunity to the homologous strain has been shown to last for up to 3½ years, but immunity to heterologous strains begins to wane after 1 month and is usually absent after a year, although the illness is often milder.[50,51] Primary infections are more often symptomatic than infections of previously immune persons.[52] Seroconversion has been observed in asymptomatic subjects and mildly ill patients, but whether owing to immune protective mechanisms or avirulent strains is not known.[53]

Experimental studies in mice have shown that T lymphocytes are critically important to immunity.[54] Antibodies to the homologous strain confer partial protection, but heterologous antibodies do not.[55] Antibodies enhance clearance of *O. tsutsugamushi* from the blood, and B-lymphocyte depletion increases the susceptibility of mice to a moderately pathogenic strain.[54] Whether antibodies inhibit attachment and entry or other host–*Orientia* interactions is not clear.[56,57] The potential importance of macrophages is suggested by the conversion of infection with a sublethal dose to a fatal infection when macrophage function is impaired by treatment with silica.[58]

A single gene that determines resistance or susceptibility of mice to *O. tsutsugamushi* is related to its role in generating an effective Th1-type cell-mediated immunity. Indeed, murine macrophages activated by IFN-γ kill *O. tsutsugamushi*, and TNF-α inhibits the growth of orientiae in human endothelial cells.[59,60] The source of protective TNF-α is likely mononuclear phagocytes, although one study reported that *O. tsutsugamushi* infection of murine macrophages does not stimulate TNF-α production, which does in fact result from stimulation of immune spleen cells with *O. tsutsugamushi* antigen.[61–63] The observation of elevated concentrations of serum IFN-γ and macrophage colony–stimulating factor in patients during the acute stage of scrub typhus suggests roles as host defenses.[64] Immune cytotoxic T lymphocytes mediate major histocompatibility complex (MHC) class I–restricted cytotoxicity against *O. tsutsugamushi*–infected target cells.[65] Immune mechanisms clearly do control rickettsial infection of peritoneal macrophages, resolve the hepatic lesions, and control the peritonitis in mice. Immune cytokines are likely very important in vivo with cytotoxic T lymphocytes and antibodies potentially also playing significant roles. The perivascular lymphohistiocytic infiltrate, the likely source of paracrine immune cytokines, may result from production of macrophage chemoattractant proteins 1 and 2, macrophage inflammatory proteins 1α, 1β, and 2, and RANTES by endothelial cells and/or macrophages.[63,66,67]

DIAGNOSIS

The diagnosis can be simple in a patient who has visited an endemic area and presents with a fever, rash, eschar, lymphadenopathy, and acute hearing loss. Unfortunately, this scenario is rarely the case. Scrub typhus is an often overlooked cause of both pyrexia and pneumonitis of undetermined cause.[25,35] The single most useful diagnostic clue is the eschar, which is virtually pathognomonic when seen by a physician experienced in diagnosing scrub typhus. However, even a typical eschar can be overlooked,[68] eschars without crusts are often misdiagnosed, and many cases of scrub typhus do not manifest an eschar.

Laboratory confirmation is difficult. The Weil-Felix test using the *Proteus* OX-K antigen is often the only diagnostic tool readily available in endemic areas, but it is unacceptably insensitive.[32] The indirect immunofluorescence and immunoperoxidase assays have been considered as the gold standard reliable serodiagnostic methods[69–71] but have technical requirements which limit their use to a small number of medical centers. Rapid diagnostic tests requiring no special equipment and reliable recombinant 56-kDa protein antigen tests have been developed. The best results have been obtained with a pool of truncated recombinant 56-kDa proteins of Karp, Kato, and Gilliam strains, which has been prepared as a dipstick test on a rapid lateral flow assay for the serodiagnosis of scrub typhus in the rural tropics where the majority of disease transmission occurs.[72–75] The introduction of tests that do not rely upon microscopy holds great promise for improving the serodiagnosis of scrub typhus, particularly in the rural tropics. The same antigens are also very appropriate for use in enzyme immunoassays in the reference diagnostic laboratories[76] for accurately testing large numbers of sera.[77]

O. tsutsugamushi can be isolated from blood or tissues. Whole blood from patients with acute scrub typhus is injected intraperitoneally into white mice, which are then observed for signs of illness or death. Organisms can be demonstrated in Giemsa-stained impression smears taken from the surface of the spleen or peritoneum.

The etiologic diagnosis can also be made by performing PCR assays on whole blood or even on dried blood dotted onto filter paper.[78–82] However, the sensitivity and specificity of PCR for diagnosing scrub typhus have not yet been determined by prospective clinical trials. Further refinements may lead to more widespread use of PCR for diagnosis of *O. tsutsugamushi* infection, but expense and technical requirements currently constrain its use to the research setting.

The differential diagnosis depends on the diseases prevalent in the area in which the illness originated. The importance of a careful search for an eschar cannot be overemphasized—its presence is virtually pathognomonic for scrub typhus in much of Asia. Tularemia, spotted fever rickettsiosis, and anthrax can cause eschars but have a different epidemiology. Eschars frequently occur in the genital region, where they often lose their crust. Thus they can be confused with the ulcers of syphilis, chancroid, or lymphogranuloma venereum. A rash that is hemorrhagic, particularly if associated with leukopenia and thrombocytopenia, suggests infection with dengue virus rather than *O. tsutsugamushi*. Marked myalgia, liver involvement, and raised serum creatinine levels suggest leptospirosis rather than scrub typhus. However, dual infections with leptospirosis and scrub typhus have been reported.[83] Typhoid fever and malaria are prominent in the differential diagnosis, but plasmodia are generally detectable in blood films from Asian patients infected with *Plasmodium* spp. and enteric fever rarely causes generalized lymphadenopathy or conjunctival suffusion. Infectious mononucleosis was the most frequent misdiagnosis in American servicemen serving in Vietnam who were infected by *O. tsutsugamushi*.[32] Febrile patients from urban areas are more likely to have murine typhus than scrub typhus, although transmission of *O. tsutsugamushi* occurs in suburban areas of Bangkok, Hong Kong, and Canton.[84,85]

TREATMENT AND PROGNOSIS

Scrub typhus is said to respond even more promptly to antibiotics than other rickettsial diseases, with patients generally becoming afebrile within 24 to 36 hours after beginning antibiotic therapy. Early antibiotic treatment shortens the disease course, reduces mortality, and accelerates convalescence. Treatment must often be presumptive, and the benefits of avoiding severe scrub typhus by early antibiotic administration generally outweigh the risks of a 1-week course of tetracycline—the treatment of choice. Either oral tetracycline (500 mg four times daily) or oral doxycycline (100 mg twice daily for 7 days) is recommended. Shorter treatment courses are often curative, but may result in relapse.[32] A 1-week course of chloramphenicol (50 to 75 mg/kg/day) is also effective although less so than tetracyclines. Parenteral therapy should be given to patients who are vomiting or have severe disease. In areas where parenteral formulations of tetracyclines are unavailable, chloramphenicol is a useful alternative for treatment of severe disease.

The susceptibility of different strains of scrub typhus to antibiotics can be determined in mice, in cell culture, and by flow cytometry.[86,87] Scrub typhus cases from northern Thailand that respond poorly to conventional therapy have been described.[88] Whether resistant strains occur elsewhere is unknown. The mechanism of resistance has not yet been elucidated. Rifampin was the only antibiotic more active than doxycycline against resistant strains of *O. tsutsugamushi* in mice and was equally effective against drug-sensitive strains. Rifampin controlled fever more rapidly than did doxycycline in a controlled, blinded treatment trial of mild scrub typhus acquired in Chiangrai Province in northern Thailand.[89] However, neither the efficacy of rifampicin for severe disease nor the optimal treatment regimen for drug-resistant scrub typhus have yet been determined. Ciprofloxacin treatment does not appear to be effective.[18]

Therapy for pregnant women and children poses several problems. Chloramphenicol is best avoided during pregnancy and cannot be given to neonates; tetracycline is contraindicated in pregnancy because of its teratogenic potential, and repeated long courses administered to young children cause staining of the permanent teeth. Newer macrolide antibiotics appear to be effective for scrub typhus. Roxithromycin treatment of children with scrub typhus yielded defervescence as promptly as doxycycline or chloramphenicol.[90] Three Japanese patients were treated successfully with clarithromycin,[91] and cases of both drug-sensitive and drug-resistant scrub typhus have been cured by azithromycin. Macrolides would be particularly useful for the treatment of *O. tsutsugamushi* infection during pregnancy and early childhood. The need for effective treatment in pregnant women and infants is underscored by recent documentation of transmission of scrub typhus from mother to fetus.[92]

Scrub typhus was a dreaded disease in the preantibiotic era. Prompt antibiotic therapy generally prevents death, but in northern Thailand up to 15% of patients still die. Deaths are attributable to a variety of factors, including late presentation, delayed diagnosis, and drug resistance. The severity of scrub typhus does not appear to be increased in patients infected with human immunodeficiency virus (HIV).[93] Surprisingly, HIV viral load falls in a substantial proportion of AIDS patients during acute scrub typhus.[94] A passive plasma transfer study showed that long-acting factors that suppress HIV appear in the blood during some acute scrub typhus infections.[95] It has been suggested that *O. tsutsugamushi*–related HIV suppression may be mediated by antibody or other pathways such as downregulation of the CCR5 coreceptor for HIV.[61] Good supportive care and early detection of complications are important in severe cases if a good outcome is to be obtained.

PREVENTION AND CONTROL

Weekly doses of 200 mg of doxycycline can prevent *O. tsutsugamushi* infection.[96,97] Weekly chloramphenicol is also effective,[98] but has unacceptable risks for use as chemoprophylaxis. Daily doxycycline prevents malaria, but its ability to prevent scrub typhus has not been tested; daily chloramphenicol is not protective.[98] Chemoprophylaxis should be considered for nonimmune persons sent to an endemic area to perform work that places them at high risk of acquiring scrub typhus. Soldiers and road construction crews are typical examples, but chemoprophylaxis should also be considered in high-risk travelers such as trekkers. Contact with chiggers can be reduced by applying repellent to the tops of boots, socks, and on the lower trousers and by not sitting or lying directly on the ground. Unfortunately, these measures are frequently not practiced by those exposed occupationally.

During the 1940s, attempts to protect man against scrub typhus by immunization with killed rickettsial vaccines gave uniformly discouraging results under the conditions of field exposure.[99,100] Other vaccine strategies have included gamma-irradiated organisms that were metabolically active but incapable of growth, and combined infection and antibiotic prophylaxis.[51,101] Currently there is no vaccine in use. The protection of mice with a recombinant 56-kD protein vaccine that stimulated both T- and B-lymphocyte responses sounds a note of encouragement,[102] but the existence of innumerable heterologous strains implies that a broadly effective vaccine might not be forthcoming soon.

REFERENCES

1. Fan M-Y, Walker DH, Yu S-R, et al: Epidemiology and ecology of rickettsial diseases in the People's Republic of China. Rev Infect Dis 9:823, 1987.
2. Kawamura A Jr, Tanaka H, Tamura A: Tsutsugamushi Disease. Tokyo, University of Tokyo Press, 1995, pp 1–158.
3. Nagayo M, Tamiya T, Imamura A, et al: Demonstration of the virus of tsutsugamushi disease. Trans Jpn Pathol Soc 14:193, 1924.
4. Nagayo M, Tamiya T, Mitamura T, et al: On the virus of tsutsugamushi disease and its demonstration by a new method. Trans Jpn Pathol Soc 20:556, 1930.
5. Ogata N, Unno Y: On the transfer of causative agent of tsutsugamushi disease to the rabbit testis and microorganisms appearing in the testis. (In Japanese) J Chiba Med Soc 7:1215, 1929.
6. Ogata N, Nakajima G, Kajima S: Animals employed for experimental infection by pathogenic rickettsiae in laboratory—Especially recommendation to use mouse for the detection of *Rickettsia tsutsugamushi*. (In Japanese) Tokyo Med J 2760:155, 1932.
7. Tamura A, Ohashi N, Urakami H, et al: Classification of *Rickettsia tsutsugamushi* in a new genus, *Orientia* gen. nov. as *Orientia tsutsugamushi* comb. nov. Int J Syst Bacteriol 45:589, 1995.
8. Silverman DJ, Wisseman CL Jr: Comparative ultrastructural study on the cell envelopes of *Rickettsia prowazekii, Rickettsia rickettsii,* and *Rickettsia tsutsugamushi.* Infect Immun 21:1020, 1978.
9. Ohashi N, Nashimoto H, Ikeda H, et al: Diversity of immunodominant 56-kDa type-specific antigen (TSA) of *Rickettsia tsutsugamushi*: Sequence and comparative analyses of the genes encoding TSA homologues from four antigenic variants. J Biol Chem 267:12728, 1992.
10. Qiang Y, Tamura A, Urakami H, et al: Phylogenetic characterization of *Orientia tsutsugamushi* isolated in Taiwan according to the sequence homologies of 56kDa type-specific antigen genes. Microbiol Immunol 47:577, 2003.
11. Ohashi N, Koyama Y, Urakami H, et.al: Demonstration of antigenic and genotypic variation in *Orientia tsutsugamushi* which were isolated in Japan, and their classification into type and subtype. Microbiol Immunol 40:627, 1996.
12. Oaks EV, Rice RM, Kelly DJ, et al: Antigenic and genetic relatedness of eight *Rickettsia tsutsugamushi* antigens. Infect Immun 57:3116, 1989.
13. Park C-S, Kim I-C, Lee J-B, et al: Analysis of antigenic characteristics of *Rickettsia tsutsugamushi* Boryong strain and antigenic heterogeneity of *Rickettsia tsutsugamushi* using monoclonal antibodies. J Korean Med Sci 8:319, 1993.
14. Stover CK, Marana DP, Dasch GA, et al: Molecular cloning and sequence analysis of the Sta58 major antigen gene of *Rickettsia tsutsugamushi*: Sequence homology and antigenic comparison of Sta58 to the 60-kilodalton family of stress proteins. Infect Immun 58:1360, 1990.
15. Dasch GA, Strickman D, Watt G, et al: Measuring genetic variability in *Orientia tsutsugamushi* by PCR/RFLP analysis: A new approach to questions about its epidemiology, evolution, and ecology. In Kazar J, Toman R (eds): Rickettsiae and Rickettsial Disease, Bratislava, Slovakia, Slovak Academy of Sciences, 1996, p 79.
16. Burgdorfer W: Ecological and epidemiological considerations of Rocky Mountain spotted fever and scrub typhus. In Walker DH (ed): Biology of Rickettsial Diseases, Boca Raton, FL, CRC Press, 1988, p 33.
17. Traub R, Wisseman CL Jr: The ecology of chigger-borne rickettsiosis (scrub typhus). J Med Entomol 11:237, 1974.
18. Mathai E, Rolain JM, Verghese GM, et al: Outbreak of scrub typhus in southern India during the cooler months. Ann NY Acad Sci 990:359, 2003.
19. Kularatne SA, Edirisingha JS, Gawarammana IB, et al: Emerging rickettsial infections in Sri Lanka: The pattern in the hilly central province. Trop Med Int Health 8:803–811, 2003.
20. Roberts LW, Robinson DM: Efficiency of transovarial transmission of *Rickettsia tsutsugamushi* in *Leptotrombidium arenicola* (Acari: Trombiculidae). J Med Entomol 13:493, 1977.
21. Shirai A, Saunders JP, Dohany AL, et al: Transmission of scrub typhus to human volunteers by laboratory-reared chiggers. Jpn J Med Sci Biol 35:9, 1982.
22. Kollars TM, Kengluecha A, Khlaimanee N, et al: Temporal changes in prevalence of scrub typhus rickettsia (*Orientia tsutsugamushi*) infecting the eggs of *Leptotrombidium imphalum* (Acari: Trombiculidae). J Med Entomol 38:108, 2001.
23. Ogawa M, Hagiwara T, Kishimoto T, et al: Scrub typhus in Japan: epidemiology and clinical features of cases reported in 1998. Am J Trop Med Hyg 67:162, 2002.
24. Takahashi M, Urakami H, Yoshida Y, et al: Occurrence of high ratio of males after introduction of minocycline in a colony of *Leptotrombidium fletcheri* infected with *Orientia tsutsugamushi*. Eur J Epidemiol 13:79, 1997.
25. Brown GW, Robinson DM, Huxsoll DL, et al: Scrub typhus: A common cause of illness in indigenous populations. Trans R Soc Trop Med Hyg 70:444, 1976.
26. Brown GW, Robinson DM, Huxsoll DL: Serological evidence for a high incidence of transmission of *Rickettsia tsutsugamushi* in two Orang Asli settlements in peninsular Malaysia. Am J Trop Med Hyg 27:121, 1978.
27. Corwin A, Soderquist R, Suwanabun N, et al: Scrub typhus and military operations in Indochina. Clin Infect Dis 29:940, 1999.
28. Blake FG, Maxcy KF, Sadusk JF Jr, et al: Studies on tsutsugamushi disease (scrub typhus, mite-borne typhus) in New Guinea and adjacent islands: Epidemiology, clinical observations and etiology in the Dobadura area. Am J Hyg 41:243, 1945.
29. Maxcy KF: Scrub typhus (tsutsugamushi disease) in the U.S. Army during World War II. In Moulton FR (ed): Rickettsial Diseases of Man. Boston, Thomas, Adams & Davis, 1946, p 36.
30. Sayen JJ, Pond HS, Forrester JS, et al: Scrub typhus in Assam and Burma. Medicine (Baltimore) 25:155, 1946.
31. Noad KB, Haymaker W: The neurological features of tsutsugamushi fever, with special reference to deafness. Brain 76:113, 1953.
32. Berman SJ, Kundin WD: Scrub typhus in South Vietnam. Ann Intern Med 79:26, 1973.
33. Kim SJ, Chung IK, Chung IS, et al: The clinical significance of upper gastrointestinal endoscopy in gastrointestinal vasculitis related to scrub typhus. Endoscopy 32:950, 2000.
34. Nagaki Y, Hayasaka S, Kadoi C, et al: Branch retinal vein occlusion in the right eye and retinal hemorrhage in the left in a patient with classical tsutsugamushi disease. Jpn J Ophthalmol 45:103, 2001.
35. Chaykul P, Panich V, Silpapojakul K: Scrub typhus pneumonitis: an entity which is frequently missed. Q J Med 256:595, 1988.
36. Tsay RW, Chang FY: Acute respiratory distress syndrome in scrub typhus. (Letter) QJ Med 95:126, 2002.
37. Aronoff DM, Watt G: Prevalence of relative bradycardia in *Orientia tsutsugamushi* infection. Am J Trop Med Hyg 68:477, 2003.
38. Watt G, Kantipong P, Jirajarus K: Acute scrub typhus in Northern Thailand: EKG changes. Southeast Asian J Trop Med Public Health 33:312, 2002.
39. Silpapojakul K, Ukkachoke C, Krisman S, et al: Rickettsial meningitis and encephalitis. Arch Intern Med 151:1753, 1991.

40. Kim DE, Lee SH, Park KI, et al: Scrub typhus encephalomyelitis with prominent focal neurologic signs. Arch Neurol 57:1770, 2000.
41. Settle EB, Pinkerton H, Corbett AJ: A pathologic study of tsutsugamushi disease (scrub typhus) with notes on clinicopathologic correlation. J Lab Clin Med 30:639, 1945.
42. Allen AC, Spitz S: A comparative study of the pathology of scrub typhus (tsutsugamushi disease) and other rickettsial diseases. Am J Pathol 21:603, 1945.
43. Murata M, Sudo K, Suzuki K, et al: Proliferating sites of *Rickettsia tsutsugamushi* in mice by different routes of inoculation evidenced with immunofluorescence. Jpn J Exp Med 55:193, 1985.
44. Park JH, Hart MS: The pathology of scrub typhus. Am J Clin Pathol 16:139, 1946.
45. Levine HD: Pathologic study of thirty-one cases of scrub typhus fever with especial reference to the cardiovascular system. Am Heart J 31:314, 1946.
46. Ewing EP Jr, Takeuchi A, Shirai A, et al: Experimental infection of mouse peritoneal mesothelium with scrub typhus rickettsiae: An ultrastructural study. Infect Immun 19:1068, 1978.
47. Ihn K-S, Han S-H, Kim M-S, et al: Cellular invasion of *Orientia tsutsugamushi* requires initial interaction with cell surface heparan sulfate. Microbial Pathogenesis 28:227, 2000.
48. Kim DE, Lee SH, Park K-J, et al: Scrub typhus encephalomyelitis with prominent focal neurologic signs. Arch Neurol 57:1770, 2000.
49. Kee S-H, Cho K-A, Kim B-U, et al: Disassembly of focal adhesions during apoptosis of endothelial cell kine ECV304 infected with *Orientia tsutsugamushi*. Microb Pathog 27:265, 2002.
50. Smadel JE, Ley HL Jr, Diercks FH, et al: Immunity in scrub typhus: Resistance to induced reinfection. Arch Pathol 50:847, 1950.
51. Smadel JE, Ley HL Jr, Diercks FH, et al: Immunization against scrub typhus: Duration of immunity in volunteers following combined living vaccine and chemoprophylaxis. Am J Trop Med Hyg 1:87, 1952.
52. Olson JG, Bourgeois AL: *Rickettsia tsutsugamushi* infection and scrub typhus incidence among Chinese military personnel in the Pescadores Islands. Am J Epidemiol 106:172, 1977.
53. Brown GW, Shirai A, Groves MG: Development of antibody to *Rickettsia tsutsugamushi* in soldiers in Malaysia. Trans R Soc Trop Med Hyg 77:225, 1983.
54. Jerrells TR: Mechanisms of immunity to *Rickettsia* species and *Coxiella burnetii*. In Walker DH (ed): Biology of Rickettsial Diseases. Boca Raton, FL, CRC Press, 1988, p 79.
55. Shirai A, Catanzaro PJ, Phillips SM, et al: Host defenses in experimental scrub typhus: Role of cellular immunity in heterologous protection. Infect Immun 14:39, 1976.
56. Hanson BA: Effect of immune serum on infectivity of *Rickettsia tsutsugamushi*. Infect Immun 42:341, 1983.
57. Tamura A: Invasion and intracellular growth of *Rickettsia tsutsugamushi*. Microbiol Sci 5:228, 1988.
58. Jerrells TR, Osterman JV: Role of macrophages in innate and acquired host resistance to experimental scrub typhus infection of inbred mice. Infect Immun 37:1066, 1982.
59. Hanson B: Susceptibility of *Rickettsia tsutsugamushi* Gilliam to gamma interferon in cultured mouse cells. Infect Immun 59:4125, 1991.
60. Geng P-Q, Jerrells TR: The role of tumor necrosis factor in host defense against scrub typhus rickettsiae. I. Inhibition of growth of *Rickettsia tsutsugamushi,* Karp strain, in cultured murine embryonic cells and macrophages by recombinant tumor necrosis factor-alpha. Microbiol Immunol 38:703, 1994.
61. Jerrells TR, Geng P-Q: The role of tumor necrosis factor in host defense against scrub typhus rickettsiae. II. Differential induction of tumor necrosis factor-alpha production by *Rickettsia tsutsugamushi* and *Rickettsia conorii*. Microbiol Immunol 38:713, 1994.
62. Kim MK, Kang JS: *Orientia tsutsugamushi* suppresses the production of inflammatory cytokines induced by its own heat-stable component in murine macrophages. Microb Pathog 31:145, 2001.
63. Moriuchi M, Tamura A, Moriuchi H: In vitro reactivation of human immunodeficiency virus-1 upon stimulation with scrub typhus rickettsial infection. Am J Trop Med Hyg 68:557, 2003.
64. Iwasaki H, Takada N, Nakamura T, et al: Increased levels of macrophage colony-stimulating factor, gamma interferon, and tumor necrosis factor alpha in sera of patients with *Orientia tsutsugamushi* infection. J Clin Microbiol 35:3320, 1997.
65. Rollwagen FM, Dasch GA, Jerrells TR: Mechanisms of immunity to rickettsial infection: Characterization of a cytotoxic effector cell. J Immunol 136:1418, 1986.
66. Cho N-H, Seong S-Y, Huh M-S, et al: Expression of chemokine genes in murine macrophages infected with *Orientia tsutsugamushi*. Infect Immun 68:594, 2000.
67. Cho N-H, Seong S-Y, Huh M-S, et al: Induction of the gene encoding macrophage chemoattractant protein 1 by *Orientia tsutsugamushi* in human endothelial cells involves activation of transcription factor activator protein 1. Infect Immun 70:4841, 2002.
68. Watt G, Strickman D: Life-threatening scrub typhus in a traveler returning from Thailand. Clin Infect Dis 18:624, 1994.
69. Brown GB, Shirai A, Rogers C, et al: Diagnostic criteria for scrub typhus: Probability values for immunofluorescent antibody and *Proteus* OXK agglutinin titers. Am J Trop Med Hyg 32:1101, 1983.
70. Bozeman FM, Elisberg BL: Serological diagnosis of scrub typhus by indirect immunofluorescence. Proc Soc Exp Biol Med 32:568, 1963.
71. Kelly DJ, Wong PW, Gan E, et al: Comparative evaluation of the indirect immunoperoxidase test for the serodiagnosis of rickettsial disease. Am J Trop Med Hyg 38:400, 1988.
72. Weddle JR, Chan TC, Thompson K, et al: Effectiveness of a dot-blot immunoassay of anti-*Rickettsia tsutsugamushi* antibodies for serologic analysis of scrub typhus. Am J Trop Med Hyg 53:43, 1995.
73. Coleman RE, Sangkasuwan V, Suwanabun N, et al: Comparative evaluation of selected diagnostic assays for the detection of IgG and IgM antibody to *Orientia tsutsugamushi* in Thailand. Am J Trop Med Hyg 67:497, 2002.
74. Jiang J, Marienau KJ, May LA, et al: Laboratory diagnosis of two scrub typhus outbreaks at Camp Fuji, Japan in 2000 and 2001 by enzyme-linked immunosorbent assay, rapid flow assay, and western blot assay using outer membrane 56 KD recombinant proteins. Am J Trop Med Hyg 69:60, 2003.
75. Wilkinson R, Rowland D, Ching W-M: Development of an improved rapid lateral flow assay for the detection of *Orientia tsutsugamushi*–specific IgM/IgM antibodies. Ann NY Acad Sci 990:386, 2003.
76. Jang W-J, Huh M-S, Park K-H, et al: Evaluation of an immunoglobulin M capture enzyme-linked immunosorbent assay for diagnosis of *Orientia tsutsugamushi* infection. Clin Diagn Lab Immunol 10:394, 2003.
77. Suwanabun N, Chouriyagune C, Eamsila C, et al: Evaluation of an enzyme-linked immunosorbent assay in Thai scrub typhus patients. Am J Trop Med Hyg 56:38, 1997.
78. Kelly DJ, Marana DP, Stover CK, et al: Detection of *Rickettsia tsutsugamushi* by gene amplification using polymerase chain reaction techniques. Ann NY Acad Sci 590:564, 1990.
79. Murai K, Tachibana N, Okayama A, et al: Sensitivity of polymerase chain reaction assay for *Rickettsia tsutsugamushi* in patients' blood samples. Microbiol Immunol 36:1145, 1992.
80. Furuya Y, Yoshida Y, Katayama T, et al: Serotype-specific amplification of *Rickettsia tsutsugamushi* DNA by nested polymerase chain reaction. J Clin Microbiol 31:1637, 1993.
81. Kawamori F, Akiyama M, Sugieda M, et al: Two-step polymerase chain reaction for diagnosis of scrub typhus and identification of antigenic variants of *Rickettsia tsutsugamushi*. J Vet Med Sci 55:749, 1993.
82. Sugita Y, Yamakawa Y, Takahashi K, et al: A polymerase chain reaction system for rapid diagnosis of scrub typhus within six hours. Am J Trop Med Hyg 49:636, 1993.
83. Watt G, Jongsakul K, Chouriyagune C, et al: Differentiating dengue virus infection from scrub typhus in Thai adults with fever. Am J Trop Med Hyg 68:536, 2003.
84. Strickman D, Tanskul P, Eamsila C, et al: Prevalence of antibodies to rickettsiae in the human population of suburban Bangkok. Am J Trop Med Hyg 51:149, 1994.
85. Heap BJ: Scrub typhus in Hong Kong. J Trop Med Hyg 94:97, 1991.
86. Kelly DJ, Salata KF, Strickman D, et al: *Rickettsia tsutsugamushi* infection in cell culture: Antibiotic susceptibility determined by flow cytometry. Am J Trop Med Hyg 53:602, 1995.
87. McClain JB, Joshi B, Rice R: Chloramphenicol, gentamicin, and ciprofloxacin against murine scrub typhus. Antimicrob Agents Chemother 32:285, 1988.
88. Watt G, Chouriyagune C, Ruangweerayud R, et al: Scrub typhus infections poorly responsive to antibiotics in Northern Thailand. Lancet 348:86, 1996.
89. Watt G, Kantipong P, Jongsakul K, et al: Doxycycline and rifampicin for mild scrub-typhus infections in northern Thailand: A randomized trial. Lancet. 356:1057, 2000.
90. Lee K-Y, Lee H-S, Hong J-H, et al: Roxithromycin treatment of scrub typhus (tsutsugamushi disease) in children. Pediatr Infect Dis J 22:130, 2003.

91. Miura N, Kudoh Y, Osabe M, et al: Three cases of tsutsugamushi disease successfully treated with clarithromycin. Acta Med Nagaski 40:44, 1995.
92. Wang C-L, Yang KD, Cheung S-N, et al: Neonatal scrub typhus: A case report. Pediatrics 89:965, 1992.
93. Kantipong P, Watt G, Jongsakul K, et al: HIV infection does not influence the clinical severity of scrub typhus. Clin Infect Dis 23:1168, 1996.
94. Watt G, Kantipong P, de Souza M, et al: HIV-1 suppression during acute scrub typhus infection. Lancet 356:475, 2003.
95. Watt G, Kantipong P, Jongsakul K, et al: Passive transfer of scrub typhus plasma to patients with AIDS: A descriptive clinical study. QJ Med 599, 2001.
96. Olson JG, Bourgeois AL, Fang RCY, et al: Prevention of scrub typhus. Prophylactic administration of doxycycline in a randomized double blind trial. Am J Trop Med Hyg 29:989, 1980.
97. Twartz JC, Shirai A, Selvaraju G, et al: Doxycycline prophylaxis for human scrub typhus. J Infect Dis 146:811, 1982.
98. Smadel JE, Traub R, Ley HL: Chloramphenicol (Chloromycetin) in the chemoprophylaxis of scrub typhus (tsutsugamushi disease). II. Results with volunteers exposed in hyperendemic areas of scrub typhus. Am J Med 50:75, 1949.
99. Card WI, Walker JM: Scrub typhus vaccine. Field trial in Southeast Asia. Lancet 1:481, 1947.
100. Berge TO, Gauld RL, Kitaoka M: A field trial of a vaccine prepared from the Volner strain of *Rickettsia tsutsugamushi*. Am J Hyg 50:377, 1949.
101. Eisenberg GHG Jr, Osterman JV: Gamma-irradiated scrub typhus immunogens: Broad-spectrum immunity with combinations of rickettsial strains. Infect Immun 26:131, 1979.
102. Seong SY, Huh MS, Jang WJ, et al: Induction of homologous immune response to *Rickettsia tsutsugamushi* Boryong with a partial 56-kilodalton recombinant antigen fused with the maltose-binding protein MBP-BOR56. Infect Immun 65:1541, 1997.

53

Ehrlichioses and Anaplasmosis

J. STEPHEN DUMLER
DAVID H. WALKER

INTRODUCTION

As human habitats increasingly overlap those of ticks and their hosts, exposure to previously unrecognized microbes that have evolved within mammalian–tick enzootic cycles occurs, and significant new human pathogens have emerged. Important examples of this process include obligately intracellular bacteria related to the genus *Rickettsia* that are in the family Anaplasmataceae and the genera *Ehrlichia* and *Anaplasma*.[1,2] *Neorickettsia* (*Ehrlichia*) *sennetsu* was identified as a cause of a mononucleosis-like illness in Japan in 1954, and since 1986, at least four new distinct species in the family Anaplasmataceae have been identified as tick-borne human pathogens.[1–5]

AGENTS

Anaplasmataceae are classified based on similarities in *rrs* (16S ribosomal RNA genes), *gro*ESL, *rpo*B, and *glt*A. A recent reclassification resulted in the current scheme for Anaplasmataceae, including the genera *Ehrlichia*, *Anaplasma*, *Neorickettsia*, and *Wolbachia*.[2,6,7] *N. sennetsu* infects mostly mononuclear phagocytes, has never been identified in humans outside of the Far East, and is likely transmitted by ingestion of trematode-infested fish. *Ehrlichia chaffeensis* infects peripheral blood monocytes and tissue macrophages and is the major cause of human monocytotropic ehrlichiosis (HME) in the United States.[1,5,8,9] With the recent taxonomic reorganization, the former *E. phagocytophila* or human granulocytic ehrlichiosis (HGE) agent that infects neutrophils is now called *Anaplasma phagocytophilum*.[2,10,11] *Ehrlichia ewingii*, a pathogen of neutrophils, has also been identified as a significant human pathogen in the United States, particularly among immunocompromised patients.[4,12] A role for *Wolbachia* spp. that infect filarial nematodes has been proposed in complicating human filariasis based upon exacerbation of inflammation by the symbiont's components.[13] Finally, a single person with asymptomatic persistent *Ehrlichia canis* infection was identified in Venezuela.[3] It must be remembered that, until recently, Anaplasmataceae were considered only as pathogens of animals or as benign symbiotic bacteria. Moreover, a number of Anaplasmataceae cause diseases in animals in tropical locations. Given the propensity for some to infect potentially both animals and humans, it would not be surprising to discover that previously or newly identified Anaplasmataceae beyond *Wolbachia* spp. are significant causes of human disease in tropical regions.

With the exception of *Wolbachia* spp. (which will be separately considered), each of the Anaplasmataceae pathogenic for humans lives within professional phagocytic cells in vivo in an endosome.[14,15] Although not proved for all species, these intracellular bacteria attach to ligands on phagocytic cells, are engulfed, and then subvert intracellular endosomal trafficking to avoid lysosomal fusion and to allow replication within the vacuole.[16,17] Another common theme among these organisms is the ability to generate a changing variety of surface immunogenic proteins, which probably contributes to immune evasion in persistently infected reservoir hosts but could also allow infection of new niches among alternative hosts such as humans.[18–20] The closely related genera *Ehrlichia* and *Anaplasma* are tick-transmitted, whereas *Neorickettsia* spp. rely on infection of trematode stages and their hosts, and *Wolbachia* symbionts of *Brugia*, *Onchocerca*, and other filarial nematodes are passed transovarially.[21–24] The mechanisms of cell injury are not known, although increasing data suggest the induction of immunopathologic responses such as overproduction of tumor necrosis factor–α (TNF-α).[25–27]

In vitro cultivation was a major limitation in the study of *Ehrlichia* spp. and the diseases they cause. However, recent investigations have led to the development of methods for cultivation in specific host cell lines. Such developments as the growth of *Ehrlichia canis* and *E. chaffeensis* in the canine DH82 or human THP-1 macrophage cell line,[9,28,29] *A. phagocytophilum* in human HL-60 promyelocyte cells,[30] and the growth of several species in tick cell cultures[31] allow more comprehensive investigation and development of reproducible diagnostic tools. Remarkably, the genome sequences of *E. chaffeensis*, *E. canis*, *Ehrlichia ruminantium*, *A. phagocytophilum*, *N. sennetsu*, *Anaplasma marginale*, *Wolbachia pipientis*, and several other *Wolbachia* spp. are nearing completion and should propel fundamental and translational research on infections caused by these agents.

Human Monocytotropic Ehrlichiosis (HME)

AGENT: *EHRLICHIA CHAFFEENSIS*

E. chaffeensis cells have a wide range of ultrastructural appearances.[32] In general, two types of ehrlichial cells are observed within the vacuoles of host cells: ehrlichiae with a central condensation of ribosomes and DNA fibrils, called *dense-core cells*, and ehrlichiae in which these components are evenly distributed throughout the bacterium, called *reticulate cells*. While both forms have been observed in replication, the gp120 that is implicated as an adhesin of *E. chaffeensis* is differentially expressed on dense-core cells, analogous to the situation in *Chlamydia*.[33]

The antigenic constituents of *E. chaffeensis* have been examined in some detail. Protein immunoblots of *E. chaffeensis* with experimentally prepared antisera and sera from convalescent human patients reveal the presence of dominant antigens at 200, 120, 66, 55, 44, 29, 28, and 22 kD.[34,35] However, analysis of additional isolates of *E. chaffeensis* has indicated

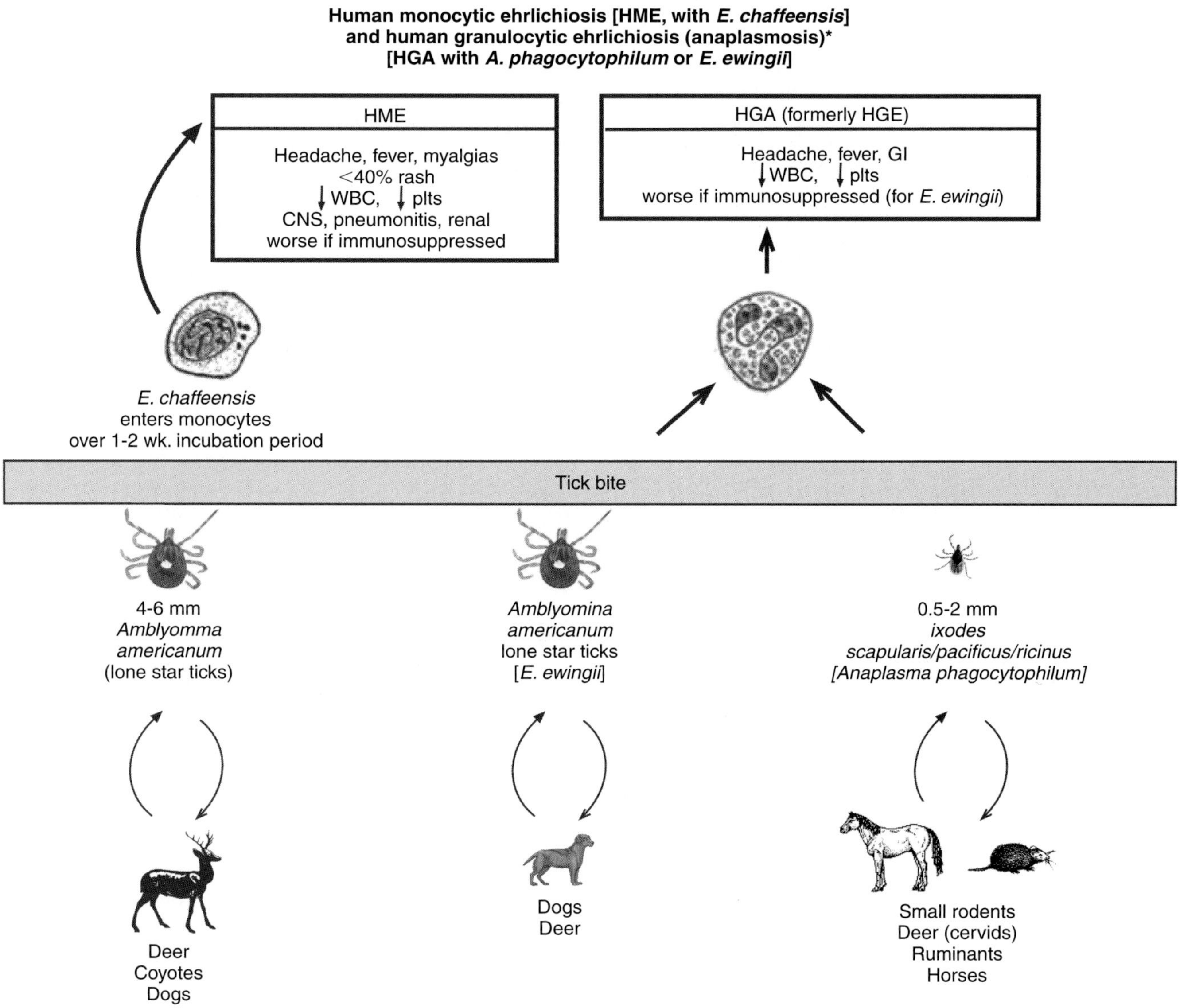

a degree of variation in structure and specific epitopes.[36] The immunodominant p28 family of proteins in *Ehrlichia* is encoded by at least 22 paralogs that are present contiguously in a locus and can be independently transcribed.[37] The 120-kD protein appears to function in some degree as an adhesin.[33] Both the 120-kD protein and another surface-exposed protein called VLPT contain variable numbers of tandem repeats.[38] Components of a type IV secretion mechanism expressed by *E. chaffeensis* are found in the parasitophorous vacuoles of infected macrophages.[39] Their presence suggests the potential for direct introduction of cell-regulating bacterial proteins and components that may directly or indirectly influence the recognized changes in host gene transcription with infection.[40]

EPIDEMIOLOGY

HME was identified because of clinical and geographic similarities to Rocky Mountain spotted fever (RMSF).[1,5,41] Onset is associated with tick exposure and bites, and the major vector is *Amblyomma americanum,* the Lone Star tick.[1,5,21] Lone Star ticks are found across areas of the south-central and southeastern United States, coinciding generally with areas where HME is found. All stages of *A. americanum* readily feed on deer, which are the major reservoir.[42] Deer experimentally inoculated with *E. chaffeensis* become persistently infected in the absence of disease.[43] White-tailed deer (*Odocoileus virginianus*) in regions of the southeastern and central United States have been reported to be infected or to have serologic evidence of infection.[42] White-tailed deer in areas devoid of Lone Star ticks show an absence of exposure to *E. chaffeensis* until Lone Star ticks spread into those regions and serologic evidence of infection emerges in deer.[44] Many canids have serologic evidence of infection with *Ehrlichia* infections, and dogs can be persistently infected subclinically with *E. chaffeensis*.[45–47]

The incidence and prevalence of HME are poorly documented. Prior investigations indicate that the infection occurs at a rate similar to or greater than that of RMSF, and recent studies based upon active, prospective identification in southeastern Missouri suggest that HME occurs at least at rates of 2 to 5 per 100,000 population—figures that are 10-fold higher than reported in investigations by passive reporting and are possibly more than an order of magnitude even higher.[1,5,48–50] Serologic studies suggest that infection with *E. chaffeensis* or an antigenically related organism also occurs in Europe, Africa, Asia, and Latin America.[3,51–55] Asymptomatic seroconversion may confound seroprevalence and diagnostic studies[56]; moreover, milder infection with *E. ewingii* or the presence in ticks of *Ehrlichia* spp. that are nonpathogenic to humans may account for some serologic reactions in tick-exposed populations.[57] Most infections occur from April through September, with a peak in July, when the ticks are active.[1,5]

DISEASE

Most individuals with HME have an undifferentiated febrile illness within 1 to 4 weeks after tick exposure or bite.[1,5,50,58] The mean age is 48 years, although infections also occur in children, for whom the age-adjusted seroprevalence in the south central and eastern United States varies between 2% and 22%.[59] Although most patients reside in rural areas, rural zip codes and seroprevalence are not correlated.[59] Frequent findings include headache, myalgias, and malaise, while gastrointestinal, respiratory, or central nervous system (CNS) abnormalities, or rash is present in fewer than 40% of patients (Table 53-1). Laboratory features often include leukopenia, thrombocytopenia, and mild-to-moderate elevations in serum hepatic transaminase activities (Table 53-2). Severe manifestations include meningoencephalitis, a toxic shock–like syndrome, respiratory insufficiency, acute renal failure, severe hepatitis, myocarditis, and prolonged fever of undetermined origin.[26,60–66] The case-fatality rate is 3%, and immunosuppressed persons (e.g., human immunodeficiency virus–infected, organ transplant recipients, or corticosteroid-treated) are at risk of overwhelming infection that is often fatal.[12,66-68] Early diagnosis and treatment are important to prevent severe disease.[1,5] Pathologic features include perivascular lymphohistiocytic infiltrates without vasculitis, small noncaseating granulomas in hyperplastic bone marrow, and evidence of macrophage activation. Bone marrow is generally hypercellular or normocellular, indicating that pancytopenia, leukopenia, and thrombocytopenia occur as a result of peripheral sequestration or consumption of blood cells. Hepatocellular apoptosis and, in severe cases, necrosis of liver, spleen, and lymph nodes has been observed.[26,64,68–70] Except in immunocompromised patients, the presence of *E. chaffeensis* in lesions is scanty, suggesting that disease may be partly mediated by host factors.[70]

Table 53-1 *Percentage of Ehrlichiosis Patients with Specific Symptoms or Signs at Any Time During the Course of Illness*

Symptom or Sign	Monocytotropic Ehrlichiosis[58] (n = 156–211)	Granulocytotropic Anaplasmosis[87,105] (n = 18–41)
Fever	97	94–100
Myalgia	68	78–98
Headache	81	61–85
Malaise	84	98
Nausea	68	39
Vomiting	37	34
Diarrhea	25	22
Cough	26	29
Arthralgias	41	27–78
Rash	36	2–11
Stiff neck	NA	22
Confusion	20	17

NA, not available.

Table 53-2 *Percentage of Ehrlichiosis Patients with Specific Abnormal Laboratory Findings at Any Time During the Course of Illness*

Laboratory Abnormality	Monocytotropic Ehrlichiosis[58] (n = 156–211)	Granulocytotropic Anaplasmosis[87,105] (n = 18–41)
Leukopenia	60–74	50–59
Thrombocytopenia	72	59–92
Anemia	50	6–50
Elevated serum aspartate transaminase	86–88	69–91
Elevated serum creatinine	24	0–70

PATHOGENESIS AND IMMUNITY

The pathogenesis of infection caused by *E. chaffeensis* is not well understood. Entry of *E. chaffeensis* into macrophages is mediated by binding of glycoprotein (gp) 120 and possibly other adhesins to host cell E- and L-selectin, probably at cholesterol-rich membrane lipid rafts or caveolae and glycosylphosphatidylinositol (GPI)-anchored proteins.[39,71] Binding of a heat-sensitive protein on *E. chaffeensis* initiates host cell phospholipase C and tyrosine kinase activation and mobilizes cytosolic free calcium in association with bacterial entry.[39,73] Entry is receptor-mediated and is impeded by transglutaminase inhibitors, but clathrin binding is not involved. Once internalized, *E. chaffeensis* alters the parasitophorous vacuole, leading to its accumulation of cellular transferrin receptors after activation of iron-responsive protein-1 that inhibits degradation of transferrin mRNA transcripts.[17] This effect leads to iron availability for bacterial growth and to redirection of the parasitophorous vacuole into a receptor salvage pathway that avoids lysosomal fusion. Genes involved in iron acquisition by *E. chaffeensis* are not regulated by an operon system, a situation that is evolutionarily divergent from other gram-negative bacteria. However, ferric (Fe III) iron is bound by a functionally conserved protein of the ferric binding protein (Fbp) family found extracellularly on dense-cored ehrlichiae that shares structural homology and iron binding capacity with Fbps of other gram-negative bacteria.[73] Down-regulation of host RAB5A, SNAP23, and STX16 with *E. chaffeensis* infection may underlie the altered endosomal trafficking and inhibition of its fusion with lysosomes.[74] The precise mechanism by which *E. chaffeensis* alters host gene transcription is not clear. Treatment with deferoxamine diminishes ehrlichial growth probably because the iron is utilized as a cofactor in oxidative phosphorylation, a critical metabolic pathway for some *Ehrlichia* spp. that apparently cannot utilize glucose or glucose 6-phosphate as energy sources.[17,75]

Infection of macrophages with *E. chaffeensis* results in production of the cytokines interleukin (IL)-1β, IL-8, and IL-10, but not TNF-α, IL-6, or granulocyte macrophage colony–stimulating factor (GM-CSF), a profile that suggests a relative lack of proinflammatory induction signals and the potential for immunosuppression.[76] Inflammatory chemokines IL-8, MCP-1, and MIP-1α are produced in response to *E. chaffeensis* and glycoproteins gp120 and gp200 through interactions with pattern recognition receptors. The cytokine response appears to be stimulated by *E. chaffeensis* carbohydrates, since periodation diminishes cytokine secretion. However, typical lipopolysaccharide-CD14 interaction does not account for the cytokine responses, since IL-1β induction by *E. chaffeensis* is not inhibited by monoclonal antibodies to CD14. When bound to immunoglobulin, macrophage-Fc receptor binding stimulates a strong proinflammatory response that could underlie local tissue injury with mounting immunity. Moreover, *E. chaffeensis* inhibits the expression of mRNA of IL-12, IL-15, and IL-18, cytokines that are key to the development of effective Th1 cellular immunity, and *E. chaffeensis* contains neither lipopolysaccharides or peptidoglycan pathogen associated molecular patterns associated with Toll-like receptor activation. Notably, downregulation of TLR2 and TLR4 genes in *E. chaffeensis*-infected cells occurs as a result of inhibition of p38 MAPK leading to reduced transcription factor PU.1 activity.[40] Furthermore, ehrlichiae down-regulate the expression of major histocompatibility complex (MHC) class II on infected cells, a potential mechanism of evading innate and acquired immune responses.[77] Animal models of monocytotropic *Ehrlichia* indicate that the humoral immune response, particularly to an epitope on the first hypervariable region of P28-19, a strong response by interferon-γ (IFN-γ)-producing CD4 Th1 cells, synergistic activity of IFN-γ and TNF-α, and CD8 cytotoxic T lymphocytes act together to control ehrlichial infections.[27,78–83]

The mechanisms by which *E. chaffeensis* damage infected host cells in vitro and in vivo is unknown. Clearly, in vitro infection causes cytolysis of infected macrophages, macrophage-like cell lines, endothelial cell lines, some fibroblast cell lines, and human embryonic lung cells.[9,29,84–86] Some of these cells contain many *E. chaffeensis* morulae, suggesting that simple mechanical lysis may be involved. The in vivo correlate is significant necrosis associated with abundant *E. chaffeensis* organisms that are found in spleen, liver, and other mononuclear phagocyte–rich tissues of immunocompromised patients who become infected.[26,68] In contrast, most immunocompetent patients do not develop tissue necrosis, and *E. chaffeensis* can be difficult or impossible to identify in pathologic lesions including perivascular lymphohistiocytic infiltrates, granulomas, apoptotic hepatocytes, and apoptotic γ/δ T lymphocytes in blood during early convalescence.[26,70,87] It is these latter pathologic findings in the absence of significant quantities of *E. chaffeensis* that suggest the contribution of host responses in the disease process.

DIAGNOSIS

Diagnosis is most often based on serologic studies,[1,5,48] which should include both *E. chaffeensis* and *A. phagocytophilum* antigens, since there is clinical similarity and serologic cross-reactivity occurs in some cases.[50,88] Seroconversion, fourfold rise in antibody titer to greater than or equal to 128, or a single serum titer greater than or equal to 256 in a patient with a consistent illness provides evidence of infection.[50] The development of recombinant antigens from *E. chaffeensis* holds promise for highly specific and sensitive serologic assays that may be useful in field conditions.[57,89] Peripheral blood smears should be examined for ehrlichial morulae (Fig. 53-1) in leukocytes, but except in immunocompromised patients, these are helpful in less than 10% of cases.[1,5,90] Polymerase chain reaction (PCR) amplification of *E. chaffeensis* DNA from acute-phase blood is between 56% and 95% sensitive, is highly specific, and provides timely information.[50,90,91] *E. chaffeensis* may be cultured from clinical samples in various cell lines, but the method is neither sensitive nor timely.[9,36,50,90]

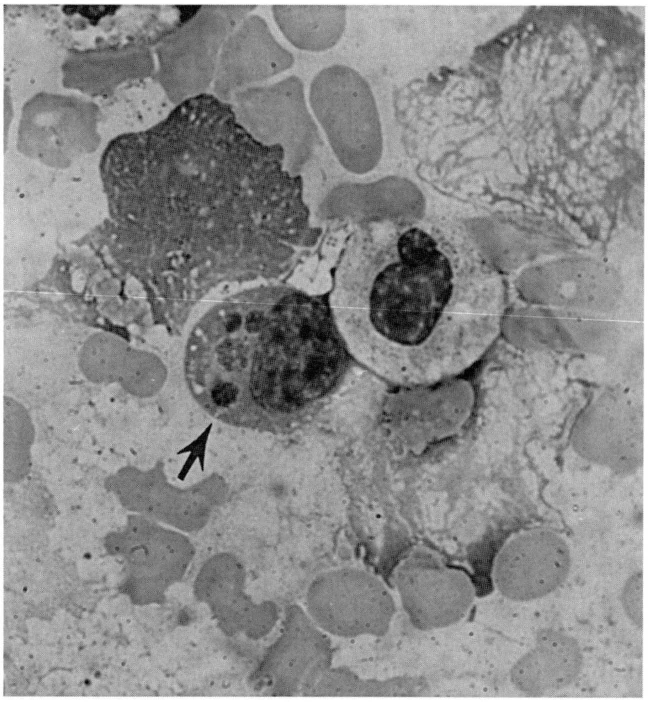

FIGURE 53-1 Peripheral blood mononuclear cell with intracytoplasmic aggregate (morulae) of *Ehrlichia chaffeensis* (*arrow*). (Wright stain; original magnification ×1000.)

AGENT: *EHRLICHIA EWINGII*

Known as a canine pathogen of neutrophils since the 1960s, *E. ewingii* was recently recognized as another cause of undifferentiated febrile illness following tick bites in geographic regions that overlap the distribution of HME and RMSF.[4,12] To avoid confusion with older nomenclature, it is prudent to avoid the term *human granulocytic ehrlichiosis* to refer to infection by *E. ewingii*. Despite its neutrophil host, the bacterium is more closely related to and shares more antigens with *E. chaffeensis* than with *A. phagocytophilum*.[2,12,57] It is presumed that a proportion of patients with a serologic diagnosis of HME actually have *E. ewingii*. This is in part based upon the known serologic cross-reactions and because 10%

of a cohort of suspected HME patients in Missouri were discovered to have *E. ewingii* instead.[4] *E. ewingii* is transmitted by *A. americanum* tick bites, although *Dermacentor variabilis* ticks may be naturally infected as well.[92,93] Similar to *E. chaffeensis*, white-tailed deer are persistently infected with *E. ewingii* in nature and are likely to be the most important reservoir, although a role for dogs as reservoirs has also been suggested.[94,95] Although only a small number of infected individuals has been described, the infection is most often recognized in immunocompromised persons, including those with HIV or with organ transplants.[4,12] In general, the infection is similar to HME, but it is milder and associated with fewer complications and no deaths. As the bacterium has not yet been cultivated in vitro, no specific serologic test is available and serodiagnosis cannot be reliably achieved using surrogate *E. chaffeensis* testing. Although infected neutrophils may occasionally be observed in peripheral blood, definitive identification currently depends on identification of *E. ewingii* nucleic acids in clinical samples.[4,96]

Human Granulocytotropic Anaplasmosis (HGA)

AGENT: *ANAPLASMA PHAGOCYTOPHILUM*

A. phagocytophilum contains a number of protein antigens, and the immunodominant major surface protein-2 (Msp2) 44-kD proteins are encoded by at least 22 paralogs that appear to be individually transcribed and expressed within a single bacterial cell.[19,97,98] With time, recombination by gene conversion or more complicated combinatorial mechanisms generates antigenic variants that may promote persistence in reservoir hosts by immune evasion. In hosts that develop significant clinical signs, including humans, persistent infection is not documented. Msp2 complexes in *A. phagocytophilum* are also involved in adhesion to fucosylated surface proteins of neutrophils, including platelet selectin glycoprotein ligand (PSGL)-1.[99–101] After binding, the bacteria are internalized within endosomes that do not acquire any markers of maturation but contain bacterial proteins, some presumably related to a type IV secretion mechanism encoded in the genome.[39] A 155-kD protein called AnkA of unknown function is secreted by the bacterium, enters into the host cell nucleus, and complexes with host cell chromatin.[102]

EPIDEMIOLOGY

Human granulocytotropic anaplasmosis (HGA; formerly, human granulocytotropic ehrlichiosis, HGE) was first identified in febrile patients who reported tick bites.[10,11,103] *Ixodes persulcatus*–complex ticks, including *Ixodes scapularis*, *Ixodes pacificus*, *Ixodes ricinus*, and *Ixodes persulcatus*, are naturally infected and except for *I. persulcatus*, each is proved competent for transmission of *A. phagocytophilum*.[22–24,104,105] Small rodents appear to be a major reservoir, but cervids, ruminants, raccoons, and rabbits, among many other animals, are infected in nature and may be important reservoirs as well.[105–109] Ticks are important hosts, but the lack of transovarial transmission emphasizes the critical role of the mammal–tick–mammal transmission cycle that is facilitated by *Anaplasma* persistence in mammalian reservoirs.[22] HGA is most frequently recognized in the upper Midwest and northeastern United States and occasionally in northern California, areas that have a high incidence of *Ixodes* tick–related diseases,[11,88,110] including coinfections with Lyme disease and babesiosis.[111–114] Passive case collection reveals incidences as high as 58 and 51 cases per 100,000 population in the upper Midwest and Connecticut, respectively.[88,115,116] A worldwide high seroprevalence rate indicates that HGA probably is widely distributed and significantly underdiagnosed.[117–120] Most cases occur in May through July, when nymphal-stage ticks are active, although infections may be recognized even during winter months.[88]

On a worldwide basis, a high percentage of *Ixodes* spp. ticks, particularly those in the *I. persulcatus* complex, harbor *A. phagocytophilum*. The highest proportions of infected ticks are *I. scapularis,* found in the northeastern and upper midwestern United States, where infection may be found in up to 50% (median ≈11%).[104,121,122] Up to 7% (median 2%) of *I. pacificus* in California, and up to 33% of *I. persulcatus* and *I. ricinus* in Asia and Europe (median 5% and 4%, respectively) are infected.[123–125] Infection has also been demonstrated in *Dermacentor* ticks (*D. variabilis* and *D. occidentalis* in California), in Korean *Haemaphysalis longicornis*, and in several *Ixodes* spp. that seldom bite humans (*I. dentatus, I. trianguliceps*).[107,124,126,127] The anaplasmae spread from the tick's gut to the salivary gland and are inoculated into the dermis during tick feeding.[24] Transovarial transmission of *A. phagocytophilum* has not been demonstrated.[22,23]

DISEASE

HGA is usually an undifferentiated febrile illness accompanied by headache, myalgias, rigors, and malaise; gastrointestinal, respiratory, and CNS abnormalities occur in a minority of patients[88,110,128] (see Table 53-1). Rash is rare. The median age is between 43 and 60 years with up to a 2:1 male predominance. Leukopenia (50% to 59% of patients), thrombocytopenia (59% to 92%), and elevations in serum hepatic transaminases (69% to 91%) are often present [88,110,128] (see Table 53-2). The manifestations of severe illness may include prolonged fever, shock, confusion, seizures, pneumonitis, acute renal failure, rhabdomyolysis, acute abdomen, hemorrhage, opportunistic infections, and death;[88,110,129–133] misdiagnosis and late therapy contribute to severe morbidity. CNS infection and cerebrospinal fluid pleocytosis are rare, but reported complications include VIIth cranial nerve palsy, brachial plexopathy, and demyelinating polyneuropathy.[134–136] The case fatality rate is probably less than 0.5%, but 50% or more of infected patients require hospitalization, even in Europe, where disease is considered to be milder.[88,103] Opportunistic infections, including disseminated candidiasis, herpetic esophagitis, cryptococcal pneumonitis, and invasive pulmonary aspergillosis, are major causes of death and occur in patients with and without prior immunocompromise.[88,129,137]

PATHOGENESIS AND IMMUNITY

The pathogenesis of HGA is not well understood but appears to be related to inadequate control of inflammation triggered by *A. phagocytophilum* infection.[25,137] Limited pathologic examinations of human tissue samples show changes associated with macrophage activation, similar to those in *E. chaffeensis* infection, except lacking granulomas.[88,129,137] Neutrophil infection by *A. phagocytophilum* yields activation of host chemokine expression, motility, and degranulation but deactivation of endothelial cell adhesion and transcytosis, respiratory burst, and apoptosis.[138–142] Such changes allow longer persistence of infected cells in blood that can be ingested by biting ticks. However, the persistent activation may contribute to increasing inflammation and bystander cell injury accompanied by reduced ability to control other infections. Infection mediates early responses by interaction with macrophage Toll-like receptor–2 but not Toll-like receptor–4.[143] These interactions also promote specific immunity that incites production of Th1 proinflammatory cytokines, which are responsible for most inflammatory tissue injury in animal models.[25]

DIAGNOSIS

Retrospective diagnosis is mostly by serologic tests using indirect fluorescent antibody and one of several *A. phagocytophilum* strains.[103,144,145] Occasional serologic cross-reactions to *E. chaffeensis* occur, but the homologous titer is usually higher.[103,146] A fourfold increase, seroconversion, or a high single antibody titer (usually ≥64) in a patient with a consistent illness is confirmatory. Careful examination of Giemsa- or Wright-stained peripheral blood smears (Fig. 53-2) may be diagnostic during the acute phase in 18% to 80% of patients.[103] PCR diagnosis is rapid and relatively sensitive, whereas culture is not timely.[30,147]

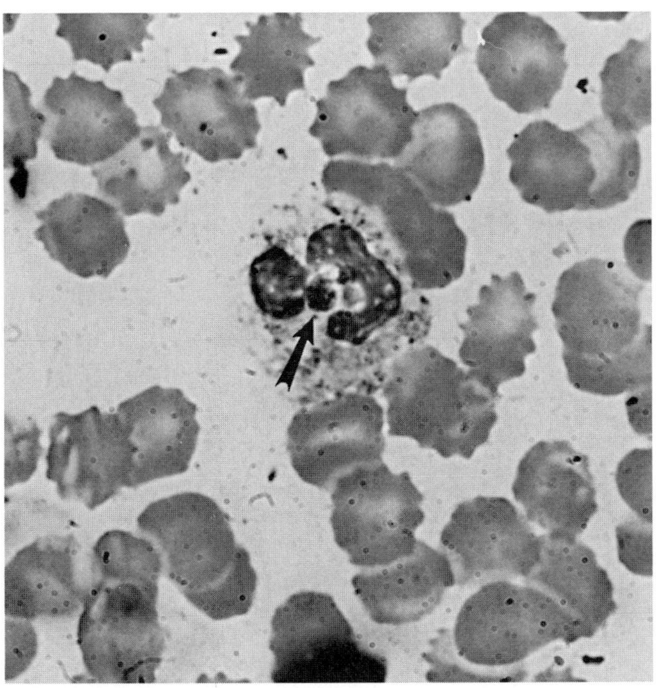

FIGURE 53-2 Peripheral blood neutrophil with intracytoplasmic aggregate (*arrow*) of ehrlichiae in a patient with human granulocytic ehrlichiosis. (Wright stain; original magnification ×1000.)

Neorickettsiosis

AGENT: *NEORICKETTSIA SENNETSU*

Originally recognized as an illness mimicking infectious mononucleosis in Japan, *N. sennetsu* infections have subsequently been documented in Malaysia and might occur unrecognized in other areas of Asia where raw or undercooked fish are eaten.[148,149] Recent investigations have identified complex cycles of bacterial infection of trematodes, the cercariae of which may infect snails and aquatic insects.[150] These are in turn ingested by a variety of animals, including fish, mammals, and birds, that may be reservoirs.[151] The infection has never been reported to cause fatal disease. Diagnosis by serology or culture is available in very few laboratories.

TREATMENT

Because severity of HME and HGA may result from therapeutic delays, patients should be treated empirically. Most patients defervesce within 24 to 48 hours after starting doxycycline or tetracycline treatment.[1,58,103] Chloramphenicol should not be used, since in vitro minimal inhibitory concentrations cannot be effectively achieved in vivo.[152–154] The preferred adult regimen is oral doxycycline 100 mg twice daily or tetracycline 250 to 500 mg every 6 hours. For children, doxycycline 4.4 mg/kg in two divided doses per day or tetracycline 25 to 50 mg/kg/day in four divided doses is recommended. Therapy is administered for at least 3 days after defervescence, and some physicians treat for 14 to 21 days. *N. sennetsu* ehrlichiosis also responds to treatment with tetracycline. Some evidence suggests efficacy of rifampin.[152–156] Resistance to fluoroquinolones in *Ehrlichia* is mediated by an amino acid change in GyrA, suggesting the potential for resistance in *A. phagocytophilum* as well.[157]

PREVENTION AND CONTROL

Simple precautions aimed at reducing tick exposure, including avoiding tick-infested habitats, wearing appropriate barrier clothing, using tick repellents, and removing attached ticks carefully and early, will lower the risk of disease acquisition. Conflicting data exist regarding a "grace period" during which transfer of the infectious agents is delayed immediately after tick attachment for HME and HGA. Some studies suggest a significant reduction in transmission if ticks are removed within 36 hours,[158,159] whereas others show a high transmission rate within 24 hours,[160] suggesting that daily tick removal may not be sufficient to prevent *A. phagocytophilum* transmission.

WOLBACHIA-RELATED COMPLICATIONS OF FILARIASIS

Wolbachia spp. are endocytoplasmic bacteria that are diversely spread throughout the world of insects, arthropods, helminths, and crustaceans.[161] These bacteria have diverse effects on the population dynamics of their hosts, usually leading to feminization of gender ratios associated with bacterial survival only in females. Examples that distort gender ratio include cytoplasmic incompatibility between infected and uninfected parents, parthenogenesis, and feminization of genetic males, among others. In addition, endosymbiont bacteria of helminths can influence the survival of larval instars.

The inflammatory complications of lymphatic filariasis and river blindness are part of the pathogenesis of these infections.[162] These inflammatory processes are associated more often with death of the nematodes, whether naturally or by therapeutic intervention. Much of the subsequent inflammation can be attributed to innate responses of the host toward endosymbiont bacterial components, in part through CD14, Toll-like receptor–4, or other innate immune receptors.[162] Clinical trials to assess the effect of doxycycline treatment in lymphatic filariasis have demonstrated depletion of *Wolbachia* bacteria from adult worms and microfilariae, inhibition of embryogenesis, declining microfilariae quantities, and reduced spermatozoa present in female genital tracts.[163,164] Further assessment is required to show whether bacterial endosymbiont elimination will provide additional benefit for patients with lymphatic filariasis or river blindness.

REFERENCES

1. Olano JP, Walker DH: Human ehrlichioses. Med Clin North Am 86:375, 2002.
2. Dumler JS, Barbet AF, Bekker CP, et al: Reorganization of genera in the families Rickettsiaceae and Anaplasmataceae in the order Rickettsiales: unification of some species of *Ehrlichia* with *Anaplasma*, *Cowdria* with *Ehrlichia* and *Ehrlichia* with *Neorickettsia*, descriptions of six new species combinations and designation of *Ehrlichia equi* and HGE agent as subjective synonyms of *Ehrlichia phagocytophila*. Int J Syst Evol Microbiol 51:2145, 2001.
3. Perez M, Rikihisa Y, Wen B: *Ehrlichia canis*–like agent isolated from a man in Venezuela: antigenic and genetic characterization. J Clin Microbiol 34:2133, 1996.
4. Buller RS, Arens M, Hmiel SP, et al: *Ehrlichia ewingii*, a newly recognized agent of human ehrlichiosis. N Engl J Med 341:148, 1999.
5. Paddock CD, Childs JE: *Ehrlichia chaffeensis*: a prototypical emerging pathogen. Clin Microbiol Rev 16:37, 2003.
6. Inokuma H, Brouqui P, Drancourt M, et al: Citrate synthase gene sequence: a new tool for phylogenetic analysis and identification of *Ehrlichia*. J Clin Microbiol 39:3031, 2001.
7. Taillardat-Bisch AV, Raoult D, Drancourt M: RNA polymerase beta-subunit-based phylogeny of *Ehrlichia* spp., *Anaplasma* spp., *Neorickettsia* spp. and *Wolbachia pipientis*. Int J Syst Evol Microbiol 53:455, 2003.
8. Anderson BE, Dawson JE, Jones DC, et al: *Ehrlichia chaffeensis,* a new species associated with human ehrlichiosis. J Clin Microbiol 29:2838, 1991.
9. Dawson JE, Anderson BE, Fishbein DB, et al: Isolation and characterization of an *Ehrlichia* from a patient diagnosed with human ehrlichiosis. J Clin Microbiol 29:2741, 1991.
10. Chen S-M, Dumler JS, Bakken JS, et al: Identification of a granulocytotropic *Ehrlichia* species as the etiologic agent of human disease. J Clin Microbiol 32:589, 1994.
11. Bakken JS, Dumler JS, Chen SM, et al: Human granulocytic ehrlichiosis in the upper midwest United States: a new species emerging? JAMA 272:212, 1994.
12. Paddock CD, Folk SM, Shore GM, et al: Infections with *Ehrlichia chaffeensis* and *Ehrlichia ewingii* in persons coinfected with human immunodeficiency virus. Clin Infect Dis 33:1586, 2001.
13. Taylor MJ, Cross HF, Bilo K: Inflammatory responses induced by the filarial nematode *Brugia malayi* are mediated by lipopolysaccharide-like activity from endosymbiotic *Wolbachia* bacteria. J Exp Med 191:1429, 2000.
14. Barnewall RE, Rikihisa Y, Lee EH: *Ehrlichia chaffeensis* inclusions are early endosomes which selectively accumulate transferrin receptor. Infect Immun 65:1455, 1997.
15. Webster P, IJdo JW, Chicoine LM, et al: The agent of human granulocytic ehrlichiosis resides in an endosomal compartment. J Clin Invest 101:1932, 1998.
16. Wells MY, Rikihisa Y: Lack of lysosomal fusion with phagosomes containing *Ehrlichia risticii* in P388D1 cells: abrogration of inhibition with oxytetracycline. Infect Immun 56:3209, 1985.
17. Barnewall RE, Ohashi N, Rikihisa Y: *Ehrlichia chaffeensis* and *E. sennetsu*, but not the human granulocytic ehrlichiosis agent, colocalize with transferrin receptor and up-regulate transferrin receptor mRNA by activating iron-responsive protein 1. Infect Immun 67:2258, 1999.
18. Brayton KA, Knowles DP, McGuire TC, et al: Efficient use of a small genome to generate antigenic diversity in tick-borne ehrlichial pathogens. Proc Natl Acad Sci USA 98:4130, 2001.
19. Scorpio DG, Caspersen K, Ogata H, et al: Restricted changes in major surface protein-2 (*msp2*) transcription after prolonged in vitro passage of *Anaplasma phagocytophilum*. BMC Microbiol 4:1, 2004.
20. Long SW, Zhang XF, Qi H, et al: Antigenic variation of *Ehrlichia chaffeensis* resulting from differential expression of the 28-kilodalton protein gene family. Infect Immun 70:1824, 2002.
21. Anderson BE, Sims KG, Olson JG, et al: *Amblyomma americanum*: a potential vector of human ehrlichiosis. Am J Trop Med Hyg 49:239, 1994.
22. MacLeod JR, Gordon WS: Studies in tick-borne fever of sheep. 1. Transmission by the tick, *Ixodes ricinus,* with a description of the disease produced. Parasitology 25:273, 1933.
23. Richter PJ, Kimsey RB, Madigan JE, et al: *Ixodes pacificus* as a vector of *Ehrlichia equi*. J Med Entomol 33:1, 1996.
24. Telford SR III, Dawson JE, Katavolos P, et al: Perpetuation of the agent of human granulocytic ehrlichiosis in a deer tick–rodent cycle. Proc Natl Acad Sci USA 93:6209, 1996.
25. Martin ME, Caspersen K, Dumler JS: Immunopathology and ehrlichial propagation are regulated by interferon-gamma and interleukin-10 in a murine model of human granulocytic ehrlichiosis. Am J Pathol 158:1881, 2001.
26. Sehdev AE, Dumler JS; Hepatic pathology in human monocytic ehrlichiosis: *Ehrlichia chaffeensis* infection. Am J Clin Pathol 119:859, 2003.
27. Ismail N, Soong L, McBride JW, et al: Overproduction of TNF-α by $CD8^+$ type 1 cells and down-regulation of IFN-γ production by $CD4^+$ Th1 cells contribute to toxic shock-like syndrome in an animal model of fatal monocytotropic ehrlichiosis. J Immunol 172:1786–1800, 2004.
28. Dawson JE, Fishbein DB, Eng TR, et al: Diagnosis of human ehrlichiosis with the indirect fluorescent antibody test: kinetics and specificity. J Infect Dis 162:91, 1990.
29. Barnewall RE, Rikihisa Y: Abrogation of gamma interferon–induced inhibition of *Ehrlichia chaffeensis* infection in human monocytes with iron transferrin. Infect Immun 62:4804, 1994.
30. Goodman JL, Nelson C, Vitale B, et al: Direct cultivation of the causative agent of human granulocytic ehrlichiosis. N Engl J Med 334:262, 1996.
31. Munderloh UG, Tate CM, Lynch MJ, et al: Isolation of an *Anaplasma* sp. organism from white-tailed deer by tick cell culture. J Clin Microbiol 41:4328, 2003.
32. Popov VL, Han VC, Chen SM, et al: Ultrastructural differentiation of the genogroups in the genus *Ehrlichia*. J Med Microbiol 47:235, 1998.
33. Popov VL, Yu X, Walker DH: The 120 kDa outer membrane protein of *Ehrlichia chaffeensis*: preferential expression on dense-core cells and gene expression in *Escherichia coli* associated with attachment and entry. Microb Pathog 28:71, 2000.
34. Chen S-M, Dumler JS, Feng H-M, et al: Identification of the antigenic constituents of *Ehrlichia chaffeensis*. Am J Trop Med Hyg 50:52, 1994.
35. Rikihisa Y, Ewing SA, Fox JC: Western immunoblot analysis of *Ehrlichia chaffeensis, E. canis,* or *E. ewingii* infections in dogs and humans. J Clin Microbiol 32:2107, 1994.
36. Chen S-M, Popov VL, Westerman EL, et al: Genetic and antigenic diversity of *Ehrlichia chaffeensis*: comparative analysis of a novel human strain from Oklahoma and previously isolated strains. J Infect Dis 175:856, 1997.
37. Long SW, Zhang XF, Qi H, et al: Antigenic variation of *Ehrlichia chaffeensis* resulting from differential expression of the 28-kilodalton protein gene family. Infect Immun 70:1824, 2002.
38. Yabsley MJ, Little SE, Sims EJ, et al: Molecular variation in the variable-length PCR target and 120-kilodalton antigen genes of *Ehrlichia chaffeensis* from white-tailed deer (*Odocoileus virginianus*). J Clin Microbiol 41:5202, 2003.
39. Lin M, Rikihisa Y: Obligatory intracellular parasitism by *Ehrlichia chaffeensis* and *Anaplasma phagocytophilum* involves caveolae and glycosylphosphatidylinositol-anchored proteins. Cell Microbiol 5:809, 2003.

40. Lin M, Rikihisa Y: *Ehrlichia chaffeensis* downregulates surface Toll-like receptors 2/4, CD14 and transcription factors PU.1 and inhibits lipopolysaccharide activation of NF-kappaB, ERK 1/2 and p38 MAPK in host monocytes. Cell Microbiol 6:175, 2004.
41. Maeda K, Markowitz N, Hawley RC, et al: Human infection with *Ehrlichia canis,* a leukocytic rickettsia. N Engl J Med 316:853, 1987.
42. Dawson JE, Childs JE, Biggie KL, et al: White-tailed deer as a potential reservoir of *Ehrlichia* spp. J Wildl Dis 30:162, 1994.
43. Dawson JE, Stallknecht DE, Howerth EW, et al: Susceptibility of white-tailed deer (*Odocoileus virginianus*) to infection with *Ehrlichia chaffeensis,* the etiologic agent of human ehrlichiosis. J Clin Microbiol 32:2725, 1994.
44. Lockhart JM, Davidson WR, Dawson JE, et al: Temporal association of *Amblyomma americanum* with the presence of *Ehrlichia chaffeensis* reactive antibodies in white-tailed deer. J Wildl Dis 31:119, 1995.
45. Dawson JE, Ewing SA: Susceptibility of dogs to infection with *Ehrlichia chaffeensis,* causative agent of human ehrlichiosis. Am J Vet Res 53:1322, 1992.
46. Dawson JE, Biggie KL, Warner CK, et al: Polymerase chain reaction evidence of *Ehrlichia chaffeensis,* an etiologic agent of human ehrlichiosis, in dogs from southeast Virginia. Am J Vet Res 57:1175, 1996.
47. Breitschwerdt EB, Hegarty BC, Hancock SI: Sequential evaluation of dogs naturally infected with *Ehrlichia canis*, *Ehrlichia chaffeensis*, *Ehrlichia equi*, *Ehrlichia ewingii*, or *Bartonella vinsonii*. J Clin Microbiol 36:2645, 1998.
48. Fishbein DB, Kemp A, Dawson JE, et al: Human ehrlichiosis: prospective active surveillance in febrile hospitalized patients. J Infect Dis 160:803, 1989.
49. Carpenter CF, Gandhi TK, Kong LK, et al: The incidence of ehrlichial and rickettsial infection in patients with unexplained fever and recent history of tick bite in central North Carolina. J Infect Dis 180:900, 1999.
50. Olano JP, Masters E, Hogrefe W, et al: Human monocytotropic ehrlichiosis, Missouri. Emerg Infect Dis 9:1579, 2003.
51. Brouqui P, Le Cam C, Kelly PJ, et al: Serologic evidence for human ehrlichiosis in Africa. Eur J Epidemiol 10:695, 1994.
52. Morais JD, Dawson JE, Greene C, et al: First European case of ehrlichiosis. Lancet 338:633, 1991.
53. Uhaa IJ, MacLean JD, Greene CR, et al: A case of human ehrlichiosis acquired in Mali: clinical and laboratory findings. Am J Trop Med Hyg 46:161, 1992.
54. Ravyn MD, Korenberg EI, Oeding JA, et al: Monocytic *Ehrlichia* in *Ixodes persulcatus* ticks from Perm, Russia. Lancet 353:722, 1999.
55. Park JH, Heo EJ, Choi KS, et al: Detection of antibodies to *Anaplasma phagocytophilum* and *Ehrlichia chaffeensis* antigens in sera of Korean patients by western immunoblotting and indirect immunofluorescence assays. Clin Diagn Lab Immunol 10:1059, 2003.
56. Yevich SJ, Sanchez JL, DeFraites RF, et al: Seroepidemiology of infections due to spotted fever group rickettsiae and *Ehrlichia* species in military personnel exposed in areas of the United States where such infections are endemic. J Infect Dis 175:1266, 1995.
57. Unver A, Rikihisa Y, Ohashi N, et al: Western and dot blotting analyses of *Ehrlichia chaffeensis* indirect fluorescent-antibody assay-positive and -negative human sera by using native and recombinant *E. chaffeensis* and *E. canis* antigens. J Clin Microbiol 37:3888, 1999.
58. Fishbein DB, Dawson JE, Robinson LE: Human ehrlichiosis in the United States, 1985 to 1990. Ann Intern Med 120:736, 1994.
59. Marshall GS, Jacobs RF, Schutze GE, et al: Tick-Borne Infections in Children Study Group: *Ehrlichia chaffeensis* seroprevalence among children in the southeast and south-central regions of the United States. Arch Pediatr Adolesc Med 156:166, 2002.
60. Dunn BE, Monson TP, Dumler JS, et al: Identification of *Ehrlichia chaffeensis* morulae in cerebrospinal fluid mononuclear cells. J Clin Microbiol 30:2207, 1992.
61. Dimmitt DC, Fishbein DB, Dawson JE: Human ehrlichiosis associated with cerebrospinal fluid pleocytosis. Am J Med 87:677, 1989.
62. Ratnasamy N, Everett ED, Roland WE, et al: Central nervous system manifestations of human ehrlichiosis. Clin Infect Dis 23:314, 1996.
63. Fichtenbaum CJ, Peterson LR, Weil GJ: Ehrlichiosis presenting as a life-threatening illness with features of the toxic shock syndrome. Am J Med 95:351, 1993.
64. Dumler JS, Sutker WL, Walker DH: Persistent infection with *Ehrlichia chaffeensis*. Clin Infect Dis 17:903, 1994.
65. Smith Sehdev AE, Sehdev PS, Jacobs R, et al: Human monocytic ehrlichiosis presenting as acute appendicitis during pregnancy. Clin Infect Dis 35:e99, 2002.
66. Safdar N, Love RB, Maki DG: Severe *Ehrlichia chaffeensis* infection in a lung transplant recipient: a review of ehrlichiosis in the immunocompromised patient. Emerg Infect Dis 8:320, 2002.
67. Tan HP, Dumler JS, Maley WR, et al: Human monocytic ehrlichiosis: an emerging pathogen in transplantation. Transplantation 71:1678, 2001.
68. Marty AM, Dumler JS, Imes G, et al: Ehrlichiosis mimicking thrombotic thrombocytopenic purpura: case report and pathological correlation. Hum Pathol 26:920, 1995.
69. Walker DH, Dumler JS: Human monocytic and granulocytic ehrlichioses: discovery and diagnosis of emerging tick-borne infections and the critical role of the pathologist. Arch Pathol Lab Med 121:785, 1997.
70. Dumler JS, Dawson JE, Walker DH: Human ehrlichiosis: hematopathology and immunohistologic detection of *Ehrlichia chaffeensis*. Hum Pathol 24:391, 1993.
71. Zhang JZ, McBride JW, Yu XJ: L-selectin and E-selectin expressed on monocytes mediating *Ehrlichia chaffeensis* attachment onto host cells. FEMS Microbiol Lett 227:303, 2003.
72. Lin M, Zhu MX, Rikihisa Y: Rapid activation of protein tyrosine kinase and phospholipase C-γ_2 and increase in cytosolic free calcium are required by *Ehrlichia chaffeensis* for internalization and growth in THP-1 cells. Infect Immun 70:889, 2002.
73. Doyle C, Zhang ZF, Popov VL, et al: An immunoreactive 38-kDa protein of *Ehrlichia canis* shares structural homology and iron-binding capacity with the ferric binding protein family. Infect Immun 73:62, 2005.
74. Zhang JZ, Sinha M, Luxon BA, et al: Survival strategy of obligately intracellular *Ehrlichia chaffeensis*: novel modulation of immune response and host cell cycles. Infect Immun 72:498, 2004.
75. Park J, Rikihisa Y: L-Arginine-dependent killing of intracellular *Ehrlichia risticii* by macrophages treated with gamma interferon. Infect Immun 60:3504, 1992.
76. Lee EH, Rikihisa Y: Absence of tumor necrosis factor alpha, interleukin-6 (IL-6), and granulocyte-macrophage colony-stimulating factor expression but presence of IL-1β, IL-8, and IL-10 expression in human monocytes exposed to viable or killed *Ehrlichia chaffeensis*. Infect Immun 64:4211, 1996.
77. Harrus S, Waner T, Friedmann-Morvinski D, et al: Down-regulation of MHC class II receptors of DH82 cells, following infection with *Ehrlichia canis*. Vet Immunol Immunopathol 96:239–243, 2003.
78. Ganta RR, Wilkerson MJ, Cheng C, et al: Persistent *Ehrlichia chaffeensis* infection occurs in the absence of functional major histocompatibility complex class II genes. Infect Immun 70:380, 2002.
79. Winslow GM, Yager E, Shilo K, et al: Antibody-mediated elimination of the obligate intracellular bacterial pathogen *Ehrlichia chaffeensis* during active infection. Infect Immun 68:2187, 2000.
80. Li JS, Chu F, Reilly A, et al: Antibodies highly effective in SCID mice during infection by the intracellular bacterium *Ehrlichia chaffeensis* are of picomolar affinity and exhibit preferential epitope and isotype utilization. J Immunol 169:1419, 2002.
81. Byrom B, Barbet AF, Obwolo M, et al: $CD8^+$ T cell knockout mice are less susceptible to *Cowdria ruminantium* infection than athymic, $CD4^+$ T cell knockout, and normal C57BL/6 mice. Vet Parasitol 93:159, 2000.
82. Byrom B, Obwolo M, Barbet AF, et al: A polarized Th1 type immune response to *Cowdria ruminantium* infection is detected in immune DBA/2 mice. J Parasitol 86:983, 2000.
83. Li JS, Yager E, Reilly M, et al: Outer membrane protein-specific monoclonal antibodies protect SCID mice from fatal infection by the obligate intracellular bacterial pathogen *Enrlichia chaffeensis*. J Immunol 166:1855, 2001.
84. Dawson JE, Candal FJ, George VG, et al: Human endothelial cells as an alternative to DH82 cells for isolation of *Ehrlichia chaffeensis, E. canis,* and *Rickettsia rickettsii*. Pathobiology 61:293, 1993.
85. Brouqui P, Birg ML, Raoult D: Cytopathic effect, plaque formation, and lysis of *Ehrlichia chaffeensis* grown on continuous cell lines. Infect Immun 62:405, 1994.
86. Chen S-M, Popov VL, Feng H-M, et al: Cultivation of *Ehrlichia chaffeensis* in mouse embryo, Vero, BGM, and L929 cells and study of *Ehrlichia*-induced cytopathic effect and plaque formation. Infect Immun 63:647, 1995.
87. Caldwell CW, Everett ED, McDonald G, et al: Apoptosis of γ/δ T cells in human ehrlichiosis. Am J Clin Pathol 105:640, 1996.
88. Bakken JS, Krueth J, Wilson-Nordskog C, et al: Clinical and laboratory characteristics of human granulocytic ehrlichiosis. JAMA 275:199, 1996.

89. Yu X-J, Crocquet-Valdes P, Cullman LC, et al: The recombinant 120-kilodalton protein of *Ehrlichia chaffeensis,* a potential diagnostic tool. J Clin Microbiol 34:2853, 1996.
90. Standaert SM, Yu T, Scott MA, et al: Primary isolation of *Ehrlichia chaffeensis* from patients with febrile illnesses: clinical and molecular characteristics. J Infect Dis 181:1082, 2000.
91. Everett ED, Evans KA, Henry RB, et al: Human ehrlichiosis in adults after tick exposure: diagnosis using polymerase chain reaction. Ann Intern Med 120:730, 1994.
92. Steiert JG, Gilfoy F: Infection rates of *Amblyomma americanum* and *Dermacentor variabilis* by *Ehrlichia chaffeensis* and *Ehrlichia ewingii* in southwest Missouri. Vector Borne Zoonotic Dis 2:53, 2002.
93. Anziani OS, Ewing SA, Barker RW: Experimental transmission of a granulocytic form of the tribe *Ehrlichieae* by *Dermacentor variabilis* and *Amblyomma americanum* to dogs. Am J Vet Res 51:929, 1990.
94. Yabsley MJ, Varela AS, Tate CM, et al: *Ehrlichia ewingii* infection in white-tailed deer (*Odocoileus virginianus*). Emerg Infect Dis 8:668, 2002.
95. Liddell AM, Stockham SL, Scott MA, et al: Predominance of *Ehrlichia ewingii* in Missouri dogs. J Clin Microbiol 41:4617, 2003.
96. Gusa AA, Buller RS, Storch GA, et al: Identification of a p28 gene in *Ehrlichia ewingii*: evaluation of gene for use as a target for a species-specific PCR diagnostic assay. J Clin Microbiol 39:3871, 2001.
97. Zhi N, Ohashi N, Tajima T, et al: Transcript heterogeneity of the p44 multigene family in a human granulocytic ehrlichiosis agent transmitted by ticks. Infect Immun 70:1175, 2002.
98. Barbet AF, Meeus PF, Belanger M, et al: Expression of multiple outer membrane protein sequence variants from a single genomic locus of *Anaplasma phagocytophilum*. Infect Immun 71:1706, 2003.
99. Park J, Choi KS, Dumler JS: Major surface protein 2 of *Anaplasma phagocytophilum* facilitates adherence to granulocytes. Infect Immun 71:4018, 2003.
100. Herron MJ, Nelson CM, Larson J, et al: Intracellular parasitism by the human granulocytic ehrlichiosis bacterium through the P-selectin ligand, PSGL-1. Science 288:1653, 2000.
101. Carlyon JA, Akkoyunlu M, Xia L, et al: Murine neutrophils require alpha1,3-fucosylation but not PSGL-1 for productive infection with *Anaplasma phagocytophilum*. Blood 102:3387, 2003.
102. Caturegli P, Asanovich KM, Walls JJ, et al: *ankA*: an *Ehrlichia phagocytophila* group gene encoding a cytoplasmic protein antigen with ankyrin repeats. Infect Immun 68:5277, 2000.
103. Bakken JS, Dumler JS: Human granulocytic ehrlichiosis. Clin Infect Dis 31:554, 2000.
104. Pancholi P, Kolbert CP, Mitchell PD, et al: *Ixodes dammini* as a potential vector of human granulocytic ehrlichiosis. J Infect Dis 172:1007, 1995.
105. Magnarelli LA, Stafford KC, Mather TN, et al: Hemocytic rickettsia-like organisms in ticks: serologic reactivity with antisera to ehrlichiae and detection of DNA of agent of human granulocytic ehrlichiosis by PCR. J Clin Microbiol 33:2710, 1995.
106. Walls JJ, Greig B, Neitzel DS, et al: Natural infection of small mammal species in Minnesota with the agent of human granulocytic ehrlichiosis. J Clin Microbiol 35:853, 1997.
107. Goethert HK, Telford SR III: Enzootic transmission of the agent of human granulocytic ehrlichiosis among cottontail rabbits. Am J Trop Med Hyg 68:633, 2003.
108. Levin ML, Nicholson WL, Massung RF, et al: Comparison of the reservoir competence of medium-sized mammals and *Peromyscus leucopus* for *Anaplasma phagocytophilum* in Connecticut. Vector Borne Zoonotic Dis 2:125, 2002.
109. Alberdi MP, Walker AR, Urquhart KA: Field evidence that roe deer (*Capreolus capreolus*) are a natural host for *Ehrlichia phagocytophila*. Epidemiol Infect 124:315, 2000.
110. Aguero-Rosenfeld ME, Horowitz HW, Wormser GP, et al: Human granulocytic ehrlichiosis (HGE): a case series from a single medical center in New York State. Ann Intern Med 125:904, 1996.
111. Nadelman RB, Horowitz HW, Hsieh TC, et al: Simultaneous human granulocytic ehrlichiosis and Lyme borreliosis. N Engl J Med 337:27, 1997.
112. Moss WJ, Dumler JS: Simultaneous infection with *Borrelia burgdorferi* and human granulocytic ehrlichiosis. Pediatr Infect Dis J 22:91, 2003.
113. Bjoersdorff A, Wittesjo B, Berglun J, et al: Human granulocytic ehrlichiosis as a common cause of tick-associated fever in Southeast Sweden: report from a prospective clinical study. Scand J Infect Dis 34:187, 2002.
114. Thompson C, Spielman A, Krause PJ: Coinfecting deer-associated zoonoses: Lyme disease, babesiosis, and ehrlichiosis. Clin Infect Dis 33:676, 2001.
115. Ijdo JW, Meek JI, Cartter ML, et al: The emergence of another tickborne infection in the 12-town area around Lyme, Connecticut: human granulocytic ehrlichiosis. J Infect Dis 181:1388, 2000.
116. Gardner SL, Holman RC, Krebs JW, et al: National surveillance for the human ehrlichioses in the United States, 1997–2001, and proposed methods for evaluation of data quality. Ann NY Acad Sci 990:80, 2003.
117. Bakken JS, Goellner P, Van Etten M, et al: Seroprevalence of human granulocytic ehrlichiosis among permanent residents of northwestern Wisconsin. Clin Infect Dis 27:1491, 1998.
118. Aguero-Rosenfeld ME, Donnarumma L, Zentmaier L, et al: Seroprevalence of antibodies that react with *Anaplasma phagocytophila*, the agent of human granulocytic ehrlichiosis, in different populations in Westchester County, New York. J Clin Microbiol 40:2612, 2002.
119. Cizman M, Avsic-Zupanc T, Petrovec M, et al: Seroprevalence of ehrlichiosis, Lyme borreliosis and tick-borne encephalitis infections in children and young adults in Slovenia. Wien Klin Wochenschr 112:842, 2000.
120. Walder G, Tiwald G, Dierich MP, et al: Serological evidence for human granulocytic ehrlichiosis in Western Austria. Eur J Clin Microbiol Infect Dis 22:543, 2003.
121. Courtney JW, Dryden RL, Montgomery J, et al: Molecular characterization of *Anaplasma phagocytophilum* and *Borrelia burgdorferi* in *Ixodes scapularis* ticks from Pennsylvania. J Clin Microbiol 41:1569, 2003.
122. Chang YF, Novosel V, Chang CF, et al: Detection of human granulocytic ehrlichiosis agent and *Borrelia burgdorferi* in ticks by polymerase chain reaction. J Vet Diagn Invest 10:56, 1998.
123. Kramer VL, Randolph MP, Hui LT, et al: Detection of the agents of human ehrlichioses in ixodid ticks from California. Am J Trop Med Hyg 60:62, 1999.
124. Kim CM, Kim MS, Park MS, et al: Identification of *Ehrlichia chaffeensis*, *Anaplasma phagocytophilum*, and *A. bovis* in *Haemaphysalis longicornis* and *Ixodes persulcatus* ticks from Korea. Vector Borne Zoonotic Dis 3:17, 2003.
125. Christova I, Schouls L, van De Pol I, et al: High prevalence of granulocytic ehrlichiae and *Borrelia burgdorferi* sensu lato in *Ixodes ricinus* ticks from Bulgaria. J Clin Microbiol 39:4172, 2001.
126. Holden K, Boothby JT, Anand S, et al: Detection of *Borrelia burgdorferi*, *Ehrlichia chaffeensis*, and *Anaplasma phagocytophilum* in ticks (Acari: Ixodidae) from a coastal region of California. J Med Entomol 40:534, 2003.
127. Bown KJ, Begon M, Bennett M, et al: Seasonal dynamics of *Anaplasma phagocytophila* in a rodent-tick (*Ixodes trianguliceps*) system, United Kingdom. Emerg Infect Dis 9:63, 2003.
128. Blanco JR, Oteo JA: Human granulocytic ehrlichiosis in Europe. Clin Microbiol Infect 8:763, 2002.
129. Hardalo C, Quagliarello V, Dumler JS: Human granulocytic ehrlichiosis in Connecticut: report of a fatal case. Clin Infect Dis 21:910, 1995.
130. Wong S, Grady LJ: *Ehrlichia* infection as a cause of severe respiratory distress (letter). N Engl J Med 334:273, 1996.
131. Shea KW, Calio AJ, Klein NC, et al: Rhabdomyolysis associated with *Ehrlichia chaffeensis* infection. Clin Infect Dis 21:2056, 1995 [see correction Clin Infect Dis 22:605, 1996].
132. Low A, Turett G: Human granulocytic ehrlichiosis presenting as acute abdomen in an adult. Clin Infect Dis 37:139, 2003.
133. Gershel JC: Human granulocytic ehrlichiosis presenting as abdominal pain. Pediatrics 106:602, 2000.
134. Lee FS, Chu FK, Tackley M, et al: Human granulocytic ehrlichiosis presenting as facial diplegia in a 42-year-old woman. Clin Infect Dis 31:1288, 2000.
135. Horowitz HW, Marks SJ, Weintraub M, et al: Brachial plexopathy associated with human granulocytic ehrlichiosis. Neurology 46:1026, 1996.
136. Bakken JS, Erlemeyer SA, Kanoff RJ, et al: Demyelinating polyneuropathy associated with human granulocytic ehrlichiosis. Clin Infect Dis 27:1323, 1998.
137. Lepidi H, Bunnell JE, Martin ME, et al: Comparative pathology, and immunohistology associated with clinical illness after *Ehrlichia phagocytophila*-group infections. Am J Trop Med Hyg 62:29, 2000.

138. Klein MB, Hu S, Chao CC, et al: The agent of human granulocytic ehrlichiosis induces the production of myelosuppressing chemokines without induction of proinflammatory cytokines. J Infect Dis 182:200, 2000.
139. Park J, Choi KS, Grab DJ, et al: Divergent interactions of *Ehrlichia chaffeensis*- and *Anaplasma phagocytophilum*-infected leukocytes with endothelial cell barriers. Infect Immun 71:6728, 2003.
140. Choi KS, Garyu J, Park J, et al: Diminished adhesion of *Anaplasma phagocytophilum*–infected neutrophils to endothelial cells is associated with reduced expression of leukocyte surface selectin. Infect Immun 71:4586, 2003.
141. Banerjee R, Anguita J, Roos D, et al: Cutting edge: infection by the agent of human granulocytic ehrlichiosis prevents the respiratory burst by down-regulating $gp91^{phox}$. J Immunol 164:3946, 2000.
142. Yoshiie K, Kim HY, Mott J, et al: Intracellular infection by the human granulocytic ehrlichiosis agent inhibits human neutrophil apoptosis. Infect Immun 68:1125, 2000.
143. Choi KS, Scorpio DG, Dumler JS: *Anaplasma phagocytophilum* ligation to TLR2 but not TLR4 activates macrophages for NF-kB nuclear translocation. Infect Immun 189:1921, 2004.
144. Bakken JS, Haller I, Riddell D, et al: The serological response of patients infected with the agent of human granulocytic ehrlichiosis. Clin Infect Dis 34:22, 2002.
145. Aguero-Rosenfeld ME: Diagnosis of human granulocytic ehrlichiosis: state of the art. Vector Borne Zoonotic Dis 2:233, 2002.
146. Walls JJ, Aguero-Rosenfeld M, Bakken JS, et al: Inter- and intralaboratory comparison of *Ehrlichia equi* and human granulocytic ehrlichiosis (HGE) agent strains for serodiagnosis of HGE by the immunofluorescent-antibody test. J Clin Microbiol 37:2968, 1999.
147. Edelman DC, Dumler JS: Evaluation of an improved PCR diagnostic assay for human granulocytic ehrlichiosis. Mol Diag 1:41, 1996.
148. Misao T, Kobayashi Y: Studies on infectious mononucleosis (glandular fever): isolation of etiologic agent from blood, bone marrow, and lymph node of patients with infectious mononucleosis by using mice. Tokyo Iji Shinshi 71:683, 1955.
149. Tachibana N: Sennetsu fever: the disease, diagnosis, and treatment. In Lieve L (ed): Microbiology—1986. Washington, DC, American Society for Microbiology, 1986, p. 205.
150. Madigan JE, Pusterla N, Johnson E, et al: Transmission of *Ehrlichia risticii*, the agent of Potomac horse fever, using naturally infected aquatic insects and helminth vectors: preliminary report. Equine Vet J 32:275, 2000.
151. Pusterla N, Johnson EM, Chae JS, et al: Digenetic trematodes, *Acanthatrium* sp. and *Lecithodendrium* sp., as vectors of *Neorickettsia risticii*, the agent of Potomac horse fever. J Helminthol 77:335, 2003.
152. Brouqui P, Raoult D: In vitro antibiotic susceptibility of the newly recognized agent of ehrlichiosis in humans, *Ehrlichia chaffeensis*. Antimicrob Agents Chemother 36:2799, 1992.
153. Klein MB, Nelson CM, Goodman JL: Antibiotic susceptibility of the newly cultivated agent of human granulocytic ehrlichiosis: promising activity of quinolones and rifamycins. Antimicrob Agents Chemother 41:76, 1997.
154. Maurin M, Bakken JS, Dumler JS: Antibiotic susceptibilities of *Anaplasma (Ehrlichia) phagocytophilum* strains from various geographic areas in the United States. Antimicrob Agents Chemother 47:413, 2003.
155. Buitrago MI, Ijdo JW, Rinaudo P, et al: Human granulocytic ehrlichiosis during pregnancy treated successfully with rifampin. Clin Infect Dis 27:213, 1998.
156. Krause PJ, Corrow CL, Bakken JS: Successful treatment of human granulocytic ehrlichiosis in children using rifampin. Pediatrics 112:e252, 2003.
157. Maurin M, Abergel C, Raoult D: DNA gyrase–mediated natural resistance to fluoroquinolones in *Ehrlichia* spp. Antimicrob Agents Chemother 45:2098, 2001.
158. Katavolos P, Armstrong PM, Dawson JE, et al: Duration of tick attachment required for transmission of granulocytic ehrlichiosis. J Infect Dis 177:1422, 1998.
159. Hodzic E, Fish D, Maretzki CM, et al: Acquisition and transmission of the agent of human granulocytic ehrlichiosis by *Ixodes scapularis* ticks. J Clin Microbiol 36:3574, 1998.
160. des Vignes F, Piesman J, Heffernan R, et al: Effect of tick removal on transmission of *Borrelia burgdorferi* and *Ehrlichia phagocytophila* by *Ixodes scapularis* nymphs. J Infect Dis 183:773, 2001.
161. Charlat S, Hurst GD, Mercot H: Evolutionary consequences of *Wolbachia* infections. Trends Genet 19:217, 2003.
162. Taylor MJ: *Wolbachia* in the inflammatory pathogenesis of human filariasis. Ann NY Acad Sci 990:444, 2003.
163. Hoerauf A, Volkmann L, Hamelmann C, et al: Endosymbiotic bacteria in worms as targets for a novel chemotherapy in filariasis. Lancet 355:1242, 2000.
164. Hoerauf A, Mand S, Volkmann L, et al: Doxycycline in the treatment of human onchocerciasis: Kinetics of *Wolbachia* endobacteria reduction and of inhibition of embryogenesis in female *Onchocerca* worms. Microbes Infect 5:261, 2003.

54

Q Fever

THOMAS J. MARRIE

INTRODUCTION

Q fever is a disease that results from infection with the microorganism *Coxiella burnetii.* It was described by Dr. E.H. Derrick in August 1935, at which time he investigated an outbreak of undiagnosed febrile illness among workers at the Canon Hill Abattoir in Brisbane, Australia.[1] Shortly thereafter the organism responsible for this outbreak was isolated and eventually was named *Coxiella burnetii* in honour of Dr. Herald Rae Cox and Sir Frank Macfarlane Burnet, two scientists who contributed so much to our knowledge of this disease.[2]

AGENT

C. burnetii is the sole species of its genus, and on the basis of 16S ribosomal RNA (rRNA) phylogeny it has been placed in the γ subdivision of Proteobacteria, with a specific but distant relationship to *Legionella.* It is an obligate phagolysosomal parasite of eukaryotes and measures $0.3 \times 1.0\ \mu m$ (Fig. 54-1).[3] It forms spores and has survived for 586 days in tick feces at room temperature, for longer than 160 days in water, for 30 to 40 days in dried cheese made from contaminated milk, and for up to 150 days in soil. In nature and in laboratory animals, it exists in the phase I state. Repeated passage of phase I organisms in embryonated chicken eggs leads to conversion to phase II avirulent forms.[4] This is accompanied by the loss of the methylated sugars virenose and dihydrohydroxystreptose, as well as a large number of other sugar components of the O-antigen side chain and some components of the outer core of the lipopolysaccharide.[5]

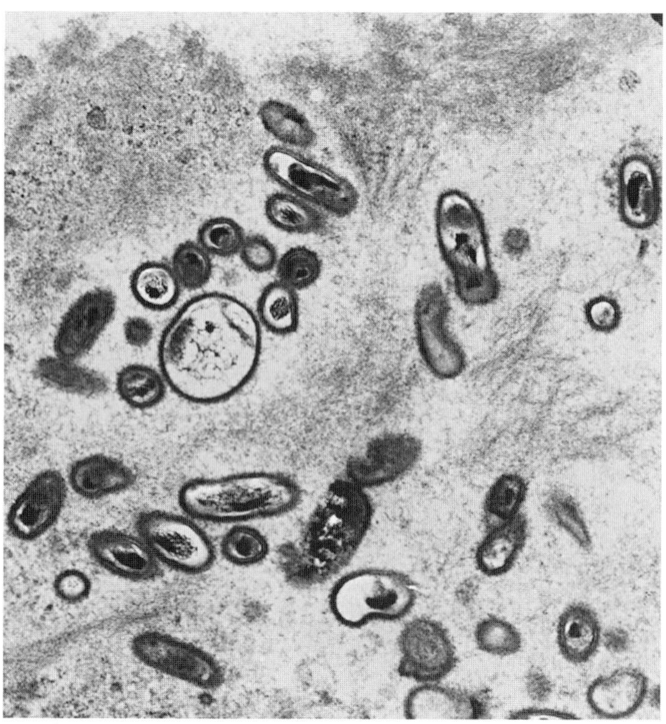

FIGURE 54-1 Transmission electron micrograph of a cardiac vegetation from a patient with *Coxiella burnetii* endocarditis showing *C. burnetii* cells. (Magnification ×23,335.)

For some time, *Coxiella burnetii* has been viewed as a potential bioterrorism weapon. It is easy to disperse, extremely infectious with, for the most part, self-limiting infection, and does not damage the environment.

The 1,995,275 base pair genome and 37,393 base pair plasmid of *C. burnetii* phase I, Nine Mile strain, have been sequenced.[6] It possesses 2134 encoded proteins, 29 insertion sequence elements, 83 pseudogenes, and 13 proteins containing ankyrin repeat units. It contains homologues of *L. pneumophila.*

EPIDEMIOLOGY

Q fever is found worldwide, including tropical countries, with the exception of New Zealand (no data are available about prevalence in Greenland and northernmost North America). In 1955, a review of the geographic distribution of Q fever indicated that it was found in Algeria, Belgian Congo (now Congo), the Cameroons (Cameroon), Egypt, Ubangi Shari (Central African Republic), Kenya, Libya, Madagascar, Rhodesia (now Zimbabwe), and South Africa.[7] More recent studies indicate that Q fever is endemic in Zimbabwe, Tunisia, and Northeast Africa.[8–10] Q fever is a zoonosis. There is an extensive wildlife and arthropod (mainly ticks) reservoir of *C. burnetii.*[11] Cattle, sheep, and goats are the animals that usually are the source of transmission of this microorganism to humans.[11] However, cats, dogs, and rabbits are also important in this regard. *C. burnetii* localizes to the uterus and mammary glands in female mammals. During pregnancy, reactivation occurs (although primary infection can occur as well), and the organism multiplies in the placenta, reaching 10^9 guinea pig infective doses per gram of tissue. These organisms are shed into the environment at the time of parturition. Man becomes infected after inhaling organisms aerosolized at the time of parturition or later when organisms in dust are stirred up on a windy day. Infected animals can shed *C. burnetii* in milk or feces for months. Outbreaks of abortion due to *C. burnetii* have been reported in goats and sheep but not in cattle. We have noted that the stillbirth rate among *C. burnetii*–infected cats is high—about 70%, compared with 10% for control cats.

DISEASE

In most instances, humans become infected with *C. burnetii* following inhalation of contaminated aerosols.[12] In Nova Scotia entire families have developed Q fever pneumonia following exposure to infected parturient cats. Usually the cat gives birth in the house, and the person who cleans up the products of conception develops symptoms a day or two earlier than the remaining members of the family and is more severely ill. Certain occupational groups are at high risk of *C. burnetii* infection; these include abattoir workers

Q fever *(Coxiella burnetii)*

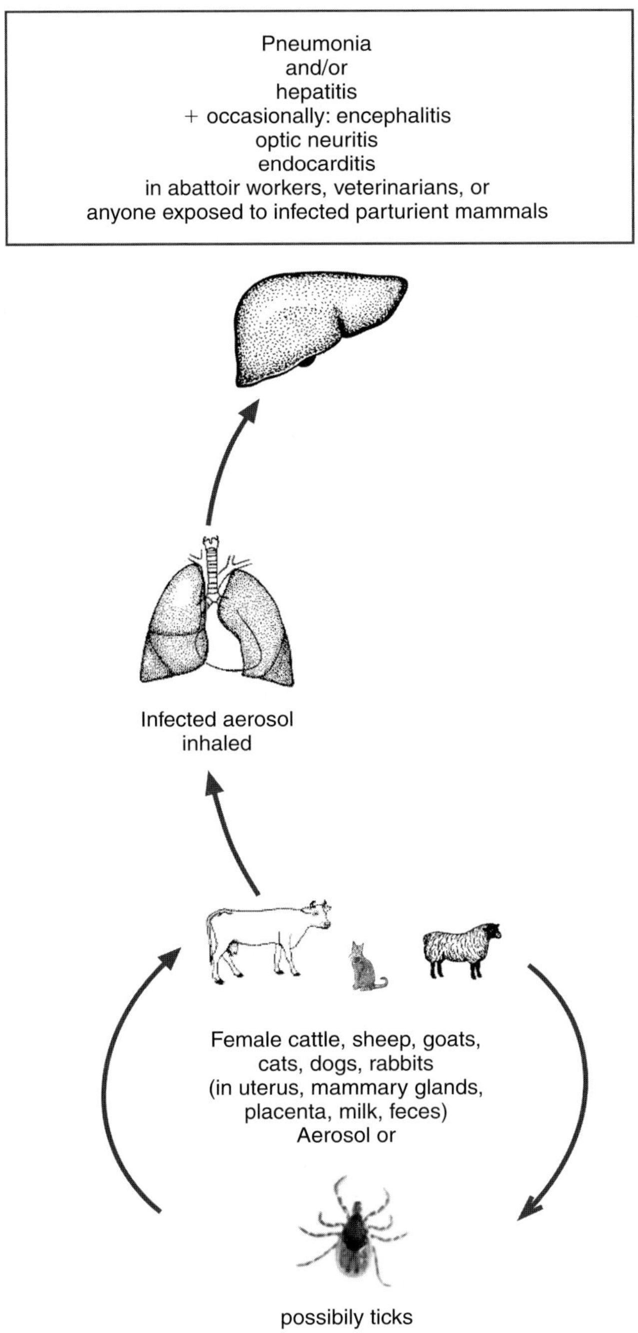

and veterinarians. Those who live in the vicinity of farms with infected animals are also at high risk of infection. High winds can disperse *C. burnetii*–contaminated dust 10 or more kilometers from these farms.[13,14]

It is likely that ingestion of *C. burnetii*–contaminated milk also causes infection, although the experimental evidence for this in humans is inconclusive. We have postulated that the route of infection determines whether or not one develops hepatitis or pneumonia following exposure to *C. burnetii*. It is our contention that ingestion of *C. burnetii* results in hepatitis, whereas inhalation of the organism results in pneumonia. In a mouse model that imperfectly mimicked these routes of infection, we were able to show that intraperitoneal injection of *C. burnetii* resulted in hepatitis, whereas inhalation of *C. burnetii* resulted in pneumonia and no hepatitis. Experimental infection of humans by aerosol, however, has resulted in the development of hepatic granulomas.

Rarely, infection has occurred via the percutaneous route following crushing of infected ticks between the fingers or as a result of transfusion of contaminated blood. Vertical transmission from mother to infant can occur, and person-to-person transmission at the time of autopsy has rarely been reported. Recently, sexual transmission of Q fever has been documented, but this also seems to be very uncommon.

Several outbreaks of *C. burnetii* have occurred in institutions using pregnant sheep for research. These infected pregnant sheep were usually transported along crowded corridors, and a large number of employees in these institutions developed Q fever. It is now a universal recommendation that facilities that work with pregnant sheep must ensure that they are not infected with *C. burnetii* before they are brought into the facility.

The incubation period for Q fever in humans is about 2 weeks with a range of 2 to 29 days. A dose-response effect has been demonstrated both experimentally and clinically. *C. burnetii* is one of the most infectious agents known to man, as a single microorganism is capable of initiating infection. The resulting illness in humans can be divided into acute and chronic varieties.

Acute Q Fever

Self-Limited Illness

Self-limited illness is the most common manifestation of Q fever. In areas where Q fever is endemic, 12% or more of the population have antibodies to *C. burnetii*, and most of these infections are subclinical or undiagnosed. A study from the south of Spain found that 108 of 505 adults (21%) who had fever for more than 1 week and less than 3 weeks had Q fever. All of these patients had normal chest radiographs.

Pneumonia

This illness is more severe than the self-limited febrile illness. The major manifestations are fever; severe headache, often with retro-orbital pain; and cough. Surprisingly, a large number of patients with Q fever pneumonia may not have cough. In our studies in Nova Scotia of 51 patients with radiographically documented Q fever pneumonia, only 14 (27%) had cough.[12] This cough is usually nonproductive. In most instances the pneumonia is of mild to moderate severity and can be treated on an outpatient basis. However, occasionally the pneumonia can be severe and rapidly progressive, resulting in respiratory failure requiring assisted ventilation. Nausea, vomiting, and diarrhea occur in 10% to 30% of patients with Q fever pneumonia. The most common physical finding is inspiratory crackles. About 5% of Q fever patients with pneumonia have splenomegaly.

The radiographic features of Q fever pneumonia are variable. Subsegmental and segmental pleural-based opacities are common. Multiple rounded opacities are suggestive of this illness, especially the variety that follows exposure to parturient cats (Fig. 54-2). Pleural effusions occur in about one-third of patients. Hilar lymphadenopathy may also be present.

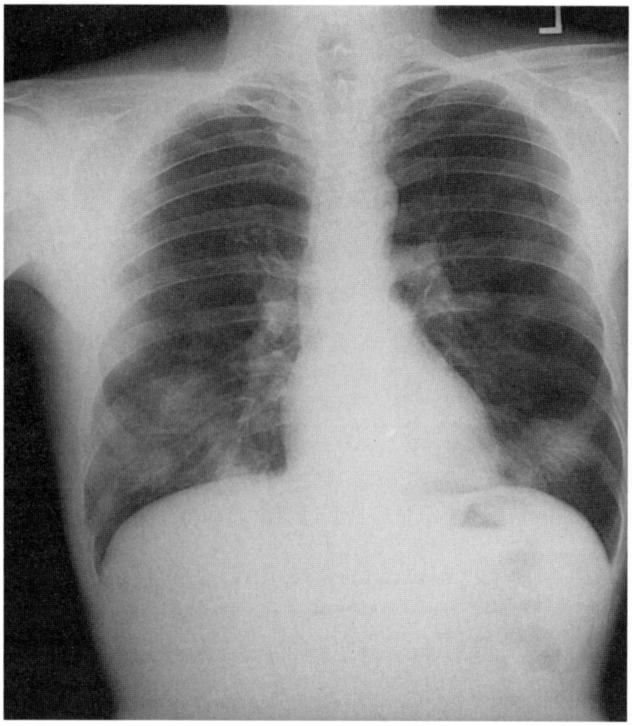

FIGURE 54-2 Chest radiograph of a young man who developed Q fever pneumonia following exposure to the products of conception of an infected parturient cat. Note the multiple rounded pulmonary opacities.

Pulmonary tissue has been examined in only a small number of patients with Q fever pneumonia. In these instances the bronchial epithelial lining has been abnormal, and the interstitial space has contained edema along with infiltration by lymphocytes and macrophages. The alveolar spaces are filled with macrophages. We studied one patient with a pseudotumor due to *C. burnetii.* In this instance the lung mass was composed of a mixture of macrophages, multinucleate giant cells, plasma cells, and lymphocytes.

The white blood cell count is usually normal, although one-third of patients have leukocytosis. A slight elevation in hepatic transaminase levels occurs in almost all of these patients.

Hepatitis

There are three presentations of Q fever hepatitis: (1) pyrexia of unknown origin with mild to moderate elevation of hepatic enzymes; (2) a hepatitis-like picture; (3) incidental hepatitis. Liver biopsy reveals distinctive "doughnut" granulomas, that is, a granuloma with a central lipid vacuole and fibrin deposits.

Neurologic Manifestations

Aseptic meningitis or encephalitis complicates up to 1% of cases of Q fever. In some geographic areas the neurologic manifestations of Q fever are much more common than in others. In a study from Plymouth, England, Reilly and co-workers reported a 22% incidence of neurologic manifestations among 103 patients with Q fever.[15] These manifestations included residual weakness, recurrent meningitis, blurred vision, paresthesias, and sensory loss involving the left leg. Other neurologic manifestations of Q fever have included hallucinations, dysphagia, and hemifacial pain suggestive of trigeminal neuralgia. The much higher rate of neurologic involvement in studies from the United Kingdom suggests that a neurotropic strain of *C. burnetii* may be circulating in that country. Rarely, behavioral disturbances, cerebellar signs and symptoms, cranial nerve palsies, extrapyramidal disease, Miller-Fisher syndrome, and demyelinating polyradiculoneuritis have been reported in Q fever.

Chronic Q Fever

The usual manifestation of chronic Q fever is culture-negative endocarditis. Most of these patients have fever, and nearly all have abnormal native heart valves or prosthetic heart valves. Hepatomegaly or splenomegaly, or both, occur in about half of patients with Q fever endocarditis, and one-third have marked clubbing of the digits. Marked hyperglobulinemia (≥70 g/L) is common and is a useful clue to diagnosis.[16] Microscopic hematuria is usually present. Arterial emboli complicate the clinical course of about one-third of patients with Q fever endocarditis.

In Q fever endocarditis, the vegetation is quite smooth and may form nodules on the valve. Microscopically, there is subacute and chronic inflammatory cell infiltrate, and many large foamy macrophages full of characteristic microorganisms are readily seen by electron microscopy (see Fig. 54-1).

Q Fever in the Immunocompromised Host and During Pregnancy

Two recently recognized manifestations of Q fever include fever in immunocompromised patients and Q fever during pregnancy. The latter has been infrequently recognized but is a growing problem, especially in southern France and Israel. A recent study of 66 human immunodeficiency virus type 1 (HIV-1) seropositive persons living in Bangui, Central Africa Republic, found that 11 (16.7%) were also seropositive for *C. burnetii.* Two of the seven HIV-infected patients for whom clinical data were available had a history compatible with symptomatic Q fever.[17] Investigators in France found that 10.4% of 500 HIV-positive persons in Marseilles had Q fever antibodies at a titer equal to or greater than 1:225 compared with 4.1% of 925 healthy blood donors. They also found that 5 of 63 patients hospitalized with Q fever from 1987 to 1989 in Marseilles were HIV-positive. In France, 20% of patients with chronic Q fever were immunocompromised. These patients had cancer, chronic myeloid leukemia, acquired immunodeficiency syndrome (AIDS), renal transplantation, chronic alcoholism, or were receiving corticosteroid therapy or renal dialysis. Q fever has caused fatal interstitial pneumonia in an 11-year-old boy with the genetic condition, chronic granulomatous disease of childhood.

PATHOGENESIS AND IMMUNITY

Over the past few years a considerable amount has been learned about the pathogenesis of *C. burnetii* infection. The attachment of virulent forms of *C. burnetii* to monocytes is mediated by αv $\beta 3$ integrin only[18] whereas the interaction of the avirulent form with monocytes requires αv $\beta 3$ and complement receptor 3 (CR3) integrins.[18] It is likely that the virulent variant inhibits the internalization mediated by CR3 through the impairment of cross talk between these two integrins.[18] *C. burnetii* avoids phagocytosis by interfering with the spatial distribution of complement receptor 3 on the surface of phagocytes.[19] Interferon γ mediates intracellular killing of *C. burnetii* by promoting apoptosis of infected monocytes through activation of caspase-3.[20] Interleukin-4 enables monocytes to support *C. burnetii* replication.[21] *C. burnetii* is not eradicated by the T-cell dependent immune response, and subsequent immunosuppression can lead to relapse.[22,23] Indeed, *C. burnetii* DNA persists in monocytes and bone marrow years after acute Q fever.[24] *C. burnetii* survives in monocytes from patients with chronic infection but not in monocytes from patients with acute Q fever or from seronegative control subjects.[25] This defect, which disappears when the patients are cured, is related to dysregulation of the cytokine network.[26] The secretion of soluble TNF receptor (TNF R75) is increased in these patients and may be responsible for the microbicidal defect,[27] which is also associated with IL-10 overproduction.[28] Furthermore, anti-IL-10 antibodies restore the microbial activity of the monocytes in vitro.[28] The complexity of the host-microorganism interaction is illustrated by investigators who used DNA microarray analysis and found that a total of 335 genes in the *C. burnetii*–infected human monocytic leukemia cell line THP-1 were up-or-down-regulated at least twofold.[29]

TREATMENT AND PROGNOSIS

The prognosis is excellent in acute Q fever, with mortality being extremely rare. Fluoroquinolones and rifampin are the most active agents against *C. burnetii* in vitro. A 10-day course of tetracycline, doxycycline, or a fluoroquinolone will adequately treat acute Q fever. Macrolides have also been used to treat acute Q fever; however, some strains of *C. burnetii* are resistant to macrolides. Chronic Q fever should be treated with two antimicrobial agents for at least 3 years.[30] Some authorities recommend lifelong therapy for chronic Q fever. We currently use rifampin (300 mg twice daily) and ciprofloxacin (750 mg twice daily) as the agents of first choice in the treatment of chronic Q fever. Another regimen is doxycycline and hydroxychloroquine. The hydroxychloroquine alkalinizes the phagolysosome rendering doxycycline bactericidal.[31] In treating this condition, antibody titers should be measured every 3 months for the first 2 years. A progressive decline in antibody titer reflects successful therapy of chronic Q fever.

PREVENTION AND CONTROL

A formalin-inactivated *C. burnetii* whole-cell vaccine protects against infection and has a 1% rate of induration developing at the inoculation site. The use of only seronegative pregnant sheep in research facilities and control of ectoparasites on livestock are measures that can reduce Q fever infection.

REFERENCES

1. Derrick EH: “Q” fever, a new fever entity: Clinical features, diagnosis and laboratory investigation. Med J Aust 2:281, 1937.
2. McDade JE: Historical aspects of Q fever. In Marrie TJ (ed): Q Fever: The Disease, Boca Raton, FL, CRC Press, 1990, p 5.
3. McCaul TF, Williams JC: Development cycle of *Coxiella burnetii*: Structure and morphogenesis of vegetative and sporogenic differentiations. J Bacteriol 147:1063, 1981.
4. Stoker MG, Fiset P: Phase variation of the nine mile and other strains of *Rickettsia burnetii*. Can J Microbiol 2:310, 1956.
5. Thomson HA, Hoover TA, Vodkin MH: Do chromosomal deletions in the lipopolysaccharide biosynthetic regions explain all cases of phase variation in *Coxiella burnetii* strains? Ann NY Aca Sci 990:664, 2003.
6. Seshadri R, Paulsen IT, Eisen JA, et al: Complete genome sequence of the Q-fever pathogen *Coxiella burnetii*. PNAS 100:5455, 2003.
7. Kaplan MM, Bertagna P: The geographical distribution of Q fever. Bull World Health Organ 13:829, 1995.
8. Kelly PJ, Matthewman LA, Mason PR, et al: Q fever in Zimbabwe. S Afr Med J 83:21, 1993.
9. Letaiéf AD, Yacoub S, Dupont HT, et al: Seroepidemiological survey of rickettsial infections among blood donors in central Tunisia. Trans R Soc Trop Med Hyg 89:266, 1995.
10. Botros BA, Soliman AK, Salib AW, et al: *Coxiella burnetii* antibody prevalence among human populations in north-east Africa determined by enzyme immunoassay. J Trop Med Hyg 98:173, 1995.
11. Babudieri B: Q fever: A zoonosis. Adv Vet Sci 5:81, 1959.
12. Marrie TJ: *Coxiella burnetii* (Q fever) pneumonia. Clin Infect Dis 21(Suppl 3):S253, 1995.
13. Hawker JI, Ayres JG, Blair MR, et al: A large outbreak of Q fever in the West Midlands: windborne spread into a metropolitan area. Commun Dis Public Health 1:180, 1998.
14. Tissot-Dupont H, Torres S, Nezri M, et al: Hyperendemic focus of Q fever related to sheep and wind. Am J Epidemiol 150:67, 1999.
15. Reilly S, Northwood JL, Caul EO: Q fever in Plymouth, 1972–1988. A review with particular reference to neurological manifestations. Epidemiol Infect 105:391, 1990.
16. Levy PY, Drancourt M, Etienne J, et al: Comparison of different antibiotic regimens for therapy of 32 cases of Q fever endocarditis. Antimicrob Agents Chemother 35:533, 1991.
17. Bélec L, Grésenguet G, Ekala MT, et al: *Coxiella burnetii* infection among subjects infected with HIV type 1 in the Central African Republic. Eur J Microbiol Infect Dis 12:775, 1993.
18. Capo C, Lindberg FP, Meconi S, et al: Subversion of monocyte functions by *Coxiella burnetii*: impairment of the cross-talk between $\alpha_v\beta_3$ integrin and CR3. J Immunol 163: 6078, 1999.
19. Capo C, Moynault A, Collette Y, et al: *Coxiella burnetii* avoids macrophage phagocytosis by interfering with spatial distribution of complement receptor 3. J Immunol 170:4217, 2003.
20. Dellacasagrande J, Ghigo E, Raoult D, et al: IFN-induced apoptosis and microbicidal activity in monocytes harboring the intracellular bacterium *Coxiella burnetii* require membrane TNF and homotypic cell adherence. J Immunol 169:6309, 2002.
21. Ghigo E, Imbert G, Capo C, et al: Interleukin-4 induces *Coxiella burnetii* replication in human monocytes but not in macrophages. Ann NY Acad Sci 990:450, 2003.
22. Sidwell RW, Thorpe BD, Gebhardt LP: Studies of latent Q fever infections. I. Effects of whole body X irradiation upon latently infected guinea pigs, white mice and deer mice. Am J Hyg 79:113, 1964.
23. Sidwell RW, Thorpe BD, Gebhardt LP: Studies of latent Q fever infections. II. Effects of multiple cortisone injections. Am J Hyg 79:320, 1964.
24. Harris RJ, Storm PA, Lloyd A, et al: Long-term persistence of *Coxiella burnetii* in the host after primary Q fever. Epidemiol Infect 124:543, 2000.
25. Dellacasagrande J, Ghigo E, Capo C, et al: *Coxiella burnetii* survives in monocytes from patients with Q fever endocarditis: Involvement of tumor necrosis factor. Infect Immun 68:160, 2000.
26. Honstettre A, Imber G, Ghigo E, et al: Dysregulation of cytokines in acute Q fever: Role of interleukin-10 and tumor necrosis factor in chronic evolution of Q fever. Clin Infect Dis 187:956, 2003.
27. Ghigo E, Capo C, Amirayan N, et al: The 75-kD tumour necrosis factor (TNF) receptor is specifically up-regulated in monocytes during Q fever endocarditis. Clin Exp Immunol 121:295, 2000.
28. Ghigo E, Capo C, Raoult D, et al: Il-10 stimulates *Coxiella burnetii* replication in human monocytes through TNF down-modulation: Role in microbicidal defect of Q fever. Infect Immun 69:2345, 2001.
29. Ren Q, Robertson SJ, Howe D, et al: Comparative DNA microarray analysis of host cell transcriptional responses to infection by *Coxiella burnetii* or *Chlamydia trachomatis*. Ann NY Acad Sci 990:701, 2003.
30. Raoult D, Marrie T: Q fever. Clin Infect Dis 20:489, 1995.
31. Raoult D, Houpikian P, Tissot-Dupont, et al: Treatment of Q fever endocarditis: Comparison of two regimens containing doxycycline and ofloxacin or hydroxychloroquine. Arch Intern Med 159:167, 1999.

E. VIRAL INFECTIONS

55

Measles

CIRO A. DE QUADROS
BRADLEY S. HERSH
JON KIM ANDRUS

INTRODUCTION

Measles is the most infectious virus known to humans.[1] Despite the availability of an effective preventive measure (live measles vaccine), measles continues to cause more deaths than any other single infectious agent.[2] The World Health Organization (WHO) estimates that in 2003 there were more than 30 million measles cases worldwide and about 530,000 measles-related deaths.[3] Most measles deaths occur among children living in developing countries. Globally, the disease accounts for approximately 4% of deaths among children younger than 5 years of age, and it is especially lethal in infants younger than 1 year of age. Children may die from acute measles infection or from its sequelae, including encephalitis, pneumonia, diarrhea, and malnutrition. The disease thrives in cities, especially in deprived urban areas where crowding, poor sanitation, and low measles vaccination coverage ensure the ongoing circulation of the virus.

AGENT

Measles is caused by an RNA virus of the genus *Morbillivirus* of the Paramyxoviridae family.[4] The virus is antigenically stable and is quite sensitive to ultraviolet light, heat, and drying.

EPIDEMIOLOGY

Measles occurs in most areas of the world. In temperate climates, it occurs more often in late winter and early spring. In tropical climates, transmission appears to increase after the rainy season. In the absence of measles vaccination, epidemics often occur every 2 or 3 years and usually last between 2 and 3 months, although the duration varies according to population size, crowding, and population immunity. Where measles is common, most children will have been infected by the time they are 10 years old. Countries with relatively high vaccination coverage levels usually have 5- to 7-year periods with low measles incidence. However, as pools of susceptible hosts build up and become large enough to sustain widespread transmission, explosive outbreaks may occur.

The incubation period of measles is approximately 10 days (range, 8 to 13 days) from the time of exposure until the onset of fever and approximately 14 days until the rash appears. Measles is most communicable 1 to 3 days before the onset of fever and cough, and transmission efficiency is high. Secondary attack rates among susceptible household contacts are reported to be more than 80%.[5] Outbreaks have been reported in populations in which only 3% to 7% of the individuals were susceptible.[6–8] There is a marked reduction in communicability of the virus following the appearance of the rash.

DISEASE

The disease begins with a prodrome of fever, malaise, cough, and a runny nose. Conjunctivitis and bronchitis are commonly present. A harsh, nonproductive cough is present throughout the febrile period, persists for 1 or 2 weeks in uncomplicated cases, and is often the last symptom to disappear. Generalized lymphadenopathy commonly occurs in young children. Older children may complain of photophobia and arthralgias.

Within 2 to 4 days after the prodrome, symptoms begin; a characteristic red maculopapular (often referred to as "blotchy") rash usually appears behind the ears and on the face. In dark-skinned children the rash may not be as evident. The rash peaks in 2 or 3 days and is most concentrated on the trunk and upper extremities. The rash lasts from 3 to 7 days and may be followed by a brawny or fine desquamation (Fig. 55-1). Some children develop severe exfoliation, especially if they are severely malnourished.

Frequent complications from measles in developing countries include pneumonia, diarrhea, and otitis media.[9] Lower respiratory tract infections are the most important cause of significant morbidity and mortality in children with measles.[10] Pneumonia may be due to the measles virus alone or, more commonly, due to secondary infection with other viral agents or bacteria. Many infants and children may develop chronic diarrhea after acute measles illness.[11] Diarrhea is one of the major factors contributing to the adverse impact of measles on the nutritional status of children.[12]

Measles is more severe in malnourished children.[13] Additionally, measles may exacerbate malnutrition because of decreased food intake due to malaise, increased metabolic requirements in the presence of fever, or because parents and health practitioners inappropriately withhold food during an acute illness. Undernutrition may in turn lead to vitamin A deficiency and keratitis, resulting in a high incidence of childhood blindness in measles outbreaks.[14]

The most common neurologic manifestation of measles infection is febrile convulsions. Encephalitis or postinfectious encephalopathy occurs in approximately 1 in 1000 infected children. Subacute sclerosing panencephalitis is a rare chronic, degenerative neurologic disorder associated with the persistent infection of the central nervous system with a defective measles virus.[15] It may develop several years after a measles infection.

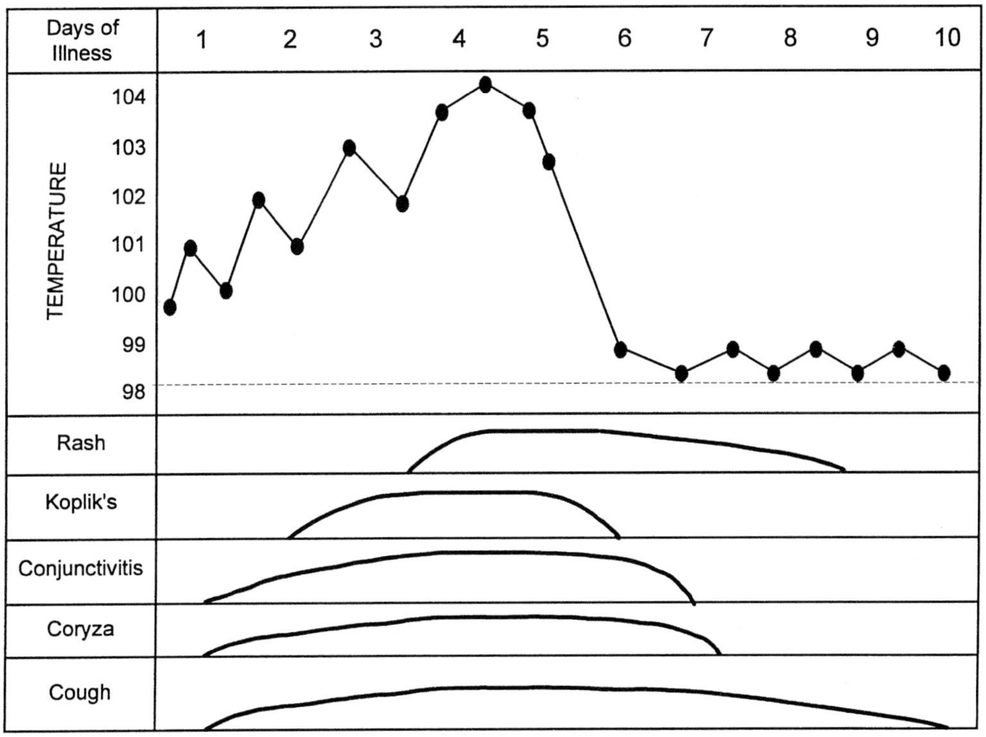

FIGURE 55-1 Schematic clinical course of a typical case of measles. (From Krugman S, Katz SL, Gershon A, et al [eds]: Infectious Diseases in Children, 9th ed. St. Louis, Mosby-Year Book, 1992, p 224.)

PATHOGENESIS

Measles virus is transmitted from person to person via respiratory droplets or airborne spray to mucous membranes in the upper respiratory tract or the conjunctiva. Common-source outbreaks associated with airborne transmission have been documented. Humans are the only reservoir for the virus. Although monkeys in captivity may become infected, measles transmission among them in the wild does not appear to be an important means for the virus to persist in nature.

Following exposure of a susceptible host, measles virus replicates in the respiratory tract, spreads and becomes amplified in local lymphatic tissues, and results in generalized infection via primary viremia.[16] Many tissues and organs of the body can be infected, including lymphoid tissue, skin, gastrointestinal tract, lungs, and liver. Measles infection has been shown to cause a suppression of the immune system which can persist several months after acute infection.[17] This immunosuppression is thought to account for the increased susceptibility of measles patients to secondary bacterial and viral infections that result in pneumonia and gastroenteritis.

DIAGNOSIS

In countries where measles transmission is endemic and the disease is frequent, measles can be diagnosed with reasonable accuracy on clinical grounds alone. Koplik's spots may be seen on the buccal mucosa in more than 80% of the cases if careful daily examinations are performed soon before the rash appears.[18] Their presence is said to be pathognomonic of measles infection.

However, in areas where measles is no longer endemic due to high vaccination coverage, the large number of rashlike illnesses occurring in childhood makes laboratory confirmation the key to definitive diagnosis. Many illnesses are accompanied by a rash and a variety of nonspecific symptoms. When examining for measles, it is important to consider rubella, scarlet fever, roseola, dengue fever, and the early stages of chickenpox in the differential diagnosis. Other diseases and conditions that may present in a similar form include Kawasaki syndrome, toxic shock syndrome, enterovirus and adenovirus infections, rickettsial diseases, and drug hypersensitivity rashes.

Measles virus isolation remains the "gold standard" for the laboratory confirmation of a suspected measles case.[4,19] However, due to the technical difficulties in isolating measles virus, this procedure is only performed in specialized laboratories. More commonly, measles infection is confirmed in the laboratory by documenting a serologic response to the measles virus in the host.

Measles-specific antibodies can be detected at onset of the rash and generally reach their peak approximately 1 month following infection. Immunoglobulin M (IgM) antibodies usually fall below the limits of detection by 6 weeks following infection, whereas IgG antibodies persist for many years after infection. Classically, the documentation of increasing titers of measles-specific antibody from acute to convalescent paired sera using complement fixation, the neutralization test, and hemaglutination inhibition assays was used to confirm acute measles infection.[20] In recent years, various enzyme immunoassays (EIAs) have been used to detect both measles-specific IgG and IgM antibodies.[21–23]

Testing serum for the presence of IgM antibodies via EIA to confirm clinical measles diagnosis is increasingly being used by many laboratories. A major advantage of using the IgM assays over previous approaches is that usually only a single serum specimen is needed for measles confirmation. The measles IgM capture assay developed by the Centers for Disease Control and Prevention (CDC) has been found to be highly sensitive and specific for confirming measles infection when compared with traditional methods such as neutralization and hemagglutination inhibition.[24,25] Several commercial indirect measles IgM assays are available. The major advantage of these tests is that they are easy to perform and produce results in 2 or 3 hours versus 6 or 7 hours for the capture assay.[22,26] However, there are major differences between individual commercial assays. Some compare well with the IgM capture assay, whereas other tests have produced a significant number of false-positive and false-negative results.[27]

TREATMENT AND PROGNOSIS

Other than supportive care, including fluids (such as oral rehydration solution), antipyretics, and nutritional therapy, there is no specific treatment for uncomplicated measles infection. However, antibiotics may be indicated for treatment of secondary bacterial infections, such as pneumonia. Moreover, the administration of vitamin A to hospitalized children with acute measles infections has been demonstrated to significantly reduce the risk of dying from measles. WHO recommends that vitamin A be given to all children with acute measles infection in areas that have experienced high measles mortality rates.[28] Many children require 4 to 8 weeks to recover their premeasles nutritional status.

In developed countries the case-fatality rate for measles tends to be low (between 0.1 and 1.0 per 1000 cases).[29] In developing countries, however, the overall case-fatality rate has been estimated at between 3% and 6% with the highest case-fatality rate occurring in infants 6 to 11 months of age.[30] In certain high-risk populations, case-fatality rates as high as 20% or 30% have been reported in infants under 1 year of age.[31] Moreover, extremely high measles mortality rates have been reported among infants and children living in refugee camps.[32]

PREVENTION AND CONTROL

The original measles vaccines approved for use in children in 1963 were attenuated, live, and inactivated vaccines and are no longer used. The vaccines currently in use in most countries are further attenuated live measles virus vaccines. These are generally derived from the original Edmonston measles vaccine virus strain. The Moraten strain vaccine is used principally in the United States, whereas the Schwarz vaccine has been the strain most commonly used in other countries.[33–35] By 1982, virtually all countries in the world had incorporated measles vaccine into their routine vaccination schedules, and since then coverage has increased substantially. By 1990, the estimated overall global coverage for children by 2 years of age was approximately 80%.

Immunization with live measles vaccine has been demonstrated to be protective for more than 20 years, and immunity is thought to be lifelong.[36] Vaccine effectiveness is estimated to be between 90% and 95%.[37] The vaccine, however, does not provide protection in the presence of passively acquired maternal antibodies, which tend to wane between 6 and 9 months of age. Vaccine effectiveness increases steadily after this age, reaching its maximum between the ages of 9 and 12 months. The development and persistence of serum antibodies following measles vaccination are lower but parallel to the response following natural measles infection. Peak antibody responses occur 6 to 8 weeks after infection or vaccination.

There are very few absolute contraindications to receiving measles vaccine. Measles vaccine should not be given to people with the following conditions or characteristics: severe immunosuppression, pregnancy, history of anaphylactic reaction to neomycin, or history of recent receipt of immunoglobulin or other blood products.[38] Vaccine can be administrated safely and effectively to children with mild acute illnesses. Malnutrition should be considered an indication to vaccinate, not a contraindication. If a malnourished child becomes infected, the disease may aggravate his or her nutritional status and increase the chances of complications or death. Similarly, asymptomatic infection with the human immunodeficiency virus should not be considered a contraindication to measles vaccination.[39]

At the standard-dose, further attenuated measles vaccine is considered to be one of the safest vaccines available.[40] Approximately 5% to 15% of infants vaccinated with measles vaccine may develop a mild fever, and approximately 5% develop a generalized rash that lasts for 1 to 3 days. These symptoms may arise 5 to 10 days after vaccination and are generally mild and well tolerated.[41] Febrile convulsions have been reported to occur in approximately 1 in 1000 children following measles vaccination.[42] Severe neurologic events following measles vaccination, such as encephalitis and encephalopathy, are estimated to occur in less than 1 in 1 million vaccinees.[43]

Before the widespread use of measles vaccine, measles was a universal disease. Large epidemics tended to occur every 2 or 3 years. With the widespread use of measles vaccine, the interval between epidemics has increased, and the magnitude of outbreaks has decreased.[44,45] The vaccination strategy currently used to control measles in most developing countries has been to immunize infants through the routine health services delivery system, administering a single dose of measles vaccine between 9 and 12 months of age.

Most countries that have achieved and maintained high vaccine coverage with measles vaccine have reported a 90% or more reduction in the incidence of measles and measles-related deaths compared to the prevaccine era.[46–49] In a review of cost-effective health measures, the World Bank evaluated measles immunization as being one of the most cost-effective public health interventions currently available.[50]

Although measles vaccine coverage has markedly increased, measles outbreaks have continued to occur. Typically, several years of low measles incidence have been followed by gradually increasing measles activity, which culminates in the occurrence of a large measles outbreak. Even in areas where high coverage rates have been achieved and maintained, outbreaks have been reported.[51]

In the United States and other developed countries that have maintained relatively high levels of immunization coverage for several years, two distinct patterns of measles transmission have been observed. Outbreaks have been reported among populations of highly vaccinated school-age children as well as among unvaccinated preschool-age children living in densely populated, poor, urban areas.[52] The outbreaks among vaccinated school-age children have tended to be small and self-limited, whereas those among unvaccinated preschool-age children have frequently been quite large and difficult to control.[53]

Large measles outbreaks have been reported in developing countries that have failed to achieve and maintain high levels of vaccination coverage.[54,55] Moreover, outbreaks have been reported from countries that have developed strong systems for vaccine delivery and have achieved high measles vaccination coverage.[56–59] Factors that have been implicated in these outbreaks include the failure to achieve and maintain sufficiently high levels of vaccination coverage, the occurrence of primary vaccination failure (the failure to seroconvert following vaccination) in 5% to 10% of vaccinated children, and the accumulation of susceptible children over time.

Efforts to control measles transmission, once an outbreak has started, have proved to be frustrating and often ineffective.[60–62] Due to the very high communicability of measles, many susceptible people have already been infected before the outbreak is recognized and control activities implemented. Given the difficulties in controlling measles outbreaks, increased efforts should be made to prevent them. This goal is accomplished by achieving and maintaining very high levels of measles immunity among infants and children.

There is a wide variation in estimates among mathematical modelers on what level of population immunity is necessary to stop or prevent circulation of measles virus.[63] This situation is understandable considering the large number of variables that affect measles transmission, including population density, living patterns, humidity, and the large number of assumptions that must be made in constructing an epidemiologic model. Nevertheless, it is clear that the efficiency of transmission is very high, and outbreaks have been reported in highly vaccinated populations.[64,65]

During the mid-1980s, measles virus continued to circulate and remained an important cause of morbidity and mortality, even in areas with relatively high measles vaccination coverage. This stimulated discussions of and research into improved mechanisms for measles control. In order to prevent the occurrence of measles outbreaks among highly vaccinated school-age children, some countries, including Chile, Denmark, Israel, Norway, Sweden, and the United States, instituted a routine two-dose measles vaccination schedule.[66] Moreover, increased efforts have been made to raise measles vaccination coverage among preschool-age children living in impoverished inner-city areas.[67]

To improve measles control in developing countries where, despite the presence of moderate to high vaccination coverage, measles virus was continuing to circulate and cause significant morbidity and mortality among infants and young children, work was conducted on developing and testing a higher potency measles vaccine that could provide measles immunity, in the presence of maternally acquired measles antibodies, to children younger than 9 months of age. Several studies found that a high-titer preparation of the Edmonston–Zagreb further attenuated live measles vaccine could stimulate high rates of seroconversion in 6-month-old infants.[68–70] Based on these results, the WHO recommended that high-titer Edmonston–Zagreb vaccine be used to vaccinate infants starting at 6 months of age in areas experiencing high-level measles mortality in infants and children.[71] Data from studies in Senegal, however, suggested that girls vaccinated at 5 or 6 months of age with high-titer measles vaccine were, for an unexplained reason, at a higher risk of dying (late mortality from causes other than measles) than girls vaccinated at 9 or 10 months of age.[72,73] Based on these concerns, these vaccines are no longer recommended.[74]

An early success in interrupting measles transmission occurred in The Gambia, a country of approximately 1 million people located on the Atlantic coast near the western tip of Africa. Annual national measles immunization campaigns were begun in The Gambia starting in 1967.[75] The campaign strategy included village-by-village programs carried out by mobile vaccination teams. Initially, children 6 months to 6 years of age were immunized. Subsequent campaigns targeted young children not previously immunized. Measles transmission was interrupted within 1 year after the program began, and the country remained free of measles during the period 1968 to 1970.[76] Soon thereafter, the program was discontinued due to lack of financial support; measles virus was introduced from neighboring countries, and transmission was reestablished.[77,78] The Gambia, however, was the first developing country to interrupt measles transmission and to demonstrate that measles elimination was technically feasible.

In 1986, Cuba, based largely on the measles elimination experience of The Gambia as well as its own successful experience with polio eradication, developed a new national measles vaccination strategy using standard-titer, further attenuated measles vaccine. A mass measles vaccination campaign was conducted targeting all children 1 to 14 years of age, regardless of measles disease history or vaccination status. During a 6-month period, nearly 2.5 million children were vaccinated, resulting in a coverage of approximately 98%. Following the campaign, measles surveillance was strengthened, and the reported number of confirmed measles cases rapidly decreased to record low levels. Between 1989 and 1992, fewer than 20 confirmed measles cases were reported annually. Because of the accumulation of susceptible preschool-age children since the prior campaign, a repeat mass measles vaccination campaign was conducted in November 1993 targeting all children 2 to 6 years of age, regardless of prior vaccination or measles disease history. More than 880,000 children were vaccinated during this campaign, resulting in a 98% coverage. The last serologically confirmed case in Cuba occurred in June 1993.

After reviewing the measles elimination experiences of several countries, particularly The Gambia and Cuba, the Pan American Health Organization (PAHO) developed a regional measles elimination strategy that continues to evolve as additional experience accumulates[79] and which shares similarities to the highly successful PAHO polio eradication strategy that is currently being implemented throughout the world.[80] The strategy aims to rapidly interrupt measles transmission and to maintain the interruption in measles virus circulation by sustaining high population immunity. Measles case surveillance and measles virus surveillance are other key elements of the strategy.

The PAHO measles elimination strategy has three main vaccination components. First, a one-time-only "catch-up" measles vaccination is conducted. Attempts are made to vaccinate all children 9 months to 14 years of age, regardless of measles disease history or vaccination status. The goal is to rapidly interrupt measles virus circulation through the achievement of high levels of measles immunity across a wide age cohort where most measles transmission is occurring.

Following the catch-up campaign, efforts are directed at strengthening infant immunization through routine vaccination services to slow down the accumulation of susceptible children and to help maintain the interruption of measles virus circulation. This component of the strategy is referred to as "keep-up" vaccination. Since the risk of an infant being exposed to circulating measles virus is low, the age of routine measles vaccination can be safely increased from 9 months to 12 months of age, thus providing an increase in measles vaccine effectiveness. Efforts are made to achieve 90% coverage in each successive birth cohort in every district.

Since measles vaccine is less than 100% effective and universal vaccination coverage is rarely achieved, by definition there will be an accumulation of susceptible infants and children over time, thus increasing the risk of a measles outbreak should the virus be reintroduced. To reduce the number of susceptible preschool-age children to low levels, periodic "follow-up" vaccination campaigns are conducted targeting all children 1 through 4 years of age, regardless of vaccination status or disease history. In addition to raising the level of measles immunity among previously immunized children, these campaigns provide measles vaccination to previously unvaccinated children and to those children who were vaccinated but who, for some reason, failed to respond to the vaccine. Through these periodic vaccination campaigns, which supplement vaccination coverage obtained through routine vaccination services, the strategy aims to achieve and maintain high measles population immunity in preschool-age and school-age children.

The interval between follow-up campaigns is determined by the vaccination coverage obtained through routine vaccination services. Campaigns are conducted when the estimated number of accumulated susceptible preschool-age children approaches the number of infants in an average birth cohort. In practice, these campaigns will need to be conducted every 3 to 5 years.

By the end of 1995, all countries of Latin America and the English-speaking Caribbean had conducted catch-up measles vaccination campaigns (Fig. 55-2). The combined regional 1- to 14-year-old measles vaccination coverage is estimated to be 93%. The catch-up measles vaccination campaigns had an immediate impact in reducing measles incidence in the region (Fig. 55-3). The 2106 total confirmed measles cases reported during 1996 from Latin America and Caribbean countries is the lowest number ever reported up until that time and represents a 99% reduction compared with the cases reported in 1990, only 6 years earlier. Measles is now a rare infection in Latin America and the Caribbean. Surveillance evaluations conducted during 1995 and 1996 in Mexico, El Salvador, and Nicaragua did not detect any evidence of measles virus circulation.

Following the catch-up campaign in the English-speaking Caribbean in 1991, it has been more than 14 years since the last indigenous laboratory-confirmed case was reported from those countries. Similarly, it has been more than 16 years since the last laboratory-confirmed measles case was detected in Cuba. In other Latin American and Caribbean countries, measles transmission is occurring at extremely low levels, if at all. Most laboratory-confirmed cases have been sporadic and isolated in terms of time and place.

As a direct result of these successes, as well as the eradication of poliomyelitis from the Americas, in September 1994 the Ministers of Health of the Region of the Americas unanimously established the goal of measles eradication from the Western Hemisphere by 2000.[81]

The PAHO encourages countries to conduct follow-up campaigns every 4 years and to maintain high routine immunization coverage by targeting poor performing districts for additional support in order to protect against large outbreaks when importations occur. After essentially eliminating

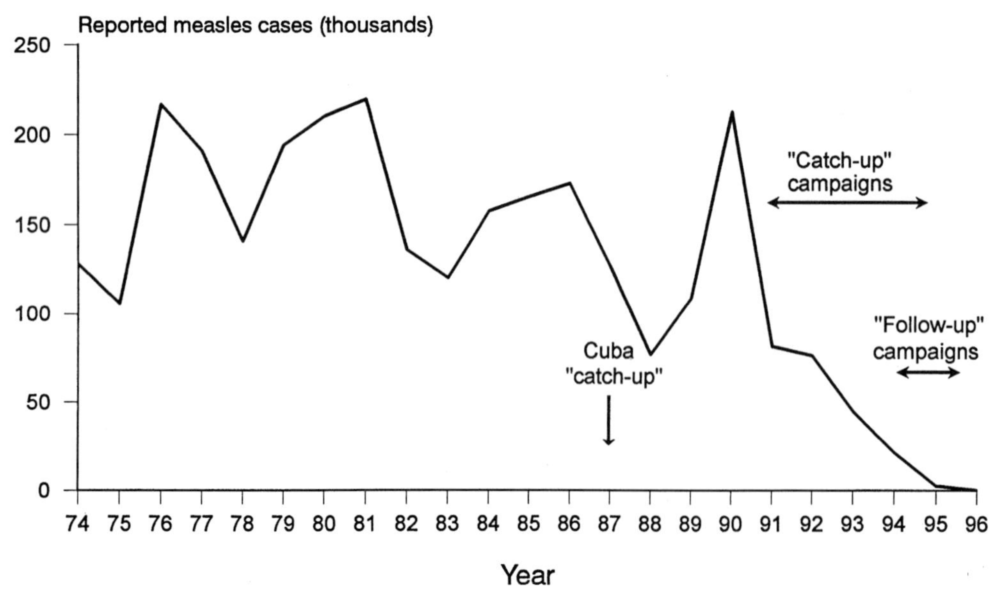

FIGURE 55-2 Annual reported measles cases in Latin American and Caribbean countries, 1974 through September 1996. (Data from the Pan-American Health Organization, Washington, DC.)

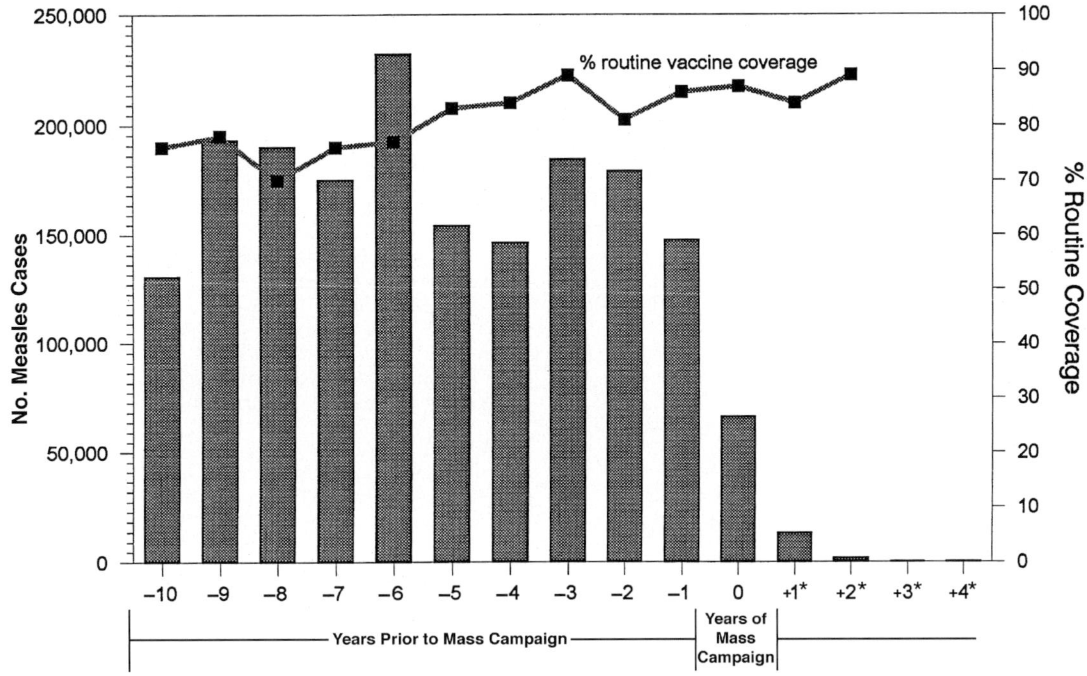

FIGURE 55-3 Impact of a mass campaign on measles cases in the Americas, 1991–1995. In categories −10 to 0, data from 45 countries; +1, 44 countries; +2, 42 countries; +3, 26 countries; and +4, 23 countries. (Data from the Pan-American Health Organization Epidemiology Surveillance System, Washington, DC.)

endemic disease, in 2001–2002 a huge measles outbreak occurred in Colombia and Venezuela, resulting from an initial measles virus importation into Colombia. The virus genotype was D9 and transmission was stopped with supplemental immunization campaigns in November 2002. This most likely represents the last endemic transmission in the region. During this outbreak, Colombia reported 139 and Venezuela 2501 measles cases, respectively.

Beginning in 2003, Mexico also experienced an outbreak resulting from importation of measles virus. The virus genotype was Hl and was considered to be an importation because it had never been isolated previously in the Americas. Hl genotype is quite common in the Far East. Because population immunity was high, the outbreak remained relatively small and contained. During the outbreak period (April 2003 to July 2004) a total of 108 measles cases were reported. All but 2 cases occurred in the contiguous two states and Federal District of Mexico City.

These last outbreaks in the region highlight the fact that importations are to be expected if endemic transmission is still occurring in other parts of the world. The PAHO strategy has clearly demonstrated that regional measles eradication is indeed possible (Fig. 55-4), particularly when the strategies are implemented well.

The challenge for regions embarking on the PAHO strategy will be to maintain high population immunity with excellent immunization coverage and high-quality surveillance, especially to deal with importations. In addition, as Figure 55-4 demonstrates, implementation of measles elimination strategies should uncover the "hidden" disease burden of rubella and congenital rubella syndrome (CRS).

To that end, in September 2003, the Directing Council of PAHO adopted the initiative to eliminate rubella and CRS by the year 2010. Integrating the elimination of measles with the elimination of rubella will greatly enhance the capacity of countries to sustain progress. In addition, countries are encountering new opportunities to expand the benefits of disease control and elimination activities to other aspects of public health, most importantly in improving health care for women and reducing inequities in health care in the poorest countries.[82,83] It is expected that the adoption of similar strategies in countries worldwide will achieve global eradication of measles in the first decade of the twenty-first century.[84,85]

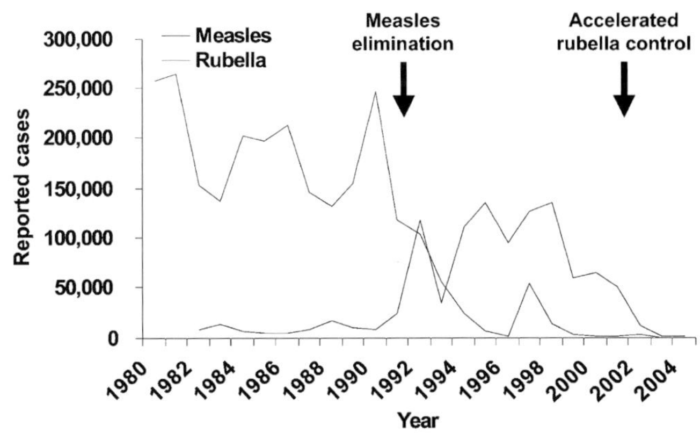

FIGURE 55-4 Trends in reported measles and rubella cases in the Americas, 1980–2004. (From the Pan American Health Organization Epidemiology Surveillance System, Washington, DC.)

REFERENCES

1. Black FL: Measles. In Evans AS (ed): Viral Infections of Humans. Epidemiology and Control, 3rd ed. New York, Plenum, 1989, pp 451–465.
2. World Bank: World Development Report 1993: Investing in Health. New York, Oxford University Press, 1993.
3. World Health Organization: The World Health Report—1998. Geneva, World Health Organization, 1998.
4. Bellini WJ, Rota JS, Rota PA: Virology of measles virus. J Infect Dis 170(Suppl 1):S15–S23, 1994.
5. Hope-Simpson RE: Infectiousness of communicable diseases in the household. Lancet 2:549–554, 1952.
6. Shasby DM, Shope TC, Downs H, et al: Epidemic measles in a highly vaccinated population. N Engl J Med 296:585–589, 1977.
7. Nkowane BM, Bart SW, Orenstein WA, et al: Measles outbreak in a vaccinated school population: Epidemiology, chains of transmission and the role of vaccine failures. Am J Public Health 77:434–438, 1987.
8. Gustafson TL, Lievens AW, Brunell PA, et al: Measles outbreak in a fully immunized secondary school population. N Engl J Med 316:771–774, 1987.
9. Morley D, Woodland M, Martin WJ: Measles in Nigerian children. A study of the disease in West Africa, and its manifestations in England and other countries during difficult epochs. J Hyg (Camb) 61:115–134, 1963.
10. Morley DC: Measles in the developing world. Proc R Soc Med 67:1112–1115, 1974.
11. Greenberg BL, Sack RB, Salazar-Lindo E, et al: Measles associated diarrhea in hospitalized children in Lima, Peru: Pathogenic agents and impact on growth. J Infect Dis 164:495–502, 1991.
12. Sarker SA, Wahed MA, Rahaman MM, et al: Persistent protein losing enteropathy in post measles diarrhoea. Arch Dis Child 61:739–743, 1986.
13. Koster F, Curlin G, Aziz KMA, et al: Synergistic impact of measles and diarrhea in nutrition and mortality in Bangladesh. Bull World Health Organ 59:901–908, 1981.
14. Reddy V, Bhaskaram P, Raghuramulu N, et al: Relationship between measles, malnutrition, and blindness: A prospective study in Indian children. Am J Clin Nutr 44:924–930, 1986.
15. Modlin JF, Halsey NA, Eddins DL, et al: Epidemiology of subacute sclerosing panencephalitis. J Pediatr 94:231–236, 1979.
16. Griffin DE, Ward BJ, Esolen LM: Pathogenesis of measles virus infection: An hypothesis for altered immune responses. J Infect Dis 170 (Suppl 1):S24–31, 1994.
17. McChesney MB, Oldstone BA: Virus-induced immunosuppression: Infections with measles virus and human immunodeficiency virus. Adv Immunol 45:335–380, 1989.
18. Koplik H: The diagnosis of the invasion of measles from a study of the exanthema as it appears on the buccal mucous membrane. Arch Pediatr 13:918–922, 1896.
19. Gershon AA, Krugman S: Measles virus. In Lennette EH, Schmidt NJ (eds): Diagnostic Procedures for Viral, Rickettsial and Chlamydial Infectious Diseases, 5th ed. Washington DC, American Public Health Association, 1979, pp 665–693.
20. Cutchins EC: A comparison of the hemagglutination-inhibition, neutralization and complement fixation tests in the assay of antibody to measles. J Immunol 88:788–795, 1962.
21. Boteler WL, Luiperbeck PM, Fuccillo DA, et al: Enzyme-linked immunosorbent assay for detection of measles antibody. J Clin Microbiol 17:814–818, 1983.
22. Lievens AW, Brunell PA: Specific immunoglobulin M enzyme-linked immunosorbent assay for confirming the diagnosis of measles. J Clin Microbiol 24:291–394, 1986.
23. Rossier E, Miller H, McCulloch B, et al: Comparison of immunofluorescence and enzyme immunoassay for detection of measles-specific immunoglobulin M antibody. J Clin Microbiol 29:1069–1071, 1991.
24. Erdman DD, Anderson LJ, Adams DR, et al: Evaluation of monoclonal antibody-based capture enzyme immunoassays for detection of specific antibodies to measles virus. J Clin Microbiol 29:1466–1471, 1991.
25. Hummel KB, Erdman DD, Heath J, et al: Baculovirus expression of the nucleoprotein gene of measles virus and the utility of the recombinant protein in diagnostic enzyme immunoassays. J Clin Microbiol 30:2874–2880, 1992.
26. Ozanne G, D'Halewyn MA: Performance and reliability of the Enzygnost measles enzyme-linked immunosorbent assay for detection of measles virus–specific immunoglobulin M antibody during a large measles epidemic. J Clin Microbiol 30:564–569, 1992.
27. Arista S, Ferraro D, Cascio A, et al: Detection of IgM antibodies specific for measles virus by capture and indirect enzyme immunoassays. Res Virol 146:225–232, 1995.
28. Expanded Programme on Immunization: Programme for the Prevention of Blindness. Joint WHO/UNICEF statement: Vitamin A for measles. Wkly Epidemiol Rec 62:133–134, 1987.
29. Englehandt SF, Halsey NA, Eddins DL, et al: Measles mortality in the United States 1971–1975. Am J Public Health 70:1166–1169, 1980.
30. Assaad F: Measles: Summary of worldwide impact. Rev Infect Dis 5:452–459, 1983.
31. Hull HF, Williams PJ, Oldfield F: Measles mortality and vaccine efficacy in rural West Africa. Lancet 1:972–975, 1983.
32. Toole MJ, Waldman RJ: Prevention of excess mortality in refugee and displaced populations in developing countries. JAMA 263:3296–3302, 1990.
33. Schwarz AJF, Anderson JT, Ramos-Alvarez M, et al: Extensive clinical evaluations of a highly attenuated live measles vaccine. JAMA 199:84–88, 1967.
34. Hilleman MR, Buynak EB, Weibel RE: Development and evaluation of the Moraten measles virus vaccine. JAMA 206:587–590, 1968.
35. Krugman S, Constantinidis P, Medovy H, et al: Comparison of two further attenuated live measles-virus vaccines. Am J Dis Child 117:137–138, 1969.
36. Markowitz LE, Preblud SR, Fine PEM, et al: Duration of measles vaccine-induced immunity. Pediatr Infect Dis J 9:101–110, 1990.
37. Krugman S, Giles JP, Jacobs AM, et al: Studies with a further attenuated live measles-virus vaccine. Pediatrics 31:919–928, 1963.
38. Markowitz LE, Katz SL: Measles vaccine. In Plotkin SA, Mortimer EA (eds): Vaccines, 2nd ed. Philadelphia, WB Saunders, 1994, pp 229–276.
39. Onorato IM, Markowitz LE, Oxtoby MJ: Childhood immunization, vaccine-preventable diseases and infection with human immunodeficiency virus. Pediatr Infect Dis J 7.588–595, 1988.
40. Fine PEM: Safety of measles vaccines. In Kurstak E (ed): Measles and Poliomyelitis—Vaccines, Immunization and Control. Vienna, Springer-Verlag, 1993, pp 63–73.
41. Peltola H, Heinonen OP: Frequency of true adverse reactions to measles–mumps–rubella vaccine. A double-blind placebo-controlled trial in twins. Lancet 1:939–942, 1986.
42. Miller CL: Surveillance after measles vaccination in children. Practitioner 226:535–537, 1982.
43. Landrigan PJ, Witte JJ: Neurologic disorders following live measles-virus vaccination. JAMA 223:1459–1462, 1973.
44. Fine PEM, Clarkson JA: Measles in England and Wales—I: An analysis of factors underlying seasonal patterns. Int J Epidemiol 11:5–14, 1982.
45. Mclean AR, Anderson RM: Measles in developing countries. Part I: Epidemiological parameters and patterns. Epidemiol Infect 100:111–133, 1988.
46. Bloch AB, Orenstein WA, Stetler HC, et al: Health impact of measles vaccination in the United States. Pediatrics 76:524–532, 1985.
47. Clemens JD, Stanton B, Chakraborty J, et al: Measles vaccination and childhood mortality in rural Bangladesh. Am J Epidemiol 128:1330–1333, 1988.
48. Holt EA, Boulos R, Halsey NA, et al: Childhood survival in Haiti: Protective effect of measles vaccination. Pediatrics 85:188–194, 1990.
49. Clements CJ, Cutts FT: The epidemiology of measles: Thirty years of vaccination. Curr Top Microbiol Immunol 191:13–33, 1995.
50. World Bank: World Development Report 1993: Investing in health. New York, Oxford University Press, 1993, pp 60–64.
51. Cutts FT, Markowitz LE: Successes and failures in measles control. J Infect Dis 170(Suppl 1):S32–S41, 1994.
52. Markowitz LE, Preblud SR, Orenstein WA, et al: Patterns of transmission in measles outbreaks in the United States, 1985–1986. N Engl J Med 320:75–81, 1989.
53. Hersh BS, Markowitz LE, Maes EF, et al: The geographic distribution of measles in the United States, 1980–1989. JAMA 267:1936–1941,1992.
54. Dabis F, Sow A, Waldman RJ, et al: The epidemiology of measles in a partially vaccinated population in an African city: Implications for immunization programs. Am J Epidemiol 127:171–178, 1988.

55. Ndikuyeze A, Cook A, Cutts FT, et al: Priorities in global measles control: Report of an outbreak in N'Djamena, Chad. Epidemiol Infect 115:309–314, 1995.
56. Taylor WR, Mambu RK, Ma-Disu W, et al: Measles control effort in urban Africa complicated by high incidence of measles in the first year of life. Am J Epidemiol 27:788–794, 1988.
57. Kambarami RA, Nathoo KJ, Nkrumah FK, et al: Measles epidemic in Harare, Zimbabwe, despite high measles immunization coverage rates. Bull World Health Organ 169:213–219, 1991.
58. Foster SO, McFarland DA, John AM: Measles. In Jamison DT, Mosley WH, Measham AR, et al (eds): Disease Control Priorities in Developing Countries. New York, Oxford University Press, 1993, pp 161–188.
59. Chen RT, Weierbach R, Bisoffi Z, et al: A post-honeymoon period measles outbreak in Muyinga Province, Burundi. Int J Epidemiol 23:185–193, 1994.
60. Wassilak SGF, Orenstein WA, Strickland PL, et al: Continuing measles transmission in students despite a school based outbreak control program. Am J Epidemiol 122:208–217, 1985.
61. Davis RM, Whitman ED, Orenstein WA, et al: A persistent outbreak of measles despite appropriate prevention and control measures. Am J Epidemiol 126:438–449, 1987.
62. Robertson SE, Markowitz LE, Berry DA, et al: A million dollar measles outbreak: Epidemiology, risk factors and a selective revaccination strategy. Public Health Rep 107:24–31, 1992.
63. Fine PEM: Herd immunity: History, theory, practice. Epidemiol Rev 15:265–302, 1993.
64. Chen RT, Goldbaum GM, Wassilak SGF, et al: An explosive point-source outbreak in a highly vaccinated population. Am J Epidemiol 129:173–182, 1989.
65. Hersh BS, Markowitz LE, Hoffman RE, et al: A measles outbreak at a college with a prematriculation immunization requirement. Am J Public Health 81:360–364, 1991.
66. Rosenthal SR, Clements CJ: Two-dose measles vaccination schedules. Bull World Health Organ 71:421–428, 1993.
67. National Vaccine Advisory Committee: The measles epidemic: The problems, barriers and recommendations. JAMA 266:1547–1552,1991.
68. Markowitz LE, Sepulveda J, Diaz-Ortega JL, et al: Immunization of six-month-old infants with different doses of Edmonston–Zagreb and Schwarz measles vaccines. N Engl J Med 322:580–587, 1990.
69. Whittle HC, Campbell H, Rahman S, et al: Antibody persistence in Gambian children after high-dose Edmonston–Zagreb measles vaccine. Lancet 336:1046–1048, 1990.
70. Job JS, Halsey NA, Boulos R, et al: Successful immunization of infants at 6 months of age with high dose Edmonston–Zagreb measles vaccine. Pediatr Infect Dis J 10:303–311, 1991.
71. Expanded Programme on Immunization: Measles immunization before 9 months of age. Wkly Epidemiol Rec 2:8, 1990.
72. Garenne M, Leroy J, Beau FP, et al: I. Child mortality after high-titre measles vaccines: Prospective study in Senegal. Lancet 338:903–920, 1991.
73. Aaby P, Samb B, Simondon F, et al: Divergent mortality for male and female recipients of low-titer and high-titer measles vaccines in rural Senegal. Am J Epidemiol 138:746–755, 1993.
74. Expanded Programme on Immunization: Safety of high titre measles vaccines. Wkly Epidem Rec 67:357–361, 1992.
75. Foster SO, Pifer JM: Mass measles control in west and central Africa. Afr J Med Med Sci 2:151–158, 1971.
76. Foege WH: Measles vaccination in Africa. In Proceedings of the International Conference on the Application of Vaccines against Viral, Rickettsial, and Bacterial Diseases of Man, Scientific Publication No. 226. Washington, DC, Pan American Health Organization, 1971, pp 207–212.
77. Williams PJ, Hull HF: Status of measles in The Gambia, 1981. Rev Infect Dis 5:391–394, 1983.
78. Thacker SB, Millar JD: Mathematical modeling and attempts to eliminate measles: A tribute to the late Professor George Macdonald. Am J Epidemiol 133:517–525, 1991.
79. de Quadros CA, Olivé JM, Hersh BS, et al: Measles elimination in the Americas—Evolving strategies. JAMA 275:224–229, 1996.
80. de Quadros CA, Andrus JK, Olivé JM, et al: Polio eradication from the Western Hemisphere. Annu Rev Public Health 13:239–252, 1992.
81. Pan American Health Organization: Measles elimination by the year 2000. EPI Newslett 16:1–2, 1994.
82. Castillo-Solorzano C, Andrus JK: Rubella elimination and improving health care for women. Emerg Infect Dis 10:2017–2021, 2004.
83. Andrus JK, Roses Periago M: Elimination of rubella and congenital rubella syndrome in the Americas: Another opportunity to address inequities in health. Pan Amer J Public Health 15:145–146, 2004.
84. Hopkins DR, Koplan JP, Hinman AR, et al: The case for global measles eradication. Lancet 1:1396–1398, 1982.
85. Expanded Program on Immunization: Meeting on advances in measles elimination: Conclusions and recommendations. Wkly Epidemiol Rec 71:305–309, 1996.

56

Nipah and Hendra Viral Infections

RAMON FLICK
PRAMILA WALPITA
MARKUS CZUB

INTRODUCTION

Over the past decade, outbreaks of severe diseases in humans, sea mammals, and Serengeti lions emerged and were in part attributed to infections with previously unknown paramyxoviruses. Of these, Hendra (HeV), Nipah (NiV), and Menangle viruses,[1–3] the previously unknown causative agents of diseases in humans and livestock in Australia and Malaysia, clearly merit the term emerging. Additionally, other novel paramyxoviruses have been isolated from bats,[4] tree shrews,[5] horses,[6] rodents, and humans[7]; however, infection with these viruses has not been associated with overt clinical disease. Only HeV and NiV are unusual among the paramyxoviruses in that they cause potentially fatal disease in a number of host species, including humans. Both viruses are designated as biosafety level (BSL)-4 agents.

In 1994, HeV caused an explosive outbreak of respiratory disease, claiming the lives of 14 horses and 2 humans in Australia.[2,8] In horses and cats,[9] natural and experimental infection with HeV is characterized by pulmonary lesions, including pulmonary edema and congestion, as well as hydrothorax and enlarged local lymph nodes.[2,8,10,11] Histologically, necrosis of alveolar walls and damage to small blood vessels in major organs are observed. In experimentally infected guinea pigs, there is generalized vascular disease; however, with only limited pulmonary pathology. The two human cases showed severe lung lesions and meningitis, respectively.[12]

NiV infections were first diagnosed in 1998–1999 in Malaysia.[13–17] Of 265 human cases of encephalitis, there were 105 fatalities.[16,18–20] The disease was initially attributed to Japanese encephalitis (JE), which is endemic in the region. However, epidemiologic considerations ruled out the possibility because JE virus is mosquito-borne and has no occupational association.[21] Moreover, JE virus vaccination drives were not effective in controlling the outbreak. Studies leading to isolation of the new agent were performed relatively rapidly. Infection with NiV leads to neurologic syndromes in humans and occasionally in pigs, although the latter show primarily mild respiratory disease.[13,22] The key histopathologic features in humans are systemic endothelial infection, vasculitis, thrombosis, ischemia, and necrosis. These changes are most pronounced in the central nervous system (CNS). In pigs, lesions are found in the brain or lungs. In the respiratory tract, lesions consist of tracheitis and both suppurative and nonsuppurative bronchopneumonia and interstitial pneumonia. As a consequence of NiV infection in pigs, more than a million animals were culled.[13,16,19,23,24]

AGENTS

Classification

HeV and NiV belong to the family Paramyxoviridae of the order Mononegavirales. These viruses share similar genome organization and replication strategy. HeV and NiV have been proposed to form a new genus, *Henipavirus*, within the subfamily Paramyxovirinae.[25,26] Like other paramyxoviruses, henipaviruses have a single-stranded RNA genome with negative orientation. Unique features of henipaviruses within the subfamily Paramyxovirinae are their larger genomes (18.2 kb vs. 15.1 to 15.9 kb), longer untranslated regions, mostly at the 3' end, in each of the six transcription units, and a P protein that is more than 100 amino acids longer than any other known phosphoprotein in the family.[26] The nucleic acid sequence homology between HeV and NiV ranges from 70% to 85% for the coding regions and from 40% to 45% for the noncoding regions.[27] Homologies to other members of the paramyxovirus subfamily are less than 45%.[13]

Biologic and Virologic Properties

The biologic properties of NiV and HeV are similar to those of other Paramyxovirinae in many respects, but quite distinct in several others. NiV and HeV grow to high titers in cell cultures derived from different organs of many species.[2,8,27,28] Both viruses induce a strong cytopathic effect in the form of syncytia.[28–30] The extent of diversity of the paramyxoviruses is further underscored by the fact that unlike the other paramyxoviruses, NiV and HeV are able to cause infection, disease, and death in a wide range of species including humans, pigs, horses, cats, and dogs. These findings raise questions about the evolutionary relationships with members of the order Mononegavirales. Electron microscopic studies of NiV and HeV show classical morphologic features of viruses belonging to the family Paramyxoviridae. They are pleomorphic enveloped viruses of variable diameter (120 to 500 nm), and in infected cells, they have helical filamentous nucleocapsids with the typical "herringbone" appearance. The HeV envelopes are covered with projections that give them a distinct "double fringed" appearance, while NiV envelopes are "single fringed."[11,31] An additional unusual feature of NiV-infected cells, and to a lesser extent of HeV-infected cells, is the presence of tubule-like structures that are present at the cell periphery and in association with the endoplasmic reticulum and that appear to be involved in viral assembly and budding.[11]

Replication

Recent evidence suggests that both NiV and HeV bind to the same glycoprotein receptor by a mechanism that is independent of sialic acid mediation.[32] Cleavage of HeV and NiV fusion protein precursor F_0 into disulfide-linked F_1 and F_2 subunits is a prerequisite for infectivity and is achieved by mechanisms unlike those of other paramyxoviruses.[33,34] Recent minigenome-based studies indicate that the sequence elements that control NiV and

HeV replication reside in the noncoding genomic and antigenomic promoter nucleotides.[35] Minigenome-based experiments and comparison with other paramyxoviruses suggest that during viral infection full-length genome copies are made via replication intermediate strands called the antigenome and that genomic and antigenomic RNAs serve as functional templates for transcription and replication only when they are encapsidated with the N protein. For the majority of paramyxoviruses including NiV, functional nucleocapsid formation requires that the total number of nucleotides in the genome length RNA be divisible by six (i.e., it obeys the *rule of six*).[35–37]

EPIDEMIOLOGY

NiV and HeV are contagious, highly virulent, and capable of infecting several mammalian species. Subsequent to the outbreak in Malaysia and Singapore, there were smaller outbreaks of human NiV infection in Bangladesh in 2003–2004.[38]

Seroepidemiologic data indicate that fruit bats are a natural host for both NiV and HeV.[9,39–43] These animals roost in large groups in trees. It is possible that infected bats shed virus via saliva or urine and infect other animals and humans, although the exact mode of virus transmission is yet to be determined.[44,45] Data from the recent outbreak in Bangladesh suggest that human-to-human transmission of NiV is possible when close contact occurs.[38,46]

Under experimental conditions, NiV is able to infect cats, pigs, guinea pigs, and hamsters, while HeV infects horses, cats, and bats. Additional animal species may also be susceptible to infection. The natural disease in pigs is called porcine respiratory and encephalitis syndrome.[22] Although NiV did spread very rapidly among pigs under the farming conditions in Malaysia, a large percentage of the pigs remained asymptomatic, and the majority (85% to 95%) of the diseased pigs recovered.[22] Pigs transmit NiV to other pigs, other animals, and humans by an uncharacterized mechanism[44,45]; 93% of the afflicted humans in Malaysia had close occupational contact with infected pigs. Epidemiologic observations and laboratory findings indicate that porcine body fluids such as saliva, blood, and urine contain the virus. Subsequently, pig farmers and abattoir workers are at high risk for infection with NiV when exposed to NiV-infected pigs (or other animals).[44]

Under experimental conditions, HeV does not appear to be very contagious. Similarly, exposure of health-care workers to NiV-infected individuals during the Malaysian outbreak did not result in person-to-person transmission of infection.[44,45] On the basis of these and further epidemiologic data, it is speculated that transmission of HeV and NiVs occurs via aerosols or droplets and that humans are infected with low efficiency.[47] However, it is possible that natural infections are promoted by as yet unknown factors such as virus amplification in other hosts. Fruit bats, which have a high prevalence of antibodies to HeV, NiV, and other paramyxoviruses, might serve as an reservoir for further emerging paramyxoviruses.[4,9,40–43]

DISEASES

Nipah Virus Infection

Human NiV disease is a febrile encephalitis. Subclinical infection with NiV seems infrequent in humans; 75% of those who seroconverted developed disease.[19,20] The incubation period based on the time of exposure until onset of fever ranged from a few days to 2 weeks with a mean incubation period of 10 days.[18,19] Initial symptoms were often described as influenza-like with sore throat, fever, headache, and myalgia. Clinical manifestations of encephalitic disease were dizziness, headache, vomiting, convulsions, reduced level of consciousness, and coma.[16,18–20] Late onset or relapse of NiV encephalitis occurred in 12 (7.5%) of those who survived the acute phase, and of these, 17% died. Respiratory tract involvement was present in 14% to 24% of patients in the Malaysian outbreak and manifested as nonproductive cough, fever, and myalgia. None had primary lung disease.[20] In contrast, pneumonitis was present in 3 of the 11 patients in the Singapore outbreak.[16]

Hendra Virus Infection

The incubation period of HeV infection in humans is 4 to 18 days. Symptoms at onset are of severe influenza-like illness with high fever, headache, and myalgia. The first two human patients with HeV infection had respiratory symptoms; one died of respiratory failure and pneumonia, and the other recovered slowly 6 weeks after onset.[17] The second patient who died had neurologic disease that ran a protracted course; the initial illness was a mild meningoencephalitis. The patient continued to suffer from fatigue, developed epileptic seizures, and finally became comatose and died 13 months after exposure to HeV.[10,12]

PATHOGENESIS

Nipah Virus Infection

Postmortem studies of culture-confirmed NiV patients showed marked multiorgan vasculitis with endothelial damage in the arterioles, venules, and capillaries. In some cases, endothelial cells had lysed and sloughed into the lumen of the blood vessels; multinucleated giant cells, which are characteristic of paramyxoviral infections, were observed by light and electron microscopy.[11,13] The brain was the most severely affected organ.[13,48] In one study, evaluation at autopsy of microscopic features in the CNS showed necrotic lesions, perivascular cuffing, thrombosis, and vasculitis in 80% to 90% of the 30 cases examined; endothelial syncytia were present in 27% and meningitis in 57% of the patients.[20] The severity of the CNS pathology was demonstrated also by magnetic resonance imaging (MRI) analysis of 31 encephalitis patients in the Malaysian outbreak.[49] Other affected organs were the kidney, lung, and heart.[13,20]

Illness of pigs was largely due to respiratory disease and included a loud and distinctive cough and neurologic symptoms. The nature of the disease depended on the age of the pig. In sows and boars, symptoms of acute febrile respiratory illness predominated. Neurologic symptoms, when present, included spasms, seizures, head pressing, and pharyngeal muscle paralysis. Abortions occurred in diseased pregnant sows. In suckling pigs, mortality was higher, and the symptoms were a combination of respiratory and neurologic disease.[13] In pigs, respiratory tract involvement was the most common feature at postmortem examination. Giant cell pneumonia was present with multinucleated syncytial cells in the lung. NiV antigen was identified in the giant cells, the epithelial lining, the necrotic areas of the upper and lower respiratory tract, and renal tubular cells.[50,51]

Hendra Virus Infection

The horse trainer who died of HeV infection had interstitial pneumonia. The second human who developed fatal disease died of encephalitis with histopathologic and MRI evidence of CNS lesions.[10,12]

In horses, the incubation period is between 8 and 11 days. An acute febrile respiratory or neurologic illness of short duration (1 to 3 days) results in death; symptoms include fever, rapid and shallow breathing, congested mucous membranes, ataxia, and head pressing.[2,8,10] The major pathologic changes in equines are in the lungs; the virus replicates in endothelial cells, apparently leading to endothelial damage, pulmonary edema, congestion, consolidation, and hemorrhage.[10,11]

DIAGNOSIS

Clinical history of the patient is an important consideration in the choice of laboratory investigations and in the differential diagnosis. Since initial presentation of NiV disease is often nonspecific, the geographic location, clinical history, and occupational exposure are important clues in the differential diagnosis. NiV should be an important consideration if the patient has been the endemic regions and JE is excluded.[21] MRI is useful in excluding JE because of the distinct difference in the appearance and distribution of brain lesions between NiV encephalitis and JE.[21,49] In the Malaysian and Singapore outbreaks, NiV disease showed abnormal cerebrospinal fluid (CSF) in 75% of the patients and abnormal liver function tests in 50%[18,19,24]; thrombocytopenia and leukopenia were also noted.[16] Serology provides an etiologic diagnosis[52,53]: NiV-specific immunoglobulin M (IgM) and IgG levels were detected by enzyme immunoassays in 100% of the patients by day 12 and day 25, respectively.

Virus isolation is of limited availability because NiV is a BSL-4 agent. However, when biocontainment facilities are available, virus can be isolated from urine, CSF, throat and nasal secretions[47,54] and tissues from various organs of the body.[28] A variety of cells are permissive for NiV cultivation although Vero (green monkey kidney) cells are used most frequently.[26–28] Virus isolates showing classical syncytial cytopathic effect[1,28] should be confirmed by immunostaining of virus-specific antigen. A real-time reverse transcription–polymerase chain reaction (RT-PCR) assay provides a sensitive and specific means to detect virus and to measure the virus load.[55] However, caution has to be taken with negative PCR results because the source of tissue and the time of sampling may determine a negative result despite an ongoing infection.

The biocontainment requirements also limit the use of virus isolation for HeV diagnosis. Nevertheless, a variety of cell lines are permissive for HeV propagation. Vero cells are generally used for cell culture,[2,8,13,27] and when infected show marked syncytial cytopathic effect that is distinct from that produced by NiV.[1,28] Immunostaining demonstrates viral antigen in formalin-fixed, paraffin-embedded tissues. Electron microscopic studies identify the classical morphology of the virus with its double-fringed envelope.[11,31] A variety of tests are available for serodiagnosis of HeV, including enzyme immunoassay (EIA), blocking EIA, neutralization assay, indirect immunofluorescence, and immunoblotting.[52,53] RT-PCR can detect HeV in formalin-fixed tissues.[52,53,55]

TREATMENT AND PROGNOSIS

No specific treatment is available for NiV or HeV infection. Whether ribavirin might be of value in the treatment of NiV infection remains unclear and requires blinded, randomized, controlled trials.

Thus, treatment of infected humans is supportive and designed to sustain life and relieve symptoms. Prognosis is poor, since the case-fatality rate is high (around 40% with NiV in humans[16,18–20]). Survivors of encephalitis may suffer lifelong disabilities.

PREVENTION AND CONTROL

In an outbreak, the source of infection needs to be identified and prevented from further transmitting the infection. Preventive measures include clinical care in an isolation ward and culling of infected animals. Experimental vaccines against NiV show promising results in animals; however, it is doubtful whether these vaccines will become available for humans.

REFERENCES

1. Chua KB, Goh KJ, Wong KT, et al: Fatal encephalitis due to Nipah virus among pig-farmers in Malaysia. Lancet 354:1257–1259, 1999.
2. Murray K, Selleck P, Hooper P, et al: A morbillivirus that caused fatal disease in horses and humans. Science 268:94–97, 1995.
3. Philbey AW, Kirkland PD, Ross AD, et al: An apparently new virus (family Paramyxoviridae) infectious for pigs, humans, and fruit bats. Emerg Infect Dis 4:269–271, 1998.
4. Chua KB, Wang LF, Lam SK, et al: Tioman virus, a novel paramyxovirus isolated from fruit bats in Malaysia. Virology 283:215–229, 2001.
5. Tidona CA, Kurz HW, Gelderblom HR, et al: Isolation and molecular characterization of a novel cytopathogenic paramyxovirus from tree shrews. Virology 258:425–434, 1999.
6. Renshaw RW, Glaser AL, Van Campen H, et al: Identification and phylogenetic comparison of Salem virus, a novel paramyxovirus of horses. Virology 270:417–429, 2000.
7. van den Hoogen BG, de Jong JC, Groen J, et al: A newly discovered human pneumovirus isolated from young children with respiratory tract disease. Nat Med 7:719–724, 2001.
8. Murray K, Rogers R, Selvey L, et al: A novel morbillivirus pneumonia of horses and its transmission to humans. Emerg Infect Dis 1:31–33, 1995.
9. Williamson MM, Hooper PT, Selleck PW, et al: Transmission studies of Hendra virus (equine morbillivirus) in fruit bats, horses and cats. Aust Vet J 76:813–818, 1998.
10. Barclay AJ, Paton DJ: Hendra (equine morbillivirus). Vet J 160:169–176, 2000.
11. Hyatt AD, Zaki SR, Goldsmith CS, et al: Ultrastructure of Hendra virus and Nipah virus within cultured cells and host animals. Microbes Infect 3:297–306, 2001.
12. O'Sullivan JD, Allworth AM, Paterson DL, et al: Fatal encephalitis due to novel paramyxovirus transmitted from horses. Lancet 349:93–95, 1997.
13. Chua KB, Bellini WJ, Rota PA, et al: Nipah virus: A recently emergent deadly paramyxovirus. Science 288:1432–1435, 2000.
14. Halpin K, Young PL, Field H, et al: Newly discovered viruses of flying foxes. Vet Microbiol 68:83–87, 1999.
15. Parashar UD, Sunn LM, Ong F, et al: Case-control study of risk factors for human infection with a new zoonotic paramyxovirus, Nipah virus, during a 1998–1999 outbreak of severe encephalitis in Malaysia. J Infect Dis 181:1755–1759, 2000.
16. Paton NI, Leo YS, Zaki SR, et al: Outbreak of Nipah-virus infection among abattoir workers in Singapore. Lancet 354:1253–1256, 1999.
17. Selvey LA, Wells RM, McCormack JG, et al: Infection of humans and horses by a newly described morbillivirus. Med J Aust 162:642–645, 1995.
18. Chong HT, Kunjapan SR, Thayaparan T, et al: Nipah encephalitis outbreak in Malaysia, clinical features in patients from Seremban. Can J Neurol Sci 29:83–87, 2002.

19. Goh KJ, Tan CT, Chew NK, et al: Clinical features of Nipah virus encephalitis among pig farmers in Malaysia. N Engl J Med 342:1229–1235, 2000.
20. Wong KT, Shieh WJ, Kumar S, et al: Nipah virus infection: Pathology and pathogenesis of an emerging paramyxoviral zoonosis. Am J Pathol 161:2153–2167, 2002.
21. Lim CC, Sitoh YY, Hui F, et al: Nipah viral encephalitis or Japanese encephalitis? MR findings in a new zoonotic disease. Am J Neuroradiol 21:455–461, 2000.
22. Mohd Nor MN, Gan CH, Ong BL: Nipah virus infection of pigs in peninsular Malaysia. Rev Sci Tech 19:160–165, 2000.
23. Garner MG, Whan IF, Gard GP, et al: The expected economic impact of selected exotic diseases on the pig industry of Australia. Rev Sci Tech 20:671–685, 2001.
24. Lee KE, Umapathi T, Tan CB, et al: The neurological manifestations of Nipah virus encephalitis, a novel paramyxovirus. Ann Neurol 46:428–432, 1999.
25. Chan YP, Chua KB, Koh CL, et al: Complete nucleotide sequences of Nipah virus isolates from Malaysia. J Gen Virol 82:2151–2155, 2001.
26. Wang LF, Yu M, Hansson E, et al: The exceptionally large genome of Hendra virus: Support for creation of a new genus within the family Paramyxoviridae. J Virol 74:9972–9979, 2000.
27. Wang L, Harcourt BH, Yu M, et al: Molecular biology of Hendra and Nipah viruses. Microbes Infect 3:279–287, 2001.
28. Daniels P, Ksiazek T, Eaton BT: Laboratory diagnosis of Nipah and Hendra virus infections. Microbes Infect 3:289–295, 2001.
29. Westbury HA: Hendra virus disease in horses. Rev Sci Tech 19:151–159, 2000.
30. Westbury HA, Hooper PT, Selleck PW, et al: Equine morbillivirus pneumonia: Susceptibility of laboratory animals to the virus. Aust Vet J 72:278–279, 1995.
31. Hyatt AD, Selleck PW: Ultrastructure of equine morbillivirus. Virus Res 43:1–15, 1996.
32. Eaton BT, Wright PJ, Wang LF, et al: Henipaviruses: recent observations on regulation of transcription and the nature of the cell receptor. Arch Virol Suppl 122–131, 2004.
33. Michalski WP, Crameri G, Wang L, et al: The cleavage activation and sites of glycosylation in the fusion protein of Hendra virus. Virus Res 69:83–93, 2000.
34. Moll M, Diederich S, Klenk HD, et al: Ubiquitous activation of the Nipah virus fusion protein does not require a basic amino acid at the cleavage site. J Virol 78:9705–9712, 2004.
35. Halpin K, Bankamp B, Harcourt BH, et al: Nipah virus conforms to the rule of six in a minigenome replication assay. J Gen Virol 85:701–707, 2004.
36. Calain P, Roux L: The rule of six, a basic feature for efficient replication of Sendai virus defective interfering RNA. J Virol 67:4822–4830, 1993.
37. Kolakofsky D, Pelet T, Garcin D, et al: Paramyxovirus RNA synthesis and the requirement for hexamer genome length: The rule of six revisited. J Virol 72:891–899, 1998.
38. Enserink M: Emerging infectious diseases: Nipah virus (or a cousin) strikes again. Science 303:1121, 2004.
39. Chua KB: Nipah virus outbreak in Malaysia. J Clin Virol 26:265–275, 2003.
40. Chua KB, Koh CL, Hooi PS, et al: Isolation of Nipah virus from Malaysian Island flying-foxes. Microbes Infect 4:145–151, 2002.
41. Field H, Mackenzie J, Daszak P: Novel viral encephalitides associated with bats (Chiroptera)—host management strategies. Arch Virol Suppl 113–121, 2004.
42. Mackenzie JS, Field HE: Emerging encephalitogenic viruses: Lyssaviruses and henipaviruses transmitted by frugivorous bats. Arch Virol Suppl 97–111, 2004.
43. Williamson MM, Hooper PT, Selleck PW, et al: Experimental Hendra virus infection in pregnant guinea-pigs and fruit bats (*Pteropus poliocephalus*). J Comp Pathol 122:201–207, 2000.
44. Chan KP, Rollin PE, Ksiazek TG, et al: A survey of Nipah virus infection among various risk groups in Singapore. Epidemiol Infect 128:93–98, 2002.
45. Mounts AW, Kaur H, Parashar UD, et al: A cohort study of health care workers to assess nosocomial transmissibility of Nipah virus, Malaysia, 1999. J Infect Dis 183:810–813, 2001.
46. Butler D: Fatal fruit bat virus sparks epidemics in southern Asia. Nature 429:7, 2004.
47. Chua KB, Lam SK, Goh KJ, et al: The presence of Nipah virus in respiratory secretions and urine of patients during an outbreak of Nipah virus encephalitis in Malaysia. J Infect 42:40–43, 2001.
48. Lam SK and Chua KB: Nipah virus encephalitis outbreak in Malaysia. Clin Infect Dis 34(Suppl 2):S48–S51, 2002.
49. Sarji SA, Abdullah BJ, Goh KJ, et al: MR imaging features of Nipah encephalitis. Am J Roentgenol 175:437–442, 2000.
50. Hooper P, Zaki S, Daniels P, et al: Comparative pathology of the diseases caused by Hendra and Nipah viruses. Microbes Infect 3:315–322, 2001.
51. Tanimura N, Imada T, Kashiwazaki Y, et al: Monoclonal antibody-based immunohistochemical diagnosis of Malaysian Nipah virus infection in pigs. J Comp Pathol 131:199–206, 2004.
52. Crameri G, Wang LF, Morrissy C, et al: A rapid immune plaque assay for the detection of Hendra and Nipah viruses and anti-virus antibodies. J Virol Methods 99:41–51, 2002.
53. Kashiwazaki Y, Na YN, Tanimura N, et al: A solid-phase blocking ELISA for detection of antibodies to Nipah virus. J Virol Methods 121:259–261, 2004.
54. Chua KB, Lam SK, Tan CT, et al: High mortality in Nipah encephalitis is associated with presence of virus in cerebrospinal fluid. Ann Neurol 48:802–805, 2000.
55. Guillaume V, Lefeuvre A, Faure C, et al: Specific detection of Nipah virus using real-time RT-PCR (TaqMan). J Virol Methods 120:229–237, 2004.

57

Human Herpesvirus Infections

S. DAVID HUDNALL
LAWRENCE R. STANBERRY

INTRODUCTION

There are currently nine herpesviruses known to afflict humans—in eight cases, the human is the only known host, while in one case the human rarely plays accidental host to a simian virus. All herpesviruses share certain genetic structural and biologic characteristics, yet exhibit a bewildering range of clinical disease manifestations (Table 57-1). All herpesviruses have relatively large and complex double-stranded DNA genomes ranging in size from 125 kbp to 229 kbp with large (greater than 100 bp) reiterated sequences called terminal repeats present at the end(s) of the linear genome. The herpesvirus genome encodes more than 60 genes, including many involved in nucleic acid metabolism and DNA synthesis. The herpes virion is a 120-nm to 800-nm particle composed of an estimated 30 to 35 proteins and consisting of an electron-dense toroidal core containing a linear double-stranded DNA molecule enclosed sequentially by a 100-nm icosadeltahedral nucleocapsid with 162 capsomers, an amorphous tegument layer, and a trilaminar lipid envelope. The envelope is largely derived from host cell nuclear membrane but contains viral glycoproteins important in target cell binding and as targets for neutralizing antibodies. These shared physical properties explain the remarkable ultrastructural similarity of all herpesviruses. After fusion with the target cell, the unenveloped virion migrates to the cell nucleus where the capsid is lost and the linear DNA molecule circularizes in the terminal repeat region(s) to form the closed circular (episomal) form characteristic of the latent cycle. The episomal form replicates during the latent cycle in synchrony with the host genome during S (synthesis) phase through the action of host cell DNA polymerase, while in the lytic cycle replication is driven by viral DNA polymerase. Replication proceeds by a rolling circle mechanism which yields end-to-end concatamers, which are then cleaved at the terminal repeats into monomers. Integration of viral DNA into the host genome does sometimes occur but apparently does not contribute significantly to virus persistence or viral-induced cell transformation.

All herpesviruses exhibit two distinct cycles of infection—the latent and lytic cycles. The latent cycle is characterized by gene expression limited to a few regulatory genes, the products of which are presumably required for maintenance of intranuclear episomal DNA. All viral gene expression is mediated by host cell RNA polymerase II. The latently infected host cell provides a means for virus persistence by remaining viable and serving as a poor target for the host immune system, while retaining the capability of producing infectious virus after switching into the lytic cycle. The lytic cycle is characterized by activation of a large number of viral genes involved in viral DNA replication and virion assembly, most often leading to inhibition of host cell macromolecular synthesis, release of infectious virus, and host cell death. The latent and lytic cycles play complementary roles for the herpesvirus—latency allows for viral persistence while lysis allows for viral spread. However, the factors which govern the balance between the latent and lytic states are poorly understood. Further details of viral replication are available in several excellent texts.[1–5]

The herpesviruses are currently classified on the basis of biologic characteristics by the Herpesvirus Study Group of the International Committee on the Taxonomy of Viruses into three subfamilies—the alpha-, beta-, and gammaherpesviruses. The alphaherpesviruses—herpes simplex virus (HSV), varicella-zoster virus (VZV), cercopithecine virus 1 (CHV-1)—have high reproductive rates with rapid spread and lethal lysis of infected cells in vitro. Although mucocutaneous epithelia are initially infected, latency is established in the neurons of sensory ganglia. The betaherpesviruses—cytomegalovirus (CMV), human herpesviruses 6 and 7 (HHV-6, HHV-7)—have low reproductive rates with slow spread and nonlethal cytomegalia of infected cells in vitro. Infection may be widespread while latency is likely established in secretory epithelial tissues and leukocytes. The gammaherpesviruses—Epstein-Barr virus (EBV), human herpesvirus 8 (HHV-8)—infect lymphocytes, epithelial tissues, and mesenchymal cells, while latency is likely established in B lymphocytes. The gammaherpesviruses are distinct from the other herpesvirus subfamilies in being causally linked to malignant lymphoid, epithelial, and mesenchymal tumors in humans.

The human herpesviruses are distributed throughout the world with no significant geographic variation. In many developing areas, including the tropics, children appear to acquire most herpesvirus infections, with the exception of VZV, at an earlier age than in developed countries, presumably due to greater transmissibility and exposure from overcrowding and poor general hygiene. In most cases, primary infection is acquired in early childhood and, with the exception of VZV (varicella), is usually asymptomatic. Symptomatic primary infections with the alphaherpesviruses usually present as mucocutaneous vesicular eruptions—HSV-1 most often localized to the oral region, HSV-2 localized to the genital region, while VZV is most often generalized to cutaneous areas. Primary symptomatic CMV and EBV infections commonly present in young adults as mononucleosis syndromes with pharyngitis and adenopathy, while HHV-6 infection usually presents with fever and a characteristic macular rash. Little is known of the clinical characteristics of primary HHV-7 and HHV-8 infection. Human infection with CHV-1 usually leads to HSV-like vesicular lesions at the site of inoculation (animal bite) followed rapidly by neurologic symptoms. Those at greatest risk of serious herpesvirus infection include the very young (fetus, newborn) and the immunocompromised (malnourished, persons with acquired immunodeficiency syndrome [AIDS], organ transplant recipients, and

Table 57-1 *Clinical Characteristics of Human Herpesvirus Infection*

Virus	Congenital/Neonatal Infection	Primary Infection	Recurrent Infection	Ocular Disease	Skin Disease	CNS Disease
HSV-1	Rare	Gingivostomatitis, usually in childhood	Herpes labialis	Keratoconjunctivitis, keratitis; most common cause of ulcerative eye infection	Oral mucocutaneous vesicular eruption; intraoral ulcers	Most common sporadic acute viral encephalitis in adults
HSV-2	Congenital infection uncommon; systemic infection in neonate	Herpes genitalis, usually in young adults; a common ulcerative genital infection	Herpes genitalis; usually very mild	Rare	Genital mucocutaneous vesicular eruption	Rare; encephalitis in neonates
VZV	Rare congenital syndrome with skin/autonomic defects; neonatal infection with typical rash	Varicella (chickenpox), usually mild in childhood; adult onset in tropics more severe	Zoster (shingles), usually in older adults	Ophthalmic zoster; rare in varicella	Vesicular eruption; generalized in varicella; dermatomal distribution in zoster	Rarely in elderly with cranial nerve zoster (Ramsay-Hunt syndrome)
CMV	Growth and mental retardation (cytomegalic inclusion disease)	Often asymptomatic in childhood; mono-nucleosis usually in adults	Rare; pneumonia and colitis in immunodeficient	Retinitis in congenital infection	Rare ulcerative perineal eruption in immunodeficient	Encephalitis in congenital infection
EBV	Rare	Often symptomatic in childhood; mononucleosis usually in adolescents/young adults	Burkitt's lymphoma; AIDS lymphoma; posttransplant lymphoma; nasopharyngeal carcinoma	Not reported	Rare maculopapular eruption of trunk and arms	Rare
HHV-6	Rare	Exanthem subitum, in young children	Unknown	Not reported	Maculopapular eruption of trunk and neck	Rare
HHV-7	Rare	? HHV-6-negative exanthem subitum	Unknown	Not reported	? Maculopapular eruption of trunk and neck	Not reported
HHV-8	Not reported	Not reported	Kaposi's sarcoma; primary effusion-based B-cell lymphoma; ? lymphoma; ? Castleman's disease	Not reported	Multifocal macules, plaques, or nodules (Kaposi's sarcoma)	Not reported
CHV-1	Not reported	Vesicular dermatitis at bite site with paresthesia	Not reported	Not reported	Painful vesicular eruption at bite	Severe encephalitis

CHV-1, cercopithecine virus 1; CMV, cytomegalovirus; EBV, Epstein-Barr virus; HHV-6-8, human herpesviruses 6-8; HSV-1, herpes simplex virus type 1; HSV-2, herpes simplex virus type 2; VZV, varicella-zoster virus.

cancer patients), who have either immature or deficient immune systems. In these cases, dissemination to visceral organs and the central nervous system (CNS) often leads to a poor outcome.

In most cases, following primary infection herpesviruses persist in the host in a latent state with no recurrence of clinical symptoms. However, a significant number of healthy seropositive persons (20% for EBV) will continue to shed infectious virus intermittently and contribute to the ubiquitous distribution of the herpesviruses. Clinical recurrence in most cases is the result of reactivation of latent infection rather than reinfection. In some cases (e.g., HSV-2), recurrence leads to a clinical illness closely resembling that of the primary presentation but usually of lesser severity (herpes genitalis), whereas in other cases (e.g., VZV) recurrence leads to a clinical illness which does not resemble the primary presentation and is often of greater clinical severity (herpes zoster). Reactivation may be induced by a variety of stimuli, including sunlight, emotional stress, menses, poor nutritional status, severe illness, trauma, or immunosuppression—all perhaps leading to a transient period of immune suppression. The herpesviruses are susceptible to nucleoside analogues such as vidarabine, trifluridine, penciclovir, acyclovir, ganciclovir, famciclovir, and valacyclovir, as well as the viral DNA polymerase inhibitors foscarnet and cidofovir.[6,7] Antiviral drug resistance to both nucleoside analogues and DNA polymerase inhibitors is of increasing concern.[8] Prevention of VZV infection is now attainable by use of a Food and Drug Administration (FDA)–approved live attenuated varicella vaccine (Varivax). Subunit vaccines against CMV and EBV are under development.

Herpes Simplex Viruses

AGENT

The infectious nature of HSV was first demonstrated by induction of typical dendritic corneal lesions in rabbits from material obtained from human herpes keratitis and herpes labialis lesions.[9] The distinction between the two virus strains, HSV-1 (above-the-belt lesions) and HSV-2 (below-the-belt lesions), was first made in 1968,[10] although it is now recognized that either virus strain can cause comparable primary infection at any anatomic site.[11] HSV virions contain 150 kbp of linear, double-stranded DNA encoding at least 84 proteins.[12] HSV gene expression may be temporally classified into three distinct phases termed alpha (immediate early), beta (early), and gamma (late). Alpha genes are expressed without prior protein synthesis and are largely involved in transcriptional transactivation. Beta genes are dependent upon prior alpha gene expression and encode proteins required for DNA replication. Gamma genes are dependent upon prior DNA replication and encode virion structural proteins. Beta and gamma gene expression is accompanied by inhibition of cellular DNA, RNA, and protein synthesis and by cell death.[13] At least 12 glycoproteins are embedded in the viral envelope; some of these glycoproteins are important in viral infectivity and also as targets of the immune system.[14] The antigenic difference between glycoprotein G (gG) from HSV-1 (gG-1) and HSV-2 (gG-2) is the basis for serologic distinction of the two HSV types.[15] In culture, HSV inhibits host cell macromolecular synthesis and causes rapid cell lysis of a number of cell types.[16,17]

EPIDEMIOLOGY

The two strains of the herpes simplex virus, HSV-1 and HSV-2, differ not only in genetic sequence (with approximately 50% sequence homology) but also in biologic and clinical behavior. Both strains are found worldwide with high seroprevalence and with no seasonal variation or epidemics. HSV-1 infection is primarily acquired during childhood and adolescence and is more widespread than HSV-2 infection, which is usually acquired during adolescence and early adulthood. HSV-1 seroprevalence exhibits marked geographic variation with relatively low rates (less than 70%) in France, Japan, the United States, and Sweden, and relatively high rates (greater than 95%) in Spain, Italy, Africa, China, and Latin America. Seroprevalence is higher in low socioeconomic groups and in developing regions—by adolescence, up to 80% have anti-HSV-1 antibodies in the developing world, while by the third decade only 60% are seropositive in the developed world.[18] HSV-2 seroprevalence is generally highest in Africa and South America, intermediate in northern Europe and North America, lower in western and southern Europe, and lowest in Asia.[19] Age-specific HSV-2 prevalence is higher in women than men and in populations with higher-risk sexual behaviors. HSV-1 infection is most often acquired through oral transmission following direct contact with either an acutely infected person or a healthy individual who is asymptomatically shedding virus. Primary or initial HSV-1 infection is most often asymptomatic.[20] Asymptomatic oral viral shedding is common in children (20%) while less common (3%) in adults.[21,22] However, unlike varicella, there is no apparent increase in transmission in day-care environments.[23]

DISEASE

Symptomatic primary infection follows an incubation period of 2 to 20 days and is characterized by fever, sore throat, cervical lymphadenopathy, and a vesicular rash in the oral cavity termed *gingivostomatitis*.[24] In adolescents and adults, symptomatic primary HSV-1 infection is most often characterized by a mononucleosis syndrome with pharyngitis, cervical lymphadenopathy, and fever.[25] Acute HSV-1 keratoconjunctivitis is a common cause of viral eye infection in adults in developed countries and presumably in the tropics and in most cases heals without corneal scarring. Recurrent herpes (HSV-1) keratitis manifests as a corneal ulcer with a characteristic dendritic branching pattern which may progress and lead to corneal scarring and loss of vision. Necrotizing herpetic retinopathies are rare, potentially blinding retinal disorders resulting from ocular infections with HSV-1 or HSV-2, varicella-zoster virus, or cytomegalovirus.[26] Herpetic dermatitis may be seen in athletes (herpes gladiatorium or scrumpox) from person-to-person abrasion, in health-care workers on their unprotected fingers (herpetic whitlow), and in patients with eczema in which herpetic superinfection leads to a severe disseminated form termed *Kaposi's varicelliform eruption*.[27–29] Although rare, HSV-1 encephalitis is the most common cause of acute sporadic viral encephalitis beyond the neonatal period. The early onset of seizures and localizing signs indicating temporal or frontal lobe involvement are characteristic.[30] Disseminated HSV infections outside the neonatal period are rare but can occur in immunocompromised patients and occasionally in the pregnant woman. Infection in these patients may disseminate by direct extension from the upper oral cavity to involve the trachea and lungs and/or the esophagus and gastrointestinal tract, or dissemination may occur via viremia to involve visceral organs and the central nervous system.[31,32] HSV-1 is also a common cause of genital herpes.[33–37]

Latent HSV-1 in cervical and trigeminal sensory ganglia may reactivate to cause recurrent infections; it is estimated that 20% to 40% of primary infections are followed by at least one symptomatic recurrence. The most common recurrent HSV-1 infection is herpes labialis (fever blisters or cold sores).[38,39] It is characterized by a vesicular eruption on or about the lips (Plate 57-1A; Fig. 57-1). Recurrent HSV-1 infections may also be asymptomatic or take the form of keratoconjunctivitis, keratitis, retinitis, whitlow, cutaneous lesions (gladiatorium), encephalitis, erythema multiforme, duodenal ulcer, or genital herpes, although HSV-1 tends to cause fewer episodes of recurrent genital herpes than does HSV-2.[35,36] HSV-2 infection is most often acquired by sexual transmission in adolescents or young adults.[40] It is estimated that 80% to 90% of HSV-2 infections are asymptomatic, but asymptomatically infected individuals shed virus from genital sites and may transmit virus to sexual partners or newborn infants.[41–44] The most common presentation of HSV-2 infection in adults is herpes genitalis, which is also the most common cause of genital ulcers in the developed world. The classical presentation of genital herpes is a painful vesicular eruption of the female vulva (Plate 57-1B), vagina, cervix, urethra, and perineum, and of the male glans, preputium, and shaft of the penis. The vesicular lesions typically progress to form shallow painful ulcers, which eventually crust and heal without scarring. Anorectal involvement and cutaneous lesions on the buttocks and thighs are relatively common and may result from anogenital sex or from zosteriform spread of virus from genital to rectal or other adjacent cutaneous sites. Primary infection is often complicated by aseptic meningitis and urinary retention and rarely by transverse myelitis and autonomic dysfunction. Recurrent HSV-2 genital herpes is quite common, and more than 50% of persons with symptomatic primary infection experience recurrences, typically four to five outbreaks in the first year. Recurrent HSV-1 genital herpes is relatively uncommon, and the patients that experience recurrences following a primary infection typically experience only a single outbreak annually. Symptomatic recurrent genital herpes tends to be considerably less severe than the initial outbreak. Subclinical HSV-2 genital infections (asymptomatic shedding) are very common following initial infection in both patients who have experienced symptomatic initial infection and those that are asymptomatically infected. HSV shedding, as detected by culture, occurs on about 3% of days for immunocompetent men and women, and more frequently if measured by polymerase chain reaction (PCR) methods or if the individual is HIV-infected.[42,45–47]

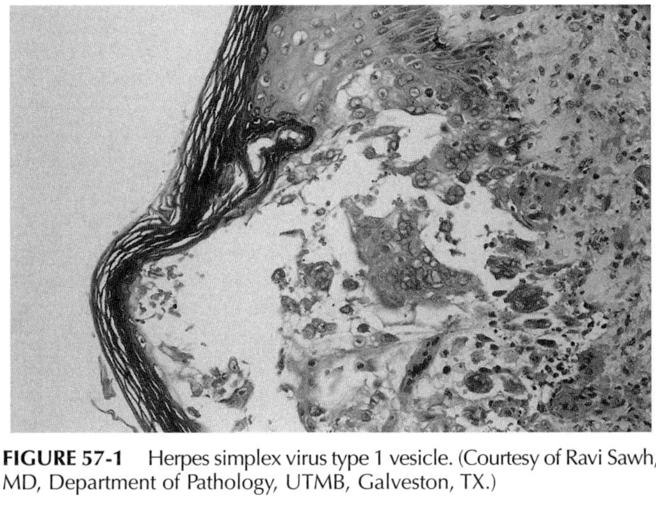

FIGURE 57-1 Herpes simplex virus type 1 vesicle. (Courtesy of Ravi Sawh, MD, Department of Pathology, UTMB, Galveston, TX.)

HSV infection of the fetus or newborn is referred to as neonatal herpes. Most cases occur as a consequence of spread of virus from a mother with genital HSV infection to her infant at the time of delivery, although cases of intrauterine transmission and postpartum acquisition have been documented.[44,48,49] Intrauterine infection early in gestation is a rare cause of intrauterine death and spontaneous abortion.[50] Perinatally acquired neonatal herpes, as with maternal genital herpes, may be due to either HSV-1 or HSV-2. The risk of maternal-infant transmission is greatest (approaching 50%) for women experiencing primary genital infection near term, while the risk of transmission for women with a history of genital herpes prior to pregnancy is less than 2%. The difference in risk of transmission probably relates to the presence or absence of HSV-specific maternally derived antibodies that afford the infant some protection against infection and the amount of virus present in the genital tract (high concentrations during the initial infection and several logs less virus during recurrent infections).[51] Most cases of neonatal herpes result from unrecognized or asymptomatic maternal genital herpes.[44] Unlike other HSV infections, asymptomatic neonatal herpes probably does not occur. Infection is initiated at a portal of entry: the conjunctival sac of the eye, the nasopharynx, or at a site where the skin is abraded such as occurs with the use of a scalp electrode. Infection that remains localized to the portal of entry results in skin, eye, or mouth (SEM) disease. Without treatment, SEM disease typically progresses to more severe forms of the infection through direct extension to the lungs to produce a necrotizing pneumonitis, via intraneuronal spread to cause CNS disease or through viremic spread to visceral organs resulting in disseminated infection.[51] There is approximately an equal distribution of cases in the SEM, CNS, and disseminated disease categories, but outcome, while generally good for infants with SEM disease, is very poor for infants with disseminated infection with mortality approaching 50% despite antiviral therapy. Infants with CNS disease are likely to survive, but those with HSV-2 infection are very likely to suffer neurological sequelae.[52]

PATHOGENESIS AND IMMUNITY

In vivo, primary infection begins with replication of virus in epithelial cells, which results in cell death. Virus gains entry to sensory nerve fibers that innervate the portal of entry and move via a retrograde axoplasmic transport process to the neuron cell body located in sensory ganglia, cervical and trigeminal ganglia in the case of oral infection, and sacral ganglia in the case of genital infection. Once the virus enters the neuronal nuclei, one of two events occur: Either the virus replicates producing progeny virus which moves back to the periphery via anterograde transport process where it is released at the nerve ending to infect epithelial cells, or the virus establishes a nonreplicating persistent state referred to as latency.[53] In latently infected neurons the virus remains largely quiescent, except for transcription of a small region of the genome that encodes an mRNA referred to as the latency associated transcript, or LAT.[54,55] Recurrent HSV infections occur when the latent virus periodically reactivates, resulting in viral production and transport to the periphery where the progeny virus are released from the nerve endings to replicate further in epithelial cells.[53,56] Both the primary and recurrent infections can be symptomatic, characterized by the development of typical herpetic vesicles and ulcers, but more often the recurrent infections are asymptomatic, with virus replication in epithelial cells causing no apparent disease but resulting in virus shedding, which can be transmitted to a susceptible host.[57,58] While it is recognized that LAT is involved in the reactivation from latency, the mechanisms responsible for the establishment, maintenance, and reactivation from latency are unknown. Reactivation from the latent state and the development of recurrent infections occur despite the presence of a full range of humoral and cellular immune responses that develop following the primary infection. The development of recurrent infections is probably facilitated by a variety of immune evasion genes encoded by the virus, including a virus-encoded Fc receptor that leads to resistance to antibody-dependent cell-mediated cytotoxicity (ADCC) and an ICP47 gene product that inhibits human leukocyte antigen (HLA)–mediated viral peptide expression and recognition by cytotoxic T cells.[59–63]

DIAGNOSIS

With the possible exception of herpes labialis, the clinical diagnosis of most HSV infections should be confirmed by laboratory testing. While most clinicians feel confident that they can accurately diagnose common HSV infections such as genital herpes, recent studies have shown that the accuracy of clinical diagnoses is poor even for experienced clinicians.[64,65] Four types of laboratory tests are available to help confirm the diagnosis, including viral culture, viral antigen detection, viral nucleic acid detection, and viral serology. For three of the four laboratory tests (culture, antigen detection, and nucleic acid detection), a lesion must be present in order to obtain the test sample. Serology may be useful in some cases when patients are evaluated after lesions have resolved. The gold standard for HSV diagnosis remains viral isolation by cell culture. Inoculation of fibroblast cell cultures with vesicular or cerebrospinal fluid (CSF) leads to rapid cytopathic change (24 to 48 hours) indicative of alphaherpesvirus infection (HSV-1, HSV-2, VZV). In general, HSV infection leads more consistently and rapidly to cytopathic change than does VZV. However, clear distinctions among HSV-1, HSV-2, and VZV can be made by the use of direct immunofluorescence using commercially available fluorescent-labeled virus-specific antibodies. Results of positive tests are typically available within five days and negative results within six days.[66] Detection of HSV antigen by enzyme immunoassay (EIA) is a less sensitive alternative to viral culture and nucleic acid detection, with sensitivities in the range of 65% to 81% compared to culture and PCR.[67,68] The Tzanck test, the cytologic examination of Wright-Giemsa–stained smears of scrapings from the vesicle base to detect multinucleated giant cells with intranuclear inclusions, should not be used due to its poor sensitivity.[69] Detection of HSV DNA by PCR is not widely available but is the preferred method for examining cerebrospinal fluid and is finding increasing use for the diagnosis of mucocutaneous HSV infections. In addition to greater sensitivity, test results may be available within 24 to 48 hours.[66,68,70–72] Serology may be useful in confirming the clinical diagnosis of a recent illness when lesions are no longer present. Serologic detection of HSV-specific immunoglobulin M (IgM) is generally not useful. The tests are insensitive, and recurrent HSV infection can result in an anamnestic IgM response. For the HSV-seronegative patient, seroconversion by comparison of paired acute and convalescent serum samples is evidence of a recent infection. Increasing titers of virus-specific IgG are not useful in establishing the diagnosis of a recent infection as titers can vary widely in response to recurrent infections. Detection of HSV-2-antibodies in an adolescent or adult is a biomarker for genital herpes. Cases of suspected genital herpes can be confirmed by detection of HSV-2-specific antibodies using type-specific serological tests that have recently become available commercially. One caveat to remember is that many cases of genital herpes are due to HSV-1, and hence the HSV-2 type-specific serological tests will not be useful in these cases. Clinicians need to be aware that several FDA-approved HSV antibody tests claim to be type-specific but are remarkably inaccurate. The only type-specific serological tests with acceptable performance characteristics are those based on differences in the HSV-1 and HSV-2 glycoprotein G.[73,74]

TREATMENT AND PROGNOSIS

Several drugs have proven effective in the treatment of various herpes simplex virus infections.[75] Intravenous acyclovir is the drug of choice for life-threatening HSV infections and HSV encephalitis. Oral herpes infections in the immunocompetent host have been successfully treated with oral acyclovir and its more bioavailable prodrug, valaciclovir, as well as a related nucleoside analog, famciclovir. Recurrent herpes labialis can also be treated with topical acyclovir and penciclovir and *N*-docosanol, an over-the-counter treatment. A variety of topical preparations have been used in the management of ocular herpes including acyclovir, trifluridine, idoxuridine, and vidarabine. Acyclovir-resistant strains of HSV have been documented in immunocompromised patients but are very rare in patients with an intact immune system.[76] Foscarnet and cidofovir have been successfully used in treatment of acyclovir-resistant HSV disease.[77] However, foscarnet-resistant HSV has been documented in patients with AIDS.[78] Antiviral drugs are useful in the treatment of primary and recurrent HSV infections, and daily suppressive use has proven effective in preventing recurrent oral and genital HSV infections. Latent infection is not altered by treatment with any currently available drug, and when suppressive therapy is discontinued most patients return to a pretreatment recurrence pattern. All life-threatening HSV infections require treatment, and most experts feel that all first episode cases of genital herpes should be treated with an oral antiviral drug.

PREVENTION AND CONTROL

Unfortunately, because of the high rate of clinically inapparent infections and healthy carrier states, hygienic measures are not very effective in prevention of HSV infections. However, patients with extensive mucocutaneous disease should be isolated as secretions and contact with lesions may result in transmission. Condom use has been shown to reduce, but not eliminate, the risk of genital HSV transmission.[79,80] A recent landmark study has shown that suppressive oral valaciclovir therapy (500 mg daily) can also significantly reduce, but not eliminate, the risk of transmission of genital HSV-2 infection among monogamous heterosexual couples.[81] Evidence suggests that cesarean delivery will reduce but not eliminate the risk of maternal-fetal transmission for women with active genital herpes at term.[82] This strategy is not without its consequences since it is estimated that four mothers die from cesarean-related complications for every seven babies prevented from developing fatal neonatal HSV infection.[83] An alternative but as yet unproven strategy is the use of an oral anti-HSV drug by women with a history of genital herpes for the final four weeks of gestation. The rationale is to prevent symptomatic recurrences and asymptomatic shedding at term and thereby reduce the risk of maternal-infant transmission. This strategy has been shown to reduce symptomatic and subclinical recurrences in the pregnant woman and to reduce the need for cesarean delivery for active genital herpes. The safety of such therapy in the fetus/newborn and its effectiveness in preventing neonatal herpes has not been established.[84–86] While there have been unsuccessful attempts to develop an effective HSV vaccine for over 60 years,[87] the recent success of an HSV glycoprotein vaccine in protecting women against acquiring genital herpes suggests that the development of a safe and effective HSV vaccine is feasible.[88] Further development of the HSV-2 glycoprotein D vaccine is under way.

Varicella-Zoster Virus

AGENT

The transmissible agent was demonstrated first in the vesicle fluid of varicella.[89] The connection between varicella and zoster was made by noting varicella among children exposed to family members with zoster.[90] Varicella was induced in susceptible children by inoculation with fluid from zoster lesions.[91] Viruses isolated from varicella and zoster were later shown to be identical biologically, antigenically, and genetically.[92,93] The VZV genome is the smallest of the known human herpesviruses and consists of double-stranded DNA 125 kb in size with approximately 70 genes.[94] Large portions of the genome are colinear with the HSV-1 genome.[95] The three most abundant viral envelope glycoproteins, gB, gE, and gH, likely are involved in infectivity since they are major targets of neutralizing antibodies. Antigenic similarity between HSV-1 gB and VZV gB leads to serologic cross-reactivity.[96]

EPIDEMIOLOGY

Humans are the only known natural host for VZV, which is associated with two forms of illness—a primary form known as varicella (chickenpox) and a secondary form known as herpes zoster (shingles). VZV is a highly contagious infection spread usually from airborne infectious oral or respiratory secretions or sometimes through direct transfer from skin lesions or via maternal-fetal transmission. Secondary attack rates in susceptible household contacts exceed 85%.[97] In temperate climates, infection rates show a marked seasonal variation, with epidemics in late winter and early spring. In contrast, no seasonal variation is seen in tropical climates. The reasons for this marked difference are not clear, although it has been suggested that heat, humidity, and lack of increased exposure to virus within confined spaces during the winter months may account for some of the difference. In rural India, despite close quarters, unexpectedly low rates of household transmission were documented.[98] In Singapore, varicella has occurred in two very large epidemics separated by 23 years.[99] Although asymptomatic primary infection is rare, serologic studies suggest that subclinical reinfection is common.[100] Rarely, immunocompetent patients may experience second episodes of varicella.[101] Varicella in temperate climates most often presents in preschool and school-age children less than 10 years of age with the highest incidence in the 3- to 6-year-old group.[102] Despite the prevalence of varicella in childhood, some people in temperate climates do reach adulthood without exposure: A study of military recruits in the United States in the prevaccine era showed that 8% of recruits are seronegative, with a slightly higher seronegative rate in nonwhites and a much higher seronegative rate (20%) in recruits enlisting from outside the United States.[103]

DISEASE

Following a 10- to 21-day (typically 14- to 16-day) incubation period, a prodrome of fever, headache, and malaise is followed 24 to 36 hours later by a diffuse maculopapular rash (Plate 57-1C). In the very young, the prodrome is often unrecognized. The rash is progressive, with successive crops at different stages occurring over a 2- to 7-day period, followed by complete healing within 20 days. The stages of the lesions are successively as follows: macular, papular, vesicular, pustular, and crusting. A hallmark of varicella is the simultaneous presence of lesions at various stages. The rash preferentially involves the trunk, with relative sparing and later involvement of the face and extremities. Oropharyngeal lesions may be seen. In normal, previously healthy children, the disease is generally benign and self-limiting, with the most common complication being secondary bacterial infection of skin lesions. Scarring is another common complication. Neurologic complications include encephalitis and acute cerebellar ataxia.[104] Varicella encephalitis with an incidence of 0.1% typically presents with headaches, seizures, altered thought patterns, and vomiting, with a mortality rate of 5% to 20%. Acute cerebellar ataxia is less common (0.025% incidence) than encephalitis and typically presents within 1 week of the rash with ataxia, vomiting, altered speech, vertigo, and/or tremor, with resolution within 2 to 4 weeks.

In immunodeficient or malnourished children not treated with intravenous acyclovir, the mortality rate ranges from 15% to 18%.[105] These cases are characterized by dissemination, with pneumonia, myocarditis, arthritis, hepatitis, hemorrhage, and encephalopathy (cerebellar ataxia is most common). Superinfection of skin lesions with *Staphylococcus aureus* or *Streptococcus pyogenes* may lead to pyoderma, impetigo, erysipelas, nephritis, gangrene, or sepsis. In the Central American tropics, varicella in young, malnourished children may be complicated by severe diarrhea.

Adults tend to have more severe disease than children, with a 15-fold increase in mortality. Adult-onset varicella is more often complicated by pneumonitis and encephalitis, with clinically significant pneumonitis in up to 15% of cases. In the prevaccine era, approximately 4% of normal adults in the United States (temperate climate) were VZV seronegative and therefore susceptible to adult-onset varicella.[106] In contrast, in the tropics a much higher percentage of adults is VZV seronegative and therefore susceptible to adult-onset varicella. Persons from tropical areas who relocate to temperate areas are at risk of developing adult-onset varicella, especially if in contact with young children. Maternal varicella in early gestation leads rarely to the congenital varicella syndrome characterized by skin defects, atrophy of extremities, and autonomic nervous system dysfunction.[107,108] Maternal varicella in late gestation may lead to neonatal varicella, with a mortality rate as high as 30% in untreated infants.[109,110]

Recurrent VZV infection is manifest as herpes zoster (shingles), a disease usually seen in adults over 50 years of age. Data suggest racial differences in the risk of developing zoster, with white elderly more at risk than black elderly.[111] Zoster may also rarely occur in childhood. Zoster in immunocompromised patients may be quite protracted and severe. The increased incidence of zoster in the aged as well as in immunocompromised patients is likely due to decreased anti-VZV cell-mediated immunity.[112,113] Interestingly, there is evidence that exposure of at-risk seropositive persons to varicella protects against development of zoster, presumably by boosting their immune response.[114] After primary infection, VZV (like HSV) persists in the latent state within spinal and cranial nerve ganglia. Nonspecific stimuli such as stress, immunodeficiency, or malignancy may induce activation of latent virus with involvement of the skin in the nerve distribution supplied by the affected ganglion. Herpes zoster presents after a 3- to 4-day prodrome of fever, malaise, and gastrointestinal disturbance as a painful cutaneous vesicular eruption in a dermatomal distribution (Plate 57-1D). The rash is usually unilateral and along one dermatome only. In severe cases, the eruption may be more generalized and varicelliform. The vesicles heal within 5 days, but postherpetic neuralgia may commence. Postherpetic neuralgia, seen in up to 50% of patients over 50 years old, is defined as constant or intermittent debilitating pain of more than one month's duration in the area of the involved dermatome. Infection of the eye, ear, and throat may occur if ophthalmic, trigeminal, or geniculate ganglia are involved. Herpes zoster ophthalmicus is a particularly serious condition, which if untreated may lead to blindness. The Ramsay-Hunt syndrome is defined as a triad of involvement of the external auditory meatus, loss of taste in the tongue, and ipsilateral facial palsy. Involvement of the spinal cord may lead to weakness or cranial nerve palsy. The risk of encephalitis is increased in the elderly with cranial nerve involvement and in AIDS patients. Postzoster encephalitis may present in one of three forms: infarcts due to large-vessel vasculitis, multifocal leukoencephalopathy, and ventriculitis.[115]

PATHOGENESIS AND IMMUNITY

As is characteristic of alphaherpesviruses, VZV replicates rapidly in a restricted range of cells in vitro with rapid cell death. VZV replicates best in human diploid fibroblasts but also infects primary human keratinocytes.[116] A live attenuated vaccine strain (OKa) is propagated in WI-38 and MRC-5 diploid fibroblast lines. In cell culture, the virus remains largely cell associated with little release of infectious virus.[117] However, cell-free virus can be obtained by sonication of infected cultures. Infection induces the formation of multinucleated cells with eosinophilic intranuclear inclusions seen both in vitro and in vivo. Transmission occurs mainly through respiratory spread, and viremia disseminates the virus to mucocutaneous sites, visceral organs, and the peripheral nervous system. Latent infection is established in cranial, dorsal root, and autonomic ganglia.[118–124] The cell specificity of latent virus was previously controversial, but it is now widely agreed that latent VZV primarily resides in neurons and to a much lesser extent in non-neuronal satellite cells.[125] Evidence suggests that at least five viral genes are transcribed during latency, and unlike HSV latency, transcription from the latent VZV genome results in viral protein expression.[126] Like HSV, latent VZV can reactivate, albeit very rarely, to cause recurrent infection (e.g., zoster or shingles). Unlike HSV, reactivation of VZV can result in neuronal injury that causes a prolonged pain syndrome referred to as postherpetic neuralgia.[127]

DIAGNOSIS

The clinical diagnosis of varicella in childhood, now that variola (smallpox) has been eradicated, is not usually difficult. The rash is quite characteristic and only rarely needs to be differentiated from enteroviral exanthem, *S. aureus* infection, drug reactions, contact dermatitis, and disseminated HSV-1 infection. Diagnosis by culture of vesicle fluid is less sensitive than for HSV or CMV and may take 7 days. This method has been supplanted by the more rapid and sensitive shell vial method, which gives results in 1 to 3 days. Very rapid, sensitive, and specific detection may supplant culture-based systems in the near future as multiplex PCR assays become more widely available.[128] Scrapings of the base of the vesicles reveal multinucleated giant cells with intranuclear inclusions, which cannot reliably be differentiated from HSV. However, immunofluorescence on cultures or scrapings utilizing virus-specific antibodies can differentiate between HSV-1, HSV-2, and VZV. Serologic detection of IgM and a high titer or greater than fourfold rise in IgG anti-VZV antibody may be useful in some cases. Detection of IgM may signify primary infection (chickenpox), while either a high titer or fourfold rise in IgG titer indicates recurrence. However, increased IgM may also be seen in recurrence. The clinical diagnosis of herpes zoster in adults is also not usually difficult given the characteristic dermatomal pattern of involvement.

TREATMENT AND PROGNOSIS

Although vidarabine and interferon-α have been used in the treatment of severe VZV infection, acyclovir is the drug of choice.[129] Acyclovir is most effective in severe VZV infection if administered intravenously (IV) within 24 hours after the rash develops.[130] Oral acyclovir treatment of otherwise healthy children with chickenpox should be considered, particularly in adolescents and secondary household contacts, although the benefit is modest.[131–134] Due to the detection of acyclovir-resistant strains in patients with AIDS, foscarnet therapy should be considered for severe infection in this setting.[135,136] For herpes zoster, the drugs of choice are famciclovir and valacyclovir. Early treatment of zoster has been shown to both shorten the course of cutaneous disease and reduce the duration and severity of postherpetic neuralgia.[137] Topical steroids may also be useful in herpetic uveitis and keratitis. Painful zoster may be treated with wet compresses and analgesics containing codeine. Gabapentin, a structural analogue of the neurotransmitter gamma-aminobutyric acid, is useful in the management of postherpetic neuralgia.[138] Antihistamines may be useful to ameliorate the intense pruritus of varicella in childhood. A live attenuated vaccine (OKa) is licensed in the United States for routine use in children and susceptible adults.[139] The vaccine has been shown to be safe and effective, and its widespread use has resulted in a decline in varicella cases in the United States.[140] The vaccine virus may induce mild varicella and is capable of reactivation with development of herpes zoster.[141,142] In some cases, as in patients with leukemia, two doses of vaccine are required to achieve 95% seroconversion rates.[143] As with other vaccines, immunization with the VZV vaccine does not always result in protection, as evidenced by numerous reports of vaccine failure.[144]

PREVENTION AND CONTROL

Owing to the high prevalence of the infection in the prevaccine era, its high transmissibility, and the fact that infected persons are contagious 24 to 48 hours before clinical signs occur, it is difficult to prevent infection by isolation. However, reverse isolation is recommended for hospitalized patients with varicella and for children or immunocompromised adults with herpes zoster. Patients with varicella should be bathed often to prevent staphylococcal and streptococcal superinfection. Immunocompromised children, neonates born to mothers who present with varicella during the week prior to and a few days after birth, and seronegative pregnant females should be treated with varicella-zoster immune globulin (VZIG) within 96 hours of exposure.[145] VZIG, however, has no effect on the course of herpes zoster or on risk of reactivation.

Human Cytomegalovirus

AGENT

Human CMV is classified as a betaherpesvirus by virtue of tropism for salivary glands; high species specificity (no natural host other than humans); and slow, nonlethal growth in cell culture.[146] Of the human herpesviruses, CMV is most closely related genetically to HHV-6.[147] CMV virions range from 150 nm to 200 nm in diameter and may be distinguished from other herpesviruses by having a more pleomorphic envelope.[148] CMV has the largest genome of all herpesviruses at 230 kbp, with a large-scale genomic arrangement similar to that of HSV-1.[149,150] The human CMV genome has been completely sequenced and contains approximately 200 open reading frames (ORFs) and an unusually large number of repeat units.[151] Purified virions contain at least 30 polypeptides, including the major capsid protein (MCP, pUL86), which, unlike capsid proteins from other herpesviruses, is poorly immunogenic.[152,153] The major envelope glycoprotein of CMV (gB, gpUL55), which is involved in cell penetration and fusion, is the major target of neutralizing antibody, as well as an important target of the cellular immune system.[154–156] Sequence variation in gB has been used to define four CMV gB subtypes.[157] gB type 1 CMV may be more often associated with clinically significant disease in bone marrow transplant recipients.[158]

EPIDEMIOLOGY

CMV is ubiquitous, with seroprevalence rates of 40% to 80% in young adults in the Western world, while in some tropical regions, such as Barbados and Tanzania, the rate approaches 100%.[159] No seasonal variations are described.[159] The vast majority of CMV infections are subclinical, but in infancy infection is often followed by a prolonged period of viral shedding.[160,161] Those at risk of serious infection include the fetus, the newborn, the elderly, the debilitated, and the immunocompromised. Primary infection most often occurs in young children. Low socioeconomic status, breastfeeding, and increased exposure to young children is associated with an increased rate of early childhood infection. Up to 60% of infants acquire CMV infection during the first 6 months. Perhaps the most common mode of transmission in infants is by breastfeeding.[162,163] At least 30% of seropositive women excrete CMV in breast milk during the first year postpartum.[164] Young children who attend day care and are in close contact with other children are much more likely to acquire CMV infection than children who stay home (80% vs. 20%).[165] Seroprevalence again increases in adolescence and young adulthood with sexual activity. Infection in this age group may be manifest as a mononucleosis syndrome with fever, fatigue, and myalgia mimicking that caused by EBV.[166,167] However, in contrast to EBV-induced mononucleosis, adenopathy, pharyngitis, and tonsillitis are not pronounced, and the heterophile antibody test is negative.

DISEASE

Following primary infection, viral excretion from many sites, including saliva and urine, is prolonged, thus leading to a vast reservoir of infectious virus. However, probably owing to its unstable nature, CMV transmission requires intimate contact, as has been described in children in day-care settings or in overcrowded or unsanitary areas. CMV has also been implicated in some cases of recurrent aphthous ulcers and Behçet's disease.[168] However, those most at risk of serious CMV infection are neonates and immunocompromised (post-transplant, AIDS) patients. In the United States, 1% of newborns shed CMV in the urine, thus making CMV infection the most common congenital infection. Congenital CMV infection most often follows primary maternal infection. The risk to the fetus is much less in the case of reactivated maternal infection due to the presence of a preexisting maternal immune response. Given the very high seropositivity rates in the developing world, congenital CMV is probably less common in the tropics. Approximately 1% of CMV-seronegative pregnant females will acquire a primary infection during pregnancy with a fetal infection rate of 40%, while approximately 10% of CMV-seropositive pregnant females will have a recurrent CMV infection during pregnancy with a fetal infection rate of 10%. Approximately 20% of the time, primary maternal infection leads to clinically apparent disease in the newborn, with a mortality rate of 20% to 30%. Early congenital infection often leads to fetal death or permanent neurologic damage. In fact, more than 90% of infants born with symptomatic congenital infection and up to 20% of those with asymptomatic infection later prove to be permanently neurologically impaired. The most severe form of congenital infection, cytomegalic inclusion disease (CID), is characterized by disseminated infection leading to hepatosplenomegaly, microcephaly, mental retardation, nerve deafness, thrombocytopenic purpura, and hemolytic anemia. The seriousness of congenital CMV infection is underscored by the fact that in the United States and England 0.1% of all newborns have CMV-associated residual defects (hearing loss, psychomotor retardation, blindness). Hearing loss is by far the most common neurologic deficit and is the most common cause of acquired hearing loss in U.S. children, while chorioretinitis leading to loss of vision is the second most common CMV-induced neurologic deficit.[169,170] Children with CID may excrete CMV in body fluids for years and therefore serve as reservoirs of infection.[171] Postnatal infection may follow transmission from an infected mother's cervicovaginal secretions, urine, saliva, or breast milk. Although usually asymptomatic, postnatally infected infants serve as sources of infection of children and adults. Seronegative pregnant mothers are at risk of infection from toddlers attending preschool since up to 80% may be excreting virus in saliva and urine.[165] Given the high rate of the CMV carrier state, CMV may also be transmitted through blood transfusion, which in the premature infant may lead to a respiratory distress syndrome and in seronegative adults to a mononucleosis syndrome. In immunocompromised patients (organ transplant, malignancy, AIDS), CMV infection may lead to severe multisystem disease with fever, pneumonitis, leukopenia, arthritis, hepatitis, retinitis, ulcerative gastrointestinal disease, and encephalitis. CMV is probably the most common post-transplant infection, with viral shedding in nearly 100% of all patients.[172] The role of CMV infection in transplant rejection is unclear; although it has been implicated as a cofactor in chronic liver allograft rejection, it apparently plays no role in acute cardiac transplant rejection.[173,174] CMV has been implicated in chemotherapy-induced neutropenic fevers of unknown origin.[175] CMV has also been implicated as a cofactor in the clinical progression of AIDS.[176] Recent reports of the presence of CMV within atherosclerotic vascular lesions has led to suggestions that CMV may be a cofactor in the pathogenesis of atherosclerosis.[177,178]

PATHOGENESIS AND IMMUNITY

CMV gene expression can be temporally classified into three distinct phases, termed alpha (immediate early), beta (delayed early), and gamma (late). Alpha genes are expressed without prior protein synthesis and are largely involved in transcriptional transactivation. Beta genes are dependent upon prior alpha gene expression and encode proteins required for DNA replication. Gamma genes are dependent upon prior DNA replication and encode virion structural proteins. CMV replication is slow, with 42 to 72 hours required before progeny virus is recovered.[179] Like all betaherpesviruses, CMV exhibits a highly restricted host cell range in vitro. Primary fibroblasts from skin and lung are most permissive, while undifferentiated or transformed cells are nonpermissive.[180] Unlike the alphaherpesviruses, CMV stimulates cellular molecular synthesis and cell enlargement (cytomegalia).[181,182] Large characteristic nucleocapsid inclusions form within the nucleus and the cytoplasm.[183] In primary infection and in healthy carriers, CMV appears to replicate in salivary gland epithelium and may also be found in renal tubular cells and peripheral blood monocytes.[184–187] However, in the immunocompromised host (fetus, newborn, AIDS patients, transplant recipients), CMV may replicate in virtually any organ.

DIAGNOSIS

Congenital CMV infection should be differentiated from congenital toxoplasmosis, rubella, herpes simplex, and syphilis. Clinically, congenital toxoplasmosis closely resembles CID, but unlike CMV the cerebral calcifications are usually scattered rather than confined to the periventricular areas. Since the introduction of the rubella vaccine in 1969, congenital rubella has become rare in the developed world, yet remains a problem in the tropics. Congenital rubella is more often associated with glaucoma, cataracts, microphthalmia, and cardiac malformations (especially patent ductus arteriosus). Congenital herpes simplex is rare and probably leads in most cases to fetal demise. Neonatal disease is most often acquired at birth from mothers with herpes genitalis and usually, but not always, presents with a characteristic vesicular rash. Detection of virus-specific IgM in the affected neonate is usually sufficient to confirm the diagnosis. Newborns with congenital syphilis commonly present with a characteristic complex of rhinitis, diffuse maculopapular desquamative rash, and osteochondritis. CMV mononucleosis in older children and young adults may be differentiated from EBV mononucleosis by a combination of clinical features (higher fever, absent or mild pharyngitis, and adenopathy) and a negative heterophile antibody test. Although more specific, viral serology for mononucleosis is seldom required. CMV hepatitis is usually milder than disease due to hepatitis A, B, or C. Elevated CMV-specific IgM or a fourfold rise in IgG titers using paired acute and convalescent serum samples are useful in normal adults to detect active CMV infection. CMV culture is most useful in cases in which serology is unreliable, that is, in congenital infection and in the post-transplant and AIDS setting. Amniotic fluid culture may be appropriate in some circumstances. Culture of CMV on human embryonic fibroblasts is sensitive and specific but is not a rapid test—the characteristic cytopathic effect (CPE) may take up to 2 to 5 weeks

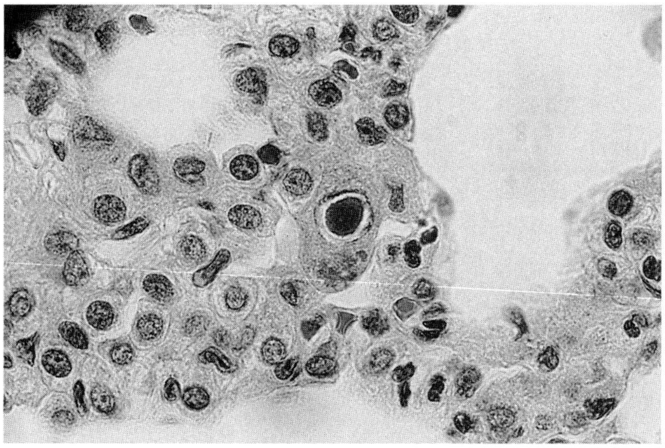

FIGURE 57-2 Cytomegalovirus pneumonitis. (Courtesy of Vicki Schnadig, MD, Department of Pathology, UTMB, Galveston, TX.)

to become apparent. More rapid diagnosis is obtained with the use of shell vial cultures in which the sample is centrifuged onto a fibroblast culture and is stained on day 1 or 2 with CMV early antigen (EA)–specific fluorescein-conjugated antiserum. The shell vial assay has been shown to be more sensitive than serology in the diagnosis of infection in the neonate and immunodeficient patient.[188] However, because of the high rate of asymptomatic viral shedding and reactivation, interpretation of culture and serology results must be carefully evaluated in each specific clinical setting. PCR-based tests provide very rapid, sensitive, and specific detection and will likely eventually supplant culture-based systems. PCR was shown to be more sensitive in detection of CMV from urine than either conventional or shell vial culture.[189] However, the detection of CMV DNA by PCR does not correlate well with CMV disease—in one study, the positive predictive value of CMV PCR for disease in transplant patients was only 27.8%.[190] It is likely that serial quantitative PCR assays in susceptible populations will lead to improvements in the positive predictive value of the test. Although CMV has been classified by gene sequence analysis of the CMV major envelope glycoprotein gB into four subtypes, a recent PCR study failed to detect subtype differences in clinical outcome or viral load in renal transplant patients.[191] CMV infection in tissue is characterized by the presence of large intranuclear inclusions in infected cells (Fig. 57-2).

TREATMENT AND PROGNOSIS

Ganciclovir and foscarnet have been used both as CMV prophylaxis and as treatment of severe infection in the post-transplant and AIDS settings. The renal toxicity of foscarnet and the myelotoxicity of ganciclovir sometimes limit their use. In CMV retinitis, both foscarnet and cidofovir are effective. Ganciclovir, cidofovir, and foscarnet resistance has been shown to be due both to viral DNA polymerase mutations, and, in the case of ganciclovir, also to poor phosphorylation.[192–195]

PREVENTION AND CONTROL

The importance of prevention of primary CMV infection in pregnant women is difficult to overemphasize. CMV is probably the most common congenital infection worldwide. Seronegative pregnant women exposed to toddlers, especially those with a high level of contact with other toddlers, as in the day-care setting, are at risk of acquiring primary CMV infection with fetal transmission and development of congenital CMV disease, a serious disease which leads in most cases to either fetal loss or a child with permanent neurologic damage. Simple behavioral changes by pregnant women in contact with toddlers, such as frequent handwashing and use of disposable diapers and gloves, may be quite effective in preventing infection.[196] In seronegative newborns and allograft recipients, the risk of post-transfusion CMV infection can be markedly reduced by administration of either leukocyte-reduced blood products or CMV-seronegative donor blood products. Subunit vaccines using the CMV major envelope glycoprotein gB and other proteins are currently under development.[197]

Epstein-Barr Virus

AGENT

EBV is a human herpesvirus of the gammaherpesvirus subfamily and genus *Lymphocryptovirus*. Humans are the only known natural host for EBV, although all Old World primate species have closely related lymphocryptoviruses.[198] EBV was first identified as a typical herpesvirus by electron microscopy from a biopsy of endemic African Burkitt's lymphoma.[199] EBV was also shown to cause most cases of infectious mononucleosis.[200] Permanent transformed cell lines harboring EBV can be obtained from infectious mononucleosis blood and from Burkitt's lymphoma tissue.[201] Subsequently, the virus was shown to also be associated with a number of other human diseases, including undifferentiated nasopharyngeal carcinoma (NPC) and other lymphocyte-rich carcinomas, oral hairy leukoplakia in AIDS patients, malignant lymphoma of both B- and T-cell types, and Hodgkin's disease (HD).[202–210] Although in vitro only B cells appear to be efficiently infected and transformed, in vivo it appears as though the host cell range for EBV is not as restricted—not only B cells but in some cases T cells, epithelial cells, and mesenchymal cells may harbor EBV. EBV gains access to the B lymphocyte through the C3d receptor (CR2, CD21).[211] An EBV strain obtained from a patient with mononucleosis and used to transform marmoset B cells (B95–8) has been cloned and sequenced.[212] EBV DNA is 172 kb in size with several sets of repeat elements separated by unique regions containing more than 100 ORFs. Given the importance of the phenomenon of B-cell latency, a great deal of attention has been devoted to the latent genes which encode six nuclear proteins (*EBNA1–6*), three membrane proteins (*LMP1, 2A, 2B*), and two highly abundant nonpolyadenylated nuclear RNAs (*EBER1-2*). Also, there are some EBV genes with homology to human genes, including *BHRF1* (*bcl2*-like), *BCRF1* (*IL10*-like), and *BZLF1* (*jun/fos*-like).[213–215] It has been suggested that these genes may have been appropriated from the primate genome to provide a survival advantage to EBV-infected cells.[198]

EPIDEMIOLOGY

There appear to be two distinct strains of EBV, type 1 (or A type) and type 2 (or B type), which differ in geographic distribution, biologic properties, and genetic sequences.[216,217] The strains differ genetically mostly in the *EBNA2, EBNA3,* and *EBER* genes. Type 2 isolates transform B cells in vitro with much lower efficiency than type 1 isolates.[218] Although type 2 isolates are more commonly isolated from Asia, Africa, and AIDS patients, they may be recovered not infrequently from the oropharynx of normal persons from the developed world.[216] Although type 1 isolates are more commonly isolated from tumors, no clear difference in pathogenicity of type 1 vs. type 2 EBV is established.

DISEASE

EBV is a human gammaherpesvirus that establishes transient lytic infection of the oropharyngeal mucosal epithelium and chronic latent infection of B lymphocytes. Infection most often occurs following contact with infectious saliva of healthy carriers or patients with infectious mononucleosis. EBV, like the other herpesviruses, has a ubiquitous distribution with an overall adult seroprevalence exceeding 90%. The high rate of seroprevalence is maintained by a large population of healthy carriers—up to 20% of healthy seropositive people in the developed world and 45% of African children excrete virus intermittently in saliva. Unlike CMV, EBV is not recognized as a common congenital or neonatal infection and has not clearly been shown to be transmitted through the genital tract. In the developing world and especially in subequatorial areas of Africa endemic for Burkitt's lymphoma, early childhood infection is the rule and is nearly always asymptomatic. Even in developed countries, many, if not most, primary infections occur in childhood and are subclinical. Primary infection as it occurs in adolescents and young adults classically presents as infectious mononucleosis. Because of the high rate of childhood infection in the tropics, infectious mononucleosis is seldom encountered. Although EBV accounts for the majority of cases of infectious mononucleosis, similar syndromes are caused by CMV, *Toxoplasma,* and viral hepatitis. EBV-associated mononucleosis typically follows an incubation period of 1 to 2 months and is characterized by several weeks of fever, pharyngitis, malaise, headache, and posterior cervical lymphadenopathy. Laboratory features include atypical lymphocytosis, positive heterophile antibody test (which may be negative in children), positive IgM anti–viral capsid antigen (VCA), and elevated IgG anti-VCA. Most of the atypical lymphocytes in peripheral blood express an immunophenotype consistent with activated CD8-positive cytotoxic T cells, with a lesser increase in natural killer (NK) cells.[219] Other manifestations include mild hepatitis, splenomegaly, encephalitis, polyneuritis, pneumonia, ampicillin-induced rash, and a variety of autoimmune phenomena. In the vast majority of cases, complete spontaneous recovery without recurrence follows. Rarely, however, probably associated with immunodeficiency, either a fatal hemophagocytic syndrome with marrow failure or malignant B-cell lymphoma may intervene. EBV, unlike the other human herpesviruses, with the possible exception of HHV-8, is clearly oncogenic and as such is classically associated with at least three human malignancies—endemic Burkitt's B-cell lymphoma, post-transplant B-cell lymphoma, and NPC—and more loosely associated with other human malignancies—HD, lymphocyte-rich carcinoma, gastric adenocarcinoma,[220,221] smooth muscle tumors,[222,223] some T-cell lymphomas, and other B-cell lymphomas (AIDS-associated, sporadic nonendemic Burkitt's, primary CNS lymphoma).[224] EBV is also associated with Duncan's disease, a fatal infectious mononucleosis–like illness in boys with the rare X-linked lymphoproliferative syndrome.[225] HIV-positive patients and rarely post-transplant patients develop a benign wartlike lesion on the lateral borders of the tongue called oral hairy leukoplakia, which is productively infected with EBV.[206]

Endemic Burkitt's lymphoma is the most common childhood malignancy in the central equatorial regions of Africa in areas ravaged by holoendemic falciparum malaria.[226] Endemic Burkitt's lymphoma is also found in coastal Papua New Guinea, another area ravaged by holoendemic falciparum malaria.[201] It usually presents as a rapidly enlarging tumor of the jaw or abdomen in children. The tumor is very aggressive and fatal without treatment. However, due to the rapid growth rate, the tumor is exquisitely sensitive to chemotherapy. Treatment with cyclophosphamide, vincristine, cytarabine, and intrathecal methotrexate leads to a 93% clinical remission rate and 63% 2-year disease-free survival rate. Prospective serologic studies indicate that children who develop Burkitt's lymphoma have elevated EBV antibody titers (higher than age-matched controls) months to years prior to tumor development. The tumor has a highly characteristic "starry-sky" histologic appearance with monotonous sheets of mitotically active lymphoblasts interspersed with debris-laden phagocytic histiocytes (Fig. 57-3). The tumor cells invariably contain a chromosome translocation involving the c-*myc* gene on chromosome 8 and an immunoglobulin gene on chromosome 2, 14, or 22: t(8;14), t(2;8), or t(8;22). Sporadic Burkitt's lymphoma is a tumor that usually presents as an abdominal mass in older children and adults in nonendemic areas. Despite sharing an identical histologic appearance and similar c-*myc* translocations with endemic Burkitt's lymphoma, sporadic Burkitt's is uncommonly (approximately 20%) associated with EBV.[227] The c-*myc* breakpoints seen in endemic Burkitt's are most often found far upstream of *c-myc,* while those seen in sporadic Burkitt's lymphoma are most often found within, or close to, the c-*myc* gene.[228]

NPC is a disease of adults with a peak incidence at age 50 to 54 years and a male predominance (3:1). NPC is one of the

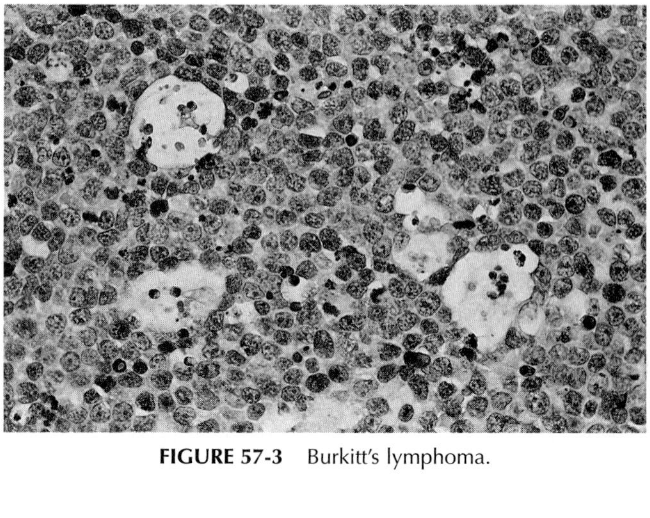

FIGURE 57-3 Burkitt's lymphoma.

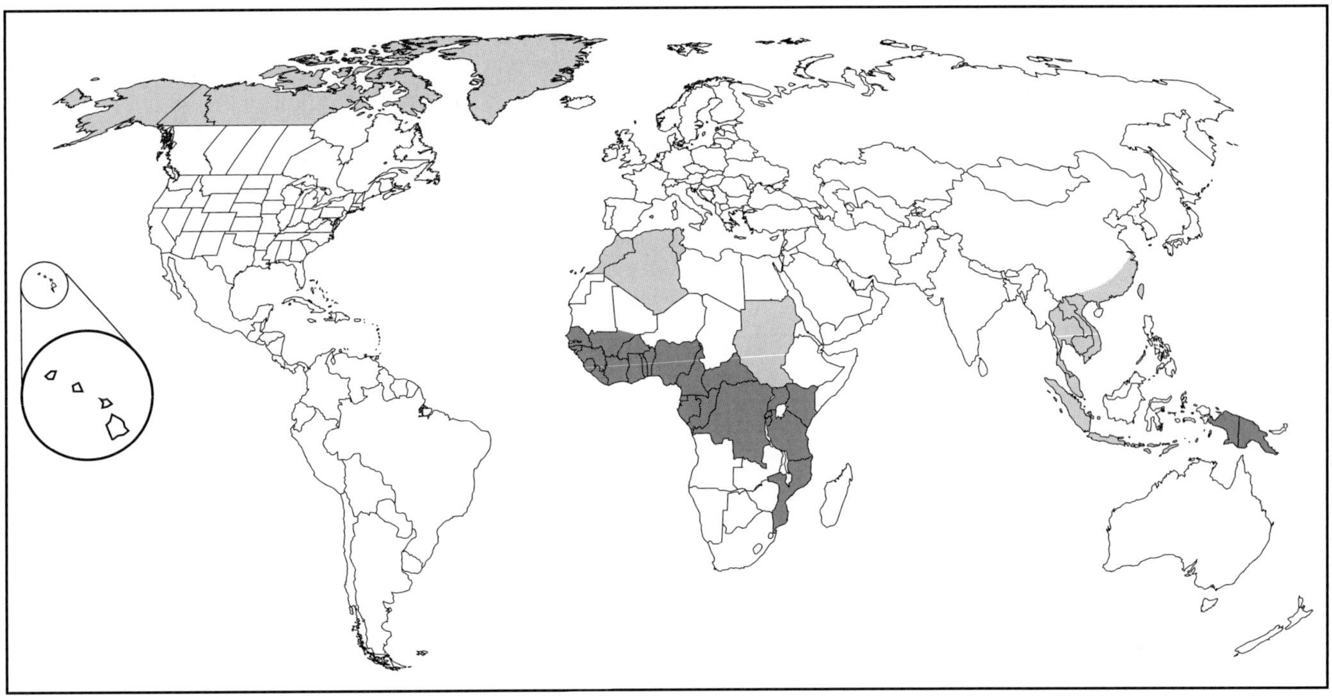

Nasopharyngeal Carcinoma and Endemic African Burkitt's Lymphoma

■ Endemic African Burkitt's Lymphoma

□ Nasopharyngeal Carcinoma

most common malignant tumors in the southern Chinese, especially Cantonese, and has a lower incidence in North African Arabs and in Aleuts. The endemic nature of NPC suggests that either genetic or environmental factors may influence risk. Genetic studies of the Singapore Chinese population have suggested linkage to HLA haplotypes A2Bw46 and A19B17.[229] Environmental studies have suggested an increased risk with consumption of salted fish during infancy and occupational exposure to smoke or dust.[230–233] Salted fish from southern China and Greenland, as well as preserved foods from Tunisia, all areas with endemic NPC, contain a significant amount of volatile nitrosamines.[234] The role of environmental factors is underscored by the fact that the incidence of NPC in second-generation immigrant Chinese in North America is lower than in the first generation.[235] Patients may present with nasal stuffiness, nosebleeds, ear pain, hearing loss, facial pain, difficulty swallowing, taste changes, and cervical adenopathy. There are three histologic subtypes of NPC: well-differentiated squamous cell carcinoma, nonkeratinizing carcinoma, and lymphocyte-rich undifferentiated carcinoma with EBV in situ positive tumor cells (Plate 57-2). The lymphocyte-rich undifferentiated form of NPC is both the most common (80% of cases) and the most consistently EBV-associated subtype (100% of cases) (see Plate 57-2), whether occurring in endemic areas or not.[204,236] EBV gene expression is limited to *EBER1/2, EBNA1, LMP1/2,* and unusual transcripts from the *Bam A* region.[222,237] *LMP1* gene expression has been shown to induce phenotypic changes and transformation in epithelial cells and is therefore likely to play a role in NPC pathogenesis.[238–241] Analysis of DNA from NPC has revealed deletions on the short arm of chromosome 3, which may be sites of tumor suppressor genes.[242] Overexpression of wild-type *p53* and *bcl-2* in NPC cells also suggests a role for these cellular genes in NPC pathogenesis.[243,244] EBV is also associated in NPC-endemic areas, especially Southeast Asia, with carcinomas with undifferentiated NPC-like histologic features arising in the thymus, salivary glands, and lung. However, unlike NPC, similar tumors arising in nonendemic areas are seldom EBV associated.

Organ transplant patients are at increased risk for the development of EBV-associated post-transplant B-cell lymphoproliferative disorders (PTLDs).[245,246] The risk varies with the organ transplanted, with the highest risk associated with HLA-mismatched T cell–depleted bone marrow transplants (24%) and the lowest risk associated with undepleted bone marrow and renal transplants (1%). This organ-specific risk is likely a reflection of the various degrees of induced immunosuppression required to prevent graft rejection.[247] Another important risk factor for PTLD is EBV serologic status, with EBV-seronegative patients at a 76-fold increased risk compared with EBV-seropositive patients.[248,249] The increased risk of PTLD in the pediatric age group reflects the relatively low seropositivity rate of children in the developed world. The clinical presentation of PTLD is highly variable but may present in the early post-transplant period, particularly in seronegative patients, as an infectious mononucleosis–like illness with fever, lymphadenopathy, and fatigue; in the late post-transplant period as a solid tumor, often extranodal, with involvement of the gastrointestinal tract, CNS, or allograft; and in heavily immunosuppressed patients as a fulminant sepsis-like presentation with multiorgan involvement.[250] Pathologically, PTLD is heterogeneous and ranges from diffuse polymorphous lymphoid hyperplasia to monomorphic large B-cell lymphoma (Fig. 57-4). B-cell clonality studies indicate heterogeneity with polyclonal, oligoclonal, and monoclonal B-cell populations.[251,252] The EBV gene expression pattern is very similar to that seen in vitro in lymphoblastoid cells with limited lytic activity.[253,254] Although limited cytogenetic studies have failed to identify a characteristic chromosomal abnormality in most cases, some monomorphic cases do contain Burkitt-like c-*myc* rearrangements.[254] PTLD has been subclassified into three clinicopathologic types—a polyclonal plasmacytic type without cytogenetic abnormalities, which regresses following immunorestoration; a monoclonal polymorphic type without cytogenetic abnormalities, which regresses following either immunorestoration or chemotherapy; and a monoclonal immunoblastic lymphoma or myeloma with mutations of c-*myc*, *N-ras*, or *p*53, which does not respond to therapy.[255]

HD is a common malignant lymphoproliferative disease with a worldwide distribution. First described by Thomas Hodgkin from postmortem records of adults with massive peripheral lymphadenopathy, the disease continues to confound efforts to fully understand the process.[256] The incidence of HD is bimodal, with an early peak in the developed world in late adolescents and early adults that is shifted to childhood in the developing world and a late peak beyond the age of 50 years.[257] This pattern of incidence, as well as other epidemiologic data, had suggested that an infectious agent is involved. HD usually presents with peripheral lymphadenopathy often confined to the neck and sometimes accompanied by a mediastinal mass or splenomegaly, or both. Patients may also present with a variety of nonspecific systemic findings including fever, weight loss, anemia, and malaise. Unlike the non-Hodgkin's lymphomas, HD rarely involves extranodal sites other than the spleen and bone marrow.

Prognosis and treatment of HD are heavily dependent on determination of the stage of the disease. The Ann Arbor staging system comprises stages I to IV based on anatomical extent, followed by an A (without) or B (with) for the presence of systemic findings.[258] Treatment ranges from surgical excision and limited radiotherapy in stage I disease to combination radiotherapy and multiagent chemotherapy in stage IV disease. HD is usually classified as one of four histologic types— nodular sclerosis, mixed cellularity, lymphocyte predominant, and lymphocyte depleted—which differ not only in the composition of the reactive background but also in the type of Reed-Sternberg (RS) cells.[259] Although there is some association of histologic type with prognosis, this association may not be independent of stage. The histology of HD is puzzling—like no other malignant tumor, the malignant RS cells are usually in the distinct minority, while most of the cells within the tumor are not malignant and include T cells, histiocytes, granulocytes, and fibrous stromal cells (Fig. 57-5). The RS cell itself is also a mystery. Unlike the cells of most tumors these cells do not morphologically resemble any known normal cell. The lack of resemblance is more than morphological—the immunophenotype and genotype of the classic RS cell do not correspond to those of any known normal cell. The RS cell characteristic of lymphocyte-predominant HD, the L&H or popcorn cell, has been shown to have the phenotypic and genotypic characteristics of a B lymphocyte, while the classic RS cells characteristic of the other histologic types of HD remain uncertain. While PCR analysis of single RS cells has led to varied results, in one report clonal immunoglobulin rearrangements consistent with a monoclonal B-cell origin for the RS cells were found in three of three patients tested.[260–262]

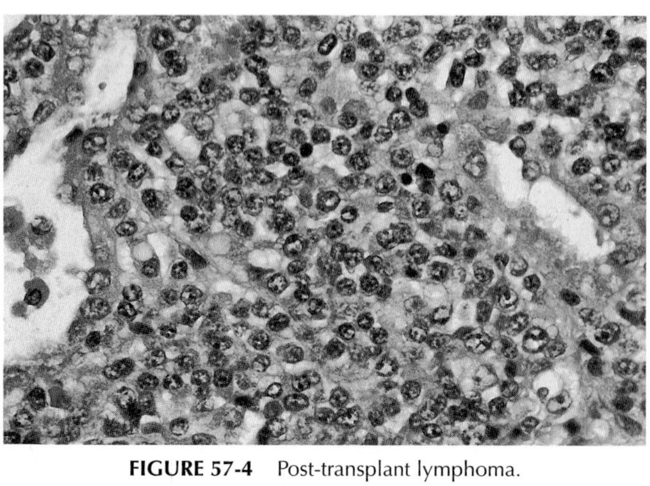

FIGURE 57-4 Post-transplant lymphoma.

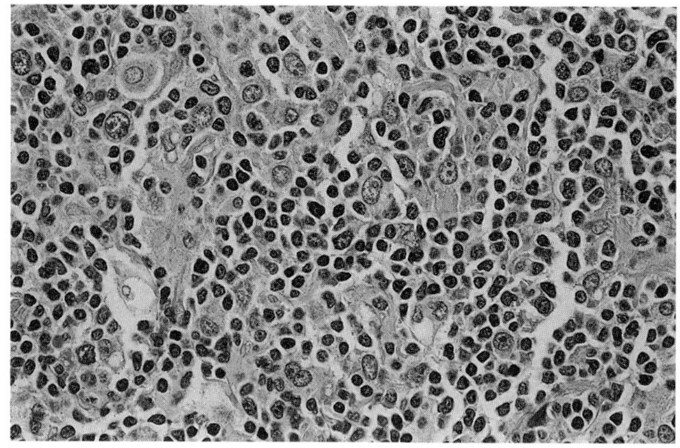

FIGURE 57-5 Hodgkin's disease.

EBV has been associated with most cases of non–lymphocyte-predominant HD by PCR and shown to be localized within the RS cells by in situ hybridization.[207] As EBV primarily infects B cells, it is curious that it is the classic RS cells rather than the B-cell L&H RS cells of lymphocyte-predominant HD which are EBV-positive. This may be explained by the fact that EBV infection of B cells is associated with downregulation of the expression of the B-cell antigen CD20 commonly used in tissue sections to detect B-cell phenotype.[263] The fact that EBV within a given case is clonal supports the notion that the virus is not merely a passenger virus but is playing an important role in growth of the RS cells.[208,264] EBV gene expression in RS cells is restricted to *EBER1/2*, *LMP1*, and *EBNA1*, an EBV latency pattern termed type II shared with that of NPC. A 30-bp deletion within the EBV *LMP1* gene, which is present in a high percentage of EBV-positive HD cases, was suggested to be of pathogenetic significance.[265] However, further studies have cast doubt on this hypothesis since the deletion may also be found in EBV isolates from normal persons.[266] EBV is clearly not essential to the development of all cases of classic HD because up to 40% of these cases are EBV negative.[267] The association of EBV with HD varies with age, geographic location, and histologic subtype. HD is more strongly associated with EBV before the age of 15 and after the age of 50 years.[268,269] The EBV association is stronger in the developing world than in the Western world and is more commonly associated with mixed cellularity type and less commonly with the nodular sclerosis type.[270,271] Also, EBV does not play an important role in the rare familial form of HD.[272] The role of EBV does appear to be magnified in cases in which the host is immunocompromised, since HD in the setting of AIDS is nearly always EBV positive, suggesting that poor control of EBV infection may allow EBV to play a role. Although the risk of developing HD is significantly increased in patients with a past history of infectious mononucleosis, more recent studies indicate that those HD patients with a history of infectious mononucleosis were paradoxically less likely to develop EBV-associated HD.[273,274] Another puzzle is that no EBV-specific cellular immune response is seen in EBV-positive HD tissues from presumably immunocompetent persons, while intact responses are seen in EBV-negative cases.[275] It has been suggested that inhibitory cytokines such as interleukin-10 (IL-10) secreted by the RS cells actively inhibit the cellular immune response.[263] Although EBV probably acts as an important cofactor in a multistep process leading to HD, it is likely that cellular genetic changes also play an important role since RS cells have cytogenetic abnormalities.[276] In fact, the EBV status of HD does not appear to impact clinical prognosis.[277] EBV is also found in certain forms of T-cell lymphoma.[278] Nasal-type angiocentric T/NK (T/natural killer)-cell lymphomas, which are prevalent in China, initially present with local involvement of the nose, skin, lung, or gastrointestinal tract, but often disseminate and run an aggressive course.[279] Angioimmunoblastic lymphadenopathy (AILD)–like T-cell lymphoma (Fig. 57-6) usually presents with fever, rash, dysgammaglobulinemia, hepatosplenomegaly, and lymphadenopathy.[280] Node-based T-immunoblastic lymphomas often have Hodgkin-like or anaplastic large cell features and in young persons may present with an infectious mononucleosis–like illness.[281] Some peripheral T-cell lymphomas may either develop or present with an often rapidly fatal hemophagocytic syndrome characterized by pancytopenia, a disseminated intravascular coagulation–like coagulopathy, hepatosplenomegaly, and pulmonary involvement.[282]

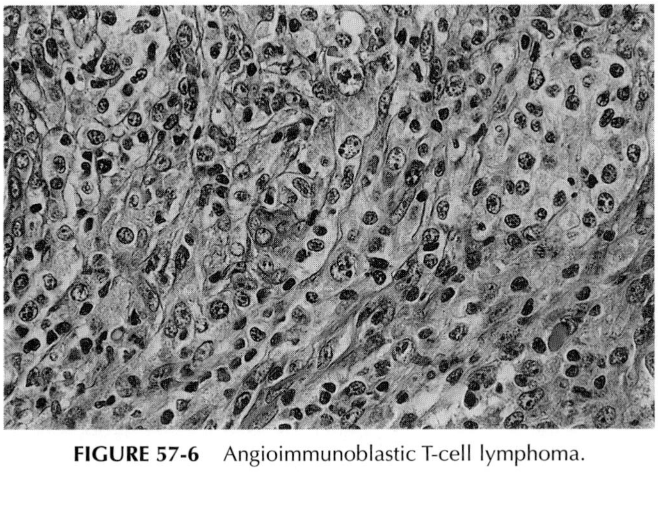

FIGURE 57-6 Angioimmunoblastic T-cell lymphoma.

Peripheral lymphadenopathy in hemophagocytic syndrome is often unremarkable. An unusual EBV-associated syndrome described as hypersensitivity to mosquito bites has been described in Japan.[283,284] In these cases, EBV is found within clonal NK cells in the skin lesions as well as in blood.

PATHOGENESIS AND IMMUNITY

Like the other herpesviruses, EBV may exist in either a latent or lytic state. However, the predominant mode of B-cell infection appears to lead to latency. Owing to the consistency of patterns of latent EBV gene expression seen in different cell types, these patterns have been categorized into type I typical of African Burkitt's lymphoma with *EBER1–2* and *EBNA1* expression, type II seen in NPC and HD with *EBER1–2* and *LMP1/2* expression, and type III seen in latent-transformed B cells with *EBER1–2, EBNA1–6,* and *LMP1/2* expression.[285] As noted previously, at least 10 latent EBV genes are active in EBV-transformed B cells, yet only a few are required for B-cell transformation.[198] Of the latent genes, *LMP1* is the only one that has been clearly shown to exhibit transforming function.[286] Although EBV-transformed B cells grow continuously in cell culture, they are normal diploid cells and unable to form tumors in nude mice and are therefore not considered malignant. African Burkitt's lymphoma cells, on the other hand, are not only EBV infected but also have a chromosomal translocation involving the c-*myc* gene on chromosome 8 and one of the immunoglobulin genes on chromosome 2 (κ light chain), 14 (heavy chain), or 22 (λ light chain). These translocations lead to production of excessive amounts of myc protein, a protein important in cell cycle progression.[287,288] The consistent presence of c-*myc* translocations in all cases of Burkitt's lymphoma, whether EBV positive or EBV negative, emphasizes the dominant role of the c-*myc* gene translocation in the genesis of Burkitt's lymphoma. The primacy of c-*myc* activation has also been shown in vitro by inducing proliferation of EBV-transformed B cells independent of *EBNA2* and *LMP1* activity.[289] However, the finding of single-sized fused EBV terminal repeats most consistent with monoclonal virus within tumors has led to the suggestion that EBV is not simply a passenger but is playing an important role in growth of the tumor.[290] The set of latent EBV genes (type II) active in NPC differs from that seen in transformed B cells and includes unusual complementary strand transcripts from the *Bam A* fragment.[291] However, advances in this area have been hampered by lack of simple in vitro systems for analysis of EBV effects on normal human epithelial cells in culture. Interestingly, the latency type II NPC pattern rather than the latency type III lymphoblastoid B-cell gene expression pattern is typical of the malignant RS cells of HD, cells which are likely B lymphoid in origin.[292]

DIAGNOSIS

Infectious mononucleosis due to EBV may be difficult to differentiate from other infectious diseases without serologic testing for heterophile antibody and in heterophile-negative cases (in young children) for specific EBV antibody (anti-VCA). In most cases, the clinical presentation of a rapidly growing jaw or abdominal mass in a child in an endemic area is virtually diagnostic of Burkitt's lymphoma. Because of the rapid and specific clinical presentation of endemic Burkitt's lymphoma, EBV serology has not proved useful in the diagnosis of Burkitt's lymphoma. On the other hand, the predominance of nonspecific findings (nasal stuffiness and nosebleeds) in the early stages of NPC may delay the clinical diagnosis. Fortunately, large-scale screening in susceptible populations for elevated anti-VCA or anti-EA IgA antibody titers has proved very useful in early detection of the disease and the recurrence of NPC. Recent efforts have focused on the use of BZLF1 IgG, EA IgG, and ADCC tests in prognosis.[293] The clinical diagnosis of post-transplant lymphoproliferative disease should be suspected if fever, lymphadenopathy, tonsillar enlargement, allograft failure, or abdominal mass is detected. Given the high rate of EBV seropositivity and viral reactivation in the transplant populations, serologic studies generally are not useful. An increase in EBV load, as assessed by quantitative EBV PCR of peripheral blood, has been shown to herald the emergence of PTLD.[294–296] EBV may be detected rapidly in tumor cells from tissue biopsies by immunostaining for the EBV LMP1 protein, by in situ hybridization for highly abundant EBV EBER-1 or EBER-2 RNA, or by detection of EBV DNA by PCR. Cell culture isolation of EBV is technically difficult and is therefore not routinely performed in the clinical laboratory.

TREATMENT AND PROGNOSIS

Treatment of Burkitt's lymphoma and NPC with antiviral drugs is not effective—instead these malignant tumors require standard antineoplastic therapy. For NPC, radiotherapy alone often leads to 5-year survival rates of 50% to 60%.[297,298] Although the addition of chemotherapy leads to higher initial remission rates, no improvement in survival has been shown.[299] In the post-transplant setting, prophylaxis in seronegative patients with hyperimmune globulin may be useful. The nucleoside analogue acyclovir has been used in some cases to inhibit EBV replication and blunt disease, but is incapable of eradicating latent virus. In patients with severe acute complications of EBV infection, such as airway obstruction from tonsillar enlargement, corticosteroids may be useful. Appropriate treatment of PTLD should be individualized to the specific case. Options include reduction of immunosuppressive medication, interferon-α, intravenous immune globulin, acyclovir, localized radiotherapy, and conventional chemotherapy. Reduction of immunosuppressive therapy in the early stages of PTLD often leads to clinical remission and cure but should be carefully titrated to prevent organ transplant rejection.[300] Immunosuppressive withdrawal may be accompanied by acyclovir therapy, which, although ineffective in inhibiting tumor cell growth, should prevent further active viral infection. Interferon alpha-2b with intravenous immune globulin may induce remissions in both polyclonal and monoclonal PTLD and may be considered in those in whom immunosuppressive withdrawal has failed.[301,302] Radiotherapy should probably be limited to treatment of unresectable highly localized processes. Cytotoxic chemotherapy should probably be limited, as a last resort, to refractory cases owing to the severe life-threatening complications.[303] More experimental approaches with some promise include donor leukocyte transfusion and transfusion of in vitro expanded autologous EBV-specific cytotoxic T cells in bone marrow transplant recipients.[304,305] Oral hairy leukoplakia is effectively treated with high-dose oral acyclovir or desciclovir, although recurrence following cessation of therapy is common.[306,307] Recent in vitro results suggest that vidarabine and foscarnet may be useful in treatment of EBV-positive NK large granular lymphocyte (LGL) disorders.[308]

PREVENTION AND CONTROL

As with the other herpesviruses, hygienic measures are not very effective in preventing EBV infection. The large number of healthy seropositive viral excreters in the population provides a constant source of infectious virus, and measures to minimize contact with infectious saliva are impractical. Since congenital EBV infection is not a clinical problem, isolation of seronegative mothers from seropositive excreters is not warranted. Although unproven, measures to curb holoendemic malaria may be useful in prevention of Burkitt's lymphoma in central Africa, and avoidance of salted fish in southern China may be useful in prevention of NPC.[231,235] Ultimately, the development of an EBV vaccine may lead to decreased rates of Burkitt's lymphoma and NPC if administered to seronegative children in the endemic areas. Vaccine development has focused on the 350-kDa, major envelope glycoprotein (gp350), which is the major target of neutralizing antibodies in vivo.[309] Gp350 subunit vaccines, as well as vaccinia and adenovirus recombinant gp350 vaccines, are undergoing evaluation.[310]

Human Herpesvirus 6

AGENT

HHV-6 was first identified as a herpesvirus growing from primary lymphocyte cultures of patients with AIDS-associated lymphoproliferative disease.[311] The virus has subsequently been isolated from adults with AIDS[312,313] and children with a febrile illness called exanthem subitum (or roseola infantum, pseudorubella, or sixth disease).[314] The electron microscopic appearance of the virus is typical of herpesviruses with a prominent tegument.[315] Within 3 to 5 days of culture, infected lymphocytes display a characteristic CPE with ballooning enlargement somewhat similar to that seen with CMV.[316] Although the in vitro host cell range differs among different isolates, most can be propagated in normal T cells and T-cell lines, while some isolates have been shown to infect the fibroblast cell line MRC-5 and EBV-infected B cells.[317–320] In vivo, the major target cell in peripheral blood appears to be the $CD4^+$ $CD8^-$ T lymphocyte.[321] The animal host range of the virus has not been clearly established. Serologic studies in nonhuman primates have yielded mixed results, with one study detecting serologic positivity in 8 of 10 species, whereas others detected no positivity in any species tested.[311,322,323]

The HHV-6 genome is 160 kb to 170 kb in length with a long unique region flanked on both ends by terminal repeats.[324–326] Sequence analysis demonstrates that HHV-6 is a betaherpesvirus with closest homology to HHV-7 and CMV and likely encodes 80 to 100 proteins.[327] Genetic, serologic, and biologic evidence suggests two distinct subtypes termed HHV-6A (represented by prototype strains GS and U1102) and HHV-6B (represented by prototype strain Z29).[328,329] The U1102 strain genome contains an interesting gene encoding a protein with close homology to the transregulatory rep 68/78 protein of the human parvovirus AAV-2 strain.[330] Transfection of NIH3T3 cells with HHV-6 DNA induces phenotypic changes associated with cell transformation, including the ability of these transfected cells to grow as tumors in nude mice.[331] Although a transmissible virus-like agent was demonstrated in children with exanthem subitum as early as 1950,[332] it was not until 1988 that HHV-6 was shown to be the cause of the disease.[314] It was subsequently shown that exanthem subitum is associated in almost all cases with the HHV-6B subtype.[190,328,333,334]

EPIDEMIOLOGY

Like the other herpesviruses, HHV-6 is ubiquitous with greater than 80% seropositivity in U.S. adults detected with a sensitive enzyme-linked immunosorbent assay (ELISA).[335] Primary infection most often occurs in early childhood with seroprevalence rates exceeding 80% by 2 years of age in Japan, Italy, and Thailand.[336–338] HHV-6, like HHV-7, appears to persistently infect the salivary glands where it is shed into the saliva.[339,340] Although high rates of HHV-6 positivity in saliva from healthy adults have been reported by some researchers, others have reported much lower rates.[341–346] It has been suggested that the high rates of salivary HHV-6 reported in some studies may be complicated by the cross-reactivity of some reagents and assays with HHV-7.[347] Intrauterine infection appears to be fairly common, with nearly 30% of healthy newborns positive for HHV-6 DNA in blood. Sexual and perinatal transmission is also likely to be common given that up to 30% of uterine cervical secretions are HHV-6 DNA positive.[348] Primary infection in children less than 2 years old is often characterized by a syndrome of high fever and evanescent rash (exanthem subitum; Plate 57-1E). Indeed, exanthem subitum is the most common exanthem in children less than 2 years of age. Nearly half of all first febrile episodes after birth and up to 40% of all pediatric emergency room admissions for febrile illness may be due to HHV-6 infection. In one recent study, 10% of all febrile episodes in infants were due to either HHV-6A or HHV-6B infection.[349] In a tropical Brazilian study, primary HHV-6 and HHV-7 infections in children were often misdiagnosed as measles.[350]

DISEASE

A high fever for 4 to 5 days is followed in up to 70% of cases by a diffuse evanescent (less than 2 days) maculopapular rash on the chest and abdomen with relative sparing of the face and extremities. Febrile convulsions, splenomegaly, and cervical lymphadenopathy are common. Complications may include hepatitis, thrombocytopenia, hemophagocytic syndrome, meningitis, and encephalitis. An association with a specific form of massive cervical lymphadenopathy of childhood, sinus histiocytosis with massive lymphadenopathy, has been reported.[351] Symptomatic primary infection in adults is neither common nor well described but may present as heterophile-negative mononucleosis or hepatitis.[352,353] Although HHV-6 has been suggested as a possible factor in chronic fatigue syndrome, a prospective study was unable to establish any correlation between HHV-6 seropositivity and chronic fatigue syndrome.[354] HHV-6 has been implicated in some cases of idiopathic acute liver failure.[355] In the post-transplant setting, serologic evidence of reactivation is commonly observed and may be associated with a variety of symptoms, including fever, rash, hepatitis, pneumonitis, neurologic dysfunction, and marrow suppression.[321] Although HHV-6 DNA has been detected in some cases of lymphoproliferative disease,[356–358] the lack of consistent positivity in any specific type of lymphoproliferative disease would argue against a causal link. HHV-6 has also recently been directly implicated in the pathogenesis of multiple sclerosis.[359,360]

DIAGNOSIS

Clinical diagnosis of classic roseola infantum in childhood is not usually difficult and does not require serologic confirmation. Due to the high seroprevalence, single-point IgG titers are not useful. Diagnosis of active infection serologically requires either detection of increased IgM or a greater than fourfold rise in IgG titers from paired acute and convalescent serum specimens using indirect immunofluorescence (IFA), anticomplement immunofluorescence, or ELISA. Virus culture systems have been described. However, caution in interpretation of positive results is warranted owing to the high rate of viral isolation from the normal population. Given the availability of HHV-6 DNA sequence information, the most rapid and sensitive assays for direct detection of HHV-6 are PCR-based assays, which can distinguish between HHV-6A and HHV-6B strains.[333,361]

TREATMENT AND PROGNOSIS

The susceptibility of HHV-6 to antiviral drugs is likely similar to that of the related herpesvirus CMV. The nucleoside analogue, ganciclovir, and viral DNA polymerase inhibitors, cidofovir and foscarnet, may be useful in severe infection, as in the post-transplant setting, but have not been tested in a controlled manner. Although uncomplicated primary infection in childhood is self-limited, infection in immunocompromised patients such as organ transplant may lead to life-threatening complications.

PREVENTION AND CONTROL

Given the high infection rate in infancy and childhood and the high rate of asymptomatic oral shedding, preventive measures are unlikely to be effective.

Human Herpesvirus 7

AGENT

HHV-7 (strain RK) was first isolated from peripheral blood CD4+ T lymphocytes of a healthy 26-year-old subject during attempts to isolate and propagate HHV-6.[362] Several additional isolates were obtained from normal healthy persons.[363] Another strain (JI) was isolated from a patient with chronic fatigue syndrome.[364] The ultrastructural appearance of the virus is characteristic of a typical human herpesvirus with a very prominent tegument similar to that seen with HHV-6. The HHV-7 genome is 145 kbp in size with sequence homology to other betaherpesviruses HHV-6 and CMV.[365,366] Antigenically, HHV-7 is similar to HHV-6 since both serologic[367,368] and T cell–mediated[369] cross-reactivity have been described. HHV-7 appears to preferentially infect CD4-positive T cells, although infection of CD8-positive lymphocytes has also been demonstrated.[364] Virus is present not only in peripheral blood but also in saliva, salivary glands, and uterine cervical secretions. Transmission likely occurs most commonly through the oral route, but may also occur via the genital tract.

EPIDEMIOLOGY

HHV-7 infection is very common, with adult seroprevalence ranging from over 80% in western Europe and the United States to 60% in Japan.[337,364,367,370] The virus actively replicates in the oral region with salivary isolation rates of 55% to 96% of normal healthy adults.[336,342,346,347,371] Primary infection is common in early childhood—42% of children are seropositive by 2 years of age and 82% by 4 years of age—but appears to occur later than primary HHV-6 infection.[338,372]

DISEASE

Primary HHV-7 infection in children is a febrile illness that may be complicated by seizures.[373] HHV-7 has been isolated from some patients with exanthem subitum, chronic fatigue syndrome, chronic mononucleosis, hepatitis, and CMV-like disease in the post-transplant setting.[371–378] It has been suggested both from in vitro and clinical observations that under some conditions, such as post-transplant or AIDS settings, HHV-7 may act to exacerbate other betaherpesvirus infections (CMV and HHV-6) by reactivation from latency.[378,379]

DIAGNOSIS

Serologic, culture, immunohistologic, PCR, and in situ hybridization techniques for the detection of HHV-7 infection have been described but are not widely available for clinical use. However, given the high prevalence of virus infection in the normal population and the absence of clearly defined clinical disease associations, the clinical utility of viral detection or antibody titer is unclear. Assays should certainly be carefully designed and tested to avoid cross-reactivity with the related betaherpesviruses HHV-6 and CMV.

TREATMENT AND PROGNOSIS

Although controlled studies are unavailable, it is likely that HHV-7 infection, like the betaherpesvirus CMV, will respond to treatment with the nucleoside analogue ganciclovir as well as the viral DNA polymerase inhibitors foscarnet and cidofovir.

PREVENTION AND CONTROL

It is likely that, like HHV-6, the high infection rate in childhood and high rate of asymptomatic oral shedding in adults will preclude effective preventive measures.

Human Herpesvirus 8

AGENT

Infectious virus recovered from both the EBV-positive primary effusion lymphoma (PEL) cell line BC-1 and from a Kaposi's sarcoma (KS) biopsy specimen have been cloned and sequenced.[380,381] Although the virus was originally reported as 250 kb to 270 kb in size, a more recent estimate is 150 kb to 160 kb.[382,383] DNA sequence analysis has revealed close sequence homology to the gammaherpesviruses, herpesvirus saimiri and EBV.[380,384] A striking feature of the viral genome is the presence of genes with homology to cell cycle regulatory and signaling proteins including complement binding proteins, *bcl*-2, IL-6, IL-8 receptor, nerve cell adhesion molecule (N-CAM) family protein, macrophage inflammatory proteins (MIP-I, MIP-II), cyclin D, and interferon regulatory factor 1, some of which may be important in cell transformation.[380–385] No genes with homology to the known transforming genes of EBV (*EBNA, LMP*) or herpesvirus saimiri (*ORF1*) are present. However, it is interesting to note that EBV infection of B cells induces increased expression of some of the same cellular genes (cyclin D, complement receptor 2, *bcl*-2, IL-8 receptor–like protein, and IL-6) for which HHV-8 encodes a homologue.[381] This suggests that both gammaherpesviruses use the same strategy for successful infection, but in the case of EBV the elements of the program remain within the human host cell while with HHV-8 the program has been acquired by the virus from the host cell.

EPIDEMIOLOGY

PEL cell lines have been utilized as targets for the development of IFA and ELISA assays for detection of anti-HHV-8 antibodies in human serum. Assay variations have included IFA on unstimulated cells, phorbol ester or *N*-butyric acid–stimulated cells for more sensitive detection of antibody to lytic antigens,[386–389] isolated cell nuclei for detection of antibody to nuclear antigens,[386,390,391] and ELISA using recombinant antigens.[391] As expected, nearly all patients with KS are seropositive using any of the preceding methods. Also, not surprisingly, a variable proportion of AIDS patients without KS are seropositive. Both seroconversion and detection of HHV-8 DNA by PCR were shown to precede development of KS in HIV-positive patients.[390,392,393]

Immunosuppressed renal transplant recipients exhibit both serologic and molecular evidence of HHV-8 activation,[394] a phenomenon that may be at least partially due to steroid effects on viral replication.[395] Transmission of HHV-8 in transplant recipients may occur by blood transfusion or by allograft transmission.[396,397] Tremendous geographic variation in HHV-8 seroprevalence has been noted. In central Africa, the seroprevalence is approximately 50%, while in southern Europe it ranges up to 20% and is about 5% in northern Europe and in the United States.[398] Seroprevalence rates reported from different laboratories on normal healthy controls from nonendemic regions have varied tremendously (0 to 24%).[387–391]

Although some variations in results may be due to real geographic or demographic differences, some variability is also likely due to differences in the sensitivity of assay signal detection and the selection of antigen substrate.[399] Seroprevalence studies designed to detect the age of infection have revealed that as contrasted with an early age of infection in Africa,[400] in the United States infection appears to be delayed until adolescence.[401]

DISEASE

The clinical characteristics of primary HHV-8 infection have not yet been described. In addition to KS, HHV-8 has also been detected by PCR in high-grade large B-cell lymphomas arising in body cavities, that is, primary effusion lymphoma,[402–404] multicentric Castleman's disease,[405] AILD,[406] non-KS skin tumors in allograft transplant recipients,[407] angiosarcoma,[408] and multiple myeloma.[409]

KS was first described by Kaposi as an indolent tumor of the lower extremity in elderly males of Mediterranean or eastern European descent.[410] KS is a dermal spindle cell neoplasm, likely of endothelial cell origin, which in the skin is manifest as irregular discolored patches, plaques, nodules, or umbilicated tumors (Plate 57-1F). Although most investigators regard KS as a malignant disease, the indolent behavior of classic KS with spontaneous regression seen in some cases has led some to suggest a reactive process.[411,412] Analysis of DNA of KS lesions has yielded inconsistent results, with some studies suggestive of a nonclonal process and other studies suggestive of a clonal process.[413,414] Pathologically, the early lesion (the patch stage) consists of irregular branching ectatic vascular channels in the upper dermis lined by plump relatively normal-appearing endothelium (Fig. 57-7). At this stage, the pathologic changes may be subtle, and distinction from hemangioma or granulation tissue difficult. The late lesion (the plaque stage) consists of an irregular nodular spindle cell proliferation with mitotic figures in both the upper and lower dermis, vascular slits, extravasated erythrocytes, hemosiderin deposition, so-called hyaline bodies, and admixed inflammatory cells. At this stage, the pathologic changes are quite characteristic, although in some cases distinction from angiosarcoma may be difficult. KS has been described in four different clinical settings—classic Mediterranean, endemic African, epidemic AIDS associated, and iatrogenic.[415] Classic KS presents as a chronic, generally indolent, cutaneous disease of the lower extremity, most often in elderly white males (male-to-female ratio, 3:1; mean age, 68 years) of Mediterranean, eastern European, or Jewish ancestry.[410] Interestingly, up to 35% of these persons may develop second tumors, especially malignant lymphoma. Endemic African KS occurs in the sub-Saharan equatorial regions and presents most often in young adult black males (male-to-female ratio, 14:1; mean age, 35 years) with either a florid form (40%), a benign nodular form (25%), or an aggressive form (15%), as well as in young black male children (mean age, 3 years) with a lymphadenopathic form.[416] Endemic KS is often an aggressive disease with a fatal outcome. Iatrogenic KS occurs in persons following chronic treatment with drugs with immunosuppressive effects administered for solid organ transplantation,[246,417] autoimmune disease,[418] and malignancy. Iatrogenic KS is a generally indolent disease with complete remission in up to 24% of cases following immune restoration. Epidemic AIDS–associated KS is the most common malignant neoplasm in AIDS patients in the Western world.[419] The risk of development of KS in AIDS appears to be directly related to the degree of immunodeficiency and is strongly inversely correlated with the absolute CD4 count. Sexual transmission of HHV-8 is suggested by the much higher incidence of KS in HIV-positive homosexual or bisexual males than in other risk groups such as HIV-positive females and IV drug users. AIDS-associated KS is an aggressive disease closely resembling endemic African KS, with widespread dissemination to lymph nodes and viscera.

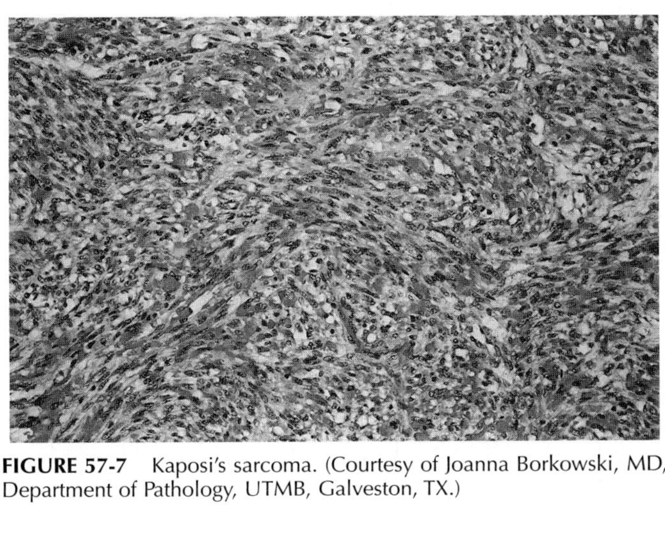

FIGURE 57-7 Kaposi's sarcoma. (Courtesy of Joanna Borkowski, MD, Department of Pathology, UTMB, Galveston, TX.)

Although HHV-8 is nearly always detected in KS lesions within the KS spindle cells, the role HHV-8 plays in the pathogenesis of KS is unclear. Prior to the discovery of HHV-8, work was presented implicating CMV as the causative agent of KS.[420–422] Also, inflammatory cytokines (basic fibroblast growth factor, oncostatin M, and IL-6) from activated T cells and the HIV-1 tat protein have been shown to induce KS-like spindle cell transformation of normal endothelium both in vitro and in vivo.[423–429] Results of DNA analysis of KS spindle cells are not consistent, with some reporting diploidy and others aneuploidy.[429–432] Although no consistent KS-specific chromosomal abnormality has been described, chromosome X inactivation analysis reveals that AIDS KS is a monoclonal tumor.[433] Analysis of HHV-8 terminal repeats by Southern blotting in a KS biopsy are consistent with monoclonal virus, a finding most consistent with tumor cell monoclonality, as would be expected if KS were a malignant neoplasm.[380] Despite these findings, the absence of HHV-8 in spindle cell cultures derived from KS biopsies is puzzling.[434,435] Perhaps HHV-8 is lost from cells after serial passage in vitro.

Castleman's disease is a peculiar lymphoproliferative disorder which presents either as a solitary or multicentric form.[436,437] The more common solitary form usually presents asymptomatically as an anterior mediastinal or neck mass with hyaline vascular histology. The less common multicentric form usually presents with fever, anemia, and generalized lymphadenopathy with plasma cell histology. Patients with the solitary form have an excellent prognosis and in fact are often cured of disease by surgical excision of the mass. On the other hand, patients with the multicentric form have a poor prognosis. Lymph node biopsies of multicentric Castleman's disease may contain HHV-8 DNA by PCR.[405] However, the significance of these findings is unclear since only a minority of cases contain viral DNA.[438] Regarding non-KS vascular lesions, in one PCR study of 155 vascular lesions (including 17 cases of KS and 15 cases of angiosarcoma), HHV-8 DNA

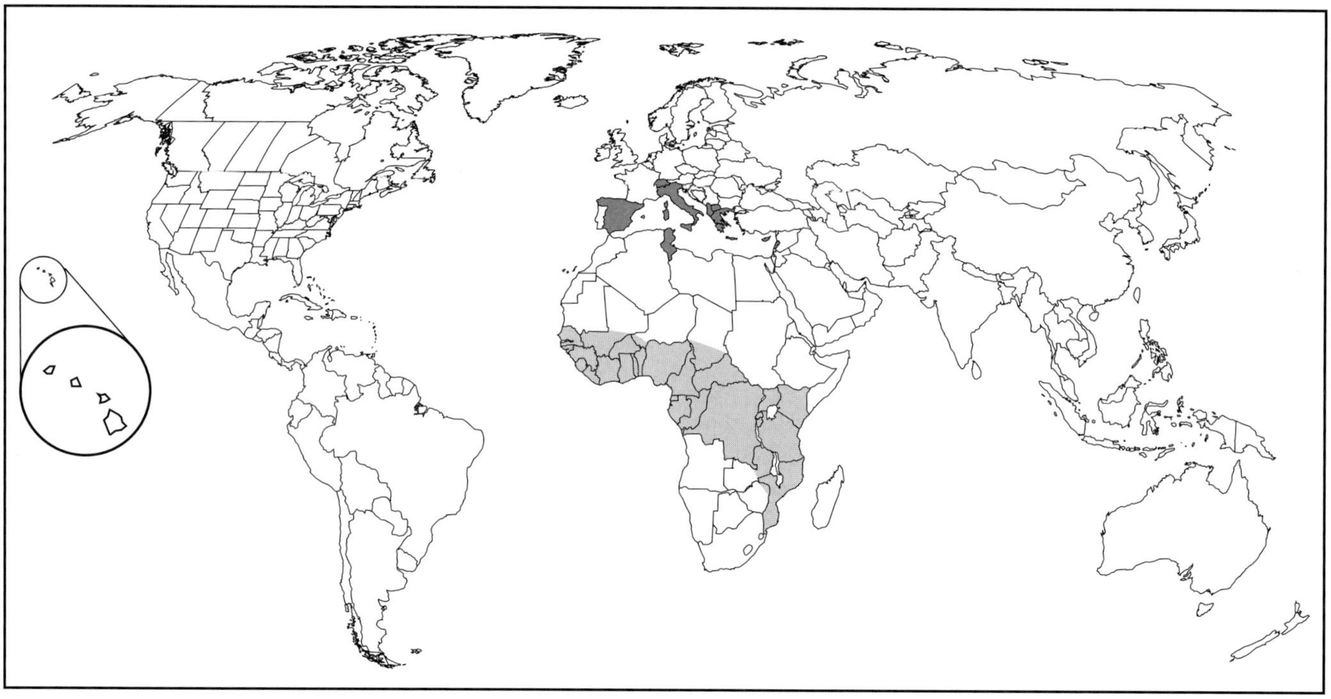

Kaposi's Sarcoma
- Classic Mediterranean Kaposi's Sarcoma
- Endemic African Kaposi's Sarcoma

was present only in the KS cases, while in another study HHV-8 was found in angiosarcoma (7 of 24) and hemangioma (1 of 20).[408,439] The significance of these findings is unclear since only a minority of cases contain viral DNA.

PEL is a high-grade malignant lymphoma most often seen in homosexual males with AIDS.[255,403,404,440,441] The tumor presents as a malignant effusion of pleural, pericardial, or peritoneal cavities and tends not to disseminate but to remain confined to the body cavity. Despite the lack of dissemination, these patients do not tolerate chemotherapy well and succumb within a few months of diagnosis. The malignancy is composed of large anaplastic cells with a null cell immunophenotype (negative B- and T-cell markers, CD30-positive) and a B-cell genotype (Jh rearranged) and are usually coinfected with both EBV and HHV-8.[401] Interestingly, up to one third of PEL cases may be associated with KS.[442] Although usually seen in males with AIDS, rare HHV-8-positive PELs have been described in HIV-negative males and females.[404,442,443]

Multiple myeloma, a malignant plasma cell neoplasm which arises in the bone marrow, is the second most common malignancy of the blood in the United States.[444] Monoclonal gammopathy of undetermined significance (MGUS) is an even more common related condition characterized by a monoclonal proliferation of plasma cells but accompanied by much less severe clinical findings. However, up to 25% of patients with MGUS progress to multiple myeloma.[445] Although HHV-8 DNA had previously been shown to be absent from myeloma cells, HHV-8 DNA was recently reported within the dendritic cell compartment of the bone marrow of 15 of 15 patients with myeloma and two of eight patients with MGUS, while absent from 10 normal bone marrow samples and 16 samples from patients with other malignancies.[409,446] The authors suggest that the role of the infected dendritic cells may be in stimulating growth of the abnormal plasma cells by elaboration of HHV-8 vIL-6, a factor shown to support the growth of a murine plasmacytoma cell line.[382]

PATHOGENESIS AND IMMUNITY

HHV-8 was first detected as a unique DNA sequence from an AIDS KS skin biopsy using PCR-based representational difference analysis.[447] Subsequently, this DNA sequence was detected by PCR in nearly all lesional skin biopsies from patients with all forms of KS—classic, endemic African, iatrogenic, and epidemic AIDS associated.[447–451] Virus has been localized within the KS tumor cells by in situ hybridization.[452,453] However, viral DNA has also been detected in other tissues as well, including nonlesional skin,[385] non-KS skin tumors,[407] peripheral blood,[454] lymphoid tissue,[455] saliva,[456–458] sensory ganglia,[459] semen,[460,461] and prostate tissue. However, some of these findings have been disputed by others.[451,462,463] HHV-8 DNA has been found not only in KS patients but also in human immunodeficiency virus (HIV)–positive persons without KS as well as HIV-negative healthy controls. Within the blood, the virus has been localized largely to the CD19 B-cell compartment, although it may also be found in some T cells.[464] HHV-8 DNA has also been detected in some cases of AIDS-associated primary effusion B-cell lymphoma (PEL) where it may be accompanied by EBV.[402,438,465] Infectious virus obtained from the PEL cell line BC-1 has been shown in vitro to infect normal peripheral blood B cells.[466] HHV-8 DNA has been detected in biopsy material from non-KS skin lesions (squamous cell carcinoma, basal cell carcinoma, actinic keratosis, Bowen's disease) and also from normal skin of HIV-negative persons.[467] HHV-8 has also been found in some cases of AIDS-associated multicentric Castleman's disease.[405] In another study, HHV-8 DNA was detected by PCR only occasionally in biopsy material from patients with HIV-negative reactive lymphadenopathy (4 of 23 patients), HIV-negative angioimmunoblastic lymphadenopathy (3 of 15), lymphoma (1 of 43), multicentric Castleman's disease (0 of 5), and Hodgkin's disease (0 of 45).[406] The HHV-8-positive reactive lymphadenopathy changes were characterized by florid follicular hyperplasia with increased vascularity resembling HIV-related lymphadenopathy and multicentric Castleman's disease. Normal healthy controls have also been shown to harbor HHV-8 DNA albeit at a lower rate.[406,461] In one study, HHV-8 DNA was found in 6% of normal skin tissues, in 7% of peripheral blood samples, in 44% of prostate tissues, and in 91% of semen samples from healthy immunocompetent Italian males.[468] It has been reported that not only HHV-8 but also EBV and CMV may be detected in African KS biopsies, and CMV, HHV-6, HHV-7, and human papillomavirus in AIDS KS biopsies.[469–471] However, the lack of consistent positive results in these studies argues against these other viruses playing an etiologic role. The increasing number of reports of HHV-8 PCR positivity in normal and abnormal tissues from patients without KS strongly suggests that viral infection may not be strictly limited to persons with KS. It is possible that HHV-8, like the related gammaherpesvirus EBV, will prove to be present not only in patients with virus-associated neoplasms but also in normal persons and serve as an important cofactor in human tumorigenesis, especially in a setting of immunodeficiency.

Coculture of KS spindle cells with a variety of endothelial and epithelial cell lines led to lytic infection of approximately 1% of the cells of the embryonal kidney epithelial cell line 293 from which virus could be serially passaged.[472] Interestingly, virus obtained from an HHV-8-positive, body cavity–based lymphoma cell line did not induce any evidence of infection. Infection of primary microvascular endothelial cells by HHV-8 has been reported and in two cases was associated with cellular transformation.[473–475] Like all herpesviruses, the virus appears to reside within infected cells either in the latent state as a circular episomal form or in the lytic state as a linear form. In one report, it was shown that linear lytic virus is found in the peripheral blood, whereas only episomal latent virus is present within the KS skin lesion itself.[454]

DIAGNOSIS

Because of the very strong correlation of HHV-8 positivity with KS, diagnosis of KS is presumptive evidence of HHV-8 infection. Rapid and specific confirmation of HHV-8 infection, however, may be accomplished by both qualitative and quantitative PCR methods performed on DNA isolated from body fluids or tissue.[447,476] Serologic assays (IFA nuclear antigen assay, IFA lytic antigen assay, ELISA recombinant antigen assay) are currently under development and will likely prove very useful in seroprevalence studies, in characterization of the immune response, and in detection of primary infection (IgM-specific assays). Although an in vitro culture method has recently been described, the technical complexity of the method in its current form makes it unlikely to be useful in the clinical laboratory setting.[472]

TREATMENT AND PROGNOSIS

Although HHV-8 infection may not respond to treatment with the nucleoside analogues acyclovir and ganciclovir as well as the other herpesviruses, long-term remission of KS has been reported following treatment with foscarnet,[477] and HIV-positive patients treated with foscarnet or ganciclovir have a decreased risk of KS development.[478] Also, clearance of HHV-8 DNA from the peripheral blood of an HIV-positive patient following treatment with the HIV protease inhibitor indinavir has been reported.[479] The use of highly active antiretroviral therapy (HAART) in AIDS-related KS is associated with a dramatic clinical response. Local therapy of KS has included cryotherapy, surgical excision, intralesional vinblastine, vincristine, or interferon-α, and radiotherapy. Systemic therapy has included both single- and multiple-agent chemotherapy and interferon-α.[480] Anti-neoplastic agents such as liposomal anthracyclines and paclitaxel, as well as antiangiogenic agents such as retinoic acids, AGM 1470 (TNP 470), thalidomide, and glufanide disodium (IM 862) have shown some promise in patients with KS.[481]

PREVENTION AND CONTROL

At this time there is no specific information regarding methods of prevention or control of HHV-8 infection. However, the best prevention advice is to reinforce the more general safe sex practices that have been promoted to prevent human immunodeficiency virus and other sexually transmitted diseases.

Cercopithecine Herpesvirus 1

AGENT

CHV-1, or B virus, is a simian herpesvirus indigenous to Asian monkeys of the genus *Macaca,* including rhesus and cynomolgus species. The virus was first isolated from the first reported human case in a laboratory worker in 1932,[482,483] and it was not until 1954 that the virus was isolated from the spinal cord of a rhesus monkey that was being used in poliovirus research.[484] Nucleotide sequence analysis indicates that of the human herpesviruses HSV-1 is most similar to CHV-1.[485,486] The genome is larger than that of HSV-1 and is composed of a long and short unique region, each flanked by inverted repeat sequences like that of HSV-1. The complete 157-kbp nucleotide sequence of strain E2490 was recently completed.[487] Unexpectedly, the virus apparently lacks a homolog of the HSV-1 34.5 gene encoding a neurovirulence factor. Serologic cross-reactivity between CHV-1 and HSV-1 often leads to serious difficulties in the interpretation of assay results.

EPIDEMIOLOGY

CHV-1 is the only nonhuman primate herpesvirus that has been shown to infect humans. Monkeys of the genus

Macaca, including rhesus and cynomolgus species native to Asia and northern Africa, have adult seroprevalence rates of greater than 80%.[488] However, only 2% to 3% of seropositive monkeys shed virus at any particular time.[489] Although no other Old World or New World monkeys are known to naturally harbor virus, the virus can induce fatal disease in non-macaque primates, including man. Clinically apparent infection in housed monkeys is usually manifest as a self-limited oropharyngeal and mucocutaneous infection that resembles human HSV-1 infection. However, cases of disseminated infection with interstitial pneumonitis, hepatitis, gastrointestinal involvement, and a high mortality rate have been reported. A prospective 16-month study of 157 housed rhesus monkeys detected nine symptomatic infections—eight recurrent and one primary infection.[490] The risk of infection increased with age, and transmission occurred only during the breeding season. Virus could be isolated from both oral and genital tissues. Like HSV in man, CHV-1 remains latent within sensory ganglia of monkeys following primary infection.[489]

DISEASE

Human infection with CHV-1 is rare—fewer than 40 cases have been described.[491] A serologic study of 321 primate handlers revealed no cases of asymptomatic infection.[492] Humans are infected in most cases by animal bite, but transmission has also occurred following direct inoculation of the eye or respiratory tract with monkey body fluids. Person-to-person transmission from intimate contact with vesicular lesions has been documented in a single case in Florida. In most cases, after an incubation period of 3 to 5 days, a localized vesicular eruption at the site of inoculation is accompanied by fever, myalgia, headache, or nausea. The vesicular eruption is clinically and pathologically similar to that caused by HSV. Neurologic symptoms follow 3 to 7 days after development of the vesicular eruption. Paresthesia or hyperesthesia of the affected limb is followed rapidly by weakness and paralysis. Transverse myelitis may be followed by signs of encephalitis and neurologic death. At least one case has been described without bite or scratch wounds and with only nonspecific symptoms followed 5 days later by neurologic symptoms. Although uncommon, respiratory transmission followed by fever, pneumonitis, and neurologic symptoms has also been reported.

DIAGNOSIS

The clinical diagnosis of CHV-1 infection in man should be suspected in persons with fever, myalgia, and neurologic complaints in close contact with monkeys of the *Macaca* genus, particularly in confined animals with HSV-1-like vesicular oropharyngeal lesions. CHV-1 infection should be differentiated from the much more common HSV-1 infection. The vesicular eruption of HSV infection is virtually indistinguishable both clinically and pathologically from CHV-1 infection. However, given the clinical settings in which humans come into contact with CHV-1, this distinction should in most cases not be difficult. Although the high degree of antigenic cross-reactivity of HSV and CHV-1 make serologic distinction difficult,[493] serologic tests which apparently do not cross-react with HSV have been recently described.[492,494,495] Specific diagnosis can also be made by viral culture[492] or PCR.[496,497]

TREATMENT AND PROGNOSIS

All bites or scratches should be immediately cleaned vigorously with soap or detergent, and eyes and mucous membranes should be vigorously rinsed with sterile saline. The cleaning and rinsing procedures are followed immediately by collection of a swab of the wound or scratch for culture and a serum sample for baseline "acute" serology. Serum is collected again after 3 weeks for "convalescent" serology. Following risk assessment, postexposure prophylaxis with a 14-day course of oral valacyclovir or acyclovir is recommended. For B virus disease, treatment with intravenous acyclovir or ganciclovir is recommended until all symptoms resolve and two consecutive virus cultures are reported negative.[498] Immune globulin has not been shown to be efficacious.[499] The monkey should be isolated, examined, and treated, if appropriate, by a veterinarian. Human infection often leads to a rapidly ascending encephalomyelitis with historical overall mortality rate of 70%—a rate similar to untreated HSV encephalitis.[500] However, more recently the case-fatality rate has declined, probably owing to more rapid therapeutic intervention.

PREVENTION AND CONTROL

CHV-1 infection in humans will most effectively be prevented by establishment of virus-free colonies of macaques. Certainly, all persons who are in contact with Asian macaque monkeys should be trained to recognize the herpes simplex–like mucocutaneous lesions characteristic of infection in monkeys. These animals should be isolated and treated accordingly. A meeting cosponsored by the Centers for Disease Control and Prevention (CDC) and Emory University in Atlanta first put forth recommendations regarding prevention and treatment of CHV-1 infections in 1995.[501] These recommendations were recently updated in 2002.[498] All macaques should be presumed to be infectious at all times and handled accordingly.

ACKNOWLEDGMENTS

Our sincere appreciation to Ruthie Williams and Linda Beachey of the University of Texas Medical Branch (UTMB) Hematopathology Division for their secretarial assistance, and to Dr. Stephen Tyring of the UTMB Departments of Dermatology and Microbiology and Immunology for his expert information regarding antiviral therapy and dermatologic manifestations of herpesvirus infections.

REFERENCES

1. Fields BN, Knipe DM, Howley PM (eds): Fields' Virology, 3rd ed. Philadelphia, Lippincott-Raven, 1996.
2. Mandell GL, Bennett JE, Dolin R (eds): Principles and Practice of Infectious Diseases, 4th ed. New York, Churchill Livingstone, 1995.
3. Webster RG, Granoff A: Encyclopedia of Virology. San Diego, Academic Press, 1994.
4. Roizman B, Whitley RJ, Lopez C: The Human Herpesviruses. New York, Raven Press, 1993.
5. Evans AS: Viral Infections of Humans—Epidemiology and Control, 3rd ed. New York, Plenum Press, 1989.

6. Tyring SK: Infections involving the skin. In Richman DD, Whitley RJ, Hayden FG (eds): Clinical Dermatology. New York, Churchill Livingston, 1997, p 127.
7. Tyring SK: Newer aspects of herpesvirus infections. Curr Opin Dermatol 4:42, 1997.
8. Reusser P: Herpesvirus resistance to antiviral drugs: A review of the mechanisms, clinical importance and therapeutic options. J Hosp Infect 33:235, 1996.
9. Lowenstein A: Aetiologische Untersuchungen Über den fieberhaften Herpes. Munch Med Wochenschr 66:769, 1919.
10. Nahmias AJ, Dowdle WR: Antigenic and biologic differences in herpesvirus hominis. Prog Med Virol 10:110, 1968.
11. Yoshikawa T, Hill JM, Stanberry LR, et al: The characteristic site-specific reactivation phenotypes of HSV-1 and HSV-2 depend upon the latency-associated transcript region. J Exp Med 184:659, 1996.
12. Roizman B, Knipe DM: Herpes simplex viruses and their replication. In Knipe DM, Howley PM (eds): Fields' Virology. Philadelphia, Lippincott Williams & Wilkins, 2001, p 2399.
13. Read GS, Frenkel N: Herpes simplex virus mutants defective in the virion associated shut-off of host polypeptide synthesis and exhibiting abnormal synthesis of α (immediate early) viral polypeptides. J Virol 46:498, 1983.
14. Spear PG, Longnecker R: Herpesvirus entry: An update. J Virol 77:10179, 2003.
15. Bergstrom T, Trybala E: Antigenic differences between HSV-1 and HSV-2 glycoproteins and their importance for type-specific serology. Intervirology 39:176, 1996.
16. Roizman B, Roane PR Jr: Multiplication of herpes simplex virus. II. The relationship between protein synthesis and the duplication of viral DNA in infected Hep-2 cells. Virology 22:262, 1964.
17. Roizman B, Borman GS, Kamali-Rousta M: Macromolecular synthesis in cells infected with herpes simplex virus. Nature 206:1374, 1965.
18. Whitley RJ, Gnann JW: The epidemiology and clinical manifestations of herpes simplex virus infections. In Roizman B, Whitley RJ, Lopez C (eds): The Human Herpesviruses. New York, Raven Press, 1993, p 69.
19. Smith JS, Robinson NJ: Age-specific prevalence of infection with herpes simplex virus types 2 and 1: A global review. J Infect Dis 186(Suppl 1):S3, 2002.
20. Cesario TC, Poland JD, Wulff H, et al: Six years experiences with herpes simplex virus in a children's home. Am J Epidemiol 90:416, 1969.
21. Buddingh GH, Schrum DI, Lanier JC, et al: Studies of the natural history of herpes simplex infections. Pediatrics 11:595, 1953.
22. DeGiordana HM, Banza CA, Russi JC, et al: Prevalence of herpes simplex virus infection. Arch Pediatr Uruguay 41:107, 1970.
23. Schmitt DL, Johnson DW, Henderson FW: Herpes simplex type 1 infections in group day care. Pediatr Infect Dis J 10:729, 1991.
24. Scott TF, Steigman AJ, Convey JH: Acute infectious gingivostomatitis: Etiology, epidemiology, and clinical pictures of a common disorder caused by the virus of herpes simplex. JAMA 117:999, 1941.
25. McMillan JA, Weiner LB, Higgins AM, et al: Pharyngitis associated with herpes simplex virus in college students. Pediatr Infect Dis 12:280, 1993.
26. Guex-Crosier Y, Rochat C, Herbort CP: Necrotizing herpetic retinopathies. A spectrum of herpes virus-induced diseases determined by the immune state of the host. Ocul Immunol Inflamm 5:259, 1997.
27. Wollenberg A, Zoch C, Wetzel S, et al: Predisposing factors and clinical features of eczema herpeticum: A retrospective analysis of 100 cases. J Am Acad Dermatol 49:198, 2003.
28. Dworkin MS, Shoemaker PC, Spitters C, et al: Endemic spread of herpes simplex virus type 1 among adolescent wrestlers and their coaches. Pediatr Infect Dis J 18:1108, 1999.
29. Avitzur Y, Amir J: Herpetic whitlow infection in a general pediatrician—An occupational hazard. Infection 30:234, 2002.
30. Kimberlin DW: Herpes simplex virus infections of the central nervous system. Semin Pediatr Infect Dis 14:83, 2003.
31. Devine SM, Wingard JR: Viral infections in severely immunocompromised cancer patients. Support Care Cancer 2:355, 1994.
32. Kang AH, Graves CR: Herpes simplex hepatitis in pregnancy: A case report and review of the literature. Obstet Gynecol Surv 54:463, 1999.
33. Kalinyak JE, Fleagle G, Docherty JJ: Incidence and distribution of herpes simplex virus types 1 and 2 from genital lesions in college women. J Med Virol 1:173, 1977.
34. Wolontis S, Jeansson S: Correlation of herpes simplex virus types 1 and 2 with clinical features of infection. J Infect Dis 135:28, 1977.
35. Reeves WC, Corey L, Adams HG, et al: Risk of recurrence after first episodes of genital herpes: Relation to HSV type and antibody response. N Engl J Med 305:315, 1981.
36. Corey L, Adams H, Brown A, et al: Genital herpes simplex virus infections: Clinical manifestations, course and complications. Ann Intern Med 98:958, 1983.
37. Mertz GJ, Rosenthal SL, Stanberry LR: Is herpes simplex virus type 1 (HSV-1) now more common than HSV-2 in first episodes of genital herpes? Sex Transm Dis 30:801, 2003.
38. Ship II, Morris AL, Durocher RT, et al: Recurrent aphthous ulcerations and recurrent herpes labialis in a professional school student population. I. Experience. Oral Surg Oral Med Oral Pathol Radiol Endod 13:1191, 1960.
39. Ship II, Morris AL, Durocher RT, et al: Recurrent aphthous ulcerations and recurrent labialis in a professional school student population. IV. Twelve month study of natural disease patterns. Oral Surg Oral Med Oral Pathol 14:39, 1961.
40. Josey WE, Nahmias AJ, Naib ZM: The epidemiology of type-2 (genital) herpes simplex virus infections. Obstet Gynecol Surg 27:295, 1972.
41. Fleming DT, McQuillan GM, Johnson RE, et al: Herpes simplex virus type 2 in the United States, 1976 to 1994. N Engl J Med 337:1105, 1997.
42. Wald A, Zeh J, Selke S, et al: Reactivation of genital herpes simplex virus type 2 infection in asymptomatic seropositive persons. N Engl J Med 342:844, 2000.
43. Yeager AS, Arvin AM: Reasons for the absence of a history of recurrent genital infections in mothers of neonates infected with herpes simplex virus. Pediatrics 73:188, 1984.
44. Brown ZA, Benedetti J, Ashley R, et al: Neonatal herpes simplex virus infection in relation to asymptomatic maternal infection at the time of labor. N Engl J Med 324:1247, 1991.
45. Schacker T, Zeh J, Hu HL, et al: Frequency of symptomatic and asymptomatic herpes simplex virus type 2 reactivations among human immunodeficiency virus-infected men. J Infect Dis 178:1616, 1998.
46. Augenbraun M, Corey L, Reichelderfer P, et al: Herpes simplex virus shedding and plasma human immunodeficiency virus RNA levels in coinfected women. Clin Infect Dis 33:885, 2001.
47. Koelle DM, Wald A: Herpes simplex virus: The importance of asymptomatic shedding. J Antimicrob Chemother 45(Suppl T3):1, 2000.
48. Chatterjee A, Chartrand SA, Harrison CJ, et al: Severe intrauterine herpes simplex disease with placentitis in a newborn of a mother with recurrent genital infection at delivery. J Perinatol 21:559, 2001.
49. Francis DP, Herrmann KL, MacMahon JR, et al: Nosocomial and maternally acquired herpesvirus hominis infections. A report of four fatal cases in neonates. Am J Dis Child 129:889, 1975.
50. Hutto C, Arvin A, Jacobs R, et al: Intrauterine herpes simplex virus infections. J Pediatr 110:97, 1987.
51. Stanberry LR: The pathogenesis of herpes simplex virus infections. In Stanberry LR (ed): Genital and Neonatal Herpes. London, John Wiley and Sons, 1996, pp 31–48.
52. Kimberlin DW, Lin CY, Jacobs RF, et al: Natural history of neonatal herpes simplex virus infections in the acyclovir era. Pediatrics 108:223, 2001.
53. Stanberry LR: The pathogenesis of herpes simplex virus infections. In Stanberry LR (ed): Genital and Neonatal Herpes. London, John Wiley and Sons, 1996, p 31.
54. Stevens JG, Wagner EK, Devi-Rao GB, et al: RNA complementary to a herpesvirus alpha gene mRNA is prominent in latently infected neurons. Science 235:1056, 1987.
55. Croen KD, Ostrove JM, Dragovic LJ, et al: Latent herpes simplex virus in human trigeminal ganglia. Detection of an immediate early gene "anti-sense" transcript by in situ hybridization. N Engl J Med 317:1427, 1987.
56. Cook ML, Stevens JG: Pathogenesis of herpetic neuritis and ganglionitis in mice: Evidence of intra-axonal transport of infection. Infect Immun 7:272, 1973.
57. Wald A, Zeh J, Selke S, et al: Reactivation of genital herpes simplex virus type 2 infection in asymptomatic seropositive persons. N Engl J Med 342:844, 2000.
58. Esmann J: The many challenges of facial herpes simplex virus infection. J Antimicrob Chemother 47(Suppl T1):17, 2001.

59. York IA, Roop C, Andrew DW, et al: A cytosolic herpes simplex virus protein inhibits antigen presentation to CD8– T lymphocytes. Cell 77:525, 1994.
60. Hill A, Jugovic P, York I, et al: Herpes simplex virus turns off the TAP to evade host immunity. Nature 375:411, 1995.
61. Nagashunmugam T, Lubinski J, Wang L, et al: In vivo immune evasion mediated by the herpes simplex virus type 1 immunoglobulin G Fc receptor. J Virol 72:5351, 1998.
62. Favoreel HW, Nauwynck HJ, Pensaert MB: Immunological hiding of herpesvirus-infected cells. Arch Virol 145:1269, 2000.
63. Friedman HM: Immune evasion by herpes simplex virus type 1, strategies for virus survival. Trans Am Clin Climatol Assoc 114:103, 2003.
64. Koutsky LA, Stevens CE, Holmes KK, et al: Underdiagnosis of genital herpes by current clinical and viral-isolation procedures. N Engl J Med 326:1533, 1992.
65. Langenberg AG, Corey L, Ashley RL, et al: A prospective study of new infections with herpes simplex virus type 1 and type 2. Chiron HSV Vaccine Study Group. N Engl J Med 341:1432, 1999.
66. Marshall DS, Linfert DR, Draghi A, et al: Identification of herpes simplex virus genital infection: Comparison of a multiplex PCR assay and traditional viral isolation techniques. Mod Pathol 14:152, 2001.
67. Verano L, Michalski FJ: Comparison of a direct antigen enzyme immunoassay, Herpchek, with cell culture for detection of herpes simplex virus from clinical specimens. J Clin Microbiol 33:1378, 1995.
68. Slomka MJ, Emery L, Munday PE, et al: A comparison of PCR with virus isolation and direct antigen detection for diagnosis and typing of genital herpes. J Med Virol 55:177, 1998.
69. Bagg J, Mannings A, Munro J, et al: Rapid diagnosis of oral herpes simplex or zoster virus infections by immunofluorescence: Comparison with Tzanck cell preparations and viral culture. Br Dent J 167:235, 1989.
70. Aurelius E, Johansson B, Skoldenberg B, et al: Rapid diagnosis of herpes simplex encephalitis by nested polymerase chain reaction assay of cerebrospinal fluid. Lancet 337:189, 1991.
71. Domingues RB, Lakeman FD, Mayo MS, et al: Application of competitive PCR to cerebrospinal fluid samples from patients with herpes simplex encephalitis. J Clin Microbiol 36:2229, 1998.
72. Koenig M, Reynolds KS, Aldous W, et al: Comparison of Light-Cycler PCR, enzyme immunoassay, and tissue culture for detection of herpes simplex virus. Diagn Microbiol Infect Dis 40:107, 2001.
73. Ashley RL: Performance and use of HSV type-specific serology test kits. Herpes 9:38, 2002.
74. Ashley RL: Sorting out the new HSV type specific antibody tests. Sex Transm Infect 77:232, 2001.
75. Villarreal EC: Current and potential therapies for the treatment of herpes-virus infections. Prog Drug Res 60:263, 2003.
76. Bacon TH, Levin MJ, Leary JJ, et al: Herpes simplex virus resistance to acyclovir and penciclovir after two decades of antiviral therapy. Clin Microbiol Rev 16:114, 2003.
77. Chilukuri S, Rosen T: Management of acyclovir-resistant herpes simplex virus. Dermatol Clin 21:311, 2003.
78. Safrin S, Kemmerly S, Plotkin B, et al: Foscarnet-resistant herpes simplex virus infection in patients with AIDS. J Infect Dis 169:193, 1994.
79. Wald A, Langenberg AG, Link K, et al: Effect of condoms on reducing the transmission of herpes simplex virus type 2 from men to women. JAMA 285:3100, 2001.
80. Casper C, Wald A: Condom use and the prevention of genital herpes acquisition. Herpes 9:10, 2002.
81. Corey L, Wald A, Patel R, et al: Once-daily valaciclovir to reduce the risk of transmission of genital herpes. New Engl J Med 350:11, 2004.
82. Brown ZA, Wald A, Morrow RA, et al: Effect of serologic status and cesarean delivery on transmission rates of herpes simplex virus from mother to infant. JAMA 289:203, 2003.
83. Randolph AG, Washington AE, Prober CG: Cesarean delivery for women presenting with genital herpes lesions. Efficacy, risks, and costs. JAMA 270:77, 1993.
84. Scott LL, Sanchez PJ, Jackson GL, et al: Acyclovir suppression to prevent cesarean delivery after first-episode genital herpes. Obstet Gynecol 87:69, 1996.
85. Braig S, Luton D, Sibony O, et al: Acyclovir prophylaxis in late pregnancy prevents recurrent genital herpes and viral shedding. Eur J Obstet Gynecol Reprod Biol 96:55, 2001.
86. Watts DH, Brown ZA, Money D, et al: A double-blind, randomized, placebo-controlled trial of acyclovir in late pregnancy for the reduction of herpes simplex virus shedding and cesarean delivery. Am J Obstet Gynecol 188:836, 2003.
87. Stanberry LR, Cunningham AL, Mindel A, et al: Prospects for control of herpes simplex virus disease through immunization. Clin Infect Dis 30:549, 2000.
88. Stanberry LR, Spruance SL, Cunningham AL, et al: Glycoprotein-D-adjuvant vaccine to prevent genital herpes. N Engl J Med 347:1652, 2002.
89. Steiner P: Zu Inokulation der Varicellen. Wien Med Wochenschr 25:306, 1875.
90. von Bakay J: Über den aetiologischen Zusammenhang der Varizelllen met gewissen Fällen von Herpes zoster. Wien Klin Wochenschr 22:1323, 1909.
91. Kundratitz K: Experimentelle Übertagungen von Herpes zoster auf Menschen and die Beziehungen von Herpes zoster zu Varizellen. Z Kinderheilkol 39:379, 1925.
92. Weller TH, Witton HM, Bell EJ: The etiologic agents of varicella and herpes zoster. J Exp Med 108:843, 1958.
93. Straus SE, Reinhold W, Smith HA, et al: Endonuclease analysis of viral DNAs from varicella and subsequent zoster infections in the same patient. N Engl J Med 311:1362, 1984.
94. Davison AJ, Scott J: The complete DNA sequence of varicella-zoster virus. J Gen Virol 67:1759, 1986.
95. Davison AJ, Wilkie NM: Location and orientation of homologous sequences in the genomes of five herpesviruses. J Gen Virol 64:1927, 1983.
96. Grose C: Glycoproteins of varicella-zoster virus and their herpes simplex virus homologs. Rev Infect Dis 13:S960, 1991.
97. Hope-Simpson RE: Infectiousness of communicable diseases in the household (measles, chickenpox, and mumps). Lancet 2:549, 1952.
98. Sinha DP: Chickenpox—A disease predominantly affecting adults in rural West Bengal, India. Int J Epidemiol 5:367, 1976.
99. Ooi PL, Goh KT, Doraisingham S, et al: Prevalence of varicella-zoster virus infection in Singapore. Southeast Asian J Trop Med Public Health 23:22, 1992.
100. Arvin AM, Koropchak CM, Wittek AM: Immunologic evidence for reinfection with varicella-zoster virus. J Infect Dis 148:200, 1983.
101. Junker AK, Angus E, Thomas EE: Recurrent varicella-zoster virus infections in apparently immunocompetent children. Pediatr Infect Dis J 10:569, 1991.
102. Finger R, Hughes JP, Meade BJ, et al: Age-specific incidence of chickenpox. Public Health Rep 109:750, 1994.
103. Struewing JP, Hyams KC, Tueller JE, et al: The risk of measles, mumps and varicella among young adults: A serosurvey of U.S. Navy and Marine Corps recruits. Am J Public Health 83:1717, 1993.
104. Johnson R, Milbourne PE: Central nervous system manifestations of chickenpox. Can Med Assoc J 102:831, 1970.
105. Feldman S, Hughes WT, Daniel CB: Varicella in children with cancer. Pediatrics 56:388, 1975.
106. van Loon F, Markowitz L, McQuillan G, et al: Varicella seroprevalence in U.S. population. In Program and Abstracts of the 33rd Interscience Conference on Antimicrobial Agents and Chemotherapy, New Orleans, September 1993.
107. Paryani SG, Arvin AM: Intrauterine infection with varicella zoster virus after maternal varicella. N Engl J Med 314:1542, 1986.
108. Harger JH, Ernest JM, Thurnau GR, et al: Frequency of congenital varicella syndrome in a prospective cohort of 347 pregnant women. Obstet Gynecol 100:260, 2002.
109. Preblud SR, Bregman DJ, Vernon LL: Deaths from varicella in infants. Pediatr Infect Dis 4:503, 1985.
110. Brunell PA: Placental transfer of varicella-zoster antibody. Pediatrics 38:1034, 1966.
111. Schmader K, George LK, Burchett BM, et al: Racial differences in the occurrence of herpes zoster. J Infect Dis 171:701, 1995.
112. Berger R, Florent G, Just M: Decrease of the lymphoproliferative response to varicella zoster virus antigen in the aged. Infect Immun 32:24, 1981.
113. Levin MJ, Smith JG, Kaufhold RM, et al: Decline in varicella-zoster virus (VZV)-specific cell-mediated immunity with increasing age and boosting with a high-hose VZV vaccine. J Infect Dis 188:1336, 2003.
114. Gershon AA, LaRussa P, Steinberg S, et al: The protective effect of immunologic boosting against zoster: An analysis in leukemic

children who were vaccinated against chickenpox. J Infect Dis 173:450, 1996.
115. Kleinschmidt-DeMasters BK, Amlie-Lefond C, et al: The patterns of varicella-zoster virus encephalitis. Hum Pathol 27:927, 1996.
116. Sexton CJ, Navsaria HA, Leigh IM, et al: Replication of varicella-zoster virus in primary human keratinocytes. J Med Virol 38:260, 1992.
117. Weller TH: Serial propagation in vitro of agents producing inclusion bodies derived from varicella and herpes zoster. Proc Soc Exp Biol Med 83:340, 1953.
118. Croen KD, Ostrove JM, Dragovic LJ, et al: Patterns of gene expression and sites of latency in human nerve ganglia are different for varicella-zoster and herpes simplex viruses. Proc Natl Acad Sci USA 85:9773, 1988.
119. Vafai A, Wroblewska Z, Mahalingham R, et al: Recognition of similar epitopes on varicella-zoster virus gpl and gpIV by monoclonal antibodies. J Virol 62:2544, 1988.
120. Mahalingham R, Wellish M, Wolf W, et al: Latent varicella-zoster virus DNA in human trigeminal and thoracic ganglia. N Engl J Med 323:627, 1990.
121. Mahalingham R, Wellish MC, Dueland AN, et al: Localization of herpes simplex virus and varicella-zoster virus DNA in human ganglia. Ann Neurol 31:444, 1992.
122. Furuta Y, Takasu T, Fukuda S, et al: Detection of varicella-zoster virus DNA in human geniculate ganglia by polymerase chain reaction. J Infect Dis 166:1157, 1992.
123. Liedtke W, Opalka B, Zimmermann CW, et al: Age distribution of latent herpes simplex virus I and varicella-zoster virus genome in human nervous tissue. J Neurol Sci 116:6, 1993.
124. Meier JL, Holman RP, Croen KD, et al: Varicella-zoster virus transcription in human trigeminal ganglia. Virology 193:193, 1993.
125. Kennedy PG: Key issues in varicella-zoster virus latency. J Neurovirol 8(Suppl 2):80, 2002.
126. Kennedy PG: Varicella-zoster virus latency in human ganglia. Rev Med Virol 12:327, 2002.
127. Gilden DH, Cohrs RJ, Mahalingam R: Clinical and molecular pathogenesis of varicella virus infection. Viral Immunol 16:243, 2003.
128. Stocher M, Leb V, Bozic M, et al: Parallel detection of five human herpes virus DNAs by a set of real-time polymerase chain reactions in a single run. J Clin Virol 26:85, 2003.
129. Arvin AM: Antiviral therapy for varicella and herpes zoster. Semin Pediatr Infect Dis 13:12, 2002.
130. Shepp D, Dandliker PS, Meyers JD: Treatment of varicella-zoster virus in severely immunocompromised patients: A randomized comparison of acyclovir and vidarabine. N Engl J Med 314:208, 1987.
131. Balfour HH Jr, Rotbart HA, Feldman S, et al: Acyclovir treatment of varicella in otherwise healthy adolescents. The Collaborative Acyclovir Varicella Study Group. J Pediatr 120:627, 1992.
132. Dunkle LM, Arvin AM, Whitley RJ, et al: A controlled trial of acyclovir for chickenpox in normal children. N Engl J Med 325:1539, 1991.
133. Enright AM, Prober C: Antiviral therapy in children with varicella zoster virus and herpes simplex virus infections. Herpes 10:32, 2003.
134. Klassen TP, Belseck EM, Wiebe N, et al: Acyclovir for treating varicella in otherwise healthy children and adolescents: a systematic review of randomised controlled trials. BMC Pediatr 2:9, 2002.
135. Jacobson MA, Berger TG, Fikrig S, et al: Acyclovir-resistant varicella-zoster virus infection after chronic oral acyclovir therapy in patients with the acquired immunodeficiency syndrome (AIDS). Ann Intern Med 112:187, 1990.
136. Gershon AA: Prevention and treatment of VZV infections in patients with HIV. Herpes 8:32, 2001.
137. Johnson RW, Dworkin RH: Treatment of herpes zoster and postherpetic neuralgia. BMJ 26:748, 2003.
138. Curran MP, Wagstaff AJ: Gabapentin: in postherpetic neuralgia. CNS Drugs 17:975, 2003.
139. Arvin AM, Gershon AA: Live attenuated varicella vaccine. Annu Rev Microbiol 50:59, 1996.
140. Centers for Disease Control and Prevention (CDC): Decline in annual incidence of varicella—Selected states, 1990–2001. MMWR 52:884, 2003.
141. Plotkin SA, Starr SE, Connor K, et al: Zoster in normal children after varicella vaccine. J Infect Dis 159:1000, 1989.
142. Watson BM, Piercy SA, Plotkin SA, et al: Modified chickenpox in children immunized with the Oka/Merck varicella vaccine. Pediatrics 91:17, 1993.
143. Gershon AA, Steinger SP, LaRussa P, et al: Immunization of healthy adults with live attenuated varicella vaccine. J Infect Dis 158:132, 1988.
144. Galil K, Lee B, Strine T, et al: Outbreak of varicella at a day-care center despite vaccination. N Engl J Med 347:1909, 2002.
145. Gershon AA: Symposium on infectious complications of neoplastic disease (Part II). Immunoprophylaxis of varicella-zoster infections. Am J Med 76:672, 1984.
146. Roizman B, Carmichael LE, Deinhardt F, et al: Herpesviridae. Definition, provisional nomenclature, and taxonomy. Intervirology 16:201, 1981.
147. Karlin S, Mocarski ES, Schachtel GA: Molecular evolution of herpesviruses: Genomic and protein sequence comparisons. J Virol 68:1886, 1994.
148. Wright HT Jr, Goodheart CR, Lielausis A: Human cytomegalovirus. Morphology by negative staining. Virology 23:419, 1964.
149. Geelen JL, Walig C, Wertheim P, et al: Human cytomegalovirus DNA. I. Molecular weight and infectivity. J Virol 26:813, 1978.
150. Lakeman AD, Osborn JE: Size of infectious DNA from human and murine cytomegaloviruses. J Virol 30:414, 1979.
151. Chee MS, Bankier AT, Beck S, et al: Analysis of the protein-coding content of the sequence of human cytomegalovirus stain AD169. Curr Top Microbiol Immunol 154:125, 1990.
152. Kim KS, Sapienza VJ, Carp RI, et al: Analysis of structural polypeptides of purified human cytomegalovirus. J Virol 20:604, 1976.
153. Jahn G, Mach M: Human cytomegalovirus phosphoproteins and glycoproteins and their coding regions. Curr Top Microbiol Immunol 154:171, 1990.
154. Gibson W: Protein counterparts of human and simian cytomegaloviruses. Virology 128:391, 1983.
155. Rasmussen L, Resta S, Merigan T: Human cytomegalovirus glycoprotein-receptor interactions. Transplant Proc 23:60, 1991.
156. Borysiewicz LK, Hickling JK, Graham S, et al: Human cytomegalovirus-specific cytotoxic T cells. Relative frequency of stage-specific CTL recognizing the 72-kD immediate early protein and glycoprotein B expressed by recombinant vaccinia virus. J Exp Med 168:919, 1988.
157. Chou S: Comparative analysis of sequence variation in gp116 and gp55 components of glycoprotein B of human cytomegalovirus. Virology 188:388, 1992.
158. Fries BC, Chou S, Boeckh M, et al: Frequency distribution of cytomegalovirus envelope glycoprotein genotypes in bone marrow transplant recipients. J Infect Dis 169:769, 1994.
159. Gold E, Nankervis GA. Cytomegalovirus. In Evans AS (ed): Viral Infections of Humans: Epidemiology and Control, 2nd ed. New York, Plenum Press, 1982, p 167.
160. Kumar ML, Nankervis GA, Gold E: Inapparent congenital cytomegalovirus infection: A follow-up study. N Engl J Med 288:1377, 1973.
161. Alford CA, Stagno S, Pass RF, et al: Epidemiology of cytomegalovirus. In Nahmais A, Dowdle W, Schinazi R (eds): The Human Herpesviruses: An Interdisciplinary Perspective. New York, Elsevier, 1981, p 159.
162. Reynolds DW, Stagno S, Hosty TS, et al: Maternal cytomegalovirus excretion and perinatal infection. N Engl J Med 289:1, 1973.
163. Stagno S, Reynolds DW, Pass RF, et al: Breast milk and the risk of cytomegalovirus infection. N Engl J Med 302:1073, 1980.
164. Dworsky M, Yow M, Stagno S, et al: Cytomegalovirus infection of breast milk and transmission in infancy. Pediatrics 72:295, 1983.
165. Pass RF, Hutto C, Reynolds DW, et al: Increased frequency of cytomegalovirus in children in group day care. Pediatrics 74:121, 1984.
166. Horwitz CA, Henle W, Henle G: Diagnostic aspects of the cytomegalovirus mononucleosis syndrome in previously healthy persons. Postgrad Med 66:153, 1979.
167. Klemola E, Kaariainen L: Cytomegalovirus as a possible cause of a disease resembling infectious mononucleosis. BMJ 2:1099, 1965.
168. Sun A, Chang JG, Kao CL, et al: Human cytomegalovirus as a potential etiologic agent in recurrent aphthous ulcers and Behçet's disease. J Oral Pathol Med 25:212, 1996.
169. Boppana SB, Pass RF, Britt WJ, et al: Symptomatic congenital cytomegalovirus infection: Neonatal morbidity and mortality. Pediatr Infect Dis 11:93, 1992.

170. Hicks T, Fowler K, Richardson M, et al: Congenital cytomegalovirus infections and neonatal auditory screening. J Pediatr 123:779, 1993.
171. Stagno S, Reynolds DW, Tsiantos A, et al: Comparative, serial virologic and serologic studies of symptomatic and subclinical congenital and naturally acquired cytomegalovirus infection. J Infect Dis 132:568, 1975.
172. Pollard AB: Cytomegalovirus infections in renal, heart, heart-lung and liver transplantation. Pediatr Infect Dis J 7:97, 1988.
173. Lautenschlager I, Hockerstedt K, Jalanko H, et al: Persistent cytomegalovirus in liver allografts with chronic rejection. Hepatology 25:190, 1997.
174. Boriskin YS, Booth JC, Corbishley CM, et al: Human cytomegalovirus and acute rejection after heart transplantation are not directly associated. J Med Virol 50:59, 1996.
175. Persson L, Dahl H, Linde A, et al: Human cytomegalovirus, human herpesvirus-6 and human herpesvirus-7 in neutropenic patients with fever of unknown origin. Clin Microbiol Infect 9:640, 2003.
176. Webster A: Cytomegalovirus as a possible cofactor in HIV disease progression. J Acquir Immune Defic Syndr Hum Retrovirol 4:S47, 1991.
177. Shi Y, Tokunaga O: Herpesvirus (HSV-1, EBV and CMV) infections in atherosclerotic compared with non-atherosclerotic aortic tissue. Pathol Int 52:31, 2002.
178. Lin TM, Chen WJ, Chen HY, et al: Increased incidence of cytomegalovirus but not *Chlamydia pneumoniae* in atherosclerotic lesions of arteries of lower extremities from patients with diabetes mellitus undergoing amputation. J Clin Pathol 56:429, 2003.
179. Stinski MF: Molecular biology of cytomegaloviruses. In Roizman B (ed): The Herpesviruses. New York, Plenum Press, 1983, p 67.
180. Rowe WP, Hartley JW, Waterman S, et al: Cytopathogenic agent resembling human salivary gland virus recovered from tissue cultures of human adenoids. Proc Soc Exp Biol Med 92:418, 1956.
181. Tanaka S, Furukawa T, Plotkin SA: Human cytomegalovirus simulates host cell RNA synthesis. J Virol 15:297, 1975.
182. Furukawa T, Sakuma S, Plotkin SA: Human cytomegalovirus infection of WI-38 cells stimulates mitochondrial DNA synthesis. Nature 262:414, 1976.
183. Fons MP, Graves K, Cavallo T, et al: Human cytomegalovirus: Development and progression of nuclear inclusions by primary clinical isolates and laboratory-adapted stains. Proc Soc Exp Biol Med 181:416, 1986.
184. Fetterman GH, Sherman FE, Fabizio NS, et al: Generalized cytomegalic inclusion disease of the newborn: Localization of inclusions in the kidney. Arch Pathol 86:86, 1968.
185. Myerson D, Hackman RC, Nelson JA, et al: Widespread presence of histologically occult cytomegalovirus. Hum Pathol 15:430, 1984.
186. Taylor-Wiedeman J, Sissons JG, Borysiewicz LK, et al: Monocytes are a major site of persistence of human cytomegalovirus in peripheral blood mononuclear cells. J Gen Virol 72:2059, 1991.
187. Taylor-Wiedeman J, Hayhurst GP, Sissons JG, et al: Polymorphonuclear cells are not sites of persistence of human cytomegalovirus in healthy individuals. J Gen Virol 74:265, 1993.
188. Weber B, Opp M, Born HJ, et al: Laboratory diagnosis of congenital human cytomegalovirus infection using polymerase chain reaction and shell vial culture. Infection 20:155, 1992.
189. Carter IW, Cloonan MJ: Comparison between three PCR methods for detection of human cytomegalovirus DNA. Pathology 27:161, 1995.
190. Barber L, Egan JJ, Lomax J, et al: Comparative study of three PCR assays with antigenaemia and serology for the diagnosis of HCMV infection in thoracic transplant recipients. J Med Virol 49:137, 1996.
191. Vogelberg C, Meyer-Konig U, Hufert FT, et al: Human cytomegalovirus glycoprotein B genotypes in renal transplant recipients. J Med Virol 50:31, 1996.
192. Lurain NS, Thompson KD, Holmes EW, et al: Point mutations in the DNA polymerase gene of human cytomegalovirus that result in resistance to antiviral agents. J Virol 66:7146, 1992.
193. Stanat SC, Reardon JE, Eric A, et al: Ganciclovir-resistant cytomegalovirus clinical isolates: Mode of resistance to ganciclovir. Antimicrob Agents Chemother 35:2191, 1991.
194. Sullivan V, Biron KK, Talarico C, et al: A point mutation in the human cytomegalovirus DNA polymerase gene confers resistance to ganciclovir and phosphonylmethoxyalkyl derivatives. Antimicrob Agents Chemother 37:19, 1993.
195. Chou S, Lurain NS, Thompson KD, et al: Viral DNA polymerase mutations associated with drug resistance in human cytomegalovirus. J Infect Dis 188:32, 2003.
196. Adler SP, Finney JW, Manganello AM, et al: Prevention of child-to-mother transmission of cytomegalovirus by changing behaviors: A randomized controlled trial. Pediatr Infect Dis J 15:240, 1996.
197. Britt WJ: Vaccines against human cytomegalovirus: Time to test. Trends Microbiol 4:34, 1996.
198. Kieff E: Epstein-Barr virus and its replication. In Fields BN, Knipe DM, Howley PM (eds): Fields' Virology, 3rd ed. Philadelphia, Lippincott-Raven, 1996, p 2343.
199. Epstein MA, Achong BG, Barr YM: Virus particles in cultured lymphoblasts from Burkitt's lymphoma. Lancet 1:7203, 1964.
200. Henle W, Diehl V, Kohn G, et al: Herpes-type virus and chromosome marker in normal leukocytes after growth with irradiated Burkitt cells. Science 157:1064, 1967.
201. Pope JH, Achong BG, Epstein MA: Burkitt lymphoma in New Guinea: Establishment of a line of lymphoblasts in vitro and description of their fine structure. J Natl Cancer Inst 39:933, 1967.
202. Henle G, Henle W, Hiehl V: Relation of Burkitt's tumor–associated herpes-type virus to infectious mononucleosis. Proc Natl Acad Sci USA 59:94, 1968.
203. Zur Hausen H, Schule-Holthausen H, Klein G, et al: EBV DNA in biopsies of Burkitt tumours and anaplastic carcinomas of the nasopharynx. Nature 228:1056, 1970.
204. Wolf H, zur Hasen H, Becker V: EBV viral genomes in epithelial nasopharyngeal carcinoma cells. Nature 244:245, 1973.
205. Nonoyama M, Huang CH, Pagano JS, et al: DNA of Epstein-Barr virus detected in tissue of Burkitt's lymphoma and nasopharyngeal carcinoma. Proc Natl Acad Sci USA 70:3265, 1973.
206. Greenspan JS, Greenspan D, Lennette ET, et al: Replication of Epstein-Barr virus within the epithelial cells of oral "hairy" leukoplakia, an AIDS-associated lesion. N Engl J Med 313:1564, 1985.
207. Weiss LM, Strickler JG, Warnke RA, et al: Epstein-Barr viral DNA in tissues of Hodgkin's disease. Am J Pathol 129:86, 1987.
208. Weiss LM, Movahed LA, Butler AE, et al: Analysis of lymphoepithelioma and lymphoepithelioma-like carcinomas for Epstein-Barr virus by in situ hybridization. Am J Surg Pathol 13:625, 1989.
209. Harabuchi Y, Yamanaka N, Kataura A, et al: Epstein-Barr virus in nasal T-cell lymphomas in patients with lethal midline granuloma. Lancet 335:128, 1990.
210. Su IJ, Hsieh HC, Lin KH, et al: Aggressive peripheral T-cell lymphoma containing Epstein-Barr viral DNA: A clinicopathological and molecular analysis. Blood 68:1954, 1991.
211. Fingeroth JD, Weiss JJ, Teddr TF, et al: Epstein-Barr virus receptor of human B lymphocytes is the C3d receptor CR2. Proc Natl Acad Sci USA 81:45610, 1984.
212. Baer R, Bankier AT, Biggin MD, et al: DNA sequence and expression of the B95-8 Epstein-Barr virus genome. Nature 310:207, 1984.
213. Pearson G, Luka J, Petti L, et al: Identification of an Epstein-Barr virus early gene encoding for a second component of the restricted early antigen complex. Virology 160:151, 1987.
214. Moore KW, Vieira P, Fiorentino DF, et al: Homology of cytokine synthesis inhibitory factor (IL-10) to the Epstein-Barr virus gene BCRFI. Science 248:1230, 1990.
215. Packham G, Economou A, Rooney CM, et al: Structure and function of the Epstein-Barr virus BZLF1 protein. J Virol 64:2110, 1990.
216. Sixbey JW, Shirley P, Chesney PJ, et al: Detection of a second widespread strain of Epstein-Barr virus. Lancet 2:761, 1989.
217. Apolloni A, Sculley TB: Detection of A-type and B-type Epstein-Barr virus in throat washings and lymphocytes. Virology 202:978, 1994.
218. Rickinson AB, Young LS, Rowe M: Influence of the Epstein-Barr virus nuclear antigen EBNA 2 on the growth phenotype of virus-transformed B cells. J Virol 61:1310, 1987.
219. Hudnall SD, Patel J, Schwab H, et al: Comparative immunophenotypic features of EBV-positive and EBV-negative atypical lymphocytosis. Clin Cytometry 55B:22–28, 2003.
220. Shibata D, Weiss LM: Epstein-Barr virus–associated gastric adenocarcinoma. Am J Pathol 140:769, 1992.
221. Imai S, Koizumi S, Sugiura M, et al: Gastric carcinoma: Monoclonal epithelial malignant cells expressing Epstein-Barr virus latent infection protein. Proc Natl Acad Sci USA 91:9131, 1994.

222. Kingma DW, Shad A, Tsokos M, et al: Epstein-Barr virus (EBV)–associated smooth-muscle tumor arising in a post-transplant patient treated successfully for two PT-EBV–associated large-cell lymphomas. Case report. Am J Surg Pathol 20:1511, 1996.
223. McClain KL, Leach CT, Jenson HB, et al: Association of Epstein-Barr virus with leiomyosarcomas in children with AIDS. N Engl J Med 332:12, 1995.
224. Anagnostopoulos I, Hummel M: Epstein-Barr virus in tumours. Histopathology 29:297, 1996.
225. Purtilo DT, Cassel C, Yang JSP, et al: X-linked recessive progressive combined variable immunodeficiency (Duncan's disease). Lancet 1:935, 1975.
226. Burkitt D: A children's cancer dependent upon climatic factors. Nature 194:232, 1962.
227. Andersson M, Klein G, Zigler JL, et al: Association of Epstein-Barr viral genomes with American Burkitt lymphoma. Nature 260:357, 1976.
228. Shiramizu B, Barriga F, Neequaye J, et al: Patterns of chromosomal breakpoint locations in Burkitt's lymphoma: Relevant to geography and EBV association. Blood 77:1516, 1991.
229. Chan SH, Day NE, Kunaratnam N, et al: HLA and nasopharyngeal carcinoma in Chinese—A further study. Int J Cancer 32:171, 1983.
230. Yu MC, Ho JHC, Lai SH, et al: Cantonese-style salted fish as a cause of nasopharyngeal carcinoma: Report of a case-control study in Hong Kong. Cancer Res 46:956, 1986.
231. Yu MC, Huang TB, Henderson BE: Diet and nasopharyngeal carcinoma: A case-control study in Guangzhou, China. Int J Cancer 43:1077, 1989.
232. Armstrong RW, Armstrong MJ, Jay MC, et al: Salted fish and inhalants as risk factors for carcinoma in Malaysian Chinese. Cancer Res 43:2697, 1983.
233. West S, Hildesheim A, Dosemeci M: Non-viral risk factors for nasopharyngeal carcinoma in the Philippines: Result from a case-control study. Int J Cancer 55:722, 1993.
234. Poirier S, Ohshiima H, de The G, et al: Volatile nitrosamine levels in common foods from Tunisia, South China and Greenland, high risk areas for nasopharyngeal carcinoma (NPC). Int J Cancer 39:293, 1987.
235. Levine PH, Conelly R: Epidemiology of nasopharyngeal cancer. In Wittes RE (ed): Head and Neck Cancer. New York, Wiley, 1985, p 13.
236. Niedobitek G, Hansmann ML, Herbst H, et al: Esptein-Barr virus and carcinomas: Undifferentiated carcinomas but not squamous cell carcinomas of the nasopharynx are regularly associated with the virus. J Pathol 165:17, 1991.
237. Young LS, Dawson CW, Clark D, et al: Epstein-Barr virus gene expression in nasopharyngeal carcinoma. J Gen Virol 69:1051, 1988.
238. Wang D, Liebowitz D, Kieff E: The truncated form of the Epstein-Barr virus latent-infection membrane protein expressed in virus replication does not transform rodent fibroblasts. J Virol 62:2337, 1988.
239. Wang F, Gregory CD, Rowe M, et al: Epstein-Barr virus nuclear antigen 2 specifically induces expression of the B-cell activation antigen CD23. Proc Natl Acad Sci USA 83:3452, 1987.
240. Dawson CW, Rickinson AB, Young LS: Epstein-Barr virus latent membrane protein inhibits human epithelial cell differentiation. Nature 344:777, 1990.
241. Niedobitek G, Herbst H, Young LS, et al: Patterns of Epstein-Barr virus infection in non-neoplastic lymphoid tissue. Blood 79:2520, 1992.
242. Choi PHK, Seven MWM, Haung DP, et al: Nasopharyngeal carcinoma: Genetic changes, Epstein-Barr virus infection, or both. A clinical and molecular study of 36 patients. Cancer 72:2873, 1993.
243. Niedobitek G, Rowlands DC, Young LS, et al: Overexpression of p53 in Hodgkin's disease: Lack of correlation with Epstein-Barr virus infection. J Pathol 169:207, 1993.
244. Lu QL, Elia G, Lucas S, et al: Bcl-2 proto-oncogene expression in Epstein-Barr virus–associated nasopharyngeal carcinoma. Int J Cancer 53:29, 1993.
245. Starzl TE, Penn I, Halgrimson CG: Immunosuppression and malignant neoplasms. N Engl J Med 283:934, 1970.
246. Penn I: Cancer is a complication of severe immunosuppression. Surg Gynecol Obstet 162:603, 1986.
247. Swinnen LJ: Lymphoproliferative disorders following organ transplantation: Clinical syndromes and treatment options. EBV Rep 3:141, 1996.
248. Ho M, Jaffe R, Miller G, et al: The frequency of Epstein-Barr virus infection and associated lymphoproliferative syndrome after transplantation and its manifestations in children. Transplantation 45:719, 1988.
249. Walker RC, Paya CV, Marshall WF, et al: Pretransplantation seronegative Eptein-Barr virus status is the primary risk factor for posttransplantation lymphoproliferative disorder in adult heart, lung, and other solid organ transplantation. J Heart Lung Transplant 14:214, 1995.
250. Morrison VA, Dunn DL, Manivel JC, et al: Clinical characteristics of post-transplant lymphoproliferative disorders. Am J Med 97:14, 1994.
251. Cleary ML, Warnke R, Sklar J: Monoclonality of lymphoproliferative lesions in cardiac-transplant recipients. Clonal analysis based on immunoglobulin-gene rearrangements. N Engl J Med 310:488, 1984.
252. Hanto DW, Birkenbach M, Frizzera G, et al: Confirmation of the heterogeneity of posttransplant Epstein-Barr virus–associated B cell proliferations by immunoglobulin gene rearrangement analyses. Transplantation 47:458, 1989.
253. Katz BZ, Raab-Traub N, Miller G: Latent and replicating forms of Epstein-Barr virus DNA in lymphomas and lymphoproliferative disease. J Infect Dis 160:589, 1989.
254. Locker J, Nalesnik M: Molecular genetic analysis of lymphoid tumours arising after organ transplantation. Am J Pathol 235:977, 1989.
255. Knowles DM, Cesarman E, Chadburn A, et al: Correlative morphologic and molecular genetic analysis demonstrates three distinct categories of post-transplantation lymphoproliferative disorders. Blood 85:552, 1995.
256. Hodgkin T: On some morbid appearance of the absorbent glands and spleen. Med Chir Trans 17:68, 1832.
257. Gutensohn N, Cole P: Epidemiology of Hodgkin's disease. Semin Oncol 7:92, 1980.
258. Carbone P, Kaplan H, Musshoff K, et al: Report of the committee on Hodgkin's disease staging. Cancer Res 31:1860, 1971.
259. Lukes R, Craver L, Hall T, et al: Report of the nomenclature committee. Cancer Res 26:1311, 1966.
260. Trumper LH, Brady G, Bragg A, et al: Single-cell analysis of Hodgkin and Reed-Sternberg cells: Molecular heterogeneity of gene expression and p53 mutations. Blood 81:3097, 1993.
261. Roth G, Curiel T, Lacy J: Epstein-Barr viral nuclear antigen 1 antisense oligodeoxynucleotide inhibits proliferation of Epstein-Barr virus–immortalized B cells. Blood 84:582, 1994.
262. Kupper R, Rajewsky K, Zhao M, et al: Hodgkin disease: Hodgkin and Reed-Sternberg cells picked from histological sections show clonal immunoglobulin gene rearrangements and appear to be derived from B cells at various stages of development. Proc Natl Acad Sci USA 91:10962, 1994.
263. Niedobitek G: The role of Epstein-Barr virus in the pathogenesis of Hodgkin's disease. Ann Oncol 4:S11, 1996.
264. Anagnostopouos I, Herbst H, Niedobitek G, et al: Demonstration of monoclonal EBV genomes in Hodgkin's disease and Ki-1-positive anaplastic large cell lymphoma by combined Southern blot and in situ hybridization. Blood 74:810, 1989.
265. Knecht H, Brousset P, Bachmann E, et al: Latent membrane protein 1: A key oncogene in EBV-related carcinogenesis? Acta Haematol 90:167, 1993.
266. Sandvej K, Munch M, Hamilton-Dutoit S: Mutations in the Epstein-Barr virus latent membrane protein-1 (BNLF-1) gene in spontaneous lymphoblastoid cell lines—Effect on in vitro transformation associated parameters and tumorigenicity in scid and nude mice. JCP Clin Mol Pathol 49:290, 1996.
267. Hummel M, Anagnostopoulos I, Dallengach F, et al: EBV infection patterns in Hodgkin's disease and normal lymphoid tissue: Expression and cellular localization of EBV gene products. Br J Haematol 82:689, 1992.
268. Jarrett RF, Gallagher A, Jones DB, et al: Detection of Epstein-Barr virus genomes in Hodgkin's disease: Relation to age. J Clin Pathol 44:844, 1991.
269. Khan G, Norton AJ, Slavin G: Epstein-Barr virus in Hodgkin disease. Relation to age and subtype. Cancer 71:3124, 1993.
270. Ambinder RF, Browning PJ, Loren ZI, et al: Epstein-Barr virus and childhood Hodgkin's disease in Honduras and the United States. Blood 81:462, 1993.
271. Jarrett AF, Armstrong AA, Alexander E: Epidemiology of EBV and Hodgkin's lymphoma. Ann Oncol 7:5, 1996.

272. Lin AY, Kingma DW, Lennette ET, et al: Epstein-Barr virus and familial Hodgkin's disease. Blood 88:3160, 1996.
273. Miller G, Lipman M: Release of infectious Epstein-Barr virus by transformed marmoset leukocytes. Proc Natl Acad Sci USA 70:190, 1973.
274. Mueller NE: Epstein-Barr virus and Hodgkin's disease: An epidemiological paradox. EBV 4:1, 1997.
275. Frisan T, Sjoberg J, Dolcetti R, et al: Local suppression of Epstein-Barr virus (EBV)–specific cytotoxicity in biopsies of EBV-positive Hodgkin's disease. Blood 86:1493, 1995.
276. Popperma S, Kaleta J, Hepperle B: Chromosomal abnormalities in patients with Hodgkin's disease: Evidence for frequent involvement of the 14q chromosomal region but infrequent bcl-2 gene rearrangement in Reed-Sternberg cells. J Natl Cancer Inst 84:1789, 1992.
277. Fellbaum C, Hansmann ML, Niedermeyer H, et al: Influence of Epstein-Barr virus genomes on patient survival in Hodgkin's disease. Am J Clin Pathol 98:319, 1992.
278. Su IJ: Epstein-Barr virus and T cell lymphomas. EBV Rep 3:1, 1996.
279. Su IJ, Hsieh HC, Lin KH, et al: Aggressive peripheral T-cell lymphomas containing Epstein-Barr viral DNA: A clinicopathologic and molecular analysis. Blood 77:799, 1991.
280. Anagnostopoulos I, Hummel M, Finn T, et al: Heterogeneous Epstein-Barr virus infection patterns in peripheral T-cell lymphoma of angioimmunoblastic lymphadenopathy type. Blood 80:1804, 1992.
281. Kanavaros P, Jiwa NM, de Bruin PC, et al: High incidence of EBV genome in CD30-positive non-Hodgkin's lymphomas. J Pathol 168:307, 1992.
282. Su IJ, Hsu YH, Liu MT, et al: Epstein-Barr virus–containing T-cell lymphoma presents with hemophagocytic syndrome mimicking malignant histiocytosis. Cancer 72:2019, 1993.
283. Ishihara S, Ohshima K, Tokura Y, et al: Hypersensitivity to mosquito bites conceals clonal lymphoproliferation of Epstein-Barr viral DNA-positive natural killer cells. Jpn J Cancer Res 88:82, 1997.
284. Yachie A, Kanegane H, Kasahara Y: Epstein-Barr virus–associated T-/natural killer cell lymphoproliferative diseases. Semin Hematol 40:124, 2003.
285. Rowe M, Lear AL, Croom Carter D, et al: Three pathways of Epstein Barr virus gene activation from EBNA1 positive latency in B lymphocytes. J Virol 66:122, 1992.
286. Wang D, Liebowitz D, Kieff E: An EBV membrane protein expressed in immortalized lymphocytes transforms established rodent cells. Cell 43:831, 1985.
287. Dalla Favera R, Martinotti S, Gallo RC, et al: Translocation and rearrangements of the c-myc oncogene locus in human undifferentiated B-cell lymphomas. Science 219:963, 1983.
288. Marcu KB, Harris LJ, Stantnon LW, et al: Transcriptionally active c-myc oncogene is contained within NIARD, a DNA sequence associated with chromosome translocations in B-cell neoplasia. Proc Natl Acad Sci USA 80:519, 1983.
289. Polack A, Hortnagel K, Pajic A, et al: c-myc activation renders proliferation of Epstein-Barr virus (EBV)–transformed cells independent of EBV nuclear antigen 2 and latent membrane protein 1. Proc Natl Acad Sci USA 93:10411, 1996.
290. Raab-Traub N, Flynn K: The structure of the termini of the Epstein-Barr virus as a marker of clonal cellular proliferation. Cell 47:883, 1986.
291. Gilligan K, Rajadurai P, Lin JC, et al: Expression of the Epstein-Barr virus BamHI A fragment in nasopharyngeal carcinoma: Evidence for a viral protein expressed in vivo. J Virol 65:6252, 1991.
292. Pallesen G, Hamilton-Dutoit SJ, Rowe M, et al: Expression of Epstein-Barr virus latent gene products in tumour cells of Hodgkin's disease. Lancet 337:320, 1991.
293. Yip TC, Lau WH, Ngan RKC, et al: Role of Epstein-Barr virus serology in the present and the future. EBV Rep 3:25, 1996.
294. Riddler SA, Breinig MC, McKnight JLC: Increased levels of circulating Epstein-Barr virus (EBV)–infected lymphocytes and decreased EBV nuclear antigen antibody responses are associated with the development of post-transplant lymphoproliferative disease in solid-organ transplant recipients. Blood 84:972, 1994.
295. Savoie A, Perpete C, Carpentier L, et al: Direct correlation between the load of Epstein-Barr virus–infected lymphocytes in the peripheral blood of pediatric transplant patients and risk of lymphoproliferative disease. Blood 83:2715, 1994.
296. Rooney CM, Loftin SK, Holladay MS, et al: Early identification of Epstein-Barr virus–associated post-transplantation lymphoproliferative disease. Br J Haematol 89:98, 1995.
297. Ho JHC: Nasopharynx. In Halnan KE, Boak JL, Crowther D, et al (eds): Treatment of Cancer. London, Chapman & Hall, 1982, p 249.
298. Huang SC, Chu GL: Nasopharyngeal cancer: Study II. Int J Radiat Oncol Biol Phys 7:713, 1981.
299. Chan ATC, Teo PML, Leung TWT, et al: A prospective randomized study of chemotherapy adjunctive to definitive radiotherapy in advanced nasopharyngeal carcinoma. Int J Radiat Oncol Biol Phys 33:569, 1995.
300. Starzl TE, Nalesnik MA, Porter KA, et al: Reversibility of lymphomas and lymphoproliferative lesions developing under cyclosporin A–steroid therapy. Lancet 1:583, 1984.
301. Shapiro RS, Chauvenet A, McGuire W, et al: Treatment of B-cell lymphoproliferative disorders with interferon alpha and intravenous gamma globulin. N Engl J Med 318:1334, 1988.
302. Filipovich AH, Mathur A, Kamat D, et al: Lymphoproliferative disorders and other tumors complicating immunodeficiencies. Immunodeficiency 5:91, 1994.
303. Leblond V, Sutton L, Dorent R, et al: Lymphoproliferative disorders after organ transplantation: A report of 24 cases observed in a single center. J Clin Oncol 13:961, 1995.
304. Papadopoulos EB, Ladanyi M, Emanuel D, et al: Infusion of donor leukocytes to treat Epstein-Barr virus–associated lymphoproliferative disorders after allogeneic bone marrow transplantation. N Engl J Med 330:1185, 1994.
305. Rooney CM, Smith CA, Breener MK, et al: Prophylaxis and treatment of Epstein-Barr virus lymphoproliferative disease using genetically modified cytotoxic T lymphocytes. Lancet 345:9, 1995.
306. Resnick L, Herbst JS, Ablashi DV, et al: Regression of oral hairy leukoplakia after orally administered acyclovir therapy. JAMA 259:384, 1988.
307. Greenspan D, DeSouza YG, Conant MA, et al: Efficacy of desciclovir in the treatment of Epstein-Barr virus infection in oral hairy leukoplakia. AIDS 3:571, 1990.
308. Ishii M, Yamaguchi N, Ohshima S, et al: Possibility of preventive treatment for EBV-associated NK cell-lineage proliferative disorders. Intern Med 42:250, 2003.
309. Thorley-Lawson DA, Geilinger K: Monoclonal antibodies against the major glycoprotein (gp 350/220) of Epstein-Barr virus neutralize infectivity. Proc Natl Acad Sci USA 77:5308, 1980.
310. Morgan AJ: Epstein-Barr virus vaccines. Vaccine 10:563, 1992.
311. Salahuddin SZ, Ablashi DV, Markham PD, et al: Isolation of a new virus, HBLV, in patients with lymphoproliferative disorders. Science 243:596, 1986.
312. Downing RG, Sewankambo N, Serwadda D, et al: Isolation of human lymphotropic herpesviruses from Uganda. Lancet 2:390, 1987.
313. Lopez C, Pellett P, Stewart J, et al: Characteristics of human herpes virus-6. J Infect Dis 157:1271, 1988.
314. Yamanishi K, Okuno T, Shiraki K, et al: Identification of human herpesvirus-6 as a causal agent for exanthem subitum. Lancet 1:1065, 1988.
315. Biberfeld P, Kramarsky B, Salahuddin SZ, et al: Ultrastructural characterization of a new human B lymphotropic DNA virus (HBLV) isolated from patients with lymphoproliferative disease. J Natl Cancer Inst 79:933, 1987.
316. Wyatt LS, Balachandran N, Frenkel N: Variations in the replication and antigenic properties of human herpesvirus 6 strains. J Infect Dis 162:852, 1990.
317. Ablashi DV, Lusso P, Hung C: Utilization of human hematopoietic cell lines for the propagation and characterization of HBLV (human herpesvirus 6). Int J Cancer 42:787, 1988.
318. Ablashi DV, Lusso P, Hung C, et al: Utilization of human hematopoietic cell lines for the propagation and characterization of HBLV (human herpesvirus 6). Dev Biol Stand 70:139, 1989.
319. Black JB, Sanderlin KC, Goldsmith CS, et al: Growth properties of human herpesvirus-6 strain Z29. J Virol Methods 26:133, 1989.
320. Luka J, Okano M, Thiele G: Isolation of human herpesvirus-6 from clinical specimens using human fibroblast cultures. J Clin Lab Anal 4:483, 1990.
321. Takahashi K, Sonoda S, Higashi K, et al: Predominant CD4 T-lymphocyte tropism of human herpesvirus 6–related virus. J Virol 63:3161, 1989.
322. Higashi K, Asada H, Kurata T, et al: Presence of antibody to human herpesvirus 6 in monkeys. J Gen Virol 70:3171, 1989.

58

Smallpox and Monkeypox

DONALD A. HENDERSON
LUCIANA L. BORIO

INTRODUCTION

Smallpox, although now eradicated, poses a potential threat to all countries should strains of the virus be accidentally released or deliberately disseminated as an act of biological terrorism. Smallpox was once by far the most serious of all infectious diseases, killing 25% to 30% of unvaccinated persons who became infected.[1] Under the aegis of the World Health Organization (WHO), eradication was achieved during a 10-year program culminating in the occurrence of the last case on October 26, 1977.[1] In 1980, vaccination was stopped in all countries except for workers in *Orthopoxvirus* research laboratories and some military services. Two laboratories, one in the United States and one in Russia, have been authorized officially by the World Health Assembly to retain stocks of the virus. However, other stocks may be present in Russia or other countries at unpublicized sites. Should the virus be released, either deliberately or accidentally, a global calamity could result because population immunity is now very low, reserve supplies of vaccine are limited, and only a few producers have a capacity to manufacture more. For these reasons, the occurrence of a suspected case of smallpox, wherever found, is a public health emergency, warranting immediate and thorough investigation by national and international authorities.

Monkeypox, the only other member of the *Orthopoxvirus* genus to cause serious systemic human infection, induces an illness that may be all but indistinguishable clinically from smallpox but is associated with a lower person-to-person transmission rate and has case-fatality rates of 10% to 15%.[2] First detected in 1970 in the Democratic Republic of the Congo (renamed Zaire between 1971 and 1997), cases subsequently have been found scattered across tropical rain forest areas of Africa extending from Congo to the Ivory Coast. Most cases, however, have been found in Congo. In contradistinction to smallpox, monkeypox has a zoonotic reservoir, including African ground squirrels and perhaps other rodents, and in the past has spread infrequently from person to person. In 1996 to 1997, however, outbreaks of more than 300 cases of monkeypox were reported from one area in Congo with epidemiologic characteristics suggesting the possibility that monkeypox might be able to spread more widely in a now largely unvaccinated population.[3] The fact, however, that major outbreaks of varicella were occurring concomitantly (M. Szczeniowski, personal communication, 1998) has confused the epidemiologic picture. Special studies are continuing.

In the summer of 2003, an outbreak of monkeypox affected 72 persons in the midwestern United States who had contact with infected prairie dogs from a single distributor. This was the first outbreak of monkeypox in the Western Hemisphere. In this outbreak, no cases of monkeypox could be attributed exclusively to person-to-person transmission. This outbreak led the Centers for Disease Control and Prevention (CDC) and the Food and Drug Administration (FDA) to ban the importation, sale, distribution, transport, and release into the environment of prairie dogs and several other African rodent species.[4]

AGENTS

History of Smallpox

Because smallpox has no animal reservoir and no human carrier state, it is assumed to have emerged from an animal reservoir sometime after the first agricultural settlements, about 10,000 BC,[5] when populations were large enough to sustain human-to-human transmission of the virus. The first certain evidence of smallpox in the ancient world comes from mummified remains of the Eighteenth Egyptian Dynasty (1580–1350 BC) and of the better known Ramses V (1157 BC).[6] Written descriptions of the disease, however, did not appear until the fourth century AD in China[7] and the tenth century in southwestern Asia.[8]

From northeastern Africa, smallpox was probably carried by Egyptian traders to India during the first millennium BC,[1] where it became established as an endemic infection. Although epidemics of disease are described in the Bible and in Greek and Roman literature, descriptions of clinical signs are sparse and there is no original Greek or Latin word for smallpox despite its distinctive rash.[9] From the populated endemic areas of Asia and perhaps Africa, smallpox spread with increasing frequency into less populous areas of these continents and into Europe, becoming established as an endemic infection when populations increased sufficiently in number.

The name "variola" was first used during the sixth century by Bishop Marius of Avenches (Switzerland), the word being derived from the Latin *varius* ("spotted") or *varus* ("pimple").[10] There is little doubt that smallpox was already endemic in some areas of Europe by this time.[7] In the Anglo-Saxon world of the tenth century, the word *poc* or *pocca,* a bag or pouch, described an exanthematous disease, possibly smallpox, and English accounts began to use the word *pockes.* With the appearance of syphilis in Europe in the late fifteenth century, writers began to use the prefix *small-* to distinguish variola, the smallpox, from syphilis, the great pox.[11]

In the early sixteenth century, smallpox began to be imported into the Western Hemisphere. Catastrophic epidemics followed, which decimated Amerindian tribes and resulted in the collapse of both the Aztec and Incan empires.[5] Central and southern Africa probably became endemic for smallpox about this time or soon thereafter.

The impact of smallpox on history and human affairs was profound.[7] Deities to smallpox became a part of the cultures of India, China, and parts of Africa. In Europe, as of the end of the eighteenth century, an estimated 400,000 persons died annually from smallpox, and survivors accounted for one-third of all cases of blindness. During the eighteenth century alone, five reigning European monarchs died of smallpox, and the Austrian Hapsburg line of succession shifted four times in four generations.

A method of protection against naturally acquired smallpox infection appears to have been discovered in India sometime before AD 1000.[12,13] There it became the practice to deliberately inoculate, either into the skin or by nasal insufflation, scabs or pustular material from lesions of patients. This practice resulted in an infection that was usually less severe than an infection acquired naturally. From India, the practice spread to China, western Asia, and Africa, and finally, in the early eighteenth century, to Europe and North America.[14] Case-fatality rates associated with variolation, as it was called, were about one-tenth as great as when infection was naturally acquired, but those infected in this manner were capable of transmitting smallpox to others. After cowpox began to be used as a protective vaccine, the practice of variolation diminished. Even as recently as the 1960s and 1970s, however, variolation continued to be performed among remote populations in some parts of Ethiopia, western Africa, Afghanistan, and Pakistan.[1] In 1796, Edward Jenner demonstrated that material could be taken from a human pustular lesion caused by cowpox virus (i.e., an *Orthopoxvirus* species closely related to smallpox virus) and inoculated into the skin of another person, producing a superficial infection with few symptoms.[15] He showed that the individual, after recovery, was protected from inoculation with smallpox. He called the material *vaccine,* from the Latin *vacca* ("cow"), and the process *vaccination.* Pasteur,[16] in recognition of Jenner's discovery, later broadened the term to denote preventive inoculation with other agents. Jenner's discovery was immediately recognized for its significance. Within 5 years, his paper had been translated into six languages,[17] and the vaccine had begun to be employed widely in many countries of Europe; within a decade, it had been transported to countries throughout the world.[18]

As the nineteenth century progressed, however, the initial wave of enthusiasm for vaccination subsided as difficulties were experienced in sustaining the virus through arm-to-arm inoculation and it was found that, on some occasions, syphilis was transmitted in the process.[19,20] Although vaccination material, dried on threads or ivory points, could be transported over long distances, it was often found, on receipt, to be noninfectious. When fresh material was sought, problems occurred because the cowpox disease was found only in Europe and was only sporadically present.[21] In some areas, significant opposition to vaccination was voiced by religious leaders and antivaccinationist societies who opposed, on principle, infecting humans with an animal disease.[22]

Growth of the virus on the flank of a calf offered the prospect for provision of an adequate and safer supply of vaccine material. Although this approach was employed in Italy as early as 1805,[23] it appears to have been largely unknown elsewhere until it was more widely publicized at a medical congress in 1864.[24] Thereafter, the practice was gradually adopted in other countries, although arm-to-arm vaccination in England, for example, continued until it was finally banned in 1898.[25] With an assured source of vaccine, the numbers of vaccinations increased, and the incidence of smallpox in the more industrialized countries diminished rapidly. However, not until after World War I did most of Europe become smallpox-free, and not until after World War II was transmission stopped throughout Europe and North America.

In most other parts of the world, especially in tropical and semitropical areas and in the developing countries, smallpox continued largely unabated until the middle of the twentieth century. In these countries, continuing difficulties were experienced in sustaining the virus through arm-to-arm inoculation. After calves began to be used for vaccine production, the harvested vaccine remained viable for only 1 or 2 days at ambient temperatures, thus limiting its widespread application. The only control programs that were notably successful were those in Indonesia and in certain of the French colonies, which, in the 1920s, began using a specially prepared and more stable air-dried[26] or freeze-dried[27] vaccine.

In the late 1940s, a commercially feasible process for large-scale production of a highly heat-stable freeze-dried vaccine was perfected.[28] This process offered vastly better possibilities for smallpox control. Recognizing the value of such a vaccine, the Pan American Sanitary Organization[29] decided, in 1950, to undertake a hemisphere-wide eradication program and by 1967 succeeded in eliminating smallpox from all countries of the Americas except Brazil. Meanwhile, in 1958, the U.S.S.R. proposed to the World Health Assembly that a global smallpox eradication program be undertaken,[30] and this was so decided the following year.[31] Some progress was made during the period from 1959 to 1966, but the results overall were disappointing. Finally, in 1966, the World Health Assembly decided to intensify the eradication program by providing additional funds specifically for this effort.[32]

During 1967, the year the Intensified Global Eradication Program began, an estimated 10 to 15 million smallpox cases[33] occurred in 31 countries in which the disease was endemic. The campaign was based on a twofold strategy: (1) mass vaccination campaigns that would reach at least 80% of the population using vaccine of assured potency and stability and that would be assessed by independent teams, and (2) development of a system to detect and contain cases and outbreaks.[34] Numerous problems had to be surmounted, including deficient supervision and discipline in national health services, epidemic smallpox among refugees fleeing areas stricken by civil war and famine, shortages of funds and vaccine, and a host of other problems posed by difficult terrain, climate, and cultural beliefs.[35–37] Despite the problems, steady progress was made, and on October 26, 1977, the last known naturally occurring case of smallpox was recorded in Merka, Somalia.[38] Two further cases occurred in 1978 as a result of a laboratory infection in Birmingham, England,[39] but these cases were the last. Detailed accounts of national programs are provided in books dealing with those in India,[40,41] Bangladesh,[42] Ethiopia,[43] and Somalia.[44]

An extensively illustrated volume entitled *Smallpox and Its Eradication*[1] provides a detailed account of the eradication campaign, as well as an overall account of progress in smallpox control through history. It also gives a description of the virology, the clinical features, and the pathogenesis of the disease. Complementing this text is a historical record of smallpox, *The Greatest Killer: Smallpox in History*, by Donald R. Hopkins.[7]

History of Monkeypox

Monkeypox was first described in 1959 as a primate infection in a Danish laboratory[45] and subsequently was determined to be the cause of eight additional laboratory outbreaks between 1958 and 1968.[46] In August 1970, the first human case was identified in a tropical rain forest village in Equateur province, Democratic Republic of the Congo.[47] Clinically, the disease closely resembles smallpox. Most patients, however, exhibit cervical, axillary, and sometimes inguinal lymphadenopathy, which are almost never observed with smallpox. It is assumed that the disease was prevalent for many years, not being identified as such until smallpox transmission was interrupted throughout the rain forest areas and surveillance for smallpox-like diseases was greatly enhanced.

Between 1970 and 1995, more than 400 human cases of monkeypox were detected, mainly in Zaire. The cases were scattered, primarily occurring as single cases in a village, but in some few instances it was clear that human-to-human transmission could occur. Investigations revealed that the virus had a natural reservoir in ground squirrels and possibly other rodents, man and monkeys being only incidental hosts. An outbreak in 1996 to 1997 of more than 300 possible cases of monkeypox in central Zaire raised the question at first as to whether human-to-human transfer of virus might occur more frequently than had been thought[3] (Fig. 58-1). However, a simultaneous outbreak of varicella was found to be occurring in the same region, and it was clear that a substantial number of the suspected monkeypox cases were actually varicella cases.[48] In the U.S. outbreak of 2003, most patients with monkeypox reported exposure to wild or exotic mammals (including prairie dogs), and some patients were also household contacts of affected people. However, no cases of monkeypox could be attributed exclusively to person-to-person contact.[49]

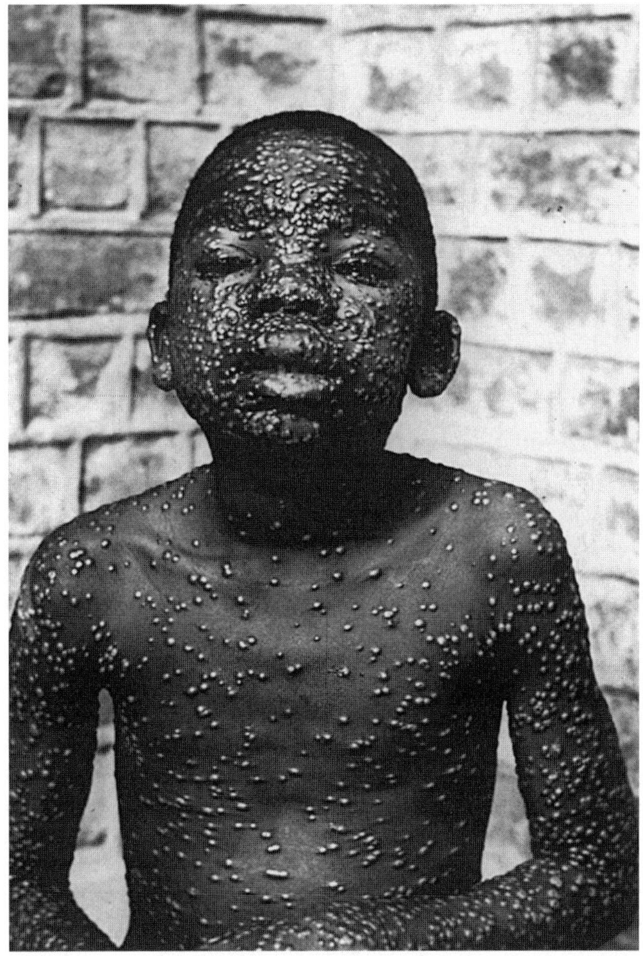

FIGURE 58-1 Congolese boy showing the typical rash of monkeypox. Although the causal virus is different from smallpox virus, the rash is indistinguishable from clinical smallpox. (Courtesy of the World Health Organization, Geneva.)

Taxonomy

Variola and monkeypox viruses belong to the genus *Orthopoxvirus,* subfamily Chordopoxvirinae, family Poxviridae. Two other members of this genus, vaccinia and cowpox, also can infect humans, causing cutaneous lesions, but those viruses are seldom transmitted from person to person. The poxviruses are the largest and most complex of all viruses. The virion is a brick-shaped structure with a diameter of about 200 nm.[50] An outer membrane of tubular lipoprotein subunits, arranged irregularly, encloses a dumbbell-shaped core and two "lateral bodies" of unknown nature. The core contains the viral DNA and associated proteins. There is an envelope that contains cellular lipids and several virus-specific polypeptides.

Restriction endonuclease maps of the genome definitively identify the species of the *Orthopoxvirus* genus. Smallpox and monkeypox are most closely related and have more than 95% homology. There are more than 100 polypeptides in the virion. The core proteins include a transcriptase, several other enzymes, and numerous antigens recognizable by immunodiffusion. The lipoprotein outer membrane of the virion is synthesized de novo; the envelope, when present, is derived from membranes of the Golgi apparatus but contains several virus-specific polypeptides. Most proteins are common to all members of the genus, and there is extensive cross-protection and cross-neutralization among them.

Cell Cycle

A specific cell-surface receptor for smallpox virus has not been identified.[51] Once inside the cell, replication of the poxviruses occurs in the host cell's cytoplasm.[50] Unlike other DNA viruses, the poxviruses encode the dozens of enzymes required for transcription and replication of the viral genome. The viral core is released into the cytoplasm after fusion of the virion with the plasma membrane. Transcription is initiated by the viral transcriptase. A transcription factor, capping and methylating enzymes, and a poly (A) polymerase enable functional capped and polyadenylated messenger RNAs (mRNAs) to be produced, without splicing, within minutes after infection. The polypeptides produced by translation of these mRNAs complete the uncoating of the core. Transcription of about 100 genes, distributed throughout the genome, occurs before viral DNA synthesis begins. Early proteins include DNA polymerase, thymidine kinase, and other enzymes required for genome replication.

Transcription of intermediate and late genes is controlled by the binding of specific viral proteins to characteristic promoter sequences. Virion assembly occurs in circumscribed areas of the cytoplasm. Intracellular mature virus moves to the vicinity of the *trans*-Golgi network or early endosomes on microtubules and acquire a double membrane. This intracellular enveloped virus moves to the cell surface on microtubules, where the outermost membrane fuses with the plasma membrane, and the virus is released from the cell by exocytosis. Most particles, however, are not enveloped and are later released by cell disruption. Both types of particles are infectious, but the enveloped particles, which are more rapidly taken up by cells, appear to be the more important in spread of the virus throughout the body.

EPIDEMIOLOGY

Smallpox

Smallpox was once worldwide in scope, persisting as an endemic disease in areas where susceptible populations were sufficiently large to permit year-round transmission. In more remote or isolated areas, epidemics occurred only sporadically following introduction of the disease. Transmission eventually ceased when the number of susceptible contacts diminished to very low numbers because infection resulted in essentially permanent immunity. Before vaccination was practiced, almost everyone eventually contracted the disease.

The seasonal occurrence of smallpox was similar to that of varicella and measles, its incidence being highest during winter and spring. This factor was consonant with the observation that the duration of survival of the virus in the aerosolized form was inversely proportional to both temperature and humidity.[52] Such seasonal variation was undoubtedly amplified in many countries by social events, such as the congregation of large numbers of people during the dry season at festivals and marriage parties, and the movement of nomads during this period. Where there was less variation in temperature and humidity, as in equatorial areas of Indonesia and Congo, there was little discernible fluctuation in incidence throughout the year.

There were also longer-term trends in incidence in the endemic areas, which resulted in major epidemics at intervals of 4 to 7 years,[1,53] presumably relating to the pace of accumulation of susceptible people.

Within the household, smallpox was as infectious as chickenpox but less infectious than measles.[54–56] With few exceptions, however, smallpox spread less widely and rapidly than these diseases. This finding can be accounted for by the fact that transmission of smallpox virus did not occur until onset of rash, as attested by numerous epidemiologic observations. By then most patients were already confined to bed because of the high fever and malaise of the prodromal illness; secondary cases were usually restricted to the few who came in contact with them, usually in the household or hospital. On average, a given case of smallpox seldom resulted in more than two to five cases in a subsequent generation, most of whom were relatives or friends. For this reason, smallpox outbreaks tended to be clustered in a segment of a town or village and in localized areas of a province or district.[57–60] Most outbreaks, therefore, could be contained successfully by vaccination of a comparatively small number of residents in and near the houses in which patients lived.

The age distribution of smallpox cases depended on the acquired immunity of the population, whether by vaccination or by infection. Cases among adults were regularly found, however, even as recently as 1974 to 1975 in India, where vaccination had been widely practiced and where smallpox was endemic. During this period, 21% of a carefully documented series of 23,546 patients were older than 20 years of age, and 2% were older than 50 years of age.[61] In western Africa from 1967 to 1969, most cases were in rural villages, and the age distribution of cases approximated the age profile of the population.[62] In all countries, males and females were equally affected.

Where the Asian form of variola major was prevalent, case-fatality rates among the unvaccinated were about 25% to 30% overall (Table 58-1), but for those younger than 1 year of age, they ranged from 40% to 50%. Variola major in Africa was a milder disease, with case-fatality rates of about 5% to 15%. Variola minor, which after 1967 was present only in Brazil and southern and eastern Africa, resulted in case-fatality rates of 1% or less.

Transmission of variola virus, with few exceptions, resulted from virus-containing droplets expressed by a patient from the oral, nasal, or pharyngeal mucosa that were inhaled by susceptible persons in close contact with the patient. Such transmission was possible from the time of onset of rash and was most frequent during the first week of the exanthem. Virus was also present in high titer in scabs that had separated from the skin lesions.[63] Epidemiologic evidence, however, showed that infected scabs played a negligible role in transmission of infection, presumably because the virus was tightly

Table 58-1 Smallpox Case-Fatality (CF) Rates by Vaccination Status, India 1974–1975

	Vaccinated			*Unvaccinated*		
Age (yr)	**Cases**	**Deaths**	**CF Rates**	**Cases**	**Deaths**	**CF Rates**
0–4	114	12	10.5	725	331	45.7
5–9	174	6	3.4	605	94	15.5
10–14	103	8	7.8	292	17	5.8
15–19	70	4	5.7	72	11	15.3
20–49	337	16	4.7	232	56	24.1
50+	57	7	12.2	45	13	28.9
Totals	855	53	6.2	1971	522	26.5

From Basu RN, Jezek Z, Ward NA: The eradication of smallpox from India. In History of International Public Health, No. 2. New Delhi, World Health Organization, Southeast Asia Regional Office, 1979.

bound in its fibrin matrix. It was standard practice, nevertheless, during the global eradication program, to isolate patients until all scabs had separated from the skin. Airborne infection over longer distances was uncommon, although two outbreaks within hospitals demonstrated this to be possible.[61,64] The infection of persons such as laundry workers who handled linen from patients has also been repeatedly documented.[9] However, various older accounts that purport to document transmission over great distances on other fomites, such as carpets, letters, and cotton rags, are suspect because the virus does not survive for long periods at customary ambient temperatures.[65]

Monkeypox

Monkeypox was first identified as the cause of illness in captive monkeys in a research facility in Copenhagen in 1958.[66] The first human cases were identified in 1970. The epidemiology of monkeypox differs substantially from that of smallpox. Until 2003, when the first outbreak of monkeypox occurred in the Western Hemisphere, the disease caused only sporadic cases in central and western Africa and one outbreak of uncertain size in the Democratic Republic of the Congo.

Between 1970, when the first human cases of monkeypox were identified, and 1981, national surveillance programs detected 67 cases of monkeypox in six countries: Cameroon (2), Ivory Coast (2), Liberia (4), Nigeria (3), Sierra Leone (1), and Congo/Zaire.[55] Concerned as to whether monkeypox could possibly be sustained by direct human-to-human transmission, WHO and Zaire staff undertook a greatly intensified surveillance program between 1981 and 1986 to better define the epidemiology of the disease. In all, 338 additional cases were detected in Zaire, and during this period 6 cases occurred in the Central African Republic (Fig. 58-2).

The studies in Zaire revealed that there was a natural reservoir host for the virus in ground squirrels (genera *Funisciurus* and *Heliosciurus*) and perhaps other rodents and that humans and monkeys were incidental victims and did not readily transmit infection to others.[67] With the cessation of these studies, surveillance activities decreased sharply, and only occasional suspect cases were subsequently reported until 1996.

As yet, the most reliable and comprehensive epidemiologic data derive from the 1981 to 1986 field studies conducted in 17 health zones of three regions of Zaire (Equateur, Bandundu, and Kasai Oriental).[2] Seventy percent of the patients lived within 100 m of the edge of the rain forest. There was no apparent seasonal trend.

The 338 cases (of a total of 404 recognized in Africa during this period) occurred in 203 separate outbreaks, of which 132 were single cases only. The other cases occurred in outbreaks of between 2 and 7 cases. An animal source of infection was suspected for 245 cases, 42 of which were coprimaries.

Apparent human-to-human spread of infection occurred much less frequently than with smallpox. In all, there were 69 second-generation cases, 19 in the third generation, and 5 fourth- and fifth-generation cases. All were close contacts: 71 household contacts, 10 relatives or neighbors living nearby, and 12 others living in neighboring villages. Only 40 (10%) of 431 unvaccinated household contacts who lived in the confined, poorly ventilated huts developed monkeypox (Table 58-2). Most patients were unvaccinated young children. Forty-three who had been previously vaccinated developed disease, of whom 60% developed "mild" or "moderate" disease in contrast with 26% of the unvaccinated[3] (Table 58-3). Contacts between patients and wild animals within the 2 to 3 weeks preceding illness were frequent and diverse and included several species of monkeys, rodents, and antelope. However, based on extensive ecological studies in different areas of Zaire, it appears that the primary reservoir is ground squirrels. Indeed, wherever cases of monkeypox were documented, the residents normally trapped and consumed squirrels, and in a southern study area where rodents were seldom eaten, monkeypox cases were rare.

The active surveillance program ended in 1986. Between 1986 and 1992, only 13 cases of human monkeypox were reported in Africa; no cases were reported between 1993 and 1995.[48]

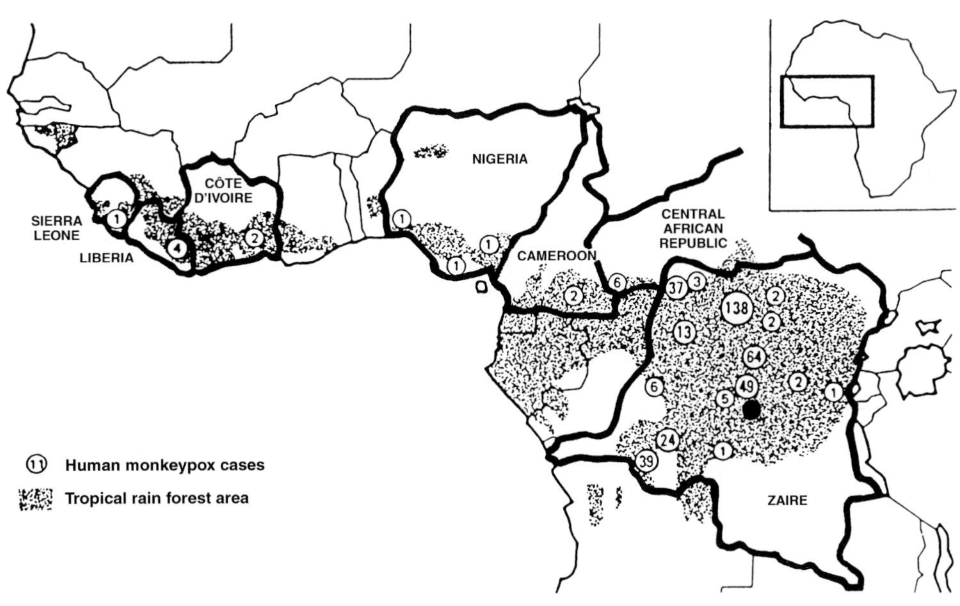

FIGURE 58-2 Map showing location of the 404 reported cases of human monkeypox, 1971–1986. The black dot indicates the locale of the 1996 and 1997 epidemics. (Courtesy of the World Health Organization, Geneva. From Jezek Z, Fenner F: Human monkeypox. In Melnick JL [ed]: Monographs in Virology, No. 17. Basel, Karger, 1988.)

Table 58-2 Monkeypox Cases in Zaire by Generation of Infection and Year

Primary and Coprimary Cases		Subsequent Cases by Generation				
Year		Second	Third	Fourth	Fifth	Total
1981	6	1	—	—	—	7
1982	24	13	3	—	—	40
1983	58	19	3	3	1	84
1984	62	18	6	—	—	86
1985	47	11	4	—	—	62
1986	42	7	3	1	—	59
Totals	245	69	19	4	1	338

From Jezek Z, Fenner F: Human monkeypox. In Melnick JL (ed): Monographs in Virology, No. 17. Basel, Karger, 1988.

In July 1996, a sizable outbreak of monkeypox was reported from the Katano-Kombe health zone, Kasai Oriental region in central Zaire.[3] Initial investigations by WHO, the Congolese, and international teams discovered 92 possible cases in 12 villages, with onsets between February 1996 and February 1997. Three persons died. Studies, however, had to be interrupted because of civil disorder. How many of the cases were caused by monkeypox virus infection and how many were caused by varicella is uncertain. Comparatively few cases were seen during the acute phase of illness, and few specimens were tested. There was general concern, however, that monkeypox might spread with greater facility in a population where vaccination had ceased in the 1970s. In October 1997 an additional 419 cases of vesiculopustular disease were detected.[68] The low case-fatality rate (1.5%) and the high secondary transmission rate (78%) sharply distinguish these most recent outbreaks from those prior to this time. Given the facts that varicella spreads readily from person to person and is associated with a low case-fatality rate, the observations are best explained as a mixed epidemic composed primarily of varicella cases with a scattering of monkeypox infections.

In the spring of 2003, monkeypox emerged for the first time in the Western Hemisphere. The outbreak affected 72 persons (37 were laboratory confirmed) in the central United States (http://www.cdc.gov/od/oc/media/mpv/cases.htm). People developed a febrile rash illness after close contact with sick pet prairie dogs and other mammals. No one died. The probable introduction of monkeypox into the United States occurred during a shipment of small mammals (which included African rodents) from Ghana to Texas.[49] Sick animals were subsequently transported to a Chicago area pet distributor via an Iowa animal vendor. In Chicago, sick animals were cohoused with prairie dogs that were subsequently transported to a vendor in Wisconsin and sold to the index patient and others. All cases appear to have resulted from close contact with infected prairie dogs. Although some patients were also household contacts of affected people, no cases of monkeypox could be attributed exclusively to person-to-person contact. There were no secondary cases in this outbreak. However, strict infection control measures were undertaken, which included pre- and postexposure vaccination of potentially exposed people with smallpox vaccine. In all, 30 persons received smallpox vaccine; 7 preexposure and 23 postexposure.[69]

Table 58-3 Monkeypox Cases in Zaire, 1981–1986, by Age of Primary and Secondary Cases

Age (yr)	Primary Cases (%)	Secondary Cases (%)
0–1	16 (6)	11 (12)
1–4	114 (46)	34 (37)
5–9	85 (35)	31 (33)
10–14	21 (9)	3 (3)
15+	9 (4)	14 (15)
Totals	245 (100)	93 (100)

From Jezek Z, Fenner F: Human monkeypox. In Melnick JL (ed): Monographs in Virology, No. 17. Basel, Karger, 1988.

DISEASES

Smallpox and monkeypox have an incubation period of about 12 days, with a range of 7 to 17 days. A 2- to 5-day period of high fever, malaise, and prostration with headache and backache is followed by the development of a maculopapular rash. The rash appears first on the mucosa of the mouth and pharynx, the face, and the forearms, and spreads to the trunk and legs. Within 1 to 2 days, the rash becomes vesicular and then pustular. The pustules are characteristically round, tense, and deeply embedded in the dermis; crusts begin to form about the eighth or ninth day. When they separate, they leave pigment-free skin and, eventually, pitted scars. The eruption is characteristically more extensive on the face and distal parts of the arms and legs, and lesions are occasionally found on the palms and soles (Figs. 58-3 and 58-4).

Illness caused by variola major was generally more severe, with a more extensive rash, a higher fever, and a greater degree of prostration than illness caused by variola minor. A milder form of disease was also seen among those who had previously been vaccinated, the rash in such persons tending to be more scant and atypical and the evolution of lesions more rapid.

Cases of smallpox among pregnant women often resulted in spontaneous abortion of the fetus or a stillborn infant with evidence of lesions on the skin. One congenital monkeypox infection has been reported: a child born in the seventh month of pregnancy with generalized skin lesions. The child recovered from infection but died of malnutrition at 7 weeks of age.[2] The principal distinguishing characteristic of monkeypox is the temporary enlargement of lymph nodes seen in African patients in 86% of unvaccinated patients and 54% of those previously vaccinated.[2] In the U.S. outbreak of 2003, lymphadenopathy was present in approximately 47% of the first 30 cases reported.[70] Most cases exhibit generalized lymphadenopathy; about a fourth exhibit lymphadenopathy only in one or two areas—in the submaxillary, cervical, axillary, or inguinal regions. The lymphadenopathy typically develops coincident with or shortly after the onset of the prodromal fever, occasionally 1 or 2 days after the onset of rash. The nodes are 1 to 2 cm in diameter and are firm, tender, and occasionally painful. In most cases, there is edema of the surrounding subcutaneous tissue. Abscess formation occurs in a few cases.

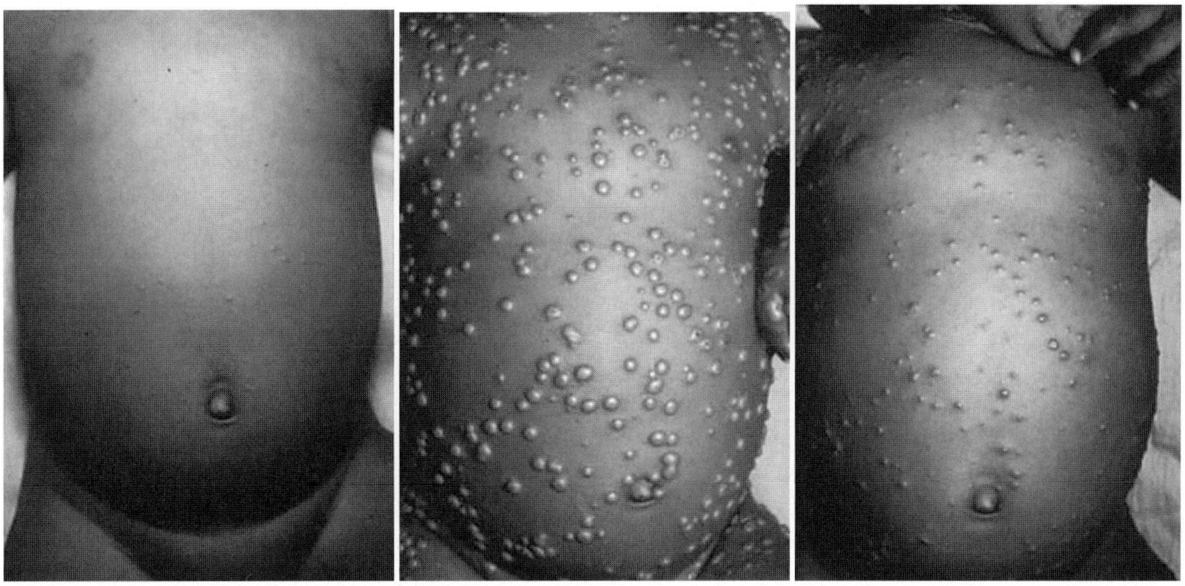

FIGURE 58-3 *A*, Smallpox day 2: papules in the same stage of development. Papules are usually seen first on the face and subsequently on the body and extremities; they eventually form vesicles. *B*, Smallpox day 5: the fluid in the vesicles becomes cloudy and looks like pus. At this stage, the pocks are called pustules. *C*, Smallpox day 8: around day 8 of rash, the pustules are firm to the touch and deeply embedded in the skin. Pustules gradually dry up and form scabs that eventually fall off. (Courtesy of the World Health Organization, Geneva. Available at http://www.who.int/emc/diseases/smallpox/slideset/.)

Of the 338 monkeypox cases observed during the Zaire studies, complications occurred in 122, almost all among the unvaccinated.[2] Sixteen percent of the unvaccinated patients experienced secondary infection of their lesions with boils, cutaneous or subcutaneous abscesses, and septic dermatitis. Pulmonary distress and bronchopneumonia occurred late in the course of illness in 34 patients (10%), of whom 19 died. Vomiting and diarrhea leading to severe dehydration occurred in 8% and corneal ulceration in 4% of patients.

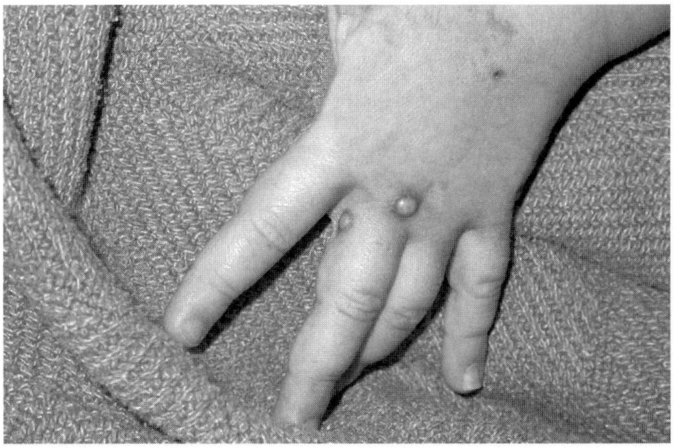

FIGURE 58-4 Monkeypox. Disseminated monkeypox skin lesions. As in smallpox, these lesions evolve from papules to vesiculopustules, which crust and detach. (Courtesy of Drs. E. Stratman, K. Reed, and J. Melski, Marshfield Clinic, Marshfield, WI.)

Death as a result of smallpox virus infection usually occurs late in the first week or during the second week of the illness and is commonly due to the effects of an overwhelming viremia. Occasionally with smallpox, a severe and always fatal hemorrhagic form occurs, with extensive bleeding into the skin and gastrointestinal tract, followed by death within a few days. Such hemorrhagic cases have not been observed with monkeypox. Among the 338 monkeypox cases in the 1981 to 1986 Zaire study, there were 33 deaths, a case-fatality rate of 9.8%. All were unvaccinated children between 3 months and 8 years of age. There were no deaths among the 72 cases in the U.S. outbreak of 2003.

PATHOGENESIS AND IMMUNITY

It is presumed that in humans the pathogenetic and immune responses to smallpox and monkeypox are essentially the same. Natural infection occurs following implantation of the virus on the oropharyngeal or respiratory mucosa.[1] Virions in droplets expressed from nasal and oropharyngeal secretions are far more infectious than those bound in the fibrin mesh of scabs. After migration to and multiplication in regional lymph nodes, an asymptomatic viremia develops around the third or fourth day, followed by multiplication of virus in the spleen, bone marrow, and lymph nodes. A secondary viremia begins around the eighth day, accompanied by fever and toxemia. The virus, contained in leukocytes, then localizes in small blood vessels of the dermis and beneath the oral and pharyngeal epithelium and subsequently infects adjacent cells. In the skin, this process results in the characteristic maculopapular lesions and, later, the vesicular and pustular lesions, which, for reasons unknown, are more extensive on the face and distal extremities. Lesions in the mouth and pharynx ulcerate quickly because of the absence of a stratum corneum, releasing large amounts of virus into the saliva about the time the cutaneous rash first becomes visible. Virus titers in saliva are highest during the first week of illness, corresponding to the period during which patients are most infectious.

Hemagglutinin-inhibiting (HI) and neutralizing antibodies can be detected beginning around the sixth day of illness, or about 18 days after infection, and complement-fixing (CF) antibodies approximately 2 days later.[71–73] Neutralizing antibodies are long-lasting, whereas HI antibodies decline to low levels within 5 years, and CF antibodies rarely persist for longer than 6 months. Little is known about the development of cell-mediated immunity.

The genome of variola virus revealed DNA sequences that would not have been understood at the time of the eradication of smallpox. Numerous viral proteins resemble cytokine receptors or binding proteins that antagonize the effects of gamma interferon, tumor necrosis factor-α (TNF-α), interleukin (IL)-1β, IL-18, and CC chemokines. The theme of viral inhibition of host immunity is also evident in variola proteins that bind C4a and C3b and inhibit complement activation, bind double-stranded RNA preventing activation of protein kinase PKR and 2.5A synthetase, and inhibit caspase-mediated TNF- and Fas-induced apoptosis.

Except for the lesions in the skin and mucous membranes and lymphoid hyperplasia, other organs are seldom involved. Secondary bacterial infection is not common, and death, when it occurs, probably results from the toxemia associated with circulating immunocomplexes and soluble variola antigens.[74,75] With smallpox, encephalitis sometimes ensues that is indistinguishable from the acute perivascular demyelination observed as a complication of infection due to vaccinia, measles, and varicella.

As the patient recovers, the scabs separate and the characteristic pitted scarring gradually develops. The scars are most evident over the face and result from the destruction of sebaceous glands followed by contraction of granulation tissue and fibrosis.

DIAGNOSIS

Most cases of smallpox and monkeypox can be diagnosed readily by the appearance of the typical deep-seated rash, the centrifugal distribution of lesions, and the fact that, on any given area of the body, all lesions are at the same stage of development. With smallpox, hemorrhagic cases were often initially misdiagnosed as meningococcemia, acute leukemia, or drug toxicity, but their identity was soon established by examining other patients who were the source of infection or to whom disease had been transmitted. Varicella was by far the most frequent disease to be confused with smallpox or monkeypox. Patients who had previously been vaccinated and those with variola minor sometimes exhibited a sparse and atypical rash with minimal systemic symptoms that resembled varicella; some severe cases of varicella in adults with extensive rash were also mistaken for smallpox.[76]

The methodology for the laboratory diagnosis of poxvirus infections has recently been reviewed by Damon and Esposito.[77] Diagnosis of poxvirus infection is confirmed rapidly by electron microscopic identification of virus particles in vesicular or pustular fluid or scabs. A suspected case of smallpox or monkeypox should be immediately reported to the relevant public health agency. All *Orthopoxvirus* virions have the same appearance, a distinctive brick-shaped knobby morphology, one which is shared by the virions of molluscum contagiosum and tanapox. The orthopoxviruses grow and produce a cytoplasmic effect in cultured cells derived from many species, although they generally grow best in cells from humans and other primates. The four orthopoxviruses that infect humans (variola, vaccinia, cowpox, and monkeypox), however, cannot be differentiated readily from one another in most cell cultures. For diagnostic purposes, they are customarily grown on the chorioallantoic membrane (CAM) of 10- to 12-day-old chick embryos on which they produce pocks characteristic of their species. Other biologic assay methods include reproductive ceiling temperatures in cell cultures or on CAM, and lethality or infectivity for various animals or animal tissues.

Each species of *Orthopoxvirus* has a distinctive DNA map demonstrable by polymerase chain reaction (PCR) amplification of various genome DNA segments followed by restriction endonuclease assays of the amplicons. Another PCR method uses primers targeting the gene sequence encoding the hemagglutinin glycoprotein, since this locus is unique to the orthopoxviruses.[78] Yet other PCR methods target the gene for the A-type inclusion body protein. In addition, DNA oligonucleotide microarray using the *crmB* (cytokine response modifier—a TNF receptor homologue produced by orthopoxviruses) gene as the target has been reported as a method for the identification of orthopoxviruses at the species level, since orthopoxviruses contain either a full-length or a truncated form of this gene.[79] A random amplified polymorphic DNA fragment length polymorphism method has also been reported.[80]

Recovered patients exhibit high titers of neutralizing, HI, and CF orthopoxvirus antibodies, but within a given genus, poxviruses are so closely related antigenically that it is difficult to identify the species utilizing virus neutralization tests with hyperimmune reference sera. Characteristic residual facial scars are most useful in documenting prior cases of variola major or monkeypox,[1] but such scars were too infrequent to be of value in identifying recovered cases of variola minor.[81]

TREATMENT

There is no specific treatment for smallpox or monkeypox. In experimental studies of the action of various antiviral drugs against two strains of variola major virus, one strain of variola minor virus, monkeypox, and other poxviruses in tissue culture, three compounds showed significant inhibition patterns—cidofovir (hydroxypropyl methylcellulose phthalate, HPMPC), its cyclic derivative (cyclic HPMPC), and ribavirin.[82] The first two compounds inhibit DNA polymerase, and ribavirin inhibits inosine monophosphate dehydrogenase. Cidofovir is licensed for the treatment of cytomegalovirus retinitis in patients with acquired immunodeficiency syndrome; ribavirin is licensed for the treatment of chronic hepatitis C and respiratory syncytial virus infections. There is a single reported case of the successful use of ribavirin in the treatment of progressive vaccinia; however, it is not possible to judge the efficacy of the drug, since it was combined with vaccinia immunoglobulin.[83] Mouse models of *Orthopoxvirus* infection have shown that systemic delivery of cidofovir before onset of disease can prevent a fatal outcome.[84–86] Unfortunately, drug administration after disease onset has proved disappointing (P. Jahrling, personal communication, 2003). Further studies are in progress at the U.S. Army Medical Research Institute of Infectious Diseases and the CDC. The CDC currently holds an investigational new drug protocol for the use of cidofovir in the treatment of smallpox, certain vaccinia complications (i.e., severe generalized vaccinia, eczema vaccinatum, or progressive vaccinia) (http://www.bt.cdc.gov/agent/smallpox/vaccination/cidofovir.asp), and severe monkeypox infection (http://www.cdc.gov/ncidod/monkeypox/treatmentguidelines.htm). The drug must be administered intravenously and is associated with considerable toxicity. An orally available formulation is under development.[87]

Supportive therapy, maintenance of fluids and nutrition, and good nursing care are the best that can be offered to most patients. Such care for suspect smallpox patients could most safely be provided by people who have recovered from smallpox (as smallpox reinfections are virtually unknown), but few such individuals are now available. Note that health-care workers can be protected from disease even when vaccinated two to three days after exposure and protected from a fatal outcome when vaccinated as long as four to five days after. Thus, all who care for patients should be vaccinated or revaccinated before exposure to patients or as soon thereafter as possible. Those who bear a scar from previous vaccination are preferred because of the more rapid development of protective immunity after revaccination. Similar precautions in providing care for monkeypox cases are probably called for but are less essential given the diminished likelihood of human-to-human transmission of monkeypox.

The skin lesions, although pustular, do not usually contain bacteria, and in fact, secondary bacterial infections are uncommon under most circumstances.[9] To accelerate the clearing of skin lesions and to minimize scarring, all manner of treatments have been devised ranging from physical abrading of the pustules to painting of the skin with gentian violet. None proved useful.

PREVENTION AND CONTROL

General Preventive Measures

With smallpox eradication confirmed and no cases for more than 25 years, preventive measures against smallpox should not be needed. However, an increase in international terrorism and the growing threat of biological weapons pose special problems with respect to smallpox. Likewise, preventive measures against monkeypox have been deemed unnecessary given the fact that cases have been few and that the 1980s studies in Zaire showed that the virus spread only with difficulty from person to person. Recent events, however, have challenged both positions.

Of special concern is the possibility that smallpox virus might be disseminated deliberately and so have the opportunity to reestablish itself. So far as is known, stocks of smallpox virus are presently retained at only two WHO-authorized laboratories: in the United States at the CDC, Atlanta; and in Russia, at Vektor Laboratories, Koltsovo, Novosibirsk. However, it is impossible to state with certainty that no other stocks exist either in Russia or in other countries. Destruction of the authorized stocks of virus had been recommended by a WHO Expert Advisory Panel,[88] was endorsed by a number of international and national microbiological societies and advisory groups, and at one time, approved by the World Health Assembly (WHA) to take place in June 1999. However, continuing debate by those favoring and those opposing this action resulted in a decision to postpone destruction of the virus pending further studies, which some have believed might eventuate in an improved vaccine or antiviral therapy.[89,90] Meanwhile, the WHA has approved studies of the virus only in the two WHO-designated laboratories, both of which are to be regularly visited by international teams to assure biological security; protocols for all studies are to be reviewed by a WHO expert group.

Should smallpox cases once again occur, the potential for epidemic spread is great. Because vaccination programs ceased in 1980, there are very large numbers of people who have never been vaccinated and large numbers of adults with waning immunity. Thus, the early detection of suspect smallpox cases represents a major public health emergency requiring immediate and thorough investigation by national and international authorities. National health authorities and WHO should be notified promptly, specimens of pustular fluid and scabs should be collected in screw cap glass bottles, and patients should be isolated in their houses or in special isolation facilities set aside for this purpose. Special attention should be paid to severely ill patients who experience bleeding into the skin such as one might see with severe meningococcemia. Such patients will not have the typical smallpox rash but may be experiencing the highly transmissible, always fatal, hemorrhagic form of smallpox and should be isolated with particular care.

Specimens from patients need to be processed at specially equipped laboratories whose proficiency has been certified by WHO. Should vaccine be required, limited supplies could be obtained from the WHO stockpile or one of several national stockpiles. However, the quantities of vaccine available are limited and would need to be used with discretion.

The question of appropriate preventive measures against monkeypox is being kept under review. Based on the information available to date, the WHO Expert Committee on Smallpox has advised that no special preventive measures be taken with respect to vaccination in the enzootic areas. However, continuing surveillance and investigation of outbreaks has been advised as the virus is transmissible from person to person, and levels of vaccine-induced protective immunity are declining. Balancing the possible benefits of protective vaccination are several factors: the very low incidence of monkeypox; the possibility of adverse reactions to smallpox vaccine; and difficulties in conducting a vaccination program throughout the large, sparsely populated rain forest areas where roads are few and often impassable.

Smallpox Vaccine

Smallpox vaccine (vaccinia virus, an *Orthopoxvirus*) provides durable protection against infection due to the other principal orthopoxviruses to which humans are susceptible, notably, variola, monkeypox, and cowpox. Although the vaccine virus is generally assumed to be a descendent of one or more cowpox strains used by Jenner at the turn of the nineteenth century, the vaccinia virus strains today are clearly a species of *Orthopoxvirus* with distinctive DNA maps that are similar to each other but very different from both cowpox and variola. That the vaccinia strains are not mutants of variola virus seems certain,[91] but where the present vaccinia species arose is unknown. It is possible that the species represents a laboratory survivor of a now naturally extinct species of *Orthopoxvirus*, perhaps horsepox.[92]

Many strains of vaccinia, known by different names, have been used by different producers during this and the past century, but little is known about their origins or passage histories. Characterization of strains is further complicated by the fact that a seed lot system for vaccine production was not used until the 1960s. Thus, even those strains with common names and ancestors have different passage histories, having been passed sequentially through a variety of vaccinifers, such as cows, sheep, and water buffalo, with periodic passages through rabbits, horses, and even humans. Most of the existing stocks of vaccine derive from one of four strains: (1) the Lister strain from the Lister Institute, England, which during the 1960s and 1970s was used for production by most producers except those in the Americas, China, and India; (2) the New York Board of Health (NYBOH) strain, which was used throughout the Americas; (3) the Temple of Heaven strain used in China; and (4) the Patwadanger strain used in India.[1] However, there are today only a few manufacturers now capable of producing smallpox vaccine on a commercial scale.

Smallpox vaccine traditionally was grown on the skin of a calf and harvested after sacrifice of the animal. The vaccine was purified by the addition of fluorocarbon and differential centrifugation, and its bacterial content was reduced by the addition of phenol. Peptone was added as a stabilizing agent, and the vaccine was freeze-dried. Because of its source, the vaccine inevitably contained some bacteria, but the number of bacteria was usually 10 or less per milliliter. Microbiological examination routinely confirmed that none is a human pathogen. For reconstitution of the vaccine, a solution of 50% (v/v) glycerin in McIlvaine solution is used.

Three cell culture vaccines have been produced and tested, one in the Netherlands, one in Japan, and one in the United States. The Netherlands vaccine developed in the 1970s consisted of Lister strain vaccinia grown in primary rabbit kidney cell cultures.[93,94] In studies of 45,000 Indonesian children, the vaccine compared favorably with the standard Lister strain calf lymph vaccine.[95] This remained an experimental vaccine and is not available today. In Japan, Hashizume and others, also in the 1970s, attenuated the Lister strain through multiple low-temperature passages and produced this vaccine in rabbit kidney cells.[96,97] This strain, called the LC16m8, was found to be satisfactorily immunogenic and less reactogenic than standard strains when tested in 40,000 Japanese children. Further studies of this vaccine are now in progress in Japan and the United States. In the United States, the NYBOH strain was plaque-purified and grown in Vero cells culture. Phase I and II studies, as well as animal-challenge studies using monkeypox, indicate that the vaccine is equivalent in immunogenicity to the NYBOH strain and has comparable reactogenicity. Licensure in the United States is projected in 2005. Meanwhile, several hundred million doses have been produced and are available for use in an emergency.

Freeze-dried smallpox vaccine is the most stable of currently available vaccines. The vaccine can be preserved almost indefinitely at −20°C, and most batches can be preserved for years at 4°C. International standards require that the vaccine in its freeze-dried form maintain full potency when incubated at 37°C for one month.[98] Studies of vaccine produced at the Lister Institute, however, demonstrated that the vaccine retained full potency for 64 weeks when incubated at temperatures of up to 45°C and for 104 weeks at 37°C.[99] After reconstitution, the vaccine is much more sensitive to temperature and to exposure to direct light. During the eradication program, unused reconstituted vaccine was routinely discarded at the end of each day, although it could be preserved in this form for at least 4 weeks at 4°C.

The vaccine is inoculated intradermally using a bifurcated needle. Vaccine, as reconstituted for use, is required to have a titer of not less than 10^8 pock-forming units per milliliter when assayed on the CAMs of 12-day-old chick embryos. Approximately 0.0025 mL of vaccine adheres by capillarity to the tines of the bifurcated needle when it is dipped into the vaccine. The needle is positioned vertically to the skin surface, usually the lateral surface of the upper arm, and 15 rapid strokes are made. These strokes should be sufficiently vigorous so that within 20 to 30 seconds, a trace of blood appears at the vaccination site.

Results of Vaccination

Successful primary vaccination results in virus proliferation in the basal cells of the epidermis, producing the typical Jennerian vesicle. A papule with surrounding erythema develops in 3 to 5 days, rapidly becoming a vesicle and later a pustule. It reaches its maximum size after 8 to 12 days. A scab forms that separates at 14 to 30 days, leaving a typical vaccination scar. A low-grade fever usually accompanies the development of the pustule, and swelling of the draining lymph nodes, associated with tenderness, is often observed. Viremia may occasionally occur[100] between the third and tenth days, and vaccinia virus can sometimes be isolated from tonsillar swabs.[101]

An individual's response to revaccination depends on the level of immunity. Erythema typically develops within 24 to 48 hours as a classic delayed hypersensitivity reaction. As Benenson[102] has shown, this reaction can be elicited with both live and inactivated vaccine. People with some residual cell-mediated immunity, but not enough to inhibit viral replication, evidence erythema at the site and development of a vesicle and sometimes a pustule that evolve in a sequence more rapid than that in a primary vaccination reaction. The presence of erythema at the vaccination site 6 to 8 days after vaccination is evidence that viral proliferation has taken place and that the revaccination was successful. Those with substantial immunity may experience no more than the hypersensitivity reaction.

Because it is impossible to distinguish between a hypersensitivity reaction due to the use of impotent vaccine and a similar reaction due to a high level of immunity, the WHO Expert Committee on Smallpox[103] recommended that such a response be termed an *equivocal reaction*. Repeat vaccinations were advised for people with equivocal reactions.

Following primary vaccination, neutralizing and HI antibodies develop by the tenth day and are present in almost all people by the end of 2 weeks; CF antibodies develop in fewer than half of the vaccinees.[72] Because the antibody response following primary vaccination usually occurs 4 to 8 days earlier than the response after naturally acquired smallpox infection,[104] primary vaccination even after exposure could modify or abort an attack of smallpox. The neutralizing antibodies are most persistent and may be detected for 20 years or more; HI and CF antibodies, however, are usually not detectable beyond 6 months. Antibody response after revaccination is more rapid, usually within 7 days, and antibody titers are generally higher. However, some people who exhibit a substantial rise in neutralizing antibody titer after revaccination fail to exhibit a rise in either HI or CF antibody levels.

Little is known about the cell-mediated immunity that is induced. Pincus and Flick[105] demonstrated the beginning development of delayed hypersensitivity, an index of cell-mediated immunity, as early a 2 days after vaccination. In a trial designed to evaluate the immunogenicity of undiluted and diluted smallpox vaccine in primary vaccinees, the development of a vesicle after vaccination correlated with the development of vaccinia virus-specific cytotoxic T-cell responses.[106] Conversely, the absence of a primary skin vesicle after primary vaccination was associated with the lack of T- or B-cell responses.

Reliable data are surprisingly sparse concerning the efficacy and durability of protection afforded by vaccination. A study conducted in 2003 measured antibody and T-cell mediated immune responses to vaccinia in volunteers examined 1 month to 75 years after vaccination.[107] In that study, vaccinia-specific T-cell memory declined slowly, with an estimated half-life of 8 to 15 years; vaccinia-specific antibody responses were maintained in the same range as that observed between 1 and 7 years after vaccination. The authors concluded that vaccine protection is more substantial and long-lasting than previously believed. Unfortunately, specific correlates of immunity to variola are not known because sophisticated laboratory methods to study them were not available during the time in which the disease was endemic.

Before 1967, when the intensified global eradication program began, revaccination every 3 to 10 years was considered essential to ensure protection. In part, this practice was based on early data largely from the United Kingdom, such as those provided by Hanna,[108] and on more recent data from India,[109] which compared the frequency of cases among those with and without vaccination scars. However, the vaccine in use in the populations studied was far lower in titer than that used after 1967. Moreover, most of the vaccine was heavily contaminated with bacteria and even in the absence of virus could induce infection and a scar resembling that following successful vaccination. Another observation suggesting that protection might persist for no more than 3 to 5 years was the increasing proportion of people who exhibited a major reaction to revaccination beginning about this time. Mistakenly, resistance to intradermal inoculation with vaccinia virus was equated with resistance to variola virus acquired by droplet inhalation.

From studies conducted after 1967, it became apparent that vaccinial immunity was far more durable than most investigators believed. It was found that with the available higher-titer vaccines, major reactions could be induced in people successfully vaccinated as recently as 3 to 6 months before and, indeed, in almost all of those who had experienced smallpox only 1 year previously.[110] Because natural infection effectively confers permanent immunity, it was apparent that the ability of vaccinia virus to proliferate when inoculated into the basal cells of the dermis correlated poorly with the level of protection afforded against natural infection. Moreover, in most countries, 90% or more of cases were people without vaccination scars. This finding led to surveys in the endemic countries that disclosed vaccine-efficacy ratios of 80% or more among those vaccinated 20 years previously. Heiner and colleagues,[56] however, showed that this protection could not be attributed solely to the vaccine. They discovered that previously vaccinated persons often developed inapparent infection with substantial increases in antibody levels. Immunity in the endemic countries was thus a composite of past experiences with both vaccinia and variola infections. Data from countries where smallpox was introduced after an absence of many years provide insufficient information to permit calculation of vaccine-efficacy ratios, but they do indicate that the vaccine provides substantial long-term protection against a fatal outcome.[111]

It has been shown that smallpox vaccine can be administered at the same time as a number of other antigens, usually at a different site, with levels of safety and efficacy comparable to those observed when the vaccines are given separately.[112–119]

Complications of Vaccination

Skin Reactions

After vaccination, three types of abnormal skin reactions may occur, as follows: (1) eczema vaccinatum and (2) progressive vaccinia, which are both associated with abnormal host reactions; and (3) generalized vaccinia. Vaccinia virus from a lesion may also be accidentally inoculated at other sites on the body or transferred to other persons. The approximate frequency of such complications and rates per million vaccinees are shown in Table 58-4, based on a national survey by Lane and colleagues[120] in the United States, the only country in which comprehensive studies of this type were undertaken. More detailed prospective studies in 10 states[121] revealed higher rates for eczema vaccinatum, generalized vaccinia, and accidental infection, as well as for other complications; the higher rates resulted from the detection of more minor complications.

Eczema Vaccinatum. Eczema vaccinatum occurs in both vaccinated people and their unvaccinated contacts who have active or quiescent eczema. Either concurrent with or shortly after the development of the local vaccinial lesion, or after an incubation period of 5 days in an unvaccinated eczematous contact, a vaccinial eruption occurs at sites that are eczematous or that had previously been so. The areas become intensely inflamed, and the eruption sometimes spreads to normal skin. Constitutional symptoms are usually severe, with high temperature and generalized lymphadenopathy. Treatment with vaccinia immunoglobulin (available from the CDC) appears to reduce mortality.[122]

Progressive Vaccinia. Progressive vaccinia occurs in people who suffer from deficient immunomechanisms, such as agammaglobulinemia, defective cell-mediated immunity, or

*Table 58-4 Complications of Smallpox Vaccination in the United States, 1968**

Vaccination Status and Age (yr)	Estimated No. of Vaccinations	Postvaccinal Encephalitis	Progressive Vaccinia	Eczema Vaccinatum	Generalized Vaccinia	Accidental Infection	Other
Primary vaccinations							
<1	614,000	4 (3)	—	5	43	7	10
1–4	2,733,000	6	6	31	47	91	40
5–9	1,553,000	5 (1)	1 (1)	11	20	32	8
10–19	406,000	—	1 (1)	3	5	3	1
20+	288,000	1	2	7	13	4	5
Unknown		—	—	1	3	5	2
Total	5,594,000	16 (4)	10 (2)	58	131	142	66
Revaccinations							
<1	—	—	—	—	—	—	—
1–4	478,000	—	—	1	—	1	1
5–9	1,643,000	—	1 (1)	4	1	3	2
10–19	2,657,000	—	1	3	—	—	—
20+	3,796,000	—	4 (1)	—	9	3	6
Total	8,574,000	—	6 (2)	8	10	7	9
Unvaccinated contacts		—	—	60 (1)	2	44	8
Total	14,168,000	16 (4)	16 (4)	126 (1)	143	193	83

*Number of reported cases (deaths in parentheses).
From Lane JM, Ruben FL, Neff JM, et al: Complications of smallpox vaccination, 1968: National surveillance in the United States. N Engl J Med 281: 1220–1224, 1969.

immunodeficiency associated with tumors of the reticuloendothelial system or the use of immunosuppressive drugs. In such patients, the vaccinia lesion fails to heal; secondary lesions sometimes appear elsewhere on the body and then gradually spread. Methisazone (*N*-methylisatin β-thiosemicarbazone), an antiviral substance which inhibits protein synthesis, was believed to be partially effective in treatment,[123] but is no longer available. A recent case was treated successfully with ribavirin 20 mg/kg day in three divided doses for 5 days and vaccinia immunoglobulin.[83]

Generalized Vaccinia. With generalized vaccinia, one to many lesions develop in 6 to 9 days after vaccination at locations other than the vaccination site in otherwise healthy people. The evolution of these lesions follows the same temporal course as that of the vaccination lesion itself. Although patients may experience high fever and malaise, an uneventful recovery without the need for specific therapy is usual.

Accidental Inoculation

Accidental inoculation of vaccinia virus, transferred from the lesion at the vaccination site, is by far the most common, although innocuous, complication. The most common sites for inoculation are the eyelids, vulva, and perineum. Such lesions evolve rapidly and heal at the same time as the primary lesion. Accidental infection of normal contacts may also occur.

Postvaccinal Encephalopathy and Encephalitis

Among those without known contraindications to vaccination, postvaccinal encephalopathy and encephalitis are the most serious complications. The incidence of these related complications was substantially higher in Europe following the use of strains in common use at that time[124] than in the United States, where the NYBOH strain was employed. Illness usually begins between 11 and 15 days after vaccination and is accompanied by fever, vomiting, headache, malaise, and anorexia, followed by disorientation and drowsiness and sometimes convulsions and coma. Death occurs in 10% to 35% of cases, usually within a week. Some survivors have residual paralysis or mental impairment. Paralysis, when present, tends to be of the upper motor neuron type. Among those patients who recover fully, symptoms and signs resolve within 2 weeks.

Many reports document the frequency of cases of postvaccinal encephalopathy and encephalitis in Europe and the United States, but comparison of rates is difficult because of differing criteria for diagnosis and variability in the completeness of reporting. The usual levels of incidence, such as those reported from the Netherlands,[125–127] Germany,[126,128,129] and Austria,[130] were higher than those in the United Kingdom,[126] and these rates in turn were higher than those in the United States.[101,102,114] Whatever the criteria and methods, differences between the rates caused a number of countries to begin using the Lister strain, then in use in the United Kingdom. A dramatic reduction in the incidence of postvaccinal encephalitis subsequently occurred.[125,131]

Myopericarditis

Because of the threat of smallpox being used as a biological weapon, vaccination of U.S. military personnel and some health-care workers began in 2002. From December 2002 to

May 2003, approximately 450,000 military personnel were vaccinated against smallpox, of whom 37 experienced acute myopericarditis. Eighty-seven percent were men, 70.5% were primary vaccinees, and the median age was 26 years. Beginning between 7 and 19 days postvaccination, some vaccinees developed chest pain and signs of myopericarditis, including typical electrocardiographic changes, elevated cardiac enzymes, and/or depressed cardiac function on imaging studies. Only one patient developed severe heart failure, and there were no deaths.[132,133] The findings paralleled those reported in 1983 by Finnish investigators. Finnish military personnel given the Finnish strain of vaccine are reported to have developed myopericarditis at a rate of approximately 100 per million vaccinees.[134] In the U.S. civilian smallpox vaccination program, there were 15 cases of myopericarditis among approximately 36,000 vaccinated. In contrast to the military program, 90% were revaccinees, 71% were female, and the median age was 48 years. Again, no fatalities were reported.

Other Types of Heart Disease

Nine cases of heart-related incidents, such as angina and myocardial infarction, among health-care workers vaccinated in the United States in 2003 were reported. However, there is no evidence that any were causally related. Six of the nine reported having a history of ischemic heart disease prior to vaccination, and only one had no recognized cardiac disease risk factor prior to vaccination.[135] Further studies are in progress. Meanwhile, people with known heart disease or with three or more cardiac risk factors have been asked to defer vaccination for the present time.

Indications for Vaccination

In endemic countries, which, until after World War I, consisted of most of the world, vaccination was recommended for everyone, with revaccination every 3 to 10 years. The only exceptions were infants, for whom primary vaccination was customarily delayed until 3 to 12 months of age, mainly because of more frequent vaccination failures at an earlier age. As higher-titer vaccines became available in the 1920s, French and then German physicians showed that a high proportion of successful vaccinations could be achieved at birth, and in some hospitals, this became routine practice,[136] as it did in some parts of the United States.[137]

As time passed and the incidence of smallpox declined, it became increasingly common for smallpox-free countries to delay primary vaccination until children were older. This resulted in part from the demonstration that maternal antibody inhibited virus proliferation[137] and in part from the belief that older children could better cope with the fever and systemic symptoms of vaccinial infection.

Vaccination at a later age was also less likely to be associated mistakenly with other events, such as sudden infant death syndrome, which might be temporally but not causally related. Some European countries recommended that vaccination be delayed until the second year of life to avoid postvaccinal encephalopathy, and the United States adopted the practice of vaccinating at 12 months of age, when studies suggested a higher frequency of postvaccinal encephalitis among those vaccinated at less than 1 year of age than among those vaccinated between 1 and 4 years of age.[120] What these changes in policy may have achieved, however, is unknown, because no studies were performed to validate that complications were subsequently less frequent.

As a rule, most vaccination practices in the developing countries tended to parallel those in Europe and North America, and as of 1967 most countries, even those with endemic smallpox, delayed vaccination until the child was 3 to 9 months of age. Notable exceptions were Hong Kong,[114] where neonatal vaccination had been traditional at least since World War II, and Madras, India,[109] where neonatal vaccination was introduced in the late 1950s. During the late 1960s, it became apparent that vaccines that met international standards of potency consistently resulted in high levels of vaccination "takes" in newborns. Thus, newborn vaccination was recommended for all countries, although not all countries followed the practice.

Primary vaccination was provided for adults if required, although many workers considered it to be associated with a substantially higher incidence of postvaccinal encephalitis. Earlier European data suggest this to be the case,[124] but this was not borne out in studies conducted in the United States.[120,138] A review of U.S. military medical records between 1946 and 1962, conducted by the CDC, revealed no cases of central nervous system complications among an estimated 2 million recruits who were given primary vaccinations.

Since 1980 routine vaccination of the general population has ceased in all countries. Vaccination is still recommended for those working in laboratories where orthopoxviruses are used. A few countries now provide vaccination to military forces as a protection in case variola virus is used as a biological warfare agent. In addition, several countries, including the United States, the United Kingdom, and Israel, have resumed vaccination of selected members of the population, such as health-care workers, public health practitioners, and emergency first responders, who might be at higher risk of coming in contact with a smallpox patient by virtue of their professions if the virus were used as a bioterrorism agent. Since 2003, the United States has vaccinated approximately 39,500 such persons in the first phase of its smallpox vaccination program. The effort to vaccinate additional healthcare workers has waned because of concerns about possible complications from prospective vaccines.

Contraindications to Vaccination

During campaigns in areas that were endemic for smallpox, WHO recognized no contraindications to vaccination for two reasons: (1) the risk associated with smallpox infection was significantly greater than the risk of complications, and (2) most vaccinations were performed by people without medical training who could not be expected to recognize conditions such as eczema or to identify patients with immunodeficiency syndromes. In nonendemic areas, four conditions were generally accepted as contraindications:

1. Immune disorders included agammaglobulinemia, hypogammaglobulinemia, neoplasms affecting the reticuloendothelial system, and compromised immune status associated with the use of immunosuppressive drugs. People with such disorders, if vaccinated, were at substantial risk of developing the frequently fatal progressive vaccinia.

2. People with active eczema or a past history of eczema were at special risk of developing eczema vaccinatum, a serious and sometimes fatal complication. Because family members with eczema were also at risk of contact spread of vaccinia, it was recommended that either the healthy vaccinee or the eczematous family member live apart from the family until the lesion had fully scabbed over.
3. Pregnant women were not vaccinated on the general principle that immunization of any sort should be avoided during pregnancy and because of the rare risk of fetal vaccinia.
4. Many countries recognized as contraindications disorders of the central nervous system in potential vaccinees and sometimes their families, hoping in so doing to minimize the risk of postvaccinal encephalitis. However, there is no evidence that the exclusion of such persons affected the incidence of that complication.

ACKNOWLEDGMENT

The material pertaining to smallpox and vaccinia is derived in large part from the chapter Smallpox and Vaccinia by D. A. Henderson, Luciana Borio, and Michael Lane in *Vaccines*, edited by S. Plotkin and W. Orenstein, published by WB Saunders in 2004. The material is reproduced with the permission of Saunders.

REFERENCES

1. Fenner F, Henderson DA, Arita I, et al: Smallpox and Its Eradication. Geneva: World Health Organization, 1988.
2. Jezek Z, Fenner F: Human monkeypox. In Melnick J, (ed): Monographs in Virology. Vol. 17. Basel, Switzerland, Karger, 1988.
3. Human monkeypox in Kasai Oriental, Zaire (1996–1997). Wkly Epidemiol Rec 72:101–104, 1997.
4. Reed KD, Melski JW, Graham MB, et al: The detection of monkeypox in humans in the Western Hemisphere. N Engl J Med 350:342–350, 2004.
5. McNeill WH: Plagues and Peoples. New York, Anchor Books/Doubleday, 1998, p 365.
6. Ruffer MA: Pathological note on the royal mummies of the Cairo Museum. In Moodie RL (ed): Studies in the Palaeopathology of Egypt. Chicago, IL, University of Chicago Press, 1921, pp 175–176.
7. Hopkins DR: The Greatest Killer: Smallpox in History. Chicago, IL, University of Chicago Press, 2002.
8. Rhazes (Al-Razi, Abu Bakr Muhammad ibn Zakariya): De variolis et morbillis commentarius. London, G Bowyer, 1766 [On smallpox and measles, Med Classics 4:22–84, 1939].
9. Dixon CW: Smallpox. London, J & A Churchill, Ltd, 1962, p 1460.
10. Moore J: The History of the Smallpox. London, Longman, Hurst, Rees, Orme & Brown, 1815.
11. Creighton C: History of Epidemics in Britain. Cambridge, UK, Cambridge University Press, 1894 [reprint, London, Cass, 1965].
12. Macgowan DJ: Report on the health of Wenchow for the half-year ended 31 March 1884. China, Imperial Maritime Customs Medical Reports 27:9–18, 1884.
13. Needham J: China and the origins of immunology. Centre of Asian Studies occasional papers and monographs, No. 41. Hong Kong, Centre of Asian Studies, University of Hong Kong, 1980.
14. Miller G: Putting Lady Mary in her place: a discussion of historical causation. Bull Hist Med 55:2–16, 1981.
15. Jenner E: An inquiry into the causes and effects of the variolae vaccinae, a disease discovered in some of the western counties of England, particularly Gloucestershire and known by the name of the cow pox. London, 1798 [reprinted in Camac CNB (ed): Classics of Medicine and Surgery. New York, Dover, 1959].
16. Pasteur L: Vaccination in relation to chicken-cholera and splenic fever. In Transactions of the International Medical Congress, Seventh Session, London, August 2–9, 1881, Vol 1, pp 85–90 [Reprinted in Vallery-Radot P (ed): Oeuvres de Pasteur, Vol 6. Paris, Masson, pp 370–378, 1933].
17. FeFanu W: A Bio-Bibliography of Edward Jenner 1749–1823. London, Harvey & Blythe, 1951.
18. Bowers JZ: The odyssey of smallpox vaccination. Bull Hist Med 55:17–33, 1981.
19. Nott JC: Smallpox epidemic in Mobile during the winter of 1865–6.Nashville J Med Surg 2:372–380, 1867.
20. Creighton C: The Natural History of Cow-Pox and Vaccinal Syphilis. London, Cassell, 1887.
21. Baxby D: The origins of vaccinia virus. J Infect Dis 136:453–455, 1977.
22. The History of Inoculation and Vaccination. London, Burroughs, Wellcome, 1913.
23. Galbiati: Memoria sulla inoculazione vaccina coll'umore ricavato immediatement dalla vacca precedentemente inoculata Naples, 1810.
24. Congrès Medical de Lyon: Compte-rendu des travaux et des discussions. Gazette Med Lyon: 19:449–471, 1864.
25. Dudgeon JA: Development of smallpox vaccine in England in the eighteenth and nineteenth centuries. Br Med J 1:1367–1372, 1963.
26. Otten L: Trockenlymphe. Z Hyg Infektionskrankheiten 107:677–696, 1927.
27. Fasquelle R, Fasquelle A: [History of smallpox control in French speaking African countries]. Bull Soc Pathol Exot Filiales 64:734–756, 1971.
28. Collier LH: The development of a stable smallpox vaccine. J Hyg (Lond) 53:76–101, 1955.
29. Final Reports of the First, Second and Third Meetings of the Directing Council, publication No. 247. Washington, DC, Pan American Sanitary Organization, 1950.
30. Eradication of Smallpox. Official Records of the World Health Organization, No. 87. Geneva, World Health Organization, 1958, pp 263–264, 508–512.
31. Smallpox Eradication. Official Records of the World Health Organization, No. 95. Geneva, World Health Organization, 1959, pp 572–588.
32. Official Records of the World Health Organization, No. 152. Geneva, World Health Organization, 1966, p 291.
33. The global eradication of smallpox. Final report of the global commission for the certification of smallpox eradication. In History of International Public Health, No. 4. Geneva, World Health Organization, 1980.
34. Handbook for Smallpox Eradication in Endemic Areas. Geneva, World Health Organization, 1967.
35. Henderson DA: The eradication of smallpox. Sci Am 235:25–33, 1976.
36. Henderson DA: Smallpox eradication. Proc R Soc Lond B Biol Sci 199:83–97, 1977.
37. Henderson DA: The deliberate extinction of a species. Proc Am Philos Soc 126:461–471, 1982.
38. Deria A, Jezek Z, Markvart K, et al: The world's last endemic case of smallpox: surveillance and containment measures. Bull World Health Organ 58:279–283, 1980.
39. Shooter RA: Report of the Investigation into the Cause of the 1978 Birmingham Smallpox Occurrence. London, HMSO, 1980.
40. Basu RN, Jezek Z, Ward NA: The eradication of smallpox from India. In History of International Public Health, No.2. New Delhi, World Health Organization, South-East Asia Regional Office, 1979.
41. Brilliant LB: The Management of Smallpox Eradication in India. Ann Arbor, University of Michigan Press, 1985.
42. Joarder AK, Tarantola D, Tulloch J: The eradication of smallpox from Bangladesh. WHO regional publications. South-East Asia series; No. 8. New Delhi: World Health Organization South-East Asia Regional Office, 1980.
43. Tekeste Y, Hailu A, do Amaral C, et al: Smallpox Eradication in Ethiopia. Brazzaville, Geneva, World Health Organization, 1948.
44. Jezek Z, Al Aghbari M, Hatfield R, et al: Smallpox Eradication in Somalia. Alexandria, Egypt, World Health Organization Eastern Mediterranean Regional Office and Ministry of Health, Somali Democratic Republic, 1981.
45. Von Magnus P, Andersen EK, Petersen KB, et al: A pox-like disease in cynomolgus monkeys. Acta Pathol Microbiol Scand 46:156–176, 1959.
46. Arita I, Gispen R, Kalter SS, et al: Outbreaks of monkeypox and serological surveys in nonhuman primates. Bull World Health Organ 46:625–31, 1972.
47. Ladnyi ID, Ziegler P, Kima A: A human infection caused by monkeypox virus in Basankusu Territory, Democratic Republic of the Congo. Bull World Health Organ 46:633–639, 1972.

48. Heymann DL, Szczeniowski M, Esteves K: Re-emergence of monkeypox in Africa: a review of the past six years. Br Med Bull 54:693–702, 1998.
49. Update: multistate outbreak of monkeypox—Illinois, Indiana, Kansas, Missouri, Ohio, and Wisconsin, 2003. MMWR 52:616–618, 2003.
50. White DO, Fenner FJ: Medical Virology. San Diego, Academic Press, 1994.
51. Bray M, Buller M. Looking back at smallpox. Clin Infect Dis 38:882–889, 2004.
52. Harper GJ: Airborne micro-organisms: survival test with four viruses. J Hyg (Lond) 59:479–486, 1961.
53. Rogers L: Smallpox and vaccination in British India during the last seventy years. Proc R Soc Lond B Biol Sci 38:135–139, 1944.
54. Hope Simpson RE: Infectiousness of communicable diseases in the household (measles, chickenpox and mumps). Lancet 2:549–554, 1952.
55. Carvalho Filho ES de, Morris L, Lavigne de Lemos A, et al: Smallpox eradication in Brazil, 1967–69. Bull World Health Organ 43:797–808, 1970.
56. Heiner GG, Fatima N, Daniel RW, et al: A study of inapparent infection in smallpox. Am J Epidemiol 94:252–268, 1971.
57. Henderson RH, Yekpe M: Smallpox transmission in Southern Dahomey: a study of a village outbreak. Am J Epidemiol 90:423–428, 1969.
58. Thomas DB, McCormack WM, Arita I, et al: Endemic smallpox in rural East Pakistan. 1. Methodology, clinical and epidemiologic characteristics of cases, and intervillage transmission. Am J Epidemiol 93:361–372, 1971.
59. Thomas DB, Arita I, McCormack WM, et al: Endemic smallpox in rural East Pakistan. 2. Intervillage transmission and infectiousness. Am J Epidemiol 93:373–383, 1971.
60. Thomas DB, Mack TM, Ali A, et al: Epidemiology of smallpox in West Pakistan. 3. Outbreak detection and interlocality transmission. Am J Epidemiol 95:178–189, 1972.
61. Anders W, Posch J: Die Pockenausbruche 1961/62 in Nordrhein-Westfalen. Bundesgesunheitbl 17:265–269, 1962.
62. Foege WH, Millar JD, Henderson DA: Smallpox eradication in West and Central Africa. Bull World Health Organ 52:209–222, 1975.
63. Mitra AC, Sarkar JK, Mukherjee MK: Virus content of smallpox scabs. Bull World Health Organ 51:106–107, 1974.
64. Wehrle PF, Posch J, Richter KH, et al: An airborne outbreak of smallpox in a German hospital and its significance with respect to other recent outbreaks in Europe. Bull World Health Organ 43:669–679, 1970.
65. Huq F: Effect of temperature and relative humidity on variola virus in crusts. Bull World Health Organ 54:710–712, 1976.
66. Von Magnus P, Anderson EK, Petersen KB, et al: A pox-like disease in cynomolgus monkeys. Acta Pathol Microbiol Scand 46:156–176, 1959.
67. Khodakevich L, Szczeniowski M, Manbu ma D, et al: The role of squirrels in sustaining monkeypox virus transmission. Trop Geogr Med 39:115–122, 1987.
68. Human monkeypox—Kasai Oriental, Democratic Republic of Congo, February 1996–October 1997. MMWR 46:1168–1171, 1997.
69. Update: multistate outbreak of monkeypox—Illinois, Indiana, Kansas, Missouri, Ohio, and Wisconsin, 2003. MMWR 52:642–646, 2003.
70. Multistate outbreak of monkeypox—Illinois, Indiana, and Wisconsin, 2003. MMWR 52:537–540, 2003.
71. Downie AW, Saint Vincent L, Rao AR, et al: Antibody response following smallpox vaccination and revaccination. J Hyg (Lond) 67:603–608, 1969.
72. Downie AW, Saint Vincent L, Goldstein L, et al: Antibody response in non-haemorrhagic smallpox patients. J Hyg (Lond) 67:609–618, 1969.
73. McCarthy K, Downie AW, Bradley WH: The antibody response in man following infection with viruses of the pox group. 2. Antibody response following vaccination. J Hyg (Lond) 56:466–478, 1958.
74. Downie AW, McCarthy K, Macdonald A, et al: Virus and virus antigen in the blood of smallpox patients: their significance in early diagnosis and prognosis. Lancet 265:164–166, 1953.
75. Martin DB: The cause of death in smallpox: an examination of the pathology record. Mil Med 167:546–551, 2002.
76. White E: Chickenpox in Kerala. Indian J Public Health 22:141–151, 1978.
77. Damon IK, Esposito JJ: Poxviruses that infect humans. In Murray PR, Baron EJ, Jorgensen JH, et al (eds): Manual of Clinical Microbiology, 8th ed. Washington DC, ASM Press, 2003, pp 1583–1591.
78. Ropp SL, Jin Q, Knight JC, et al: PCR strategy for identification and differentiation of small pox and other orthopoxviruses. J Clin Microbiol 33:2069–2076, 1995.
79. Lapa S, Mikheev M, Shchelkunov S, et al: Species-level identification of orthopoxviruses with an oligonucleotide microchip. J Clin Microbiol 40:753–757, 2002.
80. Stemmler M, Neubauer H, Meyer H: Comparison of closely related orthopoxvirus isolates by random amplified polymorphic DNA and restriction fragment length polymorphism analysis. J Vet Med B Infect Dis Vet Public Health 48:647–654, 2001.
81. Jezek Z, Hardjotanojo W: Residual skin changes in patients who have recovered from variola minor. Bull World Health Organ 58:139–140, 1980.
82. Baker RO, Bray M, Huggins JW: Potential antiviral therapeutics for smallpox, monkeypox and other orthopoxvirus infections. Antiviral Res 57:13–23, 2003.
83. Kesson AM, Ferguson JK, Rawlinson WD, et al: Progressive vaccinia treated with ribavirin and vaccinia immune globulin. Clin Infect Dis 25:911–914, 1997.
84. Bray M, Martinez M, Smee DF, et al: Cidofovir protects mice against lethal aerosol or intranasal cowpox virus challenge. J Infect Dis 181:10–19, 2000.
85. Smee DF, Bailey KW, Wong M, et al: Intranasal treatment of cowpox virus respiratory infections in mice with cidofovir. Antiviral Res 47:171–177, 2000.
86. Smee DF, Bailey KW, Sidwell RW: Treatment of lethal vaccinia virus respiratory infections in mice with cidofovir. Antivir Chem Chemother 12:71–76, 2001.
87. Ciesla SL, Trahan J, Wan WB, et al: Esterification of cidofovir with alkoxyalkanols increases oral bioavailability and diminishes drug accumulation in kidney. Antiviral Res 59:163–171, 2000.
88. Report of the Ad Hoc Committee on Orthopoxvirus Infections. Executive Board Report EB 95/33, 10 October 1994. Geneva, World Health Organization, 1994.
89. Mahy BW, Almond JW, Berns KI, et al: The remaining stocks of smallpox virus should be destroyed. Science 262:1223–1224, 1993.
90. Roizman B, Joklik W, Fields B, et al: The destruction of smallpox virus stocks in national repositories: a grave mistake and a bad precedent. Infect Agents Dis 3:215–217, 1994.
91. Herrlich A, Mayr A, Mahnel H, et al: Experimental studies on transformation of the variola virus into the vaccinia virus. Arch Gesamte Virusforsch 12:579–599, 1963.
92. Baxby D: Jenner's smallpox vaccine: the riddle of vaccinia virus and its origin. London, Heinemann Educational Books, 1981.
93. Hekker AC, Bos JM, Smith L: A stable freeze-dried smallpox vaccine make in monolayer cultures of primary rabbit kidney cells. J Biol Stand 1:21–32, 1973.
94. Hekker AC, Huisman J, Polak MF, et al: Field work with a stable freeze-dried vaccine prepared in monolayers of rabbit kidney cells. In International Symposium of Smallpox Vaccine. Symposia Series in Immunobiological Standardization, No. 19, 1973, pp 187–195.
95. Hekker AC, Bos JM, Kumara R, et al: Large-scale use of freeze-dried vaccine prepared in primary cultures of rabbit kidney cells. Bull World Health Organ 54:279–284, 1976.
96. Hashizume S, Yoshizawa H, Morita M, et al: Properties of attenuated mutant of vaccinia virus, LC 16m8, derived from Lister strain. In Quinna GV Jr (ed): Vaccinia Viruses as Vectors for Vaccine Antigens. New York, Elsevier, 1985, pp 87–99.
97. Japan, Ministry of Health: Report of Committee on Smallpox Vaccination. Investigation of treatment of complications caused by smallpox vaccination (in Japanese). J Clin Virol 3:269–278, 1975.
98. WHO Expert Committee on Smallpox Eradication: Second Report. World Health Organ Tech Rep Ser 493, 1972.
99. Cross RM, Kaplan C, McClean D: The heat resistance of dried smallpox vaccine. Lancet 272:446–448, 1957.
100. Blattner RJ, Norman JO, Heys FM, et al: Antibody response to cutaneous inoculation with vaccinia virus: viremia and viruria in vaccinated children. J Pediatr 64:839–852, 1964.
101. Gins HA, Hackenthal H, Kamentzewa N: Experimentelle Untersuchungen uber die Generalisierung des Vaccine-virus beim Menschen und Versuchstier. Z Hyg Infektionskrankheit 110:429–441, 1929.
102. Benenson AS: Immediate (so-called immune) reaction to smallpox vaccination. JAMA 143:1238–1249, 1950.

103. WHO Expert Committee on Smallpox: First report. World Health Organ Tech Rep Ser 283, 1964.
104. Downie AW, McCarthy K: The antibody response in man following infection with viruses of the pox group. 3. Antibody response in smallpox. J Hyg (Lond) 56:479–487, 1958.
105. Pincus WB, Flick JA: The role of hypersensitivity in the pathogenesis of vaccinia virus infection in humans. J Pediatr 62:57–62, 1963.
106. Frey SE, Couch RB, Tacket CO, et al: Clinical responses to undiluted and diluted smallpox vaccine. N Engl J Med 346:1265–1274, 2002.
107. Hammarlund E, Lewis MW, Hansen SG, et al: Duration of antiviral immunity after smallpox vaccination. Nat Med 9:1131–1137, 2003.
108. Hanna W: Studies in Smallpox and Vaccination. Bristol, UK, Wright, 1913.
109. Rao AR: Smallpox. Vol. 281. Bombay, India: Kothari Book Depot, 1972.
110. Zikmund V, Das N, Krishnayengar R, et al: Contribution to the problem of challenge vaccination: observations on vaccination of cured smallpox cases in India in 1971, 1972 and 1973. Indian J Public Health 22:102–106, 1978.
111. Mack TM: Smallpox in Europe, 1950–1971. J Infect Dis 125:161–169, 1972.
112. Winter PA, Mason JH, Kuhr E, et al: Combined immunization against poliomyelitis, diphtheria, whooping cough, tetanus and smallpox. S Afr Med J 37:513–515, 1963.
113. Karchmer AW, Friedman JP, Casey HL, et al: Simultaneous administration of live virus vaccines: measles, mumps, poliomyelitis, and smallpox. Am J Dis Child 121:382–328, 1971.
114. Lin HT: A study of the effect of simultaneous vaccination with BCG and smallpox vaccine in newborn infants. Bull World Health Organ 33:3213–36, 1965.
115. Meers PD: Further observations on 17D-yellow fever vaccination by scarification, with and without simultaneous smallpox vaccination. Transfusion (Paris) 54:493–501, 1960.
116. Breman JG, Coffi E, Bomba-Ire R, et al: Evaluation of a measles-smallpox vaccination campaign by a sero-epidemiologic method. Am J Epidemiol 102:564–571, 1975.
117. Meyer HM, Jr., Hostetler DD, Jr., Bernhein BC, et al: Response of Volta children to jet inoculation of combined live measles, smallpox and yellow fever vaccines. Bull World Health Organ 30:783–794, 1964.
118. Ruben FL, Smith EA, Foster SO, et al: Simultaneous administration of smallpox, measles, yellow fever, and diphtheria-pertussis-tetanus antigens to Nigerian children. Bull World Health Organ 48:175–181, 1973.
119. Foege WH, Foster SO: Multiple antigen vaccine strategies in developing countries. Am J Trop Med Hyg 23:685–689, 1974.
120. Lane JM, Ruben FL, Neff JM, et al: Complications of smallpox vaccination, 1968: national surveillance in the United States. N Engl J Med 281:1201–1208, 1969.
121. Lane JM, Ruben FL, Neff JM, et al: Complications of smallpox vaccination, 1968: results of ten statewide surveys. J Infect Dis 122:303–309, 1970.
122. Kempe CH: Studies smallpox and complications of smallpox vaccination. Pediatrics 26:176–189, 1960.
123. Brainerd HD, Hanna L, Jawetz E: Methisazone in progressive vaccinia. N Engl J Med 276:620–622, 1967.
124. Wilson GS: The Hazards of Immunization. London, Athlone Press, 1967.
125. Polak MF: Complications of smallpox vaccination in the Netherlands, 1959–1970. In International Symposium on Smallpox Vaccine. Symposia Series in Immunobiological Standardization, Vol 19. Basel, Switzerland, Karger, 1973, pp 235–242.
126. Stuart G: Memorandum on post-vaccinal encephalitis. Bull World Health Organ 1:36–53, 1947–1948.
127. van den Berg CA: L'encephalite post-vaccinale aux Pays-Bas. Bull Office Intern Hyg Publique 38:847–848, 1946.
128. Femmer J, cited by Wilson GS: The Hazards of Immunization. London, Athlone Press, 1967.
129. Seeleman K: Zerebrale Komplikationen nach Pockenschutzimpfungen mit besonderer Berucksichtigung der Alterdisposition in Hamburg 1939 bis 1958. Dtsch Med Wechenschr 85:1081–1089, 1960.
130. Berger K, Putigam F: Ueber die Erkrankungshaufigkeit verschiedener Altersklassen von Erstimpfungen an postvakzinaler Enzephalitis nach subkutaner Pockenschutzimpfung. Wien Med Wechenschr 104:487–492, 1954.
131. Berger K, Heinrich W: Decrease in postvaccinal deaths in Austria after introducing a less pathogenic virus strain. In International Symposium on Smallpox Vaccine. Symposia Series in Immunobiological Standardization, Vol 19. Basel, Switzerland, Karger, 1973, pp 199–203.
132. Halsell JS, Riddle JR, Atwood JE, et al: Myopericarditis following smallpox vaccination among vaccinia-naive US military personnel. JAMA 289:3283–3289, 2003.
133. Grabenstein JD, Winkenwerder W Jr: US military smallpox vaccination program experience. JAMA 289:3278–3282, 2003.
134. Karjalainen J, Heikkila J, Nieminen MS, et al: Etiology of mild acute infectious myocarditis: relation to clinical features. Acta Med Scand 213:65–73, 1983.
135. Update: cardiac-related events during the civilian smallpox vaccination program—United States, 2003. MMWR 52:492–496, 2003.
136. Urner JA: Some observations of the vaccination of pregnant women and newborn infants. Am J Obstet Gynecol 13:70–76, 1927.
137. Lieberman BL: Vaccination of pregnant women and newborn infants. Am J Obstet Gynecol 14:217–220, 1927.
138. Neff JM, Lane JM, Pert JH, et al: Complications of smallpox vaccination. 1. National survey in the United States, 1963. N Engl J Med 276:125–132, 1967.

immunofluorescence of monolayers of MDCK cells inoculated by centrifugation (shell-vial).[33] Conserved influenza antigens (M or NP) directly in clinical samples can be detected by one of several techniques (e.g., immunofluorescence [IF], enzyme immunoassay [EIA]), and multiple point-of-care kits are commercially available with turnaround time of 15 to 30 minutes. One commercial assay is based on detection of influenza-specific NA activity. The sensitivities of these assays are higher in children (up to 90%) than in adults (generally 50% to 70%) and depend on duration of illness and sample type.[20]

Several formats of reverse transcription–polymerase chain reaction (RT-PCR) assays have been used for the detection of influenza A and B RNAs in clinical samples, with the advantage of detecting genomes of noninfectious virus.[20] The time to perform RT-PCR is longer but the cost may be lower than for commercial rapid antigen detection kits, especially in developing countries. Real-time RT-PCR has enabled the development of assays that provide rapid quantitative detection of influenza A and B with high sensitivity.[34,35] These assays have great potential to replace other methods, because they are simultaneously rapid, highly sensitive, quantitative, and amenable to being used in multiplex format, which might include probes for several different respiratory pathogens.[35] However, the costs are still prohibitive for most laboratories in developing nations. Serologic diagnosis of influenza using paired acute and convalescent serum can be done retrospectively by a variety of techniques but mainly for serologic survey purposes.[20]

TREATMENT

Amantadine and rimantadine are M2 ion channel blockers that inhibit influenza A virus replication at the uncoating step.[20] In uncomplicated influenza A in adults without underlying diseases, treatment with either drug can reduce the duration of influenza illness by approximately 1 to 2 days if started early, within 48 hours from the onset of symptoms. Amantadine is excreted in an unchanged state in the urine, while rimantadine is extensively metabolized after absorption and less than 10% of the dose is excreted unchanged in the urine. Elderly persons need only half the dose to achieve similar plasma levels. Amantadine or rimantadine may cause gastrointestinal upset and central nervous system side effects. Central nervous system (CNS) intolerance is more common with amantadine and, when severe, can be manifested as agitation, psychosis, seizures, and coma. Mild complaints including insomnia, dizziness, anxiety, dry mouth, anorexia, and nausea are reversible upon discontinuation. Amantadine and rimantadine are marketed as 100-mg tablets and 10-mg/mL syrup. The recommended dose is 100 mg twice daily for adults older than 65 years of age (100 mg/day for patients ≥65 years of age). For children under age 10 years, a rimantadine dose of 5 mg/kg/day (maximum, 150 mg/day) has been suggested.[20] Dose reductions proportional to the creatinine clearance (ClCr) are suggested for patients with renal insufficiency (amantadine for ClCr <60 to 80 mL/min/1.73 m^2; rimantadine for ClCr <10 to 20 mL/min/1.73 m^2). Influenza virus resistant to amantadine-rimantadine emerges in approximately one third of treated patients; such viruses are transmissible to close contacts and cause typical influenza illness. Resistance to these drugs renders them ineffective and is sometimes present naturally, including in recent human isolates of H5N1 virus.[20]

The neuraminidase inhibitors zanamivir and oseltamivir inhibit both influenza A and B viruses by blocking the active site of the enzyme for cleavage of sialic acid, thus inhibiting virus release from infected cells and spread within the respiratory tract.[36] In adults and children older than 5 years, inhaled zanamivir (10 mg twice daily for 5 days) provides 1- to 2.5-day reduction in illness[37] and reduces antibiotic use for lower respiratory complications by 40%. Zanamivir is generally well tolerated but may uncommonly induce bronchospasm, particularly in those with influenza and pre-existing airway disease.[20] Oseltamivir (75 mg orally twice daily for 5 days) reduces illness severity, time to resumption of daily activities by 1 to 3 days, and rates of complications leading to antibiotic prescription and hospitalization by about 50% in adults. In children 1 to 12 years of age, oseltamivir reduces the frequency of otitis media and, consequently, antibiotic prescriptions. Side effects include mild-to-moderate nausea or emesis. Dosage of neuraminidase inhibitors does not need to be adjusted for the elderly.[20] Resistance emergence is uncommon with both drugs,[20] although a recent study of children treated with oseltamivir detected drug-resistant viruses in 18%, often in association with prolonged viral excretion, and showed that children can be a source of viral transmission, even after 5 days of treatment.[38]

Antipyretic-analgesic drugs may be used for influenza-induced fever and aches. Aspirin should be avoided because of its association with Reye's syndrome.

PREVENTION AND CONTROL

Immunization with formalin-inactivated or live-attenuated multivalent influenza virus vaccines and chemoprophylaxis for influenza virus A are the methods available for preventing influenza. Influenza vaccine is used prior to the influenza season and currently includes one strain of influenza B and two strains of subtypes H3N2 and H1N1 of influenza A virus, chosen by the World Health Organization (WHO) surveillance network among the viruses most likely to circulate in the next influenza season.[20,39] The inactivated vaccine has an approximate 70% to 90% efficacy in preventing illness in healthy children and adults.[39] It also reduces influenza-related hospitalizations and mortality in elderly and high-risk patients. The Centers for Disease Control and Prevention (CDC) recommends the immunization of persons aged 50 years and older; residents of nursing homes; children and adults with chronic cardiovascular or pulmonary disease, including asthma; persons chronically ill with diabetes mellitus, renal dysfunction, or hemoglobinopathies; immunosuppressed patients including those with HIV infection; children and adolescents on chronic aspirin therapy who may develop postinfluenza Reye's syndrome; women who will be pregnant during the influenza season; children aged 6 to 23 months; those who can transmit influenza to persons at high risk, such as health-care workers and household contacts of those at high risk including children 0 to 23 months of age; crew members of cruise ships; providers of essential services; and unimmunized travelers to areas where influenza may be circulating, including the tropics, the southern hemisphere between April and September, and those traveling in large organized tourist groups. In addition, vaccine is made available to anyone interested in reducing the likelihood of becoming ill with influenza.[20,39] The inactivated vaccine, administered as a single intramuscular (IM) dose shortly before influenza season (two doses in previously unimmunized children <9 years of age), is safe during pregnancy but should be avoided in persons with history of anaphylactic reactions to eggs.[39] Vaccine safety and efficacy in children has been extensively evaluated and has shown a favorable safety profile with efficacy in 1- to 15-year-old children of 77% to 91%. Inactivated vaccine is not currently recommended for children younger than 6 months, but vaccination of household contacts and caregivers should reduce the risk of these high-risk children contracting influenza. Healthy people aged 5 to 49 years who are not contacts of immunosuppressed patients can receive either inactivated or intranasal live-attenuated vaccines.[39]

Influenza inactivated vaccine has been recently introduced in many tropical areas of the world, with a composition based on influenza viruses circulating in the southern hemisphere. The vaccine is given prior to the influenza season, which for most countries in the southern hemisphere is between May and July.[40] In South America, annual vaccination of the elderly has reduced hospitalizations and mortality for respiratory diseases.[41] Continuous surveillance has already shown that regional variations of circulating influenza virus strains should be taken in consideration in the formulation of influenza vaccines with compositions more appropriate for South America.[42]

Live-attenuated, cold adapted vaccines administered intranasally are well tolerated, genetically stable, and rarely transmissible and have the advantage of inducing local secretory immunoglobulin A (IgA) responses. Because of potential interference between components, two doses may be required in young children.[20] This vaccine was licensed in the United States in 2003, where it has become an option for healthy persons aged 5 to 49 years, including those in close contact with groups at high risk and those wanting to avoid influenza.[39] This vaccine is not recommended for persons with asthma and other chronic disorders of the pulmonary or cardiovascular systems; persons with underlying medical conditions, including diabetes, renal dysfunction, and hemoglobinopathies; persons with known or suspected immunodeficiency diseases or who are receiving immunosuppressive therapies; children or adolescents receiving aspirin or other salicylates; persons with a history of Guillain-Barré syndrome; pregnant women; and persons with a history of hypersensitivity to eggs.[39] Cold-adapted trivalent influenza vaccine is highly effective (92% in phase 3 studies) in preventing culture-confirmed influenza in healthy children and has provided protection against drift variant strains in some studies. In young and middle-aged adults, efficacy is generally comparable to that of inactivated vaccine.[39]

Other investigational approaches have been explored in influenza vaccine development, including recombinant HA produced in insect cells, virosomes incorporating surface glycoproteins, M2 protein conjugated with hepatitis B virus core, and naked DNA encoding influenza virus nucleoprotein or HA.[20] Cell culture–based vaccines (MDCK, Vero) have been approved in Europe and may offer an alternative to the limitations of the current egg-grown vaccines. The technique of reverse genetics has been used to rapidly produce candidate vaccines against potential pandemic threat viruses.

Amantadine and rimantadine are approved for use, and are 70% to 90% effective in the prophylaxis of influenza A during outbreaks. Unvaccinated elderly persons, immunodeficient patients, patients in chronic care institutions experiencing outbreaks, persons who could not be vaccinated, and those who received a vaccine strain different from the outbreak strain may receive prophylaxis with amantadine or rimantadine. Prophylaxis should be started as early as possible at doses equivalent to those used for therapy, and continued until 1 week after the end of the outbreak for a total of at least 2 weeks.[39] Amantadine- and rimantadine-resistant mutants of influenza A virus occur in up to 30% of treated patients and may be associated with failure of drug prophylaxis.[43] Both oseltamivir (75 mg twice daily) and inhaled zanamivir (10 mg/dose twice daily) are more than 80% effective in the prophylaxis of influenza during outbreaks, but only oseltamivir has been approved for this indication in the United States.[20,39]

Antiviral agents, especially the neuraminidase inhibitors, could significantly help in the control of a future influenza pandemic by reducing lower respiratory complications and hospitalizations as well as potentially person-to-person transmission. However, supply limitations[44] pose a real difficulty. Therefore, policies to ensure a reasonable supply of these drugs, as well as directions to optimize the use of limited supplies, are important issues to be considered.[18]

Respiratory Syncytial Virus

Respiratory syncytial virus (RSV) is the single most important viral cause of lower respiratory disease and a major cause of morbidity and mortality in children worldwide. RSV is the leading cause of hospitalization in young children in developed and developing countries.[45] In tropical areas, RSV has been the most frequently isolated virus in hospital-based ARI studies of children.[5]

AGENT

RSV, the only known human pathogen of the genus *Pneumovirus* in the family Paramyxoviridae, is a pleomorphic RNA virus with helical nucleocapsid and lipid-containing envelope. Antigenic differences in the surface glycoprotein G permit the classification of RSV into groups A and B, each with antigenic subgroups.[46] The interaction of RSV envelope glycoprotein G with glycosaminoglycans enables adherence to the cell surface. However, G protein–independent mechanisms of attachment must exist, since mutants devoid of G protein can also enter host cells. RSV enters the cell by fusion of viral envelope with cell membranes, a process mediated by binding of the viral F protein to the cell GTPase RhoA.[46] The syncytia resulting from fusion of the infected cells to adjacent ones are the major feature of the cytopathic effect of paramyxoviruses. Once in the cytoplasm, the negative-strand RNA is transcribed by viral transcriptase into mRNAs, which then direct viral protein synthesis. An intermediate positive-strand full-length cRNA serves as a template for the synthesis of progeny negative-strand RNA. As they bud through the cell membrane, the virions acquire a glycoprotein-containing envelope.[46] RSV causes asymptomatic infection in a variety of experimental animals, but natural infection occurs only in humans and chimpanzees.[47] RSV grows well in several human heteroploid cell lines, such as HEp-2, HeLa, and A549, and is sensitive to ether, chloroform, detergents, and a pH less than 5. RSV is inactivated at 55°C, survives poorly on porous surfaces, and loses infectivity significantly by slow freezing and storage at temperatures above 4°C.[46]

EPIDEMIOLOGY

RSV occurs worldwide and causes annual outbreaks in temperate climates in the winter and early spring, with sporadic cases throughout the year.[47] In tropical regions, where temperature fluctuations are smaller and the only significant seasonal variable is often rainfall, RSV outbreaks tend to occur in the rainy seasons. Such has been the case in Malaysia, Hong Kong, India, Papua New Guinea, Colombia, Kenya, and The Gambia.[12] Interestingly, in Singapore RSV peak activity occurs from March to August, a period of higher temperature, higher day-to-day temperature variation, and lower relative humidity.[48] In southeast Brazil, RSV occurs seasonally, within a broader range of months from February through July, after the rainy season and when temperatures tend to be cooler, with slight variations from year to year.[49] In regions where average winter temperatures are colder, such as in São Paulo city and the southernmost parts of Brazil, as well as in Argentina, RSV peak activity tends to occur in July and August.[50–52]

Most children have specific serum RSV antibody by age 2 years, but reinfections occur throughout life. More than one subtype of either RSV group may cocirculate in one season, with group predominance changing from year to year, without apparent correlation with clinical or epidemiologic characteristics of the illness they cause.[49,53] RSV transmission requires close contact and occurs either by large-particle aerosols or by contamination of hands and inoculation into the eye or nose. Secondary infections in family contacts of an index case are common, after an average incubation period ranging from 2 to 8 days.[45]

It is estimated that 30% of all infants will have RSV infection that requires medical attention and that 2% of them will be hospitalized.[45] An estimated 10% of children will have bronchiolitis in their first year of life, with 60% to 90% of those infections caused by RSV.[54] In southeast Brazil, RSV is the leading cause of lower respiratory tract infections in children younger than 1 year of age and is responsible for up to 85% of hospitalizations in this age group during peak months.[52]

CLINICAL FEATURES

The spectrum of illnesses caused by RSV ranges from mild URI to severe LRI, including pneumonia, bronchiolitis, tracheobronchitis, and croup.[45] In infants and young children, URI with fever and otitis media is common. During outbreaks, RSV RNA has been detected in up to 75% of middle ear effusions in children with RSV infection and acute otitis media.[55]

The most frequent LRI caused by RSV in infants is bronchiolitis, usually preceded by 2 to 3 days of URI symptoms, and progressing to lower respiratory tract involvement characterized by tachypnea, dyspnea, cough, expiratory wheezing, air trapping, and in more severe cases, intercostal muscle retractions and cyanosis. Fever is present in only 50% of infants. Chest radiographs may show hyperaeration of the lungs and sometimes segmented atelectasis.[45] Blood counts usually show lymphocytosis, and an increase in neutrophils with a left shift could be associated with bacterial superinfection. The most frequent bacterial superinfection in children with RSV infections is acute otitis media, which may be found in up to 60% of children with brochiolitis.[56] However, more serious bacterial infections that may require sepsis work-up is uncommon in previously healthy infants with RSV infections.[57] This may be different, however, in developing tropical areas, where RSV frequently causes infections in children previously debilitated by other diseases and malnutrition.

Infants with congenital heart disease, premature infants, or infants with underlying pulmonary conditions, such as cystic fibrosis and bronchopulmonary dysplasia, as well as immunocompromised hosts of any age, are at risk for severe and fatal RSV infections. HIV-infected children with RSV infections have a higher rate of pneumonia and prolonged illness and virus shedding, but the general severity of the RSV disease is not increased.[45] Differential diagnosis of acute bronchiolitis includes asthma, pneumonia, congenital heart and lung diseases, and cystic fibrosis. Particular clinical signs are generally not accurate predictors of specific viral causes, but in a study conducted in the Philippines, wheezing was a significant predictor of viral LRI, while manifestations of higher severity, such as chest indrawing and cyanosis, were more often associated with bacterial LRI.[58] The most frequent RSV illness in children over 3 years of age and adults is URI with coryza and cough, sore throat, and hoarseness, often accompanied by low-grade fever. Exacerbations of chronic pulmonary diseases and wheezing can also be seen in adults with RSV infection.[45]

The role of RSV infections in causing wheezing and asthma exacerbations in infants is well established in studies conducted in temperate areas.[59] Similar observations have been made in an emergency room study conducted in Southeast Brazil, which found that infection with respiratory viruses, especially RSV, and a family history of allergy were independently associated with wheezing.[60] Similar findings have been observed in urban Nigerian preschool children.[61]

RSV has been increasingly recognized as a cause of LRI in the elderly, mainly characterized by interstitial pneumonia, prolonged cough, and dyspnea in persons with chronic pulmonary conditions, and it should be considered in the differential diagnosis of flulike illnesses.[62]

PATHOGENESIS AND IMMUNITY

RSV replicates in respiratory epithelium to reach titers as high as 10^6 $TCID_{50}$/mL in nasal secretions of infected babies, and virus shedding may be as prolonged as 3 weeks after the symptoms disappear.[46] RSV spreads from cell to cell and may involve the entire respiratory tree, reaching bronchioles in 1 to 3 days after the onset of rhinorrhea. Replication in the bronchiolar epithelium causes necrosis of ciliated cells, syncytia formation, peribronchiolar inflammation with abundant lymphocytes and macrophages, and impairment of secretion clearance, resulting in small airway obstruction and the hyperinflation characteristic of bronchiolitis. Pneumonia frequently coexists, evidenced by interstitial mononuclear infiltrate, eosinophilic cytoplasmic inclusions in epithelial cells, and multinucleated giant cells. The most severe RSV disease occurs in young babies, whose immature airways may be unable to compensate for the pathologic changes.[46]

Naturally acquired immunity to RSV is incomplete and short-lived, but the severity of illness tends to decrease with reinfections. Local secretory IgA correlates better with protection than does serum antibody level and age, and pre-existing virus-specific maternal antibodies influence the development of neutralizing antibodies. Cell-mediated immune response is central to recovery from RSV infection, and patients with suppressed cell-mediated immune response are at risk of severe RSV pulmonary disease and fatal outcome.[45,46]

The type of immune response to the virus is probably a major factor in the development of wheezing and asthma exacerbations. A bias toward a Th2 cytokine response seems to be associated with more severe disease, whereas a Th1 response leads to effective viral clearance and milder illness. The virus itself generally triggers a Th1 response, but a pre-existing Th1 deficiency may be associated with disease severity in some children. It has been suggested that RSV bronchiolitis may be a marker of predisposition to wheezing or asthma later in life.[46,63]

Children vaccinated with a formalin-inactivated RSV vaccine developed in the 1960s had severe disease when exposed to natural infection, apparently as a consequence of an imbalance between protective and immunopathologic T-cell responses elicited by previous parenteral immunization with inactivated RSV. This would favor a CD4+ Th2 cytokine pattern in response to subsequent RSV infections, whereas a previous natural infection would favor a CD4+ Th1 pattern in response to reinfection.[64]

DIAGNOSIS

Nasopharyngeal aspirates or swabs, nasal washings, and lower respiratory samples are all appropriate specimens for RSV isolation. This is usually accomplished in cultures of HEp-2 cell line, in which RSV induces syncytia in 3 to 5 days. RSV antigen detection by EIA, including membrane-based EIA, is sensitive and specific and requires virtually no equipment, making it ideal for field studies. Rapid RSV detection by IF of exfoliated respiratory cells may be even more sensitive than EIA-based methods.[45,46]

The increasing use of rapid tests has facilitated the assessment of RSV in tropical areas.[1] Ideally, a combination of a rapid method with viral isolation should be used for maximal RSV detection, but the cost may still be prohibitive for the meager resources available in some tropical areas. Detection of RSV RNA by conventional RT-PCR has shown suboptimal sensitivity, especially when compared with easy-to-perform, more sensitive rapid methods.[45] However, more recently developed assays based on real-time RT-PCR are proving to be more sensitive than conventional RT-PCR assays, with the added conveniences of being rapid, quantitative, and amenable to simultaneous detection and subtyping of RSV directly from clinical specimens.[65] RSV serology has limited value for case management but may be useful for epidemiologic surveys.[45]

TREATMENT

URI caused by RSV requires no specific treatment, and antibiotics are needed only when bacterial otitis media or sinusitis are present.[45] The supportive treatment of infants with RSV bronchiolitis consists basically in preventing hypoxemia and electrolyte imbalance, in addition to aerosolized bronchodilators. The lack of obvious correlation between radiologic findings and disease severity suggests that a chest film should be recommended only for severely ill or deteriorating infants.[54] To prevent hypoxemia, requirements may vary from simple removal of respiratory secretions and proper positioning of the infant to mechanical respiratory assistance and even extracorporeal membrane oxygenation (ECMO). Pulse oximetry has been advocated to assess oxygen needs, but in tropical developing areas, where oximeters may not be available, serial clinical assessment is essential to monitor disease progression. For this purpose, crackles and cyanosis seem to correlate better with hypoxemia than tachypnea and intercostal retraction.[54] Correction of hypoxemia can be accomplished with 40% or lower oxygen concentrations.[45] Oxygen should be humidified with saline and delivered by mask if head boxes or tents are unavailable. The role of corticosteroids remains unclear with some evidence that they are not beneficial.[54]

The only antiviral drug currently approved for the treatment of infants with RSV is the synthetic nucleoside ribavirin, delivered by small-particle aerosol via a mist tent, mask, oxygen hood, or ventilator. It is recommended only for infants and young children with an underlying condition, such as congenital heart disease, cystic fibrosis, or immunosuppression. Premature infants, infants younger than 6 weeks of age, and severely ill infants may also be considered for therapy.[66] Aerosolized ribavirin is well tolerated, but it is expensive and its prolonged administration requires facilities that may not be available in impoverished tropical areas. Passive immunotherapy with RSV immunoglobulin, in combination with aerosolized ribavirin, improved the outcome of RSV pneumonia in bone marrow transplant patients.[67] The use of RSV-intravenous immunoglobulin (IVIG) or humanized monoclonal antibody against RSV has shown no benefit for the treatment of RSV infections in infants.[45]

PREVENTION AND CONTROL

No vaccine is currently available for RSV prophylaxis. The disease enhancement caused by formalin-inactivated vaccine in the 1960s plus results of more recent unsuccessful trials of live-attenuated vaccines, have significantly slowed progress toward an RSV vaccine.[2] Purified fusion protein vaccine has been tested for safety and immunogenicity in seropositive children older than 18 months, and was associated with reduction of lower respiratory tract illness, but not of RSV infection rates, in children with cystic fibrosis.[45] These and other candidate subunit vaccines, as well as intranasal live-attenuated vaccines, should be tested in high-risk children with underlying bronchopulmonary diseases.

Passive immunization of high-risk infants with monthly infusions of RSV immunoglobulin during the RSV season reduced the incidence and severity of RSV infections in high-risk children.[68] This costly intervention is the only available means of protecting high-risk children against serious RSV LRI. Monthly intramuscular injections of humanized monoclonal antibody should be considered for passive immunoprophylaxis during RSV season for high-risk infants such as preterm infants less than 6 months old, children with congenital heart disease, and children less than 2 years of age with bronchopulmonary dysplasia.[45]

Hospitalized infants with RSV infection should be isolated or grouped to prevent cross-infection. Hand washing; use of eye-nose goggles, gowns, and gloves; and decontamination of surfaces and fomites are additional nosocomial infection control measures.[45]

Human Parainfluenza Viruses

Human parainfluenza viruses (HPIVs) are the single most frequent cause of croup in infants and children worldwide and are second only to RSV as cause of LRI in infants.[45,69] Little is known about the epidemiology of HPIVs in tropical countries, but these viruses have been detected in up to 13% of children in hospital-based ARI studies in developing countries.[5,21]

AGENTS

HPIVs are distributed in two genera of the family Paramyxoviridae, sharing the structural and biological characteristics already mentioned in the RSV section. HPIVs are classified antigenically into types 1 to 4, and HPIV-4 has subtypes A and B. HPIV types 1 and 3 are classified in the genus *Respirovirus*, while HPIV types 2 and 4 are in the genus *Rubulavirus*. HPIV-1 and -3 are the types most frequently associated with LRI in children, the immunocompromised, the chronically ill, and the elderly, whereas PIV-4 causes mostly URI in both children and adults.[69]

Binding of HPIV to sialic acid in the cell membrane is mediated by the glycoprotein HN, which contains hemagglutinin and neuraminidase activities. Fusion of viral and cell membranes is mediated by the viral F protein, which is cleaved by cellular proteolytic enzymes.[45] Once inside the cell, the cycle is similar to other Paramyxoviridae, as summarized in the RSV section. HPIVs can be propagated in primary simian or human kidney cells and in several cell lines, such as HEp-2, Vero, MDCK, LLC-MK2, BHK, and HeLa.[69] A variety of experimental animals undergo asymptomatic infection with PIV, but only higher primates develop symptoms.[45,69]

EPIDEMIOLOGY

Primary HPIV infection occurs early in childhood, and by age 5 virtually all children are seropositive.[19] An estimated one third of all viral LRIs in children in the United States are caused by HPIV-1 and -3.[69,70]

In most temperate regions, HPIV-1 and -2 cause epidemics in the fall of alternate years, either in co-circulation or alternating with one another. The biennial pattern of HPIV-1 is found in both hemispheres.[69] HPIV-1 causes most croup epidemics, whereas HPIV-2 more frequently causes illness with milder manifestations, although it can also cause croup.[69] HPIV-3 occurs endemically throughout the year, with sporadic spring outbreaks mainly among infants, and HPIV-4 occurs sporadically throughout the year in children and adults.[45,69,70] In tropical areas HPIVs may account for up to 15% of child hospital admissions due to LRI.[21] Community-based ARI studies in children under age 5 years show higher HPIV activity during rainy seasons in tropical countries.[3,24] HPIVs were the most frequent viruses detected in school-aged children with bronchial asthma exacerbations in urban Nigeria.[61]

HPIVs spread mainly within families and closed communities, such as nurseries, day-care centers, and pediatric wards, with high secondary attack rates. In a longitudinal study conducted with children less than 2 years of age with ARI in a day-care center for low-income families in Northeast Brazil, HPIVs represented 11% of the viruses detected.[11]

The virus does not persist long in the environment and is transmitted mainly by large droplets and fomites.[45] Viral shedding usually lasts 3 to 10 days, but shedding of HPIV for months has been reported in very young children and immunosuppressed hosts.[71]

CLINICAL FEATURES

Primary HPIV infection may cause rhinitis, pharyngitis, laryngotracheobronchitis (croup), bronchiolitis, or pneumonia. Approximately two thirds of all PIV infections in children result in febrile URI with associated otitis media in 10% to 34%. The remaining one third of PIV infections are cases of croup, bronchiolitis, or pneumonia.[61,63] HPIVs, mainly of types 1 and 2, cause up to 74% of all cases of croup.[69]

Croup is the most striking clinical presentation of HPIV infection and is most common between the ages of 6 and 36 months.[72] Croup is manifested by inspiratory stridor, barking cough, and hoarseness caused by subglottic edema, preceded by rhinorrhea, mild cough, and low-grade fever.[45,72] Most children recover in 2 to 5 days, but some may develop bronchiolitis and pneumonia and present with a bronchopneumonia-croup syndrome.[45,69,72]

Since immunity to HPIVs is incomplete, infections tend to occur throughout life, but little is known about HPIV infections in adults. In general, adults have only nonspecific URI, commonly with hoarseness.[45]

HPIVs can cause particularly severe diseases in immunocompromised hosts, especially children with severe combined immunodeficiency and bone marrow transplant patients. Mortality in bone marrow transplant patients with HPIV infection varies from 10% to 20% in most series.[45,69]

PATHOGENESIS AND IMMUNITY

HPIVs replicate in ciliated epithelial cells, causing cytolysis of the respiratory mucosa. The infection begins in the upper respiratory tract and tends to disseminate down the respiratory tree. The larynx and trachea are mostly involved in the croup syndrome, and extensive involvement of the lower respiratory tree may be present in tracheobronchitis, bronchopneumonia, and bronchiolitis.[69,71,72]

Similar to influenza, factors determining the extent of HPIV infection include the susceptibility of the viral F protein to be cleaved and tissue-specific differences in the production of proteases to cleave it.[45]

Host immunity is largely mediated by humoral immunity to the two surface proteins HN and F. Virtually all children by the age of 3 years will have seroconverted to HPIVs, generally first to HPIV-3 but later also to HPIV-1 and -2. At school age, a significant proportion of children will have seroconverted also to HPIV-4. Secretory antibody targeted to the HN glycoprotein is the best marker of protection against PIV,[71] but the protection conferred by antibodies is limited, and repeated infections will develop. T-cell immune response seems to be involved in the clearance of virus and additionally in the development of inflammatory infiltrate, edema, and excess mucus secretion,[69] and immunocompromised hosts may develop progressive and even lethal disease.[73]

Like RSV, PIVs cause mononuclear interstitial infiltrate, epithelial necrosis, inflammatory exudate into the alveoli, and hyaline membrane formation in the lungs.[45]

DIAGNOSIS

PIV is present in respiratory secretions until about 8 days from the onset of symptoms and can be isolated in monkey kidney primary cells and several continuous cell lines. Virus can be detected in the monolayers by hemadsorption with guinea pig erythrocytes in around 3 days after inoculation and confirmed by IF.[69,71] Shell-vial assays have been developed for HPIV detection but with mixed results.[69] IF of exfoliated respiratory epithelial cells has produced conflicting and sometimes disappointing results, with most studies reporting sensitivities between 50% and 75% at best.[69] Detection of viral RNA by RT-PCR, including commercially available multiplex assays for several respiratory viruses, has enhanced the sensitivity of detection of HPIV from clinical samples.[69,74] Real-time PCR for respiratory viruses in multiplex format is sensitive and specific for HPIV.[35]

TREATMENT

At present, only supportive and symptomatic treatment is available for PIV infections. Management of croup includes supplemental oxygen and racemic epinephrine nebulization in hospitalized patients. Mist therapy, although traditional, has no proven value.[72] Short-term, high-dose systemic corticosteroids may reduce the need for intubation, and nebulized budesonide has a rapid effect and is as safe and efficacious as nebulized epinephrine in moderately severe croup.[72] Several antiviral agents have in vitro activity against HPIVs, but none has reached clinical testing.[69] There have been anecdotal reports of reduced HPIV shedding in immunocompromised patients treated with ribavirin, but this finding has not resisted scrutiny.[69] Future possibilities include the BCX 2798 and BCX 2855 compounds, whose design is based on the three-dimensional structure of the HN protein, which inhibit the hemagglutinin and neuraminidase activities of the protein and were effective in vitro and in an animal model against HPIV-1, -2 and -3.[75]

PREVENTION AND CONTROL

No interventions are available for the prevention of HPIV infections. Early trials with inactivated HPIV vaccine in the 1960s were unsuccessful.[69] Recently, a live-attenuated, cold-adapted HPIV-3 vaccine was found to be immunogenic for children as young as 1 month of age and holds promise for further development.[69] The same vaccine was tested in combination with a live-attenuated RSV vaccine candidate, showing that this approach is feasible and deserves further study.[76] Characterization of HPIV proteins HN and F has led to development of subunit immunogens that showed efficacy in animal models.[69]

Rhinoviruses

Human rhinoviruses (HRVs) are the most frequent respiratory pathogens of humans.[77] They were the most frequently isolated viruses in children under 5 years of age with ARI in an urban slum in northeast Brazil.[3]

AGENTS

Human rhinoviruses are small, nonenveloped, positive-strand RNA viruses in the family Picornaviridae, with over 100 identified serotypes.[77]

HRV serotypes have been classified according to receptor-specificity into three groups. The major group includes 91 serotypes whose receptor is intercellular adhesion molecule–1 (ICAM-1); the minor group contains 10 serotypes whose receptor is the low-density lipoprotein receptor (LDLR); and the remaining serotype, HRV-87, utilizes a sialoprotein as cell receptor. Unlike other picornaviruses, HRVs are acid-labile, a property that distinguishes them from enteroviruses.[77]

The HRV genome is a monocistronic single-stranded RNA, packed in an icosahedral capsid composed of 12 pentamers. Surrounding the fivefold vertex, each pentamer contains a 1.2- to 3.0-nm-wide canyon that contains the receptor binding site. Following receptor binding, the viral positive-strand RNA is released into the cytoplasm and directs the synthesis of a polyprotein, whose cleavage products include an RNA polymerase. This enzyme will produce an expanding pool of positive-strand RNA using as a template an intermediate negative-strand RNA. The positive-strand RNA can be either translated into virion proteins or packaged as a genome into newly assembled virions. The HRV replication cycle takes place in the cytoplasm, and mature virions are released when the host cell is lysed.[77]

HRVs are resistant to ethanol, ether, chloroform, and nonionic detergent but are sensitive to UV light; to pH lower than 5 and higher than 9; and to halogens such as chlorine, bromine, iodine, and phenolic disinfectants. They are stable for days on environmental surfaces and for years at minus 70°C.[77]

HRV infects only higher primates and causes illness only in humans. Several cell lines of primate origin support HRV propagation, but certain strains of HeLa cells and human embryonic fibroblasts provide higher sensitivity for HRV isolation from clinical specimens.[78] The optimal growth temperature for HRV is 33°C to 35°C.[77]

EPIDEMIOLOGY

HRV infections occur in people from all continents, including remotely located population groups, such as Bushmen from the Kalahari Desert, native Alaskans, and an isolated Amazon Indian tribe.[79] HRV has been estimated to cause up to 80% of all autumn colds in temperate climates.[80] In tropical countries, very few community-based studies of viral ARI have used adequate HRV detection methods,[5] and this has limited the assessment of the actual impact of HRV in those areas. However, available evidence indicates that HRV is frequently associated with ARI in children in Brazil. In Fortaleza, a city in northeast Brazil, HRV detected by isolation in cell culture represented 46% of the viruses in children under 5 years of age with ARI.[3] In Salvador, another city in the same region, HRV represented 52% of the viruses detected by RT-PCR in association with ARI in children younger than 2 years of age attending a day-care center for the underprivileged.[11] Data on the frequency of HRV among adults in tropical countries are even more scarce. In Singapore, HRV was detected in 20% of the samples obtained from adults with ARI symptoms attending primary care centers.[81]

HRV transmission requires close exposure and occurs mainly by hand-to-hand contact, followed by self-inoculation into the eye or nose, but also by airborne spread. Once HRV reaches the nasal cavity, infection occurs in virtually 100% of susceptible subjects, and approximately 75% of those infected develop illness after a 1- to 2-day incubation.[77] Children play a central role in spreading the virus in the household.

Evidence suggests that indoor HRV transmission is favored by high relative humidity and crowding of young children, as occurs in the United States at the beginning of the school term, which may explain the autumn seasonal peak of HRV.[77] In tropical northeastern Brazil, however, where relative humidity remains above 70% reaching 90% during the rainy season, longitudinal studies have found no obvious HRV seasonality.[3,11]

CLINICAL FEATURES

HRV colds are indistinguishable from colds of other viral causes and consist of nasal discharge, nasal obstruction, sneezing, sore or scratchy throat, hoarseness, cough, and headache. Facial and ear pressure may be present. Fever and malaise are uncommon. These symptoms last approximately 7 days but may persist for up to 2 weeks in 25% of cases. Infants and toddlers may display only nasal discharge and be otherwise asymptomatic.[77] The majority of patients have obstruction and mucosal abnormalities of the sinus cavities, eustachian tubes, and middle ear, which predispose to secondary bacterial sinusitis and otitis media, each complication found in approximately 2% of all colds.[82] HRV RNA may be detected by RT-PCR in maxillary sinus brushings in 40% of adults presenting with acute sinusitis,[83] and in 24% of the samples of middle ear fluid from children less than 7 years of age with diagnosis of acute otitis media.[84]

HRV is frequently associated with exacerbations of chronic obstructive pulmonary disease and asthma attacks in children over 2 years of age and in adults.[59,77,85]

PATHOGENESIS AND IMMUNITY

HRV replication is restricted to the respiratory epithelium, taking place in scattered ciliated cells of the nose and in nonciliated cells of the nasopharynx.[86] This tropism seems to be a consequence of receptor availability. Infection of a limited number of cells triggers the release of cytokines, chemokines, and inflammatory mediators, which together with stimulation of the local parasympathetic nerve endings, results in the cold symptoms. Kinins, prostaglandins, and proinflammatory cytokines and chemokines may contribute to vasodilation, increased vascular permeability, influx of polymorphonuclear leukocytes, exocrine gland secretion, and nerve ending stimulation, resulting in nasal obstruction, rhinorrhea, sneezing, cough, and sore throat.[77]

Serotype-specific neutralizing IgM, IgG, and IgA antibodies develop in most infected persons in 7 to 21 days and persist for years. Protection from infection is partially attributed to the presence of IgA antibody in nasal secretions, and recovery from illness is more dependent on cell-mediated immunity. HRV-induced blastogenesis, natural killer cell activity, mitogen-stimulated cell production of IL-2 and IFN-γ have been documented during HRV infection.[77,87] HRV induces the expression of human β-defensin 2 (HBD-2) in the respiratory epithelium, which supports a role for HBD-2 in host defense to HRV infection.[88]

DIAGNOSIS

HRV can be detected in respiratory secretions by isolation in cultures of susceptible cell lines.[78] HRV shedding peaks around 48 hours after infection and declines rapidly, but may remain at low levels for up to 3 weeks.[77] Cultures should be kept at 33°C to 35°C in a roller drum and examined for 10 to 14 days. The presence of HRV, indicated by the typical CPE, is confirmed by the acid sensitivity of the isolate. Rapid immunocytochemical methods are not available because of the large number of serotypes. RT-PCR in clinical samples is more sensitive and less tedious than HRV isolation,[83] and the recently introduced real-time PCR-based assay is more sensitive than conventional RT-PCR.[89] PCR-based assays have been useful in studies to assess the impact of HRV in different settings. The homotypic nature of HRV antibodies restricts serology to experimental settings.[77]

TREATMENT

Trials of antiviral agents for HRV have been conducted, but no specific treatment suitable for routine use has yet been identified, mainly because of lack of potency, untoward side effects, and drug delivery problems.[90] Ruprintrivir, a selective inhibitor of HRV 3C protease, has potent, broad-spectrum anti-HRV activity in vitro. A double-blind, placebo-controlled clinical trial of intranasal ruprintrivir in experimental HRV infection reduced symptoms by 33% and also decreased viral titers and nasal discharge.[91]

Symptomatic relief from cold symptoms can be obtained with a broad variety of nonprescription medications. Systemic sympathomimetic decongestants, such as pseudoephedrine, may reduce nasal obstruction, first-generation antihistamines may reduce sneezing and rhinorrhea, and nonsteroidal anti-inflammatory drugs such as naproxen or ibuprofen may reduce headache, cough, and systemic symptoms.[77]

PREVENTION AND CONTROL

The large number of HRV serotypes with minimal cross-antigenicity has hampered the development of an HRV vaccine.

It may be possible to reduce exposure to HRV by hand washing after contact with a cold sufferer or after handling objects that may have been contaminated with respiratory secretions.[77] Studies in experimentally infected volunteers show that application of the virucidal agents salicylic acid or pyroglutamic acid to the hands reduced recovery of rhinovirus from the hand skin of treated persons as compared with controls.[92] This result suggests that rhinovirus transmission can be prevented by virucidal hand treatments.

Short-term, postexposure prophylaxis by intranasal IFN-α significantly reduced the incidence of HRV colds in household contacts of an index case.[93] However, the cost and difficulty of making the drug available to homes in a timely fashion reduce the utility of this approach for extended use by populations, especially in tropical countries.

Ruprintrivir has also been evaluated for prophylaxis of HRV colds starting 6 hours prior to inoculation of human volunteers. This approach reduced the proportion of subjects with positive viral cultures and viral titers but did not affect the frequency of colds.[91]

Respiratory Adenoviruses

Respiratory infections caused by adenoviruses are among the most frequent illnesses that these viruses cause, particularly in children under age 5 years.[94] Adenoviruses have been frequently isolated in ARI studies in tropical countries.[5] In the south cone of South America, adenoviruses were the second most frequent virus recovered from children hospitalized for ARI.[95]

AGENTS

Adenoviruses are nonenveloped, icosahedral DNA viruses of the genus *Mastadenovirus* in the family Adenoviridae.[94] Adenoviruses are distinguished antigenically by group-specific (A through F) and type-specific (1 through 49) antigens and by genomic subtypes identified by restriction site mapping.[93,94]

The adenovirus capsid consists of three morphologically, antigenically, and functionally distinct types of capsomers: hexons, penton bases, and fibers that project from the penton bases. The hexon and penton bases contain complement-fixing, group-specific antigens common to all human adenoviruses, whereas the fibers have primarily neutralizing and hemagglutination-inhibiting, type-specific antigens. Adenoviruses are commonly accompanied by small, single-stranded DNA parvoviruses known as adenoassociated viruses, which do not seem to cause any specific disease. Most people have antibodies to at least one of the four serotypes of adenoassociated virus by age 10 years.[96]

The fiber protein binds to the host cell, through the protein coxsackie and adenovirus receptor (CAR) of the immunoglobulin superfamily, which serves as a high-affinity receptor for adenoviruses. The class I major histocompatibility complex (MHC) also may serve as receptor for adenovirus 5.[94] Ligand-receptor interaction facilitates interaction of the penton base with cell surface integrins, which triggers entry. After endocytosis, the double-stranded linear genomic DNA is transported to the nucleus, where "early" and "late" sets of viral genes are transcribed, resulting in mRNAs coding for structural and nonstructural proteins. Virus assembly takes place in the nucleus, and the infectious cycle is completed by the release of up to 1 million virions upon cell lysis.[94]

Adenoviruses replicate well in continuous cell lines of epithelial origin, such as HEp-2, HeLa, and A549, and can be adapted to grow in human embryonic lung fibroblasts. They are stable over a wide pH range (5 to 9), resistant to isopropyl alcohol, ether, and chloroform, stable for weeks at room temperature and for years at approximately 20°C or colder, and can be lyophilized. They are inactivated by sodium hypochlorite and a temperature of 60°C for 2 minutes.[97]

EPIDEMIOLOGY

Respiratory transmission of adenoviruses occurs at all ages but is of prime importance during epidemics among military recruits. Ocular transmission has been associated with swimming pools and physician offices where sterilization or hand washing has been inadequate. Asymptomatic infection and a prolonged carrier state are common.[94]

Low-number adenovirus serotypes (1, 2, 3, and 5) are more frequent before age 5 years and account for 5% to 20% of cases of URI and approximately 5% of cases of LRI in children.[98] In adults, adenoviruses occur sporadically and cause mostly URI. Infections by adenoviruses types 4 and 7 are usually epidemic, with attack rates of 6% to 16% per week in newly assembled military recruits, whose adenovirus carriage rate may be as high as 18%.[94] In this group, the adenoviral syndromes vary from mild colds to severe LRI, but overall attack rates may reach 80%, with 20% to 40% of the individuals needing hospitalization.[94]

In temperate climates, adenoviral infections are more frequent in late winter, spring, and early summer, whereas in northeast Brazil they seem to occur year-round.[5] In Salvador, also in northeast Brazil, adenoviruses were detected in 11% of children younger than age 2 years with ARI in a day-care center.[11] In tropical areas the incidence of adenovirus infections in military recruits is lower, and different serotypes may be involved.[98]

Pharyngoconjunctival fever, commonly caused by adenoviruses types 3 and 7, may be epidemic or endemic among children during the summer in temperate climates. Inadequate chlorination or filtration of swimming pools and lakes has been associated with epidemics.[99] The incubation period of adenovirus infections averages 10 days.[98]

CLINICAL FEATURES

Adenovirus respiratory diseases may involve all parts of the respiratory tract, and up to 50% of nonepidemic infections are asymptomatic. In fact, adenoviruses were discovered because of their propensity for latency in adenoidal tissue.[94,98] In southeast Brazil, adenoviruses were detected with equal frequency in wheezing young children and asymptomatic controls.[60]

Most adenoviral illnesses consist of febrile colds, and in children the fever may be high and long-lasting. Pharyngitis is common and may be associated with fever, pharyngeal exudate, granular appearance of the mucosa, and anterior cervical adenopathy, similarly to streptococcal pharyngitis.[94] Adenoviruses can be recovered from up to 20% of cases of pharyngitis in small children. Pharyngitis may be concurrent with pharyngoconjunctival fever, a syndrome caused by adenovirus types 3 and 7 and characterized by conjunctivitis, frequently unilateral, which may last for 1 to 2 weeks, preauricular adenopathy, cough, rhinitis, malaise, and fever.[99] The most frequent complication of adenoviral colds is acute otitis media, which occurs in up to 30% of cases.[100]

Adenovirus LRIs consist mainly of bronchitis and pneumonia, and may make up over 10% of childhood LRIs in temperate areas.[101] Adenoviruses may cause permanent lung parenchymal damage, especially when concurrent with measles.[101] Epidemic adenoviral infections in military recruits have a spectrum of clinical manifestation ranging from colds to severe pneumonia. Typically, however, the manifestations are fever, pharyngeal symptoms, cough, chest pain, headache, and malaise.[98]

Overwhelming pneumonitis may be part of disseminated adenoviral infections in newborn infants and patients with immunodeficiencies, including acquired immunodeficiency syndrome (AIDS). However, the frequent concomitance of other respiratory pathogens in AIDS patients and the high prevalence of asymptomatic adenovirus infection shed doubt on the causal role of the adenovirus in these patients.[102] Adenoviruses are also an important cause of epidemic keratoconjunctivitis.[94,98]

While most adenoviral ARIs are self-limited and uncommonly associated with death or permanent sequelae,[94] adenoviruses alone or associated with other pathogens have been recovered from 20% of fatal cases of LRI in Argentina.[103]

PATHOGENESIS AND IMMUNITY

Adenoviral respiratory disease results from necrosis of cells of airway epithelia, and viremia may result in disseminated infection in immunocompromised persons. Bronchiolitis, interstitial pneumonitis, and mononuclear cell infiltrates are part of the inflammatory process in the lungs. It remains unclear why certain strains are more virulent than others. For example, the genomic variant B7h was associated with the majority of fatal lower respiratory disease in South America.[95]

In addition to lytic infection, adenoviruses may become latent in epithelial and lymphoid cells, which is probably important to maintaining the virus in populations.[94] A possible role of latent adenovirus in the pathogenesis of chronic airway inflammation has been suggested.[94,96,104]

Protection from adenovirus infection and disease is mainly due to type-specific neutralizing antibody, but reinfections, mostly asymptomatic, may occur. A long-lived T-cell immune response develops in most infected immunocompetent persons and is not only responsible for recovery but also is involved in tissue pathologic changes.[94]

DIAGNOSIS

Adenoviruses can be detected in respiratory, ocular, or ear secretions, but clinical correlation is required, because asymptomatic virus shedding is common. Isolation of adenoviruses in cell culture with identification by IF constitutes the standard diagnostic method, but direct detection of viral antigens or viral DNA by PCR in clinical samples is an attractive rapid alternative.[94] Rapid antigen detection by immunochromatography is around 95% sensitive in comparison with cell culture, and easily can be used in point-of-care diagnosis of adenovirus. However, both conventional and real-time PCR are more sensitive than cell culture is.[105] Positive results by PCR should be interpreted with caution, given the propensity of adenoviruses to cause latency.

Adenoviruses cause a characteristic CPE in a variety of cell lines of human origin, and maintenance of cultures for 2 weeks combined with blind passage (i.e., passage of cells even without obvious CPE to see if it develops after passage) may increase adenovirus recovery.[3,94] Inoculation of cells by centrifugation followed by immunostaining may shorten the detection time.[106]

Several serologic tests can detect antibodies to the common hexon antigen.[94] However, their clinical utility is restricted.

TREATMENT

At present, there is no routine effective antiviral treatment for adenovirus infections. Successful therapy of severe adenoviral infections in immunocompromised patients with IV ribavirin has been reported.[107] Cidofovir has shown some efficacy in the rabbit ocular model of adenoviral infection. Iododeoxyuridine and adenine arabinoside were unsuccessful in the treatment of adenoviral keratoconjunctivitis.[94]

PREVENTION AND CONTROL

A live vaccine consisting of wild-type adenovirus packaged in enteric-coated capsules induces immunity by ensuring enteric infection without infection of the respiratory tree. This approach has been used successfully to vaccinate military recruits against adenoviruses types 4 and 7.[98] Proper sterilization, hand washing, and chlorination can prevent adenovirus spread via tonometers, hands, and swimming pools.

Coronaviruses

Coronaviruses are enveloped viruses with distinct virion morphology, displaying widely spaced, long petal-shaped spikes at the surface, that confer a crownlike appearance, the origin of the name *corona*. The envelope contains a long helical nucleocapsid with single, positive-stranded RNA, 27 to 32 kb in size, which is the largest known viral RNA genome.[108] Until very recently, only three human coronaviruses (HCoVs) were known to exist: HCoV-229E, HCoV-OC43, and the CoV associated with severe acute respiratory syndrome (SARS-CoV). Recently, two groups in The Netherlands almost simultaneously published studies that resulted in the identification of two new strains of HCoV: HCoV-NL63[109] and HCoV-NL.[110] In addition, PCR primers directed to conserved replicase 1a sequences of animal CoVs led to the identification of yet another HCoV detected in 8.8% of children from New Haven, Connecticut with symptoms of ARI. This agent was designated HCoV-NH and is likely to represent the same species of HCoV-NL and -NL63.[111] On the basis of antigenic and genetic studies, the known human coronaviruses are distributed in three of the four coronavirus groups so far identified. HCoV-229E, -NH, -NL, and -NL63 belong to group I, HCoV-OC43 belongs to group II, and SARS-CoV is the only known constituent of group IV, while group III contains no known human viruses and consists only of the avian infectious bronchitis virus.

Coronavirus RNA synthesis occurs in the cytoplasm via a negative-strand RNA intermediate. The viral RNA possesses a 5′ cap followed by a leader sequence and an untranslated region, with another 3′ terminal untranslated region followed by a poly(A) tail. The genome is polycistronic and the synthesis of subgenomic negative-sense RNAs is done by discontinuous transcription to originate a nested set of subgenomic mRNAs that share the 5′ leader sequence and overlap at the 3′ end. The envelope contains the structural proteins S (spike), M (membrane), E (envelope), and only in the case of some group II coronaviruses, HA (hemagglutinin). The S glycoprotein contains neutralizing and T-cell epitopes and functions as the cell receptor ligand, thereby determining tissue tropism. The M protein is embedded in the envelope and interacts with the N (nucleocapsid) protein during maturation. In addition to the nucleocapsid and envelope proteins, a replicase is present in cells infected by all coronaviruses. New virions assemble by budding through intracellular membranes and are released through vesicles of the secretory pathway.[108]

HUMAN CORONAVIRUSES UNRELATED TO SARS

HCoV-229E and -OC43 are considered to be second only to rhinoviruses as agents of common colds, causing infections with variable frequency, depending mainly on the detection method and season of the study. Up to 35% of mild upper respiratory tract infections in adults have been attributed to HCoV-229E.[112] While HCoV-229E and -OC43 are documented causes of colds in temperate regions, their impact as causes of respiratory infections in tropical regions has not been defined.

AGENTS

Human coronaviruses were first isolated in England, almost 40 years ago, in human organ cultures of tracheal and nasal tissues. There have been relatively few field studies based on HCoV isolation in cell culture, likely because these viruses are too fastidious to be propagated, but most respiratory isolates obtained so far have been antigenically similar to either HCoV-229E or -OC43.[112] These agents have the same structural features as the other members of the family. The S protein of HCoV-229E binds to the metalloprotease human aminopeptidase N at the cell surface, and entry is independent of enzymatic activity of the receptor. The hemagglutinin of HCoV-OC43 binds to sialic acid present in glycoproteins on the cell surface and this interaction facilitates infection, but to the best of our knowledge, a specific receptor has not been identified for this agent.[108]

EPIDEMIOLOGY

HCoVs have been found throughout the world and are considered to be the second most frequent cause of common cold, accounting for an average rate of 15% of respiratory illnesses in the general population in the United States. However, the rates may be quite variable from year to year, ranging from 1% to 35% in years of peak activity. HCoV infections occur mainly in the winter and spring months, but summer activity has also been documented. During the autumn peak of rhinovirus activity, 8% of the adults with a cold negative for rhinovirus were positive for HCoV by RT-PCR in Charlottesville, VA.[80]

HCoV-229E has caused well-documented winter outbreaks at 2- to 4-year intervals in temperate regions.[112,113] Similarly, winter outbreak of HCoV-OC43 has also been detected in Europe.[114] In contrast, little is known about the prevalence of HCoV-229E and -OC43 in tropical countries. In Brazil, the activity of HCoV-229E as cause of respiratory infections in nonhospitalized children was first documented by serology in the early 1970s, with a seropositivity rate of 26% in adults by complement fixation assay.[115]

CLINICAL FEATURES

The usual manifestations of HCoV infection are typical common colds. The incubation period tends to be 1 day longer that that for rhinovirus colds, with illness duration of 6 to 7 days. Low-grade fever may occur in up to 20% of the patients, and in addition to nasal symptoms, cough and sore throat occur frequently. More serious infections of the lower respiratory tract caused by HCoV have also been documented, either sporadically in infants with pneumonia and immunocompromised patients, or in up to 33% of previously healthy Marine Corps recruits with pneumonia.[112,113] In addition, HCoV-229E and -OC43 have been recognized in association with influenza-like illnesses in frail elderly patients. Eight of 100 (8%) nasopharyngeal swabs from older patients hospitalized for cardiopulmonary illnesses during the influenza seasonal outbreak in Rochester, N.Y., were positive for HCoV (five for HCoV-229E).[116]

Respiratory HCoV infections have been associated with exacerbations of asthma, chronic bronchitis, and recurrent wheezing in children.[112,113] HCoV was detected by RT-PCR in 38 of 292 (13%) episodes of asthma in children 9 to 11 years old in England.[117] In Brazil, HCoV was detected in respiratory samples from 3 (2 OC43 and 1 229E) of 73 (4%) children younger than 2 years of age who came to the ER with wheezing.[60]

Similarly to HRV, HCoV infections have been frequently recognized in association with otitis media and maxillary sinusitis in children and adults. HCoV was detected by RT-PCR in the middle ear effusion or nasopharyngeal aspirate from 16 of 92 (17%) children with acute otitis media in Finland[84] and in nasal swabs from 3 of 20 adults with acute maxillary sinusitis.[83]

PATHOGENESIS AND IMMUNITY

There is no convenient small animal model to study the pathogenesis of HCoV, and humans naturally or experimentally infected are the only source of information obtained in vivo.

HCoVs are transmitted by the respiratory route, and experimentally infected volunteers shed virus for approximately 5 days, beginning 48 hours after infection, which is approximately the time of onset of symptoms.[112,113] The peak of symptoms occurs 2 to 4 days postinoculation.[112] HCoV-229E is known to infect airway epithelial cells from the apical surface, where the receptor is constitutively expressed, and to exit productively infected cells through the same route.[118] Ultrastructural studies of nasal epithelium of volunteers experimentally infected with HCoV-229E revealed significantly greater epithelial cell damage, ciliary loss, and cytolysis in virus-inoculated subjects than in sham-inoculated ones on day 3 postinfection.[119]

In the United States, seropositivity to HCoV-OC43 and -229E rises during the first 5 years of life, and around 40% of adults are seropositive. Symptomatic reinfections are possible, despite the presence of antibodies, suggesting rapidly waning immune response or circulation of closely related but antigenically different viruses.[113,120] Several studies indicate that respiratory HCoVs are able to reach the central nervous system.[112,113,120] The recently reported temporal association between HCoV-NH infection and Kawaski disease[121] awaits confirmation.

DIAGNOSIS

Laboratory diagnosis in clinical samples by isolation is tedious, because the two best characterized strains of HCoV are difficult to grow in routine cell cultures. Since primers can be developed for relatively constant parts of the genome, RT-PCR–based assays for HCoV-229E and -OC43 have recently become the best alternative to other methods of detection.[80] More recently, a quantitative real-time PCR-based assay for HCoVs has been developed, providing a faster means for detection and determination of viral load with potential applications in clinical studies.[122] Serologic diagnosis of HCoV by EIA is sensitive and specific and has been useful in epidemiologic surveys.[113]

TREATMENT AND PREVENTION

Intranasal interferon protects against experimental infection with HCoV-229E,[123] but no specific antiviral therapy is available, and treatment of HCoV-induced colds remains largely symptomatic. No vaccines are currently available for HCoV.

SARS-CORONAVIRUS

SARS was first reported to WHO by Carlo Urbani, a physician working in Hanoi, Vietnam, in February 2003. Retrospective analysis revealed that cases compatible with the new disease had occurred in China starting in November 2002. SARS is caused by a newly recognized coronavirus that emerged in China, subsequently spreading to several other countries in Asia, the Americas, and Europe.[124] Isolation and characterization of the agent was accomplished in record time after the 2002–2003 outbreak started, by four research groups in the WHO laboratory network.[124] In February 2003 a single infected person from the province of Guangdong, China, spent 1 day at a hotel in Hong Kong and transmitted the virus to 16 other people, who in turn seeded outbreaks of SARS in other countries in Asia and in Canada. In a matter of weeks, SARS had affected thousands of people in 25 countries in all continents, causing enormous global impact and intense media coverage, fueled by fast spread via international travel by newly infected individuals.[125] At the time of this writing, no current cases of SARS are registered, and there have been 8117 reported cases of SARS, of which 775 were fatal.[126]

AGENT

The HCoV that fulfills Koch`s postulates as the causative agent of SARS[127] shares structural features and genome organization of the family Coronaviridae (Fig. 59-1). The prompt recognition of the peculiar morphology of a coronavirus in the electron microscopic studies of Vero E6 cells inoculated with oropharyngeal material from a patient was the initial finding that resulted in the identification of SARS-CoV.[128] The viral genome is 29,727 nucleotides in length, with more than 11 open reading frames coding for 23 putative proteins, some of which have unknown functions. SARS-CoV is phylogenetically different and equidistant from all previously known coronaviruses, but isolates from different origins are relatively homogeneous genetically. Genome analysis reveals that SARS-CoV is neither a host-range mutant nor a recombinant of

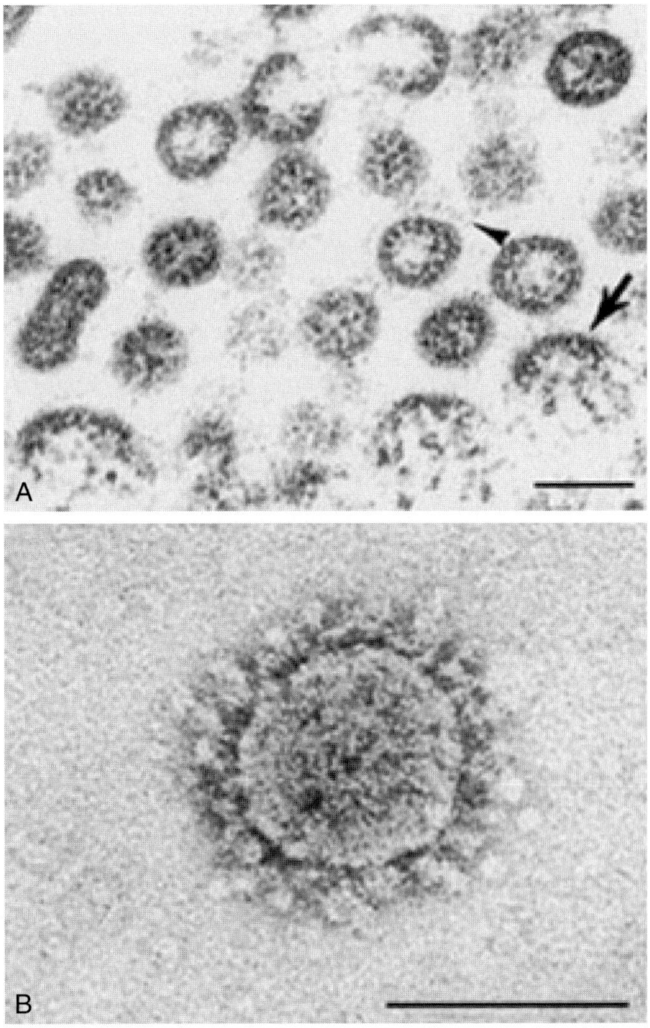

FIGURE 59-1 Ultrastructural features of SARS-CoV in Vero E6 cells. *A*, Thin-section electron microscopic view of SARS-CoV nucleocapsids aligned along the membrane of the rough endoplasmic reticulum (*arrow*) during budding of particles into the cisternae and coronavirus surface projections (*arrowhead*). *B*, Electron microscopic picture of a negatively stained extracellular particle of SARS-CoV, with the typical club-shaped surface projections. Bars represent 100 nm. (From Ksiazek TG, Erdman D, Goldsmith CS, et al: A novel coronavirus associated with severe acute respiratory syndrome. N Engl J Med 348:1953–1966, 2003.)

previously known coronaviruses but rather an independently emerged virus. SARS-CoV seems to have evolved from an animal SARS-like virus, acquiring greater fitness in humans during the course of the outbreaks, probably through the appearance of nucleotide deletions in open reading frame 8.[129] It is also noteworthy that genetic signatures present in the genomes allow for differentiation of isolates obtained from different clusters.[129] The replicative cycle of SARS-CoV is thought to follow the same main steps as other coronaviruses.

EPIDEMIOLOGY

SARS coronavirus (SARS-CoV) probably emerged around November 2002 in the province of Guangdong, China, where there was no serologic evidence of infection caused by this virus in sera of healthy humans sampled prior to that time.[130] At the beginning of the outbreak, many affected individuals in Guangdong were directly or indirectly involved with game trade, and indeed, palm civets and raccoon dogs from wild-game markets in the area were later found to harbor a CoV 99% homologous to SARS-CoV at the nucleotide level. This suggests that animal-to-human interspecies transmission was involved in the outbreak, providing the source of an agent that later adapted to efficient human-to-human transmission.[131,132] Interestingly, shortly after the lifting of a wildlife trade ban that originally had been imposed to control the SARS outbreak, new cases were again detected in Guangdong, all of them caused by viruses newly introduced from animals. Since the ban was reinstalled, there have been no further naturally acquired human cases of SARS in Guangdong.[131]

Remarkably, 1.8% of 938 serum samples from adults recruited in 2001 in Hong Kong tested positive for SARS-CoV antibodies, suggesting that a small proportion of healthy people from Hong Kong, as opposed to Guangdong, China, had been exposed to SARS-related viruses at least 2 years before the outbreak.[133] It is probable that SARS-CoV precursors previously crossed the species barrier and may even have caused subclinical human infection, but perhaps only occasionally this event generated strains adapted to successful human-to-human transmission.[131]

SARS-CoV is mainly transmitted between humans by the deposition of infected droplets or aerosols on the respiratory epithelium. The number of confirmed secondary cases generated by one index case of SARS is relatively low, ranging from 2.2 to 3.7, suggesting relatively inefficient transmission. In addition, transmission is infrequent during the first 5 days of illness, partly because of the low viral load in respiratory secretions during that phase. For reasons not completely understood, some SARS patients, identified as superspreaders, disproportionately contribute to the generation of a high number of secondary cases.[131] Excretion of SARS-CoV in sputa and stools may average 21 and 27 days, respectively, after symptom onset, but an excretion period as prolonged as 126 days has been documented in stools.[134] Such prolonged shedding of virus in feces raises the possibility of oral-fecal transmission and, in fact, one outbreak of SARS was attributed to a faulty sewage system.[131]

Case-fatality rates estimated based on cases admitted to hospital have been around 13% for patients younger than age 60 and 43% for those older than age 60 years. However, it is likely that case-fatality rates based on all infections occurring in the community would be lower.[135]

Transmission of SARS-CoV among health-care workers and between patients in the hospital setting played a pivotal role in outbreak propagation. Analysis of data from initial outbreaks indicates that close contact is the most important factor leading to nosocomial transmission of this agent. Despite the lack of complete studies on the sensitivity of SARS-CoV to different environmental conditions, there have been reports of SARS-CoV persisting for up to 2 days on environmental surfaces and 4 days in diarrheal stools.[136]

CLINICAL FEATURES

The median incubation period of SARS is 4 to 6 days. Clinical symptoms and signs of SARS appear 2 to 10 days after exposure, and systemic symptoms, such as fever, chills, myalgia, and malaise, usually appear first. Respiratory symptoms appear 2 to 7 days later, represented most frequently by nonproductive cough, dyspnea, chest pain, headache, and sore throat. Diarrhea and vomiting may occur. Chest radiograms frequently reveal infiltrates consistent with viral pneumonitis, consisting mostly of consolidations and ground-glass opacifications. Computed tomography (CT) scans in patients with normal or equivocal chest radiograms may show unilobar or multilobar abnormalities. Fever generally subsides in 48 hours, but one or two relapses within 8 to 15 days are frequently observed. Lymphopenia with reduction of both CD4+ and CD8+ cells, slight decrease in platelet counts, prolonged coagulation profile, and elevated serum enzymes (lactic dehydrogenase [LDH], creatinine kinase [CK], and C-reactive protein [CRP]) are often observed. Around one third of patients may have CD4+ lymphocyte counts below 200 cells/mm^3 and higher susceptibility to secondary infections. Watery diarrhea with an average of six evacuations per day is common.[130,131,137]

Radiologic worsening of the pulmonary lesions seen at admission, with or without appearance of new lesions, is a frequent observation, with development of diffuse ground-glass changes frequently heralding the development of acute respiratory distress syndrome (ARDS). Hypoxemia is noted in approximately half of the patients at around 9 days after the onset of symptoms, and a high proportion of those admitted to the intensive care unit (ICU), especially older males, require mechanical ventilation around day 13. Development of spontaneous pneumomediastinum during follow-up is not uncommon, probably as a consequence of ruptured peripheral lung lesions into the pleural space.[130]

Prognosis is related to the level of viral replication in tissues, and patients with high viral loads in serum, nasopharyngeal aspirates, or feces, as well as those in whom virus can be detected from multiple sites, tend to have poor clinical outcome.[131] In addition to old age and severe underlying diseases, CK and CRP levels have been identified as predictors of poor outcome.[138]

PATHOGENESIS AND IMMUNITY

The N-terminal portion of the spike glycoprotein is needed for virus attachment to the virus receptor, identified as the metallopeptidase angiotensin-converting enzyme homolog (ACE-2),[139] but it is unclear whether the mechanism of entry is contingent on pH-dependent endocytosis.[131] Some inconsistencies between ACE-2 and SARS-CoV tissue distribution suggest that ACE-2 may not be the only receptor, or that a coreceptor molecule may be needed for cell infection.

SARS-CoV spike protein can also bind the dendritic cell-specific C-type lectin intercellular adhesion molecule 3–grabbing nonintegrin (DC-SIGN), which does not result in dendritic cell infection by the agent but allows for SARS-CoV to be transported to susceptible target cells elsewhere.[140]

SARS-CoV has been detected in studies using different combinations of immunohistochemistry, in situ hybridization, and electron microscopy in pneumocytes and on the apical surface of enterocytes. Marked inflammatory infiltrates and mucosal atrophy have not been observed in the intestine, and the pathogenesis of the SARS-CoV–related diarrhea remains largely unknown.[131]

SARS-CoV viral load in the upper airways is low in the 4 initial days, with the peak at day 10 of illness. Quantitative RT-PCR for SARS-CoV in nasopharyngeal aspirates from patients who tested positive at admission revealed viral loads around 10^5 copies/mL on days 5 and 15 after clinical onset, and peak 10^7 copies/mL on day 10.[130] Higher viral loads can be detected in the lower respiratory tract than in the upper airways. Pulmonary tissue shows diffuse alveolar damage, mixed infiltrate, lung edema, hyaline membrane, abundant macrophages in alveoli and interstitium, and syncytia formation.

Besides respiratory secretions and stools, SARS-CoV can be detected in urine in up to 30% of patients, with titers averaging $10^{4.4}$ copies/mL, in association with abnormal urinalysis results.[141]

The effect of SARS-CoV infection on the immune system is highlighted by pronounced T-cell lymphopenia and elevation of several inflammatory cytokines (IL-1β, IL-6, and IL-12) and chemokines (MCP-1 and IP-10) observed in SARS patients. While MCP-1 is likely to be involved in the lung monocytic/macrophagic infiltrate, its role is not firmly established, since other viral diseases that are associated with elevated MCP-1, such as influenza, do not include such prominent histologic features. In addition, since immunologic markers in the peripheral blood may not reflect what happens in the microenvironment of the lung, the pathogenic importance of these findings is not clear. Co-inheritance of HLA-B*0703 and -B60 is higher among SARS patients than in the general population, favoring a role for the genetic background in susceptibility to SARS-CoV.[131] The pathogenesis of the T-cell lymphopenia remains unknown.

Seroconversion has been documented in 93% of the patients at around 20 days and the rise in IgG titers correlates with decrease in viral load.[130] Paradoxically, clinical worsening also occurs during this phase, suggesting that, rather than unchecked viral replication, immunopathologic factors may be responsible for the lung lesions.[130]

While infection in experimental animals, such as cynomolgus macaques, ferrets, cats, golden Syrian hamsters, mice, and African green monkeys, does not induce disease that mimics that in humans, these models are important for studies of pathogenesis and development of vaccines and therapy.[129] In addition, the development of an infectious cDNA clone of SARS-CoV should permit reverse genetics experiments and may help elucidate determinants of viral pathogenesis.[142]

DIAGNOSIS

Low viral loads in the upper respiratory tract in the first few days of illness account for the relatively poor sensitivity (35% to 65%) of first-generation RT-PCR for diagnosis in that period. SARS-CoV is detectable by RT-PCR in nasopharyngeal aspirates in only one third of patients at presentation and in two thirds at day 14. RT-PCR may be positive for SARS-CoV in stools from as much as 97% of patients at day 14, and in urine in 42% of samples at day 15.[130] Testing multiple nasopharyngeal, serum, and fecal samples increases the sensitivity of the diagnosis by RT-PCR.[143,144]

To overcome the low sensitivity of conventional RT-PCR, quantitative real-time PCR-based assays for SARS-CoV have been developed that improve sensitivity and turnaround time, allow for amplification and analysis to be done in a closed system, and thus reduce cross-contamination. In addition, the capability of the assay to quantitate viral load has contributed not only to understanding viral pathogenesis but also to predicting outcome, since high viral loads are associated with poor prognosis.[143]

The ability to grow SARS-CoV in Vero E6 cell cultures was critical to identifying the agent. SARS-CoV can be recovered by isolation from respiratory secretions, feces, and urine in the first 3 weeks of illness, but the overall sensitivity is relatively low and recovery is more likely to be successful from respiratory secretions than from stools and urine.[143] Recent small outbreaks of SARS-CoV originating in laboratories[143] have heightened concern about laboratory safety issues regarding SARS specimens. The WHO guidelines for biosafety in the diagnosis of SARS (updates available at the WHO web site) recommend that propagation of SARS-CoV in cell culture for isolation or for preparation of viral stocks and cell slides be performed in biosafety level 3 (BSL3) laboratories, whereas handling serum and blood specimens for routine tests and serology can be performed in BSL2 laboratories. Nucleic acid extraction procedures, inoculation of bacterial or mycologic cultures, and preparation of sample smears can be done in BSL2 laboratories, observing BSL3 work practices (use of safety cabinets, sealed centrifuges, protective equipment, 5% bleach spillage decontamination, and proper waste disposal).

Although not useful for early diagnosis, seroconversion determined by IFA or EIA remains the gold standard for confirming SARS diagnosis. IgG seroconversion is detectable in over 90% of patients at around day 28.[130] Antibody cross-reaction with other human coronaviruses, however rare, remains a possibility; therefore, confirmation of positive serology by an independent neutralization assay should be performed if available.[143]

TREATMENT

The main component of treatment of SARS patients is supportive therapy, chiefly the management of hypoxemia and ARDS. During the 2003 outbreak, treatment included a broad-spectrum antiviral agent (ribavirin) and immunosuppressive doses of corticosteroids, aimed at reducing the immunopathologic damage to the lungs. The use of high-dose steroid therapy is controversial and for the most part supported by anecdotal evidence, whereas the use of ribavirin is based on the broad antiviral spectrum of the drug. However, SARS-CoV is only modestly susceptible to ribavirin in vitro, and therapeutic doses are difficult to achieve clinically. Since it became possible to grow SARS-CoV in culture, many potential antiviral compounds have been evaluated in vitro, but just a few have been tested in animal models and even fewer are in clinical testing.[131]

Interferons (IFN-αn1/n3, leukocytic IFN-α, IFN-β) and HIV protease inhibitors were consistently active in vitro and may be considered for animal testing and clinical trials.[131]

The resolution of the structure of SARS-CoV principal protease has prompted studies of the inhibitory capacity of known anti-HIV protease inhibitors for treatment of SARS. In one open-label study, a combination of HIV protease inhibitor (lopinavir plus pharmacokinetic booster ritonavir) and ribavirin was used to treat SARS patients and the outcomes were compared with historical controls treated with ribavirin alone. At day 21 after onset of symptoms, development of ARDS or death was significantly less frequent in the group treated with the combination (2.3%) than in historical controls (28.8%). In addition, peak viral loads in respiratory samples and stools were reduced in the group treated with the combination as compared with controls.[145] However, since there were differences in outcome predictors, such as sex, platelet counts, and LDH levels, between the two groups, these results should be interpreted with caution.

A preliminary open-label study found that a restricted number of patients treated with subcutaneous interferon alfacon-1 in association with corticosteroids showed reduced oxygen-saturation impairment and faster resolution of radiographic chest findings than those treated with corticosteroids alone.[146]

Convalescent plasma has also been tested in the treatment of SARS patients. In one preliminary uncontrolled study, convalescent plasma may have reduced the frequency of poor outcome when given before 14 days of illness.[147]

PREVENTION

It is impossible to predict whether naturally reemerging SARS-CoV would be likely to cause a global outbreak. Nevertheless, a vaccine for this agent would be relevant for high-risk individuals, such as workers in laboratories, hospitals, and game-animal farming. Therefore, considerable effort has been directed at developing such a vaccine. It has been shown that SARS-CoV spike protein produced in bacteria and expressed on chimeric parainfluenza virus, as well as spike protein–encoding DNA, induced neutralizing antibodies and protected experimental animals from challenge with live virus. At present, no SARS-CoV vaccine is available for human use. Therefore, in the absence of person-to-person transmission of SARS-CoV worldwide, prevention of future outbreaks of SARS requires careful surveillance. The goal is to maximize early detection of new cases of SARS to implement control measures, thereby minimizing social disruption.[131]

To reach this goal, the CDC recommends testing for SARS-CoV in patients who require hospitalization for radiographically confirmed pneumonia or ARDS without identifiable etiology and who have one of the following risk factors in the 10 days before the onset of illness: (1) travel to mainland China, Hong Kong, or Taiwan, or close contact with an ill person with a history of recent travel to one of these areas, or (2) employment in an occupation associated with a risk for SARS-CoV exposure (e.g., health-care worker with direct patient contact; worker in a laboratory that contains live SARS-CoV), or (3) belonging to a cluster of cases of atypical pneumonia without an alternative diagnosis (updates on these recommendations are made available at the CDC web site http://www.cdc.gov/ncidod/sars).

During times of overt SARS activity, prevention of human-to-human transmission is pivotal to curtailing outbreaks. Although SARS infectiousness relative to the onset and termination of clinical symptoms has not been accurately determined, it is clear that shortening the time from onset to hospital admission and isolation reduces the risk of transmission, thus contributing substantially to curtailing of outbreaks. Identification of new cases through contact tracing played an important role in the control of the outbreaks registered so far. Stringent isolation procedures must be adopted for confirmed and suspected cases, which require a high level of alertness among health-care workers for early identification of SARS cases. The scenario may be further complicated in situations in which other diseases such as influenza and Hantavirus pulmonary infections may occur simultaneously.[135]

Rates of transmission of SARS-CoV among health-care workers vary, depending on stringency of control measures adopted, presence of so-called superspreaders in the hospital, and kind of activities carried out by personnel, especially as related to proximity to the index case. Assisting during intubation, suctioning, and manipulating ventilatory apparatuses seem to be high-risk activities. While studies conducted in different settings have produced conflicting results, one study in Toronto found that up to 25% of the nurses who cared for SARS patients in critical care units became infected.[148] The presence of severe watery diarrhea may add to the challenge for the infection control team.[130] An updated set of recommendations for health-care and laboratory personnel is available at the CDC web site (http://www.cdc.gov/ncidod/sars).

Metapneumoviruses

A new paramyxovirus was described in The Netherlands in 2001, in association with respiratory illness in children. The agent was first detected by analysis of previously unidentifiable viral isolates that induced cytopathic effect in LLC-MK2 cell cultures. The isolates were recovered over a 10-year period in respiratory secretions from 28 children with ARI occurring in the winter time. Electron microscopy of cell culture isolates revealed paramyxovirus-like particles, and RNA sequencing revealed genome sequences and organization consistent with a paramyxovirus of the subfamily *Pneumovirinae*, most closely related to avian pneumovirus of the genus *Metapneumovirus*. Rather than an avian virus that can also infect humans, this agent is now recognized as a primarily human pathogen, and thus has been named human metapneumovirus (HMPV).[156,157] HMPV antibodies detected in sera collected in 1958 in The Netherlands indicate that this agent has been in circulation for at least 4 to 5 decades.[156]

AGENT

HMPV particles are enveloped, pleomorphic, spherical, and filamentous particles, with a mean diameter of about 209 nm.[156,157] Complete genome sequences of HMPV are available and, in contrast to the genomic organization of pneumoviruses, metapneumoviruses have different positioning of the genes between M and L and lack NS1 and NS2 genes.[156,158] Similar to HRSV, genetic and antigenic studies indicate that HMPV isolates cluster into two main serotype named A and B, with N gene sequences 83% to 85% similar at the nucleotide level, each subgroup including two genetic lineages (A1, A2, B1, and B2).[156,159,160] Both are globally distributed. There have been no detailed studies of the HMPV replication cycle, but it is likely to be similar to that of other human paramyxoviruses.

EPIDEMIOLOGY

HMPV is a frequent cause of community-acquired ARI in children and adults in all continents, although with variable incidence in different settings.[157,159,161–169] In the United States, HMPV has been reported in up to 20% of lower respiratory tract illnesses whose etiology would have been unidentifiable prior to the development of assays for the detection of HMPV.[170] In Canada, during the 2001–2002 winter season, HMPV was detected in 15% of patients of all age groups from four different provinces.[167]

Similar to HRSV, HMPV infections are more frequent in the colder months in temperate regions, and different strains of both subgroups A and B cocirculate during the same year.[157,162] However, only limited knowledge is available about HMPV seasonality in more tropical climates. Peaks of HMPV activity have been documented in the spring/summer in Hong Kong,[171] while in South Africa HMPV has been detected in 6% to 9% of children with ARI admitted to hospitals in the winter season.[161,165] HMPV was detected alone or simultaneously with RSV in 24% of children younger than 3 years of age admitted to health-care facilities in Aracaju, northeast Brazil, in the months of April and May, 2002.[164] Interestingly, HMPV was not detected by the same methods in that same city, in the following year.[166] This apparent variability in HMPV incidence from year to year has also been observed in studies conducted in Argentina[168] and Italy, where HMPV frequencies varied from 7% to 43% in three consecutive annual respiratory virus seasons.[172] Long-term prospective studies will be needed to establish whether there is a seasonal pattern in HMPV circulation in tropical regions of the world.

CLINICAL FEATURES

Clinically, HMPV infections resemble closely those caused by HRSV, ranging from mild upper ARI to severe bronchiolitis and pneumonia. The median age of children hospitalized with HMPV infection is older than those with HRSV. HRSV in hospitalized infants and young children may require intensive care and mechanical ventilation,[156,173,174] and dual infection with HMPV and HRSV appears to increase the likelihood of severe illness.[175,176] The most frequent symptoms in all age groups are fever, dyspnea, cough, wheezing/stridor, rhinitis, and sore throat.[162,173] All infected children in one study had either pneumonia or bronchiolitis, frequently accompanied by otitis media.[162] HMPV may cause more serious infections in patients with comorbid or immunosuppressive conditions, as well as in the very young and the elderly.[162,167] In one study, all individuals older than 65 with lower respiratory infection caused by HMPV had at least one underlying chronic or debilitating condition, including lymphoma, leukemia, or neurologic or cardiovascular diseases.[162]

HMPV infection in adults may present as influenza-like illness, acute bronchitis, or common cold.[162] In England, in the winter of 2000–2001, HMPV was detected by RT-PCR in association with 2.2% of samples taken from patients in all age groups with influenza-like illnesses negative for HRSV and influenza viruses.[159]

HMPV has been increasingly recognized as cause of acute wheezing in children. One study conducted in Finland found HMPV in 8% of wheezing children, who presented significantly higher levels of IL-8 in nasal secretions as compared to children with HRSV-associated wheezing.[174] A study conducted in Brazil found that 47% of the children with HMPV had wheezing and 31% had chest indrawing.[164] Previous history of asthma has been more frequently associated with HMPV than with HRSV infection and HMPV-infected patients are more often treated with bronchodilators and corticosteroids than HRVS-infected patients.[173]

PATHOGENESIS AND IMMUNOLOGY

Little is known about specific mechanisms of pathogenesis and host immune response in HMPV infections. HMPV is a pathogen of both the upper and lower respiratory tracts.[162] HMPV replicates efficiently in the respiratory tract of monkeys, with virus shedding peaking between days 2 and 8 following infection.[156] Serologic data indicates that HMPV infects young individuals, and by the age of 5 virtually all children have become seropositive for the agent; reinfections at later ages are common.[156,157,159]

Interestingly, coinfection with HMPV has been reported to correlate with increased severity of HRSV infections. A study conducted in the United Kingdom found that this coinfection caused a tenfold increase in the relative risk of admission to the ICU for mechanical ventilation in children under 2 with HRSV bronchiolitis.[173] A similar finding was also reported in Germany.[176]

DIAGNOSIS

HMPV can be isolated in LLC-MK2 cells from nasal aspirates or nasopharyngeal swabs. The cytopathic effect, characteristically negative on hemadsorption testing, develops usually late after inoculation (up to 23 days).[160] Sensitive RT-PCR assays for this agent have been developed in many different laboratories and have rapidly become standard for HMPV diagnosis.[159,169] A real-time PCR assay for HMPV showed to be more sensitive than conventional RT-PCR, even when hybridization was used to increase sensitivity of the detection of amplicons generated by the conventional method.[169] Using real-time PCR, HMPV was detected in 10% of 329 samples collected from patients with ARI in Australia from March to October 2001 that were negative for other pathogens.[169]

TREATMENT, PREVENTION, AND CONTROL

Other than supportive measures, oxygen therapy, bronchodilators, corticosteroids and mechanical ventilation, there is no specific antiviral treatment for this agent.[173] Ribavirin is inhibitory for HMPV in vitro.[176] Although a HMPV vaccine is not available at this time, the demonstration that hamsters, ferrets, and African green monkeys are susceptible to infection by HMPV, and that hamsters vaccinated with serotype A were protected from challenge with either A or B HMPV serotypes opens possibilities for HMPV vaccine design.[176] Humanized neutralizing monoclonal antibody to F protein is active in experimentally infected animals.[177]

REFERENCES

1. Selwyn BJ: The epidemiology of acute respiratory tract infection in young children: Comparison of findings from several developing countries. Rev Infect Dis 12:S870, 1990.
2. McIntosh K, Halonen P, Ruuskanen O: Report of a workshop on respiratory viral infections: Epidemiology, diagnosis, treatment and prevention. Clin Infect Dis 16:151, 1993.
3. Arruda E, Hayden FG, McAuliffe JF, et al: Acute respiratory viral infections in ambulatory children of urban northeast Brazil. J Infect Dis 164:252, 1991.
4. de Romaña GL, Brown KH, Black RE, et al: Longitudinal studies of infectious diseases and physical growth of infants in Huascar, an underprivileged peri-urban community in Lima, Peru. Am J Epidemiol 129:769, 1989.
5. Arruda E, Geist FC, McAuliffe MI, et al: Viral respiratory tract illnesses in a developing tropical area. In Guerrant RL, Souza MAS, Nations MK (eds): At the edge of Development: Health Crises in a Transitional Society. Durham, NC, Carolina Academic Press 1996, p 203.
6. Berman S: Epidemiology of acute respiratory infections in children of developing countries. Rev Infect Dis 13:S454, 1991.
7. Pan American Health Organization: Acute respiratory infections in the Americas. Epidemiol Bull 16:1, 1995.
8. Garenne M, Ronsmans C, Campbell H: The magnitude of mortality from acute respiratory infections in children under 5 years in developing countries. Rapp Trimest Statist Sanit Mond 45:180, 1992.
9. Rahman M, Huq F, Sack DA, et al: Acute lower respiratory tract infections in hospitalized patients with diarrhea in Dhaka, Bangladesh. Rev Infect Dis 12:S899, 1990.
10. Anderson LJ, Parker RA, Strikas RA et al: Day-care center attendance and hospitalization for lower respiratory tract illness. Pediatrics 82:300, 1988.
11. Souza LS, Ramos EA, Carvalho FM et al: Viral respiratory infections in young children attending day care in urban Northeast Brazil. Pediatr Pulmonol 35:184, 2003.
12. Shek LP, Lee B: Epidemiology and seasonality of respiratory tract virus infections in the tropics. Pediatric Respiratory Reviews 4:105, 2003
13. Lares B, Rebhun LA, Souza MA, et al: The cultural context of breast-feeding: Perspectives on the recent decline in breast-feeding in Northeast and Northcentral Brazil. In Guerrant RL, Souza MAS, Nations MK (eds): At the Edge of Development: Health Crises in a Transitional Society. Durham, NC, Carolina Academic Press, 1996, p 335.
14. Rahmathullah L, Underwood BA, Thulasiraj RT, et al: Reduced mortality among children in Southern India receiving a small weekly dose of vitamin A. N Engl J Med 323:929, 1990.
15. Nations MK, Amaral ML: Search for a solution: Blending oral rehydration therapy (ORT) and popular medicine. In Guerrant RL, Souza MAS, Nations MK (eds): At the Edge of Development: Health Crises in a Transitional Society. Durham, NC, Carolina Academic Press, 1996, p 401.
16. Leigh MW, Carson JL, Denny FW Jr: Pathogenesis of respiratory infections due to influenza virus: Implications for developing countries. Rev Infect Dis 13:S501, 1991.
17. Peltola VT, McCullers JA: Respiratory viruses predisposing to bacterial infections: Role of neuraminidase.Pediatr Infect Dis J 23:S87, 2004.
18. Lipatov AS, Govorkova EA, Webby RJ, et al: Influenza: Emergence and control. J Virol 78:8951, 2004
19. Lamb RA, Krug RM: Orthomyxoviridae: The viruses and their replication. In Knipe DM, Howley PM, Griffin DE, et al (eds): Fields' Virology, 4th ed. Philadelphia, Lippincott Williams & Wilkins, 2001, p 1487.
20. Hayden FG, Palese P: Influenza virus. In Richman DD, Whitley RJ, Hayden FG (eds): Clinical Virology. Washington, ASM Press, 2002, p 891.
21. Steinhoff MC: Viral vaccines for the prevention of childhood pneumonia in developing nations: Priorities and prospects. Rev Infect Dis 13:S562, 1991.
22. Neuzil KM, Mellen BG, Wright PF, et al: The effect of influenza on hospitalizations, outpatient visits, and courses of antibiotics in children. N Engl J Med 342:225, 2000.
23. John J, Cherian T, Steinhoff MC, et al: Etiology of acute respiratory infections in children in tropical southern India. Rev Infect Dis 13:S463, 1991.
24. Vathanophas K, Sangchai R, Raktham S, et al: A community-based study of acute respiratory tract infection in Thai children. Rev Infect Dis 12:S957, 1990.
25. Tupasi TE, Lucero MG, Magdangal DM, et al: Etiology of acute lower respiratory tract infection in children from Alabang, Metro Manilla. Rev Infect Dis 12:S929, 1990.
26. de Paiva TM, Ishida MA, Hanashiro KA, et al: Outbreak of influenza type A (H1N1) in Iporanga, São Paulo State, Brazil. Rev Inst Med Trop Sao Paulo 43:311, 2001.
27. Pontoriero AV, Baumeister EG, Campos AM, et al: Antigenic and genomic relation between human influenza viruses that circulated in Argentina in the period 1995–1999 and the corresponding vaccine components. J Clin Virol 28:130, 2003.
28. Schoub BD, McAnerney JM, Besselaar TG: Regional perspectives on influenza surveillance in Africa. Vaccine 20(suppl 2):S45, 2002.
29. http://www.cdc.gov/flu/avian/outbreaks. Accessed January 2005.
30. Guan Y, Poon LL, Cheung CY, et al: H5N1 influenza: A protean pandemic threat. Proc Natl Acad Sci USA 101:8156, 2004.
31. Serwint JR, Miller RM, Korsch BM: Influenza type A and B infections in hospitalized pediatric patients. Am J Dis Child 145:623, 1991.
32. Rott R, Klenk HD, Nagay Y, et al: Influenza viruses, cell enzymes, and pathogenicity. Am J Resp Crit Care Med 152:S16, 1995.
33. Mills RD, Cain KJ, Woods GL: Detection of influenza virus by centrifugal inoculation of MDCK cells and staining with monoclonal antibodies. J Clin Microbiol 27:2505, 1989.
34. Stone B, Burrows J, Schepetiuk S, et al: Rapid detection and simultaneous subtype differentiation of influenza A viruses by real time PCR. J Virol Methods 117:103, 2004.
35. Templeton KE, Scheltinga SA, Beersma MF, et al: Rapid and sensitive method using multiplex real-time PCR for diagnosis of infections by influenza A and influenza B viruses, respiratory syncytial virus, and parainfluenza viruses 1, 2, 3, and 4. J Clin Microbiol 42:1564, 2004.
36. Von Itzstein M, Wu WY, Kok GB, et al: Rational design of potent sialidase-based inhibitors of influenza virus replication. Nature 363:418, 1993.
37. Hayden FG, Osterhaus AD, Treanor JJ, et al: Efficacy and safety of the neuraminidase inhibitor zanamivir in the treatment of influenzavirus infections. N Engl J Med 337:874, 1997.
38. Kiso M, Mitamura K, Sakai-Tagawa Y, et al: Resistant influenza A viruses in children treated with oseltamivir: Descriptive study. Lancet 364:759, 2004.
39. Centers for Disease Control and Prevention: Prevention and Control of Influenza: Recommendations of the Advisory Committee on Immunization Practices (ACIP). MMWR 53:1, 2004.
40. van Essen GA, Palache AM, Forleo E, et al: Influenza vaccination in 2000: Recommendations and vaccine use in 50 developed and rapidly developing countries. Vaccine 21:1780, 2003.
41. Stamboulian D, Bonvehí PE, Nacinovich FM, et al: Immunization against influenza in the elderly: The Argentinian experience, 1993–1997. Vaccine 17(suppl 1):S53, 1999.
42. Savy V: Regional perspectives on influenza surveillance in South America. Vaccine 20:S47, 2002.
43. Hayden FG, Couch RB: Clinical and epidemiologic importance of influenza A viruses resistant to amantadine and rimantadine. Rev Med Virol 2:89, 1992.
44. Hayden FG: Pandemic influenza: Is an antiviral response realistic? Pediatr Infect Dis J 23:S262, 2004.
45. Piedra PA, Englund JA, Glezen WP: Respiratory syncytial virus and parainfluenza viruses. In Richman DD, Whitley RJ, Hayden FG (eds): Clinical Virology. Washington, ASM Press, 2002, p 763.
46. Collins PL, Chanock RM, Murphy BR: Respiratory syncytial virus. In Knipe DM, Howley PM, Griffin DE, et al (eds): Fields' Virology, 4th ed. Philadelphia, Lippincott Williams & Wilkins, 2001, p 1443.
47. Centers for Disease Control and Prevention: Brief report: Respiratory syncytial virus activity–United States, 2003–2004. MMWR 53:1159, 2004.
48. Chew FT, Doraisingham S, Ling AE, et al: Seasonal trends of viral respiratory tract infections in the tropics. Epidemiol Infect 121:121, 1998.
49. Cintra OA, Owa MA, Machado AA, et al: Occurrence and severity of infections caused by subgroup A and B respiratory syncytial virus in children in southeast Brazil. J Med Virol 65:408, 2001.

50. Straliotto SM, Siqueira MM, Muller RL, et al: Viral etiology of acute respiratory infections among children in Porto Alegre, RS, Brazil. Rev Soc Bras Med Trop 35:283, 2002.
51. Carballal G, Videla C, Sequeira MD, et al: Respiratory syncytial virus: Changes in prevalence of subgroups A and B among Argentinian children. J Med Virol 61:275, 2000.
52. Vieira SE, Stewien KE, Queiroz DAO, et al: Clinical patterns and seasonal trends in respiratory syncytial virus hospitalizations in Sao Paulo, Brazil. Rev Inst Med Trop (Sao Paulo) 43:125, 2001.
53. Siqueira MM, Nascimento JP, Anderson LJ: Antigenic characterization of respiratory syncytial virus group A and B isolates in Rio de Janeiro, Brazil. J Clin Microbiol 29:557, 1991.
54. Rakshi K, Couriel JM: Management of acute bronchiolitis. Arch Dis Child 471:463, 1994.
55. Okamoto Y, Kudo K, Shirotori K, et al: Detection of genomic sequences of respiratory syncytial virus in otitis media with effusion in children. Ann Otol Rhinol Laryngol 101:7, 1992.
56. Andrade MA, Hoberman A, Glustein J, et al: Acute otitis media in children with bronchiolitis. Pediatrics 101:617, 1998.
57. Titus MO, Wright SW: Prevalence of serious bacterial infections in febrile infants with respiratory syncytial virus infection. Pediatrics 112:282, 2003.
58. Tupasi TE, Lucero MG, Magdangal DM, et al: Etiology of acute lower respiratory tract infection in children from Alabang, Metro Manilla. Rev Infect Dis 12:S929, 1990.
59. Rakes GP, Arruda E, Ingram JM, et al: Rhinovirus and respiratory syncytial virus in wheezing children requiring emergency care. IgE and eosinophil analyses. Am J Respir Crit Care Med 159:785, 1999.
60. Camara AA, Silva JM, Ferriani VP, et al: Risk factors for wheezing in a subtropical environment: Role of respiratory viruses and allergen sensitization. J Allergy Clin Immunol 113:551, 2004.
61. Gbadero DA, Johnson ABR, Aderele WI, et al: Microbial inciters of acute asthma in urban Nigerian children. Thorax 50:739, 1995.
62. Griffin MR, Coffey CS, Neuzil KM, et al: Winter viruses: Influenza- and respiratory syncytial virus-related morbidity in chronic lung disease. Arch Intern Med 162:1229, 2002.
63. Psarras S, Papadopoulos NG, Johnston SL: Pathogenesis of respiratory syncytial virus bronchiolitis-related wheezing. Pediatr Respir Rev 5(suppl A):S179, 2004.
64. Graham BS: Pathogenesis of respiratory syncytial virus vaccine–augmented pathology. Am J Respir Crit Care Med 152:S63, 1995.
65. Kuypers J, Wright N, Morrow R: Evaluation of quantitative and type-specific real-time RT-PCR assays for detection of respiratory syncytial virus in respiratory specimens from children. J Clin Virol 31:123, 2004.
66. American Academy of Pediatrics Committee on Infectious Diseases: Reassessment of the indications for ribavirin therapy in respiratory virus infections. Pediatrics 97:137, 1996.
67. Whimbey E, Champlin RE, Englund JA, et al: Combination therapy with aerosolized ribavirin and intravenous immunoglobulin for respiratory syncytial virus disease in adult bone marrow transplant recipients. Bone Marrow Transplant 16:393, 1995.
68. Groothuis JR: Role of antibody and use of respiratory syncytial virus (RSV) immune globulin to prevent severe RSV disease in high-risk children. J Pediatr 124:S28, 1994.
69. Henrikson KJ: Parainfluenza viruses. Clin Microbiol Rev 16:242, 2003.
70. Knott AM, Long CE, Hall CB: Parainfluenza viral infections in pediatric outpatients: Seasonal patterns and clinical characteristics. Pediatr Infect Dis J 13:269, 1994.
71. Vainionpaa R, Hyypia T: Biology of parainfluenza viruses. Clin Microbiol Rev 7:265, 1994.
72. Leung AKC, Kellner JD, Johnson DW: Viral croup: A current perspective. J Pediatr Health Care 18:297, 2004.
73. Apalsch AM, Green M, Ledesma-Medina J, et al: Parainfluenza and influenza virus infections in pediatric organ transplant recipients. Clin Infect Dis 20:394, 1995.
74. Coiras MT, Aguilar JC, Garcia ML, et al: Simultaneous detection of fourteen respiratory viruses in clinical specimens by two multiplex reverse transcription nested-PCR assays. J Med Virol 72:484, 2004.
75. Alymova IV, Taylor G, Takimoto T, et al: Efficacy of novel hemagglutinin-neuraminidase inhibitors BCX 2798 and BCX 2855 against human parainfluenza viruses in vitro and in vivo. Antimicrob Agents Chemother 48:1495, 2004.
76. Belshe RB, Newman FK, Anderson EL, et al: Evaluation of combined live, attenuated respiratory syncytial virus and parainfluenza 3 virus vaccines in infants and young children. J Infect Dis 190:2096, 2004.
77. Gwaltney JM Jr, Heinz BA: Rhinovirus. In Richman DD, Whitley RJ, Hayden FG (eds): Clinical Virology. Washington, ASM Press, 2002, p 995.
78. Arruda E, Crump CE, Rollins BS, et al: Comparative susceptibilities of human embryonic fibroblasts and HeLa cells for isolation of human rhinoviruses. J Clin Microbiol 34:1277, 1996.
79. Thwing CJ, Arruda E, Vieira Filho JP, et al: Rhinovirus antibodies in an isolated Amazon Indian tribe. Am J Trop Med Hyg 48:771, 1993.
80. Arruda E, Pitkaranta A, Witek TJ Jr, et al: Frequency and natural history of rhinovirus infections in adults during autumn. J Clin Microbiol 35:2864, 1997.
81. Hong CY, Lin RT, Tan ES, et al:Acute respiratory symptoms in adults in general practice. Fam Pract 21:317, 2004.
82. Gwaltney JM, Phillips CD, Miller RD, et al: Computed tomographic study of the common cold. N Engl J Med 330:25, 1994.
83. Pitkaranta A, Arruda E, Malmberg H, et al: Detection of rhinovirus in sinus brushings of patients with acute community-acquired sinusitis by reverse transcription–PCR. J Clin Microbiol 35:1791, 1997.
84. Pitkaranta A, Virolainen A, Jero J, et al: Detection of rhinovirus, respiratory syncytial virus, and coronavirus infections in acute otitis media by reverse transcriptase polymerase chain reaction. Pediatrics 102:291, 1998.
85. Heymann PW, Carper HT, Murphy DD, et al: Viral infections in relation to age, atopy, and season of admission among children hospitalized for wheezing. J Allergy Clin Immunol 114:239, 2004.
86. Arruda E, Boyle TR, Winther B, et al: Localization of human rhinovirus replication in the upper respiratory tract by in situ hybridization. J Infect Dis 171:1329, 1995.
87. Hsia J, Goldstein AL, Simon GL, et al: Peripheral blood mononuclear cells interleukin-2 and interferon-g production, cytotoxicity, and antigen-stimulated blastogenesis during experimental rhinovirus infection. J Infect Dis 162:591, 1990.
88. Proud D, Sanders SP, Wiehler S: Human rhinovirus infection induces airway epithelial cell production of human beta-defensin 2 both in vitro and in vivo. J Immunol 172:4637, 2004.
89. Dagher H, Donninger H, Hutchinson P, et al: Rhinovirus detection: Comparison of real-time and conventional PCR. J Virol Methods 117:113, 2004.
90. Arruda E, Hayden FG: Clinical studies of antiviral agents for picornaviral infections. In Jeffries DJ, De Clercq E (eds): Antiviral Chemotherapy. London, Wiley, 1995, p 321.
91. Hayden FG, Turner RB, Gwaltney JM, et al: Phase II, randomized, double-blind, placebo-controlled studies of ruprintrivir nasal spray 2-percent suspension for prevention and treatment of experimentally induced rhinovirus colds in healthy volunteers. Antimicrob Agents Chemother 47:3907, 2003.
92. Turner RB, Biedermann KA, Morgan JM, et al: Efficacy of organic acids in hand cleansers for prevention of rhinovirus infections. Antimicrob Agents Chemother 48:2595, 2004.
93. Hayden FG, Albrecht JK, Kaiser DL, et al: Prevention of natural colds by contact prophylaxis with intranasal alpha2-interferon. N Engl J Med 314:71, 1986.
94. Horwitz MS: Adenoviruses. In Knipe DM, Howley PM, Griffin DE, et al (eds): Fields' Virology, 4th ed. Philadelphia, Lippincott Williams & Wilkins, 2001, p 2301.
95. Kajon AE, Mistchenko AS, Videla C, et al: Molecular epidemiology of adenovirus acute lower respiratory infections of children in the south cone of South America (1991–1994). J Med Virol 48:151, 1996.
96. Hogg JC: Latent viral infections in airway epithelium. Chest 101:81S, 1992.
97. Hierholzer JC: Adenoviruses. In Schmidt NJ, Emmons RW (eds): Diagnostic Procedures for Viral, Rickettsial and Chlamydial Infections, 6th ed. Washington, DC, American Public Health Association, 1989, p 218.
98. Foy HM: Adenoviruses. In Evans AS (ed): Viral Infections of Humans, 4th ed. New York, Plenum Press, 1997, p 119.
99. Centers for Disease Control and Prevention: Outbreak of pharyngoconjunctival fever at a summer camp—North Carolina, 1991. MMWR 41:342, 1992.
100. Ruuskanen O, Arola M, Putto-Laurila A, et al: Acute otitis media and respiratory virus infection. Pediatr Infect Dis J 8:94, 1989.

101. Ruuskanen O, Nohynek H, Ziegler T, et al: Pneumonias in childhood: Etiology and response to antimicrobial therapy. Eur J Clin Microbiol Infect Dis 11:217, 1992.
102. Khoo SH, Bailey AS, de Jong JC, et al: Adenovirus infections in human immunodeficiency virus–positive patients: Clinical features and molecular epidemiology. J Infect Dis 172:629, 1995.
103. Carballal G, Siminovich M, Murtagh P, et al: Etiologic, clinical and pathologic analysis of 31 fatal cases of acute respiratory tract infections in Argentinian children under 5 years of age. Rev Infect Dis 12:S1074, 1990.
104. Matsuse T, Hayashi S, Kuwano K, et al: Latent adenoviral infection in the pathogenesis of chronic airway obstruction. Am Rev Respir Dis 146:177, 1992.
105. Fujimoto T, Okafuji T, Okafuji T, et al: Evaluation of a bedside immunochromatographic test for detection of adenovirus in respiratory samples, by comparison to virus isolation, PCR and real-time PCR. J Clin Microbiol 42:5489, 2004.
106. Rabalais GP, Stout GG, Ladd KL, et al: Rapid diagnosis of respiratory viral infections by using a shell vial assay and monoclonal antibody pool. J Clin Microbiol 30:505, 1992.
107. McCarthy AJ, Bergin M, DeSilva LM, et al: Intravenous ribavirin therapy for disseminated adenovirus infection. Pediatr Infect Dis J 14:1003, 1995.
108. Lai MMC, Holmes KV: Coronaviridae: The viruses and their replication. In Knipe DM, Howley PM, Griffin DE (eds): Fields' Virology. Lippincott Williams & Wilkins, Philadelphia, 2001, p 1163.
109. Van der Hoek, Pyrc K, Jebbink MF, et al: Identification of a new human coronavirus. Nat Med 4:368, 2004.
110. Fouchier RAM, Hartwig NG, Bestebroer TM, et al: A previously undescribed coronavirus associated with respiratory disease in humans. PNAS 101:6212, 2004.
111. Esper F, Weibel C, Ferguson D, et al: Evidence of a novel human coronavirus that is associated with respiratory tract disease in infants and young children. J Infect Dis 191:492, 2005.
112. McIntosh K: Coronaviruses. In Richman DD, Whitley RJ, Hayden FG (eds): Clinical Virology, 2nd ed. ASM Press, Washington, DC, 2002, p 1087.
113. Monto AS: Coronaviruses. In Evans AS, Kaslow RA (eds): Viral Infection of Humans, 4th ed. Plenum Medical, New York, 1997, p 211.
114. Vabret A, Mourez T, Gouarin S, et al: An outbreak of coronavirus OC43 respiratory infection in Normandy, France. Clin Infect Dis 36:985, 2003.
115. Candeias JA, Carvalho RP, Antonacio F: Seroepidemiologic study of coronavirus infection in Brazilian children and civilian adults. Rev Inst Med Trop (Sao Paulo) 14:121, 1972.
116. Falsey AR, Walsh EE, Hayden FG: Rhinovirus and coronavirus infection-associated hospitalizations among older adults. J Infect Dis 185:1338, 2002.
117. Johnston SL, Pattemore PK, Sanderson G, et al: Community study of role of viral infections in exacerbations of asthma in 9–11 year old children. BMJ 310:1225, 1995.
118. Wang G, Deering C, Macke M, et al: Human coronavirus 229E infects polarized airway epithelia from the apical surface. J Virol 74: 9234, 2000.
119. Chilvers MA, McKean M, Rutman A, et al: The effects of coronavirus on human nasal ciliated respiratory epithelium. Eur Respir J 18:965, 2001.
120. Holmes KV, Coronaviruses. In Knipe DM, Howley PM, Griffin DE (eds): Fields' Virology. Philadelphia, Lippincott Williams & Wilkins, 2001, p 1187.
121. Esper F, Shapiro ED, Weibel C, et al: Association between a novel human coronavirus and Kawasaki disease. J Infect Dis 191:499, 2005.
122. Van Elden LJ, van Loon AM, van Alphen, et al: Frequent detection of human coronaviruses in clinical specimens from patients with respiratory tract infections by use of a novel real-time reverse-transcriptase polymerase chain reaction. J Infect Dis 189:652, 2004.
123. Higgins PG, Phillpotts RJ, Scott GM, et al: Intranasal interferon as protection against experimental respiratory coronavirus infection in volunteers. Antimicrob Agents Chemother 24:713, 1983.
124. Drosten C, Preiser W, Günther S, et al: Severe acute respiratory syndrome: Identification of the etiological agent. Trends Mol Med 9:325, 2003.
125. Centers for Disease Control and Prevention: Update: Outbreak of severe acute respiratory syndrome worldwide, 2003. MMWR 52:241, 2003.
126. http://www.cdc.gov/ncidod/sars/
127. Fouchier RAM, Kuiken T, Schutten M, et al: Koch's postulates fulfilled for SARS virus. Nature 423:240, 2003.
128. Ksiazek TG, Erdman D, Goldsmith CS, et al: A novel coronavirus associated with severe acute respiratory syndrome. N Engl J Med 348:1953, 2003.
129. Ruan Y, Wi CL, Ee LA, et al: Comparative full-length genome sequence analysis of 14 SARS coronavirus isolates and commom mutations associated with putative origins of infection. Lancet 361:1779, 2003.
130. Peiris JSM, Chu CM, Cheng VCC, et al: Clinical Progression and viral load in a community outbreak of coronavirus-associated SARS pneumonia: A prospective study. Lancet 361:1767, 2003.
131. Peiris JSM, Guan Y, Yuen KY: Severe acute respiratory syndrome. Nat Med 10:S88, 2004.
132. Guan Y, Zheng BJ, He YQ, et al: Isolation and characterisation of viruses related to SARS coronavirus from animals in Southern China. Science 302:276, 2003.
133. Zheng BJ, Guan Y, Wong KH, et al: SARS-related virus predating SARS outbreak, Hong-Kong. Emerging Infect Dis 10: 176, 2004.
134. Liu W, Tang F, Fontanet A, et al: Long-term SARS coronavirus excretion from patient cohort, China. Emerg Infect Dis 10:1841, 2004.
135. Donnelly CA, Ghani AC, Leung GM, et al: Epidemiological determinants of spread of causal agent of severe acute respiratory syndrome in Hong Kong. Lancet 361:1761, 2003.
136. Tambyah PA: SARS: Responding to an unknown virus. Eur J Clin Microbiol Infect Dis 23:589, 2004.
137. http://www.cdc.gov/ncidod/sars/absenceofsars.htm. Accessed January 2005.
138. Wang JT, Sheng WH, Fang CT, et al: Clinical manifestations, laboratory findings, and treatment outcomes of SARS patients. Emerging Infect Dis 10:818, 2004.
139. Li W, Moore MJ, Vasilieva N, et al: Angiotensin-converting enzyme 2 is a functional receptor for the SARS coronavirus. Nature 426: 450, 2003.
140. Yang ZY, Huang Y, Ganesh L, et al: pH-dependent entry of severe acute respiratory syndrome coronavirus is mediated by the spike glycoprotein and enhanced by dentritic cell transfer through DC SIGN. J Virol 78:5642, 2004.
141. Hung IF, Cheng VC, Wu AK, et al: Viral loads in clinical specimens and SARS manifestations. Emerg Infect Dis 10:1550, 2004.
142. Yount B, Curtis KM, Fritz EA, et al: Reverse genetics with a full-length infectious cDNA clone of severe acute respiratory syndrome coronavirus. Proc Natl Acad Sci USA 100:12995, 2003.
143. Poon LLM, Guan Y, Nicholls JM, et al: The aetiology, origins, and diagnosis of severe acute respiratory syndrome. Lancet Infect Dis 4:663, 2004.
144. Yam WC, Chan KH, Poon CLL, et al: Evaluation of reverse transcription-PCR assays for repid diagnosis of severe respiratory syndrome associated with a novel coronavirus. J Clin Microbiol 41:4521, 2003.
145. Chu CM, Cheng VCC, Hung IFN, et al: Role of lopinavir/ritonavir in the treatment of SARS: Initial virological and clinical finings. Thorax 59:252, 2004.
146. Loutfy MR, Blatt LM, Siminovitch KA, et al: Interferon alfacon-1 plus corticosteroids in severe acute respiratory syndrome. JAMA 290:3251, 2003.
147. Cheng Y, Wong R, Soo YO, et al: Use of convalescent plasma therapy in SARS patients in Hong Kong. Eur J Clin Microbiol Infect Dis 24:44, 2005.
148. Loeb M, McGeer A, Henry B, et al: SARS among critical care nurses, Toronto. Emerg Infect Dis 10:251, 2004.
149. Borrero HI, Fajardo L, Bedoya A, et al: Acute respiratory tract infections among a birth cohort of children from Cali, Colombia, who were studied through 17 months of age. Rev Infect Dis 12:S950, 1990.
150. Forgie IM, Campbell H, Lloyd-Evans N, et al: Etiology of acute lower respiratory tract infections in children in a rural community in The Gambia. Pediatr Infect Dis J 11:466, 1992.
151. Ong SB, Lam KL, Lam SK: Viral agents of acute respiratory infections in young children in Kuala Lampur. Bull World Health Organ 60:137, 1982.
152. Hazlett DT, Bell TM, Turkei PM, et al: Viral etiology and epidemiology of acute respiratory infections in children in Nairobi, Kenya. Am J Trop Med Hyg 39:632, 1988.

153. Ghafoor A, Nomani NK, Ishaq Z, et al: Diagnoses of acute lower respiratory tract infections in children in Rawalpindi and Islamabad, Pakistan. Rev Infect Dis 12:S907, 1990.
154. Suwanjutha S, Chantarojanasiri T, Watthana-Kasetr S, et al: A study of nonbacterial agents of acute lower respiratory tract infection in Thai children. Rev Infect Dis 12:S923, 1990.
155. Tupasi TE, de Leon LE, Lupisan S, et al: Patterns of acute respiratory tract infection in children: A longitudinal study in a depressed community in Metro Manila. Rev Infect Dis 12:S940, 1990.
156. van den Hoogen BG, de Jong JC, Groen J, et al: A newly discovered human pneumovirus isolated from young children with respiratory tract disease. Nat Med 7:719, 2001.
157. Peret TC, Boivin G, Li Y, et al: Characterization of human metapneumoviruses isolated from patients in North America. J Infect Dis 185:1660, 2002.
158. van den Hoogen BG, Bestebroer TM, Osterhaus AD, et al: Analysis of the genome sequence of a human metapneumovirus. Virology 295:119, 2002.
159. Stockton J, Stephenson I, Fleming D, et al: Human metapneumovirus as a cause of community-acquired respiratory illness. Emerg Infect Dis 8:897, 2002.
160. van den Hoogen BG, Herfst S, Sprong L, et al: Antigenic and genetic variability of human metapneumoviruses. Emerg Infect Dis 10:658, 2004.
161. Madhi SA, Ludewick H, Abed Y, et al: Human metapneumovirus-associated lower respiratory tract infections among hospitalized human immunodeficiency virus type 1 (HIV-1)-infected and HIV-1-uninfected African infants. Clin Infect Dis 37:1705, 2003.
162. Boivin G, Abed Y, Pelletier G, et al: Virological features and clinical manifestations associated with human metapneumovirus: A new paramyxovirus responsible for acute respiratory infections in all age groups. J Infect Dis 186:1330, 2002.
163. Xepapadaki P, Psarras S, Bossios A, et al: Human metapneumovirus as a causative agent of acute bronchiolitis in infants. J Clin Virol 30:267, 2004.
164. Cuevas LE, Ben Nasser AM, Dove W, et al: Human metapneumovirus and respiratory syncytial virus, Brazil. Emerg Infect Dis 9:1626, 2003.
165. Ijpma FF, Beekhuis D, Cotton MF, et al: Human metapneumovirus infection in hospital referred South African children. J Med Virol 73:486, 2004.
166. Serafino RL, Gurgel RQ, Dove W, et al: Respiratory syncytial virus and metapneumovirus in children over two seasons with a high incidence of respiratory infections in Brazil. Ann Trop Paediatr 24:213, 2004.
167. Bastien N, Ward D, Caeseele PV, et al: Human metapneumovirus infections in the Canadian population. J Clin Microbiol 41:4642, 2003.
168. Galiano M, Videla C, Puch SS, et al: Evidence of human metapneumovirus in children in Argentina. J Med Virol 72:299, 2004.
169. Mackay IM, Jacob KC, Woolhouse D, et al: Molecular assays for detection of human metapneumovirus. J Clin Microbiol 41:100, 2003.
170. Williams JV, Harris PA, Tollefson SJ, et al: Human metapneumovirus in lower respiratory tract disease in otherwise healthy infants and children. New Engl J Med 350:443, 2004.
171. Peiris JS, Tang WH, Chan KH, et al: Children with respiratory disease associated with metapneumovirus in Hong Kong. Emerg Infect Dis 9:628, 2003.
172. Maggi F, Pifferi M, Vatteroni M, et al: Human metapneumovirus associated with respiratory tract infections in a 3-year study of nasal swabs from infants in Italy. J Clin Microbiol 41:2987, 2003.
173. van den Hoogen BG, van Doornum GJ, Fockens JC, et al: Prevalence and clinical symptoms of human metapneumovirus infection in hospitalized patients. J Infect Dis 188:1571, 2003.
174. Jartti T, van den Hoogen B, Garofalo RP, et al: Metapneumovirus and acute wheezing in children. Lancet 360:1393, 2002.
175. Semple MG, Cowell A, Dove W, et al: Dual infection of infants by human metapneumovirus and human respiratory syncytial virus is strongly associated with severe bronchiolitis. J Infect Dis 191:382, 2004.
176. Konig B, Konig W, Arnold R, et al: Prospective study of human metapneumovirus infection in children less than 3 years of age. J Clin Microbiol 42:4632, 2004.
177. MacPhail M, Schickli JH, Tang RS, et al: Identification of small animal and primate models for evaluation of vaccine candidates for human metapneumovirus (HMPV) and implications for HMPV design. J Gen Virol 85:1655, 2004.

60

Enterovirus Infections, Including Poliomyelitis

MARK A. PALLANSCH
HAMID JAFARI

INTRODUCTION

Enteroviruses are among the most common of human viruses, possibly infecting a billion or more persons annually worldwide. Most infections are largely inapparent, but enteroviruses may cause a wide spectrum of acute disease, including mild upper respiratory illness (common cold), febrile rash (hand-foot and-mouth disease and herpangina), conjunctivitis, aseptic meningitis, pleurodynia, myocarditis, encephalitis, acute flaccid paralysis (paralytic poliomyelitis), and neonatal sepsis-like disease.[1,2] Enterovirus infections result in hundreds of thousands of hospitalizations per year in the developed world, with aseptic meningitis accounting for the vast majority of these cases. The disease burden in the developing world of the tropics is poorly estimated, with the exception of poliomyelitis. Enterovirus infections are more common in most developing countries, so it is reasonable to assume that significant morbidity can be attributed to these viruses globally.

Poliomyelitis is the best described enterovirus disease found in the tropics and is probably a disease of antiquity. It was only by the mid-19th century, however, when the Industrial Revolution brought increased urbanization to Europe and North America that larger and more frequent outbreaks of poliomyelitis began in these regions. From the late 1800s, outbreaks were occurring in several European countries and in the United States, and they remained a dominant public health problem in the developed world for the first half of the 20th century. It was only much later that the disease burden due to polio in the developing world, particularly the tropics, was fully appreciated. At the time that the polio vaccines first became available in the 1960s, it is possible that more than 500,000 children a year were paralyzed by poliovirus infection every year, mostly in the developing countries of the tropics.

The knowledge gained about the nature of enteroviruses and the spectrum of clinical disease largely has followed the progress made with studies of polioviruses. Despite this progress, much remains to be learned about the differences found in the tropics that affect the epidemiology and disease burden in these areas.

AGENTS

Enteroviruses are members of the genus *Enterovirus* in the family Picornaviridae and are among the simplest viruses in terms of genetic complexity and size.[3] All are small, round, 30-nm particles with icosahedral symmetry and no lipid envelope. The infectious particles are relatively heat-resistant, resistant to acid pH (which distinguishes them from rhinoviruses), and also resistant to many common detergents and disinfectants, including most soaps, nonionic detergents, ethanol, ether, chloroform, and other lipid solvents. The virus is stable for weeks or more at 4°C and for days at room temperature; however, the virus is readily inactivated by desiccation, ultraviolet light, heat, formaldehyde, and free chlorine.[4,5] The genomic RNA is infectious and serves as messenger RNA for viral protein synthesis. The RNA is translated in a single open reading frame into one large polyprotein, which is then processed through proteolytic cleavage by two distinct virus-encoded proteases into the functional viral proteins.[6]

Historically, the classification of enteroviruses into the subgroups of polioviruses, coxsackieviruses A and B, and echoviruses was based on the empirical observations of their association with some clinical syndromes, susceptibility to infection or disease, tissue tropism, nature of disease in suckling mice, growth in certain specific cell cultures, and in some cases antigenic similarities.[7] Using these criteria, 64 different serotypes were recognized and classified, despite the fact that several antigenically related viruses had different pathogenic properties in mice. This last discrepancy eventually led to the last four viruses being designated only as enterovirus 68–71.[8] A more satisfactory resolution and a completely new classification followed from the advent of comprehensive genetic studies. The complete RNA genetic sequences for all the recognized enteroviruses have been determined,[9] which has allowed a more detailed description and comparison among these viruses.[10] From these new data and to avoid the inconsistencies of the previous classification scheme, the human enteroviruses have been reclassified into five species: A–D and poliovirus.[11] More recent characterization of previously unidentified enteroviruses and increased emphasis on genetic relationships rather than clinical disease has resulted in the proposal that the three polioviruses be reclassified as members of human enterovirus species C.[12] The new classification is given in Table 60-1.

Continued characterization of enterovirus clinical isolates has also identified many new members of the genus, with the naming continuing from enterovirus 73 sequentially.[13–16] These have been assigned to one of the four species and are included in Table 60-1 for reference. At this time, very little is known about any distinctive clinical or epidemiologic features of these new viruses, but it is clear that there are likely to be many more of these described with the wider application of sequencing studies to viruses from the developing world. Also as a part of these studies, it was demonstrated that echoviruses 22 and 23 are genetically distinct from the enteroviruses,[17] and they have been reclassified as members of the new picornavirus genus, *Parechovirus,* and renamed human parechoviruses 1 and 2, respectively. In addition to the members of the genera *Enterovirus* and *Parechovirus*, at least three more genera in this virus family have members that infect humans: *Rhinovirus, Kobuvirus,* and *Hepatovirus* (hepatitis A virus).

Table 60-1 Proposed Species Taxonomy for Genus Enterovirus

Species	Serotypes
Enterovirus A (EV-A)	CAV2–8, 10, 12, 14, 16 EV71, 76, 89–92
Enterovirus B (EV-B)	CAV9, CBV1–6 E1–7, 9, 11–21, 24–27, 29–33 EV69, 73–75, 77–88, 93–95
Enterovirus C (EV-C)	CAV1, 11, 13, 17, 19–22, 24 EV96 PV1–3*
Enterovirus D (EV-D)	EV68, 70

CAV, coxsackievirus A; CBV, coxsackievirus B; E, echovirus; EV, enterovirus; PV, poliovirus.
*Proposed.

The genetic diversity and groupings evident from genomic sequence analysis are also correlated with the antigenic properties of the viruses. These antigenic groupings, which form the basis of the serotype definition for these viruses, are the primary means of distinguishing different enterovirus isolates and are also important for issues of immunity and disease protection. Antisera to each of the viruses raised in animals are usually type specific and provide reference reagents for the serotype determination of the enterovirus isolates.[18] Antigenic differences among isolates in the same serotype can be very complex, but variation at one or several epitopes does not change the serotype as determined by polyclonal antibodies or host response. It should be emphasized that the great diversity of serotypes of enteroviruses presents considerable problems for laboratory diagnosis and epidemiologic investigations, but the serotype usually has minimal importance to the diagnosis and clinical management of an individual patient.

EPIDEMIOLOGY

The patterns of virus shedding and routes of transmission for enteroviruses are consistent with only a few exceptions.[19] The virus is isolated in the highest titer and for the longest time, often several weeks, in stool specimens but can also be isolated from respiratory secretions. Therefore, both fecal-oral transmission and spread by contact with respiratory secretions (person-to-person, fomites, and large-particle aerosol) are considered the most important modes of transmission for these viruses. The relative importance of the different modes probably varies with the virus and the environmental setting. In addition, enteroviruses that cause a vesicular exanthem can, presumably, be spread by direct or indirect contact with vesicular fluid that contains infectious virus. Another exception to the usual modes of enterovirus transmission are the agents of acute hemorrhagic conjunctivitis: enterovirus 70 (EV70) and coxsackievirus A24 variant (CAV24). These two viruses are seldom isolated from respiratory tract or stool specimens and are probably spread primarily by direct or indirect contact with eye secretions, including fomites.[20] Enteroviruses are efficiently amplified and transmitted among humans without intermediaries such as arthropods or other animals. Although several species of nonhuman primates may become experimentally or even naturally infected with some human enteroviruses,[21] including poliovirus, there is no evidence that they play any significant role in virus circulation or constitute an effective animal reservoir.

In tropical regions, especially where sanitation is poor, the efficiency of transmission is high. Consequently, not only is the overall prevalence of enterovirus infections higher, but also the average age of infection is younger. During infancy and preschool age, children get frequent infections with many enteroviruses.[22–24] It is not uncommon in these areas to detect two or three simultaneous infections of different enterovirus serotypes, often causing no disease. Since children likely become infected with nearly all enteroviruses in the tropics, most adults are immune and nearly all babies are born with maternal antibodies to most enteroviruses.[25,26] Normally, neonates not protected by maternal antibodies are at risk for serious illness when infected by enteroviruses. Because of the protective maternal antibodies, neonatal enterovirus disease is extremely rare in the tropics, despite the high prevalence of enterovirus infections in older children. In contrast, in temperate regions where the overall prevalence of enterovirus infections and maternal antibodies are much lower, neonatal enterovirus diseases are relatively more common.[27]

It is important to note that shedding may be intermittent and is affected by the immune status of the individual. Past natural infection with the same enterovirus serotype, and immunization in the case of poliovirus, serves to significantly reduce the extent and duration of virus shedding.[28,29] Immunity will protect against disease but does not form an absolute block that will prevent future infection. Therefore, immune individuals can also contribute to virus transmission, while not being at risk for significant disease. This makes it difficult to track the extent of virus transmission by only observing disease incidence.

Enteroviruses are prevalent worldwide, but in communities with clean food and water, good hygiene, and safe disposal of excreta, the transmission is much less intense; therefore, the incidence is lower, and infections occur over a broader age range, including adults.[2] In temperate regions a seasonal pattern is prominent, with increased prevalence in summer and autumn and low prevalence in winter and spring. In the tropics the prevalence is also much higher during the warm and wet seasons than in the cooler months; however, seasonal differences are less prominent and infections are prevalent throughout the year.[22,23,30,31]

An important concept in understanding the epidemiology of the enteroviruses is variation: by serotype, by time, by geographic location, and by disease. This concept is illustrated in surveillance studies of nonpolio enterovirus infections.[19] There are two primary patterns of enterovirus prevalence: endemic and epidemic. The epidemic pattern is characterized by sharp peaks in numbers of isolations followed by periods with few isolations. Individual peaks of activity may be a single year or a few years. By contrast, viruses that show an endemic pattern are isolated in about the same numbers every year, with only rare peaks observed. Where surveillance data exist, similar endemic and epidemic patterns are seen for most enteroviruses, but are often not reflected in changes of disease incidence.

Many studies have examined the prevalence of antibodies to the enteroviruses in specific populations.[32,33] Several important conclusions can be drawn from these serosurveys. First, the number of persons who have neutralizing antibody to any given enterovirus is large, indicating a high incidence of past infection. Second, infections with one serotype of enterovirus can boost the antibody titers to other enterovirus serotypes as measured by either immunoglobulin M (IgM) or neutralization. The pattern of the heterotypic response varies by serotype and among individuals. Third, the pattern of antibody prevalence by serotype varies by geographic location, by time, and by age. Thus, prevalence data from different years and locations are not directly comparable.

The epidemiology of poliovirus infection has been radically altered by the widespread use of both inactivated polio vaccine (IPV) and oral polio vaccine (OPV). The recent activities of the Polio Eradication Initiative have eliminated endemic poliovirus from most of the world.[34] Since 1988, poliomyelitis from wild poliovirus has declined dramatically and in the year 2004 remains endemic in only six countries in Africa, the Middle East, and Southern Asia (Fig. 60-1). Three regions of the world—the Americas, the Western Pacific, and Europe—have been certified to be free of endemic poliovirus transmission.[35] It is also highly likely that one of the three serotypes of wild poliovirus (type 2) has already been eliminated from the entire world.[36] The only remaining wild type 2 viruses are now found in laboratories and vaccine manufacturing facilities.

Even in areas that are no longer endemic, poliomyelitis can still be observed associated with exposure to OPV, either among vaccine recipients (usually with the first dose) or their contacts.[37–39] The incidence of disease associated with use of OPV is estimated to be 1 case for every 750,000 doses among first-dose recipients and 1 case for every 6.4 million doses (all doses) among contacts.[40] Many developed countries have switched to IPV to eliminate these few remaining cases of vaccine-associated paralytic poliomyelitis.

Recently, five outbreaks of poliomyelitis have been documented that were caused by Sabin OPV strains that had acquired the capacity to cause paralysis and be transmitted among human populations (see later discussion under Polio Eradication). These events are extremely rare and occur only in populations with low immunization coverage. Polio-free countries that have populations with low OPV immunization rates are at risk of importation and spread of wild poliovirus strains as well as emergence of circulating vaccine-derived polioviruses.

Any area with endemic wild polioviruses can serve as a reservoir for reintroduction of poliovirus to areas that have no endemic poliovirus circulation.[41] In addition to several documented long-range importations over the past 25 years, wild poliovirus recently spread from an endemic reservoir in Nigeria to cause cases in 12 additional countries during 2004 and re-establish virus circulation in six of these.[42] The frequency and ease of international travel probably results in frequent introduction of wild poliovirus into all regions of the world. High rates of polio vaccine coverage are necessary to prevent poliomyelitis epidemics.

A powerful tool for tracking the circulation of wild poliovirus strains is the genomic sequence characterization of poliovirus isolates. By comparing the genetic changes among poliovirus isolates, their geographic and temporal origins can be determined. For example, sequence analysis has traced the circulation of a particular poliovirus strain throughout endemic countries, elucidated pathways of transmission during outbreaks, and documented importations from endemic regions into polio-free countries.[43–46] The WHO Poliovirus Laboratory Network of 145 formally accredited poliovirus laboratories provides critical information about wild poliovirus circulation, allowing immunization efforts to be targeted to the virus reservoir areas.[47] In addition, improved sequencing technology has facilitated the analysis of complete genomes of circulating polioviruses. This approach has expanded the understanding of the types of mutations that occur in human populations, including the frequent exchange of genetic material between poliovirus and other enteroviruses.[44,48,49] Similar studies, although with less comprehensive surveillance activities, are now also being applied to nonpolio enterovirus outbreaks as well.[50,51] The result of this molecular epidemiology is a more refined understanding of the complexities of enterovirus transmission and epidemiology.

CLINICAL SYNDROMES CAUSED BY ENTEROVIRUSES

Enterovirus infections can result in a wide variety of disease syndromes. The most common result of enterovirus infection is either no symptoms or mild upper respiratory tract symptoms.[2,19] Other mild enteroviral illness, consisting of fever, headache, malaise, and occasionally mild gastrointestinal symptoms, may also occur. The gastrointestinal symptoms may be the effect of local infection without viremia. Much less frequently, serious illness brings the patient to the attention of a physician.

It is important to remember that the link between an enterovirus infection and a disease syndrome should be made with caution. Inapparent infections and prolonged excretion of virus, especially in stools, are common. A definitive link cannot be made between infection and disease based solely on isolating virus from the stool of an individual patient. A link can be inferred if the virus is isolated from a site that corresponds to the clinical symptoms and if that site is normally sterile. Most associations between enterovirus infection and disease have been made from studies of outbreaks in which a large number of persons with the same clinical signs and symptoms have evidence of infection with the same serotype. Such studies have clearly demonstrated that enterovirus infection can cause aseptic meningitis, pericarditis, pleurodynia, myocarditis, acute hemorrhagic conjunctivitis (AHC), and encephalitis. When an individual patient has a disease syndrome shown clearly to be associated with enterovirus infection and there is no evidence of involvement by another agent, infection implies probable causation.

The most commonly recognized serious manifestation of enterovirus infection is central nervous system (CNS) disease, usually aseptic meningitis, but sometimes encephalitis or paralysis.[2,19] Although the association between myocarditis and pericarditis and enterovirus infection is clearly established, it is not yet clear how often enterovirus infections are responsible for the disease syndromes. Several studies suggest, but do not clearly show, that enterovirus infection may be associated with a large fraction of cases of acute myocarditis.[52,53] By contrast, different studies have failed to show conclusive evidence for significant involvement of enterovirus infection in idiopathic dilated cardiomyopathies.[54]

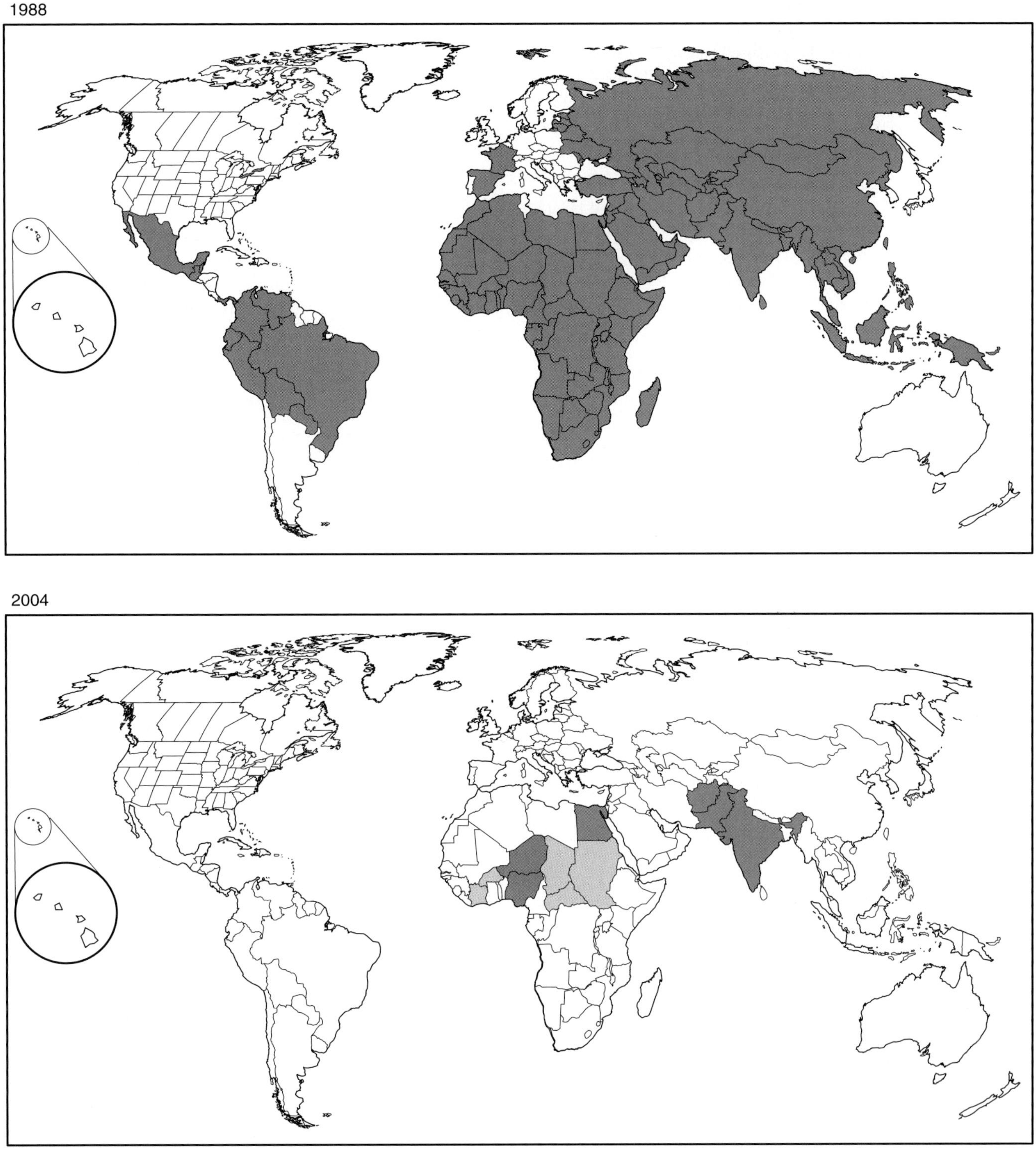

FIGURE 60-1 Global distribution of wild polioviruses and progress in eradication. The maps indicate (*shading*) which countries were endemic for wild poliovirus circulation in the year indicated. In 2004, several countries (*light shading*) that were polio-free for at least 3 years suffered importations of wild poliovirus and circulation was reestablished for a period of at least 6 months.

It is neither necessary nor practical to enumerate all diseases caused by each of the enterovirus serotypes. A limited number of viruses cause a few clinically distinct diseases (e.g., poliomyelitis, AHC, and herpangina). They are relatively easily recognized, and etiologic confirmation by laboratory tests, if required, can be directed at a few specific enteroviruses. Certain syndromes have varied causes, including some enteroviruses. In such cases etiologic diagnosis is important for giving appropriate treatment or avoiding inappropriate treatment (e.g., meningitis, encephalitis, and myocarditis).

In general, with some notable exceptions, most enteroviruses are capable of causing a variety of clinical disease, and for any specific disease it is difficult to predict the serotype from signs and symptoms alone.

Poliomyelitis

The term *poliomyelitis* refers to the inflammatory damage (due to infection) of the anterior horn cells of the spinal cord, recognized clinically as acute-onset lower motor neuron paralysis (or paresis) of one or more muscles. When its viral cause was recognized, the agent was called poliovirus, thereby redefining poliomyelitis as spinal cord disease caused specifically by one or another poliovirus serotype. Polioviruses may cause other diseases, but muscle paralysis due to myelitis is the commonest. Until poliovirus infections were controlled by immunization, they were the most common cause of acute flaccid paralysis (AFP). This is no longer the case in most countries.

Poliomyelitis may vary widely in severity, from paresis of one or a few muscles, or paralysis of one or more limbs, to quadriplegia and paralysis of the muscles of respiration (diaphragm, intercostal muscles). In infants and young children, severe paraspinal muscle weakness (head lag) and localized abdominal muscle paralysis causing a bulge (pseudohernia) when the child cries are diagnostic features in many cases, irrespective of the severity. Tendon reflexes of the affected limbs are lost; in others they may be sluggish. The illness usually starts with fever and myalgia, which may last up to a week, followed by the sudden onset of paralysis that progresses to its maximum within 4 days, and is typically asymmetric. Cerebral functions are not altered usually, unless hypoxia occurs. In such cases, drowsiness and occasionally mild muscle rigidity or an extensor plantar response in the unparalyzed limbs may be mistaken for upper motor neuron involvement. These signs disappear with oxygen therapy or assisted ventilation. During the acute phase of illness, the cerebrospinal fluid (CSF) shows predominantly lymphocytic pleocytosis with moderate elevation of protein. Nerve conduction studies show lower motor neuron involvement without sensory neuropathy.

Most children recover from the acute illness, but some 70% continue to have some residual motor weakness, which may vary from mild impairment to complete flaccid paralysis. The permanent loss of motor neurons results in denervation atrophy of the affected muscles. With growth, relative shortening of the limb and deformities such as talipes equinus or equinovarus develop. If the paraspinal muscles are paralyzed, severe scoliosis may develop.

During the acute illness, cranial nerve nuclei of the medulla or higher levels may be involved, manifesting clinically as paralysis of the muscles of deglutition or central paralysis of respiration. This condition is called *bulbar poliomyelitis.* When spinal muscle paralysis and bulbar disease occur together, the term *bulbospinal poliomyelitis* is applied. Occasionally facial (seventh cranial nerve) paralysis may occur, either isolated or in combination with spinal or bulbar poliomyelitis. While the vast majority of poliovirus infections are either asymptomatic or associated with nonspecific febrile illnesses, the case-fatality rate of those who develop poliomyelitis is 2% to 5% and in epidemics as high as 10%. Death is most often due to respiratory paralysis or arrest in children with bulbar poliomyelitis.

Poliomyelitis should be considered in all cases of pure motor paralysis and is usually associated with a normal or slightly elevated value for protein, normal sugar value, and moderate mononuclear pleocytosis in CSF. Early in the illness polymorphonuclear cells may predominate in the CSF, followed by a shift to mononuclear cells. Defects in the ventral horns of the spinal cord can be observed by magnetic resonance imaging (MRI). The MRI lesion corresponds to the innervation pattern of the affected extremity. Electromyography and nerve conduction velocities (NCVs) generally fail to show evidence of a conduction block.

The differential diagnosis includes spinal cord compression, stroke, neuropathy, and Guillain-Barré syndrome (GBS). Spinal cord compression is unlikely in the absence of central involvement in neural imaging. Lack of sensory involvement would exclude neuropathies. For stroke in the setting of meningoencephalitis, flaccid paralysis sometimes occurs, but the classic spasticity of upper motor lesions should follow. In GBS, protein concentration is markedly elevated in the CSF and pleocytosis is mild or absent. Fever is usually absent, and paralysis is usually symmetric and ascending with evidence of conduction block by NCV.

Delayed progression of neuromuscular symptoms (postpolio syndrome) may occur 20 years or longer after the initial paralysis due to poliovirus.[55] Postpolio syndrome is characterized by new muscle weakness associated with dysfunction of surviving motor neurons. The illness is usually associated with deterioration of those nerves involved in reinnervation during recovery from the original poliovirus infection. Inflammation is sometimes present in association with degenerating neurons.[56] It is believed that the life span of these nerves has been shortened by the process of reinnervation. This syndrome is not a form of amyotrophic lateral sclerosis. It does not appear that reactivation or replication of poliovirus is involved, but current data are inconclusive.[57,58]

Paralytic Myelitis Caused by Other Enteroviruses

A clinical syndrome of AFP may be caused infrequently by certain enteroviruses other than polioviruses. In children, EV71 may cause AFP either sporadically or in small outbreaks. Several other enteroviruses have been found to be associated with AFP on rare occasions. The clinical picture is usually one of a mild disease, occasionally with paralysis of a single muscle such as the deltoid, and often with complete recovery. In a few cases, particularly adults, EV70 has been associated with meningomyelitis and AFP affecting one or more limbs.[59] Although most patients recover completely, some may continue to have residual paralysis, as in poliomyelitis.

Viral Meningitis

Fever, headache, and nuchal rigidity, often with Brudzinski's sign, are characteristic of meningitis in children and adults. The CSF is usually clear and under normal or mildly to moderately increased pressure and with mild-to-moderate pleocytosis (usual range, 100 to 1000 cells per microliter). Although on the first or second day of illness, CSF cells may be predominantly neutrophils, they are predominantly lymphocytes when evaluated 1 or 2 days later. Enteroviral meningitis usually occurs sporadically while other children are infected with the same virus without neurologic disease or even asymptomatically. Occasionally it may occur as small outbreaks. Enteroviruses are by far the most frequent cause of viral meningitis in most locations.

In the tropics, enteroviral meningitis occurs almost exclusively in children less than 10 years of age, similarly to poliomyelitis. In temperate regions, it may occur in children or adults, reflecting the delayed age pattern of enterovirus infections in general. The onset is usually sudden, with fever. Sometimes the fever may be biphasic—a short (1 or 2 days) febrile period accompanied by few or no other signs and symptoms and then, after a day or two, the typical features of meningitis. In older children and adults, headache is common, along with photophobia in some. In infants and young children, febrile convulsions may occur at the onset, in which case careful examination is necessary to rule out encephalitis or other CNS disease. Vomiting, anorexia, skin rash, cough, pharyngitis, diarrhea, and myalgia are also frequently present. Before its closure, the anterior fontanel may bulge as a sign of raised intracranial pressure.

Many other viruses may cause viral meningitis, such as mumps, herpes simplex, Epstein-Barr virus, arenavirus, and several arboviruses. The clinical picture and the laboratory findings on CSF examination lead to a diagnosis of aseptic meningitis. Viral isolation in cell culture or suckling mice from CSF is successful only early in the course of illness. Virus isolation and detection by molecular methods are the only definitive agent-specific diagnostic results.

Treatment is essentially supportive, and the course of illness is nearly always benign, usually lasting less than a week. Complete recovery is the rule. Although some data suggest that neurologic, cognitive, or development or language abnormalities may follow enteroviral meningitis in infancy, other studies indicate that the prognosis is more benign.

Encephalitis

Infection of the brain parenchyma is a relatively rare manifestation of enteroviral infection. The encephalitis may be global or focal. It is probably more common in children than in adults in both tropical and temperate regions. The illness starts with fever and constitutional symptoms. After a few days, confusion, irritability, lethargy, or drowsiness develops and usually progresses rapidly to generalized convulsions and coma. In some children, focal encephalitis is characterized by focal seizures, very much as in herpes simplex virus encephalitis. Other clinical manifestations are usually related to elevated intracranial pressure and to cranial nerve or cerebellar involvement. Occasionally myelitis may also occur, with lower motor neuron paralysis of muscles.

More recently, a syndrome of fatal brain stem encephalitis has been described in several countries of Southeast Asia that is associated with EV71 infection.[60,61] Although sporadic cases of infection with this virus have been described since the virus was first recognized in 1971, the deaths occurred in the context of widespread hand-foot-and-mouth disease (HFMD) outbreaks. The fatal outcome had few clinical predictive symptoms but was specifically associated with young children, mostly less than 2 years of age. The onset of neurologic symptoms was particularly rapid, and death occurred often within 24 hours as a result of cardiopulmonary failure, presumably neurogenic.[62]

The CSF is usually clear with mild, predominantly lymphocytic pleocytosis in the usual range of 5 to 200 cells per microliter. The CSF protein concentration is normal or slightly elevated, and the glucose concentration is normal or slightly decreased. As a rule, CSF culture does not yield an enterovirus. Brain tissue is seldom obtained by biopsy for virus isolation. It is generally believed that herpes simplex virus, several arthropod-transmitted viruses, and enteroviruses are the most common causes of viral encephalitis.

Acute Myocarditis and Pericarditis and Chronic Sequelae

Acute myocarditis with or without pericarditis caused by several EVs can occur in infants, children, adolescents, and young adults. The most common serotypes implicated with acute myocarditis are the coxsackie B viruses.[63] Myocarditis usually starts with fever and mild symptoms followed after a short interval by palpitations, chest pain, shortness of breath, and congestive cardiac failure. Occasionally, arrhythmia may be the only manifestation. Pericarditis may accompany myocarditis; often a pericardial rub is heard, but occasionally there is frank pericardial effusion. Investigation usually confirms cardiomegaly and electrocardiographic evidence of myocarditis. The case-fatality rate is high enough to warrant caution in predicting prognosis.

Treatment is supportive. Most patients recover; however, sequelae have been recognized, including chronic myocarditis, dilated cardiomyopathy, and chronic relapsing or constrictive pericarditis.[64,65]

Acute Hemorrhagic Conjunctivitis

Mild conjunctival hyperemia is noted with many EV diseases. However, a severe form of conjunctivitis, usually occurring in rapidly spreading epidemics and characterized by subconjunctival hemorrhage in nearly half the subjects is caused by two enterovirus serotypes. This disease is different from other enteroviral illnesses, having occurred in global pandemics since its introduction around 1969, when both EV70 and CVA24v emerged as causes of acute hemorrhagic conjunctivitis (AHC).[66,67] AHC epidemics have recurred in many regions at periodic intervals, with several years in between. To date they have occurred largely in the tropical and subtropical countries of Asia, Africa, and Latin America. Only sporadic cases or small outbreaks have occurred in temperate climates.

The illness has a sudden onset. The incubation period for these agents is shorter than for other enteroviruses (24 to 72 hours), systemic illness much less common, and conjunctival replication of virus is the rule. Spread is mainly through direct contact, via fingers or fomites. Eye pain, photophobia, excessive lacrimation, and congestion of the conjunctiva are almost always present. In most cases, the ocular discharge is nonpurulent but may be mucoid in severe cases. The characteristic subconjunctival hemorrhage in a proportion of cases in the epidemic is an important diagnostic feature. The disease is usually bilateral. Adults and school-age children are more affected than infants and preschool children, although household spread is efficient regardless of age. After a few days, symptoms abate, but the hemorrhage resolves slowly. Soothing eye drops, such as sterile saline or mild decongestants, are used to ameliorate the symptoms. Recovery is complete in 5 to 10 days.

During EV70 epidemics, a small proportion of subjects develop acute paralysis of muscle groups of one or more limbs, usually within a few days after the onset of eye disease, resembling poliomyelitis, but in reality a radiculomeningomyelitis.[59] Other than this, the only common complication is secondary bacterial infection.

Pleurodynia (Bornholm Disease)

A distinct illness with mild or high fever of short duration and chest pain located on either side of the sternum or retrosternally may occur sporadically or in outbreaks. The pain is usually intermittent or spasmodic and sometimes excruciating, often exacerbated by deep breathing. Intercostal muscle tenderness and a pleural rub, when present, are important signs distinguishing the illness from myocardial infarction, which is often suspected in adults. The chest radiograph and electrocardiogram are normal. Symptoms usually last for a few days to more than 2 weeks, with occasional relapses. In children severe abdominal pain, apparently arising from the diaphragm, may occur.

This syndrome has primarily been associated with coxsackie B viruses,[68] particularly CVB3 and CVB5, although sporadic cases may be caused by other enteroviruses. Rarely, pleurodynia may be accompanied by another clinical manifestation of enterovirus infection, such as aseptic meningitis, or even myocarditis.

Hand-Foot-and-Mouth Disease

The distinguishing feature of this illness is the vesicular eruption of the hands and feet and in the mouth. The oral lesions, mostly on the buccal mucosa, become shallow ulcers. Coxsackievirus A16 is the most frequent etiologic agent, occasionally causing outbreaks. Other enteroviruses, especially coxsackieviruses A10 and EV 71, may also cause HFMD outbreaks. The etiologic agent can be isolated from the vesicles and from the throat and feces. Occasionally, HFMD may occur with other enterovirus involvement such as meningitis.

Herpangina

This illness is characterized by a typical crop of vesicles on the soft palate, uvula, other parts of the oropharynx, or the tongue. Each vesicle is about 1 to 2 mm in diameter, with a surrounding red areola. It occurs usually only in children younger than 10 years old. Fever and sore throat are the common symptoms. Careful examination of the oropharynx reveals 1 to 10 or 12 discrete lesions, which usually subside without ulcerating.

Short Fever with Maculopapular Rash

Many enteroviruses may cause a short febrile illness with a maculopapular rash resembling rubella or mild measles, particularly in infants and very young children. The distribution of the rash on the face, neck, and chest, and occasionally on the arms and thighs may mimic other well-recognized exanthems. Sometimes there may be mild upper respiratory symptoms, adding to the difficulty of accurate clinical diagnosis. Outbreaks of enterovirus exanthem have also been called Boston exanthem.

Diarrhea

Mild diarrhea is a common accompanying symptom in many enteroviral diseases. However, occasionally enteroviruses may cause a short diarrheal illness. Although occasional outbreaks of diarrhea without other typical enterovirus symptoms have been attributed to enterovirus infections, these are very uncommon.

Neonatal Enterovirus Diseases

Neonates are more vulnerable to invasive enterovirus diseases than are older children and adults. In the tropics, where most adults are immune to enteroviruses, neonates are protected by maternal antibodies. Therefore, paradoxically, neonatal enteroviral diseases are more common where the general transmission potential is less intense than in the tropics. Infection may occur in utero or, more commonly, perinatally.

Many of the clinical features described previously in relatively distinct and self-limited illness, as well as the more sinister lesions in the CNS or the heart, may cluster together in the sick neonate.[69,70] Such illnesses very much resemble other severe systemic infectious disease such as bacterial septicemia. Thus, the infant may present with lethargy, feeding difficulty, vomiting, tachycardia, dyspnea, cyanosis, jaundice, and diarrhea, with or without fever. Clinical evidence for aseptic meningitis, encephalitis, myocarditis, hepatitis, or pneumonia may be present in any combination. The case-fatality rate is high. Sometimes death may occur rapidly.

PATHOGENESIS

Enteroviruses are cytopathic, and much of the associated disease presumably results from tissue-specific cell destruction. Some disease manifestations, enteroviral exanthems and myocarditis, for example, are thought to result from the host immune response to the infection.[2] The actual mechanisms of virus-induced disease, however, have not been well characterized. Typically, the primary site of infection is the epithelial cells of the respiratory or gastrointestinal tract and in the lymphoid follicles of the small intestine, followed by a viremia that may lead to a secondary site of tissue infection. Secondary infection of the CNS results in aseptic meningitis or, rarely, encephalitis or paralysis. Other tissue-specific infection can result in pleurodynia or myocarditis. Disseminated infection can lead to exanthems, nonspecific myalgias, or severe multiple-organ disease in neonates.

Virus infection is dependent on the presence of specific receptors. Five distinct receptors for different nonpolio enteroviruses have been identified from human cells, two different integrins, decay-accelerating factor (DAF), the "coxsackievirus-adenovirus receptor" (CAR), and intracellular adhesion molecule 1 (ICAM-1). The receptor for poliovirus (PVR; CD155) is a member of the immunoglobulin superfamily. Some enteroviruses are able to use more than one receptor, and other unidentified receptors for this group of viruses may also exist. These host receptors may also contribute to host specificity, although studies comparing receptor homologs in resistant hosts are still in progress. Studies of the virus-receptor interactions should improve our understanding of the pathogenesis of enteroviral disease and, possibly, help develop prevention or treatment strategies.[71]

Once attached to the host cell, the virions are thought to be transferred into the cell by pinocytosis. Poliovirus is also endocytosed by M cells in the gut, and this may also be true for other enteroviruses. After virus entry into the host cell, the virus genome is released into the cytoplasm where it then functions as a messenger RNA. Translation leads to the synthesis of viral structural proteins, two proteases and the viral replicase. The sites of viral replication are cytoplasmic membranes that are increased during the infection.[72] Along with the newly formed capsid proteins, the replicated genomic RNA is assembled into progeny virus particles, which are released from the cell by cell lysis or apoptosis.[73] A single virion is thus replicated to generate tens of thousands of progeny virions within a few hours.

The sequence of events following virus infection of the host is generalized from experimental infection of polioviruses in chimpanzees and monkeys, partially corroborated by fragmentary data in sick children. After multiplication at and near the primary site of entry, virus reaches the adjacent lymphoid follicles and draining lymph nodes. Viral multiplication may continue at these sites, and virus is shed into the pharyngeal and intestinal lumina for many days to several weeks. Transient viremia occurs, at least in some cases. When such primary viremia disseminates the infection to distant sites, other susceptible organs may become infected. A second amplification resulting from infection and release of virus from these sites may result in a more intense secondary viremia and further widespread dissemination. Disease may manifest following the primary or secondary viremia. Primary viremia starts 1 to 3 days after virus inoculation and lasts for 1 to 5 days. Secondary viremia starts soon thereafter and may also last for a few days. The appearance of virus-neutralizing antibody in blood coincides with, and may be responsible for, cessation of the viremia, although other factors may also limit the viremia period in the absence of antibody.

The exact pathway taken by enteroviruses to reach the CNS is not clearly understood. Viremic spread across the blood-brain barrier or entry via peripheral nerves are two possibilities.[74,75] The relatively broad range of the incubation period (5 to 30 days) suggests that one pathway may operate in some cases and the other pathway may be taken in others. It is possible that the route of viral spread may, at least in part, determine the site of lesions and the consequent nature of disease. It is also possible that the second pathway is only used by poliovirus among the enteroviruses. For reasons that are not clear, there is a predilection to poliovirus infection and neuronal damage in the lumbar enlargement of the spinal cord leading to lower limb paralysis in a majority of cases.

Polioviruses exhibit the greatest neurovirulence among the enteroviruses; all others have varied but lower neurovirulence. Neurotropism and neurovirulence are at least, in part, two genetically determined properties of the virus. The specific neurotropism related to poliomyelitis is correlated with the use of the specific poliovirus receptor by the virus.[76,77] The RNA sequences of neurovirulent and attenuated vaccine strains of polioviruses show only a very limited number of base changes and indirectly suggest viral determinants affecting neurovirulence. Sequence similarities within the 5′ noncoding region between polioviruses and other enteroviruses that are the result of recombination suggest that the potential neurovirulence of some of the other enteroviruses may be greater than previously recognized,[12] or that vaccine attenuation is a distinct process. Regardless, the reason CNS disease is not more common among infected children is not clear.

In myelitis caused by polioviruses, neurons of the anterior horn region are infected. While many cells are killed and removed by neuronophagia, others recover and regain their function. Paralysis is due to damage to many motor neurons. Neuronal recovery is also reflected in the recovery of muscle function. It is not generally appreciated that a large number of scattered neurons may be destroyed without resulting paralysis. Perivascular lymphocytic cuffing and interstitial microglial infiltration are usually also observed.

There is a marked increase in the risk of developing paralysis when intramuscular injections are given during the incubation period.[78] This "provocation poliomyelitis" may be explained by possible enhancement of virus entry into the peripheral nerves via the nerve endings in the injected muscle.[79] In such cases the limb in which the injection was given is significantly more frequently affected by paralysis. In experimental animals, poliovirus injection into the ulnar nerve has consistently caused AFP, clinically closely resembling the human disease.

IMMUNITY

Infection with enteroviruses elicits a strong humoral immune response. Infection with one serotype provides long-term protection from infection by that serotype but usually little protection from infection by other serotypes. Often this response is heterotypic; that is, infection with one serotype induces an immune response to several other serotypes.[80,81] Young children develop a more homotypic antibody response, whereas older children and adults develop a more heterotypic response. This age difference in the specificity of the antibody response to an enterovirus infection probably reflects exposure to a greater number of serotypes with advancing age. The basis of this heterotypic response is not known, but it may reflect shared epitopes present in multiple serotypes.

Although both humoral and cell-mediated responses occur, the former is probably more important and certainly better investigated and understood. It is not clear what role may be played by cell-mediated immunity in recovery or protection, other than supporting the humoral response. Antibodies are usually detected and quantitated using the property of virus neutralization, by which infectious virus is rendered noninfectious following antibody binding. Virus-binding antibody can be detected and quantitated by enzyme-linked immunoassay (EIA). This method is easily adapted to detecting and measuring class-specific (IgM, IgG, and IgA) antibodies. Although antibody has to bind to the virus for neutralization, only antibodies directed at certain specific surface epitopes will render the virus noninfectious. Antibodies directed at many other non-neutralizing sites are also detected by EIA. While neutralizing antibodies are highly serotype-specific, antibodies detected by EIA are usually more broadly reactive and less specific.

Within 7 to 10 days after primary infection, IgM antibodies appear in the blood, subsequently rise in titer, and persist for up to 3 to 6 months. IgG antibodies appear shortly thereafter, rise in titer over 2 to 3 weeks, and remain at relatively high levels for a few years; they persist at detectable levels for one or more decades. IgA antibody appears after 2 to 4 weeks, both systemically and at mucosal surfaces. Local immunity, which inhibits reinfection, is due partly to mucosal IgA and partly to serum IgG transudate. Humoral immunity is believed to be the major factor in recovery from and clearance of enterovirus infection, as well as protection from disease upon reinfection or from reinfection itself on re-exposure. In the case of polioviruses, vaccine-induced humoral immunity protects against invasive disease and to a lesser extent against reinfection and amplification. Children with agammaglobulinemia do not develop antibodies; hence, they are highly susceptible to disease and chronic infection with prolonged virus shedding. Despite widespread transmission of wild poliovirus and extensive use of oral poliovirus vaccine (OPV) in areas with high incidence of HIV infection, surveillance data do not suggest that persons with HIV infection or AIDS are at higher risk of poliomyelitis or prolonged excretion of polioviruses. One study found that HIV-infected children were more likely than HIV-negative children to shed enteroviruses; however, two other studies in Africa did not detect prolonged excretion of poliovirus among children or adults with HIV infection or AIDS.[82–84]

Like other gastrointestinal infections, the local immunity is neither absolute nor long lasting. Reinfections do occur, but the duration of viral shedding is shortened. There is no risk of disease in reinfection, since systemic immunity prevents viral dissemination, even long after primary infection. In other words, the risk of invasive infection and disease occurs only with the primary infection. However, such reinfections can contribute to continued circulation of polioviruses in spite of high immunization coverage in regions with high force of transmission.

DIAGNOSIS

The key to laboratory confirmation of enterovirus infection is the collection of appropriate clinical specimens for direct detection by molecular methods, virus isolation, or serologic studies.[85] Enterovirus infection cannot be inferred from the clinical syndrome alone, since many other infectious agents can cause similar illness. In the case of poliovirus, isolation also makes it possible to determine whether the virus is wild or vaccine-related.[86] In areas considered to be free of wild poliovirus, this information may be important to public health officials, who must decide whether intervention is needed to prevent further cases of poliomyelitis.

Enterovirus isolation is accomplished by inoculation of appropriate specimens onto susceptible cultured cells. The best specimens for isolation of virus, in order of sensitivity for detection, are stool specimens or rectal swabs, throat swabs or washings, and CSF. Fecal specimens should always be obtained, since virus is excreted longest and in the highest titer from the intestinal tract. Throat swabs or washings and CSF are most likely to yield virus isolates if they are obtained early in the acute phase of the illness. For cases of acute hemorrhagic conjunctivitis, the best specimens, in order of sensitivity, are conjunctival swabs and tears. The virus is detected in cell culture by its cytopathic effect and classically identified as a specific enterovirus by neutralization with type-specific antisera,[87] but serotyping remains a time-consuming and expensive procedure.[85]

For cases of poliomyelitis, WHO has established a standard procedure for investigation, and it is applied to all cases of AFP, not only suspected poliomyelitis. Most countries of the world have adopted this standard approach, referred to as AFP surveillance.[88] The laboratory procedures are extensively documented and implemented in all 145 laboratories that make up the Global Poliovirus Laboratory Network. Stool specimens from any child can be sent to one of these laboratories to be tested for the presence of poliovirus. In addition, this information is then shared immediately with public health officials for an appropriate response (see later discussion).

The use of the polymerase chain reaction (PCR) to detect enterovirus genomes in cell culture, clinical specimens, and tissues promises to significantly improve the detection of enteroviruses.[89,90] This technique is more rapid than isolation and has the potential for providing diagnostic answers in a timely way for clinical patient management. Molecular serotyping systems offer many advantages and may eventually supplant antigenic typing as global stocks of serotype-specific antisera are depleted.[91] Methods have been developed using the PCR assay for rapid detection and characterization of polioviruses, including determination of the virus serotype.[92] Nucleic acid probes, PCR, enzyme-linked immunosorbent assay (ELISA), and monoclonal antibodies can be employed to determine whether the isolate is vaccine-derived or wild poliovirus. The different methods have different sensitivities and specificities for the different strains of viruses.[86]

Serologic studies can be used in certain circumstances for detecting infection. Classically, infection has been demonstrated by a rise in titers of neutralizing antibody between acute and convalescent serum pairs. Poliovirus infection may occasionally be confirmed by demonstrating a rise in titers of neutralizing antibody to one of the poliovirus serotypes, but because of widespread use of vaccine this is often compromised. Enzyme immunoassays have been developed, such as those to detect CVB-specific IgM antibodies.[93] In most cases, the IgM antibody tests are not serotype specific. Depending on the configuration and sensitivity of the test, from 10% to nearly 70% of serum samples show a heterotypic response due to other enterovirus infections. A positive result with this method indicates recent enteroviral infection, although with IgM assays the infecting serotype may not be the same one determined by the assay. In general, serology is more valuable as an epidemiologic tool than for clinical diagnosis.

A general diagnostic caveat, however, is shared among enteroviruses and other ubiquitous pathogens. Since enterovirus infections are quite common, especially in childhood, and since most infections are noninvasive and prolonged, the detected enterovirus infection need not be the cause of the illness under investigation. It is an issue of probabilities. If the clinical syndrome is already known to be associated with the detected agent, then infection is taken as reasonable evidence of causation. If the presence of the agent is found in diseased tissue or a relevant body fluid (such as CSF), that constitutes concrete evidence of invasion, hence causation.

TREATMENT

Since no antiviral therapy is presently available for enterovirus infections, treatment is directed toward alleviating symptoms. Drugs have been identified that exhibit antiviral activity against several enteroviruses including poliovirus in

61

Rotavirus Infections

MARIA C. JAIMES
JUANITA ANGEL
MANUEL A. FRANCO
JASON ROSÉ
HARRY B. GREENBERG

INTRODUCTION

Rotaviruses are the most important cause of severe dehydrating diarrhea in young children in both developed and less developed countries (Box 61-1). In tropical countries (mostly developing countries), rotavirus (RV) infection has several unique characteristics. First, it is a major public health problem, responsible for approximately 1200 deaths in children each day.[1] This presumably occurs because of inadequate access to timely rehydration therapy. Second, in countries within 10 degrees of the equator, rotavirus infection occurs throughout the year, as opposed to countries with more temperate climates where it presents as a seasonal disease, occurring from late fall to early spring.[2] An explanation for this observation is not available. Third, in tropical countries simultaneous infections with multiple RVs is not uncommon, children become infected with RVs at a somewhat earlier age, and the serotypes of the RV strains circulating in tropical settings seem to differ to some degree from what is seen in North America, Western Europe, Japan, and Australia.[3,4]

AGENTS

Rotaviruses belong to the family Reoviridae. Viruses in this family are icosahedral, nonenveloped, with a segmented double-stranded RNA genome and a multiple-layered protein coat.[5]

Rotaviruses are classified into groups (A through G), depending on the presence of cross-reactive antigenic epitopes and on the overall genetic similarity of their genomes. This chapter focuses on the most thoroughly studied group of RVs, group A, which are the principal pathogen of humans and many other species. Group B and C RVs also infect humans and animals, whereas groups D through G have only been documented in animals. The group B RVs have been associated with annual epidemics of diarrhea in adult humans in China[6] and have been detected sporadically in adults and children in India.[7] Group C RVs have been detected occasionally in diarrheal samples from children worldwide, and seroepidemiological studies show that infection with this virus can be quite high (up to 50%) in children older than 3 years and adults.[8]

Detailed structural analysis of the viral particle has been performed by cryoelectron microscopy and several viral proteins have been crystallized.[5] The complete 1000 Å viral particles consist of three protein layers with spike structures extending beyond the outer layer. Each particle has 11 RNA segments surrounded by the innermost protein layer. Each RNA segment is monocistronic with the possible exception of genes 9 and 11.[5] The gene coding assignments and many of the properties of the 11 genome segments of RV have been extensively studied. The virus has eight structural proteins designated by the prefix VP and five nonstructural proteins designated by the prefix NSP. The outer viral layer is composed of a major structural glycoprotein, VP7, and a spike protein, VP4. The latter protein is cleaved in vivo by trypsin into VP5 and VP8, a process that greatly enhances infectivity in vitro and in vivo. The middle viral layer is composed of VP6 and the inner layer is composed of VP2. On the inner side of VP2, VP1, the viral polymerase, and VP3, the guanyl transferase, are associated with the viral RNA. It has been shown that antibodies against VP7 and VP4 can neutralize RV growth in vitro, and the presence of these neutralizing antibodies has been used to evaluate the effectiveness of vaccination strategies. This finding has led to the further classification of RVs into G (glycoprotein, VP7) and P (protease-sensitive, VP4) serotypes.

Viral replication appears to be generally restricted in vivo to the enterocytes on the tips of intestinal villi, except in immunodeficient children, in whom infection of the liver and kidney has also been documented.[9] Recent studies, however, appear to indicate that viremia is more common than previously believed, which may signify that replication is more widespread than previously imagined.[10] In vivo and in vitro

Box 61-1 Key Features of Rotaviruses

Virus

Icosahedral, nonenveloped, with triple-layered protein coat
Genome consists of 11 RNA segments
Purified rotavirus RNA is not infectious
Gene reassortment during mixed viral infections

Epidemiology and Seasonality

Principal cause of severe dehydrating diarrhea in infants worldwide
Causes 352,000 to 592,000 infant deaths annually in developing countries
Year-round infection in countries within 10 degrees of the equator
Winter peaks in all other regions of the world
Important host range restriction

Disease

Viral infection mostly limited to the enterocyte
Diarrhea affects principally children age 2 to 24 months
Asymptomatic infection and reinfection common
Diagnosis and treatment
Rapid diagnosis by viral antigen detection in stool by solid phase immunoassay
Treatment is supportive, aimed at preventing dehydration
Jennerian and human attenuated vaccines of acceptable efficacy should be available in the near future

Data modified from Kapikian AZ, Hoshino Y, Chanock RM: Rotaviruses. In Fields BN, Knipe DM, Howley PM (eds): Fields Virology, vol. 2. Philadelphia, Lippincott Williams & Wilkins, 2001, p 1787.

viral attachment to the host cell is mediated primarily by VP4.[5] The process of entry of the virus into the cell is not completely elucidated and is preceded by interaction with several putative binding and postbinding receptors.[11] Replication occurs in the cell cytoplasm following partial uncoating of parental viral particles. The cellular genes activated by viral infection have been studied using microarrays.[5] Assembly of new viral particles is a multistep process in which unique transient enveloped particles are present inside the endoplasmic reticulum of the infected cell. Mature virions, without an envelope, can be liberated from infected live cells by exocytosis or after cell lysis.[5]

Transfected purified genomic RV RNA is not infectious. This feature has hampered molecular manipulation of the RV genome.[5] The RV genome, because of its segmented nature, is capable of undergoing gene reassortment at high frequency during mixed viral infections. The ability to isolate genetic reassortants has been exploited to make gene coding assignments for the virus. In addition, genetic reassortants have been used to develop "modified jennerian" vaccine candidates in which attenuated animal viruses carry one or two human RV genes encoding the RV surface proteins.

EPIDEMIOLOGY

Diarrhea accounts for 2.5 million deaths per year in children younger than 5 years old in developing countries,[12] and of these RV is estimated to be responsible for 14% to 20% (352,000 to 592,000 deaths annually).[1] Although the mortality caused by RV is very low in developed countries, the incidence of rotaviral disease is similar in children in both developed and developing countries, suggesting that common public health measures will not replace the need for an effective vaccine.[1] Moreover, in developed countries RV is still a very important public health problem and has an enormous health cost impact.[13] In the United States, for example, in children aged 1 month through 4 years, 13.5% of hospitalizations are associated with diarrhea, and RV accounts for 16.5% to 30% of cases.[14]

In the temperate zones of the world, rotaviral infection occurs primarily during epidemic peaks in the cooler months of the year.[2] This pattern is not seen in countries within 10 degrees of the equator, where infection occurs in an endemic fashion year-round.[2] In the United States, a yearly wave of rotaviral illness spreads throughout the country, originating in the southwest in November and ending in the northeast in March.[15] A similar pattern of distribution has been reported in Europe.[16] A clear explanation has not been provided for this interesting phenomenon.

Rotaviruses are usually transmitted by the fecal–oral route, but indirect evidence suggests that they may also be transmitted by the respiratory route.[15] A study has shown that feces from asymptomatic adults may provide a vehicle for the transmission of RV.[17] Water-borne outbreaks of RV are probably rare due to the relative instability of RV at high relative humidity.[5] Food-borne outbreaks are also rare, although it has been reported that oyster and mussel samples can be heavily contaminated by RV.[18] Although animal and human group A RVs can reassort in vitro, substantial host range restriction barriers inhibit widespread intraspecies transmission and reassortment in vivo. However, some studies have shown that strains isolated from India, Brazil, and Malawi are reassortants between human and animal strains.[3,19,20]

Worldwide, most human infections are caused by RV group A of four serotypes: P[8]G1 is by far the most common (53% of strains), followed by P[8]G3, P[4]G2, and P[8]G4.[21,22] Nonetheless, in the past 10 years G9 has been recognized as a very important emerging serotype, being detected at significant rates in developing and developed countries.[21,23–25] Other unusual strains currently circulate and can arise sporadically in both developed and developing countries, but

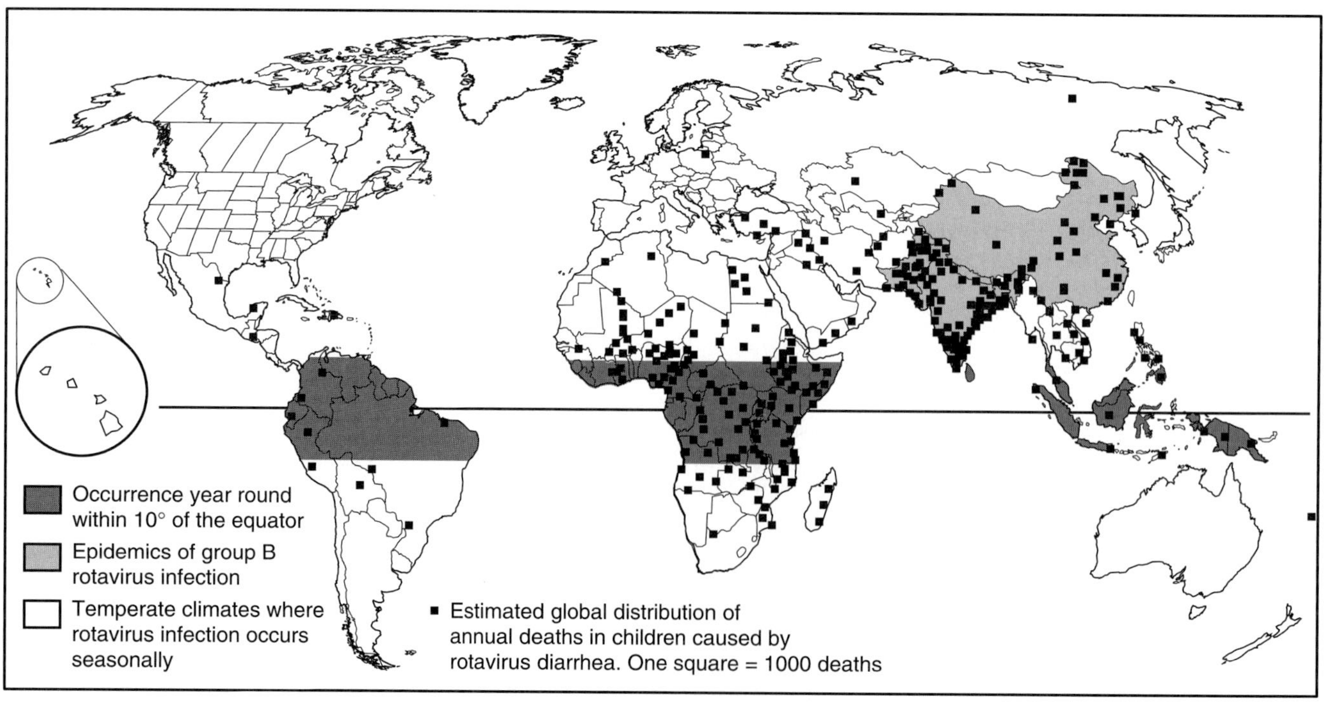

especially in the latter[23,26]: In India, strains of genotype P[6] account for 43% of typeable strains[21]; in Brazil, G5 strains are commonly found in children with diarrhea[21]; and in The Netherlands, a major outbreak of diarrhea among neonates was reported to be due to a P[6],G9 virus.[26] Whether these unusual serotypes will emerge as major causes of disease in large areas of the world remains to be determined. Also, although generally most RV infections are caused by only one virus, the number of mixed infections reported has increased, mostly in developing countries.[24,25]

DISEASE

The pathophysiology of human RV-induced diarrhea has not been fully elucidated.[27] The pathologic changes in the intestines of children with severe RV infection include shortening and atrophy of the villi, mononuclear infiltration in the lamina propria, and distention of the cisternae of the endoplasmic reticulum.[28] A direct relationship between the extent of intestinal histopathology and disease has not been demonstrated either in humans[29] or in mice.[5] This discrepancy between histopathology and disease may be explained by the fact that RV can cause diarrhea by multiple mechanisms at different times after infection.[27] During the initial phases of the disease, secretory,[30,31] altered intestinal motility and altered paracellular permeability components may all play important roles in the pathophysiology of diarrhea. Late in the disease a malabsorption component due to destruction of enterocytes or defective turnover of microvillar membrane disaccharidases may cause an osmotic diarrhea.[27] Rotaviral NSP4 was the first viral enterotoxin[30] described and has been proposed to mediate (at least partially) all of the mechanisms mentioned previously. It has been postulated that viral infection (NSP4 being implicated or not) induces secretory diarrhea and probably increases intestinal motility by stimulating the enteric nervous system.[31,32] Whether the toxic effect of NSP4 is physiologically and clinically relevant in children or other animals besides mice remains to be determined.

The factors that determine viral virulence seem to be multiple and depend on both viral and host elements: Studies in mice using reassortants between a murine virus and a simian virus concluded that NSP1 was important in determining viral virulence, whereas VP4 and VP7 were not.[5] Studies in pigs with virus reassortants have implicated VP4, VP3, VP7, and NSP4 but not NSP1 in affecting viral virulence.[5] In a study in Mexico, the severity of RV-associated diarrhea was related to different P serotypes rather than to G serotypes.[33]

The peak incidence of rotaviral illness in children occurs between 2 months and 2 years of age and occurs at a younger age in developing than in developed countries.[34] Rotavirus infection is frequently asymptomatic in neonates, suggesting infection with specific attenuated strains during the neonatal period and/or protective maternal immune effects.[35,36] In adults, infection is generally asymptomatic, and disease is seen occasionally in the elderly and in personnel who take care of sick children.[37,38]

The clinical features of RV illness are not distinguishable from other enteric infections and do not permit a diagnosis based only on physical examination and history.[5] Typically, RV-induced diarrhea is watery, lasts for approximately 5 days, is preceded by the sudden onset of vomiting, and is frequently accompanied by fever and dehydration.[39] The incubation period of RV has been estimated to be less than 48 hours. Viral excretion in feces lasts 10 days in the majority of children and up to 57 days in small subgroups.[40]

Although in all species examined to date, RV infection appears to be highly restricted to the mature villus tip cells of the small intestine, there is increasing evidence of extraintestinal spread of the virus, and viremia, in humans and other species.[9,10] The role of extraintestinal RV spread, especially in fatal cases, is unclear.[41] Seizures have been reported in association with RV infection and the virus has been detected in cerebrospinal fluid samples by polymerase chain reaction (PCR).[42] Electrolyte abnormalities and fever associated with infection may also explain some of the seizures, and a firm conclusion concerning the mechanism of seizures cannot currently be drawn.

Many innate mechanisms participate in the host's defense against RV: Age-dependent gastric inactivation of heterologous RV has been shown in mice[43] and has been invoked as one of the factors that determine the age restriction of RV-induced diarrhea in mice. Intestinal mucins, certain cytokines, and chemokines have also been proposed as innate intestinal factors that may play a role in modulating RV infection.[5]

The immune system has been shown to be crucial for eliminating RV infection, since immunodeficient mice and children do not resolve primary infection and become chronically infected.[9] Studies in mice have shown that both antibody and cytotoxic T cells can mediate viral clearance and protection from RV reinfection. Cytotoxic T lymphocytes are probably the initial effector mechanism that mediates viral clearance, whereas antibodies are the principal mechanism of protection from reinfection.[5]

The observation that children infected with RV as neonates were later protected against severe RV disease as well as the fact that in animal models primary infection protects against reinfection indicated that vaccination against RV was feasible.[35] It has been shown that natural RV infection can protect against reinfection. Recurrent episodes of RV disease are less severe than the first episode: One episode of RV infection had a protective efficacy of 77% against RV-induced diarrhea and two RV infections, either symptomatic or asymptomatic, completely protected against moderate to severe disease.[44]

One explanation for recurrent RV infection after primary infection is that protection from reinfection is mediated by intestinal RV-specific IgA, which is not long-lasting.[45] Secondary infections will generally boost the fecal IgA response and in many but not all children induce protective fecal anti-RV IgA levels.[45] A second explanation for recurrent illness is that protective antibodies are primarily directed at serotype-specific regions on the rotaviral proteins VP4 and VP7, the two proteins of the outer viral layer.[5] According to this hypothesis, people become reinfected if they encounter a second RV with VP4 or VP7 proteins of different serotypes from the virus that caused their first infection. This possibility has been supported by some animal and clinical studies[46,47] but not by others.[48]

Based on the hypothesis that protective immunity is specific for the VP7 or VP4 serotypes, a major effort has been devoted to characterizing the serologic variability of the two outer RV proteins. However, protective efficacy following human and murine vaccination has not been strictly dependent on the serotype of the vaccine strain, nor has it correlated well with the titer of serotype-specific serum antibody,[48] and currently there is no precise and reliable marker of protection induced by vaccination. These observations suggest that local antibody levels may be the critical determinant of protection or that antibody levels to non-serotype-specific regions of VP4, VP7, or other proteins may play an important role in immunity. It is interesting to note that in mice, nonneutralizing antibodies to VP6 (an antigenically conserved protein making up the middle layer of the virion) can also protect against RV reinfection,[49] probably by inhibiting intracellular viral transcription. In addition, suckling pups nursed by dams vaccinated with an NSP4-derived peptide can be partially protected from heterologous RV diarrhea.[30]

DIAGNOSIS

Diagnosis of RV infection in the clinical setting is not strictly essential when diarrhea is of mild or moderate intensity. During the RV "season" in developed countries, well over 50% of the moderate to severe diarrheal episodes in young children will be due to RV. In tropical countries, because of the presence of other enteric pathogens and the absence of seasonal occurrence of rotaviral disease, it is more difficult, without a diagnostic assay, to determine which diarrheal episode is caused by RV. There are several sensitive, specific, and rapid diagnostic assays for RV; probably the simplest and fastest are solid phase immunoassays that detect RV antigen in stool samples.[50] A second simple and inexpensive method of detecting and characterizing RVs is silver staining of electrophoretically separated viral RNA extracted from stool samples. This technique (used as a component of molecular epidemiological studies of RVs) has the disadvantage that very similar electropherotypes can correspond to very different serotypes.[51] Tissue culture of human RVs has also become a relatively efficient way to identify RVs since RVs grow well in tissue culture when trypsin is added to the culture medium.[5] However, this detection technique is time-consuming and, like electron microscopy, requires specialized expensive equipment and/or reagents. Finally, the use of PCR has increased the sensitivity of assays for detecting RV and has permitted typing of viruses by gene sequence without the laborious process of culturing viruses or the use of less sensitive monoclonal antibody-based typing assays.[52] Microarray methods have been proposed for genotyping the virus.[53]

TREATMENT AND PROGNOSIS

An excellent review on the treatment of gastroenteritis in children has been performed by a Centers for Disease Control and Prevention team[54] and is available at http://www.cdc.gov/mmwr/preview/mmwrhtml/rr5216a1.htm. The recommendations of the American Academy of Pediatrics, which include a useful management algorithm, are available at http://www.aap.org/policy/gastro.htm.

Because RV disease resolves within 1 or 2 weeks without treatment, the basic therapeutic goal is to prevent dehydration. The oral hydration solution until recently recommended by the World Health Organization (WHO) was derived from the formula initially created to treat secretory cholera diarrhea and thus had a high sodium concentration and an osmolarity of 331 mmol/L. After a detailed analysis that indicated that the high sodium concentration formula was associated with an increased incidence of transient, asymptomatic hypernatremia, and that rehydration formulas with reduced osmolarity (245 mmol/L) were equally as effective as those with high osmolarity for the treatment of children with cholera diarrhea, WHO changed its recommendation to a lower osmolarity ORS for the general treatment of dehydration.

After rehydration, rapid age-appropriate refeeding is recommended.[54] Rotavirus disease has been shown to induce self-limited intestinal lactase deficiency.[55] Nevertheless, many studies indicate that withholding lactose-containing products, particularly maternal milk, is not warranted.[54,56]

Several studies have indicated that passive oral immunotherapy can shorten the duration of RV infection in animals and humans.[57] This strategy will probably only be economically feasible for special cases, such as the treatment and prevention of RV infection in immunodeficient patients[58] or low-birth-weight infants in whom the newer preparations of antirotaviral immunoglobulins (bovine colostrum and egg yolk immunoglobulins) have not been tested.[59] Recent studies (including a large multicenter European study[60] and a meta-analysis[61]) suggest that Lactobacillus (the bacteria present in yogurt) is safe and effective as a treatment for children with acute infectious diarrhea. However, the potential exists for great variability among different preparations of lactobacilli and a general recommendation on their use has not been issued.[54] Although several studies in developing countries have shown that zinc supplementation is useful for the treatment and prevention of diarrhea,[62] further studies are needed to determine if this is the case for nourished children from developed countries. No pharmacological treatment of RV diarrhea is recommended: Racecadotril, an enkephalinase inhibitor that acts on the enteric nervous system, has been shown to be useful as an adjunct to treat RV diarrhea.[63] Ondansetron, a serotonin antagonist, was effective in reducing the emesis from gastroenteritis during the phase of oral rehydration.[64] More studies are needed before these preparations can be recommended for treatment of RV diarrhea.

Acute or chronic complications of RV disease other than dehydration are very rare. Malnutrition, low birth weight, and prematurity are all predisposing factors for the severe, life-threatening dehydration associated with RV disease.[65,66] In developing countries, diarrhea is directly related to linear growth retardation during childhood, a determinant of short stature, and impaired capacities in adults.[67] Associations of RV infection with necrotizing enterocolitis, hemorrhagic gastroenteritis of neonates, and pneumatosis intestinalis in infancy have been reported, but a causal relationship has not been established.[5] HIV-infected children do not seem to be more susceptible to RV, and it will probably be safe to give them the live RV vaccines currently being developed.[20] Although several reports have suggested that group A and C RVs may be implicated in extrahepatic biliary atresia of children, evidence suggests that this is not the case.[68]

Soon after the discovery of RVs, the feasibility of a RV vaccine was established.[69] Studies of the cost-effectiveness of a RV vaccine have clearly established the potential usefulness of this approach.[13] Since RV reinfection occurs even after natural infection, the primary aim of anti-RV vaccination strategies is to prevent severe RV disease rather than prevent RV infection or mild illness. Based on the observation that animal RVs appear to be substantially restricted for growth, pathogenicity, and transmission in humans (host range restriction), the most studied strategy for vaccination of children has been a jennerian or modified jennerian approach using bovine or simian viruses or reassortants as vaccines. In some cases of strict jennerian vaccine failure, the vaccine and the wild-type human strain did not share G serotype specificities.[46] Therefore, the jennerian strategy was modified to include animal virus reassortants that contained the four genes encoding the most common VP7 (G) serotypes. A vaccine of this type, the quadrivalent rhesus vaccine (RotaShield), was the first licensed for use in the United States and showed efficacy against moderate to severe diarrhea in the 70% to 90% range. This vaccine was subsequently withdrawn from the market because of its association with intussusception within the first 1 or 2 weeks following vaccination.[70] However, the impact of this RV vaccine on the total attributable risk of intussusception remains highly controversial.[70,71] Nonetheless, it seems unlikely that this vaccine will ever be reconsidered for widespread use in the United States. The RotaShield experience did show that this oral vaccine could be administered concurrently with oral poliovirus and breast-feeding and that an oral vaccine could greatly reduce severe RV disease.[72,73]

The jennerian vaccine approach is currently being pursued in China, where an attenuated lamb RV vaccine has been licensed since 2000.[74] A modified jennerian pentavalent vaccine made of bovine virus reassortants containing human G1, G2, G3, G4 (VP7), and P[8] (VP4) is being studied in a large, multicenter trial.[75] A challenge for this vaccine and perhaps other formulations is the increasing number of pathogenic strains with different G serotypes emerging worldwide. Another approach under investigation is based on the excellent protection induced by natural human primary RV infection[35,44,76]: Two different tissue culture-adapted human viruses are being tested as vaccine candidates. An early phase II trial with the neonatal strain RV3 (P[6]G3)[77] showed rather modest immunogenicity and protective efficacy. Better immunogenicity and protective efficacy have been obtained with the 89-12 (P[8]G1) vaccine candidate currently being tested in a large worldwide trial.[78] It remains to be demonstrated, however, whether a vaccine based on a single human strain is able to induce broad immune responses across commonly and newly circulating serotypes. Protection rates provided by the human 89-12 and bovine pentavalent vaccine have varied from 70% to 80% against any RV disease to 90% and 100% against severe gastroenteritis and are similar to protection rates afforded by the discontinued tetravalent rhesus vaccine.[75,76,79]

Promising strategies to improve vaccine efficacy include vaccination with recombinant virus-like particles,[80] microencapsulating the heterologous RVs to improve their immunogenicity after oral administration,[81] or administering recombinant viral proteins produced in vegetables.[82] Based on the observation that maternally derived milk antibodies can protect animals against infection by RV, several investigators have also advocated immunization of pregnant women with RV as a strategy to protect the newborn against RV diarrhea.[83] This strategy is controversial because milk antibodies in humans seem to have a low protective efficacy against RV infection.[84]

Because of the high excretion rate and very efficient spread of RVs, it is unlikely that disease transmission will be affected substantially by traditional hygiene and public health interventions. Decontamination of surfaces thought to be contaminated with RV should be done with care because RVs have been shown to be highly resistant to many commonly used disinfectants.[85] A spray composed of 0.1% *o*-phenylphenol and 79% ethanol has been shown to be highly effective at decontaminating such surfaces.[86]

ACKNOWLEDGMENTS

This work was supported by the Pontificia Universidad Javeriana and grants FIRCA TWO5647-02 and NIH R37 AI21362-20.

REFERENCES

1. Parashar UD, Hummelman EG, Bresee JS, et al: Global illness and deaths caused by rotavirus disease in children. Emerg Infect Dis 9:565, 2003.
2. Cook SM, Glass RI, LeBaron CW, et al: Global seasonality of rotavirus infections. Bull World Health Organ 68:171, 1990.
3. Gulati BR, Nakagomi O, Koshimura Y, et al: Relative frequencies of G and P types among rotaviruses from Indian diarrheic cow and buffalo calves. J Clin Microbiol 37:2074, 1999.
4. Unicomb LE, Podder G, Gentsch JR, et al: Evidence of high-frequency genomic reassortment of group A rotavirus strains in Bangladesh: Emergence of type G9 in 1995. J Clin Microbiol 37:1885, 1999.
5. Kapikian AZ, Hoshino Y, Chanock RM: Rotaviruses. In Fields BN, Knipe DM, Howley PM (eds): Fields Virology, vol. 2. Philadelphia, Lippincott-Raven, 2001, p 1787.
6. Penaranda ME, Ho MS, Fang ZY, et al: Seroepidemiology of adult diarrhea rotavirus in China, 1977 to 1987. J Clin Microbiol 27:2180, 1989.
7. Sanekata T, Ahmed MU, Kader A, et al: Human group B rotavirus infections cause severe diarrhea in children and adults in Bangladesh. J Clin Microbiol 41:2187, 2003.
8. Kuzuya M, Fujii R, Hamano M, et al: Seroepidemiology of human group C rotavirus in Japan based on a blocking enzyme-linked immunosorbent assay. Clin Diagn Lab Immunol 8:161, 2001.
9. Gilger MA, Matson DO, Conner ME, et al: Extraintestinal rotavirus infections in children with immunodeficiency. J Pediatr 120:912, 1992.
10. Blutt SE, Kirkwood CD, Parreno V, et al: Rotavirus antigenaemia and viraemia: A common event? Lancet 362:1445, 2003.
11. López S, Arias CF: Attachment and post-attachment receptors for rotavirus. In Desselberger U, Gray J (eds): Viral Gastroenteritis: Perspectives in Medical Virology, vol. 9. Amsterdam, Elsevier, 2003, p 143.
12. Kosek M, Bern C, Guerrant RL: The global burden of diarrhoeal disease, as estimated from studies published between 1992 and 2000. Bull World Health Organ 81:197, 2003.
13. Tucker AW, Haddix AC, Bresee JS, et al: Cost-effectiveness analysis of a rotavirus immunization program for the United States. JAMA 279:1371, 1998.
14. Parashar UD, Holman RC, Clarke MJ, et al: Hospitalizations associated with rotavirus diarrhea in the United States, 1993 through 1995: Surveillance based on the new ICD-9-CM rotavirus-specific diagnostic code. J Infect Dis 177:13, 1998.
15. LeBaron CW, Lew J, Glass RI, et al: Annual rotavirus epidemic patterns in North America. Results of a 5-year retrospective survey of 88 centers in Canada, Mexico, and the United States. Rotavirus Study Group. JAMA 264:983, 1990.
16. Koopmans M, Brown D: Seasonality and diversity of group A rotaviruses in Europe. Acta Paediatr Suppl 88:14, 1999.
17. Barnes GL, Callaghan SL, Kirkwood CD, et al: Excretion of serotype G1 rotavirus strains by asymptomatic staff: A possible source of nosocomial infection. J Pediatr 142:722, 2003.
18. Le Guyader F, Haugarreau L, Miossec L, et al: Three-year study to assess human enteric viruses in shellfish. Appl Environ Microbiol 66:3241, 2000.

19. Santos N, Lima RC, Nozawa CM, et al: Detection of porcine rotavirus type G9 and of a mixture of types G1 and G5 associated with Wa-like VP4 specificity: Evidence for natural human–porcine genetic reassortment. J Clin Microbiol 37:2734, 1999.
20. Cunliffe NA, Gondwe JS, Kirkwood CD, et al: Effect of concomitant HIV infection on presentation and outcome of rotavirus gastroenteritis in Malawian children. Lancet 358:550, 2001.
21. Gentsch JR, Woods PA, Ramachandran M, et al: Review of G and P typing results from a global collection of rotavirus strains: Implications for vaccine development. J Infect Dis 174(Suppl 1):S30, 1996.
22. Koshimura Y, Nakagomi T, Nakagomi O: The relative frequencies of G serotypes of rotaviruses recovered from hospitalized children with diarrhea: A 10-year survey (1987–1996) in Japan with a review of globally collected data. Microbiol Immunol 44:499, 2000.
23. Griffin DD, Kirkwood CD, Parashar UD, et al: Surveillance of rotavirus strains in the United States: Identification of unusual strains. The National Rotavirus Strain Surveillance System collaborating laboratories. J Clin Microbiol 38:2784, 2000.
24. Fischer TK, Page NA, Griffin DD, et al: Characterization of incompletely typed rotavirus strains from Guinea-Bissau: Identification of G8 and G9 types and a high frequency of mixed infections. Virology 311:125, 2003.
25. Jain V, Das BK, Bhan MK, et al: Great diversity of group A rotavirus strains and high prevalence of mixed rotavirus infections in India. J Clin Microbiol 39:3524, 2001.
26. Widdowson MA, van Doornum GJ, van der Poel WH, et al: Emerging group-A rotavirus and a nosocomial outbreak of diarrhoea. Lancet 356:1161, 2000.
27. Michelangeli F, Ruiz MC: Physiology and pathophysiology of the gut in relation to viral diarrhea. In Desselberger U, Gray J (eds): Viral Gastroenteritis: Perspectives in Medical Virology, vol. 9. Amsterdam, Elsevier, 2003, p 23.
28. Greenberg HB, Clark HF, Offit PA: Rotavirus pathology and pathophysiology. Curr Top Microbiol Immunol 185:255, 1994.
29. Kohler T, Erben U, Wiedersberg H, et al: Histological findings of the small intestinal mucosa in rotavirus infections in infants and young children. Kinderarztl Prax 58:323, 1990.
30. Ball JM, Tian P, Zeng CQ-Y, et al: Age-dependent diarrhea induced by a rotaviral nonstructural glycoprotein. Science 272:101, 1996.
31. Lundgren O, Peregrin AT, Persson K, et al: Role of the enteric nervous system in the fluid and electrolyte secretion of rotavirus diarrhea [see comments]. Science 287:491, 2000.
32. Lundgren O, Svensson L: The enteric nervous system and infectious diarrhea. In Desselberger U, Gray J (eds): Viral Gastroenteritis: Perspectives in Medical Virology, vol. 9. Amsterdam, Elsevier, 2003, p 51.
33. Mota-Hernandez F, Calva JJ, Gutierrez-Camacho C, et al: Rotavirus diarrhea severity is related to the VP4 type in Mexican children. J Clin Microbiol 41:3158, 2003.
34. Bresee JS, Glass RI, Ivanoff B, et al: Current status and future priorities for rotavirus vaccine development, evaluation and implementation in developing countries. Vaccine 17:2207, 1999.
35. Bishop RF, Barnes GL, Cipriani E, et al: Clinical immunity after neonatal rotavirus infection. A prospective longitudinal study in young children. N Engl J Med 309:72, 1983.
36. Vial PA, Kotloff KL, Losonsky GA: Molecular epidemiology of rotavirus infection in a room for convalescing newborns. J Infect Dis 157:668, 1988.
37. Rodriguez WJ, Kim HW, Brandt CD, et al: Longitudinal study of rotavirus infection and gastroenteritis in families served by a pediatric medical practice: Clinical and epidemiologic observations. Pediatr Infect Dis J 6:170, 1987.
38. Marshall J, Botes J, Gorrie G, et al: Rotavirus detection and characterization in outbreaks of gastroenteritis in aged-care facilities. J Clin Virol 28:331, 2003.
39. Uhnoo I, Olding SE, Kreuger A: Clinical features of acute gastroenteritis associated with rotavirus, enteric adenoviruses, and bacteria. Arch Dis Child 61:732, 1986.
40. Richardson S, Grimwood K, Gorrell R, et al: Extended excretion of rotavirus after severe diarrhoea in young children. Lancet 351:1844, 1998.
41. Lynch M, Shieh WJ, Tatti K, et al: The pathology of rotavirus-associated deaths, using new molecular diagnostics. Clin Infect Dis 37:1327, 2003.
42. Iturriza-Gomara M, Auchterlonie IA, Zaw W, et al: Rotavirus gastroenteritis and central nervous system (CNS) infection: Characterization of the VP7 and VP4 genes of rotavirus strains isolated from paired fecal and cerebrospinal fluid samples from a child with CNS disease. J Clin Microbiol 40:4797, 2002.
43. Bass DM, Baylor R, Broom R, et al: Molecular basis of age-dependent gastric inactivation of rhesus rotavirus in the mouse. J Clin Invest 89:1741, 1992.
44. Velazques RF, Matson DO, Calva JJ, et al: Rotavirus infection in infants as protection against subsequent infections. N Engl J Med 335:1022, 1996.
45. Coulson BS, Grimwood K, Hudson IL, et al: Role of coproantibody in clinical protection of children during reinfection with rotavirus. J Clin Microbiol 30:1678, 1992.
46. Green KY, Taniguchi K, Mackow ER, et al: Homotypic and heterotypic epitope-specific antibody responses in adult and infant rotavirus vaccines: Implications for vaccine development. J Infect Dis 161:667, 1990.
47. Chiba S, Nakata S, Ukae S, et al: Virological and serological aspects of immune resistance to rotavirus gastroenteritis. Clin Infect Dis 16(Suppl 2):S117, 1993.
48. Ward RL, Bernstein DI: Lack of correlation between serum rotavirus antibody titers and protection following vaccination with reassortant RRV vaccine. Vaccine 13:1226, 1995.
49. Burns JW, Siadat PM, Krishnaney AA, et al: Protective effect of rotavirus VP6-specific IgA monoclonal antibodies that lack neutralizing activity [see comments]. Science 272:104, 1996.
50. Gilchrist MJ, Bretl TS, Moultney K, et al: Comparison of seven kits for detection of rotavirus in fecal specimens with a sensitive, specific enzyme immunoassay. Diagn Microbiol Infect Dis 8:221, 1987.
51. Nakagomi T, Gentsch JR, Das BK, et al: Molecular characterization of serotype G2 and G3 human rotavirus strains that have an apparently identical electropherotype of the short RNA pattern. Arch Virol 147:2187, 2002.
52. Iturriza-Gomara M, Green J, Brown DW, et al: Comparison of specific and random priming in the reverse transcriptase polymerase chain reaction for genotyping group A rotaviruses. J Virol Methods 78:93, 1999.
53. Lovmar L, Fock C, Espinoza F, et al: Microarrays for genotyping human group a rotavirus by multiplex capture and type-specific primer extension. J Clin Microbiol 41:5153, 2003.
54. King CK, Glass R, Bresee JS, et al: Managing acute gastroenteritis among children: Oral rehydration, maintenance, and nutritional therapy. MMWR Recomm Rep 52:1, 2003.
55. Noone C, Menzies IS, Banatvala JE, et al: Intestinal permeability and lactose hydrolysis in human rotaviral gastroenteritis assessed simultaneously by non-invasive differential sugar permeation. Eur J Clin Invest 16:217, 1986.
56. Haffejee IE: Cow's milk-based formula, human milk, and soya feeds in acute infantile diarrhea: A therapeutic trial. J Pediatr Gastroenterol Nutr 10:193, 1990.
57. Sarker SA, Casswall TH, Juneja LR, et al: Randomized, placebo-controlled, clinical trial of hyperimmunized chicken egg yolk immunoglobulin in children with rotavirus diarrhea. J Pediatr Gastroenterol Nutr 32:19, 2001.
58. Losonsky GA, Johnson JP, Winkelstein JA, et al: Oral administration of human serum immunoglobulin in immunodeficient patients with viral gastroenteritis. A pharmacokinetic and functional analysis. J Clin Invest 76:2362, 1985.
59. Mohan P, Haque K: Oral immunoglobulin for the prevention of rotavirus infection in low birth weight infants. Cochrane Database Syst Rev: CD003740, 2003.
60. Guandalini S, Pensabene L, Zikri MA, et al: Lactobacillus GG administered in oral rehydration solution to children with acute diarrhea: A multicenter European trial. J Pediatr Gastroenterol Nutr 30:54, 2000.
61. Van Niel CW, Feudtner C, Garrison MM, et al: Lactobacillus therapy for acute infectious diarrhea in children: A meta-analysis. Pediatrics 109:678, 2002.
62. Strand TA, Chandyo RK, Bahl R, et al: Effectiveness and efficacy of zinc for the treatment of acute diarrhea in young children. Pediatrics 109:898, 2002.
63. Cezard JP, Duhamel JF, Meyer M, et al: Efficacy and tolerability of racecadotril in acute diarrhea in children. Gastroenterology 120:799, 2001.
64. Ramsook C, Sahagun-Carreon I, Kozinetz CA, et al: A randomized clinical trial comparing oral ondansetron with placebo in children with vomiting from acute gastroenteritis. Ann Emerg Med 39:397, 2002.

65. Checkley W, Gilman RH, Black RE, et al: Effects of nutritional status on diarrhea in Peruvian children. J Pediatr 140:210, 2002.
66. Newman RD, Grupp-Phelan J, Shay DK, et al: Perinatal risk factors for infant hospitalization with viral gastroenteritis. Pediatrics 103:E3, 1999.
67. Checkley W, Epstein LD, Gilman RH, et al: Effects of acute diarrhea on linear growth in Peruvian children. Am J Epidemiol 157:166, 2003.
68. Schweizer P, Petersen M, Jeszberger N, et al: Immunohistochemical and molecular biological investigations regarding the pathogenesis of extrahepatic biliary atresia. Part 1: Immunohistochemical studies. Eur J Pediatr Surg 13:7, 2003.
69. Wyatt RG, Mebus CA, Yolken RH, et al: Rotaviral immunity in gnotobiotic calves: Heterologous resistance to human virus induced by bovine virus. Science 203:548, 1979.
70. Murphy BR, Morens DM, Simonsen L, et al: Reappraisal of the association of intussusception with the licensed live rotavirus vaccine challenges initial conclusions. J Infect Dis 187:1301, 2003.
71. Murphy TV, Smith PJ, Gargiullo PM, et al: The first rotavirus vaccine and intussusception: Epidemiological studies and policy decisions. J Infect Dis 187:1309, 2003.
72. Rennels MB, Ward RL, Mack ME, et al: Concurrent oral poliovirus and rhesus–human reassortant rotavirus vaccination: Effects on immune responses to both vaccines and on efficacy of rotavirus vaccines. The US Rotavirus Vaccine Efficacy Group. J Infect Dis 173:306, 1996.
73. Rennels MB, Wasserman SS, Glass RI, et al: Comparison of immunogenicity and efficacy of rhesus rotavirus reassortant vaccines in breastfed and nonbreastfed children. US Rotavirus Vaccine Efficacy Group. Pediatrics 96:1132, 1995.
74. Mohan KV, Kulkarni S, Glass RI, et al: A human vaccine strain of lamb rotavirus (Chinese) NSP4 gene: Complete nucleotide sequence and phylogenetic analyses. Virus Genes 26:185, 2003.
75. Heaton PM, Clark HF, Ward R, et al: Bovine–human reassortant rotavirus vaccine: Development history and program status, 8th international symposium on double stranded RNA viruses, Castelvecchio Pascoli, Italy, 2003. Abstract RT.5.
76. Bernstein DI, Sack DA, Rothstein E, et al: Efficacy of live, attenuated, human rotavirus vaccine 89-12 in infants: A randomised placebo-controlled trial. Lancet 3547:287, 1999.
77. Barnes GL, Lund JS, Mitchell SV, et al: Early phase II trial of human rotavirus vaccine candidate RV3. Vaccine 20:2950, 2002.
78. De Vos B, Hardt K, Linhares AC, et al: Efficacy of two doses of a human monovalent rotavirus vaccin, RotarixTM in preventing gastroenteritis due to G1 and non G1 rotavirus in Brazil, Mexico and Venezuela, 8th international symposium on double stranded RNA viruses, Castelvecchio Pascoli, Italy, 2003. Abstract RT.4.
79. Rennels MB, Glass RI, Dennehy PH, et al: Safety and efficacy of high-dose rhesus–human reassortant rotavirus vaccines—Report of the National Multicenter Trial. United States Rotavirus Vaccine Efficacy Group. Pediatrics 97:7, 1996.
80. Bertolotti-Ciarlet A, Ciarlet M, Crawford SE, et al: Immunogenicity and protective efficacy of rotavirus 2/6-virus-like particles produced by a dual baculovirus expression vector and administered intramuscularly, intranasally, or orally to mice. Vaccine 21:3885, 2003.
81. Brubaker JO, Macartney KK, Speaker TJ, et al: Specific attachment of aqueous-based microcapsules to macrophages, B cells, and dendritic cells in vitro. J Microencapsul 19:213, 2002.
82. Wu YZ, Li JT, Mou ZR, et al: Oral immunization with rotavirus VP7 expressed in transgenic potatoes induced high titers of mucosal neutralizing IgA. Virology 313:337, 2003.
83. Pickering LK, Morrow AL, Herrera I, et al: Effect of maternal rotavirus immunization on milk and serum antibody titers. J Infect Dis 172:723, 1995.
84. Glass RI, Ing DJ, Stoll BJ, et al: Immune response to rotavirus vaccines among breast-fed and nonbreast-fed children. Adv Exp Med Biol 310:249, 1991.
85. Lloyd EN, Springthorpe VS, Sattar SA: Chemical disinfection of human rotavirus-contaminated inanimate surfaces. J Hyg (London) 97:163, 1986.
86. Ward RL, Bernstein DI, Knowlton DR, et al: Prevention of surface-to-human transmission of rotaviruses by treatment with disinfectant spray. J Clin Microbiol 29:1991, 1991.

62

Calicivirus Infections

MARC-ALAIN WIDDOWSON
STEPHAN S. MONROE

INTRODUCTION

The illness caused by human caliciviruses was first described in the medical literature in 1929 as "winter vomiting disease."[1] In 1972, Norwalk virus was identified by immune electron microscopy (IEM) of fecal specimens from an outbreak at a school in Norwalk, Ohio.[2] This marked the first identification of a viral agent as a cause of gastroenteritis, and the event was closely followed by the identification of rotavirus (a reovirus) in 1973 as another viral cause of gastroenteritis.[3] In 1976, human viruses with surface features similar to those of established animal caliciviruses were identified by electron microscopy in stools from young children in the United Kingdom[4] and Sapporo, Japan. With the cloning of the Norwalk virus genome in 1990[5] and with the ensuing development of reverse transcription–polymerase chain reaction (RT-PCR), many related but antigenically diverse viruses were identified and placed into provisionally termed groups called "Norwalk-like viruses" and "Sapporo-like viruses." These groups subsequently were defined as separate genera in the family *Caliciviridae* and, in 2001, they were given the official genus names of *Norovirus* and *Sapovirus,* respectively.

Human caliciviruses are now acknowledged as one of the most frequent causes of gastroenteritis in both temperate and tropical countries and in persons of all ages. Although illness is often short-lived, symptoms can be debilitating, leading to dehydration and attendant complications, and may be a particular problem in water-stressed or poorly nourished persons who live in the tropics.

AGENTS

The human caliciviruses, like other members of the family Caliciviridae, are small (approximately 27 nm), nonenveloped RNA viruses with a single major capsid protein. The name *calicivirus* refers to the cup-shaped indentations often seen on the surface of particles visualized by electron microscopy. Viruses now classified as sapoviruses often exhibit the typical calicivirus morphology and were frequently called "classic human caliciviruses." Viruses now classified as noroviruses often lack the distinct surface depressions and were frequently called small, round-structured viruses (SRSV; Fig. 62-1). Individual strains have historically been assigned names based on the location of the outbreak of gastroenteritis with which they were associated (e.g., Norwalk, Hawaii, Snow Mountain, Southampton, Sapporo).

The RNA genome of Norwalk virus, the prototype norovirus, contains 7654 nucleotides, excluding the poly(A) tail, and is organized into three open reading frames (ORFs).[5,6] The first ORF encodes a nonstructural polyprotein that is processed in infected cells to generate several proteins, including the viral helicase, VPg, protease, and RNA-dependent RNA polymerase. The second ORF encodes the major capsid protein, VP1, and the third encodes a small, basic protein, VP2, that is present in virus particles but whose precise function remains unknown.[7] The genomic organization of sapoviruses is slightly different, with the nonstructural polyprotein and major capsid protein both encoded in ORF1 and the small basic protein encoded in ORF2.[8]

Much has been learned about the structure and antigenicity of noroviruses by studying virus-like particles (VLPs) produced by expression of the capsid protein, using recombinant systems.[9] The precise structure of the VLPs of Norwalk virus has been determined, originally by electron cryomicroscopy[10] and subsequently by x-ray crystallography.[11] These VLPs have also been used as antigens for detecting antibodies and as immunogens for generating specific antisera.[12–16]

Human caliciviruses cannot be grown in cell culture nor passaged in small animals, so it is difficult to characterize the antigenic relationships among virus strains. Cross-challenge studies in humans and IEM findings indicated that there are multiple antigenic types.[17–19] The cloning and sequencing of Norwalk virus[5,6] and several other strains[20,21] in the early 1990s allowed for the classification of human calicivirus strains by genetic analysis. Analyses of the predicted amino acids of the complete capsid protein genes (ORF2) has allowed for classification of noroviruses into five major genetic groups or genogroups (GI–GV), three of which (GI, GII, and GIV) contain viruses detected in humans.[22–25] These genogroups can be further subdivided into more than 29 clusters. Sapoviruses can be similarly classified into five genogroups, four of which contain viruses detected in humans.[26] The precise antigenic relationships among strains within and between genogroups

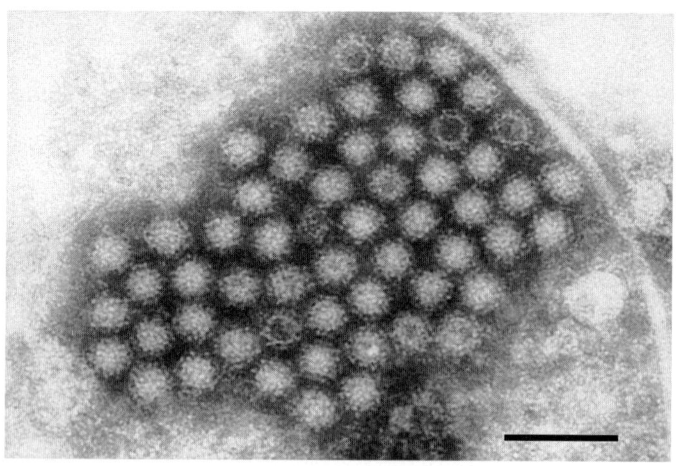

FIGURE 62-1 Negative stain electron micrograph of norovirus particles found in the stool of an ill resident during an outbreak of gastroenteritis in a nursing home, August 1999. (Courtesy of Charles Humphrey, Centers for Disease Control and Prevention, Atlanta, GA.)

remain to be established. Noroviruses also have been found in cows, pigs, and mice.[27,28] These strains have not been found in human infections, but recent serologic evidence suggests that zoonotic transmission may occur.[29]

EPIDEMIOLOGY

The cloning of the norovirus genome in the early 1990s led to the development of sensitive antigen and antibody detection assays that did not require human reagents. These assays have allowed for better understanding of the epidemiology of noroviruses through more complete outbreak investigations, community-based incidence studies, and cross-sectional serosurveys throughout the world.

Norovirus disease often presents as large outbreaks of acute gastroenteritis of short duration in persons of all ages in a variety of settings. Investigations of these outbreaks have been conducted almost exclusively in more developed countries but have proved valuable in elucidating mechanisms of virus transmission (Table 62-1). Noroviruses are highly infectious and are transmitted primarily through the fecal-oral route either by consumption of contaminated food or water or by direct person-to-person spread. Moreover, aerosolization of vomitus droplets has been documented as a mode of transmission[30] and evidence now strongly suggests an important role for environmental contamination and fomites as a source of continuing infection.[31,32]

Attack rates in outbreaks can be over 50%, and there is often substantial secondary spread to contacts of cases. Outbreaks occur year-round, but are particularly common and protracted in the colder months in closed (e.g., nursing homes) or semi-closed (e.g., hotels) settings where transmission is predominantly from person to person. From July 1997 to June 2000, 39% of 264 norovirus outbreaks confirmed by the Centers for Disease Control and Prevention were associated with restaurants or catered events, 25% with nursing homes and hospitals, 13% with schools and day-care centers, 10% with vacation settings (e.g., cruise ships), and 12% with other settings.[33] Outbreaks of norovirus gastroenteritis have been recently reported as a particular problem on cruise ships.[23] Sapoviruses have rarely been reported to cause outbreaks.

Foodborne outbreaks of norovirus are often associated with salads, sandwiches, bakery products, and other foods that are handled and contaminated just before serving by infected foodhandlers. Contaminated oysters have been frequently associated with widespread outbreaks of norovirus gastroenteritis.[34] Contamination of fresh produce at the source also has been documented[35] and may be an under-recognized cause of norovirus infection. Waterborne outbreaks of norovirus gastroenteritis in developed countries have been associated with recreational water[36] and with sewage contamination of drinking water. Both groundwater well sources[37] and municipal water systems have been implicated,[38] the latter usually with an accompanying chlorination failure. The waterborne route of infection may be more important in tropical countries where poor water quality is a problem.

Recently conducted prospective population- or physician-based studies have used RT-PCR to better characterize the epidemiology of endemic norovirus illness in adults and children. A Dutch study found norovirus in 16% of persons of all ages with gastroenteritis,[39] and a recent Australian study, also population-based, reported a comparable estimate of 11%,[40] suggesting that noroviruses are the most common cause of acute gastroenteritis of adults.

Studies in both developed and developing settings have also led to an increasing appreciation that noroviruses are an important cause of acute gastroenteritis among young children, though they remain second to rotaviruses. In Finland, a prospective study of children under two years of age detected rotavirus in 29% of 832 episodes of gastroenteritis, noroviruses in 20%, and sapoviruses in 9%.[41] Rotavirus gastroenteritis was on average more severe than that of norovirus, while sapovirus infection was associated with still milder symptoms. Similarly, a study of children under five years of age hospitalized with nonbacterial gastroenteritis in urban Indonesia found rotavirus in stools of 47% of cases and norovirus in 24%.[42]

Molecular analysis of norovirus detected in outbreaks and sporadic cases suggests that infections with GII strains are several-fold more common than those of GI strains. Certain GII strains have become predominant for a brief time, both globally and nationally,[43] although specific biologic properties that led to this predominance have not yet been defined.

Table 62-1 Characteristics of Noroviruses That Facilitate Spread

Characteristic	Observation	Consequences
Low infectious dose	Less than 100 particles	Permits multiple modes of spread; person to person, via airborne droplets of vomitus, food, water, and environmental contamination
Prolonged asymptomatic shedding	Up to 2 weeks	Increased secondary spread and poses difficulties in implementing control measures
Environmental stability	Resists chlorine, heating, freezing, and desiccation	A contaminated environment can act as a source of infection for several weeks
Substantial strain diversity	Multiple genetic and antigenic types	Require composite diagnostics; repeat infections by different strains
Lack of lasting immunity	Disease can recur with reinfection by same strain	Childhood infection does not protect from disease in adulthood; difficult to develop vaccine with long-lasting immunity

Modified from Parashan U, Quiroz ES, Mountas AW, et al: "Norwalk-like viruses." Public health consequences and outbreak management. MMWR Recomm Rep 50:1–17, 2001.

Nonetheless, seroprevalence studies using recombinant antigens of viruses from GI (Norwalk virus) and GII (Mexico virus) demonstrate that infections with both groups of viruses are extremely common throughout the world, including among isolated groups of Amazonian Indians.[44] A study of over 2000 sera from persons in 11 different sites in 4 countries in southern Africa found an overall seroprevalence of antibodies to both Norwalk virus and Mexico virus of greater than 90%, even in children of 5 years of age.[45] However, there is some suggestion that in developed countries, antibodies to GI strains may be acquired later in childhood and remain at a slightly lower seroprevalence in adults than antibodies to GII strains.[46,47] Low socioeconomic status has been associated with increased seroprevalence of norovirus antibodies in Canada and Chile.[48,49] Studies in northeast Brazil have documented 0.7 seroconversions per child per year, maximum in the second year of life, with 8 different genotypes (5 in group I; 3 in group II) among 12 children.[50,51]

The few studies that have looked at norovirus infections among HIV-infected persons in developed and developing countries have not found evidence to support a major pathogenic role for caliciviruses in this population, although increased viral shedding has been weakly associated with immunodeficiency.[52,53]

DISEASE

The incubation period for norovirus-associated gastroenteritis in humans is usually between 24 and 48 hours (median in outbreaks is 33 to 36 hours), but illness can occur within 12 hours of exposure.

Norovirus gastroenteritis usually presents as acute-onset vomiting, watery nonbloody diarrhea, with accompanying symptoms of abdominal cramps, nausea, headache, malaise, and, in some cases, a low-grade fever. Symptoms last 24 to 60 hours but can be quite severe, with as many as 20 vomiting episodes in a 24-hour period reported. A high proportion of cases with vomiting (over 50%) is one of the characteristics that help differentiate outbreaks of norovirus from those of bacterial etiology. Dehydration and ensuing problems are the most common complications of infection, especially among the very young and elderly, and may require medical attention or hospitalization. Fatalities are rare. Recovery is usually complete with no evidence of any serious long-term sequelae. Norovirus disease among young children is usually less severe than rotavirus disease, although the number of daily episodes of vomiting may be similar.[54]

Studies with volunteers given stool filtrates from norovirus-infected persons have shown that as many as 30% of infections may be asymptomatic, and a Dutch study found 5% of well controls with evidence of norovirus in stool by RT-PCR.[39]

PATHOGENESIS AND IMMUNOLOGY

As few as 10 to 100 ingested norovirus particles are thought to be sufficient to initiate infection in humans, and shedding of virus in the stool generally begins along with onset of symptoms.

Use of molecular detection methods in volunteers fed stool filtrates has indicated that virus antigens can be found in stools for up to two weeks after recovery.[55] Examination by light microscopy of biopsies of the proximal small intestine of norovirus-infected volunteers has shown blunting and broadening of the intestinal villi, vacuolation of the villus epithelial cells, mononuclear cell infiltration into the lamina propria, but an intact mucosa.[56] Histological lesions have not been found in biopsies of the colonic and gastric mucosa.[57] This suggests that replication of virus is limited to the small intestine; however, since no biopsies from areas of small bowel other than the jejunum have been examined, the extent of small-intestinal involvement and sites of viral replication remain unknown. Diarrhea is thought to be caused by several mechanisms, including reduced absorptive capacity of the disrupted epithelium, proliferation of the secretory crypt cells, and reduced expression of certain digestive enzymes, such as sucrase, which leads to an increased osmotic pull of accumulated carbohydrates in the gut lumen. Nausea and vomiting are probably induced by disrupted gastric motor function and a pronounced delay in the emptying of gastric contents into the small intestine.[58]

Mechanisms of immunity to norovirus infection remain unclear. Volunteer studies originally showed that some subjects developed a short-lived immunity of 6 to 14 weeks, which correlated with a rise in serum antibody levels. Yet these same individuals were susceptible to illness again when rechallenged with the same strain over three years later.[59] Immunity appears to be strain specific, and given the genetic variability in circulating noroviruses, individuals are likely to be repeatedly infected with noroviruses during their lifetime. Interestingly, in challenge studies, individuals with high levels of pre-existing serum antibody paradoxically seemed predisposed to illness, while a proportion of individuals remained asymptomatic with low antibody titers despite repeated challenge.[55,60] Multiple exposures to the same strain may eventually induce improved immunity,[60] an observation that gives hope to the development of a future vaccine. Host genetic factors are now recognized as important determinants of susceptibility to infection and may explain many of the apparent paradoxes from earlier studies. Human ABH histo-blood group antigens are expressed on the surface of gut epithelial cells and are thought to act as receptor sites for noroviruses. One of the first studies of the role of these antigens found that volunteers of blood group O were more susceptible to infection with Norwalk virus and more likely to be symptomatic once infected than were persons with blood group B.[61] Investigations of the binding of different norovirus strains with different carbohydrate moieties have found that particular antigens—H type 1 and Lewis^b—bind strongly to Norwalk virus VLPs. Individuals who are secretors (Se^+) express *FUT2* fucosyltransferase that makes H type 1 and Lewis^b antigens, and therefore these persons are more susceptible to infection with Norwalk virus than are nonsecretors (Se^-).[62] Different norovirus strains may have specific binding properties to different blood group antigens.[63] Since ABH histo-blood group antigen expression varies among different populations around the world, it is possible that the distribution of circulating norovirus strains may vary in different parts of the world.

DIAGNOSIS

Norwalk virus was initially identified by IEM,[2] and although electron microscopy is still occasionally used today, it is generally too cumbersome for routine use. Direct detection of viral antigen in stools was historically done using reagents derived from human volunteers.[64] These assays suffered from low sensitivity and high levels of background reactivity. More recently, antigen detection assays based on reagents derived from recombinant-expressed capsid proteins have been shown to be sensitive and specific for detecting a variety of norovirus strains.[65,66]

The current state-of-the-art tool for diagnosing noroviruses and sapoviruses, using stool samples, is RT-PCR. Since the original description of an RT-PCR assay for detecting Norwalk virus,[67] dozens of assays have been described that use primers targeted to conserved regions of the RNA-dependent RNA polymerase gene,[67–70] with direct comparisons indicating that no single assay is best for detecting all known strains.[71] More recently, assays using primers targeted to the capsid protein gene have been used to detect and type norovirus strains.[24,72] The latest advance in detection of noroviruses is the use of real-time RT-PCR assays, which employ fluorogenic probes or dyes.[73–76] These highly sensitive assays offer great promise for improved detection of virus in stool samples collected after the resolution of symptoms, when the level of viral shedding is low.

Serologic diagnosis of norovirus infection was initially performed by using IEM or assays utilizing reagents from human volunteers.[77–80] The availability of recombinant-expressed norovirus capsid proteins has allowed for the development of highly sensitive and specific assays for detecting historic exposure (seroprevalence) and recent exposure (seroconversion) to noroviruses.[72,81–84] The frequent occurrence of cross-reactive antibody responses in infected individuals limits the usefulness of these assays for determining the subtype of the infecting strain.

TREATMENT AND PROGNOSIS

Calicivirus gastroenteritis is self-limiting, and patients usually make a rapid and full recovery. No specific antiviral treatment exists. Rehydration therapy and treatment to correct electrolyte disturbances may be necessary, usually via oral administration, but in some cases administration of intravenous fluids is required. In some cases of severe vomiting, antiemetic drugs may be of use. In experimentally infected adults, oral administration of bismuth subsalicylate reduced the severity of abdominal cramps and the duration of gastrointestinal symptoms[85]; however, the American Association of Pediatrics does not recommend the use of such pharmacologic agents in children.[86]

PREVENTION AND CONTROL

Standard hygienic precautions, including frequent hand washing and care in the disposal or cleaning of materials soiled with feces or vomitus, will help prevent calicivirus infection. Due to the lack of a cell-culture system for human caliciviruses, studies to determine the efficacy of disinfectants to inactivate noroviruses have not been performed. However, prompt use of chlorine solutions at a concentration of 1000 parts per million on hard surfaces is recommended in the United Kingdom to help control outbreaks in hospitals.[87]

Correct handling of ready-to-eat foods and exclusion from work of ill foodhandlers until at least 24 hours after resolution of symptoms (encouraged by provision of paid sick leave) will likely reduce foodborne transmission of noroviruses. Although viral antigens have been detected in stools 13 days after virus challenge in volunteers,[88] the public health significance of prolonged shedding remains unclear. Noroviruses may be able to survive chlorine levels in excess of those routinely present in public water systems.[89] Water treatment processes aimed at providing safe water in poorer countries may not be fully effective against caliciviruses.

The antigenic diversity of norovirus strains and the apparent lack of long-term immunity have challenged the development of a vaccine. Nonetheless, early development of norovirus vaccines has begun with use of recombinantly expressed VLPs. These VLPs have proved immunogenic in humans[90] and have been administered orally using transgenic potatoes,[91] raising the interesting possibility of an edible vaccine.

REFERENCES

1. Zahorsky J: Hyperemesis hiemis or the winter vomiting disease. Arch Pediatr 46:391–395, 1929.
2. Kapikian AZ, Wyatt RG, Dolin R, et al: Visualization by immune electron microscopy of a 27-nm particle associated with acute infectious nonbacterial gastroenteritis. J Virol 10:1075–1081, 1972.
3. Bishop RF, Davidson GP, Holmes IH, et al: Detection of a new virus by electron microscopy of faecal extracts from children with acute gastroenteritis. Lancet 1:149–151, 1974.
4. Madeley CR, Cosgrove BP: Caliciviruses in man (letter). Lancet 1:199–200, 1976.
5. Xi JN, Graham DY, Wang KN, et al: Norwalk virus genome cloning and characterization. Science 250:1580–1583, 1990.
6. Jiang X, Wang M, Wang K, et al: Sequence and genomic organization of Norwalk virus. Virology 195:51–61, 1993.
7. Glass PJ, White LJ, Ball JM,et al: Norwalk virus open reading frame 3 encodes a minor structural protein. J Virol 74:6581–6591, 2000.
8. Liu BL, Clarke IN, Caul EO, et al: Human enteric caliciviruses have a unique genome structure and are distinct from the Norwalk-like viruses. Arch Virol 140:1345–1356, 1995.
9. Jiang X, Wang M, Graham DY, et al: Expression, self-assembly, and antigenicity of the Norwalk virus capsid protein. J Virol 66:6527–6532, 1992.
10. Prasad BV, Rothnagel R, Jiang X, et al: Three-dimensional structure of baculovirus-expressed Norwalk virus capsids. J Virol 68:5117–5125, 1994.
11. Prasad BV, Hardy ME, Dokland T, et al: X-ray crystallographic structure of the Norwalk virus capsid. Science 286:287–290, 1999.
12. Jiang X, Zhong WM, Farkas T, et al: Baculovirus expression and antigenic characterization of the capsid proteins of three Norwalk-like viruses. Arch Virol 147:119–130, 2002.
13. Jiang X, Matson DO, Ruiz-Palacios GM, et al: Expression, self-assembly, and antigenicity of a snow mountain agent-like calicivirus capsid protein. J Clin Microbiol 33:1452–1455, 1995.
14. Herrmann JE, Nowak NA, Blacklow NR: Detection of Norwalk virus in stools by enzyme immunoassay. J Med Virol 17:127–133, 1985.
15. Belliot G, Noel JS, Li JF, et al: Characterization of capsid genes, expressed in the baculovirus system, of three new genetically distinct strains of "Norwalk-like viruses." J Clin Microbiol 39:4288–4295, 2001.
16. Leite JP, Ando T, Noel JS, et al: Characterization of Toronto virus capsid protein expressed in baculovirus. Arch Virol 141:865–875, 1996.
17. Wyatt RG, Dolin R, Blacklow NR, et al: Comparison of three agents of acute infectious nonbacterial gastroenteritis by cross-challenge in volunteers. J Infect Dis 129:709–714, 1974.
18. Okada S, Sekine S, Ando T, et al: Antigenic characterization of small, round-structured viruses by immune electron microscopy. J Clin Microbiol 28:1244–1248, 1990.
19. Lewis D: Norwalk agent and other small-round structured viruses in the U.K. J Infect 23:220–222, 1991.
20. Lambden PR, Caul EO, Ashley CR, et al: Sequence and genome organization of a human small round-structured (Norwalk-like) virus. Science 259:516–519, 1993.

21. Lew JF, Kapikian AZ, Valdesuso J, et al: Molecular characterization of Hawaii virus and other Norwalk-like viruses: Evidence for genetic polymorphism among human caliciviruses. J Infect Dis 170:535–542, 1994.
22. Chakravarty S, Hutson AM, Estes MK, et al: Evolutionary trace residues in noroviruses: Importance in receptor binding, antigenicity, virion assembly, and strain diversity. J Virol 79:554–568, 2005.
23. Widdowson M-A, Cramer EH, Hadley L, et al: Outbreaks of acute gastroenteritis on cruise ships and on land: Identification of a predominant circulating strain of norovirus—United States, 2002. J Infect Dis 190:27–36, 2004.
24. Vinje J, Hamidjaja RA, Sobsey MD: Development and application of a capsid VP1 (region D) based reverse transcription PCR assay for genotyping of genogroup I and II noroviruses. J Virol Methods 116:109–117, 2004.
25. Kageyama T, Shinohara M, Uchida K, et al: Coexistence of multiple genotypes, including newly identified genotypes, in outbreaks of gastroenteritis due to Norovirus in Japan. J Clin Microbiol 42:2988–2995, 2004.
26. Farkas T, Zhong WM, Jing Y, et al: Genetic diversity among sapoviruses. Arch Virol 149:1309–1323, 2004.
27. van Der Poel WH, Vinje J, van Der Heide R, et al: Norwalk-like calicivirus genes in farm animals. Emerg Infect Dis 6:36–41, 2000.
28. Karst SM, Wobus CE, Lay M, et al: STAT1-dependent innate immunity to a Norwalk-like virus. Science 299:1575–1578, 2003.
29. Widdowson M-A, Rockx B, Schepp R, et al: Detection of serum antibodies to bovine norovirus in veterinarians and the general population in the Netherlands. J Med Virol 76:119–128, 2005.
30. Marks PJ, Vipond IB, Carlisle D, et al: Evidence for airborne transmission of Norwalk-like virus (NLV) in a hotel restaurant. Epidemiol Infect 124:481–487, 2000.
31. Evans MR, Meldrum R, Lane W, et al: An outbreak of viral gastroenteritis following environmental contamination at a concert hall. Epidemiol Infect 129:355–360, 2002.
32. Cheesbrough JS, Green J, Gallimore CI, et al: Widespread environmental contamination with Norwalk-like viruses (NLV) detected in a prolonged hotel outbreak of gastroenteritis. Epidemiol Infect 125:93–98, 2000.
33. Fankhauser RL, Monroe SS, Noel JS, et al: Epidemiologic and molecular trends of "Norwalk-like viruses" associated with outbreaks of gastroenteritis in the United States. J Infect Dis 186:1–7, 2002.
34. Dowell SF, Groves C, Kirkland KB, et al: A multistate outbreak of oyster-associated gastrenteritis: Implications for interstate tracing of contaminated shellfish. J Infect Dis 171:1497–1503, 1995.
35. Ponka A, Maunula L, von Bonsdorff CH, et al: An outbreak of calicivirus associated with consumption of frozen raspberries. Epidemiol Infect 123:469–474, 1999.
36. Kappus KD, Marks JS, Holman RC, et al: An outbreak of Norwalk gastroenteritis associated with swimming in a pool and secondary person-to-person transmission. Am J Epidemiol 116:834–839, 1982.
37. Beller M, Ellis A, Lee SH, et al: Outbreak of viral gastroenteritis due to a contaminated well. International consequences. JAMA 278:563–568, 1997.
38. Kukkula M, Maunula L, Silvennoinen E, et al: Outbreak of viral gastroenteritis due to drinking water contaminated by Norwalk-like viruses. J Infect Dis 180:1771–1776, 1999.
39. de Wit MA, Koopmans MP, Kortbeek LM, et al: Sensor, a population-based cohort study on gastroenteritis in the Netherlands: Incidence and etiology. Am J Epidemiol 154:666–674, 2001.
40. Marshall JA, Hellard ME, Sinclair MI, et al: Incidence and characteristics of endemic Norwalk-like virus-associated gastroenteritis. J Med Virol 69:568–578, 2003.
41. Lew JF, Valdesuso J, Vesikari T, et al: Detection of Norwalk virus or Norwalk-like virus infections in Finnish infants and young children. J Infect Dis 169:1364–1367, 1994.
42. Subekti D, Lesmana M, Tjaniadi P, et al: Incidence of Norwalk-like viruses, rotavirus and adenovirus infection in patients with acute gastroenteritis in Jakarta, Indonesia. FEMS Immunol Med Microbiol 33:27–33, 2002.
43. Noel JS, Fankhauser RL, Ando T, et al: Identification of a distinct common strain of "Norwalk-like viruses" having a global distribution. J Infect Dis 179:1334–1344, 1999.
44. Gabbay YB, Glass RI, Monroe SS, et al: Prevalence of antibodies to Norwalk virus among Amerindians in isolated Amazonian communities. Am J Epidemiol 139:728–733, 1994.
45. Smit TK, Bos P, Peenze I, et al: Seroepidemiological study of genogroup I and II calicivirus infections in South and southern Africa. J Med Virol 59:227–231, 1999.
46. Pelosi E, Lambden PR, Caul EO, et al: The seroepidemiology of genogroup 1 and genogroup 2 Norwalk-like viruses in Italy. J Med Virol 58:93–99, 1999.
47. Gray JJ, Jiang X, Morgan-Capner P, et al: Prevalence of antibodies to Norwalk virus in England: Detection by enzyme-linked immunosorbent assay using baculovirus-expressed Norwalk virus capsid antigen. J Clin Microbiol 31:1022–1025, 1993.
48. Gurwith M, Wenman W, Gurwith D, et al: Diarrhea among infants and young children in Canada: A longitudinal study in three northern communities. J Infect Dis 147:685–692, 1983.
49. O'Ryan ML, Vial PA, Mamani N, et al: Seroprevalence of Norwalk virus and Mexico virus in Chilean individuals: Assessment of independent risk factors for antibody acquisition. Clin Infect Dis 27:789–795, 1998.
50. Talal AH, Moe CL, Lima A, et al: Seroprevalence and seroincidence of Norwalk-like virus infections among Brazilian infants and children. J Med Virol 61:117–124, 2000.
51. Parks CG, Moe CL, Rhodes D, et al: Genomic diversity of "Norwalk-like viruses" (NLVs): Pediatric infections in a Brazilian shantytown. J Med Virol 58:426–434, 1999.
52. Grohmann GS, Glass RI, Pereira HG, et al: Enteric viruses and diarrhea in HIV-infected patients. Enteric Opportunistic Infections Working Group. N Engl J Med 329:14–20, 1993.
53. Levett PN, Gu M, Luan B, et al: Longitudinal study of molecular epidemiology of small round-structured viruses in a pediatric population. J Clin Microbiol 34:1497–1501, 1996.
54. Pang XL, Joensuu J, Vesikari T: Human calicivirus-associated sporadic gastroenteritis in Finnish children less than two years of age followed prospectively during a rotavirus vaccine trial. Ped Infect Dis J 18:420–426, 1999.
55. Graham DY, Jiang X, Tanaka T, et al: Norwalk virus infection of volunteers: New insights based on improved assays. J Infect Dis 170:34–43, 1994.
56. Agus SG, Dolin R, Wyatt RG, et al: Acute infectious nonbacterial gastroenteritis: Intestinal histopathology. Histologic and enzymatic alterations during illness produced by the Norwalk agent in man. Ann Intern Med 79:18-25, 1973.
57. Widerlite L, Trier JS, Blacklow NR, et al: Structure of the gastric mucosa in acute infectious bacterial gastroenteritis. Gastroenterology 68:425–430, 1975.
58. Meeroff JC, Schreiber DS, Trier JS, et al: Abnormal gastric motor function in viral gastroenteritis. Ann Intern Med 92:370–373, 1980.
59. Parrino TA, Schreiber DS, Trier JS, et al: Clinical immunity in acute gastroenteritis caused by Norwalk agent. N Engl J Med 297:86–89, 1977.
60. Johnson PC, Mathewson JJ, DuPont HL, et al: Multiple-challenge study of host susceptibility to Norwalk gastroenteritis in US adults. J Infect Dis 161:18–21, 1990.
61. Hutson AM, Atmar RL, Graham DY, et al: Norwalk virus infection and disease is associated with ABO histo-blood group type. J Infect Dis 185:1335–1337, 2002.
62. Lindesmith L, Moe C, Marionneau S, et al: Human susceptibility and resistance to Norwalk virus infection. Nat Med 9:548–553, 2003.
63. Hutson AM, Atmar RL, Estes MK: Norovirus disease: Changing epidemiology and host susceptibility factors. Trends Microbiol 12:279–287, 2004.
64. Greenberg HB, Kapikian AZ: Detection of Norwalk agent antibody and antigen by solid-phase radioimmunoassay and immune adherence hemagglutination assay. J Am Vet Med Assoc 173:620–623, 1978.
65. Burton-MacLeod JA, Kane EM, Beard RS, et al: Evaluation and comparison of two commercial enzyme-linked immunosorbent assay kits for detection of antigenically diverse human noroviruses in stool samples. J Clin Microbiol 42:2587–2595, 2004.
66. Richards AF, Lopman B, Gunn A, et al: Evaluation of a commercial ELISA for detecting Norwalk-like virus antigen in faeces. Journal of Clin Virol 26:109–115, 2003.
67. Jiang X, Wang J, Graham DY, et al: Detection of Norwalk virus in stool by polymerase chain reaction. J Clin Microbiol 30:2529–2534, 1992.
68. Vinje J, Koopmans MP: Molecular detection and epidemiology of small round-structured viruses in outbreaks of gastroenteritis in the Netherlands. J Infect Dis 174:610–615, 1996.

69. Ando T, Monroe SS, Gentsch JR, et al: Detection and differentiation of antigenically distinct small round-structured viruses (Norwalk-like viruses) by reverse transcription–PCR and Southern hybridization. J Clin Microbiol 33:64–71, 1995.
70. Moe CL, Gentsch J, Ando T, et al: Application of PCR to detect Norwalk virus in fecal specimens from outbreaks of gastroenteritis. J Clin Microbiol 32:642–648, 1994.
71. Vinje J, Vennema H, Maunula L, et al: International collaborative study to compare reverse transcriptase PCR assays for detection and genotyping of noroviruses. J Clin Microbiol 41:1423–1433, 2003.
72. Noel JS, Ando T, Leite JP, et al: Correlation of patient immune responses with genetically characterized small round-structured viruses involved in outbreaks of nonbacterial acute gastroenteritis in the United States, 1990 to 1995. J Med Virol 53:372–383, 1997.
73. Kageyama T, Kojima S, Shinohara M, et al: Broadly reactive and highly sensitive assay for Norwalk-like viruses based on real-time quantitative reverse transcription–PCR. J Clin Microbiol 41:1548–1557, 2003.
74. Hohne M, Schreier E: Detection and characterization of norovirus outbreaks in Germany: Application of a one-tube RT-PCR using a fluorogenic real-time detection system. J Med Virol 72:312-319, 2004.
75. Pang X, Lee B, Chui L, et al: Evaluation and validation of real-time reverse transcription–PCR assay using the LightCycler system for detection and quantitation of norovirus. J Clin Microbiol 42:4679–4685, 2004.
76. Richards GP, Watson MA, Kingsley DH: A SYBR green, real-time RT-PCR method to detect and quantitate Norwalk virus in stools. J Virol Methods 116:63–70, 2004.
77. Kapikian AZ, Greenberg HB, Cline WL, et al: Prevalence of antibody to the Norwalk agent by a newly developed immune adherence hemagglutination assay. J Med Virol 2:281–294, 1978.
78. Dolin R, Reichman RC, Roessner KD, et al: Detection by immune electron microscopy of the Snow Mountain agent of acute viral gastroenteritis. J Infect Dis 146:184–189, 1982.
79. Gary GW, Jr., Kaplan JE, Stine SE, et al: Detection of Norwalk virus antibodies and antigen with a biotin-avidin immunoassay. J Clin Microbiol 22:274–278, 1985.
80. Cubitt WD, Blacklow NR, Herrmann JE, et al: Antigenic relationships between human caliciviruses and Norwalk virus. J Infect Dis 156:806–814, 1987.
81. Farkas T, Thornton SA, Wilton N, et al: Homologous versus heterologous immune responses to Norwalk-like viruses among crew members after acute gastroenteritis outbreaks on 2 US Navy vessels. J Infect Dis 187:187–193, 2003.
82. Jiang X, Matson DO, Cubitt WD, et al: Genetic and antigenic diversity of human caliciviruses (HuCVs) using RT-PCR and new EIAs. Arch Virol 12:251–262, 1996.
83. Monroe SS, Stine SE, Jiang X, et al: Detection of antibody to recombinant Norwalk virus antigen in specimens from outbreaks of gastroenteritis. J Clin Microbiol 31:2866–2872, 1993.
84. Treanor JJ, Jiang X, Madore HP, et al: Subclass-specific serum antibody responses to recombinant Norwalk virus capsid antigen (rNV) in adults infected with Norwalk, Snow Mountain, or Hawaii virus. J Clin Microbiol 31:1630–1634, 1993.
85. Steinhoff MC, Douglas RG, Jr., Greenberg HB, et al: Bismuth subsalicylate therapy of viral gastroenteritis. Gastroenterology 78:1495–1499, 1980.
86. American Academy of Pediatrics: Practice parameter: The management of acute gastroenteritis in young children. Provisional Committee on Quality Improvement, Subcommittee on Acute Gastroenteritis. Pediatrics 97:424–435, 1996.
87. Chadwick PR, Beards G, Brown D, et al: Management of hospital outbreaks of gastro-enteritis due to small round structured viruses. J Hosp Infect 45:1–10, 2000.
88. Okhuysen PC, Jiang X, Ye L, et al: Viral shedding and fecal IgA response after Norwalk virus infection. J Infect Dis 171:566–569, 1995.
89. Keswick BH, Satterwhite TK, Johnson PC, et al: Inactivation of Norwalk virus in drinking water by chlorine. Appl Environ Microbiol 50:261–264, 1985.
90. Ball JM, Graham DY, Opekun AR, et al: Recombinant Norwalk virus-like particles given orally to volunteers: Phase I study. Gastroenterology 117:40–48, 1999.
91. Tacket CO, Mason HS, Losonsky G, et al: Human immune responses to a novel Norwalk virus vaccine delivered in transgenic potatoes. J Infect Dis 182:302–305, 2000.

63

Astroviruses, Enteric Adenoviruses, and Other Gastroenteritis Viruses

JOSEPH S. BRESEE
ROGER I. GLASS

INTRODUCTION

Diarrheal disease remains one of the most common causes of morbidity and mortality in developing countries. The problem is particularly acute among young children, who will have an estimated 15 episodes of diarrhea in the first five years of life[1] and among whom 2.5 million deaths will occur each year.[2] For up to half of all episodes, an etiologic agent cannot be found. The importance of viral agents as causes of diarrheal disease has been increasingly appreciated, beginning with the discovery of rotavirus[3] and caliciviruses[4] in the 1970s. More recently, advances in detection methods for some other viruses, such as astroviruses and enteric adenoviruses, have led us to appreciate their role as causes of diarrheal disease. In addition, a variety of other viruses, such as picobirnaviruses, coronaviruses, and toroviruses, have been associated with gastroenteritis, but their clinical and public health importance remains unclear (Table 63-1). Many of these viruses may be responsible for the fraction of illness for which a pathogen cannot be found and a better understanding of their epidemiology will have implications for programs to decrease morbidity and mortality in developing countries.

Astroviruses

AGENTS

Astroviruses were first identified in 1975[5,6] and named based on a characteristic 5- or 6-pointed appearance noted by electron microscopy (EM). Since 1990, improvements in diagnostic methods, including the adaptation of astrovirus to grow in continuous cell lines[7]; sequencing and elucidation of the structure of the genome[8–10]; and development of improved methods of detection, including enzyme immumoassays and reverse-transcription polymerase chain reaction,[11–14] have led to new insights into the role of astrovirus in human disease. It is now clear that astroviruses are a common cause of sporadic gastroenteritis among children, possibly second only to rotavirus, and may be associated with large-scale outbreaks of diarrhea as well.

Astroviruses are 28- to 30-nm, spherical, nonenveloped viruses with a positive sense ssRNA genome and have been classified in their own family, Astroviridae.[15] Eight serotypes of human astroviruses have been identified.[16,17] Of these, type 1 is predominant in most studies, accounting for more than half of strains isolated[16,18,19]; types 2, 3, and 4 each account for 10% to 16% of astrovirus detections; and types 5, 6, 7, and 8 are less uncommonly detected.[16,17] The relative distribution of types seems to vary by geographic location and by year,[20] and more variability may be found in developing countries.[21,22]

EPIDEMIOLOGY

Gastroenteritis associated with astroviruses has been reported worldwide, both as sporadic disease and as outbreaks. Cases of astrovirus-associated gastroenteritis are most common among children less than 2 years of age,[19,23–32] and are less frequent among older children and adults.[33,34] In volunteer studies, most adults neither became infected nor developed diarrhea.[33,35] However, in a large outbreak among schoolchildren,[36,37] teachers became ill as well, perhaps as a result of a large dose of virus in this type of setting or a different mechanism of spread. In addition, outbreaks have been reported among the elderly, probably due to waning immunity with increasing age.[38–40]

Gastroenteritis associated with astrovirus, like rotavirus, occurs in both developed[19,23,24,27–30,41–43] and developing countries,[32,44–48] suggesting that improvements in water and sanitation are unlikely to decrease disease incidence. In temperate climates, astrovirus diarrhea cases peak in winter,[17,19,24,29,31] whereas the seasonality is less clear in tropical settings.[32,44,46] With improvements in detection methods, astrovirus represents an important cause of community-acquired and nosocomial illness and may be the most common viral cause of gastroenteritis in children after rotavirus and possibly Norwalk-like viruses.[19] In developing countries, astroviruses have generally been detected in less than 10% of young children treated for gastroenteritis in outpatient clinics or in hospitals, and the lower proportions reported from some studies (<1%–3%) may reflect insensitive detection methods rather than true prevalence.[19,21,42,45,47–50] Even so, one study in rural Mexico has found astrovirus to be the most common cause of diarrhea in the first three years of life, causing 26% of diarrheal episodes in a prospectively followed cohort.[32] Outbreaks of astrovirus gastroenteritis have been reported in schools,[36,37] day-care centers,[25,51,52] hospitals,[26,29,39,53,54] nursing homes,[38,40] and households.[32,55] Nosocomial spread of astroviruses may be common.[56] While the modes of transmission are still unknown, the primary mode of spread of virus is likely to be through fecal–oral contamination via person-to-person contact,[33,35,36,53] although the stability of the virus in water may indicate that waterborne spread is possible.[57]

DISEASE

Astroviruses cause a syndrome characterized by 2 to 5 days of watery diarrhea, often accompanied by vomiting and less often by high fever, abdominal pain, and other constitutional symptoms.[23,29,44,46] It is generally milder than rotavirus, less commonly resulting in dehydration,[19,23,26,39,44] and rarely

Table 63-1 Summary of Virologic and Epidemiologic Features of Certain Viruses Associated with Gastroenteritis

Virus	Family	Taxonomy	Detection	Epidemiology	Comment
Astrovirus	Astroviridae	28–30nm, ssRNA, N-env;10% have 5–6 point star appearance; 8 serotypes	EM, IEM, EIA, RT-PCR	Endemic, most disease in children <2 years; epidemic, children and adults, including elderly; daycare, schools, hospitals	No clear seasonality in tropical countries; fairly common cause of viral diarrhea in children; less severe than rotavirus
Enteric adenovirus	Adenoviridae	70–80nm, dsRNA, icosahedral, N-env; 2 main serotypes	EIA, EM, IEM, RT-PCR, culture, DNA probes, hybridization	Endemic disease in children <2 years;	No clear seasonality; disease as severe as rotavirus, but less common
Picobirnavirus	Birnaviridae	35nm, dsRNA, bisegmented genome	EM, PAGE, RT-PCR	Associated with diarrhea in HIV infected adults; no clear association with diarrhea in healthy persons	Possible association with *Cryptosporidium* infection.
Coronavirus	Coronaviridae	60–200nm, ssRNA, pleomorphic, env, with club-shaped projections give a halo appearance	EM	Not known	May cause diarrhea in children and adults; possible association with tropical sprue and NEC
Torovirus	Coronaviridae	100–150nm, ssRNA pleomorphic, env, with club-shaped projections	EM	Not known	Possible cause of diarrhea in humans

EIA, enzyme immunoassay; EM, electron microscopy; env, enveloped; IEM, immune electron microscopy; N-env, nonenveloped; RT-PCR, reverse transcriptase–polymerase chain reaction.

associated with death.[45] Lactose intolerance[43,58] and poor weight gain[46] have been reported following astrovirus infection, and children with poor nutritional status may develop more severe disease[46] or chronic diarrhea.[50] Illness among adults is generally mild and of short duration.[33,35,39] However, in studies of immunocompromised persons, astrovirus is often the most common virus detected in persons with diarrhea and associated with prolonged shedding of virus.[59–61] HIV infection was associated with more severe astrovirus disease in children with HIV in Malawi.[21] Indirect evidence suggests that immunity to astrovirus develops early in life.[25,33,35]

Astrovirus infects intestinal epithelial cells. The incubation period is 3 to 4 days,[33,35] but may be shorter in outbreak settings.[37] Children may shed virus 1 to 2 days prior to illness and for 4 to 5 days following illness,[25,29,51] but shedding for 3 weeks has been reported when more sensitive detection methods have been used. Since most illness with astroviruses is found in young children and elderly persons, it is assumed that protection from illness is conferred by infection, and that the protection is relatively durable. Like many other enteric viruses, the immunologic correlates of protection are poorly understood for astroviruses.

DIAGNOSIS

Until recently, electron microscopy was the only method to detect astrovirus in fecal specimens, but was relatively insensitive.[9,24,26,31,36,37,40,47,53,58,62,63] Enzyme immunoassays have been developed,[11,42] which were more sensitive, easier, and less expensive to use.[23,25,30,36,42,44,46,64] Molecular diagnostic methods including reverse transcriptase–polymerase chain reaction and probes, as well as virus cultivation, are available in research laboratories.[65]

TREATMENT, PROGNOSIS, AND PREVENTION

Therapy for astrovirus diarrhea includes rehydration with oral or intravenous fluids. Illness is generally mild and self-limited, but malabsorption and lactose intolerance have been reported following infection. Death associated with astroviruses is rare.[43,45,58]

In outbreaks, identification of the source of infection, such as food or contact with ill persons, may be helpful in preventing further illness. Sporadic cases are common in children and no methods of prevention have been identified. Since the infection may be spread though close personal contact, enteric precautions including appropriate hand-washing practices and isolation of ill persons may be advisable.

Enteric Adenovirus

AGENTS

When adenoviruses were first identified in fecal specimens of children with diarrhea, their etiologic role was questioned because adenoviruses are common causes of other illnesses (e.g., URIs) in children and are excreted in the stool. But unlike the common respiratory adenoviruses, enteric adenoviruses were difficult to grow and were therefore distinguished as the fastidious enteric adenoviruses (FEAs). Eventually, these FEAs were placed in their own group and found to belong to two predominant serotypes, 40 and 41. Besides these serotypes, only serotype 31 has occasionally been causally associated with gastroenteritis. Like astroviruses, the development of rapid, sensitive diagnostic assays for the detection of EAs has increased our appreciation of their role as causes of diarrhea in children.

Adenoviruses are members of the family Adenoviridae and of the genus *Mastadenovirus*. The 47 defined serotypes are divided into 6 subgroups (A–F); serotypes 40 and 41 are the only members of subgroup F (called enteric adenoviruses because they have been associated with gastroenteritis in humans).[66,67] Enteric adenoviruses are nonenveloped, icosahedral, double-stranded DNA viruses, and are 70 to 80 nm in size.

EPIDEMIOLOGY

Like rotavirus and astrovirus diarrhea, diarrhea associated with enteric adenoviruses occurs primarily among children less than 2 years of age. Infection is probably universal, and the age-specific incidence does not appear to differ between temperate and tropical countries, suggesting that improvements in water and sanitation will not decrease the incidence of disease.

Compared to other viral agents in developing countries, EAs appear to account for a smaller proportion of diarrheal disease than in developed countries. Enteric adenoviruses generally have been detected in 1% to 4% of children with diarrhea in many studies,[19,49] although they have been detected commonly in some studies. Enteric adenoviruses were more common than rotavirus in a rural outpatient setting in Guatemala (14% of children with diarrhea had EA detected in stool compared to 5% with rotavirus), and were associated with 31% of hospital admissions for diarrhea.[68] In two South African studies, 6.5% to 13.2% of hospital admissions for diarrhea were associated with EAs[69,70]; in one study,[70] EAs were detected as often as rotaviruses. In the few studies that have examined the role of EAs in an adult population, they appear to be less important causes of gastroenteritis than in children. No seasonality of EA infections was apparent in studies in temperate[31,71–73] or tropical countries,[68,74] but few studies have reviewed multiple seasons.

DISEASE

Infections with EA can range from being mild or asymptomatic to producing profuse, nonbloody, watery diarrhea and vomiting.[71,72,75–79] Children often have 6 to 10 stools per day, and the mean duration of illness is 5 to 9 days.[68,71,72,75–78] Abdominal pain[71,76] and 2 to 3 days of low-grade fever (<38.5°C) are also frequently present, whereas temperatures *greater than or equal to* 39°C occur in less than 10% to 25% of children.[71,75] Mild isotonic dehydration may occur in 15% to 50% of children,[71,72,76] and only severe cases require hospitalization. Respiratory symptoms, including pneumonia, have been associated with EA infections but are present less commonly than with other adenoviruses.[72,75,77] Asymptomatic infections have been documented in 8% and 17% of children in day-care center studies.[23,68,71,72] Serum electrolytes are usually normal, and a slight leukocytosis may be present in a minority of children.[71]

Gastroenteritis associated with EAs has a similar presentation among patients in developed and developing countries. However, enteric adenoviruses may be associated with chronic diarrhea and less common serotypes in HIV-infected subjects.[59,80–84] Deaths from EA gastroenteritis are uncommon, but have been reported, particularly among immunocompromised children.[75,85,86] Long-term complications appear to be rare, but lactose intolerance[71] and malabsorption[87] have been reported and may exacerbate disease among children in developing countries where malnutrition is prevalent.

Differentation of EA-associated gastroenteritis from other causes of viral gastroenteritis is difficult. EA-associated diarrhea may be more severe and prolonged than viral gastroenteritis caused by other agents[71,72,88] and is commonly associated with a high fever and dehydration similar to rotavirus.[71,88]

Like other viral agents of gastroenteritis, the exact mode of transmission is unknown. EAs are probably transmitted by fecal–oral spread, by person-to-person contact, or by respiratory droplets. No foodborne or waterborne outbreaks have been described.[89]

The incubation period of the disease is 7 to 10 days,[77,78,90] and viral shedding may persist for 10 to 14 days.[90] Mechanisms of diarrhea and immunity associated with EA are poorly understood. Type 40- and 41-specific antibodies develop following infection[71,91,92] and can be detected in the absence of recent diarrheal illness.[69,92] Children can become ill when reinfected with EA.[93] However, illness among adults is uncommon, even in outbreak settings where they have a high likelihood of exposure.

DIAGNOSIS

Electron microscopy (EM) was first used to detect enteric adenoviruses in fecal specimens when they are shed in large amounts (as many as 10^{11} particles/gram of feces). Since EM cannot distinguish EAs from nonenteric serotypes,[94] immune electron microscopy (IEM) can enhance sensitivity and specificity of EA detection.[95–98] Enzyme immunoassays using monoclonal antibodies to types 40 and 41 and to the adenovirus hexon common to all serotypes have been developed.[98–102] These are the easiest, most rapid methods for detection[103] and have proven to be highly sensitive and specific compared to IEM.[98] There are currently no commercial kits using DNA detection methods. Enteric adenoviruses grow in Graham 293 cells, a cell line transformed by adenovirus type 5.[104] Viruses can then be identified using one of the preceding methods or by use of restriction enzyme analysis.

TREATMENT, PROGNOSIS, AND PREVENTION

No specific therapy is available for EA gastroenteritis, so treatment is directed toward prevention and treatment of dehydration. Oral rehydration solutions are effective in treating diarrhea with mild and moderate dehydration, and severe dehydration may require use of intravenous fluids.

Prevention of illness is currently not possible due to lack of understanding of risk factors for transmission. Attention to good hand washing when caring for ill persons seems reasonable.

Novel Viruses Associated with Gastroenteritis

PICOBIRNAVIRUS

First identified in 1985,[105] picobirnaviruses (PBVs) have since been detected in a variety of animals.[106–111] The virus has since been detected in human fecal specimens from patients with and without diarrhea,[59,112–115] but has been associated with disease only in a study of HIV-infected adults in the United States[59] and Argentina.[116]

Picobirnaviruses are small (pico), bisegmented (bi-RNA) viruses that are members of the family Birnaviridae. Atypical picobirnaviruses have been detected with three segments of RNA.[112] On electron miscroscopy, the virus is a 35-nm, discreet virus with no distinctive surface structure.

Little is known about the distribution or incidence of picobirnaviruses. In two studies, PBVs have been detected from diarrheic stools of adults with coexistent *Cryptosporidium* infection, and in one study, HIV-infected patients with chronic diarrhea excreted the virus for seven months.[59,113] The geographic or temporal distribution of picobirnaviruses is unknown, although viruses have been isolated from humans in several countries.

No serologic immune response, measured by IEM, was detected in a group of adults with HIV,[59] although serum antibody has been detected by solid-phase IEM in infected rabbits.[110]

Although PBVs may be seen by EM, the most sensitive and specific methods of detection involves identification of two segments of RNA by polyacrylamide electrophoresis from a stool specimen.[59]

CORONAVIRUSES

Coronaviruses were first reported in association with diarrhea in adults[117] and tropical sprue among children and adults in India in 1975.[118] While subsequent reports documented detection of coronavirus-like particles (CVLPs) in stools of persons with diarrhea, they could not associate CVLPs with diarrhea.[119,120]

Coronoviruses are pleomorphic, 60 to 200 nm, ssRNA viruses that belong to the family Coronaviridae. Because of their pleomorphic appearance, misdiagnosis is problematic and no confirmatory test is available. Consequently, the prevalence of human enteric coronaviruses (HECVs) is unknown, and while they have been detected in studies in several countries,[16,24,45,62,121–129] they are not clearly associated with disease. In studies that have compared rates of HECV detection in stools from patients with diarrhea versus controls, the results are mixed. Because of the long duration of shedding and the possibility for asymptomatic infection, the pathogenicity of HECVs may be difficult to prove by comparing rates of detection between well and ill persons. Many studies have reported the majority of viral detections among young children and infants,[24,121,126–128,130] but detections among adults are common.[24,84,119,127,131] With some exceptions,[45,126,130] most studies have reported no differences in detection by time of year.[127] Mode of spread of HECVs is unknown.

Illness descriptions from outbreaks thought to be associated with coronaviruses have included the occurrence of vomiting and diarrhea of short duration, often accompanied by fever.[117,130] Besides gastroenteritis, HECVs have been reported in association with other gastrointestinal diseases including necrotizing enterocolitis,[132,133] and neonatal diarrhea[122] in infants, and tropical sprue.[118,134] In several reports of clinical signs and symptoms associated with the new severe acute respiratory syndrome (SARS)-associated coronavirus, diarrhea has been a common symptom, reported in around a quarter of patients[135,136] It is not clear whether patients with the SARS coronavirus can have diarrhea without respiratory symptoms.

HECVs may be identified with EM by their distinctive 20-nm, clublike projections.[137] Enteric coronaviruses are distinct from respiratory coronaviruses and do not cross-react by enzyme-linked immunosorbent assay (ELISA) or immunoblots, although there is cross-reactivity on IEM.[129]

TOROVIRUSES

Toroviruses are members of the family Coronaviridae and the genus *Torovirus*. They are pleomorphic, 100- to 150-nm, ssRNA viruses with 20-nm, clublike projections extending from the capsid.[138–140]

The epidemiology of these infections remains unclear. Toroviruses have been detected in stools of children and adults with diarrhea in developed countries.[49,140–142] However, in these studies there was no epidemiologic association with illness, and the detections could not be confirmed using additional tests. In an EM survey of diarrhea among children in Toronto, torovirus-like particles were detected in 224 (8%) of 3800 stool specimens. The particles in some of these stools were later confirmed as torovirus by an ELISA incorporating bovine and human antibodies.[143]

A serum response to infection can be measured in infected cows, which develop IgM and IgG following gastrointestinal infection,[144] but no serum immune response has been reported in humans. Electron microscopists can identify torovirus-like particles in human specimens but cannot confirm the detection.[145] Several additional methods including ELISA,[144,146] cDNA probes for hybridization,[142] and RT-PCR[143] have been used successfully in animals and hold promise for detection of human disease.

OTHER VIRUSES

A variety of other viruses have been implicated in gastroenteritis to some degree including parvoviruses, enteroviruses, reoviruses, and pestiviruses, and have been reviewed in detail elsewhere. Parvoviruses, reoviruses, and pestiviruses may cause diarrhea in nonhumans, and there are reports of human cases of gastrointestinal illnesses.[147–153] However, the data are inconclusive, and they are not currently thought to be causes of gastroenteritis in humans.

REFERENCES

1. Glass RI, Bresee JS, Parashar U: The global burden of dehydrating disease. In Farthing MJG, Mahalanabis D (eds): The Control of Food and Fluid Intake in Health and Disease, Vol. 51. Philadelphia, Lippincott Williams and Wilkins, 2003, pp 17–31.
2. Kosek M, Bern C, Guerrant RI: The global burden of diarrhoeal disease, as estimated from studies published between 1992 and 2000. Bull WHO 81:197–204, 2003.
3. Bishop RF, Davidson GP, Holmes IH, et al: Virus particles in epithelial cells of duodenal mucosa from children with viral gastroenteritis. Lancet 1:1281–1283, 1973.
4. Kapikian AZ, Wyatt RG, Dolin R, et al: Visualization by immune electron microscopy of a 27 nm particle associated with acute infectious nonbacterial gastroenteritis. J Virol 10:1075–1081, 1972.
5. Appleton H, Buckley M, Thom BT, et al: Virus-like particles in winter vomiting disease. Lancet 1:1297, 1975.
6. Madeley CR, Cosgrove BP: Viruses in infantile gastroenteritis. (Letter) Lancet 2:124, 1975.
7. Willcocks MM, Carter MJ, Laidler FR, et al: Growth and characterisation of human faecal astrovirus in a continuous cell line. Arch Virol 113:73–81, 1990.
8. Jiang B, Monroe SS, Koonin EV, et al: RNA sequence of astrovirus: Distinctive genomic organization and a putative retrovirus-like ribosomal frameshifting signal that directs the viral replicase synthesis. PNAS USA 90:10539–10543, 1993.
9. Lewis TL, Greenberg HB, Herrmann JE, et al: Analysis of astrovirus serotype 1 RNA, identification of the viral RNA-dependent RNA polymerase motif, and expression of a viral structural protein. J Virol 68:77–83, 1994.
10. Willcocks MM, Brown TDK, Madeley CR, et al: The complete sequence of a human astrovirus. J Gen Virol 75:1785–1788, 1994.
11. Herrmann JE, Nowak NA, Perron-Henry DM, et al: Diagnosis of astrovirus gastroenteritis by antigen detection with monoclonal antibodies. J Infect Dis 161:226–229, 1990.
12. Herrmann JE, Hudson RW, Perron-Henry DM, et al. Antigenic characterization of cell-cultivated serotypes and development of astrovirus-specific monoclonal antibodies. J Infect Dis 158:182–185, 1988.
13. Taniguchi K, Urasawa T, Morita Y, et al: Direct serotyping of human rotavirus in stools using serotype 1-, 2-, 3-, and 4-specific monoclonal antibodies to VP7. J Infect Dis 155:1159–1166, 1987.
14. Jonasson TO, Kjeldsberg E, Grinde B: Detection of human astrovirus serotype 1 by the polymerase chain reaction. J Virological Methods 44:83–88, 1993.
15. Monroe SS, Jiang B, Stine SE, et al: Subgenomic RNA sequence of human astrovirus supports classification of Astroviridae as a new family of RNA viruses. J Virol 67:3611–3614, 1993.
16. Noel JS, Lee TW, Kurtz JB, et al: Typing of human astroviruses from clinical isolates by enzyme immunoassay and nucleotide sequencing. J Clin Microbiol 33:797–801, 1995.
17. Lee TW, Kurtz JB: Prevalence of human astrovirus serotypes in the Oxford region 1976–1992, with evidence for two new serotypes. Epidemiol Infect 112:187–193, 1994.
18. Noel J, Mansoor A, Thaker U, et al: Identification of adenoviruses in faeces from patients with diarrhoea at the Hospitals for Sick Children, London, 1989–1992. J Med Virol 43:84–90, 1994.
19. Dennehy PH, Nelson SM, Spangenberger S, et al: A prospective case-control study of the role of astrovirus in acute diarrhea among hospitalized young children. J Infect Dis 184:10–15, 2001.
20. Willcocks MM, Kurtz JB, Lee TW, et al: Prevalence of human astrovirus serotype 4: Capsid protein sequence and comparison with other strains. Epidemiol Infect 114:385–391, 1995.
21. Cunliffe NA, Dove W, Gondwe JS, et al: Detection and characterization of human astroviruses in children with acute gastroenteritis in Blantyre, Malawai. J Med Virol 67:563–566, 2002.
22. Guerrero ML, Noel JS, Mitchell DK, et al: A prospective study of astrovirus diarrhea of infancy in Mexico City. Pediatr Infect Dis J 17:723–727, 1998.
23. Lew JF, Moe CL, Monroe SS, et al: Astrovirus and adenovirus associated with diarrhea in children in day care settings. J Infect Dis 164:673–678, 1991.
24. Monroe SS, Glass RI, Noah N, et al: Electron microscopic reporting of gastrointestinal viruses in the United Kingdom, 1985–87. J Med Virol 33:193–198, 1991.
25. Mitchell DK, Van R, Morrow AL, et al: Outbreaks of astrovirus gastroenteritis in day care centers. J Pediatr 123:725–732, 1993.
26. Kurtz JB, Lee TW, Pickering D: Astrovirus associated gastroenteritis in a children's ward. J Clin Pathol 30:948–952, 1977.
27. Madeley CR, Cosgrove BP, Bell EJ, et al: Stool viruses in babies in Glasgow: 1. Hospital admissions with diarrhoea. J Hygiene 78:261–273, 1977.
28. Riepenhoff-Talty M, Saif LJ, Barret HJ, et al: Potential spectrum of etiological agents of viral enteritis in hospitalized infants. J Clin Microbiol 17:352–356, 1982.
29. Esahli H, Breback K, Bennet R, et al: Astroviruses as a cause of nosocomial outbreaks of infant diarrhea. Pediatr Infect Dis J 10:511–515, 1991.
30. Kotloff KL, Herrmann JE, Blacklow NR, et al: The frequency of astrovirus as a cause of diarrhea in Baltimore children. Pediatr Infect Dis J 11:587–589, 1992.
31. Bates PR, Bailey AS, Wood DJ, et al: Comparative epidemiology of rotavirus, subgenus F (Types 40 and 41) adenovirus, and astrovirus gastroenteritis in children. J Med Virol 39:224–228, 1993.
32. Maldonado Y, Cantwell M, Old M, et al: Population-based prevalence of symptomatic and asmptomatic astrovirus infection in rural Mayan infants. J Infect Dis 178:334–339, 1998.
33. Midthun K, Greenberg HB, Kurtz JB, et al: Characterization and seroepidemiology of a type 5 astrovirus associated with an outbreak of gastroenteritis in Marin County, California. J Clin Microbiol 31:955–962, 1993.
34. Pager C, Steele A: Astrovirus-associated diarreha in South African Adults. Clin Infect Dis 35:1452–1453, 2002.
35. Kurtz JB, Lee TW, Craig JW, et al: Astrovirus infection in volunteers. J Med Virol 3:221–230, 1979.
36. Oishi I, Yamazaki K, Kimoto T, et al: A large outbreak of acute gastroenteritis associated with astrovirus among students and teachers in Osaka, Japan. J Infect Dis 170:439–443, 1994.
37. Konno T, Suzuki H, Ishida N, et al: Astrovirus-associated epidemic gastroenteritis in Japan. J Med Virol 9:11–17, 1982.
38. Gray JJ, Wreghitt TG, Cubitt WD, et al: An outbreak of gastroenteritis in a home for the elderly associated with astrovirus type 1 and human calicivirus. J Med Virol 23:377–381, 1987.
39. Lewis DC, Lightfoot NF, Cubitt WD, et al: Outbreaks of astrovirus type 1 and rotavirus gastroenteritis in a geriatric in-patient population. J Hosp Infect 14:9–14, 1989.
40. Oshiro LS, Haley CE, Roberto RR, et al: A 27-nm virus isolated during an outbreak of acute infectious nonbacterial gastroenteritis in a convalescent hospital: A possible new serotype. J Infect Dis 143:791–795, 1981.
41. Eshali H, Breback K, Bennet R, et al: Astroviruses as a cause of nosocomial outbreaks of infant diarrhea. Pediatr Infect Dis J 10:511–515, 1991.
42. Moe CL, Allen JR, Monroe SS, et al: Detection of astrovirus in pediatric stool samples by immunoassay and RNA probe. J Clin Microbiol 29:2390–2395, 1991.
43. Donelli G, Ruggeri FM, Tinari A, et al: A three-year diagnostic and epidemiological study on viral infantile diarrhoea in Rome. Epidemiol Infect 100:311–320, 1988.
44. Herrmann JE, Taylor DN, Echeverria P, et al: Astroviruses as a cause of gastroenteritis in children. N Engl J Med 324:1757-1760, 1991.
45. Singh PB, Sreenivasan MA, Pavri KM: Viruses in acute gastroenteritis in children in Pune, India. Epidemiol Infect 102:345–353, 1989.
46. Cruz JR, Bartlett AV, Herrmann JE, et al: Astrovirus-associated diarrhea among Guatemalan ambulatory rural children. J Clin Microbiol 30:1140–1144, 1992.
47. Pavone R, Schinaia N, Hart CA, et al: Viral gastro-enteritis in children in Malawi. Ann Tropic Paediatr 10:15–20, 1990.
48. Avery RM, Shelton AP, Beards GM, et al: Viral agents associated with infantile gastroenteritis in Nigeria: Relative prevalence of adenovirus serotypes 40 and 41, astrovirus, and rotavirus serotypes 1 to 4. J Diarrhoeal Dis Res 10:105–108, 1992.

49. Waters V, Ford-Jones EL, Petric M, et al: Etiology of community-acquired pediatric viral diarrhea: a prospective longitudinal study in hospitals, emergency departments, pediatric practices and child care centers during the winter rotavirus outbreak, 1997–1998. Pediatr Infect Dis J 19:843–848, 2000.
50. Unicomb LE, Banu NN, Azim T, et al: Astrovirus infection in association with acute persistent and nosocomial diarrhea in Bangladesh. Pediatr Infect Dis J 17:605–611, 1998.
51. Mitchell DK, Monroe SS, Jiang X, et al: Virologic features of an astrovirus diarrhea outbreak in a day care center revealed by reverse transcription-polymerase chain reaction. J Infect Dis 172:1437–1444, 1995.
52. Silva A, Leite E, Assis R, et al: An outbreak of gastroenteritis associated with astrovirus serotype 1 in a day care center in Rio de Janeiro, Brazil. Memorias Institut Oswaldo Cruz 96:1069-1073, 2001.
53. Ashley CR, Caul EO, Paver WK: Astrovirus-associated gastroenteritis in children. J Clin Pathol 31:939–943, 1978.
54. Ford-Jones EL, Mindorff CM, Gold R, et al: The incidence of viral-associated diarrhea after admission to a pediatric hospital. Am J Epidemiol 131:711–718, 1990.
55. Tanaka H, Kisielius JJ, Ueda M, et al: Intrafamilial outbreak of astrovirus gastroenteritis in Sao Paulo, Brazil. J Diarrhoeal Dis Res 12:219–221, 1994.
56. Rodriguez-Baez N, O'Brien R, Qiu SQ, et al: Astrovirus, adenovirus, and rotavirus in hospitalized children: prevalence and association with gastroenteritis. J Pediatr Gastroenterol Nutr 35:64–68, 2002.
57. Abad FX, Pinto RM, Villena C, et al: Astrovirus survival in drinking water. Appl Environ Microbiol 63:3119–3122, 1997.
58. Nazar H, Rice S, Walker-Smith JA: Clinical associations of stool astrovirus in childhood. J Pediatr Gastroenterol Nutr 1:555–558, 1982.
59. Grohmann GS, Glass RI, Pereira HG, et al: Enteric viruses and diarrhea in HIV-infected patients. N Engl J Med 329:14–20, 1993.
60. Cox GJ, Matsui SM, Lo RS, et al: Etiology and outcome of diarrhea after marrow transplantation: A prospective study. Gastroenterol 107:1398–1407, 1994.
61. Cubitt WD, Mitchell DK, Carter MJ, et al: Application of electronmicroscopy, enzyme immunoassay, and RT-PCR to monitor an outbreak of astrovirus type 1 in a paediatric bone marrow transplant unit. J Med Virol 57:313–321, 1999.
62. Lew JF, Glass RI, Petric M: Six-year retrospective surveillance of gastroenteritis viruses indentified at ten electron microscopy centers in the U.S. and Canada. Pediatr Infect Dis J 9:709–714, 1991.
63. Madeley CR, Cosgrove BP: 28 nm particles in faeces in infantile gastroenteritis. Lancet 2:451–452, 1975.
64. Utagawa ET, Nishizawa S, Sekine S, et al: Astrovirus as a cause of gastroenteritis in Japan. J Clin Microbiol 32:1841–1845, 1994.
65. Glass RI, Noel JS, Mitchell D, et al: The changing epidemiology of astrovirus-associated gastroenteritis: a review. Arch Virol 12 (suppl):287–300, 1996.
66. Gary GW Jr., Hierholzer JC, Black RE: Characteristics of noncultivable adenoviruses associated with diarrhea in infants: a new subgroup of human adenoviruses. J Clin Microbiol 10:96–103, 1979.
67. DeJong JC, Wigand R, Kidd AH, et al: Candidate adenoviruses 40 and 41: Fastidious adenoviruses from human infant stool. J Med Virol 11:215–231, 1983.
68. Cruz JR, Caceres P, Cano F, et al: Adenovirus types 40 and 41 and rotaviruses associated with diarrhea in children from Guatemala. J Clin Microbiol 28:1780–1784, 1990.
69. Kidd AH, Banatvala JE, de Jong JC: Antibodies to fastidious faecal adenoviruses (species 40 and 41) sera from children. J Med Virol 11:333–341, 1983.
70. Tiemessen CT, Wegerhoff FO, Erasmus MJ, et al: Infection by enteric adenoviruses, rotaviruses, and other agents in a rural African environment. J Med Virol 28:176–182, 1989.
71. Uhnoo I, Wadell G, Svensson L, et al: Importance of enteric adenoviruses 40 and 41 in acute gastroenteritis in infants and young children. J Clin Microbiol 20:365–372, 1984.
72. Kotloff KL, Losonsky GA, Morris JG Jr, et al: Enteric adenovirus infection and childhood diarrhea: an epidemiologic study in three clinical settings. Pediatrics 84:219–225, 1989.
73. Kim K-H, Yang J-M, Joo S-I, et al: Importance of rotavirus and adenovirus types 40 and 41 in acute gastroenteritis in Korean children. J Clin Microbiol 28:2279–2284, 1990.
74. Herrmann JE, Blacklow NR, Perron-Henry DM, et al: Incidence of enteric adenoviruses among children in Thailand and the significance of these viruses in gastroenteritis. J Clin Microbiol 26:1783–1786, 1988.
75. Krajden M, Brown M, Petrasek A, et al: Clinical features of adenovirus enteritis: A review of 127 cases. Pediatr Infect Dis J 9:636–641, 1990.
76. Jarecki-Khan K, Tzipori SR, Unicomb LE: Enteric adenovirus infection among infants with diarrhea in rural Bangladesh. J Clin Microbiol 31:484–489, 1993.
77. Yolken RH, Lawrence F, Leister F, et al: Gastroenteritis associated with enteric type adenovirus in hospitalized infants. J Pediatr 101:21–26, 1982.
78. Richmond SJ, Caul EO, Dunn SM, et al: An outbreak of gastroenteritis in young children caused by adenoviruses. Lancet 1:1178–1181, 1979.
79. Saderi H, Roustai MH, Sabahi F, et al: Incidence of enteric adenovirus gastroenteritis in Iranian children. J Clin Virol 24:1–5, 2002.
80. Cevenini R, Mazzaarachio R, Rumpianesi F, et al: Prevalence of enteric adenovirus from acute gastroenteritis: A five year study. Eur J Epidemiol 3:147–150, 1987.
81. Janoff EN, Orenstein JM, Manischewitz JF, et al: Adenovirus colitis in the acquired immunodeficiency syndrome. Gastroenterol 100:976–979, 1991.
82. Hierholzer JC, Wigand R, Anderson LJ, et al: Adenoviruses from patients with AIDS: A plethora of serotypes and a description of five new serotypes of subgenus D (types 43–47). J Infect Dis 158:804–813, 1988.
83. Smith PD: Gastrointestinal infections in AIDS. Ann Intern Med 116:63–77, 1992.
84. Thomas PD, Pollok RC, Gazzard BG: Enteric viral infections as a cause of diarrhoea in the acquired immunodeficiency syndrome. HIV Med 1:19–24, 1999.
85. Krilov LR, Rubin LG, Frogel M, et al: Disseminated adenovirus infection with hepatic necrosis in patients with human immunodeficiency virus infection and other immunodeficiency states. Rev Infect Dis 12:303–307, 1990.
86. Yolken RH, Bishop CA, Townsend TR: Infectious gastroenteritis in bone-marrow transplant recipients. N Engl J Med 306:1009–1012, 1982.
87. Mavromichalis J, Evans N, McNeish A, et al: Intestinal damage in rotavirus and adenovirus gatroenteritis assessed by D-xylose malabsorption. Arch Dis Childhood 52:589–591, 1977.
88. Grimwood K, Carzino R, Barnes G, et al: Patients with enteric adenovirus gastroenteritis admitted to an Australian teaching hospital from 1981 to 1992. J Clin Microbiol 33:131–136, 1995.
89. Centers for Disease Control: Viral agents of gastroenteritis: Public health importance and outbreak management. MMWR 39:1–24, 1990.
90. Uhnoo I, Olding-Stenkvist E, Kreuger A: Clinical features of acute gastroenteritis associated with rotavirus, enteric adenoviruses, and bacteria. Arch Dis Childhood 61:732–738, 1986.
91. Chiba S, Nakata S, Nakamura I, et al: Outbreak of infantile gastroenteritis due to type 40 adenovirus. Lancet 2:954–957, 1983.
92. Shinozaki T, Araki K, Ushijima H, et al: Antibody response to enteric adenovirus types 40 and 41 in sera from people in various age groups. J Clin Microbiol 25:1679–1682, 1987.
93. Unicomb LE, Jarecki-Khan K, Hall A, et al: Previous enteric adenovirus infection does not protect against subsequent symptomatic infection: Longitudinal follow-up of eight infants. Microbiol Immunol 40:161–168, 1996.
94. Brandt CD, Rodrigues WJ, Kim HW, et al: Rapid presumptive recognition of diarrhea-associated adenoviruses. J Clin Microbiol 20:1008–1009, 1984.
95. Leite JPG, Pereira HG, Azeredo RS, et al: Adenovirus in faeces of children with acute gastroenteritis in Rio de Janeiro, Brazil. J Med Virol 15:203–209, 1985.
96. Wood DJ, Bailey AS: Detection of adenovirus types 40 and 41 in stool specimens by immune electron microscopy. J Med Virol 21:191–199, 1987.
97. Svensson L, von Bonsdorff CH: Solid-phase immune electron microscopy (SPIEM) by use of protein A and its application for characterization of selected adenovirus serotypes. J Med Virol 10:242–253, 1982.

98. Wood DJ, Bijlsma K, Dejong JC, et al: Evaluation of a commercial monoclonal antibody-based enzyme immunoassay for detection of adenovirus types 40 and 41 in stool specimens. J Clin Microbiol 27:1155–1158, 1989.
99. Singh-Naz N, Rodriguez WJ, Kidd AH, et al: Monoclonal antibody enzyme-linked immunosorbent assay for specific identification and typing of subgroup F adenoviruses. J Clin Microbiol 26:297–300, 1988.
100. Johansson ME, Uhnoo I, Kidd AH, et al: Direct identification of enteric adenovirus, a candidate new serotype, associated with infantile gastroenteritis. J Clin Microbiol 12:95–100, 1980.
101. Herrman JE, Perron-Henry DM, Blacklow NR: Antigen detection with monoclonal antibodies for the diagnosis of adenovirus gastroenteritis. J Infect Dis 155:1167–1171, 1987.
102. August MJ, Warford AL: Evaluation of a commercial monoclonal antibody for detection of adenovirus antigen. J Clin Microbiol 25:2233–2235, 1987.
103. Ahluwalia G, Scott-Taylor T, Klisko B, et al: Compmarison of detection methods for adenovirus from enteric clinical specimens. Diagn Microbiol Infect Dis 18:161–166, 1994.
104. Takiff HE, Stauss SE, Garon CF: Propagation and in vitro studies of previously non-cultivatable enteral adenoviruses in 293 cells. Lancet 2:832–834, 1981.
105. Pereira HG, Flewett TH, Candeias JN, et al: A virus with bisegmented double-stranded RNA genome in rat (*Oryzomys nigripes*) intestines. J Gen Virol 69:2749–2754, 1988.
106. Pereira HG, de Araujo HP, Fialho AM, et al: A virus with bisegmented double-stranded RNA genome in guinea pig intestines. Memorias Instit Oswald Cruz 84:137–140, 1989.
107. Gatti MSV, Pestana de Castro AF, Ferraz MMG, et al: Viruses with bisegmented double-stranded RNA in pig faeces. Res Veter Sci 47:397–398, 1989.
108. Chasey D: Porcine picobirnavirus in UK? Veterin Record 126:465, 1990.
109. Vanopdenbosch E, Wellemans G: Bovine birna type virus: A new etiological agent of neonatal calf diarrhoea? Vlaams Diergeneeskd Tijdschr 59:1–4, 1990.
110. Gallimore C, Lewis D, Brown D: Detection and characterization of a novel bisegmented double-stranded RNA virus (picobirnavirus) from rabbit faeces. Arch Virol 133:63–73, 1993.
111. Leite JPG, Monteiro SP, Fialho AM, et al: A novel avian virus with trisegmented double-stranded RNA and further observations on previously described similar viruses with bisegmented genome. Virus Res 16:119–126, 1990.
112. Ludert JE, Liprandi F: Identification of viruses with bi- and trisegmented double-stranded RNA genome in faeces of children with gastroenteritis. Institut Pasteur/Elsevier 144:219–224, 1993.
113. Gallimore C, Green J, Casemore D, et al: Detection of picobirnavirus associated with *Cryptosporidium* positive stools from humans. Arch Virol 140:1275–1278, 1995.
114. Pereira HG, Fialho AM, Flewett TH, et al: Novel viruses in human feces. Lancet 2:103–104, 1988.
115. Banyai K, Jakab F, Reuter G, et al: Sequence heterogeneity among human picobirnaviruses detected in a gastroenteritis outbreak. Arch Virol 148:2281–2291, 2003.
116. Giordano MO, Martinez LC, Rinaldi D, et al: Diarrhea and enteric emerging viruses in HIV-infected patients. AIDS Res Hum Retroviruses 15:1427–1432, 1999.
117. Caul EO, Paver WK, Clarke SK: Coronavirus particles in faeces from patients with gastroenteritis (letter). Lancet 1:1192, 1975.
118. Mathan M, Mathan VI, Swaminathan SP, et al: Pleomorphic virus-like particles in human faeces. Lancet 1:1068–1069, 1975.
119. Clarke SK, Caul EO, Egglestone SI: The human enteric coronaviruses. Postgrad Med J 55:135–142, 1979.
120. Macnaughton MR, Davies HA: Human enteric coronaviruses. Arch Virol 70:301–313, 1981.
121. Schnagl RD, Morey R, Homes IH: Rotavirus and coronavirus-like particles in aboriginal and non-aboriginal neonates in Kalgoorlie and Alice Springs. Med J Aust 2:178, 1979.
122. Vaucher YE, Ray CG, Minnich LL, et al: Pleomorphic, enveloped, virus-like particles associated with gastrointestinal illness in neonates. J Infect Dis 145:27, 1982.
123. Yognian H, Wang N, Lo H, et al: A finding of coronavirus particles in feces of patients with diarrhea. Chin J Epidemiol 8:25, 1987.
124. Bennett PH, Gust ID: Coronavirus-like particles and other agents in the faeces of children in Efate, Vanuatu. J Trop Med Hyg 85:213, 1982.
125. Simhon A, Mata L: Fecal rotaviruses, adenoviruses, coronavirus-like particles, and small round viruses in a cohort of rural Costa Rican children. Am J Trop Med Hyg 34:931–936, 1985.
126. Sitbon M: Human-enteric-coronavirus-like particles (CVLP) with differnet epidemiological characteristics. J Med Virol 16:67, 1985.
127. Payne CM, Ray CG, Bourdin V, et al: An eight-year study of the viral agents of acute gastroenteritis in humans: Ultrastructural observations and seasonal distribution with a major emphasis on coronavirus-like particles. Diagn Microbiol Infect Dis 5:39–54, 1986.
128. Kidd A, Esrey S, Ujfalusi M: Shedding of coronavirus-like particles by children in Lesotho. J Med Virol 27:164–169, 1989.
129. Gerna G, Passarani N, Battaglia M, et al: Coronaviruses and gastroenteritis: Evidence of antigenic relatedness between human enteric coronavirus strains and human coronavirus OC43. Microbiol Rev 7:315, 1984.
130. Mortensen ML, Ray CG, Payne CM, et al: Coronavirus-like particles in human gastrointestinal disease. Am J Dis Child 139:928, 1985.
131. Noel J, Cubitt D: Identification of astrovirus serotypes from children treated at the Hospitals for Sick Children, London 1981–93. Epidemiol Infect 113:153–159, 1994.
132. Chany C, Moscovici O, Lebon P, et al: Association of coronavirus-like infection with neonatal necrotizing enterocolitis. Pediatr 69:209–214, 1982.
133. Rousset S, Moscovici O, Lebon P, et al: Intestinal lesions containing coronavirus-like particles in neonatal necrotizing enterocolitis: an ultrastructural analysis. Pediatr 73:413–422, 1984.
134. Baker SJ, Mathan M, Mathan VI, et al: Chronic enterocyte infection with coronavirus: One possible cause of the syndrome of tropical sprue? Digest Dis Sci 27:1039–1043, 1982.
135. Lee N, Hui D, Wu A, et al: A major outbreak of severe acute respiratory syndrome in Hong Kong. N Engl J Med 358:1986–1994, 2003.
136. Wang J-T, Sheng W-H, Fang C-T, et al: Clinical manifestations, laboratory findings and treatment outcomes of SAS patients. Emerg Infect 10:818–831, 2004.
137. Lai M, Holmes K: Coronaviridae: The viruses and their replication. In D. Knipe PH (ed): Fields Virology, Vol. 1, 4th ed. Philadelphia, Lippincott, Williams and Wilkins, 2001, pp 1163–1186.
138. Weiss M, Horzinek M: The proposed family Toroviridae: Agents of enteric infections. Arch Virol 92:1–15, 1987.
139. Koopmans M, Horzinek M: Toroviruses of animals and humans (a review). Adv Virus Res 43:233–273, 1994.
140. Koopmans MPG, Goosen ESM, Lima AAM, et al: Association of torovirus with acute and persistent diarrhea in children. Pediatr Infect Dis J 16:504-507, 1997.
141. Beards GM, Green J, Hall C, et al: An enveloped virus in stools of children and adults with gastroenteritis that resembles the Breda virus of calves. Lancet 1:1050–1052, 1984.
142. Koopmans M, Snijder EJ, Horzinek MC: cDNA probes for the detection of bovine torovirus (Breda virus) infections. J Clin Microbiol 29:493–497, 1991.
143. Koopmans M, Petric M, Glass RI, Monroe SS: Enzyme-linked immunosorbent assay reactivity of torovirus-like particles in fecal specimens from humans with diarrhea. J Clin Microbiol 31:2738–2744, 1993.
144. Koopmans M, van den Boom U, Woode G, Horzinek MC: Seroepidemiology of Breda virus in cattle using ELISA. Veter Microbiol 19:223–243, 1989.
145. Fagerland JA, Pohlenz JFL, Woode GN: A morphologic study of the replication of Breda virus (proposed family Toroviridae) in bovine intestinal cells. J Gen Virol 67:1293–1304, 1986.
146. Brown DWG, Beards GM, Flewett TH: Detection of Breda virus antigen and antibody in humans and animals by enzyme immunoassay. J Clin Microbiol 24:637–640, 1987.
147. Appleton H, Higgins PG: Viruses and gastroenteritis in infants (letter). Lancet 1:1297, 1975.
148. Gomez J, Estes MK, Matson DO, et al: Serotyping of human rotaviruses in Argentina by ELISA with monoclonal antibodies. Arch Viro 112:249–259, 1990.

149. Appleton H: Small round viruses: Classification and role in food-borne infections. In Ciba Foundation Symposium, Bock G, Whelan J (eds): Novel diarrhoea viruses. New York, John Wiley & Sons, 1987, pp 108–125.
150. Ramos-Alvarez M: Cytopathogenic enteric viruses associated with undifferentiated diarrheal syndromes in early childhood. Ann NY Acad Sci 67:326–331, 1957.
151. Ramos-Alvarez M, Sabin AB: Enteropathogenic viruses and bacteria. Role in summer diarrheal diseases of infancy and early childhood. JAMA 167:147–156, 1958.
152. Rosen L, Hovis JF, Mastrota FM, et al: An outbreak of infection with a type 1 reovirus among children in an institution. Am J Hygiene 71:266–274, 1960.
153. Yolken R, Dubovi E, Leister F, et al: Infantile gastroenteritis associated with excretion of pestivirus antigens. Lancet 1:517–520, 1989.

64

Viral Hepatitis

MARTIN TAGLE
STANLEY M. LEMON
EUGENE R. SCHIFF

INTRODUCTION

Viral hepatitis is an important cause of morbidity and mortality worldwide, particularly in the tropics. It is caused by no fewer than five distinct viruses, each with unique molecular characteristics and replication cycles but sharing a common tropism for the liver and overlapping clinical patterns of disease. In most tropical areas, clinically apparent acute viral hepatitis is uncommon among local people, since infection is acquired early in life and most often is subclinical. On the other hand, sporadic cases are frequent among visitors, and outbreaks of the enterically transmitted viruses have occasionally been reported when food or water becomes contaminated with human feces.[1] The general characteristics of the different hepatitis viruses are shown in Table 64-1.

Hepatitis A

Hepatitis A is endemic in most tropical and subtropical regions of the world but is seldom diagnosed, since most infections are anicteric and acquired during childhood.[1] Outbreaks of hepatitis were described in Europe in the 17th and 18th centuries.[2] Epidemiologic analysis that led to the differentiation between hepatitis A ("infectious hepatitis") and hepatitis B ("serum hepatitis") came from studies done among troops during World War II.[2,3] The hepatitis A virus was isolated in cell culture for the first time in 1979.

AGENT

Hepatitis A virus (HAV) belongs to the family Picornaviridae, which includes the enteroviruses and rhinoviruses. HAV is a nonenveloped, single-stranded RNA virus, measuring approximately 27 to 28 nm in diameter. The linear genome (Fig. 64-1) is of positive or mRNA polarity and has a poly(A) tail at its 3′ end.[4] The virus genome serves as the RNA message for translation of virus-specific proteins, which begins immediately after penetration of the cell and uncoating and is not dependent on virus replication or RNA transcription. HAV is relatively heat-stable and is inactivated by autoclaving, ultraviolet radiation, formalin. and iodine. HAV is destroyed by boiling within 5 minutes, but steaming of shellfish may not be sufficient to destroy infectivity.[5]

EPIDEMIOLOGY

HAV is found in high titers in stools of infected persons, and the principal mode of transmission is fecal-oral. Person-to-person contact with infected family members remains one of the most important mechanisms of HAV transmission. Food-borne or waterborne transmission is promoted by the high stability of the virion in the environment and can occur when food or water is contaminated with HAV and ingested by susceptible persons. Some of the vehicles involved in outbreaks of HAV include raw or partially cooked shellfish, milk, salad, and hamburgers. Recently, an outbreak of hepatitis A involving 555 persons was reported, associated with consumption of green onions at a restaurant in Pennsylvania.[6] There were three deaths due to fulminant hepatitis. Green onions and other selected produce items (e.g., strawberries) may be more vulnerable to contamination because plant surfaces are particularly complex or prone to adherence of viral or fecal particles.[7] In addition, such produce is frequently imported unprocessed into the United States from Mexico and other countries with high HAV endemicity.

HAV is highly endemic in less developed countries, where most persons acquire the infection in early childhood.[2,8]

Table 64-1 Characteristics of the Hepatitis Viruses

	Hepatitis A (HAV)	Hepatitis B (HBV)	Hepatitis C (HCV)	Hepatitis D (HDV)	Hepatitis E (HEV)
Nucleic acid	RNA	DNA	RNA	RNA	RNA
Antigens (Ag)	HAV Ag	HBsAg, HBcAg, HBeAg	Core, E2, NS3	HDV Ag	HEV Ag
Antibodies	IgM anti-HAV IgG anti-HAV	Anti-HBs Anti-HBc Anti-HBe	Anti-HCV	IgM anti-HDV IgG anti-HDV	Anti-HEV
Mode of transmission	Fecal-oral	Percutaneous, sexual, vertical	Percutaneous, ?sexual, ?perinatal	Percutaneous, sexual	Fecal-oral
Risk of chronicity	No	Yes	Yes	Yes	No
Vaccine available	Yes	Yes	No	No	No
Incubation period (days)	15–60	30–160	15–180	21–160	15–60

HBcAg, hepatitis B core antigen; HBeAg, hepatitis B e antigen; HBsAg, hepatitis B surface antigen.

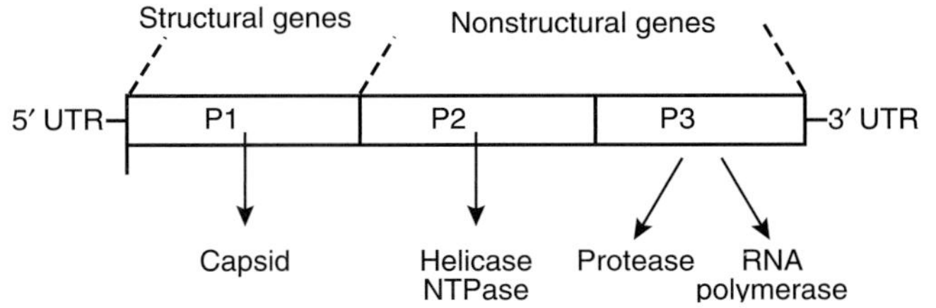

FIGURE 64-1 Hepatitis A genome. The boxed region represents the polyprotein coding segment. NTPase, nucleoside 5′-triphosphatase; UTR, untranslated RNA.

Areas of high endemicity, where travelers are particularly susceptible to acquire the infection, include most of Africa, Asia, and Central and South America. In some parts of the world with lower endemicity, such as Eastern Europe, the former Soviet Union, and parts of Asia, children may escape infection during childhood, but reported rates of hepatitis A can be paradoxically higher owing to transmission to older age persons, who are more likely to have clinically overt disease. A gradient from northern to southern Europe exists, in which hepatitis A is almost nonexistent in Scandinavian countries but relatively prevalent in Mediterranean countries.[2] The rates of hepatitis A in the United States have been decreasing gradually over the past several decades, probably as a result of improvement in water supplies, sewage disposal, and reduced crowding.[8]

Occasionally, large foodborne outbreaks occur, such as in Shanghai in 1988, associated with ingestion of raw shellfish.[9] In the early 1980s, an increase in the number of injection-drug users with hepatitis A was observed in the United States. This increase reached a peak in 1986, when 19% of reported cases of hepatitis A were associated with intravenous drug abuse[10] and likely reflects parenteral transmission of the virus. In 1991, there was a marked increase in the number of cases of hepatitis A reported among homosexual men in the United States, Canada, and Australia, probably related to sexual practices.[11] The mechanism of transmission of hepatitis A in this setting is likely due to oral-anal contact.[9] In serologic surveys, anti-HAV-positive persons reported more frequent oral-anal contact, longer duration of homosexual activity, and a larger number of sexual partners than persons without serologic evidence of HAV infection.[12,13] Outbreaks of hepatitis A have been reported in health care personnel working in a burn unit[14] and in neonatal intensive care units.[15] Transmission of HAV by blood transfusion is rare, but donors in the prodromal phase of infection have been shown to transmit the virus by this route.[15–17] Approximately 50% of patients do not have a source identified for their infection.[18] In the United States, anti-HAV prevalence varies directly with age: Among persons 6 to 11 years of age, the prevalence is 9%; 20 to 29 years of age, 19%; 40 to 49 years of age, 33%; and greater than 70 years of age, 75%.[19] Anti-HAV prevalence is inversely related to income and household size.[19] In developing countries, the disease is hyperendemic, and most infections occur early in childhood.[8,20] Different patterns of antibody prevalence may be seen in populations belonging to high and low socioeconomic status from the same developing country.

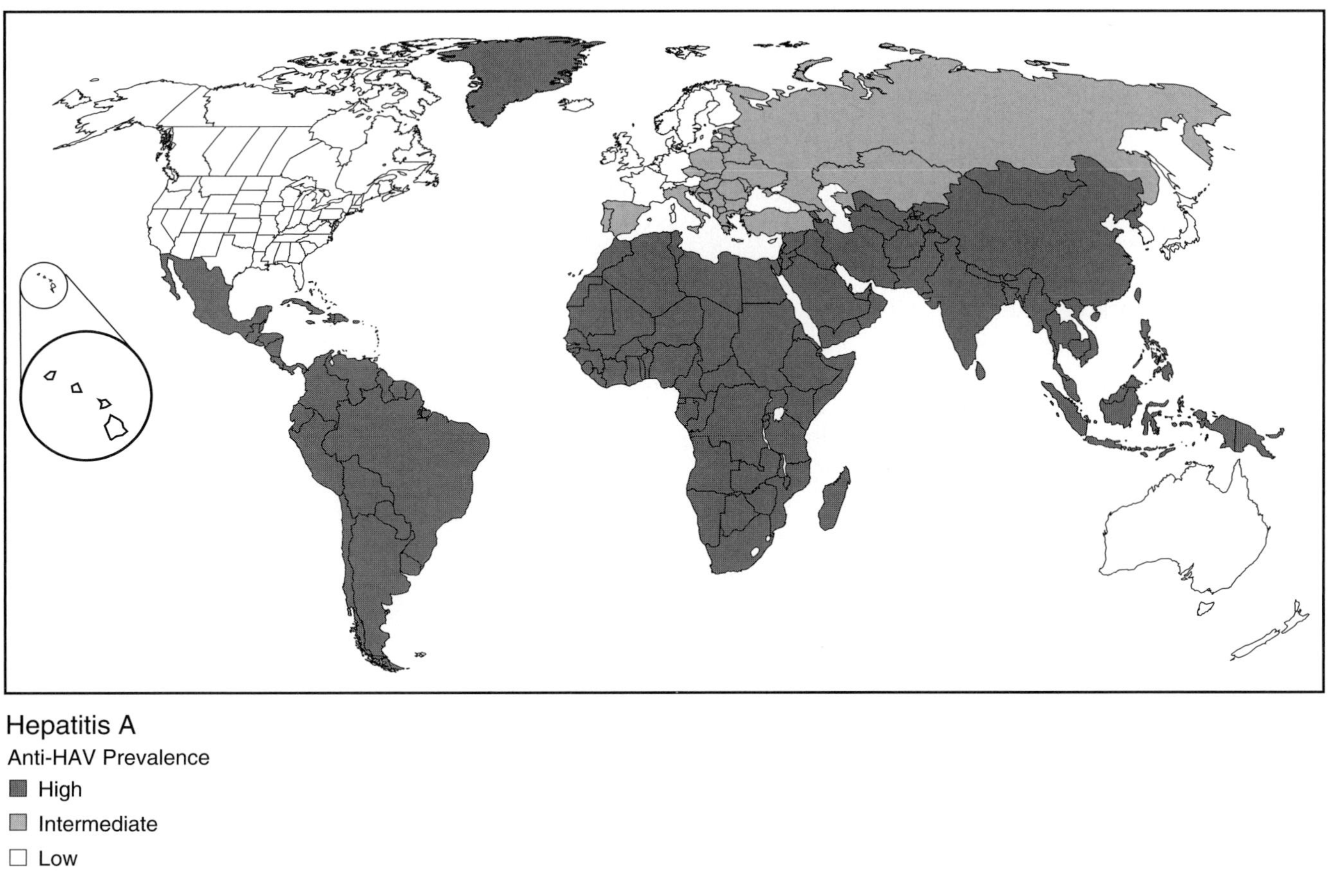

DISEASE

Hepatitis A is very often a subclinical infection of the liver, usually running an anicteric course, particularly in children. The likelihood of having symptoms with HAV infection is related to the person's age. In children less than 6 years of age, most (70%) infections are asymptomatic; if illness does occur, it is not usually accompanied by jaundice. Among older children and adults, infection is usually symptomatic, with jaundice occurring in greater than 70% of patients.[21] Most cases occur 2 to 6 weeks following exposure to the virus (incubation period). HAV has been documented in stool samples 2 to 3 weeks prior to the development of symptoms. The disease course is usually benign, starting with a mild prodromal phase appearing 1 to 7 days prior to the onset of dark urine,[17] including flulike symptoms, fever, malaise, anorexia, and nausea induced by fatty foods or tobacco. Most patients seek medical attention when they experience dark urine (choluria), which is followed by light-colored stools and jaundice. On physical examination, tender hepatomegaly may be present, and splenomegaly can be detected in about 15% of cases. In a significant proportion of patients, the appearance of jaundice is associated with rapid resolution of symptoms. The duration of illness is variable but usually lasts about 3 weeks. Prematurely born infants have been reported to shed HAV for longer periods than adults, possibly up to several months after the onset of illness.[22] Hepatitis A may run a protracted course, and in some cases, jaundice can last 12 to 18 weeks, with marked pruritus and fever (cholestatic hepatitis),[23] but recovery is the rule, and there are no chronic sequelae in the liver.[24] Relapsing hepatitis A can occur, in which exacerbations of symptoms and liver test abnormalities are found weeks to months after the onset of acute illness, but complete resolution is anticipated as well. Chronic shedding of HAV in feces does not occur; however, shedding can occur in persons who have relapsing illness.[25] Extrahepatic manifestations of hepatitis A are uncommon. Cutaneous vasculitis with IgM deposits,[26] cryoglobulinemia,[27] and cholecystitis[28] have been reported, along with neurologic syndromes such as Guillain-Barré, myelopathy, mononeuritis, meningoencephalitis, or exacerbation of pre-existing multiple sclerosis.[29] Hepatitis A infection can also behave as a triggering factor for autoimmune hepatitis, which should be suspected in patients with persistently elevated aminotransferase levels months after the resolution of the icteric phase.[30] The age at the time of diagnosis is an important determinant of prognosis.[31,32] Infection in the very young is associated with an asymptomatic or mild infection, although fulminant cases occur in very young children, whereas infection in adults older than 50 years of age is more likely to be associated with a fulminant course. Warning signs of this complication include irritability, changes in sleep pattern, and confusion. Although not at increased risk for HAV infection, persons who have chronic liver disease of any etiology are at increased risk for fulminant hepatitis A[33,34] should they become infected.

PATHOGENESIS AND IMMUNITY

HAV is transmitted by the fecal-oral route, possibly replicating initially in the epithelial cells of the small intestine, after which it reaches the liver through the portal circulation. The liver is the major site of replication, which occurs in the hepatocyte.[35] After intrahepatocyte replication, the virus is shed into the sinusoids and biliary canaliculi, passing into the intestine and then being eliminated in feces. Extrahepatic sites of replication such as the oropharynx have been postulated,[36] but the disease is essentially confined to the liver. In cell culture, most HAV isolates are not cytopathic; thus the liver injury is most likely due to a cell-mediated immune response.[31,37] During acute HAV infection, viremia and fecal shedding of virus occur within days of infection and typically persist until the appearance of symptoms. Initially IgM is produced, followed by IgG, and they both function as neutralizing antibodies in vitro.[31] Anti-HAV IgG persists throughout life and confers complete protection against reinfection with HAV.

DIAGNOSIS

Elevation of aminotransferase levels (ALT, AST) is a sensitive, although nonspecific, indicator of parenchymal liver damage. However, there is no correlation between clinical severity and degree of transaminase elevation. Prothrombin time prolongation is a sign of severity, especially when associated with changes in mental status. High levels of alkaline phosphatase are seen in cholestatic hepatitis. Serologic diagnosis requires measurement of immunoglobulin M to the HAV particle (IgM anti-HAV), which usually is present during the acute phase of illness, declining and becoming undetectable 3 to 6 months after the infection (Fig. 64-2). IgG anti-HAV becomes detectable during the acute phase, reaching high titers during convalescence, persisting for life and conferring permanent immunity. HAV RNA can be detected in the blood and stool of most persons during the acute phase of infection by use of nucleic acid amplification methods, and nucleic acid sequencing has been used to determine the relatedness of HAV isolates. However, these methods, available in only a limited number of research laboratories, generally are not used for diagnostic purposes.[7]

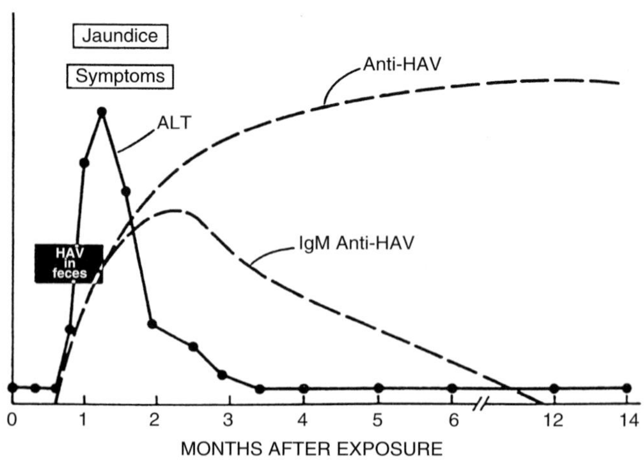

FIGURE 64-2 Serologic diagnosis of hepatitis A. ALT, alanine transaminase; HAV, hepatitis A virus; anti-HAV, antibody to HAV. (From Hoofnagle JH, Di Bisceglie AM: Serologic diagnosis of acute and chronic viral hepatitis. Semin Liver Dis 11:73, 1991.)

TREATMENT AND PROGNOSIS

There is no specific therapy for HAV infection, and management is essentially supportive. The identification of patients requiring liver transplantation becomes critical when there is development of hepatic encephalopathy, although even in fulminant cases spontaneous recovery occurs more frequently than in hepatitis B. With careful selection, the survival rate for fulminant hepatitis A patients after transplantation is 80%.[38] In uncomplicated cases of hepatitis A, there is no indication for admission to the hospital, and no data support prolonged bed rest or dietary restriction as measures that favorably affect the clinical course.

PREVENTION AND CONTROL

Good hygiene practices, especially for persons who work in the food industry, are important. Travelers to endemic areas should be advised against eating raw and uncooked food, with particular emphasis on vegetables, shellfish, and impure drinking water. Immunoglobulin (IG) provides protection against hepatitis A through passive transfer of antibody. IG for both intramuscular administration (IGIM) and intravenous administration (IGIV) contains anti-HAV, but IGIM is the product used for the prevention of HAV infection. The only generally accepted indication for passive immunization with immunoglobulin before exposure (pre-exposure immunoprophylaxis) of hepatitis A is travel to endemic areas.[39] Serum levels of neutralizing antibodies persist for approximately 18 weeks. Whenever possible, immunoglobulin should be administered 2 weeks before departure. When used for pre-exposure prophylaxis, a dose of IG (0.02 mL/kg) administered intramuscularly (IM) confers protection for about 3 months, and a dose of 0.06 mL/kg IG administered IM confers protection for about 5 months. When administered within 2 weeks following an exposure to HAV (0.02 mL/kg IM), IG is greater than 85% effective in preventing hepatitis A.[40] Efficacy is greatest when IG is administered early in the incubation period; when administered later in the incubation period, IG often only attenuates the clinical expression of HAV infection.[40] Postexposure prophylaxis is recommended especially for close personal contacts such as household and sexual partners, regardless of the age of the contact. Immunoglobulin prophylaxis is not recommended for casual contacts of hepatitis A patients (i.e., at school or work). The recommended dose is 0.02 mL/kg IM within 2 weeks of exposure. No transmission of hepatitis B virus, HIV, HCV, or other viruses has been reported from IGIM.

In 1995, an inactivated hepatitis A vaccine (Havrix) was licensed by the Food and Drug Administration (FDA) in the United Stated for use in persons aged more than 2 years to prevent HAV infection.[41] Hepatitis A vaccine is not approved for use in children younger than 2 years of age because of concern that children who have passively acquired maternal antibodies will have a diminished response to vaccine.[42] It is recommended for travelers to endemic areas and other high-risk groups. Each milliliter of the Havrix vaccine for adults contains 1440 ELU (ELISA units) of viral antigen. The recommended dose for adults is 1 mL IM in the deltoid muscle, plus a 1-mL booster dose 6 to 12 months later.[41] Protective levels of specific humoral antibodies are detectable in 80% to 98% of adult recipients 15 days after the first dose and in 96% after 1 month.[43] Another inactivated hepatitis A vaccine

Table 64-2 Hepatitis A Vaccines

	Havrix	VAQTA
Recommended dose	2–18 yr: 720 ELU >19 yr: 1440 ELU (1 mL)	2–17 yr: 25 units* >18 yr: 50 units
Approved schedule of administration	0, 6–12 mo (adults and children)	0, 6 mo (adults) 0, 6–18 mo (children)
Injection site	Deltoid	Deltoid
Duration of immunity	10–20 yr	10–20 yr

ELU, enzyme-linked immunosorbent assay units.
*1 unit = 1 ng hepatitis A virus antigen.

(VAQTA) has been licensed in the United States, and comparative features of these two vaccines, which are similar with respect to their clinical attributes, are shown in Table 64-2.

Both licensed vaccines are highly immunogenic in persons aged 18 years of age or older when administered according to the recommended schedules.[44,45] Protective antibody levels develop in 94% to 100% of adults 1 month after the first dose. After the second dose, all persons have protective levels of antibody. On the other hand, in some studies, administration of hepatitis A vaccine to persons with HIV infection resulted in lower seroconversion rates and antibody concentrations.[46,47] Among HIV-infected men, those who respond to hepatitis A vaccination have significantly more $CD4^+$ T lymphocytes at baseline (540/μL) compared with those who do not respond (280/μL).[47] Estimates of antibody persistence derived from kinetic models of antibody decline indicate that protective levels of anti-HAV could be present for 20 years or longer.[48] Immunization policy should be tailored to the specific population. Persons at high risk for HAV infection, including homosexually active men, persons with multiple sexual contacts, and travelers to endemic regions, should consider immunization, as well as those at risk for severe disease if infected, such as those with chronic hepatitis C.[49] Prevaccination screening for anti-HAV might be cost effective in high and intermediate endemic regions, but costs of testing and availability of vaccine should be taken into account.

In May 2001, the FDA licensed a combined hepatitis A and B vaccine (Twinrix) for use in persons aged 18 years or older.[50] Twinrix contains the antigenic components used in Havrix and Engerix-B. The antigenic components in Twinrix have been used routinely in separate single-antigen vaccines in the United States since 1995 and 1989 as hepatitis A and B vaccines, respectively (Table 64-3; see also Prevention of hepatitis B, in the following section). The efficacy of Twinrix is expected to be comparable to that of existing single-antigen hepatitis vaccines. The persistence of anti-HAV and anti-HBs following Twinrix administration is similar to that following single-antigen hepatitis A and B vaccine administration at 4 years' follow-up (unpublished data, GlaxoSmithKline Biologicals, 2001).

Hepatitis B

Human hepatitis B infection is still a major health problem throughout the world. It may evolve into chronic hepatitis and is a common cause of cirrhosis and hepatocellular carcinoma.

Table 64-3 Doses and Recommended Schedule for Combined Hepatitis A and B Vaccine

Vaccine	Age Group	Antigens Used	Volume	No. of Doses	Schedule
Twinrix	18 years and older	Havrix (720 ELU) combined with Engerix-B (20 mg)	1.0 mL	3	0, 1, and 6 mo

Hepatitis B ("serum hepatitis") emerged in importance in the first half of the 20th century with the increased use of syringes and needles for the treatment of syphilis and administration of insulin in diabetics.[2] Large epidemics of bloodborne hepatitis followed the administration of yellow fever vaccines containing human serum. The association of hepatitis B specifically with blood and blood products was recognized as distinct from hepatitis A in volunteer studies, and the agent was first transmitted to chimpanzees in the 1970s.

AGENT

Hepatitis B virus (HBV) is a member of the family Hepadnaviridae, genus *Orthohepadnavirus*. Other hepadnaviruses have been described in the woodchuck, ground squirrel, tree squirrel, and domestic duck. The hepadnaviruses are a family of hepatotropic, DNA-containing viruses that share several features. Morphologically, the intact virions are 42 nm in diameter and frequently found in association with 20-nm, DNA-free, spherical and tubular particles containing the surface glycoprotein (HBsAg).[51] Humans cannot be infected by the nonhuman hepadnaviruses. There is an inner nucleocapsid, composed mainly of a phosphoprotein, hepatitis B core antigen (HBcAg), which forms active complexes with the viral polymerase that generates the mature double-stranded DNA genome. HBcAg also plays a role in packaging pregenomic RNA. The HBV genome is composed of circular DNA (Fig. 64-3) that is only partially double-stranded.[52] Based on comparisons of nucleotide sequences, the HBV sequences have been classified into eight genotypes at present, named A through H, with important geographic and clinical differences[53–55] (see Epidemiology).

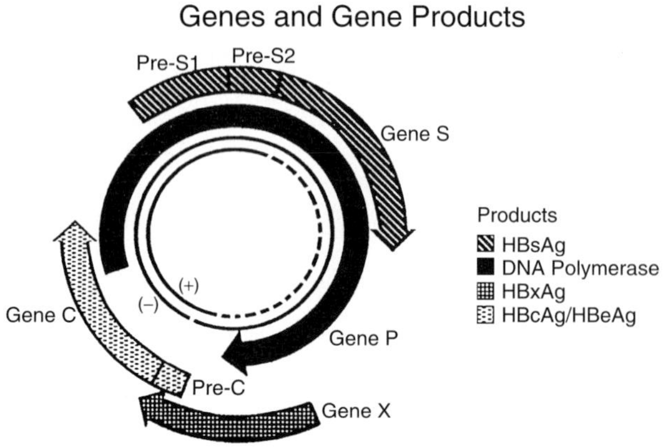

FIGURE 64-3 Hepatitis B genome. HBsAg, hepatitis B surface antigen; HBxAg, hepatitis B x antigen; HBcAg/HBeAg, hepatitis B core antigen/hepatitis B e antigen. (From Koff RS, Dienstag GL, Riely CA, et al: AGA Clinical Teaching Project, Unit 3, Viral Hepatitis, 2nd ed. Timonium, Md., Milner-Fenwick, 1994.)

One DNA strand is complete except for a small nick (the minus strand), while the other is incomplete (the plus strand). Minus-strand DNA is synthesized from an RNA template, the "pregenome," by reverse transcription, while plus-strand DNA is transcribed within the nascent virus particle from packaged minus-strand DNA. Both reactions are catalyzed by the same virally encoded enzyme, the HBV DNA polymerase, which is packaged within virus particles. Transcription of plus-strand DNA is terminated upon exit of the virus particle from the cell and completed only upon entry into a new cell at the beginning of the virus life cycle. Minus-strand DNA directs the transcription of messenger sense RNAs containing four overlapping reading frames that encode the structural proteins (the surface, or envelope, protein and the core protein), the polymerase (pol), and a protein of uncertain function (X). Carefully regulated expression of the core protein reading frame leads to two distinct proteins:[51,56] the core protein itself (HBcAg) and a closely related polypeptide called hepatitis B e antigen (HBeAg). HBeAg is a soluble nonstructural protein with an ill-defined function, although its presence correlates with circulating HBV DNA in serum. The precore region of the core reading frame can undergo a G-to-A mutation, resulting in the formation of a stop codon at nt 1896 that abolishes the synthesis of HBeAg (precore mutant).[54] Expression of the surface protein reading frame (S) is similarly complex. The S reading frame includes an upstream pre-S region, which encodes two minor surface protein species, pre-S1 and pre-S2, that share a common carboxyl terminus with the major surface protein, HBsAg. These proteins are likely to contain sites for the binding of the HBV to hepatocytes and are highly immunogenic. There are data suggesting that the pre-S proteins appear in serum coincidentally with the period of active HBV replication and disappear when viral replication diminishes.[57] A third reading frame encodes the DNA polymerase, pol, which also has reverse transcriptase activity. A fourth reading frame, X, encodes the hepatitis B x antigen (HBxAg),[55,58] which in cell culture is a transcriptional transactivator capable of upregulating the expression of a number of genes.[59] HBxAg has been proposed to be an important factor in the tumorigenic potential of HBV, since it has been shown to exist in an integrated form within the genome of patients with chronic hepatitis B who develop hepatocellular carcinoma.[59]

The replication of the HBV genome involves four major steps[51]:

1. After viral entry, completion of plus-strand DNA synthesis and the formation of a fully double-stranded, covalently closed, circular DNA molecule (cccDNA)
2. Transcription of cccDNA into a slightly greater than genome-length RNA, the "pregenome," by host RNA polymerase, as well as four to five shorter messenger

RNAs encoding the various proteins expressed by the virus
3. Synthesis of new minus-strand DNA by reverse transcription of the RNA pregenome RNA
4. Synthesis of new plus-strand DNA utilizing minus-strand DNA as a template, commencing after particle assembly but prior to release of the newly replicated particle from the cell

HBV infection begins with the attachment of the virion to the surface of the hepatocyte.[60] Subsequently, the cccDNA generated within the host cell nucleus is transcribed to pregenomic and subgenomic viral RNAs by host RNA polymerase. Translation of this pregenomic RNA leads to the production of pol and core proteins.[60] This pregenomic RNA is encapsidated into viral nucleocapsid core particles. The encapsidation mechanism is highly selective for genomic RNA, and depends on a region located near the 5′ end of the genome called the ε signal.[61] The ε region at the 5′ end of the pregenomic RNA interacts with the pol protein.[62] This pol-ε interaction is stabilized by the host's heat shock protein 90 (Hsp 90). The core proteins dimerize around the pregenomic RNA pol complex and form the viral nucleocapsids. Once the pregenomic RNA is packed into a nucleocapsid, it serves as a template for reverse transcription and minus-strand DNA synthesis. The pol protein is bound to the 5′-ε end and starts synthesizing the first three nucleotides of the minus-strand DNA. This nascent DNA chain is in turn translocated to the 3′ end of the pregenomic RNA, binding to a 12-nucleotide complementary region called direct repeat 1 (DR1). Subsequently, minus-strand DNA synthesis continues, and the template pregenomic RNA is degraded by the RNaseH activity of the pol protein except for the last few nucleotides.[63] These RNA oligomers are translocated to the 3′ copies of another 12-nucleotide segment called direct repeat 2 (DR2), from which the synthesis of the plus strand DNA is initiated. The nucleocapsid containing the partially double-stranded DNA is directed to the endoplasmic reticulum and Golgi apparatus for virion assembly. The characteristic partially double-stranded genome (with a large gap in the plus strand) results from premature termination of plus-strand synthesis by the pol protein.

Mutations are introduced into the viral genome probably as a result of errors during reverse transcription during replication. An unusual serologic pattern, clinically characterized by rapidly progressive liver failure, was described for the first time by Chu and associates in 1987.[64] These investigators reported on patients who had measurable HBV DNA in serum in the absence of detectable HBeAg. The term anti-HBe antigen-negative hepatitis B is currently used to describe this special category of infection with HBV, which typically results from mutation in the precore region of the genome (see Epidemiology and Disease).

EPIDEMIOLOGY

The prevalence of HBV varies widely in different parts of the world. Approximately 350 million people are chronic

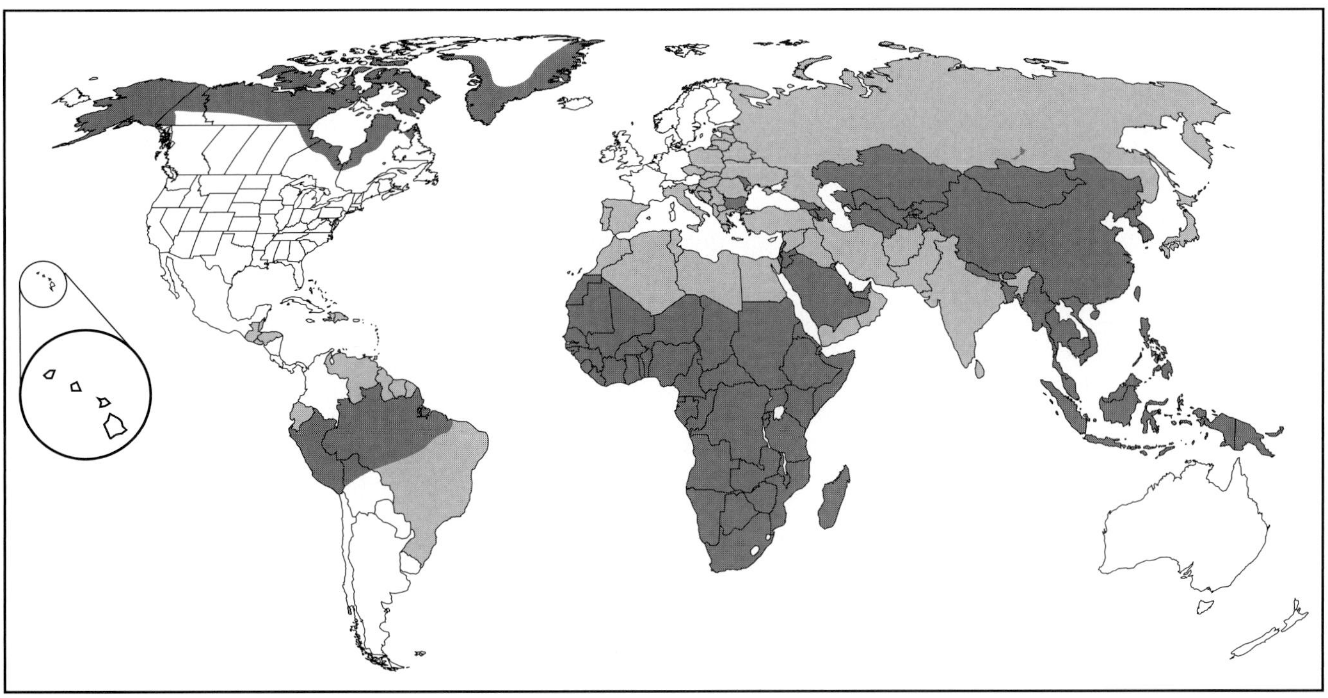

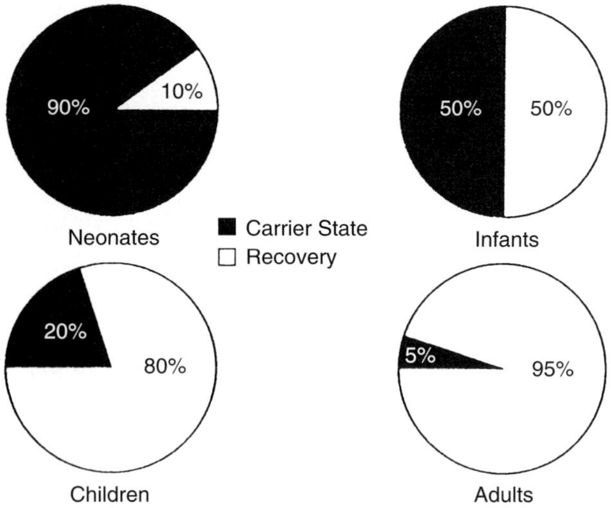

FIGURE 64-4 Risk of developing chronic hepatitis B virus (HBV) infection in relationship to age at the time of HBV infection. The highest risk occurs early in life. (From Koff RS: Viral hepatitis. In Schiff L, Schiff ER [eds]: Diseases of the Liver, 7th ed. Philadelphia, JB Lippincott, 1993, p 537.)

carriers of the virus, and about three quarters of these live in Asia.[1,65] Chronic HBV infection is found in 6% to 10% of adults with evidence of infection, approximately 25% of infected children aged 1 to 5 years, and 70% to 90% of infected infants[66,67] (Fig. 64-4). This reflects a greater proportion of acute infection progressing to persistence among the very young. Generally speaking, probably less than 1% of new infections in healthy adults result in viral persistence for more than 6 months. Transmission of HBV from an infected mother to her infant during birth (perinatal or vertical transmission) results in the highest rate of persistent infection. In Asia perinatal infection accounts for about 15% to 20% of chronic HBV infections in adults, and this correlates well with the prevalence of HBsAg-positive mothers. Perinatal transmission is known to occur at a lower rate in HBeAg-negative mothers.[68,69]

Horizontal transmission among young children is common in highly endemic regions, while sexual transmission of HBV dominates in well-developed countries with lower overall prevalence of the infection. Bloodborne infection is also common among illicit injection drug users. HBsAg has been found in blood and various body fluids, such as saliva, menstrual and vaginal discharges, seminal fluid, colostrum, breast milk, and serous exudates, and these have been implicated as vehicles of transmission of the infection.[70] A cross-sectional seroprevalence study conducted to assess the frequency of HBV infection among children born in the United States to Southeast Asian refugees showed that about 7% of the young children of HBsAg-negative mothers were infected with HBV, suggesting that child-to-child transmission remains an important route of infection among this group.[71] Among Alaskan Eskimos, the highest incidence of HBV infection occurs during the first 5 years of life,[72] and chronic infection rates can range from 5% to 10%, a phenomenon similar to that described in the Middle East.[73] In the United States, the incidence of hepatitis B reached a plateau and began to decrease after the mid-1980s, probably as a result of intensive efforts to control the spread of human immunodeficiency virus (HIV) in the same high-risk populations.[2] An epidemiologic study conducted in the United States between 1981 and 1988 showed that the proportions of hepatitis B cases accounted for by homosexual activity decreased by 62%, whereas the proportion of cases acquired by heterosexual exposure increased by 38%.[66] In another study conducted on attendees at a sexually transmitted disease clinic and college students, the risk of acquiring HBV infection was increased with increasing number of sexual partners. The prevalence of HBV infection was 6% for those with fewer than five recent partners (in the past 4 months) versus 21% for those with five or more partners.[67]

The proportion of hepatitis B patients with a history of parenteral drug use increased by 80% in the United States between 1981 and 1988.[66] In the same study, a decline of 75% in the number of health care workers reported with hepatitis B reflects the positive impact of HBV immunization and implementation of universal blood precautions. Additional possible risk factors for the transmission of HBV infection include traditional tattooing, bloodletting, and ritual circumcision. Results of investigations on the role of biting insects do not support a significant role in viral transmission. Even though HBsAg has been detected in some mosquito species and other arthropods, no convincing evidence for replication of HBV in insects has been obtained.[70] HBV is not transmitted by the fecal-oral route, and urine is not infectious unless contaminated with blood. There is no evidence that airborne infections occur.

Table 64-4 summarizes the prevalence of serologic markers for HBV among well-defined population groups at risk. They should be screened for HBV infection and immunized if seronegative.[74]

High rates of infection occur in northern Africa, sub-Saharan Africa, the Arabic Middle East, Southeast Asia, the Philippines, Polynesia, Indonesia, Eskimo populations throughout the Arctic,[68] and the Amazonian Basin of South America.[75] In South America, the prevalence of HBsAg increases from south to north, from 0.5% to 1.1% in Chile, Argentina, Uruguay, and southeastern Brazil to moderate rates (1.5% to 3%) in mid and northeastern Brazil.[75] A remarkably high prevalence has been noticed in the central Amazonian region (5% to 15%) as well as some areas in Colombia, Peru, and Venezuela. In Central America the prevalence of HBsAg

Table 64-4 Prevalence of HBV Serologic Markers in Population Groups That Should Be Screened for HBV infection

Population	Prevalence of HBV Serologic Markers (%)	
	HBsAg	**All Markers**
Persons born in endemic areas	13	70–85
Men who have sex with men	6	35–80
Injecting drug users	7	60–80
Dialysis patients	3–10	20–80
HIV-infected patients	8–11	89–90
Pregnant women (USA)	0.4–1.5	
Family/household and sexual contacts	3–6	30–60

of an RNA intermediate to relaxed, circular, partially double-stranded DNA (see the preceding Agent section), its DNA polymerase functions as a reverse transcriptase. The polymerase (P) gene is the largest, encoding a protein of 832 amino acids.[124] Within the active site of the polymerase lies a highly conserved amino acid motif consisting of the sequence Tyr-Met-Asp-Asp (YMDD). This motif is essential for nucleotide binding and for polymerase activity, and mutations in this region may confer resistance to lamivudine and thus have important therapeutic and prognostic implications. Pooled data from three clinical trials involving 731 treatment-naïve patients who received lamivudine (100 mg/day) for 1 year demonstrated that HBeAg seroconversion (defined as loss of HBeAg, detection of anti-HBe, and loss of HBV DNA) occurred in 16% to 18% of patients compared with as few as 6% of untreated controls.[125,126] Follow-up reports of the Asian study on lamivudine showed that the HBeAg seroconversion rates increased with time, from 17% at 1 year to 27%, 33%, and 47% at 2, 3, and 4 years, respectively.[127]

However, the selection of lamivudine-resistant mutants during therapy is a major concern. The most common mutation affects the YMDD motif of the HBV DNA polymerase (methionine to valine or isoleucine). Lamivudine resistance is usually manifested by the reappearance of HBV DNA in serum after its initial disappearance. In the Asian study, lamivudine resistance increased from 14% at 1 year to 38%, 49%, and 66% after 2, 3, and 4 years of treatment, respectively.[127] However, HBeAg seroconversion has been maintained in 25% of patients who continued treatment after the detection of mutants.[128] Dienstag and colleagues studied histologic and clinical outcome after 3 years of lamivudine therapy in 63 patients who received 100 mg daily.[129] Most patients showed improvement (56%) or no change (33%) in the necroinflammatory score compared with baseline (median follow-up, 3.5 years). The proportion of patients showing histologic improvement overall was higher in the subgroup of subjects without YMDD mutation compared with the group with the YMDD variant, but even in the latter group there were patients whose histologic activity scores decreased. Five patients showed improvement of cirrhosis by the end of treatment, and one reverted almost completely. The authors concluded that although the emergence of YMDD mutations can diminish histologic benefit, these patients do not experience rapid deterioration and instead benefit from continued treatment.

Durability of response after HBeAg seroconversion with lamivudine treatment is variable. HBeAg seroconversion durability is reported in 77% of western patients[130] after 3 years, in contrast with a much lower response in Asian studies.[131,132] A study in Taiwan conducted on 82 HBeAg-positive patients with chronic hepatitis on liver biopsy showed a sustained response (seroconversion of HBeAg to anti-HBe, clearance of HBV DNA, and normalization of ALT for 1 year after 12 months of lamivudine therapy) in 52% of patients.[133] Patients with genotype B had a much higher rate of sustained response than those with genotype C (61% vs. 25%, respectively).

Lamivudine should be administered for at least 1 year,[122] but the benefit of prolonged therapy should be balanced against the risk of resistant mutants. The recommended dose for adults is 100 mg daily, and it should be reduced in patients with renal insufficiency. Two thirds of patients with HBeAg-negative chronic HBV infection can achieve an initial response (clearance of HBV DNA)[134]; however, the relapse rate after stopping therapy is even higher than with IFN treatment in this particular group of patients.[135] The incidence of YMDD mutants in HBeAg-negative patients increases with time, as occurs in HBeAg-positive chronic hepatitis B.[134]

Lamivudine is well tolerated in patients with decompensated cirrhosis and may even result in clinical improvement and reduction of the Child-Pugh score.[136–138] However, the potential selection of lamivudine-resistant mutations might be a drawback for prolonged therapy in patients with cirrhosis undergoing orthotopic liver transplantation.[139] Lok and coworkers[140] analyzed retrospectively data for nearly 1000 patients from clinical trials performed on all five continents among HBeAg-positive subjects with chronic hepatitis B who were treated with lamivudine for up to 6 years. This cohort was compared with a group of 200 patients who received placebo for 1 year. The median duration of lamivudine treatment was 4 years. The most common adverse events were hepatitis flares occurring in 21% of patients receiving lamivudine in year 5, most of them related to HBeAg seroconversion and emergence of lamivudine-resistant mutations, but overall fewer than 1% had liver-related adverse side effects or decompensation. Patients who had lamivudine-resistant mutants for more than 4 years tended to have more adverse events, leading these experts to suggest that HBeAg-positive patients with compensated liver disease may remain stable during the first 1 to 3 years after the emergence of lamivudine-resistant mutations, but more prolonged therapy may be associated with clinical worsening. The emergence of lamivudine-resistant mutations signals the time when alternative treatments for chronic hepatitis B should be contemplated.

Adefovir Dipivoxil

Adefovir dipivoxil, an antiviral drug recently approved by FDA for the therapy of chronic hepatitis B, is an oral prodrug of adefovir, an analog of adenosine monophosphate. Adefovir diphosphate, the active metabolite, effectively inhibits HBV DNA polymerase intracellularly. Marcellin and colleagues[141] conducted a study on 515 HBeAg-positive patients with chronic hepatitis B receiving adefovir dipivoxil 10 mg/day, 30 mg/day, or placebo for 48 weeks. Histologic improvement, HBeAg seroconversion, normalization of ALT, and clearance of HBV DNA were observed in a much higher proportion of adefovir dipivoxil-treated patients compared with those who received placebo. The safety profile of the 10 mg dose was similar to that of placebo, whereas the 30 mg dose was associated with a higher frequency of adverse events and renal function abnormalities. No adefovir-resistant mutants were identified in the HBV DNA polymerase gene. Hadziyannis and colleagues studied the impact of adefovir dipivoxil in 185 patients with HBeAg-negative chronic hepatitis B in a multicenter, double-blind, placebo-controlled trial.[142] Patients received adefovir dipivoxil 10 mg daily or placebo for 48 weeks. Fifty-one percent of patients in the adefovir dipivoxil group reduced their HBV DNA levels to fewer than 400 copies per milliliter, compared with 0 patients in the placebo group. Histologic improvement and normalization in ALT levels were significantly more frequent in the adefovir dipivoxil group. No mutations in the HBV DNA polymerase associated with resistance to the drug were observed. The absence of adefovir-resistant mutations in the two trials was confirmed in a sophisticated virologic substudy conducted by Westland and associates.[143] However, Angus and colleagues reported the first case of the occurrence of both virologic and clinical resistance to adefovir dipivoxil therapy in a patient who developed breakthrough during a 96-week course of adefovir dipivoxil.[144] Comparing pretreatment and post-treatment HBV DNA by PCR sequencing, an asparagine to threonine mutation was identified at residue 236 in domain D of the HBV polymerase, causing a marked reduction in the susceptibility to adefovir. The patient responded to lamivudine "rescue" therapy, achieving normalization of ALT and significant decrease in HBV DNA. Despite data suggesting that resistance to adefovir dipivoxil is significantly less common than for lamivudine, the clinician treating patients with chronic hepatitis B should take into consideration the fact that drug resistance is likely to emerge to any antiviral drug during prolonged monotherapy.[141] In the near future, combination antiviral therapy may provide the best chance of long-term suppression of viral replication and prevention of disease progression.[145] Combination therapy with lamivudine and adefovir dipivoxil has recently been proved safe and effective in both compensated and decompensated patients with chronic hepatitis B in two well-designed, randomized clinical trials.[146,147]

Table 64-5 Hepatitis B Vaccines

	Recombivax HB Dose		***Engerix-B Dose***	
	μg	**mL**	**μg**	**mL**
Infants born to HBsAg-positive mothers	5	0.5	10	0.5
Infants born to HBsAg-negative mothers and children <11 yr	2.5	0.5*	10	0.5
Children and adolescents 11–19 yr	5	0.5	20	1
Adults >20 yr	10	1	20	1
Dialysis patients and other immunocompromised persons	40	1†	40	2‡
Licensed schedule of administration	0, 1, and 6 mo		0, 1, and 6 mo or 0, 1, 2, and 12 mo	

HBsAg, hepatitis B surface antigen.
*New pediatric formulation.
†Special formulation.
‡Two 1-mL doses administered at one site at 0, 1, 2, and 6 months.

Other Antiviral Agents

Entecavir is a deoxyguanine nucleoside analog. It is a selective inhibitor of the replication of HBV, capable of causing pronounced reduction in HBV DNA levels in short-term studies[148] with almost no side effects. Long-term clinical trials are needed to establish the efficacy of this antiviral agent.

Famciclovir is the oral prodrug of penciclovir. It is less efficacious than lamivudine, and famciclovir-resistant mutants have been reported.[149] It has to be administered three times a day. For these reasons, it seems unlikely that famciclovir will be part of the therapeutic regimes against chronic hepatitis B.[122]

PREVENTION AND CONTROL

The initial strategy for vaccination against hepatitis B was targeted against high-risk groups such as sexual and close contacts of patients with hepatitis B, homosexual men, infants born to infected mothers, IVDUs, hemodialysis patients, sexually active heterosexuals, and health care personnel. However, this strategy failed to have a significant impact on the disease prevalence and incidence because many of these individuals were infected with HBV before vaccination.[66] Since about 30% of all cases of acute hepatitis B occur in persons who do not have an identifiable risk factor, control of hepatitis B in western societies requires routine screening of all pregnant women and routine immunization of all infants,[2,66] which would lead to disease prevention by providing immunity before persons engage in high-risk activities. For these reasons, it is now recommended to incorporate hepatitis B immunization into the standard childhood vaccination programs (see later discussion). Control in less developed regions rests on infant immunization. The original plasma-derived vaccine (Heptavax-B), widely used among health care workers and other high-risk groups in the early 1980s,[150] is no longer being manufactured in the United States. Two vaccines produced by recombinant DNA technology, Recombivax-HB and Engerix-B, are currently available. The doses and recommended schedules are shown in Table 64-5. The adult vaccination schedule is a series of three doses given by IM injection in the deltoid muscle at 0, 1, and 6 months. Engerix-B is now licensed for use on a four-dose schedule with doses at 0, 1, 2, and 12 months. For adult patients lacking antibodies against hepatitis A, Twinrix is a suitable alternative (see Prevention and Control for hepatitis A virus).

A rapid immunization schedule using Engerix-B given at 0, 1, and 2 months was compared with the standard schedule (0, 1, and 6 months) in a prospective, randomized fashion.[151] The accelerated schedule provided seroconversion rates identical to those offered by the standard schedule. The importance of vaccination among health care workers cannot be overemphasized and is well exemplified in a report describing the transmission of HBV from an unvaccinated thoracic surgeon to 19 patients in 1 year.[152] Protection lasts at least as long as measurable antibody to HBsAg (anti-HBs) persists in the circulation.[122] Five years after vaccination, about 80% of vaccinated persons have antibody levels considered protective (≥10 mIU/mL).[153] The Advisory Committee for Immunization Practices (ACIP) and the American Academy of Pediatrics currently recommend that all infants be vaccinated against HBV.[122] There are two dosing options: (1) at birth, 1 to 2 months of age, and 6 to 18 months of age; or (2) 1 to 2 months of age, 4 months, and 6 to 18 months. The loss of detectable anti-HBs after vaccination does not necessarily mean a lack of protection. Intact immunologic memory B cells may persist in hepatitis B vaccine responders who have low (<10 mIU/mL) anti-HBs levels 7 to 8 years after immunization.[154] A European Consensus Group on hepatitis B immunity noted that there are no data to support the need for booster doses in immunocompetent individuals responding to a primary course.[155] Patients undergoing hemodialysis represent a special group, since their response rate to hepatitis B vaccine is only around 60%, and hepatitis B can occur even in patients thought to have an antibody

Table 64-6 Recommendations for Hepatitis B Prophylaxis Following Percutaneous Exposure

	Exposed Person	
Source	**Unvaccinated**	**Vaccinated**
HBsAg-positive	1. HBIG × 1 immediately* 2. Initiate HB vaccine† series	1. Test exposed person for anti-HBs‡ 2. If inadequate antibody,§ HBIG × 1 immediately plus HB vaccine booster dose
Known source		
High risk HBsAg-positive	1. Initiate HB vaccine series 2. Test source for HBsAg. If positive, HBIG × 1	Test source for HBsAg only if exposed person is vaccine nonresponder; if source is HBsAg- positive, give HBIG × 1 immediately plus HB vaccine booster dose
Low risk HBsAg-positive	Initiate HB vaccine series	Nothing required
Unknown source	Initiate HB vaccine series	Nothing required

HB, hepatitis B; HBIG, hepatitis B immune globulin; HBsAg, hepatitis B surface antigen.
*HBIG dose 0.06 mL/kg intravascularly (IM).
†HB vaccine dose 20 μg IM for adults, 10 μg IM for infants or children under 10 years of age. First dose within 1 week; second and third doses, 1 and 6 months later, respectively.
‡See text for details.
§Less than 10 SRU by RIA, negative EIA.
Data from Protection against viral hepatitis: Recommendations of the Immunization Practices Advisory Committee (ACIP). MMWR 39:1, 1990.

response to the vaccine.[156] Hemodialysis patients represent the only group in which booster immunization is recommended when anti-HBs levels fall below 10 mIU/mL.[157] Other immunocompromised patients such as organ transplant recipients also have a low response rate to hepatitis B vaccination.[158] Among native residents in areas endemic for HBV such as the Peruvian Amazonian region, the response rate after the administration of three doses of Engerix-B was 73.5%.[159] In this study, the third dose was administered 14 months after the first in 16% of the natives, with no difference in the rate of seroconversion when compared with the 32% that received the recommended 0, 1, and 6 months regimen. This has practical implications for vaccination programs in rural areas of difficult access, where flexibility in the vaccination schedule is required.

Reports of multiple sclerosis following HBV vaccination caused concern regarding the safety of this vaccine. However, a large case-control study performed in nurses from the United States showed no association between HBV vaccination and this neurologic disease.[160] A recombinant vaccine, Hepacare, contains pre-S1 and pre-S2 antigens in addition to HBsAg and appears to provide equivalent seroprotection to a standard three-dose regimen with Engerix-B within 6 months.[161] It has been suggested that the inclusion of the pre-S antigens in this novel vaccine may enhance its immunogenicity and possibly offer advantages for adults at risk for suboptimal serologic response to conventional recombinant vaccines, such as older adults or immunosuppressed persons.[162]

Postexposure prophylaxis is indicated in unvaccinated persons who are exposed to HBV. Infants born to HBsAg-positive mothers should receive hepatitis B immunoglobulin (HBIG) 0.5 mL IM and hepatitis B vaccine within 12 hours of birth and two more doses of vaccine at 1 and 6 months of age. For sexual contacts, HBIG 0.06 mL/kg IM within 2 weeks of exposure and simultaneous hepatitis B vaccination series are recommended.[122] The HBV vaccine and HBIG should be administered at different sites. If the exposed person has previously been vaccinated against HBV, serum anti-HBs titers should be determined immediately, and a new vaccine series is recommended for individuals with antibody levels less than 10 mIU/mL. Health care workers who have a percutaneous exposure should follow the same guidelines as patients exposed by sexual contact. General guidelines for hepatitis B prophylaxis after percutaneous or mucosal exposure are shown in Table 64-6.

Hepatitis C

When stored samples of prospectively studied cases of transfusion-associated hepatitis in 1975 revealed that most cases were not associated with hepatitis A or B viruses, the term "non-A, non-B" (NANB) hepatitis was adopted.[163] The infectious nature of NANB hepatitis was demonstrated a few years later when it was transmitted to chimpanzees, and in 1989 a short segment of the viral RNA was reverse-transcribed, cloned, and sequenced, identifying the agent, which was named hepatitis C virus (HCV).[164]

AGENT

HCV is a single-stranded RNA virus with a genome length of approximately 9.5 kb and a mean diameter of approximately 55 nm, classified in the family approximately Flaviviridae (with yellow fever, dengue, and Japanese encephalitis viruses), and is the only member of the genus *Hepacivirus*. The genome of HCV (Fig. 64-7) contains a single large open reading frame (ORF) with an upstream 5′ nontranslated region that plays a role in translation of the viral proteins and replication of the viral RNA. The ORF encodes a large polyprotein that is cleaved into structural and nonstructural proteins by host and virus proteases.[165] Approximately 30% of the ORF adjacent to the 5′ end encodes the structural proteins which include the nucleocapsid protein, core (C), with RNA binding activity, two envelope proteins, E1 and E2, and possibly a small "viroporin," p7, that forms an ion channel in membranes.

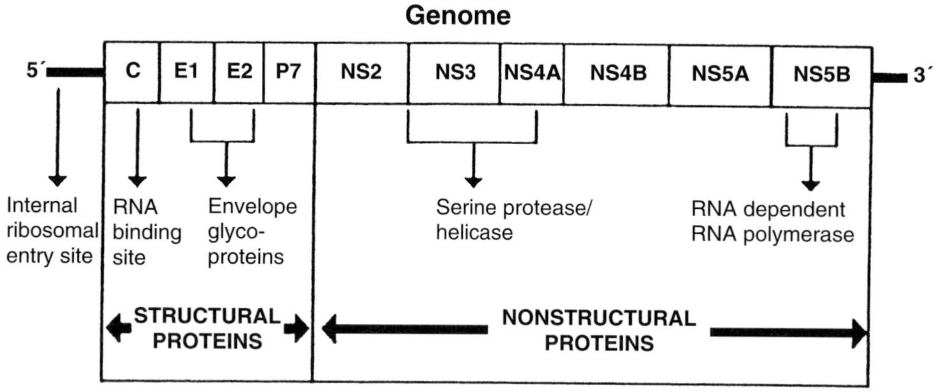

FIGURE 64-7 Hepatitis C genome. (From Koff RS, Dienstag JL, Riely CA, et al: AGA Clinical Teaching Project, Unit 3, Viral Hepatitis, 2nd ed. Timonium, Md., Milner-Fenwick, 1994.)

The 5′ nontranslated RNA (NTR) acts as an internal ribosome entry site (IRES), and its structure has been visualized by cryoelectron microscopy.[166] The nonstructural proteins are involved in polyprotein processing and viral RNA replication and include two viral proteases (activities associated with NS2/NS3 and NS3/4A) and an RNA-dependent RNA polymerase (NS5B) adjacent to the 3′ end. NS3 has both helicase and protease activity. Six distinct genotypes of HCV have been identified. There appear to be differences among genotypes regarding virulence, geographic distribution, and response to therapy with IFN. HCV is characterized by its genetic variability, undergoing a high rate of mutation.[167] These mutations are more frequently identified in the hypervariable region of the genome, located in the E2 region. An infected individual typically has multiple related HCV-RNA sequences in the blood and liver simultaneously, termed *quasispecies*.[168] These arise as a result of the tendency of the viral polymerase to be error-prone and because of multiple selective forces including immune pressure exerted by the host. This concept may explain in part the enormous difficulties encountered in efforts to develop an effective vaccine against HCV. The 5′NTR is highly conserved, however, and is utilized in the detection of HCV-RNA by the reverse transcriptase–PCR (RT-PCR) method.

EPIDEMIOLOGY

The worldwide prevalence of HCV infection, based on immunoassays for antibodies to HCV (anti-HCV), approximates 1% to 2%.[169] In the United States, 1.8% of the population is positive for anti-HCV antibodies.[169] Seroprevalence using second-generation assays is around 0.3% in Australia; 1.5% to 3% in the Philippines, Indonesia, Thailand, and Vietnam; 1% in Taiwan and China; and as high as 3% to 4% in Japan.[170] The prevalence is approximately 7% in sub-Saharan Africa,[171] and the highest reported prevalence is in Egypt, where 6% to 28% (average, 22%) have antibodies against HCV, presumably owing to spread by contaminated needles during parenteral antischistosomal treatment.[172] The prevalent genotype in Europe is 1b (47%), followed by 1a (17%) and 3 (16%).[173] In the United States, about 57% of cases have genotype 1a, 17% genotype 1b, 14% genotype 2, and 7% genotype 3.[174] The great majority of hemophiliacs who received blood products during the 1980s became infected with HCV.[175] The risk of acquiring HCV from a blood transfusion in the United States was previously about 1 in 103,000 transfused units,[176] probably due to blood donations in the 12-week period before development of anti-HCV in the infected donor. This interval may be shortened to 3 weeks using RT-PCR to detect HCV RNA.[177]

HCV infection is also common among IVDUs, acquired by sharing contaminated needles. The prevalence of anti-HCV in this population ranges from 50% to 90%.[178,179] In other areas of the world, the intravenous route is also important, with a prevalence of HCV among IVDUs around 70% in New Zealand, Hong Kong, and Taiwan.

Transmission of HCV to health care workers by needle sticks is well documented,[180,181] and the 2% to 4% seroconversion rate reported after percutaneous accidental exposure falls between the 15% to 30% risk for HBV and the 0.3% for human immunodeficiency virus (HIV).[182,183] However, using RT-PCR for the detection of HCV-RNA, Mitsui and colleagues reported a rate of 10% following a single accidental percutaneous exposure.[181] Cardiothoracic surgery is associated with a high risk of glove perforation occurring during wire sternotomy closure,[182] leading to contact of the surgeon's blood with the patient's open wound. Hepatitis C has been transmitted nosocomially during colonoscopy or general surgery, although such infections appear to be unusual.[182,184] Health care workers are usually at much greater risk of infection from their patients than vice versa. Patients on chronic hemodialysis are considered a high-risk population, and studies using RT-PCR for the detection of HCV-RNA show a high prevalence of HCV among these patients, which can be underestimated when only anti-HCV tests are utilized.[185]

Perinatal transmission of HCV is uncommon. HCV-RNA detection is preferable to antibody detection methods,[186] since the passive acquisition of maternal anti-HCV has been found in 72% to 86% of infants, which is lost between the second and twelfth months after birth.[187] The risk of transmission of HCV from mother to infant is increased if the mother is coinfected with HIV.[188,189] A hypothetical explanation for this phenomenon is the high HCV titers in these mothers as a consequence of HIV-related immunosuppression.[187] The likelihood of sexual transmission of HCV is similarly low although not negligible.[190] In a study of Japanese sex workers, the prevalence of HCV was 6.2%,[191] significantly higher than in the general population.

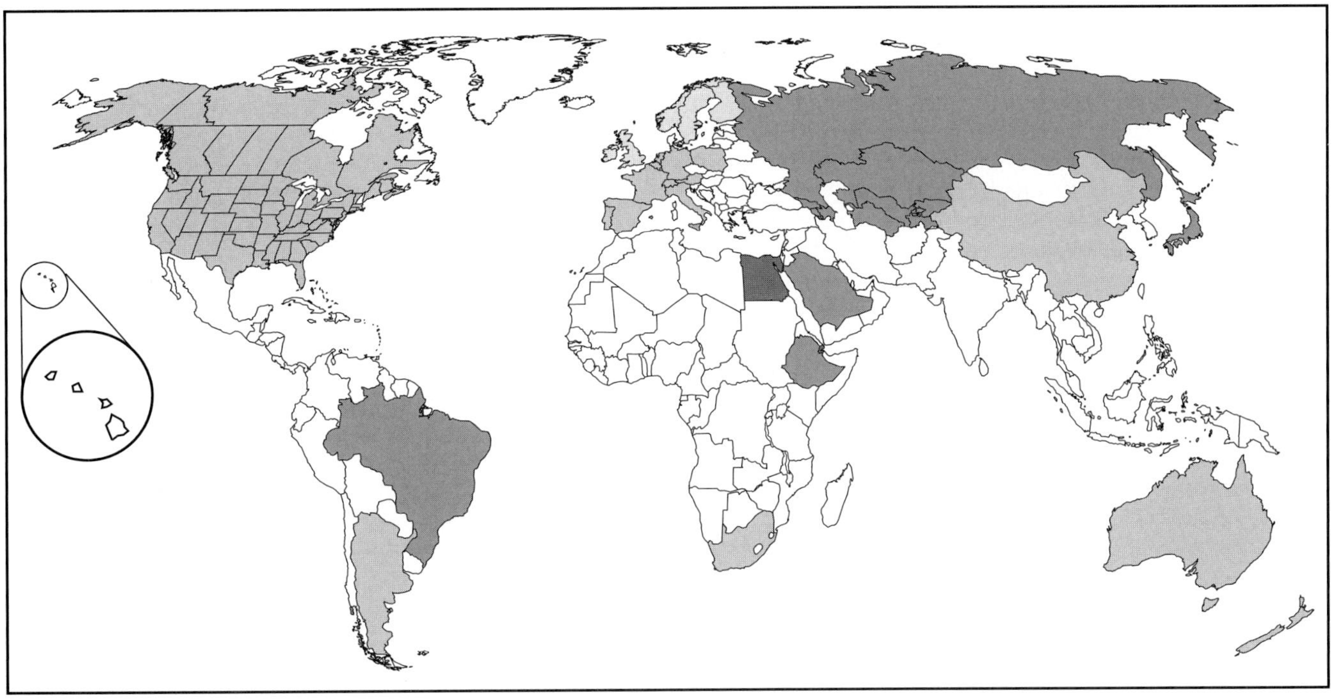

Hepatitis C

Anti-HCV Prevalence

- ■ >5%—High
- ■ 1.1%-5%—Intermediate
- ■ 0.2%-1%—Low
- ■ ≤0.1%—Very Low
- □ Unknown

The incidence of anti-HCV antibodies is only minimally increased in male homosexuals, in comparison to the high prevalence of HBV and HIV infection. Wright and colleagues retrospectively evaluated more than 500 HIV-positive male homosexuals without a history of blood transfusion or IV drug use and found that the prevalence of anti-HCV as determined by second-generation antibody testing was 11.7%, several times higher than the rate reported in volunteer blood donors.[192] Among stable heterosexual partners of HCV-infected, HIV-negative persons, the median rate of anti-HCV positivity is 1% in North America, 6% in southern Europe, and 11% in Southeast Asia.[193] Importantly, the use of genotyping to evaluate anti-HCV concordant couples may lead to overestimation of HCV sexual transmission, since HCV genotypes that are prevalent in the population may be present in partners with different sources of infection. Rather, sequence analysis should be used for this purpose.[193]

DISEASE

The clinical presentation of acute HCV infection is indistinguishable from other acute viral hepatitides. The incubation period averages about 6 weeks, based on transfusion-related acquired acute cases,[194] which is intermediate between that for hepatitis A and hepatitis B. Symptoms are usually very mild, characterized by malaise and fever and with elevations of aminotransferase activity that are usually less pronounced than in hepatitis B. Acute hepatitis C accounts for around 16% of cases of acute hepatitis in the United States.[195] The vast majority of cases has an anicteric course and may go unnoticed if laboratory tests are not monitored. Although some investigators have found cases of fulminant hepatitis and the presence of HCV in blood,[196,197] there is little evidence that HCV has a fulminant course in the United States, although this has been more commonly reported in Japan.

Probably the most remarkable aspect of HCV infection from a clinical standpoint is its ability to become chronic, as occurs in more than 50% to 85% of patients.[198] A Japanese study of the natural history of HCV disease suggests that approximately 20 years are required to develop cirrhosis, and 30 years for hepatocellular carcinoma, but some cases appear to extend over a 60-year period.[199] Once HCV infection is established, chronicity is the rule, and histologic progression evolves insidiously. However, many patients remain without significant liver disease for decades or even for life. The rate of progression of fibrosis seems to be related to the age of acquisition of the infection. Children seem to be more likely to clear the infection spontaneously than adults, for unknown reasons.[200,201] Factors accelerating the progression to fibrosis include alcohol, male sex, advanced age at acquisition, smoking, and coinfection with HIV or HBV.[202–206] Community-based cohort studies are more accurate than post-transfusion cohorts, blood banks, or liver clinics for estimating disease progression at a population level because they avoid selection bias.

The estimated rate of progression to cirrhosis after 20 years of chronic HCV infection is between 4% and 10% in community-based cohorts.[207]

As a rule, clinically apparent disease is uncommon, and patients often come in late in the course of the disease with manifestations of end-stage liver disease. A large proportion of cases of chronic hepatitis C are identified incidentally during biochemical screening at routine examinations or in the course of screening for blood donation. Patients with chronic HCV infection typically have nonspecific symptoms such as fatigue and malaise. Serum alanine aminotransferse (ALT) levels fluctuate and may even be normal, making ALT an unreliable marker of disease activity or recovery. Many extrahepatic manifestations have been associated with chronic HCV infections. Essential mixed cryoglobulinemia is characterized by circulating mixed cryoprecipitable globulins and can be accompanied by arthritis, generalized vasculitis, and cutaneous purpura.[208] Successful interferon treatment is associated with a decrease in "cryocrit" and improvement in the clinical manifestations of essential mixed cryoglobulinemia.[209] Porphyria cutanea tarda (PCT) is characterized by the development of skin hypersensitivity to sun, formation of vesicles and bullae, hyperpigmentation, and hypertrichosis, associated with iron overload and chronic liver disease.[209] Anti-HCV was found in 82% of Italian patients and in 79% of Spanish patients with PCT by second-generation immunoassays.[210,211]

A subset of HCV-infected patients may have membranoproliferative glomerulonephritis as a consequence of deposition of HCV antigen-antibody complexes in glomeruli.[212] Proteinuria and glomerular deposition of IgG, IgM, and C3 have been demonstrated, as well as HCV-RNA–containing cryoprecipitates and antibodies to nucleocapsid proteins. Lymphocytic sialoadenitis and capillaritis are frequent findings in salivary gland and labial mucosal biopsy specimems, resembling those seen in Sjögren's syndrome.[213,214] Other extrahepatic manifestations of HCV include corneal ulcers,[215] erythema nodosum,[216] and polyarteritis nodosa.[217] HCV RNA has been detected in peripheral lymphocytes and in biopsy samples of lymphoma tissue, although its significance is uncertain.[218] Gisbert and colleagues published a meta-analysis evaluating the prevalence of hepatitis C infection in patients with B-cell non-Hodgkin lymphoma (NHL).[219] They found a prevalence of HCV in patients with NHL of 15%, higher than that reported in the general population.

A significant proportion of patients with HCC have HCV infection, detected not only by anti-HCV tests but also by HCV-RNA levels.[220,221] Time elapsed since acquiring HCV infection and the development of cirrhosis seems to be the main factor for the development of HCC. A median of 30 years is the time frame in which most HCC begins to appear.[222] The strongest correlation between the presence of HCV infection and HCC is seen in Japan, Spain, and Italy, while HCV is less commonly found in patients with HCC in the United States and southern Africa.[223,224] HCV was present in 26% of 1930 patients with HCC in the absence of HBV markers.[225] In the United States, there was a twofold increase in HCC between 1975 and 1998, and a shift in incidence from elderly patients to relatively younger patients between 40 and 60 years of age has been observed.[222]

Despite the strong epidemiologic association between HCV and HCC, little is known about the mechanism by which chronic hepatitis C results in HCC. Although HCC has been described in noncirrhotic livers,[226] cirrhosis is present in the majority of patients with HCV-related HCC. There is no evidence that the HCV genome can become integrated within the genome of the hepatocytes as occurs in chronic HBV infection.[227] However, transgenic mice expressing HCV proteins (core protein or the entire polyprotein) have been shown to be at risk for HCC despite the absence of inflammation or cirrhosis in these animals. As with HBV-associated HCC, chronic inflammation, oxidative stress, and attendant host chromosomal DNA damage may all contribute to carcinogenesis.

PATHOGENESIS AND IMMUNITY

Recent depletion experiments in chimpanzees have defined important roles for both $CD4^+$ and $CD8^+$ T lymphocytes in protection against HCV infection but have not resolved longstanding questions concerning the mechanisms exploited by the virus in establishing persistent infections. HCV-specific $CD4^+$ T cells are detected both in the liver and peripheral blood of HCV-infected patients.[228] The $CD4^+$ T cell response to HCV is sustained and vigorous in patients with acute, self-limited HCV infection, and is weak and delayed in patients who become chronically infected.[229] The potential protective role of HCV-specific CD4 T cells is suggested by studies showing accelerated liver disease progression in patients co-infected with HIV, who have generalized impairment in $CD4^+$ T cells.[230] $CD4^+$ T cell help is required for the development of an effective $CD8^+$ response, and it has been suggested that interferon-γ–secreting $CD8^+$ T cells play an important role in clearance of the virus from from liver. However, the $CD8^+$ T-cell response in HCV infection demonstrates several puzzling features. HCV-specific $CD8^+$ T cells are present and activated within the liver in patients with chronic hepatitis C, but they are incapable of eliminating the infection. In some patients, they appear to have a "stunned" phenotype, and do not secrete interferon-γ in response to antigen stimulation. The HCV-specific $CD8^+$ T-cell response is remarkably variable, and more work is needed to characterize these responses in chronic HCV infection.[231]

It appears that the antibody response is of limited importance in clearing HCV. Two studies seem to exclude a critical role for antibodies in the resolution of infection.[232,233] However, more studies are needed to define the role of antibody in immunity. The quasispecies nature of the virus confers a survival advantage, allowing rapid selection of mutants that are capable of escaping antibody-mediated neutralization.[234]

Finally, recent evidence suggests that HCV is capable of disrupting important innate immune responses that not only have direct intracellular antiviral effects but also play a role in shaping subsequent adaptive T-cell immunity. The NS3/4A protease acts to disrupt the signaling pathways that lead to induction of endogenous interferon synthesis in response to virus infection, by blocking the virus-induced activation of interferon-regulatory factor 3 (IRF-3).[235,236] Moreover, the NS5A protein appears to block one of the interferon-mediated effector mechanisms by binding to protein kinase R (PKR) near its catalytic site, and preventing the dsRNA-activated PKR-mediated shutdown of viral and cellular protein translation.[237] The disruption of innate immune responses to the infection may thus be very important in determining persistence of the infection, while also perhaps contributing to resistance to interferon therapy.

DIAGNOSIS

Indirect Tests: Antibody Assays

The detection of anti-HCV antibodies is the most common and practical means of diagnosing HCV infection. Second- or third-generation enzyme immunoassays (EIAs) are used to detect mixtures of antibodies against various HCV epitopes of the core, NS3, NS4, and (in third-generation assays) NS5 proteins.[238] Current EIAs have a specificity of 99% and are positive in more than 99% of immunocompetent patients with detectable HCV RNA.[239] EIAs can be negative in hemodialysis patients or in profoundly immunodepressed patients. The presence of elevated aminotransferases in a patient with EIA-positive anti-HCV is almost diagnostic of active HCV infection, although in some cases it requires confirmation with molecular HCV RNA detection. Immunoblot (RIBA) tests have been used as confimatory tests, but currently there is no role for them in the clinical setting except for the low-risk patient who tests positive for anti-HCV and has negative HCV RNA.[238]

Direct Tests

Detection of HCV RNA

Qualitative HCV RNA detection assays are useful because they are much more sensitive than quantitative assays. They are based on target amplification, by either RT-PCR or transcription-mediated amplification (TMA).[240] The World Health Organization (WHO) has established an international standard for HCV RNA units.[241] One international unit (IU) represents a certain amount of HCV RNA rather than the number of viral particles (copies per milliliter); this standard should be universally adopted. The detection cutoff of the two commercially available assays is 50 IU of HCV RNA per milliliter. The manual TMA assay is more sensitive (10 IU/mL), but both assays are 98% to 99% specific.[240] For quantification of HCV RNA, the detection limits of current assays vary from 30 IU/mL to 615 IU/mL, and the upper limit of linear quantification is between 500,000 IU/mL and 7,700,000 IU/mL. Samples above the upper limit of normal must be diluted 1/10 or 1/100 and have a specificity of 98% to 99%.[240] Three commercial tests are currently available to quantify HCV viremia: a branched-chain DNA assay (Quantiplex HCV RNA, version 2.0) and two assays involving RT-PCR (Cobas Amplicor HCV monitor, version 2.0 and HCV Superquant). All are reliable although not easily comparable.[242] Future assays will be predominantly real-time RT-PCR.

Even with the most sensitive technique, however, HCV-RNA may be sporadically undetectable in serum, and a single negative HCV-RNA determination should not be interpreted as absolute evidence of absence of HCV infection.

HCV Core Antigen

Total HCV core antigen can be detected and quantified with an EIA assay. The HCV core antigen correlates closely with the HCV RNA level[243]; however, the assay does not detect HCV core antigen when the HCV RNA level is below 20,000 IU/mL.

Clinical Applications

HCV RNA positivity in an anti-HCV-negative patient is highly suggestive of acute hepatitis C. Subjects with anti-HCV antibodies but with no HCV RNA may have cleared HCV RNA spontaneously in the past.[238] It is advisable to test such patients for HCV RNA a few months later, since HCV RNA levels may fluctuate somewhat. Symptomatic patients with both anti-HCV and HCV RNA may have acute hepatitis C or exacerbation of chronic hepatitis C. HCV RNA becomes detectable in serum between 1 and 2 weeks following occupational exposure. It is recommended that the source and the exposed individual be tested for antibody to HCV RNA. If the source individual is HCV EIA-positive, HCV RNA, anti-HCV, and ALT should be tested in the exposed individual at exposure and again between 2 and 8 weeks later. If seroconversion occurs, the exposed individual should be referred to a specialist for consideration of therapy, as early treatment with IFN may be efficacious in this setting (see later discussion). Infants born to HCV-positive mothers should be tested for HCV infection by HCV RNA tests on two occasions between the ages of 2 and 6 months or be tested for anti-HCV after 15 months, since passive transplacental transfer of antibodies from the mother may be present.[244]

Liver Biopsy

Testing for ALT is not accurate in determining the severity of liver disease. The levels may be normal or fluctuate, and a single normal value does not rule out active infection, advanced disease, or cirrhosis[169] (Fig. 64-8). Liver biopsy is frequently recommended in the initial evaluation of patients with chronic hepatitis C with abnormal levels of ALT.[245] The typical histologic findings in chronic hepatitis C include hepatocellular necrosis and inflammation (grade) and fibrosis (stage).[246] Assessment of the stage and rapidity of progression of fibrosis is helpful in determining the prognosis and need for therapy in an individual patient. Liver biopsy is the gold standard to assess fibrosis. The most frequently used staging

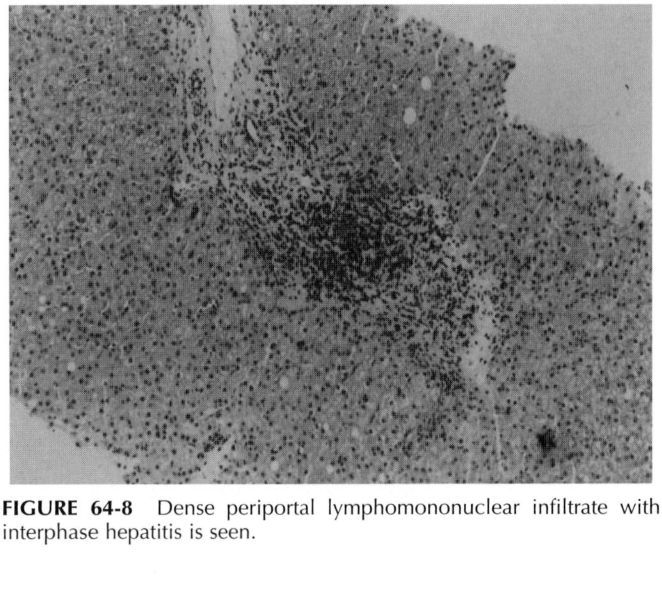

FIGURE 64-8 Dense periportal lymphomononuclear infiltrate with interphase hepatitis is seen.

systems are the Histologic Activity Index (HAI or Knodell Score) and the METAVIR.[247] These scoring systems have potential limitations. Hepatic fibrosis may not be homogeneous throught the liver, and in some cases fibrosis may be underestimated and cirrhosis missed. There are no clinical, biochemical, or virologic tests to accurately predict progression of fibrosis.[248] Patients with minimal or no fibrosis can be assured of a favorable outcome and even defer antiviral therapy.[245] Additionally, liver biopsy can provide information regarding the contribution of iron, concurrent alcohol use, and steatosis. There is a significant association between steatosis and inflammation and fibrosis score on liver biopsy.[249,250] Genotype 3a is consistently linked to steatosis more strongly than other genotypes.[250] Accumulating evidence suggests that steatosis contributes to the progression in HCV-related disease, probably owing to oxidative stress and cytokine-mediated injury.[251] Because a favorable response to antiviral therapy occurs in 80% of patients infected with genotype 2 or 3, it may not be always necessary to perform liver biopsy in these patients to make a decision to treat.[245]

TREATMENT AND PROGNOSIS

Since a large proportion of patients with chronic HCV infection develop progressive chronic hepatitis, cirrhosis, and sometimes HCC, the main rationale for treatment of chronic hepatitis C is to prevent these complications, render the patient noninfectious, and eventually ameliorate the symptoms. The decision to treat patients should be based on solid diagnostic grounds, ideally with histologic evaluation.

In 1991, recombinant IFN-α was approved for the treatment of patients with chronic hepatitis C with persistently elevated serum aminotransferases and biopsy-proved chronic active hepatitis. Two important preliminary trials published in 1989,[252,253] which involved the adminstration of IFN to patients with chronic HCV infection, showed complete biochemical resolution in roughly 50% of patients, with simultaneous histologic improvement after 6 months of therapy. Aminotransferases were at baseline levels in nearly 50% of responders 1 year after discontinuation of therapy. The success of clinical trials has been evaluated in terms of response (i.e, clearance of HCV RNA) at the end of therapy (*end of treatment response, ETR*), and 6 months after cessation of therapy (*sustained virologic response, SVR*). Long-term follow up of patients with SVR shows a high probability of maintaining virologic and histologic remission over the years.[254] The patient with acute hepatitis C represents a special and controversial situation regarding therapy. Jaeckel and associates[255] treated 44 acutely infected patients with a 24-week course of IFN-α monotherapy, and 98% achieved a sustained biochemical and virologic response. More recently, Gerlach and coworkers[256] identified 60 individuals with acute hepatitis C as part of a prospective observational study investigating the outcome of the natural course of infection in patients with acute hepatitis C. Six patients received immediate antiviral therapy, and 54 were left untreated. Of the 37 (68%) of 54 patients who initially cleared virus spontaneously, 13 relapsed and remained virus-positive, while 24 (44%) remained persistently virus-negative. Those with self-limited disease were more likely to have symptomatic onset of illness, whereas no patient with asymptomatic presentation cleared HCV RNA without treatment. Importantly, antiviral therapy was begun 3 to 6 months after onset of symptoms, and in 21 (81%) of 26 a sustained response was achieved. Therefore, this and other studies[257] support the concept that a significant proportion of patients with acute hepatitis C will clear virus spontaneously and not require immediate therapy. A prudent period of observation with serial viral load determinations following acute symptomatic hepatitis C infection is a reasonable management strategy for this subgroup.

Regarding chronic hepatitis C, only a subgroup of patients have a clear indication for therapy. Patients with detectable HCV RNA, persistently elevated ALT, and moderate necrosis, inflammation, and fibrosis on liver biopsy should be offered therapy if there are no contraindications, since they are at high risk for disease progression.[245,258] Patients with normal or near-normal ALT, or no fibrosis and minimal necroinflammatory changes on liver biopsy, may not need treatment and should be monitored periodically,[245] but decisions to treat such patients should be carefully individualized, and the patient's desire to eliminate the virus should be considered. Several variables have been consistently associated with a higher likelihood of SVR in different clinical trials: HCV genotype other than 1, lower baseline viral load, absence of bridging necrosis/cirrhosis, low body mass, female sex, and adherence to the regimen.[259–265] Persons with decompensated cirrhosis are unlikely to have a response and may deteriorate with therapy.

Monotherapy with IFN shows an SVR of less than 20%, but the addition of ribavirin to IFN improves the SVR to 44%.[259,260] The attachment of polyethylene glycol to IFN-α (pegylated IFN, PEG IFN) extends the half-life and duration of therapeutic action of IFN-α. In contrast to IFN-α, which is administered three times a week, PEG IFN is given only once a week. Two PEG IFN formulations are currently available for use as once weekly therapy for hepatitis C: 40 kD PEG chain form of IFN-α-2a and 12 kD chain form of IFN-α-2b. The former is supplied as a ready-to-use formulation, independent of body weight, whereas the latter is supplied as a lyophilized powder that requires reconstitution before use and is formulated by body weight, expressed in μg/kg/wk. The former is cleared primarily by the liver, whereas 30% of the PEG IFN-α-2b is cleared by the kidney. Clinical trials comparing PEG IFN monotherapy to standard IFN have been performed with both PEG IFNs, showing SVR of 25% (at 1.5 μg/kg/wk) with PEG IFN-α-2b versus 12% for standard IFN at 3 mU three times weekly.[263] In another study, PEG IFN-α-2a at a dose of 180 μg once weekly for 48 weeks was compared with IFN-α-2a at a dose of 6 mU three times weekly for 12 weeks and then 3 mU three times weekly for 36 weeks.[261] The SVR in the PEG IFN-α-2a group was 39% compared with 19% in the standard IFN group. Pegylated interferon plus ribavirin has thus become the new standard of care for the treatment of chronic hepatitis C.[245] In two large trials in which ribavirin was given in combination with PEG IFN or standard IFN, the overall rate of SVR was 54% for PEG IFN-α-2b versus 47% for standard IFN-α-2b,[264] and 56% for PEG IFN-α-2a versus 45% for standard IFN-α-2a.[265] Patients with genotypes 2 and 3 deserve special consideration. Sustained virologic responses with standard IFN and ribavirin were comparable to those with PEG IFN and ribavirin; therefore, standard IFN could be used in treating patients with these genotypes. Twenty-four weeks of therapy at an 800-mg daily dose of ribavirin seems sufficient for persons with genotypes 2 and 3, while patients with genotype 1 need 48 weeks of treatment and 1000 to 1200 mg/day ribavirin.[245,264,265] In recent trials of PEG IFN and ribavirin, retrospective analysis yielded important information with significant impact on the management of patients with chronic HCV. Early virologic response (EVR) was defined as loss of HCV RNA or a decrease in HCV RNA by at least two log–fold compared with baseline values. By week 12 of therapy, 86% of patients treated with PEG IFN-α-2a plus ribavirin had achieved EVR. Of these, 65% subsequently achieved SVR. In contrast, among the 14% of patients without EVR by week 12, only 3% went on to SVR, resulting in a negative predictive value of 97%.[266] Similar findings are reported more recently in a study utilizing PEG IFN-α-2b and ribavirin.[267] Thus, in the absence of EVR, discontinuation of therapy should be considered.

Another important aspect to consider with therapy against HCV is histologic response. Poynard and colleagues compared 10 different regimes of PEG IFN-α-2b and conventional IFN with and without ribavirin and found that 24% of patients who received PEG IFN-α-2b (1.5 g/kg/wk) plus ribavirin achieved histologic response compared with only 16% on IFN monotherapy.[268] Camma and colleagues performed a meta-analysis of three studies on more than 1000 previously untreated patients with pretreatment and post-treatment liver biopsies to assess the differences between PEG IFN-α-2a and standard IFN-α-2a in terms of histologic improvement.[269] PEG IFN-α-2a induced a marked reduction in grade and stage in patients who achieved SVR, and no histologic benefit was seen for nonresponders after 24 to 48 weeks. Nonobese patients (body mass index <30 kg/m^2) and those with high pretreatment ALT levels had the greatest probability of histologic response. Currently, the outcome for patients with advanced fibrosis is uncertain. The HALT-C (hepatitis C antiviral long-term treatment against cirrhosis) trial is a multicenter, randomized, controlled study sponsored by the NIH currently conducted at 11 centers in the United States, designed to determine whether long-term treatment with PEG IFN in previous nonresponders with advanced fibrosis can prevent or even reverse cirrhosis and reduce the risk of developing end-stage liver disease and HCC.[270] The results of this trial are eagerly awaited.

Patients with chronic hepatitis C and concurrent HIV infection may have an accelerated course of HCV disease.[271] Treatment with PEG IFN has not been evaluated in large-scale studies, but it should be offered to this special group of patients on a case-by-case basis.[272] Despite great advances in therapy of chronic hepatitis C in the last 15 years, 50% of patients still do not respond to therapy. Thus, there is a need for more effective therapies. Based on current knowledge of the HCV-encoded enzymes required for viral replication, many pharmaceutical manufacturers are pursuing the development of compounds that specifically inhibit enzymes critical to the HCV life cycle. Some potential targets are the HCV NS3/4A protease, the NS5B polymerase, and the viral IRES. Ribozymes designed to cleave the HCV IRES RNA have entered phase II clinical trials.[273] Histamine, acting via H_2 receptors on phagocytic cells, suppresses the activity of a key enzyme in oxygen radical formation, the NADPH oxidase.[274] By this mechanism, histamine protects NK cells and T cells against oxygen radical–induced dysfunction, reversing immunosuppression caused by HCV-induced oxidative stress in the liver. Ongoing trials are evaluating the safety and efficacy of the triple combination of PEG IFN, ribavirin, and histamine in HCV-infected patients.[274] In the next few years new agents may be used alone or in combination with PEG IFN and ribavirin for the management of chronic hepatitis C.

PREVENTION AND CONTROL

A major feature of HCV of great concern for vaccine development is the heterogeneity of its genome. The existence of quasispecies is one feature of HCV that helps it to evade host surveillance. There is also considerable heterogeneity in the nucleotide sequences, and likely antigenic characteristics of different strains and genotypes of HCV. While the cellular immune response seems to play an important role in the control of HCV infection, the existence and efficacy of neutralizing antibodies are less clear. A study performed in humans argues against a critical role of such antibodies in the resolution of infection.[275] However, no good test for neutralizing antibodies exists.

Currently no vaccine is available for the prevention of hepatitis C. Most of the focus to date is on the development of vaccines capable of inducing strong and long-lasting cell-mediated responses.[276] Progress in the understanding of the genomic organization of some viral agents has resulted in the production of recombinant vectors to deliver vaccine antigens and allow their endogenous expression by cells of the immunized host. Bruna-Romero and colleagues vaccinated mice with a recombinant adenovirus containing core and E1 genes of HCV.[277] Induction of a strong and long-lasting (up to 100 days) specific CTL response targeted against six different epitopes could be demonstrated. However, it is difficult to predict whether specific CTL responses in chronic HCV patients will exacerbate or control CTL-mediated liver injury.[276] Certainly, the vaccine developers face a great challenge. In the meantime, preventive measures directed at maximizing universal precautions, education of the population regarding high-risk behaviors, and careful screening of blood and organ donors are the only ways to prevent the transmission of this disease.

Hepatitis D

Hepatitis D virus (HDV) infection is caused by an RNA satellite virus, called delta (δ) hepatitis virus, that requires the presence of HBV for its complete life cycle. The HDV agent was discovered in 1977 by Rizzetto and associates[278] when a previously unrecognized antigen was seen by immunofluorescence in the nuclei of the hepatocytes of HBV-infected patients. In 1980 HDV transmission to HBV-infected chimpanzees established HDV as a distinct infectious agent.[279]

AGENT

HDV is unique because it does not resemble any other animal virus and has not been formally classified.[2] A relationship of HDV to viroids, plant satellite viruses, and simple infectious RNA molecules has been proposed.[280] The HDV genome is the smallest among the human hepatitis viruses and is 1.68 kb in length. It is a single-stranded, circular RNA

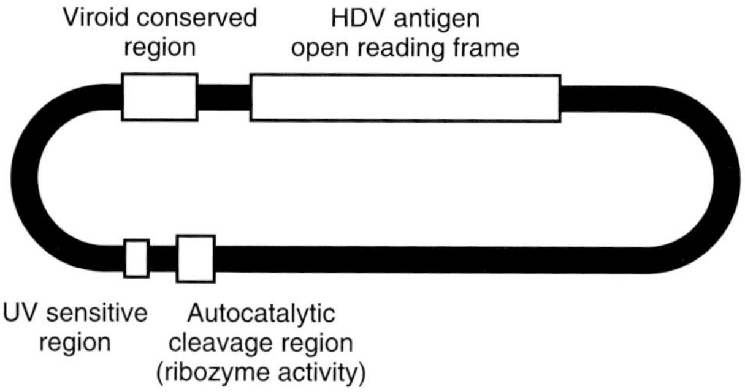

FIGURE 64-9 Hepatitis D anti-genome. UV, ultraviolet light. (From Koff RS, Dienstag JL, Riely CA, et al: AGA Clinical Teaching Project, Unit 3, Viral Hepatitis, 2nd ed. Timonium, Md., Milner-Fenwick, 1994.)

molecule (Fig. 64-9). The virion particles have an envelope composed of HBsAg that encloses the RNA genome along with the hepatitis delta antigen (HDAg). It is a negative-stranded RNA virus, since only the negative-strand RNA is packaged and found in the serum of infected patients. There is variability in the nucleotide sequence, and studies of the HDV genome in African patients suggest the existence of more than three genotypes of HDV.[281] Both the genome and the antigenome RNA contain autocatalytic cleavage sites with ribozyme activity, while the positive-sense antigenome contains an open reading frame for HDAg. HDV replication is regulated by two types of HDV antigens—the large form and the small form—which have identical sequences but differ in length by 19 amino acids owing to a C-terminal extension in the large delta antigen.[282] The longer protein inhibits HDV replication and participates in its packaging. The smaller HDAg protein promotes HDV RNA replication. Remarkably, these closely related proteins are the only proteins expressed by the virus. The key point for the clinician to understand, however, is that HDV replication is dependent on active expression of the HBV envelope protein, HBsAg, for packaging of the genome and completion of the HDV life cycle.

The RNA replication occurs in the hepatocyte nucleus, and extrahepatic sites have never been documented. The genomic RNA is copied by a rolling circle mechanism. An antigenomic strand is synthesized from the genome, and these antigenomic molecules self-cleave to form genome unit length fragments that self-ligate to a circular configuration. The new circle is used as a template to create new copies of the original molecule.[51] Interestingly, and in contrast with the other human hepatitis viruses, the viral RNA has enzymatic properties (ribozymes) that cleave and religate the viral RNA during the process of RNA replication; these ribozymes resemble those that occur in plant satellite viruses.[51]

EPIDEMIOLOGY

HDV infection is found only in HBV-infected persons, but the prevalence of the two is not necessarily parallel. For instance, in southern Africa, where the prevalence of HBsAg carriers is around 15%, HDV is not found. Overall, HDV affects approximately 5% of HBV carriers worldwide.[283] In Italy, where HDV was originally described, its prevalence has decreased substantially in the past decade.[2] Other areas of high prevalence are the Middle East, West Africa, and the Pacific Islands[284] as well as Eastern Europe.[285] In areas of low prevalence of HBV infection, infection with HDV affects mainly high-risk groups.[278] In the United States the prevalence of HDV among HBsAg-positive blood donors is low (1.4% to 8%) but is higher in HBsAg-positive IVDUs (20% to 53%) and hemophiliacs (48% to 80%).[7] The first report of HDV infection in South America occurred among Yupca Indians of Venezuela, who exhibited an HBsAg prevalence of 70%.[286] A form of fulminant hepatitis known for several decades in northern Colombia has been named "hepatitis of the Sierra Nevada de Santa Marta." Up to 60% of HBsAg carriers in one village of this endemic area had antibody to hepatitis D antigen.[287] There is also a high incidence of HBV and HDV serologic markers among the residents of the Peruvian and Brazilian Amazon Basin.[288–290] Ten percent of Peruvian jungle residents (where the prevalence of HBsAg was 22.7%) had antibody to delta antigen,[289] and the foreign missionaries who worked in this area had a higher incidence of serologic markers for hepatitis B and D than did blood donors from the Peruvian coast.

HDV infection is transmitted by the parenteral route through contact with blood or body secretions. Direct parenteral inoculation is the most efficient route, accounting for the epidemic dissemination of the HDV agent among IVDUs.[291] Post-transfusion HDV infection is a rare event, but the risk is higher in carriers of HBsAg[292] and in patients receiving multiple blood transfusions or blood products, as occurs in hemophiliacs. Sexual transmission of HDV is not so efficient as it is in HBV, and perinatal transmission has never been reported in the United States.[10] On the other hand, researchers have described seven groups of Brazilian Indians from the Amazon region, in whom sexual transmission was suggested as the most important mechanism of dissemination of HDV.[293]

DISEASE

HDV infection can either occur simultaneously with HBV infection (coinfection) or as a superinfection in a person with chronic HBV infection. It is difficult, if not impossible, to differentiate hepatitis D from other types of viral hepatitis on clinical grounds alone. There is a wide spectrum of disease, from asymptomatic to end-stage liver disease. However, when compared with asymptomatic individuals having the HBsAg carrier state alone, subjects with HBsAg and anti-HDV antibodies have a fourfold risk of developing severe liver damage.[294] In some acute cases, a biphasic pattern of illness can be seen, in which the patient can have a second peak of ALT and a "flare" approximately 2 weeks after the presentation. This occurred in 23% of patients in a prospective study[295] and may be the only clinical clue to the presence of dual infection.

Patients with chronic hepatitis D may be asymptomatic or have nonspecific symptoms such as fatigue or vague right upper quadrant discomfort. Approximately 25% may have well-established cirrhosis at presentation.[296] Coinfection with HDV and HBV follows the natural history of acute uncomplicated hepatitis B, with a rate of chronicity of less than 5%. This is probably due to the inability of HDV to continue to replicate without HBV. In a prospective study of IVDUs with HBV-HDV coinfection, only 2.4% developed chronicity.[297]

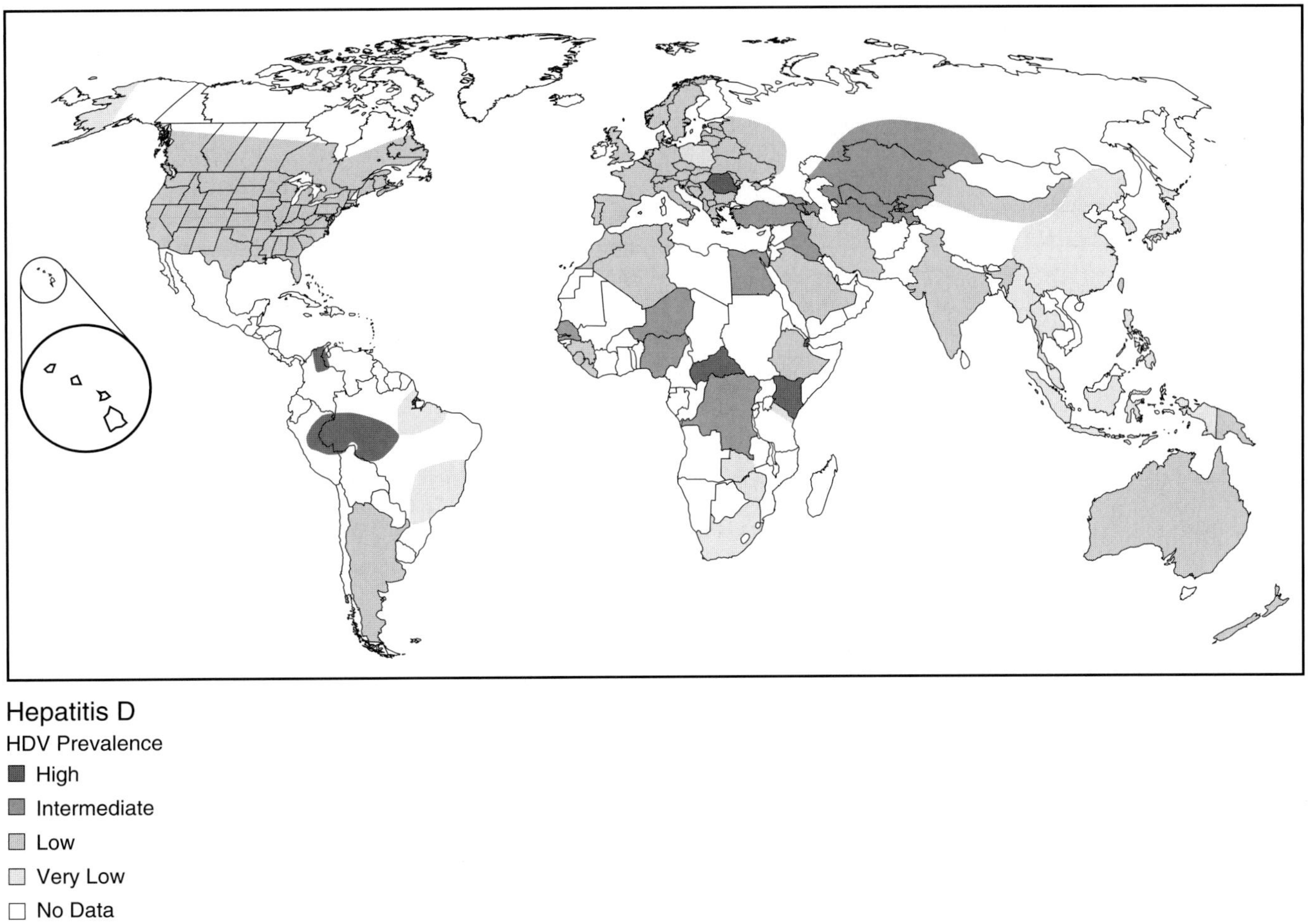

On the other hand, with superinfection, chronicity is the rule, and up to 70% of patients develop cirrhosis at some point. There is, however, a possible variability in the biologic behavior of HDV between different geographic areas. For instance, in a Chinese study involving follow-up for 8 years in patients with superinfection, the rate of progression to cirrhosis was not statistically different from that of HBsAg carriers.[298]

Besides accelerating the course of HBV-related chronic liver disease, HDV is highly associated with fulminant hepatitis,[299] which is more commonly seen with superinfection than with coinfection.[295] Additionally, mortality of patients with fulminant hepatitis is higher in patients with superinfection.

The association between HDV infection and HCC is controversial. Verme and coworkers[300] showed that patients with HDV and HCC were younger than HBV carriers with negative markers for HDV, suggesting that the dual infection triggers a more severe necroinflammatory reaction that leads to neoplastic transformation.

PATHOGENESIS AND IMMUNITY

HDV is absolutely dependent on HBV for its replication and pathogenicity, since the HDV RNA is packaged by the HBV envelope protein, HBsAg. Because of its dependence on HBV, HDV can only infect a person who is already a carrier of HBV (superinfection) or who is simultaneously being infected with HBV (coinfection). In superinfection, HDV replication suppresses HBV replication, seemingly at the transcriptional level.[301] Therefore, superinfection with HDV may be associated with a reduction in intrahepatic levels of HBsAg, HBeAg, and HBV DNA.[302] According to some studies, the pathogenesis of HDV can be explained by two mechanisms: by direct cytopathic action of HDV expressing HDV antigen in the hepatocyte membrane or by replication of HDV RNA and subsequent cellular destruction.[303] Autoimmunity has been described in HDV infection, with the documentation of antiliver, -kidney, and -microsomal (LKM) antibodies.[278]

HDV RNA and HDV antigen (HDAg) are detected early, concurrent with the detection of HBsAg. As HBsAg disappears, HDAg is also cleared and anti-HDV antibodies appear, initially IgM and later IgG. These antibodies are usually detectable late and not at the onset of symptoms. Sometimes the early appearance of isolated IgM anti-HDV or the presence of convalescent titers of IgG anti-HDV may be the only serologic evidence of HDV infection.

In the case of superinfection, HDAg and HDV RNA usually remain detectable in serum, along with high titers of IgM and IgG anti-HDV.[304] The course of HDV infection might be modified by multiple factors, such as acute HDV infection in carriers of mutant variants of HBV.[305] In this scenario, replication of HDV occurs with less efficiency owing to less functional HBV, leading to a more benign course. Not much is known about the cellular response of the immune system in the setting of HDV infection.

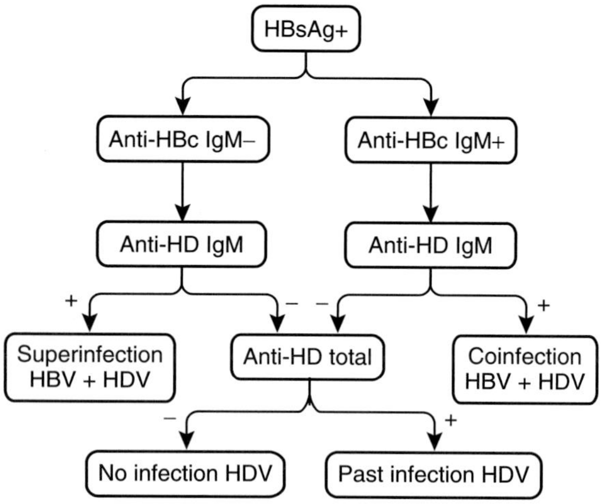

FIGURE 64-10 Algorithm for the evaluation of a patient infected with hepatitis D. HBsAG, hepatitis B surface antigen; HBc, hepatitis B core antigen; HBV, hepatitis B virus; HD, hepatitis D; HDV, hepatitis D virus.

DIAGNOSIS

The serodiagnosis of HDV coinfection and superinfection is slightly different (see Pathogenesis and Immunity). An algorithm shows the interpretation of the different clinical scenarios of HBV/HDV interactions (Fig. 64-10). The hallmark of the diagnosis in both situations is the presence of anti-HDV, which can be measured by radioimmunoassay (RIA) and enzyme-linked immunosorbant assay (ELISA). The serologic response to HDV is not so strong or consistent as occurs with hepatitis A or B. The IgM and IgG responses are usually strong in superinfected HBsAg carriers developing chronic HDV infection.[306] In the case of coinfection, some patients may express only IgM or IgG or may have both the primary IgM and secondary IgG responses. The most important diagnostic marker for hepatitis D is IgM anti-HDV, and its presence correlates with ongoing liver inflammation and predicts progression to cirrhosis.[307] Therefore, unlike in hepatitis A and B, in HDV infection the presence of IgM antibody is not necessarily diagnostic of acute infection.

HDAg can be detected in serum, although only in the early stages of infection before the appearance of anti-HDV, because the antigen forms complexes with antibody becoming masked, owing to the usually high titers of antibody.[308] The more sensitive Western blot analysis allows detection of lower levels of HD antigenemia. This technique involves ultracentrifugation and detergent treatment of viral particles, followed by electrophoresis and detection of the antigen by a radiolabeled antibody. Viremia can also be demonstrated by direct detection of HDV RNA using RT-PCR[309] or molecular hybridization assays.[310]

Performance of a liver biopsy is indicated to assess disease stage and prognosis, but no histologic features are pathognomonic for HDV.[311] The presence of intrahepatic HDAg can be visualized by immunofluorescence of the tissue sample, appearing as nuclear staining in hepatocytes,[312] and this is considered the "gold standard" by many authorities.

TREATMENT AND PROGNOSIS

There is no effective therapy for acute hepatitis D, and treatment is essentially directed to patients with chronic HDV infection. Rosina and colleagues conducted a 12-month randomized controlled trial with IFN in 61 Italian patients with chronic delta hepatitis.[313] The patients were randomly assigned to receive either IFN 5 mU/m^2 three times daily for the first 4 months and then 3 mU/m^2 three times daily for the remaining 8 months or no treatment. Despite a greater reduction of ALT levels in the treated group, the serum HDV RNA, intrahepatic HDAg, and histologic activity index scores were not statistically different between treatment and control groups at any given time. Another study compared IFN in doses of 9 mU or 3 mU three times daily versus no treatment for 48 weeks.[314] Fifty percent of the patients treated with the higher dose regimen had a complete response (defined as complete normalization of ALT and undetectable HDV RNA) compared with only 21% of those who received the lower dose regimen and none of the controls. In addition, there was significant histologic improvement in the group that received the higher dose compared with the other two groups. Remarkably, despite the high dosage and prolonged treatment period, all patients completed the 48-week course of therapy.

Agents developed to treat chronic hepatitis B, such as the nucleoside analog lamivudine or adefovir dipivoxil, may prove to be useful in managing chronic delta hepatitis by inhibiting HBV replication, but there are currently no published trials assessing the efficacy of these drugs in the setting of HDV infection. These agents rarely result in termination of HBsAg expression, which is the HBV protein that provides the necessary helper function to HDV. Potential targets for HDV therapy in the future may include inhibitors of HDAg phosphorylation, HBsAg glycosylation, or inhibitors of HDV RNA ribozyme activity.[315] The serious nature of chronic delta hepatitis is a challenge requiring development of novel therapeutic approaches.

PREVENTION AND CONTROL

Since the HDV RNA is packaged by the HBV envelope protein, HBsAg, antibodies to HBsAg are protective against HDV infection. Thus, immunization against HBV also provides protection against HDV in HBV-naïve individuals. However, for HBV carriers, no effective vaccine is available to specifically protect against HDV. A study utilizing preparations of HDAg to vaccinate woodchucks with chronic woodchuck hepatitis virus infection against HDV infection failed to show a protective effect of the vaccine.[316] Patients already infected with HBV should be strongly advised against using contaminated needles or engaging in high-risk sexual practices to avoid superinfection with HDV. The annual incidence of HDV infection seems to be steadily falling worldwide.

Hepatitis E

Hepatitis E is an enterically transmitted form of viral hepatitis that appears to be common in tropical and subtropical areas, and epidemics have been reported in Asia, Africa, the Middle East, and Central America.[1] It is a distinct agent that has been associated with fulminant hepatic failure among pregnant women but has no known chronic sequelae.

An extensive outbreak of waterborne hepatitis was reported in India in 1955. In further retrospective analysis 25 years later, all stored serum samples were found to have

108. Peters M: Mechanism of action of interferons. Semin Liver Dis 9:235, 1989.
109. Wong DK, Cheung AM, O'Rourke K, et al: Effect of alpha-interferon treatment in patients with hepatitis B e antigen-positive chronic hepatitis B. A meta-analysis. Ann Intern Med 119:312, 1993.
110. Wong DK, Heathcote J: The role of interferon in the treatment of viral hepatitis. Pharmacol Ther 63:177, 1994.
111. Perrillo RP, Tamburro C, Regenstein F, et al: Low-dose titratable interferon alpha in decompensated liver disease caused by chronic infection with hepatitis B virus. Gastroenterology 109:908, 1995.
112. Perrillo RP, Schiff ER, Davis GL, et al: A randomized, controlled trial of interferon alpha-2b alone and after prednisone withdrawal for the treatment of chronic hepatitis B. N Engl J Med 323:295, 1990.
113. Perrillo RP, Regenstein F, Peters MG, et al: Prednisone withdrawal followed by recombinant alpha interferon in the treatment of chronic type B hepatitis: A randomized controlled trial. Ann Intern Med 109:95, 1988.
114. Khalili M, Perrillo RP: Interferon therapy of hepatitis B. Clin Liver Dis 3:363, 1999.
115. Lin SM, Sheen IS, Chien RN, et al: Long-term beneficial effect of interferon therapy in patients with chronic hepatitis B virus infection. Hepatology 29:971, 1999.
116. Lau DT, Everhart J, Kleiner DE, et al: Long-term follow-up of patients with chronic hepatitis B treated with interferon alpha. Gastroenterology 113:1660, 1997.
117. Fong TL, Di Bisceglie AM, Gerber MA, et al: Persistence of hepatitis B virus DNA in the liver after loss of HBsAg in chronic hepatitis B. Hepatology 18:1313, 1993.
118. Cohard M, Poynard T, Mathurin P, et al: Prednisone-interferon combination in the treatment of chronic hepatitis B: Direct and indirect meta-analysis. Hepatology 20:1390, 1994.
119. Hadziyannis SJ, Vassilopoulos D: Hepatitis B e antigen-negative chronic hepatitis B: From clinical recognition to pathogenesis and treatment. Viral Hepat Rev 1:7, 1995.
120. Olivieri F, Santantonio T, Bellati G, et al: Long term response to therapy of chronic anti-HBe positive hepatitis B is poor independent of type and schedule of interferon. Am J Gastroenterol 94:1366, 1999.
121. Lok AS, Wu PC, Lai CL, et al: A controlled trial of interferon with or without prednisone priming for chronic hepatitis B. Gastroenterology 102:2091, 1992.
122. Lok AS, McMahon BJ: Chronic hepatitis B. AASLD practice guidelines. Hepatology 34:1225, 2001.
123. Benhamou Y, Dohin E, Lunel-Fabiani F, et al: Efficacy of lamivudine on replication of hepatitis B virus in HIV-infected patients. Lancet 345:396, 1995.
124. Lee WM: Hepatitis B virus infection. N Engl J Med 337:1733, 1997.
125. Dienstag JL, Schiff ER, Wright TL, et al: Lamivudine as initial treatment for chronic hepatitis B in the United States. N Engl J Med 341:1256, 1999.
126. Lai CL, Chien RN, Leung NW, et al: A one-year trial of lamivudine for chronic hepatitis B. Asia Hepatitis Lamivudine Study Group. N Engl J Med 339:61, 1998.
127. Leung NW, Lai CL, Chang TT, et al: Extended lamivudine treatment in patients with chronic hepatitis B enhances hepatitis B e antigen seroconversion rates: results after three years of therapy. Hepatology 33:1527, 2001.
128. Liaw YF, Chien RN, Yeh CT, et al: Acute exacerbation and hepatitis B virus clearance after emergence of YMDD motif mutation during lamivudine therapy. Hepatology 30:567, 1999.
129. Dienstag JL, Goldin RD, Heathcote EJ, et al: Histological outcome during long-term lamivudine therapy. Gastroenterology 124:105, 2003.
130. Dienstag JL, Cianciara J, Karayalcin S, et al: Durability of serologic response after lamivudine treatment of chronic hepatitis B. Hepatology 37:748, 2003.
131. Song BC, Duh DJ, Lee HC, et al: Hepatitis B e antigen seroconversion after lamivudine therapy is not durable in patients with chronic hepatitis B in Korea. Hepatology 32:803, 2000.
132. Lee KM, Cho SW, Kim SW, et al: Effect on virological response on post-treatment durability of lamivudine-induced HBeAg seroconversion. J Viral Hepat 9:208, 2002.
133. Chien RN, Yeh CT, Tsai SL, et al: Determinants for sustained HBeAg response to lamivudine therapy. Hepatology 38:1267, 2003.
134. Hadziyannis SJ, Papatheodoridis GV, Dimou E, et al: Efficacy of long-term lamivudine monotherapy in patients with hepatitis B e antigen-negative chronic hepatitis B. Hepatology 32:847, 2000.
135. Santantonio T, Mazzola M, Iacovazzi T, et al: Long-term follow-up of patients with anti-HBe/HBV DNA-positive chronic hepatitis B treated for 12 months with lamivudine. J Hepatol 32:300, 2000.
136. Perrillo RP, Wright T, Rakela J, et al: A multicenter United States–Canadian trial to assess lamivudine monotherapy before and after liver transplantation for chronic hepatitis B. Hepatology 33:424, 2001.
137. Villenueve JP, Condreay LD, Willems B, et al: Lamivudine treatment for decompensated cirrhosis resulting from chronic hepatitis B. Hepatology 31:207, 2000.
138. Yao FY, Bass NM: Lamivudine treatment in patients with severely decompensated cirrhosis due to replicating hepatitis B infection. J Hepatol 33:301, 2000.
139. Steinmuller T, Seehofer D, Rayes N, et al: Increasing applicability of liver transplantation for patients with hepatitis B-related liver disease. Hepatology 35:1528, 2002.
140. Lok AS, Lai CL, Leung N, et al: Long-term safety of lamivudine treatment in patients with chronic hepatitis B. Gastroenterology 125:1714, 2003.
141. Marcellin P, Chang TT, Lim SG, et al: Adefovir dipivoxil for the treatment of hepatitis B e antigen–positive chronic hepatitis B. N Engl J Med 348:808, 2003.
142. Hadziyannis SJ, Tassopoulos NC, Heathcote EJ, et al: Adefovir dipivoxil for the treatment of hepatitis B e antigen-negative chronic hepatitis B. N Engl J Med 348:800, 2003.
143. Westland CE, Yang H, Delaney WE, et al: Week 48 resistance surveillance in two phase 3 clinical studies of adefovir dipivoxil for chronic hepatitis B. Hepatology 38:96, 2003.
144. Angus P, Vaughan R, Xiong S, et al: Resistance to adefovir dipivoxil therapy associated with the selection of a novel mutation in the HBV polymerase. Gastroenterology 125:292, 2003.
145. Shaw T, Locarnini S: Combination chemotherapy for hepatitis B virus: The final solution? Hepatology 32:430, 2000.
146. Perrillo R, Hann HW, Mutimer D, et al: Adefovir dipivoxil added to ongoing lamivudine in chronic hepatitis B with YMDD mutant hepatitis B virus. Gastroenterology 126:81, 2004.
147. Peters MG, Hann HW, Martin P, et al: Adefovir dipivoxil alone or in combination with lamivudine in patients with lamivudine-resistant chronic hepatitis B. Gastroenterology 126:91, 2004.
148. de Man RA, Wolters LM, Nevens F, et al: Safety and efficacy of oral entecavir given for 28 days in patients with chronic hepatitis B virus infection. Hepatology 34:578, 2001.
149. Aye TT, Bartholomeusz A, Shaw T, et al: Hepatitis B virus polymerase mutations during antiviral therapy in a patient following liver transplantation. J Hepatol 26:1148, 1997.
150. Dienstag JL, Werner BG, Polk F, et al: Hepatitis B vaccine in health care personnel: Safety, immunogenicity, and indicators of efficacy. Ann Intern Med 101:34, 1984.
151. Marsano LS, Greenberg RN, Kirkpatrick RB, et al: Comparison of a rapid hepatitis B immunization schedule to the standard schedule for adults. Am J Gastroenterol 91:111, 1996.
152. Harpaz R, Von Seidlein L, Averhoff FM, et al: Transmission of hepatitis B virus to multiple patients from a surgeon without evidence of inadequate infection control. N Engl J Med 334:549, 1996.
153. Hadler SF, Maynard J: Long-term immunogenicity and efficacy of hepatitis B vaccine in homosexual men. N Engl J Med 315:209, 1986.
154. vanHattum J, Maikoe T, Poel J, et al: Persistence of immune memory in responders to hepatitis B vaccination who subsequently lost anti-HBs titer. Hepatology 12:885, 1990.
155. Banatvala JE, Van Damme P: Hepatitis B vaccine: Do we need boosters? J Viral Hepat 10:1, 2003.
156. Stevens CE, Alter HJ, Taylor PE, et al: Hepatitis B vaccine in patients receiving hemodialysis. Immunogenicity and efficacy. N Engl J Med 311:496, 1984.
157. Centers for Disease Control: Protection against viral hepatitis: Recommendations of the Immunization Practices Advisory Committee (ACIP). MMWR 39:1, 1990.
158. Jacobson IM, Jaffers G, Dienstag JL, et al: Immunogenicity of hepatitis B vaccine in renal transplant recipients. Transplantation 39:393, 1985.
159. Colichon A, Vildosola H, Sjögren M, et al: Respuesta serologica a una vacuna DNA recombinante en nativos residentes de dos areas hiperendemicas a hepatitis B en la amazonia peruana. Rev Gastroenterol Peru 13:78, 1993.
160. Ascherio A, Zhang SM, Hernan MA, et al: Hepatitis B vaccination and the risk of multiple sclerosis. N Engl J Med 344:327, 2001.

161. Young MD, Schneider DL, Zuckermann AJ, et al: Adult hepatitis B vaccination using a novel triple antigen recombinant vaccine. Hepatology 34:372, 2001.
162. Zuckerman JN, Zuckerman AJ, Symington I, et al: Evaluation of a new hepatitis B triple-antigen vaccine in inadequate responders to current vaccines. Hepatology 34:798, 2001.
163. Feinstone SM, Kapikian AZ, Purcell RH, et al: Transfusion-associated hepatitis not due to viral hepatitis type A or B. N Engl J Med 292:767, 1975.
164. Choo-QL, Kuo G, Weiner AJ, et al: Isolation of a cDNA clone derived from a blood-borne non-A, non-B viral hepatitis genome. Science 244:359, 1989.
165. Grakoui A, McCourt DW, Wychowski C, et al: Characterization of the hepatitis C virus-encoded serine protease: Determination of proteinase-dependent polyprotein cleavage site. J Virol 67:2832, 1993.
166. Spahn CM, Kieft JS, Grassucci RA, et al: Hepatitis C virus IRES RNA-induced changes in the conformation of the 40S ribosomal subunit. Science 291:1959, 2001.
167. Okamoto H, Kojima M, Okada SI, et al: Genetic drift of hepatitis C virus during an 8.2-year infection in a chimpanzee: Variability and stability. Virology 190:894, 1992.
168. Martell M, Esteban JI, Quer J, et al: Hepatitis C virus (HCV) circulates as a population of different but closely related genomes: Quasispecies nature of HCV genome distribution. J Virol 66:3225, 1992.
169. Lauer GM, Walker BD: Hepatitis C virus infection. N Engl J Med 345:41, 2001.
170. Mansell CJ, Locarnini SA: Epidemiology of hepatitis C in the East. Semin Liver Dis 15:15, 1995.
171. Frommel D, Tekle-Haimanot R, Berthe N, et al: A survey of antibodies to hepatitis C virus in Ethiopia. Am J Trop Med Hyg 49:435, 1993.
172. Frank C, Mohamed MK, Strickland GT, et al: The role of parenteral antischistosomal therapy in the spread of hepatitis C virus in Egypt. Lancet 355:887, 2000.
173. Bellentani S, Miglioli L, Masutti F, et al: Epidemiology of hepatitis C virus infection in Italy: The slowly unraveling mystery. Microbes Infect 2:1757, 2000.
174. Wasley A, Alter MJ: Epidemiology of hepatitis C: Geographic differences and temporal trends. Semin Liver Dis 20:1, 2000.
175. Rumi MG, Colombo M, Gringeri A, et al: High prevalence or antibody to hepatitis C virus in multi-transfused hemophiliacs with normal transaminase levels. Ann Intern Med 112:379, 1990.
176. Legler TJ, Riggert J, Simson G, et al: Testing of individual blood donations for HCV RNA reduces the residual risk of transfusion-transmitted HCV infection. Transfusion 40:1192, 2000.
177. Beld M, Habibuw MR, Rebers SP, Boom R, et al: Evaluation of automated RNA-extraction technology and a qualitative HCV assay for sensitivity and detection of HCV RNA in pool-screening systems. Transfusion 40:575, 2000.
178. Esteban JI, Esteban R, Viladomiu L, et al: Hepatitis C virus antibodies among risk groups in Spain. Lancet 2:294, 1989.
179. van den Hoek JAR, van Haarstrecht HJA, Goudsmit J, et al: Prevalence, incidence, and risk factors of hepatitis C virus infection among drug users in Amsterdam. J Infect Dis 162:823, 1990.
180. Seeff LB: Hepatitis C from a needlestick injury. Ann Intern Med 115:411, 1991.
181. Mitsui T, Iwano K, Masuko K, et al: Hepatitis C virus infection in medical personnel after needlestick accident. Hepatology 16:1109, 1992.
182. Schiff ER: Hepatitis C among health care providers: Risk factors and possible prophylaxis. Hepatology 16:1300, 1992.
183. Centers for Disease Control and Prevention: Recommendations for preventing transmission of human immunodeficiency virus and hepatitis B virus to patients during exposure-prone invasive procedures. MMWR 40:1, 1991.
184. Ross RS, Viazov S, Gross T, et al: Transmission of hepatitis C virus from a patient to an anesthesiology assistant to five patients. N Engl J Med 343:1851, 2000.
185. Katsoulidou A, Paraskevis D, Kalapothaki V, et al: Molecular epidemiology of a hepatitis C virus outbreak in a haemodialysis unit. Multicentre Haemodialysis Cohort Study on Viral Hepatitis. Nephrol Dial Transplant 14:1188, 1999.
186. Westjal R, Widell A, Mansson AS, et al: Mother-to-infant transmission of hepatitis C virus. Ann Intern Med 117:887, 1992.
187. Rall CJN, Dienstag JL: Epidemiology of hepatitis C virus infection. Semin Gastrointest Dis 6:3, 1995.
188. Thaler MM, Park CK, Landers DV, et al: Vertical transmission of hepatitis C virus. Lancet 338:17, 1991.
189. Yeung LT, King SM, Roberts EA: Mother-to-infant transmission of hepatitis C virus. Hepatology 34:223, 2001.
190. Everhart JE, Di Biscegie AM, Murray LM, et al: Risk for non-A, non-B (type C) hepatitis through sexual or household contacts with chronic carriers. Ann Intern Med 112:544, 1990.
191. Nakashima K, Kashiwagi S, Hayashi J, et al: Sexual transmission of hepatitis C virus among female prostitutes and patients with sexually transmitted disease in Fukuoka, Kyushu, Japan. Am J Epidemiol 136:1132, 1992.
192. Wright TL, Hollander H, Pu X, et al: Hepatitis C in HIV-infected patients with and without AIDS: Prevalence and relationship to patient survival. Hepatology 17:1152, 1994.
193. Zylberberg H, Thiers V, Lagorce D, et al: Epidemiological and virological analysis of couples infected with hepatitis C virus. Gut 45:112, 1999.
194. Aach RD, Stevens CE, Hollinger FB, et al: Hepatitis C virus in post-transfusion hepatitis: An analysis with first and second-generation assays. N Engl J Med 325:1325, 1991.
195. Williams I: Epidemiology of hepatitis C in the United States. Am J Med 107(suppl):2, 1999.
196. Yanagi M, Kaneko S, Unoura M, et al: Hepatitis C virus in fulminant hepatic failure. N Engl J Med 324:1895, 1991.
197. Farci P, Alter HJ, Shimoda A, et al: Hepatitis C virus-associated fulminant hepatic failure. N Engl J Med 335:631, 1996.
198. Alter H, Seef L: Recovery, persistence and sequelae in hepatitis C virus infection: A perspective on long-term outcome. Semin Liver Dis 20:17, 2000.
199. Kiyosawa K, Sodeyama T, Tanaka E, et al: Interrelationship of blood transfusion, non-A, non-B hepatitis and hepatocellular carcinoma: Analysis by detection of antibody to hepatitis C. Hepatology 12:671, 1990.
200. Vogt M, Lang T, Frosner D, et al: Prevalence and clinical outcome of hepatitis C infection in children who underwent cardiac surgery after implementation of blood-donor screening. N Engl J Med 341:866, 1999.
201. Thomas DL, Astemborski J, Rai A, et al: The natural history of hepatitis C virus infection: host, viral and environmental factors. JAMA 284:450, 2000.
202. Wiley TE, McCarthy M, Breidi L, et al: Impact of alcohol on the histological and clinical progression of hepatitis C infection. Hepatology 28:805, 1998.
203. Ostapowicz G, Watson KJR, Locarnini SA, Desmond PV: Role of alcohol in the progression of liver disease caused by hepatitis C virus infection. Hepatology 27:1730, 1998.
204. Peters MG, Terrault NA: Alcohol use and hepatitis C. Hepatology 36:S220, 2002.
205. Poynard T, Bedossa P, Opolon P: Natural history of liver fibrosis progression in patients with chronic hepatitis C: The OBSVIRC, METAVIR, CLINIVIR and DOSVIRC groups. Lancet 349:825, 1997.
206. Di Martino V, Rufat P, Boyer N, et al: The influence of human immunodeficiency virus coinfection on chronic hepatitis C in injection drug users: A long-term retrospective cohort study. Hepatology 34:1193, 2001.
207. Ghany MG, Kleiner DE, Alter H, et al: Progression of fibrosis in chronic hepatitis C. Gastroenterology 124:97, 2003.
208. Marcelin P, Descamps V, Martinot-Peignoux M, et al: Cryoglobulinemia with vasculitis associated with hepatitis C virus infection. Gastroenterology 104:272, 1993.
209. Koff RS, Dienstag JL: Extrahepatic manifestations of hepatitis C and the association with alcoholic liver disease. Semin Liver Dis 15:101, 1995.
210. Fargion S, Piperno A, Cappellini MD, et al: Hepatitis C virus and porphyria cutanea tarda: Evidence of a strong association. Hepatology 16:1322, 1992.
211. Herrero C, Vicente A, Bruguera M et al: Is hepatitis C virus infection a trigger of porphyria cutanea tarda? Lancet 341:788, 1993.
212. Johnson RJ, Gretch DR, Yamabe H, et al: Membranoproliferative glomerulonephritis associated with hepatitis C virus infection. N Engl J Med 328:465, 1993.
213. Pawlostky JM, Ben Yahia M, Andre C, et al: Immunological disorders in C virus chronic active hepatitis: A prospective case-control study. Hepatology 19:841, 1994.
214. Haddad J, Deny P, Munz-Gotheil C, et al: Lymphocytic sialadenitis of Sjögren's syndrome associated with chronic hepatitis C virus liver disease. Lancet 339:321, 1992.

215. Wilson SE, Lee WM, Murakami C, et al: Mooren-type hepatitis C virus–associated corneal ulceration. Ophthalmology 101:736, 1994.
216. Domingo P, Ris J, Martinez E, et al: Erythema nodosum and hepatitis C (letter). Lancet 336:1377, 1990.
217. Cacoub P, Lunel-Fabiani F, Du LTH: Polyarteritis nodosa and hepatitis C virus infection (letter). Ann Intern Med 116:605, 1992.
218. Gasparotto D, De Re V, Biocchi M: Hepatitis C virus: B-cell proliferation and lymphomas. Leuk Lymphoma 43:747, 2002.
219. Gisbert JP, Garcia-Buey L, Pajares JM, Moreno-Otero R: Prevalence of hepatitis C virus infection in B-cell non-Hodgkin's lymphoma: Systematic review and meta-analysis. Gastroenterology 125:1723, 2003.
220. Di Bisceglie AM: Hepatitis C and hepatocellular carcinoma. Semin Liver Dis 15:64, 1995.
221. Mangia A, Vallari D, Di Bisceglie AM: Use of confirmatory tests for hepatitis C viral infection in patients with hepatocellular carcinoma. J Med Virol 43:125, 1994.
222. El-Serag HB, Mason AC: Rising incidence of hepatocellular carcinoma in the United States. N Engl J Med 340:745, 1999.
223. Di Bisceglie AM, Order SE, Klein JL, et al: The role of chronic viral hepatitis in hepatocellular carcinoma in the United States. Am J Gastroenterol 86:335, 1991.
224. Kew MC, Houghton M, Choo QL, et al: Hepatitis C virus antibodies in southern African blacks with hepatocellular carcinoma. Lancet 335:873, 1990.
225. Resnick RH, Koff R: Hepatitis C–related hepatocellular carcinoma: Prevalence and significance. Arch Intern Med 153:1672, 1993.
226. Herr W, Gerken G, Poralla T, et al: Hepatitis C virus associated primary hepatocellular carcinoma in a noncirrhotic liver. Clin Invest 71:49, 1993.
227. Fong TL, Shindo M, Feinstone SM, et al: Detection of replicative intermediates of hepatitis C viral RNA in liver and serum of patients with chronic hepatitis C. J Clin Invest 88:1058, 1991.
228. Chang KM: Immunopathogenesis of hepatitis C virus infection. Clin Liver Dis 7:89, 2003.
229. Missale G, Bertoni R, Lamonaca V, et al: Different clinical behaviors of acute hepatitis C virus infection are associated with different vigor of the anti-viral cell-mediated immune response. J Clin Invest 98:706, 1996.
230. Puoti M, Bonacini M, Spinetti A, et al: Liver fibrosis progression is related to CD4 cell depletion in patients coinfected with hepatitis C virus and human immunodeficiency virus. J Infect Dis 183:134, 2001.
231. Lauer GM, Ouchi K, Chung RT, et al: Comprehensive analysis of CD8(+)–T cell responses against hepatitis C virus reveals multiple unpredicted specificities. J Virol 76:6104, 2002.
232. Cooper S, Erickson AL, Adams EJ, et al: Analysis of a successful immune response against hepatitis C virus. Immunity 10:439, 1999.
233. Takaki A, Wiese M, Maertens G, et al: Cellular immune responses persist and humoral responses decrease two decades after recovery from a single-source outbreak of hepatitis C. Nat Med 6:578, 2000.
234. Pawlotsky JM: Hepatitis C virus genetic variability: Pathogenic and clinical implications. Clin Liver Dis 7:45, 2003.
235. Foy E, Li K, Wang C, et al: Regulation of interferon regulatory factor-3 by the hepatitis C virus serine protease. Science 300:1145, 2003.
236. Li K, Foy E, Ferreon JC, et al: Immune evasion by hepatitis C virus NS3/4A protease-mediated cleavage of the TLR3 adaptor protein TRIF. Proc Natl Acad Sci USA 102:2992, 2005.
237. Gale MJ Jr, Korth MJ, Tang NM, et al: Evidence that hepatitis C virus resistance to interferon is mediated through repression of the PKR protein kinase by the nonstructural 5A protein. Virology 230:217, 1997.
238. Pawlotsky JM: Use and interpretation of hepatitis C virus diagnostic assays. Clin Liver Dis 7:127, 2003.
239. Colin C, Lanoir D, Touzet S, et al: Sensitivity and specificity of third-generation hepatitis C virus antibody detection assays: An analysis of the literature. J Viral Hepat 8:87, 2001.
240. Pawlotsky JM: Molecular diagnosis of viral hepatitis. Gastroenterology 122:1554, 2002.
241. Pawlotsky JM, Bouvier-Alias M, Hezode C, et al: Standardization of hepatitis C virus RNA quantification. Hepatology 32:654, 2000.
242. Martinot-Peignoux M, Boyer N, Le Breton V, et al: A new step toward standardization of serum hepatitis C virus RNA quantification in patients with chronic hepatitis C. Hepatology 31:726, 2000.
243. Haber MM, West AB, Haber AD, et al: Relationship of aminotransferases to liver histological status in chronic hepatitis C. Am J Gastroenterol 90:1250, 1995.
244. Ohto H, Terazawa S, Sasaki N, et al: Transmission of hepatitis C virus from mothers to infants. N Engl J Med 330:744, 1994.
245. National Institutes of Health Consensus Development Conference Statement: Mangement of hepatitis C—2002. Hepatology 36:S3, 2002.
246. McCormick SE, Goodman ZD, Maydonovitch CL, et al: Evaluation of liver histology, ALT elevation, and HCV RNA titer in patients with chronic hepatitis C. Am J Gastroenterol 91:1516, 1996.
247. Williams AL, Hoofnagle JH: Ratio of serum aspartate to alanine aminotransferase in chronic hepatitis: relationship to cirrhosis. Gastroenterology 95:734, 1988.
248. Hourigan LF, Macdonald GA, Purdie D, et al: Fibrosis in chronic hepatitis C correlates significantly with body mass index and steatosis. Hepatology 29:1215, 1999.
249. Adinolfi LE, Gambardella L, Andreana A, et al: Steatosis accelerates the progression of liver damage of chronic hepatitis C patients and correlates with specific HCV genotype and visceral obesity. Hepatology 33:1358, 2001.
250. Monto A, Alonzo J, Watson JJ, et al: Steatosis in chronic hepatitis C: Relative contributions of obesity, diabetes mellitus and alcohol. Hepatology 36:729, 2002.
251. Leonardo A, Adinolfi LE, Loria P, et al: Steatosis and hepatitis C virus: Mechanisms and significance for hepatic and extrahepatic disease. Gastroenterology 126:586, 2004.
252. Di Bisceglie AM, Martin P, Kassianides C, et al: Recombinant interferon alpha therapy for chronic hepatitis C: A randomized, double-blind, placebo-controlled trial. N Engl J Med 321:1506, 1989.
253. Davis GL, Balart LA, Schiff ER, et al: Treatment of chronic hepatitis C with recombinant interferon alpha: A multicenter randomized, controlled trial. Hepatitis Interventional Therapy Group. N Engl J Med 321:1501, 1989.
254. Reichard O, Glaumann H, Fryden A, et al: Long-term follow-up of chronic hepatitis C patients with sustained virological response to alpha-interferon. J Hepatol 30:783, 1999.
255. Jaeckel E, Comberg M, Wedemeyer H, et al: Treatment of acute hepatitis C with interferon alpha-2b. N Engl J Med 345:1452, 2001.
256. Gerlach JT, Diepolder HM, Zachoval R, et al: Acute hepatitis C: High rate of both spontaneous and treatment-induced viral clearance. Gastroenterology 125:80, 2003.
257. Hofer H, Watkins-Riedel T, Janata O, et al: Spontaneous viral clearance in patients with acute hepatitis C can be predicted by repeated measurements of serum viral load. Hepatology 37:60, 2003.
258. EASL International Consensus Conference on Hepatitis C: Paris, 26–28 February 1999, consensus statement. J Hepatol 30:956, 1999.
259. Poynard T, Marcellin P, Lee SS, et al: Randomised trial of interferon alpha-2b plus ribavirin for 48 weeks or for 24 weeks versus interferon alpha-2b plus placebo for 48 weeks for treatment of chronic infection with hepatitis C virus. International Hepatitis Interventional Therapy Group (IHIT). Lancet 352:1426, 1998.
260. McHutchison JG, Gordon SC, Schiff ER, et al: Interferon alpha-2b alone or in combination with ribavirin as initial treatment for chronic hepatitis C. N Engl J Med 339:1485, 1998.
261. Zeuzem S, Feinman V, Rasenak J, et al: Peginterferon alpha-2a in patients with chronic hepatitis C. N Engl J Med 343:1666, 2000.
262. Heathcote EJ, Shiffman ML, Cooksley WGE, et al: Peginterferon alpha-2a in patients with chronic hepatitis C and cirrhosis. N Engl J Med 343:1673, 2000.
263. Lindsay KL, Trepo C, Heintges T, et al: A randomized, double-blind trial comparing pegylated interferon alpha-2b to interferon alpha-2b as initial treatment for chronic hepatitis C. Hepatology 34:395, 2001.
264. Manns MP, McHutchison JG, Gordon SC, et al : Peginterferon alpha-2b plus ribavirin compared with interferon alpha-2b plus ribavirin for initial treatment of chronic hepatitis C: A randomized trial. Lancet 358:958, 2001.
265. Fried MW, Shiffman ML, Reddy RK, et al: Pegylated (40 kDa) interferon alpha 2-a (PEGASYS) in combination with ribavirin: Efficacy and safety results from a phase III, randomized, actively-controlled, multicenter study. Gastroenterology 120:288, 2001.
266. Fried MW, Shiffman ML, Reddy KR, et al: Combination of peginterferon alpha-2a plus ribavirin in patients with chronic hepatitis C virus infection. N Engl J Med 347:975, 2002.
267. Davis GL, Wong JB, McHutchison JG, et al: Early virologic response to treatment with peginterferon alpha-2b plus ribavirin in patients with chronic hepatitis C. Hepatology 38:645, 2003.

268. Poynard T, McHutchison JG, Manns M, et al: Impact of pegylated interferon alpha-2b and ribavirin on liver fibrosis in patients with chronic hepatitis C. Gastroenterology 122:1303, 2002.
269. Camma C, Di Bona D, Schepis F, et al: Effect of peginterferon alpha-2a on liver histology in chronic hepatitis C: A meta-analysis of individual patient data. Hepatology 39:333, 2004.
270. National Institutes of Health: HALT-C trial. Hepatology 36:792, 2002.
271. Sanchez-Quijano A, Leal M, Lissen E: Hepatitis cronica por virus C en pacientes coinfectados por el virus de la inmunodeficiencia humana. Gastroenterol Hepatol 25:423, 2002.
272. Graham CS, Baden LR, Yu E, et al: Influence of human immunodeficiency virus infection on the course of hepatitis C virus infection: A meta-analysis. Clin Infect Dis 33:562, 2001.
273. Di Bisceglie AM, McHutchison JG, Rice CM : New therapeutic strategies for hepatitis C. Hepatology 35:224, 2002.
274. De Francesco R, Rice CM: New therapies on the horizon for hepatitis C: Are we close? Clin Liver Dis 7:211, 2003.
275. Cooper S, Erickson AL, Adams EJ, et al: Analysis of a successful immune response against hepatitis C virus. Immunity 10:439, 1999.
276. Inchauspe G, Feinstone S: Development of a hepatitis C virus vaccine. Clin Liver Dis 7:243, 2003.
277. Bruna-Romero O, Lasarte JJ, Wilkinson G, et al: Induction of cytotoxic T-cell response against hepatitis C virus structural antigens using a defective recombinant adenovirus. Hepatology 25:470, 1997.
278. Rizzetto M, Canese MG, Arico S, et al: Immunofluorescence detection of new antigen-antibody system (δ/antiδ) associated to hepatitis B virus in liver and serum of HBsAg carriers. Gut 18:997, 1977.
279. Rizzetto M, Canese MG, Gerin JI, et al: Transmission of hepatitis B virus–related delta agent to chimpanzees. J Infect Dis 141:590, 1980.
280. Elena SF, Dopazo J, Flores R, et al: Phylogeny of viroids, viroidlike satellite RNAs, and the viroidlike domain of hepatitis D virus RNA. Proc Natl Acad Sci USA 88:5631, 1991.
281. Radjef N, Ivannuishina V, Anais P, et al: Hepatitis D virus (HDV) genome analysis from Africa suggests the existence of more than three world-wide genotypes. J Hepatol 34S:120, 2001.
282. Lazinski DW, Taylor JM: Relating structure to function in the hepatitis delta virus antigen. J Virol 67:2672, 1993.
283. Rizzetto M, Hadziyannis S, Hanson BG, et al: Hepatitis delta virus infection in the world: Epidemiological patterns and clinical expression. Gastroenterol Int 5:18, 1992.
284. Dimitrakakis M, Crowe S, Gust I: Prevalence of delta infection in the Western Pacific region. J Med Virol 18:335, 1986.
285. Tapalaga D, Forzani B, Hele C, et al: Prevalence of the hepatitis delta virus in Romania. Hepatogastroenterology 33:238, 1986.
286. Hadler SC, De Monzon M, Ponzetto A, et al: Delta virus infection and severe hepatitis: An epidemic in the Yupca Indians of Venezuela. Ann Intern Med 100:339, 1984.
287. Ljunggren KE, Patarroyo ME, Engle R, et al: Viral hepatitis in Colombia: A study of the "Hepatitis of the Sierra Nevada de Santa Marta." Hepatology 5:299, 1985.
288. Ruiz-Chavez RA, Jaimes Hidalgo A, Montejo JG, et al: Marcadores serologicos de hepatitis viral en la region amazonica del Peru: Estudio de una poblacion representativa. Diagnostico 24:5, 1989.
289. Colichon AA, Sjögren MH, Galvez JD, et al: Hepatitis B and delta hepatitis in inhabitants of the Peruvian Amazon Basin. In Zuckerman AJ (ed): Viral Hepatitis and Liver Disease. New York, Alan R. Liss, 1988, p 425.
290. Bensabath G, Hadler SC, Pereira Soares MC, et al: Epidemiologic and serologic studies of acute viral hepatitis in Brazil's Amazon Basin. Bull Pan Am Health Organ 21:16, 1987.
291. Lettau LA, McCarthy JG, Smith MH, et al: Outbreak of severe hepatitis due to delta and hepatitis B virus in parenteral drug abusers and their contacts. N Engl J Med 317:1256, 1987.
292. Rosina F, Saracco G, Rizzetto M: Risk of post-transfusion infection with the hepatitis delta virus: A multicenter study. N Engl J Med 312:1488, 1985.
293. Braga WSM, Brasil LM, Souza RAB, et al: Ocorrencia da infeccao pelo virus da hepatite B (VHB) e delta (VHD) em sete grupos indígenas do estado de Amazonas. Rev Soc Bras Med Trop 34:349, 2001.
294. Arico S, Rizzetto M, Zanetti A, et al: Clinical significance of antibody to the hepatitis delta virus in symptomless HBsAg carriers. Lancet 2:356, 1985.
295. De Cock KM, Govindarajan S, Chin KP, et al: Delta hepatitis in the Los Angeles area: A report of 126 cases. Ann Intern Med 105:108, 1986.
296. Rizzetto M, Verme G, Recchia S, et al: Chronic hepatitis in carriers of hepatitis B surface antigen, with intrahepatic expression of the delta antigen. Ann Intern Med 98:437, 1983.
297. Carredda F, Antinori S, Re T, et al: Course and prognosis of acute HDV hepatitis. Prog Clin Biol Res 364:267, 1987.
298. Lin H-H, Liaw Y-F, Chen T-J, et al: Natural course of patients with chronic type B hepatitis following acute hepatitis delta virus infection. Liver 9:129, 1989.
299. Govindarajan S, Chin KP, Redeker AG, et al: Fulminant B viral hepatitis: Role of delta agent. Gastroenterology 86:1417, 1984.
300. Verme G, Brunetto MR, Oliveri F, et al: Role of hepatitis delta virus infection in hepatocellular carcinoma. Dig Dis Sci 36:1134, 1991.
301. Chen PJ, Yang PM, Chen CR, et al: Characterization of the transcripts of hepatitis D and B viruses in infected human livers. J Infect Dis 160:944, 1989.
302. Rizzetto M: Transmission of hepatitis B virus–associated delta antigen to chimpanzees. J Infect Dis 121:590, 1980.
303. Oliviero S, D'adamio L, Chiarberge E, et al: Characterization of hepatitis delta antigen gene of a highly pathogenic strain of hepatitis delta virus. Prog Clin Biol Res 364:321, 1991.
304. Govindarajan S, Gupta S, Valinluck B, et al: Correlation of IgM anti-hepatitis D virus (HDV) to HDV RNA in sera of chronic HDV. Hepatology 10:34, 1989.
305. Brunetto MR, Stemler M, Bonino F, et al: A new hepatitis B virus strain in patients with severe anti-HBe positive chronic hepatitis B. J Hepatol 10:258, 1990.
306. Aragona M, Caredda F, Lavarini C, et al: Serological response to the hepatitis delta virus in hepatitis D. Lancet 3:478, 1987.
307. Farci P, Aragona M, Crivelli O, et al: Diagnostic and prognostic significance of the IgM antibody to the hepatitis delta virus. JAMA 255:1443, 1986.
308. Buti M, Esteban R, Jardi R, et al: Chronic delta hepatitis: detection of hepatitis delta virus antigen in serum by immunoblot and correlation with other markers of delta viral replication. Hepatology 10:907, 1989.
309. Battegay M, Simpson LH, Hoofnagle JH, et al: Elimination of hepatitis delta virus infection after loss of hepatitis B surface antigen in patients with chronic delta hepatitis. J Med Virol 44:389, 1994.
310. Smedile A, Rizzetto M, Denniston K, et al: Type D hepatitis: The clinical significance of hepatitis D virus RNA in serum as detected by a hybridization-based assay. Hepatology 6:1297, 1986.
311. Verme G, Amoroso P, Lettieri G, et al: A histological study of hepatitis delta virus liver disease. Hepatology 6:1303, 1986.
312. Stocklin F, Gudat F, Krey G, et al: Delta antigen in hepatitis B: Immunohistology of frozen and paraffin-embedded liver biopsies and relation to HBV infection. Hepatology 1:238, 1981.
313. Rosina F, Pintus C, Meschievitz C, et al: A randomized controlled trial of a 12-month course of recombinant human interferon-α in chronic delta (type D) hepatitis: a multicenter Italian study. Hepatology 13:1052, 1991.
314. Farci P, Mandas A, Coiana A, et al: Treatment of chronic hepatitis D with interferon alpha-2a. N Engl J Med 330:88, 1994.
315. Chen P-J, Wu H-L, Wang C-H, et al: Molecular biology of hepatitis D virus: Research and potential for application. J Gastroenterol Hepatol 12:S188, 1997.
316. Karayiannis P, Saldanha J, Monjardino J, et al: Immunization of woodchucks with recombinant hepatitis delta agent does not protect against hepatitis delta virus infection. Hepatology 12:1125, 1990.
317. Wong DC, Purcell RH, Sreenivasan MA, et al: Epidemic and enteric hepatitis in India: Evidence for non-A, non-B etiology. Lancet 2:876, 1980.
318. Myint H, Soe MM, Khin T, et al: A clinical and epidemiological study of an epidemic of non-A, non-B hepatitis in Rangoon. Am J Trop Med Hyg 34:1183, 1985.
319. Reyes GR, Purdy MA, Kim PJ, et al: Isolation of a cDNA from the virus responsible for enterically transmitted non-A, non-B hepatitis. Science 247:1335, 1990.
320. Bradley DW: Hepatitis E virus: A brief review of the biology, molecular virology, and immunology of a novel virus. J Hepatology 22:140, 1995.
321. Tam AW, Smith MM, Guerra ME, et al: Hepatitis E virus (HEV): Molecular cloning and sequencing of the full-length viral genome. Virology 185:120, 1991.
322. Schlauder GG, Frider B, Sookian S, et al: Identification of two novel isolates of hepatitis E virus in Argentina. J Infect Dis 182:294, 2000.

323. Worm HC, Schlauder GG, Wurzer H, Mushawas IK: Identification of a novel variant of hepatitis E virus in Austria: Sequence, phylogenetic and serological analysis. J Gen Virol 81:2885, 2000.
324. Meng J, Pillot J, Dai X, Fields HA: Neutralization of different geographic strains of the hepatitis E virus with anti-hepatitis E virus positive serum samples obtained from different sources. Virology 249:316, 1998.
325. Wong DC, Purcell RH, Sreenivasan MA, et al: Epidemic and enteric hepatitis in India: Evidence for non-A, non-B etiology. Lancet 2:876, 1980.
326. Myint H, Soe MM, Khin T, et al: A clinical and epidemiological study of an epidemic of non-A, non-B hepatitis in Rangoon. Am J Trop Med Hyg 34:1183, 1985.
327. Wald A: Hepatitis E. Adv Pediatr Infect Dis 10:157, 1995.
328. Kane MA, Bradley DW, Shrestha SM, et al: Epidemic non-A, non-B hepatitis in Nepal. JAMA 252:3140, 1984.
329. DeCock KM, Bradley DW, Sanford NL, et al: Epidemic non-A, non-B hepatitis in patients from Pakistan. Ann Intern Med 106:227, 1987.
330. Velasquez O, Stetler HC, Avila C, et al: Epidemic transmission of enterically transmitted non-A, non-B hepatitis in Mexico, 1986–1987. JAMA 263:3281, 1990.
331. Paul DA, Knigge MF, Ritter A, et al: Determination of hepatitis E virus seroprevalence by using recombinant fusion proteins and synthetic peptides. J Infect Dis 169:801, 1994.
332. Kwo PY, Schlauder GG, Carpenter HA, et al: Acute hepatitis E by a new isolate acquired in the United States. Mayo Clin Proc 72:1133, 1997.
333. Clemente-Casares P, Pina S, Buti M, et al: Hepatitis E virus epidemiology in industrializad countries. Emerg Infect Dis 9:448, 2003.
334. Parana R, Cotrim H, Cortney-Boennec MI, et al: Prevalence of hepatitis E virus IgG in patients from a referral center of liver disease in Salvador-Bahia, Brazil. Am J Trop Med Hyg 1:60, 1997.
335. Fix AD, Abdel-Hamid M, Purcell RH, et al: Prevalence of antibodies to hepatitis E in two rural Egyptian communities. Am J Trop Med Hyg 62:519, 2000.
336. Ooi WW, Gawoski JM, Yarbough PO, Pankey GA: Hepatitis E seroconversion in United States travelers abroad. Am J Trop Med Hyg 61:822, 1999.
337. Van der Poel WHM, Verschoor F, Van der Heide R, et al: Hepatitis E virus sequences in swine related to sequences in humans, the Netherlands. Emerg Infect Dis 7:970, 2001.
338. Kabrane-Lazizi Y, Fine JB, Elm J, et al: Evidence for widespread infection of wild rats with hepatitis E virus in the United States. Am J Trop Med Hyg 61:331, 1999.
339. Tien N-T, Claysson HT, Khiem HB, et al: Detection of immunoglobulin G to hepatitis E virus among several animal species in Vietnam. Am J Trop Med Hyg 57:211, 1997.
340. Meng XJ, Wiseman B, Elvinger F, et al: Prevalence of antibodies to hepatitis E virus in veterinarians working with swine and in normal blood donors in the United States and other countries. J Clin Microbiol 40:117, 2002.
341. Robson SC, Adams S, Brink N, et al: Hospital outbreak of hepatitis E. Lancet 339:1424, 1992.
342. Chauhan A, Jameel S, Dilawari JB, et al: Hepatitis E virus transmission to a volunteer. Lancet 341:149–150, 1993.
343. Belabbes E-H, Bougermouh A, Benatallah A, et al: Epidemic non-A, non-B viral hepatitis in Algeria: Strong evidence for its spreading by water. J Med Virol 16:257, 1985.
344. Sheikh A, Sugitani M, Kinukawa N, et al: Hepatitis E virus infection in fulminant hepatitis patients and an apparently healthy population in Bangladesh. Am J Trop Med Hyg 66:721, 2002.
345. Bradley DW: Enterically-transmitted non-A, non-B hepatitis. Br Med Bull 46:442, 1990.
346. Favorov MO, Fields HA, Purdy MA, et al: Serologic identification of hepatitis E virus infections in epidemic and endemic settings. J Med Virol 36:246, 1992.
347. Bradley DW: Hepatitis E virus: a brief review of the biology, molecular virology, and immunology of a novel virus. J Hepatol 22:140, 1995.
348. Hyams KC, Purdy MA, Kaur M, et al: Acute sporadic hepatitis E in Sudanese children: Analysis based on a new Western blot assay. J Infect Dis 165:1001, 1992.
349. Krawczynski K, Bradley DW: Enterically transmitted non-A, non-B hepatitis: Identification of virus-associated antigen in experimentally infected cynomolgus monkeys. J Infect Dis 159:1042, 1989.
350. Chau KH, Dawson GJ, Bile KM, et al: Detection of IgA class antibody to hepatitis E virus in serum samples from patients with hepatitis E virus infection. J Med Virol 40:334, 1993.
351. Jameel S, Durgapal H, Habibullah CM, et al: Enteric non-A, non-B hepatitis: Epidemics, animal transmission and hepatitis E virus detection by the polymerase chain reaction. J Med Virol 37:263, 1992.
352. Drabick JJ, Gambel JM, Gouvea VS, et al: A cluster of acute hepatitis E infection in United Nations Bangladeshi peace keepers in Haiti. Am J Trop Med Hyg 57:449, 1997.
353. Purdy MA, McCaustland KA, Krawczynski K, et al: Preliminary evidence that a trpE-HEV fusion protein protects cynomolgus macaques against challenge with wild-type hepatitis E virus (HEV). J Med Virol 41:90, 1993.

65

Overview of Viral Hemorrhagic Fevers

C. J. PETERS
SHERIF R. ZAKI

INTRODUCTION

Several viruses regularly cause a syndrome that is referred to as hemorrhagic fever (HF). They belong to four different families of RNA viruses, but all are lipid enveloped and zoonotic in their maintenance strategies. The taxonomy is helpful in understanding their natural history and pathogenesis but does not accurately predict the clinical syndromes following infection with a given family member. For example, virtually all the arenaviruses are maintained by chronic infection of a single rodent host and spread to humans by aerosols of rodent excreta and related mechanisms, with the details of the human epidemiology mainly predictable by rodent dynamics and human behavior. However, Tamiami and Whitewater Arroyo viruses are North American arenaviruses not associated with any disease, and the best known American arenavirus is lymphocytic choriomeningitis virus, which came to the Americas when the common house mouse, *Mus musculus*, was introduced in post-Columbian times. Lymphocytic choriomeningitis virus infection of humans mainly causes subclinical infection, acute undifferentiated febrile disease, and febrile central nervous system illnesses such as aseptic meningitis, but two cases have resembled the HF syndrome.

AGENT

The HF viruses occur worldwide (Table 65-1) and the geographic site of infection is an important determinant of the risk to an individual patient. The geography and knowledge of the incubation period are important in suspecting an exported viral HF. The syndrome characteristically begins with fever, myalgia, and malaise, which then progress to prostration, gastrointestinal and other system involvement, and signs of vascular damage. Involvement of the vascular system is usually manifest by vascular dysregulation (mild hypotension, postural hypotension, flushing, and injected conjunctivae), vascular damage (nondependent edema and organ dysfunction), and hemorrhage. Hemorrhage is usually diffuse in microvascular beds throughout the body and occurs particularly in patients with thrombocytopenia or marked platelet dysfunction. Many patients have little or no bleeding, but some present with extensive cutaneous and mucosal hemorrhage. Severe cases will have shock, central nervous system involvement, or extensive hemorrhagic phenomena. The clinical findings in the different HFs vary in a characteristic way for each virus, but any individual patient is difficult to classify without virologic diagnosis (Tables 65-2 and 65-3). The detailed manifestations of each VHF are often based on fragmentary clinical observations and lack proper appreciation of the entire spectrum, which in some cases includes such manifestations as pancreatitis.

PATHOGENESIS

Although there are common themes, the different viruses also differ in their pathology and pathogenesis (Table 65-4). Usually, hemorrhages are present in many organs, and effusions are commonly found in serous cavities, but they may be minimal or absent in some patients. There is widespread necrosis, which may be present in any organ system and that varies from modest and focal to massive in extent. Liver and lymphoid systems are usually extensively involved, and the lung regularly has varying degrees of interstitial pneumonitis, diffuse alveolar damage, and hemorrhage. Acute tubular necrosis and microvascular thrombosis may also be seen. The inflammatory response is usually minimal. These changes, which may be a direct effect of viral infection or a consequence of cytokine secretion, have considerable variation among the different viruses (see Table 65-4).

DIAGNOSIS

Correct diagnosis in most of the diseases depends on demonstration of the infecting virus or one of its products in acute serum samples. Viral antigens are readily demonstrable, and often an antigen detection enzyme-linked immunosorbent assay (ELISA) is the best test for identifying patients because of its rapidity and robustness; it is particularly likely to be positive in the more severely ill patient, who is in greatest need of therapy and who may provide the greatest risk of dissemination. Reverse transcription-polymerase chain reaction (RT-PCR) is usually more sensitive but also more subject to artifact and contamination. RT-PCR has a unique role in providing an amplicon that can be sequenced for genetic analysis, although this very genetic variation may be a source of difficulty in ensuring that appropriate primers are applied to unknown samples. In general, viremia and antigenemia are readily detected during the acute phase and disappear as the patient improves. RT-PCR is usually positive during the same period and perhaps 1 or 2 days longer. IgM antibodies may be detectable during illness and usually appear early in convalescence, providing a sensitive, specific method of diagnosis, particularly if they are measured by an IgM capture ELISA technique. Diagnosis of initial patients in any outbreak, particularly if there are unusual features, benefits from study of virus isolates and classic serologic responses, particularly the neutralization test, animal pathogenesis, and genomic analysis. Most of the viruses are hazardous and should only be isolated or studied under BSL4 containment. Hantaviruses are an exception to the generalizations: The patients typically present with an ongoing immune response and are best diagnosed with the IgM capture ELISA; virus isolation is difficult, but RT-PCR on acute blood clot may give valuable genetic information about the infecting virus.

Table 65-1 *Geography and Epidemiology of Hemorrhagic Fever Viruses*

Virus	Disease	Geography	Vector/Reservoir	Human Infection
Arenaviridae				
Junin	Argentine HF	Argentine pampas	Chronic infection of small field rodent, *Calomys musculinus*.	Infects agricultural workers disproportionately. Major transmission in fall: Aerosol transmission to humans.
Machupo	Bolivian HF	Beni Department, Bolivia	Chronic infection of small field rodent, *Calomys callosus*.	Rural residents and farmers main target; rodent can invade towns to cause epidemics. Aerosol transmission to humans. Interhuman transmission not usual, but occurs.
Guanarito	Venezuelan HF	Portuguesa state, Venezuela	Chronic infection of field rodent, *Zygodontomys brevicauda*.	Rural residents in recently developed area with small farms.
Sabia	Brazilian HF	Rural area near Saõ Paulo, Brazil	Presumably chronic infection of unidentified rodents.	Single infection observed in nature: little information on epidemiologic potential.
Lassa	Lassa fever	West Africa	Chronic infection of rodents of the genus *Mastomys*.	The reservoir rodent is very common in Africa, and the disease is a major cause of severe febrile illness in West Africa. Spread to man occurs by aerosols and by capturing the rodent for consumption, as well as person-to-person transmission. Lassa fever is the most commonly exported HF.
Bunyaviridae				
Rift Valley fever	Rift Valley fever	Sub-Saharan Africa	Vertical infection of floodwater *Aedes* mosquitoes. Epidemics occur from horizontal transmission by many different mosquito species between domestic animals, particularly sheep and cattle.	Humans acquire virus by mosquito bite; contact with blood of infected sheep, cattle, or goats; and aerosols generated from infected domestic animal blood. No interhuman transmission observed.
Crimean-Congo HF	Crimean-Congo HF	Africa, Middle East, Balkans, southern Russia, western China	Tick–mammal–tick infection. Vertical infection occurs in ticks. *Hyalomma* ticks are thought to be the natural reservoir, but other genera may become infected and transmit.	Tick bite; squashing ticks; and exposure to aerosols or fomites from slaughtered cattle and sheep. (Domestic animals do not show illness but may become infected when transported to market or when held in pens for slaughter.) Nosocomial epidemics observed on numerous occasions.
Hantaan, Seoul, Puumala, and others	Hemorrhagic fever with renal syndrome (HFRS)	Worldwide depending on rodent reservoirs	Horizontal infection in a single rodent genus or species typical of the virus. Viruses associated with HFRS have been obtained from Muridae (subfamilies Murinae or Avicolinae) rodents (rats, mice, and voles).	Aerosols from freshly shed urine of infected rodents. Some infections may be acquired from secondary aerosols or droplets from previously shed rodent excreta and secreta or from rodent bites. Interhuman transmission never documented.

Continued

Table 65-1 *Geography and Epidemiology of Hemorrhagic Fever Viruses—cont'd*

Virus	Disease	Geography	Vector/Reservoir	Human Infection
Sin Nombre, Black Creek Canal, Bayou, and others	Hantavirus pulmonary syndrome (HPS)	Americas	As for hantaviruses causing HFRS. All viruses associated with HPS have come from Muridae (subfamily Sigmodontinae) rodents, if the reservoir is known.	As for hantaviruses causing HFRS. Entering abandoned, closed buildings may be a particular risk in some settings. Interhuman transmission rarely observed with Andes virus
Filoviridae				
Marburg, Ebola	Marburg HF Ebola HF	Africa, ?Philippines	Unknown	Infection of index case occurs from unknown source. Infected nonhuman primates sometimes provide link to humans. Later spread among human or nonhuman primates by close contact with another case. Aerosol transmission suspected in one captive monkey outbreak.
Flaviridae				
Yellow fever	Yellow fever	Africa, South America	Mosquito–monkey–mosquito maintenance with occasional human infection when unvaccinated humans enter forest. Large epidemics among humans with *Aedes aegypti* as mosquito vector.	Mosquito infection of humans entering forest and encountering infected sylvatic vector. Emergence of epidemics into African savannas via specific *Aedes* mosquito vectors. In cities or villages, interhuman transmission by *Ae. aegypti*. Fully developed cases are no longer viremic and direct interhuman transmission not believed to be a problem although the virus is highly infectious (including aerosols) in the laboratory.
Dengue (types 1–4)	Dengue HF (DHF), dengue shock syndrome (DSS)	Tropics and subtropics worldwide	Maintained by *Ae. aegypti*–human–*Ae. aegypti* transmission with frequent geographic transport of viruses by travelers.	DHF/DSS is a problem in areas where multiple dengue viruses are being transmitted. With the increased worldwide distribution of *Ae. aegypti* and movement of dengue viruses in travelers, this zone is enlarging. The disease was first noted in Southeast Asia but is now common in the Americas and the Caribbean, as well as the Pacific rim countries.
Kyasanur Forest disease (KFD)	KFD	Karnataka state, India	Tick–vertebrate–tick	Most infections occur from tickbite acquired in rural areas of the endemic zone. Monkey die offs may accompany increased virus activity.
Omsk HF (OHF)	OHF	Western Siberia	Poorly understood cycle involving ticks, voles, muskrats, and possibly water-borne and mosquito transmission.	Few cases in recent years.
Al Kumrah		Middle East? Africa?	Unknown. Surmised to involve tick–domestic livestock–tick cycle by analogy to genetically related tick-borne flaviviruses.	Transmitted to humans working in livestock-related occupations by unknown route. Genetically related to KFD virus.

HF, Hemorrhagic fever.

Table 65-2 Clinical Features of the Viral Hemorrhagic Fevers

Disease	Incubation Period (Days)	Case Infection Ratio	Case Fatality	Characteristic Features
Arenaviridae				
South American HF	7–14	Most (>1/2) result in disease	15%–30%	Typical cases have hypotension, shock, obvious bleeding, and neurologic symptoms such as dysarthria and intention tremor. Some cases have virtually pure neurologic syndrome.
Lassa fever	5–16	Mild infections probably common	2%–15%	Prostration and shock; fewer hemorrhagic or neurologic manifestations than South American HF except in severe cases. Thrombocytopenia less common and less severe. Deafness develops in convalescence in 20%.
Bunyaviridae				
Rift Valley fever	2–5*	≈1%	≈50%	Severe disease associated with bleeding, shock, anuria, and icterus. Encephalitis and retinal vasculitis also occur, but without overlap with HF syndrome.
Crimean-Congo HF	3–12	20%–100%	15%–30%	Most severe bleeding and ecchymoses of all the HFs.
HF with renal syndrome	9–35	>3/4 Hantaan virus 1/20 Puumala virus	5%–15% Hantaan virus <1% Puumala virus	Febrile stage followed by shock and renal failure. Bleeding during febrile stage, shock, and renal failure. Puumala virus infections have a similar course but are much milder.
Hantavirus pulmonary syndrome	7–28	Very high	40%–50%	Febrile stage followed by acute pulmonary edema and shock. Manifestations largely limited to thoracic cavity.
Filoviridae				
Marburg or Ebola HF	3–16	High (particularly Zaire subtype of Ebola)	25%–90%	Most severe of the HFs. Marked weight loss and prostration. Maculopapular rash common. Patients have had late sequelae (hepatitis, uveitis, orchitis) often with virus isolation from biopsy or aspiration.
Flaviviridae				
Yellow fever	3–6	50% of nonimmune <5% of heterologous flavivirus immune	20%–50%	Acute febrile period with defervescence accompanied in severe cases by jaundice and renal failure.
Dengue HF (DHF), dengue shock syndrome (DSS)	3–15*	0.007% of nonimmune and 1.0% of heterologous immune	Untreated, 10%–15% Treated, <1%	High fever for 3–5 days with the development of shock lasting 1–2 days. DHF is not equated to DSS. DSS is the most dangerous manifestation and is due to an acute vascular leak. Attack rates, mortality quite variable with epidemic virus strain and surveillance.
Kyasanur Forest disease (KFD) Omsk HF	3–8	Variable	0.5%–9.0%	Typical biphasic disease with a febrile or hemorrhagic period often followed by CNS involvement. Similar to tick-borne encephalitis except hemorrhagic manifestations are not characteristic of first phase of tick-borne encephalitis.

HF, Hemorrhagic fever.
*Uncomplicated disease; incubation for HF may differ.

Table 65-3 *Specific Clinical Findings in Different Hemorrhagic Fevers*

Disease	Hemorrhage	Thrombocytopenia	Leukocyte Count	Rash	Icterus	Renal Disease	Pulmonary Disease	Tremor, Dysarthria	Encephalopathy	Deafness	Eye Lesions
Arenaviridae											
South American HF	+++	+++	⇓⇓⇓	0	0	0	+	+++	++	0	0
Lassa fever	+/S	+	N	++	0	0	+	+	+/S	++	0
Bunyaviridae											
Rift Valley fever	+++	+++	⇓⇓/⇑⇑	0	++	+	0	0	E	0	Retina
Crimean-Congo HF	+++	+++	⇓⇓/⇑	0	++	0	+	0	+	0	0
HFRS	+++	+++	⇑⇑⇑	0	0	+++	+	0	+	0	0
HPS	+	++	⇑⇑	0	0	+	+++	0	+	0	0
Filoviridae											
Marburg and Ebola HFs	++	+++		+++	++	0	+	0	++	+	Uveitis
Flaviviridae											
Yellow fever	+++	++	N/⇓⇓	0	+++	++	+	0	++	0	0
DHF, DSS	++	+++	⇑⇑	+++	+	0	+	0	+	0	0
KFD, OHF	++	++	⇓⇓	0	0	0	++	0	E	0	Retina

DHF, dengue hemorrhagic fever; DSS, dengue shock syndrome; E, develop true encephalitis either after HF (KFD, Omsk) or in other patients (Rift Valley fever); HF, hemorrhagic fever; HFRS, hemorrhagic fever with renal syndrome; HPS, Hantavirus pulmonary syndrome; KFD, Kyasanur Forest disease; N, normal; OHF, Omsk hemorrhagic fever; S, characteristic, seen in severe case; +, occasional or mild; ++, commonly seen, may be severe; +++, characteristic and usually marked; ⇑, occasionally or mildly increased; ⇓⇓, decreased; ⇑⇑, commonly increased, may be marked; ⇑⇑⇑, characteristically increased and usually marked; 0, absent.

Table 65-4 Viral Tropism and Pathologic Features of Viral Hemorrhagic Fevers

Disease	Pathologic Features*
Arenaviridae	
Argentine HF Bolivian HF Venezuelan HF Lassa fever	Multifocal hepatocellular necrosis with minimal inflammatory response, interstitial pneumonitis, myocarditis, and lymphoid depletion; extensive parenchymal cell and reticuloendothelial infection, more than morphologic lesions would suggest.
Bunyaviridae	
Rift Valley fever (RVF)	Widespread hepatocellular necrosis and hemorrhage, sometimes with midzonal distribution, minimal inflammatory response, disseminated intravascular coagulation, lymphoid depletion; RVF antigens in few individual hepatocytes; encephalitis and retinal vasculitis also seen.
Crimean-Congo HF	Widespread hepatocellular necrosis and hemorrhage with minimal or no inflammatory cell response and lymphoid depletion; hepatic and endothelial cell infection and damage.
Hemorrhagic fever with renal syndrome (HFRS)	Retroperitoneal edema in severe HFRS, mild to severe renal pathologic changes; congestion and hemorrhagic necrosis of renal medulla, right atrium of the heart, and anterior pituitary; extensive endothelial infection mainly in renal and cardiac microvasculature.
Hantavirus pulmonary syndrome (HPS)	Large bilateral pleural effusions and severely edematous lungs, mild to moderate interstitial pneumonitis, immunoblasts, and atypical lymphocytes in lymphoid tissues and peripheral blood; extensive infection of endothelial cells in pulmonary microvasculature.
Filoviridae	
Ebola HF	Extensive and disseminated infection and necrosis in major organs such as liver, spleen, lung, kidney, skin, and gonads; extensive hepatocellular necrosis associated with formation of characteristic intracytoplasmic viral inclusions; lymphoid depletion, microvascular infection, and injury.
Marburg HF	Similar to Ebola HF.
Flaviviridae	
Yellow fever	Midzonal hepatocellular necrosis; minimal inflammatory response; Councilman bodies and microvesicular fatty change; hepatocellular and Kupffer cell infection; lymphoid necrosis (nodes, spleen); focal myocarditis; acute renal tubular necrosis.
Dengue HF, dengue shock syndrome	Centrilobular and midzonal hepatocellular necrosis with minimal inflammatory response; Councilman bodies and microvesicular fatty change; hyperplasia of mononuclear phagocytic cells in lymphoid tissues and atypical lymphocytes in peripheral blood; widespread infection of mononuclear phagocytic and endothelial cells.
Kyasanur Forest disease (KFD)	Focal hepatocellular degeneration, fatty change, and necrosis; pulmonary hemorrhage, depletion of malpighian follicles, sinus histiocytosis, erythrophagocytosis, mild myocarditis, and encephalitis.
Omsk HF	Little known; scattered focal hemorrhage, interstitial pneumonia, and normal lymphoid tissues.

HF, Hemorrhagic fever.
*These features represent the characteristic pathologic findings in the different viral HFs. More general findings seen to variable degrees in all HFs are not listed.

Ideally, blood samples from HF patients should be collected early in the course of illness, and both serum and blood clot should be frozen as soon as possible. A second sample should be obtained before discharge or death for comparative serology, and this can be supplemented by a later follow-up blood sample. In fatal cases, a full autopsy should be performed with a complete set of organs collected in formalin for diagnostic studies; spleen, liver, and lymph nodes should be collected frozen for virus isolation. Classic histopathology is often useful in suspecting yellow fever, Rift Valley fever, or a filovirus infection and in diagnosing some of the confounding diseases. Immunohistochemistry on fixed tissues can usually make a definitive diagnosis possible. Precautions appropriate to each virus should be taken to prevent infection while processing samples or performing a necropsy. Frozen samples should be appropriately packed and, whenever possible, shipped on dry ice, although diagnoses can sometimes be made on mishandled specimens. The receiving laboratory should be advised of the shipment, its estimated time of arrival, and the waybill number to allow for tracing the materials if, as often happens, there is a delay en route. Diagnostic expertise and consultation are available from several laboratories.

TREATMENT AND PREVENTION

Approaches to the prevention and treatment of the viral HFs vary with the infecting virus (Table 65-5). Barrier nursing and avoidance of parenteral exposures of hospital staff are important in management of all these diseases, but they are particularly important in Crimean-Congo HF and the filovirus diseases because of the regularity with which nosocomial transmission has been seen. The general principles of therapy are similar for all the HFs and require rapid atraumatic hospitalization, careful maintenance of fluid balance to avoid overhydration in the face of fragile systemic and pulmonary capillary beds, as well as probable myocardial compromise, management of the bleeding diathesis according to the usual principles, and the specific therapy appropriate to each disease (see Table 65-5). It is extremely important to exclude or empirically treat the conditions that may be most

Table 65-5 Prevention and Treatment of Viral Hemorrhagic Fevers

Disease	Prevention	Treatment
Arenaviridae		
Argentine HF	Safe, effective vaccine used for high-risk residents of endemic area.	Infusion of convalescent plasma during first 8 days of illness reduces mortality from 15%–30% to <1%.
Bolivian HF	Elimination of specific reservoir rodents from towns practical and effective; sporadic cases due to exposure outside towns, person-to-person transmission in families and institutions cannot be prevented; Argentine HF vaccine protects experimental animals against Bolivian virus.	Ribavirin likely to be effective and should be used in this and other arenavirus diseases unless proven effective alternative therapy available.
Lassa fever	None; intensive village-based rodent control may reduce risk.	Ribavirin effective in reducing mortality; use in higher risk patients, e.g., if aspartate transaminase >150 U/L.
Bunyaviridae		
Rift Valley fever	Vaccination of domestic livestock prevents epizootics/epidemics but not sporadic, endemic infections of humans; human vaccine safe and effective but limited supply; veterinarians and virology workers in sub-Saharan Africa candidates for vaccine.	Ribavirin and antibody therapy should be tried in HF patients based on studies in experimental animals.
Crimean-Congo HF	Tick avoidance; no slaughter of acutely infected animals (healthy but viremic and therefore an undetected threat); barrier nursing of suspected patients particularly important.	Ribavirin should be used based on in vitro sensitivity and on uncontrolled South African experience.
HF with renal syndrome (HFRS)	Rodent control and avoidance impractical in most cases; investigational vaccines deserve further evaluation.	Early diagnosis and supportive care lifesaving; ribavirin has positive effect during initial 4 days illness and should be used in severe HFRS if available.
Hantavirus pulmonary syndrome	Rodent avoidance useful; care should be taken before entering or cleaning closed buildings with potential rodent infestations.	Early diagnosis and supportive care potentially lifesaving; avoidance of hypoxia and excessive hydration coupled with careful management of shock.
Filoviridae		
Ebola/Marburg HF	Barrier nursing and needle sterilization in African hospitals particularly important; avoid close contact with suspected patients; do careful evaluation of sick nonhuman primates.	None other than supportive, which may be of limited utility; antiviral therapies urgently needed.
Flaviviridae		
Yellow fever	Vaccine is probably the safest and most effective in the world; control of *Aedes aegypti* would eliminate urban transmission but sylvatic transmission remains.	None other than supportive.
Dengue HF	Reduction of dengue transmission by *A. aegypti* control; investigational vaccines will probably be available soon; possibly useful in travelers but may be limited in solving hyperendemic dengue transmission that leads to dengue HF.	Supportive care effective and greatly reduces mortality.
Tick-borne flaviviruses	Avoidance of ticks; vaccination; postexposure prophylaxis with virus-specific IgG.	Supportive care.

HF, Hemorrhagic fever.

important in the differential diagnosis, particularly malaria, rickettsial infections, leptospirosis, relapsing fever, typhoid, and shigellosis.

SUGGESTED READING

Hemorrhagic Fevers

Management of patients with suspected viral hemorrhagic fever. MMWR 37:1–15, 1988.
Peters, CJ: Pathogenesis of viral hemorrhagic fevers. In Nathanson N, Ahmed R, Gonzalez-Scarano F, et al (eds): Viral Pathogenesis. Philadelphia, Lippincott-Raven, 1996.
Peters CJ, Jahrling PB, Khan AS: Management of patients infected with high-hazard viruses. Arch Virol 11(suppl):1–28, 1996.
Peters, CJ, Zaki SR, Rollin PE: Viral hemorrhagic fevers. In Mandell GL (ed): Atlas of Infectious Diseases, vol 8, Fekety R (ed). Philadelphia, Current Medicine, 1997, pp 10.1–10.26.
Smorodintsev AA, Kazbintsev LI, Chudakov VG: Virus Hemorrhagic Fevers. Jerusalem, Israel Program for Scientific Translations, 1964.
Update: Management of patients with suspected viral hemorrhagic fever—United States. MMWR 44:475–479, 1995.
Zaki SR, Peters CJ: Viral hemorrhagic fevers. In Connor DH, Schwartz DA, Chandler FW (eds): Diagnostic Pathology of Infectious Diseases. Norwalk, Conn, Appleton & Lange, 1997, pp 347–364.

Arenaviridae

Barry M, Russi M, Armstrong L, et al: Brief report: Treatment of a laboratory-acquired Sabiá virus infection. N Engl J Med 333:294–296, 1995.
Enria D, Maiztegui JI: Antiviral treatment of Argentine hemorrhagic fever. Antiviral Res 23:23–31, 1994.
Fulhorst, C, Ksiazek TG, Mills, JN, et al: Venezuelan hemorrhagic fever: Clinical and epidemiologic studies of 165 cases. Clin Infect Dis 26:308–313, 1998.
Johnson KM, Halstead SB, Cohen SN: Hemorrhagic fevers of Southeast Asia and South America: A comparative appraisal. Prog Med Virol 9:105–158, 1967.
Johnson KM, McCormick JB, Webb PA, et al: Clinical virology of Lassa fever in hospitalized patients. J Infect Dis 155:456–464, 1987.
McCormick JB, King IJ, Webb PA, et al: A case–control study of the clinical diagnosis and course of Lassa fever. J Infect Dis 155:445–455, 1987.
Molinas FC, de Bracco MME, Maiztegui JI: Hemostasis and the complement system in Argentine hemorrhagic fever. Rev Infect Dis 11(suppl 4): 762–767, 1989.
Peters CJ: Arenaviruses. In Richman DD, Whitley RJ, Hayden FG (eds): Clinical Virology. Washington, DC, ASM Press, 2002, pp 949–969.
Peters CJ, Kuehne RW, Mercado RR, et al: Hemorrhagic fever in Cochabamba, Bolivia. Am J Epidemiol 99:425–433, 1971.

Bunyaviridae

Al Hazmi M, Ayoola EA, Abdurahman M, et al: Epidemic Rift Valley fever in Saudi Arabia: A clinical study of severe illness in humans. Clin Infect Dis 36:245–252, 2003.
Bruno P, Hassell LH, Brown J, et al: The protean manifestations of hemorrhagic fever with renal syndrome. A retrospective review of 26 cases from Korea. Ann Intern Med 113:385–391, 1990.
Bui-Mansfield LT, Torrington KG, Kim T: Acute pancreatitis in patients with hemorrhagic fever with renal syndrome. Military Med 166:167–170, 2001.
Duchin JS, Koster F, Peters CJ, et al: Hantavirus pulmonary syndrome: A clinical description of 17 patients with a newly recognized disease. N Engl J Med 330:949–955, 1994.
Huggins JW, Hsiang CM, Cosgriff TM, et al: Prospective, double-blind, concurrent, placebo controlled clinical trial of intravenous ribavirin therapy of hemorrhagic fever with renal syndrome. J Infect Dis 164:1119–1127, 1991.
Ketai LH, Williamson MR, Telepak RJ, et al: Hantavirus pulmonary syndrome (HPS): Radiographic findings in 16 patients. Radiology 191:665–668, 1994.
Laughlin LW, Meegan JM, Strausbaugh LJ, et al: Epidemic Rift Valley fever in Egypt: Observations of the spectrum of human illness. Trans R Soc Trop Med Hyg 73:630–633, 1979.
Peters CJ, Khan AS: Hantavirus pulmonary syndrome: The new American hemorrhagic fever. Clin Infect Dis 34:1224–1231, 2002.
Peters CJ, LeDuc JW: Bunyaviridae: Bunyaviruses, phleboviruses, and related viruses. In Belshe R (ed): Textbook of Human Virology, ed 2. St. Louis, Mo, Mosby-Year Book, 1991, pp 571–614.
Swanepoel R, Gill DE, Shepherd AJ, et al: The clinical pathology of Crimean-Congo hemorrhagic fever. Rev Infect Dis 11(suppl 4): S794–S800, 1989.
Swanepoel R, Shepard AJ, Leman PA, et al: Epidemiologic and clinical features of Crimean-Congo hemorrhagic fever in South Africa. Am J Trop Med Hyg 6:120–132, 1987.
Symposium on Epidemic Hemorrhagic Fever, May 1954. Am J Med 16:617–709, 1954.
Zaki SR: Hantavirus-associated diseases. In Connor DH, Schwartz DA, Chandler FW (eds): Diagnostic Pathology of Infectious Diseases. Norwalk, Conn, Appleton & Lange, 1997, pp 347–364.
Zaki SR, Greer PW, Coffield LM, et al: Hantavirus pulmonary syndrome: Pathogenesis of an emerging infectious disease. Am J Pathol 146:552–579, 1995.

Filoviridae

Ebola haemorrhagic fever in Zaire, 1976. Report of an international commission. Bull World Health Organ 56:271–293, 1978.
Martini GA, Siegert R (eds): Marburg Virus Diseases. Berlin, Springer-Verlag, 1971.
Pattyn SR (ed): Ebola Virus Haemorrhagic Fever. Amsterdam, Elsevier/North-Holland, 1978. http://www.itg.be/ebola.
Peters CJ, Leduc JW: An introduction to Ebola: The virus and the disease and articles in the supplement. J Infect Dis 179(suppl 1), 1999. http://www.journals/uchicago.edu/JID/journal/contents/v179nS1.html.
WHO/International Study Team: Ebola hemorrhagic fever in Sudan, 1976. Bull World Health Organ 56:247–270, 1978.

Flaviviridae

Burke DS, Monath TP: Flaviviruses. In Knipe DM, Howley PM (eds): Fields' Virology, 4th ed. Philadelphia, Lippincott Williams & Wilkins, 2001, pp 1043–1126.
Halstead SB: Antibody, macrophages, dengue virus infection, shock, and hemorrhage: A pathogenic cascade. Rev Infect Dis 11(suppl 4): S830–S839, 1989.
Halstead SB: Dengue and dengue hemorrhagic fever. In Feigin RD, Cherry JD (eds): Textbook of Pediatric Infectious Disease. Philadelphia, Saunders, 1987, pp 1510–1521.
Kerr JA: The clinical aspects and diagnosis of yellow fever. In Strode GR (ed): Yellow Fever. New York, McGraw-Hill, 1951, pp 385–425.
Touatre J: Yellow fever. Clinical notes (C Chassaignac, trans). New Orleans Med Surg J, 1898.

66

Arenavirus Infections

DELIA ENRIA
JAMES N. MILLS
RAMON FLICK
MICHAEL D. BOWEN
DAN BAUSCH
WUN-JU SHIEH
C. J. PETERS

INTRODUCTION

Arenaviruses are rodent-borne pathogens that are important causes of hemorrhagic fever (HF) in Africa and South America. Lymphocytic choriomeningitis (LCM) virus occurs in Europe, the Americas, and elsewhere, causing febrile disease, sometimes with central nervous system (CNS) involvement, and congenital infections. Several South American viruses result in HF, but the geographic distribution of each disease is limited. In Africa, the only identified HF is Lassa fever, found only in West Africa. There are many arenaviruses in Africa and the Americas that are not associated with human disease. Arenaviruses cause chronic, inapparent infections of their rodent host, sometimes with prolonged or lifelong viremia and vertical transmission. Human epidemiology is determined by the distribution of infected rodents and their contact with humans, although in some cases interhuman infection has occurred. Thus these diseases occur in rural environments where humans and rodents come into particularly close contact. Their aerosol infectivity and stability have put them in the first rank of bioterrorist threats.[1] Overt cell damage by arenaviruses is minimal or modest, but they alter cell function and induce mediators of shock, directly or by immunopathologic mechanisms. They are sensitive to the antiviral drug ribavirin, and there is a safe, effective vaccine against Argentine HF.

AGENTS

There are currently 20 recognized members of the Arenaviridae. They are shown in Figure 66-1 along with their known distribution and putative hosts. Their associated diseases are described in Table 66-1.

Virion Morphology and Structure

Arenaviruses derive their name from the Latin *arenosus* (sandy) from the granular or sandy appearance of virions when viewed by thin-section electron microscopy.[2] Virions are spherical to pleomorphic, have a mean diameter of 110 nm to 130 nm (range 50–300 nm), and are enveloped in a lipid bilayer derived from cell membranes (Fig. 66-2). Embedded in the lipid bilayer are club-shaped projections, 8 nm to 10 nm in length, which are composed of the viral glycoproteins, GP1 (molecular weight, 40–64 kD) and GP2 (35–44 kD).[3] A GP1 tetramer forms the head of the spike, whereas a GP2 tetramer forms the stalk.[4] GP1 and GP2 are derived by postranslational cleavage of a precursor molecule, GPC. The most abundant viral protein is the nucleoprotein, NP (63–78 kD), which associates with genomic RNA in circular nucleocapsid structures.[3,5] The viral L protein (200–250 kD) has transcriptase and replicase activity and is a minor component of nucleocapsids.[6,7] The Z protein (10–14 kD) is a small structural protein with a zinc-binding domain (RING finger motif).[8,9] By interacting with the viral polymerase, it inhibits transcription and replication.[10] Furthermore, it serves as a counterpart of the matrix protein found in other negative sense RNA viruses and is necessary for the generation of virus-like particles.[11] The electron-dense granules that give arenaviruses their sandy appearance have been identified as host cell ribosomes.[3] The function of these ribosomes has yet to be determined.

The lipid envelope of arenavirions makes them susceptible to organic solvents and detergents. Virus infectivity can also be inactivated by exposure to temperatures above 55°C, acidic or basic pH, ultraviolet light, and gamma irradiation.[12] Disinfectants containing phenolic compounds, hypochlorite, or quaternary amines effectively inactivate arenaviruses.[13]

Genomic Organization

The arenavirus genome consists of two single-stranded RNA molecules designated S (small) and L (large), the lengths of which are approximately 3.4 kb and 7.2 kb, respectively. Two genes are encoded on each RNA in an ambisense orientation. The NP gene is encoded at the 3′ end of the S RNA in the complementary sense, whereas the glycoprotein precursor (GPC) gene is encoded at the 5′ end of the S RNA in message sense. In a similar manner, the L protein is encoded at the 3′ end of the L RNA and the Z protein gene is found at the 5′ end of the L RNA. The 19 nucleotides at the 3′ end of each genomic segment are similar in all arenaviruses and are partial inverted complements to the 19 nucleotides at the 5′ end of each RNA. This sequence complementarity allows genomic RNAs to form a circular conformation with short base paired "panhandle" structures necessary for efficient RNA synthesis.[14] The conserved sequences at the ends of each genomic RNA speculatively function as a binding site for the L protein. The genes on each viral RNA segment are separated by noncoding intergenic regions in both S and L segments. These intergenic regions have the potential to form several distinct stem-loop structures that are thought to play a role in transcriptional termination.[5]

Replication

Arenaviruses gain entry into cells by attachment of the GP1 glycoprotein to one or more cellular receptors. One of these has been partially characterized as a 120- to 140-kD protein (alpha dystroglycan) found on primate and rodent cells.[15] Virus is then taken into large, smooth-walled vesicles where, in an acid environment, the GP2 glycoprotein mediates

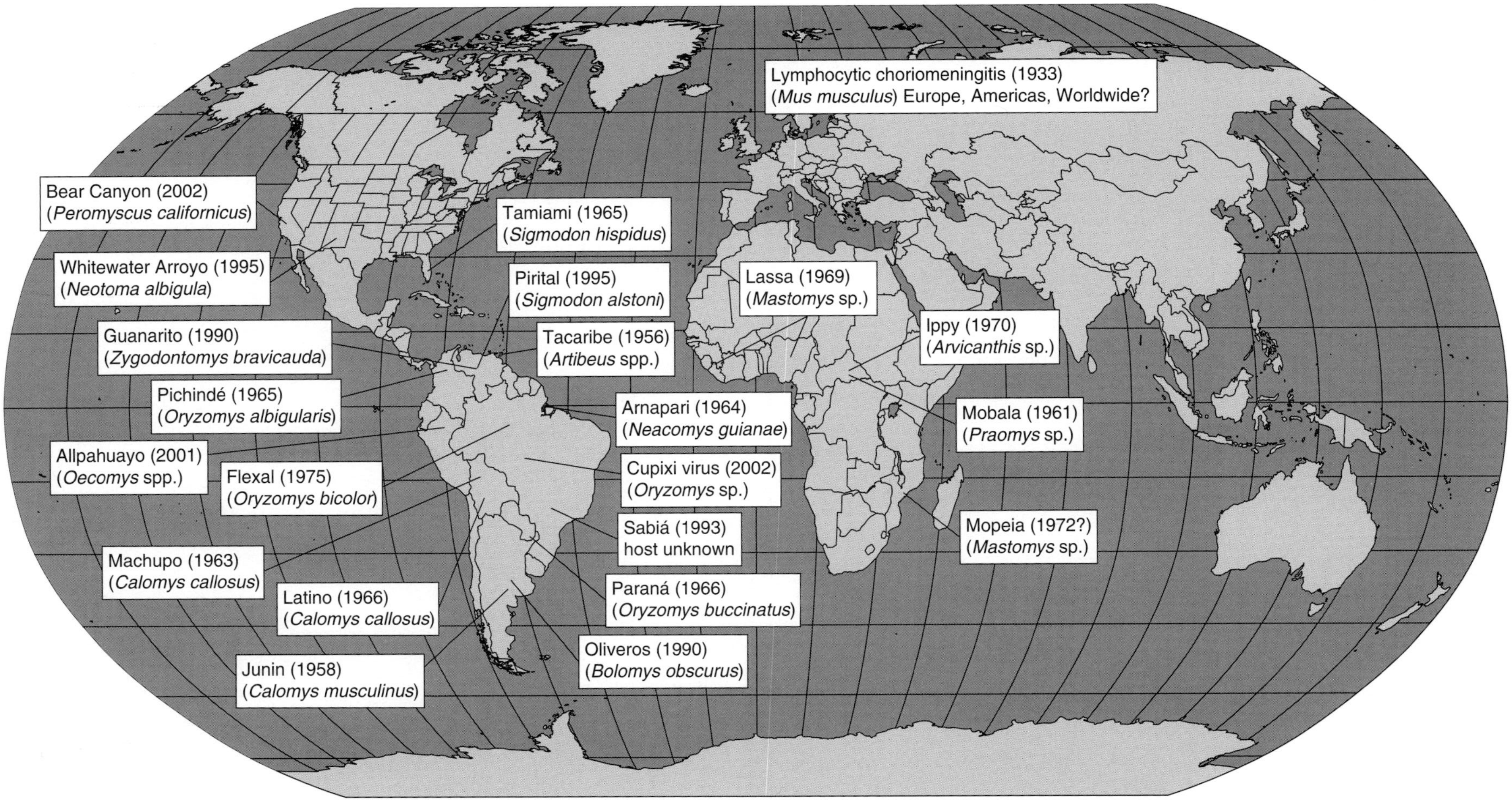

FIGURE 66-1 Recognized arenaviruses and their geographic distribution. Reservoirs are shown below the viruses in *italics*.

Table 66-1 Arenaviruses and Their Diseases

Virus	Disease	Clinical Manifestations
New World Viruses or Tacaribe Complex		
Junin	Argentine HF	Severe systemic disease with hemorrhage, prominent neurologic manifestations
Machupo	Bolivian HF	Resembles Argentine HF
Guanarito	Venezuelan HF	Resembles Argentine HF
Sabia	—	Limited experience suggests resemblance to Argentine HF but one case with prominent liver necrosis as well
Flexal	—	Two symptomatic laboratory infections observed; disease spectrum not defined
Pichinde	—	Asymptomatic
Amapari, Pirital, and others	—	Human infections not yet identified, pathogenicity unknown
Old World Viruses		
LCM	LCM	Acute febrile illness with thrombocytopenia and leukopenia; sometimes associated with orchitis; aseptic meningitis often follows the initial febrile period Encephalitis rarely occurs; maternal infection may result in fetal hydrocephalus and chorioretinitis
Lassa	Lassa fever	Severe systemic illness; hemorrhagic manifestations or neurologic involvement sometimes seen
Mopeia, Mobala	—	Human infection never observed, but laboratory animal studies suggest less pathogenic than Lassa virus
Unnamed new isolates	—	Human infection never observed

HF, hemorrhagic fever; LCM, lymphocytic choriomeningitis.

fusion between the virion membrane and the endosomal membrane. This process releases nucleocapsids into the cytoplasm where replication takes place.[5]

The ambisense arrangement of arenavirus genes appears to provide a unique mechanism for regulating gene transcription, with genes lying at the 3′ end of each genomic vRNA (i.e., NP, L) being expressed first. Genes residing at the 5′ end of each genomic segment (i.e., GPC, Z) cannot be expressed in the absence of protein synthesis.[16] To initiate gene expression, the viral L protein, which has RNA-dependent RNA polymerase activity and possibly endonuclease activity, is thought to cleave the cap and one to seven bases from cellular messenger RNAs (mRNAs) and use these primers to initiate transcription of subgenomic mRNAs ("cap snatching").[17,18]

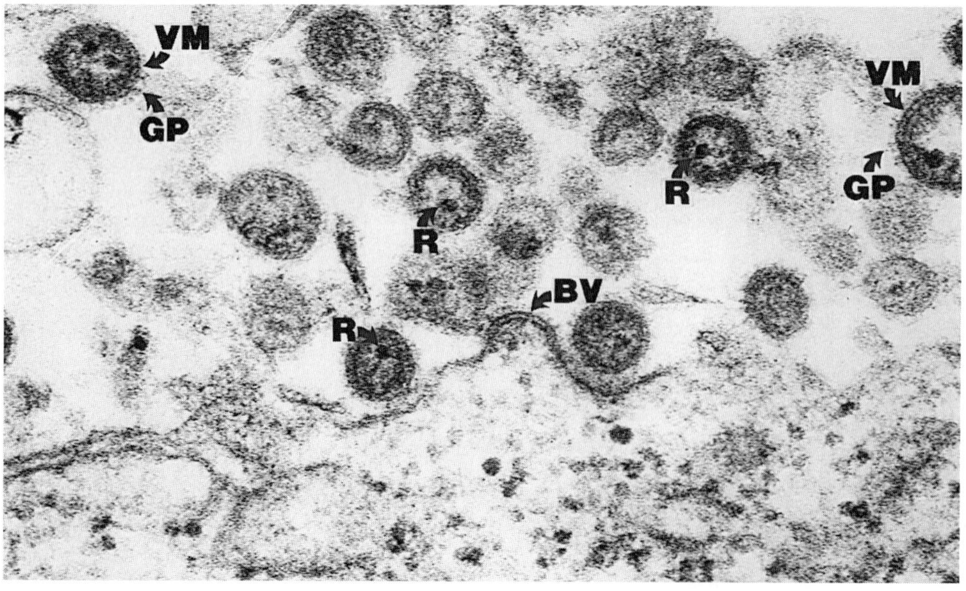

FIGURE 66-2 Electron micrograph of Machupo virions. Glycoprotein spikes (GP) are embedded in the virion membrane (VM). Electron-dense ribosomes (R) are present in the interior of the virions. A virion budding from a cell membrane (BV) is visible. (Courtesy of C. Goldsmith, Atlanta, GA; S. Zaki, Atlanta, GA; and F. Murphy, Davis, CA.)

of Guanarito virus genotypes (some closely matching genotypes from case patients in the disease-endemic area) in host populations over a wide area of the Venezuelan llanos, including areas in five states up to several hundred kilometers from the disease-endemic area.

Lassa fever is a West African disease. The countries most often associated with it are Sierra Leone, Guinea, Liberia, and Nigeria. The extent of Lassa fever transmission in the intervening countries is not known with certainty, but there is evidence to suggest its presence in Côte d'Ivoire, Burkina Faso, and Senegal.[91–93] This broad geographic distribution in an area that enjoys considerable tourism from the United Kingdom and other developed areas make Lassa fever the most exported of the viral hemorrhagic fevers.[94] Lassa virus is carried by rodents of the *Mastomys* species complex.[95,96] At least eight species occur in Africa south of the Sahara, and their systematics and distribution are complex and poorly understood.[97] Two species of multimammate rats are frequently associated with Lassa virus infection. Although morphologically very similar, *Mastomys huberti* and *Mastomys erythroleucus* are distinguished by karyotyping. *M. huberti,* the 32-chromosome species, tends to be found in houses and villages; *M. erythroleucus* has 38 chromosomes and is found more frequently in "bush" areas.[98,99] Although infection in *Mastomys* populations is focal, both species may have a high prevalence of antibody (near 30%).[96]

Several other Old World arenaviruses are known from African rodents (see Table 66-1 and Fig. 66-3), but their distribution and pathogenicity for humans are not understood. It seems likely that with further research the patterns seen with the several African viruses will come to resemble those of their American relatives.

LCM virus has a broad distribution wherever the common house mouse *(Mus musculus)* is found, including Europe, the Americas, Australia, and Japan.[69,100–104] Both *Mus m. domesticus* and *M. m. musculus* have yielded virus. The phylogenetic relationships of the viruses and the possible infection of other subspecies of *Mus* are unknown.

Transmission to Humans

Argentine Hemorrhagic Fever

Epidemics occur predominantly during the major harvesting season in Argentina, with a peak incidence in the month of May. The disease is four times as prevalent in males as in females, and is more prevalent among rural workers than in urban populations. Children under 14 years of age constitute about 10% of cases annually, but disease is uncommon in those less than 4 years old and exceptional in those less than 2 years of age. The seasonal distribution of the illness and the prevalence in male rural workers reflect occupational exposure of humans and the habits of the rodent host of Junin virus. Annual incidence within the endemic area may be as low as 1 in 100,000, but in the areas of highest activity it reaches 140 per 100,000 population and 355 per 100,000 adult males.

The Argentine HF endemic area is largely a patchwork of crop fields, which is crisscrossed by linear islands of relatively stable border habitats (roadsides, fence lines, and railroad rights of way). The primary host for Junin virus, the drylands vesper mouse *(C. musculinus),* is a habitat generalist.[105] Although it is most frequently captured in stable border habitats, it ventures into mature and postharvest crop fields where it supplements its diet with grain from corn and soybeans.[106] The drylands vesper mouse is rarely captured in or around human dwellings, although it may enter parklands and undeveloped areas adjacent to the surrounding pampas. In the early years of Argentine HF, the men affected worked in close contact with the land and harvested crops by hand. Later, mechanized agricultural practices became common, but the workers in the field, especially tractor drivers, have continued to become infected. Cases may be associated with the inhalation of infectious aerosols generated during the mechanized harvesting process, or with exposure to primary aerosols of rodent urine or contact with contaminated nesting materials in border habitats. The annual incidence of Argentine HF is positively correlated with local population densities of the reservoir.[107] This epidemiologic pattern is being further modified through vaccination of high-risk populations (see Fig. 66-5).

Argentine HF is not usually contagious, although person-to-person transmission can occur. A special situation is represented by a small number of women who are thought to have acquired the disease from their convalescent spouses through intimate contact.[108]

Bolivian Hemorrhagic Fever

The reservoir for Machupo virus is a species of the genus *Calomys* closely related but not identical to *C. callosus.* The host species resides in habitats where grassland intergrades into forest and, unlike *C. musculinus,* thrives in villages and near human habitations, which are found on high ground in seasonally inundated areas of the Beni Department. Bolivian HF tends to be a seasonal disease, with more cases occurring in the dry season, at the peak of agricultural activity. Most sporadic cases have involved adult men in rural areas, probably via contact with the rodent host in agricultural settings or in isolated small cottages.

However, family and community clusters of Bolivian HF cases affecting both sexes and all age groups have been centered around towns or hospitals. Epidemics in towns may occur during epizootic conditions when rodent densities reach unusually high levels and rodents invade towns or villages. In 1963–1964, a Bolivian HF epidemic occurred in the village of San Joaquin that resulted in 637 cases and 113 deaths among the town's 3000 residents.[82] The outbreak ended abruptly after two weeks of continuous trapping in homes, during which 3000 *C. callosus* rodents were captured.[109] Transmission to humans under these conditions is likely from inhalation of infectious aerosols concentrated within confined spaces of houses and outbuildings, but direct contact of broken skin or mucous membranes with rodent excreta or contaminated fomites such as food is also a consideration.

Person-to-person transmission, likely via direct contact with infectious body fluids, may occur in familial or nosocomial settings. For example, five health-care workers who were exposed to the index case or a secondary case contracted Bolivian HF in a hospital in Cochabamba in 1971,[110] and in 1994 a farm worker transmitted fatal Bolivian HF to six of eight family members.[111] Transmission by intimate contact during convalesence is also possible.[112]

Venezuelan Hemorrhagic Fever

In 1989, a severe HF was recognized by clinicians in the municipality of Guanarito, Guanarito State, Venezuela. At first, efforts toward laboratory diagnosis centered on dengue viruses, but the causative agent was soon isolated, shown to be an arenavirus, and named Guanarito virus.[113] Guanarito virus is specifically associated with *Z. brevicauda,* while a second arenavirus, Pirital virus, is associated with co-occurring *S. alstoni*.[114] Within the Venezuelan HF endemic area, both rodent species are commonly captured in crop fields, borders, and roadside habitats, and they are only rarely captured in the peridomestic environment.

While cases have been observed throughout the year, epidemics appear to have a seasonal peak in November to January, coinciding with maximum agricultural activity in the endemic region. Although children and adults of both sexes suffer disease, the highest risk is among adult male agricultural workers.[83] Thus transmission to humans likely occurs most frequently outside the home and may be related to agricultural activities. Person-to-person transmission or nosocomial infection has not been observed in spite of the fact that Venezuelan HF patients, like other South American HF patients, are usually admitted to open wards with minimal isolation precautions.

Lymphocytic Choriomeningitis

The natural rodent reservoir of the virus is the cosmopolitan house mouse, *M. musculus,* although outbreaks of human disease have also been traced to pet hamsters *(Mesocricetus auratus)* in the United States,[115] Germany,[102] and France.[116] As its name implies, the house mouse is frequently found living in close association with humans within homes and other man-made structures in both rural and urban situations. Infection with LCM virus in house mouse populations can be highly focal. In inner-city Baltimore, antibody-positive mice were clustered within residential blocks[117]; infection varied from 0% (0/753) to 27% (214/594) of mice on four farms in California.[118]

The incidence of human disease peaks in the fall and winter, presumably reflecting the seasonal invasion of homes by mice. As expected, human disease is associated with the regional prevalence of mouse infection and can vary by region or even by house.[102,119] Risk of infection is higher among rural dwellers and, in the United States, in low-income groups.[120] Human seroprevalence to LCM virus has often been found to range from 5% to 10% in the United States and elsewhere.[69,102,120,121] An antibody survey using hospital patients in Birmingham, Alabama, showed a prevalence of IgG antibody to LCM virus that was much lower in younger patients than in patients over 30 years of age, although it was not known whether this represented a secular decrease in risk of infection in recent decades or a lesser risk in children.[120] The number of acute LCM cases annually is not known because diagnostic testing is not commonly performed; during the period 1941 to 1958, LCM was the confirmed diagnosis in about 10% of patients with febrile CNS disease admitted to a tertiary care hospital in Washington, D.C.[122,123]

Lassa Fever

Lassa fever is an extremely common infection among adults in endemic areas of West Africa. In a heavily affected region such as Sierra Leone's Eastern Province, the disease may be responsible for more than one-fourth of medical admissions and of medical deaths.[96] In the same area it is also common among pediatric admissions.[124] Because of the similar incidence of disease among men and women and the frequent involvement of children, peridomestic exposure is likely to be important.[125] Indeed, rodent density may be higher in houses than in the surrounding agricultural or bush areas.[96] In this setting, transmission to humans may occur via inhalation of primary aerosols from rodent urine, by contact with contaminated fomites, or by ingestion of contaminated food. Human infection is also enhanced by the practice of hunting and consuming rodents as a food source, as well as the high levels of rodent infestation, open food storage, and closed shutters during the day—a practice that favors prolonged rodent activity.[96] These factors are exacerbated in the diamond-mining areas of Sierra Leone and during civil disruption. In Guinea, cases were clustered during the dry season and early part of the rainy season, coinciding with the period of maximum infection in *Mastomys* populations.[73,125]

Interhuman transmission of Lassa fever occurs but it is difficult to quantitate because of the frequent presence of infected *Mastomys* in houses.[126] At least one outbreak provided evidence of person-to-person transmission of Lassa virus without confounding infected rodents or reported needle use.[127] Although rare,[128] devastating hospital outbreaks have occurred and have been attributed to aerosols[129] or to lack of sterilization of parenteral injection equipment.[130]

Maintenance of the Virus in Rodent Host Populations

Argentine Hemorrhagic Fever

Junin virus is likely maintained in *C. musculinus* reservoir populations primarily via horizontal transmission. When transmitted vertically, the virus may have important deleterious effects on fitness. Newborn *C. musculinus* infected with Junin virus in the laboratory have high mortality (70%), and survivors show stunting and greatly reduced fecundity.[131] Animals infected in the laboratory as adults showed a split response. Half of the animals developed antibody and cleared virus; the remainder had chronic viremia and persistent shedding of virus in urine and saliva; there was no obvious deleterious effect on these chronically infected adults.[132] Field studies of natural populations demonstrated that infection with Junin virus among wild *C. musculinus* was more frequent among males than females and was positively correlated with age and the presence of wounds or scars.[68] These data suggest that aggressive encounters between adult males may be an important mechanism of transmission within reservoir populations.

Bolivian Hemorrhagic Fever

As with Junin virus, vertical transmission of Machupo virus would have a severe effect on host reproductive fitness of its reservoir rodent. In the laboratory, females inoculated at birth were chronically infected and sterile.[133] Also, as was later shown to be the case with Junin virus and *C. musculinus*, colonized *Calomys* rodents infected with Machupo virus as adults showed a split response: 50% of the animals developed antibody and cleared viral infection, while 50% showed chronic viremia and viruria. Longitudinal field studies are needed to assess the mechanisms of transmission of Machupo virus in natural populations.

Venezuelan Hemorrhagic Fever

Laboratory experiments indicate that the maintenance pattern for Guanarito virus in *Z. brevicauda* may be different from either the Junin or Machupo models.[134] Newborn *Z. brevicauda* inoculated subcutaneously with Guanarito virus developed a chronic infection with persistent shedding of virus in urine and saliva. There was no detectable effect of infection on growth of these animals (after 3 weeks). Subcutaneous inoculation of adult animals resulted in a split response. Four of 12 animals showed only transient viremia, followed by the development of high-titer neutralizing and immunofluorescent antibody. The remainder showed chronic viremia and persistent shedding of virus in urine and saliva. Eleven females that had been inoculated with Guanarito virus as adults had only two apparently normal litters after being paired with males, while 11 sham-inoculated females had 10 litters. Thus, horizontal transmission of virus has an apparent negative effect on reproductive fitness. The presence of virus in the blood of one of three pups born to an infected female indicates that vertical transmission is possible, but the fecundity of females infected as newborns has not been studied.[135]

Lassa Fever and Lymphocytic Choriomeningitis

In contrast to the pattern with the New World arenaviruses, LCM and Lassa viruses are thought to be maintained by vertical transmission within reservoir populations. All pups born to chronically infected females are themselves chronically infected (perhaps transovarially).[136] Conversely, inoculation of adult hosts with LCM or Lassa virus results in an immunizing infection[64,67,70,71]; young born to immunized animals are also protected by maternal antibody. This pattern was observed in field studies of Lassa virus in Guinea; most animals trapped were naïve, or chronically infected, with only occasional antibody-positive rodents.[73] Thus, strict horizontal transmission of virus within host populations would likely result in its rapid extinction.

DISEASES

Clinical Manifestations

The South American HFs resemble one another, and Argentine HF is the best described. Lassa fever has a similar pathogenesis, but neurologic involvement, thrombocytopenia, leukopenia, and bleeding manifestations are less prominent.

Argentine Hemorrhagic Fever

The incubation period is usually 6 to 14 days with outer limits of 4 to 21 days. The onset of illness is insidious, with chills, malaise, anorexia, headache, myalgias, and moderate hyperthermia (38°C to 39°C). After several days, this gives way to further constitutional, gastrointestinal, neurologic, and cardiovascular signs and symptoms. Low backache, retro-orbital pain, nausea or vomiting, epigastric pain, photophobia, dizziness, and constipation or mild diarrhea are common symptoms. An almost constant absence of productive cough, sore throat, or nasal congestion is helpful in distinguishing the initial symptoms of Argentine HF from those of influenza or other acute respiratory infections.

During the first week of illness, physical examination reveals flushing of the face, neck, and upper chest. Conjunctival congestion and periorbital edema may also occur. The oropharyngeal membranes are congested, and there is congestion of the vessels bordering the gums, which may bleed spontaneously or under slight pressure. An enanthem characterized by petechiae and small vesicles is almost invariably found over the soft palate if carefully sought.[137] Most patients have cutaneous petechiae in the axillary regions, upper chest, and arms. Lymph nodes become enlarged, particularly in the lateral cervical regions. There are no signs of pulmonary abnormalities. Relative bradycardia and orthostatic hypotension are common. Generally, there is no hepatomegaly or splenomegaly, and jaundice is very rare.

At the end of the first week of evolution, oliguria and different degrees of dehydration occur. Neurologic signs are very common. The patient may be irritable and lethargic, with a fine tremor of the hand and tongue. Moderate ataxia, cutaneous hyperesthesia, and a decrease in deep tendon reflexes and muscular tonicity are present. In females, mild to moderate metrorrhagia is constantly present and, in some cases, is the first sign of the disease.

During the second week of illness, 70% to 80% of the patients begin to improve. In the remaining 20% to 30%, severe hemorrhagic or neurologic manifestations, shock, and superimposed bacterial infections appear between 8 and 12 days after the onset of symptoms. Profuse bleeding may occur in the form of hematemesis, melena, hemoptysis, epistaxis, hematomas, metrorrhagia, or hematuria. The severe neurologic manifestations generally begin with mental confusion, marked ataxia, increased irritability, and intention tremors; these are followed by delirium, generalized convulsions, and coma. Acute renal failure is uncommon, but may occur in terminal cases or after prolonged periods of shock, and is secondary to acute tubular necrosis. Superimposed bacterial infections such as pneumonia and septicemia or thrush can also complicate the clinical course.

Patients begin to improve by the third week of illness and experience a prolonged convalescence. Temporary hair loss is common. Many patients have asthenia, irritability, and memory changes, but these disappear gradually over a period of 1 to 3 months. During convalescence, 10% of Argentine HF patients treated with immune plasma develop a late neurologic syndrome. This late neurologic syndrome appears after a period of 7 to 80 days (mean, 20 days) free of symptoms, differs from the neurologic manifestations of the acute period of Argentine HF, and is characterized by febrile symptoms and cerebellar signs as well as cranial nerve palsies.[138,139]

Clinical laboratory studies are quite helpful in establishing an early clinical diagnosis in South American HF. During the acute phase, there is progressive leukopenia and thrombocytopenia, with counts falling to 1000 to 2000 white blood cells (WBCs) and 50,000 to 100,000 platelets per microliter.

The sedimentation rate is normal or decreased. Almost invariably, there is proteinuria and a urinary sediment containing hyaline-granular casts and red blood cells. Round cells with cytoplasmic inclusions are also found, but are not diagnostic. Serum creatinine and urea are normal or increased in proportion to dehydration and shock in the severely ill patient. In Argentine HF, aspartate transaminase (AST), creatine phosphokinase (CPK), and lactate dehydrogenase (LDH) elevations are common but mild, and hyperbilirubinemia or hyperamylasemia is rare. During the acute illness, cerebrospinal fluid (CSF) is normal, even in patients with severe neurologic disease. However, during the late neurologic syndrome following immune plasma therapy, the CSF may have tens to hundreds of cells with normal sugar and normal or slightly increased protein.

Argentine HF during pregnancy is uncommon, but in the last trimester more than half of patients die, at least in part due to tardy recognition of the disease and failure to administer specific treatment. Congenital malformations, fetal death, and death of neonates has also been seen.[140] Children tend to have a milder clinical course, but severe and even fatal disease has been seen.

Other South American Hemorrhagic Fevers

Bolivian HF[82,112,141] and Venezuelan HF[83,113] have clinical characteristics similar to those of Argentine HF. Bolivian HF cases from a nosocomial outbreak occurring at high altitude had jaundice and a high mortality, but the reason was not determined.[110] Patients with Venezuelan HF frequently complain of sore throat among their initial symptoms, and hearing loss in convalescence has been reported.

Only a single naturally acquired infection with Sabia virus has been identified, and it resembled other South American HFs except for extensive liver necrosis and jaundice.[142] One laboratory infection appeared to be a mild case of HF,[143] and a second was treated, apparently successfully, with ribavirin and developed only mild disease.[144]

Lassa Fever

Lassa fever is seen in both sexes and all age groups. Typically, after an incubation period of about 10 days (range, 3 to 21 days), the patient notes the insidious onset of fever, headache, generalized weakness, and malaise.[125,145–150] Within a few days, these may be followed by sore throat with or without visible pharyngitis, cough, retrosternal chest pain, conjunctivitis, abdominal pain, and a variety of other generalized symptoms. The minority of patients with florid Lassa fever may then manifest facial and neck swelling, subconjunctival hemorrhage, and bleeding.[137] The bleeding is typically a mild oozing from the nose, mouth, or genitourinary or gastrointestinal tract and, with the exception of vaginal bleeding in pregnant women, is unlikely to be hemodynamically significant. Maculopapular or petechial rashes have been observed in white-skinned, but not black-skinned patients. Whether this difference reflects ease of observation or different manifestations of Lassa fever based on genetic makeup is uncertain.

Elevated respiratory rates, with or without mild rales on lung auscultation, are frequently noted. Hypotension and tachycardia may be present, especially in more severe cases. Pleural effusions are common, and pericardial effusions are occasionally seen late in the course of the disease, particularly in males. A variety of encephalopathic and other neurologic manifestations have been noted in severely ill patients, but it is not clear to what extent these represent direct effects of Lassa virus on the CNS, secondary immune-mediated effects, or nonspecific metabolic ones common to any critically ill patient.[151,152]

Surviving patients generally begin to defervesce within approximately 10 days of onset. With the exception of sensorineural deafness (see following discussion), recovery is usually complete. Conversely, patients with severe illness may deteriorate rapidly, progressing to shock, delirium, respiratory distress, coma, seizures, and death.[125,149] The contribution of poor fluid balance, nutritional status, and patient monitoring in this setting of limited resources is unknown. Other underlying health problems such as malnutrition, tuberculosis, and acquired immunodeficiency syndrome (AIDS), as well as nosocomial infections, may affect the clinical course of Lassa fever as well.

Lassa fever in pregnant women carries a significantly elevated risk for both the mother and the fetus.[95,153] Maternal mortality is particularly elevated during the third trimester, when fetal death approaches 100%.[153]

Pediatric Lassa fever is less well described but produces a spectrum of disease ranging from undifferentiated febrile illness to severe Lassa fever.[124,154,155] A "swollen baby syndrome" comprised of anasarca, abdominal distention, and bleeding with a high mortality has been described in several Liberian infants.[154] Whether this syndrome is a general feature of Lassa virus infection of infants or related to other concomitant health risks or therapies specific to the area of study is not clear.

Abnormalities in clinical laboratory measurements are usually mild to moderate. Thrombocytopenia, usually not less than 100,000/μL, may be seen. Although often normal, a mild diminution in the WBC count with lymphopenia may occur.[146,149,156] Severely ill patients are more likely to be thrombocytopenic, are usually lymphopenic, and may have an elevated WBC count with neutrophilia. Moderate hemoconcentration and proteinuria are usually present with an elevated blood urea nitrogen (BUN).[146–148,150] These are likely a result of capillary leak, fever, and decreased fluid intake resulting in loss of intravascular volume. The AST is often elevated, and higher values are predictive of a poor prognosis, as is the level of viremia.[157] The disproportionate elevation in AST compared to the alanine transaminase (ALT) value suggests that its source is not solely the liver but rather may result from diffuse ischemic end-organ damage. Disseminated intravascular coagulation (DIC) is not part of the pathogenesis of Lassa fever. A variety of nonspecific electrocardiographic changes have been reported.[158] Based on limited observations, radiographic studies are usually nonspecific and correlate with the physical exam.[159]

Sensorineural deafness is the major chronic sequela of Lassa fever and may occur in up to one-fourth of those infected. Typically, the deafness presents during convalescence. There is no correlation with the severity of the acute febrile illness, level of viremia, or AST. It may be uni- or bilateral and is permanent in approximately two-thirds of cases.[160] Depression and cerebellar ataxia have been reported during recovery, but are relatively uncommon.[152] Lassa virus can often be isolated from CSF; however, a systematic correlation with any of the neurologic manifestations of the disease is not available.[151,160]

Although a broad range of case-fatality rates from Lassa fever have been reported, about 15% is a good estimate in the patient seeking medical treatment. Nigerian outbreaks have often been associated with a higher mortality than those in countries further west in Africa. Community investigations conducted in Sierra Leone found milder infections to be common but the role of preexisting immunity is unresolved.[96] The presence of bleeding, high viremia or antigenemia, and elevated AST independently confer a poor prognosis.[145,149]

Lymphocytic Choriomeningitis

Typical LCM is characterized by two phases, a period of fever and viremia followed by a CNS phase in which virus no longer circulates, antibodies are found in serum, but virus is still present in the CNS[78,79,116,121–123,161–163] (reviewed in Lehmann-Grube[69] and Peters[164,165]). Neurologic disease is presumed to be immunopathologic and mediated by CD8+ T cells, as is the process seen in the intracranially infected adult mouse.[5,37,166] Immunosuppressed patients inoculated with LCM virus did not develop CNS signs, although virus grew in the brain.[167] A substantial proportion of infections are subclinical, some of the remainder consist of fever alone, and others show both the initial febrile phase and the CNS disease, often with a short afebrile remission between the two.

The disease may begin with abrupt onset of fever, malaise, and myalgia with additional weakness, gastrointestinal symptoms, and occasionally sore throat or cough. Arthralgia, testicular pain, parotid pain, or even frank inflammation may occur. During this phase, which may last from a few days to 2 to 3 weeks, leukopenia, lymphopenia, thrombocytopenia, and elevation of LDH and AST are seen.[78,161,163]

The neurologic phase begins with aseptic meningitis, usually after a short period of defervescence but possibly continuous with the initial febrile stage or even without preceding fever. The findings are those of aseptic meningitis, but headache may be severe and disturbances of consciousness may be seen. Signs of nervous system involvement may last 1 to 4 weeks and virtually always resolve without sequelae. Rarely, LCM may present as encephalitis[122,123] with a very occasional fatal outcome; in the latter case, cerebral neuronal invasion can be demonstrated.[168] The CSF may have normal or low glucose, and cell counts often reach hundreds to thousands of lymphocytes per microliter.

Convalescence may be delayed for several weeks with asthenia, febrile sensations, difficulties in memory, poor cognitive function, headaches, or arthralgia.

Occasionally, LCM virus infection has been associated with ascending paralysis, Parkinson's syndrome, transverse myelitis, or myocarditis, but a causal link remains to be established. Deafness has rarely been reported with LCM[169,170] and may be a feature, based on the similarity to Lassa fever. Rarely, LCM virus has caused a syndrome resembling viral HF.[171]

As in other arenavirus infections, LCM virus can cross the placenta, with fetal infection or death.[78,172,173] The most common manifestation identified has been hydrocephalus with chorioretinitis. This was first reported from Lithuania[174,175] but has been confirmed in Germany,[172] France,[176] and more recently by several cases in the United States.[177–180] This is probably a much more common problem than appreciated.

Pathology

Animal Models

Natural and experimental infection of different animals, including guinea pigs, rats, hamsters, and nonhuman primates, have provided useful information on the comparative pathology of arenavirus infections. Lassa virus infection of rhesus monkeys, squirrel monkeys, and guinea pigs demonstrated a wide spectrum of organ tropism involving liver, spleen, lymph nodes, heart, lungs, pancreas, kidneys, and adrenal glands at early stages of infection. The common pathologic findings include hepatocellular necrosis and regeneration, lymphoid necrosis in spleen and lymph nodes, myocarditis, focal arteritis, renal tubular necrosis, and late mononuclear choriomeningoencephalitis.[181–184]

LCM virus infection of marmosets and tamarins can induce a highly fatal disease (callitrichid hepatitis). The histopathologic lesions are similar to those in human Lassa fever and consistently show focal necrosis in the liver, spleen, lymph nodes, adrenal glands, intestine, and pancreas.[185] In addition, LCM virus causes a viral HF syndrome in rhesus monkeys,[31] so it is not surprising that rarely human infection by LCM virus may also produce manifestations resembling HF.[171]

Machupo virus infection of rhesus and African green monkeys causes hemorrhage and necrosis in multiple organs. The hemorrhages are present in the skin, heart, brain, and nasal mucosa; necrosis is observed in the liver, adrenal cortex, myocardium, gastrointestinal mucosa, lymphoid tissue, and epithelial cells of the tongue, mouth, esophagus, and skin. Animals that die late in the course of Machupo virus infection frequently have meningoencephalitis and bronchopneumonia.[186]

Junin virus infection of rhesus monkeys, marmosets, and guinea pigs produces lesions similar to reported human cases of Argentine HF. The common findings include hemorrhage, bone marrow necrosis, mild hepatocellular necrosis, polioencephalomyelitis, and autonomic ganglioneuritis.[187]

Guanarito virus infection of guinea pigs results in focal epithelial cell necrosis of the gastrointestinal tract, interstitial pneumonia, and lymphoid and hematopoietic cell necrosis. Viral antigen is present in lymphoid tissues, macrophages, endothelial cells of multiple organs, pulmonary epithelium, epithelium of the gastrointestinal tract, and other tissues. Intact virions and typical arenavirus inclusions are visualized by immune electron microscopy in these same tissues.[188]

Human Pathology

Pathologic descriptions of arenavirus infections in humans are limited to a few necropsy series.[182,183,189–191] Gross and microscopic pathologic findings in these human cases are generally similar among different arenavirus infections.[192] Common gross findings at postmortem examinations include ecchymoses and petechial hemorrhages involving skin, conjunctivae, mucous membranes, and internal organs. The degree of hemorrhage varies, and sometimes can be minimal or absent. Conjunctival suffusion, pleural effusion, pericardial effusion, and ascites are frequently present.

Microscopically, congestion and variable degrees of necrosis are usually observed in multiple organ systems. Necrosis is most prominent in the liver (Fig. 66-6) and spleen, but is also

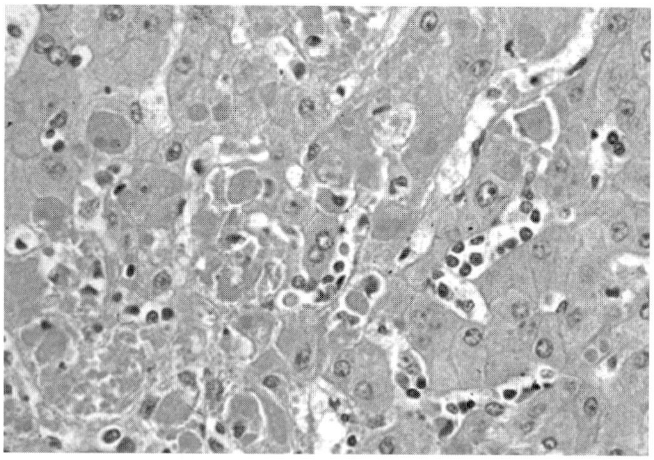

FIGURE 66-6 Lassa virus infection in the liver, showing multifocal hepatocellular necrosis with cytoplasmic eosinophilia, nuclear pyknosis, cytolysis, and fatty metamorphosis. (Hematoxylin and eosin stain.)

frequently found in adrenal gland, kidney, and gastrointestinal mucosa. The most consistent histopathologic feature is seen in the liver and comprises multifocal hepatocellular necrosis with cytoplasmic eosinophilia, Councilman body formation, nuclear pyknosis, cytolysis, and fatty metamorphosis. Inflammatory cell infiltrates in necrotic areas are usually minimal and, when present, consist of a mixture of mononuclear cells and neutrophils. The spleen usually shows depletion of follicles and focal necrosis. Other pathologic features that may be present in arenavirus infections include mild interstitial pneumonitis, diffuse alveolar damage, myocardial necrosis, and acute renal tubular necrosis.

Because none of these pathologic features are specific, a confirmatory assay such as immunohistochemistry or in situ hybridization is essential to establish a definitive tissue diagnosis, and such assays can also delineate the spectrum of tissue tropism as well as elucidate possible pathogenic mechanisms.

In Lassa fever, the localization of viral antigens can be summarized as: (1) hepatocytes, especially those in the areas of necrosis (Fig. 66-7); (2) cells of the mononuclear phagocytic system such as Kupffer cells in hepatic sinusoids, alveolar macrophages, and endothelial cells; (3) mesothelial cells lining the pericardium, pleura, peritoneum, and serosal surfaces of other organs; and (4) specialized cells involved in hormone secretion, including those in the adrenal gland, ovary, uterus, placenta, and breast.[184]

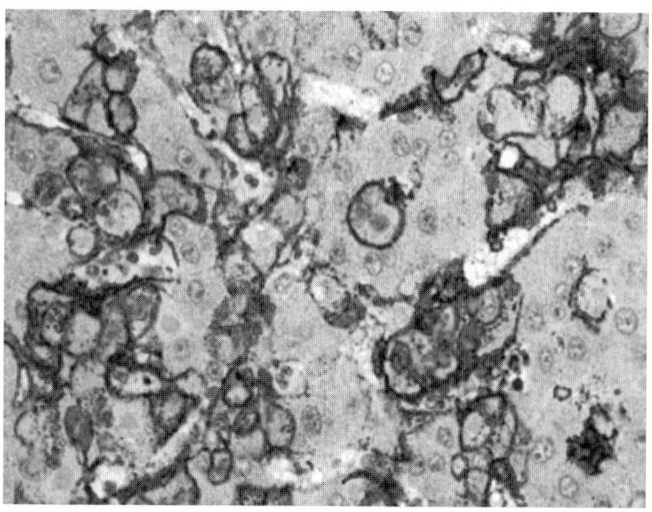

FIGURE 66-7 Antigens of Lassa virus are present in hepatocytes and sinusoidal lining cells, including Kupffer cells and endothelial cells. (Immunoalkaline phosphatase staining, Naphthol fast red substrate with light hematoxylin counterstain.)

In Argentine HF, ultrastructural and immunohistochemical studies reveal characteristic intracellular viral inclusions that are more prominent in lymphoid tissues, coincident with the presence of Junin virus antigens. Macrophages are usually the cell type involved, although there is often necrosis in adjacent lymphocytes.[193] In the kidney, a large number of virus-like intracytoplasmic particles are found in distal and collecting tubules coincident with severe tissue necrosis and large quantities of Junin virus antigen as demonstrated by immunofluorescence.[194] Morphologic studies of the bone marrow indicate that an acute and transient arrest of hemopoiesis occurs, with bone marrow hypocellularity, but without permanent hematologic sequelae in survivors.[195]

Although further study is needed, some possible pathogenetic mechanisms in arenavirus infections can be suggested from these findings.

1. The presence of abundant Lassa virus antigens in or adjacent to the necrotic hepatocytes and Junin virus particles near necrotic foci in the kidney suggests that cellular necrosis can be a consequence of direct viral infection. Although hepatocellular necrosis is the most consistent histopathologic feature in arenavirus infections, it alone is insufficient to explain the fatal outcome in most instances.
2. Lymphoid tissues are the main sites of viral replication, as evidenced by the large amount of viral antigen present, high virus titers when determined, and the presence of lymphocytopenia and lymphocyte depletion in spleen and lymph nodes.
3. The widespread hemorrhages in arenavirus infections do not appear to be a result of DIC or clotting factor abnormalities; instead, the interactions of viral antigens with platelets, inflammatory cells, macrophages, and endothelial cells may play a more critical role in pathogenesis. The demonstrated infection of macrophages and endothelial cells may induce secretion of physiologically active substances, including cytokines and other inflammatory mediators, and subsequently cause microvascular instability leading to capillary leak syndrome.
4. The involvement of mesothelial cells can explain serous effusions commonly seen in patients with arenavirus infections.
5. The presence of viral antigens in hormone-secreting cells suggests that an interaction between arenaviruses and hormone receptors may exist. This interaction may further enhance the pathogenicity of the virus and cause more severe pathophysiologic effects. These effects might contribute to the higher mortality of pregnant women with Lassa fever and Argentine HF.

PATHOGENESIS AND IMMUNITY

The paucity of histologic lesions to explain disordered organ function and death is a common characteristic of all arenavirus infections, particularly arenaviral HFs. Studies of LCM virus have shown that the infected cell may have altered function without morphologic changes, but this has not been examined in the HFs. In South American HF, the altered pathophysiology seems to be the result of direct viral action in contrast to the more well-known and well-studied mouse models of LCM virus infection in which immunopathologic T-cell action causes acute encephalitis, and B-cell products result in chronic immune complex disease.[37,39] Several studies failed to demonstrate immune complexes, complement activation, or DIC as relevant pathogenic mechanisms in Argentine HF.[196,197] Immunosuppression of the Junin virus–infected guinea pig or the hamster undergoing systemic LCM virus infection failed to ameliorate disease.[198,199] Mediators released or activated as a result of the virus-cell interactions, such as lymphokines, vasoactive mediators, and proteolytic enzymes, may also explain some of the alterations.

In Argentine HF, bleeding itself seems to be a joint outcome of thrombocytopenia, abnormal platelet function induced by a plasma component,[200] and alterations in blood coagulation with activation of fibrinolysis. Hemostatic abnormalities include prolongation of activated partial thromboplastin time (APTT); low levels of factors VIII and IX; increased values of factor V, von Willebrand factor, and fibrinogen; and mild decreases in antithrombin III as well as plasminogen. Endothelial cell involvement is also suspected considering that Junin virus replicates well in cultured endothelial cells, a feature supported in human disease by increased levels of von Willebrand factor.[197,201]

Argentine HF is also characterized by an acute transitory immunodeficiency. There is a lag in the humoral immune response, with antibodies appearing during the second week of illness, coincident with the recovery of the patients.[196] During the acute phase, cell-mediated immunity is also depressed as measured by delayed-type hypersensitivity to nonviral recall antigens and lymphocyte proliferation stimulated by mitogens, as well as marked changes in the T-cell subpopulations; all return to normal values in early convalescence.[202,203] Both cellular immunity and antibody are important in recovery by Junin virus–infected guinea pigs[204] and in protection of vaccinees.[205,206]

Very high titers of endogenous interferon (IFN) have been demonstrated in serum samples of Argentine HF patients during the acute period of the disease and are significantly higher in fatal cases.[207] The levels of IFN-α decreased after the transfusion of immune plasma. Tumor necrosis factor-α (TNF-α) levels are also markedly elevated, particularly in fatal cases.[208] Another study suggested an association between histocompatibility antigens and the severity of Argentine HF.[209] Lassa fever probably has a similar pathogenesis as South American HF. Major differences are the less severe thrombocytopenia, the minor neurologic involvement, and the mechanism of recovery from acute disease. Although platelet counts do not fall to the low levels found in South American HF, there are soluble serum factors that mediate a profound but reversible inhibition of platelet aggregation,[200] and extensive inhibition is associated with clinical bleeding. Signs of neurologic disease are less frequent in Lassa fever, but may have been underestimated; indeed, Lassa virus has been isolated from CSF on several occasions, in contrast to Argentine HF in which virus has never been isolated from CSF or CNS tissues in spite of the frequent appearance of brain dysfunction. Cytokine activation is also present in Lassa fever.[210] In humans and in animal models, recovery from Lassa fever is not mediated by antibody, as judged by the low, late, and variable levels of in vitro neutralization by convalescent serum and the lack of protection in passive transfer experiments.[31,211] Spleen cell transfers in strain 13 guinea pigs suggest that cellular immunity is responsible for clearing viremia and survival.

The role of cellular immunity in recovery may also be relevant to the severity of Lassa fever in pregnant women. The placenta does not express maternal major histocompatibility complex (MHC) antigens,[212] but in Lassa fever it is highly infected (W-J Shieh, unpublished data); by analogy with the situation that holds for LCM virus–infected neurons, which do not express class I major histocompatibility complex (MHC) and cannot be lysed by host CD8+ T lymphocytes,[213] it seems likely that maternal T cells cannot control placental infection.

The Pichinde guinea pig model has been explored in detail as a model of severe arenavirus infection, and results suggest that many of the same mediators activated in septic shock are involved in the pathogenesis of Lassa fever.[31,214] Sulfidopeptide leukotrienes, catecholamines, platelet activating factor, endorphins, and TNF-α[215–217] are all activated. Excessive sodium loss occurs in the face of extensive infection of the mineralocorticoid-secreting zones of the adrenal cortex, although serum corticosteroid levels are somewhat elevated. One potentially important finding is the decrease in cardiac index and increase in peripheral vascular resistance seen from the outset, and the poor response to fluid infusion. This resembles the situation in hantavirus diseases but contrasts with the usual situation in septic shock. These results, combined with the pulmonary infection and interstitial infiltrates seen in humans and animal models, recommend that fluids be used with caution in supporting the circulation.

Although little is known about the pathogenesis of sensorineural deafness, its occurrence during convalescence, as well as lack of association with severity of the acute febrile illness, peak AST level, or antiviral therapy, suggests a possible immune-mediated injury.[213] Auditory patterns resemble idiopathic nerve deafness. [218]

DIAGNOSIS

Differential Diagnosis

During the first week of illness, the clinical manifestations of South American HF are nonspecific and can be confused with several acute febrile conditions. Among the infectious diseases, the differential diagnosis includes typhoid fever, hepatitis, infectious mononucleosis, leptospirosis, hantavirus pulmonary syndrome, dengue, dengue HF, and rickettsioses. Malaria should also be considered in endemic areas. Diseases presenting with hematologic or neurologic alterations such as intoxications, rheumatic diseases, and blood dyscrasias may also be mistaken. In the respective endemic areas or in patients with a history of travel to the specific geographic regions, a febrile syndrome with leukopenia and thrombocytopenia is suspicious of one of the South American HFs.

As with the South American diseases, the initial presentation of Lassa fever is often very nonspecific, and the differential diagnosis includes most febrile illnesses found in West Africa (see Chapter 65). Malaria, typhoid, and bacillary dysentery are important conditions to rule out or treat empirically.

Combinations of clinical variables have been examined to facilitate determination of both clinical diagnosis and outcome of patients with Lassa virus infection.[149] Although statistically significant positive predictive values can be obtained, they apply only to areas of high prevalence (41% of all adult febrile hospital admissions in this example), a condition unlikely to be met except in selected epidemic settings or in relatively uncommon areas of intense endemic transmission. The pharyngitis often seen in Lassa fever can be a confusing feature.

LCM virus infection should be suspected in any acute febrile disease associated with myalgia, thrombocytopenia, and leukopenia. Orchitis may occur, and CNS manifestations sometimes develop later. The classic presentation of LCM virus infection is aseptic meningitis occurring in the fall, particularly if an initial prodromal period of fever, perhaps with a remission, occurs before the CNS phase. High lymphocyte counts and low glucose values may be found in the CSF, leading to confusion with granulomatous meningitis. History of mouse or hamster contact may also be elicited but is often not present. If TORCH (*to*xoplasma, *r*ubella, *c*ytomegalovirus, and *h*erpesvirus) testing is negative or doubtful in cases of neonatal hydrocephalus or chorioretinitis, LCM virus testing should be done.

Laboratory Diagnosis

In the arenaviral HFs, viremia occurs throughout the acute febrile period, and the viruses can readily be isolated from blood and from lymphoid tissues of fatal cases.[219] Isolation is usually performed in Vero cells. The presence of virus can also be detected by ELISA for viral antigen or reverse transcription–polymerase chain reaction (RT-PCR). Fatal cases can also be diagnosed by immunohistochemistry on fixed tissues. Antibodies are usually measured by IFA[52] or increasingly by ELISA. Neutralization tests are extremely valuable for confirming specificity of reactions provided the arenavirus species is sensitively neutralized by convalescent serum.[31]

In Argentine HF, cocultivation of peripheral blood mononuclear cells improves the sensitivity of virus recovery.[220] Viral isolations can also be performed in guinea pigs or suckling mice. The ELISA is the method of choice for serologic diagnosis. RT-PCR has been successfully applied and can play a role in establishing etiologic diagnosis in patients dying before the appearance of the specific antibodies.

Recent Bolivian HF cases[111] have been diagnosed by antigen detection ELISA and immunoglobulin M (IgM) ELISA, although the classic approach employs suckling hamster inoculation for virus isolation and IFA with confirmatory neutralization tests for serology.[52]

In Africa, acute Lassa fever is best diagnosed by the combined ELISA for Lassa IgM antibody and antigen, which yields a sensitivity over 90% within 48 hours of admission.[221,222] Sensitive RT-PCR assays exist, but even in developed countries strain variation and problems of cross-contamination pose practical problems.[223,224] Lassa antigen is usually present in blood within a few days of infection and becomes undetectable after the appearance of IgM ELISA antibody, which typically appears a few days after the onset of illness and peaks by about 10 to 12 days. IgG ELISA antibodies typically take longer to develop, but are present in almost all patients by approximately 3 weeks and last for a period of years. It is unclear whether reinfection takes place, although its occurrence is suggested by the finding of significant sharp IgG IFA titer elevations in individuals previously shown positive, sometimes in association with mild febrile disease.[149] Lassa virus can be isolated from serum early in the disease course in about two-thirds of surviving and virtually all fatal cases. In survivors, this viremia is typically cleared by about 2 weeks. Conversely, in fatal cases, viremia persists unabated until death. Virus has also been isolated from serous effusions and a wide array of body tissues.[147,157,183]

Other serologic tests may be applied to Lassa fever, including IFA, which, like the IgM ELISA, may detect antibodies while patients are still acutely ill.[157] In contrast, neutralizing antibodies appear late in Lassa fever, often several weeks after disease resolves.[211] Furthermore, the final response is low in titer, best seen with a constant serum-varying virus test, and intensely complement dependent. It has been clearly shown in monkeys and guinea pigs that this neutralizing titer correlates with the ability to transfer protection (reviewed in Peters and associates).[31]

LCM virus circulates in the blood before the onset of CNS symptoms and later can be isolated from CSF by inoculation of adult mice intracranially or by use of Vero cells.[13,69,225] After the onset of CNS disease, ELISA IgM capture antibody tests in serum and CSF should be positive[226] (also T.G. Ksiazek, unpublished observations). The LCM virus antibody response resembles that to Lassa virus in that the neutralizing antibody response is greatly delayed, complement dependent, and of poor quality.[222,227] An RT-PCR procedure with sufficient sensitivity to detect LCM virus in clinical samples has been described, simplifying future viral diagnosis.[228]

TREATMENT

General Supportive Treatment

Supportive treatment consists of adequate hydration, symptomatic measures, and proper management of the neurologic alterations, blood losses, shock, and superimposed infections. There is no indication for the use of steroids or alpha interferon. Medication should be given by the oral or intravenous route. Intramuscular and subcutaneous injections are contraindicated because of the risk of hematomas.

In the Argentine HF–endemic area, several observations have been made: Pneumonia is the most common secondary bacterial infection and is often accompanied by radiographic changes and an increase in fever but not by leukocytosis; it usually responds to antibiotics. Platelet transfusions have been used, but the complex nature of the coagulopathy and clinical experience suggest they are not useful. Strategies such as desmopressin or activated factor VII have not been evaluated. Transfusions are needed occasionally, but most of the severe forms are neurologic. It is useful to sedate agitated patients with diphenhydramine or diazepam; diazepam also gives some protection against seizures. Cerebral edema may require both steroids and mannitol.

Virus-Specific Therapy

For Argentine HF, a specific treatment is available: the transfusion of immune plasma within the first 8 days of onset of symptoms.[138,203] This treatment reduces the case-fatality rate, from 15%–30% to less than 1%, and is now standardized based on the amount of neutralizing antibodies to Junin virus infused. Immune plasma is of no benefit to patients when it is initiated after 8 days of illness.

For the other South American HFs, the specific treatment suggested is ultravenous ribavirin, which should be considered for off-label use unless a proven alternative effective therapy is available.[144,229] Ribavirin may also prove useful in the treatment of Argentine HF patients[203]; this may be increasingly important as human immunodeficiency virus (HIV) and hepatitis C infections increase in the pampas, making donor selection more difficult, and because plasma-treated patients develop lower titers in convalesence, requiring more plasma for effective therapy of subsequent patients.[203]

Lassa fever can be treated effectively with the nucleoside analogue ribavirin. The drug was found to be highly effective in vitro and in a monkey model, leading to trials in West Africa that established its utility in human Lassa fever.[230,231] Patients with poor prognostic indicators (e.g., AST >150 units/mL) should be treated with intravenous ribavirin given in a dose of 30 mg/kg initially, 15 mg/kg every 6 hours for 4 days, and 7.5 mg/kg every 8 hours for 6 more days (this is not a licensed drug). The drug should be diluted in 150 mL of 0.9% saline and slowly infused[232] over a 30-minute period. Modest anemia should be expected, both from hemolysis and from a fully reversible normoblastic maturation arrest.

Uterine evacuation appears to improve survival significantly in pregnant women with Lassa fever.[153] Although contraindicated in pregnancy, the elevated maternal mortality rate, along with the almost universal fetal loss, suggests that ribavirin could be used as well, especially in the third trimester when maternal mortality is particularly high.

Neutralizing antibodies have been effective in laboratory models of Lassa fever, but this therapy should not be used unless the infused material is standardized by laboratory assays. Only supportive management is available for LCM.

PREVENTION

Containment of Patients

Acutely ill patients with South American HF or with Lassa fever are viremic during the acute phase of their illness, and the viruses are infectious by parenteral inoculation. Needle precautions should be emphasized, and transmission of Lassa fever within hospitals by inadequate parenteral precautions has caused serious epidemics in African hospitals.[130] Person-to-person transmission of Lassa fever is uncommon in the medical care setting,[128] but has occurred in the hospital as well as in the community so that barrier nursing precautions should be strictly enforced. Airborne transmission of Lassa fever has not been suspected to be a problem except in a single hospital epidemic in Nigeria.[129]

The South American HFs have not been regarded as highly contagious in the endemic areas where they occur, and person-to-person transmission is uncommon. Nevertheless, there are unusual patients who have disseminated both Junin (J.I. Maiztegui, unpublished observations) and Machupo viruses[110–112] to hospital staff and to families, in some instances suggesting aerosol transmission. Although the major focus should be on the proper patient care using basic precautions that will prevent parenteral and droplet exposure to blood and body fluids, the authors believe that, when possible, it is prudent to implement small-particle aerosol precautions once patients with arenavirus HFs are identified.[144,233–236]

Clinically well patients leaving the hospital are not generally contagious. HF patients have transmitted virus to spouses in convalesence so that intimate contact should be cautious and condoms should be used during sex for 2 to 3 months. Lassa virus has been isolated from urine for several weeks, and the use of disinfectant in the toilet bowl before voiding is advised. Breastfeeding is thought to be a risk factor for transmission from mother to infant and should be temporarily avoided unless there is no other way to support the baby.

It is not known if arenaviruses could adapt to rodents outside the endemic area. The striking rodent species-specificity of arenaviruses seen to date would argue that this is unlikely, but the ability of LCM virus to maintain itself within hamster colonies[13] and of Lassa virus to chronically infect newborn laboratory mice[164] suggests that precautions should be taken to minimize the discharge of exotic arenaviruses to the environment. For these reasons, we also recommend the sterilization of all materials leaving a patient's room in nonendemic areas, including adding disinfectant to toilets before use.

Barrier nursing in African hospitals should be emphasized, both because of the possibility of transmission and the potential presence of other viral HF. Locally applicable methods for such activities have been developed.[237]

Rodent Control

Rodent control has been successful in the control of Bolivian HF epidemics occurring in towns of the Beni Department,[238] but sporadic cases still occur after rural exposure or contact with a case.[111] For Argentine HF, rodent control or the control of human contact with infected rodent populations is impractical.

The fecundity and ubiquity of the *Mastomys* species complex across West Africa make widespread elimination of rodents unfeasible as a control measure for Lassa fever. Intense trapping in towns may be indicated during epidemics, although care should be taken to ensure that disposal of the trapped rodent does not inadvertently lead to exposure to potentially Lassa virus–infected blood, urine, or feces. Educational campaigns to appropriately store foodstuffs and avoid rodents as a food source, a practice common in some areas of West Africa, may have some impact.

LCM prevention depends on the exclusion of wild mice from dwellings, workplaces, and areas where colonized rodents are housed. The last is particularly important because of the risk of dissemination of infected animals to the pet trade or to laboratories. The occult infection of mouse colonies has been a recurring theme ever since LCM virus was first recognized.[13,239,240] In addition, the virus can be maintained in colonies of hamsters and possibly other rodents, and pet rodents could be infected if wild mice gain access. Pregnant women, in particular, must be protected from infection because of the risk of fetal damage.[180]

Vaccination

A live attenuated Junin virus vaccine (Candid #1)[86] with proven safety, immunogenicity, and efficacy in preventing Argentine HF is now available for use in high-risk populations.[206] Application of 175,000 doses targeted to the maximum risk groups has resulted in a major reduction in morbidity and mortality from Argentine HF (see Fig. 66-5). With sufficient supplies of vaccine to protect the whole population at risk, Argentine HF would be definitively controlled. Candid #1 may also be effective in the prevention of Bolivian HF, as suggested by preclinical studies, but the vaccine does not cross-protect against infection with Guanarito or Sabia viruses in experimental studies (P. B. Jahrling, personal communication, 1995).

Definitive control of Lassa fever in Africa urgently requires an effective vaccine. Immunization with the vaccinia-vectored GP gene of Lassa virus has spared nonhuman primates from death and given partial protection from disease and viremia, suggesting the feasibility of a Lassa vaccine.[241] Other approaches have also protected laboratory animals, but the use of killed vaccines has not generally been successful in preventing arenavirus disease (reviewed in Clegg and Sanchez).[242]

Bibliographic note: Many original references have been omitted in favor of reviews, particularly in the area of basic virology. The interested reader should consult standard texts[5,219] or recent reviews.[243,244]

REFERENCES

1. Peters CJ: Viral hemorrhagic fevers as bioterrorist threats. In Mandell GL, Bennett JE, Dolin R (eds): Mandell's and Bennett's Principles and Practice of Infectious Diseases. Philadelphia, Churchill Livingstone, 2004, pp 3626–3629.
2. Rowe WP, Murphy FA, Bergold GH, et al: Arenoviruses: Proposed name for a newly defined virus group. J Virol 5:651–652, 1970.
3. Pedersen IR: Structural components and replication of arenaviruses. [Review.] Adv Virus Res 24:277–330, 1979.
4. Burns J, Buchmeier M: Glycoproteins of the arenaviruses. In Salvato M (ed): The Arenaviridae. New York, Plenum Press, 1993, pp 17–35.
5. Buchmeier MJ, Bowen MDPCJ: Arenaviridae: The viruses and their replication. In Knipe DM, Howley PM (eds): Fields' Virology, 4th ed. Philadelphia, Lippincott, Williams, and Wilkins, 2001, pp 1635–1668.
6. Buchmeier MJ, Parekh BS: Protein structure and expression among arenaviruses. [Review.] Curr Top Microbiol Immunol 133:41–57, 1987.
7. Lukashevich IS, Djavani M, Shapiro K, Sanchez A, et al: The Lassa fever virus L gene: Nucleotide sequence, comparison, and precipitation of a predicted 250 kDa protein with monospecific antiserum. J Gen Virol 78(Pt 3):547–551, 1997.
8. Iapalucci S, Lopez N, Rey O, et al: The 5′ region of Tacaribe virus L RNA encodes a protein with a potential metal binding domain. Virology 173:357–361, 1989.
9. Salvato MS, Schweighofer KJ, Burns J, et al: Biochemical and immunological evidence that the 11 kDa zinc-binding protein of lymphocytic choriomeningitis virus is a structural component of the virus. Virus Res 22:185–198, 1992.
10. Jacamo R, Lopez N, Wilda M, et al: Tacaribe virus Z protein interacts with the L polymerase protein to inhibit viral RNA synthesis. J Virol 77:10383–10393, 2003.
11. Lee KJ, Perez M, Pinschewer DD, et al: Identification of the lymphocytic choriomeningitis virus (LCMV) proteins required to rescue LCMV RNA analogs into LCMV-like particles. J Virol 76:6393–6397, 2002.
12. Buchmeier M, Clegg J, Franze-Fernandez M, et al: Virus taxonomy: Sixth report of the International Committee on Taxonomy of Viruses. In Fauquet F, Fauquet C, Bishop D, et al (eds): Family *Arenaviridae*. New York, Springer-Verlag, 1995, pp 319–323.
13. Peters C: Viral infections of vertebrates, virus infections of rodents and lagomorphs. In Horzinek M, Osterhaus A (eds): Arenaviruses. Amsterdam, Elsevier, 1994, pp 321–341.
14. Lee KJ, Perez M, Pinschewer DD, et al: Identification of the lymphocytic choriomeningitis virus (LCMV) proteins required to rescue LCMV RNA analogs into LCMV-like particles. J Virol 76:6393–6397, 2002.
15. Cao W, Henry MD, Borrow P, et al: Identification of alpha-dystroglycan as a receptor for lymphocytic choriomeningitis virus and Lassa fever virus. Science 282(5396):2079–2081, 1998.
16. Bishop D: Arenaviridae and their replication. In Fields B, Knipe D, Howley P, et al. (eds): Virology, 2nd ed. New York, Raven Press, 1990, pp 1231–1243.
17. Meyer BJ, Southern PJ: Concurrent sequence analysis of 5' and 3' RNA termini by intramolecular circularization reveals 5' nontemplated bases and 3' terminal heterogeneity for lymphocytic choriomeningitis virus mRNAs. J Virol 67:2621–2627, 1993.
18. Garcin D, Kolakofsky D: Tacaribe arenavirus RNA synthesis in vitro is primer dependent and suggests an unusual model for the initiation of genome replication. J Virol 66:1370–1376, 1992.
19. Garcin D, Kolakofsky D: A novel mechanism for the initiation of Tacaribe arenavirus genome replication. J Virol 64:6196–6203, 1990.
20. Salvato MS, Shimomaye EM: The completed sequence of lymphocytic choriomeningitis virus reveals a unique RNA structure and a gene for a zinc finger protein. Virology 173:1–10, 1989.
21. Borden KL, Campbell Dwyer EJ, Salvato MS: An arenavirus RING (zinc-binding) protein binds the oncoprotein promyelocyte leukemia protein (PML) and relocates PML nuclear bodies to the cytoplasm. J Virol 72:758–766, 1998.
22. Garcin D, Rochat S, Kolakofsky D: The Tacaribe arenavirus small zinc finger protein is required for both mRNA synthesis and genome replication. J Virol 67:807–812, 1993.
23. Perez M, de la Torre JC: Characterization of the genomic promoter of the prototypic arenavirus lymphocytic choriomeningitis virus. J Virol 77:1184–1194, 2003.
24. Eichler R, Strecker T, Kolesnikova L, et al: Characterization of the Lassa virus matrix protein Z: Electron microscopic study of virus-like particles and interaction with the nucleoprotein (NP). Virus Res 100:249–255, 2004.
25. Dalton AJ, Rowe WP, Smith GH, et al: Morphological and cytochemical studies on lymphocytic choriomeningitis virus. J Virol 2:1465–1478, 1968.
26. Wright KE, Salvato MS, Buchmeier MJ: Neutralizing epitopes of lymphocytic choriomeningitis virus are conformational and require both glycosylation and disulfide bonds for expression. Virology 171:417–426, 1989.
27. Wright KE, Spiro RC, Burns JW, et al: Post-translational processing of the glycoproteins of lymphocytic choriomeningitis virus. Virology 177:175–183, 1990.
28. Burns JW, Buchmeier MJ: Protein-protein interactions in lymphocytic choriomeningitis virus. Virology 183:620–629, 1991.
29. McKee KT, Jr., Mahlandt BG, Maiztegui JI, et al: Experimental Argentine hemorrhagic fever in rhesus macaques: Viral strain-dependent clinical response. J Infect Dis 152:218–221, 1985.
30. Kenyon RH, Green DE, Maiztegui JI, et al: Viral strain dependent differences in experimental Argentine hemorrhagic fever (Junin virus) infection of guinea pigs. Intervirology 29:133–143, 1988.
31. Peters CJ, Jahrling PB, Liu CT, et al: Experimental studies of arenaviral hemorrhagic fevers. Curr Top Microbiol Immunol 134:5–68, 1987.
32. Borden E, Nathanson N: Tacaribe virus infection of the mouse: An immunopathologic disease model. Lab Invest 30:465–473, 1974.
33. Coto C, Leon M: Susceptibilidad exacerbada del raton de la dias a la infeccion con arenavirus. Medicina (B Aires) 38:281–289, 1978.
34. Martinez PL, Coto C, Weissenbacher M: The Tacaribe complex: The close relationship between a pathogenic (Junin) and a nonpathogenic (Tacaribe) arenavirus. In Salvato M (ed): The Arenaviridae. New York, Plenum Press, 1993, pp 81–298.
35. Webb PA, Justines G, Johnson KM: Infection of wild and laboratory animals with Machupo and Latino viruses. Bull World Health Organ 52:493–499, 1975.
36. Rowe W: Studies on pathogenesis and immunity in lymphocytic choriomeningitis infection of the mouse. Naval Medical Research Institute NNMC 12:167–220, 1954.

37. Buchmeier MJ, Welsh RM, Dutko FJ, et al: The virology and immunobiology of lymphocytic choriomeningitis virus infection. [Review.] Adv Immunol 30:275–331, 1980.
38. Ahmed R, Salmi A, Butler LD, et al: Selection of genetic variants of lymphocytic choriomeningitis virus in spleens of persistently infected mice. Role in suppression of cytotoxic T lymphocyte response and viral persistence. J Exp Med 160:521–540, 1984.
39. Oldstone MB, Tishon A, Buchmeier MJ: Virus-induced immune complex disease: Genetic control of C1q binding complexes in the circulation of mice persistently infected with lymphocytic choriomeningitis virus. J Immunol 130:912–918, 1983.
40. Hotchin J: Transient virus infection: Spontaneous recovery mechanism of lymphocytic choriomeningitis virus-infected cells. Nat New Biol 241:270–272, 1973.
41. Welsh RM, Jr., Buchmeier MJ: Protein analysis of defective interfering lymphocytic choriomeningitis virus and persistently infected cells. Virology 96:503–515, 1979.
42. Oldstone MB, Buchmeier MJ: Restricted expression of viral glycoprotein in cells of persistently infected mice. Nature 300:360–362, 1982.
43. Francis SJ, Southern PJ: Molecular analysis of viral RNAs in mice persistently infected with lymphocytic choriomeningitis virus. J Virol 62:1251–1257, 1988.
44. Bruns M, Kratzberg T, Zeller W, et al: Mode of replication of lymphocytic choriomeningitis virus in persistently infected cultivated mouse L cells. Virology 177:615–624, 1990.
45. Stocker C, Martinez PL, Kratzberg T, et al: Characterization of a virus variant produced by L cells persistently infected with lymphocytic choriomeningitis virus. J Gen Virol 75:3431–3439, 1994.
46. Meyer BJ, Southern PJ: A novel type of defective viral genome suggests a unique strategy to establish and maintain persistent lymphocytic choriomeningitis virus infections. J Virol 71:6757–6764, 1997.
47. Oldstone MB, Rodriguez M, Daughaday WH, et al: Viral perturbation of endocrine function: Disordered cell function leads to disturbed homeostasis and disease. Nature 307:278–281, 1984.
48. Klavinskis LS, Oldstone MB: Lymphocytic choriomeningitis virus can persistently infect thyroid epithelial cells and perturb thyroid hormone production. J Gen Virol 68:1867–1873, 1987.
49. Welsh RM, Lampert PW, Oldstone MB: Prevention of virus-induced cerebellar diseases by defective-interfering lymphocytic choriomeningitis virus. J Infect Dis 136:391–399, 1997.
50. Johnson K, Wiebenga N, MacKenzie R, et al: Virus isolations from human cases of hemorrhagic fever in Bolivia. Proc Soc Exp Biol Med 118:113–118, 1965.
51. Rowe WP, Pugh WE, Webb PA, et al: Serological relationship of the Tacaribe complex of viruses to lymphocytic choriomeningitis virus. J Virol 5:289–292, 1970.
52. Peters CJ, Webb PA, Johnson KM: Measurement of antibodies to Machupo virus by the indirect fluorescent technique. Proc Soc Exp Biol Med 142:526–531, 1973.
53. Wulff H, Lange J, Webb P: Interrelationships among arenaviruses measured by indirect immunofluorescence. Intervirology 9:344–350, 1978.
54. Sanchez A, Pifat DY, Kenyon RH, et al: Junin virus monoclonal antibodies: Characterization and cross-reactivity with other arenaviruses. J Gen Virol 70:1125–1132, 1989.
55. Fulhorst CF, Bowen MD, Ksiazek TG, et al: Isolation and characterization of Whitewater Arroyo virus, a novel North American arenavirus. Virology 224:114–120, 1996.
56. Buchmeier MJ, Lewicki HA, Tomori O, et al: Monoclonal antibodies to lymphocytic choriomeningitis and pichinde viruses: Generation, characterization, and cross-reactivity with other arenaviruses. Virology 113:73–85, 1981.
57. Ruo SL, Mitchell SW, Kiley MP, et al: Antigenic relatedness between arenaviruses defined at the epitope level by monoclonal antibodies. J Gen Virol 72:549–555, 1991.
58. Wozniak A: Comparison of New World arenaviruses, including those causing hemorrhagic fever, by serological, biological, and biochemical methods. University of North Carolina at Chapel Hill, 1988.
59. Allison L, Salter M, Buchmeier M, et al: Neutralization of arenaviruses: Reaction of Tacaribe virus and variants with monoclonal antibodies. In Compans R, Bishop D (eds): Segmented Negative Strand Viruses. Orlando, FL, Academic Press, 1984, pp 209–216.
60. Gonzalez JP, McCormick JB, Saluzzo JF, et al: An arenavirus isolated from wild-caught rodents (*Pramys* species) in the Central African Republic. Intervirology 19:105–112, 1983.
61. Swanepoel R, Leman PA, Shepherd AJ, et al: Identification of Ippy as a Lassa-fever-related virus. Lancet 1:639, 1985.
62. Bowen MD, Peters CJ, Nichol ST: The phylogeny of New World (Tacaribe complex) arenaviruses. Virology 219:285–290, 1996.
63. Bowen MD, Peters CJ, Nichol ST: Phylogenetic analysis of the Arenaviridae: Patterns of virus evolution and evidence for cospeciation between arenaviruses and their rodent hosts. Mol Phylogenet Evol 8:301–316, 1997.
64. Childs J, Peters C: Ecology and epidemiology of arenaviruses and their hosts. In Salvato M (ed): The Arenaviridae. New York, Plenum Press, 1993, pp 331–373.
65. Sabattini M, Gonzales de Rios L, Diaz G, et al: Infeccion natural y experimental de roedores con virus Junin. Medicina (B Aires) 37:149–161, 1977.
66. Sabattini M, Contigiani M: Ecological and biological factors influencing the maintenance of arenaviruses in nature, with special reference to the agent of Argentinean haemorrhagic fever. International Symposium on Tropical Arboviruses and Haemorrhagic Fevers, Belem, Brazil, April 14–18, 1980. Rio de Janeiro, Academia Brasileria de Ciencias, 1982, pp 251–262.
67. Traub E: Epidemiology of lymphocytic choriomeningitis in a mouse stock observed for four years. J Exp Med 69:801–817, 1939.
68. Mills JN, Ellis BA, Childs JE, et al: Prevalence of infection with Junin virus in rodent populations in the epidemic area of Argentine hemorrhagic fever. Am J Trop Med Hyg 51:554–562, 1994.
69. Lehmann-Grube F: Lymphocytic Choriomeningitis Virus. Virology Monographs. New York, Springer-Verlag, 1971.
70. Traub E: The epidemiology of lymphocytic choriomeningitis in white mice. J Exp Med 64:183–200, 1936.
71. Murphy F, Walker D: Arenaviruses: Persistent infection and viral survival in reservoir hosts. In Kurstak E, Maramorosch K (eds): Virus and Environment. New York, Academic Press, 1978, pp 155–180.
72. Mims CA: Effect on the fetus of maternal infection with lymphocytic choriomeningitis (LCM) virus. J Infect Dis 120:582–597, 1969.
73. Demby AH, Inapogui A, Kargbo K, et al: Lassa fever in Guinea: II. Distribution and prevalence of Lassa virus infection in small mammals. Vector Borne Zoonotic Dis 1:283–297, 2001.
74. Danes L, Benda R, Fuchsova M: Experimental inhalation infection with the lymphocytic choriomeningitis virus (WE strain) of the monkeys of the *Macacus cynomolgus* and *Macacus rhesus* species. Bratisl Lek Listy 43:21–34, 1963.
75. Stephenson EH, Larson EW, Dominik JW: Effect of environmental factors on aerosol-induced Lassa virus infection. J Med Virol 14:295–303, 1984.
76. Kenyon RH, McKee KT, Jr., Zack PM, et al: Aerosol infection of rhesus macaques with Junin virus. Intervirology 33:23–31, 1992.
77. Hinman AR, Fraser DW, Douglas RG, et al: Outbreak of lymphocytic choriomeningitis virus infections in medical center personnel. Am J Epidemiol 101:103–110, 1975.
78. Biggar R, Woodall J, Walter P, et al: Lymphocytic choriomeningitis outbreak associated with pet hamsters: Fifty-seven cases from New York State. JAMA 232:494–500, 1975.
79. Baum SG, Lewis AM, Jr., Rowe WP, et al: Epidemic nonmeningitic lymphocytic-choriomeningitis-virus infection. An outbreak in a population of laboratory personnel. N Engl J Med 274:934–936, 1996.
80. Rai SK, Micales BK, Wu MS, et al: Timed appearance of lymphocytic choriomeningitis virus after gastric inoculation of mice. Am J Pathol 151:633–639, 1997.
81. Skinner HH, Knight EH: Epidermal tissue as a primary site of replication of lymphocytic choriomeningitis virus in small experimental hosts. J Hyg 82:21–30, 1979.
82. Johnson K, Halstead S, Cohen S: Hemorrhagic fevers of South-east Asia and South America: A comparative appraisal. Prog Med Virol 9:105–158, 1967.
83. de Manzione Nuris, Salas R, Paredes H, et al: Venezuelan hemorrhagic fever: Clinical and epidemiologic studies of 165 cases. Clin Infect Dis 26:308–313, 1998.
84. Redford K, Eisenberg J: Mammals of the Neotropics: The Southern Cone. Chicago, Chicago Press, 1992.
85. Maiztegui J, Feuillade M, Briggiler A: Progressive extension of the endemic area and changing incidence of Argentine hemorrhagic fever. Med Microbiol Immunol 175:149–152, 1986.
86. Enria DA, Barrera Oro JG: Junin virus vaccines. [Review.] Curr Top Microbiol Immunol 263:239–261, 2002.

87. Garcia J, Calderron G, Sabattini M, et al: Infeccion por virus Junin de *Calomys musculinus* en areas con diferente situacion epidemiologica para la fiebre hemorrhagica Argentina. Medicina (B Aires) 56:624, 1996.
88. Musser G, Carleton M: Family Muridae. In Wilson E, Reeder D (eds): Mammal Species of the World, A Taxonomic and Geographic Reference. Washington, DC, Smithsonian Institution, 1993, pp 501–755.
89. Salazar-Bravo J, Dragoo JW, Bowen MD, et al: Natural nidality in Bolivian hemorrhagic fever and the systematics of the reservoir species. Infect Genet Evol 1:191–199, 2002.
90. Weaver SC, Salas RA, de Manzione N, et al: Guanarito virus (Arenaviridae) isolates from endemic and outlying localities in Venezuela: Sequence comparisons among and within strains isolated from Venezuelan hemorrhagic fever patients and rodents. Virology 266:189–195, 2000.
91. Gunter S, Emmerich P, Laue T, et al: Imported Lassa fever in Germany: Molecular characterization of a new Lassa virus strain. Emerg Infect Dis 6:466–476, 2000.
92. Saluzzo JF, Adam F, McCormick JB, et al: Lassa fever virus in Senegal. J Infect Dis 157:605, 1998.
93. van der Heide RM: [A patient with Lassa fever from the Upper Volta, diagnosed in the Netherlands]. [Dutch.] Nederl Tijdschr Geneeskunde 126:566–569, 1982.
94. Centers for Disease Control and Prevention: Imported Lassa fever—New Jersey, 2004. MMWR 53:894–897.
95. Monath TP, Newhouse VF, Kemp GE, et al: Lassa virus isolation from *Mastomys natalensis* rodents during an epidemic in Sierra Leone. Science 185:263–265, 1974.
96. McCormick JB, Webb PA, Krebs JW, et al: A prospective study of the epidemiology and ecology of Lassa fever. J Infect Dis 155:437–444, 1987.
97. Robbins C, Van Der Straeten E: Comments on the systematics of *Mastomys* Thomas 1915 with the description of a new West African species. Senckenbergiana Biol 69:1–14, 1989.
98. Robbins CB, Krebs JW, Jr., Johnson KM: *Mastomys* (rodentia: muridae) species distinguished by hemoglobin pattern differences. Am J Trop Med Hyg 32:624–630, 1983.
99. Happold D: The Mammals of Nigeria. New York, Clarendon Press, 1987, p 402.
100. Smith AL, Singleton GR, Hansen GM, et al: A serologic survey for viruses and *Mycoplasma pulmonis* among wild house mice (*Mus domesticus*) in southeastern Australia. J Wildl Dis 29:219–229, 1993.
101. Morita C, Matsuura Y, Fujii H, et al: Isolation of lymphocytic choriomeningitis virus from wild house mice (*Mus musculus*) in Osaka Port, Japan. J Vet Med Sci 53:889–892, 1991.
102. Ackermann R: Epidemiologic aspects of lymphocytic choriomeningitis in man. In Lehmann-Grube F (ed): Lymphocytic Choriomeningitis Virus and Other Arenaviruses. Berlin, Springer-Verlag, 1973, pp 233–237.
103. Ambrosio AM, Feuillade MR, Gamboa GS, et al: Prevalence of lymphocytic choriomeningitis virus infection in a human population of Argentina. Am J Trop Med Hyg 50:381–386, 1994.
104. Boursot P, Auffray J-C, Britton-Davidian J, et al: The evolution of house mice. Annu Rev Ecol Syst 24:119–152, 1993.
105. Mills JN, Ellis BA, McKee KT, Jr., et al: Junin virus activity in rodents from endemic and nonendemic loci in central Argentina. Am J Trop Med Hyg 44:589–597, 1991.
106. Ellis B, Mills J, Childs J, et al: Structure and floristics of habitats associated with five rodent species in an agroecosystem in central Argentina. J Zool 243:437–460, 1997.
107. Mills JN, Ellis BA, McKee KT, Jr., et al: A longitudinal study of Junin virus activity in the rodent reservoir of Argentine hemorrhagic fever. Am J Trop Med Hyg 47:749–763, 1992.
108. Briggiler A, Enria D, Feuillade M, et al: Contagio interhumano e infeccion inaparente por virus Junin on matrimonios del area endemica de fiebre hemorragica argentina. Medicina (B Aires) 47:565, 1987.
109. Kuns ML: Epidemiology of Machupo virus infection. II. Ecological and control studies of hemorrhagic fever. Am J Trop Med Hyg 14:813–816, 1965.
110. Peters C, Kuehne R, Mercado R, et al: Hemorrhagic fever in Cochabama, Bolivia. Am J Epidemiol 99:425–433, 1974.
111. Kilgore PE, Peters CJ, Mills JN, et al: Prospects for the control of Bolivian hemorrhagic fever. Emerg Infect Dis 1:97–100, 1995.
112. Douglas R, Wiebenga N, Couch R: Bolivian hemorrhagic fever probably transmitted by personal contact. Am J Epidemiol 82:85–91, 1965.
113. Salas R, de Manzione N, Tesh RB, et al: Venezuelan haemorrhagic fever. Lancet 338:1033–1036, 1991.
114. Fulhorst CF, Bowen MD, Salas RA, et al: Natural rodent host associations of Guanarito and pirital viruses (family Arenaviridae) in central Venezuela. Am J Trop Med Hyg 61:325–330, 1999.
115. Gregg M: Recent outbreaks of lymphocytic choriomeningitis in the United States of America. Bull World Health Organ 52:549–554, 1975.
116. Brouqui P, Rousseau MC, Saron MF, et al: Meningitis due to lymphocytic choriomeningitis virus: Four cases in France. Clin Infect Dis 20:1082–1083, 1995.
117. Childs JE, Glass GE, Ksiazek TG, et al: Human-rodent contact and infection with lymphocytic choriomeningitis and Seoul viruses in an inner-city population. Am J Trop Med Hyg 44:117–121, 1991.
118. Gardner M, Henderson B, Estes J, et al: Unusually high incidence of spontaneous lymphomas in wild house mice. J Natl Cancer Inst 50:1571–1579, 1973.
119. Blumenthal W, Ackermann R, Scheid W: [Distribution of the lymphocytic choriomeningitis virus in an endemic area]. [German] Deutsche Med Wochenschr 93:944–948, 1968.
120. Park JY, Peters CJ, Rollin PE, et al: Age distribution of lymphocytic choriomeningitis virus serum antibody in Birmingham, Alabama: Evidence of a decreased risk of infection. Am J Trop Med Hyg 57:37–41, 1997.
121. Armstrong C: Studies on choriomeningitis and poliomyelitis. Bull NY Acad Med 17:295–318, 1941.
122. Adair C, Gauld R, Smadel J: Aseptic meningitis, a disease of diverse etiology: Clinical and etiologic studies on 854 cases. Ann Intern Med 39:675–704, 1953.
123. Meyer H, Johnson R, Crawford E, et al: Central nervous system syndromes of "viral" etiology. A study of 713 cases. Am J Med 29:334–347, 1960.
124. Webb PA, McCormick JB, King IJ, et al: Lassa fever in children in Sierra Leone, West Africa. Trans R Soc Trop Med Hyg 80:577–582, 1986.
125. Bausch DG, Demby AH, Coulibaly M, et al: Lassa fever in Guinea: I. Epidemiology of human disease and clinical observations. Vector Borne Zoonotic Dis 1:269–281, 2001.
126. Keenlyside RA, McCormick JB, Webb PA, et al: Case-control study of *Mastomys natalensis* and humans in Lassa virus–infected households in Sierra Leone. Am J Trop Med Hyg 32:829–837, 1983.
127. Lassa fever outbreak in Plateau State 1992–1993. Nigeria Bull Epidemiol 3:2–9, 1993.
128. Helmick CG, Webb PA, Scribner CL, et al: No evidence for increased risk of Lassa fever infection in hospital staff. Lancet 2:1202–1205, 1986.
129. Carey DE, Kemp GE, White HA, et al: Lassa fever. Epidemiological aspects of the 1970 epidemic, Jos, Nigeria. Trans R Soc Trop Med Hyg 66:402–408, 1972.
130. Fisher-Hoch SP, Tomori O, Nasidi A, et al: Review of cases of nosocomial Lassa fever in Nigeria: The high price of poor medical practice. BMJ 311:857–859, 1995.
131. Vitullo AD, Hodara VL, Merani MS: Effect of persistent infection with Junin virus on growth and reproduction of its natural reservoir, *Calomys musculinus*. Am J Trop Med Hyg 37:663–669, 1987.
132. Vitullo AD, Merani MS: Vertical transmission of Junin virus in experimentally infected adult *Calomys musculinus*. Intervirology 31:339–344, 1990.
133. Johnson K: Arenaviruses. In Fields B, Knipe K (eds): Virology. New York, Raven Press, 1985, pp 1033–1053.
134. Fulhorst CF, Ksiazek TG, Peters CJ, et al: Experimental infection of the cane mouse *Zygodontomys brevicauda* (family Muridae) with Guanarito virus (Arenaviridae), the etiologic agent of Venezuelan hemorrhagic fever. J Infect Dis 180:966–969, 1999.
135. Experimental infection of the cane mouse *Zygodontomys brevicauda* with Guanarito virus (Arenaviridae). Presented at the 43rd Annual Meeting of the Amerian Society of Tropical Medicine and Hygiene, Cincinnati, OH, November 13, 1994.
136. Mims CA, Tosolini FA: Pathogenesis of lesions in lymphoid tissue of mice infected with lymphocytic choriomeningitis (LCM) virus. Br J Exp Pathol 50:584–592, 1969.
137. Peters C, Zaki S, Rollin P: Viral hemorrhagic fevers. In Mandell G (ed): Atlas of Infectious Diseases, External Manifestations of Systemic Infections. Philadelphia, Current Medicine, 1997, pp 10.1–10.26.

138. Maiztegui JI, Fernandez NJ, de Damilano AJ: Efficacy of immune plasma in treatment of Argentine haemorrhagic fever and association between treatment and a late neurological syndrome. Lancet 2:1216–1217, 1979.
139. Enria D, Damilano Ad, Briggiler A, et al: Sindrome neurologico tardio en enfermos de fiebre hemorragica Argentina tratados con plasma immune. Medicina (B Aires) 45:615–620, 1985.
140. Briggiler A, Lewis S, Enria D, et al: Argentine hemorrhagic fever in pregnant women. Medicina (B Aires) 50:443, 1990.
141. Stinebaugh B, Schloeder F, Johnson K, et al: Bolivian hemorrhagic fever. A report of four cases. Am J Med 40:217–230, 1966.
142. Lisieux T, Coimbra M, Nassar ES, Burattini MN, et al: New arenavirus isolated in Brazil. Lancet 343:391-392, 1994.
143. Vasconcelos PF, Travassos da Rosa AP, Rodrigues SG, et al: [Laboratory-acquired human infection with SP H 114202 virus (Arenavirus: Arenaviridae family): Clinical and laboratory aspects]. [Portuguese.] Revista Instit Med Trop Sao Paulo 35:521–525, 1993.
144. Barry M, Russi M, Armstrong L, et al: Brief report: Treatment of a laboratory-acquired Sabia virus infection [see comment]. N Engl J Med 333:294–296, 1995.
145. Frame JD, Baldwin JM, Jr., Gocke DJ, et al: Lassa fever, a new virus disease of man from West Africa. I. Clinical description and pathological findings. Am J Trop Med Hyg 19:670–676, 1970.
145. Mertens P, Patton R, Baum J, et al: Clinical presentation of Lassa fever cases during the hospital epidemic at Zorzor, Liberia, March–April 1972. Am J Trop Med Hyg 22:780–784, 1973.
147. Monath TP, Maher M, Casals J, et al: Lassa fever in the Eastern Province of Sierra Leone, 1970-1972. II. Clinical observations and virological studies on selected hospital cases. Am J Trop Med Hyg 23:1140–1149, 1974.
148. Monson MH, Frame JD, Jahrling PB, et al: Endemic Lassa fever in Liberia. I. Clinical and epidemiological aspects at Curran Lutheran Hospital, Zorzor, Liberia. Trans R Soc Trop Med Hyg 78:549–553, 1984.
149. McCormick JB, King IJ, Webb PA, et al: A case-control study of the clinical diagnosis and course of Lassa fever. J Infect Dis 155:445–455, 1987.
150. Frame JD: Clinical features of Lassa fever in Liberia. Rev Infect Dis 11(Suppl 4):S783–S789, 1989.
151. Solbrig M, McCormick J: Lassa fever: Central nervous system manifestations. J Trop Geogr Neurol 1:23–30, 1991.
152. Solbrig M: Lassa virus and central nervous system diseases. In Salvato M (ed): The Arenaviridae. New York, Plenum Press, 1993, pp 325–330.
153. Price ME, Fisher-Hoch SP, Craven RB, et al: A prospective study of maternal and fetal outcome in acute Lassa fever infection during pregnancy. BMJ 297:584–587, 1988.
154. Monson MH, Cole AK, Frame JD, et al: Pediatric Lassa fever: A review of 33 Liberian cases. Am J Trop Med Hyg 36:408–415, 1987.
155. Monath TP: Lassa fever: Review of epidemiology and epizootiology. [Review.] Bull World Health Organ 52:577–592, 1975.
156. Fisher-Hoch S, McCormick JB, Sasso D, et al: Hematologic dysfunction in Lassa fever. J Med Virol 26:127-135, 1998.
157. Johnson KM, McCormick JB, Webb PA, Smith ES, et al: Clinical virology of Lassa fever in hospitalized patients. J Infect Dis 155:456–464, 1987.
158. Cummins D, Bennett D, Fisher-Hoch SP, et al: Electrocardiographic abnormalities in patients with Lassa fever. J Trop Med Hyg 92:350–355, 1989.
159. Ketai L, Alrahji AA, Hart B, et al: Radiologic manifestations of potential bioterrorist agents of infection. Am J Roentgenol 180:565–575, 2003.
160. Cummins D, McCormick JB, Bennett D, et al: Acute sensorineural deafness in Lassa fever [see comment]. JAMA 264:2093–2096, 1990.
161. Vanzee BE, Douglas RG, Betts RF, et al: Lymphocytic choriomeningitis in university hospital personnel. Clinical features. Am J Med 58:803–809, 1975.
162. Farmer T, Janeway C: Infections with the virus of lymphocytic choriomeningitis. Medicine (Baltimore) 21:1–64, 1942.
163. Lewis JM, Utz JP: Orchitis, parotitis and meningoencephalitis due to lymphocytic-choriomeningitis virus. N Engl J Med 265:776–780, 1961.
164. Peters C: Arenaviruses. In Belshe R (ed): Textbook of Human Virology. St. Louis, Mosby–Year Book, 1991, pp 541–570.
165. Peters C: Arenavirus diseases. In Porterfield J (ed): Kass Handbook of Infectious Diseases. Exotic Viral Infections. New York, Chapman and Hall, 1995, pp 227–246.
166. Cole GA, Nathanson N, Prendergast RA: Requirement for theta-bearing cells in lymphocytic choriomeningitis virus-induced central nervous system disease. Nature 238:335–337, 1972.
167. Horton J, Hotchin JE, Olson KB, et al: The effects of MP virus infection in lymphoma. Cancer Res 31:1066–1068, 1971.
168. Warkel RL, Rinaldi CF, Bancroft WH, et al: Fatal acute meningoencephalitis due to lymphocytic choriomeningitis virus. Neurology 23:198–203, 1973.
169. Hirsch E: Sensorineural deafness and labyrinth damage due to lymphocytic choriomeningitis. Report of a case. Arch Otolaryngol 102:499–500, 1976.
170. Hetil O: Lymphocytic choriomeningitis causing unilateral deafness. Sci J Organ Health Workers 30:761–812, 1989.
171. Smadel JE, Green RH, Paltauf RF, et al: Lymphocytic choriomeningitis: Two human fatalities following an unusual febrile illness. Proc Soc Exp Biol Med 49:683–686, 1942.
172. Ackermann R: Lymphozytare choriomeningitis: Diaplazentare ubertragung. Munch Med Wochenschr 118:689–690, 1976.
173. Komrower G, Williams B, Stones P: Lymphocytic choriomeningitis in the newborn. Lancet 1:697–698, 1955.
174. Sheinbergas MM: Hydrocephalus due to prenatal infection with the lymphocytic choriomeningitis virus. Infection 4:185–191, 1976.
175. Sheinbergas MM, Ptashekas RS, Pikelite RL, et al: [Clinical and pathomorphologic findings in hydrocephalus caused by prenatal infection with lymphocytic choriomeningitis virus]. [Russian.] Zhurn Nevropatol Psikhiatr Imeni S-S-Korsakova 77:1004–1007, 1977.
176. Chastel C, Bosshard S, Le Goff F, et al: Transplacental infection by lymphocytic choriomeningitis virus. Results of a retrospective serological study in France. [French.] Nouv Presse Med 7:1089–1092, 1978.
177. Barton LL, Budd SC, Morfitt WS, et al: Congenital lymphocytic choriomeningitis virus infection in twins. Pediatr Infect Dis J 12:942–946, 1993.
178. Larsen PD, Chartrand SA, Tomashek KM, et al: Hydrocephalus complicating lymphocytic choriomeningitis virus infection. Pediatr Infect Dis J 12:528–531, 1993.
179. Barton LL, Peters CJ, Ksiazek TG: Lymphocytic choriomeningitis virus: An unrecognized teratogenic pathogen. Emerg Infect Dis 1:152–153, 1995.
180. Barton LL, Mets MB, Beauchamp CL: Lymphocytic choriomeningitis virus: Emerging fetal teratogen. Am J Obstet Gynecol 187:1715–1716, 2002.
181. Walker DH, Johnson KM, Lange JV, et al: Experimental infection of rhesus monkeys with Lassa virus and a closely related arenavirus, Mozambique virus. J Infect Dis 146:360–368, 1982.
182. Walker DH, Murphy FA: Pathology and pathogenesis of arenavirus infections. [Review.] Curr Top Microbiol Immunol 33:89–113, 1987.
183. Walker DH, McCormick JB, Johnson KM, et al: Pathologic and virologic study of fatal Lassa fever in man. Am J Pathol 107:349–356, 1982.
184. Shieh WJ, Greer PW, Ruo SL: Lassa fever: An immunopathologic study with pathogenetic and diagnostic implications. Lab Invest 76:141A, 1997.
185. Montali RJ, Connolly BM, Armstrong DL, et al: Pathology and immunohistochemistry of callitrichid hepatitis, an emerging disease of captive New World primates caused by lymphocytic choriomeningitis virus. Am J Pathol 147:1441–1449, 1995.
186. McLeod CG, Jr., Stookey JL, White JD, et al: Pathology of Bolivian hemorrhagic fever in the African green monkey. Am J Trop Med Hyg 27:822–826, 1978.
187. Green DE, Mahlandt BG, McKee KT, Jr: Experimental Argentine hemorrhagic fever in rhesus macaques: Virus-specific variations in pathology. J Med Virol 22:113–133, 1987.
188. Hall WC, Geisbert TW, Huggins JW, et al: Experimental infection of guinea pigs with Venezuelan hemorrhagic fever virus (Guanarito): A model of human disease. Am J Trop Med Hyg 55:81–88, 1966.
189. Elsner B, Schwarz E, Mando O, et al: Pathology of 12 fatal cases of Argentine hemorrhagic fever. Am J Trop Med Hyg 22:229–236, 1973.
190. Child PL, MacKenzie RB, Valverde LR, et al: Bolivian hemorrhagic fever. A pathologic description. Arch Pathol 83:434–445, 1967.

191. Maiztegui JI, Laguens RP, Cossio PM, et al: Ultrastructural and immunohistochemical studies in five cases of Argentine hemorrhagic fever. J Infect Dis 132:35–53, 1975.
192. Zaki SR, Peters CJ: Viral Hemorrhagic Fevers. Norwalk, CT, Appleton & Lange, 1997.
193. Gonzalez PH, Cossio PM, Arana R, et al: Lymphatic tissue in Argentine hemorrhagic fever. Pathologic features. Arch Pathol Lab Med 104:250–254, 1980.
194. Cossio P, Laguens R, Arana R, et al: Ultrastructural and immunohistochemical study of the human kidney in Argentine haemorrhagic fever. Virchows Archiv A Pathol Anat Histol 368:1–9, 1975.
195. Ponzinibbio C, Gonzalez PH, Maiztegui J, et al: [Morphological study of human bone marrow in Argentinian hemorrhagic fever]. [Spanish.] Medicina 39:441–446, 1979.
196. de Bracco MM, Rimoldi MT, Cossio PM, et al: Argentine hemorrhagic fever. Alterations of the complement system and anti-Junin-virus humoral response. N Engl J Med 299:216–221, 1978.
197. Heller MV, Marta RF, Sturk A, et al: Early markers of blood coagulation and fibrinolysis activation in Argentine hemorrhagic fever. Thromb Haemost 73:368–373, 1995.
198. Kenyon RH, Green DE, Peters CJ: Effect of immunosuppression on experimental Argentine hemorrhagic fever in guinea pigs. J Virol 53:75–80, 1985.
199. Genovesi EV, Peters CJ: Immunosuppression-induced susceptibility of inbred hamsters (*Mesocricetus auratus*) to lethal-disease by lymphocytic choriomeningitis virus infection. Arch Virol 97:61–76, 1987.
200. Cummins D, Fisher-Hoch SP, Walshe KJ, et al: A plasma inhibitor of platelet aggregation in patients with Lassa fever. Br J Haematol 72:543–548, 1989.
201. Andrews BS, Theofilopoulos AN, Peters CJ, et al: Replication of dengue and junin viruses in cultured rabbit and human endothelial cells. Infect Immun 20:776–781, 1978.
202. Vallejos DA, Ambrosio AM, Feuillade MR, et al: Lymphocyte subsets alteration in patients with Argentine hemorrhagic fever. J Med Virol 27:160–163, 1989.
203. Enria DA, Maiztegui JI: Antiviral treatment of Argentine hemorrhagic fever. Antiviral Res 23:23–31, 1994.
204. Kenyon RH, Condie RM, Jahrling PB, et al: Protection of guinea pigs against experimental Argentine hemorrhagic fever by purified human IgG: Importance of elimination of infected cells. Microb Pathogen 9:219–226, 1990.
205. Peters CJ, Kenyon RH, Barrera-Oro JG, et al: Assays of cell-mediated immunity in recipients of a live, attenuated Junin virus vaccine. 40th Annual Meeting of the American Society of Tropical Medicine and Hygiene, Boston, MA, December 1–5, 1991.
206. Maiztegui JI, McKee KT, Jr., Barrera Oro JG, et al: Protective efficacy of a live attenuated vaccine against Argentine hemorrhagic fever. AHF Study Group. J Infect Dis 177:277–283, 1998.
207. Levis SC, Saavedra MC, Ceccoli C, et al: Correlation between endogenous interferon and the clinical evolution of patients with Argentine hemorrhagic fever. J Interferon Res 5:383–389, 1985.
208. Heller MV, Saavedra MC, Falcoff R, et al: Increased tumor necrosis factor-alpha levels in Argentine hemorrhagic fever. J Infect Dis 166:1203–1204, 1992.
209. Saavedra M, Feuillade M, Levis S, et al: Antigenos de histocompatibilidad en la fiebre hemorrhagica Argentina. Medicina (B Aires) 45:342, 1985.
210. Mahanty S, Bausch DG, Thomas RL, et al: Low levels of interleukin-8 and interferon-inducible protein-10 in serum are associated with fatal infections in acute Lassa fever. J Infect Dis 183:1713–1721, 2001.
211. Jahrling PB, Frame JD, Rhoderick JB, et al: Endemic Lassa fever in Liberia. IV. Selection of optimally effective plasma for treatment by passive immunization. Trans R Soc Trop Med Hyg 79:380–384, 1985.
212. Hunt J, Orr H: HLA and maternal-fetal recognition. FASEB J 6: 2344–2348, 1992.
213. Joly E, Mucke L, Oldstone MB: Viral persistence in neurons explained by lack of major histocompatibility class I expression. Science 253:1283–1285, 1991.
214. Peters C: Pathogenesis of viral hemorrhagic fevers. In Nathanson N, Ahmed R, Gonzalez-Scarano F, et al (eds): Viral Pathogenesis. Philadelphia, Lippincott-Raven, 1997, pp 779–799.
215. Aronson JF, Herzog NK, Jerrells TR: Tumor necrosis factor and the pathogenesis of Pichinde virus infection in guinea pigs. Am J Trop Med Hyg 52:262–269, 1995.
216. Fennewald SM, Aronson JF, Zhang L, et al: Alterations in NF-kappaB and RBP-Jkappa by arenavirus infection of macrophages in vitro and in vivo. J Virol 76:1154–1162, 2002.
217. Cummins D, Molinas FC, Lerer G, et al: A plasma inhibitor of platelet aggregation in patients with Argentine hemorrhagic fever. Am J Trop Med Hyg 42:470–475, 1990.
218. Liao BS, Byl FM, Adour KK: Audiometric comparison of Lassa fever hearing loss and idiopathic sudden hearing loss: Evidence for viral cause [see comment]. Otolaryngol Head Neck Surg 106:226–229, 1992.
219. Peters CJ: Arenaviruses. In Richman DD, Whitley RJ, Haydon FG (eds): Clinical Virology. Washington, DC, ASM Press, 2002, pp 949–969.
220. Ambrosio AM, Enria DA, Maiztegui JI: Junin virus isolation from lympho-mononuclear cells of patients with Argentine hemorrhagic fever. Intervirology 25:97–102, 1986.
221. Niklasson BS, Jahrling PB, Peters CJ: Detection of Lassa virus antigens and Lassa virus-specific immunoglobulins G and M by enzyme-linked immunosorbent assay. J Clin Microbiol 20:239–244, 1984.
222. Bausch DG, Rollin PE, Demby AH, et al: Diagnosis and clinical virology of Lassa fever as evaluated by enzyme-linked immunosorbent assay, indirect fluorescent-antibody test, and virus isolation. J Clin Microbiol 38:2670–2677, 2000.
223. Demby AH, Chamberlain J, Brown DW, et al: Early diagnosis of Lassa fever by reverse transcription–PCR. J Clin Microbiol 32:2898–2903, 1994.
224. Trappier SG, Conaty AL, Farrar BB, et al: Evaluation of the polymerase chain reaction for diagnosis of Lassa virus infection. Am J Trop Med Hyg 49:214–221, 1993.
225. de Souza M, Smith AL: Comparison of isolation in cell culture with conventional and modified mouse antibody production tests for detection of murine viruses. J Clin Microbiol 27:185–187, 1989.
226. Deibel R, Schryver GD: Viral antibody in the cerebrospinal fluid of patients with acute central nervous system infections. J Clin Microbiol 3:397–401, 1976.
227. Lehmann-Grube F, Kallay M, Ibscher B, et al: Serologic diagnosis of human infections with lymphocytic choriomeningitis virus: Comparative evaluation of seven methods. J Med Virol 4:125–136, 1979.
228. Park JY, Peters CJ, Rollin PE, et al: Development of a reverse transcription–polymerase chain reaction assay for diagnosis of lymphocytic choriomeningitis virus infection and its use in a prospective surveillance study. J Med Virol 51:107–114, 1997.
229. Kilgore PE, Ksiazek TG, Rollin PE, et al: Treatment of Bolivian hemorrhagic fever with intravenous ribavirin. Clin Infect Dis 24:718–722, 1997.
230. Jahrling PB, Hesse RA, Eddy GA, et al: Lassa virus infection of rhesus monkeys: Pathogenesis and treatment with ribavirin. J Infect Dis 141:580–589, 1980.
231. McCormick JB, Walker DH, King IJ, et al: Lassa virus hepatitis: A study of fatal Lassa fever in humans. Am J Trop Med Hyg 35:401–407, 1986.
232. Fisher-Hoch SP, Gborie S, Parker L, et al: Unexpected adverse reactions during a clinical trial in rural West Africa. Antiviral Res 19:139–147, 1992.
233. Armstrong LR, Dembry LM, Rainey PM, et al: Management of a Sabia virus–infected patients in a US hospital. Infect Control Hosp Epidemiol 20:176–182, 1999.
234. Peters CJ, Jahrling PB, Khan AS: Patients infected with high-hazard viruses: Scientific basis for infection control. [Review.] Arch Virol Suppl 11:141–168, 1996.
235. Centers for Disease Control and Prevention: Viral hemorrhagic fever: Initial management of suspected and confirmed cases. MMWR 32(Suppl 2):27S–38S, 1983.
236. Centers for Disease Control and Prevention: Update: Management of patients with suspected viral hemorrhagic fever—United States. JAMA 274:374–375, 1995.
237. Peters CJ; Centers for Disease Control and Prevention and World Health Organization: Infection Control for Viral Hemorrhagic Fevers in the African Health Care Setting. Atlanta, GA, CDC, 1998. Accessed at http://www.cdc.gov/ncidod/dvrd/spb/mnpages/vhfmanual.htm.
238. Mercado R: Rodent control programmes in areas affected by Bolivian haemorrhagic fever. Bull World Health Organ 52:691–696, 1975.
239. Smith AL, Paturzo FX, Gardner EP, et al: Two epizootics of lymphocytic choriomeningitis virus occurring in laboratory mice despite intensive monitoring programs. Can J Comp Med 48:335–337, 1984.

240. Hotchin J: The contamination of laboratory animals with lymphocytic choriomeningitis virus. Am J Pathol 64:747–769, 1971.
241. Auperin D: Construction and evaluation of recombinant virus vaccines for Lassa fever. In Salvato M (ed): The Arenaviridae. New York, Plenum Press, 1993, pp 259–280.
242. Clegg J, Sanchez A: Vaccines against arenaviruses and filoviruses. In Levine M, Woodrow G, Kaper J, et al. (eds): New Generation Vaccines, 2nd ed. New York, Marcel Dekker, 1997, pp 749–765.
243. Oldstone MB: Arenaviruses. I: The epidemiology molecular and cell biology of arenaviruses. Introduction. [Review.] Curr Top Microbiol Immunol 262:1–197, 2002.
244. Oldstone MB: Arenaviruses. II. The molecular pathogenesis of arenavirus infections. Introduction. [Review.] Curr Top Microbiol Immunol 263:1–268, 2002.

67

Bunyaviral Fevers: Rift Valley Fever and Crimean-Congo Hemorrhagic Fever

DOUGLAS M. WATTS
RAMON FLICK
C.J. PETERS
ROBERT E. SHOPE

AGENTS

Viruses of the family Bunyaviridae are classified into five genera: *Orthobunyavirus, Phlebovirus, Hantavirus, Nairovirus,* and *Tospovirus*. Member viruses of these genera contain negative sense, trisegmented, single-stranded RNA. The viruses replicate in the cytoplasm and mature in association with the Golgi apparatus. The virions are spherical, approximately 90 nm in diameter with a lipid envelope into which are inserted spike-like structures containing two surface glycoproteins responsible for attachment and induction of neutralizing antibody. Each RNA segment consists of one or more genes: the small (S) segment codes for the nucleocapsid protein; the middle-sized (M) segment for the glycoprotein precursor, which is posttranslationally cleaved into the two mature glycoproteins; and the large (L) segment for the polymerase. The S and M segments of some viruses encode additional nonstructural proteins (NS_S and NS_M, respectively).[1]

Bunyaviral fevers are commonly encountered in the tropics, but the cause is usually undiagnosed because laboratory diagnostic capabilities are lacking. The clinician by default may treat the patient for malaria or another commonly suspected febrile illness. The family Bunyaviridae contains at least 41 tropical viruses that cause fever and sometimes rash.[2] A few of these viruses also cause meningoencephalitis, hemorrhage, arthritis, or retinitis. Two important bunyavirus infections found in tropical Africa and elsewhere are associated with hemorrhage and are sometimes fatal; these are Rift Valley fever, caused by a *Phlebovirus*, and Crimean-Congo hemorrhagic fever, caused by a *Nairovirus*.

EPIDEMIOLOGY

Rift Valley Fever

Rift Valley fever (RVF) virus is a mosquito-borne agent serologically related to the sandfly fever viruses.[3] The virus infects domestic ruminants, primarily sheep, cattle, and goats, and on occasion causes explosive and devastating outbreaks among these animals and humans. RVF virus was first isolated in 1930 during an outbreak of hepatitis and abortion in sheep in the Rift Valley of Kenya.[4] The disease was for many years thought to be localized in the Rift Valley of Africa, where it regularly appears in sheep and cattle during periods of heavy rain, but the virus has now been demonstrated to be enzootic in most countries of sub-Saharan Africa. In 1977, RVF virus was transported out of the tropics north to Egypt, where it caused a "virgin soil" epidemic in an estimated 200,000 people, with 598 reported deaths in the Nile delta.[5] In 1987, an epidemic involving about 1200 persons in Mauritania was linked to the opening of the Diama Dam near the mouth of the Senegal River.[6] RVF was again detected in Mauritania in 1998, and in Egypt during 1993 and 1997, after an absence of 13 years.[7–9] In 2000, an outbreak of RVF occurred on the Red Sea Coast of Saudi Arabia and Yemen and represented the first documented cases outside of Africa and Madagascar.[10] Irrigation farming and accumulation of water in depressions that supported large numbers of mosquitoes were correlated with many of the human cases in the Arabian Peninsula. Continued surveillance is required to determine whether an enzootic cycle of RVF virus is established in Egypt and on the Arabian Peninsula.

Several species of *Culex* and *Aedes* mosquitoes have been implicated as vectors during epizootics and epidemics of RVF. The enzootic maintenance and transmission cycle is not fully understood; however, studies in Kenya showed that RVF virus was maintained over dry seasons in the eggs of flood-water *Aedes* mosquitoes.[11] The infected eggs remain dormant in the dambos (depressions) of East Africa. After heavy rains, the eggs hatch and are believed to give rise to a new batch of infected mosquitoes that initiate mosquito-livestock-mosquito cycles involving several different species as vectors. RVF transmission also results from direct and aerosol exposure to blood and amniotic fluids of infected sheep and cattle as an occupational disease in butchers, veterinarians, and farmers. Person-to-person transmission has not been reported.

Crimean-Congo Hemorrhagic Fever

Crimean-Congo hemorrhagic fever (CCHF) virus is a tick-borne agent that was first definitively recognized in the Crimea at the end of World War II when Soviet troops returned to assist in cultivation of tick-infested land left fallow during the war.[12,13] The agent was named Crimean hemorrhagic fever virus and was subsequently found to be indistinguishable from a virus isolated in 1956 from a febrile child in Stanleyville (now Kisangani), Democratic Republic of the Congo, leading to the current designation of CCHF virus.[14] Since the discovery of this disease, the virus or serologic evidence of infection has been found in tropical Africa and temperate Europe and Asia as far east as western China.[15,16]

CCHF virus is serologically related to two other nairoviruses—Dugbe and Nairobi sheep disease viruses—that cause febrile disease in humans.[17] CCHF virus distribution coincides with that of its primary vector, *Hyalomma* ticks. These ticks in the immature stages feed on rodents and ground birds, and in the adult stage on cattle and other large mammals.[15] The wild vertebrate and domestic animal

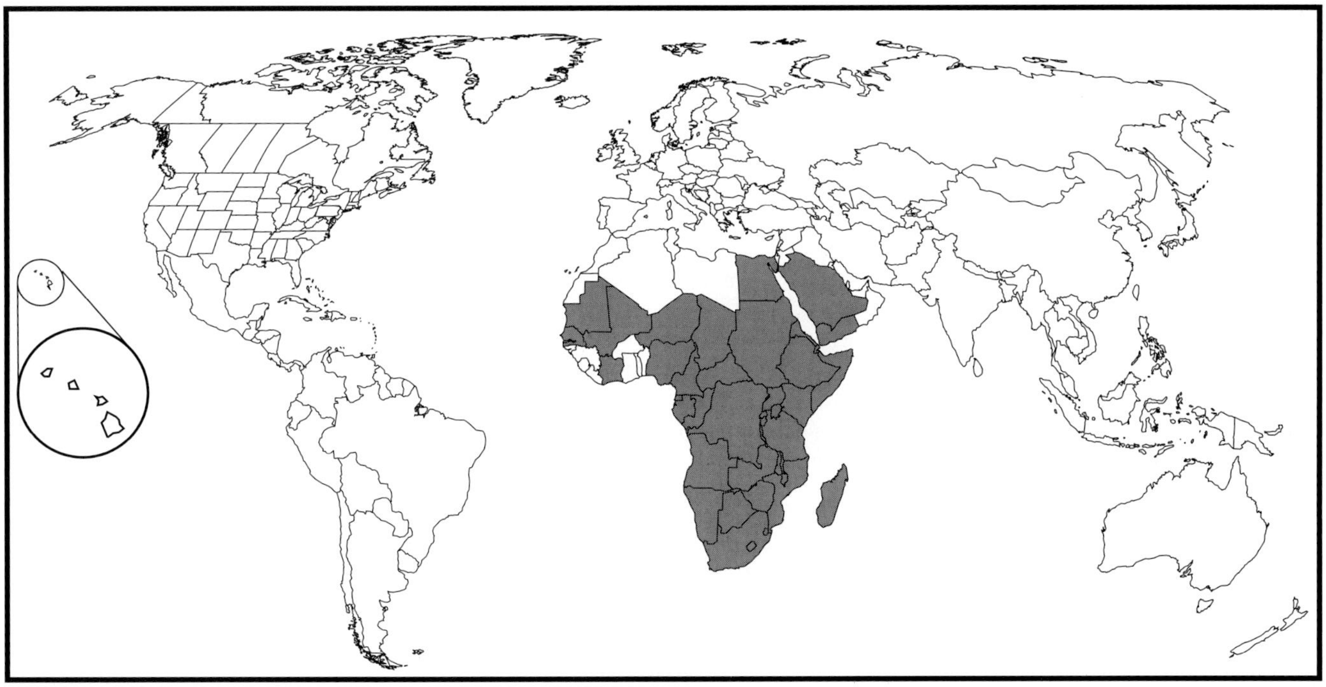

Rift Valley Fever Virus and Antibody

hosts do not become sick. Humans contract CCHF through the bite of an infected tick, squashing an infected tick, aerosols, or contact with blood or tissue from infected animals, or via the nosocomial route. Outbreaks are usually small, fewer than 100 cases, and more commonly involve agricultural workers, especially abattoir workers; military personnel or campers; and medical care workers.[15,16,18–20] Nosocomial spread among hospital staff is common, and strict universal precautions should be taken with hospitalized cases of CCHF.[21]

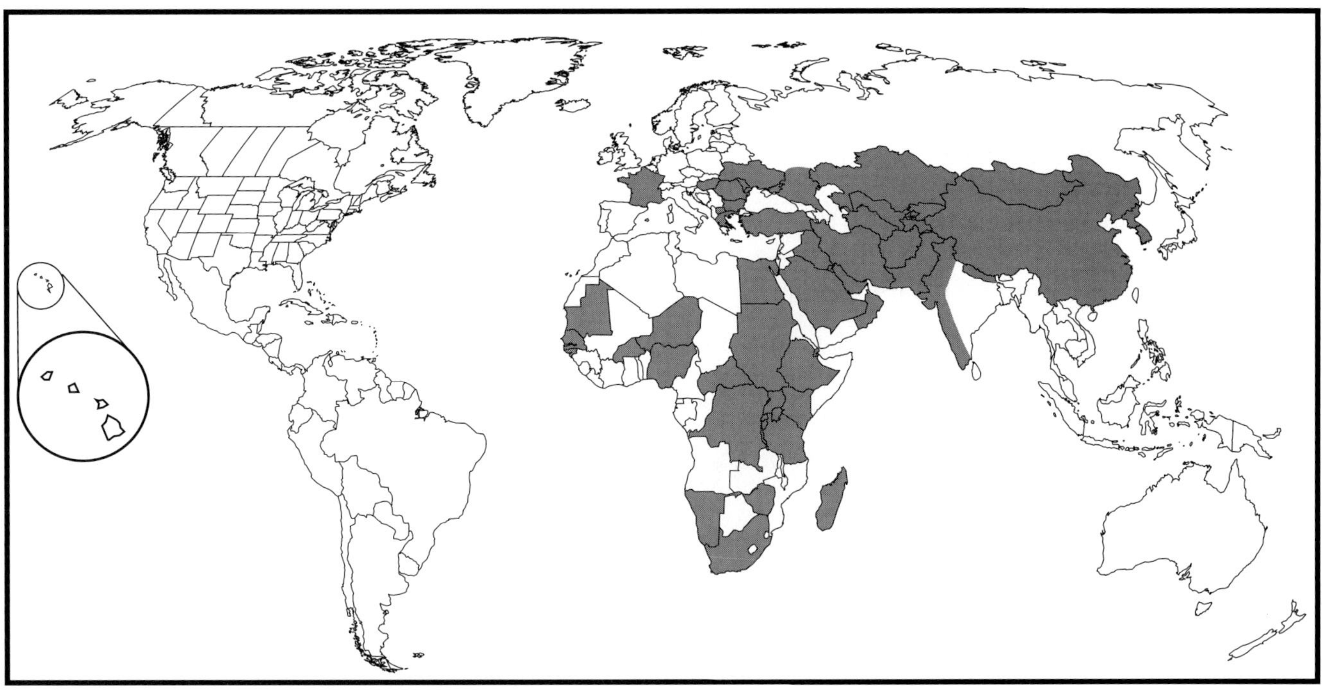

Crimean-Congo Hemorrhagic Fever Virus and Antibody

DISEASES

Rift Valley Fever

Human infections with RVF are usually associated with a brief, self-limited febrile illness.[3,22] The incubation period is typically 2 to 6 days. Most patients have a sudden onset of fever, malaise, severe myalgia with lower backache, chills, headache, retro-orbital pain, photophobia, and anorexia. Fever usually lasts for 4 days. In a minority of patients, fever returns after 2 or 3 days, accompanied by return of symptoms, flushed face, nausea, vomiting, and injected conjunctivae. Most persons infected with RVF virus recover without sequelae, although convalescence may take 2 or 3 weeks.

In about 1% of cases, RVFV infection is associated with two severe complications.[3,5–7,22–24] *Hemorrhagic fever* is manifested as epistaxis, hematemesis, melena, and ecchymoses at sites of inoculations. Onset is usually early in the course of illness, and the syndrome carries a poor prognosis. The illness progresses to disseminated intravascular coagulation (DIC), anemia, leukopenia, thrombocytopenia, renal impairment or failure, and hepatitis as evidenced by abnormal liver transaminases, prolonged prothrombin time (PT) and partial thromboplastin time (PTT), and fibrin degradation products. Jaundice is manifested early in the course. Death follows massive gastrointestinal hemorrhage, oliguria, or anuria, associated with fibrin deposition in glomeruli and damage to proximal tubules. Myocardial necrosis occurs in some fatal cases. Death occurs within 3 to 6 days; survivors recover slowly. *Encephalitis* may develop a week or more after the febrile phase as severe headache, meningismus, confusion, and vertigo with cerebrospinal fluid (CSF) pleocytosis. The patient's condition may deteriorate with stupor or coma, and survivors may have residual brain damage.[7]

In 1% to 10% of survivors, retinopathy presents about 7 to 20 days after the primary fever. The patient has decreased visual acuity in one or both eyes. Retinitis with macular cotton wool exudates and edema appears in one or both eyes. Lesions may resolve, but severe defects become permanent with loss of central vision.

Crimean-Congo Hemorrhagic Fever

The incubation period of CCHF is 3 to 6 days in nosocomial outbreaks and 2 to 12 days in other situations.[15,25] Outbreaks of CCHF are focal in nature. The clinical spectrum ranges from fever, malaise, and prostration to severe and fatal hemorrhagic disease. The case fatality rate has varied from 10% to more than 50%, with most deaths occurring 5 to 14 days after onset. Illness begins with sudden onset of symptoms, including dizziness, neck pain and stiffness, myalgia, especially in the lower back, headache, eye pain and photophobia, arthralgias, chills, anorexia, sore throat, nausea and vomiting, and abdominal pain. Patients may develop altered consciousness progressing to aggressive behavior and unconsciousness. The face is flushed, as are the neck and upper chest. Conjunctival injection and congestion of the pharynx and soft palate are also observed. About 50% of patients develop hepatomegaly. In moderately severe illness, fever lasts 5 to 20 days (average 9 days). The illness may be biphasic with fever followed by one to two afebrile days, then return of fever associated with epistaxis, petechiae, purpura, and thrombocytopenia. Some patients develop jaundice. Hemorrhage often begins with blood leakage at sites of needlesticks, and may become profuse. Shock ensues in severe cases and may be accompanied by liver failure, cerebral hemorrhage, anemia, dehydration, diarrhea, myocardial infarction, pulmonary edema, DIC, and pleural effusions. Defervescence occurs between days 7 and 20 with cessation of bleeding and general improvement. Convalescence is prolonged, usually 2 to 4 months, and is characterized by weakness, confusion, asthenia, alopecia, and neuralgias.

PATHOGENESIS AND IMMUNITY

Rift Valley Fever

RVFV infections, like those of other phleboviruses, are regulated primarily by interferon and neutralizing antibodies, with cellular immunity occupying a much lesser role.[26] Reconstructing the human disease based on available information and animal models, we suppose that mosquito or aerosol infections lead to a viremic phase. An early interferon response protects endothelium and hepatocyte targets.[27] If extensive target cell infection occurs, the acutely cytolytic RVFV infection results in extensive hepatitis and also initiates DIC, a lethal combination that may be tilted toward either pathogenic mechanism.[23] The extensive DIC can result in renal failure in the monkey model.[28,29] In rodents, the host genotype is an important determinant of the type of disease resulting from infection.[30] The encephalitis observed in a minority of humans appears to be a consequence of a lytic viral process.[31] In rodent models, there is a multifocal, acutely necrotic process,[30,32] which also is seen in intracranially inoculated nonhuman primates.[33] The pathogenesis of the retinal disease is not well understood, although some data suggest that it is a consequence of a retinal vasculitis.[34]

Viremia and either hemorrhagic fever or uncomplicated disease from RVFV end with the appearance of the neutralizing antibody response.[26,27] The critical phases of disease occur before host cellular effector mechanisms come into play. In the case of late encephalitis, histologic study shows an acute suppurative lesion that does not have the lymphocytic infiltrates characteristic of T cell–mediated immunopathologic disease. The protective mechanisms of vaccines are thought to be based almost entirely on a neutralizing antibody response.[26,35]

Crimean-Congo Hemorrhagic Fever

Clinicopathologic studies indicate that all patients present with abnormal clinical laboratory test results, but the changes are moderate in nonfatal infections and marked in patients with fatal outcomes.[36–38] The course of infection is characterized by a transient leukopenia. Creatine kinase (CK) levels are increased early during the first week of disease, and then decline and subsequently increase markedly in fatal cases. The elevated CK coincides with elevated blood urea levels. In addition, serum aspartate aminotransferase (AST) and alanine aminotransferase (ALT) levels increase during the latter half of the first week. The elevated levels of CK, AST, and ALT are accompanied by an increase in alkaline phosphatase, γ-glutamyltransferase, and lactate dehydrogenase. Patients have proteinuria during the first week of illness, and the total serum protein and albumin levels are decreased during the first and second week in severely ill patients, despite corrective therapy.

Thrombocytopenia is a prominent feature of CCHF viral infection. Platelet counts are extremely low during the early phase of illness among fatal cases, and decrease to thrombocytopenic levels for all patients by the end of the first week of illness. The more prominent findings for CCHF patients are the grossly abnormal prothrombin ratio (PR), activated partial prothrombin time (APPT), thrombin time (TT), fibrinogen, and fibrin degradation products values recorded during the course of fatal infections. Most patients show a decline in hemoglobin during the second week of illness, even patients who do not have hemorrhagic manifestations. In summary, the occurrence during the first 5 days of illness of leukocyte counts $\geq 10 \times 10^9$/L, platelet counts $\leq 20 \times 10^9$/L, AST ≥200 U/L, ALT ≥150 U/L, PTT ≥60 seconds or fibrinogen ≤110 mg/dL are ≥90% predictive of fatal outcomes.

Knowledge of the pathogenesis of CCHF is based primarily on descriptions of autopsied tissue and therefore limited to changes that occur in the terminal stages of disease.[37,39] Immunohistochemical and in situ hybridization studies on formalin-fixed human tissues indicate that the main targets of CCHF viral infection are mononuclear phagocytes, endothelial cells, and hepatocytes, accompanied by parenchymal necrosis in the liver. Viral antigen and viral RNA were present within cells lining hepatic sinusoids, including Kupffer and endothelial cells, as well as in endothelial cells of other tissues and lymphoreticular cells of the spleen. The presence of virus in the mononuclear phagocytes and endothelial cells is believed to reflect phagocytic and immunologic activities related to virus clearance, or these cells may support the replication and shedding of virus back into circulation. While evidence of necrosis is not readily demonstrated in the mononuclear phagocytes and endothelial cells, necrosis and depletion of lymphoid cells are prominent in splenic tissue. The absence of necrosis in infected mononuclear phagocytes and the depletion of lymphoid cells may protect the virus from phagocytosis and suppress the immune response, thereby allowing the virus to replicate and spread in CCHF patients. In addition, infection of mononuclear phagocytes and endothelial cells could play a role in the pathogenesis of CCHF by causing secretion of cytokines and other inflammatory mediators.

Viremia and uncomplicated disease associated with CCHF viral infection end with the onset of the neutralizing antibody response. In nonfatal CCHF cases, IgM and IgG antibody can be demonstrated as early as day 7 to 9 after the onset of illness. In contrast, an antibody response is usually not demonstrable among fatal cases, suggesting that the humoral immune response is important for recovery.

DIAGNOSIS

Several classical and molecular techniques can be used to diagnose CCHF[15,16,37–42] and RVF[24,42–45] viral infections. The viruses are easily isolated by intracerebral inoculation of blood or organs in baby mice or by inoculation of Vero cell culture (Fig. 67-1). Other vertebrate cell cultures are also susceptible. Mice sicken and the virus is identified in brain or liver by immunofluorescence or by reverse transcription–polymerase chain reaction (RT-PCR). Nucleic acid sequences of RVF and CCHF virus may be detected directly in patients' viremic blood by RT-PCR, although caution is warranted when using this technique for CCHF virus because variation in nucleotide sequences among strains may require more than a single primer pair to detect all viruses. The use of PCR or the slower virus isolation techniques is essential for diagnosing fatal CCHF cases because these patients usually fail to develop detectable antibody. The antigen-capture enzyme-linked immunosorbent assay (ELISA) can be used to detect viral antigen in the patient's acute serum in 5 to 6 hours, as compared with days for the classical virus isolation method, but is less sensitive. However, the assay is of value for the more severe CCHF cases because of the higher titer and prolonged viremia.

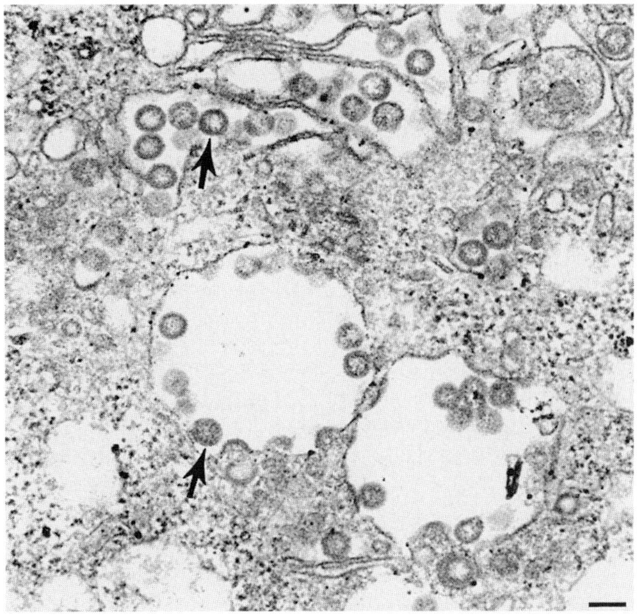

FIGURE 67-1 Electron micrograph of Rift Valley fever virus grown in BHK-21 cells, showing virus particles *(arrows)* maturing within the Golgi apparatus and cytoplasmic vesicles. Bar = 100 nm. (Courtesy of Dr. F.A. Murphy, Davis, CA.)

In convalescing patients, ELISA is used to detect IgM in serum and CSF (RVF) and to detect a rise in IgG level in paired acute and convalescent sera. In the case of RVF, the neutralization test is the most specific for detecting virus-specific antibody. The results of each or a combination of these laboratory tests can be supported by immunohistochemistry and in situ hybridization analysis of autopsied tissues, preferably mononuclear phagocytes, endothelial cells, and hepatocytes. The laboratory should be notified that specimens originate from a hemorrhagic fever patient, so that appropriate biosafety measures can be taken.

TREATMENT AND PROGNOSIS

Usually, treatment of a patient with hemorrhagic fever must be initiated before an etiologic diagnosis is made.[46]

There is no established treatment for RVF, although in experimental animals ribavirin and passive antibody can be protective.[47] In addition, recombinant or lymphoblastoid human IFN-α

doses of 5×10^3 units/kg body weight daily for 5 days suppresses RVF viremia and disease in rhesus monkeys.[48]

Ribavirin is effective for inhibiting CCHF viral replication in cell culture and in animal models.[38,39,49–51] It is believed to be helpful in treatment of human disease, but clinical trials have not been done.[19,52,53] Limited studies suggest that CCHF immune serum is beneficial when administered intravenously in a dose of 250 mL over 1 to 2 hours on successive days, and when given early in infection.[54,55] The evidence is based on observed clinical improvement, but the study did not include placebo control patients.

If viral hemorrhagic fever is suspected in the tropics and laboratory confirmation is not available, it would be reasonable to use intravenous ribavirin at 30 mg/kg body weight for one dose, then 16 mg/kg every 6 hours for 4 days, then 8 mg/kg every 8 hours for 6 days.[56,57] High-risk contacts who develop fever could be treated promptly with ribavirin. Intravenous and oral ribavirin can be obtained in the United States from ICN Pharmaceuticals, Inc. (Costa Mesa, CA) after an Investigational New Drug (IND) application number has been secured from the Food and Drug Administration, Division of Antiviral Drug Products (301-827-2335, or after hours, 202-857-8400). Although there are promising therapeutic candidates, the only measures that are routinely administered for hemorrhagic cases are supportive therapies focused on hematologic and fluid imbalances.

PREVENTION AND CONTROL

Nosocomial spread of CCHF is prevented by maintaining hemorrhagic fever patients in isolation and using universal precautions.

All patients should be assumed to have a communicable disease until proved otherwise. Local and national health authorities should be notified immediately. Patients should be placed in isolation and universal precautions used by medical and nursing staff, including gown, foot covers, mask, double gloves, and needle precautions. The health-care workers should use respirators if this protection is available.

Inactivated and live attenuated vaccines for RVF have been developed by the U. S. Department of Defense for human use. Most experience has been with the inactivated vaccine, which has been nonreactogenic, induces neutralizing antibodies, and protects laboratory workers.[35] The live-attenuated vaccine that has been inoculated into 60 humans seems to be safe and induces neutralizing antibodies, although the database is obviously small. However, neither of these vaccines is currently available.

Prevention and control of RVF entails vaccination of sheep and cattle in enzootic areas. Livestock serve as amplifying hosts, and their immunization is the key to the prevention of amplification and transmission. Both inactivated and attenuated RVF vaccines have been used in livestock. There is limited availability of most vaccines except two South African products: the live Smithburn neurotropic strain is poorly immunogenic in cattle and causes abortion and fetal abnormalities in pregnant ewes. The manufacturer recommends the inactivated vaccine for cattle. A mouse brain–derived vaccine for CCHF is used in Bulgaria but is not available outside that country.[15] During epizootics, to avoid exposure to virus in the blood, farmers should not slaughter and butcher sick animals, and dead animals should be buried. Control of mosquitoes is usually impractical, but personal protective measures may be helpful. The epidemic of 1987 in Mauritania was predicted and illustrates the risk of new dam construction with subsequent flooding of large areas in RVF epizootic regions.

Prevention and control of CCHF are achieved by control of *Hyalomma* ticks. Farmers, soldiers, campers, and abattoir workers should be taught to remove ticks in a timely fashion and without crushing them. In endemic areas, a measure of tick control has been achieved by environmental sanitation of underbrush habitats. Acaricides may be useful on domestic animals to control CCHF-infected ticks if used 10 to 14 days prior to slaughter or export of animals from enzootic regions. The use of gloves by abattoir workers has been suggested in order to prevent direct contact of skin with viremic blood of sheep and cattle, but may be difficult to institute in practice.

REFERENCES

1. Schmaljohn CS, Hooper JW: Bunyaviridae: the viruses and their replication. In Knipe DM, Howley PM (eds), with Griffin DE, Lamb RA, Martin MA, et al: Fields' Virology, 4th ed. Philadelphia, Lippincott, Williams and Wilkins, 2001, p. 1581.
2. Chin J (ed): Control of Communicable Diseases Manual, 17th ed. Washington, DC, American Public Health Association, 2000, p. 33.
3. Peters CJ, Linthicum KJ: Rift Valley fever. In Beran GW (ed): Handbook Series of Zoonoses, Section B: Viral Zoonoses, 2nd ed. Boca Raton, FL, CRC Press, 1994, p. 125.
4. Daubney R, Hudson JR, Garnham PC: Enzootic hepatitis or Rift Valley fever: an undescribed virus disease of sheep, cattle and man from East Africa. J Pathol 34:545, 1931.
5. Meegan JM, Shope RE: Emerging concepts on Rift Valley fever. Perspect Virol 11:267, 1981.
6. Digoutte JP, Peters CJ: General aspects of the 1987 Rift Valley fever epidemic in Mauritania. Res Virol 140:27, 1989.
7. Peters CJ: Emergence of Rift Valley fever. In Saluzzo JF, Dodet B (eds): Factors in the Emergence of Arbovirus Diseases. Paris, Elsevier, 1997, p. 253.
8. Arthur R, El-Sharkawy MS, Cope SE, et al: Recurrence of Rift Valley fever in Egypt. Lancet 342:1149, 1993.
9. Abd el-Rahim IH, Abd el-Hakim U, Hussein M: An epizootic of Rift Valley fever in Egypt in 1997. Rev Sci Tech 18:741, 1999.
10. Fagbo, SF: The evolving transmission pattern of Rift Valley fever in the Arabian Peninsula. Ann NY Acad Sci 969:201, 2002.
11. Linthicum KJ, Davies FG, Kairo A, et al: Rift Valley fever virus (family Bunyaviridae, genus *Phlebovirus*): Isolations from Diptera collected during an inter-epizootic period in Kenya. J Hyg 95:197, 1985.
12. Chumakov, MP: Contribution to 30 years of investigation of Crimean haemorrhagic fever. Med Virol 22:5, 1974.
13. Leshchinskaya EV: Clinical picture of Crimean hemorrhagic fever (in Russian). Trudy Inst Polio Virusn Entsefalitov Akad Med Nauk SSSR 7:226 (in English: NAMRU3-1856), 1965.
14. Casals J: Antigenic similarities between the virus causing Crimean hemorrhagic fever and Congo virus. Proc Soc Exp Biol Med 131:233, 1969.
15. Hoogstraal H: The epidemiology of tick-borne Crimean-Congo haemorrhagic fever in Asia, Europe and Africa. J Med Entomol 15:307, 1979.
16. Watts DM, Ksiazek TG, Linthicum KJ, et al: Crimean-Congo hemorrhagic fever. In Monath TG (ed): The Arboviruses: Epidemiology and Ecology, Vol II. Boca Raton, FL, CRC Press, 1989, p. 177.
17. Casals J, Tignor GH: The *Nairovirus* genus: serological relationships. Intervirology 14:144, 1980.
18. Scrimgeour EM: Crimean-Congo haemorrhagic fever in Oman. Lancet 347:692, 1996.
19. Mardani M, Jahromi MK, Naieni KH, et al: The efficacy of oral ribavirin in the treatment of Crimean-Congo hemorrhagic fever in Iran. Clin Infect Dis 36:1613, 2003.

20. Khan AS, Maupin GO, Rollin PE, et al: An outbreak of Crimean-Congo hemorrhagic fever in the United Arab Emirates, 1994–1995. Am J Trop Med Hyg 57:519, 1997.
21. Bumey MI, Ghafoor A, Saleen M, et al: Nosocomial outbreak of viral hemorrhagic fever caused by Crimean hemorrhagic fever–Congo virus in Pakistan. Am J Trop Med Hyg 29:941, 1976.
22. Laughlin LW, Watten RH: Epidemic of Rift Valley fever in Egypt: observations on the spectrum of human illness. Trans R Soc Trop Med Hyg 76:630, 1979.
23. Al Hazmi M, Ayoola EA, Abduraham M, et al: Epidemic of Rift Valley fever in Saudi Arabia: a clinical study of severe illness in humans. Clin Infect Dis 36:245, 2003.
24. Madani TA, Al-Mazrou YY, Al-Jeffri MH, et al: Rift Valley fever epidemic in Saudi Arabia: epidemiological, clinical, and laboratory characteristics. Clin Infect Dis 37:1084, 2003.
25. Swanepoel R, Shepherd AJ, Leman PA, et al: Epidemiologic and clinical features of Crimean-Congo hemorrhagic fever in southern Africa. Am J Trop Med Hyg 36:120, 1987.
26. Peters CJ: Viral hemorrhagic fevers. In Nathanson N, Ahmed R, Gonzales-Scarano F, et al: Viral Pathogenesis. Philadelphia, Lippincott-Raven, 1997, p. 799.
27. Morrill JC, Jennings GB, Johnson AJ, et al: Pathogenesis of Rift Valley fever in rhesus monkeys: role of interferon response. Arch Virol 110:195, 1990.
28. Cosgriff TM, Morrill JC, Jennings GB, et al: Hemostatic derangement produced by Rift Valley fever virus in rhesus monkeys. Rev Infect Dis 11(Suppl 4):S807, 1989.
29. Peters CJ, Jones D, Trotter R, et al: Experimental Rift Valley fever in rhesus macaques. Arch Virol 99:31, 1988.
30. Anderson GW Jr, Slone TW Jr, Peters CJ: Pathogenesis of Rift Valley fever virus (RVFV) in inbred rats. Microbiol Pathog 2:283, 1987.
31. van Velden DJ, Meyer JD, Olivier J, et al: Rift Valley fever affecting humans in South Africa: a clinicopathological study. S Afr Med J 51:867, 1977.
32. Anderson GW Jr, Slone TW Jr: Peters CJ: The gerbil, *Meriones unguiculatus*, a model for Rift Valley fever viral encephalitis. Arch Virol 102:187, 1988.
33. Morrill JC, Peters CJ: Pathogenicity and neurovirulence studies of a mutagen-attenuated Rift Valley fever vaccine in rhesus monkeys. Vaccine 21:2994, 2003.
34. Cohen C, Luntz MH: Rift Valley fever and rickettsial retinitis including fluorescein (author's transl). [German]. Klin Monatsbl Augenheilkd 169:685, 1976.
35. Pittman PR, Liu CT, Cannon RS, et al: Immunogenicity of an inactivated Rift Valley fever vaccine in humans: a 12-year experience. Vaccine 18:181, 1999.
36. Swanepoel R, Gill DE, Shepherd AJ, et al: The clinical pathology of Crimean-Congo hemorrhagic fever. Rev Infect Dis 11:S794, 1989.
37. Gear JHS: Crimean-Congo hemorrhagic fever. In Gear JHS (ed): CRC Handbook of Viral and Rickettsial Hemorrhagic Fevers. Boca Raton, FL, CRC Press, 1986, p. 121.
38. Burt FJ, Leman PA, Smith JF, et al: The use of a reverse transcription-polymerase chain reaction for the detection of viral nucleic acid in the diagnosis of Crimean-Congo haemorrhagic fever. J Virol Methods 70:129, 1998.
39. Burt FJ, Swanepoel R, Shieh W-J, et al: Immunohistochemical and in situ localization of Crimean-Congo hemorrhagic fever (CCHF) virus in human tissues and implications for CCHF pathogenesis. Arch Pathol Lab Med 121:839, 1997.
40. Schwarz TF, Nitschko H, Jager G, et al: Crimean-Congo haemorrhagic fever in Oman. Lancet 346:1230, 1995.
41. Shepherd AJ, Swanepoel R, Leman PA: Antibody response in Crimean-Congo hemorrhagic fever. Rev Infect Dis 11(Suppl 4):801, 1989.
42. Drosten CS, Gottig S, Schilling M, et al: Rapid detection and quantification of RNA of Ebola and Marburg viruses, Lassa virus, Crimean-Congo hemorrhagic fever virus, Rift Valley fever virus, dengue virus, and yellow fever virus by real-time reverse transcription-PCR. J Clin Microbiol 40:2323, 2002.
43. Garcia S, Crance JM, Billecocq A, et al: Quantitative real-time PCR detection of Rift Valley fever virus and its application to evaluation of antiviral compounds. J Clin Microbiol 39:4456, 2001.
44. Swanepoel R, Struthers JK, Erasmus M J, et al: Comparison of techniques for demonstrating antibodies to Rift Valley fever virus. J Hyg 97:317, 1986.
45. Paweska JT, Burt FJ, Anthony F, et al: IgG-sandwich and IgM-capture enzyme-linked immunosorbent assay for the detection of antibody to Rift Valley fever virus in domestic ruminants. J Virol Methods 113:103, 2003.
46. Dykewicz CA, Shope RE: Viral hemorrhagic fevers. In Schlossberg D (ed): Current Therapy of Infectious Disease. St. Louis, Mosby-Year Book, 1996, p. 515.
47. Peters CJ, Reynolds JA, Slone TW, et al: Prophylaxis of Rift Valley fever with antiviral drugs, immune serum, an interferon inducer, and a macrophage activator. Antiviral Res 6:285, 1986.
48. Morrill JC, Jennings GB, Cosgriff TM, et al: Prevention of Rift Valley fever in rhesus monkeys with interferon-alpha. Rev Infect Dis 11(Suppl 4):S815, 1989.
49. Watts DM, Ussery MA, Nash D, et al: Inhibition of Crimean-Congo hemorrhagic fever viral infectivity yields in vitro by ribavirin. Am J Trop Med Hyg 41:591–595, 1989.
50. Paragas J, Whitehouse CA, Endy TP, et al: A simple assay for determining antiviral activity against Crimean-Congo hemorrhagic fever virus. Antiviral Res 62:21, 2004.
51. Tignor GH, Hanham CA: Ribavirin efficacy in an in vivo model of Crimean-Congo hemorrhagic fever virus (CCHF) infection. Antiviral Res 22:309–325, 1993.
52. Fisher-Hoch SP, Khan JA, Rehman S, et al: Crimean Congo-haemorrhagic fever treated with oral ribavirin. Lancet 346:472, 1995.
53. Papa A, Bozovi B, Pavlidou V, et al: Genetic detection and isolation of Crimean-Congo hemorrhagic fever virus, Kosovo, Yugoslavia. Emerg Infect Dis S8: 852, 2002.
54. Vassilenko SM, Vassilev TL, Bozadjiev LG, et al: Specific intravenous immunoglobulin for Crimean-Congo haemorrhagic fever. Lancet 335:791, 1990.
55. Vassilev T, Valchev V, Kazarov G, et al: A reference preparation for human immunoglobulin against Crimean/Congo hemorrhagic fever. Biologicals 19:57, 1991.
56. Huggins JW: Prospects for treatment of viral hemorrhagic fevers with ribavirin, a broad spectrum antiviral drug. Rev Infect Dis 11:S750, 1989.
57. Centers for Disease Control and Prevention: Management of patients with suspected viral hemorrhagic fever. MMWR 37:1, 1988.

68

Hantavirus Infections

C. J. PETERS
JAMES N. MILLS
CHRISTINA SPIROPOULOU
SHERIF R. ZAKI
PIERRE E. ROLLIN

INTRODUCTION

Hantaviruses are rodent-borne agents with a broad geographic distribution in the Americas, Asia, and Europe (Table 68-1). They cause inapparent, chronic infections of rodents and spread to humans through infectious urine, saliva, or feces (Fig. 68-1). The human host suffers one of two major diseases: hemorrhagic fever with renal syndrome (HFRS) or hantavirus pulmonary syndrome (HPS). HFRS is mainly an Old World disease, and HPS to date has been encountered only in the Americas. With the exception of Andes virus in Argentina and southern Chile, interhuman transmission of hantaviruses has never been established. The viruses are virtually noncytopathic, and disease is believed to be largely immunopathologic. Prevention rests on rodent avoidance when feasible, but candidate vaccines for HFRS are being tested. Supportive management is important to survival. The viruses are sensitive to the antiviral effects of ribavirin in cell culture, and that drug is an adjunct in the therapy of severe HFRS.

AGENTS

Description

Hantaviruses were first discovered because of an interest in the presumed viral etiology of HFRS. Early work in 1930 to 1950 in Manchuria and the Soviet Union, centered on human studies, suggested a viral agent, but it was not until Hantaan virus was isolated by passage in the suspected rodent reservoir and identified with convalescent serum from HFRS patients that a reliable experimental system was obtained.[1,2] Isolation in cell culture led to the characterization of Hantaan and related viruses and the demonstration that they formed a new genus, *Hantavirus,* within the family Bunyaviridae.[3,4] The distinctive syndrome associated with several American hantaviruses was not discovered until 1993.[5]

Hantaviruses presumably originated as parasites of the order Rodentia. Their phylogeny corresponds to that of their rodent hosts, suggesting the divergence of the viruses of

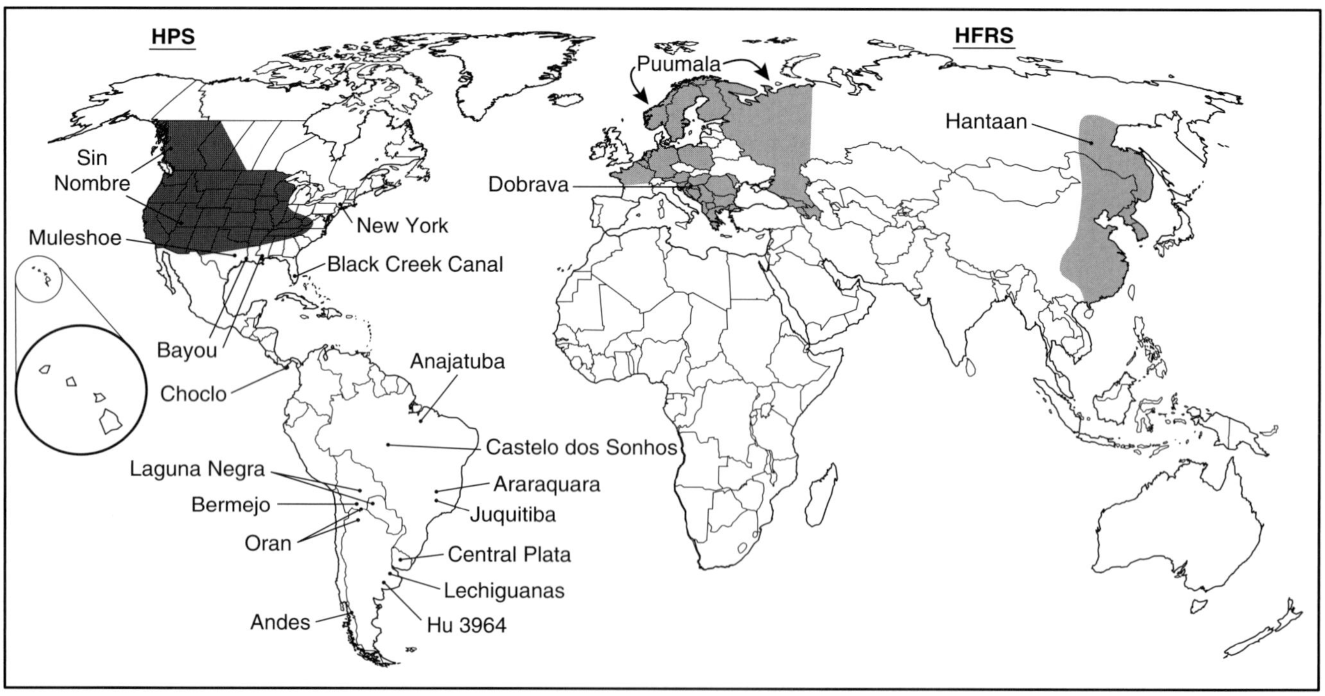

Hantaviruses

Hantavirus pulmonary syndrome (HPS)

Hemorrhagic fever with renal syndrome (HFRS)

Table 68-1 Hantaviruses, Their Reservoirs, and Hantavirus Diseases

Rodent Reservoir Subfamily	Rodent Reservoir	Virus	Disease	Disease Distribution
Murinae	*Apodemus agrarius*	Hantaan	HFRS	Asia
	Apodemus agrarius	Saaremaa	HFRS	Balkans
	Apodemus flavicollis	Dobrava	HFRS	Balkans
	Apodemus peninsulae	Amur	HFRS	Far eastern Russia
	Bandicota indicus	"Thailand"	Not known	—
	Rattus norvegicus	Seoul	HFRS	Asia, elsewhere
Arvicolinae	*Clethrionomys glareolus*	Puumala	HFRS	Europe
	Clethrionomys rufocanus	Puumala-like	Not known	—
	Lemmus sibericus	Topografov	Not known	—
	Microtus arvalis/Microtus rossiameridionalis	Tula	Not known	—
	Microtus californicus	Isla Vista	Not known	—
	Microtus fortis	Khabarovsk	Not known	—
	Microtus ochrogaster	Bloodland Lake	Not known	—
	Microtus pennsylvanicus	Prospect Hill	Not known	—
Sigmodontinae	*Bolomys obscurus*	Maciel	Not known	—
	Calomys laucha	Laguna Negra	HPS	Paraguay, Bolivia
	Oligoryzomys flavescens	Lechiguanas	HPS	Central Argentina
	Oligoryzomys longicaudatus	Andes	HPS	Southwestern Argentina
	Oligoryzomys microtis	Rio Mamore	Not known	Bolivia
	Oryzomys palustris	Bayou	HPS	Southeastern United States
	Peromyscus leucopus	New York–1	HPS	Eastern United States
	Peromyscus maniculatus	Sin Nombre	HPS	United States and western Canada
	Reithrodontomys megalotis	El Moro Canyon	Not known	—
	Reithrodontomys mexicanus	Rio Segundo	Not known	—
	Sigmodon alstoni	Cano Delgadito	Not known	—
	Sigmodon hispidus spadicipygus	Black Creek Canal	HPS	Southern Florida
	Sigmodon hispidus texianus	Muleshoe	HPS	Texas, United States
	Oligoryzomys nigripes	Juquitiba	Not known	Southeastern Brazil
	Peromyscus boylii	Limestone Canyon	Not known	Southwestern United States, Mexico
	Bolomys lasiurus	Araraquara	HPS	Southeastern Brazil
	Unknown	Castelo dos Sonhos	HPS	Central Brazil
	Oligoryzomys chacoensis	Bermejo	HPS	Northwest Argentina, Southern Bolivia
	Oligoryzomys sp.	Oran	HPS	Northwest Argentina, Southern Bolivia
	Akodon azarae	Pergamino	Not known	Central Argentina
	Oligoryzomys fornesi	Anajatuba	HPS?	Northern Brazil
	Holochilus sciureus	Rio Mearim	Not known	Northern Brazil
	Oligoryzomys flavescens	Central Plata	HPS	Southern Uruguay
	Oligoryzomys fulvescens	Choclo	HPS	Panama
	Zygodontomys brevicauda	Calabazo	Not known	Panama
	Oecomys bicolor	Maporal	Not known	Central Venezuela

HFRS, hemorrhagic fever with renal syndrome; HPS, hantavirus pulmonary syndrome.

America and Eurasia more than 20 million years ago. Little is known of the possibility of hantaviruses of other animals, although it is believed that at least one (Thottapalayam virus) may be a virus of a shrew (*Suncus murinus*, order Insectivora).[6]

Morphology

Hantavirus morphology is typical of the members of the Bunyaviridae family, with the virus particles being generally spherical although polymorphic. Elongated particles have also been observed.[7,8] Virus particle size varies from 70 to 120 nm with a dense core containing the riboprotein structures and surface glycoproteins embedded in the lipid bilayer envelope.

Replication

Hantaviruses are enveloped RNA viruses with a three-segmented negative-sense genome. The segments are designated as S (small, 1600 to 2060 nucleotides), M (medium, approximately 3700 nucleotides), and L (large, 6500 to 7000 nucleotides).[3–9] "Negative sense" signifies that the RNA genome is complementary to the messenger RNA (mRNA) coding for the viral proteins. The naked RNA genome is not infectious. An infectious virus unit requires that viral RNA be encapsidated by the nucleoprotein (N), forming the nucleocapsid core associated with the L viral polymerase protein. To form a mature virus, this unit is then enveloped by a lipid bilayer membrane derived from the host cell.

Hantaviruses

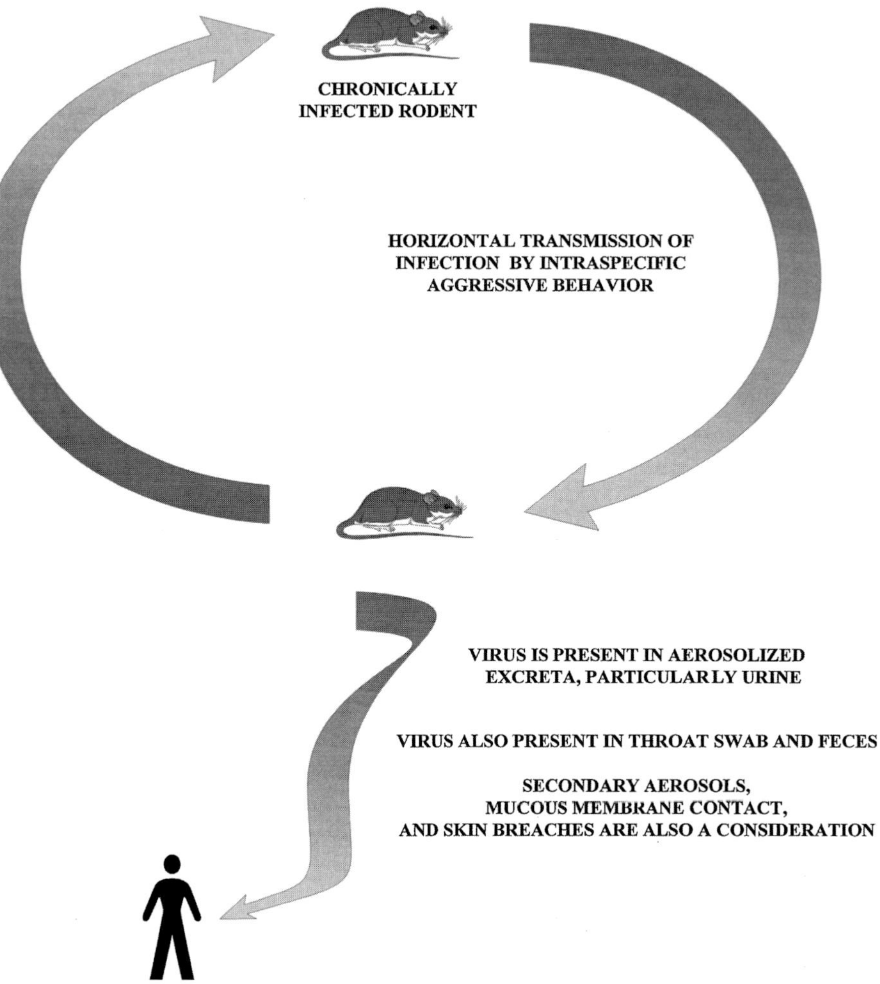

FIGURE 68-1 Transmission cycle of hantaviruses. The virus chronically infects its specific rodent host and is spread to other rodents horizontally. Virus shedding on mucosal surfaces is responsible for maintenance (usually an infected rodent bites or has other close contact with another of the same species) and for human infection (probably by aerosolization of virus-laden urine as it is shed, although other possibilities exist). Humans are a dead end in virus transmission, but a single hantavirus epidemic showed person-to-person spread. (Courtesy of K. Wagoner.)

Embedded in the membrane are the two surface glycoproteins, G1 and G2.

The coding strategy for each segment is simple. The S segment encodes the nucleocapsid N protein (molecular weight, 48 kD); the L segment, the polymerase L protein (250 kD); and the M segment, the two glycoproteins, G1 (72 kD) and G2 (54 kD). No nonstructural proteins (NSs or Nsm in analogy with other Bunyaviridae) have been detected in infected cells although there is evolutionary evidence for the existence of an NS equivalent in some hantaviruses.[10]

Infection is initiated by attachment of the virus to the cell, presumably mediated by the virus surface glycoproteins after interaction, in the case of the HPS viruses, with β-integrins.[11] Viral replication is initiated after virion uptake by the infected cells and release of the viral ribonucleoprotein cores into the cytoplasm. Each negative-strand virus RNA segment is transcribed by the virion-associated polymerase (L) to produce a functional mRNA. The relative amounts of the mRNAs synthesized are inversely proportional to their length. Thus, S mRNA is the most abundant and L mRNA the least. A simple explanation may be that the transcription elongation process is discontinuous with the polymerase pausing and possibly prematurely terminating at specific sites along the genome. The longer the gene, the higher the possibility of the presence of pausing sites. The 5′ ends of all three mRNAs are capped and contain a nontemplated guanine (G) residue. A prime-and-realign model has been proposed for the initiation of transcription of the hantaviruses.[12] The termination at the 3′ ends of the mRNAs is not the same for each template RNA segment. Hantavirus mRNAs may be stabilized by a stem-loop structure that forms at the 3′ noncoding region and initially none of the mRNAs were believed to be polyadenylated, although recent studies have reported that the Sin nombre virus (SNV) M mRNA is polyadenylated.[13] The three mRNAs are transcribed in the infected cell cytoplasm, and their translation is directly coupled to the transcription process.

The ratio of the individual virus proteins synthesized reflects the relative abundance of the virus mRNAs, with the N the most abundant protein. Two of the mRNAs, N and L, are translated on free ribosomes. The GPC mRNA is translated

rodents into contact with humans, or might be a marker for homes in which cats were kept because of the presence of rodents; studies have generally shown cats to be a risk factor or to be neutral, and there is no indication that cats become chronically infected or shed virus during acute infection.[64,99]

Studies of HPS in the southwestern United States during 1993 found rural residence and an excess of small rodents trapped by standardized methods in and around case households to be the major risk factors.[59,100] If the number of rodents found during the study was controlled for, agricultural activities and cleaning peridomestic structures were still risk factors, but reported sighting or trapping of rodents in the home was not a significant variable. Most houses were in piñon-juniper habitats, but house type or measures of environmental sanitation had no correlation. Interestingly, a history of opening and cleaning uninhabited structures, such as summer cabins, has continued to be a common activity among HPS patients.[101] Recent studies demonstrated a higher prevalence of antibody to Sin Nombre virus among peridomestic populations than among sylvatic populations of deer mice in rural areas of Montana.[102] In South America, HPS has generally been associated with rural living and agriculture.

Risks do not remain constant in a given area. In addition to previously noted changes in rodent populations over time, changing patterns have been reported from Korea and China with sustained, marked increases in the incidence of HFRS in southern Korea and areas of China.[78,103] It is not known to what extent this reflects increased disease incidence, increased reporting, or both.

DISEASES

Infection of the rodent host is followed by viremia and then an immune response that terminates viremia but leaves a chronic infection with lifelong virus excretion on mucosal surfaces, all with no recognized signs of overt disease. Infection of humans, however, may lead to severe disease at the time of the immune response, but chronic infection does not occur, and virus shedding leading to interhuman transmission is unknown, except with Andes virus. The clinical syndrome that occurs in humans takes two forms: the classic HFRS and HPS.

Hemorrhagic Fever with Renal Syndrome

HFRS Following Hantaan Virus Infection

Typically severe disease has a characteristic progression beginning with fever, which gives way to a brief period of hypotension followed by renal failure and finally diuresis.[96,104–110] (Fig. 68-3). The onset is abrupt, with fever, chills, malaise, myalgia, thirst, and headache. Capillary dilation is evidenced by flushing of the face and neck and by conjunctival and pharyngeal injection. Increased capillary permeability is generalized but most characteristically results in retroperitoneal edema accompanied by severe backache. During this phase, low-grade disseminated intravascular coagulation (DIC) appears and thrombocytopenia develops[111]; the cause is unknown but may reflect endothelial infection by the virus and a hypothesized procoagulant shift in the nonwetting surface of the vessel lining.[35,112] Bleeding is commonly seen in the skin and conjunctivae. Abdominal pain, anorexia, nausea, vomiting, mild cough, hiccough, and dizziness are also frequent. Proteinuria is usually present. The white blood cell count is normal or slightly elevated, often with a left shift.

After 3 to 7 days, the high fever falls and is replaced by a low-grade fever or normal temperature, and the patient enters the hypotensive phase. There may be only a few hours of transient hypotension or 1 to 3 days of severe clinical shock; kinin activation occurs during this period and is proportional to the severity of the shock.[113] Milder cases have a relative or even absolute bradycardia, but severely affected patients show tachycardia, narrow pulse pressure, and cold moist extremities; the blood pressure may fall to undetectable levels. The patient is usually apprehensive with a clouded sensorium, and nausea and vomiting are severe problems. Proteinuria increases, as does back pain. Hemoconcentration from plasma extravasation may result in a hematocrit of 55% to 65% or higher in severe cases. The urine, which contains red blood cells, white blood cells, and casts, decreases in volume, and the specific gravity moves to 1.010. Platelets reach their nadir, usually below 70,000/μL, and white blood cells are increased, often above 30,000/μL and occasionally reaching leukemoid levels. Careful management with Trendelenburg's position, pressors, and inotropic agents usually results in survival, but some patients die in severe shock during this phase. Because of the marked increase in vascular permeability, including in the lung, large quantities of fluids can be dangerous, and human serum albumin is often given for refractory shock. Cardiovascular measurements during the Korean War showed that patients did not conform to the expected findings in septic shock but rather had a low cardiac output and a high peripheral resistance.[114] Patients in frank shock with peripheral vasoconstriction were often given one to two units of albumin with apparent improvement.

After the hypotensive phase, a period of oliguria occurs with all the complications expected from uremia and electrolyte abnormalities. Platelets begin to rise, but bleeding, including hematuria, hemoptysis, and gastrointestinal hemorrhage, is troublesome during this stage. Fluid is resorbed and the patients may be overexpanded, leading to a high-output state, hypertension, and sometimes fatal pulmonary edema. Dialysis is indicated urgently for overhydration because of the likelihood of pulmonary edema as well as intracranial hemorrhage.

After 3 to 7 days of oliguria, urine output increases and may reach several liters daily. Electrolyte abnormalities and dehydration may threaten the patient during this phase. Urine specific gravity is fixed around 1.010, and the concentrating defect may persist 3 weeks to 3 months.

Other clinical laboratory tests can be useful. The aspartate transaminase (AST) level is usually elevated but not massively except in occasional cases of Seoul virus infection. Electrocardiograms (ECGs) are often abnormal with sinus bradycardia, low voltage, electrolyte changes, or nonspecific ST-T wave findings.[115,116] Atrial arrhythmias are not uncommon, but in spite of the right atrial lesion usually seen at autopsy, there are generally no specific findings on the ECG, although there is one report of elevation of the P-R interval in association with right atrial hemorrhage and dilation.[117] Plain films of the abdomen usually do not show the renal shadows, because of retroperitoneal edema. Magnetic resonance imaging (MRI) may suggest hemorrhage because of the low T2-weighted signal intensity along the outer medulla.[118] Pulmonary infiltrates are not common except in the face of overhydration, but occasionally pulmonary edema or effusions are present even early

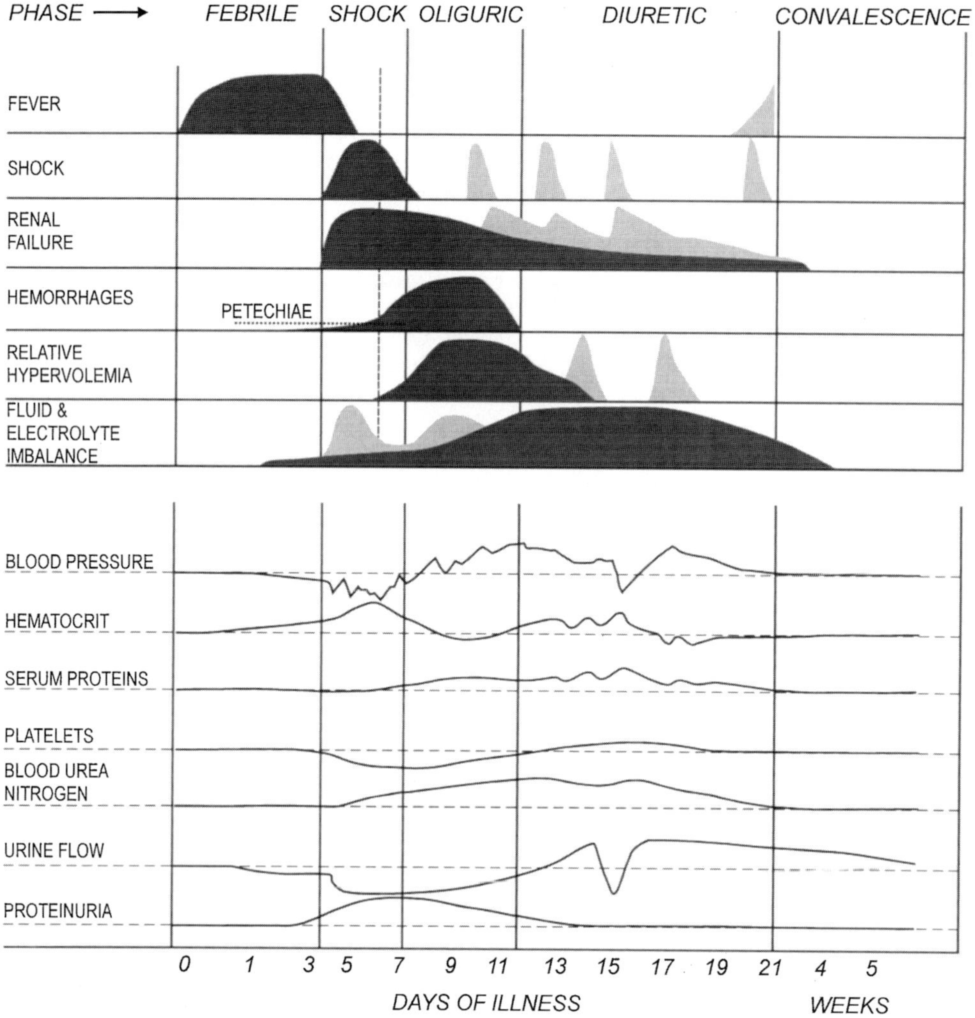

FIGURE 68-3 Schema of clinical course of severe hemorrhagic fever with renal syndrome (HFRS). (Modified from Sheedy JA, Froeb HF, Batson HA, et al: The clinical course of epidemic hemorrhagic fever. Am J Med 16:619–628, 1954.)

in disease.[116] The renogram shows patterns consistent with obstruction or tubular damage.[116]

A number of complications of HFRS have been observed. In consonance with the tightly swollen kidneys described at necropsy,[96,119] renal rupture may occur in the oliguric or early diuretic phase of illness and can respond to conservative management or require operative therapy.[120] Abdominal and back pain, signs of retroperitoneal hemorrhage, and abnormal ultrasound examination are present. Transient hypopituitarism and frank intrapituitary hemorrhage have been associated with pituitary apoplexy, abnormal anterior pituitary hormonal responses, delayed diuresis, and late appearance of Sheehan's syndrome.[121] These complications can be suspected by functional tests of the anterior pituitary and confirmed with computed tomography (CT) or MRI of the sella turcica.

Recovery is thought to be complete, but a small proportion of patients with residual abnormalities have left medical observation in all these studies. Interest in sequelae of hantaviruses is high because of an extensive study in Baltimore linking hypertensive chronic renal failure to the presence of Seoul antibodies.[81]

Description of the severe disease provides an excellent framework for understanding the pathogenesis of HFRS but is misleading in identifying the milder forms of Hantaan virus infection or of the milder renal syndromes associated with other hantaviruses. The spectrum of Hantaan virus infection includes fulminant disease with early death, patients whose clinical course "skips" one or more phases, telescoping of the phases, and very mild disease not readily identified as HFRS.[109]

HFRS Following Seoul Virus Infection

Seoul virus causes HFRS in humans and has been responsible for fatal infections in laboratory workers exposed to occultly infected rats, although the overall mortality is low, perhaps 1% or less.[69,122,123] The clinical picture of human disease acquired from wild *R. norvegicus* in Asia differs from that of Hantaan virus infection by its lesser severity and by having more prominent liver involvement.[69,77]

Mild HFRS Following Puumala Virus Infection

In Europe most cases of HFRS are caused by Puumala virus and are similar to but much milder than Hantaan virus infection.[124–128] The patient typically has fever, myalgia, malaise, and anorexia. Escalating abdominal pain, perhaps associated with nausea and vomiting, may lead to suspicion of a surgical emergency, but the onset of oliguria or the abnormal results of urinalysis usually averts operative intervention. Myopia, blurred vision, and even glaucoma have been reported in a significant proportion of patients and are very suggestive of the diagnosis.[128,129] The clinical course usually progresses rapidly through petechiae, mild hypotension, and transient oliguria with recovery. Diuresis and hyposthenuria may be notable and persist into convalescence.

In keeping with the milder clinical course, clinical laboratory abnormalities are fewer, including maximum creatinine levels. Thrombocytopenia is only present in one-half to three-fourths, leukocytosis in one-half of patients. Dialysis is required in fewer than 5% of patients, and mortality is less than 1%. As with Hantaan virus infection, sequelae are uncommon or absent, although hypertension in convalescence has been reported.[130,131]

Puumala virus is known to cause mild or asymptomatic disease based on retrospective serologic data, and some patients have had virtually asymptomatic infection or notable disease without detected renal involvement.[132–134] Occasional patients have shown a dominant neurologic picture clinically suggesting viral encephalitis or other neurologic manifestations, including Guillain–Barré syndrome.[128,135]

Infection with Other Old World Hantaviruses and Other Syndromes

As mentioned previously, Dobrava virus, associated with the rodent *A. flavicollis,* is a cause of lethal HFRS in the Balkans.[86,87] Some Southeast Asian patients, possibly infected with Seoul virus, have severe hepatitis as well as renal failure, and an initial report suggests the possibility of hantavirus infection in Chinese patients with clinical hepatitis and no markers for hepatitis A through E infection.[136,137] Some viruses from *Microtus* and other Arvicolinae species in eastern Europe and Russia are suspected to cause HFRS; no definite evidence establishes their pathogenicity or spectrum of disease.

Hantavirus Pulmonary Syndrome

The other major syndrome associated with hantavirus infection is pulmonary rather than renal and was recognized only in 1993[5,138,139] (Fig. 68-4). The pathogenesis is similar to that of HFRS in many ways, but the resultant clinical picture is distinctive (Table 68-2) and is caused by a different set of hantaviruses than HFRS (see Table 68-1).

The disease begins with the abrupt onset of fever, myalgia, and malaise, often accompanied by chills, anorexia, and headache.[138,140–142] The patient's subjective condition worsens with prostration and sometimes prominent gastrointestinal symptoms such as nausea, vomiting, abdominal pain, and diarrhea. Dizziness may be present as well.[141,143] Pharyngitis, rhinorrhea, rash, and cough usually are absent. If patients come in for medical attention because of their extreme discomfort, they usually will be sent away because of the lack of objective findings. This prodromal stage lasts 3 to 5 days (range, 1 to 10 days) before cardiorespiratory compromise supervenes.

With the onset of pulmonary edema, patients seek medical attention because of shortness of breath. They may have developed a productive or nonproductive cough by this time. Objective findings include tachypnea, fever, mild hypotension, and often surprisingly few physical signs of pulmonary edema. At this stage there is evidence of arterial desaturation

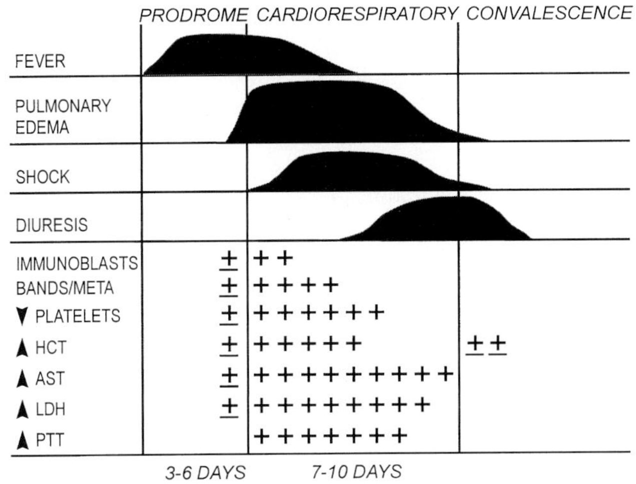

FIGURE 68-4 Schema of clinical course of severe hantavirus pulmonary syndrome (HPS). META, metamyelocytes; HCT, hematocrit; AST, aspartate transaminase; LDH, lactate dehydrogenase; PTT, partial thromboplastin time. (Prepared by Li Lien Yang.)

Table 68-2 Pathogenesis of Typical HFRS from Hantaan Virus Infection and HPS from Sin Nombre Virus Infection

HFRS	HPS
Incubation	
Typically 2–3 wk (7–42 days)	Typically 1–2 wk (1–4 wk)
Early Signs, Symptoms, and Antibody Response	
3–5 days' fever, myalgia, malaise; often gastrointestinal symptoms; flushing, conjunctival injection	3–5 days' fever, myalgia, malaise; often gastrointestinal symptoms
IgM antibody and immunoblasts already present	IgM antibody and immunoblasts already present
Disease Course	
DIC, kinin, complement activation; bleeding diathesis	Abnormal PTT, platelets
Back pain, retroperitoneal leak	Dyspnea, hypoxemia, pulmonary edema
Hypotension and shock	Hypotension and shock
Defervesence	Some continued fever
Shock lasting 12–48 hr	Shock and pulmonary edema worsening up to 24–48 hr
Recovery	
Oliguric renal failure; problems in circulatory status, bleeding, fluid balance	Pulmonary failure and shock management
Diuresis 5–10 days later	Resolution of lung lesion and shock in 3–6 days

DIC, disseminated intravascular coagulation; HFRS, hemorrhagic fever with renal syndrome; HPS, hantavirus pulmonary syndrome; PTT, partial thromboplastin time.

by oximetry or blood gas analysis. The chest radiograph usually shows subtle (peribronchial edema, Kerley B lines) or marked (alveolar pattern, pleural effusions) signs of increased pulmonary vascular permeability[140]; early on there may be a normal radiograph, a basilar pattern, or asymmetric development of edema.[141]

Several clinical laboratory abnormalities will almost always be present within a day of onset of dyspnea: thrombocytopenia, left shift (the white blood cell count may be normal, but there is often leukocytosis), and atypical lymphocytes.[33] Unfortunately these are not always present to aid in the initial diagnosis. Mildly elevated AST, prolonged partial thromboplastin time (PTT), slightly decreased serum bicarbonate, and increases in serum lactate dehydrogenase (LDH) often occur as well. Severe metabolic acidosis and increased lactate levels above 4 mmol/L are poor prognostic signs.[142] The development of DIC or a clinically significant bleeding diathesis is seen only in a minority of patients.[34,143]

The hospital course is marked by a rapid and progressive increase in hypoxemia. Some patients abruptly have arrest in the emergency ward, and others require intubation within a few hours. About a third of patients are managed successfully with careful monitoring and oxygen administration. Severely ill patients may have copious quantities of endotracheal secretions with protein values exceeding 80% of those of serum and an electrophoretic pattern resembling that of serum.[138,142] Most deaths occur within 48 hours of admission. Patients who are stabilized and survive 2 to 3 days will usually survive, although a few die later with findings of diffuse alveolar damage[34]; it is not known whether this pulmonary finding is secondary to the HPS process or a reflection of lung damage from ventilatory support and secondary bacterial infection.

Although the pulmonary findings dominate the initial presentation of the patient, there are also important independent cardiovascular effects that can be fatal even if hypoxia is properly managed.[142,144] Patients often have low cardiac output, elevated systemic vascular resistance, and a normal or even low pulmonary wedge pressure. Fluid administration and inotropic support may not reverse this picture and the final outcome can be progressive lactic acidosis and fatal shock, often terminating in electromechanical dissociation. Echocardiography in some patients has shown left ventricular contractility to be markedly reduced.

Within a few days most patients will have an improved cardiopulmonary status, and respiratory and circulatory support can be discontinued. In the absence of complications, most patients leave the hospital within 10 to 14 days. No definite sequelae beyond those of intubation and hypoxia have been identified, although emerging studies suggest that there may be prolonged respiratory compromise in some cases.

Infection with Other Sigmodontine Hantaviruses

Most HPS identified in the United States and Canada has been caused by Sin Nombre virus. Different, but related, viruses have caused HPS in the United States and elsewhere in the Americas. The disease reported with Juquitiba virus in Brazil,[145] Laguna Negra virus in Paraguay,[93] Lechiguanas virus in Argentina, and Andes virus in Argentina and Chile[92,146,147] is virtually identical to that of Sin Nombre virus. In other situations there has been a similar clinical picture with variations. A single nonfatal infection with Black Creek Canal virus in Florida showed typical HPS associated with modest renal failure (creatinine, 4.6 mg/dL) and a markedly elevated serum creatine phosphokinase (CPK).[148] In the southern United States, three cases associated with Bayou virus have been seen and were also associated with renal failure and markedly elevated serum CPK; two patients survived.[149,150] In the northern zone of Argentina near Bolivia, concomitant renal failure also seemed to be commonly found in what is thought to be infection with Oran virus.[92,147] In one Andes virus outbreak in Argentina, flushing of the facial area was noted in some patients. An outbreak caused by Andes virus in Chile had several patients with petechiae and even frank bleeding.[151] Thus, the basic Sin Nombre virus pattern will probably have many variations as the clinical syndromes associated with these other viruses are delineated.

In Paraguay and in Salta province of Argentina, substantial antibody prevalence has been found among healthy persons sampled for surveillance purposes, but it is difficult to interpret these data relative to the virulence of the viruses known to cause HPS in those areas because the hantavirus specificity of the antibodies is unknown.[93,152] The surveys were performed with an immunoglobulin G (IgG) capture enzyme-linked immunosorbent assay (ELISA) that detects antibodies from a wide variety of sigmodontine and arvicoline hantaviruses.[139] Almost all Sin Nombre virus infections are clinically evident based on studies of contacts of index cases during the 1993 epidemic in the southwestern United States,[59] intensive searches for milder disease forms in clinics,[153] and the very low incidence of antibodies found in normal populations in the United States.[154]

Pathologic Features

Pathologic lesions in both HFRS and HPS are primarily vascular with generalized capillary dilation and edema. Hantaviral antigens are present in abundance within vascular endothelia of patients with fatal HPS and HFRS. In contrast, morphologic changes of the endothelium are uncommon and, when present, consist of prominent and swollen endothelial cells, suggesting that the increased vascular permeability and edema most likely stem from dysfunctional changes in endothelial cells.

In patients with HFRS, large amounts of protein-rich gelatinous retroperitoneal edema fluid is found during the hypotensive stage of the disease. A characteristic triad is congestion and hemorrhagic necrosis of the outer renal medulla, anterior pituitary, and right atrium.[96,112,119,155,156] Microscopically, the most characteristic changes in HFRS are seen in the kidney, with variable degrees of tubular dilation, degeneration, necrosis, interstitial hemorrhage, and mononuclear inflammatory cell infiltrates. These changes are mildest in NE and most severe in Hantaan virus–associated HFRS. An interstitial pneumonitis, similar to that seen in HPS, is seen in some fatal cases.

Typical fatal HPS cases differ from HFRS in that the lesions are primarily confined to the thoracic cavity and are not usually associated with hemorrhage.[33,34,156] Pleural effusions are accompanied by diffuse interstitial and alveolar pulmonary edema. Interstitial pneumonitis is characterized by mononuclear interstitial infiltrate composed of T cells (both CD4+ and CD8+) and activated macrophages. Hyaline membranes are usually scant, and other histopathologic features of diffuse alveolar damage typically are not present. In spite of abundant pulmonary capillary endothelial viral antigen expression, there are few morphologic lesions in most cases, even at the ultrastructural level. Lymphoid tissue shows an active immune response with variable numbers of immunoblasts present within the red pulp, periarteriolar sheaths of the spleen, and sinuses of lymph nodes. Hantaviral antigens can usually be detected in follicular dendritic cells present within germinal centers.[34]

PATHOGENESIS AND IMMUNITY

Both HFRS and HPS have remarkable similarities in their pathogenesis (see Table 68-2). In both diseases, antibodies are present from their earliest clinical stages[2,139,157,158] and activated T lymphocytes are found in peripheral blood.[33,159] This, of course, suggests an immunopathologic basis for at least part of the disease syndromes.

In the case of HFRS, several clinical findings must be addressed. The fever, increase in vascular permeability, and shock can be explained by the presence of mediators of inflammation released during the immune response to the virus.[160] Elevated serum levels of cytokines such as tumor necrosis factor-α (TNF-α), interleukin (IL)-6, IL-10, interferon (IFN)-γ, and IFN-α are present,[161,162] and within the kidney endothelial adhesion molecules are increased with the concomitant presence of mononuclear cells expressing TNF-α.[162] Nitric oxide (NO) production is also increased.[163] Bradykinin is one candidate for a major mediator of shock.[113]

The renal failure of HFRS is not simply due to shock and acute tubular necrosis, because of the lack of correlation of these clinical events with the histopathologic findings.[108] It is possible that metabolically vulnerable sections of the medullary nephrons near the cortical border suffer damage when the circulation to the kidney is compromised by intrarenal factors and circulatory instability.[160] Other factors may be involved, such as the intrarenal production of mediators and the infection of renal endothelial and tubular epithelial cells.[32,164,165] The extraordinary hyposthenuria seen during and after the oliguric phase is presumably related to the location of the lesion in the renal tubule. Anterior pituitary necrosis may have a similar pathogenesis involving its portal circulation. The origin of the right atrial necrosis and hemorrhage is not known. Bleeding during the early phases of the disease is probably related to vascular infection, with Hantaan virus triggering a procoagulant state in endothelium that leads to DIC. Later, a uremic coagulopathy is superimposed.

HPS is thought to result primarily from the influx of activated T lymphocytes into the lung with subsequent secretion of mediators and activation of macrophages.[34] Direct measurement of T-cell mediators in the circulation has supported this idea.[165]

One may ask whether HPS is just a variant of acute respiratory distress syndrome (ARDS) or of HFRS. While the finding of bilateral infiltrates and hypoxemia in HPS meets the usual clinical definition of ARDS, the clinical entity of sepsis-associated ARDS differs from HPS in clinical presentation,[141] pathology,[33,34] pathogenesis (typical ARDS damage mediated by polymorphonuclear leukocyte mechanisms), radiology,[140] and the presence of multiorgan dysfunction in ARDS.

Besides pulmonary dysfunction, another factor that may contribute to the severe shock syndrome observed in HPS patients is myocardial dysfunction. In occasional patients with HPS, extensive amounts of hantaviral antigens can be found in the microvasculature of cardiac tissues, despite little histologic evidence of tissue damage or inflammatory cell infiltrate. However, it is not clear how the magnitude or extent of involvement of cardiac endothelial cells contributes to the pathophysiology of the shock syndrome.

Similar comparisons with HFRS suggest that the pulmonary syndrome caused by Sin Nombre virus infection is a distinct entity. There is massive, selective accumulation of viral antigen in pulmonary endothelial cells, with other capillary beds far less affected and other cell types inconsistently involved. In HFRS, endothelial infection is also disseminated, albeit with some concentration in the kidney.[34,112,156] Although both HPS and HFRS demonstrate activation of mediators that participate in the sepsis syndrome, the patterns of organ involvement between the two diseases and compared with the sepsis syndrome are different (see Table 68-2). Severe HFRS from Hantaan virus infection regularly has early signs of DIC,[111] early activation of kinin pathways,[113] massive retroperitoneal edema,[119] and obvious cutaneous manifestations of increased vascular permeability and vascular instability,[39,108] whereas Sin Nombre virus infection uncommonly shows DIC or hemorrhagic manifestations and has massive intrathoracic vascular "leak" manifested by pulmonary edema and pleural effusions,[36] but signs of systemic vascular leak and dilation are not seen on physical examination.[138]

There is a pulmonary lesion in both HFRS and HPS; careful conventional and CT imaging has demonstrated pulmonary infiltrates or effusions in half of Puumala virus–infected patients as well as decreased diffusion capacity and other pulmonary functions in most patients with relatively mild HFRS, so clearly there is a functional defect in the lung to match the interstitial mononuclear infiltrate seen in postmortem examination of Hantaan virus–infected patients.[166,167] However, when pulmonary edema is seen in HFRS it usually is a consequence of overhydration, although occasionally it may occur early in the disease course, suggesting massive cytokine activation.[168–170] The pathogenesis of pulmonary lesions in HFRS requires more investigation, as does the origin of the renal and hemorrhagic lesions seen in some HPS patients, particularly those infected with sigmodontine hantaviruses other than Sin Nombre virus.

Host Factors

In Puumala infection, the host major histocompatibility complex (MHC) is either protective or predictive of more severe disease, depending on the haplotype.[171] In addition, data for all hantavirus diseases suggest that children suffer less disease than expected.[172] This has not been properly studied or analyzed in terms of infection-disease ratios and risk factors. The only HPS outbreak involving a significant number of children was the epidemic in Chile in which 6 of 28 (21%) patients were less than 16 years of age, compared with only 8 of 176 (4%) of U.S. patients.[151]

DIAGNOSIS

Differential Diagnosis of Hemorrhagic Fever with Renal Syndrome

Any patient with fever, thrombocytopenia, and renal abnormalities should be suspected of having hantavirus disease.

Common diseases entering into the differential diagnosis include leptospirosis, murine or louse-borne typhus, pyelonephritis, malaria, and other hemorrhagic fevers (see Chapter 65). In addition, poststreptococcal glomerulonephritis, blood dyscrasias, glaucoma, and acute abdominal emergencies may be important in the differential diagnosis. Severe cases may resemble fulminant sepsis, and milder cases could be mistaken for influenza, hepatitis A, or streptococcal pharyngitis. The leukemoid reaction occasionally seen may suggest leukemia to the inexperienced clinician, particularly with the appearance of myelocytes and atypical lymphocytes in peripheral blood. Hemoconcentration associated with vascular leak may be mistaken for dehydration in the febrile, vomiting patient; if hypotension is present it may be attributed to the dehydration, and ensuing renal failure may be attributed to the hypotension or the effects of antibiotics given for the presumed bacterial gastroenteritis.

The clinical picture of Puumala virus infection with its milder presentation and lesser abnormalities of blood and renal function can be difficult to recognize if the diagnosis is not considered and sought. The most important consideration, also valid for Hantaan virus infection, is disease mimicking an acute abdominal emergency, which should be distinguished by routine urinalysis and blood examination.

Differential Diagnosis of Hantavirus Pulmonary Syndrome

Recognition during the prodrome is difficult, but once dyspnea is reported, the finding of thrombocytopenia, left shift (often with leukocytosis and myelocytes), or immunoblasts is common and is helpful. Hypoxemia may be present early, even with a virtually normal chest radiograph.[140] Suspicion of the diagnosis during this phase is critical because of the precipitous fall in oxygenation that may occur over the next few hours. Confusing presentations with abdominal pain and gastrointestinal symptoms may cause misdiagnosis of an acute abdominal emergency. The initial fever and myalgia may lead to consideration of influenza, but the latter typically has cough and coryza among early symptoms, whereas HPS patients rarely have respiratory symptoms until the cardiorespiratory phase. Pneumococcal and other pneumonias can be ruled out because of the symmetric findings of interstitial infiltrates progressing to alveolar pulmonary edema in HPS, although a few cases have had asymmetric findings in the early hours of disease. Misdiagnosis of pneumonia has led to excessive fluid loads associated with antibiotic administration and misinterpretation of the elevated hematocrit as due to dehydration requiring rapid infusion of intravenous fluids.

It should be kept in mind that the flushing, conjunctival injection, and hemorrhagic signs, which are usual in severe or moderate HFRS, have not been seen in North American or in most South American cases until late stages of a minority of severe cases that demonstrate DIC. Renal failure may occur with Bayou, Black Creek Canal, or some South American viruses, but most infections with sigmodontine-derived hantaviruses will have only proteinuria and perhaps mild elevation of creatinine.

Laboratory Diagnosis

The diagnosis of all known hantavirus diseases is best made by IgM capture ELISA using an infected cell lysate as antigen and employing an uninfected control for each unknown serum. This test is sensitive, specific, rapid, and inexpensive.[139,157,158,173] Positive results have been obtained with virtually every serum sample from HFRS or HPS patients, including serum drawn during the early febrile phases. The test is cross-reactive and may detect acute hantavirus infections caused by other viruses than the one used to prepare the antigen, both a blessing and a curse depending on the situation. For example, the use of the Sin Nombre virus antigen has detected all known agents of HPS in the Americas.[139,145–149,151,174–176] Other serologic tests may be employed: Western blots with recombinant New World hantavirus antigens have provided useful diagnostic reagents,[175,177,178] and indirect fluorescent antibody (IFA) tests have classically been used in diagnosis of Hantaan virus infections.[1,177] Any "sandwich" IgM method suffers from the specificity of the IgM conjugate (a serious problem with IFA tests) and from competition between IgG and IgM antibodies as well as rheumatoid factor giving false positives, and any test without a negative antigen control for each serum sample must deal with the inevitable false positives arising from nonspecific "sticky" serum, as well as the possibility of binding to nonviral components of the test antigen preparation.[179] Serologic surveys or tests on convalescent patients may require IgG antibody determinations to assess the history of infection or to identify the infecting serotype. The IgG ELISA provides a sensitive, specific, and practical test for determining seroprevalence. Such antibodies are known to persist at least from the Korean War in the early 1950s until the late 1990s, and seroprevalence in many populations is less than 0.5%, suggesting considerable specificity. In general, when attempting to ascertain the infecting virus, Hantaan virus and Seoul virus are more cross-reactive with one another and the arvicoline and sigmodontine viruses among themselves. The most specific serologic test available is the neutralization test, but even in that assay differences between close phylogenetic relatives are not necessarily large and results can be misleading.[3,89,90,139,180,181] ELISA tests with truncated recombinant antigens[182] and hemagglutination-inhibition tests[79] have shown some utility in distinguishing Hantaan virus and Seoul virus infections, but the best serologic alternative to the technically difficult neutralization test in New World hantavirus infections has been Western blot tests with selected epitopes.[4,175,180] None of these assays has been evaluated against a battery of known sera, and unfortunately such a collection does not exist. The IFA test has been useful in detecting hantavirus disease around the world and is still useful for its cross-reactivity[66,139] but apparently suffers from nonspecific reactions that are more important in interpretation of data in low-incidence populations (T. G. Ksiazek, unpublished observations).[158,183]

The use of RT-PCR has been essential to recent advances in hantavirus research. Because the viruses are difficult to isolate, that approach is inefficient.

Development of sensitive primers to apply to clinical situations and to rodent reservoirs has allowed the definitive identification of the infecting hantavirus in large numbers of patients or suspected reservoirs for the first time.[5,61,184] RT-PCR has no obvious role in acute diagnosis because of the sensitivity of the IgM ELISA, but, combined with sequencing of the amplicon, it is essential when definitive identification of the infecting virus is needed. RNA can be amplified from serum or preferably clotted blood from patients with HPS for at least

10 days of illness and from many HFRS patients.[74,185] It must be borne in mind that cross-contamination between samples either in PCR or virus isolation is easy and that many reported results have been found spurious when sequencing and genetic analysis are applied. Sequencing of viral genomes can be useful in determining the geographical site of infection if sufficient background material is available to allow an assessment of the spectrum of genetic variability and if there is sufficient viral genetic divergence.[5]

Another important diagnostic modality is immunohistochemistry on formalin-fixed, paraffin-embedded tissue. This has been widely used in HPS to confirm diagnoses and to make retrospective assessments of suspicious cases.[34,112,186] RT-PCR can also rescue genetic information from paraffin blocks, but the technique requires careful primer adjustment and shielding against cross-contamination.[187]

TREATMENT

Hemorrhagic Fever with Renal Syndrome

As for HPS and other hemorrhagic fevers, rapid hospitalization in a setting of intensive monitoring and careful supportive care is extremely important. The experience in the Korean War strongly suggested that early helicopter evacuation improved the outcome relative to prolonged transport over rough roads. Conversely, long medical evacuation flights of seriously ill patients have been associated with adverse outcomes.[110] Management of shock (see previous discussion), judicious sedation and analgesia, careful evaluation for secondary infections, and appropriately timed dialysis for uremia, hypertension, or electrolyte abnormalities should keep the mortality well below 5% as compared with the 10% seen with careful management without dialysis and the even higher rate in inexperienced hands.

Ribavirin given intravenously within 4 days of onset was shown in one carefully controlled study in China to reduce mortality, bleeding, and the duration of renal failure in a setting in which hemodialysis was not available.[188] Immunosuppression, immunostimulation, and IFN play no role in therapy. In both HFRS and HPS, passive antibody administration has no established role. Indeed, these patients already have an ongoing immune response with neutralizing antibodies present at the onset of disease so that the use of Fab or other blocking strategies might be more plausible than an antiviral antibody strategy. Under these circumstances and in the absence of an animal model of human disease, it is difficult to see how an adequate scientific rationale for such therapy could be established.

The administration of steroids was reported to have a sparing effect in the Korean War experience.[189] In a randomized study of 48 carefully selected, clinically diagnosed HFRS patients with less than 72 hours of symptoms, those treated with 1.1 g oral cortisone over 5 days had a milder course than lactose placebo recipients. The duration of proteinuria and azotemia and the severity of azotemia were judged to be statistically significantly less in steroid-treated patients. Although not statistically different, the steroid group had less fever, were thought to be less "ill," and required less analgesia. No side effects were attributed to steroids; it is interesting that the two deaths in the placebo group were from irreversible shock, whereas the steroid-treated group tended to have less shock and had no irreversible shock. The three deaths in the steroid group were from gastrointestinal hemorrhage (one case) and bronchopneumonia (two cases). It is not clear that the findings in this small study are relevant to the therapy of hantavirus diseases today, given improvements in the ability to support patients, the potency of corticosteroid dosage, and the possible side effects of steroids.

Hantavirus Pulmonary Syndrome

Early recognition and admission of the patient are crucial to survival. A small minority of patients has been identified who do not seek medical care and survive, but because of the rapidity of decompensation all patients should have careful monitoring for administration of supplemental oxygen to combat hypoxemia; the majority will require intensive cardiopulmonary support. Mortality at best is about 30% to 40%. When patients first present, hypoxemia should be managed by high concentrations of inspired oxygen through a nonrebreathing mask, and the circulation should be supported by modest use of fluids and early administration of inotropic and pressor agents. If possible, a Swan-Ganz catheter should be used for careful monitoring of the circulation, and sufficient fluid should be given to assure adequate filling pressure. Fluids should not be "pushed" without monitoring, and it should not be assumed that patients will respond as those in septic shock with its differing hemodynamic pattern.

There is no known specific therapy for HPS. Ribavirin was used in an open-label study in 1993 and 1994, with no obvious improvement compared with untreated controls, perhaps because of the immunopathologic nature of the disease and the short time available between admission and death (usually only 24 to 48 hours).[190] Ribavirin is now under careful evaluation in a double-blind, placebo-controlled trial. Extracorporeal membrane oxygenator support has resulted in survival of a gravely ill patient expected to die, as has administration of NO.[144] Until a definitive diagnosis is obtained, treatable conditions such as plague, tularemia, or rickettsial diseases, which could be confused with HPS, should stimulate appropriate antibiotic coverage.

In high-risk situations or when dealing with contacts of patients such as in the Andes virus epidemic with person-to-person transmission,[176] the use of convalescent plasma containing neutralizing antibodies could be used early, or the subject could be monitored and treated with intravenous ribavirin at the first sign of fever. Neither of these approaches is of known efficacy, and both have potential side effects so they should be undertaken with careful virologic and clinical monitoring and informed consent, if at all.

PREVENTION

Reduction of human-rodent contact is the key to prevention. Guidelines generally emphasize the denial of access to dwellings by rodent-proofing, removal of cover for rodents near dwellings, and protection of food sources within homes.[96,191] For example, it has been possible to markedly reduce entry of rodents into rustic cabins in the United States with modifications of only moderate cost.[192] Infestations of rodents should be eliminated from dwellings by snap-trapping (do not use live traps or glue boards). Simultaneous rodent proofing is important to prevent reinfestation.[193,194] Pretreatment with insecticides is important in areas where plague is endemic.[191]

Handling dead rodents and cleaning rodent nests within buildings is probably dangerous, and gloves should be used to protect skin; the rodent and surrounding detritus should be wetted with a household disinfectant or detergent. Little work has been done on the environmental stability of hantaviruses because of the difficulty in assays and the many possible variables. The viruses are lipid-enveloped and susceptible to common disinfectants and would be lysed by thorough exposure to detergents. In solution they are quite labile at acid pH (<5.0) but are relatively stable when held at neutral pH, particularly if protein is present as a buffer. Small amounts of virus can be detected after several days at 4°C to 22°C. In limited experiments with dried Hantaan virus in buffer, residual infectivity was decreased after rehydration.[195,196] It is likely that excreta exposed to drying and environmental temperature no longer contain infectious virus after 1 to 2 days. Areas inhabited by rodents should be cleaned with a wet mop or after wetting with detergent; in no case should a vacuum cleaner be used. In the particular case of infrequently occupied cabins, the structure should be opened and allowed to ventilate for an hour or more before entering and cleaning. Disturbing the environment within such structures may result in rodent activity and generation of aerosols that are protected from dissipation by breezes and from inactivation by the ultraviolet light of sunshine.[101]

Nosocomial transmission or interpersonal transmission has never even been suspected in HFRS, in spite of the large number of patients and the lack of precautions during early hemodialysis therapy in Korea.[65,66,95] When large antigen accumulations were found in lung tissue of HPS patients,[34] it became particularly important to rule out spread to medical personnel, and no clinical or serologic evidence of such infection was found among 266 exposed health-care workers.[197] It was therefore surprising to find clear epidemiologic, ecological, and molecular genetic evidence of limited interpersonal spread during a small Andes virus epidemic in Patagonia in 1996.[176] The significance of this observation is unknown, but retrospective examination of the U.S. experience failed to find any evidence suggesting nosocomial or person-to-person transmission.[198]

The need to educate at-risk populations about the true risk from rodent exposure is acute in the United States where the disease is rare but the case-fatality rate is high.[143,199] Interestingly, in Europe, where there are many more infected persons, albeit with less mortality, there is almost no public health education. In some occupations and in residents of many areas of Asia and South America, rodent avoidance is not a practical solution, and vaccination is the only practical approach.

Vaccine development for hantaviruses may be particularly difficult given the lack of an animal model for hantavirus diseases and the fact that the diseases are thought to be immunopathologic in origin. Animal models do exist for encephalitis (suckling mice) and for antigen accumulation (hamsters, rabbits, rats, natural hosts) so that passive and active protection experiments can be done. Recent development of a realistic hamster model for HPS[200] should open the way for accelerated vaccine development.[201] In vitro neutralization of hantaviruses is efficient, and passive antibody transfer of polyclonal and monoclonal neutralizing serums can prevent infection in animal models.[4,202] In the mouse, CD8+ T lymphocytes are also capable of conferring protection.[203] Several types of immunogens have blocked hantavirus infection in these animal systems, including infection with cross-reacting hantaviruses, vaccinia-vectored genes, baculovirus-expressed proteins,[204] inactivated virus preparations,[205] and DNA vaccines.[201] The relatively close genetic relationships among the American hantaviruses,[206] the cross-reaction seen in neutralizing antibodies,[180] cross-reactive T cells,[207] and cross-protective relationships suggest that there might be a basis for a relatively simple vaccine protecting against multiple HPS viruses.

In Asia, Hantaan and Seoul viruses appear to be major health problems, and it may be possible to protect against both viruses with a single vaccine because cross-neutralization, cross-reactive T cells, and cross-protection against infection can be demonstrated in rodent systems.[203] In the Americas, the number of hantaviruses causing disease is large, and the impact of any one of the viruses is relatively small. If cross-protection could be obtained, there would be a place for a vaccine to deal with local epidemics and particularly high-risk situations.

Hantaan and Seoul virus vaccines are being tested in humans with initially promising results, and it is hoped that published efficacy trials in humans will be available to permit evaluation of their place in the prevention of HFRS.[205,208–210]

REFERENCES

1. Lee H, Lee P: Korean hemorrhagic fever. 1. Demonstration of the causative antigen and antibodies. Korean J Intern Med 19:371, 1976.
2. Lee HW, Johnson KM: Isolation of the etiologic agent of Korean Hemorrhagic fever. J Infect Dis 137:298–308, 1978.
3. Schmaljohn CS, Hasty SE, Harrison SA et al: Characterization of Hantaan virions, the prototype virus of hemorrhagic fever with renal syndrome. J Infect Dis 148:1005–1012, 1983.
4. Schmaljohn CS, Hasty SE, Dalrymple JM, et al: Antigenic and genetic properties of viruses linked to hemorrhagic fever with renal syndrome. Science 227:1041–1044, 1985.
5. Nichol ST, Spiropoulou CF, Morzunov S, et al: Genetic identification of a hantavirus associated with an outbreak of acute respiratory illness. [Comment]. Science 262:914–917, 1993.
6. Carey DE, Reuben R, Panicker KN, et al: Thottapalayam virus: A presumptive arbovirus isolated from a shrew in India. Indian J Med Res 59:1758–1760, 1971.
7. White JD, Shirey FG, French GR, et al: Hantaan virus, aetiological agent of Korean haemorrhagic fever, has Bunyaviridae-like morphology. Lancet 1:768–771, 1982.
8. Goldsmith CS, Eliott LH, Peters CJ, et al: Ultrastructural characteristics of Sin Nombre virus, causative agent of hantavirus pulmonary syndrome. Arch Virol 140:2107–2122, 1995.
9. Schmaljohn CS, Hooper JW: *Bunyaviridae:* The viruses and their replication. In Fields BN, Knipe DM, Howley PM, et al (eds): Fields Virology, 4th ed. Philadelphia, Lippincott-Raven, 2001, pp 1581–1602.
10. Spiropoulou CF, Morzunov S, Feldmann H, et al: Genome structure and variability of a virus causing hantavirus pulmonary syndrome. Virology 200:715–723, 1994.
11. Gavrilovskaya IN, Shepley M, Shaw R, et al: Beta3 integrins mediate the cellular entry of hantaviruses that cause respiratory failure. Proc Nat Acad Sci USA 95:7074–7079, 1998.
12. Garcin D, Lezzi M, Dobbs SM, et al: The 5′ ends of Hantaan virus (Bunyaviridae) RNAs suggest a prime-and-realign mechanism for the initiation of RNA synthesis. J Virol 69:5754–5762, 1995.
13. Hutchinson KL, Peters CJ, Nichol ST: Sin Nombre virus mRNA synthesis. Virology 224:139–149, 1996.

14. Chizhikov VE, Spiropoulou CF, Morzunov SP, et al: Complete genetic characterization and analysis of isolation of Sin Nombre virus. J Virol 69:8132–8136, 1995.
15. Flick K, Hooper J, Schmaljohn C, et al: Rescue of Hantaan virus minigenomes. Virology 306:219–224, 2003.
16. Spiropoulou CF: Hantavirus maturation. In Schmaljohn CS, Nichol ST (eds): Hantaviruses, Current Topics in Microbiology and Immunology. New York, Springer-Verlag, 2001, pp 33–46.
17. Ravkov EV, Nichol ST, Peters CJ, et al: Role of actin microfilaments in Black Creek Canal virus morphogenesis. J Virol 72:2865–2870, 1998.
18. Spiropoulou CF, Goldsmith C, Showmaker T, et al: Sin Nombre glycoprotein trafficking. Virology 308:48–63, 2003.
19. Ravkov EV, Nichol ST, Peters CJ, et al: Role of actin microfilaments in Black Creek Canal virus morphogenesis. J Virol 72:2865–2870, 1998.
20. Rodriguez LL, Owens JH, Peters CJ, et al: Genetic reassortment among víruses causing hantavirus pulmonary syndrome. Virology 242:99–106, 1998.
21. Plyusnin A, Kukkonen SKJ, Plyusnina A, et al: Transfection-mediated generation of functionally competent Tula hantavirus with recombinant S RNA segment. EMBO J 21:1497–1503, 2002.
22. Nichol ST: Bunyavirdae. In Fields BN, Knipe DM, Howley PM, et al (eds): Fields Virology, 4th ed. Philadelphia, Lippincott-Raven, 2001, pp 1603–1633.
23. Lee HW, French GR, Lee PW, et al: Observations on natural and laboratory infection of rodents with the etiologic agent of Korean hemorrhagic fever. Am J Trop Med Hyg 30:477–482, 1981.
24. Hooper JW, Larsen T, Custer DM, et al: A lethal disease model for hantavirus pulmonary syndrome. Virology 289:6–14, 2001.
25. Milazzo ML, Eyzaquirre EJ, Molina CP, et al: Maporal viral infection in the Syrian golden hamster: A model of hantavirus pulmonary syndrome. J Infect Dis 186:1390–1395, 2002.
26. French GR, Foulke RS, Brand OA, et al: Korean hemorrhagic fever: Propagation of the etiologic agent in a cell line of human origin. Science 211:1046–1048, 1981.
27. Gavrilovskaya IN, Chumakov MP, Apekina NS, et al: Adaptation to laboratory and wild animals of the haemorrhagic fever with renal syndrome virus present in the foci of European USSR: Brief report. Arch Virol 77: 87–90, 1983.
28. Elliott LH, Ksiazek TG, Rollin PE, et al: Isolation of the causative agent of hantavirus pulmonary syndrome. Am J Trop Med Hyg 51:102–108, 1994.
29. Nemirov K, Lundkvist A, Vaheri A, et al: Adaptation of Puumala hantavirus to cell culture is associated with point mutations in the coding region of the L segment and in the noncoding regions of the S segment. J Virol 77:8793–8800, 2003.
30. Lee HW: Korean hemorrhagic fever. Prog Med Virol 28:96–113, 1982.
31. Galeno H, Mora J, Villagra E, et al: First human isolate of hantavirus (Andes virus) in the Americas. Emerg Infect Dis 8:657–661, 2002.
32. Temonen M, Vapalahti O, Holthofer H, et al: Susceptibility of human cells to Puumala virus infection. J Gen Virol 74:515–518, 1993.
33. Nolte KB, Feddersen RM, Foucar K, et al: Hantavirus pulmonary syndrome in the United States: A pathological description of a disease caused by a new agent. Hum Pathol 26:110–120, 1995.
34. Zaki SR, Greer PW, Coffield LM, et al: Hantavirus pulmonary syndrome: Pathogenesis of an emerging infectious disease. Am J Pathol 146:552–579, 1995.
35. Yanagihara R, Silverman, DJ: Experimental infection of human vascular endothelial cells by pathogenic and nonpathogenic hantaviruses. Arch Virol 111:281–286, 1990.
36. Sundstrom JB, McMullan LK, Spiropoulou CF, et al: Hantavirus infection induces the expression of RANTES and IP-10 without causing increased permeability in human lung microvascular endothelial cells. J Virol 75:6070–6085, 2001.
37. Traub R, Wisseman CL Jr : Korean hemorrhagic fever. J Infect Dis 138:267–272, 1978.
38. Lee HW, Lee PW, Baek LJ, et al: Intraspecific transmission of Hantaan virus, etiologic agent of Korean hemorrhagic fever, in the rodent *Apodemus agrarius*. Am J Trop Med Hyg 30:1106–1112, 1981.
39. Peters CJ, Zaki SR, Rollin PE: Viral hemorrhagic fevers. In Mandell GL, Fekety R (eds): Atlas of Infectious Diseases. External Manifestations of Systemic Infections, Vol. 8. Philadelphia, Churchill Livingstone, 1997.
40. Mills JN, Ksiazek TG, Ellis BA, et al: Patterns of association with host and habitat: antibody reactive with Sin Nombre virus in small mammals in the major biotic communities of the southwestern United States. Am J Trop Med Hyg 56:273–284, 1997.
41. Dohmae K, Koshimizu U, Nishimune Y: In utero and mammary transfer of hantavirus antibody from dams to infant rats. Lab Anim Sci 43:557–561, 1993.
42. Glass GE, Childs JE, Korch GW, et al: Association of intraspecific wounding with hantaviral infection in wild rats (*Rattus norvegicus*). Epidemiol Infect 101:459–472, 1988.
43. Douglass RJ, Wilson T, Semmens WJ, et al: Longitudinal studies of Sin Nombre virus in deer mouse dominated ecosystems of Montana. Am J Trop Med Hug 65:33–41, 2001.
44. Glass GE, Livingstone W, Mills JN, et al: Black Creek Canal virus infection in *Sigmodon hispidus* in Southern Florida. Am J Trop Med Hyg 59:699–703, 1999.
45. Childs JE, Korch GW, Smith GA, et al: Geographical distribution and age related prevalence of antibody to Hantaan-like virus in rat populations of Baltimore, Maryland, USA. Am J Trop Med Hyg 34:385–387, 1985.
46. Niklasson B, Hornfeldt B, Lundkvist A, et al: Temporal dynamics of Puumala virus antibody prevalence in voles and of nephropathia epidemica incidence in humans. Am J Trop Med Hyg 53:134–140, 1995.
47. Escutenaire P, Chalon R, Verhagen P, et al: Spatial and temporal dynamics of Puumala hantavirus infection in red bank vole (*Clethrionomys glareolus*) populations in Belgium. Virus Res 67:91–107, 2000.
48. Nuzum EO, Rossi CA, Stephenson EH, et al: Aerosol transmission of Hantaan and related viruses to laboratory rats. Am J Trop Med Hyg 38:636–640, 1988.
49. Krebs DJ, Myers JH: Population cycles in small mammals. Adv Ecol Res 8:267–399, 1974.
50. Hornfeldt B: Delayed density dependence as a determinant of vole cycles. Ecology 75:791–806, 1994.
51. Centers for Disease Control and Prevention: Hantavirus pulmonary syndrome—Colorado and New Mexico, 1998. MMWR 47:449–452, 1998.
52. Centers for Disease Control and Prevention: Update: hantavirus pulmonary syndrome—United States, 1999. MMWR 48:521–525, 1999.
53. Toro J, Vega JD, Khan AS, Navarrete M, et al: An outbreak of hantavirus pulmonary syndrome, Chile, 1997. Emerg Infec Dis 4:687–694, 1998.
54. Marua R, Gonzales LE, Navarrete M, et al: Efectos del florecimiento del arbusto Chusquea quila Kunth (Poaceae) sobre la demografia de poblaciones de roedores de los bosques templados frios del sur Chileno. Bol Soc Biol (Conception, Chile) 67:37, 1996.
55. Mills JN, Ksiazek TG, Peters CJ, et al: Long-term studies of hantavirus reservoir populations in the southwestern United States: A synthesis. Emerg Infect Dis 5:135–142, 1999.
56. Yates TL, Mills JN, Parmenter RR, et al: The ecology and evolutionary history of an emergent disease: Hantavirus pulmonary syndrome. Bioscience 52:989–998, 2002.
57. Bayard V, Kitsutani PT, Barria EO, et al: Outbreak of hantavirus pulmonary syndrome, Los Santos Panama, 1999–2000. Emerg Infect Dis 10:1635–1642, 2004.
58. Carroll DS, Mills JN, Montgomery JM, et al: Hantavirus pulmonary syndrome in central Bolivia: Relationships between reservoir hosts, habitats, and viral genotypes. Am J Trop Med Hyg 72:42–46, 2005.
59. Zeitz PS, Butler JC, Cheek JE, et al: A case-control study of hantavirus pulmonary syndrome during an outbreak in the southwestern United States. [See comment]. J Infect Dis 171:864–870, 1995.
60. Ahlm C, Juto P, Stegmayr B, et al: Prevalence of serum antibodies to hantaviruses in northern Sweden as measured by recombinant nucleocapsid proteins. Scand J Infect Dis 29:349–354, 1997.
61. Childs JE, Ksiazek TG, Spiropoulou C, et al: Serologic and genetic identification of *Peromyscus maniculatus* as the primary rodent reservoir for a new hantavirus in the southwestern United States. J Infect Dis 169:1271–1280, 1994.
62. Rowe JE, St Jeor SC, Riolo J, et al: Coexistence of several novel hantaviruses in rodents indigenous to North America. Virology 213:122–130, 1995.
63. Nowotny N, Weissenboeck H, Aberle S, et al: Hantavirus infection in the domestic cat. JAMA 272:1100–1101, 1994.
64. Xu ZY, Guo CS, Wu YL, et al: Epidemiological studies of hemorrhagic fever with renal syndrome: Analysis of risk factors and mode of transmission. J Infect Dis 152:137–144, 1985.
65. Tsai TF: Hemorrhagic fever with renal syndrome: mode of transmission to humans. Lab Anim Sci 37:428–430, 1987.

66. Yanagihara R: Hantavirus infection in the United States: Epizootiology and epidemiology. Rev Infect Dis 12:449–457, 1990.
67. Dixon KE: A comparison of case-crossover and case-control designs in a study of risk factors for hemorrhagic fever with renal syndrome. Epidemiology 8:243–246, 1997.
68. Dournon E, Moriniere B, Girard P, et al: HFRS after a wild rodent bite in the Haute-Savoie and risk of exposure to Hantaan-like virus in a Paris laboratory. Lancet 1:676–677, 1984.
69. Kawamata J, Yamanouchi T, Dohmae K, et al: Control of laboratory acquired hemorrhagic fever with renal syndrome (HFRS) in Japan. Lab Anim Sci 37:431–436, 1987.
70. Dimmick RL, Vogl WF, Schmidt L, et al: Potential for accidental microbial aerosol transmission in the biological laboratory. In Hellman A, Oxman MN, Pollack R (eds): Biohazards in Biological Research. Cold Spring Harbor, New York, Cold Spring Harbor Laboratory, 1973, p 246.
71. Yanagihara R, Amyx HL, Gajdusek DC, et al: Experimental infection with Puumala virus, the etiologic agent of nephropathia epidemica, in bank voles (*Clethrionomys glareolus*). J Virol 55:34–38, 1985.
72. Gavrilovskaya IN, Apekina NS, Myasnikova YA, et al: Pathogenesis of hemorrhagic fever with renal syndrome virus infection and mode of horizontal transmission of hantavirus in bank voles. Arch Virol (suppl 1):57–62, 1990.
73. Hutchinson KL, Rollin PE, Peters CJ: Pathogenesis of a North American hantavirus, Black Creek Canal virus, in experimentally infected *Sigmodon hispidus*. Am J Trop Med Hyg 59:58–65, 1998.
74. Antoniadis A, Stylianakis A, Papa A, et al: Direct genetic detection of Dobrava virus in Greek and Albanian patients with hemorrhagic fever with renal syndrome. [See comment]. J Infect Dis 174:407–410, 1996.
75. LeDuc JW, Smith GA, Childs JE, et al: Global survey of antibody to Hantaan-related viruses among peridomestic rodents. Bull World Health Organ 64:139–144, 1986.
76. Lee HW, Baek LJ, Johnson KM: Isolation of Hantaan virus, the etiologic agent of Korean hemorrhagic fever, from wild urban rats. J Infect Dis 146:638–644, 1982.
77. Park SC, Pyo HJ, Joe JB, et al: A clinical study of hemorrhagic fever with renal syndrome caused by Seoul virus infection. Korean J Intern Med 4:130–135, 1989.
78. Chen HX, Qiu FX, Dong BJ, et al: Epidemiological studies on hemorrhagic fever with renal syndrome in China. J Infect Dis 154:394–398, 1986.
79. Li YL, Ruo SL, Tong Z, et al: A serotypic study of hemorrhagic fever with renal syndrome in rural China. Am J Trop Med Hyg 52:247–251, 1995.
80. Glass GE, Watson AJ, LeDuc JW, et al: Domestic cases of hemorrhagic fever with renal syndrome in the United States. Nephron 68:48–51, 1994.
81. Glass GE, Watson AJ, LeDuc JW, et al: Infection with a ratborne hantavirus in US residents is consistently associated with hypertensive renal disease. J Infect Dis 167:614–620, 1993.
82. Kariwa H, Isegawa Y, Arikawa J, et al: Comparison of nucleotide sequences of M genome segments among Seoul virus strains isolated from eastern Asia. Virus Res 33:27–38, 1994.
83. LeDuc JW: Epidemiology of Hantaan and related viruses. Lab Anim Sci 37:413–418, 1987.
84. LeDuc JW, Smith GA, Macy M, et al: Certified cell lines of rat origin appear free of infection with hantavirus. J Infect Dis 152:1082–1083, 1985.
85. McKenna P, van der Groen G, Hoofd G, et al: Eradication of hantavirus among laboratory rats by application of caesarian section and a foster mother technique. J Infect 25:181–190, 1992.
86. Avsic-Zupanc T, Poljak M, Furlan P, et al: Isolation of a strain of a Hantaan virus from a fatal case of hemorrhagic fever with renal syndrome in Slovenia. Am J Trop Med Hyg 51:393–400, 1994.
87. Antoniadis A, Stylianakis A, Papa A, et al: Direct genetic detection of Dobrava virus in Greek and Albanian patients with hemorrhagic fever with renal syndrome. [See comment]. J Infect Dis 174:407–410, 1996.
88. Lokugamage K, Karjwa H, Hayasaka D, et al: Genetic characterization of hantaviruses transmitted by the Korean field mouse (*Apodemus peninsulae*), far east Russia. Emerg Infect Dis 8:768–776, 2002.
89. Chu YK, Rossi C, LeDuc JW, et al: Serological relationships among viruses in the Hantavirus genus, family Bunyaviridae. Virology 198:196–204, 1994.
90. Xiao SY, Leduc JW, Chu YK, et al: Phylogenetic analyses of virus isolates in the genus Hantavirus, family Bunyaviridae. Virology 198:205–217, 1994.
91. Mills JN, Ellis BA, McKee KT, et al: A longitudinal study of Junin virus activity in the rodent reservoir of Argentine hemorrhagic fever. Am J Trop Med Hyg 47:749–763, 1992.
92. Levis S, Morzunov SP, Rowe JC, et al: Genetic diversity and epidemiology of hantaviruses in Argentina. J Infect Dis 177:529–538, 1988.
93. Williams RJ, Bryan RT, Mills JN, et al: An outbreak of hantavirus pulmonary syndrome in western Paraguay. Am J Trop Med Hyg 57:274–282, 1997.
94. Mills JN, Childs JE: Ecologic studies of rodent reservoirs: their relevance for human health. Emerg Infect Dis 4:529–537, 1998.
95. Gauld RL, Craig JP: Epidemiological pattern of localized outbreaks of epidemic hemorrhagic fever. Am J Hyg 59:32–38, 1954.
96. Smorodinstev AA, Chudokov VG, et al: In Smorodinstev AA, Chudakov VG, Churilov AV (eds): Hemorrhagic Nephrosonephritis. New York, Pergamon Press, 1959.
97. Korpela H, Lahdevirta J: The role of small rodents and patterns of living in the epidemiology of nephropathia epidemica. Scand J Infect Dis 10:303–305, 1978.
98. Dixon KE, Nang RN, Kim DY, et al: A hospital-based, case-control study of risk factors for hemorrhagic fever with renal syndrome in soldiers of the armed forces of the Republic of Korea. Am J Trop Med Hyg 54:284–288, 1996.
99. Nowotny N: The domestic cat: A possible transmitter of viruses from rodents to man. [Comment]. Lancet 343:921, 1994.
100. Childs JE, Krebs JW, Ksiazek T, et al: A household-based, case-control study of environmental factors associated with hantavirus pulmonary syndrome in the southwestern United States. Am J Trop Med Hyg 52:393–397, 1995.
101. Armstrong LR, Zaki SR, Goldoft MJ, et al: Hantavirus pulmonary syndrome associated with entering or cleaning rarely used, rodent-infested structures. [Comment]. J Infect Dis 172:1166, 1995.
102. Kuenzi AJ, Douglass RJ, White D, et al: Antibody to Sin Nombre virus in rodents associated with peridomestic habitats in west central Montana. Am J Trop Med Hyg 63:137–146, 2001.
103. Kim S, Kim W, Yoon HJ, et al: Changing patterns of epidemiology and death causes on epidemic hemorrhagic fever in Korea. Korean J Infect Dis 8:58, 1976.
104. Andrew R: Epidemic haemorrhagic fever: 40 cases from Korea. BMJ 1:1063–1068, 1953.
105. Ganong WF, Zucker E, Clawson CK, et al: The early field diagnosis of epidemic hemorrhagic fever. Ann Intern Med 38:61–66, 1953.
106. Earle DP: Analysis of sequential physiologic derangements in epidemic hemorrhagic fever; with a commentary on management. Am J Med 16:690–709, 1954.
107. Powell GM: Hemorrhagic fever: a study of 300 cases. Medicine (Baltimore) 33:97–153, 1954.
108. Sheedy JA, Froeb HF, Batson HA, et al: The clinical course of epidemic hemorrhagic fever. Am J Med 16:619–628, 1954.
109. Lee JG, Cho B, Lee MC, et al: Clinical features of serologically proven Korean hemorrhagic fever patients. Seoul J Med 21:163, 1980.
110. Bruno P, Hassell LH, Quan J, et al: The protean manifestations of hemorrhagic fever with renal syndrome: A retrospective review of 26 cases from Korea. Ann Intern Med 113:385–391, 1990.
111. Lee M, Kim BK, Kim S, et al: Coagulopathy in hemorrhagic fever with renal syndrome (Korean hemorrhagic fever). Rev Infect Dis 11 (suppl 4): S877–S883, 1989.
112. Zaki SR: Hantavirus-associated diseases. In Connor DH, Chandler FW, Schwartz DA, et al (eds): The Pathology of Infectious Diseases. Norwalk, CT, Appleton & Lange, 1997, p 125.
113. Sirotin BZ, Obukhova GG, Mogila TV: [Kallikrein-kinin, coagulative and fibrinolytic blood systems in patients with hemorrhagic fever and renal syndrome]. Terapevticheskii Arkhiv 53:84–87, 1981.
114. Entwisle G, Hale E: Hemodynamic alterations in hemorrhagic fever. Circulation 15:414–425, 1957.
115. Smyth AG, Powell GM: The electrocardiogram in hemorrhagic fever. Am Heart J 47:218–240, 1954.
116. Koh C, Kim W, Lee JS, et al: Clinical study of Korean hemorrhagic fever. Korean J Med 15:757, 1972.
117. Chun PK, Godfrey LJ: Unique selective right atrial hemorrhage with epidemic (Korean) hemorrhagic fever. Am Heart J 108:410–412, 1984.
118. Kim YS, Lee JS, Ahn C, et al: Magnetic resonance imaging of the kidney in hemorrhagic fever with renal syndrome: its histopathologic correlation. Nephron 76:477–480, 1997.

119. Hullinghorst RL, Steer A: Pathology of epidemic hemorrhagic fever. Ann Intern Med 38:77–101, 1953.
120. Valiakhmetov RZ, Gafarov AI, Memkhes VS, et al: [Spontaneous rupture of the kidneys in hemorrhagic fever with renal syndrome]. Urol Nefrol 6:50–53, 1990.
121. Lee JG, Han JS, Kim S, et al: Panhypopituitarism in the acute stage of hemorrhagic fever with renal syndrome: A case report. Arch Virol (suppl 1):95, 1990.
122. Desmyter J, LeDuc JW, Johnson KM, et al: Laboratory rat associated outbreak of haemorrhagic fever with renal syndrome due to Hantaan-like virus in Belgium. Lancet 2:1445–1448, 1983.
123. Lloyd G, Bowen ET, Jones N, et al: HFRS outbreak associated with laboratory rats in UK. Lancet 1:1175–1176, 1984.
124. Lahdevirta J: Nephropathia epidemica in Finland: A clinical histological and epidemiological study. Ann Clin Res 3:1–54, 1971.
125. Niklasson B, Hornfeldt B, Mullart M, et al: An epidemiologic study of hemorrhagic fever with renal syndrome in Bashkirtostan (Russia) and Sweden. Am J Trop Med Hyg 8:670–675, 1993.
126. Mustonen J, Brummer-Korvenkontio M, Hedman K, et al: Nephropathia epidemica in Finland: A retrospective study of 126 cases. Scand J Infect Dis 26:7–13, 1994.
127. Rollin PE, Coudrier D, Sureau P, et al: Hantavirus epidemic in Europe, 1993. [See comment]. Lancet 343:115–116, 1994.
128. Colson P, Damoiseaux P, Brisbois J, et al: [Epidemic of hantavirus disease in Entre-Sambre-et-Meuse, 1992–1993: Clinical and biological aspects]. Acta Clin Belg 50:197–206, 1995.
129. Kontkanen MI, Puustjarvi TJ, Lahdevirta JK, et al: Intraocular pressure changes in nephropathia epidemica: A prospective study of 37 patients with acute systemic Puumala virus infection. Ophthalmology 102:1813–1817, 1995.
130. Kleinknecht D, Rollin PE: Hypertension after hemorrhagic fever with renal syndrome. Nephron 61:121, 1992.
131. Niklasson B, Hellsten G, LeDuc JW: Hemorrhagic fever with renal syndrome: A study of sequelae following nephropathia epidemica. Arch Virol 137:241–247, 1994.
132. Niklasson B, LeDuc J, Nystrom K, et al: Nephropathia epidemica: Incidence of clinical cases and antibody prevalence in an endemic area of Sweden. Epidemiol Infect 99:559–562, 1987.
133. Niklasson B, Jonsson M, Lundkvist A, et al: Comparison of European isolates of viruses causing hemorrhagic fever with renal syndrome by a neutralization test. Am J Trop Med Hyg 45:660–665, 1991.
134. Alexeyev OA, Baranov BA: Puumala virus infection without signs of renal involvement. Scand J Infect Dis 25:525–527, 1993.
135. Alexeyev OA, Morozov VG, Efremor AG, et al: A case of haemorrhagic fever with renal syndrome complicated by spleen haemorrhage. Scand J Infect Dis 26:491–492, 1994.
136. Chan KP, Chan YC, Doraisingham S: A severe case of hemorrhagic fever with renal syndrome in Singapore. Southeast Asian J Trop Med Public Health 27:408–410, 1996.
137. Meng G, Lan Y, Nakagawa M, et al: High prevalence of hantavirus infection in a group of Chinese patients with acute hepatitis of unknown aetiology. J Viral Hepat 4:231–234, 1997.
138. Duchin JS, Koster FT, Peters CJ, et al: Hantavirus pulmonary syndrome: A clinical description of 17 patients with a newly recognized disease. The Hantavirus Study Group. [See comment]. N Engl J Med 330:949–955, 1994.
139. Ksiazek TG, Peters CJ, Rollin PE, et al: Identification of a new North American hantavirus that causes acute pulmonary insufficiency. Am J Trop Med Hyg 52:117–123, 1995.
140. Ketai LH, Williamson MR, Telepak RJ, et al: Hantavirus pulmonary syndrome: Radiographic findings in 16 patients. Radiology 191:665–668, 1994.
141. Moolenaar RL, Dalton C, Lipman HB, et al: Clinical features that differentiate hantavirus pulmonary syndrome from three other acute respiratory illnesses. Clin Infect Dis 21:643–649, 1995.
142. Hallin GW, Simpson SQ, Crowell RE, et al: Cardiopulmonary manifestations of hantavirus pulmonary syndrome. Crit Care Med 24:252–258, 1996.
143. Khan AS, Ksiazek TG, Peters CJ: Hantavirus pulmonary syndrome. Lancet 347:739–741, 1996.
144. Levy H: Hantavirus infection. Curr Opin Infect Dis 10:103, 1997.
145. Iversson LB, da Rosa AP, Rosa MD, et al: [Human infection by hantavirus in southern and southeastern Brazil]. Rev Associacao Medica Brasileira 40:85–92, 1994.
146. Lopez N, Padula P, Rossi C, et al: Genetic identification of a new hantavirus causing severe pulmonary syndrome in Argentina. Virology 220:223–226, 1996.
147. Parisi M, Enria E, Padula P, et al: Genetic identification of a new hantavirus causing severe pulmonary syndrome in Argentina. Medicina (B Aires) 56:1, 1996.
148. Khan AS, Gaviria M, Rollin PE, et al: Hantavirus pulmonary syndrome in Florida: Association with the newly identified Black Creek Canal virus. Am J Med 100:46–48, 1996.
149. Khan AS, Spiropoulou CF, Morzunov S, et al: Fatal illness associated with a new hantavirus in Louisiana. J Med Virol 46:281–286, 1995.
150. Hjelle B, Goade D, Torres-Martinez N, et al: Hantavirus pulmonary syndrome, renal insufficiency, and myositis associated with infection by Bayou hantavirus. Clin Infect Dis 23:495–500, 1996.
151. Hantavirus pulmonary syndrome—Chile, 1997. MMWR 46:949–951, 1997.
152. Enria DA, Briggler AM, Pini N, et al: Clinical manifestations of new world hantaviruses. [Review] Curr Topmicrobiol Immunol 256:117–134, 2001.
153. Simonsen L, Dalton MJ, Breiman RF, et al: Evaluation of the magnitude of the 1993 hantavirus outbreak in the southwestern United States. J Infect Dis 172:729–733, 1995.
154. Zeitz PS, Graber JM, Voorhes RA, et al: Assessment of occupational risk for hantavirus infection in Arizona and New Mexico. J Occup Environ Med 39:463–467, 1997.
155. Forslund T, Saltevo J, Anttinen J, et al: Complications of nephropathia epidemica: three cases. J Intern Med 232:87–90, 1992.
156. Zaki SR, Peters CJ: Viral hemorrhagic fevers. In Connor DH, Chandler FW, Schwartz DA, et al (eds): The Pathology of Infectious Diseases. Norwalk, Conn., Appleton & Lange, 1997, p 347.
157. Niklasson B, Kjelsson T: Detection of nephropathia epidemica (Puumala virus)–specific immunoglobulin M by enzyme-linked immunosorbent assay. J Clin Microbiol 26:1519–1523, 1988.
158. LeDuc JW, Ksiazek TG, Rossi C, et al: A retrospective analysis of sera collected by the Hemorrhagic Fever Commission during the Korean Conflict. J Infect Dis 162:1182–1184, 1990.
159. Lewis RM, Lee HW, See AF, et al: Changes in populations of immune effector cells during the course of haemorrhagic fever with renal syndrome. Trans R Soc Trop Med Hyg 85:282–286, 1991.
160. Peters CJ: Viral hemorrhagic fever. In Nathanson N, Ahmed R, Gonzalez-Scarano F (eds): Viral Pathogenesis. Philadelphia, Lippincott-Raven, 1997, p 779.
161. Krakauer T, LeDuc JW, Morrill JC, et al: Serum levels of alpha and gamma interferons in hemorrhagic fever with renal syndrome. Viral Immunol 7:97–101, 1994.
162. Linderholm M, Ahlm C, Settergren B, et al: Elevated plasma levels of tumor necrosis factor (TNF)–alpha, soluble TNF receptors, interleukin (IL)–6, and IL-10 in patients with hemorrhagic fever with renal syndrome. J Infect Dis 173:38–43, 1996.
163. Groeneveld PH, Colson P, Kwappenberg KM, et al: Increased production of nitric oxide in patients infected with the European variant of hantavirus. Scand J Infect Dis 27:453–456, 1995.
164. Kim S, Kang ET, Kim YG, et al: Localization of Hantaan viral envelope glycoproteins by monoclonal antibodies in renal tissues from patients with Korean hemorrhagic fever. Am J Clin Pathol 100:398–403, 1993.
165. Koster FT, Simpson SQ, Feddersen KM, et al: Immunopathogenesis of hantavirus pulmonary syndrome (HPS): Role of the T cell. In US-Japan Cooperative Medical Sciences Program. Abstracts of the 29th Joint Viral Diseases Panels Meeting, Santa Fe, New Mexico, 1996.
166. Linderholm M, Billstrom A, Settergren B, et al: Pulmonary involvement in nephropathia epidemica as demonstrated by computed tomography. Infection 20:263–266, 1992.
167. Linderholm M, Sandstrom T, Rinnstrom O, et al: Impaired pulmonary function in patients with hemorrhagic fever with renal syndrome. Clin Infect Dis 25:1084–1089, 1997.
168. Kim D: Clinical analysis of 111 fatal cases of epidemic hemorrhagic fever. Am J Med 39:218–220, 1965.
169. Bruno P, Hassell LH, Quan J, et al: Hemorrhagic fever with renal syndrome imported to Hawaii from West Germany. Am J Med 89:232–234, 1990.
170. Clement J, Colson P, McKenna P: Hantavirus pulmonary syndrome in New England and Europe. [Comment]. N Engl J Med 331:545–546, 1994; author reply 331:547–548, 1994.

171. Plyusnin A, Horling J, Kanenva M, et al: Puumala hantavirus genome in patients with nephropathia epidemica: Correlation of PCR positivity with HLA haplotype and link to viral sequences in local rodents. J Clin Microbiol 35:1090–1096, 1997.
172. Khan AS, Ksiazek TG, Peters CJ, et al: Viral hemorrhagic fevers. Semin Pediatr Infect Dis 8:64, 1997.
173. Ivanov AP, Tkachenko EA, Petrov VA, et al: Enzyme immunoassay for the detection of virus specific IgG and IgM antibody in patients with haemorrhagic fever with renal syndrome. Arch Virol 100:1–7, 1988.
174. Feldmann H, Sanchez A, Monrunov S, et al: Utilization of autopsy RNA for the synthesis of the nucleocapsid antigen of a newly recognized virus associated with hantavirus pulmonary syndrome. Virus Res 30:351–367, 1993.
175. Hjelle B, Jenison S, Torrez-Martinez N, et al: Rapid and specific detection of Sin Nombre virus antibodies in patients with hantavirus pulmonary syndrome by a strip immunoblot assay suitable for field diagnosis. J Clin Microbiol 35:600–608, 1997.
176. Wells RM, Sosa Estani S, Yadon ZE, et al: An unusual hantavirus outbreak in southern Argentina: person-to-person transmission? Hantavirus Pulmonary Syndrome Study Group for Patagonia. Emerg Infect Dis 3:171–174, 1997.
177. Jenison S, Yamada T, Morris C, et al: Characterization of human antibody responses to four corners hantavirus infections among patients with hantavirus pulmonary syndrome. J Virol 68:3000–3006, 1994.
178. Elgh F, Wadell G, Juto P: Comparison of the kinetics of Puumala virus specific IgM and IgG antibody responses in nephropathia epidemica as measured by a recombinant antigen–based enzyme-linked immunosorbent assay and an immunofluorescence test. J Med Virol 45:146–150, 1995.
179. Duermeyer W, Wielaard F, van der Veen J: A new principle for the detection of specific IgM antibodies applied in an ELISA for hepatitis A. J Med Virol 4:25–32, 1979.
180. Chu YK, Jennings G, Schmaljohn A, et al: Cross-neutralization of hantaviruses with immune sera from experimentally infected animals and from hemorrhagic fever with renal syndrome and hantavirus pulmonary syndrome patients. J Infect Dis 172:1581–1584, 1995.
181. Lundkvist A, Hukic M, Horling J, et al: Puumala and Dobrava viruses cause hemorrhagic fever with renal syndrome in Bosnia-Herzegovina: Evidence of highly cross-neutralizing antibody responses in early patient sera. J Med Virol 53:51–59, 1997.
182. Wang M, Rossi C, Schmaljohn CS: Expression of non-conserved regions of the S genome segments of three hantaviruses: evaluation of the expressed polypeptides for diagnosis of haemorrhagic fever with renal syndrome. J Gen Virol 74:1115–1124, 1993.
183. Tsai TF, Bauer SP, Sasso DR, et al: Serological and virological evidence of a Hantaan virus–related enzootic in the United States. J Infect Dis 152:126–136, 1985.
184. Nichol ST, Ksiazek TG, Peters CJ: Hantavirus pulmonary syndrome and newly described hantaviruses in the United States. In Eliott RM (ed): The Bunyaviridae. New York, Plenum Press, 1996, p 269.
185. Hjelle B, Spiropoulou CF, Torres-Martinez N, et al: Detection of Muerto Canyon virus RNA in peripheral blood mononuclear cells from patients with hantavirus pulmonary syndrome. J Infect Dis 170:1013–1017, 1994.
186. Zaki SR, Khan AS, Goodman RA, et al: Retrospective diagnosis of hantavirus pulmonary syndrome, 1978–1993: Implications for emerging infectious diseases. Arch Pathol Lab Med 120:134–139, 1996.
187. Schwarz TF, Zaki SR, Morzunov S, et al: Detection and sequence confirmation of Sin Nombre virus RNA in paraffin-embedded human tissues using one-step RT-PCR. J Virol Methods 51:349–356, 1995.
188. Huggins JW, Hsiang CM, Cosgriff TM, et al: Prospective, double-blind, concurrent, placebo-controlled clinical trial of intravenous ribavirin therapy of hemorrhagic fever with renal syndrome. J Infect Dis 164:1119–1127, 1991.
189. Sayer WJ, Entwhisle G, Uyeno BT, et al: Cortisone therapy of early epidemic hemorrhagic fever: A preliminary report. Ann Intern Med 42:839–851, 1955.
190. Chapman LE, Mertz GJ, Peters CJ, et al: Intravenous ribavirin for hantavirus pulmonary syndrome: Safety and tolerance during 1 year of open-label experience. Ribavirin Study Group. Antiviral Ther 4:211–219, 1999.
191. Centers for Disease Control: Hantavirus pulmonary syndrome—United States: updated recommendations for risk reduction. MMWR 51:1–13, 2002.
192. Glass GE, Johnson JS, Hodenbach GA, et al: Experimental evaluation of rodent exclusion methods to reduce hantavirus transmission to humans in rural housing. Am J Trop Med Hyg 56:359–364, 1997.
193. Hopkins AS, Whitetail-Eagle J, Corneli AL, et al: Experimental evaluation of rodent exclusion methods to reduce hantavirus transmission to residents in a Native American community in New Mexico. Vector Borne Zoonotic Dis 2:61–68, 2002.
194. Douglass RJ, Kuenzi AJ, Williams CY, et al: Removing deer mice from buildings and the risk for human exposure to Sin Nombre virus. Emerg Infect Dis 9:390–392, 2003.
195. Lee HW, Baek LJ, Seyons YW, et al: Physiochemical properties of Hantaan virus. 2. The effect of temperature and pH on infectivity of Hantaan virus. J Korean Soc Virology 13:23–28, 1983.
196. Schmaljohn J, Huggins JW: Laboratory and field safety. In Lee HW, Calisher CH, Schmaljohn C (eds): Manual of Hemorrhagic Fever with Renal Syndrome and Hantavirus Pulmonary Syndrome. Seoul, WHO Collaborating Center for Virus Reference and Research (Hantaviruses), Asan Institute for Life Sciences, 1999, pp 192–198.
197. Vitek CR, Ksiazek TG, Peters CJ, et al: Evidence against infection with hantaviruses among forest and park workers in the southwestern United States. Clin Infect Dis 23:283–285, 1996.
198. Wells RM, Young J, Williams RJ, et al: Hantavirus transmission in the United States. Emerg Infect Dis 3:361–365, 1997.
199. Yang L, Lloyd ES: Getting the message out: Use of private-sector partner to increase public awareness of hantavirus disease prevention. In Abstracts of the 124th Annual Meeting of the American Public Health Association, New York, 1996.
200. Hooper JW, Larsen T, Custer DM, et al: A lethal disease model for hantavirus pulmonary syndrome. Virology 289:6–14, 2001.
201. Custer DM, Thompson E, Schmaljohn CS, et al: Active and passive vaccination against hantavirus pulmonary syndrome with Andes virus M genome segment-based DNA vaccine. J Virol 77:9894–9905, 2003.
202. Arikawa J, Yao JS, Yoshimatsu K, et al: Protective role of antigenic sites on the envelope protein of Hantaan virus defined by monoclonal antibodies. Arch Virol 126:271–281, 1992.
203. Asada H, Balachandra K, Tamura M, et al: Cross-reactive immunity among different serotypes of virus causing haemorrhagic fever with renal syndrome. J Gen Virol 70:819–825, 1989.
204. Schmaljohn CS, Chu YK, Schmaljohn AL, et al: Antigenic subunits of Hantaan virus expressed by baculovirus and vaccinia virus recombinants. J Virol 64:3162–3170, 1990.
205. Schmaljohn C: Prospects for vaccines to control viruses in the family Bunyaviridae. Rev Med Virol 85:240–251, 1994.
206. Monroe MC, Morzunov SP, Johnson AM, et al: Genetic diversity and distribution of *Peromyscus*-borne hantaviruses in North America.[Erratum in Emerg Infect Dis 5:314, 1999]. Emerg Infect Dis 5:75–86, 1999.
207. Ennis FA, Cruz J, Spiropoulou C, et al: Hantavirus pulmonary syndrome: CD8+ and CD4+ cytotoxic T lymphocytes to epitopes on Sin Nombre virus nucleocapsid protein isolated during acute illness. Virology 238:380–390, 1997.
208. Lee H, Ahn C, Song JW, et al: Field trial of an inactivated vaccine against hemorrhagic fever with renal syndrome in humans. Arch Virol (suppl 1):35, 1990.
209. Chen H: Cooperative Group on the ninth-five years National Medical Scientific Study 96-906-03-13. Evaluation on the efficacy of vaccines against HFRS and study on their antibody dependent immunization enhancement and immunological strategy. Chung Hua Yu Fang I Hsueh Tsa Chih (Chin J Prevent Med) 8:321, 1997.
210. McClain DJ, Summers PL, Harrison SA, et al: Clinical evaluation of a vaccinia-vectored Hantaan virus vaccine. J Med Virol 60:77–85, 2000.

69

Sandfly Fever, Oropouche Fever, and Other Bunyavirus Infections

ROBERT B. TESH

INTRODUCTION

The family Bunyaviridae includes more than 300 antigenically distinct members, most of which are transmitted by arthropods.[1] At least 41 of these viruses have been associated with human illness in the tropics. Apart from those members that produce serious and sometimes fatal disease (i.e., the hantaviruses, Rift Valley fever virus, and Crimean-Congo hemorrhagic fever virus), most of the remaining human pathogenic tropical bunyaviruses produce nonspecific febrile illnesses. Because of their nonspecific nature and the limited virus diagnostic capabilities in many tropical countries, these infections are often unrecognized or are misdiagnosed as other more common febrile illnesses such as malaria or dengue. This chapter describes some of the more common bunyavirus fevers.

PHLEBOTOMUS (SANDFLY) FEVER

Historically, phlebotomus fever (PF) has been mainly a disease of military importance, since it typically has caused epidemics when large numbers of nonimmune adults enter an area of endemic virus activity. The disease occurred in troops during the Napoleonic Wars, the Austrian occupation of the Adriatic, the British colonization of India and Pakistan, and the North African and Mediterranean campaigns in World War II.[2,3] The largest reported outbreak of PF occurred in Serbia in 1948, when over 1 million persons were affected. PF outbreaks still occur among tourists vacationing in the Mediterranean region.[4–7]

Many of the PF group of viruses appear to be maintained in their insect vectors by vertical (transovarial) virus transmission.[3] Consequently, virus activity is determined primarily by adult sandfly activity rather than by the immune status of the local human or animal populations. During periods of vector abundance (i.e., summer in subtropical or Mediterranean climates and the rainy season in drier tropical climates), phlebovirus activity is continuous. In this situation one sees little illness in the native population, most of whom are already immune, but when a group of nonimmune adults enters the area, an epidemic quickly ensues.[2]

Although more than 40 PF virus serotypes have been described,[2] three viruses (Naples, Sicilian, and Toscana) account for most of the recognized PF cases. This is probably because their sandfly vectors (*Phlebotomus papatasi, P. perniciosus,* and *P. perfiliewi*) are highly anthropophilic, readily enter houses, and have a wide geographic distribution in the Mediterranean region and central Asia.[3] In contrast, most of the New World phleboviruses and their vectors have a more focal and sylvan distribution; consequently, PF cases in this region are infrequent and occur mainly in persons who enter forested areas for work or recreation.

After an incubation period of 3 to 5 days, PF begins suddenly with fever, severe frontal headache, retroorbital pain, photophobia, malaise, anorexia, nausea, vomiting, and low back pain.[8] The face is often flushed and the conjunctivae are injected, but a true rash is absent. The disease is self-limited, and symptoms usually disappear within 2 to 3 days; however, a general feeling of weakness and depression frequently lasts for a week or more after the illness. A marked leukopenia (<4000/μL), consisting of an initial lymphopenia, followed by a protracted neutropenia, also occurs in PF.[8]

Meningitis or meningoencephalitis sometimes occurs with Toscana virus infection. Originally described in central Italy, this infection probably occurs throughout much of the Mediterranean region of Europe. These cases began as classic PF, with a nonspecific febrile illness for 2 to 4 days before the appearance of more serious symptoms, such as nuchal rigidity, positive Kernig's sign, lethargy, and mental confusion.[7] In these cases the hematologic picture is similar to that of classic PF, but the cerebrospinal fluid (CSF) may show increased pressure, pleocytosis (11 to 1400 cells/μL), and elevated protein content. The neurologic abnormalities usually resolve in a few days, and patients recover spontaneously in 1 to 2 weeks, although headache may persist.

The recovery of phleboviruses from patients with PF is uncommon, since the viremia associated with this disease is quite transient (24 to 36 hours), and most patients do not seek medical care so early. The one exception is patients with neurologic disease due to Toscana virus infection; virus can sometimes be recovered from the CSF after it has disappeared from the blood.[6] Culture in Vero cells is the isolation system of choice for most phleboviruses.[2]

A number of serologic techniques can be used for the diagnosis of PF, but each has its limitations. The IgM-capture enzyme-linked immunosorbent assay (ELISA)[9] and plaque reduction neutralization test (PRNT)[2,10] are quite specific and sensitive, but one must screen against a variety of phlebovirus serotypes because of their focal and sometimes overlapping distribution. Seroconversion can be demonstrated in paired samples by IgG ELISA and by fluorescent antibody (FA) or hemagglutination-inhibition (HI) tests, but these techniques are not serotype-specific.

Treatment of PF is symptomatic. Except for patients with neurologic symptoms, as in Toscana virus infection, hospitalization is usually unnecessary. The headache associated with PF can be severe, and narcotics are sometimes needed for relief.

PF is a self-limited, nonfatal disease, and recovery is complete. One attack of PF confers lifelong immunity against the infecting virus type but not against heterologous serotypes.[8,10] Thus, second cases of the disease can occur among persons living in regions where more than one phlebovirus is active. There are no vaccines for PF. Control measures are directed against the vector and include household spraying with residual insecticides and the use of insect repellents.[3]

OROPOUCHE FEVER

Oropouche fever is a midge-borne viral disease that has emerged during the past 40 years as an increasing public health problem in tropical America.[11,12] The causative agent, Oropouche virus, was first isolated from the blood of a febrile forest worker in Trinidad in 1955.[13] Since 1961, about 30 outbreaks of Oropouche virus have been reported from the Amazon regions of Brazil and Peru and from Panama.[12] The number of persons affected has varied with each outbreak, but the two largest recorded epidemics (Belem and Manaus, Brazil, in 1980 and 1981) each involved about 100,000 people.

It is postulated that Oropouche virus is maintained in two distinct cycles: (1) an epidemic urban cycle involving the biting midge *Culicoides paraensis* and possibly *Culex quinquefasciatus* mosquitoes; and (2) a silent maintenance cycle in which forest animals (principally sloths) are the vertebrate hosts, and a yet unidentified arthropod serves as the vector.[11] However, the epidemiology of this disease is still not fully elucidated. It is often confused with dengue and other flulike illnesses, and the true incidence is unknown.[12]

Oropouche fever is characterized by the abrupt onset of fever, chills, severe headache, generalized myalgia, arthralgia, anorexia, weakness, dizziness, and photophobia.[11] Nausea, vomiting, diarrhea, and epigastric pain may also occur. Some Oropouche fever patients exhibit brief meningitic symptoms. Rash is rarely present, but leukopenia is a common feature of this disease. The acute clinical illness usually lasts 2 to 5 days, although a period of asthenia and occasionally dizziness may persist for up to a month. A significant percentage of patients (as high as 60% in some outbreaks) have a recrudescence of their original symptoms within 2 to 10 days after they become afebrile.[11] The recurrent illness associated with Oropouche fever seems to occur more commonly in persons who quickly resume strenuous activities. No virus can be isolated from the patient's serum during the recurrent illness, and detectable humoral antibodies are usually present.

Oropouche virus can often be isolated from the patient's serum during the first 2 to 4 days of the disease. The virus can be isolated in newborn mice, adult hamsters, and a variety of mammalian cell cultures. Demonstration of virus-specific antibody can be demonstrated by ELISA, FA, HI, or the PRNT. Treatment is symptomatic. No fatalities have been reported with Oropouche fever; lifelong immunity follows recovery.

There is no vaccine against Oropouche fever. Given our limited knowledge of the maintenance cycle of Oropouche virus, vector control appears to be the best prevention and control strategy. *C. paraensis* is a daytime biter and, because of its tiny size, readily passes through window screens. Spraying in and around houses with residual insecticides seems to be the best method of control of adult peridomestic populations of this midge vector. Cleaning up rotting vegetation (banana stalks, decomposing fruit, etc.) around houses also helps to eliminate *C. paraensis* larval breeding sites.

GROUP C AND GUAMA VIRUS INFECTIONS

Group C and Guama viruses are found throughout the New World tropics and subtropics, including Florida, Central America, and the warmer regions of South America.[14] At least 25 different virus serotypes have been identified. Most of the serotypes have focal distribution which coincides with forest or forest-fringe habitats, usually in low-lying swampy areas. These viruses are maintained in a continuous sylvan cycle involving mosquitoes, mainly *Culex* of the subgenus *Melanoconion,* and small mammals such as rodents and marsupials. Humans are infected when they enter the swampy habitats where these viruses are endemic and are bitten by infected mosquitoes. Cases are usually sporadic, and because they are usually not reported, their true incidence is unknown.

Persons infected by group C and Guama group viruses develop sudden fever (38°C to 40°C), severe headache, vertigo, myalgia, arthralgia, and nausea. The fever lasts 2 to 5 days and is sometimes biphasic. Rash is absent. Patients recover with weakness and anorexia lasting 1 or 2 weeks, but without sequelae.

These viruses can be recovered from patients' serum during the acute febrile phase of the illness. They grow well in a variety of cell cultures and kill newborn mice and hamsters. Antibodies can also be detected in paired acute and convalescent serum by HI, ELISA, FA, and the PRNT. Treatment is symptomatic. The major risk factor is occupation; avoidance of swampy forest habitats or personal protection against mosquito bites is the only prevention.

BWAMBA, ILESHA, AND TATAGUINE VIRUS INFECTIONS

These three bunyaviruses have been isolated repeatedly from sick persons and mosquitoes in east, central, and west Africa.[15,16] The diseases associated with them are similar: the acute onset of fever, headache, vertigo, severe myalgia, and rash, lasting 4 to 5 days and followed by a week or more of asthenia. No deaths or serious complications have been reported. Most of the mosquito isolations of Bwamba, Ilesha, and Tataguine viruses have been made from *Anopheles* and *Aedes* species.[15] The viruses are thought to be maintained in a mosquito-wild vertebrate cycle, but little other information is available. Given their demonstrated disease potential, wide geographic distribution, and the relatively high antibody rates found in serosurveys among humans in some African countries,[14,15] it seems likely that these agents are of greater health importance to the local populations and to visitors than is currently recognized. But because of the paucity of functioning virus laboratories in Africa and the nonspecific nature of illness associated with them, most of these infections are probably never recognized or reported. Diagnosis can be made by virus isolation from blood during the febrile period or by antibody detection in paired acute and convalescent sera.

REFERENCES

1. Elliott RM, Bouloy M, Calisher CH, et al: Family Bunyaviridae. In van Regenmortel MHV, Fauquet CM, Bishop DHL, et al (eds): Virus Taxonomy. Classification and Nomenclature of Viruses. San Diego, CA, Academic Press, 2000, p 599.
2. Tesh RB: Phlebotomus fevers. In Monath TP (ed): The Arboviruses: Epidemiology and Ecology, vol. 6. Boca Raton, FL, CRC Press, 1989, p 15.
3. Tesh RB: The genus *Phlebovirus* and its vectors. Ann Rev Entomol 33:169, 1988.
4. Eitrem R, Niklasson B, Weiland O: Sandfly fever among Swedish tourists. Scand J Infect Dis 23:451, 1991.
5. Schwarz TF, Jager G, Gilch S, et al: Travel-related vector-borne virus infections in Germany. In Schwarz TF (ed): Imported Virus Infections. Vienna, Springer-Verlag, 1996, p 57.
6. Verani P, Nicoletti L: Phlebovirus infections. In Porterfield JS (ed): Exotic Viral Infections. London, Chapman & Hall, 1995, p 295.
7. Braito A, Ciufolini MG, Pippi L, et al: Phlebotomus-transmitted Toscana virus infections of the central nervous system: A seven-year experience in Tuscany. Scand J Infect Dis 30:505, 1998.
8. Bartonelli PJ, Tesh RB: Clinical and serological responses of volunteers infected with phlebotomus fever virus (Sicilian type). Am J Trop Med Hyg 25:456, 1976.
9. Eitrem R, Vene S, Niklasson B: ELISA for detection of IgM and IgG antibodies to sandfly fever Sicilian virus. Res Virol 142:387, 1991.
10. Tesh RB, Duboise SM: Viremia and immune response with sequential *Phlebovirus* infections. Am J Trop Med Hyg 36:622, 1987.
11. LeDuc JW, Pinheiro FP: Oropouche fever. In Monath TP (ed): The Arboviruses: Epidemiology and Ecology, vol. 4. Boca Raton, FL, CRC Press, 1989, p 1.
12. Tesh RB: The emerging epidemiology of Venezuelan hemorrhagic fever and Oropouche fever in tropical South America. Ann NY Acad Sci 740:129, 1994.
13. Anderson DR, Spence L, Downs WG, et al: Oropouche virus: A new human disease agent from Trinidad, West Indies. Am J Trop Med Hyg 10:574, 1961.
14. Shope RE, Woodall JP, Travassos da Rosa A: The epidemiology of diseases caused by viruses in groups C and Guama (Bunyaviridae). In Monath TP (ed): The Arboviruses: Epidemiology and Ecology, vol. 3. Boca Raton, FL, CRC Press, 1988, p 37.
15. Gonzalez JP, Georges A-J: Bunyaviral fevers: Bunyamwera, Ilesha, Germiston, Bwamba, and Tataguine. In Monath TP (ed): The Arboviruses: Epidemiology and Ecology, vol. 2. Boca Raton, FL, CRC Press, 1988, p 87.
16. Calisher CH, Nathanson N: Bunyavirus infections. In Porterfield JS (ed): Exotic Viral Infections. London, Chapman & Hall, 1995, p 247.

70

Filovirus Infections

VICTORIA WAHL-JENSEN
HEINZ FELDMANN
ANTHONY SANCHEZ
SHERIF R. ZAKI
PIERRE E. ROLLIN
C. J. PETERS

INTRODUCTION

Within the family *Filoviridae* there are two genera, *Marburgvirus* and *Ebolavirus*. The hemorrhagic fevers caused by filoviruses are among the most severe with high mortality rates. Filoviruses are considered emerging/reemerging zoonotic agents whose natural host remains unknown. The viruses are highly pathogenic in human and nonhuman primates, and the frequency of outbreaks and their impact on wildlife has been increasing in recent years. Introduction into the human population can lead to serious epidemics when inadequate sterilization of needles and lack of barrier nursing practices result in nosocomial transmission. Interhuman transmission also appears to occur in African homes by contamination through fomites and droplets. In the laboratory setting, the viruses are highly infectious by small-particle aerosols. The viruses attack endothelial cells, dendritic cells, macrophages, and other cells to produce severe hemorrhagic fever for which there is no established treatment.

AGENTS

Taxonomy

The family *Filoviridae* is currently divided into two genera, *Marburgvirus* and *Ebolavirus*.[1] Within the genus *Marburgvirus*, there is a single species *Lake Victoria marburgvirus* that is designated "MARV" and contains six strains with the prototype being strain Musoke. The genus *Ebolavirus* consists of four recognized species: *Ivory Coast ebolavirus* (ICEBOV), *Reston ebolavirus* (REBOV), *Sudan ebolavirus* (SEBOV) and *Zaire ebolavirus* (ZEBOV). The prototype virus for the genus is ZEBOV strain Mayinga.

Evolution

The phylogeny of filoviruses has been determined using GP gene sequences.[2–5] These studies indicate that the family *Filoviridae* has undergone a great deal of divergence. At the nucleotide level, Ebola and Marburg viruses differ by approximately 55%, and at the amino acid level by up to 67%. This divergence is also manifested in the GP gene organization (expression strategy), as discussed in the following sections. There is also a significant amount of variation among Ebola viruses, which differ from 37% to 40% at the nucleotide level and 34% to 43% at the amino acid level.[2] This divergence indicates that the ICEBOV, REBOV, SEBOV, and ZEBOV represent distinct clades within the phylogenetic tree and probably are distinct virus species. Despite the marked genetic divergence seen in the family, within each species of Ebola virus there is a remarkable amount of genetic stasis.[2,6,7] This stability may point to a state of extreme fitness within a given ecological niche that has not changed appreciably over the last few decades. It is anticipated that filoviruses will be found to be associated with a particular natural host,[8] and that genetic variation seen in the family reflects adaptations of these viruses to their hosts, perhaps even coevolution of virus and host. The similar replication strategy of the family *Filoviridae* to other members of the order Mononegavirales shows their common evolutionary origin from an ancient progenitor. Phylogenetic analyses of conserved polymerase amino acid sequences clearly separate families from one another, but these comparisons show filoviruses to be more closely related to paramyxoviruses than to rhabdoviruses and that pneumoviruses are more like filoviruses than are other paramyxoviruses.[9]

Virion Structure

Virions are filamentous but pleomorphic, often occurring as either long filamentous forms (with branching) that can reach 14 μm in length, and shorter forms that appear as U, 6, or circular shapes.[10,11] Electron microscopy studies of MARV and EBOV demonstrate ultrastructural differences between MARV and other filoviruses.[11] All filovirus particles have a uniform diameter of 80 nm, but MARV virions recovered from culture fluids are consistently shorter (795–828 nm) than SEBOV (974–1063 nm), ZEBOV (990–1086 nm), or REBOV (1026–1083 nm) particles. Virions are surrounded by a host cell, plasma membrane–derived lipid envelope studded with surface glycoprotein spikes approximately 7 nm in diameter and spaced 5 nm to 10 nm apart on the envelope.[11] The lipid envelope provides protection for the helical nucleocapsid (50 nm in diameter with an axial space 20 nm in diameter and a helical periodicity of 5 nm). The molecular mass of an average filoviral particle is $3–6 \times 10^8$ Da with a density in potassium tartrate of 1.14 g/cm^3.

Genome Organization and Replication

The genome of all filoviruses consists of a nonsegmented, single, negative-stranded linear RNA molecule and contributes 1.1% of the total virion mass with a molecular mass of approximately 4.0×10^6 Da. The average size of a filoviral genome is 19 kb with MARV being slightly larger then EBOV (MARV 19.1 kb; EBOV 18.9 kb). The complete nucleic acid sequence for three strains of MARV (Popp 1967, Musoke 1980, and M/S.Africa/Johannesburg/1975/Ozolin) and four EBOV strains (ZEBOV Zaire strain 1995, ZEBOV strain Mayinga, REBOV strain Pennsylvania, and REBOV strain Philippines) have been determined.[12–15]

The linear arrangement of the genes is nucleoprotein (NP), virion structural protein (VP) 35, VP40, glycoprotein (GP),

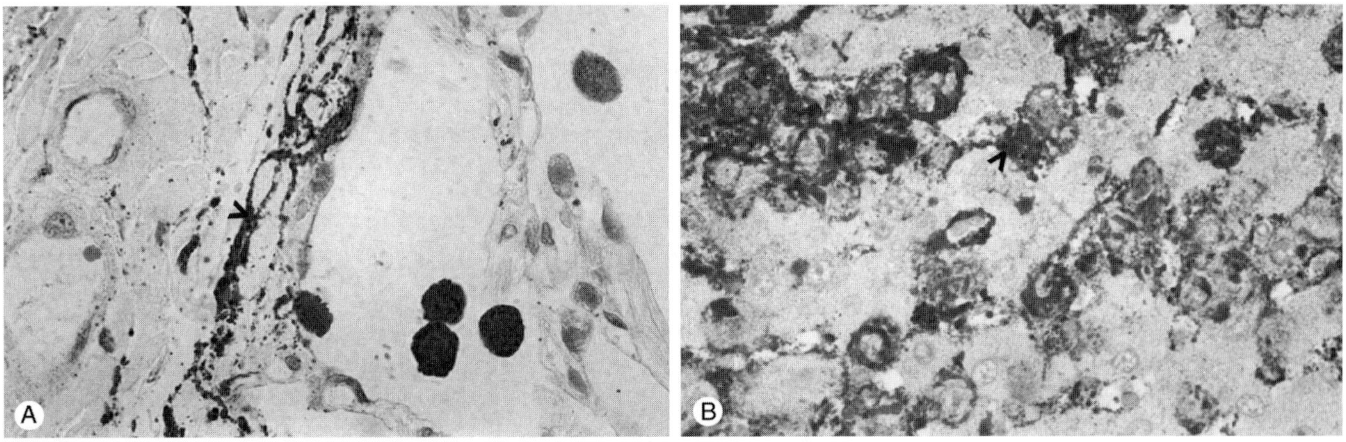

FIGURE 70-3 Ebola virus antigen–positive cells in lung and liver of an Ebola patient as determined by immunohistochemistry. *A,* Lung showing fibroblast and endothelial cell infection *(arrowhead)* as well as involvement of several alveolar macrophages. *B,* Heavy viral burden and necrosis can be seen in this section of liver immunostained for Ebola virus antigens. Viral antigens are in hepatocytes and Kupffer cells, many of which are necrotic *(arrowhead).* (Immunoalkaline phosphatase staining, naphthol-fast red substrate with light hematoxylin counterstain; *A,* ×158; *B,* ×250.)

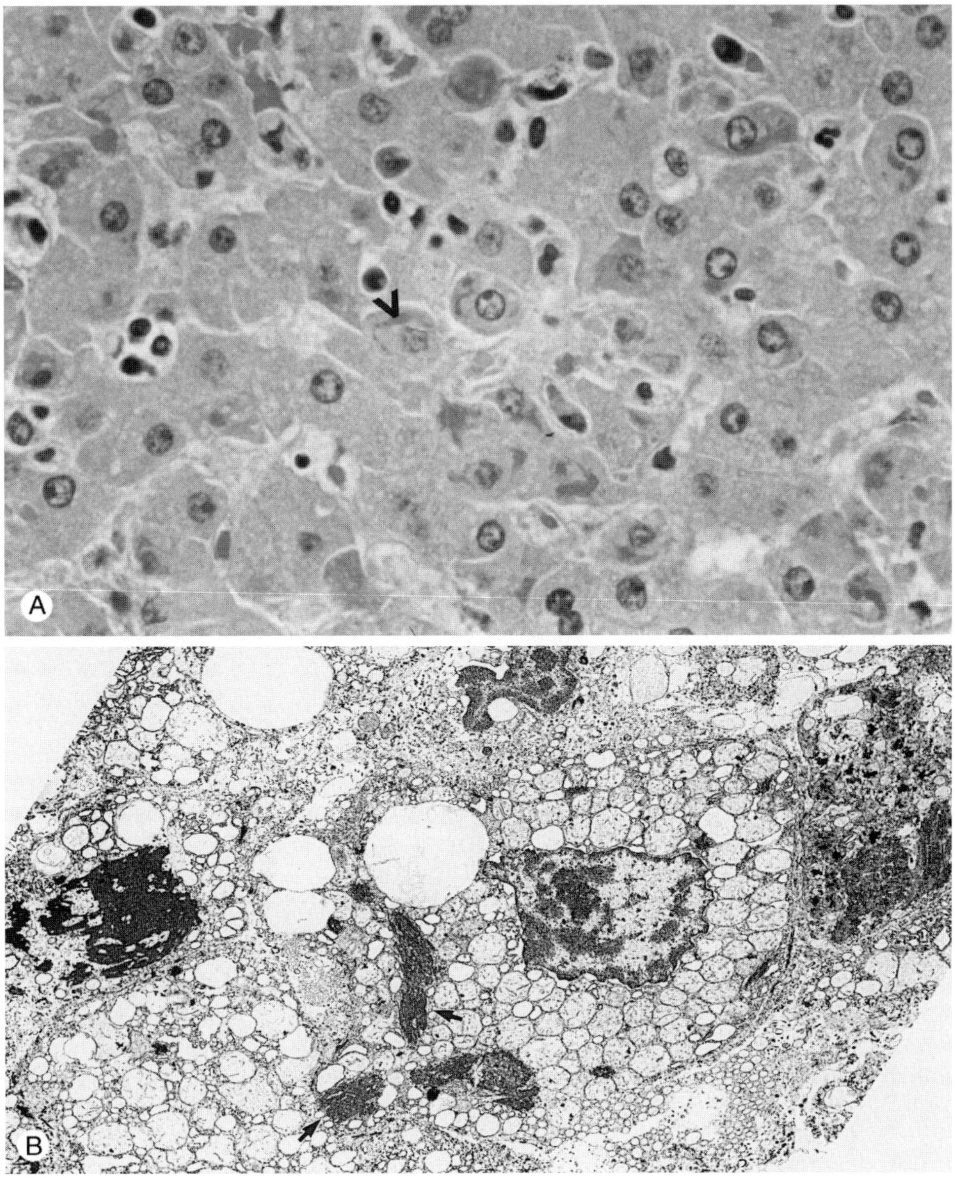

FIGURE 70-4 Liver in Ebola virus infection. *A,* Photomicrograph of liver showing hepatocellular necrosis and numerous, eosinophilic, crescent-shaped, intracytoplasmic viral inclusions typical of Ebola virus infection *(arrowhead).* (Hematoxylin and eosin, ×158.) *B,* Thin-section electron micrograph of same liver demonstrating that inclusions *(arrows)* are composed of aggregrates of viral nucleocapsid. (×7,000.)

in addition to studies using susceptible animal models (mice, guinea pigs, and nonhuman primates). The high containment setting necessary to study filoviruses, along with certain inconsistencies between animal models and human infection, have proven to be challenges in the understanding of filovirus pathogenesis. One aspect concerning animal models that should be kept in mind is that they do not always adequately reproduce EHF; specifically, there are differences in hemorrhagic manifestations, coagulopathy, and bystander apoptosis. Despite these challenges, recent studies have shed significant light on the current model of pathogenesis.

The primary mechanism for human filoviral infection is close contact with skin and secretory products from infected individuals. Virus is believed to enter via small skin lesions and mucous membranes from which it can acquire direct access to the vascular system or indirect access through the lymphatic system.[88] Monocytes/macrophages and dendritic cells (DC) are primary sites of viral replication.[97,103–105] Cells of the mononuclear phagocytic system (MPS) located in multiple organs including the liver (Kupffer cells), spleen, lymph nodes, lung (alveolar macrophages), serous cavities (pleural and peritoneal macrophages) and nervous system (microglia) are infected; however, the lymph nodes, liver, and spleen are the organs consistently preferred for filovirus replication.[89] Organ tropism may be enhanced by direct access of particles to sessile cells of the MPS without penetration of cellular or tissue barriers.[106] Subsequent to infection and replication in macrophages, viral particles gain secondary access to lymph nodes and then ultimately the vascular system, which initiates a state of viremia.[88] In addition to tissues from fatal human cases and in vitro studies, a serial sacrifice experiment of EHF in cynomolgus monkeys has given a tremendous amount of data regarding the progression of disease in the animal model that most closely resembles human infection.[103,107] Virus was shown to spread from initial infection sites by monocytes and dendritic cells to regional lymph nodes, most probably via lymphatics, and to liver and spleen via blood. Virus was then shown to infect tissue macrophages, DC, and fibroblastic reticular cells (FRC).[103] Monocytes/macrophages have been shown experimentally to be early and sustained targets of EBOV in both guinea pigs and moribund monkeys.[61,104,108,109] The recent study in cynomolgus monkeys confirmed these observations with viral RNA detected in lymphoid monocytes/macrophages as early as two days postinfection.[103] The interaction between filoviruses and DC may be critical for the outcomes of EBOV infections. The lymphoid hypoplasia and lack of a detectable immune response in fatal infections could be explained by the early infection of dendritic cells, their increased expression of the TNF-related apoptosis-inducing ligand TRAIL and bystander apoptosis of lymphocytes, the partial suppression MHC class II in EBOV-infected immature dendritic cells,[110,111] and the putatively immunosuppressive motif in the C-terminal region of $GP_{1,2}$.[2,13,112] In tandem with T-lymphocyte depletion, infected monocytes/macrophages release a host of soluble mediators including proinflammatory cytokines such as MIP-1α and MCP-1. These cytokines usually recruit additional macrophages to infected areas and in EHF could increase the number of target cells available for viral infection and further amplify an already dysregulated host response.[103] Cultured primary human monocytes/macrophages are also activated upon infection resulting in an increase of TNF-α, interleukin (IL)-1β, IL-6, and IL-8.[113,114] Infection by MARV led to a significant increase in release of TNF-α with peak values of 3 ng/mL by 12–24 hours postinfection. UV-inactivation of whole virus does not impair the activation of production of cytokines at either the transcriptional or protein level.[113] EBOV-infected patients also exhibit increased serum levels of various cytokines, and increased levels of IL-10, neopterin, and IL-1 receptor antagonist (IL-1RA) have correlated with fatal outcome, whilst presence of IL-1β and elevated concentrations of IL-6 in the plasma during the symptomatic phase have been identified as markers of nonfatal infections.[115–118]

Infected macrophages discovered in various tissues are thought to originate from infected circulating monocytes/macrophages that extravasate following infection.[104,105,114] Virus-induced cytokine release activates the endothelium and is proposed to be the trigger for extravasation. Specifically, various inflammatory mediators including TNF-α, IL-1β, and hydrogen peroxide increase the expression of various cell adhesion molecules on endothelial cells including intravascular adhesion molecule-1 (ICAM-1), vascular cell adhesion molecule-1 (VCAM-1) and E- and P-selectins.[88] In spite of the in vitro upregulation of these molecules, which mediate the binding of leukocytes to the surface of the endothelium and initiate extravasation,[119–121] there is a lack of leukocytic infiltrates in areas of focal necrosis, thereby suggesting a deficient immunoreaction of unknown mechanism.[105]

Endothelial dysfunction can lead to a multitude of vascular effects that may cause disturbances in vascular permeability or hemorrhage. During filovirus infection, the endothelium appears to be affected in two ways: directly by infection with filoviruses, leading to activation and later cell death, and indirectly by a mediator-induced inflammatory response.[90] In vitro virus-induced cytokine release leads to activation of the endothelium defined as increased expression and/or release of adhesion molecules as well as a breakdown of the endothelial barrier function.[91,122] While the molecular mechanisms for the disruption of endothelial barrier function are not completely understood, there is evidence for changes in the protein organization of the adherens junction, specifically the VE-cadherin/catenin complex.[88] Additionally, supernatants from MARV-infected macrophages increase the permeability of HUVEC monolayers, and this effect can be partially blocked by antibodies that neutralize TNF-α, suggesting a critical role for this protein in virus-induced shock.[114] A recent serial sacrifice experiment of EHF in monkeys revealed ultrastructural evidence of endothelial cell activation and disruption but attributes it to indirect mechanisms since they were unable to associate the changes with the presence of intracytoplasmic EBOV antigens. Overall, the data suggest that EBOV affects the function of endothelial cells in the early stages of infection and that EBOV-induced coagulopathy results primarily from vasculopathy induced by factors secreted by infected monocytes/macrophages and dendritic cells (including cytokines and tissue factor); whereas direct virus-induced cytolysis of endothelial cells plays a later, secondary role in hemorrhagic diathesis.[107] The fact that antigen-positive endothelial cells are a hallmark of human infection and that filoviruses readily replicate in human umbilical cord endothelial cells (HUVEC) in vitro cannot be dismissed. Whether their infection plays a major role in EBOV pathogenesis as compared to indirect effects of mediators remains to be determined. The role of EBOV-soluble glycoproteins in endothelial activation and dysfunction is unknown. EBOV sGP was suggested to play a role in immune suppression by inactivation of neutrophils, but these data have been disputed.[44,45,123] The ability of sGP to function in endothelial activation has been suggested in a model by Schnittler and colleagues as a third mechanism by which the endothelium is altered during filovirus infection.[91] Furthermore, synthesis of full length $GP_{1,2}$ was found to induce cytotoxic effects in human endothelial cells, and this ability was mapped to the mucin-like domain of the protein.[124]

DIAGNOSIS

An acute febrile illness with headache and diarrhea can be caused by a variety of different agents including other causes of viral hemorrhagic fever (see Chapter 65). Both occupational and travel history are imperative in narrowing the diagnosis. Rural travel, jungle or cave exposure, contact with sick humans, or contact with sick or dead primates should all raise concern.[10] More common causes of febrile illness that should be ruled out for travelers include rickettsioses, malaria, typhoid fever, leptospirosis, borreliosis, septicemic plague, and dysentery.[125]

An etiologic diagnosis should be sought at the earliest stages of illness. Virus, viral antigen, and viral RNA in serum or blood should be sought during the acute phase of illness.[125] The most commonly used cell line for both isolation and propagation of filoviruses is the Vero (*Cercopithecus aethiops*, African green monkey kidney) cell line, particularly the E6 clone.[19] In addition to Vero cells, both MA-104 and SW13, a human adrenal carcinoma cell line, have proven useful in primary virus isolation.[126] Filoviruses also infect primary cell cultures, particularly monocytes, macrophages, and endothelial cells.[113,114]

Virus can be demonstrated directly by electron microscopic analysis of tissue culture supernatants, blood, or serum, in addition to scanning of cell cultures for cytopathic effects and immunofluorescent staining of infected cells. Detection of viral antigen from infected patients may be accomplished by enzyme-linked immunosorbent assay (ELISA); in a minority of patients, if levels are low, a more sensitive method to detect viral RNA such as reverse transcriptase polymerase chain reaction (RT-PCR) is more appropriate. IgM-capture ELISA may only be positive during the early stages of convalescence, and patients can be followed for rising IgG levels to further increase confidence in the diagnosis.

TREATMENT

There is currently no specific antiviral therapy for filovirus HF, and patient care is supportive in nature.[10,127] Supportive treatment should include attention to fluid and electrolyte balance, particularly with respect to potassium substitution. In several outbreaks, antibiotics were administered (tetracycline, chloramphenicol, penicillin, cephalothin, and streptomycin) but did not alter the fever or course of disease. During various outbreaks and experimentally in animal models, a number of treatments were administered in an attempt to reduce severity of disease. In particular, neutralizing antibodies specific for the viral surface glycoprotein were shown to be both protective and therapeutic in rodent models.[128–130] Baboons were successfully protected from EBOV challenge, but only when large volumes of a hyperimmune horse serum were administered within 4 hours of infection with a low virus dose.[131] The use of horse serum in humans has been questioned, however, because horses produce a subclass of immunoglobulin (IgG_T) that is highly immunogenic in humans.[90] The use of convalescent sera during an outbreak in Kikwit was reported as protective; however, the data were actually not useful, because the treatment was started relatively late in disease at a stage when most patients are already destined to survive.[66,90,132] The use of convalescent sera was also reported during the MARV outbreak in Frankfurt, Germany.[127,133]

Since the coagulation cascade is dysregulated during EHF (leading to disseminated intravascular coagulation, DIC), treatments to alleviate microthrombus formation have been attempted. Heparin was used to treat two surviving MARV-infected patients.[125] Most recently it has been shown that infection with EBOV induces overexpression of the procoagulant tissue factor in primate monocytes and macrophages, suggesting that inhibition of the tissue-factor pathway could ameliorate the effects of EBOV HF.[134] In further studies, macaques were administered recombinant nematode anticoagulant protein c2 (rNAPc2), a potent inhibitor of tissue factor–initiated blood coagulation, and postexposure protection was conferred and provided a new foundation for therapeutic regimens that target the disease process rather than viral replication.[135] Treated animals had increased survival times with 33% survival rate and attenuation of the coagulation and proinflammatory responses.

PREVENTION

The first attempts to develop a vaccine for EBOV began soon after the first outbreak in 1976 and used formalin-fixed or heat-inactivated virus in an attempt to confer protection to guinea pigs and nonhuman primates.[90,136] Despite initial optimism, the protection achieved in both studies was inconsistent, and it was later demonstrated that inactivated virus did not induce sufficient immunity to reliably protect baboons against a lethal dose of virus.[137]

Since the 1990s, there has been a greater effort on vaccine development particularly for EBOV. The majority of these attempts have focused on subunit vaccines that are based on one or more of the viral structural proteins. A variety of approaches including naked DNA, adenovirus, vaccinia virus, vesicular stomatitis virus, Venezuelan equine encephalitis virus replicons and virus-like particles have been used as mechanisms to deliver $GP_{1,2}$, NP, VP24, VP30, VP35, and/or VP40.[138–145] The efficacy and specific details of these vaccine strategies have been recently reviewed in great detail.[90,145] These studies, as well as therapeutic studies, have led to an important conclusion about animal models: interventions in the mouse are most successful; success is somewhat more difficult to achieve in the guinea pig; and the primate model is most demanding. The only successful EBOV vaccine in nonhuman primates is the adenovirus-vectored GP gene. It protected guinea pigs and macaques against lethal challenge and has been inoculated into humans in a phase I trial.[139,146] The difficulty of obtaining an Ebola vaccine candidate and the adenovirus success have important implications for vaccine development against viruses that have effective escape hatches against the immune response if we can understand the mechanisms at play. There are still formidable problems to overcome in a successful human Ebola vaccine because of the difficulties in defining a target population for efficacy testing. Nevertheless, with today's hectic travel, the threat of bioterrorism, social unrest in the endemic areas, and the increase in naturally occurring epidemics, a vaccine may well be needed. Possible targets would include nonhuman primates in endemic areas, medical personnel in Africa, and research workers worldwide.[90]

REFERENCES

1. Feldmann H, Geisbert T, Jahrling PB, et al: Filoviridae. ICTVdB—The Universal Virus Database, 2004.
2. Sanchez A, Trappier SG, Mahy BW, et al: The virion glycoproteins of Ebola viruses are encoded in two reading frames and are expressed through transcriptional editing. Proc Natl Acad Sci USA 93:3602–3607, 1996.
3. Sanchez A, Trappier SG, Stroher U, et al: Variation in the glycoprotein and VP35 genes of Marburg virus strains. Virol 240:138–146, 1998.
4. Georges-Courbot MC, Sanchez A, Lu CY, et al: Isolation and phylogenetic characterization of Ebola viruses causing different outbreaks in Gabon. Emerg Infect Dis 3:59–62, 1997.
5. Suzuki Y, Gojobori T: The origin and evolution of Ebola and Marburg viruses. Mol Biol Evol 14:800–806, 1997.
6. Sanchez A, Ksiazek TG, Rollin PE, et al: Detection and molecular characterization of Ebola viruses causing disease in human and nonhuman primates. J Infect Dis 179:S164–S169, 1999.
7. Rodriguez LL, De Roo A, Guimard Y, et al: Persistence and genetic stability of Ebola virus during the outbreak in Kikwit, Democratic Republic of the Congo, 1995. J Infect Dis 179:S170–S176, 1999.
8. Murphy FA, Peters CJ: Ebola virus: Where does it come from and where is it going? In Krause RM (ed): Emerging Infections. New York, Academic Press, 1998, pp 375–410.
9. Muhlberger E, Sanchez A, Randolf A, et al: The nucleotide sequence of the L gene of Marburg virus, a filovirus: Homologies with paramyxoviruses and rhabdoviruses. Virol 187:534–547, 1992.
10. Sanchez A, Khan AS, Zaki SR, et al: Filoviridae: Marburg and Ebola viruses. In Knipe DM, Howley PM, Griffin DE, et al (eds): Fields' Virology, 4th ed. Philadelphia, Lippincott Williams & Wilkins, 2001, pp 1279–1304.
11. Geisbert TW, Jahrling PB: Differentiation of filoviruses by electron microscopy. Virus Res 39:129–150, 1995.
12. Feldmann H, Muhlberger E, Randolf A, et al: Marburg virus, a filovirus: messenger RNAs, gene order, and regulatory elements of the replication cycle. Virus Res 24:1–19, 1992.
13. Sanchez A, Kiley MP, Holloway BP, et al: Sequence analysis of the Ebola virus genome: Organization, genetic elements, and comparison with the genome of Marburg virus. Virus Res 29:215–240, 1993.
14. Groseth A, Stroher U, Theriault S, et al: Molecular characterization of an isolate from the 1989/90 epizootic of Ebola virus Reston among macaques imported into the United States. Virus Res 87:155–163, 2002.
15. Ikegami T, Calaor AB, Miranda ME, et al: Genome structure of Ebola virus subtype Reston: Differences among Ebola subtypes. Arch Virol 146:2021–2027, 2001.
16. Muhlberger E, Lotfering B, Klenek HD, et al: Three of the four nucleocapsid proteins of Marburg virus, NP, VP35, and L, are sufficient to mediate replication and transcription of Marburg virus-specific monocistronic minigenomes. J Virol 72:8756–8764, 1998.
17. Volchkov VE, Volchkova VA, Muhlberger E, et al: Recovery of infectious Ebola virus from complementary DNA: RNA editing of the GP gene and viral cytotoxicity. Science 291:1965–1969, 2001.
18. Neumann G, Feldmann H, Watanabe S, et al: Reverse genetics demonstrates that proteolytic processing of the Ebola virus glycoprotein is not essential for replication in cell culture. J Virol 76:406–410, 2002.
19. Feldmann H, Kiley MP: Classification, structure, and replication of filoviruses. Curr Top Microbiol Immunol 235:1–21, 1999.
20. Modrof J, Moritz C, Kolesnikova L, et al: Phosphorylation of Marburg virus VP30 at serines 40 and 42 is critical for its interaction with NP inclusions. Virol 287:171–182, 2001.
21. Muhlberger E, Weik M, Volchkov VE, et al: Comparison of the transcription and replication strategies of Marburg virus and Ebola virus by using artificial replication systems. J Virol 73:2333–2342, 1999.
22. Becker S, Rinne C, Hofsass U, et al: Interactions of Marburg virus nucleocapsid proteins. Virol 249:406–417, 1998.
23. Basler CF, Wang X, Muhlberger E, et al: The Ebola virus VP35 protein functions as a type I IFN antagonist. Proc Natl Acad Sci USA 97:12289–12294, 2000.
24. Basler CF, Mikulasova A, Martinez-Sobrido L, et al: The Ebola virus VP35 protein inhibits activation of interferon regulatory factor 3. J Virol 77:7945–7956, 2003.
25. Han Z, Boshra H, Sunyer JO, et al: Biochemical and functional characterization of the Ebola virus VP24 protein: Implications for a role in virus assembly and budding. J Virol 77:1793–1800, 2003.
26. Jasenosky LD, Neumann G, Lukashevich I, et al: Ebola virus VP40-induced particle formation and association with the lipid bilayer. J Virol 75:5205–5214, 2001.
27. Volchkova VA, Klenek HD, Volchkov VE: Delta-peptide is the carboxy-terminal cleavage fragment of the nonstructural small glycoprotein sGP of Ebola virus. Virol 265:164–171, 1999.
28. Volchkova VA, Feldmann H, Klenk HC, et al: The nonstructural small glycoprotein sGP of Ebola virus is secreted as an antiparallel-orientated homodimer. Virol 250:408–414, 1998.
29. Noda T, Sagara H, Suzuki E, et al: Ebola virus VP40 drives the formation of virus-like filamentous particles along with GP. J Virol 76:4855–4865, 2002.
30. Bavari S, Bosio CM, Wiegand E, et al: Lipid raft microdomains: A gateway for compartmentalized trafficking of Ebola and Marburg viruses. J Exp Med 195:593–602, 2002.
31. Huang Y, Xu L, Sun Y, et al: The assembly of Ebola virus nucleocapsid requires virion-associated proteins 35 and 24 and posttranslational modification of nucleoprotein. Mol Cell 10:307–316, 2002.
32. Volchkov VE, Chepurnov AA, Volchkova VA, et al: Molecular characterization of guinea pig-adapted variants of Ebola virus. Virol 277:147–155, 2000.
33. Volchkov VE, Feldmann H, Volchkova VA, et al: Processing of the Ebola virus glycoprotein by the proprotein convertase furin. Proc Natl Acad Sci USA 95:5762–5767, 1998.
34. Jeffers SA, Sanders DA, Sanchez A: Covalent modifications of the Ebola virus glycoprotein. J Virol 76:12463–12472, 2002.
35. Geyer H, Will C, Feldmann H, et al: Carbohydrate structure of Marburg virus glycoprotein. Glycobiology 2:299–312, 1992.
36. Will C, Muhlberger E, Linder D, et al: Marburg virus gene 4 encodes the virion membrane protein, a type I transmembrane glycoprotein. J Virol 67:1203–1210, 1993.
37. Sanchez A, Yang ZY, Xu L, et al: Biochemical analysis of the secreted and virion glycoproteins of Ebola virus. J Virol 72:6442–6447, 1998.
38. Malashkevich VN, Schneider BJ, McNally ML, et al: Core structure of the envelope glycoprotein GP2 from Ebola virus at 1.9-A resolution. Proc Natl Acad Sci USA 96:2662–2667, 1999.
39. Weissenhorn W, Carfi A, Lee KH, et al: Crystal structure of the Ebola virus membrane fusion subunit, GP2, from the envelope glycoprotein ectodomain. Mol Cell 2:605–616, 1998.
40. Weissenhorn W, Calder LJ, Wharton SA, et al: The central structural feature of the membrane fusion protein subunit from the Ebola virus glycoprotein is a long triple-stranded coiled coil. Proc Natl Acad Sci USA 95:6032–6036, 1998.
41. Ruiz-Arguello MB, Goni FM, Pereira FB, et al: Phosphatidylinositol-dependent membrane fusion induced by a putative fusogenic sequence of Ebola virus. J Virol 72:1775–1781, 1998.
42. Ito H, Watanabe S, Sanchez A, et al: Mutational analysis of the putative fusion domain of Ebola virus glycoprotein. J Virol 73:8907–8912, 1999.
43. Volchkov VE, Becker S, Volchkova VA, et al: GP mRNA of Ebola virus is edited by the Ebola virus polymerase and by T7 and vaccinia virus polymerases. Virol 214:421–430, 1995.
44. Yang Z, Delgado R, Xu L, et al: Distinct cellular interactions of secreted and transmembrane Ebola virus glycoproteins. Science 279:1034–1037, 1998.
45. Sui J, Marasco WA: Evidence against Ebola virus sGP binding to human neutrophils by a specific receptor. Virol 303:9–14, 2002.

46. Maruyama T, Buchmeier MJ, Parren PWHI, et al: Ebola virus, neutrophils, and antibody specificity. Science 282:843, 1998.
47. Hayes CG, Burans JP, Ksiazek TG, et al: Outbreak of fatal illness among captive macaques in the Philippines caused by an Ebola-related filovirus. Am J Trop Med Hyg 46:664–671, 1992.
48. Conrad JL, Issacson M, Smith EB, et al: Epidemiologic investigation of Marburg virus disease, southern Africa, 1975. Am J Trop Med Hyg 27:1210–1215, 1978.
49. Leirs H, Mills JN, Krebs JW, et al: Search for the Ebola virus reservoir in Kikwit, Democratic Republic of the Congo: Reflections on a vertebrate collection. J Infect Dis 179:S155–S163, 1999.
50. Reiter P, Turrell M, Coleman R, et al: Field investigations of an outbreak of Ebola hemorrhagic fever, Kikwit, Democratic Republic of the Congo, 1995: Arthropod studies. J Infect Dis 179:S148–S154, 1999.
51. Swanepoel R, Leman PA, Burt FJ, et al: Experimental inoculation of plants and animals with Ebola virus. Emerg Infect Dis 2:321–325, 1996.
52. van der Groen G, et al: Growth of Lassa and Ebola viruses in different cell lines. In Pattyn SR (ed): Ebola Virus Hemorrhagic Fever. Amsterdam, Elsevier, 1978, p 255.
53. WHO: Ebola haemorrhagic fever in Sudan, 1976. Bull World Health Organ, 1976.
54. WHO: Ebola haemorrhagic fever in Zaire, 1976. Report of an international commission. Bull World Health Organ, 1978.
55. Dowell SF, Mukunu R, Ksiazek TG, et al: Transmission of Ebola hemorrhagic fever: A study of risk factors in family members, Kikwit, Democratic Republic of the Congo, 1995. Commission de Lutte contre les Epidemies a Kikwit. J Infect Dis 179:S87–S91, 1999.
56. Roels TH, Bloom AS, Buffington J, et al: Ebola hemorrhagic fever, Kikwit, Democratic Republic of the Congo, 1995: Risk factors for patients without a reported exposure. J Infect Dis 179:S92–S97, 1999.
57. Khan AS, Tshioko FK, Heymann DL, et al: The reemergence of Ebola hemorrhagic fever, Democratic Republic of the Congo, 1995. Commission de Lutte contre les Epidemies a Kikwit. J Infect Dis 179:S76–S86, 1999.
58. Peters CJ, Jahrling PB, Khan AS: Patients infected with high-hazard viruses: Scientific basis for infection control. Arch Virol Suppl 11:141–168, 1996.
59. Zaki SR, Shieh WJ, Greer PW, et al: A novel immunohistochemical assay for the detection of Ebola virus in skin: Implications for diagnosis, spread, and surveillance of Ebola hemorrhagic fever. Commission de Lutte contre les Epidemies a Kikwit. J Infect Dis 179:S36–S47, 1999.
60. Pokhodiaev VA, Gonchar NI, Pshenichov VA: An experimental study of the contact transmission of the Marburg virus. Vopr Virusol 36:506–508, 1991.
61. Jaax NK, Davis KJ, Geisbert TJ, et al: Lethal experimental infection of rhesus monkeys with Ebola-Zaire (Mayinga) virus by the oral and conjunctival route of exposure. Arch Pathol Lab Med 120:140–155, 1996.
62. Kalongi Y, Mwanza K, Tshisuaka M, et al: Isolated case of Ebola hemorrhagic fever with mucormycosis complications, Kinshasa, Democratic Republic of the Congo. J Infect Dis 179:S15–S17, 1999.
63. Peters CJ, Sanchez A, Feldmann PE, et al: Filoviruses as emerging pathogens. Semin Virol 5:147, 1994.
64. Baron RC, McCormick JB, Zubeir OA: Ebola virus disease in southern Sudan: Hospital dissemination and intrafamilial spread. Bull World Health Organ 61:997–1003, 1983.
65. Francis DP, Smith DH, Hightor RB, et al: Ebola fever in Sudan, 1976: Epidemiological aspects of the disease. In Pattyn S (ed): Ebola Virus Haemorrhagic Fever. Amsterdam, Elsevier, 1978, p 129.
66. Sadek RF, Khan AS, Stevens G, et al: Ebola hemorrhagic fever, Democratic Republic of the Congo, 1995: Determinants of survival. J Infect Dis 179:S24–S27, 1999.
67. Peters CJ, Johnson ED, Jahrling PB, et al: Filoviruses. In Morse SS (ed): Emerging Viruses. New York, Oxford University Press, 1992, p 159.
68. Simpson DIH: Marburg virus: A review of laboratory studies. In Balner H, Beveridge WI (eds): Infections and Immunosuppression in Subhuman Primates. Copenhagen, Munksgaard, 1970, p 39.
69. Jaax N, Jahrling P, Geisbert T, et al: Transmission of Ebola virus (Zaire strain) to uninfected control monkeys in a biocontainment laboratory. Lancet 346:1669–1671, 1995.
70. Bazhutin NB, Belanov EF, Spiridonov VA, et al: [The effect of the methods for producing an experimental Marburg virus infection on the characteristics of the course of the disease in green monkeys.] Vopr Virusol 37:153–156, 1992.
71. Belanov EF, Muntianov VP, Kriuk VD, et al: [Survival of Marburg virus infectivity on contaminated surfaces and in aerosols.] Vop Virusol 41:32–34, 1996.
72. Chepurnov AA, Cheuv IuP, P'iankov OV, et al: [The effect of some physical and chemical factors on inactivation of the Ebola virus.] Vopr Virusol 40:74–76, 1995.
73. Johnson E, Jaax N, White J, et al: Lethal experimental infections of rhesus monkeys by aerosolized Ebola virus. Int J Exp Pathol 76:227–236, 1995.
74. DeMarcus TA, Tipple MA, Ostrowski SR: US policy for disease control among imported nonhuman primates. J Infect Dis 179:S281–S282, 1999.
75. Rollin PE, Williams RJ, Bressler DS, et al: Ebola (subtype Reston) virus among quarantined nonhuman primates recently imported from the Philippines to the United States. J Infect Dis 179:S108–S114, 1999.
76. Ksiazek TG, Rollin PE, Jahrling PB, et al: Enzyme immunosorbent assay for Ebola virus antigens in tissues of infected primates. J Clin Microbiol 30:947–950, 1992.
77. Elliott LH, Bauer SP, Perez-Oronoz G, et al: Improved specificity of testing methods for filovirus antibodies. J Virol Methods 43:85–89, 1993.
78. Ksiazek TG, West CP, Rollin PE, et al: ELISA for the detection of antibodies to Ebola viruses. J Infect Dis 179:S192–S198, 1999.
79. Le Guenno B, Formentry P, Wyers M, et al: Isolation and partial characterisation of a new strain of Ebola virus. Lancet 345:1271–1274, 1995.
80. Formenty P, Boesch C, Wyers M, et al: Ebola virus outbreak among wild chimpanzees living in a rain forest of Cote d'Ivoire. J Infect Dis 179:S120–S126, 1999.
81. Georges AJ, Leroy EM, Renaut AA, et al: Ebola hemorrhagic fever outbreaks in Gabon, 1994-1997: Epidemiologic and health control issues. J Infect Dis 179:S65–S75, 1999.
82. Leroy EM, Rouquet P, Formenty P, et al: Multiple Ebola virus transmission events and rapid decline of central African wildlife. Science 303:387–390, 2004.
83. Walsh PD, Abernethy KA, Bermejo M, et al: Catastrophic ape decline in western equatorial Africa. Nature 422:611–614, 2003.
84. WHO. Outbreak of Ebola haemorrhagic fever, Uganda, August 2000–January 2001. Weekly Epidemiol Record 76:41–46, 2001.
85. Towner JS, Rollin PE, Bausch DG, et al: Rapid diagnosis of Ebola hemorrhagic fever by reverse transcription-PCR in an outbreak setting and assessment of patient viral load as a predictor of outcome. J Virol 78:4330–4341, 2004.
86. Bausch DG, Borchert M, Grein T, et al: Risk factors for Marburg hemorrhagic fever, Democratic Republic of the Congo. Emerg Infect Dis 9:1531–1537, 2003.
87. Swanapoel R, Smit S, Burt F, et al: Multiple introduction of genetically diverse Marburg viruses into the human population during the hemorrhagic fever outbreak in Durba, Democratic Republic of Congo, 1998-2000. In Mahy BW, Kolakofsky D (eds): Eleventh International Conference on Negative Strand Viruses. Quebec City, Canada, June 24-29, 2001. 2001, abstract #172.
88. Schnittler HJ, Feldmann H: Molecular pathogenesis of filovirus infections: Role of macrophages and endothelial cells. Curr Top Microbiol Immunol 235:175–204, 1999.
89. Feldmann H, Klenk HD: Marburg and Ebola viruses. Adv Virus Res 47:1–52, 1996.
90. Feldmann H, Jones S, Klenk HD, et al: Ebola virus: From discovery to vaccine. Nat Rev Immunol 3:677–685, 2003.
91. Schnittler HJ, Feldmann H: Viral hemorrhagic fever—A vascular disease? Thromb Haemost 89:967–972, 2003.
92. Ksiazek TG, Rollin PE, Williams AJ, et al: Clinical virology of Ebola hemorrhagic fever (EHF): Virus, virus antigen, and IgG and IgM antibody findings among EHF patients in Kikwit, Democratic Republic of the Congo, 1995. J Infect Dis 179:S177–S187, 1999.
93. Rowe AK, Bertolli J, Khan AS, et al: Clinical, virologic, and immunologic follow-up of convalescent Ebola hemorrhagic fever patients and their household contacts, Kikwit, Democratic Republic of the Congo. Commission de Lutte contre les Epidemies a Kikwit. J Infect Dis 179:S28–S35, 1999.
94. Bwaka MA, Bonnet MJ, Calain P, et al: Ebola hemorrhagic fever in Kikwit, Democratic Republic of the Congo: Clinical observations in 103 patients. J Infect Dis 179:S1–S7, 1999.
95. Formenty P, Hatz C, Le Guenno B, et al: Human infection due to Ebola virus, subtype Cote d'Ivoire: Clinical and biologic presentation. J Infect Dis 179:S48–S53, 1999.

96. Martini GA, Siegert R: Marburg Virus Disease. New York, Springer-Verlag, 1971.
97. Zaki SR, Peters CJ: Viral hemorrhagic fevers. In Connor DH, et al. (eds): Pathology of Infectious Diseases. New York, Appleton and Lange, 1997, pp 347–364.
98. Zaki S, Kilmarx PH: Ebola virus hemorrhagic fever. In Horsburgh CR Jr, Nelson AM (eds): Pathology of Emerging Infections. Washington, DC, ASM Press, pp 299–310.
99. Murphy FA, Simpson DI, Whitfield SG, et al: Marburg virus infection in monkeys. Ultrastructural studies. Lab Invest 24:279–291, 1971.
100. Dietrich M: Marburg virus disease. In Pattyn S (ed): Ebola Virus Haemorrhagic Fever. Amsterdam, Elsevier, 1978, pp 271–278.
101. Fisher-Hoch SP, Brammer TL, Trappier SG, et al: Pathogenic potential of filoviruses: Role of geographic origin of primate host and virus strain. J Infect Dis 166:753–763, 1992.
102. Murphy FA: Pathology of Ebola virus infection. In Pattyn S (ed): Ebola Virus Haemorrhagic Fever. Amsterdam, Elsevier, 1978, pp 61–82.
103. Geisbert TW, Hensley LE, Larsen T, et al: Pathogenesis of Ebola hemorrhagic fever in cynomolgus macaques: Evidence that dendritic cells are early and sustained targets of infection. Am J Pathol 163:2347–2370, 2003.
104. Geisbert TW, Jahrling PB, Hanes MA, et al: Association of Ebola-related Reston virus particles and antigen with tissue lesions of monkeys imported to the United States. J Comp Pathol 106:137–152, 1992.
105. Ryabchikova E, Price BBS: Ebola and Marburg Viruses: A View of Infection Using Electron Microscopy. Columbus, OH, Batelle Press, 2003.
106. Schnittler HJ, Feldmann H: Marburg and Ebola hemorrhagic fevers: Does the primary course of infection depend on the accessibility of organ-specific macrophages? Clin Infect Dis 27:404–406, 1998.
107. Geisbert TW, Young HA, Jahrling PB, et al: Pathogenesis of Ebola hemorrhagic fever in primate models: Evidence that hemorrhage is not a direct effect of virus-induced cytolysis of endothelial cells. Am J Pathol 163:2371–2382, 2003.
108. Davis KJ, Anderson AO, Geisbert TW, et al: Pathology of experimental Ebola virus infection in African green monkeys. Involvement of fibroblastic reticular cells. Arch Pathol Lab Med 121:805–819, 1997.
109. Connolly BM, Steele KE, Davis KJ, et al: Pathogenesis of experimental Ebola virus infection in guinea pigs. J Infect Dis 179:S203–S217, 1999.
110. Hensley LE, Young HA, Jahrling PB, et al: Proinflammatory response during Ebola virus infection of primate models: Possible involvement of the tumor necrosis factor receptor superfamily. Immunol Lett 80:169–179, 2002.
111. Geisbert TW, Hensley LE, Gibb TR, et al: Apoptosis induced *in vitro* and *in vivo* during infection by Ebola and Marburg viruses. Lab Invest 80:171–186, 2000.
112. Bukreyev A, Volchkov VE, Blinov VM, et al: The GP-protein of Marburg virus contains the region similar to the "immunosuppressive domain" of oncogenic retrovirus P15E proteins. FEBS Lett 323:183–187, 1993.
113. Stroher U, West E, Bugany H, et al: Infection and activation of monocytes by Marburg and Ebola viruses. J Virol 75:11025–11033, 2001.
114. Feldmann H, Bugany H, Mahner F, et al: Filovirus-induced endothelial leakage triggered by infected monocytes/macrophages. J Virol 70:2208–2214, 1996.
115. Baize S, Leroy EM, Georges-Courbot MC, et al: Defective humoral responses and extensive intravascular apoptosis are associated with fatal outcome in Ebola virus-infected patients. Nat Med 5:423–426, 1999.
116. Villinger F, Rollin PE, Brar SS, et al: Markedly elevated levels of interferon (IFN)-gamma, IFN-alpha, interleukin (IL)-2, IL-10, and tumor necrosis factor-alpha associated with fatal Ebola virus infection. J Infect Dis 179:S188–S191, 1999.
117. Leroy EM, Baize S, Volchkov VE, et al: Human asymptomatic Ebola infection and strong inflammatory response. Lancet 355:2210–2215, 2000.
118. Baize S, Leroy EM, Georges AJ, et al: Inflammatory responses in Ebola virus-infected patients. Clin Exp Immunol 128:163–168, 2002.
119. Vestweber D: The selectins and their ligands. Curr Top Microbiol Immunol 184:65–75, 1993.
120. Vestweber D: Selectins: Cell surface lectins which mediate the binding of leukocytes to endothelial cells. Semin Cell Biol 3:211–220, 1992.
121. Lenter M, Levinovitz A, Isenmann S, et al: Monospecific and common glycoprotein ligands for E- and P-selectin on myeloid cells. J Cell Biol 125:471–481, 1994.
122. Vallet B: Bench-to-bedside review: Endothelial cell dysfunction in severe sepsis: A role in organ dysfunction? Crit Care 7:130–138, 2003.
123. Maruyama T, Rodriguez LL, Jahrling PB, et al: Ebola virus can be effectively neutralized by antibody produced in natural human infection. J Virol 73:6024–6030, 1999.
124. Yang ZY, Duckers JH, Sullivan NJ, et al: Identification of the Ebola virus glycoprotein as the main viral determinant of vascular cell cytotoxicity and injury. Nat Med 6:886–889, 2000.
125. Peters CJ, Khan AS: Filovirus diseases. Curr Top Microbiol Immunol 235:85–95, 1999.
126. McCormick JB, Bauer SP, Elliott LH, et al: Biologic differences between strains of Ebola virus from Zaire and Sudan. J Infect Dis 147:264–267, 1983.
127. Slenczka WG: The Marburg virus outbreak of 1967 and subsequent episodes. Curr Top Microbiol Immunol 235:49–75, 1999.
128. Maruyama T, Parren PW, Sanchez A, et al: Recombinant human monoclonal antibodies to Ebola virus. J Infect Dis 179:S235–S239, 1999.
129. Parren PW, Geisbert TW, Maruyama T, et al: Pre- and postexposure prophylaxis of Ebola virus infection in an animal model by passive transfer of a neutralizing human antibody. J Virol 76:6408–6412, 2002.
130. Wilson JA, Hevey M, Bakken R, et al: Epitopes involved in antibody-mediated protection from Ebola virus. Science 287:1664–1666, 2000.
131. Krasnianskii BP, Mikhailov VV, Borisevich IV, et al: [Preparation of hyperimmune horse serum against Ebola virus.] Vopr Virusol 40:138–140, 1995.
132. Mupapa K, Massamba M, Kibadi K, et al: Treatment of Ebola hemorrhagic fever with blood transfusions from convalescent patients. International Scientific and Technical Committee. J Infect Dis 179:S18–S23, 1999.
133. Stille W, Bohle E, Helm E, et al: An infectious disease transmitted by *Cercopithecus aethiops* ("Green monkey disease"). Ger Med Mon 13:470–478, 1968.
134. Geisbert TW, Young HA, Jahrling PB, et al: Mechanisms underlying coagulation abnormalities in Ebola hemorrhagic fever: Overexpression of tissue factor in primate monocytes/macrophages is a key event. J Infect Dis 188:1618–1629, 2003.
135. Geisbert TW, Hensley LE, Jahrling PB, et al: Treatment of Ebola virus infection with a recombinant inhibitor of factor VIIa/tissue factor: A study in rhesus monkeys. Lancet 362:1953–1958, 2003.
136. Mikhailov VV, Borisevich IV, Chernikova NK, et al: The evaluation in hamadryas baboons of the possibility for the specific prevention of Ebola fever. Vopr Virusol 39:82–84, 1994.
137. Chupurnov AA, Chernukhin IV, Ternovoi VA, et al: [Attempts to develop a vaccine against Ebola fever.] Vopr Virusol 40:257–260, 1995.
138. Vanderzanden L, Bray M, Fuller D, et al: DNA vaccines expressing either the GP or NP genes of Ebola virus protect mice from lethal challenge. Virol 246:134–144, 1998.
139. Xu L, Sanchez A, Yang Z, et al: Immunization for Ebola virus infection. Nat Med 4:37–42, 1998.
140. Pushko P, Bray M, Ludwig GV, et al: Recombinant RNA replicons derived from attenuated Venezuelan equine encephalitis virus protect guinea pigs and mice from Ebola hemorrhagic fever virus. Vaccine 19:142–153, 2000.
141. Wilson JA, Bray M, Bakken R, et al: Vaccine potential of Ebola virus VP24, VP30, VP35, and VP40 proteins. Virol 286:384–390, 2001.
142. Geisbert TW, Pushko P, Anderson K, et al: Evaluation in nonhuman primates of vaccines against Ebola virus. Emerg Infect Dis 8:503–507, 2002.
143. Garbutt M, Liebscher R, Wahl-Jensen V, et al: Properties of replication-competent vesicular stomatitis virus vectors expressing glycoproteins of filoviruses and arenaviruses. J Virol 78:5458–5465, 2004.
144. Warfield KL, Bosio CM, Welcher BC, et al: Ebola virus-like particles protect from lethal Ebola virus infection. Proc Natl Acad Sci USA 100:15889–15894, 2003.
145. Geisbert TW, Jahrling PB: Towards a vaccine against Ebola virus. Expert Rev Vaccines 2:777–789, 2003.
146. Sullivan NJ, Geisbert TW, Geisbert JB, et al: Accelerated vaccination for Ebola virus haemorrhagic fever in non-human primates. Nature 424:681–684, 2003.

71

Yellow Fever

ANTHONY A. MARFIN
RACHEL BARWICK EIDEX
THOMAS P. MONATH

INTRODUCTION

Yellow fever is the first-described hemorrhagic fever; in its most fulminant form, it is characterized by severe hepatic and renal injury, hemorrhage, and high mortality. Yellow fever virus, the causative agent of this illness, is the prototype member of the *Flavivirus* genus. Yellow fever virus transmission occurs only in South America and sub-Saharan Africa. Despite this restricted range, it is important for physicians worldwide to consider yellow fever because of its potential to cause large urban outbreaks in areas outside of South America and Africa, because of the risk to travelers in endemic areas, and because of serious adverse events following immunization (AEFI) with yellow fever vaccine.

AGENT

Viral Structure

Yellow fever virus is the prototype member of the genus *Flavivirus* in the family Flaviviridae that includes more than 70 small (40 to 60 nm), single-stranded, positive-sense RNA viruses, most of which are arthropod-borne. Sequence analysis of the envelope gene revealed that yellow fever virus diverged from other mosquito-borne flaviviruses (e.g., dengue virus) approximately 3000 years ago.[1]

The 10.9-kilobase (kb) genome of yellow fever is organized into a single 10.2-kb open reading frame (ORF) flanked by a short 5′ noncoding region (NCR) and a longer 3′ NCR.[2–4] Both NCRs have highly conserved, complementary sequences that are important in the formation of a circular genome after cell entry to promote replication. Mutations or deletions in these complementary sequences affect replication and virulence. In addition, there are differences in these NCRs between yellow fever virus strains. The 5′ NCR is similar for all strains, but the 3′ NCR includes imperfect repeat sequences of 42 nucleotides. South American strains have one copy of this sequence, East African strains have two, and West African strains have three. The differences in repeat sequences appear to be due to evolutionary divergence, and there is no difference in the virulence or replication efficiency associated with the different number of sequences. The ORF consists of three structural protein genes (i.e., capsid [C], premembrane [prM], and envelope [E]) followed by seven nonstructural (NS) protein genes (NS1, NS2A, NS2B, NS3, NS4A, NS4B, and NS5). These 10 genes are translated into a single polyprotein and then cleaved into individual proteins. The C, prM, and E proteins are present in the mature virion. NS proteins are not present in the mature virion but are produced immediately after infection when they are responsible for replication and polypeptide processing.

The viral envelope is a lipid bilayer derived from the host cell with E protein dimers on the surface. The E protein is responsible for the initial attachment and infection, is the principal target of the host's immune response, and is considered the primary virulence factor. A highly conserved stretch of 14 amino acids in the E protein is responsible for fusion of the virus with the lysosomal membrane of the infected cell. The rearrangement of the E proteins to expose the fusion region is absolutely required for the virus to enter the cell cytoplasm. E gene mutations, especially in the fusion domain, greatly alter these biologic functions.[5,6] In addition, because the E protein contains epitopes against which neutralizing activity is directed, anti-E antibody provides protection by interfering with attachment and fusion.[7] Theoretically, major mutations in the E gene can reduce the protective qualities of anti-E antibody acquired by previous yellow fever infections or immunization; such a mutation has not yet been reported.

NS1 is critical to intracellular virus RNA replication, is released extracellularly, and is expressed on the surface of infected cells (Table 71-1). The secreted form has both virus-specific and cross-reactive epitopes. Antibodies to NS1 do not neutralize virus infectivity but provide protection by complement-mediated lysis of infected cells that express the NS1 epitope on their surface.[8] The E, NS1, NS2A, and NS3 proteins have a dominant cytotoxic T-cell epitope; this suggests that T-lymphocyte responses to yellow fever virus play a role in long-term immunity.[9] NS2B and NS3 form a critical enzyme complex that includes a serine protease responsible for post-translational cleavage of the virus polyprotein, an RNA helicase, and an RNA triphosphatase. The NS3 gene sequence is highly conserved at the sequence level. The protein is on the host cell surface and, because NS3 contains cytotoxic T-cell epitopes, infected cells are eliminated by cell-mediated immunity.[9,10] NS4A and NS4B are hydrophobic, membrane-associated proteins that regulate RNA replication. NS5 protein is also highly conserved and functions as the RNA-dependent RNA polymerase in virus replication.

Replication

After attachment to an as yet undefined cell receptor, virus is transported intracellularly within a phagosome. The acidic environment in the phagosomes results in fusion of the virus membrane with the vesicle membrane and release of the nucleocapsid into the cytoplasm. The uncoated, positive-sense RNA (i.e., messenger sense) is immediately translated to synthesize RNA-dependent RNA polymerase, RNA helicase, and RNA triphosphatase, which replicate full-length negative RNA strands. These negative strands serve as templates for positive RNA strands that are assembled into virions in the endoplasmic reticulum (ER) and undergo exocytosis.

Genetic Variation

Based on plaque-reduction neutralization assays, the *Flavivirus* genus was divided into eight antigenic complexes

Table 71-1 Functional Description of 10 Genes/Proteins That Are Found in Yellow Fever Virus and Other Members of the Genus Flavivirus

Gene/Protein	Primary Function	Comments
Capsid (C)	With genomic RNA, forms nucleocapsid	
Premembrane (prM)	Stabilizes E protein during exocytosis	Cleaved before release to form pr and M proteins. pr released to extracellular medium, M retained in viral envelope; failure to cleave can affect antigenicity and conformation of E protein and may reduce infectivity of virus
Envelope (E)	Receptor-mediated cell attachment and cell fusion	Forms E protein dimers within lipid bilayer of viral envelope and can be inactivated with organic solvents and detergents
NS1	RNA replication	Monomers released extracellularly and form dimers to be expressed on the surface of infected cells; antibodies to NS1 do not neutralize infectivity but do provide protective immunity through complement-mediated lysis of infected cells[68]
NS2A	RNA replication	Interacts with NS3, NS5, and 3′ NCR to replicate; critical for virion assembly and release
NS2B	See NS3	Forms complex with NS3 to perform functions
NS3	Multifunction: Serine protease, RNA helicase, RNA triphosphatase	Serine protease performs post-translational cleavage of the viral polyprotein; RNA helicase and RNA triphophatase critical to RNA replication; NS3 highly conserved base sequence; target of attack for cytotoxic T cells[14,38]
NS4A	Regulate RNA replication	Hydrophobic, membrane-associated protein
NS4B	Regulate RNA replication	Hydrophobic, membrane-associated protein
NS5	RNA-dependent RNA polymerase	In addition to polymerase function, functions as a methyltransferase for 5′ cap methylation; like NS3, highly conserved base sequence

and several other antigenically unique viruses, such as yellow fever virus.[11] Gene sequencing confirmed these relationships, grouped yellow fever with nine other flaviviruses (Banzi, Bouboui, Edge Hill, Jugra, Saboya, Potiskum, Sepik, Uganda S, and Wesselsbron viruses), and showed that yellow fever is most closely related to Sepik virus from New Guinea.[12] In addition, these analyses suggest that yellow fever virus is the most distantly related mosquito-borne flavivirus.[1,12]

Seven genotypes have been distinguished by nucleotide sequencing, but they represent a single serotype. Genomic analyses support the concept that yellow fever virus arose in Africa and that East and West African genotypes diverged prior to the introduction of the virus to the Americas.[13,14] Genomic analyses identified two genotypes in West Africa and three in Central and East Africa.[15] Within each African genotype, there is little genetic variation. This is likely due to the yellow fever virus' high-fidelity RNA-dependent RNA polymerase.[16] Unlike the error-prone replication seen in other RNA viruses that results in one mutation out of every 10^4 bases replicated, yellow fever virus averages two mutations every 10^7 bases. Yellow fever virus has achieved only a modest degree of genetic variation following introduction to the Americas. In the Americas, two genotypes have arisen despite significant geographic overlap.[17] Limited genetic analyses of M, E, NS5, and the 3′ NCR comparing the South American genotypes showed that these genotypes represent divergent lineages resulting from geographic and temporal separation and infrequent recombination. There is no difference in the resulting human disease associated with these seven YF variants, but it is unknown whether the highly variable mortality in different epidemics is due to genomic variation.

EPIDEMIOLOGY

Transmission Patterns and Ecology

In Africa, three transmission cycles can be distinguished: the sylvatic, urban, and savanna cycles (Fig. 71-1). In South America, only sylvatic and urban cycles have been identified (Fig. 71-2). In all three cycles, yellow fever virus is transmitted between primates by diurnally active tree hole-breeding mosquitoes. Neither the virus nor the clinical disease differs in these three cycles, but identifying the type of transmission cycle is important for disease control. In all of these cycles, endemic and epidemic disease patterns can occur.

The sylvatic cycle is the predominant transmission cycle in equatorial rain forests in Africa and South America. The cycle is maintained among monkeys by tree hole-breeding mosquitoes. Humans are incidentally infected when they enter the forest or when viremic monkeys exit the forests and infect mosquitoes at the forest fringe. The primary sylvatic

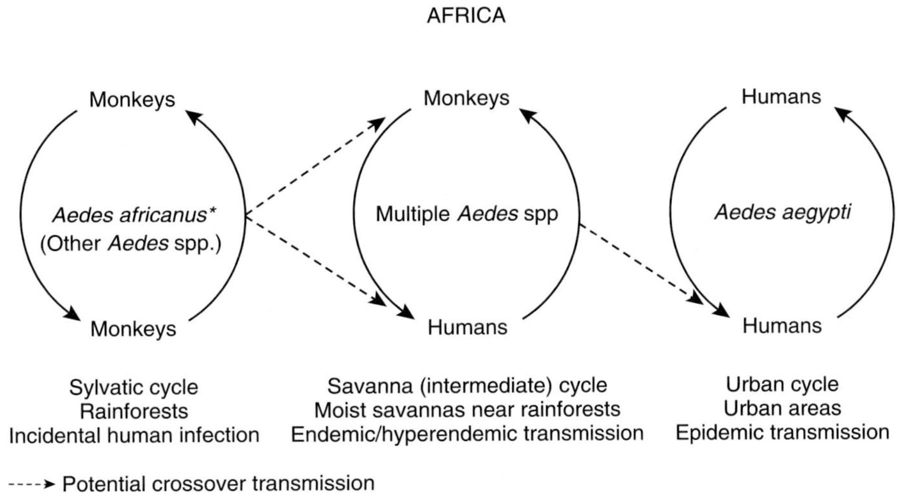

FIGURE 71-1 African transmission cycles include a sylvatic cycle, a savanna (or intermediate) cycle, and an urban cycle. In each cycle, the mosquito vectors are tree hole-breeding *Aedes* species. The urban cycle, characterized by human-to-human transmission mediated by *Aedes aegypti*, may begin when a viremic human either incidentally infected in the rain forest or infected during endemic transmission in the savanna travels to urban areas.

vectors are mosquito species that occur in tree canopies—*Aedes africanus* in Africa and *Haemagogus* species in South America. Other African mosquito species implicated in transmission include *Aedes furcifer*, *Aedes vittatus*, *Aedes luteocephalus*, and *Aedes simpsoni*; in South America, in addition to *Haemagogus* species, *Sabethes chloropterus* may be involved. Many nonhuman primate species are susceptible to yellow fever infection. Most African species do not become ill but develop viremia sufficient to infect mosquitoes; however, in South America several species develop lethal infections. Depletion of vertebrate hosts through natural immunization or death during epizootics is a factor in the cyclic disappearance of yellow fever. In many areas, deforestation and hunting have reduced monkey populations, and human beings have become the primary hosts in the transmission cycle. The sylvatic yellow fever cycle may be active but unrecognized in forested areas of countries within the yellow fever endemic zone. Evidence suggests that yellow fever virus will be maintained in one place until the amplifying primates are immune and then reemerge in areas where susceptible primates live. Disease may not be detected for years but then will reappear. Yellow fever virus is maintained through periods during which mosquitoes are absent (e.g., the dry season) by means of transovarial transmission. (i.e., vertical transmission through infected eggs). Sylvatic transmission can most effectively be prevented by vaccination of human populations at risk of exposure.

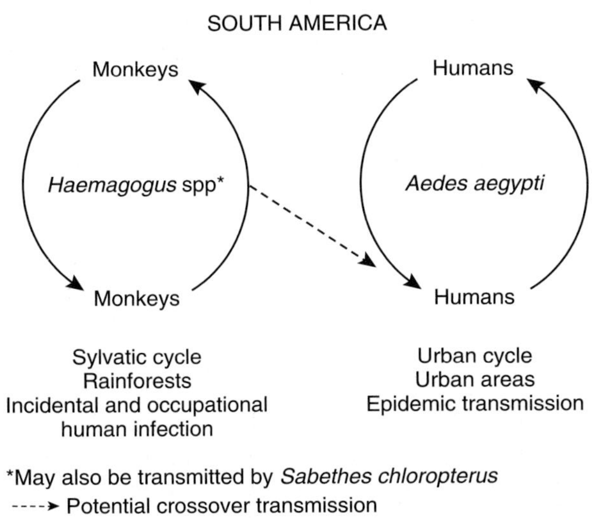

FIGURE 71-2 South American transmission cycles include a sylvatic cycle and an urban cycle. In the sylvatic cycle, the mosquito vectors are treetop feeding *Haemagogus* or *Sabethes* species. The urban cycle, characterized by human-to-human transmission mediated by *Aedes aegypti*, may begin when a viremic human either incidentally or occupationally infected in the rain forests travels to urban areas.

Urban yellow fever refers to settings in which human-to-human transmission is mediated by *Aedes aegypti*, a domestic mosquito associated with human habitation and unpolluted collections of water. In areas where *Ae. aegypti* was eliminated, urban yellow fever disappeared. In the mid-1900s, Panama, Brazil, Ecuador, Peru, Bolivia, Paraguay, Uruguay, and Argentina successfully eradicated this vector; no urban epidemics occurred. The last clearly documented *Ae. aegypti*-borne yellow fever epidemic in the Americas occurred in Trinidad in 1954. During the past 20 years, many countries that had previously eradicated *Ae. aegypti* have been reinfested.[18,19] Large urban outbreaks have not yet occurred, but *Ae. aegypti* mosquitoes were suspected as the vector during outbreaks in Bolivia in the late 1980s through the mid-1990s. In other South American countries (e.g., Venezuela, Guyana, and Surinam), eradication never occurred. These countries remain infested with *Ae. aegypti* in cities near areas with enzootic activity and have great potential for urban epidemics. In Africa, *Ae. aegypti* eradication never occurred, and yellow fever epidemics continued to occur in cities, towns, refugee camps, and rural villages where the vector is prevalent.[20,21] Because of an association between population density and the presence of *Ae. aegypti*, massive epidemics have occurred in Africa. In Nigeria in 1987, an epidemic of an

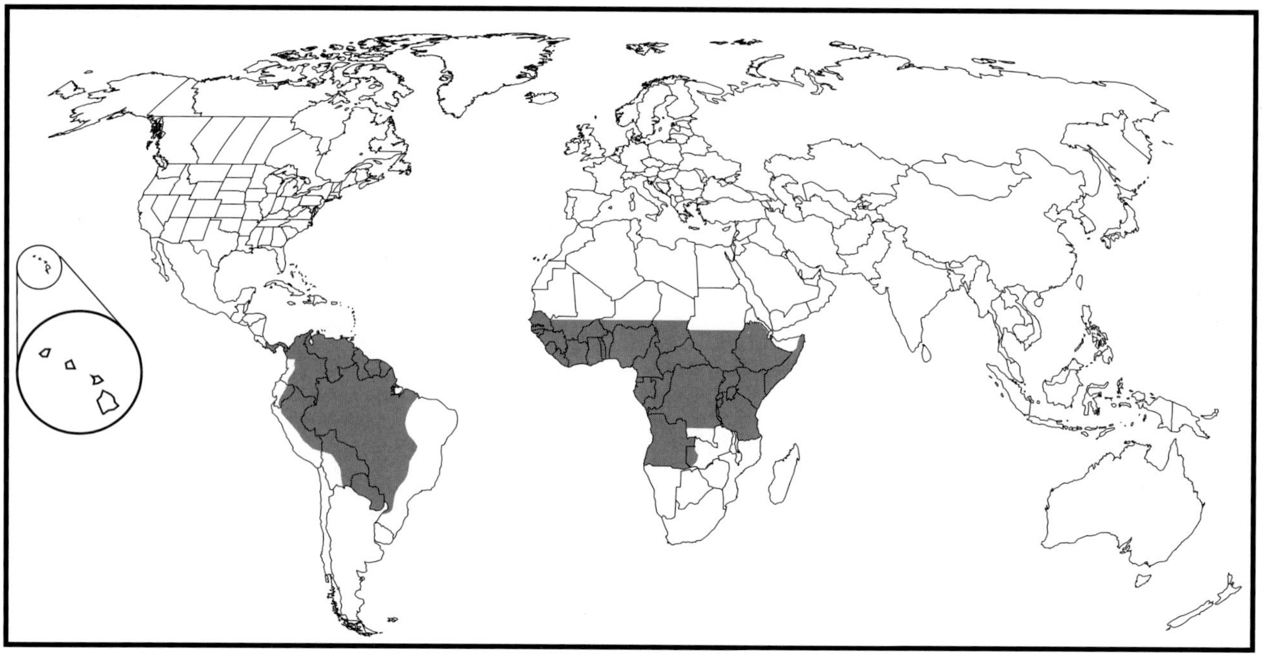

Yellow Fever

■ *Yellow Fever*

Countries and regions with yellow fever virus transmission. Shading is based on recent reports of human yellow fever infections or on the continued presence of ecological factors associated with yellow fever virus transmission in areas with historical reports of human yellow fever infections (Adapted by Jodi Udd. From the Centers for Disease Control and Prevention: Health Information for International Travelers, 2005–2006[Yellow Book]. A frequently updated version of the CDC's Yellow Book can be found at http://www.cdc.gov/travel/yb/index.htm and should be used to determine a person's actual need for yellow fever immunization.)

estimated 39,000 cases and 8400 deaths occurred in urban areas. Other major *Ae. aegypti*-borne epidemics occurred in 1965 and 1979 in Senegal and in 1971 in Angola.

Because of the mobility of potentially viremic humans, urban yellow fever outbreaks may occur in cities that are remote from sylvatic areas. When considering the potential for large urban yellow fever epidemics in South America, one can point to previous outbreaks of dengue, a flaviviral disease transmitted by *Ae. aegypti*. To eradicate *Ae. aegypti* again will be difficult because of insecticide resistance, human population growth, and the high cost. Thus, the scene is set for large urban outbreaks in the Americas. Without reduction of *Ae. aegypti*, urban yellow fever can only be prevented by vaccinating at-risk human populations.

In Africa, a savanna cycle is recognized in areas where humans live in moist grasslands bordering African rain forests where *Aedes* mosquitoes feed on both humans and monkeys. This is sometimes called the intermediate zone because it serves as a link between primates in the deep forest and people in adjacent African villages. In West Africa, the principal vectors in this zone include *Ae. furcifer*, *Ae. vittatus*, *Ae. luteocephalus*, and *Ae. africanus*. In East Africa, *Ae. africanus* and *Ae. simpsoni* are the principal vectors. During the wet and early dry seasons, high vector density occurs and mosquitoes readily enter houses. During these periods, virus transmission rates far exceed that found in sylvatic zones.

Mosquito Vectors

Tree hole-breeding mosquitoes are the primary vectors involved in the replication of virus and transmission between vertebrate hosts. Uninfected female mosquitoes become infected when they feed on an infected host with a viremia of at least 10^4 pfu/mL. After a 7- to 14-day incubation period in the mosquito, high virus titers are present in the salivary glands. During subsequent blood meals, virus is transmitted to a new vertebrate host. In addition, yellow fever virus can be transmitted transovarially, allowing viral survival in the absence of adult mosquitoes. Some populations of mosquitoes transmit yellow fever virus more efficiently than others. In the laboratory, the ability of *Ae. aegypti* to infect mice is variable and low, between 30% and 80%. Field studies during large African epidemics have shown that *Ae. aegypti* is an inefficient vector even during epidemics.[22] Despite the inefficiency, the anthropophilic nature of the vector and the high densities of the mosquito in urban areas make it an excellent vector for human-to-human transmission. It has been suggested that such inefficiency of mosquito vector strains selects greater virus virulence. For example, the low transmission efficiency of *Ae. aegypti* may select viruses that achieve higher viremia, thus increasing the pathogenicity of the virus strain.

Vertebrate Hosts

Primates are the only vertebrate hosts implicated in the yellow fever transmission cycle. In general, viremia is short (i.e., 2 to 5 days), although it can be 9 days in colobus monkeys. Infected primates either die or develop lifelong protective immunity. Except for the galago (*Galago senegalensis*), African monkeys generally become viremic but do not develop illness. Primates support the natural transmission cycle, but yellow fever virus can infect nonprimate species.

Viscerotropic disease (infection of liver, heart, and kidneys) occurs in primates, hedgehogs, and golden hamsters. In these species, the liver is primarily involved, and the virus does not cause encephalitis. Yellow fever virus does cause encephalitis in mice, hamsters, and guinea pigs after intracerebral inoculation. A number of vertebrates (e.g., sloths) have been found to have antibodies against yellow fever virus, but because of their low viremia they are unlikely to be important in maintaining virus transmission.

Geographic Distribution and Incidence

From 1985 to 1999, 25,846 yellow fever cases were reported to the World Health Organization (WHO); of these, 22,952 (89%) were reported from sub-Saharan Africa, where it affects 34 countries, and the remainder from 14 countries in tropical South America. In Africa, the number of reported cases varied from 0 to 5000 per year and suggests significant inconsistencies in surveillance and reporting. In South America, up to 300 cases per year have been reported to WHO. Case fatality is highly variable but usually approximately 20%; higher rates have been reported. Because most yellow fever cases are not reported, WHO estimated that the true incidence may be 200,000 cases and 30,000 deaths annually.[23,24] In addition to underreporting "classic" yellow fever cases, the number of yellow fever viral infections is not known but believed to be much higher. The ratio of classic yellow fever cases to the number of infections is estimated to be approximately 1:10, but this may vary greatly.

In Africa, of the 22,952 cases reported from 1985 to 1999, 5357 (23%) were fatal. The majority of outbreaks have been reported from West Africa; fewer outbreaks have been reported from Central and East Africa. This is due to a combination of factors, including higher densities of humans and *Ae. aegypti*, creating greater potential for human-to-human transmission in the west. Within Africa, Nigeria has the largest number of reported cases due to a series of epidemics from 1986 to 1994. Since 1990, outbreaks have occurred in many West African countries, including Cameroon (1990), Ghana (1993–1994, 1996), Liberia (1995, 1998, 2004), Gabon (1994), Senegal (1995–1996, 2002), Benin (1996), Guinea (2000–2001), Cote d'Ivoire (2001), and Burkina Faso (2004). During West African outbreaks, up to 3% of the population may develop yellow fever and 20% is infected. Because the population is regularly exposed in and around villages, children without naturally acquired immunity are at highest risk of infection and illness.

In East Africa, outbreaks are less frequent but have been reported from Sudan in 1940, 1959, and 2004; Ethiopia in 1960 and 1966; and Kenya in 1936 and 1992–1993. Although no human disease was reported in the intervening years, low-level virus transmission occurs. In East African countries where serosurveys were performed between outbreaks, people acquired yellow fever virus-specific antibody, showing that inapparent or mild infections occurred in the absence of recognized disease. Nonetheless, East African transmission is likely also lower due to the low vector competence of *Ae. aegypti* and *Ae. simpsoni* subpopulations.

In South America, most yellow fever cases are reported from the Orinoco, Amazon, and Araguaia river basins and contiguous grasslands. Between 1985 and 1999, 2894 cases were reported; of these, 1761 (61%) were fatal. This high fatality rate is likely due to the increased confirmation of fatal cases using histopathologic examination of liver tissue rather than greater virus virulence or poorer medical treatment. This has led to speculation that the true incidence of yellow fever in South America may be 10-fold greater than reported numbers of cases. Peru and Bolivia had the highest incidence; this is attributed to low vaccination coverage. In South America, yellow fever virus is transmitted in sparsely populated forested areas rather than urban areas. As a result, the highest incidence is among males aged 15 to 45 years who are agricultural and forest workers. In Brazil, most cases are reported from the Amazon and western Brazil; however, cases have been reported from Sao Paulo, Bahia, Tocantins, and Goias states. Also, in 1998, the first cases of yellow fever were reported in French Guiana since 1902.[25] In addition to the increased number of cases in recent years, *Ae. aegypti* has reinfested many urban centers in South America, and there is now the potential that urban yellow fever will return to the Americas.

Yellow fever has never emerged in Asia. Because urban areas in Asia have *Ae. aegypti* that is capable of transmitting yellow fever virus and a large susceptible human population, Asia is vulnerable to the introduction of the virus. As a result, India and other Asian nations require vaccination of travelers from yellow fever-endemic regions. Possible explanations for the absence of yellow fever virus in Asia include immunologic cross-protection provided by previous dengue virus infections, low vector competence of local *Ae. aegypti* populations, or the occurrence of yellow fever in remote African and South American areas populated by people who do not travel by air and are unlikely to spread infection.

Seasonality

The ecology of yellow fever virus is complex, and many factors contribute to yellow fever virus transmission. In general, virus activity increases when temperature, humidity, and rainfall increase through effects on mosquito abundance. In South America, yellow fever incidence is highest during months of high rainfall, humidity, and temperature (January to May). This corresponds to periods of increased activity and reproduction of *Haemagogus* mosquitoes, a mosquito dependent on accumulated water in tree hole-breeding sites. During this time, human exposure to potentially infected mosquitoes is also increased during agricultural activities.

In the savanna zone of West Africa, yellow fever cases begin to appear during the midrainy season (August). Peak occurs during the early dry season (October), a period that corresponds to the period of maximum longevity of mosquito vectors. Because *Ae. aegypti* breeds in receptacles used for water storage, its activity and reproduction patterns are less dependent on rainfall. As a result, when *Ae. aegypti* is involved in virus transmission, yellow fever may also occur in the dry season in both rural and urban areas.

Disease Susceptibility and Risk Factors for Human Infection

Age, sex, and occupation affect the distribution of yellow fever cases and differ in Africa and South America. In South America, *Haemagogus* mosquitoes that previously fed on viremic monkeys in the rain forest canopy transmit virus to humans. Human infection is linked to occupational activities such as forest clearing, lumbering, and road construction; up to 90% of yellow fever cases are young men. In these settings, virus-specific antibody is 2.5 to 7.5 times more common in males than females.[26] The age and sex distribution of sylvatic yellow fever cases differs from that observed during the *Ae. aegypti*-borne epidemics in South America in the early 20th century. During these epidemics, because *Ae. aegypti* breeds around houses, a higher prevalence of infection occurred among children and women.

In Africa, sylvatic *Aedes* species reach high densities in the moist savanna and enter villages. In these settings, the prevalence of infection is higher in children and women, and the prevalence of naturally acquired immunity increases with age. During outbreaks, children are at highest risk for infection and disease. A high attack rate in children (>70%) typifies areas where older people are protected by pre-existing immunity from naturally acquired infections or yellow fever vaccination campaigns.

DISEASE

Clinical manifestations of yellow fever viral infection are broad and include asymptomatic infection; abortive infection with nonspecific symptoms of viral illness (i.e., low-grade fever, myalgia, and headache); and classic yellow fever, a clinical syndrome of multiple organ system failure (MOSF) with hemorrhage, liver failure, and renal failure (Fig. 71-3). These variable manifestations make the diagnosis of less severe and sporadic infections difficult, resulting in an underestimate of morbidity and an overestimate of case fatality rates.

Triphasic Disease

After a 3- to 6-day incubation, it is estimated that 15% to 50% of infected people develop illness, beginning with the abrupt onset of fever, chills, and headache. Of those who develop any illness, approximately 75% to 85% will abort their infection and recover without developing classic yellow fever. The remaining 15% to 25% who become ill develop the syndrome known as yellow fever.[26] Following incubation, classic yellow fever is characterized by three clinical illness stages: infection, remission, and intoxication (see Fig. 71-3).

The first clinical period, the period of infection, lasts 3 or 4 days and is characterized by viremia and the pathophysiologic response to this viremia. Illness onset is abrupt, with fever of 39°C or higher, chills, malaise, headache, low back and knee pain, generalized myalgia, nausea, and dizziness. On examination, the patient has a heart rate lower than would

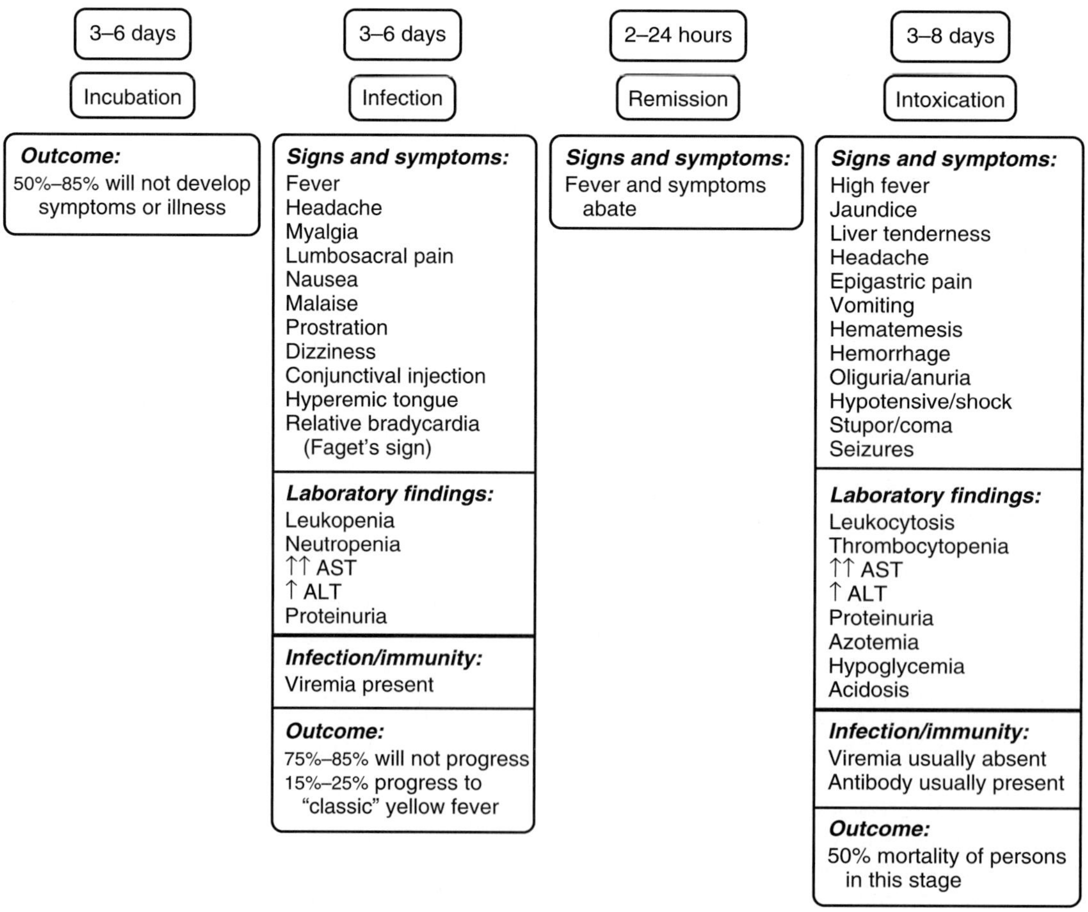

FIGURE 71-3 Stages of yellow fever infection showing the duration, major clinical and laboratory findings, and outcome of each stage. (Modified from Monath TP: Yellow fever: An update. Lancet Infect Dis 1:11–20, 2001)

be expected for the degree of fever (Faget's sign) and congestion and erythema of the conjunctivae, tongue, and face. Temperatures up to 40.5°C are associated with severe illness and poor outcome. Children 5 years old or younger may experience febrile convulsions. Laboratory abnormalities include leukopenia (1.5 to 2.5 × $10^3/\mu L$) with a relative neutropenia. Jaundice or hepatocellular enzyme elevation are rarely present during this period but may begin 2 or 3 days after illness onset. [27] In addition, proteinuria may be severe and is one of the few specific clinical findings during this early phase. Peak viremia occurs on the second or third day of illness, and infected people may serve as a source of infection for mosquitoes that poses a public health risk.[28]

The period of infection may be followed by a distinct period of remission when fever and other constitutional symptoms abate for up to 48 hours. Viremia may still be present during this period but is usually waning. Most patients will go on to recovery from the acute illness. Because they remain anicteric and the specificity of these early clinical signs are poor, it is difficult to diagnose these milder yellow fever viral infections clinically. In patients who do not abort their infection, fever will reappear and the patients will progress to the more fulminant period of intoxication.

Approximately 15% to 25% of people who develop any clinical symptoms (or 10% of all infected people) progress to the period of intoxication. This generally occurs 3 to 6 days after illness onset and lasts for approximately 3 to 8 days. During this period, viremia disappears, antibodies appear, and the signs of classic yellow fever (jaundice, renal failure, and hemorrhage) appear. It is heralded by the return of fever, relative bradycardia, nausea, and vomiting. In addition, patients develop epigastric pain, jaundice, oliguria, and hemorrhagic signs and rapidly progress to MOSF dominated by hepatic, renal, hematologic, and cardiovascular involvement. Serum concentrations of hepatocellular enzymes, aspartate aminotransferase (AST) and alanine aminotransferase (ALT), peak early in this phase. In yellow fever, AST levels are generally greater than ALT levels, in contrast to viral hepatitis, in which the reverse is true. In fatal yellow fever cases, the AST and ALT levels are usually greater than 2700 and 600 U, respectively. Direct bilirubin levels are typically between 5 and 10 mg/dL and higher in fatal cases compared to nonfatal cases.[29,30]

Renal dysfunction is characterized by albuminuria, microscopic hematuria, reduced urine output, and rising blood urea nitrogen and creatinine. As a result of increased glomerular permeability, albumin concentrations in the urine are typically in the nephrotic range (3 to 5 g/L) and may reach 20 g/L. Serum creatinine levels are three to eight times normal. Despite the severity of the renal disease and albuminuria, the extravascular fluid accumulations that accompany many hemorrhagic fever viruses (i.e., edema, ascites, and pleural effusion) are not seen in yellow fever. Also, despite the apparent severity of renal failure, dialysis is not usually needed.[31]

In addition to the pathologic changes in the liver and the kidneys, there are widespread petechiae and hemorrhages on mucosal surfaces, in the skin, and within other organs. The hemorrhagic signs include hematemesis (coffee grounds emesis), melena, hematuria, metrorrhagia, petechiae, ecchymoses, epistaxis, and oozing of blood from the gums and needle puncture sites. Laboratory findings reflect the marked dysfunction of the hematologic system and coagulation cascade that contributes to the hemorrhagic signs. These include thrombocytopenia, prolonged clotting and prothrombin times, and reductions in clotting factors synthesized by the liver (factors II, V, VII, IX, and X). Some patients develop disseminated intravascular coagulation (DIC) marked by diminished fibrinogen and factor VIII and the presence of fibrin split products.

Myocarditis occurs in many patients and undoubtedly contributes to cardiovascular dysfunction. The electrocardiogram may show sinus bradycardia without conduction defects and ST-T abnormalities presumably due to virus replication and direct viral injury to the myocardium. Bradycardia may contribute to the physiologic decompensation associated with shock and metabolic acidosis in severe cases.

Although central nervous system (CNS) signs, such as delirium, seizures, and coma, may be present, there is little to suggest direct viral invasion of the CNS. In the most severe cases, no pleocytosis is present, although there may be modest elevations of protein in the cerebrospinal fluid (CSF). In pathologic examinations, no inflammatory changes are present in the brain. Because true encephalitis is rare, it is likely that the CNS signs are the result of poor cerebral perfusion, cerebral edema, cytokine dysregulation, or metabolic abnormality.

Risk Factors for Illness

Older people and males are at risk for a more severe clinical course. Studies of the clinical course among immunosuppressed people are not available. Protein-calorie malnutrition has been associated with failure to respond immunologically to yellow fever vaccine, but there are no reports that malnourished people have more severe disease caused by wild-type yellow fever virus. Similarly, the immune response to yellow fever vaccine is significantly impaired in pregnant women compared to nonpregnant women.[32] This difference has been attributed to the immunosuppression associated with pregnancy, but pregnancy has not been reported as a risk factor for more severe disease. Human immunodeficiency virus (HIV) infection may be an important risk factor for increased yellow fever viremia following infection, disease severity, and risk for AEFI after yellow fever vaccination. A poor immune response has been noted following yellow fever 17D vaccination of HIV-infected travelers and children,[33] but there has been only a single published report of a severe AEFI in an HIV-infected person.[34]

Mortality

Nearly 50% of patients who develop hepatic and renal failure and anuria die. Disease severity and mortality are highest in older adults.[35] Death is preceded by profound hypotension and shock that is difficult to manage with fluids and vasopressors. This condition appears to be due to an outpouring of proinflammatory cytokines that are produced by infected and injured macrophages and lymphocytes rather than extravascular fluid loss. In addition to hypotension, worsening jaundice, and acute renal failure, signs of cerebral edema (e.g., hypothermia, coma, and Cheyne–Stokes respirations) are associated with impending death. Other signs include hypoglycemia, uncorrectable acidosis, leukocytosis, hyperkalemia, agitated delirium, intractable hiccups, and seizures.

Complications of yellow fever among survivors include superimposed bacterial pneumonia, parotitis, and sepsis. Late deaths during convalescence have been attributed to myocarditis, arrhythmia, or heart failure. Convalescence may be associated with weakness and fatigability lasting weeks, but healing of the liver and kidney is typically complete without postnecrotic fibrosis. In some cases, jaundice and elevated hepatocellular enzymes may persist for months.

PATHOGENESIS AND IMMUNITY

Pathogenesis and Pathophysiology

Although yellow fever has features in common with other hemorrhagic fever or hepatitis viruses, the type and severity of hepatic injury and accompanying renal injury are pathologically distinct.[36,37] Kidney, liver, and myocardial damage is due to the direct injury of viral replication. In addition to the viral-induced pathologic changes in the liver and kidneys, there are profound ischemic changes in other organs resulting from widespread hemorrhages and the resulting profound shock. In addition, there may be mitochondrial damage that results in increased membrane permeability and apoptotic cell death. Interestingly, most of this injury occurs during the period of intoxication, when yellow fever viremia is usually absent and virus-specific antibodies are developing.

Pathogenesis of Hepatic Failure

Unlike hepatitis, in which ballooning necrosis and cell-mediated inflammation are the primary cause of cell damage, the liver destruction of yellow fever results from apoptosis and is not associated with significant inflammation. Nevertheless, markers of hepatic dysfunction, such as elevated bilirubin and hepatocellular enzymes, correlate directly with disease severity and prognosis. The five central features of yellow fever liver pathology are eosinophilic degeneration of hepatocytes and Kupffer cells, midzonal (zone 2) hepatocellular degeneration, the absence of inflammation, microvesicular fatty change, and retention of the reticulin structure with return to normal histology in survivors. A unique feature of hepatic injury in yellow fever is the midzonal distribution with sparing of cells around the central vein and portal tracts. Although this unique distribution may be the result of poor tissue perfusion of this region and ischemia, yellow fever virus antigen and RNA have been observed disproportionately in the hepatocytes in the midzone, suggesting that these cells are more susceptible to virus replication.[37,38] Although, on average, up to 80% of hepatocytes may be destroyed, the livers of survivors heal without postnecrotic fibrosis.

Pathogenesis of Renal Failure

The pathogenesis of renal injury in humans is poorly understood but appears multifactorial. In studies of nonhuman primates, although viral antigen can be detected in the kidney parenchyma, the initial oliguria does not appear to be due to direct renal injury by the virus.[38] Instead, the initial injury appears to be due to renal ischemia that is out of proportion to the degree of hypovolemia that is present and more likely attributable to tumor necrosis factor (TNF) and other proinflammatory cytokines. At death, immunohistochemistry (IHC) can detect antigen in glomeruli and renal tubular cells, suggesting a role for direct viral injury. In addition, renal failure may be due to the severe hepatic injury (i.e., hepatorenal syndrome) that alters salt and water regulation and can be present in the absence of renal pathology. Prior to death, oliguria worsens and is often accompanied by proteinuria, azotemia, acidosis, shock, hyperkalemia, and severe tubular necrosis.

Pathogenesis of Myocardial Injury

Myocardial injury in yellow fever appears to be due to viral replication within the myocardial cells, where viral antigen can be demonstrated by IHC. Myocardial cells undergo similar apoptotic changes as seen in liver and kidney, as well as microsteatosis. As in other organs, damage may be patchy, and there is no significant inflammatory response. As in the liver, the reticulin structure is preserved, and no fibrosis occurs after recovery. Lesions have been noted in the conduction system. These changes often result in conduction and other rhythm disturbance abnormalities. When bradycardia is present, it may contribute to the physiologic decompensation associated with hypotension, reduced perfusion, and metabolic acidosis in severe cases. The pathological changes in these major conduction pathways suggest a physiologic basis for late deaths attributed to cardiac arrhythmias.

Coagulation Defects

Coagulopathy is the result of two processes—decreased hepatic synthesis of coagulation factors and the presence of DIC, a process of accelerated consumption of coagulation factors and platelets. The basis of DIC is the unregulated and excessive generation of thrombin that results in the consumption of coagulation factors such as fibrinogen and factor VIII. In addition, thrombin binds thrombin receptors on platelets to induce platelet activation and aggregation to endothelium and initiates simultaneous coagulation and fibrinolysis. Similar events occur in people with dengue hemorrhagic fever (DHF), in which liver function and synthesis of clotting factors are well maintained compared to yellow fever. In DHF, the events are mediated through the intrinsic coagulation pathway and activated by cytokines, particularly TNF, interleukin (IL)-6, and IL-1. It is not known whether the same mechanisms are operating in yellow fever. In studies of yellow fever virus-infected monkeys, severely ill animals have depressed levels of all clotting factors, particularly fibrinogen and factors V, VII, VIII, and X. This situation suggests that yellow fever does not specifically activate the intrinsic pathway, and that the major cause of bleeding is decreased synthesis of clotting factors.

Other Hematologic Abnormalities

Leukopenia, particularly neutropenia, is an early finding in yellow fever infection. IFN may contribute to leukopenia and thrombocytopenia by bone marrow suppression and induction of a wide array of cytokines. Neutropenia and thrombocytopenia also may be caused more directly by cytokines such as TNF, IL-1, or IL-6 released during the initial infection. The spleen and lymph nodes undergo profound changes in yellow fever infection, characterized by the appearance of large mononuclear or histiocytic cells and the disappearance of small lymphocytes.

Hypotension and Shock

Infection of the endothelium may play a central role in the pathogenesis of many hemorrhagic fevers. In dengue, infected endothelial cells release large amounts of proinflammatory cytokines (IL-6 and IL-8) and oxygen free radicals that trigger coagulation, fibrinolysis, plasma leakage, and hypotension. Endothelial infection and injury have not been specifically studied in yellow fever, but it is likely that these are important factors in pathogenesis.

Encephalopathy

In the terminal stage of infection, humans and nonhuman primates develop stupor and coma, which is probably metabolic in origin. Contributing factors include hypoglycemia (due to the liver's impaired gluconeogenesis), decreased perfusion, and acidosis. Changes in tissue concentrations of water and electrolytes in various compartments of the CNS have been described, including intracellular dehydration of medulla, cerebellum, and spinal cord. In addition, the encephalopathy appears to be partially due to the hepatorenal syndrome that frequently accompanies fatal cases of yellow fever. CNS invasion by yellow fever virus is rare. Even in fatal cases, in which seizures and coma are present, inflammatory changes in the brain are not seen.

Innate Immunity

Although there are few yellow fever-specific studies, it is assumed that the first line of host defense is a nonspecific, innate immune response. This includes the natural killer cell response and other resistance factors that interfere with virus replication before the appearance of virus-specific cytotoxic T cells and antibodies. Many studies of dengue show the importance of type-1 interferons (IFNs) in this nonspecific, innate immune response to flavivirus infection. IFN activates several host defense mechanisms, including increasing natural killer (NK) cells, CD14-bearing monocyte/macrophages, major histocompatibility complex class I (MHC-I) proteins on the host cell surface, Th1-dependent immunoglobulin synthesis, and cytotoxic T-lymphocyte activity.[39–41] Monkeys treated with IFN had lower yellow fever viremia and liver injury,[42] and IFN knockout mice showed poor yellow fever viral clearance and a poor cellular inflammatory response after intracerebral inoculation compared to parental mice.[43] It is uncertain whether these effects were due to a direct antiviral effect, immunomodulation by IFN, or induction of other cytokines. In addition to IFN, a variety of other proinflammatory cytokines and markers of T-cell activation have been found during the viremic period after yellow fever vaccination in humans, including TNF, IL-1, neopterin, β_2-microglobulin, and circulating CD8+ T cells.[44,45] It is likely that similar responses occur in people infected with wild-type yellow fever virus.

The genetic constitution of the host is one of the most important factors influencing the outcome of viral infection. This has been investigated using inbred strains of mice that differed in their resistance to flaviviruses including yellow fever virus.[46] In some cases, resistant mice appeared to be more susceptible to the antiviral action of IFN, although at least one resistance gene (*flv*) confers flavivirus-specific resistance by an IFN-independent mechanism.[47] In general, susceptibility to disease correlated with increased levels of viral replication in tissues. IFN-dependent activation of 2′,5′-oligoadenylate synthetase is under genetic control and determines susceptibility to flavivirus infections in mice. It is uncertain whether this mechanism contributes to the severe AEFI with yellow fever 17D.

Since approximately 10% of infected people develop classic yellow fever, it is clear that the innate immune system or other mechanisms may fail to protect the host. This may be due to viral mechanisms that reduce immune clearance by NK cells. Unlike many viruses that decrease the density of MHC-I proteins on the infected cell surface, flaviviruses increase their density through the increased supply of related peptides to the ER through the action of IFN.[48] Since MHC-I proteins protect cells against attack by NK cells, flavivirus-infected cells avoid clearance by the innate activity of NK cells.

Adaptive Immune Response

Up to 10^4 yellow fever virions are inoculated into extravascular tissues during probing by an infected female mosquito. In an immune host, virus first encounters yellow fever virus-specific neutralizing antibodies in the extracellular transudate and lymph. It is believed that most virions are neutralized, but it is unclear if the entire inoculum is neutralized or whether some portion is processed in the dendritic cell as in the nonimmune host.[37,49] Assuming that yellow fever virus is processed like dengue and other flaviviruses, non-neutralized virus infects epidermal dendritic cells and undergoes replication ("productive infection").

The nonspecific, innate immune response is followed by a specific immune response characterized by the development of neutralizing antibodies and cytotoxic T cells. In addition, cytolytic antibodies against viral proteins on the surface of infected cells and antibody-dependent, cell-mediated cytotoxicity contribute to viral clearance. The humoral response to yellow fever virus is characterized by the appearance of IgM antibodies in the first 7 or 8 days following infection (i.e., 4 or 5 days after illness onset). IgM levels peak 7 to 14 days after illness onset and decline rapidly over 30 to 60 days but may persist for years at low levels. Neutralizing antibodies persist for many years, if not lifelong, after natural yellow fever infection and provide complete protection against disease on reexposure to the virus. No documented case of a second clinical yellow fever infection has been reported. Complement-fixing (CF) antibodies against NS1 expressed on the infected cell surface lead to complement-mediated cytolysis and clearance of infected cells early in recovery. It is not known whether this anti-NS1 CF antibody protects against reinfection or only plays a role in virus clearance during recovery from infection.

People with pre-existing antibody to other flaviviruses (i.e., heterologous antibody) develop broadly cross-reactive antibody responses following yellow fever virus infection. In contrast to dengue, in which such heterologous antibody may enhance disease, this antibody protects against yellow fever. Nonhuman primates actively immunized with Zika, Wesselsbron, or dengue viruses are protected against a subsequent yellow fever virus challenge.[50,51] Other studies show that humans with broadly reactive antibody to unspecified African flaviviruses have a lower incidence of yellow fever disease than people with primary yellow fever infections.[52]

Although little is known about the human cellular immune responses to yellow fever, it is likely that cytotoxic T lymphocytes kill flavivirus-infected cells and contribute to viral clearance and recovery from primary infection. In studies of yellow fever viral encephalitis in T and B cell knockout mice, CD4+ cells are important for protection.[43] There are no data on human cellular responses to wild-type yellow fever virus.

DIAGNOSIS

The differential diagnosis of classic yellow fever includes severe malaria with rapid hemolysis, severe hepatitis E in pregnancy, hepatitis D superinfection, other viral hemorrhagic fevers that may rarely have jaundice (e.g., dengue hemorrhagic fever and Crimean–Congo hemorrhagic fever), leptospirosis, and relapsing fever due to *Borrelia recurrentis*. Most hemorrhagic fever viruses, such as Marburg, Ebola, and Lassa fever viruses, are not usually associated with jaundice but may still cause diagnostic confusion. Milder clinical cases or people in the early, anicteric phase of yellow fever resemble people with many other febrile illnesses.

Specific laboratory diagnosis relies on serology or, during the early, anicteric phase, on detection of virus, viral antigens, or viral RNA in blood. None of these methods are commercially available. In clinical samples, yellow fever virus-specific real-time quantitative reverse transcriptase polymerase chain reaction (rtPCR) assays can detect titers as low as 0.1 PFU/mL and much lower than standard rtPCR (lower limit, 1 PFU/mL) or virus isolation in cell culture (lower limit, 10 PFU/mL).[53] In addition to increased sensitivity, both PCR methods give a definitive result in a much shorter time than virus isolation in any system. Because clinical suspicion of yellow fever is low during the early, anicteric phase of infection when viremia is present, isolation, genomic amplification, and antigen detection have played a minor role in yellow fever diagnosis to date.

Serology is the most important diagnostic test, and yellow fever virus-specific IgM enzyme-linked immunosorbent assay (ELISA) is the most widely used serological method. The presence of IgM antibodies in a single serum sample taken on or after day 7 of clinical illness or during the early recovery phase provides a presumptive diagnosis, and demonstration of a fourfold increase in antibody titer in paired sera (using ELISA, neutralization, or HI assays) is confirmatory. The specificity of IgM ELISA is high in primary infections and in most secondary flavivirus infection. Despite this high specificity, cross-reactions between yellow fever and other flaviviruses frequently complicate serological diagnosis, especially in people who live in areas where other flaviviruses are endemic, and confirmation by the more specific neutralization assays may be necessary. When testing a person with the signs and symptoms of yellow fever during a documented yellow fever outbreak, confirmation should not be necessary.

In fatal cases, the characteristic histopathologic liver changes (e.g., midzonal necrosis and Councilman's bodies) are diagnostic. IHC with poly- or monoclonal antibodies to yellow fever virus to detect yellow fever antigen in tissue is diagnostic and more specific than standard histopathology. Despite the high potential for a specific diagnosis, liver biopsies in living patients should not be performed because fatal hemorrhage may occur.

TREATMENT AND PROGNOSIS

The management of patients with yellow fever has not been optimized because disease occurs in areas with rudimentary medical services and the hemodynamic instability of these patients often precludes transport. Because there is no yellow fever virus-specific therapy, intensive supportive care to maximize tissue perfusion, reduce hemorrhagic complications, maintain adequate glucose levels, and provide nutritional maintenance is necessary to reduce the mortality of yellow fever. In addition, the following has been recommended: nasogastric suction to prevent gastric distension and aspiration, intravenous agents to reduce gastric acidity and prevent gastric bleeding, fluid replacement with normal saline or Ringer's lactate, vasopressors if needed, administration of oxygen, correction of metabolic acidosis, treatment of bleeding with fresh-frozen plasma, and treatment of secondary infections with antibiotics. Unfortunately, patients with yellow fever do not respond dramatically to fluid replacement or vasopressors; this is likely due to irreversible pathophysiologic processes and the unchecked effect of TNF or other cytokines.[36] Heparin should only be used to treat DIC when there has been documented consumption of clotting factors and activation of fibrinolytic mechanisms and when there is adequate laboratory support to monitor heparin's effects. If available and needed, dialysis should be used in cases of renal failure or anuria. Other medical considerations may include orthotopic liver transplantation or the use of extracorporeal support systems.[54] Although these are beyond the capacity of developing nations, they may be potential interventions for Western travelers who develop yellow fever following travel or who develop MOSF as an adverse effect after yellow fever immunization. In the future, other possible nonspecific treatments may include anticytokine therapies or cytokine receptor blockers to prevent cell apoptosis.

There is no specific antiviral treatment. Although ribavirin has activity against yellow fever virus at high (potentially cytotoxic) concentrations in vitro,[55] ribavirin monotherapy has failed in animal studies. Passive antibody, IFN, and IFN inducers are only effective if given before infection or during incubation. There is no current indication for their use, and passive antibody protection should only be considered in the setting of postexposure prophylaxis (i.e., after known infection and before illness onset), such as in a laboratory exposure. Corticosteroids have not been evaluated for the treatment of yellow fever.

PREVENTION AND CONTROL

Yellow Fever Vaccine

During the 1930s, both wild-type yellow fever virus strains, Asibi and French, were attenuated to derive live vaccines known as 17D and the French neurotropic vaccine, respectively.[56] Currently, 17D is the only strain of yellow fever virus used for vaccination. During vaccine production from 1937 to 1941, two different 17D substrains, 17D-204 and 17-DD, were developed in parallel; these are used for current vaccine production. Although they differ with respect to 17D substrain and other production qualities, they are both produced in embryonated eggs and meet the same WHO standards for safety and potency. In addition, their biologic performance is similar with respect to seroconversion rate, quality of the immune response, durability of immunity, safety, and tolerability. 17D vaccines are a heterogeneous mixtures of multiple virus subpopulations. Not surprisingly, differences have been found in plaque size, oligonucleotide fingerprints, and nucleotide sequencing. There is no evidence that such variations affect safety or efficacy.

Three manufacturers in Brazil, France, and Senegal produce vaccine for the Expanded Programme of Immunization (EPI) and mass vaccination campaigns. Sanofi Pasteur and Evans (a Chiron affiliate) export vaccine for the traveler's market. Approximately 55 million doses are produced annually by these sources.

Immune Response

More than 95% of vaccinated people develop neutralizing antibodies within 10 to 14 days of immunization. Race does not appear to influence response rates. In one study, males had lower antibody titers than females.[57] In the majority of cases, antibody titers following vaccination are lower, and their appearance is delayed compared to natural yellow fever virus infections. This is likely due to less virus replication and antigen expression by the 17D strain. The minimal protective level of neutralizing antibodies induced by 17D vaccine has been estimated by dose-response studies in rhesus monkeys that are subsequently challenged after immunization with virulent yellow fever virus. In such studies, log neutralization index[58] (LNI; measured by plaque reduction) of 0.7 or greater measured 20 weeks after immunization was strongly associated with protection. Human clinical trials of 17D vaccine have shown geometric mean LNI values of 2.1 or greater measured within 1 month after vaccination.[57] The International Health Regulations stipulate that the vaccination certificate for yellow fever is valid 10 days after administration of 17D vaccine, corresponding to the time at which the majority of vaccinees are demonstrably immune. Immunity following 17D vaccination is remarkably durable and may be lifelong. Although the yellow fever immunization certificate for international travel is valid for 10 years, this interval was based on published studies showing that neutralizing antibodies were present in more than 90% of people 16 to 19 years after vaccination. Later studies of U.S. military veterans from World War II tested 30 to 35 years after a single dose of 17D vaccine showed that slightly more than 80% had neutralizing antibody, and in some subgroups more than 95% had it.[56]

Adventitious Viruses

In 1966, yellow fever 17D vaccines were found to be contaminated with avian leukosis virus (ALV), a retrovirus with a high prevalence in chicken embryos. New ALV-free seeds were prepared in the 1970s, and all international manufacturers now use ALV-free seeds as stipulated by WHO. WHO still permits some local manufacturers to use ALV-contaminated embryos. Although the presence of ALV in yellow fever vaccine is undesirable because of the possible insertion of ALV oncogenes, there is no evidence to implicate ALV in human disease. This was addressed in a retrospective study of cancer deaths in World War II veterans in which the incidence of all cancers, lymphoma, and leukemia was not significantly different in people vaccinated 5 to 22 years previously with 17D vaccine than in those not vaccinated.

During the original formulation and early use of 17D vaccines, pooled human serum was used as a vaccine stabilizer. This resulted in vaccine contamination with hepatitis B virus and a massive outbreak of jaundice and hepatitis in yellow fever vaccine recipients. Human serum was eliminated from yellow fever vaccines by 1942, and current vaccines are not contaminated with human hepatitis viruses.

Vaccine Dose, Route of Administration, and Preparations

A 17D vaccine dose contains approximately 10^5 PFU in 0.5 mL and is given subcutaneously, usually in the upper arm. All yellow fever vaccines are prepared as lyophilized powder but vary with respect to stabilizer additives and salt content. Some contain sodium chloride and buffer salts and are reconstituted with sterile water, whereas others are reconstituted with saline. Because there is no preservative in the vaccine and because the vaccine rapidly loses potency after reconstitution, it must be refrigerated at the point of use and held on ice and used soon after reconstitution. In the United States, reconstituted vaccine must be discarded within 1 hour; in EPI systems, it must be discarded within 4 hours. Vaccine is supplied in single- and multiple-dose containers. Although combination vaccines have been tested clinically (e.g., yellow fever–measles and yellow fever–typhoid), no such products are available.

Viremia Following 17D Vaccination

Wild-type yellow fever virus causes higher viremia than the 17D vaccine strains in monkeys and humans. Most adult vaccinees have virus titers less than 100 PFU/mL, which is far below the 4 or 5 logs of virus titer needed to infect mosquitoes. The low viremia following 17D vaccine may explain the apparent low risk of transplacental transmission in women immunized during pregnancy. Viremia begins 3 or 4 days after vaccination and lasts 1 to 3 days.[56] Thus, the incubation period and duration of viremia are similar to those of wild-type yellow fever virus. Like naturally acquired infections, viremia disappears when neutralizing antibodies develop 8 or 9 days after immunization. There are no data on viremia levels in infants or children given 17D vaccine or in people who are immunosuppressed.

Genetic Stability during Replication in the Vaccinated Host

The 17D vaccine is not clonal. It is a heterogeneous mixture of virus variants with varying antigenic, genetic, and biological properties. Despite this, it is considered one of the safest vaccines in use today and thought to have very little potential for reversion to wild-type or emergence of pathogenic strains. Isolation of a strain that was more virulent than the parental 17D vaccine strain has been documented only once following routine vaccination. In one fatal human encephalitis case, the viral isolate from the brain had higher neurovirulence in mice than the 17D-204 strain. This isolate caused encephalitis in nonhuman primates, reacted with a wild-type virus-specific monoclonal antibody, and had two amino acid changes in the E protein and one in NS4B. Other studies indicate a high degree of genetic stability of 17D virus during in vivo replication. Vaccine virus strains isolated from the sera of people vaccinated with the 17D-204 vaccine contained no mutations in the structural genes and a few mutations in the nonstructural protein genes, especially the NS5 protein gene.[59] Other studies have supported the finding that mutations in yellow fever virus tend to accumulate at a significantly lower rate than expected for an RNA virus.[16]

Revaccination

Revaccination or vaccination of people with naturally acquired immunity is followed by a booster antibody response in most vaccinees, although the rise in titer is less than that seen in primary vaccination. This suggests that there is decreased virus replication due to the pre-existing immunity. A stronger antibody response following revaccination is more likely in individuals with a low neutralizing antibody titer prior to vaccination. The response is characterized by a large and rapid increase in IgG antibodies, indicating a memory response resulting from prior sensitization.

Immunization in People with Prior Flavivirus Immunity

Because of cross-reactive antigenic determinants, the primary immune response to 17D vaccine may be qualitatively different in people with preexisting heterologous immunity. Several studies have shown that naturally acquired dengue immunity reduces seroconversion and blunts the immune response to 17D vaccine, whereas preexisting immunity to flaviviruses in the Japanese encephalitis complex does not. There is no clear evidence that prior flavivirus immunity enhances replication of yellow fever 17D virus or the immune response to 17D virus.

Similarly, people with preexisting immunity to the yellow fever 17D vaccine have a qualitatively different immune response to immunization with vaccines against heterologous flaviviruses. In yellow fever-immune individuals, vaccinated with an experimental, attenuated dengue vaccine, the antibody response was greater in magnitude and duration than in nonimmune individuals, suggesting that cross-reactive antibodies may be associated with enhanced dengue virus replication in vivo. A different mechanism, the anamnestic responses to cross-reactive determinants, explains the higher response in recipients of inactivated vaccines (e.g., tick-borne encephalitis vaccine).

People with heterologous flavivirus immunity broadly respond to 17D vaccination with both homologous and hetero-logous neutralizing antibodies. The phenomenon of “original antigenic sin” has been noted in people previously vaccinated with 17D virus and subsequently infected with another flavivirus. In such cases, an anamnestic response leads to a rapid rise in yellow fever antibodies, but the antibody response to the more recent heterologous infection is delayed and diminished. This phenomenon may lead to diagnostic confusion in patients with clinical syndromes resembling naturally acquired yellow fever.

Yellow Fever Vaccine Efficacy in Humans

The efficacy of yellow fever vaccine has never been tested in controlled human clinical trials. Numerous studies in nonhuman primates have demonstrated that vaccination protects vaccine recipients and that protection is strongly correlated with the development and titers of neutralizing antibody. The importance of neutralizing antibody has been shown by the protection of animals by passive immunization (infusion of serum containing yellow fever virus-specific neutralizing antibody) before or soon after challenge with virulent yellow fever virus.

Several primary observations support yellow fever vaccination as being protective in humans, including the reduction of laboratory-associated infections in vaccinated workers; the fact that in Brazil and other South American countries, yellow fever only occurs in unvaccinated people; and the rapid disappearance of cases during campaign-style vaccination programs initiated during epidemics. One of the greater testaments to the effectiveness of yellow fever vaccination is the disappearance of yellow fever from French-speaking West Africa after institution of mandatory yellow fever immunization with the French neurotropic vaccine in the 1940s. High vaccine coverage was followed by a marked reduction in disease despite continued human exposure to the enzootic cycle. Unpublished reports comparing the yellow fever incidence among the vaccinated and unvaccinated populations during a 1986 epidemic in Nigeria estimate the effectiveness to be approximately 85%.[56] Because there is an effective vaccine available that is now considered the standard of care, it is highly unlikely that a placebo-controlled trial of the 17D or any newer yellow fever vaccines will be performed. Given these constraints, licensure of any new yellow fever vaccines would likely have to be granted based on a combination of animal safety data and studies using immunologic surrogates.

Vaccine Failure

Rarely, healthy people fail to develop neutralizing antibodies following 17D vaccination. This is not an absolute refractoriness; people who fail to develop antibody after their first vaccination may develop antibody upon revaccination. More rarely, a person who was previously vaccinated may develop clinical yellow fever. Although it is uncertain whether all of these people were properly vaccinated with appropriately handled 17D vaccine, there have been five reports of vaccine recipients who developed yellow fever since development of the yellow fever vaccine.[56]

Three host factors (malnutrition, HIV infection, and pregnancy) have been associated with failure to respond immunologically to 17D vaccine. Further studies are required to assess the relevance of these findings to the use of 17D vaccine in EPI in Africa, particularly where these conditions may frequently result in vaccine failure. In one study, only approximately 40% of pregnant women seroconverted after vaccination compared to 82% to 94% among nonpregnant females of childbearing age, male students, and the general population. This difference was attributed to the immunosuppression associated with pregnancy and emphasizes the need to reimmunize at-risk women who were inadvertently vaccinated during pregnancy.

HIV infection has been associated with a reduced immunologic response to a number of inactivated and live, attenuated vaccines. Some case reports have suggested that vaccinating HIV-infected people without immunosuppression results in seroconversion. However, when 17D vaccine was administered to a small number of adult, HIV-infected travelers with CD4+ counts of 200 or more cells/μL, only 70% seroconverted within 1 month of vaccination.[56] Among HIV-infected infants in developing nations, only 17% developed neutralizing antibodies within 10 months of 17D vaccination compared to 74% of HIV-uninfected controls matched for age and nutritional status.[33] The mechanisms for this diminished response are uncertain. Although an encephalitis case has been reported in an HIV-infected Thai man following yellow fever vaccination, the number of HIV-infected people vaccinated with 17D vaccine is too small to assess safety.[34]

Yellow Fever Vaccine Safety

Preventing infection by vaccination or reducing the abundance of *Ae. aegypti* are the only two effective strategies to reduce yellow fever morbidity and mortality. 17D vaccine, the currently approved yellow fever vaccine, has been available since 1937 and widely used during outbreaks in Africa and South America and by the military and travelers operating in or visiting endemic countries.[49,60] In many affected countries, the need for yellow fever vaccination remains and, in fact, may be increasing.[19,20,61] Because of the vaccine's safety profile, its effectiveness in preventing yellow fever, the lack of virus-specific treatment, and the high mortality of yellow fever, vaccination is an integral strategy for preventing yellow fever-associated mortality and morbidity. In addition, travelers to areas where yellow fever is zoonotic, endemic, or epidemic should be vaccinated if they are at increased risk for infection based on their daily activities or living conditions.[60,62,63]

General Adverse Events

Reactions to 17D yellow fever vaccine are typically mild. After vaccination, vaccinees often report mild headaches, myalgia, low-grade fevers, or other minor symptoms for 5 to 10 days. Reactogenicity of 17D vaccine has been monitored in 12 clinical trials conducted from 1953 to 2002. In trials in which vaccinees were actively followed, incidence rates of 18% to 50% were detected. In one large study, the most common systemic side effects (which did not differ across treatment groups) were headache (~33% of subjects), myalgia (~25%), malaise (~19%), fever (~15%), and chills (~11%).[57] These were generally mild, and few vaccinees curtailed their regular activities. No placebo controls were included in these trials, making interpretation of causality of the AEFIs difficult. Immediate hypersensitivity reactions, characterized by rash, urticaria, or asthma, occur principally among people with histories of allergies to egg or other substances and are estimated to occur in 1 out of 131,000 vaccinations.[64] Gelatin, used as a stabilizer in yellow fever vaccine, has been implicated as a cause of allergic reactions to other vaccines and may play a role in reactions to yellow fever vaccine.

Yellow Fever Vaccine-Associated Viscerotropic Disease

Increasingly frequent reports of yellow fever vaccine-associated viscerotropic disease (YEL-AVD), a syndrome of MOSF following 17D vaccination that pathologically and clinically resembles naturally acquired yellow fever, have raised concern about the safety of this vaccine.[65,68] A total of 29 cases of YEL-AVD have been reported internationally.

From 1996 through 2004, the CDC received reports of 11 recipients of 17D-204 vaccine who developed this newly recognized syndrome in the United States (M. Russell, personal communication, 2005).[62,65,67,68] Ten of these cases were in civilians vaccinated in anticipation of travel, and one was in the military. All 11 people (median age, 64 years; range, 22 to 79 years) became ill within 2 to 5 days of vaccination and developed MOSF requiring intensive care; six died (case fatality rate, 55%).[67,68] In addition to fever, hypotension, and respiratory failure, these people had markedly elevated hepatocellular enzymes and bilirubin, lymphocytopenia, and thrombocytopenia. Vaccine-type yellow fever virus was isolated from the blood of two people on the seventh and eighth days after vaccination. Using IHC, yellow fever antigen was identified in the liver in one person and in multiple tissues (including lung, lymph node, spleen, heart, liver, and muscle) in two fatal cases. Two people with YEL-AVD also had evidence of neuroinvasive infection.

In addition to the 11 U.S. cases, 18 international cases of YEL-AVD have been reported in the literature, at scientific meetings, or to vaccine manufacturers.[62,66–70] The first three international cases from Australia and Brazil were reported simultaneously with the first U.S. cases. They were clinically similar to the U.S. cases except that younger people were affected. In these cases, histopathologic changes characteristic of wild-type yellow fever were noted in the liver. Using IHC and electron microscopy, yellow fever antigen and flavivirus-like particles were found to be present in the areas of mid-zonal necrosis. Vaccine-type virus was isolated from all three people. The isolated viruses retained their vaccine phenotype when placed into experimental animals. No genomic changes previously associated with reversion to virulence were detected. Within months of these reports, other cases of hospitalized people with fever, elevated hepatocellular enzymes, and renal abnormalities were identified, suggesting that, like naturally acquired infections, there may be a spectrum of AEFI.[69,71,72] These international cases occurred among recipients of 17D-204 and 17DD vaccine.

All but of these 29 cases of YEL-AVD have occurred since 1996.[68] One case occurred in 1975 and was identified retrospectively in Brazil. It is not known whether additional cases occurred between 1975 and 1996 but were unrecognized or whether YEL-AVD has newly emerged. No comparable cases were identified in a retrospective review of VAERS reports from 1990 to 1996 (M. Cetron, personal communication, 2004). The true incidence of YEL-AVD is also unknown, but attempts to quantify the risk and identify risk factors continue.[67,68,73]

Yellow Fever Vaccine–Associated Neurotropic Disease

The 17D strain of yellow fever virus has retained some of its neurovirulence as demonstrated by intracerebral inoculation of mice and nonhuman primates. In the first decade of vaccine use, vaccine-associated neurotopic disease (postvaccinal encephalitis), primarily among infants, was the most common serious AEFI. From 1945 through 1991, 21 well-documented cases were reported worldwide. Of these, 16 (76%) occurred in infants aged 9 months or younger.[56] Estimates of the yellow fever vaccine-associated neurotropic disease (YEL-AND) rate among children aged 12 months or younger were elevated and ranged from 0.5 to 4 per 1000 doses. As a result, it was recommended that vaccinating infants younger than 9 months old should be avoided because of the encephalitis risk.[62] A decision to administer vaccine to infants younger than 9 months of age should be based on the risk of exposure to natural infection, but the vaccine should not be administered to infants aged 6 months or younger. The only YEL-AND case in the United States from 1945 to 1991 involved a 3-year-old child who died in 1965.[74]

From the mid-1990s through the mid-2000s, unlike earlier reports, most reported cases of YEL-AND have occurred in adults. In a retrospective review of VAERS data from 1990 to 2002 and through prospective investigation of suspected cases of YEL-AND from 2000 to 2004 reported to VAERS, a total of 15 cases of YEL-AND have been identified among U.S. citizens.[68] The first four were reported and prospectively investigated in 2001 and 2002.[75] A retrospective review of 1995 to 2002 VAERS data identified four more people; all developed Guillain–Barré (GBS) syndrome following vaccination. Since 2002, seven more cases have been prospectively identified among U.S. residents; four had acute demyelinating disease; two had GBS; and one had encephalitis (M. Russell, CDC, personal communication 2005). Like all YEL-AVD cases, all 15 of these people became ill after their first yellow fever vaccination. In addition to these U.S. cases, five international cases have been reported to vaccine manufacturers from 1991 through 2001.[34,73] Of these, three were cases of encephalitis (including one fatal case); one was a case of GBS and one was a case of bulbar palsy. In one series the YEL-AND incidence was estimated to be 3.3 per 1 milliion doses.

In children, YEL-AND was characterized by the onset of fever and seizures, obtundation, meningismus, and paresis 7 to 21 days after immunization. In adults, symptoms included severe headache, confusion, and aphasia. Illness onset in adults varied from 4 to 23 days postvaccination, was similar to that in children, and was longer than that seen with YEL-AVD.[75] In both groups, CSF contains up to 500 cells/μL (predominantly lymphocytic) and elevated protein.

The clinical course is generally brief, recovery is complete, and mortality is low. Of the 15 reported U.S. civilians who developed YEL-AND from 1992 to 2003, all were hospitalized but none died. Similarly, of 21 people who developed YEL-AND from 1945 through 1991, only 1 (5%) died; none of the 16 infants aged 9 months or younger died.[56] Although the risk of death is believed to be low with this syndrome, certain groups of vaccine recipients may be at greater risk of death. In 2002, a fatal case of YEL-AND involving a 53-year-old man with previously unrecognized HIV infection was reported in Thailand.[34]

Risk Factors for YEL-AVD and YEL-AND

Two passive reporting surveillance systems have been used to estimate the frequency of these events: VAERS and a manufacturer's postmarketing safety surveillance system.[67,71,76] Increasing age is a risk factor for serious AEFI. Analyses of 1990 to 2003 VAERS data have demonstrated that people aged 60 years or older are at increased risk for both YEL-AVD and YEL-AND.[67,76] During this period, the all-ages incidence for YEL-AVD in the United States was estimated to be four cases per 1 million civilian doses sold. For vaccine recipients aged 61 to 70 years and those aged 71 years or older, the incidence was 23 and 19 cases per 1 million doses sold, respectively. Using these same data, the all-ages incidence for YEL-AND was estimated to be five cases per 1 million civilian doses sold. For vaccine recipients aged 61 to 70 years and those aged 71 years or older, the reported incidence was 18 and 19 cases per 1 million doses sold, respectively.

Thymus Disease as a Risk Factor

Although not as defined as age, it appears that removal of the thymus or conditions associated with thymomas are risk factors for YEL-AVD. Of 29 people with YEL-AVD identified worldwide through 2003, 4 (14%) had undergone thymectomy 2 to 20 years prior to receiving yellow fever vaccination.[68] Because the incidence of thymomas is low,[77] this observation suggests that a history of thymectomy or conditions associated with thymomas (e.g., myasthenia gravis and hypogammaglobulinemia) may be risk factors for YEL-AVD. Thymomas have been associated with decreased antibody levels, abnormal T-lymphocyte maturation, and several autoimmune conditions.

Risk Assessment

The specific mechanisms underlying serious AEFI after yellow fever vaccination are unknown. As a result, defining at-risk groups whose risk from vaccination is greater than their benefit is difficult. Notably, all reported YEL-AVD and YEL-AND cases occurred in people who were receiving their first yellow fever vaccination. No such cases of people receiving a booster dose have been reported. People receiving booster doses may have lower levels of viremia, significant differences in cytokine response, or a more profound neutralizing antibody response to check viral proliferation compared to primary recipients.

Increasing age, thymoma, and primary vaccination account for some of the increased number of cases; systematic changes in vaccine administration should also be considered. For example, before 1996, immune serum globulin (ISG) was often given as part of travel immunizations to reduce the risk of hepatitis A. Laboratory studies have shown that ISG used in the United States contains significant titers of neutralizing antibody to yellow fever due to the number of plasma donors previously vaccinated while in the military. Whether introduction of hepatitis A vaccine in 1996, which eliminated the need for ISG, may have inadvertently reduced the number of vaccinees receiving passive antibody protection is unknown.

Yellow fever vaccine has been considered one of the safest live-virus vaccines. Reports of serious AEFI after 17D vaccination require reassessment of vaccine use among travelers, and possibly among residents of endemic areas.[49] Yellow fever remains a serious and potentially fatal disease without an efficacious treatment. As a result, the need to vaccinate travelers and residents of endemic areas remains. Categorically refusing an older person vaccine on the basis of age without assessing his or her true risk for disease is not acceptable. Still, the association of increased AEFI risk with age emphasizes the importance of carefully screening travel itineraries of older travelers, travelers with a history of thymoma, or first-time vaccine recipients and only vaccinating those traveling in yellow fever-endemic areas. For travelers whose risk of serious AEFI is great and administration of vaccine is not considered an option, alternative means of prevention, such as personal protection (e.g., use of insect repellants containing *N,N*-diethyl-meta-toluamide or permethrins, wearing long sleeves and pants, using bed nets at night, or staying in air-conditioned or well-screened quarters) may be considered.

Vaccine-Associated Adverse Events in Persons Infected with HIV

Yellow fever is endemic across sub-Saharan Africa, where there is a high prevalence of HIV infection. This region has been the site of numerous vaccination campaigns to control yellow fever epidemics. During emergency vaccination campaigns, AEFI surveillance was established in Kenya in 1993 (passive surveillance) and in Cote d'Ivoire in 2001 (active surveillance.) (D. Gubler, personal communication, 2002). Surveillance was population based and not restricted to case investigations among HIV-infected people. Four encephalitis cases (only one of which was an HIV-infected person) were identified in Kenya,[56] and none were identified in Cote d'Ivoire; no cases of viscerotropic disease were identified during either vaccine campaign. Further studies (e.g., cohort studies of HIV-infected people and case–control studies of the general population) and AEFI surveillance during campaigns in countries with high HIV prevalence are needed to define the risk of serious AEFI in HIV-infected people.

CONCLUSIONS

Yellow fever remains a major public health concern in sub-Saharan Africa and tropical South America despite the availability of an effective vaccine that can have tremendous impact on disease control. Because yellow fever is an epizootic disease, the potential for human outbreaks will always remain when vaccination programs are not maintained. Unfortunately, efforts to control disease have decreased, and proposals to integrate yellow fever vaccine into EPI and routine vaccination activities have been largely replaced by a policy of emergency vaccination campaigns after an outbreak is identified.

Despite the restricted range of endemic virus transmission, it is important for all physicians to be aware of the clinical manifestations and epidemiology of yellow fever because of its potential to cause large urban outbreaks in areas outside of South America and Africa, because of the risk of travelers to these endemic areas, and because of serious adverse events associated with yellow fever vaccination. Because air travel enables anicteric, viremic travelers to return to their homes from any area of the world in less than 24 hours and because of the possibility that the traveler's home has a potential mosquito vector, there is potential for large urban outbreaks of human disease in new areas.

REFERENCES

1. Zanotto PM, Gould EA, Gao GF, et al: Population dynamics of flaviviruses revealed by molecular phylogenies. Proc Natl Acad Sci USA 93:548–553, 1996.
2. Burke DS: Flaviviruses. In Knipe DM, Howley PM (eds): Fields' Virology, 4th ed. Philadelphia, Lippincott Williams & Wilkins, 2001, pp 1043–1125.
3. Corver J, Lenches E, Smith K, et al: Fine mapping of a cis-acting sequence element in yellow fever virus RNA that is required for RNA replication and cyclization. J Virol 77:2265–2270, 2003.
4. Lindenbach BD, Rice CM: Flaviviridae: The viruses and their replication. In Knipe DM, Howley PM (eds): Fields' Virology, 4th ed. Philadelphia, Lippincott Williams & Wilkins, 2001, pp 991–1041.
5. Heinz FX, Allison SL: Flavivirus structure and membrane fusion. In Chambers TJ, Monath TP (eds): The Flaviviruses: Structure, Replication and Evolution, vol. 59. San Diego, Elsevier Academic Press, 2003, pp 63–97.
6. Hurrelbrink RJ, McMinn PC: Molecular determinants of virulence: The structural and functional basis for flavivirus attenuation. In Chambers TJ, Monath TP (eds): The Flaviviruses: Pathogenesis and Immunity, vol. 60. San Diego, Elsevier Academic Press, 2003, pp 1–42.
7. Roehrig JT: Antigenic structure of flavivirus proteins. In Chambers TJ, Monath TP (eds): The Flaviviruses: Structure, Replication and Evolution, vol. 59. San Diego, Elsevier Academic Press, 2003, pp 141–176.
8. Schlesinger JJ, Brandriss MW, Putnak JR, et al: Cell surface expression of yellow fever virus non-structural glycoprotein NS1: Consequences of interaction with antibody. J Gen Virol 71(Pt 3):593–599, 1990.
9. Co MD, Terajima M, Cruz J, et al: Human cytotoxic T lymphocyte responses to live attenuated 17D yellow fever vaccine: Identification of HLA-B35-restricted CTL epitopes on nonstructural proteins NS1, NS2b, NS3, and the structural protein E. Virology 293:151–163, 2002.
10. Lobigs M, Arthur CE, Mullbacher A, et al: The flavivirus nonstructural protein NS3 is a dominant source of cytotoxic T cell peptide determinants. Virology 202:195–201, 1994.
11. Calisher CH, Karabatsos N, Dalrymple JM, et al: Antigenic relationships between flaviviruses as determined by cross-neutralization tests with polyclonal antisera. J Gen Virol 70:37–43, 1989.
12. Kuno G, Chang JG, Tsuchiya KR, et al: Phylogeny of the genus *Flavivirus*. J Virol 72:73–83, 1998.
13. Chang GJ, Cropp BC, Kinney RM, et al: Nucleotide sequence variation of the envelope protein gene identifies two distinct genotypes of yellow fever virus. J Virol 69:5773–5780, 1995.
14. Wang E, Weaver SC, Shope RE, et al: Genetic variation in yellow fever virus: Duplication in the 3′ noncoding region of strains from Africa. Virology 225:274–281, 1996.
15. Mutebi JP, Wang H, Li L, et al: Phylogenetic and evolutionary relationships among yellow fever virus isolates in Africa. J Virol 75:6999–7008, 2001.
16. Pugachev KV, Guirakhoo F, Ocran SW, et al: High fidelity of yellow fever virus RNA polymerase. J Virol 78:1032–1038, 2004.
17. Bryant JE, Barrett AD: Comparative phylogenies of yellow fever isolates from Peru and Brazil. FEMS Immunol Med Microbiol 39:103–118, 2003.
18. Vainio J, Cutts F: World Health Organization Report: Yellow Fever. Global Programme for Vaccines and Immunization. Geneva, World Health Organization, 1998.
19. Van der Stuyft P, Gianella A, Pirard M, et al: Urbanisation of yellow fever in Santa Cruz, Bolivia. Lancet 353:1558–1562, 1999.
20. Monath TP: Facing up to re-emergence of urban yellow fever. Lancet 353:1541, 1999.
21. Nasidi A, Monath TP, DeCock K, et al: Urban yellow fever epidemic in western Nigeria, 1987. Trans R Soc Trop Med Hyg 83:401–406, 1989.
22. Miller BR, Monath TP, Tabachnick WJ, et al: Epidemic yellow fever caused by an incompetent mosquito vector. Trop Med Parasitol 40:396–399, 1989.
23. Robertson SE, Hull BP, Tomori O, et al: Yellow fever: A decade of reemergence. JAMA 276:1157–1162, 1996.
24. World Health Organization: Communicable Disease Surveillance and Response Web site, http://www.who.int/csr/disease/yellowfev/impact/en. Accessed August 8, 2004.

25. Heraud JM, Hommel D, Hulin A, et al: First case of yellow fever in French Guiana since 1902. Emerg Infect Dis 5:429–432, 1999.
26. Monath TP: Yellow fever: An update. Lancet Infect Dis 1:11–20, 2001.
27. Nassar Eda S, Chamelet EL, Coimbra TL, et al: Jungle yellow fever: Clinical and laboratorial studies emphasizing viremia on a human case. Rev Inst Med Trop Sao Paulo 37:337–341, 1995.
28. MacNamara FN: A clinico-pathological study of yellow fever in Nigeria. West Afr Med J 6:137–146, 1957.
29. Elton NW, Romero A, Trejos A: Clinical pathology of yellow fever. Am J Clin Pathol 25:135–146, 1955.
30. Oudart JL, Rey M: Proteinuria, proteinaemia, and serum transaminase activity in 23 confirmed cases of yellow fever. Bull World Health Organ 42:95–102, 1970.
31. Boulos M, Segurado AA, Shiroma M: Severe yellow fever with 23-day survival. Trop Geogr Med 40:356–358, 1988.
32. Nasidi A, Monath TP, Vandenberg J, et al: Yellow fever vaccination and pregnancy: A four-year prospective study. Trans R Soc Trop Med Hyg 87:337–339, 1993.
33. Sibailly TS, Wiktor SZ, Tsai TF, et al: Poor antibody response to yellow fever vaccination in children infected with human immunodeficiency virus type 1. Pediatr Infect Dis J 16:1177–1179, 1997.
34. Kengsakul K, Sathirapongsasuti K, Punyagupta S: Fatal myeloencephalitis following yellow fever vaccination in a case with HIV infection. J Med Assoc Thai 85:131–134, 2002.
35. Jones EM, Wilson DC: Clinical features of yellow fever cases at Vom Christian Hospital during the 1969 epidemic on the Jos Plateau, Nigeria. Bull World Health Organ 46:653–657, 1972.
36. Monath TP, Ballinger ME, Miller BR, et al: Detection of yellow fever viral RNA by nucleic acid hybridization and viral antigen by immunocytochemistry in fixed human liver. Am J Trop Med Hyg 40:663–668, 1989.
37. Monath TP, Barrett AD: Pathogenesis and pathophysiology of yellow fever. Adv Virus Res 60:343–395, 2003.
38. Monath TP, Brinker KR, Chandler FW, et al: Pathophysiologic correlations in a rhesus monkey model of yellow fever with special observations on the acute necrosis of B cell areas of lymphoid tissues. Am J Trop Med Hyg 30:431–443, 1981.
39. Kurane I, Brinton MA, Samson AL, et al: Dengue virus-specific, human CD4+ CD8- cytotoxic T-cell clones: Multiple patterns of virus cross-reactivity recognized by NS3-specific T-cell clones. J Virol 65:1823–1828, 1991.
40. Kurane I, Janus J, Ennis FA: Dengue virus infection of human skin fibroblasts in vitro production of IFN-beta, IL-6 and GM-CSF. Arch Virol 124:21–30, 1992.
41. Kurane I, Okamoto Y, Dai LC, et al: Flavivirus-cross-reactive, HLA-DR15-restricted epitope on NS3 recognized by human CD4+ CD8- cytotoxic T lymphocyte clones. J Gen Virol 76(Pt 9):2243–2249, 1995.
42. Arroyo JI, Apperson SA, Cropp CB, et al: Effect of human gamma interferon on yellow fever virus infection. Am J Trop Med Hyg 38:647–650, 1988.
43. Liu T, Chambers TJ: Yellow fever virus encephalitis: Properties of the brain-associated T-cell response during virus clearance in normal and gamma interferon-deficient mice and requirement for CD4+ lymphocytes. J Virol 75:2107–2118, 2001.
44. Hacker UT, Erhardt S, Tschop K, et al: Influence of the IL-1Ra gene polymorphism on in vivo synthesis of IL-1Ra and IL-1beta after live yellow fever vaccination. Clin Exp Immunol 125:465–469, 2001.
45. Hacker UT, Jelinek T, Erhardt S, et al: In vivo synthesis of tumor necrosis factor-alpha in healthy humans after live yellow fever vaccination. J Infect Dis 177:774–778, 1998.
46. Darnell MB, Koprowski H, Lagerspetz K: Genetically determined resistance to infection with group B arboviruses. I. Distribution of the resistance gene among various mouse populations and characteristics of gene expression in vivo. J Infect Dis 129:240–247, 1974.
47. Samuel CE: Host genetic variability and West Nile virus susceptibility. Proc Natl Acad Sci USA 99:11555–11557, 2002.
48. Regner M, Lobigs M, Blanden RV, et al: Antiviral cytotoxic T cells cross-reactively recognize disparate peptide determinants from related viruses but ignore more similar self- and foreign determinants. J Immunol 166:3820–3828, 2001.
49. Monath TP, Cetron MS: Prevention of yellow fever in persons traveling to the tropics. Clin Infect Dis 34:1369–1378, 2002.
50. Henderson BE, Cheshire PP, Kirya GB, et al: Immunologic studies with yellow fever and selected African group B arboviruses in rhesus and vervet monkeys. Am J Trop Med Hyg 19:110–118, 1970.
51. Theiler M, Anderson CR: The relative resistance of dengue-immune monkeys to yellow fever virus. Am J Trop Med Hyg 24:115–117, 1975.
52. Monath TP, Craven RB, Adjukiewicz A, et al: Yellow fever in the Gambia, 1978–1979: Epidemiologic aspects with observations on the occurrence of orungo virus infections. Am J Trop Med Hyg 29:912–928, 1980.
53. Lanciotti RS: Molecular amplification assays for the detection of flaviviruses. Adv Virus Res 61:67–99, 2003.
54. Sen S, Williams R: New liver support devices in acute liver failure: A critical evaluation. Semin Liver Dis 23:283–284, 2003.
55. Crance JM, Scaramozzino N, Jouan A, et al: Interferon, ribavirin, 6-azauridine and glycyrrhizin: Antiviral compounds active against pathogenic flaviviruses. Antiviral Res 58:73–79, 2003.
56. Monath TP: Yellow fever vaccine. In Plotkin SA, Orenstein WA (eds): Vaccines, 4th ed. Philadelphia, Saunders, 2004, pp 1095–1176.
57. Monath TP, Nichols R, Archambault WT, et al: Comparative safety and immunogenicity of two yellow fever 17D vaccines (ARILVAX and YF-VAX) in a phase III multicenter, double-blind clinical trial. Am J Trop Med Hyg 66:533–541, 2002.
58. Spector S, Tauraso NM: Yellow fever virus. I. Development and evaluation of a plaque neutralization test. Appl Microbiol 16:1770–1775, 1968.
59. Xie H, Cass AR, Barrett AD: Yellow fever 17D vaccine virus isolated from healthy vaccinees accumulates very few mutations. Virus Res 55:93–99, 1998.
60. Marianneau P, Georges-Courbot M, Deubel V: Rarity of adverse effects after 17D yellow-fever vaccination. Lancet 358:84–85, 2001.
61. Gubler DJ: The global emergence/resurgence of arboviral diseases as public health problems. Arch Med Res 33:330–342, 2002.
62. Cetron MS, Marfin AA, Julian KG, et al: Yellow fever vaccine. Recommendations of the Advisory Committee on Immunization Practices (ACIP), 2002. MMWR 51:1–11; quiz CE1–CE4, 2002.
63. McFarland JM, Baddour LM, Nelson JE, et al: Imported yellow fever in a United States citizen. Clin Infect Dis 25:1143–1147, 1997.
64. Kelso JM, Mootrey GT, Tsai TF: Anaphylaxis from yellow fever vaccine. J Allergy Clin Immunol 103:698–701, 1999.
65. Martin M, Tsai TF, Cropp B, et al: Fever and multisystem organ failure associated with 17D-204 yellow fever vaccination: A report of four cases. Lancet 358:98–104, 2001.
66. Vasconcelos PF, Luna EJ, Galler R, et al: Serious adverse events associated with yellow fever 17DD vaccine in Brazil: A report of two cases. Lancet 358:91–97, 2001.
67. Barwick RS, Marfin AA, Cetron MS: Yellow fever vaccine-associated disease, In Scheld WM, Murray BE, Hughes JM (eds): Emerging Infections, 6th ed. Washington, DC, ASM Press, 2004, pp 25–34.
68. Marfin AA, Eidex RS, Kozarsky PE, et al: Yellow fever and Japanese encephalitis vaccines: Indications and complications. Infect Dis Clin North Am 19:151–168, 2005.
69. Werfel U, Popp W: Effects of yellow fever vaccination. Lancet 358:1909, 2001.
70. Chan RC, Penney DJ, Little D, et al: Hepatitis and death following vaccination with 17D-204 yellow fever vaccine. Lancet 358:121–122, 2001.
71. Adhiyaman V, Oke A, Cefai C, et al: Effects of yellow fever vaccination. Lancet 358:1907–1908, 2001.
72. Troillet N, Laurencet F: Effects of yellow fever vaccination. Lancet 358:1908–1909, 2001.
73. Kitchener S: Viscerotropic and neurotropic disease following vaccination with the 17D yellow fever vaccine, ARILVAX®. Vaccine 22:2103–2105, 2004.
74. Anonymous: Fatal viral encephalitis following 17D yellow fever vaccine inoculation. Report of a case in a 3-year-old child. JAMA 198:671–672, 1966.
75. Centers for Disease Control and Prevention: Adverse events associated with 17D-derived yellow fever vaccination—United States, 2001–2002. MMWR 51:989–993, 2002.
76. Martin M, Weld LH, Tsai TF, et al: Advanced age a risk factor for illness temporally associated with yellow fever vaccination. Emerg Infect Dis 7:945–951, 2001.
77. Engels EA, Pfeiffer RM: Malignant thymoma in the United States: Demographic patterns in incidence and associations with subsequent malignancies. Int J Cancer 105:546–551, 2003.

72

Dengue and Dengue Hemorrhagic Fever

DUANE J. GUBLER

INTRODUCTION

The first reports of major epidemics of an illness thought to possibly be dengue occurred on three continents (Asia, Africa, and North America) in 1779 and 1780.[1–4] However, reports of illnesses compatible with dengue fever occurred even earlier. The earliest record found to date was in a Chinese "encyclopedia of disease symptoms and remedies," first published during the Chin Dynasty (265 to 420 AD) and formally edited in 610 AD (Tang Dynasty) and again in 992 AD during the Northern Sung Dynasty.[5] The disease was called "water poison" by the Chinese and was thought to be somehow connected with flying insects associated with water. Outbreaks of illness in the French West Indies in 1635 and in Panama in 1699 could also have been dengue.[4,6] Thus, dengue or a very similar illness had a wide geographic distribution before the 18th century, when the first known pandemic of dengue-like illness began. It is uncertain that the epidemics in Batavia (Jakarta), Indonesia, and Cairo, Egypt, in 1779 were dengue.[7]

At some point in the past, probably with the clearing of the forests and development of human settlements, dengue viruses moved out of the jungle and into a rural environment, where they were, and still are, transmitted to humans by peridomestic mosquitoes such as *Aedes albopictus.* Migration of people and commerce ultimately moved the viruses into the villages, towns, and cities of tropical Asia, where the viruses were most likely transmitted sporadically by *Aedes albopictus* and other closely related peridomestic *Stegomyia* species.

The slave trade between West Africa and the Americas and the resulting commerce were responsible for the introduction and the widespread geographic distribution of an African mosquito, *Aedes aegypti,* in the New World during the 17th, 18th, and 19th centuries. This species became highly adapted to humans and urban environments and was spread throughout the tropics of the world by sailing ships. The species first infested port cities and then moved inland as urbanization expanded. Because *Ae. aegypti* had evolved to become intimately associated with humans, preferring to feed on them and to share their dwellings, this species became a very efficient epidemic vector of dengue and yellow fever viruses. Therefore, when these viruses were introduced into port cities infested with *Ae. aegypti,* epidemics occurred. It was in this setting that major pandemics of dengue fever occurred during the 18th, 19th, and early 20th centuries, as the global shipping industry developed and port cities were urbanized in response to increased commerce and ocean traffic. The last major pandemic began during World War II and continues through the present.[8]

The earliest known use of the word *dengue* to describe an illness was in Spain in 1801.[9] However, the most likely origin of the word is from Swahili.[10,11] In both the 1823 and 1870 epidemics of dengue-like illness in Zanzibar and the East African coast, the disease was called *Ki-Dinga pepo.* From this came the name *dinga* or *denga,* which was used to describe the illness in both epidemics. Christie[10,11] speculates that the name *denga* was taken via the slave trade to the New World, where it was called "Dandy fever" or "The Dandy" in the St. Thomas epidemic of 1827. The illness was first called *dunga* in Cuba during the 1828 epidemic, but later changed to dengue, the name by which it has been known ever since.[12] Most likely, the Spanish recognized the disease in Cuba as the same one that was called dengue in Spain in 1801. If the word *dengue* did originate in East Africa from *dinga* or *denga,* this suggests the disease was occurring before the 1823 epidemics described by Christie. This is not unlikely since epidemics were reported in Africa, the Middle East, and Spain in the late 1700s.

With documentation that yellow fever was transmitted by mosquitoes, many early workers suspected that dengue fever was also mosquito-borne. In the previrology era, work was slow and relied on use of human volunteers. Work done by Graham (1903),[13] Bancroft (1906),[14] and Cleland and colleagues (1918)[15] documented dengue transmission by mosquitoes.

Although it had been shown that dengue fever was caused by a filterable agent,[16,17] the first dengue viruses were not isolated until the 1940s, during World War II.[18–21] Dengue fever was a major cause of morbidity among Allied and Japanese soldiers in the Pacific and Asian theaters. Sabin and his group were able to show that some virus strains from three geographic locations (Hawaii, New Guinea, and India) were antigenically similar.[20,21] This virus was called dengue 1 (DENV-1), and the Hawaii virus was designated as the prototype strain (Haw-DENV-1). Another antigenically distinct virus strain isolated from New Guinea was called dengue 2 (DENV-2), and the New Guinea C strain (NGC-DENV-2) was designated the prototype. The Japanese virus isolated by Kimura and Hotta[18,19] was subsequently shown to be DENV-1 as well. Two more serotypes, dengue 3 (DENV-3) and dengue 4 (DENV-4), were later isolated from patients with a hemorrhagic disease during an epidemic in Manila in 1956.[22] Since these original isolates were made, thousands of dengue viruses have been isolated from all parts of the tropics; all have fit into the four-serotype classification.

The occurrence of severe and fatal hemorrhagic disease associated with dengue infections is not unique to the 20th century. Patients with disease clinically compatible with dengue hemorrhagic fever (DHF) have been reported sporadically since 1780, when such cases were observed in the Philadelphia epidemic.[1] Significant numbers of cases of hemorrhagic disease were associated with several subsequent epidemics, including Charters Towers, Australia, in 1897, Beirut in 1910, Taiwan in 1916, Greece in 1928, and Taiwan in 1931.[23–29] However, epidemic occurrences such as these were relatively rare, and the long intervals between them made each a unique event that was not considered important in terms of a long-term, continuous public health problem. Understanding the emergence of dengue and DHF as a global public health problem in the last half of the 20th century requires a review of the ecological and demographic changes that occurred in the Asian and American tropics during this period. The detailed history of dengue has been recently reviewed.[30]

AGENTS

There are four dengue virus serotypes: DENV-1, DENV-2, DENV-3, and DENV-4. They belong to the genus *Flavivirus,* family *Flaviviridae* (of which yellow fever virus is the type species), which contains approximately 70 viruses.[31] The flaviviruses are relatively small (40–50 nm) and spherical with a lipid envelope. The flavivirus genome is approximately 11,000 bases and is made up of three structural and seven nonstructural proteins. There are three major subgroups within this family: tick-borne, mosquito-borne, and viruses with no known arthropod vector. The dengue viruses form a complex within the mosquito-borne subgroup. All flaviviruses have common group epitopes on the envelope protein that result in extensive cross-reactions in serologic tests. These make unequivocal serologic diagnosis of flavivirus infections difficult. This is especially true of the four dengue viruses. Infection with one dengue serotype provides lifelong immunity to that virus, but there is no cross-protective immunity to the other serotypes. Thus, persons living in an endemic area can be infected with three, and probably four, dengue serotypes during their lifetime.

EPIDEMIOLOGY

Natural History

Humans are infected with dengue viruses by the bite of an infective *Ae. aegypti* mosquito.[32] *Ae. aegypti* is a small, black-and-white, highly domesticated urban mosquito that prefers to lay its eggs in artificial containers commonly found in and around homes in the tropics, for example, flower vases, old automobile tires, buckets that collect rainwater, and trash in general. Containers used for water storage, especially 55-gallon drums and cement cisterns, are especially important in producing large numbers of adult mosquitoes in close proximity to dwellings where people live and work. The adult mosquitoes prefer to rest indoors, are unobtrusive, and prefer to feed on humans during daylight hours. The female mosquitoes are very nervous feeders, disrupting the feeding process at the slightest movement, only to return to the same or a different person to continue feeding moments later. Because of this behavior, *Ae. aegypti* females will often feed on several persons during a single blood meal and, if infective, may transmit dengue virus to multiple persons in a short period of time even if they only probe without taking blood.[33] It is not uncommon to see several members of the same household become ill with dengue fever within a 24- to 36-hour time frame, suggesting transmission by a single infective mosquito (D.J. Gubler, unpublished data). It is this behavior that makes *Ae. aegypti* such an efficient epidemic vector. Inhabitants of dwellings in the tropics are rarely aware of the presence of this mosquito, making its control difficult.

After a person is bitten by an infective mosquito, the virus undergoes an incubation period of 3 to 14 days (average, 4 to 7 days), after which the person may experience acute onset of fever accompanied by a variety of nonspecific signs and symptoms. During this acute febrile period, which may be as short as 2 days and as long as 10 days, dengue viruses may circulate in the peripheral blood. If other *Ae. aegypti* mosquitoes bite the ill person during this febrile viremic stage, those mosquitoes may become infected and subsequently transmit the virus to other uninfected persons, after an extrinsic incubation period of 8 to 12 days.[32]

Changing Disease Patterns

The disease pattern associated with dengue, which was characterized by relatively infrequent epidemics until the 1940s, changed with the ecological disruptions in Southeast Asia during and after World War II. Ideal conditions for increased transmission of mosquito-borne diseases were created, and in this setting a global pandemic of dengue began. With increased epidemic transmission, hyperendemicity (the cocirculation of multiple dengue virus serotypes) developed in Southeast Asian cities, and epidemic DHF, a newly described disease, emerged.[34,35] The first known epidemic of DHF occurred in Manila, in 1953–1954, but within 20 years the disease had spread throughout Southeast Asia. By the mid-1970s, DHF had become a leading cause of hospitalization and death among children in the region.[36] In the 1980s and 1990s, dengue transmission in Asia further intensified; epidemic DHF increased in incidence and expanded geographically west into India, Pakistan, Sri Lanka, and the Maldives, and east into China.[34,35] At the same time, the geographic distribution of epidemic DHF was expanding into new regions—the Pacific islands in the 1970s and 1980s and the American tropics in the 1980s and 1990s.[8,34,35,37–42]

Epidemiologic changes in the Americas have been the most dramatic. In the 1960s and most of the 1970s, epidemic dengue was rare in the American region because the principal mosquito vector, *Ae. aegypti,* had been eradicated from most of Central and South America.[41,42] The eradication program was discontinued in the early 1970s, and this species then began to reinvade those countries from which it had been eradicated. By the 1990s, *Ae. aegypti* had regained the geographic distribution it had before eradication was initiated (Fig. 72-1). Epidemic dengue invariably followed after reinfestation of a country by *Ae. aegypti.* By the 1980s, the American region was experiencing major epidemics of dengue in countries that had been free of the disease for 35 to 130 years.[34,41,42] With increased epidemic activity came the development of hyperendemicity and the emergence of epidemic DHF, much as had occurred in Southeast Asia 25 years earlier.[41,43] From 1981 to 2005, 28 American countries reported laboratory-confirmed DHF[34,35,42,44] (Fig. 72-2).

While Africa has not yet had a major epidemic of DHF, sporadic cases of severe disease have occurred as epidemic dengue fever has increased markedly in the past 15 years. Before the 1980s, little was known of the distribution of dengue viruses in Africa. Since then, however, major epidemics caused by all four serotypes have occurred in both East and West Africa.[34,35] Recent epidemics include Djibouti in 1991 and Jeddah, Saudi Arabia, in 1994, both of which were the first outbreaks in those countries in over 50 years.[34,35,45]

In 2005, dengue viruses and *Ae. aegypti* mosquitoes have a worldwide distribution in the tropics with over 2.5 billion

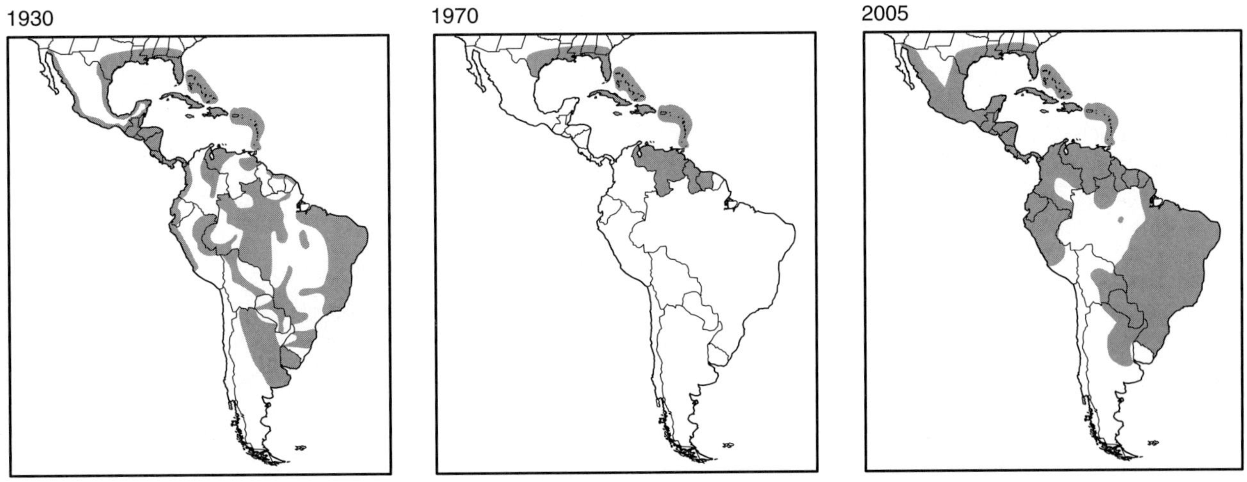

FIGURE 72-1 *Aedes aegypti:* Distribution in the Americas, 1930s, 1970, and 2005.

people living in dengue-endemic areas.[8,34,35,44] Currently, dengue fever causes more illness and death than any other arboviral disease of humans. Each year, an estimated 50 to 100 million dengue infections and several hundred thousand cases of DHF occur, depending on epidemic activity.[35,44,46,47] DHF is a leading cause of hospitalization and death among children in many Southeast Asian countries.[36]

Factors Responsible for Increased Incidence

The emergence of epidemic dengue and DHF as a global public health problem in the past 25 years is closely associated with demographic and societal changes that have occurred over the past 50 years.[34,35] A major factor has been the unprecedented population growth and, with that, unplanned and uncontrolled urbanization, especially in tropical developing countries. The substandard housing and the deterioration in water, sewer, and waste management systems associated with unplanned urbanization have created ideal conditions for increased transmission of mosquito-borne diseases in tropical urban centers.

A second major factor has been the lack of effective mosquito control in dengue-endemic areas.[34,35] Emphasis during the past 30 years has been on space spraying with insecticides to kill adult mosquitoes; this has not been effective[48,49] and, in fact, has been detrimental to prevention and control efforts by giving citizens of the community and government officials a false sense of security.[48] Additionally, the geographic distribution and population densities of *Ae. aegypti* have increased, especially in urban areas of the tropics, because of increased numbers of mosquito larval habitats in the domestic environment. The latter include nonbiodegradable plastics and used automobile tires, both of which have increased dramatically during this same period of time.

Another major factor in the global emergence of dengue and DHF is increased air travel by humans, which provides

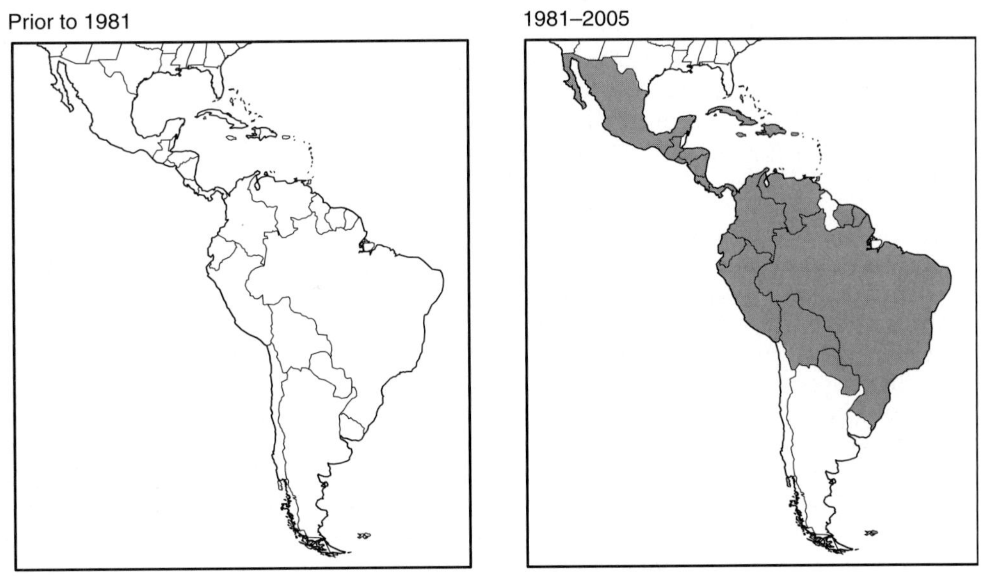

FIGURE 72-2 Dengue hemorrhagic fever in the Americas prior to 1981 and from 1981 to present.

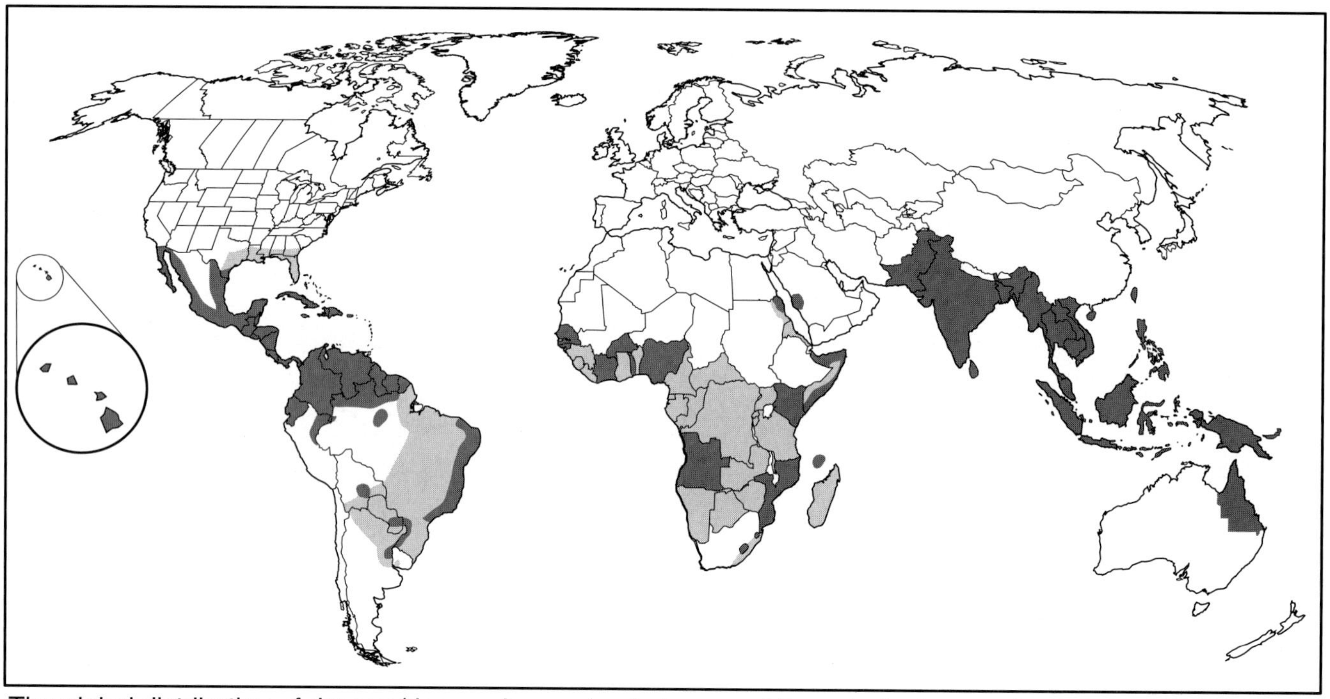

The global distribution of dengue/dengue hemorrhagic fever and the principal mosquito vector, *Aedes aegypyti*, 2005.

the ideal mechanism for the transport of dengue and other urban pathogens between population centers of the world.[34,35] For instance, in 1994, an estimated 40 million persons departed the United States by air, 51% of whom traveled for business or holiday to tropical dengue-endemic countries.[50] Many travelers become infected while visiting tropical areas, but become ill after returning home, resulting in a constant movement of dengue viruses in infected humans to all areas of the world and ensuring repeated introductions of new dengue virus strains and serotypes into areas where the mosquito vectors occur. The result is increased epidemic activity, the development of hyperendemicity, and the emergence of epidemic DHF.

The United States is not immune to the introduction of dengue viruses. Each year for the past 25 years, imported dengue cases have been documented by the Centers for Disease Control and Prevention (CDC; unpublished data, 2004).[50,51] These cases represent introductions of all four virus serotypes from all tropical regions of the world. Most dengue introductions into the United States come from the American and Asian tropics and reflect the increased number of Americans traveling to those areas. Overall, from 1976 to 2003, 3697 suspected cases of imported dengue were reported to the CDC (CDC, unpublished data, 2004).[50,51] Although adequate blood samples were received from only a portion of these patients, 875 (24%) have been confirmed as dengue.

These cases represent only the tip of the iceberg because most physicians in the United States have a low index of suspicion for dengue, which is often not included in the differential diagnosis, even if the patient recently traveled to a tropical country. As a result, many imported dengue cases are never reported. It is important to increase awareness of dengue and DHF among physicians in temperate areas, however, because the disease can be life-threatening. For example, two cases of the severe form of DHF, dengue shock syndrome (DSS), were described in Swedish tourists returning from holiday in Asia.[52] In the United States, severe disease does occur among imported cases of dengue.[53] It is important, therefore, that physicians in the United States consider dengue in the differential diagnosis of viral syndrome in all patients with a travel history to any tropical area.

The potential for epidemic dengue transmission in the United States still exists. On seven occasions in the past 25 years (in 1980 after an absence of 35 years, and in 1986, 1995, 1997, 1998, 1999, and 2001), autochthonous transmission occurred secondary to importation of the virus in humans (Table 72-1). Of interest was the 2001 Hawaii outbreak, which was the first dengue transmission in that state in 56 years[54] caused by DENV-1 virus introduced from Tahiti where a major

***Table 72-1** Autochthonous Cases of Dengue Fever in the United States, 1945–2004**

Year	Location	No. of Cases	Virus Serotype
1945	Louisiana	143	?
1980	Texas	27	DENV-1
1986	Texas	9	DENV-1
1995	Texas	7	DENV-2
1997	Texas	3	DENV-2
1998	Texas	1	DENV-2
1999	Texas	17	DENV-3
2001	Hawaii	122	DENV-1

*Reported cases in 1945. Cases in 1980, 1986, 1995, 1997, 1998, 1999, and 2001 were laboratory-confirmed.

epidemic of DHF was occurring.[55] Transmission in Hawaii was sporadic and illness mild; 122 cases were confirmed.[54] Although the outbreaks in the United States have been small, they underscore the potential for dengue transmission in areas where two competent mosquito vectors occur.[34] *Ae. aegypti,* the most important and efficient epidemic vector of dengue viruses, has been in the United States for over 200 years and has been responsible for transmitting major epidemics in the past.[56] Currently, this species is found only in the Gulf Coast states from Texas to Florida, although several foci have recently been reported in Arizona. *Ae. albopictus,* another, but less efficient epidemic vector of dengue viruses, was introduced to the continental United States in the early 1980s and has since become widespread in the eastern half of the country. Although the CDC has ceased surveillance, at last count it occurred in 1044 counties in 36 of the continental states (C.G. Moore, Colorado State University, personal communication, 2004); this species has also been found in Hawaii for over 90 years. Both *Ae. aegypti* and *Ae. albopictus* can transmit dengue viruses to humans, and their presence in the United States increases the risk of autochthonous dengue transmission secondary to imported cases.[32,50]

DISEASE

Dengue virus infection in humans causes a spectrum of illness, ranging from unapparent or mild febrile illness to severe and fatal hemorrhagic disease. Infection with all four serotypes causes a similar clinical presentation that may vary in frequency and severity. The incubation period varies from 3 to 14 days (average, 4 to 7 days). In dengue-endemic areas, dengue infections are often clinically nonspecific, especially in children, with symptoms of a viral syndrome that has a variety of local names. Important risk factors influencing the proportion of patients who have severe disease during epidemic transmission include the strain and serotype of the infecting virus, the immune status of the individual, the age of the patient, and the genetic background of the human host.[32,36–40,57–59]

Dengue Fever

Classic dengue fever is primarily a disease of older children and adults. It is characterized by sudden onset of fever and a variety of nonspecific signs and symptoms, including frontal headache, retro-orbital pain, body aches, nausea and vomiting, joint pains, weakness, and rash.[17,21,60,61] Patients may be anorectic, have altered taste sensation, and mild sore throat. Constipation is occasionally reported; diarrhea and respiratory symptoms are infrequently reported and may be due to concurrent infections.

The initial temperature may rise to 102°F to 105°F and last for 2 to 7 days. The fever may drop after a few days only to rebound 12 to 24 hours later (saddleback). Relative bradycardia may be noted despite the fever. The conjunctivae may be injected and the pharynx inflamed. Lymphadenopathy is common. Rash is variable, but occurs in up to 50% of patients as either early or late eruptions. Facial flushing or erythematous mottling may occur coincident with or slightly before onset of fever and disappear 1 to 2 days after onset of symptoms. A second rash, varying in form from scarlatiniform to maculopapular, may appear between days 2 and 6 of illness.

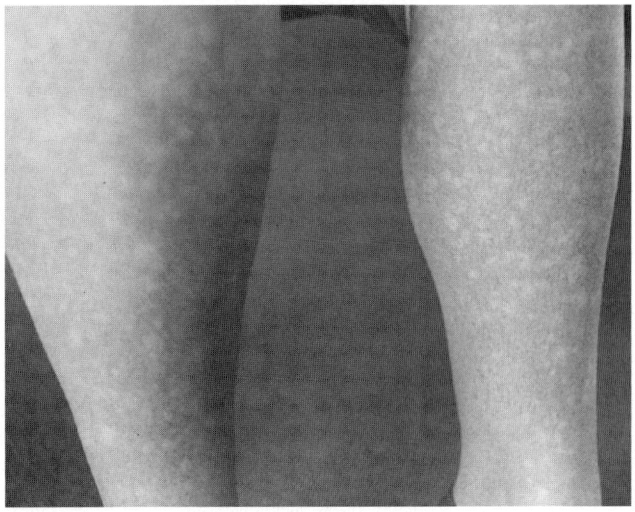

FIGURE 72-3 Rash associated with dengue infection: Islands of normal skin are surrounded by a confluent rash.

The rash usually begins on the trunk and spreads to the face and extremities. In some cases, an intense erythematous pattern with islands of normal skin may be observed (Fig. 72-3). The average duration of the second rash is 2 to 3 days. Toward the end of the febrile phase of illness or after the temperature reverts to normal, petechiae may appear; these may be scattered or confluent. Intense pruritus may occur followed by desquamation on the palms of the hands and soles of the feet.

Hemorrhagic manifestations in dengue fever patients are not uncommon and may range from mild to severe. Skin hemorrhages are the most common, including petechiae and purpura, as well as gum bleeding, epistaxis, menorrhagia, and gastrointestinal hemorrhage. Hematuria occurs infrequently, and jaundice is rare.

Clinical laboratory findings associated with dengue fever include neutropenia followed by lymphocytosis, often marked by atypical lymphocytes. Liver enzymes in the serum may be elevated; this is usually a mild elevation but, in some patients, alanine transaminase and aspartate transaminase levels may reach 500 to 1000 units/L. In one epidemic of DEN-4, 54% of confirmed patients with data had elevated liver enzymes.[62] Thrombocytopenia is also common in dengue fever; in the preceding epidemic, 34% of confirmed dengue fever patients who were tested had platelet counts of less than 100,000/μL.[62]

Dengue fever is generally self-limited and rarely fatal. The acute phase of illness lasts for 3 to 7 days, but the convalescent phase may be prolonged for weeks and may be associated with weakness and depression. No permanent sequelae are known to be associated with this infection.

Dengue Hemmorhagic Fever

DHF is primarily a disease of children under the age of 15 years, although it may also occur in adults.[36] It is characterized by sudden onset of fever, usually of 2 to 7 days' duration, and a variety of nonspecific signs and symptoms. During the acute phase of illness, it is difficult to distinguish DHF from dengue fever and other illnesses found in tropical

Table 72-2 Signs and Symptoms Associated with Laboratory-Confirmed Dengue Hemorrhagic Fever Cases, Jakarta, Indonesia, 1975–1977

Sign or Symptom	No.	Percent
Hepatomegaly	297/601*	49
Abdominal pain	281/619	45
Vomiting	279/619	45
Cough	142/619	23
Constipation	101/619	16
Nausea	90/618*	15
Headache	82/619	13
Sore throat	53/619	9
Rhinitis	50/619	8
Diarrhea	50/619	8
Chills	30/619	5
Myalgia	24/619	4
Joint pain	15/619	2
Stiff neck	15/619	2
Backache	12/619	2
Conjunctivitis	6/619	1
Pruritus	4/619	1
Paresthesias	1/619	1

*Data not available on all patients.

areas (Table 72-2). The differential diagnosis during the acute phase of illness should include measles, rubella, influenza, typhoid, leptospirosis, malaria, viral hemorrhagic fevers, and any other disease that may present in the acute phase as a nonspecific viral syndrome. Children frequently have concurrent infections with other viruses and bacteria causing upper respiratory symptoms. There is no pathognomonic sign or symptom for DHF (see Table 72-2).

The critical stage in DHF occurs most frequently from about 24 hours before to 24 hours after the temperature falls to normal or below.[36] During this time, hemorrhagic manifestations and, more importantly, signs of circulatory failure usually occur. Blood tests will usually show that the patient has thrombocytopenia (platelet count of <100,000/μL) and evidence of a vascular leak syndrome.

Common hemorrhagic manifestations include skin hemorrhages such as petechiae, purpuric lesions, and ecchymoses. Epistaxis, bleeding gums, gastrointestinal hemorrhage, and hematuria occur less frequently. The tourniquet test may be diagnostically helpful. This is done by inflating the blood pressure cuff to the midpoint between the systolic and diastolic pressures for 5 minutes and then releasing the pressure.[36] In persons with increased capillary fragility, a "shower" of petechiae will appear below the cuff. The test is positive if 20 or more petechiae per square inch are observed. Some uninfected persons may have a positive tourniquet test, however, so it does not mean that a person has DHF when the test is positive. Rather, positive results indicate that the patient has increased capillary fragility and that the physician should do further clinical laboratory tests.

Scattered petechiae are the most common hemorrhagic manifestation observed; they appear most often on the extremities, but also on the trunk, other parts of the body, and on the face in severe cases of DSS. Purpuric lesions may appear on various parts of the body but are most common at the site of venipuncture. In some patients, large ecchymotic lesions develop on the trunk and extremities, and other patients bleed actively at the site of venipuncture, some profusely. More severely ill patients have gastrointestinal hemorrhage, which is manifested by hematemesis or melena or both. Classic hematemesis and melena usually occur after prolonged shock, but patients may develop massive, frank upper gastrointestinal hemorrhage as well, often before the onset of shock. Without early diagnosis and proper management, some patients experience shock from blood loss, which may be mild or severe.[63–65] More commonly, shock is caused by plasma leakage; it may be mild and transient or progress to profound shock with undetectable pulse and blood pressure.[36] Children with profound shock are often somnolent, exhibit petechiae on the face, and have perioral cyanosis.

It is convenient for both clinicians and epidemiologists to classify DHF into four grades of illness based on severity[36] (Box 72-1). Grade I DHF is mild; the only hemorrhagic manifestations are scattered petechiae or a positive tourniquet test. Grade II DHF is more severe, with one or more overt hemorrhagic manifestations such as those mentioned previously. Grades III and IV represent more severe forms of disease (DSS). Grade III illness is characterized by mild shock with signs of circulatory failure; the patient may be lethargic or restless and have cold extremities, clammy skin, a rapid but weak pulse, narrowing of pulse pressure to 20 mm Hg or less, or hypotension. Grade IV, the most severe form of DHF or DSS, is characterized by profound shock with undetectable pulse and blood pressure.

In severe cases of DHF and DSS, fever and nonspecific constitutional signs and symptoms of a few days' duration are followed by the sudden deterioration of the patient's condition. During or shortly before or after the fall in temperature, the patient's skin may become cool, blotchy, and congested; circumoral cyanosis is frequently observed, and the pulse becomes rapid and weak. Although some patients appear lethargic at first, they become restless and then rapidly pass into a critical stage of shock. They frequently experience acute abdominal pain shortly before the onset of shock.[36,63,65]

In mild cases of DHF, all signs and symptoms abate shortly after the fever subsides. Lysis of fever, however, may be accompanied by profuse sweating and mild changes in pulse rate and blood pressure, together with coolness of extremities and skin congestion. These changes reflect mild and transient

Box 72-1 World Health Organization Classification of Dengue Hemorrhagic Fever

Grade I: Fever accompanied by nonspecific constitutional symptoms, with a positive tourniquet test or scattered petechiae as the only hemorrhagic manifestation
Grade II: The same as grade I, but with spontaneous hemorrhagic manifestations
Grade III: Circulatory failure manifested by rapid, weak pulse; narrowing of pulse pressure (≤20 mm Hg); or hypotension
Grade IV: Profound shock with undetectable pulse and blood pressure

From World Health Organization: Dengue Hemorrhagic Fever: Diagnosis, Treatment and Control, Geneva, 2nd ed. World Health Organization, 1997.

circulatory disturbances as a result of plasma leakage. Patients usually recover spontaneously or after fluid and electrolyte therapy.[36] Patients in shock are in danger of dying without appropriate management. The duration of shock is usually short; the patient may die within 8 to 24 hours or recover rapidly following antishock therapy. Convalescence for patients with DHF, with or without shock, is usually short and uneventful. Even in patients with undetectable pulse and blood pressure, once the shock is overcome surviving patients usually recover within 2 to 3 days.

As with dengue fever, leukopenia is common; thrombocytopenia and hemoconcentration are constant findings in DHF and DSS. A platelet count of less than 100,000/μL is usually found between the third and eighth day of illness. Hemoconcentration, indicating plasma leakage, is almost always present in classic DHF, but is more severe in patients with shock. Hepatomegaly is a common, but not a constant, finding.[63–65] In some countries, most patients with confirmed DHF or DSS have been found to have an enlarged liver. In other countries, however, hepatomegaly varies from one epidemic to another, suggesting that the strain or serotype of virus may influence liver involvement.[64] Elevated liver enzymes are common.

The primary pathophysiologic abnormality seen in DHF and DSS is an acute increase in vascular permeability that leads to leakage of plasma into the extravascular compartment, resulting in hemoconcentration and decreased blood pressure.[36] Plasma volume studies have shown a reduction of more than 20% in severe cases. Supporting evidence of plasma leakage includes serous effusion found post mortem, pleural effusion on radiograph, hemoconcentration, and hypoproteinemia. There are no apparent destructive vascular lesions, suggesting that the transient functional vascular changes are due to a short-acting chemical mediator.[36]

Hemostatic changes in DHF and DSS involve three factors: vascular changes, thrombocytopenia, and coagulation disorders.[36] Almost all DHF patients have increased vascular fragility and thrombocytopenia, and many have abnormal coagulograms, suggesting disseminated intravascular coagulation, which is also evidenced by concomitant thrombocytopenia, prolonged partial thromboplastin time, decreased fibrinogen level, and increased fibrin(ogen) degradation products. Gastrointestinal hemorrhage is found at autopsy in the majority of patients who die.

Atypical Dengue Infection

Some cases of severe hemorrhagic disease do not fit the preceding classification and may have a different pathogenesis.[32,65] These patients generally present with similar signs and symptoms during the acute phase of illness, but develop frank upper gastrointestinal bleeding without evidence of plasma leakage (hemoconcentration) or circulatory failure as seen in patients with classic DHF or DSS. Generally, the upper gastrointestinal bleeding occurs 3 to 5 days after onset of illness and is often the reason the patient is brought to the hospital. All such patients have significant thrombocytopenia. In many cases, bleeding may be severe enough to cause shock from blood loss rather than plasma leakage. In one study in Indonesia, 30% of patients with virologically confirmed fatal DHF had this type of severe upper gastrointestinal hemorrhaging.[65] Blood transfusions are always indicated for these patients, whose disease is generally more difficult to manage than classic DSS.[65]

Finally, some patients with dengue infection may present with neurologic disorders such as convulsions, spastic paresis, and change in consciousness, with or without hemorrhagic manifestations.[65,66] These patients, who may be admitted to the neurologic ward with a diagnosis of viral encephalitis, may subsequently develop hemorrhagic manifestations and shock. Cerebrospinal fluid findings are normal, and most evidence suggests that the virus does not cross the blood-brain barrier, although recent studies suggest that this may occur in some patients.[67–69] Further studies are necessary to identify what factors contribute to these unusual manifestations.

PATHOGENESIS AND IMMUNITY

The pathogenesis of DHF and DSS is still controversial. Two theories, which are not mutually exclusive, are frequently cited to explain the pathogenic changes that occur in DHF and DSS. The theory most commonly accepted is known as the secondary infection, or immune enhancement, hypothesis.[36,37,57] This hypothesis implies that patients experiencing a second infection with a heterologous dengue virus serotype have a significantly higher risk of developing DHF or DSS. Pre-existing heterologous dengue antibody recognizes the infecting virus and forms an antigen-antibody complex which is then phagocytosed by macrophages. Because the antibody is heterologous, however, the virus is not neutralized and is free to replicate once inside the macrophage. Thus, it is hypothesized that prior infection enhances the infection of cells of the mononuclear cell lineage by a virus that is not inactivated by neutralizing antibody. Infection of these cells initiates an immunologic cascade of events that produces cytotoxins and other vasoactive mediators, ultimately leading to increased vascular permeability, leakage, hypovolemia, shock/and death, if not corrected.[70]

The other hypothesis assumes that dengue viruses, like all animal viruses, vary and change genetically as they move through human or mosquito populations, and that there are some virus strains that have greater pathologic potential.[58,59,71] Data suggest that genetic changes in the virus genome occur randomly as the viruses are passed in nature. Some of these genetic changes are advantageous and are propagated through natural selection, resulting in viruses that have increased virus replication and higher viral load, greater epidemic potential, and increased virulence. There is epidemiologic and laboratory evidence to support both of these hypotheses, a discussion of which is beyond the scope of this chapter; most likely, both are valid. While immune enhancement may occur and may be an important factor in the pathophysiologic changes that occur in DHF and DSS, it appears that only certain strains of virus may be involved in producing severe disease by immune enhancement.

DIAGNOSIS

A definitive diagnosis of dengue infection can be made only in the laboratory and depends on isolating the virus, detecting dengue virus specific RNA sequences by nucleotide amplification test, or detecting specific antibodies in the patient's serum.[72–74] An acute-phase blood sample should always be taken as soon as possible after onset of illness, and a convalescent-phase sample should be taken 2 to 3 weeks later. Because it is frequently difficult to obtain convalescent-phase samples, however, a second blood sample should always be taken from hospitalized patients on the day of discharge from hospital.

Virus can often be isolated from acute-phase blood samples taken in the first 5 days of illness.[72–74] Viral RNA can often be detected by polymerase chain reaction (PCR) in serum or tissues[74,75] or antigen by immunohistochemistry in tissues.[76] Two serologic tests are used to detect antibodies. The IgM capture enzyme-linked immunosorbent assay (ELISA) detects IgM antibody, which usually appears by day five after onset and persists for 2 to 3 months.[72–74,77–79] The hemagglutination-inhibition test and an IgG ELISA detect IgG antibody, which appears simultaneously or shortly after IgM but persists for life. For this reason, diagnosis using IgG requires paired acute- and convalescent-phase blood samples to demonstrate a fourfold or greater rise in specific antibody, which should be confirmed by neutralization test.[72,73]

TREATMENT

There is no specific chemotherapy for DHF/DSS. However, early and effective fluid replacement of lost plasma with electrolyte solutions, plasma, or plasma expanders usually results in a favorable outcome.[36] With adequate fluid administration, DSS is reversible. Rapid replacement of fluid will usually prevent disseminated intravascular coagulation. Prognosis depends on early recognition of shock, based on careful monitoring.

In dengue-endemic areas, it is often not possible or necessary to hospitalize all patients with suspected DHF or DSS, since shock may develop in only about one-third of the patients.[36] A decrease in the platelet count, which usually precedes the rise in hematocrit, is of great diagnostic and prognostic value. In order to be able to recognize the early signs of shock and thus take preventive action, parents or family members should be advised to bring the patient back for repeat platelet and hematocrit determinations every 24 hours. They should also be instructed to keep a careful watch for any signs of clinical deterioration or warning signs of shock, such as restlessness, lethargy, acute abdominal pain, cold extremities, skin congestion, or oliguria, usually on or after the third day of illness. Patients with mild DHF can usually be rehydrated orally. An antipyretic drug may be all that is needed. Salicylates should be avoided.

Patients should be hospitalized and treated immediately if they have any signs or symptoms of shock, such as restlessness; lethargy; cold extremities; circumoral cyanosis; rapid, weak pulse; narrowing of pulse pressure to 20 mm Hg or less; hypotension; a sudden rise in hematocrit; or continuously elevated hematocrit despite the administration of intravenous fluids.[36] Frequent recording of vital signs and hematocrit determinations and monitoring of urine output are important in evaluating the results of treatment. Blood transfusions are contraindicated in patients with severe plasma leakage in the absence of hemorrhage and, if given, may cause pulmonary edema; however, they may be indicated for patients with significant clinical bleeding. It may be difficult to recognize internal bleeding in the presence of hemoconcentration. A drop in hematocrit of 10% with no clinical improvement, despite adequate fluid administration, suggests significant internal hemorrhage.[36] Transfusion of fresh whole blood is preferable; fresh frozen plasma or concentrated platelets may be indicated in some cases when consumptive coagulopathy causes massive bleeding.

Some controversy surrounds the use of steroids, but the consensus is that they have no beneficial effect in management of severe DHF or DSS. Although some physicians still use steroids in the treatment of shock cases, two double-blind studies, in Thailand and Indonesia, have shown no increase in survival rates of patients with grade IV DSS who were administered steroids.[36]

PREVENTION

Prevention and control of dengue fever/DHF currently depends on controlling the mosquito vector, *Ae. aegypti*, in and around the home where most transmission occurs. Space sprays with insecticides to kill adult mosquitoes are usually ineffective, unless they are sprayed indoors where the mosquitoes are resting. The most effective way to control the mosquitoes that transmit dengue is larval control, including eliminating, cleaning, or chemically treating water-holding containers that serve as the larval habitats for *Ae. aegypti* in the domestic environment.[47–49,80] At present, there is no vaccine for dengue viruses, although several candidates are at various stages of development.[81–83] To be effective, a dengue vaccine must protect against all four virus serotypes, i.e., be a tetravalent formulation. For use in dengue endemic countries, a dengue vaccine must be safe for use in children 9 to 12 months of age, must be economical, and should provide long lasting protective immunity (ideally more than 10 years).

Several approaches are being used to develop dengue vaccines. A live attenuated vaccine (LAV) is thought to provide the most complete and lasting immunity. At present, there are three LAV candidates under development.[81–86] Several groups have also constructed chimeric viruses using various infectious clones as backbones.[87–89] All of these chimeric candidate vaccines look very promising in primate studies. The 17-D yellow fever chimeras have recently undergone a Phase I trial in humans, but results are not yet available.

In summary, there are at least six tetravalent candidate dengue vaccines that are in or near clinical trials in humans. The Pediatric Dengue Vaccine Initiative, funded by the Bill and Melinda Gates Foundation, was founded to facilitate bringing one or more of these promising candidate vaccines to fruition.[90]

There is no completely effective method of preventing dengue infection in travelers to tropical areas. The risk of infection can be significantly reduced, however, by understanding the basic behavior and habits of the mosquito vector and by taking a few simple precautions, such as using aerosol bomb insecticides to kill adult mosquitoes indoors, using a repellent containing diethyltoluamide (DEET) on exposed skin, and wearing protective clothing treated with a similar repellant. The risk of exposure may be lower in modern, air-conditioned hotels with well-kept grounds, and in rural areas.

REFERENCES

1. Rush AB: An account of the bilious remitting fever, as it appeared in Philadelphia in the summer and autumn of the year 1780. In: Medical Inquiries and Observation. Philadelphia, Prichard & Hall, 1789, p 104.

2. Hirsch A: Dengue, a comparatively new disease: Its symptoms. In: Handbook of Geographical and Historical Pathology, vol. 1. London, Sydenham Society, 1883, p 55.
3. Pepper OHP: A note on David Bylon and dengue. Ann Med Hist Ser 33:363, 1941.
4. Howe GM: A World Geography of Human Diseases. New York, Academic Press, 1977, p 302.
5. Nobuchi H: The symptoms of a dengue-like illness recorded in a Chinese Medical Encyclopedia (in Japanese). Kanpo no Rinsho 26:422, 1979.
6. McSherry JA: Some medical aspects of the Darien scheme: Was it dengue? Scott Med J 27:183, 1982.
7. Carey DE: Chikungunya and dengue: A case of mistaken identity? J Hist Med Allied Sci 26:243, 1971.
8. Halstead SB: The XXth century dengue pandemic: Need for surveillance and research. Rapport Trimestriel Stat Sanit Mondiales 45:292, 1992.
9. Soler B, Pascual P, Petinto P: La Duquesa De Alba y Su Tiempo. Madrid, Ediciones y Publicaciones Españoles, 1949.
10. Christie J: Remarks on "Kidinga Pepo": A peculiar form of exanthematous disease. BMJ 577, 1872.
11. Christie J: On epidemics of dengue fever: Their diffusion and etiology. Glasgow Med J 16:161, 1881.
12. Munoz JA: Memoria Sobre la Epidemia que Ha Sufrido Esta Ciudad, Nombrada Vulgarmente al Dengue. Havana, Oficina del Gobierno y Capitania General, 1828.
13. Graham H: The dengue. A study of its pathology and mode of propagation. J Trop Med (London) 6:209, 1903.
14. Bancroft TL: On the aetiology of dengue fever. Aust Med Gazette 25:17, 1906.
15. Cleland JB, Bradley B, McDonald W: Dengue fever in Australia. Its history and clinical course, its experimental transmission by *Stegomyia fasciata,* and the results of inoculation and other experiments. J Hyg 16:317, 1918.
16. Ashborne PM, Craig CF: Experimental investigations regarding the etiology of dengue fever. J Infect Dis 4:440, 1907.
17. Siler JF, Hall MW, Hitchens AP: Dengue, its history, epidemiology, mechanism of transmission, etiology, clinical manifestations, immunity and prevention. Philippine J Sci 29:1, 1926.
18. Kimura R, Hotta S: Studies on dengue fever (VI). On the inoculation of dengue virus into mice (in Japanese). Nippon Igaku 3379:629, 1944.
19. Hotta S, Kimura R: Experimental studies on dengue 1. Isolation, identification and modification of the virus. J Infect Dis 90:1, 1952.
20. Sabin AB, Schlesinger RW: Production of immunity to dengue with virus modified by propagation in mice. Science 101:640, 1945.
21. Sabin AB: Research on dengue during World War II. Am J Trop Med Hyg 1:30, 1952.
22. Hammon W, Rudnick A, Sather G, et al: New hemorrhagic fevers of children in the Philippines and Thailand. Trans Assoc Am Physicians 73:140, 1960.
23. Hare FE: The 1897 epidemic of dengue in North Queensland. Aust Med Gazette 17:98, 1898.
24. Koizumi M, Yamaguchi K, Tonomura K: Dengue fever. Nisshin Igaku 6:955, 1916.
25. The dengue epidemic in Greece. League Nations Monthly Epidemiol Rep 7:335, 1928.
26. Copanaris P: L'epidemie de dengue in Grèce au cours de l'été. Office Int Hyg Public Bull 20:1590, 1928.
27. Akashi K: A dengue epidemic in the Tainan District of Taiwan in 1931 (in Japanese). Taiwan No Ikai 31:767, 1932.
28. Halstead SB, Papaevangelou G: Transmission of dengue 1 and 2 viruses in Greece in 1928. Am J Trop Med Hyg 29:635, 1980.
29. Rosen L: Dengue in Greece in 1927 and 1928 and the pathogenesis of dengue hemorrhagic fever: New data and a different conclusion. Am J Trop Med Hyg 35:642, 1986.
30. Gubler DJ: Dengue and dengue haemorrhagic fever: Its history and resurgence as a global public health problem. In Gubler DJ, Kuno G (eds): Dengue and Dengue Hemorrhagic Fever. London, CAB International, 1997.
31. Westaway EG, Blok J: Taxonomy and evolutionary relationships of flaviviruses. In Gubler DJ, Kuno G (eds): Dengue and Dengue Hemorrhagic Fever. London, CAB International, 1997.
32. Gubler DJ: Dengue. In Monath TP (ed): Epidemiology of Arthropod-Borne Viral Diseases. Boca Raton, FL, CRC Press, 1988.
33. Gubler DJ, Rosen L: A simple technique for demonstrating transmission of dengue viruses by mosquitoes without the use of vertebrate hosts. Am J Trop Med Hyg 25:146, 1976.
34. Gubler DJ, Trent DW: Emergence of epidemic dengue/dengue hemorrhagic fever as a public health problem in the Americas. Infect Agents Dis 2:383, 1994.
35. Gubler DJ, Clark GG: Dengue/dengue hemorrhagic fever: The emergence of a global health problem. Emerg Infect Dis 1:55, 1995.
36. World Health Organization: Dengue Hemorrhagic Fever: Diagnosis, Treatment and Control, 2nd ed. Geneva, World Health Organization, 1997.
37. Halstead SB: Dengue hemorrhagic fever—Public health problem and a field for research. Bull World Health Org 58:1, 1980.
38. Rosen L: Dengue—An overview. In Mackenzie JS (ed): Viral Diseases in Southeast Asia and the Western Pacific. Sydney, Australia, Academic Press, 1982, p 484.
39. Barnes WJS, Rosen L: Fatal hemorrhagic disease and shock associated with primary dengue infection on a Pacific island. Am J Trop Med Hyg 23:495, 1974.
40. Guzman MG, Kouri GP, Bravo J, et al: Dengue hemorrhagic fever in Cuba. II. Clinical investigations. Trans Soc Trop Med Hyg 78:239, 1984.
41. Gubler DJ: Dengue and dengue hemorrhagic fever in the Americas. In Thoncharoen P (ed): Dengue Hemorrhagic Fever. World Health Organization Monograph, Regional Publication, SEARO, No. 22. New Delhi, 1993.
42. Pinheiro FP: Dengue in the Americas, 1980–1987. Epidemiol Bull 10:1, 1989.
43. Gubler DJ: Dengue and dengue hemorrhagic fever in the Americas. PR Health Sci J 6:107, 1987.
44. Gubler, DJ: Epidemic dengue/dengue hemorrhagic fever as a public health, social and economic problem in the 21st century. Trends Micriobiol 10:100, 2002.
45. Rodier G, Gubler DJ, Cope SE, et al: Epidemic dengue 2 in the city of Djibouti, Horn of Africa, 1991–1992. Trans Soc Trop Med Hyg 90:237, 1996.
46. Monath TP: Dengue: The risk to developed and developing countries. Proc Natl Acad Sci USA 91:2395, 1994.
47. World Health Organization: Strengthening implementation of the global strategy for dengue fever/dengue haemorrhagic fever prevention and control. Report of the Informal Consultation, World Health Organization, October 18–20, 1999, Geneva, 2000.
48. Gubler DJ: *Aedes aegypti* and *Aedes aegypti*–borne disease control in the 1990s: Top down or bottom up. Am J Trop Med Hyg 40:571, 1989.
49. Newton EAC, Rieter P: A model of the transmission of dengue fever with an evolution of the impact of ultra–low volume (ULV) insecticide application on dengue epidemics. Am J Trop Med Hyg 47:709, 1992.
50. Gubler DJ: Arboviruses as imported disease agents: The need for increased awareness. Arch Virol 11:21, 1996.
51. Rigau-Pérez JG, Gubler DJ, Vorndam AV, et al: Dengue surveillance—United States, 1986–1992. MMWR 43:7, 1994.
52. Wittesjo B, Eitrem R, Niklasson B: Dengue fever among Swedish tourists. Scand J Infect Dis 25:699, 1993.
53. Imported dengue—United States, 1993 and 1994. MMWR 44:353, 1995.
54. Effler, P, Pang L, Kitsutani P, et al: Dengue fever outbreak in Hawaii, 2001–2002. Am J Trop Med Hyg, 2005 (in press).
55. Laille M, Institute Malarde, Papeete, Tahiti. Personal communication, 2004.
56. Ehrankramz NJ, Ventura AK, Guadrado RR, et al: Pandemic dengue in Caribbean countries and the southern United States: Past, present and potential problems. N Engl J Med 285:1460, 1971.
57. Halstead SB: Observations related to pathogenesis of dengue hemorrhagic fever. VI. Hypotheses and discussion. Yale J Biol Med 42:350, 1970.
58. Rosen L: The Emperor's new clothes revisited, or reflections on the pathogenesis of dengue hemorrhagic fever. Am J Trop Med Hyg 26:337, 1977.
59. Gubler DJ: Dengue and dengue hemorrhagic fever. Clin Microbiol Rev 11:480, 1998.
60. Waterman SH, Gubler DJ: Dengue fever. Clin Dermatol 7:117, 1989.
61. Hayes EB, Gubler DJ: Dengue and dengue hemorrhagic fever. Pediatr Infect Dis J 11:311, 1992.
62. Dietz V, Gubler DJ, Ortiz S, et al: The 1986 dengue and dengue hemorrhagic fever epidemic in Puerto Rico: Epidemiologic and clinical observations. PR Health Sci J 15:201, 1996.

63. Sumarmo SPS: Demam berdarah dengue pada anak di Jakarta. PhD thesis, University of Indonesia, Jakarta, 1983.
64. Eram S, Setyabudi Y, Sadono TI, et al: Epidemic dengue hemorrhagic fever in rural Indonesia. II. Clinical studies. Am J Trop Med Hyg 28:711, 1979.
65. Sumarmo SPS, Wulur H, Jahja E, et al: Clinical observations on virologically confirmed fatal dengue infections in Jakarta, Indonesia. Bull World Health Org 61:693, 1983.
66. Gubler DJ, Kuno G, Waterman SH: Neurologic disorders associated with dengue infection. In Pang T, Pathmanathan R (eds): Proceedings of International Conference on Dengue and Dengue Hemorrhagic Fever, Kuala Lumpur, Malaysia, September 1983. Kuala Lumpur, University of Malaysia Press, 1983, p 290.
67. Rosen L, Khin MM, U Tin: Recovery of virus from the liver of children with fatal dengue: Reflections on the pathogenesis of the disease and its possible analogy with that of yellow fever. Res Virol 140:351, 1989.
68. Row D, Weinstein P, Murray-Smith S: Dengue fever with encephalopathy in Australia. Am J Trop Med Hyg 54:253, 1996.
69. Lum LCS, Lam SK, Choy YS, et al: Dengue encephalitis: A true entity? Am J Trop Med Hyg 54:256, 1996.
70. Kurane I, Ennis FA: Immunopathogenesis of dengue virus infections. In Gubler DJ, Kuno G (eds): Dengue and Dengue Hemorrhagic Fever. London, CAB International, 1997, p 273.
71. Gubler DJ, Reed D, Rosen L, et al: Epidemiologic, clinical and virological observations on dengue in the Kingdom of Tonga. Am J Trop Med Hyg 27:581, 1978.
72. Gubler DJ, Sather GE: Laboratory diagnosis of dengue and dengue hemorrhagic fever. In Proceedings of International Symposium on Yellow Fever and Dengue, Rio de Janeiro, Brazil, May 1990, p 411.
73. Kuno G: Serodiagnosis of flaviviral infections and vaccinations in humans. Adv Virus Res 61:3, 2004.
74. Guzman MG, Kouri G: Dengue diagnosis, advances and challenges. Int J Infect Dis 8:69, 2004.
75. Lanciotti RS, Calisher CH, Gubler DJ, et al: Rapid detection and typing of dengue viruses from clinical samples using reverse transcriptase chain reaction. J Clin Microbiol 30:545, 1992.
76. Hall WC, Crowell TP, Watts DM, et al: Demonstration of yellow fever and dengue antigens in formalin-fixed paraffin embedded human liver by immunohistochemical analysis. Am J Trop Med Hyg 45:408, 1991.
77. Kuno G, Gomez I, Gubler DJ: An ELISA procedure for the diagnosis of dengue infections. J Virol Methods 33:101, 1991.
78. Burke DS, Nisalak A, Ussery MA: Antibody capture immunoassay detection of Japanese encephalitis virus immunoglobulin M and G antibodies in cerebrospinal fluid. J Clin Microbiol 15:1034, 1982.
79. Miagostovich MP, Nogueira RM, dos Santos FB, et al: Evaluation of an IgG enzyme-linked immunosorbent assay for dengue diagnosis. J Clin Virol 14:183, 1999.
80. Reiter P, Gubler DJ: Surveillance and control of urban dengue vectors. In Gubler DJ, Kuno G (eds): Dengue and Dengue Hemorrhagic Fever. London, CAB International, 1997, p 425.
81. Kinney RM, Huang CYH: Development of new vaccines against dengue fever and Japanese encephalitis. Intervirology 44:176, 2001.
82. Halstead SB, Deen J: The future of dengue vaccines. Lancet 360:1243, 2002.
83. Chang GJ, Kuno G, Purdy ED, et al: Recent advancement in flavivirus vaccine development. Expert Rev Vaccines 3:199, 2004.
84. Bhamarapravati N, Yoksan S: Live attenuated tetravalent dengue vaccine. Vaccine (suppl 2):44, 2000.
85. Sun W, Edelman R, Kanesa-Thasah N, et al: Vaccination of human volunteers with monovalent and tetravalent live-attenuated dengue vaccine candidates. Am J Trop Med Hyg 69(6 Suppl):24, 2003.
86. Whitehead SS, Falgout B, Hanley KA, et al: A live attenuated dengue virus type 1 vaccine candidate with a 30-nucleotide deletion in the 3′ untranslated region is highly attentuated and immunogenetic in monkeys. J Virol 77:1653, 2003.
87. Guirakoo F, Arroya J, Pugachev KV, et al: Construction, safety and immunogenicity in nonhuman primates of chimeric yellow fever-dengue virus tetravalent vaccine. J Virol 75:7290, 2001.
88. Huang CYH, Butrapet S, Pierro DJ, et al: Chimeric dengue type 2 (vaccine strain PDK-53)/Dengue type 1 virus as a potential candidate dengue type 1 virus vaccine. J Virol 74:3020, 2000.
89. Whitehead SS, Hanley KA, Blaney JE, et al: Substitution of the structural genes of dengue virus type 4 with those of type 2 results in chimeric vaccine candidates which are attenuated for mosquitoes, mice and rhesus monkeys. Vaccine 21:4307, 2003.
90. Accelerating the Development and Introduction of a Dengue Vaccine for Poor Children. Conference hosted by Children's Hospital No. 1 and Pasteur Institute of Ho Chi Minh City, Ho Chi Minh City, Vietnam, December 5–8, 2001.

73

Japanese Encephalitis and West Nile and Other Flavivirus Infections

DOUGLAS M. WATTS
BRUNO P. GRANWEHR
ROBERT E. SHOPE
TOM SOLOMON
ROBERT B. TESH

INTRODUCTION

Four mosquito-transmitted flaviviral diseases are of significant public health importance in tropical and subtropical regions of the world: dengue, yellow fever, Japanese encephalitis, and West Nile virus infection. Other chapters in this book address dengue and yellow fever; this chapter focuses on disease caused by Japanese encephalitis (JE) and West Nile (WN) viruses. Among the other tropical flaviviruses that cause human disease (Tables 73-1 and 73-2), Murray Valley encephalitis (MVE), Rocio, Kyasanur Forest disease (KFD), and Zika viruses will be described very briefly. Kunjin is not included because it is a subtype of WN virus and is not a frequent cause of human disease.[1] St. Louis encephalitis (SLE) virus has been isolated sporadically from patients in the tropics, but will not be described because epidemics are limited to temperate regions.

*Table 73-1 Tropical Flaviviruses Causing Encephalitis**

Virus	Distribution	Frequency of Disease
Japanese encephalitis	Asia, Pacific Islands	>10,000/yr; most epidemics in temperate region
West Nile	Africa, Asia, Europe, U.S.	Uncommon in tropics
Ilheus	South America	Uncommon
Kunjin	Australia	Uncommon
Murray Valley encephalitis	Australia	0–50/yr; uncommon in tropics
Rocio	São Paulo, Brazil	971 cases 1975–1976; last diagnosed in 1980
St. Louis encephalitis	Americas	Epidemics in the United States; uncommon in tropics

*The viruses causing these diseases have a natural cycle involving *Culex* or *Aedes* mosquitoes and birds.

*Table 73-2 Tropical Flaviviruses Associated Primarily with Fever**

Virus	Distribution	Associated Clinical Syndrome
Banzi	Africa	—
Bussuquara	South and Central America	Arthralgia
Edge Hill	Australia	Arthritis
Kokobera	Australia	Rash
Koutango	Africa	Rash
Rio Bravo	North America, Trinidad	—
Sepik	Papua New Guinea	—
Spondweni	Africa	—
Usutu	Africa	Rash
Wesselsbron	Africa, Southeast Asia	—
Zika	Africa, Southeast Asia	Rash

*These diseases are uncommon; 12 or fewer cases of each are described. Not listed is Kyasanur Forest disease virus, which causes hemorrhagic disease in India.

AGENTS

Both JE and WN viruses are members of the Japanese encephalitis serocomplex of the genus *Flavivirus*, family Flaviviridae.[2] These viruses measure about 50 nanometers in diameter and are enveloped, icosahedral virions with single-stranded, positive-sense RNA genomes of approximately 11,000 nucleotides. The three main structural proteins are the envelope (E), matrix (M), and the capsid (C) proteins. The E protein in the lipid envelope comprises the major surface protein that is thought to be responsible for virulence by mediating viral entry into cells, tissue tropism, and host range. The M proteins are responsible for the maturation of virions, and the C protein is an essential component of the virion nucleocapsids. Virus replicates in the cytoplasm, and viral assembly and maturation occur in the lumen of the endoplasmic reticulum preceding release from the host cell.

EPIDEMIOLOGY

Japanese Encephalitis Virus

JE virus is enzootic in rural agricultural areas throughout much of eastern and southern Asia and the Pacific Islands.[3–5] The principal enzootic transmission cycle involves various species of *Culex* mosquitoes and vertebrates, with *Culex tritaeniorhynchus* being the most important vector of human infections. These mosquitoes breed in rural areas, especially in flooded rice paddies, and are predominantly exophilic and zoophitic, preferring to feed on swine and birds and to a lesser extent on humans. Domestic swine and ardeid birds, such as herons and other waterfowl are the most important virus-amplifying hosts. However, the most important source of human infections is linked to the mosquito–swine transmission cycle. JE virus infection in avians does not normally cause any apparent illness, but abortions occur in infected pregnant sows. Human and equines are believed to be dead-end hosts because their infection does not produce viremia of sufficient magnitude to infect the mosquito vectors. While several other domestic and feral animals are infected in nature, their roles in the transmission cycle are unknown.

JE virus is a leading cause of viral encephalitis in tropical Asia, where it causes an estimated 35,000 to 50,000 clinical cases and 15,000 deaths annually.[6,7] Human infection and/or disease in temperate zones and the northern region of the tropical zone (northern Thailand, northern Vietnam, China, Korea, Japan, Taiwan, Nepal and northern India) is seasonal, and the incidence varies depending on vaccination practices and climatic conditions. The most common pattern of infection in northern (temperate) regions of Asia is summer epidemics; whereas, in southern (tropical) regions of Asia (southern Thailand, southern Vietnam, Malaysia, Singapore, Indonesia, the Philippines, Sri Lanka, and southern India), an endemic pattern of infection occurs with sporadic cases throughout the year and peak case rates appearing after the beginning of the rainy season.[8] In some countries, such as Japan, Taiwan, Korea, and China, the number of JE cases has been markedly reduced by the implementation of childhood immunizations.[9] However, over the past four decades, the incidence of JE has increased dramatically in central and northern India, Nepal, and the northern region of Southeast Asia. JE virus has also expanded its range into other areas of Southeast Asia and eastward to the Australasian zoogeographic region.[10] The expanding distribution of JE is not fully understood, but may be associated with changes in agricultural practices that provide suitable breeding habitat for mosquitoes or an increase in swine production.

The risk of JE infection is highest among individuals who travel or live in rural areas where rice is grown and swine are raised in close proximity to human dwellings.[3–5,8] In endemic areas, the annual infection rate is about 10% among the susceptible populations, with about 85% of the cases occurring among children under 15 years of age.[11] Most JE virus infections are silent; the ratio of symptomatic to asymptomatic infections varies from about one in 25 to one in 1000.[4] The lower incidence among adults in Asia has been attributed to high rates of immunity. The case-fatality rate among JE patients admitted to the hospital is about 25% to 30%; about half of the survivors experience severe neuropsychiatric sequelae.[3,7] In contrast to the situation in endemic regions, all age groups are affected during epidemics in nonimmune populations.[12] Similarly, when nonimmune individuals (travelers, or military personnel) visit endemic areas they too are at risk.

West Nile Virus

West Nile virus (WNV) is enzootic in most of Africa, southern Europe, the Middle East, western Asia, Australia, and North America.[13–15] The basic transmission cycle of the virus is similar throughout its range, involving mainly *Culex* mosquitoes as the primary vector and a variety of passerine birds as the major amplifying hosts. Infection of avians is usually benign in most species; however, epizootics with high mortality have been documented among certain species of birds (crows, jays, geese) during epidemics of WN in the United States, Canada, and Israel. While infection of other vertebrates, including humans and equines, is common, they are considered to be dead-end hosts because the level of viremia is thought to be insufficient to infect mosquito vectors. WNV has been isolated from a wide variety of other mosquito species, at least 40 species in Africa, Europe, and Asia and 37 species in North America. Recovery of WNV from mosquito species other than *Culex,* such as *Aedes* and *Ochlerotatus,* suggests that they might act as bridging vectors to transmit virus to humans and birds.[16,17] Experimental studies suggest that vertical transmission by infected mosquitoes and the overwintering of infected adult mosquitos may be important in the maintenance and transmission cycle of WNV. While the primary source of human infections is the bite of infected mosquitoes, observations during outbreaks in the United States in 2002 indicated that WNV could also be transmitted by other routes,[17] including transplanted organs, transfusion of blood products, transplacental spread, possibly breast milk, and accidental laboratory exposure. Estimates in the United States indicated that the risk of blood transfusion transmission was as high as 21 per 10,000 blood donations during the peak of the 2002 WN epidemic. However, screening of blood donations since 2003 has greatly reduced the risk of infection via blood products.

WNV is the cause of sporadic infections and outbreaks among humans, equines, and certain avian populations.[13,15,18] Until the mid-1990s, WNV was usually associated with sporadic cases and infrequent outbreaks of a febrile illness (fever, arthralgia, and rash), with occasional central nervous system disease. Recently, the epidemiology has changed to a pattern of more frequent and widespread outbreaks, with a marked increase in the incidence of human neurologic disease. Some of the better documented examples of this changing pattern were epidemics in Algeria during 1994, Romania in 1996 and 1997, Tunisia and the Czech Republic in 1997, Congo in 1998, Russia in 1998 and 1999, Israel in 1999 and 2000, and annually in the United States from 1999 through 2003. These epidemics and epizootics affected both urban and rural populations. The most surprising spread of WNV was to the New York City metropolitan area during 1999.[19] Although the mechanism of introduction is unknown, nucleotide sequence data revealed that the New York strain is closely related to a viral strain isolated from a goose in Israel the year before.[20] Since 1999, WNV has spread throughout the continental United States, southern Canada, Mexico, and the Caribbean.[17,21–23] The pattern of spread has been rapid and extensive; 62 human cases were documented in the United States during 1999 and 66 in 2001. However, more than 4000 cases were reported in 2002, primarily in the Ohio and Mississippi River basins. Also during the same year, the first cases were diagnosed in at least 5 provinces of Canada, including 400 cases in Ontario and Quebec. In 2003, a total of 9100 WN cases and 222 deaths were reported from 45 states and the District of Colombia in the United States.

It is assumed that the virus will continue its move southward from Central America into South America. However, the risk of severe disease among persons living in tropical America may be less because of the high prevalence of heterologous flavivirus immunity. Experimental studies in animals suggest that prior infection with dengue, St. Louis encephalitis, or the yellow fever 17-D vaccine virus provides protection against severe disease and death upon challenge with WNV.[24,25]

About 20% of WNV-infected persons during the epidemic in New York developed symptoms, and less than 1% of infections resulted in severe life-threatening neurologic illness, with the most commonly reported severe syndromes being encephalitis, meningitis, and meningoencephalitis.[26] The ratio of clinical to subclinical infection in Romania during the 1996 outbreak was lower, ranging from 1:140 to 1:320.[27] While the age-specific rates of WN infection are similar, the risk of illness among those over 50 years old is 10 times greater than among those 0 to 19 years of age.[19,21] Severe disease can occur at any age, but the elderly, young adolescent, and immunocompromised individuals are at greater risk for the severe neurologic syndromes.[19,27,28] The impact of severe disease among the elderly was reported during an outbreak in Israel during 2000.[28] Among 50 patients admitted to one hospital, 32 (64%) were age 65 or older and 22% died, all of them aged 78 years or older. During the 1996 outbreak in Romania, among 352 cases of acute central nervous system infections, 40% presented with meningitis, 44% with meningoencephalitis, and 16% had encephalitis.[27] The overall mortality rate was 5%, and all of the fatal cases were greater than 50 years of age. In the 1999 outbreak in New York, the median age of 62 hospitalized cases was 71 years, ranging from 5 to 90 years, with 88% being at least 50 years old. Sixty-three percent presented with encephalitis, 29% with meningitis, and 8% had a febrile illness. In these outbreaks, the average fatality rate for severe cases of WN was between 4% and 18%, with rates as high as 21% and 29% reported among the elderly in the United States and Israel, respectively.[22,29]

WN disease in pediatric populations is less frequent and not as severe as in adults. However, the disease spectrum ranges from a nonspecific febrile illness to severe cases involving the central nervous system. In the United States, 5% (11/225) of cases in 2002 involved individuals 18 years old and younger. Of these patients, seven (64%) required hospitalization, five for meningitis and two for encephalitis, and the other four were diagnosed with WN fever at an outpatient clinic.[21,30]

DISEASES

Japanese Encephalitis Virus

JE virus infection can begin as a mild febrile illness or aseptic meningitis, but by far the most common presentation to hospital in humans is due to acute meningomyeloencephalitis. After an incubation period of 1 to 2 weeks, patients typically present with a history of 1 to 3 days of fever, headache, stupor, and, especially in children, generalized motor seizures. Physical findings at this time may be limited to a depressed state of consciousness, but evidence of local motor impairment of limbs or cranial nerve palsy is not infrequent. Some patients have a rapid recovery, but most will develop a variety of neurologic manifestations. The case-fatality rate can be as high as 30%. In some instances, abnormal behavior is the only presenting symptom, without fever, weakness, diarrhea, vomiting, confusion, and rigors. Upper motor neuron weakness is noted in 30% to 50% of patients[31] in contrast with poliomyelitis-like flaccid paralysis occurring in up to 15% of patients.[32] This poliomyelitis-like syndrome may present with an altered level of consciousness progressing to encephalitis and respiratory paralysis in 20% to 60%, with poor prognosis for recovery.[7,31] A parkinsonian syndrome is seen in up to 25% of patients, typified by cogwheel rigidity, mask-like facies, and bradykinesia. Other movement disorders consist of myoclonic jerks and haunting orofacial dyskinesias (grimacing, chewing, and lip smacking) noted in up to a third of patients during recovery and also seen with WNV infection.[33]

Seizures occur in 85% of children and 10% of adults.[31] Uncontrolled seizures and elevated intracranial pressure demonstrated by opening pressure of greater than 25 mm Hg during lumbar puncture are predictive of poor outcome.[34] In fact, the mortality rate in patients with such findings, as well as prolonged illness, was 62% compared with 14% overall in one study including adults and children.[34] The long-term outcome of JE is grim, with survivors sharing a variety of deficits including 20% with severe cognitive and language impairment, 20% with subsequent seizures, 30% with flexion or extension contractures, and learning/behavioral disorders.[7] Other unfortunate complications, such as decubitus ulcers and pneumonia, are due to the disability caused by the virus rather than direct viral damage.[35]

Bilateral lesions in the thalamus, basal ganglia, and brainstem on brain MRI and CT scan correlate with the clinical manifestations.[36,37] Hyponatremia is presumably caused by inappropriate release of antidiuretic hormone.

Pathology

Virus is found in lungs, liver, kidneys, and myocardium as well as various regions of gray matter such as the thalamus, basal ganglia, and midbrain. A distinguishing feature of JE is predominant gray matter infection that spares white matter, unlike WN.[7,36,38] Prolonged viremia may occasionally occur for weeks to months,[39] a phenomenon recently noted in WNV infection as well, and postulated to lead to rare chronic progressive CNS infection.

West Nile Virus

After exposure to WNV, the incubation period usually ranges from 2 to 6 days, but may extend to 14 days, and as long as 21 days, for patients following organ transplantation.[22,30,40] WN fever is typically a mild illness, lasting 3 to 6 days. Infected individuals develop a sudden onset of high fever with chills, rash, malaise, headache, backache, arthralgia, myalgia, and eye pain. Other nonspecific manifestations may include nausea, vomiting, anorexia, diarrhea, rhinorrhea, sore throat, and cough. In some patients, there is generalized lymphadenopathy, and an erythematous macular, papular, or morbilliform eruption involves the entire body. A biphasic fever may occur that is similar to dengue fever.

Meningitis, encephalitis, and/or acute flaccid paralysis develop in less than 1% of WNV-infected individuals.[22,26,27] Patients with neurologic disease typically have a febrile prodrome of 1 to 7 days, which may be biphasic before they develop neurologic symptoms. While the prodrome phase is usually nonspecific, 15% to 20% of the patients may have features characteristic of WN fever, including ocular pain, facial congestion, or a rash, and less than 5% have lymphadenopathy. Typically, most patients present with a fever, stiff neck, headache, muscle weakness, gastrointestinal symptoms, disorientation, tremors, convulsions, and paralysis.

While about 30% of patients have been reported to have convulsions, the rates were much lower during outbreaks in Romania and New York. Patients with encephalitis have altered mental status or cortical signs. Other neurologic manifestations associated with WNV infection include cranial neuropathies, optic neuritis, ataxia, and seizures. Stiffness, rigidity, spasms, and tremors have been associated with basal ganglia damage during WN encephalitis. Ocular manifestations, myocarditis, pancreatitis, and fulminant hepatitis may also occur.

Pathology

Fatal cases reveal variable amounts of neuronal necrosis in the gray matter, microglial nodules, polymorphonuclear leukocytes, perivascular and leptomeningeal chronic inflammation, and neuronophagia.[38] Viral antigens are present in neurons, neuronal processes, and areas of necrosis in the brain and spinal cord, but not in the lung, liver, spleen, and kidney.

PATHOGENESIS

The pathogenesis of JE and WNV infection is similar with interplay between direct viral damage and the pathologic effects of the host immune response.[41] Infection is believed to begin with the replication of virus in the skin and regional lymph nodes to produce a primary viremia, which leads to infection of the reticuloendothelial system.[29,42] A secondary viremia follows, that may result in a systemic infection involving other organs and the central nervous system. Observations on patients who died after inoculation with WNV during cancer treatment studies suggested that the virus replicated in the spleen, lymph nodes, liver, and lungs, similar to studies in laboratory animals. WN viremia is transient, lasting only for a few days, and then ceases with the onset of symptoms and concurrent development of IgM and IgG antibodies. Immunocompromised individuals may have prolonged viremia and delayed development of symptoms and IgM antibody. The increased incidence and higher mortality rate of WN encephalitis in the elderly and immunocompromised individuals suggest that host factors are important determinants of the outcome of infection, such as immune senescence or changes in the blood-brain barrier.[29] The associations between neurocysticercosis in JE[41] and hypertension in WNV infection suggest a potential role for factors that make the blood-brain barrier vulnerable to invasion.[38] The capability to mount an early immune response plays a critical role in containing viral replication and dissemination in the CNS of mice.[43] The use of viral mutations to study viral virulence indicates that the major determinants for neuroinvasiveness are on the WN virion E protein, similar to other flaviviruses.

DIAGNOSIS

The etiologic diagnosis of a flaviviral infection cannot be determined clinically. A high index of suspicion, however, can be gleaned from the geographic area of exposure, history of arthropod abundance, and season of the year. In addition, specific clinical features, such as flaccid paralysis, unusual movement disorders, or subtle motor seizures may provide an additional clue. Leukopenia, when present, may be an indication of a viral illness. Encephalitis cases usually have pleocytosis between 5/μL and greater than 1000/μL, and initially this may be characterized by polymorphonuclear cells, but subsequently lymphocytes predominate; there is usually a normal cerebrospinal fluid to plasma glucose ratio, and an increased concentration of protein in the cerebrospinal fluid.[44]

The laboratory diagnosis of a febrile or neurologic case of JE or WN infection can be made by a variety of tests. Blood samples should be obtained as early as possible from suspected cases and tested for virus in cell culture or for genomic sequences by the PCR assay. In most cases of encephalitis, the period of viremia has ceased by the time the patient seeks medical care, and virus isolation from the blood will not be possible.[44] However, attempts should be made to isolate virus from the cerebrospinal fluid in cases of JE, WN, and other suspected flavivirus encephalitides in 1- to 3-day-old mice by intracerebral inoculation, or in cell culture such as Vero (African green monkey kidney) cells. Infected mice become sick and die in 3 to 10 days, and cell culture shows cytopathic effect during a similar period, indicating the possible presence of an infectious agent that can be identified antigenically. Isolation of virus from cerebrospinal fluid signifies a poor prognosis.[3] A serologic diagnosis can be made by showing a fourfold rise or fall in IgM and/or IgG antibody titer between acute serum and a convalescent sample collected one or two weeks after the onset of illness by neutralization, hemagglutination inhibition, immunofluorescence, or enzyme-linked immunosorbent assay (ELISA). The IgM capture ELISA is especially useful because flavivirus-specific IgM is usually present at the time the patient seeks care for encephalitis; antibody can be detected both in the serum and the cerebrospinal fluid.[45,46] IgM capture ELISA detection of antibodies on a single specimen generally indicates a recent infection, usually within the prior 6 weeks. In case of a negative IgM capture ELISA, a second test should be done a week later. However, caution must be exercised in the interpretation of IgM antibody results for WN infection because IgM antibody may persist in the serum for longer than 500 days.[47] Therefore, detection of IgM antibody in a single sample or in the absence of a rise in titer may be unrelated to the current illness. The cerebrospinal fluid IgM is oligoclonal and relatively specific and produces a stronger ELISA optical density signal than that of serum antibody. Diagnosis can also be established by virus isolation or by immunostaining of brain collected at biopsy or postmortem examination. The differential diagnosis includes other viral encephalitides caused by entero-, herpes-, alpha-, and rabies viruses, as well as tuberculosis, cerebral malaria, cerebrovascular accidents, toxins, and rickettsial infections.

Interpretation of serologic results is complicated by flavivirus cross-reacting antibody.[48] A second flavivirus infection leads to an anamnestic response that is characterized by the rapid development of antibody that is so cross-reactive among flaviviruses that it may not be possible to determine the specific infecting flavivirus.[49] In fact, the antibody titer to the first infecting flavivirus may be higher than the titer of antibodies to the more recent agent. Attempts to isolate virus from these patients is often unsuccessful. The use of reverse transcription–polymerase chain reaction (RT-PCR) to detect flavivirus RNA[50] employs consensus primers to amplify conserved regions of the genome. As a second step, primers specific for each flavivirus are used, and the resulting complementary DNA (cDNA) can be sequenced or detected by DNA-DNA hybridization. This technique is highly specific and can be completed in 1 or 2 days.

TREATMENT AND PROGNOSIS

Treatment is nonspecific and supportive for WN and JE infections. Supportive treatment of encephalitis cases includes intravenous fluid, electrolyte management, assisted respiration if needed, anticonvulsants, management of cerebral edema, prevention of secondary bacterial infections, and nursing care.[22,51] Physical and psychological rehabilitation is important in surviving patients, because sequelae are common and can result in major disability. Studies have assessed ribavirin, interferon, osmotic agents, gamma globulins, and steroids for treatment of WN in open trials, but more definitive evidence is needed to determine their efficacy, if any. For example, although interferon-alpha was shown to be the most promising treatment drug in small open trials for JE, a double-blind, placebo-controlled trial showed that it did not affect disease outcome in children.[7] Also, studies on WNV infection are being conducted, employing an open labeled–trial to assess the efficacy of interferon-alpha2b, and a placebo-controlled, double-blind, multicenter trial is being conducted to evaluate the efficacy of pooled human immunoglobulin for treatment of naturally occurring cases in the United States.[52,53] Interest in the use of anti-WNV human immunoglobulin has increased because open trials suggested that WN CNS infection was aborted in at least two human cases.[52] In addition, several studies showed varying degrees of efficacy for anti-WNV human immunoglobulin or mouse immune serum in mouse models of WNV infection.[52] However, the relevance of these animal studies for the prevention and/or treatment of human disease must be interpreted with caution.

Some of the risk factors predictive of a poor outcome and possibly death for WN neurologic cases include profound weakness, deep coma, lack of production of IgM antibody, immunosuppression, diabetes, and hypertension. Neurologic sequelae are common; for example, in one study in the United States, half of the patients had functional deficit when discharged from the hospital, and only one-third had fully recovered after one year. More recent findings indicate that the frequency and type of seizures and status epilepticus are important predictors of a poor outcome of JE in children.[54] Importantly, in many children, subtle motor seizures, such as twitching of a digit or eyebrow, were the only signs of status epilepticus that could be confirmed by electroencephalography. Awareness, appropriate attention, and management of these manifestations may lead to a better outcome.

PREVENTION AND CONTROL

Japanese Encephalitis Virus

A formalin-inactivated JE vaccine is licensed for human use in the United States and in countries of Asia. It is safe, efficacious, and has been available for many years, but is too expensive for use in most Asian countries.[11] In the United States it is used primarily for military personnel and tourists visiting Asia. This vaccine is produced in Japan, Taiwan, Korea, and Thailand in adult mouse brain and is purified by protamine sulfate precipitation and ultracentrifugation to remove myelin basic protein. In Japan (one of the main suppliers to the Western market), manufacture of this mouse-brain derived vaccine is currently being replaced with a Vero-cell derived vaccine. Vaccine made with the Beijing-1 strain of JE virus is distributed in Japan and Asia, and another vaccine made in Japan with the Nakayama strain is produced for export to the United States and Europe. A field trial in Thailand demonstrated greater than 91% efficacy after two inoculations.[11] Vaccination of U.S. nationals showed that three inoculations more effectively induced neutralizing antibodies than two.[55] Although no serious side effects were noted in the trials, some late-onset hypersensitivity reactions have been observed since. Currently, three inoculations are recommended in the United States.[56]

A JE formalin-inactivated vaccine is produced in China in primary hamster kidney cells.[57] This inexpensive vaccine has been used for decades to immunize school children, but is not available outside of China. A JE formalin-inactivated vaccine produced in Vero cells is undergoing phase III clinical trials in Japan and is likely to replace the mouse-brain derived vaccine in the near future. More recently, the SA14-14-2 live attenuated JE vaccine, produced by serial passage in mice, hamsters, and primary hamster kidney cell culture, has been widely used in China. Efficacy is 80% after one dose, but antibody wanes rapidly, and a booster dose at 12 months is recommended to achieve effective protection of 97.5% of recipients.[58] However when administered just before the start of the JE season, the efficacy of a single dose of vaccine was 99%.[59] Until recently, the use of this vaccine outside of China has been restricted by regulatory concerns over its production. The World Health Organization has recently described guidelines for the production of live attenuated JE vaccines, which will facilitate SA14-14-2's wider use in the future. The SA14-14-2 vaccine is undergoing further clinical trials in Korea.

Among the more promising novel JE candidates is a live attenuated vaccine, ChimeriVax-JE, which was prepared by replacing the prM-E genes of yellow fever 17D vaccine with the corresponding JE virus genes.[60] A recently completed randomized, double-blind, placebo-controlled phase II clinical trial showed that the vaccine was well tolerated with no adverse side effects.[61] In addition, the vaccine elicited high neutralizing antibody in more than 90% of the 87 volunteers within 30 days following a single inoculation of a range of doses. If further clinical trials are successful, this vaccine offers an advantage over inactivated vaccines that require multiple doses.

While the control of JE can be achieved by vaccination of humans,[62] vaccination will not interrupt the transmission cycles in nature. Therefore, an effective live attenuated vaccine was developed to immunize pigs, the amplifying host of JE virus.[63] These vaccines, however, have met with limited success for at least three reasons. Farmers are not prone to invest in public health, pigs in Japan are marketed at less than 1 year of age, which presents a limited window of time for immunization, and the numbers of pigs are so great that the cost of annual vaccinations is prohibitive.

Until a vaccine is available that can be administered to those at greatest risk, such as children, efforts should be made to avoid exposure to the vector mosquitoes during hours of biting or to use repellants. Vector control measures should be targeted at immature and adult vector species using larvacides and adulticides. Also, swine should be vaccinated or housed away from living quarters.

West Nile Virus

The rapidly growing global threat of WNV to human and animal health has led to numerous studies aimed at the development of vaccines using both traditional and novel approaches.[64] Veterinary vaccine development has targeted protecting equines and other domestic animals. In the United States, a formalin-inactivated vaccine was licensed for equines during 2002, and an inactivated vaccine that protected mice, geese, and equines against a lethal challenge was approved for veterinary use during 2004 in Israel. A canarypox-vectored vaccine with *prm* and E genes of WNV has recently been licensed in the United States for use in equines.[23] Several candidate vaccines for humans have been developed and are under evaluation. These include a recombinant subunit vaccine derived by expressing WNV E protein in transfected insect cells that protected hamsters from lethal challenge with WNV.[65] Also, a subunit vaccine derived by expressing the WNV E protein fused to maltose-binding protein in *Escherichia coli* induced antibody and protected mice from challenge with 10 plaque-forming units of virus, but not from higher challenge doses.[64] A DNA vaccine is under development that utilizes the optimal signal sequence from JEV for the processing of prM and E proteins to produce viral-like particles is under development. This vaccine candidate has been shown to induce antibody that protects mice and equines.[64] Among several attenuated vaccines under development, a live yellow fever virus–WN (WN-YF) chimera induced antibody that protects mice, hamsters, and monkeys against a lethal challenge with WNV.[25,66] Furthermore, the NIH has developed a live dengue virus–WN (DEN-WNV) chimera that protects mice and monkeys against a virulent strain of WNV.[64] Other strategies for developing WN vaccines include a DNA construct that produces infectious Kunjin virus in vivo capable of inducing antibody that protects mice against a lethal challenge of a New York strain of WNV.[64] Studies conducted to evaluate cross-protection against WNV induced by heterologous flaviviruses have also shown promising results.[64] While all of these preclinical studies are promising, the public health utility will depend on the eventual outcome of safety and efficacy trials that will need to be conducted in human volunteers for consideration of approval and selection for large-scale manufacture and distribution.

While a safe and effective vaccine is needed, it is not likely that vaccination of a large component of the population will be feasible and cost effective. Therefore, an effective therapeutic agent is needed for treatment of WN viral infection among those at an increased risk of severe disease, such as the immunocompromised and the elderly.[21]

In the meantime, until vaccines are available, any efforts to prevent WN disease should be targeted at reducing the risk to humans exposed to infected mosquitoes by using personal protective measures and by instituting appropriate surveillance and vector control measures.[67]

Other Flaviviruses

MVE virus, also closely related to the JE and WN viruses, is limited to Australia where it causes severe encephalitis and is maintained by *Culex* mosquitoes in the resident bird populations.[68]

Rocio virus is the cause of São Paulo encephalitis, a disease localized to the area near São Paulo, Brazil. A total of 971 cases were first recorded in 1975 in an explosive outbreak that continued through 1976.[69] A single additional fatal case was diagnosed serologically in 1980, and the disease has not been seen since. Clinically, the disease resembled St. Louis encephalitis, with about 20% of the patients having CNS sequelae and a mortality rate of 4% among hospitalized patients. The incidence during the 1975 outbreak was highest among young adult males involved in outdoor activities in agricultural areas. *Aedes* mosquitoes and wild birds were suspected as the reservoir on epidemiologic grounds. Since the initial outbreak, serologic evidence of Rocio infection in other parts of Brazil has been reported, and public health authorities are concerned about a return of Rocio outbreaks in Brazil.[70]

KFD virus is the cause of a hemorrhagic disease localized to six small forest foci in Karnataka state, India.[71] Since the disease was first recognized in 1957, about 400 to 500 cases have been reported each year, with a mortality rate of 3% to 5%. The virus belongs to the tick-borne encephalitis serocomplex. The cycle in the forest is maintained in *Haemaphysalis* ticks and small mammals and birds. KFD virus is readily isolated from monkeys that are often found sick or dead in the enzootic foci. KFD is clinically and virologically similar to Omsk hemorrhagic fever, a disease of the temperate regions of Omsk and Novosibirsk oblasts of Russia. The risk of infection is greatest among individuals who are in close contact with forested areas during the dry season. Clinically, patients present with a febrile syndrome accompanied by hemorrhages.[72] Some patients experience a biphasic course with signs of meningoencephalitis.

Zika virus has been diagnosed in 12 naturally acquired cases that occurred in Nigeria, Senegal, Central African Republic, and Indonesia.[73] Antibody prevalence of 50% or more in many African populations suggests that Zika virus infection is probably much more common than recognized. Patients have a self-limited disease characterized by fever, malaise, headache, and rash. The virus is maintained in a cycle involving *Aedes* mosquitoes and forest primates.

A formalin-inactivated vaccine for Kyasanur Forest disease (KFD) has been used in India.[74] There are no vaccines for St. Louis encephalitis, Murray Valley encephalitis (MVE), Rocio, and Ilheus viruses, and vaccines for these diseases are not likely to find commercial backing because of the small demand.

REFERENCES

1. Hall RA, Scherret JH, Mackenzie JS: Kunjin virus: An Australian variant of West Nile. Ann NY Acad Sci 951:153–160, 2001.
2. Mackenzie JS, Barrett AD, Deubel V: The Japanese encephalitis serological group of flaviviruses: A brief introduction to the group. Curr Top Microbiol Immunol 267:1–10, 2002.
3. Burke DS, Leake CJ: Japanese encephalitis. In Monath TP (ed): The Arboviruses: Epidemiology and Ecology, vol. 3. Boca Raton, FL, CRC Press, 1988, pp 68, 83.

Attachment, Penetration, and Uncoating

When a free virion comes into contact with a cell surface, the first specific attachment is made between a specific region of the HIV gp120 surface envelop glycoprotein and the 58-kD cell-surface CD4 molecule.[58] The CD4 molecule is a member of the immunoglobulin superfamily that is expressed on the surface of T lymphocytes (and at lower levels on other cells) and normally serves as a corecognition factor for major histocompatibility complex (MHC) class II in antigen presentation. The gp120-CD4 interaction initiates conformational changes in gp120, which then permit interaction of gp120 with a second cell surface receptor, the CXCR4 chemokine receptor molecule (on T lymphocytes) or the similar CCR5 molecule on macrophages.[59] Fusion of the viral lipid bilayer membrane with the cell membrane is mediated by a specific hydrophobic region fusion domain of the viral gp41 transmembrane protein. Sequential binding of gp120 to CD4 and CXCR4 (or CCR5) is thought to trigger gp41 to "harpoon" the cell membrane lipid bilayer. The process then repeats with many virion gp120 molecules interacting with the cellular receptors until fusion is complete. Fusion can proceed at neutral pH typical of extracellular fluids.

DNA Synthesis, Nuclear Transport, and Integration

Once the virus has inserted itself into the cytoplasm, the reverse transcriptase becomes activated and DNA proviral synthesis begins.[60–62] The initial event in reverse transcription—copying of virion RNA into DNA—is primed by cellular lysine transfer RNA (tRNA) (other retroviruses use other tRNA primers). The HIV reverse transcriptase molecule carries out three distinct enzymatic functions: (1) synthesis of a complete DNA negative strand using the virion RNA template, (2) degradation of the virion RNA template as the DNA strand is synthesized, and (3) synthesis of a DNA positive strand using the newly synthesized complete DNA negative strand. The net product is double-stranded DNA synthesized from an RNA template.

The sequences of the virion RNA and the proviral DNA are identical in their mid genome (protein coding regions) but differ in the arrangement of repeat and unique noncoding sequences at their terminals. In viral RNA, the order is repeat, 5′ unique, *gag-pol-env,* 3′ unique, repeat. As a consequence of a somewhat complicated series of head-to-tail jumps of the transcriptase that occur in synthesis of both the negative and positive DNA strands, this order becomes altered such that in the final double-stranded DNA provirus it becomes unique 3′, repeat, unique 5′, *gag-pol-env,* unique 3′, repeat, unique 5′. The U3-R-U5 sequence at both terminals is called the long terminal repeat, or LTR. When viral RNA is forward-transcribed, the outer unique regions of the proviral LTR DNA are not copied. This overall schema is thought to be necessary to provide for efficient priming and complete copying of both terminals. Occasionally aberrant reverse transcription occurs leading to covalently closed DNA circles containing either one or two LTRs, but these forms are dead-end.

In contrast to other retroviruses, HIV and the lentiviruses do not require that the newly infected cell undergo mitosis for integration to occur. The synthesized double-stranded DNA copy of the viral sequences is transported to the nucleus as a preintegration complex (PIC) probably through microtubules. The nucleophilic behavior of PIC is thought to be influenced by import signals under the control of integrase, viral protein R (vpr), the DNA flap, and the p17 matrix protein.[63–65]

Integration is not site-specific in the host cell chromosome; apparently it can occur anywhere. However, chromosomal sites that are transcriptionally active are more likely, presumably because the chromatin structure is more open and accessible. Proviral integration is catalyzed by the viral integrase and involves 3′ end processing of both viral DNA strands, and strand transfer of both host cell DNA strands to the activated 3′ proviral ends.[66,67] Because the activated 3′ viral DNA strands invade the host cell DNA strands at sites a few nucleotides apart, there is a characteristic short duplication of host cell sequence flanking both ends of the newly integrated provirus.

Gene Expression

The LTRs are organized such that the integrated provirus has a built-in 5′ promoter-enhancer and a 3′ polyadenylation site. The key activator on the HIV-1 5′ LTR promoter is the NF-kB binding site. Since NF-kB serves as an important cell activation factor, HIV transcription is unregulated concurrently with cell activation. The virus-encoded tat protein also increases viral transcription by binding to the tar RNA secondary structure in the 5′ LTR promoter region. An important consequence of this feedback loop is that HIV transcription is autocatalytic.[68–70] HIV transcripts are typically spliced into a large number of RNAs of different lengths. Spliced RNAs are efficiently transported from the nucleus and translated. However, long and unspliced RNAs (those containing the mid-env "rev responsive element," or RRE) are not transported unless the early viral protein rev is present in abundance.[71,72] Transport is mediated by rev binding to the RNA secondary structure formed by the RRE sequence.

Particle Assembly and Budding

Uncleaved gag precursor protein molecules and a much smaller number (5%) of gag-pol read-through proteins are targeted to the interior surface of the cell membrane by their myristoylated *N*-terminals. Viral core proteins are thereby aligned from outermost to innermost according to their position in the polyprotein: p17 matrix, p24 capsid, and nucleocapsid from the gag precursor, and then protease, reverse transcriptase, and integrase from the pol precursor. Cleavages are self-catalyzed by the viral encoded protease.[73] HIV protease is an aspartic protease which is active only as a dimer; virion assembly is thought to activate the protease. The nucleocapsid protein, the innermost of the gag proteins, interacts directly with a packaging site on full-length viral RNA via a complex of cystine residues (similar to a zinc finger motif in DNA binding proteins) and thereby guides genome encapsidation.[74] Independently, full-length gp160 envelope protein is oligomerized, glycosylated, and cleaved by cellular protease in the endoplasmic reticulum (ER) and Golgi apparatus into gp120 and gp41.[75,76] Envelope protein on the outer cell surface interacts with the p17 matrix (gag) protein via an internal cytoplasmic region of the gp41 transmembrane protein.

Genetic Organization of Human Lentiviruses from Tropical Regions

The genetic structures of HIV-1, HIV-2, and HIV-O strains thus far studied are quite similar. The most obvious difference is that *p*16 *vpu* is found only in HIV-1, while *p*16 *vpx* is found only in HIV-2 (and primate SIV strains). These two genes (of uncertain function) are present in different locations in the mid-genomic accessory gene region. Among the HIV-1 strains the genomic structure is highly conserved despite substantial nucleotide sequence variation. Potentially significant variations between HIV-1 strains have been observed in the number of SP-1 and NF-kB binding sites in the LTR promoter regions, particularly among non–B clade viruses, but these have not been systematically studied. Few attempts have been made to compare the molecular biology of clades, and no clear differences have been found.

Cell Tropism

Human and primate lentiviruses can infect a variety of cell types in vitro under relatively artificial laboratory conditions, but there is no convincing evidence that any cells except those of the mononuclear leukocyte lineages are infected in vivo. CD4- T lymphocytes were the first cells found to be infected (hence the originally proposed name HTLV-III), but a variety of macrophage-related cells (blood monocytes, skin Langerhans' cells, lymph node dendritic cells) also appear to be infected.[77,78] The presence of the two receptors—CD4 and CXCR4 (or CCR5)—appears to define the population of human cells that are permissive to HIV infection.

HIV-1 strains collected from blood early in infection are genetically homogeneous and uniformly display a characteristic "macrophage-tropic" envelope sequence.[79,80] As infection progresses over months and years, genetic variation in the blood increases so that the viral population becomes a quasispecies of genomes that may differ by 5% or more in their nucleotide sequences. Variation occurs in all genes, including the envelope, where mutations occur that change the affected virions from a macrophage-tropic to a "T cell–tropic syncytium-inducing" phenotype. The reason for this change in phenotype is not very clear, though it could be attributed to changes in the V-3 loop and V-2 region of the envelope protein, since these regions appear to determine coreceptor usage.[81,82] However, these altered viruses could as well be vertically transmitted.[83] The importance of CCR5 as a coreceptor is highlighted in the high degree of resistance to HIV-1 infection by certain individuals who show a 32-base-pair deletion in the CCR5 gene. The prevalence of this mutation is estimated to be about 16% in Caucasians, and 1% are homozygous for this trait.[84] Because most new infection initiates with a macrophage-tropic variant, these observations are consistent with a viral life cycle in which macrophage-tropic viruses are the person-to-person transmissible forms and T cell–tropic viruses are the immunologically destructive forms. This suggests a "queen-drone" relationship between the transmission-competent macrophage-tropic genomes and the host-confined T cell–tropic genomes. Based on the type of HIV-1 target cells, the cytopathic effect produced, and the coreceptor preferred, the majority of HIV-1 strains could be classified as three types of viruses: CCR5 viruses (R5) that use CCR5 as coreceptor, infect macrophages, and do not cause syncytia; CXCR4 viruses (R4) that use CXCR4 as coreceptor, infect T cells, and cause syncytia, and CCR5/CXCR4 viruses (R5X4) that are dual tropic.[85,86] M-tropic viruses predominate at the onset of infection and throughout the asymptomatic and symptomatic phases. However, evidence suggests a switch from CCR5 usage to CXCR4 for certain viruses in some individuals in the late symptomatic phase of HIV-1 infection (AIDS). As a result, there is a pool of R5, X4, and R5X4 viruses.[87,88]

Evolvability of Lentiviruses: Mutation and "Sexual" Recombination

HIV is highly evolvable through its combined properties of a high mutation rate and frequent recombination. Because HIV reverse transcriptase (like all RNA-dependent viral polymerases) lacks a proofreading and error-correcting mechanism, the nucleotide misincorporation rate is high, typically about 1 error per 10,000 nucleotides, or about one misincorporation per new genome. With its high replication rate, HIV rapidly generates a swarm of related sequences, essentially all of which differ from each other by varying degrees, from at least one nucleotide somewhere along the genome to as many as 500 nucleotides (5%). Most of these new mutations do not improve the genome fitness, and many are lethal. However, many mutations are near neutral in survival value and others may confer a slight advantage.

HIV, like all retroviruses, is "diploid," in that each virion contains two complete, replication-competent RNA strands. No other viral families are diploid (some, like the reoviruses, are, of course, double-stranded; with complementary plus- and minus-strands). If a cell becomes coinfected with two different HIV strains, progeny virions may be "heterozygous," with one strand from each parent. Recombination occurs when such a heterozygous virion subsequently infects a new cell. Because the two strands are held in close proximity through a 5′ RNA dimerization sequence, the reverse transcriptase can jump back and forth across strands giving rise to "copy choice" recombination. In some ways, this aspect of the viral life cycle is "sexual" in that parental genomic information is copackaged and recombined, with progeny showing genetic features of both parents. The observation that a high proportion of HIV-1 strains from equatorial Africa are recombinant between clades suggests that recombination occurs readily in vivo in infected humans. It seems likely that when new selective pressures are applied on HIV in vivo (such as antiviral drugs), recombination will be an important mechanism for evolution of maximally fit variants.[89]

OTHER HUMAN RETROVIRUSES (INCLUDING HUMAN T-CELL LYMPHOTROPIC VIRUSES TYPES I AND II)

Transposable Elements and Endogenous Retroviruses

The normal eukaryotic genome is studded with a large number of genetic elements that show similarity to retroviruses.[90] These "normal" mobile genomic regions, called transposons or retrotransposons (depending on whether they encode a reverse transcriptase), can undergo limited replication and reinsertion within the genome but cannot be transmitted from one host cell to another. Other genomic elements show even closer homology to full retroviruses and are thought to represent defective remnants of retroviruses that became stably integrated into the genome in the recent evolutionary past. These endogenous retroviruses can rarely become activated, or they can recombine with other related retroviruses to yield replication-competent chimeric progeny retroviruses. Transposable elements and endogenous retroviruses are thought to be the cause of a number of genetic abnormalities, malignancies, and autoimmune diseases.[91–93]

Primate Retroviruses

Some retrovirus genera have been found in primate species but not in humans.[94] These include the simian sarcoma virus; a mammalian C-type, oncogene-containing, replication-competent virus; and the Mason-Pfizer virus, a D-type replication-competent virus that can cause a fatal immunodeficiency disease in monkeys (simian AIDS, or SAIDS).[95] Human infections with these viruses have not been reported, but it is not known whether exposed humans are susceptible to infection. Other retrovirus genera are known to infect both nonhuman primates and humans, such as the human and simian foamy viruses. The foamy viruses, so named for their cytopathic effect on cells in culture, are also called spumaretroviruses.[96] They can exist as exogenous replication-competent viruses but apparently are benign.

HTLV-I and HTLV-II

The first isolation of HTLV-I was reported in 1980 in a T-cell line from a patient with a T-cell leukemia/lymphoma. The viruses were found to be similar in morphology and genomic organization to the bovine leukemia virus, a retrovirus that causes B-cell lymphomas in cattle.[97] Shortly thereafter, another related virus, HTLV-II, was identified in a T-cell line from a patient with hairy cell leukemia. These and related viruses are now collectively classified as the HTLV-BLV group. HTLV-I and -II have an overall genomic structure typical of retroviruses, with LTRs and *gag*, *pol*, and *env* genes. The HTLV-BLV group viruses are similar to the lentiviruses in that they are complex retroviruses with specific viral-encoded mechanisms for transactivation and RNA transport; the *tax* and *rex* genes of HTLV-I and -II are analogs of the HIV *tat* and *rev* genes. HTLV-I and -II share about 65% similarity in their nucleotide sequences. Within HTLV-I, strains from different parts of the world are genetically much less diverse than are HIV-1 strains, showing only about 7% sequence divergence. Clade or subtype systems have been proposed for HTLV-I and for HTLV-II in a manner similar to HIV. It is often possible to reconstruct the epidemiologic spread of HTLV-I epidemics using genetic sequence data.[98]

HTLV-I is proved to be causally associated with adult T-cell leukemia (ATL) and neurologic diseases of spinal cord known in the Caribbean as tropical spastic paraparesis (TSP) and in Japan as HTLV-associated myelopathy (HAM).[99,100] There have been clinical reports of HTLV-I and -II associated with chronic arthropathy and with uveitis, but a causal relationship remains unproved. HTLV-I can present at a variety of stages: asymptomatic, with no symptoms, signs, or laboratory evidence of disease; "smoldering" or chronic T-cell leukemia, with an elevated percentage of abnormal lymphocytes; and full-blown ATL, with an elevated white blood cell count, anemia, and hypercalcemia. The overall natural history of disease in HTLV-I infection is slow, with an average of 20 to 30 years from the time of infection to the onset of ATL. Although less common, TSP and HAM can develop within a few years after infection. Although HTLV-II has been detected in a number of patients with lymphomas and other malignancies, it is still uncertain whether HTLV-II causes significant disease.

The prevalence of HTLV varies substantially in different parts of the world.[101] Highest prevalence, on the order of 35%, has been reported from Okinawa.[102] HTLV-I is also endemic in East Asia, Papua New Guinea, the Caribbean, and equatorial Africa, where prevalence of 1% to 10% is common. As with other chronic blood-borne infections, HTLV can be transmitted from males to females or to other males by sexual intercourse, from mother to infant at the time of birth, and by blood transfusion or the use of contaminated needles.[103] High prevalence of HTLV-I and -II has been found in populations of IV drug users in the United States and Europe.[104] A variety of promising antiviral agents have activity against HTLV-I and -II in vitro, but none has proved beneficial in ATL, TSP, or HAM. Treatment of ATL is directed at induction of leukemia remission, and for TSP and HAM it is largely supportive.

MAGNITUDE OF THE HIV PANDEMIC

In 2004, 4.9 million people became infected with HIV. Globally, 40 million people are currently living with HIV, and women now represent 50% of all infections and 57% of cases in sub-Saharan Africa due to increasing heterosexual transmission in both the developing and developed world[11,105,106] (Figs. 76-4 and 76-5). The number of deaths due to AIDS continues to grow yearly with an estimated 3.1 million people dying of AIDS in 2004.[11] In many countries, AIDS is erasing decades of progress in improving life expectancy. In sub-Saharan Africa, life expectancy is now 47 years instead of the 62 years expected without AIDS (Fig. 76-6). In this setting, the death toll continues to rise with an estimated 68 million people dying earlier than they would have in the absence of AIDS in the 45 most affected countries. AIDS has a particularly strong impact on under–5 year mortality with most children who are infected at birth or through breastfeeding dying of AIDS before age 5. The majority of newly infected adults are under 25 years of age, and 90% of all new infections are occurring in developing countries. With an associated mortality rate greater than 90% and with the current lack of vaccine or curative drug, it is clear from these estimates that the HIV pandemic will continue to escalate worldwide and have an enormous impact on public health over the next several decades.[10]

Currently, the largest number of HIV-infected persons is in sub-Saharan Africa, totaling 25.4 million, and in Asia and the Pacific, totaling 8.2 million[11,12] (see Fig. 76-4). The epidemic in South Asia continues to be dominated by India, where an estimated 5.1 million infections were noted as of October 2003.[107] Although there is uncertainty about the future spread of HIV and its ultimate global dimensions, some short-term projections indicate that the incidence of HIV will increase by

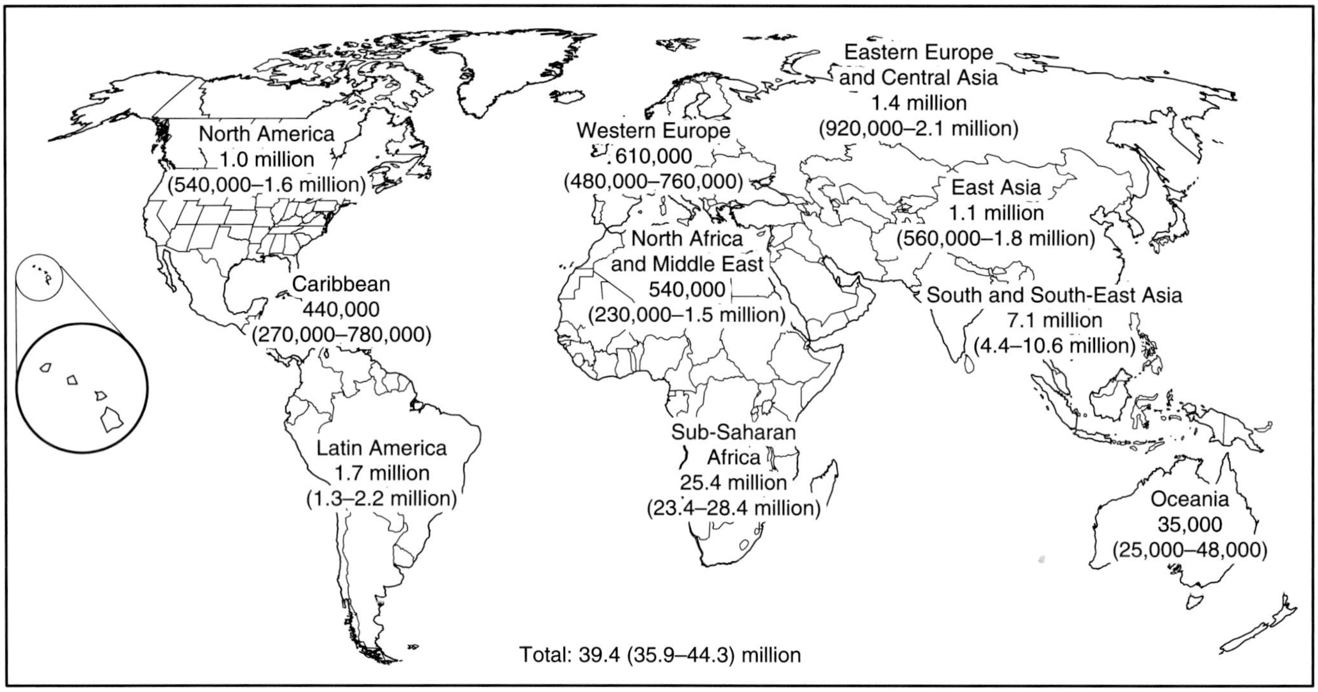

FIGURE 76-4 Estimated number of adults and children living with HIV as of the end of 2004. (Data from UNAIDS Program.)

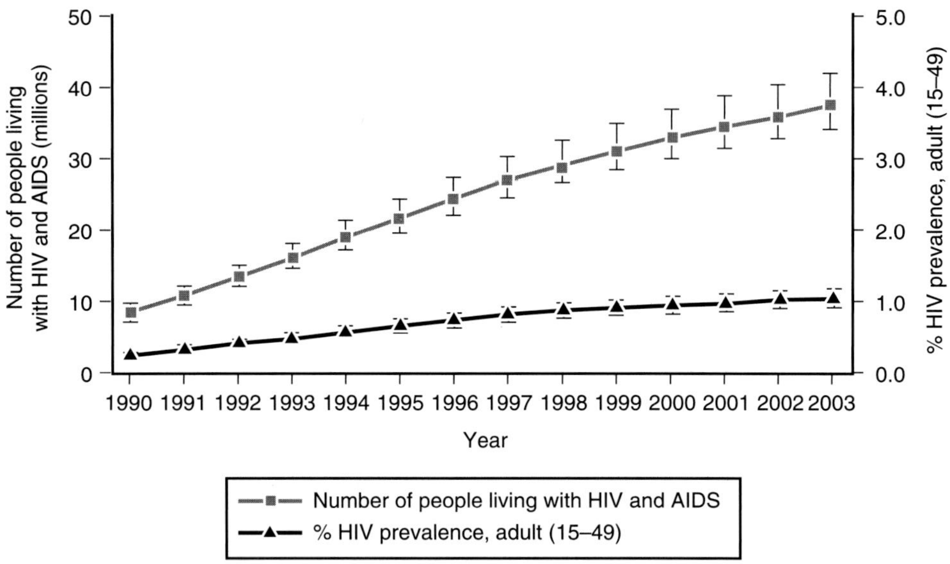

FIGURE 76-5 Growth of the global AIDS epidemic between 1990 and 2003 by prevalence and by number of people living with HIV/AIDS. (Data from UNAIDS Program.)

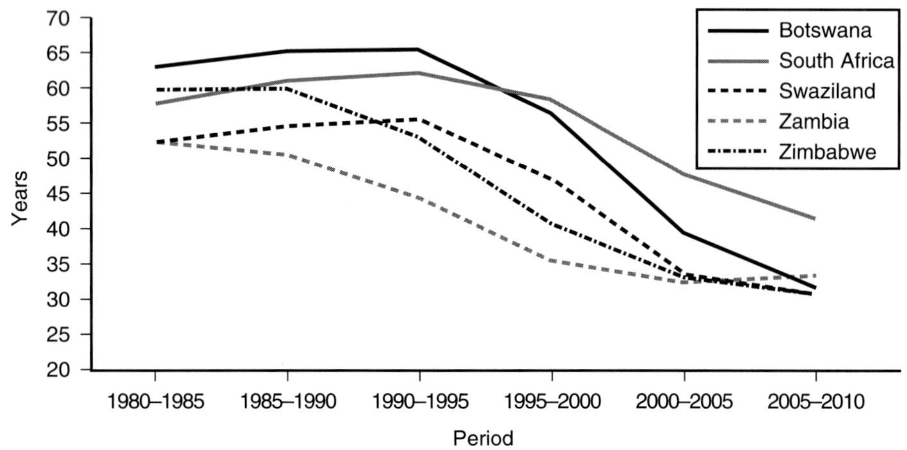

FIGURE 76-6 Impact of HIV on life expectancy in selected countries between 1980–1985 and 2005–2010. (Data from UNAIDS Program.)

4.1% in pregnant women attending urban antenatal clinics.[164] However, in view of the political events of 1996 and 1999 and the fact that DRC, with a population of 50 million, is one of the largest African countries, the HIV epidemic in that country may change rapidly with unpredictable and disastrous consequences.[163]

AIDS has emerged as the leading cause of death worldwide, surpassing tuberculosis for the first time in 1999. In 1998, 19% of all deaths in Africa were due to AIDS.[177–180] Excess deaths attributable to HIV infection are highest in 25- to 35-year-olds, an age group that usually has a low mortality. Nearly 90% of deaths in this age group were in excess of background rates and were attributable to HIV infection. The fact that many AIDS deaths occur in children and young adults has resulted in a substantial reduction in life expectancy, by more than 20 years in several countries (see Fig. 76-6). It is projected that population growth will decline more rapidly than expected and the size of the African population in the year 2025 will certainly be smaller than it would have been without AIDS.[164,169] However, because many adults bear children (often without AIDS, thus destined to be orphaned) before dying of AIDS, the population growth continues at an alarming 2% to 3% per year (i.e., doubling every 29 years or so). The increasing number of HIV infections and AIDS cases have already overwhelmed the capacity of urban health systems in some countries. In this regard, it is estimated that 80% of hospital beds in an infectious disease hospital in Abidjan, Côte d'Ivoire, and 50% in a hospital in Kampala, Uganda, are occupied by people with HIV infection. Demands for care will increasingly fall on poorly equipped and under-funded rural services, households, and individuals.

Demographic surveys in several countries have already noted significant increases in infant and child mortality.[181–183] Projections for Zambia and Zimbabwe indicate that AIDS may increase child mortality rates nearly threefold by the year 2010.[169] Owing to high levels of fertility, populations will generally continue to grow, but the critical deficits will be seen in the economically active ages. In countries where 8% of the adult population is HIV-infected, surveys have measured a doubling of mortality due to HIV and a decrease of at least 5 years in life expectancy. In 1995, UNAIDS examined the demographic impact of HIV infection and AIDS in 15 sub-Saharan African countries with a prevalence of HIV infection of more than 1% of the adult population.[108] Below that level of prevalence, the epidemic's impact on the national demographic picture is insignificant. In the 15 countries analyzed, the combined population was estimated to be 2 million people smaller than expected. In the year 2005 it will be 11.6 million smaller (291.8 million vs. 303.4 million). As a result of the high fatality rate due to HIV infection and AIDS, life expectancy at birth decreased in these 15 countries from 52.8 to 49.6 years. In the 45 most affected countries, it is projected that by 2020, 68 million people will die earlier than they would have in the absence of AIDS.[164] Average life expectancy in sub-Saharan Africa has fallen to 47 years compared to an expected 62 years in the absence of AIDS. These HIV epidemics will have severe effects on the population age structure, indenting the population pyramid in the main contributors to social and economic development, namely, young adults. Since AIDS kills people in their most productive years, it ranks as the leading cause of potential healthy life-years lost in sub-Saharan Africa.[177] In Abidjan, Côte d'Ivoire, it was estimated that 15% of adult male deaths and 17% of male years of potential life lost (YPLL) resulted from AIDS, whereas in women AIDS accounted for 13% of deaths and 12% of female YPLL.[178] In two community-based rural studies in the Masaka and Rakai districts of Uganda, mortality among HIV-infected adults was over 100 per 1000 person-years of observation (PYO), an order of magnitude higher than among adults not infected with HIV.[179,180] In both districts, the adult prevalence of HIV infection was 8% and 13%, respectively, and HIV infection was found to be the leading cause of death. In this regard, more than 80% of deaths in the 20- to 29-year-old age group occurred among those who were HIV-infected. As a result, AIDS will double or triple the adult mortality rate in sub-Saharan African countries from levels that were already eight times higher than in developed countries. In countries such as Uganda, with an estimated 1.3 million infected persons out of a total population of 17 million, AIDS looms as the predominant health problem of the entire population.

With regard to children, it is estimated that the HIV pandemic resulted in 500,000 childhood deaths in 2003.[163] Additionally, as of the year 2001, more than 14 million children under age 15 years have been orphaned as a result of the premature death of HIV-infected parents.[163] In a recent survey of child mortality in 10 central and eastern African countries, the death toll from AIDS in children under 5 years of age was found to be likely to rise from 159 to 189 per 1000 by the year 2000. Even for those children who escaped perinatal infection, survival rates will decrease because of the loss of one or both parents to AIDS. For each woman dying of AIDS in Africa, an average of two children are orphaned. Overall, infant and child mortality rates have increased by as much as 30% more than previously projected as a direct consequence of perinatal HIV infection. Consequently, pediatric AIDS is now threatening much of the progress that has been made in child survival in developing countries during the past 20 years.[181]

Care of and support for children orphaned by AIDS will be a growing concern throughout the region, and the social, economic, and demographic impact of AIDS will be enormous. For a country with a current prevalence of HIV infection of 8%, the expected increased demand for health care services ranges from 2.3% to 9.3%, depending on the state of development of its health care sector.[182,183] The strong association of HIV with a burgeoning tuberculosis epidemic combined with the excess mortality associated with HIV infection underscores the critical importance of the HIV epidemic in Africa.[184]

North Africa and the Middle East

This region represents 20 countries, with an estimated 480,000 individuals living with HIV.[11] Information on HIV infection in this region is limited, particularly among high-risk groups such as IV drug users. The highest prevalence of HIV infection in this region has been observed in Sudan, with 2.6% HIV prevalence representing almost 90% of the infections in this region.[164] The majority of infections in this regions appear to be focused on injection drug users, although there is concern that HIV may be spreading undetected among men who have sex with men, as homosexuality is highly condemned and illegal in many places. The future size and trends of the epidemic in this region are difficult to predict because of several factors: recent introduction of the virus, the status and disempowerment of women in society with associated decreased access to health care, the highly stigmatizing nature of STDs and the difficulties in their diagnosis and treatment, and the difficulty of conducting effective sexual health programs, often because of religious beliefs.

Asia

Asia, where HIV has more recently been introduced, is in the early phases of an explosive HIV infection and AIDS epidemic. Since more than 60% of the world's population lives in Asia, the HIV epidemic could affect more people in this region than in any other area of the world.[21,22] For example, despite the fact that HIV was introduced into this region in the late 1980s, there are already 7.6 million adults living with HIV infection or AIDS.[164] The overall adult prevalence of HIV infection, however, is less than 1.0% because of the large population of these countries.[164] Thus, on a per population basis, although more people may actually be infected with HIV in Asia, AIDS may still have a greater impact in sub-Saharan Africa. The epidemic, however, is spreading rapidly in Asia with sharp increases in new infections in China, Indonesia, and Vietnam and an estimated 1.1 million new infections occurring in the region in 2003.[11] Countries such as the Philippines, Singapore, North Korea, and South Korea have had only limited spread to date and the rate of growth appears to be substantially lower.[10]

The pattern of HIV spread in Asia appears to be mainly concentrated among injection drug users (IDUs), men who have sex with men, sex workers, clients of sex workers, and their immediate partners. HIV infection was initially noted among IDUs in Thailand and in Manipur, northeastern India; seroprevalence rose from 55% to 80% in IDUs.[185–189] Recent data in the Yunnan province of China bordering Burma and Laos and considered part of the "golden triangle" of heroin exportation also demonstrate an alarming prevalence of HIV infection of 43% to 82% in IDUs.[190] Data from Malaysia and Vietnam show similar increases in IDUs. Concomitant with this rise of HIV infection among IDUs, HIV infection was noted among female sex workers; although highly variable by region, prevalence rates of 30% to 65% have been reported among female sex workers in various cities of Thailand and India.[189,191] Successive waves of heterosexual transmission from these sex workers to their male clients, and subsequently to other sex partners, including spouses, have resulted in the rapid spread of HIV to the general population.[185,186] Across Asia, effective prevention efforts have been hampered partly because of stigma and discrimination of the affected groups. HIV seroprevalence in India is high in the south and west. For example, in Bombay, prevalence increased from 2% in STD clinic attendees before 1990 to 36% in 1994.[189] The prevalence in sex workers rose from 1% to 51% between 1987 and 1993, and 2% of women attending antenatal clinics were positive in 1994.[163] In Pune, the overall HIV seroprevalence in 2800 STD clinic attendees was 23.4%.[192] Among initially seronegative persons, the subsequent incidence of HIV infection was 26.1 per 100 PYO for female sex workers, 9.4% for men, and 8.4% for women who were predominantly spouses of the men attending these clinics.[193] Recently, unsafe sex between male-male sex partners has emerged as an additional important risk factor in the Indian epidemic.[194] As in Africa, recurrent genital ulcer disease, urethritis, or cervicitis was independently associated with an increased risk of seroconversion.

There is great geographic variation of HIV infection in India. Studies among sex workers in Calcutta have consistently demonstrated a low prevalence of 1.2%; in Vellore, women attending antenatal clinics have a prevalence of 0.1%. Many factors, including the prevailing sexual practices, a large population of HIV-infected female sex workers, the low social status of women, male patronage of sex workers, high rates of STDs, low rates of condom use, and the high number of IDUs in the north, make it likely that HIV will continue to spread in India and Thailand, as well as in many other populous countries.[10] India has the highest burden of infection in Asia, with an estimated 5.1 million adults and children infected with HIV, making it second only to South Africa in terms of absolute burden of infections.[107] As in Africa, the HIV epidemic is strongly associated with increasing spread of tuberculosis.[195–198] In India an estimated 1 to 2 million cases of tuberculosis occur every year. In Bombay 10% of the patients presenting with tuberculosis are now HIV-positive. Tuberculosis is also the presenting symptom of AIDS in more than 60% of AIDS cases. In Thailand public health authorities have noticed a marked increase in tuberculosis cases compared with a steady decline in previous years.[199]

HIV was introduced in Cambodia in the early 1990s and is predominantly occurring among heterosexuals with multiple sexual partners. To date there has been little evidence of a significant problem of injecting drugs in Cambodia. Levels among blood donors in Phnom Penh have risen, though, from less than 0.1% in 1991 to 10% in 1995. Dramatic rises have also been seen in sex workers, the military, STD patients, and pregnant women. Thailand and Cambodia have shown that early large-scale prevention efforts can change the natural course of the epidemic. Among pregnant women in major urban areas in Cambodia, the HIV prevalence declined from 3.2% in 1996 to 2.7% at the end of 2000.[164] The Cambodian government has implemented a multifaceted prevention program including a 100%-condom-use program and steps to counter stigma.

The epidemic in Myanmar is one of the more serious in the region. Although controversial and disputed by the government, estimates of prevalence rates as high as 3.46% (687,000 infected) have been reported.[200] This epidemic began primarily among IDUs in the late 1980s with a prevalence of HIV infection of 60% to 70% in 1992. HIV prevalence in sex workers, as in India and Thailand, has also steadily risen, from 4.3% in 1992 to 18% in 1995. In Malaysia, HIV infection levels in IDUs have also grown rapidly, from 0.1% in 1988 to 20% in 1994. Similarly, in female sex workers the rates have increased from 0.3% in 1989 to 10% in 1994. In Vietnam, HIV rates increased from 9% to 38% between 1992 and 1995. High levels have also been demonstrated in IDUs in treatment (32% in 1992–1995).

The epidemic in China has raised alarm, since it appears to be spreading into new groups of the population. Despite sketchy surveillance data, it is estimated that 850,000 Chinese were living with HIV/AIDS in 2001.[164] Several localized HIV epidemics are being observed among certain population groups across China, highlighting the need for swift action if a more serious epidemic is to be prevented. The majority of early reported HIV infections have been among IDUs in Yunnan province (about 70%).[191] However, China is currently in what has been termed the expansive phase of its epidemic with infections spreading to partners of IDUs and blood donors and a steady rise in rates observed among sex workers.[201] Men who have sex with men, ignored in the official statistics, have also emerged as a high-risk group for HIV transmission. The number of infections in China more than doubled between 1999 and 2002.

DISEASE

Pathogenesis and Natural History

After many years of debate on the hypothesis that AIDS is fundamentally an autoimmune disease, it is now clear that autoimmunity is not an essential component of the pathogenesis (Fig. 76-9). Instead, disease progression is a direct reflection of virus replication.[202,203] In the absence of active viral replication, or when viral replication is low (blood viremia levels less than 100 genome copies per milliliter), HIV infection does not progress to clinical immunodeficiency. Conversely, when viral replication is rapid (viremia greater than 100,000 genome copies per milliliter), disease progression is correspondingly rapid. Treatments with antiviral drugs slow disease progression in proportion to their effect in lowering viremia levels. The course of HIV infection can be quite variable. The initial infection is followed by an eclipse phase in which neither viremia nor an antibody response can be found. A virologic "primary infection" with high levels of viremia then appears and persists for several weeks.[204] Up to 30% of HIV-infected persons are reported to experience a mononucleosis-like syndrome of fever, pharyngitis, rash, and depressed CD4+ cell counts during this primary infection. However, in many careful studies the proportion showing symptoms during primary infection is much lower than this.[205,206] There are no published studies on symptomatic primary infections with HIV strains in tropical countries or with genotypes other than clade B.

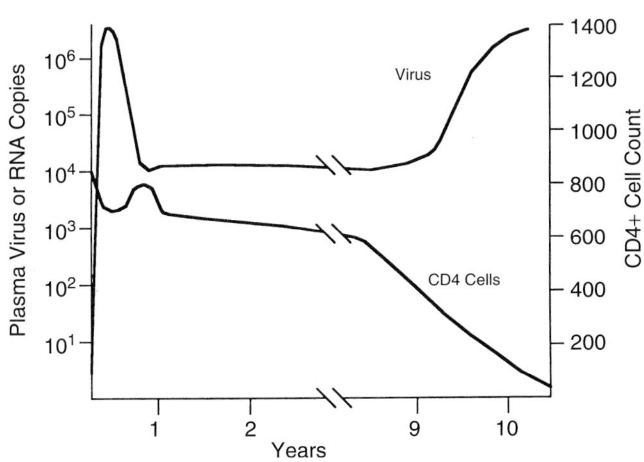

FIGURE 76-9 Diagram of the natural history of HIV infection in a "typical" case showing changes in the CD4+ cell count and the plasma RNA copy number over a span of 10 years.

Among HIV-infected patients studied in the United States and Europe, most progress from infection to AIDS in 5 to 15 years. A fraction of patients, about 5% to 10%, progress more rapidly (rapid progressors), and another fraction, perhaps 5%, show no evidence of progression over many years (nonprogressors).[207–209] In HIV-1–HIV-2 studies, HIV-2 infection invariably produces a lower viremia than does HIV-1 and HIV-2 also shows a much higher proportion of nonprogressors. Few rigorous natural history studies have been done in tropical countries or in regions where HIV-1 genotypes other than clade B predominate. One study of HIV-1 infections among commercial sex workers in Kenya showed rapid progression to AIDS (within 5 years) in 50%.[210] It is uncertain whether the high proportion of rapid progressors in this study in Africa can be attributed to the prevalent viral genotypes (probably clade A and clade D), to the high prevalence of aggressive opportunistic infection (e.g., tuberculosis), to the lack of optimal medical care, or to poor nutrition or other host factors.

There is no evidence that the virus in rapid progressors is more virulent than average. Instead, natural history studies suggest that rapid progressors mount an inadequate immune response. Most patients show low or absent antibodies or cellular responses. Rarely, rapid progressors have been described who appear to be completely but selectively unresponsive to HIV antigens. Because these patients lack HIV antibodies, they can pose a diagnostic challenge.

Nonprogressors typically have low plasma viral titers. In some nonprogressors, low viral titers are due to infection with grossly replication-defective virus, but in most patients it is uncertain whether low viral titers reflect viral factors (poor replication), host genetic factors, or an unusually strong immune response.[211] Nonprogressors do routinely show strong immune responses to HIV proteins, including antibody and cellular responses, but it is unclear if this is cause or effect.

Mechanism of Immune Dysfunction

Depletion of CD4+ T lymphocytes is the central mechanism of immune dysfunction by HIV. Progressive depletion is a consequence of a furious rate of viral replication in these cells. The turnover rate of CD4+ T lymphocytes—their destruction and replenishment—is correspondingly turbulent. Each day in an infected patient, up to 10^9 new virions are made and about 10^9 CD4+ T lymphocytes are killed and replaced.[212,213] Loss of CD4+ T cells results in a loss of recognition of antigens that are presented on class II MHC molecules. Th1 function is especially damaged with loss of cell-mediated immune functions. Th2 functions are impaired as well with gradual loss of humoral responsiveness to newly presented foreign antigens. Loss of in vivo delayed-type hypersensitivity skin test reactivity to recall antigens such as *Candida,* mumps, and tetanus parallels the loss of cell-mediated immunity and the appearance of opportunistic infections.

Three major mechanisms of CD4+ T-lymphocyte killing by HIV have been suggested: direct virus-mediated cytolysis, virus-induced apoptosis, and indirect killing through immune effector mechanisms. Direct virus-mediated cytolysis has been demonstrated in vitro. Syncytium formation may accelerate the cytolytic process. Syncytium-inducing isolates appear in blood in the late stages of illness and are a poor prognostic sign when present in earlier stages. However, the presence of syncytium-inducing virus isolates strongly co-varies with blood viral titer, so cause-and-effect relationships remain uncertain. Apoptosis may also contribute to cell destruction in vivo.[214,215] CD4+ T lymphocytes from infected patients undergo apoptotic death when stimulated in vitro. However, uninfected CD8+ as well as CD4+ cells from HIV-infected patients show increased apoptotic death. Apoptosis probably reflects the high rate of ongoing immune activation in HIV-infected persons and probably is not a principal cause of immune depletion. Immune destruction of infected cells also is not likely to be a central mechanism of CD4+ T-lymphocyte depletion: persons with weak immune responses show more rapid depletion and more rapid clinical disease progression. Other pathogenic mechanisms have been proposed, including induction of anergy by circulating soluble gp120 or by superantigen stimulation of lymphocytes, and autoimmunity induced by HIV antigens cross-reactive with normal cell proteins.[216] These in vitro mechanisms have not been established to be important in vivo.

Anti-HIV Immunity

Unlike in other infectious diseases, there is as yet no direct evidence that humans can become "immune"—in the classic sense—to HIV. Infection becomes chronic in everyone infected; no adults have spontaneously cleared their infection. Also, there is as yet no direct evidence that any candidate HIV vaccine can render a person protected against subsequent challenge. Most HIV-infected adults do mount a vigorous antibody and cellular immune response to HIV. It is thought that this immune response, while insufficient to clear infection, is nonetheless sufficient to impede viral replication.

Serum antibodies to env, gag, pol, and nef appear in the blood of most HIV-infected patients within a few weeks to months after exposure to infection. Antibodies to tat, rev, and the other accessory proteins are also detectable in a variable proportion of patients. Antibody titers to all viral proteins fall as disease develops, and low anti-HIV antibody titer is a poor prognostic sign. In vitro, antibodies can block HIV replication through ADCC (antibody-dependent cellular cytotoxicity), killing of infected cells, or virus neutralization.[217] HIV neutralizing antibody activity can be measured by mixing dilutions of serum with a small dose of virus, then monitoring viral replication when the mixtures are inoculated into cultures of CD4+ T lymphocytes. HIV anti-envelope antibodies effectively neutralize viral growth. Neutralization serotypes of HIV-1 strains have been described, and these correspond to the genotypic clusters. Paradoxically, anti-HIV serum antibodies can increase the replication of HIV-1 in cultures of macrophages and other Fc receptor–bearing cells by facilitating the initial viral binding to the cell surface. It is uncertain whether this "antibody-dependent enhancement" of HIV-1 growth has in vivo significance.[218,219]

HIV-reactive lymphocytes are present in the blood of essentially all infected patients. Cultured patient CD4+ T lymphocytes proliferate when exposed in vitro to HIV envelope or gag proteins. The vigor of proliferation is maximal in the early, asymptomatic stages of infection and decreases as disease progresses. CD8+ anti-HIV class I MHC–restricted cytotoxic T lymphocytes (CTLs) with activity against HIV core, envelope, polymerase, and nef proteins are also present in blood. Class II–restricted CTLs are also found. Appearance of CD8+ blood CTL activity correlates temporally with the initial fall of viremia, so it is thought that CTLs are important in control of replication through killing of infected cells.[220–222] CD8+ cells also release soluble factors that inhibit HIV replication through noncytolytic mechanisms.

Once established, HIV infection never spontaneously disappears completely in adults. However, spontaneous "cures" have been reported in a few infected infants.[223] It is hypothesized that passively acquired maternal immunity was important in partially suppressing the infection in these infants. Self-curing abortive and suppressed infections have also been observed in SIV-vaccinated and -challenged monkeys.[224]

Clinical Manifestations

A substantial proportion of patients with acute primary HIV infection (up to one half) may experience a mononucleosis-like illness characterized by fever, pharyngitis, and a slight morbilliform rash. Rarely, patients experience neurologic manifestations. In 80% to 90% of patients, the illness is so mild that medical care is not sought. Primary HIV infection is rarely seen in medical care facilities in tropical countries.

The early stage of chronic HIV infection is usually asymptomatic, with the CD4+ cell count remaining above 500 cells/mL. About half of patients have modest generalized lymphadenopathy. Autopsies on early-stage HIV-infected patients who die of non–HIV-related causes (e.g., automobile accidents) show HIV-1–infected cells in lymphatic tissues throughout the body.[225] At this stage a number of dermatologic conditions of uncertain cause may be present, especially seborrheic dermatitis, psoriasis, and folliculitis.[226]

Intermediate HIV disease, defined by CD4+ counts between 200 and 500 cells/mL, is also usually asymptomatic or at least without serious manifestations. Skin and mucosal opportunistic infections are common, including herpes zoster (shingles), herpes simplex, oral or vaginal candidiasis, oral hairy leukoplakia, and cervical dysplasia.[227,228] Bacterial infections caused by common respiratory tract organisms such as *Streptococcus pneumoniae* are increased, as is pelvic inflammatory disease. Patients may begin to experience fever, diarrhea, and weight loss. The occurrence of these intermediate manifestations, but without an AIDS-defining opportunistic infection or cancer, has historically been referred to as "AIDS-related complex," or ARC.

Late-stage HIV disease, AIDS, is defined by a CD4 cell count below 200 cells/mL. The list of AIDS-defining conditions issued jointly in 1993 by the Centers for Disease Control and Prevention (CDC) and WHO is shown in Box 76-1.[229] This revision included three new AIDS-defining conditions that are more common in heterosexual patients, including recurrent bacterial pneumonia, cervical carcinoma, and pulmonary tuberculosis. This listing, while an improvement, still omits several HIV-related infections that are more prevalent in tropical countries. These include parasites (*Cryptosporidium*, microsporidia, *Cyclospora*, *Leishmania donovani*, and *Trypanosoma cruzi*); fungi (*Penicillium marneffei*); and bacteria (*Bartonella*, *Rhodococcus*). The issue is not merely academic, for in many countries the availability of social benefits and access to medical care depend on a diagnosis of an AIDS-defining illness.[230]

Box 76-1 1993 U. S. Centers for Disease Control–World Health Organization Classification of AIDS-Defining Conditions

- CD4 cell count <200/μL
- Candidiasis, pulmonary or esophageal
- Cervical cancer
- Coccidioidomycosis
- Cryptosporidiosis
- Cytomegalovirus infection
- Herpes esophagitis
- HIV encephalopathy
- Histoplasmosis
- Isosporiasis
- Kaposi's sarcoma
- Lymphoma
- Mycobacterial disease
- *Pneumocystis carinii* infection
- Pneumonia, bacterial
- Progressive multifocal leukoencephalopathy (polyomavirus)
- Salmonellosis

Many common tropical infections, including malaria, schistosomiasis, filariasis, onchocerciasis, cholera, yellow fever, and dengue have not been identified as HIV-related opportunistic infections. Two very prevalent diseases, malaria and African trypanosomiasis, have been studied and shown to have no relationship.[231,232] Nonetheless, the range of HIV-related opportunistic infections does vary in different regions of the world. Certain AIDS-defining infections common in the United States are diagnosed much less frequently in Africa and Asia, particularly *Pneumocystis carinii* pneumonia (PCP), *Mycobacterium avium-intracellulare* (MAI), and cytomegalovirus (CMV) disease. Other infections are more common in tropical countries, depending on the locally prevalent microbes.

In sub-Saharan Africa, diarrhea from cryptosporidiosis, isosporiasis, or microsporidiosis is common. In Latin America, cerebral toxoplasmosis, cryptosporidiosis and isosporiasis, Chagas' disease, and cutaneous and visceral leishmaniasis are common. Cases of HIV-associated disseminated strongyloidiasis and paracoccidiomycosis have also been reported. In Southeast Asia, disseminated infections with the dimorphic fungus *P. marneffei* are common.[233]

Mycobacterium tuberculosis (MTB) is the most common serious opportunistic infection worldwide. Clinically apparent tuberculosis can occur at any stage of HIV infection, but the risk increases with immunoincompetence. Five percent to 10% of persons co-infected with HIV and MTB develop active tuberculosis each year. The prevalence of tuberculosis in persons with AIDS in Latin America has been reported to be 17% to 30%; in Africa, 25% to 44%; and in Asia, 23% to 68%. Almost half of patients with the end-stage HIV wasting syndrome (slim disease) in Africa are shown at autopsy to have disseminated MTB.[234]

DIAGNOSIS AND PROGNOSIS

Disease from HIV becomes clinically apparent only after years of asymptomatic infection and clinical signs, when they do occur, are usually unspecific. Consequently, laboratory assays are essential to diagnosing HIV infection.

HIV Antibody Assays

HIV antibody assays on blood serum or plasma are used to establish a diagnosis. The most common test is the ELISA. A variety of configurations have been developed and marketed, but plastic microtiter plates or beads are most often used as the solid-phase surface for adsorption of viral antigens. Patient antibodies that bind to viral antigens are detected with antihuman immunoglobulins tagged with enzymes. Readouts are obtained by color changes in a substrate fluid catalyzed by the enzyme.

Antibodies to HIV-2 and HIV-O are only partially cross-reactive with HIV-1 in most commercial ELISAs.[235,236] Although HIV-2 and HIV-O infections are rare outside certain well-described regions of the world, concerns about undetected HIV-2 among blood donors in the United States and Europe were sufficient to lead most manufacturers to develop and market HIV-1–HIV-2 combination ELISAs. Many current ELISAs also contain HIV-1-O antigens.

Specificities and sensitivities for most commercial ELISAs are said to exceed 99%. However, the positive predictive value of a repeatedly reactive ELISA on a single serum specimen will vary markedly depending on the true prevalence of HIV infection in the tested population. When used in a hospital laboratory in an HIV-endemic region, over 99% of repeatedly reactive specimens might be true positives. However, if exactly the same test kit was used for blood bank screening in a low-prevalence region, only 10% of repeatedly reactive specimens might be true positives.

The most effective strategy to deal with the problem of imperfect specificity of ELISAs is to confirm all positive ELISA results by testing repeatedly reactive specimens with a second assay of completely different design. Immunofluorescent assays and radioimmunoprecipitation assays have been used for this purpose, but the Western blot is most commonly used.[237] Western blot strips are prepared by electrophoresis of lysed HIV-1 viral particles through a polyacrylamide gel and blotting of the resultant viral protein bands of different molecular weights onto nitrocellulose paper. Anti-HIV antibodies in a specimen are detected with enzyme-tagged antihuman immunoglobulins. Western blots are read according to which viral bands show bound patient antibodies. Serum from HIV-infected patients usually has antibodies to all viral proteins, and interpretation of the blot is not difficult. However, incomplete banding patterns do occur and can lead to diagnostic difficulty.[238,239] Since 1989 blot interpretation criteria adopted by the CDC are most widely employed.[240] These criteria define a blot as reactive if antibodies are present to at least two of three of the following HIV structural proteins: the capsid p24 protein, the transmembrane envelope gp41 protein, and the surface envelope gp120 or gp160 protein.

Several rapid and simple HIV antibody assays have been developed that are intended for use outside laboratory settings. There are a variety of configurations, including agglutination of latex beads or red blood cells, or dot-blots on dipsticks. Antibodies are also present in body fluids other than blood serum, but at lower titers, and test kits have been developed and marketed that use urine or saliva. The sensitivity and specificity of these alternative assays can be quite good but are generally below those of serum ELISA testing.

HIV antibody testing is most effective when an algorithm for assay use is thoughtfully designed and scrupulously followed. A variety of algorithms have been proposed, each appropriate for a particular health care setting. Optimal algorithm design will vary according to many local factors: the true prevalence of HIV infection in the population to be tested, the expected ratio of HIV-1 to HIV-2 infections, the availability of laboratory facilities, speed requirements, and cost constraints. Most algorithms include the following steps: (1) a screening assay, (2) repeat testing of specimens with positive screening assay results on the same specimen, and (3) supplemental testing with a second assay of different design. In very low prevalence populations, it is advisable to verify results by obtaining and testing a new serum specimen before a diagnosis is considered established. To avoid confusion, it has been customary to describe individual assay results as "nonreactive" or "reactive" and to reserve the terms "negative" and "positive" for the algorithm bottom-line conclusion.

Diagnosis of HIV infection in infants presents special problems owing to the presence of passively acquired maternal antibodies. One approach is to wait until maternal antibodies have waned (1 year) and then test for antibodies. Another is to test directly for HIV virus, antigens, or genome with viral cultures, p24 antigen assays, or DNA polymerase chain reaction (PCR).

HIV Culture and p24 Antigen Detection

HIV can be isolated from blood plasma, peripheral blood mononuclear leukocytes (PBMLs), and lymphoid tissues in virtually all patients. The isolation rate is directly related to viral titer. The technique is expensive, labor-intensive, and relatively slow. Isolation is essential to certain types of laboratory research, such as measurement of antiviral drug sensitivity patterns. In the conventional isolation technique, normal healthy human donor PBMLs are stimulated with phytohemagglutinin and used as the culture substrate.[241] Patient specimens are co-cultivated with normal stimulated cells, and culture supernatants are monitored for up to 1 month for viral antigens (p24) or reverse transcriptase activity.[242]

HIV antigens also circulate in the blood of infected patients.[243,244] Commercial kits are available for measurement of HIV p24 capsid protein levels, which range from 50 pg/mL to 100 ng/mL. Much of the circulating HIV p24 antigen may be complexed with anti-p24 antibodies, so an immunocomplex acid dissociation step is necessary to improve sensitivity.[245,246] Serum p24 assays have been suggested as screening tests to detect HIV-infected, but antibody-negative, donated blood units. Because the antibody-negative "window" period following seroconversion is so short relative to the total duration of HIV infection, in most settings p24 antigen testing of specimens from adults adds little to antibody testing for purposes of detecting HIV infection. However, measurement of HIV p24 levels can give prognostic information. Serum p24 antigen levels are correlated with plasma viral titers and with serum genomic RNA levels. High serum p24 antigen levels portend a poor prognosis, and p24 antigen levels fall with effective antiretroviral therapy. HIV p24 antigen testing is rapidly being supplanted by detection and quantitation of HIV nucleic acids.

Measurement of HIV Nucleic Acids

The PCR, in which strands of nucleic acid are amplified exponentially one strand to two, then four, then eight, and so on has revolutionized the diagnostic approach to the HIV infected patient. PCR can be used to amplify HIV sequences from cellular proviral DNA, from cellular RNA, or from HIV virions.

DNA PCR is useful in establishing a diagnosis of HIV infection in situations in which antibody testing gives ambiguous results.[247] Testing of infants of infected mothers (all of whom passively acquire maternal antibodies) is the most important use. DNA PCR can also be used to confirm HIV infection in persons with indeterminate Western blot results.

HIV RNA measurement with PCR requires an initial conversion of the viral RNA sequences to complementary DNA (cDNA). This is done by addition of exogenous reverse transcriptase (RT), followed by PCR amplification and then quantification of the specific DNA product.[248,249] Because errors can be magnified exponentially, RT-PCR must be carefully standardized and controlled. Measured quantities of control nucleotide sequences can be added directly into each test specimen tube, as in quantitative competitive RT-PCR, or controls can be run in parallel in separate tubes in each run. Both approaches have been optimized. Commercial RT-PCR test kits are designed to quantitate genomic HIV RNA in plasma, but the technique can be modified in research laboratories to measure various splice-classes of HIV RNA in cells or to measure HIV RNA in other fluids such as semen or cervical secretions.

The branch-chain DNA (bDNA) technique is an alternative non-PCR method of RNA detection.[250] In the bDNA assay, viral RNA is pulled out of a sample by HIV-specific DNA capture sequences onto a solid phase. Captured HIV RNA is detected by binding of DNA probe sequences, which in effect have long, branched DNA tails that are enzyme-tagged. Results are read by enzyme-catalyzed substrate changes.

Both RT-PCR and bDNA assays are expensive, about U.S. $100 per assay. The bDNA assay is somewhat simpler to perform, but the RT-PCR method is more sensitive. In vivo HIV genomic RNA levels range from 10 to over 1 million copies per milliliter of plasma. The RT-PCR can approach this lower limit, but the bDNA assay can detect only down to 10,000 copies per milliliter. The RT-PCR technique is also preferred for many research purposes because a large quantity of amplified cDNA is produced.

The plasma HIV RNA level is a direct measure of in vivo HIV replication and is therefore a powerful prognostic tool. For any given untreated patient, the plasma viremia level remains relatively constant, or increases slightly, over several years. It appears that the "virologic script" for the disease course is "writ" very early after primary infection.[251,252] Patients with low viremia levels (100 to 1000 genome copies per milliliter) after seroconversion do well and are often nonprogressors, whereas patients with high viremia levels (100,000 or greater) do poorly and are often rapid progressors. Levels are typically quite low in HIV-2-infected patients compared with HIV-1-infected patients. There are as yet no reports of plasma RNA levels in developing countries where HIV-1 genotypes other than clade B predominate.

Nucleic acid amplification and detection techniques all require that the "quarry genome" sequence be known. Reagent nucleotide sequences (primer sequences and probe sequences in RT-PCR, or capture sequences and probe sequences in the bDNA assay) must be highly homologous to the quarry genome sequence for the techniques to work at all. This is not a serious problem in the United States, where essentially all HIV strains are of the B clade. However, it has proved difficult to construct a single assay that can be used worldwide, including in other countries where other genotypes predominate.

Immunologic Assessment of HIV-Infected Patients

The CD4+ T-lymphocyte count is the most widely used measure of HIV-induced damage to the immune system. In the United States, absolute counts of less than 200 cells/mL or a CD4+ percentage of less than 14% is strongly associated with an increased risk of opportunistic infections and is now accepted as definitional for AIDS.[253,254]

The CD4+ count can be performed manually and read visually, but usually it is done with an automated fluorescence-activated flow cytometer. CD4+ cell counts are vulnerable to biologic and technical errors. The main biologic error in CD4+ cell counts is attributable to a pronounced diurnal variation that can be up to 150 cells/mL in healthy adults but is usually less in patients with lower T-cell counts. This effect can be minimized by performing counts at a fixed time of day. Another common contributor to inaccurate CD4+ cell counts is simple errors in measuring the percentage of lymphocytes on a standard differential white blood cell count. Normal values for total CD4 cell counts, the percentage of lymphocytes that are CD4+-cells, and CD4+/CD8+ count ratios may differ among adults in different countries. Ideally, every clinician managing HIV-infected patients should know the local laboratory CD4+ count standard values and variability.

Delayed-type hypersensitivity skin testing is another method of assessing immune impairment. Healthy uninfected controls in the United States respond to a variety of common skin test antigens, including *Trichophyton*, mumps, tetanus, and *Candida*.[255] As HIV disease progresses, normal skin test reactivity to these common antigens is lost. Loss of skin test reactivity to *Candida* antigens correlates strongly with the appearance of clinical candidiasis. Skin testing with these antigens also provides a control for the tuberculin skin test response. The tuberculin skin test result interpretation may vary according to local prevalence. In countries where prevalence among healthy persons is high, a negative tuberculin response in an HIV-infected patient probably signifies anergy and a high risk of tuberculosis. Where possible, skin testing with control antigens should also be done in parallel with tuberculin testing. *Candida* reactivity is probably prevalent in healthy populations worldwide, but this has not been established, and antigens are not widely available. Local control antigens and values may be required.

Other markers of disease progression include serum β_2-microglobulin and neopterin levels, but these assays have relatively little clinical utility. Several staging and classification systems have been used in clinical patient management. The Walter Reed system uses CD4+ counts, skin test results, and clinical signs to define six stages with distinctive prognostic significance. The CDC (1993 revision) uses CD4+ counts and clinical signs to define nine categories. However, it now seems clear that patient prognosis and management can best be achieved with (1) a CD4+ cell count, which is the best marker of immune damage, (2) a quantitative plasma viral RNA measurement, which is the best marker of active viral replication, and (3) clinical signs and symptoms.

TREATMENT

Optimal medical management of the HIV-infected patient includes therapy with antiretroviral agents, prevention of opportunistic infections and cancers, and treatment of complications as they arise. Complete medical care includes counseling of patients and their families.

Antiretroviral Therapies

The first class of drugs proved to have clinically significant anti-HIV activity were the nucleoside analog reverse transcriptase inhibitors (NRTIs): zidovudine (AZT), didanosine (DDI), zalcitabine (DDC), stavudine (d4T), lamivudine (3TC), and abacavir (ABC) (listed here in order of their approval by the U.S. Food and Drug Administration [FDA]).[256,257] These drugs are phosphorylated by cellular enzymes to their respective triphosphate forms, which block reverse transcriptase by substrate competition with natural nucleosides and by chain termination of the growing DNA strand. As monotherapy these drugs show only modest clinical and antiviral effects. Major problems include prompt emergence of drug resistance and significant toxicities.[258]

The second major class of anti-HIV drugs are the non-nucleoside reverse transcriptase inhibitors (NNRTIs) such as nevirapine, delavirdine, efavirenz. Added to this list are tenofovir and Emtricitabine, nucleotide RT inhibitors. These drugs do not require modification by cellular enzymes but act by direct binding to sites on the reverse transcriptase. As monotherapy the NNRTIs show the same problems as the nucleoside analogs.[259] Clinical trials have shown that combinations of therapies—two or three nucleoside analogs or NNRTIs, or both—give more potent and lasting effects. Disease progression is slowed, but only on average by 1 or 2 years.[260]

The third class of antiretrovirals, the inhibitors of HIV protease, (saquinavir, indinavir, ritonavir, nelfinavir, amprenavir, lopinavir/ritonavir, atazanavir) have demonstrated clinical efficacy.[261–264] These drugs act by binding to and blocking the HIV protease enzyme that is essential to cleaving the gag-pol polyprotein. Combination therapy, usually referred to as highly active antiretroviral therapy (HAART), of reverse transcriptase inhibitors and protease inhibitors is synergistic, and some combinations have lowered plasma HIV RNA levels to undetectable levels. A newer drug, enfuvirtide (Fuzeon), in the class of fusion inhibitors (FIs), is now in use.[265]

Most studies of antiretroviral therapy of HIV have been done in industrialized countries, particularly North America and Europe. Limited in vitro screening of HIV isolates from other countries, and in particular genotypes other than clade B, has not found any obvious patterns of naturally occurring resistant viruses within the major group of HIV-1. Nevertheless, strains of HIV-1 group 0 and HIV-2 are naturally resistant to most NNRTIs. However, the price of chronic therapy with antiretrovirals with proven efficacy is high but falling worldwide, making the introduction of life-saving antiretroviral treatment programs possible in many resource-limited settings. The search for effective low-cost antiretroviral therapies must continue and be intensified in all countries.

As with other antibiotics, low or intermittent dosing with antiretrovirals as a cost-saving measure is to be discouraged because it has no therapeutic benefit and may lead to community spread of resistant virus. Short-term administration of antiretroviral drugs is warranted only for certain, clearly defined prophylactic indications, such as prevention of maternal-fetal transmission or prevention of needlestick infection in health care workers.

Experimental Therapies

Experimental drug therapies in various stages of clinical development include integrase inhibitors, tat inhibitors, and zinc finger encapsulation inhibitors. A variety of gene therapy approaches, in which DNA is introduced into cells, are being explored, including transdominant mutant viral proteins that interfere with normal viral replication steps, or intracellular synthesis of antiviral antibodies that can bind to viral proteins.

"Vaccine therapy" trials have been conducted in which candidate vaccines are administered to infected patients in an attempt to improve the anti-HIV immune response through antigen-specific immunotherapy. Although new antibody and cellular immune responses to HIV proteins can be stimulated, there has been no clinical benefit.[266]

Cytokines can also be used to treat HIV-infected patients. The first cytokine use was gamma interferon (IFN-γ). Although the antiretroviral effects of parenterally administered IFN-γ are modest, the effects on Kaposi's sarcoma were sufficiently striking that the drug was approved for this specific indication.[266,267] The mechanism of action is uncertain. Initial reports of encouraging results with oral low-dose IFN-γ were not confirmed by the findings of controlled trials sponsored by WHO.

Interleukin-2 (IL-2), a cytokine that stimulates proliferation of lymphocytes, has been shown in clinical trials to produce a marked increase in circulating CD4+ cell counts.[268] Fears that IL-2 treatment would increase in vivo HIV replication rates have not been realized. Controlled trials are under way to determine whether the rise in CD4+ cell counts provoked by IL-2 therapy has therapeutic benefit proportional to the rise in cell count. Finally, malabsorption of antiretroviral drugs may be a problem in patients with diarrhea or enteric infections, and new approaches for treating such patients are under study.[269]

Specific Antiretroviral Recommendations: Who, When, and How

Rapid advances in HIV/AIDS research continue to modify and refine the guidelines for whom to treat, when during the course of infection treatment should be begun, and which therapeutic regimen should be used. Recent recommendations are presented here.[270]

- Who? The International AIDS Society–USA panel recommends therapy for any patient with established HIV infection who is committed to the complex, long-term therapy.
- When? Therapy is usually begun when the CD4+ cell count drops below 200 cells/μL (with consideration at higher CD4+ levels and symptomatic disease) or when the plasma HIV-1 RNA level is greater than 100,000 copies/mL.
- How? Initial therapy should be with a combination of antiretroviral drugs, usually a minimum of three drugs. Nucleoside or nucleotide reverse transcriptase inhibitors (AZT, DDI, DDC, d4T, 3TC, fenovir, FTC) are used in combination with NNRTIs (nevirapine, efavirenz) and/or protease inhibitors (ritonavir, indinavir, nelfinavir, saquinavir, lopinavir/ritonavir).

As new results become available, these recommendations will be modified.

Drug Resistance

HIV rapidly develops resistance to antiretroviral drugs in vivo. Drug-resistant variants have been found in blood after monotherapy with every antiretroviral thus far evaluated.[271,272] Emergence of resistance does not require patient exposure to an exogenous source of resistant virus; mutation and natural selection can evolve a population of resistant viruses within a single patient in a matter of weeks or months. Resistant HIV can be subsequently transmitted to uninfected persons. Resistance to an antiviral drug is typically generated through mutations affecting amino acids in the HIV target enzyme that are near the drug active site. Many different mutations can lead to resistance to a single drug, and these different mutations are often synergistic in conferring resistance.

Two biochemical mechanisms abrogate the incorporation of triphosphorylated NRTIs, thus leading to drug resistance. The first mechanism is mediated by a mutation that allows reverse transcriptase to discriminate against NRTI during DNA synthesis, as a result preventing their addition to the primer DNA chain. The second mechanism is meditated by mutations in the enzyme that increase the rate of hydrolytic removal of the chain terminating NRTI and to enable the continuous synthesis of viral DNA.[273,274] The NNRTIs, which bind to a hydrophobic pocket in reverse transcriptase, close to, but not contiguous with, the active site, inhibit HIV-1 replication allosterically by displacing the catalytic aspartate residues relative to the polymerase binding site. A single mutation in the hydrophobic pocket can result in high-level resistance to one or more NNRTIs. Resistance to NNRTIs appear to emerge by the selection of a pre-existing population of mutant viruses in an individual. This is linked to the fact that resistance rapidly develops when NNRTIs are administered as monotherapy or in the presence of incomplete virus suppression. Resistance to PIs is mediated by structural changes that reduce binding affinity between the inhibitor and the mutant protease molecule. Resistance to protease has also been attributed to mutations at the cleavage sites.[275–277] Mutations occurring outside the active site appear to induce resistance by other mechanisms such as alterations in enzyme catalysis, effects on dimer stability, alterations in inhibitor binding kinetics, or active site reshaping through extensive structural disturbances.[278,279]

In any given patient, the rapidity with which resistance emerges is directly related to the viral replication rate: a high replication rate generates mutants at a high rate. Combination therapies of two or three antiretroviral drugs with different mechanisms of action may lower the replication rate sufficiently to retard the breakthrough of drug-resistant variants.

Although this has yet to be proved, early results are encouraging. Recent reports that combinations of antiretrovirals can sterilize blood and perhaps lymphoid tissue of detectable virus have raised hopes that HIV infection may not just be treatable but curable. Studies are under way to determine whether long-term combination chemotherapy of HIV can lead to cure just as long-term combination chemotherapy of MTB can lead to cure of tuberculosis.

Drug resistance can be monitored at three levels: clinical, phenotypic, and genotypic. Clinical unresponsiveness to therapy suggests resistance. For example, a rapid fall in the CD4+ count with a rise in the plasma HIV RNA level strongly suggests emergence of resistance in a treated patient. This can be verified by virus isolation followed by drug sensitivity testing in virus-infected cell cultures, but this process is complicated and expensive. For those drugs where the principal resistance mutations are well characterized, PCR amplification and screening of the viral genome can detect common mutation patterns.

Prevention of Opportunistic Infections and Cancers

Prevention of opportunistic infections (OIs) in HIV-infected patients can be accomplished in three ways: (1) preventing exposure to pathogens in the environment, (2) preventing an initial episode of disease through chemoprophylaxis or vaccination, and (3) preventing disease recurrence through chemoprophylaxis. Opportunistic cancers can be prevented by screening and treatment of precancerous lesions.

Prevention of exposure to opportunistic pathogens requires knowledge of their environmental sources. For many common OIs, e.g., PCP, the exact environmental sources are still uncertain. In some, such as *P. marneffei* infection, the sources (thought to be moldy sugar cane or bamboo) are unique to certain geographic regions.[280] Some universal practical measures include avoidance of contact with known tuberculous patients in health care facilities; avoidance of raw or uncooked eggs, poultry, or dairy products that might harbor *Salmonella;* and avoidance of undercooked meat that may be a source of *Toxoplasma.* Some water-borne OIs, such as intestinal parasites and possibly MAI, may be difficult to avoid, but where possible only clean water sources should be used.

Chemoprophylaxis with trimethoprim-sulfamethoxazole (TMP-SMX) with one double-strength tablet daily has been proved to reduce the occurrence of PCP and to prolong survival in HIV-infected patients in North America.[281] In South America and Asia, where PCP appears to be a common OI, daily TMP-SMX prophylaxis is recommended for patients with advanced infection. Recent studies from Uganda and Zambia in HIV-infected adults and children, respectively, have shown a marked reduction in morbidity and mortality following the introduction of TMP-SMX.[282,283] The incidence of other OIs is also reduced, including cerebral toxoplasmosis and some bacterial infections.[284] Daily TMP-SMX costs about U.S. $60 per year.

Chemoprophylaxis with isoniazid (INH) has been proved to prevent clinical tuberculosis in HIV-infected persons.[285] Ideally, prophylaxis should be used in HIV-infected persons who are shown to be tuberculin skin test–positive but without active tuberculosis. However, the reality in many developing countries is that many HIV-infected patients are already anergic at the time of diagnosis. Furthermore, in many countries skin test reactivity may reflect childhood bacille Calmette-Guérin (BCG) immunization. Consequently, some have suggested that in regions where MTB prevalence is high, INH prophylaxis should be considered for all HIV-infected patients who do not have active tuberculosis.[286] WHO and the International Union Against Tuberculosis recommend that prophylaxis be given for 6 to 12 months. This costs about U.S. $60 per year. Several studies of prophylaxis against tuberculosis are currently under way in Africa and Asia.

Bacterial infections, particularly *Streptococcus pneumoniae,* are an important cause of morbidity and mortality among HIV-infected patients in developing countries. The polyvalent pneumococcal vaccine costs U.S. $10 and should be considered.

Human papillomaviruses play an etiologic role in cervical cancers in women and penile and anal cancers in men. Routine screening of HIV-infected patients for perineal and genital dysplasias and precancers with treatment of early lesions is suggested.

Treatment of Opportunistic Infections

Management of the clinically ill, late-stage HIV patient is difficult in any setting, but it is particularly challenging in developing countries where diagnostic and therapeutic options are limited. Experienced physicians often use syndrome-based diagnoses to choose therapies from locally available alternatives. The approach to patients with tropical infectious disease complications of HIV infection is presented in Chapter 133.

Counseling of Patients and Families

A diagnosis of HIV/AIDS can be a devastating psychological blow. In all societies, patients require ongoing emotional support and access to factual, up-to-date information. This can be provided by medical professionals or, alternatively, by trained paraprofessionals or volunteers. Information about prognosis and treatment options is the most obvious need. However, HIV-infected patients usually need assistance with a variety of important life decisions: whom to inform about their illness; how to avoid transmitting infection to others; childbearing options; coping strategies; and custody and death planning, to name a few.

PREVENTION AND CONTROL

HIV prevention efforts can focus either on reducing transmission from already infected patients or on reducing risk in uninfected persons.

HIV Testing as a Public Health Tool

One approach to HIV epidemic control is test-linked interventions: HIV testing coupled with efforts to reduce transmission by those found to be infected.[287–289] This approach reflects the traditional public health philosophy of communicable disease control. During the 1980s a vigorous international debate ensued over the potential benefits of HIV testing, reporting, contact tracing, and quarantine versus the negative impact of such steps on human rights. When aggressive HIV testing systems were implemented in several countries, WHO became concerned about the threat of stigmatization and discrimination and led a laudable international movement to ensure that nondiscrimination was an integral part of global HIV/AIDS control. WHO also condemned mandatory HIV control programs and put a low priority on testing and counseling. The WHO campaign to minimize discrimination appears to have been successful. Public health programs in which HIV testing is linked to treatment and behavioral counseling to reduce transmitting behaviors should also be considered to slow the global spread of HIV.

In at least one specific setting, test-linked interventions to reduce transmission do have near-universal support. This is in maternal-infant transmission. Chemoprophylaxis with AZT around the time of delivery is proved to substantially reduce the risk of maternal-to-infant transmission. Pregnant women are advised to be HIV-tested, and there have been calls for mandatory testing in this setting.

Among certain groups of at-risk adults, test-linked interventions may be the only practical way to prevent infection. For example, the common public health recommendation to limit the number of sexual partners is irrelevant advice for a monogamous spouse, although use of condoms may not be. In high-incidence regions where infection of males by commercial sex workers is common, the only way a monogamous married woman may reduce her own risk is to find out if her husband is infected and make difficult—but informed—choices.

Although the ethical issues are complex, test-linked public health programs can be considered if the following conditions apply: (1) testing is accurate, (2) medical treatment is available, (3) legal rights are secure, and (4) cost-benefit calculations are favorable.

Behavioral Prevention in At-Risk Populations

Public health efforts to change human behavior are never simple.[290] In the words of a highly regarded Ugandan HIV training video, "it's not easy." Health education—conveying a knowledge of the facts—is just one step toward behavior change.[291] The full sequence of steps to reach behavior change is often abbreviated as KABP—for knowledge, attitude, belief, and practice. Many persons become HIV-infected even though they have substantial knowledge about what HIV is, how it is transmitted, and how it can be prevented. A receptive attitude is crucial. Unless the subject believes that this is an issue of personal importance and that the changes can be of personal value and is willing to put into practice risk-avoidance skills, then knowledge alone is insufficient.

Behavioral interventions intended to prevent sexually transmitted HIV infections can be designed to reach one at-risk person at a time, small groups of at-risk persons, or larger community or societal groups. Interventions targeted at individuals or small groups permit focusing of resources to those most at risk and minimize political reaction by restricting discussions of sensitive issues and avoiding public forums. However, they are highly personnel-intensive and expensive. Individual counseling has been recommended for persons who seek HIV testing. Community- and societal-level interventions through mass media can be highly effective in reaching many people at once, but the heterogeneity of risks in large groups means that only the most basic messages enjoy widespread public acceptance. Public discussions of "safe sex" have been vigorously opposed in some quarters.

Efforts to control HIV in populations of injection drug users have reconfirmed the lesson that knowledge-only programs are not very effective in bringing about long-term behavior change. Changes in attitudes and beliefs typically require a social change process, so newer control efforts have targeted the social settings for drug use.[292] Peer influence is an important factor in social change, and two-way programs that involve current drug users are more effective than one-way, top-down policies. Providing the means for safe injection practices is another proven control method. Data from several countries suggest that over-the-counter sale of needles and syringes reduces the use of contaminated injection "works," and reduces HIV transmission. However, this approach has encountered intense political resistance.

Progress Toward an HIV Vaccine

There is no HIV vaccine with proven protective efficacy. Given the current state of progress and level of effort, a globally available and affordable HIV vaccine is at least a decade away. More than two dozen HIV candidate vaccines have been tested in phase I clinical trials in humans, primarily in the United States and Europe. However, only two of these have been carried forward to phase II trials, and there are currently no plans anywhere in the world for large-scale phase III efficacy trials.[293] Some of the scientific, political, and economic obstacles to global HIV vaccine development are reviewed here.[294]

Scientific Obstacles

The key unsolved scientific problem in HIV vaccine research is the mechanism of immunity. Although vaccine-induced protection has been demonstrated in SIV analog vaccine models, there is uncertainty whether protection is primarily humoral or cellular and which epitopes are crucial. A parallel problem is how to measure correlates of immunity in vaccine trials. For example, many candidate vaccines induce HIV-neutralizing antibodies but only against selected laboratory-adapted viruses, not against fresh "street virus" isolates.

Political Obstacles

Most incident HIV infections today occur in developing countries, where the prevalent HIV strains differ from those in candidate vaccines. Regrettably, there has been no coordinated international effort to produce candidate vaccines that would be suitable for testing in developing countries. Furthermore, vaccine testing capabilities in many regions are still suboptimal despite serious efforts by WHO to strengthen research infrastructures. Concern about exploitation (the "guinea-pig issue") is one example of a host of important political issues that must be overcome.

Economic Obstacles

Vaccines in general are not a highly profitable venture for industry, especially compared to therapeutics. Liability is an ever-present threat. Other economic disincentives that are unique to private-sector HIV vaccine research and development include the following: vaccine demand is greatest in populations least able to pay; different vaccine types may be necessary for developing countries; and calls for "distributive justice" by activists may force price ceilings.

With global cooperation, none of these obstacles is insurmountable. A new effort under the sponsorship of the Rockefeller Foundation called the International AIDS Vaccine Initiative has begun to build global partnerships that directly involve all parties: scientists, manufacturers, at-risk populations, developing and industrialized countries, and international organizations.

TURNING THE TIDE ON THE AIDS PANDEMIC

The provision of antiretroviral (ARV) therapy treatment for AIDS in resource limited settings has become a reality in recent years thanks to increases in donor support, political will, and a gradual reduction in the cost of antiretroviral drugs. Despite this optimism, only 7% of individuals needing ARVs in resource-limited settings were receiving treatment at the end of 2003.[11] (Fig. 76-10). Resource-limited countries affected by the AIDS pandemic face tremendous challenges to implement ARV programs that are sustainable and can meet the tremendous demands that will be placed on existing health-care institutions.

Global HIV/AIDS Funding

The amount of global AIDS funding has increased 15-fold from U.S. $300 million in 1996 to U.S. $5 billion in 2003.[11] Unfortunately, the funding gap has grown substantially as more money is made available, and this amount represents roughly half of what will be required for resource-limited countries by 2005. Costing estimates for 2007 indicate that $20 billion will be required for HIV prevention and care in low- and middle-income countries. This amount will not be met with current domestic and international development agendas and represents an enormous challenge to donor countries.

Several key milestones have occurred in response to the AIDS pandemic, making the possibility of ARV treatment a reality in resource-limited settings. The Global Fund to Fight AIDS, Tuberculosis and Malaria (GFATM) was created to increase the global resources available to combat these major killers affecting developing countries. GFATM has now gone through four rounds of funding and more than $1.6 billion has been allocated over 2 years for HIV/AIDS projects in 94 countries.[295] The GFATM money will allow for 700,000 individuals to receive life-saving ARV treatment through its various programs.[11] In the State of the Union address of January 2003, President George W. Bush announced an unprecedented 5-year, $15-billion Emergency Plan for AIDS Relief (PEPFAR) to provide HIV care, prevention, and treatment in 15 countries severely affected by the HIV/AIDS pandemic.[296] Currently 15 countries supported through the PEPFAR program are implementing programs focused on ARV treatment, prevention of mother-to-child transmission (PMTCT), HIV prevention, and support for orphans and vulnerable children. The ambitious goal of this program is to treat 2 million people with ARVs, prevent 7 million infections, and care for 10 million HIV-infected individuals by 2007. WHO also has embarked on an ambitious plan to mobilize support for the treatment of 3 million HIV-infected individuals with ARVs by 2005 with a focus on urgency, equity, and sustainability. Support from the World Bank's Multi-country AIDS Program (MAP) is delivering $1 billion to Africa for HIV care and $155 million to the Caribbean. Increasing support from these agencies coupled with the growing private sector involvement has provided a platform for universal access to HIV care in many countries, a goal that was seemingly impossible only 5 years ago. Most countries worst hit by the HIV pandemic have now developed national AIDS plans incorporating ARV treatment and basic HIV care. Several countries in Latin America and the Caribbean now offer universal ARV coverage. Brazil was the first developing country to implement a universal HIV/AIDS treatment policy, and currently 141,000 patients receive ARVs free through the public health system. The Brazilian government estimates that from 1997 to 2003, more than 60,000 new AIDS cases, 90,000 deaths, and 633,200 AIDS-related hospital admissions have been avoided.[297] The overall cost savings from this program is estimated at U.S. $200 million, not taking into account the social benefit of this program. The Brazilian experience has demonstrated that with government political will and the involvement of other key players in health delivery, it is possible to turn the tide on the AIDS pandemic.

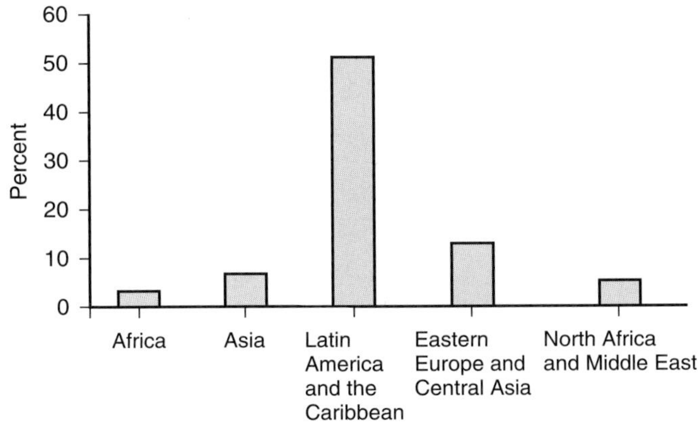

FIGURE 76-10 Percentage of the estimated 6 to 8 million HIV-infected patients who should be on antiretroviral therapy who are receiving antiretroviral drugs by 2004 by region. Only 400,000 had access to antiretroviral drugs, equaling coverage of only 7%. (Data from UNAIDS Program.)

The Challenges Ahead

The complexity of HIV care warrants a dramatic effort to strengthen human capacity to deliver ARVs. Twenty antiretroviral drugs are now approved by the FDA for the treatment of HIV infection and have an array of potentially serious side effects and drug interactions.[298] Decisions about which drugs to start with, when to start, and when to change therapy have become increasingly complex as the number of available choices increases. The training demands imposed by the complexity of HIV treatment is magnified by the reality of the scarcity of health workers in many resource-limited settings. In many settings, the current health work force must triple or quadruple to achieve the ambitious goal of universal ARV coverage. In countries most affected by AIDS, vacancy rates remain high, Malawi for example has only been able to fill half of its public sector nursing posts in recent years.[11]

Table 76-2 WHO Recommendations for Initiating Antiretroviral Therapy in Adults and Adolescents with Documented HIV Infection and Possible First-Line ARV Regimens

- WHO stage IV disease, irrespective of CD4
- WHO stage II disease, including but not restricted to HIV wasting, chronic diarrhea of unknown etiology, prolonged fever of unknown etiology, recurrent invasive bacterial infections, or recurrent/persistent mucosal candidiasis, with consideration of CD4 cell count <350/mm³ in decision-making
- WHO stage I or II disease with CD4 cell counts <200

In settings where CD4 testing is unavailable:
- WHO stage III or IV disease irrespective of total lymphocyte count
- WHO stage II disease with total lymphocyte count <1200/mm³

ARV Regimen	Major Potential Toxicities	Usage in Women (of Childbearing Age or Pregnant)
D4T/3TC/NVP	D4T-related neuropathy, pancreatitis and lipoatrophy NVP-related hepatotoxicity and severe rash	Yes
AZT/3TC/NVP	AZT-related GI intolerance, anemia, and neutropenia NVP-related hepatotoxicity and severe rash	Yes
D4T/3TC/EFV	D4T-related neuropathy, pancreatitis, and lipoatrophy EFV-related CNS toxicity and potential for teratogenicity	No*
AZT/3TC/EFV	AZT-related GI intolerance, anemia and neutropenia EFV-related CNS toxicity and potential for teratogenicity	No*

AZT, zidovudine; D4T, stavudine; EFV, efavirenz; NVP, nevirapine; 3TC, lamivudine.

*For women in whom effective contraception can be assured, EFV remains a viable option.

From Scaling up antiretroviral therapy in resource-limited settings: Treatment guidelines for a public health approach. Available at http://www.who.int/hiv/pub/prev_care/en/arvrevision2003en.pdf. Accessed 12/01/05.

As countries expand HIV care programs to meet the current expanded access goals, training and recruitment of health sector workers will be necessary to provide the platform to build sustainable programs.

Current North American and European clinical care guidelines incorporate measurements of plasma HIV viral load and CD4+ T lymphocytes as essential tools in managing patients on HAART.[298] In addition, testing for viral resistance has become a key tool in managing patients with evidence of virologic failure on HAART. Many countries faced with the challenge of delivering ARVs in resource-limited settings lack the laboratory infrastructure and trained technicians to perform the routine chemistry and hematology assays necessary to monitor patients receiving HAART. The more sophisticated virologic tests that have become standard of care in the North American and European settings remain prohibitively expensive for most countries developing HIV treatment programs. The WHO has responded to this challenge by publishing treatment guidelines aimed at resource limited settings (Table 76-2 and Box 76-2). Alternative, low-cost methods for monitoring patients receiving HAART have become a public health priority, but early results have failed to reveal a low-cost alternative that performs as well as the more expensive immunologic and virologic tests.[299]

The threat of antiretroviral resistance looms over the many countries scaling up ARV delivery programs. ARV resistance

Box 76-2 World Health Organization Classification System for HIV Infection

Clinical Stage 1

1. Asymptomatic infection
2. Persistent generalized lymphadenopathy
3. Acute retroviral infection
   Performance stage 1: asymptomatic, normal activity level

Clinical Stage 2

4. Unintentional weight loss <10% body weight
5. Minor mucocutaneous manifestations (e.g., dermatitis, prurigo, fungal nail infections, angular cheilitis)
6. Herpes zoster within previous 5 years
7. Recurrent upper respiratory tract infections
   Performance stage 2: symptomatic but nearly fully ambulatory

Clinical Stage 3

8. Unintentional weight loss >10% body weight
9. Chronic diarrhea >1 month
10. Prolonged fever >1 month (constant or intermittent)
11. Oral candidiasis
12. Oral hairy leukoplakia
13. Pulmonary tuberculosis within the previous year
14. Severe bacterial infections
15. Vulvovaginal candidiasis
    Performance stage 3: in bed more than usual but <50% of daytime during the previous month

Clinical Stage 4

16. HIV wasting syndrome
17. *Pneumocystis carinii* pneumonia
18. Toxoplasmosis of brain
19. Cryptosporidiosis with diarrhea >1 month
20. Isosporiasis with diarrhea >1 month
21. Cryptococcosis, extrapulmonary
22. Cytomegalovirus disease of an organ other than liver, spleen, or lymph node
23. Herpes simplex virus infection, mucocutaneous
24. Progressive multifocal leukoencephalopathy
25. Any disseminated endemic mycosis (e.g., histoplasmosis)
26. Candidiasis of the esophagus, trachea, bronchus, or lung
27. Atypical mycobacteriosis, disseminated
28. Non-typhoid *Salmonella* septicemia
29. Extrapulmonary tuberculosis
30. Lymphoma
31. Kaposi's sarcoma
32. HIV encephalopathy
    Performance stage 4: in bed >50% of daytime during previous month

could be devastating to resource-limited countries, resulting in early treatment failure and potentially abrogating the effectiveness of zidovudine, lamivudine, and nevirapine for the prevention of mother-to-child transmission of HIV. Countries embarking on ARV treatment programs need to ensure sustainable drug supplies in order to avoid the early pitfalls seen in the Ivory Coast, Gabon, and Uganda, where erratic therapy resulted in high levels of drug resistance.[300–302] Effective adherence strategies combined with stable drug supply in resource-limited settings has been shown to result in high levels of viral suppression, which hopefully will avoid widespread development of ARV resistance.[303]

The current expansion of ARV delivery to some areas hardest hit by the HIV pandemic provides hope and optimism for the future. The experiences of Brazil, Haiti, Thailand, Uganda, Senegal, and South Africa provide a wealth of information to design high-quality HIV treatment programs to greatly improve the health of nations facing the current HIV pandemic.[304–308] We have learned about secondary benefits of these programs from the findings in South Africa that HAART reduced the incidence of tuberculosis associated with HIV by 80%.[309] It is clear from evidence from North America, Europe, and Australia that adherence to therapy is difficult, and suboptimal antiretroviral regimens that are not as effective as HAART may result in the rapid development of drug resistance. As access to HAART expands, it is imperative that programs be supported with the necessary infrastructure to ensure high levels of adherence to build on the success demonstrated in the early treatment programs.

Enthusiasm over the expansion of ARV treatment programs throughout resource-limited settings should not overshadow the importance of basic HIV care and HIV prevention. Basic care and prophylaxis for the prevention of opportunistic infections remain low-cost interventions having the potential to greatly reduce morbidity and mortality among HIV-infected individuals.[283] Efforts to provide access to HAART that do not incorporate other low-cost interventions into a primary care plan could limit the potential effect of these programs on reducing morbidity and mortality among HIV-infected patients in resource-limited settings. Finally, prevention methods must be emphasized as treatment programs expand, to limit the number of new HIV infections and avoid any potential risk disinhibition that could result from the introduction of HAART into communities.

REFERENCES

1. Gottlieb MS, Schroff R, Schranker HM, et al: *Pneumocystis carinii* pneumonia and mucosal candidiasis in previously healthy homosexual men. N Engl J Med 305:1430, 1981.
2. Masur H, Michelis MA, Greene JB, et al: An outbreak of community-acquired *Pneumocystis carinii* pneumonia: initial manifestation of cellular immune dysfunction. N Engl J Med 305:1431, 1981.
3. Siegal FP, Lopez C, Hammer GS, et al: Severe acquired immunodeficiency in male homosexuals, manifested by chronic perianal ulcerative herpes simplex lesions. N Engl J Med 305:1444, 1981.
4. Pape JW, Liautaud B, Thomas F, et al: Characteristics of the acquired immunodeficiency syndrome in Haiti. Ann Intern Med 103:674, 1985.
5. Piot P, Quinn TC, Taelman H, et al: Acquired immunodeficiency syndrome in a heterosexual population in Zaire. Lancet 2:65, 1984.
6. Quinn TC, Mann JM, Curran JW, et al: AIDS in Africa: an epidemiologic paradigm. Science 234:955, 1986.
7. Barre-Sinoussi F, Chermann JC, Rey F, et al: Isolation of a T-lymphotropic retrovirus from a patient at risk for acquired immune deficiency syndrome (AIDS). Science 220:868, 1983.
8. Gallo RC, Salahuddin SZ, Popovic M, et al: Frequent detection and isolation of cytopathic retroviruses (HTLV-III) from patients with AIDS and at risk for AIDS. Science 224:500, 1984.
9. Mann JM, Chin J, Piot P, et al: The international epidemiology of AIDS. Sci Am 10:82, 1988.
10. Quinn TC: The global burden of the HIV pandemic. Lancet 348:99, 1996.
11. UNAIDS: 2004 Report on the global AIDS epidemic. Geneva, UNAIDS, 2004.
12. Kaplan JE, Hu DJ, Holmes KK, et al: Preventing opportunistic infections in human immunodeficiency virus–infected persons: implications for the developing world. Am J Trop Med Hyg 55:1, 1996.
13. Grant AD, Kaplan JE, DeCock KM: Preventing opportunistic infections among human immunodeficiency virus–infected adults in African countries. Am J Trop Med Hyg 65:810, 2001.
14. Barre-Sinoussi F, Cherman J-C, Ray F, et al: Isolation of a T-lymphotropic retrovirus from a patient at risk for acquired immune deficiency syndrome (AIDS). Science 224:868, 1993.
15. Gallo RC, Salahuddin SZ, Popovic M, et al: Frequent detection and isolation of cytopathic retroviruses (HTLV-III) from patients with AIDS and at risk for AIDS. Science 224:500, 1984.
16. Froland SS, Jenum P, Lindboe CF, et al: HIV-1 infection in a Norwegian family before 1970. Lancet 1:1344, 1988.
17. Bryceson A, Tomkins A, Ridley D, et al: HIV-2–associated AIDS in the 1970s. Lancet 2:221, 1988.
18. Nahmias AJ, Weiss J, Yao X, et al: Evidence for human infection with an HTLV III/LAV-like virus in Central Africa: 1959. Lancet 1:1279, 1986.
19. Getchell JP, Hicks DR, Svinivasan A, et al: Human immunodeficiency virus isolated from a serum sample collected in 1976 in Central Africa. J Infect Dis 156:833, 1987.
20. Nzilambi N, DeCock KM, Forthal DN, et al: The prevalence of infection with human immunodeficiency virus over a 10-year period in rural Zaire. N Engl J Med 318:276, 1988.
21. Srinivasan A, York D, Butler D, et al: Molecular characterization of HIV-1 isolated from a serum collected in 1976: nucleotide sequence comparison to recent isolates and generation of hybrid HIV. AIDS Res Hum Retroviruses 5:121, 1989.
22. Meyers G, Pavlakis GN: Evolutionary potential of complex retroviruses. In Levy J (ed): The Retroviridae. New York, Plenum Press, 1992.
23. English RV, Nelson P, Johnson CM, et al: Development of clinical disease in cats experimentally infected with feline immunodeficiency virus. J Infect Dis 170:543, 1994.
24. Gonda MA, Luther DG, Fong SE, et al: Bovine immunodeficiency virus: molecular biology and virus-host interactions. Virus Res 32:155, 1994.
25. Zink MC, Johnson LK: Pathobiology of lentivirus infections in sheep and goats. Virus Res 32:139, 1994.
26. Sellon DC, Fuller FJ, McGuire TC: The immunopathogenesis of equine infectious anemia virus. Virus Res 32:111, 1994.
27. Issel CJ, Foil LD: Studies on equine infectious anemia virus transmission by insects. J Am Vet Med Assoc 184:293, 1984.
28. Hirsch VM, Dapolito GA, Goldstein S, et al: A distinct African lentivirus from Sykes' monkeys. J Virol 67:1517, 1993.
29. Jin MJ, Hui H, Robertson DL, et al: Mosaic genome structure of simian immunodeficiency virus from West African green monkeys. EMBO J 14:2935, 1994.
30. Daniel MD, Letvin NL, King NW, et al: Isolation of a T-cell tropic HTLV-III-like retrovirus from macaques. Science 228:1201, 1985.
31. Kanki PJ, McLane MF, King NW, et al: Serologic identification and characterization of a macaque T-lymphotropic retrovirus closely related to HTLV-III. Science 228:1199, 1985.
32. Gurtler LG, Hauser PH, Eberle J, et al: A new subtype of human immunodeficiency virus type 1 (MVP-5180) from Cameroon. J Virol 68:1581, 1994.
33. Vanden Haesevelde M, DeCourt J-L, De Leys RJ, et al: Genomic cloning and complete sequence analysis of a highly divergent African human immunodeficiency virus isolate. J Virol 68:1586, 1994.
34. Simon F, Mauclere P, Roques P, et al: Identification of a new human immunodeficiency virus type 1 distinct from group M and O. Nature Med 4:1032, 1998.
35. Roques P, Robertson DL, Souquière S, et al: Phylogenetic characteristics of three new HIV-1 N strains and implications for the origin of group N. AIDS 18:1371, 2004.

36. Huet T, Cheynier R, Meyerhans A, et al: Genetic organization of a chimpanzee lentivirus related to HIV-1. Nature 345:356, 1990.
37. Louwagie J, McCutchan FE, Peeters M, et al: Phylogenetic analysis of gag genes from 70 international HIV-1 isolates provides evidence for multiple genotypes. AIDS 7:769, 1993.
38. Louwagie J, Janssens W, Mascola J, et al: Genetic diversity of the envelope glycoprotein from HIV-1 isolates of African origin. J Virol 69:263, 1995.
39. Roques P, Menu E, Narwa R, et al: An unusual HIV type 1*env* sequence embedded in a mosaic virus from Cameroon: identification of a new clade. European Network on the study of in utero transmission of HIV-1. AIDS Res Hum Retroviruses 15:1585, 1999.
40. Robertson DL, Anderson JP, Bradac JA, et al: HIV-1 nomenclature proposal. Science 288:56, 2000.
41. Sharp PM, Robertson DL, Gao F, et al: Origins and diversity of human immunodeficiency viruses. AIDS 8(suppl):S27, 1994.
42. Gao F, Robertson DL, Morrison SG, et al: The heterosexual human immunodeficiency virus type 1 in Thailand is caused by an intersubtype (A/E) recombinant of African origin. J Virol 70:7013, 1996.
43. Kostrikis LG, Bagdades E, Cao Y, et al: Genetic analysis of human immunodeficiency virus type 1 strains from patients in Cyprus: identification of a new subtype designated I. J Virol 71:7088, 1995.
44. Gao F, Robertson DL, Carruthers CD, et al: An isolate of human immunodeficiency virus type 1 originally classified as subtype I represents a complex mosaic comprising three different group M subtypes (A, G and I). J Virol 72:10234, 1998.
45. Nasioulas G, Paraskovis D, Magiorkinis E, et al: Molecular analysis of the full-length genome of HIV type 1 subtype I: evidence of A/G/I recombination. AIDS Res Hum Retroviruses 15:745, 1999.
46. Carr JK, Salimen MO, Albert J, et al: Full genome sequences of human immunodeficiency virus type 1 subtypes G and A/G intersubtype recombinants. Virology 247:22, 1998.
47. Carr JK, Salimen MO, Koch C, et al: Full-length sequence and mosaic structure of a human immunodeficiency virus type 1 isolate from Thailand. J Virol 70:5935, 1999.
48. Liitsola K, Tashikinova I, Laukkenen T, et al: HIV-1 genetic subtype A/B recombinant strain causing an explosive epidemic in injecting drug users in Kaliningrad. AIDS 12:1907, 1998.
49. Morrow JW, Homsy J, Eichberg JW, et al: Long-term observation of baboons, rhesus monkeys, and chimpanzees inoculated with HIV and given periodic immunosuppressive treatments. AIDS Res Hum Retroviruses 5:233, 1989.
50. Otten RA, Brown BG, Simon M, et al: Differential replication and pathogenic effects of HIV-1 and HIV-2 in Macaca nemestrina. AIDS 8:297, 1994.
51. Gartner S, Liu Y, Polonis V, et al: Adaptation of HIV-1 to pigtailed macaques. J Med Primatol 23:155, 1994.
52. Letvin N, Li J, Halloran M, et al: Prior infection with a nonpathogenic chimeric simian-human immunodeficiency virus does not efficiently protect macaques against challenge with simian immunodeficiency virus. J Virol 69:4569, 1995.
53. Johnston JB, Power C: Feline immunodeficiency virus xenoinfection: the role of chemokine receptors and envelop diversity. J Virol 76:3626, 2000.
54. Hahn BH, Shaw GM, de Cock KM, et al: AIDS as a zoonosis: scientific and public health implications. Science 287:607, 2000.
55. Robertson DL, Sharp PM, McCutchan FE, et al: Recombination in HIV-1 (letter). Nature 374:124, 1995.
56. Meyers GB, Korber BH, Hahn K-T: Human Retroviruses and AIDS: A Compilation and Analysis of Nucleic Acid and Amino Acid Sequences. Los Alamos, N.M., Los Alamos National Laboratory, 1995.
57. Cullen BR: Human immunodeficiency virus as a prototypic complex retrovirus. J Virol 65:1053, 1991.
58. Lasky LA, Nakamura G, Smith DH, et al: Delineation of a region of the human immunodeficiency virus type 1 gp120 glycoprotein critical for interaction with the CD4 receptor. Cell 50:975, 1987.
59. Doranz BJ, Berson JF, Rucker J, et al: Chemokine receptors as fusion cofactors for human immunodeficiency virus type 1 (HIV-1). Immunol Res 16:15, 1997.
60. Ji J, Loeb LA: Fidelity of HIV-1 reverse transcriptase copying RNA in vitro. Biochemistry 31:954, 1992.
61. Bukrinsky MI, Sharova N, McDonald TL, et al: Association of integrase, matrix, and reverse transcriptase antigens of human immunodeficiency virus type 1 with viral nucleic acids following acute infection. Proc Natl Acad Sci USA 90:6125, 1993.
62. Mak J, Jiang M, Wainberg MA, et al: Role of Pr160$^{gag\text{-}pol}$ in mediating the selective incorporation of tRNA (Lys) into human immunodeficiency virus type 1 particles. J Virol 68:2065, 1994.
63. Dvorin JD, Bell P, Maul GG, et al: Reassessment of the roles of integrase and the central DNA flap in human immunodeficiency virus type 1 nuclear import. J Virol 76:12087, 2002.
64. Sherman MP, Greene WC: Slipping through the door: HIV entry into the nucleus. Microbes Infect 4:67, 2002.
65. Sherman MP, DeNoronha CMC, Williams SA, et al: Insights into the biology of HIV-1 viral protein r. DNA Cell Biol 21:679, 2002.
66. Wiskerchen M, Muesing MA: Human immunodeficiency virus type 1 integrase: effects of mutations on viral ability to integrate, direct viral gene expression from unintegrated viral DNA templates, and sustain viral propagation in primary cells. J Virol 69:379, 1995.
67. Shiramizu B, Herndier BG, McCrath MS: Identification of a common clonal human immunodeficiency virus integration site in human immunodeficiency virus–associated lymphomas. Cancer Res 54:2069, 1994.
68. Bielinska A, Krasnow S, Nabel GJ: NF-kB-mediated activation of the human immunodeficiency virus enhancer: site of transcriptional initiation is independent of the TATA box. J Virol 63:4097, 1989.
69. Lu Y, Stenzel M, Sodroski JG, Haseltine WA: Effects of long terminal repeat mutations on human immunodeficiency virus type 1 replication. J Virol 63:4115, 1989.
70. Olsen HS, Rowen CA: Contribution of the TATA motif to tat-mediated transcriptional activation of human immunodeficiency virus gene expression. J Virol 66:5594, 1992.
71. Malim MH, Tiley L, McCarn D, et al: HIV-1 structural gene expression required binding of the Rev trans-activator to its RNA target sequence. Cell 60:675, 1990.
72. Malim MH, Bohnlein S, Hauber J, et al: Functional dissection of the HIV-1 rev trans-activator: derivation of a *trans*-dominant repressor of rev function. Cell 58:205, 1989.
73. Dorfman T, Burkovsky A, Ohagen A, et al: Functional domains of the capsid protein of human immunodeficiency virus type 1. J Virol 68:8180, 1994.
74. South TL, Blake PR, Sowder RC, et al: The nucleocapsid protein isolated from HIV-1 particles binds zinc and forms retroviral-type zinc fingers. Biochemistry 29:7786, 1990.
75. Earl PL, Doms RW, Moss B: Oligomeric structure of the human immunodeficiency virus type 1 envelope glycoproteins. Proc Natl Acad Sci USA 87:648, 1990.
76. Poumbourios P, el Ahmar W, McPhee DA, et al: Determinants of human immunodeficiency virus type 1 envelope glycoprotein oligomeric structure. J Virol 69:1209, 1995.
77. Pantaleo G, Fauci AS: New concepts in the immunopathogenesis of HIV infection. Annu Rev Immunol 13:487, 1995.
78. Pantaleo G, Graziosi C, Demarest JF, et al: HIV infection is active and progressive in lymphoid tissue during the clinically latent stage of disease. Nature 362:355, 1993.
79. Sullivan N, Sun Y, Li J, et al: Replicative function and neutralization sensitivity of envelope glycoproteins from primary and T-cell line-passaged human immunodeficiency virus type 1 isolates. J Virol 69:4413, 1995.
80. More JP: Back to primary school. Nature 376:115, 1995.
81. Milich L, Margolin BH, Swanstrom R: Patterns of amino acid variability in NSI-like and SI-like V3 sequences and a linked change in the CD4-binding domain of HIV-1 env protein. Virology 239:108, 1997.
82. Jansson M, Backstrom E, Scarlatti G, et al: Length variation of glycoprotein 120 V2 region in relation to biological phenotypes and coreceptor usage of primary HIV type 1 isolates. AIDS Res Hum Retroviruses 17:1405, 2001.
83. Salvatori F, Scarlatti G: HIV type 1 chemokine receptor usage in mother-to-child transmission. AIDS Res Hum Retroviruses 17:925, 2001.
84. Libert F, Cochaux P, Beckman G, et al: The δccr5 mutation conferring protection against HIV-1 in caucasian populations has a single and recent origin in North-eastern Europe. Hum Mol Genet 7:399, 1998.
85. Berger EA, Murphy PM, Farber JM: Chemokine receptors as HIV-1 coreceptors: roles in viral entry, tropism and disease. Ann Rev Immunol 17:657, 1999.
86. Moore JP, Kitchen SG, Pugach P, et al: The CCR5 and CXCR4 coreceptors—central to understanding the transmission and pathogenesis of human immunodeficiency virus type 1 infection. AIDS Res Hum Retroviruses 20:111, 2004.

87. Lopalco L, Barassi C, Pastori C, et al: CCR5-reactive antibodies in seronegative partners of HIV-seropositive individuals down modulate surface CCR5 in vivo and neutralize the infectivity of R5 strains of HIV-1 in vitro. J Immunol 164:3426, 2000.
88. Cullen BR: A new entry route for HIV. Nature Med 7:20, 2001.
89. Robertson DL, Hahn BH, Sharp PM: Recombination of AIDS viruses. J Mol Evol 40:249, 1995.
90. Lozovskaya ER, Hartl DL, Petrov DA: Genomic regulation of transposable elements in Drosophila. Curr Opin Genet Dev 5:768, 1995.
91. Leib-Mösch C, Seifarth W: Evolution and biological significance of human retroelements. Virus Genes 11:133, 1995.
92. Mountz JD, Talal N: Retroviruses, apoptosis and autogenes. Immunol Today 14:532, 1993.
93. Nakagawa K, Harrison LC: The potential roles of endogenous retroviruses in autoimmunity. Immunol Rev 152:193, 1996.
94. Franchini G, Reitz MS Jr: Phylogenesis and genetic complexity of the nonhuman primate retroviridae. AIDS Res Hum Retroviruses 10:1047, 1994.
95. Gardner MB: The history of simian AIDS. J Med Primatol 25:148, 1996.
96. Aguzzi A: The foamy virus family: molecular biology, epidemiology and neuropathology. Biochim Biophys Acta 1155:1, 1993.
97. Doolittle RF, Feng DF, McClure MA, et al: Retrovirus phylogeny and evolution. Curr Top Microbiol Immunol 157:1, 1990.
98. Gessain A, de Thé G: Geographic and molecular epidemiology of primate T lymphotropic retroviruses: HTLV-I, HTLV-II, STLV-I, STLV-PP, and PTLV-L. Adv Virus Res 47:377, 1996.
99. Uchiyama T: ATL and HTLV-I: in vivo cell growth of ATL cells. J Clin Immunol 16:305, 1996.
100. Ijichi S, Nakagawa M, Umehara F, et al: HAM/TSP: Recent perspectives in Japan. J Acquir Immune Defic Syndr Hum Retrovirol 13(suppl 1):S26, 1996.
101. Yamashita M, Ido E, Miura T, et al: Molecular epidemiology of HTLV-I in the world. J Acquir Immune Defic Syndr Hum Retrovirol 13(suppl 1):S124, 1996.
102. Yamaguchi K: Human T-lymphotropic virus type I in Japan. Lancet 343:213, 1994.
103. Ruff AJ: Breastmilk, breastfeeding, and transmission of viruses to the neonate. Semin Perinatol 18:510, 1994.
104. Taylor GP: The epidemiology of HTLV-I in Europe. J Acquir Immune Defic Syndr Hum Retrovirol 13(suppl 1):S8, 1996.
105. Piot P, Plummer FS, Mhalu JL, et al: AIDS: an international perspective. Science 239:573, 1988.
106. Haverkos HW, Quinn TC: The third wave: HIV infection among heterosexuals in the United States and Europe. Int J STD AIDS 6:227, 1995.
107. Available at http://www.nacoonline.org/factsnfigures/hivestimates2003.pdf. Accessed 9/20/04.
108. UNAIDS: The status and trends of the global HIV/AIDS pandemic. Geneva, UNAIDS, July 5–6, 1996.
109. 24. Mann J, Tarantola D: The state of the pandemic and its impact. In Mann J, Tarantola D (eds): AIDS in the World, vol 2. London, Oxford University Press, 1996.
110. Padian NS: Heterosexual transmission of acquired immunodeficiency syndrome: international perspectives and national projections. Rev Infect Dis 9:947, 1987.
111. Piot P, Goeman J, Laga M: The epidemiology of HIV and AIDS in Africa. In Essex M, Mboup S, Kanki P, et al (eds): AIDS in Africa. New York, Raven Press, 1994, p 157.
112. Piot P, Kreiss JK, Ndinya-Achola JO, et al: Heterosexual transmission of HIV. AIDS 2:1, 1988.
113. Quinn TC, Fauci AS: The changing demography of AIDS: emergence of heterosexual transmission. In Isselbacher KJ, Braunwald E, Wilson JD, et al (eds): Harrison's Principles of Internal Medicine, 13th ed. New York, McGraw-Hill, 1994, p 1.
114. Quinn TC: Population migration and the spread of types 1 and 2 human immunodeficiency viruses. Proc Natl Acad Sci USA 91:2407, 1994.
115. Flemming DT, Wasserheit JN: From epidemiological synergy to public health policy and practice: the contribution of other sexually transmitted diseases to sexual transmission of HIV infection. Sex Transm Infect 75:3, 1999.
116. Latif AS, Katzenstein DA, Bassett MT, et al: Genital ulcers and transmission of HIV among couples in Zimbabwe. AIDS 3:519, 1989.
117. Laga M, Manoka A, Kivuvu M, et al: Non-ulcerative sexually transmitted diseases as risk factors for HIV-1 transmission in women: results from a cohort study. AIDS 7:95, 1993.
118. Laga M, Diallo MO, Buve A: Inter-relationship of sexually transmitted diseases and HIV: where are we now? AIDS 8(suppl 1):S119, 1994.
119. Quinn TC, Glasser D, Cannon RO, et al: Human immunodeficiency virus infection among patients attending clinics for sexually transmitted diseases. N Engl J Med 318:197, 1988.
120. Otten M, Zaidi AA, Peterman TA, et al: High rate of HIV seroconversion among patients attending urban sexually transmitted disease clinics. AIDS 8:549, 1994.
121. Quinn TC: Association of sexually transmitted diseases and infection with the human immunodeficiency virus: biological cofactors and markers of behavioural interventions. Int J STD AIDS 7:17, 1996.
122. Reynolds SJ, Risbud AR, Shepherd ME, et al: Recent herpes simplex virus type 2 infection and the risk of human immunodeficiency virus type 1 acquisition in India. J Infect Dis 187:1513, 2003.
123. Global Programme on AIDS: An Overview of Selected Curable Sexually Transmitted Diseases. Geneva, World Health Organization, 1995.
124. Peckham C, Gibb D: Mother-to-child transmission of the human immunodeficiency virus. N Engl J Med 333:298, 1995.
125. U.S. Bureau of Census: Trends and Patterns of HIV and AIDS Infection in Selected Developing Countries. Research Note No. 14: Country Profiles. Washington, D.C., Department of State, June 1994.
126. The Working Group on Mother-to-Child Transmission of HIV: Rates of mother-to-child transmission of HIV-1 in Africa, America, and Europe: Results from 13 perinatal studies. J Acquir Immune Defic Syndr Hum Retrovirol 8:1495, 1995.
127. St Louis M, Kamenga M, Brown C, et al: Risk for perinatal HIV-1 transmission according to maternal immunologic, virologic, and placental factors. JAMA 269:2853, 1993.
128. Burns DN, Landesman S, Muenz LR, et al: Cigarette smoking, premature rupture of membranes, and vertical transmission of HIV-1 among women with low CD4- levels. J Acquir Immune Defic Syndr Hum Retrovirol 7:718, 1994.
129. Weisner B, Nachman S, Tropper P, et al: Quantitation of human immunodeficiency virus type 1 during pregnancy: relationship of viral titer to mother-to-child transmission and stability of viral load. Proc Natl Acad Sci USA 91:8037, 1994.
130. Semba RLD, Miotti PG, Chiphangwi JD, et al: Maternal vitamin A deficiency and mother-to-child transmission of HIV-1. Lancet 343:1593, 1994.
131. Brahmbhatt H, Kigozi G, Wabwire-Mengen F, et al: The effects of placental malaria on mother-to-child HIV transmission in Rakai, Uganda. AIDS 17:2539, 2003.
132. Dunn DT, Newell ML, Ades AE, et al: Risk of human immunodeficiency virus type 1 transmission through breastfeeding. Lancet 340:585, 1992.
133. World Health Organization: Global Programme on AIDS: Consensus statement from the WHO/UNICEF consultation on HIV transmission and breast-feeding. Wkly Epidemiol Rec 7:177, 1992.
134. Des Jarlais DC, Friedman SR, Choopanya K, et al: International epidemiology of HIV and AIDS among injecting drug users. AIDS 6:1053, 1992.
135. Francis HL, Quinn TC: Bloodborne transmission of HIVs in Africa. In Essex M, Mboup S, Kanki PJ, et al (eds): AIDS in Africa. New York, Raven Press, 1994, p 237.
136. Foster S, Buve A: Benefits of HIV screening of blood transfusions in Zambia. Lancet 346:225, 1995.
137. Greenberg AE, Nguyen-Dinh P, Mann JM, et al: The association between malaria, blood transfusions, and HIV seropositivity in a pediatric population in Kinshasa, Zaire. JAMA 259:545, 1988.
138. World Health Organization: The risk of transmission of AIDS and other blood-related diseases during routine malaria activities. Wkly Epidemiol Rec 65:345, 1990.
139. Gerberding JL: Management of occupational exposures to blood-borne viruses. N Engl J Med 332:444, 1995.
140. Guidelines for prevention of transmission of human immunodeficiency virus and hepatitis B virus to health-care and public-safety workers. MMWR 38(suppl 6):1, 1989.
141. Human immunodeficiency virus transmission in household settings—U.S. MMWR 43:347, 1994.

142. Friedland GH, Klein RS: Transmission of the human immunodeficiency virus. N Engl J Med 317:1125, 1987.
143. Mann JM, Quinn TC, Francis H, et al: Prevalence of HTLV-III/LAV in household contacts of confirmed AIDS patients and controls in Kinshasa, Zaire. JAMA 256:721, 1986.
144. Clerici M, Giorgi JV, Chou C-C, et al: Cell-mediated immune response to human immunodeficiency virus (HIV) type 1 in seronegative homosexual men with recent sexual exposure to HIV-1. J Infect Dis 165:1012, 1992.
145. Rowland-Jones S, Sutton J, Ariyoshi K, et al: GIV-specific CTL in HIV-exposed but uninfected Cambodian women. Nature Med 1:59, 1995.
146. Phillips DM, Zacharopoulos VR, Tan X, et al: Mechanisms of sexual transmission of HIV: does HIV infect intact epithelia? Trends Microbiol 2:454, 1994.
147. Miller CJ, Alexander NJ, Sutjipto S, et al: Genital mucosal transmission of simian immunodeficiency virus: animal model for heterosexual transmission of human immunodeficiency virus. J Virol 63:4277, 1989.
148. Kreiss JK, Coombs R, Plummer F, et al: Isolation of human immunodeficiency virus from genital ulcers in Nairobi prostitutes. J Infect Dis 160:380, 1989.
149. Cook LS, Koutsky LA, Holmes KK: Circumcision and sexually transmitted diseases. Am J Public Health 84:197, 1994.
150. Osmond D, Bacchetti P, Chaisson RE, et al: Time of exposure and risk of HIV infection in homosexual partners of men with AIDS. Am J Public Health 78:944, 1988.
151. Wolinsky SM, Wike CM, Korber BTM, et al: Selective transmission of human immunodeficiency virus type-1 variants from mothers to infants. Science 255:1134, 1992.
152. Laga M, Taelman H, Van der Stuyft P, et al: Advanced immunodeficiency as a risk factor for heterosexual transmission of HIV. AIDS 3:361, 1989.
153. Wolfs TFW, Zwart G, Bakker M, et al: HIV-1 genomic RNA diversification following sexual and parenteral virus transmission. Virology 189:103, 1992.
154. DeCock KM, Adjorlolo G, Ekepni E, et al: Epidemiology of HIV-2: why there is no HIV-2 pandemic. JAMA 270:2083, 1993.
155. Robertson DL, Sharp PM, McCutchan FE, et al: Recombination in HIV-1. Nature 374:125, 1995.
156. Sharp PM, Robertson DL, Hahn BH: Cross-species transmission and recombination of AIDS viruses. Philos Trans R Soc Lond B Biol Sci 349:41, 1995.
157. Travers K, Mboup S, Marlink R, et al: Natural protection against HIV-1 infection provided by HIV-2. Science 268:1612, 1995.
158. Soto-Ramirez LE, Renjifo B, McLane MF, et al: HIV-1 Langerhans cell tropism associated with heterosexual transmission of HIV. Science 271:1291, 1996.
159. Kunanusont C, Foy HM, Kreiss JK, et al: HIV-1 subtypes and male-to-female transmission in Thailand. Lancet 345:1078, 1995.
160. Decosas J, Kane F, Anarfi JK, et al: Migration and AIDS. Lancet 346:826, 1995.
161. Cameron DW, Simonsen JN, D'Costa LJ, et al: Female-to-male transmission of human immunodeficiency virus type 1: risk factors for seroconversion in men. Lancet 2:403, 1989.
162. Bongaarts J, Reining P, Way P, et al: The relationship between male circumcision and HIV infection in African populations. AIDS 3:373, 1989.
163. UNAIDS: AIDS Epidemic Update December 2003. Geneva, UNAIDS, 2003.
164. UNAIDS: Report on the global HIV/AIDS epidemic 2002. Geneva, UNAIDS, 2002.
165. Reynolds SJ, Shepherd ME, Risbud AR, et al: Male circumcision and risk of HIV-1 and other sexually transmitted infections in India. Lancet 363:1039, 2004.
166. Gray RH, Wawer MJ, Brookmeyer R, et al: Probability of HIV-1 transmission per coital act in monogamous, heterosexual, HIV-1-discordant couples in Rakai, Uganda. Lancet 357:1149, 2001.
167. Gray RH, Kiwanuka N, Quinn TC, et al: Male circumcision and HIV acquisition and transmission: cohort studies in Rakai, Uganda. Rakai Project Team. AIDS 14:2371, 2000.
168. Quinn TC: Epidemiology of the HIV/AIDS epidemic. In Cohen B, Trussell J (eds): Preventing and Mitigating AIDS in Sub-Saharan Africa. Washington, D.C., National Academy Press, 1996, p 269.
169. Workshop on the Status and Trends of the HIV/AIDS Epidemics in Africa: Final Report. Cosponsored by AIDS Control and Prevention (AIDSCAP) Project of Family Health International and the Francois-Xavier Bagnoud Center for Health and Human Rights of the Harvard School of Public Health. Cambridge, Mass., Harvard School of Public Health, 1996.
170. Marlink R: Biology and epidemiology of HIV-2 In Essex M, Kalengaly M, Kanki P, et al (eds): AIDS in Africa. New York, Raven Press, 1994, p 47.
171. Markovitz DM: Infection with the human immunodeficiency virus type 2. Ann Intern Med 118:211, 1993.
172. DeCock KM, Brun-Vezinet F: Epidemiology of HIV-2 infection. AIDS 3(suppl 1):S89, 1989.
173. Kanki P: Biologic features of HIV-2: an update. AIDS Clin Rev 17, 1991.
174. Jaffar S, Grant AD, Whitworth J, et al: The natural history of HIV-1 and HIV-2 infections in adults in Africa: a review of the literature. Bull WHO 82:462, 2004.
175. Kanki PJ, Travers KU, Mboup S, et al: Slower heterosexual spread of HIV-2 than HIV-1. Lancet 343:943, 1994.
176. Adjorlolo-Johnson G, DeCock KM, Ekpini E, et al: Prospective comparison of mother-to-child transmission of HIV-1 and HIV-2 in Abidjan, Ivory Coast. JAMA 272:462, 1994.
177. Chaisson RE: HIV becomes world's leading infectious cause of death. Hopkins HIV Rep 11:1, 1999.
178. DeCock KM, Barrere B, Diaby L, et al: AIDS—The leading cause of adult death in the West African city of Abidjan, Ivory Coast. Science 1249:793, 1990.
179. Mulder DW, Nunn AJ, Kamali A: Two-year HIV-1-associated mortality in a Ugandan rural population. Lancet 343:1021, 1994.
180. Sewankambo NK, Wawer MJ, Gray RH, et al: Demographic impact of HIV infection in rural Rakai District, Uganda: results of a population-based cohort study. AIDS 8:170, 1994.
181. Chin HJ: Current and future dimensions of the HIV/AIDS pandemic in women and children. Lancet 336:221, 1990.
182. Dondero TJ, Curran JW: Excess deaths in Africa from HIV: confirmed and quantified. Lancet 343:989, 1995.
183. Preble EA: Impact of HIV/AIDS on African children. Soc Sci Med 31:671, 1990.
184. DeCock KM, Soro B, Coulibaly I-M, et al: Tuberculosis and HIV infection in sub-Saharan Africa. JAMA 268:1581, 1992.
185. Brown T, Sittirai W, Vanichseni S, et al: The recent epidemiology of HIV and AIDS in Thailand. AIDS 8(suppl 2):S131, 1994.
186. Gangakhedkar RR, Bentley ME, Divikar AD, et al: Spread of HIV infection in married monogamous women in India. JAMA 278:2090, 1997.
187. Kitayaporn D, Uneklabh C, Weniger BG, et al: HIV-1 incidence determined retrospectively among drug users in Bangkok, Thailand. AIDS 8:1443, 1994.
188. Naik TN, Sarkar S, Singh HL, et al: Intravenous drug users: a new high-risk group for HIV infection in India. AIDS 5:117, 1991.
189. Bollinger RC, Tripathy SP, Quinn TC: The human immunodeficiency virus epidemic in India. Medicine (Baltimore) 74:97, 1995.
190. Cheng H, Zhang J, Capizzi J, et al: Introduction of HIV-1 subtype E into Yunnan, China. Lancet 344:953, 1994.
191. Weniger BG, Takebe Y, Ou C-Y, et al: The molecular epidemiology of HIV in Asia. AIDS 8(suppl 2): S13, 1994.
192. Rodrigues JJ, Mehendale SM, Shepherd ME, et al: The biological and behavioral risk factors for prevalent HIV infection in sexually transmitted disease clinics in India. BMJ 311:283, 1995.
193. Mehendale SM, Rodrigues JJ, Brookmeyer RS, et al: Incidence and predictors of human immunodeficiency virus type 1 seroconversion in patients attending sexually transmitted diseases clinics in India. J Infect Dis 172:1486, 1995.
194. Go VF, Srikrishnan AK, Savaram S, et al: High HIV prevalence and risk behaviors in men who have sex with men in Chennai, India. J Acquir Immune Defic Syndr 35:314, 2004.
195. Harries AD: Tuberculosis and human immunodeficiency virus infection in developing countries. Lancet 335:387, 1990.
196. Jain MK, John TJ, Keusch GT: A review of human immunodeficiency virus infection in India. J Acquir Immune Defic Syndr Hum Retrovirol 7:1185, 1994.
197. Kaur A, Babu PG, Jacob M, et al: Clinical and laboratory profile of AIDS in India. J Acquir Immune Defic Syndr Hum Retrovirol 5:883, 1992.

198. Tripathy SP: Tuberculosis and AIDS. Indian J Tuberc 38:49, 1991.
199. Swasdisevi A: Clinical study of HIV disease in the lower area of northern Thailand in 1994. J Med Assoc Thai 77:440, 1994.
200. Cohen J: HIV in Asia: Myanmar. Science 301:5640, 2003.
201. Cohen J: HIV/AIDS in China. Science 304:5676, 2004.
202. Wei X, Chosh SK, Taylor ME, et al: Viral dynamics in human immunodeficiency virus type 1 infection. Nature 373:117, 1995.
203. Ho DD, Neumann AU, Perelson AS, et al: Rapid turnover of plasma virions and CD4 lymphocytes in HIV-1 infection. Nature 373:123, 1995.
204. Graziosi C, Pantaleo G, Butini L, et al: Kinetics of HIV DNA and RNA synthesis during primary HIV-1 infection. Proc Natl Acad Sci USA 90:6505, 1993.
205. Cooper DA, Gold JA, MacLean P, et al: Acute retrovirus infection: definition of a clinical illness associated with seroconversion. Lancet 1:137, 1985.
206. Tindall B, Barker S, Donovan B, et al: Characterization of the acute clinical illness associated with human immunodeficiency virus infection. Arch Intern Med 148:945, 1988.
207. Pantaleo G, Menzo S, Vaccarezza M, et al: Studies in subjects with long-term nonprogressive human immunodeficiency virus infection. N Engl J Med 332:209, 1995.
208. Baltimore D: Lessons from people with nonprogressive HIV infection. N Engl J Med 322:259, 1995.
209. Cao Y, Qin L, Zhang L, et al: Virologic and immunologic characterization of long-term survivors of human immunodeficiency virus type 1 infection. N Engl J Med 322:201, 1995.
210. Anzala OA, Nagelkerke NJ, Bwayo JJ, et al: Rapid progression to disease in African sex workers with human immunodeficiency virus type 1 infection. J Infect Dis 171:686, 1995.
211. Korchhoff F, Greenough TC, Brettler DB, et al: Brief report: absence of intact nef sequences in a long-term survivor with nonprogressive HIV-1 infection. N Engl J Med 332:228, 1995.
212. Saal F, Sidibe S, Alves-Cardoso E, et al: Anti-HIV-2 serological screening in Portuguese populations native from or having had close contact with Africa. AIDS Res Hum Retroviruses 3:341, 1987.
213. Hu DJ, Dondero TJ, Rayfield MA, et al: The emerging genetic diversity of HIV. JAMA 275:210, 1996.
214. Ameisen JC, Capron A: Cell dysfunction and depletion in AIDS: the programmed cell death hypothesis. Immunol Today 12:102, 1991.
215. Groux H, Torpier G, Monte D, et al: Activation-induced death by apoptosis I CD4- cells from human immunodeficiency virus–infected asymptomatic individuals. J Exp Med 175:331, 1992.
216. Sheppard HW, Ascher MS, McRae B, et al: The initial immune response to HIV and immune system activation determine the outcome of HIV disease. J Acquir Immune Defic Syndr Hum Retrovirol 4:704, 1991.
217. Haynes BF, Panteleo G, Fauci AS: Towards an understanding of the correlates of protective and immunity to HIV infection. Science 271:324, 1996.
218. Burke DS: Human HIV vaccine trials: does antibody-dependent enhancement pose a genuine risk? Perspect Biol Med 35:511, 1992.
219. Mascola JR, Mathieson BJ, Zack PH, et al: Summary report: workshop on the potential risks of antibody-dependent enhancement in human HIV vaccine trials. AIDS Res Hum Retroviruses 9:1175, 1993.
220. Koup RA, Safrit JT, Cao Y, et al: Temporal association of cellular immune responses with the initial control of viremia in primary human immunodeficiency virus type 1 syndrome. J Virol 68:4650, 1994.
221. Borrow P, Lewicki H, Hahn BH, et al: Virus-specific CD8- cytotoxic T-lymphocyte activity associated with control of viremia in primary human immunodeficiency virus type 1 infection. J Virol 68:6103, 1994.
222. Paul WE: Can the immune response control HIV infection? Cell 82:177, 1995.
223. Bryson YJ, Pang S, Wei LS, et al: Clearance of HIV infection in a perinatally infected infant. N Engl J Med 332:833, 1995.
224. Shafferman A, Jahrling PB, Benveniste RE, et al: Protection of macaques with a simian immunodeficiency virus envelope peptide vaccine based on conserved human immunodeficiency virus type 1 sequences. Proc Natl Acad Sci USA 88:7126, 1991.
225. Embretson J, Zupancic M, Ribas JL, et al: Massive covert infection of helper T lymphocytes and macrophages by HIV during the incubation period of AIDS. Nature 362:359, 1993.
226. Smith KJ, Skelton HG, Yeager J, et al: Clinical features of inflammatory dermatoses in human immunodeficiency virus type 1 disease and their correlation with Walter Reed stage. J Am Acad Dermatol 28:167, 1993.
227. Valle S-L: Dermatologic findings related to human immunodeficiency virus infection in high-risk individuals. J Am Acad Dermatol 17:951, 1987.
228. Feigal DW, Katz MH, Greenspan D, et al: The prevalence of oral lesions in HIV-infected homosexual and bisexual men: three San Francisco epidemiology cohorts. AIDS 5:519, 1991.
229. 1993 revised classification system for HIV infection and expanded surveillance case definition for AIDS among adolescents and adults. MMWR 41:1, 1992.
230. Albrecht H: Redefining AIDS: Towards a modification of the current AIDS case definition. Clin Infect Dis 24:64, 1997.
231. Greenberg AE, Nsa W, Ryder RW, et al: *Plasmodium falciparum* malaria and perinatally acquired human immunodeficiency virus type 1 infection in Kinshasa, Zaire: A prospective, longitudinal cohort study of 587 children. N Engl J Med 325:105, 1991.
232. Pepin J, Ethier L, Kazadi C, et al: The impact of human immunodeficiency virus infection on the epidemiology and treatment of *Trypanosoma brucei gambiense* sleeping sickness in Nioki, Zaire. Am J Trop Med Hyg 47:133, 1992.
233. Kaplan JE, Hu DJ, Holmes HK, et al: Preventing opportunistic infections in HIV infected persons: implications for the developing world. Am J Trop Med Hyg 55:1, 1996.
234. Lucas SB, DeCock KM, Hounnou A, et al: Contribution of tuberculosis to slim disease in Africa. BMJ 308:1531, 1994.
235. Loussert-Ajakka I, Ly TD, Chaix ML, et al: HIV-1/HIV-2 seronegativity in HIV-1 subtype O infected patients. Lancet 343:1393, 1994.
236. Schable C, Zekeng L, Pau C-P, et al: Sensitivity of United States HIV antibody tests for detection of HIV-1 group O infections. Lancet 344:1333, 1994.
237. Interpretation and use of the Western blot assay for serodiagnosis of human immunodeficiency virus type 1 infections. MMWR 38:1, 1989.
238. Midthun K, Garrison L, Clements ML, et al: Frequency of indeterminate Western blot tests in healthy adults at low risk for human immunodeficiency virus infection. J Infect Dis 162:1379, 1990.
239. Genesca J, Shih JW, Jett B, et al: What do Western blot indeterminate patterns for human immunodeficiency virus mean in EIA-negative blood donors? Lancet 2:1023, 1989.
240. Hausler WJ Jr: Report of the Third Consensus Conference on HIV Testing sponsored by the Association of State and Territorial Public Health Laboratory Directors. Infect Control Hosp Epidemiol 9:345, 1988.
241. Burke DS, Fowler AK, Redfield RR, et al: Isolation of HIV-1 from the blood of seropositive adults: patient stage of illness and sample inoculum size are major determinants of positive culture. AIDS 3:1159, 1990.
242. Dewar RL, Sarmiento MD, Lawton ES, et al: Isolation of HIV-1 from plasma of infected individuals: an analysis of experimental conditions affecting successful virus propagation. J Acquir Immune Defic Syndr Hum Retrovirol 5:822, 1992.
243. Eyster ME, Ballard JO, Gail MH, et al: Predictive markers for the acquired immunodeficiency syndrome (AIDS) in hemophiliacs: persistence of p24 antigen and low T4 cell count. Ann Intern Med 110:963, 1989.
244. Hofmann B, Bygbjerg I, Dickmeiss E, et al: Prognostic value of immunologic abnormalities and HIV antigenemia in asymptomatic HIV-infected individuals: proposal of immunologic staging. Scand J Infect Dis 21:633, 1989.
245. Nishanian P, Huskins KR, Stehn S, et al: A simple method for improved assay demonstrates that HIV p24 antigen is present as immune complexes in most sera from HIV-infected individuals. J Infect Dis 162:21, 1990.
246. Kestens L, Hoofd G, Gigase PI, et al: HIV antigen detection in circulating immune complexes. J Virol Methods 31:67, 1991.
247. Ou CY, Kwok S, Mitchell SW, et al: DNA amplification for direct detection of HIV-1 in DNA of peripheral blood mononuclear cells. Science 239:295, 1988.
248. Bagnarelli P, Menzo S, Manzin A, et al: Detection of human immunodeficiency virus type 1 genomic RNA in plasma samples by reverse transcription–polymerase chain reaction. J Med Virol 34:89, 1991.

249. Menzo S, Bagnarelli P, Giacca M, et al: Alsolute quantitation of viremia in human immunodeficiency virus infection by competitive reverse transcription and polymerase chain reaction. J Clin Microbiol 30:1752, 1992.
250. Dewar RL, Highbarger HC, Sarmiento MD, et al: Application of branched DNA signal amplification to monitor human immunodeficiency virus type 1 burden in human plasma. J Infect Dis 170:1172, 1994.
251. Wong MT, Dolan MJ, Kozlow E, et al: Patterns of virus burden and T-cell phenotype are established early and are correlated with the rate of disease progression in human immunodeficiency virus type 1–infected persons. J Infect Dis 173:877, 1996.
252. Lin HJ, Myers LE, Yen-Leiberman E, et al: Multicenter evaluation of quantification methods for plasma human immunodeficiency virus type 1 RNA. J Infect Dis 170:553, 1994.
253. Moss AR, Bacchetti P, Osmond D, et al: Seropositivity for HIV and the development of AIDS or AIDS-related condition: three year follow up of the San Francisco General Hospital Cohort. BMJ 296:745, 1988.
254. Goedert JJ, Kessler CM, Aledort LM, et al: A prospective study of human immunodeficiency virus type 1 infection and the development of AIDS in subjects with hemophilia. N Engl J Med 321:1141, 1989.
255. Redfield RR, Wright DC, Tramont EC: The Walter Reed staging system for HTLV-III/LAV infection. N Engl J Med 31:314, 1986.
256. McLeod G, Hammer S: Zidovudine: Five years later. Ann Intern Med 117:487, 1992.
257. Volberding PA, Lagakos SW, Koch MA, et al: Zidovudine in asymptomatic human immunodeficiency virus infection: a controlled trial in persons with fewer than 500 CD4 positive cells per cubic millimeter. N Engl J Med 322:941, 1990.
258. Johnson V: Nucleoside reverse transcriptase inhibitors and resistance of human immunodeficiency virus type 1. J Infect Dis 17(suppl):S140, 1995.
259. Saag M, Emini E, Laskin O, et al: A short-term clinical evaluation of L-697,661, a non-nucleoside inhibitor of HIV-1 reverse transcriptase. N Engl J Med 329:1065, 1993.
260. Sande M, Carpenter C, Cobbs C, et al: Antiretroviral therapy for adult HIV infected patients: recommendations from a state-of-the-art conference. JAMA 271:1830, 1994.
261. Miller M, Jaskolski M, Rao JKM, et al: Crystal structure of a retroviral protease proves relationship to aspartic protease family. Nature 337:576, 1989.
262. Wlodawer A, Erickson JW: Structure based inhibitors of HIV-1 protease. Annu Rev Biochem 62:543, 1993.
263. Raguin G, Chene G, Mourand-Joubert L, et al, for the Puzzle 1 Study Group: Salvage therapy with amprenavir, lopinavir, and ritonavir 200 mg/d or 400 mg/d in HIV-infected patients in virological failure. Antivir Ther 9:615, 2004.
264. Johnson M, Grinsztejn B, Rodriguez C, et al: Atazanavir plus ritonavir or saquinavir, and lopinavir/ritonavir in patients experiencing multiple virological failures. AIDS 19:685, 2005.
265. Pomerantz RJ, Horn DL: Twenty years of therapy for HIV-1 infection. Nature Med 9:867, 2003.
266. Lane HC, Davey V, Kovacs JA, et al: Interferon-alpha in patients with asymptomatic human immunodeficiency virus (HIV) infection: a randomized, placebo-controlled trial. Ann Intern Med 112:805, 1990.
267. Groopman JE, Gottlieb MS, Goodman J, et al: Recombinant alpha-2 interferon therapy for Kaposi's sarcoma associated with the acquired immunodeficiency syndrome. Ann Intern Med 100:671, 1984.
268. Kovacs JA, Baseler M, Dewar RJ, et al: Increases in CD4 T lymphocytes with intermittent courses of interleukin-2 in patients with human immunodeficiency virus infection: a preliminary study. N Engl J Med 332:567, 1995.
269. Yeni PG, Hammer SM, Hirsch MS, et al: Treatment for adult HIV infection: 2004 recommendations of the International AIDS Society—USA panel. JAMA 292:2, 2004.
270. Carpenter CJ, Fishl MA, Hammer SM, et al: Antiretroviral therapy for HIV infection in 1998: updated recommendations of the International AIDS Society—USA panel. JAMA 280:78, 1998.
271. Richman DD: Resistance of clinical isolates of human immunodeficiency virus to antiretroviral agents. Antimicrob Agents Chemother 37:1207, 1993.
272. Condra JH, Schleif WA, Blahy OM, et al: In vivo emergence of HIV-1 variants resistant to multiple protease inhibitors. Nature 374:569, 1995.
273. Huang H, Chopra R, Verdine GL, Harrison SC: Structure of a covalently trapped catalytic complex of HIV-1 reverse transcriptase: implications for drug resistance. Science 282:1669, 1998.
274. Sarafianos SG, Das K, Clark AD, et al: Lamivudine (3TC) resistance in HIV-1 reverse transcriptase involves steric hindrance with beta-branched amino acids. Proc Natl Acad Sci USA 96:10027, 1999.
275. Doyon L, Croteau G, Thibeault D, et al: Second locus involved in human immunodeficiency virus type 1 resistance to protease inhibitors. J Virol 70:3763, 1996.
276. Zhang YM, Imamichi H, Imamichi T, et al: Drug resistance during indinavir therapy is caused by mutations in the protease gene and in its Gag substrate cleavage sites. J Virol 71:6662, 1997.
277. Cote HC, Brumme ZL, Harrigan PR: Human immunodeficiency virus type 1: protease cleavage site mutations associated with protease inhibitor cross-resistance selected by indinavir, ritonavir, and/or saquinavir. J Virol 75:589, 2001.
278. Erickson JW, Gulnik SV, Markowitz M: Protease inhibitors: resistance, cross-resistance, fitness and the choice of initial and salvage therapies. AIDS 13(suppl A):S189, 1999.
279. Miller V: Resistance to protease inhibitors. J Acquir Immune Defic Syndr 26(suppl 1):S34, 2001.
280. Deng Z, Ribas JL, Gibson DW, et al: Infections caused by *Penicillium marneffei* in China and Southeast Asia: review of eighteen published cases and report of four more Chinese cases. Rev Infect Dis 10:640, 1988.
281. Fischl MA, Dickinson GM, LaVoie L: Safety and efficacy of sulfamethoxazole and trimethoprim chemoprophylaxis for *Pneumocystis carinii* pneumonia in AIDS. JAMA 259:1185, 1988.
282. Chintu C, Bhat GJ, Walker AS, et al: Co-trimoxazole as prophylaxis against opportunistic infections in HIV-infected Zambian children (CHAP): a double-blind randomised placebo-controlled trial. Lancet 365:749, 2005.
283. Mermin J, Lule J, Ekwaru JP, et al: Effect of co-trimoxazole prophylaxis on morbidity, mortality, CD4-cell count, and viral load in HIV infection in rural Uganda. Lancet 364:1428, 2004.
284 Masur H, Kaplan JE, Holmes KK: USPHS/IDSA guidelines for preventing opportunistic infections—2002. Recommendations of the US Public Health Service and the Infectious Disease Society of America. Ann Intern Med 137:435, 2002.
285. Pape JW, Jean SS, Ho JL, et al: Effect of isoniazid prophylaxis on incidence of active tuberculosis and progression of HIV infection. Lancet 342:268, 1993.
286. DeCock KM, Grant A, Porter JD: Preventive therapy for tuberculosis in HIV-infected persons: international recommendations, research, and practice. Lancet 345:833, 1995.
287. Higgins DL, Galavotti C, O'Reilly KR, et al: Evidence for the effects of HIV antibody counseling and testing on risk behaviors. JAMA 266:2419, 1991.
288. McCusker J, Stoddard AM, Mayer KH, et al: Effects of HIV antibody test knowledge on subsequent sexual behaviors in a cohort of homosexually active men. Am J Public Health 78:462, 1988.
289. Otten MW, Zaida AA, Wroten JE, et al: Changes in sexually transmitted disease rates after HIV testing and posttest counseling, Miami, 1988 to 1989. Am J Public Health 83:529, 1993.
290. Kelly JA, Murphy DA, Sikkema KJ, et al: Psychological interventions to prevent HIV infection are urgently needed: new priorities for behavioral research in the second decade of AIDS. Am Psychol 48:1023, 1993.
291. Kelly JA, St. Lawrence JS, Hood HV, et al: Behavioral intervention to reduce AIDS risk activities. J Consult Clin Psychol 57:60, 1989.
292. Des Jarlais DC, Friedman SR: AIDS and the use of injected drugs. Sci Am 270:82, 1994.
293. Walker MC, Fast PE, Graham B, et al: Phase I/II preventive vaccine trials. AIDS Res Hum Retroviruses 11:1279, 1995.
294. Burke DS: Review: Human trials of experimental HIV vaccines. AIDS 9(suppl):S171, 1995.
295. Funds Committed and Dispersed. Geneva, Global Fund to Fight AIDS, Tuberculosis and Malaria, 2004. Available at http://www.theglobalfund.org.
296. Bush GW: State of the Union address, January 28, 2003. Available at http://www.whitehouse.gov/news/releases/2003/01/20030128-19.html. Accessed 10/04/04.
297. Teixeira PR, Vitoria MA, Barcarolo J: Antiretroviral treatment in resource-poor settings: the Brazilian experience. AIDS 18(suppl 3): S5, 2004.

298. Guidelines for the use of antiretroviral agents in HIV-1-infected adults and adolescents. Rockville, Md., Department of Health and Human Services, October 29, 2004. Available at http://www.aidsinfo.nih.gov/guidelines/adult/AA_102904.pdf. Accessed 11/01/04.
299. Florence E, Dreezen C, Schrooten W, et al: The role of non-viral load surrogate markers in HIV-positive patient monitoring during antiviral treatment. Int J STD AIDS. 8:538, 2004.
300. Adje C, Cheingson R, Roels TH, et al: High prevalence of genotypic and phenotypic HIV-1 drug-resistant strains among patients receiving antiretroviral therapy in Abidjan, Côte d'Ivoire. J Acquir Immune Defic Syndr 26:501, 2001.
301. Vergne L, Malonga-Mouellet G, Mistoul I, et al: Resistance to antiretroviral treatment in Gabon: need for implementation of guidelines on antiretroviral therapy use and HIV-1 drug resistance monitoring in developing countries. J Acquir Immune Defic Syndr 29:165, 2002.
302. Richard N, Juntilla M, Abraha A, et al: High prevalence of antiretroviral resistance in treated Ugandans infected with non-subtype B human immunodeficiency virus type 1. AIDS Res Hum Retroviruses 20:355, 2004.
303. Koenig SP, Leandre F, Farmer PE, et al: Scaling-up HIV treatment programmes in resource-limited settings: the rural Haiti experience. AIDS 18(suppl 3):S21, 2004.
304. Teixeira PR, Vitoria MA, Barcarolo J: Antiretroviral treatment in resource-poor settings: the Brazilian experience. AIDS 18(suppl 3):S5.
305. Praphan P: Antiretroviral treatment in resource-poor settings: what can we learn from the existing programs in Thailand? AIDS 18(suppl 3):S33, 2004.
306. Weidle PJ, Malamba S, Mwebaze R, et al: Asessment of a pilot antiretroviral drug therapy programme in Uganda: patients' response, survival, and drug resistance. Lancet 360:34, 2002.
307. Laurent C, Diakhate N, Gueye NF, et al: The Senegalese government's highly active antiretroviral therapy initiative: an 18-month follow-up study. AIDS 16:1363, 2002.
308. Coetzee D, Boulle A, Hildebrand K, et al: Promoting adherence to antiretroviral therapy: the experience from a primary care setting in Khayelitsha, South Africa. AIDS 18(suppl 3):S27, 2004.
309. Badri M, Wilson D, Wood R: Effect of highly active antiretroviral therapy on incidence of tuberculosis in South Africa: a cohort study. Lancet 2002;359:2059.

Q

R

U

V

Tropical Infectious Diseases

Tropical Infectious Diseases

Principles, Pathogens, & Practice

SECOND EDITION

Richard L. Guerrant, MD

Thomas H. Hunter Professor of International Medicine
Director, Center for Global Health
Division of Infectious Diseases and International Health
University of Virginia School of Medicine
Charlottesville, Virginia

David H. Walker, MD

Carmage and Martha Walls Distinguished Chair of Tropical Diseases
Professor and Chairman, Department of Pathology
Director, WHO Collaborating Center for Tropical Diseases
Executive Director
Center for Biodefense and Emerging Infectious Diseases
University of Texas Medical Branch
Galveston, Texas

Peter F. Weller, MD

Professor of Medicine
Harvard Medical School
Co-Chief, Infectious Disease Division
Vice Chair of Research
Department of Medicine
Beth Israel Deaconess Medical Center
Boston, Massachusetts

CHURCHILL LIVINGSTONE

ELSEVIER

ELSEVIER
CHURCHILL
LIVINGSTONE

1600 John F. Kennedy Boulevard
Suite 1800
Philadelphia, PA 19103-2899

TROPICAL INFECTIOUS DISEASES
Principles, Pathogens, & Practice
Second Edition

ISBN 13: 9780443066689
ISBN 10: 0-443-06668-X
Volume 1 Part Number: 9996003310
Volume 2 Part Number: 999600337X

Notice

Knowledge and best practice in this field are constantly changing. As new research and experience broaden our knowledge, changes in practice, treatment and drug therapy may become necessary or appropriate. Readers are advised to check the most current information provided (i) on procedures featured or (ii) by the manufacturer of each product to be administered, to verify the recommended dose or formula, the method and duration of administration, and contraindications. It is the responsibility of the practitioner, relying on his or her own experience and knowledge of the patient, to make diagnoses, to determine dosages and the best treatment for each individual patient, and to take all appropriate safety precautions. To the fullest extent of the law, neither the publisher nor the Editors assume any liability for any injury and/or damage to persons or property arising out or related to any use of the material contained in this book.

Previous edition copyrighted 1999.

ISBN 13: 9780443066689
ISBN 10: 0-443-06668-X

Acquisitions Editor: Tom Hartman
Developmental Editor: Ann Ruzycka Anderson
Project Manager: Cecelia Bayruns
Design Direction: Ellen Zanolle
Cover Designer: Andy Chapman
Marketing Manager: Megan Carr

Printed in the United States of America.

Last digit is the print number: 9 8 7 6 5 4 3 2

CONTRIBUTORS

Saad H. Abdalla, Mb,Bs (Khartoum); LRCP, MRCS, FRCPath
Senior Lecturer, Department of Haematology, Imperial College London; Honorary Consultant, Department of Haematology, St. Mary's Hospital, London, United Kingdom
Approach to the Patient in the Tropics with Anemia

Ban Mishu Allos, MD
Assistant Professor of Medicine and Preventive Medicine, Division of Infectious Diseases, Department of Medicine; Assistant Professor, Department of Preventive Medicine, Vanderbilt University School of Medicine, Nashville, TN
Campylobacter *Infections*

Jon Kim Andrus, MD
Chief, Immunization Unit, Family and Community Health, Pan American Health Organization, Washington, DC
Measles

Juanita Angel, MD, PhD
Associate Professor, Instituto de Genética Humana, Pontificia Universidad Javeriana, Bogotá, Columbia
Rotavirus Infections

Gregory M. Anstead, MD, PhD
Assistant Professor, Department of Medicine, University of Texas Health Science Center; Staff Physician, Department of Medicine, University Health System; Staff Physician, Department of Medicine, South Texas Veterans Healthcare System, San Antonio, TX
Histoplasmosis, Blastomycosis, Coccidioidomycosis, and Cryptococcosis; Paracoccidioidomycosis; Penicillioisis Marneffei

Eurico Arruda, MD, PhD
Professor of Microbiology, Department of Cell and Molecular Biology, University of Sao Paulo School of Medicine, Ribeirao Preto, Sao Paulo, Brazil
Respiratory Tract Viral Infections

Ray R. Arthur, PhD
Associate Director for Global Health, National Center for Infectious Diseases, National Centers for Disease Control and Prevention, Atlanta, GA
Surveillance for Emerging Infectious Diseases and Bioterrorism Threats

Paul S. Auerbach, MD, MS, FACEP
Clinical Professor of Surgery, Division of Emergency Medicine, Department of Surgery; Attending Physician, Emergency Medicine, Stanford University Medical Center, Stanford, CA
Animal Poisons in the Tropics; Travel-Related Health Concerns Associated with Extremes of Environment

Ronald C. Ballard, MIBiol, PhD
Chief, Laboratory Reference and Research Branch, Division of STD Prevention, Centers for Disease Control and Prevention, Atlanta, GA
Chlamydia trachomatis *Infections of the Gential Tract (Oculogenital Infections and Lymphogranuloma Venerum)*

Alan G. Barbour, MD
Professor of Medicine and Microbiology and Molecular Genetics, Department of Microbiology and Molecular Genetics and Medicine, University of California at Irvine, Irvine, CA
Relapsing Fever and Other Borrelia *Diseases*

Michele Barry, MD, FACP
Professor of Medicine and Global Health, Department of Medicine and Epidemiology and Public Health, Yale University; Firm Chief, Generalist Firm, Yale–New Haven Hospital, New Haven, CT
Ascariasis

Dan Bausch, MD, MPH&TM
Associate Professor, Department of Tropical Medicine, Tulane School of Public Health and Tropical Medicine; Associate Professor, Department of Medicine, Section of Infectious Diseases, Tulane University Medical Center, New Orleans, LA
Arenavirus Infections

John E. Bennett, MD, MACP
Head, Clinical Mycology Section, Laboratory of Clinical Investigation, National Institute of Allergy and Infectious Diseases; Clinical Center, National Institutes of Health, Bethesda, MD
Entomophthoramycosis, Lobomycosis, Rhinosporidiosis, and Sporotrichosis

Steven L. Berk, MD
Professor of Medicine/Family Medicine and Mirick-Myers Endowed Chair in Geriatric Medicine, Regional Dean, School of Medicine; Internal Medicine and Family Medicine, Texas Tech University Health Sciences Center, Amarillo, TX
Strongyloidiasis

Pascal O. Bessong, BSc (Hons), MSc, PhD
Lecturer, Department of Microbiology, University of Venda for Science and Technology, Thohoyandou, Limpopo Province, South Africa; Research Fellow, Center for Global Health and Myles H. Thaler Center for AIDS and Human Retrovirus Research, University of Virginia, Charlottesville, VA
Human Retroviral Infections in the Tropics

Frank J. Bia, MD, MPH, FACP
Professor of Medicine and Laboratory Medicine, Co-Director, International Health Program, Department of Medicine, Yale School of Medicine, New Haven, CT
Neurologic Disease

Robert E. Black, MD, MPH
Edgar Berman Professor and Chair, Department of International Health, Johns Hopkins University, Baltimore, MD
Nutrition and Miconutrients in Tropical Infectious Diseases

Martin J. Blaser, MD, MACP
Frederick H. King Professor and Chair, Department of Medicine, New York University School of Medicine; Director, Medical Service, Bellevue Hospital Center; Director, Medical Service, Tisch Hospital (NYU Medical Center); Staff Physician, Medical Service, New York Harbor Veterans Affairs Medical Center, New York, NY
Campylobacter *Infections*

Thomas P. Bleck, MD, FACP, FCCM, FCCP, FIDSA, FAAN
The Louise Nerancy Eminent Scholar in Neurology and Professor of Neurology, Neurological Surgery, and Internal Medicine; Director, Neuroscience Intensive Care Unit, Department of Neurology, University of Virginia, Charlottesville, VA
Tetanus; Rabies; Neurologic Disease

David A. Bobak, MD
Associate Professor of Medicine, Division of Infectious Diseases, Department of Medicine, Case Western Reserve University School of Medicine; Staff Physician and Director, Traveler's Healthcare Clinic, Department of Medicine, Case Medical Center/University Hospitals of Cleveland; Staff Physician, Department of Medicine, Louis B. Stokes VA Medical Center, Cleveland, OH
Enteric Clostridium *Infections; Travel-Related Health Concerns Associated with Extremes of Environment*

Luciana L. Borio, MD
Assistant Professor, Department of Medicine, University of Pittsburgh, Pittsburgh, PA; Assistant Professor, Department of Medicine, Johns Hopkins University; Center for Biosecurity of the University of Pittsburgh Medical Center, Baltimore, MD
Smallpox and Monkeypox

Michael D. Bowen, MSc, PhD
Microbiologist, Bioterrorism Rapid Response and Advanced Technology Laboratory, Bioterrorism Preparedness and Response Program, National Center for Infectious Diseases, Centers for Disease Control and Prevention, Atlanta, GA
Arenavirus Infections

Joseph S. Bresee, MD, FAAP
Assistant Professor, Department of Family and Preventive Medicine, Emory University School of Medicine; Lead, Epidemiology Team, Respiratory and Enteric Virus Branch, Division of Viral and Rickettsial Diseases, National Center for Infectious Diseases, Centers for Disease Control and Prevention, Atlanta, GA
Astrovirus, Enteric Adenovirus, and Other Gastroenteritis Viruses

Enrico Brunetti, MD
Assistant Professor, Division of Infectious and Tropical Diseases, Pavia University; Attending Physician, Division of Infectious and Tropical Diseases, IRCCS S. Matteo, Pavia, Italy
Echinococcosis

Fabrizio Bruschi, MD
Professor of Parasitology, Department of Experimental Pathology, MBIE, Università di Pisa, Pisa, Italy
Trichinellosis

Oluma Yoseph Bushen, MD
Fellow, Infectious Disease, Center for Global Health, Division of Infectious Diseases and International Health, University of Virginia, Charlottesville, VA
Cryptosporidiosis

Carlos C. Campbell, MD
Director, Arizona Area Health Education Center, Health Sciences Center, University of Arizona, Tucson, AZ
Malaria

Martin S. Cetron, MD
Director, Department of Global Migration and Quarantine, Centers for Disease Control and Prevention; Adjunct Associate Professor of Medicine, Division of Infectious Diseases, Department of Medicine, Emory University School of Medicine; Adjunct Assistant Professor of Epidemiology, Department of Epidemiology, Rollins School of Public Health, Emory University, Atlanta, GA
Migrant, Immigrant, and Refugee Health

Thomas Cherian, MB, BS, DCH, MD
Scientist, Initiative for Vaccine Research, World Health Organization, Geneva, Switzerland
Haemophilus influenzae *(Including* H. aegyptius*) Infection*

Otavio L. Cintra, MD
Department of Pediatrics, University of Sao Paulo School of Medicine at Ribeirao Preto, Ribeirao Preto, Sao Paulo, Brazil
Respiratory Tract Viral Infections

Richard F. Clark, MD, FACEP, FACMT
Professor, Department of Medicine, University of California at San Diego; Director, Division of Medical Toxicology, UCSD Medical Center; Medical Director, San Diego Division, California Poison Control System, San Diego, CA
Plant Toxins in the Tropics

Myron S. Cohen, MD
J. Herbert Bate Distinguished Professor of Medicine, Microbiology, Immunology and Public Health, Chief, Infectious Diseases, Director, Center for Infectious Diseases, Department of Medicine, University of North Carolina at Chapel Hill; UNC Health Care Systems, Chapel Hill, NC
Sexually Transmitted and Urinary Tract Infections

Robert Colebunders, MD, PhD
Professor of Tropical Diseases, Department of Clinical Sciences, Institute of Tropical Medicine; Professor of Infectious Diseases, Department of Medicine, University of Antwerp, Antwerp, Belgium
Approach to the Patient with HIV and Coinfecting Tropical Infectious Diseases

Ed Cooper, MD, FRCP, FAAP
Clinical Consultant, Partnership for Child Development, Department of Infectious Disease Epidemiology, Imperial College of Science, Technology and Medicine, London, United Kingdom
Trichuriasis

Christina M. Coyle, MD, MS
Associate Professor of Medicine, Department of Medicine, Albert Einstein College of Medicine; Director of Clinical Infectious Disease, Department of Medicine, Jacobi Hospital, Bronx, NY
Cysticercosis

D.W.T. Crompton, OBE, MA, ScD, FRSE
Professor, Institute of Biomedical and Life Sciences, University of Glasgow, Glasgow, Scotland, United Kingdom
Ascariasis

John H. Cross, PhD
Professor, Department of Preventive Medicine and Biometrics, Uniformed Services University of the Health Sciences, Bethesda, MD
Liver, Lung, and Intestinal Fluke Infections

Markus Czub, DVM, PhD
Adjunct Professor, Department of Medical Microbiology, University of Manitoba; Canadian Science Centre for Human and Animal Health, Winnipeg, Manitoba, Canada
Nipah and Hendra Viral Infections

Johanna P. Daily, MD
Harvard School of Public Health, Boston, MA
Hepatobiliary Disease

David Allan Brett Dance, HB, CLB, MSc, FRCPath
Consultant Microbiologist, Derriford Hospital; Regional Microbiologist (Southwest), Health Protection Agency, Plymouth, Devon, United Kingdom
Melioidosis

Mustapha A. Danesi, MB, FRCPI, FMCP, FWACP
Professor, Department of Medicine, College of Medicine, University of Lagos; Consultant Physician and Neurologist, Clinical Department of Medicine, Lagos University Teaching Hospital, Lagos, Lagos State, Nigeria
Neurologic Disease

Chandler R. Dawson, MD
Professor, F.I. Proctor Foundation, Professor, Department of Ophthalmology, University of California, San Francisco, San Francisco, CA
Trachoma

Catherine de Martel, MD, MS
Department of Health Research and Policy, Stanford University School of Medicine, Stanford, CA
Tropical Infectious Diseases and Malignancy

David T. Dennis, MD, MPH, DCMT
Faculty Affiliate, Department of Microbiology, Immunology, and Pathology, Colorado State University; Guest Researcher, Consultant, Division of Vector-Borne Infectious Diseases, Centers for Disease Control and Prevention, Fort Collins, CO
Plague

Ciro A. de Quadros, MD, MPH
Director, International Programs, Albert B. Sabin Vaccine Institute, Washington, DC
Measles

Rebecca Dillingham, MD
Fellow, Center for Global Health, Division of Infectious Disease and International Medicine, University of Virginia Health System, Charlottesville, VA
Social and Cultural Factors in Tropical Medicine: Reframing Our Understanding of Disease; Cyclospora, Isospora, *and* Sarcosystis *Infections*

John E. Donelson, PhD
Professor, Department of Biochemistry, University of Iowa, Iowa City, IA
African Trypanosomiasis (Sleeping Sickness)

J. Stephen Dumler, MD
Professor of Pathology, Division of Medical Microbiology, Department of Pathology, Professor, Cellular and Molecular Medicine Program, The Johns Hopkins University School of Medicine; Associate Director, Division of Medical Microbiology, Department of Pathology, The Johns Hopkins Hospital; Professor, Department of Molecular Microbiology and Immunology, The Johns Hopkins University Bloomberg School of Public Health, Baltimore, MD
Ehrlichioses and Anaplasmosis

Herbert L. DuPont, MD, FACP
Professor of Epidemiology, Department of Epidemiology, University of Texas, School of Public Health; Director, Center for Infectious Disease, University of Texas–Houston,

School of Public Health; Clinical Professor, Department of Medicine, Baylor College of Medicine; Chief, Internal Medicine, Department of Internal Medicine, St. Luke's Episcopal Hospital, Houston, TX
Gastrointestinal Symptoms

Marlene Durand, MD
Assistant Professor, Department of Medicine, Harvard Medical School; Associate Physician, Infectious Disease Unit, Department of Medicine, Massachusetts General Hospital; Director, Infectious Disease Service, Massachusetts Eye and Ear Infirmary, Boston, MA
Ocular Disease

Mark L. Eberhard, PhD
Director, Division of Parasitic Diseases, Centers for Disease Control, Atlanta, GA
Zoonotic Filariasis

Charles Edwards, MB, BS, FRCPC, FACP
Department Head, Department of Medicine, Queen Elizabeth Hospital, St. Michael, Barbados
Leptospirosis

Rachel Barwick Eidex, PhD
Epidemiologist, Division of Global Migration and Quarantine, Centers for Disease Control and Prevention, Atlanta, GA
Yellow Fever

Jerrold J. Ellner, MD, FACP
Professor and Chair, Department of Medicine, University of Medicine and Dentistry of New Jersey/New Jersey Medical School; Professor and Chair, Department of Medicine, University Hospitals, Newark, NJ
Tuberculosis and Atypical Myobacterial Infections

Delia A. Enria, MD, MPH
Director, Instituto Nacional de Enfermedades Virales Humanas, Pergamino, Argentina
Arenavirus Infections

Judith E. Epstein, MD
Assistant Professor, Department of Pediatrics, Uniformed Services University of the Health Sciences; Affiliate Staff, Pediatric Infectious Diseases, National Naval Medical Center, Bethesda, MD; Affiliate Staff, Pediatric Infectious Diseases, Walter Reed Army Medical Center; Director, Malaria Program Clinical Trials, Naval Medical Research Center, Silver Spring, MD
Typhoid Fever

Paul E. Farmer, MD, PhD
Presley Professor of Medical Anthropology, Department of Social Medicine, Harvard Medical School; Chief, Division of Social Medicine and Health Inequalities, Brigham and Women's Hospital; Founding Director, Partners in Health, Boston, MA
Social and Cultural Factors in Tropical Medicine: Reframing Our Understanding of Disease

Heinz Feldmann, MD
Associate Professor, Department of Medical Microbiology, University of Manitoba; Head, Special Pathogens Program, Public Health Agency of Canada, Winnipeg, Manitoba, Canada
Filovirus Infections

Ramon Flick, PhD
Assistant Professor, Center for Biodefense and Emerging Infectious Diseases and WHO Collaborating Center for Tropical Diseases, Department of Pathology, University of Texas Medical Branch, Galveston, TX
Nipah and Hendra Viral Infections; Arenavirus Infections; Bunyaviral Fevers: Rift Valley Fever and Crimean-Congo Hemorrhagic Fever

Kimberley K. Fox, MD, MPH
Adjunct Assistant Professor, Department of Medicine, Emory University, Atlanta, GA; Chief, Asia Regional Activities, Global AIDS Program, US Centers for Disease Control and Prevention, Bangkok, Thailand
Sexually Transmitted and Urinary Tract Infections

Manuel Franco, MD, PhD
Associate Professor, Instituto de Genética Humana, Pontificia Universidad Javeriana, Bogotá, Colombia
Rotavirus Infections

David O. Freedman, MD
Professor of Medicine and Public Health, Division of Geographic Medicine, University of Alabama at Birmingham; Director, UAB Travelers Health Clinic, UAB Health System; Director, Gorgas Course in Clinical Tropical Medicine in Lima, Peru, Gorgas Memorial Institute, Birmingham, AL
Onchocerciasis

Hector H. Garcia, MD, PhD
Associate Professor, Department of Microbiology, Universidad Peruana Cayetano Heredia; Head, Cysticercosis Unit, Instituto de Ciencias Neurologicas, Lima, Peru
Cysticercosis

Robert M. Genta, MD, DTM&H, FACG
Professor and Chair, Department of Pathology, University of Geneva School of Medicine, Geneva, Switzerland
Strongyloidiasis

Robert H. Gilman, MD, DTM&H
Professor, Department of International Health, Johns Hopkins University, Baltimore, MD
Helicobacter pylori *Infections*

Roger I. Glass, MD, PhD
Chief, Viral Gastroenteritis Section, Centers for Disease Control and Prevention, Atlanta, GA
Astrovirus, Enteric Adenovirus, and Other Gastroenteritis Viruses

Jerome Goddard, PhD
Assistant Professor of Medicine, Department of Medicine, The University of Mississippi Medical Center; State Medical Entomologist, General Environmental Services, Mississippi Department of Health, Jackson, MS
Arthropods, Tongue Worms, Leeches, and Arthropod-borne Diseases

Eduardo Gotuzzo, MD, FACP
Director, Instituto de Medicina Tropical "Alexander von Humboldt," Universidad Peruana Cayetano Heredia; Chief, Department of Infectious Diseases, Tropical Medicine and Dermatology, Hospital Nacional Cayetano Heredia, Lima, Peru
Cholera Infections; Brucellosis; Gastrointestinal Symptoms; Tropical Infectious Disease Concerns in Pregnancy

Bruno P. Granwehr, MD
Fellow, Division of Infectious Diseases, Department of Internal Medicine, University of Texas Medical Branch; Masters Student, Clinical Science Graduate Program, Department of Preventive Medicine and Community Health, Graduate School of Biomedical Sciences, University of Texas Medical Branch, Galveston, TX
Japanese Encephalitis and West Nile and Other Flavivirus Infections

John R. Graybill, MD
Professor and Chief, Division of Infectious Diseases, Department of Medicine, University of Texas Health Science Center at San Antonio, San Antonio, TX
Histoplasmosis, Blastomycosis, Coccidioidomycosis, and Cryptococcosis; Paracoccidioidomycosis; Penicillioisis Marneffei

Harry B. Greenberg, MD, FACP
Professor, Departments of Medicine, Microbiology and Immunology, Stanford University School of Medicine, Stanford, CA; Staff Physician, Department of Medicine, Division of Gastroenterology, Veterans Affairs Palo Alto Health Care System, Palo Alto, CA
Rotavirus Infections

Duane J. Gubler, MS, ScD
Director, Asia-Pacific Institute of Tropical Medicine and Infectious Diseases, Chair, Department of Tropical Medicine, Medical Microbiology and Pharmacology, John A. Burns School of Medicine, University of Hawaii, Honolulu, HI
Dengue and Dengue Hemorrhagic Fever

Richard L. Guerrant, MD, FACP
Thomas H. Hunter Professor of International Medicine, Director, Center for Global Health, University of Virginia; Division of Infectious Diseases and International Health, Department of Medicine, University of Virginia Hospital, Charlottesville, VA
Principles of Parasitism: Host–Parasite Interactions; Chemotherapy of Parasitic Diseases; Chemotherapy of Bacterial, Fungal, and Viral Diseases; Enteric Escherichia coli *Infections; Cryptosporidiosis;* Cyclospora, Isospora, *and* Sarcosystis *Infections*

Yezid Gutierrez, MD, MPH&TM, PhD
Adjunct Staff, Department of Laboratory Medicine, The Cleveland Clinic Educational Foundation, Cleveland, OH
Other Tissue Nematode Infections

Frederick G. Hayden, MD
Professor of Internal Medicine and Pathology, Department of Internal Medicine, University of Virginia School of Medicine; Physician, Department of Internal Medicine/Infectious Diseases, University of Virginia Health System, Charlottesville, VA
Respiratory Tract Viral Infections

Donald A. Henderson, MD, MPH
Professor of Medicine and Public Health, Department of Internal Medicine, University of Pittsburgh; Resident Scholar, University of Pittsburgh Medical Center, Center for Biosecurity, Baltimore, MD
Disease Eradication and Control; Smallpox and Monkeypox

Bradley S. Hersh, MD, MPH
Medical Officer, Department of Immunization, Vaccines and Biologicals, World Health Organization, Geneva, Switzerland
Measles

Barbara L. Herwaldt, MD, MPH
Medical Epidemiologist, Division of Parasitic Diseases, Centers for Disease Control and Prevention, Atlanta, GA
Cyclospora, Isospora, *and* Sarcosystis *Infections*

Erik L. Hewlett, MD
Professor, Department of Medicine and Pharmacology, University of Virginia School of Medicine; Attending Physician, Department of Internal Medicine, University of Virginia Hospital, Charlottesville, VA
Pertussis

David R. Hill, MD, DTM&H
Honorary Professor, Department of Infectious and Tropical Diseases, London School of Hygiene and Tropical Medicine; Director, National Travel Health Network and Centre, London, United Kingdom
Intestinal Flagellate and Ciliate Infections

Paul Hoffman, PhD
Associate Professor, Division of Infectious Diseases and International Health, Department of Internal Medicine, University of Virginia Health System, Charlottesville, VA
Legionellosis

Stephen L. Hoffman, MD, DTMH
Chief Executive Officer, Sanaria Inc., Rockville, MD; Adjunct Professor, Department of Preventive Medicine and Biometrics, Uniformed Services University of the Health Sciences, Bethesda, MD
Typhoid Fever; Malaria

Edward W. Hook, III, MD, FACP
Professor of Medicine, Epidemiology, and Microbiology, University of Alabama at Birmingham; Medical Director, STD Control Program, Jefferson County Department of Health, Birmingham, AL
Treponemal Infections

Donald R. Hopkins, MD, MPH
Associate Executive Director, The Carter Center, Atlanta, GA
Dracunculiasis

Duane R. Hospenthal, MD, PhD, FACP, FIDSA, Lt. Col., US Army
Associate Professor of Medicine, Department of Medicine, F. Edward Hébert School of Medicine, Uniformed Services University of the Health Sciences, Bethesda, MD; Chief, Infectious Disease Service, Department of Medicine, Brooke Army Medical Center, Fort Sam Houston, TX; Clinical Associate Professor, Department of Medicine, University of Texas Health Sciences Center at San Antonio, San Antonio, TX
Entomophthoramycosis, Lobomycosis, Rhinosporidiosis, and Sporotrichosis

Peter J. Hotez, MD, PhD
Professor and Chair, Department of Microbiology and Tropical Medicine, The George Washington University, Washington, DC
Hookworm Infections

S. David Hudnall, MD
Professor, Department of Pathology and Laboratory Medicine, The University of Texas Medical Branch, Galveston, TX
Human Herpesvirus Infections

James M. Hughes, MD, FACP
Director, Program in Global Infectious Diseases; Associate Director, Southeastern Center for Emerging Biologic Threats, Emory University School of Medicine; Director, Center for Global Safe Water, Rollins School of Public Health, Atlanta, GA
Surveillance for Emerging Infectious Diseases and Bioterrorism Threats

Raul E. Isturiz, MD, FACP
Chief, Infectious Diseases Section, Centro Medico de Caracas; Chief, Infectious Diseases Section, Centro Medico Docente la Tunidad, Caracas, Venezuela
Tropical Infectious Disease Concerns in Pregnancy

Hamid Jafari, MBBS
Director, Global Immunization Division, National Immunization Program, Centers for Disease Control and Prevention, Atlanta, GA
Enterovirus Infections, Including Poliomyelitis

Maria C. Jaimes, MD
Postdoctoral Fellow, Departments of Medicine, Microbiology and Immunology, Stanford University School of Medicine, Stanford, CA
Rotavirus Infections

Selma M.B. Jeronimo, MD, PhD
Department of Biochemistry, Bioscience Center, Universidade Federal do Rio Grande do Norte, Natal, RN, Brazil
Leishmaniasis

John L. Johnson, MD, FACP
Associate Professor of Medicine and International Health, Division of Infectious Diseases, Department of Medicine, Case Western Reserve University School of Medicine; Staff Physician, Division of Pulmonary and Critical Care Medicine, University Hospitals of Cleveland, Cleveland, OH
Tuberculosis and Atypical Myobacterial Infections

Christopher L. Karp, MD
Boomer Esiason Professor of Pediatrics, Director, Division of Molecular Immunology, Cincinnati Children's Hospital Medical Center, Cincinnati, OH
Approach to the Patient with HIV and Coinfecting Tropical Infectious Diseases

James W. Kazura, MD
Professor, Center for Global Health and Diseases, Case School of Medicine, Case Western Reserve University; Professor, Department of Medicine, University Hospitals of Cleveland, Cleveland, OH
Filariasis

Peter Kern, MD, DTM&H (Hamburg)
Professor of Medicine and Infectious Diseases, Division of Infectious Diseases and Clinical Immunology, University Hospital and Medical Center, Ulm, Germany
Echinococcosis

Gerald T. Keusch, MD
Assistant Provost and Associate Dean for Global Health, Boston University Medical Campus and School of Public Health, Boston, MA
Nutrition and Miconutrients in Tropical Infectious Diseases; Shigellosis

Jay S. Keystone, MD, MSc(CTM), FRCPC
Professor, Department of Medicine, University of Toronto; Staff Physician, Tropical Disease Unit, Toronto General Hospital, Toronto, Ontario, Canada
Health Advice for International Travel; Delusional Parasitosis

Charles H. King, MD, MS, FACP
Associate Professor of International Health, Center for Global Health and Diseases, Case Western Reserve University; Attending Physician, Department of Medicine, University Hospitals of Cleveland, Cleveland, OH
Schistosomiasis

Louis V. Kirchhoff, MD, MPH
Professor, Department of Internal Medicine (Infectious Diseases) and Epidemiology, University of Iowa; Staff Physician, Medical Service, Department of Veterans Affairs Medical Center, Iowa City, IA
American Trypanosomiasis (Chagas' Disease)

Amy D. Klion, MD
Staff Clinician, Laboratory of Parasitic Diseases, National Institute of Allergy and Infectious Disease, National Institutes of Health, Bethesda, MD
Loiasis and Mansonella *Infection*

Keith P. Klugman, MD, PhD
Professor, Department of International Health, Rollins School of Public Health, Professor, Division of Infectious Diseases, School of Medicine, Emory University, Atlanta, GA; Director, Respiratory and Meningeal Pathogens Research Unit, University of the Witwatersrand, Medical Research Council, National Institute for Communicable Diseases, Johannesburg, South Africa
Pneumococcal Infections

Dennis J. Kopecko, PhD
Chief, Laboratory of Enteric and Sexually Transmitted Diseases, Food and Drug Administration, Center for Biologics Evaluation and Research, Bethesda, MD
Shigellosis

Margaret Kosek, MD
Assistant Scientist, Department of International Health, Johns Hopkins Bloomberg School of Public Health, Baltimore, MD
Nutrition and Miconutrients in Tropical Infectious Diseases

Phyllis E. Kozarsky, MD
Professor of Medicine, Department of Medicine/Infectious Diseases; Chief, Geographic Medicine and Travelers' Health Section, Department of Medicine, Emory Unversity School of Medicine, Atlanta, GA
Health Advice for International Travel

Tim Kuberski, MD
Consultant in Infectious Diseases and Tropical Medicine, Private Practice, Glendale, AZ
Angiostrongyliasis

James L. Larson, Jr., MD, FACEP
Assistant Professor, Department of Emergency Medicine, University of North Carolina, Chapel Hill, Chapel Hill, NC
Plant Toxins in the Tropics

James W. Leduc, PhD
Director, Division of Viral and Rickettsial Diseases, National Center for Infectious Diseases, National Centers for Disease Control and Prevention, Atlanta, GA
Surveillance for Emerging Infectious Diseases and Bioterrorism Threats

Stanley M. Lemon, MD
John Sealy Distinguished University Chair and Director, Institute for Human Infections and Immunity, University of Texas Medical Branch at Galveston, Galveston, TX
Viral Hepatitis

Peter Leone, MD
Associate Professor of Medicine, Department of Medicine/Infectious Diseases, University of North Carolina; Medical Director, HIV/STD Prevention and Care Branch, North Carolina Department of Health and Human Services, Chapel Hill, NC
Gonococcal and Other Neisserial Infections

Paul N. Levett, PhD, ABMM, FCCM
Assistant Clinical Director, Provincial Laboratory, Saskatchewan Health, Regina, Saskatchewan, Canada
Leptospirosis

Michael Levin, PhD, FRCP, FRCPCH, F MED SCi
Professor, Department of Paediatrics, Imperial College London; Consultant in Paediatric Infectious Diseases, Department of Paediatrics, St. Mary's Hospital NHS Trust, Paddington, London, United Kingdom
Host Genetics and Susceptibility to Infection

Myron M. Levine, MD, DTPH, FAAP, FACPM
Professor, Departments of Medicine and Pediatrics, Director, Center for Vaccine Development, University of Maryland School of Medicine, Baltimore, MD
Cholera Infections

Aldo A. M. Lima, MD, PhD
Professor, Clinical Research Unit and Institute of Biomedicine/Center for Global Health, Faculty of Medicine; University Hospital, Clinical Research Unit and Institute of Biomedicine, Faculty of Medicine; Pharmacology, Department of Physiology and Pharmacology, Federal University of Ceará, Fortaleza, Ceará, Brasil
Cryptosporidiosis

David L. Longworth, MD
Deputy Chairman, Department of Medicine, Tufts University School of Medicine, Boston, MA; Chairman, Department of Medicine, Baystate Medical Center, Springfield, MA
Cutaneous Lesions

J. Dick MacLean, MD, FRCPC, MRCP(UK), DCMT(Lond)
Professor of Medicine, Director, Department of Medicine, McGill Centre for Tropical Diseases, McGill University; Senior Physician, Department of Medicine, Division of Tropical Diseases, Montreal General Hospital, Montreal, Quebec, Canada
Liver, Lung, and Intestinal Fluke Infections

Alan J. Magill, MD, FACP (COL, MCUSA)
Associate Professor, Department of Preventive Medicine and Biometrics, Uniformed Services University of the Health Sciences, Bethesda, MD; Attending Physician, Infectious Disease Service, Walter Reed Army Medical Center, Washington, DC; Science Director, Walter Reed Army Institute of Research, Silver Spring, MD
Infectious Diseases in Modern Military Forces

Ciro Maguiña, MD
Director, Adjunto del IMT-AVH-UPCH, Departamento de Medicina, Universidad Peruana Cayetano Heredia; Medico Infectologo Tropicalista, Departamento de Medicina Tropical, Hospital Nacional Cayetano Heredia, Lima, Peru
Bartonelloses

James H. Maguire, MD, MPH
Professor and Head, International Health Division, University of Maryland School of Medicine, Baltimore, MD
Babesiosis; Pathogenic and Opportunistic Free-Living Amebas: Acanthamoeba *spp.,* Balamuthia mandrillaris, Naegleria fowleri, *and* Sappina diploidia; *Systemic Coccidia (Toxoplasmosis); Hepatobiliary Disease*

Siddhartha Mahanty, MBBS, MPH
Staff Physician, Malaria Vaccine Development Branch, National Institute of Allergy and Infectious Diseases, National Institutes of Health, Rockville, MD
Liver, Lung, and Intestinal Fluke Infections

El-Sheikh Mahgoub, MD, PhD, FRCPath
Professor of Microbiology, Department of Medical Microbiology and Parasitology, Faculty of Medicine, University of Khartoum; Professor of Medical Education and Research, Sudan Medical Specialisation Board, Khartoum, Sudan
Mycetoma

Susan A. Maloney, MD, MHSc, FAAP
Acting Chief, Immigrant, Refugee, and Migrant Health Branch, Division of Global Migration and Quarantine, Centers for Disease Control and Prevention, Atlanta, GA
Migrant, Immigrant, and Refugee Health

Anthony A. Marfin, MD, MPH, MA
Quarantine Medical Officer, San Francisco Quarantine Station, Division of Global Migration and Quarantine, Centers for Disease Control and Prevention, San Francisco, CA
Yellow Fever

Thomas J. Marrie, MD
Dean of Faculty of Medicine and Dentistry, University of Alberta; University of Alberta Hospital, Edmonton, Alberta, Canada
Legionellosis; Psittacosis; Q Fever

Barry J. Marshall, FRACP, FRS, FAA
NHMRC Senior Principal Research Fellow, Department of Microbiology, University of Western Australia; Consultant Gastroenterologist, Department of Gastroenterology, Sir Charles Gairdner Hospital, Perth, Western Australia, Australia
Helicobacter pylori *Infections*

Gregory J. Martin, MD, FACP, Captain, Medical Corps, US Navy
Associate Professor of Medicine, Department of Internal Medicine, Uniformed Services University, Bethesda, MD; Officer in Charge, US Naval Medical Research Center Detachment, Lima, Lima, Peru
Approach to the Patient in the Tropics with Pulmonary Disease

Tadahiko Matsumoto, MD, DMSc
Clinical Professor, Department of Dermatology, Juntendo University School of Medicine; Clinical Professor, Department of Dermatology, Keio University School of Medicine; Director, Department of Dermatology, Toshiba Hospital, Tokyo, Japan; Clinical Professor, Department of Dermatology, Kurume University School of Medicine, Kurume, Japan; Adjunct Professor, Department of Pathology, Kitasato University School of Medicine, Sagamihara, Japan
Chromoblastomycosis and Phaeohyphomycosis

Steven D. Mawhorter, MD, DTMH
Staff Physician, Department of Infectious Diseases, Cleveland Clinic Foundation, Cleveland, OH; Clinical Assistant Professor, Pennsylvania State University School of Medicine, Hershey, PA
Cutaneous Lesions

James S. McCarthy, MD, FRACP, DH&TM
Associate Professor of Tropical Medicine and Infectious Diseases, School of Population Health, University of Queensland; Staff Specialist, Department of Infectious Diseases, Royal Brisbane and Women's Hospital; Senior Research Fellow, Infectious Diseases and Immunology, Queensland Institute for Medical Research, Herston, Australia
Toxocariasis and Larva Migrans Syndromes; Enterobiasis

Michael R. McGinnis, PhD
Professor, Department of Pathology, University of Texas Medical Branch, Galveston, TX
Dermatophytosis

Paul S. Mead, MD, MPH
Chief, Epidemiology, Molecular Biology and Diagnostic Activity, Bacterial Zoonoses Branch, Division of Vector-Borne Infectious Diseases, National Center for Infectious Diseases, Centers for Disease Control and Prevention, Fort Collins, CO
Plague

Wayne M. Meyers, MD, PhD, DSc (Hon)
Chief, Mycobacteriology, Department of Infectious and Parasitic Disease Pathology, Armed Forces Institute of Pathology, Washington, DC; Research Affiliate, Tulane Regional Primate Research Center, Tulane University, New Orleans, LA
Mycobacterium ulcerans *Infection (Buruli Ulcer); Leprosy*

Samuel I. Miller, MD
Professor, Department of Medicine, Microbiology, and Genome Sciences; Professor, Department of Medicine, University of Washington, Seattle, WA
Nontyphoidal Salmonellosis

James N. Mills, PhD
Chief, Medical Ecology Unit, Division of Viral and Rickettsial Diseases, National Center for Infectious Diseases, Centers for Disease Control and Prevention, Atlanta, GA
Arenavirus Infections; Hantavirus Infections

Michael Minnick, PhD
Professor of Microbiology, Assistant Dean, Division of Biological Sciences, The University of Montana, Missoula, MT
Bartonelloses

Thomas P. Monath, MD, FACP
Chief Scientific Officer, Acambis Inc., Cambridge, MA; Adjunct Professor, Department of Molecular Biology and Immunology, Harvard School of Public Health, Boston, MA
Yellow Fever

Stephan S. Monroe, PhD
Division of Viral and Rickettsial Diseases, National Center for Infectious Diseases, Centers for Disease Control and Prevention, Atlanta, GA
Calicivirus Infections

Thomas A. Moore, MD, FACP
Clinical Associate Professor, Department of Internal Medicine, University of Kansas School of Medicine–Wichita, Wichita, KS
Toxocariasis and Larva Migrans Syndromes; Enterobiasis

Jonathan P. Moorman, MD, PhD
Associate Professor, Department of Internal Medicine, James H. Quillen College of Medicine, East Tennessee State University, Johnson City, TN; Section Chief, Department of Infectious Diseases, James H. Quillen VA Medical Center, Mountain Home, TN
Enteric Clostridium *Infections*

J. Glenn Morris, Jr., MD, MPH&TM
Professor and Chairman, Department of Epidemiology and Preventive Medicine, Professor of Medicine (Infectious Diseases), Professor of Microbiology and Immunology, University of Maryland School of Medicine, Baltimore, MD
"Noncholera" Vibrio *Infections*

Megan Murray, MD, ScD
Assistant Professor, Department of Epidemiology, Harvard School of Public Health; Instructor, Infectious Disease Unit, Massachusetts General Hospital; Instructor, Division of Social Medicine and Health Inequalities, Brigham and Women's Hospital, Boston, MA; Associate Member, Broad Institute, Cambridge, MA
Epidemiology and Biostatistics

K. Darwin Murrell, PhD
Senior Scientist, Centre for Experimental Parasitology, Royal Veterinary and Agricultural University, Copenhagen, Denmark; Adjunct Professor, Department of Preventive Medicine and Biostatistics, Uniformed Services University of the Health Sciences, Bethesda, MD
Trichinellosis

G. Balakrish Nair, PhD, FNA, FNASc
Director, Laboratory Sciences Division, International Centre for Diarrhoeal Diseases Research, Bangladesh, Mohakhali, Dhaka, Bangladesh
"Noncholera" Vibrio *Infections*

Theodore E. Nash, MD
Head, Gastrointestinal Parasites Section, Laboratory of Parasitic Diseases, National Institutes of Allergy and Infectious Diseases, National Institutes of Health, Bethesda, MD
Intestinal Flagellate and Ciliate Infections

Barnett R. Nathan, MD
Assistant Professor, Department of Neurology, University of Virginia, Charlottesville, VA
Tetanus

Anne Nicholson-Weller, MD
Professor of Medicine, Harvard Medical School; Physician in Medicine, Divisions of Infectious Disease and Allergy and Inflammation, Department of Medicine, Beth Israel Deaconess Medical Center, Boston, MA
Immunology, Host Defense, Immunodeficiencies, and Vaccines

Robert L. Norris, MD, FACEP
Associate Professor, Department of Surgery, Stanford University Medical Center; Chief, Department of Emergency Medicine, Stanford Hospital and Clinics, Stanford, CA
Animal Poisons in the Tropics

Thomas B. Nutman, MD
Head, Helminth Immunology Section and Head, Clinical Parasitology Unit, Laboratory of Parasitic Diseases, National Institutes of Health, Bethesda, MD
Filariasis; Loiasis and Mansonella *Infection*

Nigel O'Farrell, MSc, MD, MRCP
Pasteur Suite, Ealing Hospital, London, United Kingdom
Calymmatobacterium granulomatis *Infection (Donovanosis)*

Michael E. Ohl, MD
Research Fellow, Division of Infectious Diseases, Department of Internal Medicine, University of Missouri, Columbia, MO; Research Fellow, Department of Medicine, University of Missouri Medical Center, Seattle, WA
Nontyphoidal Salmonellosis

Juan P. Olano, MD
Associate Professor, Director, Residency Training Program, Department of Pathology, University of Texas Medical Branch, Galveston, TX
Principles of Parasitism: Host–Parasite Interactions; Distinguishing Tropical Infectious Diseases from Bioterrorism

Luis S. Ortega, MD, MPH
Medical Epidemiologist, Division of Global Migration and Quarantine, Centers for Disease Control and Prevention, Atlanta, GA
Migrant, Immigrant, and Refugee Health

Mark A. Pallansch, PhD
Distinguished Consultant, Respiratory and Enteric Viruses Branch, Division of Viral and Rickettsial Diseases, Centers for Disease Control and Prevention, Atlanta, GA
Enterovirus Infections, Including Poliomyelitis

Jean W. Pape, MD
Professor, Department of Medicine, Weill Medical College of Cornell University, New York, NY; Director, GHESKIO Centres, Port-au-Prince, Haiti
Cyclospora, Isospora, *and* Sarcosystis *Infections*

John R. Papp, PhD
Laboratory Reference and Research Branch, Division of STD Prevention, Centers for Disease Control and Prevention, Atlanta, GA
Chlamydia trachomatis *Infections of the Gential Tract (Ocuolgenital Infections and Lymphogranuloma Venerum)*

Julie Parsonnet, MD
Associate Professor, Department of Medicine, and Health Research and Policy, Stanford University School of Medicine, Stanford, CA
Tropical Infectious Diseases and Malignancy

Geoffrey Pasvol, MA, MB ChB, DPhil, FRCP, FRCPE
Professor, Department of Infection and Tropical Medicine, Director, Wellcome Centre for Clinical Tropical Medicine, Imperial College London; Professor, Infection and Tropical Medicine, Northwick Park Hospital, London, United Kingdom
Host Genetics and Susceptibility to Infection; Approach to the Patient in the Tropics with Anemia

Richard D. Pearson, MD, FACP
Professor of Medicine and Pathology, Senior Associate Dean for Medical Education, Departments of Medicine and Pathology, University of Virginia School of Medicine; Professor of Medicine and Pathology, Department of Internal Medicine, University of Virginia Health System, Charlottesville, VA
Chemotherapy of Parasitic Diseases; Chemotherapy of Bacterial, Fungal, and Viral Diseases; Leishmaniasis; Fever and Systemic Symptoms

David A. Pegues, MD
Professor of Clinical Medicine, Division of Infectious Diseases, David Geffen School of Medicine at UCLA; Hospital Epidemiologist, UCLA Healthcare, Los Angeles, CA
Nontyphoidal Salmonellosis

Jacques Pépin, MD, MSc, FRCPC
Professor, Microbiology and Infectious Diseases, Director, Center for International Health, University of Sherbrooke, Sherbrooke, Quebec, Canada
African Trypanosomiasis (Sleeping Sickness)

C. J. Peters, MD
Professor of Pathology and Microbiology, Center for Biodefense and Emerging Infectious Diseases and WHO Collaborating Center for Tropical Diseases, University of Texas Medical Branch, Galveston, TX
Overview of Viral Hemorrhagic Fevers; Arenavirus Infections; Bunyaviral Fevers: Rift Valley Fever and Crimean-Congo Hemorrhagic Fever; Hantavirus Infections; Filovirus Infections; Distinguishing Tropical Infectious Diseases from Bioterrorism

William A. Petri, Jr., MD, PhD, FACP
Wade Hampton Frost Professor of Epidemiology, Professor of Medicine, Microbiology and Pathology, Chief, Division of Infectious Diseases and International Health, Department of Internal Medicine, University of Virginia School of Medicine; Attending Physician, University of Virginia Hospitals, Charlottesville, VA
Enteric Amebiasis

Françoise Portaels, PhD
Professor and Head, Mycobacteriology Unit, Department of Microbiology, Institute of Tropical Medicine, Antwerp, Belgium
Mycobacterium ulcerans *Infection (Buruli Ulcer)*

Thomas C. Quinn, MD, FACP
Professor, Department of Medicine, The Johns Hopkins University, Baltimore, MD; Senior Investigator and Head, International HIV/STD Research Laboratory, Laboratory of Immunoregulation, National Institute of Allergy and Infectious Diseases, National Institutes of Health, Bethesda, MD
Human Retroviral Infections in the Tropics

Didier Raoult, MD, PhD
Professor and Director, Unité des rickettsies, Faculté de Médecine, Marseille, France
Typhus Group Rickettsioses

Steven J. Reynolds, MD, MPH, DTM&H, FRCPC
Assistant Professor, Division of Infectious Diseases, Johns Hopkins School of Medicine; Staff Clinician, National Institute of Allergy and Infectious Diseases, National Institutes of Health, Bethesda, MD;

Scientific Director, NIAID/NIH International Center of Excellence in Research Program, Uganda
Human Retroviral Infections in the Tropics

José M. C. Ribeiro, MD, PhD
Senior Scientist and Section Head, Laboratory of Malaria and Vector Research, National Institute of Allergy and Infectious Diseases, Bethesda, MD
Vector Biology

Pierre E. Rollin, MD
Special Pathogens Branch, Centers for Disease Control and Prevention, Atlanta, GA
Hantavirus Infections; Filovirus Infections

Allan Ronald, MD, MACP
Professor Emeritus, Department of Medicine and Community Health Sciences, University of Manitoba, Winnipeg, Manitoba, Canada
Haemophilus ducreyi *Infections; Sexually Transmitted and Urinary Tract Infections*

Jason Rosé, PhD
Chair, Science Department, Kings Academy High School, Sunnyvale, CA
Rotavirus Infections

Ernesto Ruiz-Tiben, BS, MS, PhD
Technical Director, Dracunculiasis Eradication, The Carter Center, Atlanta, GA
Dracunculiasis

Edward T. Ryan, MD, DTM&H, FACP
Assistant Professor, Department of Medicine, Harvard Medical School; Director, Tropical and Geographic Medicine Center, Division of Infectious Diseases, Massachusetts General Hospital; Assistant Professor, Immunology and Infectious Diseases, Harvard School of Public Health, Boston, MA
Epidemiology and Biostatistics; Ocular Disease

Anthony Sanchez, PhD
Public Health Service Officer, Special Pathogens Branch, Division of Viral and Rickettsial Diseases, Centers for Disease Control and Prevention, Atlanta, GA
Filovirus Infections

Julius Schachter, PhD
Professor of Laboratory Medicine, Department of Laboratory Medicine, University of California, San Francisco, San Francisco, CA
Trachoma

Peter M. Schantz, VMD, PhD
Epidemiologist, Division of Parasitic Diseases, National Center for Infectious Diseases, Centers for Disease Control and Prevention, Atlanta, GA
Echinococcosis

W. Michael Scheld, MD, FACP
Bayer-Gerald L. Mandell Professor of Infectious Diseases, Professor of Internal Medicine, Clinical Professor of Neurosurgery, Director, Pfizer Initiative in International Health, Department of Infectious Diseases and International Health, University of Virginia, Charlottesville, VA
Meningococcal Infections

Eugene R. Schiff, MD, MACP, FRCP, MACG
Professor and Chief, Division of Hepatology, Director, Center for Liver Disease, University of Miami School of Medicine; Jackson Memorial Hospital; Consultant, The Veterans Administration; Cedars Medical Center, Miami, FL
Viral Hepatitis

David A. Schwartz, MD, MS Hyg, FCAP
Visiting Professor, Department of Pathology, Vanderbilt University, Nashville, TN; Guest Scientist, Centers for Disease Control and Prevention, Atlanta, GA
Microsporidiosis

Joseph D. Schwartzman, MD, FAAM
Professor of Pathology, Department of Pathology, Dartmouth Medical School, Hanover, NH; Medical Director of Microbiology and Serology, Department of Pathology, Dartmouth-Hitchcock Medical Center, Lebanon, NH
Systemic Coccidia (Toxoplasmosis)

Elyse G. Seltzer, MD
Senior Director, Clinical Research and Medical Affairs, Vicuron Pharmaceuticals, Inc., King of Prussia, PA
Ascariasis

Arlene C. Seña, MD, MPH
Assistant Professor of Medicine, Department of Medicine, University of North Carolina at Chapel Hill; UNC Health Care Systems, Chapel Hill, NC; Medical Director, Durham County Health Department, Durham, NC
Sexually Transmitted and Urinary Tract Infections

Daniel J. Sexton, MD, FACP
Professor, Department of Medicine, Division of Infectious Diseases, Duke University Medical School; Director, Infection Control Unit, Duke University Medical Center, Durham, NC
Spotted Fever Group Rickettsioses

Trueman W. Sharp, MD, MPH (Capt, MCUSN)
Commanding Officer, US Naval Medical Medical Research Unit No. 3, Cairo, Egypt
Infectious Diseases in Modern Military Forces

Wun-Ju Shieh, MD, MPH, PhD
Medical Officer, Infectious Disease Pathology Activity, Centers for Disease Control and Prevention, Atlanta, GA
Leptospirosis; Arenavirus Infections

Shmuel Shoham, MD
Special Volunteer, Pediatric Oncology Branch of the National Cancer Institute, National Institutes of Health; Assistant Professor, Department of Medicine, Uniformed Services University of the Health Sciences, Bethesda, MD; Attending Physician, Department of Medicine, Washington Hospital Center, Washington, DC
Mucocutaneous and Deeply Invasive Candidiasis

Robert E. Shope, MD (*Deceased*)
Professor of Pathology, Center for Biodefense and Emerging Infectious Diseases and WHO Collaborating Center for Tropical Diseases, Department of Pathology, University of Texas Medical Branch, Galveston, TX
Factors Influencing Geographic Distribution and Incidence of Tropical Infectious Diseases; Bunyaviral Fevers: Rift Valley Fever and Crimean-Congo Hemorrhagic Fever; Japanese Encephalitis and West Nile and Other Flavivirus Infections; Alphavirus Infections

H. H. Shugart, PhD
W.W. Corcoran Professor, Department of Environmental Sciences and Department of Biology, University of Virginia, Charlottesville, VA
Factors Influencing Geographic Distribution and Incidence of Tropical Infectious Diseases

Afzal A. Siddiqui, MPhil, PhD
Associate Professor of Medicine, Department of Internal Medicine, Texas Tech University Health Sciences Center; Health Research Scientist, Thomas E. Creek Veterans Affairs Medical Center, Amarillo, TX
Strongyloidiasis

Upinder Singh, MD
Assistant Professor, Department of Internal Medicine, Stanford University, Stanford, CA
Enteric Amebiasis

Michael B. Smith, MD, MS
Director, Division of Clinical Microbiology, Department of Pathology, University of Texas Medical Branch, Galveston, TX
Dermatophytosis

Bonnie L. Smoak, MD, PhD, MPH (Col, MCUSA)
Associate Professor, Department of Preventive Medicine and Biometrics, Uniformed Services University of the Health Sciences, Bethesda, MD; Director, Division of Preventive Medicine, Walter Reed Army Institute of Research, Silver Spring, MD
Infectious Diseases in Modern Military Forces

Tom Solomon, BA, BM, MRCP, DCH, DTMH, PhD
Senior Lecturer in Neurology, Department of Neurological Science, Senior Lecturer in Medical Microbiology and Tropical Medicine, Department of Medical Microbiology and Genitourinary Medicine, University of Liverpool; Honorary Consultant Neurologist, Walton Centre for Neurology and Neurosurgery; Honorary Consultant Neurologist, Royal Liverpool University Hospital, Liverpool, United Kingdom
Japanese Encephalitis and West Nile and Other Flavivirus Infections; Neurologic Disease

Anastacio de Queiroz Sousa, MD
Associate Professor, Department of Clinical Medicine, Director, Núcleo de Medicina Tropical, Federal University of Ceará; Physician, Hospital São José for Infectious Diseases, Fortaleza, Ceará, Brazil
Meningococcal Infections; Leishmaniasis

Samba O. Sow, MD, MS
Coordinator, Centre pour le Développement des Vaccins–Mali, Centre National d'Appui à la lutte contre la Maladie, Ministry of Health, Bamako, Mali
Cholera Infections

Christina Spiropoulou, PhD
Adjunct Assistant Professor, Department of Microbiology and Immunology, School of Medicine, Emory University; Special Pathogens Branch, Division of Viral and Rickettsial Diseases, Centers for Disease Control and Prevention, Atlanta, GA
Hantavirus Infections

Lawrence R. Stanberry, MD, PhD
John Sealy Distinguished Chair in Pediatrics, Chairman, Department of Pediatrics, Director, Sealy Center for Vaccine Development, Department of Pediatrics, University of Texas Medical Branch, Galveston, TX
Human Herpesvirus Infections

Robert Steffen, MD
Professor of Travel Medicine, Division of Epidemiology and Prevention of Communicable Diseases, Institute of Social and Preventive Medicine, University of Zurich; Director, World Health Organization Collaborating Centre for Travellers' Health, Zurich, Switzerland
Health Advice for International Travel

Theodore S. Steiner, MD, RRCPC
Assistant Professor, Department of Medicine, University of British Columbia, Vancouver, British Columbia, Canada
Enteric Escherichia coli *Infections; Intestinal Coccidia Infection*

Mark C. Steinhoff, MD
Professor, Department of International Health, Johns Hopkins University; Physician, Department of Pediatrics, Johns Hopkins Hospital, Baltimore, MD
Haemophilus influenzae *(Including* H. aegyptius*) Infection*

Dennis L. Stevens, MD, PhD, FACP
Professor, Department of Medicine, University of Washington School of Medicine, Seattle, WA; Chief, Infectious Diseases, Department of Medicine, Veterans Affairs Medical Center, Boise, ID
Streptococcal and Staphylococcal Infections

Kathryn N. Suh, MD, FRCPC
Assistant Professor, Department of Pediatrics, University of Ottawa; Attending Physician, Division of Infectious Diseases, Children's Hospital of Eastern Ontario, Ottawa, Ontario, Canada
Delusional Parasitosis

Martin Tagle, MD
Associate Professor of Medicine, Department of Gastroenterology and Hepatology, Universidad Peruana Cayetano Heredia; Staff Gastroenterologist and Hepatologist, Clinica Anglo-Americana, Lima, Peru
Viral Hepatitis

Tropical Infectious Diseases

G. FUNGAL INFECTIONS

77

Dermatophytosis

MICHAEL B. SMITH
MICHAEL R. MCGINNIS

INTRODUCTION

Dermatophytosis is a term used to describe mycotic infections caused by a group of fungi that usually remain localized to the superficial layers of the skin, hair, or nails. This disease is one of the most common infectious maladies worldwide. Despite their propensity to infect the exterior aspects of the host, the dermatophytes prefer a warm, moist environment for growth. As these conditions are prevalent in the environment of the tropics, it is no surprise that dermatophyte infections, while occurring in all parts of the world, are especially common in tropical regions.[1] Dermatophyte infection of the skin and hair of the scalp (tinea capitis) is exceedingly common in Africa, with a prevalence of 14% to 86% in children, depending on geographic location and the method of making the diagnosis.[1] In many tropical regions, dermatophyte infection of the glabrous skin (tinea corporis) is the most common skin disease found.[1] The rate of infection for those not native to a tropical area is usually higher than that of the indigenous population and can reach epidemic proportions. Both United States combat forces in Vietnam during the 1960s and British forces several decades earlier in Malaysia and Hong Kong experienced epidemic rates of dermatophyte infections. In Vietnam, 73% of U.S. combat infantrymen suffered from dermatophyte infections.[2] These infections were disabling enough that the soldiers were unable to capably perform in the field, and the deleterious effect on U.S. combat capability was sufficient to warrant the creation of a special medical research team by the military to address the problem.[2]

AGENTS

Dermatophytes are a closely related homogeneous clade of keratinophilic filamentous fungi[3–6] that are associated with the stratum corneum of the skin, as well as hair and nails on the living host. They possess similar appearance, physiology, antigenicity, growth requirements, infectivity, and pathology. These fungi are classified in the anamorphic genera *Epidermophyton, Keratinomyces, Microsporum,* and *Trichophyton.* Some dermatophytes may reproduce sexually when the opposite mating types are crossed with each other. The single ascomycete genus *Arthroderma* accommodates the known sexual forms of all of the dermatophytes.[7]

Even though the term *dermatophytosis* refers to an infection caused by a dermatophyte, not all dermatophytes may cause infection. The fungus colonizes the stratum corneum and then grows in a radial manner without penetrating viable tissue. Invasion of hair, which is nonliving tissue, is an example of colonization. If the fungus enters viable tissue and continues to grow, then infection is present. Majocchi's granuloma (a nodular perifolliculitis due to dermatophytes) and pseudomycetoma are examples of fungal invasion of viable tissue. Colonization or infection may result in disease if there is structural or functional harm. These may be evident as damaged or destroyed hair and nails, hyperhidrosis, pruritus, inflammation, or alopecia. Contamination, the presence of nonreplicating dermatophytes on keratinized tissue, does not occur.

In addition to dermatophytes, other species of fungi that do not colonize or invade the stratum corneum, hair, and nails on the living host are classified in the same anamorphic genera owing to their similar microscopic and colonial characteristics. Some of these species may break down keratin in substrates such as feathers and hooves, but these are no longer on the living host. These keratinophilic species are not dermatophytes. The term *dermatomycosis*[8] is parallel to dermatophytosis, but differs in that it encompasses colonization and infection of keratinized tissue by fungi not classified in the genera *Epidermophyton, Keratinomyces, Microsporum,* and *Trichophyton.* In addition, when their sexual forms are known, they are classified in genera other than *Arthroderma.*

EPIDEMIOLOGY

Based on their principal ecologic niches, dermatophytes are categorized as either anthropophilic (people-loving), geophilic (soil-loving), or zoophilic (animal-loving). Several dermatophytes may be associated with more than one ecological niche. The major advantage of this classification scheme resides in determining the source of the dermatophyte causing an infection. Clinically, geophilic and zoophilic dermatophytes typically cause more severe, self-limiting lesions. In contrast, anthropophilic species cause lesions having little inflammation that persist for long periods of time.

Transmission of dermatophytes occurs through contact with hyphal fragments and arthroconidia, usually associated with skin scales or hair fragments deposited on fomites such as combs, towels, etc. Arthroconidia are airborne propagules that can easily disseminate from one host to another. They are formed by the fragmentation of hyphae. Animal studies have shown that arthroconidia are more infective for transmission than macro- and microconidia.[9] These propagules, whether airborne or associated with fomites, are probably the primary inoculum that causes new infections. Arthroconidia can remain viable for several years on skin scales or hair shed into the environment.[10]

There is variability with respect to geographical distribution of individual species (Table 77-1). Some species are

Tinea Infections and AIDS

While early in the AIDS epidemic the prevalence of tinea infections did appear to be increased in this patient population, with the advent of improved antiretroviral therapy, this no longer appears to be the case. Approximately 20% of AIDS patients with CD4 counts less than or equal to 200/μl have either tinea pedis or onychomycosis, a rate not dissimilar to the immunocompetent population.[20] Although the number of tinea infections seen in AIDS patients approximates that seen in non-AIDS patients, the severity of infections and the variability of clinical presentation are increased.

Generalized infection can occur, often in patients with low CD4 counts, and while many times the disease is responsive to therapy, prolonged treatment, usually with oral therapy, is required, and in some cases the patients are unable to clear the infection.[21,22] Occasionally, infection with unusual species or infection by a species not commonly associated with a particular anatomic site, such as cases of *M. canis* tinea capitis or onychomycosis, is seen.[22,23]

Tissue invasion by dermatophytes in these patients is often sudden in onset, not necessarily associated with a hair follicle, encompasses larger areas, and extends deeper into tissue than with localized invasive lesions seen occasionally in immunocompetent persons (i.e., Majocchi's granuloma). Systemic invasion with a fatal outcome in AIDS patients has been reported, but appears to be infrequent.[24]

It should be noted that the medical literature addressing dermatophyte infections and AIDS originates primarily from the developed world, and that reports and studies addressing this subject in developing nations, where the AIDS epidemic is ravaging the population, and where tinea infections are common, are lacking.

PATHOGENESIS AND IMMUNITY

Dermatophyte infection is initiated by adherence of arthroconidia to corneocytes, with a subsequent rapid germination and production of germ tubes (within 4–6 hours), which grow through layers of keratin in both a horizontal and vertical direction.[10] These pathogens are able to produce and secrete keratinases, lipases, proteases, and phosphatases, all of which aid the spread of the developing hyphae through the keratin layer.

Host resistance is a combination of nonspecific, innate immune mechanisms and an acquired immune response. The intact keratin layer inhibits penetration into deeper layers of the epidermis, at least initially, and allows exposure of the fungus to lethal UV light in some anatomic locations. The skin surface has a low moisture content and a relatively high temperature, which are not ideal conditions for fungal proliferation. Transferrin in serum may compete with the fungus for iron. Cytokine production in keratinocytes is stimulated by dermatophytes, and the release of factors such as interleukin-8 by keratinocytes results not only in an influx of neutrophils, but also stimulates increased proliferation of epidermal cells and increased keratinization, which encourages shedding of the fungi.[25] Dermatophytes have been shown to activate complement, with a resultant release of chemotactic factors.[25] Unsaturated fatty acids and lipids present in adult sebum are fungistatic and may serve as a primary resistance mechanism against dermatophytes.[26] This may explain, in part, the resolution of many cases of dermatophytosis at puberty when the composition of lipids in sebum changes.

Dermatophytes are not, however, without their own defense mechanisms. The rapid germination time of these fungi makes elimination by rapid epidermal turnover less effective. Some species of dermatophytes can destroy complement-derived chemotactic factors.[25] Mannan, a cell-wall glycoprotein of fungi, not only inhibits the proliferation of keratinocytes, but, most importantly, has been demonstrated to inhibit the development of cell-mediated immunity against the infecting dermatophyte.[20] While antibody classes directed against different antigens present in dermatophytes occur in all infected patients, they are not thought to play any role in clearing an infection, and development of cell-mediated immunity appears to be the most important host factor in clearing an infection.

Infected individuals who are able to produce a decisive delayed-type hypersensitivity are able to clear their infections. The clinical course of a dermatophyte infection is related, at least in part, to the relative proportions of CD4 (T-helper) lymphocytes and CD8 (T-suppressor) lymphocytes generated in the immune response. Those patients who have decreased CD4 lymphocytes relative to CD8 lymphocytes tend to develop chronic dermatophyte infections.[10] Because 10% to 20% of the "immunocompetent" world population are thought to have chronic dermatophytosis, a selective cell-mediated immunodeficiency to dermatophytes in the population appears to be relatively common. The exact nature of this immunodeficiency and whether it is innate or acquired is yet to be completely described.

DIAGNOSIS

The clinical differential diagnosis is extensive.[13] Tinea capitis must be distinguished from seborrheic dermatitis, psoriasis, lupus erythematosus, lupus vulgaris, alopecia areata, pseudopelade, impetigo, trichotillomania, staphylococcal pyoderma, folliculitis decalvans, and secondary syphilis. Tinea corporis may be confused with psoriasis, pityriasis rosea, nummular eczema, granuloma annulare, annular secondary syphilis, lichen planus, seborrheic dermatitis, discoid lupus erythematosus, fixed drug eruption, pityriasis versicolor, candidiasis, and erythema annulare. Tinea cruris must be differentiated from candidiasis, erythrasma, seborrheic dermatitis, psoriasis, lichen planus chronicus, and contact dermatitis; and onychomycosis can be confused with various nail abnormalities such as nonmycotic leukonychia, clubbing, Beau's lines, pachyonychia congenita, contact irritants, and other skin diseases that cause dystrophic nails. In clinical material, dermatophytes must be distinguished from other filamentous hyaline hyphae formed by *Aspergillus, Scopulariopsis, Fusarium,* and *Scytalidium* species. Isolation of the fungus is the only accurate way to identify the etiologic agent.

The diagnosis of dermatophytosis is based on the clinical presentation and the demonstration of hyaline, septate, branching hyphae in the stratum corneum, nail, or hair. The demonstration of dermatophyte hyphae in clinical specimens is accomplished by mounting the material in 10% to 20% potassium hydroxide, allowing the specimen to become clear, and observing the hyphae with a microscope. The production of blue-green fluorescence when lesions are exposed to UV light with a Wood's lamp indicates the presence of *Microsporum* species.

The identification of dermatophytes is based on their colonial characteristics when grown on Sabouraud glucose agar, microscopic structures, temperature ranges for growth, a few limited nutritional tests, and their resistance to cycloheximide. Conidia and their anatomy are the principal microscopic structures used to speciate dermatophytes.[27] Even though DNA probes and polymerase chain reaction (PCR) have been developed, they are not currently a practical method of identifying dermatophyte species in the clinical laboratory.[28]

There are no distinctive histopathologic changes associated with dermatophytes. The fungi are hyaline and form hyphae that may have associated arthroconidia. The epidermis may appear unaffected to mildly hyperkeratotic with patchy parakeratosis. Acute lesions may be spongiotic, whereas inflammatory lesions contain accumulating neutrophils in microabscesses accompanied by hyperkeratosis. A mild to intense perivascular infiltrate with lymphocytes and plasma cells may be present in the dermis. In tinea capitis, the hair follicle contains large numbers of neutrophils. The fungus does not grow below the keratinizing zone of the hair. Spongiosis, dermal abscesses, and colonized hair shafts result in severely inflamed kerions.

TREATMENT

Topical antifungal drugs are the most commonly recommended treatment for most dermatophytosis, excluding tinea capitis and onychomycosis, although oral agents are often necessary in difficult cases. The major compounds include the imidazoles, triazoles, morpholines, and allylamines.

The imidazoles (clotrimazole, econazole, ketoconazole, and miconazole) and triazoles (fluconazole, itraconazole) inhibit the ergosterol biosynthetic pathway by binding to the fungal cytochrome P-450–dependent 14α-demethylase, which results in the accumulation of lanosterol and toxic metabolites in the fungal cell. Morpholines (amorolfine) result in the formation of ignosterol rather than ergosterol, which is required in the fungal plasma membrane. Allylamines (naftifine and terbinafine) inhibit squalene epoxidase, which transforms squalene to squalene epoxide, which is needed to form lanosterol and subsequently ergosterol.

Tinea capitis must be treated with oral antifungals because topical agents are unable to penetrate the hair shaft. Griseofulvin, because of its efficacy, safety, and low cost, is still considered by many to be the drug of choice.[29] The long course of treatment (8–12 weeks) required is a disadvantage, particularly where compliance is a concern. Additionally, increased doses over those required several decades ago are now necessary, and dose and duration of therapy are also dependent on species of the infecting dermatophyte, with *M. canis* requiring more therapy than *T. tonsurans*.[30] Cure rates with this drug are 70% to 100%. Pulse therapy, with periods of treatment alternating with periods of no treatment, have been used to address issues related to cost, compliance, and side effects.[30] Terbinafine is considered the second choice, except if the infection is caused by *M. canis*, for which it appears relatively ineffective (although it appears to be more effective for *T. tonsurans* than griseofulvin).[29,30] Itraconazole is efficient but expensive, and ketoconazole does not appear to be useful compared to other options.[29] Adjuvant topical therapy with either 2% ketoconazole or 1% selenium sulfide shampoo is recommended to reduce infectivity.[29]

Griseofulvin is relatively poor in eradicating onychomycosis with only a 50% cure rate after 12 months of therapy.[31] Terbinafine, itraconazole, and fluconazole have all shown utility, although long-term follow-up has suggested that terbinafine may be superior in preventing relapse and that cure with fluconazole may not occur until up to one year after completion of therapy.[31] Chemical, surgical, or laser ablation of the nail may be necessary in addition to antifungal therapy.

For tinea cruris, tinea corporis, and tinea pedis, topical antifungals for 1 to 6 weeks are usually curative. Patients with the moccasin foot form of tinea pedis, widespread disease, disease that does not respond to topical therapy, or recurrent disease require oral therapy. There have been many clinical trials that have evaluated the comparative effectiveness of allylamines and azoles, with the allylamines overall appearing more effective, and with no detectable difference between individual allylamines or azoles.[32]

Treatment of dermatophytosis in the setting of AIDS is made more difficult not only by the problem of treating a patient that is severely immunocompromised, but also by the frequency of drug interactions between antifungals and the other medications these patients must take. For example, some of the azoles interact with protease inhibitors.[20] Antilipemics, necessary in conjunction with protease inhibitor therapy, preclude the use of itraconazole.[20] Finally, some aspects of the AIDS syndrome itself can interfere with effective therapy. Oral itraconazole, which requires an acidic environment for maximal absorption, may not achieve therapeutic serum levels at normal dosage due to the hypochlorhydria found in advanced AIDS.[20] Oral terbinafine appears to be helpful in many cases and is associated with fewer side effects than many other antifungals in this setting.[20]

PREVENTION AND CONTROL

Prevention of tinea capitis requires good hygiene because most etiologic agents are anthropophilic dermatophytes. These are easily transmitted from one person to another. Tinea corporis prevention depends upon whether the dermatophyte is anthropophilic or zoophilic. When anthropophilic species are involved, clothing, towels, and bedding should not be shared. The animal source of zoophilic fungi such as *M. canis* needs to be located and treated. Tinea cruris often has a high recurrence rate. The groin area should be dried with a towel, using an absorbent powder to remove excess moisture and avoiding the use of occlusive garments. Tinea pedis relapse is very common. Antifungal powder placed on the feet and inside socks and shoes may be helpful. Daily bathing of feet and careful drying of the interdigital spaces, avoiding occlusive footwear, and not going barefoot in public facilities are appropriate preventive measures. Other than the use of antifungal lacquers, onychomycosis is difficult to prevent.

Effective vaccines against dermatophytes have been developed and used in the cattle industry.[33] LTF-130, a live vaccine against *T. verrucosum*, has been used successfully to reduce infections in cattle herds in Europe.[34] Immunity appears to be dermatophyte species–specific, and live attenuated vaccines appear necessary, as an inactivated vaccine against *M. canis* studied in cats did not prevent disease.[35] No effective vaccines for dermatophytes are currently available for humans.

REFERENCES

1. Schrum JP, Milliken LE, Bataineh O: Superficial fungal infections in the tropics. Dermatol Clin 12:687, 1994.
2. Allen AM, Taplin D: Epidemic *Trichophyton mentagrophytes* infections in servicemen: Source of infection, role of environment, host factors, and susceptibility. JAMA 226:864, 1973.
3. Kawasaki M, Masanori A, Ishizaki H, et al: Phylogeny of *Epidermophyton floccosum* and other dermatophytes. Mycopathologia 134:121, 1996.
4. Guillamón JM, Cano J, Ramón D, et al: Molecular differentiation of *Keratinomyces (Trichophyton)* species. Antonie van Leeuwenhoek 69:223, 1996.
5. Harmsen D, Schwinn A, Weig M, et al: Phylogeny and dating of some pathogenic keratinophilic fungi using small subunit ribosomal RNA. J Med Vet Mycol 33:299, 1995.
6. Leclerc MC, Philippe H, Guého E: Phylogeny of dermatophytes and dimorphic fungi based on large subunit ribosomal RNA sequence comparisons. J Med Vet Mycol 32:331, 1994.
7. Weitzman I, McGinnis MR, Padhye AA, et al: The genus *Arthroderma* and its later synonym *Nannizzia*. Mycotaxon 25:505, 1986.
8. McGinnis MR, Ajello L, Schell WA: Mycotic diseases, a proposed nomenclature. Int J Dermatol 24:9, 1985.
9. Fujita S, Matsuyama T: Experimental tinea pedis induced by non-abrasive inoculation of *Trichophyton mentagrophytes* arthrospores on the plantar part of a guinea pig foot. J Med Vet Mycol 25:203, 1987.
10. Hawranek T: Cutaneous mycology. Chem Immunol 81:129, 2002.
11. Al Sogair S, Hay RJ: Fungal infection in children: Tinea capitis. Clin Dermatol 18:679, 2000.
12. Aly R, Hay RJ, Del Palacio A, et al: Epidemiology of tinea capitis. Med Mycol 38(Suppl 1):183, 2000.
13. Rippon JW: Medical Mycology, the Pathogenic Fungi and the Pathogenic Actinomycetes, ed 3. Philadelphia, WB Saunders, 1988.
14. Kwon-Chung KJ, Bennett JE: Medical Mycology. Philadelphia, Lea & Febiger, 1992.
15. Weitzman I, Summerbell RC: The dermatophytes. Clin Microbiol Rev 8:240, 1995.
16. Leyden JJ, Aly R: Tinea pedis. Semin Dermatol 12:280, 1993.
17. Serjeantson S, Lawrence G: Autosomal recessive inheritance of susceptibility to tinea imbricata. Lancet 1:13, 1977.
18. Elewski BE, Hay RJ: Update on the management of onychomycosis: Highlights of the Third Annual International Summit on Cutaneous Antifungal Therapy. Clin Infect Dis 23:305, 1996.
19. Dompmartin D, Dompmartin A, Deluol AM, et al: Onychomycosis and AIDS: Clinical and laboratory findings in 62 patients. Int J Dermatol 29:337, 1990.
20. Burkhart CN, Chang H, Gottwald L: Tinea corporis in human immunodeficiency virus-positive patients: Case report and assessment of oral therapy. Int J Dermatol 42:839, 2003.
21. Wright DC, Lennox JL, James WD, et al: Generalized chronic dermatophytosis in patients with human immunodeficiency virus type 1 infection and CD4 depletion. Arch Dermatol 127:265, 1991.
22. Porro AM, Yoshioka MCN, Kaminski SK, et al: Disseminated dermatophytosis caused by *Microsporum gypseum* in two patients with the acquired immunodeficiency syndrome. Mycopathologia 137:9, 1997.
23. Bournerias I, De Chauvin MF, Datry A, et al: Unusual *Microsporum canis* infections in adult HIV patients. J Am Acad Dermatol 35:808, 1996.
24. Hironaga M, Okazaki N, Saito K, et al: *Trichophyton mentagrophytes* granulomas: Unique systemic dissemination to lymph nodes, testes, vertebrae, and brain. Arch Dermatol 119:482, 1983.
25. Ogawa H, Summerbell RC, Clemons KV, et al: Dermatophytes and host defense in cutaneous mycoses. Med Mycol 36(Suppl 1):166, 1998.
26. Bibel DJ, Aly R, Shah S, et al: Sphingosines: Antimicrobial barriers of the skin. Acta Dermatol Venereol 73:407, 1993.
27. McGinnis MR, Aly R: Laboratory mycology. In Aly R, Maibach H (eds): Atlas of Infections of the Skin. London, Churchill Livingstone, 1998, p 1.
28. Liu D, Coloe S, Pederson J, et al: Use of arbitrarily primed polymerase chain reaction to differentiate *Trichophyton* dermatophytes. FEMS Microbiol Lett 136:147, 1996.
29. Bennett M, Fleischer AB, Loveless JW, et al: Oral griseofulvin remains the treatment of choice for tinea capitis in children. Pediatr Dermatol 17:304, 2000.
30. Chan YC, Friedlander SF: New treatments for tinea capitis. Curr Opin Infect Dis 17:97, 2004.
31. Cribier BJ, Paul C: Long-term efficacy of antifungals in toenail onychomycosis: A critical review. Br J Dermatol 145:446, 2001.
32. Hart R, Bell-Syer SEM, Crawford F, et al: Systemic review of topical treatments for fungal infections of the skin and nails of the feet. BMJ 319:79, 1999.
33. Rybnikar A, Vrzal V, Chumela J, et al: Vaccination of cattle against trichophytosis using the Czech vaccines. J Mycol Med 6:93, 1996.
34. Gordon PJ, Bond R: Efficacy of a live attenuated *Trichophyton verrucosum* vaccine for control of bovine dermatophytosis. Vet Rec 139:395, 1996.
35. DeBoer DJ, Moriello KA, Blum JL, et al: Safety and immunologic effects after inoculation of inactivated and combined live-inactivated dermatophytosis vaccines in cats. Am J Vet Res 63:1532, 2002.

78

Mycetoma

EL-SHEIKH MAHGOUB

INTRODUCTION

Mycetoma is a subcutaneous, firm, commonly painless swelling, often characterized by the appearance of sinuses through which extrude grains or granules that are aggregations of the causative organism.[1]

These clinical symptoms are caused by an array of diverse microorganisms that have been placed into two groups: (1) aerobic actinomycetes, which are higher filamentous bacteria, and (2) true fungi. Mycetoma caused by the former is called *actinomycetoma* and that caused by the latter, *eumycetoma* (or *maduromycetoma*).

To differentiate between these two types is crucial for deciding on the line of treatment. A common mistake is to give the antibiotic treatment of actinomycetoma to patients with eumycetoma, or vice versa, simply because of their clinical similarities. Presumptive identification of the type of mycetoma can be established from the clinical picture, radiologic appearance of cavities in bones, color, and consistency of grains.

Mycetoma is a relatively frequent tropical fungal infection,[2,3] now being imported to northern countries by immigration and worldwide travel.[4,5] The causal agents of eumycetoma and their morphologic characteristics are shown in Table 78-1 and those of actinomycetoma in Table 78-2.

Mycetoma agents are soil saprophytes.[6,7] They gain entry into human tissue through a thorn prick, wood splinter, or stone cut.

Table 78-1 Morphologic Characteristics of Grains of Organisms Causing Eumycetoma

Organism	Color	Consistency
Madurella mycetomatis	Black	Hard
Madurella grisea	Black	Hard
Leptosphaeria senegalensis	Black	Hard
Exophiala jeanselmei	Black	Hard
Pyrenochaeta romeroi	Black	Hard
Curvularia spp.	Black	Hard
Phialophora verrucosa	Black	Hard
Acremonium spp.	White or yellowish	Soft
Aspergillus flavus	White or yellowish	Soft
Aspergillus nidulans	White or yellowish	Soft
Fusarium spp.	White or yellowish	Soft
Neotestudina rosatii	White or yellowish	Soft
Pseudoallescheria boydii	White or yellowish	Soft

Table 78-2 Characteristics of Grains Containing the Agents of Actinomycetoma

Organism	Color	Size
Actinomadura madurae	White	Large
Actinomadura pelletieri	Red	Small
Nocardia asteroides	Beige or orange	Minute
Nocardia brasiliensis	Beige or orange	Minute
Nocardia transvalensis	Beige or orange	Minute
Streptomyces somaliensis	Yellow	Small

EPIDEMIOLOGY

Mycetoma is endemic in tropical and subtropical parts of the world. Most mycetomas in South and Central America are caused by *Nocardia* spp. and *Madurella grisea;* in the United States and Europe, by *Pseudallescheria boydii, Scedosporium apiospermum,*[8] and *Cephalosporium* spp.; in West Africa, by *Leptosphaeria senegalensis;* and in East Africa, by *Streptomyces somaliensis.* However, *Madurella mycetomatis* is found worldwide. Distribution of mycetoma cases is influenced by rainfall. In dry parts of the tropics where there are about 3 months of rainfall and a long dry season, *M. mycetomatis, S. somaliensis,* and *Actinomadura madurae* are encountered, while in wet parts with a much longer rainy season, *Nocardia* spp. and *Actinomadura pelletieri* are found.[1]

Mycetoma is primarily a human infection, though natural infection in animals has been reported.[9] The infection cycle, however, is always from soil to humans. Mycetoma patients are usually young adults between 20 and 40 years of age and male more than female in a ratio of 5:1. This ratio is reported from many countries and is not merely due to outdoor activities of men.

DISEASE

The first lesion that the patient notices is a painless nodule the size of a peanut that slowly increases in size. In one fifth of cases, pain is the main complaint for which the patient seeks medical advice. As the mycetoma progresses, sinuses open, discharging pus and grains or granules the color and consistency of which depend on the causal organism (see Tables 78-1 and 78-2). A sinus may close but will open in a neighboring site. The clinical triad of a well-developed mycetoma, therefore, is painless swelling, sinuses, and grains. On the other hand, small intact tumors without sinuses are seen in endemic areas.

The lower limb—in most cases starting on the sole of the foot (Fig. 78-1)—is involved in more than 75% of cases, the hand in about 10% to 12%, followed by the back and other parts of the body (Plate 78-1 and Fig. 78-2).

Infection with mycetoma starts in the skin and underlying subcutaneous tissue, followed by bone, which in some cases may be the only site of infection. Mycetoma does not seem to affect muscles, though granules have been found among muscle fibers during surgical operations. Similarly, neither tendons nor nerves are involved, which may explain the absence of pain in many cases. The lesion spreads to neighboring parts through fascial planes. No hematogenous spread has been reported, but lymphatic spread is noted in about 2% of cases.[10]

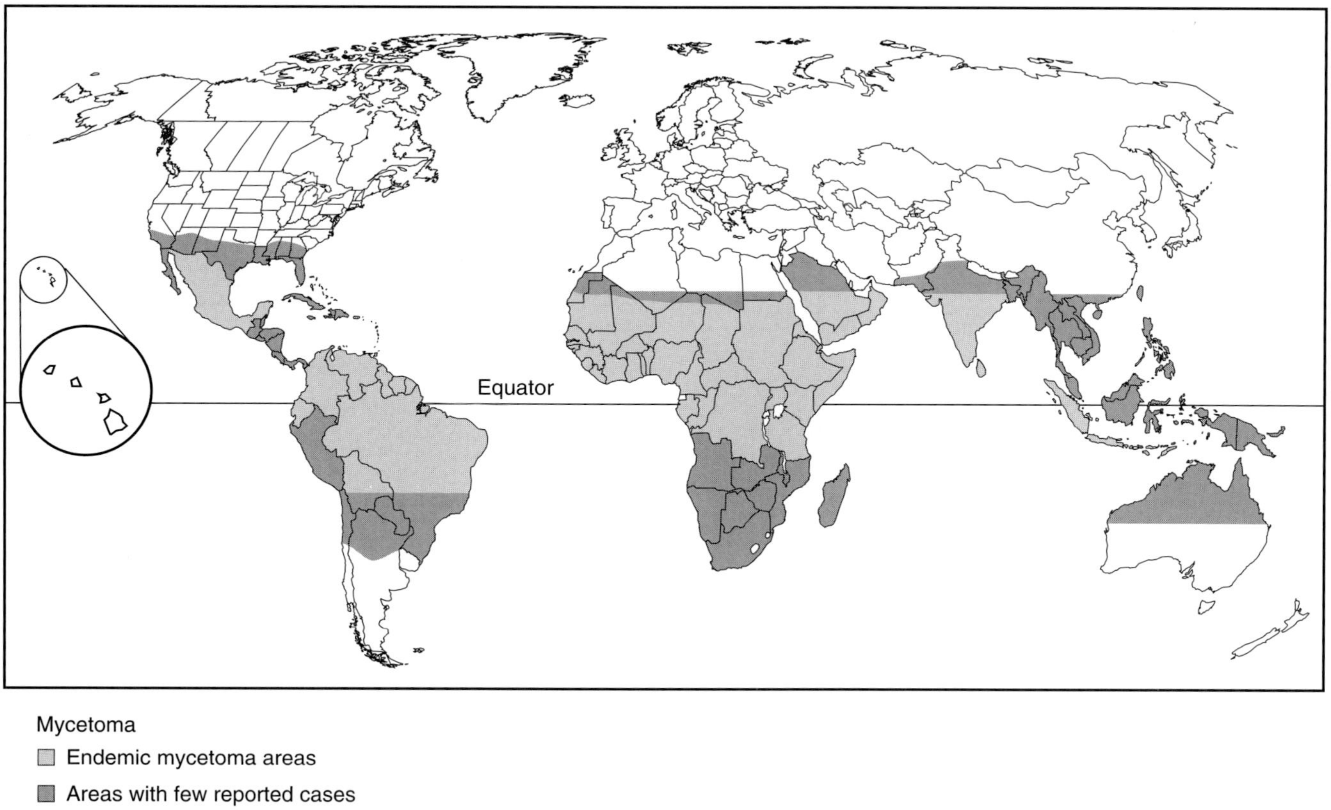

Involvement of internal organs is usually an extension from a subcutaneous lesion, for example, cutaneo-pleuro-bronchial fistulae leading to expectoration of mycetoma grains.[11] In two cases of intraspinal mycetoma, the grains appeared within an artery neighboring the dorsal spine. This may be the first report of hematogenous spread of mycetoma.[12]

The skin is often sweaty over the mycetoma and appears smooth, shiny, punctated with old healed and new sinuses, fixed to the underlying tissue, and possibly hypo- or hyperpigmented. The swelling is firm, rarely nodular, well encapsulated, and mobile in eumycetoma but with ill-defined margins and merging with surrounding tissue in actinomycetoma. The regional lymph nodes (inguinal or axillary) are usually small and shotty except when they are invaded by the mycetoma agent; then they become enlarged and firm or may even discharge pus and grains through sinuses.

PATHOGENESIS AND IMMUNITY

Immune mechanisms attempt to engulf and kill the infecting fungi or actinomycetes. Chemotactic factors attract polymorphonuclear leukocytes and multinucleated giant cells to the site of infection[13] but are ineffective because organisms continue to grow and transform to grains. The filaments forming these grains are cemented together by a hard substance in *Madurella* spp. and *S. somaliensis*.

Three types of inflammatory reaction to mycetoma agents have been identified.[14] In type I, neutrophils degranulate and

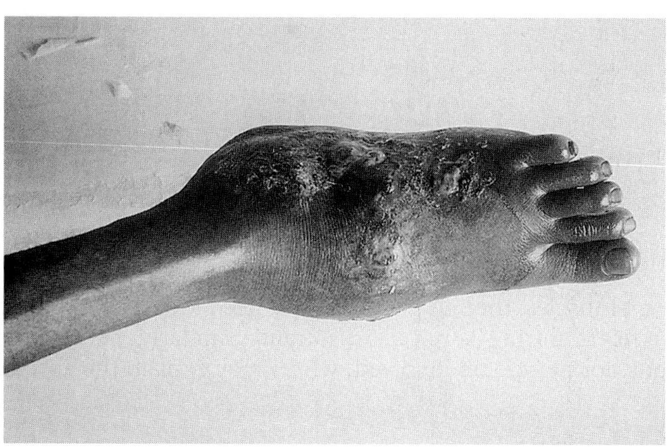

FIGURE 78-1 Mycetoma of the foot.

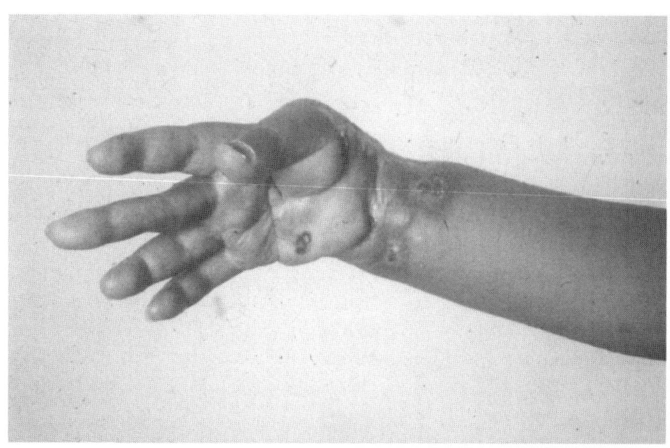

FIGURE 78-2 Mycetoma of the hand and wrist.

become adherent to the surface of the grain, causing disintegration of the grain matrix and destruction of hyphae. This binding of neutrophils to the grains is observed in the presence of immunoglobulins, which are seen on the surface. However, the presence of immunoglobulins may also be nonspecific and result from their exudation together with other plasma proteins. In the type II response, neutrophils are largely absent, and macrophages are observed engulfing fragmented grain material and dead neutrophils. In the type III response, there is a well-developed epithelioid granuloma with Langhans giant cells. Most probably this represents a delayed-type hypersensitivity reaction.

Early experiments to produce mycetoma in immunocompetent animals failed, but typical mycetoma lesions containing well-developed grains with a surrounding polymorphonuclear reaction are produced in athymic nude mice with deficient cell-mediated immunity (CMI).[15] More recently, both immunocompetent male mice and immunocompromised female mice were infected with *M. mycetomatis.*[16] Similarly, studies of mycetoma patients demonstrate some deficiency of CMI.[17] Their lymphocytes fail to transform to lymphoblasts when challenged with phytohemagglutinin. They also fail to react when sensitized and challenged by dinitrochlorobenzene. On the other hand, all types of immunoglobulins were produced in abundance, although they were not protective. Antigenic relationships between *M. mycetomatis* strains causing mycetoma in Sudanese patients showed that there was little genetic variation among them and that different manifestations of mycetoma are due to host factors rather than to the various strains.[18]

DIAGNOSIS

In endemic areas any subcutaneous swelling is considered a mycetoma until proven otherwise. The differential diagnosis includes neurofibroma, Kaposi sarcoma, fibrolipoma, malignant melanoma, osteomyelitis, and osteogenic sarcoma.

The diagnostic feature of a mycetoma in a radiograph is the presence of cavities. These are usually large in eumycetoma and mycetoma caused by *A. madurae* and are small and multiple in actinomycetoma (Fig. 78-3). These cavities contain hard grains with cement substance binding together *M. mycetomatis* or *S. somaliensis*. Spontaneous fracture does not occur. Periosteal erosion due to invasion from outside is seen in metatarsal or metacarpal bones. Bony changes in the skull are sclerotic, with dense bone formation. However, osteoporosis frequently is seen in bones of the limbs owing to either pressure on the blood supply or disuse atrophy or both.

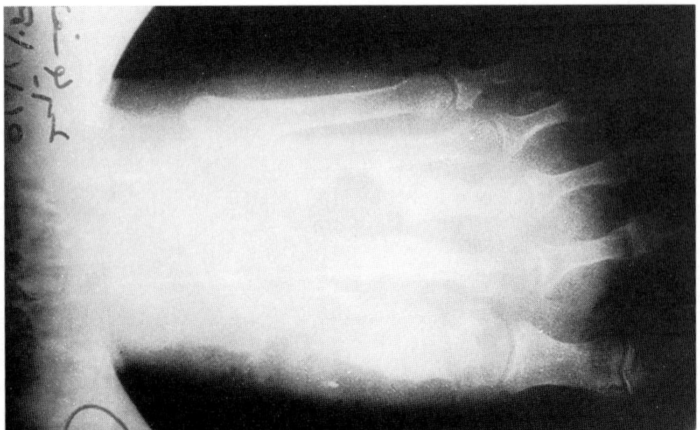

FIGURE 78-3 Mycetoma. Radiograph of the foot. Note the bone change.

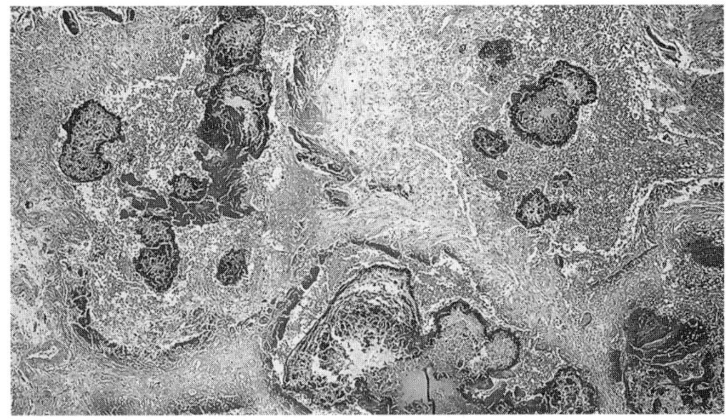

FIGURE 78-4 Histopathologic section stained with H&E. Note mycetoma grains of *M. mycetomatis.*

A presumptive diagnosis of mycetoma can be made on clinical grounds, but a definitive diagnosis can be made only by culture of the organism, histopathology, or serology.

Although grains extruded through sinuses could be cultured, a deep-seated biopsy is preferred for both culture and histopathologic studies because grains coming through sinuses are often contaminated with bacteria and may not be viable. Grains are given a quick rinse in 70% alcohol and saline. Those of actinomycetoma are planted on Löwenstein-Jensen medium, and those of eumycetoma on ordinary blood agar or any other rich medium, for example, brain-heart infusion agar, and incubated at 37°C. Subcultures are made on glucose-peptone agar for identification. Colonies formed by bacterial or fungal growth have a special configuration, often retain the color of the grains, and some of them, particularly *M. mycetomatis,* secrete a diffusible pigment in the culture medium.[1]

The biopsy specimen for histologic diagnosis is transferred to the laboratory in 10% buffered formalin. Diagnosis can be made only when grains are seen in the section because their shape, size, and affinity for the stains are quite characteristic (Fig. 78-4).

Ultrastructural studies of mycetoma grains[19,20] show closely packed filaments with an electron-dense matrix between the filaments in some areas. Individual filaments show septation, and their wall consists largely of electron-dense, finely granular material. Some filaments show cytoplasmic organelles, while others appear empty. Neutrophils are closely adherent to the surface of the grain.

Cytoplasmic extracts are refined, dried, reconstituted, and titrated as antigens for serologic diagnosis. Serum is collected from patients and tested for diagnosis or follow-up of treatment.[21] Although enzyme-linked immunosorbent assay (ELISA) has been attempted,[22–24] counterimmunoelectrophoresis remains the serologic test of choice. Precipitation lines in agar develop after 2 hours' incubation at 30°C. They are assessed for their number and intensity of color after staining with naphthalene black.[25] In attempting to improve the diagnosis of mycetoma, specific oligonucleotide primers encoding the fungal ribosomal RNA of *M. mycetomatis* were developed for use in the polymerase chain reaction (PCR). The test is highly specific and is recommended for species identification of black-grain mycetomas.[26]

TREATMENT

Prior to starting medical treatment, it is absolutely necessary to determine whether the causal organism of the mycetoma is a bacterium (actinomycetoma) or a fungus (eumycetoma); many cases of treatment failure are attributed to giving the treatment of one to the other. It is worth noting that surgical reduction of a bulky swelling without performing amputation or other drastic surgery will certainly reduce the length of treatment.

Whenever possible, depending on the availability of sophisticated laboratory facilities, in vitro sensitivity of organisms causing mycetoma to antibiotics and chemotherapeutic agents should be assessed.[27] There can be a great difference in the susceptibility of different strains of the same organism to one drug or another. In vitro testing will help select the best possible drug for the treatment of mycetoma.

Actinomycetoma

The standard treatment for actinomycetoma is a combination of streptomycin sulfate and co-trimoxazole, but if there is no response after 3 weeks, a combination of streptomycin with one of the following drugs is given: diaminodiphenyl sulfone (dapsone), sulfadoxine-pyrimethamine (Fansidar), or rifampicin.[28] Injections of streptomycin sulfate are given intramuscularly (IM) at 14 mg/kg/d for the first month and on alternate days thereafter. Each tablet of co-trimoxazole contains 400 mg of sulfamethoxazole and 80 mg of trimethoprim. The usual daily dose is 23 mg/kg/d of sulfamethoxazole and 4.6 mg/kg/d of trimethoprim given in two divided doses. The dose is halved if there is a reduction in either hemoglobin or white blood cell count. Dapsone tablets of 100 mg are given, usually at 1.5 mg/kg morning and evening; in the few cases in which anemia or leukopenia appears, 0.7 mg/kg is given twice daily. Tablets containing 500 mg of sulfadoxine and 25 mg of pyrimethamine are given at 7.5 mg/kg twice weekly. After clinical cure is achieved or when an effect on the bone marrow is noted, the dosage is reduced to 7.5 mg/kg once per week. The dose of rifampicin is 4.3 mg/kg morning and evening.

Amikacin alone and in combination with co-trimoxazole has been used for actinomycetoma patients who have no response to the first-line treatments or have a potentially hazardous site of infection; it is contraindicated when there is hepatic, hearing, or renal impairment.[3,29] The therapy is given in cycles. A *cycle* is defined as the period of simultaneous administration of amikacin 15 mg/kg/d divided into two daily doses for 3 weeks and co-trimoxazole (35 mg sulfamethoxazole and 7 mg trimethoprim per kilogram per day) for 5 weeks. Twenty-six patients in Mexico have been treated with this therapy. Twenty-one needed one or two cycles of treatment (5 to 10 weeks), and only five needed three cycles (15 weeks). After the treatment was completed, the patients were asymptomatic and remained without further medication. All patients have been evaluated for periods of between 6 months and 7 years. Side effects were minimal with no gastrointestinal disturbances and normal creatinine clearance rates.

The combination of amoxicillin and clavulanic acid has been reported to be effective for treatment of mycetoma due to *Nocardia brasiliensis* when there is resistance to drugs commonly used, when there is bone or visceral involvement, and in the case of side effects to sulfones or aminoglycosides.[30] β-Lactam resistance in *N. brasiliensis* is mediated by β-lactamase and is reversed in the presence of clavulanic acid.

Eumycetoma

It would be appropriate to select an antimycotic agent after isolation of the causative fungus if antimycotic testing is available.[5] However, in the case of eumycetoma due to *M. mycetomatis* and *M. grisea,* which constitute the major causative agents in tropical and subtropical Africa, Asia, and South America, the drug of choice is ketoconazole[31,32] at a dose of 200 mg twice daily; no significant side effects or biochemical abnormalities are seen. Ketoconazole, however, may not be as effective in mycetoma caused by *P. boydii.* Liver function tests should be performed regularly every month during treatment in patients treated with an imidazole.

Itraconazole was not effective in the treatment of mycetoma due to *M. mycetomatis* in early reports, but recent studies in Sudan (unpublished data) have shown some success. A successful outcome of treating mycetoma due to *Aspergillus flavus* with itraconazole was reported from the United States.[33] Mycetoma due to *Scedosporium apiospermum* has been treated with voriconazole.[8]

Mycetoma is a chronic infection, and likewise treatment must be continued for a long time. In all cases, treatment should continue for not less than 10 months and may have to be extended for 2 years, depending on the tolerance of the patient for the drug used. Medical treatment of an actinomycetoma can have a favorable result (Figs. 78-5 and 78-6).

Treatment Follow-up

Patients can be treated at home and be followed in clinic every 2 to 3 weeks. The size of the swelling is measured by tape at the same anatomic point to assess progressive decreases in size, sinuses are counted, and color and free movement of the skin over the swelling are assessed, but an objective response is determined by the number and intensity of precipitating antibodies in the serum by means of counterimmunoelectrophoresis.[25] As recovery progresses, precipitation arcs become fewer and change from strong to faint in appearance until finally they disappear. Actinomycetoma patients should be monitored by determination of the total white cell count and hemoglobin concentration every month.

PREVENTION AND CONTROL

There is no vaccine against mycetoma agents. Since entry of the causal organisms is often associated with a skin-penetrating injury such as a thorn prick, it was suggested to encourage those exposed to infection, such as field laborers and animal herders, to wear shoes. However, the most effective method of control, at present, is to detect early cases

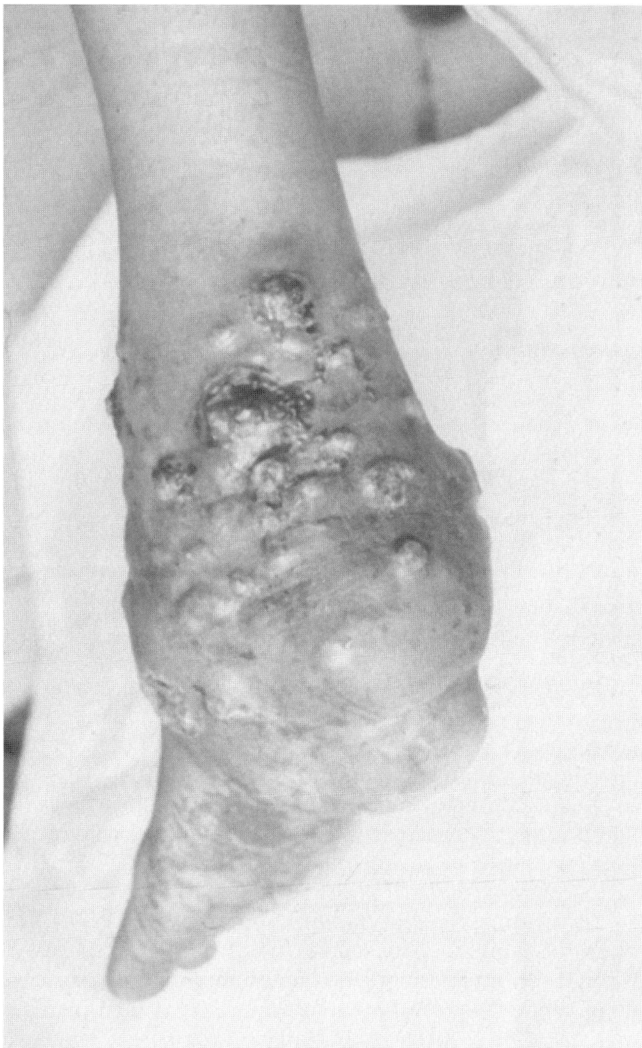

A

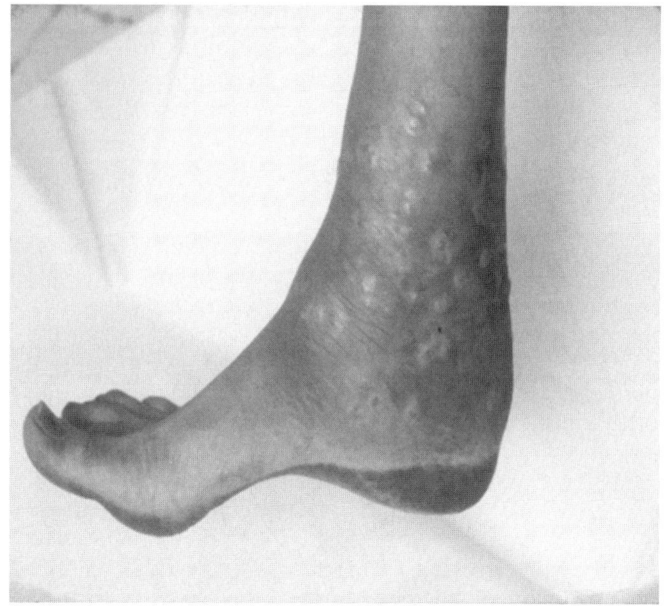

B

FIGURE 78-5 Patient with *S. somaliensis* mycetoma before (*A*) and after (*B*) treatment with streptomycin and dapsone.

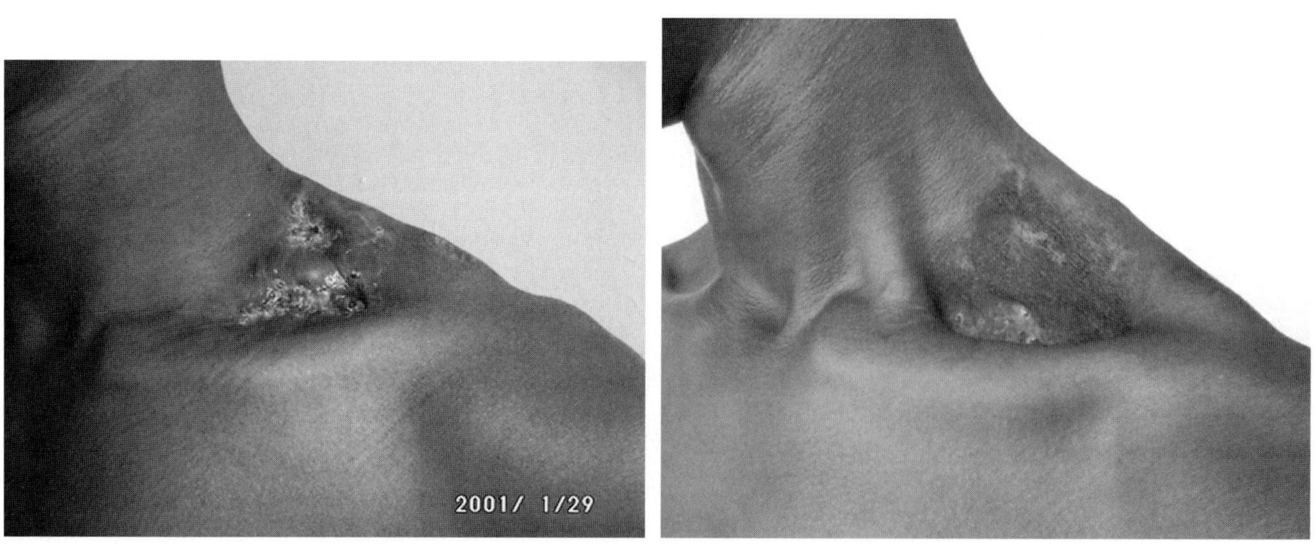

A B

FIGURE 78-6 Patient with *M. mycetomatis* eumycetoma treated with ketoconazole before (*A*) and after (*B*) treatment.

when swellings are small, excise them, and give concurrent medical treatment to prevent recurrence. In endemic areas, awareness of the disease and its complications should be increased through health education.

REFERENCES

1. Mahgoub ES: Tropical Mycoses. Beerse, Belgium, Janssen Research Council, 1989, p 57.
2. Mahgoub ES, Murray IG: Mycetoma. London, Heinemann, 1973.
3. Welch O: Mycetoma. Semin Dermatol 12:290, 1993.
4. Hay RJ, Mackenzie DWR: Mycetoma (Madura foot) in the United Kingdom: A survey of forty-four cases. Clin Exp Dermatol 8:553, 1983.
5. Hoog GS, Buiting A, Tan CS, et al: Diagnostic problems with imported cases of mycetoma in the Netherlands. Mycoses 36:81, 1993.
6. Ahmed A, Adelmann D, Fahal A, et al: Environmental occurrence of *Madurella mycetomatis,* the major agent of human eumycetoma in Sudan. J Clin Microbiol 40:1031, 2002.
7. Ajello G, Brown J, Maghoub ES, et al: A note on the isolation of pathogenic aerobic actinomycetes from Sudanese soils. Curr Microbiol 2:25, 1979.
8. Bosma F, van Hamersvelt HW, de Sevaux RG, et al: Two cases of subcutaneous *Scedosporium apiospermum* infection treated with voriconazole. Clin Microbiol Infect 9:750, 2003.
9. Gumaa SA, Mohamed FHA, Mahgoub ES, et al: Mycetoma in goats. Sabouraudia 16:217, 1978.
10. El Hassan AM, Mahgoub ES: Lymph node involvement in mycetoma. Trans R Soc Trop Med Hyg 66:165, 1972.
11. Fahal AH, Sharfi AR, Sheik HE, et al: Internal fistula formation: an unusual complication of mycetoma. Trans R Soc Trop Med Hyg 90:550, 1996.
12. Arbab MAR, Elhag IA, Abdul Gadir AF, Siddik HER: Intraspinal mycetoma: Report of two cases. Am J Trop Med Hyg 56:27–29, 1997.
13. Yousif MA, Hay RJ: Leucocyte chemotaxis to mycetoma agents. Trans R Soc Trop Med Hyg 81:319, 1987.
14. Fahal AH, El Toum EA, El Hassan AM, et al: The host tissue reaction to *Madurella mycetomatis:* New classification. J Med Vet Mycol 33:15, 1995.
15. Mahgoub ES: Experimental infection of athymic nude New Zealand mice "nu nu" strain with mycetoma agents. Sabouraudia 16:211, 1978.
16. Ahmed AO, van Vianen W, ten Kate MT, et al: A murine model of *Madurella mycetomatis* eumycetoma. FEMS Immunol Med Microbiol 37:29, 2003.
17. Mahgoub ES, Gumaa SA, El Hassan AM: Immunological status of mycetoma patients. Bull Soc Pathol Exot 70:48, 1977.
18. Ahmed A, van de Sande W, Verbrugh H, et al: *Madurella mycetomatis* strains from mycetoma lesions in Sudanese patients are clonal. J Clin Microbiol 41:1, 2003.
19. Wethered DB, Markey MA, Hay RJ, et al: Ultrastructural and immunogenic changes in the formation of mycetoma grains. J Med Vet Mycol 25:39, 1986.
20. Nasher M, Wethered DB, Hay RJ, et al: The ultrastructure of mycetoma grains caused by *Streptomyces somaliensis* . Am J Trop Med Hyg 37:174, 1987.
21. Mahgoub ES. Mycetoma. In Diamond RD, Mandel GL (eds): Atlas of Infectious Diseases. Philadelphia, Current Medicine, 2000, p 181.
22. Mc Laren M, Mahgoub ES, Georgakopoulos E: Preliminary investigation on use of ELISA in serodiagnosis of mycetoma. Sabouraudia 16:25, 1978.
23. Wethered DB, Markey MA, Hay RJ, et al: Humoral immune responses to mycetoma organisms: characterization of specific antibodies by the use of enzyme-linked immunosorbent assay and immuno-blotting. Trans R Soc Trop Med Hyg 82:918, 1988.
24. Salinas-Carmona MC, Welsh O, Casillas SM: Enzyme-linked immunosorbent assay for serological diagnosis of *Nocardia brasiliensis* and clinical correlation with mycetoma infections. J Clin Microbiol 31:2901, 1993.
25. Gumaa SA, Mahgoub ES: Counterimmunoelectrophoresis in the diagnosis of mycetoma and its sensitivity as compared to immunodiffusion. Sabouraudia 13:309, 1975.
26. Ahmed A, Mukhtar MM, Kools-Sijmons M, Fahal AH, et al: Development of a species-specific PCR-restriction fragment length polymorphism analysis procedure for identification of *Madurella mycetomatis.* J Clin Microbiol 37:3175, 1999.
27. Venugopal PV, Venugopal TV, Ramakrishna ES, et al: Antimycotic susceptibility testing of agents of black grain eumycetoma. J Med Vet Mycol 31:161, 1993.
28. Mahgoub ES: Medical management of mycetoma. Bull World Health Organ 54:303, 1976.
29. Wortman PD: Treatment of a *Nocardia brasiliensis* mycetoma with sulfamethoxazole and trimethoprim, amikacin and amoxicillin and clavulanate. Arch Dermatol 129:564, 1993.
30. Gomez A, Saul A, Bonifaz A, et al: Amoxicillin and clavulanic acid in the treatment of actinomycetoma. Int J Dermatol 32:218, 1993.
31. Mahgoub ES, Gumaa SA: Ketoconazole in the treatment of eumycetoma due to *Madurella mycetomi.* Trans R Soc Trop Med Hyg 78:376, 1984.
32. Venugopal PV, Venugopal TV: Treatment of eumycetoma with ketoconazole. Aust J Dermatol 34:27, 1993.
33. Witzig RS, Greer DL, Hyslop JR: *Aspergillus flavus* mycetoma and epidural abscess successfully treated with itraconazole. J Med Vet Mycol 34:133, 1996.

79

Chromoblastomycosis and Phaeohyphomycosis

TADAHIKO MATSUMOTO

INTRODUCTION

Human and animal infections caused by fungi whose mycelia or cells in tissue are dark-colored (dark brown, olive, or black) can be separated into four categories: superficial, cutaneous, subcutaneous, and systemic diseases. The term dematiaceous, which had been used to describe dark-colored fungi, was found to be epistemologically incorrect and has been replaced by "phaeoid" (Gr. *phaios,* dusky).[1]

In most cases, the pigment in the cell walls of the hyphae or conidia is melanin, and specifically dihydroxynaphthalene (DHN) melanin appears to be common to most of the medically important phaeoid fungi. In comparison with what is known about the role of fungal melanins in phytopathogenic fungi, current knowledge of their role in infections of humans and lower animals is at an early stage of development. However, recent investigation of the possible effects of fungal melanins in the pathogenesis of the phaeoid fungi has already yielded some interesting results.[2,3] Definitive proof of the involvement of melanin in the virulence of phaeoid fungi awaits further molecular biological studies that specifically alter the DHN-melanin biosynthesis pathway by gene disruption.

The cutaneous and subcutaneous mycoses with etiologic agents that have phaeoid invasive forms are chromoblastomycosis, eumycotic mycetoma (in part; see Chapter 78), and phaeohyphomycosis. Visceral or systemic infections also occur as disseminated cases of phaeohyphomycosis of the internal organs. Phaeoid fungal infections have a broad spectrum of clinical features, ranging in severity from superficial and mild to deep-seated, serious, and fatal.[4]

Chromoblastomycosis

Chromoblastomycosis is a mycotic infection of cutaneous and subcutaneous tissues characterized by the development in tissue of phaeoid muriform cells by its etiologic agents. The term sclerotic cells, as used for the characteristic cells seen in tissue in chromoblastomycosis, has been replaced by "muriform cells."[5]

AGENTS

The principal etiologic agents of chromoblastomycosis are *Cladophialophora* (formerly *Cladosporium*) *carrionii, Fonsecaea compactum, Fonsecaea pedrosoi, Phialophora verrucosa,* and *Rhinocladiella aquaspersa.* Among them, *F. pedrosoi* is the most frequent agent, followed by *C. carrionii* and *P. verrucosa. F. pedrosoi* is predominant in warm and humid areas, whereas *C. carrionii* occurs in arid and semiarid zones. *F. pedrosoi* and *P. verrucosa* have been reported as etiologic agents of phaeohyphomycosis as well, the latter also as an etiologic agent of black grain mycetomas. *Fonsecaea compactum* is sometimes considered as a dysgonic strain or variety of *F. pedrosoi*. These fungi are present in soil, decaying wood, and decomposing vegetation.[4,6]

In culture, all these species produce similar dark colonies with short aerial hyphae and gray, green, brown, or black velvety surfaces. These agents are differentiated by their microscopic morphology, physiology, serology (exoantigen tests), and molecular biology.[4,7,8]

EPIDEMIOLOGY

Although most cases of chromoblastomycosis have occurred predominantly in tropical and subtropical areas, the disease has been reported from the temperate zones of every continent in the world. Brazil and Madagascar are the countries with the highest prevalence. The highest incidence of chromoblastomycosis has occurred in Costa Rica.[9,10] However, partially because of the gradually and steadily rising global temperature and marked increase of immigration and travel, the reported cases of chromoblastomycosis have been spreading from tropical and subtropical areas to temperate areas. Generally it affects the exposed areas of the skin, mostly the distal part of the legs of male outdoor laborers who often work barefooted.

DISEASE

The primary lesion is a small, pink, scaly papule that occurs at the site of inoculation of the etiologic fungus. The traumatic injury could be very minor or it could have occurred many years previously, more than two decades in some cases, and subsequently forgotten. The papule gradually enlarges to form a superficial erythematous or purplish plaque. The lesion at first may be scaly or verrucous in appearance, but as it progresses it becomes a verrucous nodule. Occasionally, the lesion is pruritic, and when a secondary bacterial infection appears, the patient may complain of pain. Satellite lesions may develop by way of the superficial lymphatics, or by autoinoculation through scratching. New lesions resemble the primary ones and transform themselves into the types of lesions just described. They frequently merge to form a verrucous, sometimes cauliflower-like mass. On the surface, hemopurulent black dots are often observed. Ulceration may occur when a secondary infection or a localized injury to the lesions coexists. Secondary infections also lead to lymphatic stasis, which may result in elephantiasis. Scars may be formed in the center of the lesions when they enlarge centrifugally (Fig. 79-1).

PATHOGENESIS AND IMMUNITY

Although, in general, chromoblastomycosis is localized at the site of the primary inoculation, the etiologic fungus can break through cutaneous tissue, metastasize to subcutaneous lymphatics or muscle tissue, and disseminate to other organs, including the central nervous system. Early diagnosis of

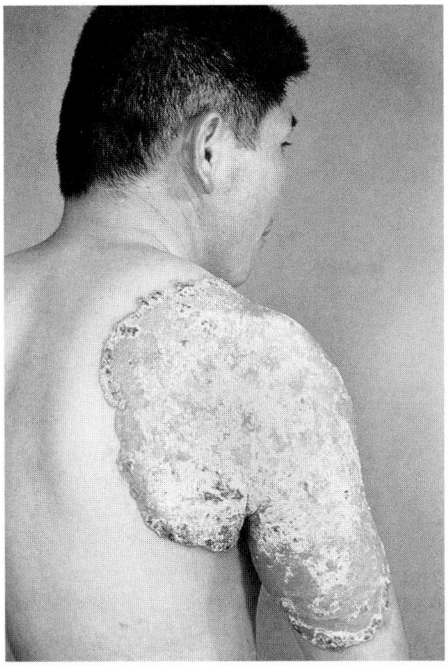

FIGURE 79-1 Chromoblastomycosis caused by *Fonsecaea pedrosoi.*

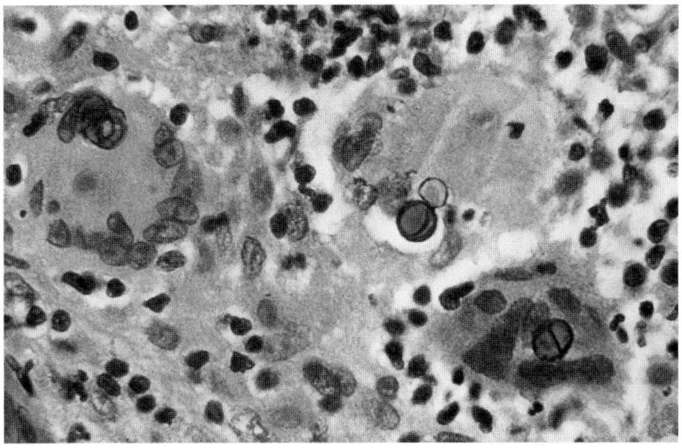

FIGURE 79-2 Phaeoid muriform cells in chromoblastomycosis caused by *Fonsecaea pedrosoi* (periodic acid–Schiff stain).

metastasis is of utmost importance in treatment. The tissue response in chromoblastomycosis is not specific for establishing a histopathologic diagnosis. Fundamentally, it is a mixed purulent and granulomatous inflammatory reaction, which may also occur in other mycoses.

The small granulomatous nodules, consisting of epithelioid cells and multinucleated giant cells, are found in the dermis or in subcutaneous tissues. Wood splinters are occasionally encountered in situ. The granulomas may have microabscesses containing polymorphonuclear leukocytes and necrotic debris. The surrounding stroma, infiltrated with lymphocytes, plasma cells, macrophages, and polymorphonuclear leukocytes, may show marked fibrosis, especially in older lesions. In the epidermis, either acanthosis or pseudoepitheliomatous hyperplasia or both are recognized. The hyperplastic epidermis may extend into the affected dermis, forming lips around the necrotic tissue. The stratum corneum is frequently distorted and shows hyperkeratosis and parakeratosis. Cellular infiltrates in the epidermis, consisting of polymorphonuclear leukocytes, may occasionally form keratolytic microabscesses.

In tissue, the phaeoid, round to polygonal, thick-walled, and multicellular muriform cells are the characteristic and diagnostic features of chromoblastomycosis. The muriform cells represent an intermediate vegetative form arrested between yeast and hyphal formation. The muriform cells occur free in tissues or may be contained in giant cells or in microabscesses, as well as in the epidermis, and even in the stratum corneum (Fig. 79-2).

The wide distribution of muriform cells could be explained, in part, by a phenomenon called "transepidermal (or transepithelial) elimination." This phenomenon causes foreign material (e.g., fungus cells) in the dermis to be eliminated via transepidermal passage without causing any major structural alteration or epidermal degeneration.[11]

A morphologic study of the host-parasite interaction in chromoblastomycosis revealed that some of the phagocytosed fungal cells are damaged but that intracellular killing of the fungus is rare. These findings suggested that the tissue form of the etiologic agents of chromoblastomycosis resisted the fungicidal activity of the cutaneous macrophages that possessed the ultrastructural features of stimulated phagocytes.[12]

DIAGNOSIS

Diagnosis is based on the characteristic clinical appearance of chromoblastomycosis, by the presence of phaeoid muriform cells in tissue, and by the isolation and identification of the etiologic fungi (Fig. 79-3).

The exoantigen test is applicable to identification of cultures in some species; however, none of the reagents are commercially available. Molecular probes are being developed for the phaeoid fungi, but their application is currently limited to taxonomic purposes (see Phaeohyphomycosis).

TREATMENT AND PROGNOSIS

The treatment of choice is surgical excision of small lesions and antifungal chemotherapy with flucytosine with or

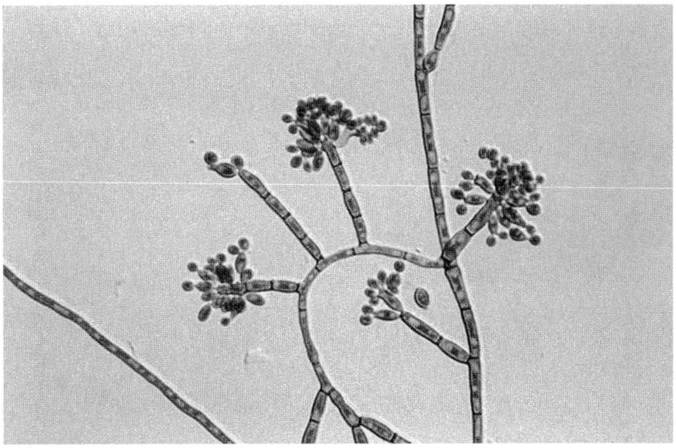

FIGURE 79-3 In vitro micromorphology of *Fonsecaea pedrosoi.*

without intravenous amphotericin B. As long-term therapy, itraconazole 200 to 400 mg/day effectively controls the disease, although in limited trials saperconazole was reported to be more effective and required shorter treatment courses than itraconazole.[6] The efficacy of fluconazole (100 to 400 mg/day) has not been satisfactory.[13] A recent report from Madagascar on terbinafine (500 mg/day for 6 to 12 months) in the treatment of the 42 Malagasy patients with chromoblastomycosis described promising and encouraging results (a global efficacy of about 75%).[14] Alternate week and combination therapy with itraconazole and terbinafine was effective for some cases of chromoblastomycosis in which patients demonstrated minimal to poor response to monotherapy with oral itraconazole or terbinafine. Flucytosine (100 to 200 mg/kg/day) is effective when combined with itraconazole. Resistance to flucytosine may develop if it is used alone. Antifungal agents under development may play an important role in the treatment of chromoblastomycosis. Agents of chromoblastomycosis are sensitive in vitro to the new triazoles, voriconazole and posaconazole, and also to some of the echinocandins.

Local heat therapy, using a pocket warmer or an electric pad, has been used successfully in cases of chromoblastomycosis. A study of the mechanisms underlying the effectiveness of topical heat therapy suggested that heat killing of the causative organism is unlikely to have been the sole reason for the effectiveness of this modality.[15,16]

Chromoblastomycosis is still notoriously resistant to treatment, with the result that management is extremely frustrating. Clinical type, etiologic species, duration of disease, site of infection, underlying condition of the patient, and experience of the physician are primary factors dictating the type of treatment and the patient's outcome.

PREVENTION AND CONTROL

The incidence of chromoblastomycosis would be reduced through education, economic development, and early diagnosis and treatment. The low incidence of infections does not justify the development of vaccines, assuming such an approach were feasible.[17]

Phaeohyphomycosis

Phaeohyphomycosis is an infection of humans and other animals caused by a number of phaeoid fungi, characterized by the basic development of dark-colored filamentous hyphae in invaded tissues. The term phaeohyphomycosis encompasses distinct mycotic infections regardless of the site of the lesion, pattern of tissue response (granuloma or abscess), or taxonomic classification of the etiologic agents.[18]

AGENTS

Along with the increasing number of immunocompromised patients, the number of genera and species of fungi causing phaeohyphomycosis has been growing. As of 1998, the phaeoid fungi, verified as causing phaeohyphomycosis, comprised 109 species classified in 60 genera, and still growing. Among them, *Exophiala jeanselmei* and *Wangiella dermatitidis* were the most common species, followed by such phaeoid fungus species as *Alternaria alternata, Bipolaris spicifera, Curvularia lunata, Exophiala moniliae, Exophiala spinifera, Exserohilum rostratum, Phaeoacremonium parasiticum, Phialemonium obovatum,* and *Phialophora repens.*[19]

EPIDEMIOLOGY

In contrast to chromoblastomycosis, cases of phaeohyphomycosis occur with equal frequency in tropical, subtropical, and temperate areas, partly because of the opportunistic nature of its etiologic agents. Previously, the distribution of the pathogenic phaeoid fungi was generally believed to be limited to tropical and subtropical areas. However, there have been several reports of the isolation of potentially pathogenic phaeoid fungi from nonclinical sources. They have provided new ecologic insights into the global distribution of this particular group of fungi.[4]

DISEASE

Phaeohyphomycosis is a cosmopolitan disease. The patients are usually adults, about half of whom seem to be immunologically compromised by such associated underlying diseases as diabetes mellitus, tuberculosis, leprosy, acquired immunodeficiency syndrome (AIDS), lymphoma, and leukemia. Some patients appear to be locally compromised because of the application of topical corticosteroids. The lesions may occur in almost any part of the body, often in exposed parts, especially the upper arms. Inoculation of the agent is considered to be caused by wounds made by contaminated plant materials, so that occasionally patients can recall the history of an injury at the site of the lesion.

The most common and typical lesions are cutaneous or subcutaneous cysts or abscesses, frequently caused by *E. jeanselmei.* The primary lesion occurs as a single, discrete, asymptomatic small nodule. This is palpable under the smooth and slightly elevated skin. The nodule gradually evolves to become an encapsulated, fluctuant abscess with a liquefied center (Fig. 79-4). The overlying epidermis is hardly affected, but, exceptionally, formation of a sinus tract or ulceration is observed. Occasionally, a granulomatous, slightly elevated plaque may appear when the main site of the lesion is in the epidermis and dermis. Less frequently, it is manifested as a small verrucous nodule, or a

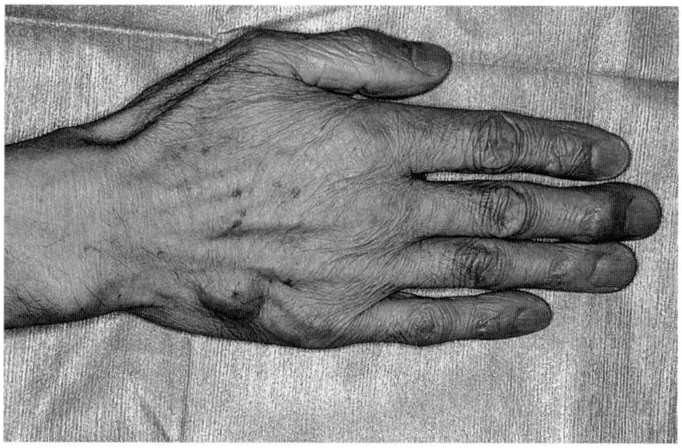

FIGURE 79-4 Subcutaneous phaeohyphomycosis caused by *Exophiala jeanselmei.*

verrucous plaque consisting of coalesced nodules, which resembles the clinical appearance of chromoblastomycosis.

Lymph node involvement and dissemination are rare. However, phaeohyphomycosis may occur in the central nervous system or other internal organs, such as the liver, lungs, or pancreas. It may appear as a hematogenous metastasis from cutaneous or subcutaneous infections, or without any visible lesions. Human infections caused by *W. dermatitidis* have been equally distributed between cutaneous and subcutaneous infections, and systemic involvement. *W. dermatitidis* should be regarded as a dermotropic and neurotropic pathogen.[5,20]

PATHOGENESIS

Cyst or abscess formation is mainly confined to the dermis and adjacent subcutaneous tissue. Three stages have been described: (1) a tuberculoid phase, (2) a stellate abscess, and (3) a fluctuant abscess. In the primary lesion, a hypercellular tubercle composed mainly of epithelioid cells and foreign body giant cells is formed. Scattered foci of necrosis follow, accompanied by acute and chronic cellular infiltrations, and stellate abscesses develop. The stellate abscesses coalesce to transform themselves into a fluctuant abscess.[21]

The abscess is surrounded by a thick wall. The inner layer is made up of a combination of epithelioid cells, macrophages, giant cells of foreign body and Langhans types, and neutrophils. The middle layer is composed predominantly of vascularized scar tissue surrounded by an outer layer of hyalinized fibrous tissue. The center of the abscess contains necrotic debris mixed with polymorphonuclear leukocytes. Foreign plant material, as in chromoblastomycosis, may be present. The granulomatous lesions in the middle to upper dermis mainly consist of epithelioid and giant cells that are covered by the necrotic epidermis. Pseudoepitheliomatous hyperplasia, hyperkeratosis, parakeratosis, and acanthosis overlying the upper dermal granuloma are recognized in phaeohyphomycosis. These appear clinically as verrucous plaques resembling chromoblastomycosis.

The pigmented fungal elements show a variety of morphologies in the tissue of phaeohyphomycosis. They may be dark-walled, short, septate, branched or unbranched hyphal elements, catenulate spherical cells (toruloid or moniliform hyphae), isolated spherical cells that have divided by budding or by septation in a single plane, or various combinations of any of these (Fig. 79-5). The spherical yeastlike cells occasionally resemble the muriform cells of chromoblastomycosis, but differ by having thinner cell walls, septation in only one plane, and frequently a catenulate morphology. It is important to note that mycoses caused by phaeoid fungi are variable and that a single fungus species may cause more than one type of disease. Chromoblastomycosis and phaeohyphomycosis represent extremes of a continuum of infections caused by phaeoid fungi.[17]

The brown color of the fungal elements, generally easily observable in hematoxylin and eosin–stained tissue slides, is lighter than that of chromoblastomycosis and is often overlooked. Periodic acid–Schiff, Gomori's methenamine silver, or other stains for fungi may be required to detect the fungal elements in such a case. If questions should arise concerning the pigmentation of the mycelium in tissue sections, the Fontana-Masson silver stain, specific for melanin, may be used to advantage. Mycelium that appears to be hyaline in hematoxylin and eosin–stained sections may give a positive reaction for melanin.[22]

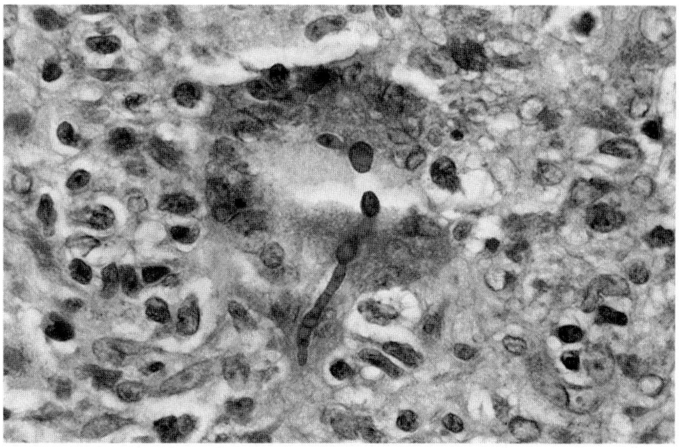

FIGURE 79-5 Septate mycelium in cutaneous phaeohyphomycosis caused by *Wangiella dermatitidis* (periodic acid–Schiff stain).

DIAGNOSIS

Diagnosis of phaeohyphomycosis is based on the presence of phaeoid hyphae in tissue and by the isolation and identification of compatible etiologic fungi (Fig. 79-6). The exoantigen test is applicable to identification of cultures in some phaeoid fungi; however, none of the reagents are commercially available. Molecular probes are also being developed for some of the agents of phaeohyphomycosis, but their application is currently limited to taxonomic purposes.

Many physicians regard molecular diagnosis as infallible, and several groups advocate use of the 18S rRNA gene locus as the sole PCR target necessary for fungal diagnostics. However, molecular identification of medically important fungi should be confirmed by sequence analysis of an additional rRNA gene locus, such as the internal transcribed spacer (ITS) region(s). For example, the molecular interrelationships of one group of phaeoid molds and yeasts, *Exophiala spinifera* clade, were studied using sequences of the small-subunit (SSU) and ITS domains of ribosomal DNA. The resulting proposals were three new species, including *E. oligosperma*, redefinition of *E. jeanselmei*, and two new combinations: *E. exophialae* and *E. heteromorpha*.[23]

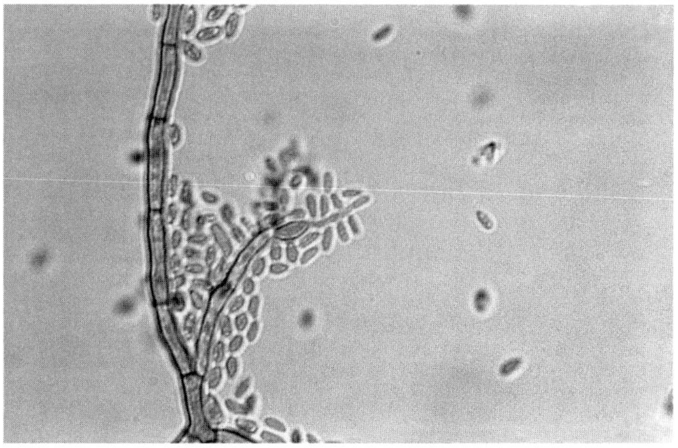

FIGURE 79-6 In vitro micromorphology of *Exophiala moniliae*.

TREATMENT AND PROGNOSIS

Successful treatment of cutaneous and subcutaneous phaeohyphomycosis is achieved by simple surgical excision. However, cases of systemic and disseminated phaeohyphomycosis are serious and have a high rate of mortality. Antifungal chemotherapy with either amphotericin B or flucytosine or combination therapy with these agents should be attempted. Treatment with fluconazole, itraconazole, ketoconazole, or terbinafine has been reported with mixed results.[19,24] Clinical responses were well correlated with in vitro susceptibility test results; however, resistance did not preclude clinical response.

As in the case of chromoblastomycosis, antifungal agents under development may play an important role in the treatment of phaeohyphomycosis. Some of the fungi causing phaeohyphomycosis are sensitive in vitro to the new triazoles, voriconazole and posaconazole, and also to some of the echinocandins.

Local heat therapy, using a pocket warmer or an electric pad, may also be applied to cutaneous and subcutaneous phaeohyphomycosis, even though some of the etiologic fungi possess considerable thermotolerance.[15,16]

PREVENTION AND CONTROL

Prevention and control are not practical for phaeohyphomycosis. Owing to the cosmopolitan, ubiquitous nature of the fungi causing phaeohyphomycosis, it is not feasible to attempt their eradication.[17]

ACKNOWLEDGMENT

Dr. Libero Ajello, former Director of the Division of Mycotic Diseases and now a Guest Researcher of the Mycotic Diseases Branch, Division of Bacterial and Mycotic Diseases, National Center for Infectious Diseases, Centers for Disease Control and Prevention, Atlanta, Georgia, provided helpful suggestions and revision of the manuscript.

REFERENCES

1. Pappagianis D, Ajello L: Dematiaceous—a mycologic misnomer? J Med Vet Mycol 32:319, 1994.
2. Dixon DM, Migliozzi J, Cooper CR, et al: Melanized and non-melanized multicellular-form mutants of *Wangiella dermatitidis* in mice: mortality and histopathology studies. Mycoses 35:17, 1992.
3. Polak, A, Dixon DM: Pathogenicity of *Wangiella dermatitidis*. In Vanden Bossche H, Odds FC, Kerridge D (eds): Dimorphic Fungi in Biology and Medicine. New York, Plenum Press, 1993, p. 307.
4. Matsumoto T, Ajello L: Agents of phaeohyphomycosis. In Collier L, Balows A, Sussman M (eds): Topley and Wilson's Microbiology and Microbial Infections, 9th ed. Vol 4. London, Arnold, 1998, p. 503.
5. Matsumoto T, Padhye AA, Ajello L, et al: Critical review of human isolates of *Wangiella dermatitidis*. Mycologia 76:232, 1984.
6. Restrepo A: Treatment of tropical mycoses. J Am Acad Dermatol 31(Suppl):S91, 1994.
7. De Hoog GS: On the potentially pathogenic dematiaceous hyphomycetes. In Howard DH (ed): Fungi Pathogenic for Humans and Animals. Pt A: Biology. New York, Marcel Dekker, 1983, p. 149.
8. Dixon DM, Polak-Wyss A: The medically important dematiaceous fungi and their identification. Mycoses 34:1, 1991.
9. Al-Doory Y: Chromomycosis. Missoula, MT, Mountain Press, 1972.
10. Ocampo FA: Chromomycosis. Puebla, Mexico, Editorial Cientifico Cultural, 1977.
11. Batres E, Wolf JE, Rudolph AH, et al: Transepithelial elimination of cutaneous chromomycosis. Arch Dermatol 114:1231, 1977.
12. Walter P, Garin Y, Richard-Lenoble D: Chromoblastomycosis: a morphological investigation of the host-parasite interaction. Virchows Archiv 397:203, 1982.
13. Diaz M, Negroni R, Montero-Gei F, et al: A Pan-American 5-year study of fluconazole therapy for deep mycoses in the immunocompetent host. Clin Infect Dis 14(Suppl 1):S68, 1992.
14. Esterre P, Raharisolo C, Inzan CK, et al: From tropical mycology to a public health approach: chromoblastomycosis in Madagascar (in French). J Mycol Med 13:133, 2003.
15. Tagami H, Ginoza M, Imaizumi S, et al: Successful treatment of chromoblastomycosis with topical heat therapy. J Am Acad Dermatol 10:615, 1984.
16. Tagami H, Ohi M, Aoshima T, et al: Topical heat therapy for cutaneous chromomycosis. Arch Dermatol 115:740, 1979.
17. McGinnis MR: Black fungi: A model for understanding tropical mycoses. In Walker DH (ed): Global Infectious Diseases: Prevention, Control, and Eradication. Vienna, Springer-Verlag, 1992, p. 129.
18. Ajello L: Hyalohyphomycosis and phaeohyphomycosis: two global disease entities of public health importance. Eur J Epidemiol 2:243, 1986.
19. Matsumoto T, Ajello L: Dematiaceous fungi potentially pathogenic to humans and lower animals. In Arora DK, Ajello L, Mukerji KG (eds): Handbook of Applied Mycology. Vol 2: Humans, Animals, and Insects. New York, Marcel Dekker 1991, p. 117.
20. Matsumoto T, Matsuda T, McGinnis MR, et al: Clinical and mycological spectra of *Wangiella dermatitidis* infections. Mycoses 36:145, 1993.
21. Ichinose H: Subcutaneous abscesses due to brown fungi. In Baker RD (ed): The Pathologic Anatomy of Mycoses. Berlin, Springer-Verlag, 1971, p. 719.
22. Wood C, Russel-Bell B: Characterization of pigmented fungi by melanin staining. Am J Dermatopathol 5:71, 1983.
23. De Hoog GS, Vicente V, Caligiorne RB, et al: Species diversity and polymorphism in the *Exophila spinifera* clade containing opportunistic black yeast-like fungi. J Clin Microbiol 41:4767, 2003.
24. Sharkey PK, Graybill JR, Rinaldi MG, et al: Itraconazole treatment of phaeohyphomycosis. J Am Acad Dermatol 23:577, 1990.

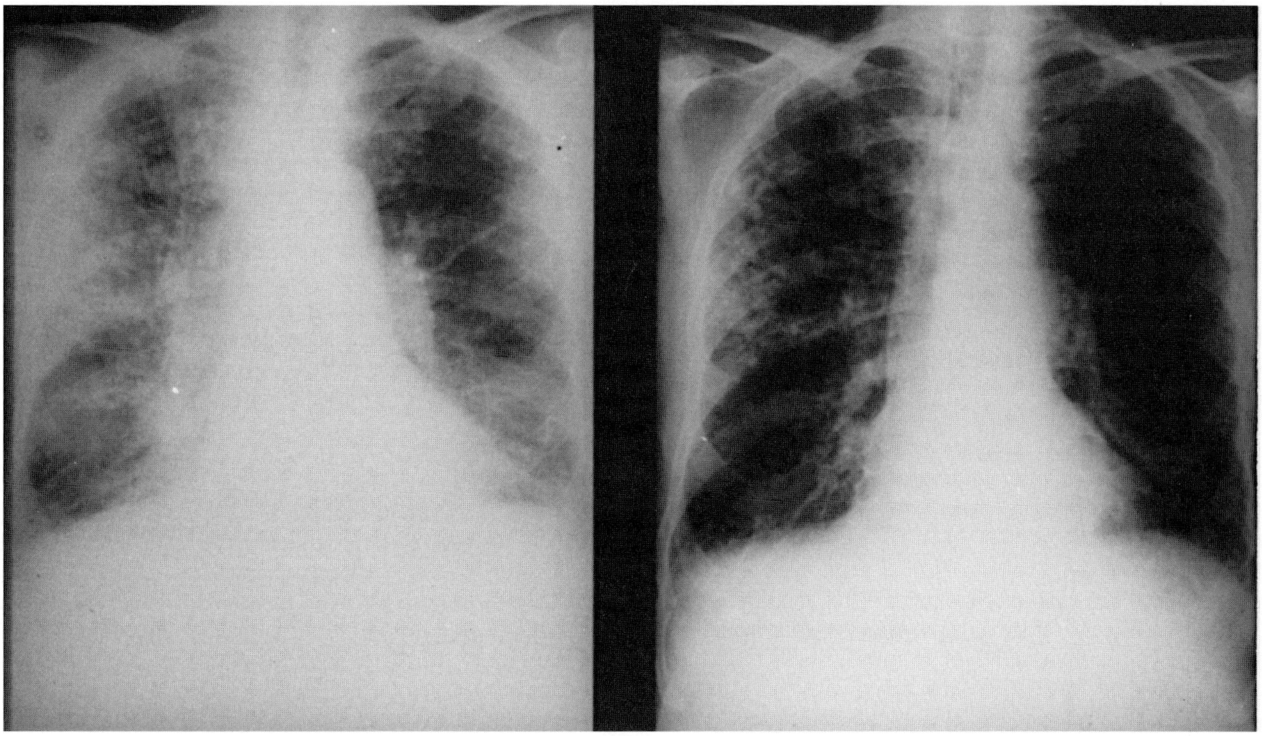

FIGURE 80-2 Chronic pulmonary coccidioidomycosis before (*left*) and after (*right*) treatment with ketoconazole.

thin-walled residual cavities, nodules, abscesses, or infiltrates, which may wax and wane. The course and rate of evolution from primary disease are highly variable. Pulmonary foci may coalesce into nodules that persist, resolve slowly, or undergo necrosis to form cavities. Cavities may persist for months or even years, may slowly resolve (Fig. 80-2), or may rupture into the pleural space, causing pneumothorax, empyema, or both.[83] Hemoptysis or, rarely, severe hemorrhage may also occur. In a case–control study conducted in Kern County, California, risk factors for severe pulmonary disease were diabetes, recent history of smoking, low income, and older age.[84]

Dissemination, when it occurs, often presents within a few months of the primary infection. Pregnancy, particularly the third trimester, poses a hazard for dissemination.[85] Filipinos, African Americans, and Hispanics are also at increased risk of dissemination (Fig. 80-3). Patients with poorly developed cell-mediated immune response may have miliary pulmonary infiltrates and widespread extrapulmonary infection with abscesses draining purulent material and many spherules, neutrophils, and few lymphocytes seen in the lesions. This disseminated infection is associated with a negative skin test and high complement fixation antibody titer. In contrast, the patient with partially competent cell-mediated immunity may have a few granulomas in the skin or scattered lung foci, with a few spherules seen trapped within multinucleated giant cells. In patients with AIDS, the infection has a more aggressive course, which correlates inversely with the CD4 lymphocyte count.[78] Focal pulmonary lesions are the most easily treated, whereas diffuse pulmonary disease occurs in those with the lowest CD4 counts and has the shortest survival time—a median of 1 month. Pulmonary cavitation is rather uncommon in patients with AIDS and coccidioidomycosis.[86] For HIV patients on HAART, one may anticipate a much more benign course , but few data are available.

Coccidioidal meningitis is a chronic lymphocytic meningitis, with low glucose, elevated protein, and culture-positive cerebrospinal fluid (CSF) in up to half of patients.[87]

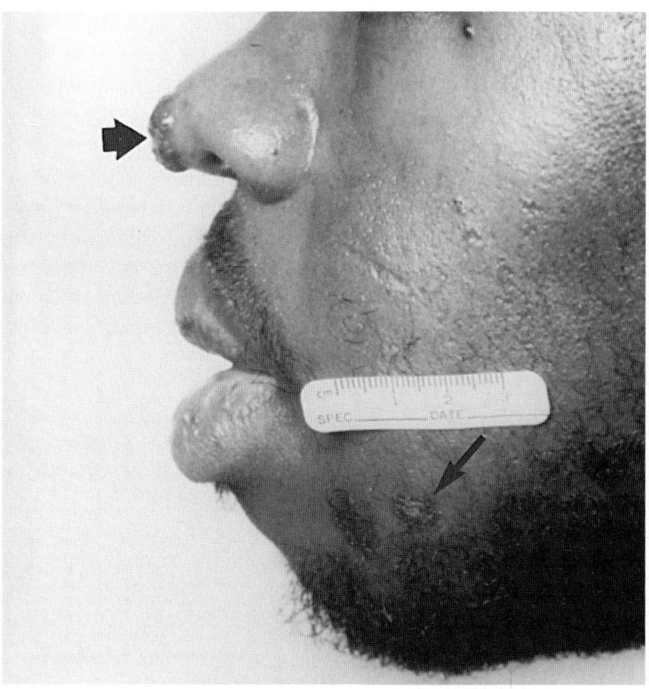

FIGURE 80-3 Facial lesions of chronic coccidioidomycosis (*arrows*).

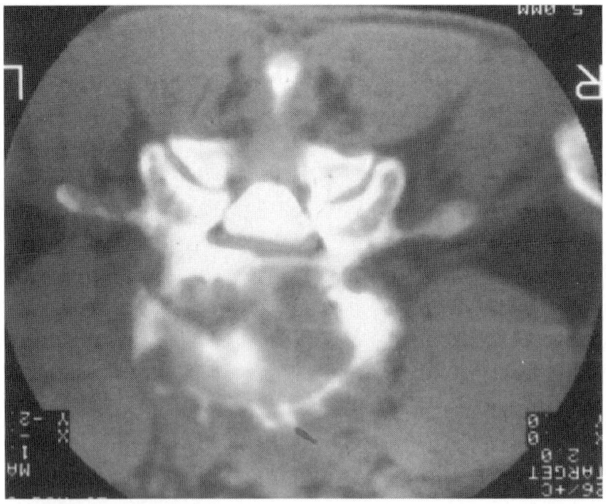

FIGURE 80-4 Dissemination of coccidioidomycosis to the bones, resulting in destruction of the L4–L5 vertebrae.

Eosinophilia may occur in the CSF of up to 70% of patients with coccidioidal meningitis.[88] There is associated focal vasculitis, but some series report remarkably few clinically apparent focal lesions. In one series of 15 patients autopsied with disseminated disease, 8 had CNS involvement. Of these, 8 had meningitis, 7 had encephalitis, 5 had parenchymal abscesses and granulomas, 4 had endarteritis obliterans, 2 had infarcts, and 1 had radiculitis. Associated clinical findings included headache, confusion, seizures, and nuchal rigidity, each in a minority of patients; none had focal neurologic findings.[89] A larger series of 25 patients, collected from 1955 through 1958, identified headache, vomiting, and meningismus in multiple patients, but none had focal neurologic deficits. Fourteen died within 8 months of diagnosis, and 4 survived (with no treatment) for more than 55 months.[90] Other series of patients with coccidioidal CNS infection reported clinical consequences of focal vasculitis and recommended that corticosteroids be considered as emergency therapy.[91] Banuelos and coworkers[92] reported 6 patients with brain abscesses. Approximately one-third of patients with brain abscesses have no associated meningitis, and these patients may have negative CSF serology, thus increasing the difficulty of making a diagnosis.

Dissemination to the bones occurs most often in the vertebrae and other weight-bearing joints, such as the knee (Fig. 80-4). Arthritis is associated with synovial thickening and fluid accumulation. Paraspinous abscesses may occur. If the infection is untreated, the course is quite variable and may wax and wane over many years. On the other hand, coccidioidal meningitis is usually lethal within 1 year if not treated.

DIAGNOSIS

Serodiagnosis is a major indirect method for diagnosis. Acute primary coccidioidomycosis is associated with positive IgM primary tube precipitin [or immunodiffusion tube precipitin (IDTP)] tests. This test is not titered and usually reverts to negative within a few months of infection. The complement fixation [or immunodiffusion complement fixation (IDCF)] test measures IgG antibody, converts to positive later than the IDTP test, and generally remains positive for months. Rising titers are associated with progressive disease, whereas declining titers are associated with resolution.[93] In the CSF, a positive IDCF of any titer is considered diagnostic of coccidioidal meningitis. ELISA tests are replacing these older procedures. The polymerase chain reaction has been advocated for early diagnosis (prior to serologic conversion) using serum or CSF as the specimen. However, this method is not sufficiently sensitive to be useful in clinical practice.[94] Skin test antigens are not available.

The most specific methods to document coccidioidomycosis are culture or histopathologic evaluation. Bronchial lavage and pulmonary biopsy may be diagnostic when routine sputum cultures are nonrevealing.[95] Needle biopsy of lung nodules may also yield the diagnosis.[96] Tissue biopsies showing the characteristic spherule (Fig. 80-5) are pathognomonic. Mycelial forms of *Coccidioides* may also occur in cytologic and histologic specimens.[97] Obtaining positive cultures of *C. immitis* from clinical specimens is usually not difficult. The organism converts to the mycelial form and grows readily on most culture media, appearing within 7 to 10 days. Recovery of organisms from the CSF is less predictable, although McGinnis[98] has noted that 76% of cases have positive cultures and 8% may have spherules identified. The mold may not produce characteristic arthroconidia for some time. Careless handling of cultures has caused a number of human infections in laboratory workers. *Coccidioides immitis* was declared a "select agent" due to concerns about its use in bioterrorism. The scientific basis for this classification is probably unwarranted.[99] Nevertheless, cultures

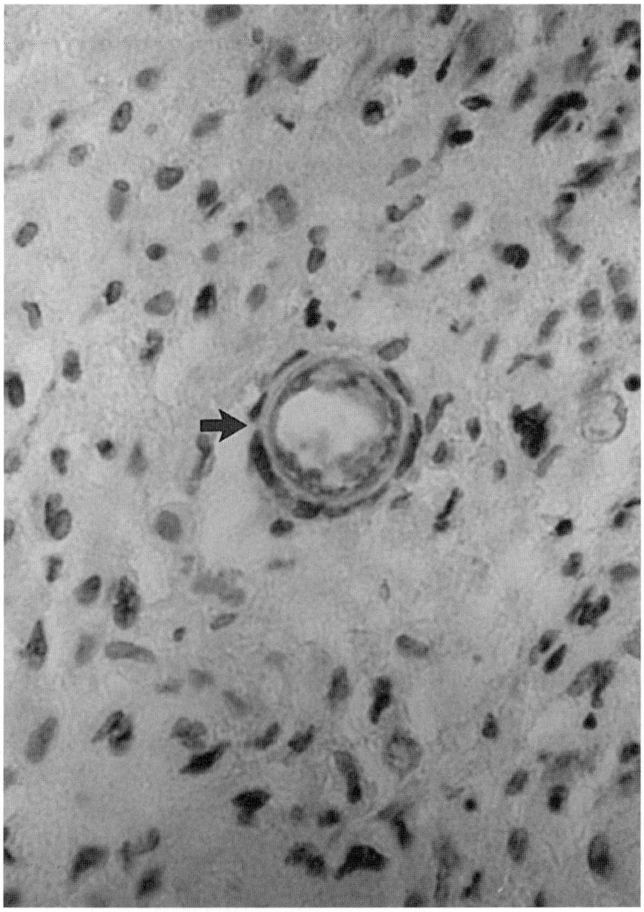

FIGURE 80-5 *Coccidioides immitis* spherule in skin lesion. Note large size of the spherule (*arrow*), double wall, and inner contents (endospores).

must be handled expeditiously, the organism must be destroyed following identification, and reports must be generated and promptly sent to the appropriate state authorities.

TREATMENT AND PROGNOSIS

Coccidioides immitis has one remarkable distinction from most other fungal pathogens. This organism tests susceptible in vitro to most antifungals. However, clinical responses are often very slow, incomplete, or nonexistent. Relapses occur (sometimes after years of remission) in approximately 30% of patients after treatment with antifungal agents is stopped. Therefore, terms such as "remission" and "disease-free interval," rather than "cure," should be used with regard to treatment results for coccidioidomycosis.

Practice guidelines for the treatment of coccidioidomycosis were published in 2000.[100] Approximately half of exposed people remain asymptomatic. The management of patients with primary pulmonary disease is uncertain. For most immunocompetent people, the disease will resolve without antifungals. Patients with concurrent risk factors (immunosuppression, pregnancy in the third trimester, or immediate postpartum status) should be treated. Nonpregnant patients with primary infection with *C. immitis* are treated with itraconazole or fluconazole (400 mg/day) orally for several months. There are no controlled studies, and efficacy is unclear. Amphotericin B is reserved for seriously ill patients with diffuse pneumonia and pregnant patients (in whom the azoles may be teratogenic for the fetus). Amphotericin B has a 50% to 75% response rate. People of Filipino or African American descent have a higher risk for dissemination, and this factor should be considered in the decision to treat.[100]

Ketoconazole produces less than a 40% response rate, as assessed using a global point-counting system developed by the Mycoses Study Group. Better responses are obtained with itraconazole at 400 mg/day (57%) and fluconazole (65%), given at 400 mg/day, for up to 2 years.[101,102] A study comparing oral fluconazole (400 mg per day) versus itraconazole (200 mg twice a day) in the treatment of nonmeningeal coccidioidomycosis found equivalency; however, there was a trend toward greater efficacy with itraconazole. Furthermore, itraconazole showed superior efficacy in skeletal infections.[103] Treatment of coccidioidal vertebral disease usually requires surgical stabilization in addition to medical therapy. In all patients with invasive disease, the treatment of coccidioidomycosis should be prolonged, perhaps for several years. Fluconazole relapse rates (37%) are higher than those for itraconazole (16%).

The potent triazoles, voriconazole and posaconazole, have been used to treat coccidioidomycosis. In a murine model of coccidioidomycosis, posaconazole was more effective than itraconazole.[104] Although numbers of patients are limited, responses have been excellent with posaconazole, even in patients failing other antifungals.[105] Posaconazole has the potential of becoming a first-line drug for the treatment of coccidioidomycosis. Caspofungin has proven effective in mice,[106] and there is emerging a very small clinical experience with the drug. However, no general conclusions can be made regarding the efficacy of the echinocandins in the treatment of coccidioidomycosis.

For patients with disseminated coccidioidomycosis, high-dose fluconazole is recommended.[100] Coccidioidal meningitis used to be considered the worst form of coccidioidomycosis, with only 40% to 50% response rate to intrathecal amphotericin B in follow-up evaluations continued for many years.[87] Recently, fluconazole has proved to be a more effective and well-tolerated treatment for coccidioidal meningitis, with favorable responses in 79% in a Mycoses Study Group investigation of 47 patients.[107] Also in this series, 9 patients had AIDS, of whom 6 achieved a clinical response and survived 9 to 26 months, ultimately succumbing to other causes. Thus, coccidioidal meningitis responds similarly to fluconazole in the presence or absence of AIDS. In this series, symptoms responded more rapidly than resolution of CSF abnormalities, being largely resolved by 4 months of therapy; however, 9 patients had more than 10 leukocytes per microliter in CSF after 20 months of treatment. Responses were similar in patients treated for the first time and in patients who had relapsed after prior therapy. Ten patients failed to respond to 400 mg/day of fluconazole, and some investigators have recommended doses up to 800 mg/day. Fluconazole, with a loading dose of 800 mg/day for several days, followed by fluconazole at 400 mg/day, is the current regimen of choice for coccidioidal meningitis. Itraconazole has also been used for treatment of coccidioidal meningitis, but the experience is limited.[108] In a rabbit model of coccidioidal meningitis, fluconazole and itraconazole had equal efficacies, but fluconazole led to more rapid responses. Neither drug was able to eliminate the fungus from CNS tissues.[109] Whether in AIDS or immunocompetent patients, once azole therapy has been initiated for coccidioidal meningitis, it should be continued lifelong. In a review of 18 patients, 14 patients treated for up to 8 years relapsed when treatment was stopped.[110]

Intravenous amphotericin B is not effective in coccidioidal meningitis, and intrathecal amphotericin B has been given by multiple methods, including Ommaya reservoirs.[111] Intrathecal amphotericin was previously the treatment of choice for coccidioidal meningitis, but should now be reserved for those who fail aggressive azole therapy. In some patients, doses up to 1.5 mg of amphotericin B were administered intrathecally (with hydrocortisone or methylprednisone) with a goal to administer 12 mg/month for 2 months.[112] Treatment averaged 45 months in these patients. Although effective in many patients, response rates were never much higher than 50% despite treatment for years, and complications of intrathecal amphotericin B were many, related to both inflammation caused by the drug and secondary infections caused by the injections.[113]

In AIDS, coccidioidomycosis typically presents toward the later phases of immunodeficiency. Diffuse pulmonary disease is common and is the worst manifestation, with a median survival of only 1 month, and no clearly superior treatment regimens have been identified. Meningitis and focal pulmonary disease are associated with a higher CD4 count and also with better responses to therapy.[78] Posaconazole has been used successfully in patients with AIDS.[105] With HAART, there is the potential of discontinuing chronic suppression when the CD4 counts have risen and the viral load has declined. However, there are no specific recommendations, and any discontinuation should be approached with caution.

PREVENTION AND CONTROL

There is no effective vaccine or other preventive measure. A vaccine consisting of formalin-killed spherules was tested in a large study in the San Joaquin Valley in California.[114] Although the vaccine caused seroconversion in 17% of recipients vs. 1% of placebo recipients, there were no differences in the incidence of suspected cases among vaccine recipients and placebo recipients. There are ongoing preclinical studies of coccidioidal vaccines prepared from specific antigens.[115] Using an expression library immunization approach, a protective antigen termed ELI-Ag1 was discovered that protects mice from lethal challenge with *C. immitis* arthroconidia.[116] Studies have suggested that immunization with a potential vaccine against coccidioidomycosis in endemic areas would be cost-effective.[117] Guidelines have been published for field workers in endemic areas to decrease their risk of acquiring coccidioidomycosis.[72]

Cryptococcosis

AGENT

Cryptococcus neoformans is the only encapsulated fungus, appears as spherical or ellipsoid yeast-like cells, reproduces by budding, and is ubiquitous in soil and avian guano.[118] The organism can transform to a mycelial form (*Filobasidiella neoformans*) and mate sexually.[119] There are two subspecies, *C. neoformans* var. *neoformans* and *C. neoformans* var. *gattii*. Five serotypes of *C. neoformans*, A through D and AD, have been recognized based on the antigenic specificity of the capsule.[120] *C. neoformans* var. *neoformans* (serotypes A and D) has a worldwide distribution and can infect both immunocompetent and immunodeficient subjects. Serotype A is the cause of most cases of cryptococcosis in patients with AIDS. *C. neoformans* var. *gattii* (serotypes B and C) is found as a mycelium on *Eucalyptus camaldulensis*, a tree native to Australia, where it causes severe pneumonia and meningitis in immunocompetent patients; it is less commonly seen in AIDS patients. Cryptococcosis caused by *C. neoformans* var. *gattii* has also been reported from areas in which *E. camaldulensis* trees have been imported.[121] Other tree species have been found that also harbor *C. neoformans* var. *gatti*.[122] The varietal status of serotype AD is uncertain.[120]

EPIDEMIOLOGY

The incidence of cryptococcosis has increased in many areas corresponding with the pandemic of AIDS and is a major cause of morbidity and mortality among these patients.[123] India, with its burgeoning AIDS epidemic, has seen a sizeable increase in the number of cases of cryptococcosis.[124] In both Rwanda and Cambodia, *Cryptococcus* is the leading cause of meningitis in people with AIDS.[125,126] In developing countries without access to antifungal drugs and HAART, cryptoccocal meningitis is often rapidly fatal. In a cohort of AIDS patients from Uganda, cryptococcosis accounted for 17% of the mortality, with a median survival of only 26 days after diagnosis.[127] In a study from Zimbabwe conducted in 1995, cryptococcosis was the AIDS-defining illness in 88% of AIDS patients admitted to two tertiary care hospitals; the median survival from time of diagnosis was 14 days.[128]

In Brazil, cryptococcosis is a significant problem in the AIDS population as well.[129] Fortunately, the incidence of cryptococcosis has diminished by greater than 80% since the advent of HAART in the United States and Europe. Furthermore, in the HAART era patients tend to present with cryptococcosis as the first manifestation of an opportunistic infection, whereas in prior years it was one of many such infections throughout the course of AIDS.[130] Cryptococcosis remains a major threat to life in developing nations, where access to HAART is limited. Cryptococcosis also occurs in people with other conditions causing defects in cell-mediated immunity, such as lymphoma, chronic leukemia, organ transplant, cirrhosis of the liver, and chronic steroid use.

DISEASE AND PATHOGENESIS AND IMMUNITY

Host defenses, virulence, and inoculum size determine the likelihood of development of clinical disease caused by *C. neoformans*. In the Bronx, New York, serological testing indicates that the majority of children (70%) have been exposed to the fungus, but very few children have symptomatic disease.[131] Depressed cell-mediated immunity is the major risk factor for development of cryptococcosis. Depressed phagocytosis, opsonization, and complement activity are also important contributors.[132] Anticryptococcal antibodies have been shown to be protective in experimentally inoculated animals.[133] An initial small clinical experience has shown that therapeutic monoclonal antibodies are benign, but efficacy has not been tested. Cryptococci are inhaled and, in most people, are contained and killed by neutrophils and alveolar macrophages. In an effective immune response to *C. neoformans*, murine models indicate that IL-12 and IL-18 act synergistically to stimulate early interferon-γ production by natural killer cells and γδ T cells, which stimulates macrophage destruction of intracellular cryptococci. This effect decreases fungal burdens in the lung and brain.[134] In a murine model of pulmonary and disseminated disease, a Th1-type immune response is necessary to control the infection.[135] Thereby, granulomas form in the lung or brain to control the infection.[120] Humoral immunity also contributes to host defense against *Cryptococcus* by providing opsonins for effective phagocytosis, enhanced natural killer cell function, and clearance of capsular polysaccharides.[120] However, under conditions of defective cell-mediated immunity, there are defective granuloma formation and fewer intracellular yeast, and extracellular fungal masses are present.[120]

The most important virulence factor of *C. neoformans* is its polysaccharide capsule. The principal capsular component, glucuronoxylomannan, displays a number of immunomodulatory activities: reduction of the anticryptococcal activity of neutrophils[136]; induction of IL-10 production by monocytes, which inhibits a Th1-type immune response[137]; and disruption of dendritic cell maturation and activation.[138] *C. neoformans* is able to produce melanin using various phenolic substrates that are found in human brain tissue.[139] The melanin protects the fungus from phagocytosis, nitrogen- and oxygen-derived oxidants, and amphotericin B. Superoxide dismutase and thiol peroxidase also protect the fungus from host-derived oxidants.[140,141] *C. neoformans* also displays phenotypic switching, in which variant colonies are produced that differ in morphology, virulence, and capsular characteristics, which in turn alters the immune response.[142]

Table 80-2 Clinical Manifestations of Cryptococcosis

Site	Clinical Findings
Pulmonary	Cough, chest pain, sputum production, fever, nodules, hilar adenopathy, focal or diffuse infiltrates, pleural effusion
Central nervous system	Meningitis: subacute: headache, meningismus, nausea and vomiting, mental changes, photophobia; focal: cryptococcoma
Skin	Acneiform lesions, papules, purpura, vesicles, nodules, ulcers, molluscum-like lesions, cellulitis
Others	Eye, prostate, adrenal, liver, heart, bone, lymph node, joint, kidney

In immunosuppressed patients, the organisms prevail to cause either pneumonia or disseminate to reach the meninges, skin, and bones. Primary cryptococcal pneumonia has been very well described in immunocompetent as well as immunosuppressed people. In immunocompetent hosts, chest infection is usually relatively mild, with productive cough, pleuritic chest pain, and fever as the main manifestations. Chest radiographs show single or multiple lung nodules, mediastinal lymphadenopathy, and occasionally pleural effusion. Dissemination is exceedingly rare.[143] However, in the immunocompromised host, cryptococcal pneumonia is more severe, with prominent alveolar and interstitial infiltrates; moreover, nodules and cavitation can be seen. In these patients, dissemination to the CNS is common, especially in those with AIDS.[144]

Cryptococcal meningitis is the most frequent presentation of cryptococcosis in the immunocompromised host. It occurs almost exclusively in immunocompromised patients. Typically, cryptococcal meningitis is subacute, manifested by progressive headache, fever, lethargy, personality changes, or memory loss. Variable presentations, either acute or chronic, have been described. Signs of meningeal irritation are usually absent.[145] Skin involvement in cryptococcosis is not uncommon, particularly with disseminated disease. A wide variety of skin lesions have been reported, including papules, acneiform rash, cellulitis, abscesses, ulcers, molluscum contagiosum-like lesions, vesicles, and nodules.[145] Bone, eye, and the prostate gland are other sites involved in *C. neoformans* infection. The prostate is a potentially protected sanctuary during treatment, a situation that might result in relapse.[146] Clinical manifestations of cryptococcosis are summarized in Table 80-2.

In contrast, *C. neoformans* var. *gatti* causes disease primarily in immunocompetent people and has increased propensity to form cryptococcomas in the brain and lungs. It produces greater neurologic morbidity and is less responsive to treatment than var. *neoformans*.[147]

DIAGNOSIS

Demonstration of *C. neoformans* in tissue or normally sterile body fluids, through cultures or special stains, is the basis for the diagnosis of cryptococcosis. GMS stain demonstrates yeast nonspecifically, whereas mucicarmine stain is specific in staining the capsule. The India ink preparation or nigrosin stain can be rapidly performed and is very useful in demonstrating the encapsulated yeast in tissues and body fluids. *C. neoformans* can be commensal in the mouth and sputum, which makes sputum cultures less useful in the diagnosis of cryptococcal pneumonia. *C. neoformans* grows well in Sabouraud agar and routine laboratory media, with white to cream-colored colonies developing in 36 to 72 hours.

Detection of the capsular polysaccharide antigen is both sensitive and specific. Two methods have been developed with comparable sensitivity and specificity—the latex agglutination test and enzyme immunoassay.[148] These techniques are more sensitive (95%) than India ink preparation (50%) and cultures (75%). Antigen detection is very helpful in promptly detecting relapse. A titer of more than 1:8 is indicative of active disease in the less severely immunosuppressed patient, and if it is detected in the CSF, it makes the diagnosis of cryptococcal meningitis highly likely. Titers in the CSF and serum are commonly greater than 500 in patients with AIDS and cryptococcosis. When cryptococcal meningitis is suspected, lumbar puncture is essential. Opening pressure should be measured, and CSF should be examined by the India ink method, cryptococcal antigen assay, and culture.

TREATMENT AND PROGNOSIS

Practice guidelines for the treatment of cryptococcosis were published in 2000.[149] In CNS disease in non-HIV patients, an induction/consolidation approach is used; amphotericin B (0.7 to 1 mg/kg/day) combined with 5-flucytosine (5-FC) (25 mg/kg every 6 hours) for 2 weeks, followed by fluconazole (400 mg/day) for 10 weeks, is recommended. Combined treatment with amphotericin and 5-FC clears cryptococci from the CSF faster than amphotericin B alone.[150] Liposomal amphotericin B, which is less toxic than conventional amphotericin B, can be used for treatment of cryptococcal meningitis at doses of 3 to 6 mg/kg/day. Fluconazole and itraconazole are active against *C. neoformans* and can be used to treat pulmonary disease in both HIV and non-HIV patients with mild-to-moderate pulmonary disease; non-HIV patients should be treated for 6 to 12 months, but HIV patients may require lifelong therapy, depending on the response to antiretroviral therapy. Severe pulmonary disease in the non-HIV patient should be treated like CNS disease. In HIV patients with CNS disease, a similar induction/consolidation approach can be used as in the non-HIV patient, but after the 10-week period of fluconazole, maintenance therapy with fluconazole at 200 to 400 mg per day is necessary.[149] If fluconazole is used as initial treatment for cryptococcal meningitis, doses of 400 to 800 mg/day are indicated; however, it sterilizes the CSF more slowly than amphotericin B.[151] In cases of AIDS, suppressive therapy with fluconazole (200 mg/day) should be continued until the CD4 count has risen to greater than 100 cells/μL, at which time treatment may be discontinued.[152] Some patients have had months of HAART with CD4 greater than 100 cells/μL, whereas others have stopped relatively soon after the CD4 count reached 100 cells/μL. Four relapses occurred among 100 patients in this setting.

In some patients, rapid rise of CD4 and decline in HIV titers have been associated with increasing headache and signs of meningitis.[153] This may occur as soon as 11 days after

HAART, and it may occur with very little change in total CD4 counts. Typically, the CSF shows an inflammatory response with lymphocytes and a stable or lower antigen concentration. Organisms may be seen on India ink examination, but cultures are negative. This is a form of "immune reconstitution disease." This syndrome is managed by continuing the antifungal drug suppression and often limited courses of corticosteroids to reduce the exuberant host inflammatory response.

In recent years, in vitro resistance to fluconazole (MIC >16 μg/mL) and clinical relapse have been seen with cryptococcal meningitis in AIDS patients.[154] Mutations of the target lanosterol 14-α demethylase may account for clinically relevant resistance.[155] Some resistance to voriconazole has also been noted.[156] For patients with infection with fluconazole-resistant isolates, both voriconazole and posaconazole may be acceptable alternatives. Response to each has been reported in approximately 50% of patients.[157] Nevertheless, in the United States, surveillance through 1998 indicates that resistance of *C. neoformans* to azole antifungal agents is rare.[158] Caspofungin has no role in the management of cryptococcosis because the target 1,3-β-D-glucans are not present in *C. neoformans*.

Because increased intracranial pressure (ICP) to more than 25 cm of water has been observed to be associated with acute mortality, it is important to maintain normal ICP by frequent lumbar punctures or CSF shunting if required.[159] In one series of 10 patients shunted, 9 improved.[160] In another series of 27 patients, placement of shunts was not uniformly helpful, with poor outcome in 10, perhaps because of delays in surgery. Coma indicated a poor prognosis.[161]

The prognosis in cryptococcosis is variable, being determined by many factors. Limited disease such as cryptococcal pneumonia carries a better prognosis than disseminated disease with meningitis. The degree of immunosuppression of the host and the effectiveness of antifungal therapy are the main prognostic factors. In non-HIV-associated cases of cryptococcal meningitis, a poor outcome is associated with a high burden of organisms (positive India ink or high CSF or serum cryptococcal antigen concentration), poor inflammatory response (CSF white blood cell count less than 20/μL), low CSF glucose, high CSF opening pressure, and altered mental status.[162] In HIV-infected patients, low serum albumin, low CD4 count, and high CSF antigen titers (>11,024, reflecting heavy fungal burden) are pretreatment indicators that correlate with poor outcome.[163] Likewise, rising CSF antigen titers suggest that the infection is not resolving. In a study of untreated cryptococcal meningitis from Zimbabwe, severely impaired mental status and hyponatremia at presentation were associated with death within 3 days, whereas a low CSF glucose level was associated with survival greater than 14 days.[128]

PREVENTION AND CONTROL

There are no vaccines for *C. neoformans*. Because the organism is widely distributed in nature, there is no way to prevent contact with *C. neoformans*. No human-to-human transmission is known to occur, except with organ transplantation. Transmission from pet psittacine birds has been reported. Thus, it may be prudent to advise immunocompromised patients to avoid birds and their guano.[164] Studies have shown fluconazole at 200 mg/day to be effective but costly for primary prophylaxis against cryptococcal meningitis in AIDS patients.[165] A lower dose of 100 mg three times per week may be effective and is less costly.

REFERENCES

1. Ajello L: Relationship of *Histoplasma capsulatum* to avian habitats. Public Health Rep 79:266, 1964.
2. Keath EJ, Kobayashi GS, Medoff G: Classification of *Histoplasma capsulatum* by restriction fragment length polymorphisms in a nuclear gene. J Clin Microbiol 30:2104, 1992.
3. Goodwin RA, Lloyd JE, DesPrez RM: Histoplasmosis in normal host. Medicine (Baltimore) 60:231, 1981.
4. Wheat J: Endemic mycoses in AIDS: A clinical review. Clin Microbiol Rev 8:146, 1995.
5. Hajjeh RA, Pappas PG, Henderson H, et al: Multi-center case–control study of risk factors for histoplasmosis in human immunodeficiency virus-infected persons. Clin Infect Dis 32:1215, 2001.
6. Wallis RS, Broder MS, Wong JY, et al: Granulomatous infectious diseases associated with tumor necrosis factor antagonists. Clin Infect Dis 38:1261, 2004.
7. Adderson EE: Histoplasmosis in a pediatric oncology center. J Pediatr 144:100, 2004.
8. Whitt SP, Koch GA, Fender B, et al: Histoplasmosis in pregnancy: Case series and report of transplacental transmission. Arch Intern Med 164:454, 2004.
9. Panackal AA, Hajjeh RA, Cetron MS, et al: Fungal infections among returning travelers. Clin Infect Dis 35:1088, 2002.
10. Gugnani HC, Muotoe-Okafor FA, Kaufman L, et al: A natural focus of *Histoplasma capsulatum* var. *duboisii* is a bat cave. Mycopathologia 127:151, 1994.
11. Chandler FW, Ajello L: *Histoplasmosis duboisii*. In Connor DH, Chandler FW, Manz HJ, et al (eds): Pathology of Infectious Diseases. Stamford, Conn, Appleton & Lange, 1997, p 1017.
12. Wheat LJ, Connolly-Stringfield PA, Baker RL, et al: Disseminated histoplasmosis in the acquired immune deficiency syndrome: Clinical findings, diagnosis and treatment and review of the literature. Medicine (Baltimore) 69:361, 1990.
13. Kataria YP, Campbell PB, Burlingham BT: Acute pulmonary histoplasmosis presenting as ARDS: Effect of therapy on clinical and laboratory features. South Med J 74:534, 1981.
14. Goodwin RA, Owens FT, Snell JD, et al: Chronic pulmonary histoplasmosis. Medicine (Baltimore) 55:413, 1976.
15. Wheat LJ, Slama TG, Kohler RB, et al: Cavitary histoplasmosis occurring during two large urban outbreaks: Analysis of clinical, epidemiologic, roentgenographic and laboratory features. Medicine (Baltimore) 63:201, 1984.
16. Davis AM, Pierson RN, Loyd JE: Mediastinal fibrosis. Sem Resp Infect 16:119, 2001.
17. Balthazar EJ, Megibow AJ, Barry M, et al: Histoplasmosis of the colon in patient with AIDS: Imaging findings in four cases. Am J Roentgenol 161:585, 1993.
18. Karimi K, Wheat LJ, Connolly P, et al: Differences in histoplasmosis in patients with acquired immunodeficiency syndrome in the United States and Brazil. J Infect Dis 186:1655, 2002.
19. Kanawaty DS, Stalker MJ, Munt PW: Nonsurgical treatment of histoplasma endocarditis involving a bioprosthetic valve. Chest 99:253, 1991.
20. Wheat LJ, Batteiger BE, Sathapatayavongs B: *Histoplasma capsulatum* infections of the central nervous system: A clinical review. Medicine (Baltimore) 69:244, 1990.
21. Corcoran GR, Al-Abdely H, Flanders CD, et al: Markedly elevated serum lactate dehydrogenase levels are a clue to the diagnosis of disseminated histoplasmosis in patients with AIDS. Clin Infect Dis 24:942, 1997.
22. Wheat LJ, Chetchotisakd P, Williams B, et al: Factors associated with severe manifestations of histoplasmosis in AIDS. Clin Infect Dis 30:877, 2000.
23. Fleming AF: Opportunistic infections in AIDS in developed and developing countries. Trans R Soc Trop Med Hyg 84(suppl 1):1, 1990.
24. Woods JP, Heinecke EL, Luecke JW, et al: Pathogenesis of *Histoplasma capsulatum*. Sem Respir Infect 16:91, 2001.

25. Newman SL, Gootee L, Gabay J: Human neutrophil-mediated fungistasis against *Histoplasma capsulatum*. Localization of fungistatic activity to azurophil granules. J Clin Invest 92:624, 1993.
26. Newman SL, Gootee L, Morris R, et al: Digestion of *Histoplasma capsulatum* yeasts by human macrophages. J Immunol 149:574, 1992.
27. Newman SL: Cell-mediated immunity to *Histoplasma capsulatum*. Sem Respir Infect 16:102, 2001.
28. Deepe GS: Role of CD8 T-cells in host resistance to systemic infection with *Histoplasma capsulatum* in mice. J Immunol 152:3491, 1994.
29. Allendoerfer R, Magee DM, Deepe GS, et al: Transfer of protective immunity in murine histoplasmosis by a CD4 T-cell clone. Infect Immun 61:714, 1993.
30. Sarosi GA, Johnson PC: Disseminated histoplasmosis in HIV infected patients. Clin Infect Dis 14:560, 1992.
31. George RB, Lambert RS: Significance of serum antibodies to *Histoplasma capsulatum* in endemic areas. South Med J 77:161, 1984.
32. Wheat LJ, Kohler RB, Tewari RP: Diagnosis of disseminated histoplasmosis by detection of *Histoplasma capsulatum* antigen in serum and urine specimens. N Engl J Med 314:83, 1986.
33. Wheat LJ: Laboratory diagnosis of histoplasmosis: Update 2000. Sem Respir Infect 16:131, 2001.
34. Rickerts V, Bialek R, Tintelnot K, et al: Rapid PCR-based diagnosis of disseminated histoplasmosis in an AIDS patient. Eur J Clin Microbiol Infect Dis 21:821, 2002.
35. Wheat J, Sarosi G, McKinsey D, et al: Practice guidelines for the management of patients with histoplasmosis. Clin Infect Dis 30:688, 2000.
36. Wheat J: Histoplasmosis: Recognition and treatment. Clin Infect Dis 19(suppl 1):S19, 1994.
37. Dismukes WE, Bradsher RW, Cloud GC, et al: Itraconazole therapy for blastomycosis and histoplasmosis. Am J Med 93:489, 1992.
38. Wheat J, Marichal P, van den Bossche H: Hypothesis on the mechanism of resistance to fluconazole in *Histoplasma capsulatum*. Antimicrob Agents Chemother 41:410, 1997.
39. Wheat LJ, Connolly P, Smedema M, et al: Emergence of resistance to fluconazole as a cause of failure during treatment of histoplasmosis in patients with acquired immunodeficiency syndrome. Clin Infect Dis 33:1910, 2001.
40. Wheat LJ, Cloud G, Johnson P: Clearance of fungal burden during treatment of disseminated histoplasmosis with liposomal amphotericin B versus itraconazole. Antimicrob Agents Chemother 45:2354, 2001.
41. Johnson PC, Wheat LJ, Cloud GA, et al: Safety and efficacy of liposomal amphotericin B compared with conventional amphotericin B for induction therapy of histoplasmosis in patients with AIDS. Ann Intern Med 137:105, 2002.
42. Connolly P, Wheat LJ, Schnizlein-Bick C, et al: Comparison of a new triazole, posaconazole, with itraconazole and amphotericin B for treatment of histoplasmosis following pulmonary challenge in immunocompromised mice. Antimicrob Agents Chemother 44:2604, 2000.
43. Goldman M, Zackin R, Fichtenbaum CJ: Safety of discontinuation of maintenance therapy for disseminated histoplasmosis after immunologic response to anti-retroviral therapy. Clin Infect Dis 38:1486, 2004.
44. Couppié P, Sobesky M, Aznar C, et al: Histoplasmosis and acquired immunodeficiency syndrome: A study of prognostic factors. Clin Infect Dis 38:134, 2004.
45. McKinsey DS, Wheat LJ, Cloud GA, et al: Itraconazole prophylaxis for fungal infections in patients with advanced human immunodeficiency virus infection: Randomized, placebo-controlled, double-blind study. National Institute of Allergy and Infectious Diseases Mycoses Study Group. Clin Infect Dis 28:1049, 1999.
46. Klein BS, Vergeront JM, DiSalvo AF, et al: Two outbreaks of blastomycosis along rivers in Wisconsin. Am Rev Respir Dis 136:1333, 1987.
47. Cano MV, Ponce-de-Leon GF, Tippen S, et al: Blastomycosis in Missouri: Epidemiology and risk factors for endemic disease. Epidemiol Infect 131:907, 2003.
48. Klein BS, Vergeront JM, Weeks RJ, et al: Isolation of *Blastomyces dermatitidis* in soil associated with a large outbreak of blastomycosis in Wisconsin. N Engl J Med 314:529, 1986.
49. Bradshear RW: Water and blastomycosis: Don't blame beaver. Am Rev Respir Dis 136:1324, 1987.
50. Baumgardner DJ, Burdick JS: An outbreak of human and canine blastomycosis. Rev Infect Dis 13:898, 1990.
51. Gnann JW, Bressler GS, Bodet CA III, et al: Human blastomycosis after a dog bite. Ann Intern Med 98:48, 1983.
52. Baily G, Robertson VJ, Neill P, et al: Blastomycosis in Africa: Clinical features, diagnosis and treatment. Rev Infect Dis 13:1005, 1991.
53. Bradsher RW: Blastomycosis. Clin Infect Dis 14(suppl 1):S82, 1992.
54. Sugar AM, Picard M, Wagner R, et al: Interactions between human bronchoalveolar macrophages and *Blastomyces dermatitidis* conidia: Demonstrations of fungicidal and fungistatic effects. J Infect Dis 171:1559, 1995.
55. Brummer E, Sugar AM, Stevens DA: Enhanced oxidative burst in immunologically activated but not elicited polymorphonuclear leukocytes correlates with fungicidal activity. Infect Immun 49:396, 1985.
56. Frey CL, DeMarsh PL, Drutz DJ: Divergent patterns of pulmonary blastomycosis induced by conidia and yeasts in athymic and euthymic mice. Am Rev Respir Dis 140:1218, 1989.
57. Fraser VJ, Keath EJ, Powderly WG: Two cases of blastomycosis from a common source: Use of DNA restriction analysis to identify strains. J Infect Dis 163:1378, 1991.
58. Pappas P, Bradsher RW, Powderly WG, et al: Blastomycosis in patients with acquired immunodeficiency syndrome. Ann Intern Med 116:847, 1992.
59. Lemos LB, Baliaga M, Guo M: Blastomycosis: The great pretender can also be an opportunist. Initial clinical diagnosis and underlying diseases in 123 patients. Ann Diagn Pathol 6:194, 2002.
60. Klein BS: Molecular basis of pathogenicity in *Blastomyces dermatitidis*; The importance of adhesion. Curr Opin Microbiol 3:339, 2000.
61. Finkel-Jimenez B, Wüthrich M, Klein BS: BAD1, an essential virulence factor of *Blastomyces dermatitidis*, suppresses host TNF-α production through TGF-β-dependent and -independent mechanisms. J Immunol 168:5746, 2002.
62. Lemos LB, Guo M, Baliga M: Blastomycosis: Organ involvement and etiologic diagnosis. A review of 123 patients from Mississippi. Ann Diagn Pathol 4:391, 2000.
63. Soufleris AJ, Klein BS, Courtney BT, et al: Utility of anti-WI-1 serological testing in the diagnosis of blastomycosis in Wisconsin residents. Clin Infect Dis 19:87, 1994.
64. Klein BS, Vergeront JM, Kaufman L, et al: Serological test for blastomycosis: Assessments during a large point-source outbreak in Wisconsin. J Infect Dis 155:262, 1987.
65. Klein BS, Jones JM: Purification and characterization of the major antigen WI-1 from *Blastomyces dermatititis* yeasts and immunological comparison with A antigen. Infect Immun 62:3890, 1994.
66. Chapman SW, Bradsher RW Jr, Campbell GD Jr, et al: Practice guidelines for the management of patients with blastomycosis. Clin Infect Dis 30:679, 2000.
67. Dismukes W, Bradsher RW, Cloud GC, et al: Itraconazole for blastomycosis and histoplasmosis. Am J Med 93:489, 1992.
68. Yancey RW Jr, Perlino CA, Kaufman L: Asymptomatic blastomycosis in the central nervous system with progression in patients given ketoconazole therapy: A report of two cases. J Infect Dis 164:807, 1991.
69. Pappas PG, Bradsher RW, Chapman SW, et al: Treatment of blastomycosis with fluconazole: A pilot study. Clin Infect Dis 20:267, 1995.
70. Crampton TL, Light RB, Berg GM, et al: Epidemiology and clinical spectrum of blastomycosis diagnosed at Manitoba hospitals. Clin Infect Dis 34:1310, 2002.
71. Stevens DA: Current concepts: Coccidioidomycosis. N Engl J Med 332:1077, 1995.
72. Fisher FS, Bultman MW, Pappagianis D: Operational guidelines for geological fieldwork in areas endemic for coccidioidomycosis (Valley fever) [open-file report 00-348]. Reston, VA: U.S. Geological Survey, 2000. Available at http://geopubs.wr.usgs.gov/open-file/of00-348/of00-348.pdf; Accessed October 2001.
73. Kolivras KN, Comrie AC: Modeling valley fever (coccidioidomycosis) incidence on the basis of climate conditions. Int J Biometeorol 47:87, 2003.
74. Centers for Disease Control and Prevention: Coccidioidomycosis in workers at an archeologic site—Dinosaur National Monument, Utah, June–July 2001. MMWR 50:1005, 2001.
75. Chiller TM, Galgiani JN, Stevens DA: Coccidioidomycosis. Infect Dis Clin North Am 17:41, 2003.
76. Schneider E, Hajjeh RA, Spiegel RA, et al: A coccidioidomycosis outbreak following the Northridge, Calif, earthquake. JAMA 277:904, 1997.

77. Galgiani J: *Coccidioides immitis*. In Mandel GL, Bennett JE, Dolin R (eds): Principles and Practice of Infectious Diseases, 5th ed. New York, Churchill Livingstone, 2000, p 2746.
78. Fish DG, Ampel NM, Galgiani JN, et al: Coccidioidomycosis during human immunodeficiency virus infection. Medicine (Baltimore) 69:394, 1990.
79. Ampel NM, Dols CL, Galgiani JN: Coccidioidomycosis during human immunodeficiency virus infection: Results of a prospective study in a coccidioidal endemic area. Am J Med 94:235, 1993.
80. Wright PW, Pappagianis D, Wilson M, et al: Donor-related coccidioidomycosis in organ transplant recipients. Clin Infect Dis 37:1265, 2003.
81. Bialek R, Kern J, Herrmann T, et al: PCR assays for identification of *Coccidioides posadasii* based on the nucleotide sequence of the antigen 2/proline-rich antigen. J Clin Microbiol 42:778, 2004.
82. Drutz DJ: Coccidioidal pneumonia. In Pennington J (ed): Respiratory Infections: Diagnosis and Management. New York, Raven Press, 1983, p 353.
83. Hyde L: Coccidioidal pulmonary cavitation. Dis Chest 54(suppl 1):17, 1968.
84. Rosenstein NE, Emery KW, Werner SB, et al: Risk factors for severe pulmonary and disseminated coccidioidomycosis: Kern County, California, 1995–1996. Clin Infect Dis 32:708, 2001.
85. Peterson CM, Schuppert K, Kelly P, et al: Coccidioidomycosis and pregnancy. Obstet Gynecol Surv 48:149, 1993.
86. Gallant JE, Ko AH: Cavitary pulmonary lesions in patients infected with human immunodeficiency virus. Clin Infect Dis 22:671, 1996.
87. Kelly PC: Coccidioidal meningitis. In Stevens DA (ed): Coccidioidomycosis: A Text. New York, Plenum Press, 1980, p 163.
88. Ragland AS, Arsura E, Ismail Y, et al: Eosinophilic pleocytosis in coccidioidal meningitis: Frequency and significance. Am J Med 95:254, 1993.
89. Mischel PS, Vinters HV: Coccidioidomycosis of the central nervous system: Neuropathological and vasculopathic manifestations and clinical correlates. Clin Infect Dis 20:400, 1995.
90. Vincent T, Galgiani JN, Huppert M, et al: The natural history of coccidioidal meningitis: VA–Armed Forces cooperative studies 1955–1958. Clin Infect Dis 16:247, 1993.
91. Williams PL, Johnson R, Pappagianis D, et al: Vasculitis and encephalitic complications associated with *Coccidioides immitis* infection of the central nervous system in humans: Report of 10 cases and review. Clin Infect Dis 14:673, 1992.
92. Banuelos AF, Williams PL, Johnson RGH, et al: Central nervous system abscesses due to *Coccidioides* species. Clin Infect Dis 22:240, 1996.
93. Smith CE, Saito MT, Simons SA: Pattern of 39,500 serologic tests in coccidioidomycosis. JAMA 160:546, 1956.
94. Johnson SM, Simmons KA, Pappagianis D: Amplification of coccidioidal DNA in clinical specimens by PCR. J Clin Microbiol 42:1982, 2004.
95. Wallace JM, Catanzaro A, Moser KM, et al: Flexible fiberoptic bronchoscopy for diagnosing pulmonary coccidioidomycosis. Am Rev Respir Dis 123:286, 1981.
96. Forseth J, Rohwedder BE, Levine BE, et al: Experience with needle biopsy for coccidioidal lung nodules. Arch Intern Med 146:319, 1986.
97. Muñoz B, Castañn LR, Calderon I, et al: Parasitic mycelial forms of *Coccidioides* species in Mexican patients. J Clin Microbiol 42:1247, 2004.
98. McGinnis MR: Detection of fungi in cerebrospinal fluid. Am J Med 75(1B):129, 1983.
99. Deresinski S: *Coccidioides immitis* as a potential bioweapon. Sem Respir Infect 18:216, 2003.
100. Galgiani JN, Ampel NM, Catanzaro A, et al: Practice guidelines for the treatment of coccidioidomycosis. Clin Infect Dis 30:658, 2000.
101. Graybill JR, Stevens DA, Galgiani JN, et al: Itraconazole treatment of coccidioidomycosis. Am J Med 89:292, 1990.
102. Catanzaro A, Galgiani JN, Levine BE, et al: Fluconazole therapy for coccidioidal meningitis. Am J Med 98:249, 1995.
103. Galgiani JN, Catanazaro A, Cloud GA, et al: Comparison of oral fluconazole and itraconazole for progressive, nonmeningeal coccidioidomycosis. Ann Intern Med 133:676, 2000.
104. González GM, Tejerina R, Najvar LK, et al: In vitro and in vivo activities of posaconazole against *Coccidioides immitis*. Antimicrob Agents Chemother 46:1352, 2002.
105. Anstead G, Corcoran G, Lewis J, et al: Posaconazole in the treatment of coccidioidomycosis: A case series. Abstract #143, Infectious Diseases Society of America Annual Meeting, San Diego, CA, October 2003.
106. González GM, Tijerina R, Najvar LK, et al: Correlation between antifungal susceptibilities of *Coccidioides immitis* in vitro and antifungal treatment with caspofungin in a mouse model. Antimicrob Agents Chemother 45:1854, 2001.
107. Galgiani JN, Catanzaro A, Cloud GA, et al: Fluconazole therapy for coccidioidal meningitis. Ann Intern Med 119:28, 1993.
108. Tucker RM, Denning DW, Dupont B, et al: Itraconazole for chronic coccidioidal meningitis. Ann Intern Med 112:108, 1990.
109. Sorensen KN, Sobel RA, Clemons KV, et al: Comparison of fluconazole and itraconazole in a rabbit model of coccidioidal meningitis. Antimicrob Agents Chemother 44:1512, 2000.
110. Dewsnup DH, Galgiani JN, Graybill JR, et al: Is it ever safe to stop azole therapy for *Coccidioides immitis* meningitis? Ann Intern Med 124:305, 1996.
111. Stevens DA, Shatsky SA: Intrathecal amphotericin in the management of coccidioidal meningitis. Sem Respir Infect 16:263, 2001.
112. Witorsch P, Williams T Jr, Ommaya AK, et al: Intraventricular administration of amphotericin B. JAMA 194:700, 1965.
113. Labadie JL, Hamilton RH: Survival improvement in coccidioidal meningitis with high-dose intrathecal amphotericin B. Arch Intern Med 146:2013, 1986.
114. Pappagianis D: Evaluation of the protective efficacy of the killed *Coccidioides immitis* spherule vaccine in humans. Am Rev Respir Dis 148:656, 1993.
115. Pappagianis D: Seeking a vaccine against *Coccidioides immitis* and serologic studies: Expectations and realities. Fungal Genet Biol 32:1, 2001.
116. Ivey FD, Magee DM, Woitaske MD, et al: Identification of a protective antigen of *Coccidioides immitis* by expression library immunization. Vaccine 21:4359, 2003.
117. Barnato A, Sanders GD, Owens DK: Cost-effectiveness of a potential vaccine for *Coccidioides immitis*. Emerg Infect Dis 7:797, 2001.
118. Levitz SM: The ecology of *Cryptococcus neoformans* and the epidemiology of cryptococcosis. Rev Infect Dis 13:1163, 1991.
119. Kwon-Chung KJ: Morphogenesis of *Filobasidella neoformans*, the sexual state of *Cryptococcus neoformans*. Mycologia 68:821, 1976.
120. Perfect JR, Casadevall A: Cryptococcosis. Infect Dis Clin North Am 16:837, 2002.
121. Ellis DH, Pfeiffer TJ: Natural habitat of *Cryptococcus neoformans* var. *gattii*. J Clin Microbiol 28:1642, 1990.
122. Lazera MS, Salmito Cavalcanti MA, Londero AT, et al: Possible primary ecological niche of *Cryptococcus neoformans*. Med Mycol 38:379, 2000.
123. Chuck SL, Sande MA: Infections with *Cryptococcus neoformans* in the acquired immunodeficiency syndrome. N Engl J Med 321:794, 1989.
124. Banerjee U, Datta K, Majumdar T, et al: Cryptococcosis in India: The awakening of a sleeping giant. Med Mycol 39:51, 2001.
125. Bogaerts J, Rouvroy D, Taelman H, et al: AIDS-associated cryptococcal meningitis in Rwanda (1983–1992): Epidemiologic and diagnostic features. J Infect 39:32, 1997.
126. Chhin S, Rozycki G, Pugatch D, et al: Aetiology of meningitis in HIV-infected patients in a referral hospital in Phnom Penh, Cambodia. Int J STD AIDS 15:48, 2004.
127. French N, Gray K, Watera C, et al: Cryptococcal infection in a cohort of HIV-1-infected Ugandan adults. AIDS 16:1031, 2002.
128. Heyderman RS, Gangaidozo IT, Hakim JG, et al: Cryptococcal meningitis in human immunodeficiency virus-infected patients in Harare, Zimbabwe. Clin Infect Dis 26:284, 1998.
129. Pappalardo MC, Melhem MS: Cryptococcosis: A review of the Brazilian experience for the disease. Rev Institut Med Trop Sao Paulo 45:299, 2003.
130. Mirza SA, Phelan M, Rimland D, et al: The changing epidemiology of cryptococcosis: An update from population-based active surveillance in 2 large metropolitan areas, 1992–2000. Clin Infect Dis 36:789, 2003.
131. Goldman DL, Khine H, Abadi J, et al: Serologic evidence for *Cryptococcus neoformans* infection. Pediatrics 107:EE66, 2001.
132. Mitchell TG, Perfect JR: Cryptococcosis in the era of AIDS—100 years after the discovery of *Cryptococcus neoformans*. Clin Microbiol Rev 8:515, 1995.

133. Dromer F, Chareire J, Contrepois A, et al: Protection of mice against experimental cryptococcosis by anti-*Cryptococcus neoformans* monoclonal antibody. Infect Immun 55:749, 1987.
134. Qureshi MH, Zhang T, Koguchi Y, et al: Combined effects of IL-12 and IL-18 on the clinical course and local cytokine production in murine pulmonary infection with *Cryptococcus neoformans*. Eur J Immunol 29:643, 1999.
135. Koguchi Y, Kawakami K: Cryptococcal infection and Th1–Th2 cytokine balance. Int Rev Immunol 21:423, 2002.
136. Monari C, Retini C, Casadevall A, et al: Differences in outcome of the interaction between *Cryptococcus neoformans* glucuronoxylomannan and human monocytes and neutrophils. Eur J Immunol 33:1041, 2003.
137. Retini C, Kozel TR, Pietrella D, et al: Interdependency of interleukin-10 and interleukin-12 in regulation of T-cell differentiation and effector function of monocytes in response to stimulation with *Cryptococcus neoformans*. Infect Immun 69:6064, 2001.
138. Vecchiarelli A, Pietrella D, Lupo P, et al: The polysaccharide capsule of *Cryptococcus neoformans* interferes with human dendritic cell maturation and activation. J Leukocyte Biol 74:370, 2003.
139. Gomez BL, Nosanchuk JD: Melanin and fungi. Curr Opin Infect Dis 16:91, 2003.
140. Cox GM, Harrison TS, McDade HC, et al: Superoxide dismutase influences the virulence of *Cryptococcus neoformans* by affecting growth within macrophages. Infect Immun 71:173, 2003.
141. Missall TA, Pusateri ME, Lodge JK: Thiol peroxidase is critical for virulence and resistance to nitric oxide and peroxide in the fungal pathogen *Cryptococcus neoformans*. Mol Microbiol 51:1447, 2004.
142. Pietrella D, Fries B, Lupo P, et al: Phenotypic switching of *Cryptococcus neoformans* can influence the outcome of the immune response. Cell Microbiol 5:513, 2003.
143. Campbell GD: Primary pulmonary cryptococcosis. Am Rev Respir Dis 94:236, 1966.
144. Kerkering TM, Duma RJ, Shadomy S: The evolution of pulmonary cryptococcosis: Clinical implications from a study of 41 patients with and without compromising host factors. Ann Intern Med 111:125, 1989.
145. Pema K, Diaz J, Guerra LG, et al: Disseminated cutaneous cryptococcosis: Comparison of clinical manifestations in the pre-AIDS and AIDS eras. Arch Intern Med 154:1032, 1994.
146. Larsen RA, Bozzette SA, McCutchan JA, et al: Persistent *Cryptococcus neoformans* infection of the prostate after successful treatment of meningitis. Ann Intern Med 111:125, 1989.
147. Sorrell TC: *Cryptococcus neoformans* variety *gattii*. Med Mycol 39:155, 2001.
148. Frank UK, Nishimura SL, Li NS, et al: Evaluation of an enzyme immunoassay for detection of cryptococcal capsular polysaccharide antigen in serum and cerebrospinal fluid. J Clin Microbiol 31:97, 1993.
149. Saag MS, Graybill RJ, Larsen RA, et al: Practice guidelines for the management of cryptococcal disease. Clin Infect Dis 30:710, 2000.
150. Van der Horst CM, Saag MS, Cloud GA, et al: Treatment of cryptococcal meningitis associated with the immunodeficiency syndrome. N Engl J Med 337:15, 1997.
151. Saag MS, Powderly WG, Cloud GA: Comparison of amphotericin B with fluconazole in the treatment of AIDS-associated cryptococcal meningitis. N Engl J Med 326:83, 1992.
152. Mussini C, Pezzotti P, Miro JM, et al: Discontinuation of maintenance therapy for cryptococcal meningitis in patients with AIDS treated with highly active antiretroviral therapy: An international observational study. Clin Infect Dis 38:565, 2004.
153. Cheng VC, Yuen K-Y, Chan, W-M: Immunorestitution disease involving the innate and adaptive response. Clin Infect Dis 30:882, 2000.
154. Aller AI, Matrin-Mazualos E, Lozano F: Correlation of fluconazole MICs with clinical outcome in cryptococcal meningitis. Antimicrob Agents Chemother 44:1544, 2000.
155. Rodero L, Mellado E, Rodriguez AC: G484S amino acid substitution in lanosterol 14-alpha demethylase (ERG11) is related to fluconazole resistance in a recurrent *Cryptococcus neoformans* clinical isolate. Antimicrob Agents Chemother 47:3653, 2003.
156. Mondon P, Petter R, Amalfitano G: Heteroresistance to fluconazole and voriconazole in *Cryptococcus neoformans*. Antimicrob Agents Chemother 43:1856, 1999.
157. Pitisuttithum T, Gaona-Flores V, Negroni R, et al: Efficacy of posaconazole (POS) in treatment of central nervous system (CNS) fungal infections: Results of an open label study. Abstract M-978, 43rd Interscience Conference on Antimicrobial Agents and Chemotherapy, Chicago, 2003.
158. Brandt ME, Pfaller MA, Hajjeh RA, et al: Trends in antifungal susceptibility of *Cryptococcus neoformans* isolates in the United States: 1992–1994 and 1996–1998. Antimicrob Agents Chemother 45:3065, 2001.
159. Denning DW, Armstrong RW, Stevens DA: Elevated cerebrospinal fluid pressure in patients with cryptococcal meningitis and acquired immunodeficiency syndrome. Am J Med 91:267, 1991.
160. Park MK, Hospenthal DR, Bennett JE: Treatment of hydrocephalus secondary to cryptococcal meningitis by use of shunting. Clin Infect Dis 28:629, 1999.
161. Liliang P-C, Liang C-L, Chang W-N: Shunt surgery for hydrocephalus complicating cryptococcal meningitis in human immunodeficiency virus-negative patients. Clin Infect Dis 37:673, 2003.
162. Diamond RD, Bennett JE: Prognostic factors in cryptococcal meningitis: A study in 111 cases. Ann Intern Med 80:176, 1974.
163. Robinson PA, Bauer M, Leal MAE: Early mycological treatment failure in AIDS-associated cryptococcal meningitis. Clin Infect Dis 28:82, 1999.
164. Nosanchuk JD, Shoham S, Fries BC, et al: Evidence of zoonotic transmission of *Cryptococcus neoformans* from a pet cockatoo to an immunocompromised patient. Ann Intern Med 132:205, 2000.
165. Powderly WG, Finkelstein D, Feinberg J, et al: A randomized trial comparing fluconazole with clotrimazole troches for the prevention of fungal infections in patients with advanced HIV infection. N Engl J Med 332:700, 1995.

81

Paracoccidioido-mycosis

GREGORY M. ANSTEAD
JOHN R. GRAYBILL

INTRODUCTION

Paracoccidioidomycosis is a systemic mycotic infection caused by the dimorphic fungus *Paracoccidioides brasiliensis.*[1] *Paracoccidioides brasiliensis* is restricted to the tropical Americas, from Mexico to Argentina. Approximately 80% of cases occur in Brazil, followed by Colombia and Venezuela. There have been virtually no cases reported from the Caribbean islands, Guyana, Suriname, or Chile. Cases are not randomly distributed within each country but are concentrated in areas with abundant forests and waterways, 90 to 180 cm of rainfall per year, short winters, and rainy summers.[2] *Paracoccidioides brasiliensis* has been isolated from the nine-banded armadillo (*Dasypus novemcinctus*). Infected armadillos were found more frequently in areas of disturbed vegetation, in artificial eucalyptus or pine forests, at altitudes below 800 m, near water sources, and in areas with sandy, acidic soil.[3]

AGENT

The free-living form of the fungus is presumed to be the mycelium. The mold can be grown at 18°C to 26°C, and it forms white to tan colonies with short mycelia. Hyphae are thin, septate, and generate pedunculated or single-cell arthroconidia that bud off the mycelium. When conidia are cultured in rich media at 37°C, they convert to and multiply as yeast-like cells. The cells vary from 4 to 30 µm in size and give rise to multiple narrow-based, elongated daughter cells budding from the "mother" cell. This gives a characteristic "Mickey Mouse" or "pilot wheel" appearance, similar to that seen in tissue biopsies (Fig. 81-1). *Paracoccidioides brasiliensis* is quite hardy and can multiply at 4°C in water.[2]

EPIDEMIOLOGY

All of the few cases reported outside of the endemic area occurred in patients who had traveled within the endemic regions. In these cases, the mean latency period between exposure and disease was 15 years, indicating that the fungus undergoes a characteristic long dormancy before producing the disease.[1,2] Because of the long latency, and because there have been no epidemics, the natural habitat of the fungus is unclear. Male rural workers, particularly woodcutters, are at highest risk. There are occasional cases in children (3%) and young adults (10%), but most commonly, patients are between 20 and 40 years old.[1] The rural predominance may be one reason why paracoccidioidomycosis has rarely been reported in patients with acquired immunodeficiency syndrome (AIDS).

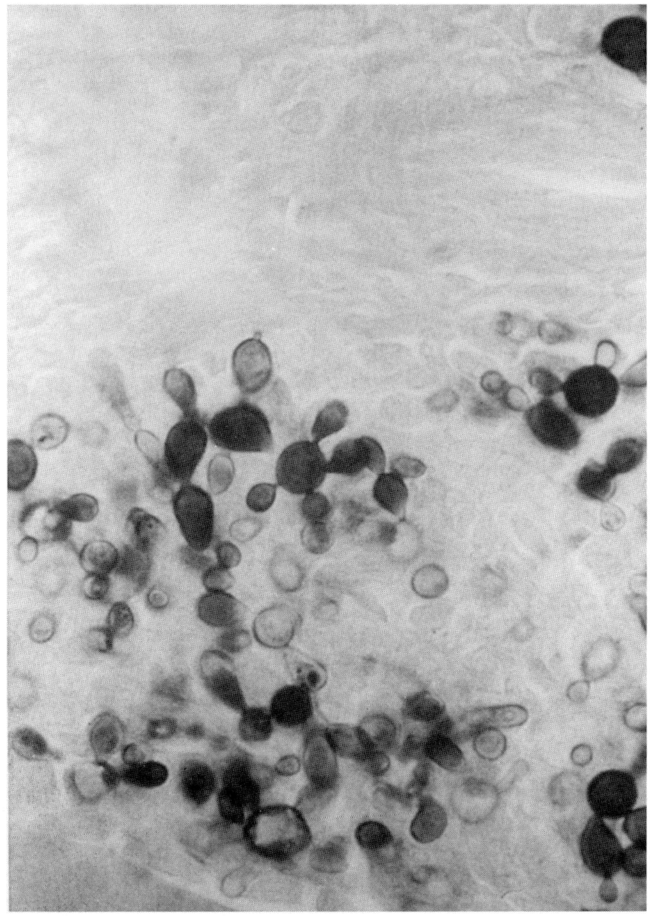

FIGURE 81-1 Gomori's methenamine silver stain of *Paracoccidioides brasiliensis* in tissue biopsy.

DISEASE

Paracoccidioidomycosis takes one of two forms: the acute (juvenile) disease or the adult chronic form.[1] Unlike the adult form, the juvenile form, which occurs primarily in children and adolescents, has no gender predilection. Juvenile paracoccidioidomycosis reflects only 3% to 5% of cases and is characterized by blood-borne dissemination to multiple sites, predominantly in the reticuloendothelial system (spleen, liver, lymph nodes, lungs, and bone marrow). Pneumonia, lymphadenopathy, hepatosplenomegaly, mucosal and skin ulceration, adrenal insufficiency, and cachexia all mark this form of the disease. Many replicating fungal cells are seen, with little granuloma formation and no fibrosis. Lymphadenopathy and hepatosplenomegaly may suggest lymphoma rather than infection. Mesenteric adenopathy may cause bowel obstruction. Central nervous system (CNS) involvement has been described.[4] In a series of 173 cases of paracoccidioidiomycosis, 13.9% had CNS involvement, typically revealed as multiple

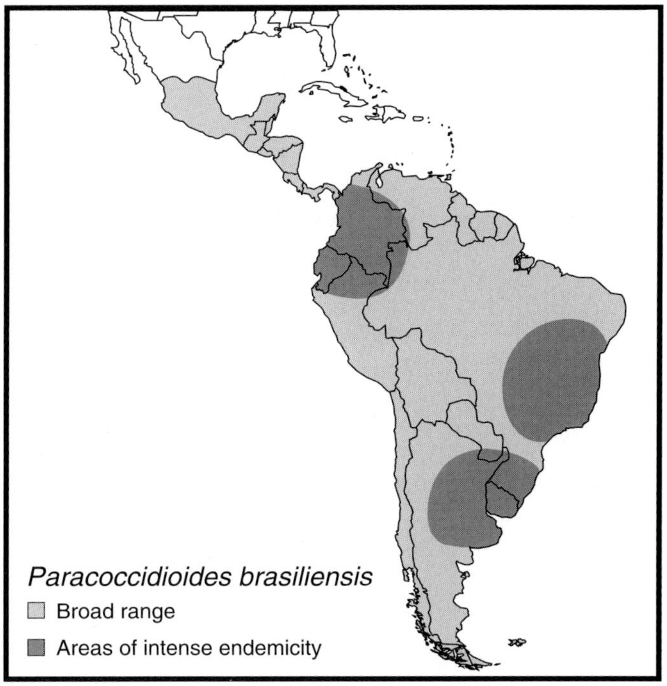

hypodense lesions with annular or nodular enhancement in the cerebral hemispheres; meningitis and spinal cord involvement are much less common. In this series, seizures were the most frequent neurologic presentation.[4] Chronic meningitis is also a common neurologic manifestation.[5] If the disease is untreated, mortality is high.

In contrast, the adult form of the disease occurs usually in males, progresses over months to years, and represents more than 90% of cases. Progressive pulmonary lesions are the hallmark, and in 25% of patients the lungs are the only organ involved. Symptoms are nonspecific and include cough, sputum production, weight loss, and dyspnea. In other patients, lymphadenopathy, hepatosplenomegaly, or skin and mucosal ulcerations may prompt the patient to seek medical attention (Fig. 81-2; Table 81-1; see also Plate 126-2E). Gallium scanning may reveal clinically unsuspected foci.[6] Chest radiographs typically show dense bilateral nodular, fibrotic, and cavitary lesions. The lesions may appear quite similar to those of tuberculosis, except for the propensity to involve the central or basilar lung fields and to spare the apices.[1] The process is destructive, and the nodular lesions may be associated with caseation and dense fibrosis.[1] Pulmonary function abnormalities may be relatively mild compared with the radiographic findings and are usually obstructive. With healing, chronic dyspnea, dysphonia, microstomia, glottic and tracheal stenosis, and adrenal insufficiency may occur. Healing occurs in association with dense fibrosis of affected tissues, and in some cases fibrosis may lead to cor pulmonale.[7] Despite efficacious therapy with azole antifungal agents, the fibrotic sequelae persist.[8,9]

In recent years, paracoccidioidomycosis has been recognized as an AIDS-associated opportunistic infection.[10,11] A review in 1995 included only 27 reported cases. This form of disease resembles the juvenile acute form and presents with aggressive pulmonary and widespread disseminated

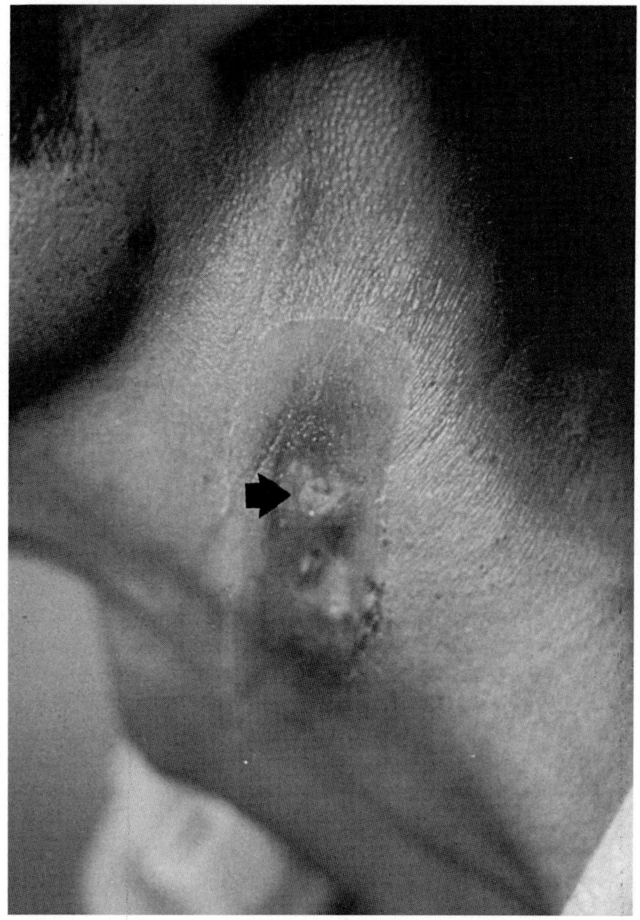

FIGURE 81-2 Ulcerative lesion on the neck of a patient with paracoccidioidomycosis *(arrow)*. (Courtesy of Dr. Angela Restrepo, CIB, Medellin, Colombia.)

disease (see Table 81-1). Meningeal involvement is more common in the AIDS patient, compared with less than 5% incidence in a series of non-AIDS patients.[1] It is of interest that AIDS-associated histoplasmosis is much more common than paracoccidioidomycosis. The reasons for this are unclear

Table 81-1 Organ Involvement in Paracoccidioidomycosis

Organ	Nonimmunocompromised Patients ($n=352$)	Patients with AIDS ($n=27$)
Lungs	77%	63%
Mucous membranes	63%	15%
Skin	12%	48%
Lymph nodes	13%	37%
Spleen, liver	5%	19%
Adrenals	3%	4%
Other	2%	15% (including 2 central nervous system, 1 bone marrow, and 1 blood)

From Brummer E, Castañeda E, Restrepo A: Paracoccidioidomycosis: An update. Clin Microbiol Rev 6:89–117, 1993.

and may relate to less contact of rural people with the human immunodeficiency virus (HIV) or the use of trimethoprim–sulfamethoxazole (which is effective against *P. brasiliensis*) as prophylaxis against *Pneumocystis*. In the series of Goldani and Sugar,[10] 12 of 13 patients with AIDS and paracoccidioidomycosis had not received trimethoprim–sulfamethoxazole prophylaxis for pneumocystosis.

PATHOGENESIS AND IMMUNITY

The pathogenesis, although not precisely defined, probably follows inhalation of conidia and subsequent transformation of the conidia into yeast cells within alveolar macrophages.[1] In the majority of immunocompetent patients, fungal growth is halted in these initial foci, and the infection is subclinical. Some patients become symptomatic years after they leave the endemic area. Therefore, some yeast cells must persist after the initial infection and reactivate later in more permissive circumstances. Markers of virulence are not well defined. Older cultures are less virulent in mice than are recent clinical isolates.[12] Mammalian female sex hormones, such as estradiol, alter mycelial band patterns and block synthesis of proteins needed for transformation to the yeast phase.[13] In vitro studies clearly show that estradiol inhibits transformation from the mycelium to the yeast. Estrogen binding proteins have been found in cytosol of both conidia and yeast cells. If estradiol is added to mycelium before the temperature is raised, novel proteins are produced. However, in vivo studies in rats found that females were highly susceptible to infection; castration, which should lower hormones and increase susceptibility, actually reduced it.[14] However, these studies were done with yeast cells, which are less susceptible than conidia[13] to hormone influences in vitro. In another study that used inhaled conidia as the infecting inoculum, in normal male mice there was progressive transformation of the conidia into tissue-form yeast cells in the first 96 hours of infection, whereas in the normal female mice no conida transformation occurred.[15]

The role of estradiol in altering the pathogenesis of paracoccidioidomycosis was definitively demonstrated in a study by Aristizabal and colleagues.[16] In this experiment, using inhaled conidia as the infecting inoculum, normal male mice suffered progressive disease, whereas normal females resisted disease progression. Castrated male mice that received exogenous estradiol initially resisted disease but ultimately had disease progression. Castrated female mice treated with testosterone were unable to control the infection.[16] Thus, estradiol inhibits transformation of the mycelia to the yeast form and promotes resistance to disease progression.

Skin tests from healthy subjects in endemic areas do not show male predominance, and male cases do not predominate among children. This situation again suggests that female sex hormones are active in suppressing symptomatic disease in women but have no influence on primary infection. Skin tests have not been useful in delineating hyperendemic areas where the fungus could be identified in its natural ecological niche.[17] The juvenile form can be reproduced in athymic mice and is relatively common in the few AIDS patients who have been reported to have paracoccidioidomycosis.[10,11] Competent cell-mediated immunity is thought to be the key to recovery.[1,2,5,18,19]

DIAGNOSIS

The endemic zone of paracoccidioidomycosis overlaps that of histoplasmosis in South America, and both the juvenile forms and the chronic pulmonary and disseminated forms of these two fungal diseases are quite similar. Therefore, a major diagnostic consideration in these areas of geographic overlap is histoplasmosis versus paracoccidioidomycosis because the diseases may be treated with different agents. Hepatosplenomegaly and bone marrow involvement are more prominent in disseminated histoplasmosis. Mucocutaneous lesions and adrenal insufficiency may occur in both diseases. In addition, approximately 10% of patients with paracoccidioidomycosis have coexistent tuberculosis, so this potential copathogen must be evaluated in each patient.[2]

On histopathologic stains of tissue biopsies, the fungal elements are pathognomonic. Potassium hydroxide preparations or calcofluor stain of sputum may also show thick-walled mother cells with multiple narrow-based budding daughter cells. Methenamine silver stain of sputum may be more sensitive than the KOH preparation. A mixed pyogranulomatous host response with neutrophils, mononuclear cells, and macrophages is usually present. Culture on Sabouraud agar at room temperature yields slowly growing (20 to 30 days) mycelia with the appearance of "white mouse hair." The identity can be confirmed by subculture at 37°C, with conversion to the more rapidly growing yeast form.

The complement fixation test has been used since 1916 for the diagnosis of paracoccidioidomycosis. Approximately 90% of patients have specific antibodies demonstrable by complement fixation, latex agglutination, immunofluorescence, tube precipitation, enzyme-linked immunosorbent assay, or other methods. Immunoblotting has been described as a highly sensitive method for the diagnosis of paracoccidioidomycosis.[20] When multiple tests are done on the same patients, results may be conflicting, and Restrepo[21] advises using only one test and using it consistently. IgG antibodies are elevated during the first year after infection but may be absent in patients with severe immunosuppression, such as AIDS.[2] In patients with progressive disease and depressed cell-mediated immunity, IgE antibodies rise later. Tests vary among different manufacturers, and there may be extensive cross-reaction of some antibodies with *Candida*, *Blastomyces dermatitidis*, *Histoplasma capsulatum*, or other fungal pathogens. Therefore, a positive serologic test does not in itself confirm active paracoccidioidomycosis.[1] Antigenemia has been detected in patients with paracoccidioidomycosis and offers a diagnostic alternative in those with severe immunodeficiencies. However, there may be false-positive reactions in patients with other mycoses.[22] Skin testing with paracoccidioidin may be useful epidemiologically, and in the individual patient it may be helpful in that conversion from anergy to a positive reaction is associated with a good prognosis.

TREATMENT AND PROGNOSIS

Paracoccidioidomycosis is one of the first major mycoses for which effective treatment became available; in 1940, Ribeiro found sulfonamide to be effective. Sulfadiazine (6 g/day) and trimethoprim–sulfamethoxazole, because of low cost, are still the mainstay of treatment. Because of the high relapse rate (as high as 25%), it is necessary to continue treatment with sulfonamides for as long as 5 years or at least 1 year after antibody titers have resolved or stabilized at a low titer.[1,2] Amphotericin B is beneficial, but the indications are not clear. Absence of symptoms for 2 years after cessation of therapy is considered by some to represent a clinical cure.[1] Three mycologically negative specimens are also considered by some to represent a cure.[1] Relapses may occur in as many as 38% of patients[2] and may be preceded by a rise in antibody titers.[1] Ketoconazole, at 200 mg/day, has been recommended for 6 to 12 months and, with 92% responses and 11% relapses, is more efficacious than sulfonamides.[23] Fluconazole is also effective, but high doses of 400 mg/day may be required.[24] The drug of choice is itraconazole (100 mg/day) for only 3 to 6 months, with 95% responses and 3.5% relapses.[25] Currently, the greatest unresolved problem with therapy is prevention of the severe fibrosis that accompanies healing, no matter what therapeutic agent is used.

Patients with AIDS have severe disseminated disease. Treatment is complex and in a review included multiple and serial drug regimens.[10] Of 27 patients, 21 (78%) were treated. Of the 15 patients who received a sulfonamide preparation, 10 survived, 3 died, and the outcome was unknown in 3 other patients. Of the 11 who received amphotericin B, 5 survived and 6 died. Of the 10 who received ketoconazole, 5 survived, 4 died, and the outcome was unknown in 1 patient. One cannot use such data to attribute drug efficacy because the patients were not similarly ill, patients clearly received multiple drugs, and those who were more seriously ill or who failed other drugs were given amphotericin B. Overall mortality was 30% of the 21 patients to whom specific antifungal therapy was given. This fatality rate is much higher than that for non-AIDS patients. When disease responds to initial treatment, lifelong suppressive therapy may be required, preferably using an azole antifungal. Histoplasmosis and cryptococcosis tend to remain in remission when treatment is discontinued in patients who have responded well to highly active antiretroviral therapy (HAART) with a sustained rise in CD4 T cells. Perhaps in the future this will be documented as well for paracoccidioidomycosis.

For additional information on paracoccidioidomycosis, the readers are referred to Restrepo-Moreno.[5]

REFERENCES

1. Franco M, Poncio-Mendes R, Moscardi-Bacchi M, et al: Paracoccidioidomycosis. Balliere's Clin Trop Med Commun Dis 4:185, 1989.
2. Brummer E, Castañeda E, Restrepo A: Paracoccidioidomycosis: An update. Clin Microbiol Rev 6:89, 1993.
3. Bagagli E, Franco M, Bosco S de M, et al: High frequency of *Paracoccidioides brasiliensis* infection in armadillos (*Dasypus novemcinctus*): An ecological study. Med Mycol 41:217, 2003.
4. de Almeida SM, Queroz-Telles F, Teive HA, et al: Central nervous system paracoccidioidomycosis: Clinical features and laboratory findings. J Infect 48:193, 2004.
5. Restrepo-Moreno A: Paracoccidioidomycosis. In Dismukes WE, Pappas PG, Sobel JD (eds): Clinical Mycology. Oxford, UK, Oxford University Press, 2003, p 328.
6. Giorgi MCP, Camargo EE, Pinto WP, et al: Gallium-67 imaging in the diagnosis of blastomycosis. Eur J Nucl Med 13:300, 1987.
7. Campos EP, Padovani CR, Cataneo AMJ: Paracoccidioidomycose: Estudie radiologico e pulmonar de 58 casos. Rev Inst Med Trop São Paulo 33:267, 1991.
8. Naranjo MS, Trujillo M, Munera MI, et al: Treatment of paracoccidioidomycosis with itraconazole. J Med Vet Mycol 28:67, 1990.
9. Lemle A, Wanke B, Miranda JL, et al: Pulmonary function in paracoccidioidomycosis (South American blastomycosis). Chest 83:827, 1983.
10. Goldani LZ, Sugar AM: Paracoccidioidomycosis and AIDS: An overview. Clin Infect Dis 21:127, 1995.
11. Silva-Vergara ML, Teixeria AC, Curi VG, et al: Paracoccidioidomycosis associated with human immunodeficiency virus infection. Report of ten cases. Med Mycol 41:259, 2003.
12. Brummer E, Restrepo A, Hanson LH, et al: Virulence of *Paracoccidioides brasiliensis:* The influence of in vitro passage and storage. Mycopathologia 109:13, 1990.
13. Restrepo A, Salazar ME, Cano LE, et al: Estrogens inhibit mycelium-to-yeast transformation in the fungus *Paracoccidioides brasiliensis:* Implications for resistance of females to parcoccidioidomycosis. Infect Immun 46:346, 1984.
14. Kerr IB, Schaeffer GV, Miranda DS: Sex hormones and susceptibility of the rat with paracoccidioidomycosis. Mycopathologia 88:149, 1984.
15. Aristizabal BH, Clemons KV, Stevens DA, et al: Morphologic transition of *Paracoccidioides brasiliensis* conidia to yeast cells: In vivo inhibition in females. Infect Immun 66:5587, 1998.
16. Aristizabal BH, Clemons KV, Cock AM, et al: Experimental *Paracoccidioides brasiliensis* infection in mice: Influence of hormonal status of the host on tissue responses. Med Mycol 40:169, 2002.
17. Restrepo A: The ecology of *Paracoccidioides brasiliensis:* A puzzle still unsolved. J Med Vet Mycol 23:323, 1985.
18. Souto JT, Figueiredo F, Furlanetto A, et al: Interferon-gamma and tumor necrosis factor-alpha determine resistance to *Paracoccidioides brasiliensis* infection in mice. Am J Pathol 156:1811, 2000.
19. Borges-Walmsley MI, Chen D, Shu X, et al: The pathobiology of *Paracoccidioides brasiliensis*. Trends Microbiol 10:80, 2002.
20. do Valle AC, Costa RL, Fialho Moneiro PC, et al: Interpretation and clinical correlation of serologic tests in paracoccidioidomycosis. Med Mycol 39:373, 2001.
21. Restrepo A: Procedimientos serologicos en la paracoccidioidomicosis. Adel Microbiol Enferm Infecc 3:182, 1984.
22. Freitas-Silva G, Roque-Arrera MC: Antigenemia in paracoccidioidomycosis. J Clin Microbiol 30:381, 1992.
23. Negroni R, Robles AM, Arechavala A, et al: Ketoconazole in the treatment of paracoccidioidomycosis and histoplasmosis. Rev Infect Dis 2:643, 1980.
24. Diaz M, Negroni R, Montero-Gei F, et al: A Pan-American 5-year study of fluconazole therapy for deep mycoses in the immunocompetent host. Pan-American Study. Clin Infect Dis 14(suppl 1):S68, 1992.
25. Negroni R, Robles AM, Arechavala A, et al: Resultados del tratamiento con itraconazole por via oral en la paracoccidioidomicosis. Rev Argent Microbiol 19(suppl):27, 1987.

82

Penicilliosis Marneffei

GREGORY M. ANSTEAD
JOHN R. GRAYBILL

INTRODUCTION

Penicillium species are fungi widely distributed in nature, found mainly in the soil and decomposing organic matter, and are considered to be common laboratory culture contaminants. *Penicillium marneffei* is by far the species that most commonly causes human disease. It was first reported as an animal pathogen in the bamboo rat *Rhizomys sinensis* in Vietnam by Capponi and associates in 1956.[1] Segretain[2] described the fungus and in 1959 named it in honor of Dr. Marneffe, the director of the Pasteur Institute of Indochina. Segretain was the first to note acquisition of the infection after accidental inoculation of his finger, which caused a local infection that resolved spontaneously. The first naturally occurring infection was reported by DiSalvo and colleagues[3] in 1973 in an American with Hodgkin's lymphoma who had traveled to Southeast Asia. The second human infection was not reported until 1984.[4] Since then, an increasing number of reports have been published. In recent years, there has been an enormous increase in the incidence of this infection in endemic areas, corresponding to the increase in acquired immunodeficiency syndrome (AIDS) cases.[5] The first case of penicilliosis marneffei in a patient with AIDS was reported in 1988.[6] Currently, penicilliosis marneffei is the fourth most common opportunistic infection, after tuberculosis, pneumocystosis, and cryptococcosis, in AIDS patients in Thailand.[7,8]

AGENT

Penicillium marneffei is the only species of the genus *Penicillium* known to be thermally dimorphic, growing in mycelial form at 25°C and in yeastlike form at 37°C and dividing by binary fission. The dimorphism of this fungus has been proposed as a factor in its greater pathogenicity compared to other members of the genus *Penicillium*.[9]

EPIDEMIOLOGY

All cases are from Southeast Asia (Thailand, Vietnam, Myanmar, Hong Kong, Indonesia, Laos, Malaysia, Singapore, Taiwan, the Manipur state of India, and the Guangxi province of China) or in people who traveled to these areas.[5,10,11] The natural reservoir of the fungus has not been identified. The organism has been isolated from the viscera of four species of bamboo rats and from the soil in areas where the rats live; the excrement of these fossorial rats may promote the growth of the fungus.[12]

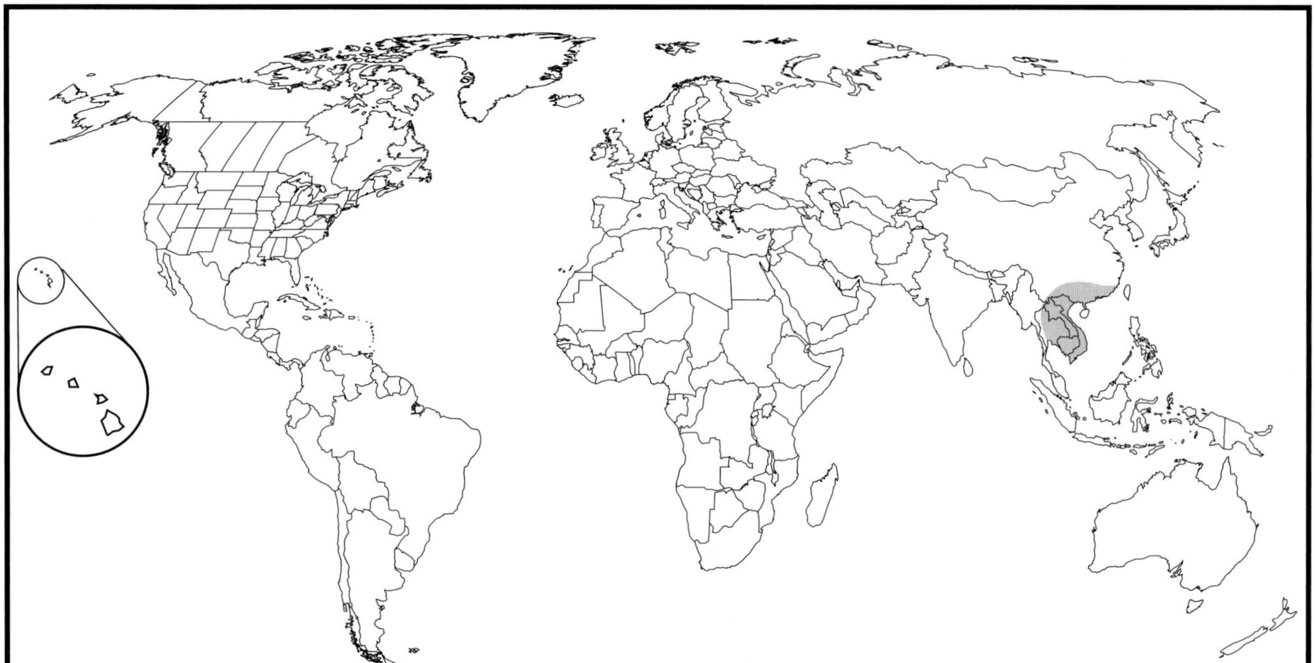

Penicillium marneffei

■ *Penicillium marneffei*

Table 82-1 Clinical Features of 80 Human Immunodeficiency Virus–Infected Patients with Disseminated Penicillium marneffei *Infection*

Symptoms and Signs	No. (%)
Fever	74 (93)
Skin lesions	54 (68)
Cough	39 (49)
Diarrhea	25 (31)
Temperature >38.3°C	79 (99)
Weight loss	61 (76)
Anemia	62 (78)
Jaundice	6 (8)
Generalized lymphadenopathy	46 (58)
Hepatomegaly	41 (51)
Splenomegaly	13 (16)
Skin lesions	57 (71)
Genital ulcer	5 (6)

Modified from Supparatpinyo K, Khamwan C, Baosoung V, et al: Disseminated *Penicillium marneffei* infection in Southeast Asia. Lancet 344:110, 1994.

The main risk factor for infection is occupational soil exposure during the rainy season. Contact with or consumption of the bamboo rats does not appear to be a risk factor.[13]

DISEASE

Clinical manifestations of penicilliosis marneffei are nonspecific. They usually develop over weeks but may be more acute, manifested by fever, chills, prostration, weight loss, and anemia. Reticuloendothelial involvement presents as generalized lymphadenopathy and hepatomegaly (Table 82-1). Liver injury may be manifested by high transaminases and alkaline phosphatase, and the blood leukocyte count is variable.

In the HIV-infected patient, there frequently are diffuse papular skin lesions with central necrosis or umbilication resembling *molluscum contagiosum*[7,14] (Fig. 82-1). Other cutaneous signs include maculopapular rash, pustules, and subcutaneous nodules. Mucocutaneous ulcers, including genital sites, can be chronic and recurrent. Respiratory complaints include cough and dyspnea. Chest radiographic findings include diffuse reticulonodular, localized interstitial, or alveolar infiltrates. One case of upper airway obstruction due to retropharyngeal abscess has been reported.[15] Osteolytic bone lesions, usually multiple, have been described. Arthritis can be monoarticular or polyarticular, with no specific joint predominance.[16] Clinical evidence of central nervous system involvement is rare. The differential diagnosis of penicilliosis marneffei includes tuberculosis, histoplasmosis, cryptococcosis, *Mycobacterium avium–intracellulare* complex infection, and lymphoid malignancies.

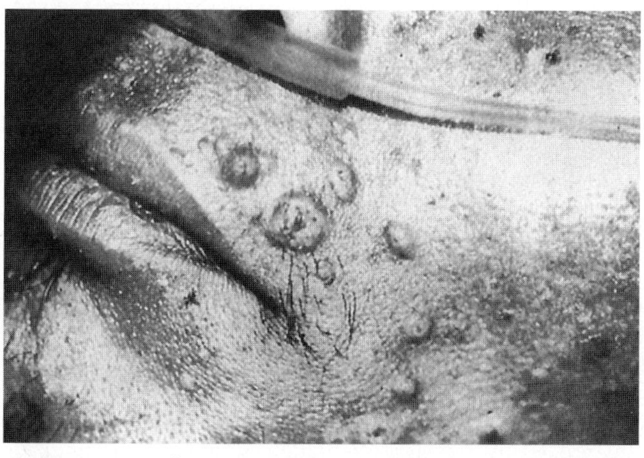

FIGURE 82-1 Molluscum contagiosum–like lesions in a patient with penicilliosis marneffei. (From Supparatpinyo K, Khamwan C, Baosoung V, et al: Disseminated *Penicillium marneffei* infection in Southeast Asia. Lancet 344:110, 1994.)

PATHOGENESIS AND IMMUNITY

The pathogenesis of penicilliosis marneffei has been poorly studied. Although the disease can be localized, it is more likely to be disseminated in both normal and immunocompromised hosts. Infection is thought to occur through inhalation of the spores or possibly through cutaneous inoculation. The organisms are engulfed by macrophages, in which they multiply intracellularly and transform into yeasts. Dissemination of infection occurs through the lymphatics or hematogenously. The reticuloendothelial system is predominantly involved. The infection can remain dormant and reactivate later, as evidenced by patients having the disease years after leaving the endemic area. In the immunocompetent host, the cell-mediated immune response is prominent with the formation of epithelioid granulomas that are indistinguishable from tuberculous granulomas.[10] In a murine model of infection, wild-type mice controlled the infection with granuloma formation and the elaboration of a classic Th1 immune response (high levels of interferon-γ and interleukin-12). Conversely, interferon-γ knockout mice suffered rapid death; the spleen and liver showed abundant yeast forms and an absence of granuloma formation.[17] There is no evidence for a role of humoral immunity in the resolution of penicilliosis marneffei infection. A suppurative reaction has been described rarely in immunocompetent patients.[10] In patients with HIV infection, the histopathologic features depend on the degree of immunosuppression.[18] At lower CD4 cell counts, the disease tends to be more invasive, with a blunted immune response reflected by the absence of granulomas and extensive proliferation of extracellular yeast and intracellular forms within foamy macrophages. Yeast forms can occasionally be demonstrated in peripheral blood.[18,19]

DIAGNOSIS

A history of travel or residence in the endemic region is essential information to facilitate a diagnosis. In disseminated disease, microbiologic diagnosis through cultures of the organism from several body sites has been highly sensitive, approaching 100% from bone marrow and lymph nodes. In HIV patients infected with *P. marneffei*, the organism has been recovered from blood cultures in 76% of cases.[7] Other sites that have yielded positive cultures include skin, liver, bone, joints, lung, and occasionally urine. Sabouraud dextrose agar is the culture medium of choice. The fungus grows rapidly

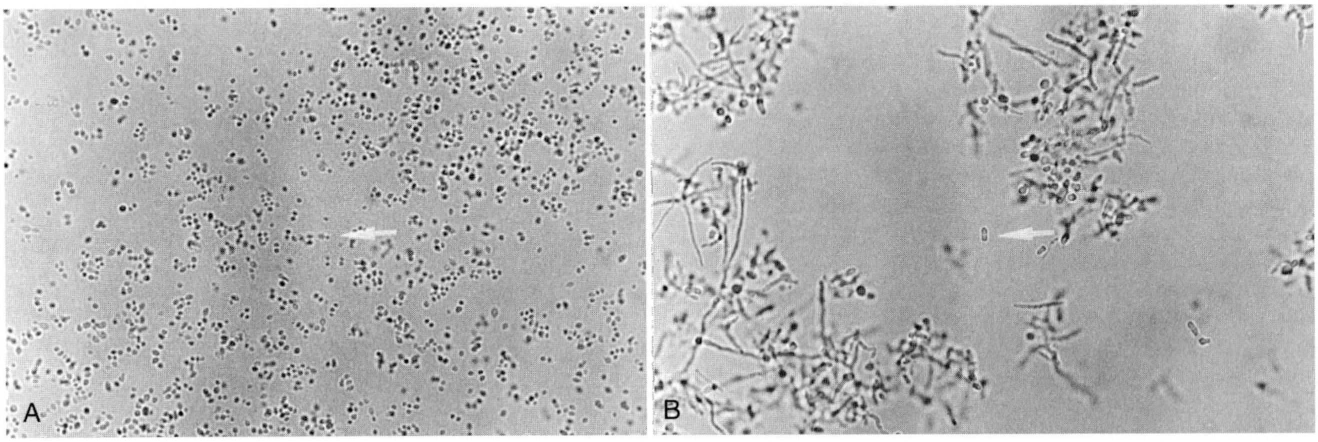

FIGURE 82-2 *A,* Small budding yeast of *Histoplasma capsulatum (arrow). B,* Larger elongated yeastlike form of *Penicillium marneffei* with central septum *(arrow).*

within 2 to 5 days in its mycelial form, producing gray colonies and a characteristic red pigment that diffuses throughout the agar.

Pathologic diagnosis can be more difficult in immunocompetent patients in whom granulomatous inflammation may be the only finding, with negative fungal stains. In immunosuppressed patients (mainly with HIV), there is more extensive disease, and numerous organisms are demonstrated by Gomori's methenamine silver or periodic acid–Schiff stains.[5,7] Wright-stained specimens from skin lesions, bone marrow, or, occasionally, peripheral blood may show yeast cells.[11,20] *Penicillium marneffei* bears a morphologic resemblance to *Histoplasma capsulatum*, and it can be difficult to distinguish between them. However, *P. marneffei* tends to form more elongated yeast cells with no budding and divides by central septate fission rather than budding (Fig. 82-2).

Specific fluorescent antibody examination of tissue samples has been described.[21] A few serodiagnostic techniques have been described, including immunodiffusion for antibody detection and an indirect immunofluorescent antibody test; however, these tests need further evaluation to be used in clinical practice.[22,23]

Rapid antigen detection assays with high sensitivity and specificity have been developed.[24,25] Sensitive polymerase chain reaction–based assays of clinical samples for the rapid diagnosis of penicilliosis marneffei have also been described.[26]

TREATMENT AND PROGNOSIS

If untreated, penicilliosis marneffei is fatal. Amphotericin B, with or without 5-flucytosine, has been successful in treating penicilliosis marneffei infection. In vitro testing shows only moderate activity of amphotericin against *P. marneffei*.[27] Azoles, particularly itraconazole and ketoconazole, are very active against *P. marneffei*, both clinically and in vitro. Fluconazole is the least active in vitro of the currently available azoles, and it has been associated with more failures than the other azoles. The echinocandin anidulofungin shows in vitro activity, but there is no reported clinical experience.[28] In one case series of penicilliosis marneffei in HIV-infected patients, amphotericin B had a response rate of 77% compared with 75% and 30% with itraconazole and fluconazole, respectively.[27] In an open-label trial of the treatment of HIV-infected people with penicilliosis marneffei, amphotericin B was given at 0.6 mg/kg/day for 2 weeks, followed by itraconazole at 400 mg/day; 97.3% of patients responded.[29] Treatment options are determined by the clinical status of the patient and the availability and cost of the drugs. For severely ill patients, amphotericin B (0.5 to 0.7 mg/kg/day) is the drug of choice. For patients with less severe illness, itraconazole (400 mg/day) is indicated. Ketoconazole, given in a 400 mg/day dose, can be an effective and much less expensive alternative to itraconazole. The duration of treatment is determined by the immune status of the patient. For HIV patients, lifelong suppressive therapy with azoles may be needed because 30% of patients relapse after cessation of therapy. For immunocompetent patients, there are not enough data to support a specific duration of treatment; however, 2 or 3 months has typically been associated with clinical resolution.[10] Clinical improvement is expected within 2 weeks of the institution of appropriate therapy.

If penicilliosis marneffei is not properly treated, the prognosis is poor, with high mortality in both HIV- and non-HIV-infected patients. Most HIV-infected patients who present with penicilliosis marneffei have a CD4 cell count of less than 50/μL as well as a history of other opportunistic infections.

PREVENTION AND CONTROL

There is no evidence of human-to-human transmission. Itraconazole (200 mg/day) has been shown to prevent penicilliosis marneffei in AIDS patients in a highly endemic area of Thailand. However, overall survival was not improved.[30] Several vaccine technologies based on the secreted cell wall antigen Mp1p (DNA by intramuscular administration, DNA vaccine delivered orally via live attenuated *Salmonella typhimurium*, and recombinant protein administered by intraperitoneal injection) were shown to be protective in a murine model of penicilliosis marneffei.[31]

REFERENCES

1. Capponi PM, Sureau P, Segretain G: Penicillose de *Rhizomys sinesis*. Bull Soc Pathol Exot 49:418, 1956.
2. Segretain G: Description d'une nouvelle espèce de penicillium: *Penicillium marneffei*. Bull Soc Mycol Fr 75:412, 1959.
3. DiSalvo AF, Fickling AM, Ajello L: Infection caused by *Penicillium marneffei*: Description of the first natural infection in man. Am J Clin Pathol 59:259, 1973.
4. Pautler KB, Padhye AA, Ajello L: Imported penicilliosis marneffei in the United States: Report of a second human infection. Sabouraudia 22:433, 1984.
5. Hilmarsdottir I, Meynard JL, Rogeaux O, et al: Disseminated *Penicillium marneffei* infection associated with human immunodeficiency virus: A report of two cases and review of 35 published cases. J Acquir Immune Defic Syndr Hum Retrovirol 6:466, 1993.
6. Piehl MR, Kaplan RL, Harber MH: Disseminated penicilliosis in a patient with acquired immunodeficiency syndrome. Arch Pathol Lab Med 112:1262, 1988.
7. Supparatpinyo K, Khamwan C, Baosoung V, et al: Disseminated *Penicillium marneffei* infection in Southeast Asia. Lancet 344:110, 1994.
8. Chariyalertsak S, Sirisanthana T, Saengwonloey O, et al: Clinical presentation and risk behaviors of patients with acquired immunodeficiency syndrome in Thailand, 1994–1998: Regional variation and temporal trends. Clin Infect Dis 32:955, 2001.
9. Cooper CR Jr, Haycocks NG: *Penicillium marneffei*: An insurgent species among the penicillia. J Eukaryotic Microbiol 47:24, 2000.
10. Deng Z, Ribas JL, Gibson DW: Infections caused by *Penicillium marneffei* in China and Southeast Asia: Review of eighteen reported cases and report of four more Chinese cases. Rev Infect Dis 10:640, 1988.
11. Ranjana KH, Priyokamar K, Singh TJ, et al: Disseminated *Penicillium marneffei* infection among HIV-infected patients in Manipur State, India. J Infect 45:268, 2002.
12. Bradsher RW. Geographic, travel, and occupational fungal infections. In Anaissie EJ, McGinnis MR, Pfaller MA (eds): Clinical Mycology. New York, Churchill Livingstone, 2003, p 583.
13. Chariyalertsak S, Sirisanthana T, Supparatpinyo K, et al: A case control study of risk factors for *P. marneffei* infections in human immunodeficiency virus-infected patients in northern Thailand. Clin Infect Dis 24:1080, 1997.
14. Borradori L, Schmit JC, Stetzkowski M, et al: *Penicilliosis marneffei* in AIDS. J Am Acad Dermatol 31:843, 1994.
15. Kwai FK: Retropharyngeal abscess caused by *Penicillium marneffei*: An unusual case of upper airway obstruction. Otolaryngol Head Neck Surg 110:445, 1994.
16. Louthrenoo W, Thamprasert K, Sirisanthana T: Osteoarticular penicilliosis marneffei: A report of eight cases and review of the literature. Br J Rheumatol 33:1145, 1994.
17. Sisto F, Miluzio A, Leopardi O, et al: Differential cytokine pattern in the spleens and livers of BALB/c mice infected with *Penicillium marneffei*: Protective role of interferon-gamma. Infect Immun 71:465, 2003.
18. Yousukh A, Jutavijittum P, Pisetpongsa P, et al: Clinicopathologic study of hepatic *Penicillium marneffei* in northern Thailand. Arch Pathol Lab Med 128:191, 2004.
19. Tsui WM, Ma KF, Tsang DN: Disseminated *Penicillium marneffei* infection in HIV-infected subjects. Histopathology 20:287, 1992.
20. Supparatpinyo K, Sirisanthana T: Disseminated *Penicillium marneffei* infection diagnosed on examination of a peripheral blood smear of a patient with human immunodeficiency virus infection. Clin Infect Dis 18:246, 1994.
21. Kaufman L, Standard PG, Anderson SA, et al: Development of specific fluorescent-antibody test for tissue form of *Penicillium marneffei*. J Clin Microbiol 33:2136, 1995.
22. Sekhon AS, Li JSK, Grag AK: Penicilliosis marneffei: Serological and exoantigens studies. Mycopathologia 77:51, 1982.
23. Yuen K, Wong SS, Tsang DN, et al: Serodiagnosis of *Penicillium marneffei*. Lancet 344:444, 1994.
24. Desakorn V, Simpson AJ, Wuthiekanun V, et al: Development and evaluation of rapid urinary antigen detection tests for the diagnosis of penicilliosis marneffei. J Clin Microbiol 40:3179, 2002.
25. Chaiyaroj SC, Chawengkirttikul R, Sirisinha S, et al: Antigen detection assay for identification of *Penicillium marneffei* infection. J Clin Microbiol 41:432, 2003.
26. Prariyachatigul C, Chaiprasert A, Geenkajorn K, et al: Development and evaluation of a one-tube seminested PCR assay for the detection and identification of *Penicillium marneffei*. Mycoses 46:447, 2003.
27. Supparatpinyo K, Nelson KE, Merz WG, et al: Response to anti-fungal therapy by human immunodeficiency virus-infected patients with disseminated *Penicillium marneffei* infection and in vitro susceptibilities of isolates from clinical specimens. Antimicrob Agents Chemother 37:2407, 1993.
28. Odabasi Z, Paetznick VL, Rodriguez JR, et al: In vitro activity of anidulafungin against selected clinically important mold isolates. Antimicrob Agents Chemother 48:1912, 2004.
29. Sirisanthana T, Supparatpinyo K, Perriens J, et al: Amphotericin B and itraconazole for treatment of disseminated *Penicillium marneffei* infection in human immunodeficiency virus-infected patients. Clin Infect Dis 26:107, 1998.
30. Chariyalertsak S, Supparatpinyo K, Sirisanthana T, et al: A controlled trial of itraconazole as primary prophylaxis for systemic fungal infection in patients with advanced human immunodeficiency virus infection in Thailand. Clin Infect Dis 34:277, 2002.
31. Wong LP, Woo PC, Wu AY, et al: DNA immunization using a secreted cell wall antigen Mp1p is protective against *Penicillium marneffei* infection. Vaccine 20:2878, 2002.

83

Mucocutaneous and Deeply Invasive Candidiasis

SHMUEL SHOHAM
THOMAS J. WALSH

INTRODUCTION AND EPIDEMIOLOGY

Candidal infections are an important cause of illness worldwide. *Candida* spp., particularly *Candida albicans,* are frequent human commensals, but a diverse range of infections can occur when host defenses break down or are breached. Mucocutaneous infections are common in all climates. In hot, humid, tropical regions, macerated skin often becomes infected, resulting in cutaneous candidiasis. Mucosal candidiasis can involve the lower genital tract, oropharynx, or esophagus. Vulvovaginal candidiasis is one of the most common genital problems of women in both industrialized and developing countries. Extensive use of antibiotics, development of human immunodeficiency virus (HIV) infection, the advent of diabetes mellitus as a global health problem, and local genital immune factors are all contributors to the widespread prevalence of vulvovaginal candidiasis. Oropharyngeal and esophageal candidiasis are typically encountered in association with local mucosal injury or as a result of defects in cell-mediated immunity. In many countries, the major driving force for these illnesses is the HIV pandemic. Moreover, with the advent of globalization, illnesses previously associated with wealthier societies can be expected to assume an increasingly important role in developing nations. In that regard, in newly industrialized countries, deeply invasive candidiasis occurring in the setting of or, as a consequence of, medical progress will likely emerge as a new challenge. Examples of such illnesses include oropharyngeal and esophageal candidiasis among recipients of cytotoxic therapies, bloodstream infection in persons with indwelling vascular devices, and disseminated candidiasis in highly compromised hosts such as neonates and transplant recipients. Expansion of populations at risk, changes in distribution of colonizing and infecting species, and the impact of widespread use of antifungal agents on the evolution of resistant organisms are now experienced in an increasing number of regions worldwide. Studies designed to optimize use of existing antifungals and to aid in the development of novel agents continue to be crucial in meeting these challenges. Perhaps even more important is expansion of our knowledge of regional and global epidemiologic patterns, candidal pathogenesis and host defenses, and the translation of this information into a better understanding of the fungus as it relates to patients in a diversity of environments.

AGENTS

The genus *Candida* encompasses more than 150 species, but only a small number are human pathogens. In nature, *Candida* spp. are principally associated with plants and rotting vegetation. Most are unable to grow at temperatures of 37°C and require vitamins produced mainly in plant materials.[1,2] Of the species known to cause human disease, *Candida albicans, Candida glabrata, Candida parapsilosis, Candida tropicalis, Candida krusei, Candida lusitaniae,* and *Candida guilliermondii* are the most commonly encountered pathogens.[3–6] Other species implicated in human disease include *Candida catenulata, Candida famata, Candida haemulonii, Candida inconspicua, Candida kefyr, Candida lambica, Candida lipolytica, Candida norvegensis, Candida pelliculosa, Candida pulcherrima, Candida rugosa, Candida sake, Candida utilis, Candida wiswanathii,* and *Candida zeylanoides*. Recently, *Candida dubliniensis* has been identified as a novel species that is increasingly being reported as a human pathogen.[7,8] Because *C. dubliniensis* shares many characteristics with *C. albicans,* it may be misidentified as *C. albicans* in clinical specimens.[9]

Laboratory identification of *Candida* spp. is achieved by assessment of a combination of morphologic and biochemical features of the fungus. *Candida* spp. grow as ovoid-shaped yeasts (blastoconidia), typically 4 to 6 μm in diameter, that reproduce by budding. Most species of *Candida* also produce filamentous growth in the form of pseudohyphae. *C. albicans* and *C. dubliniensis* are capable of producing both pseudohyphae and true hyphae.[2] Microscopic examination of yeast, hyphae, and pseudohyphae from clinical specimens is facilitated by the addition of 10% potassium hydroxide (KOH), which digests epithelial cells. Fluorescent microscopy of specimens stained with calcofluor white and the Gram method (*Candida* spp. stain gram-positive) are also useful diagnostic tools.

Phase transition from yeast to filamentous forms may be an important virulence factor in vivo. Germination can be induced under various conditions including the presence of serum, specific carbon sources, hemin, temperatures over 35°C, and pH of 6.5 to 7.0 or slightly alkaline. Conversely, lower temperatures and an acid environment favor yeast growth.[2,10] During hyphal formation, an outgrowth develops from the yeast cells termed a germ tube. Diagnostic mycology laboratories commonly test for the presence or absence of a germ tube in order to differentiate *C. albicans* and *C. dubliniensis* from other *Candida* spp. Development of a germ tube is highly suggestive but not absolutely diagnostic for these two species. Additionally, *C. albicans* and *C. dubliniensis* can produce large (8 to 12 μm), thick-walled cells termed chlamydospores. Chlamydospores are occasionally encountered in host tissue and can be induced by various culture media including corn meal agar, rice extract agar, chlamydospore agar, PCB, Tween 80-oxgall-caffeic acid, and diluted milk.[2,11,12]

Clinically important species of *Candida* grow well in routine blood culture systems and on common mycologic and bacteriologic media including Sabouraud glucose agar, sheep blood agar, and horse blood agar.[13] When grown at 25°C to 37°C on Sabouraud agar, *Candida* spp. form white-to-beige colonies that are smooth-to-wrinkled in texture. Media containing chromogenic compounds such as CHROMagar can differentiate *Candida* spp. based on the formation of various colored colonies with different morphologies, which result from the cleavage of chromogenic substrates by species-specific enzymes. CHROMagar *Candida* medium (CCM) can be used for presumptive identification of *C. albicans*, *C. tropicalis*, and *C. krusei*.[14] In a study exploring the usefulness of CCM in a developing country, more than 90% of isolates from clinical specimens were identified to species level within 48 hours, and the assay was determined to be cost effective in a resource-poor environment.[15] CCM can be used to distinguish *C. albicans* from *C. dubliniensis*. Upon primary plating of the clinical specimen on CCM, *C. dubliniensis* produces dark-green colonies, whereas *C. albicans* appears light blue-green.[13] Definitive identification of *Candida* spp. can be facilitated by metabolic tests. Commercial kits are now available that provide standardized identification of most *Candida* spp. within several days. In addition to the use of CHROMagar as described previously, *C. albicans* can be differentiated from *C. dubliniensis* by the latter's inability to grow at 45°C and by use of species-specific DNA fingerprinting probes.[16,17]

PATHOGENESIS AND IMMUNITY

Candida spp., particularly *C. albicans*, colonize the human gastrointestinal, respiratory, and reproductive tracts and the skin. Invasive disease occurs when host defenses break down or are breached. A variety of adhesins facilitate attachment of the fungus to epithelial and endothelial surfaces.[18] The ability of *Candida* spp. to form biofilms on surfaces such as catheters has contributed to the emergence of these fungi as major pathogens of patients with indwelling medical devices. Biofilm-associated infections are frequently refractory to antifungal therapy. This resistance could be due in part to changes in candidal sterol composition and upregulation of drug efflux pumps.[19,20] Production of hydrolytic enzymes including secreted aspartic proteinases, phospholipases, and lipases have all been linked to virulence of *C. albicans*.[21] Secreted aspartyl proteinases digest molecules for nutrient acquisition, disrupt host cell membranes to facilitate adhesion and tissue invasion, and break up cells and molecules of the immune system, thereby contributing to the infectious process.[22] Phospholipases promote fungal virulence through host cell damage and lysis.[23] Morphologic transitions among yeast, pseudohyphal, and hyphal forms and the phenomenon of phenotype switching are also thought to contribute to virulence in *C. albicans*.[24,25] Other virulence factors include production of a hemolytic factor that facilitates acquisition of iron by the pathogen and expression of complement receptors that act to inhibit phagocytosis.[26,27]

Clinical disease can be broadly divided into two categories: mucosal and systemic candidiasis. Innate immunity is the dominant protective mechanism against disseminated disease. Neutrophils, monocytes, endothelial cells, dendritic cells, platelets, opsonins, cytokines, chemokines, and complement all participate in protection against systemic infection.[28,29] The role of cell-mediated immunity and antibodies in disseminated disease is less clear. Cell-mediated immunity is the predominant protective mechanism against nongenital mucosal candidiasis. Clinically, patients with abnormal cell-mediated immune responses as a consequence of HIV infection or corticosteroid use are at increased risk for mucosal infections. In the lower genital tract, locally acquired mucosal immunity appears to be more important than systemic cell-mediated immunity against *C. albicans* infection, and the majority of women with candidal vaginitis do not have a discernible systemic immune defect.[30,31]

ANTIFUNGAL SUSCEPTIBILITY

Antifungal agents belonging to four major classes—azoles, polyenes, echinocandins, and pyrimidine analogs—are used to treat most candidal infections. This section describes the mechanisms of action of drugs belonging to these classes, means by which *Candida* spp. have developed resistance, and epidemiologic patterns of antifungal susceptibility.

The antifungal compounds belonging to the azole class target ergosterol biosynthesis by inhibiting the fungal cytochrome P-450–dependent enzyme lanosterol 14α-demethylase. This inhibition interrupts the conversion of lanosterol to ergosterol, which leads to accumulation of aberrant 14α-methylsterols and depletion of ergosterol in the fungal cell membrane. This interruption alters the fungal cell membrane properties and functions and, depending on organism and compound, may lead to fungal cell death or inhibition of cell growth and replication. In addition, the azoles also inhibit cytochrome P-450–dependent enzymes of the fungal respiration chain.[32] Resistance to azoles may be intrinsic, as in the case of some isolates of C. *krusei*, or acquired. Several mechanisms of azole resistance have been described in *Candida* spp. Factors contributing to decreased azole susceptibility include reduced affinity of 14α-demethylase to fluconazole, enhanced 14α-demethylation (related increased expression of *erg 11*, which allows the organism to overcome enzymatic inhibition, alteration of the ergosterol biosynthetic pathway, and upregulation of multidrug efflux transporters.[33–36] These mechanisms frequently operate simultaneously to exert antifungal resistance. Genetic analyses in *C. albicans* have demonstrated that under antifungal pressure clinical isolates can undergo minor genetic alterations that over time lead to gradual development of azole resistance through the accumulation of different molecular mechanisms.[37]

C. albicans is the most common *Candida* sp. recovered from mucocutaneous candidiasis. Most isolates are susceptible to all antifungal agents; however, emergence of resistance to azoles may be common in isolates of *C. albicans*. The most common *Candida* spp. encountered in clinical settings of bloodstream infection are *C. albicans, C. glabrata, C. parapsilosis, C. tropicalis,* and *C. krusei*. Although *C. albicans, C. tropicalis,* and *C. parapsilosis,* which account for more than two thirds of bloodstream infections, remain susceptible to fluconazole and itraconazole, resistance among *C. glabrata* and *C. krusei* has emerged as an issue with clinically relevant implications.[38] A breakpoint for fluconazole susceptibility has been set when the minimum inhibitory concentrations (MICs) are less than or equal to 8 μg/mL. Isolates for which the MIC of fluconazole is between 16 to 32 μg/mL are considered susceptible dependent upon dose (S-DD) and resistant when the MIC is greater than or equal to 64 μg/mL.[39] S-DD isolates may be treated successfully with higher dosages of fluconazole.

In a 10-year study assessing the antifungal susceptibilities of *Candida* spp. collected from 250 medical centers in 32 nations, more than 90% of *C. albicans, C. tropicalis,* and *C. parapsilosis* were found to be susceptible to fluconazole.[5] In a recent survey, 1.2% of *C. albicans* isolates were resistant to fluconazole compared with 6% of *C. tropicalis* isolates.[38] *C. glabrata* has emerged as a major cause of invasive candidiasis. In a study involving more than 200 medical centers worldwide, 60% of *C. glabrata* isolates were susceptible to fluconazole, 32% were S-DD, and 8% were resistant.[40] In that study, only 5% of *C. krusei* isolates were susceptible to fluconazole, 50% were S-DD, and 45% were resistant. Whereas *C. albicans, C. tropicalis,* and *C. parapsilosis* have generally remained sensitive to itraconazole, in an international study more than one third of *C. glabrata* and *C. krusei* isolates were found to have decreased susceptibility to that agent.[41] In vitro, nearly all isolates of *C. krusei* are susceptible to voriconazole (MIC <1 μg/mL), irrespective of their level of resistance to fluconazole.[40] However, fluconazole-resistant isolates of *C. albicans* and *C. glabrata* can have substantial in vitro cross-resistance to voriconazole.

Amphotericin B primarily acts by binding to ergosterol, the principal sterol in the cell membrane of most fungi, leading to the formation of ion channels and concentration-dependent cell death. These pores, composed of amphotericin B multimers, form most readily when ergosterol is present in the cell membrane.[42,43] Resistance to polyenes (amphotericin B and nystatin) has been reported in *Candida* spp. including *C. lusitaniae, C. tropicalis, C. glabrata,* and *C. albicans*.[35,44,45] Mechanisms of resistance include loss or marked depression of ergosterol in the cell membrane and increased catalase activity with resultant protection against polyene-induced oxidative damage.[45,46] Clinical isolates of *C. albicans* with mutations in the δ-5,6-sterol desaturase gene with associated alteration in the ergosterol biosynthetic pathway have been described. These fluconazole-resistant isolates lack ergosterol in the cytoplasmic membrane and thereby also demonstrate reduced susceptibility to amphotericin B.[47] In epidemiologic studies, the majority of *Candida* spp. remain sensitive to amphotericin B, but reduced susceptibility has been noted as described previously.[40,48]

The echinocandins are a novel class of semisynthetic amphophilic lipopeptides composed of a cyclic hexapeptide core linked to a variably configured lipid side chain. The echinocandins act by noncompetitive inhibition of the synthesis of 1,3-β-glucan, a polysaccharide in the cell wall of many pathogenic fungi. Together with chitin, the ropelike glucan fibrils are responsible for the cell wall's strength and shape, are important in maintaining the osmotic integrity of the fungal cell, and play a key role in cell division and cell growth.[49,50] Echinocandin-resistant mutants of *C. albicans* have been created under laboratory conditions.[51] Although there are currently no established interpretive breakpoints for susceptibility, in a recent study caspofungin showed excellent in vitro activity against *Candida* spp.[48] The MICs of caspofungin for *C. parapsilosis* tend to be higher, but the clinical significance of this observation is unknown at this time.

Flucytosine (5-fluorocytosine; 5-FC) is a low-molecular-weight, water-soluble, synthetic, fluorinated analog of cytosine. 5-FC has no antifungal activity of its own. It is taken up by the fungus-specific enzyme cytosine permease and converted in the cytoplasm by cytosine deaminase to 5-fluorouracil, which causes RNA miscoding and inhibits DNA synthesis.[52] Resistance to 5-FC may occur as a result of decreased cellular uptake as occurs in *C. glabrata* isolates with a defect in cytosine permease.[53] Resistance may also occur as a result of failure to metabolize 5-FC to intracellularly active metabolites such as 5-fluorouridylic acid (FUMP).[36] Primary resistance to 5-FC is uncommon among most clinically relevant *Candida* spp. In a study of more than 8800 clinical isolates from over 200 centers worldwide, 95% were sensitive (MIC ≤4 μg/mL), 2% intermediate (MIC 8 to 16 μg/mL), and 3% resistant (MIC ≥32 μg/mL) In that same study, however, primary resistance was frequently observed among isolates of *C. krusei* (5% S, 67% I, and 28% R).[54] Acquired resistance to 5-FC is far more prevalent. Because such resistance can occur during monotherapy, 5-FC generally is used in combination with other antifungal agents.

Infections of Skin and Nails

CLINICAL MANIFESTATIONS

Candida spp., particularly *C. albicans* and *C. parapsilosis,* are frequent colonizers of skin. The skin of up to one third of healthy adults may be colonized with *C. parapsilosis*.[55] Factors associated with colonization include antibiotic therapy, parenteral nutrition, low birth body mass in infants, endotracheal intubation, duration of stay for hospitalized patients, indwelling intravenous catheters, malignancies, diabetes mellitus, surgery, aging, and obesity.[56,57] Superficial infections due to *Candida* spp. regularly involve intertriginous or occluded areas, glabrous skin, and the nails.[58] *Candida* spp. frequently cause infections at large skin folds. Warm, moist surfaces and macerated skin favor superficial candidal infection. Affected sites include the groin and perianal regions, skin under pendulous breasts or large abdominal folds, and the axilla. Environmental conditions such as hot, humid weather, crowding, and poor personal hygiene predispose to candidal intertrigo.[59] Diabetes mellitus is a major risk factor for superficial candidiasis and has emerged as a problem in some tropical regions.[60] Additional host factors such as obesity, receipt of antibiotics or steroids, inflammatory skin diseases, and infections with HIV and human T-lymphotropic virus type 1 (HTLV-1) also predispose to cutaneous candidiasis.[61–63]

These cutaneous lesions consist of pruritic and sometimes painful, moist, erythematous plaques or macules. The involved skin may be eroded, and whitish scaling is often seen at the borders of lesions. Erythematous vesiculopapular or pustular satellite lesions are common. The latter may coalesce to extend the infection. *C. albicans* originating from the gastrointestinal tract plays a major role in diaper dermatitis.[64,65] Candidal diaper dermatitis is more common when nondisposable diapers are used. The warm, moist, occlusive environment beneath the diaper facilitates infection. The rash, which typically presents as a sharply marginated area of erythema, starts at the perianal region but may extend to involve the anterior thighs, genital creases, abdomen, and genitalia.[66] *Candida* miliaria, which starts out with vesiculopustular lesions, affects the backs of bedridden patients, particularly those who are sweating profusely.[67] *Candida* spp. have been reported to cause painful cutaneous and perhaps ductal infection of the mammary gland in lactating women and may be a cause of premature weaning among lactating mothers.[68] Angular cheilitis presents with macerated skin, pain, erythema, and fissures at the angles of the mouth. It can be unilateral or bilateral and often is caused by *C. albicans*.[69] *Candida* spp. may infect hair follicles. Predisposing factors for candidal folliculitis include use of steroids and antibiotics; however, these need not be present.[70,71] Infection may involve the beard area (folliculitis barbae candidomycetica) and present as erythematous plaques, papules, or pustules.

Candidal interdigital infections (erosio interdigitalis blastomycetica) and paronychia are common in the tropics. These conditions occur most commonly following prolonged immersion of hands in water or wearing of occlusive gloves. Dishwashers, laundry workers, and gardeners are at risk.[72] The clinical appearance of interdigital infection consists of a painful, erythematous, eroded area between the fingers or toes. Paronychia presents with redness, swelling, and tenderness at the nail fold that may extend beneath the nail. The infection can progress to involve the nail itself. However, candidal onychomycosis may occur without antecedent paronychia. *Candida* spp. play a relatively minor role in toenail onychomycosis but are frequently found in fingernail infections.[73,74] *C. albicans* and *C. parapsilosis* are the predominant species of *Candida* causing onychomycosis.[75,76]

Cutaneous candidal infections generally respond well to topical nystatin or imidazole derivatives.[77,78] Measures that promote dryness are important, and in that regard nystatin and miconazole in a powder vehicle are useful options. Topical corticosteroids are commonly added to the regimen and can provide rapid relief of symptoms.[79,80] In cases of extensive skin involvement, systemic therapy may be required. Infections of the nail fold can usually be managed with modification of the predisposing occupational factors, drainage, and topical antifungals. In recalcitrant cases or when the nail itself is involved, systemic therapy should be employed.[81] Candidal onychomycosis responds well to oral itraconazole.[82]

CONGENITAL CUTANEOUS CANDIDIASIS

Congenital cutaneous candidiasis presents at birth or soon thereafter. The syndrome is likely secondary to contamination of skin from a maternal source. Typically there is a generalized eruption of erythematous macules, papules, or pustules that sometimes evolve to vesicles and bullae. Involvement of the palms and soles is frequent. Very low-birth-weight infants may develop desquamating or erosive dermatitis. There often is evidence of an intrauterine infection with *Candida*.[83] Topical therapy with either nystatin or imidazole derivatives is generally sufficient.[84,85] Some infants may present with respiratory distress or clinical signs of sepsis during the first 2 days of life.[86] Such patients should be treated with systemic antifungals. Systemically disseminated candidiasis is far more common in neonates weighing less than 1000 g. Consequently, low-birth-weight neonates or infants with prolonged rupture of membranes who demonstrate clinical findings of disseminated neonatal cutaneous candidiasis should be treated with systemic antifungals.[87,88] Invasive fungal dermatitis is a newly described clinical entity characterized by erosive, crusting lesions that develop 1 to 2 weeks after birth in extremely low-birth-weight neonates. *C. albicans* is the most commonly implicated pathogen, and dissemination is common.[89]

CHRONIC MUCOCUTANEOUS CANDIDIASIS

Chronic mucocutaneous candidiasis (CMC) is a group of disorders that typically present during childhood and is characterized by recurrent and persistent candidal infections, which may involve the skin, nails, and mucosal surfaces. Patients with CMC have impaired cell-mediated responses to *Candida* spp. and subsequently are unable to effectively clear these organisms. In patients with CMC, candidal antigens trigger a predominantly Th2 instead of a Th1 cytokine response.[90–92] Additional immune defects that have been described in patients with CMC are subtle alterations in antibody responses to bacteria and fungi and impaired granulocyte and natural killer cell function.[93–95] Severity and distribution of candidal infections vary. In some patients, infections are limited to the nails, whereas in others the candidiasis is extensive and disfiguring. The initial presentation is typically oral candidiasis or diaper dermatitis. Angular cheilitis, lip fissures, paronychia, and onychia are common manifestations. Cutaneous findings include erythematous skin lesions with serpiginous borders. Local or diffuse dermatophytosis may coexist with cutaneous candidiasis.[96] *Candida* granuloma in CMC is characterized by highly disfiguring hyperkeratotic, well-demarcated lesions of the face, eyelids, scalp, lips, or acral areas that may grow to several centimeters and take a hornlike appearance.[67] Mucosal manifestations of CMC include vulvovaginitis and infections of the oropharynx, larynx, and esophagus. Oral, laryngeal, and esophageal candidiasis may occur together or independently. Symptoms include hoarseness, dysphagia, and rarely hemoptysis. The signs and symptoms of laryngitis or esophagitis can be minimal or absent, but esophageal strictures can arise from chronic inflammation.[97] CMC occurs in isolation and in association with a variety of endocrine, autoimmune, and infectious disorders. These include endocrinopathies such as hypoparathyroidism, thyroid abnormalities and Addison's disease, dental enamel dysplasia, interstitial keratitis, vitiligo, and alopecia totalis.[98] Deeply invasive candidiasis is rare in CMC. Recurrent and severe noncandidal infections are common and include septicemia, bacterial pneumonia, bronchiectasis, and opportunistic infections, including cryptococcal meningitis and disseminated histoplasmosis.[99–101] An adult form of CMC that typically presents after the third decade of life is associated with thymoma, myasthenia gravis, hypogammaglobulinemia, and abnormalities of the bone marrow and circulating blood elements.[102] CMC can occur sporadically or as a familial disease with either autosomal dominant or recessive patterns of inheritance. Treatment requires systemic antifungal therapy. The advent of azole antifungals has revolutionized the care of these patients. Clinical responses may be slow, and infections often require months of treatment to clear. Long-term therapy should be individualized, and most patients require intermittent treatment or chronic suppression to remain in remission. Relapses while on treatment and acquisition of resistance to azole antifungals can occur.[103–108] Patients with early manifestations of CMC should be evaluated for HIV infection.

CUTANEOUS PRESENTATION OF DISSEMINATED CANDIDIASIS

Hematogenously disseminated candidiasis can present with cutaneous manifestations.[109–112] The characteristic lesions consist of single or multiple 0.5- to 1-cm erythematous or purpuric papulonodules with pale centers. In highly compromised hosts, these lesions may be the initial manifestation of candidemia. A syndrome of disseminated candidiasis with extensive folliculitis has been described in injection heroin abusers.[113,114] Less commonly, disseminated infection presents as ecthyma gangrenosum or purpura fulminans.[115–117] Histologic evaluation of specimens obtained by skin biopsy are extremely useful and often establish the diagnosis of disseminated candidiasis prior to growth of the organism in blood cultures.[118] Management of systemic infection is described elsewhere in this chapter.

Oropharyngeal Candidiasis

EPIDEMIOLOGY AND PATHOGENESIS

Oropharyngeal candidiasis (OPC) is the most common mycotic infection of the oral cavity. *Candida* spp. frequently colonize the oral cavity. Multiple factors affect colonization, including HIV status and levels of serum HIV RNA, increasing age, use of dentures, receipt of antibiotics, malnutrition, and oral hygiene.[119–127] The most common colonizing species is *C. albicans*, although non-*albicans* species of *Candida* are increasingly identified. The development of infection depends upon both systemic and local determinants. Extremes in age, diabetes mellitus (particularly when glycemic control is poor), nutritional deficiencies, and immunosuppression (especially of cell-mediated immunity) are all systemic risk factors for oral candidiasis. Local factors that promote infection include the presence of dentures (especially when fit is inadequate), salivary abnormalities such as Sjögren's disease, treatment with inhaled steroids, and destruction of natural mucosal barriers with radiotherapy for head and neck cancers or cytotoxic chemotherapy.[128–135] HIV infection, which has become endemic in many regions, is one of the most important predisposing conditions worldwide. Oropharyngeal colonization with *Candida* spp. is more prevalent among seropositive persons and correlates with serum HIV-1 RNA levels.[125,136] In HIV-infected individuals, OPC is a leading cause of oral disease and is significantly associated with lower median CD4 lymphocyte counts, especially below 200/μL.[137–139] Unless antiretroviral therapy is initiated, the presence of oral candidiasis predicts the development of other serious opportunistic infections of AIDS.[140,141] Therapy with highly active antiretroviral therapy (HAART) is associated with significant decreases in the prevalence of OPC. This effect may be due to a combination of factors including immune reconstitution, decreased viral load, and antagonism of candidal virulence factors by protease inhibitors.[142–144]

AGENTS

The etiologic agent in OPC is almost always *C. albicans*; however, non-*albicans* species of *Candida* have emerged as both colonizing and infecting species in recipients of radiotherapy for head and neck malignancies, in patients with HIV, and in those with extensive past antifungal exposure.[145–149] *C. dubliniensis*, which has recently been differentiated from *C. albicans*, is increasingly recognized in OPC. This organism may be misidentified as *C. albicans,* and some isolates of *C. dubliniensis* have decreased susceptibility to azole antifungals.[150–152] *C. albicans* with reduced susceptibility to fluconazole can colonize or infect severely immunosuppressed individuals, especially when there has been extensive exposure to azoles, and such isolates may be transmitted by person-to-person spread.[149,153,154] In mucosal candidiasis refractory to clotrimazole, strains of *C. albicans* with cross-resistance to other azoles have been observed.[155]

CLINICAL MANIFESTATIONS

The clinical manifestations of OPC are diverse, and multiple forms frequently present concurrently. Pseudomembranous candidiasis, or thrush, is the most commonly encountered type. The condition is characterized by curdlike, white patches on the buccal mucosa, gingiva, palate, and tongue. The pseudomembranes may be scraped off to leave a raw, erythematous undersurface. The patches consist of desquamated epithelium, inflammatory cells, bacteria, fungal elements, keratin, and food debris. The diagnosis is suggested by the characteristic appearance of the lesions. Microscopically, yeast forms, hyphae, and pseudohyphae are evident on KOH smear or Gram stain. Erythematous candidiasis (acute atrophic candidiasis) occurs by itself or in association with the pseudomembranes.[141,156] In some cases, erythematous candidiasis occurs as a result of sloughing of the pseudomembranes. The flat, red, occasionally painful lesions are typically present on the dorsal surface of the tongue. The erythematous form of candidiasis is more difficult to recognize and is likely underdiagnosed. Median rhomboid glossitis, which presents as a smooth, sometimes raised, erythematous lesion at the midline of the dorsal surface of the tongue, was previously thought to be a developmental abnormality, but is now recognized as a manifestation of infection by *Candida*. Chronic atrophic candidiasis, which presents with mucosal erythema and edema, affects areas of persistent local trauma due to denture wear. A related condition, *Candida*-associated palatal papillary hyperplasia has been described in HIV-infected patients.[157] Angular cheilitis, inflammation at the angles of the mouth, can be precipitated by a number of causes including candidal infection. The lesions of chronic hyperplastic candidiasis (candidal leukoplakia) typically present as adherent, firm, elevated white patches on the buccal mucosa or tongue. This condition can be resistant to treatment and on rare occasions may develop into carcinoma.[158] *C. albicans* is associated with black hairy tongue, which is characterized by hypertrophy of the filiform papillae on the surface of the tongue. Black hairy tongue typically occurs following antibiotic use. Patients may complain of a tickling sensation, and treatment consists of physical débridement and good oral hygiene.[67]

TREATMENT

The major therapeutic options available for treating oral candidiasis are topical azoles (clotrimazole troches), oral azoles (fluconazole, ketoconazole, or itraconazole), oral polyenes (nystatin or amphotericin B), intravenous amphotericin B, and intravenous echinocandins (caspofungin).[88] Most patients respond to either topical or oral systemic therapy as initial treatment of OPC. Topical therapy with five times daily clotrimazole troches (10 mg) or four times daily nystatin (500,000 units in suspension or pastille form) is generally effective. However, systemic therapy may be advantageous in certain circumstances. In a comparative study of patients with HIV-associated OPC, the clinical efficacy of 14 days of fluconazole (100 mg daily) was equivalent to clotrimazole (10 mg five times daily) (98% vs. 94%; P = NS).[159] In that patient population, however, fluconazole has been associated with higher rates of mycologic eradication and fewer relapses.[139,159] In another study of patients with HIV-associated OPC, the clinical efficacy of liquid suspension fluconazole (100 mg once daily for 14 days) was superior to that of liquid nystatin (500,000 units four times daily for 14 days) (87% vs. 52%).[160] Additionally, there were fewer relapses among those patients receiving fluconazole.

Fluconazole appears to be more efficacious than ketoconazole in OPC. The rate of clinical cure of HIV-associated OPC with fluconazole (50 mg daily) was 100% compared with 75% for ketoconazole (200 mg daily).[161] In a study of children with HIV-associated OPC, oral fluconazole (3 mg/kg/d) and ketoconazole (7 mg/kg/d) had comparable safety and relapse rates. In that study, patients treated with fluconazole had higher clinical and mycologic cure rates at the end of therapy (88% and 71%, respectively) than those treated with ketoconazole (81% and 57%, respectively).[162] Itraconazole cyclodextrin solution achieves higher serum itraconazole concentrations than the capsule formulation and, if available, is the preferred form.[163] Itraconazole oral solution at 100 and 200 mg daily is well tolerated and as effective as fluconazole 100 mg tablets.[164,165] In a study of children over 5 years of age and adolescents with HIV-associated OPC, itraconazole cyclodextrin oral solution (2.5 mg/kg twice daily) was well tolerated and efficacious.[166] In that study, all patients with fluconazole-resistant isolates responded to treatment with the itraconazole solution. Furthermore, there was no clear correlation between in vitro susceptibilities to itraconazole and response to therapy.

In the 1990s, fluconazole-refractory OPC emerged as problem in HIV-infected patients.[167–170] In a cohort of persons with advanced HIV, this condition was identified in approximately 4% of patients and was associated with a poor overall prognosis (median survival after diagnosis, 32.6 weeks).[171] In most cases the infecting organism was *C. albicans,* and isolation of non-*albicans Candida* spp. remains uncommon. Profound immunosuppression and exposure to fluconazole have been recognized as risk factors, and many of the isolates have reduced in vitro susceptibility to fluconazole.[172–174] Various therapeutic options are available. Fluconazole may be given in "swish and swallow" formulation as topical therapy in cases refractory to the tablet form.[175] For OPC due to fluconazole-resistant or dose-dependent susceptible strains of *Candida*, increasing the dose of fluconazole up to a maximum of 800 mg daily and treating with longer courses of therapy are often successful.[176] As indicated previously, itraconazole oral solution (100 to 200 mg twice daily in adults and 2.5 mg/kg twice daily in children) can be effective in fluconazole-unresponsive OPC.[166,177] Additional options for recalcitrant infections include oral amphotericin B, intravenous caspofungin, combination therapy with fluconazole and terbinafine (250 mg/d) or sargramostim (GM-CSF 2.5 μg/kg/d).[178–182] Amphotericin B oral suspension, although well tolerated, has limited efficacy for the treatment of fluconazole-refractory oral candidiasis.[174]

Prophylactic antifungal therapy may be employed in patients at high risk for infection and in cases of recurrent disease. Oral clotrimazole is effective as prophylaxis in cancer patients and solid organ transplant recipients.[183–185] Fluconazole at 100 or 200 mg daily significantly reduces colonization and infection in high-risk patients, but resistance can develop on therapy.[186–188]

Some regions in developing countries with limited resources may not have access to standard antifungal therapy for treatment of oropharyngeal candidiasis. In such settings, gentian violet may be as effective as nystatin or ketoconazole.[189] A randomized, open label study of the treatment of oropharyngeal and esophageal candidiasis was conducted in Kinshasa (Zaire) among 141 inpatients with AIDS and oropharyngeal candidiasis, 136 of whom also had esophageal candidiasis. The study compared the efficacy of gentian violet mouth washes (1.5 mL 0.5% aqueous solution twice daily), oral ketoconazole (200 mg/d, after a meal), and nystatin mouth washes (200,000 units oral suspension four times daily). Patients enrolled in this study had a very high mortality (probability of death, 41.6% after 14 days). After 14 days, 72 patients could be evaluated. At that time, oropharyngeal lesions had disappeared in similar proportions of patients treated with gentian violet (11/26, 42%) and ketoconazole (10/23, 43%) and in a lower proportion of patients treated with nystatin (2/23, 9%; $P < 0.05$) In esophageal candidiasis, ketoconazole seemed more efficient than both other treatments. This study suggests that gentian violet is an effective and relatively inexpensive (0.5 US$/treatment course in Kinshasa) alternative for treatment of oropharyngeal candidiasis.

Esophageal Candidiasis

CLINICAL MANIFESTATIONS

Candida is a frequent colonizer of the esophagus. *C. albicans* is the major colonizing and infecting species.[190,191] Factors associated with esophageal candidiasis include HIV infection, organ transplantation, alcoholic liver disease, receipt of antibiotics, treatment with proton pump inhibitors, and defects in cell-mediated immunity.[192–196] Local factors such as receipt of inhaled steroids and esophageal carcinoma also predispose to esophageal candidiasis.[197–198] In HIV-infected patients with upper digestive symptoms, esophageal candidiasis is the most common cause, although sometimes multiple concurrent opportunistic infections including CMV and HSV exist. In this population, development of esophageal candidiasis is associated with low CD4 counts, high serum HIV RNA levels, antibiotic use, and concurrent or previous oropharyngeal candidiasis.[199,200]

Symptoms typically include odynophagia, dysphagia, and retrosternal pain, although esophageal candidiasis can be asymptomatic and discovered only on endoscopy. Infection is generally limited to the mucosa, but in highly compromised hosts transmural necrosis leading to perforation and invasion into deeper mediastinal structures may occur.[201] Esophageal strictures leading to stenosis can also complicate the course of patients with esophageal candidiasis.[202]

DIAGNOSIS

Radiologic studies can assist in the evaluation of patients. Typical early-stage findings include edematous esophageal folds with subsequent development of plaques and diffuse ulceration.[203] Less common radiologic manifestations are discrete ulcers, which may be mistaken for viral esophagitis, or innumerable, tiny (1- to 3-mm), round lucencies that take on the appearance of a layer of foam (foamy esophagus).[204,205]

Although it is more invasive, endoscopy offers the advantage of direct examination of the esophagus for the characteristic findings of candidal esophagitis. Furthermore, cytologic brushing or biopsy can be performed for the purpose of microbiological and histopathologic evaluation. The most common endoscopic findings are white mucosal plaques, which consist of desquamated epithelium and inflammatory cells with infiltration by fungal elements and superinfecting bacteria. With increasing severity, the scattered mucosal plaques coalesce to form circumferential disease and ultimately can cause luminal impingement.[206] The presence of white plaques in HIV-infected patients with dysphagia and odynophagia is highly predictive of esophageal candidiasis.[207]

TREATMENT

A strategy whereby empirical fluconazole is given to HIV-infected patients with esophageal symptoms has been found to be safe and cost effective. However, clinical responses need to be monitored closely, and endoscopy should be pursued for establishment of diagnosis in patients who do not improve promptly.[208–210] This approach may be very attractive in resource-poor settings. Fluconazole is the mainstay of therapy for esophageal candidiasis, and response rates are typically greater than 80%.[211,212] Fluconazole (100 mg/d for 2 to 3 weeks) is highly effective in most cases. In comparative trials, fluconazole was superior to ketoconazole, flucytosine, and itraconazole capsules.[213–215] The efficacy of itraconazole capsules and flucytosine (100 mg/kg daily orally) in combination was found to be comparable to fluconazole.[216] Voriconazole (200 mg twice daily) is as effective as fluconazole and may have a role in fluconazole-resistant infections but is associated with more adverse reactions.[217]

Itraconazole oral solution has comparable efficacy with fluconazole, and at doses of 200 to 800 mg/d has been used successfully as salvage therapy in fluconazole-resistant cases.[218,219] For azole-refractory cases, intravenous amphotericin B is commonly used. Recently, antifungals of the echinocandin class have emerged as additional options.[178,220] In a trial of adults with candidal esophagitis, intravenous caspofungin at 50 or 70 mg daily was effective in 74% and 89% of cases, respectively.[220] In that same study, intravenous amphotericin B (0.5 mg/kg daily) was effective in 63% of cases. In a trial comparing intravenous caspofungin (50 mg/d) and fluconazole (200 mg/d), the efficacy of the two agents was comparable (81% and 85%, respectively).[212] Esophageal candidiasis generally responds well to antifungal therapy. However, in persons with AIDS in the absence of immune reconstitution, recurrences are common, usually occurring within 2 to 3 months.[221] Prophylactic fluconazole (100 mg/d) is effective in preventing recurrences.[222]

Vulvovaginal Candidiasis

Candida spp. commonly colonize the lower genital tract of girls and women.[223,224] The rates of colonization decline with age.[225] The vast majority of isolated yeasts are *C. albicans*. Whereas most often these represent asymptomatic vaginal colonization, host factors such as receipt of antibiotics, diabetes mellitus, pregnancy, wearing of poorly ventilated clothing, and possibly the use of oral contraceptives can facilitate transformation to symptomatic vaginitis.[226–228] Most women will have at least one attack of vulvovaginal candidiasis in their lifetime. Vulvovaginal candidiasis is most common in women before menopause but rarely occurs before menarche. The relationship of HIV status to vulvovaginal candidiasis is far less established than for oropharyngeal infection. HIV seropositivity is associated with increased rates of vaginal colonization by *Candida*. However, the incidence of candidal vaginitis is not significantly elevated in HIV-seropositive women when compared with matched HIV-seronegative controls.[138] Clinical findings in vulvovaginal candidiasis consist of irritation, pruritus, erythema, edema, fissures, dysuria, and dyspareunia. The inflammation may extend throughout the vulva and into the perineum. A discharge, which can be thick, is often but not invariably present. Often the patient will make a self-diagnosis of "yeast" vaginitis. However, this may be unreliable and can lead to overuse of topical antifungal agents. In a patient with vaginitis, the presence of hyphae, pseudohyphae, and blastospores on microscopic evaluation of a sample treated with 10% KOH is highly suggestive of candidiasis. Estimation of the pH, the amine test, and saline microscopy are not sensitive or specific for vulvovaginal candidiasis but are useful in suggesting an alternative or concomitant cause for the symptoms. Vaginal cultures do not distinguish colonization from infection and are not commonly needed. Vaginal yeast cultures are valuable in confirming negative diagnoses, detecting false negatives on microscopy, and identifying non-*albicans* isolates.[229] In most patients, sporadic mild-to-moderate disease responds to short courses of treatment with topical azole or nystatin preparations. Alternatively, oral therapy with fluconazole in a single 150 mg dose, itraconazole (200 mg for 3 days), or ketoconazole (200 mg twice daily for 5 days) can be used effectively.[230–233] In severe cases and in persons with diabetes with poor glycemic control, a week or more of topical therapy or two sequential 150-mg doses of fluconazole given 3 days apart may be necessary to achieve an adequate clinical response.[88,234] Boric acid solution or gentian violet solution may also be useful in management of vulvovaginal candidiasis.

Some women develop recurrent vulvovaginal candidiasis. With the exception of persons with diabetes with poor glycemic control, these patients rarely have recognizable precipitating or causal factors. This condition likely occurs as a result of a local immunodeficiency state that permits uncontrolled proliferation of yeast within the vagina and hence repeated clinically evident attacks.[235] The vast majority of recurrent infections are caused by azole-sensitive *C. albicans* even in the setting of long-term exposure to azoles.[236] In a minority of cases, the infection is due to non-*albicans* isolates of *Candida*. *C. glabrata* is the most common non-*albicans* species isolated from the vagina. Patients with vaginitis due to non-*albicans* species of *Candida* have significantly reduced clinical and mycologic responses to azoles.[234] Otherwise, the clinical syndromes caused by these organisms are generally indistinguishable from *C. albicans* infections.[237] Some patients develop recurrent and often chronic *C. glabrata* vaginitis unresponsive to conventional therapy.[238] Topical boric acid (600 mg daily for 14 days) and topical flucytosine cream are options for such cases.[239,240] Boric acid treatment has also been useful in cases due to *C. krusei*.[241] Although no definitive cure for recurrent candidal vaginitis exists, long-term maintenance regimens with oral or topical azoles can effectively control symptomatic infection in some but not all patients.[235] However, before initiating a prolonged course of antifungals for management of recurrent vulvovaginal candidiasis, the diagnosis should be confirmed.

Candida Balanitis

Candida spp. are the most common infectious cause of balanitis and account for approximately one third of all cases.[67,242] The lesions start as small papules and papulopustules that may slough off, leaving erythematous erosions with associated whitish scales. The infection can spread to involve the scrotum and inguinal areas. There is often pruritus and burning, particularly following sexual intercourse.[243] In persons with diabetes or immunosuppressed patients, extensive cutaneous invasion can occur with severe edema and ulceration.[67,244] The presence of refractory *Candida* balanitis may be the harbinger of HIV infection or diabetes mellitus.

Topical therapy with azole antifungals is generally effective. In a trial involving 148 patients with candidal balanitis, 91% of men were asymptomatic after 7 days, and 98% were asymptomatic after 3 weeks of treatment with topical clotrimazole (1% cream).[245] In an open-label study, treatment with a single 150-mg dose of fluconazole was comparable in efficacy and safety to clotrimazole cream applied topically for 7 days.[246]

Respiratory Tract Infection

Candida frequently colonizes the respiratory tract.[247–251] Lower respiratory tract infection is uncommon and overdiagnosed. Pneumonia may be secondary to aspiration or due to hematogenous spread and occurs in patients with malignancies with and without severe neutropenia, lung transplant recipients, and neonates.[250,252,253] With hematogenous spread, involvement is often observed in multiple other organs as well. In lung transplant recipients, infection can occur at the bronchial anastomotic site with dehiscence of the anastomosis.[254] Among very low-birth-weight neonates, infection may be acquired postnatally or antenatally due to chorioamnionitis.[255,256]

The radiographic manifestations of candidal pneumonia include disseminated nodules in cases due to hematogenous spread and nonspecific patchy infiltrates in endobronchial infection.[250,257] Isolation of even a large number of organisms on bronchoscopic specimen does not necessarily reflect infection, and the only accepted criterion for definitive diagnosis is histologic demonstration of the fungus in lung tissue. Mortality due to actual candidal pneumonia is high and may exceed 80%.[250] *Candida* has been reported to cause epiglottitis and laryngitis in immunocompromised patients.[258–260] Laryngitis can be diagnosed by fiberoptic or indirect laryngoscopy; untreated, it can lead to airway obstruction and respiratory compromise. Invasive respiratory tract candidiasis should be treated with systemic antifungals. *Candida* spp. also frequently colonize voice prostheses and can lead to early deterioration of these devices.[261,262] Prophylactic miconazole has been shown to decrease colonization of voice prostheses and increase device lifetime.[263]

Endocarditis

Candida spp. are the most common cause of fungal endocarditis; *C. albicans, C. parapsilosis, C. glabrata,* and *C. tropicalis* account for most cases.[264,265] Risks for candidal endocarditis include injection drug use, indwelling vascular devices, prosthetic cardiac valves, pre-existing valve disease, antibiotic use, and immunosuppression.[266,267] Prosthetic valve endocarditis typically occurs in the first year after surgery but may present years later.[268] The large, friable vegetations have a propensity to produce systemic emboli, and patients regularly have peripheral arterial or central nervous system embolic events.[269–272]

Echocardiography is an important tool in the evaluation of candidal endocarditis. Large, dense heterogeneous vegetations are typical. Transthoracic echocardiography may be adequate, but transesophageal echocardiography has superior sensitivity for prosthetic valve endocarditis and allows for optimal assessment of the valvular and paravalvular structures.[269,273] Owing to the high risk for devastating embolic events, poor response to medical therapy alone, and frequent recurrence, valve replacement generally is necessary.[274] With a combined medical and surgical approach, in-hospital survival is greater than 80%, but relapses can occur.[269,275,276] A commonly used initial regimen is amphotericin B with or without flucytosine. The appropriate duration of antifungal therapy after surgery is not known, but a minimum of 6 weeks and possibly much longer has been advocated.[88] To prevent recurrences, long-term oral antifungal therapy is frequently used. In many patients, valve replacement is not an option. The optimal management of such patients is not known, but amphotericin B followed by long-term fluconazole has been used with success.[277,278]

Candidal endocarditis may extend to involve the myocardium. In a series of patients with candidal endocarditis, a hyperechogenic, heterogeneous myocardial texture observed on echocardiography was associated with extensive myocardial damage at surgery.[273]

Candidal myocarditis occurring in the setting of disseminated candidiasis but without concurrent valvular infection has been reported. Arrhythmias and conduction abnormalities may develop as a consequence of myocardial invasion.

Candidal pericarditis is a rare disease usually seen in association with cardiothoracic surgery, disseminated candidiasis, and immunocompromise. Unexplained fever, an increasing cardiac shadow on chest roentgenogram, or development of cardiac tamponade may suggest the diagnosis. Untreated, it is uniformly fatal. Pericardiocentesis followed by operative drainage and antifungal agents is the usual treatment.[279–282]

Mechanical cardiac assistance has recently emerged as an option for patients with severe heart failure. Several ventricular circulatory assist devices (VADs) are currently available for support of patients while they are waiting for improvement in cardiac function or heart transplantation. Infection in the postoperative period is the most serious complication. Fungal infections associated with VADs include device-related bloodstream infections and less commonly endocarditis.[283,284] In addition to treatment with antifungals, removal of the device generally is necessary for clearance of the infection. Implantable defibrillators and pacemakers are increasingly employed in patients with or at risk for arrhythmia. There have been several reports of infections in such devices including endocarditis due to *C. tropicalis, C. glabrata,* and *C. albicans*.[285–287] Complete device explantation and prolonged antifungal therapy are the treatment for this complication.

Urinary Tract Infection

EPIDEMIOLOGY

Candida spp. are frequent colonizers of the lower urinary tract. *C. albicans* represents approximately half of the fungal isolates in urine. Non-*albicans* species of *Candida* including *C. glabrata*, *C. tropicalis,* and *C. krusei* may also cause funguria, especially in patients previously treated with antifungal agents.[288–290] Of particular concern is the use of fluconazole in hospitalized patients. It has recently been suggested that indiscriminate use of fluconazole may lead to the emergence of fungal resistance. In a retrospective comparative study of patients admitted to medical and surgical intensive care units (ICUs), an emergence of *Candida* non-*albicans* tolerant to fluconazole was observed in fluconazole-treated patients. The same study also reported an increase in bacterial antibiotic resistance after fluconazole administration.[291]

Factors predisposing to candiduria include diabetes mellitus, urinary tract abnormalities, and malignancy.[288,292] Receipt of antimicrobial agents and presence of urinary tract drainage devices are important risk factors. In a case control study, development of candiduria was correlated with increasing duration of urinary catheterization (12 vs. 6 days), length of time on multiple antibiotics (16 vs. 7 days), and length of total hospitalization.[293] In an ICU surveillance study, candiduria developed in 22% of patients admitted for more than 7 days.[294] In that same study, independent risk factors for candiduria included age greater than 65 years, female sex, length of hospital stay before ICU admission, diabetes mellitus, total parenteral nutrition, mechanical ventilation, and previous antimicrobial use. In a neonatal ICU study, *Candida* spp. were identified in 42% of urinary tract infections, and more than half these patients had associated candidemia.[295] *C. parapsilosis* and *C. tropicalis* (25% and 13%, respectively) were the most frequent non-*albicans* species isolated in neonates with urinary tract infections in the neonatal ICU.

CLINICAL MANIFESTATIONS

In adults, candidemia rarely complicates candiduria.[288] In a study defining the risks for candidemia secondary to a urinary tract source, 88% had urinary tract abnormalities, predominantly with obstruction, and 73% had undergone urinary tract procedures before the onset of bloodstream infection.[296] Conversely, in patients with systemic candidiasis, hematogenous dissemination of fungus to the kidney may result in formation of cortical abscesses or obstructive intrarenal masses termed "fungal balls," usually at the ureteropelvic junction.[297,298] Up to a third of neonates with candidal urinary tract infections have renal pelvis fungus balls by ultrasound studies, but these may only develop weeks after the discovery of candiduria.[295,299] Other complications of candidal urinary tract infection include papillary necrosis, emphysematous pyelonephritis, and emphysematous cystitis.[300–303]

DIAGNOSIS

The diagnosis of fungal urinary tract infection represents a challenge to the clinician. The presence of *Candida* spp. in urine does not necessarily signify true infection and may instead merely represent colonization or even contamination of the urinary sample. The lack of specific signs and symptoms complicates the process of diagnosing fungal urinary tract infection, and some patients with infection are asymptomatic.[304,305] The presence of pyuria and colony counts of 10,000 to 15,000 *Candida* spp. per milliliter of urine may suggest infection; however, the predictive value of these findings when urinary catheters are in place is not known.[306,307] Indeed, studies in experimental renal candidiasis demonstrate that colony-forming units are not a reliable predictor of renal candidiasis.[308]

TREATMENT

There are various options for management of candiduria. In the absence of an underlying chronic medical condition, the identification of *Candida* spp. in the urine may represent colonization or low-grade infection that often resolves without specific therapy or with removal of the urinary catheter. All indwelling urinary instrumentation should be removed if possible. Candiduria should be treated in symptomatic patients, low-birth-weight infants, patients with neutropenia, and persons expected to undergo urinary tract instrumentation. Antifungal therapy should be given for 7 to 14 days.[88] Oral fluconazole (200 mg) was compared with placebo daily for 14 days in asymptomatic or minimally symptomatic candiduric hospitalized patients. Clearance with fluconazole was significantly higher among those patients receiving fluconazole (50% vs. 29%); however, recurrences were common, and long-term candiduria rates among treated and untreated patients were similar.[309] Systemic amphotericin B at various doses has been used successfully in candidal urinary tract infection. In patients with intact renal function, flucytosine (25 mg/kg/d) may be an option, although resistance can develop rapidly when this agent is used as monotherapy.[310,311]

Amphotericin B bladder irrigation (50 mg/L over 24 hours or 50 mg/L for 7 days) has been used for candiduria. Short-term eradication rates with this type of therapy are comparable with fluconazole, but the technique is cumbersome, and patients may complain of bladder fullness.[88,312]

Meningitis

CLINICAL MANIFESTATIONS

Candida spp. are an uncommon cause of meningitis. Infection can be secondary to hematogenous dissemination or direct inoculation. Neurosurgery, recent antibiotic therapy, and corticosteroid administration are predisposing factors. Fever, meningismus, elevated cerebrospinal fluid (CSF) pressures, and localizing neurologic signs are commonly noted. Mortality rates for patients receiving inadequate or no antifungal therapy exceed 90%. Delays in diagnosis, hypoglycorrhea, intracranial hypertension, and focal neurologic deficits are all associated with a poor prognosis.[313,314] In a series of patients with ventriculoperitoneal shunts, recent bacterial meningitis or neurosurgery (different from the shunt placement) and abdominal complications were associated with the development of candidal meningitis. The clinical manifestations in that series included hydrocephalus in 36%, fever in 31%, meningoencephalitis in 21%, and abdominal symptoms in 10%.[315] The CSF may show neutrophilic pleocytosis that is indistinguishable from bacterial meningitis or a predominance of lymphocytes. In certain circumstances, the clinical significance of *Candida* spp. isolates from cerebrospinal fluid of patients with shunts is difficult to assess. A retrospective analysis of patients with *Candida* spp. isolated from CSF following neurosurgery indicated that the diagnosis of candidal meningitis should be established by repeated cultures from both the indwelling device and lumbar puncture.[316] However, delay of potentially lifesaving therapy while waiting for a confirmatory CSF culture is potentially hazardous, and we do not advocate such an approach. Candidal meningitis may present as a subacute illness characterized by fever and headache of several weeks' duration and lymphocytic pleocytosis. Neurologic manifestations are diverse and can range from normal neurologic evaluation to signs of CNS infarcts or hydrocephalus.[317–319] Candidal infection may also present as an intense granulomatous and necrotizing basal meningitis that can lead to cranial neuropathies or basilar artery thrombosis with resultant brainstem and temporo-occipital infarction.[320,321]

Candidal meningoencephalitis frequently is associated with systemic candidiasis in premature neonates.[322,323] In a retrospective review of systemic candidiasis, more than a fifth of neonates with systemic candidiasis had candidal meningitis (0.4% of admissions to the neonatal ICU).[324] This complication is associated with very low birth weight and delivery at early gestational age. In a study of meningitis in very low-birth-weight (<1.5 kg) infants, *Candida* spp. were responsible for 20% of episodes.[325] The initial clinical features of candidal meningitis are indistinguishable from those of other causes of systemic infection in premature neonates. Analysis of CSF commonly shows hypoglycorrhachia, but pleocytosis is inconsistent, and Gram staining of CSF generally fails to detect the agent. Therefore, normal CSF parameters do not exclude meningitis.

TREATMENT

When infection is present, successful treatment generally requires systemic antifungal therapy and removal of the infected shunt.[315] Therapy with amphotericin B with and without 5-fluorocytosine has been used with success in children and adults.[324,326,327] In a series of 17 patients with candidal meningitis, the combination of amphotericin B and 5-fluorocytosine led to cure in 14 patients.[328] Because of its superior safety profile relative to conventional amphotericin B but comparable antifungal efficacy in animal models of candidal meningitis, liposomal amphotericin B is an attractive therapeutic option.[329] Liposomal amphotericin B was successful in five of six preterm infants with candidal meningitis.[330] *C. lusitaniae* can be resistant to amphotericin B, and fluconazole has been used successfully in two children with meningitis due to that pathogen.[331]

Joint Infection

CLINICAL MANIFESTATIONS

Candida spp. are an uncommon cause of infectious arthritis. Infection occurs following direct inoculation of fungus or as a result of hematogenously disseminated disease. The most commonly involved joint is the knee.[332] Infection has been reported following intra-articular injections into the knee of an unimmunocompromised man.[333] Cases of candidal arthritis have been described in association with prosthetic joints, solid organ transplantation, and hematologic malignancies and following the use of intravenous antibiotics and may be the first sign of disseminated candidiasis in a compromised host.[334–336] Deep-seated candidal infections can complicate injection drug use. In one series, osteoarticular involvement (vertebrae, costal cartilage, knees, and sacroiliac) was noted in more than a quarter of injection heroin users treated for systemic candidiasis.[337] Costochondral infection is a complication of disseminated candidiasis in users of brown heroin.[338] The clinical findings are of a mass appearing in the anterior region of the thorax. Histopathology of the lesions shows perichondritis, sometimes with associated myositis and osteomyelitis.[339] Nearly a fifth of hospital-acquired arthritis in the neonatal period is due to *Candida* spp.[340] In children, candidal arthritis typically occurs in association with disseminated candidiasis.[341] The arthritis is generally seen concomitant with or shortly after fungemia but in some cases may not manifest until weeks to months later.[342,343]

TREATMENT

Treatment consists of aspiration of the joint, systemic antifungal therapy, and in cases of prosthetic joint infection, removal of the infected hardware if feasible.[344–346] Fluconazole at doses of 200 to 800 mg daily for months to years has been used successfully.[347] Lipid formulations of amphotericin B have been successfully used in children and adults with *Candida* arthritis.[348–350] Intra-articular administration of amphotericin B has been utilized in refractory cases and may be a useful adjunct to systemic antifungal therapy.[351]

Osteomyelitis

CLINICAL MANIFESTATIONS

Candida spp. rarely cause osteomyelitis. Similarly to candidal arthritis, infection may occur following direct inoculation of the fungus or as a result of hematogenously disseminated disease.[352] Candidal mediastinitis has emerged as a complication in patients who have undergone sternotomy for thoracic surgery.[353] Common clinical manifestations are chest wall erythema, drainage, fever, and sternal instability. In one series, the onset of infection for most patients was within 28 days of surgery, but for others it was several months after the procedure. The infections were characterized by a chronic indolent course requiring prolonged therapy with an antifungal agent. Approximately a third of the patients relapsed and required a second course of treatment.[354] Surgical débridement and removal of sternotomy wires often are required.

A single strain of *C. albicans* was reported to cause postlaminectomy deep-wound infections in a cluster that involved three patients. The infections were indolent and developed weeks to months after the initial procedure. The source of the outbreak was traced to a technician who had worn artificial nails.[355] *C. tropicalis* vertebral osteomyelitis has also been reported to have complicated epidural catheterization in a patient with diabetes.[356] Spondylodiscitis and vertebral osteomyelitis can occur in association with disseminated candidiasis.[357,358] A recent review of the published literature found *C. albicans* responsible for 62% of cases, *C. tropicalis* for 19%, and *C. glabrata* for 14%. Almost all cases involved the lower thoracic or lumbar spine. Risk factors for candidal vertebral osteomyelitis included the presence of a central venous catheter, antibiotic use, immunosuppression, and injection drug use. Most patients had with back pain for more than 1 month, highlighting the indolent yet progressive course of this infection.[359] Delayed-onset osteomyelitis has been reported in two patients who developed *C. tropicalis* vertebral infections 5 and 14 months after experiencing transient fungemia.[360]

TREATMENT

Treatment of candidal osteomyelitis often requires a combined medical and surgical approach. Abscesses should be drained and devitalized tissue debrided.[361] Amphotericin B has been used with success,[359,362] as have prolonged courses of fluconazole.[363–366] The latter is an attractive option given the relative safety and oral formulation of this agent. A treatment plan consisting of surgical debridement and an initial course of amphotericin B for 2 to 3 weeks followed by fluconazole, for a total duration of therapy of 6 to 12 months has been advocated for candidal osteomyelitis.[88]

Endophthalmitis

CLINICAL MANIFESTATIONS

Candida spp. may cause intraocular infections with devastating consequences. Endogenous candidal endophthalmitis occurs in association with disseminated candidiasis and may be the initial manifestation of candidemia. In addition to the typical risk factors for disseminated candidiasis, endogenous endophthalmitis has been reported in the postpartum period and in association with induced abortions.[367,368] Patients with candidal endophthalmitis often complain of eye pain and may have blurred vision or spots in their visual fields. On examination there can be inflammation in the anterior chamber as indicated by the presence of a hypopyon. On examination of dilated pupils with an ophthalmoscope, one or more creamy-white, well-circumscribed lesions of the choroid and retina are characteristically observed. These are often accompanied by inflammatory infiltrates in the vitreous.[369] In endogenous endophthalmitis, the infection likely begins in the choroid and progresses anteriorly to the retinal layers.[369] In a rabbit model of hematogenous candidal endophthalmitis, the ocular lesions were focal chorioretinitis characterized by a combination of granulomatous and acute suppurative reactions.[370] In a study of enucleated globes from patients with candidal endophthalmitis, the vitreous was the primary focus of infection.[371]

Studies evaluating candidemic patients have reported widely varying rates for lesions consistent with candidal endophthalmitis. Recent reports have shown a decline in the percentage of cases of candidemia-associated endophthalmitis from nearly 30% in 1989 to less than 2% in 2002.[372–376] The reasons for the disparities in the studies are not clear but may be related to differences in the stringency of definitions of the ocular lesions of candidal endophthalmitis. Observation of the pathognomonic three-dimensional retina-based vitreal inflammatory lesion is uncommon, whereas nonspecific findings that may or may not be due candidal endophthalmitis (such as cotton wool spots, retinal hemorrhages, and Roth spots) are frequent.[377] Alternative explanations for the decline are the more aggressive antifungal therapies currently in use and the changing epidemiology of candidal bloodstream infections. Of note, in an experimental rabbit model of endogenous endophthalmitis, ocular tissues were found to have increased resistance to hematogenous infections with species other than *C. albicans*.[378] Because endogenous candidal endophthalmitis can lead to significant visual loss or blindness, it is reasonable to assess patients with disseminated candidiasis for ocular involvement by performing a funduscopic examination on pupils that have been dilated.

Infection of the cornea and the intraocular structures as a result of direct inoculation of the organism during trauma or surgery has been described.[369] In a series of 44 cases of postkeratoplasty candidal endophthalmitis, 40 (91%) had evidence of donor-to-host transmission of the organism.[379] An outbreak of postsurgical *C. parapsilosis* endophthalmitis was traced to a contaminated lot of irrigating solution.[380]

TREATMENT

Treatment of intraocular candidiasis depends on the extent of infection. When infection is limited to choroiditis or very minimal endophthalmitis, systemic antifungal treatment may be effective; however, if symptoms of vitreitis persist or progress, vitrectomy may be necessary.[381] Systemic therapy with amphotericin B or fluconazole in conjunction with vitrectomy (with or without intravitreal amphotericin B) has been used successfully in cases of advanced endogenous *Candida* endophthalmitis.[382,383] In one reported series, success was achieved following the administration of oral fluconazole (100 to 200 mg/d) for approximately 2 months.[384] In that report, four patients were also successfully treated with pars plana vitrectomy for moderate-to-severe vitreitis. In a series of intravenous brown heroin users with *C. albicans* endophthalmitis, favorable responses without complications were seen in all seven patients who underwent early vitrectomy (within 1 week) after the diagnosis of vitreitis. In that same series, two of three patients who underwent late vitrectomy developed blindness or scotoma. Blindness was also described in two patients with vitreitis who did not undergo vitrectomy.[385] Regardless of the therapy used, final visual acuity outcome depends most on the site of initial choroiditis, such that if the macula is spared and preretinal membranes can be effectively removed, visual acuity outcome can be good.[381]

Intra-abdominal Infections

Candidal peritonitis is most commonly seen as a complication of continuous ambulatory peritoneal dialysis (CAPD) or as a consequence of bowel injury. Rarely, spontaneous infections occur in association with chronic liver failure and ascites. CAPD has emerged as an acceptable form of renal replacement therapy in some developing countries.[386,387] In several series involving more than 2600 episodes of CAPD-associated peritonitis, 2.5% to 6% of cases were due to *Candida* spp.[388–393] Infecting organisms included *C. albicans*, *C. parapsilosis*, *C. tropicalis,* and *C. guilliermondii*. Risk factors for the development of candidal peritonitis include frequent recurrences of bacterial peritonitis and antibiotic exposure.[390–393] Clusters of candidal CAPD peritonitis have been described. An outbreak of *C. tropicalis* peritonitis was traced to infected water baths for several patients.[394] Initial clinical findings include abdominal pain and fever. The dialysate is cloudy in appearance, and fluid white cell count is typically elevated with a predominance of neutrophils.[395,396] Treatment of CAPD-associated candidal peritonitis with systemic antifungals is rarely adequate by itself. Cure rates with fluconazole alone are approximately 10%, and resolution of infection usually depends on removal of the infected catheter.[392,397,398] Failure to remove the catheter has been associated with increased mortality.[399] In a large cohort of children, *Candida* spp. accounted for approximately 2% of CAPD-associated peritonitis. As in adults, successful therapy of CAPD-associated candidal peritonitis in the pediatric age group generally requires a combination of antifungal therapy and dialysis catheter removal.[400]

Candida spp. may be isolated from the peritoneal fluid of patients with spontaneous perforation or a surgical opening of the gastrointestinal tract and rarely in association with appendicitis.[401,402] The presence of *Candida* spp. in the peritoneum, however, does not necessarily indicate infection. In a series of patients with *Candida* spp. isolated from the peritoneum, less than 40% had evidence of infection (intra-abdominal abscess or peritonitis).[403] In the neonatal population, *Candida* spp. may be seen at the site of intestinal perforation (candidal enteritis of the newborn) or in the peritoneum in necrotizing enterocolitis.[402,404–407] Peritonitis caused by *Candida* spp. has been described in patients with decompensated liver disease and ascites. The infection may be spontaneous in origin or may reflect gastrointestinal perforation.[408–410] Pancreatic abscesses due to *Candida* spp. can occur in association with pancreatitis, with pancreatic pseudocysts, and as a complication of endoscopic retrograde choledochopancreatography (ERCP).[411–413]

Chronic Disseminated Candidiasis

The syndrome of chronic disseminated candidiasis (CDC) has emerged as a problem in neutropenic patients, particularly those receiving therapy for acute leukemia. In a series of 500 adult patients with acute leukemia who received chemotherapy, CDC was diagnosed in 37 (7.4%).[414] This condition is often referred to as hepatosplenic candidiasis, but the term chronic disseminated candidiasis is more accurate, since multiple organs, including the lungs and kidneys, can be involved. The diagnosis is typically made after resolution of the neutropenia. Clinical and laboratory features include fever, abdominal pain, hepatomegaly, and elevated serum alkaline phosphatase levels. In a series of patients with CDC, abdominal ultrasonography was positive in 96% of patients,[27,28] abdominal computed tomography (CT) scan was positive in 21/21 patients (100%), and liver biopsy was positive in 10/15 patients (67%).[415] CT shows low-density lesions of the liver, spleen, and kidneys; hepatomegaly; and hepatosplenomegaly.[416] Magnetic resonance imaging (MRI) has emerged as a technique with high diagnostic accuracy and can help in distinguishing acute, subacute treated, and chronic healed CDC.[417–419] Laparoscopy typically shows yellowish nodules, and the diagnosis can be established by targeting these macroscopic lesions for biopsy.[420] Histopathologic studies may show large granulomas with yeasts and pseudohyphae.[421] Systemic treatment with amphotericin B, caspofungin, or fluconazole has been successful but needs to be prolonged, sometimes for months, until resolution of the lesions.[414,417,422–424] The presence of CDC does not preclude further chemotherapy and does not constitute a contraindication to marrow transplantation provided that antifungal therapy is continued.[425,426]

Bloodstream Infections

EPIDEMIOLOGY AND PATHOGENESIS

Candida spp. constitute an important pathogen in bloodstream infections. The vast majority of cases of candidemia occur in hospitalized patients, and approximately 25% to 50% are associated with ICUs.[427,428] Such units in particular have numerous risk factors and increased incidence of nosocomial fungal infections. In an analysis of more than 30,000 fungal infections, the highest number of nosocomial fungal infections/1000 discharges was reported from the burn/trauma service.[429] As a whole, *Candida* spp. are the fourth most common cause of nosocomial bloodstream infections in children and adults.[304,430] Crude and attributable mortality rates of approximately 60% and 40%, respectively, have been reported for nosocomial candidemia.[431,432]

C. albicans constitutes, by far, the most commonly isolated species in nosocomial candidemia, but nearly half of cases are now due to species other than *C. albicans*.[41,433] There has been a recent increase of clusters and outbreaks of bloodstream infections due to *Candida* spp. in high-risk settings such as neonatal and surgical ICUs.[434–439] The high rate of fungemia in this population is associated with several factors. Transmission of yeast between patients and health-care workers can occur via unwashed hands of hospital personnel working in ICUs.[437] Autoinfection after previous colonization with *Candida* spp. of gastrointestinal tract origin has also been demonstrated.[440] Invasive diagnostic and therapeutic interventions, such as percutaneous intravenous lines, drains, and intracranial pressure monitors that breach the protective layer of the dermis and serve as conduits for pathogenic organisms to enter the bloodstream are also likely contributors to the development of candidemia.

Other factors linked to the increased rate of *Candida* bloodstream infections rely on the use of broad-spectrum antibiotics. The empiric treatment of critically ill patients with sepsis is generally prescribed before the results of the cultures are known. In an observational study, the increased use of cephalosporins in an ICU was associated with a rise in candidemia.[441] Changes in the gut microflora associated with broad-spectrum antibiotics may play a role in bacterial translocation and overgrowth of *Candida* in the intestinal lumen with further vascular invasion.

Propofol in an emulsion preparation (Diprivan) is a lipid-based anesthetic agent that has been implicated in several outbreaks of postoperative infections due to extrinsic transmission by anesthesia staff.[442] The first outbreak occurred in 1990 when the Centers for Disease Control received reports of five outbreaks of postoperative bloodstream infection or acute febrile illness that involved *Candida* spp. In one cluster, four patients developed endogenous *Candida* endophthalmitis.[443]

Pressure-monitoring devices (transducers) are used regularly in critically ill patients for hemodynamic monitoring and can provide a portal of entry for systemic infections. Intravascular pressure monitor devices used in conjunction with arterial catheters have been implicated in several outbreaks of nosocomial bacterial and fungal bloodstream infections. Several outbreaks of infections due to the contamination of pressure monitoring with *Candida* have been reported.[444–446] The mechanism of infection was attributed to the lack of proper disinfection of reusable transducers, particularly the chamber domes, which served as a reservoir for the organism. No further outbreaks have been reported since the use of disposable systems.

Nosocomial infections result in considerable morbidity and mortality among neonates, especially those in neonatal ICUs (NICUs) The incidence of nosocomial *Candida* infections, including outbreaks, has been increasing.[434–436,439,447–450] Traditionally it has been thought that the acquisition of *C. albicans* by neonates occurs via mother-neonate transmission or from endogenous flora of colonized patients.[451] Recent epidemiologic studies, assisted by molecular typing, have demonstrated that exogenous infections due to the administration of contaminated fluids, cross-infection, and the colonized hands of health-care workers are also important contributors for the transmission of *Candida* spp. in NICUs.[435,436,438,439,452] Risk factors for fungal bloodstream infections in neonates include prematurity, especially very low-birth-weight neonates; use of broad-spectrum antibiotics; prolonged mechanical ventilation; coagulopathy; parenteral nutrition; catheterization of central vessels; H_2 blocker therapy; and prolonged hospitalization in NICUs.[453] A recent case-control study characterized the clinical aspects of 49 neonates with *Candida* bloodstream infections in the NICU.[454] The most common manifestation of *Candida* spp. bloodstream infections identified in neonates is abdominal distention (49%), followed by poor peripheral perfusion (46%) and fever (43%). Among *Candida* spp. pathogenic to humans, *C. albicans* remains the species most frequently associated with neonatal bloodstream infections in the NICU; however, recent trends toward an increase in non-*albicans* species have been reported.[439,454,455] Recent reports suggest an increasing number of infections attributable to *C. parapsilosis* in NICUs. In general, clinical reports suggest that *C. parapsilosis* is a less virulent organism than *C. albicans*. However, a comparative study of bloodstream infections due to these organisms in neonates demonstrated no significant difference in fungal eradication rate, and the overall mortality rate was comparable for both groups.[456,457] The increased morbidity of candidal bloodstream infections in neonates in NICUs mandates a high index of suspicion for this infectious complication and institution of early antifungal treatment. New and more effective strategies must be developed for prevention of transmission in the intensive care setting.

DIAGNOSIS

Blood culture is the main test for establishing the diagnosis of candidal bloodstream infection. However, such cultures are often negative despite disseminated disease. In an autopsy controlled study of the sensitivity of blood cultures for detection of tissue-proved invasive candidiasis, *Candida* spp. were isolated from blood in 11 of 19 patients (58%) with disseminated infection.[458] All *Candida* spp. isolated from blood cultures should be considered significant unless proved otherwise.[13] Since many cases of invasive candidiasis are missed by standard microbiologic methods, nonculture-based diagnostic tests are urgently needed. Such assays, including tests for D-arabinitol, mannans, glucans, anticandidal antibodies, and polymerase chain reaction (PCR) are in development.

TREATMENT

Fungal infections, particularly invasive candidiasis, are among the most serious infections acquired by critically ill patients requiring intensive care. Comorbid conditions and the increased severity of illness in patients hospitalized in ICUs mandate a high index of suspicion and early initiation of antifungal therapy for improved patient outcome. As described earlier, *Candida* spp. cause a broad range of invasive infections that require different therapeutic strategies. In addition, the choice of therapy will be directed by weighing the greater activity of amphotericin B for azole-resistant *Candida* spp. against the lesser toxicity of the azole and echinocandin antifungal agents. Treatment of invasive candidiasis due to non-*albicans* species may be guided by in vitro susceptibility testing, particularly in those patients previously treated with

154. Muller FM, Kasai M, Francesconi A, et al: Transmission of an azole-resistant isogenic strain of *Candida albicans* among human immunodeficiency virus-infected family members with oropharyngeal candidiasis. J Clin Microbiol 37:3405–3408, 1999.
155. Pelletier R, Peter J, Antin C, et al: Emergence of resistance of *Candida albicans* to clotrimazole in human immunodeficiency virus-infected children: In vitro and clinical correlations. J Clin Microbiol 38:1563–1568, 2000.
156. Silverman S Jr., Gallo JW, McKnight ML, et al: Clinical characteristics and management responses in 85 HIV-infected patients with oral candidiasis. Oral Surg Oral Med Oral Pathol Oral Radiol Endod 82:402–407, 1996.
157. Reichart PA, Schmidt-Westhausen A, Samaranayake LP, et al: *Candida*-associated palatal papillary hyperplasia in HIV infection. J Oral Pathol Med 23:403–405, 1994.
158. Sitheeque MA, Samaranayake LP: Chronic hyperplastic candidosis/candidiasis (candidal leukoplakia). Crit Rev Oral Biol Med 14:253–267, 2003.
159. Pons V, Greenspan D, Debruin M: Therapy for oropharyngeal candidiasis in HIV-infected patients: A randomized, prospective multicenter study of oral fluconazole versus clotrimazole troches. The Multicenter Study Group. J Acquir Immune Defic Syndr 6:1311–1316, 1993.
160. Pons V, Greenspan D, Lozada-Nur F, et al: Oropharyngeal candidiasis in patients with AIDS: randomized comparison of fluconazole versus nystatin oral suspensions. Clin Infect Dis 24:1204–1207, 1997.
161. De Wit S, Weerts D, Goossens H, et al: Comparison of fluconazole and ketoconazole for oropharyngeal candidiasis in AIDS. Lancet 1:746–748, 1989.
162. Hernandez-Sampelayo T: Fluconazole versus ketoconazole in the treatment of oropharyngeal candidiasis in HIV-infected children. Multicentre Study Group. Eur J Clin Microbiol Infect Dis 13:340–344, 1994.
163. Cartledge JD, Midgely J, Gazzard BG: Itraconazole solution: Higher serum drug concentrations and better clinical response rates than the capsule formulation in acquired immunodeficiency syndrome patients with candidosis. J Clin Pathol 50:477–480, 1997.
164. Graybill JR, Vazquez J, Darouiche RO, et al: Randomized trial of itraconazole oral solution for oropharyngeal candidiasis in HIV/AIDS patients. Am J Med 104:33–39, 1998.
165. Phillips P, De Beule K, Frechette G, et al: A double-blind comparison of itraconazole oral solution and fluconazole capsules for the treatment of oropharyngeal candidiasis in patients with AIDS. Clin Infect Dis 26:1368–1373, 1998.
166. Groll AH, Wood L, Roden M, et al: Safety, pharmacokinetics, and pharmacodynamics of cyclodextrin itraconazole in pediatric patients with oropharyngeal candidiasis. Antimicrob Agents Chemother 46:2554–2563, 2002.
167. Newman SL, Flanigan TP, Fisher A, et al: Clinically significant mucosal candidiasis resistant to fluconazole treatment in patients with AIDS. Clin Infect Dis 19:684–686, 1994.
168. Baily GG, Perry FM, Denning DW, et al: Fluconazole-resistant candidosis in an HIV cohort. AIDS 8:787–792, 1994.
169. Sanguineti A, Carmichael JK, Campbell K: Fluconazole-resistant *Candida albicans* after long-term suppressive therapy. Arch Intern Med 153:1122–1124, 1993.
170. Boken DJ, Swindells S, Rinaldi MG: Fluconazole-resistant *Candida albicans*. Clin Infect Dis 17:1018–1021, 1993.
171. Fichtenbaum CJ, Koletar S, Yiannoutsos C, et al: Refractory mucosal candidiasis in advanced human immunodeficiency virus infection. Clin Infect Dis 30:749–756, 2000.
172. Cameron ML, Schell WA, Bruch S, et al: Correlation of in vitro fluconazole resistance of *Candida* isolates in relation to therapy and symptoms of individuals seropositive for human immunodeficiency virus type 1. Antimicrob Agents Chemother 37:2449–2453, 1993.
173. Maenza JR, Keruly JC, Moore RD, et al: Risk factors for fluconazole-resistant candidiasis in human immunodeficiency virus-infected patients. J Infect Dis 173:219–25, 1996.
174. Fichtenbaum CJ, Zackin R, Rajicic N, et al: Amphotericin B oral suspension for fluconazole-refractory oral candidiasis in persons with HIV infection. Adult AIDS Clinical Trials Group Study Team 295. AIDS 14:845–852, 2000.
175. Martins MD, Rex JH: Fluconazole suspension for oropharyngeal candidiasis unresponsive to tablets. Ann Intern Med 126:332–333, 1997.
176. Revankar SG, Dib OP, Kirkpatrick WR, et al: Clinical evaluation and microbiology of oropharyngeal infection due to fluconazole-resistant *Candida* in human immunodeficiency virus-infected patients. Clin Infect Dis 26:960–963, 1998.
177. Saag MS, Fessel WJ, Kaufman CA, et al: Treatment of fluconazole-refractory oropharyngeal candidiasis with itraconazole oral solution in HIV-positive patients. AIDS Res Hum Retroviruses 15:1413–1417, 1999.
178. Kartsonis NA, Saah A, Lipka CJ, et al: Second-line therapy with caspofungin for mucosal or invasive candidiasis: Results from the caspofungin compassionate-use study. J Antimicrob Chemother 53:878–881, 2004.
179. Ghannoum MA, Elewski B: Successful treatment of fluconazole-resistant oropharyngeal candidiasis by a combination of fluconazole and terbinafine. Clin Diagn Lab Immunol 6:921–923, 1999.
180. Arathoon EG, Gotuzzo E, Noriega LM, et al: Randomized, double-blind, multicenter study of caspofungin versus amphotericin B for treatment of oropharyngeal and esophageal candidiases. Antimicrob Agents Chemother 46:451–457, 2002.
181. Dewsnup DH, Stevens DA: Efficacy of oral amphotericin B in AIDS patients with thrush clinically resistant to fluconazole. J Med Vet Mycol 32:389–393, 1994.
182. Vazquez JA, Hidalgo JA, De Bono S: Use of sargramostim (rh-GM-CSF) as adjunctive treatment of fluconazole-refractory oropharyngeal candidiasis in patients with AIDS: A pilot study. HIV Clin Trials 1:23–29, 2000.
183. Yeo E, Alvarado T, Fainstein V, et al: Prophylaxis of oropharyngeal candidiasis with clotrimazole. J Clin Oncol 3:1668–1671, 1985.
184. Owens NJ, Nightingale CH, Schweizer RT, et al: Prophylaxis of oral candidiasis with clotrimazole troches. Arch Intern Med 144:290–293, 1984.
185. Cuttner J, Troy KM, Funaro L, et al: Clotrimazole treatment for prevention of oral candidiasis in patients with acute leukemia undergoing chemotherapy: Results of a double-blind study. Am J Med 81:771–774, 1986.
186. Revankar SG, Kirkpatrick WR, McAtee RK, et al: A randomized trial of continuous or intermittent therapy with fluconazole for oropharyngeal candidiasis in HIV-infected patients: Clinical outcomes and development of fluconazole resistance. Am J Med 105:7–11, 1998.
187. Stevens DA, Greene SI, Lang OS: Thrush can be prevented in patients with acquired immunodeficiency syndrome and the acquired immunodeficiency syndrome-related complex: randomized, double-blind, placebo-controlled study of 100-mg oral fluconazole daily. Arch Intern Med 151:2458–2464, 1991.
188. Powderly WG, Finkelstein D, Feinberg J, et al: A randomized trial comparing fluconazole with clotrimazole troches for the prevention of fungal infections in patients with advanced human immunodeficiency virus infection. NIAID AIDS Clinical Trials Group. N Engl J Med 332:700–705, 1995.
189. Nyst MJ, Perriens JH, Kimputu L, et al: Gentian violet, ketoconazole and nystatin in oropharyngeal and esophageal candidiasis in Zairian AIDS patients. Ann Soc Belg Med Trop 72:45–52, 1992.
190. Peter Z, Zala J, Szabo O, et al: Fungal colonization of the esophagus in alcoholic liver disease. Z Gastroenterol 38:821–825, 2000.
191. Andersen LI, Frederiksen HJ, Appleyard M: Prevalence of esophageal *Candida* colonization in a Danish population: special reference to esophageal symptoms, benign esophageal disorders, and pulmonary disease. J Infect Dis 165:389–392, 1992.
192. Lopez-Dupla M, Mora Sanz P, Pintado Garcia V, et al: Clinical, endoscopic, immunologic, and therapeutic aspects of oropharyngeal and esophageal candidiasis in HIV-infected patients: a survey of 114 cases. Am J Gastroenterol 87:1771–1776, 1992.
193. Lingelbach A, Seidl HP, Frimberger E, et al: [Chronic mucocutaneous candidosis with severe esophageal stricture.] Mycoses 46(Suppl 1):15–18, 2003.
194. Gupta KL, Ghosh AK, Kochhar R, et al: Esophageal candidiasis after renal transplantation: Comparative study in patients on different immunosuppressive protocols. Am J Gastroenterol 89:1062–1065, 1994.
195. Chocarro Martinez A, Galindo Tobal F, Ruiz-Irastorza G, et al: Risk factors for esophageal candidiasis. Eur J Clin Microbiol Infect Dis 19:96–100, 2000.

196. Gundry SR, Borkon AM, McIntosh CL, et al: *Candida* esophagitis following cardiac operation and short-term antibiotic prophylaxis. J Thorac Cardiovasc Surg 80:661–668, 1980.
197. Simon MR, Houser WL, Smith KA, et al: Esophageal candidiasis as a complication of inhaled corticosteroids. Ann Allergy Asthma Immunol 79:333–338, 1997.
198. Bhatia V, Kochhar R, Talwar P, et al: Association of *Candida* with carcinoma of esophagus. Indian J Gastroenterol 8:171–172, 1989.
199. Chiou CC, Groll AH, Mavrogiorgos N, et al: Esophageal candidiasis in human immunodeficiency virus-infected pediatric patients after the introduction of highly active antiretroviral therapy. Pediatr Infect Dis J 21:388–392, 2002.
200. Chiou CC, Groll AH, Gonzalez CE, et al: Esophageal candidiasis in pediatric acquired immunodeficiency syndrome: Clinical manifestations and risk factors. Pediatr Infect Dis J 19:729–734, 2000.
201. Gaissert HA, Breuer CK, Weissburg A, et al: Surgical management of necrotizing *Candida* esophagitis. Ann Thorac Surg 67:231–233, 1999.
202. Orringer MB, Sloan H: Monilial esophagitis: An increasingly frequent cause of esophageal stenosis? Ann Thorac Surg 26:364–374, 1978.
203. Diotallevi P, Montella F, Di Sora F, et al: [Double-contrast esophagography in the diagnosis of esophagitis due to *Candida*. A study on HIV-seropositive patients.] Radiol Med (Torino) 84:59–63, 1992.
204. Sam JW, Levine MS, Rubesin SE, et al: The "foamy" esophagus: A radiographic sign of *Candida* esophagitis. Am J Roentgenol 174:999–1002, 2000.
205. Glick SN: Barium studies in patients with *Candida* esophagitis: Pseudoulcerations simulating viral esophagitis. Am J Roentgenol 163:349–352, 1994.
206. Wilcox CM, Schwartz DA: Endoscopic-pathologic correlates of *Candida* esophagitis in acquired immunodeficiency syndrome. Dig Dis Sci 41:1337–1345, 1996.
207. Narvarte G, Bussalleu A, Echevarria J, et al: [Endoscopic findings in HIV-infected patients with esophageal symptoms: experience at the Cayetano Heredia National Hospital.] Rev Gastroenterol Peru 21:287–299, 2001.
208. Wilcox CM, Alexander LN, Clark WS, et al: Fluconazole compared with endoscopy for human immunodeficiency virus-infected patients with esophageal symptoms. Gastroenterology 110:1803–1809, 1996.
209. Wilcox CM, Straub RF, Alexander LN, et al: Etiology of esophageal disease in human immunodeficiency virus-infected patients who fail antifungal therapy. Am J Med 101:599–604, 1996.
210. Rabeneck L, Laine L: Esophageal candidiasis in patients infected with the human immunodeficiency virus: A decision analysis to assess cost-effectiveness of alternative management strategies. Arch Intern Med 154:2705–2710, 1994.
211. Laine L, Dretler RH, Conteas CN, et al: Fluconazole compared with ketoconazole for the treatment of *Candida* esophagitis in AIDS: A randomized trial. Ann Intern Med 117:655–660, 1992.
212. Villanueva A, Gotuzzo E, Arathoon EG, et al: A randomized double-blind study of caspofungin versus fluconazole for the treatment of esophageal candidiasis. Am J Med 113:294–299, 2002.
213. Barbaro G, Barbarini G, Calderon W, et al: Fluconazole versus itraconazole for candida esophagitis in acquired immunodeficiency syndrome: *Candida* esophagitis. Gastroenterology 111:1169–1177, 1996.
214. Barbaro G, Barbarini G, Di Lorenzo G: Fluconazole vs. flucytosine in the treatment of esophageal candidiasis in AIDS patients: A double-blind, placebo-controlled study. Endoscopy 27:377–383, 1995.
215. Barbaro G, Barbarini G, Di Lorenzo G: Fluconazole compared with itraconazole in the treatment of esophageal candidiasis in AIDS patients: A double-blind, randomized, controlled clinical study. Scand J Infect Dis 27:613–617, 1995.
216. Barbaro G, Barbarini G, Di Lorenzo G: Fluconazole vs itraconazole-flucytosine association in the treatment of esophageal candidiasis in AIDS patients: A double-blind, multicenter placebo-controlled study. The *Candida* Esophagitis Multicenter Italian Study (CEMIS) Group. Chest 110:1507–1514, 1996.
217. Ally R, Schurmann D, Kreisel W, et al: A randomized, double-blind, double-dummy, multicenter trial of voriconazole and fluconazole in the treatment of esophageal candidiasis in immunocompromised patients. Clin Infect Dis 33:1447–1454, 2001.
218. Eichel M, Just-Nubling G, Helm EB, et al: [Itraconazole suspension in the treatment of HIV-infected patients with fluconazole-resistant oropharyngeal candidiasis and esophagitis.] Mycoses 39(Suppl 1): 102–106, 1996.
219. Wilcox CM, Darouiche RO, Laine L, et al: A randomized, double-blind comparison of itraconazole oral solution and fluconazole tablets in the treatment of esophageal candidiasis. J Infect Dis 176:227–232, 1997.
220. Kartsonis N, DiNubile MJ, Bartizal K, et al: Efficacy of caspofungin in the treatment of esophageal candidiasis resistant to fluconazole. J Acquir Immune Defic Syndr 31:183–187, 2002.
221. Laine L: The natural history of esophageal candidiasis after successful treatment in patients with AIDS. Gastroenterology 107:744–746, 1994.
222. Agresti MG, de Bernardis F, Mondello F, et al: Clinical and mycological evaluation of fluconazole in the secondary prophylaxis of esophageal candidiasis in AIDS patients: An open, multicenter study. Eur J Epidemiol 10:17–22, 1994.
223. Hammerschlag MR, Alpert S, Rosner I, et al: Microbiology of the vagina in children: Normal and potentially pathogenic organisms. Pediatrics 62:57–62, 1978.
224. Ribeiro MA, Dietze R, Paula CR, et al: Susceptibility profile of vaginal yeast isolates from Brazil. Mycopathologia 151:5–1510, 2001.
225. Hillier SL, Lau RJ: Vaginal microflora in postmenopausal women who have not received estrogen replacement therapy. Clin Infect Dis 25(Suppl 2):S23–126, 1997.
226. Sobel JD: Pathogenesis of *Candida* vulvovaginitis. Curr Top Med Mycol 3:86–108, 1989.
227. Leegaard M: The incidence of *Candida albicans* in the vagina of "healthy young women": How often do they have symptoms?—Possible etiological factors. Acta Obstet Gynecol Scand 63:85–89, 1984.
228. Lopez-Martinez R, Ruiz-Sanchez D, Vertiz-Chavez E: Vaginal candidosis: Opportunistic factors and clinical correlation in 600 patients. Mycopathologia 85:167–170, 1984.
229. Geiger AM, Foxman B, Sobel JD: Chronic vulvovaginal candidiasis: Characteristics of women with *Candida albicans*, *C. glabrata* and no candida. Genitourin Med 71:304–307, 1995.
230. Kutzer E, Oittner R, Leodolter S, et al: A comparison of fluconazole and ketoconazole in the oral treatment of vaginal candidiasis: Report of a double-blind multicentre trial. Eur J Obstet Gynecol Reprod Biol 29:305–313, 1988.
231. Multicentre Study Group: Treatment of vaginal candidiasis with a single oral dose of fluconazole. Eur J Clin Microbiol Infect Dis 7:364–367, 1988.
232. Report of an international multicentre trial: A comparison of single-dose oral fluconazole with 3-day intravaginal clotrimazole in the treatment of vaginal candidiasis. Br J Obstet Gynaecol 96:226–232, 1989.
233. Mikamo H, Kawazoe K, Sato Y, et al: Comparative study on the effectiveness of antifungal agents in different regimens against vaginal candidiasis. Chemotherapy 44:364–368, 1998.
234. Sobel JD, Kapernick PS, Zervos M, et al: Treatment of complicated *Candida* vaginitis: Comparison of single and sequential doses of fluconazole. Am J Obstet Gynecol 185:363–369, 2001.
235. Sobel JD: Pathogenesis and treatment of recurrent vulvovaginal candidiasis. Clin Infect Dis 14(Suppl 1):S148–S153, 1992.
236. Lynch ME, Sobel JD, Fidel PL Jr: Role of antifungal drug resistance in the pathogenesis of recurrent vulvovaginal candidiasis. J Med Vet Mycol 34:337–339, 1996.
237. Nyirjesy P, Seeney SM, Grody MH, et al: Chronic fungal vaginitis: The value of cultures. Am J Obstet Gynecol 173:820–823, 1995.
238. Redondo-Lopez V, Lynch M, Schmitt C, et al: *Torulopsis glabrata* vaginitis: Clinical aspects and susceptibility to antifungal agents. Obstet Gynecol 76:651–655, 1990.
239. Sobel JD, Chaim W, Nagappan V, et al: Treatment of vaginitis caused by *Candida glabrata*: Use of topical boric acid and flucytosine. Am J Obstet Gynecol 189:1297–1300, 2003.
240. Sobel JD, Chaim W: Treatment of *Torulopsis glabrata* vaginitis: Retrospective review of boric acid therapy. Clin Infect Dis 24:649–652, 1997.
241. Singh S, Sobel JD, Bhargava P, et al: Vaginitis due to *Candida krusei*: Epidemiology, clinical aspects, and therapy. Clin Infect Dis 35:1066–1070, 2002.

242. Abdullah AN, Drake SM, Wade AA, et al: Balanitis (balanoposthitis) in patients attending a department of genitourinary medicine. Int J STD AIDS 3:128–129, 1992.
243. David LM, Walzman M, Rajamanoharan S: Genital colonisation and infection with candida in heterosexual and homosexual males. Genitourin Med 73:394–396, 1997.
244. Morrissey R, Xavier A, Nguyen N, et al: Invasive candidal balanitis due to a condom catheter in a neutropenic patient. South Med J 78:1247–1249, 1985.
245. Waugh MA, Evans EG, Nayyar KC, et al: Clotrimazole (Canesten) in the treatment of candidal balanitis in men: With incidental observations on diabetic candidal balanoposthitis. Br J Vener Dis 54:184–186, 1978.
246. Stary A, Soeltz-Szoets J, Ziegler C, et al: Comparison of the efficacy and safety of oral fluconazole and topical clotrimazole in patients with candida balanitis. Genitourin Med 72:98–102, 1996.
247. el-Ebiary M, Torres A, Fabregas N, et al: Significance of the isolation of *Candida* species from respiratory samples in critically ill, non-neutropenic patients: An immediate postmortem histologic study. Am J Respir Crit Care Med 156:583–590, 1997.
248. Palabiyikoglu I, Oral M, Tulunay M: *Candida* colonization in mechanically ventilated patients. J Hosp Infect 47:239–242, 2001.
249. Rello J, Esandi ME, Diaz E, et al: The role of *Candida* sp isolated from bronchoscopic samples in nonneutropenic patients. Chest 114:146–149, 1998.
250. Haron E, Vartivarian S, Anaissie E, et al: Primary *Candida* pneumonia: Experience at a large cancer center and review of the literature. Medicine (Baltimore) 72:137–142, 1993.
251. Petrocheilou-Paschou V, Georgilis K, Kontoyannis D, et al: Pneumonia due to *Candida krusei*. Clin Microbiol Infect 8:806–809, 2002.
252. Rose HD, Sheth NK: Pulmonary candidiasis: A clinical and pathological correlation. Arch Intern Med 138:964–965, 1978.
253. Masur H, Rosen PP, Armstrong D: Pulmonary disease caused by *Candida* species. Am J Med 63:914–925, 1977.
254. Horvath J, Dummer S, Loyd J, et al: Infection in the transplanted and native lung after single lung transplantation. Chest 104:681–685, 1993.
255. Loke HL, Verber I, Szymonowicz W, et al: Systemic candidiasis and pneumonia in preterm infants: Aust Paediatr J 24:138–142, 1988.
256. Whyte RK, Hussain Z, deSa D: Antenatal infections with *Candida* species. Arch Dis Child 57:528–535, 1982.
257. Dubois PJ, Myerowitz RL, Allen CM: Pathoradiologic correlation of pulmonary candidiasis in immunosuppressed patients. Cancer 40:1026–1036, 1977.
258. Walsh TJ, Gray WC: *Candida* epiglottitis in immunocompromised patients. Chest 91:482–485, 1987.
259. Makitie AA, Back L, Aaltonen LM, et al: Fungal infection of the epiglottis simulating a clinical malignancy. Arch Otolaryngol Head Neck Surg 129:124–126, 2003.
260. Zhang S, Farmer TL, Frable MA, et al: Adult herpetic laryngitis with concurrent candidal infection: A case report and literature review. Arch Otolaryngol Head Neck Surg 126:672–674, 2000.
261. Bauters TG, Moerman M, Vermeersch H, et al: Colonization of voice prostheses by *albicans* and non-*albicans Candida* species. Laryngoscope 112:708–712, 2002.
262. van Weissenbruch R, Albers FW, Bouckaert S, et al: Deterioration of the Provox silicone tracheoesophageal voice prosthesis: Microbial aspects and structural changes. Acta Otolaryngol 117:452–458, 1997.
263. van Weissenbruch R, Bouckaert S, Remon JP, et al: Chemoprophylaxis of fungal deterioration of the Provox silicone tracheoesophageal prosthesis in postlaryngectomy patients. Ann Otol Rhinol Laryngol 106:329–337, 1997.
264. Ellis ME, Al-Abdely H, Sandridge A, et al: Fungal endocarditis: evidence in the world literature, 1965–1995. Clin Infect Dis 32:50–62, 2001.
265. Pierrotti LC, Baddour LM: Fungal endocarditis, 1995–2000. Chest 122:302–310, 2002.
266. Walsh TJ, Hutchins GM, Bulkley BH, et al: Fungal infections of the heart: An analysis of 51 autopsied patients. Am J Cardiol 45:357–366, 1980.
267. Rubinstein E, Noriega ER, Simberkoff MS, et al: Fungal endocarditis: Analysis of 24 cases and review of the literature. Medicine (Baltimore) 54:331–334, 1975.
268. Nasser RM, Melgar GR, Longworth DL, et al: Incidence and risk of developing fungal prosthetic valve endocarditis after nosocomial candidemia. Am J Med 103:25–32, 1997.
269. Melgar GR, Nasser RM, Gordon SM, et al: Fungal prosthetic valve endocarditis in 16 patients: An 11-year experience in a tertiary care hospital. Medicine (Baltimore) 76:94–103, 1997.
270. Veraldi GF, Guglielmi A, Genna M, et al: Occlusion of the common iliac artery secondary of fungal endocarditis: Report of a case. Surg Today 30:291–293, 2000.
271. Vo NM, Russell JC, Becker DR: Mycotic emboli of the peripheral vessels: Analysis of forty-four cases. Surgery 90:541–545, 1981.
272. Marrie TJ, Cooper JH, Costerton JW: Ultrastructure of *Candida parapsilosis* endocarditis. Infect Immun 45:390–398, 1984.
273. Donal E, Abgueguen P, Coisne D, et al: Echocardiographic features of *Candida* species endocarditis: 12 cases and a review of published reports. Heart 86:179–182, 2001.
274. Utley JR, Mills J, Roe BB: The role of valve replacement in the treatment of fungal endocarditis. J Thorac Cardiovasc Surg 69:255–258, 1975.
275. Muehrcke DD, Lytle BW, Cosgrove DM III: Surgical and long-term antifungal therapy for fungal prosthetic valve endocarditis. Ann Thorac Surg 60:538–543, 1995.
276. Johnston PG, Lee J, Domanski M, et al: Late recurrent *Candida* endocarditis. Chest 99:1531–1533, 1991.
277. Aaron L, Therby A, Viard JP, et al: Successful medical treatment of *Candida albicans* in mechanical prosthetic valve endocarditis. Scand J Infect Dis 35:351–352, 2003.
278. Lejko-Zupanc T, Kozelj M: A case of recurrent *Candida parapsilosis* prosthetic valve endocarditis: Cure by medical treatment alone. J Infect 35:81–82, 1997.
279. Rabinovici R, Szewczyk D, Ovadia P, et al: *Candida* pericarditis: Clinical profile and treatment. Ann Thorac Surg 63:1200–1204, 1997.
280. Gronemeyer PS, Weissfeld AS, Sonnenwirth AC: Purulent pericarditis complicating systemic infection with *Candida tropicalis*. Am J Clin Pathol 77:471–475, 1982.
281. Neughebauer B, Alvarez V, Harb T, et al: Constrictive pericarditis caused by *Candida glabrata* in an immunocompetent patient: Case report and review of literature. Scand J Infect Dis 34:615–619, 2002.
282. Schrank JH Jr, Dooley DP: Purulent pericarditis caused by *Candida* species: Case report and review. Clin Infect Dis 21:182–187, 1995.
283. Fischer SA, Trenholme GM, Costanzo MR, et al: Infectious complications in left ventricular assist device recipients. Clin Infect Dis 24:18–23, 1997.
284. Gordon SM, Schmitt SK, Jacobs M, et al: Nosocomial bloodstream infections in patients with implantable left ventricular assist devices. Ann Thorac Surg 72:725–30, 2001.
285. Kurup A, Janardhan MN, Seng TY: *Candida tropicalis* pacemaker endocarditis. J Infect 41:275–276, 2000.
286. Brown LA, Baddley JW, Sanchez JE, et al: Implantable cardioverter-defibrillator endocarditis secondary to *Candida albicans*. Am J Med Sci 322:160–162, 2001.
287. Roger PM, Boissy C, Gari-Toussaint M, et al: Medical treatment of a pacemaker endocarditis due to *Candida albicans* and to *Candida glabrata*. J Infect 41:176–178, 2000.
288. Kauffman CA, Vazquez JA, Sobel JD, et al: Prospective multicenter surveillance study of funguria in hospitalized patients. The National Institute for Allergy and Infectious Diseases (NIAID) Mycoses Study Group. Clin Infect Dis 30:14–18, 2000.
289. Alvarez-Lerma F, Palomar M, Leon C, et al: [Fungal colonization and/or infection in intensive care units. Multicenter study of 1,562 patients.] Med Clin (Barc) 121:161–166, 2003.
290. Febre N, Silva V, Medeiros EA, et al: Microbiological characteristics of yeasts isolated from urinary tracts of intensive care unit patients undergoing urinary catheterization. J Clin Microbiol 37:1584–1586, 1999.
291. Rocco TR, Reinert SE, Simms HH: Effects of fluconazole administration in critically ill patients: Analysis of bacterial and fungal resistance. Arch Surg 135:160–165, 2000.
292. Rivett AG, Perry JA, Cohen J: Urinary candidiasis: A prospective study in hospital patients. Urol Res 14:183–186, 1986.
293. Hamory BH, Wenzel RP: Hospital-associated candiduria: Predisposing factors and review of the literature. J Urol 120:444–448, 1978.

294. Alvarez-Lerma F, Nolla-Salas J, Leon C, et al: Candiduria in critically ill patients admitted to intensive care medical units. Intensive Care Med 29:1069–1076, 2003.
295. Phillips JR, Karlowicz MG: Prevalence of *Candida* species in hospital-acquired urinary tract infections in a neonatal intensive care unit. Pediatr Infect Dis J 16:190–194, 1997.
296. Ang BS, Telenti A, King B, et al: Candidemia from a urinary tract source: Microbiological aspects and clinical significance. Clin Infect Dis 17:662–666, 1993.
297. Kale H, Narlawar RS, Rathod K: Renal fungal ball: An unusual sonographic finding. J Clin Ultrasound 30:178–180, 2002.
298. Baetz-Greenwalt B, Debaz B, Kumar ML: Bladder fungus ball: A reversible cause of neonatal obstructive uropathy. Pediatrics 81:826–829, 1988.
299. Bryant K, Maxfield C, Rabalais G: Renal candidiasis in neonates with candiduria. Pediatr Infect Dis J 18:959–963, 1999.
300. Sultana SR, McNeill SA, Phillips G, et al: Candidal urinary tract infection as a cause of pneumaturia. J R Coll Surg Edinb 43:198–199, 1998.
301. Singh CR, Lytle WF Jr: Cystitis emphysematosa caused by *Candida albicans*. J Urol 130:1171–1173, 1983.
302. Hildebrand TS, Nibbe L, Frei U, et al: Bilateral emphysematous pyelonephritis caused by *Candida* infection. Am J Kidney Dis 33:E10, 1999.
303. Vordermark JS II, Modarelli RO, Buck AS: Torulopsis pyelonephritis associated with papillary necrosis: A case report. J Urol 123:96–97, 1980.
304. Richards MJ, Edwards JR, Culver DH, et al: Nosocomial infections in medical intensive care units in the United States. National Nosocomial Infections Surveillance System. Crit Care Med 27:887–892, 1999.
305. Carvalho M, Guimaraes CM, Mayer JR Jr, et al: Hospital-associated funguria: Analysis of risk factors, clinical presentation and outcome. Braz J Infect Dis 5:313–318, 2001.
306. Kozinin PJ, Taschdjian CL, Goldberg PK, et al: Advances in the diagnosis of renal candidiasis. J Urol 119:184–187, 1978.
307. Kauffman CA: Candiduria: Diagnostic and treatment conundrums. Curr Treatment Options Infect Dis 4:513–519, 2002.
308. Navarro E, Almario, JS, Schaufele RL, et al: Quantitative urine cultures do not reliably detect renal candidiasis in rabbits with experimental renal candidiasis. J Clin Microbiol 35:3292–3297, 1997.
309. Sobel JD, Kauffman CA, McKinsey D, et al: Candiduria: A randomized, double-blind study of treatment with fluconazole and placebo. The National Institute of Allergy and Infectious Diseases (NIAID) Mycoses Study Group. Clin Infect Dis 30:19–24, 2000.
310. Wise GJ, Kozinn PJ, Goldberg P: Flucytosine in the management of genitourinary candidiasis: 5 years of experience. J Urol 124:70–72, 1980.
311. Francis P, Walsh TJ: Evolving role of flucytosine in immunocompromised patients: New insights into safety, pharmacokinetics, and antifungal therapy. Clin Infect Dis 15:1003–1018, 1992.
312. Fan-Havard P, O'Donovan C, Smith SM, et al: Oral fluconazole versus amphotericin B bladder irrigation for treatment of candidal funguria. Clin Infect Dis 21:960–965, 1995.
313. Bayer AS, Edwards JE Jr, Seidel JS, et al: *Candida* meningitis: Report of seven cases and review of the English literature. Medicine (Baltimore) 55:477–486, 1976.
314. Nguyen MH, Yu VL: Meningitis caused by *Candida* species: An emerging problem in neurosurgical patients. Clin Infect Dis 21:323–327, 1995.
315. Sanchez-Portocarrero J, Martin-Rabadan P, Saldana CJ, et al: *Candida* cerebrospinal fluid shunt infection: Report of two new cases and review of the literature. Diagn Microbiol Infect Dis 20:33–40, 1994.
316. Geers TA, Gordon SM: Clinical significance of *Candida* species isolated from cerebrospinal fluid following neurosurgery. Clin Infect Dis 28:1139–1147, 1999.
317. Sanchez-Portocarrero J, Perez-Cecilia E, Roca V, et al: [*Candida albicans* meningitis in 2 parenteral drug addicts: Review of the literature.] Enferm Infecc Microbiol Clin 11:244–249, 1993.
318. Casado JL, Quereda C, Oliva J, et al: Candidal meningitis in HIV-infected patients: Analysis of 14 cases. Clin Infect Dis 25:673–676, 1997.
319. Voice RA, Bradley SF, Sangeorzan JA, et al: Chronic candidal meningitis: An uncommon manifestation of candidiasis. Clin Infect Dis 19:60–66, 1994.
320. Grimes DA, Lach B, Bourque PR: Vasculitic basilar artery thrombosis in chronic *Candida albicans* meningitis. Can J Neurol Sci 25:76–78, 1998.
321. Gorell JM, Palutke WA, Chason JL: *Candida* pachymeningitis with multiple cranial nerve pareses. Arch Neurol 36:719–720, 1979.
322. Chen JY: Neonatal candidiasis associated with meningitis and endophthalmitis. Acta Paediatr Jpn 36:261–265, 1994.
323. Aydin M, Kucukoduk S, Yalin T, et al: Amphotericin B in the treatment of candida meningitis in three neonates. Turk J Pediatr 37:247–252, 1995.
324. Fernandez M, Moylett EH, Noyola DE, et al: Candidal meningitis in neonates: A 10-year review. Clin Infect Dis 31:458–463, 2000.
325. Doctor BA, Newman N, Minich NM, et al: Clinical outcomes of neonatal meningitis in very-low birth-weight infants. Clin Pediatr (Phila) 40:473–480, 2001.
326. Lilien LD, Ramamurthy RS, Pildes RS: *Candida albicans* meningitis in a premature neonate successfully treated with 5-fluorocytosine and amphotericin B: A case report and review of the literature. Pediatrics 61:57–61, 1978.
327. Chesney PJ, Teets KC, Mulvihill JJ, et al: Successful treatment of *Candida* meningitis with amphotericin B and 5-fluorocytosine in combination. J Pediatr 89:1017–1019, 1976.
328. Smego RA Jr, Perfect JR, Durack DT: Combined therapy with amphotericin B and 5-fluorocytosine for *Candida* meningitis. Rev Infect Dis 6:791–801, 1984.
329. Groll AH, Giri N, Petraitis V, et al: Comparative efficacy and distribution of lipid formulations of amphotericin B in experimental *Candida albicans* infection of the central nervous system. J Infect Dis 182:274–282, 2000.
330. Scarcella A, Pasquariello MB, Giugliano B, et al: Liposomal amphotericin B treatment for neonatal fungal infections. Pediatr Infect Dis J 17:146–148, 1998.
331. Hawkins JL, Baddour LM: *Candida lusitaniae* infections in the era of fluconazole availability. Clin Infect Dis 36:e14–e18, 2003.
332. Fainstein V, Gilmore C, Hopfer RL, et al: Septic arthritis due to *Candida* species on patients with cancer: report of five cases and review of the literature. Rev Infect Dis 4:78–85, 1982.
333. Christensson B, Ryd L, Dahlberg L, et al: *Candida albicans* arthritis in a nonimmunocompromised patient. Complication of placebo intraarticular injections. Acta Orthop Scand 64:695–698, 1993.
334. Cuende E, Barbadillo C, E-Mazzucchelli R, et al: *Candida* arthritis in adult patients who are not intravenous drug addicts: report of three cases and review of the literature. Semin Arthritis Rheum 22:224–241, 1993.
335. Weers-Pothoff G, Havermans JF, Kamphuis J, et al: *Candida tropicalis* arthritis in a patient with acute myeloid leukemia successfully treated with fluconazole: Case report and review of the literature. Infection 25:109–111, 1997.
336. Vicari P, Feitosa Pinheiro R, Chauffaille Mde L, et al: Septic arthritis as the first sign of *Candida tropicalis* fungaemia in an acute lymphoid leukemia patient. Braz J Infect Dis 7:426–428, 2003.
337. Dupont B, Drouhet E: Cutaneous, ocular, and osteoarticular candidiasis in heroin addicts: New clinical and therapeutic aspects in 38 patients. J Infect Dis 152:577–591, 1985.
338. Bisbe J, Miro JM, Latorre X, et al: Disseminated candidiasis in addicts who use brown heroin: Report of 83 cases and review. Clin Infect Dis 15:910–923, 1992.
339. Miro JM, Brancos MA, Abello R, et al: Costochondral involvement in systemic candidiasis in heroin addicts: Clinical, scintigraphic, and histologic features in 26 patients. Arthritis Rheum 31:793–797, 1988.
340. Dan M: Septic arthritis in young infants: Clinical and microbiologic correlations and therapeutic implications. Rev Infect Dis 6:147–155, 1984.
341. Merchant RH, Sanghvi KP, Sridhar N, et al: Nursery outbreak of neonatal fungal arthritis treated with fluconazole. J Trop Pediatr 43:106–108, 1997.
342. Weigl JA: *Candida* arthritis in a premature infant treated successfully with oral fluconazole for six months. Ann Acad Med Singapore 29:253–255, 2000.
343. Swanson H, Hughes PA, Messer SA, et al: *Candida albicans* arthritis one year after successful treatment of fungemia in a healthy infant. J Pediatr 129:688–694, 1996.
344. Lazzarini L, Manfrin V, De Lalla F: Candidal prosthetic hip infection in a patient with previous candidal septic arthritis. J Arthroplasty 19:248–252, 2004.

345. Lerch K, Kalteis T, Schubert T, et al: Prosthetic joint infections with osteomyelitis due to *Candida albicans*. Mycoses 46:462–466, 2003.
346. Levine M, Rehm SJ, Wilde AH: Infection with *Candida albicans* of a total knee arthroplasty: Case report and review of the literature. Clin Orthop Jan:235–239, 1988.
347. Penk A, Pittrow L: [Fungal arthritis—A rare complication of systemic candidiasis or orthopedic intervention: Review of therapeutic experience with fluconazole.] Mycoses 41(Suppl 2):45–48, 1998.
348. Turgut B, Vural O, Demir M, et al: *Candida* arthritis in a patient with chronic myelogenous leukemia (CML) in blastic transformation, unresponsive to fluconazole, but treated effectively with liposomal amphotericin B. Ann Hematol 81:529–531, 2002.
349. Azaceta G, Olave T, de los Martires LD, et al: Successful lipid-complexed amphotericin B treatment of *Candida* arthritis in a lymphoma patient. Rev Rhum Engl Ed 66:434–435, 1999.
350. Evdoridou J, Roilides E, Bibashi E, et al: Multifocal osteoarthritis due to *Candida albicans* in a neonate: Serum level monitoring of liposomal amphotericin B and literature review. Infection 25:112–116, 1997.
351. Poplack DG, Jacobs SA: *Candida* arthritis treated with amphotericin B. J Pediatr 87:989–990, 1975.
352. Rodriguez D, Pigrau C, Almirante B, et al: [Vertebral osteomyelitis due to *Candida* spp.] Enferm Infecc Microbiol Clin 21:568–570, 2003.
353. Clancy CJ, Nguyen MH, Morris AJ: Candidal mediastinitis: An emerging clinical entity. Clin Infect Dis 25:608–613, 1997.
354. Malani PN, McNeil SA, Bradley SF, et al: *Candida albicans* sternal wound infections: A chronic and recurrent complication of median sternotomy. Clin Infect Dis 35:1316–1320, 2002.
355. Parry MF, Grant B, Yukna M, et al: *Candida* osteomyelitis and diskitis after spinal surgery: An outbreak that implicates artificial nail use. Clin Infect Dis 32:352–357, 2001.
356. Eisen DP, MacGinley R, Christensson B, et al: *Candida tropicalis* vertebral osteomyelitis complicating epidural catheterisation with disease paralleled by elevated D-arabinitol/L-arabinitol ratios. Eur J Clin Microbiol Infect Dis 19:61–63, 2000.
357. Edwards JE, Turkel SB, Elder HA, et al: Hematogenous *Candida* osteomyelitis: Report of three cases and review of the literature. Am J Med 59:89–94, 1975.
358. Lafont A, Olive A, Gelman M, et al: *Candida albicans* spondylodiscitis and vertebral osteomyelitis in patients with intravenous heroin drug addiction: Report of 3 new cases. J Rheumatol 21:953–956, 1994.
359. Miller DJ, Mejicano GC: Vertebral osteomyelitis due to *Candida* species: Case report and literature review. Clin Infect Dis 33:523–530, 2001.
360. Ferra C, Doebbeling BN, Hollis RJ, et al: *Candida tropicalis* vertebral osteomyelitis: A late sequela of fungemia. Clin Infect Dis 19:697–703, 1994.
361. Seravalli L, Van Linthoudt D, Bernet C, et al: *Candida glabrata* spinal osteomyelitis involving two contiguous lumbar vertebrae: A case report and review of the literature. Diagn Microbiol Infect Dis 45:137–141, 2003.
362. Almekinders LC, Greene WB: Vertebral *Candida* infections: A case report and review of the literature. Clin Orthop June:174–178, 1991.
363. Sugar AM, Saunders C, Diamond RD: Successful treatment of *Candida* osteomyelitis with fluconazole: A noncomparative study of two patients. Diagn Microbiol Infect Dis 13:517–520, 1990.
364. El-Zaatari MM, Hulten K, Fares Y, et al: Successful treatment of *Candida albicans* osteomyelitis of the spine with fluconazole and surgical debridement: Case report. J Chemother 14:627–630, 2002.
365. Turner DL, Johnson SA, Rule SA: Successful treatment of candidal osteomyelitis with fluconazole following failure with liposomal amphotericin B. J Infect 38:51–53, 1999.
366. Tang C: Successful treatment of *Candida albicans* osteomyelitis with fluconazole. J Infect 26:89–92, 1993.
367. Chen SJ, Chung YM, Liu JH: Endogenous *Candida* endophthalmitis after induced abortion. Am J Ophthalmol 125:873–875, 1998.
368. Cantrill HL, Rodman WP, Ramsay RC, et al: Postpartum *Candida* endophthalmitis. JAMA 243:1163–1165, 1980.
369. Klotz SA, Penn CC, Negvesky GJ, et al: Fungal and parasitic infections of the eye. Clin Microbiol Rev 13:662–685, 2000.
370. Edwards JE Jr, Montgomerie JZ, Foos RY, et al: Experimental hematogenous endophthalmitis caused by *Candida albicans*. J Infect Dis 131:649–657, 1975.
371. Rao NA, Hidayat A: A comparative clinicopathologic study of endogenous mycotic endophthalmitis: Variations in clinical and histopathologic changes in candidiasis compared to aspergillosis. Trans Am Ophthalmol Soc 98:183–193, 193–194, 2000.
372. Donahue SP, Hein E, Sinatra RB: Ocular involvement in children with candidemia. Am J Ophthalmol 135:886–887, 2003.
373. Feman SS, Nichols JC, Chung SM, et al: Endophthalmitis in patients with disseminated fungal disease. Trans Am Ophthalmol Soc 100:67–70, 70–71, 2002.
374. Brooks RG: Prospective study of *Candida* endophthalmitis in hospitalized patients with candidemia. Arch Intern Med 149:2226–2228, 1989.
375. Nolla-Salas J, Sitges-Serra A, Leon C, et al: *Candida* endophthalmitis in non-neutropenic critically ill patients. Eur J Clin Microbiol Infect Dis 15:503–506, 1996.
376. Donahue SP, Greven CM, Zuravleff JJ, et al: Intraocular candidiasis in patients with candidemia: Clinical implications derived from a prospective multicenter study. Ophthalmology 101:1302–1309, 1994.
377. Rodriguez-Adrian LJ, King RT, Tamayo-Derat LG, et al: Retinal lesions as clues to disseminated bacterial and candidal infections: Frequency, natural history, and etiology. Medicine (Baltimore) 82:187–202, 2003.
378. Edwards JE Jr, Montgomerie JZ, Ishida K, et al: Experimental hematogenous endophthalmitis due to *Candida*: Species variation in ocular pathogenicity. J Infect Dis 135:294–297, 1977.
379. Merchant A, Zacks CM, Wilhelmus K, et al: Candidal endophthalmitis after keratoplasty. Cornea 20:226–229, 2001.
380. Stern WH, Tamura E, Jacobs RA, et al: Epidemic postsurgical *Candida parapsilosis* endophthalmitis: Clinical findings and management of 15 consecutive cases. Ophthalmology 92:1701–1709, 1985.
381. Smiddy WE: Treatment outcomes of endogenous fungal endophthalmitis. Curr Opin Ophthalmol 9:66–70, 1998.
382. Christmas NJ, Smiddy WE: Vitrectomy and systemic fluconazole for treatment of endogenous fungal endophthalmitis. Ophthalmic Surg Lasers 27:1012–1018, 1996.
383. Essman TF, Flynn HW Jr, Smiddy WE, et al: Treatment outcomes in a 10-year study of endogenous fungal endophthalmitis. Ophthalmic Surg Lasers 28:185-94, 1997.
384. Akler ME, Vellend H, McNeely DM, et al: Use of fluconazole in the treatment of candidal endophthalmitis. Clin Infect Dis 20:657–664, 1995.
385. Martinez-Vazquez C, Fernandez-Ulloa J, Bordon J, et al: *Candida albicans* endophthalmitis in brown heroin addicts: Response to early vitrectomy preceded and followed by antifungal therapy. Clin Infect Dis 27:1130–1133, 1998.
386. Abraham G, Mathew M, Hinduja A, et al: Continuous ambulatory peritoneal dialysis: Indian scenario. J Indian Med Assoc 100:184–187, 2002.
387. Barsoum RS: Overview: end-stage renal disease in the developing world. Artif Organs 26:737–746, 2002.
388. Bibashi E, Memmos D, Kokolina E, et al: Fungal peritonitis complicating peritoneal dialysis during an 11-year period: Report of 46 cases. Clin Infect Dis 36:927–931, 2003.
389. Manzano-Gayosso P, Hernandez-Hernandez F, Mendez-Tovar LJ, et al: Fungal peritonitis in 15 patients on continuous ambulatory peritoneal dialysis (CAPD). Mycoses 46:425–429, 2003.
390. Goldie SJ, Kiernan-Tridle L, Torres C, et al: Fungal peritonitis in a large chronic peritoneal dialysis population: A report of 55 episodes. Am J Kidney Dis 28:86–91, 1996.
391. Cheng IK, Fang GX, Chan TM, et al: Fungal peritonitis complicating peritoneal dialysis: Report of 27 cases and review of treatment. Q J Med 71:407–416, 1989.
392. Chan TM, Chan CY, Cheng SW, et al: Treatment of fungal peritonitis complicating continuous ambulatory peritoneal dialysis with oral fluconazole: A series of 21 patients. Nephrol Dial Transplant 9:539–542, 1994.
393. Michel C, Courdavault L, al Khayat R, et al: Fungal peritonitis in patients on peritoneal dialysis. Am J Nephrol 14:113–120, 1994.
394. Yuen KY, Seto WH, Ching TY, et al: An outbreak of *Candida tropicalis* peritonitis in patients on intermittent peritoneal dialysis. J Hosp Infect 22:65–72, 1992.
395. Wong PN, Mak SK, Lo KY, et al: A retrospective study of seven cases of *Candida parapsilosis* peritonitis in CAPD patients: The therapeutic implications. Perit Dial Int 20:76–79, 2000.
396. Johnson RJ, Ramsey PG, Gallagher N, et al: Fungal peritonitis in patients on peritoneal dialysis: Incidence, clinical features and prognosis. Am J Nephrol 5:169–175, 1985.

397. Hoch BS, Namboodiri NK, Banayat G, et al: The use of fluconazole in the management of *Candida* peritonitis in patients on peritoneal dialysis. Perit Dial Int 13(Suppl 2):S357–359, 1993.
398. Montenegro J, Aguirre R, Gonzalez O, et al: Fluconazole treatment of candida peritonitis with delayed removal of the peritoneal dialysis catheter. Clin Nephrol 44:60–63, 1995.
399. Prasad KN, Prasad N, Gupta A, et al: Fungal peritonitis in patients on continuous ambulatory peritoneal dialysis: A single centre Indian experience. J Infect 48:96–101, 2004.
400. Warady BA, Bashir M, Donaldson LA: Fungal peritonitis in children receiving peritoneal dialysis: A report of the NAPRTCS. Kidney Int 58:384–389, 2000.
401. Sandven P, Qvist H, Skovlund E, et al: Significance of *Candida* recovered from intraoperative specimens in patients with intra-abdominal perforations. Crit Care Med 30:541–547, 2002.
402. Mollitt DL, Tepas JJ III, Talbert JL: The microbiology of neonatal peritonitis. Arch Surg 123:176–179, 1988.
403. Calandra T, Bille J, Schneider R, et al: Clinical significance of *Candida* isolated from peritoneum in surgical patients. Lancet 2:1437–1440, 1989.
404. Bond S, Stewart DL, Bendon RW: Invasive *Candida* enteritis of the newborn. J Pediatr Surg 35:1496–1498, 2000.
405. Baley JE, Kliegman RM, Annable WL, et al: *Torulopsis glabrata* sepsis appearing as necrotizing enterocolitis and endophthalmitis. Am J Dis Child 138:965–966, 1984.
406. Robertson NJ, Kuna J, Cox PM, et al: Spontaneous intestinal perforation and *Candida* peritonitis presenting as extensive necrotizing enterocolitis. Acta Paediatr 92:258–261, 2003.
407. Kaplan M, Eidelman AI, Dollberg L, et al: Necrotizing bowel disease with candida peritonitis following severe neonatal hypothermia. Acta Paediatr Scand 79:876–879, 1990.
408. Yang C, Yeh CT, Hung CF, et al: Case report: Spontaneous peritonitis caused by *Candida albicans*. J Gastroenterol Hepatol 14:1041–1044, 1999.
409. Nair S, Kumar KS, Sachan P, et al: Spontaneous fungal peritonitis (*Candida glabrata*) in a patient with cirrhosis. J Clin Gastroenterol 32:362–364, 2001.
410. de Luis D, Aller R, Boixeda D, et al: [Spontaneous peritonitis caused by ascitic fluid with *Candida albicans*.] Rev Clin Esp 197:500–501, 1997.
411. Howard JM, Bieluch VM: Pancreatic abscess secondary to *Candida albicans*. Pancreas 4:120–122, 1989.
412. Jalan R, Jones HL, Walker RJ: Multiple pancreatic abscesses due to *Candida albicans* following ERCP. Scott Med J 39:17–18, 1994.
413. Foust RT: Infection of a pancreatic pseudocyst due to *Candida albicans*. South Med J 89:1104–1107, 1996.
414. Chen CY, Chen YC, Tang JL, et al: Hepatosplenic fungal infection in patients with acute leukemia in Taiwan: Incidence, treatment, and prognosis. Ann Hematol 82:93–97, 2003.
415. Pagano L, Mele L, Fianchi L, et al: Chronic disseminated candidiasis in patients with hematologic malignancies: Clinical features and outcome of 29 episodes. Haematologica 87:535–541, 2002.
416. Shirkhoda A: CT findings in hepatosplenic and renal candidiasis. J Comput Assist Tomogr 11:795–798, 1987.
417. Sallah S, Semelka R, Kelekis N, et al: Diagnosis and monitoring response to treatment of hepatosplenic candidiasis in patients with acute leukemia using magnetic resonance imaging. Acta Haematol 100:77–81, 1998.
418. Semelka RC, Kelekis NL, Sallah S, et al: Hepatosplenic fungal disease: Diagnostic accuracy and spectrum of appearances on MR imaging. Am J Roentgenol 169:1311–1316, 1997.
419. Anttila VJ, Lamminen AE, Bondestam S, et al: Magnetic resonance imaging is superior to computed tomography and ultrasonography in imaging infectious liver foci in acute leukaemia. Eur J Haematol 56:82–87, 1996.
420. Anttila VJ, Farkkila M, Jansson SE, et al: Diagnostic laparoscopy in patients with acute leukemia and suspected hepatic candidiasis. Eur J Clin Microbiol Infect Dis 16:637–643, 1997.
421. Blade J, Lopez-Guillermo A, Rozman C, et al: Chronic systemic candidiasis in acute leukemia. Ann Hematol 64:240–244, 1992.
422. Sora F, Chiusolo P, Piccirillo N, et al: Successful treatment with caspofungin of hepatosplenic candidiasis resistant to liposomal amphotericin B. Clin Infect Dis 35:1135–1136, 2002.
423. Flannery MT, Simmons DB, Saba H, et al: Fluconazole in the treatment of hepatosplenic candidiasis. Arch Intern Med 152:406–408, 1992.
424. Bjorkholm M, Kallberg N, Grimfors G, et al: Successful treatment of hepatosplenic candidiasis with a liposomal amphotericin B preparation. J Intern Med 230:173–177, 1991.
425. Bjerke JW, Meyers JD, Bowden RA: Hepatosplenic candidiasis—A contraindication to marrow transplantation? Blood 84:2811–2814, 1994.
426. Walsh TJ, Whitcomb PO, Revankar SG, et al: Successful treatment of hepatosplenic candidiasis through repeated cycles of chemotherapy and neutropenia. Cancer 76:2357–2362, 1995.
427. Pfaller MA, Jones RN, Doern GV, et al: International surveillance of blood stream infections due to *Candida* species in the European SENTRY Program: Species distribution and antifungal susceptibility including the investigational triazole and echinocandin agents. SENTRY Participant Group (Europe). Diagn Microbiol Infect Dis 35:19–25, 1999.
428. Pfaller MA, Jones RN, Doern GV, et al: International surveillance of bloodstream infections due to *Candida* species: Frequency of occurrence and antifungal susceptibilities of isolates collected in 1997 in the United States, Canada, and South America for the SENTRY Program. The SENTRY Participant Group. J Clin Microbiol 36:1886–1889, 1998.
429. Beck-Sague C, Jarvis WR: Secular trends in the epidemiology of nosocomial fungal infections in the United States, 1980–1990. National Nosocomial Infections Surveillance System. J Infect Dis 167:1247–1251, 1993.
430. Wisplinghoff H, Seifert H, Tallent SM, et al: Nosocomial bloodstream infections in pediatric patients in United States hospitals: Epidemiology, clinical features and susceptibilities. Pediatr Infect Dis J 22:686–691, 2003.
431. Gudlaugsson O, Gillespie S, Lee K, et al: Attributable mortality of nosocomial candidemia, revisited. Clin Infect Dis 37:1172–1177, 2003.
432. Wey SB, Mori M, Pfaller MA, et al: Hospital-acquired candidemia: The attributable mortality and excess length of stay. Arch Intern Med 148:2642–2645, 1988.
433. Diekema DJ, Messer SA, Brueggemann AB, et al: Epidemiology of candidemia: 3-year results from the emerging infections and the epidemiology of Iowa organisms study. J Clin Microbiol 40:1298–1302, 2002.
434. Finkelstein R, Reinhertz G, Hashman N, et al: Outbreak of *Candida tropicalis* fungemia in a neonatal intensive care unit. Infect Control Hosp Epidemiol 14:587–590, 1993.
435. Sherertz RJ, Gledhill KS, Hampton KD, et al: Outbreak of *Candida* bloodstream infections associated with retrograde medication administration in a neonatal intensive care unit. J Pediatr 120:455–461, 1992.
436. Huang YC, Lin TY, Leu HS, et al: Outbreak of *Candida parapsilosis* fungemia in neonatal intensive care units: Clinical implications and genotyping analysis. Infection 27:97–102, 1999.
437. Huang YC, Lin TY, Peng HL, et al: Outbreak of *Candida albicans* fungaemia in a neonatal intensive care unit. Scand J Infect Dis 30:137–142, 1998.
438. Burnie JP, Odds FC, Lee W, et al: Outbreak of systemic *Candida albicans* in intensive care unit caused by cross infection. BMJ (Clin Res Ed) 290:746–748, 1985.
439. Welbel SF, McNeil MM, Kuykendall RJ, et al: *Candida parapsilosis* bloodstream infections in neonatal intensive care unit patients: Epidemiologic and laboratory confirmation of a common source outbreak. Pediatr Infect Dis J 15:998–1002, 1996.
440. Cole GT, Halawa AA, Anaissie EJ: The role of the gastrointestinal tract in hematogenous candidiasis: From the laboratory to the bedside. Clin Infect Dis 22(Suppl 2):S73–S88, 1996.
441. Edgeworth JD, Treacher DF, Eykyn SJ: A 25-year study of nosocomial bacteremia in an adult intensive care unit. Crit Care Med 27:1421–1428, 1999.
442. Bennett SN, McNeil MM, Bland LA, et al: Postoperative infections traced to contamination of an intravenous anesthetic, propofol. N Engl J Med 333:147–154, 1995.
443. Daily MJ, Dickey JB, Packo KH: Endogenous *Candida* endophthalmitis after intravenous anesthesia with propofol. Arch Ophthalmol 109:1081–1084, 1991.

444. Solomon SL, Alexander H, Eley JW, et al: Nosocomial fungemia in neonates associated with intravascular pressure-monitoring devices. Pediatr Infect Dis 5:680–685, 1986.
445. Weems JJ Jr, Chamberland ME, Ward J, et al: *Candida parapsilosis* fungemia associated with parenteral nutrition and contaminated blood pressure transducers. J Clin Microbiol 25:1029–1032, 1987.
446. Beck-Sague CM, Jarvis WR: Epidemic bloodstream infections associated with pressure transducers: A persistent problem. Infect Control Hosp Epidemiol 10:54–59, 1989.
447. Reagan DR, Pfaller MA, Hollis RJ, et al: Evidence of nosocomial spread of *Candida albicans* causing bloodstream infection in a neonatal intensive care unit. Diagn Microbiol Infect Dis 21:191–194, 1995.
448. Vaudry WL, Tierney AJ, Wenman WM: Investigation of a cluster of systemic *Candida albicans* infections in a neonatal intensive care unit. J Infect Dis 158:1375–1379, 1988.
449. Betremieux P, Chevrier S, Quindos G, et al: Use of DNA fingerprinting and biotyping methods to study a *Candida albicans* outbreak in a neonatal intensive care unit. Pediatr Infect Dis J 13:899–905, 1994.
450. Saxen H, Virtanen M, Carlson P, et al: Neonatal *Candida parapsilosis* outbreak with a high case fatality rate. Pediatr Infect Dis J 14:776–781, 1995.
451. Waggoner-Fountain LA, Walker MW, Hollis RJ, et al: Vertical and horizontal transmission of unique *Candida* species to premature newborns. Clin Infect Dis 22:803–808, 1996.
452. Plouffe JF, Brown DG, Silva J, Jr., et al: Nosocomial outbreak of *Candida parapsilosis* fungemia related to intravenous infusions. Arch Intern Med 137:1686–1689, 1977.
453. Saiman L, Ludington E, Pfaller M, et al: Risk factors for candidemia in neonatal intensive care unit patients. The National Epidemiology of Mycosis Survey Study Group. Pediatr Infect Dis J 19:319–324, 2000.
454. Makhoul IR, Kassis I, Smolkin T, et al: Review of 49 neonates with acquired fungal sepsis: further characterization. Pediatrics 107:61–66, 2001.
455. Rangel-Frausto MS, Wiblin T, Blumberg HM, et al: National epidemiology of mycoses survey (NEMIS): Variations in rates of bloodstream infections due to *Candida* species in seven surgical intensive care units and six neonatal intensive care units. Clin Infect Dis 29:253–258, 1999.
456. Huang YC, Lin TY, Lien RI, et al: Candidaemia in special care nurseries: Comparison of *albicans* and *parapsilosis* infection. J Infect 40:171–175, 2000.
457. Benjamin DK Jr, Ross K, McKinney RE Jr, et al: When to suspect fungal infection in neonates: A clinical comparison of *Candida albicans* and *Candida parapsilosis* fungemia with coagulase-negative staphylococcal bacteremia. Pediatrics 106:712–718, 2000.
458. Berenguer J, Buck M, Witebsky F, et al: Lysis-centrifugation blood cultures in the detection of tissue-proven invasive candidiasis: Disseminated versus single-organ infection. Diagn Microbiol Infect Dis 17:103–109, 1993.
459. Rex JH, Bennett JE, Sugar AM, et al: A randomized trial comparing fluconazole with amphotericin B for the treatment of candidemia in patients without neutropenia. Candidemia Study Group and the National Institute. N Engl J Med 331:1325–1330, 1994.
460. Edwards JE Jr, Bodey GP, Bowden RA, et al: International Conference for the Development of a Consensus on the Management and Prevention of Severe Candidal Infections. Clin Infect Dis 25:43–59, 1997.
461. Mora-Duarte J, Betts R, Rotstein C, et al: Comparison of caspofungin and amphotericin B for invasive candidiasis. N Engl J Med 347:2020–2029, 2002.
462. Nguyen MH, Peacock JE Jr, Tanner DC, et al: Therapeutic approaches in patients with candidemia: Evaluation in a multicenter, prospective, observational study. Arch Intern Med 155:2429–2435, 1995.
463. Rex JH, Bennett JE, Sugar AM, et al: Intravascular catheter exchange and duration of candidemia. NIAID Mycoses Study Group and the Candidemia Study Group. Clin Infect Dis 21:994–996, 1995.
464. Karlowicz MG, Hashimoto LN, Kelly RE Jr, et al: Should central venous catheters be removed as soon as candidemia is detected in neonates? Pediatrics 106:E63, 2000.
465. Benoit JL, Carandang G, Sitrin M, et al: Intraluminal antibiotic treatment of central venous catheter infections in patients receiving parenteral nutrition at home. Clin Infect Dis 21:1286–1288, 1995.
466. Viale P, Petrosillo N, Signorini L, et al: Should lock therapy always be avoided for central venous catheter-associated fungal bloodstream infections? Clin Infect Dis 33:1947–1948; author reply 1949–1951, 2001.
467. Schinabeck MK, Long LA, Hossain MA, et al: Rabbit model of *Candida albicans* biofilm infection: Liposomal amphotericin B antifungal lock therapy. Antimicrob Agents Chemother 48:1727–1732, 2004.
468. Goodman JL, Winston DJ, Greenfield RA, et al: A controlled trial of fluconazole to prevent fungal infections in patients undergoing bone marrow transplantation. N Engl J Med 326:845–851, 1992.
469. Rotstein C, Bow EJ, Laverdiere M, et al: Randomized placebo-controlled trial of fluconazole prophylaxis for neutropenic cancer patients: Benefit based on purpose and intensity of cytotoxic therapy. The Canadian Fluconazole Prophylaxis Study Group. Clin Infect Dis 28:331–340, 1999.
470. Winston DJ, Pakrasi A, Busuttil RW: Prophylactic fluconazole in liver transplant recipients: A randomized, double-blind, placebo-controlled trial. Ann Intern Med 131:729–737, 1999.

84

Entomophthoramycosis, Lobomycosis, Rhinosporidiosis, and Sporotrichosis

DUANE R. HOSPENTHAL
JOHN E. BENNETT

INTRODUCTION

The four diseases reviewed in this chapter—entomophthoramycosis, lobomycosis, rhinosporidiosis, and sporotrichosis—are either restricted to, or occur predominantly in, the tropical regions of the world. All present most often as lesions of the skin or mucous membranes. Though all were previously believed to be mycoses, the etiologic agent of rhinosporidiosis has recently been shown to be more closely related to a group of protistan parasites. Entomophthoramycosis presents as a painless, firm, circumscribed subcutaneous mass, either involving the nose and surrounding face or a single area of the skin elsewhere. The overlying skin is usually normal, but may be reddened and shiny. Lobomycosis presents as a single, sharply circumscribed, painless verrucous cutaneous papule or plaque. Rhinosporidiosis commonly presents as a single, soft, fleshy polyp of the nasal mucosa or palpebral conjunctiva. Sporotrichosis most often presents as one or more red nodules on the exposed skin that may ulcerate or have intermittent serosanguineous drainage.

Entomophthoramycosis

Diseases caused by species of the genera *Basidiobolus* and *Conidiobolus* are recognized by many names. Together, they are most often denoted by the term *entomophthoramycosis*, reflecting the order Entomophthorales to which they belong. Alternatively, they are grouped along with other pathogens of their class Zygomycetes and called zygomycoses. Individually, disease caused by *Basidiobolus ranarum* is termed basidiobolomycosis. *Conidiobolus coronatus* infection is called conidiobolomycosis.

EPIDEMIOLOGY

Basidiobolomycosis is a subcutaneous infection that predominantly affects children and adolescents and has its highest prevalence in tropical Africa and Southeast Asia. It was first reported by Joe and colleagues[1] in 1956 in three Indonesian children. In one of the largest series, Mugerwa[2] reported 80 cases of basidiobolomycosis from Uganda. A 5:3 male-to-female predominance was noted. Although disease was observed in persons from ages 1 to 58 years, 76% of those affected were under 10 years of age (and almost half were under 5 years old). Conidiobolomycosis is a submucosal rhinosinusitis occurring most frequently in adults in the tropics (especially in the tropical rain forests of West Africa). It was first described by Emmons and Bridges[3] in 1961 as causing nasal polyps in horses. The first human case was reported in 1965 by Bras and associates.[4] Until 1992, approximately 100 human cases had been reported.[5] *B. ranarum* and *C. coronatus* are found in nature in soil, decaying vegetation, and in the intestinal tracts of amphibians, reptiles, and other animals.[6,7] Although these fungi can be recovered throughout the world, they favor warm, humid climates. *C. coronatus* has been shown to require 95% humidity to produce conidia, with maximal conidiation occurring at 100% humidity.[8]

DISEASES

While the fungi causing these diseases and their respective clinical manifestations differ, the pathologic findings in the two entomophthoramycoses are similar. Both cause indolent infection with granulomatous changes in the skin and subcutaneous tissues without bony or systemic involvement. Basidiobolomycosis presents with a solitary, asymptomatic, circumscribed, hard, subcutaneous mass usually located in the buttock or extremities. Sixty-five percent of patients in one report had disease confined to either the buttock (28 of 75) or thigh (21 of 75).[2] These lesions do not commonly involve muscle and may not involve overlying skin.

Conidiobolomycosis most frequently begins in the submucosa of the nose, spreading to involve bilateral skin of the nasal region, the paranasal sinuses, and the pharynx. The skin is firmly attached to underlying subcutaneous tissues and may appear normal, or reddened and shiny. Conidiobolomycosis may be asymptomatic or may be diagnosed after symptoms of nasal obstruction, rhinorrhea, or epistaxis. Bacterial sinusitis from obstruction of drainage may also lead to presentation. Entomophthoramycosis is most often slowly progressive, resulting only in cosmetic disfigurement. Occasionally, long-standing infection may be complicated by obstruction of the lymphatics in basidiobolomycosis or the facial structures in conidiobolomycosis. Recently, cases of basidiobolomycosis affecting and confined to the gastrointestinal tract have been increasingly reported, including from Brazil,[9] the United States[10,11] and Kuwait.[12] A handful of disseminated cases of disease caused by *Conidiobolus* species (including one due to *C. coronatus*[13]) have been reported.[14–17] Disease caused by *C. coronatus* similar to that in humans has been seen in sheep, llamas,[18] horses, mules, dolphins, and a chimpanzee. Disease caused by *Conidiobolus incongruus* has been associated with the deaths of 700 sheep in an outbreak in Australia.[19,20] *B. ranarum* also causes granulomatous skin lesions in horses.

PATHOGENESIS AND IMMUNITY

Little is known about the pathogenesis of these diseases. Both *Basidiobolus* and *Conidiobolus* possess the ability to grow in vitro at 37°C and have been shown to elicit specific antibodies in humans and animals. Their described in vitro production of extracellular proteases and lipases has been postulated to play a role in the limited virulence of these organisms.[21,22]

DIAGNOSIS

Diagnosis of entomophthoramycosis is based on biopsy with microscopic examination of tissue and culture of the etiologic agent. Clinically, basidiobolomycosis can be confused with soft-tissue sarcoma. Fibrosing panniculitis and bacterial cellulitis are almost always painful and are thus not difficult to differentiate from this disease. On microscopic examination of biopsy material, both of these organisms are seen as short, aseptate, or sparsely septated wide hyphae with surrounding eosinophilic material in subcutaneous granulomas. The surrounding material stains strongly with periodic acid–Schiff (PAS) stain in what is referred to as the Splendore-Hoeppli phenomenon (see explanation under Sporotrichosis).[23] In addition to observation in tissue sections, these fungal elements may be seen by direct observation in potassium hydroxide wet mounts. Definitive diagnosis is made by culture. Culture of these organisms is usually done on Sabouraud glucose agar containing antibacterial antibiotics at 25°C to 30°C. Both genera grow well at temperatures of 25°C to 37°C, producing mycelial growth in several days. Conidia that are forcibly discharged are characteristic of the Entomophthorales. In cultures of *B. ranarum* and *C. coronatus,* these conidia may be seen on the covers of Petri plates as the cultures mature. *B. ranarum* produces wide hyphae (8 to 20 μm), which become progressively more septate with time. Forcibly discharged conidia, adhesive conidia, and beaked thick-walled zygospores are produced by this species. *C. coronatus* produces phototropic discharged conidia, villose conidia, but no zygospores. No commercially available serologic tests are available to diagnose the entomophthoramycoses. Studies have shown that the genera induce production of a specific antibody response, which may be shown by immunodiffusion. Studies using *B. ranarum* have shown precipitin bands of antigens specific to the species as well as one shared with *C. coronatus* and *Pythium insidiosum.*[24,25]

TREATMENT

Basidiobolomycosis and conidiobolomycosis differ in their response to therapy. Limited in vitro susceptibility data have shown high MICs for amphotericin B and flucytosine for both species, obtainable MICs for the azoles against *Basidiobolus*, and mixed results for *Conidiobolus* with the azole antifungals.[26,27] Both have responded to extended therapy with potassium iodide (6 to 12 months; Table 84-1). In basidiobolomycosis, successful therapy with ketoconazole or trimethoprim-sulfamethoxazole[28] has been reported. Spontaneous resolution is occasionally seen in both diseases, but surgical excision is rarely curative in either. No consistently effective therapy for conidiobolomycosis has yet been found. Mixed results have been reported with therapies including iodide, amphotericin B, trimethoprim-sulfamethoxazole, ketoconazole, and surgery.[5,29] Both successful and unsuccessful results of therapy with ketoconazole have been reported.[30–32] Improvement of disease with fluconazole therapy has been reported in two patients.[33,34] Response to combination therapy with fluconazole and itraconazole has been reported in one person.[35]

Table 84-1 Therapy of Entomophthoramycosis, Lobomycosis, Rhinosporidiosis, and Sporotrichosis

Disease	Primary Therapy	Alternative Therapy
Entomophthoramycosis		
Basidiobolomycosis	SSKI	Ketoconazole
Conidiobolomycosis	SSKI	Ketoconazole
Lobomycosis	Surgery	None
Rhinosporidiosis	Surgery	None
Sporotrichosis		
Cutaneous	SSKI or itraconazole	Fluconazole or heat*
Osteoarticular	Amphoteicin B or itraconazole	
Pulmonary	Surgery +/− amphotericin B or itraconazole	Amphotericin B, itraconazole
Disseminated	Amphotericin B	Itraconazole

SSKI, saturated solution of potassium iodide.
*For cutaneous plaque lesions.

Lobomycosis

Lobomycosis (Lobo's disease, keloidal blastomycosis) is a chronic cutaneous disease found only in Central and South America and is caused by the fungal pathogen *Lacazia loboi.* First described by Lobo in 1931,[36] the disease was initially thought to be an atypical presentation of paracoccidioidomycosis. In describing the second reported case in 1938,[37] Fialho thought the histopathology of these first two cases was clearly different from paracoccidioidomycosis, and coined the term *Lobo's disease* to describe the new entity. Since that time, over 300 cases have been described.[38] The etiologic agent of lobomycosis, previously denoted *Loboa loboi* or *Paracoccidioides loboi*, has been renamed *Lacazia loboi.*[39] Although a recent mouse foot-pad model has been developed to study this disease,[40,41] our inability to isolate and cultivate the organism from patients and the environment using standard methods has greatly limited our understanding of its habitat and life cycle.

EPIDEMIOLOGY

Epidemiologically, the disease is limited to the tropical and subtropical forests of Central and South America, with the greatest number of cases among the Cayabi tribe of Brazil. In total, 57 cases of lobomycosis have been reported in the Cayabi.[38] Interestingly though, no disease has been noted in those members of the tribe who were born since the tribe relocated to a different region of Brazil. This disease shows no predilection for race, sex, or age, but is seen in persons who work outdoors in rural, hot, humid areas. Cutaneous trauma is thought to be the initiating event in this disease, but cases following insect stings have been reported. Apart from human disease, lobomycosis has only been seen to occur naturally in dolphins. A single zoonotic case has been reported, occurring in the attendant of a dolphin also diagnosed with the disease.[42]

DISEASE

Lobomycosis is a chronic granulomatous disease of the dermis which produces plaques, nodules, verrucoid lesions, or ulcerated lesions. Beginning as a well-circumscribed papule, the disease is otherwise asymptomatic and spreads by local extension, autoinoculation, and possibly via the lymphatic system. Common sites of initial lesions include the extremities and the ears. The lesions grow slowly for years to decades before most patients seek medical attention. Typical features include indurated lesions with sharp, lobulated margins, which are painless and not attached to underlying structures. The skin is usually shiny, discolored, and atrophic. Complications of disease, including ulceration and bacterial superinfection, are rare. Squamous cell carcinoma has been reported in extremely chronic lesions in three patients.[43]

DIAGNOSIS

Diagnosis is made by the direct observation of *L. loboi* in lesional biopsy material. Clinically, the lesions of lobomycosis may be similar to those seen in chromoblastomycosis, paracoccidioidomycosis, leishmaniasis, mycosis fungoides, dermatofibrosarcoma protuberans, Kaposi's sarcoma, and squamous cell carcinoma. Microscopically, the dermis is replaced by histiocytic granulomas that contain organisms and remnants of organisms. Disease does not extend deeper than the subcutaneous tissue. Globose to elliptic or lemon-shaped cells approximately 10 μm in diameter strung together by small tubular connections (resembling a pearl necklace) are typically seen in tissue. The cell walls of the organisms may be quite thick (up to 1 μm). These may be seen with standard hematoxylin and eosin (H&E) stain, but are often better appreciated with PAS or Gomori's methenamine silver (GMS) stain. Direct observation of biopsy material mounted in KOH may also yield the diagnosis.

TREATMENT

The only effective therapy is early wide excision of lesions. Surgical removal of chronic lesions can be effective, but recurrence is common. Medical therapy has been ineffective in the treatment of lobomycosis. The overall prognosis in this disease is very good as the mycosis spreads very slowly and is associated with limited morbidity.

Rhinosporidiosis

Rhinosporidiosis is a chronic granulomatous submucosal or subcutaneous disease seen most commonly in India and Sri Lanka. This disease was first described in an Argentinean man by Seeber in 1900.[44] In 1923, Ashworth[45] produced a classic monograph on the morphology and clinical manifestations of rhinosporidiosis. As with *L. loboi*, study of this disease has been hampered by our inability to reproducibly culture or maintain it in the laboratory. Recent studies of 18S small-subunit ribosomal DNA sequences of the organism have placed *Rhinosporidium seeberi* into a novel group of aquatic protistan parasites.[46,47]

EPIDEMIOLOGY

The ecological niche of the organism is not known, although disease has been associated with bathing in stagnant water, river diving, and rice paddy cultivation. Disease has been reported worldwide, with areas of increased incidence in India, Sri Lanka, South America, and Africa. Indigenous cases have been reported from many countries,[48–50] although the greatest numbers of cases outside India and Sri Lanka are in persons originally from those countries. Disease occurs most frequently in children and young adults (ages 15 to 40 years) with a male predominance. A 4:1 male-to-female ratio was noted in one study of 255 cases.[51] In addition to human disease, infection in the nasal passages of cats, cattle, dogs, goats, horses, mules, ducks, parrots, and swan has been described.

DISEASE

Disease most frequently presents as friable polypoid nodules in the nose, nasopharynx, or conjunctiva. Approximately 70% of rhinosporidiosis is limited to the nasal mucous membranes, with the conjunctiva being the next most common site of infection. Submucosal lesions of the lacrimal sac, larynx, trachea, ear, vagina, and rectum, as well as subcutaneous lesions of the penis,[52] scrotum, face, scalp, and other areas of the body have been described. Rarely, isolated bone lesions[53] and disseminated cutaneous lesions[54–56] have been reported. Presenting symptoms are usually those of unilateral nasal obstruction or epistaxis. Cough secondary to postnasal discharge can occur. Occasionally the disease can be complicated by bacterial sinusitis if sinus drainage becomes obstructed. Localized disease is the rule, with disseminated disease of deep organs and tissues noted in only three of several thousand reported cases.[57]

PATHOGENESIS AND IMMUNITY

Rhinosporidiosis has been shown in limited studies to elicit a cell-mediated immune response. Immunohistochemistry has shown that the cell infiltration in human infection includes suppressor lymphocytes and natural killer cells; lymphoproliferation assays have revealed the development of specific immune suppression to *R. seeberi*.[58] Specific delayed-type hypersensitivity has been demonstrated in a mouse foot-pad model.[59]

DIAGNOSIS

Rhinosporidiosis may be suspected in subjects with polypoid lesions that contain white dots on close inspection. Nasal polyps need to be differentiated from those seen in allergic disease. Vaginal and penile lesions may resemble condylomata, while rectal lesions may mimic prolapsed internal hemorrhoids. Diagnosis is based on the direct observation of the organism in tissue. Culture and serology are not currently available. Microscopic examination can be done with KOH mounts of macerated tissue or stained histologic sections of lesions.

Direct observation of biopsy material may reveal white subepithelial dots, which are the large sporangia of *R. seeberi*. These sporangia, which may contain thousands of endospores, can grow to diameters of 350 μm. Though similar in structure to the spherules of *Coccidioides immitis*, both the sporangia and endospores are larger in rhinosporidiosis. The sporangium wall of *R. seeberi* is also much thicker. Structures of the organism stain well with GMS and PAS stains, but its size allows the diagnosis to be made easily with standard H&E staining. Histopathologically, an inflammatory response with neutrophils, lymphocytes, plasma cells, and multinucleated giant cells is seen in the submucosa underlying normal columnar or squamous epithelium. Papillomatous hyperplasia and increased vascularity may also be seen in these lesions.

TREATMENT

Surgical excision is the only known effective therapy for rhinosporidiosis. Recurrence is common following surgical excision and has led to the practice of wide surgical excision of lesions followed by electrocoagulation of their bases. Medical therapy has not proved effective, although reports of success with dapsone 100 mg/day for one year have been published.[60]

Sporotrichosis

Sporotrichosis is a chronic, usually cutaneous, fungal infection caused by *Sporothrix schenckii*. Though disease is most commonly limited to cutaneous and subcutaneous tissue, osteoarticular, pulmonary, and other deep infections can occur. Cutaneous sporotrichosis is caused by inoculation during minor trauma, although the incident is often not remembered. Extracutaneous infection is thought to be initiated via inhalation of the organism with or without dissemination. Sporotrichosis was first described in 1898 by Schenck for whom the organism was later named.[61] Study of sporotrichosis in France by Beurmann and Gougerot in the early twentieth century produced the monograph *Les Sporotrichoses*,[62] and led to the use of potassium iodide as an effective therapy for this mycosis.

AGENT

S. schenckii is a temperature-dependent dimorphic fungus which is found in the environment, usually on living or decaying plants. In this niche and in culture at room temperature, *S. schenckii* is a filamentous fungus (mold). In host tissue and at 37°C in culture, the morphology of the organism is that of a yeast.

EPIDEMIOLOGY

Though worldwide in its distribution, sporotrichosis is most commonly seen in tropical and subtropical climates. This disease usually has a focal distribution, occurring endemically and in small epidemics in temperate and tropical environments. In clustered cases it has been associated with the distribution of sphagnum moss and with mine timbers. The common cutaneous form is usually seen in young adults, without predilection for sex or race. Infection occurs in immunocompetent persons, often those who work outdoors in contact with vegetation or soil. An epidemiologic survey employing skin testing has shown a higher incidence of positive delayed cutaneous hypersensitivity in plant nursery workers than in hospitalized patients or prisoners (32.3% vs. 11.2%).[63] Pulmonary disease has a male predominance and an association with alcohol dependence. Of the 66 known cases in the world in 1986,[64] the male-to-female ratio was 6:1. Thirty of 51 of these cases were seen in patients with impairment of host defenses, with 19 associated with alcohol dependence. Disseminated disease is more common in patients who are immunosuppressed.[65–67] In the unimpaired host, the incidence of disseminated disease is thought to be quite low. Lurie[68] found only five cases of disseminated disease in over 3000 cases (incidence of 0.2%) of sporotrichosis in the study of the South African mine outbreak. Sporotrichosis has also been shown to occur in armadillos, birds, camels, cats, cattle, dogs, dolphins, goats, horses, mules, and rats.[69]

DISEASE

Cutaneous disease begins as a relatively painless papule, which enlarges slowly and then drains spontaneously. Infection can remain localized or may spread slowly via the lymphatic system to involve proximal sites on an extremity. Although infection may reach the axillary or inguinal lymph nodes, hematogenous dissemination from skin inoculation has not been described. Rarely, lesions may also be solitary and fixed, presenting as plaques which wax and wane for years without resolution. Although minor (often insignificant) trauma is thought to be the common mode by which cutaneous disease is initiated, disease following or associated with insect stings, fish handling, bites or scratches of dogs, cats, parrots, and wild rodents has been reported. Of these other potential sources of infection, zoonotic transmission from cats has been best documented.[70] Pulmonary sporotrichosis typically presents in the fifth decade of life with productive cough and upper lobe chest radiographic findings.[64] Most commonly, chest radiography reveals a solitary upper lobe thin-walled cavity with surrounding parenchymal infiltrate. Untreated pulmonary sporotrichosis is usually associated with progressive disease and death. Osteoarticular sporotrichosis is an indolent disease usually involving the joints of the knee, elbow, wrist, or ankle.[71,72] Infection presents like osteoarthritis or rheumatoid arthritis with gradual onset of pain, stiffness, and decrease in range of motion. Localized swelling is often present. Laboratory studies usually show an elevated erythrocyte sedimentation rate and synovial fluid with decreased glucose, increased protein, and leukocytes. Hematogenous spread from the lungs or occult sites may lead to chronic meningitis, endophthalmitis, brain abscesses, or disseminated skin lesions.

PATHOGENESIS AND IMMUNITY

The virulence factors and pathogen-host immunity interaction of *S. schenckii* are not currently well understood. *S. schenckii* has limited pathogenicity in laboratory animals, with large inocula being required to establish infection. Virulence of strains of *S. schenckii* can be subdivided by thermotolerance as those strains which grow at 37°C are better able to cause disseminated disease. Antibody to yeast cell wall antigens is produced in some infections. The role of this antibody in containing infection is not believed to be critical, although agglutinating antibody response in a hamster model has been associated with protection against challenge.[73] Cell-mediated immunity (CMI) likely serves a more important role in host defense, especially in humans. Human neutrophils have been shown to phagocytose and kill *S. schenckii*. This killing requires halide, myeloperoxidase, and peroxide.[74] Opsonization with human serum is thought to enhance this interaction via activation of the alternative complement pathway. Athymic mice have been shown to be unable to clear an intravenous challenge of *S. schenckii* when compared with euthymic mice,[75] further supporting the role of CMI.

DIAGNOSIS

Diagnosis of cutaneous sporotrichosis is suspected with observation of typical lesions, often with supporting history of likely exposure (e.g., agriculture, gardening, or forestry). This diagnosis is then confirmed by culture or further supported by microscopic tissue examination. The differential diagnosis of cutaneous sporotrichosis includes disease caused by *Nocardia* species (especially *N. brasiliensis*), *Mycobacterium* species (*M. marinum, M. chelonae, M. fortuitum,* and *M. kansasii*), leishmaniasis, tularemia, cat-scratch disease, chromoblastomycosis, blastomycosis, and paracoccidioidomycosis. An incorrect diagnosis of squamous cell carcinoma may be made from biopsy specimens that manifest hyperkeratosis and are not cultured correctly. Pulmonary sporotrichosis should be differentiated from *Mycobacterium avium-intracellulare* (MAI) complex infection, coccidioidomycosis, tuberculosis, and histoplasmosis. In addition to chronic bacterial osteomyelitis, osteoarticular sporotrichosis should be differentiated from mycobacterial infections. Diagnosis of pulmonary disease is usually made when *S. schenckii* is cultured from sputum, bronchoalveolar lavage, or biopsy. Osteoarticular disease may be diagnosed by culture of joint fluid or fungal stain of synovium. Blood culture is not usually helpful in the diagnosis of sporotrichosis. Although both localized[76] and disseminated[77] disease has been diagnosed by blood culture, these represent only a handful of cases. *S. schenckii* is best recovered on brain-heart infusion agar incubated at 25°C to 30°C for up to 3 weeks. Histopathologic study reveals a pyogranulomatous reaction with neutrophils and necrotic debris surrounded by epithelioid cells. In more chronic lesions, pseudoepitheliomatous hyperplasia is seen. Commonly, skin lesions have a paucity of fungal organisms, making the correct diagnosis difficult to establish without culture. It is often very difficult to find *S. schenckii* in routine H&E-stained histopathologic sections in any tissue. PAS and GMS stains improve visualization of the organism in tissue. Usually seen as oval- to cigar-shaped yeasts in tissue, *S. schenckii* may also form asteroid bodies or appear as spherical yeasts with what appears to be a capsule. The asteroid body is a central rounded yeast structure with radiating eosinophilic substance in tissue. Deposition of eosinophilic material about the infecting organism was first described by Splendore in 1908 in the study of sporotrichosis,[78] and then in 1932 by Hoeppli in the study of schistosomiasis in a rabbit model.[79] Classically, the Splendore-Hoeppli phenomenon is believed to be an immune complex (antibody-antigen) deposition. Study employing electron microscopy appears to indicate that the asteroid bodies of sporotrichosis may actually be comprised of disintegrated immune cells.[80] This phenomenon has also been seen in schistosomiasis, actinomycosis, botryomycosis, entomophthoramycosis, mycetoma, and onchocerciasis. In its atypical spherical form with a PAS-positive capsular-appearing structure, *S. schenckii* may be confused with *Cryptococcus neoformans*. Serologic and immune testing is generally of limited value in the diagnosis of sporotrichosis. Although many testing formats have been developed, the availability of these tests and perceived need for them has limited their usefulness.

TREATMENT

The treatment of sporotrichosis is based on the clinical presentation of the disease.[81] Treatment of all forms of this disease has been associated with relapse. Potassium iodide in saturated solution has been the mainstay of therapy of cutaneous sporotrichosis since the beginning of this century. First used by Beurmann for the treatment of cutaneous disease, potassium iodide remains an inexpensive, effective therapy. Iodide therapy can be poorly tolerated and associated with adverse effects. It is a bitter solution, which should be slowly titrated up to treatment doses to minimize adverse effects and increase tolerance.[82] These effects include excessive tearing and salivating, parotid enlargement, acne, and gastrointestinal upset. Supersaturated solution of potassium iodide (~1 g/mL or 47 mg/drop) can be begun at a dose of 5–10 drops three times daily, usually with juice or water. The dose can be increased slowly (5 drops per dose each week) to 25–40 drops thrice daily in those under 10 years of age and 40–50 drops thrice daily in those 10 years old or older. The duration of therapy is usually 6 to 12 weeks (until lesions are flat and soft). Itraconazole is an effective, well-tolerated alternative to iodide in the therapy of cutaneous disease. Its biggest limitation in many areas of the world is its cost. In those patients with plaque sporotrichosis who cannot tolerate iodide, heat may be beneficial. Hyperthermic therapy using a variety of modalities has been used successfully in these cutaneous infections. Successes with therapies using liquid nitrogen,[83] fluconazole,[84] saperconazole,[85] and terbinafine[86] have also been reported in cutaneous disease. Interestingly, the new broad spectrum azole voriconazole was shown in one study to be less active than itraconazole against *S. schenckii*.[87] Both itraconazole and amphotericin B have been shown to be effective in osteoarticular disease.[88,89] Intra-articular injection with amphotericin B has been reported to lead to improvement in several patients with disease recurring after parenteral therapy.[72,90] Doses ranging from 0.1 mg to 10 mg of amphotericin B injected daily to every 2 weeks have been used. Pulmonary sporotrichosis has been treated with amphotericin B, iodide, ketoconazole, miconazole, and itraconazole, all with some reported successes. Unfortunately, pulmonary disease does not respond regularly to antifungal therapy and is known to relapse. This disease is best treated surgically with or without the addition of amphotericin B or itraconazole. Disseminated sporotrichosis is most often treated with parenteral amphotericin B. Itraconazole therapy has been shown in several reports to lead to a favorable response, usually in those patients not responding to amphotericin B.[88,91]

PREVENTION

Prevention of sporotrichosis is based on avoidance of traumatic inoculation of the fungus. Fungicide treatment of timbers was used to bring a halt to the epidemic of disease seen in South African gold mines in the 1940s. The U.S. outbreak involving conifer saplings packed in sphagnum moss has led to suggestions of using chipped wood or shredded paper as packing material for these plants.[92] People who work in forestry or horticulture and others who are engaged in gardening should be encouraged to wear gloves and clothing that cover their extremities, preventing scratches and other minor trauma. Similar recommendations can be made for veterinarians and others handling pets with skin lesions.

REFERENCES

1. Joe LK, Eng NIT, Pohan A, et al: *Basidiobolus ranarum* as a cause of subcutaneous mycosis in Indonesia. Arch Dermatol 74:378, 1956.
2. Mugerwa JW: Subcutaneous phycomycosis in Uganda. Br J Dermatol 94:539, 1976.
3. Emmons CW, Bridges CH: *Entomophthora coronata,* etiologic agent of phycomycosis of horses. Mycologia 53:307, 1961.
4. Bras G, Gordon GC, Emmons CW, et al: A case of phycomycosis observed in Jamaica: Infection with *Entomophthora coronata.* Am J Trop Med Hyg 14:141, 1965.
5. Gugnani HC: Entomophthoramycosis due to *Conidiobolus.* Eur J Epidemiol 8:391, 1992.
6. Clark BM: The epidemiology of phycomycosis. In Wolstenholme GEW, Porter R (eds): Systemic Mycoses. Boston, Little, Brown, 1968, p 179.
7. Zahari P, Hirst RG, Shipton WA, et al: The origin and pathogenicity of *Basidiobolus* species in northern Australia. J Med Vet Mycol 28:461, 1990.
8. Yendol WG: Factors affecting the germination of *Entomophthora coronata.* J Invert Pathol 10:111, 1968.
9. Aguiar E, Moraes WC, Londero AT: Gastrointestinal entomophthoramycosis caused by *Basidiobolus haptosporus.* Mycopathologia 72:101, 1980.
10. Lyon GM, Smilack JD, Komatsu KK, et al: Gastrointestinal basidiobolomycosis in Arizona: Clincal and epidemiological characteristics and review of the literature. Clin Infect Dis 32:1448, 2001.
11. Zavasky D, Samowitz W, Loftus T, et al: Gastrointestinal zygomycotic infection caused by *Basidiobolus ranarum*: Case report and review. Clin Infect Dis 28:1244, 1999.
12. Khan ZU, Khoursheed M, Makar R, et al: *Basidiobolus ranarum* as an etiologic agent of gastrointestinal zygomycosis. J Clin Microbiol 39:2360, 2001
13. Walker SD, Clark RV, King CT, et al: Fatal disseminated *Conidiobolus coronatus* infection in a renal transplant patient. Am J Clin Pathol 98:559, 1992.
14. Walsh TJ, Renshaw G, Andrews, J, et al: Invasive zygomycosis due to *Conidiobolus incongruus.* Clin Infect Dis 19:423, 1994.
15. Jaffey PB, Haque AK, El-Zaatari M, et al: Disseminated *Conidiobolus* infection with endocarditis in a cocaine abuser. Arch Pathol Lab Med 114:1276, 1990.
16. Busapakum R, Youngchaiyud U, Sriumpai S, et al: Disseminated infection with *Conidiobolus incongruus.* Sabouraudia 21:323, 1983.
17. Gilbert EF, Khoury GH, Pore RS: Histopathological identification of *Entomophthora* phycomycosis: Deep mycotic infection in an infant. Arch Pathol 90:583, 1970.
18. French RA, Ashworth CD: Zygomycosis caused by *Conidiobolus coronatus* in a llama (*Lama glama*). Vet Pathol 31:120, 1994.
19. Carrigan MJ, Small AC, Perry GH: Ovine nasal zygomycosis caused by *Conidiobolus incongruus.* Aust Vet J 69:237, 1992.
20. Ketterer PJ, Kelly MA, Connole MD, et al: Rhinocerebral and nasal zygomycosis in sheep caused by *Conidiobolus incongruus.* Aust Vet J 69:85, 1992.
21. Okafor JI: Purification and characterization of protease enzymes of *Basidiobolus* and *Conidiobolus* species. Mycoses 37:265, 1994.
22. Okafor JI, Gugnani HC: Lipase activity of *Basidiobolus* and *Conidiobolus* species. Mycoses 33:81,1990.
23. Bader G, Grueber HLE: Histochemical studies of tissue forms and of perifungal substance in subcutaneous phycomycosis. Path Microbiol 35:280, 1970.
24. Inwidthaya P, Srimuang S: Immunodiffusion test for diagnosing basidiobolomycosis. Mycopathologia 118:127, 1992.
25. Kaufman L, Mendoza L, Standard PG: Immunodiffusion test for serodiagnosing subcutaneous zygomycosis. J Clin Microbiol 28:1887, 1990.
26. Yangco BG, Okafor JI, TeStrake D: In vitro susceptibilities of human and wild-type isolates of *Basidiobolus* and *Conidiobolus* species. Antimicrob Agents Chemother 25:413, 1984.
27. Guarro J, Aguilar C, Pujol I: In-vitro antifungal susceptibilities of *Basidiobolus* and *Conidiobolus* spp. strains. J Antimicrob Chemother 44:557, 1999.
28. Fomufod AK, Antia AU: Successful treatment of subcutaneous phycomycosis with trimethoprim-sulphamethoxazole (Septrin). Trop Geogr Med 23:208, 1971.
29. Martinson FD: Chronic phycomycosis of the upper respiratory tract. Rhinophycomycosis entomophthorae. Am J Trop Med Hyg 20:449, 1971.
30. Towersey L, Wanke B, Estrella RR, et al: *Conidiobolus coronatus* infection treated with ketoconazole. Arch Dermatol 124:1392, 1988.
31. Drouhet E, Dupont B: Laboratory and clinical assessment of ketoconazole in deep-seated mycoses. Ketoconazole symposium. Am J Med 74(Suppl):30, 1983.
32. Hay RJ: Ketoconazole in the treatment of fungal infection ketoconazole symposium. Am J Med 74(Suppl):16, 1983.
33. Filho LG, Nico MMS, Salebian A, et al: Entomoftoromicose rinofacial por *Conidiobolus coronatus.* Registro de um caso tratado com sucesso pelo fluconazol. Rev Inst Med Trop Sao Paulo 34:483, 1992.
34. Costa AR, Porto E, Pegas JRP, et al: Rhinofacial zygomycosis caused by *Conidiobolus coronatus.* Mycopathologia 115:1, 1991.
35. Valle ACF, Wanke B, Lazera MS, et al: Entomophthoramycosis by *Conidiobolus coronatus.* Report of a case successfully treated with the combination of itraconazole and fluconazole. Rev Inst Med Trop S Paulo 43:233, 2001.
36. Lobo J: Um caso de blastomicose produzida por uma especie nova, encontrada em Recife. Rev Med Pernambucana 1:763, 1931.
37. Fialho A: Blastomicose du tipo "Jorge Lobo." O Hospital 14:903, 1938.
38. Rodriguez-Toro G: Lobomycosis. Int J Dermatol 32:324, 1993.
39. Taborda PR, Taborda VA, McGinnis MR: *Lacazia loboi* gen. nov., comb. nov., the etiologic agent of lobomycosis. J Clin Microbiol 37:2031, 1999.
40. Belone AFF, Madeira S, Rosa PS, et al: Experimental reproduction of the Jorge Lobo's disease in BALB/c mice inoculated with *Lacazia loboi* obtained from a previously infected mouse. Mycopathologia 155:191, 2001.
41. Vilani-Moreno FR, Belone AFF, Rosa PS, et al: Evaluation of the vital staining method for *Lacazia loboi* through the experimental inoculation of BALB/c mice. Med Mycol 41:211, 2003.
42. Symmers WSTC: A possible case of Lobo's disease acquired in Europe from a bottle-nosed dolphin (*Tursiops truncatus*). Bull Soc Pathol Exot 76:777, 1983.
43. Baruzzi RG, Rodriguez DA, Michalany NS, et al: Squamous-cell carcinoma and lobomycosis (Jorge Lobo's disease). Int J Dermatol 28:183, 1989.
44. Seeber GR: Un nuevo esporozoario parasito del hombre: Dos casos encontrades en polipos nasales, thesis. National University of Buenos Aires, 1900.
45. Ashworth JH: On *Rhinosporidium seeberi* (Wernicke 1903) with special reference to its sporulation and affinities. Trans R Soc Edinburgh 53:301, 1923.
46. Fredricks DN, Jolley JA, Lepp PW, et al: *Rhinosporidium seeberi*: A human pathogen from a novel group of aquatic protistan parasites. Emerg Infect Dis 6:273, 2000.
47. Herr RA, Ajello L, Taylor JW, et al: Phylogenetic analysis of *Rhinosporidium seeberi*'s 18S small-subunit ribosomal DNA groups this pathogen among members of the proctistan Mesomycetozoa clade. J Clin Microbiol 37:2750, 1999.
48. Gaines JJ, Clay JR, Chandler FW, et al: Rhinosporidiosis: Three domestic cases. South Med J 89:65, 1996.
49. van der Coer JMGI, Marres HAM, Wielinga EWJ, et al: Rhinosporidiosis in Europe. J Laryngol Otol 106:440, 1992.
50. Lasser A, Smith HW: Rhinosporidiosis. Arch Otolaryngol 102:308, 1976.
51. Satyanarayana C: Rhinosporidiosis. With a record of 255 cases. Acta Otolaryngol 51:348, 1960.

52. Sasidharan K, Subramonian P, Moni VN, et al: Urethral rhinosporidiosis. Analysis of 27 cases. Br J Urol 59:66, 1987.
53. Adiga BK, Singh N, Arora VK, et al: Rhinosporidiosis. Report of a case with an unusual presentation with bony involvement. Acta Cytol 41:889, 1997.
54. Angunawela P, DeTissera A, Dissanaike AS: Rhinosporidiosis presenting with two soft tissue tumors followed by dissemination. Pathology 31:57, 1999.
55. Gokhale S, Ohri VC, Subramanya H, et al: Subcutaneous and osteolytic rhinosporidiosis. Indian J Pathol Microbiol 40:95, 1997.
56. Thappa DM, Venkatesan S, Sirka CS, et al: Disseminated cutaneous rhinosporidiosis. J Dermatol 25:527, 1998.
57. Agrawal S, Sharma KD, Shrivastava JB: Generalized rhinosporidiosis with visceral involvement. Arch Dermatol 80:22, 1959.
58. de Silva NR, Huegel H, Atapattu DN: Cell-mediated immune responses (CMIR) in human rhinosporidiosis. Mycopathologia 152:59, 2000.
59. Jayasekera S, Arseculeratne SN, Atapattu DN: Cell-mediated immune responses (CMIR) to *Rhinosporidium seeberi* in mice. Mycopathologia 152:69, 2000.
60. Job A, Venkateswaran S, Mathan M, et al: Medical therapy of rhinosporidiosis with dapsone. J Laryngol Otol 107:809, 1993.
61. Schenck RB: On refractory subcutaneous abscesses caused by a fungus possibly related to spororichia. Bull Johns Hopkins Hosp 9:286, 1898.
62. Beurmann L, Gougerot H: Les Sporotrichoses. Paris, Felix Alcan, 1912.
63. Schneidau JD, Lamar LM, Hairston MA: Cutaneous hypersensitivity to sporotrichin in Louisiana. JAMA 188:371, 1964.
64. Pluss JL, Opal SM: Pulmonary sporotrichosis: Review of treatment and outcome. Medicine (Baltimore) 65:143, 1986.
65. Donabedian H, O'Donnell E, Olszewski C, et al: Disseminated cutaneous and meningeal sporotrichosis in an AIDS patient. Diagn Microbiol Infect Dis 18:111, 1994.
66. Heller HM, Fuhrer J: Disseminated sporotrichosis in patients with AIDS: Case report and review of the literature. AIDS 5:1243, 1991.
67. Schamroth JM, Grieve TP, Kellen P: Disseminated sporotrichosis. Int J Dermatol 27:28, 1988.
68. Lurie HI: Five unusual cases of sporotrichosis from South Africa showing lesions in muscles, bones, and viscera. Br J Surg 50:585, 1963.
69. Werner AH, Werner BE: Sporotrichosis in man and animal. Int J Dermatol 33:692, 1994.
70. Fleury RN, Tabora PR, Gupta AK, et al: Zoonotic sporotrichosis. Transmission to humans by infected domestic cat scratching: Report of four cases in Sao Paulo, Brazil. Int J Dermatol 40:318, 2001.
71. Janes PC, Mann RJ: Extracutaneous sporotrichosis. J Hand Surg [Am] 12:441, 1987.
72. Yao J, Penn RG, Ray S: Articular sporotrichosis. Clin Orthop 204:207, 1986.
73. Reiss E (ed): *Sporothrix schenckii*. In Molecular Immunology of Mycotic and Actinomycotic Infections. New York, Elsevier, 1986, p 115.
74. Cunningham KM, Bulmer GS, Rhoades ER: Phagocytosis and intracellular fate of *Sporothrix schenckii*. J Infect Dis 140:815, 1979.
75. Shiriashi A, Nakagaki K, Arai T: Experimental sporotrichosis in congenitally athymic (nude) mice. J Reticuloendothel Soc 26:333, 1979.
76. Kosinski RM, Axelrod P, Rex JH, et al: *Sporothrix schenckii* fungemia without disseminated sporotrichosis. J Clin Microbiol 30:501, 1992.
77. Aronson NE: Disseminated sporotrichosis. JAMA 268:2021, 1992.
78. Splendore A: Sobre a culture de una nova especie de cogumelo patogé nica do homen (*Sporotrichum splendore*) ou "*Sporotrichum asteroides*" n. SP Rev Soc Cien 3:62, 1908.
79. Hoeppli R: Histological observations in experimental schistosomiasis japonica. Chin Med J (Engl) 46:1179, 1932.
80. Hiruma M, Kawada A, Ishibashi A: Ultrastructure of asteroid bodies in sporotrichosis. Mycoses 34:103, 1991.
81. Kauffman CA, Hajjeh R, Chapman SW, et al: Practice guidelines for the management of patients with sporotrichosis. Clin Infect Dis 30:684, 2000.
82. Sterling JB, Heymann WR: Potassium iodide in dermatology: A 19th century drug for the 21st century—Uses, pharmacology, adverse effects, and contraindications. J Am Acad Dermatol 43:691, 2000.
83. Bargman H: Successful treatment of cutaneous sporotrichosis with liquid nitrogen: Report of three cases. Mycoses 38:285, 1995.
84. Yoshida M, Hiruma M, Tezuda T: A case of sporotrichosis treated successfully with oral fluconazole 200 mg once weekly. Mycoses 37:281, 1994.
85. Franco L, Gomez I, Restrepo A: Saperconzole in the treatment of systemic and subcutaneous mycoses. Int J Dermatol 31:725, 1992.
86. Hull PR, Vismer HF: Treatment of cutaneous sporotrichosis with terbinafine. Br J Dermatol 126 (Suppl 39):51, 1992.
87. McGinnis MR, Nordoff N, Li R: *Sporothrix schenckii* sensitivity to voriconazole, itraconazole, and amphotericin B. Med Mycol 39:369, 2001.
88. Sharkey-Mathis PK, Kauffman CA, Graybill JR, et al: Treatment of sporotrichosis with itraconazole. Am J Med 95:279, 1993.
89. Winn RE, Anderson J, Piper J, et al: Systemic sporotrichosis treated with itraconazole. Clin Infect Dis 17:210, 1993.
90. Downs NJ, Hinthorn DR, Mhatre VR, et al: Intra-articular amphotericin B treatment of *Sporothrix schenckii* arthritis. Arch Intern Med 149:954, 1989.
91. Bolao F, Podzamczer D, Ventin M, et al: Efficacy of acute phase and maintenance therapy with itraconazole in an AIDS patient with sporotrichosis. Eur J Clin Microbiol Infect Dis 13:609, 1994.
92. Coles FB, Schuchat A, Hibbs JR, et al: A multistate outbreak of sporotrichosis associated with sphagnum moss. Am J Epidemiol 136:475, 1992.

85

Pneumocystosis

PETER D. WALZER

INTRODUCTION

Pneumocystis was discovered by Chagas in 1909 during his studies of American trypanosomiasis. The organism was established as a separate genus and species a few years later by the Delanöes, who named it in honor of Dr. Carini. *Pneumocystis* is an organism of low virulence that resides in the lungs of humans and many animals in nature.

AGENTS

Although *Pneumocystis* isolates from these hosts are morphologically indistinguishable, molecular, antigenic, and experimental transmission studies have demonstrated a high degree of genetic diversity and host specificity. This information has resulted in new nomenclature that has established the following *Pneumocystis* species: *P. carinii* and *P. wakefieldii* in rats, *P. murina* in mice, and *P. jirovecii* in humans.[1–3] *Pneumocystis* was first recognized as the pathogen that caused interstitial plasma cell pneumonia in premature, malnourished infants in European orphanages following World War II. However, the disease can occur wherever these conditions exist. More recently, *Pneumocystis* has been found to be a leading cause of pneumonia in immunocompromised patients, such as those infected with the human immunodeficiency virus (HIV).

Knowledge of the basic biology of *Pneumocystis* has been limited by the lack of a continuous in vitro culture system.[4] The developmental stages that have been identified include the 5- to 8-μm cyst or spore case, which has a thick wall and contains up to eight intracystic bodies or spores; the 1- to 4-μm trophozoite or trophic form, which is the most numerous stage; and the precyst or sporocyte, an intermediate stage. A proposed life cycle is presented in Figure 85-1.[5] The cyst (spore case) is thought to develop through a sexual cycle that culminates in the release of the intracystic bodies (spores), which then become trophic forms; the trophic forms replicate asexually by binary fission. The taxonomic status of *Pneumocystis* has clearly established the organism as a member of the fungi.[4]

EPIDEMIOLOGY

Serologic studies have revealed that *Pneumocystis* has a worldwide distribution, and that exposure to the organism occurs early in life.[6,7] Evidence suggests that *Pneumocystis* remains in the lungs for limited periods of time and that people may be transiently infected at different times in their lives. The HIV pandemic changed pneumocystosis from a sporadic disease to a problem of major medical and public health importance. Although the incidence of *Pneumocystis* pneumonia has fallen with widespread chemoprophylaxis and antiretroviral therapy, the organism remains the leading cause of opportunistic infection in HIV patients in industrialized countries.[8] Evaluation of the evidence of pneumocystosis in tropical and developing countries has been hampered by lack of access to medical care and the higher frequency of more virulent infection such as tuberculosis.[9] These factors have led to an underestimate of the true frequency of this disease. Recently, a high frequency of *Pneumocystis* has been reported in pediatric HIV patients in developing countries.[10] Other factors affecting the epidemiology are geography and season of the year.[11,12]

Studies in animal models have demonstrated that *Pneumocystis* is communicable via the airborne route.[5] Young animals acquire *Pneumocystis* infection soon after birth and play an important role in spreading the infection.[13] Molecular studies in humans support the findings from these experimental models.[14] The incubation period is approximately 4 to 8 weeks.

DISEASE

Risk factors for pneumocystosis include prematurity and malnutrition; primary immunodeficiency disorders, particularly severe combined immunodeficiency disease; infection with HIV; and cytotoxic or immunosuppressive drugs for the treatment of cancer, transplantation, and collagen vascular disorders. Studies of HIV-infected and AIDS patients have documented a significant risk of pneumocystosis when CD4 lymphocyte counts fall below 200/μL; other risk factors include persistent constitutional symptoms.[15,16] Corticosteroids are by far the most commonly used immunosuppressive drugs that predispose to *Pneumocystis* pneumonia in non-HIV-infected patients.[17] Symptoms often begin after the steroid dose has been tapered.

Pneumocystis pneumonia is characterized by the triad of dyspnea, nonproductive cough, and fever.[18] Although a productive cough and chest tightness may occur, purulent sputum should raise suspicion of bacterial infection. HIV-infected patients frequently have prolonged prodromal periods with subtle clinical manifestations; other immunocompromised hosts are usually ill for 1 or 2 weeks before they seek medical attention.[19] However, the clinical picture varies in individual patients. Physical examination reveals varying degrees of respiratory distress. Lung auscultation is nonrevealing, although basilar rales may occasionally be present. On the chest radiograph, typically these are diffuse infiltrates with symmetric reticular or granular opacities emanating from the perhilar regions (Fig. 85-2).[20] Unusual manifestations include focal infiltrates, lobar consolidation, nodules, cavities, effusions, pneumatoceles, and lymphadenopathy.[21] An increased frequency of pneumothorax and apical infiltrates has been noted with the administration of aerosolized pentamidine.[22] Very early in *Pneumocystis* pneumonia, the chest radiograph may be normal.

The principal laboratory abnormality is arterial hypoxemia with an increased alveolar–arterial (PAO_2–PaO_2) gradient; this is often accompanied by respiratory alkalosis.[23]

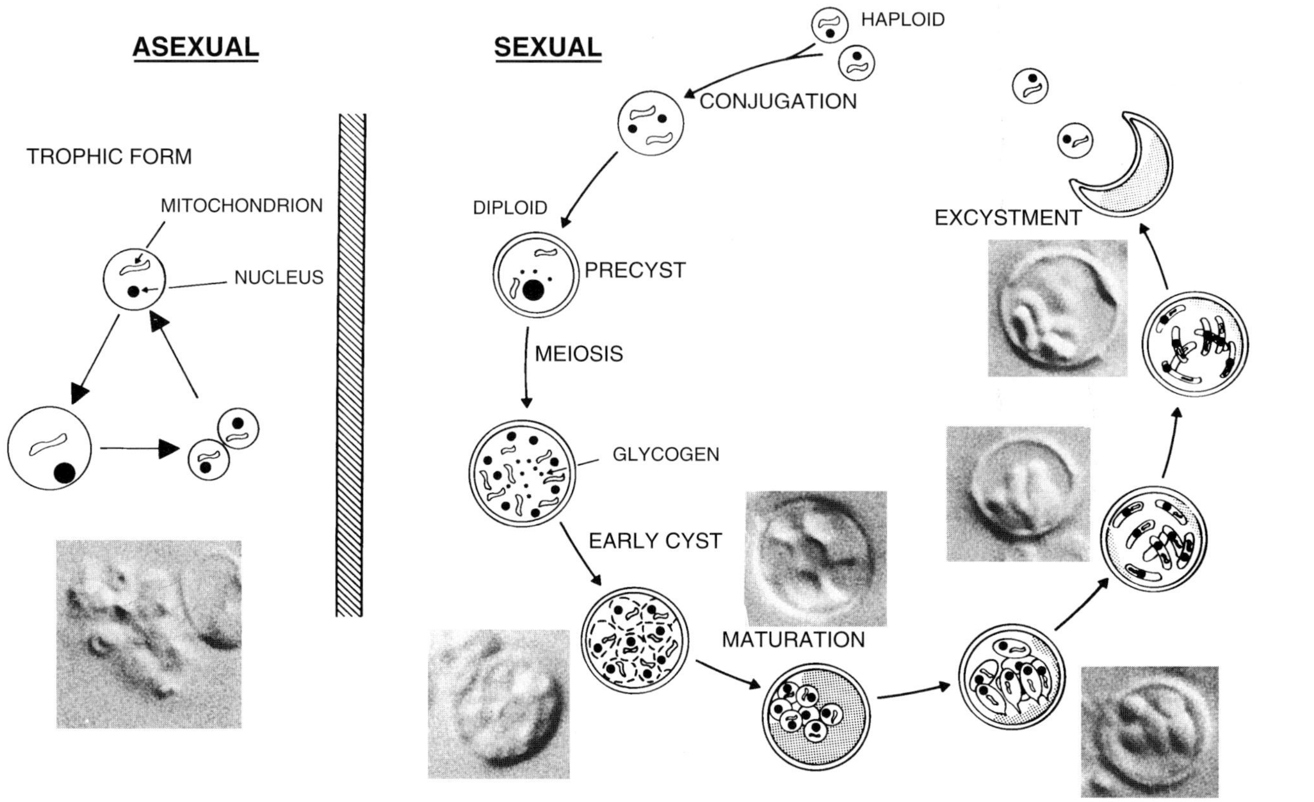

FIGURE 85-1 Proposed life cycle of *Pneumocystis carinii.* Photographs depict living trophic and cyst forms by Nomarski interference contrast microscopy. In the asexual phase, the trophic forms replicate by mitosis and cell division. In the sexual phase, the haploid trophic forms (mating types) conjugate to form a diploid zygote (early phase) that undergoes meiosis and subsequent mitosis to form eight haploid nuclei (late phase). The spores are formed by compartmentalization of nuclei and cytoplasmic organelles (e.g., mitochondria). The spores exhibit different shapes, including spherical and elongated forms. It is postulated that the elongation of the spores precedes release from the ascus. Release is thought to occur through a rent in the cell wall. After evacuation, the empty ascus usually collapses but retains some residual cytoplasm. (From Cushion M: *Pneumocystis carinii.* In Collier L, Balows A, Sussman M [eds]: Topley and Wilson's Microbiology and Microbial Infections, Vol. 4. New York, Oxford University Press, 1998, pp 645–683.)

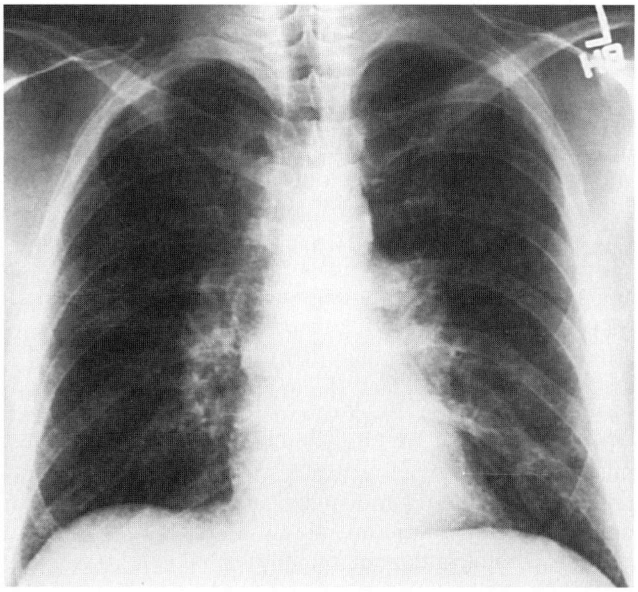

FIGURE 85-2 Chest radiograph from an HIV-infected patient with pneumocystosis. Note the typical bilateral infiltrates. (From Walzer PD, Kim CK, Cushion MT: *Pneumocystis carinii.* In Walzer PD, Genta RM [eds]: Parasitic Infections in the Compromised Host. New York, Marcel Dekker, 1989, pp 83–178.)

Blood oxygenation may be normal early in the course of pneumocystosis but will desaturate with exercise. Pulmonary function tests are characterized by alterations in lung volumes and spirometry (e.g., reversible airway obstruction and airway hyperreactivity). The diffusing capacity for carbon monoxide (DL_{CO}) has been sensitive in detecting alveolar–capillary block. Serum lactic dehydrogenase (LDH) levels, which reflect the degree of lung injury, increase with progression of pneumocystosis and decrease as the disease is treated. Imaging techniques such as the chest high-resolution computed tomograph (HRCT) may show abnormal findings (especially ground-glass opacities) but are not specific for *Pneumocystis*.[24]

The spread of *Pneumocystis* beyond the lungs is well recognized. The frequency of extrapulmonary pneumocystosis is unknown, although estimates range from uncommon to as high as 3% of cases.[25,26] Patients at highest risk are those in the late stages of HIV infection who have received aerosolized pentamidine or have not taken prophylaxis. The most common sites of extrapulmonary infection are the lymph nodes, spleen, liver, and bone marrow, although most organs in the body have been involved. Clinical features range from incidental findings at autopsy to focal involvement and systemic disease.

The natural history of untreated *Pneumocystis* pneumonia in HIV-infected and other immunocompromised patients is

86

Enteric Amebiasis

WILLIAM A. PETRI, Jr
UPINDER SINGH

INTRODUCTION

Entamoeba histolytica has been reclassified into three genetically distinct but morphologically identical species: the invasive pathogen *E. histolytica* and the noninvasive parasites *E. moshkovskii* and *E. dispar*. *E. histolytica* is the cause of amebic colitis and liver abscess. *E. dispar* is present in many asymptomatic "cyst passers" in developing countries, as well as in sexually active male homosexuals from developed countries. *E. moshkovskii* has recently been recognized to also be a prevalent infection in children in the developing world. Other amebae are less a source of diagnostic confusion as they are morphologically differentiated from the *E. histolytica/moshkovskii/dispar* group and include *Entamoeba hartmanni, Entamoeba coli, Entamoeba polecki, Entamoeba gingivalis, Iodamoeba butschlii, Endolimax nana*, and *Blastocystis hominis*. These amebae are usually nonpathogenic commensals and are reviewed briefly.

AGENT

History

A link between dysentery and liver abscess may have been first recognized in 1828 by James Annesley in his two-volume monograph *Prevalent Diseases of India*: "... hepatic disease seems to be induced by the disorder of the bowels, more particularly when this disorder is of a subacute or chronic kind." Amebae in stool were postulated to be responsible for diarrhea by Lambl in 1855, who described their appearance in the stool of a child from Prague who died of infantile diarrhea.[1,2] Fedor Lösch demonstrated amebae in the stools of a 24-year-old farmer with dysentery from his first clinic visit in November 1873 to his death in April 1874 in Saint Petersburg, Russia. Lösch described the amebae in the stool as having a "round, pear-shaped or irregular form and which are in a state of almost continuous motion." Autopsy demonstrated colonic ulcerations containing amebae. Dysentery with amebic ulcers in the colon was induced in one dog by repeated inoculations of the patient's fresh ameba-containing stool orally and rectally.[1,2]

Sir William Osler reported the first North American case of amebiasis in 1890, when he saw a young physician in Baltimore with dysentery. "Dr. B., age 29, resident in Panama for nearly six years, where he had had several attacks of dysentery, or more correctly speaking a chronic dysentery, came north in May, 1889...." On February 15, 1890, the patient was having six to eight mucoid stools with traces of blood daily, a fever of 103°F, and a tender liver extending "nearly a hand's breadth above the normal limit." Amebae were observed in the stool and abscess fluid: "The general character of the amoeba [found in the stool] correspond in every particular with those found in the liver."[3] A year later, Osler's colleagues Councilman and Lafleur proceeded through a classic investigation of 14 cases of amebic dysentery to clearly distinguish amebiasis from bacterial dysentery, and coined the terms *amebic dysentery* and *amebic liver abscess*.[4]

Piso introduced ipecac bark, used for centuries in Peru for the treatment of dysentery, to Europe in 1658. Helvetius used ipecac to successfully treat the dysentery of Louis XIV and sold it as a secret remedy to the French government. It was not until 1858 that the use of large doses of ipecac for the treatment of dysentery was promoted by the surgeon E.S. Docker, in Mauritius, who demonstrated that ipecac (60 grains two to three times a day) reduced the death rate from 10%–18% to only 2%. Unfortunately, administration of large doses of ipecac by mouth was complicated by such severe nausea and vomiting as to necessitate the coadministration of opium, chloral hydrate, or tannic acid. Leonard Rogers,[5] a professor of pathology at Calcutta, discovered that emetine, the principal alkaloid in ipecac, would kill amebae in the mucus of stools from patients with dysentery at dilutions as high as 1:100,000. In 1912, he reported the successful treatment of three patients in Calcutta, who had been unable to tolerate oral ipecac, by injection of emetine.[5]

Walker and Sellards[6] in the Philippines in 1913, in human volunteer studies, documented the cyst form of *E. histolytica* as the infective form of the parasite and the life cycle was described by Dobell in 1925. Axenic culture of *E. histolytica* was accomplished by Diamond[7] at the National Institutes of Health (NIH) in 1961, which enabled study of the cell biology and biochemistry of the parasite upon which our modern understanding of amebiasis is based.

Taxonomy

E. histolytica is a pseudopod-forming nonflagellate protozoan parasite. It is the most invasive of the *Entamoeba* group and the only *Entamoeba* to cause amebic colitis and liver abscess. Trophozoites contain a single nucleus, and nuclear division occurs without the formation of condensed metaphase chromosomes. No sexual forms of the parasite have been identified.

E. histolytica has recently been reclassified into three species that are morphologically identical but genetically distinct: *E. histolytica* (Schaudinn, 1903), an invasive disease-causing parasite, and *E. dispar* (Brumpt, 1925) and *E. moshkovskii*, both noninvasive parasites. As early as 1925, it was proposed by Brumpt[8] that two morphologically identical species of *Entamoeba*, both of which produced quadrinucleate cysts measuring 10 μm or more in diameter, infected humans. Brumpt found that only one of the species caused disease in kittens or human volunteers, and named the nonpathogenic species *Entamoeba dispar*. These studies languished in the absence of a means to distinguish the two morphologically identical parasites. It was not until Sargeaunt and colleagues[9] demonstrated in 1978 that isoenzyme typing could be used to distinguish the pathogenic from the nonpathogenic species of *Entamoeba* that the issue was reexamined.

The invasive species *E. histolytica* and the noninvasive species *E. moshkovskii* and *E. dispar* are morphologically identical but can be differentiated by isoenzyme analysis, typing by monoclonal antibodies to surface antigens, and restriction fragment length polymorphism (Box 86-1).[9–19] Earlier reports that *E. histolytica* and *E. dispar* could convert in culture[20,21] were impossible to reconcile with the genetic differences demonstrated between these two species, and were recently shown to be artifactual, with the apparent conversion due to inadvertent contamination of *E. dispar* cultures with *E. histolytica*.[22]

E. dispar and *E. moshkovskii* have never been documented to cause colitis or liver abscess. Because *E. dispar* and perhaps *E. moshkovskii* infection are more common than *E. histolytica* infection[23] and need not be treated, an important clinical advance has been the development of antigen detection tests that differentiate infection by the two amebae (see Diagnosis).

Life Cycle

The *E. histolytica* life cycle consists of an infective cyst and an invasive trophozoite form: The invasive trophozoite form is 10 to 60 μm in diameter and has a single nucleus with a central karyosome (Fig. 86-1A), while the cyst is 10 to 15 μm in diameter and contains four or fewer nuclei (Fig. 86-1B). Formation of the cyst appears to involve quorum sensing mediated in part by the parasite cell surface Gal/GalNAc lectin.[24] The quadrinucleate cyst is resistant to chlorination, gastric acidity, and desiccation and can survive in a moist environment for several weeks. Infection with *E. histolytica* occurs when cysts are ingested from fecally contaminated food or water. Excystation occurs in the intestine where a cyst undergoes nuclear followed by cytoplasmic division to form eight trophozoites. Trophozoites have the ability to colonize or invade the large bowel while cysts are never found within invaded tissues. Invasion of the intestinal mucosal barrier by

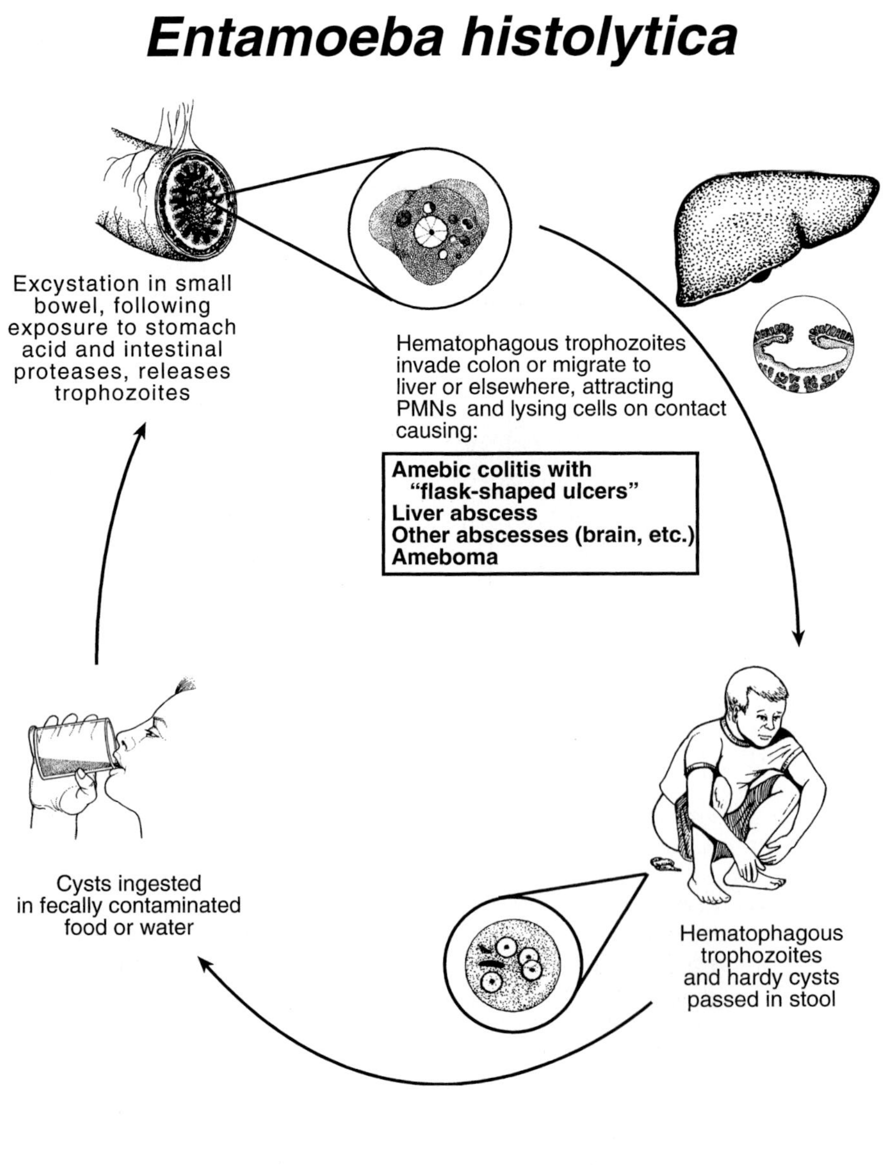

Box 86-1 Differentiation of *Entamoeba histolytica* and *Entamoeba dispar*

Biochemical Characteristics
Discrimination by isoenzyme migration
Immunologic Characteristics
Monoclonal antibodies
Genetic Characteristics
Restriction fragment pattern comparisons
Repetitive DNA sequences
Riboprinting
Clinical Characteristics
E. dispar and *E. moskkovskii* have not been associated with tissue invasion

From Petri WA Jr: Recent advances in amebiasis. Crit Rev Clin Lab Sci 33:1, 1996. Copyright Lewis Publishers, an imprint of CRC Press.

the trophozoite leads to the formation of flask-shaped colonic ulcers. Migration of colonic parasites to the liver is thought to occur via the portal vein. Whether or not infection results in colonization or invasion may be influenced by the *E. histolytica* strain and its interaction with bacterial flora; host genetic susceptibility; and factors such as malnutrition, sex, age, and immunocompetence.

Cell Biology and Biochemistry

E. histolytica is a eukaryotic organism but lacks organelles that morphologically resemble rough endoplasmic reticulum, the Golgi apparatus, or mitochondria[25–28] (Fig. 86-2; Box 86-2). The presence of nuclear-encoded mitochondrial genes, such as pyridine nucleotide transhydrogenase and *hsp*60, is consistent with *E. histolytica* having contained mitochondria at one time. Despite the lack of rough endoplasmic reticulum or Golgi apparatus, cell surface and secreted proteins contain signal sequences, and tunicamycin inhibits protein glycosylation.[26] Ribosomes form aggregated crystalline arrays in the cytoplasm of the trophozoite. Biochemical pathways differ from metazoans in the lack of glutathione and enzymes required for glutathione metabolism, the use of pyrophosphate instead of adenosine triphosphate (ATP) at several steps in glycolysis, and the inability to synthesize purine nucleotides de novo. Glucose is actively transported into the cytoplasm, where the end products of carbohydrate metabolism are ethanol, CO_2, and, under aerobic conditions, acetate.[25]

Gene Structure and Organization

E. histolytica genomic organization and promoter elements appear to be distinct from both metazoan and better-characterized protozoan organisms. The lack of mitochondria in *E. histolytica* and recombinant DNA (rDNA) sequence analysis[26] suggest that this organism is a primitive eukaryote related to *Dictyostelium*. However, phylogenetic analysis of the elongation factor 1α gene[27] and mitochondrial enzyme genes found within the *E. histolytica* genome[28] are consistent with *Entamoeba* having lost mitochondria and being more closely related to *Euglena gracilis* or *Trypanosoma cruzi*.

The sequencing of the HM1:IMSS strain of *E. histolytica* is near completion in a joint effort of the Institute for Genomic Research and the Sanger Center. Many aspects of *E. histolytica* gene organization and transcription are unusual.[29] Up to 50% of the genome is comprised of repetitive elements including

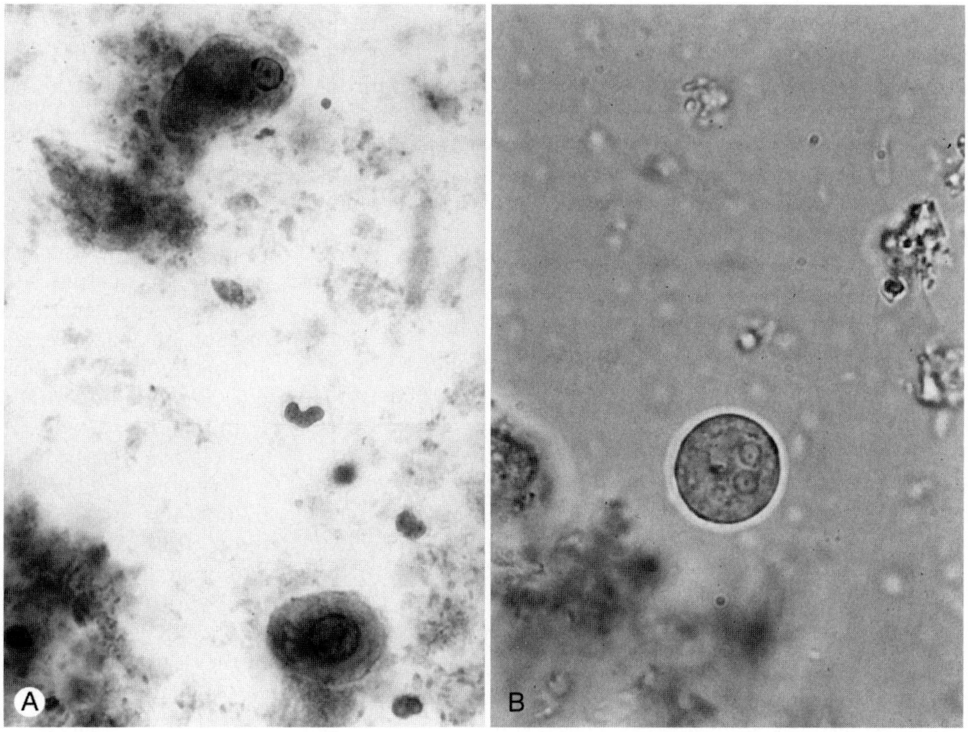

FIGURE 86-1 *Entamoeba histolytica* trophozoite and cyst. *A*, The motile and invasive trophozoite form contains a single nucleus and is 10 to 60 μm in diameter. *B*, The infectious cyst form is 10 to 15 μm in diameter and contains four nuclei. Note that it is not possible to distinguish *E. histolytica* from *E. dispar* morphologically. (Courtesy of Centers for Disease Control and Prevention, Atlanta, GA.)

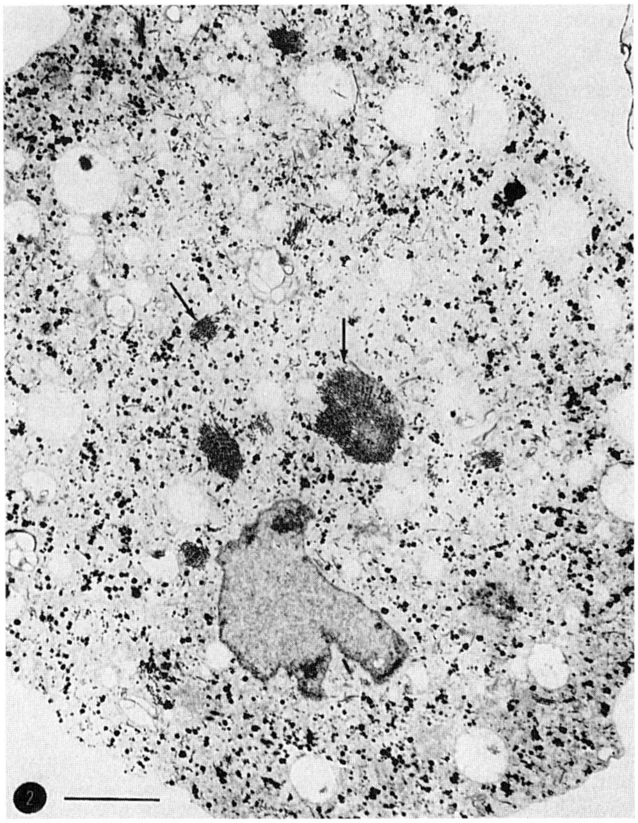

FIGURE 86-2 Electron micrograph of an *Entamoeba histolytica* trophozoite. Note the nucleus with peripheral and central chromatin, the lack of structures resembling mitochondria or rough endoplasmic reticulum, and the prominent intracytoplasmic vacuoles.

unusual tandem repeats of tRNA and 5s rRNA genes as well as retrotransposon-like elements. The genome is relatively small for a eukaryote (3.2×10^7 bp) and extremely AT-rich (67% within coding regions and 78% overall[29,30]). Transcription of protein-encoding genes is by an RNA polymerase which is resistant to 1 mg/mL α-amanitin.[31] Introns appear to be present in only 20% of genes.[32,33] There is no evidence of transplicing or polycistronic transcription.[34] However, coding regions are tightly packed, with small intergenic regions.[34] The structure of messenger RNA (mRNA) is remarkable as well, with the 5′-untranslated region having an average length of 11 bases compared to a metazoan average of 60 to 80 bases.[35] The 3′-untranslated region is also short, with an average size of only 33 bases.[34] Ribosomal RNA (rRNA) is not contained within the genome but is encoded on a circular, 24-kb DNA episome.[36]

Box 86-2 Some Unusual Features of the Cell Biology and Biochemistry of *Entamoeba histolytica*

- Lack of mitochondria, rough endoplasmic reticulum, or Golgi apparatus
- Presence of crystalline arrays of aggregated ribosomes
- Ribosomal RNA genes on multicopy circular DNA molecules
- Lack of glutathione and enzymes of glutathione metabolism
- Use of pyrophosphate instead of adenosine triphosphate at several steps in glycolysis
- Inability to synthesize purine nucleotides de novo

From Petri WA Jr: Recent advances in amebiasis. Crit Rev Clin Lab Sci 33:1, 1996. Copyright Lewis Publishers, an imprint of CRC Press.

Both transient and stable DNA-mediated transfection of *E. histolytica* with heterologous gene expression have been recently accomplished (Fig. 86-3). Deletion and replacement analysis has been conducted on the promoter of the *E. histolytica* gene encoding the heavy subunit of the *N*-acetyl-β-D-galactosamine-specific adhesin (*hgl5*).[37] Four positive upstream regulatory elements and one negative upstream regulatory element were identified in the 200 bases upstream of the start of transcription (Fig. 86-4). The transcription factors that control gene expression by these upstream regulatory elements have been identified in two cases. Both transcription factors are novel, with one containing RNA-binding motifs and the other EF-hand motifs.[38,39] Strikingly, the ability of the EF-hand containing transcription factor to bind to its cognate DNA motif is controlled by calcium.[39,40] Core promoter elements, including a TATA element at 30 bp upstream of the transcription start site, the novel conserved sequence GAAC, which is located between the TATA and initiator elements, and the conserved sequence at the transcription start site (putative initiator), have been demonstrated to regulate gene expression and control the site of transcription initiation.[41,42]

EPIDEMIOLOGY

The distribution of *E. dispar* is worldwide, while the preponderance of *E. histolytica* infection, morbidity, and mortality is experienced in Central and South America, Africa, and the Indian subcontinent. The epidemiology of amebiasis is being re-examined in light of the recently appreciated distinction between *E. histolytica, E. moshkovskii*, and *E. dispar*. Surveys that determined prevalence of infection by examining stool for parasites may have measured predominantly *E. dispar* and *E. moshkovskii* as these species are more common, while serologic surveys reflected the incidence of *E. histolytica* infection, as *E. dispar* and *E. moshkovskii* infection do not result in a positive serologic test.[43]

Two recent studies from the developing world using modern diagnostic tests have highlighted the burden of amebic disease. In Dhaka, Bangladesh, preschool children had a 2.2% annual frequency of amebic dysentery as compared to a 5.3% rate of *Shigella* dysentery during 3 years of prospective community observation.[44] An annual incidence of amebic liver abscess of 21 cases/100,000 inhabitants was observed in Hue City, Vietnam.[45] The 1987–1988 Mexican national survey of 67,668 serums (acquired by a probabilistic sampling technique from a representative cross-section of the country) demonstrated a 8.4% seropositivity for *E. histolytica* as measured with the indirect hemagglutination assay (IHA).[46] Peak seropositivity was 11% in the 5- to 9-year-old age group. In the year of the serosurvey there was an estimated 1 million cases of amebiasis and 1216 deaths due to *E. histolytica* infection in Mexico.[47]

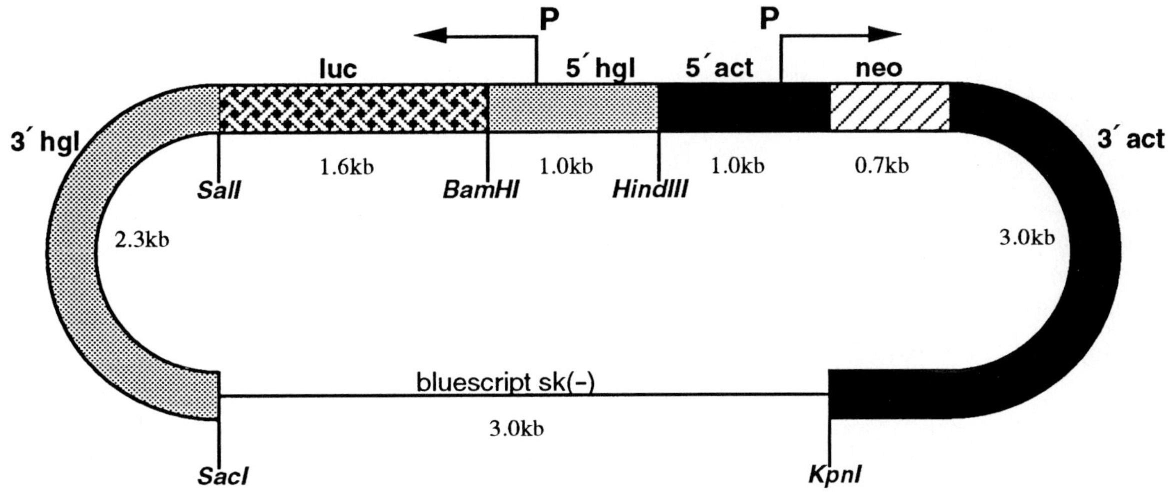

FIGURE 86-3 The two-promoter transfection vector pTCV3. The actin promoter is used to express *neo*, enabling selection of stably transfected parasites with the antibiotic G418. The lectin *hgl* promoter is used to express a gene of interest in the stably transfected amebae, which in this case is firefly luciferase.

Residents of developed nations such as the United States that are at higher risk of developing amebiasis include, most importantly, immigrants from or travelers to countries where amebiasis is endemic,[48–51] sexually active male homosexuals (who are predominantly infected with *E. dispar*[52,53]), and residents of institutions for the mentally retarded.[54] A total of 2970 cases of amebiasis in the United States were reported to the Centers for Disease Control and Prevention in 1993 (the last year that it was a reportable disease); 33% of the patients were Hispanic and 17% Asian or Pacific Islanders.[55]

Amebic liver abscess is 7 to 12 times more common in men, although in children the sex distribution is equal.[56,57] More severe disease is seen in the very young and old, the malnourished, and pregnant women.[58–61] *E. histolytica* infection in human immunodeficiency virus (HIV)–infected children was clustered in the most severely malnourished children with chronic diarrhea in a study from Tanzania.[62]

The typical patient in the United States with amebic liver abscess is a Hispanic male between the ages of 20 and 40 years. Infection with *E. histolytica* generally presents clinically within a year of immigration to the United States, although it is not rare for presentation to lag immigration by up to 12 years. Travelers to the tropics are at low but definite risk of acquiring amebic infection: one study of 2700 German citizens returning from tropical areas demonstrated a 4% incidence of *E. histolytica/E. dispar* infection.[51,63,64] Diarrhea and detection of *E. histolytica* only (no other intestinal pathogens present) occurred in 80% of travelers with pathogenic *E. histolytica*.[51]

DISEASE

Asymptomatic Colonization

Noninvasive intestinal infection is apparently the only presentation of *E. dispar* and *E. moshkovskii* infection and is also a common presentation of *E. histolytica* infection (Box 86-3). Patients may have some ill-defined gastrointestinal complaints, but for the most part tolerate the infection well. Colonization with *E. dispar* and *E. moshkovskii* does not require intervention on the part of the physician, as these amebae have never been identified as a cause of colitis or abscess. In contrast, patients colonized with *E. histolytica* are at risk of future (months to even years later) development of invasive disease and should be treated if coincidentally diagnosed.[65] Antigen detection tests to distinguish *E. histolytica*

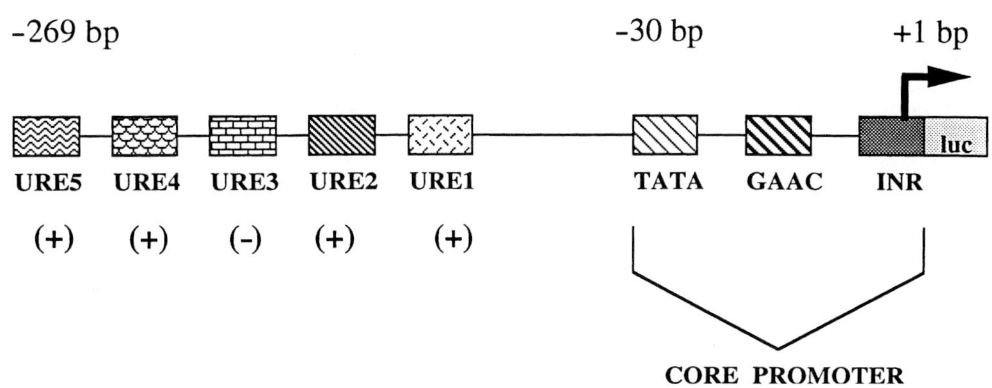

FIGURE 86-4 Structure of the promoter of the *hgl*5 gene of *Entamoeba histolytica*. Four positive and one negative upstream regulatory regions have been identified by linker scanner mutagenesis and transient transfection system using the reporter gene luciferase. Three regions have also been identified in the core promoter which appear to control gene expression.

Box 86-3 Clinical Manifestations of *Entamoeba* Infection

Asymptomatic Colonization

E. histolytica
E. dispar
E. moshkovskii

***Intestinal Amebiasis and Its Complications* (E. histolytica *Only*)**

Amebic colitis
Ameboma
Toxic megacolon
Peritonitis
Cutaneous amebiasis

***Extraintestinal Amebiasis* (E. histolytica *Only*)**

Amebic liver abscess
Splenic abscess
Brain abscess
Empyema
Pericarditis

From Petri WA Jr: Recent advances in amebiasis. Crit Rev Clin Lab Sci 33:1, 1996. Copyright Lewis Publishers, an imprint of CRC Press.

from *E. dispar* and *E. moshkovskii* infection are commercially available for clinical use (see Diagnosis).

Almost all *E. histolytica/moshkovskii/dispar* isolates from colonized homosexual males in Europe and the United States are *E. dispar*[52,65–67]; this explains the general lack of invasive amebiasis in this population at risk of HIV infection. In patients with HIV infection, no correlation has been established between the presence of *E. dispar* and gastrointestinal symptoms, and apparently antiamebic treatment is not warranted. In Japan the situation is different: 13% to 20% of homosexual men are seropositive for *E. histolytica* infection, the organism has been isolated from the stools of homosexual men, and cases of invasive amebiasis have been reported in homosexual and HIV-infected males.[68–70] This indicates the need for a more aggressive approach to the management of intestinal amebic infection in homosexual males in Japan, and demonstrates the potential for spread of pathogenic *E. histolytica* to the homosexual populations of other nations.

Dysentery and Colitis

The major concern of the physician confronted with a patient with dysentery (diarrhea that contains visible or microscopic blood) is to differentiate between infectious causes (including amebiasis, *Shigella, Salmonella, Campylobacter*, and enteroinvasive and enterohemorrhagic *Escherichia coli*) and noninfectious causes (including inflammatory bowel disease, ischemic colitis, and gastrointestinal bleeding secondary to arteriovenous malformations or diverticulitis).[70] It is at times difficult to make the diagnosis of amebic colitis, as the presentation of the illness may be insidious or chronic, bleeding may occur without diarrhea, and fever is an unusual finding. A single stool examination for parasites is insensitive, histopathologic confirmation of infection on biopsy specimens may be difficult, and serologic tests for antiamebic antibodies are not always positive in the acute setting (Table 86-1).

In a developed country such as the United States, most patients with amebiasis will be immigrants or travelers from areas with endemic amebiasis. Patients with amebic colitis typically present with a history over several weeks of gradual onset of abdominal pain and tenderness, diarrhea, and bloody stools. In one series, patients with amebic colitis had an average duration of prehospital illness of 21 days, compared with 4 days for patients with shigellosis.[71] Because of the gradual onset, weight loss is a common finding. Surprisingly, fever is present in only the minority (8% to 38%) of patients with amebic colitis.[71,72] Examination of stools reveals that they are uniformly positive for occult blood; microscopic examination of stool for *E. histolytica* cysts and trophozoites is very insensitive: A single examination is positive in only one-third to one-half of cases, with three or more examinations required in most cases to identify the organism. Stool antigen detection (the TechLab *E. histoloytica* II Test) and PCR are more sensitive than microscopy and are the only tests specific for *E. histolytica* infection.[72] Colonic lesions can vary from only mucosal thickening, to flask-shaped ulcerations, to necrosis of the intestinal wall (Fig. 86-5).

Unusual manifestations of amebic colitis include acute necrotizing colitis, ameboma (granulation tissue in colonic lumen mimicking colonic cancer in appearance), cutaneous amebiasis, and rectovaginal fistulas. Acute fulminant or necrotizing colitis is the most feared complication, occurs in about 0.5% of cases, may require surgical intervention, and has a mortality greater than 40%.[73,74] Abdominal pain, distention, and rebound tenderness are present in most patients with fulminant colitis, although frank guarding is uncommon.

Indications for surgery in fulminant amebic colitis include free extraperitoneal perforation, failure of a perforation with a localized abscess to respond to antiamebic drugs, and perhaps persistence of abdominal distention and tenderness while on antiamebic therapy. With localized colonic disease, partial colectomy with exteriorization of the ends is recommended over primary anastomosis, as anastomoses may fail due to the friable condition of the bowel wall. Better surgical results for extensive disease have been achieved with total colectomy with exteriorization of the proximal and distal ends.[73,74]

Table 86-1 *Symptoms and Signs of Amebic Colitis*

Symptoms and Signs	Percentage
Gradual onset	Most
History of symptoms >1 wk	Most
Diarrhea	94–100
Dysentery	94–100
Abdominal pain	12–80
Weight loss	44
Fever >38°C	10
Heme (+) stools	100
Male-female ratio	1:1
Immigrant from or traveler to endemic area	Most

From Petri WA Jr: Recent advances in amebiasis. Crit Rev Clin Lab Sci 33:1, 1996. Copyright Lewis Publishers, an imprint of CRC Press.

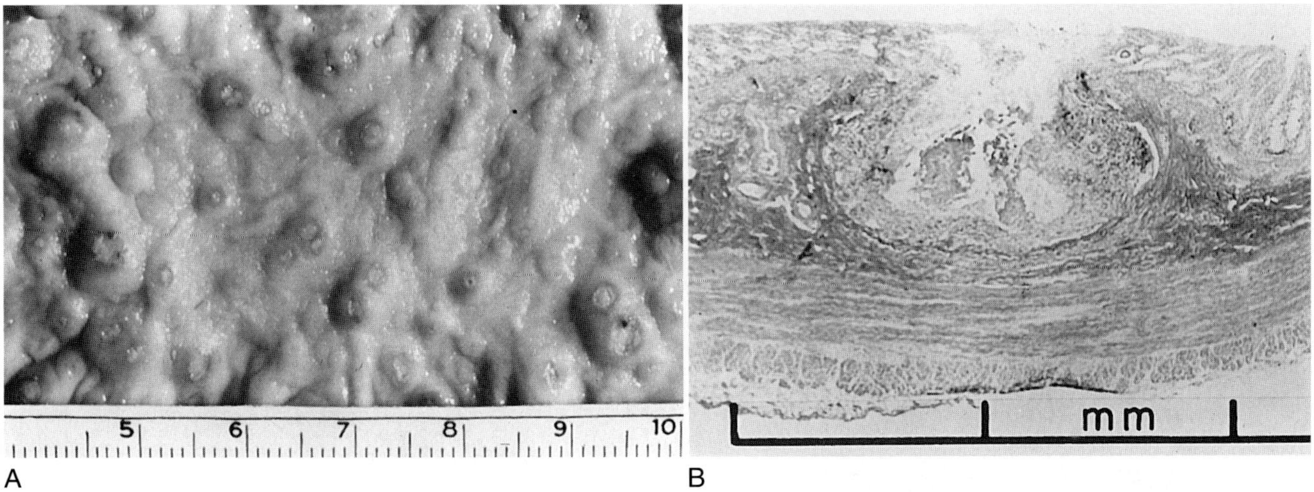

FIGURE 86-5 Amebic colitis. *A*, Multiple mucosal ulcers are visible in the resected section of the colon (the smallest division of the scale is 1 mm). *B*, Mucosal ulceration of amebic colitis, with extension of the ulcer into the submucosa. (H&E stain.) (From the collection of the late Harrison Juniper.)

Liver Abscess

A typical patient with an amebic liver abscess in the United States is an immigrant, usually a Hispanic male, 20 to 40 years old. A 1- to 2-week history of fever and abdominal pain is common. Signs of amebic liver abscess include right upper quadrant pain, fever of 38.5°C to 39.5°C, leukocytosis, abnormal serum transaminases and alkaline phosphatase, an elevated right hemidiaphragm, and a defect on hepatic imaging study[56,57,75,76] (Table 86-2; Fig. 86-6). A more chronic presentation of 2 to 12 weeks of weight loss, fever, and abdominal pain has been reported in a subset of patients with single abscesses.[57] Roughly 90% of patients with liver abscess are males, although in children (especially infants[77,78]) the sex distribution is equal. The abscess is single and in the right lobe of the liver 80% of the time. However, the most common location for a pyogenic abscess is also in the right lobe, so the location is not helpful in distinguishing the cause of an abscess.[79,80] Patients with pyogenic, as opposed to amebic, liver abscesses are more likely to be older than 50 years, present with jaundice, pruritis, sepsis, or shock, and have a palpable mass.[81]

Most patients with liver abscess do not have concurrent colitis, although a history of dysentery within the last year can sometimes be obtained. Amebae are infrequently identified microscopically in the stool (18% of cases) at the time of diagnosis of liver abscess, although they can be identified in the stool by culture in the majority of patients. Liver abscess can present acutely with fever, right upper abdominal tenderness and pain, or subacutely with prominent weight loss, fever, and abdominal pain. The peripheral white blood cell count and alkaline phosphatase level are often elevated. Chest radiograph demonstrates elevation of the right hemidiaphragm in most patients.[82,83] Early evaluation of the hepatobiliary system with ultrasound, computed tomography (CT), or magnetic resonance imaging (MRI) is essential to demonstrate the abscess in the liver.

The differential diagnosis of the lesion in the liver would include pyogenic abscess (less likely if the gallbladder and intrahepatic ducts appear normal), hepatoma, and echinococcal cyst (unlikely to present acutely with fever and abdominal pain). Aspiration of the abscess is occasionally required to diagnose amebiasis. The lack of bacterial infection in the abscess fluid is most helpful in ruling out a pyogenic abscess; amebae are rarely visualized in the pus in only the minority of cases but PCR for *E. histolytica* appears to be very sensitive. Antibodies to *E. histolytica* are present in the serum of 92% to 97% of patients on acute presentation with amebic liver abscess, and therefore are very useful diagnostically. Because a significant proportion of the population in developing countries is seropositive, antibody tests are less specific in residents or immigrants from the developing world (see Diagnosis).

Severe amebic liver abscess, defined in one study as an abscess that ruptures despite at least three days of antiamebic treatment or an abscess complicated by secondary bacterial infection, may be associated with dyspnea, elevated right hemidiaphragm and pleural effusion, jaundice, anemia, and diabetes mellitus.[83,84] Patients with findings associated with more severe disease might benefit from early drainage. Intrathoracic and intraperitoneal rupture of an amebic liver

Table 86-2 *Symptoms and Signs of Amebic Liver Abscess*

Symptoms and Signs	Range
History of symptoms >4 wk	21%–51%
Fever	85%–90%
Abdominal tenderness	84%–90%
Hepatomegaly	30%–50%
Jaundice	6%–10%
Diarrhea	20%–33%
Weight loss	33%–50%
Cough	10%–30%
Male-female ratio	9:1
Immigrant from or traveler to endemic area	Most

From Petri WA Jr: Recent advances in amebiasis. Crit Rev Clin Lab Sci 33:1, 1996. Copyright Lewis Publishers, an imprint of CRC Press.

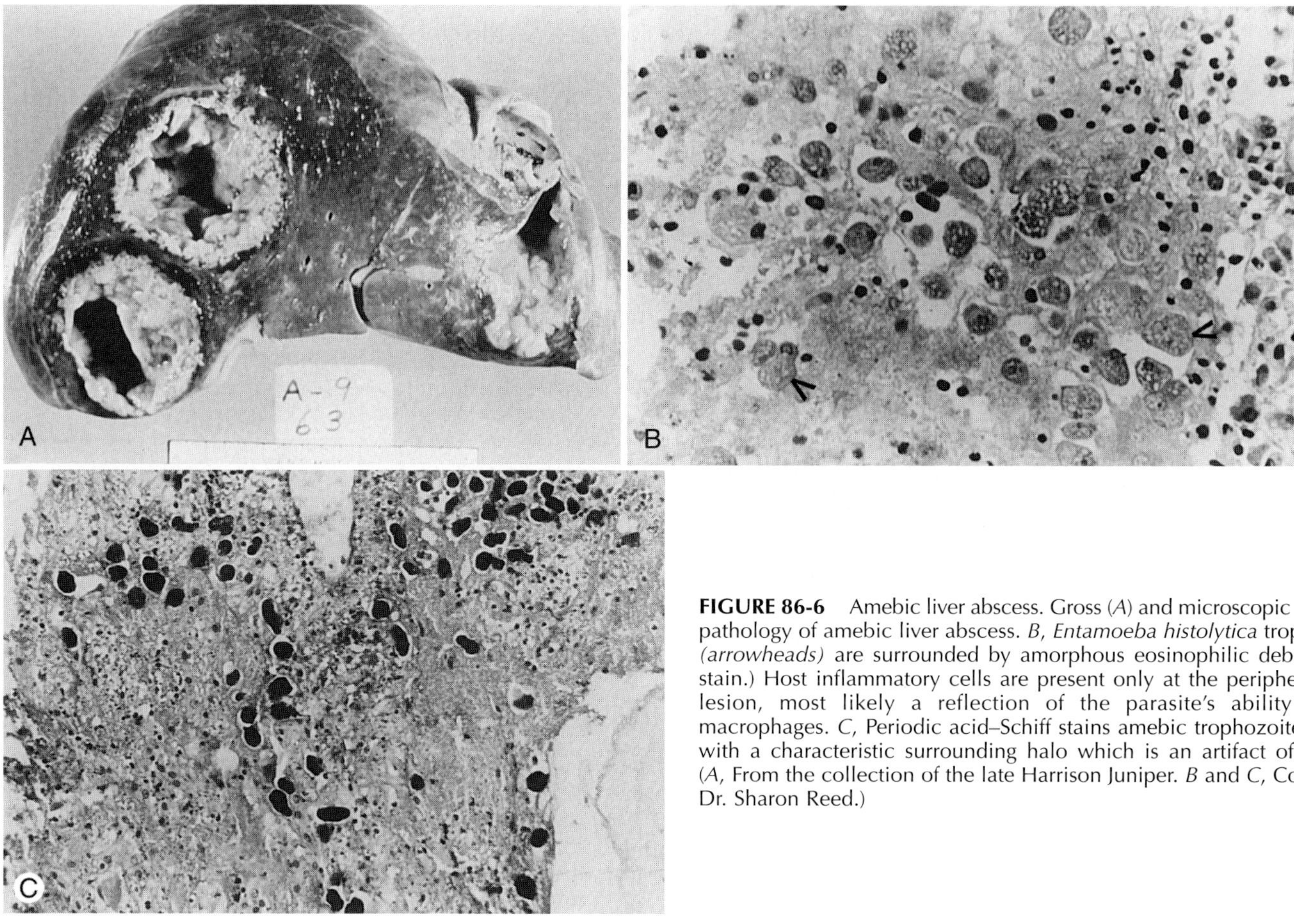

FIGURE 86-6 Amebic liver abscess. Gross (*A*) and microscopic (*B* and *C*) pathology of amebic liver abscess. *B*, *Entamoeba histolytica* trophozoites *(arrowheads)* are surrounded by amorphous eosinophilic debris. (H&E stain.) Host inflammatory cells are present only at the periphery of the lesion, most likely a reflection of the parasite's ability to lyse macrophages. *C*, Periodic acid–Schiff stains amebic trophozoites darkly, with a characteristic surrounding halo which is an artifact of fixation. (*A*, From the collection of the late Harrison Juniper. *B* and *C*, Courtesy of Dr. Sharon Reed.)

abscess can be adequately treated with antiamebic therapy without surgery if secondary bacterial infection is absent.[83]

Unusual extraintestinal manifestations of amebiasis include direct extension of the liver abscess to pleura or pericardium, brain abscess, and genitourinary amebiasis.

PATHOGENESIS

Carbohydrate-protein interactions play a key role in human infection by the *E. histolytica*.[84] Killing of host cells by *E. histolytica* trophozoites in vitro occurs only on direct contact (Fig. 86-7), which is mediated by an amebic adhesin which recognizes N- and O-linked oligosaccharides.[85–91] This amebic Gal/GalNAc lectin is a heterodimer of heavy and light subunits noncovalently associated with an intermediate subunit, all of which are encoded by multigene families designated *hgl*, *lgl*, and *igl*, respectively.[85–91] Apposition of amebic and target cell plasma membranes, as can be achieved by centrifugation of target cells and amebae into a pellet, will not lead to cytolysis if the amebic lectin is inhibited with Gal/GalNAc. This indicates that the lectin not only mediates adherence, but also participates in the cytolytic event. Antilectin monoclonal antibodies (mAbs) directed against epitope 1 of the lectin-heavy subunit block cytotoxicity but not adherence, implicating the lectin in the cytotoxic as well as adherence events. Antilectin antibodies that block cytotoxicity also cause a conformational change in the lectin, which increases carbohydrate binding capacity. One could speculate that such antibodies block cytotoxicity by preventing a second conformational change in the lectin required for cell killing.

The first receptor encountered by the lectin may be the human colonic mucin layer of the large intestine.[92] Binding of the lectin to colonic mucins is Gal/GalNAc-inhibitable and of very high affinity (dissociation constant of 8.2×10^{-11} M^{-1}). Interaction of trophozoites with colonic mucins appears to be a dynamic process, with trophozoites both inducing the secretion of, and degrading, colonic mucins.[92] The mucin layer may protect the host from contact-dependent cytotoxicity of the parasite by binding to and neutralizing the lectin, while at the same time serving as a site of attachment for the parasite to colonize the large bowel.

Invasion of the colon and hematogenous spread to the liver results in the continuous exposure of the extracellular trophozoite to the human complement system. Virulent *E. histolytica* isolated from patients with invasive amebiasis activates the alternative complement pathway but is resistant to C5b-9 complexes deposited on the membrane surface.[93] Resistance to lysis by the membrane attack complex of complement suggested the presence of a C5b-9 inhibitory molecule

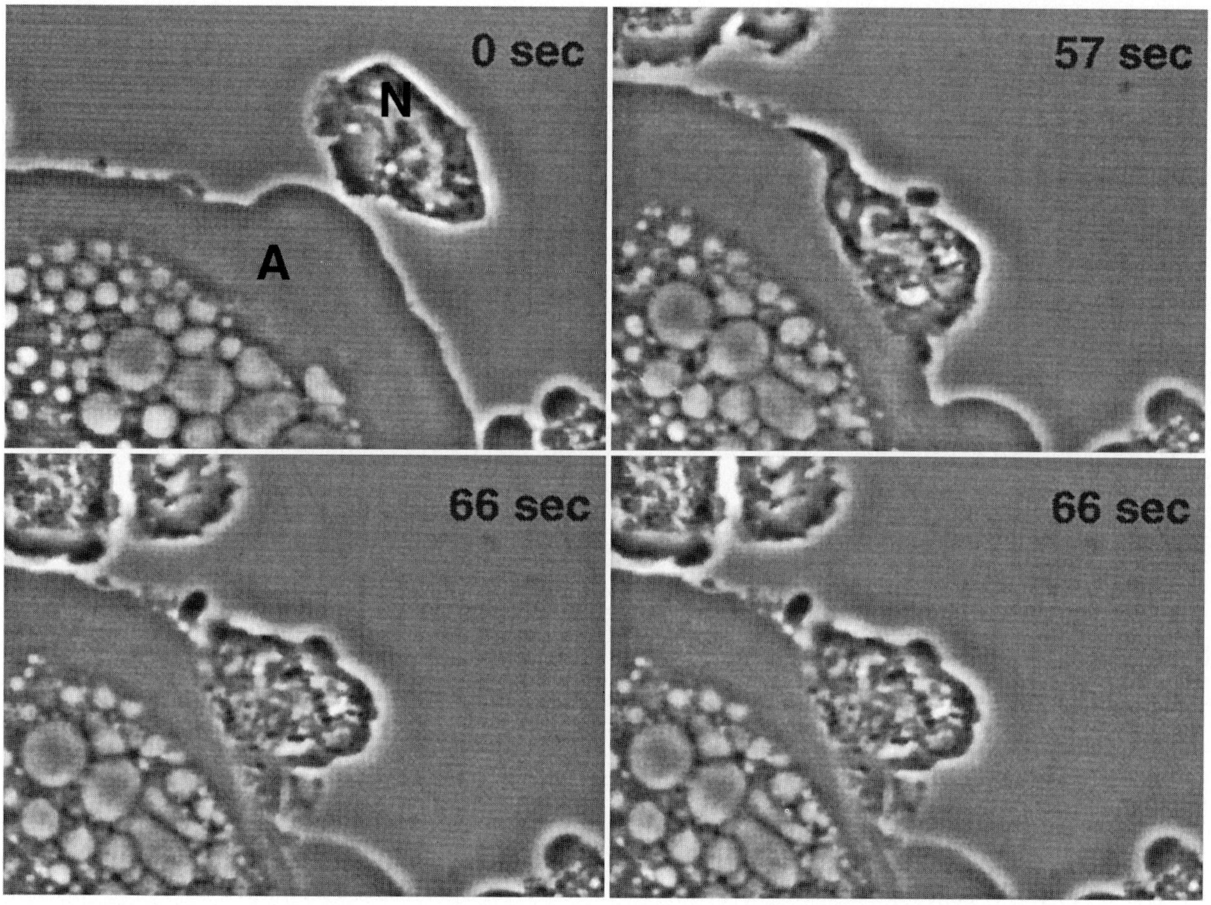

FIGURE 86-7 Killing of a human polymorphonuclear neutrophil (N) by an ameba (A). On establishing contact with the ameba, the neutrophil undergoes membrane blebbing and loss of granules and cytoplasmic integrity. (Magnification 2000×.) (From Ravdin JI, Guerrant RL: Current problems in diagnosis and treatment of amebic infections. Curr Clin Top Infect Dis 7:82–111, 1996.)

in the amebic surface. This C5b-9 inhibitory molecule was identified as the Gal/GalNAc lectin by screening for monoclonal antibodies that increased *E. histolytica* lysis by serum and purified complement.[94] Examination of the sequence of the 170-kD subunit showed limited identity with CD59, a human inhibitor of C5b-9 assembly, and the purified lectin was recognized by anti-CD59 antibodies. The lectin bound to purified human C8 and C9, and blocked assembly in the amebic membrane of the complement membrane attack complex at the steps of C8 and C9 insertion. Reconstitution of the lectin from serum-resistant into serum-sensitive amebae conferred resistance to the membrane attack complex, a direct demonstration of its C5b-9 inhibitory activity. The lectin therefore appears to function not only in adherence and host cell killing, but also in evasion of the complement system of defense via a remarkable mimicry of human CD59.[94] Recent evidence points to the cytoplasmic domain of the lectin in controlling lectin activity by inside-out signaling, through a region with homology to β_2 integrins.[95]

Contact-dependent killing by *E. histolytica*, after evasion of the colonic mucin layer, has been the subject of intensive investigation. Intracellular calcium in target cells rises approximately 20-fold within seconds of direct contact by an amebic trophozoite and is associated with membrane blebbing.[96] Cell death occurs 5 to 15 minutes after the lethal hit is delivered. Extracellular ethylenediaminetetracetate (EDTA) and treatment of the target cells with the slow sodium-calcium channel blockers verapamil and bepridil[97] significantly reduce amebic killing of target cells in suspension. Murine myeloid cells killed by *E. histolytica* undergo a process of death that morphologically resembles the programmed cell death seen with growth factor deprivation and is associated with a nucleosomal pattern of DNA fragmentation. Apoptotic death is followed by ingestion of the host cell.[98]

Isolation of an amebic pore-forming protein similar in function to pore-forming proteins of the immune system has been reported.[99] A purified 5-kD amoebapore and a synthetic peptide based on the sequence of its third amphipathic α helix have recently been shown to have cytolytic activity for nucleated cells at high concentrations (10 to 100 μM).[99] Interaction with the extracellular matrix may be mediated by fibronectin, laminin, and collagen receptors.[100,101] Proteolytic activities, such as the collagenase contained within electron-dense granules in the amebic cytoplasm, are also believed to be involved in damage to cells and the extracellular matrix of the host. Secreted amebic cysteine proteases cause a cytopathic (as opposed to cytotoxic) effect manifest by cells being released from monolayers in vitro without cell death.[102] In vivo validation of the role of the lectin, cysteine proteinases, and amebapore has recently been accomplished by reverse genetic techniques.[103-106]

IMMUNITY

Immunity to infection is associated with a mucosal IgA response against the carbohydrate recognition domain of the Gal/GalNAc lectin: children with this response had 86% fewer new infections over one year of prospective observation[107,108] (Fig. 86-8).

Several lines of evidence suggest an important role for cell-mediated immunity, via cytokine activation of macrophages and neutrophils, to kill amebae. In animal models, interventions that resulted in a depression of cellular immunity, such as neonatal thymectomy, splenectomy, steroid treatment, radiation, silica therapy, and antimacrophage or anti-lymphocyte globulin, resulted in enhanced amebic liver abscess. Lymphocytes from patients recovered from invasive amebic disease developed cell-mediated immune responses in vitro against total *E. histolytica* extracts. These responses included T-cell proliferation, amebicidal activity, and interleukin-2 (IL-2) and interferon-γ (IFN-γ) production.[109–113] Human macrophages and neutrophils, activated with IFN-γ and tumor necrosis factor-α (TNF-α), are endowed with the capability of killing *E. histolytica* trophozoites, while in the absence of IFN-γ, these effector cells were killed by the amebae. In murine macrophages, TNF-α was shown to play a central role in activating macrophages for nitric oxide–dependent cytotoxicity against *E. histolytica*. A CD4 T cell–mediated immune response may not always be protective: In the murine model of amebic colitis depeletion of CD4 T cells has been shown to ameliorate inflammation and colonic ulceration.[114]

The association of anti-parasite IgA anibody with in vivo resistance to infection, as well as the ability of pro-inflammatory cytokines to activate protective immunity in vitro suggested that MHC class II alleles could affect both the acquisition of amebiasis and its disease burden. To test this hypothesis, class II genotype frequencies were determined among a cohort of unrelated Bangladeshi children who had been followed every other day for 3 years for *E. histolytica* infection. Individuals heterozygous for the DQB1*0601/ DRB1*1501 haplotype were 10.1 times (95% CI: 2.02, 50.6) more likely not to have been infected with *E. histolytica*. Other DQB1 and DRB1 alleles (DQB1*0202, DQB1*0301, DRB1*0701) showed no evidence of association with any of the clinical outcomes related to amebiasis. This potential protective association may offer insight into why amebiasis does not occur in some children exposed to the parasite, and implicates class II restricted immune responses in protection from *E. histolytica* infection.[115]

DIAGNOSIS

See Table 86-3 for a summary of test sensitivity for amebiasis diagnosis.

Microscopy

Microscopic identification of the parasite in stool, liver abscess pus, or colonic biopsies is neither sensitive nor

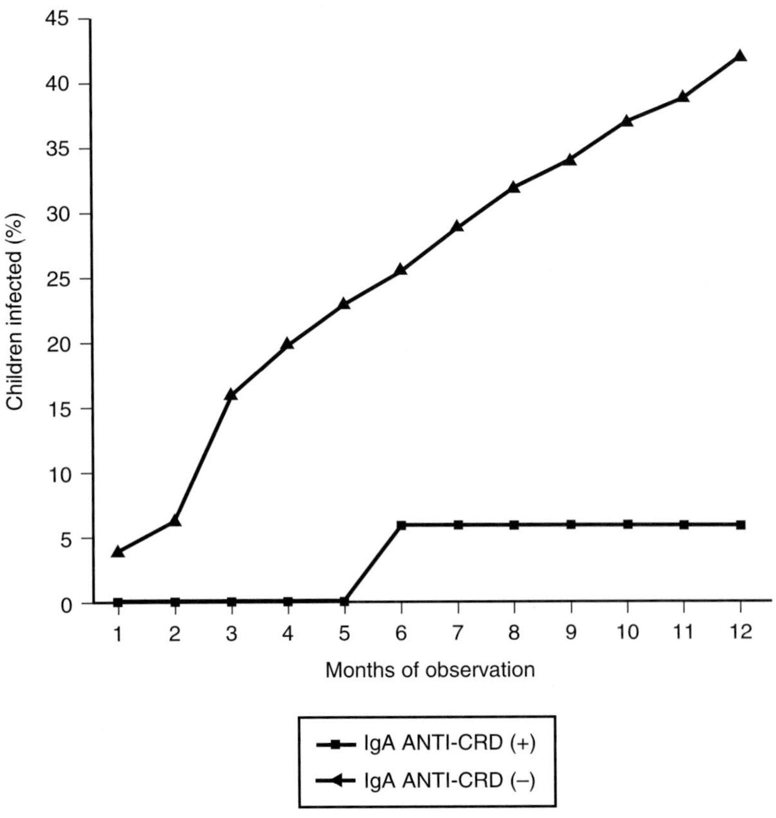

FIGURE 86-8 Acquired immunity to amebiasis in children. Children who developed stool IgA anti-CRD (Lectin Carbohydrate Recognition Domain) antibodies in the first year of the study (n = 81) had a lower incidence of new *E. histolytica* infections in the second year compared to children who remained IgA anti-CRD negative (n = 149). The two groups are statistically significantly different ($p \leq 0.04$) at every time point. (From Haque R, Duggal P, Ali IM, et al: Innate and acquired resistance to amebiasis in Bangladeshi children. J Infect Dis 186:547–552, 2002.)

Table 86-3 Sensitivity of Tests for Diagnosis of Amebiasis

Test	Colitis	Liver
Microscopy (stool)	25%–60%	10%–40%
Stool antigen detection	>90%	~40%
Serum antigen detection	65% early	~100% prior to treatment
Microscopy (abscess fluid)	N/A	≤20%
Abscess antigen detection	N/A	~40%
Serology (indirect hemagglutination)		
Acute	70%	70%–80%
Convalescent	>90%	>90%

From Haque R, Huston CD, Hughes M, et al: Current Concepts: Amebiasis. New Engl J Med 348:1565–1573, 2003.

specific and should be replaced with *E. histolytica*–specific diagnostic tests (see following discussion). Microscopic examination of a single stool specimen for amebic cysts and trophozoites in a patient with amebic colitis is no more than 33% to 50% sensitive, and in most cases is unable to distinguish pathogenic *E. histolytica* from the morphologically identical nonpathogenic *E. moshkovskii* and *E. dispar* (formerly called the nonpathogenic zymodemes of *E. histolytica*).[116] Erythrophagocytic amebae are more likely to be *E. histolytica* than *E. dispar*, but *E. dispar* trophozoites have also been found to contain ingested red blood cells. Repeated stool examinations in patients with amebic liver abscess were able to detect the parasite in only 8% to 44% of cases.[79] Identification of the parasite in aspirated pus from liver abscesses, even in the most experienced hands, is only 20% sensitive.[70]

Antigen Detection

A stool antigen detection test that is specific for *E. histolytica* is now commercially available for clinical use from TechLab, Inc. (Blacksburg, VA)[72] (Fig. 86-9). The *E. histolytica* antigen test is rapid, has improved sensitivity compared to microscopy, and is of comparable sensitivity to culture or PCR analysis. The TechLab *E. histolytica* test is based on detection of the Gal/GalNAc lectin in stool. A test to detect the Gal/GalNAc lectin in serum appears promising for the diagnosis of amebic liver abscess (a situation in which it is more difficult than amebic colitis to demonstrate the parasite in stool), with a reported sensitivity in initial tests of 67%.[72]

Polymerase Chain Reaction

Polymerase chain reaction (PCR), based on amplification of the small subunit rRNA gene, can now be used to identify *E. histolytica* in stool samples. PCR and antigen detection had comparable sensitivities when performed on fresh stool samples, identifying 87% and 85% of *E. histolytica* infections subsequently identified by isoenzyme analysis.[72] PCR detection of *E. histolytica* DNA in both stool and liver abscess pus is a sensitive test.[117–119] Use of PCR can also be used also to distinguish among isolates of *E. histolytica*, which should prove useful for epidemiologic purposes as well as in determining the virulence characteristics of different isolates.[108,120,121]

Serology

The IHA test for antiamebic antibody is 70% sensitive early in the illness, to greater than 95% sensitive on convalescence, for the diagnosis of amebic liver abscess and amebic colitis.[70] Most recent reports of series of patients with liver abscess and colitis bear these numbers out. Early in the course of amebic liver abscess the IHA test may be negative.

The major problem with current serologic tests is that they remain positive for years after an episode of amebiasis. As a result, a substantial number (between 10% and 35%) of residents of developing countries have antiamebic antibodies detected by current serologic tests.[122–124] Since the vast majority of patients with invasive amebiasis in developed countries are immigrants from developing nations, serologic tests may not be as specific as one would hope. For example, in five recent series of patients in the United States with amebic liver abscess, between 80% and 96% of patients were immigrants. Therefore current serologic tests may be inadequate for the differentiation of acute from past amebiasis, even in developed nations, and one should not make the diagnosis of amebiasis in a native of a country where amebiasis is endemic on the basis of a serologic test alone.

Colonoscopy

Colonoscopy is preferable to sigmoidoscopy because disease may be localized to the cecum or ascending colon. Cathartics or enemas should not be used to prepare the

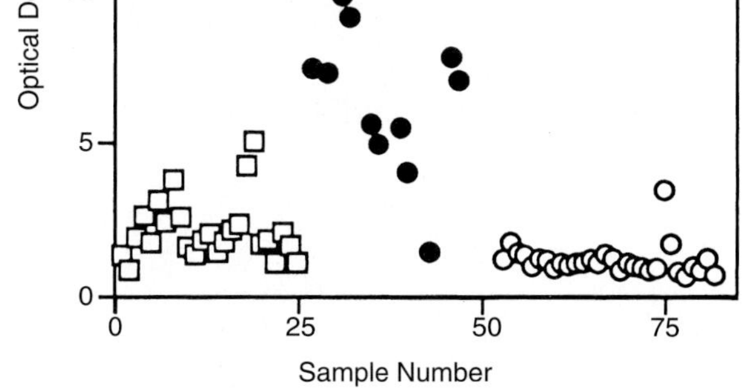

FIGURE 86-9 Antigen detection test for *Entamoeba histolytica* in stool. Stool specimens with culture-confirmed *E. dispar* (*squares*) or *E. histolytica* (*solid circles*) infection, or stools with no detectable *Entamoeba* detected by microscopy (*open circles*), were assayed using an enzyme-linked immunosorbent assay containing monoclonal antibody specific for *E. histolytica*.

patient because they will interfere with the identification of the parasite. Wet preparations of material aspirated or scraped from the base of ulcers should be examined for motile trophozoites and tested for *E. histolytica* antigen. The appearance of amebic colitis may resemble that of inflammatory bowel disease, with granular, friable, and diffusely ulcerated mucosa. Large geographic ulcers and pseudomembranes may also be present.[125–127] The detection rate of trophozoites upon histopathologic examination of colonic biopsy specimens from patients with amebic colitis varies in different reports from all to only some of the patients.[126–128] Biopsy specimens should be taken from the edge of the ulcers. Periodic acid–Schiff stains the parasites a magenta color (see Fig. 86-6), increasing the ease of detection in biopsies. *E. histolytica* has been shown to invade into carcinomas, causing diagnostic confusion.[128]

Imaging Procedures

Ultrasound, CT, and MRI studies of the liver are equally sensitive at detecting amebic abscesses (Fig. 86-10). All three techniques are incapable of differentiating an amebic from a pyogenic abscess.[129–132] At 6 months' follow-up, only one-third to two-thirds of amebic liver abscesses had disappeared upon reultrasonography.[129–132]

TREATMENT

Colonization with *E. histolytica* should be treated with a luminal agent alone; *E. dispar* and *E. moshkovskii* infection does not require treatment. Drugs effective against luminal infection include diloxanide furoate and paromomycin. Both agents are relatively well tolerated; the recommended duration of treatment with paromomycin is 7 days and with diloxanide furoate, 10 days.[133,134]

Invasive amebiasis (colitis, liver abscess, etc.) should be treated with metronidazole plus a luminal agent. The majority of patients with amebic liver abscess defervesce after 3 to 4 days' treatment with metronidazole. Metronidazole resistance has not yet been reported. Chloroquine, dehydroemetine, and percutaneous drainage of the liver abscess have all been

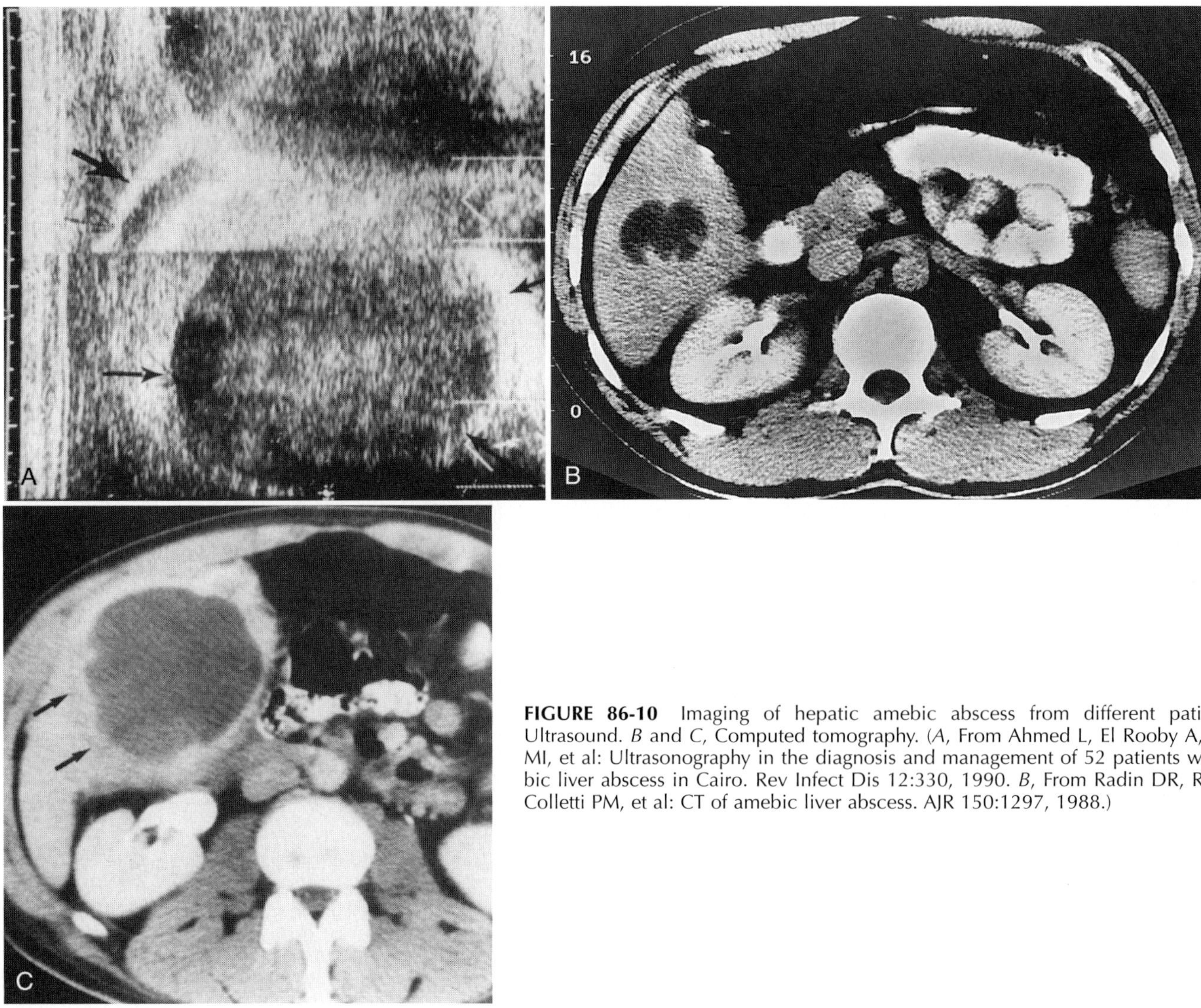

FIGURE 86-10 Imaging of hepatic amebic abscess from different patients. *A*, Ultrasound. *B* and *C*, Computed tomography. (*A*, From Ahmed L, El Rooby A, Kassem MI, et al: Ultrasonography in the diagnosis and management of 52 patients with amebic liver abscess in Cairo. Rev Infect Dis 12:330, 1990. *B*, From Radin DR, Ralls PW, Colletti PM, et al: CT of amebic liver abscess. AJR 150:1297, 1988.)

successfully added to metronidazole treatment for the rare patient not responding to metronidazole alone.[135–137] In most cases of liver abscess, percutaneous drainage is not required and does not speed recovery.[136,137] Metronidazole does not eliminate intestinal colonization in up to 50% of patients with invasive amebiasis unless therapy is prolonged for a minimum of 10 days. With shorter courses of metronidazole therapy, patients may suffer a relapse of invasive infection months later. For this reason the addition of a luminal agent is recommended.[70]

VACCINE DEVELOPMENT

Prevention of amebiasis at present requires interruption of the fecal-oral spread of the infectious cyst stage of the parasite by improved hygiene, sanitation, and water treatment. On the horizon is the development of a vaccine to prevent disease in residents of and travelers to the developing world. Both the Gal/GalNAc adherence lectin and the serine-rich antigen have proved effective in the prevention of liver abscess in the gerbil model of the disease.[138–141] Only the Gal/GalNAc lectin has been demonstrated to prevent intestinal infection with *E. histolytica*.[139] As opposed to the highly variable serine-rich antigen, the Gal/GalNAc lectin is highly conserved between isolates of *E. histolytica*.[86] Because mucosal IgA anti-Gal/GalNAc lectin antibody is a surrogate marker of the immune state in humans, vaccine design efforts are currently focused on means of mucosal immunization.[142,143]

OTHER INTESTINAL PROTOZOA

See Figure 86-11 for a summary of intestinal protozoa. *E. gingivalis* was the first parasitic ameba of humans to be described and has subsequently been isolated from a variety of human body sites, including teeth (pyorrhea alveolaris), tonsillar crypts, mucus, and vaginal and cervical smears in women with intrauterine devices.[144] It has been designated to be nonpathogenic and its presence in any of the aforementioned sites does not require treatment. Morphologically, it is identical to *E. histolytica*, with trophozoites that range from 5 to 25 μm (average 10 to 15 μm). It has a single nucleus with peripheral chromatin, and a small, well-defined karyosome that is usually centrally located. Ingested leukocytes and epithelial cells are often seen in *E. gingivalis*, which is a unique finding in that it is the only species of ameba to ingest leukocytes. No cyst form of the parasite has been identified.[145]

Entamoeba coli is a nonpathogenic protozoan with a wide human distribution. The presence of this organism in a patient's stool is a useful indication of fecal-oral exposure. The life cycle of *E. coli* is identical to that of *E. histolytica*, and the two organisms can be found concurrently in up to 10% to 30% of patients in endemic areas. However, *E. coli* is nonpathogenic and requires no specific treatment. The cysts and trophozoites of *E. coli* can be distinguished from those of the pathogenic *E. histolytica* on the basis of nuclear morphology and cyst size. Whereas *E. histolytica* cysts usually have fewer than five nuclei and are 10 to 15 μm in diameter, the cysts of *E. coli* are greater than 15 μm and often have five to eight nuclei.[146–148]

Entamoeba polecki is an intestinal protozoan that can be found in monkeys and pigs. Although in rare instances it has been reported to cause human infections, the pathogenic potential of this protozoan is at present unclear. Studies have reported that up to 19% of children in Papua, New Guinea, are colonized.[149] Although routine treatment is not currently recommended, good clinical response has been reported with metronidazole and diloxanide furoate. Most infected persons are asymptomatic, but heavy burdens with this parasite can produce nonspecific gastrointestinal symptoms such as diarrhea, cramps, anorexia, and malaise. The trophozoite form of *E. polecki* resembles that of *E. histolytica* and *E. coli* and differentiation from these and other protozoa rely on identification of the cyst stage of the organism, which is characteristically uninucleate with a large karyosome.[144–148]

Endolimax nana is a nonpathogenic commensal parasite with a worldwide distribution that commonly infects humans. It has the same life cycle as *E. histolytica* and is transmitted through oral-fecal spread and poor sanitary conditions. In the tropics it may be identified in the stool of as many as 10% to 33% of persons but requires no specific treatment. It can be distinguished from *E. histolytica* on the basis of its small size (cyst, 6 to 10 μm; trophozoite, 8 to 12 μm), vesicular nucleus, and large irregular karyosome. The cysts are often quadrinucleate.[146,147]

Iodamoeba butschlii is a nonpathogenic commensal organism. In the past it had been confused with the virulent *Naegleria* spp. It is less commonly encountered in the human gastrointestinal tract, occurring in 5% to 8% of the population in the tropics. It has a medium-sized trophozoite (9 to 20 μm) which is highly vacuolated with a large characteristic karyosome. The cysts of *I. butschlii* are uninucleate and contain a large, dense glycogen mass which stains with iodine and are thus identified as I cysts.[146,147]

Blastocystis hominis is an anaerobic protozoan that commonly inhabits the gastrointestinal tract of humans, where it resides in the cecum and large bowel.[149–161] Although it has a worldwide distribution (including infection in animals such as pigs, monkeys, rodents, and poultry), this protozoan is more commonly found in the tropics. The mode of transmission is unclear but, because of the association with unsanitary conditions, is believed to be oral-fecal spread. Prevalence rates are variable, but up to 52% of samples from homosexual males have evidence of infection with this organism in selected regions. The morphologic characteristics of *B. hominis* are its variable size (5 to 40 μm), lack of cell wall, and four morphologic forms: vacuolated, ameba-like, granular, and the recently described cyst stage. At present it is unclear whether the cyst form represents the infective form of the organism. Stool samples of persons infected with this organism typically reveal the vacuolated form, which is characterized by a large membrane-bound central body.

The pathogenicity of this organism is poorly understood, but in the last two decades there have been more frequent reports of infection with *B. hominis*. Infected persons may have gastrointestinal symptoms of diarrhea, abdominal pain, nausea, and vomiting, and systemic symptoms of anorexia and malaise. Reports of infection in immunocompetent and immunocompromised hosts are present in the literature. There is a paucity of diagnostic laboratory data (other than the identification of the vacuolated form of the parasite in stool samples stained with iron hematoxylin or trichrome stain) since stool studies typically lack fecal leukocytes, and endoscopic, histopathologic, and radiologic evaluations are

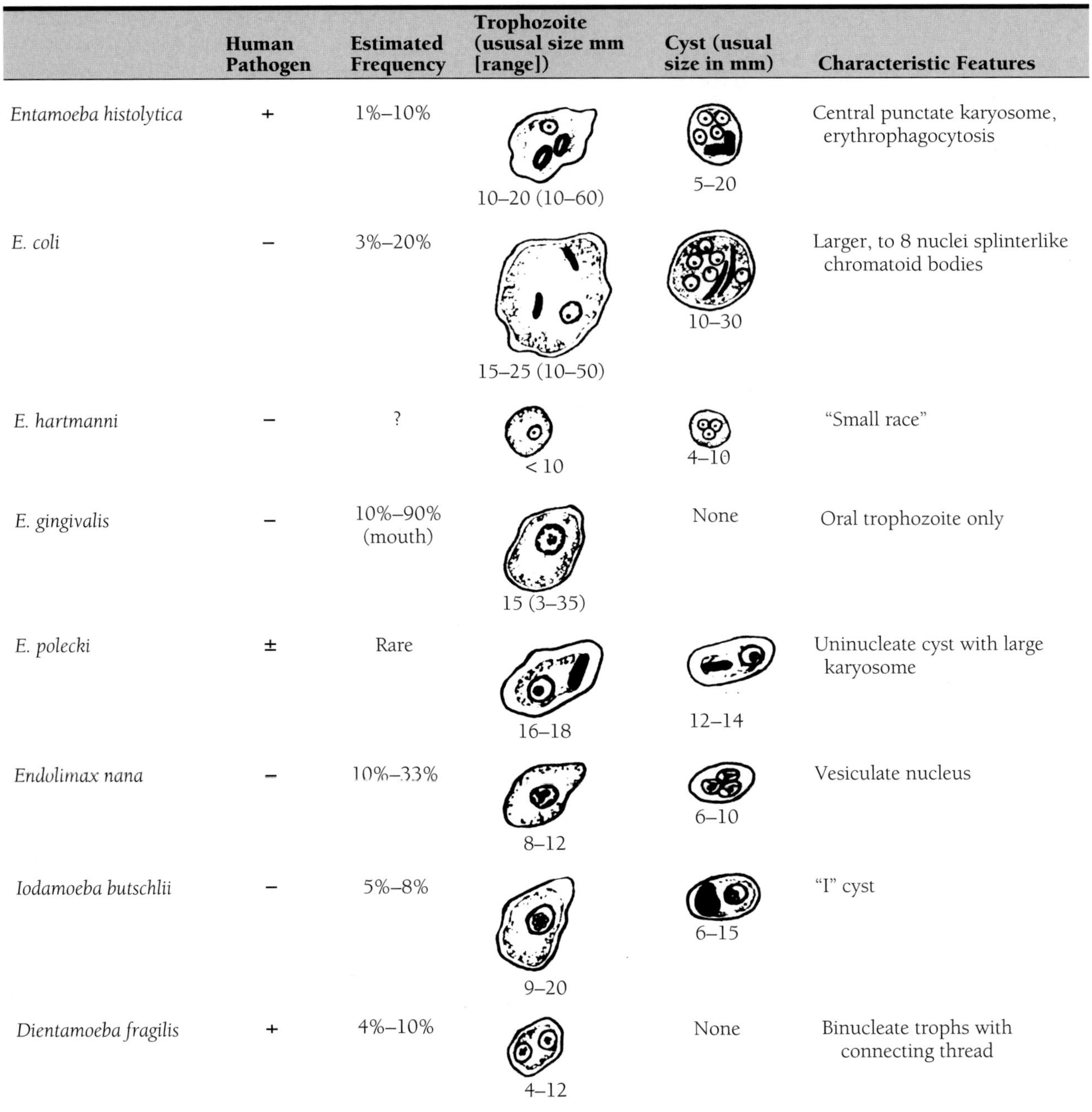

	Human Pathogen	Estimated Frequency	Trophozoite (ususal size mm [range])	Cyst (usual size in mm)	Characteristic Features
Entamoeba histolytica	+	1%–10%	10–20 (10–60)	5–20	Central punctate karyosome, erythrophagocytosis
E. coli	–	3%–20%	15–25 (10–50)	10–30	Larger, to 8 nuclei splinterlike chromatoid bodies
E. hartmanni	–	?	< 10	4–10	"Small race"
E. gingivalis	–	10%–90% (mouth)	15 (3–35)	None	Oral trophozoite only
E. polecki	±	Rare	16–18	12–14	Uninucleate cyst with large karyosome
Endolimax nana	–	10%–33%	8–12	6–10	Vesiculate nucleus
Iodamoeba butschlii	–	5%–8%	9–20	6–15	"I" cyst
Dientamoeba fragilis	+	4%–10%	4–12	None	Binucleate trophs with connecting thread

FIGURE 86-11 Amebae that infect the human gastrointestinal tract. (From Ravdin JI, Guerrant RL: Current problems in diagnosis and treatment of amebic infections. Curr Clin Top Infect Dis 7:82–111, 1986.)

usually normal. The organism has been shown to have in vitro sensitivity to a variety of agents, including emetine, metronidazole, furazolidone, co-trimoxazole, quinacrine, and pentamadine, and there are some in vivo data to support sensitivity of *B. hominis* to iodoquinol and co-trimoxazole. At present, the pathogenic potential of this protozoan parasite is unclear, its pathogenicity is poorly understood, and its role in causing human disease remains to be more clearly defined. Routine antimicrobial therapy against this organism is therefore not warranted.

Dientamoeba fragilis, once classified as an ameba, is now considered in the flagellate group and is discussed in Chapter 87.

REFERENCES

1. Stilwell GG: Amebiasis: Its early history. Gastroenterology 28:606, 1955.
2. Kean BH: A history of amebiasis. In Ravdin JI (ed): Amebiasis: Human Infection by *Entamoeba histolytica*. New York, Wiley, 1988, p 1.
3. Osler W: On the Amoeba coli in dysentery and in dysenteric liver abscess. Bull Johns Hopkins Hosp 1:53, 1890.
4. Councilman WT, Lafleur HA: Amoebic dysentery. Johns Hopkins Hosp Rep 2:395, 1891.
5. Rogers L: The rapid cure of amoebic dysentery and hepatitis by hypodermic injection of soluble salts of emetine. BMJ 1:1424, 1912.
6. Walker EL, Sellards AW: Experimental entamoebic dysentery. Philippine J Sci B Trop Med 8:253, 1913.
7. Diamond LS: Axenic cultivation of *Entamoeba histolytica*. Science 134:336, 1961.

8. Brumpt E: Étude sommaire de l, "*Entamoeba dispar*" n. sp. Amibe à kystes quadrinuclées, parasite de l'homme. Bull Acad Med (Paris) 94:943, 1925.
9. Sargeaunt PG, Williams JE, Grene JD: The differentiation of invasive and non-invasive *Entamoeba histolytica* by isoenzyme electrophoresis. Trans R Soc Trop Med Hyg 72:519, 1978.
10. Sargeaunt PG, Williams JE: Electrophoretic isoenzyme patterns of the pathogenic and non-pathogenic intestinal amoeba of man. Trans R Soc Trop Med Hyg 73:225, 1979.
11. Sargeaunt PG, Williams JE, Neal RA: A comparative study of *Entamoeba histolytica* (NIH 200, HK9 etc), "*E. histolytica* like" and other morphologically identical amoebae using isoenzyme electrophoresis. Trans R Soc Trop Med Hyg 74:469, 1980.
12. Strachan WP, Chiodini PL, Spice WM, et al: Immunologic differentiation of pathogenic and nonpathogenic isolates of *Entamoeba histolytica*. Lancet 1:561, 1988.
13. Tannich E, Horstmann RD, Knobloch J, et al: Genomic differences between pathogenic and nonpathogenic *Entamoeba histolytica*. Proc Natl Acad Sci USA 86:5118, 1989.
14. Tannich E, Burchard GD: Differentiation of pathogenic from nonpathogenic *Entamoeba histolytica* by restriction fragment analysis of a single gene amplified in vitro. J Clin Microbiol 29:250, 1991.
15. Tannich E, Scholze H, Nickel R, et al: Homologous cysteine proteinases of pathogenic and nonpathogenic *Entamoeba histolytica*. J Biol Chem 266:4798, 1991.
16. Diamond LS, Clark CG: A redescription of *Entamoeba histolytica* Shaudinn 1903 (amended Walker 1911) separating it from *Entamoeba dispar* (Brumpt 1925). J Eukaryot Microbiol 40:340, 1993.
17. Garfinkel LI, Giladid M, Huber M, et al: DNA probes specific for *Entamoeba histolytica* possessing pathogenic and nonpathogenic zymodemes. Infect Immun 57:926, 1989.
18. Edman U, Meraz MA, Rausser S, et al: Characterization of an immunodominant variable surface antigen from pathogenic and nonpathogenic *Entamoeba histolytica*. J Exp Med 172:879, 1990.
19. Clark CG, Diamond LS: Ribosomal RNA genes of "pathogenic" and "nonpathogenic" *Entamoeba histolytica* are distinct. Mol Biochem Parasitol 49:297, 1991.
20. Andrews BJ, Mentzoni L, Bjorvatn B: Zymodeme conversion of isolates of *Entamoeba histolytica*. Trans R Soc Trop Med Hyg 84:63, 1990.
21. Mirelman D, Bracha R, Wexler A, et al: Changes in isozyme patterns of a cloned culture of nonpathogenic *Entamoeba histolytica* during axenization. Infect Immun 54:827, 1986.
22. Clark CG, Diamond LS: *Entamoeba histolytica*—An explanation for the reported conversion of nonpathogenic amebae to the pathogenic form. Exp Parasitol 77:456, 1993.
23. Ali IKM., Hossain, MB, Roy, S, et al: *Entamoeba moshkovskii* infections in children, Bangladesh. Emerg Infect Dis 9:580, 2003.
24. Eichinger D: A role for a galactose lectin and its ligands during encystment of *Entamoeba*. J Eukaryot Microbiol 48:17, 2001.
25. McLaughlin J, Aley S: The biochemistry and functional morphology of the *Entamoeba*. J Protozool 32:221, 1985.
26. Mann BJ, Vedvick T, Torian B, et al: Sequence of a cysteine-rich galactose-specific lectin of *Entamoeba histolytica*. Proc Natl Acad Sci USA 88:3248, 1991.
27. Hasegawa M, Hashimoto T: Ribosomal RNA trees misleading? Nature 361:23, 1993.
28. Clark CG, Roger AJ: Direct evidence for secondary loss of mitochondria in *Entamoeba histolytica*. Proc Natl Acad Sci USA 92:6518, 1995.
29. Tannich E, Mirelman D, Petri WA Jr: Meeting report: EMBO workshop "Pathogenesis of Amoebiasis: From Genomics to Disease." Institut Pasteur, Paris, May 19–22, 2003. Protist 154:293, 2003.
30. Tannich E, Horstmann RD: Codon usage in pathogenic *Entamoeba histolytica*. J Mol Evol 34:272, 1992.
31. Lioutas C, Tannich E: Transcription of protein-coding genes in *Entamoeba histolytica* is insensitive to high concentrations of α-amanitin. Mol Biochem Parasitol 73:259, 1995.
32. Wilihoeft U, Campos-Gongora E, Touzni S,et al: Introns of *Entamoeba histolytica* and *Entamoeba dispar*. Protist 152:149, 2001.
33. Plaimauer B, Ortner S, Wiedermann G, et al: An intron-containing gene coding for a novel 39-kilodalton antigen of *Entamoeba histolytica*. Mol Biochem Parasitol 66:181, 1994.
34. Bruchhaus I, Leippe M, Lioutas C, et al: Unusual gene organization in the protozoan parasite *Entamoeba histolytica*. DNA Cell Biol 12:925, 1993.
35. Kozak, M: Compilation and analysis of sequenes upstream from the translational start site in eukaryotic mRNAs. Nucleic Acids Res 12:857, 1984.
36. Bhattacharya S, Bhattacharya A, Diamond LS, et al: Circular DNA of *Entamoeba histolytica* encodes ribosomal RNA. J Protozool 36:455, 1989.
37. Purdy JE, Pho LT, Mann BJ, et al: Upstream regulatory elements controlling expression of the *Entamoeba histolytica* lectin. Mol Biochem Parasitol 78:91, 1996.
38. Schaenman JM, Gilchrist CA, Mann BJ, et al: Identification of two *Entamoeba histolytica* sequence-specific *hgl5* enhancer-binding proteins with homology to the RNA-binding motif RRM. J Biol Chem 276:1602, 2001.
39. Gilchrist CA, Holm CF, Hughes MA, et al: Identification and characterization of an *Entamoeba histolytica* URE3 sequence-specific DNA binding protein containing EF-hand motifs. J Biol Chem 276:11838, 2001.
40. Gilchrist CA, Leo M, Line CG, et al: Calcium modulates promoter occupancy by the *Entamoeba histolytica* Ca^{2+}-binding transcription factor URE3-BP. J Biol Chem 278:4646, 2003.
41. Singh U, Rogers JB, Mann BJ, et al: Transcription initiation is controlled by three core promoter elements in the hgl5 gene of the protozoan parasite *Entamoeba histolytica*. Proc Natl Acad Sci USA 94:8812, 1997.
42. Singh U, Gilchrist CA, Schaenman JM, et al: Context-dependent roles of the *Entamoeba histolytica* core promoter element GAAC in transcriptional activation and protein complex assembly. Mol Biochem Parasitol 120:107, 2002.
43. Jackson TFHG, Gathiram V, Simjee AE: Seroepidemiologic study of antibody responses to the zymodemes of *Entamoeba histolytica*. Lancet 1:716, 1985.
44. Haque, R, Ali IM, Hossain MB, et al: Epidemiologic and clinical characteristics of acute diarrhea and endemic *E. histolytica* infections in preschool children in an urban slum of Dhaka, Bangladesh. Am J Trop Med Hyg 69:398, 2003.
45. Blessmann J, Van Linh P, Nu PA, et al: Epidemiology of amebiasis in a region of high incidence of amebic liver abscess in central Vietnam. Am J Trop Med Hyg 66:578, 2002.
46. Caballero-Salcedo A, Viveros-Rogel M, Salvatierra B, et al: Seroepidemiology of amebiasis in Mexico. Am J Trop Med Hyg 50:412, 1994.
47. Cifuentes E, Blumenthal U, Ruiz-Palacios G, et al: Escenario epidemiologico del uso agricola del agua residual: El valle del mezquital, Mexico. Salud Publica Mexico 36:3, 1994.
48. Haque R, Faruque ASG, Hahn P, et al: *Entamoeba histolytica* and *Entamoeba dispar* infection in children in Bangladesh. J Infect Dis 175:734, 1997.
49. Abuabara SF, Barrett JA, Hau T, et al: Amebic liver abscess. Arch Surg 117:239, 1982.
50. Pehrson PO: Amoebiasis in a non-endemic country. Epidemiology, presenting symptoms and diagnostic methods. Scand J Infect Dis 15:207, 1983.
51. Weinke T, Friedrich-Janicke B, Hopp P, et al: Prevalence and clinical importance of *Entamoeba histolytica* in two high-risk groups: Travelers returning from the tropics and male homosexuals. J Infect Dis 161:1029, 1990.
52. Smith PD, Lane HC, Gill VJ, et al: Intestinal infections in patients with AIDS. Ann Intern Med 108:328, 1988.
53. Krogstad DJ, Spencer MJ, Healy GR, et al: Amebiasis: Epidemiological studies in the United States, 1971–1974. Ann Intern Med 88:89, 1978.
54. Nagakura K, Tachibana H, Tanaka T, et al: An outbreak of amebiasis in an institution for the mentally retarded in Japan. Jpn J Med Sci Biol 42:63, 1989.
55. Summary of Notifiable Diseases, United States, 1993. MMWR 42:53, 1994.
56. Adams EB, MacLeod IN: Invasive amebiasis II: Amebic liver abscess and its complications. Medicine 56:325, 1977.
57. Katzenstein D, Rickerson V, Braude A: New concepts of amebic liver abscess derived from hepatic imaging, serodiagnosis, and hepatic enzymes in 67 consecutive cases in San Diego. Medicine 61:237, 1982.
58. Gathiram V, Jackson TFHG: A longitudinal study of asymptomatic carriers of pathogenic zymodemes of *Entamoeba histolytica*. S Afr Med J 72:669, 1987.
59. Tony JC, Martin TK: Profile of amebic liver abscess. Arch Med Res 23:249, 1992.

60. Armon PJ: Amoebiasis in pregnancy and the puerperium. Br J Obstet Gynaecol 85:264, 1978.
61. Wanke C, Butler T, Islam M: Epidemiologic and clinical features of invasive amebiasis in Bangladesh: A case-control comparison with other diarrheal diseases and postmortem findings. Am J Trop Med Hyg 38:335, 1988.
62. Cegielski JP, Msengi AE, Dukes CS, et al: Intestinal parasites and HIV infection in Tanzanian children with chronic diarrhea. AIDS 7:213, 1993.
63. de Lalla F, Rinaldi E, Santoro D, et al: Outbreak of *Entamoeba histolytica* and *Giardia lamblia* infections in travellers returning from the tropics. Infection 20:78, 1992.
64. Irusen EM, Jackson TFHG, Simjee AE: Asymptomatic intestinal colonization by pathogenic *Entamoeba histolytica*—Prevalence, response to therapy, and pathogenic potential. Clin Infect Dis 14:889, 1992.
65. Goldmeier D, Sargeaunt PG, Price AB, et al: Is *Entamoeba histolytica* in homosexual men a pathogen? Lancet 1:641, 1986.
66. Burchard GD, Hufert FT, Mirelman D: Characterization of 20 *Entamoeba histolytica* strains isolated from patients with HIV infection. Infection 19:164, 1990.
67. Allason-Jones E, Mindel A, Sargeaunt P, et al: *Entamoeba histolytica* as a commensal intestinal parasite in homosexual men. N Engl J Med 315:353, 1986.
68. Takeuchi T, Okuzawa E, Nozaki T, et al: High seropositivity of Japanese homosexual men for amebic infection. J Infect Dis 159:808, 1989.
69. Ohnishi K, Murata M, Okuzawa E: Symptomatic amebic colitis in a Japanese homosexual AIDS patient. Intern Med 33:120, 1994.
70. Haque R, Huston CD, Hughes M, et al: Current concepts: Amebiasis. New Engl J Med 348:1565, 2003.
71. Speelman P, McGlaughlin R, Kabir I, et al: Differential clinical features and stool findings in shigellosis and amoebic dysentery. Trans R Soc Trop Med Hyg 81:549, 1987.
72. Haque R, Mollah NU, Ali IKM, et al: Diagnosis of amebic liver abscess and intestinal infection with the Techlab *Entamoeba histolytica* II antigen detection and antibody tests. J Clin Microbiol 38:3235, 2000.
73. Ellyson JH, Bezmalinovic Z, Parks SN, et al: Necrotizing amebic colitis: A frequently fatal complication. Am J Surg 152:21, 1986.
74. Aristizabal H, Acevedo J, Botero M: Fulminant amebic colitis. World J Surg 15:216, 1991.
75. Maltz G, Knauer CM: Amebic liver abscess: A 15-year experience. Am J Gastroenterol 86:704, 1991.
76. Thompson JE, Glasser AJ: Amebic abscess of the liver. Diagnostic features. J Clin Gastroenterol 8:550, 1986.
77. Nazir Z, Moazam F: Amebic liver abscess in children. Pediatr Infect Dis J 12:929, 1993.
78. Johnson JL, Baird JS, Hulbert TV, et al: Amebic liver abscess in infancy: Case report and review. Clin Infect Dis 19:765, 1994.
79. Mehta RB, Parija SC, Chetty DV, et al: Management of 240 cases of liver abscess. Int Surg 71:91, 1986.
80. Hai AA, Singh A, Mittal VJ, et al: Amoebic liver abscess: Review of 220 cases. Int Surg 76:81, 1991.
81. Conter RL, Pitt HA, Tompkins RK, et al: Differentiation of pyogenic from amebic hepatic abscesses. Surg Gynecol Obstet 162:114, 1986.
82. Chuah SK, Chang-Chien CS, Sheen IS, et al: The prognostic factors of severe amebic liver abscess: A retrospective study of 125 cases. Am J Trop Med Hyg 46:398, 1992.
83. Greaney GC, Reynolds TB, Donovan AJ: Ruptured amebic liver abscess. Arch Surg 120:555, 1985.
84. Petri WA Jr, Mann BJ, Haque R: The bittersweet interface of parasite and host: Lectin-carbohydrate interactions during human invasion by the parasite *Entamoeba histolytica*. Ann Rev Microbiol 56:39, 2002.
85. Cheng X-J, Hughes MA, Huston CD, et al: The 150 kDa Gal/GalNAc lectin co-receptor of *Entamoeba histolytica* is a member of a gene family containing multiple CXXC sequence motifs. Infect Immun 69:5892, 2001.
86. Beck DL, Tanyuksel M, Mackey A, et al: Sequence conservation of the Gal/GalNAc lectin from clinical isolates. Exp Parasitol 101:157, 2002.
87. Ravdin JI, Guerrant RL: Role of adherence in cytopathogenic mechanisms of *Entamoeba histolytica*. Study with mammalian tissue culture cells and human erythrocytes. J Clin Invest 68:1305, 1981.
88. Guerrant RL, Brush JE, Raudin JI, et al: Interaction between *Entamoeba histolytica* and human polymorphonuclear leukocytes. J Infect Dis 143:83, 1981.
89. Ravdin JI, Croft BY, Guerrant RL: Cytopathogenic mechanisms of *Entamoeba histolytica*. J Exp Med 152:377, 1980.
90. Petri WA Jr, Smith RD, Schlesinger PH, et al: Isolation of the galactose binding adherence lectin of *Entamoeba histolytica*. J Clin Invest 80:1238, 1987.
91. Petri WA Jr: Amebiasis and the *Entamoeba histolytica* Gal/GalNAc lectin: From lab bench to bedside. J Invest Med 44:24, 1996.
92. Tse S-K, Chadee K: The interaction between intestinal mucus glycoproteins and enteric infections. Parasitol Today 7:163, 1991.
93. Reed SL, Gigli I: Lysis of complement-sensitive *Entamoeba histolytica* by activated terminal complement components. J Clin Invest 86:1815, 1990.
94. Braga LL, Ninomiya H, McCoy JJ, et al: Inhibition of the complement membrane attack complex by the galactose-specific adhesin of *Entamoeba histolytica*. J Clin Invest 90:1131, 1992.
95. Vines RR, Ramakrishnan G, Rogers JB, et al: Regulation of adherence and virulence by the *Entamoeba histolytica* lectin cytoplasmic domain which contains a β_2-integrin motif. Mol Biol Cell 9:2069, 1998.
96. Ravdin JI, Moreau F, Sullivan JA, et al: Relationship of free intracellular calcium to the cytolytic activity of *Entamoeba histolytica*. Infect Immun 56:1505, 1988.
97. Ravdin JI, Sperelakis N, Guerrant RL: Effect of ion channel inhibitors on the cytopathogenicity of *Entamoeba histolytica*. J Infect Dis 154:27, 1982.
98. Huston CD, Miller-Sims V, Petri WA Jr: Apoptotic killing and phagocytosis of host cells by the parasite *Entamoeba histolytica*. Infect Immun 71:964, 2003.
99. Leippe M, Andra J, Muller-Eberhard HJ: Cytolytic and antibacterial activity of synthetic peptides derived from amoebapore, the pore-forming peptide of *Entamoeba histolytica*. Proc Natl Acad Sci USA 91:2602, 1994.
100. Talamas-Rohana P, Meza I: Interaction between pathogenic amebas and fibronectin: Substrate degradation and changes in cytoskeleton organization. J Cell Biol 106:1787, 1988.
101. Munoz M de L, Moreno MA, Perez-Garcia JN, et al: Possible role of calmodulin in the secretion of *Entamoeba histolytica* electron-dense granules containing collagenase. Mol Microbiol 5:1707, 1991.
102. McKerrow JH, Sun E, Rosenthal PJ, et al: The proteases and pathogenicity of parasitic protozoa. Ann Rev Microbiol 47:821, 1993.
103. Vines RR, Ramakrishnan G, Rogers J, et al: Regulation of adherence and virulence by the *Entamoeba histolytica* lectin cytoplasmic domain, which contains an β2 integrin motif. Mol Biol Cell 9:2069, 1998.
104. Ankri S, Stolarsky T, Mirelman D: Antisense inhibition of expression of cysteine proteinases does not affect *Entamoeba histolytica* cytopathic or haemolytic activity but inhibits phagocytosis. Mol Microbiol 28:777, 1998.
105. Krupp IM: Antibody response in intestinal and extraintestinal amoebiasis. Am J Trop Med Hyg 19:57, 1970.
106. Zhang X, Zhang Z, Alexander D, et al: Expression of amoebapores is required for full expression of *Entamoeba histolytica* virulence in amebic liver abscess but is not necessary for the induction of inflammation or tissue damage in amebic colitis. Infect Immun 72:678, 2004.
107. Haque R, Ali IKM, Sack RB, et al: Amebiasis and mucosal IgA antibody against the *Entamoeba histolytica* adherence lectin in Bangladeshi children. J Infect Dis 183:1787, 2001.
108. Haque R, Duggal P, Ali IM, et al: Innate and acquired resistance to amebiasis in Bangladeshi children. J Infect Dis 186:547, 2002.
109. Salata RA, Pearson RD, Ravdin JI: The interaction of human leukocytes with *Entamoeba histolytica*: Killing of the virulent amebae by the activated macrophage. J Clin Invest 76:491, 1985.
110. Salata RA, Martinez-Palomo A, Murray HW, et al: Patients treated for amebic liver abscess develop cell-mediated immune responses effective in vitro against *Entamoeba histolytica*. J Immunol 136:2633, 1986.
111. Denis M, Chadee K: Human neutrophils activated by interferon-gamma and tumor necrosis factor-alpha kill *Entamoeba histolytica* trophozoites in vitro. J Leukocyte Biol 46:270, 1989.
112. Lin JY, Chadee K: Macrophage cytotoxicity against *Entamoeba histolytica* trophozoites is mediated by nitric oxide from L-arginine. J Immunol 148:3999, 1992.
113. Lin JY, Seguin R, Keller K, et al: Tumor necrosis factor alpha augments nitric oxide–dependent macrophage cytotoxicity against *Entamoeba histolytica* by enhanced expression of the nitric oxide synthase gene. Infect Immun 62:1534, 1994.

114. Houpt ER, Glembocki DJ, Obrig TG, et al: The mouse model of amebic colitis reveals mouse strain susceptibility to infection and exacerbation of disease by CD4+ T cells. J Immunol 169:4496, 2002.
115. Duggal P, Haque, R, Ali IM, et al: HLA Class II alleles influencing susceptibility to *E. histolytica* infection in Bangladeshi Children. J Infect Dis 189:520, 2004.
116. Gonzalez-Ruiz A, Haque R, Aguirre A, et al: Value of microscopy in the diagnosis of dysentery associated with invasive *Entamoeba histolytica*. J Clin Pathol 47:236, 1994.
117. Garfinkel LI, Giladi M, Huber M, et al: DNA probes specific for *Entamoeba histolytica* possessing pathogenic and nonpathogenic zymodemes. Infect Immun 57:926, 1989.
118. Tachibana H, Kobayashi S, Okuzawa E, et al: Detection of pathogenic *Entamoeba histolytica* DNA in liver abscess fluid by polymerase chain reaction. Int J Parasitol 22:1193, 1992.
119. Blessmann J, Buss H, Nu PA, et al: Real-time PCR for detection and differentiation of *Entamoeba histolytica* and *Entamoeba dispar* in fecal samples.J Clin Microbiol 40:4413, 2002.
120. Ayeh-Kumi P, Ali IKM, Lockhart L, et al: *Entamoeba histolytica*: Genetic diversity of clinical isolates from Bangladesh as demonstrated by polymorphisms in the serine-rich gene. Exp Parasitol 99:80, 2001.
121. Zaki M, Reddy SG, Jackson TFHG, et al:. Genotyping of *Entamoeba* species in South Africa: Diversity, stability, and transmission patterns within families. J Infect Dis 187:1860, 2003.
122. Caballero-Salcedo A, Viveroa-Rogel M, et al: Seroepidemiology of amebiasis in Mexico. Am J Trop Med Hyg 50:412, 1994.
123. Choudhuri G, Prakash V, Kumar A, et al: Protective immunity to *Entamoeba histolytica* infection in subjects with antiamoebic antibodies residing in a hyperendemic zone. Scand J Infect Dis 23:771, 1991.
124. Ximenez C, Leyva O, Moran P, et al: *Entamoeba histolytica*: Antibody response to recent and past invasive events. Ann Trop Med Parasitol 87:31, 1993.
125. Chun D, Chandrasoma P, Kiyabu M: Fulminant amebic colitis. A morphologic study of four cases. Dis Colon Rectum 37:535, 1994.
126. Yoon JH, Rye JG, Lee JK, et al: Atypical manifestations of amebic colitis. J Korean Med Sci 6:260, 1991.
127. Radhakrishnan S, Nakib BA, Shaikh H, et al: The value of colonoscopy in schistosomal, tuberculous and amebic colitis. Dis Colon Rectum 29:891, 1986.
128. Mhlanga BR, Lanoie LO, Norris HJ, et al: Amebiasis complicating carcinomas: A diagnositic dilemma. Am J Trop Med Hyg 46:759, 1992.
129. Sheen IS, Chien CSC, Lin DY, et al: Resolution of liver abscess: Comparison of pyogenic and amebic liver abscesses. Am J Trop Med Hyg 40:384, 1989.
130. Radin DR, Ralls PW, Colletti PM, et al: CT of amebic liver abscess. AJR 150:1297, 1988.
131. Ahmed L, El Rooby A, Kassem MI, et al: Ultrasonography in the diagnosis and management of 52 patients with amebic liver abscess in Cairo. Rev Infect Dis 12:330, 1990.
132. Elizondo G, Weissleder R, Stark DD, et al: Amebic liver abscess: Diagnosis and treatment evalution with MR imaging. Radiology 165:795, 1987.
133. McAuley JB, Herwaldt BL, Stokes SL, et al: Diloxanide furoate for treating asymptomatic *Entamoeba histolytica* cyst passers: 14 years' experience in the United States. Clin Infect Dis 15:464, 1992.
134. McAuley JB, Juranek DD: Paromomycin in the treatment of mild-to-moderate intestinal amebiasis. Clin Infect Dis 15:551, 1992.
135. Simjee AE, Gathiram V, Jackson TFHG, et al: A comparative trial of metronidazole v. tinidazole in the treatment of amoebic liver abscess. S Afr Med J 68:923, 1985.
136. van Allen RJ, Katz MD, Johnson MB, et al: Uncomplicated amebic liver abscess: Prospective evaluation of percutaneous therapeutic aspiration. Radiology 183:827, 1992.
137. Blessmann J, Binh HD, Hung DM, et al: Treatment of amoebic liver abscess with metronidazole alone or in combination with ultrasound-guided needle aspiration: A comparative, prospective and randomized study. Trop Med Int Health 8:1030, 2003.
138. Petri WA Jr, Ravdin JI: Protection of gerbils from amebic liver abscess by immunization with the galactose-specific adherence lectin of *Entamoeba histolytica*. Infect Immun 59:97, 1991.
139. Houpt E, Barroso L, Lockhart L, et al: Prevention of intestinal amebiasis by vaccination with the *Entamoeba histolytica* Gal/GalNac lectin. Vaccine 22:612, 2004.
140. Zhang T, Stanley SL Jr: Protection of gerbils from amebic liver abscess by immunization with a recombinant protein derived from the 170-kilodalton surface adhesin of *Entamoeba histolytica*. Infect Immun 62:2605, 1994.
141. Zhang T, Cieslak PR, Stanley SL Jr: Protection of gerbils from amebic liver abscess by immunization with a recombinant *Entamoeba histolytica* antigen. Infect Immun 62:1166, 1994.
142. Medina-Bolivar F, Wright R, Funk V, et al: A non-toxic lectin for antigen delivery of plant-based mucosal vaccines. Vaccine 21:997, 2003.
143. Petri WA Jr: Recent advances in amebiasis. Crit Rev Clin Lab Sci 33:1, 1996.
144. Garcia LS, Bruckner DA: Diagnostic Medical Parasitology, 3rd ed. Washington, DC, ASM Press, 1997, p 6.
145. Murray PR, Baron EJ, Pfaller MA, et al (eds): Manual of Clinical Microbiology, 6th ed. Washington, DC, ASM Press, 1995, Chapter 106.
146. Garcia LS, Bruckner DA: Diagnostic Medical Parasitology, 2nd ed. Washington, DC, American Society for Microbiology, 1993.
147. Kain KC, Keystone JS: Intestinal infection with other protozoa: Including *Isospora belli, Blastocystis hominis, Dientamoeba fragilis*. In Blaser MJ, Smith PD, Ravdin JI, et al (eds): Infections of the Gastrointestinal Tract. New York, Raven Press, 1995.
148. Wolfe MS: Miscellaneous intestinal protozoa. In Strickland GT (ed): Hunter's Tropical Medicine, 2nd ed. Philadelphia, WB Saunders, 1984.
149. Zierdt CH: *Blastocystis hominis*—Past and future. Clin Microbiol Rev 4:61, 1991.
150. Sheehan DJ, Raucher BC, McKitrick JC: Association of *Blastocystis hominis* with signs and symptoms of human disease. J Clin Microbiol 24:548, 1986.
151. Kain KC, Noble MA, Freeman HJ, et al: Epidemiology and clinical features associated with *Blastocystis hominis* infection. Diagn Microbiol Infect Dis 8:235, 1987.
152. Stenzel DJ, Boreham PF: A cyst-like stage of *Blastocystis hominis*. Int J Parasitol 21:613, 1991.
153. Stenzel DJ, Boreham PF, McDougall R: Ultrastructure of *Blastocystis hominis* in human stool samples. Int J Parasitol 21:807, 1991.
154. *Blastocystis hominis*: A commensal or pathogen? (Editorial) Lancet 337:521, 1991.
155. Jelinek T, Peyerl G, Loscher T, et al: The role of *Blastocystis hominis* as a possible intestinal pathogen in travellers. J Infect 35:63, 1997.
156. Horiki N, Maruyama M, Fujita Y, et al: Epidemiologic survey of *Blastocystis hominis* infection in Japan. Am J Trop Med Hyg 56:370, 1997.
157. Escobedo A, Nunez FA: *Blastocystis hominis* infection in Cuban AIDS patients. Memorias Instituto Oswaldo Cruz 92:321, 1997.
158. Zierdt CH: In vitro response of *Blastocystis hominis* to antiprotozoal drugs. J Protozool 30:332, 1983.
159. Taylor DN, Echeverria P, Blaser MJ, et al: Polymicrobial aetiology of traveller's diarrhea. Lancet 1:381, 1985.
160. Grossman I, Weiss LM, Simon D, et al: *Blastocystis hominis* in hospital employees. Am J Gastroenterol 87:729, 1992.
161. Schwartz E, Houston R: Effect of co-trimoxazole on stool recovery of *Blastocystis hominis*. Lancet 339:428, 1992.

87

Intestinal Flagellate and Ciliate Infections

DAVID R. HILL
THEODORE E. NASH

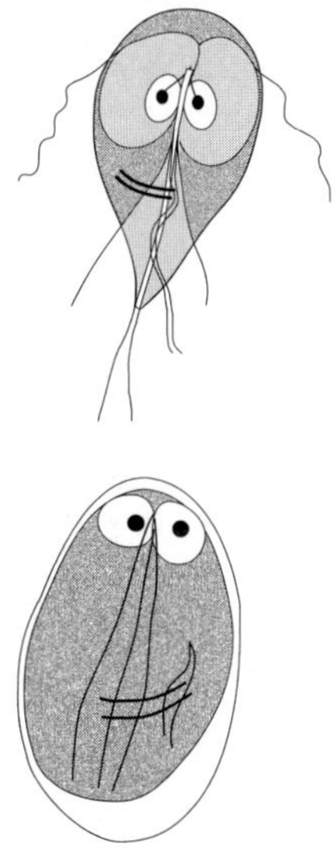

FIGURE 87-1 Schematic drawing of *Giardia lamblia* trophozoite (*top*) and cyst (*bottom*), and their key identification points.

INTRODUCTION

The most important of the many flagellates that inhabit the large and small bowel of man is *Giardia lamblia*; *Giardia* may be the most common pathogenic parasitic infection in humans. In developed countries, it is a frequent cause of endemic and epidemic diarrhea and in many developing regions of the world, where effective sanitation measures are lacking, infection is nearly universal by 2 to 3 years of age.

Of the other flagellates, only *Dientamoeba fragilis* is capable of causing enteric symptoms. *Chilomastix mesnili*, while not uncommonly seen in stool specimens, is a nonpathogen, as is *Pentatrichomonas hominis* (formerly known as *Trichomonas hominis*), and the rarely seen *Enteromonas hominis* and *Retortamonas intestinalis*. The only ciliate of man and the largest protozoan is *Balantidium coli*, a rare cause of diarrhea and dysentery, primarily in the tropics.

Giardia lamblia

AGENT

Giardia lamblia (also known as *Giardia duodenalis* or *Giardia intestinalis*) is a flagellate protozoan that inhabits the small intestine of humans and other mammals. The genus *Giardia* belongs to the category of intestinal flagellates in the division Protozoa.[1] Analysis of the 16S small ribosomal RNA (rRNA) subunit as well as analysis of other essential proteins indicates *Giardia* is among the most primitive eukaryotes.[2–4] The trophozoite form lacks a definable Golgi apparatus, classical mitochondria, and peroxisomes, organelles that are found in higher eukaryotes.[5,6] It is likely that Antony van Leeuwenhoek described the organism in his own stool in the 17th century, but Vilem Lambl is credited with describing the trophozoite in humans in 1859 and Grassi discovered the cyst form in 1879.[7]

Giardia has only two morphologic forms, the trophozoite and the cyst (Fig. 87-1). The former resides in the small intestine and is responsible for disease manifestations and the latter is the infectious, environmentally resistant form responsible for transmission. The *Giardia* that infects humans is morphologically indistinguishable from that found in a large variety of mammals. The trophozoite is 9 to 21 μm long, 5 to 15 μm wide, and 2 to 4 μm thick. When viewed from above, its shape resembles a pear or teardrop (Fig. 87-2). *Giardia* is bilaterally symmetrical, has two equal-sized nuclei that contain complete copies of the genome with a ploidy of four,[8,9] four pairs of flagella, one of which is recurrent, and possesses a ventral sucking disk which is used for adherence. Two claw-shaped median bodies consisting of microtubules conspicuously cross the middle of the parasite. These are typical of *G. lamblia* and contrast with the round median bodies in *G. muris*, a species found in some rodents.[10]

Despite the morphologic similarities among *Giardia* organisms that infect humans, analyses using a variety of complementary methodologies including isoenzyme analysis, rDNA sequence, presence of unique variant-specific surface proteins, and differences in isoenzymes or specific protein sequences indicate that *Giardia* isolates from humans vary. The human isolates fall into two major groupings that differ genetically and biologically.[6,11–21] In attempting to categorize them, there is no agreed-upon nomenclature. Groups 1/2 and Group 3, the initially described grouping,[22] are comparable to "Polish" and "Belgian" isolates and Assemblages A and B.[6,20] Assemblages have also been termed *genotypes*. Genetic differences between these two groups are so large that they are in reality different species although not officially recognized. Biological differences include variation in growth rates (T. Nash, unpublished observations), host specificity,[23] variant-specific surface protein repertoires,[24] and character of infection in animal models.[25,26] It is expected that there would be differences in virulence for humans between isolates of *Giardia*. While some studies indicate this,[27–29] others have shown clinical diversity with genetic similarity.[30] Therefore, there needs to be thorough analysis of isolates from all over the world with a careful correlation with clinical symptoms

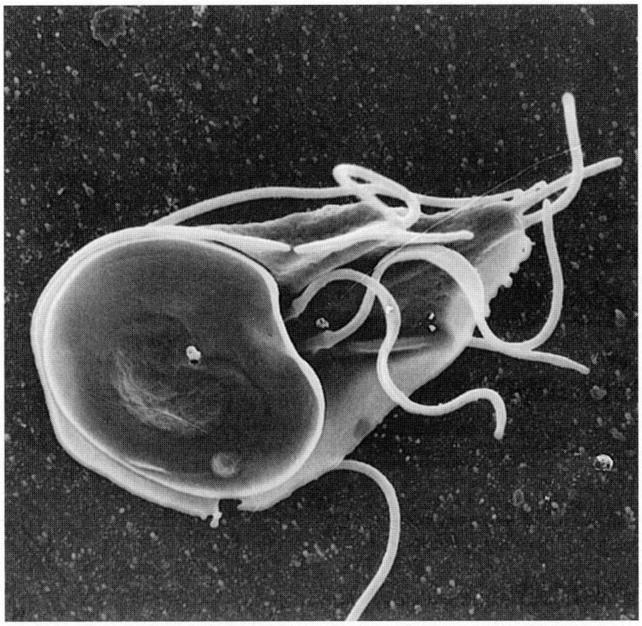

FIGURE 87-2 Scanning electron micrograph of the ventral surface of a *Giardia lamblia* trophozoite. The ventral adhesion disk and four pairs of flagella are seen. (Courtesy of D. Darwood, Rocky Mountain Laboratory, National Institute of Allergy and Infectious Diseases, National Institutes of Health, Bethesda, MD.)

before this can be resolved. In contrast, human host differences are known to contribute to the variability of clinical symptoms; patients who have common variable hypogammaglobulinemia are susceptible to severe and prolonged giardiasis.[31]

Giardia that are genetically indistinguishable from those infecting humans have been found in a wide range of animals including livestock, cats, and dogs.[20,21] In addition, *Giardia* originating from humans can experimentally infect a wide range of mammals. Although a reasonable interpretation of these data suggests cross-transmission between mammalian hosts and humans, with the exception of beavers,[15] no epidemics have implicated animals as a source of human infections. In other analyses, *Giardia* from cats, dogs, muskrats, domestic rats, and some hoofed animals such as sheep and cattle usually have distinct lineages with assignment to assemblages or genotypes with restricted enzootic potential.[6,32–34] Lastly, ongoing genetic analyses of *Giardia* found in specific animals support different species in rodents (*G. muris*), birds (*G. psittaci* and *G. ardeae*), and amphibians (*G. agilis*).[6]

Multiplication of trophozoites in the small intestine is by longitudinal binary fission with mirror image symmetry.[35] As trophozoites are swept down the intestine, they begin to form environmentally resistant, oval cysts (Fig. 87-3). These measure about 6 to 10 μm long, have four nuclei, and the anlage of two trophozoites. Although bile salts trigger encystation in vitro,[36] more recent experiments indicate that encystation occurs through cholesterol depletion and micelle destruction in vitro,[37] a process that physiologically occurs in the intestine after absorption of lipids and bile salts in the lower small bowel.

G. lamblia is the only species that can be cultured in vitro.[38] Complex nondefined media are used and the organism grows best under anaerobic or microaerophilic conditions. It utilizes glucose as a major source of carbohydrate energy, producing ethanol, alanine, acetate, and carbon dioxide, and generating ATP in the process.[6] Another potential mechanism for ATP generation is the catabolism of arginine via the arginine dihydrolase pathway.[39] Exogenous cysteine is essential to survival. Unlike most eukaryotes, *G. lamblia* is unable to synthesize purines or pyrimidines and must salvage these from the intestine. Similar to many protozoans, it is unable to produce cholesterol but can synthesize farnesyl and geranylgeranyl to isoprenylate proteins.[40] Growth is inhibited in vitro by mevinolin[40] and this pathway may become a point of chemotherapeutic intervention.

Although *Giardia lamblia* is studied because it is an important pathogen, it is also of interest because it is one of the earliest branching eukaryotes. Defining its basic biological processes leads not only to an understanding of how primitive organisms like *Giardia* function and survive, but also when essential eukaryotic cellular mechanisms appeared and how they evolved.[6] The ability to culture and harvest large numbers of trophozoites axenically, induce encystation and excystation in vitro, and the availability of a nearly complete *Giardia* genome (gmod.mbl.edu/perl/site/giardia?page=intro)[41] has allowed comparison of *Giardia* proteins, biological processes, and pathways with those of higher eukaryotes. The recent availability of molecular biology–based methods to overexpress and/or epitope tag *Giardia* or exogenous proteins or to inhibit protein synthesis through antisense or RNAi-based mechanisms[42,43] permit experimental analysis of function in vivo.

Giardia is used as a model organism to study less complex developmental processes, vesicular transport, secretion, Golgi development, cyst wall development, transcription regulation, cytoskeleton organization, and other basic mechanisms present

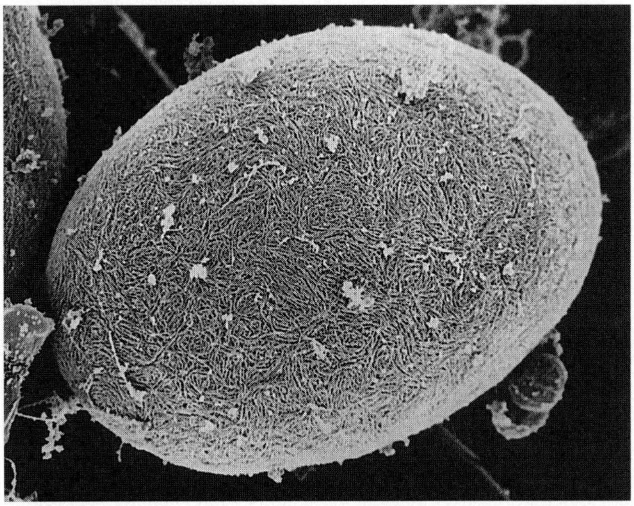

FIGURE 87-3 Scanning electron micrograph of a *Giardia lamblia* cyst (width 6.8 μm). (Courtesy of S. L. Erlandsen, Department of Cell Biology and Neuroanatomy, University of Minnesota School of Medicine, Minneapolis, MN.)

in earlier eukaryotes. The identification of residual organelles possessing remnants of mitochondrial proteins called mitosomes indicates that *Giardia* and similar eukaryotes are likely to have had mitochondria whose function has mostly been lost.[44,45] The possibility that *Giardia* had mitochondria also brings into question the evolutionary position of *Giardia*[46]; however, analysis of other essential proteins confirms its early lineage.[2–4] Other important discoveries with *Giardia* include an understanding of encystation and formation of the cyst wall as a model of an early and/or primitive developmental process as well as early secretory mechanisms,[47–54] and an understanding of novel transcription mechanisms.[55,56]

The trophozoite structure is rigid and it has its own complement of structural components, the most novel of which is a family of annexin-like proteins called giardins, some of which are immunodominant.[57,58] Vesicular transport does occur and is G protein dependent.[59] An NBD ceramide–staining structure, which is a marker for a Golgi apparatus in other eukaryotes, is not found in trophozoites but is seen in encysting organisms, suggesting that the Golgi apparatus is either formed or embellished during encystment.[59] The presence and nature of a sorting organelle is the subject of intense debate. *Giardia* possesses two equally functioning nuclei,[60] but it is not known how and if they cooperate and the manner of their communication (Fig. 87-4).

One of the most unusual features of *Giardia* is its surface, including the flagellae, which is covered by one of a family of unusual proteins (variant-specific surface proteins, VSPs) which undergo antigenic variation.[24] These change spontaneously at high rates during in vitro growth. The molecular weight of VSPs vary to a large degree and some of them have repetitive units.[61,62] These proteins are cysteine-rich (11% to 12% cysteine) occurring usually as CXXC motifs and have a conserved C terminal.[24,63] In addition, they have zinc-finger motifs,[24] bind zinc,[64,65] and one purified VSP of two studied contained zinc and iron while another showed no zinc.[64,66] The surface location of zinc fingers is highly unusual in biology.

The biologic importance of VSPs is conjectural but their differential ability to resist digestion by intestinal proteases[67] suggests that individual VSPs have unique biologic properties. Although originally discovered as an in vitro phenomenon, antigenic variation occurs in vivo in humans[68] as well as in animal model infections.[23] During experimental human infection, a *Giardia* clone (GS/H7) expressing one VSP became replaced by a mixture of other VSPs between 2 and 3 weeks after inoculation.[68] This corresponds to the time when antibody responses to the original VSP are detected. However, whether or not antigenic variation allows immunologic escape, causing chronic infections, is unknown.[24] Under experimental conditions in animals with no adaptive immune system, certain VSPs are expressed preferentially.[69] Structural similarities and particular motifs are common to VSPs, whereas other regions differ and impart unique biological characteristics that are favored by or selected against by a specific host, perhaps allowing *Giardia* to expand its host range. Therefore, the surface presence of a particular VSP appears to be the result of a combination of biological and immune selection from a repertoire of randomly expressed VSPs.

Despite these advances in understanding the biology of *Giardia,* there are important gaps in our knowledge: How does *Giardia* cause disease, what is the nature of immunity in giardiasis, what is the role of parasite antigenic variation in establishing infection and survival, and what is the true role of animals as a source of human infections?

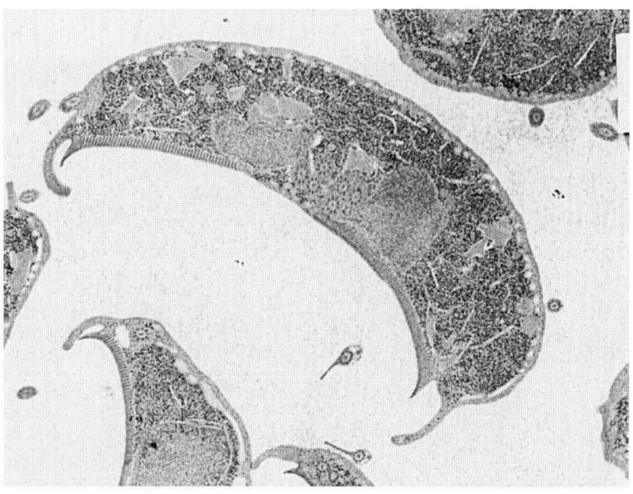

FIGURE 87-4 Transmission electron micrograph of an encysting trophozoite of *Giardia lamblia*. Two nuclei are readily seen, as well as the axonemes (intracytoplasmic projections of the flagella). Encystment-specific vesicles (ESV) are seen lining the dorsal surface. These contain cyst wall antigens. (Courtesy of B. Bowers, Laboratory of Cell Biology, National Heart and Lung Institute, National Institutes of Health, Bethesda, MD.)

EPIDEMIOLOGY

G. lamblia is one of the most widely distributed protozoan parasites, found in all climates and countries. Because transmission of *Giardia* requires oral ingestion of the cyst form of the parasite, the level of sanitation inversely correlates with the distribution of infection. Thus, poor levels of sanitation, as may be found in many developing regions, lead to fecal contamination of water and foods, accounting for high levels of childhood infection, and posing a risk to international travelers. In resource-rich regions of the world, relative resistance of the *Giardia* cyst to routine water treatment measures may allow the parasite to escape inactivation and contribute to frequent waterborne outbreaks of giardiasis. The wide distribution of *Giardia* is a major reason why it remains the most frequently found parasite in the United States, found in 4% to 7% of stools submitted to laboratories[70] and leading to an overall rate in 2002 of 7.4 cases per 100,000, with the highest rate of 23.5 in Vermont.[71]

There are three major modes of transmission—waterborne, direct fecal-oral, and foodborne. Waterborne transmission of giardiasis was first described in the 1960s from the United States,[72] and since that time has been repeatedly documented.[71,73–76] In the United States, *Giardia* remains one of the most common causes of outbreaks of diarrhea from water intended for drinking. From 1985 to 2000, it accounted for 39% of all outbreaks in which a cause was determined and affected several thousand people.[76] A frequent scenario for waterborne outbreaks is the use of *Giardia*-contaminated

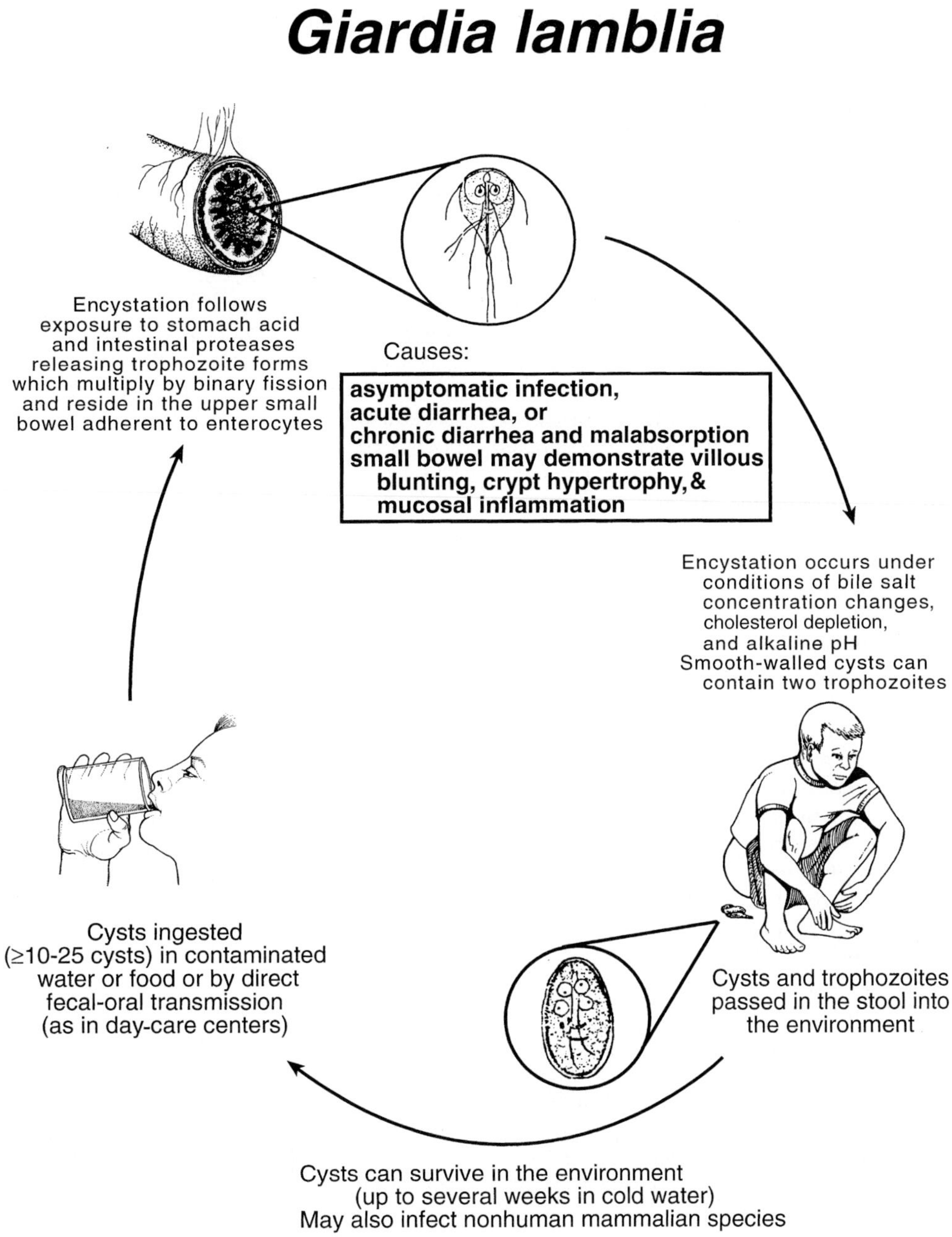

surface water that has not been subjected to flocculation, sedimentation, and filtration, as well as chlorination. In 64% of drinking water–associated outbreaks, unfiltered water was used. In a large survey of surface water supplies used for municipalities at 66 sites in the United States and Canada, 81% had *Giardia* cysts detected at a mean concentration of three cysts per liter prior to treatment,[77] and 17% had cysts after treatment.[78] Although the concentration of parasites had fallen and the species of *Giardia* and cyst viability were not determined, it emphasizes the ubiquitous presence of *Giardia*. Other waterborne outbreaks have occurred because of direct fecal contamination of the water supply when underground pipes carrying sewage and purified water mixed.[72,79]

Recreational water has also been associated with giardiasis.[71,76,80] Because of the relative resistance of *Giardia* to chlorination, swimming pool water can be a vehicle for transmission particularly when there are fecal accidents or contaminated diapers in the pool.[81] Mountainous areas of the United States and Canada have been particularly prone to waterborne outbreaks. Although it is not clear why this is the case, it may be that these areas use surface water that may be contaminated with *Giardia*, and because the water is cold, it allows cyst survival. Survival of cysts in cold lake or river water has been shown for up to 56 days.[82]

Direct fecal-oral transmission as may occur in day-care centers, custodial institutions,[83] or with anal-oral sexual practices is the second most common mode of transmission. Day-care centers throughout the world have had high infection rates, ranging from 20% to 50%.[84,85] Current surveys in Western settings are lacking. While many of the infected children may be asymptomatic, it is not uncommon for them to transmit *Giardia* to family members and thus contribute to high endemic rates of infection in a community, and even contribute to endemic rates in the United States.[86–88] A common scenario is for a mother of a young child in day care to present to a physician with complaints of diarrhea due to *G. lamblia*. Although her child is asymptomatic, when the stool is checked, it is positive. In sexually active gay men, older surveys have demonstrated prevalence rates as high as 20%.[89,90]

The third mode of transmission, food, is increasingly recognized. Given the ability of the cyst to survive outside the human host, it is surprising that foodborne outbreaks are not more frequently described. Outbreaks have occurred in restaurants, corporate offices, nursing homes, and churches. They have usually followed ingestion of foods that have not been cooked, such as salads or cold meats and fish.[91–93] Transmission may occur with as few as 10 to 25 cysts, so only low levels of contamination are necessary to establish infection.[94]

Giardiasis occurs year-round, but some epidemiologic surveys from the United States and Scotland suggest a peak incidence of giardiasis in the late summer and early fall.[71,86,95] This incidence may be due to increased recreational exposure to water or more frequent international travel during the summer months.[96,97] Acquisition of *Giardia* during international travel is increased with travel of longer than a month in duration and with travel to the Indian subcontinent.[98,99]

As has been discussed, genetically similar organisms are found in humans and a large number of mammals suggesting the potential for zoonotic transmission. However, with the exception of beavers, there are no epidemics documented from animal sources to humans. An outbreak of beaver-to-human transmission that was waterborne occurred in British Columbia.[75] *Giardia* was detected from the water supplies and from a beaver nesting in the implicated water. The human, water, and beaver isolates were identical. Despite this documented occurrence, many of the genotypes associated with animal infection (assemblages or genotypes C-G) have not been found in humans, therefore lowering their zoonotic potential.[6,32,33,100] Specifically, there is no definitive transmission from dogs or cats to humans, and screening of domestic animals is not warranted.[34,101]

Giardia is a near ubiquitous agent in developing regions. It is one of the earliest of the enteric parasites to infect infants and has prevalence rates of 10% to 30% in children less than 10 years old.[102–108] In these settings, nearly all children will become infected at some point during their childhood.

PATHOGENESIS AND IMMUNOLOGY

A hallmark of infection and disease caused by *Giardia lamblia* is clinical variability. Infections can be abortive, transient, or chronic, while accompanying disease manifestations can range from minor or none to fulminant diarrhea, severe malabsorption, and life-threatening malnutrition. Although poorly defined, both parasite and host factors are important in determining the control and susceptibility to infection and disease.

Infection follows the ingestion of as few as 10 to 25 cysts.[94] Excystation is initiated with exposure of cysts to stomach acid, intestinal proteases, and the stimulation of a parasite-derived protease.[109,110] Trophozoites that are released colonize the upper small bowel and can be present in such large numbers that they adhere to and cover a large portion of the absorptive surfaces. They may adhere via the ventral disk or possibly via specific receptor ligands.[111] It seems important that parasites are able to adhere to gut mucosa. Gerbils given a high-fiber diet had reduced rates of infection, possibly because of trapping and clearance of trophozoites in the mucous blanket,[112] and humans with asymptomatic giardiasis had decreased parasite excretion following ingestion of wheat germ agglutinin.[113]

The large number of trophozoites present in the bowel suggests a direct effect of the trophozoite on intestinal function. Thus, damage to the brush border and its enzymatic system could be a possible mechanism for some of the changes documented in clinical infection, particularly disaccharidase deficiencies. In intestinal epithelial monolayers, *Giardia* isolates have caused disruption of tight junctions, increased permeability, and have induced apoptosis.[114–116] Another possibility to account for diarrhea in giardiasis is small bowel overgrowth. While this has been documented, it may be associative rather than causative, as the presence and degree of bacterial colonization does not correlate with the development of disease in human experimental infections.[27] Mucosal invasion is rare, and there has been no evidence of a classic enterotoxin.

Biopsies of the intestine show varying degrees of mucosal inflammation with crypt hypertrophy, villous blunting, and mucosal infiltration with mononuclear inflammatory cells.[117–121] This can rarely be as severe as an entirely flattened, spruelike gut. The inflammatory response may lead to diarrhea by increasing the number of secretory crypt cells.[122] Inflammation could also initiate a cytokine reaction leading to diarrhea, which may be similar to proposed mechanisms for other adherent or minimally invasive coccidian enteric protozoa.[123] The gut may become sensitized to parasite antigen itself.[124]

Many studies have been performed on the basic biology of the trophozoite in an attempt to understand whether there are virulence differences between isolates. By a number of in vitro biochemical and molecular measures, *Giardia* organisms from humans differ (see previous discussion). Biologic differences have been noted in both animal model infections[26,125,126] and experimental human infections.[27] For instance, infections with varying isolates differed in their duration, level of cyst excretion, and ability to induce homologous or heterologous immunity. In human experimental infections, only one of two isolates was able to infect volunteers, although both originated from symptomatic donors.[68] Although correlations have been made between certain genotypes or assemblages and clinical disease,[28,29,127,128] it is premature to associate one particular isolate or genotype with increased potential to cause disease[30] until extensive controlled studies have been carried out with isolates from many regions of the world.

In part, the response of the host to *Giardia* determines the course of infection and whether there will be disease. Knowledge of the role of the immune response comes primarily from animal models of *G. lamblia* in gerbils and of *G. muris* or *G. lamblia* in mice. Relatively little data are derived directly from humans. In animals, an immune response occurs that is characterized by both the ability to self-cure and to resist rechallenge.[129,130] However, this response is both host- and parasite-dependent, and some animals are less capable of mounting an effective immune response.

In humans, the data are variable. Eighty-four percent of experimentally infected persons self-cured on average 18 days following inoculation while the remainder became chronically infected.[94] Although the evidence is indirect, epidemiologic studies in human populations suggest some acquired immunity by demonstrating decreased prevalence of infection in endemically exposed persons compared with those newly exposed.[72,131,132] In developing regions, there is increased prevalence in the young compared with adults.[102,133] However, in highly endemic populations, reinfections are common if not universal in the young,[107] and relatively high prevalence rates continue even in older populations.

The development of an immune response to *Giardia* involves both humoral and cellular mechanisms. Humans and animals produce systemic immunoglobulin G (IgG), IgM, and IgA,[27,102,120,133–140] including cytotoxic antibodies.[125,141–143] There is an important intestinal IgA response to acute infection.[68,144,145] Indirect evidence suggests a role of IgA in control of experimental infections; mouse pups are resistant to infection with *G. muris* when nursed on immune dams,[146] and infection is prolonged in anti-μ treated mice.[147] IgA-deficient mice fail to clear infection with *G. lamblia*; however, they controlled infection better than B-cell knock-out mice, suggesting B-cell dependent, IgA-independent anti-*Giardia* defenses.[148] However, conflicting data from another study of *G. lamblia* infection in B-cell knock-out mice[149] leads to the possibility that responses are dependent on the species of *Giardia* employed, model used, and stage of infection evaluated. A possible mechanism by which intestinal antibodies could prevent or help to control infection is by interfering with an important adherence step and preventing adequate colonization by *Giardia*. The production of cytotoxic intestinal IgA antibodies is plausible but as yet unproved.

Cellular immune responses are essential. Athymic, nude mice infected with *G. muris* are unable to self-cure,[150,151] but partially control the infection after the administration of immune spleen cells. This control may come at a cost, however, since following reconstitution the gut may develop inflammatory changes[150] that may be mediated through CD8+ cells.[152] Furthermore, elimination of CD4+ T cells in Peyer's patches with anti-CD4 antibodies prevents self-cure in *G. muris*–infected mice.[153] Both nude and anti-CD4-treated mice are unable to mount an intestinal IgA response,[153] suggesting that T cells are essential to the production of specific intestinal IgA. Interleukin (IL)-6-deficient mice have difficulties in the early control of *G. lamblia* infection,[154,155] as do mast cell–deficient mice.[156] It is possible this effect relates to the role IL-6 has in stimulating T helper cell–induced clonal expression of IgA-producing B cells and plasma cells.

Specific proliferative responses are found in the Peyer's patches and mesenteric lymph nodes of infected animals,[157,158] as well as in peripheral mononuclear cells from humans.[159] Macrophages and neutrophils can phagocytose *Giardia*.[160–163] Macrophages could help to process *Giardia* antigen for the development of an immune response and also could release inflammatory mediators. The role of neutrophils is undefined and natural killer cells are not essential.[164]

Patients with common variable immunodeficiency have severe and prolonged infection with *Giardia*.[31,165,166] This may be secondary to their failure to produce antibody, but is also likely related to recent findings that this immunodeficiency can be primarily a cellular-based abnormality.[167,168] Patients with X-linked agammaglobulinemia are also at increased risk.[169] Acquired immunodeficiency syndrome (AIDS) patients with severe cellular immunodeficiency may have giardiasis that is refractory to treatment.[170] Finally, local intestinal conditions including motility and microflora, and nonimmune defenses such as nitric oxide, may each play a role in whether or not *Giardia* can establish infection.[171,172]

CLINICAL MANIFESTATIONS

Clinical giardiasis is varied and ranges from asymptomatic passage of cysts to chronic diarrhea, malabsorption, and weight loss. Most symptomatic patients, however, experience a fairly characteristic syndrome of diarrhea with foul-smelling stools and gas, bloating, and abdominal cramps (Table 87-1). Following ingestion of the cyst form, there is an incubation period of approximately 1 to 2 weeks before the onset of symptoms. The incubation period may be shorter than the prepatent period (the time from ingestion of cysts to excretion of cysts in the stool), which emphasizes the importance of not eliminating giardiasis as a diagnostic possibility if a single stool specimen is negative at the onset of symptoms.[173] It can be estimated that the percentage of patients naturally infected who will develop symptoms is about 50%, 15% or more will pass cysts asymptomatically, and the remainder will show no trace of infection.

In addition to abdominal complaints in persons with symptomatic giardiasis, there is frequent malaise and anorexia. Indeed, one of the most helpful distinguishing features of giardiasis is weight loss, which occurs in over 50% of patients and averages 10 pounds. It is not clear if this weight loss is secondary to the absorptive defects seen in some patients or to the more frequent nausea and anorexia. Vomiting occurs in about one-fourth of patients and low-grade fever is uncommon. Traditional signs of inflammatory diarrhea such as tenesmus and gross blood in the stool do not occur. There has been a suggested association of

Table 87-1 Symptoms of Giardiasis

Symptom	Percentage (Range)
Diarrhea	90 (64–100)
Malaise	86 (72–97)
Flatulence	75 (35–97)
Foul-smelling, greasy stools	75 (57–87)
Abdominal cramps	71 (44–85)
Bloating	71 (42–97)
Nausea	69 (59–79)
Anorexia	66 (41–82)
Weight loss	66 (56–76)
Vomiting	23 (11–36)
Fever	15 (0–24)
Constipation	13 (0–26)
Urticaria	10 (5–14)

Data from Moore GT, Cross WM, McGuire D, et al: Epidemic giardiasis at a ski resort. N Engl J Med 281:402–407, 1969; Dykes AC, Juranek DD, Lorenz RA, et al: Municipal waterborne giardiasis: An epidemiologic investigation. Beavers implicated as a possible reservoir. Ann Intern Med 92:165–170, 1980; Shaw PK, Brodsky RE, Lyman DO, et al: A communitywide outbreak of giardiasis with evidence of transmission by a municipal water supply. Ann Intern Med 87:426–432, 1977; Mintz ED, Hudson-Wragg M, Mshar P, et al: Foodborne giardiasis in a corporate office setting. J Infect Dis 167:250–253, 1993; and reviewed in Hill DR: Giardiasis: Issues in management and treatment. Infect Dis Clin North Am 7:503–525, 1993.

giardiasis with urticaria,[174,175] Whipple disease,[176] and a reactive arthritis.[177] Although *Giardia* is generally confined to the intestine, it has been found in the stomach almost always in association with atrophic gastritis and occasionally with *Helicobacter pylori*.[178,179]

Another helpful distinguishing feature is the duration of symptoms; the course of giardiasis is frequently prolonged. In the first published study of waterborne giardiasis, illness of 10 days or more was significantly associated with infection with *Giardia*.[72] While many patients will eventually resolve infection without treatment, others will go on to a syndrome of chronic diarrhea. This may alternate with constipation or normal bowel patterns; just as the patient prepares to present to the physician with diarrhea, he or she feels better, but then relapses in several days. This pattern may continue until the patient seeks medical care or the disease resolves.

While most patients with giardiasis have a fairly benign course, reports from the United States and Scotland define the range of potentially severe giardiasis.[180,181] In the U.S. survey, hospital discharges with a diagnosis of giardiasis were reviewed. It was found that from 1979 to 1988 there were approximately 4600 persons admitted annually for giardiasis with hospital admission rates (2 per 100,000 persons) similar to those for shigellosis. Persons most frequently affected were children under the age of 5 years and women of childbearing age. Volume depletion was the most common reason for admission, and 19% of children less than 5 years old had failure to thrive. Hypokalemia has also been associated with severe infection.[182]

Malabsorption of fat, vitamins A and B_{12}, protein, and D-xylose has been documented in chronic infection.[183–186] Children who have been evaluated for failure to thrive have also been found to have giardiasis. In some cases, there is a correlation between symptoms, severity of malabsorption, and small bowel histopathologic changes, that is, inflammatory changes with villous flattening and crypt hypertrophy.[118,120] However, it is clear that some patients may have severe diarrhea without the corresponding pathologic changes, emphasizing the multiple potential mechanisms for the production of diarrhea in giardiasis. Lactose is the most common of the disaccharidases to be affected and patients who resolve infection may be lactose-intolerant for several weeks. This should be investigated in patients who "relapse" with diarrhea after treatment, before another course of therapy is empirically given.

Asymptomatic infection is most commonly seen in children. This has been best documented in day-care settings where more than 20% of children will be infected, but fewer will actually be symptomatic. In these settings, cyst passage has been documented for 6 months or more.[187,188] While children are often asymptomatic, they may introduce *Giardia* to both day-care staff and family members.[86,88] In contrast, series have documented the association of giardiasis with malabsorption, failure to thrive, and catch-up growth when *Giardia* is eliminated.[119,180,186,189]

In developing regions where children may start from a point of poor underlying nutritional status, there is ample evidence for the deleterious effect of *Giardia* upon childhood nutrition and development. Reanalysis of the classic study of diarrhea in Guatemalan children by Mata,[185] as well as other studies, indicates a role for *Giardia* in chronic diarrhea (lasting 2 to 6 weeks) and malnutrition.[102–104,190] Recent work has shown that infection with *Giardia* is associated with stunted growth in children from Ecuador[191] and Turkey,[192] increased intestinal permeability in children in Nepal,[193] low weight-for-age and height-for-age in children in Brazil,[194] and decreased cognitive function in children from Peru.[108] Catch-up growth in children treated for *Giardia* has also been documented.[195]

Therefore, *Giardia* clearly is capable of causing a chronic diarrheal syndrome in children that can be associated with malabsorption and which, in some settings, may contribute to retarded growth and nutritional deficiency. However, many children will be asymptomatically infected or coinfected with other pathogens, necessitating individual assessment of the clinical setting.

DIAGNOSIS

Because of its wide range of symptoms, giardiasis should be considered in many patients who present with diarrhea, particularly when diarrhea is prolonged and associated with weight loss. Each patient should be asked about epidemiologic risk factors of drinking water source, overseas travel, wilderness camping, day care, and sexual practices. These inquiries are especially important because the incubation period may be prolonged, and a patient may have returned from a place of exposure well before the onset of symptoms and, therefore, not associate the exposure.[98,196] Other diarrheal syndromes caused by viruses, noninvasive bacteria, parasites, and tropical sprue should be considered in the differential diagnosis. Similar syndromes, though generally more severe, are those produced by *Cryptosporidium parvum*, *Cyclospora cayetanensis*, and *Isospora belli*.[123,197,198] Since the epidemiology of *C. parvum* and *Cyclospora* are similar to that of *Giardia* and the clinical presentation and risk factors may overlap, they will need to be distinguished by stool examination.

Until recent years, the gold standard for the diagnosis of giardiasis was a stool examination for ova and parasites (O&P).[199,200] Now rapid detection of *Giardia* antigen using immunofluorescence, enzyme-linked immunosorbent assay (ELISA), and nonenzymatic assays has been employed by most commercial laboratories because of ease of use and high sensitivity and specificity. In the O&P exam, a stool is typically divided into three portions with one examined fresh, one placed in polyvinyl alcohol (PVA), and the third in 10% buffered formalin. The fresh stool can be examined under a saline wet mount or with the addition of iodine that becomes concentrated in the cysts of *Giardia*. A loose stool might yield motile trophozoites; a semi-formed or formed stool is more likely to contain only cysts. Preserved specimens can be permanently stained, usually with trichrome or iron hematoxylin and examined thoroughly. Finally, the stool can be concentrated by formalin-ether or zinc flotation techniques. Using an O&P exam, *Giardia* should be detected 50% to 70% of the time following one stool and as often as 90% following three stools.[201]

Commercial assays that detect *Giardia* antigen are more sensitive than the standard O&P. These assays are clearly an advance; however, they should not be done to the exclusion of an O&P in cases when other parasites are in the differential diagnosis. Some of the best situations in which to use antigen detection assays are in screening a population for *Giardia*, such as in an outbreak setting and children in day care, or for a test of cure. Assays that detect soluble antigen should be carefully interpreted in light of the clinical scenario, as they could be positive after a patient has stopped excreting intact, viable organisms.

Antigen detection generally utilizes polyclonal or monoclonal antibodies directed against cyst or trophozoite antigens.[202,203]

They are rapid to perform, less observer dependent than stool O&Ps, and are highly sensitive and specific. Two widely used commercial assays in the United States are the ProSpecT microplate EZ (EIA; Remel, Lenexa, KS) and the Merifluor DFA (Meridian Bioscience, Cincinnati, OH). The ProSpecT assay uses an ELISA to detect a cyst wall protein of *Giardia*[204] and has a sensitivity of 91% to 98% and a specificity of nearly 100%.[205,206] When compared directly with stool O&P, it consistently detects more positive stools. As with a stool O&P, there is increased sensitivity with three stool examinations.[207] The Merifluor immunofluorescence assay is a combination test using a monoclonal antibody to detect *Giardia* and a separate monoclonal antibody to detect *Cryptosporidium*.[206,208,209] This assay has similar sensitivity and specificity to that of the ELISA. A nonenzymatic, solid-phase assay has also been introduced, called ImmunoCard STAT! *Cryptosporidium/Giardia* Rapid Assay (Meridian Bioscience, Cincinnati, OH).[210] With low levels of parasites in the stool (≤100 cysts/10 μL), the non-immunofluorescence assays had more false negatives.[208,210] The use of genomic probes has been primarily used to detect *Giardia* cysts in water,[211] although efforts are being made to adapt it to the clinical laboratory.[212,213]

When a careful history has been taken and a stool properly tested for *Giardia*, most cases of giardiasis should be diagnosed. This lessens the need for duodenal sampling. Early studies indicated that duodenal aspiration, biopsy, or the string test had higher yields than the standard O&P.[214–217] While the new diagnostic tests have not been measured against duodenal sampling, it is likely that they are as sensitive and they are certainly less invasive and expensive for the patient. Duodenal aspirates or biopsies, however, should be used in patients for whom the diagnosis of giardiasis cannot be made by stool examinations, when there is a broad differential diagnosis, or when it is important to examine the histology of the small bowel. Small bowel biopsy may be particularly helpful in patients with human immunodeficiency virus (HIV) infection or AIDS, common variable immunodeficiency, or suspected sprue.

Serology has been reserved for seroepidemiologic studies and research settings.[102,135,136] It has not been developed for commercial use in diagnostic laboratories because of the ease and sensitivity of stool assays and because the serologic response to a noninvasive pathogen may be less reliable for individual diagnosis. Culture of human isolates has been accomplished, but is generally limited to research laboratories.[38] Duodenal isolates may be directly cultured and cysts obtained from stool may be excysted in vitro or in vivo in mice or gerbils and then cultured.[218,219]

Radiography is generally not specific and of little use in the diagnosis of giardiasis, but may reveal other lesions when there is a broader differential diagnosis. Findings on upper gastrointestinal studies have included an increased transit time and irregular thickening of the small bowel folds. Nodular lymphoid hyperplasia has been seen in patients with common variable immunodeficiency. Peripheral white blood cell counts are normal; eosinophilia is not seen. Stools should not contain inflammatory cells.

TREATMENT AND PROGNOSIS

Symptomatic patients with giardiasis should be treated (Table 87-2). Because routine culture and sensitivity testing of *Giardia* isolates is not available and in vitro results do not always correlate with the clinical picture, treatment protocols have been based on clinical experience.[220,221] Therapeutic classes

Table 87-2 *Treatment of* Giardia lamblia, Balantidium coli, *and* Dientamoeba fragilis

	Dosage	
Drug	**Adult**	**Child**
Giardiasis		
Tinidazole	2 g × 1 dose	50 mg/kg × 1 dose (max. 2 g)
Metronidazole*	250 mg tid × 5–7 days	5 mg/kg tid × 5–7 days
Nitazoxanide	500 mg bid × 3 days (≥12 years)	100 mg q12h × 3 d (age 12–47 months) 200 mg q12h × 3 d (age 4–11 years)
Alternatives		
Furazolidone	100 mg qid × 7–10 days	2 mg/kg qid × 10 days
Quinacrine†	100 mg tid × 5–7 days	2 mg/kg tid × 7 days
Paromomycin*	500 mg tid × 5–10 days	30 mg/kg/day in 3 doses × 5–10 days
Albendazole*	400 mg qd × 5 d	15 mg/kg/day × 5–7 days (max. 400 mg)
Balantidiasis		
Tetracycline*‡	500 mg qid × 10 days	10 mg/kg qid × 10 days (max. 2 g/day)
Iodoquinol*	650 mg tid × 20 days	40 mg/kg/day in 3 doses × 20 days (max. 2 g/d)
Metronidazole*	500 mg bid × 5 days	25–35 mg/kg/day in 3 doses × 5 days
Dientamoeba fragilis		
Iodoquinol*	650 mg tid × 20 days	40 mg/kg/day in 3 doses × 20 days (max. 2 g/d)
Tetracycline*‡	500 mg qd × 10 days	10 mg/kg qid × 10 days (max. 2 g/day)
Paromomycin*	500 mg tid × 7–10 days	25–30 mg/kg/day in 3 doses × 7–10 days

*Not a U.S. Food and Drug Administration–approved indication.
†No longer produced in the United States. May be obtained from certain compounding pharmacies such as Panorama Pharmacy, Panorama City, CA (800-247-9767) or Medical Center Pharmacy, New Haven, CT (203-688-6816).
‡Not recommended for use in children less than 8 years of age.

that have demonstrated both in vitro and clinical efficacy include the nitroimidazoles, nitrofurans, benzimidazoles, and a newly released agent, nitazoxanide.[220,222] The nitroimidazoles are the standard for treatment.

In 2003 and 2004, two agents were released in the United States for treatment of giardiasis: tinidazole (Tindamax, Presutti Labs) and nitazoxanide (Alinia, Romark).[222,223] These agents increase treatment options and should allow most patients with giardiasis to be successfully treated. Until the release of tinidazole in 2004, metronidazole (Flagyl) had become the drug of choice following the discontinuation of quinacrine production in the United States in 1992. Tinidazole is now the agent of choice. It has more than 3 decades of experience in the treatment of giardiasis (as well as amoebiasis and trichomoniasis) outside of the United States. From these studies, it is considered to be the most effective agent against *Giardia* and, because it has a longer half-life than metronidazole, can be given as a single dose (2 g in adults).[220,224–226]

Although metronidazole had never been approved by the U.S. Food and Drug Administration for use in giardiasis, it has proved both safe and effective from extensive clinical experience.[220] Most patients should receive metronidazole in divided doses over 5 to 7 days. Although short-course (1 or 2 days), high-dose regimens have been used, they are less effective than longer courses and may be poorly tolerated. Side effects from tinidazole and metronidazole are similar, but tinidazole may be better tolerated.[227,228] These side effects include headache, vertigo, nausea, and a metallic taste (Table 87-3). Rarely, central nervous system toxicity and a reversible neutropenia occur. The drugs should not be taken with alcohol because they may produce a disulfiram-like effect. There has been concern about potential carcinogenicity of metronidazole in children. Although the drug may be mutagenic in bacteria and carcinogenic in high doses when given to animals, these findings have never been documented in humans, and the drug has accepted use in children for the treatment of anaerobic infections and amoebiasis.[229–231] Similar concerns would apply to tinidazole. Ornidazole, a nitroimidazole not available in the United States, has excellent efficacy when given over several days or as a single dose.[220,232]

Nitazoxanide was released in the United States in 2003 for treatment of giardiasis and cryptosporidiosis in children, and then approved in 2004 for treatment of adults.[222] This drug is active against a wide variety of parasites and bacteria, including some helminths. Although there is limited experience of the drug in patients with giardiasis, it appears to be effective in 70% to 85% of cases when given over 3 days.[233–237] Its main side effect is gastrointestinal.

Furazolidone (Furozone, Roberts), a nitrofuran, has been used in children because a liquid preparation is available and the drug is generally well tolerated. However, tinidazole may be made into syrup and nitazoxanide comes in a liquid formulation. Furazolidone has an efficacy of 80% to 95% and needs to be given in four divided doses for 7 to 10 days.[220,238,239] Side effects may include gastrointestinal upset, brown discoloration of the urine, and mild hemolysis in glucose-6-phosphate dehydrogenase (G6PD)-deficient persons. Although this drug may be carcinogenic in rodents when given in high doses, this has never been established in humans and has received little attention compared with that given to metronidazole.[240]

The benzimidazoles, particularly mebendazole and albendazole, have been studied in giardiasis. Although mebendazole (Vermox, McNeil) demonstrated good activity in vitro, the results of clinical studies have been variable and generally disappointing.[220] Albendazole (Albenza, GlaxoSmithKline) is more effective than mebendazole and, when given in a single daily dose of 400 mg for 5 days, successfully treated 95% of infections in Bangladeshi children.[241] Several other clinical studies have confirmed its effectiveness, although not always at this high level.[242–245] It needs to be given for 5 days; shorter courses are less effective.[241,246] Because of albendazole's ability to kill other intestinal helminths, it is attractive when considering treatment of intestinal parasitism in resource-poor regions of the world, as is nitazoxanide.[247] Bacitracin zinc 120,000 units (USP) twice daily was effective in a trial in Tanzania, but this agent is not readily available for use and requires a 10-day course of therapy.[248]

Quinacrine is a highly effective agent, but it has not been produced in the United States since 1992. Clinical efficacy is greater then 90%.[220,249] If quinacrine can be obtained from

Table 87-3 Treatment of Giardiasis—Efficacy and Adverse Events

Drug	Efficacy	Adverse Events
Tinidazole	85%–98%	As for metronidazole
Metronidazole	80%–95%	Gastrointestinal, metallic taste, headache, disulfiram-like effect, rash; Rare: leukopenia, neuropathy, seizures ?mutagenic/carcinogenic
Nitazoxanide	70%–85%	Abdominal pain, diarrhea, vomiting, headache
Furazolidone	80%–95%	Gastrointestinal, allergic reaction, headache, disulfiram-like effect Do not take with tyramine- or tryptophan-containing food or drink, or with tricyclic antidepressants Rare: mild hemolysis in G6PD deficiency ?carcinogenic
Quinacrine	90%–95%	Gastrointestinal, headache, yellow discoloration Rare: toxic psychosis Should not be given to patients with psoriasis
Paromomycin	55%–90%	Gastrointestinal
Albendazole	85%–95%	Anorexia, constipation Rare: reversible neutropenia and elevated liver enzymes

G6PD, glucose-6-phosphate dehydrogenase.

alternative sources, it should be given for 5 to 7 days. It may not be as well tolerated as other agents, particularly in children,[239] with potential side effects of a bitter taste; nausea and vomiting; yellow discoloration of urine, skin, and sclerae; and a rare drug-induced psychosis.

Treatment of giardiasis in pregnancy has been controversial. If a woman has mild disease and is able to maintain both adequate hydration and nutrition, then treatment can be delayed until after delivery or at least until the mother has progressed beyond the first trimester. If treatment is required, the options usually considered are metronidazole or paromomycin. The safety of metronidazole has been extensively studied and information indicates that it is probably safe in the final two trimesters,[220,250–252] but it should be avoided in the first trimester.[253] Tinidazole is Pregnancy Category C and is contraindicated in the first trimester.[254] An alternative to nitroimidazoles is paromomycin, a nonabsorbable aminoglycoside. There is limited information on the treatment of *Giardia*; efficacy varies from 55% to 90% of cases.[220,255–257] It has the theoretical advantage of not being appreciably absorbed and therefore avoiding potential fetal toxicity.

Drug resistance can occur with *Giardia* and has been most completely studied with metronidazole. It appears that the mechanism of action of metronidazole in giardiasis is through covalent binding of activated drug to parasite DNA, resulting in trophozoite death.[258] The drug also inhibits parasite respiration.[259] Activation of metronidazole occurs following reduction of the nitro group by acceptance of electrons from parasite protein ferredoxins.[260,261] Resistance correlates with decreased parasite pyruvate:ferredoxin oxidoreductase.[258,260]

Patients who fail a course of treatment may do so because of drug resistance, host factors, or simply failure of a single course of treatment. For patients who fail treatment or infrequently relapse, repeat therapy with the same agent, using a drug of a different class, or combination therapy with metronidazole and quinacrine may be effective.[170,262] Nitazoxanide may also be effective in persons with resistant parasites.[263] Patients who clinically relapse should be documented to have giardiasis since many persons who have recovered have prolonged lactose intolerance that can mimic infection. Functional bowel disease has been another association with *Giardia* infection.[264] Repeated failures should be investigated for a potential immune defect such as common variable immunodeficiency.

Treatment of persons asymptomatically excreting *Giardia* cysts has been controversial, particularly when reinfection is likely to occur as in children in developing regions or in day-care settings.[107,265,266] Therefore, in each clinical setting one needs to balance the effect of *Giardia* on the host, the cost and tolerance of treatment, and the ability to obtain a sustained elimination of the parasite. If *Giardia* is contributing to nutritional abnormalities in children, a case can be made to treat. Because of the possibility of transmission in food, all food handlers should be treated.

PREVENTION AND CONTROL

The prevention of giardiasis requires the provision of potable water and adequate sewage treatment for communities and personal hygiene for individuals. Because of the wide contamination of surface water with *Giardia* cysts, treatment of water supplies needs to be adequate to remove or inactivate these relatively hardy cysts. Water should be treated by flocculation, sedimentation, filtration, and then chlorination. Most municipal water supplies use chlorine at levels of approximately 0.4 mg/L. This level of chlorination, when used alone, may not be sufficient to inactivate cysts, so it is important that the other measures are also in place.[267]

In order to purify water for personal use when camping or traveling overseas, it can be brought to a boil (or boiled for a minute if at high altitude), filtered using small-volume water filters (pore size of less than 1 μm), or halogenated with chlorine or iodine preparations.[268] Chlorine preparations may be more subject to temperature, pH, and turbidity than iodines, so some recommend iodine over chlorine.[268–270] When using halogens, it is important to increase contact time for cold water and increase the dose of the halogen for turbid water. All halogenation techniques may be inadequate for *Cryptosporidium* and therefore filtration or boiling is more reliable,[271] especially when traveling overseas where there is a higher likelihood of acquiring *Cryptosporidium* than from wilderness water in the United States.[272] The sensitivity of *Cyclospora* to halogens is likely to be similar to *Cryptosporidium*. When enteric viruses are a concern and a filter is being used, the water should also be halogenated since viruses will escape the filtration process.

Prevention of transmission in endemic foci such as day-care centers is a particular problem as it has been difficult to decrease transmission and lower prevalence rates.[187] In addition, it is possible that asymptomatic infection in some children who are otherwise well-nourished will have little deleterious effect on the child.[188,273,274] In one day-care study, a strict intervention policy with exclusion and treatment of both symptomatic and asymptomatic children did not result in better control, but incurred higher costs because of the need for parents to stay home with children.[275] The study may be flawed, however, because of the high incidence of giardiasis in the community and, therefore, the large number of children who came into day care with infection. Certainly symptomatic children, teachers, and family members should be treated. If strict hand washing, separation of diaper changing areas from play and food areas, and treatment of symptomatic children does not control the problem, then consideration can be given to treating all infected children.

Prospects for the control of giardiasis in developing regions are limited until there are both the financial resources and political and community will to provide for the proper disposal of sewage and the provision of potable water. Sanitary interventions that improve hygiene should be combined with screening and treatment of diarrheal disease, including that caused by *Giardia*. Breastfeeding has been associated with lower rates of infection in developing regions, particularly when maternal milk has contained antibody to *Giardia*.[104,276–278] Currently, there is no prospect for a vaccine against infection in humans.

Balantidium coli

Balantidium coli is the largest intestinal protozoan of man and the only ciliate (Fig. 87-5).[279] It is a rare cause of diarrhea and inflammatory colitis. The trophozoite ranges in size from 60 μm to 70 μm (it can be as long as 150–200 μm), is

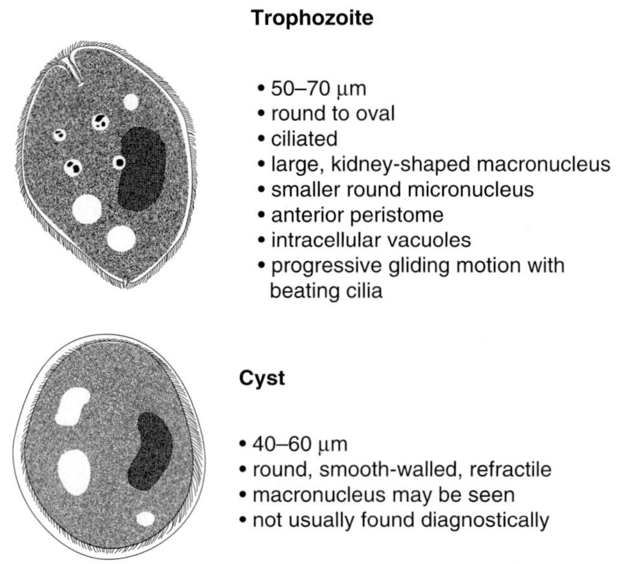

FIGURE 87-5 Schematic drawing of *Balantidium coli* trophozoite (*top*) and cyst (*bottom*), and their key identification points.

usually ovoid in shape, and has a large, kidney-shaped macronucleus with a small micronucleus often lying in its concavity (Fig. 87-6). Anteriorly it has a tunnel-shaped cytosome and posteriorly a small opening in the cell membrane called the cytopyge. Within the cytoplasm, there are numerous vacuoles and occasional intracellular erythrocytes. It is covered by longitudinal rows of cilia, which help to propel the organism. The cyst form is also large, 40 to 60 μm, round to oval, and smooth-walled. The characteristic nucleus may be visible.

Humans are an incidental host to this pathogen, which frequently inhabits the large bowel of many mammals. Pigs are likely to be one of the main sources of human infection, as they are commonly infected.[280,281] A cluster of cases of human infection in Papua New Guinea demonstrated close association of humans with pigs,[282] as did cases in a rural community in Venezuela.[283] A large outbreak of balantidiasis was reported from the Truk Islands in Micronesia, where it was postulated that the water supplies became contaminated with pig feces after a typhoon.[284] However, cases in Muslims from Iran did not have pig exposure, indicating that there are other sources of infection.[285] The parasite has been found in amphibians and insects.[286]

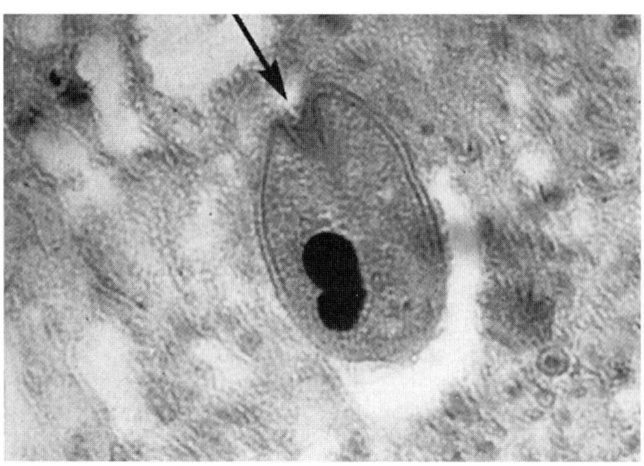

FIGURE 87-6 Trophozoite of *Balantidium coli*. The large, eccentric, kidney-shaped nucleus is readily seen. The surface is covered with short cilia. The arrow indicates the cytosome. (From Baskerville L, Ahmed Y, Ramchand S: *Balantidium* colitis. Report of a case. Dig Dis 15:727, 1970. Reproduced with permission of S. Karger AG, Basel.)

While symptomatic infection with *B. coli* has been reported from the Americas, Africa, and Latin America, it remains unusual. In the United States, it was found in less than 0.1% of stools and from only three states.[70] This low prevalence in the United States is similar to that found in other temperate climates.[286,287] Cases in captive, lowland gorillas and other primates have been described.[288,289]

Clinical infection ranges from asymptomatic, accounting for over 50% of cases, to chronic, intermittent diarrhea and weight loss, to acute dysentery in about 5% of cases.[288,290] Diarrhea is characterized by several loose stools per day, abdominal pain, and cramps, and may be associated with blood and mucus. Appendicitis, intestinal perforation with peritonitis and death, and disseminated infection to liver and lung have all been reported but are rare.[290–295] Most cases of severe extrapulmonary infection have occurred in immunocompromised hosts.[296,297]

In experimental infection, *B. coli* appears to cause disease by invasion of mucosa from the terminal ileum to rectum with subsequent inflammation.[298] These findings are borne out by sigmoidoscopic and pathologic specimens of human infection.[286,290,299] The penetration of the mucosa may be aided by the action of a hyaluronidase.[300] Most often ulcers are multiple and superficial, but they can progress to deep ulceration with perforation. The ulcers may resemble those formed by *Entamoeba histolytica*.

The diagnosis is made by demonstrating trophozoites in fresh stools or ulcer scrapings from the colon. While cysts may be found in the stool on O&P exam, it is more common to make the diagnosis by finding trophozoites.[285,286,290] *B. coli* can be grown on artificial media,[38] but this method is not readily available. Treatment is effective with tetracycline, iodoquinol, and metronidazole (see Table 87-2).[221,282,286,301,302]

Dientamoeba fragilis

Dientamoeba fragilis is an occasional intestinal protozoan of humans; its role in the causation of diarrhea has been controversial.[279] At its first description,[303] *D. fragilis* was classified as an ameba. However, immunologic and ultrastructural studies have placed it in the flagellate group, related to the *Histomonas* and *Trichomonas* genera.[304–307] Morphologically, it exists only in the trophozoite form (Fig. 87-7). It is 9 to 12 μm in size, usually has two nuclei (in arrested telophase) with a granular appearance, and frequent intracytoplasmic vacuoles. Although categorized as a flagellate, it has no flagella and does not exhibit directed motility in wet microscopy.

D. fragilis is found throughout the world. In a survey of enteric parasites in the United States, it was identified in 0.5% of stools submitted; over 50% of those identified were from California.[70] In Canada, it was found in 4% of stools from over 40,000 people[308]; in Egypt, in 13% of submitted stools[309]; and

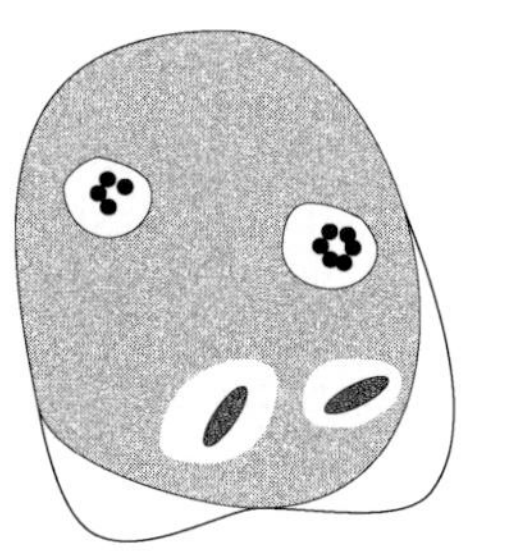

Trophozoite

- 7–12 μm
- rounded
- one or two (80%) nuclei with four to eight symmetrical chromatin granules
- intracellular vacuoles and bacteria
- best identified in permanent stains
- active psedopods, but sluggish motility

Cyst

No cyst stage

FIGURE 87-7 Schematic drawing of *Dientamoeba fragilis* trophozoite and its key identification points. *D. fragilis* has no cyst stage.

in Oman, 5% of stools.[310] Because the parasite only exists in the trophozoite form, it can be difficult to detect in stool, and thus may be missed by many laboratories unless appropriate techniques are used.[311] Thus, standard surveys may underestimate its true prevalence. In selected populations in the United States, the prevalence has been as high as 19% to 50%.[312,313] It is seen overseas, often in conjunction with other intestinal parasites, and was identified in 20% of stools of returned missionaries.[314–316]

Transmission of *D. fragilis* is presumed to be via the fecal-oral route. How it might survive stomach acid is not clear. Because of its association in some studies with *Enterobius vermicularis* (pinworm),[308,317] some investigators have proposed that the parasite is transmitted in the pinworm eggs.[318–320] This has never been formally proved.

The ability of *D. fragilis* to cause gastrointestinal symptoms has been debated through the years because the parasite is frequently seen both in conjunction with other intestinal protozoa and in asymptomatic individuals. Several studies that have surveyed patients with only *D. fragilis* in their stools have described symptoms of diarrhea, abdominal pain (frequently epigastric or lower quadrant), increased flatus, anorexia, fatigue, and malaise.[308–310,317,321–326] Abdominal symptoms may have been present for weeks.[322,324,326] A case report describes *D. fragilis* mimicking appendicitis.[327] While it appears to be confined to the large intestine, it has been detected in bile.[315] Reports of severe infection are rare.[328]

The diagnosis of *Dientamoeba* infection requires the proper handling of stools. Stools should be placed in a fixative, usually polyvinyl alcohol, and then permanently stained and examined.[308,311] A simple wet mount or iodine stain will miss many infections, and the parasite quickly disintegrates if mixed with water. Three stool examinations should increase the yield from approximately 70% to 90%.[201] Although the organism can be cultured, growth is not able to be sustained.[38,315,329,330] Detection by immunofluorescence and polymerase chain reaction (PCR) have been described but remain investigative.[331,332] An association has been the finding of peripheral eosinophilia,[333] but why this protozoan parasite should cause eosinophilia is not clear. Many of the cases of eosinophilia have been in patients in whom pinworm was also seen or in immigrant populations in whom other helminthic infections were not adequately ruled out.[311,321,322]

Successful treatment has been with metronidazole, secnidazole (a nitroimidazole not available in the United States), iodoquinol, and tetracycline[221,317,321,323,333,334] (see Table 87-2). In vitro, paromomycin is also active.[335]

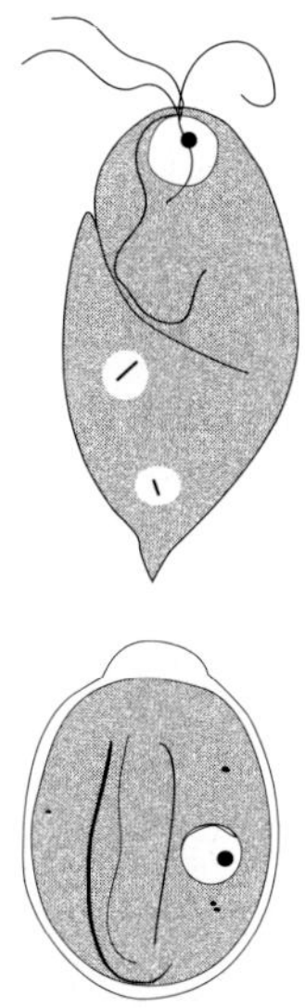

Trophozoite

- 6–10 μm × 10–20 μm
- pear shape, with posterior taper
- single anterior nucleus with small karyosome
- three anterior flagella
- spiral groove
- cytosome with curved "shepherd's crook" fibril
- irregular, jerking movement by anterior flagella

Cyst

- 6–10 μm
- unique lemon shape with anterior polar knob
- thick-walled
- single nucleus
- curved cytosomal fibril

FIGURE 87-8 Schematic drawing of *Chilomastix mesnili* trophozoite (*top*) and cyst (*bottom*), and their key identification points.

Other Flagellates

The other flagellates of humans are considered to be nonpathogens or commensals.[336,337] When they are found in the stool, they are often seen in association with other organisms and are a marker of fecal-oral contamination.[313,338] Rare clinical cases, including extra-intestinal infections, have been associated with them when other pathogens have been ruled out.[339–342] In stool surveys from the United States, *Chilomastix mesnili* (Fig. 87-8) and *Pentatrichomonas hominis* (formerly known as *Trichomonas hominis*, and named because a fifth "independent" flagellum is often seen; Fig. 87-9) were found in fewer than 0.5% of specimens.[70] However, in missionaries

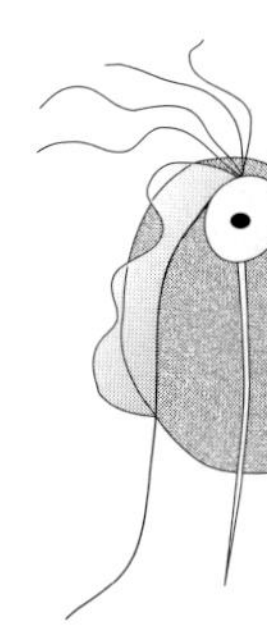

Trophozoite

- 5–8 μm × 10–15 μm
- oval or pear shape
- single anterior nucleus
- four anterior flagella
- undulating membrane with posterior projecting flagellum
- unique costa, or thin rod at attachment of body to membrane
- central axostyle with sharply pointed posterior protrusion
- rapid, jerking movement with wavelike motion of undulating membrane

Cyst

No cyst stage

FIGURE 87-9 Schematic drawing of *Pentatrichomonas hominis* trophozoite and its key identification points. *P. hominis* has no cyst stage.

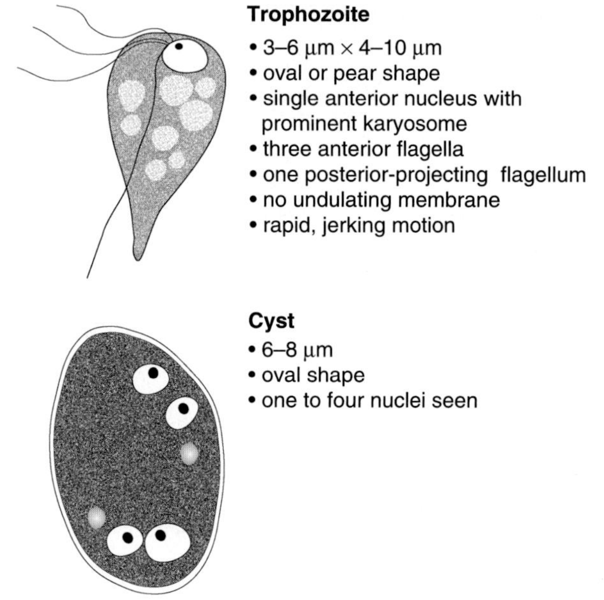

FIGURE 87-10 Schematic drawing of *Enteromonas hominis* trophozoite (*top*) and cyst (*bottom*), and their key identification points.

returning from the developing world, *C. mesnili* and *P. hominis* were seen in 3% and 2%, respectively,[314] and in a Native American population *C. mesnili* was identified in 20% of stools.[312] In stool O&P, the cyst of *C. mesnili* has a characteristic lemon-shaped cyst with an apical knob. *P. hominis*[343] has only a trophozoite stage. *Enteromonas hominis* (Fig. 87-10) and *Retortamonas intestinalis* (Fig. 87-11) are rare infections. *Trichomonas tenax* may be seen in the oral cavity; its role in causing periodontal disease is unclear.[343]

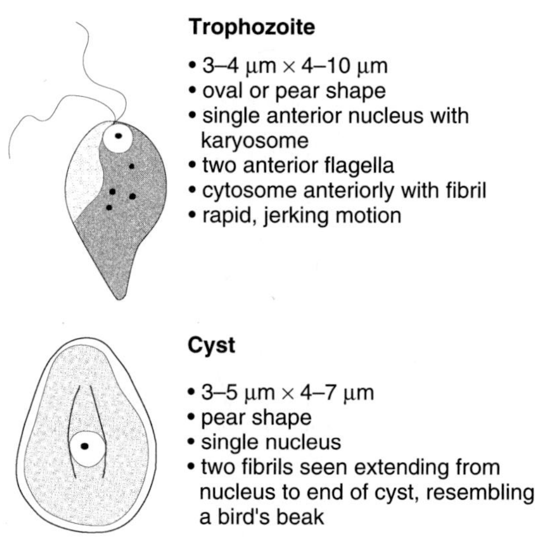

FIGURE 87-11 Schematic drawing of *Retortamonas intestinalis* trophozoite (*top*) and cyst (*bottom*), and their key identification points.

ACKNOWLEDGMENT

Parasite drawings in this chapter are by Linda Tenukas.

REFERENCES

1. Garcia LS: Classification of human parasites, vectors, and similar organisms. Clin Infect Dis 29:734–736, 1999.
2. Sogin ML, Gunderson JG, Elwood HJ, et al: Phylogenetic meaning of the kingdom concept: An unusual ribosomal RNA from *Giardia lamblia*. Science 243:75–77, 1989.
3. Best AA, Morrison HG, McArthur AG, et al: Evolution of eukaryotic transcription: insights from the genome of *Giardia lamblia*. Genome Res 14:1537–1547, 2004.
4. Triana O, Galanti N, Olea N, et al: Chromatin and histones from *Giardia lamblia*: A new puzzle in primitive eukaryotes. J Cell Biochem 82:573–582, 2001.
5. Gillin FD, Reiner DS, McCaffery JM: Cell biology of the primitive eukaryote *Giardia lamblia*. Annu Rev Microbiol 50:679–705, 1996.
6. Adam RD: Biology of *Giardia lamblia*. Clin Micro Rev 14:447–475, 2001.
7. Meyer EA: Taxonomy and nomenclature. In Meyer EA (ed): Giardiasis. The Netherlands, Elsevier Science Publications, 1990, pp 51–60.
8. Yu LZ, Birky CW Jr, Adam RD: The two nuclei of *Giardia* each have complete copies of the genome and are partitioned equationally at cytokinesis. Eukaryot Cell 1:191–199, 2002.
9. Bernander R, Palm JE, Svard SG: Genome ploidy in different stages of the *Giardia lamblia* life cycle. Cell Microbiol 3:55–62, 2001.
10. Meyer EA: Introduction. In Meyer EA (ed): Giardiasis. The Netherlands, Elsevier Science Publications, 1990, pp 1–9.
11. Nash TE, Mowatt MR: Identification and characterization of a *Giardia lamblia* group-specific gene. Exp Parasitol 75:369–378, 1992.
12. Mowatt MR, Weinbach EC, Howard TC, et al: Complementation of an *Escherichia coli* glycolysis mutant by *Giardia lamblia* triose phosphate isomerase. Exp Parasitol 78:85–92, 1994.
13. Mayrhofer G, Andrews RH, Ey PI, et al: Division of *Giardia* isolates from humans into two genetically distinct assemblages by electrophoretic analysis of enzymes encoded at 27 loci and comparison with *Giardia muris*. Parasitol 111:11–17, 1995.
14. Weiss JB, van Keulen H, Nash TE: Classification of subgroups of *Giardia lamblia* based upon ribosomal RNA gene sequence using the polymerase chain reaction. Mol Biochem Parasitol 54:73–86, 1992.
15. Baruch AC, Isaac-Renton J, Adam RD: The molecular epidemiology of *Giardia lamblia*: A sequence-based approach. J Infect Dis 174:233–236, 1996.
16. Nash TE, Keister DB: Differences in excretory-secretory products and surface antigens among 19 isolates of *Giardia*. J Infect Dis 152:1166–1171, 1985.
17. van Belkum A, Homan W, Limper L, et al: Genotyping isolates and clones of *Giardia duodenalis* by polymerase chain reaction: Implications for the detection of genetic variation among protozoan parasite species. Mol Biochem Parasitol 61:69–77, 1993.
18. Monis PT, Andrews RH, Mayrhofer G, et al: Molecular systematics of the parasitic protozoan *Giardia intestinalis*. Mol Biol Evol 16:1135–1144, 1999.
19. Homan WL, Gilsing M, Bentala H, et al: Characterization of *Giardia duodenalis* by polymerase-chain-reaction fingerprinting. Parasitol Res 84:707–714, 1998.
20. Thompson RC, Hopkins RM, Homan WL: Nomenclature and genetic groupings of *Giardia* infecting mammals. Parasitol Today 16:210–213, 2000.
21. Monis PT, Andrews RH, Mayrhofer G, et al: Genetic diversity within the morphological species *Giardia intestinalis* and its relationship to host origin. Infect Genet Evol 3:29–38, 2003.
22. Nash TE, McCutchan T, Keister D, et al: Restriction-endonuclease analysis of DNA from 15 *Giardia* isolates obtained from humans and animals. J Infect Dis 152:64–73, 1985.
23. Byrd LG, Conrad JT, Nash TE: *Giardia lamblia* infections in adult mice. Infect Immun 62:3583–3585, 1994.
24. Nash TE: Surface antigenic variation in *Giardia lamblia*. Mol Microbiol 45:585–590, 2002.
25. Aggarwal A, Bhatia A, Naik SR, et al: Variable virulence of isolates of *Giardia lamblia* in mice. Ann Trop Med Parasitol 77:163–167, 1983.
26. Aggarwal A, Nash TE: Comparison of two antigenically distinct *Giardia lamblia* isolates in gerbils. Am J Trop Med Hyg 36:325–332, 1987.

27. Nash TE, Herrington DA, Losonsky GA, et al: Experimental human infections with *Giardia lamblia*. J Infect Dis 156:974–984, 1987.
28. Homan WL, Mank TG: Human giardiasis: Genotype linked differences in clinical symptomatology. Int J Parasitol 31:822–826, 2001.
29. Thompson A: Human giardiasis: Genotype-linked differences in clinical symptomatology. Trends Parasitol 17:465, 2001.
30. Cedillo-Rivera R, Darby JM, Enciso-Moreno JA, et al: Genetic homogeneity of axenic isolates of *Giardia intestinalis* derived from acute and chronically infected individuals in Mexico. Parasitol Res 90:119–123, 2003.
31. Rosen FS, Cooper MD, Wedgwood RJP: The primary immunodeficiencies. N Engl J Med 333:431–440, 1995.
32. Thompson RC: Giardiasis as a re-emerging infectious disease and its zoonotic potential. Int J Parasitol 30:1259–1267, 2000.
33. Olson ME, O'Handley RM, Ralston BJ, et al: Update on *Cryptosporidium* and *Giardia* infections in cattle. Trends Parasitol 20:185–191, 2004.
34. Monis PT, Andrews RH, Mayrhofer G, et al: Novel lineages of *Giardia intestinalis* identified by genetic analysis of organisms isolated from dogs in Australia. Parasitol 116:7–19, 1998.
35. Benchimol M: Mitosis in *Giardia lamblia*: Multiple modes of cytokinesis. Protist 155:33–44, 2004.
36. Gillin FD, Reiner DS, Gault MJ, et al: Encystation and expression of cyst antigens by *Giardia lamblia* in vitro. Science 235:1040–1043, 1987.
37. Lujan HD, Mowatt MR, Byrd LG, et al: Cholesterol starvation induces differentiation of the intestinal parasite *Giardia lamblia*. Proc Natl Acad Sci USA 93:7628–7633, 1996.
38. Clark CG, Diamond LS: Methods for cultivation of luminal parasitic protists of clinical importance. Clin Microbiol Rev 15:329–341, 2002.
39. Edwards MR, Schofield PJ, O'Sullivan WJ, et al: Arginine metabolism during culture of *Giardia intestinalis*. Mol Biochem Parasitol 53:97–103, 1992.
40. Lujan HD, Mowatt MR, Chen GZ, et al: Isoprenylation of proteins in the protozoan *Giardia lamblia*. Mol Biochem Parasitol 72:121–127, 1995.
41. Adam RD: The *Giardia lamblia* genome. Int J Parasitol 30:475–484, 2000.
42. Touz MC, Kulakova L, Nash TE: Adaptor protein complex 1 mediates the transport of lysosomal proteins from a Golgi-like organelle to peripheral vacuoles in the primitive eukaryote *Giardia lamblia*. Mol Biol Cell 15:3053–3060, 2004.
43. Davis-Hayman SR, Nash TE: Genetic manipulation of *Giardia lamblia*. Mol Biochem Parasitol 122:1–7, 2002.
44. Lloyd D, Harris JC, Maroulis S, et al: The "primitive" microaerophile *Giardia intestinalis* (syn. *lamblia, duodenalis*) has specialized membranes with electron transport and membrane-potential-generating functions. Microbiology 148:1349–1354, 2002.
45. Tovar J, Leon-Avila G, Sanchez LB, et al: Mitochondrial remnant organelles of *Giardia* function in iron-sulphur protein maturation. Nature 426:172–176, 2003.
46. Knight J: *Giardia*: Not so special, after all? Nature 429:236–237, 2004.
47. Sun CH, McCaffery JM, Reiner DS, et al: Mining the *Giardia lamblia* genome for new cyst wall proteins. J Biol Chem 278:21701–21708, 2003.
48. Hehl AB, Marti M: Secretory protein trafficking in *Giardia intestinalis*. Mol Microbiol 53:19–28, 2004.
49. Touz MC, Lujan HD, Hayes SF, et al: Sorting of encystation-specific cysteine protease to lysosome-like peripheral vacuoles in *Giardia lamblia* requires a conserved tyrosine-based motif. J Biol Chem 278:6420–6426, 2003.
50. Chavez-Munguia B, Cedillo-Rivera R, Martinez-Palomo A: The ultrastructure of the cyst wall of *Giardia lamblia*. J Eukaryot Microbiol 51:220–226, 2004.
51. Karr CD, Jarroll EL: Cyst wall synthase: N-acetylgalactosaminyltransferase activity is induced to form the novel N-acetylgalactosamine polysaccharide in the *Giardia* cyst wall. Microbiology 150:1237–1243, 2004.
52. Lopez AB, Sener K, Jarroll EL, et al: Transcription regulation is demonstrated for five key enzymes in *Giardia intestinalis* cyst wall polysaccharide biosynthesis. Mol Biochem Parasitol 128:51–57, 2003.
53. Lujan HD, Touz MC: Protein trafficking in *Giardia lamblia*. Cell Microbiol 5:427–434, 2003.
54. Marti M, Regos A, Li Y, et al: An ancestral secretory apparatus in the protozoan parasite *Giardia intestinalis*. J Biol Chem 278:24837–24848, 2003.
55. Svard SG, Hagblom P, Palm JE: *Giardia lamblia*—A model organism for eukaryotic cell differentiation. FEMS Microbiol Lett 218:3–7, 2003.
56. Elmendorf HG, Singer SM, Nash TE: Targeting of proteins to the nuclei of *Giardia lamblia*. Mol Biochem Parasitol 106:315–319, 2000.
57. Peattie DA: The giardins of *Giardia lamblia*: Genes and proteins with promise. Parasitol Today 6:52–56, 1990.
58. Elmendorf HG, Dawson SC, McCaffery JM: The cytoskeleton of *Giardia lamblia*. Int J Parasitol 33:3–28, 2003.
59. Lujan HD, Marotta A, Mowatt MR, et al: Developmental induction of golgi structure and function in the primitive eukaryote *Giardia lamblia*. J Biol Chem 270:4612–4618, 1995.
60. Kabnick KS, Peattie DA: In situ analyses reveal that two nuclei of *Giardia lamblia* are equivalent. J Cell Sci 95:353–360, 1990.
61. Adam RD, Yang YM, Nash TE: The cysteine-rich protein gene family of *Giardia lamblia*: Loss of the CRP170 gene in an antigenic variant. Mol Cell Biol 12:1194–1201, 1992.
62. Mowatt MR, Nguyen BYT, Conrad JT, et al: Size heterogeneity among antigenically related *Giardia lamblia* variant-specific surface proteins is due to differences in tandem repeat copy number. Infect Immun 62:1213–1218, 1994.
63. Nash TE, Conrad JT, Mowatt MR: *Giardia lamblia*: Identification and characterization of a variant-specific surface protein gene family. J Eukaryot Microbiol 42:604–609, 1995.
64. Nash TE, Mowatt MR: Variant-specific surface proteins of *Giardia lamblia* are zinc-binding proteins. Proc Natl Acad Sci USA 90:5489–5493, 1993.
65. Zhang Y-Y, Aley SB, Stanley SL Jr, et al: Cysteine-dependent zinc binding by membrane proteins of *Giardia lamblia*. Infect Immun 61:520–524, 1993.
66. Papanastasiou P, McConville MJ, Ralton J, et al: The variant-specific surface protein of *Giardia*, VSP4A1, is a glycosylated and palmitoylated protein. Biochem J 322:49–56, 1997.
67. Nash TE, Merritt JW, Conrad JT: Isolate and epitope variability in susceptibility of *Giardia lamblia* to intestinal proteases. Infect Immun 59:1334–1340, 1991.
68. Nash TE, Herrington DA, Levine MM, et al: Antigenic variation of *Giardia lamblia* in experimental human infections. J Immunol 144:4362–4369, 1990.
69. Singer SM, Elmendorf HG, Conrad JT, et al: Biological selection of variant-specific surface proteins in *Giardia lamblia*. J Infect Dis 183:119–124, 2001.
70. Kappus KD, Lundgren RGJ, Juranek DD, et al: Intestinal parasitism in the United States: Update on a continuing problem. Am J Trop Med Hyg 50:705–713, 1994.
71. Hlavsa MC, Watson JC, Beach MJ: Giardiasis surveillance—United States, 1998–2002. MMWR Surv Summ 54:9–16, 2005.
72. Moore GT, Cross WM, McGuire D, et al: Epidemic giardiasis at a ski resort. N Engl J Med 281:402–407, 1969.
73. Dykes AC, Juranek DD, Lorenz RA, et al: Municipal waterborne giardiasis: An epidemiologic investigation. Beavers implicated as a possible reservoir. Ann Intern Med 92(Part 1):165–170, 1980.
74. Kent GP, Greenspan JR, Herndon JL, et al: Epidemic giardiasis caused by a contaminated public water supply. Am J Public Health 78:139–143, 1988.
75. Isaac-Renton JL, Cordeiro C, Sarafis K, et al: Characterization of *Giardia duodenalis* isolates from a waterborne outbreak. J Infect Dis 167:431–440, 1993.
76. Lee SH, Levy DA, Craun GF, et al: Surveillance for waterborne-disease outbreaks—United States, 1999–2000. MMWR 51:1–47, 2002.
77. LeChevallier MW, Norton WD, Lee RG: Occurrence of *Giardia* and *Cryptosporidium* spp. in surface water supplies. Appl Environ Microbiol 57:2610–2616, 1991.
78. LeChevallier MW, Norton WD, Lee RG: *Giardia* and *Cryptosporidium* spp. in filtered drinking water supplies. Appl Environ Microbiol 57:2617–2621, 1991.
79. Shaw PK, Brodsky RE, Lyman DO, et al: A communitywide outbreak of giardiasis with evidence of transmission by a municipal water supply. Ann Intern Med 87:426–432, 1977.
80. Stuart JM, Orr HJ, Warburton FG, et al: Risk factors for sporadic giardiasis: A case-control study in southwestern England. Emerg Infect Dis 9:229–233, 2003.
81. Porter JD, Ragassoni HP, Buchanon JD, et al: *Giardia* transmission in a swimming pool. Am J Public Health 78:659–662, 1988.

82. deRegnier DP, Cole L, Schupp DG, et al: Viability of *Giardia* cysts suspended in lake, river, and tap water. Appl Environ Microbiol 55:1223–1229, 1989.
83. Brannan DK, Greenfield RA, Owen WL, et al: Protozoal colonization of the intestinal tract in institutionalized Romanian children. Clin Infect Dis 22:456–461, 1996.
84. Thompson SC: *Giardia lamblia* in children and the child care setting: A review of the literature. J Paediatr Child Health 30:202–209, 1994.
85. Addiss DG, Stewart JM, Finton RJ, et al: *Giardia lamblia* and *Cryptosporidium* infections in child day-care centers in Fulton County, Georgia. Pediatr Infect Dis J 10:907–911, 1991.
86. Addiss DG, Davis JP, Roberts JM, et al: Epidemiology of giardiasis in Wisconsin: Increasing incidence of reported cases and unexplained seasonal trend. Am J Trop Med Hyg 47:13–19, 1992.
87. Overturf GD: Endemic giardiasis in the United States—Role of the daycare center (editorial). Clin Infect Dis 18:764–765, 1994.
88. Polis MA, Tuazon CU, Alling DW, et al: Transmission of *Giardia lamblia* from a day care center to the community. Am J Public Health 76:1142–1144, 1986.
89. Laughon BE, Druckman DA, Vernon A, et al: Prevalence of enteric pathogens in homosexual men with and without acquired immunodeficiency syndrome. Gastroenterology 94:984–993, 1988.
90. Esfandiari A, Jordan WC, Brown CP: Prevalence of enteric parasites among HIV-infected attendees of an inner city AIDS clinic. Cell Mol Biol 41(Suppl 1):S19–S23, 1995.
91. Quick R, Paugh K, Addiss D, et al: Restaurant-associated outbreak of giardiasis. J Infect Dis 166:673–676, 1992.
92. Porter JDH, Gaffney C, Heymann D, et al: Foodborne outbreak of *Giardia lamblia*. Am J Public Health 80:1259–1260, 1990.
93. Mintz ED, Hudson-Wragg M, Mshar P, et al: Foodborne giardiasis in a corporate office setting. J Infect Dis 167:250–253, 1993.
94. Rendtorff RC: The experimental transmission of human intestinal protozoan parasites: II. *Giardia lamblia* cysts given in capsules. Am J Hyg 59:209–220, 1954.
95. Flanagan PA: *Giardia*—Diagnosis, clinical course and epidemiology. A review. Epidemiol Infect 109:1–22, 1992.
96. Isaac-Renton JL, Philion JJ: Factors associated with acquiring giardiasis in British Columbia residents. Can J Public Health 83:155–158, 1992.
97. Gray SF, Gunnell DJ, Peters TJ: Risk factors for giardiasis: A case-control study in Avon and Somerset. Epidemiol Infect 113:95–102, 1995.
98. Okhuysen PC: Traveler's diarrhea due to intestinal protozoa. Clin Infect Dis 33:110–114, 2001.
99. Jelinek T, Loscher T: Epidemiology of giardiasis in German travelers. J Travel Med 7:70–73, 2000.
100. Lane S, Lloyd D: Current trends in research into the waterborne parasite *Giardia*. Crit Rev Microbiol 28:123–147, 2002.
101. Castor SB, Lindqvist KB: Canine giardiasis in Sweden: No evidence of infectivity to man. Trans R Soc Trop Med Hyg 84:249–250, 1990.
102. Gilman RH, Brown KH, Visvesvara GS, et al: Epidemiology and serology of *Giardia lamblia* in a developing country: Bangladesh. Trans R Soc Trop Med Hyg 79:469–473, 1985.
103. Farthing MJG, Mata L, Urrutia JJ, et al: Natural history of *Giardia* infection of infants and children in rural Guatemala and its impact on physical growth. Am J Clin Nutr 43:395–405, 1986.
104. Islam A, Stoll BJ, Ljungström I, et al: *Giardia lamblia* infections in a cohort of Bangladeshi mothers and infants followed for one year. J Pediatr 103:996–1000, 1983.
105. Mahmud MA, Chappell C, Hossain MM, et al: Risk factors for development of first symptomatic *Giardia* infection among infants of a birth cohort in rural Egypt. Am J Trop Med Hyg 53:84–88, 1995.
106. Fraser D, Dagan R, Naggan L, et al: Natural history of *Giardia lamblia* and *Cryptosporidium* infections in a cohort of Israeli Bedouin infants: A study of a population in transition. Am J Trop Med Hyg 57:544–549, 1997.
107. Gilman RH, Miranda E, Marquis GS, et al: Rapid reinfection by *Giardia lamblia* after treatment in a hyperendemic Third World community. Lancet 1:343–345, 1988.
108. Berkman DS, Lescano AG, Gilman RH, et al: Effects of stunting, diarrhoeal disease, and parasitic infection during infancy on cognition in late childhood: A follow-up study. Lancet 359:564–571, 2002.
109. Hetsko ML, McCaffery JM, Svard SG, et al: Cellular and transcriptional changes during excystation of *Giardia lamblia* in vitro. Exp Parasitol 88:172–183, 1998.
110. Ward W, Alvarado L, Rawlings ND, et al: A primitive enzyme for a primitive cell: The protease required for excystation of *Giardia*. Cell 89:437–444, 1997.
111. Weiland ME, Palm JE, Griffiths WJ, et al: Characterisation of alpha-1 giardin: An immunodominant *Giardia lamblia* annexin with glycosaminoglycan-binding activity. Int J Parasitol 33:1341–1351, 2003.
112. Leitch GJ, Visvesvara GS, Wahlquist SP, et al: Dietary fiber and giardiasis: dietary fiber reduces rate of intestinal infection by *Giardia lamblia* in the gerbil. Am J Trop Med Hyg 41:512–520, 1989.
113. Grant J, Mahanty S, Khadir A, et al: Wheat germ supplement reduces cyst and trophozoite passage in people with giardiasis. Am J Trop Med Hyg 65:705–710, 2001.
114. Buret AG, Mitchell K, Muench DG, et al: *Giardia lamblia* disrupts tight junctional ZO-1 and increases permeability in non-transformed human small intestinal epithelial monolayers: Effects of epidermal growth factor. Parasitol 125:11–19, 2002.
115. Scott KG, Meddings JB, Kirk DR, et al: Intestinal infection with *Giardia* spp. reduces epithelial barrier function in a myosin light chain kinase-dependent fashion. Gastroenterology 123:1179–1190, 2002.
116. Chin AC, Teoh DA, Scott KG, et al: Strain-dependent induction of enterocyte apoptosis by *Giardia lamblia* disrupts epithelial barrier function in a caspase-3-dependent manner. Infect Immun 70:3673–3680, 2002.
117. Yardley JH, Takano J, Hendrix TR: Epithelial and other mucosal lesions of the jejunum in giardiasis. Jejunal biopsy studies. Bull John Hopkins Hosp 115:389–406, 1964.
118. Duncombe VM, Bolin TD, Davis AE, et al: Histopathology in giardiasis: a correlation with diarrhea. Aust NZ J Med 8:392–396, 1978.
119. Hjelt K, Pœrregaard A, Krasilnikoff PA: Giardiasis causing chronic diarrhoea in suburban Copenhagen: Incidence, physical growth, clinical symptoms and small intestinal abnormality. Acta Paediatr 81:881–886, 1992.
120. Ridley MJ, Ridley DS: Serum antibodies and jejunal histology in giardiasis. J Clin Pathol 29:30–34, 1976.
121. Oberhuber G, Kastner N, Stolte M: Giardiasis: A histologic analysis of 567 cases. Scand J Infect Dis 32:48–51, 1997.
122. Buret A, Hardin JA, Olson ME, et al: Pathophysiology of small intestinal malabsorption in gerbils infected with *Giardia lamblia*. Gastroenterology 103:506–513, 1992.
123. Chen XM, Keithly JS, Paya CV, et al: Cryptosporidiosis. N Engl J Med 346:1723–1731, 2002.
124. Jimenez JC, Fontaine J, Grzych JM, et al: Systemic and mucosal responses to oral administration of excretory and secretory antigens from *Giardia intestinalis*. Clin Diagn Lab Immunol 11:152–160, 2004.
125. Aggarwal A, Nash TE: Antigenic variation of *Giardia lamblia* in vivo. Infect Immun 56:1420–1423, 1988.
126. Astiazaran-Garcia H, Espinosa-Cantellano M, Castanon G, et al: *Giardia lamblia*: Effect of infection with symptomatic and asymptomatic isolates on the growth of gerbils (*Meriones unguiculatus*). Exp Parasitol 95:128–135, 2000.
127. Paintlia AS, Descoteaux S, Spencer B, et al: *Giardia lamblia* groups A and B among young adults in India. Clin Infect Dis 26:190–191, 1998.
128. Read C, Walters J, Robertson ID, et al: Correlation between genotype of *Giardia duodenalis* and diarrhoea (letter). Int J Parasitol 32:229–231, 2002.
129. Roberts-Thomson IC, Stevens DP, Mahmoud AAF, et al: Giardiasis in the mouse: an animal model. Gastroenterology 71:57–61, 1976.
130. Roberts-Thomson IC, Stevens DP, Mahmoud AAF, et al: Acquired resistance to infection in an animal model of giardiasis. J Immunol 117:2036–2037, 1976.
131. Istre GR, Dunlop TS, Gaspard B, et al: Waterborne giardiasis at a mountain resort: Evidence for acquired immunity. Am J Public Health 74:602–604, 1984.
132. Isaac-Renton JL, Lewis LF, Ong CS, et al: A second community outbreak of waterborne giardiasis in Canada and serological investigation of patients. Trans R Soc Trop Med Hyg 88:395–399, 1994.
133. Miotti PG, Gilman RH, Santosham M, et al: Age-related rate of seropositivity of antibody to *Giardia lamblia* in four diverse populations. J Clin Microbiol 24:972–975, 1986.

134. Goka JAK, Mathan VI, Rolston DDK, et al: Diagnosis of giardiasis by specific IgM antibody enzyme-linked immunosorbent assay. Lancet 2:184–186, 1986.
135. Isaac-Renton J, Blatherwick J, Bowie WR, et al: Epidemic and endemic seroprevalence of antibodies to *Cryptosporidium* and *Giardia* in residents of three communities with different drinking water supplies. Am J Trop Med Hyg 60:578–583, 1999.
136. Ljungström I, Castor B: Immune response to *Giardia lamblia* in a water-borne outbreak of giardiasis in Sweden. J Med Micro 36:347–352, 1992.
137. Soliman MM, Taghi-Kilani R, Abou-Shady AF, et al: Comparison of serum antibody response to *Giardia lamblia* of symptomatic and asymptomatic patients. Am J Trop Med Hyg 58:232–239, 1998.
138. Rosales-Borjas DM, Diaz-Rivadeneyra J, Dona-Leyva A, et al: Secretory immune response to membrane antigens during *Giardia lamblia* infection in humans. Infect Immun 66:756–759, 1998.
139. Palm JE, Weiland ME, Griffiths WJ, et al: Identification of immunoreactive proteins during acute human giardiasis. J Infect Dis 187:1849–1859, 2003.
140. Rodriguez OL, Hagel I, Gonzalez Y, et al: Secretory IgA antibody responses in Venezuelan children infected with *Giardia duodenalis*. J Trop Pediatr 50:68–72, 2004.
141. Nash TE: Antigenic variation in *Giardia lamblia*. Exp Parasitol 68:238–241, 1989.
142. Hill DR, Burge JJ, Pearson RD: Susceptibility of *Giardia lamblia* trophozoites to the lethal effect of human serum. J Immunol 132:2046–2052, 1984.
143. Stager S, Felleisen R, Gottstein B, et al: *Giardia lamblia* variant surface protein H7 stimulates a heterogeneous repertoire of antibodies displaying differential cytological effects on the parasite. Mol Biochem Parasitol 85:113–124, 1997.
144. Gottstein B, Deplazes P, Tanner I: In vitro synthesized immunoglobulin A from nu/+ and reconstituted nu/nu mice against a dominant surface antigen of *Giardia lamblia*. Parasitol Res 79:644–648, 1993.
145. Snider DP, Underdown BJ: Quantitative and temporal analyses of murine antibody response in serum and gut secretions to infection with *Giardia muris*. Infect Immun 52:271–278, 1986.
146. Andrews JS, Hewlett EL: Protection against infection with *Giardia muris* by milk containing antibody to *Giardia*. J Infect Dis 143:242–246, 1981.
147. Snider DP, Gordon J, McDermott MR, et al: Chronic *Giardia muris* infection in anti-IgM-treated mice. J Immunol 134:4153–4162, 1985.
148. Langford TD, Housley MP, Boes M, et al: Central importance of immunoglobulin A in host defense against *Giardia* spp. Infect Immun 70:11–18, 2002.
149. Singer SM, Nash TE: T-cell-dependent control of acute *Giardia lamblia* infections in mice. Infect Immun 68:170–175, 2000.
150. Roberts-Thomson IC, Mitchell GF: Giardiasis in mice: I. Prolonged infections in certain mouse strains and hypothymic (nude) mice. Gastroenterology 75:42–46, 1978.
151. Stevens DP, Frank DM, Mahmoud AAF: Thymus dependency of host resistance to *Giardia muris* infection: Studies in nude mice. J Immunol 120:680–682, 1978.
152. Scott KG, Yu LC, Buret AG: Role of CD8+ and CD4+ T lymphocytes in jejunal mucosal injury during murine giardiasis. Infect Immun 72:3536–3542, 2004.
153. Heyworth MF, Carlson JR, Ermak TH: Clearance of *Giardia muris* infection requires helper/inducer T lymphocytes. J Exp Med 165:1743–1748, 1987.
154. Zhou P, Li E, Zhu N, et al: Role of interleukin-6 in the control of acute and chronic *Giardia lamblia* infections in mice. Infect Immun 71:1566–1568, 2003.
155. Bienz M, Dai WJ, Welle M, et al: Interleukin-6-deficient mice are highly susceptible to *Giardia lamblia* infection but exhibit normal intestinal immunoglobulin A responses against the parasite. Infect Immun 71:1569–1573, 2003.
156. Li E, Zhou P, Petrin Z, et al: Mast cell-dependent control of *Giardia lamblia* infections in mice. Infect Immun 72:6642–6649, 2004.
157. Gottstein B, Harriman GR, Conrad JT, et al: Antigenic variation in *Giardia lamblia*: Cellular and humoral immune response in a mouse. Parasite Immunol 12:659–673, 1990.
158. Hill DR: Lymphocyte proliferation in Peyer's patches of *Giardia muris* infected mice. Infect Immun 58:2683–2685, 1990.
159. Gottstein B, Stocks NI, Shearer GM, et al: Human cellular immune response to *Giardia lamblia*. Infection 19:421–426, 1991.
160. Smith PD, Elson CO, Keister DV, et al: Human host response to *Giardia lamblia*. I. Spontaneous killing by mononuclear leucocytes in vitro. J Immunol 128:1372–1376, 1982.
161. Owen RL, Allen CL, Stevens DP: Phagocytosis of *Giardia muris* by macrophages in Peyer's patch epithelium in mice. Infect Immun 33:591–601, 1981.
162. Hill DR, Pearson RD: Ingestion of *Giardia lamblia* trophozoites by human mononuclear phagocytes. Infect Immun 55:3155–3161, 1987.
163. Hill DR, Pohl R: Ingestion of *Giardia lamblia* trophozoites by murine Peyer's patch macrophages. Infect Immun 58:3202–3207, 1990.
164. Heyworth MF, Kung J, Eriksson EC: Clearance of *Giardia muris* infection in mice deficient in natural killer cells. Infect Immun 54:903–904, 1986.
165. Ament ME, Rubin CE: Relation of giardiasis to abnormal intestinal structure and function in gastrointestinal immunodeficiency syndromes. Gastroenterology 62:216–226, 1972.
166. Hartong WA, Gourley WK, Arvanitakis C: Giardiasis: Clinical spectrum and functional-structural abnormalities of the small intestinal mucosa. Gastroenterology 77:61–69, 1979.
167. Sneller MC: Clinical spectrum of common variable immunodeficiency. Ann Intern Med 118:720–730, 1993.
168. Bayry J, Lacroix-Desmazes S, Kazatchkine MD, et al: Common variable immunodeficiency is associated with defective functions of dendritic cells. Blood 104:2441–2443, 2004.
169. LoGalbo PR, Sampson HA, Buckley RH: Symptomatic giardiasis in three patients with X-linked agammaglobulinemia. J Pediatr 101:78–80, 1982.
170. Nash TE, Ohl CA, Thomas E, et al: Treatment of patients with refractory giardiasis. Clin Infect Dis 33:22–28, 2001.
171. Singer SM, Nash TE: The role of normal flora in *Giardia lamblia* infections in mice. J Infect Dis 181:1510–1512, 2000.
172. Eckmann L, Laurent F, Langford TD, et al: Nitric oxide production by human intestinal epithelial cells and competition for arginine as potential determinants of host defense against the lumen-dwelling pathogen *Giardia lamblia*. J Immunol 164:1478–1487, 2000.
173. Jokipii AMM, Jokipii L: Prepatency of giardiasis. Lancet 1:1095–1097, 1977.
174. Clyne CA, Eliopoulos GM: Fever and urticaria in acute giardiasis. Arch Intern Med 149:939–940, 1989.
175. Giacometti A, Cirioni O, Antonicelli L, et al: Prevalence of intestinal parasites among individuals with allergic skin diseases. J Parasitol 89:490–492, 2003.
176. Fenollar F, Lepidi H, Gerolami R, et al: Whipple disease associated with giardiasis. J Infect Dis 188:828–834, 2003.
177. Shaw RA, Stevens MB: The reactive arthritis of giardiasis. JAMA 258:2734–2735, 1987.
178. Quincey C, James PD, Steele RJ: Chronic giardiasis of the stomach. J Clin Pathol 45:1039–1041, 1992.
179. Berney DM, Rampton D, van der Walt JD: Giardiasis of the stomach. Postgrad Med J 70:237–238, 1994.
180. Lengerich EJ, Addiss DG, Juranek DD: Severe giardiasis in the United States. Clin Infect Dis 18:760–763, 1994.
181. Robertson LJ: Severe giardiasis and cryptosporidiosis in Scotland, UK. Epidemiol Infect 117:551–561, 1996.
182. Addiss DG, Lengerich EJ: Hypokalemic myopathy induced by *Giardia lamblia* (letter). N Engl J Med 330:66, 1994.
183. Solomons NW: Giardiasis: nutritional implications. Rev Infect Dis 4:859–869, 1982.
184. Gillon J: Clinical studies in adults presenting with giardiasis to a gastrointestinal unit. Scot Med J 30:89–95, 1985.
185. Mata LJ: The Children of Santa María Cauqué: A Prospective Field Study of Health and Growth. Cambridge, MA, MIT Press, 1978.
186. Burke JA: Giardiasis in childhood. Am J Dis Child 129:1304–1310, 1975.
187. Pickering LK, Woodward WE, DuPont HL, et al: Occurrence of *Giardia lamblia* in children in day care centers. J Pediatr 104: 522–526, 1984.
188. Ish-Horowicz M, Korman SH, Shapiro M, et al: Asymptomatic giardiasis in children. Pediatr Infect Dis J 8:773–779, 1989.

189. Welsh JD, Poley JR, Hensley J, et al: Intestinal disaccharidase and alkaline phosphatase activity in giardiasis. J Pediatr Gastroenterol Nutr 3:37–40, 1984.
190. Sullivan PB, Marsh MN, Phillips MB, et al: Prevalence and treatment of giardiasis in chronic diarrhoea and malnutrition. Arch Dis Child 66:304–306, 1991.
191. Sackey ME, Weigel MM, Armijos RX: Predictors and nutritional consequences of intestinal parasitic infections in rural Ecuadorian children. J Trop Pediatr 49:17–23, 2003.
192. Simsek Z, Zeyrek FY, Kurcer MA: Effect of *Giardia* infection on growth and psychomotor development of children aged 0–5 years. J Trop Pediatr 50:90–93, 2004.
193. Goto R, Panter-Brick C, Northrop-Clewes CA, et al: Poor intestinal permeability in mildly stunted Nepali children: Associations with weaning practices and *Giardia lamblia* infection. Br J Nutr 88:141–149, 2002.
194. Newman RD, Moore SR, Lima AA, et al: A longitudinal study of *Giardia lamblia* infection in north-east Brazilian children. Trop Med Int Health 6:624–634, 2001.
195. Gupta MC, Urrutia JJ: Effect of periodic antiascaris and antigiardia treatment on nutritional status of preschool children. Am J Clin Nutr 36:79–86, 1982.
196. DuPont HL, Capsuto EG: Persistent diarrhea in travelers. Clin Infect Dis 22:124–128, 1996.
197. Goodgame RW: Understanding intestinal spore-forming protozoa: Cryptosporidia, microsporidia, isospora, and cyclospora. Ann Intern Med 124:429–441, 1996.
198. Herwaldt BL: *Cyclospora cayetanensis*: A review, focusing on the outbreaks of cyclosporiasis in the 1990s. Clin Infect Dis 31:1040–1057, 2000.
199. Wolfe MS: Giardiasis. Clin Micro Rev 5:93–100, 1992.
200. Hill DR: Giardiasis: Issues in management and treatment. Infect Dis Clin North Am 7:503–525, 1993.
201. Hiatt RA, Markell EK, Ng E: How many stool examinations are necessary to detect pathogenic intestinal protozoa? Am J Trop Med Hyg 53:36–39, 1995.
202. Garcia LS, Shimizu RY: Evaluation of nine immunoassay kits (enzyme immunoassay and direct fluorescence) for detection of *Giardia lamblia* and *Cryptosporidium parvum* in human fecal specimens. J Clin Microbiol 35:1526–1529, 1997.
203. Aldeen WE, Carroll K, Robison A, et al: Comparison of nine commercially available enzyme-linked immunosorbent assays for the detection of *Giardia lamblia* in fecal specimens. J Clin Microbiol 36:1338–1340, 1998.
204. Boone JH, Wilkins TD, Nash TE, et al: TechLab and Alexon Giardia enzyme-linked immunosorbent assay kits detect cyst wall protein 1. J Clin Microbiol 37:611–614, 1999.
205. Aldeen WE, Hale D, Robison AJ, et al: Evaluation of a commercially available ELISA assay for detection of *Giardia lamblia* in fecal specimens. Diag Microbiol Infect Dis 21:77–79, 1995.
206. Zimmerman SK, Needham CA: Comparison of conventional stool concentration and preserved-smear methods with Merifluor *Cryptosporidium/Giardia* Direct Immunofluorescence Assay and ProSpecT Giardia EZ Microplate Assay for the detection of *Giardia lamblia*. J Clin Microbiol 33:1942–1943, 1995.
207. Addiss DG, Mathews HM, Stewart JM, et al: Evaluation of a commercially available enzyme-linked immunosorbent assay for *Giardia lamblia* antigen in stool. J Clin Microbiol 29:1137–1142, 1991.
208. Johnston SP, Ballard MM, Beach MJ, et al: Evaluation of three commercial assays for detection of *Giardia* and *Cryptosporidium* organisms in fecal specimens. J Clin Microbiol 41:623–626, 2003.
209. Alles AJ, Waldron MA, Sierra LS, et al: Prospective comparison of direct immunofluorescence and conventional staining methods for detection of *Giardia* and *Cryptosporidium* spp. in human fecal specimens. J Clin Microbiol 33:1632–1634, 1995.
210. Garcia LS, Shimizu RY, Novak S, et al: Commercial assay for detection of *Giardia lamblia* and *Cryptosporidium parvum* antigens in human fecal specimens by rapid solid-phase qualitative immunochromatography. J Clin Microbiol 41:209–212, 2003.
211. Guy RA, Payment P, Krull UJ, et al: Real-time PCR for quantification of *Giardia* and *Cryptosporidium* in environmental water samples and sewage. Appl Environ Microbiol 69:5178–5185, 2003.
212. Guy RA, Xiao C, Horgen PA: Real-time PCR assay for detection and genotype differentiation of *Giardia lamblia* in stool specimens. J Clin Microbiol 42:3317–3320, 2004.
213. Verweij JJ, Blange RA, Templeton K, et al: Simultaneous detection of *Entamoeba histolytica, Giardia lamblia,* and *Cryptosporidium parvum* in fecal samples by using multiplex real-time PCR. J Clin Microbiol 42:1220–1223, 2004.
214. Beal GB, Viens P, Grant RGL, et al: A new technique for sampling duodenal contents: Demonstration of upper small bowel pathogens. Am J Trop Med Hyg 19:349–352, 1970.
215. Naik SR, Rau NR, Vinayak VK: A comparative evaluation of examinations of three stool samples, jejunal aspirate and jejunal mucosal impression smears in the diagnosis of giardiasis. Ann Trop Med Parasitol 72:491–492, 1978.
216. Goka AKJ, Rolston DDK, Mathan VI, et al: The relative merits of faecal and duodenal juice microscopy in the diagnosis of giardiasis. Trans R Soc Trop Med Hyg 84:66–67, 1990.
217. Rosenthal P, Liebman WM: Comparative study of stool examinations, duodenal aspiration, and pediatric Entero-Test for giardiasis in children. J Pediatr 96:278–279, 1980.
218. Isaac-Renton JL, Shahriari H, Bowie WR: Comparison of an in vitro method and an in vivo method of *Giardia* excystation. Appl Environ Microbiol 58:1530–1533, 1992.
219. Mayrhofer G, Andrews RH, Ey PL, et al: The use of suckling mice to isolate and grow *Giardia* from mammalian faecal specimens for genetic analysis. Parasitol 105:255–263, 1992.
220. Gardner TB, Hill DR: Treatment of giardiasis. Clin Micro Rev 14:114–128, 2001.
221. Medical Letter: Drugs for parasitic infections. www.medicalletter.org/html/prm.htm Parasitic. Accessed on 2/7/05.
222. Medical Letter: Nitazoxanide (*Alinia*)—A new anti-protozoal agent. Med Lett Drug Ther 45:29–31, 2003.
223. Medical Letter: Tinidazole (Tindamax)—A new anti-protozoal drug. Med Lett Drugs Ther 46:70–72, 2004.
224. Rossignol JF, Maisonneuve H, Cho YW: Nitroimidazoles in the treatment of trichomoniasis, giardiasis, and amebiasis. Int J Clin Pharmacol Ther Toxicol 22:63–72, 1984.
225. Speelman P: Single-dose tinidazole for the treatment of giardiasis. Antimicrob Agents Chemother 27:227–229, 1985.
226. Zaat JO, Mank T, Assendelft WJ: Drugs for treating giardiasis. Cochrane Database Syst Rev:CD000217, 2000.
227. Jokipii L, Jokipii AMM: Single-dose metronidazole and tinidazole as therapy for giardiasis: Success rates, side effects, and drug absorption and elimination. J Infect Dis 140:984–988, 1979.
228. Pettersson T: Single-dose tinidazole therapy for giardiasis (letter). BMJ 1:395, 1975.
229. Beard CM, Noller KL, O'Fallon WM: Cancer after exposure to metronidazole. Mayo Clin Proc 63:147–153, 1988.
230. Falagas ME, Walker AM, Jick H, et al: Late incidence of cancer after metronidazole use: A matched metronidazole user/nonuser study. Clin Infect Dis 26:384–388, 1998.
231. Roe FJC: Safety of nitroimidazoles. Scand J Infect Dis Suppl 46:72–81, 1985.
232. Ozbilgin A, Ertan P, Yereli K, et al: Giardiasis treatment in Turkish children with a single dose of ornidazole. Scand J Infect Dis 34:918–920, 2002.
233. Bailey JM, Erramouspe J: Nitazoxanide treatment for giardiasis and cryptosporidiosis in children. Ann Pharmacother 38:634–640, 2004.
234. Gilles HM, Hoffman PS: Treatment of intestinal parasitic infections: A review of nitazoxanide. Trends in Parasitology 18:95–97, 2002.
235. Rodriguez-Garcia R, Rodriguez-Guzman LM, Cruz del Castillo AH: Eficacia y seguridad de mebendazol contra nitazoxanida en el tratamiento de *Giardia lamblia* en niños. Rev Gastroenterol Mex 64:122–126, 1999.
236. Ortiz JJ, Ayoub A, Gargala G, et al: Randomized clinical study of nitazoxanide compared to metronidazole in the treatment of symptomatic giardiasis in children from Northern Peru. Aliment Pharmacol Ther 15:1409–1415, 2001.
237. Rossignol JF, Ayoub A, Ayers MS: Treatment of diarrhea caused by *Giardia intestinalis* and *Entamoeba histolytica* or *E. dispar*: A randomized, double-blind, placebo-controlled study of nitazoxanide. J Infect Dis 184:381–384, 2001.

238. Murphy TV, Nelson JD: Five vs. ten days' therapy with furazolidone for giardiasis. Am J Dis Child 137:267–270, 1983.
239. Craft JC, Murphy T, Nelson JD: Furazolidone and quinacrine. Comparative study of therapy for giardiasis in children. Am J Dis Child 135:164–166, 1981.
240. Furoxone product information. Eatontown, NJ, Roberts Pharmaceutical Corporation, 1991.
241. Hall A, Nahar Q: Albendazole as a treatment for infections with *Giardia duodenalis* in children in Bangladesh. Trans R Soc Trop Med Hyg 87:84–86, 1993.
242. Dutta AK, Phadke MA, Bagade AC, et al: A randomised multicentre study to compare the safety and efficacy of albendazole and metronidazole in the treatment of giardiasis in children. Indian J Pediatr 61:689–693, 1994.
243. Misra PK, Kumar A, Agarwal V, et al: A comparative trial of albendazole versus metronidazole in children with giardiasis. Indian Pediatr 32:779–782, 1995.
244. Romero-Cabello R, Robert L, Muñoz-Garcia R, et al: Estudio aleatorio para comparar seguridad y eficacia de albendazol y metronidazol en el tratamiento de giardiasis en niños. Rev Latinoam Microbiol 37:315–323, 1995.
245. Yereli K, Balcioglu IC, Ertan P, et al: Albendazole as an alternative therapeutic agent for childhood giardiasis in Turkey. Clin Microbiol Infect 10:527–529, 2004.
246. Kollaritsch H, Jeschko E, Wiederman G: Albendazole is highly effective against cutaneous larva migrans but not against *Giardia* infection: Results of an open pilot trial in travellers returning from the tropics. Trans R Soc Trop Med Hyg 87:689, 1993.
247. Diaz E, Mondragon J, Ramirez E, et al: Epidemiology and control of intestinal parasites with nitazoxanide in children in Mexico. Am J Trop Med Hyg 68:384–385, 2003.
248. Andrews BJ, Panitescu D, Jipa GH, et al: Chemotherapy for giardiasis: Randomized clinical trial of bacitracin, bacitracin zinc, and a combination of bacitracin zinc with neomycin. Am J Trop Med Hyg 52:318–321, 1995.
249. Sabchareon A, Chongsuphajaisiddhi T, Attanath P: Treatment of giardiasis in children with quinacrine, metronidazole, tinidazole and ornidazole. S Asian J Trop Med Public Health 11:280–284, 1980.
250. Berget A, Weber T: Metronidazole and pregnancy. Ugeskr Laeg 134:2085–2089, 1972.
251. Burtin P, Taddio A, Ariburnu O, et al: Safety of metronidazole in pregnancy: A meta-analysis. Am J Obstet Gynecol 172:525–529, 1995.
252. Rosa FW, Baum C, Shaw M: Pregnancy outcomes after first-trimester vaginitis drug therapy. Obstet Gynecol 69:751–755, 1987.
253. Heinonen OP, Slone D, Shapiro S: Birth Defects and Drugs in Pregnancy. Littleton, MA, Publishing Sciences Group, 1977, pp 296–302.
254. Tindamax (tinidazole tablets) prescribing information. Presutti Laboratories, Inc., Arlington Heights, IL, 2004.
255. Kreutner AK, Del Bene VE, Amstey MS: Giardiasis in pregnancy. Am J Obstet Gynecol 140:895–901, 1981.
256. Rotblatt MD: Giardiasis and amebiasis in pregnancy. Drug Intell Clin Pharm 17:187–188, 1983.
257. Carter CH, Bayles A, Thompson PE: Effects of paromomycin sulfate in man against *Entamoeba histolytica* and other intestinal protozoa. Am J Trop Med Hyg 11:448–451, 1962.
258. Upcroft P, Upcroft JA: Drug targets and mechanisms of resistance in the anaerobic protozoa. Clin Micro Rev 14:150–164, 2001.
259. Paget TA, Jarroll EL, Manning P, et al: Respiration in the cysts and trophozoites of *Giardia muris*. J Gen Microbiol 135:145–154, 1989.
260. Townson SM, Upcroft JA, Upcroft P: Characterization and purification of pyruvate:ferredoxin oxidoreductase from *Giardia duodenalis*. Mol Biochem Parasitol 79:183–193, 1996.
261. Samuelson J: Why metronidazole is active against both bacteria and parasites. Antimicrob Agents Chemother 43:1533–1541, 1999.
262. Taylor GD, Wenman WM, Tyrrell DLJ: Combined metronidazole and quinacrine hydrochloride therapy for chronic giardiasis. Can Med Assoc J 136:1179–1180, 1987.
263. Abboud P, Lemee V, Gargala G, et al: Successful treatment of metronidazole- and albendazole-resistant giardiasis with nitazoxanide in a patient with acquired immunodeficiency syndrome. Clin Infect Dis 32:1792–1794, 2001.
264. D'Anchino M, Orlando D, De Feudis L: *Giardia lamblia* infections become clinically evident by eliciting symptoms of irritable bowel syndrome. J Infect 45:169–172, 2002.
265. Sullivan PS, DuPont HL, Arafat RR, et al: Illness and reservoirs associated with *Giardia lamblia* infection in rural Egypt: The case against treatment in developing world environments of high endemicity. Am J Epidemiol 127:1272–1281, 1988.
266. Addiss DG, Juranek DD, Spencer HC: Treatment of children with asymptomatic and nondiarrheal *Giardia* infection. Pediatr Infect Dis J 10:843–846, 1991.
267. Jakubowski WS: Purple burps and the filtration of drinking water supplies (editorial). Am J Public Health 78:123–125, 1988.
268. Backer H: Water disinfection for international and wilderness travelers. Clin Infect Dis 34:355–364, 2002.
269. Jarroll EL, Bingham AK, Meyer EA: Effect of chlorine on *Giardia lamblia* cyst viability. Appl Environ Microbiol 41:483–487, 1981.
270. Ongerth JE, Johnson RL, MacDonald SC, et al: Backcountry water treatment to prevent giardiasis. Am J Public Health 79:1633–1637, 1989.
271. Juranek DD: Cryptosporidiosis: Sources of infection and guidelines for prevention. Clin Infect Dis 21(Suppl 1):S57–S61, 1995.
272. Roach PD, Olson ME, Whitely G, et al: Waterborne *Giardia* cysts and *Cryptosporidium* oocysts in the Yukon, Canada. Appl Environ Microbiol 59:67–73, 1993.
273. Moya-Camarena SY, Sotelo N, Valencia ME: Effects of asymptomatic *Giardia intestinalis* infection on carbohydrate absorption in well-nourished Mexican children. Am J Trop Med Hyg 66:255–259, 2002.
274. Nunez FA, Hernandez M, Finlay CM: Longitudinal study of giardiasis in three day care centres of Havana City. Acta Trop 73:237–242, 1999.
275. Bartlett AV, Englender SJ, Jarvis BA, et al: Controlled trial of *Giardia lamblia*: Control strategies in day care centers. Am J Public Health 81:1001–1006, 1991.
276. Morrow AL, Reves RR, West MS, et al: Protection against infection with *Giardia lamblia* by breast feeding in a cohort of Mexican infants. J Pediatr 121:363–370, 1992.
277. Mahmud MA, Chappell CL, Hossain MM, et al: Impact of breast-feeding on *Giardia lamblia* infections in Bilbeis, Egypt. Am J Trop Med Hyg 65:257–260, 2001.
278. Tellez A, Winiecka-Krusnell J, Paniagua M, et al: Antibodies in mother's milk protect children against giardiasis. Scand J Infect Dis 35:322–325, 2003.
279. Weiss LM, Keohane EM: The uncommon gastrointestinal protozoa: Microsporidia, blastocystis, isospora, dientamoeba, and balantidium. Cur Clin Top Infect Dis 17:147–187, 1997.
280. Permin A, Yelifari L, Bloch P, et al: Parasites in cross-bred pigs in the Upper East region of Ghana. Vet Parasitol 87:63–71, 1999.
281. Hindsbo O, Nielsen CV, Andreassen J, et al: Age-dependent occurrence of the intestinal ciliate *Balantidium coli* in pigs at a Danish research farm. Acta Vet Scand 41:79–83, 2000.
282. Radford AJ: Balantidiasis in Papua New Guinea. Med J Aust 1:238–241, 1973.
283. Devera R, Requena I, Velasquez V, et al: Balantidiasis in a rural community from Bolivar State, Venezuela. Bol Chil Parasitol 54:7–12, 1999.
284. Walzer PD, Judson FN, Murphy KB, et al: Balantidiasis outbreak in Truk. Am J Trop Med Hyg 22:33–41, 1973.
285. McCarey AG: Balantidiasis in south Persia. BMJ 1:629–631, 1952.
286. Areán VM, Koppisch E: Balantidiasis. A review and report of cases. Am J Pathol 32:1089–1115, 1956.
287. Esteban JG, Aguirre C, Angles R, et al: Balantidiasis in Aymara children from the northern Bolivian Altiplano. Am J Trop Med Hyg 59:922–927, 1998.
288. Lee RV, Prowten AW, Anthone S, et al: Typhlitis due to *Balantidium coli* in captive lowland gorillas. Rev Infect Dis 12:1052–1059, 1990.
289. Muriuki SM, Murugu RK, Munene E, et al: Some gastro-intestinal parasites of zoonotic (public health) importance commonly observed in old world non-human primates in Kenya. Acta Trop 71:73–82, 1998.
290. Swartzwelder JC: Balantidiasis. Am J Digest Dis 17:173–179, 1950.
291. Ladas SD, Savva S, Frydas A, et al: Invasive balantidiasis presented as chronic colitis and lung involvement. Dig Dis Sci 34:1621–1623, 1989.
292. Currie AR: Human balantidiasis. A case report. S Afr J Surg 28:23–25, 1990.
293. Dodd LG: *Balantidium coli* infestation as a cause of acute appendicitis (letter). J Infect Dis 163:1392, 1991.

294. Dorfman S, Rangel O, Bravo LG: Balantidiasis: Report of a fatal case with appendicular and pulmonary involvement. Trans R Soc Trop Med Hyg 78:833–834, 1984.
295. Ferry T, Bouhour D, De Monbrison F, et al: Severe peritonitis due to *Balantidium coli* acquired in France. Eur J Clin Microbiol Infect Dis 23:393–395, 2004.
296. Anargyrou K, Petrikkos GL, Suller MT, et al: Pulmonary *Balantidium coli* infection in a leukemic patient. Am J Hematol 73:180–183, 2003.
297. Vasilakopoulou A, Dimarongona K, Samakovli A, et al: *Balantidium coli* pneumonia in an immunocompromised patient. Scand J Infect Dis 35:144–146, 2003.
298. Yang Y, Zeng L, Li M, et al: Diarrhoea in piglets and monkeys experimentally infected with *Balantidium coli* isolated from human feces. J Trop Med Hyg 98:69–72, 1995.
299. Baskerville L, Ahmed Y, Ramchand S: Balantidium colitis. Report of a case. Dig Dis 15:727–731, 1970.
300. Tempelis CH, Lysenko MG: The production of hyaluronidase by *Balantidium coli*. Exp Parasitol 6:31–36, 1957.
301. Garcia-Laverde A, de Bonilla L: Clinical trials with metronidazole in human balantidiasis. Am J Trop Med Hyg 24:781–783, 1975.
302. Knight R: Giardiasis, isosporiasis, balantidiasis. Clin Gastroenterol 7:31–47, 1978.
303. Jepps MW, Dobell C: A new intestinal amoeba from man. Parasitol 10:352–367, 1918.
304. Dwyer DM: Analysis of the antigenic relationships among *Trichomonas, Histomonas, Dientamoeba,* and *Entamoeba*. I. Quantitative fluorescent antibody methods. J Protozool 19:316–325, 1972.
305. Camp RR, Mattern CFT, Honigberg BM: Study of *Dientamoeba fragilis* Jepps & Dobell. I. Electron microscopic observations of the binucleate stages. II. Taxonomic position and revision of the genus. J Protozool 21:69–82, 1974.
306. Silberman JD, Clark CG, Sogin ML: *Dientamoeba fragilis* shares a recent common evolutionary history with the trichomonads. Mol Biochem Parasitol 76:311–314, 1996.
307. Gerbod D, Edgcomb VP, Noel C, et al: Phylogenetic position of the trichomonad parasite of turkeys, *Histomonas meleagridis* (Smith) Tyzzer, inferred from small subunit rRNA sequence. J Eukaryot Microbiol 48:498–504, 2001.
308. Yang J, Scholten T: *Dientamoeba fragilis*: A review with notes on its epidemiology, pathogenicity, mode of transmission, and diagnosis. Am J Trop Med Hyg 26:16–22, 1977.
309. Ayadi A, Bahri I: *Dientamoeba fragilis*: Pathogenic flagellate? Bull Soc Pathol Exot 92:299–301, 1999.
310. Windsor JJ, Rafay AM, Shenoy AK, et al: Incidence of *Dientamoeba fragilis* in faecal samples submitted for routine microbiological analysis. Br J Biomed Sci 55:172–175, 1998.
311. Grendon JH, Digiacomo RF, Frost FJ: *Dientamoeba fragilis* detection methods and prevalence: A survey of state public health laboratories. Pub Health Rep 106:322–325, 1991.
312. Melvin DM, Brooke MM: Parasitologic surveys on Indian reservations in Montana, South Dakota, New Mexico, Arizona, and Wisconsin. Am J Trop Med Hyg 11:765–772, 1962.
313. Millet VE, Spencer MJ, Chapin MR, et al: Intestinal protozoan infection in a semicommunal group. Am J Trop Med Hyg 32:54–60, 1983.
314. McQuay RM: Parasitologic studies in a group of furloughed missionaries. I. Intestinal protozoa. Am J Trop Med Hyg 16:154–160, 1967.
315. Talis B, Stein B, Lengy J: *Dientamoeba fragilis* in human feces and bile. Isr J Med Sci 7:1063–1069, 1971.
316. Oyofo BA, Peruski LF, Ismail TF, et al: Enteropathogens associated with diarrhea among military personnel during Operation Bright Star 96, in Alexandria, Egypt. Mil Med 162:396–400, 1997.
317. Preiss U, Ockert G, Bromme S, et al: *Dientamoeba fragilis* infection, a cause of gastrointestinal symptoms in childhood. Klin Padiatr 202:120–123, 1990.
318. Burrows RB, Swerdlow MA: *Enterobius vermicularis* as a probable vector of *Dientamoeba fragilis*. Am J Trop Med Hyg 5:258–265, 1956.
319. Ockert G: Zur epidemiologie von *Dientamoeba fragilis* Jepps et Dobell, 1918. 2. Mitteilung: versuch der übertragung der art mit Enterobius-eiern. J Hyg Epidemiol Microbiol Immunol 16:222–225, 1972.
320. Windsor JJ, Johnson EH: *Dientamoeba fragilis*: The unflagellated human flagellate. Br J Biomed Sci 56:293–306, 1999.
321. Spencer MJ, Garcia LS, Chapin MR: *Dientamoeba fragilis*. An intestinal pathogen in children? Am J Dis Child 133:390–393, 1979.
322. Spencer MJ, Chapin MR, Garcia LS: *Dientamoeba fragilis*: A gastrointestinal protozoan infection in adults. Am J Gastroenterol 77:565–569, 1982.
323. Millet V, Spencer MJ, Chapin M, et al: *Dientamoeba fragilis*, a protozoan parasite in adult members of a semicommunal group. Dig Dis Sci 28:335–339, 1983.
324. Grendon JH, DiGiacomo RF, Frost FJ: Descriptive features of *Dientamoeba fragilis* infections. J Trop Med Hyg 98:309–315, 1995.
325. Kean BH, Malloch CL: The neglected ameba: *Dientamoeba fragilis*. A report of 100 "pure" infections. Am J Digest Dis 11:735–744, 1966.
326. Norberg A, Nord CE, Evengard B: *Dientamoeba fragilis*—A protozoal infection which may cause severe bowel distress. Clin Microbiol Infect 9:65–68, 2003.
327. Schwartz MD, Nelson ME: *Dientamoeba fragilis* infection presenting to the emergency department as acute appendicitis. J Emerg Med 25:17–21, 2003.
328. Shein R, Gelb A: Colitis due to *Dientamoeba fragilis*. Am J Gastroenterol 78:634–636, 1983.
329. Sawangjaroen N, Luke R, Prociv P: Diagnosis by faecal culture of *Dientamoeba fragilis* infections in Australian patients with diarrhea. Trans R Soc Trop Med Hyg 87:163–165, 1993.
330. Windsor JJ, Macfarlane L, Hughes-Thapa G, et al: Detection of *Dientamoeba fragilis* by culture. Br J Biomed Sci 60:79–83, 2003.
331. Chan F, Stewart N, Guan M, et al: Prevalence of *Dientamoeba fragilis* antibodies in children and recognition of a 39-kDa immunodominant protein antigen of the organism. Eur J Clin Microbiol Infect Dis 15:950–954, 1996.
332. Peek R, Reedeker FR, van Gool T: Direct amplification and genotyping of *Dientamoeba fragilis* from human stool specimens. J Clin Microbiol 42:631–635, 2004.
333. Cuffari C, Oligny L, Seidman EG: *Dientamoeba fragilis* masquerading as allergic colitis. J Pediatr Gastroenterol Nutr 26:16–20, 1998.
334. Girginkardesler N, Coskun S, Cuneyt Balcioglu I, et al: *Dientamoeba fragilis*, a neglected cause of diarrhea, successfully treated with secnidazole. Clin Microbiol Infect 9:110–113, 2003.
335. Chan FT, Guan MX, Mackenzie AM, et al: Susceptibility testing of *Dientamoeba fragilis* ATC 30948 with iodoquinol, paromomycin, tetracycline, and metronidazole. Antimicrob Agents Chemother 38:1157–1160, 1994.
336. The flagellates. In Markell EK, Voge M, John DT (eds): Medical Parasitology, 6th edition. Philadelphia, WB Saunders, 1986, pp 54–67.
337. Wolfe MS: Miscellaneous intestinal protozoa. In Strickland GT (ed): Hunter's Tropical Medicine and Emerging Infectious Diseases, 8th edition. Philadelphia, WB Saunders, 2000, pp 603–610.
338. Abd-Alla MD, Wahib AA, Ravdin JI: Comparison of antigen-capture ELISA to stool-culture methods for the detection of asymptomatic *Entamoeba* species infection in Kafer Daoud, Egypt. Am J Trop Med Hyg 62:579–582, 2000.
339. Spriegel JR, Saag KG, Tsang T-K: Infectious diarrhea secondary to *Enteromonas hominis*. Am J Gastroenterol 84:1313–1314, 1989.
340. Singh S, Samantaray JC: So-called nonpathogenic intestinal parasites (letter). Am J Gastroenterol 85:764–765, 1990.
341. Jongwutiwes S, Silachamroon U, Putaporntip C: *Pentatrichomonas hominis* in empyema thoracis. Trans R Soc Trop Med Hyg 94:185–186, 2000.
342. Kawamura O, Kon Y, Naganuma A, et al: *Retortamonas intestinalis* in the pancreatic juice of a patient with small nodular lesions of the main pancreatic duct. Gastrointest Endosc 53:508–510, 2001.
343. Honigberg BM: Trichomonads found outside the urogenital tract of humans. In Honigberg BM (ed): Trichomonads Parasitic in Humans. New York, Springer-Verlag, 1990, pp 342–393.

Table 88-1 Frequency of Cryptosporidiosis among Immunocompetent Symptomatic and Asymptomatic Individuals in Developing and Developed Countries 1994–2003

Area	Patients with Diarrhea	Controls Without Diarrhea
Asia/Africa/ Latin America (n = 16)[38–53]	849/6669 (12.7%)	346/7539 (4.5%)
North America/ Europe/Australia (n = 3)[54–56]	25/1049 (2.3%)	67/5624 (1.2%)

The higher incidence of cryptosporidiosis in developing areas is thought to be due to greater exposure to the organism because of poor sanitation and crowded living conditions. Specific risk factors for acquisition in children include male sex, keeping animals in the house, and weaning.[57] In most studies breastfeeding is protective and children with cryptosporidial diarrhea are less likely to be breastfed.[58] While this may be due in part to passive transfer of immunity, it may also be due to increased exposure to potentially contaminated food and water at weaning.[59]

Those most severely affected by *Cryptosporidium* are immunocompromised patients, especially those with AIDS, in whom the disease can be fulminant and fatal. Adal and colleagues, compiling results from 22 studies published before 1993, found that 13.8% and 24% of patients with AIDS and diarrhea in developed and developing areas, respectively, had *Cryptosporidium* compared with only 0% to 5% of AIDS patients without diarrhea.[19] In five studies published with controls for 1994 through 2003 from developing countries of Africa, Asia, and Latin America, immunodeficient patients (including HIV and malignancies) have a prevalence of 16.1% in cases with diarrhea and 2.2% asymptomatic carriage of *Cryptosporidium* (Table 88-2).[60–64] Studies in immunocompromised patients with controls from developed countries since 1994 were not found.

Patients with AIDS are prone to developing debilitating disease with cryptosporidiosis. In the Nevada outbreak, 61 of the 2270 known HIV-infected patients in the area developed diarrhea, and 32 of these died within 6 months; this is similar to the high mortality in the Milwaukee outbreak, in which 48 of 82 infected patients with AIDS died within a year, with excess mortality largely attributable to the cryptosporidial illnesses.[65,66]

Table 88-2 Frequency of Cryptosporidiosis among Immunocompromised Symptomatic and Asymptomatic Individuals in Developing Countries, 1994–2003

Area	Patients with Diarrhea	Controls Without Diarrhea
Asia/Africa/ Latin America (n = 5)[60–64]	73/453 (16.1%)	7/324 (2.2%)

In developed countries, cryptosporidiosis is also sporadic. The prevalence is increased in dairy farmers and other persons who have contact with cattle.[67] Small outbreaks have been reported in day-care centers and veterinary and health-care settings. The largest outbreaks, however, have been waterborne. *Cryptosporidium* is the most common cause of recreational water outbreaks due to contaminated lakes and swimming pools. In 1999–2000, *C. parvum* accounted for the largest percentage (44%) of waterborne outbreaks involving gastroenteritis, 61% occurring in treated systems (i.e., pools).[68]

Spring is the time of peak incidence, presumably due to the propensity for heavy rains during that season to cause flooding and subsequent contamination of source water. Numerous large community-based waterborne outbreaks of *Cryptosporidium* have been reported since 1984, affecting hundreds of thousands of people.[69] By far the largest of these was the 1993 outbreak in Milwaukee, Wisconsin, in which an estimated 403,000 people developed diarrhea due to a combination of source water contamination and transient impairment of prefiltration processing. Of note, the water quality during that outbreak met all U.S. federal drinking water standards at that time.[4] The federal standards for turbidity were strengthened as a result, but a 1994 outbreak affecting over 100 people in Las Vegas, Nevada, occurred even when the water met these tougher standards (i.e., not exceeding 0.17 nephelometric turbidity units).[65]

DISEASE

Clinical Manifestations

The clinical manifestations of cryptosporidiosis are indistinguishable from those of giardiasis, isosporiasis, and cyclosporiasis. Clinical illness is characterized by watery diarrhea without red blood cells or leukocytes and may be associated with one or more nonspecific symptoms and signs, such as cramping abdominal pain, anorexia, malaise, flatulence, nausea, vomiting, and low-grade fever. When right upper quadrant pain is present in patients with AIDS, suggesting biliary tract involvement, it should point toward cryptosporidiosis, although cases of isosporiasis or cyclosporiasis with similar clinical manifestations have been reported.

The clinical manifestations of cryptosporidial infection vary according to the immune status of the host. In the immunocompetent host, the onset is usually acute, occurs after an incubation period of 2 to 14 days, and is generally self-limited. The clinical spectrum ranges from asymptomatic passage of oocysts to severe cholera-like gastroenteritis with biliary tract disease. The hallmark of cryptosporidial infection is diarrhea, which is usually described as watery, voluminous, and occasionally explosive and foul smelling. Additional symptoms seen in more than 80% of patients in the Milwaukee outbreak were abdominal cramps, fatigue, and anorexia.[4,5] In addition, more than half of patients may experience weight loss, nausea, low-grade fever (up to 38°C), chills, sweats, myalgias, and headache. The illness may be quite prolonged, lasting 10 to 14 days, with an average of 12 stools per day during the peak of the illness and often significant weight loss (median 4.5 kg in the Milwaukee outbreak). Although their HIV status is not specified, at Mulago Hospital in Kampala, Uganda, 31% of children hospitalized with persistent diarrhea and 22% with acute diarrhea (vs. 8.5% without diarrhea) had *Cryptosporidium* infections, often with wasting and stunting.[70]

Asymptomatic infection can occur in immunocompetent and immunodeficient patients. In one series, as many as 63% of childhood cryptosporidial infections in Peru were asymptomatic, although these "subclinical" infections may have lasting consequences on growth and development.[71–73] In New York, asymptomatic cryptosporidiosis was documented in 6.4% of immunocompetent and 22% of immunodeficient children.[74] Excretion of oocysts after resolution of clinical symptoms can continue for prolonged periods.[72] Relapses of cryptosporidial infection have been considered rare, although 39% of the patients infected in the Milwaukee outbreak had a brief recurrence of diarrhea after a period of normal stools.

In immunocompromised patients, cryptosporidiosis is usually much more prolonged or severe. In particular, patients with AIDS often have chronic intermittent diarrhea, with recurring 3- to 30-day episodes lasting up to 14 months. Those with low CD4 lymphocyte counts are prone to develop protracted, fulminant, and rapidly fatal diarrhea. Cryptosporidiosis in HIV-positive patients can be asymptomatic in 4%, transient in 29%, chronic in 60%, or fulminant (greater than 2 L of stool per day) in 8%. Mean survival in these HIV patients with *Cryptosporidium* co-infection was 25 weeks in the study by Blanshard and associates.[75] Patients who develop fulminant disease usually have fewer than 50 CD4 cells per microliter and sharply limited survival of only 5 weeks. Spontaneous clinical remission is associated with higher lymphocyte[76] or CD4 count.[77] In the Nevada outbreak in 1994, two-thirds of the HIV-infected patients with cryptosporidiosis developed chronic disease, with a median weight loss of 13.6 kg, and nausea, vomiting, and abdominal cramping occurred in at least 80%. Over half of these patients died within 6 months of the onset of the outbreak, of whom 60% had cryptosporidiosis listed as a cause of death on their death certificates.[65] Cryptosporidiosis has also been reported as an opportunistic pathogen in patients immunosuppressed due to cytotoxic chemotherapy or congenital immunodeficiencies.

Extraintestinal disease due to *Cryptosporidium* has been seen in immunocompromised patients, especially those in the late stages of AIDS (CD4 counts less than 50/μL). By far the most common site is the biliary tree, manifestations of which include sclerosing cholangitis and acalculous cholecystitis. Direct luminal spread of organisms from the duodenum is believed to be responsible. The hallmark symptom is right upper quadrant pain, which can resemble that of chronic or acute calculous cholecystitis. There have also been reports of respiratory cryptosporidiosis; in one study, 7 of 43 patients with AIDS and cryptosporidial diarrhea had oocysts isolated in sputum, although it was probably nonpathogenic in six.[78] One patient with AIDS had cryptosporidial sinusitis that improved during therapy with spiramycin.[79]

Pathology

Cryptosporidium is primarily a pathogen of the small bowel producing villous blunting, submucosal edema, and mononuclear inflammatory infiltrates in the lamina propria. This is often associated with evidence of malabsorption, such as abnormal D-xylose tests and evidence of intestinal barrier disruption by lactulose-mannitol permeability ratios.[80–83] In the case of *Cryptosporidium*, various life cycle forms can be seen just beneath the apical enterocyte membranes; ultrastructurally, they reside in vacuoles with specialized basal membrane folds called "feeder organelles."[83]

Complications

Cryptosporidial enteritis is usually a self-limited, nonfatal illness in normal hosts. As such, the only immediate complication of concern is volume depletion from heavy diarrhea and inadequate fluid intake, especially in young children and the elderly. This is usually treatable with oral rehydration therapy.

Cryptosporidium parvum in children has a lasting adverse effect on linear (height) growth and correlated with impaired cognitive function.[72,73] Infected children who became stunted may not catch up in either weight or height, and exhibit the deficit even 1 year after infection.[72] However, there are more subtle, long-term detrimental effects of childhood cryptosporidiosis, including both an increased overall diarrheal burden over several months following an attack and impaired growth, even with so-called asymptomatic infections.[71,72,84] As such, the public health importance of these infections in developing countries is likely to be far greater than generally recognized.

The life-threatening complications of coccidian enteritis occur most often in chronic disease, which is largely confined to immunocompromised patients. In these cases severe infection can lead to chronic malabsorption, which may be treated by total parenteral nutrition or novel approaches to enteral, glutamine-based nutrition.[85,86] Supportive therapy is especially important in cryptosporidiosis, which has no uniformly effective antimicrobial treatment at this time. Moreover, extraintestinal disease, especially of the biliary tract, can lead to substantial morbidity from chronic pain and mortality from biliary obstruction.

PATHOGENESIS AND IMMUNITY

A great mystery in the study of cryptosporidiosis is how it produces profound inflammatory and destructive pathophysiology without tissue invasion. A simple explanation would be the elaboration of an enterotoxin or cytotoxin, although thorough investigation has failed to discover such a toxin.[87] Guarino and associates[88,89] reported an enterotoxic effect of stool from infected humans or calves on intestinal strips or cells mounted in Ussing chambers, although they were unable to show that this secretagogue was parasite-derived rather than host-derived.

Most research has focused on the direct epithelial effects of infection with *Cryptosporidium*. Several observations on experimental porcine infection suggest that part of the symptomatology of cryptosporidiosis may be due to malabsorption by blunted or inflamed villi coupled with intact fluid secretion from the crypts. Prostaglandins also appear to play a role in this imbalance, but the details of this interaction are still unclear.[85,90] Two studies of intestinal epithelial cells in tissue culture have found destructive effects of *Cryptosporidium* infection, including loss of barrier integrity and moderate cell injury,[83,91] effects that are confirmed in vivo by increased lactulose-mannitol excretion ratios in patients with cryptosporidiosis.[81,82] Some of this damage may be due to release of pro-inflammatory cytokines (such as TNF-α and IL-8) induced by *Cryptosporidium* infection.[58,92] Recent work has suggested that substance P, a neuropeptide, may also play a role in mediating diarrhea in human cryptosporidiosis.[93]

The severe nature of intestinal coccidioses in patients with AIDS suggests that cell-mediated immunity is essential to clearance of these organisms. This is supported by several observations. First, humoral immune responses to *Cryptosporidium* are quite strong in patients with AIDS, perhaps even greater than those in immunocompetent individuals.[94] Second, humoral responses are not associated with clearance of infection. This has been shown in mice,[95] as well as in HIV-infected patients who develop serum and intestinal antibodies but fail to clear infections.[94,96] Third, peripheral blood mononuclear cells (PBMCs) from patients with AIDS do not have normal proliferative responses to cryptosporidial antigens even though they may respond to mitogens.[97] Finally, experimental mice become susceptible to cryptosporidial infection after depletion of functional T helper lymphocytes or treatment with dexamethasone.[98,99] On the other hand, a role for humoral immunity in the resistance to *Cryptosporidium* is suggested by the severe disease seen in patients with congenital hypo- or agammaglobulinemias but normal T-cell function.[100,101]

One hypothesis is that the cytokine interferon-γ (IFN-γ) may be required for an effective immune response to *Cryptosporidium*. IFN-γ is produced primarily by the Th1 subset of CD4 lymphocytes, which also release interleukin (IL)-2 but not IL-4, IL-5, or IL-10. Furthermore patients with advanced HIV infections are often deficient in Th1 lymphocytes.[102] Experimental mice can be rendered susceptible to cryptosporidiosis if treated with antibodies to IFN-γ, and mice immunosuppressed with dexamethasone can be protected from the organism by treatment with high doses of IFN-γ.[98,103] Gomez Morales and coworkers[97] found high amounts of IFN-γ released in response to cryptosporidial antigens by PBMCs from immunocompetent patients only if they had a history of transient cryptosporidiosis. In experimentally infected volunteers with *Cryptosporidium*, IFN-γ expression occurs in immunocompetent subjects with self-limited infection and correlates with prior exposure to *Cryptosporidium* and resistance to re-infection.[104] Finally, selective lack of IFN-γ production by lymphocytes in response to cryptosporidial antigens in an HIV-negative child was associated with chronic and ultimately fatal cryptosporidiosis; a thorough immunologic evaluation revealed no other abnormalities.[105]

Naive volunteers appear to have increased IL-15 expression in their intestinal mucosa when experimentally infected with *Cryptosporidium* and this is correlated with no or low numbers of oocyte shedding.[106] In contrast, TNF-α, IL-1β,[107] and IL-4[106] do not appear to be associated with symptoms or *Cryptosporidium* oocyst shedding in humans. In a recent study, significant elevations of fecal IL-8, IL-13, and TNF-α receptor 1 have been described in *Cryptosporidium*-infected children in Haiti,[58] and mildly increased fecal IL-8, TNF-α, and lactoferrin in some *Cryptosporidium*-infected children in Brazil.[108]

DIAGNOSIS

Cryptosporidiosis should be suspected in any patient presenting with watery diarrhea, abdominal cramps, and nausea, particularly if symptoms last more than a few days. Although persistent diarrhea (>1–2 weeks) in travelers, those with recreational water exposure, or immunocompromised individuals should raise concern for cryptosporidiosis, no obvious environmental exposure history is necessary, since the organism may be transmitted by so many different means. There are no characteristic findings on physical examination or laboratory or radiologic analysis, although volume depletion, metabolic alkalosis, and hypokalemia may be seen in more severe cases. Children in developing areas as well as patients with HIV respond to *C. parvum* with mild intestinal inflammation with detectable fecal lactoferrin (a sensitive marker for the presence of fecal leukocytes)[58,81,108] and mildly elevated IL-8 and TNF-αR1.[58] In contrast, fecal lactoferrin was not observed in healthy U.S. adults experimentally infected with *C. parvum*.[108]

In immunocompromised patients, the findings are characteristically more severe and prolonged. In addition, if the biliary tree is involved, there may be elevations in alkaline phosphatase and transaminases and irregular ductal strictures and dilations on ultrasound or endoscopic retrograde cholangiopancreatography (ERCP).[109] Pulmonary involvement can produce various infiltrates on chest radiograph.[78]

Oocyst shedding in cryptosporidiosis can be intermittent and up to three stool specimens may be needed for diagnosis.[110,111] The diagnosis can be confirmed by observation of the oocysts in stool or luminal fluids. Using a modified Kinyoun acid-fast stain, oocysts appear as red spheres 3 to 6 μm in diameter; no other organisms should be easily confused with *Cryptosporidium* based on size and appearance (Plate 88-1). Unfortunately, acid-fast staining is relatively insensitive, requiring 10,000 oocysts per gram of watery stool and 500,000 per gram of formed stool to make the diagnosis. There are several immunologic techniques, including immunofluorescence and enzyme-linked immunoassays, which are commercially available through several laboratories. These techniques have sensitivity and specificity approaching 100% for *C. parvum*; and require less technician time and experience.[112–114] Serologic testing for antibodies to cryptosporidial antigens is available for epidemiologic surveys, but is of little help in the diagnostic evaluation of patients.

While the immunoassays are adequate for clinical diagnosis of cryptosporidiosis, they are not sensitive enough to detect oocysts in environmental samples or in epidemiologic surveys of asymptomatic contacts, since the oocyte numbers are too low. Various concentration techniques including formalin–ethyl acetate sedimentation and disposable parasite concentrators have been used to increase the efficiency of oocyst recovery for immunoassays; as few as 5000 oocysts per gram of stool can be detected by these methods.[115,116] Polymerase chain reaction (PCR) testing is more sensitive, with detection of 50 to 500 oocysts per milliliter of liquid stool or less than 1 pg of DNA and less than 10 oocysts from environmental samples.[117–119]

TREATMENT AND PROGNOSIS

Cryptosporidiosis in immunocompetent patients is self-limited, and symptomatic therapy should be directed at rehydration and nutrition. Oral rehydration solution should be used as needed to prevent volume depletion. Antimotility agents (loperamide, diphenoxylate, or other opiates) may be used once more invasive conditions (e.g., bacterial enteritis, amebiasis, or pseudomembranous colitis) have been excluded. Glutamine appears to be more effective in driving electrolyte and water absorption in *Cryptosporidium*-infected porcine intestine and has the advantage of enhancing injury repair.[85,86]

The disease is much more problematic in immunocompromised patients, since it is often not self-limited and there is no acceptable antimicrobial treatment currently available. Dramatic improvements in HIV-related cryptosporidiosis after initiation of highly active antiretroviral therapy, including complete eradication of the parasite in patients, have been documented.[120,121] In a survey conducted in France from January 1995 to December 1996, there was approximately a 60% decline in the prevalence of cryptosporidiosis that coincided with the widespread use of protease inhibitors.[122] Recent data suggests that protease inhibitors, particularly indinavir, may directly interfere with the life cycle of *Cryptosporidium*.[123]

Over 100 antibacterial and antiparasitic agents have been tried to no avail. In a small double-blind, placebo-controlled trial, the nonabsorbable aminoglycoside paromomycin has been shown to reduce the frequency and intensity of diarrhea in patients with AIDS and chronic cryptosporidiosis.[124] In addition, inhaled paromomycin was associated with improvement in one reported case of respiratory cryptosporidiosis.[125] The optimal dose has not yet been established. White and coworkers[124] used 25 to 35 mg/kg/day for 14 days; larger doses (up to 50 mg/kg/day) were shown to be more effective in animal models, but vestibular toxicity has been reported at these doses in humans.[124] Maintenance therapy may be indicated in patients with AIDS and low CD4 counts to prevent relapse. A recent randomized, controlled trial has shown that paromomycin was no more effective than placebo in patients with advanced AIDS.[126]

The most promising new drug for the treatment of cryptosporidiosis is nitazoxanide, a broad-spectrum antiparasitic agent. In a double-blind, controlled study in pediatric patients with diarrhea, nitazoxanide was associated with the resolution of diarrhea in 88% of children compared to 38% on placebo.[127] In another study of malnourished children with cryptosporidial diarrhea, a significant 56% had a resolution of diarrhea and 52% had parsitological response with 3 days of treatment compared with 23% and 14%, respectively, in controls. However, no significant effect was seen in HIV-seropositive pediatric patients.[128] Nitazoxanide elixir is approved for treatment of cryptosporidiosis in children aged 1 to 11 years in the United States. In children 12-to-47 months old, a dose of 100 mg every 12 hours is used, and in older children (4 to 11 years), 200 mg every 12 hours orally is recommended.

Several other agents that have been studied include azithromycin, which at 900 to 1200 mg/day reduced the severity of diarrhea and oocyst shedding, but only in patients in whom appropriate drug levels were obtained.[129] Azithromycin at 500 mg daily was found to be ineffective compared to letrazuril and paromomycin,[130] while reduced oocyst excretion and modest clinical improvement were noted with open label combination azithromycin (600 mg qd for 4 weeks) and paramomycin (1 g bid for 8 weeks).[131] Two phase I trials of letrazuril (50–100 mg/day) have shown modest, short-lived response in 66%; however, clinical relapse and worsening diarrhea occurred in 65% of the responders.[132,133] There are reports of responses to spiramycin, including one patient with extraintestinal disease.[79] In a double-blind, placebo-controlled study of immunocompetent infants in Costa Rica, infants treated with spiramycin had significantly decreased duration of diarrhea and excretion of oocysts.[134] Bovine hyperimmune colostrum (marketed as lactobin) was reported to eradicate the organism in a child with AIDS and chronic cryptosporidiosis.[135] In another case report, a 38-year-old HIV patient with 6 to 12 L of stool/day for 3 months had resolution within 48 hours of being treated with hyperimmune bovine colostrum and remained asymptomatic for 3 months.[136] Conclusive support for the use of hyperimmune colostrum, however, has not been forthcoming.

Results of non-double-blinded therapeutic studies of cryptosporidiosis should be interpreted with caution: Immunosuppressed patients tend to have intermittent diarrhea that can improve or worsen according to the patient's CD4 count, and clinical responses do not necessarily accompany eradication of oocysts from the stools. Endpoints for successful therapy should include both the cessation of diarrhea and other clinical manifestations, as well as the absence of oocysts in the stools; relapses are frequent.

Symptomatic therapy in patients with AIDS has also been disappointing, since the profound diarrhea may be refractory to antimotility agents. Clinical improvement has been reported with the somatostatin analogue octreotide (100–300 μg subcutaneously 3 times daily), although a placebo-controlled trial found no benefit[137–140]; moreover, this agent is prohibitively expensive for widespread use. The related oral drug vapreotide was found to improve AIDS-related chronic diarrhea, but only in patients without cryptosporidiosis.[141] In biliary cryptosporidiosis, cholecystectomy or papillotomy has provided pain relief for many patients, although the operative morbidity of the former may be high.[66,109]

PREVENTION AND CONTROL

Current Approaches

The only known way to acquire any of the coccidia is to ingest infectious oocysts; the diseases can be completely prevented by elimination of oocysts from food and water and by avoidance of fecal material from infected people. However, in the case of *Cryptosporidium*, this simple-sounding goal has proved insurmountably difficult to attain. The high infectivity and ubiquitous nature of this organism make complete removal of oocysts during water treatment essential to prevent the disease, and to this day even the most technologically advanced systems cannot reliably achieve this. Since oocysts are extremely resistant to chlorination, water treatment plants must rely on mechanical means to remove them: flocculation, sedimentation, and filtration. In theory, these methods should be adequate to prevent waterborne outbreaks, and in general they are quite effective. However, the Nevada outbreak of 1994 proved that these techniques can fail even without obvious malfunction. Conversely, a massive failure of water treatment, as occurred in Washington, D.C., in 1993, may not be associated with any increase in human cases of cryptosporidiosis.[142]

The problem of inadequate elimination of *Cryptosporidium* from the water supply in developed countries is minuscule in comparison with the problems in developing areas. As noted earlier, 95% of children in some areas have serologic evidence of infection by age 2 years. Without a source of clean, filtered, or boiled water, improved sanitation, or an effective vaccine, there is no realistic way to prevent cryptosporidial infections in these areas.

Travelers to endemic areas can avoid cryptosporidiosis if they follow the maxim "boil it, cook it, peel it, or forget it." As mentioned earlier, oocysts are easily killed by heat, so hot beverages and boiled water can be considered safe. Because person-to-person transmission occurs through fecal-oral spread, travelers should probably be advised to wash their hands thoroughly before eating and after contact with young children. These precautions are especially crucial in patients with AIDS, especially those who choose to travel to developing areas during the later stages of their illness when CD4 counts are low.

Because of the ever-present risk of acquisition even in developed countries, patients with AIDS, especially those with CD4 counts less than 100/μL, should be advised of the potentially devastating impact of cryptosporidiosis. Filters that provide the greatest assurance of oocyst removal include those that operate by reverse osmosis, those labeled as absolute 1-μm filters, and those labeled as meeting National Sanitation Foundation (NSF) standard no. 53 for cyst removal. The nominal 1-μm filter rating is not standardized, and many filters in this category might not be capable of removing 99% of oocysts. Some patients may decide that the inconvenience of boiling or filtering (through "absolute" 1-μm filters) all of their drinking water is worth the benefit of protecting themselves from this disease. These patients should also be advised to avoid young farm animals, especially those with diarrhea.

Because of the threat of nosocomial spread of oocysts, strict enteric precautions should be followed when caring for any patient with possible cryptosporidiosis. This includes use of gowns and gloves when fecal soilage is possible and thorough handwashing after all contact. Potentially contaminated medical equipment should be autoclaved. The optimal cleaning compound for contaminated surfaces (e.g., mattresses, toilets) is not known.

Future Approaches

Much more recent research is devoted to *Cryptosporidium*. Several new approaches to water treatment have been explored, including ozone, ultrasonic waves, and electrochemical treatment, but these are far from ready for widespread use.[29,143] The Centers for Disease Control and Prevention (CDC) pointed to several high-priority objectives for the eventual control of cryptosporidiosis: (1) to assess the public health importance of low-level oocyst contamination of drinking water; (2) to develop guidelines and techniques for notification of the public when oocysts are detected (i.e., to know when boil-water advisories are needed); (3) to identify options for preventing cryptosporidiosis in immunocompromised patients who use the public water supply; and (4) to optimize water sampling techniques to identify *Cryptosporidium* oocysts.[28]

There is considerable interest in vaccine development against *Cryptosporidium*. However, animal models suggest that cell-mediated immunity and intact production of IFN-γ are necessary to prevent infection, so the benefit of immunization in patients with AIDS may be limited. A recent trial of a vaccine made from lyophilized oocysts was moderately protective in a bovine model; vaccinated calves had a shorter duration of diarrhea and excreted fewer oocysts.[144] There have been no vaccines tested in humans yet. A recent study in which previously infected volunteers were rechallenged with *Cryptosporidium* oocysts demonstrated only partial protection against re-infection; although fewer subjects shed oocysts after their second challenge, the rates of diarrhea were the same.[145]

Finally, glutamine, a "conditionally essential" amino acid is effective in driving electrolyte and water absorption in *Cryptosporidium*-infected porcine intestine and has the advantage of enhancing injury repair.[85,86] Clinically, glutamine and its stable derivative alanyl-glutamine have been shown to improve diarrhea and malabsorption in HIV/AIDS patients. These improvements may enhance antiretroviral drug therapy and reduce the emergence of drug resistance[146] as well as ameliorate symptoms associated with severe cryptosporidiosis.[147]

REFERENCES

1. Nime FA, Burek JD, Page DL, et al: Acute enterocolitis in a human being infected with the protozoan *Cryptosporidium*. Gastroenterology 70(4):592–598, 1976.
2. Meisel JL, Perera DR, Meligro C, et al: Overwhelming watery diarrhea associated with a *Cryptosporidium* in an immunosuppressed patient. Gastroenterology 70(6):1156–1160, 1976.
3. D'Antonio RG, Winn RE, Taylor JP, et al: A waterborne outbreak of cryptosporidiosis in normal hosts. Ann Intern Med 103(6 Part 1): 886–888, 1985.
4. MacKenzie WR, Hoxie NJ, Proctor ME, et al: A massive outbreak in Milwaukee of *Cryptosporidium* infection transmitted through the public water supply. N Engl J Med 331(3):161–167, 1994.
5. MacKenzie WR, Schell WL, Blair KA, et al: Massive outbreak of waterborne *Cryptosporidium* infection in Milwaukee, Wisconsin: Recurrence of illness and risk of secondary transmission. Clin Infect Dis 21(1):57–62, 1995.
6. Corso PS, Kramer MH, Blair KA, et al: Cost of illness in the 1993 waterborne *Cryptosporidium* outbreak, Milwaukee, Wisconsin. Emerg Infect Dis 9(4):426–431, 2003.
7. Current WL, Reese NC: A comparison of endogenous development of three isolates of *Cryptosporidium* in suckling mice. J Protozool 33(1):98–108, 1986.
8. Awad-El-Kariem FM, Robinson HA, Petry F, et al: Differentiation between human and animal isolates of *Cryptosporidium parvum* using molecular and biological markers. Parasitol Res 84(4):297–301, 1998.
9. Widmer G: Genetic heterogeneity and PCR detection of *Cryptosporidium parvum*. Adv Parasitol 40:223–239, 1998.
10. Morgan UM, Constantine CC, Forbes DA, et al: Differentiation between human and animal isolates of *Cryptosporidium parvum* using rDNA sequencing and direct PCR analysis. J Parasitol 83(5):825–830, 1997.
11. Patel S, Pedraza-Diaz S, McLauchlin J: The identification of *Cryptosporidium* species and *Cryptosporidium parvum* directly from whole faeces by analysis of a multiplex PCR of the 18S rRNA gene and by PCR/RFLP of the *Cryptosporidium* outer wall protein (COWP) gene. Int J Parasitol 29(8):1241–1247, 1999.
12. Pedraza-Diaz S, Amar C, McLauchlin J: The identification and characterisation of an unusual genotype of *Cryptosporidium* from human faeces as *Cryptosporidium meleagridis*. FEMS Microbiol Lett 189(2):189–194, 2000.
13. Pieniazek NJ, Bornay-Llinares FJ, Slemenda SB, et al: New *Cryptosporidium* genotypes in HIV-infected persons. Emerg Infect Dis 5(3):444–449, 1999.
14. Xiao L, Bern C, Limor J, et al: Identification of 5 types of *Cryptosporidium* parasites in children in Lima, Peru. J Infect Dis 183(3):492–497, 2001.
15. Mallon ME, MacLeod A, Wastling JM, et al: Multilocus genotyping of *Cryptosporidium parvum* Type 2: Population genetics and substructuring. Infect Genet Evol 3(3):207–218, 2003.
16. Xiao L, Fayer R, Ryan U, et al: *Cryptosporidium* taxonomy: Recent advances and implications for public health. Clin Microbiol Rev 17(1):72–97, 2004.
17. Katsumata T, Hosea D, Ranuh IG, et al: Short report: Possible *Cryptosporidium muris* infection in humans. Am J Trop Med Hyg 62(1):70–72, 2000.

18. Fayer R, Speer C, Dubey J: *Cryptosporidium* of man and animals. In Duley J, Speer C, Fayer R (eds): General Biology of Cryptosporidium. CRC Press, Boca Raton, FL, 1995, pp 1–29.
19. Adal K, Sterling C, Guerrnat R: *Cryptosporidium* and related species. In Blaser M, Smith P, Ravdin J, et al (eds): Infections of the Gastrointestinal Tract. New York, Raven Press, 1995, pp 1107–1128.
20. LeChevallier MW, Norton WD, Lee RG: *Giardia* and *Cryptosporidium* spp. in filtered drinking water supplies. Appl Environ Microbiol 57(9):2617–2621, 1991.
21. Dillingham RA, Lima AA, Guerrant RL: Cryptosporidiosis: Epidemiology and impact. Microbes Infect 4(10):1059–1066, 2002.
22. DuPont HL, Chappell CL, Sterling CR, et al: The infectivity of *Cryptosporidium parvum* in healthy volunteers. N Engl J Med 332(13):855–859, 1995.
23. Newman RD, Zu SX, Wuhib T, et al: Household epidemiology of *Cryptosporidium parvum* infection in an urban community in northeast Brazil. Ann Intern Med 120(6):500–505, 1994.
24. Cordell RL, Addiss DG: Cryptosporidiosis in child care settings: A review of the literature and recommendations for prevention and control. Pediatr Infect Dis J 13(4):310–317, 1994.
25. Neill MA, Rice SK, Ahmad NV, et al: Cryptosporidiosis: An unrecognized cause of diarrhea in elderly hospitalized patients. Clin Infect Dis 22(1):168–170, 1996.
26. Naumova EN, Egorov AI, Morris RD, et al: The elderly and waterborne *Cryptosporidium* infection: Gastroenteritis hospitalizations before and during the 1993 Milwaukee outbreak. Emerg Infect Dis 9(4):418–425, 2003.
27. Addiss DG, Pond RS, Remshak M, et al: Reduction of risk of watery diarrhea with point-of-use water filters during a massive outbreak of waterborne *Cryptosporidium* infection in Milwaukee, Wisconsin, 1993. Am J Trop Med Hyg 54(6):549–553, 1996.
28. Assessing the public health threat associated with waterborne cryptosporidiosis: Report of a workshop. MMWR Recomm Rep 44 (RR-6):1–19, 1995.
29. Korich DG, Mead JR, Madore MS, et al: Effects of ozone, chlorine dioxide, chlorine, and monochloramine on *Cryptosporidium parvum* oocyst viability. Appl Environ Microbiol 56(5):1423–1428, 1990.
30. Anderson BC: Moist heat inactivation of *Cryptosporidium* spp. Am J Public Health 75(12):1433–1434, 1985.
31. Peng MM, Xiao L, Freeman AR, et al: Genetic polymorphism among *Cryptosporidium parvum* isolates: Evidence of two distinct human transmission cycles. Emerg Infect Dis 3(4):567–573, 1997.
32. Sulaiman IM, Xiao L, Yang C, et al: Differentiating human from animal isolates of *Cryptosporidium parvum*. Emerg Infect Dis 4(4):681–685, 1998.
33. Quiroz ES, Bern C, MacArthur JR, et al: An outbreak of cryptosporidiosis linked to a foodhandler. J Infect Dis 181(2):695–700, 2000.
34. McLauchlin J, Amar C, Pedraza-Diaz S, et al: Molecular epidemiological analysis of *Cryptosporidium* spp. in the United Kingdom: Results of genotyping *Cryptosporidium* spp. in 1,705 fecal samples from humans and 105 fecal samples from livestock animals. J Clin Microbiol 38(11):3984–3990, 2000.
35. Fretz R, Svoboda P, Ryan UM, et al: Genotyping of *Cryptosporidium* spp. isolated from human stool samples in Switzerland. Epidemiol Infect 131(1):663–667, 2003.
36. Kuhls TL, Mosier DA, Crawford DL, et al: Seroprevalence of cryptosporidial antibodies during infancy, childhood, and adolescence. Clin Infect Dis 18(5):731–735, 1994.
37. Zu SX, Li JF, Barrett LJ, et al: Seroepidemiologic study of *Cryptosporidium* infection in children from rural communities of Anhui, China and Fortaleza, Brazil. Am J Trop Med Hyg 51(1):1–10, 1994.
38. Al Braiken FA, Amin A, Beeching NJ, et al: Detection of *Cryptosporidium* amongst diarrhoeic and asymptomatic children in Jeddah, Saudi Arabia. Ann Trop Med Parasitol 97(5):505–510, 2003.
39. Tumwine JK, Kekitiinwa A, Nabukeera N, et al: *Cryptosporidium parvum* in children with diarrhea in Mulago Hospital, Kampala, Uganda. Am J Trop Med Hyg 68(6):710–715, 2003.
40. Nunez FA, Gonzalez OM, Gonzalez I, et al: Intestinal coccidia in Cuban pediatric patients with diarrhea. Mem Inst Oswaldo Cruz 98(4):539–542, 2003.
41. Gambhir IS, Jaiswal JP, Nath G: Significance of *Cryptosporidium* as an aetiology of acute infectious diarrhoea in elderly Indians. Trop Med Int Health 8(5):415–419, 2003.
42. Menon BS, Abdullah S, Mahamud F, et al: Low prevalence of *Cryptosporidium parvum* in hospitalized children in Kota Bharu, Malaysia. Southeast Asian J Trop Med Public Health 32(2):319–322, 2001.
43. Newman RD, Sears CL, Moore SR, et al: Longitudinal study of *Cryptosporidium* infection in children in northeastern Brazil. J Infect Dis 180(1):167–175, 1999.
44. Iqbal J, Munir MA, Khan MA: *Cryptosporidium* infection in young children with diarrhea in Rawalpindi, Pakistan. Am J Trop Med Hyg 60(5):868–870, 1999.
45. Akyon Y, Erguven S, Arikan S, et al: *Cryptosporidium parvum* prevalence in a group of Turkish children. Turk J Pediatr 41(2):189–196, 1999.
46. Katsumata T, Hosea D, Wasito EB, et al: Cryptosporidiosis in Indonesia: A hospital-based study and a community-based survey. Am J Trop Med Hyg 59(4):628–632, 1998.
47. Esteban JG, Aguirre C, Flores A, et al: High *Cryptosporidium* prevalences in healthy Aymara children from the northern Bolivian Altiplano. Am J Trop Med Hyg 58(1):50–55, 1998.
48. Nacro B, Bonkoungou P, Nagalo K, et al: [Clinical profile of cryptosporidiosis in a pediatric hospital environment in Burkina Faso]. Med Trop (Mars) 58(1):47–50, 1998.
49. Okafor JI, Okunji PO: Prevalence of *Cryptosporidium* oocysts in faecal samples of some school children in Enugu State, Nigeria. J Commun Dis 28(1):49–55, 1996.
50. Nimri LF, Hijazi SS: *Cryptosporidium*. A cause of gastroenteritis in preschool children in Jordan. J Clin Gastroenterol 19(4):288–291, 1994.
51. Adam AA, Hassan HS, Shears P, et al: *Cryptosporidium* in Khartoum, Sudan. East Afr Med J 71(11):745–746, 1994.
52. Adegbola RA, Demba E, De Veer G, et al: *Cryptosporidium* infection in Gambian children less than 5 years of age. J Trop Med Hyg 97(2):103–107, 1994.
53. Chacin-Bonilla L, Bonilla MC, Soto-Torres L, et al: *Cryptosporidium parvum* in children with diarrhea in Zulia State, Venezuela. Am J Trop Med Hyg 56(4):365–369, 1997.
54. Wang KX, Li CP, Wang J, et al: Epidemiological survey of cryptosporidiosis in Anhui Province China. World J Gastroenterol 8(2):371–374, 2002.
55. Jelinek T, Lotze M, Eichenlaub S, et al: Prevalence of infection with *Cryptosporidium parvum* and *Cyclospora cayetanensis* among international travellers. Gut 41(6):801–804, 1997.
56. Lederer W, Allerberger F, Dierich MP: [*Cryptosporidia* associated gastroenteritis: Epidemiologic study of children in Tyrol and Vorarlberg.] Wien Klin Wochenschr 108(20):649–653, 1996.
57. Molbak K, Aaby P, Hojlyng N, et al: Risk factors for *Cryptosporidium* diarrhea in early childhood: A case-control study from Guinea-Bissau, West Africa. Am J Epidemiol 139(7):734–740, 1994.
58. Kirkpatrick BD, Daniels MM, Jean SS, et al: Cryptosporidiosis stimulates an inflammatory intestinal response in malnourished Haitian children. J Infect Dis 186(1):94–101, 2002.
59. Sterling CR, Gilman RH, Sinclair NA, et al: The role of breast milk in protecting urban Peruvian children against cryptosporidiosis. J Protozool 38(6):23S–25S, 1991.
60. Wuhib T, Silva TM, Newman RD, et al: Cryptosporidial and microsporidial infections in human immunodeficiency virus–infected patients in northeastern Brazil. J Infect Dis 170(2):494–497, 1994.
61. Tanyuksel M, Gun H, Doganci L: Prevalence of *Cryptosporidium* spp. in patients with neoplasia and diarrhea. Scand J Infect Dis 27(1):69–70, 1995.
62. Arikan S, Erguven S, Akyon Y, et al: Cryptosporidiosis in immunocompromised patients in a Turkish university hospital. Acta Microbiol Immunol Hung 46(1):33–40, 1999.
63. Cegielski JP, Ortega YR, McKee S, et al: *Cryptosporidium*, enterocytozoon, and *Cyclospora* infections in pediatric and adult patients with diarrhea in Tanzania. Clin Infect Dis 28(2):314–321, 1999.
64. Cranendonk RJ, Kodde CJ, Chipeta D, et al: *Cryptosporidium parvum* and *Isospora belli* infections among patients with and without diarrhoea. East Afr Med J 80(8):398–401, 2003.
65. Goldstein ST, Juranek DD, Ravenholt O, et al: Cryptosporidiosis: An outbreak associated with drinking water despite state-of-the-art water treatment. Ann Intern Med 124(5):459–468, 1996.
66. Vakil NB, Schwartz SM, Buggy BP, et al: Biliary cryptosporidiosis in HIV-infected people after the waterborne outbreak of cryptosporidiosis in Milwaukee. N Engl J Med 334(1):19–23, 1996.
67. Lengerich EJ, Addiss DG, Marx JJ, et al: Increased exposure to *Cryptosporidia* among dairy farmers in Wisconsin. J Infect Dis 167(5):1252–1255, 1993.

68. Brookhart MA, Hubbard AE, van der Laan MJ, et al: Statistical estimation of parameters in a disease transmission model: Analysis of a *Cryptosporidium* outbreak. Stat Med 21(23):3627–3638, 2002.
69. Steiner TS, Thielman NM, Guerrant RL: Protozoal agents: What are the dangers for the public water supply? Annu Rev Med 48:329–340, 1997.
70. Tumwine JK, Kekitiinwa A, Nabukeera N, et al: *Cryptosporidium parvum* in children with diarrhea in Mulago Hospital, Kampala, Uganda. Am J Trop Med Hyg 68(6):710–715, 2003.
71. Checkley W, Gilman RH, Epstein LD, et al: Asymptomatic and symptomatic cryptosporidiosis: Their acute effect on weight gain in Peruvian children. Am J Epidemiol 145(2):156–163, 1997.
72. Checkley W, Epstein LD, Gilman RH, et al: Effects of *Cryptosporidium parvum* infection in Peruvian children: Growth faltering and subsequent catch-up growth. Am J Epidemiol 148(5):497–506, 1998.
73. Guerrant DI, Moore SR, Lima AA, et al: Association of early childhood diarrhea and cryptosporidiosis with impaired physical fitness and cognitive function four–seven years later in a poor urban community in northeast Brazil. Am J Trop Med Hyg 61(5):707–713, 1999.
74. Pettoello-Mantovani M, Di Martino L, Dettori G, et al: Asymptomatic carriage of intestinal *Cryptosporidium* in immunocompetent and immunodeficient children: A prospective study. Pediatr Infect Dis J 14(12):1042–1047, 1995.
75. Blanshard C, Jackson AM, Shanson DC, et al: Cryptosporidiosis in HIV-seropositive patients. Q J Med 85(307–308):813–823, 1992.
76. McGowan I, Hawkins AS, Weller IV: The natural history of cryptosporidial diarrhoea in HIV-infected patients. AIDS 7(3):349–354, 1993.
77. Flanigan T, Whalen C, Turner J, et al: *Cryptosporidium* infection and CD4 counts. Ann Intern Med 116(10):840–842, 1992.
78. Lopez-Velez R, Tarazona R, Garcia CA, et al: Intestinal and extraintestinal cryptosporidiosis in AIDS patients. Eur J Clin Microbiol Infect Dis 14(8):677–681, 1995.
79. Davis JJ, Heyman MB: Cryptosporidiosis and sinusitis in an immunodeficient adolescent. J Infect Dis 158(3):649, 1988.
80. Modigliani R, Bories C, Le Charpentier Y, et al: Diarrhoea and malabsorption in acquired immune deficiency syndrome: A study of four cases with special emphasis on opportunistic protozoan infestations. Gut 26(2):179–187, 1985.
81. Lima AA, Silva TM, Gifoni AM, et al: Mucosal injury and disruption of intestinal barrier function in HIV-infected individuals with and without diarrhea and cryptosporidiosis in northeast Brazil. Am J Gastroenterol 92(10):1861–1866, 1997.
82. Goodgame RW, Kimball K, Ou CN, et al: Intestinal function and injury in acquired immunodeficiency syndrome–related cryptosporidiosis. Gastroenterology 108(4):1075–1082, 1995.
83. Adams RB, Guerrant RL, Zu S, et al: *Cryptosporidium parvum* infection of intestinal epithelium: Morphologic and functional studies in an in vitro model. J Infect Dis 169(1):170–177, 1994.
84. Agnew DG, Lima AA, Newman RD, et al: Cryptosporidiosis in northeastern Brazilian children: Association with increased diarrhea morbidity. J Infect Dis 177(3):754–760, 1998.
85. Argenzio RA, Rhoads JM, Armstrong M, et al: Glutamine stimulates prostaglandin-sensitive Na(+)-H+ exchange in experimental porcine cryptosporidiosis. Gastroenterology 106(6):1418–1428, 1994.
86. Carneiro-Filho BA, Bushen OY, Brito GA, et al: Glutamine analogues as adjunctive therapy for infectious diarrhea. Curr Infect Dis Rep 5(2):114–119, 2003.
87. Sears CL, Guerrant RL: Cryptosporidiosis: The complexity of intestinal pathophysiology. Gastroenterology 106(1):252–254, 1994.
88. Guarino A, Canani RB, Pozio E, et al: Enterotoxic effect of stool supernatant of *Cryptosporidium*-infected calves on human jejunum. Gastroenterology 106(1):28–34, 1994.
89. Guarino A, Canani RB, Casola A, et al: Human intestinal cryptosporidiosis: Secretory diarrhea and enterotoxic activity in Caco-2 cells. J Infect Dis 171(4):976–983, 1995.
90. Kandil HM, Berschneider HM, Argenzio RA: Tumour necrosis factor alpha changes porcine intestinal ion transport through a paracrine mechanism involving prostaglandins. Gut 35(7):934–940, 1994.
91. Griffiths JK, Moore R, Dooley S, et al: *Cryptosporidium parvum* infection of Caco-2 cell monolayers induces an apical monolayer defect, selectively increases transmonolayer permeability, and causes epithelial cell death. Infect Immun 62(10):4506–4514, 1994.
92. Seydel KB, Zhang T, Champion GA, et al: *Cryptosporidium parvum* infection of human intestinal xenografts in SCID mice induces production of human tumor necrosis factor alpha and interleukin-8. Infect Immun 66(5):2379–2382, 1998.
93. Robinson P, Okhuysen PC, Chappell CL, et al: Substance P expression correlates with severity of diarrhea in cryptosporidiosis. J Infect Dis 188(2):290–296, 2003.
94. Benhamou Y, Kapel N, Hoang C, et al: Inefficacy of intestinal secretory immune response to *Cryptosporidium* in acquired immunodeficiency syndrome. Gastroenterology 108(3):627–635, 1995.
95. Taghi-Kilani R, Sekla L, Hayglass KT: The role of humoral immunity in *Cryptosporidium* spp. infection. Studies with B cell–depleted mice. J Immunol 145(5):1571–1576, 1990.
96. Cozon G, Biron F, Jeannin M, et al: Secretory IgA antibodies to *Cryptosporidium parvum* in AIDS patients with chronic cryptosporidiosis. J Infect Dis 169(3):696–699, 1994.
97. Gomez Morales MA, Ausiello CM, Urbani F, et al: Crude extract and recombinant protein of *Cryptosporidium parvum* oocysts induce proliferation of human peripheral blood mononuclear cells in vitro. J Infect Dis 172(1):211–216, 1995.
98. Chen W, Harp JA, Harmsen AG: Requirements for CD4+ cells and gamma interferon in resolution of established *Cryptosporidium parvum* infection in mice. Infect Immun 61(9):3928–3932, 1993.
99. Rehg JE: Effect of interferon-gamma in experimental *Cryptosporidium parvum* infection. J Infect Dis 174(1):229–232, 1996.
100. Current WL, Reese NC, Ernst JV, et al: Human cryptosporidiosis in immunocompetent and immunodeficient persons. Studies of an outbreak and experimental transmission. N Engl J Med 308(21):1252–1257, 1983.
101. Lasser KH, Lewin KJ, Ryning FW: Cryptosporidial enteritis in a patient with congenital hypogammaglobulinemia. Hum Pathol 10(2):234–240, 1979.
102. Murray HW, Welte K, Jacobs JL, et al: Production of and in vitro response to interleukin 2 in the acquired immunodeficiency syndrome. J Clin Invest 76(5):1959–1964, 1985.
103. Chen W, Harp JA, Harmsen AG, et al: Gamma interferon functions in resistance to *Cryptosporidium parvum* infection in severe combined immunodeficient mice. Infect Immun 61(8):3548–3551, 1993.
104. White AC, Robinson P, Okhuysen PC, et al: Interferon-gamma expression in jejunal biopsies in experimental human cryptosporidiosis correlates with prior sensitization and control of oocyst excretion. J Infect Dis 181(2):701–709, 2000.
105. Gomez Morales MA, Ausiello CM, Guarino A, et al: Severe, protracted intestinal cryptosporidiosis associated with interferon gamma deficiency: Pediatric case report. Clin Infect Dis 22(5):848–850, 1996.
106. Robinson P, Okhuysen PC, Chappell CL, et al: Expression of IL-15 and IL-4 in IFN-gamma-independent control of experimental human *Cryptosporidium parvum* infection. Cytokine 15(1):39–46, 2001.
107. Robinson P, Okhuysen PC, Chappell CL, et al: Expression of tumor necrosis factor alpha and interleukin 1 beta in jejuna of volunteers after experimental challenge with *Cryptosporidium parvum* correlates with exposure but not with symptoms. Infect Immun 69(2):1172–1174, 2001.
108. Alcantara CS, Yang CH, Steiner TS, et al: Interleukin-8, tumor necrosis factor-alpha, and lactoferrin in immunocompetent hosts with experimental and Brazilian children with acquired cryptosporidiosis. Am J Trop Med Hyg 68(3):325–328, 2003.
109. Schneiderman DJ, Cello JP, Laing FC: Papillary stenosis and sclerosing cholangitis in the acquired immunodeficiency syndrome. Ann Intern Med 106(4):546–549, 1987.
110. Goodgame RW, Genta RM, White AC, et al: Intensity of infection in AIDS-associated cryptosporidiosis. J Infect Dis 167(3):704–709, 1993.
111. Chappell CL, Okhuysen PC, Sterling CR, et al: *Cryptosporidium parvum*: Intensity of infection and oocyst excretion patterns in healthy volunteers. J Infect Dis 173(1):232–236, 1996.
112. Garcia LS, Shimizu RY: Evaluation of nine immunoassay kits (enzyme immunoassay and direct fluorescence) for detection of *Giardia lamblia* and *Cryptosporidium parvum* in human fecal specimens. J Clin Microbiol 35(6):1526–1529, 1997.
113. Alles AJ, Waldron MA, Sierra LS, et al: Prospective comparison of direct immunofluorescence and conventional staining methods for detection of *Giardia* and *Cryptosporidium* spp. in human fecal specimens. J Clin Microbiol 33(6):1632–1634, 1995.

114. Kehl KS, Cicirello H, Havens PL: Comparison of four different methods for detection of *Cryptosporidium* species. J Clin Microbiol 33(2):416–418, 1995.
115. Perry JL, Matthews JS, Miller GR: Parasite detection efficiencies of five stool concentration systems. J Clin Microbiol 28(6):1094–1097, 1990.
116. Zierdt WS: Concentration and identification of *Cryptosporidium* spp. by use of a parasite concentrator. J Clin Microbiol 20(5):860–861, 1984.
117. Leng X, Mosier DA, Oberst RD: Simplified method for recovery and PCR detection of *Cryptosporidium* DNA from bovine feces. Appl Environ Microbiol 62(2):643–647, 1996.
118. Zhu G, Marchewka MJ, Ennis JG, et al: Direct isolation of DNA from patient stools for polymerase chain reaction detection of *Cryptosporidium parvum*. J Infect Dis 177(5):1443–1446, 1998.
119. Sturbaum GD, Reed C, Hoover PJ, et al: Species-specific, nested PCR-restriction fragment length polymorphism detection of single *Cryptosporidium parvum* oocysts. Appl Environ Microbiol 67(6): 2665–2668, 2001.
120. Foudraine NA, Weverling GJ, van Gool T, et al: Improvement of chronic diarrhoea in patients with advanced HIV-1 infection during potent antiretroviral therapy. AIDS 12(1):35–41, 1998.
121. Carr A, Marriott D, Field A, et al: Treatment of HIV-1-associated microsporidiosis and cryptosporidiosis with combination antiretroviral therapy. Lancet 351(9098):256–261, 1998.
122. Le MV, Bissuel F, Costagliola D, et al: Decreased prevalence of intestinal cryptosporidiosis in HIV-infected patients concomitant to the widespread use of protease inhibitors. AIDS 12(11):1395–1397, 1998.
123. Mele R, Gomez Morales MA, Tosini F, et al: Indinavir reduces *Cryptosporidium parvum* infection in both in vitro and in vivo models. Int J Parasitol 33(7):757–764, 2003.
124. White AC Jr, Chappell CL, Hayat CS, et al: Paromomycin for cryptosporidiosis in AIDS: A prospective, double-blind trial. J Infect Dis 170(2):419–424, 1994.
125. Scaglia M, Atzori C, Marchetti G, et al: Effectiveness of aminosidine (paromomycin) sulfate in chronic *Cryptosporidium* diarrhea in AIDS patients: An open, uncontrolled, prospective clinical trial. J Infect Dis 170(5):1349–1350, 1994.
126. Hewitt RG, Yiannoutsos CT, Higgs ES, et al: Paromomycin: No more effective than placebo for treatment of cryptosporidiosis in patients with advanced human immunodeficiency virus infection. AIDS Clinical Trial Group. Clin Infect Dis 31(4):1084–1092, 2000.
127. Rossignol JF, Ayoub A, Ayers MS: Treatment of diarrhea caused by *Cryptosporidium parvum*: A prospective randomized, double-blind, placebo-controlled study of Nitazoxanide. J Infect Dis 184(1): 103–106, 2001.
128. Amadi B, Mwiya M, Musuku J, et al: Effect of nitazoxanide on morbidity and mortality in Zambian children with cryptosporidiosis: A randomised controlled trial. Lancet 360(9343):1375–1380, 2002.
129. Soave R, Havlir D, Lancaster D: Azithromycin therapy of AIDS-related cryptosporidial diarrhea: A multi-center, placebo-controlled, double-blind study. Programs and Abstracts of the 33rd Interscience Conference on Antimicrobial Agents and Chemotherapy, New Orleans, LA, October 17, 1993.
130. Blanshard C, Shanson DC, Gazzard BG: Pilot studies of azithromycin, letrazuril and paromomycin in the treatment of cryptosporidiosis. Int J STD AIDS 8(2):124–129, 1997.
131. Smith NH, Cron S, Valdez LM, et al: Combination drug therapy for cryptosporidiosis in AIDS. J Infect Dis 178(3):900–903, 1998.
132. Loeb M, Walach C, Phillips J, et al: Treatment with letrazuril of refractory cryptosporidial diarrhea complicating AIDS. J Acquir Immune Defic Syndr Hum Retrovirol 10(1):48–53, 1995.
133. Harris M, Deutsch G, MacLean JD, et al: A phase I study of letrazuril in AIDS-related cryptosporidiosis. AIDS 8(8):1109–1113, 1994.
134. Saez-Llorens X, Odio CM, Umana MA, et al: Spiramycin vs. placebo for treatment of acute diarrhea caused by *Cryptosporidium*. Pediatr Infect Dis J 8(3):136–140, 1989.
135. Shield J, Melville C, Novelli V, et al: Bovine colostrum immunoglobulin concentrate for cryptosporidiosis in AIDS. Arch Dis Child 69(4): 451–453, 1993.
136. Ungar BL, Ward DJ, Fayer R, et al: Cessation of *Cryptosporidium*-associated diarrhea in an acquired immunodeficiency syndrome patient after treatment with hyperimmune bovine colostrum. Gastroenterology 98(2):486–489, 1990.
137. Simon DM, Cello JP, Valenzuela J, et al: Multicenter trial of octreotide in patients with refractory acquired immunodeficiency syndrome–associated diarrhea. Gastroenterology 108(6):1753–1760, 1995.
138. Garcia CD, Ramos JJ, Guzman G, et al: Octreotide therapy of large-volume refractory AIDS-associated diarrhea: A randomized controlled trial. AIDS 8(11):1563–1567, 1994.
139. Liberti A, Bisogno A, Izzo E: Octreotide treatment in secretory and cyrptosporidial diarrhea in patients with acquired immunodeficiency syndrome (AIDS): Clinical evaluation. J Chemother 4(5):303–305, 1992.
140. Kreinik G, Burstein O, Landor M, et al: Successful management of intractable cryptosporidial diarrhea with intravenous octreotide, a somatostatin analogue. AIDS 5(6):765–767, 1991.
141. Girard PM, Goldschmidt E, Vittecoq D, et al: Vapreotide, a somatostatin analogue, in cryptosporidiosis and other AIDS-related diarrhoeal diseases. AIDS 6(7):715–718, 1992.
142. Assessment of inadequately filtered public drinking water—Washington, D.C., December 1993. MMWR 43(36):661–669, 1994.
143. Owens JH, Miltner RJ, Schaefer FW III, et al: Pilot-scale ozone inactivation of *Cryptosporidium*. J Eukaryot Microbiol 41(5):56S–57S, 1994.
144. Harp JA, Goff JP: Protection of calves with a vaccine against *Cryptosporidium parvum*. J Parasitol 81(1):54–57, 1995.
145. Okhuysen PC, Chappell CL, Sterling CR, et al: Susceptibility and serologic response of healthy adults to reinfection with *Cryptosporidium parvum*. Infect Immun 66(2):441–443, 1998.
146. Bushen OY, Davenport JA, Lima AB, et al: Diarrhea and reduced levels of antiretroviral drugs improvement with glutamine or alanyl-glutamine in a randomized controlled trail in northeast Brazil. Clin Infect Dis 38(12): 1764–1770, 2004.
147. Moling O, Avi A, Rimenti G, Mian P: Glutamine supplementation for patients with severe cryptosporidiosis. Clin Infect Dis 40(5):773–774, 2005.

Isospora

AGENT AND EPIDEMIOLOGY

I. belli was first identified in U.S. troops abroad during World War I, and this association gave the species its name.[56] However, *I. belli* was not studied further until 1970 when Brandborg and colleagues[57] identified it in tissue sections from patients with malabsorptive enteritis. Since then it has been recognized primarily in residents of and travelers to developing areas, especially those with AIDS.

The oblong oocyst of *I. belli* is a larger (10–20 × 20–30 μm) and more complex structure than the oocyst of *C. cayetanensis*. It contains two sporocysts with four sporozoites in each. The asexual phase of the life cycle (from ingested oocyst through sporozoite release and meront formation) is similar to that of *C. cayetanensis*. However, *I. belli* does not form identifiable type 2 meronts; rather, the merozoites presumably can develop either into trophozoites or gametocytes. Like the oocysts of *C. cayetanensis*, the oocysts of *I. belli* are not immediately infectious when excreted in stool. Under laboratory conditions, oocysts exposed to oxygen at temperatures slightly below 37°C sporulate in 24 to 48 hours. The duration of oocyst passage has been reported to last from 21 to 120 days.[58,59]

Humans are the only known hosts for *I. belli*, although other *Isospora* spp. are found throughout the animal kingdom. *I. belli* is distributed worldwide, with highest prevalence in tropical and subtropical climates. In contrast to *Cryptosporidium* spp., *I. belli* is rarely reported as a cause of diarrhea in immunocompetent children living in developing countries. In a 2-year period, the stools of 824 infants in Haiti were examined with a modified Ziehl-Nielsen method for the presence of coccidian parasites. None of the stools contained *I. belli* oocysts, whereas 17% of the stools contained *Cryptosporidium* spp. oocysts.[60] Analysis of a community-based cohort study of children aged from 3 weeks to 2 years in Guinea that was conducted from 1996 to 1998 did suggest an association between diarrhea and *I. belli* (OR for diarrhea 3.55 [95% CI: 1.15–11.0]) although the incidence was low (11 cases/168.7 child-year at risk).[61] Outside the tropics and subtropics, isosporiasis is usually found only in patients with a history of travel to these areas.[62] In the tropics, immunosuppressed patients are particularly at risk for isosporiasis. In a 1985 study of HIV-infected patients with diarrhea in Haiti, *I. belli* was found in 15% (20/131) of stool specimens. *Cryptosporidium* spp. was the only parasitic pathogen found more frequently in that study.[63]

Acquisition of isosporiasis is thought to be due to ingestion of food or water contaminated with mature oocysts from human feces. *I. belli* oocysts are not immediately infectious, so person-to-person transmission is considered rare. In the study mentioned previously that evaluated patients in Haiti with AIDS and isosporiasis, *I. belli* oocysts were detected in none of 170 healthy household or heterosexual contacts of the patients by acid-fast stains of concentrated stool specimens.[63]

DISEASE

Isosporiasis generally produces a self-limited diarrheal illness in otherwise healthy persons. The symptoms can resemble cyclosporiasis or cryptosporidiosis, with watery diarrhea and abdominal pain usually lasting less than 1 month. However, chronic isosporiasis, with malabsorption and weight loss, has been reported in immunocompetent patients. The disease can resemble celiac sprue.[57] Two deaths due to chronic isosporiasis in otherwise healthy children under age 2 years have been reported.[58]

In immunocompromised patients, isosporiasis may be prolonged and more severe. In the 1985 Haitian case series described previously, the median duration of diarrhea was 5.8 months and the diarrhea was associated with diffuse abdominal cramps and nausea.[63] Dissemination of infection to mesenteric and tracheobronchial lymph nodes has been reported in one patient, and dissemination to lymph nodes, liver, and spleen in another.[64] Acalculous cholecystitis in patients with AIDS and *I. belli* infection also has been reported.[65,66]

When observed histopathologically, *I. belli* is found invading beyond the epithelium into the lamina propria.[57] Although the histopathologic changes are similar to those described in cyclosporiasis, infiltration of large numbers of eosinophils into the lamina propria and dilation of the lymphatics reportedly are more common with *I. belli* infection.[58]

DIAGNOSIS

Isosporiasis should be considered in residents of or travelers to tropical areas who experience persistent diarrhea, abdominal cramps, steatorrhea, weight loss, and sometimes low-grade fever. As with cryptosporidiosis and cyclosporiasis, there are no characteristic physical findings or abnormalities on routine laboratory analyses. However, peripheral eosinophilia is sometimes noted and may explain the observation of Charcot-Leyden crystals in the stool specimens of some patients with isosporiasis.[58,67] Fecal leukocytes usually are not seen.[63]

Isospora infection is diagnosed by seeing the organism in stool. The oocysts stain bright red with modified acid-fast techniques and may also be autofluorescent, and they are clearly distinguishable from *Cyclospora* or *Cryptosporidium*. *Isospora* oocysts are much larger and elliptical (10–20 × 20–30 μm). Other techniques, including lactophenol cotton blue staining, the auramine-rhodamine technique, Giemsa staining, and the heated safranin-methylene blue technique have also been used to identify *I. belli* oocysts in stool samples.[58,68] Shedding of oocysts may be intermittent. In a case series of 34 patients with AIDS and isosporiasis, diagnosis of *I. belli* infection in seven patients required examination of three stool specimens for each patient.[69] In some cases, the organism has been visualized by light microscopic examination of a small bowel biopsy specimen, a duodenal aspirate, or a mucus specimen collected by the duodenal string test.[57,58] No serologic tests for *Isospora* are commercially available. Muller and associates[70] reported the successful identification of *I. belli* DNA by a PCR assay of small bowel tissue. However, PCR has not been validated for the evaluation of stool specimens for *I. belli* and is not available commercially.

TREATMENT AND PROGNOSIS

Isosporiasis can be treated successfully in patients with or without AIDS. The regimen of choice for adults in both groups is one double-strength tablet of TMP-SMX administered orally two to four times daily for 10 days. (The higher dose, and longer treatment, may be needed for immunosuppressed patients.)[71] In a study that used this regimen for patients with AIDS and isosporiasis in Haiti in 1988, this treatment resulted in complete symptomatic relief as well as parasitologic remission for all patients. In the same study, the efficacy of various prophylactic regimens was evaluated. Relapses were common in the group that received placebo therapy for secondary prophylaxis after the initial treatment (50% within 1.6 months of completing the initial treatment). Maintenance therapy with one of two regimens—one double-strength TMP-SMX tablet three times a week or one Fansidar tablet (pyrimethamine 25 mg plus sulfadoxine 500 mg) once a week—prevented all symptomatic relapses. One asymptomatic patient who was receiving TMP-SMX prophylaxis had *I. belli* identified in a routine follow-up stool sample.[69]

For treatment of patients who are intolerant of sulfonamide-containing medications, an alternative regimen is oral pyrimethamine 50 to 75 mg/day in individual doses (+ leucovorin 10 to 25 mg/day).[71,72] Other drugs reported to be effective are roxithromycin 2.5 mg/kg every 12 hours for 15 days and diclazuril.[73,74] The therapeutic efficacy of these drugs needs to be confirmed, but these regimens are also alternatives for patients intolerant of drugs containing sulfonamides. Prevention of relapses in immunocompromised patients who are intolerant of sulfa-containing drugs can be achieved with pyrimethamine alone at 25 mg/day.[69]

Sarcocystis

AGENT

Sarcocystis spp. belong to the family Sarcocystidae. Their life cycle differs from the coccidia discussed previously in that they require two separate hosts for completion: a definitive host (in which the sexual stage develops, usually a carnivorous predator) and an intermediate host (often herbivorous prey). The cycle in the intermediate host begins with ingestion of infectious sporocysts or oocysts. These excyst in the small intestine to release sporozoites that penetrate the mucosa and develop into schizonts in the vascular endothelium. The schizonts release merozoites that enter the circulation and lodge in skeletal or cardiac muscle to form sarcocysts. When muscle that contains sarcocysts is ingested by the definitive host, the cysts rupture to release zoites (also called bradyzoites or cystozoites) that invade the intestinal epithelium and differentiate into male or female gametocytes. After fertilization, which occurs within 24 hours, zygotes undergo encystation and sporulation, and oocysts (with two sporocysts, each with four sporozoites) are excreted in the stool, and the cycle continues.

Humans can be intermediate or definitive hosts for *Sarcocystis* species. If they are intermediate hosts, the infections are considered zoonotic. However, humans are the definitive hosts for *Sarcocystis suihominis* and *Sarcocystis bovihominis* (or *Sarcocystis hominis*). The intermediate hosts are pigs and cows, respectively. Persons who ingest tissue sarcocysts of these species may develop gastrointestinal symptoms attributed to infection of the intestinal mucosa. Humans are also thought to ingest *Sarcocystis* spp. sporocysts directly, which can lead to the development of intramuscular cysts.

EPIDEMIOLOGY

Various *Sarcocystis* species are identified throughout the world, with cases of muscle sarcocystosis reported in people in Southeast Asia, India, Africa, Europe, and North and South America (including the United States). Infection may be quite common in some areas. Prevalence rates of 10% and 20% to 23% were observed in adults in rural areas

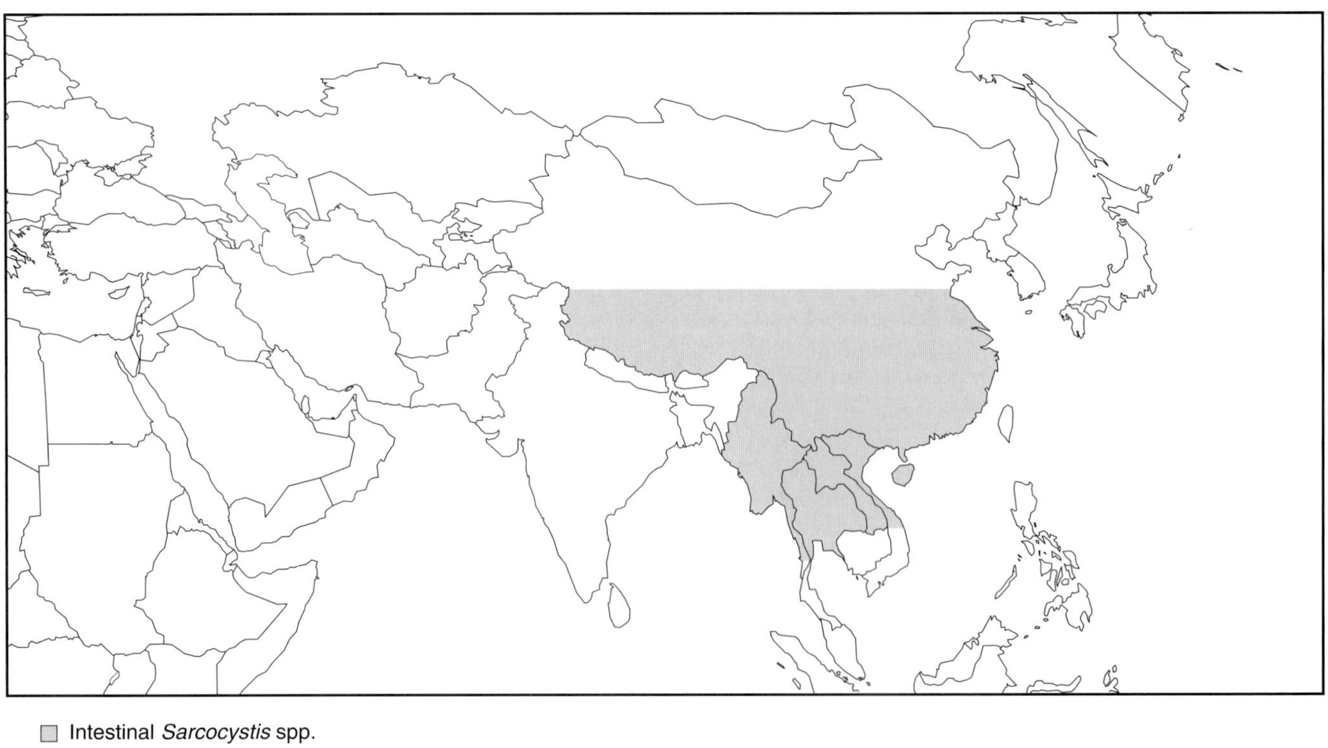

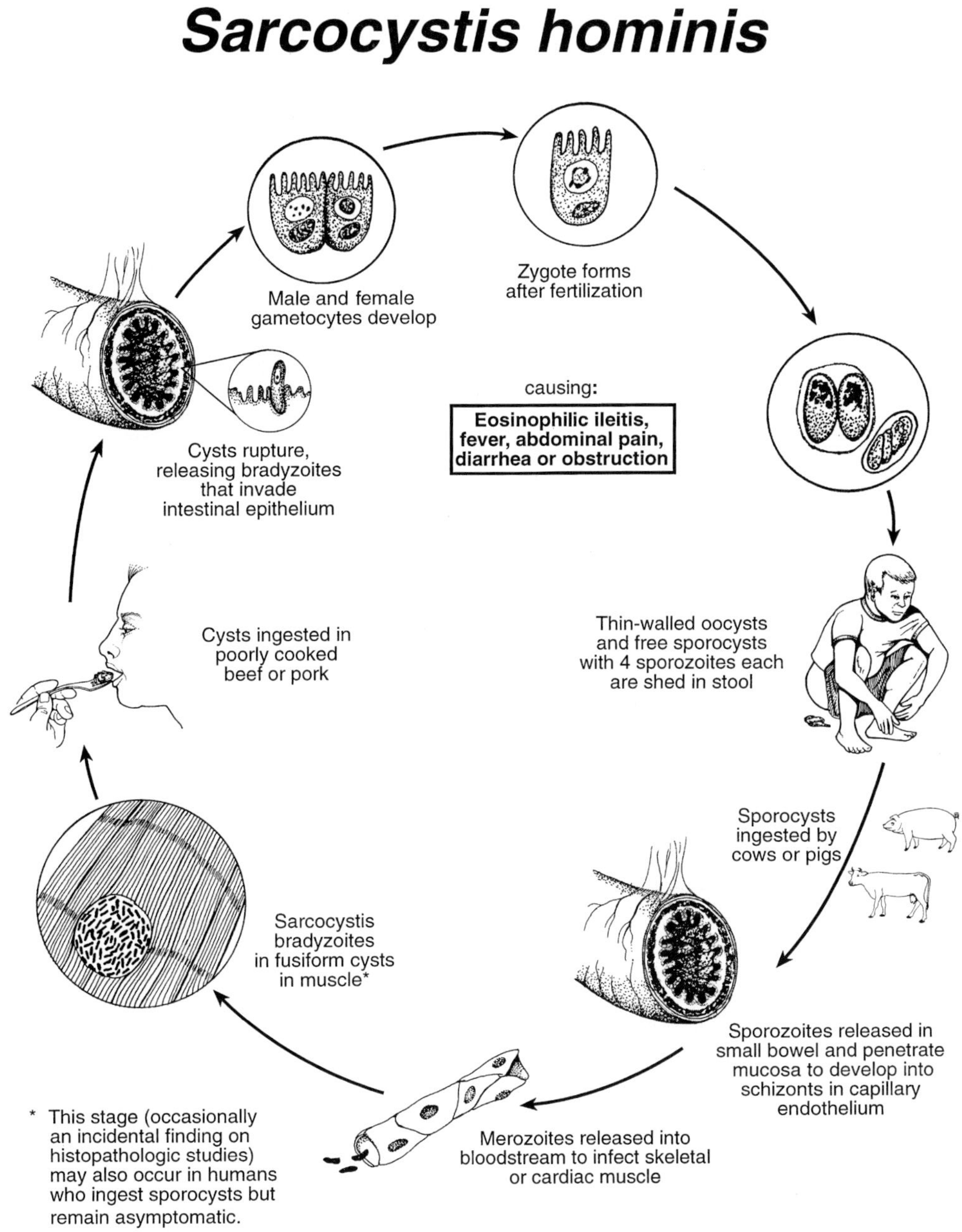

of Laos and Tibet, respectively. Most of these infections were asymptomatic.[75,76] Infection is thought to be due to consumption of undercooked beef or pork. In one case series, infections were associated with consumption of raw beef.[77]

DISEASE

Disseminated sarcocystosis is thought to result from the presence of cysts within muscle. However, sarcocysts have been found in biopsy specimens from asymptomatic persons as well as in specimens from patients with myalgias. Other patients with cysts in biopsy specimens have been found to have eosinophilia, polyarteritis nodosa, or, in one reported case, cardiomyopathy.[78] Whether the sarcocysts per se cause such manifestations has been difficult to establish.

Intestinal sarcocystosis can also result in several clinical presentations. As noted previously, most infections are asymptomatic. However, there are reports from Thailand of segmental eosinophilic or necrotizing enteritis requiring resection.[79] One volunteer who ingested 60 g of beef experimentally infected with *S. hominis* developed anemia, abdominal pain, diarrhea, fatigue, and dizziness 3 days later and shed oocysts for 42 days beginning on day 8.[79]

DIAGNOSIS AND TREATMENT

Intestinal sarcocystosis can be diagnosed by observation of sporulated sporocysts or oocysts in stool. The cysts resemble *Isospora* oocysts; they are acid-fast and contain two sporocysts. However, the thin-walled oocysts usually rupture in the bowel, releasing the sporocysts, which are not seen. Oocysts measure 15.5 × 20 μm and sporocysts 12 × 6 μm. Infection can also be diagnosed by observation of trophozoites or bradyzoites in biopsy tissue, although the organism can be mistaken for *Toxoplasma gondii* (in muscle) or *I. belli* (in the intestine).[56,77,78] Sulfadiazine, tinidazole, and acetylspiramycin have been reported to be active against intestinal *Sarcocystis* infection.[76] In cases of severe enteritis, segmental resection may be necessary. No clinical trials have been conducted to guide treatment of tissue sarcocystosis.

PREVENTION AND CONTROL

Presumably, thorough cooking of meat, especially of beef and pork, would prevent intestinal sarcocystosis. The internal temperatures required to guarantee the safety of meat are unknown, as is the effectiveness of alternative preparation techniques (e.g., curing, smoking). Regardless, raw meat should not be eaten because of the risk for infection with other known pathogens, such as cestodes, *Trichinella* spp., *T. gondii*, and enterohemorrhagic *E. coli*.

Treating animals raised for human consumption to reduce the incidence of sarcocystosis is another possible prevention strategy. However, this has proved difficult. In a survey of beef cattle in New Zealand, all the cattle tested were infected with a *Sarcocystis* species. In 80% of the cattle, the organism resembled *S. hominis*.[80] However, the human pathogen *S. hominis* cannot be distinguished by light microscopy from the related species *Sarcocystis hirsuta*. Therefore, the prevalence of *S. hominis* infection is difficult to determine.[81]

REFERENCES

1. Pieniazek NJ, Herwaldt B: Reevaluating the molecular taxonomy: is human-associated Cyclospora a mammalian Eimeria species? Emerg Infect Dis 3:381–383, 1997.
2. Relman DA, Schmidt TM, Gajadhar A, et al: Molecular phylogenetic analysis of Cyclospora, the human intestinal pathogen, suggests that it is closely related to Eimeria species. J Infect Dis 173:440–445, 1996.
3. Herwaldt BL: *Cyclospora cayetanensis:* a review, focusing on the outbreaks of cyclosporiasis in the 1990s. Clin Infect Dis 31:1040–1057, 2000.
4. Wittner M, Tanowitz HB, Weiss LM: Parasitic infections in AIDS patients: cryptosporidiosis, isosporiasis, microsporidiosis, cyclosporiasis. Infect Dis Clin North Am 7:569–586, 1993.
5. Ortega YR, Gilman RH, Sterling CR: A new coccidian parasite (Apicomplexa: Eimeriidae) from humans. J Parasitol 80:625–629, 1994.
6. Schaudinn F: Cyclospora carolytica Schaud, de Erreger der perniciosen Enteritis des Maulwurfs. Arb Kaiserl Gesundh 18:416, 1901.
7. Ortega YR, Sterling CR, Gilman RH, et al: Cyclospora species—a new protozoan pathogen of humans. N Engl J Med 328:1308–1312, 1993.
8. Ashford RW: Occurrence of an undescribed coccidian in man in Papua New Guinea. Ann Trop Med Parasitol 73:497–500, 1979.
9. Hoge CW, Shlim DR, Rajah R, et al: Epidemiology of diarrhoeal illness associated with coccidian-like organism among travellers and foreign residents in Nepal. Lancet 341:1175–1179, 1993.
10. Shlim DR, Cohen MT, Eaton M, et al: An alga-like organism associated with an outbreak of prolonged diarrhea among foreigners in Nepal. Am J Trop Med Hyg 45:383–389, 1991.
11. Fryauff DJ, Krippner R, Prodjodipuro P, et al: *Cyclospora cayetanensis* among expatriate and indigenous populations of West Java, Indonesia. Emerg Infect Dis 5:585–588, 1999.
12. Berlin OG, Novak SM, Porschen RK, et al: Recovery of Cyclospora organisms from patients with prolonged diarrhea. Clin Infect Dis 18:606–609, 1994.
13. Outbreaks of diarrheal illness associated with cyanobacteria (blue-green algae)–like bodies—Chicago and Nepal, 1989 and 1990. MMWR 40:325–327, 1991.
14. Herwaldt BL, Ackers ML: An outbreak in 1996 of cyclosporiasis associated with imported raspberries. Cyclospora Working Group. N Engl J Med 336:1548–1556, 1997.
15. Herwaldt BL, Beach MJ: The return of Cyclospora in 1997: another outbreak of cyclosporiasis in North America associated with imported raspberries. Cyclospora Working Group. Ann Intern Med 130:210–220, 1999.
16. Ortega YR, Nagle R, Gilman RH, et al: Pathologic and clinical findings in patients with cyclosporiasis and a description of intracellular parasite life-cycle stages. J Infect Dis 176:1584–1589, 1997.
17. Ashford RW, Warhurst DC, Reid GD: Human infection with cyanobacterium-like bodies. Lancet 341:1034, 1993.
18. Zerpa R, Uchima N, Huicho L: *Cyclospora cayetanensis* associated with watery diarrhoea in Peruvian patients. J Trop Med Hyg 98:325–329, 1995.
19. Soave R, Johnson WD Jr: Cyclospora: conquest of an emerging pathogen. Lancet 345:667–668, 1995.
20. Eberhard ML, Ortega YR, Hanes DE, et al: Attempts to establish experimental Cyclospora cayetanensis infection in laboratory animals. J Parasitol 86:577–582, 2000.
21. Eberhard ML, Arrowood MJ: Cyclospora spp. Curr Opin Infect Dis 15:519–522, 2002.
22. Huang P, Weber JT, Sosin DM, et al: The first reported outbreak of diarrheal illness associated with Cyclospora in the United States. Ann Intern Med 123:409–414, 1995.
23. Rabold JG, Hoge CW, Shlim DR, et al: Cyclospora outbreak associated with chlorinated drinking water. Lancet 344:1360–1361, 1994.
24. Outbreak of cyclosporiasis—northern Virginia–Washington, D.C.–Baltimore, Maryland, metropolitan area, 1997. MMWR 46: 689–691, 1997.
25. Lopez AS, Dodson DR, Arrowood MJ, et al: Outbreak of cyclosporiasis associated with basil in Missouri in 1999. Clin Infect Dis 32:1010–1017, 2001.
26. Outbreak of cyclosporiasis associated with snow peas—Pennsylvania, 2004. MMWR 53:876–878, 2004.
27. Ho AY, Lopez AS, Eberhart MG, et al: Outbreak of cyclosporiasis associated with imported raspberries, Philadelphia, Pennsylvania, 2000. Emerg Infect Dis 8:783–788, 2002.
28. Bern C, Hernandez B, Lopez MB, et al: Epidemiologic studies of *Cyclospora cayetanensis* in Guatemala. Emerg Infect Dis 5:766–774, 1999.
29. Soave R, Dubey JP, Ramos L: A new intestinal pathogen? Clin Res 34:533A, 1986.
30. Wurtz RM, Kocka FE, Peters CS, et al: Clinical characteristics of seven cases of diarrhea associated with a novel acid-fast organism in the stool. Clin Infect Dis 16:136–138, 1993.
31. Butcher AR, Lumb R, Coulter E, Nielsen DJ:Coccidian/cyanobacterium-like body associated diarrhea in an Australian traveller returning from overseas. Pathology 26:59–61, 1994.
32. Bendall RP, Lucas S, Moody A, et al: Diarrhoea associated with cyanobacterium-like bodies: a new coccidian enteritis of man. Lancet 341:590–592, 1993.
33. Taylor DN, Houston R, Shlim DR, et al: Etiology of diarrhea among travelers and foreign residents in Nepal. JAMA 260:1245–1248, 1988.
34. Eberhard ML, Nace EK, Freeman AR, et al: *Cyclospora cayetanensis* infections in Haiti: a common occurrence in the absence of watery diarrhea. Am J Trop Med Hyg 60:584–586, 1999.
35. Madico G, McDonald J, Gilman RH, et al: Epidemiology and treatment of *Cyclospora cayetanensis* infection in Peruvian children. Clin Infect Dis 24:977–981, 1997.
36. Ortega YR, Sterling CR, Gilman RH: *Cyclospora cayetanensis.* Adv Parasitol 40:399–418, 1998.
37. Shlim DR, Hoge CW, Rajah R, et al: Persistent high risk of diarrhea among foreigners in Nepal during the first 2 years of residence. Clin Infect Dis 29:613–616, 1999.
38. Hoge CW, Echeverria P, Rajah R, et al: Prevalence of Cyclospora species and other enteric pathogens among children less than 5 years of age in Nepal. J Clin Microbiol 33:3058–3060, 1995.
39. Chacin-Bonilla L, Mejia de YM, Estevez J: Prevalence and pathogenic role of *Cyclospora cayetanensis* in a Venezuelan community. Am J Trop Med Hyg 68:304–306, 2003.
40. Nunez FA, Gonzalez OM, Gonzalez I, et al: Intestinal coccidia in Cuban pediatric patients with diarrhea. Mem Inst Oswaldo Cruz 98:539–542, 2003.

of malaria in a number of countries in South and Central America, North Africa, and Asia, but with little impact in most countries of sub-Saharan Africa.[9]

In 2005 the impact of malaria in many parts of the world is similar to or greater than it was 50 years ago. *P. falciparum* has become resistant to a range of drugs, the mosquitoes have become resistant to many insecticides, and the health services infrastructure required to deliver effective malaria control measures sustainably has deteriorated or never been established. In recent years several promising new malaria control interventions have been field-tested that could, if deployed to high levels of population coverage, dramatically reduce malaria burden, especially in sub-Saharan Africa. They include interdicting contact between humans and infected mosquitoes by use of insecticide-impregnated bed nets, residual insecticide spraying, and reduction of breeding places and reducing the effects of the disease by early diagnosis and treatment and by intermittent therapy, independent of evidence of infection in pregnant women and infants. The global community has committed to reducing the health and economic impact of malaria, and funding for malaria control is being made available by international and national entities. There are substantial efforts aimed at developing vaccines, but they are years away from deployment.

AGENT

Malaria is caused by protozoa of the genus *Plasmodium*, family Plasmodiidae, suborder Haemosporidiidea, order Coccidiida. There are more than 120 *Plasmodium* species that infect mammals, birds, and reptiles. Only four species are known to consistently infect humans: *P. falciparum, P. vivax, P. malariae*, and *P. ovale*. *P. knowlesi*, a simian malaria parasite, has intermittently been reported to cause human disease.[10]

Understanding malaria is dependent on understanding the complex life cycle of the parasite in its definitive host in which sexual development occurs—the mosquito—and its intermediate host—the human (see life cycle). The life cycle of *P. falciparum* is described in the following section, the unique terminology is described in Box 90-1, and the differences among *P. falciparum* and its life cycle and that of *P. malariae, P. vivax*, and *P. ovale* are described in Table 90-1 and in the following sections.

Box 90-1 Terminology of Malariologists

Prepatent period: The time from inoculation of sporozoites until asexual erythrocytic stage parasites are demonstrated in the bloodstream.

Incubation period: The time from inoculation of sporozoites until the individual first manifests symptoms or signs of malaria.

Recurrence: Repeat infection causing malaria that is result of a relapse, recrudescence, or reinfection.

- *Relapse:* A recurrent infection caused by full development of hypnozoites from the liver. Relapses are thought to occur only with *P. vivax* or *P. ovale* infections.
- *Recrudescence:* A recurrent infection caused by full development of a blood-stage infection in which parasitaemia declined below the level of detection and then rose above the level of detection. Recrudescence occurs most commonly after inadequate treatment as a result of drug resistance, unusual pharmacokinetics, or incomplete dosage. It can also occur in immunocompromised individuals whose immune systems have been controlling an extremely low grade asexual erythrocytic stage infection for years, especially when the parasite is *P. malariae*.
- *Reinfection:* A recurrent infection caused by a new exposure to infected *Anopheles* mosquitoes.

Classification of endemnicity: This classification scheme has been used since the 1950s, but many malariologists do not currently find it useful because of the poor correlation between the number of 2- to 9-year-olds with palpable spleens and positive blood films and the intensity of malaria transmission in settings where people are fed on by more than 20 infected mosquitoes per year.

Type
Palpable Spleen (Spleen Rates)
Positive Blood Film

Holoendemic
>75% in 2- to 9-year olds, and low in adults
>75% in 2- to 9-year olds

Hyperendemic
>50% in 2- to 9-year olds, and >25% in adults
>50% in 2- to 9-year olds

Mesoendemic
11%-50% in 2- to 9-year olds
11%-50% in 2- to 9-year olds

Hypoendemic
<11% in 2- to 9-year olds
<11% in 2- to 9-year olds

Life Cycle of *P. falciparum*

When an infected female *Anopheles* spp mosquito feeds on a human (Fig. 90-1A), she is thought to inoculate an average of 5 to 10 and as many as 100 uninucleated sporozoites (approximately 1×7 μm) into the tissues or directly into the bloodstream[11] (Fig. 90-1B). The sporozoites rapidly pass through the bloodstream to the liver (probably within 2 minutes, but no more than 30 minutes).[12] In the sinusoids they penetrate and pass through Kupffer cells[13] and invade hepatocytes through a specific receptor-ligand interaction. The primary receptor is thought to be sulfated heparan glycans on the hepatocyte surface, and the parasite ligands include the thrombospondin domains of at least two sporozoite proteins—the circumsporozoite protein[14] and a protein known both as the thrombospondin-related anonymous protein (TRAP)[15] and as sporozoite surface protein 2.[16] The sporozoites may invade several hepatocytes before finding the correct hepatocyte in which to develop.[17] In the hepatocyte, host cell material is used to form a "parasitophorous" vacuole that separates the parasite from the cytoplasm of the hepatocytes. During a minimum of 5.5 days, the uninucleated *P. falciparum* sporozoite develops to a mature liver-stage schizont with an average of 30,000 and range of 10,000 to 40,000 uninucleated merozoites (see Fig. 90-1C and Table 90-1).

The mature liver-stage schizont ruptures, releasing the thousands of merozoites that are about 1.5 μm in diameter, each of which can invade a normal erythrocyte (Fig. 90-1D). There are a number of steps in this process (Fig. 90-1E), but there is unquestionably a specific interaction between receptors on the erythrocyte membrane and ligands on the merozoite surface. One of these receptor-ligand interactions is

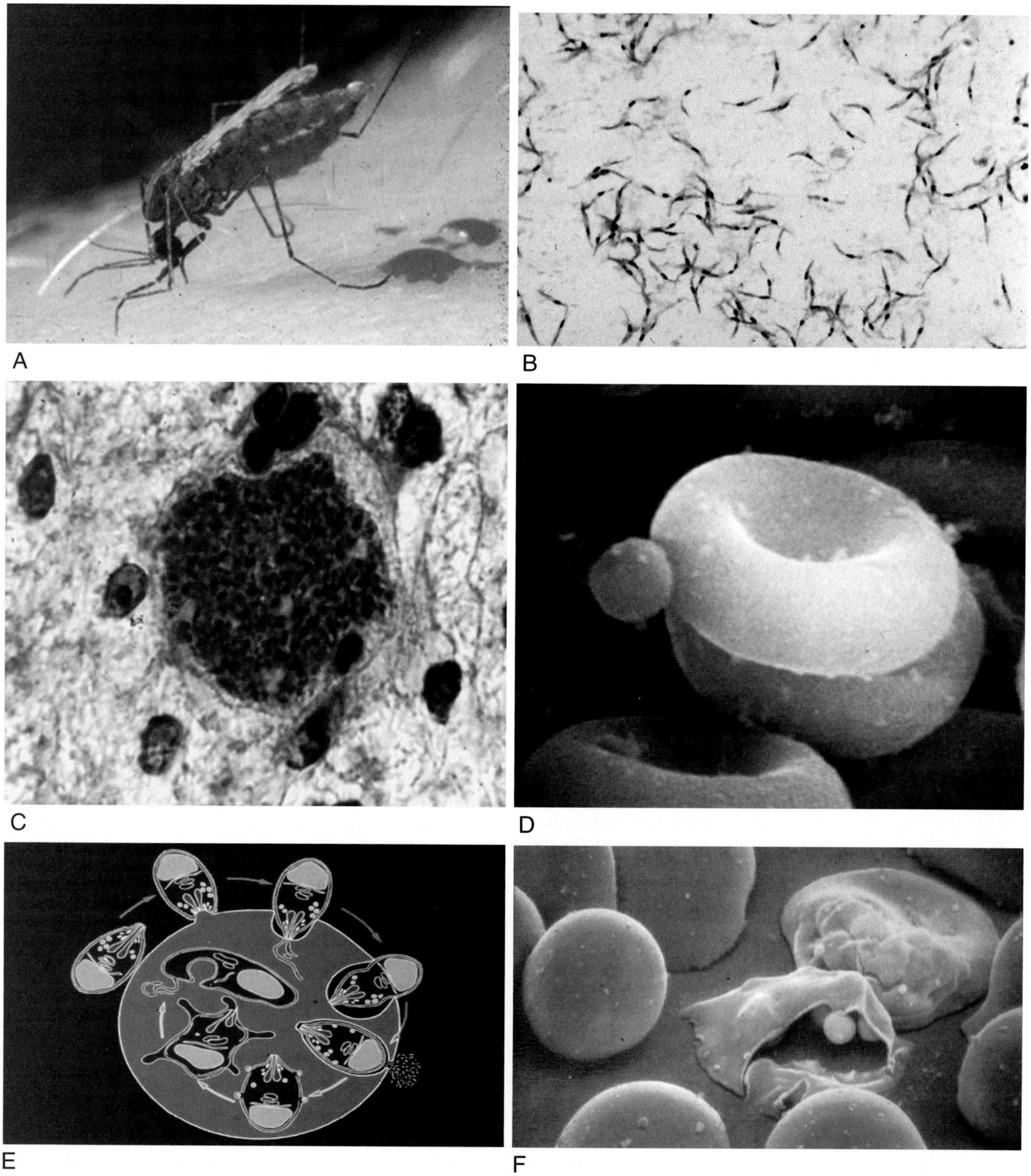

FIGURE 90-1 Vector and parasites at different stages of the life cycle. *A, Anopheles stephensi* mosquito feeding in characteristic posture. *B, P. falciparum* sporozoites in a crush preparation of a salivary gland (Giemsa stain). *C,* Mature liver-stage schizont of *P. falciparum* with thousands of merozoites (hemotoxylin and eosin stain). *D, P. falciparum* merozoite attaching to uninfected erythrocyte prior to invasion (scanning electron micrograph). *E,* Schematic of the process of a *P. falciparum* merozoite invading an erythrocyte. *F, P. falciparum* merozoites rupturing from an infected erythrocyte. Note "knobs" on the surface of the infected, unruptured erythrocyte above the rupturing erythrocyte (scanning electron micrograph).

(Continued)

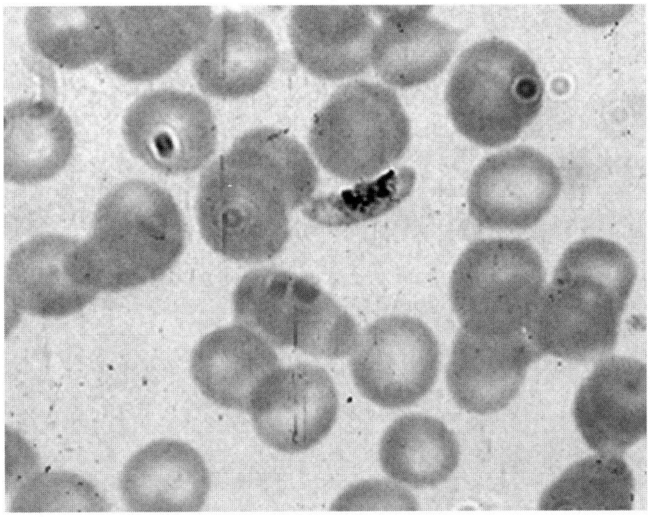

G

FIGURE 90-1—Cont'd *G, P. falciparum* gametocyte in thin blood smear (Giemsa stain). (*B,* Courtesy of © Liverpool School of Tropical Medicine, photo by A. Stich, Wellcome Trust International Health Image Collection; *C,* courtesy of Dr. P. Druilhe, Institute Pasteur, Paris, France; *D,* courtesy of © L. H. Bannister, Wellcome Trust International Health Image Collection.

between sialic acids and peptides on erythrocyte glycophorin A and the 175-kd erythrocyte-binding antigen (PfEBA175) on the merozoite.[18] In the erythrocyte, the invading merozoite develops within a parasitophorous vacuole composed of host cell material. During the next 43 to 48 hours, the uninucleated merozoite develops to maturity within the parasitophorous vacuole. First, it becomes a trophozoite and begins to secrete proteins that pass through the parasite membrane and the parasitophorous vacuole membrane and form knobs in the erythrocyte membrane (Fig. 90-1F). The proteins in the knobs, especially one called *P. falciparum* erythrocyte membrane protein 1 (PfEMP1),[19–21] bind to receptors on endothelial cells in capillaries and postcapillary venules, sequestering the infected erythrocyte in the microcirculation for the last 24 to 34 hours of its development cycle, when it changes from an immature schizont to a mature asexual erythrocytic stage schizont with an average of 16 uninucleated merozoites. It is thought that the parasite has developed this mechanism to prevent the increasingly rigid infected erythrocyte from being removed from the circulation when it passes through the spleen. When fully mature, the infected erythrocyte ruptures, releasing the merozoites (see Fig. 90-1F), which then invade normal erythrocytes, initiating the cycle of intra-erythrocytic stage development, rupture, and reinvasion that leads to a 10- to 20-fold increase in the numbers of *P. falciparum* parasites in the bloodstream every 43 to 48 hours and to all the clinical manifestations and pathology of malaria.

Alternatively, the erythrocytic stage parasites can develop to sexual stage parasites called gametocytes (Fig. 90-1G). In the gut of the mosquito, the gametocytes escape from the erythrocytes and form gametes. The male gamete fuses with the female, forming a zygote. At about 5 hours after blood-feeding, the zygote undergoes two-step meiosis. By 18 to 24 hours, the zygote has transformed into an ookinete. The ookinete traverses the midgut wall by passing through epithelial cells and comes to rest adjacent to the basal lamina. Here it begins to transform into an oocyst. From the 6th day onward, the oocyst undergoes cell division that eventually results in the formation of about 8000 daughter cells called sporozoites. By day 12, they are released into the hemocele of the mosquito and migrate to the salivary glands. In the salivary glands, they become infectious for humans and are released into the human host when the mosquito feeds.

Differences Between *P. falciparum* and Its Life Cycle and the Other Parasites That Cause Human Malaria

These differences are outlined in Table 90-1. One of the most important differences is that *P. vivax* and *P. ovale* can have prolonged (up to 3 years) liver stages. Some populations of *P. vivax* and *P. ovale* sporozoites invade hepatocytes, arrest further development, becoming hypnozoites (sleeping forms),[22,23] and then activate and initiate replication and full development a month to several years after the primary infection. When a patient who was appropriately treated for an asexual erythrocytic stage *P. vivax* or *P. ovale* infection and had elimination of clinical manifestations of the disease and all parasites from the bloodstream (clinical cure) has a recurrent case of malaria caused by development of hypnozoites, the patient is considered to have a relapse (see Box 90-1). In addition to secondary attacks caused by hypnozoites, some isolates of *P. vivax,* especially those acquired in temperate regions of the world (e.g., Korea, China) cause delayed primary infections owing to persistence in the liver that may occur up to 1 year after inoculation of sporozoites by mosquitoes. These parasites are called *P. vivax* var *hibernans*. This phenomenon of delayed primary attacks has been reported with *P. falciparum*[24] but is much less common than with *P. vivax*.

P. vivax differs from the other three parasites in that *P. vivax* merozoites cannot invade erythrocytes that lack the Duffy blood group antigen.[25] Duffy protein on the erythrocyte membrane is a receptor for a protein ligand on the merozoite surface called the Duffy binding protein or ligand (DBL).[26]

P. falciparum, P. vivax, and *P. ovale* take approximately 48 hours to complete the asexual erythrocytic stage of their life cycle (invasion, development, rupture, and reinvasion), and are called tertian (recurring every 3rd day) malarias. *P. malaria* has an approximately 72 hour cycle and is called quartan (recurring every 4th day) malaria.

Genomics of *P. falciparum*

The genomic sequence of chromosome 2 of *P. falciparum* was published in 1998,[27] and the entire genomic sequence of the 3D7 clone, which has been maintained in culture for two decades, was published in 2002.[28] The *P. vivax* genome has been partially sequenced, and while some results are available on the Internet, the results have not yet been published. Active genome projects involving over a half-dozen other rodent and simian *Plasmodium* species, as well as a *P. falciparum* isolate obtained directly from a patient, are under way. Since there is substantial evolutionary conservation among *Plasmodium* species,[29] a great deal can be inferred through comparative genomics.[30]

The *P. falciparum* genome is approximately 23 Mb in size and encodes about 5300 genes on 14 chromosomes. Fifty-four percent of the genes contain introns. On average, the coding regions of *P. falciparum* genes are longer than in other sequenced eukaryotes such as *Schizosaccharomyces pombe* (2.3 kb vs 1.4kb). The reason for this increased gene length is unknown. Fully 60% of the encoded proteins have little or no similarity to proteins in other organisms and are of unknown function. The proportion of genes encoding these so-called hypothetical proteins is higher in *P. falciparum* than in other sequenced organisms, which is probably a reflection of the greater evolutionary distance between *Plasmodium* and other well-studied eukaryotes.

Analysis of the predicted proteome provides an overview of metabolism and transport in malaria parasites.[31,32] A number of features of parasite metabolism remain unclear because of the absence of some enzymes or enzyme subunits and because the predicted subcellular localization of some enzymes differs from the known localization of the enzymes in other organisms, making it difficult to reconstruct the metabolism of the parasite with certainty. A remarkable feature of this parasite is its relative lack of transcription factors, implying that the parasite relies to a large extent on post-transcriptional control of gene function.

P. falciparum appears to have greatly reduced capacities for metabolism and for the transport of organic nutrients and ions as compared with other free-living organisms. Only 14% of the proteins encode enzymes. This is a much lower proportion than in other eukaryotes. Similarly, the *P. falciparum* genome encodes a smaller repertoire of membrane transporters in comparison with other free-living eukaryotic microbes such as *Saccharomyces cerevisiae*. The *P. falciparum* genome encodes enzymes for the complete glycolytic pathway from glucose-6 phosphate to pyruvate, and for the conversion of pyruvate to lactate. All enzymes of the tricarboxylic acid (TCA) cycle have been identified, but the function of the TCA cycle is unclear.

Other unusual features of *P. falciparum* metabolism that can be inferred from the genome sequence are the absence of gluconeogenesis and the lack of any enzymes for the biosynthesis of amino acids, apart from enzymes required for amino acid interconversions. The lack of amino acid biosynthetic pathways, and the apparent absence of clear homologs of known amino acid transporters, emphasizes the parasite's dependence on the host for amino acids, at least in the erythrocytic stages in which amino acids are obtained by the digestion of hemoglobin in the food vacuole. Overall, the metabolic and transport capabilities of *Plasmodium* are less than those of other free-living organisms, which may be a reflection of its parasitic lifestyle.

A clear difference between the genome of *P. falciparum* and other sequenced eukaryotes is the abundance of genes in the malaria parasite that are involved in immune evasion and other host-parasite interactions (3.9% and 1.3%, respectively). The 3D7 genome contains 59 *var* genes that encode highly polymorphic proteins known as *P. falciparum* erythrocyte membrane protein 1 (PfEMP1).[19–21] These proteins are expressed on the surface of infected red blood cells, mediate cytoadherence of the infected cells to host capillary endothelium, and cause sequestration of the infected cells in many organs, including the brain. The PfEMP1 proteins are thought to be the targets of protective antibody responses, but transcriptional switching between different *var* genes provides for antigenic variation and the evasion of the host immune response. The *rif* genes, of which there are 149 in the 3D7 genome, encode proteins called rifins. A third group of proteins called STEVORs (28 in the 3D7 genome) are similar in sequence to the rifins and so far, like the rifins, have no known function. Members of the PFEMP1, rifin, and STEVOR families exhibit extensive sequence diversity, and the genes encoding these proteins occur in clusters, most of which are located in subtelomeric regions in association with several kinds of repetitive sequences. The repetitive sequences are thought to facilitate recombination between different alleles of these highly polymorphic proteins and contribute to the generation of antigen diversity.

The availability of the genome sequence of *P. falciparum* has paved the way for detailed analyses of parasite biology. Technologies such as DNA microarrays[33,34] and proteomics[31,32] have provided means to assess how the parasite responds to its environment and how it functions as an organism requiring two such different hosts as humans and mosquitoes, and they may provide clues to developing new interventions against the parasite and the disease it causes.

EPIDEMIOLOGY

Malaria transmission occurs in most of Africa south of the Sahara desert; in many areas of the Indian subcontinent, Southeast Asia, and Oceania; in Central America, Haiti and the Dominican Republic; and in the Amazon basin of Brazil and contiguous countries in South America. The global distribution and prevalence of malaria infection have not changed appreciably for the past few decades. While malaria infection is widely distributed, the intensity of transmission of *Plasmodium* is greatest in Africa, where in excess of 70% of new infections globally are estimated to occur annually.

Malaria infection with the four *Plasmodium* spp that naturally infect humans is characterized by persistence of the blood stage of parasites for intervals of from months to life-long, without therapy. Consequently, in areas, notably Africa, it is difficult to characterize the incidence (of new infections) of malaria since the prevalence of infection is persistently high. It has been estimated that in the range of 300 to 800 million new malaria infections occur globally each year[1]; however, this figure is highly imprecise, particularly in areas of high levels of transmission in Africa.[35]

The major determinants of the epidemiology of malaria infection and disease relate to the *Plasmodium* spp, the transmission intensity, innate and acquired resistance of the human host, and access to and efficacy of control measures. In addition, the immunocompromised states associated with pregnancy and infection with human immunodeficiency virus (HIV) affect the epidemiology of malaria.

Plasmodium Species

The species that causes the greatest illness and death in humans, *P. falciparum*, is the predominant infection in Africa south of the Sahara, in the Amazon basin and Haiti, and many areas of Asia and Oceania. *P. vivax* is widely distributed in the Americas and Asia, and only in very circumscribed areas of Africa. The two less prevalent species, *P. malaria* and *P. ovale*, are transmitted in some areas of Africa

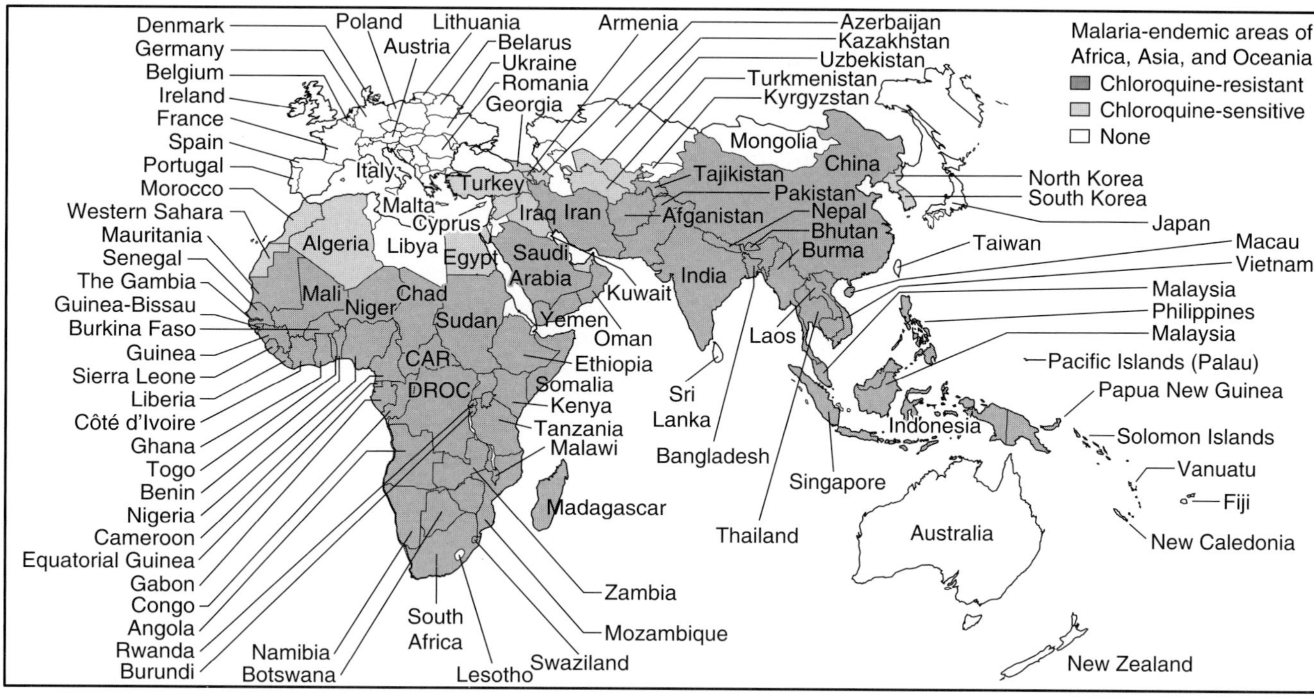

Chloroquine sensitive and resistant *P. falciparum* in Africa, Asia, and Oceania (Courtesy of Dr. M. Parise: Health Information for International Travel. Atlanta, Centers for Disease Control and Prevention, 2005–2006, in press.)

and the Amazon basin and sporadically in other parts of the world such as Oceania and Southeast Asia. As a consequence of this distribution, most illness and death attributable to malaria occurs in Africa, Asia, and the Amazon region of Brazil.

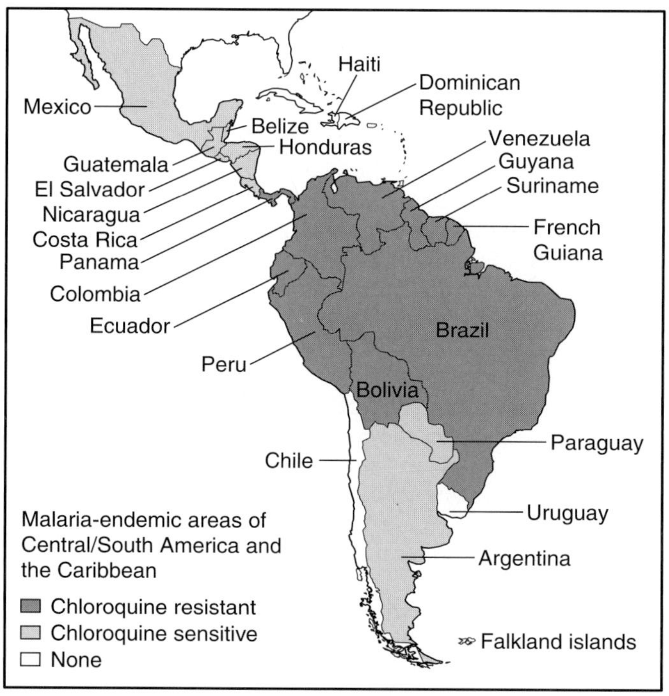

Chloroquine sensitive and resistant *P. falciparum* in Central and South America and the Caribbean (Courtesy of Dr. M. Parise: Health Information for International Travel. Atlanta, Centers for Disease Control and Prevention, 2005–2006, in press.)

Transmission Intensity

Plasmodium parasites are transmitted to humans by female mosquitoes of the *Anopheles* genus. Worldwide approximately 40 anopheline species have been documented to transmit parasites to humans. These species vary remarkably in their capacity to transmit *Plasmodium* to humans. This variability relates to basic habits, including tendency to seek out humans for a blood meal, types of water sources preferred for laying eggs, and predilection for entering human dwellings, as well as basic biologic capacity to support the development of human *Plasmodia* to development of mature infection that can be transmitted during the taking of a blood meal. Anopheline species with the greatest competence to transmit *Plasmodium* are found in the Amazon (*Anopheles darlingi*) and Africa (the species complex of *An. gambiae*).

Several identifiable factors characterize the capacity of *Anopheles* mosquitoes to transmit *Plasmodium*. The adult female mosquito can survive under ideal conditions up to 50 to 60 days. Practically, however, female anophelines survive on the average of 20 to 25 days, and consequently must be infected by malaria parasites in their early blood meals, taken every 3 to 4 days. Maturation of the parasites ingested with the blood meal requires 8 to 12 days before the mosquito has infective sporozoites in her salivary glands. Mathematical modeling of malaria transmission by MacDonald[36] and others incorporates a measure of mosquito density in a defined setting and the probability that an *Anopheles* will feed on a human during a day.

The epidemiologic measure of transmission intensity is the entomologic inoculation rate (EIR), which depends on the proportion of female anophelines with salivary glands infected with *Plasmodium* and the number of potentially infected *Anopheles* mosquitoes feeding on a person in a unit of time (day or year). There is a wide range of documented

EIRs by both time and area of the world, and even within regions of a country. In the areas of Africa with the most intense annual transmission, EIRs can reach three infected bites per day at the peak of transmission for short periods. By contrast, in most malaria endemic regions of the Americas and Asia, annual EIRs range from less than 1 up to 10 infected bites annually.

Mathematical models of malaria transmission have constructed several composite statistics to quantitate the risk of malaria transmission in defined epidemiologic settings. Vectorial capacity incorporates estimates of mosquito density and human biting rate along with daily survival (longevity) of anopheline mosquitoes to estimate the overall either receptivity or intensity of malaria parasite transmission in a defined setting. The estimation of vectorial capacity can be used to compare transmission risk in time and space, and in principle also to monitor the effect of measures used to control malaria transmission.

Black[37] developed the concept of the reproductive rate for malaria transmission that estimates the number of secondary cases of malaria that are predicted from an infected human in a population susceptible to malaria infection. A reproductive rate greater than 1.0 predicts sustaining malaria transmission in a population. Efforts to interrupt transmission must maintain the reproductive rate less than 1.0. Most of these mathematical models were developed and refined during the last century in conjunction with malaria eradication attempts and have not been refined to address malaria transmission dynamics in highly immune populations as encountered in Africa.

In Africa, transmission intensity has a major effect on the clinical manifestations of severe disease and the age at which they are encountered. For example in areas with extremely high entomologic inoculation rates (100 to 300 potentially infective bites/year) and long transmission seasons, most severe disease and malaria-associated deaths occur in infants and young children, and the primary cause of malaria-associated death is severe anemia. In areas with much less intense transmission (10 to 40 potentially infective bites/year) and more limited transmission periods, most cases of severe malaria and deaths occur in older children (e.g., 3 to 7 years of age), and cerebral malaria is responsible for a high percentage of the deaths.

Innate and Acquired Resistance

Protection from malaria can be expressed as decreased risk of being infected (developing blood-stage parasitemia) or decreased risk of developing higher density parasitemia and clinical illness due to the parasitemia (clinical immunity). This protection is mediated by innate mechanisms and by acquired adaptive immune responses. In settings of natural transmission, it has been demonstrated that humans do not acquire persisting protection from being infected by mosquito transmission but do develop immune-mediated protection against parasites and disease. It is presumed that in the field the natural variability of the *Plasmodium* parasite (antigenic variation) is the major factor responsible for persisting susceptibility to infection even after lifelong exposure.

Innate Resistance

It has often been stated that malaria has had more impact on the human genome then any other infectious agent. In settings where humans are exposed to high levels of malaria transmission, it has been documented that genetically determined traits are selected for over generations that mediate protection against either infection or the risk of clinical or severe malaria illness.

A well-characterized protective mutation is the Duffy factor, a minor erythrocyte surface antigen that, in the homozygous recessive state, is associated with complete protection against *P. vivax* infection.[25] The Duffy antigen is sterically associated with the protein required for attachment and penetration of *P. vivax* merozoites into red blood cells. The homozygous Duffy configuration is uniform in African blacks, and variable among blacks of African origin, and vivax infection does not occur in homozygous recessive individuals.

The sickle cell mutation in human hemoglobin is a balanced polymorphism that has been selected for in areas of intense *P. falciparum*, mainly in Africa. In the heterozygous state, the sickle trait affords protection against the development of higher density, life-threatening parasitemia, probably because the variant hemoglobin is a poor substrate for digestion by the parasite and because the infected cells are more easily subject to mechanical damage in the circulation.[38,39] Some studies have shown that the incidence rate of cerebral malaria is reduced by 90% in children with sickle cell trait as compared with their peers.[45] There is evidence that a number of other polymorphisms including hemoglobinopathies and erythrocyte membrane variants have evolved and afford a survival advantage to affected individuals. For example, recent studies in West Africa have demonstrated that hemoglobin (Hb) C affords protection against a range of malaria illness manifestations.[40] Other erythrocyte disorders associated with an advantage to the host include HbE, HbF, alpha- and beta-thalassemia, glucose-6-phosphate dehydrogenase (G6PD) deficiency, and red cell cytoskeleton abnormalities such as ovalocytosis. These and other red cell abnormalities effecting infection with *Plasmodium* spp parasites have been recently summarized.[38]

Reduction of Morbidity and Mortality of Malaria by Adaptive Human Immune Responses

Acquired or adaptive human immune responses occurring on the basis of an individual being exposed to infection with *Plasmodium* spp parasites can diminish the pathogenic effects of malaria parasites on the human host and also are implicated in the pathogenesis of disease. This section focuses on reduction in pathology. The role of host immune responses in pathogenesis is discussed in a subsequent section on pathogenesis.

In areas with the most intense *P. falciparum* transmission in sub-Saharan Africa, the role of host immune responses in ameliorating disease can be viewed as generally having three different stages during an individual's life.

Neonatal Period and Early Infancy. New infections, especially higher density parasitemias, and clinical manifestations of malaria are much less common in infants less than 6 months of age than in older infants and children.[35,41] Newborns have significant protection against high-density parasitemia for periods ranging to 6 months of age. This protective immunity is acquired passively across the placenta in utero, and presumably is primarily mediated by maternal antibodies.

coexisting renal impairment often compounds the acidosis, and in children ketoacidosis may also contribute. Acidotic breathing, sometimes called respiratory distress, is a poor prognostic sign. It is often followed by circulatory failure refractory to volume expansion or inotropic drugs, or by respiratory arrest. The plasma concentrations of bicarbonate or lactate are the best biochemical prognosticators in severe malaria. The prognosis of severe acidosis is poor.

Adults with severe falciparum malaria, and sometimes vivax malaria, may develop noncardiogenic pulmonary edema even after several days of antimalarial therapy. This manifestation may also rarely develop in otherwise uncomplicated vivax malaria, where recovery is usual. The pathogenesis of this variant of the adult respiratory distress syndrome is unclear. The mortality rate in falciparum malaria is high. This condition can be aggravated by overly vigorous administration of intravenous fluid.

Mild hemolytic jaundice is common in malaria. Severe jaundice is associated with *P. falciparum* infection, is more common among adults than among children, and results from hemolysis, hepatocyte injury, and cholestasis. When accompanied by other vital organ dysfunction (often renal impairment), liver dysfunction carries a poor prognosis. Hepatic dysfunction contributes to hypoglycemia, lactic acidosis, and impaired drug metabolism. Occasional patients with falciparum malaria may develop deep jaundice (with hemolytic and cholestatic components) without evidence of other viral organ dysfunction.

Renal impairment is common among adults with severe falciparum malaria but very rare among young children. The pathogenesis of renal failure is unclear but may be related to erythrocyte sequestration interfering with renal microcirculatory flow and metabolism. This results in "acute tubular necrosis" although renal cortical necrosis never develops. Acute renal failure may occur simultaneously with other vital organ dysfunction, in which case the mortality is high, or may progress as other disease manifestations resolve. In survivors, urine flow resumes in a median of 4 days, and serum creatinine levels return to normal in a mean of 17 days. Early dialysis or hemofiltration considerably enhances the likelihood of a patient's survival, particularly in acute hypercatabolic renal failure.

Anemia is a prominent feature of malaria. Anemia can develop rapidly, and transfusion is often required. In many areas of Africa, children may develop severe anemia resulting from both shortened red cell survival and masked dyserythropoiesis, as a consequence of repeated malarial infections. Anemia is a common consequence of antimalarial drug resistance, which results in repeated or continued infection.

Slight coagulation abnormalities are common in falciparum malaria, and mild thrombocytopenia is usual. Fewer than 5% of patients with severe malaria have significant bleeding with evidence of disseminated intravascular coagulation. Hematemesis, presumably from stress ulceration or acute gastric erosions, may also occur.

Aspiration pneumonia following convulsions is an important cause of death in cerebral malaria. Chest infections and catheter-induced urinary tract infections are common among patients who are unconscious for more than 3 days. Septicemia may complicate severe malaria; in endemic areas, *Salmonella* bacteremia has been associated specifically with *P. falciparum* infections.

Malaria in Pregnancy

In hyperendemic and holoendemic areas, falciparum malaria especially in primigravid and secundigravid women is associated with low birth weight (average reduction, ~170 g) and consequently increased neonatal mortality. In general, infected mothers in areas of stable transmission remain asymptomatic despite intense accumulation of parasitized erythrocytes in the placental microcirculation. Maternal HIV infection predisposes pregnant women to malaria and predisposes their newborns to congenital malaria infection and low birth weight.

In areas with unstable transmission of malaria, pregnant women are prone to severe infection and are particularly vulnerable to developing severe malaria with high-density parasitemias, anemia, hypoglycemia, and acute pulmonary edema. Fetal distress, premature labor, and stillbirth or low birth weight are common. Congenital malaria occurs in fewer than 5% of newborns whose mothers are infected and is related directly to the parasite density in maternal blood and in the placenta. *P. vivax* malaria in pregnancy is also associated with a reduction in birth weight (average, 100 g), but, in contrast with the situation in falciparum malaria, this effect is greater in multigravid than in primigravid women.

Malaria in Children

Most of the estimated 1 to 3 million persons who die of falciparum malaria each year are young African children. In endemic areas there is considerable diagnostic overlap between septicemia and severe malaria. Convulsions, coma, hypoglycemia, metabolic acidosis, and severe anemia are more common among children with severe malaria than in adults, whereas deep jaundice, acute renal failure, and acute pulmonary edema are unusual in childhood. Severely anemic children may have labored deep breathing, which in the past has been attributed incorrectly to "anemic congestive cardiac failure" but is caused by metabolic acidosis, often compounded by hypovolemia. In general, children tolerate antimalarial drugs well and respond rapidly to treatment.

Transfusion Malaria

Malaria can be transmitted by blood transfusion, needlestick injury, sharing of needles by infected drug addicts, or organ transplantation. The incubation period in these settings is often short because there is no pre-erythrocytic stage of development. The clinical features and management of these cases are the same as for naturally acquired infections. Radical chemotherapy with primaquine is unnecessary for blood-transmitted *P. vivax* and *P. ovale* infections.

Hyperreactive Malarial Splenomegaly

Chronic or repeated malarial infections produce hypergammaglobulinemia; normochromic, normocytic anemia; and, in certain situations, splenomegaly. Some residents of malaria-endemic areas of tropical Africa and Asia exhibit an abnormal immunologic response to repeated infection that is characterized by massive splenomegaly, hepatomegaly, marked elevations in serum titers of IgM and malarial antibody, hepatic sinusoidal lymphocytosis, and (in Africa) peripheral B-cell lymphocytosis. This syndrome has been associated with the production of cytotoxic IgM antibodies to suppressor (CD8+) lymphocytes, antibodies to CD4+ T cells, and an increase in the ratio of CD4+ T cells to CD8+ T cells.[56] These events may lead to uninhibited B-cell production of IgM and the formation of cryoglobulins (IgM aggregates and immunocomplexes). This immunologic process stimulates reticuloendothelial hyperplasia and clearance activity and eventually produces splenomegaly. Patients with hyperreactive malarial splenomegaly (HMS) feel an abdominal mass or a dragging sensation in the abdomen and occasional sharp abdominal pains suggesting perisplenitis. Anemia and some degree of pancytopenia are usually evident, but in many cases malarial parasites cannot be found in peripheral blood smears. Vulnerability to respiratory and skin infections is increased; many patients die of overwhelming sepsis. Persons with HMS who are living in endemic areas should receive antimalarial chemoprophylaxis; the results are usually good. In nonendemic areas, antimalarial treatment is advised. In some cases refractory to therapy, clonal lymphoproliferation may develop and then evolve to a malignant lymphoproliferative disorder.

Quartan Malarial Nephropathy

Chronic or repeated infections with *P. malariae*, and possibly other malarial species, may cause soluble immunocomplex injury to the renal glomeruli, resulting in the nephrotic syndrome. Other unidentified factors must contribute to this process, since only a small proportion of infected patients develop renal disease. The histologic appearance is that of focal or segmental glomerulonephritis with splitting of the capillary basement membrane. Subendothelial dense deposits are seen on electron microscopy, and immunofluorescence reveals deposits of complement and immunoglobulins; in samples of renal tissue from children, *P. malariae* antigens are often visible. A coarse-granular pattern of basement membrane immunofluorescent deposits (predominantly IgG3) with selective proteinuria carries a better prognosis than a fine-granular, predominantly IgG2 pattern with nonselective proteinuria. Quartan nephropathy usually responds poorly to treatment with either antimalarial agents or glucocorticoids and cytotoxic drugs.

Burkitt's Lymphoma and Epstein-Barr Virus Infection

It is possible that malaria-related immunosuppression promotes infection with lymphoma viruses. Burkitt's lymphoma is strongly associated with Epstein-Barr virus. The prevalence of this childhood tumor is high in malarious areas of Africa.

Laboratory Findings

Normochromic, normocytic anemia is usual. The leukocyte count is generally normal, although it may be raised in very severe infections. The erythrocyte sedimentation rate, plasma viscosity, and levels of C-reactive protein and other acute-phase proteins are high. The platelet count is usually reduced to approximately $10^5/\mu L$. Severe infections may be accompanied by prolonged prothrombin and partial thromboplastin times and by more severe thrombocytopenia. In uncomplicated malaria, plasma concentrations of electrolytes, blood urea nitrogen, and creatinine are usually normal. Findings in severe malaria may include metabolic acidosis, with low plasma concentrations of glucose, sodium, bicarbonate, calcium, phosphate, and albumin together with elevations in lactate, blood urea nitrogen, creatinine, urate, muscle and liver enzymes, and conjugated and unconjugated bilirubin. Hypergammaglobulinemia is usual in immune and semi-immune subjects, and urinalysis generally gives normal results. In adults and children with cerebral malaria, the mean opening pressure at lumbar puncture is approximately 160 mm of cerebrospinal fluid (CSF); the CSF is usually normal or has a slightly elevated total protein level [<1.0 g/L (100 mg/dL)] and cell count ($<20/\mu L$).

PATHOGENESIS

The pathophysiology of malaria results from destruction of erythrocytes (both infected and uninfected), the consequent liberation of parasite and erythrocyte material into the circulation, and the host reaction to these events. *P. falciparum* malaria–infected erythrocytes specifically sequester in the microcirculation of vital organs, interfering with microcirculatory flow and host tissue metabolism.

Toxicity and the Role of Cytokines

No potent malaria toxin has been identified, but malaria parasites do induce release of cytokines in much the same way as bacterial endotoxin does.[57] A glycolipid material with some similarities to bacterial endotoxin is released on schizont rupture. This is derived from the glycosylphosphatidylinositol anchor that covalently links proteins including the malaria parasite surface antigens to the cell membrane lipid bilayer. Malaria antigen–related IgE complexes also activate cytokine release. These malaria parasite products, like the endotoxin of bacteria, induce activation of the cytokine cascade, but they are *considerably* less potent than bacteria. For example, an *E.coli* bacteremia of 1 bacterium/mL carries an approximate mortality of 20%, whereas in falciparum malaria only parasitemias of well over 10^9/mL have such a lethal effect. Cells of the macrophage-monocyte series, γ/δ T cells, α/β T cells, CD14+ cells, and possibly endothelium, are stimulated to release cytokines in a mutually amplifying chain reaction. Initially, tumor necrosis factor alpha (TNF-α), which plays a pivotal role, interleukin (IL)-1, and γ-interferon are produced and in turn induce release of a cascade of other "pro-inflammatory" cytokines including IL-8, IL-12, IL-18. These are balanced by production of the "anti-inflammatory" cytokines IL-6 and IL-10. Cytokines are responsible for many symptoms and signs of the infection, particularly fever and malaise. Plasma inflammatory cytokine concentrations are elevated in both acute vivax and falciparum malaria.[58] In established vivax malaria, which tends to synchronize earlier than *P. falciparum*, a pulse release of TNF occurs at the time of schizont rupture and is followed by the characteristic symptoms and signs of the "paroxysm," i.e., shivering, cool extremities, headache, chills, a spike of fever, and sometimes rigors followed by sweating, vasodilatation, and defervescence. For a given number of parasites, *P. vivax* is a more potent inducer of

TNF release than *P. falciparum,* which may explain why it has a lower pyrogenic density.

There is a positive correlation between cytokine levels and prognosis in severe falciparum malaria and a disturbed balance between pro- and anti-inflammatory cytokines.[58] Acute malaria is associated with high levels of most cytokines, but the balance differs in relation to severity. IL-12 and TGF-β1, which may regulate the balance between pro- and anti-inflammatory cytokines, are higher in uncomplicated than in severe malaria. IL-10, a potent anti-inflammatory cytokine, increases markedly in severe malaria but, in fatal cases, does not increase sufficiently to restrain the production of TNF.[58] A reduced IL-10/TNF ratio has also been associated with childhood malarial anemia in areas of high transmission.

Does TNF play a causal role in cerebral dysfunction or death from severe malaria? Genetic studies from Africa indicate that children with the (308A) TNF2 allele, a polymorphism in the TNF promoter region, have a relative risk of 7 for death or neurologic sequelae from cerebral malaria.[59] A separate polymorphism in this region that affects gene expression was associated with a fourfold increased risk of cerebral malaria. On the other hand, the clinical studies in cerebral malaria with anti-TNF antibodies and other strategies to reduce TNF production reported to date have shown no convincing effects other than reduction in fever. Furthermore the 308 polymorphism is not associated with fatal cerebral malaria in Asian adults.[60] There is no direct evidence that systemic release of TNF or other cytokines causes coma in humans (although mechanisms involving release of nitric oxide within the central nervous system (CNS) and consequent inhibition of neurotransmission can be hypothesized). In adults with severe malaria, elevated plasma TNF concentrations have been associated specifically with renal dysfunction,[57,58] and TNF levels were actually lower in patients with pure cerebral malaria compared with those with other manifestations of severe disease. Severe malarial anemia has been associated with a different TNF promoter polymorphism (238A; odds ratio 2.5).

Cytokines are probably involved in placental dysfunction, suppression of erythropoiesis, and inhibition of gluconeogenesis, and do cause fever in malaria. Tolerance to malaria, or premunition, reflects both immune regulation of the infection and also reduced production of cytokines in response to malaria ("antitoxic immunity"). Cytokines may also be important mediators of parasite killing by activating leukocytes, and possibly other cells, to release toxic oxygen species and nitric oxide, and by generating parasiticidal lipid peroxides and causing fever. So, whereas high concentrations of cytokines may be harmful, lower levels probably promote parasite clearance and thereby benefit the host.

Sequestration and Cytoadherence

Erythrocytes containing mature forms of *P. falciparum* adhere to microvascular endothelium ("cytoadherence") and thus disappear from the circulation. This is called sequestration, and it starts at approximately 12 hours of asexual development. The process is accelerated by fever. Sequestration does not occur to a significant extent with the other three human malaria parasites. Sequestration is thought to be central to the pathophysiology of falciparum malaria, since it interferes with microcirculatory flow.[61] Once infected red cells adhere, they do not enter the circulation again, remaining stuck until they rupture at merogony (schizogony). As a consequence, whereas in the other malarias of humans, mature parasites are commonly seen on blood smears, these forms are rare in falciparum malaria and often indicate serious infection. It was thought that ring stage infected erythrocytes do not cytoadhere at all, but recent pathologic and laboratory studies show that that they do, although much less so than more mature stages. Sequestration occurs predominantly in the venules of vital organs. It is greatest in the brain, particularly in the white matter; prominent in the heart, eyes, liver, kidneys, intestines, and adipose tissue; and least frequent in the skin. Even within the brain, the distribution of sequestered erythrocytes varies markedly from vessel to vessel,[61] presumably reflecting differences in the local expression of endothelial receptors. Cytoadherence and the related phenomenon of rosetting lead to microcirculatory obstruction in falciparum malaria. The consequences of microcirculatory obstruction are activation of the vascular endothelium and reduced oxygen and substrate supply, which leads to anaerobic glycolysis, lactic acidosis, and cellular dysfunction.

Cytoadherence is mediated by several different processes. The most important parasite ligands are a family of strain-specific, high-molecular-weight, parasite-derived proteins termed *P. falciparum* erythrocyte membrane protein 1, or PfEMP1. These proteins (molecular mass 240 to 260 kd) are encoded by *var* genes, a family of over 50 genes distributed throughout the parasite's genome.[19–21] PfEMP1 is transcribed, synthesized, and stored within the parasite and, beginning at around 12 hours of development, is then exported to the surface of the infecting erythrocyte. These accretions cause humps or knobs on the surface of the red cell, and these are the points of attachment to vascular endothelium. PfEMP1 expression is greatest at the middle of the asexual cycle. PfEMP1 also appears to be a major antigenic determinant for the blood-stage parasite. As in other protozoal parasites, the immunodominant surface antigen undergoes antigenic variation to "change its coat" and avoid immune mediated attack. *P. falciparum* "switches" to a new variant of PfEMP1 at a rate of at least 2% per cycle.[62] In the chronic phase of untreated infection, this results in small waves of parasitemia approximately every 3 weeks. The central role of parasite-derived proteins in cytoadherence is not accepted by all. It has been suggested that cytoadherence is mediated by altered red cell membrane components such as a modified form of the red cell cytoskeleton protein band 3 (the major erythrocyte anion transporter, also called *Pf*alhesin). In culture, most parasites lose the ability to cytoadhere after several cycles of replication. In vivo, cytoadherence may be modulated by the spleen. In those patients who have had a splenectomy and who develop falciparum malaria, all stages of the parasite can be seen in peripheral blood smears.

Vascular Endothelial Ligands

Several different sticky proteins present on the surface of vascular endothelium have been shown to bind parasitized red cells. The interaction between these proteins and the variant surface adhesin of the parasitized red cell is complex. Probably the most important protein is the leukocyte differentiation antigen CD36[63]; nearly all freshly obtained parasites bind to CD36. Binding is increased at low pH (<7.0) and in the presence of high calcium concentrations. CD36 is constitutionally expressed on vascular endothelium and monocytes/ macrophages although usually it is not present on the surface of cerebral vessels. CD36 is expressed on platelets, and platelets may form a bridge between infected erythrocytes and vascular endothelium. The intercellular adhesion molecule (ICAM1), which is also the receptor for rhinovirus attachment, appears to be the major cytoadherence receptor in the brain.[64] Expression of ICAM1, but not CD36, is up-regulated by cytokines (notably TNF). At physiologic shear rates (i.e., those likely to be encountered in the human microcirculation) the binding forces ($\approx 10^{-10}$N) are similar for CD36 and ICAM1. Binding to the two ligands is synergistic.[65] Once stuck, the parasitized erythrocytes remain attached until schizont rupture, and then the residual ghost's membranes (sometimes with attached malaria pigment) often remain tethered within the vessel. Thrombospondin (a natural ligand to CD36) also binds to some parasitized red cells (probably to modified band 3), and recently the ubiquitous proteins VCAM, PECAM, E-selectin, and α/β integrin have also been shown to bind in some circumstances.[65] P-selectin has been shown to mediate rolling. The relative importance of these molecules and their interactions is still not clear. Chondroitin sulfate A (CSA) appears to be a major receptor for cytoadherence in the placenta.[66] Hyaluronic acid also has been proposed as a candidate for placental adhesion. Antibodies that inhibit parasitized red cell cytoadherence to CSA are generally present in multigravidae in endemic areas but not in primegravidae.[67] This may explain why the adverse effects of pregnancy on birth weight are greater in primegravidae. Other as yet unidentified vascular receptors are also present, since sequestration also occurrs in vessels expressing none of the potential ligands identified so far. Thus, ICAM1 appears to be the major vascular ligand in the brain involved in cerebral sequestration, CSA is the major ligand in the placenta, and CD36 is probably the major ligand in the other organs and also in platelet-mediated cytoadherence. Severity is related to the number of parasites in the body and distribution of cytoadherence within the vital organs. The relative importance of parasite phenotype and the various potential vascular ligands in the pathophysiology of severe falciparum malaria and the precise role of the spleen remain to be determined.

Rosetting and Aggregation

Erythrocytes containing mature parasites also adhere to uninfected erythrocytes.[68] This process leads to the formation of "rosettes" when suspensions of parasitized erythrocytes are viewed under the microscope. Rosetting shares some characteristics of cytoadherence. It starts at around 16 hours of the asexual life cycle development (slightly after cytoadherence begins) and is trypsin-sensitive. However, parasite species that do not sequester do form rosettes, and unlike cytoadherence, rosetting is inhibited by certain heparin subfractions and calcium chelators. Furthermore, whereas all fresh isolates of *P. falciparum* cytoadhere, not all rosette. Rosetting is mediated by attachment of specific domains of PfEMP1 to the complement receptor CR1, heparan sulfate, blood group A antigen, and probably other red cell surface molecules. Attachment is facilitated by serum components. Rosetting has been associated with severe malaria in some studies but not in others.[69] It has been suggested that rosetting might encourage cytoadherence by reducing flow (shear rate), which would enhance anaerobic glycolysis, reduce pH, and facilitate adherence of infected erythrocytes to venular endothelium. Rosetting tends to start in venules, and this certainly could reduce flow. The adhesive forces involved in rosetting could also impede forward flow of uninfected erythrocytes as they squeeze past sticky cytoadherent parasitized red cells in capillaries and venules. The mechanical obstruction, or "static hindrance," would be compounded by the lack of deformability of the adherent and circulating parasitized red cells. Recently, a new adherence property of parasitized red cells has been characterized and associated with disease severity in African children and Thai adults.[70] This is the platelet mediated aggregation of parasitized erythrocytes and is mediated via platelet CD36. These cells clump together in ex vivo cultures. Aggregation could also contribute to vascular occlusion.

Erythrocyte Deformability

As the parasite matures inside the erythrocyte, the normally flexible biconcave disc becomes progressively more spherical and rigid. The reduction in deformability results from reduced membrane fluidity, increasing sphericity, and the enlarging and relatively rigid intraerythrocytic parasite. Loss of uninfected red cell deformability has been recognized recently as a major contributor to disease severity and outcome. Increased erythrocyte rigidity measured at the low shear stresses encountered in capillaries and venules is correlated closely with outcome in severe malaria.[71] When assessed at the shear rates encountered on the arterial side, and importantly in the spleen, reduced red cell deformability correlates with anemia. This is a malaria-specific phenomenon, since it is not found in severe sepsis.

Immunologic Processes

It is unlikely that severe malaria, in particular cerebral malaria, results from specific immune-mediated damage. In relation to the degree of parasitized red cell sequestration, relatively few leukocytes are found in or around the cerebral vessels in fatal cases (although there are more in African children than in adults studied in Southeast Asia). Thus, there is little pathologic evidence in humans for widepread cerebral vasculitis. Indeed, fatal falciparum malaria is remarkable for the lack of extravascular pathology. Despite the enormous intravascular antigenic load in malaria, with the formation and deposition of immunocomplexes and variable complement depletion, there is little evidence of a specific immunopathologic process in severe malaria.

Acute malaria infections are associated with malaria antigen-specific unresponsiveness. This selective paresis is one of the factors contributing to the slow development of an effective and specific immune response in malaria. Acute malaria is characterized by nonspecific polyclonal B-cell activation. There is a reduction in circulating T cells with an increase in the γ/δ T-cell subset, but other T-cell proportions usually are normal. Although residents of hyperendemic or holoendemic malarious areas have hypergammaglobulinemia, most of this antibody is not directed against malaria antigens. In nonimmune individuals, the acute antibody response to infection often comprises mostly IgM or IgG_2 isotypes, which are unable to arm cytotoxic cells and thus kill asexual malaria parasites.

These observations have led to the suggestion that malaria induces an immunologic "smoke screen" with broad-spectrum and nonspecific activation that interferes with the orderly development of a specific cellular immune response. In severe malaria there is evidence of a broader immune suppression, with defects in monocyte and neutrophil chemotaxis, reduced monocytic phagocytic function, and a tendency to bacterial superinfection.

In the nephrotic syndrome associated with chronic *P. malariae* infections, malaria antigen and immunocomplexes can be eluted from the kidney, indicating a role for quartan malaria in this condition. Why some children are affected while the majority are not is unresolved.

Cerebral Malaria

In the past it was suggested that cerebral malaria resulted from an increase in cerebral capillary permeability, which led to brain swelling, coma, and death. There is evidence of a mild generalized increase in systemic vascular permeability in severe malaria. It is now clear from imaging studies that the majority of adults and children with cerebral malaria show no evidence of cerebral edema. However, the role of raised intracranial pressure in cerebral malaria remains unclear. Whereas 80% of adults have opening pressures at lumbar puncture that are in the normal range (<200 mm CSF), 80% of children have elevated opening pressures (>100 mm CSF; the normal range is lower in children), and intracranial pressure may rise transiently to very high levels. Some patients with cerebral malaria die of acute respiratory arrest with neurologic signs that are compatible with brainstem compression. However, these signs are also common and may persist for many hours in survivors.[72] The elevation in opening pressure usually is not great (in general it is much lower than in bacterial or fungal meningitis), and there is no difference between these lumbar puncture opening pressures in surviving children and fatal cases. Studies of computerized tomography (CT) or magnetic resonance imaging (MRI) generally show slight brain swelling in cerebral malaria (compatible with an increased intracerebral blood volume).[73] Immunohistochemical studies on autopsy brain tissues indicates focal disruption of endothelial junctions and endothelial activation in areas of intense sequestration, but clinical investigation have also failed to detect major alterations in blood-brain barrier permeability. Thus, raised intracranial pressure probably arises from an increase in cerebral blood volume, independent of permeability.[74] This results from the circulating blood required to maintain cerebral perfusion and a considerable sequestered static biomass of intracerebral parasites. Children may be particularly vulnerable, since after the skull sutures have fused, there is less space for cranial expansion than in adults. The possibility that a sudden rise in intracranial pressure accounts for some deaths cannot be excluded.[74]

The cause of coma in cerebral malaria is not known. Undoubtedly there is an increase in cerebral anaerobic glycolysis with cerebral blood flows that are inappropriately low for the arterial oxygen content, increased cerebral metabolic rates for lactate, and increased CSF concentrations of lactate, but these changes do not provide sufficient explanation for coma. Presumably the metabolic milieu created adjacent to the sequestered and highly metabolically active parasites and their attachment to the activated cerebral vascular endothelium interferes with endothelial and blood-brain barrier function. But how this interferes with neurotransmission is not known. Recent studies point to a disruption of axonal transport as the most likely explanation for rapidly reversible neurologic deficit. Cytokines increase production of nitric oxide, a potent inhibitor of neurotransmission, by leukocytes, smooth muscle cells, microglia, and vascular endothelium through induction of the enzyme nitric oxide synthase. Inducible nitric oxide synthase expression is increased in the brain in fatal cerebral malaria.

Renal Failure

There is renal cortical vasoconstriction and consequent hypoperfusion in severe falciparum malaria. In patients with acute renal failure (ARF), renal vascular resistance is increased. The renal injury in severe malaria results in acute tubular neurosis. The oxygen consumption of the kidneys is reduced in ARF, and it is not improved by dopamine-induced arteriolar vasodilatation and consequent increase in renal blood flow suggesting a fixed injury.[75] Acute tubular necrosis presumably results from renal microvascular obstruction and cellular injury consequent upon sequestration in the kidney and the filtration of free hemoglobin, myoglobin, and other cellular material. Significant glomerulonephritis is rare. Massive hemolysis compounds the insult in blackwater fever complicating malaria, and hemoglobinuria may itself lead to renal impairment. Mild renal impairment occurs in young children with severe malaria, but established ARF is almost confined to older children and adults.

Pulmonary Edema

Despite intense sequestration in the myocardial vessels, the heart's pump function is remarkably well preserved in severe malaria. Pulmonary edema in malaria results from a sudden increase in pulmonary capillary permeability that is not reflected in other vascular beds.[76] The pulmonary capillary wedge pressure is usually normal, and the threshold for the development of pulmonary edema is relatively low. Whereas ARF, severe metabolic acidosis, and coma are seen only in falciparum malaria, acute pulmonary edema may also occur in vivax malaria. The cause of this increase in pulmonary capillary permeability is not known.

Fluid Space and Electrolyte Changes

Following rehydration, the plasma volume is increased in moderate and severe malaria. Total body water and extracellular volume are usually normal or slightly reduced—even in children who are acidotic. Plasma renin activity, aldosterone, and antidiuretic hormone concentrations are elevated, reflecting an appropriate activation of homeostatic mechanisms to maintain adequate circulating volume in the presence of general vasodilatation and a falling hematocrit. Mild hyponatremia and hypochloremia are common in severe malaria, but serum potassium concentrations usually are normal. Occasionally hyponatremia is severe. Studies in Kenyan children indicate inappropriate antidiuretic hormone (arginine vasopressin) secretion in two thirds of cases.[77]

Anemia

The pathogenesis of anemia is multifactorial. There is obligatory destruction of red cells containing parasites at merogony, accelerated destruction of nonparasitized red cells that parallels disease severity, and bone marrow dyserythropoeisis. In severe malaria, anemia develops rapidly; the rapid hemolysis of unparasitized red cells is the major contributor to the decline in hematocrit.[78] Bone marrow dyserythropoeisis persists for days or weeks following acute malaria, and reticulocyte counts are usually low in the acute phase of the disease. The cause of the dyserythropoiesis is thought to be related to intramedullary cytokine production. Serum erythropoetin levels are usually elevated, although in some series it has been suggested that the degree of elevation was insufficient for the degree of anemia.

In falciparum malaria, the entire red cell population (i.e., both infected and uninfected red cells) becomes more rigid. This loss of deformability correlates with disease severity and outcome and, when measured at the high shear rates encountered in the spleen, with the degree of resulting anemia. The mechanism responsible has not been identified although there is evidence in acute malaria for increased oxidative damage, which might compromise red cell membrane function and deformability.

The role of antibody (i.e., Coombs'-positive hemolysis) in anemia is unresolved. The majority of studies do not show increased red cell immunoglobulin binding in malaria, but in the presence of a lowered recognition threshold for splenic clearance, this might be difficult to detect. The splenic threshold for the clearance of abnormal erythrocytes, whether because of antibody coating or reduced deformability, is lowered. Thus, the spleen removes large numbers of relatively rigid cells, resulting in shortened erythrocyte survival, particularly in severe malaria. This is unaffected by corticosteroids.

In the context of acute uncomplicated malaria, the anemia is worse in younger children and those with protracted infections. Loss of unparasitized erythrocytes accounts for approximately 90% of the acute anemia resulting from a single infection. Iron deficiency and malaria often coincide in the same patient, and in some areas routine iron supplementation following malaria promotes recovery from anemia.

Coagulopathy and Thrombocytopenia

There is accelerated coagulation cascade activity with accelerated fibrinogen turnover, consumption of antithrombin III, reduced factor XIII, and increased concentrations of fibrin degradation products in acute malaria. In severe infections, the prothrombin and partial thromboplastin times may be prolonged, and in occasional patients (<5%) bleeding may be significant. The coagulation cascade is activated via the intrinsic pathway. Intravascular thrombus formation is observed rarely at autopsy in fatal cases and fibrin deposition is sparse and platelets are strikingly unusual.

Thrombocytopenia is common to all four human malarias and is caused by increased splenic clearance. Platelet turnover is increased.[79] The role of platelet-bound antibody in malarial thrombocytopenia is controversial. There is evidence of platelet activation in some studies but not others. Erythrocytes containing mature parasites may activate the coagulation cascade directly, and cytokine release is also procoagulant. It was suggested in the past that disseminated intravascular coagulation (DIC) is important in the pathogenesis of severe malaria, but detailed prospective clinical and pathogenesis studies have refuted this. Coagulation cascade activity is directly proportional to disease severity, but hypofibrinogenemia resulting from DIC is significant in less than 5% of patients with severe malaria, and lethal hemorrhage (usually gastrointestinal) is quite unusual.

Blackwater Fever

This is a poorly understood condition in which there is massive intravascular hemolysis and the passage of Coca-Cola–colored urine. Blackwater (urine) occurs in three circumstances: (1) when patients with G6PD deficiency take oxidant drugs (e.g., primaquine or sulphonamides) irrespective of whether they have malaria, (2) occasionally when patients with G6PD deficiency have malaria and receive quinine treatment, and (3) in some patients with severe, quinine-treated falciparum malaria who have normal erythrocyte G6PD levels. How quinine causes blackwater in these last two situations is not known, since it is not an oxidant drug. G6PD-deficient red cells are particularly susceptible to oxidant stress because they are unable to synthesize adequate quantities of NADPH through the pentose shunt. This leads to low intraerythrocytic levels of reduced glutathione and both alterations in the erythrocyte membrane and increased susceptibility to organic peroxides. Blackwater fever may be associated with acute renal failure, although in most cases renal function remains normal.

The Spleen

There is considerable splenic enlargement in malaria and an increased capacity to clear red cells from the circulation both by Fc receptor–mediated (immune) mechanisms and by recognition of reduced deformability (filtration). The increased filtration of the spleen and the reduced deformability of the entire red cell population result in the rapid development of anemia in severe malaria. The spleen may also modulate cytoadherence. It plays a central role in limiting the acute expansion of the malaria infection by removing parasitized erythrocytes, and this has led to the suggestion that a failure to augment splenic clearance sufficiently rapidly may be a factor in the development of severe malaria. The spleen is capable of removing damaged intraerythrocytic parasites and returning the once infected red cells to the circulation (a process known as "pitting"),[80] where they have shortened survival. This is an important contributor to parasite clearance following antimalarial drug treatment (particularly treatment with artemisinin derivatives).

Gastrointestinal Dysfunction

Abdominal pain may be prominent in acute malaria. Minor stress ulceration of the stomach and duodenum is common in severe malaria. The pattern of malabsorption of sugars, fats, and amino acids suggests reduced splanchnic perfusion. This results from both gut sequestration and visceral vasoconstriction. Gut permeability is increased, and this may be associated with reduced local defenses against bacterial toxins or even whole bacteria in severe disease. Antimalarial drug absorption is remarkably unaffected in uncomplicated malaria, except for those drugs which have fat (i.e., food) dependent absorption (halofantrine, atovaquone, lumefantrine).

Liver Dysfunction

Jaundice is common in adults with severe malaria, and there is other evidence of hepatic dysfunction, with reduced clotting factor synthesis, reduced metabolic clearance of the antimalarial drugs, and a failure of gluconeogenesis, which contributes to lactic acidosis and hypoglycemia. Nevertheless, true liver failure (as in fulminant viral hepatitis) is unusual. There is sequestration in the hepatic microvasculature, and although many patients with acute falciparum malaria have elevated liver blood flow values, in very severe infections liver blood flow is reduced. Liver blood flow values less than 15 mL/kg/min are associated with elevated venous lactate concentrations, suggesting a flow limitation to lactate clearance and thus a contribution of liver dysfunction to lactic acidosis. Recent direct measurements of hepatic venous lactate concentrations in severe malaria confirm that the hepatosplanchnic extraction ratio is inversely correlated with mixed venous plasma lactate (i.e., hyperlactatemia is associated with reduced liver clearance of lactate). There is no relationship between liver blood flow and impairment of antimalarial drug clearance. Jaundice in malaria appears to have hemolytic and cholestatic components. Cholestatic jaundice may persist well into the recovery period.

Acidosis

Acidosis is a major cause of death in severe falciparum malaria. Recent studies indicate that the main acid (i.e., the main contributor to the anion gap) is unidentified. There is commonly a lactic acidosis, although ketoacidosis (and sometimes salicylate intoxication) may predominate in children, and the acidosis of renal failure is common in adults.[81,82] In severe malaria, the arterial, capillary, venous and CSF concentrations of lactate rise in direct proportion to disease severity. In bacterial sepsis there is hyperlactatemia, but unless there is profound shock, the lactate-pyruvate ratio is usually less than 15. This indicates that hypermetabolism is the source of lactate accumulation in sepsis. In severe malaria the pathogenesis is different; lactate-pyruvate ratios often exceed 30, reflecting tissue hypoxia and anaerobic glycolysis.

Lactic acidosis results from several discrete processes: the tissue anaerobic glycolysis consequent upon microvascular obstruction; a failure of hepatic and renal lactate clearance; and the production of lactate by the parasite. Lactate turnover in both adults and children with severe malaria is increased approximately threefold compared with values obtained in healthy adults.[83] Studies in children using stable isotope techniques indicate that increased lactate production (resulting from anaerobic glycolysis) rather than reduced clearance is the main cause of lactate accumulation although in adults reduced clearance is certainly a contributor. Hyperlactatemia is associated with hypoglycemia and is accompanied by hyperalaninemia and elevated glycerol concentrations, reflecting the impairment of gluconeogenesis through the Cori cycle. Lactate, glutamine, and alanine are the major gluconeogenic precursors. Triglyceride and free fatty acid levels are also elevated in acute malaria, and plasma concentrations of ketone bodies are raised in patients who have been unable to eat. Ketoacidosis may be prominent in children.

In severe malaria there is dysfunction of all organ systems, particularly those with obligatory high metabolic rates. The endocrine glands are no exception. Pituitary-thyroid axis abnormalities result in the "sick euthyroid" syndrome and also parathyroid dysfunction. Mild hypocalcemia is common, and hypophosphatemia may be profound in the very seriously ill. By contrast, the pituitary-adrenal axis appears normal in acute malaria.

Hypoglycemia

Hypoglycemia is associated with hyperlactatemia and shares the same pathophysiological etiology: an increased peripheral requirement for glucose consequent upon anaerobic glycolysis (the Pasteur effect), the increased metabolic demands of the febrile illness[83] and the obligatory demands of the parasites that use glucose as their major fuel (all of which increase demand), and a failure of hepatic gluconeogenesis and glycogenolysis (reduced supply).[84] Hepatic glycogen is exhausted rapidly: stores in fasting adults last approximately 2 days, but children have enough for only 12 hours. Healthy children have approximately three times higher rates of glucose turnover compared with adults, but in severe malaria turnover is increased by more than 50% (to values five times higher than those in adults with severe malaria). The net result of impaired gluconeogenesis, limited glycogen stores, and greatly increased demand results in a hypoglycemia in 20% to 30% of children with severe malaria.[85,86] In patients treated with quinine, this is compounded by quinine-stimulated pancreatic β-cell insulin secretion.[84] Hyperinsulinemia is balanced by reduced tissue sensitivity to insulin, which returns to normal as the patient improves. This probably explains why quinine-induced (hyperinsulinaemic) hypoglycemia tends to occur after the first 24 hours of treatment, whereas malaria-related hypoglycemia (with appropriate suppression of insulin secretion) is often present when the patient with severe malaria is first admitted. Hypoglycemia contributes to nervous system dysfunction, and in cerebral malaria is associated with residual neurologic deficit in survivors.

Placental Dysfunction

Pregnancy increases susceptibility to malaria. This is probably caused by a suppression of systemic and placental cell-mediated immune responses. There is intense sequestration of *P. falciparum*–infected erythrocytes in the placenta, local activation of pro-inflammatory cytokine production, and maternal anemia. This leads to placental insufficiency and fetal growth retardation. Illness close to term results in prematurity. In areas of intense transmission, a malaria attributable reduction in birth weight (≈170 g) is confined to primigravidae.[87] There is no convincing evidence that malaria causes abortion or stillbirth in this context. With lower levels of transmission (i.e., less immunity) the risk extends to other pregnancies, and there is a propensity to develop severe malaria with a high incidence of fetal death. The recent discovery that *P. vivax*, a parasite not thought to cytoadhere, also reduces birth weight (by about two thirds the amount caused by *P. falciparum*), puts into question the primary role of sequestration in the pathogenesis of placental insufficiency.[88]

Bacterial Infection

Patients with severe malaria are vulnerable to bacterial infections, particularly of the lungs and urinary tract (following catheterization). Postpartum sepsis is common. Spontaneous bacterial septicemia may also occur. It is relatively unusual in adults (probably less than 1% of cases) but is much more common in young children. In malaria-endemic areas, where parasitemia is common in children, it may be difficult to distinguish bacterial infections with *coincident* parasitemia from infections complicating malaria. *Salmonella* septicemias are an important complication of otherwise uncomplicated falciparum malaria in African children.

DIAGNOSIS

Prompt and accurate diagnosis of malaria is the key to effective disease management. Since malaria cannot be diagnosed clinically, blood must be examined either by microscopy, after staining thick and thin films (Giemsa at pH 7.2 is preferred; Wright's, Field's, or Leishman's can also be used), or by rapid antigen detection tests (RDTs). Staining of parasites with the fluorescent dye acridine orange is an alternative that allows more rapid diagnosis of malaria (but not speciation of the infection) in patients with low parasitemias.[89] Polymerase chain reaction (PCR) is more sensitive than other methods of diagnosis but is still a research tool.[90]

In many endemic areas, a high percentage of individuals (often 95% of children and 50% of adults) always have low densities of *P. falciparum* in their blood during transmission seasons. Thus, the presence of parasites does not ensure that clinical symptoms and signs such as elevated temperature are due to malaria. Furthermore, in high transmission areas, parasitemias of up to 10,000 parasites per microliter may be tolerated without symptoms or signs in partially immune individuals. In these cases, an absolute density of parasites in the blood (often 5000 to 20,000 parasites/μL blood) is used to make the clinical diagnosis of malaria, and patients with lower levels of parasitemia must be investigated for other causes of their symptoms and signs. Nonetheless, few clinicians would withhold antimalaria treatment from a patient with clinical symptoms and signs and any level of parasitemia.

Blood Films

The gold standard for diagnosis of malaria is the blood film. Thick films are optimal for diagnosis, particularly at low parasitemias, because 20 to 40 times more blood is examined. Determination of the species of parasite can often be done by an expert on a thick film but is best done on a thin film (Plate 90-1). In a patient suspected of having malaria with a negative blood film, the blood film should be examined every 12 hours for 36 to 48 hours before considering it to be negative. See Table 90-1 and Figure 90-4 for instructions on preparing blood films, comparative morphology of *P. falciparum*, *P. vivax*, *P. ovale*, and *P. malariae* in blood films, and examples of blood films in *P. falciparum* and *P. vivax*.

Estimation of Parasite Density

Since one criterion for diagnosing severe malaria is the density of parasitemia (see Box 90-2), it is important, particularly in *P. falciparum* infections, to determine the density of parasitemia. The density of parasitemia is expressed as percentage of erythrocytes parasitized, or as the numbers of parasitized erythrocytes per microliter of blood. The percent parasitemia is estimated by determining the number of parasitized erythrocytes per 1000 red cells in a thin blood film. At low densities of parasitemia percent parasitemia is extremely difficult to determine, and the number of parasites/μL blood is estimated. The number of parasites/μL blood is derived from the number of parasitized erythrocytes per 200 white blood cells (WBCs), generally in a thick blood film. If the WBC count is known, then one can calculate the parasite density per microliter. For example, if there are 100 parasites per 200 WBCs and the WBC count is 6000/μL, the parasite density is (100 parasites/200 WBCs) × 6000 WBCs/μL = 3000 parasites/μL blood. If the WBC count is not known, it is generally assumed to be 8000 WBCs/μL. The number of parasites/μL blood can also be estimated by knowing the percent parasitemia and the number of erythrocytes/μL blood. If there are 5×10^6 erythroctyes/μL blood, then a 1% parasitemia corresponds to 50,000 parasitized erythrocytes/μL blood. An expert microscopist who examines 200 fields of a thick blood film at 1000× magnification can detect approximately 5 parasitized erythroctyes/μL blood, which for an individual with 5×10^6 erythroctyes/μL blood is a percent parasitemia of 0.0001%.

In the benign malarias (where sequestration is considered not to occur), the number of parasites in the body may be estimated simply by multiplying the parasite density by the estimated blood volume. In *P. falciparum* the microscopist can see only part of the first half of the asexual life cycle. In the second half of the asexual cycle the parasitized cells are sequestered. As a consequence there may be large discrepancies between the number of parasites in the peripheral (circulating) blood and the number of parasites in the body (the parasite burden). This is the reason that in a febrile patient suspected of having malaria, negative blood smears are repeated every 12 hours for 36 to 48 hours. If all of the parasites are synchronous (at the same stage of development) and sequestered, a patient with a negative blood smear read by an inexperienced microscopist, or a low parasitemia read by an experienced microscopist, could have a high parasitemia 12 to 24 hours later.

Rapid Diagnostic Tests

Rapid, simple, sensitive, and specific antibody–based diagnostic stick or card tests (RDTs) detect *P. falciparum*–specific, histidine-rich protein (HRP) 2[91,92] or lactate dehydrogenase[93] antigens. Some of these tests incorporate a second antibody, which allows falciparum malaria to be distinguished from the less dangerous malarias. *P. falciparum* HRP2-based tests may remain positive for several weeks after acute infection. This is a disadvantage in high transmission areas where infections are highly prevalent but is of value in the diagnosis of severe malaria in patients who have taken antimalarial drugs and cleared peripheral parasitemia. Although an expert microscopist can detect as few as 5 parasites/μL blood, in general

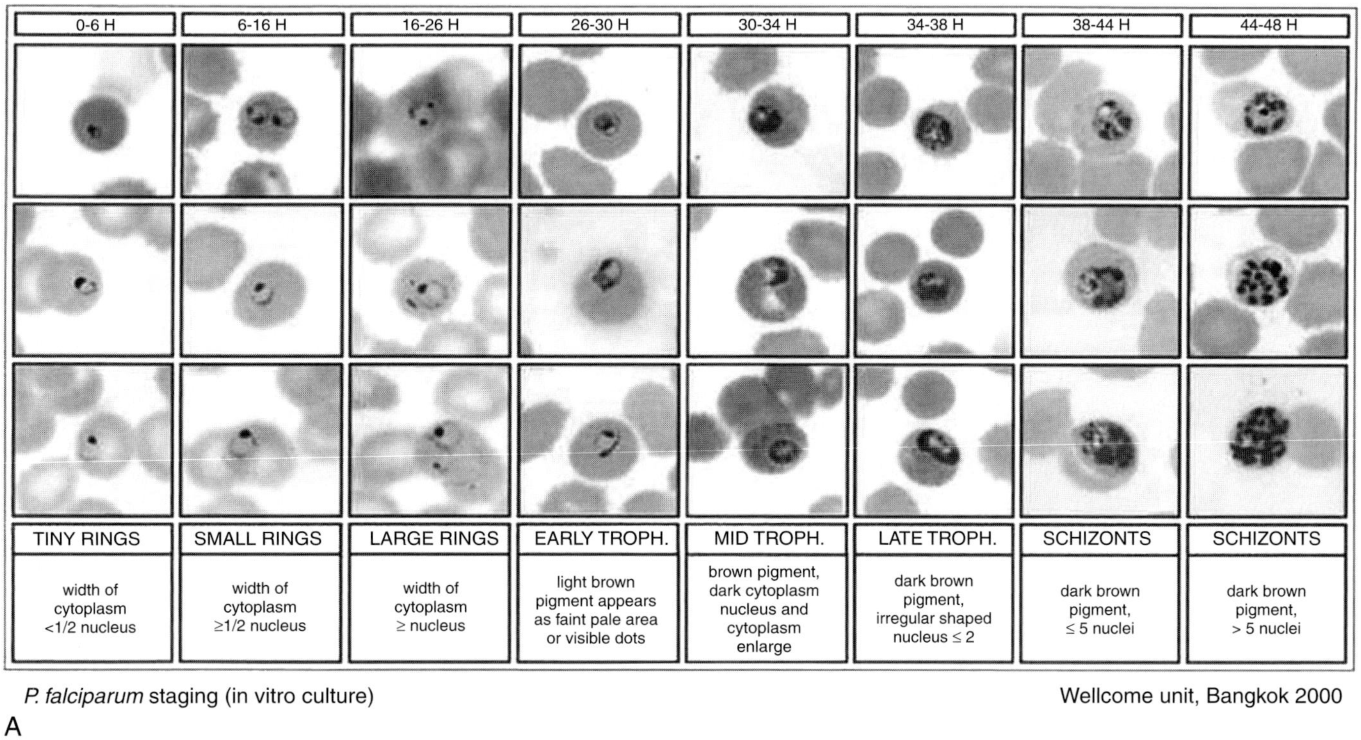

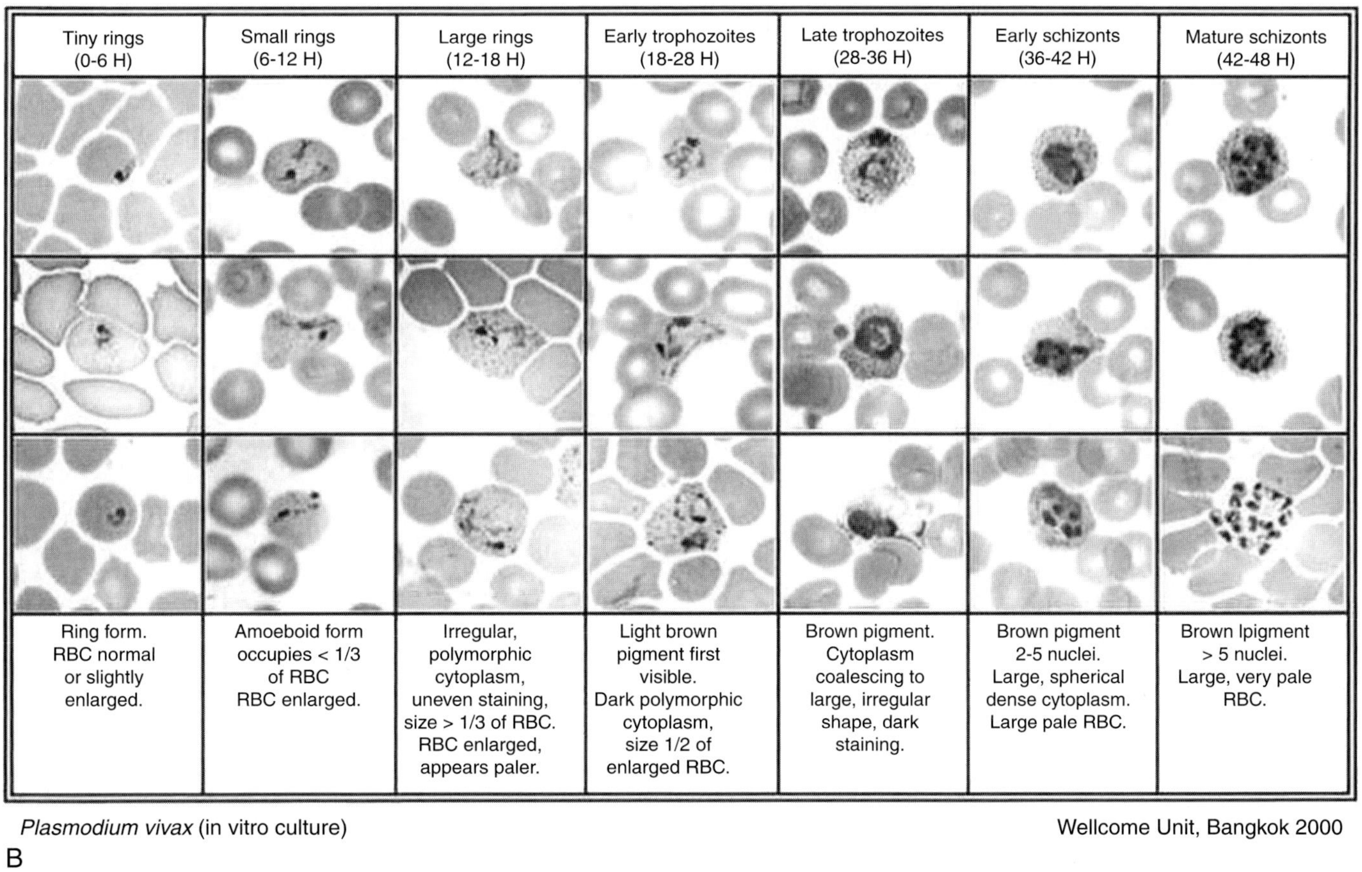

FIGURE 90-4 Characteristic features in Giemsa-stained blood smears. *A, P. falciparum. B, P. vivax.* (*A,* From Silamut K, Phu NH, Whitty C, et al: A quantitative analysis of the microvascular sequestration of malaria parasites in the human brain. Am J Pathol 155:395–410, 1999. *B,* From Chotivanich K, Silamut K, Udomsangpetch R, et al: Ex-vivo short-term culture and developmental assessment of *Plasmodium vivax*. Trans R Soc Trop Med Hyg 95:677–680, 2001.)

microscopy and RDTs have similar levels of detection at approximately 50 parasites per microliter. This also corresponds to the level at which fever develops, although many patients feel unwell for 1 or 2 days before this. A parasitemia of 50/μL corresponds to a total body parasite burden in an adult of >100 million parasites and a percent parasitemia of 0.001%.

Blood Film Findings Useful in Identifying Patients with Poor Prognoses

Parasite Density

The relationship between parasitemia and prognosis is complex. Patients with >3% parasitemia (approximately 1×10^5 parasites per microliter in a patient with anemia) are at increased risk of dying,[55,94] but individuals with a history of repeated infections (semi-immunes) may tolerate parasitemia levels many times higher with only minor symptoms, and some patients, especially nonimmunes, may die with much lower counts. The clue to the discrepancy lies both in the immune status of the host and in the stage of development of parasites on the peripheral blood smear.

Mature Parasites

A predominance of more mature parasites indicates that a greater proportion are sequestered and carries a worse prognosis for any parasitemia than does a predominance of younger forms.[95] In severe malaria, a poor prognosis is indicated by a predominance of more mature *P. falciparum* parasites (i.e., >20% of parasites with visible pigment) in the peripheral blood film (see Box 90-2).

Malaria Pigment in Polymorphonuclear Leukocytes

Another simple estimation is the number of polymorphonuclear leukocytes that contain malaria pigment.[96] This reflects the amount of recent schizont rupture. Patients with >5% neutrophils containing malaria pigment have an increased risk of dying (see Box 90-2).[96] Phagocytosed malarial pigment seen inside peripheral blood monocytes also provides a clue to recent infection if malarial parasites are not detectable. After the clearance of the parasites, malarial pigment often is evident for several days in peripheral blood phagocytes, bone marrow aspirates, or smears of fluid expressed after intradermal puncture.

Presence of Gametocyes (Sexual Erythrocytic Stage Parasites) in Blood Films

In *P. falciparum* infection, gametocytemia peaks 1 week after the peak in asexual parasites. Gametocytes are not involved in the pathogenesis of malaria. The mature gametocytes are not affected by most antimalarial drugs, so their persistence does not constitute evidence of drug resistance.

Antiparasite Antibodies

In endemic areas presence of antiparasite blood-stage antibodies is used as an epidemiologic tool but in general cannot be used to determine whether an individual is infected, because virtually all individuals have such antibodies. In the past, the presence of anti-asexual erythrocytic stage parasite antibodies was used to determine whether an individual with persistent clinical manifestations consistent with malaria, but negative blood films, might in fact have malaria. In general, the same laboratories that can assess anti-blood-stage antibodies can perform PCR, and PCR has replaced antibodies in the diagnosis of cryptic infections because it detects parasite material, not the host's immune response to the parasites.

TREATMENT

Antimalarial Drugs

The objective of treating severe malaria is to save life, and of treating uncomplicated malaria is to prevent the development of severe complications and cure the infection. In general the antimalarial drugs are more toxic than antibacterials, i.e., the therapeutic ratio is narrower, but serious adverse effects are rare. The available antimalarials fall into four broad groups:

1. *Quinoline-related or quinoline-like compounds.* The quinoline-related or quinoline-like compounds (quinine, quinidine, chloroquine, amodiaquine, mefloquine, halofantrine, lumefantrine, piperaquine, pyronaridine) chemically interfere with intraparasitic heme detoxification, preventing the dimerization process that results in the formation of hemozoin (malaria pigment). Primaquine and tafenoquine are structurally related 8-aminoquinolines that kill liver and sexual stages of *P. falciparum* and all stages of *P. vivax, P. malariae,* and *P. ovale*. These are also the only drugs that kill the persistent liver stages of *P. vivax* and *P. ovale*, but their mechanism of action is unknown.
2. *Antifols.* The antifols (pyrimethamine, cycloguanil, chlorcycloguanil, trimethoprim) competitively inhibit plasmodial dihydrofolate reductase. They are synergistic with sulfonamides and sulfones. Cycloguanil and chlorcycloguanil are the active metabolites of proguanil and chlorproguanil, respectively.
3. *Artemisinin compounds.* The artemisinin compounds (artemisinin, dihydroartemisinin, artemether, artesunate) are endoperoxides naturally extracted from the naturally occuring Artemisinin plant. They have the broadest time window of action on the asexual malarial parasites, from medium-sized rings to early schizonts, and produce the most rapid therapeutic responses. They inhibit plasmodial ATPase 6 (a calcium ATPase).
4. *Atovaquone.* Atovaquone is a potent inhibitor of cytochrome-mediated electron transport. It is synergistic with proguanil (in this case, the parent compound, not the antifol metabolite cycloguanil).

Several antibacterial drugs also have antiplasmodial activity although in general their action is slow and they are used only in combination with the antimalarial drugs. Those used are the sulfonamides and sulphones, tetracyclines, lincosamides, macrolides, and chloramphenicol. Significant resistance has been reported to the sulfonamides but not to the other classes of antibiotics. Drugs that are active against sensitive *P. falciparum* are also active against the other three malaria species. The most effective antimalarial drugs are combinations of an artemisinin derivative with a slowly eliminated antimalarial drug (artemisinin combination treatments).[97,98]

Pharmacokinetics

The antimalarial drugs vary considerably in their pharmacokinetic and pharmacodynamic properties (Table 90-3). Oral absorption ranges from good (quinine, chloroquine, amodiaquine, sulfadoxine-pyrimethamine, artemisinin derivatives, primaquine) to variable (mefloquine, lumefantrine, halofantrine, atovaquone). These are lipophilic hydrophobic compounds; oral absorption is increased by coadministration with fatty food or drinks. Acute malaria may cause reduced oral antimalarial absorption. Elimination rates also vary considerably from the artemisinin derivatives, which have terminal elimination half-lives ($t_{1/2}$) of less than an hour; quinine, proguanil, and chlorproguanil ($t_{1/2}$ <1 day); pyrimethamine, lumefantrine, and atovaquone ($t_{1/2}$ <1 week), through to mefloquine, chloroquine, and piperaquine, which have $t_{1/2}$ values of weeks. Although acute malaria may impair metabolic clearance, with the exception of quinine and quinidine in severe malaria, this does not significantly affect dosing or treatment responses.

Some antimalarial drugs have active metabolites that contribute most of the antimalarial activity. In vivo artesunate is almost completely hydrolyzed to dihydroartemisinin (DHA), which is the most potent artemisinin derivative. After oral administration, artemether and artemotil are also largely converted to DHA. Amodiaquine is almost completely converted to desethylamodiaquine, and most of the antimalarial activity of proguanil and chlorproguanil derives from their antifol triazine metabolites cycloguanil and chlorcycloguanil, respectively.

Drugs that are eliminated rapidly (artemisinins, quinine) must be given for at least 7 days to ensure high cure rates, unless they are accompanied by a more slowly eliminated partner. This why in most artemisinin combinations (ACTs), the artemisinin derivatives are partnered with slowly eliminated compounds, and the treatment course can be shortened to a total of 3 days (Fig. 90-5).[98] Shorter ACT treatment courses (i.e., 1 or 2 days) are less effective, may be more prone to resistance, and are not recommended.

Drug interactions among the antimalarials are generally inconsequential. The exception is the potentially dangerous exacerbation of halofantrine's effect in prolonging ventricular repolarization (QT prolongation) when given following mefloquine treatment. This may increase the risk of sudden death from ventricular tachyarrhthymias.[99] There is insufficient information on interactions of antimalarials with other drugs (e.g., antiretrovirals).

The global death toll from malaria is rising, and in some areas the increased death toll has been attributed to drug resistance.[100] *P. falciparum* has developed increased resistance to all classes of antimalarial drugs with the exception of the more recently introduced artemisinin derivatives. The other human malarias are generally more drug sensitive, although they have developed antifol resistance rapidly in some areas. Chloroquine resistance has now developed in *P. vivax* and in Oceania, and in parts of Indonesia is a substantial problem.[101,102] Elsewhere *P. vivax* remains generally chloroquine sensitive.[103] There has been one report of chloroquine-resistant *P. malariae*.[104]

Classification of Patients for Treatment

It is critical that the care provider determine whether a patient with malaria has uncomplicated or complicated malaria based on clinical, laboratory, or parasitologic findings (see Box 90-2).

Treatment of Uncomplicated *P. falciparum* Malaria

The goal of treatment of uncomplicated malaria is to cure the infection rapidly and reliably. This means achieving a

Table 90-3 Summary of Pharmacokinetic Properties of Antimalarial Drugs

Drug	Absorption: Time to Peak PO	IM	Oral Dose (mg/kg)	Plasma Peak Level (mg/L)	Binding (%)	V_d/f* (L/kg)	Clearance/f (mL kg^{-1} min^{-1})	$T_{1/2}\beta$† (hr)
Quinine	6	1	10	8 oral 15 IV/IM	90	0.8	1.5	16
Quinidine	1	...	10	5	85	1.3	1.7	10
Chloroquine	5	0.5	10	0.12	55	10–1000	2.0	30–60 days
Artesunate	1.5	0.5	4	0.5	...	0.15	50	0.75‡
Artemether	2	3–18	4	1.5	95	2.7	54	1
Mefloquine	17	...	25	...	>98	20	0.35	14 days
Halofantrine	15	...	8	0.9‡	>98§	...	7.5	113
Lumefantrine	6	...	9	3.5‡	>98§	2.7	3.0	86
Pyrimethamine	6	41	1.25	0.5	94	...	0.33	87
Atovaquone	6	...	15	5‡	99.5	6	2.5	30
Healthy subjects¶								
Primaquine	3	...	0.6	0.15	...	3	6	6
Proguanil (chlorguanide)	3	...	3.5	0.17	75	24	19	16
Pyrimethamine	4	...	0.3	0.35	...	2.9	0.4	85

*V_d/f is the total apparent volume of distribution divided by "f", the fraction of drug absorbed.
†$T_{1/2}$ of the active metabolite dihydroartemisinin.
‡Absorption increased significantly by fats.
§Binds to lipoproteins.
¶Pregnancy is usually associated with lower drug concentrations and higher treatment failure rates.

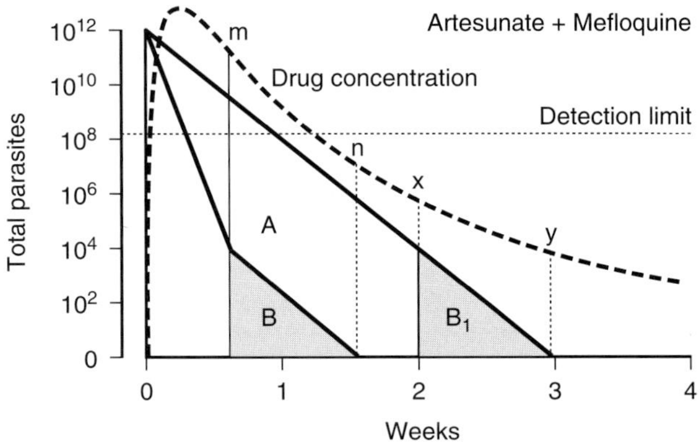

FIGURE 90-5 Pharmacodynamic rationale underlying artemisinin combination treatment (artesunate + mefloquine). Vertical axis (logarithmic scale) shows total number of parasites in the body of an adult with approximately 2% parasitemia. Artesunate given for 3 days covers two asexual cycles and reduces the parasite numbers by a factor of 10^8. Residual parasites (10^4) are killed by high concentrations of mefloquine (m to n) (B). If mefloquine alone is used, parasite numbers reduce more slowly and are not eliminated completely for approximately 3 weeks. Thus, in combination treatment, no parasite is exposed to artesunate alone, and only 0.0000001% of the original infecting biomass is exposed to mefloquine alone. (Redrawn from White NJ: Assessment of the pharmacodynamic properties of the antimalarial drugs in vivo. Antimicrob Agents Chemother 41:1413–1422, 1997.)

prompt clinical response and then preventing recrudescence. Effective treatment dramatically lowers the risk of progression to severe disease and the additional morbidity associated with treatment failure. Reduction of transmission and prevention of resistance are both important additional considerations for patients treated where malaria is transmitted. In falciparum malaria there is a continuum from mild to severe malaria. Young children with malaria may deteriorate rapidly. Many patients are intolerant of oral medication and require parenteral or rectal administration for 1 or 2 days until they can swallow and retain oral treatment reliably, even though they never show signs of severity. They should receive the same dose regimens as in severe malaria.

Patients without physical signs of severity but who on examination of the blood film are found to have a high parasitemia can be treated with oral antimalarials if their condition can be monitored closely. These patients are at increased risk of developing severe malaria and thus have an increased mortality rate. These patients should be treated with rapidly acting antimalarials such as the artemisinin derivatives or quinine and should be immediately switched to parenteral therapy if signs of severity develop.

After it has been established whether the patient has uncomplicated or complicated malaria, treatment is dependent on the care provider's estimation of how good follow-up will be, whether the patient is returning to a malaria-endemic area, and the availability of specific antimalarials. Several drugs that are recommended in tropical countries (e.g., artemisinin compounds, piperaquine) are not available in some temperate countries (e.g., the United States). Drug regimens, including single drugs, with expected cure rates of 100% are used for treating patients in whom there will be good follow-up, such as returning travelers, in nonendemic areas. In malaria-endemic areas, it is now recommended that antimalarials should be used in combinations, to augment cure rates (which should be at least 90%) and to prevent the emergence of resistance.

Combining two or more antimalarial drugs with different modes of action (and thus drug targets) provides two main advantages: (1) cure rates are usually increased, and (2) in the rare event that a mutant parasite that is resistant to one of the drugs arises de novo during the course of the infection, it will be killed by the other drug. Mutual protection prevents the emergence of resistance.[98] This is the same principle underlying the combination treatment of tuberculosis and HIV infections. Prevention of resistance is necessary to ensure that antimalarial treatment remains highly effective. Both partner drugs in a combination must be independently effective. ACTs are the most rapidly and reliably effective antimalarial drugs, and they have the advantage of inhibiting gametocyte development and thus reducing transmissibility. Artemisinin and its derivatives (artesunate, artemether, artemotil, dihydroartemisinin) produce rapid clearance of parasitemia and rapid resolution of symptoms. They reduce parasite numbers by a factor of approximately 10,000 each asexual cycle,[98] which is more than other antimalarial drugs (which reduce parasite numbers by between 100 and 1000 fold per cycle). Artemisinin is five to ten times less potent than its derivatives and has generally given way to the derivatives. When given alone or in combination with rapidly eliminated compounds (tetracyclines, clindamycin), a 7-day course of treatment with an artemisinin compound is required, but when given in combination with slowly eliminated antimalarial drugs, shorter courses of treatment (3 days) are highly effective.

The artemisinin compounds are active against all four species of malaria parasites infecting humans. There is no confirmed resistance to these drugs, but unless they are given for 1 week they cannot be expected to eliminate asexual erythrocytic stage parasites entirely. The artemisinin derivatives are also remarkably well tolerated. The only significant adverse effect to emerge from extensive clinical trials has been rare (≈1:3000) type 1 hypersensitivity reactions (manifested initially by urticaria). They also have the advantage from a public health perspective of reducing gametocyte carriage and thus the transmissibility of malaria. This contributes to malaria control.

Specific Drugs and Drug Regimens

See Table 90-4 for details.

Atovaquone-Proguanil

This combination of a naphthaquinone and biguanide is effective against all malarias, including multidrug-resistant falciparum malaria. Atovaquone-proguanil is given in a 3-day, once daily regimen. Atovaquone-proguanil is well tolerated with no serious adverse effects. The main problem is the high cost of manufacturing atovaquone. While it continues to be useful for the treatment of travelers and in prophylaxis, it is simply too expensive for large-scale deployment in endemic areas.

Mefloquine

Mefloquine alone is highly effective against *P. falciparum* from most parts of the world except specific areas of

Southeast Asia (see Table 90-4). Depending on the local sensitivity of the parasite to the drug, a dose of 15 mg base/kg to 25 mg base/kg is administered singly or in two divided doses 8 to 24 hours apart. Children metabolize mefloquine more rapidly than adults and should receive the higher dose. The principal problems with mefloquine are nausea and vomiting in young children, and CNS adverse effects (dizziness, dysphoria, nightmares, and less commonly seizures, encephalopathy, or psychosis). Gastrointestinal intolerance can be reduced by splitting the dose, as mentioned previously.

Sulfadoxine-Pyrimethamine

Although resistance to sulfadoxine-pyrimethamine (SP) has spread rapidly in recent years (see Table 90-4), compromising the efficacy of the combination, there are still some areas, notably in West Africa and Pakistan, Afghanistan, and Northwest India, where this combination is very effective. A major advantage of SP is that it is delivered as a single dose and is generally well tolerated.

Chloroquine

Chloroquine is still the treatment of choice for *P. vivax, P. ovale, P. malariae*, and the occasional monkey malaria that gets transmitted to humans, but for *P. falciparum* there are now very few places where chloroquine can be relied upon. If one is confident of the response in a locale with presumed chloroquine-sensitive *P. falciparum* (see Table 90-4), then chloroquine can be used. If uncertain, one should choose another antimalarial.

***Table 90-4** Dosage Regimens of Antimalarials for Treatment of Uncomplicated Malaria**

Type	Malaria Endemic Area	Outside Malaria Endemic Area
P. vivax, P. malariae, P. ovale, known chloroquine–sensitive *P. falciparum**	Chloroquine phosphate (1 tablet contains 250 mg salt, equivalent to 155.3 mg base). 10 mg/kg base at 0, 24 hr followed by 5 mg/kg base at 48 hr May be combined with artesunate 4 mg/kg/day for 3 days	Chloroquine phosphate (1 tablet contains 250 mg salt, equivalent to 155.3 mg base). 10 mg/kg base at 0, 24 hr followed by 5 mg/kg base at 48 hr
*P. falciparum** known to be sensitive to sulfadoxine–pyrimethamine (SP)	Oral artesunate 4 mg/kg daily for 3 days + pyrimethamine 1.25 mg/kg + sulfadoxine 25 mg/kg (single dose), 3 tablets in an adult	Pyrimethamine 1.25 mg/kg + sulfadoxine 25 mg/kg (single dose) 3 tablets in an adult
*P. falciparum** known to be sensitive to amodiaquine	Oral artesunate 4 mg/kg daily for 3 days + Amodiaquine 10 mg base/kg/day for 3 days	Amodiaquine 10 mg base/kg/day for 3 days
P. falciparum known to be sensitive to mefloquine (see Table 90-2 and preceding map for known mefloquine-resistant areas)	Combination only (see below)	Mefloquine 15–25 mg base/kg (single dose or divided into 2 doses given 8–24 hours apart)
	Treatments Effective Everywhere in the World	Treatments Effective in Infections Acquired Anywhere in the World
Chloroquine-resistant *P. vivax*† and multidrug resistant-*P. falciparum**	a. Oral artesunate 4 mg/kg daily for 3 days + mefloquine 25 mg base/kg (15 mg/kg on day 2, 10 mg/kg on day 3) b. Artemether-lumefantrine 1.5/9 mg/kg twice daily for 3 days with food	a. Atovaquone 20 mg/kg/day, proguanil 8 mg/kg/day for 3 days; this should be combined with artesunate in endemic areas b. Quinine 10 mg salt/kg 3 times daily plus doxycycline 3 mg/kg once daily or clindamycin 10 mg/kg twice daily for 7 days

*In endemic areas, only combination treatments should be used for falciparum malaria, whereas outside the endemic area highly effective monotherapies may be used.
†This refers to truly resistant infections, which are a significant problem only in Oceania and Indonesia, and should not be confused with relapses.

General Points

A. Pregnancy: Artemisinin and derivatives should not be given in the first trimester of pregnancy. Halofantrine, primaquine, and tetracycline should not be used at any time in pregnancy, and sulfadoxine should not be used very near to term. Mefloquine has been associated with an increased risk of stillbirth in one study but not in another. Atovaquone–proguanil and artemether-lumefantrine have not been evaluated adequately in pregnancy.
B. Vomiting may be less likely if the patient's temperature is lowered before oral drug administration.
C. Contraindications to mefloquine treatment include use of the drug in the previous 63 days, epilepsy or neuropsychiatric disorder, history of allergy, or following cerebral malaria.
D. Short courses of artesunate or quinine (<7 days) alone are not recommended.
E. In renal failure the dose of quinine should be reduced by one third to one half after 48 hours, and doxycycline but *not* tetracycline should be prescribed.
F. The doses of all drugs are unchanged in children and pregnant women.
G. Oral treatment of uncomplicated hyperparasitemic infections should include an artemisinin derivative and be prolonged to minimize the chance of recrudescence, e.g., artesunate loading dose of 4 mg/kg initially followed by 2 mg/kg/day on the following 6 days, in combination with mefloquine, clindamycin, or doxycycline as in the table.
H. Patients with *P. vivax* and *P. ovale* infections should also be given primaquine 0.5 mg base/kg (up to 30 mg base) daily for 14 days to prevent relapse (see Table 90-5). In mild G6PD deficiency, 0.75 mg base/kg should be given once weekly for 6 weeks.
I. Use of tetracyclines in pregnant women or children under 8 years of age is contraindicated.

Quinine

Quinine continues to have an important role in malaria treatment. Although there is reduced susceptibility to quinine in parts of Southeast Asia and South America, these reductions are not large and quinine is still effective in these areas. It is still the drug of choice for uncomplicated falciparum malaria in the first trimester of pregnancy regardless of location. Quinine may also be part of second-line treatment regimens, but it is not standard first-line treatment in endemic areas, because it must be given three times daily and is poorly tolerated (bitter taste, nausea, tinnitus, dysphoria, giddiness—a symptom complex termed cinchonism). Poor tolerance reduces adherence to the 7-day regimens needed to achieve high cure rates where there is resistance. In most cases quinine should be combined with either a tetracycline (e.g., doxycycline or tetracycline) or, in children, clindamycin. These antibiotics are given for 7 days. When treating *P. falciparum* from areas with minimal to no quinine resistance, the quinine is generally given for 3 days and the antimalarial antibiotic for 7 days. These combined regimens achieve cure rates of over 90% even in areas of high-level drug resistance. Oral quinine is also often given to complete a full 7 days of treatment following parenteral treatment for severe malaria. Serious adverse effects from oral quinine are unusual in uncomplicated malaria, although hypoglycemia may occur in late pregnancy.

Treatment with Artemisinin Derivatives and Another Antimalarial

Artesunate-Mefloquine. This 3-day combination treatment is effective against all malaria everywhere. The side effects are similar to mefloquine alone (see previous discussion), although early vomiting is reduced by the combination. Fixed-dose regimens are currently being developed that will incorporate the currently recommended doses in a single tablet—4 mg/kg artesunate and 8 mg/kg mefloquine administered daily for 3 days.

Artemether-Lumefantrine. This is a 3-day, six-dose regimen. Provided that there is adequate absorption of lumefantrine, this combination would also be expected to be effective against all malaria everywhere. The principal problem with artemether-lumefantrine is variable oral absorption of lumefantrine, which may give rise to treatment failure as a result of inadequate blood concentrations. Absorption of lumefantrine is increased by coadministration with fats (food, milk) and improves as the patient recovers from illness. The combination is remarkably well tolerated and rapidly effective.

Artesunate-Amodiaquine. Amodiaquine is more effective than chloroquine against *P. falciparum* in Africa, parts of South America, and Oceania, but not in Asia. Artesunate-amodiaquine is effective in some areas of Africa and South America, but resistance to amodiaquine is increasing. Despite being an "old" drug, there is insufficient information on the pharmacokinetics of amodiaquine, and there are still uncertainties over the true incidence of clinically significant leukopenia, agranulocytosis, and hepatitis when it is used for treatment. All three were observed when amodiaquine was used in antimalarial prophylaxis. Oral amodiaquine is considered more palatable than chloroquine by young children. The combination is generally well tolerated.

Artesunate-Sulfadoxine-Pyrimethamine. A 3-day artesunate-SP combination is well tolerated and effective where sensitivity to SP is retained.

Chlorproguanil-Dapsone. This antifol-biguanide combination is given in a 3-day, once daily regimen. It is more effective than SP against antifol-resistant *P. falciparum*, but it is not effective against parasites with the I164L mutation in *Pfdhfr*. Nearly all recent clinical trials have been conducted with 14-day follow-up, so true efficacy is uncertain. Chlorproguanil-dapsone has been well tolerated in clinical trials, although there are some concerns over an increased risk of anemia, probably resulting from dapsone-induced hemolysis. There is insufficient evidence at present to recommend this drug.

Dihydroartemisinin-Piperaquine. This fixed combination of dihydroartemisinin and piperaquine is a bisquinoline compound with structural similarities to chloroquine. The treatment course is once daily for 3 days. Piperaquine is considerably more active than chloroquine against resistant *P. falciparum*. It is eliminated slowly (terminal half-life ≈ 1 month). The combination was highly effective and well tolerated in large treatment trials in Southeast Asia. It is a promising prospect, but the combination has not yet been evaluated in Africa or the Americas.

Antibacterials with Antimalarial Activity

Many antibiotics that target protein or nucleic acid synthesis are effective against plasmodia. In general these drugs are relatively weak antimalarials that clear parasitemia slowly if used alone, so they are always combined with a specific antimalarial drug. The main exception is trimethoprim-sulfamethoxazole, which has good antimalarial activity (since trimethoprim has the same mode of action as pyrimethamine) but has to be given for 5 to 7 days. Unfortunately, resistance to SP means resistance to trimethoprim-sulfamethoxazole, and continued use of the antibacterial may also select for SP resistance. Thus, trimethoprim- sulfamethoxazole is not recommended for antimalarial use. The tetracyclines, clindamycin, and sulphonamides are all used in antimalarial treatment. Rifampicin, chloramphenicol, and azithromycin all have significant antimalarial activity. Fosmidomycin is being investigated as an antimalarial. Pending further information, these latter drugs are not recommended for general use.

In the assessment of antimalarial drug efficacy, a follow-up period of at least 28 days is required for rapidly eliminated drugs, but for drugs that are more slowly eliminated (terminal half-life >24 hours; see Table 90-3), the follow-up period should be greater than 42 days.

Treatment of Malaria Caused by *P. vivax*, *P. ovale*, or *P. malariae*

P. vivax is still generally sensitive to chloroquine although resistance is increasing in some areas, notably Oceania, Indonesia, and Peru. Resistance to pyrimethamine is prevalent in many areas, and SP is consequently ineffective. Proguanil or chlorproguanil are also ineffective in these areas. In general *P. vivax* is sensitive to all the other antimalarial drugs, is more sensitive than *P. falciparum* to the artemisinin derivatives, and is less sensitive to mefloquine (although mefloquine is still effective). In contrast to *P. falciparum*, asexual stages of *P. vivax* are susceptible to primaquine. Thus, chloroquine plus primaquine can be considered a combination treatment. The only drugs with substantial activity against the hypnozoites are the 8-aminoquinolines (primaquine, tafenaquine).[103,106] Recently simple methods for short-term culture of *P. vivax* have been developed, allowing ex vivo assessment of asexual stage drug sensitivity. In vivo assessment suggests that *P. vivax* in East Asia and Oceania is more primaquine-tolerant than elsewhere. There are few recent data on the in vivo susceptibility of *P. ovale* and *P. malariae*. Both are regarded as sensitive to chloroquine, although there is a single recent report of chloroquine resistance in *P. malariae*.[104] Experience indicates that *P. ovale* and *P. malariae* are susceptible also to amodiaquine, mefloquine, and the artemisinin derivatives. The antifol susceptibility is less certain.

For chloroquine-sensitive vivax malaria (i.e., in most places where *P. vivax* is prevalent) the traditional 25 mg base/kg dose of chloroquine is well tolerated and effective. Some have recommended lower total doses, but this is not recommended, since it may encourage the emergence of resistance. Chloroquine is given in an initial dose of 10 mg base/kg followed by either 5 mg/kg at 6, 24, and 48 hours or more commonly as 10 mg/kg on the second day and 5 mg/kg on the third day. The treatment duration can be shortened to 36 hours. It is also clear that if ACT treatment is given, then *P. vivax* will respond as well as or better than *P. falciparum*. The exception is a regimen containing SP. It appears that *P. vivax* has developed resistance to SP more rapidly than has *P. falciparum*.

There are relatively few data on treatment responses in chloroquine-resistant vivax malaria. Studies from Indonesia indicate that atovaquone-proguanil,[105] halofantrine,[103] mefloquine, and amodiaquine are efficacious. (Atovaquone-proguanil [3 doses over 3 days], mefloquine [25 mg/kg during 1 day], or amodiaquine [30 mg base/kg over 3 days] combined with primaquine should be given for chloroquine-resistant vivax malaria.)

To achieve radical cure of vivax or ovale malaria, relapse must be prevented by giving primaquine.[106] However, the frequency and pattern of relapses vary geographically. It has become clear in recent years that whereas 50% to 60% of *P. vivax* infections in Southeast Asia relapse, the frequency is lower in Indonesia (30%) and the Indian subcontinent (15% to 20%). Thus, the preventive efficacy of primaquine must be set against the prevalent relapse frequency. It appears that the total dose of 8-aminoquinoline given is the main determinant of liver-stage curative efficacy. There is no evidence that the short courses of primaquine widely recommended (such as 5 days of treatment) have any efficacy. Primaquine is given for 14 days. The usually recommended adult dose has been 15 mg base (0.25 mg/kg/day), but in Southeast Asia, particularly Indonesia, and in Oceania, higher doses (0.6 mg base/kg/day) are required, and the CDC now recommends the 0.6 mg/kg dose up to an adult dose of 30 mg base/day (Table 90-5). Primaquine causes abdominal

***Table 90-5** Drugs Used in the Prophylaxis of Malaria as Recommended by the U.S. Centers for Disease Control and Prevention*

Drug	Usage	Adult Dose	Pediatric Dose	Comments/Adverse Reactions/ Contraindications
Atovaquone/ proguanil (Malarone)	Primary prophylaxis* in areas with chloroquine-resistant or mefloquine-resistant *P. falciparum* Begin 1–2 days before entering endemic area and continue for 7 days after leaving	Adult tablets contain 250 mg atovaquone and 100 mg proguanil hydrochloride 1 adult tablet orally daily	Pediatric tablets contain 62.5 mg atovaquone and 25 mg proguanil hydrochloride 11–20 kg: 1 tablet 21–30 kg: 2 tablets 31–40 kg: 3 tablets ≥40 kg: 1 adult tablet daily (Adult tablets contain 250 mg atovaquone and 100 mg proguanil hydrochloride)	Contraindicated in persons with severe renal impairment (creatinine clearance <30 mL/min) Atovaquone/proguanil should be taken with food or a milky drink Not recommended for children <11 kg, pregnant women, and women breast-feeding infants weighing <11 kg
Chloroquine phosphate (Aralen and generic)	Primary prophylaxis* only in areas with chloroquine-sensitive *P. falciparum* Begin 1–2 weeks before entering endemic area and continue for 4 weeks after leaving	300 mg base (500 mg salt) orally once per week	5 mg/kg base (8.3 mg/kg salt) orally once per week, up to maximum adult dose of 300 mg base	May exacerbate psoriasis
Doxycycline (Many brand names and generic)	Primary prophylaxis* in areas with chloroquine-resistant or mefloquine-resistant *P. falciparum*	100 mg orally daily	≥8 years of age: 2 mg/kg up to adult dose of 100 mg/day	Contraindicated in children ≤8 years of age and pregnant women

Continued

Table 90-5 *Drugs Used in the Prophylaxis of Malaria as Recommended by the U.S. Centers for Disease Control and Prevention—Cont'd*

Drug	Usage	Adult Dose	Pediatric Dose	Comments/Adverse Reactions/ Contraindications
	Begin 1–2 days before entering endemic area and continue for 28 days after leaving			
Hydroxy-chloroquine sulfate (Plaquenil)	An alternative to chloroquine for primary prophylaxis* only in areas with chlorquine-sensitive *P. falciparum* Same schedule as chloroquine	310 mg base (400 mg salt) orally once per week	5 mg/kg base(6.5 mg/kg salt) orally once per week, up to maximum adult dose of 310 mg base	See chloroquine comment
Mefloquine (Lariam and generic)	Primary prophylaxis* in areas with chloroquine-resistant *P. falciparum* Begin at least 2 weeks before entering an endemic area and continue for 4 weeks after leaving A loading dose (1 tablet/day for 3 consecutive days) may be given if the individual is leaving immediately for an endemic area. Such individuals should be counseled and monitored closely for side effects	228 mg base (250 mg salt) orally once per week	5–10 kg: ⅛ tablet orally once/week 10–20 kg: ¼ tablet once/week 20–30 kg: ½ tablet once/week 30–45 kg: ¾ tablet once/week >45 kg: 1 tablet once/week The recommended dose of mefloquine is 5 mg/kg body weight once weekly Approximate tablet fraction is based on this dosage Exact doses for children weighing less than 10 kg should be prepared by a pharmacist	Contraindicated in persons allergic to mefloquine and in persons with active depression or a previous history of depression, generalized anxiety disorder, psychosis, schizophrenia, other major psychiatric disorders,or seizures Not recommended for persons with cardiac conduction abnormalities
Primaquine	An option for primary prophylaxis* in special circumstances Call Malaria Hotline (770-488-7788) for additional information Begin 1 or 2 days before entering an endemic area, and continue for 3–7 days after leaving	30 mg base (52.6 mg salt) orally daily	0.6 mg/kg base (1.0 mg/kg salt) up to adult dose, orally daily	Contraindicated in persons with G6PD deficiency Contraindicated during preganancy and lactation unless the infant being breast-fed has a documented normal G6PD level Use in consultation with malaria experts
Primaquine	Used for terminal prophylaxis† risk of relapses of *P. vivax* and *P. ovale*	30 mg base (52.6 mg salt) orally once daily for 14 days after departure from malarious area Note: The recommended dose of primaquine for terminal prophylaxis has been increased from 15 mg to 30 mg for adults	0.6 mg/kg base (1.0 mg/kg salt) up to adult dose orally once daily for 14 days after departure from malarious area Note: The recommended dose of primaquine for terminal prophylaxis† has been increased from 0.3 mg/kg to 0.6 mg/kg for children	Indicated for persons who have had prolonged exposure to *P. vivax* or *P. ovale,* or both Contraindicated in persons with G6PD deficiency‡ Contraindicated during pregnancy and lactation unless the infant being breast-fed has a documented normal G6PD level

**Primary prophylaxis* refers to the use of antimalarial drugs to prevent symptoms associated with blood-stage infection; these drugs are taken before, during, and for a period of time after travel in the malaria-risk area.

†*Terminal prophylaxis* refers to the use of primaquine to lower the risk of relapse from liver-stage infection with *P. vivax* or *P. ovale*. Primaquine is taken after departure from the malaria-risk area.

‡Primaquine is contraindicated in individuals with the severe G6PD deficiency (approximately 5%–10% of normal activity) found in some individuals of Mediterranean and Asian background, but can be given safely to individuals with modest G6PD deficiency (approximately 20% of normal activity) found in individuals of African background.

Available at www.cdc.gov/travel/malariadrugs2.htm.

discomfort when taken on an empty stomach; it should always be taken with food.

The inherited sex-linked deficiency of G6PD is associated with some protection against falciparum malaria but increased susceptibility to oxidant hemolysis. The prevalence of G6PD deficiency varies but can be a high as 20%. There are a large number of different genotypes, each with different levels of deficiency. Primaquine is an oxidant and causes variable hemolysis in G6PD-deficient individuals. Fortunately, primaquine is eliminated rapidly, so hemolysis is self-limiting provided no further drug is taken. Screening for G6PD deficiency is not generally available outside hospitals, although rapid stick tests are under development. Many people are unaware of their G6PD status. If a patient is known or suspected (individuals of Mediterranean and Asian descent) to be severely G6PD deficient (≈5% to 10% of normal G6PD activity), then primaquine should not be given. For the majority of patients with mild variants (≈20% of normal G6PD activity), often found in black Africans, primaquine can be given in a dose of 0.75 mg base/kg once weekly for 6 weeks. If significant hemolysis occurs on treatment, primaquine should be stopped. Primaquine is not given during pregnancy because G6PD status of the fetus is unknown. Tafenoquine is a more active and more slowly eliminated 8-aminoquinoline in development. It also causes oxidant hemolysis.

Treatment of Severe Malaria

Death from severe malaria often occurs within hours of admission to hospital or clinic, so it is essential that therapeutic concentrations of antimalarial drug be achieved as soon as safely possible. This is why a loading dose of certain drugs is essential, particularly quinine, quinidine, and artemether. Nearly all cases of severe malaria result from *P. falciparum* infection. Many patients with malaria, including those with species other than *P. falciparum*, cannot take oral medications initially because of repeated vomiting. They do not fulfil the criteria of severe malaria but do require parenteral (or rectal) administration of antimalarials. In practice if there is uncertainty the patient should be treated as having severe malaria until able to swallow medications reliably. Management of severe malaria comprises four main areas: assessment of the patient, specific antimalarial treatment, adjunctive therapy, and supportive care.[54]

Severe malaria is a medical emergency. The airway should be secured in unconscious patients and breathing and circulation assessed. The patient should be weighed or weight estimated so that drugs, including antimalarials, and fluids can be given on a body weight basis. An intravenous cannula should be inserted, and immediate measurements of blood glucose (stick test), hematocrit, parasitemia (parasite count, stage of malaria parasite development, and proportion of neutrophils containing malaria pigment), and in adults, renal function (blood urea or creatinine) should be taken. The degree of acidosis is an important determinant of outcome; the plasma bicarbonate or venous lactate should be measured if possible. If facilities are available, arterial or capillary blood pH and gases should be measured in patients who are unconscious, hyperventilating, or in shock. Blood should be taken for cross-match, and (if possible) full blood count, platelet count, clotting studies, bacterial culture, and full biochemistry. Intravenous fluids may then be started. The assessment of fluid balance is critical in severe malaria. Acidotic breathing or respiratory distress, particularly in severely anemic children, often indicates hypovolemia and requires prompt but careful rehydration and, if available, rapid blood transfusion. In adults there is a thin dividing line between overhydration, which may produce pulmonary edema, and underhydration contributing to shock and worsening acidosis and renal impairment. Careful and frequent evaluations of the jugular venous pressure, peripheral perfusion, venous filling, skin turgor, and urine output should be made. When there is uncertainty over the jugular venous pressure, and if nursing facilities permit, a central venous catheter should be inserted and the pressure (CVP) measured directly.

When these immediate measures have been completed, a more detailed clinical examination should be conducted, with particular note of the level of consciousness and record of the coma score. Several coma scales have been advocated. The Glasgow coma scale (GCS) is suitable for adults, and the simple Blantyre modification (BCS) or childrens' Glasgow Coma Scale (CGCS) for children.[107] Unconscious patients must have a diagnostic lumbar puncture to exclude bacterial meningitis. The opening pressure should be recorded and the rise and fall with respiration noted.CSF should be sent for microscopic analysis, culture, and measurement of glucose, lactate, and protein. After rapid clinical assessment and confirmation of the diagnosis of severe malaria, full doses of antimalarial treatment should be started without delay.

Specific Antimalarial Treatment of Severe Malaria

Currently four commonly used parenteral drug treatments are recommended for severe malaria: artesunate, artemether, quinine, and quinidine (Box 90-3). Artemotil is also used in some areas. Artesunate, artemether, artemisinin, and quinine have also been formulated for rectal administration. Although chloroquine is available in parenteral formulations and has been used widely in the past, it is no longer recommended because resistance is too widespread to rely on it. Even in a patient considered to need parenteral treatment for *P. vivax, P. ovale, or P. malariae* infection, it is best to treat for falciparum malaria because there may be a mixed infection. The intramuscular preparation of sulfadoxine-pyrimethamine should not be used to treat severe malaria, since resistance is widespread and responses are slow.

There have been several treatment comparisons in severe malaria, mainly between intramuscular artemether and intramuscular or intravenous quinine.[108] None of these show clear evidence of benefit in terms of survival, although the artemisinin derivatives are simpler to use and safer (principally because of the reduced risk of hypoglycemia). None of the trials was designed to detect less than a 30% reduction in mortality. In an individual patient data analysis of the largest series of prospectively studied patients with severe malaria, 1919 patients were enrolled in randomized comparisons of artemether versus quinine. The mortality in artemether recipients was 136/961 (14%) and in the quinine recipients was 164/958 (17%; $P=0.08$). In the prospectively defined subgroup analysis of adults (largely from Southeast Asia), the mortality difference in favor of artemether was statistically significant.[108] There had been concern that saving the lives of

Box 90-3 Treatment of Severe Malaria

Artesunate IV: 2.4 mg/kg stat, at 12 and 24 hours, then daily
or
Artemether IM: initial dose of 3.2 mg/kg followed by 1.6 mg/kg every 24 hours until oral medication is tolerated*
or
Quinine IV: loading dose (LD) 20 mg salt/kg given over 4 hours, then 10 mg salt/kg given 8 hours after the LD was started, followed by 10 mg salt/kg every 8 hours†
or
Quinine IM: loading dose of 20 mg salt/kg is given as two simultaneous injections in the anterior thigh (10 mg salt/kg in each) after dilution of the quinine in sterile water to a concentration of 60 to 100 mg/mL, maintenance dose of 10 mg salt/kg is given as one IM injection every 8 hours using the same dilution
or
Quinidine IV: 10 mg base/kg infused over 1–2 hours followed by 1.2 mg base/kg per hour by constant infusion.

- Electrocardiographic monitoring necessary‡
- Total treatment duration for all regimens = 7 days
- Once the patient has recovered sufficiently to tolerate oral medication reliably, the parenteral treatment can be discontinued and a second drug should be added, such as doxycyline 3 mg/kg for 7 days, clindamycin 10 mg/kg bid for 7 days, or atovaquone 20 mg/kg/day + proguanil 8 mg/kg/day for 3 days§
- SP single dose can be used if parasites are known to be sensitive

*Absorption of IM artemether may be inadequate in a subgroup of patients with shock.
†If QTc (on electrocardiogram) is greater than 25% of baseline or exceeds 600 msec or hypotension occurs temporarily reduce or stop infusion.
‡Some authorities recommend a lower dose of 6.2 mg base/kg initially over 1 hour followed by 0.012 mg base/kg/hr.
§Mefloquine should not be used because of the increased risk of post-malaria neurologic syndrome (Mai NTH, Day NPJ, Chuong LV, et al: Post-malaria neurological syndrome. Lancet 348:917–921, 1996).

patients with cerebral malaria might increase rates of neurologic sequelae, but there was no associated increase. There are fewer data for artesunate and very few trials with artemotil (also known as arteether), but since they have a common biologically active metabolite (DHA) they are likely to be at least equivalent to artemether. Indeed, the pharmacokinetic properties of artesunate are superior to those of artemether and artemotil because it is water soluble and can be given either by intravenous or intramuscular injection. Quinidine is more toxic than quinine and should be used only when none of the other effective parenteral drugs are available.[54]

Pharmacologic Considerations. In severe malaria it is essential that parasiticidal concentrations of antimalarial drug are attained as soon as safely possible.

- **Artesunate:** Parasiticidal levels are attained immediately following IV injection and within minutes of IM injection. No dose adjustments are needed in liver or renal dysfunction. Artesunate is rapidly hydrolyzed to DHA in vivo. The therapeutic range of DHA is unknown but by extrapolation from in vitro data is exceeded considerably by current dose regimens.
- **Artemether and artemotil:** These oil-based formulations are slowly and erratically absorbed following intramuscular injection (there is no intravenous formulation), and some patients may not achieve parasiticidal concentrations within the first few hours after starting treatment. Absorption is particularly poor in children and adults with poor peripheral perfusion. Artemether is also converted to DHA in vivo, but concentrations of the parent compound exceed those of DHA, so artemether contributes the majority of antimalarial effect in vivo. No dose adjustments are needed in liver or renal dysfunction.
- **Quinine:** A full loading dose (20 mg quinine dihydrochloride salt/kg) should always be given irrespective of the degree of vital organ dysfunction unless there is clear evidence that the patient has already received adequate quinine treatment (>40 mg salt/kg in the past 48 hours). For quinine there is considerable variability in apparent volume of distribution, so the full loading dose is necessary to ensure that the majority of patients do have adequate blood concentrations. In the past there was too much concern over the dangers of potential quinine toxicity and insufficient concern over the dangers of undertreatment in severe malaria. The risk-benefit ratio changes as treatment progresses. The majority of deaths from malaria occur within the first 48 hours following admission to hospital; undertreatment may have fatal consequences. In practice, quinine toxicity in the first 24 hours of treatment is rare. The maintenance dose studied in Asia has been 10 mg/kg every 8 hours, but the dose interval in Africa has sometimes been 12 hours. Currently, an 8 hour interval is recommended. After 48 hours of treatment if there is no clinical improvement in severe malaria, or if the patient is in acute renal failure, a dose reduction by 1/3 to 1/2 is recommended to avoid continued accumulation to potentially toxic concentrations. The therapeutic range has not been well defined, but total plasma concentrations of between 8 and 15 mg/L are thought to be safe and effective. Toxicity is increasingly likely with plasma concentrations over 20 mg/L (free quinine >2 mg/L).

Quinidine is more toxic than quinine. Both hypotension and prolongation of ventricular repolarization (QTc interval) are common when parenteral quinidine is used in the treatment of severe malaria. There have been only two small studies of quinidine in severe malaria so dose recommendations rest on limited information. Ideally patients receiving quinidine should have careful cardiovascular monitoring and frequent measurement of plasma concentrations to guide dosing. As with quinine, the dose should be reduced if there is no clinical improvement within 48 hours.

Where Parenteral Treatment Cannot Be Given. In most areas of the rural tropics, severe malaria occurs far from medical attention. Since delay in starting treatment can have fatal consequences, rectal formulations of artemisinin have been developed. These can be given by village health workers pending transfer to a facility where parenteral treatment and supportive can be given.[109–111]

Supportive Care

Patients with severe malaria require intensive nursing in an intensive care unit if possible. Following the initial assessment and commencement of antimalarial treatment, clinical observations should be made as frequently as possible. These should include recording of vital signs, with an accurate assessment of respiratory rate and pattern, assessment of the coma score, and urine output. The blood glucose should be checked, with rapid stick tests every 4 hours if possible, particularly in unconscious patients. Convulsions should be treated promptly with anticonvulsants such as intravenous or rectal diazepam or intramuscular paraldehyde.

Each patient's fluid requirements should be assessed individually. Adults with severe malaria are vulnerable to fluid overload and the physician treads a narrow path between underhydration, and thus worsening renal impairment, and overhydration, with the risk of precipitating pulmonary edema. If the patient becomes oliguric (<0.4 mL of urine/kg/hr) despite adequate rehydration and the blood urea or creatinine are rising or already high, fluids should be restricted to replace insensible losses only. Children, on the other hand, are more likely to be dehydrated and may respond well to a rate-controlled bolus of fluid. The fluid regimen must also be tailored around infusion of the antimalarial drugs. The CVP should be maintained between 0 and 5 cm. If the venous pressure is significantly elevated (usually because of overenthusiastic fluid administration), the patient should be nursed with the head at 45 degrees and intravenous furosemide given if necessary.

If blood glucose is less than 4 mmol/L, then a 10% glucose infusion should be started following saline replacement; if it is less than 2.2 mmol/L, then hypoglycemia should be treated immediately (0.3 to 0.5 g/kg glucose or 5 mL/kg 10% dextrose as an IV bolus). Hypoglycemia should be suspected in any patient who deteriorates suddenly. Stick tests may overestimate the frequency of hypoglycemia, so laboratory confirmation may be necessary.

Patients with acute pulmonary edema should be nursed upright and given oxygen, and the right-sided filling pressures should be reduced with whichever treatments are available (loop diuretics, opiates, venodilators, venesection, hemofiltration, dialysis). The right-sided pressure should be reduced to the lowest level compatible with an adequate cardiac output. Positive pressure ventilation should be started (if available) if the patient becomes hypoxic.

Less than 5% of patients with severe malaria develop clinically significant DIC. These patients should be given fresh blood transfusions and vitamin K. Patients with secondary pneumonia should be given empirical treatment with a third-generation cephalosporin unless admitted with clear evidence of aspiration, in which case penicillin or clindamycin is adequate. Children with persistent fever despite parasite clearance may have a systematic *Salmonella* infection, although in most cases of persistent fever after parasite clearance no other pathogen is identified. Urinary tract infections are common in catheterized patients. Antibiotic treatments should depend on likely local antibiotic sensitivity patterns.

Severe Malaria in Pregnancy

Pregnant women in the second and third trimesters are more likely to develop severe malaria than are other adults, often complicated by pulmonary edema and hypoglycemia.[54] Maternal mortality from severe malaria approximates 50%, which is higher than in nonpregnant adults. Fetal death and premature labor are common. The role of early cesarean section for the viable live fetus is unproved but is recommended by many authorities. Obstetric advice should be sought at an early stage, the pediatricians alerted, and the blood glucose checked frequently. Hypoglycemia should be expected and is often recurrent if the patient is receiving quinine. The antimalarial drugs should be given in full doses (Boxes 90-3 and 90-4). Severe malaria may also present immediately following delivery. Postpartum bacterial infection is a common complication in these cases. Falciparum malaria has also been associated with severe mid-trimester hemolytic anemia in Nigeria. This often requires transfusion in addition to antimalarial treatment and folate supplementation.

Follow-up Treatment of Severe Malaria

When the patient with severe malaria has recovered sufficiently, oral medication should be substituted. Infections resulting in severe malaria are more likely to recrudesce than milder infections. They are a potentially important source of resistance, and it is correspondingly important that a full course of curative treatment be completed. There has been only one comparative evaluation of consolidation treatments and no studies in which recrudescence rates were documented. A randomized comparison of oral quinine plus SP versus mefloquine (following parenteral artemether or quinine) was

Box 90-4 Treatment of Uncomplicated Malaria in Pregnancy

Quinine 10 mg salt/kg tid for 7 days. This should be combined with clindamycin (10 mg/kg bid) for 7 days in the second and third trimesters of pregnancy*

or if the infection is known to be from an area with SP sensitivity, pyrimethamine 1.25 mg/kg + sulfadoxine 25 mg/kg (single dose) 3 tablets in an adult

or if the infection is known to be from an area with chloroquine sensitivity to *P. falciparum* or for infections with *P. vivax*, *P. ovale*, or *P. malariae*

Chloroquine Phosphate (1 tablet contains 250 mg salt, equivalent to 155.3 mg base)* 10 mg/kg base at 0, 24 hr followed by 5 mg/kg base at 48 hr

Artemisinin derivatives should not be used in the first trimester of pregnancy. In the second and thrid trimesters of pregnancy, artesunate (2 mg/kg/day for 7 days) may be given with one of the other drugs

The role of mefloquine in the treatment of malaria in pregnancy remains uncertain; in one large study, there were no adverse effects† but in another, there was an increased risk of stillbrith‡

*Quinine has been shown to be safe in all trimesters. There is no evidence for an increased risk of abortion, stillbirth, or congenital abnormality, but in the third trimester there is an increased risk of iatrogenic hypoglycemia with quinine treatment.

†Steketee RW, Wirima JJ, Slutsker L, et al: treatment and prevention in pregnancy: Indications for use and adverse events associated with use of chloroquine or mefloquine. Am J Trop Med Hyg. 55(1 Suppl): 50–56,1996.

‡Nosten F, Vincenti M, Simpson JA, et al: The effects of mefloquine treatment in pregnancy. Clin Infect Dis, 28:808–815, 1999.

conducted in Vietnam. Mefloquine recipients had a significantly increased risk of neuropsychiatric reactions (absolute risk of 5% compared with 0.1% to 1% in uncomplicated malaria). In a nonrandomized study of doxycycline pharmacokinetics following severe malaria, it was suggested that the current dose regimen (3 to 3.5 mg/kg/day) may be insufficient.

Current practice is to continue the same drug orally as given parenterally to complete 7 days of treatment. In nonpregnant adults, doxycycline is added to either quinine, artesunate, or artemether also to complete 7 days of treatment. Doxycycline is preferred to other tetracyclines because it can be given once daily and does not accumulate in renal failure. Since doxycycline only starts when the patient has recovered sufficiently, the doxycycline course finishes after the quinine, artemether, or artesunate course. Where available and affordable, clindamycin may be substituted in children and pregnant women because doxycycline cannot be given to these groups. In areas where SP is still effective, it is often given as consolidation therapy. Although following parenteral treatment with a full course of artemisinin combination treatment (i.e., artesunate-amodiaquine, or artemether-lumefantrine) is theoretically a good alternative, this has not been evaluated in clinical trials.

PREVENTION AND CONTROL

Malaria Prevention in Visitors to Malaria-endemic Areas

Malaria poses a health risk to visitors to malaria-endemic regions. Annually millions of travelers from nonendemic countries travel to areas where there is a malaria risk. As well, many residents of nonendemic regions of countries that have areas of malaria risk are at risk of infection during short-term visits. Prevention and suppression of infection are far more effective than reliance on treatment of malaria illness in these visitors, owing to the unpredictability of the availability and quality of medical care in many settings. The prevention of infection and disease relies largely on the prophylactic use of malaria drugs, and the specific regimens are outlined in Table 90-5.

Several general principles should guide the protection of visitors to regions with risk of malaria transmission. First and foremost, individuals should be protected optimally if there is any risk, since a single infected mosquito bite may result in a fatal malaria infection. If the area to be visited has any *P. falciparum,* the choice of drug for prevention should be based on an assumption of drug resistance unless the travel is to Haiti or Central America. Finally, while the use of efficacious drugs (chemoprophylaxis) can afford a high degree of protection, it is important for visitors to use mosquito protection, including bed nets and repellents, and to be aware of how to secure safe and effective medical attention in the event of a potential malaria illness.

Malaria drugs for use in prevention among visitors have several distinct modes of action. Most drugs used for chemoprophylaxis are only blood schizonticides (only killing blood-stage parasites). These include chloroquine and other 4-aminoquinolines and mefloquine. These drugs do not prevent primary infection of the liver but kill parasites once they erupt from the liver and invade erythrocytes, thereby preventing disease progression.

A limited number of drugs have activity against parasites developing in hepatocytes and are termed tissue schizonticides and causal prophylactic drugs. The 8-aminoquinolones, primaquine[112] and the longer acting tafenaquine[113] (in development), kill liver-stage parasites. Primaquine has only modest activity against the asexual erythrocytic stages, and tafenaquine probably has more activity against blood stages. The best activity of atovaquone/proguanil,[114] tetracycline, and doxycycline is against the asexual erythrocytic stages (blood schizonticides), but they all have some activity against *P. falciparum* liver stages, and atovaquone/proguanil may have activity against *P. vivax* liver stages. Atovaquone/proguanil[114] and doxycycline are considered first-line drugs. Primaquine is now being recommended more often for chemoprophylaxis because it can be taken on the day of arrival in a malarious area and for only a few days afterward[112,115] and is much less expensive than atovaquone-proguanil, which has a similar dosing regimen. The specific recommendations of the CDC are outlined in Table 90-5.

Drug Safety and Contraindications

The risk of being infected during visits to malaria-endemic areas is highly variable but is low in the vast majority of settings. Furthermore, most travelers are healthy, and avoidance of travel and risk also is an option. Consequently, drugs used for chemoprophylaxis need to be well tolerated and should not pose a substantive health risk. The current standard chemoprophylactic drugs are within acceptable levels of safety, yet each has a spectrum of potential and non-life-threatening adverse side effects that must be appreciated by travelers and their medical advisors. The CDC[116] and WHO have excellent information on these risks and advice for special populations.

Pregnant women and young children pose special challenges in the chemoprophylactic use of drugs. For several drugs there are specific contraindications for these populations (e.g., tetracycline). Licensure of most drugs by the FDA does not generally address the safety of drugs during pregnancy and in infancy (e.g., mefloquine); consequently, their use for short-term travel needs to be considered carefully. Ancillary prevention methods (bed nets) and the delaying of travel should always be considered.

Malaria Drug Prophylaxis for Residents of Malaria-endemic Areas

The routine use of malaria drugs for suppressing malaria disease lost favor during the 1970s to 1980s due principally to the presumption that the use of drugs on a mass basis at subtherapeutic doses would foster the intensification of drug resistance to valuable therapeutic drugs, notably chloroquine.

In recent years selective use of malaria drugs in a preventive mode but at therapeutic doses (intermittent preventive treatment, or IPT) has been documented to be highly effective in controlling the risk of death and severe anemia in pregnant women and infants (see later).

Malaria Control in Malaria-endemic Areas

During the past decade there has been a renewal in the global commitment to control the enormous health and economic burden that malaria extracts. Underlying this resurgence is a highly cost-effective set of malaria control interventions that, despite technical limitations such as drug resistance, have been demonstrated to control both malaria transmission and disease. While the treatment of malaria illness remains a constant component of malaria control, prevention has become the predominant cost-effective approach. The major challenge to the control of malaria has been the development of effective program delivery systems to attain and sustain high population coverage.

Based on malaria epidemiology and the capacity of local health system infrastructures to deliver malaria control interventions, there are currently several distinct settings for malaria prevention and control efforts. In areas where malaria transmission is either highly seasonal or of low intensity, principally in the Indian subcontinent and Southeast Asia and most of the Americas, malaria control focuses around the prompt and effective treatment of malaria illness and selective use of antimosquito measures. In many of these areas there is a continuation of control methods developed during the malaria eradication programs of 1950 to 1975, with the use of the indoor spraying of residual insecticides (currently very limited use of DDT and more typically use of less environmentally threatening chemicals) to interrupt malaria transmission.

Malaria control programming and funding has in recent years focused on developing national level programs to stem the health and economic burden in Africa. Based on WHO and Roll Back Malaria guidance, the following are the key malaria control and prevention interventions advocated for the Africa region.

Insecticide-treated Nets

Based on evidence from five randomized controlled trials and population-based program effectiveness studies in different malaria transmission settings, insecticide-treated nets (ITNs) can reduce the number of under-5 deaths from all causes by about 20% and clinical episodes of malaria by about half [117] (Fig. 90-6). Since malaria causes approximately 20% of under-5 mortality in Africa, the protective efficacy of nets on malaria-specific mortality in children less than 5 years of age is probably at least 80%, in the range of the protective efficacy of most childhood vaccines.[118,119] Recent evidence shows that ITNs protect not only those who sleep under them but also those in the same dwelling and those living nearby. Current ITNs need to be re-treated after three washes, or at least once a year. ITNs are less effective in parts of Asia, where the main malaria vectors bite outdoors early in the evening.

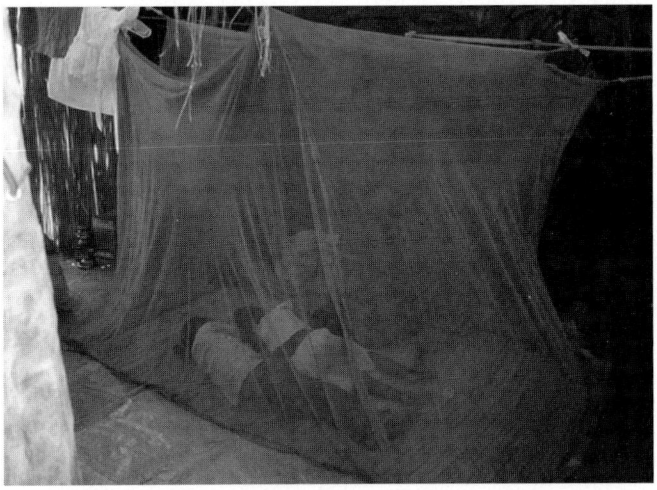

FIGURE 90-6 Children sleeping under an insecticide-impregnated bed net. (Courtesy of C. Campbell.)

Indoor Residual Spraying

Indoor residual spraying (IRS) has been a highly effective intervention in many parts of the world, and in particular in the Americas, in Asia and in Southern Africa. IRS, through its house-to-house, publicly funded and managed approach can achieve very high coverage and thus major impact on malaria disease burden. IRS programs are of limited application in most rural areas with stable malaria endemicity, especially those where there has been no tradition of managing programs of such logistic complexity. [120]

Intermittent Preventive Treatment

Intermittent preventive treatment (IPT) is the preferred approach to reduce the adverse consequences of malaria during pregnancy; it involves the administration of full curative treatment doses of an effective antimalarial drug, preferably single-dose, at predefined intervals during pregnancy, beginning in the second trimester after quickening. IPT with SP is highly effective in reducing the malaria parasite load, thus reducing severe anemia in the mother and lowering the proportion of low-birth-weight babies.[121,122] There is uncertainty how to deploy IPT in the increasing areas of SP resistance and whether IPT should be deployed in low transmission settings.

Prompt and Effective Case Management of Malaria Illness

The prompt recognition that a febrile illness could potentially be caused by malaria is the key to limiting the risk of progression to severe or fatal disease. In most of the malaria-endemic world, malaria is self-diagnosed and treated; many episodes of fever not caused by malaria are therefore self-treated with antimalarials. Standard microscopy—and increasingly, rapid diagnostic tests in certain settings—allow for a proper diagnosis of malaria and increase the chances that antimalarial drugs are used for the correct purpose and not simply in response to an unspecified fever episode.

While drug efficacy should be the principal determinant of which drugs are used to treat malaria infections, in many settings there are many drugs of variable or undocumented quality, and a majority of malaria drugs come from commercial outlets without the advice of a health care provider.

Program Goals for Malaria Control

Global eradication of malaria transmission is not a realistic goal for the foreseeable future. However, elimination of malaria transmission in some regions (mainly in areas of Asia and the Americas) could be accomplished with increased and sustained funding and political prioirty. For the Africa region, the Abuja Ministerial Summit in 2000 established malaria program targets to be obtained by the end of 2005. These program coverage targets are as follows:

- 60% of malaria patients have access to appropriate treatment within 24 hours of onset of symptoms

- 60% of children and pregnant women are protected by ITNs
- 60% of pregnant women have access to appropriate presumptive IPT for malaria.

Pilot malaria program trials have demonstrated that with integrated application of the malaria control interventions it is possible to reduce malaria deaths and economic impact by 60% to 80%.[1,2]

Development of New and More Effective Malaria Control and Prevention Tools

Although there are highly efficacious interventions for malaria control and intervention, continued emphasis on the development of new and more efficacious methods is required.

Response to Drug Resistance and the Development of New Malaria Drugs

Since the early 1960s, resistance to an increasingly broad spectrum of malaria drugs has been documented in *P. falciparum* (see Table 90-2).

Resistance has had a profound impact on malaria control and prevention efforts globally. Alternative drugs to chloroquine have proved to be considerably more expensive and have safety profiles that limit their programmatic use in some populations.

In response to the continued spread of drug resistance, WHO has developed strategies in an attempt to slow the development and spread of drug resistance. Currently it is recommended that areas affected by resistance to one or more of the standard malaria drugs should deploy combination therapy, that is, the use of two or more efficacious drugs that have distinct modes of action. Further, based on experience in Southeast Asia, artemisinin-containing combination therapy is preferred.

The cost of ACT therapy is a major challenge to broad implementation of this policy guidance, especially in Africa.

The development of novel malaria drugs has received renewed attention in recent years, notably under the guidance of several multinational initiatives such as the Medicines for Malaria Venture (www.mmv.org), a public private partnership devoted to malaria drug development, and the continued activities of institutions such as Walter Reed U.S. Army Institute of Research and WHO/TDR (www.who.int/tdr). There are promising leads, but cost and the long lead time required to move efficacious compounds to licensure remain serious impediments to the control and prevention of malaria globally.

Development of Malaria Vaccines

Malaria vaccines could benefit those living wherever there is malaria and travelers to these areas. The primary goal, however, must be to prevent the enormous numbers of deaths and cases of severe malaria in infants and young children in Africa caused by *P. falciparum*. Thus, most malaria vaccine development efforts are focused on *P. falciparum*.

There are no commercially available vaccines for human parasites. Parasites present a greater challenge than do the viruses and bacteria for which we have vaccines because they are more complex. They have much larger genomes coding for more proteins. They have multistage life cycles in which they express many different proteins at different times (Fig. 90-7). As a result, protective immune responses against the extracellular sporozoites that enter with the bite of a mosquito may have no effect on the parasites that later emerge from the liver and infect red blood cells (the asexual erythrocytic stage merozoites). The *P. falciparum* parasite in particular has enormous variability in its proteins. These characteristics are critical to the parasite's survival because they enable it to evade host immune defenses. They also mean that a vaccine containing just a single sequence of a single protein, or a few proteins, may fail to have a large, sustainable impact on the disease. A truly effective malaria vaccine may need to induce both antibody and T-cell responses. Antibodies have the potential to block sporozoites as they enter the body (see Fig. 90-7) but have to act within minutes to block entry into the liver. They can also prevent infection of red blood cells, help destroy those that are already infected, and prevent infection of mosquitoes. T cells have the potential to kill infected liver cells, thereby controlling and even eliminating infection. Both types of responses may have to be directed against multiple different proteins, at different stages of the complex parasite life cycle, and at the same time.[123–126] If so, malaria vaccine developers face a technical problem that has never been solved.

Scientists attempting to develop a malaria vaccine keep two observations in mind. The first is that most malaria-associated deaths and severe disease in sub-Saharan Africa occur in infants, young children, and pregnant women. Adolescents and adults rarely develop severe disease or die after repeated infections with *P. falciparum*. They have presumably developed natural immunity that limits parasite replication and severe forms of malaria but does not prevent infection resulting in milder symptoms.[41] Pregnant women, especially with their first child, apparently lose this immunity. This observation has led to the idea that a vaccine would be worthwhile even if it only limited the severity of disease for those most at risk without preventing infection or moderate disease. Such a vaccine would probably not be useful for travelers. The second observation is that when volunteers are exposed to more than a thousand bites from *P. falciparum*–infected *Anopheles* mosquitoes that have been irradiated to weaken the sporozoites they carry, they develop protective immunity against multiple strains of *P. falciparum*. If these volunteers are exposed to normal sporozoites, more than 93% are completely protected against developing erythrocytic stage infection.[127] This is the strongest evidence that development of a highly effective malaria vaccine is possible, and accordingly there are efforts to develop vaccines that prevent all infections with *P. falciparum* in a majority (>85%) of recipients.[128]

There are three main strategies by which it may be possible to achieve one or both of the preceding goals. The first is to create vaccines that counter sporozoites as they enter the body and invade and reproduce in the liver (pre-erythrocytic stage vaccines). These have the potential to limit or prevent infection altogether. The second is to limit parasite invasion of erythrocytes and subsequent multiplication and pathologic effects (asexual erythrocytic stage and antitoxin vaccines). Such vaccines would limit only severe disease—they would not prevent infection or mild disease. The third strategy is to prevent the spread of viable parasites to other people with "transmission-blocking vaccines." These stimulate the production of antibodies that are ingested with the parasite

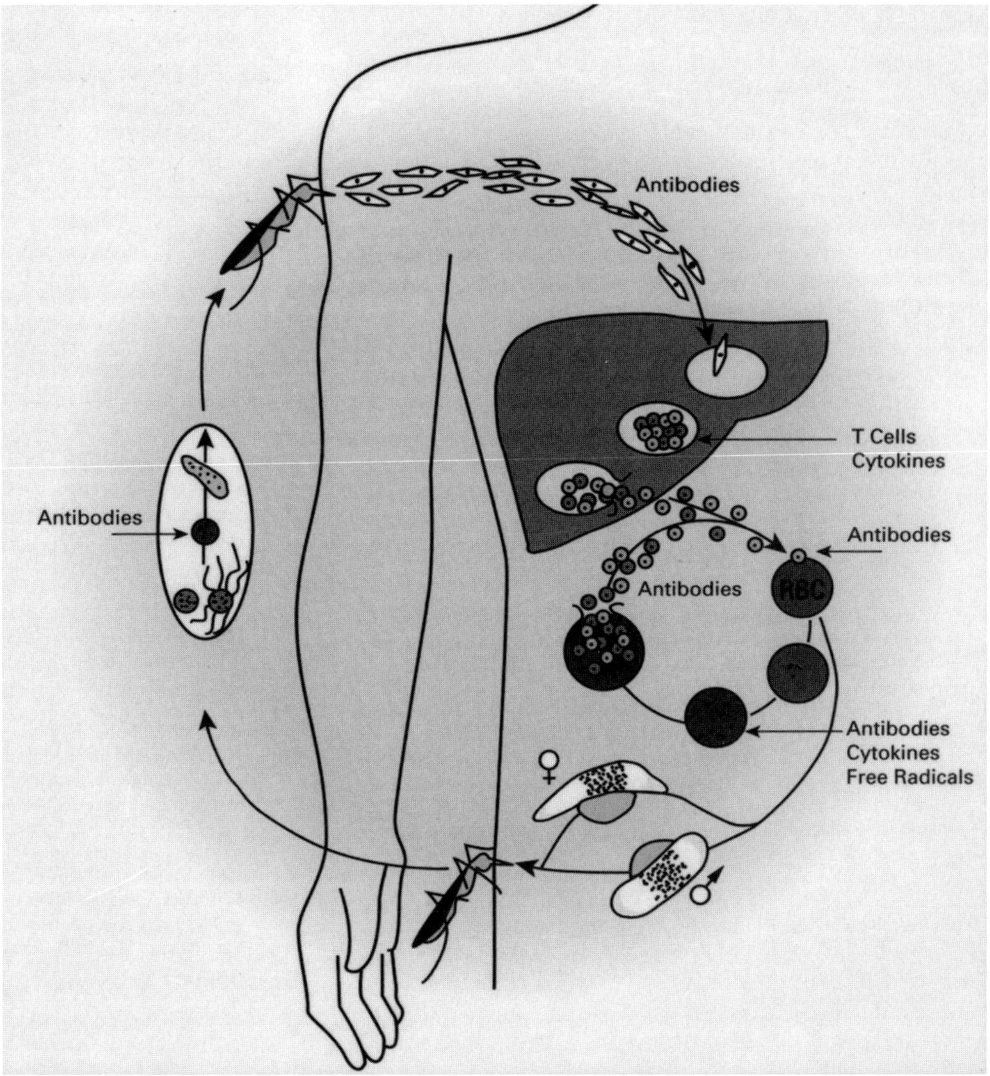

FIGURE 90-7 Schematic of the life cycle of *P. falciparum* with indication of which immune responses can affect which stage of the life cycle. (From Hoffman SL [ed]: Malaria Vaccine Development: a Multi-Immune Response Approach. Washington, DC, ASM Press, 1996. Courtesy of the American Society of Microbiology.)

and destroy the parasite within the vector's gut (see Fig. 90-7). It may be necessary to combine all three strategies to have maximum success. Current vaccine candidates in clinical trials, however, contain just one or a few proteins. In contrast, the protective immune responses elicited by natural exposure to malaria or by immunization with radiation-attenuated sporozoites could be directed at many—perhaps hundreds or even thousands—of the proteins encoded by the 5300 genes in the *P. falciparum* genome.

According to WHO in 2004 more than 70 subunit malaria vaccine candidates are in different stages of development.[129] Despite these efforts only one *P. falciparum* protein, the *P. falciparum* circumsporozoite protein (PfCSP),[130] has been repeatedly evaluated in clinical trials and shown to provide complete protection in a portion of volunteers. The protein was discovered in 1979 by the Nussezweig group, shown to be protective in mice in 1980, and first shown to protect humans as a vaccine in 1987. The lead candidate based on this protein is called RTS,S/AS02A, and it protects 40% to 45% of nonimmune volunteers against experimental challenge with *P. falciparum* for 2 to 3 weeks.[131,132] In 1- to 4-year-old children in Mozambique during 6 months it reduced the incidence of new clinical attacks of malaria by 22.6%, new *P. falciparum* infection by 10.4%, and the incidence of severe disease by 58%.[133] In addition to the modern subunit vaccine approaches, there is a major effort to develop a nonreplicating, metabolically active whole sporozoite *P. falciparum* vaccine.[128]

It currently costs $0.5 billion to $1 billion to bring a vaccine to market. There are large numbers of vaccine candidates in preclinical and clinical development, and many more candidates are likely to enter efficacy field trials in the next 5 years. Furthermore, emerging genomic and proteomic studies of *P. falciparum* will lead to the development of even more candidate vaccines.[134] It will unquestionably take creative public-private partnerships to bring a malaria vaccine to the infants who need it most. Despite the great need, it will be a number of years before a malaria vaccine is widely used to successfully prevent the morbidity and mortality of *P. falciparum* in the 20 to 25 million infants born annually in sub-Saharan Africa.

ACKNOWLEDGMENTS

The authors thank Dr. Judy Epstein of the Naval Medical Research Center and Ms. Sunena Wadhwa of Sanaria for their extensive support.

REFERENCES

1. Breman JG, Egan A, Keusch GT: The intolerable burden of malaria: a new look at the numbers. Am J Trop Med Hyg 64:iv–vii, 2001.
2. Sachs J, Malaney P: The economic and social burden of malaria. Nature 415:680–685, 2002.
3. Gilles HM: Historical outline. In Warrell DA, Gilles HM (ed): Essential Malariology, 4th ed. London, Arnold, 2002, p 7, ref 3.
4. Honigsbaum M: The Fever Trail: In Search of the Cure for Malaria. Great Britain, Macmillan, May 2001.
5. Rocco F: The Miraculous Fever Tree: Malaria and the Quest for the Cure That Changed the World. New York, HarperCollins, 2003.
6. Laveran A: Note sur un nouveau parasite trouve dans le sang de plusieurs malades atteints de fievre palustre. Bull Acad Med Ser 2, 9:1235–1236, 1880.
7. Ross R: On some peculiar pigmented cells found in two mosquitoes fed on malarial blood. BMJ 2:1786–1788, 1897.
8. Beadle C, Hoffman SL: History of Malaria in the United States Naval Forces at War: World War I through the Vietnam Conflict. Clin Infect Dis 16:320–329, 1993.
9. Najera JA: Malaria control: achievements, problems and strategies. Parassitologia 43:1–89, 2001.
10. Singh B, Sung LK, Matusop A, et al: A large focus of naturally acquired *Plasmodium knowlesi* infections in human beings. Lancet 363: 1017–1024, 2004.
11. Beier JC, Davis JR, Vaughan JA, et al: Quantitation of *Plasmodium falciparum* sporozoites transmitted in vitro by experimentally infected *Anopheles gambiae* and *Anopheles stephensi*. Am J Trop Med Hyg 44:564–570, 1991.
12. Fairley NH: Sidelights on malaria in man obtained by subinoculation experiments. Trans R Soc Trop Med Hyg 40:621–676, 1947.
13. Mota MM, Rodriguez A: Migration through host cells: the first steps of Plasmodium sporozoites in the mammalian host. Cell Microbiol 6:1113–1118, 2004.
14. Dame JB, Williams JL, McCutchan TF, et al: Structure of the gene encoding the immunodominant surface antigen on the sporozoite of the human malaria parasite *Plasmodium falciparum*. Science 225:593–599, 1984.
15. Robson KJ, Hall JR, Jennings MW, et al: A highly conserved amino acid sequence in thrombospondin, properdin and in proteins from sporozoites and blood stages of a human malaria parasite. Nature 335:79–82, 1988.
16. Rogers WO, Malik, A., Mellouk S, et al: Characterization of *Plasmodium falciparum* sporozoite surface protein 2. Proc Natl Acad Sci USA 89:9176–9180, 1992.
17. Mota MM, Hafalla JC, Rodriguez A: Migration through host cells activates plasmodium sporozoites for infection. Nat Med 8:1318–1322, 2002.
18. Sim BK, Chitnis CE, Wasniowska K, et al: Receptor and ligand domains for invasion of erythrocytes by *Plasmodium falciparum*: Science 264:1941–1944, 1994.
19. Baruch DI, Pasloske B, Singh HB, et al: Cloning the *P. falciparum* gene encoding PfEMP1, a malarial variant antigen and adherence receptor on the surface of parasitized human erythrocytes. Cell 82:77–87, 1995.
20. Su XZ, Heatwole VM, Wertheimer SP, et al: The large diverse gene family var encodes proteins involved in cytoadherence and antigenic variation of *plasmodium falciparum*–infected erythrocytes. Cell Jul 14; 82:89–100, 1995.
21. Horrocks P, Pinches R, Christodoulou Z, et al: Variable var transition rates underlie antigenic variation in malaria: Proc Natl Acad Sci USA 101:11129–11134, 2004.
22. Krotoski WA, Collins WE, Bray RS, et al: Demonstration of hypnozoites in sporozoite transmitted *Plasmodium vivax* infection. Am J Trop Med Hyg 31:1291–1293, 1982.
23. Krotoski WA: The hypnozoite and malarial relapse. Prog Clin Parasitol 1:1–19, 1989.
24. Malaria Surveillance—United States, 2002. MMWR Surveill Summ 2004 Apr 30;53:21–34, 2002.
25. Miller LH, Mason SJ, Clyde DF, et al: The resistance factor to *Plasmodium vivax* in blacks: The Duffy-Blood-Group Genotype, FyFy. N Engl J Med 295:302–304.
26. Chitnis CE, Miller LH: Identification of the erythrocyte binding domains of *Plasmodium vivax* and *Plasmodium knowlesi* proteins involved in erythrocyte invasion. J Exp Med 180:497–506, 1994.
27. Gardner MJ, Tettelin H, Carucci DJ, et al: Chromosome 2 sequence of the human malaria parasite *Plasmodium falciparum*. Science 282:1126–1132, 1998.
28. Gardner MJ, Hall N, Fung E, et al: Genome sequence of the human malaria parasite *Plasmodium falciparum*. Nature 419:498–511, 2002.
29. Carlton JM, Angiuoli SV, Suh BB, et al: Genome sequence and comparative analysis of the model rodent malaria parasite *Plasmodium yoelii yoelii*. Nature 419:512–519, 2002.
30. Gardner MJ: Parasite Genomics: Microbial Genomes. Totowa, NJ, Humana Press, 2004.
31. Florens L, Washburn MP, Raine JD, et al: A proteomic view of the *Plasmodium falciparum* life cycle. Nature 419:520–526, 2002.
32. Lasonder E, Ishihama Y, Anderson JS, et al: Analysis of the *Plasmodium falciparum* proteome by high-accuracy mass spectrometry. Nature 419:537–542, 2002.
33. Le Roch KG, Zhou Y, Blair PL, et al: Discovery of gene function by expression profiling of the malaria parasite life cycle. Science 301:1503–1508, 2003.
34. Bozdech Z, Zhu J, Joachimiak MP, et al: Expression profiling of the schizont and trophozoite stages of *Plasmodium falciparum* with a long-oligonucleotide microarray. Genome Biol 4:R9, 2003.
35. Snow RW, Craig M, Deichmann U, et al: Estimating mortality, morbidity, and disability due to malaria in Africa's non-pregnant population. Bull World Health Organ 77:624–640, 1999.
36. MacDonald G: The epidemiology and control of malaria. London/New York, Oxford University Press, 1957.
37. Black RH: Manual on epidemiology and epidemiological services in malaria programmes. Geneva, World Health Organization, 1968.
38. Nagel R: Innate resistance to malaria conferred by red cell genetic defects. In Abdalla SH, Pasvol G, Hoffman SL (eds): Malaria: A Hematological Perspective. London, Imperial College Press, 2004, pp 277–315.
39. Bayoumi RA: The sickle cell trait modifies the intensity and specificity of the immune response against *Plasmodium falciparum* malaria and leads to acquired protective immunity. Med Hypotheses 22:287–298, 1987.
40. Rihet P, Flori L, Tall F, et al: Hemoglobin C is associated with reduced *Plasmodium falciparum* parasitemia and low risk of mild malaria attack. Hum Mol Genet 13:1–6, 2004.
41. Baird JK: Age-dependent characteristics of protection v. susceptibility to *Plasmodium falciparum*. Ann Trop Med Parasitol 92:367–390, 1998.
42. Schofield L, Hewitt M, Evans K, et al: Synthetic GPI as a candidate anti-toxic vaccine in a model of malaria. Nature 418:785–789, 2002.
43. Cohen S, McGregor IA, Carrington S: Gamma-globulin and acquired immunity to human malaria. Nature (London) 192:733–737, 1961.
44. Sabchareon AD, Outtara D, Burnouf T, et al: Parasitologic and clinical human response to immunoglobulin administration in falciparum malaria. Am J Trop Med Hyg 45:297–308, 1991.
45. Hill A, Elvin J, Willis AC, et al: Molecular analysis of the association of HLA-B53 and the resistance to severe malaria. Nature (London) 360:434–439, 1992.
46. Baird JK, Owusu AS, Utz GC, et al: Seasonal malaria attack rates in infants and young children in northern Ghana. Am J Trop Med Hyg 66:280–286, 2002.
47. Owusu Agyei S, Koram KA, Baird JK, et al: Incidence of symptomatic and asymtomatic *Plasmodium falciparum* infection following curative therapy in adult residents of northern Ghana. Am J Trop Med Hyg 65:197–203, 2001.
48. Hoffman SL, Oster CN, Plowe CV, et al: Naturally acquired antibodies to sporozoites do not prevent malaria: vaccine development implications. Science 237:639–642, 1987.
49. Beier JC, Oster CN, Onyango FK, et al: *Plasmodium falciparum* incidence relative to entomologic inoculation rates at a site proposed for testing malaria vaccines in western Kenya. Am J Trop Med Hyg 50:529–536, 1994.
50. Phillips-Howard PA, Nahlen BL, Wannemuehler KA, et al: Impact of permethrin-treated bed nets on the incidence of sick child visits to peripheral health facilities. Am J Trop Med Hyg 68:38–43, 2003.
51. Zucker JR, Lackritz EM, Ruebush TK, et al: Childhood mortality during and after hospitalization in western Kenya: effect of malaria treatment regimens. Am J Trop Med Hyg 5:655–660, 1996.
52. Steketee RW, Nahlen BL, Parise ME, et al: The burden of malaria in pregnancy in sub-Saharan Africa. Am J Trop Med Hyg 641(Suppl 2): 28–35, 2001.
53. Kuile FO, Parise ME, Verhoeff FH, et al: The burden of co-infection with human immunodeficiency virus type 1 and malaria in pregnant

women in sub-Saharan Africa. Am J Trop Med Hyg 71(Suppl 2): 41–54, 2004.

54. World Health Organization: Control of Tropical Diseases: Severe and Complicated Malaria, 2nd ed. Trans R Soc Trop Med Hyg 1990; 84(Suppl 2):1–65.
55. Luxemburger C, Ricci F, Nosten F, et al: The epidemiology of severe malaria in an area of low transmission in Thailand. Trans R Soc Trop Med Hyg 91:256–262, 1997.
56. Hoffman SL, Piessens WF, Ratiwayanto S, et al: Reduction of suppressor T lymphocytes in the tropical splenomegaly syndrome. N Engl J Med 310:337–341, 1984.
57. Kwiatkowski D, Hill AVS, Sambou I, et al: TNF concentrations in fatal cerebral, non-fatal cerebral, and uncomplicated *Plasmodium falciparum* malaria. Lancet 336:1201–1204, 1990.
58. Day NPJ, Hien TT, Schollaardt, et al: The prognostic and pathophysiological role of pro- and anti-inflammatory cytokines in severe malaria. J Infect Dis 180:1288–1297, 1999.
59. McGuire W, Hill AV, Allsopp CE, et al: Variation in the TNF-alpha promoter region associated with susceptibility to cerebral malaria. Nature 371:508–510, 1994.
60. Hananantachai H, Patarapotikul J, Looareesuwan S, et al: Lack of association of -308A/G TNFA promoter and 196R/M TNFR2 polymorphisms with disease severity in Thai adult malaria patients. Am J Med Genet 102:391–392, 2001.
61. Silamut K, Phu NH, Whitty C, et al: A quantitative analysis of the microvascular sequestration of malaria parasites in the human brain. Am J Path 155:395–410, 1999.
62. Roberts DJ, Craig AG, Berendt AR, et al: Rapid switching to multiple antigenic and adhesive phenotypes in malaria. Nature 357:689–692, 1992.
63. Barnwell JW, Asch AS, Nachman RL, et al: A human 88-kD membrane glycoprotein (CD36) functions in vitro as a receptor for a cytoadherence ligand on *Plasmodium falciparum* infected erythrocytes. J Clin Invest 84:765–772, 1989.
64. Turner GDH, Morrison H, Jones M, et al: An immunohistochemical study of the pathology of fatal malaria: evidence for widespread endothelial activation and a potential role for intercellular adhesion molecule–1 in cerebral sequestration. Am J Pathol 145:1057–1069, 1994.
65. Yipp BG, Anand S, Schollaardt T, et al: Synergism of multiple adhesion molecules in mediating cytoadherence of *Plasmodium falciparum*–infected erythrocytes to microvascular endothelial cells under flow. Blood 96:2292–2298, 2000.
66. Fried M, Duffy PE: Adherence of *Plasmodium falciparum* to chondroitin sulfate A in the human placenta. Science 272:1502–1504, 1996.
67. Fried M, Nosten F, Brockman A, et al: Maternal antibodies block malaria. Nature 395:851–852, 1998.
68. Udomsangpetch R, Wahlin B, Carlson J, et al: *Plasmodium falciparum*–infected erythrocytes form spontaneous erythrocyte rosettes. J Exp Med 169:1835–1840, 1989.
69. Carlson J, Helmby H, Hill AVS, et al: Human cerebral malaria: association with erythrocyte rosetting and lack of anti-rosetting antibodies. Lancet 336:1457–1460, 1990.
70. Pain A, Ferguson DJ, Kai O, et al: Platelet-mediated clumping of *Plasmodium falciparum*–infected erythrocytes is a common adhesive phenotype and is associated with severe malaria. Proc Natl Acad Sci USA 98:1805–1810, 2001.
71. Dondorp AM, Angus BJ, Hardeman MR, et al: Prognostic significance of reduced red cell deformability in severe falciparum malaria. Am J Trop Med Hyg 57:507–511, 1997.
72. Looareesuwan S, Wilairatana P, Krishna S, et al: Magnetic resonance imaging of the brain in cerebral malaria. Clin Infect Dis 21:300–309, 1995.
73. Newton CR, Peshu N, Kendall B, et al: Brain swelling and ischaemia in Kenyans with cerebral malaria. Arch Dis Child 70:281–287; 1994.
74. Newton CR, Hien TT, White NJ: Cerebral malaria. J Neurol Neurosurg Psychiatry 69:433–441, 2000.
75. Day NP, Phu NH, Mai NT, et al: Effects of dopamine and epinephrine infusions on renal hemodynamics in severe malaria and severe sepsis. Crit Care Med 28:1353–1362, 2000.
76. Charoenpan P, Indraprasit S, Kiatboonsri S, et al: Pulmonary edema in severe falciparum malaria: hemodynamic study and clinicophysiologic correlation. Chest 9:1190–1197, 1990.
77. Sowunmi A, Newton CR, Waruiru C, et al: Arginine vasopressin secretion in Kenyan children with severe malaria. J Trop Pediatr 46:195–199, 2000.
78. Price RN, Simpson J, Nosten F, et al: Factors contributing to anemia in uncomplicated falciparum malaria. Am J Trop Med Hyg 65:614–622, 2001.
79. Skudowitz RB, Katz J, Lurie A, et al: Mechanisms of thrombocytopenia in malignant tertian malaria. BMJ 2:515–518, 1973.
80. Chotivanich K, Udomsangpetch R, Dondorp A, et al: The mechanisms of parasite clearance after antimalarial treatment of *Plasmodium falciparum* malaria. J Infect Dis 182:629–633, 2000.
81. Day NP, Phu NH, Mai NT, et al: The pathophysiologic and prognostic significance of acidosis in severe adult malaria. Crit Care Med 28:1833–1840, 2000.
82. Taylor TE, Borgstein A, Molyneux ME: Acid-base status in paediatric *Plasmodium falciparum* malaria. Q J Med 86 99–109, 1993.
83. Agbenyega T, Angus BJ, Bedu-Addo G, et al: Glucose and lactate kinetics in children with severe malaria. J Clin Endocrinol Metab 85:1569–1576, 2000.
84. White NJ, Warrell DA, Chanthavanich P, et al: Severe hypoglycaemia and hyperinsulinaemia in falciparum malaria. N Engl J Med 309:61–66, 1983.
85. White NJ, Miller KD, Marsh K, et al: Hypoglycaemia in African children with severe malaria. Lancet 1:708–711, 1987.
86. Taylor TE, Molyneux ME, Wirima JJ, et al: Blood glucose levels in Malawian children before and during the administration of intravenous quinine in severe falciparum malaria. N Engl J Med 319:1040–1047, 1988.
87. Brabin BJ: Analysis of malaria in pregnancy in Africa. Bull World Health Organ 61:1005–1016, 1983.
88. Nosten F, McGready R, Simpson JA, et al: The effects of *Plasmodium vivax* malaria in pregnancy. Lancet 354:546–549, 1999.
89. Rickman LS, Long GW, Oberst R, et al: Rapid diagnosis of malaria by acridine orange staining of centrifuged parasites. Lancet 1:68–71, 1989.
90. Schneider P, Wolters L, Schoone G, et al: Real-time nucleic acid sequence-based amplification is more convenient than real-time PCR for quantification of *Plasmodium falciparum*. J Clin Microbiol 43:402–405, 2005.
91. Shiff CJ, Minjas J, Premji Z: The ParaSight(R)-F test: a simple rapid manual dipstick test to detect *Plasmodium falciparum* infection. Parasitol Today 10:494–495, 1994.
92. Beadle C, Long GW, Weiss WR, et al: Diagnosis of malaria by detection of *Plasmodium falciparum* HRP-2 antigen with a rapid dipstick antigen-capture assay. Lancet 343:564–568, 1994.
93. Piper R, Lebras J, Wentworth L, et al: Immunocapture diagnostic assays for malaria using *Plasmodium* lactate dehydrogenase (pLDH). Am J Trop Med Hyg 60:109–118, 1999.
94. Field JW, Niven JC: A note on prognosis in relation to parasite counts in acute subtertian malaria. Trans R Soc Trop Med Hyg 30:569–574, 1939.
95. Silamut K, White NJ: The relationship of stage of parasite development to prognosis in falciparum malaria. Trans R Soc Trop Med Hyg 87:436–443, 1993.
96. Phu NH, Day NPJ, Diep TS, et al: Intraleukocytic malaria pigment and prognosis in severe malaria. Trans R Soc Trop Med Hyg 89:197–199, 1995.
97. Nosten F, van Vugt M, Price R, et al: Effects of artesunate-mefloquine combination on incidence of *Plasmodium.falciparum* malaria and mefloquine resistance in western Thailand: a prospective study Lancet 356:297–302, 2000.
98. White NJ: Assessment of the pharmacodynamic properties of the antimalarial drugs in vivo. Antimicrob Agents Chemother 41:1413–1422, 1997.
99. Nosten F, ter Kuile FO, Luxemburger C, et al: Cardiac effects of antimalarial treatment with halofantrine. Lancet 341:1054–1056, 1993.
100. Trape JF: The public health impact of chloroquine resistance in Africa. Am J Trop Med Hyg 64(Suppl 1–2):12–17, 2001.
101. Murphy GS, Basri H, Purnomo, et al: Vivax malaria resistant to treatment and prophylaxis with chloroquine. Lancet 341:96–100, 1993.
102. Baird JK, Leksana B, Masbar S, et al: Diagnosis of resistance to chloroquine by *Plasmodium vivax*: timing of recurrence and whole blood chloroquine levels. Am J Trop Med Hyg 56:621–626, 1997.
103. Baird JK, Basri H, Subianto B, et al: Treatment of chloroquine-resistant *Plasmodium vivax* with chloroquine and primaquine or halofantrine. J Infect Dis 171:1678–1682, 1995.
104. Maguire JD, Sumawinata IW, Masbar S, et al: Chloroquine-resistant *Plasmodium malariae* in south Sumatra, Indonesia. Lancet 360:58–60, 2002.

105. Lacy MD, Maguire JD, Barcus MJ, et al: Atovaquone/proguanil therapy for *Plasmodium falciparum* and *Plasmodium vivax* malaria in Indonesians who lack clinical immunity. Clin Infect Dis 35:e92–e95, 2002.
106. Baird JK, Hoffman SL: Primaquine therapy for malaria. Clin Infect Dis 39:1336–1345, 2004.
107. Newton CR, Chokwe T, Schellenberg JA, et al: Coma scales for children with severe falciparum malaria. Trans R Soc Trop Med Hyg 91:161–165, 1997.
108. Artemether–Quinine Meta-analysis Study Group: A meta-analysis using individual patient data of trials comparing artemether with quinine in the treatment of severe falciparum malaria. Trans R Soc Trop Med Hyg 95:637–650, 2001.
109. Hien TT, Arnold K, Vinh H, et al: Comparison of artemisinin suppositories with intravenous artesunate and intravenous quinine in the treatment of cerebral malaria. Trans R Soc Trop Med Hyg 86:582–583, 1992.
110. Phuong CXT, Bethell DB, Phuong PT, et al: Comparison of artemisinin suppositories, intramuscular artesunate, and intravenous quinine for the treatment of severe childhood malaria. Trans R Soc Trop Med Hyg 91:335–342, 1997.
111. Nosten F, van Vugt M, White NJ: Intrarectal artemisinin derivatives. Med Trop (Mars) 58(Suppl 3):63–64, 1998.
112. Baird JK, Fryauff DJ, Hoffman SL: Primaquine for prevention of malaria in travelers. Clin Infect Dis 37:1659–1667, 2003.
113. Hale BR, Owusu-Agyei S, Fryauff DJ, et al: A randomized, double-blind, placebo-controlled, dose-ranging trial of tafenoquine for weekly prophylaxis against *Plasmodium falciparum*. Clin Infect Dis 36:541–549, 2003.
114. Ling J, Baird JK, Fryauff DJ, et al: Randomized, placebo-controlled trial of atovaquone/proguanil for the prevention of *Plasmodium falciparum* or *Plasmodium vivax* malaria among migrants to Papua, Indonesia. Clin Infect Dis 35:825–833, 2002.
115. Fryauff DJ, Baird JK, Basri H, et al: Randomised placebo-controlled trial of primaquine for prophylaxis of falciparum and vivax malaria. Lancet 346:1190–1193, 1995.
116. National Center for Infectious Diseases: Traveler's Health. Available at http://www.cdc.gov/travel/. Accessed 5/15/05.
117. Alonso PL, Lindsay SW, Armstrong JRM, et al: The effect of insecticide-treated bed nets on mortality of Gambian children. Lancet 337:1499–1502, 1991.
118. Lengeler C: Insecticide-treated bednets and curtains for preventing malaria (Cochrane Review). In The Cochrane Library, Issue 2, 2003. Oxford: Update Sofware.
119. Roll Back Malaria Partnership: RBM Consensus Statement on Insecticide Treated Netting. March 2004. Available at http://rbm.who.int/partnership/wg/wg_itn/docs/RBMWINStatement Vector.pdf. Accessed 2/14/05.
120. Goodman CA, Coleman P, Mills A: Cost effectiveness of malaria control in sub-Saharan Africa. Lancet 354:378–385, 1999.
121. Parise ME, Ayisi JG, Nahlen BL, et al: Efficacy of sulfadoxine-pyrimethamine for prevention of placental malaria in an area of Kenya with a high prevalence of malaria and human immunodeficiency virus infection. Am J Trop Med Hyg 59:813–822, 1998.
122. Kayentao K, Kodio M, Newman RD, et al: Comparison of intermittent preventive treatment with chemoprophylaxis for the prevention of malaria during pregnancy in Mali. J Infect Dis 191:109–116, 2005.
123. Hoffman SL (ed): Malaria Vaccine Development: A Multi-Immune Response Approach. Washington, DC, ASM Press, 1996.
124. Richie TL, Saul A: Progress and challenges for malaria vaccines. Nature 415:694–701, 2002.
125. Long CA, Hoffman SL: Parasitology. Malaria—from infants to genomics to vaccines. Science 297:345–347, 2002.
126. Hoffman SL: Save the children. Nature 430:2–3, 2004.
127. Hoffman SL, Goh LM, Luke TC, et al: Protection of humans against malaria by immunization with radiation-attenuated *Plasmodium falciparum* sporozoites. J Infect Dis 185:1155–1164, 2002.
128. Luke TC, Hoffman SL: Rationale and plans for developing a non-replicating, metabolically active, radiation-attenuated *Plasmodium falciparum* sporozoite vaccine. J Exp Biol 206:3803–3808, 2003.
129. World Health Organization: Immunizations, Vaccines and Biologicals. Available at http://www.who.int/vaccines/en/aboutus.shtml. Accessed 2/14/05.
130. Dame JB, Williams JL, McCutchan TF, et al: Structure of the gene encoding the immunodominant surface antigen on the sporozoites of the human malaria parasite *Plasmodium falciparum*. Science 225:593–599, 1984.
131. Stoute JA, Slaoui M, Heppner DG, et al: A preliminary evaluation of a recombinant circumspzorozoite protein vaccine against *Plasmodium falciparum* malaria. N Engl J Med 336:86–91, 1997.
132. Kester KE, McKinney DA, Tornieporth N, et al: RTS,S Malaria Vaccine Evaluation Group. Efficacy of recombinant circumsporozoite protein vaccine regimens against experimental *Plasmodium falciparum* malaria. J Infect Dis 183:640–647, 2001.
133. Alonso P, Sacarlal J, Aponte JJ, et al: Efficacy of the RTS,S/AS02 vaccine against *Plasmodium falciparum* infection and disease in young African children: randomised controlled trial. Lancet 364:1411–1420, 2004.
134. Hoffman SL, Subramanian GM, Collins FH, Venter JC: *Plasmodium*, human and *Anopheles* genomics and malaria. Nature 415:702–709, 2002.

91

Babesiosis

SAM R. TELFORD III
JAMES H. MAGUIRE

INTRODUCTION

Babesiosis, a tick-borne malaria-like zoonosis, appears to have plagued humans since antiquity in its veterinary form. "Behold, the hand of the Lord is upon thy cattle. ... [They] shall be afflicted with a grievous murrain" (Exodus 9) may refer to red-water fever due to *Babesia bovis.* Human babesiosis has been reported mainly from Europe and the eastern or western United States and, recently, from subtropical areas such as Taiwan, the Canary Islands, and South Africa. The prevalence of babesiosis afflicting domestic animals in tropical regions suggests that human infection is not rare in the tropics and perhaps is mistaken for falciparum malaria.[1]

AGENT

History and Taxonomy

The genus *Babesia* is named after the Romanian bacteriologist Victor Babes, who in 1888 attributed "hemoglobinuric fever" of cattle to inclusions he detected within erythrocytes. Subsequently, these organisms were determined to be distinct from plasmodia and other coccidia and were assigned to the suborder Piroplasmidea on the basis of their erythrocytic localization, replication by budding rather than schizogony, and inability to produce hemozoin.[2] Currently, they are classified as apicomplexans of the order Piroplasmidora and family Babesiidae.[3] More than 100 species of *Babesia* have been described from domestic and wild mammals on the basis of morphology and life cycle.[3] Molecular taxonomic analyses suggest that there is even greater diversity than what has previously been recognized.[4–7] The powerful new methods of molecular phylogenetics will eventually stimulate the development of a new classification for the piroplasms, but such an action is currently premature inasmuch as life cycle information is lacking for a large proportion of currently recognized taxa.

Life Cycle

In 1893, Theobald Smith[8] described the life cycle of *Babesia bigemina*, the agent of bovine red-water fever, and in doing so demonstrated for the first time transmission of an infectious agent by arthropods. All piroplasms for which the life cycle has been described require a tick as the definitive host. On ingestion of infectious blood from a vertebrate host, babesiae undergo syngamy and replicate in the intestinal epithelium of the tick vector and develop further in the salivary glands, ovaries, and other tissues. Sporozoites in the salivary glands are deposited in the skin of a vertebrate host during the tick's blood meal. Because of transstadial transmission, ticks infected as larvae generally remain infected as nymphs and adults. Transovarial transmission in the tick has been documented for some species, such as *B. bigemina*, but not for others, such as *Babesia microti*; such a major life history difference has long been considered to represent a significant phylogenetic divergence.

The common belief that sporozoites enter erythrocytes directly (no pre-erythrocytic phase) has not been critically examined. Exoerythrocytic forms have been demonstrated in

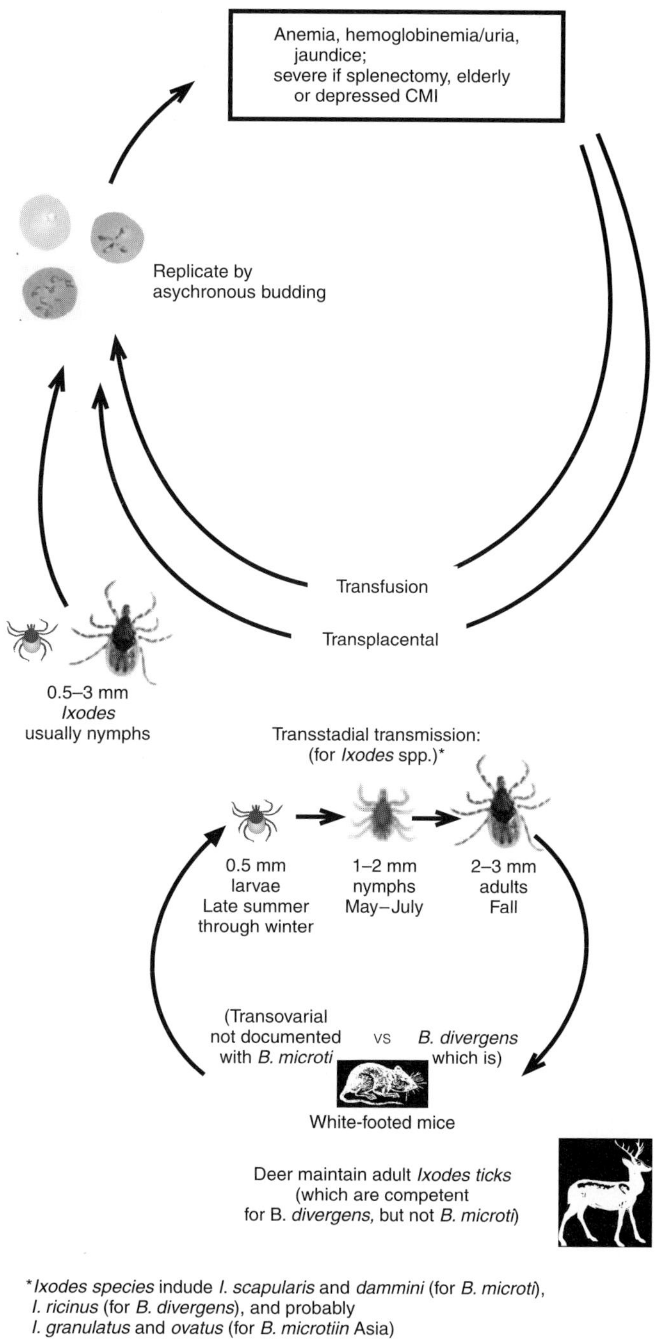

the lymphocytes with *Babesia equi* and the closely related *Theileria* species[9,10] and may occur in infections with *B. microti*.[10] The process by which the extracellular merozoite invades erythrocytes (induced endocytosis) is similar to that of the plasmodia. In the rat babesia, *Babesia rodhaini*, complement appears to facilitate invasion by modification of either the red blood cell surface or that of the merozoite.[11]

Following entry into the erythrocyte, the pear-shaped trophozoites (piroplasms) replicate by asynchronous budding rather than by schizogony, as occurs in malarial parasites. During replication, double-membraned segments develop and pinch off from the parental piroplasm, resulting in both asexually reproducing merozoites and "accordion"-like non-replicating sexual parasites (gametocytes[12]). Asexual forms appear as simple rings, pairs, or tetrads and are difficult to distinguish from sexual stages by light microscopy.

EPIDEMIOLOGY

Two major epidemiologic patterns of human babesiosis are apparent. The first involves splenectomized or otherwise compromised persons and diverse babesiae, some of which have been distinguished only by molecular phylogenetic methods. A bovine-infecting species identified as *Babesia bovis* (perhaps conspecific with *Babesia divergens*[13]) was the cause of the first convincingly documented case of human babesial infection in 1957. The patient, a 33-year-old splenectomized farmer living in Yugoslavia and who had been exposed to cattle, died as a result of hemolytic anemia, hemoglobinuria, and renal failure.[14] Since then, more than two dozen sporadic cases have been reported from Ireland, Yugoslavia, France, the British Isles, Spain, the Canary Islands, Portugal, Germany, Sweden, and Russia.[15] All were severe and many were fatal despite treatment. The vector is *Ixodes ricinus*, which also transmits Lyme disease, granulocytic ehrlichiosis, and tick-borne encephalitis; to date, the only known reservoirs of *B. divergens* other than ticks are cattle and reindeer.

In 1992, a splenectomized man living in rural Missouri and with unspecified exposure history died of infection with a parasite closely related to if not conspecific with *B. divergens*, designated MO-1.[16] A splenectomized Kentucky resident who had been exposed while hunting rabbits recovered from a similar infection in 2001[17]; sequencing of a large portion of the 18S rDNA demonstrated virtual identity (99.8%) with sequences of bovine-derived *B. divergens* and 100% identity with an agent maintained among cottontail rabbits by *Ixodes dentatus*.[18] Accordingly, this infection appears to be due to exposure to *I. dentatus* or to rabbit blood. A third case was reported in a splenectomized resident of Washington state.[19] Although the degree of DNA sequence similarity between the U.S. divergens-like parasites and the European cattle parasites is within that which might be expected due to geographic variation of a single species, the former fails to propagate by subinoculation into gerbils, whereas the latter readily does so. Accordingly, molecular phylogenetic data must be complemented with additional life history data, in particular cattle inoculation to demonstrate the development of typical bovine red water, prior to concluding identity. Although European "divergens babesiosis" has heretofore been solely attributed to infection by *B. divergens*, molecular analysis suggests that another closely related babesia, designated EU-1[20] and perhaps representing *Babesia capreoli* (an agent maintained by *I. ricinus* among red or roe deer[21,22]), also parasitizes humans and could be mistaken by inexperienced microscopists for *B. divergens* infection. Thus, it appears that divergens babesiosis may be due to diverse parasites that are geographically widespread.

A variation on this epidemiologic pattern has emerged along the Pacific Coast of the United States. The agent WA-1 is closely related by DNA sequencing to the canine pathogen *Babesia gibsoni*.[23,24] CA-type (DNA sequences designated CA-1, CA-2, etc.) agents[25] are most closely related to parasites of mule deer and bighorn sheep.[6] Both agents cause a similar disease and appear morphologically indistinguishable on blood smears, with abundant Maltese-cross forms within parasitized erythrocytes. Of seven reported cases of WA-1 or CA-type babesiosis, four occurred among people who had undergone splenectomy, and one involved an apparently healthy 41-year-old man. The others were transfusion-induced cases involving a spleen-intact elderly man with multiple medical problems[26] and a premature infant.[27] It appears that most infections are subclinical because surveys have shown a seroprevalence of 3.5% to 20% among people with exposure in rural and semirural areas of California.[28] As with *B. divergens*, splenectomized or otherwise compromised individuals appear to suffer pathology; cases are sporadic.

The second major epidemiologic pattern is that of endemic infection due to the widely distributed rodent piroplasm *B. microti*.[29] The risk of human infection with this organism is not increased in the absence of a spleen, although infected people without spleens are at high risk of becoming severely ill. The global distribution of *B. microti* parallels that of *Borrelia burgdorferi* and other agents transmitted by ticks in the *Ixodes persulcatus* species complex.[30] Human babesiosis due to *B. microti* has been reported from Taiwan and Japan.[31,32] A report of *B. microti* babesiosis in a Swiss patient[33] should be considered inconclusive: The photomicrographs from the patient's blood smear appear to demonstrate platelets as opposed to parasites, and associated laboratory tests (serology and polymerase chain reaction) were conflicting. It is likely, however, that *B. microti* is zoonotic in Europe: A mild self-limited febrile case in a German forest worker was anecdotally reported in the caption of a photomicrograph of this parasite from this patient's blood smear.[34]

In the United States, *B. microti* babesiosis remains limited to the terminal moraine islands of New York, Massachusetts, and Rhode Island and focal areas in Connecticut, New Jersey, Wisconsin, and Minnesota.[35] Because most cases are asymptomatic or mildly symptomatic, the incidence is difficult to estimate and differs from year to year due to fluctuations in the densities of the rodent reservoir and tick vectors. Although there have been only several hundred reported cases of symptomatic infection with *B. microti* since the first reported case in 1969, serologic surveys indicate that in highly endemic areas as many as 9% to 21% of people have been infected.[36] The incidence of babesiosis has been increasing in areas of southern New England since the 1990s, and on Block Island, Rhode Island, there may be as many as 900 cases per 100,000 residents per year.[37] There have been more than 40 cases of babesiosis acquired from blood products from asymptomatically infected donors,[38] most commonly packed red blood cells but also platelets and frozen-deglycerolized red blood cells,[39] and one case of vertically transmitted infection.[40]

Few cases of babesiosis have been reported outside the United States and Europe. There have been isolated case reports demonstrating active infection (publication of a photomicrograph of a blood smear) in China[41] and South Africa[42] and serosurveys suggesting human babesial infection in Latin America and West Africa. Because of the ubiquity of ticks and the diversity of *Babesia* species and animal hosts, it is likely that transmission to human beings occurs in tropical areas. Some cases of presumed chloroquine-resistant malaria infections may have represented cases of babesiosis because of the difficulty in distinguishing between immature plasmodial and babesial trophozoites in blood smears, and *Babesia* are poorly susceptible to chloroquine.[1]

Seasonality and Ecology

Human *B. divergens* cases occur mainly in cattle-raising regions during summer months when the presumed vector, *I. ricinus*, is most active and the incidence of red water fever in cattle is greatest.[15] The only known reservoir hosts for *B. divergens* are cattle and reindeer. The American *B. divergens*-like agent (MO-1) is most likely transmitted by *I. dentatus*.[18] Although long thought to be specific for rabbits and birds, this tick appears to feed on humans more frequently than appreciated.[43] Approximately 2% of host-seeking adult *I. dentatus* and 11% to 29% of rabbits were found to be infected during a 5-year study on Nantucket Island. Rabbits were more likely to be actively infected during the fall or spring months, coinciding with the activity of larvae or adults, respectively.[18] Such a pattern is suggestive of maintenance by transovarial transmission, thought to be a main mode of perpetuation for *B. divergens* in the European *I. ricinus*.[15] *Babesia capreoli* (?EU-1) is maintained by *I. ricinus*, probably with roe and red deer as amplifying hosts.[22]

The few reported cases of WA-1 and CA-type babesiosis had their onset between June and August. Vectors and reservoirs remain to be described, although canids, ungulates, and their associated ticks are suspected given the genetic relatedness of these agents to *B. gibsoni* and the mule deer or bighorn sheep babesias, respectively.[6]

In contrast, the ecology of *B. microti* has been well studied.[44] Its enzootic cycle in the northern United States depends on the interaction of subadult deer ticks, *Ixodes dammini* (thought by some to be a variant of *Ixodes scapularis*) and their main source of blood meals, the white-footed mouse (*Peromyscus leucopus*). Deer (*Odocoileus virginianus*) are the hosts on which adult ticks primarily feed, but they are incompetent reservoirs. Adult ticks feed during the autumn and lay eggs during the spring. The eggs hatch in late July, and the emergent larvae feed mainly during August and September, at which time they may acquire babesial infection from an infected mouse. Fed larvae overwinter and molt to the nymphal stage during the spring. The life cycle of the tick is complete when nymphs that have fed on a mouse or other host during the summer molt to the adult stage in the fall.

Humans become infected primarily by the nymphal ticks (Fig. 91-1) rather than adults because survival of *B. microti* during the nymphal to adult tick molt is poor.[45] In addition, people are likely to discover the large adult deer tick and remove it before the tick has fed long enough to deliver an infectious inoculum of sporozoites. Accordingly, in more than 80% of reported cases, the onset of illness occurred between May and August, when nymphs are most abundant.[46]

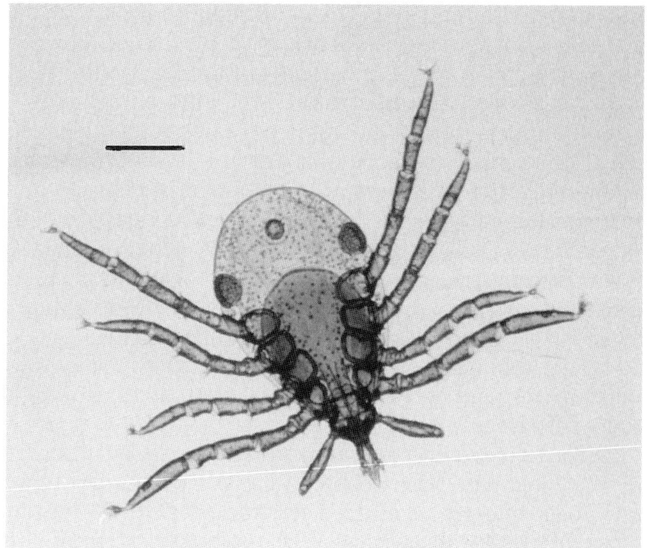

FIGURE 91-1 Nonfed nymphal deer tick, *Ixodes dammini*. (Cleared and mounted in Berlese's fluid; bar = 595 μm.)

In Taiwan and Japan, the zoonotic vectors of *B. microti* remain to be described, although *Ixodes granulatus* and *Ixodes ovatus* have been found to be infected (personal communications, C. M. Shih, National Defense University, Taipei, 2002; and Masayoshi Tsuji, Rakuno-Gakuen University, Hokkaido, 2003). Various small rodents (*Apodemus* spp. and *Rattus* spp.) are frequently parasitised.[47,48] *Babesia microti* appears to be part of a characteristic microbial assemblage with the agents of Lyme disease, granulocytic ehrlichiosis, and tick-borne encephalitis virus throughout the Holarctic, and therefore knowledge of the life cycle of any one of the assemblage provides basic information about those of the other three.[30,49]

PATHOGENESIS AND IMMUNITY

Lysis of parasitized erythrocytes leads to anemia, hemogloblinemia, hyperbilirubinemia, and, in severe cases, intense jaundice, massive hemogloblinuria, and renal shutdown. Electron microscopy shows parasite-mediated damage to the erythrocyte membrane with perforations, protrusions, and inclusions.[50,51] There is reduced deformability of infected red blood cells that enhances their removal by the spleen. In experimental *B. bovis* infections, increased peroxidation of membrane lipids appears to be responsible for a further decrease in erythrocyte survival and adherence of infected red blood cells to the endothelium of small blood vessels.[52]

In several of the European cases, autopsy showed parasites in erythrocytes in congested capillaries of various organs, especially the sinusoids of the liver.[53,54] Other findings in these cases and in fatal cases due to *B. microti* suggest a cytokine-mediated shock syndrome. Indeed, laboratory studies of rodents infected by *B. microti* or WA-1 clearly demonstrate overproduction of the proinflammatory mediators tumor necrosis factor-α (TNF-α) and interferon-γ.[55] Mice with a genetic disruption in the TNF-α pathway were less likely to die of fulminating WA-1 infection, as were CD4 and CD8 gene knockout mice, whereas in γδ T-cell knockout mice and control mice WA-1 infection terminated fatally. Thus, CD8+T cells may contribute to the WA1-induced pathology.[55] In addition, depletion of macrophages and natural killer cells seems to increase susceptibility.[56] Acute tubular necrosis, ischemic necrosis of liver, spleen, pancreas, and heart, noncardiac pulmonary edema, and swelling and congestion of the brain and other organs have been demonstrated, even in cases in which parasites had been cleared by treatment.[57] Other findings at autopsy have included hemophagocytosis, hypercellularity of the bone marrow, extramedullary hematopoiesis, and hemosiderin deposits in the Kupffer cells and the kidneys, which correspond to findings in histopathologic studies of rodent infections.[58,59]

Asplenia, advanced age, and depressed cellular immunity are associated with severe clinical illness.[60,61] The spleen traps and phagocytoses parasitized erythrocytes, thus limiting parasitemia, particularly early in the infection. Nevertheless, people with intact spleens have died of overwhelming infections, and people without spleens have recovered from babesiosis, even without specific therapy.[61] The severity of illness is greater in people older than 5 years than in younger adults, and overt illness in children seems unusual.[36] As a rule, younger people who become ill are asplenic or immunocompromised or have other underlying medical conditions.[62]

Babesia microti infections may be particularly severe in people who are infected with human immunodeficiency virus (HIV) or are receiving corticosteroids or other immunosuppressive therapy.[63] Similarly, hamsters that receive antilymphocyte serum and athymic mice experience high parasitemias and mortality when exposed to *B. microti*.[64,65] CD4 gene knockout mice sustained *B. microti* parasitemias for longer periods of time than did congeneic controls.[55] Humoral immunity appears to be less important than cellular immunity in controlling infection. Passive transfer of immune serum to immunodeficient severe combined immunodeficiency (SCID) and nude mice fails to protect them from *B. microti* infection.[66] B cell-deficient mice remain less susceptible to *B. microti* infection, whereas T-cell receptor–deficient mice are readily infected.[67] Antibody titers are generally high when *B. microti* patients present to the clinic, but the magnitude of the titer is not inversely related to parasitemia (S.R.T., unpublished results, 1997). Whether sterilizing immunity develops is questionable; premunition, first described in Theobald Smith's seminal report,[8] may be axiomatic with babesial infections. Human infection may last more than 1 year, even in the absence of underlying illness.[68] Reinfection has not been reported and would be difficult to distinguish from recrudescence of an earlier infection.

DISEASE

Depending on the species of babesia and host factors, infection can be subclinical, cause a self-limited febrile illness, produce a moderate to severe illness resembling malaria, or progress rapidly to death. Infection with *B. divergens* occurs almost always in splenectomized people and runs a fulminant and usually fatal course without treatment.[15] After an incubation period of 1 to 4 weeks, patients infected with *B. divergens* become acutely ill with high fever, prostration, rigors, diaphoresis, headache, myalgia, jaundice, and hemogloblinuria. Nausea, vomiting, and diarrhea are prominent, and the liver may be enlarged and painful. Most patients develop acute respiratory distress. Renal failure induced by intravascular hemolysis and hypotension ensues and is followed by coma and death, usually within 1 week of onset of symptoms. The three patients with the U.S. divergens-like infection, one of whom died, presented with fever, headache, and rigors; thrombocytopenia, hemoglobinuria, and proteinuria were noted.

Most infections with *B. microti* are subclinical, and available data suggest the same for babesiosis due to WA-1 or CA-1. Subclinical infections have been detected during serosurveys and investigation of blood donors following transfusion-induced cases.[26,27,69] Parasites are not seen in blood smears, but have been isolated by animal inoculation in a small percentage of asymptomatic people with positive serologic tests for antibodies to *Babesia*.[27,36] Subpatent parasitemia in the absence of symptoms may last more than 1 year.[70]

Because of the small number of reported cases, the spectrum of illness among people with clinically apparent WA-1 or CA-type infection remains to be defined. Four of seven people with symptomatic infections had been splenectomized. These included two patients who had severe disease with high parasitemia and multisystem organ failure, one of whom died.[25] The index case—a healthy, spleen-intact man—had a moderately severe illness with a 3% parasitemia, high fever, and a slow recovery.[23] A similar illness occurred in an elderly man with multiple medical problems who acquired infection from a blood transfusion.[26]

People with symptomatic *B. microti* infections typically experience an influenza-like illness 1 to 4 weeks after a tick bite or 4 to 9 weeks following transfusion. There is a gradual onset of malaise, anorexia, and fatigue followed within 1 week by sustained or intermittent fever as high as 40°C, drenching sweats, and myalgia.[69] Nausea, vomiting, headache, shaking chills, dark urine, emotional lability, and depression are not uncommon.[71] Physical examination may show mild splenomegaly and, less often, hepatomegaly. Most patients have mild to moderate anemia; thrombocytopenia; a normal or depressed white blood cell count; mildly elevated hepatic enzymes; and evidence of hemolysis, including hyperbilirubinemia, elevated serum lactic dehydrogenase, and decreased haptoglobin levels. Parasitemias may range from 1% to 20% in spleen-intact people.

After several days to several weeks, fever and more intense symptoms may resolve spontaneously, but weakness, malaise, and fatigue persist for months.[71] In other people, largely the elderly, those without spleens, and those who are immunosuppressed or have other underlying medical problems, illness can be severe, with intense hemolysis leading to jaundice, severe anemia, and renal failure. Parasitemias can reach 85% in asplenic patients.[50] Severe pancytopenia in some cases is due to hemophagocytosis.[72] Disseminated intravascular coagulation, hypotension, and adult respiratory distress syndrome have been seen in fatal cases. Noncardiac pulmonary edema, occasionally requiring mechanical ventilation, may also occur in people with less severe illness several days after beginning therapy.[73] In a series from New York State of 136 patients with babesiosis due to *B. microti*, mortality was 5% despite treatment.[60] Babesiosis in people with acquired immunodeficiency syndrome (AIDS) is characterized by its prolonged duration and frequent relapses. There have been five reports of *B. microti* infection in people with advanced HIV infection.[63,74–77] Two people who had been splenectomized had parasitemias in excess of 40% and more severe illness than the three who were spleen intact, who had up to 20% parasitemia. Recrudescences occurred in four patients and lasted as long as 400 days after the initial episode; further recurrences were prevented by continual administration of antimicrobial agents.

People with *B. microti* infection who are coinfected with *Borrelia burgdorferi* experience more symptoms and longer duration of illness than people infected with either organism alone.[78] In a fatal case of a man with coexistent babesiosis and Lyme disease, the cause of death appeared to be related to pancarditis caused by the Lyme disease spirochete.[79] Another man with coinfection developed a more severe case of transverse myelitis than that which is seen with Lyme disease alone.[80] Coinfection with *B. microti* and *Ehrlichia chaffeensis* led to multiorgan failure and death in an 85-year-old man.[81] Antibodies to *Anaplasma phagocytophilum* have been demonstrated in people with babesiosis or antibodies to *B. microti*, but it is not clear that the infections occurred simultaneously.[82] The differential diagnosis for babesiosis includes other tick-borne diseases, including Lyme disease, ehrlichiosis, typhoidal tularemia, and Rocky Mountain spotted fever, all of which may be endemic in the same region, as occurs in New England. *Borrelia burgdorferi* or the agent of human granulocytic ehrlichiosis may be carried simultaneously by a tick carrying *B. microti* and may coinfect a person with babesiosis.[83,84] Other illnesses that may be confused with babesiosis include viral hepatitis, bacterial sepsis, infectious mononucleosis, leptospirosis, malaria, and relapsing fever.

DIAGNOSIS

The nonspecific symptoms and absence of a history of a tick bite in most cases preclude the ability to make a diagnosis of babesiosis on clinical grounds alone. The definitive diagnosis usually follows demonstration of organisms parasitizing erythrocytes on conventional Giemsa-stained thin films. The small nucleus of *Babesia* can be difficult to identify on thick films, particularly when parasitemia is sparse.

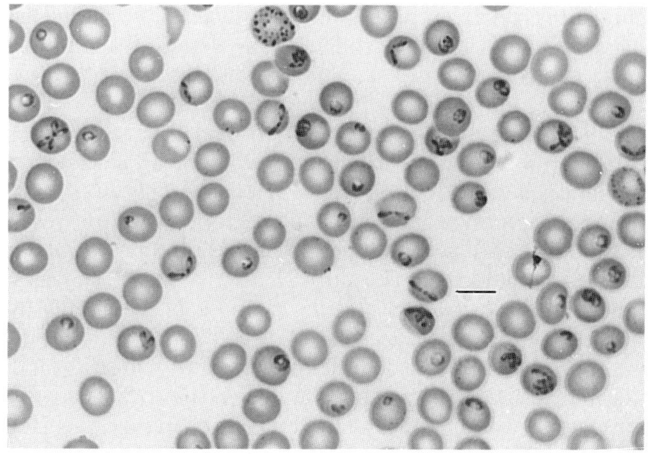

FIGURE 91-3 *Babesia divergens,* gerbil. Pyriform doublets extending across the diameter of the red blood cell, robust ring forms, and Maltese crosses may be found concurrently. (Bar = 6.7 μm.)

Sequential blood smears may be required to detect organisms when the level of parasitemia is low.

Babesia is distinguished on blood smear from *Plasmodium falciparum* by a combination of criteria, including the demonstration of basket-shaped and frequently extracellular merozoites (Fig. 91-2), red blood cells containing four or more parasites, and the presence of tetrad forms (Maltese crosses). Tetrad forms, however, are rarely encountered with *B. microti* infection, in contrast to acute *B. divergens* (Fig. 91-3) and WA-1 (Fig. 91-4) infections, in which they are frequent. The absence of hemozoin (malarial pigment) is considered diagnostic for the piroplasms, but early ring stages of the plasmodia also lack pigment. *Babesia divergens* and related infections may be identified by the presence of accole forms and paired divergent pyriforms occupying no more than 20% to 25% of the erythrocyte area, along with small single oval or round merozoites; high parasitemias are often apparent.

Serologic testing is useful, particularly in diagnosing chronic *B. microti* and WA-1 infections in which the parasitemia is subpatent. The indirect fluorescent antibody test

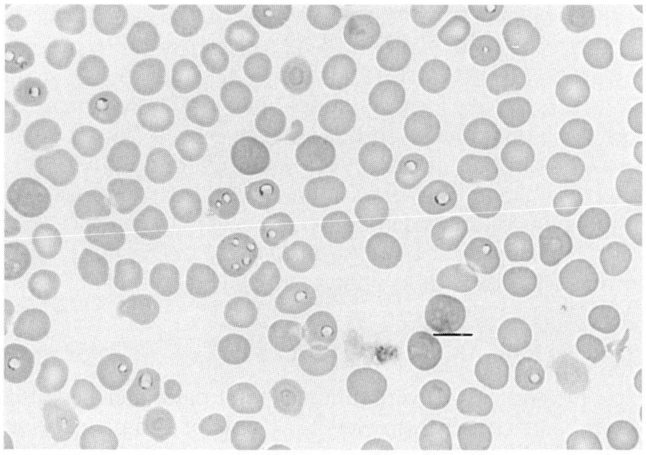

FIGURE 91-2 *Babesia microti,* hamster. Note multiple rings within single erythrocytes, incomplete closure of rings, and chromatin that extends along the margin of the ring as opposed to being distinctly punctate as in *Plasmodium falciparum.* (Bar = 9.3 μm.)

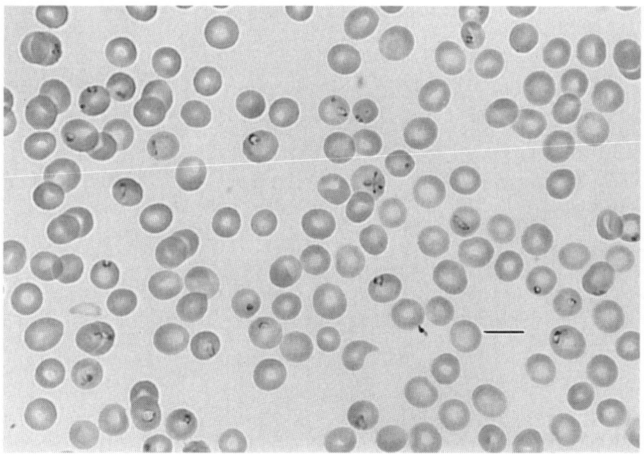

FIGURE 91-4 *Babesia gibsoni* (WA-1), hamster. Rings are smaller and more delicate than in *Babesia microti;* Maltese cross forms are commonly observed. (Bar = 7.5 μm.)

using antigen derived from infected hamster red blood cells[85] is sensitive and specific, and it is the serologic method of choice. Indeed, in cases in which parasitemia is difficult to detect, detection of specific immunoglobulin M (IgM) confirms a clinical diagnosis of babesiosis.[86] Absence or low titers of specific antibodies against *B. microti* when blood smears contain parasites suggests an infection by another *Babesia* sp. or an immunocompromised patient (splenectomy, HIV, or recent infusion of anti-B-cell antibody). Because specific antibodies do not become detectable until at least 1 week after onset of illness, serology is not reliable for diagnosis of the rapidly fulminating *B. divergens* babesiosis.[15]

Subinoculation of a sample of blood into hamsters facilitates diagnosis of *B. microti* infection when smears are negative. Approximately 300 parasites are sufficient to induce persistent parasitemia, which becomes detectable between 1 and 6 weeks following inoculation. *Babesia divergens* can be isolated by inoculation of gerbils, but this procedure is only useful for confirming the diagnosis of this rapidly progressive infection in retrospect. Polymerase chain reaction (PCR)-based assays, which can detect *Babesia* DNA corresponding to three parasites in a 100-μL sample of blood, have the advantage of yielding a diagnosis in less than 1 day.[87] In addition, sequencing of the amplification products may provide more rapid specific identification than immunological analysis or animal inoculation studies when the identity of the infecting parasite is questioned.

TREATMENT AND PROGNOSIS

The combination of quinine (650 mg orally three times daily and clindamycin either 1.2 g intravenously twice daily or 600 mg orally three times a day) can be used to treat babesiosis due to all species.[88,89] The pediatric doses are quinine 25 mg/kg/day and clindamycin 20 to 40 mg/kg/day, both in three divided doses.[88] Treatment should be continued for at least 7 days or until parasitemia remits. Although an in vitro analysis of drug efficacy against *B. divergens* suggested that quinine has poor antibabesial activity[90] and therefore clindamycin alone (which demonstrated significantly greater activity) may be used to treat cases of divergens babesiosis,[91] without experimental trials in animals confirming this assertion such a course of action cannot be recommended. In particularly severe cases of *B. divergens* babesiosis, complete blood exchange transfusion (two or three blood volumes) should be undertaken, followed by treatment with clindamycin and quinine.[92] Because *B. divergens* parasitemias increase very rapidly, any case of babesiosis acquired in Europe should be regarded as an emergency requiring prompt treatment and frequent monitoring of blood smears.

Babesiosis due to WA-1 appears to respond to the combination of quinine and clindamycin, but the small number of cases that have been treated to date does not permit strong conclusions about the efficacy of this regimen. Because illness due to *B. microti* is often mild and short-lived, not all cases require treatment. For people with *B. microti* infections that are non-life-threatening, the combination of atovaquone and azithromycin may be used. A prospective randomized trial demonstrated that patients treated with atovaquone (750 mg orally every 12 hours for 7 days) and azithromycin (500 mg orally on day 1, then 250 to 600 mg/day for 7 days) cleared parasitemia as effectively as did those receiving clindamycin and quinine, with fewer side effects,[93] Atovaquone is extremely active against both *B. microti* and *B. divergens* in rodents, but recrudescences of parasitemia occur.[94,95] Azithromycin is active against *B. microti* as well,[96] and it prevents recrudescences in animals when given along with atovaquone.[94] Combination therapy including atovaquone or azithromycin or both and also quinine or clindamycin has been used as an alternative for treating human babesiosis when other regimens have failed or patients have developed side effects while receiving standard therapy.[93,94] Quinine and clindamycin should be given if the symptoms are sufficiently severe or if the patient is elderly, splenectomized, or immunocompromised. Treatment may occasionally fail, especially in high-risk patients or in those who must discontinue quinine due to side effects such as severe tinnitus. In most patients who complete the full regimen, parasite DNA seems to become undetectable by PCR within 1 month.[68] In a minority of cases, particularly in immunocompromised patients, symptoms may resolve but parasitemia persists.[63,97] Exchange transfusion should be considered in severely ill patients with parasitemias in excess of 10% and evidence of severe hemolysis or organ failure.[98] Following treatment, patients with AIDS should remain on suppressive therapy to prevent relapses.[63] The ideal regimen and duration of suppression have not been determined, but combinations of quinine, clindamycin, and other drugs have been used for periods of 6 months or maintained for life.

A variety of other agents have been tried for treating infected humans and experimental animals. Administration of chloroquine, sulfadiazine, or pyrimethamine failed to reduce *B. microti* parasitemia in hamsters,[87] and chloroquine and cotrimoxazole did not eliminate parasites from people infected with this organism, although symptomatic improvement was seen among people who received chloroquine.[99] Pentamidine and diminazene are active in animal models, but results of treatment of infected humans with pentamidine have been mixed,[100] and a patient successfully treated with diminazene developed complications resembling Guillain–Barré syndrome.[101] High doses of tetracyclines are active against *B. microti* in rodents, and doxycycline in combination with other agents appears to have efficacy in refractory cases in people with AIDS.[63] However, patients who are treated with a tetracycline for Lyme disease (e.g., 100 mg doxycycline orally twice a day for 14 days) appear to require specific antibabesial treatment if they are coinfected (T. J. Lepore, Nantucket Cottage Hospital, Nantucket, MA, personal communication, 1997). *Babesia microti* infections in hamsters were successfully cleared by two experimental 8-aminoquinolines (WR006026 and WR238605) under evaluation as antimalarials, and it may be that these compounds will eventually provide another treatment option. Other recently developed antimalarials (mefloquine, halofantrine, and artemisinin), however, were not effective.[102]

PREVENTION AND CONTROL

Repellents or arthropod toxicants are useful for personal protection. Permethrin-based formulations applied to shoes, socks, and trousers are particularly active against ticks,[103] although ticks may attach and feed briefly before succumbing to permethrin intoxication. Commonly used DEET (diethyltoluamide) repellents will also repel most ticks but are more volatile and require frequent reapplication. Preventing ticks from crawling underneath clothing by simply tucking trouser cuffs into socks also greatly reduces the risk. Also, because delivery of an infectious inoculum usually requires more than 1 day of tick attachment, the body surface of people who have visited a site where transmission is intense should be examined daily and all ticks should be removed promptly with forceps.

Various public health strategies may be followed to protect human populations against zoonotic babesial infection. The abundance of vector ticks may be temporarily reduced by spraying acaricides. Less environmentally intrusive applications of fiber-formulated permethrin[104] interrupt transmission of *B. microti* infection when rodents carry fibers into their nests and acaricide accumulates on the coats of the rodents and in sites where ticks rest. Acaricides may be applied to presumed cattle reservoirs for *B. divergens* to reduce the prevalence of infectious ticks. In areas of *B. microti* transmission, reducing the density of deer that serve as hosts to adult ticks may greatly diminish the local populations of deer ticks.[105] Reducing the density of rodent reservoirs seems impractical.

Efforts to develop veterinary vaccines against babesiosis have had mixed success. Cattle have been successfully vaccinated with attenuated parasites or exoantigen preparations, but recombinant antigens seem less effective due to parasite strain polymorphism. In addition, the mechanisms of protective antibabesial immunity are incompletely described.[106] Crude parasite lysates have been successfully used to immunize hamsters against infection by *B. microti*,[107] but subunit immunogens have yet to be described. Two immunodominant antigens, of 37 and 58 kDa, show promise as the basis for a subunit vaccine inducing protective immunity to *B. divergens*.[108] Vaccination as a strategy for preventing babesiosis in humans therefore seems premature but not without promise. People who are at risk of developing severe infections should carefully practice personal protection measures.

REFERENCES

1. Young AS, Morzaria SP: Biology of *Babesia*. Parasitol Today 2:211, 1986.
2. Wenyon CM: Protozoology, 2 vols. New York, William Wood, 1926.
3. Levine ND: The Protozoan Phylum Apicomplexa, Vol. 2. Boca Raton, Fla, CRC Press, 1988.
4. Schnittger L, Yin H, Gubbels MJ, et al: Phylogeny of sheep and goat *Theileria* and *Babesia* parasites. Parasitol Res 91:398, 2003.
5. Allsopp MT, Cavalier-Smith T, De Waal DT, et al: Phylogeny and evolution of the piroplasms. Parasitology 108:147, 1994.
6. Kjemtrup AM, Thomford J, Robinson T, et al: Phylogenetic relationships of human and wildlife piroplasm isolates in the western United States inferred from the 18S nuclear small subunit RNA gene. Parasitology 120:487, 2000.
7. Goethert HK, Telford SR III: What is *Babesia microti*? Parasitology 127:301, 2003.
8. Smith T: Some problems in the etiology and pathology of Texas cattle fever and their bearing on the comparative study of protozoan diseases. Trans Assoc Am Physicians 8:117, 1893.
9. Schein E, Reihbein G, Voigt WP, et al: *Babesi equi* (Laveran 1901). 1. Development in horses and in lymphocyte culture. Z Parasitenkd 34:68, 1981.
10. Mehlhorn H, Schein E: The piroplasms: Lifecycle and sexual stages. Adv Parasitol 23:37, 1987.
11. Chapman WE, Ward PA: The complement profile in babesiosis. J Immunol 117:935, 1976.
12. Rudzinska MA, Spielman A, Lewengrub S, et al: Sexuality in piroplasms as revealed by electron microscopy in *Babesia microti*. Proc Natl Acad Sci USA 80:2966, 1983.
13. Hoare CA: Comparative aspects of human babesiosis. Trans R Soc Trop Med Hyg 74:143, 1980.
14. Skrabalo Z, Deanovic Z: Piroplasmosis in man: Report on a case. Trop Geogr Med 9:11, 1957.
15. Zintl A, Mulcahy G, Skerrett HE, et al: *Babesia divergens*, a bovine blood parasite of veterinary and zoonotic importance. Clin Microbiol Rev 16:622, 2003.
16. Herwaldt B, Persing DH, Précigout E, et al: A fatal case of babesiosis in Missouri: Identification of another piroplasm that infects humans. Ann Intern Med 124:643, 1996.
17. Beattie JF, Michelson ML, Holman PJ: Acute babesiosis caused by *Babesia divergens* in a resident of Kentucky. N Engl J Med 347:697, 2002.
18. Goethert HK, Telford SR III: Enzootic transmission of *Babesia divergens* among cottontail rabbits on Nantucket Island, Massachusetts. Am J Trop Med Hyg 69:455, 2003.
19. Herwaldt B, de Bruyn G, Pieniazek NJ, et al: *Babesia divergens*-like infection, Washington state. Emerg Infect Dis 10:622, 2004.
20. Herwaldt BL, Caccio S, Gherlinzoni F, et al: Molecular characterization of a non-*Babesia divergens* organism causing zoonotic babesiosis in Europe. Emerg Infect Dis 9:942, 2003.
21. Enigk K, Friedhoff K: *Babesia capreoli* n.sp. beim Reh (*Capreolus capreolus* L.). Z Tropenmed Parasitol 13:8, 1962.
22. Gray JS, Murphy TM, Waldrup KA, et al: Comparative studies of *Babesia* spp. from white-tailed and sika deer. J Wildl Dis 27:86, 1991.
23. Quick RE, Herwaldt BL, Thomford JW, et al: Babesiosis in Washington state: A new species of *Babesia*? Ann Intern Med 119:284, 1993.
24. Thomford J, Conrad PA, Telford SR III, et al: Cultivation and phylogenetic characterisation of a newly recognised human pathogen. J Infect Dis 169:1050, 1994.
25. Persing DH, Herwaldt BL, Glaser C, et al: Infection with a *Babesia*-like organism in northern California. N Engl J Med 332:298, 1995.
26. Herwaldt BL, Kjemtrup AM, Conrad PA, et al: Transfusion-transmitted babesiosis in Washington state: First reported case caused by a WA1-type parasite. J Infect Dis 175:1259, 1997.
27. Kjemtrup AM, Lee B, Fritz CL, et al: Investigation of transfusion transmission of a WA1-type babesial parasite to a premature infant in California. Transfusion 42:1482, 2002.
28. Fritz CL, Kjemtrup AM, Conrad PA, et al: Seroepidemiology of emerging tickborne infectious diseases in a northern California community. J Infect Dis 175:1432, 1997.
29. Western KA, Benson GD, Gleason NN, et al: Babesiosis in a Massachusetts resident. N Engl J Med 283:854, 1970.
30. Telford SR III, Goethert HK: Emerging tick-borne infections: Rediscovered and better characterised, or truly "new"? Parasitology 129(suppl):S301, 2004.
31. Shih CM, Liu LP, Chung WC, et al: Human babesiosis in Taiwan: Asymptomatic infection with a *Babesia microti*-like organism in a Taiwanese woman. J Clin Microbiol 35:450, 1997.
32. Saito-Ito A, Tsuji M, Wei Q, et al: Transfusion-acquired, autochthonous human babesiosis in Japan: Isolation of *Babesia microti*-like parasites with hu-RBC-SCID mice. J Clin Microbiol 38:4511, 2000.
33. Meer-Scherrer L, Adelson M, Mordechai E, et al: *Babesia microti* infection in Europe. Curr Microbiol 48:435, 2004.
34. Peters W: A Colour Atlas of Arthropods in Clinical Medicine. London, Wolfe.
35. Herwaldt BL, McGovern PC, Gerwel MP, et al: Endemic babesiosis in another eastern state: New Jersey. Emerg Infect Dis 9:184, 2003.
36. Krause PJ, Telford SR III, Pollack RJ, et al: Babesiosis: An underdiagnosed disease of children. Pediatrics 89:1045, 1992.
37. Krause PJ, McKay K, Gadbaw J, et al: Increasing burden of human babesiosis in endemic sites. Am J Trop Med Hyg 68:431, 2003.
38. Lux JZ, Weiss D, Linden JV, et al: Transfusion-associated babesiosis after heart transplant. Emerg Infect Dis 9:116, 2003.
39. Pantanowitz L, Telford SR III, Cannon ME: The impact of babesiosis on transfusion medicine. Transfus Med Rev 16:131, 2002.
40. New DL, Quinn JB, Quereshi MZ, et al: Vertically transmitted babesiosis. J Pediatr 131:163, 1997.
41. Li JF, Meng DB: The discovery of human babesiosis in China. China J Vet Med 10:19, 1984.
42. Bush JB, Isaacson M, Mohamed AS, et al: Human babesiosis: A preliminary report of 2 suspect cases in southern Africa. S Afr Med J 78:699, 1990.

43. Armstrong PM, Rosa Brunet L, Spielman A, et al: Risk of Lyme disease: Perceptions of residents of a Lone Star tick infested community. Bull WHO 79:916, 2001.
44. Spielman A, Wilson ML, Levine JF, et al: Ecology of *Ixodes dammini*-borne human babesiosis and Lyme disease. Annu Rev Entomol 30:439, 1985.
45. Piesman J, Karakshian SJ, Lewengrub S, et al: Development of *Babesia microti* sporozoites in adult *Ixodes dammini*. Int J Parasitol 16:381, 1986.
46. Piesman J, Mather TN, Dammin GJ, et al: Seasonal variation of transmission risk of Lyme disease and human babesiosis. Am J Epidemiol 126:1187, 1987.
47. Van Peenen PFD, Chang SJ, Bankneider AR, et al: Piroplasms from Taiwanese rodents. J Protozool 24:310, 1977.
48. Shiota T, Kurimoto H, Haguma N, et al: Studies on babesia first found in murine in Japan: Epidemiology, morphology, and experimental infection. Z Bakt Mikrobiol Hyg 256:347, 1984.
49. Telford SR III, Gorenflot A, Brasseur P, et al: Babesial infestations in human and wildlife. In JP Kreier (ed): Parasitic Protozoa, 2nd ed. New York, Academic Press, p 1.
50. Sun T, Tenebaum MJ, Greenspan J, et al: Morphologic and clinical observations in human infection with *Babesia microti*. J Infect Dis 148:239, 1983.
51. Krogstad DJ, Sutera SP, Boylan CW, et al: Intraerythrocytic parasites and red cell deformability: *Plasmodium berghei* and *Babesia microti*. Blood Cells 17:209, 1991.
52. Commins MA, Goodger BV, Waltisbuhl DJ, et al: *Babesia bovis*: Studies of the parameters influencing microvascular stasis of infected erythrocytes. Res Vet Sci 44:226, 1988.
53. Skrabalo Z: Babesiosis. In Marcial-Rojas RA (ed): Pathology of Protozoal and Helminthic Diseases. Baltimore, Williams & Wilkins, 1971, p 232.
54. Fitzpatrick JEP, Kennedy CC, McGeown MG, et al: Further details on third reported case of redwater (babesiosis) in man. BMJ 2:770, 1969.
55. Hemmer RM, Ferrick DA, Conrad PA: Role of T cells and cytokines in fatal and resolving experimental babesiosis: Protection in TNFRp55−/− mice infected with the human *Babesia* WA1 parasite. J Parasitol 86:736, 2000.
56. Aguilar-Delfin I, Wettstein PJ, Persing DH: Resistance to acute babesiosis is associated with interleukin-12- and gamma interferon-mediated responses and requires macrophages and natural killer cells. Infect Immun 71:2002, 2003.
57. Herwaldt BL, Springs FE, Roberts PP, et al: Babesiosis in Wisconsin: A potentially fatal disease. Am J Trop Med Hyg 53:146, 1995.
58. Cullen JM, Levine JF: Pathology of experimental *Babesia microti* infection in the Syrian hamster. Lab Anim Sci 37:640, 1983.
59. Wozniak EJ, Lowenstine LJ, Hemmer R, et al: Comparative pathogenesis of human WA-1 and *Babesia microti* isolates in a Syrian hamster model. Lab Anim Sci 46:507, 1997.
60. Meldrum SC, Birkhead GS, White DJ, et al: Human babesiosis in New York state: An epidemiologic description of 136 cases. Clin Infect Dis 15:1019, 1992.
61. Rosner F, Zarrabi MH, Benach JL, et al: Babesiosis in splenectomized adults. Am J Med 76:696, 1984.
62. Benach JL, Habicht GS: Clinical characteristics of human babesiosis. J Infect Dis 144:481, 1981.
63. Falagas ME, Klempner MS: Babesiosis in patients with AIDS: A chronic infection presenting as fever of unknown origin. Clin Infect Dis 22:809, 1996.
64. Wolf RE: Effects of antilymphocyte serum and splenectomy on resistance to *Babesia microti* infection in hamsters. Clin Immunol Immunopathol 2:381, 1974.
65. Clark IA, Allison AC: *Babesia microti* and *Plasmodium berghei yoelii* infections in nude mice. Nature 252:328, 1974.
66. Igarashi I, Suzuki R, Waki S, et al: Roles of CD4(+) T cells and gamma interferon in protective immunity against *Babesia microti* infection in mice. Infect Immun 67:4143, 1999.
67. Clawson ML, Paciorkowski N, Rajan TV, et al: Cellular immunity, but not gamma interferon, is essential for resolution of *Babesia microti* infection in BALB/c mice. Infect Immun 70:5304, 2002.
68. Krause PJ, Spielman A, Telford SR III, et al: Persistent parasitemia after acute babesiosis. N Engl J Med 339:160, 1998.
69. Ruebush TK, Juranek DD, Chisholm ES, et al: Human babesiosis on Nantucket Island: Evidence for self limited and sub-clinical infections. N Engl J Med 297:825, 1977.
70. Wittner M, Rowin KS, Tanowitz HB, et al: Successful chemotherapy for transfusion babesiosis. Ann Intern Med 96:601, 1982.
71. Golightly LM, Hirschhorn LR, Weller PF, et al: Fever and headache in a splenectomized woman. Rev Infect Dis 11:629, 1989.
72. Slovut DP, Benedetti E, Matas J: Babesiosis and hemophagocytic syndrome in an asplenic renal transplant recipient. Transplantation 62:537, 1996.
73. Boustani MR, Lepore TJ, Gelfand JA, et al: Acute respiratory failure in patients treated for babesiosis. Am J Respir Crit Care Med 149:1689, 1994.
74. Machtinger L, Telford SR III, Inducil C, et al: Treatment of babesiosis by red blood cell exchange in an HIV-positive, splenectomized patient. J Clin Apheresis 8:78, 1993.
75. Benezra D, Brown AE, Polsky G, et al: Babesiosis and infection with human immunodeficiency virus (HIV). Ann Intern Med 107:944, 1987.
76. Ong KR, Stavropoulos C, Inada Y: Babesiosis, asplenia and AIDS. Lancet 336:112, 1990.
77. Froberg MK, Dannen D, Bakken JS: Babesiosis and HIV. Lancet 363:704, 2004.
78. Krause PJ, Telford SR III, Spielman A, et al: Concurrent Lyme disease and babesiosis. Evidence for increased severity and duration of the disease. JAMA 275:1657, 1996.
79. Marcus LC, Steere AC, Duray PH, et al: Fatal pancarditis in a patient with coexistent Lyme disease and babesiosis. Demonstration of spirochetes in the myocardium. Ann Intern Med 103:374, 1985.
80. Oleson CV, Sivalingam JJ, O'Neill BJ, et al: Transverse myelitis secondary to coexistent Lyme disease and babesiosis. J Spinal Cord Med 26:168, 2003.
81. Javed MZ, Srivastava M, Zhang S, et al: Concurrent babesiosis and ehrlichiosis in an elderly host. Mayo Clinic Proc 76:563, 2001.
82. Mitchell PD, Reed KD, Hofkes JM: Immunoserologic evidence of *Borrelia burgdorferi*, *Babesia microti*, and human granulocytic ehrlichia species in residents of Wisconsin and Minnesota. J Clin Microbiol 34:724, 1996.
83. Piesman J, Mather TN, Telford SR III, et al: Concurrent *Borrelia burgdorferi* and *Babesia microti* infection in nymphal *Ixodes dammini*. J Clin Microbiol 24:446, 1986.
84. Telford SR III, Dawson JE, Katavolos P, et al: Perpetuation of the agent of human granulocytic ehrlichiosis in a deer tick–rodent cycle. Proc Natl Acad Sci USA 93:6209, 1996.
85. Krause PJ, Telford SR III, Ryan R, et al: Antibody testing for babesiosis: Standardisation of a serologic test for the diagnosis of human *Babesia microti* infection. J Infect Dis 169:923, 1994.
86. Krause PJ, Ryan R, Telford S III, et al: Efficacy of immunoglobulin M serodiagnostic test for rapid diagnosis of acute babesiosis. J Clin Microbiol 34:2014, 1996.
87. Persing DH, Mathiesen D, Marshall WF, et al: Detection of *Babesia microti* by polymerase chain reaction. J Clin Microbiol 30:2097, 1992.
88. Drugs for parasitic infections. Med Lett Drugs Ther, August 2004 (www.medletter.com/freedocs/parasitic.pdf).
89. Dammin GJ, Spielman A, Mahoney EB, et al: Clindamycin and quinine treatment for *Babesia microti* infections. MMWR 32:65, 1983.
90. Brasseur P, Lecoublet S, Kapel N, et al: In vitro evaluation of drug susceptibilities of *Babesia divergens* isolates. Antimicrob Agents Chemother 42:818, 1998.
91. Brasseur P, Lecoublet S, Kapel N, et al: Quinine in the treatment of *Babesia divergens* infections in humans. Eur J Clin Microbiol Infect Dis 15:840, 1996.
92. Gorenflot A, Bazin C, Ambroise-Thomas P: Babésioses humaines: Traitement des formes graves. Presse Med 16:1099, 1987.
93. Krause PJ, Lepore T, Sikand VK, et al: Atovaquone and azithromycin for the treatment of babesiosis. N Engl J Med 343:1454, 2000.
94. Wittner M, Lederman J, Tanowitz HB, et al: Atovaquone in the treatment of *Babesia microti* infections in hamsters. Am J Trop Med Hyg 55:219, 1996.
95. Pudney M, Gray JS: Therapeutic efficacy of atovaquone against the bovine intraerythrocytic parasite, *Babesia divergens*. J Parasitol 83:307, 1997.
96. Weiss LM, Wittner M, Wasserman S, et al: Efficacy of azithromycin for treating *Babesia microti* infection in the hamster model. J Infect Dis 168:1289, 1993.
97. Smith RP, Evans AT, Popovsky M, et al: Transfusion-acquired babesiosis and failure of antibiotic treatment. JAMA 256:2726, 1986.
98. Jacoby GA, Hunt JV, Kosinski J, et al: Treatment of transfusion-induced babesiosis by exchange transfusion. N Engl J Med 303:1098, 1980.

99. Miller LH, Neva FA, Gill F: Failure of chloroquine in human babesiosis (*Babesia microti*): Case report and chemotherapeutic trials in hamsters. Ann Intern Med 88:200, 1978.
100. Raoult D, Soulayrol L, Toga B, et al: Babesiosis, pentamidine, and cotrimoxazole. Ann Intern Med 107:944, 1987.
101. Ruebush TK, Rubin RH, Wolpow ER, et al: Neurologic complications following the treatment of human *Babesia microti* infection with diminazene aceturate. Am J Trop Med Hyg 28:184, 1979.
102. Marley SE, Eberhard ML, Steurer FJ, et al: Evaluation of selected antiprotozoal drugs in the *Babesia microti*–hamster model. Antimicrob Agents Chemother 41:91, 1997.
103. Schreck CE, Snoddy EL, Spielman A: Pressurized sprays of permethrin or DEET on military clothing for personal protection against *Ixodes dammini* (Acari:Ixodidae). J Med Entomol 23:396, 1986.
104. Mather TN, Ribeiro JMC, Spielman A: Lyme disease and babesiosis: Acaricide focused on potentially infected ticks. Am J Trop Med Hyg 36:609, 1987.
105. Wilson ML, Telford SR III, Piesman J, et al: Reduced abundance of immature *Ixodes dammini* (Acari:Ixodidae) following elimination of deer. J Med Entomol 25:224, 1988.
106. Musoke AJ, Palmer GH, McElwain TF, et al: Prospects for subunit vaccines against tickborne diseases. Br Vet J 152:621, 1996.
107. Benach JL, Habicht GS: Glucan as an adjuvant for a murine *Babesia microti* immunisation trial. Infect Immun 35:947, 1982.
108. Carcy B, Precigout E, Valentin A, et al: A 37 kilodalton glycoprotein of *Babesia divergens* is a major component of a protective fraction containing low molecular mass culture derived exoantigen. Infect Immun 63:811, 1995.

92

African Trypanosomiasis (Sleeping Sickness)

JACQUES PÉPIN
JOHN E. DONELSON

INTRODUCTION

Human African trypanosomiasis (HAT), or sleeping sickness, is a purely African disease caused by two morphologically identical subspecies of trypanosomes—*Trypanosoma brucei gambiense* and *Trypanosoma brucei rhodesiense*—transmitted to humans by tsetse flies. Clinically, *T. b. gambiense* HAT is characterized by an early stage during which trypanosomes are found in the blood or lymph node aspirates of mostly asymptomatic persons and by a late stage during which there is involvement of the central nervous system (CNS) with somnolence, other neurologic symptoms, and trypanosomes in the cerebrospinal fluid (CSF). *T. b. rhodesiense* HAT, which is sometimes seen in short-term visitors to eastern and southern Africa, is a much more acute febrile illness occurring within days of the infective bite and which, if untreated, can be fatal in a matter of weeks.

AGENT

T. b. gambiense and *T. b. rhodesiense* are morphologically identical to a third salivarian trypanosome, *Trypanosoma brucei brucei,* which infects domestic and wild animals but does not survive in humans because it is lysed by apolipoprotein L-I in the high-density lipoprotein (HDL) fraction of human serum.[1,2] This group of three subspecies is often referred to as the *T. brucei* complex. Several other African trypanosome species are important pathogens of domestic livestock and wildlife in Africa but do not infect humans and are not discussed here.

The genus *Trypanosoma* occurs within the order Kinetoplastida. The single large mitochondrion of these organisms contains an appendage called the kinetoplast that lies in close proximity to the basal body at the base of the flagellum (Fig. 92-1). In the *T. brucei* complex, the kinetoplast contains as much as 10% of the total DNA of the organism. This DNA is organized into homogeneous maxicircle DNA molecules (about 20,000 base pairs each), which are equivalent to mitochondrial DNAs of other organisms, and heterogeneous minicircle DNA molecules (about 1000 base pairs each). A unique feature of organisms in the order Kinetoplastida is that some of their kinetoplast DNA genes are transcribed into RNAs that must be extensively edited by insertions or deletions of uridine nucleotides at many locations along the messenger RNA (mRNA) molecule before the correct mitochondrial proteins can be synthesized.[3] In the *T. brucei* complex, as many as 50% of nucleotides in some kinetoplast mRNAs are added or deleted after the initial synthesis of the RNA molecule. The reasons for the existence of this kinetoplast RNA editing and, indeed, the need for the kinetoplast itself are unknown, but this distinctive property of trypanosomes and related organisms does offer an attractive target for future drug development. The sequence determination of the 3.5×10^7 base-pair DNA genome in the nucleus of *T. b. brucei* is nearing completion[4,5] and may provide the foundation for identification of potential new drug targets.

During their life cycle the members of the *T. brucei* complex cycle between the mammalian bloodstream and several species of tsetse flies of the genus *Glossina.* When a tsetse fly bites an infected person, or an animal in the case of *T. b. rhodesiense,* trypanosomes in the bloodstream can be ingested with the blood meal (see Fig. 92-1). In the fly, the infected blood moves to the lumen of the midgut, where the bloodstream trypanosomes transform during a 2- to 3-day period into the

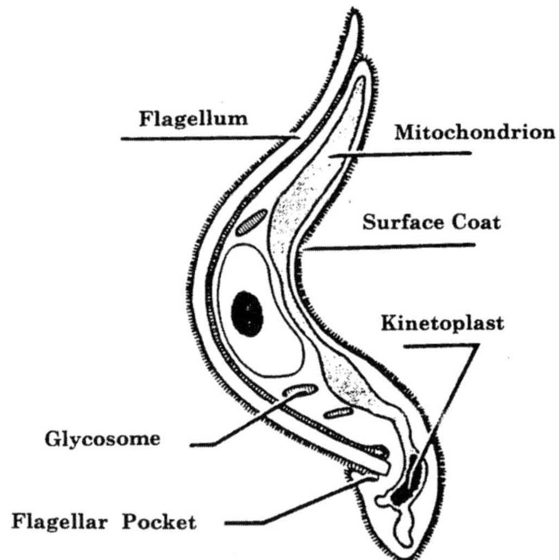

A

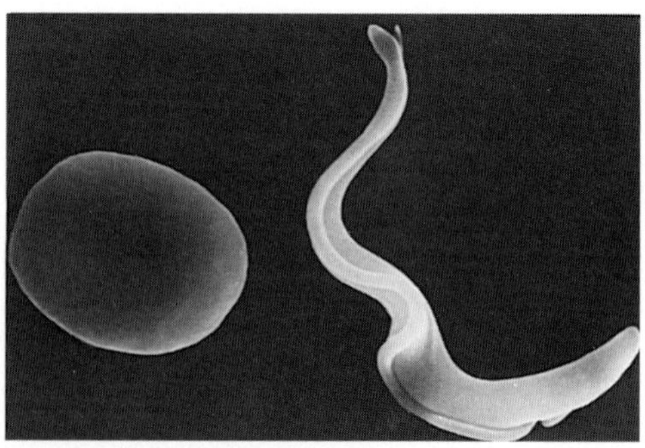
B

FIGURE 92-1 *A,* Schematic diagram of a bloodstream trypanosome showing some of its subcellular organelles and the surface location of the variant surface glycoprotein. *B,* Scanning electron micrograph of a bloodstream *Trypanosoma brucei rhodesiense* adjacent to a rat red blood cell. (×5500.)

procyclic stage. This transformation is accompanied by many developmental changes including an increase in body length, a switch from anaerobic to aerobic metabolism, and a change in the main nutritional carbon source from glucose to proline, which is also used as the predominant energy source by the tsetse fly itself during flight.[6,7] In addition, the major protein on the surface of bloodstream trypanosomes, the variant surface glycoprotein (VSG), is replaced by an invariant surface protein called procyclin. After 2 to 3 weeks of multiplication in the midgut, the procyclic trypanosomes migrate to the salivary gland, where they undergo several additional developmental changes, culminating in the formation of the mature metacyclic stage. Metacyclic trypanosomes reacquire a VSG coat and stop multiplying. An infected tsetse fly can harbor as many as 10,000 to 20,000 metacyclic trypanosomes, of which one is potentially sufficient to initiate the mammalian infection if transmitted during the fly bite. Each trypanosome of the mature metacyclic population is completely covered with about 10^7 copies of a single VSG, but the population as a whole expresses 10 to 20 different metacyclic VSGs.[8] Moreover, one study showed that these metacyclic VSGs gradually diverged over a 20-year period,[9] indicating that a vaccine directed against the metacyclic VSGs would not be successful.

The tsetse fly injects the metacyclic trypanosomes into the connective tissue of the skin, where a temporary local inflammation, called a chancre, often develops. From this initial

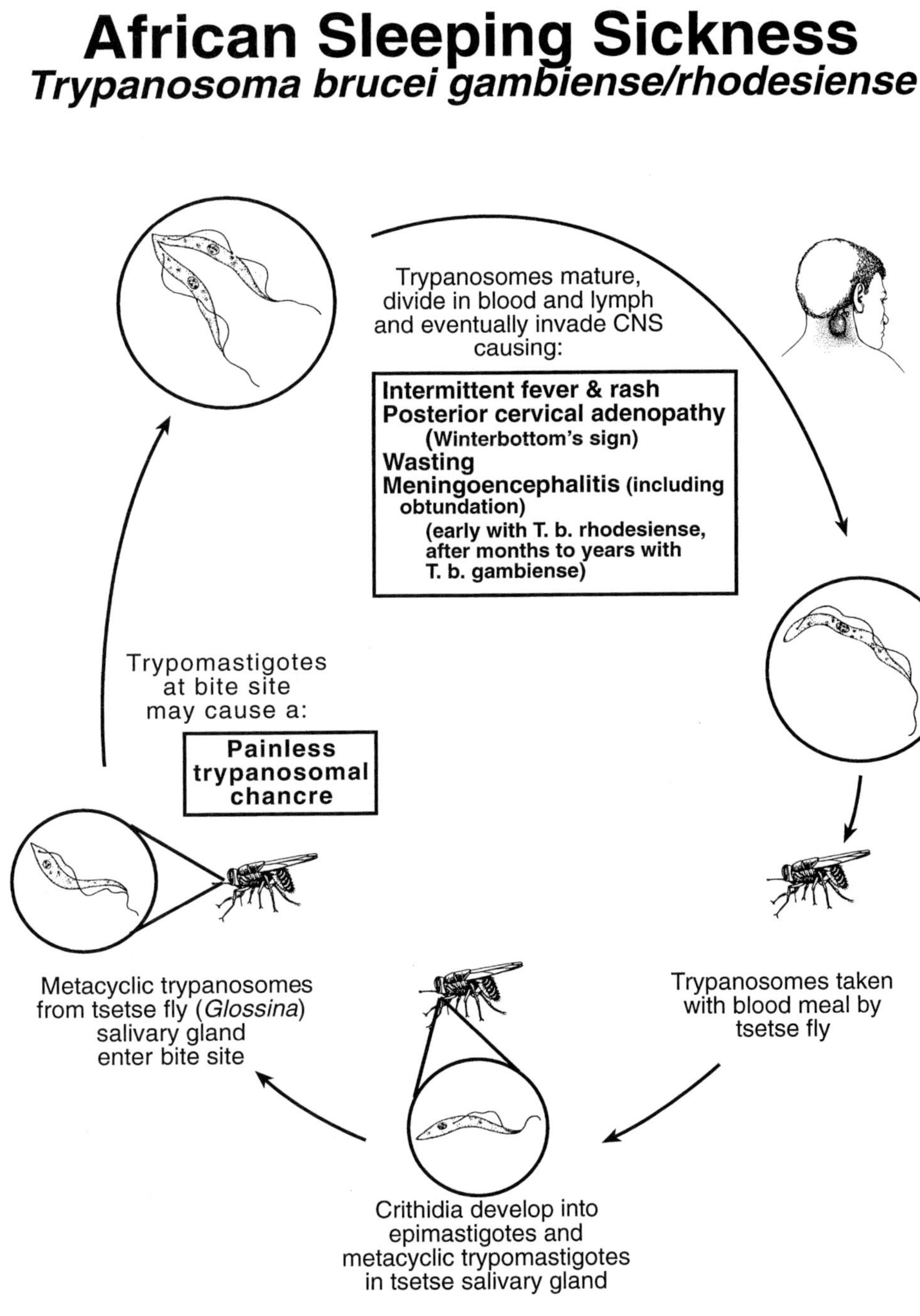

portal of entry, the parasites enter the draining lymphatics and pass into the bloodstream through the thoracic duct. They begin to multiply again by binary fission and transform back into the bloodstream form, returning to anaerobic glycolysis as the main source of adenosine triphosphate (ATP). They continue, however, to express the metacyclic VSGs on their surface for about 5 days after the initiation of infection. They then switch from the expression of metacyclic VSGs to the bloodstream VSGs, one of which is sometimes the same VSG as on the surface of trypanosomes ingested by the fly.[10] The slender bloodstream form of the parasite actively divides every 5 to 10 hours, whereas the shorter, stumpy form does not divide but has a more developed mitochondrion and is thought to be more infective to the insect. These bloodstream forms can traverse the walls of the blood and lymph capillaries to the connective tissues and eventually enter the CSF and the brain. The parasite's life cycle is completed when a tsetse fly takes up the bloodstream forms while feeding on an infected mammal.

While in the bloodstream, African trypanosomes are in constant contact with their host's immune system. As a result, they have evolved sophisticated mechanisms with which to evade immune attack. The VSG is a crucial component of one of these evasion mechanisms, a phenomenon called antigenic variation. As early as 1910, HAT was reported to be characterized by successive waves of parasites in the blood.[11] It is now well known that these peaks of parasitemia are due to trypanosomes expressing antigenically different VSGs.[12] The nuclear DNA of the *T. brucei* complex contains as many as 1000 different VSG genes. Usually each trypanosome expresses one, and only one, of these VSGs at a given instant. The 10^7 copies of a VSG on a trypanosome represent about 5% of the total protein of the organism. The major function of all this protein on the surface of the living trypanosome is to serve as a barrier to protect other invariant constituents of the organism's outer membrane from attack by the immune system.

The three-dimensional structures of two different VSGs have been shown by x-ray crystallography to be cylindrical, allowing them to pack very closely together on the parasite's surface. During an infection, antibodies are continually raised against the VSG, but the trypanosome population manages to escape total destruction because individual parasites occasionally undergo antigenic variation by switching spontaneously from the expression of one VSG to another. New antibodies must be directed against the VSG of the switched parasite and its descendants, enabling the population as a whole to stay one step ahead of this humoral (B-cell) immune response. The switch rate of the bloodstream trypanosome's antigenic variation appears to range between 10^{-2} and 10^{-6} per parasite per doubling time.[13] The switch itself is often associated with spontaneous VSG gene rearrangements that maneuver duplicated copies of silent VSG genes into special gene expression sites located near the ends of some chromosomes, where they are transcribed into mRNA. Sometimes these rearrangements result in the formation of new VSG genes that are mosaic or mutated versions of preexisting genes.[14,15] This ability to create new VSG gene versions during the DNA rearrangements likely means that bloodstream trypanosomes have the potential to express sequentially a much larger repertoire of VSG proteins than they have VSG genes. Hence, the development of a HAT vaccine directed against bloodstream VSGs is also unlikely.

The tsetse fly vector corresponds to the *Glossina* genus, found only in Africa, which contains 22 species, only a few of them being involved in the transmission of HAT: the riverine *palpalis* group (*G. palpalis, G. tachinoides,* and *G. fuscipes*) for *T. b. gambiense,* and the *morsitans* group (*G. morsitans, G. pallidipes,* and *G. swynnertoni*) for *T. b. rhodesiense.* Tsetse flies live in hot, humid, and dark ecologic niches, and their distinct requirements relate to epidemiologic differences between *gambiense* and *rhodesiense* HAT. The *palpalis* group is found mostly in forests lying on the banks of a river and humans are a variable source (10% to 40%) of their blood meals, while the more zoophilic *morsitans* group is seen in the woodland and thickets of East African savannas. Once infected with trypanosomes, tsetse flies remain infected for the rest of their lives (a few months). Less than 5% are infected in epidemic areas.

EPIDEMIOLOGY

HAT is endemic only in sub-Saharan Africa between latitudes 15 degrees north and 15 degrees south, corresponding to the distribution of its vector.[16,17] Its incidence increased considerably at the beginning of the 20th century as a consequence of population migrations brought on by colonization, when huge epidemics devastated several regions of Africa. There is some debate, however, whether this might have been initially exaggerated to cover up a genocide in the Free State of Congo.[18] Reports of control programs in the 1920s and 1930s described tens of thousands of cases detected each year in many countries. In some endemic areas HAT caused almost half of the overall mortality. Trypanosomiasis control was organized in West and Central Africa around mobile case-finding teams that regularly examined the population of endemic foci through cervical lymph node palpation and aspiration to detect and then treat infected but asymptomatic persons. In the late 1940s and 1950s, millions of people were given pentamidine "chemoprophylaxis" twice a year, but it probably corresponded more to early treatment than to prevention. Such initiatives were highly successful, and the incidence of HAT decreased dramatically. After the end of the colonial era, HAT remained at a low level ("residual endemicity") or disappeared in countries able to maintain some case-finding activities, but it increased considerably when such programs were interrupted for just a few years. As a result, the distribution of sleeping sickness today parallels that of wars or civil conflicts that have recently devastated parts of Africa, with the highest incidences occurring in the Democratic Republic of Congo (DRC), Angola, and Sudan. Underdiagnosis and underreporting are substantial. The total number of cases was recently estimated to be around 100,000 per year, with probably between one third and one half of cases remaining undetected and untreated.[16] The burden of HAT was estimated in a 2003 WHO Report to be 48,000 deaths per year and 1.5 million disability-adjusted life-years lost.[19]

Gambian HAT is endemic in western and central Africa and Rhodesian HAT in eastern and southern Africa. Uganda is the only country in which both subspecies are known to present. In West Africa, the disease has disappeared from Senegal, The Gambia, Guinea-Bissau, Sierra Leone, and Ghana for ecologic reasons that are poorly understood, since significant tsetse fly populations remain. A few hundred cases are diagnosed each year in Côte d'Ivoire, Guinea, and Nigeria. The country with

or suramin has been given for decades in the hope of reducing the risk of encephalopathy, but this remains unproved and cannot be recommended. Standard "adjuvant" drugs are anthelminthics (ivermectin, albendazole, or thiabendazole, especially if the patient has strongyloidiasis, to avoid corticosteroid-induced complications) and antimalarials. Encephalopathy should be treated with anticonvulsants (phenytoin, phenobarbital, or diazepam) and IV steroids (dexamethasone or hydrocortisone) to reduce cerebral edema. Dimercaprol (BAL), a heavy metal chelator, is useless and may even be deleterious in the treatment of encephalopathy whose pathogenesis is an immunologic reaction rather than arsenic toxicity.[58] Polyneuropathy (up to 10%) is a direct toxic effect of arsenic, which if neglected can progress to paraplegia or quadriplegia. When a patient complains of paresthesias, melarsoprol should be withheld for a while and thiamine (100 mg three times a day) administered. Tremors are sometimes seen and respond well to β-blockers. Fever can be caused by lysis of trypanosomes, but superinfections should always be sought, especially pneumonia. Cutaneous reactions (1%) can be troublesome. Phlebitis and cellulitis at the injection sites are caused by the propylene glycol solvent.

After treatment, all patients should be followed with an LP every 6 months for 2 years, or sooner if symptoms recur. A relapse is certain if trypanosomes are found in the CSF (rarely in blood or lymph nodes), but most relapses are characterized only by an elevated CSF WBC. Patients should be considered as having postmelarsoprol (or posteflornithine) relapse if their CSF WBC is greater than $50/mm^3$ and higher than the previous determination, or if it is $20/mm^3$ to $49/mm^3$ and higher than the previous measurement with attendant recurrence of symptoms. When in doubt, the LP should be repeated after 1 to 2 months. The trend in the CSF WBC is more important than the absolute value, since many genuinely cured patients have a slightly elevated CSF WBC 6 months after treatment. Patients who relapse after melarsoprol treatment should be given eflornithine (a second course of melarsoprol is usually ineffective) and vice versa. Patients with a CSF WBC greater than $20/mm^3$ after pentamidine treatment are considered to be relapsing. Those with borderline results ($6/mm^3$ to $19/mm^3$) should be retested earlier than the routine 6-month interval. Patients who relapse after having received pentamidine for early-stage Gambian HAT should be treated with eflornithine or melarsoprol. Surprisingly, the vast majority of late-stage adult patients cured by melarsoprol or eflornithine, even if comatose before treatment, have no obvious sequelae. Children display sequelae more frequently (e.g., poor performance at school).

In early-stage Rhodesian HAT, suramin is the treatment of choice and is superior to pentamidine. A test dose is initially given although anaphylaxis is rare. Several regimens are recommended,[17] but this probably does not matter given the drug's extremely long half-life of approximately 50 days. Melarsoprol would be effective but is avoided because of the risk of encephalopathy. The failure rate with suramin varies from 0% to 31%.[50] Adverse effects are fever, proteinuria, and urticaria. Suramin is 99.7% protein-bound and has no CSF penetration. *T. b. rhodesiense* is resistant to eflornithine. Melarsoprol is the only effective treatment for late-stage patients, having a 95% cure rate. Despite the lack of controlled trials, most authorities recommend starting with a small dose of melarsoprol and increasing it progressively. Pretreatment with suramin is generally advocated on the theoretical grounds that it might prevent seeding of the CSF when the LP is conducted. Several regimens are used; Table 92-1 lists one of those recommended by WHO.[17] Melarsoprol-induced encephalopathy is more common in Rhodesian (5% to 18%) than in Gambian HAT, and mortality during treatment is higher (3% to 12%). Although not studied in such patients, it seems reasonable to administer prednisolone at the same dosage as in Gambian HAT. The same adjuvant drugs should be used, and encephalopathy should be treated along the same lines. Follow-up should be as in Gambian HAT, except that LPs should be carried out every 3 months during the first year. Most patients who relapse after melarsoprol treatment of

Table 92-1 *Treatment Regimens for Gambian and Rhodesian Trypanosomiasis*

	Trypanosoma brucei gambiense	***Trypanosoma brucei rhodesiense***
Early stage	Pentamidine IM 4 mg/kg up to 300 mg/day for 7 days	Suramin IV 5 mg/kg on day 1, then 20 mg/kg IV (up to 1.0 g) on days 3, 5, 12, 19, 26
Late stage	Eflornithine IV 100 mg/kg q6h for 14 days *or* Melarsoprol IV 2.2 mg/kg daily for 10 days	Melarsoprol (dose in mg/kg): 1.80 mg/kg (day 5), 2.16 (day 6), 2.52 (days 7, 14), 2.88 (day 15), 3.24 (day 16), 2.9 (day 20), 3.6 (up to 180 mg) (days 23, 24, 25)
Relapses	Postpentamidine: melarsoprol or eflornithine as above; Postmelarsoprol: eflornithine as above; Posteflornithine: melarsoprol as above	Postsuramin: melarsoprol as above; Postmelarsoprol: second course of melarsoprol, 3 × 4 daily injections, all doses at 3.6 mg/kg (up to 180 mg)
Melarsoprol-induced encephalopathy		
Prevention	Prednisolone 1 mg/kg up to 40 mg/day, started 1–2 days before first dose of melarsoprol, continued until last dose, tapered over 3 days (30, 20, 10 mg)	As in *T. b. gambiense*
Treatment	Anticonvulsants, IV corticosteroids	As in *T. b. gambiense*
Pretreatment	None	Suramin 5 mg/kg on day 1, 20 mg/kg on day 3
Adjuvant drugs	Antimalarials, anthelminthics	As in *T. b. gambiense*

Rhodesian HAT are cured by a second course of the same drug. For those who relapse a second time, a combination of melarsoprol and nifurtimox might be considered. For Gambian HAT patients who relapse after two separate treatments with melarsoprol and eflornithine, the best option is probably the simultaneous administration of eflornithine and melarsoprol at maximal dosage.[60]

Given the lack of financial incentives, it appears unlikely that new drugs will be developed for HAT in the near future, although one possible new prodrug DB289 [2,5-bis(4-amidinophenyl)furan-bis-O-methylamidoxime] has completed Phase I clinical trials and is about to enter Phase II[49] (see also http://www.sti.ch/scih/africa1.htm). A high priority should be given to studies of combinations of drugs such as melarsoprol-eflornithine or melarsoprol-nifurtimox, which might allow shorter, less toxic, treatment.

PREVENTION AND CONTROL

For Gambian HAT, case finding remains the cornerstone of disease control. Infected individuals can remain asymptomatic and contagious for months or years before developing overt sleeping sickness, and they become less contagious when CNS involvement progresses, since trypanosomes are then found more in the CSF than in the bloodstream. The only way to break the chain of transmission is to identify and treat asymptomatic persons. Populations of endemic foci should be examined twice a year by mobile teams. Previous case-finding surveys based only on detection and aspiration of cervical lymphadenopathy gave excellent results when 95% or more of the inhabitants were present. If only 50% of the population participates, as is often the case nowadays,[61] and if only this traditional method is used, not enough carriers will be identified to modify the epidemic dynamics. However, use of the CATT to identify suspects on whom parasitologic assays are concentrated doubles the number of parasitemic persons detected (half of whom have no lymphadenopathy) and will compensate for the lower participation.

The best approach is to perform the CATT on all inhabitants. CATT-positive subjects should have blood examinations (ideally the mAECT, or at least a thick and a wet smear) and lymph node aspiration if feasible. Most control programs treat only persons in whom trypanosomes have been seen. Whether the systematic treatment of individuals with a positive CATT and negative parasitologic assays would lead to more rapid disease control is unknown, but it seems that many such individuals have merely transiently positive CATT assays as a result of infection with trypanosomes that are not pathogenic for humans.[62] Pentamidine "chemoprophylaxis" of the whole population of endemic areas would not be acceptable today because of its adverse effects and the risk of transmission of blood-borne pathogens, and certainly no traveler is at sufficiently high risk of HAT to warrant consideration of individual chemoprophylaxis.

To what extent HAT case finding can be integrated within the activities of multipurpose fixed health centers has been much debated. It is possible to improve the efficacy of passive case detection by rural health centers but not to delegate to them active case finding.[63] The subjects in most cases passively detected by health centers already have an abnormal CSF, and their treatment must have only a modest impact on transmission. Vector control by tsetse fly trapping is a useful adjuvant, but its cost is such that it is not sustainable on a large scale and should be considered only for high-incidence villages. Given the lack of commercial potential and the capacity of the parasite to undergo continuous antigenic variation, it is unlikely that an antitrypanosome vaccine will ever be developed. For Rhodesian HAT, the recent experience of the Uganda national control program showed that a major epidemic can be controlled through surveillance and case detection by sleeping sickness orderlies, combined with intensive tsetse fly trapping.[64] The performance of national control programs should be closely monitored through predetermined indicators.[65]

REFERENCES

1. Rifkin MR: Identification of the trypanocidal factor in normal human serum: High density lipoprotein. Proc Natl Acad Sci USA 75:3450, 1978.
2. Vanhamme L, Paturiaux-Hanocq F, Poelvoorde P, et al: Apolipoprotein L-I is the trypanosome lytic factor of human serum. Nature 422:83, 2003.
3. Simpson L, Sbicego S, Aphasizhev R: Uridine insertion/deletion RNA editing in trypanosome mitochondria: A complex business. RNA 9:265, 2003.
4. El-Sayed NM, Ghedin E, Song J, et al: The sequence and analysis of *Trypanosoma brucei* chromosome II. Nucleic Acids Res 31:4856, 2003.
5. Hall N, Berriman M, Lennard NJ, et al: The DNA sequence of chromosome I of an African trypanosome: Gene content, chromosome organisation, recombination and polymorphism. Nucleic Acids Res 31:4864, 2003.
6. Vickerman K: Developmental cycles and biology of pathogenic trypanosomes. Br Med Bull 41:105, 1985.
7. van Weelden SW, Fast B, Vogt A, et al: Procyclic *Trypanosoma brucei* do not use Krebs cycle activity for energy generation. J Biol Chem 278:12854, 2003.
8. Vickerman K, Barry JD: African trypanosomiasis. In Cohen S, Warren KS (eds): Immunology of Parasitic Infections. Oxford, Blackwell Scientific, 1982, p 204.
9. Barry JD, Crowe JS, Vickerman K: Instability of the *Trypanosoma brucei rhodesiense* metacyclic variable antigen repertoire. Nature 306:699, 1983.
10. Hajduk S, Vickerman K: Antigenic variation in cyclically transmitted *Trypanosoma brucei:* Variable antigen type composition in the first parasitaemia in mice bitten by trypanosome-infected *Glossina morsitans.* Parasitology 83:609, 1981.
11. Ross R, Thompson D: A case of sleeping sickness studied by precise enumerative methods: Regular periodic increase in the parasites disclosed. Proc R Soc London B Biol Sci 82:411, 1910.
12. Donelson JE: Antigenic variation and the African trypanosome genome. Acta Trop 85:391, 2003.
13. Turner CM: The rate of antigenic variation in fly-transmitted and syringe-passaged infections of *Trypanosoma brucei*. FEMS Microbiol Lett 153:227, 1997.
14. Lu Y, Hall T, Gay LS, et al: Point mutations are associated with a gene duplication leading to the bloodstream re-expression of a trypanosome metacyclic VSG. Cell 72:397, 1993.
15. Roth C, Bringaud F, Layden RE, et al: Active late-appearing variable surface antigen genes in *Trypanosoma equiperdum* are constructed entirely from pseudogenes. Proc Natl Acad Sci USA 86:9375, 1989.
16. Pépin J, Méda H: The epidemiology and control of human African trypanosomiasis. Adv Parasitol 49:71, 2001.
17. World Health Organization: Control and surveillance of African trypanosomiasis. WHO Technical Report Series No 881, Geneva, 1998.
18. Hochschild A: King Leopold's ghost: A history of greed, terror, and heroism in colonial Africa. Boston, Houghton Mifflin, 1999.
19. World Health Organization: The World Health Report 2003: Shaping the Future. Geneva, 2003.
20. Ekwanzala M, Pépin J, Khonde N, et al: In the heart of darkness: Sleeping sickness in Zaire. Lancet 348:1427, 1996.
21. Robays J, Ebeja Kadima A, Lutumba P et al: Human African trypanosomiasis amongst urban residents in Kinshasa: A case-control study. Trop Med Int Health 9:869, 2004.

22. Jelinek T, Bisoffi Z, Bonazzi L, et al: Cluster of African trypanosomiasis in travelers to Tanzanian national parks. Emerg Infect Dis 8:634, 2002.
23. Lejon V, Boelaert M, Jannin J, et al: The challenge of *Trypanosoma brucei gambiense* sleeping sickness diagnosis outside Africa. Lancet Infect Dis 3:804, 2003.
24. Khonde N, Pépin J, Niyonsenga T, et al: Epidemiological evidence for immunity following *T. b. gambiense* sleeping sickness. Trans R Soc Trop Med Hyg 89:607, 1995.
25. Khonde N, Pépin J, Niyonsenga T, et al: Familial aggregation of *Trypanosoma brucei gambiense* trypanosomiasis in a very-high incidence community. Trans R Soc Trop Med Hyg 91:521, 1997.
26. Méda HA, Doua F, Laveissière C, et al: Human immunodeficiency virus infection and human African trypanosomiasis: A case-control study in Côte d'Ivoire. Trans R Soc Trop Med Hyg 89:639, 1995.
27. Févre EM, Coleman PG, Odiit M, et al: The origins of a new *Trypanosoma brucei rhodesiense* sleeping sickness outbreak in eastern Uganda. Lancet 358:625, 2001
28. Moore AC, Ryan ET, Waldron MA: Case records of the Massachusetts General Hospital—Weekly clinicopathological exercises: Case 20-2002. N Engl J Med 346:2069, 2002.
29. Boatin BA, Wyatt GB, Wurapa FK, et al: Use of symptoms and signs for diagnosis of *Trypanosoma brucei rhodesiense* trypanosomiasis by rural health personnel. Bull World Health Organ 64:389, 1986.
30. Sanner BM, Doberauer C, Tepel M, et al: Fulminant disease simulating bacterial sepsis with disseminated intravascular coagulation after a trip to East Africa. Intens Care Med 26:646, 2000.
31. Urquhart GM, Murray M, Murray P, et al: Immunosuppression in *Trypanosoma brucei* infections in rats and mice. Trans R Soc Trop Med Hyg 67:528, 1973.
32. Sileghem M, Flynn JN, Darji A, et al: African Trypanosomiasis. In Kierszenbaum F (ed): Parasite Infections and the Immune System. San Diego, Academic Press, 1994, p 1.
33. Diffley P: Trypanosomal surface coat variant antigen causes polyclonal lymphocyte activation. J Immunol 131:1983, 1983.
34. Dempsey WA, Mansfield JM: Lymphocyte function in experimental African trypanosomiasis. 5. Role of antibody and the mononuclear phagocyte system in variant-specific immunity. J Immunol 130:405, 1983.
35. Poltera AA: Pathology of human African trypanosomiasis with reference to experimental African trypanosomiasis and infections of the central nervous system. Br Med Bull 41:169, 1985.
36. Poltera AA, Cox JN, Owor R: Pancarditis involving the conducting system and all valves in human African trypanosomiasis. Br Heart J 38:827, 1976.
37. Bentivoglio M, Grassi-Zucconi G, Olsson T, et al: *Trypanosoma brucei* and the nervous system. Trends Neurosci 17:325, 1994.
38. Lumsden WHR, Kimber CD, Strange M: *Trypanosoma brucei*: detection of low parasitemia in mice by a miniature anion-exchanger/centrifugation technique. Trans R Soc Trop Med Hyg 71:421, 1976.
39. Bailey JW, Smith DH: The quantitative buffy coat for the diagnosis of trypanosomes. Trop Doct 24:54, 1994.
40. Truc P, Aerts D, McNamara JJ, et al: Direct isolation of *Trypanosoma brucei* from man and other animals, and its potential value for the diagnosis of Gambian trypanosomiasis. Trans R Soc Trop Med Hyg 86:627, 1992.
41. Penchenier L, Simo G, Grébaut P, et al: Diagnosis of human trypanosomiasis, due to *Trypanosoma brucei gambiense* in central Africa, by the polymerase chain reaction. Trans R Soc Trop Med Hyg 94:392, 2000.
42. Cattand P, Miézan BT, de Raadt P: Human African trypanosomiasis: use of double centrifugation of CSF to detect trypanosomes. Bull World Health Organ 66:83, 1988.
43. Miézan TW, Méda HA, Doua F, et al: Single centrifugation of cerebrospinal fluid in a sealed Pasteur pipette for simple, rapid and sensitive detection of trypanosomes. Trans R Soc Trop Med Hyg 94:293, 2000.
44. Noireau F, Lemesre JL, Nzoukoudi MY, et al: Serodiagnosis of sleeping sickness in the Republic of Congo: Comparison of indirect immunofluorescent antibody test and card agglutination test. Trans R Soc Trop Med Hyg 82:237, 1988.
45. Truc P, Lejon V, Magnus E, et al: Evaluation of the micro-CATT, CATT/ *Trypanosoma brucei gambiense*, and LATEX/*T.b. gambiense* methods for serodiagnosis and surveillance of human African trypanosomiasis in West and Central Africa. Bull World Health Organ 80:882, 2002.
46. Miézan T, Doua F, Cattand P, et al: Evaluation du Testryp CATT appliqué au sang prélevé sur papier filtre et au sang dilué, dans le foyer de trypanosomiase à *Trypanosoma brucei gambiense* en Côte d'Ivoire. Bull World Health Organ 69:603, 1991.
47. Sahlas DJ, MacLean JD, Janevski J, et al: Out of Africa. N Engl J Med 347:749, 2002.
48. Sabbah P, Brosset C, Imvbert P, et al: Human African trypanosomiasis: MRI. Neuroradiology 39:708, 1997.
49. Fairlamb AH: Chemotherapy of human African trypanosomiasis: Current and future prospects. Trends Parasitol 19:488, 2003.
50. Pépin J, Milord F: The treatment of human African trypanosomiasis. Adv Parasitol 33:1, 1994.
51. World Health Organization: WHO-Aventis collaborative working group: one cornerstone of a global alliance for controlling and eliminating African sleeping sickness. TDR News 70, 12, 2003.
52. Lejon V, Reiber H, Legros D, et al: Intrathecal immune response pattern for improved diagnosis of central nervous system in trypanosomiasis. J Infect Dis 187:1475, 2003.
53. Pépin J, Khonde N, Maiso F, et al: Short-course eflornithine in Gambian trypanosomiasis: A multicentre randomized controlled trial. Bull World Health Organ 78:1284, 2000.
54. Milord F, Loko L, Ethier L, et al: Eflornithine concentrations in serum and cerebrospinal fluid of 63 patients treated for *T. b. gambiense* sleeping sickness. Trans R Soc Trop Med Hyg 87:473, 1993.
55. Khonde N, Pépin J, Mpia B: A seven-day course of eflornithine for relapsing *T. b. gambiense* trypanosomiasis. Trans R Soc Trop Med Hyg 91:212, 1997.
56. Burri C, Nkunku S, Merolle A, et al: Efficacy of a new, concise, schedule for melarsoprol in treatment of sleeping sickness caused by *Trypanosoma brucei gambiense*: A randomised trial. Lancet 355:1419, 2000.
57. Pépin J, Milord F, Guern C, et al: Trial of prednisolone for prevention of melarsoprol-induced encephalopathy in *gambiense* sleeping sickness. Lancet 333:1246, 1989.
58. Pépin J, Milord F, Khonde N, et al: Risk factors for encephalopathy and mortality during melarsoprol treatment of *T. b. gambiense* sleeping sickness. Trans R Soc Trop Med Hyg 89:92, 1995.
59. Pépin J, Milord F, Khonde N, et al: Gambiense trypanosomiasis: Frequency of, and risk factors for, failure of melarsoprol therapy. Trans R Soc Trop Med Hyg 88:447, 1994.
60. Simarro P, Asumu PN: Gambian trypanosomiasis and synergism between melarsoprol and eflornithine: First case report. Trans R Soc Trop Med Hyg 90:315, 1996.
61. Robays J, Bilengue MMC, Van der Stufyt P, et al: The effectiveness of active population screening and treatment for sleeping sickness control in the Democratic Republic of Congo. Trop Med Int Health 9:542, 2004.
62. Garcia A, Jamonneau V, Magnus E, et al: Follow-up of Card Agglutination Trypanosomiasis Test (CATT) positive but apparently aparasitaemic individuals in Côte d'Ivoire: Evidence for a complex and heterogeneous population. Trop Med Int Health 5:786, 2000.
63. Pépin J, Guern C, Milord F, et al: Intégration de la lutte contre la trypanosomiase humaine dans un réseau de centres de santé polyvalents. Bull World Health Organ 67:301, 1989.
64. Smith DH, Pépin J, Stich A: Human African trypanosomiasis: an emerging public health crisis. Br Med Bull 54:341, 1998.
65. Bouchet B, Legros D, Lee K: Key indicators for the monitoring and evaluation of control programmes of human African trypanosomiasis due to *Trypanosoma brucei gambiense*. Trop Med Int Health 3:474, 1998.

93

American Trypanosomiasis (Chagas' Disease)*

LOUIS V. KIRCHHOFF

INTRODUCTION

American trypanosomiasis (Chagas' disease) is a zoonosis caused by *Trypanosoma cruzi,* a protozoan parasite found only in the Americas. The geographic range of *T. cruzi* infection in humans and other mammalian hosts is primarily determined by the distribution of the various species of blood-sucking triatomine insects that act as its vectors. This range extends from the southern United States to Central Argentina. Although major portions of the range of *T. cruzi* lie in temperate regions, Chagas' disease is generally considered a tropical disease because the majority of infected persons live in the tropics.

AGENT

The genus *Trypanosoma* contains about 20 species, but only *T. cruzi* and the two African trypanosome subspecies, *Trypanosoma brucei gambiense* and *T. b. rhodesiense,* cause disease in humans.[1] *Trypanosoma rangeli*, which also is found only in the Americas, can be transmitted to humans, but it does not cause a persistent infection and is not pathogenic.[2] *T. cruzi* was first described in 1909 by the Brazilian physician Carlos Chagas, who saw the motile parasites while doing microscopic examinations of dissected intestines of triatomine insects.[3] The complex life cycle of *T. cruzi* involves insect vectors as well as mammalian hosts (Fig. 93-1). The vectors become infected when they ingest blood from mammals that have circulating trypomastigotes, which are nondividing but infective forms of the parasite (Fig. 93-2). Once inside the midgut of an insect host, the parasites undergo transformation to epimastigotes, which are flagellates having a distinct morphology, and these organisms then multiply extracellularly. After migration to the hindgut, epimastigotes transform into nondividing metacyclic trypomastigotes, which are then discharged with the feces around the time of a subsequent blood meal. Transmission to a second mammalian host occurs when breaks in the skin, mucous membranes, or conjunctivae are contaminated with insect feces containing the infective metacyclic forms. Inside the new host, these parasites enter a variety of host cell types and, after transformation into amastigotes, multiply intracellularly. When proliferating amastigotes fill the host cell, they differentiate into trypomastigotes and the cell ruptures. The parasites released invade adjacent tissues and spread hematogenously to distant sites where they initiate further cycles of intracellular multiplication. Thus they maintain a parasitemia infective for vectors. *T. cruzi* can also be transmitted by transfusion of blood donated by infected persons,[4] from mother to fetus,[5–7] and in laboratory accidents.[8]

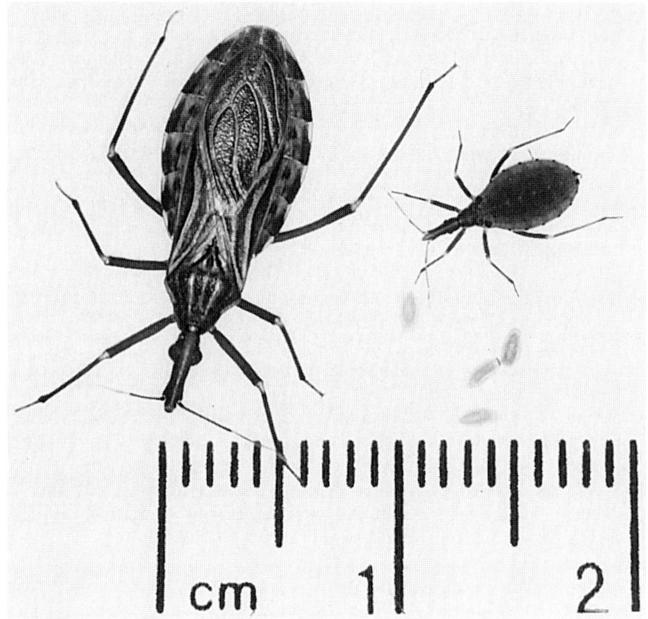

FIGURE 93-1 Eggs, second instar nymph, and adult of *Rhodnius prolixus,* a triatomine vector of *Trypanosoma cruzi.*

DISTRIBUTION OF *TRYPANOSOMA CRUZI*

Epizootiology

Infection with *T. cruzi* is a zoonosis, and involvement of humans in the cycle of transmission is not necessary for

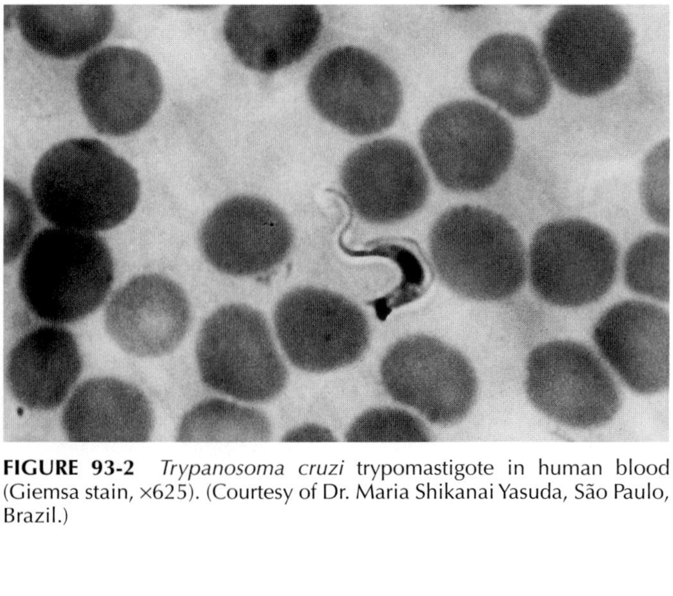

FIGURE 93-2 *Trypanosoma cruzi* trypomastigote in human blood (Giemsa stain, ×625). (Courtesy of Dr. Maria Shikanai Yasuda, São Paulo, Brazil.)

*All material in this chapter is in the public domain, with the exception of the borrowed figures.

perpetuation of the parasite in nature. *T. cruzi* is found only in the Western Hemisphere, where it primarily infects wild and domestic mammals and insects.[9,10] Triatomine vectors that transmit *T. cruzi* are found in spotty distributions, from central Argentina to the southern half of the United States.[11,12] Hollow trees, burrows, palm trees, and other animal shelters are places where transmission of *T. cruzi* occurs among infected vectors and nonhuman mammalian hosts. Piles of wood, old vegetation, and roof tiles near houses have also been found to harbor large numbers of insects.[13,14] Vector-borne transmission to humans takes place only in areas inhabited by triatomine species that defecate during or immediately after blood meals. However, this restriction does not apply to transmission to nonhuman mammalian hosts, which can become infected by eating infected insects.[15]

T. cruzi has been found in more than 100 species of domestic and wild mammals,[16] from the southern United States[10,17–20] to Central Argentina.[21,22] Opossums, wood rats, armadillos, raccoons, dogs, and cats are typical hosts, but *T. cruzi* is not a problem in livestock. Nontypical hosts can become infected when held in zoos in areas in which *T. cruzi* is enzootic.[23–25] This lack of species-specificity, combined with the fact that infected mammals have lifelong parasitemias, results in an enormous domestic and sylvatic reservoir in enzootic areas.

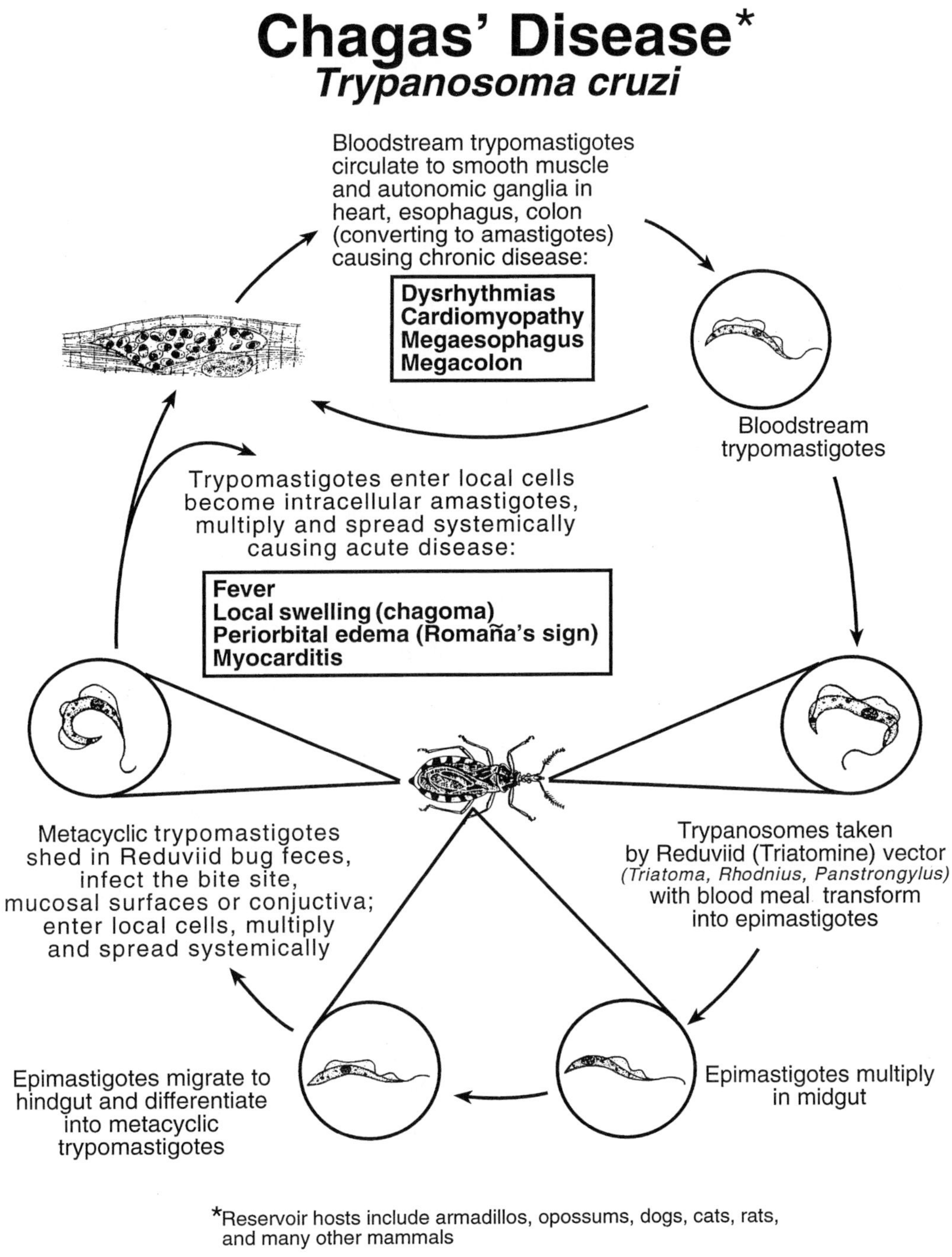

Epidemiology of Chagas' Disease in Latin America

Historically, humans have become part of the cycle of *T. cruzi* transmission as farmers and ranchers open up land in enzootic regions. When this development takes place, vectors such as *Triatoma infestans, Rhodnius prolixus,* and *Panstrongylus megistus* invade the nooks and crannies of the primitive wood, mud-walled, and stone houses that are typical of rural Latin America. In this manner the vectors become domiciliary, establishing a cycle of transmission which involves humans and peridomestic mammals and is largely independent of the sylvatic cycle.[13,26–28] For the most part, Chagas' disease has been a problem of poor people living in rural areas. In recent decades, however, large numbers of infected people have migrated to cities, thus urbanizing the disease and resulting in frequent transmission by blood transfusion prior to the implementation of effective serologic screening.[29–32]

Early reports indicated that most cases of acute Chagas' disease that came to medical attention occurred in children.[33] Prevalence data support this view, but few age-specific and geographic incidence data have been available because most cases of the acute illness go undetected due to its mild nature and the lack of access to medical care among those at highest risk. The Pan American Health Organization estimated that 10 to 12 million people are infected with *T. cruzi* and that roughly 45,000 deaths each year are attributable to Chagas' disease.[34] However, in recent years, the epidemiology of *T. cruzi* infection has improved markedly in several endemic countries, as vector and blood bank control programs have achieved considerable success. As a consequence, prevalence rates in younger age groups have been decreasing in many areas.[35–37]

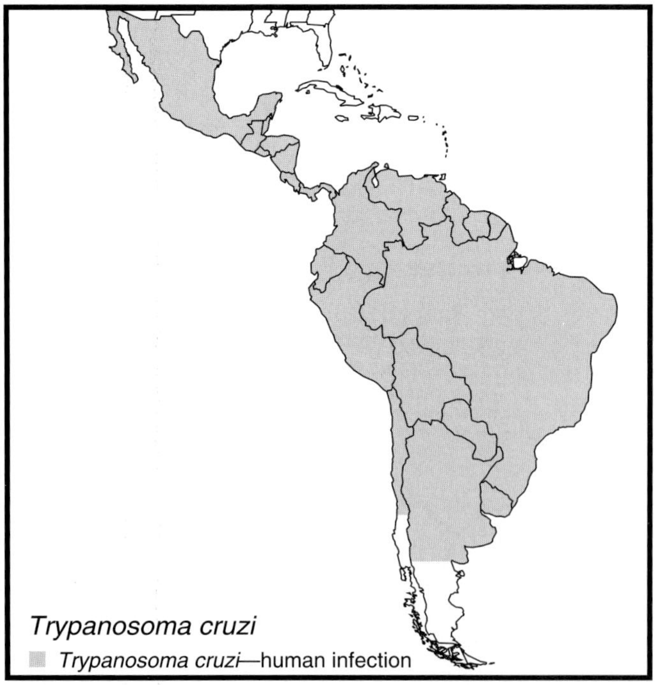

Note: The epidemiologic database in many areas is limited. Transmission of *T. cruzi* has been interrupted in many large areas in the endemic area (e.g., Argentina, Brazil, Chile, Uruguay). At least 80,000 *T. cruzi* –infected immigrants now reside in the United States.

A major international eradication program in the "Southern Cone" countries of South America (Brazil, Paraguay, Uruguay, Argentina, Chile, and Bolivia) has provided the framework for much of this progress. Uruguay and Chile were certified as transmission-free in 1997 and 1999, respectively. It appears likely that Brazil and Argentina will be certified as transmission-free in 2005 or 2006.[38,39] Similar control programs have been established recently in the Andean countries and in Central America.[40] In Mexico, legislation mandating nationwide blood donor screening is about to be passed, and this reflects a growing awareness of Chagas' disease as a public health problem there.[32,41] The obstacles hindering the elimination of *T. cruzi* transmission to humans throughout the endemic range are economic and political, and no technological advances are necessary for its completion.

The epidemiology of symptomatic chronic Chagas' disease is noteworthy. As many as 70% of persons who harbor *T. cruzi* chronically never develop associated cardiac or gastrointestinal symptoms. Among those who do develop either type of disease, the mean age of onset of symptoms is 35 to 45 years, although the age range is quite broad. In the past, the relatively high frequency of sudden death among young adults in some areas was attributed to arrhythmias due to chronic Chagas' disease, and several decades ago in one highly endemic area of Brazil chagasic cardiac disease was found to be the most frequent cause of death in adults.[42] Among Brazilian patients with chronic *T. cruzi* infection, the prevalence of megadisease has been found to range from 2.6% to 17.3%.[43,44]

Interestingly, there is considerable geographic variation in the relative prevalence of cardiac and megadisease in patients with chronic Chagas' disease. In most South American countries, megadisease is nearly as common as chagasic cardiac disease, but in Colombia, Venezuela, Central America, and Mexico megadisease is virtually unknown. It is not known if host factors or parasite strain differences cause these different patterns of clinical expression of the disease.

Epidemiology of Chagas' Disease in the United States

Despite the presence of the sylvatic cycle of *T. cruzi* in many parts of the southern and western United States, only five instances of autochthonous transmission there have been reported.[45–47] Our relatively high housing standards and low overall vector density probably underlie the rarity of transmission of *T. cruzi* to humans in the United States. In the past years, seven laboratory-acquired cases of acute Chagas' disease and nine imported infections have been reported to the Centers for Disease Control and Prevention (CDC), but none in the latter group occurred in returning tourists. Although the number of imported and autochthonous cases of acute Chagas' disease may be many times the number reported, the fact remains that the illness is rare in the United States.

In contrast, the number of persons in the United States with chronic *T. cruzi* infections has grown enormously in recent years. It is currently estimated that 12 million persons born in countries in which Chagas' disease is endemic currently live in the United States. Approximately 8 million of these individuals are from Mexico,[48,49] where the overall prevalence of *T. cruzi* infection may be 0.5% to 1.0%.[32] Moreover, a large proportion of these immigrants have come from Central

America, a region in which *T. cruzi* prevalence is high.[30,50,51] A study among Salvadorans and Nicaraguans in Washington, D.C., found a 5% prevalence rate of *T. cruzi* infection.[52] Seroprevalence studies done in a Los Angeles hospital where 50% of donors are Hispanic have shown that between 1 in 1000 and 1 in 500 donors are infected with *T. cruzi*.[53] In another study, carried out in seven blood banks in three southwestern states, roughly 1 in 600 donors with Hispanic surnames were found to be infected.[54] In a much larger study performed in Miami and Los Angeles, the *T. cruzi* prevalence rate was found to be 1 per 8800 in the general donor population and 1 per 710 among donors who had spent a month or more in an endemic area.[55,56] It can be estimated from these findings and census data that there are 80,000 to 120,000 *T. cruzi*–infected people now living in the United States. The presence of these immigrants creates a risk of transfusion-associated transmission of the parasite here, and to date seven such cases have been reported in the United States and Canada.[57] All the reported cases occurred in immunosuppressed patients in whom the diagnosis of *T. cruzi* infection was made because of the fulminant course of the illness. Since most transfusions are given to immunocompetent patients in whom acute Chagas' disease would follow a mild course, it is reasonable to infer that many other instances of transfusion-associated transmission of *T. cruzi* have occurred in the United States and have gone unnoticed. In recent years, however, the risk may have been reduced by screening prospective blood donors with questions relating to Chagas disease.[58] Finally, three recipients of transplants obtained from a *T. cruzi*–infected Central American immigrant developed acute Chagas' disease and one died of the latter illness.[59]

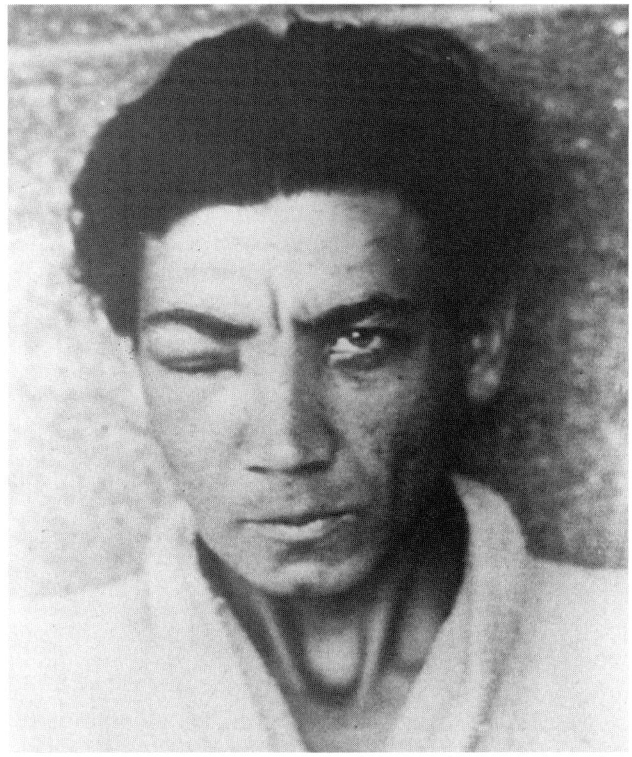

FIGURE 93-3 Romaña's sign (unilateral painless periorbital edema) in a Brazilian patient with acute Chagas' disease. (Courtesy of Dr. Mário Shiroma, São Paulo, Brazil.)

DISEASE

The clinical manifestations of acute and chronic Chagas' disease are very different and are described separately.

Acute Chagas' Disease

The first sign of acute Chagas' disease can be a chagoma, which is an erythematous and indurated lesion at the site of parasite entry that appears a week or two after transmission has occurred.[60] When the conjunctiva is the portal of entry, the patient may develop Romaña's sign, which is unilateral and painless periorbital edema (Fig. 93-3). Romaña's sign is found in only a small proportion of patients with acute *T. cruzi* infection and similar findings can be the result of several other processes.

Systemic spread of the parasites from the site of initial multiplication may be accompanied by malaise, fever, and edema of the face and lower extremities, as well as hepatosplenomegaly and generalized lymphadenopathy. A peripheral lymphocytosis may accompany the high parasitemias of acute Chagas' disease, and mild elevation of transaminases may also be present. Muscles, including the heart, can be heavily parasitized, and severe myocarditis with functional impairment occasionally causing death develops in a small proportion of patients[33,46,61] (Fig. 93-4). Nonspecific electrocardiographic (ECG) changes can occur, but the life-threatening conduction defects common in chronic cardiac Chagas' disease are usually not seen. *T. cruzi* also can invade the central nervous system,[62] but neurologic findings are not common. Rarely, meningoencephalitis develops, and it is associated with a poor prognosis.[63] In the vast majority of patients, the acute illness resolves spontaneously in 4 to 8 weeks and they then enter the *indeterminate phase* of the infection, which is characterized by a lack of symptoms, subpatent parasitemias, and generally detectable antibodies to a variety of *T. cruzi* antigens.

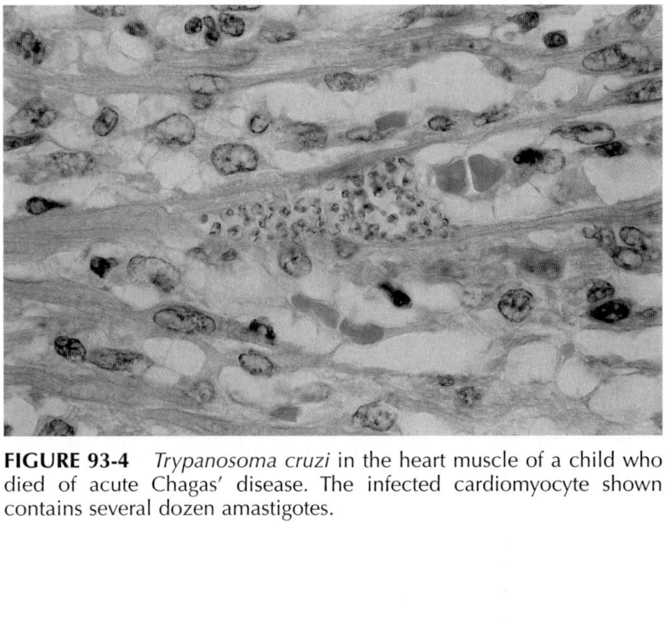

FIGURE 93-4 *Trypanosoma cruzi* in the heart muscle of a child who died of acute Chagas' disease. The infected cardiomyocyte shown contains several dozen amastigotes.

Chronic Chagas' Disease

Chronic Chagas' Cardiopathy

Although most persons with chronic *T. cruzi* infections remain in the indeterminate phase for life, approximately 10% to 30% develop symptomatic chronic Chagas' disease, usually years or even decades after the infection was initially acquired. Cardiac problems are the most frequent complications of chronic Chagas' disease.[64,65] Hearts obtained at autopsy from patients who died of chagasic heart disease usually have a global appearance due to chamber enlargement, which is often greater on the right than the left. Mural thrombi are frequently present, often in the right atrium and the apex of the left ventricle. Left ventricular apical aneurysm is typical in patients with advanced cardiac Chagas' disease. At a cellular level, the process that underlies these gross pathologic lesions is a chronic inflammation with mononuclear cell infiltration and diffuse fibrosis that affects the conduction system as well as the cardiac muscle.[66,67] Parasites are rarely seen on histological examination, but they can often be detected by polymerase chain reaction–based assays.[68] The process results in a variety of dysrhythmias, including atrial bradyarrhythmias and fibrillation; premature ventricular contractions; bundle branch blocks, often of the right bundle; and complete atrioventricular block. Most instances of sudden death in persons with chronic *T. cruzi* infection probably result from complete atrioventricular block, ventricular tachycardia, or ventricular fibrillation.

The symptoms associated with chronic cardiac Chagas' disease reflect the congestive failure, rhythm disturbances, and thromboembolism that result from the fibrosing cardiopathy.[69] The arrhythmias can cause dizziness and syncope, and sudden death is a common occurrence.[42,70] The cardiomyopathy frequently affects the right side of the heart more than the left, and thus symptoms of right-sided failure are often present. The progression of chagasic arrhythmias and cardiomyopathy is gradual, but once congestive heart failure develops, death often occurs within several months.

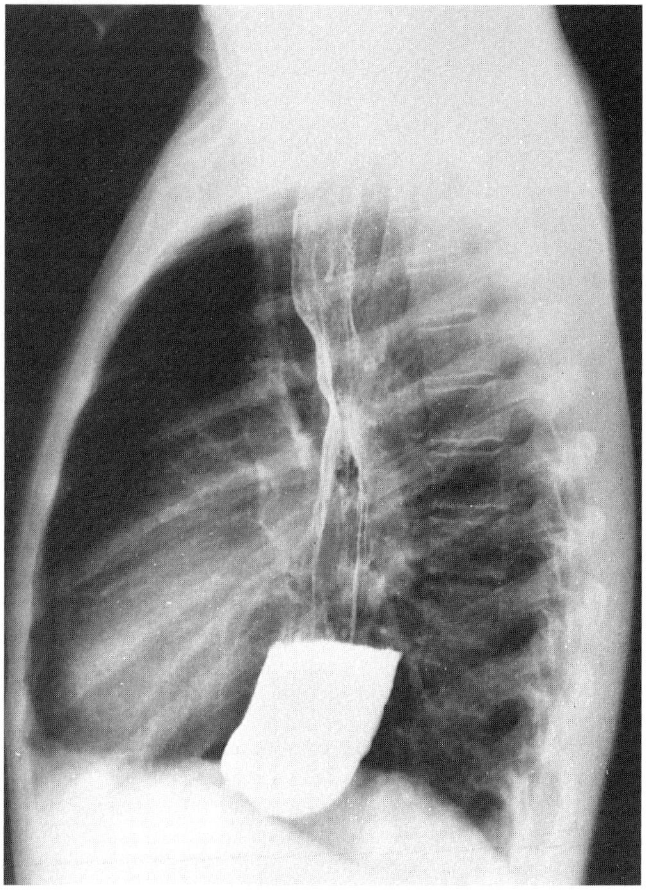

FIGURE 93-5 Barium esophagogram in a Brazilian patient with dolichomegaesophagus caused by chronic Chagas' disease. Contrast material is pooled in the distal esophagus, which is markedly enlarged. (From Neva FA, Brown HW: Basic Clinical Parasitology, 6th ed. Norwalk, CN, Appleton & Lange, 1994.)

Chronic Gastrointestinal Chagas' Disease (Megadisease)

Dysfunction of the gastrointestinal tract is the second most common consequence of chronic *T. cruzi* infection.[71,72] As in the case of chagasic cardiopathy, gastrointestinal Chagas' disease usually occurs years or even decades after infection with *T. cruzi* is acquired. Dysfunction related to megaesophagus (Fig. 93-5) is the most typical clinical manifestation, but symptoms due to megacolon (Fig. 93-6) are also frequent. Other gastrointestinal and urinary viscera can be affected as well, but this is much less common.[73] The process underlying megadisease is a loss of neurons in the gut.[74] Quantitative assessments of this degenerative process have shown that in severely affected patients as many as 85% of the neurons in the esophagus and 50% of those in the colon may be lost. The factors that determine the rate and pattern of the neuronal destruction are not known.

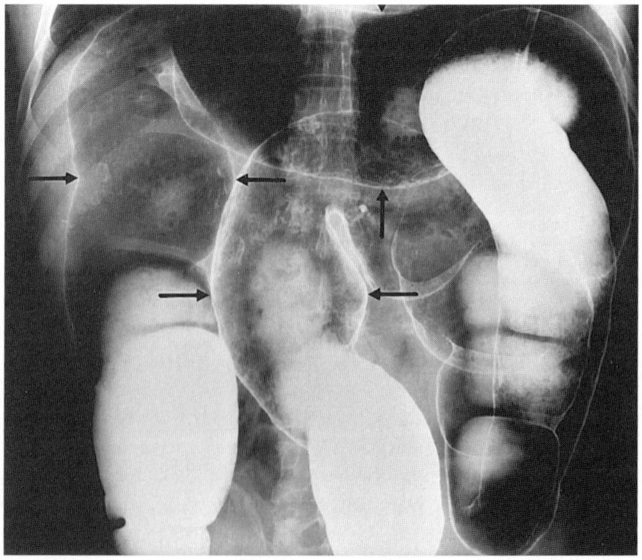

FIGURE 93-6 Barium enema examination of a patient with megacolon caused by Chagas' disease. Markedly increased diameter of the ascending, transverse, and sigmoid segments of the large bowel are marked with opposing arrows.

Pathologic examination of esophageal specimens obtained surgically or at autopsy from patients with megaesophagus have shown dilation and varying degrees of thickening of the muscular wall. As in the case of cardiac tissue, microscopic examination shows mononuclear cell infiltration and fibrosis, but finding parasites is unusual. The most common symptom associated with chagasic megaesophagus is dysphagia. Many patients experiencing this sense the accumulation of swallowed food in the esophagus and take in water or more food, or even eat in a standing position, to facilitate its passage into the stomach. Pain, typically starting in the lower substernal area and spreading upward, is also a frequent symptom in patients with megaesophagus. In patients with severe degrees of megaesophagus, regurgitation can become a problem, and if the underlying problem is not treated, it can lead to intermittent aspiration with associated chronic cough, bronchitis, and pneumonia.

As in the case of chagasic megaesophagus, colonic disease is manifested by dilation and thickening of the wall. Typically, the sigmoid colon is the most affected segment. As the disease progresses, the colon can become markedly enlarged in both length and diameter, and the thickening of the wall can become less pronounced. The pathologic changes evident on microscopic examination of affected colonic tissue are similar to those found in the esophagus. The cardinal symptom associated with Chagas' disease of the colon is constipation. As the size of the colon increases gradually over years, the frequency of bowel movements decreases, and some patients can go for several weeks without bowel movements. Pain is also a common symptom, resulting from accumulation of feces and flatus, as well as ineffective and recurrent colonic contractions.

Other organs also can be affected by chronic gastrointestinal Chagas' disease. The most common occurrence is hypertrophy of the parotid glands, which is present in as many as 25% of patients with chagasic megaesophagus. The stomach may also be affected, although much less commonly than the colon and esophagus, and affected patients usually have either megaesophagus or megacolon.[75] Hypoperistalsis, hypotonia, decreased acid secretion, and delayed emptying of the stomach have been documented in patients with megaesophagus, but dilation of the stomach is not found frequently.[76]

The pathogenesis of the cardiac and gastrointestinal lesions of chronic Chagas' disease has been debated for decades.[77–79] Recently, convincing evidence has accumulated supporting the concept that low-level presence of parasites in chronically affected cardiac tissue, detectable by molecular methods, stimulates a chronic inflammatory response that over time leads to the pathologic changes observed microscopically.[80,81]

Trypanosoma cruzi Infection in Immunosuppressed Patients

Immunosuppression of persons who chronically harbor *T. cruzi* can lead to a recrudescence of the infection, frequently with an intensity that is atypical of acute Chagas' disease in immunocompetent patients. The incidence of reactivation of *T. cruzi* in patients who become immunosuppressed is not known, and both its occurrence[82–84] and its absence[85,86] have been reported. Persons immunosuppressed by the human immunodeficiency virus (HIV) and infected with *T. cruzi* are also at risk for reactivation of the latter. To date, several dozen such cases have been described,[87–92] and it is noteworthy that many of these patients developed *T. cruzi* brain abscesses, which do not occur in immunocompetent persons with acute or chronic Chagas' disease. The diagnosis of *T. cruzi* brain abscesses in HIV-positive patients is complicated by the fact that these lesions are difficult to distinguish radiographically from those of cerebral toxoplasmosis.

DIAGNOSIS

The approaches used to diagnose acute and chronic Chagas' disease are quite different and will be considered separately.

Acute Chagas' Disease

The first step in diagnosing acute Chagas' disease is determining that the patient has a history consistent with exposure to *T. cruzi*. Risk factors include residence or a blood transfusion in an endemic country, birth to a mother known or suspected of being infected with *T. cruzi*, or a laboratory accident involving the parasite. When considering geographic risk, it is important to bear in mind that there have been no reports of imported cases among tourists returning to the United States from countries in which Chagas' disease is endemic. Two such cases in tourists returning to Europe, however, have been described.[93,94] It is also worthy of note that only five cases of autochthonous transmission of *T. cruzi* have been described here, and the most recent of these occurred in 1998.[47]

Patients with acute Chagas' disease may develop a variety of local and systemic signs, but these are usually mild. Occasionally, severe myocarditis develops, leading to nonspecific ECG changes, radiographic signs of cardiomegaly, or pericardial effusion detectable by echocardiography. Invasion of the central nervous system by the parasites can lead to abnormal cerebrospinal fluid values. The differential diagnoses of all of these clinical findings are quite broad, however, and in the absence of a parasitologic diagnosis they can only be viewed as suggestive of Chagas' disease.

A definitive diagnosis of acute Chagas' disease is made by detecting parasites, and serologic assays for *T. cruzi*–specific IgM, which are neither standardized nor widely available, are of limited importance.[95] Circulating trypomastigotes are highly motile and frequently can be seen in wet preparations of anticoagulated blood or buffy coat. The parasites often can be seen in Giemsa-stained smears as well. In immunocompetent patients with acute Chagas' disease, examination of blood preparations is the cornerstone of detecting *T. cruzi*. In immunocompromised patients suspected of having acute Chagas' disease, however, other specimens such as bone marrow, lymph node aspirates, endomyocardial tissue, skin lesion biopsies, cerebrospinal fluid, and pericardial fluid should be examined microscopically. When these methods fail to detect organisms in any patient with clinical and epidemiologic histories suggesting a diagnosis of acute Chagas' disease, as is often the case,[96,97] efforts to grow the parasites can be undertaken. This is done by culturing blood or other specimens in specialized liquid medium[98,99] or by xenodiagnosis, which is a method employing laboratory-reared insect vectors.[100] A major drawback to these approaches is the fact that they take a minimum of several weeks to complete, and this is far beyond the time at which decisions regarding drug treatment need to be made. In addition, although blood culture and xenodiagnosis are more sensitive than microscopic examination of blood and other specimens, their sensitivities in detecting *T. cruzi* in acutely infected patients have not been determined. Hemoculture for *T. cruzi* infection is available in my laboratory. Xenodiagnosis is not done in the United States.

Chronic Chagas' Disease

As mentioned previously, patients with chronic cardiac Chagas' disease can develop a variety of dysrhythmias, including right bundle branch block, which is the most representative conduction abnormality of Chagas' cardiopathy. Nonetheless, it is a nonspecific finding and especially in nonendemic countries the vast majority of persons with right bundle branch block do not have Chagas' disease. Echocardiographic and radiographic signs of chronic cardiac Chagas' disease are similar to those found in patients with heart failure due to cardiomyopathies caused by other processes. Megacolon and megaesophagus are best diagnosed by barium contrast radiographic tests. It is important to keep in mind, however, that all of these diagnostic studies are useful primarily for defining the degree of associated abnormalities in patients known to be infected with the parasite.

Chronic Chagas' disease is usually diagnosed by detecting IgG antibodies that bind specifically to parasite antigens, and isolating the organism is not of major importance. At the present time, about 30 assays for the serologic diagnosis of *T. cruzi* infection are available commercially. Most of these are based on enzyme-linked immunosorbent assay (ELISA), indirect immunofluorescence, and indirect hemagglutination formats, and they are used widely in Latin America for clinical testing and for screening donated blood.[101] Several tests are based on recombinant antigens.[102–104] Many of the assays have sensitivities and specificities that are less than ideal, and false positive reactions typically occur with samples from patients having illnesses such as leishmaniasis, syphilis, malaria, and other parasitic and nonparasitic diseases. Because of these shortcomings, most authorities recommend that samples be tested in two or three assays based on different formats before decisions regarding infection status are made. This additional testing, however, carries with it an enormous economic and logistical burden, particularly in regard to donated blood. As an example, in the largest blood donor center in São Paulo, Brazil (Hemocentro, 22,000 donations/month), two tests for antibodies to *T. cruzi* are employed and 1.1% of donated units are discarded because of reactivity in one or more of the assays (E. Sabino, São Paulo, Brazil, personal communication, 2004). As many as two thirds of these donations may have come from persons who are not infected with *T. cruzi*, but whose blood must be discarded because of inconsistent test results. Clearly more accurate tests for detecting chronic *T. cruzi* infection are needed. Some years ago a lysate-based ELISA (Chagas' Kit, Hemagen Diagnostics, Inc., Columbia, MD) was cleared by the Food and Drug Administration (FDA) for clinical testing [510(k)] but not for screening donated blood. Within the past year, an ELISA based on recombinant antigens (Chagatest ELISA Recombinante v3.0, Wiener Laboratories, Rosario, Argentina) was also cleared by the FDA for clinical testing. Two other tests have received 510(k) clearance (Chagas EIA, Abbott Laboratories, Abbott Park, IL,[105] and Chagas' IgG ELISA, Meridian Diagnostics, Inc., Cincinnati, OH[101]), but neither is currently marketed in the United States.

The possibility of using PCR assays for detecting *T. cruzi* infection has been the focus of considerable study. Although the numbers of parasites in the blood of chronically infected persons is extremely low, PCR assays have the potential for detecting their presence because they have large numbers of highly conserved nuclear and kinetoplast DNA (kDNA) sequences. Moser and coworkers[106] described a PCR assay in which a 188–base pair nuclear repetitive DNA sequence is amplified using primers called TCZ1 and TCZ2. Each parasite contains approximately 100,000 copies of this sequence, and in contrived experiments as little as 0.5% of the genome of a single organism gave a positive result. A study in mice with acute and chronic *T. cruzi* infections indicated clearly that TCZ1-TCZ2 assay is much more sensitive than microscopic examination of blood.[107] In another PCR assay, described by Sturm and coworkers,[108] a 330–base pair segment of the *T. cruzi* kinetoplast minicircle is amplified using primers S35-S36. It is estimated that each parasite has 120,000 copies of this sequence, and in mixing experiments the authors detected 0.1% of one parasite genome. To date, two head-to-head comparisons of the TCZ1-TCZ2 and S35-S36 assays have been described, and in both cases the TCZ1-TCZ2 test appeared to have a slight edge in terms of sensitivity.[107,109] PCR assays for *T. cruzi* detection based on several other primer pairs have been described but none appears to have any advantage over tests based on TCZ1-TCZ2 and S35-S36, probably because the parasite has fewer copies of the DNA sequences they amplify.

Since these two original reports were published in 1989, more than 100 articles have appeared that deal with the detection of *T. cruzi* by PCR tests. In nine key human studies published in the 1990s, the sensitivities of the PCR assays ranged from 44.7% to 100%, with most results falling a bit over 90%.[98,99,110] These disappointing results are likely the result of a sampling phenomenon in that the large numbers of amplifiable sequences are not dispersed, but rather are contained in the rare parasites that may or may not be swept up with blood drawn for testing. Clearly the level of sensitivity achieved with PCR assays for *T. cruzi* infection is not high enough to allow their use for confirmatory testing of donated blood. Nonetheless, PCR assays are potentially useful for detecting *T. cruzi* in persons with borderline serologic results, in persons suspected of having acute or congenital Chagas' disease in whom parasites are not detected microscopically, and in infected patients who have received specific treatment. In such individuals, only positive PCR results can be taken as truly indicative of infection status. No PCR test for detecting *T. cruzi* is currently available commercially.

Parasitologic diagnoses of chronic *T. cruzi* infections also can be made by xenodiagnosis and hemoculture. As noted, xenodiagnosis is not available in the United States. When done properly, hemoculture, which is available in my laboratory, may have a sensitivity as high as 70% in persons with chronic *T. cruzi* infections.[98] Its use should be limited to patients suspected of having acute or congenital *T. cruzi* infection who are negative by microscopic examination of blood and to persons who may have chronic Chagas' disease whose serologic studies are indeterminate.

TREATMENT AND PROGNOSIS

Antiparasitic Drugs

Therapy for *T. cruzi* is unsatisfactory and the need for a parasitologically curative drug regimen is the most important current challenge in Chagas' disease research. Many dozens of drugs have been tested for activity against *T. cruzi,* including those active against other parasitic protozoans, and only two have been found to be clinically useful.[111,112] The first of these is nifurtimox (Lampit, Bayer 2502), a nitrofuran derivative with which extensive clinical experience has accumulated during the three decades it has been available.[113] Its mechanism of action is not known.

In patients with acute Chagas' disease, nifurtimox reduces the severity and duration of the illness and lessens mortality. Parasitologic cures are achieved with nifurtimox only in approximately 70% of these patients. Those not cured enter the indeterminate phase of *T. cruzi* infection and are at risk of symptomatic chronic Chagas' disease. In general, cure rates are less than 20% in patients with chronic *T. cruzi* infection. Nifurtimox must be taken for long periods and can cause severe side effects, including gastrointestinal complaints such as nausea, vomiting, abdominal pain, anorexia, and weight loss.[114] Some patients taking the drug also develop neurologic symptoms, such as restlessness, insomnia, twitching, paresthesias, polyneuritis, and seizures. Treatment with nifurtimox should be initiated as early as possible in patients with acute Chagas' disease. In the case of a laboratory accident with a reasonable likelihood of transmission, therapy should be started before parasitologic or clinical signs of infection become apparent.[8,115] Nifurtimox is available in 30- and 120-mg tablets. For adults, the recommended oral dosage is 8 to 10 mg/kg body weight per day. For adolescents, the dose is 12.5 to 15 mg/kg/day, and for children 1 to 10 years of age, it is 15 to 20 mg/kg/day. The drug should be given each day in four divided doses, and treatment should be continued for 90 to 120 days. Nifurtimox can be obtained from the CDC Drug Service (770-639-3670).

The drug of choice for treating *T. cruzi* is the nitroimidazole derivative benznidazole (Radimil, Roche 7-1051).[116] Cure rates are similar to those of nifurtimox.[117] Side effects can include granulocytopenia, rash, and peripheral neuropathy. The recommended oral dosage of benznidazole is 5 mg/kg body weight per day for 60 days.

The question of whether patients in the indeterminate or chronic symptomatic phases of *T. cruzi* infection should be treated is controversial. The fact that parasitologic cure rates are so low is a central issue in this debate. Recent studies in *T. cruzi*–infected laboratory animals and humans suggest that the persistent presence of organisms in heart muscle is associated with inflammation, thus implicating the parasites in the chronic pathogenesis.[68,80,118,119] Moreover, limited studies in humans have shown that the appearance and/or progression of cardiac lesions in drug-treated patients may be less than in untreated controls.[117] After reviewing these and other studies, a panel of experts convened several years ago by the World Health Organization recommended that all persons in the indeterminate phase of *T. cruzi* infection should be given drug therapy, and that patients with symptomatic Chagas' disease, hepatic impairment, renal disease, or pregancy should not.[120] This recommendation stimulated a lot of debate and currently there is no consensus regarding the treatment of asymptomatic persons with long-standing *T. cruzi* infection.[121,122]

Some authors have pointed out that there is no convincing evidence that specific treatment affects long-term clinical outcome.[123] Recent reports of long-term studies indicating that, in adults, cure rates with nifurtimox and benznidazole are less than 10% have added fuel to the debate.[124–126] Cure rates may be considerably higher in children.[127] Finally, concern relating to these two drugs is raised by reports of experiments showing that 33% of rabbits treated with nifurtimox and 42% of those given benznidazole developed lymphomas, whereas none of the control animals developed tumors.[128,129] Although these findings should be a cause for concern, it should be kept in mind that these two drugs have been used for decades in endemic countries and no reports of an increased incidence of lymphomas have appeared.

Several other compounds merit comment. Some years ago it was shown that recombinant interferon-γ (IFN-γ) reduced the severity of acute *T. cruzi* infection in mice.[130] To my knowledge, only two patients with acute Chagas' disease have been treated with IFN-γ. The first was an immunosuppressed recipient of a contaminated blood transfusion[131] and the other acquired the infection in the laboratory. Both patients were given nifurtimox in addition to IFN-γ and recovered. The person infected in the laboratory was antibody- and PCR-negative 10 years after the incident and the infection status of the immunocompromised patient has not been assessed. Since most patients resolve the acute illness in a matter of weeks even without drug treatment, my view is that nifurtimox or benznidazole should be used alone in immunocompetent patients. Whether IFN-γ should be given in addition in immunocompromised patients remains an open question.

The activities of allopurinol and the antifungal agents itraconazole, ketoconazole, and fluconazole against *T. cruzi* have been studied extensively in laboratory animals and to a lesser extent in infected persons. None of these agents has shown a level of anti–*T. cruzi* activity that justifies its use in humans. Posaconazole, which was recently approved by the FDA for treating fungal infections, has been shown to cure *T. cruzi* infections in mice.[132] Efficacy trials in monkeys and humans infected with the parasite are being planned. Other promising drugs are being evaluated.[133–135]

Treatment of Clinical Chagas' Disease

Beyond the possible use of antiparasitic drugs, the treatment of both acute and chronic Chagas' disease is symptomatic. Patients with severe acute chagasic myocarditis should be supported, as would any patient with acute congestive cardiomyopathy. In patients with symptomatic chronic Chagas' heart disease, therapy is directed at ameliorating symptoms through the use of cardiotropic drugs and anticoagulants. Pacemakers have been shown to be useful in patients with ominous bradyarrhythmias or heart block.[70]

Cardiac transplantation is an option in patients with end-stage Chagas' heart disease, and more than 100 *T. cruzi*–infected patients have undergone the procedure in Brazil and the United States.[136,137] Reactivated acute Chagas' disease occurred often in the patients transplanted initially in Brazil due to the postoperative immunosuppression, but this has been less of a problem in the last decade or so as smaller doses of cyclosporine have been used. In addition, the fact that the usual parasitologic methods for detecting acute *T. cruzi* infection were not sensitive detectors of the reactivations and the occurrence of malignant neoplasms was an additional problem.[138] It also merits mention that patients who have had heart transplants for Chagas' disease often develop cutaneous lesions containing large numbers of parasites.[139] One such case has been observed in a *T. cruzi*–infected patient who underwent renal transplantation,[140] but interestingly lesions of this type have not been reported in co-infected persons with HIV/AIDS.[89] The efficacy and toxicity of long-term prophylaxis with either nifurtimox or benznidazole in *T. cruzi*–infected patients after cardiac transplantation have not been assessed. In spite of these problems, the long-term survival of Chagas' patients with heart transplants is greater than that of individuals receiving heart transplants for other reasons, most likely because the lesions of chronic *T. cruzi* infection are often limited to the heart.[141] The frequency with which *T. cruzi*–infected immigrants in the United States are considered for cardiac transplantation will increase over time as this group increases in size and ages.

Megaesophagus associated with Chagas' disease should be treated as is idiopathic achalasia.[73] The best relief of symptoms is achieved by balloon dilation of the lower esophageal sphincter.[142] Patients with megaesophagus who fail to respond to repeated balloon dilation may require surgical treatment.[143] The procedure most often used is wide esophagocardiomyectomy of the anterior gastroesophageal junction, combined with valvuloplasty to reduce reflux. Patients with extreme megaesophagus can be treated with esophageal resection with reconstruction using an esophagogastroplasty. In developed countries, laparoscopic myotomy is being used with increasing frequency to treat idiopathic achalasia, and this relatively simple procedure may become the method of choice for both idiopathic achalasia and Chagas' disease. A possible role for the injection of botulinum toxin is being evaluated.[144]

Patients in the early stages of colonic dysfunction associated with chronic *T. cruzi* infection can be managed with a high-fiber diet and occasional laxatives and enemas. Fecal impaction necessitating manual disimpaction may occur, as can toxic megacolon, which requires surgical intervention.[145] Volvulus is a complication of chagasic megacolon that requires immediate attention. This usually occurs when the lengthened and enlarged sigmoid colon twists and folds on itself, causing a constellation of symptoms. Endoscopic emptying can be done initially in patients without clinical, endoscopic, or radiographic signs of ischemia in the affected segment. Cases that are complicated should be treated with surgical decompression. In either case, however, surgical treatment of the megacolon is ultimately necessary because of the common recurrence of volvulus.[143,146] Several surgical procedures have been used to treat advanced chagasic megacolon, and all of them include resection of the sigmoid as well as removal of part of the rectum.

PREVENTION AND CONTROL

Since there are no vaccines or chemoprophylaxis for preventing transmission of *T. cruzi,* reducing the number of new cases in Latin America must depend on reducing contact with insect vectors and on serologic identification of infected blood donors. Elimination of domiciliary vectors is best accomplished by improving housing conditions, spraying of insecticides, and educating at-risk populations. As noted previously, major successes with these approaches have been achieved in several endemic countries.[35] Elimination of the sylvatic reservoirs is not a reasonable goal. In view of the successes of low-technology measures in reducing the transmission of *T. cruzi,* it appears unlikely that the recent major advances in understanding the molecular biology of the parasite and the pathogenesis of Chagas' disease will play a substantive role in the eventual elimination this public health problem.

Since chronic *T. cruzi* infection carries with it the risk of serious cardiac and gastrointestinal disease, I feel that in industrialized countries immigrants from endemic regions and children of infected mothers should be screened serologically. Identification of infected persons is important because pacemakers have been shown to benefit some patients who develop rhythm disturbances. Infected individuals should have ECGs done every 6 to 12 months with the goal of early detection of rhythm disturbances. The possibility of congenital transmission is another reason for screening.

Tourists from the United States who travel in areas where *T. cruzi* transmission occurs should avoid sleeping in dilapidated dwellings in rural areas and should use insect repellent and mosquito nets to reduce exposure to vectors. Nonetheless, it is important to keep in mind that the risk of acquiring *T. cruzi* infection during short-term residence in an endemic country is extremely low. As noted, a Frenchwoman was reported to have become infected with *T. cruzi* during a several-weeks stay in Colombia, and an Italian tour guide acquired the infection while traveling in Brazil.[93,94] To my knowledge, no incidents of this type have been reported among tourists returning to the United States. People traveling in endemic areas should avoid sleeping in primitive dwellings and should use bed nets and insect repellent to reduce exposure to insects.[147,148] Special precautions for people engaging in outdoor activities in the United States are not warranted. Laboratorians should wear eye protection and gloves when working with *T. cruzi,* and suitable containment should be used for infected insects.[149]

As stated previously, seven instances of transfusion-associated transmission of *T. cruzi* have been reported in the United States and Canada. In all these patients, the courses of acute Chagas' disease were particularly fulminant because of the immunosuppression they were receiving, and this certainly contributed to the definitive diagnoses. Since most transfusions are given to immunocompetent persons in whom acute *T. cruzi* infection would be a mild illness, it is reasonable to infer that many other cases have occurred here but have not been noticed. The question as to how best to avoid transmission of the parasite via transfusion in the United States has been debated since the first instance occurred in 1988. Common sense suggests that if screening is warranted in the endemic countries from which the 12 million immigrants living here have come, then they should be tested when they present for donation here. In some donor centers, prospective donors have been asked questions relating to risk for *T. cruzi* infection, with the purpose of deferring persons at high risk for harboring the parasite. The efficacy of this approach is not known, but related data obtained in the United States.[150] and Brazil[151] suggest that it may not be serving its purpose.

94

Leishmaniasis

SELMA M. B. JERONIMO
ANASTACIO DE QUEIROZ SOUSA
RICHARD D. PEARSON

INTRODUCTION

Leishmania species are members of the family Trypanosomatidae, order Kinetoplastida[1,2] (Table 94-1). They reside as intracellular amastigotes within macrophages in mammals and as extracellular promastigotes in the gut of their insect vectors, phlebotomine sand flies. The clinical manifestations of infection vary as a consequence of the virulence of the infecting *Leishmania* species and the cell-mediated immune responses of their mammalian hosts. Leishmaniasis has historically been divided into three major clinical syndromes: cutaneous, mucosal, and visceral. Each of these encompasses a spectrum of findings, and there is overlap between them. Although specific *Leishmania* species tend to cause one syndrome or another, there are frequent variations making generalizations difficult.

Leishmania species are endemic in scattered areas of every continent except Australia and Antarctica (see Table 94-1). Cutaneous leishmaniasis is a problem for residents, refugees, military personnel, and workers in endemic areas of Latin America, the Middle East, Asia, and the Indian subcontinent. Close to 700 cases due to *Leishmania major* have been reported among U.S. military personnel serving in Iraq, with additional cases reported from Afghanistan.[3–5] Many were acquired along the Iraq–Syria or Iraq–Iran borders. Mucosal leishmaniasis due to *Leishmania braziliensis* is endemic in Latin America. Major epidemics of visceral leishmaniasis have been reported in eastern India and Bangladesh,[6,7] among refugees in the Sudan,[8,9] and in cities that have expanded into endemic areas in northeastern Brazil.[10] Visceral leishmaniasis emerged as an important opportunistic disease in people with acquired immunodeficiency syndrome in Spain, southern France, and Italy,[11–16] and it occurs in people who are immunosuppressed following organ transplantation or chemotherapy.[17–19] Finally, viscerotropic leishmaniasis was identified in a group of U.S. troops infected during Operation Desert Storm with *Leishmania tropica*, a species historically associated with cutaneous leishmaniasis.[20]

AGENT

Lainson and Shaw have classified *Leishmania* species into two subgenera, *Viannia* and *Leishmania*, based on their development in the gut of the sand fly. The subgenus *Viannia* includes *L. braziliensis* and related species that develop in the hindgut before migrating to the midgut and foregut (peripylaria). The subgenus *Leishmania* includes species that occupy the midgut and foregut only (suprapylaria). Within each subgenus, speciation has historically been based on multiple factors, including geographic distribution, animal reservoir, and sand fly species. Refinements in taxonomy are likely to be made as more is learned about the genetic diversity of the parasites.

Several assays can be used to identify *Leishmania* species. Isoenzyme analysis[21–23] is used at several World Health Organization (WHO) reference laboratories. Other approaches include species-specific monoclonal antibodies,[24] restriction endonuclease digestion of kinetoplast DNA (kDNA),[25] and hybridization with species-specific kDNA probes.[26] Polymerase chain reaction (PCR) assays using species-specific oligonucleotide primers are available in research and some reference laboratories and are the method of choice for speciation.[27–33]

The life cycle is relatively simple.[34] Amastigotes are equipped to live at acid pH within parasitophorous vacuoles in macrophages.[35] They are oval or round in shape and approximately 2 or 3 μm in diameter. Amastigotes have a relatively large, eccentrically located nucleus; a specialized mitochondrial structure, the kinetoplast, which contains a substantial amount of extranuclear DNA in the form of catenated mini- and maxicircles; and a flagellar pocket and flagellum, which lie within the confines of the cell. They multiply by simple binary division. A row of subpellicular microtubules is arrayed under the plasma membrane much like the ribs of an umbrella. In the gut of the sand fly,[36] leishmania live and multiply as extracellular, flagellated promastigotes that vary morphologically from short, stumpy forms to elongated ones ranging from 10 to 15 μm in length and 2 or 3 μm in diameter. A single flagellum extends from the anterior pole. After development in the sand fly gut, which takes approximately 1 or 2 weeks depending on the *Leishmania* species, infectious metacyclic promastigotes migrate to the proboscis.[37,38]

Leishmania species are transmitted by female sand flies of the genus *Lutzomyia* in the Americas and *Phlebotomus* elsewhere. Depending on the species, sand flies live in forested areas, rodent burrows, or debris in peridomestic habitats. They are weak fliers, but they can be carried considerable distances if caught in the wind and have been dispersed more than 200 m from the original foci.[39] Sand flies probe with their proboscis to form a venous pool, from which they obtain blood by capillary action. Metacyclic promastigotes obstruct the proboscis of leishmania-infected sand flies, preventing easy aspiration of blood and stimulating the fly to probe even more. Although not well quantified, a relatively small number of promastigotes are thought to be inoculated. Sand fly saliva has been shown to enhance the infectivity of promastigotes by inhibiting the L-arginine-dependent nitric oxide killing mechanism of macrophages.[40,41]

IMMUNOLOGY

The outcome of leishmanial infection is dependent on a series of complex and only partially understood interactions between *Leishmania* species-specific virulence factors and the genetically determined cell-mediated immune responses of their mammalian hosts.[42–45] An array of cytokines secreted by

Table 94-1 *Clinical Syndromes Caused by* Leishmania *Species and Their Geographic Distribution*

Clinical Syndromes	*Leishmania* Species	Location
Visceral leishmaniasis		
Kala-azar: generalized involvement of the reticuloendothelial system (spleen, bone marrow, liver)	*L. (L.) donovani*	Indian subcontinent, northern and eastern China, Pakistan, Nepal, eastern Africa, Sudan, Kenya
	L. (L.) infantum/chagasi	Middle East, Mediterranean littoral, Balkans, central and southwestern Asia, northern and northwestern China, northern and sub-Saharan Africa, Latin America
	L. (L.) donovani (archibaldi)	Sudan, Kenya, Ethiopia
	L. (L.) spp.	Kenya, Ethiopia, Somalia
	L. (L.) chagasi	Latin America
	L. (L.) amazonensis	Brazil (Bahia State)
	L. (L.) tropica	Israel, India, and viscerotropic disease in Saudi Arabia (U.S. troops)
Post-kala-azar dermal leishmaniasis	*L. (L.) donovani*	Indian subcontinent, East Africa and Sudan
	L. (L.) spp.	Kenya, Ethiopia, Somalia
Old World cutaneous leishmaniasis		
Single or limited number of skin lesions	*L. (L.) major*	Middle East, northwestern China, northwestern India, Pakistan, Africa
	L. (L.) tropica	Mediterranean littoral, Middle East, western Asiatic area, Indian subcontinent
	L. (L.) aethiopica	Ethiopian highlands, Kenya, Yemen
	L. (L.) infantum/chagasi	Mediterranean basin
	L. (L.) donovani (archibaldi)	Sudan and East Africa
	L. (L.) spp.	Kenya, Ethiopia, Somalia
Diffuse cutaneous leishmaniasis	*L. (L.) aethiopica*	Ethiopian highlands, Kenya, Yemen
New World cutaneous leishmaniasis		
Single or limited number of skin lesions	*L. (L.) mexicana* (chiclero ulcer)	Central America, Mexico, Texas
	L. (L.) amazonensis	Amazon basin and neighboring areas, Bahia and other states in Brazil
	L. (V.) braziliensis	Multiple areas of Central and South America
	L. (V.) guyanensis (forest yaws)	Guyana, Suriname, northern Amazon basin
	L. (V.) peruviana (uta)	Peru (western Andes) and Argentinean highlands
	L. (V.) panamensis	Panama, Costa Rica, Colombia
	L. (V.) pifanoi	Venezuela
	L. (V.) garnhami	Venezuela
	L. (V.) venezuelensis	Venezuela
	L. (V.) colombiensis	Colombia and Panama
	L. (L.) infantum/chagasi	Central and South America
Diffuse cutaneous leishmaniasis	*L. (L.) amazonensis*	Amazon basin and neighboring areas, Bahia and other states in Brazil
	L. (V.) pifanoi	Venezuela
	L. (L.) mexicana	Mexico and Central America
	L. (L.) spp.	Dominican Republic
American mucocutaneous leishmaniasis	*L. (V.) braziliensis* (espundia)	Multiple areas in Latin America

(*L.*), subgenus *Leishmania*; (*V.*), subgenus *Viannia*.

Modified from Pearson RD, Sousa AQ: Clinical spectrum of leishmaniasis. *Clin Infect Dis* 22:1–13, 1996; data from Lainson R, Shaw JJ: Evolution, classification and geographic distribution. In Peters W, Killick-Kendrick R (eds): The Leishmaniases in Biology and Medicine. London, Academic Press, 1987, pp 1–120.

lymphocytes and macrophages are involved. Antileishmanial antibodies are present but alone are not protective.

Leishmania–Macrophage Interactions

The focus of leishmanial infection is the macrophage, the sole sanctuary for the parasite in mammals. In vitro studies using murine and human mononuclear phagocytes indicate that promastigotes can bind to several macrophage receptors.[46] Two surface molecules on promastigotes are known to be involved in attachment: a 63-kDa neutral protease (gp63)[47,48] and a lipophosphoglycan (LPG).[49,50] The glycosylation of these molecules varies among *Leishmania* species and with the stage of promastigote development.[37,38] The attachment of promastigotes is mediated by several different macrophage receptors, including the complement receptors

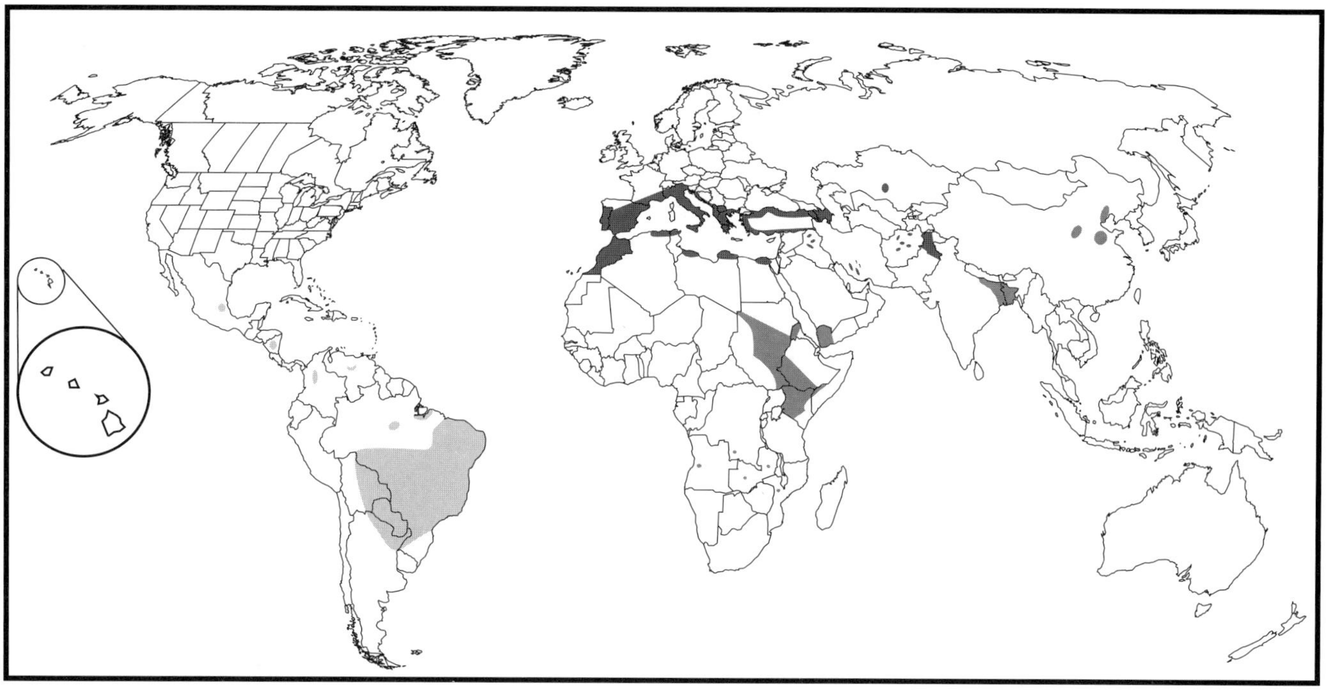

Visceral Leishmaniasis

Leishmania (L.) chagasi

Leishmania (L.) donovani

Leishmania (L.) infantum

most frequently affected, but more recent data indicate that the mean age has increased to 20 years, possibly related to a decline in herd immunity.[129] *Leishmania donovani* is also endemic in eastern Africa. It is responsible for sporadic cases of visceral leishmaniasis in Ethiopia, Somalia, Kenya, and adjacent countries, and it has caused a major epidemic of visceral leishmaniasis among refugees in the Sudan.[8,9,130] *Phlebotomus orientalis* is thought to be the vector. Rats, gerbils, ground squirrels, and small carnivores are potential reservoirs.

Leishmania infantum/chagasi is endemic in scattered areas extending from France, across the Mediterranean littoral,[131] to the Middle East and into western China.[132,133] Canine species are the major reservoirs. Most cases occur in children or immunocompromised adults. Visceral leishmaniasis has been an important opportunistic infection among people with HIV infection in southern France, Spain, and Italy.[11–13,15,16]

Leishmania infantum/chagasi is the principal cause of visceral leishmaniasis in Latin America.[73,74] It is endemic in northeastern Brazil and in other widely scattered areas of South and Central America. Children are the most commonly affected; 80% of cases occur in children younger than age 10 years. Sporadic cases occur in endemic regions, but epidemics have been reported in cities that have expanded into rural endemic areas.[10] *Lutzomyia longipalpis* and other *Lutzomyia* species are the vectors. Domestic dogs and wild foxes are thought to be the major reservoirs, although the clustering of cases in households suggests that humans may also serve as a reservoir.[74]

CLINICAL MANIFESTATIONS

A spectrum of findings is observed within each of the three major clinical syndromes: cutaneous, mucosal, and visceral leishmaniasis. Each of these syndromes is associated with more than one *Leishmania* species, and any given species is capable of producing more than one syndrome. Variations are common, particularly among people who are concurrently infected with HIV or other immunosuppressive illness.

Cutaneous Leishmaniasis

The typical lesion of cutaneous leishmaniasis develops at the site where promastigotes are inoculated by an infected sand fly. Promastigotes are taken up by mononuclear phagocytes, convert to amastigotes, and multiply within them. Additional mononuclear cells are recruited to the area, and a nodule develops. It enlarges slowly and then ulcerates. Multiple lesions may be present in the same patient. The morphology of the cutaneous lesions is quite variable, and it is not possible to make a species-specific diagnosis based on their characteristics.[127,134]

Depending on the location, Old World cutaneous leishmaniasis is known locally as Oriental sore, bouton d'Orient, bouton de Crete, bouton d'Alep, bouton de Briska, Aleppo evil, Baghdad boil, and Delhi boil. In Latin America, it is variously known as pian bois (bush yaws), uta, and Chiclero's ulcer.

There is substantial variation in the morphology of the lesions. The classic wet lesion of *L. major* is "pizza-like," with a raised outer border, granulating base, and overlying white, purulent exudate. This type of lesion is also seen with *L. braziliensis* in Latin America. In the dry lesions due to *L. tropica* in the Middle East or India, the ulcer tends to be smaller and covered with a crust. In leishmaniasis recidiva, which is associated with *L. tropica* infection in the Middle East, skin lesions on the face or extremities enlarge slowly while healing in the center. They can persist for decades. Contiguous mucosal involvement is observed in some patients. Some leishmanial lesions are papular, acneiform, nodular, or volcano-like with minimal or no ulceration. Cutaneous lesions persist for months, and in some cases years, before they heal, leaving flat, atrophic scars as evidence of disease. Once a lesion has resolved, the person is usually left with immunity against the infecting *Leishmania* species.

Biopsies of cutaneous lesions demonstrate a spectrum of findings ranging from a predominance of macrophages containing abundant intracellular amastigotes to a predominance of lymphocytes with granuloma formation and few identifiable parasites.[105,106] There appears to be a balance between protective and disease-enhancing mononuclear cell populations in the lesions,[104] but eventually protective elements dominate, amastigotes are cleared, and the lesions heal.

Peripheral lymphadenopathy is observed in some geographic locations. A subset of people infected with *L. braziliensis* develop regional adenopathy, fever, and constitutional symptoms before the skin lesion(s) appears.[135,136] The constitutional findings and the adenopathy resolve as the skin lesion enlarges. In other patients there is involvement of local lymphatics in a sporotrichoid pattern.[134,137] Old World cutaneous leishmaniasis is much less commonly associated with sporotrichoid presentations, although cases have been reported from the Middle East.[138] Necrotizing lymphadenitis has also been reported with *L. major* infection.[139]

Rarely, *L. amazonensis* or *L. braziliensis* disseminates, producing large numbers of cutaneous lesions, often in association with mucosal disease. The lesions tend to be papular or acneiform with few ulcers. This can occur in patients with no demonstrable immune defect or in patients with acquired immunodeficiency syndrome (AIDS).[140] Diffuse cutaneous dissemination of *L. major* has also been associated with AIDS.[141]

Diffuse cutaneous leishmaniasis is an uncommon, anergic variant of cutaneous leishmaniasis that is frequently associated with *L. aethiopica* infections in Africa,[142,143] *L. mexicana* or *L. amazonensis* infections in Central and South America,[144,145] and a separate *Leishmania* species in the Dominican Republic.[146] It begins with a localized lesion that does not ulcerate. Amastigotes progressively disseminate to macrophages in other areas of skin forming cutaneous nodules or plaques. Diffuse cutaneous leishmaniasis with visceral dissemination has also been reported in a patient with AIDS in the West Indies.[147]

Cutaneous leishmaniasis should be considered in the differential diagnosis of subacute or chronic skin lesions in people who have lived, worked, or traveled in endemic areas. The differential diagnosis includes cutaneous fungal infections, such as paracoccidioidomycosis, histoplasmosis, sporotrichosis, chromomycosis, lobomycosis; lupus vulgaris (*Mycobacterium tuberculosis*),[148] *Mycobacterium ulcerans*, and other atypical myobacterial infections; yaws, syphilis, and leprosy; cutaneous neoplasms; and cutaneous sarcoidosis.

Mucosal Leishmaniasis (Espundia)

A small percentage of people infected with *L. braziliensis* and occasionally with other *Leishmania* species develop mucosal lesions in the nose, mouth, pharynx, or larynx months to years after resolution of the primary skin lesion. The condition is known in Latin America as espundia.[149–154] Mucosal leishmaniasis often begins with nasal stuffiness and inflammation. Ulceration of the nasal mucosa and septum follows. The lips, cheeks, soft palate, pharynx, and larynx may eventually be involved, resulting in substantial disfigurement and, rarely, aspiration and death. Eustachian tube blockage with secondary middle ear infection has been reported,[155] as well as involvement of the genitalia.[156] Therapeutic failures and relapses are common with traditional pentavalent antimony chemotherapy.

Mucosal involvement is also observed with other *Leishmania* species, although the pathophysiology may be somewhat different. Destructive involvement of the nose and mouth has been reported with *L. tropica* in Saudi Arabia.[157] Mucosal involvement of the upper respiratory tract, larynx, or oral pharynx has been observed in patients with visceral leishmaniasis in the Sudan[158,159] before and, in some cases, following treatment. In southern Europe, mucosal involvement has been reported rarely in apparently immunocompetent people[160,161] and more frequently in those who are immunosuppressed with neoplasms[162] or AIDS.[163,164] The differential diagnosis of mucosal leishmaniasis includes paracoccidioidomycosis, histoplasmosis, syphilis, tertiary yaws, rhinosporidiosis, leprosy, sarcoidosis, basal cell carcinoma and other neoplasms, intranasal cocaine abuse, and midline granuloma.

Visceral Leishmaniasis

Visceral leishmaniasis is a spectral syndrome. The majority of infections are inapparent and self-resolving; a subset smolder with mild symptoms.[165] Only a minority progress to full-blown visceral leishmaniasis, or kala-azar, which is characterized by fever, weight loss, hepatosplenomegaly, neutropenia, and hypergammaglobulinemia.[166]

Early epidemiologic studies in Africa[72] indicated that the prevalence of positive leishmanin skin tests in endemic areas was much higher than would be predicted based on the incidence of clinically apparent disease. Subsequently, prospective studies of *L. chagasi* in hyperendemic regions of northeastern Brazil demonstrated that the ratio of inapparent to apparent infection was greater than 6.5:1 in children younger than 5 years of age, the most susceptible group, and increased to 18:1 or higher in older children and adults.[73,74]

The determinants of progressive visceral leishmaniasis remain to be defined. Genetically determined cell-mediated immune responses of the host are probably the most important, as discussed previously. Malnutrition is known to suppress cell-mediated immune responses, and it may contribute to progression to symptomatic visceral leishmaniasis,[167–169] although it did not correlate with the development of disease in one prospective study.[74]

The incubation is typically weeks to several months, but it may be as short as 10 days or as long as several years.[170] The onset of visceral leishmaniasis is usually insidious, but it can be abrupt, with high fever suggesting malaria or another acute infection. In some cases, symptoms have first become manifest in people who have become immunocompromised years after moving from endemic areas.[171]

Full-blown, progressive visceral leishmaniasis, or kala-azar, is associated with fever, abdominal enlargement, weakness, loss of appetite, and weight loss.[166] The clinical findings are similar with *L. donovani* and *L. infantum/chagasi*. Symptoms may be present for weeks to months before patients come to medical attention in rural, endemic areas. The fever pattern may be intermittent, remittent with twice-daily temperature spikes, or, less commonly, continuous. The spleen is firm, nontender, and over time becomes massively enlarged. There is hepatomegaly; the liver typically has a sharp edge and smooth consistency. Peripheral adenopathy is observed in some patients in the Sudan[9] and occasionally elsewhere.[172] Some patients in India develop hyperpigmentation leading to the name kala-azar, which means "black fever" in Hindi.

The late stages of disease are characterized by malnutrition, severe wasting, and progressive debilitation, which are probably due to secretion of cytokines such as TNF-α and IL-1 by infected macrophages.[173] Stunting, decreased height for age, is seen in children.[74] Peripheral edema may occur late in the disease. Petechiae, ecchymoses, and gingival bleeding may also be observed. Hepatic function can be affected and fulminant hepatitis has been reported.[174] Death is often associated with a secondary bacterial infection, such as pneumonia, septicemia, dysentery, or tuberculosis, or with measles or other viral infection.[175]

Laboratory findings include anemia, neutropenia, thrombocytopenia, eosinopenia, and pronounced hypergammaglobulinemia.[166] The anemia is usually normocytic, normochromic, unless there is concomitant iron deficiency. It appears to be due to a combination of factors, including hemolysis, bone marrow suppression, hemorrhage, hypersplenism, and hemodilution.[176–178] Leukopenia can be profound with white blood cell counts below 1000/mL.[166–179] Eosinopenia is the rule.[166–180] The globulin level can reach 9 or 10 g/dL and is due to polyclonal B cell activation. Circulating immune complexes and rheumatoid factors are frequently present.[181,182] Elevated liver enzymes and bilirubin are noted in some patients.[174–183]

The differential diagnosis of visceral leishmaniasis is broad. When patients present with a subacute or chronic course and splenomegaly, hepatosplenic schistosomiasis, myeloproliferative diseases, and tropical splenomegaly due to chronic malaria must be considered. Other possibilities include miliary tuberculosis, histoplasmosis, brucellosis, subacute bacterial endocarditis, infectious mononucleosis, or prolonged *Salmonella* bacteremia. Patients with more acute presentations must be differentiated from those with malaria, amebic liver abscess, acute Chagas' disease, acute schistosomiasis (Katayama fever), typhoid fever, and other acute bacterial or viral infections.

Visceral leishmaniasis in people with concurrent HIV presents in the typical manner in more than two-thirds of cases, but atypical presentations are common. Splenomegaly may be absent.[13,15,16] Amastigotes can be found in macrophages in virtually any organ. They may be seen in biopsies of the lung or pleura[14,184,185] or larynx[163]; in the mucosa of the mouth, esophagus, stomach, or small intestine[186–190]; or in skin lesions.[191] Aplastic anemia has been the presenting problem in several cases.[192] Asymptomatic leishmanial infections in patients with HIV infection have also been documented.[193] In addition, *Leishmania* species that commonly cause cutaneous disease, such as *L. braziliensis*, can disseminate in the setting of AIDS.[194]

Viscerotropic leishmaniasis was reported in a small group of U.S. military troops infected with *L. tropica* during Operation Desert Storm.[20] They presented with low-grade fever, malaise, fatigue, and, in some instances, diarrhea. Although some had enlarged spleens, none demonstrated massive hepatosplenomegaly, wasting, or the progressive deterioration observed in patients with classic kala-azar. Similar visceralizing *L. tropica* infections have been reported in civilians living in endemic regions.

Post-Kala-Azar Dermal Leishmaniasis

A subset of people with visceral leishmaniasis in India[3,195] and Africa[196,197] develop skin lesions following treatment, ranging from hyperpigmented macules to frank nodules. Skin lesions typically appear in India 1 or 2 years after treatment and may persist for as long as 20 years. In the Sudan they usually appear at the end or within 6 months of therapy and persist for only a few months to 1 year. Persistence of lesions beyond 1 year is associated with high antileishmanial antibody titers and negative leishmanial skin test responses.[197] The skin lesions contain amastigotes and are thought to be the reservoir of infection during interepidemic periods.[3] Antileishmanial treatment is indicated in Indian post-kala-azar dermal leishmaniasis. In a few instances in India, visceral leishmaniasis has recurred in patients with post-kala-azar dermal leishmaniasis. The differential diagnosis includes leprosy.[198]

DIAGNOSIS

Parasite Identification

Although genus- and species-specific molecular probes are available for use in research settings, the diagnosis of leishmaniasis is most often still confirmed in the clinical setting by identifying leishmania amastigotes in a Wright–Giemsa-stained touch preparations[199] or tissue sections or by isolating the parasite in culture. Amastigotes are seen in macrophages in tissue sections, but they may appear to be extracellular in touch preparations. They must be differentiated from the fungus *Histoplasma capsulatum*, which is of similar size but lacks a kinetoplast, and *Toxoplasma gondii*, which typically is smaller.

Leishmania can be grown as promastigotes in a number of culture systems, including Novy, MacNeal, Nicolle (NNN) medium, Schneider's insect medium,[200] and several other tissue culture media to which fetal calf serum has been added. The cultures are incubated at 24 to 26°C to approximate sand fly temperatures. In the United States culture media can be obtained from the Centers for Disease Control and Prevention.

Promastigotes can be seen in cultures within a few days if the infection is heavy, or they may take several weeks to reach detectable levels if it is light. Speciation is available through WHO reference laboratories based on isoenzyme patterns,[21,22] monoclonal antibodies,[24] or other assays. Leishmania can also be identified in tissue or culture by PCR using genus- or species-specific probes.[27–33] In cases of suspected cutaneous leishmaniasis, a biopsy should be obtained from the raised border of the skin lesion after the area is meticulously cleaned.[201] The specimen is then divided into pieces for culture, touch preparation, and histopathology. Sterile saline without a bacteriostatic agent can be injected in the margin of the lesion, aspirated, and cultured as well. Appropriate cultures and tissue studies should be performed in order to assess for the possibility of bacteria, mycobacteria, and fungi that are in the differential diagnosis.

The histopathology of cutaneous leishmaniasis is characterized by acute and chronic inflammatory changes with a predominantly mononuclear cell infiltrate consisting of macrophages, lymphocytes, and plasma cells. There may be focal necrosis of infected macrophages. Early in infection macrophages filled with intracellular amastigotes are prevalent. Over time, parasitized mononuclear cells are eliminated from the lesion and a granulomatous response with epithelioid giant cells evolves. The changes are not diagnostic unless amastigotes are identified either visually or by another assay. The sensitivity of blood cultures for cutaneous or mucosal leishmaniasis has not been fully studied but is probably low. Cultures have been positive in some cases.[136,202,203]

In patients with visceral leishmaniasis, fine-needle aspiration of the spleen for culture and touch preparation yields a diagnosis in 96% to 98% of cases.[204] Although generally safe in the hands of an experienced operator, hemorrhage can occur, particularly if the patient has a coagulopathy. Bone marrow aspiration is not as sensitive, but it is diagnostic in more than half of all cases and preferred by some physicians. In India, cultures of peripheral blood buffy coat may be positive for *L. donovani*. Occasionally, *Leishmania* species that more commonly cause cutaneous lesions are isolated from patients with typical visceral leishmaniasis.[124,128] In patients with concurrent HIV infection, the diagnosis is often made by identifying amastigotes in macrophages in biopsies of the lung or pleura, oral or intestinal mucosa, or other sites.[14,158,184,186–192] Amastigotes may also be identified in aspirates of lymph nodes if lymphadenopathy is present.[205]

Serology

Antileishmanial antibody titers are typically present in high titer in people with visceral leishmaniasis and at low titer or undetectable in those with cutaneous leishmaniasis. They can be measured by a number of assays. Enzyme-linked immunosorbent assay (ELISA), indirect immunofluorescent tests, and agglutination assays have all been used.[206–211]

The sensitivity and specificity of these tests for the diagnosis of visceral leishmaniasis depend on the infecting *Leishmania* species and the leishmanial antigen used. In general, the highest titers are obtained when the homologous *Leishmania* species is used as the antigen source. Unfortunately, the specificity with crude antigen preparations is limited. Cross-reacting antibodies can develop in patients with Chagas' disease, African trypanosomiasis, malaria, leprosy, tuberculosis, schistosomiasis, or potentially other diseases.

Recently developed assays based on recombinant leishmanial antigens provide comparable sensitivity with greater specificity. Assays using rK39, a recombinant kinesin-like antigen initially identified in *L. chagasi/infantum*, have proven to be both sensitive and specific for the diagnosis of visceral leishmaniasis throughout the world.[212] Antibodies to rK39 are typically not detectable in people with cutaneous leishmaniasis, other infections, or self-resolving *L. donovani* or *L. infantum/chagasi* infections. Both ELISA and immunochromatographic strip tests using rK39 have been reported to have sensitivities greater than 90% and specificities of 98% or higher for the diagnosis of visceral leishmaniasis due to *L. donovani* and *L. infantum/chagasi*.[213] Although antibodies are usually present in high titer in immunocompetent patients with classic visceral leishmaniasis, they are not always detectable in people with visceral leishmaniasis and AIDS, limiting their sensitivity in that setting. The lower titers of antibodies in people with cutaneous leishmaniasis and the presence of cross-reacting "natural" antibodies at low titers in the sera of people who have never been exposed to *Leishmania* species make current serological tests useless for the diagnosis of cutaneous leishmaniasis.

Skin Test

The intradermal leishmanin (Montenegro) skin test is positive in the majority of people who have asymptomatic, self-resolving *L. donovani* and *L. infantum/chagasi* infections and in people with cutaneous or mucosal leishmaniasis. The skin test is negative in people with progressive visceral leishmaniasis or diffuse cutaneous leishmaniasis, but it becomes positive in the majority of people who are successfully treated for visceral leishmaniasis. The likelihood of a positive skin test appears to be greatest when the infecting *Leishmania* species is used as a source of antigen.[214] Leishmanin skin test reagents are not approved for use in the United States.

TREATMENT

Visceral Leishmaniasis

The treatment of leishmaniasis is in a state of transition. Pentavalent antimonial compounds were considered the treatment of choice,[215] but the development of resistance and substantial untoward effects have limited their use in some areas.[216] Liposomal amphotericin B is the only drug approved by the Food and Drug Administration (FDA) for the treatment of visceral leishmaniasis in the United States.[217] The most recent addition is miltefosine, an orally administered compound, which is now used for visceral leishmaniasis in India, where resistance to pentavalent antimonial drugs has become widespread.[218–220]

Liposomal amphotericin B is generally considered the treatment choice for visceral leishmaniasis in the United States and other industrialized countries.[217] Although expensive, it is highly effective and generally well tolerated. Other lipid-associated amphotericin B preparations also appear to be effective, but they have been less extensively studied and are not FDA approved.[221–223] Amphotericin B deoxycholate has long been known to have excellent antileishmanial activity, but its use has been limited by its toxicity.[224] Liposomal and lipid-associated amphotericin B are less toxic and theoretically attractive for the treatment of leishmaniasis in that they selectively target delivery of the drug to macrophages, the sole site of leishmanial infection. The manufacturer's recommended dosage for liposomal amphotericin B in immunocompetent people is 3.0 mg/kg body weight daily on days 1 through 5, 14, and 21. Data from India suggest that a total dose of 15 mg of amphotericin B divided over five injections is 97% effective. The cure rate decreases with shorter courses and lower doses. For immunocompromised people, the manufacturer recommends 4.0 mg/kg body weight on days 1 through 5, 10, 17, 24, 31, and 38. The high cost and limited availability of liposomal amphotericin B have largely restricted its use to the United States and other industrialized countries.

For decades, pentavalent antimony (Sbv) was the treatment of choice for visceral leishmaniasis, and it is still used in many endemic areas where antimony resistance is not encountered. The response rate remains high in patients infected with *L. infantum/chagasi* in Latin America and with *L. donovani* in the Sudan.[225] As discussed previously, miltefosine has replaced pentavelent antimonials in India, where resistance is widespread among *L. donovani* isolates.[218–220] Two Sbv preparations are available: sodium stibogluconate (Pentostam) and meglumine antimonate (Glucantime).[215] Meglumine antimonate is used in Latin America and French-speaking countries, and sodium stibogluconate is used elsewhere. Although the bioavailability may vary among lots, these two compounds appear to be comparable when administered on the basis of their Sbv content. Meglumine antimonate contains approximately 8.5% (85 mg/mL) Sbv, whereas sodium stibogluconate contains approximately 10% Sbv (100 mg/mL). The recommended dose is 20 mg Sbv per kilogram body weight per day given intravenously or intramuscularly. This dose should not be exceeded. The recommended duration of treatment is 20 to 28 days.[215] Longer periods of treatment have been used for patients who respond slowly and for the treatment of post-kala-azar dermal leishmaniasis.[226,227]

Although most patients are able to complete a full course of pentavalent antimony therapy, side effects are common. They include nausea, vomiting, abdominal pain, anorexia, myalgia, arthralgia, headache, and malaise. Chemical pancreatitis with elevated amylase and lipase is observed in many patients. Severe, clinically apparent pancreatitis is well documented, particularly among patients with renal failure.[228] Sbv causes dose-dependent electrocardiographic changes that include prolonged Q-T intervals and nonspecific ST-T wave effects that resolve within 2 months after the conclusion of therapy.[229] Sudden death has been observed with doses of Sbv in excess of 20 mg/kg/day, presumably due to arrhythmias. Renal failure is a rare complication.[230]

The most exciting recent advance in the treatment of leishmaniasis has been the development of miltefosine.[218] It is licensed in India and widely used there for the treatment of visceral leishmaniasis.[231,232] Miltefosine was initially developed as an antineoplastic drug. It is a phosphocholine analogue and well absorbed after oral administration. The mechanism of its antileishmanial activity has not been defined, but it is known to interact with membrane constituents and to affect cell signaling pathways by inhibiting protein kinase C and phospholipase C. Miltefosine 100 mg daily in adults for 4 weeks has been reported to cure 97% of people with visceral leishmaniasis in India. A dose of 2.5 mg/kg/daily for 4 weeks was 95% effective in children ages 2 to 11 years. Miltefosine is associated with mild to moderate nausea, vomiting, and diarrhea and "motion sickness" at higher doses. Elevation of transaminases, BUN, and creatinine has been noted early in therapy, but typically decreases with continuation of the drug. Miltefosine has potential reproductive toxicity, and it cannot be used during pregnancy. Women taking it must use appropriate contraceptive measures. In addition, the number of people treated to date and the period of follow-up after treatment are relatively limited. Additional postmarketing surveillance is needed to exclude infrequent or delayed untoward effects. Finally, although miltesone resistance has not been a clinical problem, it has been documented in vitro.[233]

Alternative drugs for the treatment of visceral leishmaniasis include amphotericin B deoxycholate and pentamidine isethionate, but both have substantial toxicities. Amphotericin B deoxycholate 0.5 to 1.0 mg/kg body weight can be given either daily or every other day for up to 8 weeks.[234] Amphotericin B must be administered parenterally, and is frequently associated with fever, malaise, weight loss, and nephrotoxicity. Pentamidine isethionate 4 mg/kg body weight daily or every other day for 15 doses is another effective but toxic alternative. Lower doses of pentamidine, 2 mg/kg body weight daily, are in general better tolerated but less effective. Pentamidine can cause vascular collapse if infused too rapidly, and it can cause life-threatening hypoglycemia followed by diabetes mellitus due to pancreatic beta cell injury.[235] Insulin-dependent diabetes is a potentially fatal problem for impoverished populations without access to insulin or refrigeration. Pentamidine is also associated with headache, flushing, nausea, vomiting, abdominal discomfort, and reversible azotemia. It can also produce local inflammation and abscess formation when given intramuscularly.

A number of other drugs have been tried or are under investigation. Parenterally administered paromomycin (aminosidine), an aminoglycoside, has been used alone and in combination with other antileishmanial drugs. A dose of 16 mg/kg/day reportedly cured 89% of patients in one study in India.[236] Paromomycin must be administered parenterally for the treatment of visceral leishmaniasis. Side effects include ototoxicity and nephrotoxicity. The imidazole antifungals also have leishmaniacidal activity. Ketoconazole and itraconazole have been reported to be effective in some cases of visceral leishmaniasis,[237–240] but failures are also well documented.[239] Substantial interest was engendered by the development of recombinant interferon (rINF)-γ, which in vitro activates macrophages to kill intracellular amastigotes.[241–245] Unfortunately, rINF-γ was not curative when used as monotherapy.[246]

Even with effective antileishmanial chemotherapy, the death rate for people with visceral leishmaniasis approaches 10% in some series. Secondary bacterial and viral infections are common and may prove fatal. Patients should be evaluated for secondary infections and promptly treated with appropriate antibiotics. Visceral leishmaniasis can also be associated with severe malnutrition, which must be addressed. Finally, people with visceral leishmaniasis often have evidence of hypersplenism, but splenectomy is not indicated except in the rare case in which signs of hypersplenism persist following treatment.

Unfortunately, there are no rigid criteria to document cure in patients treated for visceral leishmaniasis. Improvement in temperature, sense of well-being, and hematological abnormalities and resolution of hepatosplenomegaly are typically used to assess the clinical response. Treatment does not necessarily result in sterile immunity as indicated by clinical relapses, which usually occur within 6 months of completion of therapy in immunocompetent patients. The development of a positive leishmanin skin test, which tends to occur as early as 6 months to 1 year after chemotherapy, seems to indicate immunity.

The treatment of people with concurrent visceral leishmaniasis and AIDS poses special challenges. The greatest experience to date has been in Spain, southern France, and Italy. The initial parasitiological cure rates with pentavant antimony, amphotericin B deoxycholate, and lipid-associated amphotericin B have been substantially lower than seen in immunocompetent people. Even in people who initially respond, relapse rates are high. Secondary prophylaxis with regularly administered liposomal amphotericin B, pentavalent antimony, or, possibly in the future, miltefosine, seems prudent, but data are lacking to document their efficacy or to aid in the selection of a specific regimen. Highly active antiretroviral chemotherapy has been shown to decrease the likelihood of visceral leishmaniasis developing in people with AIDS and should be initiated as soon as possible in those with concurrent AIDS and visceral leishmaniasis.

Cutaneous Leishmaniasis

The goal of treatment in cutaneous leishmaniasis is to limit tissue damage and, in the case of *L. braziliensis* and related species, to prevent the later development of American mucosal disease. The natural history of cutaneous leishmaniasis varies with *Leishmania* species. In most instances, the lesions heal spontaneously with time. In general, people with cosmetically inconsequential cutaneous lesions can be followed expectantly, provided that the infection is not due to *L. braziliensis* or related *Leishmania* species that are associated with American mucosal leishmaniasis. People with involvement of the face, those with large lesions, those with diffuse cutaneous leishmaniasis, and those infected with a *Leishmania* species that can produce mucosal leishmaniasis should be treated. Systemic therapy is recommended to prevent later mucosal disease in the latter case, but the efficacy has not been clearly demonstrated.

Pentavalent antimony drugs are used in many settings, but *Leishmania* species vary in their susceptibility. Typically, Sbv 20 mg/kg/day is given for 20 days.[215,216] Shorter courses and lower doses have been used, but they may predispose to the development of antimony resistance. Even with successful chemotherapy, lesions typically epithelialize slowly over a period of weeks. The published results are variable. Cure rates with *L. braziliensis* in residents of Brazil or Columbia have been in the range of 60% to 70%, but they were greater than 95% in U.S. troops infected with *L. panamensis* in Panama. In the case of *L. major*, 60% of placebo recipients healed within 20 weeks after seeking medical attention in one study, and 74% of those receiving pentavalent antimony healed within 30 days. A number of other drugs and approaches have been proposed. The imidazole antifungals have variable activity. Ketoconazole, itraconazole, and fluconazole have been used effectively in some but not all settings. For example, ketoconazole 400 to 600 mg/day for 4 to 8 weeks was reported to be effective in approximately 70% of people with *L. major* and *L. mexicana* infections, but it was less effective against *L. tropica*, *L. aethiopica*, and *L. braziliensis*.[247,248] Fluconazole (200 mg daily for 6 weeks) was superior to placebo in people with cutaneous leishmaniasis due to *L. major* in Saudi Arabia.[249] At the end of the treatment period, 60% of placebo recipients were cured versus 90% of the fluconazole-treated group. The published experience with miltefosine is still limited.[250] In an open-label trial in Columbia, treatment of soldiers with 50 to 100 mg per day for 21 days cured 66%; higher doses of 133 to 150 mg/day cured 94%, but 40% of recipients developed motion sickness. Vomiting and diarrhea occurred on 2% of treatment days. The results were promising, but the number of subjects treated was small. Allopurinol was reported to be effective in one study, but its use has been questioned.[251] A number of other drugs have been reported to have antileishmanial activity, but many of the studies have had relatively small sample sizes and were not done in a controlled, blinded manner. Given that spontaneous healing occurs with visceral leishmaniasis, it is impossible to formulate recommendations from uncontrolled studies.

Topical therapy has been another approach. The application of 15% paromomycin and 12% methylbenzethonium has been used successfully in a subset of patients with cutaneous leishmaniasis in Israel and Guatemala.[252,253] Intralesional injections of antimony have also been used to treat *L. major*. Typically, 0.5 to 2.0 mL (100 mg /mL) is injected around all sides of a lesion until it blanches. When 10 such injections were administered on alternative days to Egyptian patients, 85% were cured at 3-month follow-up. The cure rate with cryotherapy in the same study was 73%.

Other approaches have been tried. Immunotherapy with a combination of leishmania promastigote antigens and live bacille Calmette–Guérin (BCG) has been used effectively in Venezuela and Brazil, but the time to clinical response is relatively long.[254] Patients in Guatemala with cutaneous leishmaniasis and in the Dominican Republic with diffuse cutaneous leishmaniasis have been successfully treated with locally applied heat,[255] although the treatment requires close monitoring. In diffuse cutaneous leishmaniasis, an anergic variant that responds poorly to Sbv, combined therapy with Sbv and rINF-γ was reported to be successful.[256] Leishmaniasis recidivans is another variant that responds poorly to most forms of therapy, although some success has been achieved with intralesional injections of Sbv with or without systemic Sbv therapy.

Mucosal Leishmaniasis

Mucosal leishmaniasis due to *L. braziliensis* is usually treated with a Sbv, 20 mg/kg for 28 days, but only 60% of patients have clinical responses, and relapses are observed in up to 30% of cases in Brazil.[24,150,257,258] Amphotericin B has been used as an alternative as well as pentamidine, 2 to 4 mg/kg once or twice a week until the lesions clear.[249,259–261] Miltefosine and liposomal amphotericin B are potential future treatment possibilities, but they have not been studied in this setting. The combination of Sbv plus rINF-γ was reported to work in a limited number of cases.[262] Plastic surgery may be necessary for cosmetic purposes in people with mucosal leishmaniasis, but it should be delayed for at least 1 year after clinically apparently successful chemotherapy because skin grafts are likely to be lost if infection relapses.

PREVENTION

Leishmaniasis can be prevented by interrupting sand fly transmission or by removing or treating reservoirs of infection. It is hoped that in the future it will be prevented by immunization, but no vaccine is currently available.

The short-term visitor to an endemic area should use personal protective measures to avoid sand fly bites. Sand flies tend to bite from dusk to dawn. The application of DEET (diethyltoluamide)-containing insect repellents to exposed skin and under pant and shirt cuffs, the use of fine-mesh screens or insect nets, and the application of insecticide (usually permethrin or other pyrethroids) to clothing and bednets[263–265] decrease the risk of transmission of leishmanias as well as malaria and other diseases transmitted by sand flies and mosquitoes.[262] Unfortunately, these measures are often not practical or affordable for local residents.

Residual insecticide spraying is effective where transmission occurs in the domestic or peridomestic setting, but the use of residual insecticides has been limited by concern for the environment, cost, and potential evolution of resistance among sand flies and other arthropod vectors. It is of historical note that the use of residual DDT for malaria control following World War II was credited with dramatic reduction in the transmission of leishmaniasis in India, Bangladesh, and southern Iran.[265–267] Epidemics of visceral leishmaniasis subsequently followed the discontinuation of spraying. Residual insecticides have also been used successfully in other locations where transmission is peridomestic. One novel adaptation of this approach was the use of deltamethrin-impregnated collars for domestic dogs that serve as a reservoir for *L. chagasi/infantum*.[268,269] Residual insecticides are not useful in rural areas where wild animals serve as reservoirs and arboreal sand flies are responsible for transmission.

Reservoir control programs have also been attempted.[270] In northeastern and southeastern Brazil, where *L. infantum/chagasi* is endemic and domestic dogs are thought to be a major reservoir, large numbers of seropositive dogs have been killed, but the efficacy of dog eradication has not been clearly demonstrated.[74,271] Poisoning rodents and deep plowing have been used in Asia to reduce the reservoir density with uncertain results. In India, where humans are the reservoir of *L. donovani*, early case identification and treatment of infected patients with visceral leishmaniasis or post-kala-azar dermal leishmaniasis are potentially important elements in control.

Clinical experience in humans and studies in animals suggest that the eventual development of an effective leishmanial vaccine(s) is likely. People who have recovered from leishmaniasis develop high-level immunity against reinfection with the same *Leishmania* species. In *L. tropica* endemic areas of the Middle East, mothers have for generations exposed the bottoms of their infants to sand flies to facilitate the development of a lesion at an acceptable site and the development of immunity to protect against disfiguring lesions of the face and extremities.

In Russia and Israel, troops were "immunized" with live *L. major* promastigotes injected into the buttocks. This practice was discontinued in Israel because some of the resulting lesions were large and others healed slowly. There was also concern that parasites could persist in the skin even after clinical cure. A vaccine made of killed promastigotes from multiple strains of *Leishmania* was used in Brazil in military troops. It was shown to stimulate cellular immune responses in a subset of recipients, although its clinical efficacy in preventing cutaneous leishmaniasis was not clearly documented.[272]

These observations coupled with extensive studies of experimentally infected mice suggest that a defined vaccine(s) is feasible. Such a vaccine could be based on the use of recombinant antigens or possibly genetically altered, living *Leishmania* that could survive long enough in vivo to elicit protective immunity but bear mutations or gene knockouts that ultimately would result in their death. Such an *L. mexicana* strain was shown to provide protective immunity in mice.[273] Given the rapid advances that have been made in understanding the immunobiology of leishmaniasis, it seems that an effective vaccine will likely be developed.[274,275]

REFERENCES

1. Lainson R, Shaw JJ: Evolution, classification and geographic distribution. In Peters W, Killick-Kendrick R (eds): The Leishmaniases in Biology and Medicine. London, Academic Press, 1987, pp 1–120.
2. Peters W, Killick-Kendrick R (eds): The Leishmaniases in Biology and Medicine. London, Academic Press, 1987.
3. Centers for Disease Control and Prevention: Cutaneous leishmaniasis in U.S. military personnel—Southwest/Central Asia, 2002–2003. MMWR 52:1009–1012, 2003.
4. Centers for Disease Control and Prevention: Update: Cutaneous leishmaniasis in U.S. military personnel—Southwest/Central Asia, 2002–2004. MMWR 53:264–265, 2004.
5. Centers for Disease Control and Prevention: Two cases of visceral leishmaniasis in U.S. military personnel—Afghanistan, 2002–2004. MMWR 53:265–268, 2004.
6. Addy M, Nandy A: Ten years of kala-azar in West Bengal. Part 1. Did post-kala-azar dermal leishmaniasis initiate the outbreak in 24-Parganas? Bull World Health Organ 70:341–346, 1992.
7. Elias M, Rahman AJ, Khan NI: Visceral leishmaniasis and its control in Bangladesh. Bull World Health Organ 67:43–49, 1989.
8. de Beer P, el Harith A, Deng LL, et al: A killing disease epidemic among displaced Sudanese population identified as visceral leishmaniasis. Am J Trop Med Hyg 44:283–289, 1991.
9. Zijlstra EE, el-Hassan AM, Ismael A, et al: Endemic kala-azar in eastern Sudan: A longitudinal study on the incidence of clinical and subclinical infection and post-kala-azar dermal leishmaniasis. Am J Trop Med Hyg 51:826–836, 1994.
10. Jeronimo SMB, Oliveira S, Mackay S, et al: An urban outbreak of visceral leishmaniasis in Natal, Brazil. Trans R Soc Trop Med Hyg 88:386–388, 1994.
11. Montalban C, Calleja JL, Erice A, et al: Visceral leishmaniasis in patients with human immunodeficiency virus. Co-operative Group for the Study of Leishmaniasis in AIDS. J Infect 21:261–270, 1990.
12. Rosenthal E, Marty P, Poizot-Martin I, et al: Visceral leishmaniasis and HIV-1 co-infection in southern France. Trans R Soc Trop Med Hyg 89:159–162, 1995.
13. Berenguer J, Moreno S, Cercenado E, et al: Visceral leishmaniasis in patients infected with human immunodeficiency virus (HIV). Ann Intern Med 111:129–132, 1989.
14. Chenoweth CE, Singal S, Pearson RD, et al: Acquired immunodeficiency syndrome-related visceral leishmaniasis presenting in a pleural effusion. Chest 103:648–649, 1993.
15. Medrano FJ, Hernandez-Quero J, Jimenez E, et al: Visceral leishmaniasis in HIV-1-infected individuals: A common opportunistic infection in Spain. AIDS 6:1499–1503, 1992.

16. Peters BS, Fish D, Golden R, et al: Visceral leishmaniasis in HIV infection and AIDS: Clinical features and response to therapy. Q J Med 77:1101–1111, 1990.
17. Golino A, Duncan JM, Zeluff B, et al: Leishmaniasis in a heart transplant patient. J Heart Lung Transplant 11:820–823, 1992.
18. Moulin B, Ollier J, Bouchouareb D, et al: Leishmaniasis: A rare cause of unexplained fever in a renal graft recipient. Nephron 60:360–362, 1992.
19. Kher V, Ghosh AK, Gupta A, et al: Visceral leishmaniasis: An unusual case of fever in a renal transplant recipient. Nephrol Dial Transplant 6:736–738, 1991.
20. Magill AJ, Grogl M, Gasser RA, et al: Visceral infection caused by *Leishmania tropica* in veterans of Operation Desert Storm. N Engl J Med 328:1383–1387, 1993.
21. Gardener PJ, Chance ML, Peters W: Biochemical taxonomy of *Leishmania* II: Electrophoretic variation of malate dehydrogenase. Ann Trop Med Parasitol 68:317–325, 1974.
22. Rassam MB, Al-Mudhaffar SA, Chance ML: Isoenzyme characterization of *Leishmania* species from Iraq. Ann Trop Med Parasitol 73:527–534, 1979.
23. Schnur LF, Chance ML, Ebert F, et al: The biochemical and serological taxonomy of visceralizing *Leishmania*. Ann Trop Med Parasitol 75:131–144, 1981.
24. Pratt DM, David JR: Monoclonal antibodies that distinguish between New World species of *Leishmania*. Nature 291:581–583, 1981.
25. Arnot DE, Barker DC: Biochemical identification of cutaneous leishmanias by analysis of kinetoplast DNA. II. Sequence homologies in *Leishmania* kDNA. Mol Biochem Parasitol 3:47–56, 1981.
26. Wirth DF, Pratt DM: Rapid identification of *Leishmania* species by specific hybridization of kinetoplast DNA in cutaneous lesions. Proc Natl Acad Sci USA 79:6999–7003, 1982.
27. de Brujin MH, Labrada LA, Smyth AJ, et al: A comparative study of diagnosis by the polymerase chain reaction and by current clinical methods using biopsies from Colombian patients with suspected leishmaniasis. Trop Med Parasitol 44:201–207, 1993.
28. Lopez M, Inga R, Cangalaya M, et al: Diagnosis of *Leishmania* using the polymerase chain reaction: A simplified procedure for field work. Am J Trop Med Hyg 49:348–356, 1993.
29. Rodriguez N, Guzman B, Rodas A, et al: J. Diagnosis of cutaneous leishmaniasis and species discrimination of parasites by PCR and hybridization. J Clin Microbiol 32:2246–2252, 1994.
30. Uliana SR, Nelson K, Beverley SM, et al: Discrimination amongst *Leishmania* by polymerase chain reaction and hybridization with small subunit ribosomal DNA derived oligonucleotides. Eukaryotic Microbiol 41:324–330, 1994.
31. Ibrahim ME, Smyth AJ, Ali MH, et al: The polymerase chain reaction can reveal the occurrence of naturally mixed infections with *Leishmania* parasites. Acta Trop 57:327–332, 1994.
32. Nuzum E, White F III, Thakur C, et al: Diagnosis of symptomatic visceral leishmaniasis by use of the polymerase chain reaction on patient blood. J Infect Dis 171:751–754, 1995.
33. Laskay T, Miko TL, Negesse Y, et al: Detection of cutaneous *Leishmania* infection in paraffin-embedded skin biopsies using the polymerase chain reaction. Trans R Soc Trop Med Hyg 89:273–275, 1995.
34. Molyneux DH, Killick-Kendrick R: Morphology, ultrastructure, and life cycles. In Peters W, Killick-Kendrick R (eds): The Leishmaniases in Biology and Medicine. London, Academic Press, 1987, pp 121–176.
35. Jeronimo SMB, Pearson RD: The *Leishmania:* Protozoans adapted for intracellular survival. Subcell Biochem 18:1–37, 1992.
36. Lewis DJ, Ward RD: Transmission and vectors. In Peters W, Killick-Kendrick R (eds): The Leishmaniases in Biology and Medicine. London, Academic Press, 1987, pp 235–262.
37. Sacks DL, Perkins PV: Identification of an infective stage of *Leishmania* promastigotes. Science 223:1417–1419, 1984.
38. Sacks DL, Hienz S, Sher A: Identification of cell surface carbohydrates and antigen changes between non-infective and infective developmental stages of *Leishmania major* promastigotes. J Immunol 135:564–569, 1985.
39. Killick-Kendrick R, Rioux JA, Bailly M, et al: Ecology of leishmaniasis in the south of France. 20. Dispersal of Phlebotomus ariasi Tonnoir, 1921 as a factor in the spread of visceral leishmaniasis in the Cevennes. Ann Parasitol Hum Comp 59:555–572, 1984.
40. Theodos CM, Ribeiro JM, Titus RG: Analysis of enhancing effect of sand fly saliva on *Leishmania* infection in mice. Infect Immun 59:1592–1598, 1991.
41. Hall LR, Titus RG: Sand fly vector saliva selectively modulates macrophage functions that inhibit killing of *Leishmania major* and nitric oxide production. J Immunol 155:3501–3506, 1995.
42. Russo DM, Barral-Netto M, Barral A, et al: Human T-cell responses in *Leishmania* infections [Review]. Prog Clin Parasitol 3:119–144, 1993.
43. Reiner SL, Locksley RM: The regulation of immunity to *Leishmania major* [Review]. Annu Rev Immunol 13:151–177, 1995.
44. Scott P: Development and regulation of cell-mediated immunity in experimental leishmaniasis. Immunol Res 27:489–498, 2003.
45. Scharton-Kersten T, Scott P: The role of the innate immune response in Th1 cell development following *Leishmania major* infection. J Leukoc Biol 57:515–522, 1995.
46. Wilson ME, Donnelson JE, Pearson RD, et al: Macrophage receptors and leishmania. In Korkonen TK, Hovi T, Makela PH (eds): Molecular Recognition in Host–Parasite Interactions. New York, Plenum, 1992, pp 17–30.
47. Russell DG, Wilhelm H: The involvement of the major surface glycoprotein (gp63) of *Leishmania* promastigotes in attachment to macrophages. J Immunol 136:2613–2620, 1986.
48. Etges R, Bouvier J, Bordier C: The major surface protein of *Leishmania* promastigotes is a protease. J Biol Chem 261:9098–9101, 1986.
49. McConville MJ, Bacic A, Mitchell GF, et al: Lipophosphoglycan of *Leishmania major* that vaccinates against cutaneous leishmaniasis contains an alkylglycerophosphoinositol lipid anchor. Proc Natl Acad Sci USA 84:8941–8945, 1987.
50. King DL, Chang Y-D, Turco SJ: Cell surface lipophosphoglycan of *Leishmania donovani*. Mol Biochem Parasitol 24:47–53, 1987.
51. Blackwell JM, Ezekowitz RAB, Roberts MB, et al: Macrophage complement and lectin-like receptors bind *Leishmania* in the absence of serum. J Exp Med 162:324–331, 1985.
52. Wozencraft AO, Sayers G, Blackwell JM: Macrophage type 3 complement receptors mediate serum-independent binding of *Leishmania donovani*. J Exp Med 164:1332–1337, 1986.
53. Wilson ME, Pearson RD: Evidence that *Leishmania donovani* utilizes a mannose receptor on human mononuclear phagocytes to establish intracellular parasitism. J Immunol 136:4681–4688, 1986.
54. Wilson ME, Pearson RD: Roles of CR3 and mannose receptors in the attachment and ingestion of *Leishmania donovani* by human mononuclear phagocytes. Infect Immun 56:363–369, 1988.
55. Mosser DM, Vlassara H, Edelson PJ, et al: *Leishmania* promastigotes are recognized by the macrophage receptor for advanced glycosylation end products. J Exp Med 165:140–145, 1987.
56. Mosser DM, Edelson PJ: Activation of the alternative complement pathway by *Leishmania* promastigotes: Parasite lysis and attachment to macrophages. J Immunol 132:1501–1502, 1984.
57. Pearson RD, Steigbigel RT: Mechanism of lethal effect of human serum upon *Leishmania donovani*. J Immunol 125:2195–2201, 1980.
58. Puentes SM, Sacks DL, da Silva RP, et al: Complement binding by two developmental stages of *Leishmania major* promastigotes varying in expression of a surface lipophosphoglycan. J Exp Med 167:887–902, 1988.
59. Murray HW, Rubin BY, Rothermel CD: Killing of intracellular *Leishmania donovani* by lymphokine-stimulated human mononuclear phagocytes. Evidence that interferon-γ is the activating cytokine. J Clin Invest 72:1506–1510, 1983.
60. Squires KE, Schreiber RD, McElrath MJ, et al: Experimental visceral leishmaniasis: Role of endogenous IFN-γ in host defense and tissue granulomatous response. J Immunol 143:4255–4249, 1989.
61. Liew FY, Li Y, Moss D, et al: Resistance to *Leishmania major* infection correlates with the induction of nitric oxide synthase in murine macrophages. Eur J Immunol 21:3009–3014, 1991.
62. Green SJ, Meltzer MS, Hibbs S, et al: Activated macrophages destroy intracellular *Leishmania major* amastigotes by an L-arginine-dependent killing mechanism. J Immunol 144:278–283, 1990.
63. Evans TG, Thai L, Granger DL, et al: Effect of in vivo inhibition of nitric oxide production in murine leishmaniasis. J Immunol 151:907–915, 1993.
64. Evans TG, Reed SS, Hibbs JB Jr: Nitric oxide production in murine leishmaniasis: Correlation of progressive infection with increasing systemic synthesis of nitric oxide. Am J Trop Med Hyg 54:486–489, 1996.
65. Blackwell JM, Barton CH, White JK, et al: Genetic regulation of leishmanial and mycobacterial infections: The Lsh/Ity/Bcg gene story continues [Review]. Immunol Lett 43:99–107, 1994.

66. Sypek JP, Wyler DJ: Antileishmanial defense in macrophages triggered by tumor necrosis factor expressed on CD4+ T lymphocyte plasma membrane. J Exp Med 174:755–759, 1991.
67. Birkland TP, Sypek JP, Wyler DJ: Soluble TNF and membrane TNF expressed on CD4+ T lymphocytes differ in their ability to activate macrophage antileishmanial defense. J Leukoc Biol 51:296–299, 1992.
68. Bradley DJ, Taylor BA, Blackwell J, et al: Regulation of *Leishmania* populations within the host. III. Mapping of the locus controlling susceptibility to visceral leishmaniasis in the mouse. Clin Exp Immunol 37:7–14, 1979.
69. Plant JE, Blackwell JM, O'Brien AD, et al: Are the Lsh and Ity disease resistance genes of lone locus on mouse chromosome 1. Nature 297:510–511, 1982.
70. Formica S, Roach TJ, Blackwell JM: Interaction with extracellular matrix proteins influences Lsh/Ity/Bcg (candidate Nramp) gene regulation of macrophage priming/activation for tumour necrosis factor-α and nitrite release. Immunology 82:42–50, 1994.
71. Mulero V, Searle S, Blackwell JM, et al: Solute carrier 11a1 (Slc11a1; formerly Nramp1) regulates metabolism and release of iron acquired by phagocytic, but not transferrin-receptor-mediated, iron uptake. Biochem J 363:89–94, 2002.
72. Manson-Bahr PEC: East African kala-azar with special reference to the pathology, prophylaxis and treatment. Trans R Soc Trop Med Hyg 53:123–137, 1959.
73. Badaró R, Jones TC, Lorenco R, et al: A prospective study of visceral leishmaniasis in an endemic area of Brazil. J Infect Dis 154:639–649, 1986.
74. Evans TG, Teixeira MJ, McAuliffe IT, et al: Epidemiology of visceral leishmaniasis in northeast Brazil. J Infect Dis 166:1124–1132, 1992.
75. Scott P, Natovitz P, Coffman RL, et al: Immunoregulation of cutaneous leishmaniasis. T-cell lines that transfer protective immunity or exacerbation belong to different T helper cell subsets and respond to distinct parasite antigens. J Exp Med 168:1675–1684, 1988.
76. Heinzel FP, Sadick MD, Holaday BJ, et al: Reciprocal expression of interferon-gamma or interleukin 4 during the resolution or progression of murine leishmaniasis. Evidence for expansion of distinct helper T-cell subsets. J Exp Med 169:59–72, 1989.
77. Murray HW, Squires KE, Miralles CD, et al: Acquired resistance and granuloma formation in experimental visceral leishmaniasis. Differential T-cell and lymphokine roles in initial versus established immunity. J Immunol 148:1858–1863, 1992.
78. Reiner NE, Ng W, Wilson CB, et al: Modulation of in vitro monocyte cytokine responses to *Leishmania donovani*. Interferon-γ prevents parasite-induced inhibition of interleukin 1 production and primes monocytes to respond to *Leishmania* by producing both tumor necrosis factor-α and interleukin 1. J Clin Invest 85:1914–1924, 1990.
79. Holaday BJ, Pompeu MM, Evans T, et al: Correlates of leishmania-specific immunity in the clinical spectrum of infection with *Leishmania chagasi*. J Infect Dis 167:411–417, 1993.
80. Leal LM, Moss DW, Kuhn R, et al: Interleukin-4 transgenic mice of resistant background are susceptible to *Leishmania major* infection. Eur J Immunol 2:566–569, 1993.
81. Noben-Trauth N, Kropf P, Muller I: Susceptibility to *Leishmania major* infection in interleukin-4-deficient mice. Science 271:987–990, 1996.
82. Satoskar A, Bluethmann H, Alexander J: Disruption of the murine interleukin-4 gene inhibits disease progression during *Leishmania mexicana* infection but does not increase control of *Leishmania donovani* infection. Infect Immun 63:4894–4899, 1995.
83. Karp CL, el-Safi SH, Wynn TA, et al: In vivo cytokine profiles in patients with kala-azar. Marked elevation of both interleukin-10 and interferon-gamma. J Clin Invest 91:1644–1648, 1993.
84. Holaday BJ, Pompeu MML, Jeronimo S, et al: Potential role of interleukin-10 in the immunosuppression associated with kala-azar. J Clin Invest 92:2626–2632, 1993.
85. Heinzel FP, Schoenhaut DS, Rerko RM, et al: Recombinant interleukin 12 cures mice infected with *Leishmania major*. J Exp Med 177:1505–1509, 1993.
86. Akuffo H, Maasho K, Howe R: Natural and acquired resistance to *Leishmania:* Cellular activation by *Leishmania aethiopica* of mononuclear cells from unexposed individuals through the stimulation of natural killer (NK) cells. Clin Exp Immunol 94:516–521, 1993.
87. Campbell KA, Ovendale PJ, Kennedy MK, et al: CD40 ligand is required for protective cell-mediated immunity to *Leishmania major*. Immunity 4:283–289, 1996.
88. Padigel UM, Farrell JP: CD40–CD40 ligand costimulation is not required for initiation and maintenance of a Th1-type response to *Leishmania major* infection. Infect Immun 71:1389–1395, 2003.
89. Padigel UM, Kim N, Choi Y, et al: TRANCE–RANK costimulation is required for IL-12 production and the initiation of a Th1-type response to *Leishmania major* infection in CD40L-deficient mice. J Immunol. 171:5437–5441, 2003.
90. Barral-Netto M, Barral A, Brownell CE, et al: Transforming growth factor-β in leishmanial infection: A parasite escape mechanism. Science 247:545–548, 1992.
91. Reiner NE, Ng W, McMaster WR: Parasite–accessory cell interactions in murine leishmaniasis II. *Leishmania donovani* suppresses macrophage expression of class I and class II major histocompatibility complex gene products. J Immunol 138:1926–1932, 1987.
92. Reiner NE, Malemud CJ: Arachidonic acid metabolism by murine peritoneal macrophages infected with *Leishmania donovani:* In vitro evidence for parasite-induced alterations in cyclooxygenase and lipoxygenase pathways. J Immunol 134:556–563, 1985.
93. Milano S, Arcoleo F, Dieli M, et al: In vivo evidence for PGE2 and LTB4 involvement in cutaneous leishmaniasis: Relations with infection status and cytokine production. Parasitology 112:13–19, 1996.
94. Bretscher PA, Wei G, Menon JN, et al: Establishment of stable, cell-mediated immunity that makes "susceptible" mice resistant to *Leishmania major*. Science 257:539–542, 1992.
95. Menon JN, Bretscher PA: Characterization of the immunological memory state generated in mice susceptible to *Leishmania major* following exposure to low doses of *L. major* and resulting in resistance to a normally pathogenic challenge. Eur J Immunol 26:243–249, 1996.
96. Reiner SL, Wang ZE, Hatam F, et al: TH1 and TH2 cell antigen receptors in experimental leishmaniasis. Science 259:1457–1460, 1993.
97. Skeiky YA, Benson DR, Guderian JA, et al: Immune responses of leishmaniasis patients to heat shock proteins of *Leishmania* species and humans. Infect Immun 63:4105–4114, 1995.
98. Rossi-Bergmann B, Muller I, Godinho EB: TH1 and TH2 T-cell subsets are differentially activated by macrophages and B cells in murine leishmaniasis. Infect Immun 61:2266–2269, 1993.
99. Bacellar O, Lessa H, Schriefer A, et al: Up-regulation of Th1-type responses in mucosal leishmaniasis patients. Infect Immun 70:6734–6740, 2002.
100. Ritter U, Korner H: Divergent expression of inflammatory dermal chemokines in cutaneous leishmaniasis. Parasite Immunol 24:295–301, 2002.
101. Ghersetich I, Menchini G, Teofoli P, et al: Immune response to Leishmania infection in human skin. Clin Dermatol 17:333–338, 1999.
102. Barral A, Costa JM, Bittencourt AL, et al: Polar and subpolar diffuse cutaneous leishmaniasis in Brazil: Clinical and immunopathologic aspects. Int J Dermatol 34:474–479, 1995.
103. Carvalho EM, Correia FD, Bacellar O, et al: Characterization of the immune response in subjects with self-healing cutaneous leishmaniasis. Am J Trop Med Hyg 53:273–277, 1995.
104. Pirmez C, Yamamura M, Uyemura K, et al: Cytokine patterns in the pathogenesis of human leishmaniasis. J Clin Invest 91:1390–1395, 1993.
105. Ridley DS: The pathogenesis of cutaneous leishmaniasis. Trans R Soc Trop Med Hyg 73:150–160, 1979.
106. Ridley MJ, Ridley DS: Cutaneous leishmaniasis: Immune complex formation and necrosis in the acute phase. Br J Exp Pathol 65:336, 1984.
107. Division of Communicable Disease Prevention and Control, Communicable Disease Program, HPC/HCT, PAHO: Leishmaniasis in the Americas. Epidemiol Bull 15:8–11, 1994.
108. Desjeux P: Human leishmaniases: Epidemiology and public health aspects. World Health Stat Q 45:267–275, 1992.
109. Low GC, Cooke WE: A congenital case of kala-azar. Lancet 2:1209–1211, 1926.
110. Banerji D: Possible congenital infection of kala-azar. J Indian Med Assoc 24:433–435, 1955.
111. Chung HL, Chow HK, Lu JR: The first two cases of transfusion kala-azar. Chin Med J 66:325, 1948.
112. Andre R, Brumpt L, Dreyfuss B, et al: Leishmaniose cutanée ganglionaire et kala-azar transfusionel. Bull Mem Soc Med Hopt 25–26:584, 1957.

113. Symmers WStC: Leishmaniasis acquired by contagion. A case of marital infection in Britain. Lancet 1:127–132, 1960.
114. Evans TG, Pearson RD: Clinical and immunological responses following accidental inoculation of *Leishmania donovani*. Trans R Soc Trop Med Hyg 82:854–856, 1988.
115. Herwaldt BL, Juranek DD: Laboratory-acquired malaria, leishmaniasis, trypanosomiasis, and toxoplasmosis [Review]. Am J Trop Med Hyg 48:313–323, 1993.
116. Shaw JJ, Lainson R: Ecology and epidemiology: New world. In Peters W, Killick-Kendrick R (eds): The Leishmaniases in Biology and Medicine. London, Academic Press, 1987, pp 291–363.
117. Jones TC, Johnson WD Jr, Barretto AC, et al: Epidemiology of American cutaneous leishmaniasis due to *Leishmania braziliensis braziliensis*. J Infect Dis 156:73–83, 1987.
118. Grimaldi G Jr, Tesh RB, McMahon-Pratt DM: A review of the geographic distribution and epidemiology of leishmaniasis in the new world. Am J Trop Med Hyg 41:687–725, 1989.
119. Young DG, Arias JR: Phlebotomine sandflies of the Americas, Technical Paper 33. Washington, DC, Pan American Health Organization, 1991.
120. Hepburn NC, Tidman MJ, Hunter JA: Cutaneous leishmaniasis in British troops from Belize. Br J Dermatol 128:63–68, 1993.
121. Weigle KA, Santrich C, Martinez F, et al: Epidemiology of cutaneous leishmaniasis in Colombia: Environmental and behavioral risk factors for infection, clinical manifestations, and pathogenicity. J Infect Dis 168:709–714, 1993.
122. Simpson MH, Mullins JF, Stone OJ: Disseminated anergic cutaneous leishmaniasis. An autochthonous case in Texas and the Mexican states of Tamaulipas and Nuevo Leon. Arch Dermatol 97:301–303, 1968.
123. Nelson DA, Gustafson TL, Spielvogel RL: Clinical aspects of cutaneous leishmaniasis acquired in Texas. J Am Acad Dermatol 12:985–992, 1985.
124. Barral A, Pedral-Sampaio D, Grimaldi JG, et al: Leishmaniasis in Bahia, Brazil: Evidence that *Leishmania amazonensis* produces a wide spectrum of clinical disease. Am J Trop Med Hyg 44:536–546, 1991.
125. Sanchez JL, Diniega BM, Small JW, et al: Epidemiologic investigation of an outbreak of cutaneous leishmaniasis in a defined geographic focus of transmission. Am J Trop Med Hyg 47:47–54, 1992.
126. Ashford RW, Bettini S: Ecology and epidemiology: Old World. In Peters W, Killick-Kendrick R (eds): The Leishmaniasis in Biology and Medicine. London, Academic Press, 1987, pp 365–424.
127. Manson-Bahr PEC, Apted FIC: Leishmaniasis. In Manson-Bahr PEC, Apted FIC (eds): Manson's Tropical Diseases, 18th ed. London, Bailliere Tindall, 1982, pp 92–115.
128. Sacks DL, Kenney RT, Kreutzer RD, et al: Indian kala-azar caused by *Leishmania tropica*. Lancet 345:959–961, 1995.
129. Basu D, Mallik KK: Changes in age incidence of kala-azar in India. Indian J Public Health 39:26, 1995.
130. Ashford RW, Seaman J, Schorscher J, et al: Epidemic visceral leishmaniasis in southern Sudan: Identify and systematic position of the parasites from patients and vectors. Trans R Soc Trop Med Hyg 86:379–380, 1992.
131. Marty P, Le Fichoux Y, Pratlong F, et al: Human visceral leishmaniasis in Alpes-Maritimes, France: Epidemiological characteristics for the period 1985–1992. Trans R Soc Trop Med Hyg 88:33–34, 1994.
132. Soleimanzadeh G, Edrissian GH, Movahhed-Danesh AM, et al: Epidemiological aspects of kala-azar in Meshkin-Shahr, Iran: Human infection. Bull World Health Organ 71:759–762, 1993.
133. Lu HG, Zhong L, Guan LR, et al: Separation of Chinese *Leishmania* isolates into five genotypes by kinetoplast and chromosomal DNA heterogeneity. Am J Trop Med Hyg 50:763–770, 1994.
134. Melby PC, Kreutzer RD, McMahon-Pratt D, et al: Cutaneous leishmaniasis: Review of 59 cases seen at the National Institutes of Health [Review]. Clin Infect Dis 15:924–937, 1992.
135. Barral A, Barral-Netto M, Almeida R, et al: Lymphadenopathy associated with *Leishmania braziliensis* cutaneous infection. Am J Trop Med Hyg 47:587–592, 1992.
136. Sousa A, de Q, Parise ME, Pompeu MM, et al: Bubonic leishmaniasis: A common manifestation of *Leishmania (Viannia) braziliensis* infection in Ceara, Brazil. Am J Trop Med Hyg 53:380–385, 1995.
137. Willems JP, Schmidt SM, Greer KE, et al: Sporotrichoid cutaneous leishmaniasis in a traveler. South Med J 90:325–327, 1997.
138. Kibbi AG, Karam PG, Kurban AK: Sporotrichoid leishmaniasis in patients from Saudi Arabia: Clinical and histologic features. J Am Acad Dermatol 17:759–764, 1987.
139. Gaafar A, Ismail A, el Kadaro AY, et al: Necrotizing and suppurative lymphadenitis in *Leishmania major* infections. Trop Med Int Health 1:243–250, 1996.
140. Herrera E, Sanchez P, Bosch RJ: Disseminated cutaneous leishmaniasis in an HIV-infected patient. Int J STD AIDS 6:125–126, 1995.
141. Gillis D, Klaus S, Schnur LF, et al: Diffusely disseminated cutaneous *Leishmania major* infection in a child with acquired immunodeficiency syndrome. Pediatr Infect Dis J 14:247–249, 1995.
142. Mengistu G, Laskay T, Gemetchu T, et al: Cutaneous leishmaniasis in southwestern Ethiopia: Ocholo revisited. Trans R Soc Trop Med Hyg 86:149–153, 1992.
143. Bryceson ADM: Diffuse cutaneous leishmaniasis in Ethiopia. I. The clinical and histological features of the disease. Trans R Soc Trop Med Hyg 63:708–737, 1969.
144. Carvalho EM, Barral A, Costa JM, et al: Clinical and immunopathological aspects of disseminated cutaneous leishmaniasis. Acta Trop 56:315–325, 1994.
145. Barral A, Costa JM, Bittencourt AL, et al: Polar and subpolar diffuse cutaneous leishmaniasis in Brazil: Clinical and immunopathologic aspects. Int J Dermatol 34:474–479, 1995.
146. Zeledon R: Leishmaniasis in the Caribbean Islands. A review. Ann NY Acad Sci 653:154–160, 1992.
147. Cnudde F, Raccurt C, Boulard F, et al: Diffuse cutaneous leishmaniasis with visceral dissemination in an AIDS patient in Guadeloupe, West Indies [Letter]. AIDS 8:559–560, 1994.
148. Paksoy N, Hekim E: Comparative analysis of the clinicopathological features in cutaneous leishmaniasis and lupus vulgaris in Turkey. Trop Med Parasitol 44:37–39, 1993.
149. Walton BC, Chinel LV, Eguia y Eguia O: Onset of espundia after many years of occult infection with *Leishmania braziliensis*. Am J Trop Med Hyg 22:696–698, 1973.
150. Marsden PD: Mucosal leishmaniasis ("espundia" Escomel, 1911) [Review]. Trans R Soc Trop Med Hyg 80:859–876, 1986.
151. Zajtchuk JT, Casler JD, Netto EM, et al: Mucosal leishmaniasis in Brazil. Laryngoscope 99:925–939, 1989.
152. Bittencourt AL, Barral A: Evaluation of the histopathological classifications of American cutaneous and mucocutaneous leishmaniasis [erratum appears in Mem Inst Oswaldo Cruz 86:378, 1991]. Mem Inst Oswaldo Cruz 86:51–56, 1991.
153. Klotz O, Lindenberg H: The pathology of leishmaniosis of the nose. Am J Trop Med 3:117–141, 1923.
154. Zinneman HH, Hall WH, Wallace FG: Leishmaniasis of the larynx. Am J Med 31:654–658, 1961.
155. Lessa HA, Carvalho EM, Marsden PD: Eustachian tube blockage with consequent middle ear infection in mucosal leishmaniasis [Letter]. Rev Soc Bras Med Trop 27:103, 1994.
156. Aleixo J: Leishmaniose com localizacao genital. An Bras Dermatol Sifilolog 20:69–71, 1945.
157. Morsy TA, Khalil NM, Salama MM, et al: Mucosal leishmaniasis caused by *Leishmania tropica* in Saudi Arabia. J Egypt Soc Parasitol 25:73–79, 1995.
158. Abbas K, el Toum IA, el Hassan AM: Oral leishmaniasis associated with kala-azar. A case report. Oral Surg Oral Med Oral Pathol 73:583–584, 1992.
159. el-Hassan AM, Meredith SE, Yagi HI, et al: Sudanese mucosal leishmaniasis: Epidemiology, clinical features, diagnosis, immune responses and treatment. Trans R Soc Trop Med Hyg 89:647–652, 1995.
160. Navarro Cunchillos M, Villanueva Marcos JL, Torre-Cisneros J, et al: Isolated laryngeal leishmaniasis in an immunocompetent patient: Successful treatment with surgery. J Laryngol Otol 108:249–251, 1994.
161. Grant A, Spraggs PD, Grant HR, et al: Laryngeal leishmaniasis. J Laryngol Otol 108:1086–1088, 1994.
162. Baily GG, Pitt MA, Curry A, et al: Leishmaniasis of the tongue treated with liposomal amphotericin B. J Infect 28:327–331, 1994.
163. Canovas DL, Carbonell J, Torres J, et al: Laryngeal leishmaniasis as initial opportunistic disease in HIV infection. J Laryngol Otol 108:1089–1092, 1994.
164. Miralles ES, Nunez M, Hilara Y, et al: Mucocutaneous leishmaniasis and HIV. Dermatology 189:275–277, 1994.

165. Badaro R, Jones TC, Carvalho EM, et al: New perspectives on a subclinical form of visceral leishmaniasis. J Infect Dis 154:1003–1011, 1986.
166. Evans T, Reis MdeF, de Alencar JE, et al: American visceral leishmaniasis (kala-azar). West J Med 142:777–781, 1985.
167. Harrison LH, Naidu TG, Drew JS, et al: Reciprococal relationships between undernutrition and the parasitic disease visceral leishmaniasis. Rev Infect Dis 8:447–453, 1986.
168. Cerf BJ, Jones TC, Badaro R, et al: Malnutrition as a risk factor for severe visceral leishmaniasis. J Infect Dis 156:1030–1033, 1987.
169. Dye C, Williams BG: Malnutrition, age and the risk of parasitic disease: Visceral leishmaniasis revisited. Proc R Soc Lond B Biol Sci 254:33–39, 1993.
170. Stone HH, Tool CD, Pugsley WS: Kala-azar (visceral leishmaniasis): Report of a case with 34 month incubation period and positive Doan–Wright test. Ann Intern Med 36:686–693, 1952.
171. Badaro R, Carvalho EM, Rocha H, et al: *Leishmania donovani:* An opportunistic microbe associated with progressive disease in three immunocompromised patients. Lancet 1:647–649, 1986.
172. Morsy TA, Mangoud AM, Aly MA, et al: Lymphatic leishmaniasis. An adult case without visceral involvement from Sharkia Governorate, Egypt. J Egypt Soc Parasitol 22:533–537, 1992.
173. Pearson RD, Cox G, Jeronimo SM, et al: Visceral leishmaniasis: A model for infection-induced cachexia [Review]. Am J Trop Med Hyg 47:8–15, 1992.
174. Singh UK, Sinha RK, Sharma VK: Fulminant hepatitis in Kala-azar. Indian J Pediatr 62:571–574, 1995.
175. Andrade TM, Carvalho EM, Rocha H: Bacterial infections in patients with visceral leishmaniasis. J Infect Dis 162:1354–1359, 1990.
176. Knight R, Woodruff AW, Pettitt LE: The mechanism of anaemia in kala-azar. A study of 2 patients. Trans R Soc Trop Med Hyg 61:701–705, 1967.
177. Woodruff AW, Topley E, Knight R, et al: The anaemia of kala-azar. Br J Haematol 22:319–329, 1972.
178. Pippard MJ, Moir D, Weatherall DJ, et al: Mechanism of anaemia in resistant visceral leishmaniasis. Ann Trop Med Parasitol 80:317–323, 1986.
179. Musumeci S, D'Agata A, Schiliro G, et al: Studies of the neutropenia in kala-azar: Results in two patients. Trans R Soc Trop Med Hyg 70:500–503, 1977.
180. Jeronimo SM, Duggal P, Braz RF, et al: An emerging peri-urban pattern of infection with *Leishmania chagasi*, the protozoan causing visceral leishmaniasis in northeast Brazil. Scand J Infect Dis 36:443–449, 2004.
181. Carvalho EM, Andrews BS, Martinelli R, et al: Circulating immune complexes and rheumatoid factor in schistosomiasis and visceral leishmaniasis. Am J Trop Med Hyg 32:61–68, 1983.
182. Pearson RD, de Alencar JE, Romito R, et al: Circulating immune complexes and rheumatoid factors in visceral leishmaniasis. J Infect Dis 147:1102, 1983.
183. Hervas JA, Alberti P, Ferragut J, et al: Acute hepatitis as a presenting manifestation of kala azar. Pediatr Infect Dis J 10:409–410, 1991.
184. Matheron S, Cabie A, Parquin F, et al: Visceral leishmaniasis and HIV infection: Unusual presentation with pleuropulmonary involvement, and effect of secondary prophylaxis [Letter]. AIDS 6:238–240, 1992.
185. Duarte MI, da Matta VL, Corbett CE, et al: Interstitial pneumonitis in human visceral leishmaniasis. Trans R Soc Trop Med Hyg 83:73–76, 1989.
186. Datry A, Similowski T, Jais P, et al: AIDS-associated leishmaniasis: An unusual gastro-duodenal presentation. Trans R Soc Trop Med Hyg 84:239–240, 1990.
187. Altes J, Salas A, Llompart A, et al: Small intestinal involvement in visceral leishmaniasis [Letter]. Am J Gastroenterol 86:1283, 1991.
188. Delsedime L, Coppola F, Mazzucco G: Gastric localization of systemic leishmaniasis in a patient with AIDS. Histopathology 19:93–95, 1991.
189. Muigai R, Gatei DG, Shaunak S, et al: Jejunal function and pathology in visceral leishmaniasis. Lancet 2:476–479, 1983.
190. Sendino A, Barbado FJ, Mostaza JM, et al: Visceral leishmaniasis with malabsorption syndrome in a patient with acquired immunodeficiency syndrome. Am J Med 89:673–675, 1990.
191. Kumar PV, Sadeghi E, Torabi S: Kala azar with disseminated dermal leishmaniasis. Am J Trop Med Hyg 40:150–153, 1989.
192. Grau JM, Bosch X, Salgado AC, et al: Human immunodeficiency virus (HIV) and aplastic anemia [Letter]. Ann Intern Med 110:576–577, 1989.
193. Condom MJ, Clotet B, Sirera G, et al: Asymptomatic leishmaniasis in the acquired immunodeficiency syndrome (AIDS) [Letter]. Ann Intern Med 111:767–768, 1989.
194. Hernandez DE, Oliver M, Martinez C, et al: Visceral leishmaniasis with cutaneous and rectal dissemination due to *Leishmania braziliensis* in acquired immunodeficiency syndrome (AIDS). Int J Dermatol 34:114–115, 1995.
195. Sen Gupta PC, Bhattacharjee B: Histopathology of post-kala-azar dermal leishmaniasis. J Trop Med Hyg 56:110–116, 1953.
196. Muigai R, Gachihi GS, Oster CN, et al: Post kala-azar dermal leishmaniasis: The Kenyan experience. East Afr Med J 68:801–806, 1991.
197. el Hassan AM, Ghalib HW, Zijlstra EE, et al: Post kala-azar dermal leishmaniasis in the Sudan: Clinical features, pathology and treatment. Trans R Soc Trop Med Hyg 86:245–248, 1992.
198. Dhar S, Kaur I, Dawn G, et al: Post-kala-azar dermal leishmaniasis mimicking leprosy: Experience with 4 patients, with some unusual features in 1. Lepr Rev 66:250–256, 1995.
199. Berger RS, Perez-Figaredo RA, Spielvogel RL: Leishmaniasis: The touch preparation as a rapid means of diagnosis. J Am Acad Dermatol 16:1096–1105, 1987.
200. Hockmeyer WT, Kager PA, Rees PH, et al: The culture of *Leishmania donovani* in Schneider's insect medium: Its value in the diagnosis and management of patients with visceral leishmaniasis. Trans R Soc Trop Med Hyg 75:861–863, 1981.
201. Pearson RD, Navin TR, Sousa AQ, et al: Leishmaniasis. In Kass EH, Platt R (eds): Current Therapy in Infectious Diseases. Toronto, BC Decker, 1990, pp 384–389.
202. Nuwayri-Salti N, Mu'Atassem D, Salman S, et al: Chronic cutaneous leishmaniasis: *Leishmania* parasites in blood. Int J Dermatol 31:562–564, 1992.
203. Martinez JE, Arias AL, Escobar MA, et al: Haemoculture of *Leishmania (Viannia) braziliensis* from two cases of mucosal leishmaniasis: Re-examination of haematogenous dissemination. Trans R Soc Trop Med Hyg 86:392–394, 1992.
204. Chulay JD, Bryceson ADM: Quantitation of amastigotes of *Leishmania donovani* in smears of splenic aspirates from patients with visceral leishmaniasis. Am J Trop Med Hyg 32:475–479, 1983.
205. Tallada N, Raventos A, Martinez S, et al: *Leishmania* lymphadenitis diagnosed by fine-needle aspiration biopsy. Diagn Cytopathol 9:673–676, 1993.
206. Walton BC, Brooks WH, Arjona I: Serodiagnosis of American leishmaniasis by indirect fluorescent antibody test. Am J Trop Med Hyg 21:296–299, 1972.
207. Badaro R, Reed SG, Carvalho EM: Immunofluorescent antibody test in American visceral leishmaniasis: Sensitivity and specificity of different morphological forms of two *Leishmania* species. Am J Trop Med Hyg 32:480–484, 1983.
208. Pearson RD, Evans T, Wheeler DA, et al: Humoral factors during South American visceral leishmaniasis. Ann Trop Med Parasitol 80:465–468, 1986.
209. Zijlstra EE, Ali MS, el-Hassan AM, et al: Kala-azar: A comparative study of parasitological methods and the direct agglutination test in diagnosis. Trans R Soc Trop Med Hyg 86:505–507, 1992.
210. Scott JM, Shreffler WG, Ghalib HW, et al: A rapid and simple diagnostic test for active visceral leishmaniasis. Am J Trop Med Hyg 44:272–277, 1991.
211. Weigle KA, de Davalos M, Heredia P, et al: Diagnosis of cutaneous and mucocutaneous leishmaniasis in Colombia: A comparison of seven methods. Am J Trop Med Hyg 36:489–496, 1987.
212. Badaro R, Benson D, Eulalio MC, et al: rK39: A cloned antigen of *Leishmania chagasi* that predicts active visceral leishmaniasis. J Infect Dis 173:758–761, 1996.
213. Braz RF, Nascimento ET, Martins DR, et al: The sensitivity and specificity of *Leishmania chagasi* recombinant K39 antigen in the diagnosis of American visceral leishmaniasis and in differentiating active from subclinical infection. Am J Trop Med Hyg 67:344–348, 2002.
214. Abramson MA, Dietze R, Frucht D, et al: Comparison of New and Old World leishmanins in an endemic region of Brazil. Clin Infect Dis 20:1292–1297, 1995.
215. Herwaldt BL, Berman JD: Recommendations for treating leishmaniasis with sodium stibogluconate (Pentostam) and review of pertinent clinical studies. Am J Trop Med Hyg 46:296–306, 1992.

216. Grogl M, Thomason TN, Franke ED: Drug resistance in leishmaniasis: Its implication in systemic chemotherapy of cutaneous and mucocutaneous disease. Am J Trop Med Hyg 47:117–126, 1992.
217. Meyerhoff A: U.S. Food and Drug Administration approval of AmBisome (liposomal amphotericin B) for treatment of visceral leishmaniasis. Clin Infect Dis 28:42–48, 1999.
218. Pearson RD: The development of miltefosine for the treatment of visceral and cutaneous leishmaniasis. Curr Infect Dis Rep 6:41–42, 2003.
219. Bhattacharya SK, Jha TK, Sundar S, et al: Efficacy and tolerability of miltefosine for childhood visceral leishmaniasis in India. Clin Infect Dis 38:217–221, 2004.
220. Berman J: Current treatment approaches to leishmaniasis. Curr Opin Infect Dis 16:397–401, 2003.
221. Croft SL, Davidson RN, Thornton EA: Liposomal amphotericin B in the treatment of visceral leishmaniasis. J Antimicrob Chemother 28(suppl B):111–118, 1991.
222. Davidson RN, Croft SL, Scott A, et al: Liposomal amphotericin B in drug-resistant visceral leishmaniasis. Lancet 337:1061–1062, 1991.
223. Torre-Cisneros J, Villanueva JL, Kindelan JM, et al: Successful treatment of antimony-resistant visceral leishmaniasis with liposomal amphotericin B in patients infected with human immunodeficiency virus. Clin Infect Dis 17:625–627, 1993.
224. Berman J: Current treatment approaches to leishmaniasis. Curr Opin Infect Dis 16:397–401, 2003.
225. Chulay JD, Fleckenstein L, Smith DH: Pharmacokinetics of antimony during treatment of visceral leishmaniasis with sodium stibogluconate or meglumine antimoniate. Trans R Soc Trop Med Hyg 82:69–72, 1988.
226. Thakur CP, Kumar K, Sinha PK, et al: Treatment of post-kala-azar dermal leishmaniasis with sodium stibogluconate. BMJ 295:886–887, 1987.
227. Thakur CP, Kumar K: Efficacy of prolonged therapy with stibogluconate in post kala-azar dermal leishmaniasis. Indian J Med Res 91:144–148, 1990.
228. Gasser RA Jr, Magill AJ, Oster CN, et al: Pancreatitis induced by pentavalent antimonial agents during treatment of leishmaniasis. Clin Infect Dis 18:83–90, 1994.
229. Antezana G, Zeballos R, Mendoza C, et al: Electrocardiographic alterations during treatment of mucocutaneous leishmaniasis with meglumine antimoniate and allopurinol. Trans R Soc Trop Med Hyg 86:31–33, 1992.
230. Balzan M, Fenech F: Acute renal failure in visceral leishmaniasis treated with sodium stibogluconate. Trans R Soc Trop Med Hyg 86:515–516, 1992.
231. Jha TK, Sundar S, Thakur CP, et al: Miltefosine, an oral agent, for the treatment of Indian visceral leishmaniasis. N Engl J Med 341:1795–1800, 1999.
232. Sundar S, Makharia A, More DK: Short-course oral miltefosine for treatment of visceral leishmaniasis. Clin Infect Dis 31:1110–1113, 2000.
233. Perez-Victoria FJ, Gamarro F, Ouellette M, et al: Functional cloning of the miltefosine transporter. A novel P-type phospholipid translocase from Leishmania involved in drug resistance. J Biol Chem 278:49965–49971, 2003.
234. Mishra M, Biswas UK, Jha AM, et al: Amphotericin versus sodium stibogluconate in first-line treatment of Indian kala-azar. Lancet 344:1599–1600, 1994.
235. Wispelwey B, Pearson R: Pentamidine. A risk–benefit analysis [Review]. Drug Saf 5:212–219, 1990.
236. Thakur CP, Kanyok TP, Pandey AK, et al: A prospective randomized, comparative, open-label trial of the safety and efficacy of paromomycin (aminosidine) plus sodium stibogluconate versus sodium stibogluconate alone for the treatment of visceral leishmaniasis. Trans R Soc Trop Med Hyg 94:429–431, 2000.
237. Raffi F, Merrien D, Le Pape P, et al: Use of an itraconazole/allopurinol combination for the treatment of visceral leishmaniasis in a patient with AIDS. Clin Infect Dis 21:1338–1339, 1995.
238. Rashid JR, Wasunna KM, Gachihi GS, et al: The efficacy and safety of ketoconazole in visceral leishmaniasis. East Afr Med J 71:392–395, 1994.
239. Halim MA, Alfurayh O, Kalin ME, et al: Successful treatment of visceral leishmaniasis with allopurinol plus ketoconazole in a renal transplant recipient after the occurrence of pancreatitis due to stibogluconate. Clin Infect Dis 16:397–399, 1993.
240. Wali JP, Aggarwal P, Gupta U, et al: Ketoconazole in the treatment of antimony- and pentamidine-resistant kala-azar [Letter]. J Infect Dis 166:215–216, 1992.
241. Badaro R, Falcoff E, Badaro FS, et al: Treatment of visceral leishmaniasis with pentavalent antimony and interferon gamma. N Engl J Med 322:16–21, 1990.
242. Neva FA: Immunotherapy for parasitic disease [Editorial]. N Engl J Med 322:55–57, 1990.
243. de Gorgolas M, Castrillo JM, Fernandez Guerrero ML: Visceral leishmaniasis in patients with AIDS: Report of three cases treated with pentavalent antimony and interferon-γ. Clin Infect Dis 17:56–58, 1993.
244. Sundar S, Rosenkaimer F, Murray HW: Successful treatment of refractory visceral leishmaniasis in India using antimony plus interferon-gamma. J Infect Dis 170:659–662, 1994.
245. Lustig V, Kager PA, Meenhorst PL: Treatment of visceral leishmaniasis in a patient with AIDS with antimony and γ-interferon: Remission and prevention of relapse by maintenance therapy with weekly pentamidine. Neth J Med 47:66–69, 1995.
246. Sundar S, Murray HW: Effect of treatment with interferon-gamma alone in visceral leishmaniasis. J Infect Dis 172:1627–1629, 1995.
247. Navin TR, Arana BA, Arana FE, et al: Placebo-controlled clinical trial of sodium stibogluconate (Pentostam) versus ketoconazole for treating cutaneous leishmaniasis in Guatemala. J Infect Dis 165:528–534, 1992.
248. Weinrauch L, Livshin R, el-On J: Ketoconazole in cutaneous leishmaniasis [Letter]. Br J Dermatol 117:666–668, 1987.
249. Alrajhi AA, Ibrahim EA, De Vol EB, et al: Fluconazole for the treatment of cutaneous leishmaniasis caused by *Leishmania major*. N Engl J Med 346:891–895, 2002.
250. Soto J, Toledo J, Gutierrez P, et al: Treatment of American cutaneous leishmaniasis with miltefosine, an oral agent. Clin Infect Dis 33:E57–E61, 2001.
251. Velez I, Agudelo S, Hendrickx E, et al: Inefficacy of allopurinol as monotherapy for Colombian cutaneous leishmaniasis. A randomized, controlled trial. Ann Intern Med 126:232–236, 1997.
252. Arana BA, Mendoza CE, Rizzo NR, et al: Randomized, controlled, double-blind trial of topical treatment of cutaneous leishmaniasis with paromomycin plus methylbenzethonium chloride ointment in Guatemala. Am J Trop Med Hyg 65:466–470, 2000.
253. el-On J, Halevy S, Grunwald MH, et al: Topical treatment of Old World cutaneous leishmaniasis caused by *Leishmania major*: A double-blind control study. J Am Acad Dermatol 27:227–231, 1992.
254. Convit J, Castellanos PL, Ulrich M, et al: Immunotherapy of localized, intermediate, and diffuse forms of American cutaneous leishmaniasis. J Infect Dis 160:104–115, 1989.
255. Navin TR, Arana BA, Arana FE, et al: Placebo-controlled clinical trial of meglumine antimonate (glucantime) vs. localized controlled heat in the treatment of cutaneous leishmaniasis in Guatemala. Am J Trop Med Hyg 42:43–50, 1990.
256. Badaro R, Johnson WD Jr: The role of interferon-gamma in the treatment of visceral and diffuse cutaneous leishmaniasis [erratum appears in J Infect Dis 169:233, 1994]. J Infect Dis 167(suppl 1):513–517, 1993.
257. Franke ED, Wignall FS, Cruz ME, et al: Efficacy and toxicity of sodium stibogluconate for mucosal leishmaniasis. Ann Intern Med 113:934–940, 1990.
258. Franke ED, Llanos-Cuentas A, Echevarria J, et al: Efficacy of 28-day and 40-day regimens of sodium stibogluconate (Pentostam) in the treatment of mucosal leishmaniasis. Am J Trop Med Hyg 51:77–82, 1994.
259. Sampaio SAP, Godoy JT, Paiva L, et al: The treatment of American (mucocutaneous) leishmaniasis with amphotericin B. Arch Dermatol 82:627–635, 1960.
260. Miranda JL, Lima NDS, DaCuhna JF: A anfotericina B na terapeutic de leishmaniose tegumentar Americana. O Hospital 59:31–53, 1961.
261. Crofts MA: Use of amphotericin B in mucocutaneous leishmaniasis. J Trop Med Hyg 79:111–113, 1976.
262. Falcoff E, Taranto NJ, Remondegui CE, et al: Clinical healing of antimony-resistant cutaneous or mucocutaneous leishmaniasis following the combined administration of interferon-γ and pentavalent antimonial compounds. Trans R Soc Trop Med Hyg 88:95–97, 1994.

263. Alexander B, Cadena H, Usma MC, et al: Laboratory and field evaluations of a repellent soap containing diethyltoluamide (DEET) and permethrin against phlebotomine sand flies (Diptera: Psychodidae) in Valle del Cauca, Colombia. Am J Trop Med Hyg 52:169–173, 1995.
264. Soto J, Medina F, Dember N, et al: Efficacy of permethrin-impregnated uniforms in the prevention of malaria and leishmaniasis in Colombian soldiers. Clin Infect Dis 21:599–602, 1995.
265. Mutinga MJ, Renapurkar DM, Wachira DW, et al: A bioassay to evaluate the efficacy of permethrin-impregnated screens used against phlebotomine sandflies (Diptera: Psychodidae) in Baringo District of Kenya. East Afr Med J 70:168–170, 1993.
266. Marinkelle CJ: The control of leishmaniasis. Bull World Health Organ 58:807–818, 1980.
267. Davies CR, Llanos-Cuentas A, Canales J, et al: The fall and rise of Andean cutaneous leishmaniasis: Transient impact of the DDT campaign in Peru. Trans R Soc Trop Med Hyg 88:389–393, 1994.
268. Alexander B, Maroli M: Control of phlebotomine sandflies. Med Vet Entomol 17:1–18, 2003.
269. Gavgani AS, Hodjati MH, Mohite H, et al: Effect of insecticide-impregnated dog collars on incidence of zoonotic visceral leishmaniasis in Iranian children: A matched-cluster randomised trial. Lancet 360:374–379, 2002.
270. Tesh RB: Control of zoonotic visceral leishmaniasis: Is it time to change strategies? Am J Trop Med Hyg 52:287–292, 1995.
271. Dietze R, Barros GB, Teixeira L, et al: Effect of eliminating seropositive canines on the transmission of visceral leishmaniasis in Brazil. Clin Infect Dis 25:1240–1242, 1997.
272. Mayrink W, Antunes CMF, Da Costa CA, et al: Further trials of a vaccine against American cutaneous leishmaniasis [Letter]. Trans R Soc Trop Med Hyg 80:1001, 1986.
273. Titus RG, Gueiros-Filho FJ, de Freitas LA, et al: Development of a safe live *Leishmania* vaccine line by gene replacement. Proc Natl Acad Sci USA 92:10267–10271, 1995.
274. Scott P, Artis D, Uzonna J, et al: The development of effector and memory T cells in cutaneous leishmaniasis: The implications for vaccine development. Immunol Rev 201:318–338, 2004.
275. Reed SG, Campos-Neto A: Vaccines for parasitic and bacterial diseases. Curr Opin Immunol 15:456–460, 2003.

95

Pathogenic and Opportunistic Free-Living Amebas: Acanthamoeba *spp.*, Balamuthia mandrillaris, Naegleria fowleri, *and* Sappinia diploidea

GOVINDA S. VISVESVARA
JAMES H. MAGUIRE

INTRODUCTION

Infections caused by the pathogenic and opportunistic free-living amebas such as *Acanthamoeba, Balamuthia*, and *Naegleria* have been recorded from all parts of the world including the tropics.[1–5] Diseases caused by these amebas in tropical countries have received little attention because of more pressing health problems and the likelihood that many cases go undetected because of limited resources for diagnosis and low rates of autopsy, the method by which most infections are detected, even in industrialized countries. Because these infections occur most often in immunocompromised persons, greater numbers of cases would be expected in sub-Saharan Africa, South Asia, and other areas where the HIV epidemic is burgeoning. Limited diagnostic expertise in many developed and developing countries contributes to our lack of knowledge of the actual incidence of these infections.

AGENTS

Pathogenic and opportunistic free-living amebas of the genera *Acanthamoeba, Balamuthia, Naegleria* are mitochondria-bearing, aerobic, eukaryotic protists. Although they exist as free-living entities in nature, they cause life- and sight-threatening disease in humans and other animals.[1–37] *Acanthamoeba* and *Balamuthia* cause an insidious chronic granulomatous disease known as granulomatous amebic encephalitis (GAE) in both immunocompetent and immunosuppressed persons and animals.[1–6,8–10,15,16,23–37] *N. fowleri* produces a necrotizing, hemorrhagic meningoencephalitis, primary amebic meningoencephalitis (PAM), principally in healthy immunocompetent hosts who have a history of recent contact with fresh warm water.[1,7,13–15,17–22,26,27] Recently, *Sappinia diploidea*, a free-living ameba that normally lives in soil contaminated with feces of elk, bison, and cattle has been identified as causing encephalitis in an otherwise healthy young man.[38,39] Since all these amebas have the ability to exist as free-living organisms in nature and occasionally invade a host and live as parasites within host tissue, they have been called amphizoic amebas. In contrast to the free-living amebas, *Entamoeba histolytica* is an anaerobic ameba that lacks mitochondria, commonly causes gastrointestinal pathology, and is strictly parasitic.

Acanthamoeba Species

Although the genus *Acanthamoeba* was named by Volkonsky in 1931, Puschkarew in 1913 first isolated the ameba from dust and named it *Ameba polyphagus*. Page later redescribed the ameba and renamed it *Acanthamoeba polyphaga*.[40] Sir Aldo Castellani in 1930[41] also isolated an ameba that occurred as a contaminant in a yeast culture plate and was later named *Acanthamoeba castellanii*. In 1958, Culbertson and colleagues demonstrated the pathogenic potential of *Acanthamoeba* when they isolated an ameba, now known as *Acanthamoeba culbertsoni*, contaminating monkey kidney cell culture during production of the poliomyelitis vaccine.[42] It is now well established that several species of *Acanthamoeba* (*A. castellanii, A. culbertsoni, A. healyi, A. polyphaga, A. rhysodes*) cause GAE, an insidious disease with a protracted course and usually fatal outcome.[1] GAE usually occurs in persons with acquired immunodeficiency syndrome (HIV/AIDS) or who are otherwise immunocompromised, debilitated, or malnourished (Fig. 95-1). In addition to GAE, *Acanthamoeba* can cause a disseminated disease involving skin, sinuses, lungs, and other organs and also a painful, sight-threatening infection of the eye, *Acanthamoeba* keratitis.[1,11,12,16,43]

Life Cycle

Acanthamoeba has two stages in its life cycle: a feeding and reproducing trophozoite stage and a resistant cyst stage (Fig. 95-2). The trophozoites feed on bacteria and detritus present in the environment and multiply by binary fission. A unique and characteristic feature of *Acanthamoeba* is the presence of fine, tapering, thorn-like pseudopodia, acanthopodia, that emanate from its surface. The trophozoites range in size from 15 to 45 μm and have a single nucleus with a centrally placed, large, densely staining nucleolus. The cytoplasm is finely granular and contains numerous mitochondria, ribosomes, food vacuoles, and a contractile vacuole (see Fig. 95-2A). Cysts are double walled and range in size from 10 to 25 μm. The outer cyst wall, the ectocyst, is wrinkled with folds and ripples and contains protein and lipid. The inner cyst wall, the endocyst, contains cellulose and hence is PAS positive. It is stellate, polygonal, oval, or spherical. Pores, or ostioles, at the junction of the ectocyst and the endocyst are

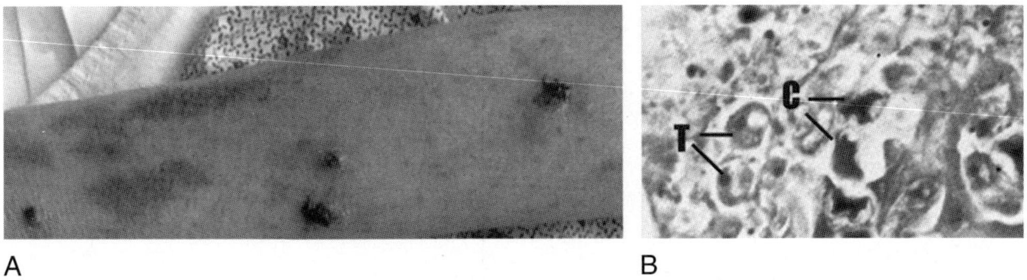

FIGURE 95-8 *A,* HIV/AIDS patient with skin ulcers caused by *Acanthamoeba. B,* A section through the ulcer showing *Acanthamoeba* trophozoites (T) and cysts (C). (H&E stain, ×1000)

AIDS, and there have been reports of osteomyelitis, otitis, endophthalmitis, and adrenalitis in immunosuppressed patients with and without AIDS. There are reports of identification of *Acanthamoeba* spp or *B. mandrillaris* in other organs, such as kidneys, lymph nodes, liver, prostate, testes, and uterus.

Pathologic Findings

The initial site of infection in GAE, due to either *Acanthamoeba* or *Balamuthia*, probably is the lower respiratory tract, skin, or sinuses, and invasion of the brain and other organs results from hematogenous spread from these sites. On gross examination, the brain is edematous and there may be evidence of uncal and tonsillar herniation. Multiple areas of meningeal softening and inflammation overlie necrotic and hemorrhagic lesions in the cortex (Figs. 95-9 and 95-10). Such lesions extend into the white matter in the brainstem, cerebral hemispheres, and cerebellum and have the appearance of hemorrhagic infarcts. Microscopic examination shows amebic trophozoites and cysts in necrotic and viable tissue within the CNS, skin, lungs, and other organs (see Fig. 95-9B). There are areas of necrosis, hemorrhage, and inflammatory infiltrates, consisting of neutrophils, mononuclear cells, and multinucleated giant cells. Trophozoites and cysts of *Acanthamoeba* are seen extracellularly or within macrophages, which also contain lipid (see Fig. 95-9B). In the case of *Balamuthia* infection, the nucleus of the trophozoites may occasionally contain two or three nucleoli (see Fig. 95-10B). The walls of blood vessels are surrounded and infiltrated with amebas, which may provoke vasculitis and thrombosis.[1,6,9,23–37] In some patients, especially those with advanced HIV disease, the inflammatory reaction is sparse and granulomas are not present.

Pathogenesis and Immunity

With a few exceptions, GAE caused by *Acanthamoeba* spp affects hosts whose metabolic, physiologic, or immunologic integrity are lost, whereas disease due to *Balamuthia* affects both healthy and immunocompromised persons. Among the commonly recognized causes of susceptibility to these infections are diseases or conditions such as AIDS, hematologic malignancies, cancer, liver disease, diabetes mellitus, pregnancy, and therapy with corticosteroids and other immunosuppressive drugs following organ transplantation.[1] The etiologic agents may enter the skin or reach the respiratory tract through aerosol or inhalation of airborne dust containing the trophic or cyst stage. The trophozoites or most likely the cysts may temporarily be contained at the site of entry by the body's immune system. However, if the immune system is impaired, or in healthy persons, for reasons not well understood, the cyst excysts and trophozoites invade tissue and gain access to the circulation, where they are carried to the brain and other organs. In an immunocompetent host, immunoglobulins and complement promote recognition of these amebas by neutrophils, macrophages, and lymphocytes. These cells,

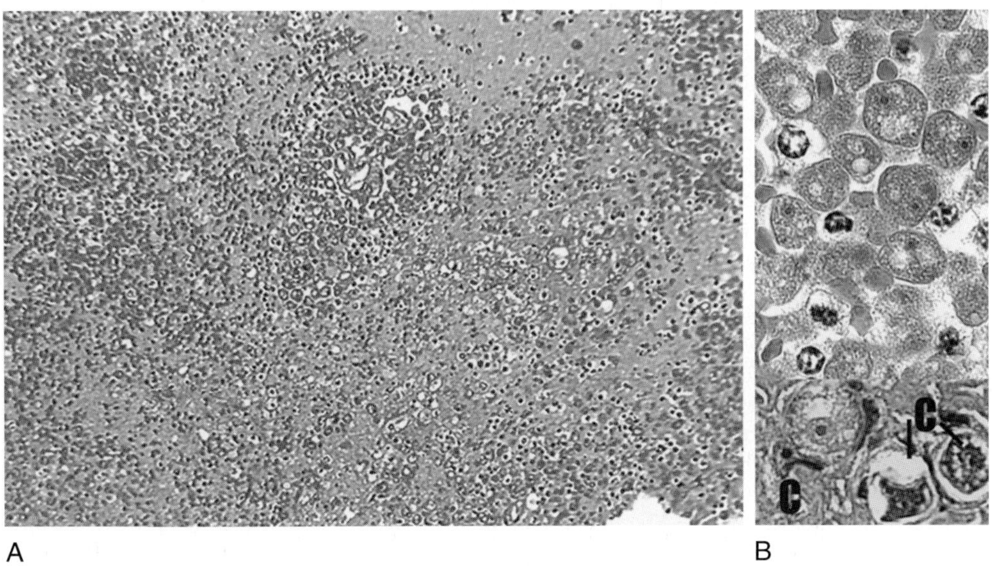

FIGURE 95-9 Brain section of a patient infected with *Acanthamoeba* (H&E stain). *A,* Low-power view of a CNS section showing chronic inflammatory changes. (magnification ×100) *B,* Higher magnification (×1000) showing the characteristic nuclear morphology of the trophozoite cysts (C) with double walls.

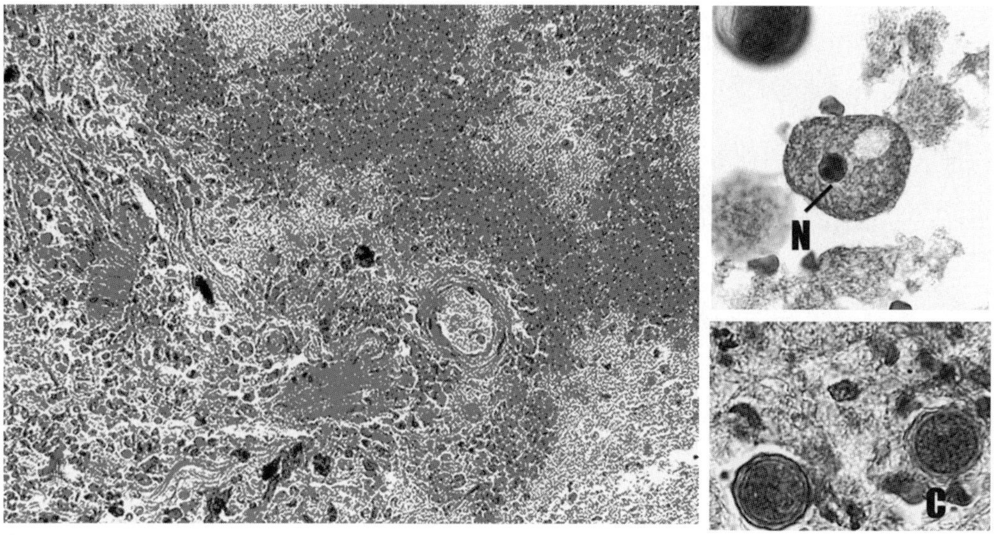

A B

FIGURE 95-10 CNS section of a patient that died of *Balamuthia mandrillaris* GAE (H&E stain). *A,* Low-power view depicting intense inflammatory reaction. (magnification ×100) *B,* Higher magnification (×1000) of the same section showing a trophozoite with multiple nucleoli (N) and cysts (C).

through the cytokines, destroy the amebas. However, in susceptible persons these elements are absent or impaired, and amebas continue to proliferate and damage host tissues.

Since *Acanthamoeba* and other small amebas are ubiquitous in nature it is reasonable to expect humans and other animals to be exposed to the amebas or their antigens and develop serum antibodies to them. Whether this natural antibody results in the development of protective immunity against infection is not known. Previous studies have shown that antibodies to *Acanthamoeba* exist in sera of healthy soldiers as well as hospitalized patients in Czechoslovakia, adults and children from New Zealand, and patients hospitalized for respiratory disorders.[1,15,16,58–60] Antibodies to *Acanthamoeba* have also been demonstrated in patients who developed GAE.[1,4,35,37] For example, a Nigerian patient from whose CSF *A. rhysodes* was repeatedly isolated exhibited an increase in titer from 256 to 1024 against *A. rhysodes* in serum samples collected 16 months apart.[4] Antibody titer for *A. castellanii* of 512 was detected in an immunocompromised patient with systemic lupus erythematosus who developed *Acanthamoeba* encephalitis.[37] High titers (256) of antibody to *A. castellanii* were also demonstrated in an acute serum sample from a renal transplant patient with cutaneous acanthamebiasis who had been taking immunosuppressive medications.[37] It is interesting to note that complement-fixing antibody to *A. culbertsoni* was demonstrated in 2 of 1000 serum samples collected randomly in the United States. Notably, one of the serum samples was from a patient with an old brain infarct. The initial serum sample had a complement fixation titer of 8 that rose to 16 and 64 in subsequent serum samples taken 1 and 2 months, respectively, after the initial sample was collected.[1,15] The patient subsequently died of cerebral hemorrhage, and amebas were demonstrated in the brain sections. Of note, in vitro studies have demonstrated that *Acanthamoeba* activates the alternative complement pathway, which is independent of antibody activation.[1,15,16,56]

Antibodies to *B. mandrillaris* have been demonstrated in sera from healthy individuals in South Australia using immunofluorescence and flow cytometry. Antibodies of the IgG and IgM classes were detected with titers ranging from 64 to 256.[61] In another study, about 3% of approximately 225 serum samples collected from patients hospitalized with encephalitis in California had titers of about 128 for anti–*B. mandrillaris* antibody by immunofluorescence testing.[62] All these patients were confirmed as having been infected with *B. mandrillaris* by specific immunostaining of biopsy sections using rabbit anti–*B. mandrillaris* serum. Two patients that survived the infection had anti–*B. mandrillaris* titers of 128 in the acute phase that decreased to 64 during convalescence.[30]

Acanthamoeba Keratitis

Acanthamoeba keratitis (AK) is a painful, sight-threatening infection of the cornea that may lead to chronic ulceration of the cornea, loss of visual acuity, and eventually blindness and enucleation (Fig. 95-11). AK generally affects healthy persons and is associated with trauma to the cornea or minor erosion of the corneal epithelium from hard or soft contact lens wear and the subsequent use of contaminated saline solution. It is characterized by corneal inflammation, severe ocular pain, photophobia, tearing, blurred vision, and refractoriness to the commonly used antibiotics and antifungal and antiviral agents. Amebas adhere to corneal epithelial cells and secrete proteinases that facilitate invasion of the cornea and later the underlying stroma.[63] Amebic trophozoites and cysts are seen between the lamellae of the cornea, and inflammatory infiltrates consisting primarily of polymorphonuclear leukocytes in the superficial and middle layers of the corneal stroma are common (see Fig. 95-11B). Infiltration of nerves causes radial keratoneuritis, and later a characteristic 360° or paracentral stromal ring infiltrate develops. Anterior uveitis is common. In late stages, AK is characterized by necrosis, ulceration, descemetocele formation, and perforation of the cornea. A nonsuppurative keratitis with recurrent ulceration and a waxing and waning clinical course is a typical history. AK is often misdiagnosed as dendritic keratitis due to herpes simplex virus.[1,11,12,15,16]

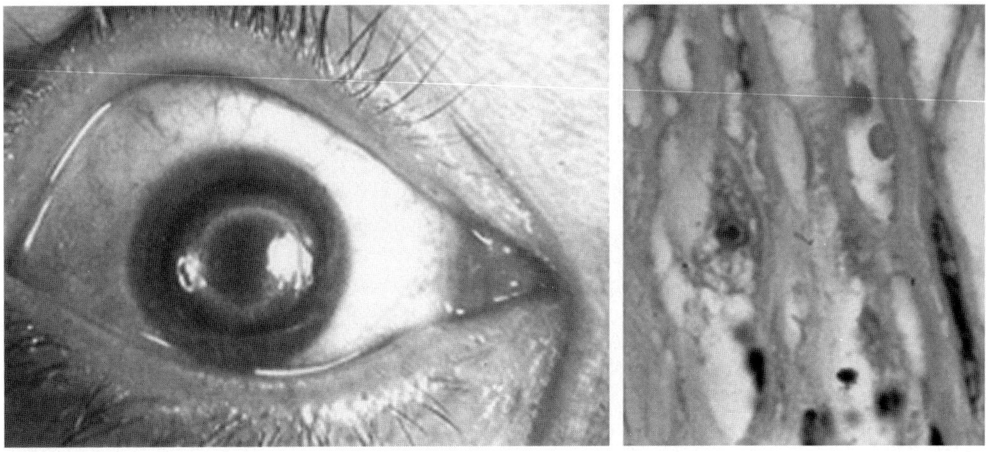

A B

FIGURE 95-11 *Acanthamoeba* keratitis. Note the concentric ring infiltrate *(A)* and a section of the cornea showing *Acanthamoeba* trophozoite in the corneal stroma *(B)*. (magnification ×1000)

Immunoblotting was used to test sera from normal individuals and keratitis patients for anti-*Acanthamoeba* antibodies and immune reactivity. Significantly, sera from keratitis patients had low levels of IgA, perhaps indicative of a greater vulnerability to AK.[1,16,60,64] In another study, immunofluorescent and precipitin antibody to *Acanthamoeba* were demonstrated in patients with *Acanthamoeba* keratitis.[1,11,12,15,16,60]

Primary Amebic Meningoencephalitis

PAM is an acute, fulminating, rapidly fatal disease that usually affects children and young adults with a history of recent contact with warm fresh water. The time from fresh water contact (swimming and diving, water skiing, or simply immersing the head in water) to onset of illness is typically 5 to 7 days. The cause of death usually is increased intracranial pressure with brain herniation leading to cardiopulmonary arrest and pulmonary edema. Early in the illness, patients may experience changes in smell or taste, but usually the first symptoms are sudden onset of bifrontal or bitemporal headaches, high fever, neck stiffness, nausea, and vomiting. Irritability, restlessness, and mental status changes are present at initial presentation, and nuchal rigidity and positive Kernig's and Brudzinski's signs can be demonstrated. Photophobia may occur late in the clinical course followed by neurologic abnormalities including lethargy, seizures, confusion, coma, diplopia, or bizarre behavior. Cranial nerve palsies (third, fourth, and sixth cranial nerves) may indicate brain herniation from brain edema and increased intracranial pressure, often in excess of 600 mm H_2O. Death occurs within a week of onset of symptoms. Cardiac rhythm abnormalities and myocardial necrosis are sometimes found. CT scan of the head without contrast is often normal or shows cerebral edema with obliteration of the cisterns surrounding the midbrain and the subarachnoid space over the cerebral hemispheres. Marked diffuse enhancement in these regions may be seen after administration of intravenous contrast medium.[56] CSF may vary in color from grayish to yellowish-white, tinged red with as few as 250/mm^3 red cells in the early stages. However, as the disease progresses the red blood cells increase in number to as high as 24,600/mm^3. CSF white blood cells, predominantly polymorphonuclear leukocytes, vary from 300 mm^3 to as high as 26,000 mm^3. CSF protein may reach 580 mg/mL or higher, and glucose levels of 10 mg/100 mL or lower are commonly seen.[1,13–15,17–22,27]

Pathologic Findings

The cerebral hemispheres are usually soft, markedly swollen, edematous, and severely congested. Uncal and tonsillar herniations are present. The leptomeninges are severely congested, diffusely hyperemic, and opaque, with limited purulent exudate within sulci, at the base of the brain, and around the brainstem and cerebellum. The olfactory bulbs are markedly hemorrhagic and necrotic and are usually surrounded by purulent exudate. The cortex shows numerous superficial hemorrhagic areas, most commonly in the base of the orbitofrontal and temporal lobes, base of the brain, hypothalamus, midbrain, pons, medulla oblongata, and upper portion of the spinal cord.[1,27]

Microscopically, the cerebral hemispheres, brainstem, cerebellum, and upper portion of the spinal cord are suffused with fibrinopurulent leptomeningeal exudate containing numerous neutrophils, some lymphocytes, and few eosinophils and macrophages. Large numbers of trophozoites, usually in pockets and without the presence of neutrophils, are seen within edematous and necrotic neural tissue (Fig. 95-12). Trophozoites also are abundant deep in Virchow-Robin spaces, usually around blood vessels, but with no inflammatory response. Amebas ranging in size from 8 to 12 μm are characterized by the presence of a large nucleus with a centrally located, deeply staining large nucleolus. Amebic cysts are conspicuously absent.[1,17,18,27]

Pathogenesis and Immunity

The portal of entry into the CNS is the olfactory neuroepithelium. It is believed that the sustentacular cells lining the olfactory neuroepithelium phagocytose the amebas that enter the nasal passages of the victims while indulging in aquatic activities. The amebic trophozoites penetrate the cribriform

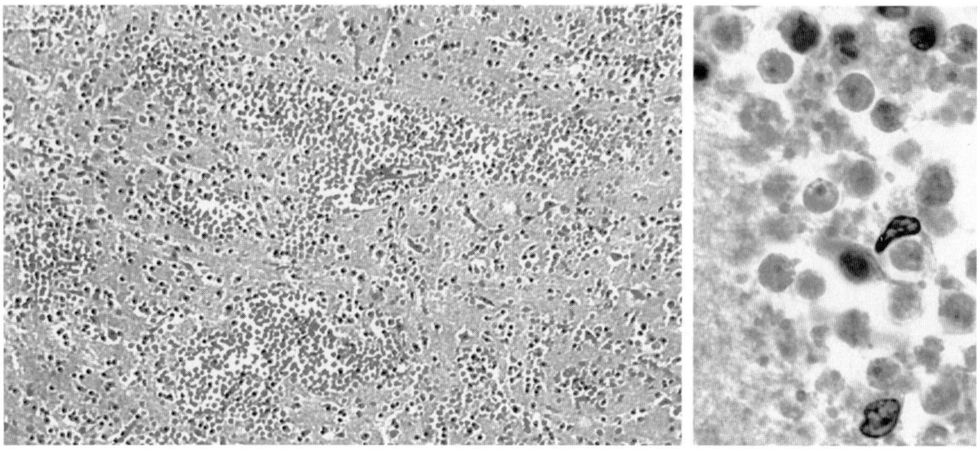

A B

FIGURE 95-12 *A,* CNS section of a patient who died of primary amebic meningoencephalitis due to *Naegleria fowleri*. (H&E stain, ×100) *B,* Higher magnification (×1000) showing numerous amebic trophozoites but no cysts.

plate of the ethmoid bone, enter the subarachnoid space, and eventually reach the brain parenchyma. *N. fowleri* trophozoites likely possess virulence factors that contribute to the dissolution and necrosis of brain tissue, such as production and secretion of a phospholipase, release of neuraminidase, creation of pores in target cell membranes, and aggressive phagocytic activity. Additionally, amebas possess amebostomes, or food cups, that are capable of pinching off bits and pieces of brain cell cytoplasm.[1,27]

The incubation period of PAM, which varies from 2 to 15 days, depends on the size of the inoculum and the virulence of the amebas. The importance of virulence is illustrated by incubation periods as long as 3 or 4 weeks in experimental infections that employed a mildly virulent strain of *N. fowleri*.[1]

Very little information exists on the antibody response to *N. fowleri* infection, probably because most patients die before serum antibodies become detectable. However, in one patient who survived PAM infection, an antibody titer of 4096 to *N. fowleri* was demonstrated by immunofluorescence in serum samples obtained at 7, 10, and 42 days of hospitalization; antibodies to *N. fowleri* were still present after 4 years.[20] There are reports of antibodies to *N. fowleri* and other *Naegleria* species in serum samples of hospitalized patients in Tennessee as well as in apparently healthy persons.[1,15,27,65,66] IgG but not IgM antibodies were detected in sera from newborn infants, indicating transplacental transfer.[62] A difference was noted in the capacity of sera from Pennsylvania residents to agglutinate *N. fowleri* and other *Naegleria* spp. when compared with sera obtained from residents of North Carolina. Sera from the southeastern area had significantly greater agglutinating ability (attributable to IgM antibodies) than those of the northeastern state, suggesting a higher degree of exposure to *N. fowleri* in persons from the warmer southern region.[66] Apparently, normal human serum, but not heat-inactivated serum, stimulates production of protein kinases in *N. fowleri*, which may be effective in destroying complement and protecting amebas from the membrane-attack complex of the complement cascade.[67]

DIAGNOSIS: CLINICAL AND LABORATORY METHODS

Granulomatous Amebic Encephalitis

Neuroimaging

CT and MRI scans of the head demonstrate the presence of single or multiple lesions but are not specific for GAE. The typical enhancing, space-occupying lesions of *Acanthamoeba* or *Balamuthia* infection can mimic brain abscess, tumor, cerebrovascular accidents, and other diseases.[1]

CSF Examination

Lumbar puncture is often contraindicated in patients with GAE and large or multiple lesions because of the risk of herniation. When CSF is obtained, analysis usually shows lymphocytic pleocytosis with mild elevation of proteins and normal glucose, but no amebas. Unlike *N. fowleri, Acanthamoeba* spp and *B. mandrillaris* are not readily found in the CSF. There have been only a few reports of isolation of *Acanthamoeba* spp.; in one case it was isolated repeatedly from the CSF of a Nigerian patient.

Brain and Skin Biopsies

Although in many cases of GAE the diagnosis was made only at autopsy, brain and skin biopsies have yielded *Acanthamoeba* spp. and *B. mandrillaris* in specimens from several patients antemortem.[1,8,15,30,31,33,34] Biopsies in a few patients were lifesaving because they permitted timely administration of specific therapy.[1,5,9,16,24,30,31,33,34] In general, *Acanthamoeba* spp. and *B. mandrillaris* are difficult to differentiate in tissue sections by light microscopy because of their similar morphology although occasionally it may be possible to identify *Balamuthia* based on the presence of multiple nucleoli within the nucleus (see Fig. 95-10B).[1,3,9,16,24–28,32] However, they can be differentiated by immunofluorescence analysis of tissue sections using rabbit anti-*Acanthamoeba or* anti–*B. mandrillaris* sera. Biopsy or autopsy tissues fixed in formalin can be deparaffinized, rehydrated, post-fixed in Karnovsky's, dehydrated, and embedded in plastic (EPON) for electron microscopic studies. Ultrastructural examination demonstrates the characteristic features of trophozoites and cysts and facilitates the identification of the specific ameba. For identification of the species of *Acanthamoeba,* it is necessary to perform immunohistochemistry (either immunoperoxidase or immunofluorescence test) on tissue specimens or amebas in culture. Unlike *Acanthamoeba* spp., *Balamuthia* cannot be easily cultured on non-nutrient agar plates seeded with bacteria. Hence biopsy specimens should be inoculated on layers of mammalian cell cultures.[24,25] Specimens for culture should be processed as soon as possible.[1,15,24]

PCR has been used widely as a means of improving on the taxonomy and understanding the phylogeny of members of the genus *Acanthamoeba* and in identification of amebas in culture.[12,68] A PCR probe consisting of a primer pair specific for *Balamuthia* has been developed from sequence data of mitochondrial 16S rRNA genes.[69] Using this specific probe a clinical isolate obtained from the brain of a child was found to be identical to an ameba isolated from flowerpot soil in the home of the child.[70] Hopefully such precise tests will become common in the future.

Acanthamoeba Keratitis

Clinical and Laboratory Diagnostic Methods

Ocular infections with *Acanthamoeba* can resemble bacterial, fungal, or viral infections, especially those caused by herpes simplex virus. A history of corneal trauma or use of potentially contaminated contact lens solution, the characteristic ring infiltrates, and failure of conventional antimicrobial agents should suggest the diagnosis.

Trophozoites and especially cysts can be recovered from corneal scrapings or biopsy specimens but not from swabs. When microscopic examination or culture of specimens is negative, culturing amebas from contact lenses, lens case, or cleaning solution lend support to a clinical diagnosis of AK. Molecular techniques are employed increasingly in the identification of the ameba in samples of corneal epithelium and tear fluid and in the identification of the genotype of *Acanthamoeba*.[1,12,16,71,72] Scanning confocal microscopy allows in vivo visualization of cysts and trophozoites in the cornea.[73]

Primary Amebic Meningoencephalitis

No distinctive clinical features differentiate PAM from acute bacterial meningitis or meningoencephalitis although failure of broad-spectrum antibiotics may alert the clinician to the possibility of a nonbacterial cause of the rapidly progressive illness. It is crucial to obtain a history of potential exposure to warm fresh water or hot springs during the past week.

CSF Examination

The CSF pressure is usually elevated (300 to >600 mm H_2O). The cerebrospinal fluid is characterized by a neutrophil-predominant pleocytosis, absence of bacteria, normal or decreased glucose concentration, and elevated protein content in the range of 100 mg/100 mL to 1000 mg/100 mL. A wet mount of the CSF should be examined immediately under the microscope for the presence of actively moving trophozoites. Smears of CSF should be stained with Giemsa or Wright stain to identify the trophozoite by delineating the nucleus with a centrally placed, large nucleolus. Gram's stain is not useful.

Neuroimaging Findings

CT scans of the head are usually done without contrast in the evaluation of cases of meningitis, and in PAM, the findings are unremarkable or show only cerebral edema. When contrast is administered, meningeal enhancement of the basilar cisterns and sulci may be seen, but these are not specific for amebic infection.[1,56]

Serologic tests usually are of no value in the diagnosis of *N. fowleri* infections, since most patients die too soon (within 5–7 days) in the disease process to mount a detectable immune response.

Molecular techniques such as PCR and nested PCR assays for the specific identification of *N. fowleri* in cultured amebas from patients and the environment as well as *N. fowleri* DNA in the environment have been developed.[74–76] Sequencing of the 5.8S rRNA gene and the internal transcribed spacers 1 and 2 (ITS1 and ITS2) of *N. fowleri* has shown that the genomic region can be used to identify specific genotypes. Epidemiologic typing of *N. fowleri* has also been done by analyzing the 5.8S rRNA gene and the ITS of clinical isolates.[74–76] For example, *N. fowleri* amebas isolated from two cases who had visited the same hot spring in California at different times belonged to the same genotype (II), and these in turn differed from genotypes of other *N. fowleri* strains examined.[63,65] Although such precise tests have not been used as yet to identify *N. fowleri* DNA in CSF or brain tissue, research is on the horizon and soon there will be PCR-based assays to identify *N. fowleri*–specific DNA in the CSF.

TREATMENT AND PROGNOSIS

Granulomatous Amebic Encephalitis

Because most cases of GAE have been diagnosed postmortem or only a few days premortem, experience with specific treatment is limited, and current recommendations are based on in vitro studies of susceptibility of isolates to different antimicrobial agents and a small number of cases of successful treatment. Treatment is more likely to succeed if the diagnosis is made early in the course of the disease and treatment is instituted before the infection disseminates, particularly to the CNS. Several patients with GAE due to *Acanthamoeba* and *Acanthamoeba* cutaneous infection without CNS involvement have been successfully treated with multidrug regimens consisting of various combinations of pentamidine isethionate, sulfadiazine, 5′ flucytosine, fluconazole or itraconazole, trimethoprim-sulfamethoxazole, and topical application of chlorhexidine gluconate for skin ulcers.[1,5,16,26,33–35] In vitro experiments suggests that azithromycin may also be of value in the treatment of *Acanthamoeba* GAE. Cure of infection in a few cases with involvement of the nasal mucosa and paranasal sinuses has included surgical debridement of diseased tissue. Three patients with GAE caused by *B. mandrillaris* also have recovered from the disease. They were treated with pentamidine isethionate, sulfadiazine, azithromycin or clarithromycin, fluconazole, and in two cases flucytosine as well.[9,30,31]

Acanthamoeba Keratitis

Unlike GAE, AK often can be cured by aggressive application of topical antimicrobial agents that achieve high tissue levels, and surgery when necessary. In early infections, debridement may remove infectious organisms or improve the penetration of antimicrobial drugs. Medical cure has been achieved with the application of either polyhexamethylene biguanide (PHMB) or chlorhexidine gluconate with or without propamidine isethionate (Brolene). When medical treatment failed, a combination of debridement and penetrating keratoplasty has been used with good results in some cases.[1,11,12,16]

Primary Amebic Meningoencephalitis

PAM is almost always fatal. Only a few patients have survived this disease. A well-studied patient, a California girl, who survived the infection was aggressively treated with intravenous and intrathecal amphotericin B, intravenous and intrathecal miconazole, and oral rifampin. At 4 years' follow-up, she was found to be completely healthy and free of neurologic deficits.[20] In vitro studies clearly indicate that amphotericin B is greater than 10 times as active as miconazole. Miconazole is not available in the United States.

PREVENTION AND CONTROL

Granulomatous Amebic Encephalitis

Diseases produced by *A. castellanii* spp. and by *B. mandrillaris* have occurred most often in hosts with weakened immune systems, and presently no clearly defined methods are available for the prevention of infection with these amebas.

Acanthamoeba Keratitis

Contact lenses, which are being used not only for vision correction but also for cosmetic purposes, are the major risk factor for AK along with use of contaminated lens solutions. Education of patients regarding the proper care of contact lenses is important in the prevention of AK. Contact lenses should not be used during swimming or while performing water-sport activities.

Primary Amebic Meningoencephalitis

N. fowleri is a thermophilic ameba and hence it proliferates when the ambient temperature increases (above 30°C). As global temperature increases because of global warming, cases of *N. fowleri* PAM may be seen in countries where it has not been recorded. Since *N. fowleri* is susceptible to chlorine at one part per million, it can be controlled readily by adequate chlorination of swimming pools, including during warm summer months. However, it is not possible to chlorinate natural bodies of water such as lakes and ponds, where *N. fowleri* may proliferate. Appropriate warnings should therefore be posted around such areas, particularly during the hot summer months.

REFERENCES

1. Martinez AJ, Visvesvara GS: Free-living amphizoic and opportunistic amebas. Brain Pathol 7:583–598, 1997.
2. Lawande RV, Macfarlane JT, Weir WRC, et al: A case of primary amebic meningoencephalitis in a Nigerian farmer. Am J Trop Med Hyg 29:21–25, 1980.
3. Rutherfoord GS: Amebic meningoencephalitis due to free-living amoeba. S Afr Med J 69:52–55, 1986.
4. Cleland PG, Lawande RV, Onyemelukwe G, et al: Chronic amebic meningoencephalitis. Arch Neurol 39:56–57, 1982.
5. Singhal T, Bajpai A, Kalra V, et al: Successful treatment of *Acanthamoeba* meningitis with combination oral antimicrobials. Pediatr Infect Dis J 20:623–627, 2001.
6. Rideout BA, Gardiner CH, Stalis IH, et al: Fatal infections with *Balamuthia mandrillaris* (a free-living amoeba) in gorillas and other old world primates. Vet Pathol 34:15–22, 1997.
7. Lozano-Alarcon F, Bradley GA, Houser BS, et al: Primary amebic meningoencephalitis due to *Naegleria fowleri* in a South American tapir. Vet Pathol 14:239–243, 1997.
8. Bakardjiev A, Azimi PH, Ashouri N, et al: Amebic encephalitis caused by *Balamuthia mandrillaris*: report of four cases. Pediatr Infect Dis 22:447–452, 2003.
9. Martinez AJ, Visvesvara GS: *Balamuthia mandrillaris* infection (editorial). J Med Microbiol 50:205–207, 2001.
10. Schuster FL, Glaser C, Honarmand S, et al: *Balamuthia* encephalitis risk, Hispanic Americans. Emerg Infect Dis 10:1510–1512, 2004.
11. Jones DB, Visvesvara GS, Robinson NM: *Acanthamoeba polyphaga* keratitis and *Acanthamoeba* uveitis associated with fatal meningoencephalitis. Trans Ophthalmol Soc UK 95:221–232, 1975.
12. Seal DV: *Acanthamoeba* keratitis update—incidence, molecular epidemiology and new drugs for treatment. Eye 17:893–905, 2003.
13. McKee T, Davis L, Blake P, et al: Primary amebic meningoencephalitis—Georgia, 2002. MMWR 52:962–964, 2003.
14. Okuda DT, Hanna HJ, Coons SW, et al: *Naegleria fowleri* hemorrhagic meningoencephalitis: report of two fatalities in children. J Child Neurol 19:231–233, 2004.
15. Visvesvara GS, Stehr-Green JK: Epidemiology of free-living ameba infections. J Protozool 37:25S–33S, 1990.
16. Marciano-Cabral F, Cabral G: *Acanthamoeba* spp as agents of disease in humans. Clin Microbiol Rev 16:273–307, 2003.
17. Fowler M, Carter RE: Acute pyogenic meningitis probably due to *Acanthamoeba* sp: a preliminary report. BMJ 2:740–774, 1965.
18. Butt CG: Primary amebic meningoencephalitis. N Engl J Med 274:1473–1476, 1966.
19. Lares-Villa F, De Jonckheere JF, De Moura H, et al: Five cases of primary amebic meningoencephalitis in Mexicali, Mexico: study of the isolates. J Clin Microbiol 31:685–688, 1993.
20. Seidel JS, Harmatz P, Visvesvara GS, et al: Successful treatment of primary amebic meningoencephalitis. N Engl J Med 306:346–348, 1982.
21. Cerva L, Novak K: Amoebic meningoencephalitis: sixteen fatalities. Science 160:92, 1968.
22. Cursons R, Sleigh J, Hood D, et al: A case of primary amoebic meningoencephalitis: North Island, New Zealand. N Z Med J 116:1187, 2003.
23. Denney CF, Iragui LD, Uber-Zak LD, et al: Amebic meningoencephalitis caused by *Balamuthia mandrillaris:* case report and review. Clin Infect Dis 25:1534–1538, 1997.
24. Visvesvara GS, Martinez AJ, Schuster FL, et al: Leptomyxid ameba, a new agent of amebic meningoencephalitis in humans and animals. J Clin Microbiol 28:2750–2756, 1990.
25. Visvesvara GS, Schuster FL, Martinez AJ: *Balamuthia mandrillaris*, N. G., N. Sp, agent of amebic meningoencephalitis in humans and other animals. J Eukaryot Microbiol 40:504–514, 1993.
26. Visvesvara GS, Stehr-Green JK: Epidemiology of free-living ameba infection. J Protozool 37:25S–33S, 1990.

27. Martinez AJ: Free-living Amebas: Natural History, Prevention, Diagnosis, Pathology and Treatment of Disease. Boca Raton, Fla., CRC Press, 1985.
28. Chimelli L, Hahn MD, Scaravilli F, et al: Granulomatous amebic encephalitis due to ptornyxid ameba: report of the first Brazilian case. Trans R Soc Trop Med 86:635, 1992.
29. Kinde H, Visvesvara GS, Barr BC, et al: Amebic meningoencephalitis caused by *Balamuthia mandrillaris* (leptomyxid ameba) in a horse. J Vet Diagn Invest 10:378–381, 1998.
30. Deetz TR, Sawyer MH, Billman G, et al: Successful treatment of *Balamuthia* amoebic encephalitis: presentation of two cases. Clin Infect Dis 37:1304–1312, 2003.
31. Jung S, Schelper RL, Visvesvara GS, et al: *Balamuthia mandrillaris* meningoencephalitis in an immunocompetent patient: an unusual clinical course and a favorable outcome. Arch Pathol Lab Med 128: 466–468, 2003.
32. Khalife GE, Pambuccian SE, Visvesvara GS, et al: Disseminated *Acanthamoeba* infection masquerading as bacillary angiornatosis in a patient with AIDS. Int J Surg Pathol 2:11–16, 1994.
33. Seijo Martinez M, Gonzalez-Mediero G, Santiago P, et al: Granulomatous amebic encephalitis in a patient with AIDS: isolation of *Acanthamoeba* sp group II from brain tissue and successful treatment with sulfadiazine and fluconazole. J Clin Microbiol 38:3892–3895, 2000.
34. Sharma PP, Gupta P, Murali MV, et al: Primary amebic meningoencephalitis caused by *Acanthamoeba*: successfully treated with cotrimoxazole. Indian Pediatr 30:1219–1222, 1993.
35. Slater CA, Sickel JZ, Visvesvara GS, et al: Brief report: successful treatment of disseminated *Acanthamoeba* infection in an immunocompromised patient. N Engl J Med 331:85–87, 1994.
36. Selby DM, Chandra RS, Rakusan TA, et al: Amebic osteomyelitis in a child with acquired immunodeficiency syndrome: a case report. Pediatr Pathol Lab Med 18:89–95, 1998.
37. Grunnet ML, Cannon GH, Kushner JP: Fulminant amebic meningoencephalitis due to *Acanthamoeba*. Neurology 31:174–176, 1981.
38. Gelman BB, Rauf SJ, Nader R, et al: Amoebic encephalitis due to *Sappinia diploidea*. JAMA 285:2450–2451, 2001.
39. Gelman BB, Popov V, Chaljub G, et al: Neuropathological and ultrastructural features of amebic encephalitis caused by *Sappinia diploidea*. J Neuropathol Exp Neurol 62:990–998, 2003.
40. Page, FC: Re-definition of the genus *Acanthamoeba* with descriptions of three species. J Protozool 14:709–724, 1967.
41. Castellani A: An amoeba found in culture of a yeast: preliminary note. Trop Med Hyg 33:160, 1930.
42. Culbertson CG, Smith JW, Minner JR: *Acanthamoeba*: observation on animal pathogenicity. Science 127:1506, 1958.
43. Kilvington S, Gray T, Dart J, et al: *Acanthamoeba* keratitis: the role of domestic tap water contamination in the United Kingdom. Invest Ophthalmol Vis Sci 45:165–169, 2004.
44. Page FC: A New Key to Freshwater and Soil Gymnamoebae. Ambleside, Cumbria, UK, Freshwater Biological Association, 1988.
45. Schuster FL: Cultivation of pathogenic and opportunistic free-living amebas. Clin Microbiol Rev 15:342–354, 2002.
46. Schuster FL, Visvesvara GS: Axenic growth and drug sensitivity studies of *Balamuthia mandrillaris*, an agent of amebic meningoencephalitis in humans and other animals. J Clin Microobiol 34:385–388, 1996.
47. Abraham SN, Lawande RV: Incidence of free-living amoebae in the nasal passages of local population in Zaria, Nigeria. J Trop Med Hyg 85:217–222, 1982.
48. Badenoch PR, Grimmond TR, Cadwgan J, et al: Nasal carriage of free-living amoebae. Microbiol Ecol Health Dis 1:209–211, 1988.
49. Michel R, Röhl R, Schneider H: Isolation of free-living amoebae from nasal mucosa of healthy individuals. Zbl Bakt Hyg I Abr Orig B 176:155–159, 1982.
50. Abd H, Johansson T, Golovliov I, et al: Survival and growth of *Francisella tularenssis* in *Acanthamoeba castellanii*. Appl Environ Microbiol 69:600–606, 1990.
51. Barker J, Humphrey TJ, Brown MW: Survival of *Escherichia coli* 0157 in a soil protozoan: implications for disease. FEMS Microbiol Lett 173:291–295, 1990.
52. Greub G, Raoult D: Microorganisms resistant to free-living amoebae. Clin Microbiol Rev 17:413–433, 2004.
53. Schuster FL, Dunnebacke TH, Booton GC, et al: Environmental isolation of *Balamuthia mandrillaris* associated with a case of amebic encephalitis. J Clin Microbiol 41:3175–3180, 2003.
54. Steinberg JP, Galindo RL, Kraus ES, et al: Disseminated acanthamebiasis in a renal transplant recipient with osteomyelitis and cutaneous lesions: case report and literature review. Clin Infect Dis 35:e43–e49, 2002.
55. Pritzker AS, Kim BK, Agrawal D, et al: Fatal granulomatous amebic encephalitis caused by *Balamuthia mandrillaris* presenting in a skin lesion. J Am Acad Dermatol 50(suppl 2):S38–S41.
56. Schumacher DJ, Tien RD, Lane KL: Neuroimaging findings in rare amebic infections of the central nervous system. AJNR 16:930–935, 1995.
57. Healy JF: *Balamuthia* amebic encephalitis: radiographic and pathologic findings. AJNR 23:486–489, 2002.
58. Cerva L: *Acanthamoeba culbertsoni* and *Naegleria fowleri*: occurrence of antibodies in man. J Hyg Epidemiol Microbiol 33:99–103, 1989.
59. Cursons RTM, Brown TJ, Keys EA, et al: Immunity to pathogenic free-living amoebae: role of humoral immunity. Infect Immun 29:401–407, 1980.
60. Ferrante A: Immunity to *Acanthamoeba*. Rev Infect Dis 13(suppl 5): S403–S409, 1991.
61. Huang ZH, Ferrante A, Carter RF: Serum antibodies to *Balamuthia mandrillaris*, a free-living amoeba recently demonstrated to cause granulomatous amoebic encephalitis. J Infect Dis 179:1305–1308, 1999.
62. Schuster FL, Glaser C, Honarmand S, et al: Testing for *Balamuthia* amebic encephalitis by indirect immunofluorescence. In Lares-Villa F, Booton GC, Marciano-Cabral F (eds): Xth International Meeting on the Biology and Pathogencity of Free-Living Amoebae: Proceedings. ITSON DIEP. Ciudad Obregón, Mexico, 2003, pp 173–178.
63. Kumar R, Lloyd D: Recent advances in treatment of *Acanthamoeba* keratitis. Clin Infect Dis 35:434–441, 2002.
64. Walochnik J, Obwaller A, Haller-Schober E-M, et al: Anti-*Acanthamoeba* IgG, IgM, and IgA immunoreactivities in correlation to strain pathogenicity. Parasitol Res 87:651–656, 2001.
65. Dubray BL, Wilhelm WE, Jennings BR: Serology of *Naegleria fowleri* and *Naegleria lovaniensis* from a hospital survey. J Protozool 34:322–327, 1987.
66. Marciano-Cabral F, Cline ML, Bradley SG: Specificity of antibodies from human sera for *Naegleria* species. J Clin Microbiol 25:692–697, 1987.
67. Chu D-MT, Ferguson TJ, Marciano-Cabral F: Protein kinase activation and protein phosphorylation in *Naegleria fowleri* amebae in response to normal human serum. J Eukaryot Microbiol 47:40–47, 2000.
68. Booton GC, Rogerson A, Bonilla TD, et al: Molecular and physiological evaluation of subtropical environmental isolates of *Acanthamoeba* spp, causal agent of *Acanthamoeba* keratitis. J Eukaryot Microbiol 51:192–200, 2004.
69. Booton GC, Carmichael JR, Visvesvara GS, et al: Identification of *Balamuthia mandrillaris* by PCR assay using the mitochondrial 16S rRNA gene as a target. J Clin Microbiol 41:453–455, 2003.
70. Booton GC, Schuster FL, Carmichael JR, et al: *Balamuthia mandrillaris*: identification of clinical and environmental isolates using genus-specific PCR. J Eukaryot Microbiol 50:508–509, 2003.
71. Pasricha G, Sharma S, Garg P, et al: Use of 18S rRNA gene-based PCR assay for diagnosis of *Acanthamoeba* keratitis in non-contact lens wearers in India. J Clin Microbiol 41:3206–3211, 2003.
72. Lehmann OJ, Green SM, Morlet N, et al: Polymerase chain reaction analysis of corneal epithelial and tear samples in the diagnosis of *Acanthamoeba* keratitis. Invest Ophth Vis Sci 39:1261–1265, 1998.
73. Pfister DR, Cameron JD, Krachmer JH, et al: Confocal microscopy findings of *Acanthamoeba* keratitis. Am J Ophthalmol 121:119–128, 1996.
74. De Jonckheere JF: A century of research on the amoeboflagellate genus *Naegleria*. Acta Protozool 41:309–342. 2002.
75. Réveiller F, Cabanes P-A, Marciano-Cabral F: Development of a nested PCR assay to detect the pathogenic free-living amoeba *Naegleria fowleri*. Parasitol Res 88:443–450, 2002.
76. Zhou L, Sriram R, Visvesvara GS, et al: Genetic variations in the internal transcribed spacer and mitochondrial small subunit rRNA gene of *Naegleria* spp. J Eukaryot Microbiol 50:522–526, 2003.

96

Microsporidiosis

LOUIS M. WEISS
DAVID A. SCHWARTZ

INTRODUCTION

Early on in the development of the field of microbiology, the Microsporidia were identified as the infectious pathogen responsible for pebrine, a disease of the economically important silkworm.[1] The Microsporidia are worldwide in distribution, with infections reported from all continents except Antarctica.[2–10] They are obligate intracellular eukaryotic parasites. As is true for many pathogens, the frequency of infection may be higher in tropical countries, as suggested by early serologic studies of travelers and residents of the tropics.[11,12] These organisms are most likely zoonotic and/or water-borne infections. The Microsporidia infect nearly every animal phyla including other protists. They are important veterinary and agricultural parasites in insects, fish, birds, laboratory rodents, rabbits, dogs, primates, and many other mammals.[13] Microsporidia have also been described in many animals kept as household pets.[13,14] Some species of Microsporidia have been used as biologic pesticides for the biologic control of destructive species of grasshoppers and locusts.[15] Microsporidia were first recognized in mammalian tissue more than 75 years ago[16] and suspected as being etiologic in human disease in 1959[17] in a child with encephalitis.

AGENTS

The class or order Microsporidia was elevated to the phylum Microspora in 1977 by Sprague and Vavra.[18] Sprague and Becnel suggested that the term Microsporidia should be used instead for the phylum; as such, the term "Microsporidia" is a proper name and should be capitalized.[19] Although traditionally believed to be "primitive" protozoa, recent molecular phylogenetic analysis has suggested that Microsporidia are related to the fungi.[20–22] Microsporidia are currently classified on the basis of ultrastructural features, including size and morphology of the spores, number of coils of the polar tube, developmental life cycle, and host-parasite relationship. Tuzet and colleagues,[23] Sprague and Vavra,[18] Larsson,[24] Issi,[25] Weiser,[26] and Sprague and associates[27] provide overviews of the history, ultrastructural and structural characteristics, and life cycle differences among taxa of Microsporidia. Sequence data of rRNA from the Microsporidia have been used to develop diagnostic polymerase chain reaction (PCR) primers and in the study of phylogenetic relationships (reviewed in Weiss and Vossbrinck[28]).

The phylum Microsporidia contains more than 1000 species distributed into 144 genera, of which the following have been demonstrated in human disease (Table 96-1)[13,27]: *Nosema* (*N. corneum* renamed *Vittaforma corneae*[29] and *N. algerae* renamed *Bracheola algerae*[30]), *Pleistophora*, *Encephalitozoon*, *Enterocytozoon*,[31] *Septata*[32] (reclassified as *Encephalitozoon*[33]), *Trachipleistophora*,[34,35] *Brachiola*,[30] and *Microsporidium*.[13] Within their hosts, Microsporidia often infect the digestive tract, but reproductive, respiratory, muscle, excretory, and nervous system infections also occur.[13,36] In the immunosuppressed host (e.g., those treated with immunosuppressive drugs or those infected with human immunodeficiency virus [HIV]), microsporidian infection can produce a wide range of clinical diseases. Reports of diarrheal syndromes in patients with acquired immunodeficiency syndrome (AIDS) due to microsporidiosis were first published in 1985.[31] In addition to gastrointestinal tract involvement, it has been recognized that Microsporidia can infect virtually any organ system, and cases of encephalitis, ocular infection, sinusitis, myositis, and disseminated infection are well described in the literature. These organisms have also been reported in immune-competent individuals. Other intestinal pathogens may occur simultaneously or sequentially with microsporidiosis.[37]

***Table 96-1** Microsporidia Identified as Pathogenic to Humans*

Genus (Species)	Reported Infections
Encephalitozoon	
Enc. cuniculi	Hepatitis, peritonitis, nephritis, encephalitis,† urethritis, cellulitis prostatitis, sinusitis, keratoconjunctivitis, cystitis, diarrhea,† disseminated infection
*Enc. hellem**	Keratoconjunctivitis, sinusitis, prostatitis, pneumonitis, nephritis, urethritis, cystitis, diarrhea, disseminated infection
*Enc. intestinalis**	Diarrhea,† intestinal perforation, keratoconjunctivitis, cholangitis, nephritis
Enterocytozoon bieneusi	Diarrhea,† wasting syndrome, cholangitis, rhinitis, bronchitis
Trachipleistophora	
*T. hominis**	Myositis, keratoconjunctivitis, sinusitis
T. anthropopthera	Encephalitis, disseminated infection
Pleistophora sp.	
P. ronneafiei	Myositis
Pleistophora sp.	Myositis†
Brachiola	
B. vesicularam	Myositis
*B.(Nosema) algerae**	Keratoconjunctivitis, myositis, skin infection
B. (Nosema) connori	Disseminated infection
Nosema	
N. ocularum	Keratoconjunctivitis†
Vittaforma	
*Vittaforma corneae**	Keratoconjunctivitis,† urinary tract infection
Microsporidium	
Microsporidium africanus	Corneal ulcer†
Microsporidium ceylonesis	Corneal ulcer†

*Organism can be grown in tissue culture.
†Cases reported in immunocompetent hosts.

The Microsporidia are eukaryotes containing a nucleus with a nuclear envelope, an intracytoplasmic membrane system, and chromosome separation on mitotic spindles, as well as vesicular golgi[38] and a mitochondrial "remnant."[39] The genome size of the Microsporidia varies from 2.3 to 19.5 Mb,[40] with that of the Encephalitizoonidae being less than 3.0 Mb (making these among the smallest eukaryotic genomes so far identified).[41] Chromosomal analysis of *Encephalitozoon cuniculi* suggests it is diploid.[42] The Microsporidia form characteristic unicellular spores (Figs. 96-1 and 96-2) that, for the human pathogenic microsporidia, range from 1.0 to 3.0 μm by 1.5 to 4.0 μm in size.[13,43] The spore coat consists of an electron-dense, proteinaceous exospore, an electron-lucent endospore composed of chitin and protein, and an inner membrane or plasmalemma.[44] A defining characteristic of all Microsporidia is an extrusion apparatus consisting of a polar tube that is attached to the inside of the anterior end of the spore by an anchoring disc and coils around the sporoplasm in the spore (Fig. 96-3). During germination, the polar tube rapidly everts forming a hollow tube that brings the sporoplasm into

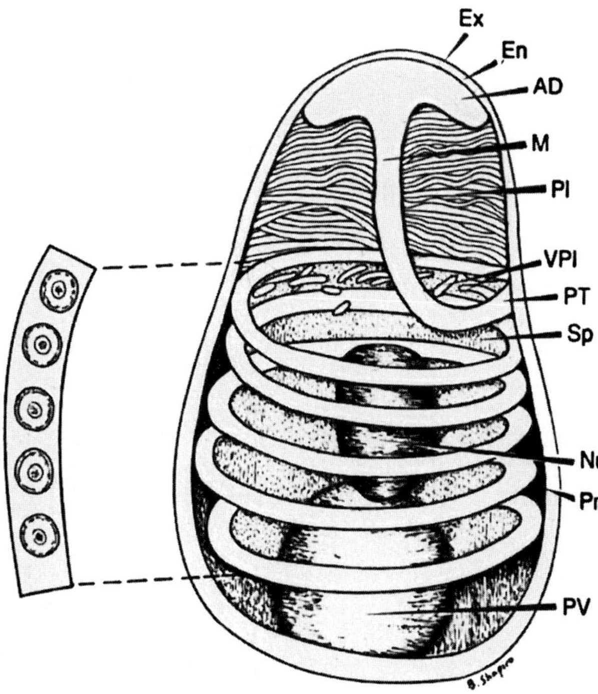

FIGURE 96-1 Structure of a microsporidian spore. Depending on the species, the size of the spore can vary from 1 to 10 μm, and the number of polar tubule coils can vary from a few to 30 or more. The extrusion apparatus consists of the polar tube (PT), vesiculotubular polaroplast (VPl), lamellar polaroplast (Pl), the anchoring disk (AD), and manubrium (M). This organelle is characteristic of the microsporidia. A cross-section of the coiled polar tube is illustrated. The nucleus (Nu) may be single (such as in encephalitozoonae and enterocytozoonae) or a pair of abutted nuclei termed a *diplokaryon* (such as in *Nosema*). The endospore (En) is an inner, thicker, electron-lucent region, and the exospore (Ex) is an outer electron-dense region. The plasma membrane (Pm) separates the spore coat from the sporoplasm (Sp), which contains ribosomes in a coiled helical array. The posterior vacuole (PV) is a membrane-bound structure. (From Wittner M, Weiss LM [eds]: The Microsporidia and Microsporidiosis. Washington, DC, ASM Press, 1999.)

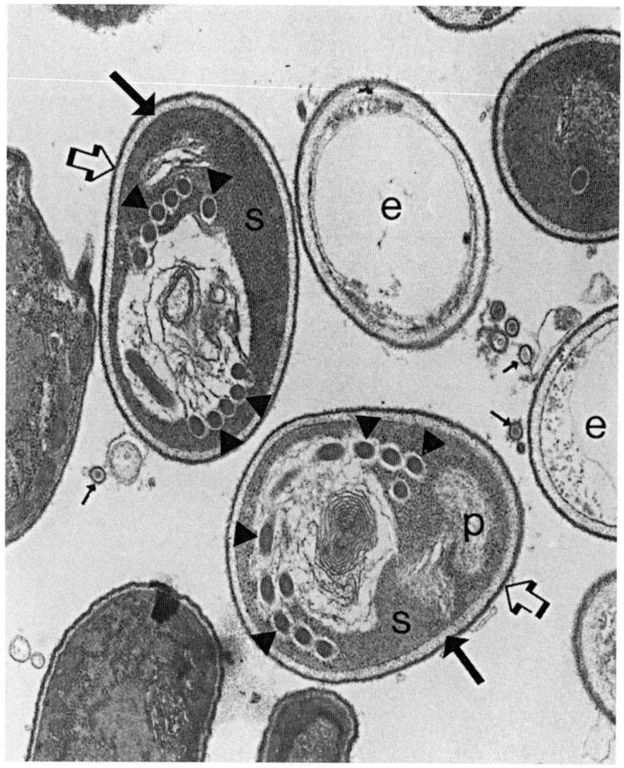

FIGURE 96-2 Transmission electron microscopy of mature spores of *Encephalitozoon hellem* in a parasitophorous vacuole. The spore wall consists of an electron-dense exospore (*open arrows*) and an electron-lucent endospore (*large solid arrows*). The characteristic coiled polar tube, also known as the polar filament, is seen in cross-section (*arrowheads*). One can also see the polaroplasts (p) within the sporoplasm (s) as well as ribosomes and rough endoplasmic reticulum. Some extruded polar tubules are seen in cross-section (*small arrows*), and empty spores (e) are also seen that have discharged their contents. (Original magnification ×7000.)

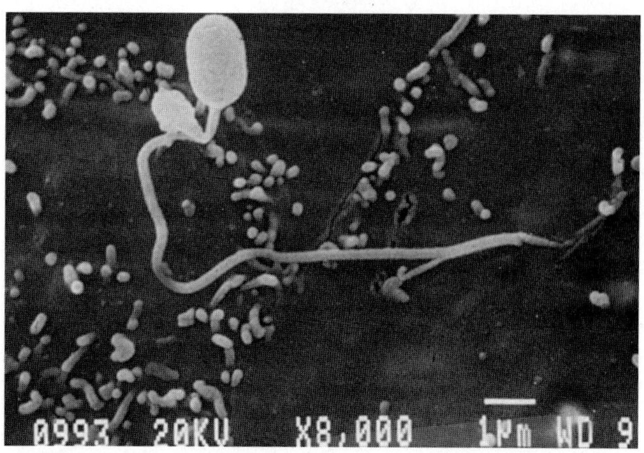

FIGURE 96-3 Scanning electron microscopy of a single mature spore of *Encephalitozoon hellem* from tissue culture demonstrating an extruded polar tube. (Original magnification ×8000.) (From Schwartz DA, Sokottka I, Leitich GJ, et al: Pathology of microsporidiosis. Emerging parasitic infections in patients with the acquired immunodeficiency syndrome. Arch Pathol Lab Med 120:173–188, 1996.)

intimate contact with the host cell. The polar tube provides a bridge to deliver the sporoplasm to the host cell. The mechanism by which the polar tube interacts with the host cell membrane is not known, but this may require the participation of the host cell.[45] If a spore is phagocytosed by a host cell, germination will occur and the polar tube can pierce the phagocytic vacuole, delivering the sporoplasm into the host cell cytoplasm. The overall process of germination and formation of the polar tube inoculates the sporoplasm directly into a host cell, functioning essentially like a hypodermic needle.[46,47]

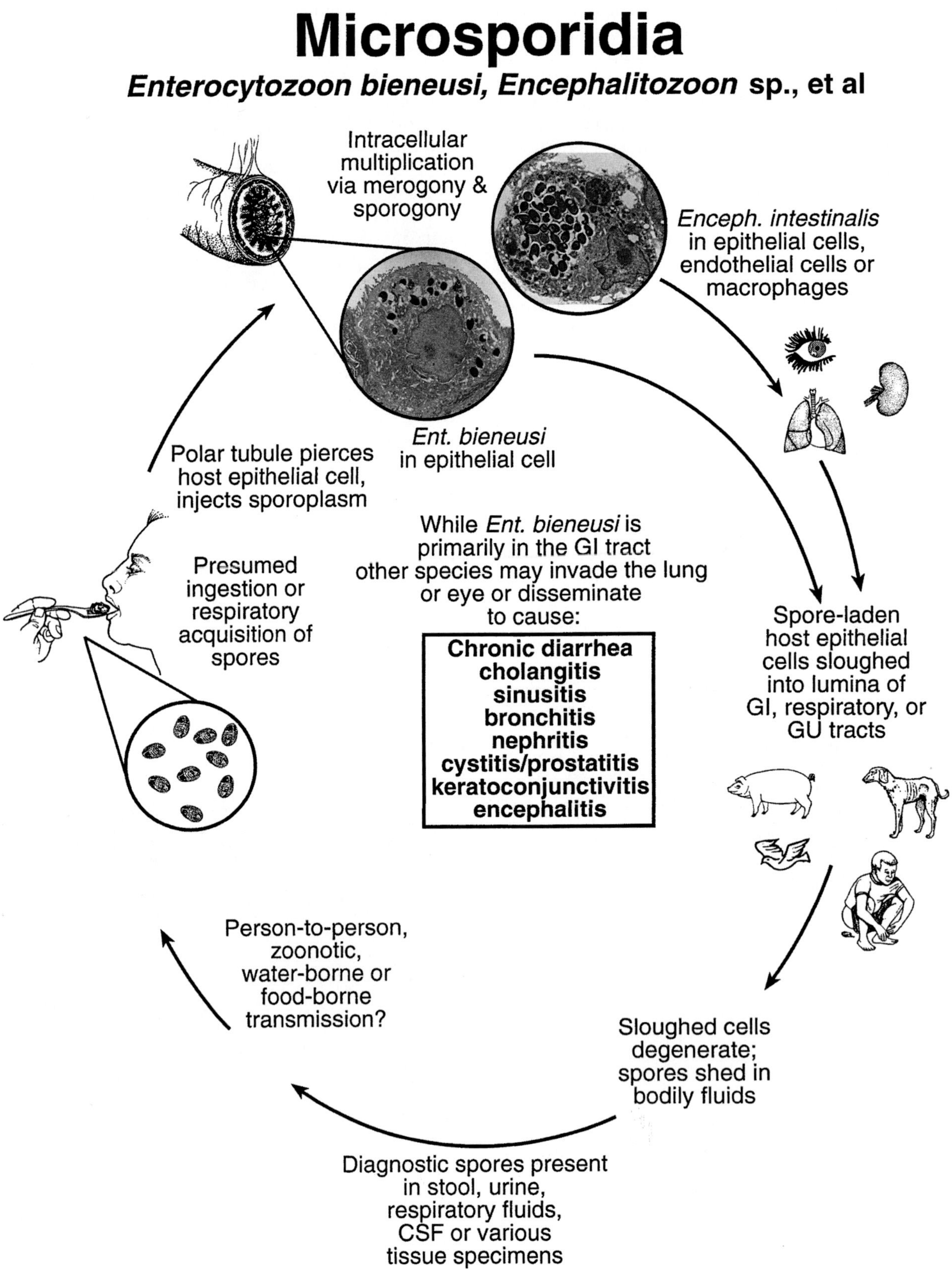

The general features of the microsporidian life cycle are as follows:

1. Spores are ingested or inhaled and then germinate, resulting in the extension of the polar tube, which injects the sporoplasm into the host cell.
2. This germination is followed by merogony, during which the injected sporoplasm develops into meronts (the proliferative stage) that multiply, depending on the species, by either binary fission or multiple fission with the formation of multinucleate plasmodial forms.
3. This stage is followed by sporogony, during which meront cell membranes thicken to form sporonts that, after subsequent division, give rise to sporoblasts that go on to form mature spores without additional multiplication. Once a host cell becomes distended with mature spores, the cell ruptures, releasing mature spores into the environment and completing its life cycle. The combination of multiplication during both merogony and sporogony results in a large number of spores being produced from a single infection and illustrates the enormous reproductive potential of these organisms.

EPIDEMIOLOGY

Microsporidia appear to be common self-limited or asymptomatic enteric pathogens in immunocompetent hosts.[10,48] There have been multiple reports of *Encephalitozoon bieneusi* in travelers and residents of tropical countries,[4,48–56] as well as reports of *Encephalitozoon intestinalis*.[57] Serosurveys in humans have demonstrated a high prevalence of antibodies to *Enc. cuniculi* and *Enc. hellem*, suggesting asymptomatic infection is common.[5,58] In HIV-positive Czech patients, 5.3% were seropositive to *Enc. cuniculi* and 1.3% to *Enc. hellem*.[59] In Slovakia, 5.1% of slaughterhouse workers were seropositive to *Encephalitozoon* spp.[60] Singh and colleagues found positive antibody titers in 8.6% of healthy adults in England, 43% of Nigerians with tuberculosis, 19% of Malaysians with filariasis, and 36% of Ghanians with malaria.[11] In another study, 12% of travelers returning from the tropics were seropositive and no control nontravelers were positive.[12] Antibodies to *Enc. intestinalis* were found among 5% of pregnant French women and 8% of Dutch blood donors.[61]

Enterocytozoon bieneusi causes the majority of infections in patients with AIDS and presents as diarrhea with wasting syndrome. Infections with *Ent. bieneusi* have been reported in liver and in heart-lung transplantation recipients, and *Encephalitozoon* spp. infections have been reported in patients with kidney, pancreas, liver, or bone marrow transplantation.[62–69] Reported prevalence rates in the 25 studies conducted on patients with HIV infection before the widespread use of highly active antiretroviral therapy (1989 to 1998) varied between 2% and 70%.[2,8–10,36,70–75] When combined, these studies identify 375 cases of *Ent. bieneusi* among 2400 patients with chronic diarrhea for a prevalence rate of 15% in this population. With immune reconstitution due to highly active antiretroviral therapy, the incidence of microsporidiosis has decreased.

Microsporidian spores are commonly found in surface water, and human pathogenic species have been found in municipal water supplies, tertiary sewage effluent, and groundwater.[51,76–78] Water contact has been found to be an independent risk factor for microsporidiosis in some studies[79,80] but not in others.[81,82] *Encephalitozoon cuniculi* spores are viable for at least 6 days in water.[83] Most microsporidian infections are transmitted

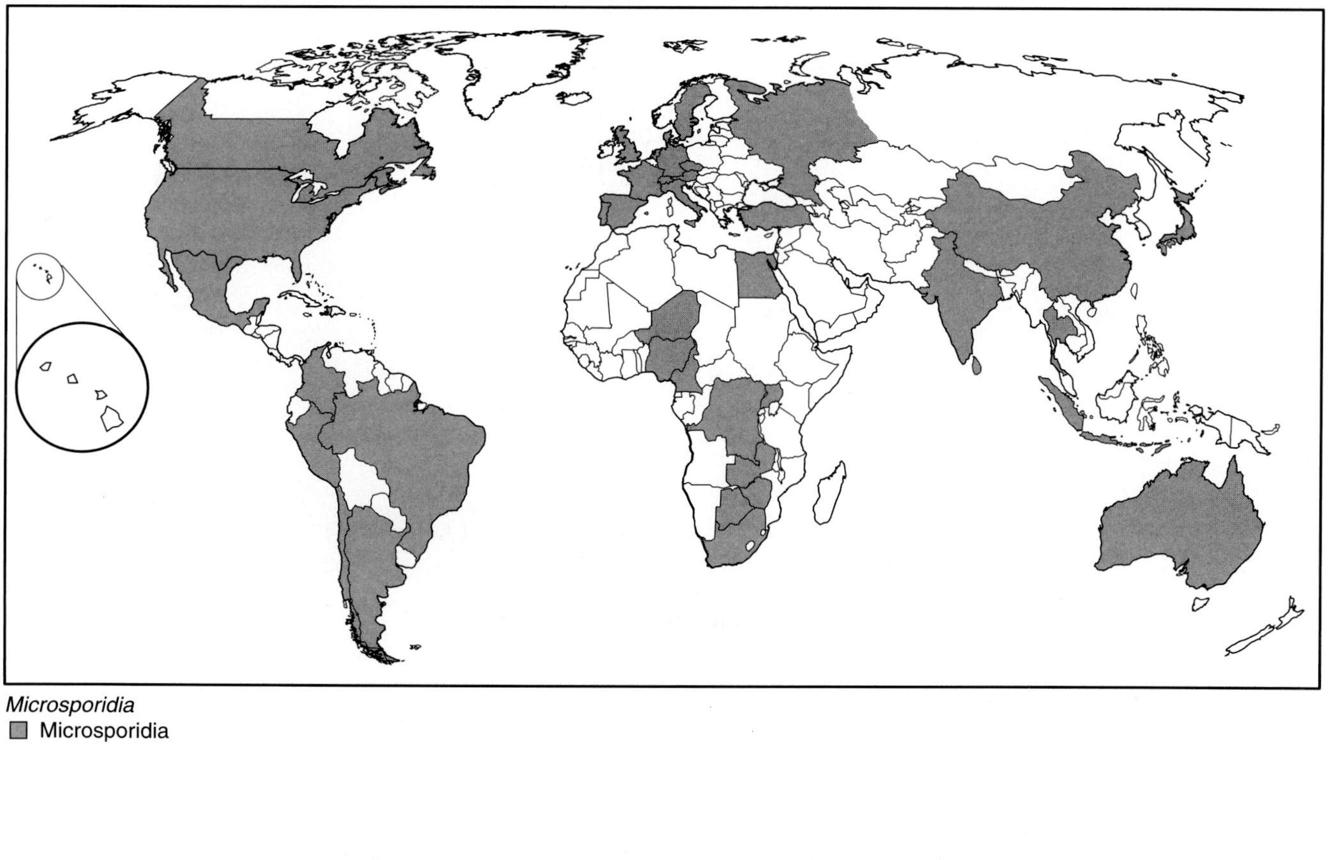

Microsporidia
■ Microsporidia

by oral ingestion of spores, with the site of initial infection being the gastrointestinal tract. Microsporidia of the genus *Encephalitozoon* are widely distributed parasites of mammals and birds,[79] and the onset of microsporidiosis has been associated with exposure to livestock, fowl, and pets,[10,14,84,85] suggesting that microsporidiosis may be a zoonosis. In Mexico, spores of *Enc. intestinalis* were identified by fluorescent antibody and PCR methods in the feces of a goat, donkey, cow, and pig.[85] *Enterocytozoon bieneusi* has been reported in pigs,[86] dogs,[87] chickens,[88] and simian immunodeficiency virus (SIV)–infected rhesus monkeys.[89,90] Viable infective spores of Microsporidia are present in multiple human body fluids (e.g., stool, urine, and respiratory secretions) during infection.[91] Person-to-person transmission is supported by concurrent infections in cohabitating homosexual men.[9] It has been possible to transmit *Encephalitozoon* spp. via rectal infection in rabbits, suggesting the possibility of sexual transmission.[92] *Encephalitozoon hellem* has been demonstrated in the respiratory mucosa, prostate, and urogenital tract of patients, raising the possibility of respiratory and sexual transmission in humans.[93,94] Although congenital transmission of *Enc. cuniculi* has been demonstrated in rabbits, mice, dogs, horses, foxes, and squirrel monkeys, it has not been demonstrated in humans.[95]

DISEASES

Microsporidian Infection in Immunosuppressed Hosts

Although the majority of reported cases of Microsporidia involve diarrhea, the spectrum of diseases caused by these organisms has expanded to include keratoconjunctivitis, disseminated disease, hepatitis, myositis, sinusitis, kidney and urogenital infection, ascites, cholangitis, and asymptomatic carriage.[13,36,96] *Encephalitozoon bieneusi* infection usually involves chronic diarrhea of 3 to 10 bowel movements per day,[36,43,97–99] anorexia, weight loss, and bloating without associated fever. It occurs more commonly in patients with AIDS having CD4+ counts less than 50 cells/mm^3. Diarrhea is often associated with malabsorption, weight loss, and wasting syndrome.[97] The mortality of patients with advanced HIV disease and chronic diarrhea with wasting has been reported to be in excess of 50%.[99,100] In patients undergoing liver and bone marrow transplantation,[62–69,101–104] clinical manifestations have included watery, nonbloody diarrhea; nausea; and diffuse abdominal pain. *Encephalitozoon bieneusi* can also invade cholangioepithelium,[100] leading to sclerosing cholangitis, AIDS cholangiopathy, and cholecystitis,[105] with associated abdominal pain, nausea, vomiting, and fever. Imaging studies (abdominal ultrasound, computed tomography, endoscopic ultrasonography, and endoscopic retrograde cholangiopancreatography) usually demonstrate dilated biliary ducts, irregularities of the bile duct wall, and gallbladder abnormalities such as thickening, distention, or the presence of sludge. Systemic dissemination is rare. There is one case report describing this organism in nasal mucosa[106] and there are two case reports of respiratory tract involvement with *Ent. bieneusi* associated with chronic diarrhea, persistent cough, dyspnea, wheezing, and chest radiographs with interstitial infiltrates.[97,107]

Encephalitozoon cuniculi, *Enc. hellem*, and *Enc. intestinalis* (previously known as *Septata intestinalis*) been associated with gastroenteritis, keratitis, sinusitis, bronchiolitis, nephritis, cystitis-ureteritis, urethritis, prostatitis, hepatitis, fulminant hepatic failure, peritonitis, and cerebritis, as well as disseminated infection.[13,43,96,108–114] An *Encephalitozoon* sp. has also been reported in a case of nodular skin lesions.[115,116] *Encephalitozoon intestinalis* most commonly causes diarrhea[117] but can also cause cholangitis,[32,118] keratoconjuctivitis, ostemyelitis of the mandible,[119] upper respiratory infections, renal failure, keratoconjunctivitis, and disseminated infection in patients with AIDS.[118–122] Elimination of this parasite from patients with diarrhea following treatment with albendazole correlates with the resolution of symptoms.[120,123] *Encephalitozoon cuniculi* has been associated with hepatitis,[124] peritonitis,[111] hepatic failure,[112] disseminated disease with fever,[113] renal insufficiency, and intractable cough.[125] Cases of encephalitis and seizures due to *Enc. cuniculi* have been reported in AIDS patients.[113,114] These infections have been reported to respond to albendazole.[108,113,114,125] *Encephalitozoon hellem* has been reported to cause disseminated disease associated with renal failure, nephritis, pneumonia, bronchitis, sinusitis, and keratoconjunctivitis.[94,126–128]

Of the reports in the literature of ocular infection due to Encephalitozoonidae, most have been attributed to *Enc. hellem*, including three cases originally classified as *Enc. cuniculi*.[129,130] Patients present with bilateral coarse punctate epithelial keratopathy and conjunctival inflammation resulting in redness, foreign body sensation, photophobia, excessive tearing, blurred vision, and changes in visual acuity. Ocular microsporidial infection in HIV-1-infected patients has been restricted to the superficial epithelium of the cornea and conjunctiva (i.e., superficial keratoconjunctivitis) and rarely progresses to corneal ulceration. Physical examination reveals conjunctival hyperemia with superficial punctate keratopathy, and slit-lamp examination usually demonstrates punctate epithelial opacities, granular epithelial cells with irregular fluorescein uptake, conjunctival injection, superficial corneal infiltrates, and a noninflaimed anterior chamber (Fig. 96-4). Ocular infection is often associated with disseminated disease,[126,131–134] and thus urine examination often demonstrates microsporidian spores.[126,131–134]

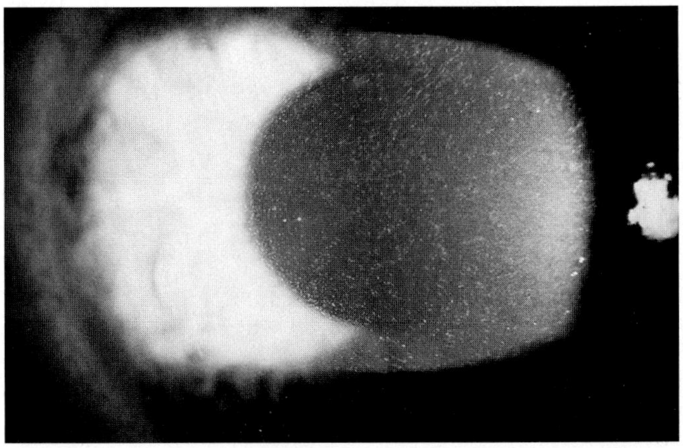

FIGURE 96-4 Slit lamp photomicrograph demonstrated punctate epithelial keratopathy in a patient with AIDS and microsporidian keratoconjunctivitis due to *Encephalitozoon hellem*. (From Schwartz DA, Visvesvara GS, Diesenhouse MC, et al: Pathologic features and immunofluorescent antibody demonstration of ocular microsporidiosis [*Encephalitozoon hellem*] in seven patients with acquired immunodeficiency syndrome. Am J Opthamol 115:285–292, 1993.)

Trachipleistophora hominis has been described in several patients with AIDS as a cause of disseminated disease,[34] with associated myositis, sinusitis, and keratoconjunctivitis. *Trachipleistophora anthropophthera* was described in several patients with AIDS having encephalitis associated with myositis and keratoconjunctivitis.[35,135] *Brachiola vesicularum* was reported as a cause of myositis,[30] as was *Pleistophora* sp (*Pleistophora ronneafiei*).[136–139] The presentation of these microsporidian myositis cases has included myalgias, weakness, elevated serum creatinine phosphokinase and aldolase levels, and abnormal electromyography consistent with inflammatory myopathy.[30,34,137,138] A fatal infection in a 4-month-old athymic male infant with severe diarrhea and malabsorption was demonstrated to be due to *Brachiola (Nosema) connori* at autopsy, where Microsporidia were seen in the lungs, stomach, small and large bowel, kidneys, adrenal glands, myocardium, liver, and diaphragm.[140] A case of urinary tract infection and prostatitis due to *Vit. corneae* has also been reported in a patient with AIDS.[141] In a child with leukemia, skin infection was due to *B. algerae* and spores were seen infecting the cellular elements of the dermis.[142]

Microsporidian Infection in Immunocompetent Hosts

In patients with or without HIV infection, the most common symptom of microsporidian infection is diarrhea.[3,4,9,49,53,57,62,63,79,143] *Encephalitozoon bieneusi* has been identified as a cause of self-limited diarrhea in immunocompetent patients and travelers[9,48,55–57,144,145] and has been found in up to 10% of African children with diarrhea.[2,146,147] *Encephalitozoon intestinalis* was found in 8% of the stools of patients in a survey for the etiology of diarrhea in Mexico[79] and has been seen in travelers with chronic diarrhea.[57] Cerebral infections due to *Enc. cuniculi* are described in several mammals but have been reported only rarely in immunocompetent humans. In a 3-year-old boy with seizures and hepatomegaly, *Encephalitozoon* infection was suggested by positive immunoglobulin G (IgG) and IgM indirect immunofluorescence assays (using *Enc. cuniculi* as the antigen).[58] Similarly, *Encephalitozoon* spp. infection was reported in a 9-year-old Japanese boy with headache, vomiting, spastic convulsions, and recurrent fever.[17] *Pleistophora* spp. have been identified in the skeletal muscle of an HIV-negative patient with myositis.[136–138,148] *Brachiola algerae* causing myositis with significant elevations in creatine phosphokinase (CPK) and muscle pain has been seen in a patient with rheumatoid arthritis treated with steroids and antibody to tumor necrosis factor-α.[149]

Ocular infections with ulcer or deep cornea stroma infection associated with eye pain have been reported in immunocompetent patients. In 1981, corneal microsporidiosis due to *Microsporidium africanus*[150] was described, and in 1973 infection due to *Microsporidium ceylonesis* was described.[151] Other cases of microsporidian keratitis have since been identified in immunocompetent hosts.[13] One of these organisms was classified as *N. ocularum*[152] and the other, which was successfully propagated in vitro, was named *N. corneum*[153] (now *V. cornea*[29]). *Brachiola algerae* infection of the cornea has also been reported.[142] In these immunocompetent patients with corneal infections, one patient required enucleation,[150] one underwent unsuccessful penetrating keratoplasty,[151] one was successfully treated with a corneal transplant,[152] and the last was maintained on a variety of topical agents without effect until keratoplasty.[154] *Encephalitozoon* spp. corneal infections have been described in contact lens wearers.[155]

PATHOGENESIS AND IMMUNITY

Infection of the epithelium of the gastrointestinal tract (small intestine and biliary epithelium) is the most frequent presentation of microsporidiosis. *Encephalitozoon bieneusi* infection does not produce active enteritis or ulceration, but infection results in variable degrees of villus blunting and crypt hyperplasia. The organism is located on the apical surface of the enterocytes of the small intestine and epithelial cells of the biliary tract and pancreas. Spores are rarely found on the basal surface or in the lamina propria.[110,156] Infection may be associated with increased intraepithelial lymphocytes and epithelial disarray. *Encephalitozoon intestinalis* and other *Encephalitozoon* spp. are invasive; spores are found in the apical and basal sides of infected intestinal enterocytes and in the lamina propria.[157] Histopathology can demonstrate areas of necrosis and mucosal erosion.

Encephalitozoon spp. infect the genitourinary system in most mammals, including humans,[48,110,120,158] in which infection discovered in any organ (eye, gastrointestinal tract, liver, central nervous system, etc.) is often associated with the shedding of spores in the urine. Granulomatous interstitial nephritis composed of plasma cells and lymphocytes is the most frequent pathologic finding. This is associated with tubular necrosis, with the lumen of the tubules containing amorphous granular material. Spores are located in the necrotic tubes and sloughing tubular epithelial cells.[64,68,102,104] As spores and infected tubular cells are shed into the bladder, they can infect other epithelial cells of the urogenital tract, causing ureteritis, prostatitis, and cystitis[110] and infection in macrophages, muscle, and supporting fibroblasts of the associated mucosa.

Lower respiratory tract infection due to Encephalitozoonidae has demonstrated erosive tracheitis, bronchitis, and bronchiolitis.[159,131] In most cases, organisms are found in intact or sloughed epithelial cells. Sinus biopsies in AIDS patients with chronic sinusitis and microsporidiosis have demonstrated spores in epithelium as well as in supporting structures.[128,160–166]

Infection with *Enc. cuniculi*, *Enc. hellem*, or *Enc. intestinalis* can result in punctate keratopathy and conjunctivitis that is characterized by multiple punctate corneal ulcers (e.g., a superficial epithelial keratitis). Microsporidian spores are present in corneal and conjunctival epithelium that can be obtained by scraping or biopsy of the lesions. The organisms do not invade the corneal stroma but remain limited to the epithelium. Inflammatory cells are rarely present.[84,91,124,167,168] Infections in immunocompetent hosts with other species of Microsporidia have usually involved deeper levels of the corneal stroma with associated necrosis and acute inflammatory cells, with some giant cells in several cases. Clinically, these patients have a corneal stromal keratitis and occasionally a uveitis.

DIAGNOSIS

Coprodiagnosis

Examination by light microscopy of stool specimens using special stains is the practical method for the diagnosis of gastrointestinal microsporidiosis. Experience is greatest with

Box 96-1 Weber's Chromotrope-Based Staining

Stain Preparation

The chromotrope-based staining solution is prepared by mixing 6.0 g of chromotrope 2R, 0.15 g of fast green, and 0.7 g of phosphotungstic acid. After standing for 30 minutes in 3 mL of glacial acetic acid, these ingredients are mixed with 100 mL of distilled water. Acid alcohol for rinsing is prepared with 4.5 mL of acetic acid and 995.5 mL of 90% ethyl alcohol. Chromotrope staining solutions are also commercially available.

Slide Preparation

Ten-microliter aliquots of a suspension of unconcentrated stool fixed in 10% formalin are spread very thinly onto a glass slide. Smears are fixed in methanol for 5 minutes and stained for 90 minutes. After staining, slides are rinsed in acid alcohol for 10 seconds and then rinsed briefly in 95% alcohol. Smears are then successively dehydrated in 95% alcohol for 5 minutes, 100% alcohol for 10 minutes, and Hemo-De (a xylene substitute) for 10 minutes. The slides are scanned at ×1000 magnification (oil immersion).

Weber's chromotrope-based stain[169] (Box 96-1). Some laboratories prefer the Ryan modification,[170] which uses aniline blue in place of fast green. Using these chromotrope 2R stains, spores appear as 1- to 3-μm ovoid light pink structures with a beltlike stripe girding them diagonally and equatorially. *Enterocytozoon* spores are smaller (0.1 × 1.5 μm) than *Encephalitozoon* spores (1.0 to 1.5 × 2.5 to 3.0 μm). The Gram-chromotrope stain (Box 96-2; Plate 96-1) combines chromotrope 2R staining with a Gram-staining step and results in violet-staining spores,[171] and it can be performed in 11 minutes. Spores can also be visualized by ultraviolet (UV) microscopy using chemofluorescent optical brightening agents such as Calcofluor white M2R (fluorescent brightener 28, Fungi-Fluor)[172] or Uvitex 2B (Fungiqual A),[173] which stain chitin in the spore wall. Chemofluorescent stains also stain fungi, but microsporidian spores can be distinguished from yeast because they have a uniform oval shape and are nonbudding. The limit of detecting Microsporidia by these light microscopy techniques appears to be 50,000 organisms/mL.[174] Overall, the sensitivity of the chemofluorescent brightener-based stains is slightly higher than that of chromotrope-based stains (especially when low numbers of spores are present in a sample); however, the specificity of the chemofluorescent stains is lower (90% vs. 100% in one study).[174] It has been reported that microsporidian spores in food can give a false-positive result, but this does not appear to be a common

Box 96-2 Description of the Quick-Hot

Gram-Chromotrope Staining Technique for Microsporidia, for Use with the Slide Stainer*

A. Prepare a thin smear of the material to be stained (e.g., feces, urine, sputum, saliva, and cell culture supernatants) and air dry.

B. Heat-fix smear (three times for 1 second each over a low flame or 5 minutes on a slide warmer at 60°C). Cool to room temperature before staining.

Note: For formalin-fixed, paraffin-embedded tissue sections, deparaffinize as usual, hydrate in a series of alcohols, and bring the slides to water before performing Gram's stain.

C. Perform Gram's stain (without the safranin step).

We followed the Gram staining procedures as described in either the Gram Stain Kit SG100 or Carr–Scarborough and Boekel Slide Stainer brochure, with slight modifications as follows:

C1. Dip slides into well containing gentian violet solution and let stand for 30 seconds.†

C2. Rinse off excess stain gently with water.

C3. Dip slides into well with Gram's iodine solution and allow to remain on the slide for 30 seconds.†

C4. Remove Gram's iodine solution by gently rinsing with decolorizer solution. Hold the slide at an angle and add the decolorizer solution dropwise until it flows off the slide colorless.‡

C5. Wash slide gently with cold water to remove excess decolorizer solution.

D. Perform chromotrope stain.

D1. Place the slide in warm (50°C to 55°C) chromotrope stain (1.0 g chromotrope 2R [Mallinckrodt], 0.15 g fast green, 0.25 g phosphotungstic acid, 3 mL acetic acid, and 100 mL distilled water) for at least 1 minute.†

D2. Rinse in 90% acid alcohol (4.5 mL acetic acid and 995.5 mL of 90% ethyl alcohol) for 1 to 3 seconds.‡

D3. Rinse in 95% ethyl alcohol for 30 seconds.

D4. Rinse twice, 30 seconds each time, in 100% ethyl alcohol placed in two different containers; let dry.§ Mount with Cytoseal 60 and examine.

*Turn on slide stainer 15 minutes before starting to stain slides.

†For formalin-fixed, paraffin-embedded tissue sections, we recommend that the staining times be prolonged for 30 seconds in each step.

‡Take extra care during the destaining process to achieve correct staining of spores.

§For formalin-fixed, paraffin-embedded tissue sections, we recommend that the slides be washed briefly in a solution of 50% ethyl alcohol/50% xylene for 15 seconds and subsequently in 100% xylene for 15 seconds before mounting with Cytoseal 60 and without letting the slide dry.

Data from Moura and colleagues.[171]

problem in the use of stool specimens for diagnosis of these infections.

Because renal involvement with shedding of spores in the urine is common in all of the species of Microsporidia that disseminate, urine specimens should be obtained whenever the diagnosis of microsporidiosis is considered. This has therapeutic implications because the Microsporidia that disseminate (e.g., *Encephalitozoon*) are usually sensitive to albendazole, but those that do not disseminate (e.g., *Ent. bieneusi*) are resistant. Definitive identification of the Microsporidia causing an infection cannot be done with light microscopy and requires either ultrastructural examination (e.g., electron microscopy) or molecular techniques (e.g., species-specific PCR). If stool examination is negative in the setting of chronic diarrhea (more than 2 months' duration), then endoscopy should be performed.

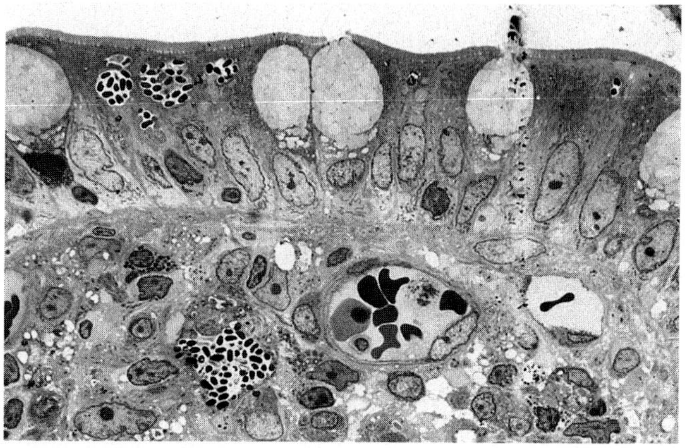

FIGURE 96-6 *Encephalitozoon intestinalis* in a duodenal biopsy plastic-embedded section stained with toluidine blue. Unlike *Enterocytozoon*, the spores of *Encephalitozoon intestinalis* develop in a vacuole, termed the parasitophorous vacuole, as shown in both superficial enterocytes and in a lamina propria macrophage. (Magnification ×1000.)

Cytologic Techniques

In body fluids other than stool (e.g., urine, cerebrospinal fluid, bile, duodenal aspirates, bronchoalveolar lavage fluid, and sputum), Microsporidia have been easily visualized using a variety of stains (e.g., Chromotrope 2R, chemofluorescent optical brightening agents, Giemsa, Brown–Hopps Gram stain, acid fast staining, and/or Warthin–Starry silver staining).[43,175,176] Since Microsporidia often infect mucosa or epithelium, cytologic preparations are useful for diagnosis.[43] Microsporidia have been easily demonstrated in intestinal and biliary epithelium, epithelium of the cornea and conjunctivae, epithelium of the sinonasal and tracheobronchial regions, renal tubular epithelium, and urothelium. Microsporidian keratitis cell samples obtained by gentle rubbing over the conjunctiva and cornea with a tissue swab usually reveal multiple, gram-positive, oval organisms within epithelial cells (Fig. 96-5).

Histologic Techniques

Using routine procedures, microsporidian spores are discernible with a modified tissue chromotrope 2R or tissue Gram stain (Brown–Hopp or Brown–Brenn) in biopsy and autopsy tissue specimens. In people with intestinobiliary infections, the jejunum and ileum (followed by the duodenum) have the greatest concentration of organisms and highest diagnostic yield (Fig. 96-6). In transbronchial biopsies, spores are best identified in bronchial or bronchiolar epithelium, but they can also be found within alveolar spaces. Microsporidia are usually gram positive and some are also acid-fast positive. Due to their thick wall, unstained spores are refractile and as such can be birefringent in unstained tissue sections. With experience, Microsporidia can also be seen on hematoxylin and eosin stain. Other stains that may be useful include periodic acid–Schiff, Giemsa, and Steiner silver stains. Biopsy or autopsy material should, if possible, also be placed in electron microscopic fixative when microsporidiosis is suspected because definitive diagnosis of species requires ultrastructural information. Although molecular methods such as PCR can be performed using formalin-fixed tissue, better results are obtained with unfixed tissue or tissue fixed in ethanol.

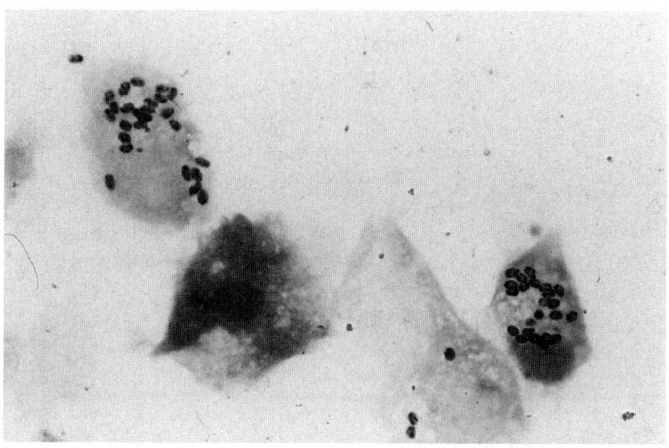

FIGURE 96-5 Conjunctival smear from a patient with AIDS and *Encephalitozoon hellem* keratoconjunctivitis stained with Gram stain. Numerous gram-positive microsporidian spores can be seen within the cytoplasm of the epithelial cells as well as outside of these cells.

Electron Microscopy, Immunofluorescence, Molecular Diagnostic Methods, Serology, and Tissue Culture

Electron microscopy is a useful technique for confirmation of microsporidian infection in patient tissues and fluids, as well as for detailed ultrastructural studies of microsporidian life cycles and host-parasite relationships that are required for the description of new species of Microsporidia (see Figs. 96-1 and 96-2). Electron microscopy should be performed on any new or atypical infections that are diagnosed as being due to Microsporidia. Fluorescent antibody reagents can be used for the species-level identification of various Microsporidia in both cytologic and tissue specimens,[177–181] but these are available only in research and reference laboratories. Serologic tests for the diagnosis of microsporidiosis have been developed and utilized for epidemiologic studies, but they have not been useful for the diagnosis of microsporidiosis in AIDS patients.[182] Molecular diagnostic techniques such as PCR are being used with increasing success and have successfully identified

Microsporidia at the species level in intestinal biopsies, stool specimens, and other tissues (for a review see Weiss and Vossbrinck[40]).[183–186] Currently, these tests are available only in reference laboratories such as the Centers for Disease Control and Prevention. The in vitro cultivation of several human-infecting Microsporidia has enhanced our understanding of these pathogens (for a review see Visvesvara[187]). *Vittaforma corneae*,[153] *Enc. cuniculi*, *Enc. hellem*,[167] *T. hominis*,[34] and *Enc. intestinalis*[188] have been cultivated in vitro, whereas *Ent. bieneusi* has not. The isolation of Microsporidia from clinical specimens is not a routine procedure and is available only in a few specialized research laboratories.

DIAGNOSIS

The Microsporidia are generally considered after the more common pathogens of the gastrointestinal, hepatobiliary, respiratory, genitourinary, ocular, musculoskeletal, and central nervous systems have been considered and ruled out. The index of suspicion for microsporidiosis should be highest in patients with severe immunosuppression, especially, but not exclusively, those infected with HIV. Intestinal microsporidiosis should be considered in any patient with chronic diarrhea or hepatobiliary disease of uncertain cause. The differential diagnosis includes other infectious agents characterized by chronic diarrhea, such as *Cryptosporidium*, *Cyclospora*, *Giardia*, or *Isospora*. Intestinal microsporidiosis should be considered in cases of presumptive traveler's diarrhea in which other routine pathogens have been excluded. A diagnosis of microsporidiosis should also be considered in cases of unexplained keratoconjunctivitis or corneal ulcers, persistent sinusitis or diffuse lower respiratory disease, unexplained renal insufficiency or abnormalities in urinary sediment, and myositis. Since dissemination can occur, microsporidiosis may affect virtually any organ system, including bone and the central nervous system. Therefore, the identification of Microsporidia in any specimen should prompt a thorough search in all other readily available sources, including stool, urine, sputum, nasal and conjunctival swabs, and possibly cerebrospinal fluid, with consideration of more invasive approaches for those patients requiring a tissue-based diagnosis (e.g., myositis).

TREATMENT AND PROGNOSIS

For a review of drugs used in microsporidiosis in humans and animals, see Costa and Weiss[189] (Table 96-2). Although albendazole has significant activity against many Microsporidia, such as the Encephalitozoonidae, it has limited efficacy for *Ent. bieneusi* infection,[190–192] with relapse of symptoms rapidly occurring with the discontinuation of therapy in patients who reported improvement of symptoms with treatment. Other studies have found that albendazole has no efficacy in *Ent. bieneusi* infection.[193] Fumagillin is used to treat honeybees infected with the microsporidian *Nosema apis* and has been used to treat microsporidiosis in aquaculture.[194,195] Fumagillin and its semisynthetic analogue, TNP-470, were found to have activity in vitro and in vivo against *Enc. cuniculi*, *Enc. hellem*, *Enc. intestinalis*, and *V. corneae*.[196–201] Fumagillin has also been demonstrated in both a dose-escalation trial and a randomized clinical trial to be effective for the treatment of human infection

Table 96-2 Treatment Options for Microsporidiosis

Organism	Drug	Dosage and Duration
All microsporidian infections	Restoration of immune function can be critical in control of infection. Patients with AIDS should have highly active antiretroviral therapy optimized.	
Enterocytozoon bieneusi	No effective commercial treatment.	
	Oral fumagillin 20 mg TID (e.g., 60 mg/day has been effective in a clinical trial.	
	Albendazole* resulted in clinical improvement in up to 50% of patients in some studies; however, it was not effective in other studies.	
Encephalitzoonidae infection (systemic, sinusitis, encephalitis, hepatitis, etc.)		
Enc. cuniculi	Albendazole	400 mg BID†
Enc. hellem	Albendazole	400 mg BID
Enc. intestinalis	Albendazole	400 mg BID
Encephalitozoonidae keratoconjunctivitis	Fumagillin solution‡ (Fumadil B 3 mg/mL)	2 drops every 2 hr for 4 days, then 2 drops 4 times a day§
	Patients may also need albendazole* if systemic infection is present.	
Trachipleistophora hominis	Albendazole	400 mg BID
Brachiola vesicularum	Albendazole	400 mg BID
	± itraconozole	400 mg QD

*Albendazole 400 mg BID.
†The duration of treatment for microsporidiosis has not been established. Relapse of infection has occurred upon stopping treatment. Patients should be maintained on treatment for at least 4 weeks and most patients should be on treatment indefinitely.
‡Fumagillin bicylohexylammonium.
§Eyedrops should be continued indefinitely; relapse is common on stopping treatment.
Adapted from Costa and Weiss.[189]

with *Ent. bieneusi* at a dose of 60 mg/day (20 mg TID).[196,197] Treatment was associated with resolution of diarrhea, clearance of spores, improvement of Karnofsky scores, and improvement in D-xylose absorption tests. The main limiting toxicity of this treatment was thrombocytopenia, which was reversible on stopping fumagillin treatment. Despite a few case reports that indicated that metronidazole was effective for *Ent. bieneusi* infection, the majority of studies have demonstrated that this drug is not effective.[158,198,202] Other medications used without success in the treatment of gastrointestinal microsporidiosis are azithromycin, paromomycin, and quinacrine. Clinical studies have demonstrated that improvement of immune function can result in clinical response with the elimination of the organism and normalization of intestinal architecture in gastrointestinal microsporidiosis.[203–207] Part of the primary treatment of microsporidiosis in the setting of AIDS is the institution of effective antiretroviral therapy.

There are numerous case reports that demonstrate the efficacy of 2 to 4 weeks of 400 mg BID of albendazole for the treatment of microsporidian infections due to *Encephalitozoon* spp. A double-blind, placebo-controlled trial of eight patients with AIDS and diarrhea due to *Enc. intestinalis* demonstrated that albendazole (400 mg BID for 3 weeks) treatment led to a resolution of the diarrhea and elimination of the organism, similar to observations in case reports.[120,121,123,158,163,208,209] In case reports of chronic sinusitis, respiratory infection, and disseminated infection due to *Enc. hellem*, treatment with 400 mg of albendazole twice daily resulted in resolution of symptoms and clearance of the organism.[210,211] In a patient with disseminated *Enc. cuniculi* infection involving the central nervous system, conjunctiva, sinuses, kidney, and lungs, clinical improvement was demonstrated with albendazole treatment.[114] The successful use of albendazole has also been reported in cases of urethritis,[212] renal failure,[213] and disseminated infection[125] due to *Encephalitozoon* spp. In addition, albendazole has been reported to have activity in the treatment of disseminated microsporidian infection with *T. hominis* and in myositis due to a *Brachiola vesicularum*.[30,34]

Ocular microsporidiosis can be treated with a solution of 3 mg/ml of Fumidil B (fumagillin bicylohexylammonium) in saline[199,214–217]; however, recurrence is known to occur when topical therapy is discontinued. Although clearance of Microsporidia from the eye can be demonstrated, the organism is still present systemically and can often be demonstrated in urine or nasal smears. The use of albendazole as a systemic agent is thus also reasonable for the treatment of ocular infection and should probably be used in addition to topical treatment. Polymyxin B, propamidine isethionate 0.1% (Brolene), gramicidin, neomycin sulfate, and tetracycline have limited efficacy and should not be used except as treatment for secondary bacterial infections. Keratoplasty provides temporary improvement in some cases, and debulking by corneal scraping may be useful in cases not responding to medical treatment. Steroids may be useful in decreasing the associated inflammatory response.

PREVENTION AND CONTROL

The presence of infective spores in various bodily fluids suggests that body substance precautions in health-care settings and general attention to hand washing and other personal hygiene measures should be useful in preventing primary infections. Hand washing may be particularly important in the prevention of ocular infections, which may occur as a result of inoculation of conjunctival surfaces by fingers contaminated with respiratory fluids or urine. Whether respiratory precautions are necessary for people with spores in sputum or other respiratory secretions is unknown. It is reasonable to screen close contacts of index cases of microsporidiosis. Spores survive and remain infective in the environment for prolonged periods of time.[83] In a typical hospital environment, *Enc. cuniculi* spores can survive and remain infectious for at least 1 month but can be rendered noninfectious by a 30-minute exposure to most common disinfectants and by the methods employed for sterilization. Therefore, the procedures used to clean most hospital rooms should be sufficient to limit infection.

It is likely that these organisms are food- or water-borne pathogens and the usual sanitary measures that prevent contamination of food and water with the urine and feces of animals should decrease the chance for infection. Existing guidelines for the prevention of opportunistic infections that address food, water, and animal contact may be useful in preventing microsporidiosis. Severely immunocompromised patients may wish to consider using bottled or filtered water in some settings. No prophylactic antiparasitic agents have been identified for these organisms. Microsporidiosis has developed in patients on trimethoprim–sulfamethoxazole prophylaxis[218] and those receiving dapsone, pyrimethamine, itraconazole, azithromycin, and/or atovaquone.[219] No studies have evaluated albendazole for prophylaxis, but given its relative lack of efficacy for *Ent. bieneusi* infections, it is unlikely to be effective for prevention. The most effective prophylaxis is a restoration of immune function in immunocompromised hosts. In AIDS patients, several studies have demonstrated that highly active antiretroviral therapy can produce remission of intestinal microsporidiosis.[203–207]

REFERENCES

1. Naegeli C: Uber die neue Krankheit der seidenraupe und verwandte Organismen. Bot Zeit 15:760–761, 1857.
2. Drobniewski F, Kelly P, Carew A, et al: Human microsporidiosis in African AIDS patients with chronic diarrhea. J Infect Dis 171:515–516, 1995.
3. Aoun K, Bouratbine A, Datry A, et al: Presence of intestinal microsporidia in Tunisia: A case report. Bull Soc Pathol Exotique 90:176, 1997.
4. Hautvast JL, Tolboom JJ, Derks TJ, et al: Asymptomatic intestinal microsporidiosis in a human immunodeficiency virus-seronegative, immunocompetent Zambian child. Pediatr Infect Dis J 16:415–416, 1997.
5. van Gool T, Luderhoff E, Nathoo KJ, et al: High prevalence of *Enterocytozoon bieneusi* infections among HIV-positive individuals with persistent diarrhoea in Harare, Zimbabwe. Trans R Soc Trop Med Hyg 89:478–480, 1995.
6. Morakote N, Siriprasert P, Piangjai S, et al: Microsporidium and Cyclospora in human stools in Chiang Mai, Thailand. Southeast Asian J Trop Med Public Health 26:799–800, 1995.
7. Brazil P, Sodre FC, Cuzzi-Maya T, et al: Intestinal microsporidiosis in HIV-positive patients with chronic unexplained diarrhea in Rio de Janeiro, Brazil: Diagnosis, clinical presentation and follow-up. Rev Inst Med Trop Sao Paulo 38:97–102, 1996.
8. Weitz JC, Botehlo R, Bryan R: Microsporidiosis in patients with chronic diarrhea and AIDS, in HIV asymptomatic patients and in patients with acute diarrhea. Rev Med Child 123:849–856, 1995.
9. Bryan RT, Schwartz DA: Epidemiology of microsporidiosis. In Weiss LM (ed): The Microsporidia and Microsporidiosis. Washington, DC, ASM Press, 1999, pp 502–516.

10. Deplazes P, Mathis A, Weber R: Epidemiology and zoonotic aspects of microsporidia of mammals and birds. Contrib Microbiol 6:236–260, 2000.
11. Singh M, Kane GJ, Mackinlay L, et al: Detection of antibodies to *Nosema cuniculi* (Protozoa: Microsporidia) in human and animal sera by the indirect fluorescent antibody technique. Southeast Asian J Trop Med Public Health 13:110–113, 1982.
12. World Health Organization: Parasitic diseases surveillance. Antibody to *Encephalitozoon cuniculi* in man. WHO Weekly Epidem Rec 58:30, 1983.
13. Wittner M, Weiss LM: The Microsporidia and Microsporidiosis. Washington, DC, ASM Press, 1999.
14. Black SS, Steinohrt LA, Bertucci DC, et al: *Encephalitozoon hellem* in budgerigars (*Melopsittacus undulatus*). Vet Pathol 34:189–198, 1997.
15. American Mosquito Control Association: Biological control of mosquitoes. In AMCA Bulletin, No. 6. Fresno, Calif, American Mosquito Control Association, 1985.
16. Levaditi C, Nicolau S, Schoen R: L'agent etiologique de l'enchalite epizootique du lapin (*Encephalitozoon cuniculi*). C R Soc Biol 89:984–986, 1923.
17. Matsubayashi H, Koide T, Mikata T, et al: A case of Encephalitozoon-like body infection in man. Arch Pathol Lab Med 67:181–185, 1959.
18. Sprague V, Vavra J: Systematics of the Microsporidia. In Bulla LA, Cheng TC (eds): Comparative Pathobiology, Vol. 2. New York, Plenum Press, 1977.
19. Sprague VV, Becnel JJ: Note on the name–author–date combination for the taxon *Microsporidies Balbiani,* 1882, when ranked as a phylum. J Invertebr Pathol 71:91–94, 1998.
20. Keeling PJ, McFadden GI: Origins of microsporidia. Trends Microbiol 6:19–23, 1998.
21. Weiss LM, Edlind TD, Vossbrinck CR, et al: Microsporidian molecular phylogeny: The fungal connection. J Eukaryot Microbiol 46:17S–18S, 1999.
22. Hirt RP, Logsdon JM Jr, Healy B, et al: Microsporidia are related to fungi: Evidence from the largest subunit of RNA polymerase II and other proteins. Proc Natl Acad Sci USA 96:580–585, 1999.
23. Tuzet O, Maurand J, Fize JA, et al: Proposition d'un nouveau cadre systematique pour les genres de Microsporidies. C R Acad Sci (Paris) 272:1268–1271, 1971.
24. Larsson JIR: Identification of microsporidian genera—A guide with comments on the taxonomy. Arch Protistenkd 136:1–37, 1988.
25. Issi IV: Microsporidia as a phylum of parasitic protozoa. [Russian] Protozoology 10:6–135, 1986.
26. Weiser J: A proposal of the basis for microsporidian taxonomy. Proc Int Congr Protozool 5:267, 1977.
27. Sprague V, Becnel JJ, Hazard EI: Taxonomy of phylum Microspora. Crit Rev Microbiol 18:285–395, 1992.
28. Weiss LM, Vossbrinck CR: Microsporidiosis: Molecular and diagnostic aspects. Adv Parasitol 40:351–395, 1998.
29. Silveira H, Canning EU: *Vittaforma corneae* n. comb. for the human microsporidium *Nosema corneum* Shadduck, Meccoli, Davis & Font, 1990, based on its ultrastructure in the liver of experimentally infected athymic mice. J Eukaryot Microbiol 42:158–165, 1995.
30. Cali A, Takvorian PM, Lewin S, et al: *Brachiola vesicularum*, n. g., n. sp., a new microsporidium associated with AIDS and myositis. J Eukaryot Microbiol 45:240–251, 1998.
31. Desportes I, Le Charpentier Y, Galian A, et al: Occurrence of a new microsporidian: *Enterocytozoon bieneusi* n. g., n. sp., in the enterocytes of a human patient with AIDS. J Protozool 32:250–245, 1985.
32. Cali A, Kotler DP, Orenstein JM: *Septata intestinalis* N. G., N. Sp., an intestinal microsporidian associated with chronic diarrhea and dissemination in AIDS patients. J Eukaryot Microbiol 40:101–112, 1993.
33. Hartskeerl RA, Van Gool T, Schuitema AR, et al: Genetic and immunological characterization of the microsporidian *Septata intestinalis* Cali, Kotler and Orenstein, 1993: Reclassification to *Encephalitozoon intestinalis*. Parasitology 110:277–285, 1995.
34. Field AS, Marriott DJ, Milliken ST, et al: Myositis associated with a newly described microsporidian, *Trachipleistophora hominis*, in a patient with AIDS. J Clin Microbiol 34:2803–2811, 1996.
35. Yachnis AT, Berg J, Martinez-Salazar A, et al: Disseminated microsporidiosis especially infecting the brain, heart, and kidneys. Report of a newly recognized pansporoblastic species in two symptomatic AIDS patients. Am J Clin Pathol 106:535–543, 1996.
36. Weber R, Bryan RT, Schwartz DA, et al: Human microsporidial infections. Clin Microbiol Rev 7:426–461, 1994.
37. Hewan-Lowe K, Furlong B, Sims M, et al: Coinfection with *Giardia lamblia* and *Enterocytozoon bieneusi* in a patient with acquired immunodeficiency syndrome and chronic diarrhea. Arch Pathol Lab Med 121:417–422, 1997.
38. Desportes-Livage I: Biology of microsporidia. Contrib Microbiol 6:140–165, 2000.
39. Williams BA, Hirt RP, Lucocq JM, et al: A mitochondrial remnant in the microsporidian *Trachipleistophora hominis*. Nature 418:865–869, 2002.
40. Weiss LM, Vossbrinck CR: Molecular biology, molecular phylogeny, and molecular diagnostic approaches to the Microsporidia. In Weiss LM (ed): The Microsporidia and Microsporidia. Washington, DC, ASM Press, 1999, pp 129–171.
41. Vivares CP, Metenier G: Towards the minimal eukaryotic parasitic genome. Curr Opin Microbiol 3:463–467, 2000.
42. Brugere JF, Cornillot E, Metenier G, et al: Occurrence of subtelomeric rearrangements in the genome of the microsporidian parasite *Encephalitozoon cuniculi*, as revealed by a new fingerprinting procedure based on two-dimensional pulsed field gel electrophoresis. Electrophoresis 21:2576–2581, 2000.
43. Weber R, Deplazes P, Schwartz D: Diagnosis and clinical aspects of human microsporidiosis. Contrib Microbiol 6:166–192, 2000.
44. Vavra J: Structure of the Microsporidia. In Bulla LA Jr, Cheng TC (eds): Comparative Pathobiology. New York, Plenum Press, 1976, pp 1–85.
45. Foucault C, Drancourt M: Actin mediates *Encephalitozoon intestinalis* entry into the human enterocyte-like cell line, Caco-2. Microb Pathogen 28:51–58, 2000.
46. Lom J: On the structure of the extruded microsporidian polar filament. Z Parasitenkd 38:200–213, 1972.
47. Weidner E: Ultrastructural study of microsporidian invasion into cells. Z Parasitenkd 40:227–242, 1972.
48. Weber R, Bryan RT: Microsporidial infections in immunodeficient and immunocompetent patients. Clin Infect Dis 19:517–521, 1994.
49. Cegielski JP, Ortega YR, McKee S, et al: *Cryptosporidium, Enterocytozoon,* and *Cyclospora* infections in pediatric and adult patients with diarrhea in Tanzania. Clin Infect Dis 28:314–321, 1999.
50. Maiga I, Doumbo O, Dembele M, et al: Human intestinal microsporidiosis in Bamako (Mali): The presence of *Enterocytozoon bieneusi* in HIV seropositive patients. Sante 7:257–262, 1997.
51. Cotte L, Rabodonirina M, Chapuis F, et al: Waterborne outbreak of intestinal microsporidiosis in persons with and without human immunodeficiency virus infection. J Infect Dis 180:2003–2008, 1999.
52. Wanke CA, DeGirolami P, Federman M: *Enterocytozoon bieneusi* infection and diarrheal disease in patients who were not infected with human immunodeficiency virus: Case report and review. Clin Infect Dis 23:816–818, 1996.
53. Gainzarain JC, Canut A, Lozano M, et al: Detection of *Enterocytozoon bieneusi* in two human immunodeficiency virus-negative patients with chronic diarrhea by polymerase chain reaction in duodenal biopsy specimens and review. Clin Infect Dis 27:394–398, 1998.
54. Albrecht H, Sobottka I: *Enterocytozoon bieneusi* infection in patients who are not infected with human immunodeficiency virus. Clin Infect Dis 25:344, 1997.
55. Sandfort J, Hannemann A, Gelderblom H, et al: *Enterocytozoon bieneusi* infection in an immunocompetent patient who had acute diarrhea and who was not infected with the human immunodeficiency virus. Clin Infect Dis 19:514–516, 1994.
56. Sobottka I, Albrecht H, Schottelius J, et al: Self-limited traveller's diarrhea due to a dual infection with *Enterocytozoon bieneusi* and *Cryptosporidium parvum* in an immunocompetent HIV-negative child. Eur J Clin Microbiol Infect Dis 14:919–920, 1995.
57. Raynaud L, Delbac F, Broussolle V, et al: Identification of *Encephalitozoon intestinalis* in travelers with chronic diarrhea by specific PCR amplification. J Clin Microbiol 36:37–40, 1998.
58. Bergquist NR, Stintzing G, Smedman L, et al: Diagnosis of encephalitozoonosis in man by serological tests. Br Med J (Clin Res Ed) 288:902, 1984.
59. Pospisilova Z, Ditrich O, Stankova M, et al: Parasitic opportunistic infections in Czech HIV-infected patients—A prospective study. Cent Eur J Public health 5:208–213, 1997.
60. Cislakova L, Prokopcakova H, Stef'kovic M, et al: *Encephalitozoon cuniculi*—Clinical and epidemiologic significance. Results of a

preliminary serologic study in humans. Epidemiol Mikrobiol Immunol 46:30–33, 1997.
61. van Gool T, Vetter JC, Weinmayr B, et al: High seroprevalence of *Encephalitozoon* species in immunocompetent subjects. J Infect Dis 175:1020–1024, 1997.
62. Rabodonirina M, Bertocchi M, Desportes-Livage I, et al: *Enterocytozoon bieneusi* as a cause of chronic diarrhea in a heart–lung transplant recipient who was seronegative for human immunodeficiency virus. Clin Infect Dis 23:114–117, 1996.
63. Sax PE, Rich JD, Pieciak WS, et al: Intestinal microsporidiosis occurring in a liver transplant recipient. Transplantation 60:617–618, 1995.
64. Gumbo T, Hobbs RE, Carlyn C, et al: Microsporidia infection in transplant patients. Transplantation 67:482–484, 1999.
65. Kelkar R, Sastry PS, Kulkarni SS, et al: Pulmonary microsporidial infection in a patient with CML undergoing allogeneic marrow transplant. Bone Marrow Transplant 19:179–182, 1997.
66. Mahmood MN, Keohane ME, Burd EM: Pathologic quiz case: A 45-year-old renal transplant recipient with persistent fever. Arch Pathol Lab Med 127:e224–e226, 2003.
67. Metge S, Van Nhieu JT, Dahmane D, et al: A case of *Enterocytozoon bieneusi* infection in an HIV-negative renal transplant recipient. Eur J Clin Microbiol Infect Dis 19:221–223, 2000.
68. Mohindra AR, Lee MW, Visvesvara G, et al: Disseminated microsporidiosis in a renal transplant recipient. Transpl Infect Dis 4:102–107, 2002.
69. Sing A, Tybus K, Heesemann J, et al: Molecular diagnosis of an *Enterocytozoon bieneusi* human genotype C infection in a moderately immunosuppressed human immunodeficiency virus seronegative liver-transplant recipient with severe chronic diarrhea. J Clin Microbiol 39:2371–2372, 2001.
70. Weiss LM: ... and now microsporidiosis. Ann Intern Med 123:954–956, 1995.
71. van Gool T, Dankert J: Human microsporidiosis: Clinical, diagnostic and therapeutic aspects of an increasing infection. Clin Microbiol Infect 1:75–85, 1995.
72. Bryan RT, Cali A, Owen RL, et al: Microsporidia: Opportunistic pathogens in patients with AIDS. Prog Clin Parasitol 2:1–26, 1991.
73. Coyle CM, Wittner M, Kotler DP, et al: Prevalence of microsporidiosis due to *Enterocytozoon bieneusi* and *Encephalitozoon (Septata) intestinalis* among patients with AIDS-related diarrhea: Determination by polymerase chain reaction to the microsporidian small-subunit rRNA gene. Clin Infect Dis 23:1002–1006, 1996.
74. Voglino MC, Donelli G, Rossi P, et al: Intestinal microsporidiosis in Italian individuals with AIDS. Ital J Gastroenterol 28:381–386, 1996.
75. Kyaw T, Curry A, Edwards-Jones V, et al: The prevalence of *Enterocytozoon bieneusi* in acquired immunodeficiency syndrome (AIDS) patients from the northwest of England: 1992–1995. Br J Biomed Sci 54:186–191, 1997.
76. Avery SW, Undeen AH: The isolation of microsporidia and other pathogens from concentrated ditch water. J Am Mosq Control Assoc 3:54–58, 1987.
77. Sparfel JM, Sarfati C, Liguory O, et al: Detection of microsporidia and identification of *Enterocytozoon bieneusi* in surface water by filtration followed by specific PCR. J Eukaryot Microbiol 44:78S, 1997.
78. Dowd SE, Gerba CP, Pepper IL: Confirmation of the human-pathogenic microsporidia *Enterocytozoon bieneusi*, *Encephalitozoon intestinalis*, and *Vittaforma corneae* in water. Appl Environ Microbiol 64:3332–3335, 1998.
79. Enriquez FJ, Taren D, Cruz-Lopez A, et al: Prevalence of intestinal encephalitozoonosis in Mexico. Clin Infect Dis 26:1227–1229, 1998.
80. Hutin YJ, Sombardier MN, Liguory O, et al: Risk factors for intestinal microsporidiosis in patients with human immunodeficiency virus infection: A case–control study. J Infect Dis 178:904–907, 1998.
81. Conteas CN, Berlin OG, Lariviere MJ, et al: Examination of the prevalence and seasonal variation of intestinal microsporidiosis in the stools of persons with chronic diarrhea and human immunodeficiency virus infection. Am J Trop Med Hyg 58:559–561, 1998.
82. Wuhib T, Silva TMJ, Newman RD, et al: Cryptosporidial and microsporidial infections in human immunodeficiency virus-infected patients in northeastern Brazil. J Infect Dis 170:494–497, 1994.
83. Waller T: Sensitivity of *Encephalitozoon cuniculi* to various temperatures, disinfectants and drugs. Lab Anim 13:227–230, 1979.
84. Yee RW, Tio FO, Martinez JA, et al: Resolution of microsporidial epithelial keratopathy in a patient with AIDS. Ophthalmology 98:196–201, 1991.
85. Bornay-Llinares FJ, da Silva AJ, Moura H, et al: Immunologic, microscopic, and molecular evidence of *Encephalitozoon intestinalis (Septata intestinalis)* infection in mammals other than humans. J Infect Dis 178:820–826, 1998.
86. Deplazes P, Mathis A, Muller C, et al: Molecular epidemiology of *Encephalitozoon cuniculi* and first detection of *Enterocytozoon bieneusi* in faecal samples of pigs. J Eukaryot Microbiol 43:93S, 1996.
87. del Aguila C, Izquierdo F, Navajas R, et al: *Enterocytozoon bieneusi* in animals: Rabbits and dogs as new hosts. J Eukaryot Microbiol 46:8S–9S, 1999.
88. Reetz J, Rinder H, Thomschke A, et al: First detection of the microsporidium *Enterocytozoon bieneusi* in non-mammalian hosts (chickens). Int J Parasitol 32:785–787, 2002.
89. Mansfield KG, Carville A, Shvetz D, et al: Identification of an *Enterocytozoon bieneusi*-like microsporidian parasite in simian immunodeficiency virus-inoculated macaques with hepatobiliary disease. Am J Pathol 150:1395–1405, 1997.
90. Schwartz DA, Anderson DC, Klumpp SA, et al: Ultrastructure of atypical (teratoid) sporogonial stages of *Enterocytozoon bieneusi* (Microsporidia) in naturally infected rhesus monkeys (*Macacca mulatta*). Arch Pathol Lab Med 122:423–429, 1998.
91. Schwartz DA, Visvesvara GS, Diesenhouse MC, et al: Pathologic features and immunofluorescent antibody demonstration of ocular microsporidiosis (*Encephalitozoon hellem*) in seven patients with acquired immunodeficiency syndrome. Am J Ophthalmol 115:285–292, 1993.
92. Fuentealba IC, Mahoney NT, Shadduck JA, et al: Hepatic lesions in rabbits infected with *Encephalitozoon cuniculi* administered per rectum. Vet Pathol 29:536–540, 1992.
93. Schwartz DA, Visvesvara G, Weber R, et al: Male genital tract microsporidiosis and AIDS: Prostatic abscess due to *Encephalitozoon hellem*. J Eukaryot Microbiol 41:61S, 1994.
94. Schwartz DA, Bryan RT, Hewanlowe KO, et al: Disseminated microsporidiosis and AIDS; Pathologic evidence for respiratory transmission of *Encephalitozoon* infection Int. Conf. AIDS, July 19–24, 1992.
95. Hunt RD, King NW, Foster HL: Encephalitozoonosis: Evidence for vertical transmission. J Infect Dis 126:212–214, 1972.
96. Franzen C, Muller A: Microsporidiosis: Human diseases and diagnosis. Microbes Infect 3:389–400, 2001.
97. Weber R, Muller A, Spycher MA, et al: Intestinal *Enterocytozoon bieneusi* microsporidiosis in an HIV-infected patient: Diagnosis by ileo-colonoscopic biopsies and long-term follow up. Clin Invest 70:1019–1023, 1992.
98. Rijpstra AC, Canning EU, Van Ketel RJ, et al: Use of light microscopy to diagnose small-intestinal microsporidiosis in patients with AIDS. J Infect Dis 157:827–831, 1988.
99. Molina JM, Sarfati C, Beauvais B, et al: Intestinal microsporidiosis in human immunodeficiency virus-infected patients with chronic unexplained diarrhea—Prevalence and clinical and biologic features. J Infect Dis 167:217–221, 1993.
100. Pol S, Romana CA, Richard S, et al: Microsporidia infection in patients with the human immunodeficiency virus and unexplained cholangitis. N Engl J Med 328:95–99, 1993.
101. Goetz M, Eichenlaub S, Pape GR, et al: Chronic diarrhea as a result of intestinal microsposidiosis in a liver transplant recipient. Transplantation 71:334–337, 2001.
102. Guerard A, Rabodonirina M, Cotte L, et al: Intestinal microsporidiosis occurring in two renal transplant recipients treated with mycophenolate mofetil. Transplantation 68:699–707, 1999.
103. Kelkar R, Sastry PSRK, Kulkarni SS, et al: Pulmonary microsporidial infection in a patient with CML undergoing allogeneic marrow transplant. Bone Marrow Transpl 19:179–182, 1997.
104. Latib MA, Pascoe MD, Duffield MS, et al: Microsporidiosis in the graft of a renal transplant recipient. Transpl Int 14:274–277, 2001.
105. Beaugerie L, Teilhac MF, Deluol AM, et al: Cholangiopathy associated with microsporidia infection of the common bile duct mucosa in a patient with HIV infection. Ann Intern Med 117:401–402, 1992.
106. Hartskeerl RA, van Gool T, Schuitema ARJ, et al: Genetic and immunological characterization of the microsporidian *Septata intestinalis* Cali, Kotler and Orenstein, 1993: Reclassification to *Encephalitozoon intestinalis*. Parasitology 110:277–285, 1995.
107. del Aguila C, Lopez-Velez R, Fenoy S, et al: Identification of *Enterocytozoon bieneusi* spores in respiratory samples from an AIDS

patient with a 2-year history of intestinal microsporidiosis. J Clin Microbiol 35:1862–1866, 1997.

108. Orenstein JM, Gaetz HP, Yachnis AT, et al: Disseminated microsporidiosis in AIDS: Are any organs spared? AIDS 11:385–386, 1997.
109. Schwartz DA, Visvesvara GS, Leitch GJ, et al: Pathology of symptomatic microsporidial (*Encephalitozoon hellem*) bronchiolitis in the acquired immunodeficiency syndrome—A new respiratory pathogen diagnosed from lung biopsy, bronchoalveolar lavage, sputum, and tissue culture. Hum Pathol 24:937–943, 1993.
110. Schwartz DA, Sobottka I, Leitch GJ, et al: Pathology of microsporidiosis: Emerging parasitic infections in patients with acquired immunodeficiency syndrome. Arch Pathol Lab Med 120:173–188, 1996.
111. Zender HO, Arrigoni E, Eckert J, et al: A case of *Encephalitozoon cuniculi* peritonitis in a patient with AIDS. Am J Clin Pathol 92:352–356, 1989.
112. Sheth SG, Bates C, Federman M, et al: Fulminant hepatic failure caused by microsporidial infection in a patient with AIDS. AIDS 11:553–554, 1997.
113. Mertens RB, Didier ES, Fishbein MC, et al: *Encephalitozoon cuniculi* microsporidiosis: Infection of the brain, heart, kidneys, trachea, adrenal glands, and urinary bladder in a patient with AIDS. Modern Pathol 10:68–77, 1997.
114. Weber R, Deplazes P, Flepp M, et al: Cerebral microsporidiosis due to *Encephalitozoon cuniculi* in a patient with human immunodeficiency virus infection. N Engl J Med 336:474–478, 1997.
115. Kester KE, Turiansky GW, McEvoy PL: Nodular cutaneous microsporidiosis in a patient with AIDS and successful treatment with long-term oral clindamycin therapy. Ann Intern Med 128:911–914, 1998.
116. Kester KE, Visvesvara GS, McEvoy P: Organism responsible for nodular cutaneous microsporidiosis in a patient with AIDS. Ann Intern Med 133:925, 2000.
117. Vangool T, Canning EU, Gilis H, et al: *Septata intestinalis* frequently isolated from stool of AIDS patients with a new cultivation method. Parasitology 109:281–289, 1994.
118. Willson R, Harrington R, Stewart B, et al: Human immunodeficiency virus 1-associated necrotizing cholangitis caused by infection with *Septata intestinalis*. Gastroenterology 108:247–251, 1995.
119. Belcher JW Jr, Guttenberg SA, Schmookler BM: Microsporidiosis of the mandible in a patient with acquired immunodeficiency syndrome. J Oral Maxillofac Surg 55:424–426, 1997.
120. Molina JM, Oksenhendler E, Beauvais B, et al: Disseminated microsporidiosis due to *Septata intestinalis* in patients with AIDS: Clinical features and response to albendazole therapy. J Infect Dis 171:245–249, 1995.
121. Dore GJ, Marriott DJ, Hing MC, et al: Disseminated microsporidiosis due to *Septata intestinalis* in nine patients infected with the human immunodeficiency virus: Response to therapy with albendazole. Clin Infect Dis 21:70–76, 1995.
122. Orenstein JM, Tenner M, Kotler DP: Localization of infection by the microsporidian *Enterocytozoon bieneusi* in the gastrointestinal tract of AIDS patients with diarrhea. AIDS 6:195–197, 1992.
123. Weber R, Sauer B, Spycher MA, et al: Detection of *Septata intestinalis* in stool specimens and coprodiagnostic monitoring of successful treatment with albendazole. Clin Infect Dis 19:342–345, 1994.
124. Terada S, Reddy KR, Jeffers LJ, et al: Microsporidian hepatitis in the acquired immunodeficiency syndrome. Ann Intern Med 107:61–62, 1987.
125. De Groote MA, Visvesvara G, Wilson ML, et al: Polymerase chain reaction and culture confirmation of disseminated *Encephalitozoon cuniculi* in a patient with AIDS: Successful therapy with albendazole. J Infect Dis 171:1375–1378, 1995.
126. Weber R, Kuster H, Visvesvara GS, et al: Disseminated microsporidiosis due to *Encephalitozoon hellem*—Pulmonary colonization, microhematuria, and mild conjunctivitis in a patient with AIDS. Clin Infect Dis 17:415–419, 1993.
127. Visvesvara GS, Leitch GJ, da Silva AJ, et al: Polyclonal and monoclonal antibody and PCR-amplified small-subunit rRNA identification of a microsporidian, *Encephalitozoon hellem*, isolated from an AIDS patient with disseminated infection. J Clin Microbiol 32:2760–2768, 1994.
128. Franzen C, Mueller A, Salzberger B, et al: Chronic rhinosinusitis in patients with AIDS: Potential role of microsporidia. AIDS (London) 10:687–688, 1996.
129. Rastrelli P, Didier E, Yee R: Microsporidial keratitis. Ophthalmol Clin North Am 7:614–635, 1994.
130. Lowder CY, Meisler DM, McMahon JT, et al: Microsporidia infection of the cornea in a man seropositive for human immunodeficiency virus. Am J Ophthalmol 109:242–244, 1990.
131. Schwartz DA, Bryan RT, Hewanlowe KO, et al: Disseminated microsporidiosis (*Encephalitozoon hellem*) and acquired immunodeficiency syndrome—Autopsy evidence for respiratory acquisition. Arch Pathol Lab Med 116:660–668, 1992.
132. Degroote MA, Visvesvara G, Wilson ML, et al: Polymerase chain reaction and culture confirmation of disseminated *Encephalitozoon cuniculi* in a patient with AIDS: Successful therapy with albendazole. J Infect Dis 171:1375–1378, 1995.
133. Lacey CJN, Clarke AMT, Fraser P, et al: Chronic microsporidian infection of the nasal mucosae, sinuses and conjunctivae in HIV disease. Genitourinary Med 68:179–181, 1992.
134. Franzen C, Schwartz DA, Visvesvara GS, et al: Immunologically confirmed disseminated, asymptomatic *Encephalitozoon cuniculi* infection of the gastrointestinal tract in a patient with AIDS. Clin Infect Dis 21:1480–1484, 1995.
135. Vavra J, Yachnis AT, Shadduck JA, et al: Microsporidia of the genus *Trachipleistophora*—Causative agents of human microsporidiosis: Description of *Trachipleistophora anthropophthera* n. sp. (Protozoa: Microsporidia). J Eukaryot Microbiol 45:273–283, 1998.
136. Cali A, Takvorian PM: Ultrastructure and development of *Pleistophora ronneafiei* n. sp., a microsporidium (Protista) in the skeletal muscle of an immune-compromised individual. J Eukaryot Microbiol 50:77–85, 2003.
137. Chupp GL, Alroy J, Adelman LS, et al: Myositis due to Pleistophora (Microsporidia) in a patient with AIDS. Clin Infect Dis 16:15–21, 1993.
138. Grau A, Valls ME, Williams JE, et al: Myositis caused by Pleistophora in a patient with AIDS. Med Clin (Barc) 107:779–781, 1996.
139. Macher AR, Neafie R, Angritt P, et al: Microsporidia myositis and the acquired immunodeficiency syndrome (AIDS): A four year follow-up. Ann Intern Med 109:343–344, 1988.
140. Margileth AM, Strano AJ, Chandra R, et al: Disseminated nosematosis in an immunologically compromised infant. Arch Pathol 95:145–150, 1973.
141. Deplazes P, Mathis A, van Saanen M, et al: Dual microsporidial infection due to *Vittaforma corneae* and *Encephalitozoon hellem* in a patient with AIDS. Clin Infect Dis 27:1521–1524, 1998.
142. Visvesvara GS, Belloso M, Moura H, et al: Isolation of *Nosema algerae* from the cornea of an immunocompetent patient. J Eukaryot Microbiol 46:10S, 1999.
143. Desportes-Livage I, Doumbo O, Pichard E, et al: Microsporidiosis in HIV-seronegative patients in Mali. Trans R Soc Trop Med Hyg 92:423–424, 1998.
144. Lopez-Velez R, Turrientes MC, Garron C, et al: Microsporidiosis in travelers with diarrhea from the tropics. J Travel Med 6:223–237, 1999.
145. Muller A, Bialek R, Kamper A, et al: Detection of microsporidia in travelers with diarrhea. J Clin Microbiol 39:1630–1632, 2001.
146. Orenstein JM, Chiang J, Steinberg W, et al: Intestinal microsporidiosis as a cause of diarrhea in human immunodeficiency virus–infected patients: A report of 20 cases. Hum Pathol 21:475–481, 1990.
147. Tumwine JK, Kekitiinwa A, Nabukeera N, et al: *Enterocytozoon bieneusi* among children with diarrhea attending Mulago Hospital in Uganda. Am J Trop Med Hyg 67:299–303, 2002.
148. Ledford DK, Overman MD, Gonzalvo A, et al: Microsporidiosis myositis in a patient with the acquired immunodeficiency syndrome. Ann Intern Med 102:628–630, 1985.
149. Coyle CM, Weiss LM, Rhodes LV 3rd, et al: Fatal myositis due to the microsporidian Brachiola algerae, a mosquito pathogen. N Engl J Med 351:42–47, 2004.
150. Pinnolis M, Egbert PR, Font RL, et al: Nosematosis of the cornea: Case report, including electron microscopic studies. Arch Ophthalmol 99:1044–1047, 1981.
151. Ashton N, Wirasinha PA: Encephalitozoonosis (nosematosis) of the cornea. Br J Ophthalmol 57:669–674, 1973.
152. Cali A, Meisler DM, Lowder CY, et al: Corneal microsporidioses: Characterization and identification. J Protozool 38:215S–217S, 1991.
153. Shadduck JA, Meccoli RA, Davis R, et al: Isolation of a microsporidian from a human patient. J Infect Dis 162:773–776, 1990.

154. Davis RM, Font RL, Keisler MS, et al: Corneal microsporidiosis. A case report including ultrastructural observations. Ophthalmology 97:953–957, 1990.
155. Chan CM, Theng JT, Li L, et al: Microsporidial keratoconjunctivitis in healthy individuals: A case series. Ophthalmology 110:1420–1425, 2003.
156. Schwartz DA, Abou-Elella A, Wilcox CM, et al: The presence of *Enterocytozoon bieneusi* spores in the lamina propria of small bowel biopsies with no evidence of disseminated microsporidiosis. Enteric Opportunistic Infections Working Group. Arch Pathol Lab Med 119:424–428, 1995.
157. Orenstein JM, Dieterich DT, Kotler DP: Systemic dissemination by a newly recognized intestinal microsporidia species in AIDS. AIDS 6:1143–1150, 1992.
158. Gunnarsson G, Hurlbut D, DeGirolami PC, et al: Multiorgan microsporidiosis: Report of five cases and review. Clin Infect Dis 21:37–44, 1995.
159. Schwartz DA, Visvesvara GS, Leitch GJ, et al: Pathology of symptomatic microsporidial (*Encephalitozoon hellem*) bronchiolitis in the acquired immunodeficiency syndrome: A new respiratory pathogen diagnosed from lung biopsy, bronchoalveolar lavage, sputum, and tissue culture. Hum Pathol 24:937–943, 1993.
160. Didier ES, Rogers LB, Orenstein JM, et al: Characterization of *Encephalitozoon (Septata) intestinalis* isolates cultured from nasal mucosa and bronchoalveolar lavage fluids of two AIDS patients. J Eukaryot Microbiol 43:34–43, 1996.
161. Dunand VA, Hammer SM, Rossi R, et al: Parasitic sinusitis and otitis in patients infected with human immunodeficiency virus: Report of five cases and review. Clin Infect Dis 25:267–272, 1997.
162. Franzen C, Muller A, Salzberger B, et al: Chronic rhinosinusitis in patients with AIDS: Potential role of microsporidia. AIDS 10:687–688, 1996.
163. Gritz DC, Holsclaw DS, Neger RE, et al: Ocular and sinus microsporidial infection cured with systemic albendazole. Am J Ophthalmol 124:241–243, 1997.
164. Josephson GD, Sarlin J, Reidy J, et al: Microsporidial rhinosinusitis: Is this the next pathogen to infect the sinuses of the immunocompromised host? Otolaryngol Head Neck Surg 114:137–139, 1996.
165. Moss RB, Beaudet LM, Wenig BM, et al: Microsporidium-associated sinusitis. Ear Nose Throat J 76:95–101, 1997.
166. Pedro-de-Lelis FJ, Sabater-Marco V, Herrera-Ballester A: Necrotizing maxillary sinus mucormycosis related to candidiasis and microsporidiosis in an AIDS patient. AIDS 9:1386–1388, 1995.
167. Didier ES, Didier PJ, Friedberg DN, et al: Isolation and characterization of a new human microsporidian, *Encephalitozoon hellem* (n. sp.) from three AIDS patients with keratoconjunctivitis. J Infect Dis 163:617–621, 1991.
168. Cali A, Meisler DM, Rutherford I, et al: Corneal microsporidiosis in a patient with AIDS. Am J Trop Med Hyg 44:463–468, 1991.
169. Weber R, Bryan RT, Owen RL, et al: Improved light-microscopal detection of microsporidia spores in stool and duodenal aspirates. N Engl J Med 326:161–166, 1992.
170. Ryan NJ, Sutherland G, Coughlan K, et al: A new trichrome-blue stain for detection of microsporidial species in urine, stool, and nasopharyngeal specimens. J Clin Microbiol 31:3264–3269, 1993.
171. Moura H, Schwartz DA, Bornay-Llinares F, et al: A new and improved "quick-hot Gram-chromotrope" technique that differentially stains microsporidian spores in clinical samples, including paraffin-embedded tissue sections. Arch Pathol Lab Med 121:888–893, 1997.
172. Vavra J, Dahbiova R, Hollister WS, et al: Staining of microsporidian spores by optical brighteners with remarks on the use of brighteners for the diagnosis of AIDS associated human microsporidioses. Folia Parasitol (Praha) 40:267–272, 1993.
173. van Gool T, Snijders F, Reiss P, et al: Diagnosis of intestinal and disseminated microsporidial infections in patients with HIV by a new rapid fluorescence technique. J Clin Pathol 46:694–699, 1993.
174. Didier ES, Orenstein JM, Aldras A, et al: Comparison of three staining methods for detecting microsporidia in fluids. J Clin Microbiol 33:3138–3145, 1995.
175. Field AS, Marriott DJ, Hing MC: The Warthin–Starry stain in the diagnosis of small intestinal microsporidiosis in HIV-infected patients. Folia Parasitol (Praha) 40:261–266, 1993.
176. Field AS: Light microscopic and electron microscopic diagnosis of gastrointestinal opportunistic infections in HIV-positive patients. Pathology 34:21–35, 2002.
177. Weiss LM, Cali A, Levee E, et al: Diagnosis of *Encephalitozoon cuniculi* infection by Western blot and the use of cross-reactive antigens for the possible detection of microsporidiosis in humans. Am J Trop Med Hyg 47:456–462, 1992.
178. Zierdt CH, Gill VJ, Zierdt WS: Detection of microsporidian spores in clinical samples by indirect fluorescent-antibody assay using whole-cell antisera to *Encephalitozoon cuniculi* and *Encephalitozoon hellem*. J Clin Microbiol 31:3071–3074, 1993.
179. Croppo GP, Visvesvara GS, Leitch GJ, et al: Identification of the microsporidian *Encephalitozoon hellem* using immunoglobulin G monoclonal antibodies. Arch Pathol Lab Med 122:182–186, 1998.
180. Beckers PJ, Derks GJ, Gool T, et al: *Encephalocytozoon intestinalis*-specific monoclonal antibodies for laboratory diagnosis of microsporidiosis. J Clin Microbiol 34:282–285, 1996.
181. Accoceberry I, Thellier M, Desportes-Livage I, et al: Production of monoclonal antibodies directed against the microsporidium *Enterocytozoon bieneusi*. J Clin Microbiol 37:4107–4112, 1999.
182. Didier ES: Immunology of microsporidiosis. Contrib Microbiol 6:193–208, 2000.
183. Katzwinkel-Wladarsch S, Deplazes P, Weber R, et al: Comparison of polymerase chain reaction with light microscopy for detection of microsporida in clinical specimens. Eur J Clin Microbiol Infect Dis 16:7–10, 1997.
184. Fedorko DP, Nelson NA, Cartwright CP: Identification of microsporidia in stool specimens by using PCR and restriction endonucleases. J Clin Microbiol 33:1739–1741, 1995.
185. Ombrouck C, Ciceron L, Biligui S, et al: Specific PCR assay for direct detection of intestinal microsporidia *Enterocytozoon bieneusi* and *Encephalitozoon intestinalis* in fecal specimens from human immunodeficiency virus-infected patients. J Clin Microbiol 35:652–655, 1997.
186. Franzen C, Muller A: Molecular techniques for detection, species differentiation, and phylogenetic analysis of microsporidia. Clin Microbiol Rev 12:243–285, 1999.
187. Visvesvara GS: In vitro cultivation of microsporidia of clinical importance. Clin Microbiol Rev 15:401–413, 2002.
188. Visvesvara GS, da Silva AJ, Croppo GP, et al: In vitro culture and serologic and molecular identification of *Septata intestinalis* isolated from urine of a patient with AIDS. J Clin Microbiol 33:930–936, 1995.
189. Costa SF, Weiss LM: Drug treatment of microsporidiosis. Drug Resist Update 3:384–399, 2000.
190. Blanshard C, Ellis DS, Tovey DG, et al: Treatment of intestinal microsporidiosis with albendazole in patients with AIDS. AIDS 6:311–313, 1992.
191. Blanshard C, Peacock C, Ellis D, et al: Treatment of intestinal microsporidiosis with Albendazole. VII International Conference on AIDS: Science Challenging AIDS, Florence, Italy, July 16–21, 1991.
192. Dieterich DT, Lew EA, Kotler DP, et al: Treatment with Albendazole for intestinal disease due to *Enterocytozoon bieneusi* in patients with AIDS. J Infect Dis 169:178–183, 1994.
193. Leder K, Ryan N, Spelman D, et al: Microsporidial disease in HIV-infected patients: A report of 42 patients and review of the literature. Scand J Infect Dis 30:331–338, 1998.
194. Kano T, Fukui H: Studies on Pleistophora infection in eel, *Anguilla japonica* I. Experimental induction of microsporidiosis and fumagillin efficacy. Fish Pathol 16:193–200, 1982.
195. Higgins MJ, Kent ML, Moran JD, et al: Efficacy of the fumagillin analog TNP-470 for *Nucleospora salmonis* and *Loma salmonae* infections in Chinook salmon *Oncorhynchus tshawytscha*. Dis Aquat Organ 34:45–49, 1998.
196. Molina JM, Goguel J, Sarfati C, et al: Trial of oral fumagillin for the treatment of intestinal microsporidiosis in patients with HIV infection. ANRS 054 Study Group. Agence Nationale de Recherche sur le SIDA. AIDS 14:1341–1348, 2000.
197. Molina JM, Tourneur M, Sarfati C, et al: Fumagillin treatment of intestinal microsporidiosis. N Engl J Med 346:1963–1969, 2002.
198. Molina JM, Goguel J, Sarfati C, et al: Potential efficacy of fumagillin in intestinal microsporidiosis due to *Enterocytozoon bieneusi* in patients with HIV infection: Results of a drug screening study. The French Microsporidiosis Study Group. AIDS 11:1603–1610, 1997.

199. Diesenhouse MC, Wilson LA, Corrent GF, et al: Treatment of microsporidial keratoconjunctivitis with topical fumagillin. Am J Ophthalmol 115:293–298, 1993.
200. Didier ES: Effects of albendazole, fumagillin, and TNP-470 on microsporidial replication in vitro. Antimicrob Agents Chemother 41:1541–1546, 1997.
201. Coyle C, Kent M, Tanowitz HB, et al: TNP-470 is an effective antimicrosporidial agent. J Infect Dis 177:515–518, 1998.
202. Eeftinck Schattenkerk JK, van Gool T, van Ketel RJ, et al: Clinical significance of small-intestinal microsporidiosis in HIV-1-infected individuals. Lancet 337:895–898, 1991.
203. Foudraine NA, Weverling GJ, van Gool T, et al: Improvement of chronic diarrhoea in patients with advanced HIV-1 infection during potent antiretroviral therapy. AIDS 12:35–41, 1998.
204. Goguel J, Katlama C, Sarfati C, et al: Remission of AIDS-associated intestinal microsporidiosis with highly active antiretroviral therapy. AIDS 11:1658–1659, 1997.
205. Maggi P, Larocca AM, Quarto M, et al: Effect of antiretroviral therapy on cryptosporidiosis and microsporidiosis in patients infected with human immunodeficiency virus type 1. Eur J Clin Microbiol Infect Dis 19:213–217, 2000.
206. Martins SA, Muccioli C, Belfort R Jr, et al: Resolution of microsporidial keratoconjunctivitis in an AIDS patient treated with highly active antiretroviral therapy. Am J Ophthalmol 131:378–379, 2001.
207. Miao YM, Awad-El-Kariem FM, Franzen C, et al: Eradication of cryptosporidia and microsporidia following successful antiretroviral therapy. J Acquir Immune Defic Syndr 25:124–129, 2000.
208. Molina JM, Chastang C, Goguel J, et al: Albendazole for treatment and prophylaxis of microsporidiosis due to *Encephalitozoon intestinalis* in patients with AIDS: A randomized double-blind controlled trial. J Infect Dis 177:1373–1377, 1998.
209. Sobottka I, Albrecht H, Schafer H, et al: Disseminated *Encephalitozoon (Septata) intestinalis* infection in a patient with AIDS: Novel diagnostic approaches and autopsy-confirmed parasitological cure following treatment with albendazole. J Clin Microbiol 33:2948–2952, 1995.
210. Lecuit M, Oksenhendler E, Sarfati C: Use of albendazole for disseminated microsporidian infection in a patient with AIDS. J Infect Dis 19:332–333, 1994.
211. Visvesvara GS, Leitch GJ, Dasilva AJ, et al: Polyclonal and monoclonal antibody and PCR-amplified small-subunit rRNA identification of a microsporidian, *Encephalitozoon hellem*, isolated from an AIDS patient with disseminated infection. J Clin Microbiol 32:2760–2768, 1994.
212. Corcoran GD, Isaacson JR, Daniels C, et al: Urethritis associated with disseminated microsporidiosis: Clinical response to albendazole. Clin Infect Dis 22:592–593, 1996.
213. Aarons EJ, Woodrow D, Hollister WS, et al: Reversible renal failure caused by a microsporidian infection. AIDS 8:1119–1121, 1994.
214. Rosberger DF, Serdarevic ON, Erlandson RA, et al: Successful treatment of microsporidial keratoconjunctivitis with topical fumagillin in a patient with AIDS. Cornea 12:261–265, 1993.
215. Wilkins JH, Joshi N, Margolis TP, et al: Microsporidial keratoconjunctivitis treated successfully with a short course of fumagillin. Eye 8:703–704, 1994.
216. Garvey MJ, Ambrose PG, Ulmer JL: Topical fumagillin in the treatment of microsporidial keratoconjunctivitis in AIDS. Ann Pharmacother 29:872–874, 1995.
217. Lowder CY, McMahon JT, Meisler DM, et al: Microsporidial keratoconjunctivitis caused by *Septata intestinalis* in a patient with acquired immunodeficiency syndrome. Am J Ophthalmol 121:715–717, 1996.
218. Albrecht H, Sobottka I, Stellbrink HJ, et al: Does the choice of *Pneumocystis carinii* prophylaxis influence the prevalence of *Enterocytozoon bieneusi* microsporidiosis in AIDS patients? AIDS 9:302–303, 1995.
219. Conteas CN, Berlin OG, Speck CE, et al: Modification of the clinical course of intestinal microsporidiosis in acquired immunodeficiency syndrome patients by immune status and anti-human immunodeficiency virus therapy. Am J Trop Med Hyg 58:555–558, 1998.

97

Systemic Coccidia (Toxoplasmosis)

JOSEPH D. SCHWARTZMAN
JAMES H. MAGUIRE

INTRODUCTION

Toxoplasma gondii is a versatile intracellular parasite that has adapted to infect many animal species and is capable of causing a wide spectrum of disease, the preponderance of which is asymptomatic.[1–3] Active invasion of host cells leads to their eventual death; a complex interplay of the host cell–mediated immune response arrests the acute infection and maintains continued suppression of the persistent encysted zoites, usually for the life of the host. The wide host range of *T. gondii* is an exception to the rule of most other members of the phylum Apicomplexa. *Toxoplasma* also has a wide geographic range: its single species is found worldwide, with the exception of a very few isolated islands. The ability to infect many species by at least two routes and its broad distribution are responsible for the high prevalence of infection in the human population; perhaps a third of the world's people are chronically infected by *T. gondii*. The spectrum of disease caused by *T. gondii* does not differ with its geographic distribution. Serious illness is unusual except among persons with deficient cell-mediated immunity and infants infected in utero. Toxoplasmosis is an economically important cause of abortion in sheep, swine, and goats.[4,5]

AGENT

History and Taxonomy

In 1908, Nicolle and Manceaux[6] in Tunis identified *T. gondii* in a laboratory rodent, the North African gondi. In the same year, Splendore[7] noted identical forms in a laboratory rabbit in Brazil. Understanding of the importance of this parasite for humans did not come until 1937 when Wolf and Cowen[8] in New York identified it as a cause of "granulomatous encephalomyelitis." Appreciation of the role of chronic infection came with the identification by Wilder[9] in the 1950s of *Toxoplasma* in eyes previously thought to have been involved with tuberculosis or syphilis. The high prevalence of the infection was only realized after the serologic dye test was developed by Sabin and Feldman[10] in 1948. Congenital toxoplasmosis in infants was recognized before either generalized disease in adults or the lymphadenitis of primary *Toxoplasma* infections in adults was appreciated.[8] The role of reactivation of latent infections in the production of disease in immunosuppressed adults was recognized at the outset of solid organ transplantation.[11] The onset of acquired immunodeficiency syndrome (AIDS) brought recognition of central nervous system (CNS) reactivation causing multifocal encephalitis.[12]

T. gondii is a genetically homogeneous single species with a clonal population structure.[13] Three genetic types make up 95% of isolates from all continents.[14,15] Type II strains, defined on the basis of extensive genotyping, are most commonly recovered from humans with both congenital and acquired toxoplasmosis.[14] Type I stains are more virulent in outbred mice, more frequent in congenital infections in some geographic areas,[16] and along with "atypical" strains (recombinant genotypes of type I and type II strains) are overrepresented in serious ocular infections.[17] Genetic evidence suggests that the clonal lineages arose approximately 10,000 years ago and spread rapidly perhaps because of concurrent acquisition of efficient oral infectivity.[18–20]

Life Cycle

The asexual stages of *T. gondii* are pathogenic for man and animals.[21] Two forms are produced, a rapidly dividing, invasive tachyzoite in all tissues, and a slowly dividing bradyzoite in cysts predominantly found in brain and muscle[1,22] (Figs. 97-1 and 97-2). Tachyzoite replication causes acute disease, while the bradyzoite cyst is long-lived, with slow turnover, and is responsible for latency and reactivation. Reservoirs of human infection are birds and rodents ingested by cats, as well as human food animals, especially pigs, goats, and sheep, which can carry orally infectious cysts in meat.[4,5,23] The sexual stage is found in the small intestinal epithelium of both wild and domestic Felidae. Oocysts, the end product of the sexual cycle, are resistant to environmental conditions, tend to float in watered soils, and thereby remain in the superficial layers where they may be ingested by contamination of vegetables or hands.[24,25] Oocysts sporulate within 12 to 24 hours to several days after passage from the cat and are thereafter infectious.

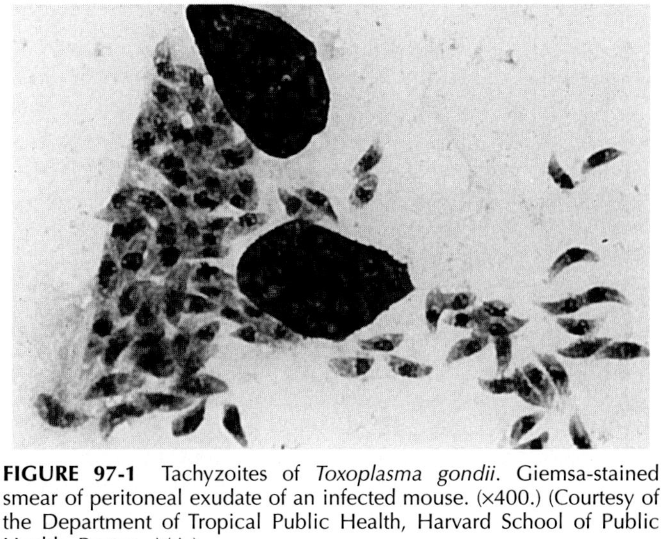

FIGURE 97-1 Tachyzoites of *Toxoplasma gondii*. Giemsa-stained smear of peritoneal exudate of an infected mouse. (×400.) (Courtesy of the Department of Tropical Public Health, Harvard School of Public Health, Boston, MA.)

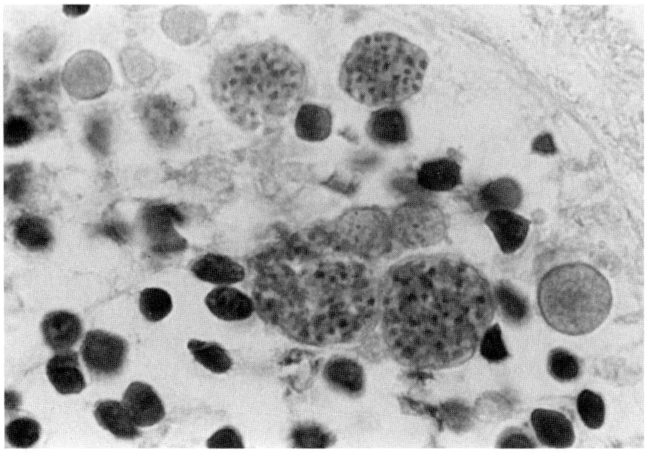

FIGURE 97-2 Congenital toxoplasmosis. Tissue cysts in uvea of human eye with numerous intracellular bradyzoites. (Hematoxylin and eosin, ×1000.) (Courtesy of the Department of Tropical Public Health, Harvard School of Public Health, Boston, MA.)

ECOLOGY, EPIDEMIOLOGY, AND DISTRIBUTION

Humans may be infected both by eating cysts in meat and by ingestion of oocysts from contaminated soil. The relative risk of infection in industrialized countries is considered to be higher from the ingestion of undercooked meat, epecially lamb and beef, but in societies with little meat in the diet, oocysts are more important.[26] Birds and rodents are important in picking up oocysts from soil and scavenging bradyzoite cysts from infected animals.[1,27] Grazing food animals (e.g., sheep) are probably infected by soil oocysts, but swine are omnivores and may also ingest infected rodents.[3–5] The prevalence of *Toxoplasma* in swine is quite variable. Bovine and fowl *Toxoplasma* levels are low, but the high consumption of beef may explain the association with acquired toxoplasmosis.[28–29] Although sexual recombination has been shown to take place in cats, it appears to be rare in nature.[17,24,25,30] The distribution of *T. gondii* is worldwide; all genotypes are found on all continents except Antarctica. Islands without *T. gondii* have been found in the Pacific, and along the coast of Central America.[26,31,32] Hot, dry climates have a lower incidence of toxoplasmosis than temperate, moist climates, and rates are low at high altitudes.[26,33,34] Geographic foci of transmission by oocysts (cat cycle) have been described in societies that do not consume meat.[35] The role of the cat in the transmission of toxoplasmosis is established, but the epidemiology of transmission includes the possible role of dogs. Dogs have been proposed as vectors of oocysts based on associations in epidemiologic surveys and their habit of rolling in cat feces or eating cat feces.[27] River water contaminated with oocysts was believed to be the source of an outbreak in a Panamanian jungle.[36] Public water supplies were implicated in an outbreak in British Columbia, and drinking unfiltered municipal and surface water were associated with a high level of endemicity in Rio de Janeiro State, Brazil.[31,32] *Toxoplasma* infection also is acquired by transplacental transmission[2] and, less commonly, through organ transplantation[11] and laboratory accident.[37] Although *Toxoplasma* DNA can be detected by polymerase chain reaction (PCR) in blood from chronically infected persons,[38] transmission of toxoplasmosis by transfusion of banked blood has not posed a public health problem.[39] Man is a dead-end host for *T. gondii*, which is of importance in the potential epidemiology of drug resistance.

Serologic surveys demonstrate prevalences of infection from less than 10% to greater than 90% in various geographic locations.[2,40–50] In parts of France, where rates of infection may exceed 90% by the fourth decade,[2,40,41] transmission appears to be related to ingestion of rare or raw meat. In contrast, rates in England and Finland are approximately 20%.[42,43] In moist tropical areas of Latin America and sub-Saharan Africa, where cats are abundant and the climate favors survival of oocysts, the prevalence may approach 90%.[26,27,44–48] In comparison, rates in hot, dry regions such as North Africa usually do not exceed 20%.[49] Rates in the United States also vary, ranging from 3% in Denver, Colorado, to 17% in Massachusetts, and to 30% in Birmingham, Alabama.[2,50] The seroprevalence of toxoplasmosis among persons aged 12 to 49 years in the United States remained stable at around 16% throughout the 1990s.[51]

PATHOGENESIS, PATHOLOGY, AND CLINICAL MANIFESTATIONS

Primary Disease

The primary route of infection is oral, with progression of the infection through the gastrointestinal tract to local lymphatics and spread to other organs documented in the mouse, but this has not been followed step by step in humans.[2,22,50,52] In mice fed bradyzoites, the first step appears to be local invasion of the small intestinal epithelium. The bradyzoite and tachyzoite are both capable of active invasion of many cell types and replicate within a parasite-modified vacuole.[52–58] Bradyzoites rapidly convert to tachyzoites in vivo. In vitro, the formation of bradyzoite cysts can be stimulated by various maneuvers that stress the infected cells.[59,60] The key step in spreading the infection from the localized initial site is likely infection of circulating monocytes in the lamina propria; this cell subset has been shown to be permissive for *T. gondii* replication in both mice and humans and may therefore be responsible for transport of the parasite widely throughout tissues.[22,52,61]

Tachyzoites are found in all organs in acute infection, most prominently in muscle, including heart, and in the liver, spleen, lymph nodes, and the CNS.[2,50,52] The initial pathologic lesion is necrosis caused by death of parasitized cells, with a vigorous acute inflammatory reaction. As the disease progresses, more lymphocytic infiltration develops, but true granulomas are not formed. If the host controls the replication of tachyzoites effectively, tissues are restored to anatomical integrity without scarring, and cysts containing the long-lived bradyzoites remain without sign of host reaction.[62] The humoral immune response is rapid and may be capable of killing extracellular tachyzoites (and is of use diagnostically), but it is not protective in the mouse model.[61] Control of the disease appears to depend on the elaboration of appropriate cytokines including interleukin (IL)-2, IL-12, and interferon-γ (INF-γ)[63–65] followed by a specific cell-mediated immunity with CD8+ helper T cells apparently the most important subgroup.[66–68] In some experimental infections, there is intense acute inflammation with few identifiable parasites and early death, which

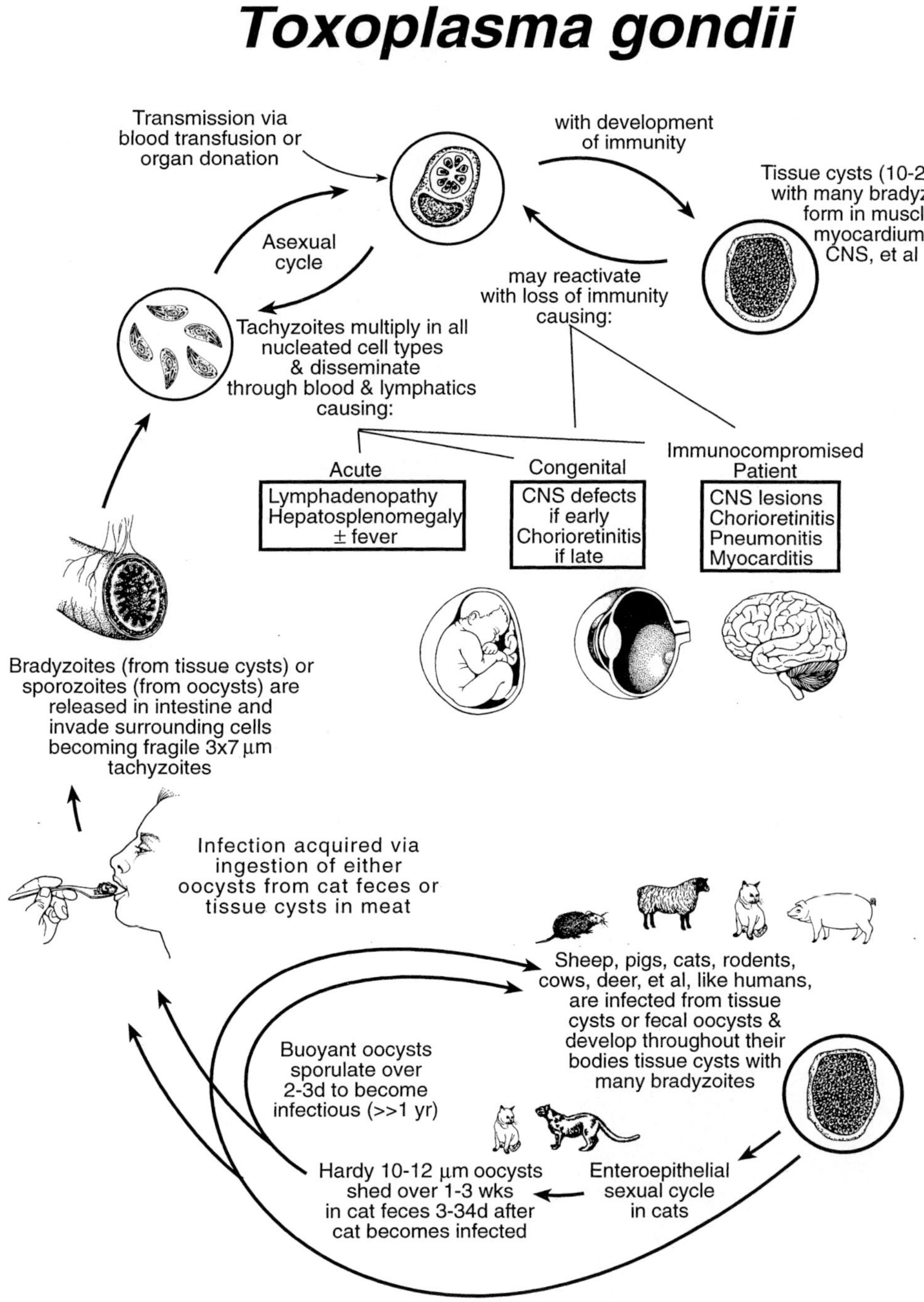

may be caused by an overly vigorous cytokine response to the infection.[69]

Subclinical or unrecognized infection is the usual outcome of primary infection in immunocompetent persons.[1,2,36,70–75] When symptoms occur, the most common manifestation is painless lymphadenopathy, with or without fever.[50,74] Usually a single cervical node is enlarged, but there may be multiple enlarged nodes at one site or generalized lymphadenopathy. Toxoplasmic lymphadenopathy may persist for 4 to 6 weeks, raising the suspicion of lymphoma.[74,76] Occasionally, a syndrome of fever, headache, malaise, myalgia, lymphadenopathy, hepatosplenomegaly, and atypical lymphocytosis develops after an incubation period of 5 to 20 days.[36,71–73] The course of illness may last weeks or months, suggesting a diagnosis of infectious mononucleosis. Pneumonitis, myocarditis, meningoencephalitis, polymyositis, and death are rare complications in otherwise healthy persons.[77,78] In Brazil and British Columbia, a high incidence of acute acquired retinochoroiditis has been described.[79,80] Retinochoroiditis in primary acute infection is more common than previously has been considered and may be associated with particular genotypes.[81]

Congenital Disease

Primary infection of the mother and infection of the placenta is the mechanism by which almost all congenital disease is transmitted.[2,34,82–84] The placenta is an imperfect barrier to infection of the fetus and allows transmission to the fetus in 30% to 50% of infections acquired during pregnancy.[2,82] Congenital infection is exceptionally rare when the mother acquires infection before gestation,[85,86] and most of the few reported cases have occurred when maternal infection occurred within 3 months of conception or in the setting of maternal immunosuppression due to human immunodeficiency virus (HIV) infection or immunosuppressive therapy.[87,88] Acute infection is apparent in fewer than 20% of mothers, but both symptomatic and asymptomatic infections place the fetus at risk. The rate of transplacental transmission and the severity of disease vary with time of gestation.[2,87] If maternal infection occurs during the first trimester, the risk of fetal infection is only around 10%, but disease is usually severe. Rates of congenital infection rise to about 65% for maternal infection during the third trimester and approach 100% at term, but neonatal infection in these instances usually is asymptomatic.[34]

Overall, fewer than 15% of infants with congenital toxoplasmosis have severe impairment of the brain or eyes, and about 80% are asymptomatic at birth or have mild disease that is not detected by routine physical examination.[82,89–92] However, more than 85% of those with asymptomatic infection will develop adverse sequelae of the CNS or eyes in subsequent years.[91,92]

Early fetal infections lead to spontaneous abortion, stillbirth, or severe neonatal disease.[2,52,84] In the brain, there are foci of necrosis, microglial nodules, and perivascular mononuclear inflammation in association with free and intracellular tachyzoites.[2,52] Vascular thrombosis may lead to large areas of coagulation necrosis. Necrosis around ventricles or the aqueduct of Sylvius may lead to hydrocephalus, and areas of necrotic brain become calcified. Neurologic sequelae include seizures, psychomotor retardation, deafness, hydrocephalus, microcephalus, and prominent intracerebral calcifications visible on radiographs (Fig. 97-3). A common feature of severe congenital toxoplasmosis is bilateral retinochoroiditis manifested by necrosis of the retina and granulomatous inflammation of the choroid.[93] Lesions are near to or in the macula, and vitritis and uveitis are frequently present. There may be micro-ophthalmia, strabismus, cataracts, glaucoma, and optic atrophy. Systemic manifestations such as fever, hypothermia, jaundice, vomiting, diarrhea, lymphadenopathy, hepatosplenomegaly, pneumonitis, myocarditis, and rash may be present.[2,90] Laboratory studies show anemia, thrombocytopenia, high cerebrospinal fluid (CSF) protein, and CSF pleocytosis.

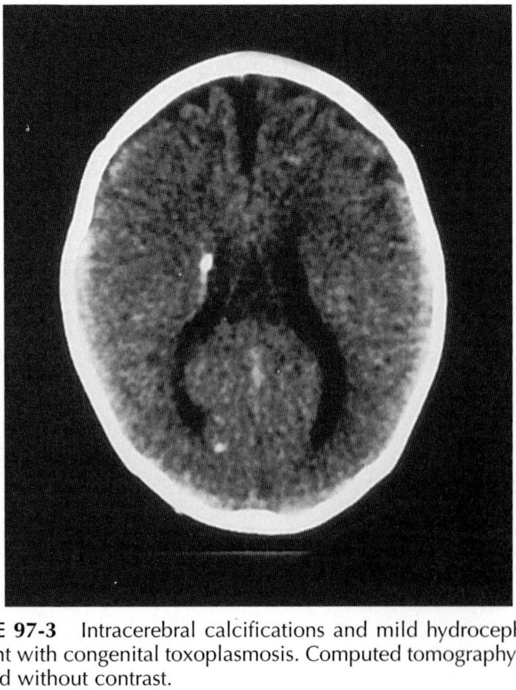

FIGURE 97-3 Intracerebral calcifications and mild hydrocephalus in an infant with congenital toxoplasmosis. Computed tomography scan of the head without contrast.

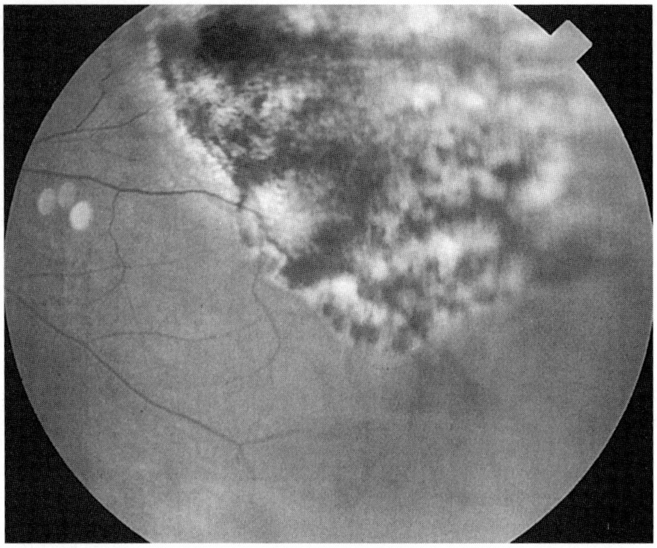

FIGURE 97-4 Healed retinochoroiditis in the periphery of the fundus of the eye of an adult who had documented congenital toxoplasmosis.

While the majority of infants who acquire infection late in pregnancy appear normal at birth, meticulous examination often shows abnormalities such as retinal scars (Fig. 97-4) or abnormal CSF.[89,90] Healthy-appearing infants occasionally develop severe CNS or ocular disease during the first months of life. More commonly, persons with asymptomatic infections at birth experience recurrent episodes of retinochoroiditis or impaired psychomotor development during the first 10 to 20 years of life.[91,92]

Ocular Disease

Toxoplasmosis may account for as many as one third of cases of retinochoroiditis.[93–95] Most cases occur in teenagers and young adults and in the past have been ascribed to reactivation of congenitally acquired infection. Population-based studies in southern Brazil and recent experience with clusters of acute disease in adults have shown that acquired infection may account for more cases of retinochoroiditis than congenital infection.[79–81,96,97] Active disease causes pain, photophobia, and blurred vision in the absence of constitutional symptoms. On funduscopic examination, the vitreous is hazy, and elevated, pale-yellow, or white cotton-like patches are seen in the retina. Healed scars are pale with distinct margins and prominent black spots of choroidal pigment. Recurrent retinochoroiditis usually occurs at the borders of scars and may lead to blindness.

Disease in Persons with AIDS and Other Causes of Immunodeficiency

Toxoplasmosis is life-threatening for persons with impaired cellular immunity, in particular those with HIV infections and CD4+ T-cell counts less than 100/μL of blood and persons receiving immunosuppressive medications.[11,12,98] Disease in these persons is more commonly due to reactivation of chronic infection than to newly acquired infection.[99,100] Historically, approximately one-third or more of AIDS patients with antibodies to *Toxoplasma* reactivated their latent infection, but with the widespread use of antimicrobial drugs to prevent *Pneumocystis jirovecii* pneumonia and highly active antiretroviral therapy (HAART), the incidence of reactivation and toxoplasmosis-associated deaths has decreased.[101,102] Because of the high prevalence of chronic *Toxoplasma* infection in tropical climates, reactivated toxoplasmosis is a more frequently observed opportunistic infection among HIV-infected immigrants from developing regions than among HIV-infected natives of industrialized countries.[103] In many tropical regions, reactivation of toxoplasmosis is less common than might be expected because of the short life expectancy of HIV-infected persons due to other causes.[104] Persons who receive chemotherapy for organ transplantation or treatment of lymphomas and leukemia are particularly susceptible to toxoplasmosis, although rates of reactivation in these persons are not as great as those among persons with AIDS.[11,105,106] Transplantation of *Toxoplasma*-infected organs (especially hearts) places antibody-negative recipients at risk of severe generalized toxoplasmosis.[107–109] Immunodeficient persons who receive leukocyte transfusions are also at risk of acquiring toxoplasmosis.[110]

The predominant manifestation of toxoplasmosis in immunocompromised persons is multifocal necrotizing encephalitis[12,98,99] (Fig. 97-5). Patients present with altered level of consciousness, headache, focal neurologic deficits, seizures, and often fever. Computed tomography (CT) and magnetic resonance (MR) scans of the head typically demonstrate multiple low-density lesions at the corticomedullary junction or in the basal ganglia that enhance following the administration of intravenous contrast (Fig. 97-6). There is often a mononuclear CSF pleocytosis and mild elevation of protein, but meningeal signs are uncommon. After the brain, the lungs and heart are the next most frequently involved organs in immunocompromised persons. Toxoplasmic myocarditis is frequently subclinical,[111] while a syndrome of rapidly progressive pulmonary infiltrates and shock may evolve when there is pulmonary infection.[112,113] Generalized toxoplasmosis is also seen in immunocompromised patients, and involvement of liver, spleen, lymph nodes, pancreas, intestines, thyroid, peritoneum, testes, retina, and spinal cord has been documented.[98,99,114–116] Without treatment, CNS toxoplasmosis and other severe forms of the disease in compromised hosts are fatal.

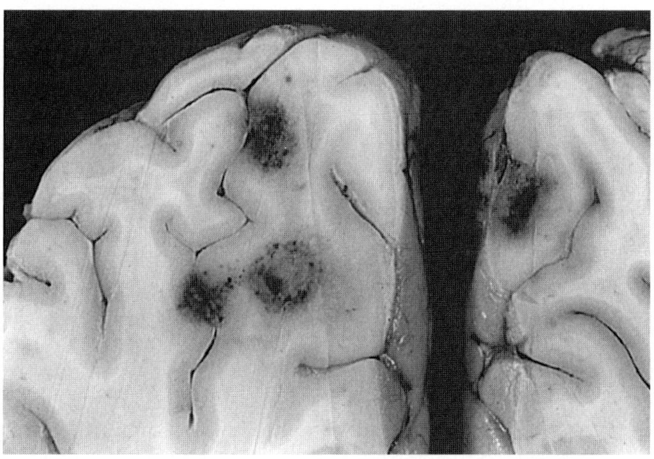

FIGURE 97-5 Section of brain showing lesions of toxoplasmosis at autopsy of a patient with acquired immunodeficiency syndrome (AIDS).

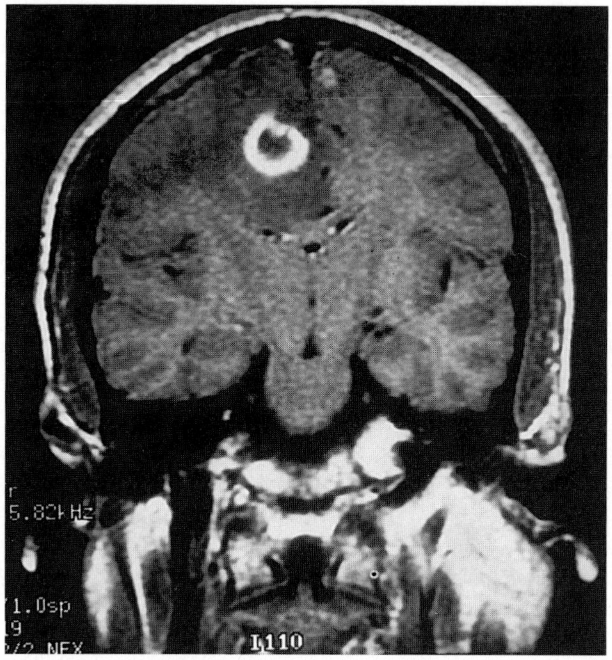

FIGURE 97-6 Magnetic resonance (MR) image of the brain showing a ring-enhancing hypodense lesion and surrounding edema in a patient with CNS toxoplasmosis and AIDS.

DIAGNOSIS

Differential Diagnosis

Because the differential diagnosis of the various forms of toxoplasmosis is broad, diagnostic confirmation in the laboratory is essential in most cases. Acute toxoplasmosis in healthy persons must be differentiated from mononucleosis due to Epstein-Barr virus or cytomegalovirus, acute HIV infection, other viral infections, cat-scratch disease, tuberculosis, fungal diseases, secondary syphilis, tularemia, African and American trypanosomiasis, visceral leishmaniasis, Hodgkin's disease, lymphoma, and sarcoidosis. The differential diagnosis of congenital toxoplasmosis includes congenital infections due to cytomegalovirus, *Herpes simplex,* rubella, *Listeria,* syphilis, *Trypanosoma cruzi,* and erythroblastosis fetalis. The clinical presentation of acute toxoplasmic retinochoroiditis can be indistinguishable from uveitis associated with syphilis, tuberculosis, leprosy, or sarcoidosis. CNS toxoplasmosis in immunocompromised persons may mimic other causes of enhancing mass lesions such as lymphoma, metastatic carcinoma, tuberculoma, and brain abscesses.

Direct Detection and Isolation of Parasites

Toxoplasma may be demonstrated on stained specimens of tissue, blood, amniotic fluid, and CSF.[117] The diagnosis of acute infection requires identification of tachyzoites, since the finding of tissue cysts does not distinguish acute from chronic infection.[52] Care is needed to distinguish *Toxoplasma* from other intracellular organisms such as *Histoplasma, Trypanosoma cruzi, Sarcocystis,* and *Leishmania*. Tachyzoites may be difficult to find in tissue sections stained with hematoxylin and eosin or other routine stains, and special techniques such as direct immunofluorescence or the peroxidase-antiperoxidase method may be necessary for their detection.[117,118] Parasites usually are not detected by microscopic examination of lymph nodes in cases of lymphadenitis, but the histopathologic changes may be sufficiently distinctive to permit a diagnosis of toxoplasmosis.[52,74]

Parasites may be recovered from both tissue cysts or tachyzoites in tissues and body fluids by inoculation into mice or tissue culture.[52,117–119] Assays based on the PCR[119] are extremely sensitive for the diagnosis of congenital toxoplasmosis when amniotic fluid is examined.[120,121] Such assays are commercially available and can also detect parasite DNA in blood,[38,122] CSF,[123] aqueous humor,[124] and fluid from bronchoalveolar lavage[125]; with variable sensitivity.

Serologic Tests

Serologic testing remains an important means of confirming infection with *Toxoplasma*. A variety of methods are sensitive and specific for the detection of IgG antibody to *T. gondii* antigens.[2,10,75,117,126–132] Thus, the serologic diagnosis of toxoplasmosis acquired in the distant past is quite reliable. The Sabin-Feldman dye test detects both IgG and IgM antibody by its ability to lyse live *T. gondii* in the presence of human complement and was for many years the gold standard.[10] Indirect fluorescent and antibody enzyme-linked immunosorbent assay (ELISA) are sensitive tests for the detection of IgG antibody and correlate well with the dye test in adults.[126] Isotype-specific ELISA for IgG, IgM, IgA, and IgE; IgM capture ELISA; immunosorbent agglutination (ISAGA); and others are available from some reference laboratories.[127–131] Results of these tests must be interpreted with age-matched populations. The IgM capture ELISA and IgM-ISAGA are sensitive for detection of specific IgM antibodies, but titers in infants less than 6 months old are lower than in adults.[129,131] While a negative IgM test nearly always rules out a recently acquired infection,[133] a positive test is less useful because commercially available tests have been reported to generate false positive results,[127,130] and specific IgM antibodies may remain detectable for greater than 1 year.[129] Determination of the functional avidity of anti-toxoplasma IgG antibody, by its ability to withstand dissociation from antigen in chaotropic salt solution, is useful in distinguishing recently acquired antibody (low avidity) from that seen in infection more than 4 months old (high avidity).[132,134,135] The IgG avidity test has become important for estimating dates of infections in pregnant women, and a commercial test based on this principal is available in Europe, but not yet in the United States. Because low-avidity results may persist for up to a year, a battery of tests including ELISA for IgM, IgA, IgE, the dye test, and differential agglutination test should be employed for interpretation of low- or equivocal avidity test results.[136] Direct agglutination of formalin- or acetone-fixed tachyzoites in the presence of 2-mercaptoethanol is thought to distinguish early antibodies (which react to acetone-fixed parasites) from those that develop later in infection (which react to formalin-fixed parasites).[136] An agglutination titer using acetone-fixed parasites that is at least one-fourth of that using formalin-fixed organisms is indicative of recent infection.

Diagnosis of Specific Syndromes

The diagnosis of suspected acute acquired toxoplasmosis usually is confirmed by demonstrating rising titers of specific IgG antibodies or by detecting specific IgM antibodies.[2] A single positive IgG test does not distinguish acute from chronic infection because antibodies to *Toxoplasma* persist indefinitely after acute infection, occasionally in high titers. Detection of specific IgM antibody in newborns by IgM-ELISA or the more sensitive IgM-ISAGA indicates congenital infection, but a negative result does not exclude the diagnosis because commonly available assays lack sensitivity to detect the low-avidity IgM antibodies synthesized by young infants.[2,89,129,131,137,138] Infants with severe toxoplasmosis at birth in particular may have negative IgM tests; in these cases, organisms usually are detected by PCR or by smears or culture of tissue, CSF, or blood.[89]

Specific IgG antibodies are nearly always present in the serum of infants with congenital toxoplasmosis. Uninfected infants born to infected mothers have specific IgG antibodies because of passive transfer of maternal IgG across the placenta, but these antibodies do not persist longer than 6 to 12 months in the absence of active infection.[138] Examination of the pattern of bands in Western blots between mothers and infants can be used to determine specific fetal antibody production.[136] In active retinochoroiditis, low titers of specific IgG antibodies are usually present, but IgM antibody in the serum is not detected.[93–95]

Immunocompromised patients with reactivation toxoplasmosis have positive specific IgG tests and negative IgM tests.[12,98] While the absence of specific IgG antibodies weighs heavily against the diagnosis of active toxoplasmosis in these patients, a positive titer does not distinguish active from latent infection. For this reason, the diagnosis of CNS toxoplasmosis in AIDS patients and other severely immunocompromised patients is usually made clinically.[12,98,138] Persons with a suggestive clinical history, positive specific IgG test, and typical radiographic findings are given a trial of anti-*Toxoplasma* chemotherapy. In cases of toxoplasmosis, clinical and radiographic improvement is seen within 7 to 10 days. A diagnostic brain biopsy is indicated if there is failure to improve within this time.[138] PCR amplification of *Toxoplasma* DNA has high predictive value, but relatively low sensitivity.[136] Brain biopsy without an antecedent therapeutic trial is indicated for immunocompromised persons with negative specific IgG tests or nonenhancing or single lesions and those who have been receiving prophylactic trimethoprim-sulfamethoxazole, because their CNS lesions are unlikely to be due to toxoplasmosis. Positron emission tomography may help distinguish

CNS lymphoma from toxoplasmosis in persons with contrast-enhancing brain lesions.[139,140]

TREATMENT

Indications and Treatment Regimens

Most immunocompetent persons with primary toxoplasmosis do not require therapy unless there is visceral disease or persistent severe symptoms.[2,141] The exception is the pregnant mother, in whom early treatment may reduce the risk of fetal infection or may reduce the severity of disease if transplacental transmission has already occurred.[2,34,121,142,143] All children with congenital toxoplasmosis should receive treatment for 1 year.[2,84,89,90,137,144] Retinochoroiditis is treated for 1 to 2 weeks after resolution of symptoms with both anti-*Toxoplasma* drugs and corticosteroids to reduce inflammation.[94,133] The frequency of recurrent episodes of retinochoroiditis may be reduced by intermittent therapy with trimethoprim-sulfamethoxazole.[145] Immunosuppressed patients require therapy to control progressive disease, and therapy must be extended for the period of cell-mediated immunosuppression to prevent relapse.[11,12,101,146]

Most drugs for treating toxoplasmosis are active only against the tachyzoite form of the parasite, although atovaquone has activity in vitro against tissue cysts as well.[147,148] Treatment even with atovaquone as a rule does not eradicate infection. Standard therapy for most indications is the combination of the oral agent pyrimethamine and a sulfonamide, which are synergistic when given together.[2,37,141,149] A loading dose of pyrimethamine 200 mg over 1 day in divided doses for adults or 2 mg/kg/day for 2 to 3 days for young children is followed by a daily dose of 1 mg/kg/day for adults or every 1 to 3 days for young children.[2,84,89,90,137,150] In immunocompromised adults with CNS toxoplasmosis or other severe disease, pyrimethamine 75 to 100 mg/day is given for 4 to 6 weeks followed by 25 to 50 mg/day for the duration of immunosuppression.[12,150,151] Sulfadiazine or triple sulfonamides are preferred over other sulfonamides, which have less activity against *T. gondii*.[2] A loading dose of 50 to 75 mg/kg for adults or 75 to 100 mg/kg for infants is followed by daily doses of 75 to 100 mg/kg/day in four divided doses for adults or 100 to 150 mg/kg/day in four divided doses for infants. Leukovorin (folinic acid) 5 to 10 mg/day should be administered simultaneously to overcome the bone marrow–suppressive effects of pyrimethamine. Persons who receive pyrimethamine should have a peripheral blood cell and platelet count at least weekly. Clindamycin 600 mg orally or intravenously four times a day in combination with pyrimethamine has been successful in the treatment of adult AIDS patients with CNS toxoplasmosis who could not tolerate sulfonamides.[151–153]

Pyrimethamine is teratogenic and should not be used during the first trimester.[2,34] The macrolide antibiotic spiramycin (3–4 g/day in divided doses) has been used safely during pregnancy.[2,34,82,142,143,154] It is not as effective as pyrimethamine and sulfonamides, but appears to reduce the rate of transplacental transmission. There is no uniformly accepted treatment regimen for congenital toxoplasmosis. Some authorities recommend standard doses of pyrimethamine and sulfonamides for 1 year, while others employ lower doses of pyrimethamine or give intermittent doses of spiramycin.[2,89,90,150,155] Other drugs that have activity against *T. gondii* include dapsone, azithromycin, clarithromycin, roxithromycin, atovaquone, minocycline, and rifabutin.[2,141]

Maintenance and Prophylactic Therapy in Immunocompromised Persons

Following treatment of active toxoplasmosis in immunocompromised patients, suppressive therapy should be continued for the duration of immunosuppression, which often is for life.[12,101,144,154,156,157] The most effective regimen is the combination of pyrimethamine 25 to 50 mg/day plus sulfadiazine 2 to 4 g/day with leukovorin 5 mg/day. This regimen also affords protection against *P. jirovecii* pneumonia. Clindamycin 300 mg to 450 mg orally three times a day has been used for persons who cannot tolerate sulfonamides.[12,151] Prophylaxis to prevent reactivation of toxoplasmosis should be given to all HIV-infected persons who have a positive serologic test for antibodies to *T. gondii* and CD4+ T-lymphocyte counts of less than 200/μL.[158,159] The combination of trimethoprim and sulfamethoxazole is effective in the same doses used to prevent *P. jirovecii* pneumonia. The combination of dapsone 50 mg/day plus pyrimethamine 50 mg/week with leukovorin 10 mg/week[157] or atovaquone 750 mg of suspension twice a day,[154] is an alternative for persons who cannot tolerate sulfonamides. The efficacy of azithromycin in preventing reactivation of toxoplasmosis is under study.[2,141] Suppressive therapy or prophylaxis for toxoplasmosis in HIV-infected patients can be safely withdrawn when the CD4+ T-lymphocyte counts has returned to greater than 200/μL and the HIV viral load has remained low for 6 months.[160]

Management of Acute Toxoplasmosis During Pregnancy

A strategy for the management of toxoplasmosis acquired by the pregnant woman has been outlined by French investigators.[2,121,132,143] When the diagnosis of acute toxoplasmosis is suspected, the mother receives spiramycin 1 g orally three or four times a day while awaiting results of confirmatory serologic tests. The purpose of spiramycin is to prevent fetal infection if this has not yet occurred. If the confirmatory studies indicate that infection may have been acquired after conception, an amniocentesis is performed as soon as possible at 17 weeks or later. Amniotic fluid is examined by a sensitive and specific PCR-based assay for *Toxoplasma*.[121] A positive assay confirms fetal infection, in which case one option is to terminate the pregnancy depending on the stage of gestation and the parents' wishes. If infection appears to have occurred late in pregnancy or if the parents wish to continue the pregnancy, pyrimethamine, sulfadiazine, and leukovorin are given until term. If the PCR assay is negative, the fetus is considered to be uninfected, and spiramycin is continued until delivery. The pregnancy is monitored closely with periodic fetal ultrasonography, and the amniocentesis is repeated if there is suspicion that fetal infection has occurred. The newborn is tested for infection at the time of delivery and treated aggressively if congenital toxoplasmosis is detected. This strategy has been shown to be effective in lowering the rate of severe congenital toxoplasmosis by identifying infections that occur early in pregnancy and that would have devastating consequences if the pregnancy were continued.[121,142,143] It is controversial whether it has otherwise achieved a significant reduction in the overall numbers of cases of congenital toxoplasmosis by reducing the rate of transplacental transmission when compared with historical data.[161,162] By identifying pregnancies in which transmission from the mother to the fetus has not occurred, it also has eliminated the need for considering termination of pregnancy on every occasion of acute maternal infection. In effect, it has spared as many as seven or eight uninfected fetuses from the possibility of therapeutic abortion for every fetus that is infected.

Variations of this strategy are practiced in countries of Europe where rates of maternal infection are high and the infrastructure exists for antenatal serologic screening of pregnant mothers to detect new infections as well as the laboratory expertise to perform accurate examination of amniotic fluid specimens. In countries such as the United States, where rates of acute maternal infection are low, this strategy is not uniformly practiced, and there is ongoing debate about its cost-effectiveness.[163–166] In several states, newborn screening for IgM antibodies to *T. gondii* is practiced to identify subclinical as well as symptomatic congenital infections soon after birth so that treatment can be given in a timely fashion to lower the risk of adverse sequelae.[50,89,131] It is not known, however, whether postnatal treatment is effective, because controlled trials have not been carried out.[167] In developing countries, where rates of maternal infections are high, the costs of antenatal screening and diagnosis or newborn screening and treatment are prohibitive.

PREVENTION AND CONTROL

Several studies have shown the efficacy of educational efforts to teach techniques for avoidance of acquisition of toxoplasmosis.[168,169] Seronegative pregnant women or immunocompromised persons should not be exposed to cat feces either in the setting of litter boxes or by digging in soils where cats have defecated.[170,171] Hands should be washed after contact with potentially contaminated soil or meat that may contain tissue cysts. Meat should be thoroughly cooked. In light of recent suggestions that dogs that roll in cat feces may carry infectious oocysts, pet grooming may be a risk factor for transmission.

One strategy for preventing human toxoplasmosis is to reduce the bradyzoite load in food animals. A commercial live vaccine is available in New Zealand and the European Union which reduces the incidence of *Toxoplasma*-induced abortion in sheep, and may reduce the load of parasites in herds under certain management schemes.[172] There is some evidence that careful husbandry practices in swine lower *Toxoplasma* burdens, including cooking feeds and excluding cats from farms.[3,5,170] A vaccine for cats that prevents oocyst shedding has been developed and tested, but is not commercially available.[173] Should it be marketed, it is not expected to have a major impact on the epidemiology of disease, but could be recommended in situations where cat owners are willing to pay to lower the risk of cat transmission. No human vaccine is available or near development.

REFERENCES

1. Frenkel JK: Transmission of toxoplasmosis and the role of immunity in limiting transmission and illness. J Am Vet Med Assoc 196:233, 1990.
2. Remington JS, McLeod R, Desmonts G: Toxoplasmosis. In Remington JS, Klein JO (eds): Infectious Diseases of the Fetus and Newborn Infant, 4th ed. Philadelphia, WB Saunders, 1995, p 140.
3. Dubey JP, Beattie CP: Toxoplasmosis in Animals and Man. Boca Raton, FL, CRC Press, 1998.
4. Dubey JP: Status of toxoplasmosis in sheep and goats in the United States. J Am Vet Med Assoc 196:259, 1990.
5. Dubey JP, Weigel RM, Siegel AM, et al: Sources and reservoirs of *Toxoplasma gondii* on 47 swine farms in Illinois. J Parasitol 81:723, 1995.
6. Nicolle C, Manceaux L: Sur une infection á corps de Leishman (ou organisme voisins) du gondi. CR Acad Sci 147:763, 1908.
7. Splendore A: Un nuovo protozoa parassite dei conigli. Incontro nelle lesioni anatomiche d'una malattia che ricorda in molti punti il kala-azar dell' unomo. Rev Soc Sci (São Paulo) 3:109, 1908.
8. Wolf A, Cowen D: Granulomatous encephalomyelitis due to an encephalitozoon (encephalitozoic encephalomyelitis). A new protozoan disease of man. Bull Neurol Inst NY 7:266, 1937.
9. Wilder HC: *Toxoplasma* chorioretinitis in adults. Arch Ophthalmol 48:127, 1952.
10. Sabin AB, Feldman HA: Dyes as microchemical indicators of a new immunity phenomenon affecting a protozoan parasite (*Toxoplasma*). Science 108:660, 1948.
11. Ruskin J, Remington JS: Toxoplasmosis in the compromised host. Ann Intern Med 84:193, 1976.
12. Luft BJ, Remington JS: Toxoplasmic encephalitis in AIDS. Clin Infect Dis 15:211, 1995.
13. Sibley LD, Boothroyd JC: Virulent strains of *Toxoplasma gondii* comprise a single clonal lineage. Nature 359:82, 1992.
14. Ajzenberg D, Cogne N, Paris L, et al: Genotype of 86 *Toxoplasma gondii* isolates associated with human congenital toxoplasmosis, and correlation with clinical findings. J Infect Dis 186:684, 2002.
15. Howe DK, Honore S, Derouin F, et al: Determination of genotypes of *Toxoplasma gondii* strains isolated from patients with toxoplasmosis. J Clin Microbiol 35:1411, 1997.
16. Fuentes E, Rubio J, Ramirez C, et al: Genotypic characterization of *Toxoplasma gondii* strains associated with human toxoplasmosis in Spain: Direct analysis from clinical samples. J Clin Microbiol 39:1566, 2001.
17. Grigg ME, Ganatra J, Boothroyd J, et al: Unusual abundance of atypical strains associated with human ocular toxoplasmosis. J Infect Dis 184:633, 2001.
18. Su C, Evans D, Cole, RH, et al: Recent expansion of *Toxoplasma* through enhanced oral transmission. Science 299:414, 2003.
19. Sibley DL: Recent origins among ancient parasites. Vet Parasitol 115:185, 2003.
20. Grigg ME, Bonnefoy S, Hehl AB, et al: Success and virulence in *Toxoplasma* as the result of sexual recombination between two distinct ancestries. Science 294:161, 2001.
21. Pfefferkorn LC, Pfefferkorn ER: *Toxoplasma gondii* genetic recombination between drug resistant mutants. Exp Parasitol 50:305, 1980.
22. Wong S-Y, Remington JS: Biology of *Toxoplasma gondii*. AIDS 7:299, 1993.
23. Dubey JP, Frenkel JK: Feline toxoplasmosis from acutely infected mice and the development of *Toxoplasma* cysts. J Protozool 23:537, 1976.
24. Frenkel JK, Dubey JP, Miller NL: *Toxoplasma gondii* in cats: Faecal stages identified as coccidian oocysts. Science 167:893, 1970.
25. Frenkel JK, Ruiz A, Chinchilla M: Soil survival of *Toxoplasma* oocysts in Kansas and Costa Rica. Am J Trop Med Hyg 24:439, 1975.
26. Etheredge GD, Frenkel JK: Human *Toxoplasma* infection in Kuna and Embera children in the Bayano and San Blas, Eastern Panama. Am J Trop Med Hyg 53:448, 1995.
27. Frenkel JK, Hassanein KM, Hassanein RS, et al: Transmission of *Toxoplasma gondii* in Panama City, Panama: A five-year prospective cohort study of children, cats, rodents, birds, and soil. Am J Trop Med Hyg 53:458, 1995.
28. Cook AJC, Gilbert RE, Buffolano W, et al: Sources of toxoplasma infection in pregnant women: European multicenter case-control study. BMJ 321:142, 2000.
29. Dubey JP: Status of toxoplasmosis in cattle and the United States. J Am Vet Med Assoc 196:257, 1992.
30. Sibley LD, LeBlanc AJ, Pfefferkorn ER, et al: Generation of a restriction fragment length polymorphism linkage map for *Toxoplasma gondii*. Genetics 132:1003, 1992.

31. Isaac-Renton J, Bowie WR, King A, et al: Detection of *Toxoplasma gondii* oocysts in drinking water. Appl Environ Microbiol 64:2278, 1998.
32. Wallace GD: Serologic and epidemiologic observations on toxoplasmosis on three Pacific atolls. Am J Epidemiol 90:103, 1969.
33. Walton BC, Arjona I, Benchoff BM: Relationship of *Toxoplasma* antibodies to altitude. Am J Trop Med Hyg 15:492, 1966.
34. Wong SY, Remington JS: Toxoplasmosis in pregnancy. Clin Infect Dis 18:853, 1994.
35. Rawal BD: Toxoplasmosis: A dye-test survey on sera from vegetarians and meat eaters in Bombay. Trans R Soc Trop Med Hyg 53:61, 1959.
36. Benenson MW, Takafuji ET, Lemon SM, et al: Oocyst-transmitted toxoplasmosis associated with ingestion of contaminated water. N Engl J Med 307:666, 1982.
37. Frenkel JK, Weber RW, Lûnde MN: Acute toxoplasmosis. Effective treatment with pyrimethamine, sulfadiazine, leucovorin calcium and yeast. JAMA 173:1471, 1960.
38. Guy EC, Joynson DH: Potential of the polymerase chain reaction in the diagnosis of active *Toxoplasma gondii* infection by detection of parasite in blood. J Infect Dis 172:319, 1995.
39. Kimball AC, Kean BH, Kellner A: The risk of transmitting toxoplasmosis by blood transfusion. Transfusion 5:447, 1965.
40. Desmonts G, Couvreur J: Toxoplasmosis in pregnancy and its transmission to the fetus. Bull NY Acad Med 50:146, 1974.
41. Thulliez P: Screening programme for congenital toxoplasmosis in France. Scand J Infect Dis Suppl 84:43, 1992.
42. Joynson DHM: Epidemiology of toxoplasmosis in the U.K. Scand J Infect Dis Suppl 84:65, 1992.
43. Koskiniemi M, Lappalainen M, Koskela P, et al: The programme for antenatal screening of toxoplasmosis in Finland: A prospective cohort study. Scand J Infect Dis Suppl 84:70, 1992.
44. Sousa OE, Saenz RE, Frenkel JK: Toxoplasmosis in Panama: A 10-year study. Am J Trop Med Hyg 38:315, 1988.
45. Gomez-Marin JE, Montoya-de-Londono MT, Castano-Osorio JC: A maternal screening program for congenital toxoplasmosis in Quindio, Colombia, and application of mathematical models to estimate incidences using age-stratified data. Am J Trop Med Hyg 57:180, 1997.
46. Doehring E, Reiter-Owana I, Bauer O, et al: *Toxoplasma gondii* antibodies in pregnant women and their newborns in Dar es Salaam, Tanzania. Am J Trop Med Hyg 52:546, 1995.
47. Bowry TR, Camargo ME, Kinyanjui M: Sero-epidemiology of *Toxoplasma gondii* infection in young children in Nairobi, Kenya. Trans R Soc Trop Med Hyg 80:439, 1986.
48. Onadeko MO, Joynson DHM, Payne RA: The prevalence of *Toxoplasma* infection among pregnant women in Ibadan, Nigeria. J Trop Med Hyg 95:143, 1992.
49. Hamadto HA, Rashid SM, el-Fakahany AF, et al: Seroepidemiological studies for toxoplasmosis among out- and inpatients in Benha University Hospitals, Qualyobia Governate. J Egypt Soc Parasitol 27:223, 1997.
50. Hoff R, Weiblen BJ, Reardon LA, et al: Screening for congenital *Toxoplasma* infection. In Bellisario R, Mizejewski GJ (eds): Transplacental Disorders: Perinatal Detection, Treatment, and Management. New York, Alan R Liss, 1990, p 169.
51. Jones JL, Kruszon-Moran D, Wilson M: Toxoplasma *gondii* infection in the United States, 1999–2000. Emerg Infect Dis 9:1371, 2003.
52. Frenkel JK: Toxoplasmosis. In Connor DH, Chandler FW, Schwartz DA, et al (eds): Pathology of Infectious Diseases. Stamford, CT, Appleton & Lange, 1997, p 1261.
53. Pfefferkorn ER: Cell biology of *Toxoplasma gondii*. In Wyler DJ (ed): Modern Parasite Biology: Cellular, Immunological, and Molecular Aspects. New York, WH Freeman, 1990, p 26.
54. Mineo JR, Kasper LH: Attachment of *Toxoplasma gondii* to host cells involves major surface protein, SAG-1 (P30). Exp Parasitol 79:11, 1994.
55. Morisaki JH, Heuser JE, Sibley LD: Invasion of *Toxoplasma gondii* occurs by active penetration of the host cell. J Cell Sci 108:2457, 1995.
56. Peterson PK, Gekker G, Hu S, et al: Intracellular survival and multiplication of *Toxoplasma gondii* in astrocytes. J Infect Dis 168:1472, 1993.
57. Saffer LD, Long Krug SA, Schwartzman JD: The role of phospholipase in host cell penetration by *Toxoplasma gondii*. Am J Trop Med Hyg 40:145, 1989.
58. Sibley LD: Interactions between *Toxoplasma gondii* and its mammalian host cells. Semin Cell Biol 4:335, 1993.
59. Schwab JC, Beckers CJ, Joiner KA: The parasitophorous vacuole membrane surrounding intracellular *Toxoplasma gondii* functions as a molecular sieve. Proc Natl Acad Sci USA 91:509, 1994.
60. Weiss LM, Laplace D, Takvorian PM, et al: A cell culture system for development of *Toxoplasma gondii* bradyzoites. J Eukaryot Microbiol 42:150, 1997.
61. Fadul CE, Channon JY, Kasper LH: Survival of immunoglobulin G-opsonized *Toxoplasma gondii* in nonadherent human monocytes. Infect Immun 63:4290, 1995.
62. Pavesio CE, Chiappino ML, Setzer PY, et al: *Toxoplasma gondii* differentiation and death of bradyzoites. Parasitol Res 78:1, 1992.
63. Gazzinelli RT, Amichay D, Sharton-Kersten T, et al: Role of macrophage-derived cytokines in the induction and regulation of cell-mediated immunity to *Toxoplasma gondii*. Curr Top Microbiol Immunol 219:127, 1996.
64. Hunter CA, Remington JS: The role of IL12 in toxoplasmosis. Res Immunol 146(Suppl):546, 1995.
65. Pfefferkorn ER: Interferon gamma blocks the growth of *Toxoplasma gondii* in human fibroblasts by inducing the host cells to degrade tryptophan. Proc Natl Acad Sci USA 81:908, 1984.
66. Denkers EY, Sher A: Role of natural killer and NK1+ T-cells in regulating cell-mediated immunity during *Toxoplasma gondii* infection. Biochem Soc Trans 25:699, 1997.
67. Peterson PK, Gekker G, Hu S, et al: Human astrocytes inhibit intracellular multiplication of *Toxoplasma gondii* by a nitric oxide–mediated mechanism. J Infect Dis 171:516, 1995.
68. Brown CR, McLeod R: Class I MHC genes and CD8+ T cells determine cyst number in *Toxoplasma gondii* infection. J Immunol 145:3438, 1990.
69. Khan IA, Schwartzman JD, Matsura T, et al: A dichotomous role for nitric oxide during acute *Toxoplasma gondii* infection in mice. Proc Natl Acad Sci USA 94:13955, 1997.
70. Krick JA, Remington JS: Toxoplasmosis in the adult—An overview. N Engl J Med 298:550, 1978.
71. Frenkel JK: Toxoplasmosis in human beings. J Am Vet Med Assoc 196:240, 1990.
72. Kean BH, Kimball AC, Christensen WN: An epidemic of acute toxoplasmosis. JAMA 208:1002, 1969.
73. Teutsch SM, Juranek DJ, Sulzer A, et al: Epidemic toxoplasmosis associated with cats. N Engl J Med 300:695, 1979.
74. McCabe RE, Brooks RG, Dorfman RF, et al: Clinical spectrum in 107 cases of toxoplasmic lymphadenopathy. Rev Infect Dis 9:754, 1987.
75. Montoya JG, Remington JS: Studies on the serodiagnosis of toxoplasmic lymphadenitis. Clin Infect Dis 20:781, 1995.
76. Sheagren JN, Lunde MN, Simon HB: Chronic lymphadenopathic toxoplasmosis. A case with marked hyperglobulinemia and impaired delayed hypersensitivity responses during active infection. Am J Med 60:300, 1976.
77. Montoya JG, Jordan R, Lingamneni S, et al: Toxoplasmic myocarditis and polymyositis in patients with acute acquired toxoplasmosis diagnosed during life. Clin Infect Dis 24:676, 1997.
78. Greenlee JE, Johnson WD, Jr., Campa JF, et al: Adult toxoplasmosis presenting as polymyositis and cerebellar ataxia. Ann Intern Med 83:367, 1975.
79. Glasner PD, Silveira C, Kruszon-Moran D, et al: An unusually high prevalence of ocular toxoplasmosis in southern Brazil. Am J Ophthalmol 114:136, 1992.
80. Bowie WR, King AS, Werker DH, et al: Outbreak of toxoplasmosis associated with municipal drinking water. The BC Toxoplasma Investigation team. Lancet 350:173, 1997.
81. Montoya JG, Remington JS: Toxoplasmic chorioretinitis in the setting of acute acquired toxoplasmosis. Clin Infect Dis 23:277, 1996.
82. Desmonts G, Couvreur J: Congenital toxoplasmosis: A study of 378 pregnancies. N Engl J Med 290:1110, 1974.
83. Kimball AC, Kean BH, Fucs F: Congenital toxopasmosis: A prospective study of 4048 obstetric patients. Am J Obstet Gynecol 111:211, 1971.
84. Lynfield R, Guerina NG: Toxoplasmosis. Pediatr Rev 18(Suppl):75, 1997.
85. Gavinet MF, Robert F, Firtion G, et al: Congenital toxoplasmosis due to maternal reinfection during pregnancy. J Clin Microbiol 35:1276, 1997.
86. Vogel N, Kirisits M, Michael E, et al: Congenital toxoplasmosis transmitted from an immunologically competent mother infected before conception. Clin Infect Dis 23:1055, 1996.
87. Minkoff H, Remington JS, Holman S, et al: Vertical transmission of toxoplasmosis by human immunodeficiency virus–infected women. Am J Obstet Gynecol 176:555, 1997.

88. Mitchell CD, Erlich SS, Mastrucci MT, et al: Congenital toxoplasmosis occurring in infants perinatally infected with human immunodeficiency virus 1. Pediatr Infect Dis J 9:512, 1990.
89. Guerina NG, Hsu HW, Meissner HC, et al: Neonatal serologic screening and early treatment for congenital *Toxoplasma gondii* infection. The New England Regional Toxoplasma Working Group. N Engl J Med 330:1858, 1994.
90. McAuley J, Boyer KM, Patel D, et al: Early and longitudinal evaluations of treated infants and children and untreated historical patients with congenital toxoplasmosis. The Chicago Collaborative Treatment Trial. Clin Infect Dis 18:38, 1994.
91. Wilson CB, Remington JS, Stagno S, et al: Development of adverse sequelae in children born with subclinical congenital *Toxoplasma* infection. Pediatrics 66:767, 1980.
92. Koppe JG, Loewer-Sieger DH, de Roever-Bonnet H: Results of 20-year follow-up of congenital toxoplasmosis. Lancet 1:254, 1986.
93. Mets MB, Holfels E, Boyer KM, et al: Eye manifestations of congenital toxoplasmosis. Am J Ophthalmol 123:1, 1997.
94. Tabbara KF: Ocular toxoplasmosis: Toxoplasmic retinochoroiditis. Int Ophthalmol Clin 35:15, 1995.
95. Pavesio CE, Lightman S: *Toxoplasma gondii* and ocular toxoplasmosis: Pathogenesis. Br J Ophthalmol 80:1099, 1996.
96. Silveira C, Belfort R, Jr., Muccioli C, et al: A follow-up study of *Toxoplasma gondii* infection ion southern Brazil. Am J Ophthalmol 131:351, 2001.
97. Holland GN: Ocular toxoplasmosis: A global reassessment. Part 1: Epidemiology and course of disease. Am J Ophthalmol 136:973, 2003.
98. Mariuz P, Bosler EM, Luff BJ: Toxoplasmosis in individuals with AIDS. Infect Dis Clin North Am 81:365, 1994.
99. Bertoli FM, Espino JR, Arosemena T, et al: A spectrum in the pathology of toxoplasmosis in patients with acquired immunodeficiency syndrome. Arch Pathol Lab Med 119:214, 1995.
100. Hunter CA, Remington JS: Immunopathogenesis of toxoplasmic encephalitis. J Infect Dis 170:1057, 1994.
101. Richards FO, Jr., Kovacs JA, Luft BJ: Preventing toxoplasmic encephalitis in persons infected with human immunodeficiency virus. Clin Infect Dis 21(Suppl 1):S49, 1995.
102. Jones JL, Sehgal M, Maguire JH: Toxoplasmosis-associated deaths among human immunodeficiency virus–infected persons in the United States, 1992–1998. Clin Infect Dis 34:1161, 2002.
103. Kreiss JK, Castro KG: Special considerations for managing suspected human immunodeficiency virus infection and AIDS in patients from developing countries. J Infect Dis 162:955, 1990.
104. Lucas SB, Honnou A, Peacock C, et al: The mortality and pathology of HIV infection in a West African city. AIDS 7:1569, 1993.
105. Israelski DM, Remington JS: Toxoplasmosis in patients with cancer. Clin Infect Dis 17(Suppl 2):S423, 1993.
106. Derouin F, Devergie A, Auber P: Toxoplasmosis in bone marrow–transplant recipients: Report of seven cases and review. Clin Infect Dis 15:267, 1992.
107. Michaels MG, Wald ER, Fricker FJ, et al: Toxoplasmosis in pediatric recipients of heart transplants. Clin Infect Dis 14:847, 1992.
108. Renoult E, Georges E, Biava MF, et al: Toxoplasmosis in kidney transplant recipients: Report of six cases and review. Clin Infect Dis 24:625, 1997.
109. Mayes JT, O'Connor BJ, Avery R, et al: Transmission of *Toxoplasma gondii* infection by liver transplantation. Clin Infect Dis 21:511, 1995.
110. Siegal SE, Lunde MN, Gelderman AH, et al: Transmission of toxoplasmosis by leukocyte transfusion. Blood 37:388, 1971.
111. Grange F, Kinney EL, Monseuz JJ, et al: Successful therapy for *Toxoplasma gondii* myocarditis in acquired immunodeficiency syndrome. Am Heart J 20:643, 1990.
112. Campagna AC: Pulmonary toxoplasmosis. Semin Respir Infect 12:98, 1997.
113. Schnapp LM, Geaghan SM, Campagna A, et al: *Toxoplasma gondii* pneumonitis in patients infected with the human immunodeficiency virus. Arch Intern Med 152:1073, 1992.
114. Albrecht H, Skorde J, Arasteh K, et al: Disseminated toxoplasmosis in AIDS patients—Report of 16 cases. Scand J Infect Dis 27:71, 1995.
115. Bonacini M, Kanel G, Alamy M: Duodenal and hepatic toxoplasmosis in a patient with HIV infection: Review of the literature. Am J Gastroenterol 91:1838, 1996.
116. Besnier JM, Verdier M, Cotty F, et al: Toxoplasmosis of the bladder in a patient with AIDS. Clin Infect Dis 21:452, 1995.
117. Garcia LS, Bruckner DA: Tissue protozoa. In Diagnostic Medical Parasitology, 3rd ed. Washington, DC, ASM Press, 1997, p 111.
118. Nash G, Kerschma RL, Herndier B, et al: The pathological manifestations of pulmonary toxoplasmosis in the acquired immunodeficiency syndrome. Hum Pathol 25:652, 1994.
119. van de Ven E, Melchers W, Galama J, et al: Identification of *Toxoplasma gondii* infections by BI gene amplification. J Clin Microbiol 29:2120, 1991.
120. Grover CM, Thulliez P, Remington JS, et al: Rapid prenatal diagnosis of congenital *Toxoplasma* infection by using polymerase chain reaction and amniotic fluid. J Clin Microbiol 28:2297, 1990.
121. Hohlfeld P, Daffos F, Costa JM, et al: Prenatal diagnosis of congenital toxoplasmosis with a polymerase-chain-reaction test on amniotic fluid. N Engl J Med 331:695, 1994.
122. Filice GA, Hitt JA, Mitchell CD, et al: Diagnosis of *Toxoplasma* parasitemia in patients with AIDS by gene detection after amplification with polymerase chain reaction. J Clin Microbiol 31:2327, 1993.
123. Lebech M, Lebech AM, Nelsing S, et al: Detection of *Toxoplasma gondii* DNA by polymerase chain reaction in cerebrospinal fluid from AIDS patients with cerebral toxoplasmosis. J Infect Dis 165:982, 1992.
124. Brezin AP, Equwuagu CG, Silveira C, et al: Analysis of aqueous humor in ocular toxoplasmosis. N Engl J Med 324:699, 1991.
125. Bretagne SJ, Costa M, Fleury-Feith J, et al: Quantitative competitive PCR with bronchoalveolar lavage fluid for diagnosis of toxoplasmosis in AIDS patients. J Clin Microbiol 33:1662, 1995.
126. Walton BC, Benchoff BM, Brooks WH: Comparison of indirect fluorescent antibody test and methylene blue dye test for detection of antibodies to *Toxoplasma gondii*. Am J Trop Med Hyg 15:149, 1966.
127. Roos T, Martius J, Gross U, et al: Systematic serologic screening for toxoplasmosis during pregnancy. Obstet Gynecol 81:243, 1993.
128. Skinner LJ, Chatterton JM, Joss AW, et al: The use of an IgM immunosorbent agglutination assay to diagnose congenital toxoplasmosis. J Med Microbiol 28:125, 1989.
129. Naot Y, Desmonts G, Remington JS, et al: IgM enzyme-linked immunosorbent assay test for the diagnosis of congenital *Toxoplasma* infection. J Pediatr 98:32, 1981.
130. Verhofstede C, Van RL, Plum J: Comparison of six commercial enzyme linked immunosorbent assays for detecting IgM antibodies against *Toxoplasma gondii*. J Clin Pathol 42:1285, 1989.
131. Hsu H-W, Grady GF, Maguire, JH, et al: Newborn screening for congenital *Toxoplasma* infection: Five years experience in Massachusetts, USA. Scand J Infect Dis Suppl 84:59, 1992.
132. Lappalainen M, Koskela P, Koskiniemi M, et al: Toxoplasmosis acquired during pregnancy: Improved serodiagnosis based on avidity of IgG. J Infect Dis 167:691, 1993.
133. Montoya JG, Lisenfeld O: Toxoplasmosis. Lancet 363:1965, 2004.
134. Jenum PA, Stray-Pedersen B, Gundersen A-G: Improved diagnosis of primary *Toxoplasma gondii* infection in early pregnancy by determination of antitoxoplasma immunoglobulin G avidity. J Clin Microbiol 35:1972, 1997.
135. Beghetto E, Buffolano W, Spadoni A, et al: Use of an immunoglobulin G avidity assay based on recombinant antigens for diagnosis of primary *Toxoplasma gondii* infection during pregnancy. J Clin Microbiol 41:5414, 2003.
136. Remington JS, Thulliez P, Montoya JG: Recent developments for diagnosis of toxoplasmosis. J Clin Microbiol 42:941, 2004.
137. Boyer KM: Diagnosis and treatment of congenital toxoplasmosis. Adv Pediatr Infect Dis 11:449, 1996.
138. Liesenfeld O, Montoya JG, Kinney S, et al: Effect of testing for IgG avididty in the diagnosis of *Toxoplasma gondii* infection in pregnant women: Experience in a US reference laboratory. J Infect Dis 183:1248, 2001.
139. Mathews C, Barba D, Fullerton SC: Early biopsy versus empiric treatment with delayed biopsy of non-responders in suspected HIV-associated cerebral toxoplasmosis: A decision analysis. AIDS 9:1243, 1995.
140. Pierce MA, Johnson MD, Maciunas RJ, et al: Evaluating contrast-enhancing brain lesions in patients with AIDS by using positron emission tomography. Ann Intern Med 123:594, 1995.
141. Georgiev VS: Management of toxoplasmosis. Drugs 48:179, 1994.
142. Desmonts G, Daffos F, Forrestier F, et al: Prenatal diagnosis of congenital toxoplasmosis. Lancet 1:500, 1985.
143. Daffos F, Forrestier F, Capella-Pavlovsky M, et al: Prenatal diagnosis of 746 pregnancies at risk for congenital toxoplasmosis. N Engl J Med 318:217, 1988.

144. Roizen N, Swisher CN, Stein MA, et al: Neurologic and developmental outcome in treated congenital toxoplasmosis. Pediatrics 95:11, 1995.
145. Silveira C, Belfort R, Jr., Muccioli C, et al: The effect of long-term intermittent trimethoprim/sulfamethoxazole treatment on recurrences of toxoplasmic retinochoroiditis. Am J Ophthalmol 134:41, 2002.
146. Fung HB, Kirschenbaum HL: Treatment regimens for patients with toxoplasmic encephalitis. Clin Ther 18:1037, 1996.
147. Gross U, Pohl F: Influence of antimicrobial agents on replication and stage conversion of *Toxoplasma gondii*. Curr Top Microbiol Immunol 219:235, 1996.
148. Araujo FG, Lin T, Remington JS: The activity of atovaquone (566c80) in murine toxoplasmosis is markedly augmented when used in combination with pyrimethamine or sulfadiazine. J Infect Dis 167:494, 1993.
149. Schoondermark-van de VE, Galama EJ, Vree T, et al: Study of treatment of congenital *Toxoplasma gondii* infection in rhesus monkeys with pyrimethamine and sulfadiazine. Antimicrob Agents Chemother 39:137, 1995.
150. Drugs for parasitic infections. Med Lett Drugs Ther. www.medletter.com, August 2004.
151. Bartlett JG: Pocket Book of Disease Therapy. Baltimore, Williams & Wilkins, 1996.
152. Rolston KV, Hoy J: Role of clindamycin in the treatment of central nervous system toxoplasmosis. Am J Med 83:551, 1987.
153. Fichera ME, Bhopale MK, Roos DS: In vitro assays elucidate peculiar kinetics of clindamycin action against *Toxoplasma gondii*. Antimicrob Agents Chemother 39:1530, 1995.
154. Torres RA, Weinberg W, Stansell J, et al: Atovaquone for salvage treatment and suppression of toxoplasmic encephalitis in patients with AIDS. Atovaquone/Toxoplasmic Encephalitis Study Group. Clin Infect Dis 24:422, 1997.
155. Chang HR, Pechere JC: Activity of spiramycin against *Toxoplasma gondii* in vitro in experimental infections and human infection. J Antimicrob Chemother 22(Suppl):87, 1988.
156. Kovacs JA: Toxoplasmosis in AIDS: Keeping the lid on. Ann Intern Med 123:230, 1995.
157. Podzamczer D, Miro JM, Bolao F, et al: Twice-weekly maintenance therapy with sulfadiazine-pyrimethamine to prevent recurrent toxoplasmic encephalitis in patients with AIDS. Spanish Toxoplasmosis Study Group. Ann Intern Med 123:175, 1995.
158. Podzamczer D, Salazar A, Jimenez J, et al: Intermittent trimethoprim-sulfamethoxazole compared with dapsone-pyrimethamine for the simultaneous primary prophylaxis of *Pneumocystis* pneumonia and toxoplasmosis in patients infected with HIV. Ann Intern Med 122:755, 1995.
159. Carr A, Tindall B, Brew BJ, et al: Low-dose trimethoprim-sulfamethoxazole prophylaxis for toxoplasmic encephalitis in patients with AIDS. Ann Intern Med 117:106, 1992.
160. Kirk O, Reiss P, Uberti-Foppa C, et al: Safe interruption of maintenance therapy against previous infection with four common HIV-associated opportunistic pathogens during potent antiretroviral therapy. Ann Intern Med 137:239, 2002.
161. Eskild A, Magnus P: Commentary: Little evidence of effective prenatal treatment against congenital toxoplasmosis—The implications for testing in pregnancy. Int J Epidemiol 30:1314, 2001.
162. Thulliez P: Commentary: Efficacy of prenatal treatment for toxoplasmosis: A possibility that cannot be ruled out. Int J Epidemiol 30:1315, 2001.
163. McCabe R, Remington JS: Toxoplasmosis: The time has come. N Engl J Med 318:313, 1988.
164. Peckham CS, Logan S: Screening for toxoplasmosis during pregnancy. Arch Dis Child 68:3, 1993.
165. Lappalainen MH, Sintonen J, Koskiniemi M, et al: Cost-benefit analysis of screening for toxoplasmosis during pregnancy. Scand J Infect Dis 27:265, 1995.
166. Eskild A, Oxman A, Magnus P, et al: Screening for toxoplasmosis in pregnancy: What is the evidence of reducing a health problem? J Med Screen 3:188, 1996.
167. Petersen E, Schmidt DR: Sulfadiazine and pyrimethamine in the postnatal treatment of congenital toxoplasmosis: What are the options? Expert Rev Anti Infect Ther 1:175, 2003.
168. Carter AO, Gelmon SB, Wells GA, et al: The effectiveness of a prenatal education programme for the prevention of congenital toxoplasmosis. Epidemiol Infect 103:539, 1989.
169. Henderson JB, Beattie CP, Hale EG, et al: The evaluation of new services: Possibilities for preventing toxoplasmosis. Int J Epidemiol 13:65, 1984.
170. Dubey JP: Strategies to reduce transmission of *Toxoplasma gondii* to animals and humans. Vet Parasitol 64:65, 1996.
171. Wilson CB, Remington JS: What can be done to prevent congenital toxoplasmosis? Am J Obstet Gynecol 138:357, 1980.
172. Buxton D, Innes EA: A commercial vaccine for ovine toxoplasmosis. Parasitology 110(Suppl):S11, 1995.
173. Choromanski L, Freyre A, Popiel R, et al: Safety and efficacy of modified live feline *Toxoplasma gondii* vaccine. Dev Biol Stand 84:269, 1995.

I. NEMATODE INFECTIONS

98 Filariasis

THOMAS B. NUTMAN
JAMES W. KAZURA

INTRODUCTION

Lymphatic filariasis is caused by infection with any of three closely related parasitic nematodes—*Wuchereria bancrofti, Brugia malayi,* or *Brugia timori.* Unlike most other helminthiases endemic in tropical areas of the world, the burden of infection and disease in lymphatic filariasis occurs primarily during adulthood and not childhood or infancy. The greater impact of lymphatic filariasis on older age groups is due to the inefficiency of transmission by the obligatory arthropod vector and the fact that infection burdens are determined by the chronicity and intensity of exposure to infective stages of the organisms, which do not multiply in the mammalian host.

Because disease due to lymphatic filariasis is characterized by disfigurement of the limbs (elephantiasis) and genitalia (hydroceles and other anatomical changes in the male genitalia), it is often perceived as having adverse economic and psychosexual effects as well as medical consequences. This is particularly evident in the developing countries of the tropics where physical labor is still the major means of earning money. According to some estimates, lymphatic filariasis is among the leading health-related impediments to economic and social development in economically disadvantaged areas of the tropics.[1]

Lymphatic filariasis can be transmitted in any region of the world where the appropriate mosquito vector breeds. It currently is a significant health problem in tropical Africa, Asia, and the Indian subcontinent, many islands of the western and southern Pacific, and focal areas of Latin America. The infection was endemic in the southern United States and Japan in the 19th and first half of the 20th century, but disappeared as breeding sites diminished with development of modern water drainage and sewage systems. In the tropics, the geographic distribution of *W. bancrofti* and *B. malayi* infections is expanding due to increased numbers of breeding sites that appear when large numbers of people migrate from rural areas to urban slums. These pessimistic epidemiologic trends contrast the recently realized appreciation that it may be possible to eradicate lymphatic filariasis by using currently available chemotherapies in a cost-effective manner.[2]

AGENTS

The existence of lymphatic filariasis has been recorded in ancient Chinese, Indian, Persian, and Arabic writings, but the causative agents and their life cycles were not described in detail until the late 19th century.[3,4] The microfilariae of *W. bancrofti,* first discovered by Demarquay in hydrocele fluid from a patient in Cuba in 1863,[5] were later identified in the urine by Wucherer in 1868[6] and in the blood by Lewis in 1872.[7] Manson described the periodicity of microfilariae in the peripheral blood[8] and also demonstrated that mosquitoes transmit the parasite.[9] Bancroft was the first to describe the adult female worm[10] and the adult male worm was later described by Bourne.[11] Bancroft in 1899[12] and Low in 1900[13] established the mode of transmission of the parasite. Lichenstein, Brug, and Buckley were primarily responsible for the identification of the brugian parasites.[14]

W. bancrofti, B. malayi, and *B. timori* are threadlike nematodes having five morphologically and biochemically distinct stages in their life cycle. Infective or third-stage larvae are transmitted to humans during blood feeding by mosquitoes. The organisms are deposited from the mouth parts of the mosquito in the vicinity of the skin puncture wound, and within several minutes make their way through the dermis to enter the local lymphatics. Several hours later, infective larvae shed their cuticle and develop a new surface (a process referred to as molting) that presents novel antigens and other molecules to the mammalian host. These fourth-stage larvae migrate centrally in lymphatic vessels and over a period of approximately 9 months develop into sexually mature adult male or female worms. Adult worms are considerably larger than larval stages (male worms are 20–40 mm in length, and female worms 40–100 mm) and have highly differentiated and complex reproductive and digestive systems. This stage of the parasite dwells primarily in the afferent lymphatics. Although all of the anatomical areas in which adult lymphatic filariae live in humans are not known with certainty, large numbers are present in the lymphatics of the lower extremities (inguinal and obturator groups), upper extremities (axillary lymph nodes), and, for *W. bancrofti,* male genitalia (epididymis, spermatic cord, testicle). Based on observations of inflammatory reactions elicited by administration of drugs that kill adult worms, it is likely that adult filariae are distributed in subcutaneous tissues more than several centimeters distant from major lymph node groups. The mean reproductive life span of adult worms is approximately 5 years.

Following copulation with male worms, fecund female parasites release large numbers (often more than 10,000 per day) of embryonic forms or first-stage larvae. These parasites are referred to as microfilariae, which distinguish their small size compared with the larger adult worm (the former are 260 mm in length and approximately 10 mm in width). Microfilariae of lymphatic filariae differ from those of other filarial nematodes that infect humans in several ways. First, *W. bancrofti* and *Brugia* microfilariae are enclosed by an acellular sheath. This chitin-containing structure is a remnant of the embryonic eggshell or vitelline membrane and is not present in microfilariae of *Onchocerca volvulus* or *Loa loa.* Microfilariae of

W. bancrofti and *B. malayi* differ morphologically from each other in the pattern of nuclei in the cephalic and caudal regions. Second, after their release from female worms, microfilariae enter the blood (presumably by passage through the thoracic duct), where they circulate in large numbers. In many endemic areas, it is not unusual for the blood of an infected person to contain more than 10,000 microfilariae per milliliter. Third, *W. bancrofti* and *Brugia* microfilariae frequently have a nocturnal periodicity whereby large numbers of the organisms are present in the peripheral circulation between midnight and 6 AM with few or none present in the circulation during the day. When absent from the peripheral circulation, microfilariae are sequestered in deep vascular beds of the lung and other organs. This peculiar behavior appears to be an example of adaptation to local ecological conditions in that the time at which peak parasitemia occurs coincides with the time when the local mosquito vectors take their blood meal.[15] In most areas of the world, this occurs during the night hours. The mechanisms that regulate microfilarial periodicity in humans are poorly understood, though the lower pH present in the pulmonary venous circulation during sleep is thought to play a role in migration of the parasites from this site.

After ingestion in a blood meal taken by a female mosquito, microfilariae exsheath within 24 hours, penetrate the chitinous gut wall of the mosquito, and migrate into the thoracic musculature. Over a period of 10 days to 2 weeks, the organisms mature to become third-stage larvae capable of infecting another human.[16] The nature of the relationship between filarial larvae and the local mosquito populations has a profound impact on local transmission efficiency. For example, if mosquitoes ingest unusually large numbers of microfilariae, the overall efficiency of transmission may be reduced by virtue of the fact that heavily infected mosquitoes have a shortened life span, precluding development of infective larvae. Conversely, in some mosquito-filarial interactions, there may be more efficient transmission at lower microfilarial densities, a phenomenon referred to as facilitation.

An interesting biologic feature of *W. bancrofti* and *Brugia* species relates to the fact that these nematodes carry the obligatory bacterial endosymbiont *Wolbachia*. Ultrastructure studies

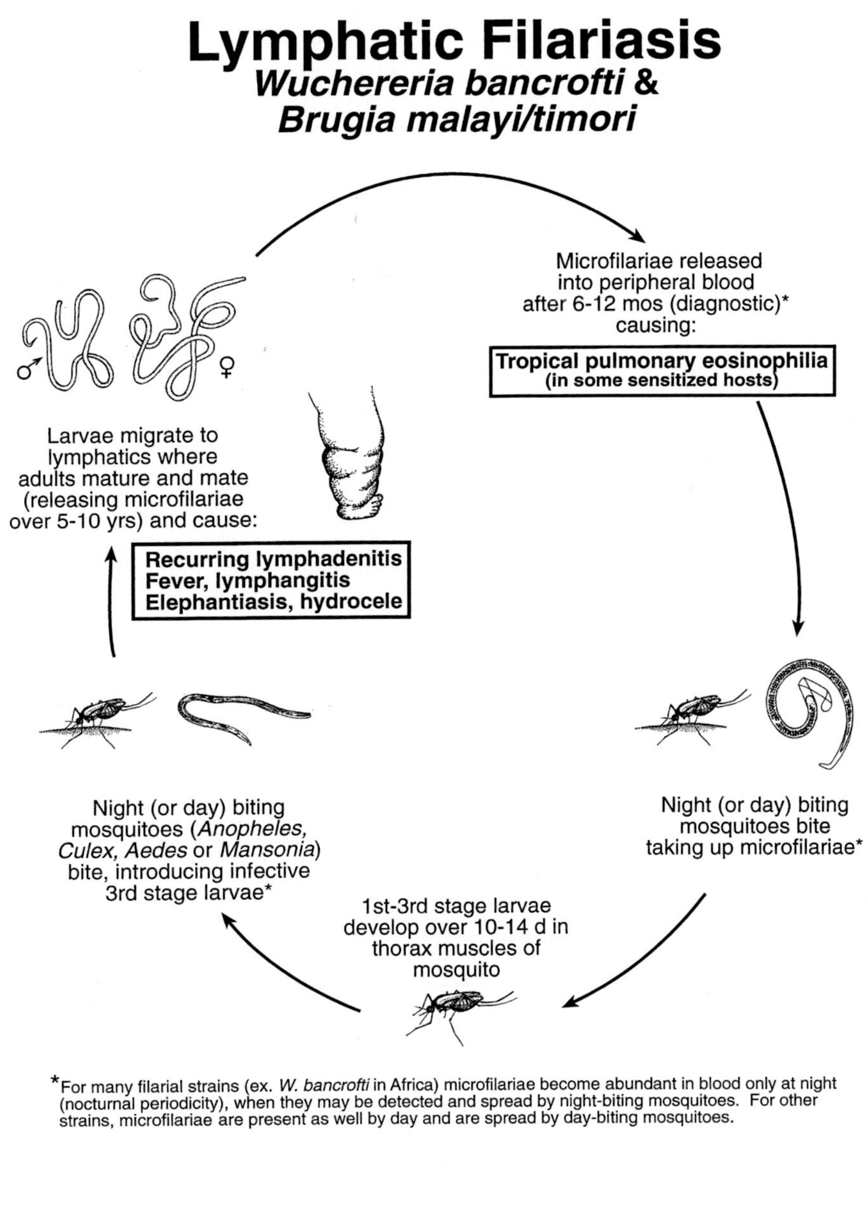

performed in the 1970s suggested the presence of intracellular bacteria in adult worms and microfilariae,[17,18] but it was not until the late 1990s when molecular probes and genome sequence data became available that *Wolbachia* were definitively identified in human filarial parasites.[19,20] These *Rickettsia*-like endosymbiotic bacteria appear to affect filariae in several ways that are pertinent to human filariasis. Incubation of *Brugia* worms with tetracycline and other antibiotics known to kill *Wolbachia* diminishes the release of microfilariae and suppresses larval molting, suggesting that the bacteria are involved in embryogenesis and regulation of the parasite life cycle.[21,22] In the context of human lymphatic filariasis, administration of doxycycline to persons with *W. bancrofti* infection prior to the microfilaricidal drug ivermectin has been observed to augment the suppression of microfilaremia.[23] In addition, acute post-treatment febrile reactions in patients with *B. malayi* infection given diethylcarbamazine have been correlated with presence of *Wolbachia* and pro-inflammatory cytokines in the blood,[24] consistent with the notion that *Wolbachia*-derived molecules with the property of bacterial endotoxins are released by dying worms and initiate inflammatory responses mediated by innate immune pathways.[25] Taken together, these findings raise the possibility that antibiotics directed against *Wolbachia* might be useful in efforts aimed at controlling and treating lymphatic filariasis (see later discussion). There is a need, however, to identify anti-*Wolbachia* agents that can be given for short periods of time (doxycycline was administered daily for 6 weeks prior to ivermectin in the study cited previously) and with broader applicability than the tetracycline antibiotics, which cannot be given to pregnant women or young children because of their effect on dentition and bone growth.

EPIDEMIOLOGY

It is estimated that 120 million people worldwide are infected with one of the three genera of lymphatic filariae.[26,27] More than 90% of infections are due to *W. bancrofti* and, of these, the greatest number of infected persons live in sub-Saharan Africa, Southeast Asia, and the western Pacific. The infection is prevalent in India, Indonesia, the Philippines, Papua New Guinea, and several Pacific countries, such as parts of Fiji and Tahiti. Up until the last decade or so, there were also more than 20 to 30 million cases in China. Bancroftian filariasis is also a significant public health problem in many countries of equatorial East Africa (e.g., Kenya and Tanzania) and West Africa (e.g., Nigeria and Ghana). Within Africa, *W. bancrofti* infection is not limited to these tropical zones since endemic foci are found as far north as the Nile delta in Egypt and Sudan. The prevalence of bancroftian filariasis has decreased markedly over the past few decades in Latin America. Endemic foci persist in several islands in the Caribbean (Haiti, Dominican Republic, Trinidad and Tobago) and coastal areas of South America (Brazil, Guyana, Suriname). There are no animal reservoirs of *W. bancrofti*.

Infection with *B. malayi* is limited to Asia (China, India, and Malaysia) and several Pacific island groups (e.g., Indonesia and the Philippines). There are fewer than 10 to 20 million persons in these areas infected with *B. malayi*, which may coexist with *W. bancrofti*. *B. malayi* infection is a zoonosis in that there are feline and primate reservoirs. *B. timori* infection is limited in its distribution to the islands of southeastern Indonesia.

Within a given geographic area, the distribution of lymphatic filariasis is highly focal such that the frequency of

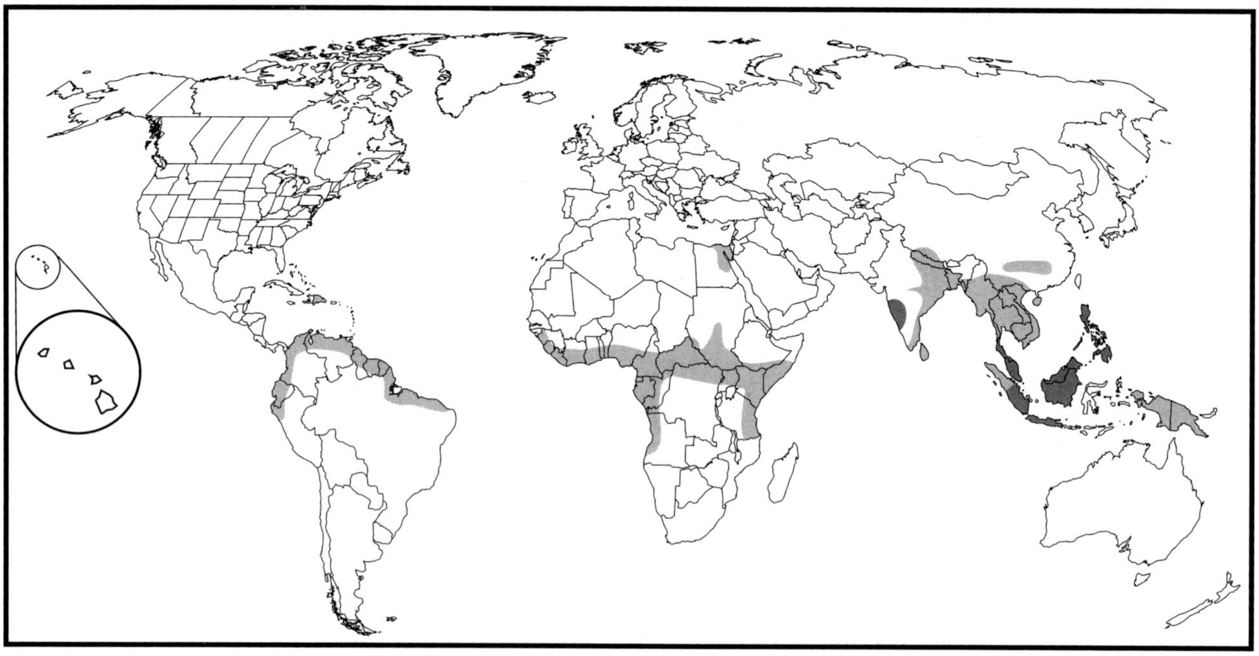

Lymphatic Filariasis

■ *Wuchereria bancrofti*

■ *Wuchereria bancrofti* and *Brugia malayi*

Note: *Brugia timori* is limited to the Timor Island of Indonesia infection in some communities is high compared with physically approximate localities. This heterogeneity of infection patterns, both at the local level and globally, is due in large part to the peculiarities of the ecological relationships between the mosquito vector, the human host, and the impact of filarial parasites on both. Unlike other common vector-borne infectious diseases of the tropics (e.g., malaria), several genera of mosquitoes are capable of transmitting lymphatic filariae. *W. bancrofti* is transmitted in many rural areas of Africa and the Pacific by *Anopheles* species.[28] The proximity of human dwellings to breeding sites increases the risk of repeated contact with mosquitoes bearing infective larvae. In many urban areas of the world, including India, *Culex* species is the major vector of *W. bancrofti* and *B. malayi*.[29] Unlike anopheline mosquitoes, larvae of these mosquitoes breed readily in small pools of water that form in discarded tires and cans. Other vectors include *Aedes aegytii* in some Pacific islands (e.g., Tahiti) and *Mansonia,* which transmits only *B. malayi*. These various genera of mosquitoes also differ in their efficiency of transmission. In general, anopheline mosquitoes are less efficient vectors of *W. bancrofti* than are culicine mosquitoes.

The age-related pattern of infection, as judged by the proportion of persons harboring microfilariae in the blood (the "microfilarial carrier rate," see later discussion), increases gradually with age up until the third or fourth decade of life, after which it remains constant or slightly decreases. This epidemiologic pattern is related to the gradual slow accumulation of adult-stage worms over time. The proportion of the entire population or a specific age group with patent infection is remarkably variable in different endemic areas. For example, the overall microfilarial carrier rates are approximately 10% in the Nile delta, 20% to 40% in parts of East Africa, and often greater than 60% in Papua New Guinea.

In addition to these differences in infection patterns, there is remarkable variation in the frequency of various disease manifestations according to age and geographic area. Lymphatic disease, manifest by persistent lymphedema of the lower extremity or genital disease in males (see later discussion), is rare in persons less than 10 years of age, and tends to increase gradually throughout life. Of the total 120 million persons estimated to be infected in all endemic areas, about one-third have some clinically overt disease. The likelihood of developing such manifestations appears to be particularly high in some areas of the world, such as India, Pacific islands such as Papua New Guinea, and equatorial Africa, whereas it is considerably lower in the Caribbean and South America. Systematic epidemiologic studies using uniform criteria for clinical diagnosis and unbiased samples of populations at risk of lymphatic disease have not, however, been performed in most endemic areas.

Recent studies have demonstrated that the local transmission conditions account in part for the striking heterogeneity of disease manifestations that may be observed within a given geographic area. In some areas of Papua New Guinea, for example, the prevalence of lymphedema of the lower extremities may vary from less than 5% to 15% in villages within 10 km of each other. Hydrocele rates in men over the age of 20 years also range from less than 1% to over 20% in geographically approximate sites.[30] Based on the fact that there is a positive correlation between the intensity of transmission[30] and disease, it is likely that cumulative exposure to infective larvae is an important risk factor for lymphatic pathology at the population level.

DISEASES

Infection with *W. bancrofti, B. malayi,* or *B. timori* can cause a wide variety of clinical manifestations, ranging from those without apparent clinical disease to those with lymphedema and/or severe disfigurement of the limbs and genitalia. From the clinical perspective, it should be stressed that there is a great deal of overlap in these symptom complexes, several of which may occur contemporaneously, and an individual may manifest each at different times during his or her lifetime.

Subclinical Patent Infection

The overwhelming majority of filarial-infected inhabitants in endemic areas have few overt clinical manifestations of their filarial infection despite large numbers of circulating microfilariae in the peripheral blood.[31] Although they may be clinically asymptomatic, virtually all persons with patent *W. bancrofti* or *B. malayi* infection (microfilaria- and/or circulating filarial antigen-positive) have some degree of subclinical disease that includes microscopic hematuria and/or proteinuria,[32] dilated (and tortuous) lymphatics (visualized by lymphoscintigraphy[33–35]), and—in men with *W. bancrofti* infection—scrotal lymphangiectasia (detectable by ultrasound).[36–38]

Moreover, population-based studies of the relationship between microfilarial carrier rates and the frequency of lymphatic disease (see later discussion) indicate that microfilaremia per se is not more common among clinically asymptomatic persons compared with those with disease.[39] Both of these findings suggest that patent infection is not necessarily a clinically benign condition.

Acute Adenolymphangitis

Acute adenolymphangitis (ADL) is often the first manifestation of lymphatic filariasis, which appears during adolescence. It is characterized by the sudden onset of high fever, painful lymph node and lymphatic inflammation (lymphangitis and lymphadenitis), and transient local edema. The lymphangitis is retrograde, extending peripherally from the lymph node draining the area where the adult parasites reside—the retrograde nature of the lymphadenitis distinguishes filarial-induced disease from bacterial-induced lymphangitis. Regional lymph nodes (e.g., inguinal, obdurator, axillary, epitrochlear) are often enlarged, and the entire lymphatic channel can become indurated and inflamed. Concomitant local thrombophlebitis can occur as well. In brugian filariasis, a single local abscess may form along the involved lymphatic tract and subsequently rupture to the surface. The lymphadenitis and lymphangitis can involve both the upper and lower extremities in both bancroftian and brugian filariasis, but involvement of the genital lymphatics occurs almost exclusively with *W. bancrofti* infection. This genital involvement can be manifested by funiculitis, epididymitis, scrotal pain, and tenderness.

In previously asymptomatic persons, the typical episode has a duration of 4 days to approximately 1 week, and may recur one to three times per year.[40] Episodes of ADL tend to be more severe and of longer duration in persons with preexisting lymphatic disease of the affected extremity.[40]

In endemic areas, another type of acute disease—dermatolymphangioadenitis (DLA)—is recognized as a syndrome that includes high fever, chills, myalgias, and headache. Edematous inflammatory plaques clearly demarcated from normal skin are seen. Vesicles, ulcers, and hyperpigmentation may also be noted. There is often a history of trauma, burns, radiation, insect bites, punctiform lesions, or chemical injury. Entry lesions, especially in the interdigital area, are common. DLA is often diagnosed as cellulitis.

Filarial Fever

Persons with filarial infection may present with an acute self-limited episode of fever in the absence of obvious inflammation of the lymphatics as described previously. These "filarial fevers" may be confused with other febrile illnesses, particularly malaria, and are often diagnosed on the basis of an appropriate epidemiologic history (i.e., chronic exposure to mosquitoes bearing infective larvae) and laboratory findings supportive of the diagnosis (see later discussion).

Lymphedema of the Arms, Legs, and Breasts

Swelling of the upper or lower extremities is the most common chronic manifestation of lymphatic filarial infection. Disease of the lower extremities is more prevalent.

Leg involvement in bancroftian filariasis may include the entire limb, whereas only the area below the knee is usually involved in brugian filariasis. The World Health Organization has developed a grading system to quantify the severity of involvement.[41] Grade I indicates pitting edema that is reversible upon elevation of the leg; grade II, nonpitting edema that does not resolve with elevation of the extremity; and grade III, an increase in the degree of swelling compared with grade II, and sclerosis with papillomatous changes in the skin. Grades II and III lymphedema are commonly referred to as elephantiasis (Fig. 98-1). Although both lower extremities may be involved, asymmetrical involvement is the rule.

In some persons with filarial-associated edema, the overlying skin may exude serous fluid suggestive of lymph. Although it is possible that this sign occurs as a result of increased hydrostatic pressure in the lymphatics draining the skin, skin turgor alone cannot reliably be used to distinguish between edema due to lymphatic disease and that from other causes, such as cardiac failure and liver disease.

Unilateral or bilateral involvement of the female breast occurs in adult residents of filarial endemic areas. This should be distinguished from chronic mastitis and other causes of chronic breast inflammation.

Disease Involving the Genitourinary System

Along with lymphatic disease of the lower extremities, disease of the male genitalia is the most common manifestation of bancroftian filariasis. Indeed, in many endemic areas, its prevalence is greater than that of lymphedema. Genital involvement is uncommon in *Brugia* infection. The prevalence of disease of the female genitalia is not known since systematic surveys have not included examination of this anatomical area. Anecdotal evidence suggests that the frequency of vulvar disfigurement is low. Genital disease is usually not experienced until the teenage years. Acute painful episodes of epididymitis or funiculitis last several days and are accompanied by fever and malaise. Involvement is most commonly unilateral.

Chronic disease of the male genitals mostly produces hydroceles, which vary in diameter from less than 5 cm to over 30 cm (Fig. 98-2). As is the case with other causes of hydrocele, the scrotal contents appear translucent when transilluminated.

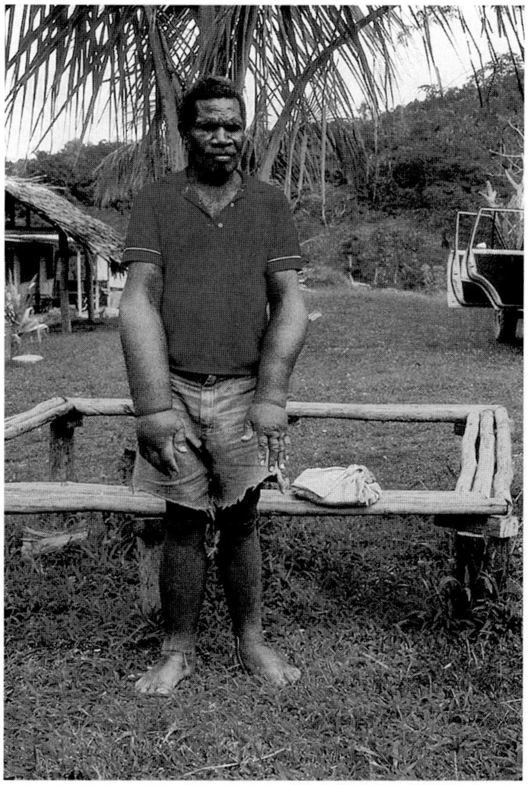

FIGURE 98-1 Lymphedema of the upper and lower extremities in a 50-year-old man. Swelling had been present for approximately 10 years, and the level of microfilaremia was 1000 parasites per milliliter of blood.

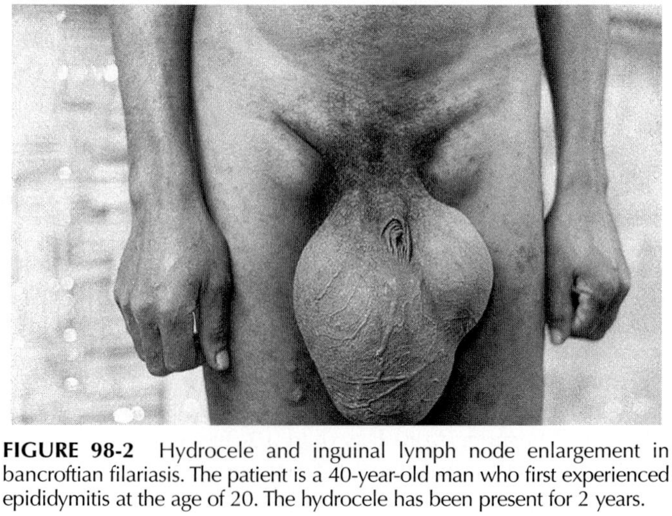

FIGURE 98-2 Hydrocele and inguinal lymph node enlargement in bancroftian filariasis. The patient is a 40-year-old man who first experienced epididymitis at the age of 20. The hydrocele has been present for 2 years.

Hydroceles are usually not painful unless they are complicated by acute epididymitis or funiculitis. Thickening of the spermatic cord commonly accompanies hydroceles. The skin of the scrotum may also be thickened and have a "brawny" character on palpation. If hydrocele fluid is drained, it is clear and straw-colored. Parasites are usually not found in this fluid. Inguinal lymph nodes and other nearby lymph nodes may also be enlarged (see Fig. 98-2).

Lymphedema of the Genitalia

Lymphedema of the genitalia involves swelling of the scrotum and/or thickened scrotal or penile skin that may have characteristic "peau d'orange" appearance.[42] In long-standing cases, verrucous lesions and lymphorrea are common. The genitals may be grossly deformed and terms such as "ram horn penis" have been used to describe the gross distortion of the penis seen in this condition.

Genital Lymphorrhea

In this condition, lymph oozes out to the exterior directly from dilated ruptured lymphatic vessels. The dermis may be normal. This frequently occurs in the scrotal wall.

Chyluria

Patients in filarial endemic areas may occasionally pass urine with a milky appearance. Upon settling, a fatty layer separates above a clear aqueous phase. This condition results from obstruction or physiologic impairment of the renal lymphatics, with passage of lymph from the lacteals draining the genitourinary tract. Chyluria may have serious nutritional consequences in that large amounts of fat and protein are lost in the urine. Its precise frequency in filarial endemic areas has not been established, but is exceedingly low compared to lymphedema of the extremities and hydroceles.

Tropical Pulmonary Eosinophilia

Tropical pulmonary eosinophilia (TPE), an asthma-like condition, is a distinct syndrome that develops in some individuals infected with either *W. bancrofti* or *B. malayi*.[43,44] This syndrome affects males and females at a ratio of 4-to-1, often during the third decade of life. The majority of cases have been reported from India, Pakistan, Sri Lanka, Brazil, Guyana, and Southeast Asia. The main clinical features include a history of residence in filarial endemic regions, paroxysmal cough and wheezing that are usually nocturnal (and probably related to the nocturnal periodicity of microfilariae), weight loss, low-grade fever, adenopathy, and pronounced blood eosinophilia (>3000 eosinophils/mL). Chest x-rays may be normal but generally show increased bronchovascular markings; diffuse miliary lesions or mottled opacities may be present in the middle and lower lung fields. Tests of pulmonary function show restrictive abnormalities in most cases and obstructive defects in half. Total serum IgE levels (10,000 to 100,000 ng/mL) and antifilarial antibody titers are characteristically elevated.

Unlike many subjects with lymphatic filariasis, those with TPE do not have microfilaremia. Administration of the antifilarial drug diethylcarbamazine (see later discussion) leads to significant symptomatic improvement with commensurate decreases in eosinophilia and serum immunoglobulin E (IgE). If patients with tropical pulmonary eosinophilia are not treated appropriately, the disease may progress to chronic restrictive lung disease with interstitial fibrosis.[45]

Lymphatic Filariasis in Expatriates

American servicemen returning from prolonged exposure to infectious mosquitoes in the South Pacific during World War II and French soldiers exposed in Indochina (now Vietnam) suffered from acute episodes of acute adenolymphangitis of the legs accompanied by eosinophilia. These acute disease manifestations were apparently caused by immune-mediated inflammatory responses to developing larvae and resolved on departure from the endemic area.[46] Progression to chronic lymphedema or elephantiasis was rare. More recent studies of Indonesian transmigrants from nonendemic to endemic regions[47] as well as studies in which volunteers were experimentally infected with infective larvae of *B. malayi*[48] provide corroboration of this process. This propensity to develop acute disease manifestations has been interpreted to be due to lack of immunological "tolerance" to filarial antigens seen commonly in those with lifelong (and early) exposure to the filarial organisms. In contrast to the preceding situation, the risk of developing acute or chronic manifestations of lymphatic filariasis for the traveler to endemic areas is extraordinarily small, given the inefficiency of transmission and the requirement for repeated contact with infected mosquitoes, although it has been seen rarely.

PATHOGENESIS AND IMMUNOLOGY

The precise and likely multiple mechanisms leading to the diverse clinical manifestations of lymphatic filariasis have not been established. However, several factors have been suggested to underlie the development of lymphedema of the legs. Some studies suggest that lack of patent infection or amicrofilaremia is associated with elephantiasis, whereas microfilaremia is more common among clinically asymptomatic persons. Because these diverse clinical conditions correlate with differences in filarial antigen-specific T-cell responses,[49] it is possible that the qualitative nature of host immunity affects the pathologic sequelae of chronic infection. Second, a variety of epidemiologic, immunologic, and parasitologic observations in humans and experimental animals suggest that prenatal sensitization and the consequent immunologic tolerance to filarial antigens influences the pathologic response to infection and the propensity to development of subclinical microfilaremia during childhood.[50,51] Third, based on studies of immunodeficient mice experimentally infected with *Brugia,* it is probable that parasite-derived molecules directly impair lymphatic function independent of the host immune system.[52] Fourth, correlations between entomologic indices of transmission and patent infection and disease rates indicate that the degree of exposure to mosquitoes harboring infective larvae is a major determinant of the frequency of microfilaremia and clinical morbidity at the population level.[53] Fifth, preexisting lymphatic dysfunction may predispose to secondary bacterial infections in persons who do not use footwear.[54] Finally, in view of the fact that susceptibility of mice to disease from a variety of helminth infections is related to the presence of genes both within and outside the major histocompatibility complex, it is possible that differences in these gene frequencies among infected persons with or without lymphatic disease is a risk factor.[55–58]

Establishing the relative importance of these diverse factors and a central unifying hypothesis to explain the pathogenesis of human lymphatic filariasis has been difficult because the onset of disease occurs over a period of years or decades and because of the marked heterogeneity in transmission and disease in various geographic areas. The immunological basis for the relative lack of pathology seen in the majority of individuals with patent infection, however, has been reasonably well-studied in both cross-sectional and longitudinal population-based studies; moreover, the development of circulating antigen assays to identify infected persons without microfilaremia (see next section) and measurements of multiple cytokines and chemokines have advanced our understanding of this immunologically complex filarial infection.[59,60] Studies in animal models and in vitro human systems have suggested that the initial immune response to infective stage larvae (L3) and to the next developmental stages (L4 and early adult stages) are dominated by pro-inflammatory and both Th1-like and Th2-like T cell responses.[61,62] With the onset of patency (when microfilariae appear in the blood), there is a marked diminution of the antigen-specific T cell responses (most notably T cell–derived interferon [IFN]-gamma).[63–69]

Clearly the inability of T cells to proliferate or produce IFN-gamma in response to parasite antigen is the hallmark of chronic, patent lymphatic filarial infection. This lack of T cell responsiveness has been shown to be primarily directed at antigen produced by microfilariae found in the circulation,[70] but secreted antigens from other parasite stages have been implicated as well. The mechanisms for this selective immune tolerance have been postulated to include: genetic predisposition,[55,56] diminished frequency of T and B cell precursors,[49] suppressor T cells or monocytes,[71,72] altered immune responses because of in utero exposure,[50] increased expression of downregulatory molecules like CTLA-4,[73] altered antigen-presenting cell function,[59,74] and the presence of regulatory cytokines such as interleukin (IL)-10 and transforming growth factor-β (TGF-β).[75] Most recently, antigen reactive cells with regulatory function (e.g., classical Th2 cells, T regulatory cells, and/or IL-10 producing antigen-presenting cells) as well as antigen nonspecific T regulatory cells have been implicated as contributors to the modulating influences of pro-inflammatory responses presumably needed to induce pathology.[59,76,77]

Examination of protective immunity against lymphatic filariasis in human populations has been extraordinarily difficult. However, population-based studies[78–80] have identified groups of individuals who appear to be infection free despite long-term exposure to the filarial parasites. On balance cells from such individuals are more likely to respond immunologically to parasite antigen than were those with patent infection. Serum from these infection-free individuals has been used to identify possible vaccine candidates, only a few of which have been tested in animal models. The best evidence, however, for the induction of protective immunity has come from studies in animals (birds, cats, ferrets) given radiation-attenuated L3 larvae; in these studies, irradiated L3s induced protection to varying degrees (from 60%–95% protection from challenge).[81–84] Attempts with subunit vaccines using recombinant antigens or DNA vaccination have been less successful, but for one antigen (Bm-ALT-1) levels of protection reached close to 60%.[85]

DIAGNOSIS

Lymphatic filariasis is diagnosed by a combination of the appropriate epidemiologic history, physical findings, and laboratory tests. In residents of endemic areas, the appearance of lymphedema of the extremities or disease of the male genitalia is most likely due to filarial infection if the patient is older than 15 years of age and there is no other obvious cause, such as trauma to the lymphatics or congestive heart failure.

A definitive diagnosis can be made only by detection of the parasites and hence can be difficult. Adult worms localized in lymphatic vessels or nodes are largely inaccessible. Examination, however, of the scrotum or the female breast using high-frequency ultrasound in conjunction with Doppler techniques may result in the identification of motile adult worms within dilated lymphatics.[86–89] Worms may be visualized in the lymphatics of the spermatic cord in up to 80% of infected men.[86] Live adult worms have a distinctive pattern of movement within the lymphatic vessels (termed the *filaria dance sign*).[36,86]

Microfilariae can be found in blood, in hydrocele fluid, or (occasionally) in other body fluids. Such fluids can be examined microscopically, either directly using a giemsa-stained thin blood smear or—for greater sensitivity—after concentration of the parasites by the passage of blood through a polycarbonate cylindrical 3- to 5-mm pore filter (Nuclepore) or by the centrifugation of fluid fixed in 2% formalin (Knott's concentration technique).[90] The timing of blood collection is critical and should be based on the periodicity of the microfilariae in the endemic region involved.

Many infected individuals do not have microfilaremia, and definitive diagnosis in such cases can be difficult. Assays for circulating antigens of *W. bancrofti* permit the diagnosis of microfilaremic and cryptic (amicrofilaremic) infection. Two tests are commercially available: one is an enzyme-linked immunosorbent assay (ELISA)[91] and the other a rapid-format immunochromatographic card test.[92] Both assays have sensitivities that range from 96% to 100% and specificities that approach 100%. There are currently no tests for circulating antigens in brugian filariasis.

Polymerase chain reaction (PCR)–based assays for DNA of *W. bancrofti* and *B. malayi* in blood have been developed.[93–98] A number of studies indicate that this diagnostic method is of equivalent or greater sensitivity compared with parasitologic methods, detecting patent infection in almost all infected subjects.

Antibody-based assays for diagnosing filarial infection have typically used crude parasite extract and have suffered from poor specificity. Improvements have been made by the use of detection of antifilarial IgG4 antibodies[99] in that they have relatively less cross-reactivity to nonfilarial helminth antigens. Specificity has also been improved by the use of species-specific recombinant antigens for both brugian and bancroftian infection[100]; indeed, a diagnostic dipstick test has been developed for use in areas endemic for brugian filariasis.[101]

In cases of suspected lymphatic filariasis, radionuclide lymphoscintigraphic imaging of the limbs reliably demonstrates widespread lymphatic abnormalities in both asymptomatic microfilaremic persons and those with clinical manifestations of lymphatic pathology. While of potential utility in the delineation of anatomic changes associated with infection, lymphoscintigraphy is unlikely to assume primacy in the diagnostic evaluation of individuals with suspected infection.

It is important to note, however, that it is not possible to exclude a diagnosis of filarial-induced disease in the absence of circulating antigens or parasites since disease may persist in persons with so-called burned-out infections. This situation may occur in persons who have received multiple courses of treatment or who have left endemic areas. Ancillary evidence consistent with the diagnosis of lymphatic filariasis includes peripheral blood eosinophilia, elevated serum IgE, and increased filarial-specific antibodies.

TREATMENT AND PROGNOSIS

Asymptomatic Lymphatic Filariasis

The optimal approach to these patients has not yet been established. However, on the basis of recent evidence demonstrating that such persons have abnormal lymphatics despite the lack of clinically overt disease, it seems advisable that a course of diethylcarbamazine be given. The drug (6 mg/kg/day) is administered two to three times daily for a total dose of 72 mg/kg body weight over a period of 10 to 14 days. In bancroftian filariasis, this results in greater than a 90% decrease in microfilaremia within one month, which persists for at least one year. The rate of lowering of *Brugia* microfilaremia is considerably slower.

Because of the possibility of acute side effects from drug therapy, such as fever, malaise, and occasionally bronchospasm (related to the release of large amounts of filarial antigens from dying parasites), the dose should ideally be limited to 3 mg/kg body weight on the first day. Fever and malaise are common in the first few days of treatment, and antipyretics such as aspirin should be given in such situations. In heavily infected patients, painful nodules in the skin, lymph node enlargement, and epididymitis may appear within a week or so of drug administration and persist for several weeks afterward. These are apparently due to inflammatory responses to dying parasites and resolve over a month or so. Management is symptomatic and should include proper hygiene to avoid secondary infections.

Recent population-based studies have established that annual single doses of diethylcarbamazine (6 mg/kg) alone or in combination with ivermectin (400 μg/kg) or albendazole (400 mg) may be as effective as a complete course in terms of lowering the level of microfilaremia.[102–105]

Acute Adenolymphangitis

At present, it is recommended that a course of diethylcarbamazine be given along with analgesics. Cellulitis due to secondary bacterial infections of the lower extremities should be treated by proper cleansing and administration of antibiotics based on results of microbiologic tests.

Hydroceles and Elephantiasis

The optimal course for management of these conditions is not entirely clear. Drainage of hydroceles provides immediate relief, though they recur in the absence of drug therapy or surgical removal of the tunica albuginea. In the case of lymphedema of the lower extremities, it seems wise at present to administer diethylcarbamazine given the fact that the parasite load will be diminished, even though fibrosis of the lymphatics may preclude establishment of normal lymphatic drainage. In severe cases of deforming elephantiasis, surgical approaches involving lymphatic-venous and nodal-venous anastomoses have been moderately successful in diminishing the degree of leg swelling.[106] The long-term effects of these expert surgical techniques are under study at the present time. In all cases, it is important that the occurrence of secondary bacterial infections be kept to a minimum by practicing proper hygiene and prompt treatment of infections that do occur.

PREVENTION AND CONTROL

Individual protection against filarial infection may be achieved by avoiding contact with infected mosquitoes. This can be done by use of bed nets, particularly those impregnated with insecticides such as permethrin. Although this approach may be useful in some circumstances, it is impractical in many areas of the world because of lack of acceptance of their use, their cost, and the fact that filarial infection is acquired over a period of 10 to 20 years. With respect to population-based approaches to control lymphatic filariasis, recent studies suggest that community-based drug therapy programs involving single annual doses of diethylcarbamazine[107] or table salt mixed with diethylcarbamazine[54] given for 4 to 6 years may be an effective means of decreasing transmission and possibly eradicating filariasis. The current strategy of the global plan to eliminate lymphatic filaraisis is based on mass treatment with single annual doses of diethylcarbamazine plus albendazole or albendazole plus ivermectin for areas where onchocerciasis coexists (diethylcarbamazine is not recommended because of its potential for diminishing visual acuity in onchocerciasis).[103,108] Information available at the end of 2003 indicates that 122 million persons in 38 countries have thus far participated. The strategy of the global plan is being refined and guided by ongoing research aimed at understanding the ecology and transmission efficiency of the various mosquito vector species and efficacy of various drug regimens combined with insecticide-impregnated bed nets being used in malaria control programs.[109]

REFERENCES

1. Evans DB, Gelband H, Vlassoff C: Social and economic factors and the control of lymphatic filariasis: A review. Acta Trop 53:1–26, 1993.
2. Ottesen EA: The global programme to eliminate lymphatic filariasis. Trop Med Int Health 5:591–594, 2000.
3. Routh HB, Bhowmik KR: History of elephantiasis. Int J Dermatol 32:913–916, 1993.
4. Rajan TV: Lymphatic filariasis: A historical perspective. In Nutman TB (ed): Lymphatic Filariasis, vol. 1. London, Imperial College Press, 2000, pp 1–4.

5. Demarquay J-N: Helminthologie. Gazette Med Paris 18:665–667, 1863.
6. Wucherer OEH: Noticia preliminar sobrevermes de uma especie ainda nao descripta, encontrados na urina de donentes de hematuria intertropical no Brazil. Gazetas Med Bahia 3:97–99, 1868.
7. Lewis TR: On a hematozoan inhabiting human blood, its relation to chyluria and other diseases. Government of India, 1872.
8. Manson P: On filarial periodicity. BMJ 2:644–646, 1899.
9. Manson P: Further observations on filaria sanguinis hominis, China imperial maritime customs. 1877.
10. Cobbold TS: Discovery of the adult representative of a microscopic Filariae. Lancet 2:70–71, 1877.
11. Bourne AG: A note on filaria *Filaria Sanguinis Hominis* (with description of a male specimen). BMJ 1:1050–1051, 1888.
12. Bancroft TL: On the metamorphosis of the young form of *Filaria bancrofti* Cobbold (*Filaria sanguinis hominis* Lewis; *Filaria nocturna* Manson) in the body of *Culex ciliaris*, the house mosquito of Australia. J Trop Med 2:91–94, 1899.
13. Low GC: A recent observation on *Filaria nocturna* in *Culex*; Probable mode of infection of man. BMJ 1:1456–1457, 1900.
14. Buckley JJ: On *Brugia* gen. nov. for *Wuchereria* spp. of the malayl' group, i.e., *W. malayi* (Brug, 1927), *W. pahangi* Buckley and Edeson, 1956, and *W. patei* Buckley, Nelson and Heisch, 1958. Ann Trop Med Parasitol 54:75–77, 1960.
15. O'Connor FW: Filarial periodicity with observations and on the mechanisms of migration of the microfilariae and from parent worm to the blood stream. PR J Public Health Trop Med 6:263, 1931.
16. Southgate BA: Intensity and efficiency of transmission and the development of microfilaraemia and disease: Their relationship in lymphatic filariasis. J Trop Med Hyg 95:1–12, 1992.
17. Kozek WJ, Marroquin HF: Intracytoplasmic bacteria in *Onchocerca volvulus*. Am J Trop Med Hyg 26:663–678, 1977.
18. McLaren DJ, Worms MJ, Laurence BR, Simpson MG: Micro-organisms in filarial larvae (Nematoda). Trans R Soc Trop Med Hyg 69:509–514, 1975.
19. Sironi M, Bandi C, Sacchi L, et al: Molecular evidence for a close relative of the arthropod endosymbiont *Wolbachia* in a filarial worm. Mol Biochem Parasitol 74:223–227, 1995.
20. Taylor MJ, Hoerauf A: *Wolbachia* bacteria of filarial nematodes. Parasitol Today 15:437–442, 1999.
21. Hise AG, Gillette-Ferguson I, Pearlman E: The role of endosymbiotic *Wolbachia* bacteria in filarial disease. Cell Microbiol 6:97–104, 2004.
22. Rajan TV: Relationship of anti-microbial activity of tetracyclines to their ability to block the L3 to L4 molt of the human filarial parasite *Brugia malayi*. Am J Trop Med Hyg 71:24–28, 2004.
23. Hoerauf A, Mand S, Volkmann L, et al: Doxycycline as a novel strategy against bancroftian filariasis-depletion of *Wolbachia* endosymbionts from *Wuchereria bancrofti* and stop of microfilaria production. Med Microbiol Immunol (Berl) 192:211–216, 2003.
24. Cross HF, Haarbrink M, Egerton G, et al: Severe reactions to filarial chemotherapy and release of *Wolbachia* endosymbionts into blood. Lancet 358:1873–1875, 2001.
25. Taylor MJ, Cross HF, Bilo K: Inflammatory responses induced by the filarial nematode *Brugia malayi* are mediated by lipopolysaccharide-like activity from endosymbiotic *Wolbachia* bacteria. J Exp Med 191:1429–1436, 2000.
26. Michael E, Bundy DA: Global mapping of lymphatic filariasis. Parasitol Today 13:472–476, 1997.
27. Michael E, Bundy DA, Grenfell BT: Re-assessing the global prevalence and distribution of lymphatic filariasis. Parasitology 112:409–428, 1996.
28. Bockarie M, Kazura J, Alexander N, et al: Transmission dynamics of *Wuchereria bancrofti* in East Sepik Province, Papua New Guinea. Am J Trop Med Hyg 54:577–581, 1996.
29. Sasa M: Human Filariasis. Baltimore, Baltimore University Press, 1976.
30. Kazura JW, Bockerie M, Alexander N, et al: Transmission intensity and its relationship to infection and disease due to *Wuchereria bancrofti* in Papua New Guinea. J Infect Dis 176:242–246, 1997.
31. Ottesen EA: Infection and disease in lymphatic filariasis—An immunological perspective. Parasitology 104:S71–S79, 1992.
32. Dreyer G, Ottesen EA, Galdino E, et al: Renal abnormalities in microfilaremic patients with bancroftian filariasis. Am J Trop Med Hyg 46:745–751, 1992.
33. Freedman DO, de Almeida Filho PJ, Besh S, et al: Lymphoscintigraphic analysis of lymphatic abnormalities in symptomatic and asymptomatic human filariasis. J Infect Dis 170:927–933, 1994.
34. Case T, Leis B, Witte M, et al: Vascular abnormalities in experimental and human lymphatic filariasis. Lymphology 24:174–183, 1991.
35. Witte MH, Jamal S, Williams WH, et al: Lymphatic abnormalities in human filariasis as depicted by lymphangioscintigraphy. Arch Intern Med 153:737–744, 1993.
36. Mand S, Marfa-Debrekyei Y, Dittrich M, et al: Animated documentation of the filaria dance sign (FDS) in bancroftian filariasis. Filaria J 2:3, 2003.
37. Noroes J, Addiss D, Santos A, et al: Ultrasonographic evidence of abnormal lymphatic vessels in young men with adult *Wuchereria bancrofti* infection in the scrotal area. J Urol 156:409–412, 1996.
38. Noroes J, Addiss D, Amaral F, et al: Occurrence of living adult *Wuchereria bancrofti* in the scrotal area of men with microfilaraemia. Trans R Soc Trop Med Hyg 90:55–56, 1996.
39. Michael E, Grenfell BT, Bundy DA: The association between microfilaraemia and disease in lymphatic filariasis. Proc R Soc Lond B Biol Sci 256:33–40, 1994.
40. Pani SP, Yuvaraj J, Vanamail D, et al: Episodic adenolymphangitis and lymphoedema in patients with bancroftian filariasis. Trans R Soc Trop Med Hyg 89:72–74, 1995.
41. Lymphatic filariasis. Fourth report of the WHO Expert Committee on Filariasis. World Health Organ Tech Rep Ser 702:3–112, 1984.
42. Dreyer G, Noroes J, Figueredo-Silva J, et al: Pathogenesis of lymphatic disease in bancroftian filariasis: A clinical perspective. Parasitol Today 16:544–548, 2000.
43. Ottesen EA, Nutman TB: Tropical pulmonary eosinophilia. Annu Rev Med 43:417–424, 1992.
44. Coutinho AD, Rocha A, Madeiros Z, et al: [Tropical filarial pulmonary eosinophilia and its differential diagnosis.] Rev Hosp Clin Fac Med Sao Paulo 53:42–51, 1998.
45. Rom WN, Vijayan VJ, Cornelius MJ, et al: Persistent lower respiratory tract inflammation associated with interstitial lung disease in patients with tropical pulmonary eosinophilia following conventional treatment with diethylcarbamazine. Am Rev Respir Dis 142:1088–1092, 1990.
46. Wartman WB: Filariasis in American armed servicemen in World War II. Medicine (Baltimore) 12:181, 1947.
47. Partono F, Pribadi PW, Soewarta A: Epidemiological and clinical features of *Brugia timori* in a newly established village. Karakuak, West Flores, Indonesia. Am J Trop Med Hyg 27:910–915, 1978.
48. Nutman TB: Experimental infection of humans with filariae. Rev Infect Dis 13:1018–1022, 1991.
49. King CL, Kumaraswami V, Poindexter RW, et al: Immunologic tolerance in lymphatic filariasis. Diminished parasite-specific T and B lymphocyte precursor frequency in the microfilaremic state. J Clin Invest 89:1403–1410, 1992.
50. Steel C, Guinea A, McCarthy JS, et al: Long-term effect of prenatal exposure to maternal microfilaraemia on immune responsiveness to filarial parasite antigens. Lancet 343:890–893, 1994.
51. Lammie PJ, Hitch WL, Walker Allen EM, et al: Maternal filarial infection as risk factor for infection in children. Lancet 337:1005–1006, 1991.
52. Nelson FK, Greiner DL, Schultz LD, et al: The immunodeficient scid mouse as a model for human lymphatic filariasis. J Exp Med 173:659–663, 1991.
53. Das PK, Srividya A, Pani SP, et al: Cumulative exposure and its relationship with chronic filarial disease in bancroftian filariasis. Southeast Asian J Trop Med Public Health 25:516–521, 1994.
54. Ottesen EA, Ramachandran CP: Lymphatic filariasis infection and disease: Control strategies. Parasitol Today 11:129, 1995.
55. Choi EH, Zimmerman PA, Fuster CB, et al: Genetic polymorphisms in molecules of innate immunity and susceptibility to infection with *Wuchereria bancrofti* in South India. Genes Immun 2:248–253, 2001.
56. Hise AG, Hazlett FE, Bockerie MJ, et al: Polymorphisms of innate immunity genes and susceptibility to lymphatic filariasis. Genes Immun 4:524–527, 2003.
57. Cuenco KT, Halloran ME, Louis-Charles J, et al: A family study of lymphedema of the leg in a lymphatic filariasis-endemic area. Am J Trop Med Hyg 70:180–184, 2004.
58. Cuenco KT, Halloran ME, Lammie PJ: Assessment of families for excess risk of lymphedema of the leg in a lymphatic filariasis-endemic area. Am J Trop Med Hyg 70:185–190, 2004.

59. Maizels RM, et al: Helminth parasites—Masters of regulation. Immunol Rev 201:89–116, 2004.
60. Maizels RM, Yazdanbakhsh M: Immune regulation by helminth parasites: Cellular and molecular mechanisms. Nat Rev Immunol 3:733–744, 2003.
61. Babu S, Nutman TB: Proinflammatory cytokines dominate the early immune response to filarial parasites. J Immunol 171:6723–6732, 2003.
62. Graham SP, Trees AJ, Collins RA, et al: Down-regulated lymphoproliferation coincides with parasite maturation and with the collapse of both gamma interferon and interleukin-4 responses in a bovine model of onchocerciasis. Infect Immun 69:4313–4319, 2001.
63. Taubert A, Zahner H: Cellular immune responses of filaria (*Litomosoides sigmodontis*) infected BALB/c mice detected on the level of cytokine transcription. Parasite Immunol 23:453–462, 2001.
64. Schreuer D, Hammerberg B: Modulation of cellular and humoral immunity, and disease manifestation during onset of patency in *Brugia pahangi*–infected dogs. Immunology 79:658–666, 1993.
65. Soboslay PT, Dreweck CM, Taylor HR, et al: Experimental onchocerciasis in chimpanzees. Cell-mediated immune responses, and production and effects of IL-1 and IL-2 with *Onchocerca volvulus* infection. J Immunol 147:346–353, 1991.
66. Nutman TB, Kumaraswami V: Regulation of the immune response in lymphatic filariasis: Perspectives on acute and chronic infection with *Wuchereria bancrofti* in South India. Parasite Immunol 23:389–399, 2001.
67. Bosshardt SC, Coleman SM, McVay CS, et al: Impact of microfilaremia on maintenance of a hyporesponsive cellular immune response in *Brugia*-infected gerbils (*Meriones unguiculatus*). Infect Immun 63:940–945, 1995.
68. Misra S, Mukherjee M, Dikshit M, et al: Cellular immune response of *Mastomys* and gerbils in experimental filariasis. Trop Med Int Health 3:124–129, 1998.
69. Rao UR, Nasarre C, Coleman SM, et al: Cellular immune responses of jirds to extracts of life cycle stages and adult excretory secretory products during the early development of *Brugia pahangi*. Exp Parasitol 82:255–266, 1996.
70. Mahanty S, Luke HE, Kumaraswami V, et al: Stage-specific induction of cytokines regulates the immune response in lymphatic filariasis. Exp Parasitol 84:282–290, 1996.
71. Piessens WF, Ratiwayanto S, Tuti S, et al: Antigen-specific suppressor cells and suppressor factors in human filariasis with *Brugia malayi*. N Engl J Med 302:833–837, 1980.
72. Piessens WF, Partono F, Hoffman SL, et al: Antigen-specific suppressor T lymphocytes in human lymphatic filariasis. N Engl J Med 307:144–148, 1982.
73. Steel C, Nutman TB: CTLA-4 in filarial infections: Implications for a role in diminished T cell reactivity. J Immunol 170:1930–1938, 2003.
74. Semnani RT, Nutman TB: Toward an understanding of the interaction between filarial parasites and host antigen-presenting cells. Immunol Rev 201:127–138, 2004.
75. King CL, Mahanty S, Abrams JS, et al: Cytokine control of parasite-specific anergy in human lymphatic filariasis. Preferential induction of a regulatory T helper type 2 lymphocyte subset. J Clin Invest 92:1667–1673, 1993.
76. Satoguina J, Mempel M, Larbi J, et al: Antigen-specific T regulatory-1 cells are associated with immunosuppression in a chronic helminth infection (onchocerciasis). Microbes Infect 4:1291–1300, 2002.
77. Hoerauf A, Brattig N: Resistance and susceptibility in human onchocerciasis—Beyond Th1 vs. Th2. Trends Parasitol 18:25–31, 2002.
78. Ravindran B, Satapathy AK, Sahoo PK, et al: Protective immunity in human lymphatic filariasis: Problems and prospects. Med Microbiol Immunol (Berl) 192:41–46, 2003.
79. Steel C, Guinea A, Ottesen EA: Evidence for protective immunity to bancroftian filariasis in the Cook Islands. J Infect Dis 174:598–605, 1996.
80. Freedman DO, Nutman TB, Ottesen EA: Protective immunity in bancroftian filariasis. Selective recognition of a 43-kD larval stage antigen by infection-free individuals in an endemic area. J Clin Invest 83:14–22, 1989.
81. Yates JA, Higashi GI: *Brugia malayi*: Vaccination of jirds with 60cobalt-attenuated infective stage larvae protects against homologous challenge. Am J Trop Med Hyg 34:1132–1137, 1985.
82. Oothuman P, Denham DA, McGreevy PB, et al: Successful vaccination of cats against *Brugia pahangi* with larvae attenuated by irradiation with 10 krad cobalt 60. Parasite Immunol 1:209–216, 1979.
83. Storey DM, Al-Mukhtar AS: Vaccination of jirds, *Meriones unguiculatus*, against *Litomosoides carinii* and *Brugia pahangi* using irradiate larvae of *L. carinii*. Tropenmed Parasitol 33:23–24, 1982.
84. Crandall R, Crandall C, Nayar J, et al: Resistance and disease in *Brugia malayi* infection of ferrets following prior infection, injection of attenuated infective larvae and injections of larval extracts. Parasite Immunol 16:425–433, 1994.
85. Gregory WF, Atmadja AK, Allen JE, et al: The abundant larval transcript-1 and -2 genes of *Brugia malayi* encode stage-specific candidate vaccine antigens for filariasis. Infect Immun 68:4174–4179, 2000.
86. Dreyer G, Santos A, Noroes J, et al: Amicrofilaraemic carriers of adult *Wuchereria bancrofti*. Trans R Soc Trop Med Hyg 90:288–289, 1996.
87. Dreyer G, Noroes J, Rocha A, et al: Detection of living adult *Wuchereria bancrofti* in a patient with tropical pulmonary eosinophilia. Braz J Med Biol Res 29:1005–1008, 1996.
88. Dreyer G, Brandao AC, Amaral F, et al: Detection by ultrasound of living adult *Wuchereria bancrofti* in the female breast. Mem Inst Oswaldo Cruz 91:95–96, 1996.
89. Dreyer G, Santos A, Noroes J, et al: Ultrasonographic detection of living adult *Wuchereria bancrofti* using a 3.5-MHz transducer. Am J Trop Med Hyg 59:399–403, 1998.
90. Eberhard ML, Lammie PJ: Laboratory diagnosis of filariasis. Clin Lab Med 11:977–1010, 1991.
91. More SJ, Copeman DB: A highly specific and sensitive monoclonal antibody-based ELISA for the detection of circulating antigen in bancroftian filariasis. Trop Med Parasitol 41:403–406, 1990.
92. Weil GJ, Lammie PJ, Weiss N: The ICT Filariasis Test: A rapid-format antigen test for diagnosis of bancroftian filariasis. Parasitol Today 13:401–404, 1997.
93. Lizotte MR, Supali T, Partono F, et al: A polymerase chain reaction assay for the detection of *Brugia malayi* in blood. Am J Trop Med Hyg 51:314–321, 1994.
94. Rao UR, Williams SA, Klei TR: Quantification of PCR amplification products of *Brugia* HhaI repeat DNA using a semiautomated Q-PCR system. Mol Cell Probes 16:13–23, 2002.
95. Kluber S, Supali T, Williams SA, et al: Rapid PCR-based detection of *Brugia malayi* DNA from blood spots by DNA Detection Test Strips. Trans R Soc Trop Med Hyg 95:169–170, 2001.
96. Rahmah N, Ashikin AN, Anuar AK, et al: PCR-ELISA for the detection of *Brugia malayi* infection using finger-prick blood. Trans R Soc Trop Med Hyg 92:404–406, 1998.
97. McCarthy JS, Zhong M, Gopinath R, et al: Evaluation of a polymerase chain reaction-based assay for diagnosis of Wuchereria bancrofti infection. J Infect Dis 173:1510–1514, 1996.
98. Nutman TB, Zimmerman PA, Kubofeik J, et al: A universally applicable diagnostic approach to filarial and other infections. Parasitol Today 10:239–243, 1994.
99. Lal RB, Ottesen EA: Enhanced diagnostic specificity in human filariasis by IgG4 antibody assessment. J Infect Dis 158:1034–1037, 1988.
100. Lammie PJ, Weil G, Noordin R, et al: Recombinant antigen-based antibody assays for the diagnosis and surveillance of lymphatic filariasis—A multicenter trial. Filaria J 3:9, 2004.
101. Rahmah N, Taniawati S, Shenoy RK, et al: Specificity and sensitivity of a rapid dipstick test (Brugia Rapid) in the detection of *Brugia malayi* infection. Trans R Soc Trop Med Hyg 95:601–604, 2001.
102. Horton J, Witt C, Ottesen EA, et al: An analysis of the safety of the single dose, two drug regimens used in programmes to eliminate lymphatic filariasis. Parasitology 121(Suppl):S147–S160, 2000.
103. Molyneux DH, Bradley M, Hoerauf A, et al: Mass drug treatment for lymphatic filariasis and onchocerciasis. Trends Parasitol 19:516–522, 2003.
104. Ottesen EA: Major progress toward eliminating lymphatic filariasis. N Engl J Med 347:1885–1886, 2002.
105. Addiss D, Critchley J, Ejere H, et al: Albendazole for lymphatic filariasis. Cochrane Database Syst Rev CD003753, 2004.

106. Jamal S: Lymphovenous anastomosis in filarial lymphedema. Lymphology 14:64–68, 1981.
107. Bockarie MJ, Alexander ND, Hyun P, et al: Randomised community-based trial of annual single-dose diethylcarbamazine with or without ivermectin against *Wuchereria bancrofti* infection in human beings and mosquitoes. Lancet 351:162–168, 1998.
108. Molyneux D: Lymphatic filariasis (elephantiasis) elimination: A public health success and development opportunity. Filaria J 2:13, 2003.
109. Soremekun S, Maxwell C, Zuwakuu M, et al: Measuring the efficacy of insecticide treated bednets: The use of DNA fingerprinting to increase the accuracy of personal protection estimates in Tanzania. Trop Med Int Health 9:664–672, 2004.

sequences, a PCR-based multiplex technique has been developed that appears to be approximately 10 times more sensitive than traditional blood filtration. Furthermore, a colorimetric detection system that can be performed at ambient temperature has simplified the readout, permitting its use in endemic areas.[98]

The differential diagnosis of Calabar swellings includes angioedema associated with C1 inhibitor deficiency, infection with other filariae (particularly *M. perstans* and *O. volvulus*), nematode and trematode infections (e.g., trichinellosis and gnathostomiasis), and hypereosinophilic syndromes. Although "eye worm" in the setting of a compatible exposure history is extremely suggestive of loiasis, subconjunctival migration of other nematodes, including *Dirofilaria repens* (a filarial parasite of dogs and cats) and *Thelazia californiensis* (deer eye worm), has been reported.[99,100] Finally, the symptoms of *L. loa* infection may sometimes be difficult to distinguish from those of onchocerciasis or bancroftian filariasis, infections that may be coendemic with loiasis.

TREATMENT AND PROGNOSIS

Diethylcarbamazine (DEC) is effective against both microfilariae and adult worms and, at a dose of 8 to 10 mg/kg/day for 21 days, remains the drug of choice for the treatment of *L. loa* infection in amicrofilaremic patients, including most long-term visitors to endemic areas.[101] Although it is curative after a single course in 45% to 50% of such patients, multiple courses are often necessary and recrudescence may occur up to 8 years post-treatment.[102] Mild side effects of treatment are common and include Calabar swellings, pruritus, arthralgias, fever, nausea, diarrhea, right upper quadrant discomfort, and a sensation of creeping under the skin.[35,103] Antihistamines or steroids may reduce the development and severity of these symptoms. Occasionally, mobile adult worms are seen under the skin following DEC treatment and may be removed with forceps through a small skin incision[103] or by excisional biopsy.[104]

More serious complications of the treatment of loiasis, including renal failure, shock, coma, and fatal encephalitis, are related to the microfilarial burden and may be provoked or exacerbated by the massive microfilarial lysis that occurs with DEC treatment.[105,106] Historically, a gradual increase in the dose of DEC and pretreatment with antihistamines and steroids have been advocated to prevent these complications; however, numerous reports have demonstrated that these interventions do not prevent encephalitis.[50] The exact number of microfilariae that presents a significant risk is unknown, but 2500/mL blood has been suggested. Alternatives for people with high levels of circulating microfilariae include no treatment, removal of circulating microfilariae by cytapheresis prior to DEC treatment,[107,108] and newer drugs, including ivermectin[109–113] and albendazole.[114]

Ivermectin, the microfilaricidal drug of choice in onchocerciasis, has been shown to reduce microfilarial levels in patients with *L. loa* infection but is ineffective against the adult worms.[109,112] In addition, side effects secondary to microfilarial lysis occur in 30% to 70% of patients with high levels of circulating microfilariae and, in rare cases, may be life-threatening.[109,110]

In uncontrolled studies, prolonged administration of high doses of the anthelminthic mebendazole has led to a decrease in the numbers of circulating microfilariae in some patients with loiasis.[115,116] The frequency of adverse effects that occur because of the high doses necessary to achieve reasonable blood levels has limited its utility. Furthermore, clearance of microfilaremia is rare, and at least one study has failed to demonstrate any effect of mebendazole on *L. loa* microfilarial levels.[117] Albendazole, a related benzimidazole with better oral bioavailability, has been shown in a double-blind, placebo-controlled study to decrease microfilarial levels in *Loa*-infected patients when used at a dose of 200 mg twice daily for 3 weeks.[114] Adverse effects were not observed, even in people with more than 50,000 microfilariae per milliliter of blood. Unfortunately, shorter, higher dose regimens do not appear effective.[118,119] The gradual decrease in blood microfilarial levels over the course of several months suggests that albendazole may have a preferential effect on the adult parasite, explaining the lack of adverse effects associated with massive microfilarial antigen release during albendazole treatment. Sequential therapy with albendazole and a microfilaricidal agent (DEC or ivermectin) may provide an alternative to pretreatment cytapheresis in patients with high microfilarial levels.

PREVENTION AND CONTROL

Weekly chemoprophylaxis with diethylcarbamazine (300 mg) is effective for prevention of loiasis in long-term travelers to endemic areas.[2] In an uncontrolled study, monthly administration of DEC 100 mg on 3 successive days each month was also suggested as a regimen that would provide effective prophylaxis.[120] Vector control programs have achieved only limited success, primarily because of the dense vegetation in endemic areas and difficulties of access to the *Chrysops* breeding sites.[40]

Mansonella Streptocerca

INTRODUCTION

Streptocerciasis, infection with the filarial nematode *M. streptocerca*, is limited to the tropical rain forests of Central Africa, although a small focus has also been found in western Uganda.[121] Although the infection can be completely asymptomatic, characteristic clinical features include a chronic, pruritic dermatitis and lymphadenopathy, often indistinguishable from onchocerciasis. Because adult male and female worms have been found in the skin of chimpanzees and because microfilariae have been found in gorillas, streptocerciasis may be a zoonosis.

AGENT

Although microfilariae of *M. streptocerca* (synonyms: *Dipetalonema streptocerca* and *Tetrapetalonema streptocerca*) were first identified in 1922 in the skin of Ghanaians by Macfie and Corson,[122] the demonstration of adult female[123] and adult male worms did not occur until 1972.[124] Infective larvae are most likely transmitted to the host by the bite of an infected midge, *Culicoides grahamii*.[125,126] Over the course of months to years, these larvae develop into white, threadlike adult worms (males, 17 or 18 mm × 40 to 50 μm; females, 27 mm × 65 to 85 μm) that live in the dermal layer of the skin. In bisexual infections, microfilariae (sheathless, 2.5 to 5.0 × 180 to 240 μm) are produced and reside in the upper dermal and collagen layers of the skin.[127] *Mansonella streptocerca* has also been found in nonhuman primates,[128] which appear to be additional definitive hosts for this parasite.

EPIDEMIOLOGY

There are no good estimates of the number of residents of endemic areas in western and central Africa infected with *M. streptocerca*.[23] *Mansonella streptocerca* has been found in the tropical rain forests of northern Angola, Cameroon, Central African Republic, People's Republic of Congo, Equatorial Guinea, Nigeria, Uganda, and the Democratic Republic of Congo. In endemic areas, 40% of people may be infected (i.e., have clinical symptoms or detectable skin-dwelling microfilariae). Detailed analyses of the seasonality and ecology of *M. streptocerca* infection have not been performed.

DISEASE

The major clinical manifestations of streptocerciasis are dermatologic[124,127] and include pruritus, papular rashes, and pigmentation changes. A chronic, pruritic dermatitis, characterized by nonanesthetic hypopigmented macules, is most common.[124] These macules may be discrete or confluent, and they are located predominantly over the shoulder girdle and thorax. Dermal thickening is often present. Papular eruptions occur relatively less frequently. Inguinal adenopathy is extremely common in streptocerciasis; in several studies the incidence of this finding was 100%.[124] Although it has been reported that massive lymphedema (elephantiasis) can occur as a result of *M. streptocerca* infection, this remains unproven. Infection is associated with peripheral blood eosinophilia without leukocytosis.[124,127]

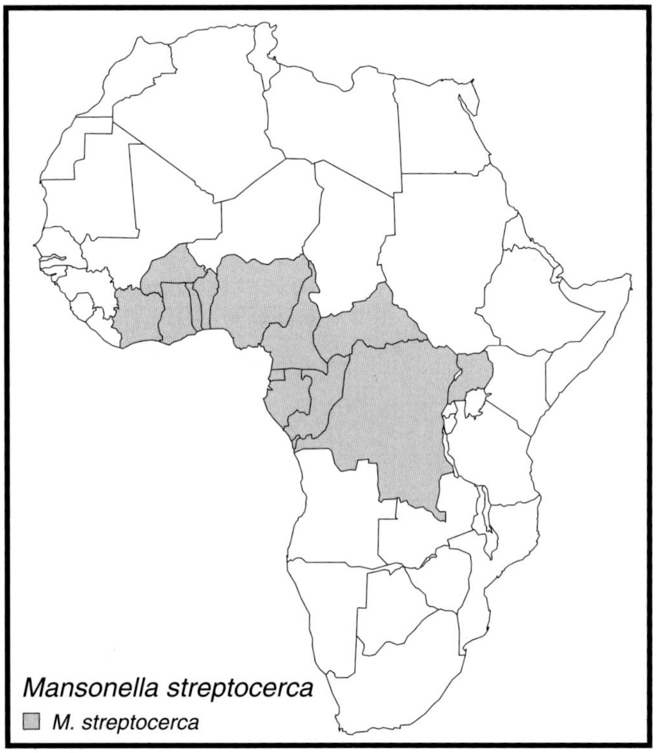

PATHOGENESIS AND IMMUNITY

Most of the pathologic changes seen in streptocerciasis are dermal and consist of sclerosis of the papillae, edema, fibrosis, and perivascular infiltration with lymphocytes and eosinophils.[124,127] Dermal lymphatics are also dilated. Similar to *O. volvulus* and many of the other filarial pathogens of humans, *M. streptocerca* is well adapted to the host and provokes little inflammatory reaction in the absence of treatment. With filaricidal treatment, however, inflammatory reactions do appear around adult worms and microfilariae, suggesting that the parasite is releasing antigens to which the host's inflammatory system responds.[124,127]

DIAGNOSIS

Streptocerciasis should be suspected in any person returning from an endemic area who presents with pruritus, a rash, or bilateral inguinal adenopathy. Definitive diagnosis is made by the identification of *M. streptocerca* microfilariae in skin snips. These are approximately 270×5 μm in size and are distinguished from the microfilariae of other species (most notably the skin-dwelling *O. volvulus*) by a characteristic tapered hook-shaped tail (shepherd's crook) and nuclei extending to the end of the tail.[124,129,130] Adult worms may be found in skin biopsies, but this is extremely uncommon. *Mansonella streptocerca* DNA can be identified in skin biopsies using a nested PCR-based assay.[131] This approach is specific and more sensitive than skin snips for the diagnosis of streptocerciasis. There is little value in serologic evaluation for this infection.

Streptocerciasis may be confused with onchocerciasis and other chronic dermatitides. If hypopigmented macules are present, these can resemble those of lepromatous leprosy. Although the nonanesthetic nature of the nodules and their location on the upper body may suggest streptocerciasis, histopathologic evaluation is often necessary to distinguish leprosy from *M. streptocerca* infection.

TREATMENT AND PROGNOSIS

DEC 6 mg/kg/day in divided doses for 14 to 21 days appears to be effective in killing both microfilariae and adults.[124,127,132,133] As in onchocerciasis, increased pruritus, urticaria, and papular eruptions along with systemic findings (arthralgias, myalgias, headaches, fever, nausea, and vomiting) may accompany treatment. Generally, these symptoms occur within 24 to 48 hours after treatment and can be treated symptomatically with antihistamines and anti-inflammatory agents. Ivermectin (150 μg/kg) appears to have a salutary microfilaricidal effect both in the short term (6 to 12 days)[134] and in the long term (1 year).[135]

PREVENTION AND CONTROL

There have been no studies of chemoprophylaxis for prevention of streptocerciasis. Control programs have not been attempted, but the microfilarial suppression seen with ivermectin suggests that mass treatment campaigns for *W. bancrofti* and *O. volvulus* control may help to dampen transmission of *M. streptocerca* as well.[135]

10-fold less intense. Thus, infected individuals in Latin America have relatively low worm burdens with the result that few people are blind from the disease. Forest-strain *O. volvulus*, found in rain-forested coastal regions of sub-Saharan Africa, uncommonly causes blindness even in relatively heavily infected persons.[29,30]

In distinct contrast, in endemic savanna regions of Africa, a direct linear relationship between a derived parameter, the community microfilarial load, and the incidence of blindness in that community exists.[29,31,32] Thus, even moderate parasite burdens in those infected with the savanna strain of *O. volvulus* may result in blindness.[33] On an individual basis, the incidence of blindness is significantly and positively associated with increasing microfilarial burden.[34] DNA probe data from excised nodules demonstrate that in villages at the savanna-forest interface, mixed strain infection can occur.

Other factors influencing the epidemiology of onchocerciasis are less well defined. No known sex differences in acquisition of infection have been described. Age is related only to cumulative exposure to infection. Vector abundance varies seasonally with precipitation patterns and with dispersal patterns. No defined genetic markers have been clearly associated with risk of either disease acquisition or disease progression in onchocerciasis.[35–37] However, children of *O. volvulus*–infected mothers have a significantly higher risk of parasite infection and they become infected at a younger age and with increased microfilaria intensity.[38]

The skin lesions and intense pruritus caused by onchodermatitis make it a leading cause of morbidity in infected areas. The resulting disfigurement results in profound psychosocial consequences and isolation by the community.

Fifty percent of all infected persons live outside of the savanna and forest/transition zone regions where blinding severe-strain parasites exist. In these regions, skin manifestations are the main complications of disease. Using standardized dermatological methodology developed over the past decade, it has become apparent that the unremitting pruritus and disfiguring skin lesions were much more important than previously appreciated. The profound psychosocial implications make onchocercal skin disease a major public health problem and more than 50% of the disability-associated life-years lost due to onchocerciasis are due, not to blindness, but to skin disease.[28,39–41] On a community basis, there is a strong correlation between prevalence of itching and *O. volvulus* endemicity in the community. In hyperendemic communities, 30% to 40% of the population has symptomatic skin disease.

A link between onchocerciasis and epilepsy (thought secondary to erosion of nodules through the skull) has often been reported[42–48] but just misses statistical significance on meta-analysis.[49,50] A proposed link to hyposexual dwarfism is similarly elusive.[42,47,49–51]

The socioeconomic consequences of onchocerciasis are profound, though the disease is not itself a direct cause of mortality.[52] *O. volvulus*–induced blindness is, however, associated with a life expectancy that is at least 10 years shorter than that of nonblinded persons in the same area.[53,54] The consequences of onchocerciasis extend beyond the individual and affect family, community, and country. The common image of young boys holding sticks to guide blind, unproductive men in their twenties and thirties attests to why entire villages become economically nonviable when blindness rates reach about 10%. Relocation of villages to healthier locales away from vector breeding sites by the rivers is an option, but the soil away from rivers may be less fertile.

DISEASE

In symptomatic persons, an inflammatory response to the microfilarial stage of the parasite causes the dermatitis, keratitis, and chorioretinitis that are the cardinal manifestations of infection. The subcutaneous nodules, which contain adult worms encased in a fibrous capsule, evoke no inflammatory response and hence few, if any, clinical symptoms.

Of particular importance to clinicians in nononchocerciasis-endemic areas is that a nonspecific dermatitis is almost always the sole clinical manifestation of disease in short-term visitors to endemic areas.[2,3] Transmission of onchocerciasis is highly inefficient when compared with other vector-borne diseases such as malaria. Infection is uncommon after a short stay of a year or less in an endemic area. In a study of infected expatriates, the median duration of exposure was 2 years (range, 20 months to 6 years). In these lightly infected persons, a median period of 18 months (range, 3 months to 3 years) from the end of exposure before the onset of symptoms then passed.

Dermatitis

The pruritus of onchocerciasis, which is secondary to tissue reaction to motile larvae as they migrate subcutaneously, is the most severe, intractable, and unresponsive to antipruritus medication that is known. In the more heavily infected persons in endemic areas, scratching and excoriation to the point of bleeding, and even suicide, occurs. An almost complete inability to sleep is common. Episodes of localized rash, erythema, and angioedema may be superimposed on the ongoing dermatologic manifestations at essentially any stage of the disease.[55]

A commonly recognized scheme categorizes skin disease into five groups. Within each group a category-specific grading for severity, activity, and distribution is included.[28,39,41] The categories are not mutually exclusive in a given patient and the clinical findings are not necessarily specific for onchodermatitis.

1. Acute papular onchodermatitis (APOD): Small pruritic papules may be scattered on limbs, shoulders, and trunk. Lesions may progress to become vesicular or pustular. Lesions may be spontaneous or occur as a reaction to ivermectin or diethylcarbamazine. Histologically, the papules are intraepidermal microabscesses; microfilariae are inconsistently present. A variable perivascular infiltrate of lymphoid origin is seen in this and most types of onchocercal skin disease. Microfilariae, when found, are in the superficial dermis and are frequently associated with lymphatics.
2. Chronic papular onchodermatitis (CPOD): Papules, which are often flat-topped, are larger but more variable in size and height than in the acute papular eruption. Dermatitis is usually symmetrical over buttocks, waist, and shoulder areas and less pruritic than in the acute eruption. Clinical hyperpigmentation and hyperkeratosis correlate histologically with epidermal acanthosis and

incontinence of pigment. This is the most common skin manifestation in hyperendemic areas.
3. Lichenified dermatitis: An intensely pruritic eruption limited to one limb, usually the leg, sowda consists of hyperpigmented papules and plaques with accompanying edema of the entire limb. Regional lymph nodes are enlarged and show prominent follicular hyperplasia suggesting that sowda is due to an aberrant humoral hyperresponsiveness in affected persons. Bacterial superinfection is common due to excoriation of the intensely pruritic lesion. Histologically, few microfilariae are found and hyperkeratosis, acanthosis, and dermal fibrosis are found. Sowda is most common in Yemen and the Sudan but is seen elsewhere in Africa.
4. Atrophy: Premature atrophy is due to degeneration of one or more of the structural elements of the skin with chronic infection. Atrophy is most common over the buttocks but can occur over limbs. Pruritus is uncommon. Clinically, fine wrinkles will appear after pushing along the skin surface with one finger. Loss of elasticity can be demonstrated by slow return to position of skin pinched between two fingers. Histologically, special stains reveal loss of elastic fibers. In order to avoid confusion with senile atrophy, the diagnosis of onchocercal atrophy should only be made in those under age 50 years.
5. Depigmentation: Areas of complete depigmentation over the anterior shin with islands of normally pigmented skin, commonly called "leopard skin," are seen in advanced onchodermatitis.

In Mexico and Guatemala, chronic skin lesions peculiar to this region are described. These include *erisipela de la costa*, a macular rash and edema of the face, and *mal morado*, a lesion associated with a reddish discoloration, particularly on the trunk and upper limbs.

Moderate to severe pruritus is the major presenting complaint in expatriates and an evanescent nonspecific maculopapular rash, which may have an urticarial component, is the main physical finding. The rash is often localized to one area of the body, usually the trunk, presumably in proximity to the few adult worms present. The long incubation period of onchocercal dermatitis and the unfamiliarity of physicians in the industrialized world with its manifestations make misdiagnosis frequent.

Subcutaneous Nodules

Asymptomatic 0.5-cm to 3.0-cm subcutaneous onchocercomas occurring most often over bony prominences are freely movable encapsulated nodules that contain coiled masses of adult worms. In Latin America, where the vector *S. ochraceum* bites high, the nodules are often located on the head and upper body, whereas in Africa where *S. damnosum* bites lower, the nodules are most often over the hips and lower limbs. Palpable subcutaneous nodules are uncommonly found in the lightly infected expatriates.

Lymphadenopathy

Lymphadenopathy is frequently found in inguinal and femoral areas. The so-called hanging groin results when lymphadenopathy occurs in inguinofemoral nodes in a sling of stretched-out atrophic abdominal skin. Lymph nodes are scarred, nontender, and fibrotic.

Eye

Involvement of all tissues of the eye has been described. Host reaction to microfilariae of *O. volvulus* as they migrate through the eye initially presents as a punctate keratitis or as snowflake corneal opacities. Individual opacities clear spontaneously to be followed by others. Free microfilariae may be visible by slit-lamp examination in the anterior chamber or aqueous humor. Long-standing infection with savanna-strain *O. volvulus* leads to sclerosing keratitis, and eventually to blindness. Sclerosing keratitis is characterized by a fibrovascular pannus and an inflammatory infiltrate at the level of Bowman's membrane. The opacity develops around the edge of the cornea and as it becomes vascularized advances toward the center. Iridocyclitis with flare and cells in the anterior chamber leads to development of synechiae, raised intraocular pressure, and secondary glaucoma. Adult *O. volvulus* does not migrate through the subconjunctiva. In contrast, the occasional subconjunctival migration of the long slender adult worm of *Loa loa*, confusingly called the eye worm, is visible to the naked eye of both the patient and the observer; lacrimation, pain, and extreme anxiety typically ensue (see Chapter 99).

Inflammatory disturbances of the retinal pigment epithelium lead to chorioretinitis, chorioretinal atrophy, and posterior ocular disease, and are thought to cause blindness in the rain forest but have also been found secondary to savanna-strain disease. The importance of optic neuritis in ocular onchocerciasis has been more appreciated recently. Optic atrophy may occur in up to 10% of the population of savanna regions. The acute phase can last for a year or more. A postneuritic optic atrophy associated with scarring and retinal pigment disturbance or with vascular sheathing of retinal vessels then ensues. Visual field loss may progress to keyhole vision or even total loss of light perception. Ophthalmologic abnormalities or intraocular microfilariae (even on slit-lamp examination) are not found in the expatriate group.

Human Immunodeficiency Virus and Onchocerciasis

Onchocerciasis patients who are human immunodeficiency virus (HIV)-positive may have more severe skin disease when compared to those who are HIV-negative.[56] Impaired immunoglobulin G (IgG) and IgM responses to *O. volvulus* antigens occurs in HIV-positive persons with onchocerciasis. However, no epidemiologic association between HIV infection and onchocerciasis has been demonstrated.[57] Both initial microfilaria densities and efficacy of ivermectin treatment are the same in HIV-positive and HIV-negative persons with onchocerciasis.[58]

PATHOGENESIS AND IMMUNITY

Systemic Immune Responses

The parasite seems to be able to modulate potentially deleterious parasite-specific immune responses in order to live in relative immunologic harmony with its host. Severe pathologic complications are seen only in a subset of infected patients.

In *O. volvulus*–infected individuals, a highly polarized immune response to specific parasite antigens occurs. There are (1) impaired production of type 1 cytokine (interferon [IFN]-γ) but brisk production of type 2 cytokines (interleukin [IL]-4 and IL-5)[59–62]; (2) production of IL-10 both spontaneously and in response to parasite antigen[1,63,64]; and (3) high serum levels of both polyclonal and specific IgE and IgG4.[1,62,65,66] A central role for the immunomodulatory action of IL-10 has been demonstrated by examining new migrants to infected areas and by the response to ivermectin treatment. Early infection is associated with vigorous cellular responses but as infections become chronic, down-regulation is effected through IL-10.[64] Continued treatment with ivermectin of nonendemic patients no longer exposed to new infection showed decreased IL-10 production at follow-up without any fundamental type 2 to type 1 shift.[1] This effect is only transient in endemic individuals with continued exposure and re-infection.[67,68] A number of in vitro and circumstantial clinical studies have demonstrated a generalized depression of cellular immune responses to nonparasite antigen in *O. volvulus*–infected persons.[61,69–73] A prospective in vivo study showed that concurrent infection with *O. volvulus* did not prevent development of a protective antitetanus response after administration of tetanus vaccine, but heavier *O. volvulus* infection was able to attenuate the magnitude of this protective response.[74] The biologic relevance of the degree of generalized immunosuppression found in onchocerciasis patients remains to be proven. Several findings have implicated seemingly unrelated autoimmune pathways in the pathogenesis of disease, with a number of putative autoantigens described, but true etiologic associations have not been shown.[75–82]

Immune Responses in Local Tissue

Sclerosing keratitis, the major cause of blindness resulting from infection with *O. volvulus*, is manifested by corneal opacification and neovascularization.[83] A biphasic recruitment of first neutrophils (see later *Wolbachia* discussion) and later eosinophils to the central cornea in response to degenerating microfilariae appears causative.[84,85] Direct evidence for this exists in rabbit, guinea pig, and mouse models of onchocercal keratitis. In these models, the predominately lymphocytic inflammatory ocular reaction is parasite antigen–specific, CD4+ dependent, and manifest only in animals presensitized with parasite antigen. Murine onchocercal keratitis has been demonstrated to be Th2 (IL-4)-dependent. Supporting data included corneal localization of IL-4 (but not IFN-γ) messenger RNA (mRNA) in both intact immunized mice and in nude mice reconstituted with immune splenocytes, as well as a failure to develop keratitis in IL-4 knockout mice. At the same time, the migration of eosinophils is IL-5-dependent as these cells are absent from the corneas of IL-5 gene knockout mice. ICAM-1 and PECAM-1 but not VCAM-1 are involved in recruitment of effectors cells to the avascular cornea.[86,87]

Corroborating studies on human tissue have not been performed to date due to the unavailability of corneal tissue from infected persons. Data on local ocular immune responses in human onchocerciasis are limited and only conjunctival and iris, but not corneal, tissue has been examined. A single study, however, indicates a predominance of IL-4-producing (vs. IL-2-producing) T cells among lymphocyte infiltrates in conjunctival biopsies from patients with ocular onchocerciasis.[88–90] A study demonstrating a Th2-like systemic immune response in humans with well-characterized onchocercal keratitis corroborates the findings in the murine model of onchocercal keratitis.[63]

Local type 2 responses have been implicated in the cutaneous pathology but the associations are generally weak.[91] Numbers of microfilariae found in the skin of individual patients are not correlated with presence or absence of skin disease. Tissue damage is most pronounced after treatment with ivermectin and diethylcarbamazine, which kills the dermal microfilariae. In these cases, pathogenesis is secondary to eosinophil recruitment and degranulation after activation of the eotaxin and RANTES pathways.[92–97]

Role of the Endosymbiont *Wolbachia*

O. volvulus uniformly harbors endosymbiotic intracellular bacteria, which are essential for fertility and reproduction.[4–6] Eradication of these bacteria, such as with doxycycline therapy,[98] not only sterilizes the adult females but may shorten their life span. In the absence of any known adulticidal drug, this finding has implications for treatment and control of *O. volvulus*. *Wolbachia* released from dying parasites after diethylcarbamazine or ivermectin treatment of infected individuals induces release of TNF and related mediators.[7] These sometimes severe post-treatment reactions (the Mazzotti reaction[99]) were until recently attributed to release of parasite antigen systemically. *Wolbachia* do not produce endotoxin, but their major surface proteins have been shown to induce the innate immune system through TLR-2 and TLR-4. In the murine model of onchocercal keratitis, *Wolbachia* have been shown capable of inducing the early neutrophilic response and causing corneal opacities.[100] A defined role for *Wolbachia* in ongoing pathogenesis in humans awaits further study.

DIAGNOSIS

Clinical Examination

O. volvulus has a quite well-defined distribution, but because of the geographic overlap with other filarial parasites, a well-taken travel or residence history by an epidemiologically cognizant physician will eliminate the need for unnecessary diagnostic investigations in those with no possible exposure. *O. volvulus*, *Loa loa*, *Mansonella perstans*, *Mansonella ozzardi*, and *Mansonella streptocerca* all may cause overlapping clinical syndromes. In suspected onchocerciasis, the history should focus on duration and intensity of exposure and its chronology with respect to an incubation period that may be 2 years or more.

A physical examination with the patient completely disrobed is necessary to detect (1) the localized dermatitis, often occurring in the buttock region, associated with either *O. volvulus* or *M. streptocerca*; (2) subcutaneous nodules; or (3) Calabar swellings of loiasis. A thorough palpation of all lymph node groups, including those in the inguinal region, will aid in the diagnosis of *Wuchereria bancrofti*, *O. volvulus*, or *M. streptocerca*. Slit-lamp examination of the eye is required to work up possible onchocerciasis, although the yield is so low in lightly infected expatriates that it is likely unnecessary. The patient should first sit for 10 minutes with the head forward and bowed to allow microfilariae located posteriorly and inferiorly to become visible. Fluorescein angiography is the most sensitive detector of early chorioretinal lesions.

Laboratory Diagnosis

Outside of research settings, definitive diagnosis is most often dependent on the relatively unsophisticated parasitologic demonstration of the 220- to 360-mm-long microfilariae in skin snips. In well-equipped clinical settings, biopsy or ultrasound demonstration of adult parasites in any nodules that are present can be diagnostic.

Skin Snips

Skin microfilariae are optimally detected utilizing skin snips taken down to the level of the dermal papillae. This type of skin biopsy employs either a razor blade to slice a thin piece of skin which has been tented up with a needle or a corneoscleral biopsy instrument to obtain 1 to 2 mg of skin bloodlessly.[101,102] The ability to use disposable materials with the former technique in areas where the risk of blood-borne pathogens is high and sophisticated sterilization is not available is a real advantage. A microscopic count of the highly motile microfilariae migrating out of six biopsies, one from over each scapula, iliac crest, and lateral aspect of each calf, is performed after incubation of the skin snips with saline in microplate wells at 37°C. In heavier infection, motile microfilariae will be visible emerging from the skin snip under low-power microscopy in 10 to 60 minutes, but negative snips should be covered to prevent evaporation and checked periodically for at least 24 hours. A heavily infected person may have more than 100 microfilariae per milligram of skin. In Africa, the highest yield will be from the iliac crest and in Latin America from over the scapula. In expatriates, the majority of infected persons do not have microfilariae in their skin and those that do have very low counts.

Deep punch biopsy of the skin is not necessary and multiple skin snips will have a higher yield than one random traumatic deep biopsy. Blood contaminating a skin snip may result in one of the blood-borne microfilaria escaping into the specimen, with *M. ozzardi* (which lives in superficial capillaries) most frequently incriminated. If the patient has been in an area endemic for *M. streptocerca,* it is then necessary to fix the skin and to stain the microfilariae for identification. In contrast to *M. streptocerca, O. volvulus* microfilariae have anterior nuclei that are side by side, a caudal space free of nuclei, and a tail tapered to a fine point. *M. streptocerca* is most often found in snips taken over the upper trunk.

Blood Examination

Because of the geographic overlap in the distribution of filarial parasites that may cause overlapping clinical syndromes, examination for circulating microfilaremia is often necessary. A properly timed and processed blood sample is thus vital (see Chapters 98 and 99).

Urine and Other Fluids

Microfilariae of *O. volvulus* have been found in the urine of some infected persons during mass epidemiologic studies in hyperendemic regions, with microfilarial counts being well correlated with skin counts.[103] Examination of the urine, however, has no utility as a general diagnostic technique and is no substitute for properly performed skin snips in the diagnostic workup of a single patient. Cerebrospinal fluid microfilariae can be seen in severe *O. volvulus* infection.

Demonstration of the Adult Parasite

A coil of hairlike white worms discovered in an excised subcutaneous or intramuscular nodule in the appropriate epidemiologic setting is diagnostic of onchocerciasis on visual inspection. Most nodules have only 3 to 5 adults in them, though nodules containing as many as 50 have been found.

Serology

Serologic testing for *O. volvulus* IgG is not generally available and when done usually utilizes a crude antigenic preparation of a nononchocercal filarial parasite. Standardization is often poor; a positive result, at best, cannot differentiate between the eight filarial species and, at worst, may cross-react with other helminthic infections like strongyloidiasis. Despite the lack of specificity, the sensitivity of this type of serology is almost 100%. Most people resident in endemic areas will have antibodies whether or not they are currently infected. Thus, serologic evaluation in filarial disease is helpful only in two situations: (1) in persons exposed to or infected with filarial parasites who are originally from nonendemic areas and were presumably seronegative initially; and (2) to detect a quantitative decrease in antibody levels that may occur as a response to definitive therapy.

Eosinophil Count

The total eosinophil count is unhelpful diagnostically as it is often but inconstantly elevated in onchocerciasis. Recently infected temporary residents may have moderately elevated eosinophil counts but counts are normal in up to 30%. Persons with chronic long-standing infection may also have normal eosinophil counts or may have eosinophilia due to parasitism with another helminth.

IgE Levels

Serum IgE levels may be elevated in onchocerciasis, but high levels are an inconstant finding and nonspecific.

Ultrasound Examination

Adult worms in suspect onchocercomata will produce a central, relatively homogeneous echogenic area containing echo-dense particles with a lateral acoustic shadow. The utility of random ultrasound examination for occult nodules has not been established.[104–107] Sequential ultrasonographic monitoring of nodules after macrofilaricidal therapy can provide information on drug effect.

Mazzotti Test

A 50-mg dose of diethylcarbamazine (DEC, Mazzotti test) can be given to a patient suspected of harboring *O. volvulus* but in whom no microfilariae can be detected after a rigorous and unfruitful search of blood, skin snips, and after a careful ophthalmologic examination. Within 15 minutes to 24 hours, but most often within 3 hours, the infected patient will develop pruritus with or without erythema over involved areas as microfilariae die in the skin.[99,108,109] Severe reactions in both skin and eye may occur in more heavily infected patients, emphasizing the importance of reserving this maneuver for very lightly infected persons. A patch test performed by applying topical DEC to a small area of skin in order to provoke a localized Mazzotti reaction[110,111] is a highly sensitive and specific diagnostic test in children under the age of 15 years, but the requisite drug and standardization materials are not readily available in the United States.

DNA Diagnosis of Individual Patients

Detection of parasite DNA in routine skin snips by PCR amplification of O-150, an *O. volvulus*–specific 150-bp repeated genomic DNA family, is recognized as the most sensitive available technique for detecting low-level infections in individual patients.[112–115] This technique, available only in the research setting, is of special importance in the diagnosis of expatriates who are typically lightly infected. A standard uncomplicated PCR protocol is applied to DNA extracted from skin snips that are fresh, frozen, or preserved in ethanol. Unanswered questions include how long parasite DNA remains in the skin after treatment or the natural death of adult worms and how extensively parasite DNA is distributed in the body in light infections.

Diagnostic Difficulties

Scabies, insect bites, hypersensitivity reactions, miliaria rubra, and contact dermatitis enter the differential diagnosis of acute pruritic disease. In expatriates, Calabar swellings (see Chapter 99), clinically similar episodes of localized rash, and mild angioedema can mimic onchodermatitis. Tuberculoid leprosy and eczema should be considered if there are chronic skin changes. Dermatomycoses, previous trauma, and yaws can also cause hypopigmented skin lesions. Onchocercal chorioretinitis must be differentiated from choroiditis due to syphilis, tuberculosis, or toxoplasmosis. Optic neuropathy in endemic areas may be due to nutritional optic atrophy, syphilis, or primary glaucoma. In expatriates with a highly suggestive clinical and epidemiologic history (i.e., being a travel partner of a skin snip–positive patient) but with negative skin snips and no nodules, presumptive diagnosis can be made on the basis of the Mazzotti test and serology if available.

TREATMENT AND PROGNOSIS

No available nontoxic agent is able to kill the long-lived (14 years) adult worms of *O. volvulus*. Because the pathologic sequelae of *O. volvulus* infection are entirely due to the microfilariae in skin and ocular tissue, repeated microfilaricidal therapy is necessary for morbidity reduction.

Ivermectin

Ivermectin, a semisynthetic macrocyclic lactone originally synthesized in the 1970s for veterinary use, is the most potent anthelminthic agent ever developed.[116] Receptor-mediated hyperpolarization of cells after an influx of negatively charged ions occurs utilizing a novel glutamate-sensitive chloride channel present in nematodes.[117] The drug is well absorbed orally, excretion is almost entirely in the feces, and the serum half-life is 12 hours.

Large field trials in Africa in the 1980s established ivermectin as the treatment of choice in a single oral microfilaricidal dose of 150 μg/kg administered every 6 to 12 months.[118,119] Skin microfilariae are killed within days though maximum reduction may not occur for up to 2 weeks. Ocular microfilariae counts do not begin to be reduced for at least 2 weeks. Further microfilarial production is suppressed for 6 months before once again reaching levels that lead to renewed transmission at about 12 months. Annual treatment, as has been practiced over the years in control programs, effectively reduces progression and rates of ocular disease including blinding and skin disease as manifest by pruritus.[31,120–123] Advanced eye disease and existing blindness is not reversed. Higher doses of ivermectin given yearly do not have enhanced effect on viability or fecundity of female adult worms and cause significant side effects.[124,125] Increasing the frequency of ivermectin administration to every 3 months decreases microfilaria production up to threefold and may permanently impair fecundity.[124–126] Effect of such regimens on total adult life span is unclear.

Pruritus in lightly infected expatriates may be refractory to annual or 6-month therapy and many clinicians find it necessary to treat more aggressively with standard doses for the first 2 years or so (Fig. 100-1).[127–129] Ivermectin administration should be titrated to symptoms and may be given as often as every 3 months. Appropriate duration of therapy in those without further exposure to transmission is not known. While annual treatment in these cases should theoretically be offered for the possible 14-year life span of the adult worm, clinical experience is that most patients stop returning after several years, so likely are failing to develop recurrent symptoms after several years of therapy.

Ivermectin by itself has no intrinsic pharmacologic effects in humans and is remarkably nontoxic in usual treatment doses. Fever, pruritus, urticaria, myalgia, painless swelling of the limbs and face, and tender lymphadenopathy are not severe and occur mostly within 1 day of treatment.[130,131] Symptomatic treatment with analgesics and antihistamines is generally sufficient. Severity is in general in proportion to the microfilarial load. Postural hypotension occurs in approximately 1 in 1000 patients but can be eliminated if patients are routinely instructed to rest in bed if dizziness occurs. Reactions are diminished on subsequent treatments of individuals or populations. Ivermectin appears to be safe in pregnancy but treatment is best postponed until after delivery.[132]

In co-infected patients with high levels of microfilaremia due to *Loa loa* infection, caution must be exercised in the use of ivermectin to avoid causing encephalopathy (see Chapter 99) due to *L. loa* microfilaria that enter the central nervous system after treatment.[133–138] In resource-rich settings, plasmapheresis may be used to reduce *L. loa* microfilaremia in co-infected

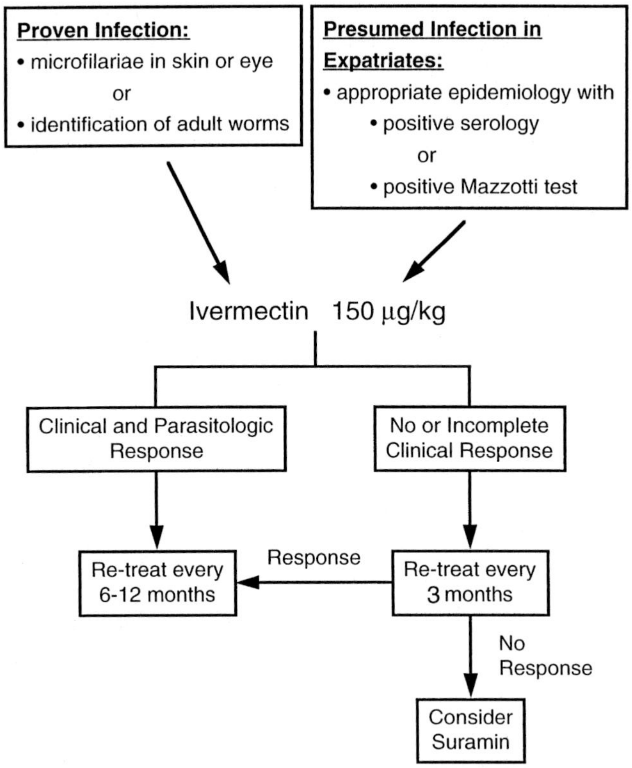

FIGURE 100-1 Treatment algorithm for individual patients.

patients prior to administration of ivermectin. Mass treatment with ivermectin for onchocerciasis is difficult in loiasis endemic areas in the absence of the ability to ascertain which individuals might be heavily infected with *L. loa*. Such co-infected areas have been avoided in the past, but rapid epidemiologic assessment tools have been developed to allow for close monitoring and rapid treatment of ivermectin-induced *L. loa* reactions after identification of a community as high risk for such occurrence.[139] Such protocols have not been field tested at this time. Ivermectin resistance has been reported in a few patients in Ghana but does not appear to be clinically important in any area of the world at present.[140]

Doxycycline

Doxycycline 100 mg/day for 6 weeks leads to death of the endosymbiotic *Wolbachia* found in *O. volvulus* worms, followed by complete cessation of early embryogenesis for at least 18 months, and thus production of transmissible microfilaria for a longer period.[98,141,142] This is in contrast to ivermectin which kills larvae during a later stage of intrauterine microfilaria production with the result that early embryos survive to become microfilaria that are transmissible again within a year or less. Higher doses of doxycycline may have longer duration of effect. Shorter duration of therapy appears ineffective. Six weeks of doxycyline is not a practical public health strategy for mass treatment programs. Nevertheless, since ivermectin therapy alone may not be able to interrupt transmission (see later discussion), combination therapy for varying periods is worthy of further investigation. In the treatment of individual patients, there is no evidence at this time to suggest that the addition of doxycycline to conventional ivermectin strategies (see previous discussion) has any benefit with respect to symptom relief or total duration of therapy.

Diethylcarbamazine

Diethylcarbamazine (DEC) is a piperazine derivative with microfilaricidal but not adulticidal activity used for over 40 years prior to the introduction of ivermectin. Due to frequent unacceptable reactions to dying microfilariae, ranging from urticaria and angioedema to hypotension and death, DEC should no longer be used for microfilaricidal treatment of this parasite. Reactions are related to microfilarial load so that the 50 mg used for the Mazzotti test in a patient with negative skin snips and a normal slit-lamp examination is thought to be safe.

Suramin

Suramin is the only available agent adulticidal to *O. volvulus* and is extremely toxic, necessitating hospitalization for several days with each dose. The original regimen of weekly 1-g doses given for 6 weeks is clearly unsafe. Toxicity includes a fatal progressive wasting syndrome, exfoliative dermatitis, progression of chorioretinitis, and development of optic atrophy. Better-tolerated weekly escalating dose regimens, which deliver 4 g or 5 g total, have been developed but are still not completely without risk and have the disadvantage that at least 34% of adult worms are viable 1 year later.[143-145] Because regular ivermectin treatment almost always controls symptoms and prevents development of disease, suramin treatment is rarely if ever undertaken nowadays. One exception may be in individuals with severe hyperreactive onchodermatitis whose symptoms cannot be controlled with repeated aggressive ivermectin therapy. Suramin is also a potent microfilaricide but with delayed effect. Skin microfilaria counts remain unchanged for at least 6 weeks.

Nodulectomy

Periodic removal of palpable nodules to reduce the microfilarial load and the ensuing pathologic changes has been pursued with success for many years in Latin America. In Africa, where nodules are deeper, more numerous, and less accessible, this strategy appears to be ineffective. Removal of a single nodule in an expatriate with no further exposure anticipated may be considered as it may represent the only nidus of infection.

Adulticidal Drugs

Despite intensive efforts at drug discovery, no nontoxic adulticides have been identified. Amocarzine and moxidectin, two recent candidates, are no longer in development.

PREVENTION AND CONTROL

Prophylaxis

There are no effective vaccines or chemoprophylactic drugs. For expatriates or others with sufficient resources, personal mosquito protection using repellents is likely of benefit.

As *Simulium* spp. are daytime biters, bednet programs in place for malaria control have no effect of onchocerciasis transmission.

In contrast to malaria or some other parasitic infections, only limited evidence exists for the development of any degree of protective immunity to *O. volvulus* in populations with long-term natural exposure to the parasite. Perhaps for this reason, efforts at development of a vaccine against onchocerciasis have been disappointing. In experimental animals, which are not naturally permissive hosts for *O. volvulus*, a protective immune response can be induced after inoculation with live radiation–attenuated L3-stage larvae. Despite the cloning and expression of several dozen *O. volvulus* recombinant antigens, none has been effective enough in animal screens to be considered for human trials.

Vector Control

The Onchocerciasis Control Program (OCP), funded by the World Health Organization (WHO), the World Bank, and the United Nations Development Program, extended from 1974–2002 over 11 countries of West Africa most affected by blinding savanna-strain *O. volvulus*.[121,146,147] A strategy of aggressive vector control using aerial larvaciding of 50,000 km rivers combined with annual ivermectin treatments (added in 1988) essentially interrupted transmission in the area under control. It is estimated that 35 million people were protected from infection, 10 million children have been born into areas that were free of disease transmission, and between 125,000 and 200,000 people have been prevented from going blind. Because rapid development of the larvae necessitates weekly treatment of the rivers, the program cost over $550 million and was unsustainable. Because infected blackflies will invade from around the perimeter of the controlled region and infected individuals will continue to migrate into controlled areas, maintenance of the success of the OCP will depend on establishment of ongoing ivermectin treatment programs.

Mass Ivermectin Distribution

Building a sustainable infrastructure for the mass community-based distribution[148,149] of the microfilaricide ivermectin has become the primary control strategy on a global basis. The Mectizan Donation Program (MDP) is a unique and generous initiative established in 1988 by Merck & Company, the manufacturer of ivermectin, to provide free drug to any governmental or nongovernmental program that can demonstrate need and capability to distribute it[150,151]; 250 million doses have been distributed to 2002.

The African Program for Onchocerciasis Control (APOC), to run from 1995 to 2009, assists 18 affected African countries outside the original OCP area in establishing sustainable national programs for ivermectin distribution with the hope that national governments will take over after 2009.[31,120,121] Directed by WHO, initial funding has come from the World Bank, but contributions from multiple other donors will be required to completely fund the initiative. Merck has committed over 400 million ivermectin tablets valued at over $200 million. The strategy is based on annual mass treatment with ivermectin to communities with greater than 40% prevalence of infection in order to break the transmission cycle by eliminating microfilariae available to vectors from the skin of infected persons. The expense and logistics of performing detailed parasitologic diagnostics in individual communities has led to the development of simplified rapid epidemiologic mapping tools for identification of high-priority areas for ivermectin distribution. There is no nonhuman reservoir of *O. volvulus;* but unfortunately current calculations that take into account expected coverage rates and the known levels of microfilaria recurring in the skin 1 year after treatment predict that transmission cannot be broken with the current strategy.[152,153] Thus, morbidity will be significantly reduced but without breaking transmission, so the treatment programs might have to be continued in perpetuity. Three-monthly ivermectin treatment does permanently affect microfilaria production and may even prove to shorten adult female life span but is likely not a sustainable strategy in the African context.[125–127] APOC distributed 25 million tablets of ivermectin in 2002.

OEPA (Onchocerciasis Elimination Programme in the Americas) is slated to run from 1991–2007 and aims to eliminate clinical onchocerciasis by 2007 as well as interrupt transmission using a strategy of biannual ivermectin treatment and 85% coverage of affected communities. Six countries are covered (Brazil, Colombia, Ecuador, Guatemala, Mexico, and Venezuela), and at least Mexico will implement 3-monthly therapy to better have a chance at interrupting transmission.

REFERENCES

1. Henry NL, Law M, Nutman TB, et al: Onchocerciasis in a nonendemic population: Clinical and immunologic assessment before treatment and at the time of presumed cure. J Infect Dis 183:512, 2001.
2. McCarthy JS, Ottesen EA, Nutman TB: Onchocerciasis in endemic and nonendemic populations: Differences in clinical presentation and immunologic findings. J Infect Dis 170:736, 1994.
3. Encarnacion CF, Giordano MF, Murray HW: Onchocerciasis in New York City. The Moa-Manhattan connection. Arch Intern Med 154:1749, 1994.
4. Hoerauf A, Buttner DW, Adjei O, et al: Onchocerciasis. BMJ 326:207, 2003.
5. Taylor MJ, Hoerauf A: *Wolbachia* bacteria of filarial nematodes. Parasitol Today 15:437, 1999.
6. Taylor MJ: *Wolbachia* in the inflammatory pathogenesis of human filariasis. Ann NY Acad Sci 990:444, 2003.
7. Keiser PB, Reynolds SM, Awadzi K, et al: Bacterial endosymbionts of *Onchocerca volvulus* in the pathogenesis of post-treatment reactions. J Infect Dis 185:805, 2002.
8. Nelson GS: Human onchocerciasis: Notes on the history, the parasite and the life cycle. Ann Trop Med Parasitol 85:83, 1991.
9. Robles R: A new disease from Guatemala. Juventud Med Guatemala 15:97, 1917.
10. Blacklock DB: The development of *Onchocerca volvulus* in *Simulium damnosum*. Ann Trop Med Parasitol 20:1, 1926.
11. Blacklock DB: The development of *Onchocerca volvulus* (Leuckart, 1893). The cause of worm nodules in man in Africa. BMJ 1:129, 1927.
12. Duke BOL: Human Onchocerciasis—An Overview of the Disease. Acta Leidensia 59:9, 1990.
13. Duke BO: The population dynamics of *Onchocerca volvulus* in the human host. Trop Med Parasitol 44:61, 1993.
14. Duke BOL, Lewis DJ, Moore PJ: *Onchocerca-Simulium* complexes I. Transmission of forest and Sudan-savannah strains of *Onchocerca volvulus*, from Cameroon, by *Simulium damnosum* from various West African bioclimatic zones. Ann Trop Med Parasitol 60:318, 1966.
15. Lobos E, Weiss N: Immunochemical comparison between worm extracts of *Onchocerca volvulus* from savanna and rain forest. Parasite Immunol 7:333, 1985.
16. Bryceson AD, van Veen KS, Oduloju AJ, et al: Antigenic diversity among *Onchocerca volvulus* in Nigeria, and immunological differences

between onchocerciasis in the savanna and forest of Cameroon. Clin Exp Immunol 24:168, 1976.

17. Flockhart HA, Cibulskis RE, Karam M, et al: *Onchocerca volvulus*: Enzyme polymorphism in relation to the differentiation of forest and savannah strains of this parasite. Trans R Soc Trop Med Hyg 80:285, 1986.
18. Erttmann KD, Meredith SE, Greene BM, et al: Isolation and characterization of form specific DNA sequences of *O. volvulus*. Acta Leiden 59:253, 1990.
19. Meredith SE, Lando G, Gbakima AA, et al: *Onchocerca volvulus*: Application of the polymerase chain reaction to identification and strain differentiation of the parasite. Exp Parasitol 73:335, 1991.
20. Zimmerman PA, Dadzie KY, De Sole G, et al: *Onchocerca volvulus* DNA probe classification correlates with epidemiologic patterns of blindness. J Infect Dis 165:964, 1992.
21. Ogunrinade A, Boakye D, Merriweather A, et al: Distribution of the blinding and nonblinding strains of *Onchocerca volvulus* in Nigeria. J Infect Dis 179:1577, 1999.
22. Higazi TB, Katholi CR, Mahmoud BM, et al: *Onchocerca volvulus*: Genetic diversity of parasite isolates from Sudan. Exp Parasitol 97:24, 2001.
23. Adjami AG, Toe L, Bissan Y, et al: The current status of onchocerciasis in the forest/savanna transition zone of Côte d'Ivoire. Parasitol 128:407, 2004.
24. Unnasch TR, Williams SA: The genomes of *Onchocerca volvulus*. Int J Parasitol 30:543, 2000.
25. Toe L, Tang J, Back C, et al: Vector-parasite transmission complexes for onchocerciasis in West Africa. Lancet 349:163, 1997.
26. Tang J, Toe L, Back C, et al: Mitochondrial alleles of *Simulium damnosum* sensu lato infected with *Onchocerca volvulus*. Int J Parasitol 25:1251, 1995.
27. Tang J, Toe L, Back C, et al: The *Simulium damnosum* species complex: Phylogenetic analysis and molecular identification based upon mitochondrially encoded gene sequences. Insect Mol Biol 4:79, 1995.
28. Kipp W, Bamhuhiiga J: Onchodermal skin disease in a hyperendemic onchocerciasis focus in western Uganda. Am J Trop Med Hyg 67:475, 2002.
29. Dadzie KY, Remme J, Rolland A, et al: Ocular onchocerciasis and intensity of infection in the community. II. West African rainforest foci of the vector *Simulium yahense*. Trop Med Parasitol 40:348, 1989.
30. Dadzie KY, Remme J, Baker RH, et al: Ocular onchocerciasis and intensity of infection in the community. III. West African rainforest foci of the vector *Simulium sanctipauli*. Trop Med Parasitol 41:376, 1990.
31. Remme JH: Research for control: The onchocerciasis experience. Trop Med Int Health 9:243, 2004.
32. Remme J, Dadzie KY, Rolland A, et al: Ocular onchocerciasis and intensity of infection in the community. I. West African savanna. Trop Med Parasitol 40:340, 1989.
33. Anderson JH, Fuglsang H, Hamilton PJS, et al: Studies on onchocerciasis in the United Cameroon Republic II. Comparison of onchocerciasis in the rain-forest and Sudan-savanna. Trans R Soc Trop Med Hyg 68:209, 1974.
34. Little MP, Basanez MG, Breitling LP, et al: Incidence of blindness during the onchocerciasis control programme in western Africa, 1971–2002. J Infect Dis 189:1932, 2004.
35. Murdoch ME, Payton A, Abiose A, et al: HLA-DQ alleles associate with cutaneous features of onchocerciasis. The Kaduna-London-Manchester Collaboration for Research on Onchocerciasis. Hum Immunol 55:46, 1997.
36. Meyer CG, Gallin M, Erttmann KD, et al: HLA-D alleles associated with generalized disease, localized disease, and putative immunity in *Onchocerca volvulus* infection. Proc Natl Acad Sci USA 91:7515, 1994.
37. Brattig NW, Tischendorf FW, Reifegerste S, et al: Differences in the distribution of HLA antigens in localized and generalized form of onchocerciasis. Trop Med Parasitol 37:271, 1986.
38. Kirch AK, Duerr HP, Boatin B, et al: Impact of parental onchocerciasis and intensity of transmission on development and persistence of *Onchocerca volvulus* infection in offspring: An 18-year follow-up study. Parasitol 127:327, 2003.
39. Murdoch ME, Hay RJ, Mackenzie CD, et al: A clinical classification and grading system of the cutaneous changes in onchocerciasis. Br J Dermatol 129:260, 1993.
40. Murdoch ME, Asuzu MC, Hagan M, et al: Onchocerciasis: The clinical and epidemiological burden of skin disease in Africa. Ann Trop Med Parasitol 96:283, 2002.
41. Hagan M: Onchocercal dermatitis: Clinical impact. Ann Trop Med Parasitol 92(Suppl 1):S85, 1998.
42. Duke BO: Onchocerciasis, epilepsy and hyposexual dwarfism. Trans R Soc Trop Med Hyg 92:236, 1998.
43. Kabore JK, Cabore JW, Melaku Z, et al: Epilepsy in a focus of onchocerciasis in Burkina Faso. Lancet 347:836, 1996.
44. Kaiser C, Asaba G, Leichsenring M, et al: High incidence of epilepsy related to onchocerciasis in West Uganda. Epilepsy Res 30:247, 1998.
45. Kamgno J, Pion SD, Boussinesq M: Demographic impact of epilepsy in Africa: Results of a 10-year cohort study in a rural area of Cameroon. Epilepsia 44:956, 2003.
46. Kipp W, Kasoro S, Burnham G: Onchocerciasis and epilepsy in Uganda [Letter]. Lancet 343:183, 1994.
47. Newell ED, Vyungimana F, Bradley JE: Epilepsy, retarded growth and onchocerciasis, in two areas of different endemicity of onchocerciasis in Burundi. Trans R Soc Trop Med Hyg 91:525, 1997.
48. Ovuga E, Kipp W, Mungherera M, et al: Epilepsy and retarded growth in a hyperendemic focus of onchocerciasis in rural western Uganda. East Afr Med J 69:554, 1992.
49. Druet-Cabanac M, Boussinesq M, Dongmo L, et al: Review of epidemiological studies searching for a relationship between onchocerciasis and epilepsy. Neuroepidemiol 23:144, 2004.
50. Twum-Danso NA: Mass treatment of onchocerciasis with ivermectin: Should people with epilepsy and/or growth-retardation syndromes be excluded? Ann Trop Med Parasitol 98:99, 2004.
51. Kipp W, Burnham G, Bamuhiiga J, et al: The Nakalanga syndrome in Kabarole District, Western Uganda. Am J Trop Med Hyg 54:80, 1996.
52. Evans DB, Gelband H, Vlassoff C: Social and economic factors and the control of lymphatic filariasis: A review. Acta Trop 53:1, 1993.
53. Kirkwood B, Smith P, Marshall T, et al: Relationships between mortality, visual acuity and microfilarial load in the area of the Onchocerciasis Control Programme. Trans R Soc Trop Med Hyg 77:862, 1983.
54. Little MP, Breitling LP, Basanez MG, et al: Association between microfilarial load and excess mortality in onchocerciasis: An epidemiological study. Lancet 363:1514, 2004.
55. Onchocerciasis and its control. Report of a WHO Expert Committee on Onchocerciasis Control. World Health Organ Tech Rep Ser 852:1, 1995.
56. Kipp W, Bamuhiiga J, Rubaale T: *Simulium neavei*–transmitted onchocerciasis: HIV infection increases severity of onchocercal skin disease in a small sample of patients. Trans R Soc Trop Med Hyg 97:310, 2003.
57. Tawill SA, Gallin M, Erttmann KD, et al: Impaired antibody responses and loss of reactivity to *Onchocerca volvulus* antigens by HIV-seropositive onchocerciasis patients. Trans R Soc Trop Med Hyg 90:85, 1996.
58. Fischer P, Kipp W, Kabwa P, et al: Onchocerciasis and human immunodeficiency virus in western Uganda: Prevalences and treatment with ivermectin. Am J Trop Med Hyg 53:171, 1995.
59. King CL, Nutman TB: Regulation of the immune response in lymphatic filariasis and onchocerciasis. Immunol Today 12:A54, 1991.
60. Gallin M, Edmonds K, Ellner JJ, et al: Cell-mediated immune responses in human infection with *Onchocerca volvulus*. J Immunol 140:1999, 1988.
61. Ward DJ, Nutman TB, Zea-Flores G, et al: Onchocerciasis and immunity in humans: Enhanced T cell responsiveness to parasite antigen in putatively immune individuals. J Infect Dis 157:536, 1988.
62. Greene BM, Gbakima AA, Albiez EJ, et al: Humoral and cellular immune responses to *Onchocerca volvulus* infection in humans. Rev Infect Dis 7:789, 1985.
63. Plier DA, Awadzi K, Freedman DO: Immunoregulation in onchocerciasis: Persons with ocular inflammatory disease produce a Th2-like response to *Onchocerca volvulus* antigen. J Infect Dis 174:380, 1996.
64. Cooper PJ, Mancero T, Espinel M, et al: Early human infection with *Onchocerca volvulus* is associated with an enhanced parasite-specific cellular immune response. J Infect Dis 183:1662, 2001.
65. Dafa'alla TH, Ghalib HW, Abdelmageed A, et al: The profile of IgG and IgG subclasses of onchocerciasis patients. Clin Exp Immunol 88:258, 1992.
66. Brattig NW, Krawietz I, Abakar AZ, et al: Strong IgG isotypic antibody response in sowdah type onchocerciasis. J Infect Dis 170:955, 1994.
67. Lee SJ, Francis HL, Awadzi K, et al: Changes in antibody profile after treatment of human onchocerciasis. J Infect Dis 162:529, 1990.

68. Steel C, Lujan-Trangay A, Gonzalez-Peralta C, et al: Immunologic responses to repeated ivermectin treatment in patients with onchocerciasis. J Infect Dis 164:581, 1991.
69. Kilian HD, Nielsen G: Cell-mediated and humoral immune response to tetanus vaccinations in onchocerciasis patients. Trop Med Parasitol 40:285, 1989.
70. Kilian HD, Nielsen G: Cell-mediated and humoral immune responses to BCG and rubella vaccinations and to recall antigens in onchocerciasis patients. Trop Med Parasitol 40:445, 1989.
71. Prost A, Nebout M, Rougemont A: Lepromatous leprosy and onchocerciasis. BMJ 1:589, 1979.
72. Rougemont A, Boisson-Pontal ME, Pontal PG, et al: Tuberculin skin tests and B.C.G. vaccination in a hyperendemic area of onchocerciasis. Lancet 1:309, 1977.
73. Greene BM, Fanning MM, Ellner JJ: Non-specific suppression of antigen-induced lymphocyte blastogenesis in *Onchocerca volvulus* infection in man. Clin Exp Immunol 52:259, 1983.
74. Cooper PJ, Espinel I, Paredes W, et al: Impaired tetanus-specific cellular and humoral responses following tetanus vaccination in human onchocerciasis: A possible role for interleukin-10. J Infect Dis 178:1133, 1998.
75. Rokeach LA, Zimmerman PA, Unnasch TR: Epitopes of the *Onchocerca volvulus* RAL1 antigen, a member of the calreticulin family of proteins, recognized by sera from patients with onchocerciasis. Infect Immun 62:3696, 1994.
76. Zhou Y, Dziak E, Unnasch TR, et al: Major retinal cell components recognized by onchocerciasis sera are associated with the cell surface and nucleoli. Invest Ophthalmol Vis Sci 35:1089, 1994.
77. McKechnie NM, Gurr W, Braun G: Immunization with the cross-reactive antigens Ov39 from *Onchocerca volvulus* and Hr44 rrom human retinal tissue induces ocular pathology and activates retinal microglia. J Infect Dis 176:1334, 1997.
78. McKechnie NM, Braun G, Connor V, et al: Immunologic cross-reactivity in the pathogenesis of ocular onchocerciasis. Invest Ophthalmol Vis Sci 34:2888, 1993.
79. Engelbrecht F, Eisenhardt G, Turner J, et al: Analysis of antibody responses directed against two *Onchocerca volvulus* antigens defined by monoclonal antibodies. Trop Med Parasitol 43:47, 1992.
80. Braun G, McKechnie NM, Gurr W: Molecular and immunological characterization of Hr44, a human ocular component immunologically cross-reactive with antigen Ov39 of *Onchocerca volvulus*. J Exp Med 182:1121, 1995.
81. Braun G, McKechnie NM, Connor V, et al: Immunological cross-reactivity between a cloned antigen of *Onchocerca volvulus* and a component of the retinal pigment epithelium. J Exp Med 14:169, 1991.
82. Lux FA, McCauliffe DP, Buttner DW, et al: Serological cross-reactivity between a human Ro/SS-A autoantigen (calreticulin) and the lambda Ral-1 antigen of *Onchocerca volvulus*. J Clin Invest 89:1945, 1992.
83. Higazi TB, Pearlman E, Whikehart DR, et al: Angiogenic activity of an *Onchocerca volvulus Ancylostoma* secreted protein homologue. Mol Biochem Parasitol 129:61, 2003.
84. Hall LR, Pearlman E: Pathogenesis of onchocercal keratitis (river blindness). Clin Microbiol Rev 12:445, 1999.
85. Pearlman E, Hall LR: Immune mechanisms in *Onchocerca volvulus*–mediated corneal disease (river blindness). Parasite Immunol 22:625, 2000.
86. Kaifi JT, Diaconu E, Pearlman E: Distinct roles for PECAM-1, ICAM-1, and VCAM-1 in recruitment of neutrophils and eosinophils to the cornea in ocular onchocerciasis (river blindness). J Immunol 166:6795, 2001.
87. Berger RB, Blackwell NM, Lass JH, et al: IL-4 and IL-13 regulation of ICAM-1 expression and eosinophil recruitment in *Onchocerca volvulus* keratitis. Invest Ophthalmol Vis Sci 43:2992, 2002.
88. Chan CC, Nussenblatt RB, Kim MK, et al: Immunopathology of ocular onchocerciasis. 2. Anti-retinal autoantibodies in serum and ocular fluids. Ophthalmology 94:439, 1987.
89. Chan CC, Ottesen EA, Awadzi K, et al: Immunopathology of ocular onchocerciasis. I. Inflammatory cells infiltrating the anterior segment. Clin Exp Immunol 77:367, 1989.
90. Chan CC, Li Q, Brezin AP, et al: Immunopathology of ocular onchocerciasis. 3. Th-2 helper T cells in the conjunctiva. Ocular Immunol 1:71, 1993.
91. Timmann C, Abraha RS, Hamelmann C, et al: Cutaneous pathology in onchocerciasis associated with pronounced systemic T-helper 2-type responses to *Onchocerca volvulus*. Br J Dermatol 149:782, 2003.
92. Ackerman SJ, Kephart GM, Francis H, et al: Eosinophil degranulation. An immunologic determinant in the pathogenesis of the Mazzotti reaction in human onchocerciasis. J Immunol 144:3961, 1990.
93. Kephart GM, Gleich GJ, Connor DH, et al: Deposition of eosinophil granule major basic protein onto microfilariae of *Onchocerca volvulus* in the skin of patients treated with diethylcarbamazine. Lab Invest 50:51, 1984.
94. Cooper PJ, Beck LA, Espinel I, et al: Eotaxin and RANTES expression by the dermal endothelium is associated with eosinophil infiltration after ivermectin treatment of onchocerciasis. Clin Immunol 95:51, 2000.
95. Cooper PJ, Awadzi K, Ottesen EA, et al: Eosinophil sequestration and activation are associated with the onset and severity of systemic adverse reactions following the treatment of onchocerciasis with ivermectin. J Infect Dis 179:738, 1999.
96. Cooper PJ, Schwartz LB, Irani AM, et al: Association of transient dermal mastocytosis and elevated plasma tryptase levels with development of adverse reactions after treatment of onchocerciasis with ivermectin. J Infect Dis 186:1307, 2002.
97. Pearlman E, To L, Boatin BA, et al: Eotaxin expression in *Onchocerca volvulus*–induced dermatitis after topical application of diethylcarbamazine. J Infect Dis 180:1394, 1999.
98. Hoerauf A, Mand S, Volkmann L, et al: Doxycycline in the treatment of human onchocerciasis: Kinetics of *Wolbachia* endobacteria reduction and of inhibition of embryogenesis in female *Onchocerca* worms. Microbes Infect 5:261, 2003.
99. Mazzotti L: The feasibility of using the allergic reactions which follow the administration of hetrazan as an auxiliary means of diagnosis in onchocerciasis. Rev Inst Salud Enfermed Trop Mex 9:935, 1948.
100. Saint Andre A, Blackwell NM, Hall LR, et al: The role of endosymbiotic *Wolbachia* bacteria in the pathogenesis of river blindness. Science 295:1892, 2002.
101. Taylor HR, Munoz B, Keyvan-Larijani E, et al: Reliability of detection of microfilariae in skin snips in the diagnosis of onchocerciasis. Am J Trop Med Hyg 41:467, 1989.
102. Taylor HR, Keyvan-Larijani E, Newland HS, et al: Sensitivity of skin snips in the diagnosis of onchocerciasis. Trop Med Parasitol 38:145, 1987.
103. Buck AA, Anderson RI, Colston JA Jr, et al: Microfilaruria in onchocerciasis. A clinical and epidemiological follow-up study in the Republic of Chad. Bull World Health Organ 45:353, 1971.
104. Homeida MA, Mackenzie CD, Williams JF, et al: The detection of onchocercal nodules by ultrasound technique. Trans R Soc Trop Med Hyg 80:570, 1986.
105. Poltera AA, Reyna O, Zea Flores G, et al: Detection of skin nodules in onchocerciasis by ultrasound scans. Lancet 1:505, 1987.
106. Poltera AA, Reyna O, Zea-Flores G, et al: Use of an ophthalmologic ultrasoundscanner in human onchocercal skin nodules for non-invasive sequential assessment during a macrofilaricidal trial with amocarzine in Guatemala. The first experiences. Trop Med Parasitol 42:303, 1991.
107. Reyna O, Flores Z, Nowell de Arevalo AM, et al: Ultrasound detection of changes in the vitreous humor of onchocerciasis patients from Guatemala. Trans R Soc Trop Med Hyg 82:606, 1988.
108. Taylor HR: Mazzotti test for onchocerciasis [Letter]. Lancet 339:1549, 1992.
109. Francis H, Awadzi K, Ottesen EA: The Mazzotti reaction following treatment of onchocerciasis with diethylcarbamazine: Clinical severity as a function of infection intensity. Am J Trop Med Hyg 34:529, 1985.
110. Kilian HD: The use of a topical Mazzotti test in the diagnosis of onchocerciasis. Trop Med Parasitol 39:235, 1988.
111. Toe L, Adjami AG, Boatin BA, et al: Topical application of diethylcarbamazine to detect onchocerciasis recrudescence in West Africa. Trans R Soc Trop Med Hyg 94:519, 2000.
112. Pischke S, Buttner DW, Liebau E, et al: An internal control for the detection of *Onchocerca volvulus* DNA by PCR-ELISA and rapid detection of specific PCR products by DNA Detection Test Strips. Trop Med Int Health 7:526, 2002.
113. Toe L, Boatin BA, Adjami A, et al: Detection of *Onchocerca volvulus* infection by O-150 polymerase chain reaction analysis of skin scratches. J Infect Dis 178:282, 1998.
114. Boatin BA, Toe L, Alley ES, et al: Detection of *Onchocerca volvulus* infection in low prevalence areas: A comparison of three diagnostic methods. Parasitology 125:545, 2002.

115. Vincent JA, Lustigman S, Zhang S, et al: A comparison of newer tests for the diagnosis of onchocerciasis. Ann Trop Med Parasitol 94:253, 2000.
116. Campbell WC: Ivermectin as an antiparasitic agent for use in humans. Annu Rev Microbiol 45:445, 1991.
117. Cully DF, Vassilatis DK, Liu KK, et al: Cloning of an avermectin-sensitive glutamate-gated chloride channel from *Caenorhabditis elegans*. Nature 371:707, 1994.
118. Greene BM, Dukuly ZD, Munoz B, et al: A comparison of 6-, 12-, and 24-monthly dosing with ivermectin for treatment of onchocerciasis. J Infect Dis 163:376, 1991.
119. Greene BM, Taylor HR, Cupp EW, et al: Comparison of ivermectin and diethylcarbamazine in the treatment of onchocerciasis. N Engl J Med 313:133, 1985.
120. Tielsch JM, Beeche A: Impact of ivermectin on illness and disability associated with onchocerciasis. Trop Med Int Health 9:A45, 2004.
121. Molyneux DH, Bradley M, Hoerauf A, et al: Mass drug treatment for lymphatic filariasis and onchocerciasis. Trends Parasitol 19:516, 2003.
122. Brieger WR, Awedoba AK, Eneanya CI, et al: The effects of ivermectin on onchocercal skin disease and severe itching: Results of a multicentre trial. Trop Med Int Health 3:951, 1998.
123. Emukah EC, Osuoha E, Miri ES, et al: A longitudinal study of impact of repeated mass ivermectin treatment on clinical manifestations of onchocerciasis in Imo State, Nigeria. Am J Trop Med Hyg 70:556, 2004.
124. Awadzi K, Attah SK, Addy ET, et al: The effects of high-dose ivermectin regimens on *Onchocerca volvulus* in onchocerciasis patients. Trans R Soc Trop Med Hyg 93:189, 1999.
125. Gardon J, Boussinesq M, Kamgno J, et al: Effects of standard and high doses of ivermectin on adult worms of *Onchocerca volvulus*: A randomised controlled trial. Lancet 360:203, 2002.
126. Unnasch TR: River blindness. Lancet 360:182, 2002.
127. Davidson RN, Godfrey-Faussett P, Bryceson AD: Adverse reactions in expatriates treated with ivermectin. Lancet 336:1005, 1990.
128. Bryan RT, Stokes SL, Spencer HC: Expatriates treated with ivermectin. Lancet 337:304, 1991.
129. Whitworth JA, Maude GH, Luty AJ: Expatriates treated with ivermectin. Lancet 337:625, 1991.
130. Pacque M, Munoz B, Greene BM, et al: Community-based treatment of onchocerciasis with ivermectin: Safety, efficacy, and acceptability of yearly treatment. J Infect Dis 163:381, 1991.
131. Chijioke CP, Okonkwo PO: Adverse events following mass ivermectin therapy for onchocerciasis. Trans R Soc Trop Med Hyg 86:284, 1992.
132. Pacque M, Munoz B, Poetschke G, et al: Pregnancy outcome after inadvertent ivermectin treatment during community-based distribution. Lancet 336:1486, 1990.
133. Twum-Danso NA, Meredith SE: Variation in incidence of serious adverse events after onchocerciasis treatment with ivermectin in areas of Cameroon co-endemic for loiasis. Trop Med Int Health 8:820, 2003.
134. Twum-Danso NA: Serious adverse events following treatment with ivermectin for onchocerciasis control: A review of reported cases. Filaria J 2(Suppl 1):S3, 2003.
135. Twum-Danso NA: *Loa loa* encephalopathy temporally related to ivermectin administration reported from onchocerciasis mass treatment programs from 1989 to 2001: Implications for the future. Filaria J 2(Suppl 1):S7, 2003.
136. Kamgno J, Gardon J, Gardon-Wendel N, et al: Adverse systemic reactions to treatment of onchocerciasis with ivermectin at normal and high doses given annually or three-monthly. Trans R Soc Trop Med Hyg 98:496, 2004.
137. Duke BO: Overview: Report of a Scientific Working Group on Serious Adverse Events following Mectizan® treatment of onchocerciasis in *Loa loa* endemic areas. Filaria J 2 (Suppl 1):S1, 2003.
138. Awadzi K: Clinical picture and outcome of serious adverse events in the treatment of onchocerciasis. Filaria J 2(Suppl 1):S6, 2003.
139. Addiss DG, Rheingans R, Twum-Danso NA, et al: A framework for decision-making for mass distribution of Mectizan® in areas endemic for *Loa loa*. Filaria J 2(Suppl 1):S9, 2003.
140. Awadzi K, Boakye DA, Edwards G, et al: An investigation of persistent microfilaridermias despite multiple treatments with ivermectin, in two onchocerciasis-endemic foci in Ghana. Ann Trop Med Parasitol 98:231, 2004.
141. Hoerauf A, Volkmann L, Hamelmann C, et al: Endosymbiotic bacteria in worms as targets for a novel chemotherapy in filariasis. Lancet 355:1242, 2000.
142. Hoerauf A, Mand S, Adjei O, et al: Depletion of *Wolbachia* endobacteria in *Onchocerca volvulus* by doxycycline and microfilaridermia after ivermectin treatment. Lancet 357:1415, 2001.
143. Awadzi K, Hero M, Opoku NO, et al: The chemotherapy of onchocerciasis XVIII. Aspects of treatment with suramin. Trop Med Parasitol 46:19, 1995.
144. Chijioke CP, Umeh RE, Mbah AU, et al: Clinical pharmacokinetics of suramin in patients with onchocerciasis. Eur J Clin Pharmacol 54:249, 1998.
145. Duke BO: Suramin and the time it takes to kill *Onchocerca volvulus*. Trop Med Parasitol 42:346, 1991.
146. Molyneux DH, Davies JB: Onchocerciasis control: Moving towards the millennium [Review]. Parasitol Today 13:418, 1997.
147. Thylefors B: Eliminating onchocerciasis as a public health problem. Trop Med Int Health 9:A1, 2004.
148. Homeida M, Braide E, Elhassan E, et al: APOC's strategy of community-directed treatment with ivermectin (CDTI) and its potential for providing additional health services to the poorest populations. African Programme for Onchocerciasis Control. Ann Trop Med Parasitol 96(Suppl 1):S93, 2002.
149. Richards FO, Jr., Miri ES, Katabarwa M, et al: The Carter Center's assistance to river blindness control programs: Establishing treatment objectives and goals for monitoring ivermectin delivery systems on two continents. Am J Trop Med Hyg 65:108, 2001.
150. Burnham G, Mebrahtu T: The delivery of ivermectin (Mectizan). Trop Med Int Health 9:A26, 2004.
151. Peters DH, Phillips T: Mectizan Donation Program: Evaluation of a public-private partnership. Trop Med Int Health 9:A4, 2004.
152. Winnen M, Plaisier AP, Alley ES, et al: Can ivermectin mass treatments eliminate onchocerciasis in Africa? Bull World Health Organ 80:384, 2002.
153. Borsboom GJ, Boatin BA, Nagelkerke NJ, et al: Impact of ivermectin on onchocerciasis transmission: Assessing the empirical evidence that repeated ivermectin mass treatments may lead to elimination/eradication in West-Africa. Filaria J 2:8, 2003.

101

Zoonotic Filariasis

MARK L. EBERHARD

INTRODUCTION

Zoonotic filariasis is human infection with a filarial parasite that normally parasitizes some other animal host. As is typical of filariae, obligate development occurs in an appropriate arthropod intermediate host and transmission is through the bite of an infected vector. In this regard, transmission of filariasis, including zoonotic infections, has a greater likelihood of occurring in tropical or subtropical climates. This may be due, in part, to a wider diversity of species and greater number of biting insects throughout the year, hence a transmission season that may be year-round. However, as a general rule, a far greater number and range of types of zoonotic infections occur in temperate than in tropical regions. Any unique aspects of zoonotic filarial infections limited to the tropics is a reflection only of the geographic distribution of a particular species of parasite involved. Zoonotic filarial infections, therefore, are neither restricted nor unique to the tropics.

AGENT

The first well-recognized report of human infection with a zoonotic filaria is attributed to Addario[1] in 1885, who described a case from Italy and called the parasite *Filaria conjunctivae*. It was Desportes,[2] working in Paris in 1939 and 1940, who correctly recognized that *F. conjunctivae* infection was actually caused by species of *Dirofilaria*, and he applied the name *Dirofilaria conjunctivae* to these zoonotic infections. Although these subcutaneous infections were seen in various anatomic locations, the term *conjunctivae* was applied because of the marked periorbital involvement in many cases. It was not until 1965, however, that Orihel and Beaver[3] concluded that *D. conjunctivae* infection in the United States is most often caused by *Dirofilaria tenuis*, a parasite of raccoons (*Procyon lotor*), whereas in Europe, the former USSR, Africa, Southeast Asia, and elsewhere, these infections are commonly caused by *Dirofilaria repens*, a natural parasite of dogs and other mammals in those areas. Since then, several additional species of *Dirofilaria* have been recognized as causes of subcutaneous infection in humans.[4] Subcutaneous infections caused by members of the genus *Dirofilaria* probably constitute the most commonly recognized zoonotic filarial infections in humans.[5–7]

The second most commonly encountered form of zoonotic filarial infection, that caused by the dog heartworm, *Dirofilaria immitis*, was first reported by Faust and coworkers[8] in 1941 from the vena cava of a woman in New Orleans. Infections with *D. immitis* most frequently result in a well-circumscribed lesion in a lobe of the lung and are commonly referred to as coin lesions.[4] These infections are widely reported from around the world, and large series of cases have been described.[9]

More recently, several other genera of filariae have been recognized with some frequency as causes of zoonotic infections. These include *Dipetalonema*-like worms,[10–16] *Onchocerca*,[17–26] and *Brugia*.[27–41] These infections have involved recovery of adult worms in tissue biopsy or surgically excised specimens, although occasionally worms have been recovered free from the surrounding tissues.

On occasion, microfilariae that did not correspond to known human species have been found in skin or blood. These include *Brugia* species,[34] *Mansonella rhodhaini*,[42] *Meningonema peruzzii*,[43,44] *Microfilaria semiclarum*,[45] *Microfilaria bolivarensis*,[46] *Dirofilaria*-like,[47] and *Dipetalonema*-like species.[48] The presence of microfilariae in skin, blood, or cerebrospinal fluid (CSF) indicates the presence of adult male and female worms somewhere in the host tissues.

Of the six or seven genera of filariae most often recognized as causing zoonotic infections, including *Dirofilaria, Brugia, Onchocerca, Mansonella, Meningonema, Loaina*, and *Dipetalonema*-like, all are in the family Onchocercidae (superfamily Filarioidea, order Spirurida),[49] and, with one exception, belong to one of two subfamilies, Dirofilariinae or Onchocerciinae. The exception, *Meningonema peruzzii*, is in the subfamily Splendidofilaria (family Onchocercidae). Although human infections have been reported with filariae from a wide range of mammalian hosts, as far as is known no avian, reptilian, or amphibian filariae have caused human infection.

For ease of review, zoonotic filariae are discussed according to the tissue or organ that they infect in the human host. This information is summarized in Table 101-1.

EPIDEMIOLOGY

The actual, and potential, distribution of zoonotic filariasis is worldwide, depending on the species of filaria. The potential for any given individual to acquire a zoonotic filarial infection is quite low. It would seem that spending an appreciable amount of time outdoors exposed to insect bites is the greatest risk factor. However, there must be other factors besides exposure to infective bites that contribute to infection, since it is likely that nearly everyone who spends time outdoors occasionally will be bitten by an infected insect and exposed to infective filarial larvae. However, in the majority of people, these infective larvae apparently do not survive to undergo development.

Regardless of the type, all zoonotic filariae are transmitted to humans through the bite of infected arthropods. As far as is known, transmission of most zoonotic filarial infections has been through mosquito bites, although *Culicoides* and *Simulium* are undoubtedly responsible for transmitting zoonotic *Onchocerca* and *Mansonella* infections. Other known filarial vectors, such as mites, ticks, and tabanid flies, also could be responsible for transmitting infections to humans, although no human infections due to filariae transmitted by these vectors are recognized to have occurred.

Table 101-1 Summary of Major Zoonotic Filarial Infections Reported to Cause Infection in Humans

Site	Parasite	Natural Host	Geographic Distribution in Natural Host	Geographic Distribution of Reported Human Cases
Lung	*Dirofilaria immitis*	Dog	Cosmopolitan	North and South America, Australia, Japan, Europe
Skin, subcutaneous tissue	*Dirofilaria tenuis*	Raccoon	North America	North America
	Dirofilaria repens	Dog	Europe, Russia, Middle East, Africa, Southeast Asia	Europe, Russia, Middle East, Africa, Southeast Asia
	Dirofilaria ursi	Bear	North America, Japan	North America, Japan
	D. immitis	Dog	Cosmopolitan	North America, Japan
	Dirofilaria striata	Bobcat, wildcats	North and South America	United States
	Onchocerca spp.	Ungulates	Cosmopolitan	North America, Europe, Russia, Japan
	Mansonella rhodhaini	Chimpanzee	Africa (Gabon)	Africa (Gabon)
Eye	*D. tenuis*	Raccoon	North America	North America
	D. repens	Dog	Europe, Russia, Africa, Southeast Asia	Europe, Russia, Africa, Southeast Asia
	D. immitis	Dog	Cosmopolitan	Australia, Southeast Asia
	Loaina spp.	Rabbit, kangaroo	North America, Australia	South America, Australia
	Dipetalonema-like	?	?	North America
	Onchocerca spp.	Ungulates	Cosmopolitan	United States, Hungary
	Brugia ceylonensis	Dog	Sri Lanka	Sri Lanka
Lymphatics	*Brugia* spp.	Rodents, carnivores	North America, Africa, Southeast Asia	North and South America, Africa
Blood	*Microfilaria bolivarensis*	?	South America (Venezuela)	South America (Venezuela)
	Dipetalonema semiclarum	?	Africa (Congo)	Africa (Congo)

The geographic distribution of the filariae that are recognized as causes of zoonotic infections is, for the most part, poorly defined, and the distribution of human infections is even more patchy. More zoonotic infections are detected and identified in North America and Europe than in Latin America, Africa, or Southeast Asia. This is illustrated by the number of zoonotic *Brugia* infections reported from the United States[28,30–32,34,35,38–40] and the large series of zoonotic *D. repens* cases documented by Pampiglione and co-workers[50–53] from Italy. However, this in no way implies that the true incidence of zoonotic infections is higher in temperate than in tropical regions. This disparate distribution of known cases undoubtedly reflects better access to health care and a much different level of health-related concerns on the part of both patient and clinician.

Equally poorly defined are other factors that may contribute to filarial infections. There may well be seasonality to the transmission potential, and this would be more marked in temperate than in tropical areas. Mosquito-transmitted zoonotic infections are almost certainly acquired during the warmer summer months in the northern United States and Canada, for instance, than during the winter months. In the tropics, other factors, such as rainfall, availability of breeding sites, and so on, are probably more important in determining the likelihood of transmission than is temperature. Proximity to the natural definitive host also may play an important role in acquisition of infection. In the case of zoonotic infection with *D. immitis* or *D. repens*, both natural infections of dogs, having an infected dog in the household or in the neighborhood probably increases the risk of exposure to infected mosquito bites. Numerous wild animals, such as raccoons and rabbits, which harbor *D. tenuis* and *Brugia leporis*, respectively, commonly live in residential areas and persons who "never travel to the country" may be exposed in their own backyard or community park.

Unfortunately, there is no way to estimate the number of zoonotic filarial infections acquired each year, nor is it possible to gauge the percentage of infections that are detected and diagnosed each year. Many of these zoonotic infections, especially those caused by species of *Dirofilaria*, are now becoming more widely recognized by clinicians and pathologists, and unless there is something unusual about the case, they are not routinely reported in the literature. The more unusual infections, such as those caused by *Brugia* or *Onchocerca*, when recognized, still hold enough interest to merit publication. Overall, however, it is probably safe to say that hundreds of zoonotic infections are attributable to various *Dirofilaria* species each year. On the other hand, the author is aware of no more than about 30 reported cases of zoonotic *Brugia* infections, all but one or two occurring in the Western Hemisphere. The possibility of zoonotic *Brugia* infections, especially in Southeast Asia, would seem to be high, especially after Edeson and others were able to demonstrate experimental infections in humans with *Brugia pahangi*.[27] However, it would be nearly impossible to recognize and distinguish a zoonotic *B. pahangi* infection from a *Brugia malayi* infection based on the morphologic aspects of either microfilariae in blood smears or adults in lymphatic tissues. Some zoonotic filarial infections have been recognized on only several occasions. These include 10 reported cases of *Onchocerca*,[17–26] several cases of *Dipetalonema*-like worms,[10–16] three observations of a *Loaina*-like worm,[54,55] and one instance of *Macacanema*.[56]

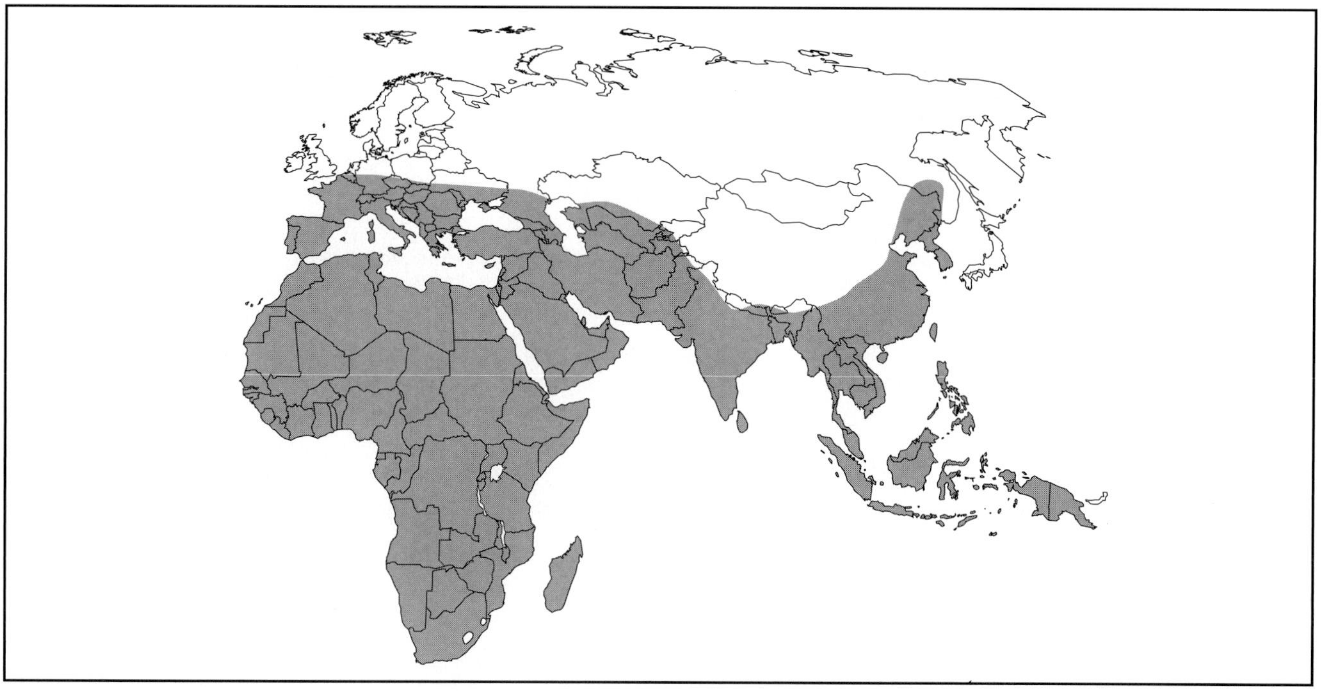

Dirofilaria repens in Dogs and Other Carnivores

■ Approximate distribution

Note: The actual distribution may extend farther northward into the Scandinavian countries and also be more extensive in central Asia. The parasite is not recognized to occur in the Western Hemisphere, nor in Australia. Zoonotic human cases have been reported from virtually all recognized endemic areas.

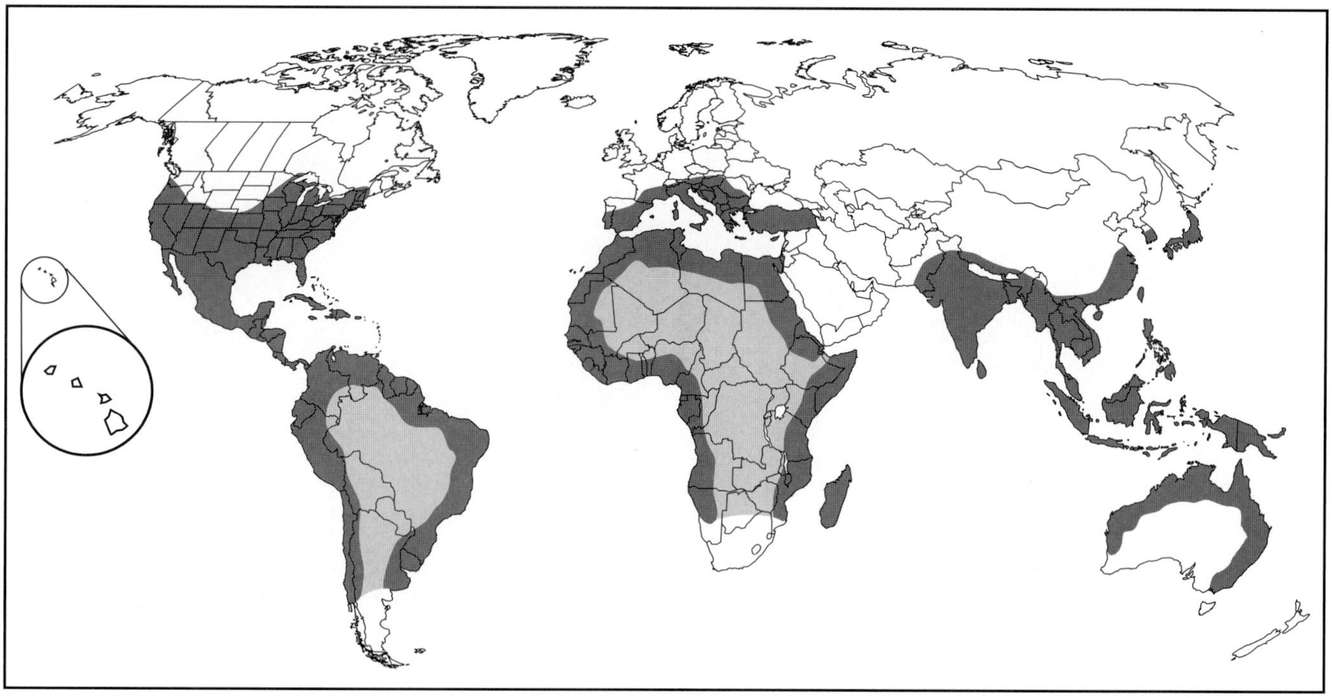

Dirofilaria immitis in Dogs

■ Areas of known distribution

□ Areas of possible distribution

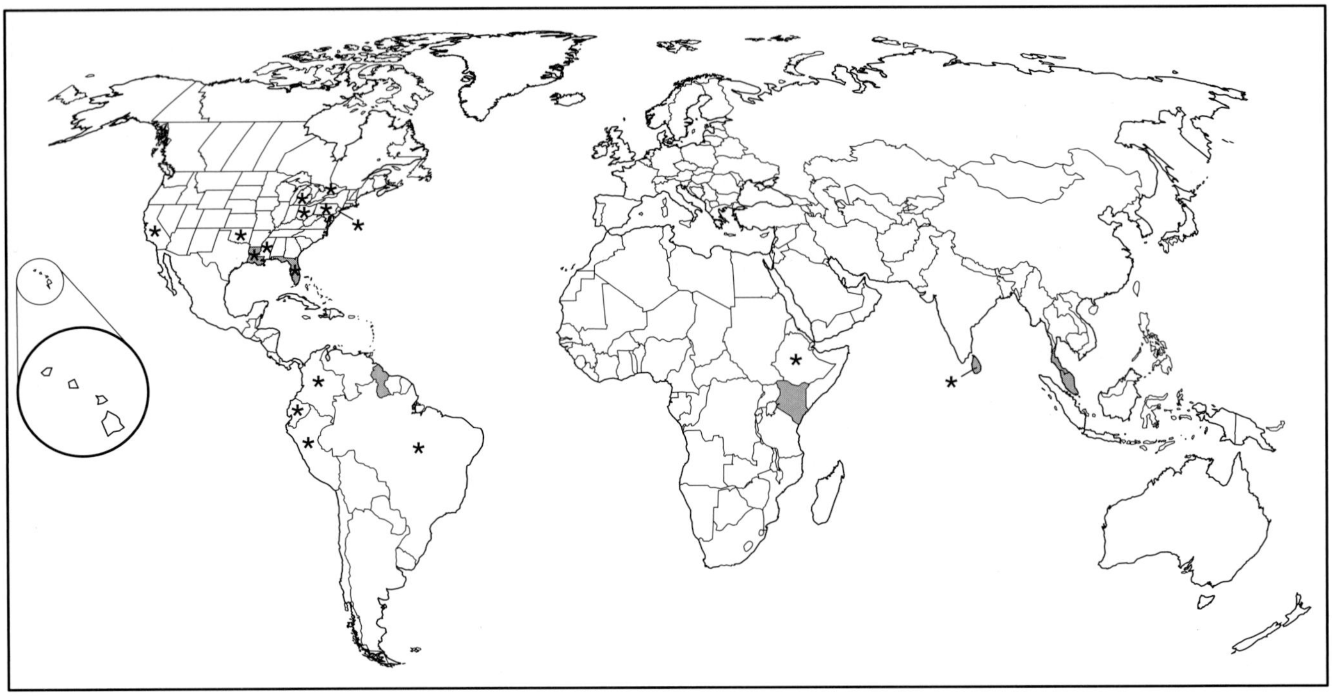

Brugia spp.
■ Approximate geographic distribution
* Distribution of recognized zoonotic cases

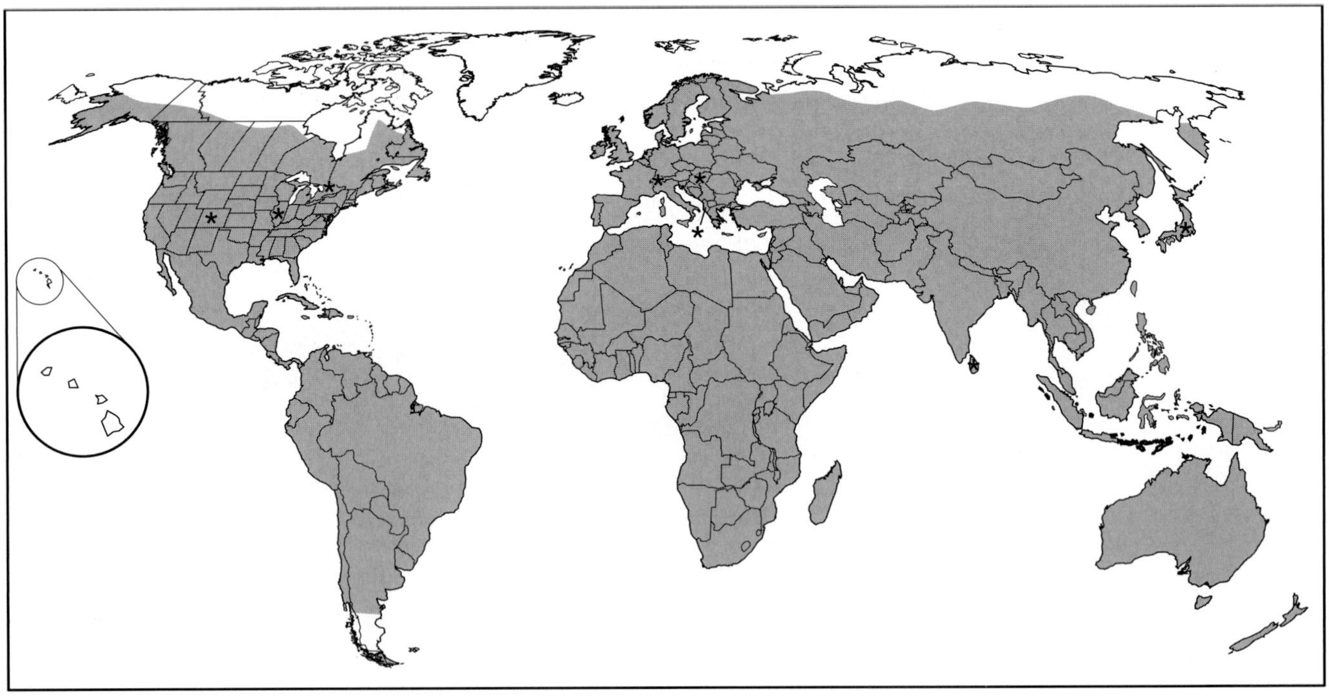

Onchocerca spp.
■ Geographic distribution
* Known human cases

Although most often caused by a single, infertile worm, zoonotic filarial infections occasionally are recognized to be caused by more than one worm. This has been most evident in cases in which gravid female worms were observed or in which microfilariae were detected. Both instances require not only the presence of a male worm but also that both worms survive long enough to reach sexual maturity and mate. This situation has been reported at least four times in the case of *Dirofilaria* infections,[57–60] three times in *Brugia* infections,[34,35,37] and once in a *Dipetalonema*-like infection.[48] Orihel and colleagues[61] have described a different situation in which two *D. repens* worms, both female and both unmated, were recovered from the same person about 10 months apart. The authors concluded that the worms were from the same inoculum but appeared in the conjunctiva at different times. Female worms, at least in the case of *Dirofilaria*, are recorded about three times more often than male worms, although there is no biologic basis for this difference. Again, Orihel and colleagues raised the possibility that infection with male worms occurs as frequently but goes unrecognized more often.[61]

DISEASE

The disease, its clinical manifestations, and pathologic findings are reflected in the anatomic site of infection and can, for ease of discussion, be broken into four major categories of lesions: subcutaneous, lung, eye, and lymphatic.

Subcutaneous Infections

Several different filarial parasites cause subcutaneous or connective tissue infections, including species of *Dirofilaria*, *Onchocerca*, and *Dipetalonema*-like. The vast majority of skin and subcutaneous lesions are caused by one of several species of *Dirofilaria*. In Europe, Africa, and Southeast Asia, *D. repens* is most often incriminated as the etiologic agent and would be at the top of the list of suspected species. In the United States and Canada, *D. tenuis* is most frequently involved, although, in decreasing order, *D. ursi* of bears (or *D. subdermata* of porcupines), *D. striata* of bobcats, and *D. immitis* of dogs are also recognized to cause human infection. Subcutaneous infection due to one of these *Dirofilaria* species most commonly results in the appearance of a small (0.5 to 1.5 cm), discrete nodule that is noticed by the patient anywhere from several days to several weeks prior to surgical removal.[4,62] On sectioning, one or more sections of encased filarial worm are evident (Fig. 101-1). These nodules can be either painless or painful and with or without signs of local inflammation. Occasionally, there has been some sensation that a moving worm was present, and in these cases, there tends to be more generalized edema and swelling and a less discrete nodule. These later cases likely represent worms that are beginning to reach the end of their sojourn in the human body but have not yet become fully enclosed in a granulomatous nodule. There is little systemic sign of infection, although some patients may have an elevated eosinophilia; generally, the presentation is otherwise unremarkable. Zoonotic *Dirofilaria* infections can be expected to occur in almost any anatomic location, but some of the more unusual locations include the bladder,[63] spermatic cord[64–68] or epididymis,[69] liver,[70] and mouth.[71]

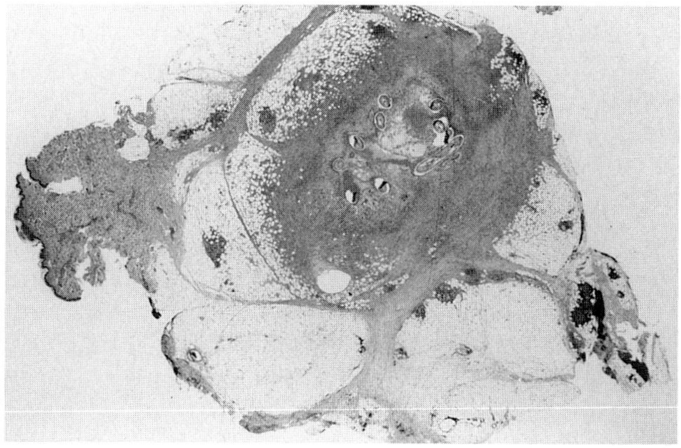

FIGURE 101-1 A subcutaneous nodule caused by a zoonotic filarial infection due to *Dirofilaria tenuis* from a case in South Carolina. Note the proximity of the nodule to the skin surface and the numerous sections of a single parasite encased in the nodule, which measured approximately 8 mm in diameter. (H&E stain.)

Eye Infections

A report of a worm in, on, or near the eye of a patient (Fig. 101-2) is always a dramatic occurrence for both patient and clinician. Patients frequently report the sensation of "movement of an object" in or near the eye, and the physician

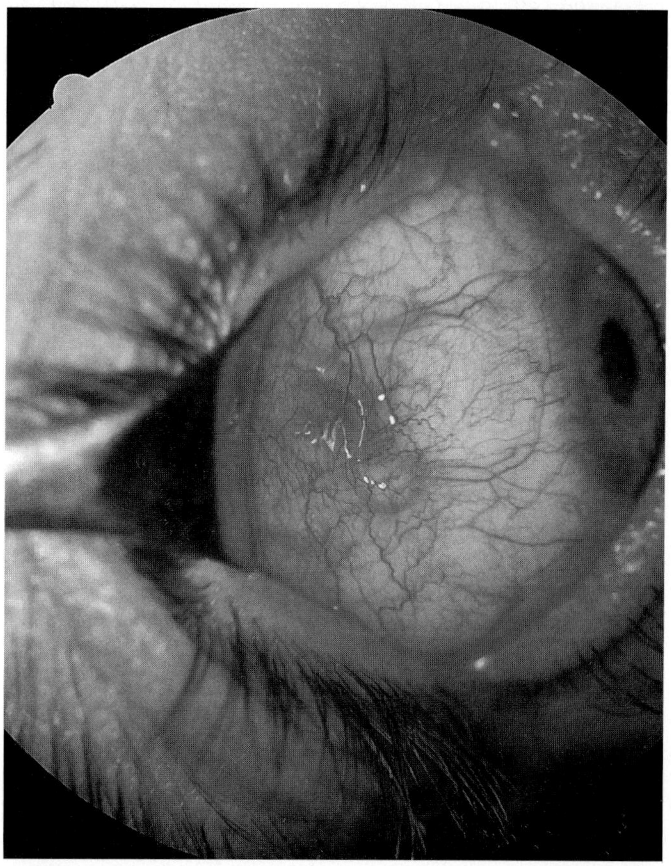

FIGURE 101-2 Clinical photograph of coiled *Dirofilaria repens* on the conjunctiva. (From Pampiglione S, Canestri Trotti G, Rivasi F: Human dirofilariasis due to *Dirofilaria* [*Nochtiella*] *repens*: A review of world literature. Parassitologia 37:149–193, 1995.)

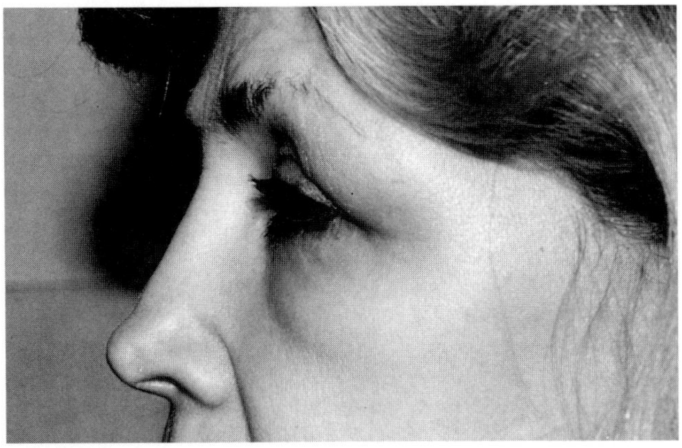

FIGURE 101-3 Clinical photograph of facial edema in a patient with periorbital soft tissue swelling due to *Dirofilaria tenuis* infection. (From Kersten RC, Locastro AJ, Eberhard ML, et al: Periorbital dirofilariasis. Ophthalmic Plast Reconstr Surg 10:293–296, 1994.)

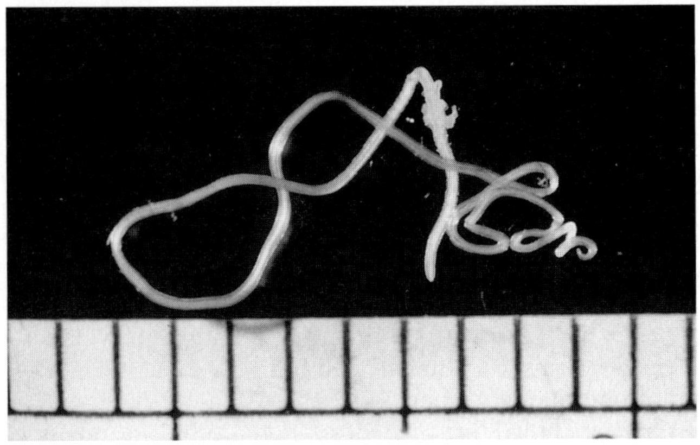

FIGURE 101-5 Male *Dirofilaria tenuis* worm removed intact from the conjunctiva of a patient in the United States. Scale is in millimeters.

can occasionally see the worm in the conjunctiva, on the eye itself, or in the anterior and posterior chambers.[4,62] The presence of a worm in or around the eye is frequently accompanied by swelling or edema of the eyelid and face (Figs. 101-3 and 101-4) and a sharp stinging or burning sensation. Worms located in the retina and anterior or posterior chamber of the eye are frequently recognized by the patient because of blurred vision and pain in or behind the eye. In some cases, there is no inflammation, blurred vision, or swollen lids. In general, reports of a worm in the connective tissues around the eye have been diagnosed as *Loa loa* or a zoonotic *Dirofilaria* species. Reports of a worm in the chamber of the eye often have been attributed to natural human filariae such as *Wuchereria bancrofti*, *L. loa*, or *Brugia malayi*. However, zoonotic infections due to *Dirofilaria* (*D. repens*, *D. immitis*), *Loaina*, *Dipetalonema*-like worms, *Brugia ceylonensis*, and *Onchocerca* have been described.[23,41,55] Many times, worms around or in the eye are recovered free from the tissues (Fig. 101-5), while occasionally those in the eye can either be extracted by irrigation-aspiration[72] or destroyed in situ using photocoagulation.[73]

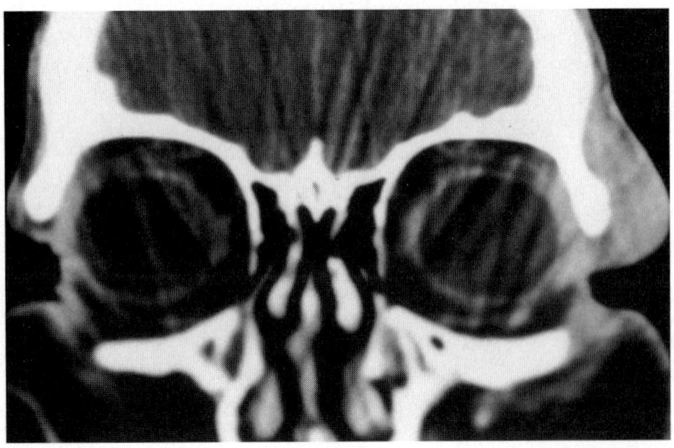

FIGURE 101-4 Coronal CT scan of the same patient as in Figure 101-3, demonstrating a discrete soft tissue mass without bony or intraorbital involvement. (From Kersten RC, Locastro AJ, Eberhard ML, et al: Periorbital dirofilariasis. Ophthalmic Plast Reconstr Surg 10:293–296, 1994.)

Lung Infections

The second most common finding associated with zoonotic filarial infections is discrete lesions in the lung parenchyma resulting in very well-circumscribed, circular nodules (Figs. 101-6 through 101-8) that on radiographs appear as coin lesions.[4,62] These lesions are due most often to *D. immitis* but can be caused by *Brugia*-like worms.[15] There is a tendency for these nodules to be solitary and somewhat larger than those due to subcutaneous dirofilariasis. There are cases of multiple nodules[74] as well as reports of transient nodules, suggesting that human infections are much more common than thought.[75] Occasionally, these nodules are reported to be calcified.[76] Again, as in the case of subcutaneous dirofilariasis, patients with a lung nodule due to *D. immitis* are generally not in bad health, and it is not unusual for the lesions

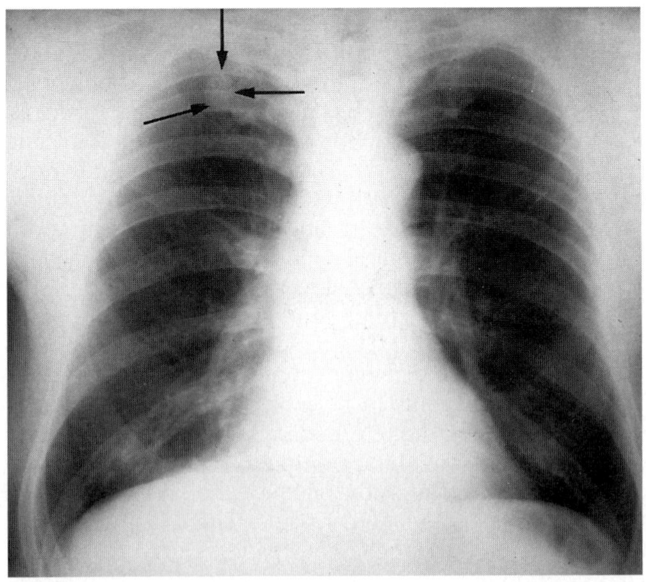

FIGURE 101-6 Radiograph showing a solitary, subpleural nodule (coin lesion) of the upper lobe of the right lung due to *Dirofilaria* infections. (From Pampiglione S, Canestri Trotti G, Rivasi F: Human dirofilariasis due to *Dirofilaria* [*Nochtiella*] *repens*: A review of world literature. Parassitologia 37:149–193, 1995.)

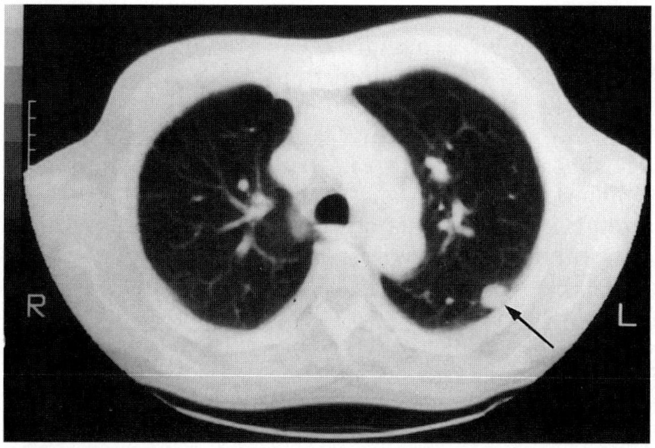

FIGURE 101-7 CT scan of a solitary nodule in the left lung due to *Dirofilaria* infection. (From Pampiglione S, Canestri Trotti G, Rivasi F: Human dirofilariasis due to *Dirofilaria* [*Nochtiella*] *repens*: A review of world literature. Parassitologia 37:149–193, 1995.)

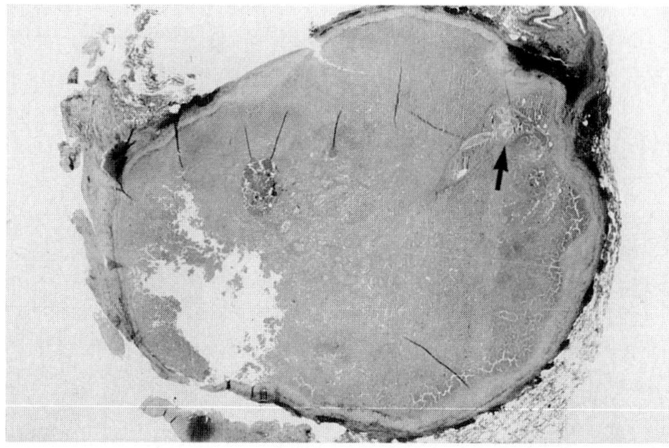

FIGURE 101-9 Panoramic view of a histologic section of a classic coin lesion in the lung caused by *Dirofilaria immitis* infection. Some normal lung tissue is evident at the lower right-hand corner of the section, and several sections of a worm are evident (*arrow*). Note the well-circumscribed nature of this lesion, which measures approximately 12 mm in diameter. (H&E stain.)

to be detected on chest film as part of a routine physical examination. Over 50% of these patients are asymptomatic, although there are some reports of chest pain, low-grade fever, cough, and malaise. Eosinophilia may or may not be a remarkable clinical feature. In direct contrast to subcutaneous dirofilariasis, pulmonary dirofilariasis is almost always confused initially with a malignancy. A large number of reports have addressed the problem of zoonotic filarial infections mimicking pseudotumor or carcinomas, and issues related to differential diagnosis.[77–83] Once the lesion is removed, histologic examination reveals its true nature (Fig. 101-9), and the concern of both clinician and patient can be allayed.

Lymphatic Infections

The location of zoonotic filariae in the lymphatics leads to the classic presentation of a tender, swollen lymph node (Fig. 101-10). Although zoonotic *Brugia* infections have been reported from a variety of anatomic locations, the three most common sites are the neck region, groin, and axillary region. These sites and others, such as the breast, reflect the prominent lymph nodes and channels that are found in these sites. The main presenting symptom is an enlarged, painful regional node of one to several weeks' duration. This finding frequently leads to an initial diagnosis of lymphoma or other malignancy. Eosinophilia may or may not be a presenting feature, and occasionally the enlarged node may not be tender. Histologically, the overall presentation is one of a hyperplastic node with a focal granulomatous reaction. The location of worms in a patent lymph channel is occasionally evident (Fig. 101-11), but in more advanced cases, the normal structural architecture of the lymph canal is lost in the inflammatory reaction (Fig. 101-12). These differences undoubtedly reflect

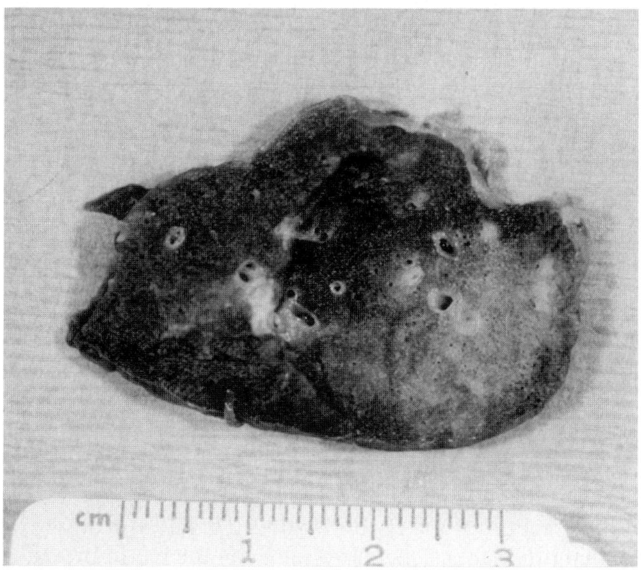

FIGURE 101-8 Infarcted lesion in the lung (coin lesion) due to *Dirofilaria immitis* infection.

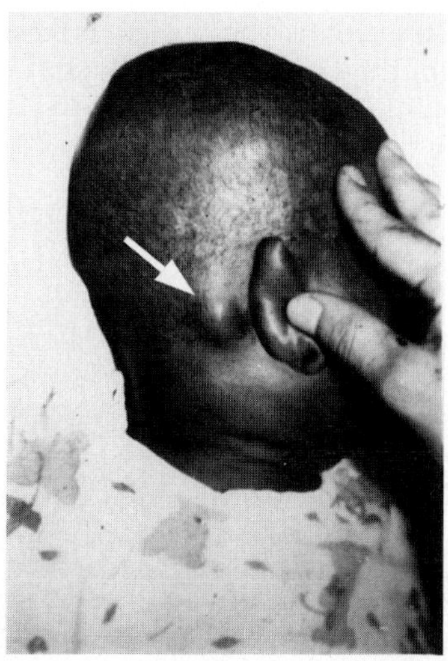

FIGURE 101-10 Clinical photograph of an enlarged retroauricular lymph node (*arrow*) in a patient with a zoonotic *Brugia* infection. (From Kozek WJ, Reyes MA, Ehrman J, et al: Enzootic *Brugia* infection in a two-year-old Colombian girl. Am J Trop Med Hyg 33:65–69, 1984.)

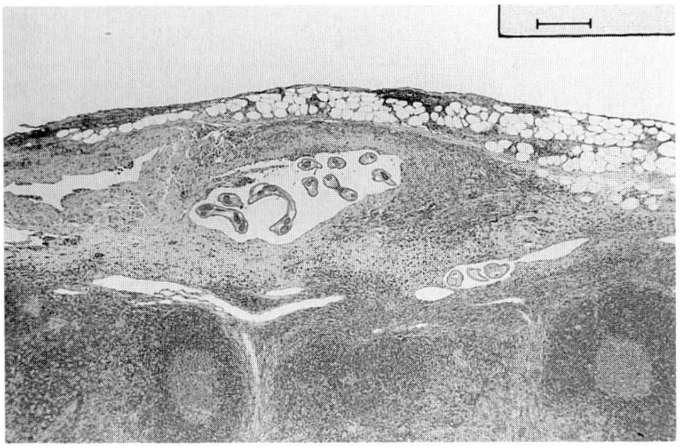

FIGURE 101-11 Histologic section of a lymph node from a case of zoonotic *Brugia* infection illustrating multiple sections of a worm in lymph channels. Scale bar = 200 μm. (H&E stain.) (From Eberhard ML, DeMeester LJ, Martin BW, et al: Zoonotic *Brugia* infection in western Michigan. Am J Surg Pathol 17:1058–1061, 1993.)

both the condition of the worm (i.e., alive or dead) and the duration of the host response. Some nodules are removed in a much more acute stage than others. Because of the small size of these worms, it may be necessary to examine numerous sections before the worm is encountered.

Microfilarial Infections

The detection of microfilariae ascribed to zoonotic filarial infections has not been correlated with clinical symptoms or signs in most cases, although there was clear central nervous system (CNS) involvement in human cases of *Meningonema peruzzii*,[43] and classic signs of lymphatic filariasis, including lymphedema, were noted in a case of zoonotic *Brugia* infection.[34]

PATHOGENESIS AND IMMUNITY

The pathogenesis of zoonotic filariasis is one of localized foreign body reaction around a dead or dying parasite. On the basis of the size of worms seen in these cases and our understanding of the life history of some of these filariae in their natural or experimental hosts, these represent infections of a month to many months' duration. More often than not, these infections are asymptomatic until just prior to the detection of the inflammatory nodule surrounding the worm. Some zoonotic infections, especially those caused by *Dirofilaria* and *Onchocerca*, may represent 6 months or more of asymptomatic growth and wandering by the developing worm. It is believed that only upon the impending death of the worm does a marked tissue reaction occur (an exception may be seen in worms that make their way to the tissues surrounding the eyes). Whether the host's response precedes and is responsible for killing the worm, or whether the worm dies because of physiologic incompatibility followed by host reaction to a moribund parasite, is unclear. The fact that many of these zoonotic infections persist asymptomatically for appreciable periods of time suggests that the latter is the case.

Limited studies indicate that the human host produces antibodies directed at the parasite, and that these antifilarial antibodies can be detected in serum samples. In several cases of zoonotic *Brugia* infections, isotype-specific, antifilarial antibodies, as determined by an enzyme-linked immunosorbent assay (ELISA) using adult *Brugia* antigens, have demonstrated elevated responses that markedly diminish by 3 months postsurgery.[39,40] Various serologic assays have also been developed to detect *Dirofilaria* infections.[84–90] These assays, although frequently not able to distinguish between different types of infections, could clearly be helpful in suspected cases when no worm was observed in the biopsy but a suggestive granulomatous reaction was present, and in conducting seroepidemiologic surveys. It has been suggested that zoonotic filarial infections result in immunopathologic reactions, such as arthritis.[91]

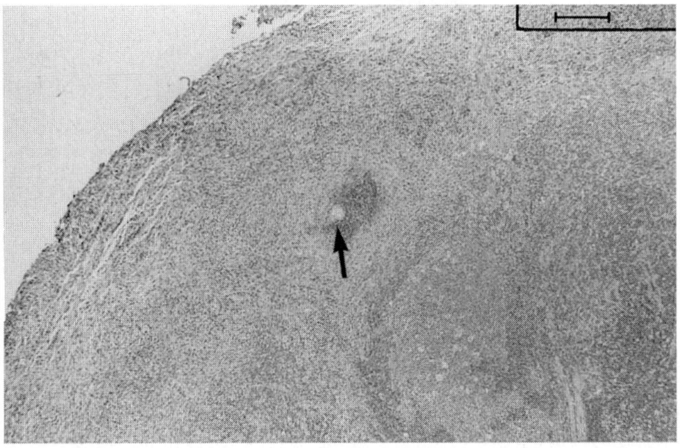

FIGURE 101-12 Histologic section of a lymph node from a zoonotic *Brugia* infection in which the lymph channel has been obliterated around the worm (*arrow*). Scale bar = 200 μm. (H&E stain.)

DIAGNOSIS

The diagnosis of zoonotic filarial infections, for the foreseeable future, will continue to be the recognition and accurate identification of these parasites in excisioned or biopsy histologic sections.[92] This is not to say that good serologic assays would not play a vital role in diagnosis and management. However, because zoonotic filarial infections are constituted of any number of different species, serologic assays that are genus-specific rather than species-specific would be much more valuable as screening tools.

Diagnosis of the genus (and species) of filaria causing the infection is best accomplished by study of the morphologic features seen in tissue sections. Occasionally, intact worms are removed, particularly from in or around the eye, and these can usually be tentatively identified based on comparison with recognized species found in the area where the patient is believed to have acquired the infection.

Location of the lesion containing the worm can frequently provide some guidance in identifying the worm. For instance, a worm associated with the lymphatic system has a high probability of being a zoonotic *Brugia* infection, while the location of a worm in a coin lesion in the lung is likely to be *D. immitis*. However, diagnosing zoonotic filarial infections based solely on the location of the lesion is sure to result in many incorrect determinations. The morphology of the worm provides a much greater degree of accuracy (sensitivity) than does the location of the lesion and ensures that a worm in an unusual location is not misdiagnosed.

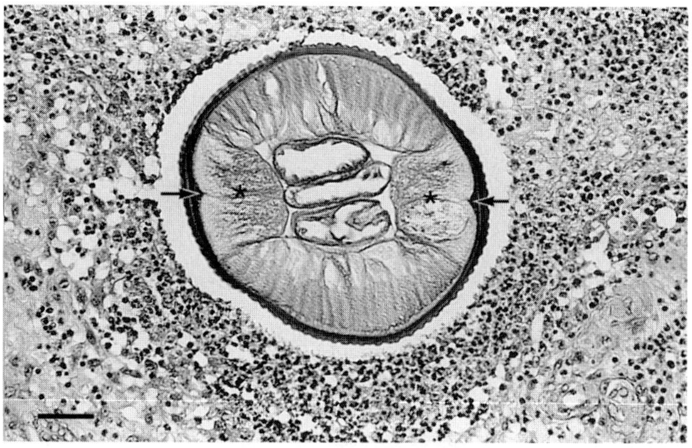

FIGURE 101-13 High-power photomicrograph of a section of a female *Dirofilaria tenuis* from the same case as illustrated in Figure 101-1. This section clearly illustrates the nature of the thick cuticle with numerous external ridges and two internal lateral ridges (*arrows*) in the region of the lateral chords. Tall, heavy musculature, prominent lateral chords (*asterisks*), two uterine tubes, and a section of intestine are also evident. Scale bar = 50 μm. (H&E stain.)

The diagnosis of zoonotic filarial infections is almost always made from stained tissue sections, and there are morphologic features that allow placement of worms into several broad groups.[62,93,94] These are discussed briefly in the following sections.

Dirofilaria

By far the most common zoonotic infections encountered are caused by species of *Dirofilaria*. Three species are believed to account for the vast majority of recognized cases. *D. immitis*, the dog heartworm, has a nearly cosmopolitan distribution that is continuing to expand; *D. repens* infects dogs and cats in Europe, Africa, Southeast Asia, and possibly elsewhere; and *D. tenuis* is a natural parasite of raccoons in North America. Other species reported from humans include *D. striata* of wildcats in North and South America, and *D. ursi*, which parasitizes bears in North America and Japan. A vast number of other dirofilariae exist, and all probably hold zoonotic potential.

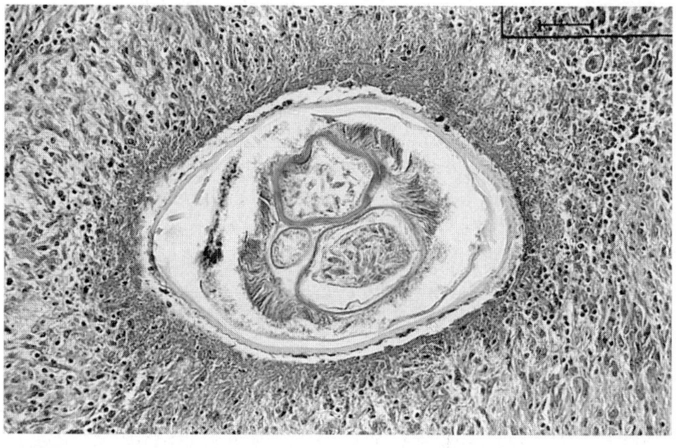

FIGURE 101-14 High-power photomicrograph of a section of a female *Dirofilaria tenuis* from the case illustrated in Figure 101-3. Although this worm is moribund and has undergone considerable degeneration, the thick cuticle with external ridging, heavy musculature, two uterine reproductive tubes, and a single digestive tube are still evident. Scale bar = 50 μm. (H&E stain.)

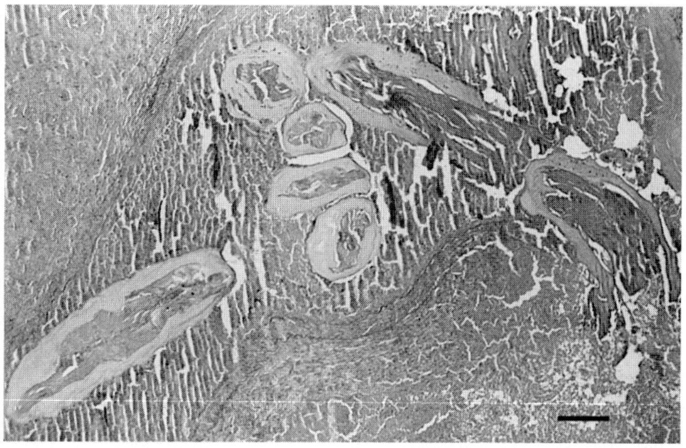

FIGURE 101-15 Photomicrograph of the coiled *Dirofilaria immitis* worm seen in Figure 101-9. At this magnification, several features of the worm are evident, including the thick cuticle and heavy musculature. Scale bar = 200 μm. (H&E stain.)

Dirofilaria worms have several consistent features that are recognizable in sections. Generally, they are relatively large worms, up to 400 or 500 mm in diameter; they have a thick cuticle, which, with the exception of *D. immitis* and *D. striata*, has prominent longitudinal ridges; and the musculature is prominent, with numerous muscle cells that extend far into the body cavity (Figs. 101-13 through 101-18). The number

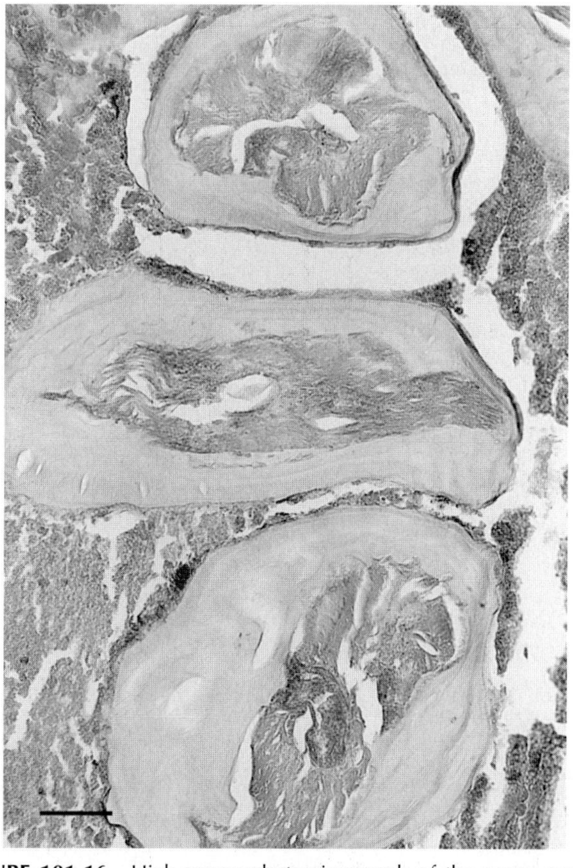

FIGURE 101-16 High-power photomicrograph of the worm seen in Figure 101-15. At this higher magnification, it is evident that the worm is moribund and has undergone considerable degeneration. The cuticle is considerably swollen and thickened and has a smooth outer surface, and remnants of the heavy musculature are evident. Scale bar = 50 μm. (H&E stain.)

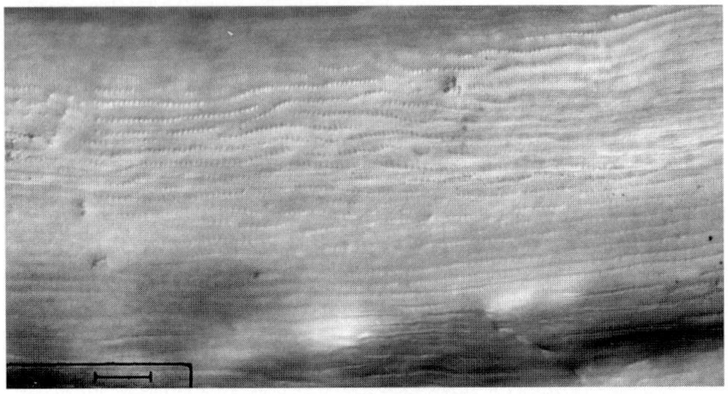

FIGURE 101-17 Low-power view of the cuticular surface of a *Dirofilaria repens* removed intact from the tissues, illustrating the beaded ridges that run longitudinally along the worm. Scale bar = 50 µm.

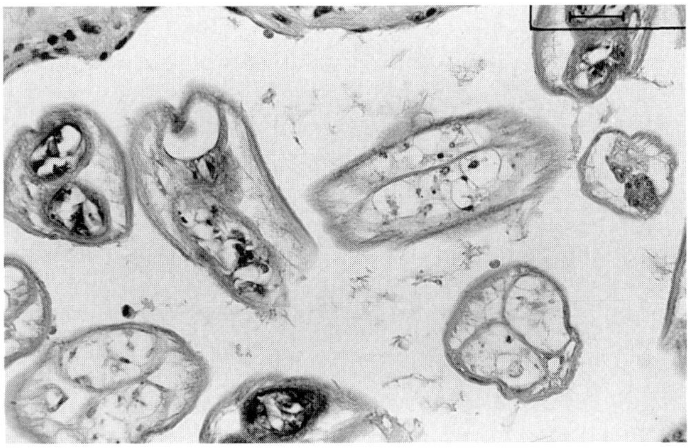

FIGURE 101-19 High-power view of a coiled female Brugia worm in a lymph channel, illustrating the small size of the worm, the thin cuticle, and the small number of low muscle cells per quadrant. Scale bar = 25 µm. (H&E stain.)

and shape of the cuticular ridging can be useful in separating species, as can the absence of ridges. It should be noted here, although true for all zoonotic filarial infections, that size can be a very useful feature in the determination of possible species. However, one must also use caution, as many of the worms removed in these cases represent immature worms, which makes size comparisons difficult. There are also notable exceptions, such as *D. ursi*–like worms, which, when seen in human tissue, are much smaller than other dirofilariae but still have typical *Dirofilaria* features (ridged cuticle, etc.).

Brugia

The recognition of small filariae in close association with lymph nodes or lymph vessels, or on rare occasions the eye, would be suggestive of infection with a zoonotic *Brugia* species (see Figs. 101-10 through 101-12). The species involved in the reported human cases have not been established. A number of species have been described from various animals; in the United States we recognize two species, *B. beaveri* of the raccoon and *B. leporis* of rabbits; from South America, *B. guyanensis* of the coatimundi; *B. tupaie* of tree shrews and *B. pahangi* in dogs, cats, slow loris, leaf monkeys, and wildcats from Malaysia; *B. patei* of dogs, cats, wildcats, and bush babies from Africa; and *B. ceylonensis* from dogs and *B. buckleyi* from hares in Sri Lanka.

In section, zoonotic *Brugia* are small worms, almost always less than 150 µm and occasionally less than 50 µm in diameter. The cuticle is relatively thin but frequently thickens over the

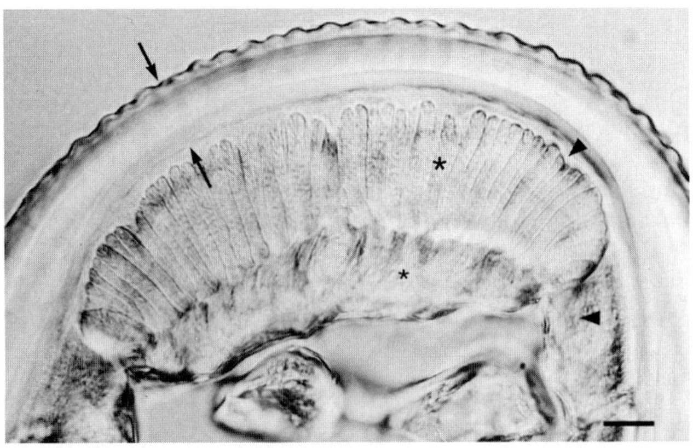

FIGURE 101-18 Cross section of an unstained *Dirofilaria repens* (in glycerin), illustrating the typical *Dirofilaria* anatomy. Evident is the thick, multilayered cuticle with external ridging (*arrows*), the thin inconspicuous hypodermal tissue that greatly expands in the area of the lateral chords (*arrowheads*), and the tall, heavy muscle cells that are composed of a narrow, basal, fibrillar, contractile portion (*large asterisk*) and a shorter cytoplasmic portion (*small asterisk*). Scale bar = 50 µm.

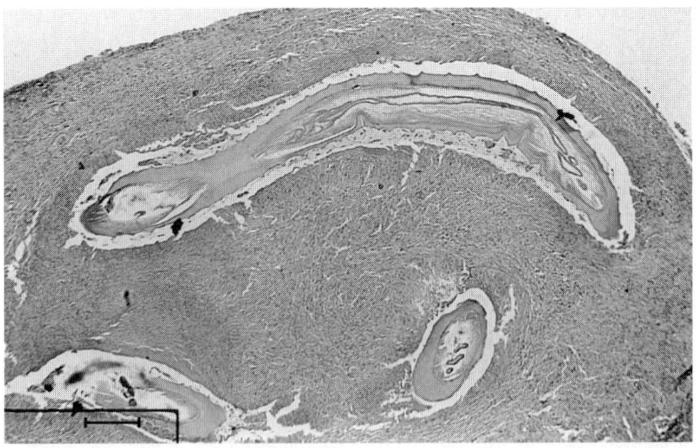

FIGURE 101-20 Low-power view of connective tissue containing three sections of a female *Onchocerca* species from a case of zoonotic human infection. The coiled nature of the worm, the thick cuticle, and ridging on the surface of the cuticle are evident. Scale bar = 200 µm. (H&E stain.) (From Ali-Khan Z: Tissue pathology and comparative microanatomy of *Onchocerca* from a resident of Ontario and other enzootic *Onchocerca* species from Canada and the U.S.A. Ann Trop Med Parasitol 71:470–482, 1977.)

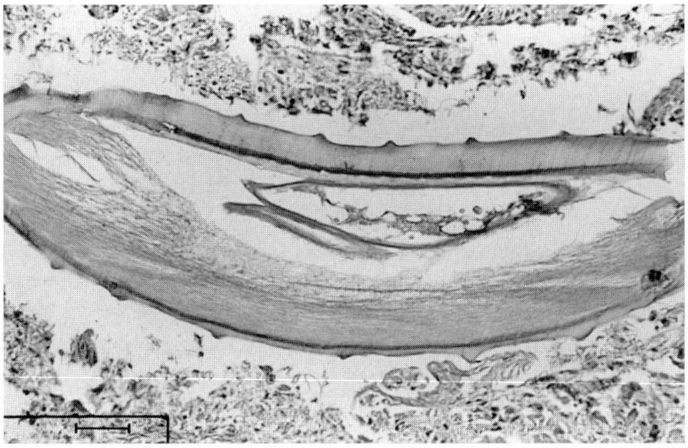

FIGURE 101-21 Higher magnification of the worm seen in Figure 101-20, illustrating the nature of the cuticle, including external ridges, internal striae, and uneven thickness. Scale bar = 50 µm. (H&E stain.) (From Ali-Khan Z: Tissue pathology and comparative microanatomy of *Onchocerca* from a resident of Ontario and other enzootic *Onchocerca* species from Canada and the U.S.A. Ann Trop Med Parasitol 71:470–482, 1977.)

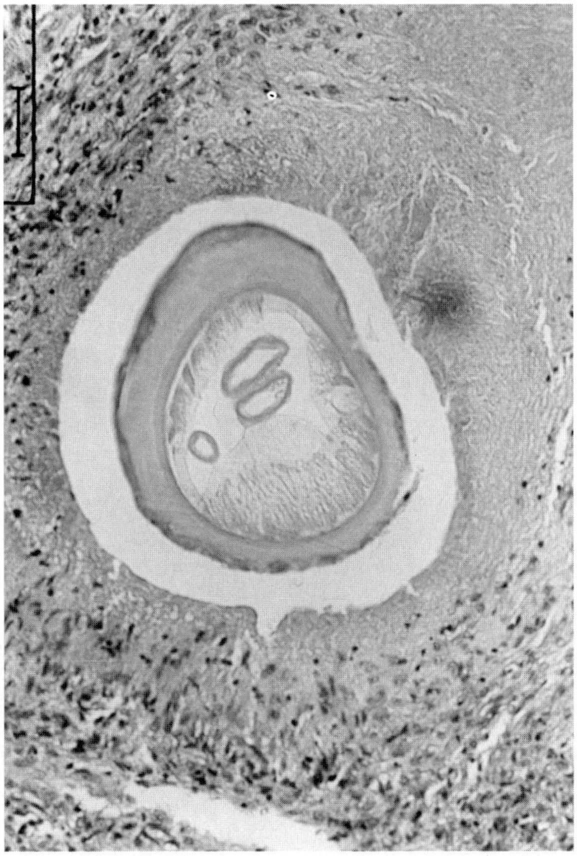

FIGURE 101-22 Higher magnification of a cross section of the female *Onchocerca* species seen in Figure 101–20, illustrating the typical features seen in zoonotic infections. The cuticle is thick throughout, but much thicker over the upper part of the worm as a result of an outer ridge. The muscle cells are few per quadrant and weak in nature; they are appreciably taller in the ventral hemisphere, seen here in the lower half of the worm. The hypodermal tissue is most evident in the region of the lateral chords. Two paired uteri are evident, as is the small intestine, which lies to the left. Scale bar = 50 µm. (H&E stain.) (From Ali-Khan Z: Tissue pathology and comparative microanatomy of *Onchocerca* from a resident of Ontario and other enzootic *Onchocerca* species from Canada and the U.S.A. Ann Trop Med Parasitol 71:470–482, 1977.)

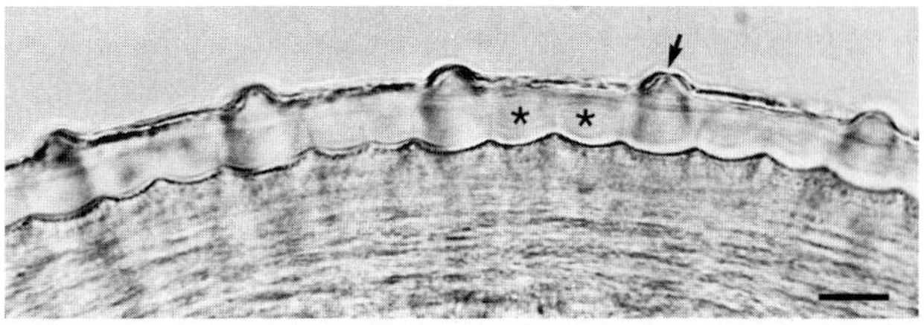

FIGURE 101-23 Unstained, cleared section of body wall of *Onchocerca stilesi*, a natural parasite of the ligaments of the legs of cattle in the United States, illustrating the external ridging (*arrow*) and internal striae (*asterisks*) in the cuticle. Compare the stained section illustrated in Figure 101-24. Scale bar = 15 µm.

lateral chords, and the muscle cells are few in number, flat, and broad, and do not extend far into the body cavity (Fig. 101-19).

Onchocerca

The number of described *Onchocerca* species that might result in zoonotic infections in humans is too great to list here, but the genus is cosmopolitan, and normal animal hosts include a wide range of ungulates, including cattle, horses, camels, various antelope, deer, and sheep. *Onchocerca* species have a predilection for residing in or near connective tissues in their natural hosts, and this has been the case in the majority of zoonotic infections as well. Two cases involving the eye have been reported,[23,26] and there is at least one additional unpublished case of *Onchocerca* being recovered from the eye.

In sections (Figs. 101-20 through 101-24), *Onchocerca* have several prominent features including, in longitudinal section, a cuticle that bears external ridges and internal striae, and in transverse section, a thick cuticle that is often unevenly thickened; prominent hypodermal tissue not restricted to the lateral chords; and few muscle cells per quadrant that are distinctive in appearance, being atrophied and wispy. Because of the extreme length of female worms and their characteristic coiling, it is not unusual to see multiple sections of worm in a single tissue section.

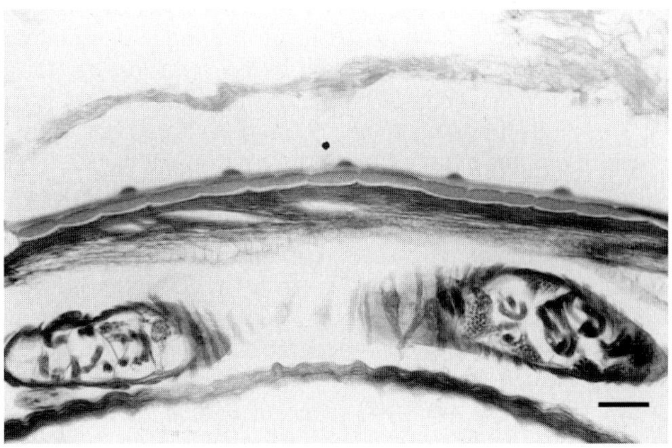

FIGURE 101-24 High-power photomicrograph of a longitudinal section of a female *Onchocerca stilesi*. This trichrome-stained section illustrates the characteristic features of the cuticle useful in identifying zoonotic onchocercal infections. The outer ridges and inner striae illustrated in Figure 101-23 are evident. Sections of uterus with developing microfilariae also are evident. Scale bar = 15 µm.

Dipetalonema-like

Zoonotic filarial infections that do not readily fall into the preceding categories are frequently referred to as *Dipetalonema*-like. Generally, these worms are small and have been reported from several anatomic locations, including the eye and subcutaneous tissue. A number of these cases have resulted in recovery of nearly intact worms from the eye.[55] The morphologic features of *Dipetalonema*-like worms in tissue are nondescript and include small size, the presence of a relatively thin, smooth cuticle, and weak musculature (see Fig. 101-20). Assigning a definitive identification to these specimens has been difficult owing in part to their immature state of development and further complicated by the large number of described species and the recognition that there may be a great number of as yet unrecognized species. This process is confounded by our lack of recognition of distinctive morphologic features of many worms in histologic section.

Interestingly, one report described recovery of microfilariae similar to *Mansonella interstitium* of squirrels from the blood of a 12-year-old child from Alabama, indicating that at least one adult male and female worm were present.[48]

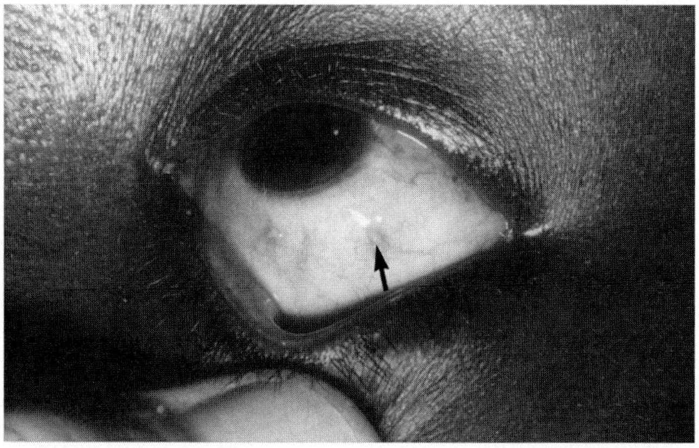

FIGURE 101-25 Photograph showing three small nodules (*arrow*) in the conjunctiva of a Ugandan, typical of those seen in cases of bung-eye. (From Baird JK, Neafie RC, Connor DH, et al: Nodules in the conjunctiva, bung-eye, and bulge-eye in Africa caused by *Mansonella perstans*. Am J Trop Med Hyg 38:553–557, 1988.)

Zoonotic Filariae of Uncertain Origin (or Incompletely Described Zoonotic Infections)

There are numerous other reports of zoonotic filarial infections in humans, some of which represent single case reports, while in others only microfilariae have been recovered with no description of the accompanying adult worm. These are briefly discussed as follows:

In 1932, Owen and Hennessey[95] first noted the occurrence of 33 cases of an unusual presentation of filariae located on the conjunctiva of persons living in Uganda. This account reported the presence of small (approximately 2 mm in diameter), yellow nodules in which were remnants of dead filarial worms. The authors referred to these cases as "bung-eye" or "bulge-eye." In 1973, Poltera[96] reviewed an additional 40 cases and provided further epidemiologic and clinical information, and he concluded that the worms were *Loa*. However, morphology of the worms does not support the diagnosis of loiasis. Baird and colleagues[97] reviewed eight cases of bung-eye (Fig. 101-25) collected from several countries in Africa, and concluded that the majority of cases were caused by aberrant localization of *Mansonella perstans* (Fig. 101-26). This determination suggests that these infections were not zoonotic but rather common human infections in an uncommon location. However, a final decision on the identity of these worms awaits a better understanding of the microanatomy of the genus *Mansonella*, which contains a number of species that infect humans as well as animals. Whether bung-eye is truly a zoonotic infection cannot be established at this time. What is clearer now is that bung-eye is not restricted geographically to Uganda but occurs in a much wider area that, for all practical considerations, appears to overlap with the range of several of the human filariae, including *M. perstans* and *M. streptocerca*.

In 1968, Dukes and colleagues[43] described two cases of microfilariae in the CSF from residents of then Rhodesia (now Zambia and Zimbabwe). The authors attributed the infections to *M. perstans* and provided detailed clinical descriptions. In 1973, Orihel and Esslinger[98] described a new filarial parasite, *Meningonema peruzzii*, from the CNS of African monkeys. The microfilariae of *M. peruzzii*, although sheathed, resemble *Mansonella perstans* microfilariae to a great extent. In that same year, Orihel,[44] who reviewed original material from the previous human cases reported by Dukes and associates was able to demonstrate a sheath on the microfilariae, and concluded that these constituted zoonotic infections due to *M. peruzzii*. Because of the anatomic location of the adult worms in the subarachnoid spaces associated with the meninges, it is highly unlikely that these worms will be encountered routinely in tissue sections. However, clinicians and laboratorians must be alert to the presence of microfilariae in CSF (and possibly blood) and to the morphologic features

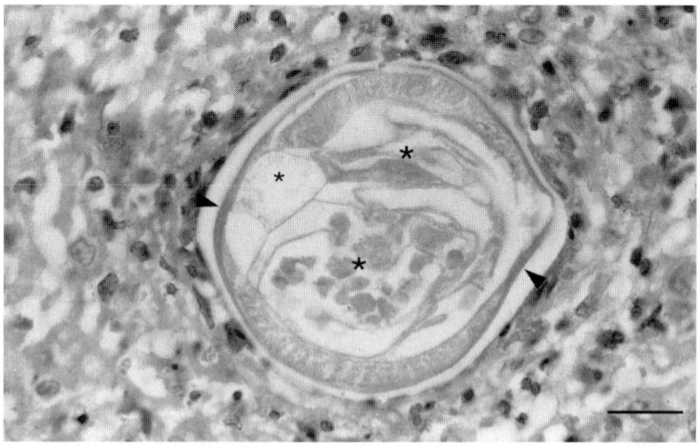

FIGURE 101-26 High-power photomicrograph of a worm, identified as *Mansonella perstans*, seen in sections of a nodule removed from a case of bung-eye in Uganda. The morphologic features of the parasite include a thin cuticle, which is thicker over the lateral chords (*arrowheads*); numerous muscle cells, which are low and do not extend far into the body cavity; paired uteri (*large asterisks*); and a very thin walled intestine (*small asterisk*). Scale bar = 20 µm. (H&E stain.) (From Baird JK, Neafie RC, Connor DH, et al: Nodules in the conjunctiva, bung-eye, and bulge-eye in Africa caused by *Mansonella perstans*. Am J Trop Med Hyg 38:553–557, 1988.)

of the parasite, including the presence of a sheath. A report of this filaria in humans further confirms its zoonotic potential and suggests that additional cases will be uncovered.[99]

An unusual microfilaria with a marked clear region in the posterior body was described by Fain[45] in 1974 from some 52 inhabitants of several villages in Zaire; the microfilaria was named *Dipetalonema semiclarum*.[45] *D. semiclarum* resembles *M. perstans* but differs by having, in addition to the clear space in the posterior half of the body, a much longer cephalic space. The adult stage has not been recovered and described, but the microfilaria does not correspond to any recognized species reported from animals of that region of Africa.

In 1980, an unrecognized microfilaria was reported from the blood of American Indians living in the Orinoco River basin in Venezuela.[46] I was given the name *Microfilaria bolivarensis*. The microfilaria superficially resembles that of *Onchocerca volvulus* but is smaller and stouter and has a shorter cephalic space and less compact nuclear column. Infections were commonly mixed with *Mansonella ozzardi*, which occurs frequently in that area. The microfilaria has not been reported since.

Richard-Lenoble and colleagues[42] reported in 1982 the occurrence of microfilariae indistinguishable from *Mansonella rhodhaini* in 14 inhabitants of Gabon. This is a natural parasite of chimpanzees, and the microfilariae measure more than 300 μm in length by only 2 to 3 μm in diameter, making them clearly distinct from either *Onchocerca volvulus* or *Mansonella streptocerca*.

TREATMENT AND PROGNOSIS

Treatment of zoonotic filarial infections almost always involves surgical removal of the worm or lesion containing the parasite. Frequently, the correct diagnosis is not made until after examination of the specimen or histologic section reveals the identification. However, since the most cases appear to involve only a single worm, surgical removal is curative. Although generally not indicated, a course of diethylcarbamazine or ivermectin would seem to offer the greatest likelihood of symptomatic treatment.

The prognosis in most cases is good. Many worms probably die and are absorbed without any clinical signs or symptoms. In those cases in which a marked tissue reaction draws attention to the presence of a foreign body, the lesion, as noted, is frequently removed surgically. If the host tissue reaction were left to run its course without surgical intervention, the parasite would eventually die and be resolved and the inflammatory lesion would subside over time. This scenario would be true for worms in almost all locations, except worms inside the eye (anterior or posterior chamber, retina). In this location, the physical damage caused by the worm itself, as well as a pronounced inflammatory reaction, could result in serious, permanent damage and loss of visual acuity.

PREVENTION AND CONTROL

Prevention and control of zoonotic filarial infections are difficult tasks, further complicated by the insect intermediate host. The surest way to prevent zoonotic filarial infections is to protect oneself from the bite of potentially infected insect vectors. This is easier stated than accomplished, especially given the wide range of potential vectors. Because the majority of filariae that are known to cause zoonotic infections are transmitted by various mosquito species, the greatest risk is through mosquito bites. Protective clothing, use of insect repellents, household screening, and behavior modification geared toward avoidance of insect bites would provide some degree of protection.

Control of zoonotic filarial infections is even more challenging. Clearly, efforts directed at reducing mosquito or other biting insect populations would significantly reduce the risk of exposure. Because of flight ranges, however, these efforts would need to be coordinated and sustained at the community level or higher. Local government efforts directed at mosquito abatement probably indirectly reduce the overall risk of zoonotic filarial infection. Of the species of filariae that are recognized to cause zoonotic infections, only the dog heartworm, *D. immitis*, occurs exclusively in a domestic pet population (although *D. repens* can be a common infection in dogs as well). Putting a household pet dog on heartworm preventive treatment may well reduce the likelihood of acquiring infection from one's own pet, but unless every dog (and wild canid) in the area is treated, a potential risk still exists. However, until there is better understanding of why some individuals exposed to zoonotic filariae develop infection while most others do not, it will be difficult to develop comprehensive prevention and control strategies.

REFERENCES

1. Addario C: Su un nematode dell'occhio umano. Ann Ottalmol 13:134, 1885.
2. Desportes C: *Filaria conjunctivae* Addario, 1885, parasite accidental de l'homme, est un *Dirofilaria*. Ann Parasitol 17:380, 1939–1940.
3. Orihel TC, Beaver PC: Morphology and relationship of *Dirofilaria tenuis* and *Dirofilaria conjunctivae*. Am J Trop Med Hyg 14:1030, 1965.
4. Beaver PC, Jung RC, Cupp EW: Clinical Parasitology, 9th ed. Philadelphia, Lea & Febiger, 1984.
5. Muro A, Genchi C, Cordero M, et al: Human dirofilariasis in the European Union. Parasitol Today 15:386, 1999.
6. Rodrigues R, Moura H, Dreyer G, et al: Human pulmonary dirofilariasis: A review. Rev Inst Med Trop Sao Paulo 37:523, 1995.
7. Pampiglione S, Rivasi F: Human dirofilariasis due to *Dirofilaria (Nochtiella) repens*: An update of world literature from 1995 to 2000. Parassitologia 42:231, 2000.
8. Faust EC, Thomas EP, Jones J: Discovery of human heartworm infection in New Orleans. Parasitology 27:115, 1941.
9. Asimacopoulos PJ, Katras A, Christie B: Pulmonary dirofilariasis: The largest single-hospital experience. Chest 102:851, 1992.
10. Cooke CT: Nematode in the anterior chamber of the eye. Trans Pacific Coast Otoophthalmol Soc 23:141, 1938.
11. Jones LT, Jordan LW, Sullivan NP: Intraocular nematode worms—report of a case and review of the literature. Arch Ophthalmol 20:1006, 1938.
12. Burns RP, Helzman R, Gerhardt N, et al: Intraocular filariasis (a motion picture). Trans Am Acad Ophthalmol Otolaryngol 70:OP745, 1975.
13. Dissanaike AS, Ramalingam S, Fong A, et al: Filaria in the vitreous of the eye of man in peninsular Malaysia. Am J Trop Med Hyg 26:1143, 1977.
14. Beaver PC, Meyer AE, Jarroll EL, et al: *Dipetalonema* from the eye of a man in Oregon, USA. Am J Trop Med Hyg 29:369, 1980.
15. Beaver PC, Brenes R, Solano GV: Zoonotic filaria in a subcutaneous artery of a child in Costa Rica. Am J Trop Med Hyg 33:583, 1984.
16. Ando K, Beaver PC, Soga T, et al: Zoonotic subcutaneous filaria of undetermined classification. Am J Trop Med Hyg 34:1138, 1985.
17. Azarova NS, Miretskij OY, Sonin MD: The first discovered case of nematode parasitism in the USSR in a human being (genus *Onchocerca* Diesing, 1841) (in Russian). Med Parazitol (Mosk) 34:156, 1965.
18. Siegenthaler R, Gubler R: Paraartikuläres Nematodengranulom (einheimische *Onchocerca*). Schweiz Med Wochenschr 95:1102, 1965.
19. Beaver PC, Horner GS, Bilos JZ: Zoonotic onchocercosis in a resident of Illinois and observations on the identification of *Onchocerca* species. Am J Trop Med Hyg 23:595, 1974.

20. Ali-Khan Z: Tissue pathology and comparative microanatomy of *Onchocerca* from a resident of Ontario and other enzootic *Onchocerca* species from Canada and the USA. Ann Trop Med Parasitol 71:469, 1977.
21. Beaver PC, Yoshimura H, Takayasu S, et al: Zoonotic *Onchocerca* in a Japanese child. Am J Trop Med Hyg 40:298, 1989.
22. Takaoka H, Bain O, Tajimi S, et al: Second case of zoonotic *Onchocerca* infection in a resident of Oita in Japan. Parasite 3:179, 1996.
23. Burr WE, Brown MF, Eberhard ML: Zoonotic *Onchocerca* (Nematoda:Filarioidea) in the cornea of a Colorado resident. Ophthalmology 105:1494, 1998.
24. Pampiglione S, Vakalis N, Lyssimachou A, et al: Subconjunctival zoonotic *Onchocerca* in an Albanian man. Ann Trop Med Parasitol 95:827, 2001.
25. Wright RW, Neafie RC, McLean M, et al: Zoonotic onchocerciasis of the shoulder: a case report. Bone Joint Surg Am 84-A:627, 2002.
26. Sallo F, Eberhard M, Fok E, et al: Zoonotic intravitreal *Onchocerca* in Hungary. Ophthalmology 112:502, 2005.
27. Edeson JFB, Wilson T, Wharton RH, et al: Experimental transmission of *Brugia malayi* and *B. pahangi* to man. Trans R Soc Trop Med Hyg 54:229, 1960.
28. Rosenblatt P, Beaver PC, Orihel TC: A filarial infection apparently acquired in New York City. Am J Trop Med Hyg 11:641, 1962.
29. Beaver PC, Fallon M, Smith GH: Pulmonary nodule caused by a living *Brugia malayi*–like filaria in an artery. Am J Trop Med Hyg 20:661, 1971.
30. Schlesinger JJ, Dubois JG, Beaver PC: *Brugia*-like filarial infection acquired in the United States. Am J Trop Med Hyg 26:204, 1977.
31. Coolidge C, Weller PF, Ramsey PG, et al: Zoonotic *Brugia* filariasis in New England. Ann Intern Med 90:341, 1979.
32. Gutierrez Y, Petras RE: *Brugia* infection in northern Ohio. Am J Trop Med Hyg 31:1128, 1982.
33. Kozek WJ, Reyes MA, Ehrman J, et al: Enzootic *Brugia* infection in a two-year-old Colombian girl. Am J Trop Med Hyg 33:65, 1984.
34. Simmons CF, Winter HS, Berde C, et al: Zoonotic filariasis with lymphedema in an immunodeficient infant. N Engl J Med 310:1243, 1984.
35. Baird JK, Alpert LI, Friedman R, et al: North American brugian filariasis: report of nine infections of humans. Am J Trop Med Hyg 35:1205, 1986.
36. Baird KJ, Neafie RC: South American brugian filariasis: report of a human infection acquired in Peru. Am J Trop Med Hyg 39:185, 1988.
37. Menendez MC, Bouza M: *Brugia* species in a man from western Ethiopia. Am J Trop Med Hyg 39:189, 1988.
38. Orihel TC, Beaver PC: Zoonotic *Brugia* infections in North and South America. Am J Trop Med Hyg 40:638, 1989.
39. Eberhard ML, DeMeester LJ, Martin BW, et al: Zoonotic *Brugia* infection in Western Michigan. Am J Surg Pathol 17:1058, 1993.
40. Elenitoba-Johnson KSJ, Eberhard ML, Dauphinais RM, et al: Zoonotic brugian lymhadenitis: An unusual case with florid monocytic B-cell proliferation. Am J Clin Pathol 105:384, 1996.
41. Dissanaike AS, Bandara CD, Padmini HH, et al: Recovery of a species of *Brugia*, probably *B. ceylonensis*, from the conjunctiva of a patient in Sri Lanka. Ann Trop Med Parasitol 94:83, 2000.
42. Richard-Lenoble D, Kombila M, Bain O: Foyer de filariose humaine au Gabon à microfilaire dermique indifférenciable de *Microfilaria rodhaini*. Ann Parasitol 57:506, 1982.
43. Dukes DC, Gelfand M, Gadd KG, et al: Cerebral filariasis caused by *Acanthocheilonema perstans*. Cent Afr J Med 14:21, 1968.
44. Orihel TC: Cerebral filariasis in Rhodesia—a zoonotic infection? Am J Trop Med Hyg 22:596, 1973.
45. Fain A: *Dipetalonema semiclarum* sp. nov. from the blood of man in the Republic of Zaire (Nematoda:Filarioidea). Ann Soc Belg Med Trop 54:195, 1974.
46. Godoy GA, Orihel TC, Volcan GS: *Microfilaria bolivarensis*: a new species of filaria from man in Venezuela. Am J Trop Med Hyg 29:545, 1980.
47. Petrocheilou V, Theodorakis M, Williams J, et al: Microfilaremia from a *Dirofilaria*-like parasite in Greece: Case report. APMIS 106:315, 1998.
48. Greene BM, Otto GF, Greenough WB III: Circulating non-human microfilaria in a patient with systemic lupus erythematosus. Am J Trop Med Hyg 27:905, 1978.
49. Anderson RC, Bain O: No. 3 Keys to genera of the Order Spirurida.3. Diplotriaenoidea, Aproctidea and Filarioidea. In Anderson RC, Chabaud AG, Willmott S (eds): CIH Keys to the Nematode Parasites of Vertebrates. Farnham Royal, Bucks, England, CAB, 1974, p 59.
50. Pampiglione S, Arlotta MR, Carla TG, et al: Human dirofilariasis in southern Italy. 1. The Puglia region. Pathologica 86:528, 1994.
51. Pampiglione S, Gallippi G, Gianotta G, et al: Human dirofilariasis in southern Italy. 2. The Calabria region. Pathologica 86:533, 1994.
52. Pampiglione S, Canestri Trotti G, De Santolo GP, et al: Human subcutaneous dirofilariasis: 8 new cases in northern Italy. Pathologica 86:396, 1994.
53. Pampiglione S, Villani M, Fioravanti ML, et al: Human dirofilariasis in southern Italy. 3. The Molise region. Pathologica 87:139, 1995.
54. Botero D, Aguledo LM, Uribe FJ, et al: Intraocular filaria, a *Loaina* species, from man in Colombia. Am J Trop Med Hyg 33:578, 1984.
55. Beaver PC: Intraocular filariasis: A brief review. Am J Trop Med Hyg 40:40, 1989.
56. Lau LI, Lee FL, Hsu WM, et al: Human subconjunctival infection of *Macacanema formosana*: The first case of human infection reported worldwide. Arch Ophthalmol 120:643, 2002.
57. Jung RC, Espenan PH: A case of infection in man with *Dirofilaria*. Am J Trop Med Hyg 16:172, 1967.
58. Pacheco G, Schofield HL Jr: *Dirofilaria tenuis* containing microfilariae in man. Am J Trop Med Hyg 14:180, 1968.
59. Pampiglione S, Schmid C, Montaperto C: Human dirofilariasis: Discovery of a gravid female of *Dirofilaria repens* in a subcutaneous nodule. Pathologica 84:77, 1992.
60. Nozais JP, Bain O, Gentilini M: A case of subcutaneous *Dirofilaria (Nochtiella) repens* with microfilaremia originating in Corsica. Bull Soc Pathol Exot 87:183, 1994.
61. Orihel TC, Helentjaris D, Alger J: Subcutaneous dirofilariasis: Single inoculum, multiple worms. Am J Trop Med Hyg 56:452, 1997.
62. Gutierrez Y: Diagnostic Pathology of Parasitic Infections with Clinical Correlations. Philadelphia, Lea & Febiger, 1990.
63. Nelson RP, Thomason WB: Human dirofilariasis of the bladder. J Urol 133:677, 1985.
64. Fini M, Perrone A, Vagliani G, et al: A case of human dirofilariasis (*D. repens*) of the spermatic cord. Minerva Urol Nefrol 44:129, 1992.
65. Pampiglione S, Montevecchi R, Lorenzini P, Puccetti M: *Dirofilaria (Nochtiella) repens* in the spermatic cord: A new human case in Italy. Bull Soc Pathol Exot 90:22, 1997.
66. Pampiglione S, Elek G, Palfi P, et al: Human *Dirofilaria repens* infection in Hungary: A case in the spermatic cord and review of the literature. Acta Vet Hung 47:77, 1999.
67. Theis JH, Gilson A, Simon GE, et al: Case report: Unusual location of *Dirofilaria immitis* in a 28-year old man necessitating orchiectomy. Am J Trop Med Hyg 64:317, 2001.
68. Pampiglioine S, Fioravanti ML, Piccolotti, et al: Human dirofilariasis in Italy: a new case in the spermatic cord. Parassitologia 44:93, 2002.
69. Marty P, Gari-Toussaint M, Le Fichoux Y, et al: Epididymal dirofilariasis mimicking testicular torsion in an adolescent. Presse Med 21:1872, 1992.
70. Kim MK, Kim CH, Yeom BW, et al: The first human case of hepatic dirofilariasis. J Korean Med Sci 17:686, 2002.
71. Tilakaratne WM, Pitakotuwage TN: Intra-oral *Dirofilaria repens* infection: Report of seven cases. J Oral Pathol Med 32:502, 2003.
72. Samples JR, Beaver PC, Fraunfelder FT, et al: A technique for removal of filariasis of the anterior chamber. Ophthalmic Surg Lasers 19:124, 1988.
73. Raymond LA, Gutierrez Y, Strong LE, et al: Living nematode (filaria-like) destroyed with photocoagulation. Ophthalmology 85:944, 1978.
74. Bradham RR, Locklair PR Jr, Grimball A: Bilateral pulmonary nodules caused by *Dirofilaria immitis*. Ann Thorac Surg 50:312, 1990.
75. Cordero M, Muro A, Simon F: Are transient pulmonary solitary nodules a common event in human dirofilariasis? Clin Invest 70:437, 1992.
76. Cordero M, Munoz MR, Muro A, et al: Small calcified nodule: An undescribed radiologic manifestation of human pulmonary dirofilariasis. J Infect Dis 165:398, 1992.
77. Ro JY, Tsakalakis PJ, White VA, et al: Pulmonary dirofilariasis: The great imitator of primary or metastatic lung tumor—a clinicopathologic analysis of seven cases and a review of the literature. Hum Pathol 20:69, 1989.

78. Roussel F, Delaville A, Campos H, et al: Fine needle aspiration of retroperitoneal human dirofilariasis with a pseudotumoral presentation. Acta Cytol 34:533, 1990.
79. MacDougall LT, Magoon CC, Fritsche TR: *Dirofilaria repens* manifesting as a breast nodule: Diagnostic problems and epidemiologic considerations. Am J Clin Pathol 97:625, 1992.
80. Frouge C, Vanel D, Tristant H: Dirofilariasis of the breast mimicking carcinoma on mammography. Am J Roentgenol 159:220, 1992.
81. Saida Y, Miyakawa E, Kon Y, et al: CT of pulmonary dirofilariasis—differential diagnosis from lung cancer. Nippon Acta Radiol 52:1273, 1992.
82. Akaogi E, Ishibashi O, Mitsui K, et al: Pulmonary dirofilariasis cytologically mimicking lung cancer: A case report. Acta Cytol 37:531, 1993.
83. Roussel F, Delaville A, Campos H, et al: Retroperitoneal human dirofilariasis with pseudotumoral presentation (Comments). Acta Cytol 37:980, 1993.
84. Muro A, Cordero M, Ramos A, et al: Seasonal changes in the levels of anti-*Dirofilaria immitis* antibodies in an exposed human population. Trop Med Parasitol 42:371, 1991.
85. Sun S, Sugane K: Immunodiagnosis of human dirofilariasis by enzyme-linked imunosorbent assay using recombinant DNA-derived fusion protein. J Helminthol 66:220, 1992.
86. Espinoza E, Cordero M, Muro A, et al: Anti-*Dirofilaria* immitis IgE: Seroepidemiology and seasonal variation in an exposed human population. Trop Med Parasitol 44:172, 1993.
87. Villanueva EJ, Rodriguez-Perez J: Immunodiagnosis of human dirofilariasis in Puerto Rico. Am J Trop Med Hyg 48:536, 1993.
88. Perera L, Muro A, Cordero M, et al: Evaluation of a 22 kDa *Dirofilaria immitis* antigen for the immunodiagnosis of human pulmonary dirofilariasis. Trop Med Parasitol 45:249, 1994.
89. Santamaria B, Cordero M, Muro A, et al: Evaluation of *Dirofilaria immitis* excretory/secretory products for seroepidemiological studies on human dirofilariosis. Parasite 2:269, 1995.
90. Wilson M, Schantz P, Nutman T, et al: Clinical immunoparasitology. In Rose NR, Hamilton RG, Detrick B (eds): Manual of Clinical Laboratory Immunology, 6th ed. Washington, DC, American Society for Microbiology, 2002.
91. Langer HE, Bialek R, Mielke H, et al: Human dirofilariasis with reactive arthritis—a case report and review of the literature. Klin Wochensch 65:746, 1987.
92. Orihel TC, Eberhard ML: Zoonotic filariasis. Clin Microbiol Rev 11:366, 1998.
93. Gutierrez Y: Diagnostic features of zoonotic filariae in tissue sections. Hum Pathol 15:514, 1984.
94. Orihel TC, Ash LR: Parasites in Human Tissues. Chicago, American Society of Clinical Pathologists, 1995.
95. Owen HB, Hennessey RSF: A note on some ocular manifestations of helminthic origin occurring in natives of Uganda. Trans R Soc Trop Med Hyg 25:267, 1932.
96. Poltera AA: The histopathology of ocular loiasis in Uganda. Trans R Soc Trop Med Hyg 67:819, 1973.
97. Baird JK, Neafie RC, Connor DH: Nodules in the conjunctiva, bung-eye, and bulge-eye in Africa caused by *Mansonella perstans*. Am J Trop Med Hyg 38:553, 1988.
98. Orihel TC, Esslinger JH: *Meningonema peruzzii* gen. et sp. n. (Nematoda:Filarioidea) from the central nervous system of African monkeys. J Parasitol 59:437, 1973.
99. Boussinesq M, Bain O, Chabaud AG, et al: A new zoonosis of the cerebrospinal fluid of man probably caused by *Menningonema peruzzii*, filaria of the central nervous system of Cercopithecidae. Parasite 3:173, 1995.

102

Dracunculiasis

ERNESTO RUIZ-TIBEN
DONALD R. HOPKINS

INTRODUCTION

Guinea worm disease (dracunculiasis), caused by the nematode parasite *Dracunculus medinensis*, is a disabling disease of rural people in parts of 11 countries in Africa.[1,2] Other synonyms for the infection include dracontiasis and dracunculosis. Salient characteristics of this infection are that it manifests by 2-to-3 foot (~1 meter) long worms emerging directly through a lesion on the skin and has an enormous adverse impact on school attendance and agricultural production. It is also close to being completely eradicated.

AGENT

Dracunculus medinensis has been known since at least ancient Egypt. Because differentiation between species of *Dracunculus* requires morphological examination of adult male worms (which are seldom available), efforts are underway to map the genome of the Guinea worm's DNA in order to ascertain this parasite's species more precisely and reliably. Although there are several known zoonotic species of *Dracunculus*, only *medinensis* is specific to humans. The life cycle of the parasite was first fully described by Alexei Fedechenko in 1870.[3]

EPIDEMIOLOGY

During the 19th and 20th centuries, dracunculiasis was common in much of southern Asia, and in North, West, and East Africa. When the Dracunculiasis Eradication Program was getting underway in 1986, an estimated 3.5 million cases still occurred in India, Pakistan, Yemen, and 17 African countries.[4] By 2004, fewer than 16,000 cases were reported in the 11 remaining endemic countries of East and West Africa; Asia was already free of the disease.

People become infected when they drink water containing tiny freshwater crustaceans called copepods or "water fleas," which act as intermediate hosts and harbor infective larvae.[5] When the ingested copepods are killed by the digestive juices in the stomach, the larvae are released and move to the small intestine, where they penetrate the intestinal wall and migrate to the connective tissues of the thorax.[5] Male and female larvae mature and mate 60 to 90 days after infection. Over the next 10 to 14 months, gravid female worms mature, reaching lengths of 70 to 100 centimeters (2–3 feet), and slowly migrate to the surface of the body. On contact with fresh water, powerful contractions cause a loop of the worm's uterus to break and discharge a swarm of motile larvae. Contraction of the worm and discharge of larvae may be repeated if the lesion is again submerged in water, until the entire brood of larvae is discharged. Motile free-swimming larvae are ingested by copepods and mature in the body cavity in about 2 weeks.

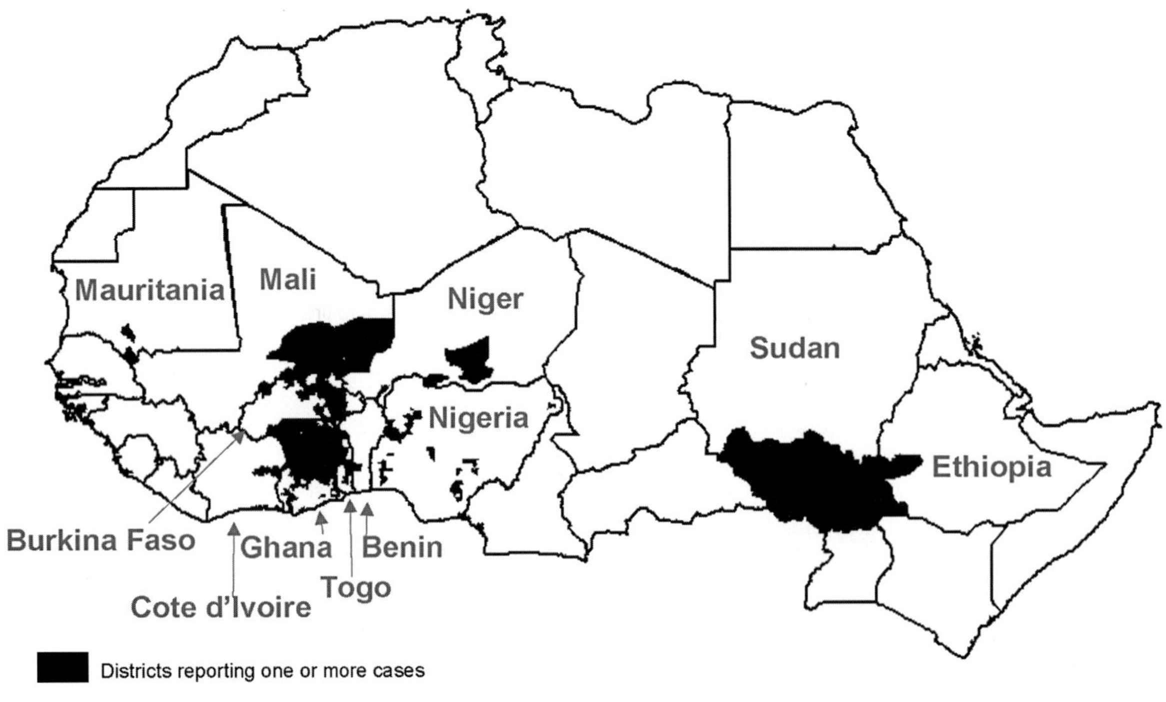

Distribution of cases of dracunculiasis (Guinea worm disease) East and West Africa, January—November 2004 (provisional)

Stagnant sources of drinking water such as ponds, cisterns, pools in dried-up river beds, and shallow unprotected hand-dug wells commonly harbor populations of copepods and are the usual sites where infection is transmitted.

The disease's seasonality varies according to location. In endemic areas just below the Sahara Desert (e.g., Mauritania, Mali, Niger, Burkina Faso, southern Sudan, and Ethiopia), transmission usually peaks during the rainy season at mid-year (May to September). This is because stagnant surface sources of water are only present during the relatively brief rainy season in such areas. In areas near the Gulf of Guinea (e.g., Côte d'Ivoire, Ghana, Togo, Benin, and Nigeria), the disease peaks during the dry season, from October to March, when surface sources of drinking water are scarcest and most concentrated, in contrast to abundant surface water sources during the rest of the year. The seasonal emergence of the worm often coincides with harvest or planting seasons, and thus significantly affects agricultural productivity and school attendance.

DISEASE

Infected persons remain asymptomatic for approximately a year after infection, when the mature female worm approaches the skin and forms a painful papule in the dermis. This papule can become a blister within 24 hours or may enlarge for several days before becoming a blister (Fig. 102-1A). Eventually the blister ruptures, exposing the worm (Fig. 102-1B). Shortly before the skin lesion forms, systemic symptoms may occur, including local erythema and urticarial rash with intense pruritus, nausea, diarrhea, and dizziness. Worms usually emerge from the lower extremities, but they can also emerge from any part of the body, including the head, upper extremities, buttocks, and genitalia. As the worm emerges through the skin lesion, the affected person pulls it out slowly and carefully (because of inflammation and pain), usually by winding a few centimeters of the worm each day on a small stick. This very painful process may last many weeks. Pain and other symptoms may lessen with the rupture of the blister, but at this

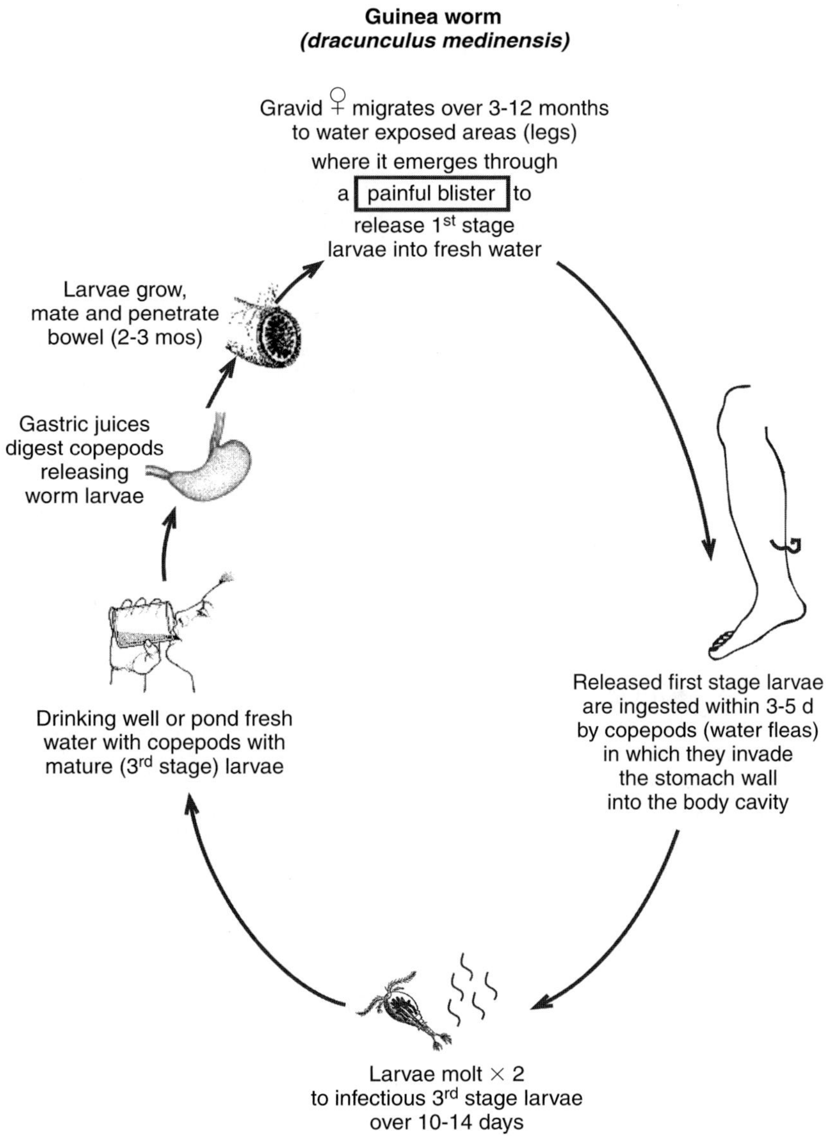

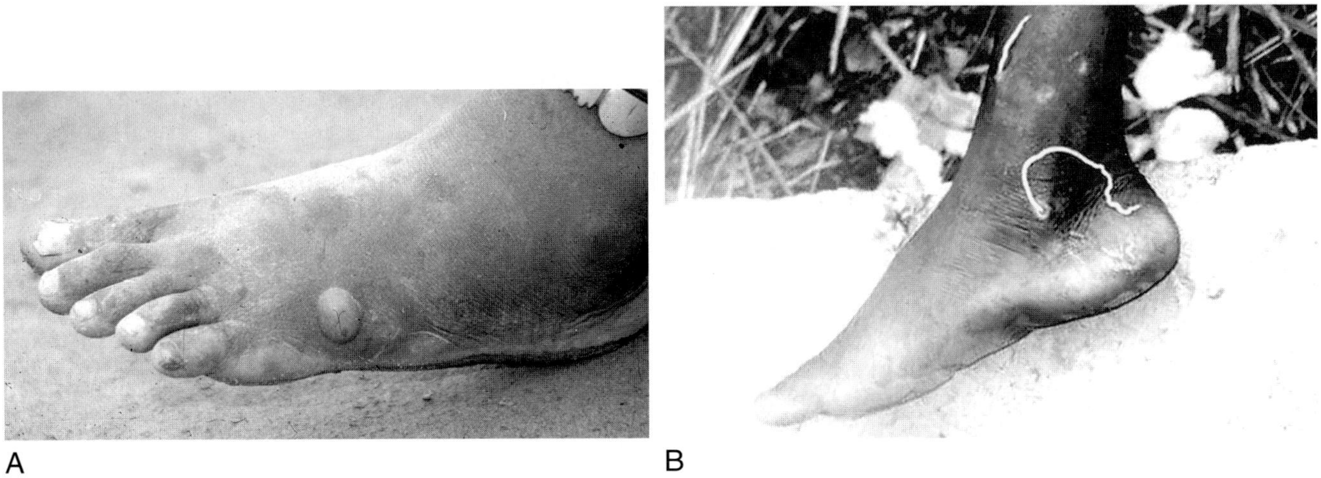

FIGURE 102-1 *A,* Blister caused by emerging nematode parasite *Dracunculus medinensis. B,* After the blister ruptures, the worm is exposed. (*A,* Courtesy of Stephen Fitzgerald; *B,* Courtesy of WHO Collaborating Center for Research, Training, and Eradication at the Centers for Disease Control and Prevention.)

time pyogenic organisms invariably invade the superficial lesion and worm tract and aggravate the condition (Fig. 102-2). If the worm breaks during extraction, an intense inflammatory reaction occurs, with pain, swelling, and cellulitis along the worm tract. The reported period of incapacitation ranges from 2 to 16 weeks (average 8.5 weeks)[6–18] and more than half of a village's population may be affected at the same time. In addition to the blisters and skin lesions, the secondary bacterial infections usually exacerbate local inflammation and often lead to sepsis, abscesses, septic arthritis, contracture of muscles near joints, or even tetanus.

PATHOGENESIS AND IMMUNITY

The symptoms produced by *Dracunculus* vary in the acute or chronic phases of the infection. The acute manifestations begin about 1 year after infection and are related to the release of the larvae into the water. The initial blister in the skin is accompanied by redness and induration and is usually preceded by slight fever and allergic symptoms. The lesion is found in 85% to 90% of cases on the lower extremities, including the ankle, or foot. The blistering lesion produces intense irritation and burning, inducing the patient to seek relief by immersing the affected limb in water, where the blister breaks, allowing the adult worm to discharge larvae into the water. The chronic manifestations are due to inflammation of the joints with clinical symptoms and signs of arthritis,[19] synovitis,[20] and muscle and tendon contractures with resultant ankylosis of the limb.[21] Migration of the worms to the retroperitoneum and from the retroperitoneum to the subcutaneous tissue in the leg sometimes results in aberrant (ectopic) locations of the worm such as in the pancreas,[22] lung,[23] periorbital tissues,[24,25] testis,[26] pericardium,[27] and the spinal cord, producing compression[28,29] as well as focal abscess formation.[30] Infected persons do not develop immunity.

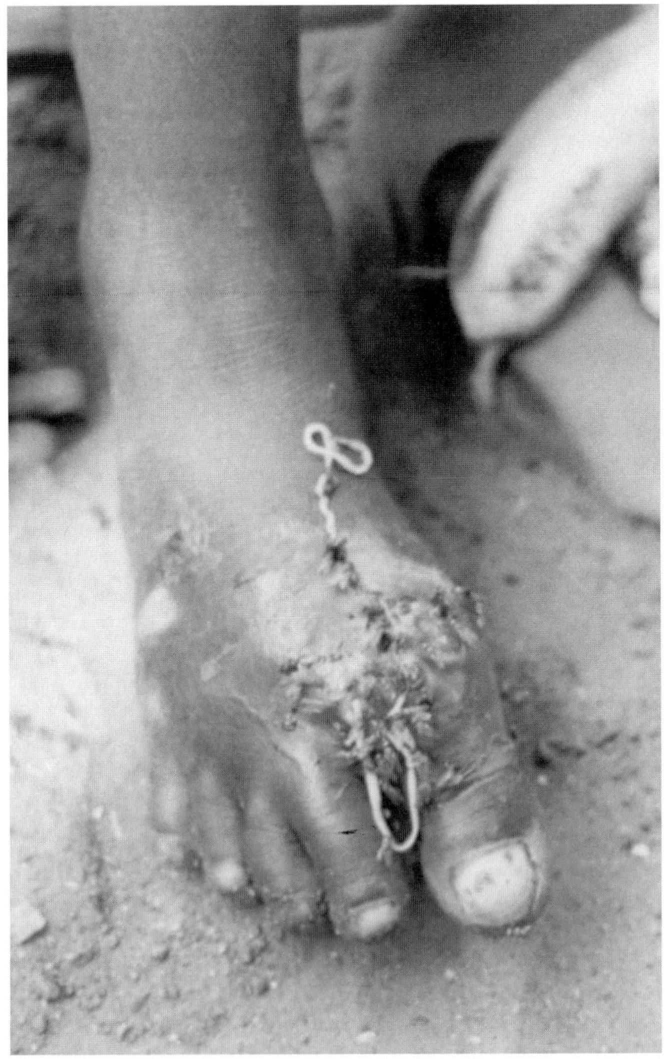

FIGURE 102-2 Pyogenic organisms invade the superficial lesion and worm tract, aggravating the condition. (Courtesy of WHO Collaborating Center for Research, Training, and Eradication at the Centers for Disease Control and Prevention.)

DIAGNOSIS AND TREATMENT

The diagnosis is indicated by the formation of the typical skin blister and emergence of the adult female worm. There is no curative drug or vaccine against dracunculiasis. Applying wet compresses to the lesion may relieve pain during the worm's emergence. Placing an occlusive bandage on the wound keeps it clean and may help prevent the patient from contaminating sources of drinking water. Oral medications to alleviate the associated pain and inflammation, and topical antiseptics or antibiotic ointment to minimize the risk of secondary bacterial infections, also help reduce inflammation and may permit removal of the worm by gentle traction over a number of days.

CONTROL AND ERADICATION

Transmission of dracunculiasis is prevented by educating people about the origin of the disease, teaching them to filter drinking water through cloth to remove the copepods, and to never enter a source of drinking water (or allowing anyone else to do it) when a Guinea worm is emerging. The ideal means of prevention is the provision of safe sources of drinking water. Applications of ABATE larvicide in selected unsafe sources of drinking water to control copepod populations is another means of controlling transmission of the disease.

The global Dracunculiasis Eradication Program (DEP) began in 1981, when the Centers for Disease Control and Prevention (CDC)[31] proposed that eradication of dracunculiasis was an ideal indicator with which to measure the success of the International Drinking Water Supply and Sanitation Decade (1981–1990), since this disease is only transmitted via drinking water. That same year, the steering committee of the Decade adopted dracunculiasis eradication as a sub-goal of their efforts. The African ministers of health passed a resolution in 1988 calling for the eradication of dracunculiasis by 1995, and the World Health Assembly endorsed that mandate in 1991.[32] Since 1988, a growing number of agencies, organizations, companies, and other institutions have assisted national programs with their efforts to eradicate dracunculiasis. India began its own independent national dracunculiasis eradication program in 1983.

The strategy for dracunculiasis eradication includes three phases.[33] During Phase I, national programs conducted nationwide or areawide case searches to determine the locations of villages with endemic transmission and the numbers of cases, organized a national secretariat and a program structure at district and village levels, and developed a national plan of action. In Phase II, program staff and village-based health workers (village volunteers) were trained to implement interventions against transmission of the disease, conduct active village-based surveillance using case registers, provided health education to mobilize communities to action, provided cloth filters, and educated villagers on their care and proper use. During Phase III, when the incidence of disease has been reduced to fewer cases per year and halting transmission is imminent, surveillance is intensified to rapidly detect all persons with emerging worms (preferably before or within 24 hours of worm emergence) and to contain transmission from each case by providing care for the wounds, applying occlusive bandages, and counseling the patient not to enter sources of drinking water. In 2001, most national programs began offering persons with dracunculiasis the option of medical care at "case containment centers." When patients voluntarily attend such case containment centers, they are provided a small monetary or in-kind incentive for agreeing to stay at the center until each Guinea worm is successfully pulled out, medical care, food, sanitation, and shelter. Care of the last cases of dracunculiasis at case containment centers or at established public health clinics permits patients to recover from their incapacitation much faster and allows the program to contain transmission from each emerging worm much more effectively. All other broad-based interventions continue to be employed until transmission is halted.

Attainment of eradication is not certified until the national program requests the World Health Organization (WHO) to validate the claim that no cases have occurred during 3 years since the last indigenous case, and an international certification team confirms that the surveillance system is sensitive and has not detected indigenous cases during the required 3-year period. An International Commission for the Certification of Dracunculiasis Eradication reviews the findings of the certification team and recommends to the WHO whether or not to certify the country free of dracunculiasis.[34]

As of 2004, the total number of reported cases of dracunculiasis had been reduced by more than 99% since 3.5 million cases were estimated in 1986. Nine of the 20 endemic countries have interrupted transmission of dracunculiasis, and 5 of the remaining countries with endemic disease reported less than 100 cases each. The number of villages reporting one or more cases outside of Sudan has dropped from greater than 23,000 to less than 2000. So far, India, Pakistan, Yemen, and Senegal are the only recently endemic countries that have been certified as dracunculiasis-free by WHO, in addition to 164 other countries.

The Sudan Guinea Worm Eradication Program began in 1992–1993 with a village-by-village search for cases in areas accessible to the government of Sudan. Many endemic areas of southern Sudan were inaccessible to the program because of the then 10-year-old civil war. The program accelerated its progress in 1995, including in rebel-held areas, under a 6-month "Guinea Worm Cease-Fire" that was negotiated between the two sides in the war by former U.S. President Jimmy Carter.[35] Sudan reported 50% or more of all cases of the disease each year from 1995 to 2003. Transmission of the disease has been interrupted in the northern states of Sudan; all of Sudan's cases are now in the southern states, where most of the fighting has occurred. A political settlement of the war was signed in January 2005. This will allow the global DEP to complete the eradication of the disease, which should be possible to achieve within about 5 years after the war ends.[36] Sudan is believed to have up to 8000 endemic villages, of which the national program had access to 6400 at the end of 2003.

REFERENCES

1. Progress towards global eradication of dracunculiasis, January-June 2003. MMWR 52:881, 2003.
2. Hopkins D, Ruiz-Tiben E, Diallo N et al: Dracunculiasis eradication: And now Sudan. Am J Trop Med Hyg 67:415, 2002.
3. Fedchenko AP: Concerning the structure and reproduction of the Guinea worm (*Filaria medinensis* L.). Proceedings of the Imperial Society of the Friends of Natural Sciences, Anthropology, and Ethnography, Vol. 8 (in Russian), 1870. Reprinted in Am J Trop Med Hyg 20:511, 1971.
4. Watts SJ: Dracunculiasis in Africa: Its geographical extent, incidence, and at-risk population. Am J Trop Med Hyg 37:121, 1987.
5. Muller R: Dracunculus and dracunculiasis. Adv Parasitol 6:73, 1971.
6. Kale OO: The clinico-epidemiological profile of Guinea worm in the Ibadan District of Nigeria. Am J Trop Med Hyg 26:208, 1977.

7. Belcher DW, Wurapa FK, Ward WB, et al: Guinea worm in southern Ghana: Its epidemiology and impact on agricultural productivity. Am J Trop Med Hyg 24:243, 1975.
8. Nwosu ABC, Ifeluze EO, Anya AO: Endemic dracontiasis in Anambra State of Nigeria. Geographic distribution, clinical features, and socio-economic impact. Ann Trop Med Parasitol 76:187, 1982.
9. Edungbola LD: Babana Parasitic Disease Project II. Prevalence and impact of dracontiasis in Babana District, Kwara State, Nigeria. Trans R Soc Trop Med Hyg 77:310, 1983.
10. Khan HD, Aminuddin M, Shah CH: Epidemiology and socio-economic implications of dracunculiasis in eleven rural communities of District Bannu (Pakistan). J Pakistani Med Assoc 36:233, 1986.
11. Smith GS, Blum D, Huttley SRA: Disability from dracunculiasis: Effect on mobility. Ann Trop Med Parasitol 83:151, 1989.
12. Sueleiman MM, Abdullahi K: Guinea worm infection in Kiri-Manai village, Sokoto. Nigerian J Parasitol 9–11:13, 1989–1990.
13. Watts SJ: Guinea worm: An in-depth study of what happens to mothers, families, and communities. Soc Sci Med 29:1043, 1989.
14. Adeyeba OA, Kale OO: Epidemiology of dracunculiasis and its socio-economic impact in a village in south-west Nigeria. West Afr J Med 10:208, 1991.
15. Ilegbodu VA, Ilegbodu AE, Wise RA, et al: Clinical manifestations, disability, and use of folk medicine in dracunculiasis in Nigeria. J Trop Med Hyg 94:35, 1991.
16. Chippaux JP, Benzou A, Agbede K: Social and economic impact of dracunculiasis: A longitudinal study carried out in two villages in Benin. Bull World Health Org 70:73, 1992.
17. Rhode JE, Sharma BL, Patto H, et al: Surgical extraction of Guinea worm: Disability reduction and contribution to disease control. Am J Trop Med Hyg 48:71, 1993.
18. Adeyeba OA: Secondary infections in dracunculiasis: Bacteria and morbidity. Int J Zoonoses 12:147, 1985.
19. Robineau M, Sereni D: Arthrite aiguë du genou avec presence intra-articulaire de microfilaires de D. medinensis. Évolutions clinique et immunologique compares. A propos d'un cas. Bull Soc Pathol Exot 71:85, 1978.
20. Sivaramappa M, Reddy CR, Devi CS, et al: Acute Guinea-worm synovitis of the knee joint. J Bone Joint Surg Am 41:1324, 1969.
21. el Garf A: Parasitic rheumatism: Rheumatic manifestations associated with calcified Guinea worm. J Rheumtol 12:976, 1985.
22. Sastry SC, Jaya KK: Dracunculus of pancreas: A case report. Indian J Pathol Microbiol 21:81, 1978.
23. Gentilini M, Carme B, Smith M, et al: A case of eosinophilic pleurisy due to *Dracunculus medinensis* infection. Trans R Soc Trop Med Hyg 72:540, 1978.
24. Verma AK: Ocular dracunculosis. J Indian Med Assoc 47:188, 1966.
25. Burnier M Jr, Hidayat AA, Neafie RC: Dracunculiasis of the orbit and eyelid. Light and electron microscopic observations of two cases. Ophthalmology 98:919, 1991.
26. Pendse AK, Sharma AK, Mewara PC: Dracunculus orchitis: A case report. J Trop Med Hyg 90:153, 1987.
27. Kinare SG, Parulkar GB, Sen PK: Constrictive pericarditis resulting from dracunculosis. BMJ 1:845, 1962.
28. Odaibo SK, Agowun IA, Oshagbemi K: Paraplegia complicating dracontiasis. J R Coll Surg 31:376, 1986.
29. Mathur PPS, Dharker SR, Hiram S, et al: Lumbar extradural compression by Guinea worm infestation. Surg Neurol 17:127, 1981.
30. Donaldson JR, Angelo TA: Quadriplegia due to Guinea-worm abcess. J Bone Joint Surg Br 197:198, 1961.
31. Hopkins DR, Foege WH: Guinea worm disease. Science 212:495, 1981.
32. Dracunculiasis: Global surveillance summary, 1991. World Health Org Wkly Epidemiol Rec 67:121, 1992.
33. Hopkins DR, Ruiz-Tiben E: Strategies for dracunculiasis eradication. Bull World Health Org 69:533, 1991.
34. International Commission for the Certification of Dracunculiasis Eradication. Third Meeting, Report and Recommendations. Geneva, WHO, 1998.
35. Implementation of health initiatives during a cease-fire—Sudan, 1995. MMWR 44:433, 1995.
36. Hopkins DR, Withers PC: Sudan's war and eradication of dracunculiasis. Lancet 360(Suppl):S21, 2002.

103

Toxocariasis and Larva Migrans Syndromes

THOMAS A. MOORE
JAMES S. McCARTHY

INTRODUCTION

Toxocariasis is the clinical term used to describe human infection with either the dog ascarid *Toxocara canis* or the feline ascarid *Toxocara cati*. As with other helminthic zoonoses, the infective larvae of these *Toxocara* species cannot mature into adults in the human host. Instead, the worms wander through tissues and organs in a vain attempt to find that which they need to mature into adults. The migration of these immature nematode larvae causes local and systemic inflammation, resulting in the "larva migrans" syndromes. Although human toxocariasis has been studied more intensively in Western countries, the disease has a global distribution, occurring in areas wherever dogs coexist with humans.

The clinical manifestations of toxocariasis (Table 103-1) are divided into visceral larva migrans (VLM) and ocular larva migrans (OLM). Subclinical infection is often referred to as covert toxocariasis. Cutaneous larva migrans, on the other hand, is most often caused by hookworms of domestic animals and is a widespread and well-recognized dermatologic problem in the tropics.

This chapter covers toxocariasis (including visceral and ocular larva migrans) and cutaneous larva migrans. Other helminthic zoonoses that cause similar larva migrans syndromes (e.g., gnathostomiasis, angiostrongyliasis, and anisakiasis) are discussed elsewhere (see Chapters 105 and 106).

AGENTS

Toxocara species are nematodes, taxonomically included within the order and family Ascaridida. The morphology of the adult worms resembles that of *Ascaris lumbricoides*, only they are much smaller: the males measure 4 to 6 cm long, females 6.5 to 10.0 cm long. The brown-colored eggs are almost spherical, with superficial pits, and are larger than *A. lumbricoides*, measuring 85 μm × 75 μm.

In the dog, the life cycle of *T. canis* is similar to that of *A. lumbricoides* in humans, but with two important differences: The parasite can undergo developmental arrest within the definitive host, and vertical transmission occurs from infected pregnant bitches to their pups.[1]

Gravid adult female worms, which are generally found only in young puppies and lactating bitches, excrete up to 200,000 eggs per day in the feces of an infected dog. Freshly passed eggs are unembryonated and develop into infective, embryonated eggs over several weeks at optimum temperature (10°C to 35°C). Lower temperatures delay embryonation. Like other ascarid eggs, *Toxocara* eggs are hardy and relatively resistant to freezing, moisture, and extremes of pH[2] and retain their infectivity for months.[3] Unembryonated eggs shed in the winter can lie dormant until temperatures rise in the spring.

On the ground, the infective first-stage larvae within these unembryonated eggs molt twice to become third-stage juveniles. However, they do not shed their second-stage cuticle until after ingestion. Infection begins when these now-embryonated eggs are ingested. The eggs hatch in the duodenum; the larvae penetrate the intestinal wall and eventually reach the liver where they increase in size but do not molt. From the liver, the larvae travel to the heart and then to the lungs, where they molt into the fourth stage. In young dogs (under 6 months), the larvae travel from the lungs into the trachea where they are swallowed. The larvae undergo an additional molt in the stomach before maturing into adults in the intestine. Mating then results in release of unembryonated eggs, making the infection patent 60 to 90 days after egg ingestion. In older dogs (6 or more months), most infective juveniles do not go from lungs to the trachea but are transported from the lungs

Table 103-1 Clinical Syndromes of Human Toxocariasis

Syndrome	Clinical Findings	Average Age	Infectious Dose	Incubation Period	Laboratory Findings	Toxocara Antibody Titer (ELISA)
Visceral larva migrans	Fever, hepatomegaly, asthma	5 yr	Moderate to high	Weeks to months	Eosinophilia, leukocytosis, elevated IgE	High
Ocular larva migrans	Visual disturbances, endophthalmitis, retinal granuloma	12 yr	Low	Months to years	Usually none	Low
Covert toxocariasis	Abdominal pain, gastrointestinal symptoms, weakness, pruritus	School age to adult	Low to moderate	Weeks to years	Eosinophilia and/or elevated IgE may be present	Low to moderate

Adapted from Glickman LT, Schantz PM: Epidemiology and pathogenesis of zoonotic toxocariasis. Epidemiol Rev 3:230–250, 1981.

to somatic tissues hematogenously. In adult dogs, none of the juveniles return to the intestine, but go to somatic tissues and remain in a state of arrested development for as long as 6 months. This migration to somatic tissue creates the conditions for transplacental and transmammary transmission to pups; latent somatic larvae are reactivated during each pregnancy and migrate either across the placenta to the fetal liver after the 45th day of gestation or to the mammary gland.[4] Larvae acquired in utero by the puppies remain as third-stage juveniles until birth, when they mature in the intestine of the pups. Puppies born with a patent infection shed large numbers of eggs from birth. In contrast, adult dogs excrete few eggs. Dogs born without infection can acquire the infection later by ingesting eggs from the soil or by ingesting embryonated eggs carried by transport hosts such as earthworms, ants, and other soil-dwelling invertebrates.

A wide variety of animals, including humans, can become infected with *T. canis* by ingesting embryonated eggs from contaminated soil, hands, or fomites. In these paratenic, or transport, hosts, the larvae follow a similar sequence of events as in an older, nonpregnant dog. The larvae do not develop to maturity, but migrate for months throughout host tissues before lodging within host tissues in a state of arrested development. The larvae do not encyst but remain exposed to the host environment, absorbing nutrients across the nematode cuticle. The larvae can survive in tissue for several years despite vigorous host immunologic responses to parasite antigens.[5]

Humans are paratenic hosts for *T. canis*. Paratenic hosts are transport hosts in which the larvae never develop into adult worms. The infection is acquired by ingesting *T. canis* embryonated eggs. Sources of these eggs are areas where dogs defecate, such as public parks.[6] Infections acquired by ingestion of raw snails and raw lamb have also been reported.

The cat roundworm, *T. cati*, has a life cycle similar to that of *T. canis* except that vertical transmission is due to lactation more than transplacental transmission. One report documents four cases of adult *T. cati* intestinal infection in children,[7] but in most cases humans are paratenic hosts. *T. cati* causes fewer cases of human infection than *T. canis*, probably because of the defecation patterns of cats, which make environmental infestation less frequent. Although other zoonotic nematodes may be responsible for some cases of visceral larva migrans, *Toxocara leonina*, another ascarid parasite of dogs and cats, has not been associated with human disease.

EPIDEMIOLOGY

The ascarids *T. canis* and *T. cati* are ubiquitous parasites of dogs and cats, respectively, and occur in both temperate and warm climates. These parasites appear to have caused disease for millennia.[8] *T. canis* infection of dogs has been reported worldwide, and canine infection rates vary widely. Not surprisingly, environmental contamination of public grounds with *T. canis* eggs is also widespread.[9–17] Infected rodents may constitute a significant reservoir of *Toxocara* larvae.[18]

Toxocariasis in man is presumed to be contracted through the ingestion of eggs from contaminated soil; children with geophagia (pica) and contact with a litter of puppies appear to be particularly vulnerable.[19] Recent data suggest that dogs infected with *T. canis* may infect people by direct contact.[20] Additional risk factors include mental retardation requiring institutionalization[21] and ingestion of infected meat[22] and raw liver from lamb[23] or chicken.[24]

Because toxocariasis does not become patent in humans, estimates of prevalence in humans depend on immunosurveys. These seroepidemiologic studies show wide differences depending on the population tested. The seroprevalence of toxocariasis in children aged 1 to 11 years in the United States, as measured by enzyme-linked immunosorbent assay, varies from approximately 4% to 8%,[25] with higher rates in Puerto Rico and the southeastern United States.[26] Even higher infection rates of 16% to 30% have been reported among socioeconomically disadvantaged African-American[25] and Hispanic[27] children. Similar rates have been reported in Europe.[28,29] The prevalence of human toxocariasis in the tropics is not well known, but is assumed to be significant since canine infection with *T. canis* is commonly found in these areas[30,31] and veterinary care is rare. Substantial rates of toxocariasis have been found among rural and jungle populations in tropical South America,[32,33] the Caribbean,[34] Southeast Asia,[35] and India.[36]

DISEASE

Visceral Larva Migrans

In 1952, Beaver and colleagues reported a series of children who presented with high circulating eosinophilia and suffered from severe, long-term, multisystem disease.[37] Examination of biopsy tissue revealed the causative agents as larvae of either *T. canis* or *T. cati*.

As classically described, the syndrome of VLM is characterized by eosinophilia, fever, and hepatomegaly.[38] It is most commonly seen in toddlers with a history of pica and an association with puppies. However, the spectrum of VLM also includes cough, wheezing, bronchopneumonia, and anemia. Although almost any organ can be affected, the liver is the most frequently involved, and hepatomegaly is a common finding. Occasionally the lesions may be mistaken for neoplastic metastases.[39] A minority of patients can develop splenomegaly or lymphadenopathy. Urticaria and subcutaneous nodules have been reported. Wheezing is a common presentation of VLM,[40] and severe asthma and hypereosinophilia can develop in intense infections.[41] Pulmonary infiltrates occur on chest radiographs, and toxocariasis can produce acute or chronic eosinophilic pneumonia,[42,43] occasionally progressing to respiratory failure.[44] Monoarthritis, panniculitis, and other rheumatologic manifestations can develop.[45]

Albeit rare, direct invasion of the central nervous system by *T. canis* larvae can occur, resulting in a variety of neurologic disorders including eosinophilic meningitis,[46] meningoencephalitis,[47,48] seizures,[49] static encephalopathy,[50] arachnoiditis,[51] solitary brain lesions,[52] and myelitis.[53,54] Cardiac involvement with *T. canis* rarely occurs, but can be serious.[55,56]

Ocular Larva Migrans

Nematode endophthalmitis was first recognized in 1950 in a series of eyes enucleated for presumed neuroblastoma.[57] Ocular involvement with *T. canis* larvae results in the clinically distinct syndrome OLM. Patients with OLM tend to be older

Visceral larva migrans
*(Toxocara canis)**

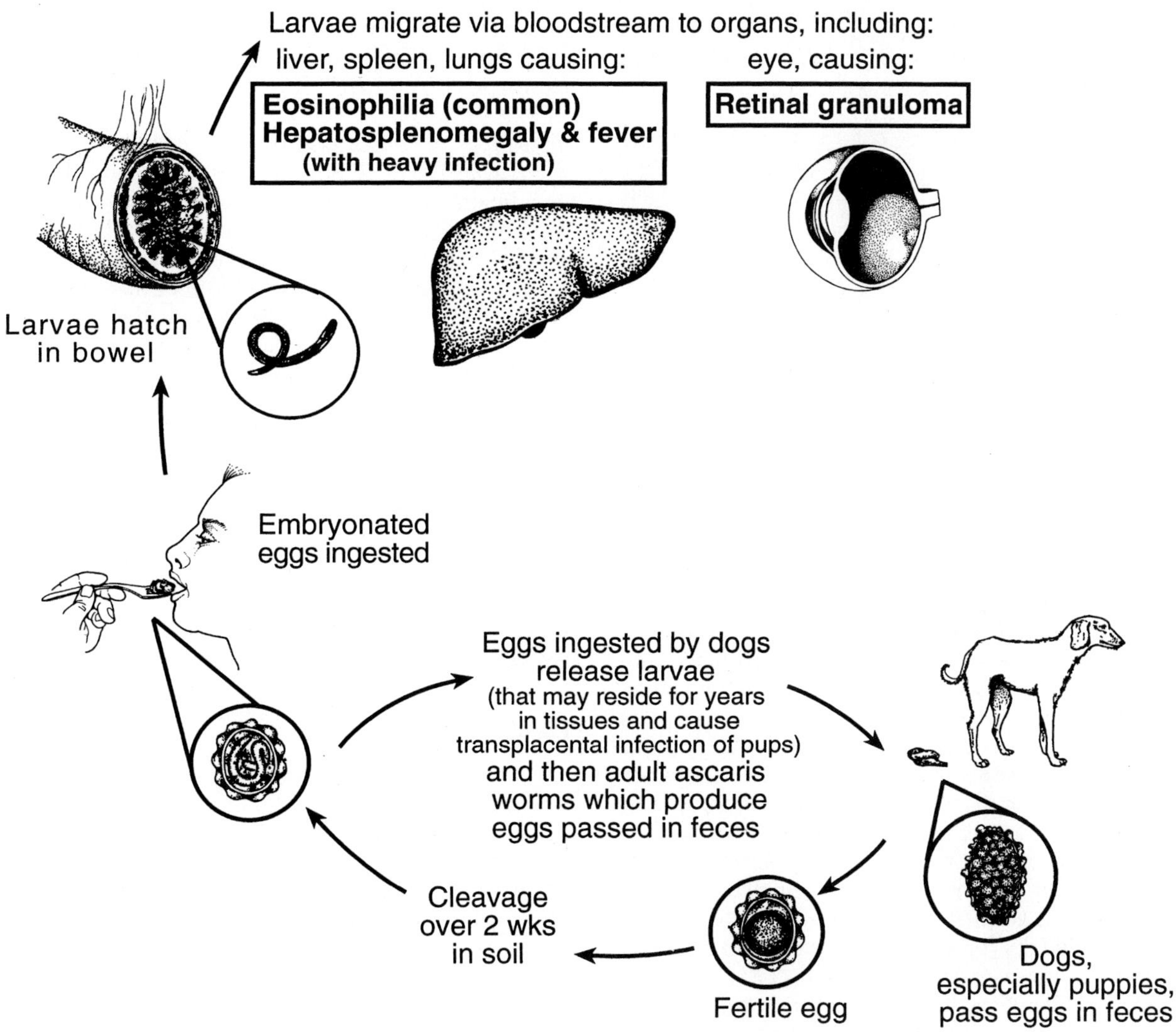

* Although VLM is characteristic for *T. canis*, it may occur with *T. cati* from cats and the general term “larva migrans” has referred to other non-human nematodes infecting humans, such as, *Baylisascaris procyonis*, a raccoon ascarid whose larvae migrate to brain and cause eosinophilic meningoencephalitis in young children.

children without evidence of other organ involvement, suggesting an alternative pathogenesis.[5] *T. canis* larvae that migrate to the eye become trapped, resulting in an eosinophilic inflammatory mass. The syndrome takes several weeks to become clinically apparent, but the patients are typically older children that present with unilateral visual deficits, ocular pain, leukocoria, or strabismus.[58] The retinal lesion most commonly presents as a solid tumor often at or near the macula. In the early stages, it is raised above the level of the retina and closely mimics a retinoblastoma (Fig. 103-1). After the acute phase has subsided, the lesion remains a well-defined circumscribed area of retinal degeneration. Strabismus due to macular damage is often the presenting symptom. Low-grade iridocyclitis with posterior synechiae may develop and progress to endophthalmitis and retinal detachment.[59] Posterior and peripheral retinochoroiditis as well as optic papillitis have also been reported.[60] The inflammatory response created by ocular involvement may result in epiretinal membrane

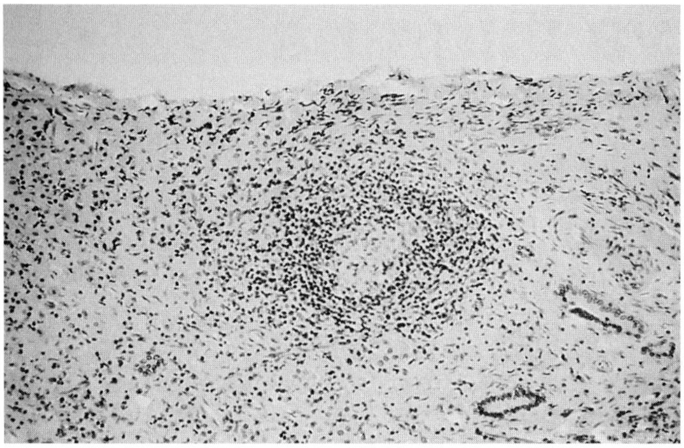

FIGURE 103-1 Granulomatous lesion of the liver due to visceral larva migrans.

formation and traction retinal detachment. In contrast to VLM, hypereosinophilia, hepatomegaly, and pulmonary symptoms are typically absent in OLM.

Covert Toxocariasis

Patients with serologic evidence of toxocariasis who have mild or no symptoms of infection fall into the category "covert" or "occult" toxocariasis. The development and commercial availability of serologic tests for toxocariasis has facilitated the identification of these individuals.[27] To minimize confusion, a new category has been recently proposed for patients with asymptomatic infection.[61] Children with hepatomegaly, cough, sleep disturbance, abdominal pain, and headache are more likely to have elevated toxocaral antibody titers.[62] Eosinophilia was identified in only a slight majority of the cases and, when present, was mild. Recurrent abdominal pain is often the sole presenting complaint.[63] Less common findings include anorexia, fever, and cervical adenitis. Covert toxocariasis occurs in adults as well, as noted in an endemic focus in the French Pyrenees: Patients demonstrated nonspecific manifestations of weakness, pruritus, rash, difficulty breathing, and abdominal pain.[64] An apparently robust association exists between *Toxocara* seropositivity and allergic asthma and recurrent bronchitis,[65] although this correlation has not been verified in other settings.[66] The impact of VLM on behavior and learning disorders is unknown but a link has been suggested in murine models[67] and evidence points to a correlation.[19]

The prevalence of *Toxocara* seropositivity suggests that most human infections are asymptomatic. Indeed, most children with mild eosinophilia and antibodies to *T. canis* do not appear to develop clinically apparent sequelae when evaluated for up to 7 years.[68]

PATHOGENESIS AND IMMUNOLOGY

The mucinous surface coat of *T. canis* larvae is a dynamic structure that turns over quite rapidly and generates large quantities of glycosylated excretory-secretory proteins.[69,70] Many of these proteins constitute a family of highly antigenic mucins[71] that, like most other tissue helminth antigens, induce a Th2-type CD4+ cellular immune response characterized by the production of interleukin (IL)-4 that promotes eosinophilia and the production of immunoglobulin E (IgE).[72] However, the recruited eosinophils adhere to a membranous layer that is frequently detached from the larval epicuticle, allowing the larvae to largely evade the immune response elicited by these antigens.[73] In murine models of infection, the dominant cytokine produced is IL-5,[74] which plays a major role in the induction of eosinophilia; however, overproduction of IL-5 in transgenic mice does not significantly inhibit the life cycle of *T. canis* larvae, suggesting an alternative method by which the parasites are cleared.[75] Investigation into other molecular aspects of the parasite promise further insight into the pathophysiology of toxocariasis.[76]

T. canis larvae elicit both a humoral and cellular response in humans. Tissue damage is due to the host inflammatory reaction more than the infection itself. In both experimental and natural infections, *Toxocara* larval antigens induce granulomatous inflammation with eosinophils, histiocytes, and fibrous tissue (Fig. 103-2). Although the granulomas commonly develop where the larvae have come to rest, they do not always contain the larvae themselves. The granulomas are found most often in the liver, but they may be found in any tissue, including the lungs, brain, and eyes. These eosinophil-mediated granulomatous responses are almost exclusively responsible for the clinical manifestations of toxocariasis; however, it is not clear what factors are responsible for the development of OLM, VLM, or covert toxocariasis. It has been proposed[5] that parasite load is the key determinant of disease severity. Specifically, ingestion of lower doses of infective eggs is more likely to result in OLM or asymptomatic infection, whereas VLM is associated with a larger inoculum.

DIAGNOSIS

Like most parasitic diseases, the diagnosis of toxocariasis is made initially on clinical grounds, with confirmatory testing playing a secondary role. The diagnosis should be entertained when a child is found to have eosinophilia (absolute eosinophil count greater than 450 eosinophils/mm^3) and leukocytosis, especially when accompanied by hepatomegaly, fever, or wheezing. Exposure to dogs, particularly puppies, is an additional clue to the diagnosis. In the absence of hepatomegaly,

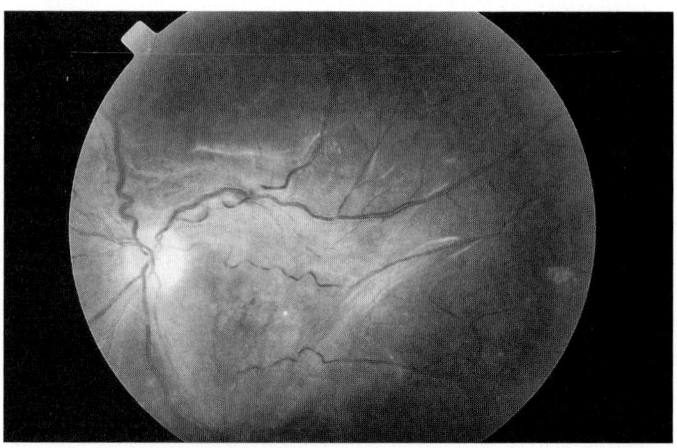

FIGURE 103-2 Retinal lesion of ocular larva migrans.

the symptoms and signs of VLM mimic tropical pulmonary eosinophilia, as well as the larva migrans syndromes seen with ascariasis, hookworm infection, and strongyloidiasis (see Chapters 109–111).

Other laboratory findings include hypergammaglobulinemia and elevated isohemagglutinin titers to A and B blood group antigens. The latter develop as a result of cross-reaction to parasite antigens. Radiographic imaging of involved organs using ultrasound, computed tomography (CT), or magnetic resonance imaging (MRI) can identify focal lesions. If biopsied, these lesions will show granulomatous inflammation; however, larvae are not always found within the granulomas. Biopsy is not recommended to establish the histopathologic diagnosis of toxocariasis.

The diagnosis is most often established by confirmatory serologic testing using an enzyme-linked immunosorbent assay (ELISA). Excretory-secretory (E-S) proteins from second-stage *T. canis* larvae maintained in vitro form the substrate for the ELISA.[77] The sensitivity has been estimated to be approximately 78%, with a specificity of approximately 92% at a cutoff dilution value of 1:32.[78,79] Limited data indicate no significant cross-reactivity in individuals infected with common helminth infections.[34,80] An ELISA based on IgE-subclass antibodies appears to be comparably sensitive for detection and post-treatment follow-up of human toxocariasis.[81] A Western blot using toxocaral E-S antigens is more specific,[82] but is more labor-intensive. More recently, an immunoblot assay has been developed using a recombinant E-S antigen.[83] Unfortunately, none of these serologic tests can distinguish between past and current infection. An antigen capture test using a monoclonal antibody to toxocaral excretory-secretory antigen offers the ability to distinguish current infection. Preliminary data indicate the test is more than 50% sensitive; however, there is a false positive rate of 25% in patients with filariasis and schistosomiasis.[84]

The diagnosis of OLM is based on typical clinical findings of a retinal or peripheral granuloma or endophthalmitis, plus an elevated antibody titer to *T. canis* larval antigens. Identification of characteristic CT or ultrasonographic findings can facilitate diagnosis.[85,86] Although the finding of elevated *Toxocara* antibodies helps to establish the diagnosis of OLM, patients can sometimes have low or even negative titers.[87,88] Finding elevated *Toxocara* antibodies in the vitreous and aqueous humor can also facilitate the diagnosis.[89,90] Other nematode infections of the eye (e.g., cysticercosis, onchocerciasis, and diffuse unilateral subacute neuroretinitis) have to be carefully considered in the differential diagnosis.[91]

Covert toxocariasis should be considered in individuals of any age who present with chronic weakness, abdominal pain, or allergic signs accompanied by elevated IgE levels and eosinophilia. Finding antitoxocaral antibodies in serum does not necessarily establish the diagnosis but, in the absence of response to skin or pulmonary allergens, would certainly support it.

TREATMENT AND PROGNOSIS

The majority of patients with toxocariasis do not require treatment, since the disease is usually self-limited; nevertheless, the disease can be fatal in severe cases. Treatment is generally reserved for patients with severe disease, although this remains a controversial point.

Acute VLM in children and adults is usually treated either symptomatically or with specific antihelminthic therapy, depending on the severity of clinical disease. Patients with either mild visceral larva migrans or covert toxocariasis and peripheral eosinophilia are often treated conservatively, since these forms of the disease are usually self-limited. Asymptomatic subjects with eosinophilia and those with covert toxocariasis in the absence of eosinophilia do not normally require any specific therapy.

Generalized treatment recommendations are limited by a paucity of controlled clinical data. Thiabendazole, mebendazole, diethylcarbamazine (DEC), albendazole, and ivermectin have been examined as treatments for VLM. Thiabendazole appears to be ineffective in asymptomatic children with toxocariasis, as measured by serial eosinophil counts and antitoxocaral antibody titers.[68] In patients with clinical illness, thiabendazole (15 mg/kg/day) appeared to be effective; however, a similar course of albendazole resulted in more frequent clinical cure and a measurable decrease in eosinophil counts.[92] A dose of 400 mg of albendazole twice a day for 5 days is the currently recommended therapy.[93] Alternatively, a 21-day course of mebendazole (20–25 mg/kg/d) has also been shown to be effective.[94] For those with severe symptoms treated with either albendazole or mebendazole, corticosteroids are often administered concomitantly (prednisone 0.5–1.0 mg/kg/d). Several small studies have demonstrated that a 21-day course of DEC (~6 mg/kg/d) results in resolution of clinical symptoms and a decline in antitoxocaral antibody titers, although patients experienced a significantly higher rate of adverse reactions.[94] In the United States, DEC is only available through the Centers for Disease Control and Prevention (CDC) Drug Service.

Albendazole has been found to be effective in OLM, but higher doses (adults, 800 mg bid; children, 400 mg bid) have been used in these clinical studies.[95] Albendazole should be administered for 4 weeks, with concomitant glucocorticoids (prednisone 0.5–1.0 mg/kg/d) for 2 to 4 weeks. Despite the promise of medical therapy, surgery is still sometimes required to treat OLM.[96]

PREVENTION AND CONTROL

An association with dogs has been identified as a substantial risk factor for the development of toxocariasis.[20,97] While the prevalence of dog ownership varies throughout the world, most of the world's population shares its environment with *T. canis*–infected dogs. Thus, exposure to canine ascarids is likely to be widespread. In the United States, an estimated 53 million dogs are distributed among 31 million households.[98] This number is not expected to decline for the foreseeable future.[99] While the true incidence of toxocariasis is unknown in the United States, one would assume a significant portion of these animals are infected given the cosmopolitan distribution of the parasite.

While discouraging geophagia in children is a laudable goal, such behavior modification in this age group is essentially unrealistic. Instead, measures that prevent infected dog feces from contaminating the environment are of paramount importance. These measures include keeping dogs on a leash and excluding pet animals from playgrounds and sandboxes where geophagia occurs. Placing a vinyl covering over sandboxes at night has been shown to reduce the viability of *T. canis* eggs.[100]

An education campaign to highlight the risk to humans would be a logical component of any control program.

An effective surveillance and control program would require attention to potentially infected animals. However, pups and kittens are frequently not brought to veterinarians until they are at least 6 weeks old, by which time exposure to environments with extensive contamination with *Toxocara* eggs may have already occurred. Despite this obstacle, the prevalence of canine infection with *T. canis* has declined as a result of animal control measures and the widespread veterinary use of broad-spectrum anthelminthics effective against the adult worms.[101] Using subcutaneous ivermectin,[102] topical selamectin (a macrocyclic lactone similar to ivermectin),[103] or oral fenbendazole[104] at scheduled intervals during pregnancy dramatically reduced the worm burden carried by puppies. As of this writing, there is no available vaccine; however, potential candidates have been identified.[105]

Cutaneous Larva Migrans

Cutaneous larva migrans (CLM), also known as creeping eruption, is a zoonosis caused by animal hookworms, most often that of the dog (*Ancylostoma caninum*) or cat (*Ancylostoma braziliense*).

Infected animals shed eggs in the stool that subsequently hatch, yielding first-stage larvae that mature into infective third-stage larvae in the soil. As with human hookworms, the infection starts when the worm enters the skin from contaminated soil that is protected from desiccation and temperature extremes, such as on beaches and under houses. As in toxocariasis, the worm cannot complete the infective cycle, so it continues to burrow through the subcutaneous tissues, resulting in the characteristic serpiginous, erythematous, elevated, and pruritic skin lesion (Fig. 103-3). The pruritus is sometimes incapacitating. The infection is often seen in travelers who have walked barefoot on beaches frequented by roaming cats and dogs. CLM is the most common dermatologic problem to affect Westerners after travel to tropical countries.[106] Almost one-third of travelers had symptoms for more than 4 weeks before the diagnosis was properly established.[107] In European travelers, the lesions are very few in number and most commonly involve the feet and buttocks. In contrast, a recent study of CLM in an endemic area indicates the clinical presentation is different from that reported in travelers.[108] Lesions were more frequent and spared the feet, most often occurring on the trunk, legs, and arms.

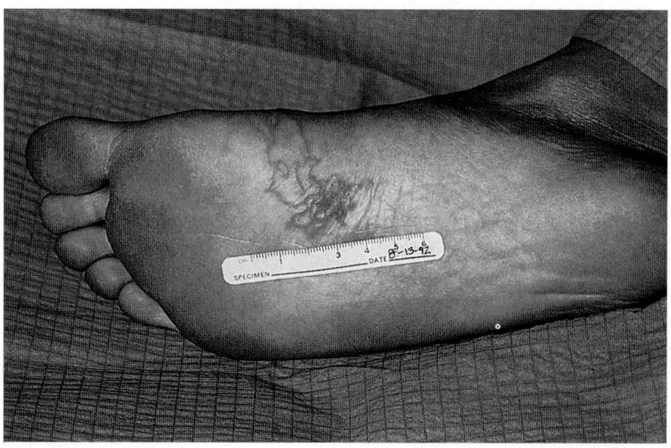

FIGURE 103-3 Typical lesion of cutaneous larva migrans involving the foot.

Systemic symptoms and eosinophilia are rare. The diagnosis is made solely on clinical grounds; skin biopsy is of negligible value. Other diagnoses to be considered include larva currens due to *Strongyloides stercoralis*, jellyfish stings, phytophotodermatitis, and myiasis. As with many other tropical diseases presenting in industrialized nations, physicians' lack of familiarity with this entity results in a significant delay in diagnosis and effective treatment. Even without treatment the lesions resolve spontaneously in 2 to 8 weeks, although longer periods of infection have been occasionally reported,[109] and the patients are often miserable due to pruritus.

Albendazole is well tolerated and quite effective, resolving the infection within 1 week[110]; however, clinical trials have yielded conflicting results with respect to the optimal dosage. It would appear that travelers with CLM should be treated with 400 to 800 mg/d for 3 to 5 days.[111] A single dose of ivermectin (200 µg/kg on an empty stomach) is well tolerated and curative in 77% of patients; 97% were cured with one or two supplemental doses, if necessary.[112] The median time required for pruritus and lesions to disappear was 3 and 7 days, respectively.

Topical cryotherapy is not recommended because it does not work and is potentially harmful to the patient.[111] Topical application of a 10% to 15% thiabendazole solution/ointment to the affected area effects a cure within 10 days in 98% of patients. Thiabendazole is also effective against CLM when given orally, although less so; 89% of patients are cured after 4 weekly doses. The side effects of oral thiabendazole make topical treatment attractive; however, this treatment has limited value for multiple lesions. Topical thiabendazole preparations are not commercially available in the United States.

ACKNOWLEDGMENT

The contributions of Leo X. Liu, MD, to the earlier edition of this chapter are gratefully acknowledged.

REFERENCES

1. Shoop WL: Vertical transmission of helminths: Hypobiosis and amphiparatenesis. Parasitol Today 7:51, 1991.
2. O'Lorcain P: The effects of freezing on the viability of *Toxocara canis* and *T. cati* embryonated eggs. J Helminthol 69:169, 1995.
3. Fan CK, Lin YH, Du WY, et al: Infectivity and pathogenicity of 14-month-cultured embryonated eggs of *Toxocara canis* in mice. Vet Parasitol 113:145, 2003.
4. Burke TM, Roberson EL: Prenatal and lactational transmission of *Toxocara canis* and *Ancylostoma caninum*: Experimental infection of the bitch at mid-pregnancy and at parturition. Int J Parasitol 15:485, 1985.
5. Schantz PM: Toxocara larva migrans now. Am J Trop Med Hyg 41(3 Suppl):21, 1989.
6. Snow KR, Ball SJ, Bewick JA: Prevalence of *Toxocara* species eggs in the soil of five east London parks. Vet Rec 120:66, 1987.
7. Eberhard ML, Alfano E: Adult *Toxocara cati* infections in U.S. children: Report of four cases. Am J Trop Med Hyg 59:404, 1998.
8. Bouchet F, Araujo A, Harter S, et al: *Toxocara canis* (Werner, 1782) eggs in the Pleistocene site of Menez-Dregan, France (300,000–500,000 years before present). Mem Inst Oswaldo Cruz 98(Suppl 1):137, 2003.
9. Ahmad B, Bhatti G, Thokar MA, et al: Human toxocariasis and ascariasis: Concomitant parasitism in Srinagar, Kashmir, India. Indian J Pathol Microbiol 45:315, 2002.

10. Habluetzel A, Traldi G, Ruggieri S, et al: An estimation of *Toxocara canis* prevalence in dogs, environmental egg contamination and risk of human infection in the Marche region of Italy. Vet Parasitol 113:243, 2003.
11. Carden SM, Meusemann R, Walker J, et al: *Toxocara canis*: Egg presence in Melbourne parks and disease incidence in Victoria. Clin Experiment Ophthalmol 31:143, 2003.
12. Anaruma-Filho F, Chieffi PP, Correa CR, et al: Human toxocariasis: A seroepidemiological survey in the municipality of Campinas (SP), Brazil. Rev Inst Med Trop Sao Paulo 44:303, 2002.
13. Shimizu T: Prevalence of *Toxocara* eggs in sandpits in Tokushima city and its outskirts. J Vet Med Sci 55:807, 1993.
14. Richards DT, Harris S, Lewis JW: Epidemiology of *Toxocara canis* in red foxes (*Vulpes vulpes*) from urban areas of Bristol. Parasitology 107:167, 1993.
15. Umeche N: Helminth ova in soil from children's playgrounds in Calabar, Nigeria. Cent Afr J Med 35:432, 1989.
16. O'Lorcain P: Prevalence of *Toxocara canis* ova in public playgrounds in the Dublin area of Ireland. J Helminthol 68:237, 1994.
17. Dada BJ, Lindquist WD: Prevalence of *Toxocara* spp. eggs in some public grounds and highway rest areas in Kansas. J Helminthol 53:145, 1979.
18. Dubinsky P, Havasiova-Reiterova K, Petko B, et al: Role of small mammals in the epidemiology of toxocariasis. Parasitology 110:187, 1995.
19. Marmor M, Glickman L, Shofer F, et al: *Toxocara canis* infection of children: Epidemiologic and neuropsychologic findings. Am J Public Health 77:554, 1987.
20. Wolfe A, Wright IP: Human toxocariasis and direct contact with dogs. Vet Rec 152:419, 2003.
21. Huminer D, Symon K, Groskopf I, et al: Seroepidemiologic study of toxocariasis and strongyloidiasis in institutionalized mentally retarded adults. Am J Trop Med Hyg 46:278, 1992.
22. Sturchler D, Weiss N, Gassner M: Transmission of toxocariasis. J Infect Dis 162:571, 1990.
23. Salem G, Schantz P: Toxocaral visceral larva migrans after ingestion of raw lamb liver. Clin Infect Dis 15:743, 1992.
24. Nagakura K, Tachibana H, Kaneda Y, et al: Toxocariasis possibly caused by ingesting raw chicken. J Infect Dis 160:735, 1989.
25. Herrmann N, Glickman LT, Schantz PM, et al: Seroprevalence of zoonotic toxocariasis in the United States: 1971–1973. Am J Epidemiol 122:890, 1985.
26. Glickman LT, Schantz PM: Epidemiology and pathogenesis of zoonotic toxocariasis. Epidemiol Rev 3:230, 1981.
27. Bass JL, Mehta KA, Glickman LT, et al: Clinically inapparent *Toxocara* infection in children. N Engl J Med 308:723, 1983.
28. Van Gemund JJ, Buijs J, Van Dongen PA, et al: Seroprevalence of *Toxocara* infection in young children in the city of The Hague. Trop Geogr Med 41:294, 1989.
29. Holland CV, O'Lorcain P, Taylor MR, et al: Sero-epidemiology of toxocariasis in school children. Parasitology 110:535, 1995.
30. Wiseman RA, Woodruff AW: Toxocariasis in Africa and Malta. The frequency of infection in host animals and its incidence and distribution in humans as revealed by skin sensitivity tests. Trans R Soc Trop Med Hyg 65:439, 1971.
31. Styles TJ: Incidence of *Toxocara canis* and other helminth parasites of dogs in Mexico City. J Parasitol 53:822, 1967.
32. Lynch NR, Eddy K, Hodgen AN, et al: Seroprevalence of *Toxocara canis* infection in tropical Venezuela. Trans R Soc Trop Med Hyg 82:275, 1988.
33. Agudelo C, Villareal E, Caceres E, et al: Human and dogs *Toxocara canis* infection in a poor neighborhood in Bogotá. Mem Inst Oswaldo Cruz 85:75, 1990.
34. Thompson DE, Bundy DA, Cooper ES, et al: Epidemiological characteristics of *Toxocara canis* zoonotic infection of children in a Caribbean community. Bull World Health Organ 64:283, 1986.
35. Hakim SL, Mak JW, Lam PL, et al: Seroprevalence of *Toxocara canis* antibodies among Orang Asli (aborigines) in Peninsular Malaysia. Southeast Asian J Trop Med Public Health 23:493, 1992.
36. Malla N, Aggarwal AK, Mahajan RC: A serological study of human toxocariasis in north India. Natl Med J India 15:145, 2002.
37. Beaver PC, Snyde CH, Carrera GM: Chronic eosinophilia due to visceral larva migrans. Pediatrics 9:7, 1952.
38. Beaver PC: The nature of visceral larva migrans. J Parasitol 55:3, 1969.
39. Almeida MT, Ribeiro RC, Kauffman WM, et al: Toxocariasis simulating hepatic recurrence in a patient with Wilms' tumor. Med Pediatr Oncol 22:211, 1994.
40. Desowitz RS, Rudoy R, Barnwell JW: Antibodies to canine helminth parasites in asthmatic and nonasthmatic children. Int Arch Allergy Appl Immunol 65:361, 1981.
41. Feldman GJ, Parker HW: Visceral larva migrans associated with the hypereosinophilic syndrome and the onset of severe asthma. Ann Intern Med 116:838, 1992.
42. Roig J, Romeu J, Riera C, et al: Acute eosinophilic pneumonia due to toxocariasis with bronchoalveolar lavage findings. Chest 102:294, 1992.
43. Inoue K, Inoue Y, Arai T, et al: Chronic eosinophilic pneumonia due to visceral larva migrans. Intern Med 41:478, 2002.
44. Bartelink AK, Kortbeek LM, Huidekoper HJ, et al: Acute respiratory failure due to *Toxocara* infection. Lancet 342:1234, 1993.
45. Kraus A, Valencia X, Cabral AR, et al: Visceral larva migrans mimicking rheumatic diseases. J Rheumatol 22:497, 1995.
46. Gould IM, Newell S, Green SH, et al: Toxocariasis and eosinophilic meningitis. Br Med J (Clin Res Ed) 291:1239, 1985.
47. Vidal JE, Sztajnbok J, Seguro AC: Eosinophilic meningoencephalitis due to *Toxocara canis*: Case report and review of the literature. Am J Trop Med Hyg 69:341, 2003.
48. Moreira-Silva SF, Rodrigues MG, Pimenta JL, et al: Toxocariasis of the central nervous system: With report of two cases. Rev Soc Bras Med Trop 37:169, 2004.
49. Bachli H, Minet JC, Gratzl O: Cerebral toxocariasis: A possible cause of epileptic seizure in children. Childs Nerv Syst (May 12, 2004: electronic publication prior to print edition).
50. Fortenberry JD, Kenney RD, Younger J: Visceral larva migrans producing static encephalopathy in an infant. Pediatr Infect Dis J 10:403, 1991.
51. Villano M, Cerillo A, Narciso N, et al: A rare case of *Toxocara canis* arachnoidea. J Neurosurg Sci 36:67, 1992.
52. Xinou E, Lefkopoulos A, Gelagoti M, et al: CT and MR imaging findings in cerebral toxocaral disease. Am J Neuroradiol 24:714, 2003.
53. Goffette S, Jeanjean AP, Duprez TP, et al: Eosinophilic pleocytosis and myelitis related to *Toxocara canis* infection. Eur J Neurol 7:703, 2000.
54. Duprez TP, Bigaignon G, Delgrange E, et al: MRI of cervical cord lesions and their resolution in *Toxocara canis* myelopathy. Neuroradiology 38:792, 1996.
55. Boschetti A, Kasznica J: Visceral larva migrans induced eosinophilic cardiac pseudotumor: A cause of sudden death in a child. J Forensic Sci 40:1097, 1995.
56. De Cock C, Lemaitre J, Deuvaert FE: Loeffler endomyocarditis: A clinical presentation as right ventricular tumor. J Heart Valve Dis 7:668, 1998.
57. Wilder HC: Nematode endophthalmitis. Trans Am Acad Ophthalmol Otolaryngol 51:99, 1950.
58. Zinkham WH: Visceral larva migrans. A review and reassessment indicating two forms of clinical expression: Visceral and ocular. Am J Dis Child 132:627, 1978.
59. Lamparielle DA, Primo SA: Ocular toxocariasis. J Am Optometric Assoc 70:245, 1999.
60. Sabrosa NA, de Souza EC: Nematode infections of the eye: Toxocariasis and diffuse unilateral subacute neuroretinitis. Curr Opin Ophthalmol 12:450, 2001.
61. Pawlowski Z: Toxocariasis in humans: Clinical expression and treatment dilemma. J Helminthol 75:299, 2001.
62. Taylor MR, Keane CT, O'Connor P, et al: Clinical features of covert toxocariasis. Scand J Infect Dis 19:693, 1987.
63. Nathwani D, Laing RB, Currie PF: Covert toxocariasis—A cause of recurrent abdominal pain in childhood. Br J Clin Pract 46:271, 1992.
64. Glickman LT, Magnaval JF, Domanski LM, et al: Visceral larva migrans in French adults: A new disease syndrome? Am J Epidemiol 125:1019, 1987.
65. Buijs J, Borsboom G, Renting M, et al: Relationship between allergic manifestations and *Toxocara* seropositivity: A cross-sectional study among elementary school children. Eur Respir J 10:1467, 1997.
66. Sharghi N, Schantz PM, Caramico L, et al: Environmental exposure to *Toxocara* as a possible risk factor for asthma: A clinic-based case-control study. Clin Infect Dis 32:E111, 2001.
67. Cox DM, Holland CV: Relationship between three intensity levels of *Toxocara canis* larvae in the brain and effects on exploration, anxiety, learning and memory in the murine host. J Helminthol 75:33, 2001.

68. Bass JL, Mehta KA, Glickman LT, et al: Asymptomatic toxocariasis in children. A prospective study and treatment trial. Clin Pediatr (Phila) 26:441, 1987.
69. Kayes SG: Human toxocariasis and the visceral larva migrans syndrome: Correlative immunopathology. Chem Immunol 66:99, 1997.
70. Page AP, Rudin W, Fluri E, et al: *Toxocara canis*: A labile antigenic coat overlying the epicuticle of infective larvae. Exp Parasitol 75:72, 2000.
71. Doedens A, Loukas A, Maizels RM: A cDNA encoding TcMUC-5, a mucin from *Toxocara canis* larvae identified by expression screening. Acta Trop 79:211, 2001.
72. Del Prete GF, De Carli M, Mastromauro C, et al: Purified protein derivative of *Mycobacterium tuberculosis* and excretory-secretory antigen(s) of *Toxocara canis* expand in vitro human T cells with stable and opposite (type 1 T helper or type 2 T helper) profile of cytokine production. J Clin Invest 88:346, 1991.
73. Badley JE, Grieve RB, Rockey JH, et al: Immune-mediated adherence of eosinophils to *Toxocara canis* infective larvae: The role of excretory-secretory antigens. Parasite Immunol 9:133, 1987.
74. Takamoto M, Kusama Y, Takatsu K, et al: Occurrence of interleukin-5 production by CD4- CD8- (double-negative) T cells in lungs of both normal and congenitally athymic nude mice infected with *Toxocara canis*. Immunology 85:285, 1995.
75. Dent LA, Daly C, Geddes A, et al: Immune responses of IL-5 transgenic mice to parasites and aeroallergens. Mem Inst Oswaldo Cruz 92(Suppl 2):45, 1997.
76. Despommier D: Toxocariasis: Clinical aspects, epidemiology, medical ecology, and molecular aspects. Clin Micro Rev 16:265, 2003.
77. de Savigny DH, Voller A, Woodruff AW: Toxocariasis: Serological diagnosis by enzyme immunoassay. J Clin Pathol 32:284, 1979.
78. Glickman L, Schantz P, Dombroske R, et al: Evaluation of serodiagnostic tests for visceral larva migrans. Am J Trop Med Hyg 27:492, 1978.
79. Jacquier P, Gottstein B, Stingelin Y, et al: Immunodiagnosis of toxocarosis in humans: Evaluation of a new enzyme-linked immunosorbent assay kit. J Clin Microbiol 29:1831, 1991.
80. Lynch NR, Hagel I, Vargas V, et al: Comparable seropositivity for ascariasis and toxocariasis in tropical slum children. Parasitol Res 79:547, 1993.
81. Magnaval JF, Fabre R, Maurieres P, et al: Evaluation of an immunoenzymatic assay detecting specific anti-*Toxocara* immunoglobulin E for diagnosis and posttreatment follow-up of human toxocariasis. J Clin Microbiol 30:2269, 1992.
82. Magnaval JF, Fabre R, Maurieres P, et al: Application of the Western blotting procedure for the immunodiagnosis of human toxocariasis. Parasitol Res 77:697, 1991.
83. Fong MY, Lau YL, Init I, et al: Recombinant expression of *Toxocara canis* excretory-secretory antigen TES-120 in *Escherichia coli*. Southeast Asian J Trop Med Public Health 34:723, 2003.
84. Gillespie SH, Bidwell D, Voller A, et al: Diagnosis of human toxocariasis by antigen capture enzyme linked immunosorbent assay. J Clin Pathol 46:551, 1993.
85. Templeton PA, Rao KC: Computed tomography of *Toxocara canis* endophthalmitis. J Comput Tomogr 11:99, 1987.
86. Wan WL, Cano MR, Pince KJ, et al: Echographic characteristics of ocular toxocariasis. Ophthalmology 98:28, 1991.
87. Schantz PM, Meyer D, Glickman LT: Clinical, serologic, and epidemiologic characteristics of ocular toxocariasis. Am J Trop Med Hyg 28:24, 1979.
88. Sharkey JA, McKay PS: Ocular toxocariasis in a patient with repeatedly negative ELISA titre to *Toxocara canis*. Br J Ophthalmol 77:253, 1993.
89. Biglan AW, Glickman LT, Lobes LA, Jr.: Serum and vitreous *Toxocara* antibody in nematode endophthalmitis. Am J Ophthalmol 88:898, 1979.
90. Benitez del Castillo JM, Herreros G, Guillen JL, et al: Bilateral ocular toxocariasis demonstrated by aqueous humor enzyme-linked immunosorbent assay. Am J Ophthalmol 119:514, 1995.
91. Sabrosa NA, Zajdenweber M: Nematode infections of the eye: Toxocariasis, onchocerciasis, diffuse unilateral subacute neuroretinitis, and cysticercosis. Ophthalmol Clin North Am 15:351, 2002.
92. Sturchler D, Schubarth P, Gualzata M, et al: Thiabendazole vs. albendazole in treatment of toxocariasis: A clinical trial. Ann Trop Med Parasitol 83:473, 1989.
93. Drugs for parasitic infections. Med Lett Drugs Ther August 2004. www.medicalletter.org
94. Magnaval JF: Comparative efficacy of diethylcarbamazine and mebendazole for the treatment of human toxocariasis. Parasitology 110:529, 1995.
95. Barisani-Asenbauer T, Maca SM, Hauff W, et al: Treatment of ocular toxocariasis with albendazole. J Ocul Pharmacol Ther 17:287, 2001.
96. Small KW, McCuen BW, De Juan E, et al: Surgical management of retinal retraction caused by toxocariasis. Am. J Ophthalmol 108:10, 1989.
97. Schantz PM, Weis PE, Pollard ZF, et al: Risk factors for toxocaral ocular larva migrans: A case-control study. Am J Public Health 70:1269, 1980.
98. Gehrke BC: Results of the 1997 AVMA survey of US pet-owning households regarding use of veterinary services and expenditures. J Am Vet Med Assoc 211:417, 1997.
99. Brown JP, Silverman JD: The current and future market for veterinarians and veterinary medical services in the US. J Am Vet Med Assoc 215:161, 1999.
100. Uga S, Kataoka N: Measures to control *Toxocara* egg contamination in sandpits of public parks. Am J Trop Med Hyg 52:21, 1995.
101. Clark JN, Daurio CP, Plue RE, et al: Efficacy of ivermectin and pyrantel pamoate combined in a chewable formulation against heartworm, hookworm, and ascarid infections in dogs. Am J Vet Res 53:517, 1992.
102. Payne PA, Ridley RK: Strategic use of ivermectin during pregnancy to control *Toxocara canis* in greyhound puppies. Vet Parasitol 85:305, 1999.
103. Payne-Johnson M, Maitland TP, Sherington J, et al: Efficacy of selamectin administered topically to pregnant and lactating female dogs in the treatment and prevention of adult roundworm (*Toxocara canis*) infections and flea (*Ctenocephalides felis felis*) infestations in the dams and their pups. Vet Parasitol 91:347, 2000.
104. Burke TM, Roberson EL: Fenbendazole treatment of pregnant bitches to reduce prenatal and lactogenic infections of *Toxocara canis* and *Ancylostoma caninum* in pups. J Am Vet Med Assoc 183:987, 1983.
105. Obwaller A, Duchene M, Bruhn H: Recombinant dissection of myosin heavy chain of *Toxocara canis* shows strong clustering of antigenic regions. Parasitol Res 87:383, 2001.
106. Caumes E, Carriere J, Guermonprez G, et al: Dermatoses associated with travel to tropical countries: A prospective study of the diagnosis and management of 269 patients presenting to a tropical disease unit. Clin Infect Dis 20:542, 1995.
107. Jelinek T, Maiwald H, Northdurft HD, et al: Cutaneous larva migrans in travelers: Synopsis of histories, symptoms and treatment of 98 patients. Clin Infect Dis 19:1062, 1994.
108. Heukelbach J, Wilcke T, Feldmeier H: Cutaneous larva migrans (creeping eruption) in an urban slum in Brazil. Int J Dermatol 43:511, 2004.
109. Richey TK, Gentry RH, Fitzpatrick JE, et al: Persistent cutaneous larva migrans due to *Ancylostoma* species. South Med J 89:609, 1996.
110. Caumes E, Carriere J, Datry A, et al: A randomized trial of ivermectin versus albendazole for the treatment of cutaneous larva migrans. Am J Trop Med Hyg 49:641, 1993.
111. Caumes E: Treatment of cutaneous larva migrans. Clin Infect Dis 30:811, 2000.
112. Bouchaud O, Houze S, Schiemann R, et al: Cutaneous larva migrans in travelers: A prospective study, with assessment of therapy with ivermectin. Clin Infect Dis 31:493, 2000.

104

Trichinellosis

FABRIZIO BRUSCHI
K. DARWIN MURRELL

INTRODUCTION

Trichinellosis, the proper term for trichinosis or trichiniasis, results from infection by a parasitic nematode belonging to the genus *Trichinella*. Trichinellosis has been an important, though often unrecognized, disease for thousands of years. Species of *Trichinella* responsible for the infection are widely distributed, including the Arctic, temperate lands, and the tropics.[1] Virtually all mammals are susceptible to infection; however, humans appear to be especially prone to developing clinical disease. Infection with various species of *Trichinella* is far more common than is generally recognized. Although the incidence of human trichinellosis is low worldwide, the parasite remains an important food-borne zoonosis because of its epizootic nature and the economic burden associated with preventing its incursion into the human food chain.[2] The prevalence of swine trichinellosis and the incidence of human trichinellosis appear to be greater in developing countries, such as China, Thailand, Mexico, Argentina, and Bolivia, and in some central European countries.[3]

Until recently, the epidemiology and systematics of this parasitic zoonosis were considered relatively simple and straightforward.[1] Human trichinellosis was believed to involve one species, *Trichinella spiralis* (Owen, 1835). During the past two decades, major changes in the understanding of this epidemiology have occurred, yielding a transmission pattern that may involve domestic swine, horses, and wild animals. Furthermore, new molecular genetic data have led to the creation of a new taxonomy for *Trichinella* that includes eight species rather than one[1] (Table 104-1). This revised taxonomy is yielding a greater comprehension of the clinical course of the disease caused by the different *Trichinella* species.[4] Although this parasite was first described more than 155 years ago, both its biology and its complete control remain an unfinished story.

AGENT

The parasite's discovery resulted from the microscopic examination of cadaver muscle in London in 1835, and it was named *Trichina spiralis* by Owen. During the mid-19th century, the life cycle and etiology of human–swine trichinellosis were elucidated by German scientists, along with its basic epidemiology. Over the succeeding 150 years, the domestic pork–human trichinellosis cycle was reported from many countries. In some regions, especially in Europe and the former Soviet Union, the problem of trichinellosis was so severe that mandatory inspection of all pork for muscle larvae (trichinae) was instituted. These measures have been effective and in countries with mandatory meat inspection, trichinellosis has become a low-incidence disease.

The classic and most frequent cause of human trichinellosis, *T. spiralis*, is normally derived from domestic pork; the pig–man epidemiologic pattern is usually referred to as the synanthropic or domestic cycle. All species of *Trichinella* are morphologically difficult to distinguish from one another, but all have a direct life cycle with complete development in a single host; there is a degree of host specificity, but the complete host range for each species is not completely known. The host capsule surrounding the infective larvae is a modified striated muscle structure called a nurse cell, which is digested away in the stomach when the infected muscle is ingested by the next host.[5] The free larvae (L1 stage) then move into the upper small intestine and invade the columnar epithelial intestinal cells. Within 30 hours, the larvae undergo four molts to reach the mature adult stages, as males and females. After mating, the female (Fig. 104-1) begins shedding live newborn larvae (NBL), approximately 5 days postinfection; the NBL are early developmental forms of the L1 stage.[3] The persistence of adult worms in the intestine of humans may last for several weeks.[4,5] The NBL migrate throughout the body via the blood and lymph circulatory system. Although the NBL may attempt to invade many different tissues, they are successful only if they can enter striated skeletal muscle cells.[6,7] The NBL continue to grow and develop during the first 2 weeks of intracellular life until they reach the fully developed L1 infective stage. The longevity of the nurse cell–L1 complex (encapsulated) appears to vary by parasite and host species, but it generally persists for 1 to several years before calcification and death occur.[8] The life cycle is completed when the host's infected muscle is ingested by a suitable host. A host capsule does not develop around *T. pseudospiralis*, *T. papuae*, and *T. zimbabwensis* muscle larvae.[8]

EPIDEMIOLOGY

The most salient feature of this parasite group's epidemiology is its obligatory transmission by ingestion of meat. A second cardinal feature is its existence in two normally

***Table 104-1** Biologic and Zoogeographic Features of* Trichinella *Species*

Species	Distribution	Major Hosts	Reported from Humans
T. spiralis	Cosmopolitan	Domestic pigs, wild mammals	Yes
T. britovi	Eurasia	Wild mammals	Yes
T. murrelli	North America	Wild mammals	Yes
T. nativa	Arctic	Bears, foxes	Yes
T. nelsoni	Equatorial Africa	Hyenas, felids	Yes
*T. pseudospiralis**	Cosmopolitan	Wild mammals, birds	Yes
*T. papuae**	Papua New Guinea	Domestic/feral pigs	No
*T. zimbabwensis**	Tanzania	Crocodiles	No

*Nonencapsulaing species.

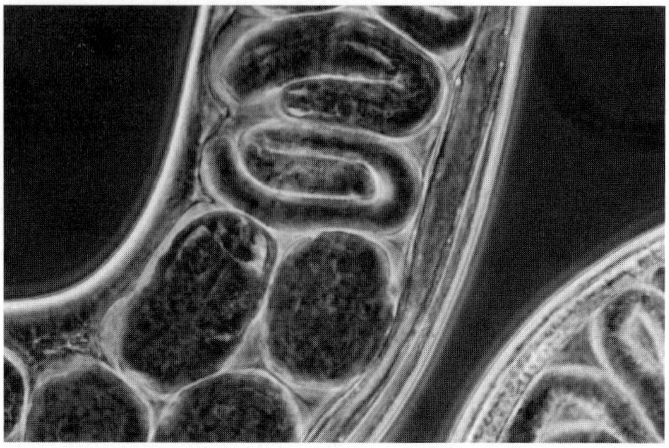

FIGURE 104-1 Living female adult worm of *Trichinella britovi*, isolated from the intestine of a rat at 6 days of infection. At this magnification it is possible to observe the embryos in the uterus cavity. (Phase contrast; original magnification × 1000.)

separate ecological systems, the sylvatic and the domestic. In certain circumstances, the two biotopes are linked through man's activities, resulting in the exposure of humans to *Trichinella* species normally confined to sylvatic animals. The species most frequently associated with human infection is *T. spiralis*, the species that is normally found in domestic pigs but frequently detected in rodents and wild mammals.[4] The domestic cycle of *T. spiralis* involves a complex set of potential routes.[4] Transmission on a farm may result from predation on or scavenging other animals (e.g., rodents), hog cannibalism, and the feeding of uncooked meat scraps. The importance of wild animal reservoirs is often underappreciated, although the frequency of transmission from infected game animals is significant.[8]

The worldwide incidence of human trichinellosis has declined substantially during the past few decades, but outbreaks are still frequent, especially in developing regions[3] (Table 104-2). In developed countries, the epidemiology of human trichinellosis is typified by urban common-source outbreaks.[4] In the United States, the largest human outbreaks

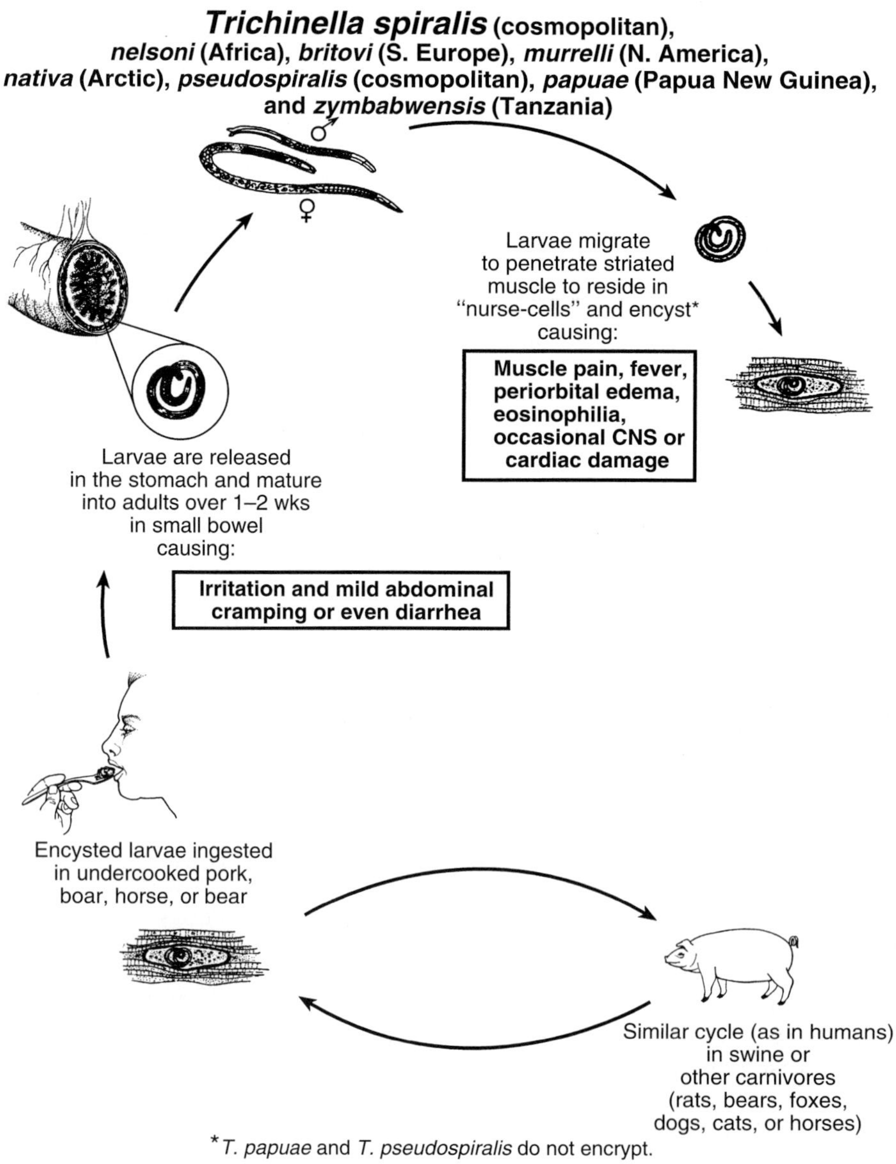

Table 104-2 Examples of Recent Human Trichinellosis Cases in Different Countries

Country	Period	No. of Cases	Sources
United States	1991–1996	230	Pork, game
Mexico	1991–1998	280	Pork
Argentina	1990–1999	5,217	Pork, game
Bulgaria	1993–2000	5,683	Pork, game
Croatia	1997–2000	1,047	Pork
Serbia	1995–2001	3,925	Pork
Romania	1990–1999	16,712	Pork
France	1995–1997	27	Game, horse
Italy	1999–2001	164	Pork, horse, game
Spain	1993–1998	290	Pork, game
China	1964–1999	23,004	Pork, dogs, game, mutton
Thailand	1994–1996	104	Pork, game

have occurred among ethnic groups with preferences for raw or only partially cooked pork. Infected meat is typically purchased from local supermarkets, butcher shops, or other commercial outlets. However, in recent years, nearly one-third or more of human infections in the United States have been derived from wild animal meat.[3,4] In Europe, where the safeguard of pork inspection is mandatory, most recent outbreaks have resulted from infected horse or wild boar meat.[2,9] The resurgence of trichinellosis in central Europe appears to result from increased transmission from both pork and wild game. In Latin America[10] and Asia, however, domestic pork appears to be the main source of infection.

Surprisingly, during the past 20 years, Europe has experienced six large outbreaks due to infected horse meat, a heretofore unrecognized source of infection.[4,8,9] Three outbreaks occurred in France in 1976 (125 patients) and two in 1985 (400 and 980 patients). Three outbreaks occurred in Italy—one in 1976 (96 patients), one in 1984 (13 patients), and one in 1986 (300 patients). Four of the outbreaks were shown to be due to *T. britovi*, one to *T. nativa*, and one to *T. spiralis*.[9]

Foreign travelers also account for some cases of human trichinellosis; 26 cases occurred from 1975 to 1989 in the United States, most of them after travel to Mexico or Asia. Globally, the prevalence of *T. spiralis* in domestic swine ranges from less than 0.001% (United States) to 25% or more (e.g., some regions of China). The global rise in consumer demand for greater food quality assurance also makes eradication of *T. spiralis* from pork an unavoidable responsibility of both producers and governments.

DISEASE

The clinical course of the acute period of infection is characterized by two phases: *enteral* (the parasite alters intestinal function) and *parenteral*, associated with an inflammatory and allergic response to muscle invasion by the larval parasites.[11] Gastrointestinal signs appear first, a result of mucosal invasion by the first-generation (ingested) larvae. These signs typically last 2 to 7 days but may persist for weeks. Subsequently, fever, myalgia, periorbital edema, and eosinophilia, which together constitute the so-called trichinellotic syndrome or general trichinellosis syndrome, begin.[12,13] However, the acute phase, lasting 1 to 8 weeks, is commonly asymptomatic, especially when the number of ingested larvae is low.

The severity of the clinical course depends on the parasite and host factors,[12] such as immune status; this is particularly evident in patients treated with immunosuppressive drugs for kidney transplantation. [14] In experimental infections, steroids and immunosuppressive treatments delay the worm expulsion,[15] and this probably also occurs in humans.[11] Furthermore, the prolonged diarrhea in the absence of myalgia, reported in elderly Inuit people, may be due to previously acquired immunity against the enteral and parenteral stages of the parasite.[16,17] The incubation period ranges from 7 to 30 days, depending on the severity of infection. When the course of infection is severe, the incubation period is brief, although death may also occur with a longer incubation period.[12]

The clinical course may be abortive (symptomatology not complete), mild (complete even if mild), moderate, or severe (often with complications).[13] Malaise, anorexia, nausea, vomiting, abdominal pain, fever, diarrhea, or constipation may occur. Diarrhea is more persistent than vomiting, lasting up to 3 months, and, when excessive, causes dehydration; this, together with enteritis, is an occasional cause of death. Variations in this pattern occur. For example, in outbreaks in the Canadian Arctic caused by the Arctic species *T. nativa*, trichinellosis occurred in two forms: the classic myopathic form and a clinical syndrome featuring prolonged diarrhea without fever and only a brief period of myalgia, affecting primarily elderly patients.[16,17]

Muscles are mainly affected during the parenteral phase, but other organs, such as the myocardium, central nervous system (CNS), lungs, kidney, and skin, may also be involved. The trichinellotic syndrome is characterized by facial edema; muscle pain and swelling; weakness; and, frequently, fever; anorexia, headache, conjunctivitis, and urticaria occur less frequently. Fever, usually remittent, generally begins at 2 weeks and peaks after 4, with temperatures as high as 40 or 41°C in severe cases. Despite fever, patients may appear in good condition. Ocular signs at this time may help in diagnosis, in particular edema of the eyelids, chemosis, conjunctivitis, conjunctival hemorrhages, disturbed vision, and ocular pain. Periorbital edema is peculiar to trichinellosis, ranging from 17% to 100% in more than 2100 trichinellosis cases reviewed.[18] The mechanisms responsible for this edema are not clear, but an allergic phenomenon is probably responsible.[18]

The entire face may also be involved, giving patients a characteristic aspect, often rendering them unrecognizable. At this time, the muscles of the rest of the body usually become painful. Extraocular muscles, masseters, tongue and larynx muscles, diaphragm, neck muscles, and intercostal muscles are most frequently infected. The pain may be so severe as to limit function of the arms and legs, inhibiting walking, speaking, moving the tongue, breathing, and swallowing. Weakness is also a consequence of the muscle involvement. The muscles become stiff, hard, and edematous; the edema may be so intense as to simulate hypertrophy.[19] Edema lasts 1 or 2 weeks and disappears with increased diuresis. In an outbreak in Thailand due to *T. pseudospiralis* myalgia and asthenia lasted more than 4 months.[20]

Gastrointestinal symptoms, such as vomiting and diarrhea, may also extend into this phase.[12] Dyspnea (even ventilatory failure),[21] coughing, and hoarseness may also be present. Dyspnea is caused primarily by parasite invasion and consequent inflammation of respiratory muscles such as the diaphragm (the most heavily infected muscle in experimental animal infections[22]). Bronchopneumonia and infarction may also be responsible. The cough begins in correspondence with the passage of the larvae through the capillary bed of the lungs approximately 1 week after infection.[23]

Neurologic manifestations, more common in severe infections, occur in 10% to 24% of cases.[24,25] In 55 patients affected by neurotrichinosis (involvement of the CNS), meningoencephalitic signs were observed in almost all cases. Less frequent signs are focal paralysis or paresis, delirium, and psychosis.[25] Headache is very common in trichinellosis, being exacerbated by movements of the head. Myocarditis is the most frequent cardiovascular complication. It is sometimes responsible for heart failure or bronchopneumonia; in some cases, death occurs between the fourth and the eighth week of infection, although sudden death may occur even earlier.[12] Arrhythmias, secondary to myocarditis, may also occur. In one case, it was necessary to use a pacemaker for 1 year to maintain normal cardiac rhythm.[21] Electrocardiographic alterations (premature contractions, prolongation of the P-R interval, small QRS complexes with intraventricular block, and flattening or inversion of the T waves, especially lead II and precordial leads) may be present from the second week and may persist up to the third or fourth week. Blood pressure may be low during the early phase of infection and also during convalescence. Edema due to heart failure has been observed, generally in the later phase of the infection when edema due to myositis has almost disappeared. Vascular signs such as epistaxis, hemoptysis, hemorrhages from the bowel, thrombosis of the femoral or pulmonary artery, and embolism are less common. In one fatal case, the arterioles of different organs were affected by disseminated intravascular coagulation with platelet-fibrin thrombi.[26] Less frequent are petechial hemorrhages, mainly subungual resembling bacterial endocarditis, and roseola and maculopapular exanthems, resembling measles.[23] After the acute period, convalescence follows (lasting from months to years), usually with a complete recovery. During the first few years, muscle larvae are slowly but completely destroyed, followed by calcification.[27] Although this is true for *T. spiralis* infections, the calcification process in infections with other species may occur earlier.[28]

The existence of chronic trichinellosis[29] or "persisting sequelae"[30] (the persistence of myalgia, early fatigability, ocular signs, and headache for decades) is somewhat controversial and requires investigation. Some studies have confirmed the occurrence of these sequelae for periods up to 10 years after clinical recovery.[31,32]

Although death is now rare in trichinellosis, owing to improved therapy, it may result from congestive heart failure due to myocarditis, encephalitis, pneumonitis, hypokalemia, or adrenal gland insufficiency.[12,23] In the United States, during the period 1991 to 1996, in 230 cases of trichinellosis reported to the Centers for Disease Control and Prevention, only 3 were fatal.[33] During an outbreak in Thailand caused by *T. pseudospiralis*, one fatality was reported in 59 patients and it was attributed to the high number of larvae ingested rather than to pathogenicity of the *Trichinella* species involved.[20]

PATHOGENESIS AND IMMUNITY

The early phase of infection, associated with the presence of the parasite in the gastrointestinal tract, induces a type 1 hypersensitivity reaction, a result of Th2 cell activation, leading to increased levels of parasite-specific IgE and eosinophils. A clear role for IgE in protective intestinal immunity has been documented in rodent models that show that parasite-specific IgE, transfused together with thoracic duct cells from immune animals, induces rapid intestinal worm expulsion during a primary infection.[34] However, the mechanisms regulating the response to a primary infection, especially in human hosts, are not clear. The prolonged diarrhea observed in the outbreaks in the Canadian Arctic[16,17] suggests adult worms persist in the intestine of people with frequent exposure to infection, a circumstance that arises from possible downregulation of the intestinal immune response, a premunition state, or a downregulation of gut physiology.

Recently, it has been shown in infected mast cell-depleted animals as well as in interleukin-9 (IL-9) transgenic mice (mast cell overproduced) that mast cells are responsible for the modifications of the intestinal epithelial barrier, including production of a mucosal chymase, occurring during *T. spiralis* infection, which lead to an increased mucosal leakiness.[35] The effect of this protease, increasing gut permeability, could facilitate the passage of antibodies to the lumen.

The parenteral phase is associated with inflammatory and allergic responses to invasion of the muscles by the migrating larvae. This invasion can directly damage the muscle cells or indirectly stimulate the infiltration of inflammatory cells, primarily eosinophils. These cells may damage the muscle tissue.[36] Neurotrichinosis arises mainly from vascular perturbations, such as vasculitis and granulomatous inflammatory reactions that surround invading larvae. The larvae tend to wander, causing damage before reentering the bloodstream, or they remain trapped and are destroyed by the provoked granulomatous reaction.[37] Neural cells may also be damaged by eosinophil degranulation products such as eosinophil-derived neurotoxin and major basic protein (MBP).[38,39] Myocarditis results initially from invasion by the migrating larvae, followed by immunopathologic processes such as eosinophil infiltration and mast cell degranulation, according to results obtained in experimental infection.[40]

The mechanisms responsible for the pronounced eosinophilia, so characteristic of trichinellosis, are not well understood. The involvement of factors specific for eosinophils such as cytokines, including IL-5[41,42] produced by the Th2 subset of $CD4^+$ T cells,[43] may be involved. The role of IgE in inducing the eosinophilia is controversial.[44,45] Eosinophils are cytotoxic for newborn larvae in vitro in both animal[46,47] and human antibody-dependent cellular cytotoxicity in vitro reactions[48,49]; they release products such as MBP,[50] peroxidase,[51] or products derived from oxidative metabolism.[52] However, their actual role in vivo is not understood. Interestingly, suppression of eosinophilia by an IL-5-specific monoclonal antibody in vivo does not modify either primary or secondary *Trichinella* infections in mice.[53]

DIAGNOSIS

The issue of whether trichinellosis is a low-prevalence disease or one that is frequently misdiagnosed cannot be adequately resolved. Diagnosis is difficult in low-level, sporadic infections because the resulting clinical manifestations are common to many other diseases,[23] including chronic fatigue syndrome.[54] Trichinellosis should be considered in the differential diagnosis of myositis in patients with human immunodeficiency virus (HIV) infection.[55] When the infection occurs in epizootic or outbreak form its diagnosis is easier. Special care must be taken when developing clinical histories, giving particular attention to eating habits during the weeks before the onset of symptoms. Ingestion of infected meat (raw or undercooked); the presence of gastroenteritis, myalgia, facial edema, subungual or conjunctival hemorrhages; and an increase in eosinophils should suggest trichinellosis.[12] Electromyography (EMG) may help in the diagnosis of moderate and severe infections during the acute period, even if the muscle changes are not pathognomonic.[12] With clinical improvement, EMG changes generally disappear within 2 or 3 months[56] but may persist for 1 to 8 years,[57] or more.[58]

A definitive diagnosis may be made when L1 stage larvae are found in a muscle biopsy, generally performed in the more accessible deltoid muscle. Biopsy is recommended only in rare and difficult cases, particularly when serology is not clear. If the result is negative, however, a low-level infection cannot be excluded.[12] Artificial digestion (1% pepsin-HCl) of a muscle sample is more sensitive than direct microscopic observation of the tissue specimen, but, importantly, larvae cannot be isolated from muscle before 17 to 21 days of infection because of their sensitivity to digestion.[59] A muscle biopsy may help, however, not only in diagnosis but also in evaluating the level of infection, the pathologic changes in the muscle tissue, and the infection duration and in the isolation of the parasite and its subsequent genetic typing by molecular techniques[60]; this is important when the source of infection is unknown or no longer available. This technique allowed for the first time the identification of *T. pseudospiralis* in a human trichinellosis case.[61] All such information is useful in deciding on therapeutic strategies.[12]

The histologic examination may reveal modifications of skeletal muscles, including at first a basophilic degeneration of the fibers, fatty metamorphosis, hyaline or hydropical degeneration or both, and interstitial inflammation; sometimes it is possible to observe dead nonencapsulated parasites. Small hemorrhages, the accumulation of inflammatory cells (myositis) such as eosinophils, lymphocytes, and macrophages, among the muscle cells are also visible. Inflammatory cells invade the muscle cells when the sarcolemma is damaged. Vascularity increases near muscle fibers.[62,63] The process of encapsulation of the parasite, with the exception of *T. pseudospiralis*, *T. papuae*, and *T. zimbabwensis*, begins at approximately 2 weeks and is usually completed at 5 weeks of infection, depending on the *Trichinella* species involved.[28] In humans, calcification begins approximately 5 months after infection and is usually completed after 18 months.

As previously mentioned, the diagnosis of trichinellosis is difficult in sporadic cases, but it is even more difficult when CNS involvement is present. Neurotrichinosis is sometimes accompanied by multifocal CNS lesions, nodular or ringlike, with a diameter of 3 to 8 mm, and, in most cases, showing contrast enhancement.[39,64] However, in cases with neurologic manifestations of trichinosis, computed tomography images of the brain have been reported to be normal.[64,65]

Eosinophilia, leukocytosis, serum muscle enzyme-level increases, and increased immunoglobulin levels, especially total IgE, are the most characteristic laboratory findings in this disease. Eosinophil levels increase dramatically during trichinellosis (up to 8700/μL).[11] Eosinophilia (based on the absolute number rather than the percentage) occurs in all cases of trichinellosis, even the subclinical; the exception may be very severe infection with eosinopenia, which has a fatal course.[66] Eosinophilia may also be absent when bacterial infections complicate the disease. After steroid therapy, eosinophil levels also decrease.[12] Leukocytosis, up to 24,000/μL,[67] occurs in very severe infections, usually early in the infection.

Increased creatine phosphokinase (CPK), lactate dehydrogenase (LDH), aldolase, and aminotransferase levels reflect skeletal muscle damage, helping in the diagnosis.[12] Serum CPK levels can increase up to more than 17,000 U/L. CPK isoenzyme profiles, however, are not very helpful. An increased level of the CPK isoenzyme MB, generally ascribed to myocardial damage, has been observed in 35% of trichinellosis patients examined with no cardiologic symptoms, suggesting a release of this isoenzyme from damaged skeletal muscle cells.[68] LDH should be evaluated together with CPK, even if the former is less specific. When high levels of CPK and LDH are present, a differential diagnosis with myopathies is necessary. Before antibody levels increase, the level of total serum LDH and of the isoenzymatic forms LD_4 and LD_5 may increase in approximately 50% of patients.[69]

Hypoalbuminemia is observed mainly in severe cases, in which the amounts of this serum protein can reach 2.5 g/dL.[13]

Immunoglobulin level changes may also occur, the most characteristic being an increase in total IgE. However, an increase in total IgE levels is not a consistent phenomenon, and it is not possible to exclude trichinellosis by its absence.[12] A poor correlation with specific IgE has been observed for both *T. spiralis*[70] and *T. britovi*[71] infections.

Many serologic tests are available for diagnosis.[12,59] There are three objectives in immunodiagnosis: (1) recognizing the acute infection to allow early anthelminthic treatment, (2) making a retrospective diagnosis, and (3) adding information to the epidemiology of the infection.[72]

Seroconversion usually occurs between the third and fifth week of infection and serum may remain positive up to 1 year or more after cessation of clinical symptoms. Antibodies have been detected, however, up to 19 years after the end of the acute phase of infection.[12] Antibody levels do not correlate with the severity of the clinical course[69] or with a particular clinical course.[73]

Indirect hemagglutination, bentonite flocculation, indirect immunofluorescence (IFA), latex agglutination, and enzyme-linked immunosorbent assay (ELISA) are the more commonly used tests, the last of which is the most sensitive.[12] Factors such as sensitivity, specificity, convenience, simplicity, cost, and commercial availability must be considered when choosing a test. However, a diagnostic laboratory should have at least two or more tests available to ensure a correct diagnosis: one to detect the response against a soluble antigen and another for antibodies that react with parasite surface antigens.[72] For the latter, the IFA is performed with whole L1 stage larvae killed with formalin[74] or with unfixed frozen sections of infected muscles[75]; the latter is more sensitive. With this test, all specific immunoglobulins can be evaluated. The ELISA method,[76] using excretory–secretory antigens, is preferable to that which uses crude extracts of *T. spiralis* muscle larvae for soluble antigen because it is more specific. This is particularly important in tropical regions where cross-reactions with other helminth parasites can give false-positive results.[77,78] Cross-reactions with *Trichinella* antigens were observed in patients with autoimmune diseases.[79] It is necessary to standardize as much as possible the antigens used for diagnostic purposes.[80,81] Recombinant[82] or synthetic[83] antigens are now available for diagnostic purposes. The ELISA can also be used for the evaluation of the different specific Ig classes (IgA and IgM)[84,85] or IgG subclasses,[86] but the sensitivity of these tests is lower than that of the ELISA IgG. The data on specific IgE are contradictory,[77,84,85] however, and this test cannot yet be recommended. The detection of circulating antigens has also not been completely satisfactory compared to IFA or a competitive inhibition assay.[87] However, it is worthwhile because it may demonstrate early the actual presence of the parasite and may represent an alternative to muscle biopsy.

The study of the cellular immune response in humans[88] is important for research purposes but of little value for diagnosis. Immunoelectrotransfer blot assay[89,90] can be used as a primary or confirmatory test. When ES antigens are used, it is quite specific and useful for follow-up studies.[61] In accordance with the International Commission on Trichinellosis, the serum reactivity for the TSL-1 antigen family (40 to 70 kDa in the reduced form) should be considered diagnostic.[81]

TREATMENT AND PROGNOSIS

It is difficult to differentiate the efficacy of drug therapy from natural recovery of infection in mild to moderate cases. Factors such as the *Trichinella* species involved, intensity and length of infection, and host response can aid in deciding on the treatment course.[12] Symptomatic treatment[66] includes analgesic and antipyretic drugs, bed rest, and corticosteroids (prednisolone at 50 mg/day), especially in severe infections to prevent shocklike symptoms. Specific treatment[66] is performed with mebendazole, which should be administered in adults at a daily dose of 5 mg/kg in two doses for 10 to 15 days (the treatment cycle may be repeated after 5 days) or with albendazole. In adults, this latter drug should be administered at a dose of 15 mg/kg/day in two doses for 10 to 15 days; in children older than 2 years, the drug is given at 10 mg/kg/day. For severe infection, the treatment may be repeated after 5 days. Blood cell counts and liver function should be regularly monitored. Albendazole in pregnant women is contraindicated and in children younger than 2 years is not recommended. Thiabendazole is no longer used because of its side effects.[66] Pyrantel has been proposed for children and pregnant women, but its efficacy is doubtful.[56] This treatment is recommended for intestinal and muscle stages, but light infections do not require treatment. The treatment goal for the very early infection phase is to limit muscle invasion by larvae; when this has already occurred, the goal is to reduce muscle damage, which is responsible for the major clinical manifestations. Therapeutic plasma levels of the drug should be maintained for an extended period rather than high levels for short periods. The success of treatment is evident from clinical improvement of the patient's symptomatology.

As previously mentioned, the prognosis *quoad vitam* is usually good with the exception of rare, heavily infected cases. That *quoad valetudinem* depends on the number of ingested larvae and on the time passed before the diagnosis has been made and treatment begins.

PREVENTION AND CONTROL

Control of swine trichinellosis and prevention of infection in humans have both direct and indirect aspects. Mandatory inspection of pork at slaughter, although common in developed countries, especially Europe,[91] is not required in the United States. In developing countries, testing for trichinellosis as part of routine inspection is rare. Instead, emphasis is placed on educating the consumer on safe handling and cooking of pork and wild game. The U.S. Department of Agriculture has established recommended procedures[92] for devitalizing any muscle larvae present in these meats by cooking or freezing. For example, the consumer should cook pork until all pink color has disappeared, which normally occurs at approximately 137°F; to allow for a margin of error, however, it is recommended that the internal temperature of meat should uniformly reach 160°F throughout, whether by conventional cooking or by microwaving. Care must be taken to avoid cold spots with the latter method.

Fresh pork less than 6 inches thick can be rendered safe if frozen to 5°F (−17°C) for 20 days, −10°F (−23°C) for 10 days, or −20°F (−29°C) for 6 days. Because of the freeze resistance shown by sylvatic species of *Trichinella*, particularly *T. nativa*, freezing of meat from game is not completely reliable. Infection from wild animal meat accounts for an important proportion of human trichinellosis; therefore, the inspection of wild game muscle is recommended and is mandatory in some European countries. Consumers should also be warned of the danger and advised on proper meat handling and preparation procedures.

The control of trichinellosis in swine relies on good general management practices.[92] For example, pork producers are encouraged to observe federal garbage feeding regulations in those states where this practice is allowed, to practice stringent rodent control, to avoid exposing pigs to dead animal carcasses of any kind, to ensure that hog carcasses are properly disposed of, and to try to establish effective barriers between domestic swine and wild and domestic animals.

A modest amount of research has been carried out on the development of a vaccine. Unlike rodents, the typical experimental host, pigs do not develop strong intestinal immunity[93]; hence, L1 stage stichocyte antigens are insufficient for a vaccine. However, the antigens of the NBL have proved highly effective in pigs, and a protovaccine has been developed.[94]

REFERENCES

1. Murrell KD, Lichtenfels RJ, Zarlenga, DS et al: The systematics of the genus *Trichinella* with a key to species. Vet Parasitol 93:293, 2000.
2. Dupouy-Camet J: Trichinellosis: A worldwide zoonosis. Vet Parasitol 93:191, 2000.
3. Murrell KD, Pozio E: Trichinellosis: The zoonosis that won't go quietly. Int J Parasitol 30:1339, 2000.
4. Bruschi F, Murrell KD: New aspects of human trichinellosis: The impact of new *Trichinella* species. Postgrad Med J 78:15, 2002.
5. Despommier DD: How does *Trichinella spiralis* make itself at home? Parasitol Today 14:318, 1998.
6. Stewart GL: Biochemistry. In Campbell WC (ed): *Trichinella* and Trichinosis. New York, Plenum Press, 1983, p 153.
7. Gould SE: Anatomic pathology. In Gould SE (ed): Trichinosis in Man and Animals. Springfield, Ill., Charles C Thomas, 1970, p 147.
8. Pozio E: New patterns of *Trichinella* infection. Vet Parasitol 98: 133, 2001.
9. Boireau P, Valle I, Roman T, et al: *Trichinella* in horses: A low frequency infection with high human risk. Vet Parasitol 93:309, 2000.
10. Ortega-Pierres MG, Arriaga C, Yepez-Mulia L: Epidemiology of trichinellosis in Mexico, Central America and South America. Vet Parasitol 93:201, 2000.
11. Capo V, Despommier DD: Clinical aspects of infection with *Trichinella* spp. Clin Microbiol Rev 9:47, 1996.

12. Murrell KD, Bruschi F: Clinical trichinellosis. In Sun T (ed): Progress in Clinical Parasitology. Boca Raton, Fla, CRC Press, 1994, p 117.
13. Kassur B, Januszkiewicz J, Poznanska H: Clinic of trichinellosis. In Kim CW, Pawlowski ZS (eds): Trichinellosis. Hanover, NH, University Press of New England, 1978, p 27.
14. Doby JM, Couatarmanac'h A, Campion JP, et al: Trichinose humaine et immuno-dépression. Un cas chez un greffé rénal. Med Mal Infect 14:293, 1984.
15. Bell RG: *T. spiralis*: Differences between "early" and "late" rapid expulsion evident from inhibition studies using cortisone and irradiation. Exp Parasitol 64:385, 1987.
16. MacLean JP, Viallet J, Law C, et al: Trichinosis in the Canadian Arctic: Report of five outbreaks and a new clinical syndrome. J Infect Dis 160:513, 1989.
17. Viallet J, MacLean JD, Goresky LA, et al: Arctic trichinosis presenting as prolonged diarrhea. Gastroenterology 91:938, 1986.
18. Tassi C, Pozio E, Pelliccia D, et al: Evaluation of some immunological parameters in trichinellosis patients with periorbital oedema. Clin Chem Enzymol Comm 4:1, 1991.
19. Aldrige FC: An outbreak of trichinosis in Pennsylvania. Am J Med Sci 181:312, 1931.
20. Jongwutiwes S, Chantachum N, Kraivichian P, et al: First outbreak of human trichinellosis caused by *Trichinella pseudospiralis*. Clin Infect Dis 26:111, 1998.
21. Compton SJ, Celum LC, Thompson D, et al: Trichinosis with ventilatory failure and persistent myocarditis. Clin Infect Dis 16:500, 1993.
22. Olsen BS, Villella JB, Gould SE: Distribution of *Trichinella spiralis* in muscles of experimentally infected swine. J Parasitol 50:489, 1964.
23. Gould SE: Clinical manifestations, a symptomatology. In Gould SE (ed): Trichinosis in Man and Animals. Springfield, Ill., Charles C Thomas, 1970, p 269.
24. Kramer MD, Aita JF: Trichinosis. In Vinken BJ, Bruyn GW (eds): Infections of the Central Nervous System, Vol. 35. Handbook of Clinical Neurology. Amsterdam, North Holland, 1978, p 267.
25. Dalessio DJ, Wolff HG: *Trichinella spiralis* infection of the central nervous system. Arch Neurol 4:407, 1961.
26. Ursell PC, Habib A, Babchick O, et al: Myocarditis caused by *Trichinella spiralis*. Arch Pathol Lab Med 108:4, 1984.
27. Gerwel C, Kociecka W, Pawlowski Z: Parasitologic examination of muscles several years after trichinosis. Epidemiol Rev 24:262, 1970.
28. Pozio E, La Rosa G, Rossi P, et al: Comparative studies on *Trichinella* isolates from various host species and geographical regions: Biological characterizations. J Parasitol 78:654, 1992.
29. Fröscher W, Gullotta F, Saathoff M, et al: Chronic trichinosis. Clinical, bioptic, serological and electromyographic observations. Eur Neurol 28:221, 1988.
30. Kassur B, Januskiewicz J, Poznanska H: Controversial aspects in human trichinellosis. In Kim CW, Ruitenberg EJ, Teppema JS (eds): Trichinellosis. Chertsey, UK, Reedbooks, 1981, p 245.
31. Feldmeier H, Biensle U, Janssen-Rosseck R, et al: Sequelae after infection with *Trichinella spiralis*: A prospective cohort study. Wien Klin Wochenschr 103:111, 1991.
32. Harms GP, Binz H, Feldmeier K, et al: Trichinosis: A prospective controlled study of patients 10 years after acute infection. Clin Infect Dis 17:637, 1993.
33. Moorhead A, Grunewald PE, Dietz VJ, et al: Trichinellosis in the United States, 1991–1996: Declining but not gone. Am J Trop Med Hyg 60:66, 1999.
34. Ahmad A, Wang CH, Bell RG: A role for IgE in intestinal immunity. Expression of rapid expulsion of *Trichinella spiralis* in rats transfused with IgE and thoracic duct lymphocytes. J Immunol 146:3563, 1991.
35. McDermott JR, Bartram RE, Knight PA, et al: Mast cells disrupt epithelial barrier function during enteric nematode infection. Proc Natl Acad Sci USA 100:7761, 2003.
36. Ferraccioli GF, Mercadanti M, Salaffi F, et al: Prospective rheumatological study of muscle and joint symptoms during *Trichinella nelsoni* infection. Q J Med 260:973, 1988.
37. Katz M, Despommier DD, Gwadz RW: *Trichinella spiralis*. In Parasitic Diseases. New York, Springer-Verlag, 1989, p 28.
38. Durack DT, Sumi SM, Klebanoff SJ: Neurotoxicity of human eosinophils. Proc Natl Acad Sci USA 76:1443, 1979.
39. Mawhorter SD, Kazura JW: Trichinosis of the central nervous system. Semin Neurol 13:148, 1993.
40. Paolocci N, Sironi M, Bettini M, et al: Immunopathological mechanisms underlying the time course of *Trichinella spiralis* cardiomyopathy in rats. Virchows Arch 432:261, 1998.
41. Haig DM, Miller HRP: Differentiation of bone marrow cells into effector cells. In Behnke JM (ed): Parasites: Immunity and Pathology. London, Taylor & Francis, 1990, p 42.
42. Finkelman FD, Shea-Donohue T, Goldhill J, et al: Cytokine regulation of host defense against parasitic gastrointestinal hematodes. Lessons from studies with rodent models. Annu Rev Immunol 15:505, 1997.
43. Maizels RM, Yazdanbakhsh M: Immune regulation by helminth parasites: Cellular and molecular mechanisms. Nature Rev Immunol 3:733, 2003.
44. Dessein AJ, Parker WL, James SL, et al: IgE antibody and resistance to infection. I. Selective suppression of the IgE antibody response in rats diminishes the resistance and the eosinophil response to *Trichinella* infection. J Exp Med 153:423, 1981.
45. Watanabe N, Katakura K, Kobayashi A, et al: Protective immunity and eosinophilia in IgE-deficient SJA/9 mice infected with *Nippostrongylus brasiliensis* and *Trichinella spiralis*. Proc Natl Acad Sci USA 85:4460, 1988.
46. Kazura JW: Immunology of *Trichinella spiralis* infection. In Cohen S, Warren K (eds): Immunity to Parasitic Infections. Oxford, Blackwell, 1982, p 654.
47. Gansmüller A, Anteunis A, Venturiello SM, et al: Antibody-dependent "in vitro" cytotoxicity of newborn *Trichinella spiralis* larvae. Nature of the cells involved. Parasite Immunol 9:281, 1987.
48. Kazura JW: Host defense mechanisms against nematode parasites: Destruction of newborn *Trichinella spiralis* larvae by human antibodies and granulocytes. J Infect Dis 143:712, 1981.
49. Venturiello SM, Giambartolomei GH, Costantino SN: Immune killing of newborn *Trichinella* larvae by human leukocytes. Parasite Immunol 15:559, 1993.
50. Wassom DL, Gleich GJ: Damage to *Trichinella spiralis* newborn larvae by eosinophil major basic protein. Am J Trop Med Hyg 28:860, 1979.
51. Ruitenberg EJ: Killing of newborn larvae of *Trichinella spiralis* by eosinophil peroxidase in vitro. Eur J Immunol 11:843, 1981.
52. Bass DA, Szejda P: Mechanisms of killing of newborn larvae of *Trichinella spiralis* by neutrophils and eosinophils: Killing by generators of hydrogen peroxide in vitro. J Clin Invest 64:1558, 1979.
53. Herndon FJ, Kayes SG: Depletion of eosinophils by IL-5 monoclonal antibody treatment of mice infected with *Trichinella spiralis* does not alter parasite burden or immunologic resistance to reinfection. J Immunol 149:3642, 1992.
54. Komaroff A, Buchwald D: Symptoms and sign of chronic fatigue syndrome, Rev Infect Dis 13(suppl):S8, 1991.
55. Louthrenoo W, Mahanuphab P, Sanguanmitra P, et al: Trichinosis mimicking polymyositis in a patient with human immunodeficiency virus infection. Br J Rheumatol 32:1025, 1993.
56. Kociecka W: Trichinellosis: Human disease, diagnosis and treatment. Vet Parasitol 93:365, 2000.
57. Kociecka W, Kaczmarek J, Stachowski B: Electromyographic studies in persons with trichinellosis history. Wiad Parazytol 21:721, 1975.
58. Piergili-Fioretti D, Cestegne B, Frangills RF, et al: Re-evaluation after 15 years of patients involved in a trichinellosis outbreak caused by *Trichinella brikovi*. Vet Parasitol, 2005, in press.
59. Despommier DD: Trichinellosis. In Walls KW, Schantz PM (eds): Immunodiagnosis of Parasitic Diseases, Vol. 1. Helminthic Diseases. New York, Academic Press, 1986.
60. Zarlesge DS, La Rosa G: Molecular and biochemical methods for parasite differentiation within the genus *Trichinella*. Vet Parasitol 93:279, 2000.
61. Andrews JRH, Bandi C, Pozio E, et al: Identification of *Trichinella pseudospiralis* from a human case using random amplified polymorphic DNA. Am J Trop Med Hyg 53:185, 1995.
62. Weatherly NF: Anatomical pathology. In Campbell WC (ed): *Trichinella* and Trichinosis. New York, Plenum Press, 1983, p 173.
63. Gutierrez Y: Trichinelloidea: *Trichuris, Trichinella* and *Capillaria*-Dioctophymatoidea: *Dioctophyma*. In Diagnostic Pathology of Parasitic Infections with Clinical Correlations. Philadelphia, Lea & Febiger, 1990, p 336.
64. Ellrodt A, Halfon P, Le Bras P, et al: Multifocal central nervous system lesions on three patients with trichinosis. Arch Neurol 44:432, 1987.
65. Rycsak M, Sober WA, Kandora TF, et al: Difficulties in diagnosing *Trichinella* encephalitis. Am J Trop Med Hyg 36:573, 1987.
66. Dupouy-Camet J, Kociecka W, Bruschi F, et al: Opinion on the diagnosis and treatment of human trichinellosis. Expert Opin Pharmacother 3:1117, 2002.

67. Kociecka W, Gabryel P, Leszyk A, et al: A case of fatal trichinellosis with early renal insufficiency and central nervous system involvement. Wiad Parazytol 33:545, 1987.
68. Tassi C, Materazzi L, Pozio E, et al: Creatine kinase isoenzymes in human trichinellosis. Clin Chim Acta 239:197, 1995.
69. Boczon K, Winiecka W, Kociecka W, et al: The diagnostic value of enzymatic and immunological test in human trichinellosis. Tropenmed Parasitol 32:109, 1981.
70. Patterson R, Roberts M, Slonka G, et al: Studies of immunoglobulins, bentonite flocculation and IgE, IgG and IgM antibodies in serum from patients with trichinosis. Am J Med 58:787, 1975.
71. Tassi C, Sparvoli N, Bruschi F: Specific and total IgE in human trichinellosis infection. Use of an amplified ELISA system. Clin Chem Enzymol Comm 3:81, 1990.
72. Ljungström I: Immunodiagnosis in man. In Campbell WC (ed): *Trichinella* and Trichinosis. New York, Plenum Press, 1983, p 403.
73. Dupouy-Camet J, van Knapen F, Ancelle T, et al: Etude des immunoglobulines specifiques (totales, IgG, IgM, IgA, IgE) en immunofluorescence indirecte et en ELISA chez quarante malades trichinés suivis pendant neuf mois. Pathol Biol (Paris) 36:803, 1988.
74. Brzosko W, Gancarz Z, Nowoslawski A: Immunofluorescence in the serological diagnosis of *Trichinella spiralis* infection. Exp Med Microbiol 17:355, 1965.
75. Ljungström I: Antibody response to *Trichinella spiralis*. In Kim C (ed): Trichinellosis. New York, Intext, 1974, p 449.
76. Engvall E, Ljungström I: Detection of human antibodies to *Trichinella spiralis* by enzyme-linked immunosorbent assay (ELISA). Acta Pathol Microbiol Scand 83:231, 1975.
77. Au ACS, Ko RC, Simon JW, et al: Study of acute trichinosis in Ghurkas: Specificity and sensitivity of enzyme-linked immunosorbent assays for IgM and IgE antibodies to *Trichinella* larval antigens in diagnosis. Trans R Soc Trop Med Hyg 77:412, 1983.
78. Mahannop P, Setasuban P, Mokarote N, et al: Immunodiagnosis of human trichinellosis and identification of specific antigen for *Trichinella spiralis*. Int J Parasitol 25:87, 1995.
79. Robert F, Weil B, Kassis N, et al: Investigation of immunofluorescence cross-reactions against *Trichinella spiralis* by Western blot (Immunoblot) analysis. Clin Diagn Lab Immunol 3:575, 1996.
80. Ortega-Pierres G, Ypez-Mulia L, Homan W, et al: Workshop on a detailed characterization of *Trichinella spiralis* antigens: A platform for future studies on antigens and antibodies to this parasite. Parasite Immunol 18:273, 1996.
81. Gamble R, Pozio E, Bruschi F, et al: International Commission on Trichinellosis: Recommendations on the use of serological tests for the detection of *Trichinella* infection in animals and man. Parasite 11:3, 2004.
82. Zarlenga D, Gamble HR: Molecular cloning and expression of an immunodominant 53-KDa excretory–secretory antigen from *Trichinella spiralis* muscle larvae. Mol Biochem Parasitol 42:165, 1990.
83. Bruschi F., Moretti A., Wassom D, et al: Use of a synthetic antigen for the serological diagnosis of human trichinellosis. Parasite 8:S141, 2001.
84. van Knapen F, Franchimont JH, Verdonk AR, et al: Detection of specific immunoglobulins (IgG, IgM, IgA, IgE) and total IgE levels in human trichinosis by means of the enzyme-linked immunosorbent assay (ELISA). Am J Trop Med Hyg 31:973, 1982.
85. Bruschi F, Tassi C, Pozio E: Parasite-specific antibody response in *Trichinella* sp. 3 human infection: A one year follow up. Am J Trop Med Hyg 43:186, 1990.
86. Ljungström I, Hammarström L, Kociecka W, et al: The sequential appearance of IgG subclasses and IgE during the course of *Trichinella spiralis* infection. Clin Exp Immunol 74:230, 1988.
87. Ivanoska D, Cuperlovic K, Gamble HR, et al: Comparative efficacy of antigen and antibody detection tests for human trichinellosis. J Parasitol 75:38, 1989.
88. Morales MA, Mele R, Sanchez M, et al: Increased CD8(+)-T-cell expression and a type 2 cytokine pattern during the muscular phase of *Trichinella* infection in humans. Infect Immun 70:233, 2002.
89. Pozio E, Varese P, Gomez Morales MA, et al: Comparison of human trichinellosis caused by *Trichinella spiralis* and *Trichinella britovi*. Am J Trop Med Hyg 48:568, 1993.
90. Yera H, Andiva S, Perret C, et al: Development and evaluation of a Western blot kit for diagnosis of human trichinellosis. Clin Diagn Lab Immunol 10:793, 2003.
91. Noeckler K, Pozio E, Voigt WP, et al: Detection of *Trichinella* infection in food animals. Vet Parasitol 93:335, 2000.
92. Gamble HR, Bessonov AS, Cuperlovic K, et al: International Commission on Trichinellosis: Recommendations on methods for the control of *Trichinella* in domestic and wild animals intended for human consumption. Vet Parasitol 93:393, 2000.
93. Murrell KD: *Trichinella spiralis*: Acquired immunity in swine. Exp Parasitol 59:347, 1985.
94. Marti HP, Murrell KD, Gamble HR: *Trichinella spiralis*: Immunization of pigs with newborn larval antigens. Exp Parasitol 63:68, 1987.

105

Angiostrongyliasis

TIM KUBERSKI

INTRODUCTION

Two species of *Angiostrongylus* cause two distinct diseases of importance. Their geographic distribution and clinical syndromes are different so they will be discussed separately. *Angiostrongylus cantonensis* causes a meningoencephalitis characterized by a high number of eosinophils in the cerebrospinal fluid (CSF). The disease is most commonly called eosinophilic meningitis and is prevalent in Southeast Asia and certain tropical Pacific islands. *Angiostrongylus costaricensis* causes an eosinophilic inflammation of the gastrointestinal tract that can mimic appendicitis and is found mainly in Central and South America.

Angiostrongylus cantonensis

AGENT

A. cantonensis was first described from China in 1935.[1] It is also known as the rat lungworm, living as an adult in the pulmonary arteries of the rat. The life cycle involves rats and mollusks, with humans being incidental hosts. The first human infection was reported from Taiwan in 1945.[2] In rats, adult worms in the pulmonary arteries produce fertilized eggs that develop into first-stage larvae.[3] These larvae penetrate the lung arterioles and move into the respiratory tract. They are then coughed up, swallowed, and passed in the feces. The larvae remain viable in the feces for variable periods, depending on moisture. They can remain infectious for several weeks in freshwater.[4] The life cycle can be completed only if these larvae are consumed by an appropriate mollusk intermediate host, usually land snails or slugs.[3] The larvae then mature into infectious third-stage larvae that remain infectious for the life of the mollusk. When a rat consumes a mollusk with viable larvae, the larvae penetrate its intestinal wall and enter the bloodstream. It is neurotropic and migrates preferentially to the central nervous system (CNS). In the CNS of the rat, the larvae mature into the fifth stage (young adults) and make their way from the subarachnoid space and sinusoids of the CNS into the pulmonary arteries, completing the life cycle. If a human consumes a mollusk with viable larvae, the larvae migrate

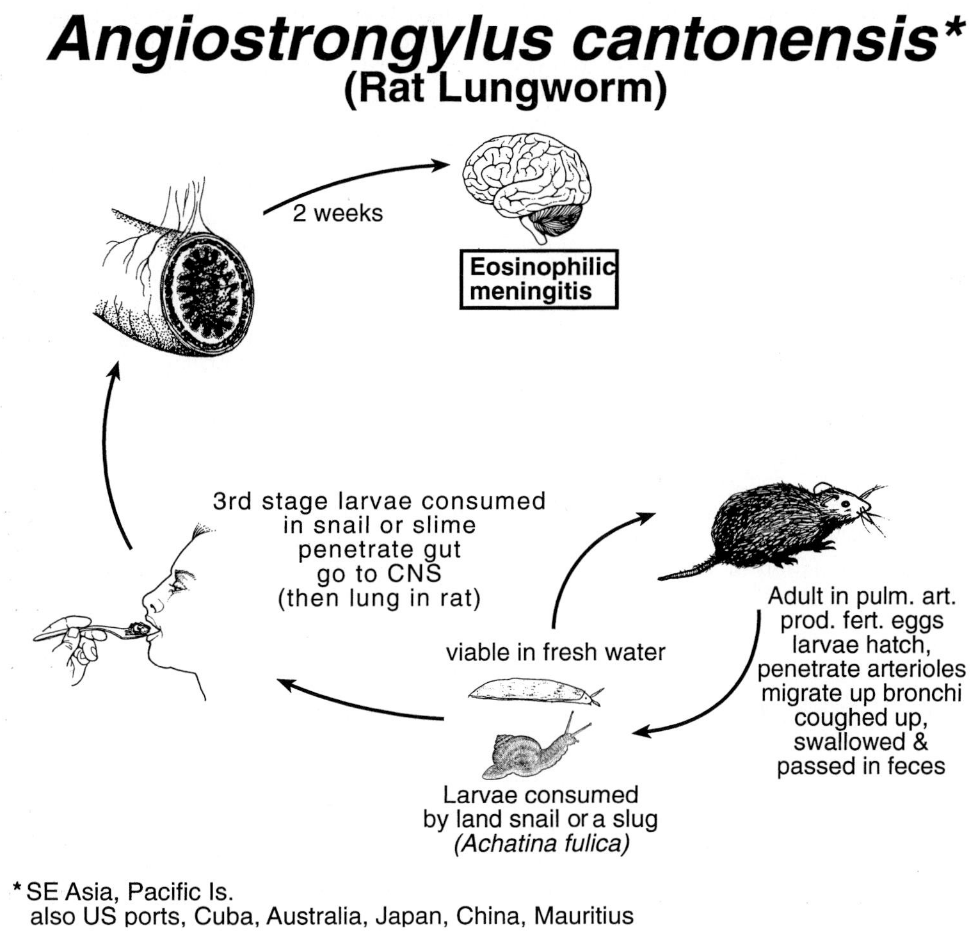

to the CNS. However, because the human is an abnormal host, the parasite is unable to complete its life cycle and dies in the CNS.[3,5]

EPIDEMIOLOGY

A. cantonensis is enzootic in Southeast Asia and on many tropical Pacific islands.[6] The first epidemic outbreaks of eosinophilic meningitis were reported from Ponape, Caroline Islands.[7] Many of the earliest reports of eosinophilic meningitis were from French Polynesia,[8–10] New Caledonia,[9] and Hawaii.[9–11] More recently, human cases have been described in Louisiana,[12] Australia,[13] Japan,[14] Vanuatu,[15] Fiji,[16] mainland China,[17] American Samoa,[18] Jamaica,[19] and in the Indian Ocean, Reunion and Mauritius.[20] Southeast Asia, Thailand,[21] and Taiwan[22] report the most cases. The parasite, and a few cases of human disease, have been reported from Africa.[6] Parasites without known human disease have been reported from Egypt, the Bahamas, and Puerto Rico.[6] The spread of this parasite is probably related to infected rats being transported to various places aboard ships or the introduction of mollusks such as the giant African snail *(Achatina fulica)*, which is capable of carrying many parasites.[6,22,23]

Purposeful or inadvertent ingestion of uncooked or marinated snails is one of the most important pieces of historical information from patients. In Thailand, eosinophilic meningitis may be related to the ingestion of sliced, pickled *Pila* snails, which are eaten as a delicacy.[21] Outbreaks of eosinophilic meningitis have been associated with consumption of raw snails, *Achatina fulica*.[24] However, there are many sporadic cases in which there is no obvious exposure to mollusks. Since cases of eosinophilic meningitis have been reported in vegetarians,[25] it is postulated that larvae can remain viable in the slime of snails or slugs and cause infection when contaminated, unwashed vegetables are eaten.[26] Many cases in young children are attributed to the unobserved ingestion of a contaminated snail or slug.[11]

A cold-blooded predator or scavenger (paratenic host) can be an incidental carrier of larvae if it has ingested an infected mollusk.[26] Thus, freshwater shrimp or crabs could carry larvae capable of causing infection if eaten raw.[27] Infectious larvae have been shown to be viable for long periods of time in such hosts, many of which are eaten raw in many tropical cultures.[26–28] These larvae are not capable of completing their life cycle, but can remain viable for long periods of time. Water in wells or cisterns could also be a source of viable larvae, becoming contaminated when released from drowned terrestrial mollusks.[9] Contamination of fingers with larvae during the collection and preparation of snails for eating is another potential source of infection.[22]

DISEASE

The incubation period is about two weeks.[21] Travel to an endemic area or exposure to mollusks is useful for establishing the time of exposure. The most common presentation is that of a nonbacterial meningitis.[29] Patients present with headache, nausea, vomiting, and neck stiffness.[21,29,30] Fever may not be a common finding in adults.[11] The main, and occasionally only, complaint is a headache, which is usually global and severe. The duration of illness ranges from 2 to 8 weeks.[21,29,30]

Paresthesias are a distinctive complaint; they are asymmetrical and usually noted on the extremities.[21,29,30] They are a complaint that may not be of obvious significance until the diagnosis of eosinophilic meningitis is considered. Paresthesias can separate this form of meningitis from others. The paresthesias can be persistent, lasting months after resolution of the illness.[29,31] Transient cranial nerve palsies, especially of the facial nerve, can occur, but serious neurologic sequelae are unusual.[21,29,30] Papilledema seems to be more common in children.[32] Most cases resolve spontaneously with complete recovery. However, serious complications and death do occur, probably resulting from larger numbers of migrating larvae or migration of larvae into critical parts of the brain.[22,29]

PATHOGENESIS AND IMMUNOLOGY

The hallmark of this infection is an eosinophilic CSF pleocytosis. This is the result of larvae migrating through the CNS. Death of the parasite in the CNS also may contribute to the eosinophilic response. Since the human is not a normal host, it is extremely rare for an adult worm to be found in the lungs of humans.[33] An episode of infection does not confer immunity.[9]

DIAGNOSIS

Finding high numbers of eosinophils in the CSF and travel to an endemic area should suggest eosinophilic meningitis (see Chapter 125). Low numbers of eosinophils can be seen in a variety of conditions, but finding greater than 10% eosinophils in the CSF should suggest this disease.[34] Typically, the CSF shows 100 to 5000 leukocytes per microliter, 10% to 90% of which are eosinophils.[29] The CSF protein is usually elevated, but the glucose is normal or mildly lowered.[29] A peripheral eosinophilia is not a consistent finding.

The differential diagnosis of eosinophils in the CSF should include other helminthic diseases, in particular gnathostomiasis and cysticercosis.[34] *Gnathostoma spinigerum* is also a cause of eosinophilic CSF pleocytosis in areas of Southeast Asia that are endemic for *A. cantonensis* (see Chapter 106).[35] *G. spinigerum* is not specifically neurotropic like *A. cantonensis*, involving the nervous system by random migration. The disease produced is characterized by nerve root pain, paraplegia, spinal cord lesions, xanthochromic CSF, and a much higher mortality rate. In addition, an ascarid parasite of raccoons, *Baylisascaris procyonis*, has rarely been the cause of eosinophilic meningoencephalitis in humans.[36] Certain nonparasitic agents, such as coccidioidomycosis and lymphomas of the CNS, can also be associated with an eosinophilic pleocytosis.[34]

Since paresthesias are common in eosinophilic meningitis, other illnesses causing paresthesias in the tropics need to be considered. Poisonings due to certain insecticides and ingestion of toxic fish or shellfish (e.g., ciguatera) can produce paresthesias.[29] The latter agents would generally not cause a classic aseptic meningitis picture.

Headaches frequently will improve dramatically after a lumbar puncture.[29] Ventricular dilation can occasionally be seen and is probably due to a transient communicating hydrocephalus caused by inflammation of the arachnoid decreasing the resorption of CSF. It is rare, but *A. cantonensis* larvae have been observed in the eye[37] and CSF.[23,38] A larger-bore needle used for spinal taps is thought to account for the increased number of larvae recovered from the CSF of patients in Taiwan.[23] A computed tomography (CT) scan of the brain in eosinophilic meningitis is generally nonspecific.[39,40] However, magnetic resonance imaging (MRI) with contrast dye can show meningeal enhancement as well as punctate areas of enhancement in the brain.[41] The usual absence of focal lesions on the CT scan helps distinguish eosinophilic meningitis from the focal lesions observed with neurocysticercosis and gnathostomiasis.[42] Patchy pulmonary infiltrates in the lower lung fields can occasionally be observed on the chest radiograph and presumably are due to migrating parasites.[43] Serology has been hampered by a lack of specificity and by cross-reactivity with other helminths.[44] Purification of antigens and defining the immunoglobulin G subclass antibody response have improved accuracy,[45] but the serodiagnosis of angiostrongyliasis is not routinely available. Elevated levels of immunoglobulin E in serum have been reported.[46]

TREATMENT

There is no specific treatment.[40] Anthelmintics and corticosteroids have been tried, but it is difficult to assess efficacy when there are no controlled studies and the disease is self-limited. Anthelmintics that cross the blood-brain barrier, such as praziquantel or albendazole, should theoretically work in this disease, but a systemic response to dying worms might make the condition worse.[15,21] Adjunctive corticosteroids or corticosteroids alone in severe cases (i.e., severe encephalitis or cranial nerve damage) might be a consideration since in such settings the inflammatory response might be contributing to the disease. Corticosteroids are not believed to alter the course of uncomplicated disease.[21]

PREVENTION AND CONTROL

Prevention is by educating travelers or persons in endemic areas that snails, slugs, freshwater shrimp, and crabs must be cooked, not simply marinated or refrigerated, before they are eaten. Vegetables must be washed if eaten uncooked. Commonly infected mollusks like the giant African land snail *A. fulica* should be handled carefully to avoid contamination of the fingers with larvae. Control of mollusks and planarians and reducing the number of rats are also important measures.

Angiostrongylus costaricensis

AGENT

A. costaricensis was first described from Costa Rica in 1971[47] and has a life cycle similar to *A. cantonensis* in that rodents are the definitive host and mollusks are intermediate hosts.[48] *A. costaricensis*, however, develops into its adult form in the mesenteric arteries of rats. The most important rat is the cotton rat (*Sigmodon hispidus*).[48] Humans are abnormal hosts; thus, the parasite is unable to complete its life cycle, dying in the gastrointestinal tract.[47]

EPIDEMIOLOGY

Human infection occurs predominantly from southern Mexico to Argentina and in Costa Rica. The clinical disease

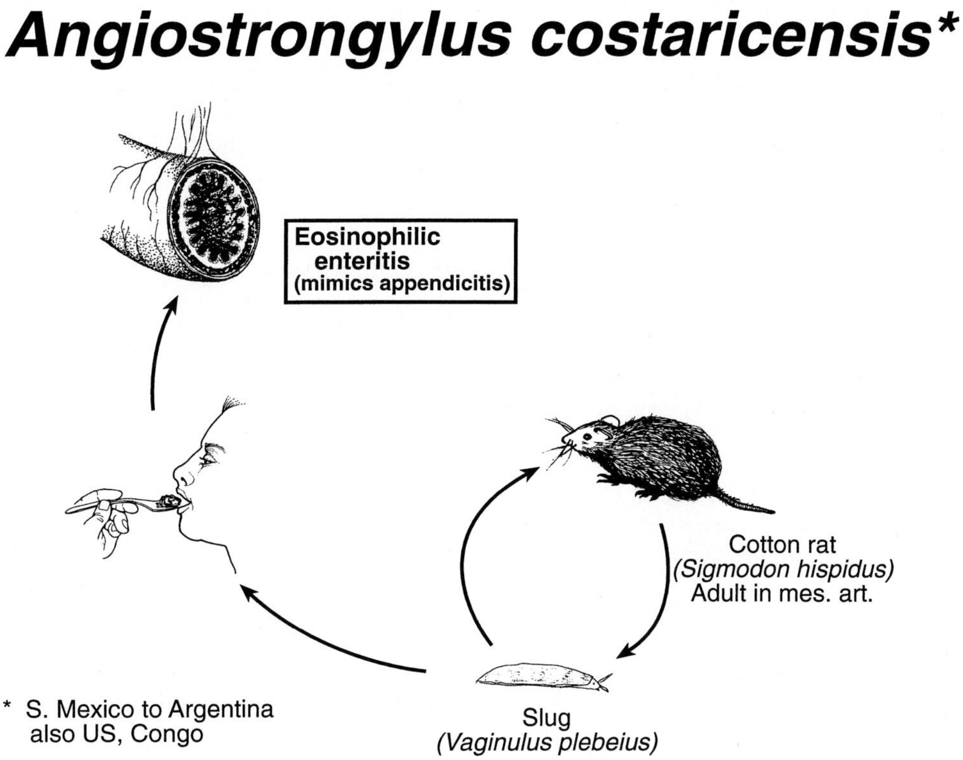

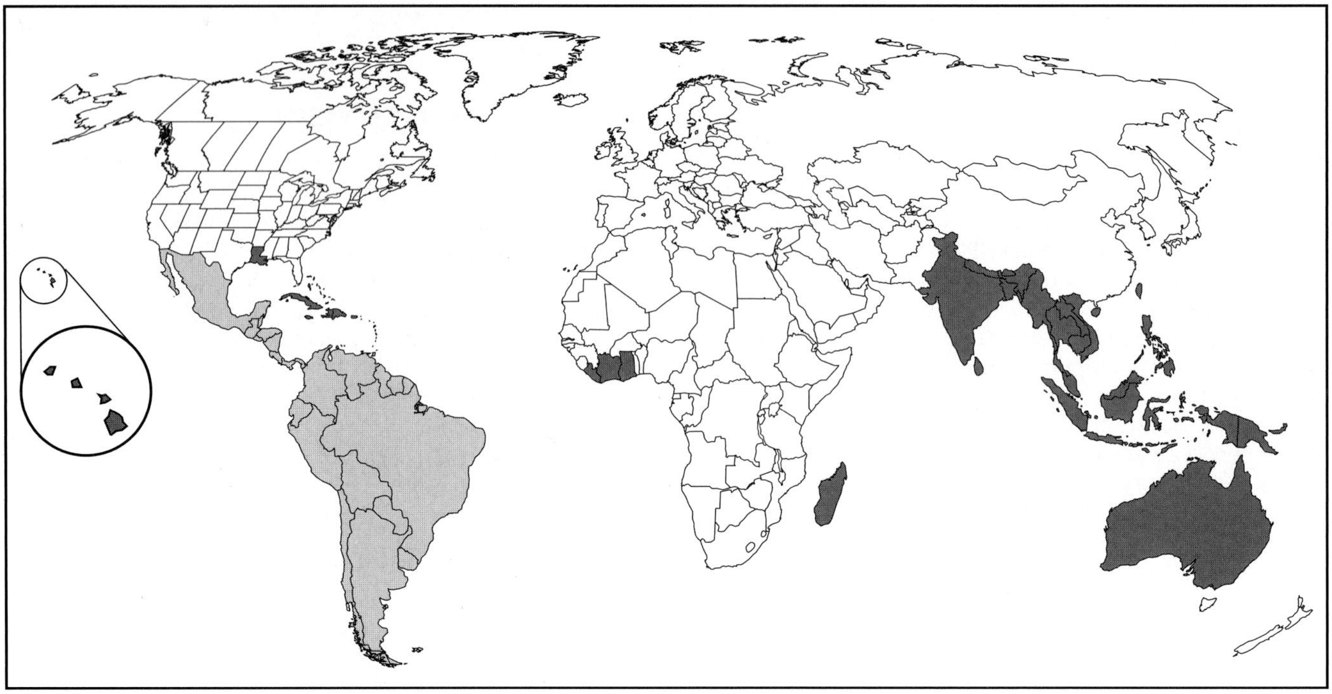

Angiostrongylus spp.
■ *Angiostrongylus costaricensis*
■ *Angiostrongylus cantonensis*

had been recognized in Costa Rica in the 1950s before *A. costaricensis* was described. Following its description in 1971,[47] abdominal angiostrongyliasis has been reported from Honduras, Mexico, Venezuela,[48] Martinique, Dominican Republic, Puerto Rico,[49] Argentina, Brazil,[50] Nicaragua,[51] and the United States.[52] A few apparently autochthonous cases have been reported from the United States (Los Angeles)[52] and Africa (Congo).[53] Parasites have been found in rodents in Colombia[54] and Panama[55] without reports of human cases.

At least 12 species of rat and one coati have been shown to be naturally infected.[56] The rat passes first-stage larvae in its feces for up to 8 months.[48] A mollusk intermediate host feeds on the feces of the rat and the larvae transform into infectious third-stage larvae in the mollusk. The mode of transmission to humans is not established. It is assumed that infectious larvae from a molluscan intermediate host, such as the slug *Vaginulus plebeius*, contaminate water or vegetation with infectious larvae, which are inadvertently consumed by humans.[48] Although this particular slug is not indigenous to the continental United States, it has been found on imported produce and flowers.[52] Most human cases have been described in children between the ages of 6 and 13 years.[57] Higher, rather than lower, socioeconomic status is more common.[57] In general, males outnumber females by 2:1.

DISEASE

The incubation period for abdominal angiostrongyliasis is not known, but is estimated to be 3 to 4 weeks.[52] Clinical findings tend to mimic those of appendicitis[57] or an inflamed Meckel's diverticulum.[52] Patients have fever, nausea, vomiting, and abdominal pain. The abdominal pain is frequently localized to the right lower quadrant.[56] Occasionally a painful mass in the right lower quadrant can be noted on rectal examination.[57] The symptoms are generally more indolent than those typical of acute appendicitis. Patients tend to have recurrent episodes over several months. Surgical exploration on the suspicion of appendicitis is frequently observed. Complications can be abscess formation, obstruction, and infarction of the bowel.[49] A few deaths have been reported.[57] Occasionally, the testicular artery can be involved, but this diagnosis is generally not made before surgery, which is usually done for a suspected torsion.[57,58]

PATHOGENESIS

In humans, the parasite usually confines itself to the abdominal cavity; it is rare for parasites to be found outside the gastrointestinal tract. Inadvertent ingestion of slugs, either chopped up in salads or on vegetation contaminated with their mucous secretions, can accidentally allow infectious third-stage larvae into the gastrointestinal tract of humans. The larvae eventually enter the mesenteric arteries where they mature into adults. The adult parasite in the mesenteric arteries can cause arteritis, thrombosis, infarction, and gastrointestinal hemorrhage.[59] Eggs from adults can lodge in capillaries, producing an inflammatory reaction within the intestinal wall. The eggs do not hatch, but degenerate and cause an eosinophilic granulomatous reaction.[60] The resultant histopathologic changes could be suggestive of an allergic granulomatous angiitis (Churg-Strauss vasculitis).[49] Transmission between humans does not take place. The parts of the intestinal tract usually involved are the terminal ileum and appendix, but other parts of the intestine and occasionally the regional lymph nodes can be involved.[47,57,60]

DIAGNOSIS

There are no diagnostic tests other than to demonstrate the parasite or its eggs in tissue. Most patients have a leukocytosis, an observation also common in appendicitis, but suspicion of this parasite should be raised when there is an associated eosinophilia on the peripheral blood smear. The eosinophilia can range from 11% to 82% with a leukocytosis of 10,000 to 50,000 white blood cells per microliter.[48,57] The worms usually localize to the mesenteric arteries of the ileocecal region, and radiologic examination of the gastrointestinal tract may show bowel edema and spasticity in that area.[56,57] Stool examination will reveal no forms of *A. costaricensis*. However, a stool examination for parasites is reasonable since *Enterobius vermicularis* could cause similar changes.[52] Human anisakiasis or visceral larva migrans due to *Toxocara* spp. could also mimic abdominal angiostrongyliasis.[61] Several serologic tests have been described, but they are not readily available and not of much clinical use.[62]

TREATMENT

No specific medical treatment is known. Surgical treatment for acute intestinal inflammation may be necessary. The use of anthelmintics has not been systematically studied, but thiabendazole or diethylcarbamazine has been suggested.[57] Acute episodes can be uncomplicated and resolve spontaneously. The prognosis is generally good.

PREVENTION AND CONTROL

Avoidance of slugs and the ingestion of raw food and water that might be contaminated by imperceptible slugs or slime from slugs are the cornerstones of prevention and control. Control of rats is important in preventing the spread of this parasite.

REFERENCES

1. Chen HT: Un nouveau nematode pulmonaire *Pulmonema cantonensis* n.g.n. sp., des rats de Canton. Ann Parasitol Hum Comp 13:312, 1935.
2. Beaver PC, Rosen L: Memorandum on the first report of *Angiostrongylus* in man, by Nomura and Lin, 1945. Am J Trop Med Hyg 13:589, 1964.
3. Mackerras MJ, Sandars DF: The life history of the rat lung-worm, *Angiostrongylus cantonensis* (Chen) (Nematoda: Metastrongylidae). Aust J Zool 3:1, 1955.
4. Richards CS, Merritt JW: Studies on *Angiostrongylus cantonensis* in molluscan intermediate hosts. J Parasitol 53:382, 1967.
5. Sonakul D: Pathologic findings in four cases of human angiostrongyliasis. Southeast Asian J Trop Med Public Health 9:220, 1978.
6. Kliks MM, Palumbo NE: Eosinophilic meningitis beyond the Pacific Basin: The global dispersal of a peridomestic zoonosis caused by *Angiostrongylus cantonensis*, the nematode lungworm of rats. Soc Sci Med 34:199, 1992.
7. Bailey CA: An Epidemic of Eosinophilic Meningitis, a Previously Undescribed Disease, Occurring on Ponape, Eastern Carolines. Bethesda, MD, U.S. Naval Medical Research Institute, Project NM 005 007, Report No. 7, October 14, 1948.
8. Rosen L, Laigret J, Bories S: Observations on an outbreak of eosinophilic meningitis on Tahiti, French Polynesia. Am J Hyg 74:26, 1961.
9. Rosen L, Loison G, Laigret J, et al: Studies on eosinophilic meningitis. 3. Epidemiologic and clinical observations on Pacific islands and the possible etiologic role of *Angiostrongylus cantonensis*. Am J Epidemiol 85:17, 1967.
10. Rosen L, Chappell R, Laqueur GL, et al: Eosinophilic meningoencephalitis caused by a metastrongylid lung-worm of rats. JAMA 179:620, 1962.
11. Char DFB, Rosen L: Eosinophilic meningitis among children in Hawaii. J Pediatr 70:28, 1967.
12. New D, Little MD, Cross J: *Angiostrongylus cantonensis* infection from eating raw snails. N Engl J Med 332:1105, 1995.
13. Heaton DC, Gutteridge BH: Angiostrongyliasis in Australia. Aust NZ J Med 10:255, 1980.
14. Kojima S, Hata H, Kobayashi M, et al: Eosinophilic meningitis: A suspected case of angiostrongylosis found in Shizuoka Prefecture, Honshu, Japan. Am J Trop Med Hyg 28:36, 1979.
15. Bowden DK: Eosinophilic meningitis in the New Hebrides: Two outbreaks and two deaths. Am J Trop Med Hyg 30:1141, 1981.
16. Uchikawa R, Takagi M, Matayoshi S, et al: The presence of *Angiostrongylus cantonensis* on Vitu Levu, Fiji. J Helminthol 58:231, 1984.
17. Yang SQ, Yu BW, Chen YS, et al: The first case of angiostrongylus cantonensis in the mainland of China. Chin Med J 101:783, 1988.
18. Beck MJ, Cardina TM, Alicata JE: Eosinophilic meningitis due to *Angiostrongyliasis cantonensis* in American Samoa. Hawaii Med J 39:254, 1980.
19. Slom TJ, Cortese MM, Gerber SI, et al: An outbreak of eosinophilic meningitis caused by *Angiostrongylus cantonensis* in travelers returning from the Caribbean. N Engl J Med 346:668, 2002.
20. Petithory J, Jay M, Sister Colette: Premier cas de méningite à éosinophiles à la Reunion probablement dû à *Angiostrongylus*. Bull Soc Pathol Exot Filiales 70:151, 1977.
21. Punyagupta S, Juttijudata P, Bunnag T: Eosinophilic meningitis in Thailand. Clinical studies of 484 typical cases probably caused by *Angiostrongylus cantonensis*. Am J Trop Med Hyg 24:921, 1975.
22. Yii CY, Chen CY, Chen ER, et al: Epidemiologic studies of eosinophilic meningitis in southern Taiwan. Am J Trop Med Hyg 24:447, 1975.
23. Wallace GD, Rosen L: Studies on eosinophilic meningitis. V. Molluscan hosts of *Angiostrongylus cantonensis* on Pacific Islands. Am J Trop Med Hyg 18:206, 1969.
24. Kliks MM, Kroenke K, Hardman JM: Eosinophilic radiculomyeloencephalitis: An angiostrongyloidiasis outbreak in American Samoa related to ingestion of *Achatina fulica* snails. Am J Trop Med Hyg 31:1114, 1982.
25. Fuller AJ, Munckhof W, Kiers L, et al: Eosinophilic meningitis due to *Angiostrongylus cantonensis*. West J Med 159:78, 1993.
26. Wallace GD, Rosen L: Studies on eosinophilic meningitis. VI. Experimental infection of rats and other homoiothermic vertebrates with *Angiostrongylus cantonensis*. Am J Epidemiol 89:331, 1969.
27. Wallace GD, Rosen L: Studies on eosinophilic meningitis. 2. Experimental infection of shrimp and crabs with *Angiostrongylus cantonensis*. Am J Epidemiol 84:120, 1966.
28. Wallace GD, Rosen L: Studies on eosinophilic meningitis. IV. Experimental infection of fresh-water and marine fish with *Angiostrongylus cantonensis*. Am J Epidemiol 85:395, 1967.
29. Kuberski T, Wallace GD: Clinical manifestations of eosinophilic meningitis due to *Angiostrongylus cantonensis*. Neurology 29:1566, 1979.
30. Yii CY: Clinical observations on eosinophilic meningitis and meningoencephalitis caused by *Angiostrongylus cantonensis* on Taiwan. Am J Trop Med Hyg 25:233, 1976.
31. Clouston PD, Corbett AJ, Pryor DS, et al: Eosinophilic meningitis: Cause of a chronic pain syndrome. J Neurol Neurosurg Psychiatry 53:778, 1990.
32. Hwang KP, Chen ER: Clinical studies on *Angiostrongyliasis cantonensis* among children in Taiwan. Southeast Asian J Trop Med Public Health 22:194, 1991.
33. Pirisi M, Gutierrez Y, Minini C, et al: Fatal human pulmonary infection caused by an *Angiostrongylus*-like nematode. Clin Infect Dis 20:59, 1995.
34. Kuberski T: Eosinophils in the cerebrospinal fluid. Ann Intern Med 91:70, 1979.
35. Punyagupta S, Bunnag T, Juttijudata P: Eosinophilic meningitis in Thailand. Clinical and epidemiological characteristics of 162 patients with myeloencephalitis probably caused by *Gnathostoma spingerum*. J Neurol Sci 96:241, 1990.

36. Huff DS, Neafie RC, Binder MJ: Case 4. The first fatal *Baylisascaris* infection in humans; An infant with eosinophilic meningoencephalitis. Pediatr Pathol 2:345, 1984.
37. Prommindaroj K, Leelawongs N, Pradatsundarasar A: Human angiostrongyliasis of the eye in Bangkok. Am J Trop Med Hyg 1:759, 1962.
38. Kuberski T, Bart RD, Briley JM, et al: Recovery of *Angiostrongylus cantonensis* from cerebrospinal fluid of a child with eosinophilic meningitis. J Clin Microbiol 9:629, 1979.
39. Ko RC, Chiu MC, Kum W, et al: First report of human angiostrongyliasis in Hong Kong diagnosed by computerized axial tomography (CAT) and enzyme linked immunosorbent assay. Trans R Soc Trop Med Hyg 78:354, 1984.
40. Koo J, Pien F, Kliks MM: *Angiostrongylus (Parastrongylus)* eosinophilic meningitis. Rev Infect Dis 10:1155, 1988.
41. Hsu WY, Chen JY, Chien CT, et al: Eosinophilic meningitis caused by *Angiostrongylus cantonensis*. Pediatr Infect Dis J 9:443, 1990.
42. Weller PF, Liu LX: Eosinophilic meningitis. Semin Neurol 13:161, 1993.
43. Shih SL, Hsu CH, Huang FY, et al: *Angiostrongylus cantonensis* infection in infants and young children. Pediatr Infect Dis J 11:1064, 1992.
44. Welch JS, Dobson C, Campbell GR: Immunodiagnosis and seroepidemiology of *Angiostrongylus cantonensis* zoonoses in man. Trans R Soc Trop Med Hyg 74:614, 1980.
45. Intapan PM, Maleewong W, Sawanyawisuth K, et al: Evaluation of human IgG subclass antibodies in the serodiagnosis of angiostrongyliasis. Parasitol Res 89:425, 2003.
46. Tsai HC, Liu YC, Kunin CM, et al: Eosinophilic meningitis caused by *Angiostrongylus cantonensis*: Report of 17 cases. Am J Med 111:109, 2001.
47. Morera P, Cespedes R: Angiostrongylosis abdominal. Una nueva parasitosis humana. Acta Medica Costaricense 14:159, 1971.
48. Morera P: Life history and redescription of *Angiostrongylus costaricensis* Morera and Cespedes, 1971. Am J Trop Med Hyg 22:613, 1973.
49. Vazquez JJ, Boils PL, Sola JJ, et al: Angiostrongyliasis in a European patient: A rare cause of gangrenous ischemic enterocolitis. Gastroenterology 105:1544, 1993.
50. Graeff-Teixeira C, Camillo-Coura L, Lenzi HL: Clinical and epidemiological aspects of abdominal angiostrongyliasis in southern Brazil. Rev Inst Med Trop São Paulo 33:373, 1991.
51. Duarte Z, Morera P, Vuong PN: Abdominal angiostrongyliasis in Nicaragua: A clinicopathological study on a series of 12 case reports. Ann Parasitol Hum Comp 66:259, 1991.
52. Hulbert TV, Larsen RA, Chandrasoma PT: Abdominal angiostrongyliasis mimicking acute appendicitis and Meckel's diverticulum: Report of a case in the United States and review. Clin Infect Dis 14:836, 1992.
53. Baird JK, Neafie RC, Lanoie L, et al: Abdominal angiostrongylosis in an African man: Case study. Am J Trop Med Hyg 37:353, 1987.
54. Malek EA: Presence of *Angiostrongylus costaricensis* Morera and Cespedes 1971 in Columbia. Am J Trop Med Hyg 30:81, 1981.
55. Tesh RB, Ackermam LJ, Dietz WH, et al: *Angiostrongylus costaricensis* in Panama: Prevalence and pathologic findings in wild rodents infected with the parasite. Am J Trop Med Hyg 22:348, 1973.
56. Morera P: Abdominal angiostrongyliasis. In Strickland GT (ed): Hunter's Tropical Medicine, 7th ed. Philadelphia, WB Saunders, 1991, p 771.
57. Loria-Cortes R, Lobo-Sanahuja JF: Clinical abdominal angiostrongylosis. A study of 116 children with intestinal eosinophilic granuloma caused by *Angiostrongylus costaricensis*. Am J Trop Med Hyg 29:538, 1980.
58. Ruiz PJ, Morera P: Spermatic artery obstruction caused by *Angiostrongylus costaricensis* Morera and Cespedes, 1971. Am J Trop Med Hyg 32:1458, 1983.
59. Silvera CT, Ghali VS, Roven S, et al: Angiostrongyliasis: A rare cause of gastrointestinal hemorrhage. Am J Gastroenterol 84:329, 1989.
60. Frenkel JK: *Angiostrongylus cantonensis* infections. In Binford CH, Connor DH (eds): Pathology of Tropical and Extraordinary Diseases, vol. 2. Washington, DC, Armed Forces Institute of Pathology, 1976, p 452.
61. Ash LR: Human anisakiasis misdiagnosed as abdominal angiostrongyliasis. Clin Infect Dis 16:332, 1993.
62. Sauerbrey M: A precipitin test for the diagnosis of human abdominal angiostrongyliasis. Am J Trop Med Hyg 26:1156, 1977.

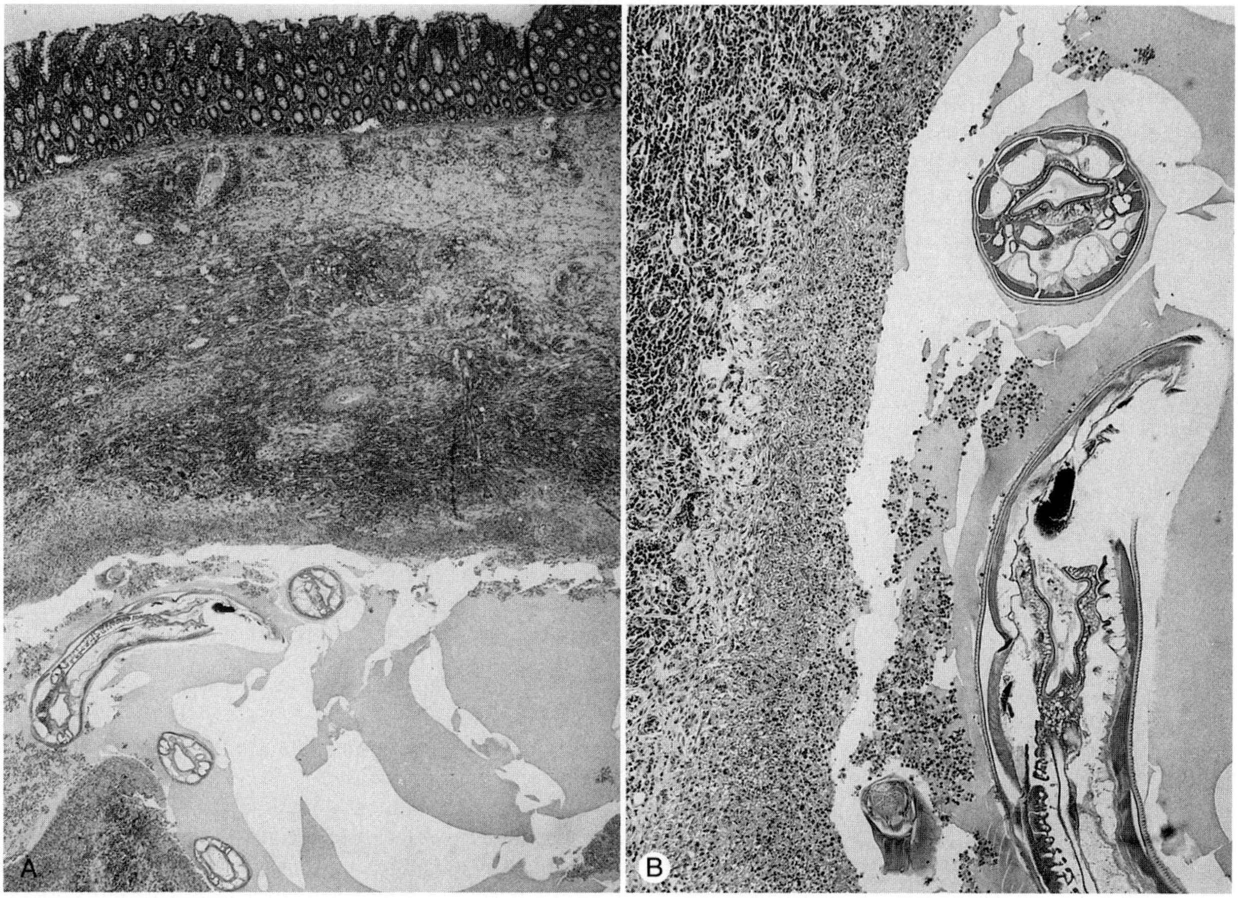

FIGURE 106-5 *Oesophagostomum* sp. in human colon. *A,* View of abscess in the wall of the colon, showing sections of the parasite. (H&E stain, ×22.) *B,* The wall of the abscess and sections of the worm. (H&E stain, ×70.)

from those of hookworms.[57] An enzyme-linked immunosorbent assay (ELISA) produced much cross-reactivity with other parasites, but if made specific for detection of IgG_4 it gave a 95% positivity.[58] A PCR assay for specific amplification of DNA of *O. bifurcum* gave better results.[59] Albendazole, used in the cases from Togo and Ghana, was found effective in mixed infections with hookworms against both parasites.[60,61] Pyrantel pamoate was effective against *Oesophagostomum* but not against the hookworms.[61]

Ternidens

One species of this genus, *Ternidens deminutus*, has been implicated in human infections.[62] This parasite has many similarities with *Oesophagostomum*, both morphologically and biologically: it also inhabits the colon where ulcerations and nodular lesions are seen, although a cause-effect relationship between the worms and the lesions remains obscure.[63] The life cycle of *T. deminutus* is mostly unknown, and the mode of infection in humans and animals remains a mystery. Experiments in humans with penetration of larvae through the skin have failed, and thus the existence of an arthropod intermediate host has been postulated.[63] *Ternidens* is usually a parasite of monkeys in Africa, India, and Indonesia; human infections have been recorded only in southeastern Africa,[64] especially Zambia and Zimbabwe, where most of the studies on this parasite have been carried out. The prevalence in the general population in Zambia and Zimbabwe is variable depending on the area studied, with the highest incidence being 87%.[64]

The symptoms produced by *Ternidens* are not well characterized, and it seems that most patients are asymptomatic. Intestinal blood loss is slight, and anemia does not develop; eosinophilia has not been detected, and although diarrhea has been observed in animals, it has not occurred in humans.[64] The lack of symptoms is likely due to the low number of worms present in the colon: eight worms in a few cases, most harboring three to five. Thiabendazole and pyrantel pamoate have been used to treat patients, curing about 90% of infections.[65,66] The diagnosis is made in stool samples by recognition of the eggs, which are easily mistaken for hookworm eggs; careful measurement of the eggs allows proper identification.

ASCARIDINA

Anisakis, Pseudoterranova, Baylisascaris, and *Lagochilascaris*

The Ascaridinae are one of the largest groups of nematodes, with one to several species found in each vertebrate species. Many genera are known in this group including *Ascaris lumbricoides* (see Chapter 109) and species of

Toxocara (see Chapter 103).[1] Other species of the Ascaridinae produce zoonotic infections in humans, such as *Anisakis, Pseudoterranova, Baylisascaris*, and *Lagochilascaris*, some of which—the anisakids—are of paramount importance in certain geographic areas.[67,68]

In general, members of the Ascaridinae are large parasites, for example, species of *Ascaris*, which can be about 35 cm long and inhabits the small intestine of humans and other animals. Most species have direct life cycles: Eggs are evacuated with the fecal mass of the host, and the eggs mature in soil to infective stages. After ingestion of infective eggs by a new host, the eggs release larvae that migrate to the lungs and back to the intestine, where they develop into adults.[1] Other species have indirect cycles: *Anisakis* and *Pseudoterranova*, parasites of marine mammals, have squid and fish as intermediate hosts[69]; and species of *Baylisascaris*, nematodes found in the intestine of raccoons, skunks, bears, martens, and other carnivores, have small rodents, birds, and many other small vertebrates as their intermediate hosts.

Anisakis and *Pseudoterranova*

Anisakiasis ("herring worm disease") and pseudoterranoviasis ("cod worm disease") generally present clinically in a manner that is indistinguishable from one another, and thus they are referred to simply as "anisakiasis." An apparent confusion in the medical literature has occurred because the names of the parasites have changed several times as knowledge of their relationships has increased and their classification improved.[70] The genus *Anisakis* has two important species, *A. simplex* and *A. physeteris*, previously known in their larval stages recovered from human infections, as *Anisakis* larva types I and II, respectively.[69] They are parasites of whales (Cetacea), seals, sea lions, walruses, and other Pinnipediae. The genus *Pseudoterranova* (known in the past as *Ascaris, Porracecum, Terranova*, and *Phocanema*) has one important species complex, *P. decipiens*, which consists of seven species impossible to differentiate based on the morphology of their larval stages.[71] This genus is parasitic exclusively of members of the Pinnipediae.[69,71] Since all these names are found in medical journals and textbooks, they are mentioned here only for clarification. Specific names should be used for the parasite, or for the disease, only when the larva recovered from humans is conclusively identified by competent taxonomists. Pathologists should use the generic "anisakid" to be precise and *Anisakis* or *Pseudoterranova* only when they identify either genus in tissue sections or on the recovered larva. In tissue sections, the larva is rarely cut in such a manner that it reveals structures that make separation of these two genera possible.[1] Clinicians studying patients suspected of suffering from anisakiasis based on serologic or skin tests using larval antigens should never refer to the patient as having a specific disease or infection (e.g., anisakiasis due to *Anisakis simplex*). There is too much serologic cross-reactivity among the different species of larvae and even much more uncertainty as to the real culprit for the reaction to an applied allergen.

As stated, anisakid worms inhabit the stomach of their final hosts, where they bury the anterior portion of their bodies into the gastric mucosa and grow attached to it. Eggs are produced and evacuated with feces into seawater where they mature, and each develops a larva that hatches to become part of the zooplankton. Larvae are ingested by squid and several other species of macro-invertebrates, where they develop into infective larvae. Ingestion of these infected intermediate hosts by smaller fish allows the larvae to grow further and remain in the infective stage. Ingestion of infected squid, macro-invertebrates, or fish by the final hosts produces the infection in the stomach.[1] Humans become infected by ingestion of raw marine fish in delicacies such as sushi, sashimi, oka, poisson cru, ceviche, and so on.[70] The infection is thus more important in Japan, where the number of cases reported is in the thousands, because raw marine fish is a daily staple.[67,68] The infection is found sporadically in other places where consumption of raw fish has been become fashionable, or where fish is a large part of the diet and occasional larvae are not killed in undercooked dishes. A small number of cases have been diagnosed in the United States[72–74] and South America.[75] A larger number in Europe,[76] especially in the Netherlands, where the infection was first recognized in the early 1960s, was traced to the consumption of raw herring[77–79]; public health measures have controlled the infection. In Spain, the disease was recognized in the early 1990s[80] and some cases reported are clinically and pathologically similar to the experience in Japan. However, in Spain an inordinate number of patients with allergies have been considered to have *Anisakis* infection based on serologic tests, IgE determination, skin tests with extracts of *Anisakis simplex* larvae, or antecedents of consumption of raw fish.[81–84] This needs further verification.

Anisakiasis is mostly an infection of the gastrointestinal tract; sometimes ectopic locations are encountered, such as the peritoneal cavity and its organs[67,68] and once the lungs.[85] In the majority of cases, the infection is produced by a single larva, uncommonly by two and rarely by several.[1] The lesion in humans is dictated by the biologic behavior of the parasite, which buries its anterior portion in the gastrointestinal mucosa and tries to develop into an adult.[69] Because humans are abnormal hosts, the parasite does not become an adult, dies as a larva, and elicits an abscess with marked inflammation, edema, and tissue eosinophilia[1] (Fig. 106-6). This abscess may be of sufficient size to be clinically palpated or seen on radiographs as a mass. The lesion is found anywhere in the esophagus, stomach, or small or large intestine. Sometimes the larva perforates the viscus wall and enters the peritoneal cavity, where it dies, producing the abscess (tumor), mostly in the omentum and only occasionally on the surface of the viscera.[67,68] Larvae have been recovered from the peritoneum by surgeons during exploratory laparotomies and in one patient under dialysis in the effluent.[86] Some persons have symptoms of itching or of a scratchy sensation in the mouth or throat during or soon after a meal of raw or insufficiently cooked fish.[74] A sensation of a foreign element (the worm) in the oral cavity makes the person retch and recover the bothersome worm, or expectorate it after a paroxysm of coughing. A good number of the cases of anisakiasis reported in the United States have presented in this manner, produced by *Pseudoterranova*, a worm that apparently has a lesser capacity for tissue invasion.[74] The recovered larva is often submitted to the physician, who should reassure the patient of the benign nature of the condition. In other cases in the United States, a larva has been found in histologic sections of the intestinal wall and correctly diagnosed as *Anisakis*.[72]

Clinically, for diagnostic and therapeutic purposes, anisakiasis is classified as gastric, intestinal, or extraintestinal.[69]

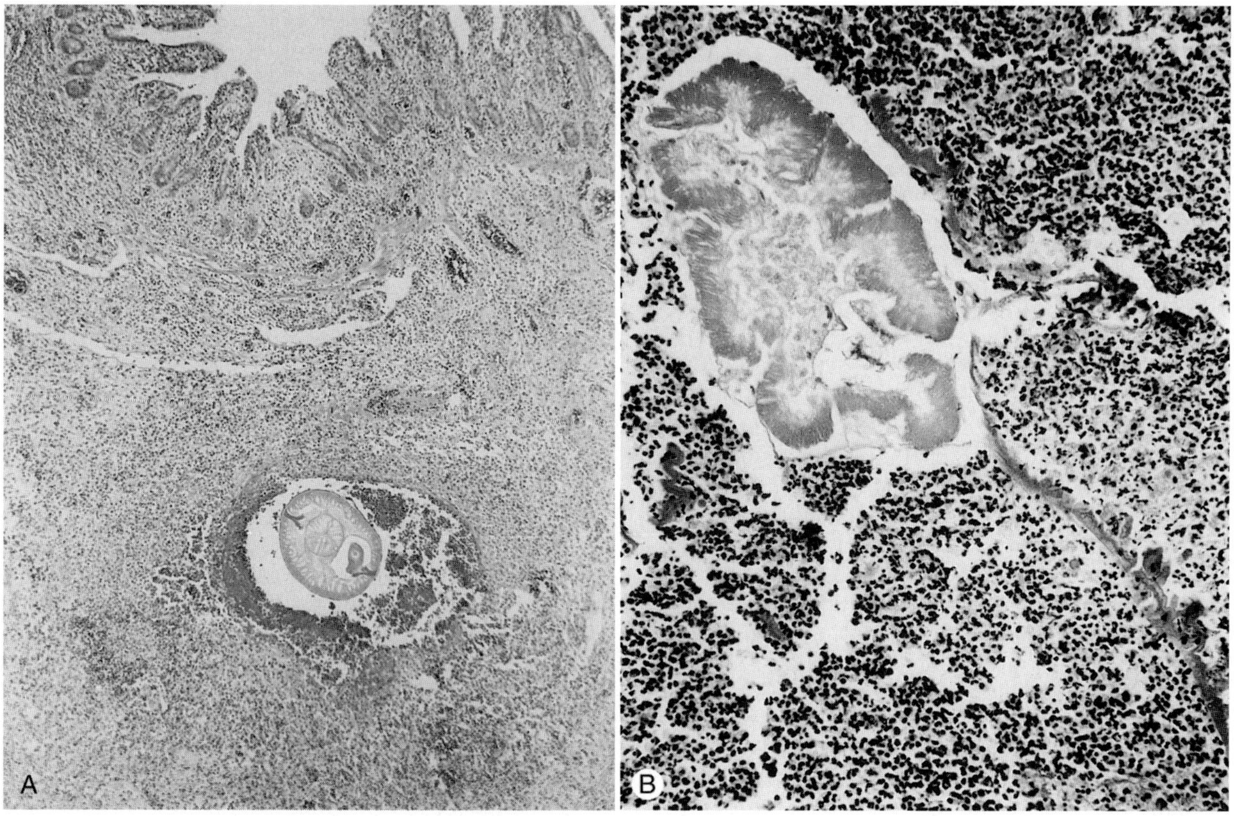

FIGURE 106-6 *Anisakis* in intestinal wall. *A,* View of the lesion showing a section of a well-preserved worm. (H&E stain, ×55.) *B,* Another patient with a similar lesion, but a markedly degenerated worm. (H&E stain, ×200.)

Often, the clinical presentation is acute; in some it has an indolent course. The main symptoms are abdominal with epigastric pain accompanied by nausea and vomiting. Sometimes the parasite is recovered with the vomitus. Abdominal distention and other clinical and radiographic signs and symptoms of intestinal obstruction may be evident.[69] These are accompanied by diarrhea, followed by normal stools or constipation, and blood and mucus in the stools. A movable, discrete mass may be palpated; and if contrast radiographs are obtained, the mass is easily seen as a defect of the intestinal wall. The mass and the symptoms resolve spontaneously in some instances, the so-called evanescent tumor of the stomach, in places where it has been observed more commonly. Mild fever, leukocytosis, and eosinophilia are almost always present, as is some amount of peritoneal fluid, which is rich in leukocytes and eosinophils. Endoscopic examination of the stomach and duodenum may reveal a red, bleeding, often ulcerated lesion, sometimes with the worm at the center with its anterior portion embedded in the mucosa and the rest of the body extending into the lumen. If the worm is detected, it can be pulled out with forceps; this usually suffices as treatment of the condition.[67,68] In radiographs the worm may be also seen as a negative image in the contrast media, in spite of the relatively small size of the parasite, 2.0 to 3.5 cm × 1 to 2 mm. Worms in the intestine are more difficult to retrieve endoscopically, and depending on how acute the symptoms are, the patient is often operated on for removal of the segment of inflamed bowel. The pathologist may find the worm on the open bowel segment grossly or sometimes on microscopic examination.[1]

Extraintestinal anisakiasis is difficult to diagnose clinically and usually requires exploratory surgery for treatment and pathologic diagnosis. The inflammatory mass is usually less than 4 cm in diameter and located anywhere in the abdominal cavity, from where it should be removed. Ectopic anisakiasis (those cases in which the worm is found outside the intestine) is rare. At least three cases diagnosed presumptively or based on Western blot have been reported in Japan.[85] The clinical diagnosis is difficult, especially since *Paragonimus, Gnathostoma, Fasciola,* and *Sparganum* produce similar syndromes. No medical treatment is available or used, since the disease resolves with removal of the worm.

Baylisascaris

Several species of *Baylisascaris* are known throughout the world as intestinal parasites of many lower vertebrates. These ascarids are common in raccoons *(B. procyonis)*, skunks *(B. columnaris)*, martens *(B. devosi)*, bears *(B. laevis)*, and other vertebrates; they necessitate an intermediate host, usually small rodents, birds, and many others, for their development.[1] Eggs evacuated with the feces of the final host mature in soil to become infective; following ingestion of eggs by the intermediate host, the larvae are freed in the intestine to produce an infection in all the tissues. The parasites eventually encapsulate after producing severe tissue damage and a high mortality in these hosts owing to central nervous system involvement.[1]

To date, about a dozen human infections have been reported, mostly in infants, five residing in the northern United States.[87–92] In two of the infants, a 10-month-old and an 18-month-old with Down syndrome, the infection was fatal. The disease in both started with a mild upper respiratory illness, but each soon developed symptoms of CNS involvement as a result of damage produced by the migrating larvae in the brain substance. The 10-month-old infant was lethargic, irritable, obtunded, with lack of spontaneous movements, and practically semicomatose when he was brought to the hospital. The other child also presented with CNS involvement, though of a lesser degree. The laboratory data showed moderate leukocytosis, with 37% and 27% eosinophilia, respectively; the spinal fluid contained 5 and 92 cells, respectively, without pathogenic organisms isolated. One child died 6 days after hospitalization; the other went home in a decompensated CNS state and died 14 months later. The other four infants were brought to the hospital because of several neurologic complaints and were diagnosed as having baylisascariasis based on serologic tests with *B. procyonis* larval antigens in the serum and spinal fluid.[90–92] These patients were treated with thiabendazole, albendazole, ivermectin, and prednisone in different combinations with some response. All four patients left the hospital with severe neurologic sequelae.[90–92] Another case was reported as *Baylisascaris* based on study of a presumably necrotic larva, too degenerated for identification. The presumed larva was eliciting an eosinophilic pseudotumor in the left myocardium that protruded into the left ventricle and resulted in the sudden death of a 10-year-old boy in Massachusetts.[93]

Examination of the tissues recovered at autopsy of fatal cases shows extensive CNS damage (Fig. 106-7), acute in the infant who died in the hospital and chronic in the infant who died at home. Microscopically, larvae with morphology similar to that of *Baylisascaris* larvae were found, encapsulated in every tissue examined.[1] Although based mostly on circumstantial and epidemiologic evidence the parasite has been called *B. procyonis* in these reports; the true species of *Baylisascaris* responsible for human and most animal infections remains to be determined. Identification of *Baylisascaris* larvae in tissues is based on morphologic characteristics, but the species of *Baylisascaris* is impossible to determine; the best possible interpretation in all cases where sections of the larvae are found in tissues is the generic *Baylisascaris* sp.[1]

Many patients suffering from diffuse unilateral subacute neuroretinitis (DUSN), with or without nematode larva observed in the retina, are said to be suffering from ocular baylisascariasis. Although this may well be the case, there is no direct confirmation for this idea and especially for labeling the parasite specifically as *B. procyonis*. This statement is made despite indirect evidence in animals where production of retinitis occurs in experimental infections with *B. procyonis*. In most of the reported patients, a nematode larva has been visualized in the retina with the slit lamp, and as well as it can be determined, the nematode has a size range consistent with the size of *Baylisascaris* larvae. Since identification of worms based on size alone is not a valid criterion to give a specific name, the role of *Baylisascaris* in the production of diffuse

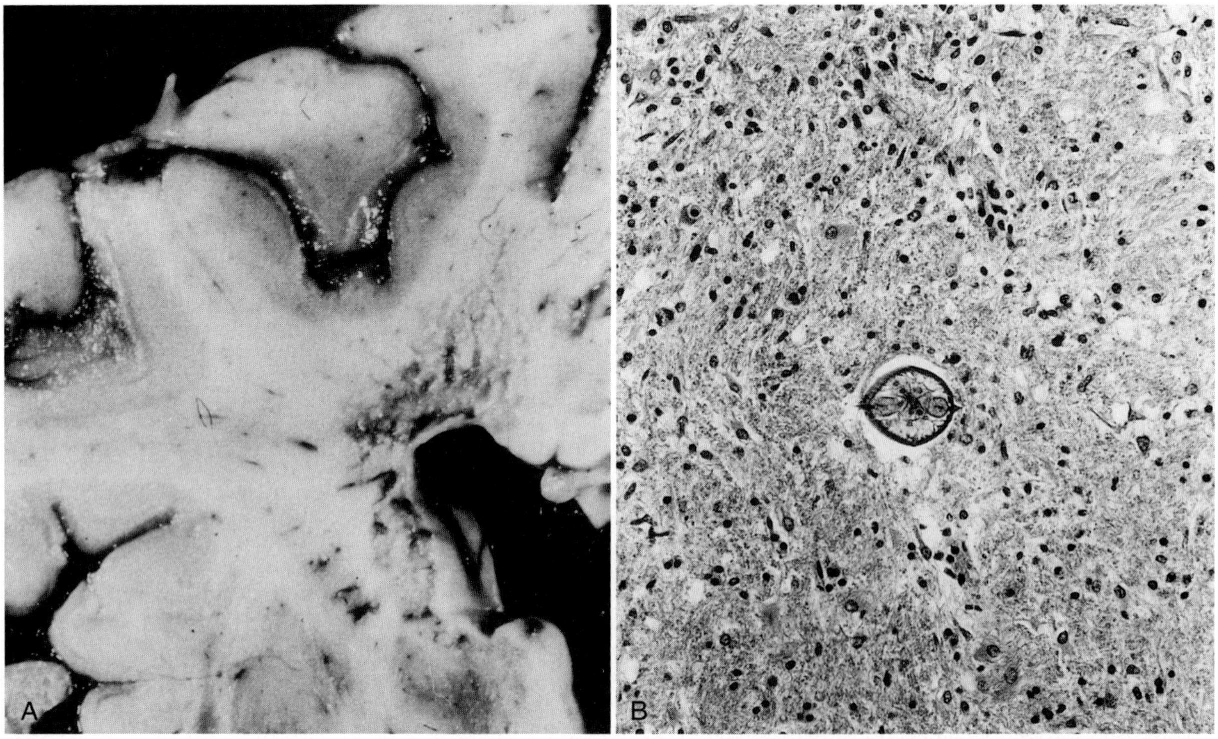

FIGURE 106-7 *Baylisascaris* sp. in human brain. *A*, Gross lesion, consisting of areas of necrosis. *B*, View of a section of the larva. (H&E stain, ×180.) (Courtesy of NS Gould, MD, Department of Pathology, Michael Reese Hospital and Medical Center, Chicago. Case reported in Fox AS, Kazacos KR, Gould NS, et al: Fatal eosinophilic meningoencephalitis and visceral larva migrans caused by the raccoon ascarid *Baylisascaris procyonis*. N Engl J Med 312:1619, 1985.)

unilateral subacute neuroretinitis remains likely but unproven.[1,94]

Lagochilascaris

Fewer than 50 infections in humans due to *Lagochilascaris* are known, and all of them are in Central and South America.[95–99] The species implicated in all known human cases is *L. minor*, the life cycle of which is now partially known, but the manner in which human infections are acquired remains obscure. A related species found in North America, *L. sprenti*, is known to reside in the stomach wall of opossums. Eggs passed with the feces become infective and are ingested by intermediate hosts where the larvae encapsulate. In some instances, the parasites develop into adults in the tissues in which they produce eggs that are evacuated through sinus tracts from the subcutaneous tissues into the skin.[100] Studies with *L. minor* of human origin have demonstrated the existence of an intermediate host.[101–103]

L. minor has been found to reside in animals in the upper airways and the oropharynx, and the disease it produces in humans parallels this location and the known development in the animal tissues. The infection is mostly characterized by marked chronic inflammation, edema, and numerous sinus tracts in the neck, face, tonsils (Fig. 106-8), throat, and mastoid and paranasal sinuses.[104] The appearance of the lesion is that of a large tumor mass. Fever and pain are absent, and the condition usually progresses for several months before the patient seeks medical help. Some complain mostly of sinusitis and cough and sometimes expectorate or pass the worms through the mouth.[105–107] Eggs are usually found in the discharged pus from the sinuses and sometimes in stool samples, where their recognition is difficult because they resemble *Ascaris* eggs.[97] At least two fatal cases have resulted from migration of the worms to the brain, causing encephalitis, and to the lungs, producing abscesses.[108,109] No studies of drugs for treatment of the infection in humans have been carried out. Treatment of one case with surgical drainage of the abscesses and administration of cambendazole and levamisole did not improve the patient's condition, whereas a course with ivermectin resulted in complete remission.[110] Another patient treated with thiabendazole was cured.[97]

SPIRURIDA

Gnathostoma, Thelazia, and *Gongylonema*

The Spirurida is a large group of nematodes characterized by having intermediate hosts in their life cycles. The largest superfamily of the Spirurida is the Filarioidea, which comprises

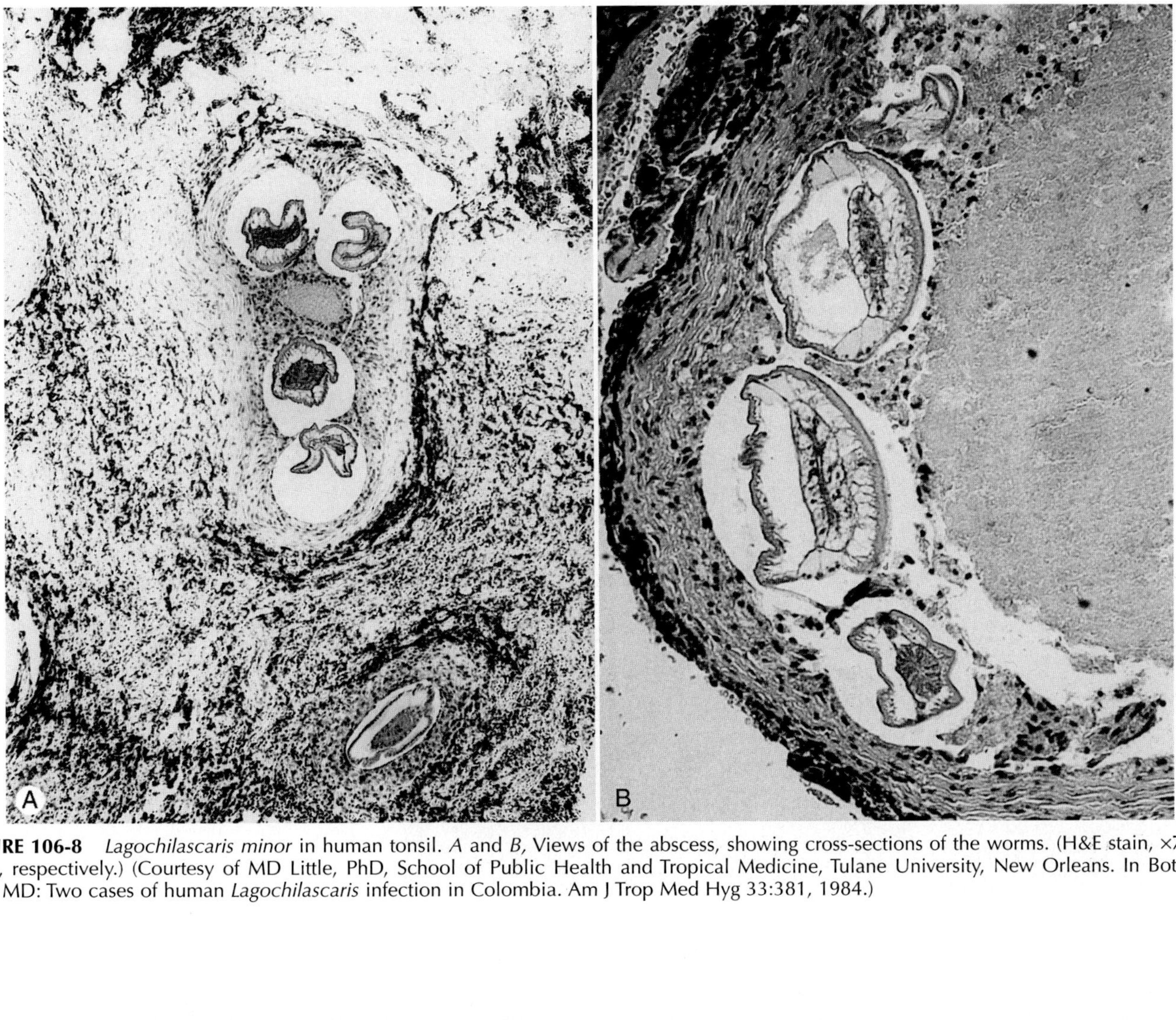

FIGURE 106-8 *Lagochilascaris minor* in human tonsil. *A* and *B,* Views of the abscess, showing cross-sections of the worms. (H&E stain, ×70 and ×180, respectively.) (Courtesy of MD Little, PhD, School of Public Health and Tropical Medicine, Tulane University, New Orleans. In Botero D, Little MD: Two cases of human *Lagochilascaris* infection in Colombia. Am J Trop Med Hyg 33:381, 1984.)

all filarial worms, some of which produce important diseases in humans (see Chapters 98–101). The intermediate hosts of those species important to humans are arthropods for filarial worms, and *Thelazia*, and fresh water fish for *Gnathostoma*. The Filarioidea has some species exclusively parasitic in humans, but the majority of the species in this group occur naturally in animals, producing zoonotic infections in humans. Infections with *Gnathostoma* are becoming more common in some geographic areas as awareness of the disease increases. *Thelazia* and *Gongylonema* infections are rare, but they continue being reported.[1]

Gnathostoma

More than 10 species of *Gnathostoma* are known as parasites of wild and domestic cats and other carnivores worldwide, each with its own geographic area of distribution. The species causing most human infections is *G. spinigerum*; rare cases due to *G. hispidum*,[111] *G. doloresi*,[112] and *G. nipponicum* are known in Southeast Asia. In Mexico and Ecuador the species is thought to be *G. binucleatum*,[113,114] and a case apparently produced by *G. malaysiae* was reported recently.[115] Gnathostomiasis is an infection that occurs in populations with a taste for raw freshwater fish in their diet. Thus, Japan and Southeast Asia in the Old World and Mexico and Ecuador in the Americas are the main foci of infection. Imported cases occur in the United States, Europe, and elsewhere. Isolated cases are known in other parts of the world.

In their natural hosts, the parasites are coiled in tumors formed in the stomach wall; eggs are evacuated with the feces and in water produce larvae that are ingested by small crustaceans, *Cyclops*, where the larvae develop further. The infected crustaceans are ingested by small freshwater fishes, frogs, snakes, and other vertebrates, where the larvae become infective and locate in the muscles. An inappropriate definitive host ingesting an infected animal will harbor the larva in its tissues and thus act as paratenic hosts. Ingestion of any of these hosts by carnivorous definitive hosts produces the infection in the stomach. If humans, not natural hosts, ingest the infective larvae, the larvae do not develop into adults (paratenism) but rather remain as larvae and migrate through the tissues, producing larva migrans, either cutaneous or visceral, depending on their location. Thus, any organ can be compromised, and the result can be devastating clinical syndromes, some of which are fatal.[1]

The distribution of human gnathostomiasis is mainly Thailand, India, Japan, China, Malaysia, the Philippines, and Vietnam.[116] Cases in Sri Lanka,[117] Zambia,[118] Bangladesh,[119] and Vietnam[120] have been recorded recently. Many cases in several foci are now known in Mexico[114,121] and Ecuador[122]; the cases seen in the United States have occurred mostly in Southeast Asian immigrants.[123–126] In humans, the symptoms and signs produced by the worms are protean and difficult to diagnose clinically, because they can compromise any organ system.[1] The larvae probably first reach the liver from the stomach soon after ingestion, and from the liver migrate to almost any other organ.

The symptoms of infection begin after ingestion of a single larva, rarely two or more, and consist of epigastric pain, nausea, and vomiting lasting sometimes 2 to 3 weeks, consistent with penetration of the intestinal wall and migration of the worm. A larva located in the subcutaneous tissues (Fig. 106-9) produces edema and inflammation,[127] seen and felt as an indurated, pruritic, erythematous lesion, sometimes known as Yangtze edema or Shanghai rheumatism, and in the United States as nodular eosinophilic migratory panniculitis. The swelling may resolve, but it will reappear in another location because of the proclivity of the larva for migration in the tissues. If the larva reaches the superficial squamous epithelium, it manifests as cutaneous larva migrans (see Chapter 103).[128] Because of the large size of the parasite, the larva is visible in the skin and can be recovered easily with slight scarification of the stratum corneum.

The most important manifestation of gnathostomiasis is produced by its migration through the CNS, resulting in often fatal syndromes[129] such as radiculomyelitis,[130]

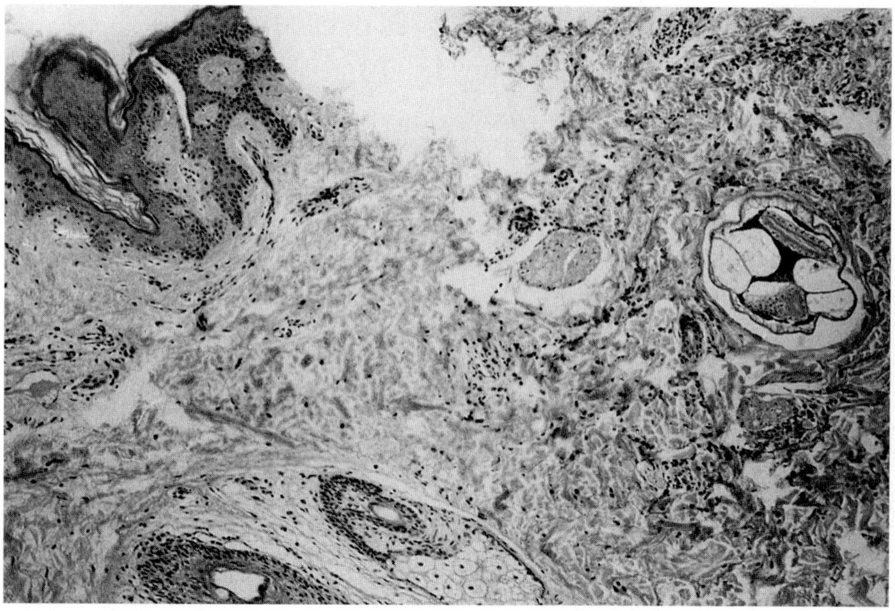

FIGURE 106-9 *Gnathostoma* sp. in section of human skin, showing the inflammatory reaction and a section of the worm in the subcutaneous tissues. (H&E stain, ×70.)

radiculomyeloencephalitis,[131] and subarachnoid hemorrhage.[132] Marked radicular pain is the result of migration of the larva through the spinal root nerves on its way to the spinal canal and brain. The pain lasts 1 to 5 days[129,131] and often is accompanied by paralysis of one or more extremities; paraplegia is often seen, sometimes followed by triplegia and quadriplegia. In the brain, the encephalitis manifests with cranial nerve symptoms, such as palsies, nystagmus, and meningeal irritation. The main clinical characteristic of *Gnathostoma* encephalitis is the migratory nature of the neurologic symptoms. Disappearance and reappearance of symptoms is common and considered characteristic[129]; the laboratory data are usually not helpful. The spinal fluid is often hemorrhagic or xanthochromic and its pressure elevated. Spinal fluid eosinophilia is present in all cases, the number of cells reaching about 500/mm^3; peripheral eosinophilia is sometimes present.

The other sites where *Gnathostoma* produces disease, in order of importance, are the eye,[126,133,134] lungs,[135,136] and gastrointestinal tract,[137] but almost every organ can be compromised.[1] In endemic areas, the clinical diagnosis is suspected by physicians accustomed to dealing with the infection; in other areas it is difficult. Confirmation of the clinical diagnosis is made by recovery of the larva and study of its morphologic characteristics. Larvae recovered from humans have measured from 2.5 to 12.5 mm in length by 0.4 to 1.2 mm in width. In histologic sections of biopsy specimens, the parasite can be recognized easily to the generic level based on its internal anatomy. More careful studies of the anatomy of the larva in good sections may allow identification of the species on the basis of the size and the nuclei of the intestinal cells.[138]

Serology is often used in the clinical practice to "corroborate" a clinical diagnosis, and various tests are available for the purpose. These tests do not, however, provide definitive proof of the infection,[139] and never do they identify the species involved because all species of *Gnathostoma* cross-react with each other.[140] Ribosomal DNA sequencing is a more promising tool for speciation of parasites.[113]

Thelazia

A few infections with *Thelazia callipaeda* in China,[141,142] Japan,[143] Korea,[144] India,[145] Russia, Taiwan,[146] and Thailand[147] have been recorded. *Thelazia californiensis* has also produced human infection in California.[148,149] The parasite is a common finding in the conjunctival sac of dogs, rabbits, and other animals. The mode of transmission to humans is unknown, but given that the eggs of the worm are discharged with tears of the infected animals, and that flies are the intermediate hosts, flies must play a role. The symptoms are lacrimation and feeling a foreign body in the conjunctiva. Careful examination of the eye reveals the worms, which can easily be retrieved.[148]

Gongylonema

Gongylonema is a parasite of ruminants that occasionally causes accidental zoonotic human infections reported in Europe,[150,151] China,[152] Morocco,[153] Russia,[154] New Zealand,[155] Sri Lanka,[156] and the United States.[157,158] In animals, the worms are located in superficial tunnels buried in the epithelium of the esophagus, the tongue (Fig. 106-10), or other places in the oral cavity; in humans worms have been recovered mainly from similar tunnels in the buccal epithelium, mainly the lips, gums, tonsils, hard and soft palates, and jaw. The worms are seen as small, migrating, threadlike structures under the superficial layers of the squamous epithelium. Humans become infected probably by accidental ingestion of the intermediate host, the cockroach. The eggs of the worm have once been found in the stools of an infected Japanese person in Thailand.[159]

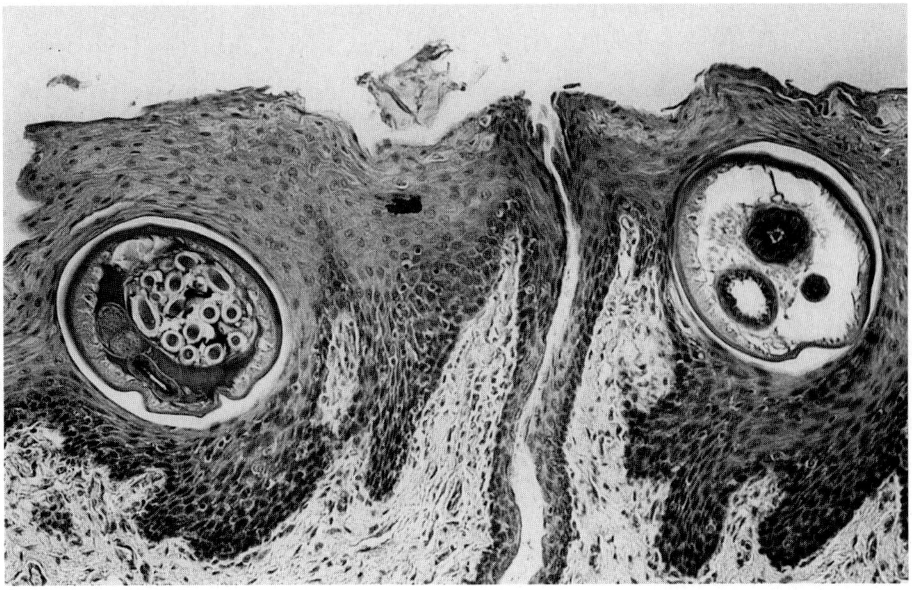

FIGURE 106-10 *Gongylonema* sp. in section of tongue of infected animal. (H&E stain, ×140.)

ENOPLIDA CAPILLARIDS

Calodium hepaticum (Capillaria hepatica) and *Paracapillaria philippinensis (Capillaria philippinensis)*

The capillarids, common parasites of animals, may cause human infection, occurring sporadically, occasionally in clusters, and rarely in large numbers (*P. philippinensis*). The capillarids belong to a larger group, the Trichinelloidea, which includes important parasites of humans such as *Trichinella spiralis* (see Chapter 104) and *Trichuris trichiura* (see Chapter 108). Their distinctive morphologic characteristic is the structure of their esophagus, which is made up of gland-like cells.

Calodium hepaticum

This worldwide parasite of small rodents, prairie dogs, monkeys, and other animals, produces a type of cirrhosis known as parasitic cirrhosis. The adult male and female worms live in the liver, where they produce eggs that elicit a marked granulomatous reaction (fibrosis) that eventually destroys the worms. The eggs survive; when by predation the host is ingested by a carnivore, the eggs in the liver are digested and evacuated with the feces of the carnivore. In the soil, the eggs become infective for the final hosts, or accidentally for humans; ingested eggs in the new host produce larvae that locate in the liver and mature into adults.

Human infections, totaling fewer than 30 worldwide, have been reported in the continental United States,[160–162] Hawaii,[163] England,[164,165] India,[166] Turkey,[167] Nigeria, South Africa,[168] Mexico,[169,170] Brazil,[171] Italy,[172] Switzerland,[173] Korea,[174] Kosovo,[175] and the former Czechoslovakia.[176] The clinical symptoms are variable, acute or subacute, with manifestations of acute hepatitis that evolve into a picture indistinguishable from visceral larva migrans (see Chapter 103). The only clinical difference with visceral larva migrans is the greater enlargement of the liver in capillariasis, about 2 to 3 cm below the costal margin, compared with 1 cm in visceral larva migrans. The only positive laboratory sign is the marked peripheral eosinophilia.[177] Liver biopsy or autopsy specimens show histologically different patterns of disease, depending on the stage of evolution of the infection. Early, immature worms (Fig. 106-11A), granulomas, and extensive eosinophilic infiltration are present. Later, the adult worms can be identified mixed with numerous eggs, all producing marked granulomatous inflammation and tissue eosinophilia (Fig. 106-11B). The latter stages are characterized by the lack of adult worms, the presence of viable eggs, and marked fibrosis.[1] The outcome of the infection apparently depends on the worm load, with some cases progressing rapidly to severe liver disease and death, others following a chronic course, and still others having remission. At least seven patients have survived. With the triad of leukocytosis, peripheral eosinophilia, and enlargement of the liver disproportionate for *Toxocara* infections, the diagnosis

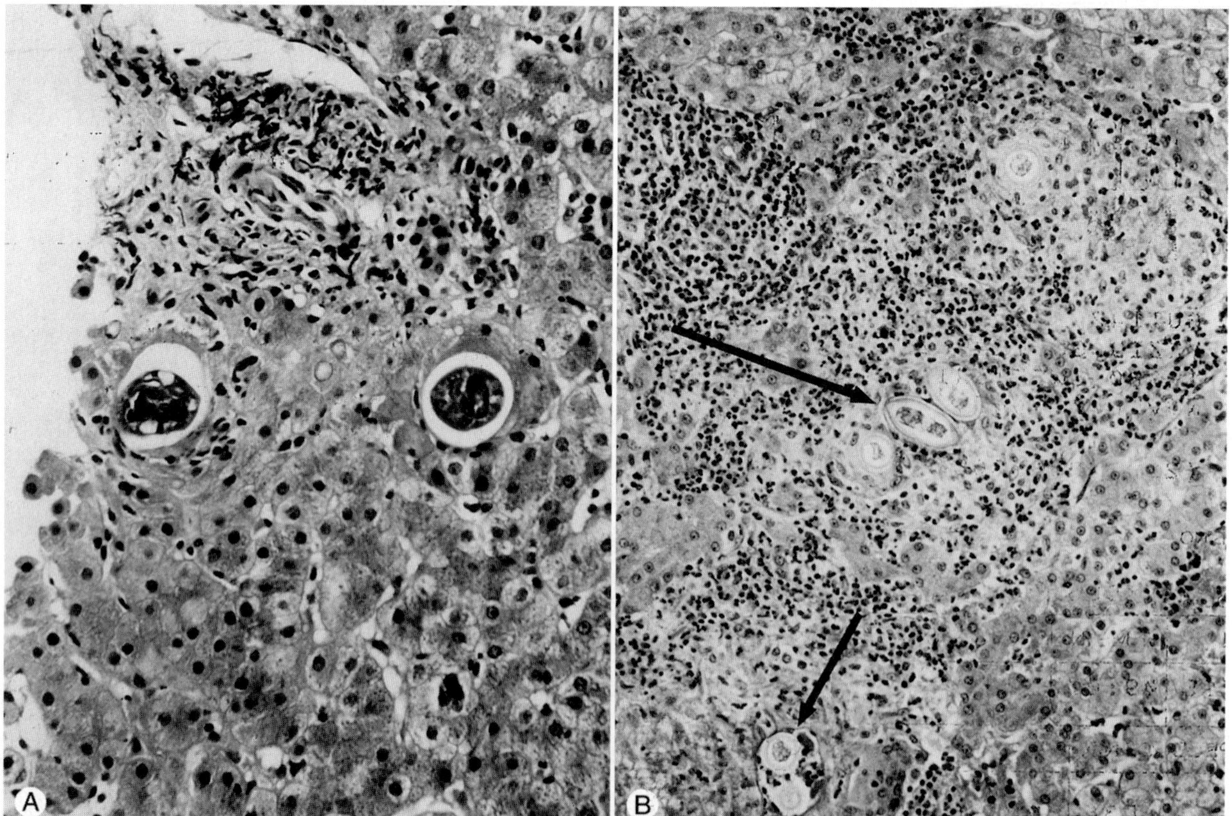

FIGURE 106-11 *Capillaria hepatica* in human liver. *A,* View of section of liver biopsy specimen showing sections of immature worms. Note the scant inflammation at this stage. (H&E, ×200.) *B,* Liver section from another patient with advanced disease. Note the granulomatous inflammation and the presence of eggs *(arrows)*. (H&E stain, ×180.)

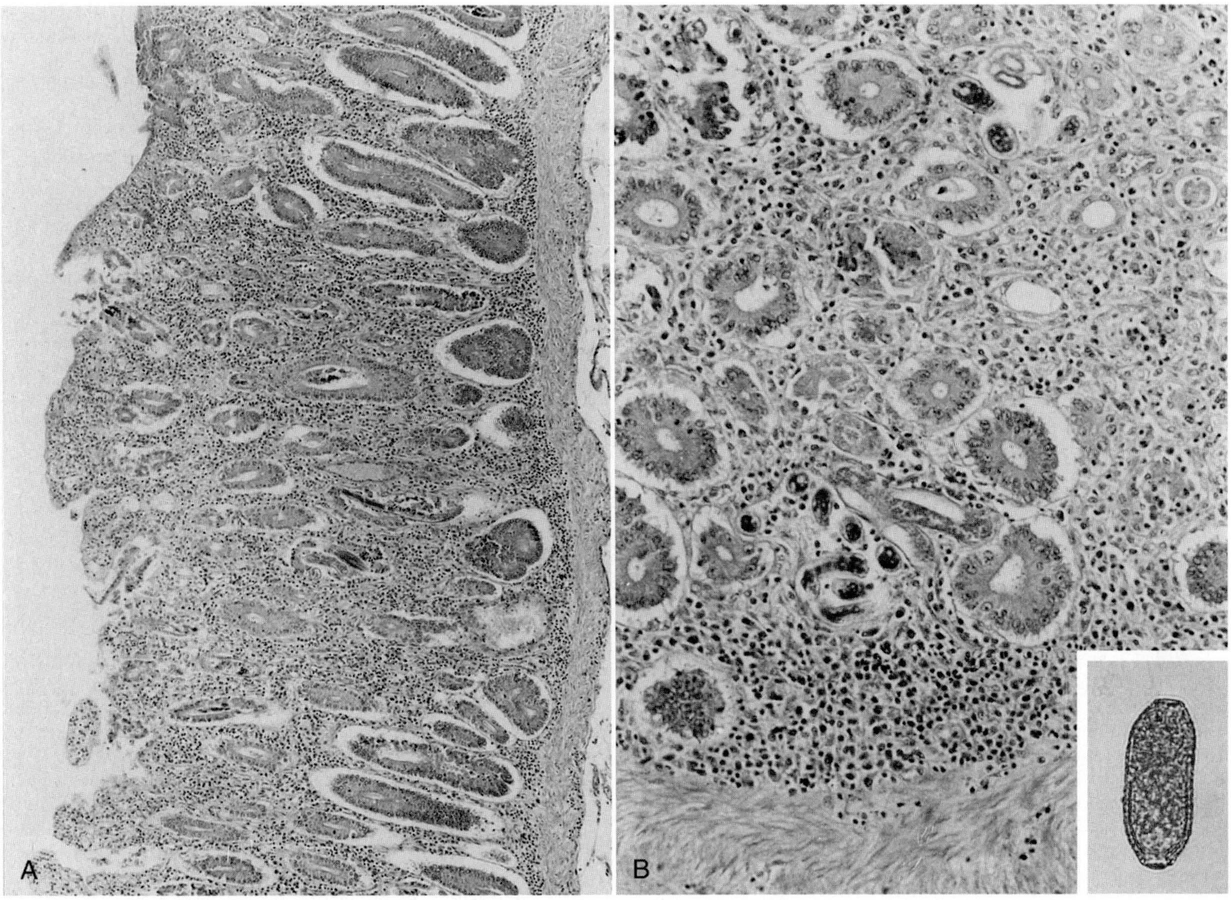

FIGURE 106-12 *Capillaria philippinensis* in human intestines. *A,* View of section of small intestine showing diffuse inflammatory infiltrate and sections of worms. (H&E stain, ×70.) *B,* The inflammatory infiltrate and the worms. (H&E, ×180). *Inset*: Egg in unstained stool sample. (H&E stain, ×450.)

may be difficult clinically, but needle liver biopsy specimens[173,174] or open biopsies[178] provide rapid and accurate identification of the problem in children and sometimes in adults. Two recent cases have been treated with thiabendazole: One patient recovered completely[173]; the other, with more severe disease, developed IgA nephropathy, and 2 years later his condition was stable, though still with severe liver damage.[174]

An important aspect of hepatic calodiasis in humans is the possibility of misdiagnosed spurious infections. If humans ingest liver of infected animals, noninfectious eggs will pass the alimentary canal and can be detected in stool samples.[179] Such ingested and passed eggs cannot be distinguished morphologically from eggs produced during active human infection. In each case in which *C. hepaticum* eggs are found in humans, a second fecal sample should be taken and examined within a few days. Finding eggs in both samples will confirm that there is indeed active infection,[1] not simply intestinal passage of ingested eggs. An immunofluorescent assay for diagnosis, using frozen sections of infected mice liver, has been described.[180]

Paracapillaria philippinensis

The agent of intestinal capillariasis is *P. philippinensis*, a nematode first described in the Philippines in 1964 during an epidemic of gastrointestinal disease that resulted in many deaths. Later the parasite was placed tentatively in the genus *Aonchoteca*[181] and more recently in the genus *Paracapillaria*.[182] The infection is found in other countries, including Thailand,[183] Iran,[184] Japan,[185] Egypt,[186] Indonesia,[187,188] Korea,[189] India,[190] and Taiwan[191] and in Spain in a traveling Colombian who probably acquired the infection in Colombia.[192] The geographic distribution of intestinal capillariasis is likely to be much larger than is presently known, and infections are probably not being diagnosed because the eggs of *P. philippinensis* are mistakenly identified as *Trichuris* eggs (Fig. 106-12, inset). In autopsy material recovered from patients dying in the Philippines' epidemic, the parasites found buried in the small intestinal mucosa (see Fig. 106-12) were recovered, enabling their recognition as a then new species.[193] The life cycle of the parasite involves small freshwater fish intermediate hosts, which upon ingestion release larvae that grow to adults in the human intestine. Some females lay eggs that mature rapidly in the intestine, produce larvae that enter the mucosa (internal autoinfection),[194] and develop into adults, explaining the large number of worms in infected persons. Other females lay eggs that are evacuated with the feces, and in water become infective and are ingested by the fish intermediate host.[195]

The clinical manifestation of infection is watery diarrhea that does not respond to customary treatment. The patient is usually a 20- to 50-year-old man who becomes infected while working in the fields, eating raw fish. The patient usually presents days after the beginning of his illness, when the symptoms are more sprue-like. Weight loss due to malabsorption of fats, vitamins, proteins, and carbohydrates is common. Abdominal pain, slight fever, and anorexia are also found, together with emaciation and dehydration.[196,197] Laboratory tests may show slight leukocytosis and eosinophilia; examination of the stools demonstrates the typical eggs, larvae, and sometimes adult worms.[198]

REFERENCES

1. Gutierrez Y: Diagnostic Pathology of Parasitic Infections with Clinical Correlations. New York, Oxford University Press, 2000, p 769.
2. Hoogstraten J, Young WG: Meningo-encephalomyelitis due to the saprophagous nematode *Micronema deletrix* Can J Neurol Sci 2:121, 1975.
3. Shadduck JA, Ubelaker J, Telford VQ: *Micronema deletrix* meningo-encephalitis in an adult man. Am J Clin Pathol 72:640, 1979.
4. Gardiner CH, Koh DS, Cardella TA: *Micronema* in man: Third fatal infection. Am J Trop Med Hyg 30:586, 1981.
5. Anderson RC, Linder KE, Peregrine AS: *Halicephalobus gingivalis* (Stefanski 1954) from a fatal infection in a horse in Ontario, Canada, with comments on the validity of *H deletrix* and a review of the genus. Parasite 5:255, 1998.
6. Ahn YK: *Rhabditis* sp infected cases in rural school children. Korean J Parasitol 23:1, 1985.
7. Goldsmid JM: *Rhabditis* (*Rhabditella*) *axei* in the urine of an African in Rhodesia. J Helminthol 305, 1967.
8. Goldsmid JM: Spurious parasites recovered from stools and urines in Rhodesia. Cent Afr J Med 173, 1970.
9. Eldridge B: Human urinary tract infection caused by *Rhabditis* sp. Microbiol Digest 10:202, 1993.
10. Campos DM, Araujo JL, Vieira MC, et al: Um caso de parasitismo por Rhabditis sp em cranca de Goiania Goias Brazil. Revista Da Sociedade Brasileira de Medicina Tropical 35:519, 2002.
11. Pasyk K: Dermatitis rhabditidosa in an 11-year-old girl: A new cutaneous parasitic disease of man. Br J Dermatol 98:107, 1978.
12. Ginsburg B, Beaver PC, Wilson ER, et al: Dermatitis due to larvae of a soil nematode *Pelodera strongyloides*. Pediatr Dermatol 2:33, 1984.
13. Jones CC, Rosen T, Greenberg C: Cutaneous larva migrans due to *Pelodera strongyloides*. Cutis 48:123, 1991.
14. Smith ME: *Strongyloides*-like worms in vaginal smears (letter). Am J Clin Pathol 38:208, 1962.
15. Caballero YCE: Un caso de parasitismo accidental por *Rhabditis pellio* en Mexico. Ann Inst Biol Univ Mex 8:393, 1937.
16. Chandler AC: *Diploscapter coronata* as a facultative parasite of man with a general review of vertebrate parasitism by rhabditoid worms. Semin Respir Infect 30:44, 1938.
17. Yokogawa S: A human case of accidental parasitism of *Diploscapter coronata* (Cobb 1893) Cobb 1913. Zool Mag Tokyo 48:507, 1936.
18. Boreham RE, McCowan MJ, Ryan AE, et al: Human trichostrongyliasis in Queensland. Pathology 27:182, 1995.
19. Wallace L, Henkin R, Mathies AW: *Trichostrongylus* infestation with profound eosinophilia. Ann Intern Med 45:146, 1956.
20. Torres P, Figueroa L, Navarrete N: Trichostrongylosis en la Provincia de Valdivia Chile. Bol Chil Parasitol 27:52, 1972.
21. Sahba GH, Arfaa F, Bijan H: Intestinal helminthiasis in the rural area of Khuzestan south-west Iran. Ann Trop Med Parasitol 61:351, 1967.
22. Otsuru M: *Trichostrongylus brevis* sp nov from man (Nematoda: Trichostrongylidae). Acta Med Biol 9:273, 1962.
23. Watson JM: Human trichostrongylosis and its relationship to ancylostomiasis in southern Iraq with comments on world incidence. Semin Respir Infect 43:102, 1953.
24. Magambo JK, Zeyhle E, Wachira TM: Prevalence of intestinal parasites among children in southern Sudan. East Afr Med J 75:288, 1998.
25. Arakawa H: A study on fecal blood loss associated with *Ancylostoma duodenale, Necator americanus,* and *Trichostrongylus orientalis* infections. Niigata Igakkai Zasshi 75:1068, 1961.
26. Correa-de-Lara TT-A, Aparecida Barbosa M, Rodrigues de Oliveira M, et al: Human syngamosis: Two cases of chronic cough caused by *Mammomonogamus laryngeus*. Chest 103:264, 1993.
27. Dufat R, Sang HT, Herrenschmidt JL, et al: A propos d'un nouveau cas de syngamose bronchique humaine en provenance de la Martinique. J Fr Med Chir Thorac 25:547, 1971.
28. Font JH: *Syngamus laryngeus* in man: Report on three additional cases from Puerto Rico. Bol Asoc Med Pto Rico 35:331, 1943.
29. Cunnac M, Magnaval JF, Cayarci D, et al: A propos de 3 cas de syngamose humaine en Guadeloupe. Revue de Pneumologie Clinique 44:140, 1988.
30. Nosanchuk JS, Wade SE, Landolf M: Case report of and description of parasite *Mammomonogamus laryngeus* (human syngamosis) infection. J Clin Microbiol 33:998, 1995.
31. Kim HY, Lee SM, Joo JE, et al: Human syngamosis: The first case in Korea. Thorax 53:717, 1998.
32. Weinstein LP, Molavi A: *Syngamus laryngeus* infection (syngamosis) with chronic cough. Ann Intern Med 74:577, 1971.
33. Timmons RF, Bowers RE, Price DL: Infection of the respiratory tracts with *Mammomanogamus* (*Syngamus*) *laryngeus*: A new case in Largo, Florida, and a summary of previously reported cases. Am Rev Respir Dis 128:566, 1983.
34. Birrell DJ, Moorhouse DE, Gardner MAH, et al: Chronic cough and haemoptysis due to a nematode "*Syngamus laryngeus*." Aust NZ J Med 8:168, 1978.
35. Leers WD, Sarin MK, Arthurs K: Syngamosis an unusual cause of asthma: The first reported case in Canada. Can Med Assoc J 132:269, 1985.
36. Gardiner CH, Schantz PM: *Mammomonogamus* infection in a human: Report of a case. Am J Trop Med Hyg 32:995, 1983.
37. Machado de Mendonca J, Davidson S, Loures JDC: Mais um caso brasileiro de singamose humana. Atas Soc Biol Rio Jan 6:18, 1962.
38. Pit DS, Rijcken FE, Raspoort EC, et al: Geographic distribution and epidemiology of *Oesophagostomum bifurcum* and hookworm infections in humans in Togo. Am J Trop Med Hyg 61:951, 1999.
39. Storey PA, Faile G, Hewitt E, et al: Clinical epidemiology and classification of human oesophagostomiasis. Trans R Soc Trop Med Hyg 94:177, 2000.
40. Anthony PP, McAdam IWJ: Helminthic pseudotumours of the bowel: Thirty-four cases of helminthoma. Gut 13:8, 1972.
41. Kaminsky RG, Ndinya-Achola JO: *Oesophagostomum* sp from Kenya: Identification through tissue sections. E Afr Med J 54:296, 1977.
42. Baylet RJ, Paillet RJ: Abces musculaire par *Oesophagostomum* (Dakar). Bull Soc Pathol Exot 32, 1959.
43. Leoutsakos B, Agnadi N, Kolisiatis S: Rectal bleeding due to *Oesophagostomum brumpti*: Report of a case. Dis Colon Rectum 20:632, 1977.
44. Jacques JE, Lynch JB: Massive oesophagostomiasis of the colon. Gut 5:80, 1964.
45. Henry A, Joyeux C: Contribution a la faune helminthologique de la Haute-Guinee Francaise. Bull Soc Pathol Exot 176, 1920.
46. Leiper RT: The occurrence of *Oesophagostomum apiostomum* as an intestinal parasite of man in Nigeria. J Trop Med Hyg 14:116, 1911.
47. Pit DS, Polderman AM, Baeta S, et al: Parasite-specific antibody and cellular immune responses in human infected with *Necator americanus* and *Oesophagostomum bifurcum*. Parasitol Res 87:722, 2001.
48. Polderman AM, Krepel HP, Baeta S, et al: Oesophagostomiasis: A common infection of man in northern Togo and Ghana. Am J Trop Med Hyg 44:336, 1991.
49. Ross RA, Gibson DI, Harris EA: Cutaneous oesophagostomiasis in man. J Helminthol 63:261, 1989.
50. Karim N, Yang CO: Oesophagostomiasis in man: Report of the first Malaysian case with emphasis on its pathology. Malays J Pathol 14:19, 1992.
51. Kwo EH: Parasitic infection in man in North Sumatra, Indonesia. Yonsei Rep Trop Med 3:23. 1972.
52. Thomas HW: The pathological report of a case of oesophagostomiasis in man. Ann Trop Med Parasitol 4:57, 1910.
53. Embil JA, Salisbury S, Meerovitch E: Familial infection with *Oesophagostomum venulosum*. In Mueller M, Gutteridge W, Koehler P: Proceeding of the 5th International Congress of Parasitology. Toronto, Amsterdam, Elsevier Biochemical Press Suppl, 5:289, 1982.
54. Storey PA, Spannbrucker N, Yelifari L, et al: Ultrasonographic detection and assessment of preclinical *Oesophagostomum bifurcum*-induced colonic pathology. Clin Infect Dis 33:166, 2001.
55. Storey PA, Faile G, Crawley D, et al: Ultrasound appearance of preclinical *Oesophagostomum bifurcum* induced colonic pathology. Gut 48:565, 2001.

56. Storey PA, Anemana S, van Oostayen JA, et al: Ultrasound diagnosis of oesophagostomiasis. Br J Radiol 73:328, 2000.
57. Krepel HP, van der Velde EA, Baeta S, et al: Quantitative interpretation of coprocultures in a population infected with *Oesophagostomum bifurcum*. Trop Geogr Med 47:157, 1995.
58. Polderman AM, Krepel HP, Verweij JJ, et al: Serological diagnosis of *Oesophagostomum* infections. Trans R Soc Trop Med Hyg 87:433, 1993.
59. Verweij JJ, Polderman AM, Wimmenhove MC, et al: PCR assay for the specific amplification of *Oesophagostomum bifurcum* DNA from human faeces. Int J Parasitol 30:137, 2000.
60. Storey PA, Bugri S, Magnussen P, et al: The effect of albendazole on *Oesophagostomum bifurcum* infection and pathology in children from rural northern Ghana. Ann Trop Med Parasitol 95:87, 2001.
61. Krepel HP, Haring R, Baeta S, et al: Treatment of mixed *Oesophagostomum* and hookworm infection: Effect of albendazole, pyrantel pamoate, levamisole, and thiabendazole. Trans R Soc Trop Med Hyg 87:87, 1993.
62. MacDonald F, Goldsmid JM: Intestinal helminth infections in the Burma Valley area of Rhodesia. Cent Afr J Med 19:113, 1973.
63. Goldsmid JM *Ternidens deminutus*: A parasitological enigma in Rhodesia. Fac Med Res Lect Ser No 4, University College of Rhodesia, Salisbury, April 30, 1970, 20 pp., 1971.
64. Goldsmid JM: *Ternidens deminutus* Railliet and Henry (Nematoda): A diagnostic problem in Rhodesia. Cent Afr J Med 13:54, 1967.
65. Goldsmid JM, McCabe RJ: Preliminary studies on the use of phenylene-diisothiocyanate-(1 4) in the treatment of hookworm and *Ternidens deminutus* infections in Rhodesia. Cent Afr J Med 227, 1972.
66. Goldsmid JM: *Ternidens deminutus* (Railliet and Henry 1909) and hookworm in Rhodesia and a review of the treatment of human infections with *T deminutus*. Cent Afr J Med 18(suppl):1, 1972.
67. Ishikura H, Namiki M: Gastric *Anisakiasis* in Japan: Epidemiology, Diagnosis, Treatment. Tokyo, Springer-Verlag, 1989.
68. Ishikura H, Kikuchi K: Intestinal *Anisakiasis* in Japan. Tokyo, Springer-Verlag, 1990, p 265.
69. Ishikura H, Kikuchi K, Nagasawa K, et al: Anisakidae and anisakidosis. Prog Clin Parasitol 3:43, 1992.
70. Oshima T: Anisakiasis: Is the sushi bar guilty? Parasitol Today 3:44, 1987.
71. McClelland G: *Terranova decipiens* (Nematoda: Anisakinae): Course of infection and pathology in seal hosts. Trans Am Microsc Soc 265, 1976.
72. Sakanari JA, Loinaz HM, Deardorff TL, et al: Intestinal anisakiasis: A case diagnosed by morphologic and immunologic methods. Am J Clin Pathol 90:107, 1988.
73. Deardorff TL, Altman J, Nolan CM: Human anisakiasis: Two case reports from the state of Washington. Proc Helminthol Soc Wash 54:274, 1987.
74. Kliks M M: Anisakiasis in the western United States: Four new case reports from California.Am J Trop Med Hyg 32:526, 1983.
75. Apt W, Hisamoto T, Llorens P, et al: Anisakiasis gastrica en Chile. Rev Med Chile 825, 1980.
76. Hubert B, Bacou J, Belveze H: Epidemiology of human anisakiasis: Incidence and source in France. Am J Trop Med Hyg 40:301, 1989.
77. Van Thiel PH, Kuipers FC, Roskam RTH: A nematode parasitic to herring causing acute abdominal syndromes in man. Trop Geogr Med 12:97, 1960.
78. Voorhuis FJ, Eijlers W: An inflammatory tumour of the stomach due probably to a herring parasite. Ned Tijdschr Geneeskd 105:2542, 1961.
79. Kuipers FC, Rodenburg W, Wielinga WJ, et al: Eosinophilic phlegmon of the alimentary canal caused by a worm. Lancet 2:1171, 1960.
80. Gutierrez-Ramos R, Guillen-Bueno R, Madero-Jarabo R, et al: Digestive haemorrhage in patients with anti-*Anisakis* antibodies. Eur J Gastroenterol Hepatol 12:337, 2000.
81. Armentia A, Lombardero M, Callejo A, et al: Occupational asthma by *Anisakis simplex*. J Allerg Clin Immunol 102:831, 1998.
82. Daschner A, Alonso-Gomez A, Caballero T, et al: Gastric anisakiasis: An underestimated cause of acute urticaria and angio-oedema? Br J Dermatol 139:822, 1998.
83. Jimenez-Saenz M, Torres GJ, Hernandez-Duran M, et al: Es la anisakiasis intestinal una infestation frecuente? Revista Espanola de Enfermedades Digestivas 95:239, 2003.
84. Pichler WJ: Anisakiasis: immunity allergy or both? Lessons on the natural role of immunoglobulin E from a nematode infestation. Clin Exp Allerg 29:1161, 1999.
85. Matsuoka H, Nakama T, Kisanuki H, et al: A case report of serologically diagnosed pulmonary anisakiasis with pleural effusion and multiple lesions. Am J Trop Med Hyg 51:819, 1994.
86. Yeum CH, Ma SK, Kim SW, et al: Incidental detection of an *Anisakis* larva in continuous ambulatory peritoneal dialysis effluent. Nephrol Dial Transplant 17:1522, 2002.
87. Murray NJ, Kazacos KR: Raccoon roundworm encephalitis. Clin Inf Dis 39:1484, 2004.
88. Huff DS, Neafie RC, Binder MJ, et al: The first fatal *Baylisascaris* infection in man: An infant with eosinophilic meningo-encephalitis. Pediatr Pathol 2:345, 1984.
89. Fox AS, Kazacos KR, Gould NS, et al: Fatal eosinophilic meningoencephalitis and visceral larva migrans caused by the raccoon ascarid *Baylisascaris procyonis*. N Engl J Med 312:1619, 1985.
90. Cunningham CK, Kazacos KR, McMillan JA, et al: Diagnosis and management of *Baylisascaris procyonis* infection in an infant with nonfatal meningoencephalitis. Clin Infect Dis 18:868, 1994.
91. Park SY, Glaser C, Murray WJ, et al: Raccoon roundworm (*Baylisascaris procyonis*) encephalitis: Case report and field investigation. Pediatrics 106:E56, 2000.
92. Gavin PJ, Kazacos KR, Tan TQ, et al: Neural larva migrans caused by the raccoon roundworm *Baylisascaris procyonis*. Pediatr Infect Dis J 21:971, 2002.
93. Boschetti A, Kasznica J: Visceral larva migrans induced eosinophilic cardiac pseudotumor: A cause of sudden death in a child. J Forensic Sci 40:1097, 1995.
94. Goldberg MA, Kazacos KR, Boyce WM, et al: Diffuse unilateral subacute neuroretinitis: Morphometric serologic and epidemiologic suppport for *Baylisascaris* as a causative agent. Ophthalmology 100:1695, 1993.
95. Costa HM, da Silva AV, Costa PR, et al: *Lagochilascaris minor* Leiper 1909 (Nematoda-Ascaridae) of human origin. Rev Inst Med Trop Sao Paulo 28:126, 1986.
96. Botero D, Little MD: Two cases of human *Lagochilascaris* infection in Colombia. Am J Trop Med Hyg 33:381, 1984.
97. Volcan GS, Ochoa FR, Medrano CE, et al: *Lagochilascaris minor* infection in Venezuela: Report of a case. Am J Trop Med Hyg 31:1111, 1982.
98. Brenes-Madrigal RR, Brenes AF: Lagochilascariasis humana en Costa Rica Programa General y Resumenes de Trabajos de el Congreso Latinoamericano y Nacional de Microbiologia, Ciudad Universitaria, Costa Rica, Diciembre 10–17, p. 35, 1961.
99. Vargas-Ocampo F, Alvarado-Aleman FJ: Infestation from *Lagochilascaris minor* in Mexico. Int J Dermatol 36:56, 1997.
100. Smith JL, Bowman DD, Little MD: Life cycle and development of *Lagochilascaris sprenti* (Nematoda: Ascarididae) from opossums (Marsupialia: Didelphidae) in Louisiana. J Parasitol 69:736, 1983.
101. Campos DM, Freire Filha LG, Vieira MA, et al: Experimental life cycle of *Lagochilascaris minor* Leiper, 1909. Rev Inst Med Trop Sao Paulo 34:277, 1992.
102. Paco JM, Campos DM, Oliveira JA: Wild rodents as experimental intermediate hosts of *Lagochilascaris minor* Leiper, 1909. Memorias do Instituto Oswaldo Cruz 94:441, 1999.
103. Pena HF, Kasai N, Gennari SM: Experimental life cycle of *Lagochilascaris major* Leiper, 1910 (Nematoda: Ascarididae) in cats (Felis domesticus). J Parasitol 88:1143, 2002.
104. Moraes MAP, Arnaud MVC, De Lima PE: Novos casos de infeccao humana por *Lagochilascaris minor* Leiper, 1909, encontrados no Estado do Para Brasil. Rev Inst Med Trop Sao Paulo 25:139, 1983.
105. Draper JW: Infection with *Lagochilascaris minor*. Br Med J 1:931, 1963.
106. Leao RNQd, Leao Filho J, Braga-Dias L, et al: Infeccao humana pelo *Lagochilascaris minor* Leiper, 1909, Registro de um caso observado no Estado do Para (Brasil). Rev Inst Med Trop Sao Paulo 20:300, 1978.
107. Artigas PDT, Araujo P, Romiti N, et al: Sobre un caso de parasitismo humano por *Lagochilascaris minor* Leiper, 1909, no estado de Sao Paulo, Brasil. Rev Inst Med Trop Sao Paulo 10:78, 1968.
108. Moraes MAP, Arnaud MVC, MacEdo RC, et al: Infeccao pulmonar fatal por *Lagochilascaris* sp provavelmente *Lagochilascaris minor* Leiper, 1909. Rev Inst Med Trop Sao Paulo 27:46, 1985.
109. Rosemberg S, Lopez MBS, Mazuda Z, et al: Fatal encephalopathy due to *Lagochilascaris minor* infection. Am J Trop Med Hyg 35:575, 1986.

110. Bento RF, Mazza CDC, Motti EF, et al: Human lagochilascariasis treated successfully with ivermectin: A case report. Rev Inst Med Trop Sao Paulo 35:373, 1993.
111. Taniguchi Y, Ando K: Human gnathostomiasis: Successful removal of *Gnathostoma hispidum*. Int J Dermatol 31:175, 1992.
112. Nawa Y, Imai JI, Ogata K, et al: The first record of a confirmed human case of *Gnathostoma doloresi* infection. J Parasitol 75:166, 1989.
113. Almeyda-Artigas RJ, Bargues MD, Mas-Coma S: ITS-2 rDNA sequencing of *Gnathostoma* species (Nematoda) and elucidation of the species causing human gnathostomiasis in the Americas. J Parasitol 86:537, 2000.
114. Leon-Regagnon V, Osorio-Sarabia D, Garcia-Prieto L, et al: Study of the ethiological agent of gnathostomosis in Nayarit, Mexico. Parasitol Int 51:201, 2002.
115. Nomura Y, Nagakura K, Kagei N, et al: Gnathostomiasis possibly caused by *Gnathostoma malaysiae*. Tokai J Exp Clin Med 25:1, 2000.
116. Daengsvang S: A monograph on the genus *Gnathostoma* and gnathostomiasis in Thailand.Tokyo, Southeast Asian Medical Information Center, 1980.
117. Samarasinghe S, Perera BJ, Ratnasena BG: First two cases of gnathostomiasis in Sri Lanka. Ceylon Med J 47:96, 2002.
118. Hale DC, Blumberg L, Frean J: Case report: Gnathostomiasis in two travelers to Zambia. Am J Trop Med Hyg 68:707, 2003.
119. Grobusch MP, Bergmann F, Teichmann D, et al: Cutaneous gnathostomiasis in a woman from Bangladesh. Int J Infect Dis 4:51, 2000.
120. Xuan lT, Rojekittikhun W, Punpoowong B, et al: Case report: Intraocular gnathostomiasis in Vietnam. Southeast Asian J Trop Med Public Health 33:485, 2002.
121. Diaz Camacho SP, Zazueta RM, Ponce TE, et al: Clinical manifestations and immunodiagnosis of gnathostomiasis in Culiacan, Mexico. Am J Trop Med Hyg 59:908, 1998.
122. Ollague W, Eduardo Gomez L, Manuel Briones I: Infeccion natural de peces de agua dulce con el tercer estado larvario de *Gnathostoma spinigerum* y su dinamica de transmision al hombre Primer reporte en Ecuador y America. Med Cutan Iber Lat Am 16:291, 1988.
123. Rusnak JM, Lucey DR: Clinical gnathostomiasis: Case report and review of the English-language literature. Clin Infect Dis 16:33, 1993.
124. Horohoe JJ, Ritterson AL, Chessin LN: Urinary gnathostomiasis. JAMA 251:255, 1984.
125. Kagen CN, Vance JC, Simpson M: Gnathostomiasis: Infestation in an Asian immigrant. Arch Dermatol 120:508, 1984.
126. Bathrick ME, Mango CA, Mueller JF: Intraocular gnathostomiasis. Am Acad Ophthalmol 88:1293, 1981.
127. Daengsvang S: Gnathostomiasis in Southeast Asia. Southeast Asian J Trop Med Public Health 12:319, 1981.
128. Pinkus H, Fan J, Degiusti D: Creeping eruption due to *Gnathostoma spinigerum* in a Taiwanese patient. Int J Dermatol 20:46, 1981.
129. Boongird P, Phanpradit P, Siridej N, et al: Neurological manifestations of gnathostomiasis. J Neurol Sci 31:279, 1977.
130. Schmutzhard E, Boongird P, Vejjajiva A: Eosinophilic meningitis and radiculomyelitis in Thailand caused by CNS invasion of *Gnathostoma spinigerum* and *Angiostrongylus cantonensis*. J Neurol Neurosurg Psychiatry 51:80, 1988.
131. Punyagupta S, Limtrakul C, Vichipanthu P, et al: Radiculomyeloencephalitis associated with eosinophilic pleocytosis: Report of nine cases. Am J Trop Med Hyg 17:551, 1968.
132. Visudhiphan P, Chiemchanya S, Somburanasim RA: Causes of spontaneous subarachnoid hemorrhage in Thai infants and children. J Neurosurg 53:185, 1980.
133. Kittiponghansa S, Prabriputaloong A, Pariyanonda S, et al: Intracameral gnathostomiasis: a cause of anterior uveitis and secondary glaucoma. Br J Ophthalmol 71:618, 1987.
134. Tansuphasiri P: Corneal perforation from *Gnathostoma spinigerum:* A case report [in Thai, English summary]. Siriraj Hosp Gaz 26:2111, 1974.
135. Vibulseth S, Leelarasamee A: A case of pulmonary gnathostomiasis. Siriraj Hosp Gaz 32:23, 1980.
136. Virasak S, Bovornkitti S, Jaroonvesama N: Gnathostomal pleurisy. Siriraj Hosp Gaz 25:1335, 1973.
137. Arromdee C, Thongprengsree S, Thirakhupt P: Intestinal gnastosomiasis. Vajira Med J 16:138, 1973.
138. Akahane H, Sano M, Mako T: Morphological difference in cross sections of the advanced third-stage larvae of *Gnathostoma spinigerum, G hispidum,* and *G doloresi*. Jpn J Parasitol 35:465, 1986.
139. Saksirisampant W, Chawengkiattikul R, Kraivichain K, et al: Specific IgE antibody responses to somatic and excretory-secretory antigens of third stage *G spinigerum* larvae in human gnathostomiasis. J Med Assoc Thai 84(suppl 1):S173, 2001.
140. Ishiwata K, Camacho SP, Ogata K, et al: Evaluation of the antigenic similarities of adult-worm extracts from three *Gnathostoma* species using sera from Mexican and Japanese patients with *Gnathostoma infections*. Ann Trop Med Parasitol 97:629, 2003.
141. Shi YE, Han JJ, Yang WY, et al: *Thelazia callipaeda* (Nematoda: Spirurida): Transmission by flies from dogs to children in Hubei, China. Trans R Soc Trop Med Hyg 82:627, 1988.
142. Zakir R, Zhong-Xia Z, Chioddini P, et al: Intraocular infestation with the worm *Thelazia callipaeda*. Br J Ophthalmol 83:1194, 1999.
143. Koyama Y, Ohira A, Kono T, et al: Five cases of thelaziasis. Br J Ophthalmol 84:441, 2000.
144. Hong ST, Park YK, Lee SK, et al: Two human cases of *Thelazia callipaeda* infection in Korea. Korean J Parasitol 33:139, 1995.
145. Mukherjee PK, Sushma V, Agrawal S: Intraocular *Thelazia* (a case report). Indian J Ophthalmol 25:41, 1978.
146. Cheung WK, Lu HJ, Liang CH, et al: Conjunctivitis caused by *Thelazia callipaeda* infestation in a woman. J Formosan Med Assoc 97:425, 1998.
147. Bhaibulaya M, Prasertsilpa S, Vajrasthira S: *Thelazia callipaeda* Railliet and Henry, 1910 in man and dog in Thailand. Am J Trop Med Hyg 19:476, 1970.
148. Kirschner BI, Dunn JP, Ostler HB: Conjunctivitis caused by *Thelazia californiensis* (letter). Am J Ophthalmol 110:573, 1990.
149. Chiapella KJ, Weinman C, Roberto R: Thelaziasis. Calif Morb Mortal Weekly Rep 25:367, 1976.
150. Illescas-Gomez MP, Rodriguez Osorio M, Gomez Garcia V, et al: Human *Gongylonema* infection in Spain. Am J Trop Med Hyg 38:363, 1988.
151. Weber G, MacHe K: Uber Hauterscheinungen bei *Gongylonema pulchrum* seine Erstbeobachtung in Deutschland beim Menschen. Hautarzt 24:286, 1973.
152. Feng LC, Tung MS, Su SC: Two Chinese cases of *Gongylonema* infection: A morphological study of the parasite and clinical study of the cases. Chin Med J 73:149, 1955.
153. Gaud J: A propos de la filariose humaine du Maroc. C R Seanc Mens Soc Sci Nat Phys Maroc 19:69, 1953.
154. Maionova VI: A case of *Gongylonema pulchrum* in man. Med Parasitol 44:111, 1975.
155. Johnston TH: A note on the occurrence of the nematode *Gongylonema pulchrum* in man in New Zealand. NZ Med J 35:172, 1936.
156. Crusz H, Sivalingam V: A note on the occurrence of *Gongylonema pulchrum* Molin, 1857, in man in Ceylon. J Parasitol 36:25, 1950.
157. Eberhard ML, Busillo C: Human *Gongylonema* infection in a resident of New York City. Am J Trop Med Hyg 61:51, 1999.
158. Wilson ME, Lorente CA, Allen JE, et al: *Gongylonema* infection of the mouth in a resident of Cambridge, Massachusetts. Clin Infect Dis 32:1378, 2001.
159. Wilde H, Suankratay C, Thongkam C, et al: Human *Gongylonema* infection in Southeast Asia. J Travel Med 8:204, 2001.
160. Ward RL, Dent JH: *Capillaria hepatica* infection in a child. Bull Tulane Med Fac 19:27, 1959.
161. Otto GF, Berthrong M, Appleby RE, et al: Eosinophilia and hepatomegaly due to *Capillaria hepatica* infection. Bull Johns Hopkins Hosp 94:319, 1954.
162. McQuown AL: *Capillaria hepatica*: A report of genuine and spurious cases. Am J Trop Med 30:761, 1950.
163. Ewing GM, Tilden IL: *Capillaria hepatica:* report of fourth case of true human infestation. J Pediatr 48:341, 1956.
164. Sumner D, Tinsley EGF: Encephalopathy due to visceral larva migrans. J Neurol Neurosurg Psychiatry 30:580, 1967.
165. Slais J: Notes on the differentiation of *Capillaria hepatica* and visceral larva migrans. Folia Parasitol 21:95, 1974.
166. Mac Arthur WP: A case of infestation of human liver with *Hepaticola hepatica* (Bancroft 1893) Hall 1916; with sections from the liver. Proc R Soc Med 83, 1924.
167. Turhan B, Unat EK, Yenermen M, et al: Human case of *Capillaria hepatica* (Bancroft 1893) Travassos, 1915. Mikrobiol Derg 7:149, 1954.
168. Silverman NH, Katz JS, Levin SE: *Capillaria hepatica* infestation in a child. S Afr Med J 47:219, 1973.

169. Romero Garcia F, Mendiola J, Biagi FF: Eosinofilia elevada con manifestacoines viscerales IV Primer caso de infeccion por *Capillaria hepatica* en Mexico. Bol Med Hosp Infant Mexico 19:473, 1962.
170. Gonzalez BD, Pelaez D, Jaramillo RY, et al: Tercer caso de capilariasis hepatica humana en Mexico. Rev Invest Clin 48:301, 1996.
171. Sawamura R, Fernandes MI, Peres LC, et al: Hepatic capillariasis in children: report of 3 cases in Brazil. Am J Trop Med Hyg 61:642, 1999.
172. Cislaghi F, Radice C: Infection by *Capillaria hepatica:* First case report in Italy. Helv Paediatr Acta 6:647, 1970.
173. Berger T, Degremont A, Gebbers JO, et al: Hepatic capillariasis in a 1-year-old child. Eur J Pediatr 149:333, 1990.
174. Choe G, Lee HS, Seo JK, et al: Hepatic capillariasis: First case report in the Republic of Korea. Am J Trop Med Hyg 48:610, 1993.
175. Terrier P, Hack I, Hatz C, et al: Hepatic capillariasis in a 2-year-old boy. J Pediatr Gastroenterol Nutr 28:338, 1999.
176. Slais J: The finding and identification of solitary *Capillaria hepatica* (Bancroft 1893) in man from Europe. Folia Parasitol 20:149, 1973.
177. Cochrane JC, Sagorin L, Wilcocks MG: *Capillaria hepatica* infection in man: A syndrome of extreme eosinophilia hepatomegaly and hyperglobulinaemia. S Afr Med J 31:751, 1957.
178. Yfanti G, Andreadis E, Spiliadou C, et al: A woman with fever and a jejunal stricture: case report. Lancet 347:802, 1996.
179. Pampiglione S, Najera E, Ricciardi ML, et al: Parasitological survey on Pygmies in Central Africa. 3. Bambuti group (Zaire). Riv Parassitol 40:187, 1979.
180. Juncker-Voss M, Prosl H, Lussy H, et al: Serological detection of *Capillaria hepatica* by indirect immunofluorescence assay. J Clin Microbiol 38:431, 2000.
181. Moravec F: Proposal of a new systematic arrangement of nematodes of the family Capillariidae. Folia Parasitologica 29:119, 1982.
182. Moravec F: Redescription and systematic status of *Capillaria philippinensis,* an intestinal parasite of human beings. J Parasitol 87:161, 2001.
183. Pradatsundarasar A, Pecharanond K, Chintanawongs C, et al: The first case of intestinal capillariasis in Thailand. Southeast Asian J Trop Med Public Health 4:131, 1973.
184. Hoghooghi-Rad N, Maraghi S, Narenj-Zadeh A: *Capillaria philippinensis* infection in Khoozestan Province, Iran: Case report Am J Trop Med Hyg 37:135, 1987.
185. Nawa Y, Imai JI, Abe T, et al: A case report of intestinal capillariasis: The second case found in Japan. Jpn J Parasitol 37:113, 1988.
186. Youssef FG, Mikhail EM, Mansour NS: Intestinal capillariasis in Egypt: A case report. Am J Trop Med Hyg 40:195, 1989.
187. Chichino G, Bernuzzi AM, Bruno A, et al: Intestinal capillariasis (*Capillaria philippinensis*) acquired in Indonesia: A case report. Am J Trop Med Hyg 47:10, 1992.
188. Bangs MJ, Purnomo, Andersen EM: A case of capillariasis in a highland community of Irian Jaya, Indonesia. Ann Trop Med Parasitol 88:685, 1994.
189. Lee SH, Hong ST, Chai JY, et al: A case of intestinal capillariasis in the Republic of Korea. Am J Trop Med Hyg 48:542, 1993.
190. Kang G, Mathan M, Ramakrishna BS, et al: Human intestinal capillariasis: First report from India. Trans R Soc Trop Med Hyg 88:204, 1994.
191. Hwang KP: Human intestinal capillariasis (*Capillaria philippinensis*) in Taiwan. Chung-Hua Min Kuo Hsiao Erh Ko i Hsueh Hui Tsa Chih 39:82, 1998.
192. Dronda F, Chaves F, Sanz A, et al: Human intestinal capillariasis in an area of nonendemicity: Case report and review. Clin Infect Dis 17:909, 1993.
193. Chitwood MB, Velasquez C, Salazar NG: *Capillaria philippinensis* sp. n. (Nematoda: Trichinellida), from the intestine of man in the Philippines. J Parasitol 54:368, 1968.
194. Cross JH, Banzon T, Clarke MD, et al: Studies on the experimental transmission of *Capillaria philippinensis* in monkeys. Trans R Soc Trop Med Hyg 66:819, 1972.
195. Bhaibulaya M, Indra-Ngarm S, Ananthapruti M: Freshwater fishes of Thailand as experimental intermediate hosts for *Capillaria philippinensis.* Int J Parasitol 9:105, 1979.
196. Dauz U, Cabrera BD, Canlas B Jr: Human intestinal capillariasis. 1. Clinical features. Acta Med Philipp 4:72, 1967.
197. Watten RH, Beckner WM, Cross JH, et al: Clinical studies on capillariasis *philippinensis.* Trans R Soc Trop Med Hyg 66:828, 1972.
198. Cabrera BD, Canlas BJ, Dauz U: Human intestinal capillariasis. 3. Parasitological features and management. Acta Med Philipp 4:92, 1967.

107

Enterobiasis

JAMES S. McCARTHY
THOMAS A. MOORE

INTRODUCTION

Enterobius vermicularis, commonly known as pinworm, is one of the most prevalent intestinal nematodes of humankind. Unlike the other common intestinal nematodes of humans, it does not disproportionately affect residents of tropical climates or populations with poor hygiene or low socioeconomic status. In addition, unlike most other human helminth parasites, the eggs that are deposited on the anal skin are immediately infective and do not require a period in the environment to embryonate. Thus, transmission is largely from person to person. Infection generally results in irritating but not life-threatening perianal pruritus.

AGENT

E. vermicularis is a member of the Oxyuridae class of nematodes. It has recently been proposed that it should be placed in a subfamily of oxyurid parasites, the Enterobiinae, a group that includes the pinworm parasites of primates and some rodents. The status of a new species proposed to infect humans, *Enterobius gregorii*,[1] remains controversial. Some authors suggest that the distinctive morphologic appearance reported to differentiate this species may instead represent transitional life cycle stages of *E. vermicularis*.[2] Further, no molecular genetic studies have yet established that this separate species indeed exists.

The adult female *E. vermicularis* worm appears as a small, white roundworm, measuring 9 to 12 mm in length and 0.5 mm in width (Fig. 107-1A). It possess a double-bulbed esophagus and a mouth with a cuticular expansion. It has a long, pointed tail and a slit-like vulva on the ventral surface about one third of the distance from the anterior end. The adult male is rarely seen in clinical practice, since it has a much shorter life span and is significantly smaller, measuring 2.5 mm in length and 0.2 mm in width. It is curved along its posterior third and has a blunt caudal excretory-copulatory spicule. A detailed morphologic description of the parasite is available.[3] Parasite eggs are the life cycle stage most readily identified for diagnosis. The characteristic eggs are ovoid and measure 50 × 25 μm. The eggs are flattened on one side, giving them the classical bean shape (Fig. 107-1B).

Life Cycle

Adult worms inhabit the lumen of the cecum and appendix. The life span of the adult female is estimated to be between 4 and 10 weeks, while the adult male's is estimated to be only about 2 weeks. Following fertilization, the gravid adult female migrates from the large intestine onto the perianal skin (Fig. 107-2), where she deposits up to 11,000 eggs by uterine contraction and rupture. The sticky eggs adhere to the anal skin and embryonate rapidly over about 6 hours to reach the infective L3 larval stage, still inside the eggshell. The intense pruritus induced by the adult female and the eggs facilitates fecal-oral transfer of eggs. Alternate modes of transmission of infective-stage eggs include fomites and sexual transmission. The minimal interval between egg ingestion and the next egg deposition is between 3 and 4 weeks. The role of retroinfection (migration of newly hatched larvae from the anal skin back into the large intestine) remains to be established.

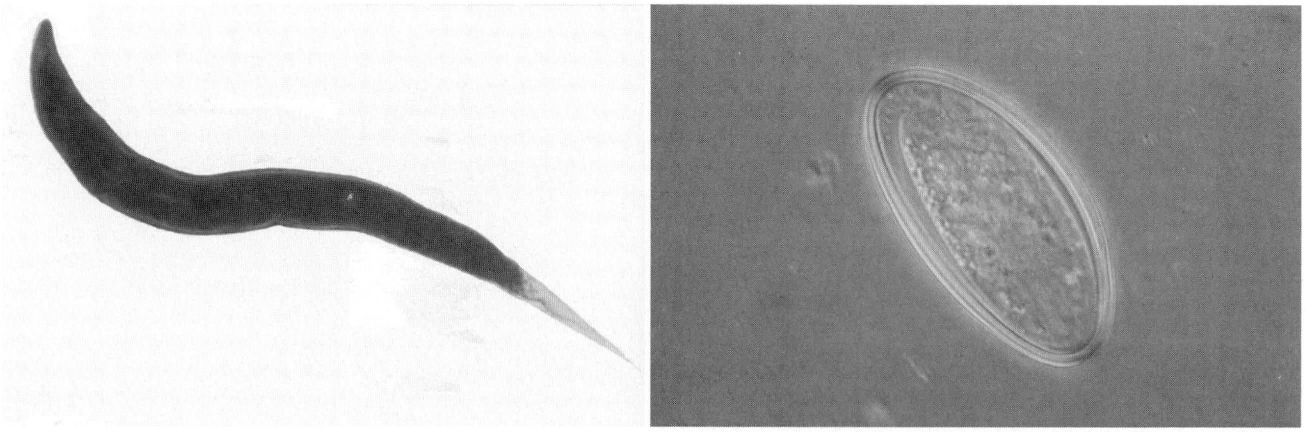

A B

FIGURE 107-1 *A,* The adult female *Enterobius vermicularis* worm appears as a small white roundworm, measuring 9 to 12 mm in length and 0.5 mm in width. *B,* The characteristic eggs are ovoid in shape and measure 50 × 25 μm. The eggs are flattened on one side, giving them the classical bean shape appearance. (Courtesy of John Walker, PhD, Westmead Hospital, Westmead, Australia.)

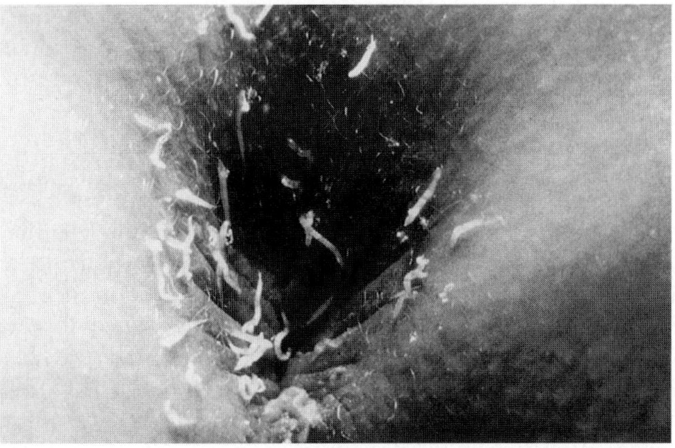

FIGURE 107-2 Adult *Enterobius vermicularis* worms in the perianal region. (From Weber M: Pinworms. N Engl J Med 328:927, 1993.)

EPIDEMIOLOGY

Pinworm eggs have been identified in coprolites (fossilized feces) from North and South America dating back as far as around 7800 BC,[4] from Han Dynasty China (206 BC to 220 AD),[5] and from ancient Egyptian mummies (30 BC to 395 AD).[6] Contemporary epidemiologic surveys have documented infection in all populations studied. However, there is a paucity of recent large-scale studies in which the prevalence and intensity of infection has been documented. Furthermore, no recent longitudinal studies have been undertaken to systematically evaluate changes in epidemiology. In a survey of results of 216,275 stool parasitologic examinations undertaken in state diagnostic laboratories in the United States in 1987, 9597 cellotape test results from 35 states were reported with a rate of 11.4% positive results for pinworm being documented.[7] In a number of reports, however, the prevalence of infection in

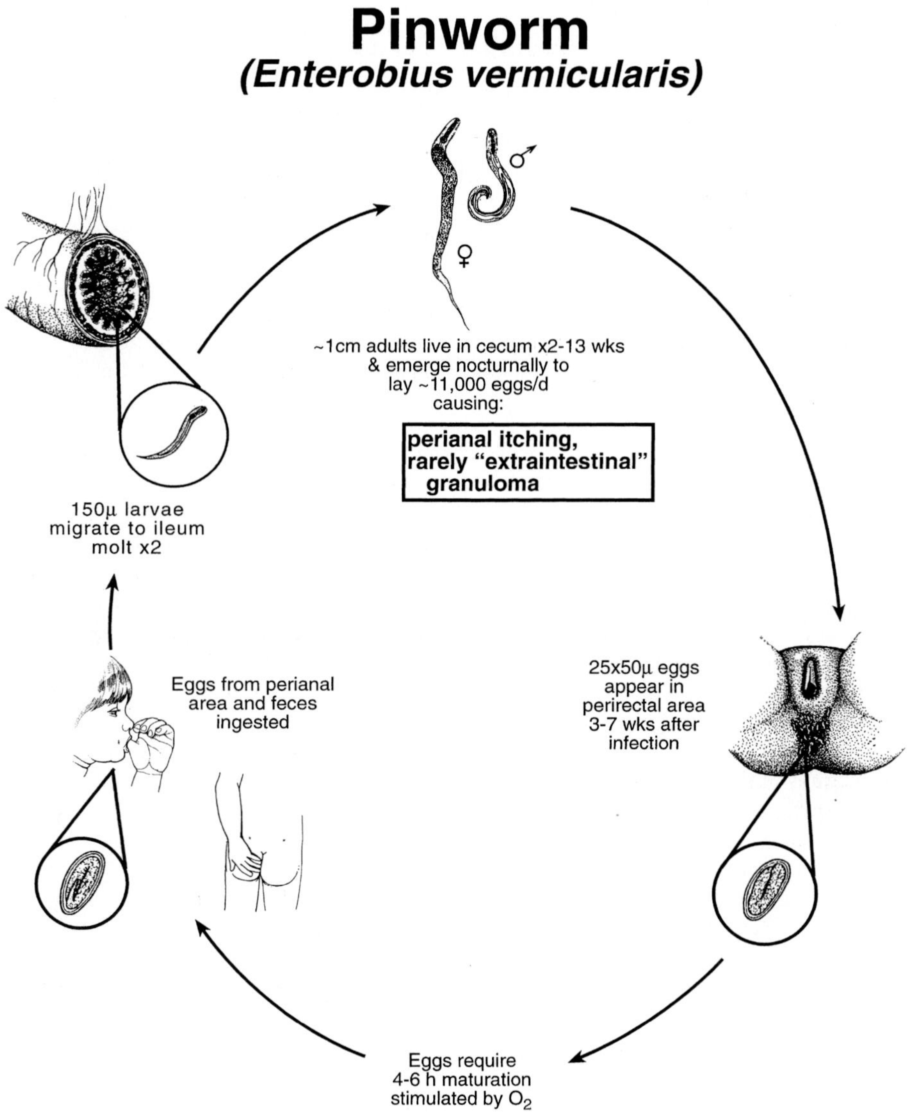

well-recognized at-risk groups such as residents of orphanages and homes for the intellectually disabled appears to be in decline.[7,8] This likely reflects improved sanitation and living standards in such institutions. Likewise in a report of cellotape test results from a large hospital in New York City in the interval from 1971 to 1986, a decline was observed in both the number of tests undertaken annually, from 248 in 1971 to 38 in 1986, and the frequency of positive tests, from 57 (23%) to 0 (0%), respectively.[9] Whether such results reflect a true decrease in prevalence remains to be conclusively established.

Although it is commonly held that enterobiasis, in contrast to other intestinal helminth infections, is more prevalent in temperate than tropical climates, there is a paucity of contemporary data to support this view. Certainly the parasite has been found throughout the developing and developed world when appropriate diagnostic testing has been undertaken. Like other intestinal helminths, the intensity of infection is overdispersed (aggregated); that is, a small proportion of the population carries a disproportionate worm burden. For example, in one study undertaken in a fishing village in southern India the most heavily infected 25% of study subjects harbored more than 90% of the parasites.[10] In this study, a significant aggregation of infection in household units was also observed. As has also been seen with other intestinal helminths, individuals with heavy infection tend to reacquire a disproportionately high parasite burden after curative treatment.[11]

Well-recognized cofactors for increased risk of *Enterobius* infection include overcrowding, poor sanitation, and lack of water for bathing and washing of hands and clothes. While sexual transmission of the parasite also occurs,[12] this route of transmission is likely to be of low significance. Likewise, although eggs have been identified in household dust, the relative role of fomites in transmission remains to be established. While the potential for nosocomial transmission of the parasite exists, such an occurrence is unlikely in hospital environments where good standards of hygiene prevail.[13]

DISEASE

The most common clinical manifestation of *E. vermicularis* infection is *pruritus ani*. This is attributable to the expulsion of eggs by gravid females onto the skin of the anus. When very heavy infection is present, an eczematous reaction with bacterial superinfection may occur. While these symptoms certainly favor spread of infection, the mechanism by which egg deposition causes irritation remains unknown. Other clinical manifestations associated with infection include teeth grinding, enuresis, insomnia, nausea, abdominal pain, vomiting, and appendicitis. The association of these manifestations with pinworm infection is unknown, since no well-performed case-control studies have been undertaken. Likewise, the incidence of asymptomatic infection remains unknown. While appendiceal pinworms have been identified in up to 4% of surgical specimens, appendiceal inflammation is not universal in their presence.[14] Furthermore, the role of pinworms in the pathogenesis of appendicitis remains to be defined. Infection of the female genital tract has been well reported, with manifestations including vulvar and cervical granulomas, salpingitis, oophoritis, tubo-ovarian abscess, and peritonitis. Eosinophilic colitis has also been reported and appears to occur early in infection, since only larvae rather than eggs have been identified in such cases.[15] Rare cases of ectopic infection involving other organs, including the breast, liver, and epididymis, and inguinal hernia have been reported.

DIAGNOSIS

A diagnosis of *E. vermicularis* infection is almost universally established by demonstrating parasite eggs using the cellotape (unfrosted Scotch tape) test. Although commercially produced tests are available, the test in essence involves preparing a wooden tongue depressor or swab stick with clear adhesive tape, with the sticky side facing outward. This is then applied to the anal skin, the tape removed and placed sticky side down on a glass slide. The slide is then examined under a microscope to identify the characteristic eggs (see Fig. 107-1B). As for other parasite infections, the collection of multiple samples has been reported to significantly improve diagnostic sensitivity.[16] Testing at night or first thing in the morning is reported to improve sensitivity. Eggs or adult parasites are rarely seen in fecal samples collected for diagnosis of other intestinal helminth infections such as ascariasis or whipworm or hookworm infections. Adult pinworms can sometimes be seen on the perianal skin (see Fig. 107-2) or in the anal canal during proctoscopy. Likewise, adult worms may occasionally be identified on toilet paper, diapers, or underwear. Infection does not generally result in eosinophilia; no serologic test is available.

TREATMENT

Although several effective anthelminthics are available, the benzimidazole anthelminthic mebendazole is the most widely used drug showing useful efficacy. It is generally administered as a single dose of 100 mg, for which a cure rate in excess of 90% is expected.[17] Alternatives include the other widely used benzimidazole drug, albendazole, also as a single dose of 400 mg, and pyrantel pamoate as a single dose of 11 mg/kg (up to a maximum dose of 1.0 g). The more recently approved broad-spectrum anthelminthic ivermectin also shows useful activity, with a single oral dose ranging from 50 to 200 μg/kg resulting in a cure rate of 85%.[18] Older drugs that are now less widely available or used but still are effective include pyrvinium pamoate 5 mg/kg up to a maximal dose of 250 mg and piperazine in a dose of 65 mg/kg for 7 days. A second course of therapy should be readministered 1 to 2 weeks after the first dose to cover for auto- or reinfection. Likewise, all individuals sharing a household where the index case is a child should be given empiric treatment.

Infection in pregnancy poses a significant clinical dilemma, with some patients suffering great discomfort. Unfortunately, the safety in pregnancy of most agents has yet to be established, and some drugs have shown teratogenic effects in animal models when administered in high dose. However, in a number of retrospective surveys of women who took mebendazole in the first trimester of pregnancy, the rate of congenital abnormalities, fetal loss, or neonatal death has not been found to be significantly higher than in the general population.[19,20] In a large World Health Organization (WHO)-sponsored study of over 7000 Sri Lankan women who took mebendazole during pregnancy a beneficial effect was observed overall, with a significantly lower rate of stillbirth and perinatal death observed in those who took the drug in comparison to those who did not, likely reflecting improved iron status due to cure of hookworm infection.[21] However, among those who took the drug contrary to advice during the first trimester there was a trend toward a higher incidence of major congenital defects, with a rate of 2.5% observed in those who took the drug versus 1.5% among those who did not (odds ratio of 1.66; 95% confidence interval, 0.81–3.56). Studies of single-dose albendazole therapy in pregnant women undertaken in Sierra Leone did not demonstrate any observed increase in frequency of fetal loss or malformation.[22] In a recent review of 49 cases of albendazole administration to women in the first trimester of pregnancy, no cases of congenital abnormalities were reported.[23] In the two cases studied where neonatal death ensued, the deaths were not likely attributable to the albendazole exposure. Nonetheless, prudence should be observed in the administration of these drugs to pregnant or potentially pregnant women, especially in the first trimester of pregnancy.

PREVENTION AND CONTROL

As mentioned previously, reinfection in household and institutional environments is common, and repeated group treatment, usually with single-dose mebendazole, is advised. Other advisable measures include careful attention to hand hygiene, trimming of fingernails, and washing of bedclothes and underwear. Regular vacuuming of house dust has also been advised, despite the lack of evidence supporting a significant role of fomites in transmission. Little is known about host immunity, and vaccine development has not been pursued. Among intestinal helminths, this parasite has not assumed a large place in public health programs in developed or developing countries.

REFERENCES

1. Hugot JP: *Enterobius gregorii* (Oxyuridae, Nematoda), a new human parasite. Ann Parasitol Hum Comp 58:403–404, 1983.
2. Hasegawa H, Takao Y, Nakao M, et al: Is *Enterobius gregorii* Hugot, 1983 (Nematoda: Oxyuridae) a distinct species? J Parasitol 84:131–134, 1998.
3. Hugot JP, Gardner SL, Morand S: The Enterobiinae subfam. Nov. (Nematoda, Oxyurida) pinworm parasites of primates and rodents. Int J Parasitol 26:147–159, 1996.
4. Fry GF, Moore JG: *Enterobius vermicularis*: 10,000-year-old human infection. Science 166:1620, 1969.
5. Wei O: Internal organs of a 2100-year-old female corpse. Lancet 2:1198, 1973.
6. Horne PD: First evidence of enterobiasis in ancient Egypt. J Parasitol 88:1019–1021, 2002.
7. Kappus KK, Juranek DD, Roberts JM: Results of testing for intestinal parasites by state diagnostic laboratories, United States, 1987. MMWR CDC Surveill Summ 40:25–45, 1991.
8. Gatti S, Lopes R, Cevini C, et al: Intestinal parasitic infections in an institution for the mentally retarded. Ann Trop Med Parasitol 94:453–460, 2000.
9. Vermund SH, MacLeod S: Is pinworm a vanishing infection? Laboratory surveillance in a New York City medical center from 1971 to 1986. Am J Dis Child 142:566–568, 1988.
10. Haswell-Elkins MR, Elkins DB, Manjula K, et al: The distribution and abundance of *Enterobius vermicularis* in a South Indian fishing community. Parasitology 95:339–354, 1987.
11. Haswell-Elkins MR, Elkins DB, Anderson RM: Evidence for predisposition in humans to infection with Ascaris, hookworm, Enterobius and Trichuris in a South Indian fishing community. Parasitology 95:323–337, 1987.
12. Harris JR, Morton RS: Sexual transmission of intestinal parasites. Br J Vener Dis 49:393, 1973.
13. Ashford RW, Hart CA, Williams RG: *Enterobius vermicularis* infection in a children's ward. J Hosp Infect 12:221–224, 1988.
14. Arca MJ, Gates RL, Groner JI, et al: Clinical manifestations of appendiceal pinworms in children: An institutional experience and a review of the literature. Pediatr Surg Int 20:372–375, 2004.
15. Liu LX, Chi J, Upton MP, Ash LR: Eosinophilic colitis associated with larvae of the pinworm *Enterobius vermicularis*. Lancet 346:410–412, 1995.
16. Fan PC, Chan CH: Consecutive examinations by scotch-tape perianal swabs in diagnosis of enterobiasis. Gaoxiong Yi Xue Ke Xue Za Zhi 6:647–652, 1990.
17. St Georgiev V: Chemotherapy of enterobiasis (oxyuriasis). Expert Opin Pharmacother 2:267–275, 2001.
18. Naquira C, Jimenez G, Guerra JG, et al: Ivermectin for human strongyloidiasis and other intestinal helminths. Am J Trop Med Hyg 40:304–309, 1989.
19. Cowden J, Hotez P: Mebendazole and albendazole treatment of geohelminth infections in children and pregnant women. Pediatr Infect Dis J 19:659–660, 2000.
20. Diav-Citrin O, Shechtman S, Arnon J, et al: Pregnancy outcome after gestational exposure to mebendazole: A prospective controlled cohort study. Am J Obstet Gynecol 188:282–285, 2003.
21. de Silva NR, Sirisena JL, Gunasekera DP, et al: Effect of mebendazole therapy during pregnancy on birth outcome. Lancet 353:1145–1149, 1999.
22. Torlesse H, Hodges M: Anthelminthic treatment and haemoglobin concentrations during pregnancy. Lancet 356:1083, 2000.
23. Bradley M, Horton J: Assessing the risk of benzimidazole therapy during pregnancy. Trans R Soc Trop Med Hyg 95:72–73, 2001.

108

Tric huriasis

ED COOPER

INTRODUCTION

Members of *Trichuris* species are successful nematode parasites of mammalian bowel and *Trichuris trichiura* has had much opportunity to coevolve with man. The *T. Trichuris* species itself is a parasite of both Old World and New World monkeys and apes.[1] Its human presence is associated with poor hygiene rather than a specifically tropical environment, although warmth and moisture in the soil enhance transmission through promotion of the viability of the infective stages. Until about 30 years ago, four things led to the underestimation of *T. trichiura* as a pathogen.

1. Low-intensity infections, which are by far the most common, are asymptomatic.
2. *Trichuris* is seldom found as the only pathogen, but is commonly just one of multiple health and environmental threats.
3. The onset of significant symptoms is often too slow to alarm the family.
4. It produces a transient, although prolonged, disease of the developing child while seldom causing disability to adults.

However, severe infections of children are amenable to treatment with highly effective drugs with minimal side effects; and this makes case-detection and treatment most rewarding and population-based prevention most productive. In the last decade, there has been a steady increase in reports on all aspects of trichuriasis, with publications reported by Medline now approaching 40 per year.

AGENT

Trichuris trichiura is a member of the nematode superfamily Trichuroidea and is related to *Trichinella spiralis*. The genus was previously often called *Trichocephalus*, logically enough since the hairlike part (tricho-) is in fact the head end (cephalus). However, the original name given by Linnaeus (1771), in the mistaken belief that the hairlike part was the tail (uris), is the official name. Whipworm is a commonly used unofficial name. The adult is shaped like a whip, with the handle representing the wider posterior section containing the reproductive organs and the intestine, while the long, fine anterior part, called the stichosome, contains the long pharynx. The whole is about 4 cm long. The male has a curled posterior end. The eggs are thick-walled and barrel-shaped, about 50 mm long, with a plug at each pole.

Eggs, passed in the feces, contain a zygote and are not infective until embryonation, which takes place in the soil over 2 to 4 weeks. The egg now contains the L1 larva. Following human ingestion, the larva is released in the stomach and passes into the intestine. It penetrates the epithelium in the mucosal crypts of the cecum.[2] The larva develops by molting, and the adult develops from the L4 stage, by now having migrated with the epithelial cells up the sides of the crypts. The anterior part of the adult lies in a tunnel within the epithelium between the mouths of the crypts, while the posterior part is free in the lumen. The stichosome is surrounded by a syncytium and debris of the epithelium. Each female produces up to 20,000 eggs per day; the life expectancy of a worm within the host has been estimated at 1 to 3 years,[2] which would imply that some adults live far longer.

EPIDEMIOLOGY AND ECOLOGY

Up to a quarter of humanity carries *T. trichiura* as an intestinal parasite. An estimate for the number of Chinese infected (212 million)[3] has brought the world estimate to over 1 billion infected human hosts. However, all parasitic infections have an aggregated ("clumped") distribution among their hosts. This is extreme in trichuriasis, where over 90% of a community may be infected but only 10% or fewer have intense, symptomatic infections.[4] There is as yet no clear evidence on any factor making the intensely infected hosts especially susceptible, apart from the obvious one of environmental exposure related to hygienic practices. Familial aggregation occurs.[5] After treatment, there is a tendency for the most heavily infected to become the most heavily re-infected, but there is much crossing over between light and heavy strata too.[6] The role of domestic pigs in transmission is unknown, although passage of the life cycle through the pig is possible.[7] Warm, damp soil provides the best medium for transmission once it is fecally contaminated. *T. trichiura* is found in humid, tropical environments but also in temperate climates including Northern Europe and South Africa. Although transmission occurs in cool climates, hyperendemicity is correlated with higher temperatures and lower altitudes.[8] The nematode is the predominant intestinal parasite in many communities in Africa and the Americas.

DISEASE

Most infections are asymptomatic. In heavy infections (many adult worms, see next section), stools become loose and frequent and there is tenesmus. Frequency can exceed 12 stools per 24 hours and nocturnal stooling is especially characteristic. Stools consist largely of mucus but may also be watery. There is a characteristic acrid smell. Frank blood is common. Trichuriasis is one of the most frequently identified causes of recurrent rectal prolapse and the worms may be seen on the prolapsed mucosa. Children with this degree of symptomatic infection are almost invariably severely anemic and growth-retarded.[9] They are also geophagic and much of their stool may consist of ingested earth or even small stones. Finger-clubbing is common, correlated in prevalence and severity with the number of adult worms harbored.[10]

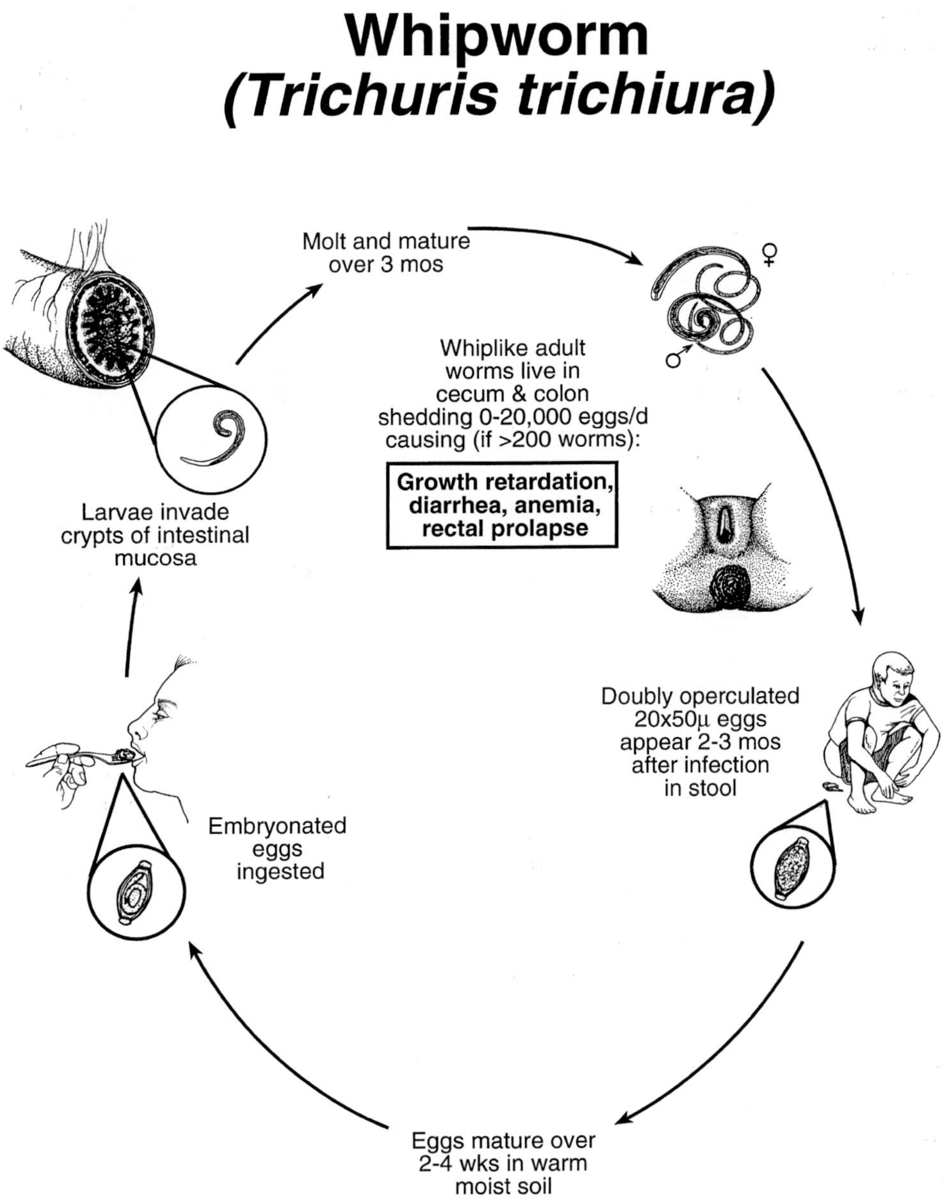

PATHOGENESIS AND IMMUNITY

Light infections (20 adult worms or fewer) are not associated with any discernible morbidity. Heavy infections (200 adult worms or more) are associated consistently with the clear-cut syndrome described previously, which has both colonic and systemic features. The difference is not only one of parasite biomass (in which a 10-fold increase may scarcely be significant clinically), but perhaps more importantly of the site affected: In light infections, the worms are confined to the cecum and the ascending colon, whereas in heavy infections there are adult worms in the distal colon and rectum, and also often in the terminal ileum. The mucosa at these latter sites may have a greater tendency to a local hypersensitivity reaction to *T. trichiura*.

In the inflamed areas, especially the rectum, the mucosa is edematous. At the cellular level, the most significant abnormalities are distended goblet cells, an increased concentration of superficial mast cells, which are degranulating, and an increase in the lamina propria of calprotectin-secreting cells, presumed to be monocytes.[11] Increased tumor necrosis factor (TNF)-α is both produced by lamina propria cells and found circulating in the peripheral blood.[11,12] Bloody mucus commonly exudes from the mucosal surface.

The systemic consequences are anemia and impaired growth.[13] The former is presumed to follow from direct loss from the gut of red blood cells followed by iron deficiency. The mechanism for the impaired growth is not clear but could involve both substrate-limited and substrate-wasting pathways. In support of the former is the finding of protein-losing enteropathy proportional to the worm burden,[13] and of the latter increased circulating TNF-α, which may inhibit appetite as well as having direct effects on cell division and metabolism. Plasma insulin-like growth factor-I (IGF-I) concentration is found to be correspondingly reduced during the *Trichuris* dysentery syndrome (TDS), although it returns to a similar level to that of comparable children from the same community within a month of worm expulsion.[14] The increase in plasma IGF-I after treatment accompanies a fall in plasma TNF-α, an increase in collagen synthesis as shown by rising plasma pro-collagen type 1, and an acceleration in physical growth. Although it had been suggested that the beneficial effect of mebendazole on child growth might be due to some systemic effect other than through worm expulsion, a quite specific worm effect has now been shown.[15]

The elevation of acute phase proteins[16] is further evidence of a systemic component in the response to heavy *Trichuris* infection. Plasma viscosity[16] is also moderately elevated and declines slowly over a period of months, despite the rapid resolution of symptoms after anthelminthic treatment.

Concentrations of immunoglobulin A (IgA), IgM, and IgG antibody to *T. trichiura* are correlated with the host's current worm burden.[17,18] Specific responses of IgG1, IgG4, IgA, and IgE have been shown.[12] As with *Ascaris*, multiple reinfections with *Trichuris* are to be expected,[19] implying that protective immunity must be incomplete. Epidemiological data combined with serology can be interpreted as consistent with an increase in immunity with age, and as suggesting that both IgA[17] and IgE[12] may be mediators of this. Some genetic polymorphism in susceptibility[20,21] has been shown but, if this is so, it is all the more remarkable that prevalence of infection can approach 100% in large and diverse communities.[22] Evidence has been sought in humans[12,23] for the divergence in immune response seen in mice,[24,25] where a Th1 cytokine response has been associated with chronic infection and a Th2 response with parasite expulsion. The human responses have been diverse and inconsistent.[12] The most striking evidence for the converse, that chronic infection induces a Th2 response that inhibits the Th1 response, has come from the remarkable experiment of deliberately infecting patients suffering from Crohn's disease or ulcerative colitis with *T. suis* eggs as anti-Th1, and therefore anti-inflammatory, therapy. Preliminary results have been encouraging.[26]

Cytokine expression in human colonic mucosa biopsied as part of investigation of *Trichuris* dysentery syndrome suggests that both interferon-γ (Th1) and interleukin-4 (Th2) may be strongly expressed in the mucosa of children with heavy and chronic infections with *T. trichiura*. This corresponds with recent data from peripheral blood.[27] It excludes T-cell anergy as an explanation for these exceptionally intense infections. In humans, downstream of T-cell recognition, some component of the immune response that leads to worm expulsion in mice appears to be either missing or attenuated.[23] Eosinophilia is often associated with trichuriasis, but its lack by no means excludes the diagnosis in any individual.

There may be neuropsychological effects of intense trichuriasis, manifest by impaired cognitive function[28] and especially locomotor development.[29] These effects are too subtle to present as a clear part of the clinical picture, unless the child is already suffering from severe social deprivation or cognitive disorder and so is more likely to have geophagia leading to the secondary acquisition of this heavy worm burden. The systemic inflammation, especially increased circulating TNF-α, is a possible mediator between the parasitized intestine and impairment of higher brain function.

DIAGNOSIS

The differential diagnosis is from other causes of infective dysentery or idiopathic colitis. A stool specimen may be

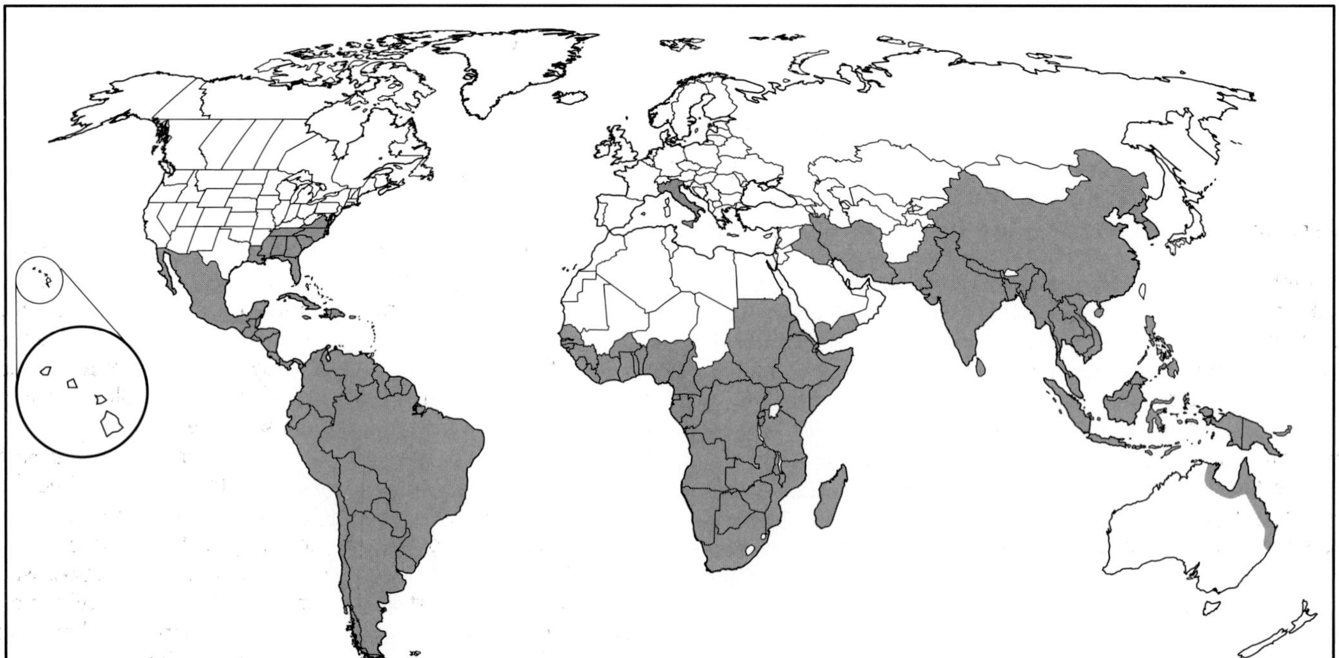

Trichuris trichiura

examined by any of the techniques for parasites, but the Kato-Katz preparation is recommended for simplicity, reliability, and quantification. Although from a population perspective a count of eggs per gram (epg) of feces is well correlated with adult worm burden, this cannot be applied to the individual. With less than 1000 epg clinically significant trichuriasis is unlikely and with over 10,000 epg it is likely, but severe cases occur with absent eggs on a single stool specimen and some lightly infected children have over 10,000 epg. Proctoscopy showing worms on the rectal mucosa is more reliable evidence of *Trichuris* colitis,[29] and this can be used in the clinic. Colonoscopy sometimes reveals an intense colonic infection, either in a research setting or if the diagnosis has not been made before the procedure. It cannot be justified as a diagnostic procedure: Presumptive treatment or a trial of treatment is fully justified in a busy clinic setting.

TREATMENT AND PROGNOSIS

Many anthelminthics effective against *Ascaris* fail against *Trichuris*, and to these must now be added ivermectin.[30,31] Mebendazole (Janssen's Vermox or generic) or albendazole (Zentel, Smith-Kline-Beecham) by mouth are effective and recommended. Single doses (mebendazole 100 mg to 500 mg; albendazole 400 mg) give a good chance of cure in light infections and are worthwhile in mass campaigns, but increasing probability of complete worm expulsion is a function of increasing exposure to the drug. For clinically significant infections, mebendazole 200 mg per day on 3 successive days is recommended, or albendazole 400 mg per day for 3 days. These drugs are contraindicated in pregnancy and not recommended for infants, but clinical judgment must be used in the event of symptomatic infection. Worm expulsion will be followed by clinical cure, but if the environment is unchanged re-infection is likely and re-treatment every 3 months,[19] or at least every year,[32] is well justified.

PREVENTION AND CONTROL

Satisfactory fecal disposal using water-seal toilets or good pit-latrines completely interrupts the life cycle of these geohelminths. Hand washing and washing of any vegetables grown in fecally contaminated soil is also useful. In the real-life situation of crowded, poor dwellings, scarce piped water and heavily contaminated soil, mass chemotherapy with cyclical repetition is highly effective.[32] The children of preschool and school age should be targeted.[2] In regions where periodic mass treatments are being used to control lymphatic filariasis, single-dose treatments with albendazole together with ivermectin have proven more efficacious in diminishing *Trichuris* infections than single-dose treatments with albendazole alone or with albendazole combined with diethylcarbamazine.[33,34]

REFERENCES

1. Ooi HK, Tenora F, Itoh K, et al: Comparative study of *Trichuris trichura* from non-human primates and from man, and their difference with *T. suis*. J Vet Med Sci (Japan) 55:363, 1993.
2. Bundy DAP, Cooper ES: *Trichuris* and trichuriasis in humans. Adv Parasitol 28:107, 1989.
3. Xu LQ, Yu SH, Jiang ZX, et al: Soil-transmitted helminthiasis: Nationwide survey in China. Bull World Health Org 73:507, 1995.
4. Bundy DAP: Epidemiological aspects of *Trichuris* and trichuriasis in Caribbean communities. Trans R Soc Trop Med Hyg 80:702, 1986.
5. Forrester JE, Scott ME, Bundy DAP, et al: Clustering of *Ascaris lumbricoides* and *Trichuris trichiura* infections within households. Trans R Soc Trop Med Hyg 82:282, 1988.
6. Bundy DAP, Cooper ES, Thompson DE, et al: Predisposition to *Trichuris trichiura* in humans. Epidemiol Infect 98:65, 1987.
7. Beer RJS: The relationship between *Trichuris trichiura* (Linnaeus 1758) of man and *Trichuris suis* (Schrank 1788) of the pig. Res Vet Sci 20:47, 1976.
8. Appleton CC, Gouws E: The distribution of common intestinal nematodes along an altitudinal transect in KwaZulu-Natal, South Africa. Ann Trop Med Parasitol 90:181, 1996.
9. Cooper ES, Bundy DAP: Trichuriasis. Clin Trop Med Comm Dis 2:629, 1987.
10. Cooper ES: Trichuriasis. In Farthing MJG, Keusch GT, Wakelin D (eds): Enteric Infection: Mechanisms, Manifestations and Management, Vol. 2. Intestinal Helminths. London, Chapman & Hall, 1995, p 201.
11. MacDonald TT, Spencer J, Murch SH, et al: Mucosal macrophages and cytokine production in the colon of children with *Trichuris trichiura* dysentery. Trans R Soc Trop Med Hyg 88:265, 1994.
12. Faulkner H, Turner J, Kamgno J, et al: Age- and infection intensity-dependent cytokine and antibody production in human trichuriasis: The importance of IgE. J Infect Dis 185:665, 2002.
13. Cooper ES, Whyte-Alleng CAM, Finzi-Smith JS, et al: Intestinal nematode infections in children: The pathophysiological price paid. Parasitology 104(Suppl):S91, 1992.
14. Stephenson LS, Holland CV, Cooper ES: The public health significance of *Trichuris trichiura*. Parasitology 121(Suppl):73, 2000.
15. Garg R, Lee LA, Beach MJ, et al: Evaluation of the Integrated Management of Childhood Illness guidelines for treatment of intestinal helminth infections among sick children aged 2–4 years in western Kenya. Trans R Soc Trop Med Hyg 96:543, 2002.
16. Cooper ES, Ramdath DD, Whyte-Alleng C, et al: Plasma proteins in children with the Trichuris Dysentery Syndrome. J Clin Pathol 50:236, 1997.
17. Lillywhite JE, Bundy DAP, Didier JM, et al: Humoral immune responses in human infection with the whipworm *Trichuris trichiura*. Parasite Immunol 131:491, 1991.
18. Needham CS, Lillywhite JE: Immunological correlates with patterns of *Trichuris* infection. Trans R Soc Trop Med Hyg 88:262, 1994.
19. Callender JEM, Grantham-McGregor SM, Walker SP, et al: Treatment effects in *Trichuris* dysentery syndrome. Acta Paediatr 83:1182, 1994.
20. Bundy DAP: Population ecology of intestinal helminth infections in human communities. Philo Trans R Soc London, Series B 321:405, 1988.
21. Brown CJ, McCloskey DJ, Bundy DA, et al: Parasitic infection with *Trichuris trichiura* influences plasma levels of soluble HLA class 1. Hum Immunol 60:1067, 1999.
22. Ratard RC, Kouemeni LE, Ekani Bessala MM, et al: Ascariasis and trichuriasis in Cameroon. Trans R Soc Trop Med Hyg 85:84, 1991.
23. Cooper ES, Spencer J, Whyte-Alleng CAM, et al: Immediate hypersensitivity in the colon of children with chronic T*richuris trichiura* dysentery. Lancet 338:1104, 1991.
24. Else KJ, Finkelman FD, Maliszewski CR, et al: Cytokine-mediated regulation of chronic intestinal helminth infection. J Exp Med 179:374, 1994.
25. Artis D, Shapira S, Mason N, et al: Differential requirement for NF-kappa B family members in control of helminth infection and intestinal infection. J Immunol 169:4481, 2002.
26. Summers RW, Elliott DE, Qadir K, et al: *Trichuris suis* seems to be safe and possibly effective in the treatment of inflammatory bowel disease. Am J Gastroenterol 98:2034, 2003.
27. Geiger SM, Massara CL, Bethony J, et al: Cellular responses and cytokine profiles in *Ascaris lumbricoides* and *Trichuris trichiura* infected patients. Parasite Immunol 24:499, 2002.
28. Nokes C, Grantham-McGregor SM, Sawyer AW, et al: Moderate to heavy infections of *Trichuris trichiura* affect cognitive function in Jamaican school children. Parasitology 104:539, 1992.
29. Gilman RH, Chong YH, Davis C, et al: The adverse consequences of heavy *Trichuris* infection. Trans R Soc Trop Med Hyg 77:432, 1983.

30. Marti H, Haji HJ, Savioli L, et al: A comparative trial of a single-dose ivermectin versus three days of albendazole for treatment of *Strongyloides stercoralis* and other soil-transmitted helminth infections in children. Am J Trop Med Hyg 55:477, 1996.
31. Ranque S, Chippaux JP, Garcia A, et al: Follow-up of *Ascaris lumbricoides* and *Trichuris trichiura* infections in children living in a community treated with ivermectin at 3-monthly intervals. Ann Trop Parasitol 95:389, 2001.
32. Zani LC, Favre TC, Pieri OS, et al: Impact of antihelminthic treatment on infection by *Ascaris lumbricoides, Trichuris trichiura* and hookworms in Covas, a rural community of Pernambuco, Brazil. Rev Inst Med Trop Sao Paulo 46:63, 2004.
33. Ismail MM, Jayakody RL: Efficacy of albendazole and its combinations with ivermectin or diethylcarbamazine (DEC) in the treatment of *Trichuris trichiura* infections in Sri Lanka. Ann Trop Med Parasitol 93:501, 1999.
34. Belizario VY, Amarillo ME, de Leon WU, et al: A comparison of the efficacy of single doses of albendazole, ivermectin, and diethylcarbamazine alone or in combinations against *Ascaris* and *Trichuris* spp. Bull World Health Org 81:35, 2003.

109

Ascariasis

ELYSE SELTZER
MICHELE BARRY
D.W.T. CROMPTON

INTRODUCTION

Ascaris lumbricoides, one of four species of nematodes that are soil-transmitted helminths, is among the most prevalent of parasitic infections in humans.[1,2] About a fifth of the world's population is estimated to be infected. *Ascaris* infections in people living in developed countries may also be due to *A. suum*, which is commonly found in domestic swine reared under conditions of poor hygiene. Taxonomists have yet to agree as to whether *A. lumbricoides* and *A. suum* are separate species.[2] However, identification to the generic level is all that clinicians require for case management and treatment. The high prevalence and diverse geographic spread of *A. lumbricoides* can be attributed to a number of factors, including the properties of its eggs in a variety of environmental conditions, the high number of eggs produced per female worm, and poor socioeconomic conditions that facilitate spread of the organism. *Ascaris* persists wherever fecal sanitation is inadequate or lacking; indiscriminate defecation by infected people contaminates the social environment and guarantees transmission. Two separate populations of *A. lumbricoides* exist: (1) juvenile and adult worms that live predominantly within the human intestine, and (2) eggs that contaminate the environment. Infection is usually transmitted via ingestion of eggs from contaminated foodstuffs, although in regions with extremely high egg burdens, infection may occasionally occur via inhalation of eggs and swallowing infected respiratory secretions. Many infections are asymptomatic, but *Ascaris* infections can be causes of morbidity by contributing in endemic areas to impaired growth and development and of morbidity and mortality due to complications caused by adult worms. While the complication rate of *Ascaris* infection is low, the high worldwide prevalence of infections makes the overall number of complications (primarily intestinal obstruction) from *Ascaris* infection fairly high, with mortality from ascariasis perhaps as high as 10,000 to 100,000 deaths per year.[3–5]

AGENT

A. lumbricoides is a nematode that has been recognized as a pathogen since ancient times, in part because of its extremely large size. Scientific description of the anatomy and clinical manifestations of *A. lumbricoides* was published by Tyson in 1683.[6] The female roundworm can reach lengths of up to 400 mm (Fig. 109-1) and the male roundworm up to 350 mm, with diameters of 30 mm to 60 mm and a yellow-white or pinkish-grey color. Female worms produce up to 200,000 eggs per day while living in the human host for about a year; these eggs are passed in feces.[2] Eggs are oval in shape, measure approximately 60 μm to 70 μm in length, and are a yellow-brown color (Fig. 109-2). Fertilized eggs tend to be shorter and wider than unfertilized eggs.

One of the factors accounting for the high prevalence of *Ascaris* infections is the ability of eggs to survive for long periods in the right climate, even under a variety of environmental conditions. The egg shell has several layers that are protective against environmental factors. The outside of the egg is coated with a sticky layer of mucopolysaccharide, which facilitates adherence to fruit, vegetables, fingers, door knobs, and so on. Fertilized eggs contain embryos that require moisture, warmth, oxygen, and shade if they are to develop to the juvenile worm infective to humans. UV light disrupts this developmental process (embryonation), the rate of which is temperature-dependent.[2,7]

Once eggs are passed in the stool, they may take 2 to 4 weeks to fully embryonate and become infective. After these eggs are ingested by a human, infective juveniles escape from their egg shells in the small intestines of susceptible hosts. They penetrate the intestinal wall and migrate to the liver via the hepatic portal system. After about 4 days in the liver, survivors move on to the lungs, where they remain for 10 more days before moving up the trachea to be swallowed and so to become established in the small intestine where they live for up to a year.[8] Egg release by mature, inseminated female worms is estimated to begin about 70 days after the ingestion of infective eggs.[2] Fluoroscopic studies have revealed that the jejunum is the worms' optimum site but they may be found elsewhere in the small bowel and stomach, sometimes in the

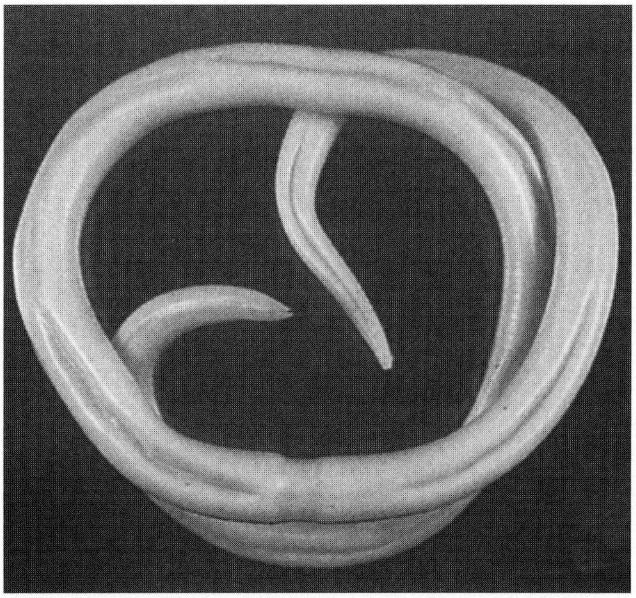

FIGURE 109-1 Female *Ascaris lumbricoides* adult worm. (From Zaman V: Atlas of Medical Parasitology, 3rd ed. Singapore, Singapore University Press, 1992.)

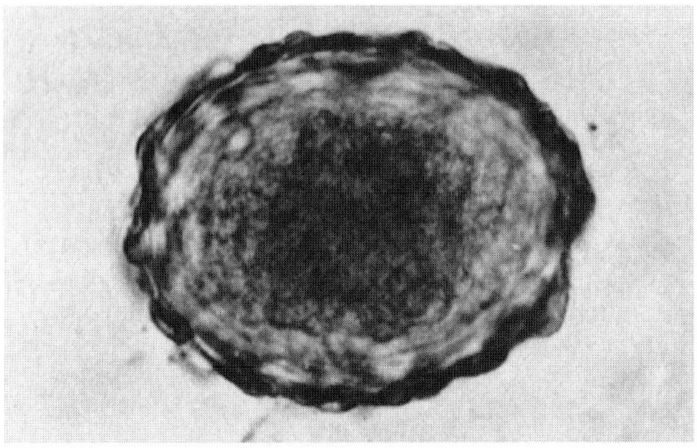

FIGURE 109-2 *Ascaris lumbricoides* egg. (From Despommier D, Gwadz R, Hotez P: Parasitic Disease, 3rd ed. New York, Springer-Verlag, 1994.)

biliary system, and more rarely in a variety of sites unconnected with the gastrointestinal tract.[3,9]

EPIDEMIOLOGY

Geographic prevalence and distribution of *A. lumbricoides* are influenced largely by climate, sanitation provision and practices, literacy rates, socioeconomic conditions, cultural habits, and the availability of, and access to, health care. A number of epidemiologic studies of *Ascaris* have demonstrated its widespread worldwide distribution.[10,11]

Insight into the population biology and transmission dynamics can be understood by reference to a mathematical framework summarized by Anderson and May.[12] This work demonstrated that host-parasite relationships between humans and *Ascaris* depend on the intensity of infection or worm burden per person. Worm burden explains the severity of disease, the success or otherwise of transmission, and the persistence of the infection in various groups in the community. Prevalence data account for the extent of *Ascaris* in a region while intensity data indicate the health risks for individuals and populations.

Modes of transmission of *A. lumbricoides* vary according to the type of community under examination. In a closed community, for example, within a small village or a family, infection is largely endemic and eggs are unlikely transferred from the outside. In a more open community, from either a rural or an urban locale, eggs can be transferred out of the community via sewage or contaminated soil but can be reintroduced into the community via contaminated produce. Finally, in a community formed under social conditions, for example, a school, factory, or some other closely knit social group, transmission will also occur.[13] *A. lumbricoides* infection has been believed to occur more in rural than in urban areas. However, as urbanization increases in many developing countries, so does the urbanization of *A. lumbricoides* increase. In general, children are infected more frequently than adults, perhaps reflecting increased soil contact from play and poorer hygiene. On the other hand, protective immunity may be weaker in children than adults.[2] Interestingly, *Ascaris* is regularly demonstrated to occur in familial clusters.[14]

Socioeconomic factors, particularly sanitation, play a large role in determining the degree of contamination of the human environment with fertile eggs. The prevalence of infection is increased where poor sanitation occurs and where the population is heavily involved with subsistence agriculture, particularly if raw human feces are used as fertilizer. High illiteracy

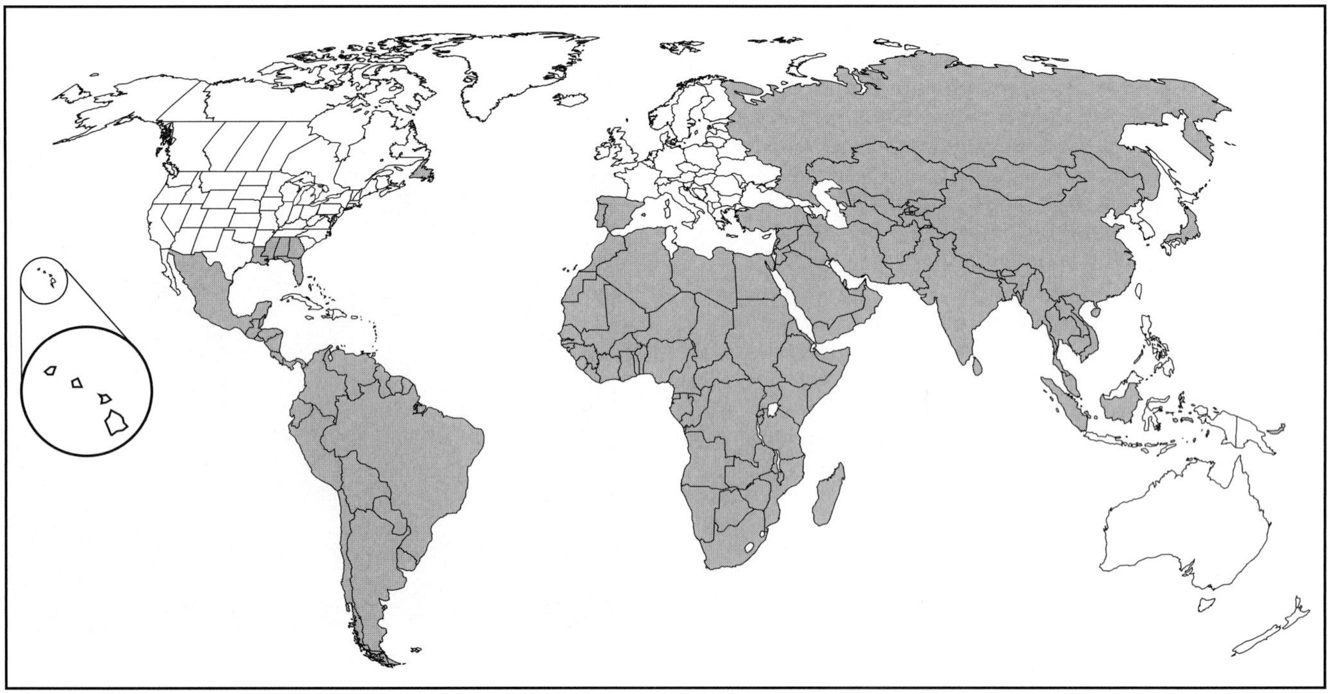

Ascaris lumbricoides

Ascaris lumbricoides

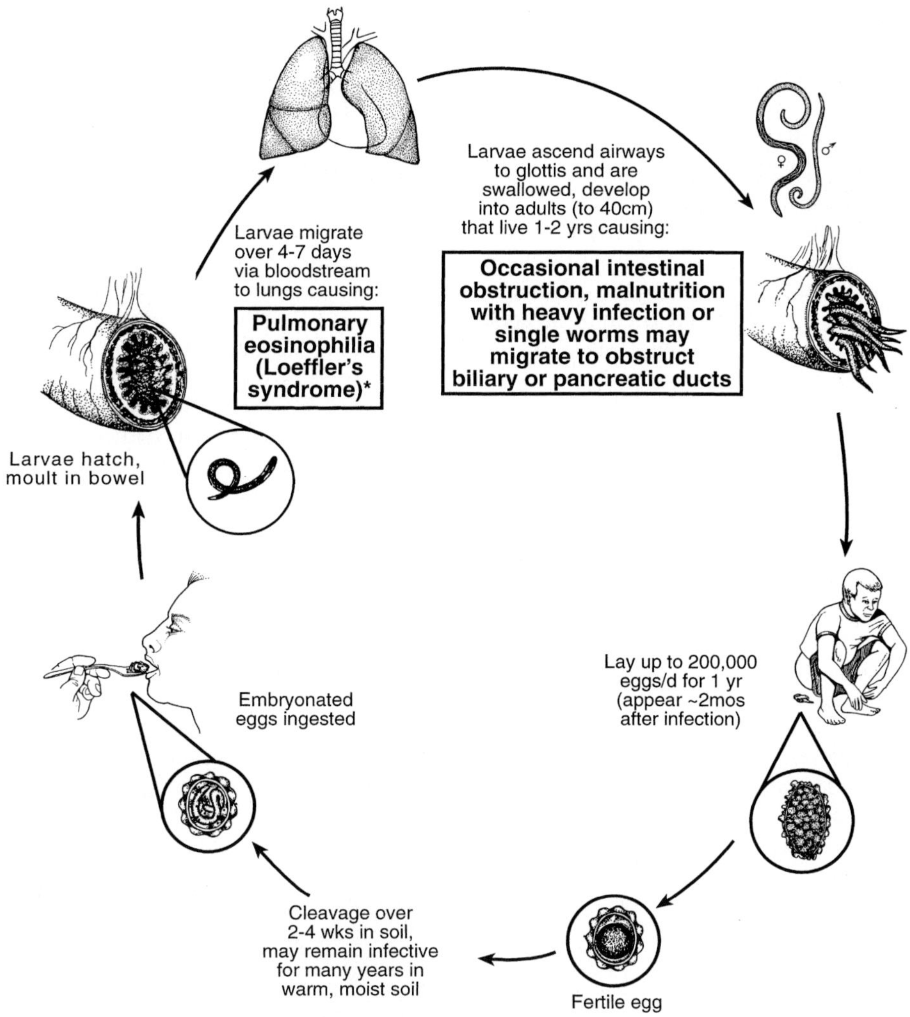

rates and particular cultural habits, such as using "night soil" (human excrement) as fertilizer and children playing in unsanitized soil, enhance transmission. Certain soils are more suited to egg survival.

Climate has a large influence on the pattern of *A. lumbricoides* infection in a particular region, in terms of the severity and character of symptoms as well as the seasonal pattern of disease. For example, in Africa, prevalence is higher in countries with warm, wet climates than in those with more arid climates.[15,16] A national study of *A. lumbricoides* infections in schoolchildren in Cameroon surveyed 22,000 children from 512 schools from various climatic zones and found a marked variability in prevalence rates, with low rates (5%) in the northern tropical zones, which were described as having a short rainy season and a long dry season, and rates up to 70% in the southern equatorial zones, characterized by abundant rainfall with few brief dry periods.[17] There were no differences within individual climatic zones in prevalence rates between rural and urban populations or between low- and high-altitude regions.[17] In Saudi Arabia, where the pattern of transmission is seasonal, pulmonary symptoms from migrating *Ascaris* predominate over intestinal symptoms and occur from March to May, after the rainy season optimizes conditions for embryonation.[18]

Numerous studies have been done on the prevalence of *Ascaris* infection in a variety of populations and locales. In China, surveys have indicated that 531 million people are infected with *Ascaris* (47% prevalence rate) compared with 212 million and 194 million infected, respectively, with *Trichuris* and hookworm.[19] A study of schoolchildren in Lagos State, Nigeria, found that in 810 fecal samples, 74% demonstrated *A. lumbricoides*, with a mean egg load of 2544 eggs per gram (epg) of stool.[20] This high prevalence was associated with customs of indiscriminate defecation, eating contaminated produce, and poor hand washing.[20] In a village in rural Burma (now Myanmar), 77% of 783 people examined were infected with *Ascaris,* with age-specific prevalences that reached a maximum of 92% from 5 to 9 years of age and a minimum of 65% from 50 years and older.[21] In an epidemiologic study of intestinal nematodes in children in the Ranomafana rain forest in southeastern Madagascar, examination of stool samples from 1292 children from birth to 10 years of age demonstrated a prevalence of *Ascaris* infection of 78%, with a prevalence of 34% by 6 to 12 months of age and 100% by 10 years of age.[22] As judged from fecal egg excretion densities (epg), the intensity of *Ascaris* infections, like those with *Trichuris trichiura*, typically are greatest in the early years of life, peaking at about 10 years of age and then declining.[23] This contrasts with hookworm infections, in which intensities do not peak until 20 to 25 years of age.[23] The greater intensities of *Ascaris* infections in young children make them at greatest risk for the clinical effects of *Ascaris* infections.

CLINICAL MANIFESTATIONS

Most infections with *A. lumbricoides* are asymptomatic.[3–5] The spectrum of symptomatic disease from ascariasis is broad, ranging from mild abdominal discomfort to mild pulmonary symptoms to abdominal catastrophes resulting in death. Particular symptoms reflect the migration of larvae or adult worms in the involved organ system, and the intensity of symptoms generally relates to the worm burden of each host. Thus, children, who usually have the highest intensity of infection, tend to have more severe clinical presentations. The most common clinical syndromes of ascariasis are pneumonitis, intestinal obstruction, biliary obstruction, and pancreatic obstruction.[2,24] The most widespread manifestation of ascariasis is its adverse effect on the growth, development, and nutritional status of children.[25,26] Other rarer consequences of *Ascaris* infection, such as the presence of the worms in the brain, kidney, and placenta, have also been reported.[2]

The migration of developing larvae through the lungs are responsible for the pulmonary manifestations of *Ascaris* infections; and hence lung involvement is due to new infections acquired via eggs ingested in the antecedent weeks and not due to any established intraintestinal adult worms. Clinical syndromes result from both the physical disruption elicited by larvae as they cross from blood vessels into the airways and immune-mediated hypersensitivity reactions to the presence of larvae. *Ascaris* antigens are allergenic and there is conflicting data about their role as a cause of asthma.[27–30] Symptoms range from mild cough, with no radiologic changes, to a Löffler's syndrome with transient pulmonary infiltrates, dyspnea, severe cough, and eosinophilia (see Chapter 125). The severity of symptoms is a reflection of the larval burden. Given the life cycle of *A. lumbricoides*, stool samples may be negative until 2 to 3 months after the pulmonary symptoms occur, unless the patient was already harboring a patent infection. In countries where transmission of *Ascaris* is seasonal (e.g., Saudi Arabia), seasonal outbreaks of pneumonitis are typical,[18] while in countries with continuous transmission pulmonary disease is uncommon.

The large adult worms can elicit the intestinal symptoms of ascariasis. These may be referable to small bowel obstruction due to a large bolus of worms or to the migration of one or a few worms from their usual intraluminal locales. Symptoms relating to the presence of worms in the small intestine tend to be nonspecific and include generalized abdominal pain, dyspepsia, appetite changes, or occasionally vomiting or diarrhea. The range of potentially serious intestinal manifestations of ascariasis is evident in series from a number of centers worldwide. For instance, in a review of abdominal ascariasis in children in Cape Town from 1958 to 1974, 528 presentations of acute abdominal symptoms were recorded, with a peak incidence in children from 4 to 8 years of age. In this series, 66% of the cases were intestinal obstruction, 25% were biliary obstruction, and 5% were pancreatitis.[31] In a review of 500 patients from India with hepatobiliary and pancreatic disease from *A. lumbricoides*, 274 patients presented with duodenal ascariasis, 171 with biliary ascariasis, 40 with hepatic ascariasis, 8 with gallbladder ascariasis, and 7 with pancreatic ascariasis.[32] The most common clinical presentation was that of biliary colic; patients presenting with acute cholangitis were the second most common.[32]

Intestinal obstruction can occur from a bolus of worms in the lumen of the intestine (Fig. 109-3). Children are at greater risk than adults, perhaps because of the smaller diameters of their intestines and their potential for greater worm burdens.[24] The numbers of worms needed to cause obstruction have been estimated to be greater than 60, with worm burdens being about 10-fold higher in fatal cases.[33] Complications of

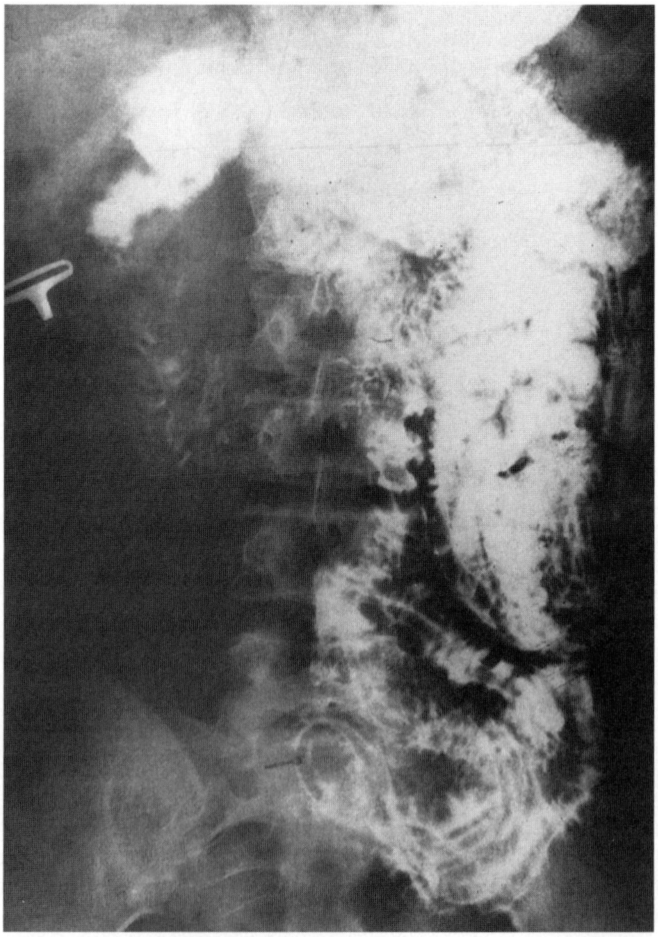

FIGURE 109-3 A bolus of worms causing intestinal obstruction. (From Zaman V: Atlas of Medical Parasitology, 2nd ed. Australia, ADIS Health Science Press, 1984.)

intestinal obstruction include bowel perforation with bacterial peritonitis due to seeding with gut bacterial flora as well as granulomatous peritonitis due to seeding with adult *Ascaris* worms and eggs.[34]

Biliary obstruction results from the presence of a worm or worms that have entered the biliary tree, where the flow of bile may be impaired, where spasms of the sphincter of Oddi may occur, or where stone formation may result.[35] Adult worms may migrate into the gallbladder,[36] sometimes becoming evident only after cholecystectomy.[37] Worms may also ascend the biliary tree to cause hepatic abscesses.[38] Pancreatitis, which occurs less frequently than biliary disease during ascariasis, can have a variety of clinical manifestations, ranging from abdominal pain and elevated serum amylase, to pancreatic calcifications, pseudocysts, or death.[39] As with intestinal obstruction, worms may be passed in stool or vomitus.

Ascaris infection affects the nutritional status of developing children and has been shown by some authors to directly decrease protein utilization, fat absorption, and increase lactose intolerance and vitamin A deficiency.[25,26,40,41] Not all authors have demonstrated a direct correlation between specific nutritional deficiencies and ascariasis.[42–44] There is agreement that *Ascaris* infection may contribute to or exacerbate poor nutritional status when there is a large worm burden present in persons who live in regions with other causes of malnutrition, such as other parasitic infections, poverty, poor living conditions, and poor diet. Careful studies have demonstrated improvement in growth and development in children treated for ascariasis.[45,46]

PATHOGENESIS AND IMMUNITY

The pathology of *A. lumbricoides* infection is related to the human host response to the presence of larvae, eggs, or adult worms in a specific tissue or organ lumen. When the larvae migrate in human tissues, cells undergo mechanical trauma as well as lysis caused by larval enzymes. In various tissues, invading larvae can induce granuloma formation from surrounding eosinophils, neutrophils, and macrophages. Particularly, the presence of *A. lumbricoides* larvae in pulmonary parenchyma induces a hypersensitivity reaction that includes increased mucus production in the bronchi, peribronchial inflammation, and bronchial spasm.[11] Human infections with *Ascaris* lead to the development of immune responses polarized to the production of Th2 cytokines.[47]

The pathophysiologic consequences of *A. lumbricoides* in the gastrointestinal tract result from the physical presence of worms in the lumen of the small intestine or wherever worms may migrate. Although, in general, the intensity of symptoms is proportional to the worm burden, in an individual, a single worm may cause significant morbidity by migrating into a particular sphincter or duct and producing an obstructive clinical syndrome. For example, a single worm that migrates into the common bile duct can produce biliary obstruction.There is controversy as to whether production of antibodies to *A. lumbricoides* is protective or merely indicative of prior or current infection. Serology is rarely needed to diagnose *Ascaris* infection and is used more frequently in epidemiologic studies of ascariasis and of host responses to various intensities of infection. *Ascaris* infection produces both specific and nonspecific increases in circulating immunoglobulin E (IgE).

Studies have examined what protective role antibodies induced by *A. lumbricoides* may have in relation to re-infection. A case-control study of Bangladeshi children with different intensities of infection suggested that antibody response to infection mirrors intensity of infection and may have no protective role.[48] However, another study that examined total and *A. lumbricoides*–specific IgE levels in serum of children with documented infection with *A. lumbricoides*, who were treated and became re-infected multiple times, found that while subjects with high pretreatment total IgE levels had higher re-infection rates, subjects with higher pretreatment anti–*A. lumbricoides* IgE levels had lower re-infection rates. The authors suggested that specific IgE antibody may be protective against *A. lumbricoides* infection and that polyclonal stimulation of IgE may reduce the effectiveness of this protective response.[49]

DIAGNOSIS

The parasitological diagnosis of *Ascaris* infection in the intestine is usually made by examining stool samples for eggs. A common method of examining a stool sample is the direct method, which involves mixing a small stool sample with a drop of 0.85% NaCl and examining the mixture on a slide under a microscope. Alternatively, much experience indicates that the Kato Katz method is the best available system. This method consists of 50 mg of fresh stool pressed under cellophane into a thin film on a slide, and then identifying and counting the eggs by microscopy. Other less commonly used techniques include the lactophenol cotton blue stain for wet mount stool preparation[50] and the Merthiolate Iodine Formalin (MIF) fecal technique.[51] Egg counts (epg) can measure both intensity of infection in an individual and prevalence of infection in a community.[3] The major deficiency of using egg counts to diagnose ascariasis or to measure intensity or prevalence of ascariasis is that it will miss infection with all male, all female, or juvenile worms. The other method of measuring intensity and prevalence of infection, although it is not generally used as a diagnostic tool, is to count the number of worms passed after anthelminthic chemotherapy.

A clinical diagnosis of *Ascaris* pneumonia is made in a patient with a recent potential exposure to infectious *Ascaris* eggs who presents with dyspnea, dry cough, fever, and eosinophilia. Examination of chest radiographs usually reveals fleeting pulmonary infiltrates and examination of the sputum may reveal Charcot-Leyden crystals (see Chapter 125). Because of the life cycle of *A. lumbricoides*, stool samples for eggs may be negative at the time of the clinical presentation of pneumonia.

Intestinal or biliary obstruction from *A. lumbricoides* should be considered in the appropriate clinical setting in someone from an *Ascaris* endemic region. Increasingly, radiographic and especially ultrasonographic techniques have been used with success to diagnose intestinal and biliary ascariasis. In intestinal ascariasis, ultrasound has reliably detected diagnostic linear echogenic images of adult worms.[52,53] In intra- and extrahepatic biliary ascariasis, ultrasonography has also proven sensitive in detecting worms in the liver, biliary tract, gallbladder, and pancreas.[53,54] Thus, when available, contemporary noninvasive ultrasound imaging can be a valuable adjunct in ascertaining whether adult *Ascaris* worms are underlying intestinal or hepatopancreatobiliary tract clinical presentations.

With the administration of oral contrast material, adult ascarid worms can be visualized by CT scans and upper GI series as tubular filling defects at times with a thread of contrast material within their own intestinal tracts.[55,56]

TREATMENT

The decisions to treat patients with ascariasis rest on several conditions, including a consideration of the potential of individuals to become readily reinfected and the resources available. In patients with uncomplicated intestinal ascariasis who reside in areas in which they are not likely to be reinfected, anthelminthic therapy is very much indicated to prevent any of the potentially serious consequences attributable to intestinal obstruction or the complications of biliary ascariasis. In regions where sanitation is poor, reinfections are likely. Thus, therapy needs to be balanced between the benefits of preventing later complications and potentially improving growth and development and any limitations on the availability of medical resources. In regions where lymphatic filariasis is present, ongoing mass treatment campaigns using periodic administrations of albendazole with ivermectin or diethylcarbamazine (see Chapter 98) can also help diminish the prevalence and intensity of *Ascaris* infections.[57]

The mainstays of drug therapy for the treatment of gastrointestinal ascariasis are the benzimadazoles (mebendazole and albendazole), levamisole, and pyrantel.[58,59] Benzimadazoles impair phosphorylation and glucose uptake in the parasite. Mebendazole and albendazole have been compared in differing doses and formulations[60,61] and for *Ascaris* infection are equally effective and well tolerated. Studies using single-dose regimens (300–500 mg of mebendazole or 400 mg of albendazole) have produced cure rates of 100%, although mebendazole may also be given as 100 mg twice a day for 3 days.[58] Informal consultations have concluded that WHO-recommended anthelminthic drugs[59] of proven quality may be given in appropriate doses to pregnant women, adolescent girls, women of reproductive age, and children aged at least 12 months, despite pregnancy Category B status. The members of the consultations advised that anthelminthic treatment should be avoided if possible during the first trimester of a pregnancy. Details covering all aspects of this matter including pharmacokinetics, safety, toxicology, and embryo toxicity are available in a series of reports.[62–65] None of the advice contradicts or undermines the judgments a physician must make on a case-by-case basis.

Pulmonary manifestations of recent *Ascaris* infections are self-limited and are not generally treated, except for supportive measures. It is unknown if anthelminthic therapy would be effective against lung-stage larvae and whether any larval death might heighten pulmonary inflammation. Although there are no published data to support this, it seems reasonable to screen carefully for gastrointestinal *A. lumbricoides* infection following pulmonary disease and to treat if evidence of *A. lumbricoides* is found in order to eradicate *A. lumbricoides* from the host.

While surgical interventions have conventionally been employed to treat the complications of intestinal ascariasis, with the heightened ability of ultrasonography to diagnose and localize adult *Ascaris* worms, increasingly there have been greater applications of nonsurgical approaches. In intestinal obstructions, medical management with anthelminthics can be successful. In one series from India, 68 patients who presented with intestinal obstruction and no signs of peritonitis were successfully treated medically with anthelminthics and intravenous fluids, whereas 24 presenting with peritonitis required surgery and had a mortality of 50%.[66] Others likewise have reported series of intestinal obstructions successfully managed medically.[67]

For those with biliary tract complications of ascariasis, nonsurgical approaches are being successfully used. A report from Ecuador of 69 patients found that treatment with 800 mg albendazole orally and analgesics and antispasmodics obviated surgical intervention for all but one patient.[68] Duodenoscopy was done in 30 patients and extracted worms from the ampulla of Vater in 10 of these without a need for sphincterotomy. Thus, in 97% of their patients, *Ascaris* was treated sucessfully with medical therapy alone or with duodenoscopy.[68] Successful endoscopic approaches to the treatment of biliary ascariasis are increasingly being reported.[69–72]

PREVENTION AND CONTROL

Prospects for the prevention of ascariasis will remain intractable in countries where *A. lumbricoides* infections are endemic until poverty is relieved, education and health awareness are strengthened, affordable and appropriate sanitation becomes widely available, and populations have access to essential drugs. Recently, good quality, generic versions of benzimidazoles have become available; one effective dose of a broad-spectrum anthelminthic drug such as albendazole is now priced at $0.02.[73] This means that in areas endemic for ascariasis access to essential drugs[59] to control morbidity and relieve the burden of suffering can become a reality.[63] When anthelminthic chemotherapy is used on a community-wide basis, transmission is reduced because fewer eggs are released to contaminate the environment.[74–77] The problem of using the limited range of anthelminthic drugs is that drug resistance may emerge.[63] Accordingly, measures to control morbidity due to ascariasis will require careful planning based on the best available epidemiological information.[12] Ascariasis was once highly prevalent in Europe.[6] Its prevention was ensured when sanitation and sewage treatment systems were installed.

REFERENCES

1. Crompton DWT: How much human helminthiasis is there in the world? J Parasitol 85:397, 1999.
2. Crompton DWT: *Ascaris* and ascariasis. Adv Parasitol 48:285, 2001.
3. Crompton DWT: *Ascaris lumbricoides*. In Scott ME (ed): Parasitic and Infectious Diseases, 1st ed. San Diego, Academic Press, 1994, p 175.
4. de Silva NR, Chan MS, Bundy DAP: Morbidity and mortality due to ascariasis: Re-estimation and sensitivity analysis of global numbers at risk. Trop Med Int Health 2:519, 1997
5. Pawlowski ZS, Davis A: Morbidity and mortality in ascariasis. In Crompton DWT, Nesheim MC, Pawlowski ZS (eds): Ascariasis and Its Prevention and Control. London, Taylor & Francis, 1989, p 71.
6. Tyson E: *Lumbricus teres*, or some anatomical observations on the round worm bred in human bodies. Philos Trans 13:153, 1683.
7. Wharton DA: *Ascaris* sp: Water loss during desiccation of embryonating eggs. Exp Parasitol 48:398, 1979.
8. Crompton DWT: Biology of *Ascaris lumbricoides*. In Crompton DWT (ed): Ascariasis and Its Prevention and Control. London, Taylor & Francis, 1989, p 175.
9. Makidino J: Observations on *Ascaris* during fluoroscopy. Am J Trop Med Hyg 5:699, 1956.

10. Chan MS, Medley GF, Jamison D, et al: The evaluation of potential global morbidity attributable to intestinal nematode infections. Parasitology 109:373, 1994.
11. Pawlowski ZS: Ascariasis. In Pawlowski ZS (ed): Intestinal Helminth Infections. London, Baillière Tindall, 1987, p 595.
12. Anderson RM, May RM: Infectious Diseases of Humans. London, Oxford University Press, 1992.
13. Morishita K: Studies on epidemiological aspects of ascariasis in Japan and basic knowledge concerning its control. In Morishita K, Yoshitaka K, Hisakichi M (eds): Progress of Medical Parasitology in Japan, Vol. 4. Tokyo, Meguro Parasitological Museum, 1972, p 3.
14. Williams D, Burke G, Henley JO: Ascariasis: A family disease. J Pediatr 84:853, 1974.
15. Crompton DWT, Tulley JJ: How much ascariasis is there in Africa? Parsitol Today 3:123, 1987.
16. Prost A: L'ascaridiose en Afrique de l'ouest. Revue épidémiologique. Ann Parasitol Hum Comp 62:434, 1987.
17. Ratard RC, Kouemeni LE, Bessala MM, et al: Ascariasis and *Trichuris* in Cameroon. Trans R Soc Trop Med Hyg 85:84, 1991.
18. Spillman RK: Pulmonary ascariasis in tropical communities. Am J Trop Med Hyg 24:791, 1974.
19. Xu LQ, Yu SH, Jiang ZX, et al: Soil-transmitted helminthiases: Nationwide survey in China. Bull World Health Org 73:507, 1995.
20. Ejezie GC: The parasitic diseases of school children in Lagos State, Nigeria. Acta Trop 38:79, 1981.
21. Hlaing T, Than S, Htay A, et al: Epidemiology and transmission dynamics of *Ascaris lumbricoides* in Okpo village, rural Burma. Trans R Soc Trop Med Hyg 78:497, 1984.
22. Kightlinger LK, Seed JR, Kighlinger MB: The epidemiology of *Ascaris lumbricoides, Trichuris trichiura* and hookworm in children in the Ranomafana rainforest, Madagascar. J Parasitol 81:159, 1995.
23. Awasthi S, Bundy DAP, Savioli L: Helminthic infections. BMJ 327:431, 2003.
24. De Silva N, Guyatt H, Bundy D: Morbidity and mortality due to *Ascaris*-induced intestinal obstruction. Trans R Soc Trop Med Hyg 91:31, 1997.
25. Crompton DWT, Nesheim MC: Nutritional impact of intestinal helminthiasis during the human life cycle. Ann Rev Nutr 22:35, 2002.
26. O'Lorcain P, Holland CV: The public health importance of *Ascaris lumbricoides*. Parasitology 121:S51, 2000.
27. Lynch NR, Palenque M, Hagel I, et al: Clinical improvement of asthma after anthelminthic treatment in a tropical situation. Am J Respir Crit Care Med 156:50, 1997.
28. Palmer LJ, Celedon JC, Weiss ST, et al: *Ascaris lumbricoides* infection is associated with increased risk of childhood asthma and atopy in rural China. Am J Respir Crit Care Med 165:1489, 2002.
29. van den Biggelaar AH, Rodrigues LC, van Ree R, et al: Long-term treatment of intestinal helminths increases mite skin-test reactivity in Gabonese schoolchildren. J Infect Dis 189:892, 2004.
30. Cooper PJ, Chico ME, Rodrigues LC, et al: Reduced risk of atopy among school-age children infected with geohelminth parasites in a rural area of the tropics. J Allergy Clin Immunol 111:995, 2003.
31. Loun JH: Biliary ascariasis in childhood. S Afr J Surg 12:219, 1974.
32. Khuroo MS, Zargar SA, Mahajan R: Hepatobiliary and pancreatic ascariasis in India. Lancet 335:1503, 1990.
33. de Silva NR, Guyatt HL, Bundy DA: Worm burden in intestinal obstruction caused by *Ascaris lumbricoides*. Trop Med Int Health 2:189, 1997.
34. Mello CM, Briggs M do C, Venancio ES, et al: Granulomatous peritonitis by *Ascaris*. J Pediatr Surg 27:1229, 1992.
35. Gonzalez AH, Regalado VC, Van den Ende J: Non-invasive management of *Ascaris lumbricoides* biliary tact migration: A prospective study in 69 patients from Ecuador. Trop Med Int Health 6:146, 2001.
36. Javid G, Wani N, Gulzar GM, et al: Gallbladder ascariasis: Presentation and management. Br J Surg 86:1526, 1999.
37. Shah OJ, Dar MA, Wani NA, et al: Biliary ascariasis as a cause of post-cholecystectomy syndrome in an endemic area. Dig Surg 21:108, 2004.
38. Javid G, Wani NA, Gulzar GM, et al: *Ascaris*-induced liver abscess. World J Surg 23:1191, 1999.
39. Maddern GJ, Dennison AR, Blumgart LH: Fatal *Ascaris* pancreatitis: An uncommon problem in the west. Gut 33:402, 1992.
40. Stephenson LS: Helminth parasites, a major factor in malnutrition. World Health Forum 15:169, 1994.
41. Blumenthal DS, Schultz MG: Effects of *Ascaris* infection on nutritional status in children. Am J Trop Med Hyg 25:682, 1976.
42. Meakins RH, Harland PSEG, Carswell F: A preliminary survey of malnutrition and helminthiasis among school children in one mountain and one lowland Ujumaa village in northern Tanzania. Trans R Soc Trop Med Hyg 75:731, 1981.
43. Gendrel D, Richard-Lenobile D, Kombila M, et al: Influence of intestinal parasitism on lactose absorption in well-nourished Africa children. Am J Trop Med Hyg 46:137, 1992.
44. Rousham EK, Mascie-Taylor CG: An 18 month study of the effect of periodic anthelminthic treatementon the growth and nutritional status of pre-school children in Bangladesh. Ann Hum Biol 21:315, 1994.
45. Hlaing T: Ascariasis and childhood malnutrition. Parasitology 107(Suppl):S512, 1993.
46. Chan MS: The global burden of intestinal nematode infections—Fifty years on. Parasitol Today 13:438, 1997.
47. Cooper PJ, Chico ME, Sandoval C, et al: Human infection with *Ascaris lumbricoides* is associated with a polarized cytokine response. J Infect Dis 182:1207, 2000.
48. Palmer DR, Hall A, Haque R, et al: Antibody isotype responses to antigens of *Ascaris lumbricoides* in a case control study of persistently heavily infected Bangladeshi children. Parasitology 111:385, 1995.
49. Hagel I, Lynch NR, DiPrisco ML, et al: *Ascaris* reinfection of slum children: Relation with the IgE response. Clin Exp Immunol 94:80, 1993.
50. Parija SC, Prabhaker PK: Evaluation of lacto-phenol cotton blue for wet mount preparation of feces. J Clin Microbiol 33:1019, 1995.
51. Bawden MP: Improvement of the merthiolate-iodine-formalin (MIF) fecal technique for hookworm, *Trichuris trichiuria* and *Ascaris lumbricoides* eggs. J Parasitol 80:474, 1994.
52. Mahmood T, Mansoor N, Quraishy S, et al: Ultrasonographic appearance of *Ascaris lumbricoides* in the small bowel. J Ultrasound Med 20:269, 2001.
53. Ferreyra NP, Cerri GG: Ascariasis of the alimentary tract, liver, pancreas and biliary system: Its diagnosis by ultrasonography. Hepatogastroenterology 45:932, 1998.
54. Schulman A: Ultrasound appearances of intra- and extrahepatic biliary ascariasis. Abdom Imaging 23:60, 1998.
55. Beitia AO, Haller JO, Kantor A: CT findings in pediatric gastrointestinal ascariasis. Comput Med Imaging Graph 21:47, 1997.
56. Reeder MM: The radiological and ultrasound evaluation of ascariasis of the gastrointestinal, biliary, and respiratory tracts. Semin Roentgenol 33:57, 1998.
57. Belizario VY, Amarillo ME, de Leon WU, et al: A comparison of the efficacy of single doses of albendazole, ivermectin, and diethylcarbamazine alone or in combinations against *Ascaris* and *Trichuris* spp. Bull World Health Org 81:35, 2003.
58. Drugs for parasitic infections. Med Lett Drugs Ther August 2004; www.medicalletter.org.
59. WHO: Model Formulary. Geneva, World Health Organization, 2002.
60. Jongsuksuntiful P, Jeradit C, Pornpattanakul S, et al: A comparative study on the efficacy of albendazole and mebendazole in the treatment of ascariasis, hookworm infection and trichuriasis. Southeast Asia J Trop Med Public Health 22:618, 1991.
61. Albonico M, Smith PG, Ercole E, et al: Rate of reinfection with intestinal nematodes after treatment of children with mebendazole or albendazole in a highly endemic area. Trans R Soc Trop Med Hyg 89:538, 1995.
62. WHO: Report of the WHO Informal Consultation on Hookworm Infection and Anaemia in Girls and Women. Geneva, World Health Organization, 1996.
63. WHO: Report of the WHO Informal Consultation on the Use of Chemotherapy for the Control of Morbidity Due to Soil-Transmitted Nematodes in Humans. Geneva, World Health Organization, 1996.
64. WHO: Prevention and Control of Schistosomiasis and Soil-Transmitted Helminthiasis. Technical Report Series 912. Geneva, World Health Organization, 2002.
65. WHO: Report of the WHO Informal Consultation on the Use of Praziquantel During Pregnancy/Lactation and Albendazole/ Mebendazole in Children Under 24 Months. Geneva, World Health Organization, 2003.
66. Wasadikar PP, Kulkarni AB: Intestinal obstruction due to ascariasis. Br J Surg 84:410, 1997.
67. Soomro MA, Akhtar J: Non-operative management of intestinal obstruction due to *Ascaris lumbricoides*. J Coll Physicians Surg Pak 13:86, 2003.

68. Gonzalez AH, Regalado VC, Van den Ende J: Non-invasive management of *Ascaris lumbricoides* biliary tract migration: A prospective study in 69 patients from Ecuador. Trop Med Int Health 6:146, 2001.
69. Misra SP, Dwivedi M: Clinical features and management of biliary ascariasis in a non-endemic area. Postgrad Med J 76:29, 2000.
70. Kamiya T, Justiniano M, Duran A, et al: Biliopancreatic ascariasis: Endoscopic approach. J Gastroenterol 37(Suppl 13):97, 2002.
71. Osman M, Lausten SB, El-Sefi T, et al: Biliary parasites. Dig Surg 15:287, 1998.
72. Sandouk F, Haffar S, Zada MM, et al: Pancreatic-biliary ascariasis: Experience of 300 cases. Am J Gastroenterol 92:2264, 1997.
73. Albonico M, Engels D, Montresor A, et al: Progress in the prevention and control of schistosomiasis ans soil-transmitted helminthiasis. Gio Ital Med Trop 7:11, 2002.
74. Asaolu SO, Holland CV, Crompton DWT: Community control of *Ascaris lumbricoides* in rural Oyo State Nigeria: Mass targeted and selective treatment with levamisole. Parasitology 103:291, 1991.
75. Hall A, Anwar KS, Tompkins AM: Intensity of reinfection with *Ascaris lumbricoides* and its implications for parasite control. Lancet 339:1253, 1992.
76. Hlaing T, Saw T, Kyin ML: The impact of 3 monthly age targeted chemotherapy on *Ascaris lumbricoides* infection. Trans R Soc Trop Med Hyg 85:519, 1991.
77. Hlaing T, Saw T, Kyin ML: Control of ascariasis through age-targeted chemotherapy. Impact of 6-monthly chemotherapeutic regimens. Bull World Health Org 58:747, 1990.

110

Hookworm Infections

PETER J. HOTEZ

INTRODUCTION

Hookworms are nematode endoparasites that cause intestinal blood loss during a part of their life cycle. An estimated 740 million people are infected with *Ancylostoma duodenale*, *Necator americanus*, or both.[1] *Necator americanus* is the predominant hookworm worldwide. Moderate and heavy worm burdens can result in hookworm disease, which is characterized by blood loss sufficient to produce iron deficiency and anemia in the human host. Children and women of reproductive age are particularly vulnerable to the effects of hookworm anemia.[2,3] For that reason, there is an increasing awareness of hookworm disease as a problem affecting maternal–child health.[4]

Perhaps more than any other nematode parasite, the life cycle of hookworms is intimately connected to rural poverty in warm climates. Hookworm infection is endemic in most developing areas of the subtropics and tropics where sanitation is poor and the environmental conditions, especially adequate moisture and sandy soils, support the survival and hatching of parasite eggs and then the subsequent migrations of larvae. Therefore, unlike *Ascaris* and *Trichuris* infections, hookworm is not usually a public health threat in urban slums. Instead, hookworm occurs primarily in impoverished tropical coastal communities and in areas of intense agricultural activity. In these high-transmission areas, hookworm infection remains endemic even when populations are routinely treated with anthelmintic drugs. In this setting, hookworm reinfection routinely occurs, and the prevalence and intensity of hookworm infection return to pretreatment levels within months.[5] Ultimately, the adequate control of hookworm may depend on new advances in biotechnology for the development of a first-generation hookworm vaccine.[6]

AGENT

Hookworms are classically identified as adult nematode worms having a buccal capsule armed with teeth or cutting plates. The two major human parasitic species, *A. duodenale* and *N. americanus*, and the minor human zoonotic parasites, *Ancylostoma ceylanicum*, *Ancylostoma caninum*, and *Ancylostoma braziliense*, are members of the family Ancylostomatidae, superfamily Strongyloidea (Table 110-1). Although most clinicians usually consider the major species as generic "hookworms," there are, in fact, important differences between them[7] (Table 110-2). The clinical features of each hookworm infection are also distinct.[8]

Necator americanus ("American murderer") was probably discovered by Charles W. Stiles,[9] who identified the parasite as the principal cause of hookworm anemia in the rural southeastern United States. Many historians also credit Bailey K. Ashford of the U.S. Army Medical Corps, who encountered hyperendemic hookworm infection in Puerto Rico at the end of the Spanish–American War.[10] Adult *N. americanus* hookworms are relatively small compared to *A. duodenale*. The males are typically between 7 and 9 mm, and the females are between 9 and 11 mm in length. They live attached via cutting plates to the mucosa and submucosa of the small intestine, where they can live for 3 to 5 years. The blood loss caused by each *N. americanus* has been estimated by ^{51}Cr-labeled red blood cell measurements to be 0.01 to 0.04 mL per worm per day[11]; in general, it is much less than *A. duodenale*-associated blood loss. *Necator americanus* is therefore considered better adapted to human parasitism.[7] Each gravid female worm produces 5000 to 10,000 eggs per day, which exit from the host in feces. The eggs are thin-shelled, hyaline, and ovoid, measuring approximately 60 × 40 μm. Further development of the eggs depends on suitable external environmental conditions. These are usually met by adequate moisture and shade at temperatures of 20 to 30°C.[12,13] Egg hatching gives rise to a first-stage (L1) rhabditiform larva approximately 250 to 300 μm in length with a characteristic flask-shaped muscular esophagus. The L1 larva presumably feeds on bacteria and other organic debris prior to undergoing two spontaneous molts over the next week. Transformation to the infective third-stage larva (L3) is accompanied by a number of developmental changes, including elongation to a length of approximately 600 μm and cessation of feeding as a consequence of mouth closure and the buildup of an electron-dense "plug" in the buccal capsule. The infective larva is developmentally arrested and will remain so until it enters a suitable definitive host.[14,15] *Necator americanus* infects humans only through the skin. The L3 larvae increase their chances of finding a definitive host by a characteristic questing behavior. The infectious process of all hookworm larvae is intimately linked to the developmental biology of the parasite because host entry is accompanied by the resumption of hookworm larval development.[15] Developing L3 larvae enter into host venules and lymphatics, where they are swept into

Table 110-1 Human Hookworms

Hookworm	Animal Reservoir Host	Disease
Necator americanus	None	Anemia
Ancylostoma duodenale	None	Anemia
Ancylostoma ceylanicum	Dogs, cats	Enteritis
Ancylostoma caninum	Dogs	Eosinophilic enteritis
Ancylostoma braziliense	Dogs, cats	Cutaneous larval migrans
Uncinaria stenocephala	Dogs	Cutaneous larval migrans

Table 110-2 Properties of the Major Species of Hookworm

Property	*Ancylostoma duodenale*	*Necator americanus*
Size of adult (female slightly larger than male)	0.3–0.5 in.	0.2–0.4 in.
No. of eggs produced daily per worm	10,000–30,000	5000–10,000
Estimated amount of blood removed daily per worm	~0.2 mL (greater draw makes this species more virulent)	~0.02 mL
Mouthparts	Teeth	Cutting plates
Natural adult life span	1 yr	3–5 yr
Ability to produce infection if ingested	Yes	No
Ability of larvae to lie dormant	Yes	No

Data from Hoagland KE, Schad GA: *Necator americanus* and *Ancylostoma duodenale*: Life history parameters and epidemiological implications of two sympatric hookworms on humans. Exp Parasitol 44:36–49, 1978; and Hotez P: Human hookworm infection. In Farthing MJG, Keusch GT, Wakelin D (eds): Enteric Infection 2: Intestinal Helminths. London, Chapman & Hall, 1995, pp 129–150.

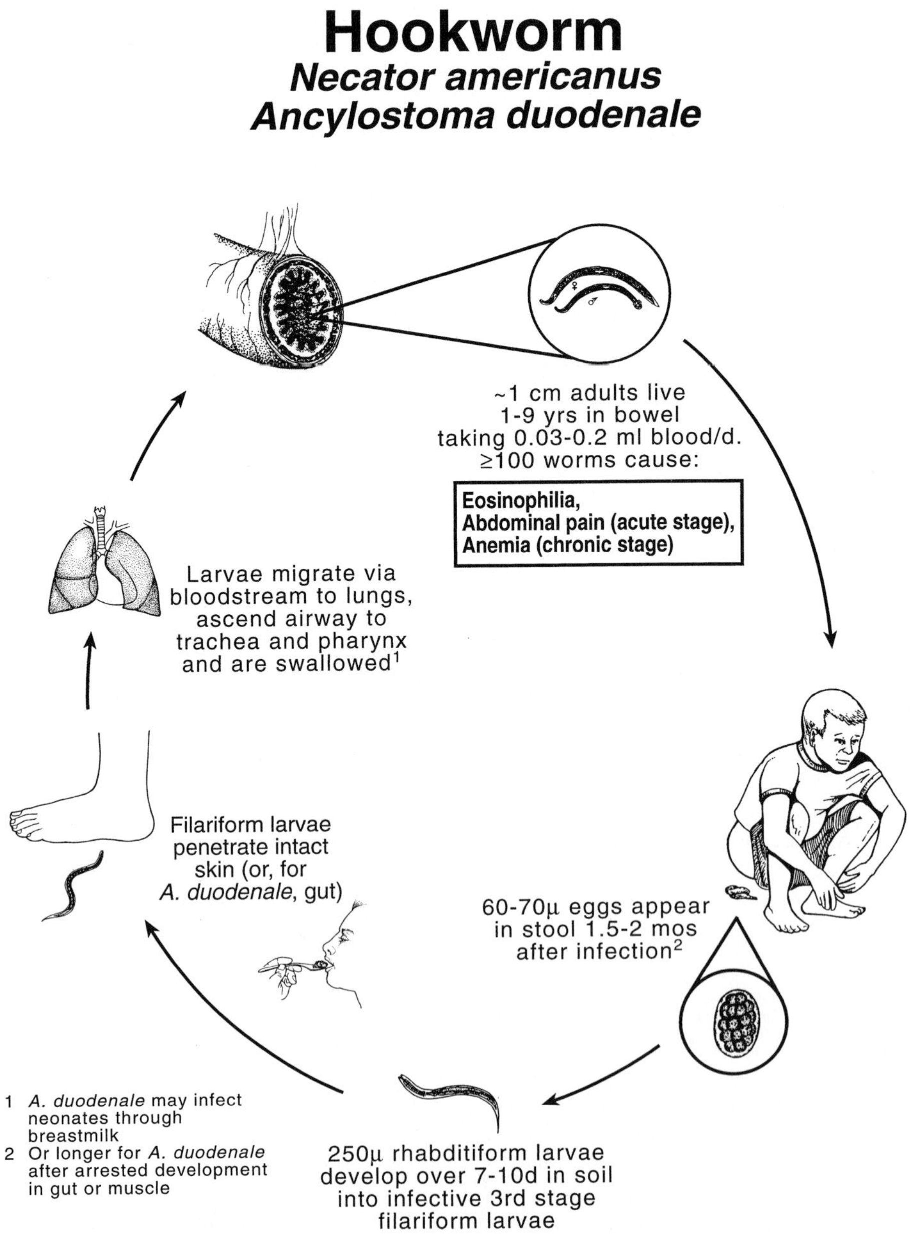

the pulmonary vasculature. The larvae migrate into the lungs and ascend the respiratory tree and epiglottis before entering the gastrointestinal tract. Entry into the small intestine stimulates the molting of L3 larvae to the L4 stage and then the adult stage. Approximately 49 to 56 days elapse from the time *N. americanus* L3 larvae enter the host until the adult female hookworm releases eggs.[7,8]

Ancylostoma duodenale was first identified from the intestine of an Italian woman in 1843 by Dubini. Its life cycle was largely elucidated by a series of impressive investigations in Egypt conducted by Looss.[16] The distinct features of the life cycle and life history stages of *A. duodenale* were a result of human investigations by G. A. Schad and colleagues working in rural West Bengal, India, in the late 1960s and early 1970s.[7,13,17–23] The adult *A. duodenale* is larger and more robust than *N. americanus*. Each adult male is 8 to 11 mm, whereas each adult female is 10 to 13 mm in length. Adult *A. duodenale* hookworms live only approximately 1 year in the small intestine. However, during that time they cause greater blood loss (0.05 to 0.30 mL per worm per day) and produce more eggs (10,000 to 30,000 eggs per day) than *N. americanus*.[7,11] Egg hatching of *A. duodenale* is faster than that of *N. americanus*.[13] *Ancylostoma duodenale* L3 larvae are infective via the oral route in addition to percutaneous entry.[7,20] In some endemic areas, oral ingestion of L3 larvae may be the predominant route of infection. Moreover, *A. duodenale* L3 larvae can remain in a developmentally arrested state, even after host entry.[17,23] Larval hypobiosis is considered evolutionarily adaptive because it allows the prolonged survival of the parasite in the host during times when the environment is unfavorable to larval development. For instance, *A. duodenale* L3 larvae probably remain arrested in the host during the hot and dry months of the year in some areas, only to resume development to egg-laying adult hookworms during or soon before the monsoon rains.[17] Arrested development may even explain how *A. duodenale* arrived with prehistoric humans during their early migrations into North America.[24] Arrested *A. duodenale* L3 larvae in maternal somatic tissues may also enter the mammary glands.[23] This phenomenon may account for vertical transmission of human ancylostomiasis to infants.[2,23,25]

Human intestinal infection with *A. ceylanicum* is probably a zoonosis transmitted by L3 larvae from eggs in either dog or cat feces and does not result in host blood loss and therefore is not considered clinically significant. However, zoonotic intestinal infection from the dog hookworm *A. caninum* can occasionally result in a severe eosinophilic enteritis syndrome.[26–31] Nonintestinal cutaneous larva migrans (CLM; "creeping eruption") occurs when L3 larvae of the dog and cat hookworm *A. braziliense* enter the skin but subsequently abort the infection (see Chapter 103).

EPIDEMIOLOGY

As noted in the Introduction, hookworm infections are common throughout the rural areas of the tropics and subtropics. Hookworm is intimately associated with the agrarian practices of societies in developing countries and is one of the most prevalent infections of humans. Coastal communities in the tropics typically have the highest intensity hookworm infections; presumably this observation reflects the mild humid climate and sandy soils in these regions, which are favorable to transmission.[32] Overall, the highest prevalence and intensity of hookworm occur in sub-Saharan Africa, followed by China and Southeast Asia.[1] China boasts the most accurate prevalence estimates because of an unusual thorough nationwide survey in which fecal examinations were performed on 1,477,742 people.[33] An estimated 194 million Chinese (17% prevalence) are infected with hookworms. Whether hookworm infection in any given endemic area is due to *A. duodenale* or *N. americanus* is often unknown because differentiation between the two species is not routinely performed in the parasite diagnostic laboratory. Often, endemic hookworm is reported as either "ancylostomiasis" or "uncinariasis" (necatoriasis) when, in reality, no efforts were made to investigate the actual etiologic agent. Worldwide, *Necator* infections are more common than ancylostoma infections. However, when the worm burdens in a given community are similar, *A. duodenale* infections produce greater blood loss and endemic hookworm anemia than *N. americanus* infections.[34]

Infections with *N. americanus* are found predominantly between the tropics of Cancer and Capricorn. *N. americanus* is the predominant hookworm in Central and South America, hence the designation New World hookworm. *Necator* infections still occur in North America, especially in southern Mexico; rare pockets may even remain in the southeastern United States, although it is no longer a significant public health threat there. Hookworm was reported from rural Georgia in the early 1970s[35] and, more recently, from east Texas. *N. americanus* is the predominant hookworm of sub-Saharan Africa, southern China, southern India, and Southeast Asia. Infections with *A. duodenale* frequently overlap *N. americanus* infections in areas of Africa, India, and China. However, they also occur as either the exclusive or predominant hookworm of northern India and China and North Africa. Possibly, the ability of *A. duodenale* to undergo arrested development in the host allows the parasite to survive in climatic conditions that are unfavorable for *N. americanus*. Arrested development also accounts for the seasonality of ancylostomiasis. In rural West Bengal, India, and presumably elsewhere, the premonsoon rise in human fecal egg excretion occurs as a consequence of arrested hookworm larvae entering the intestine and developing into adult hookworms.[17,23] Some endemic ancylostomiasis still occurs in Brazil, Paraguay, northern Argentina, and Peru, although it is gradually being displaced by *Necator* infections.[36] *Ancylostoma ceylanicum* is a minor hookworm species of India and Southeast Asia.[8] *Ancylostoma caninum* has been identified as the cause of an emerging zoonotic eosinophilic enteritis syndrome in Australia.[26–31] Eosinophilic enteritis from *A. caninum* has been reported recently in Louisiana. CLM from *A. braziliense* is found in many areas of the tropics and subtropics, including the Gulf Coast, and southern regions of that Atlantic seaboard. It also occurs commonly in Caribbean tropical beach resorts and is thus a common problem seen in the travel medicine clinic.[37]

Hookworm infection is prevalent in almost all age classes in an endemic area. The characteristic pattern of age prevalence is one of an initial rise in childhood to a stable asymptote in early adulthood.[2] Rarely, because of infantile disease from vertical transmission, *A. duodenale* infections can also be found in children younger than 1 year of age.[25] Similar to other soil-transmitted helminths (STHs), hookworm exhibits

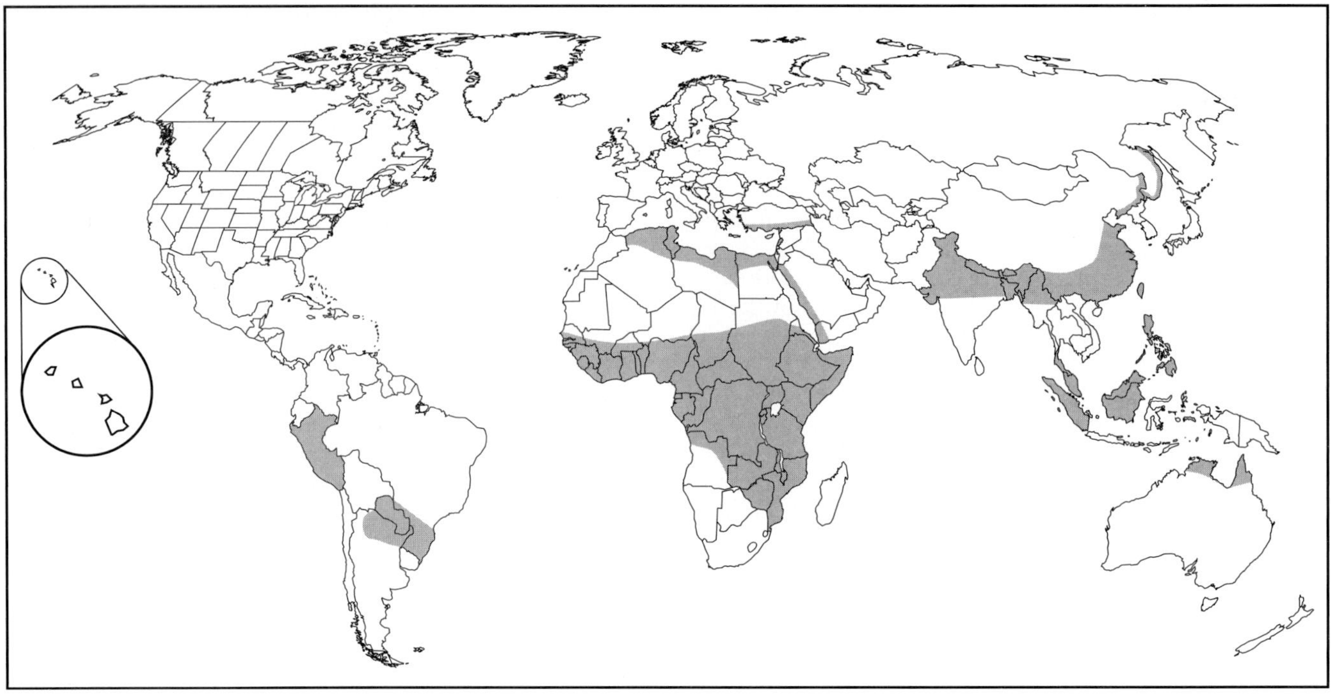

Ancylostoma duodenale

(In many regions, information on prevalence and speciation is limited.)

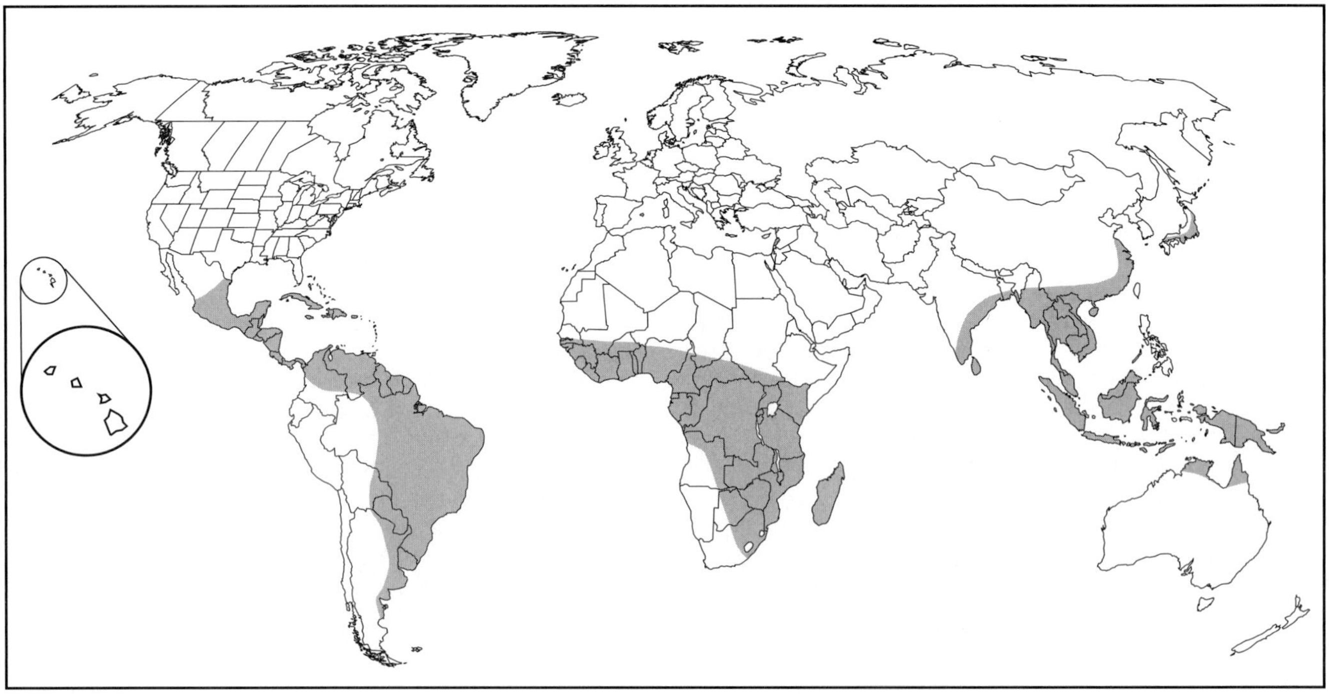

Necator americanus

(In many regions, information on prevalence and speciation is limited.)

an overdispersed distribution, with the majority (usually between 65% and 85%) of infected individuals in an endemic community exhibiting low-intensity infections, and a minority (usually between 15% and 35%) exhibiting moderate- and heavy-intensity infections. In contrast, there are marked differences in the age-dependent intensity patterns for hookworm compared with other STH infections.[2] Whereas worm burdens with *Ascaris* or *Trichuris* are often heaviest in children older than 2 years of age and then decline in adolescence, the worm burdens associated with hookworm infection do not exhibit such a clearcut pattern. It is not uncommon, for instance, for hookworm intensities to decline only slightly in adulthood or even to plateau or increase.[2,38] Studies from several different endemic areas suggest that humans are predisposed to acquire certain hookworm infection intensities so that people who are heavily infected prior to specific anthelminthic drug therapy will often reacquire heavy infections when left in the same environment.[22] Increasing evidence indicates a genetic basis for hookworm predisposition.

DISEASE

Repeated percutaneous exposure to infective hookworm larvae of either *A. duodenale* or *N. americanus* results in a papulovesicular dermatitis sometimes referred to as "ground itch." The pruritus and burning associated with ground itch typically are most intense at the site of host entry, usually on the hands and feet, and last less than 1 week. Some species of animal hookworms, including *A. braziliense*, will migrate laterally in the epidermis and give rise to local inflammation that follows the serpiginous migratory pathways of the larvae. This condition, CLM, presents commonly on the lower extremities or buttocks, usually within 2 weeks to several months after exposure to *A. braziliense* L3 larvae. Approximately 20% of patients with CLM will have eosinophilia, and some will develop pulmonary infiltrates (see Chapter 103).[37]

A second, urticarial rash can subsequently occur with the onset of *A. duodenale* or *N. americanus* larval migrations through the lungs. Hookworm pneumonitis occurs as the L3 larvae enter the alveoli and ascend the respiratory tree; it is commonly associated with wheezing, dyspnea, and a nonproductive cough. Hookworm pneumonitis is less severe than other verminous pneumonias caused by *Ascaris* or *Toxocara*. Eosinophilia can begin during the larval migratory phase, but it typically peaks when the L3 enter the small intestine. Oral ingestion of large numbers of *A. duodenale* L3 larvae results 1 or a few days later in a syndrome (Wakana disease) consisting of nausea, vomiting, cough, dyspnea, and eosinophilia.

Attachment and tissue invasion of adult *A. duodenale* and *N. americanus* hookworms to the intestinal mucosa and submucosa is accompanied by mild abdominal pain, nausea, and anorexia. The gastrointestinal symptoms are more pronounced in patients with eosinophilic enteritis from zoonotic *A. caninum* infection. Intestinal parasitism by hookworms begins approximately 1.5 to 3 months after host entry by the L3 larvae. The prepatent period can last up to 1 year or possibly even longer if the L3 larvae of *A. duodenale* first undergo a period of arrested development.[18] Hookworm-associated blood loss results from the parasite-mediated destruction of capillaries in the intestinal mucosa. The degree of iron deficiency or anemia is dependent on a number of variables, including (1) worm burden; (2) type of hookworm—*A. duodenale* causes more blood loss than *N. americanus*; (3) iron reserves and diet of the host; and (4) overall host nutritional status.[8] In very heavy infections, hookworm anemia will cause signs and symptoms of iron-deficiency anemia: fatigue, exertional dyspnea, poor concentration, koilonychia (spoon nail deformity), pale sclerae, and heart murmurs. In addition to presenting with profound iron deficiency, people with heavy hookworm burdens can develop protein malnutrition from chronic plasma protein loss and even the signs and symptoms of kwashiorkor.[8] Some of these patients will develop a pasty and sallow appearance, a condition known as chlorosis.[39] During pregnancy, the anemia resulting from hookworm disease has been linked to increased maternal mortality and several adverse neonatal outcomes, including low birth weight and increased morbidity and mortality.[2,3]

An extreme form of hookworm anemia, with high mortality, occurs in infants heavily infected with *A. duodenale*, who exhibit melena, diarrhea, pallor, and failure to thrive.[25] Most of the cases of infantile ancylostomiasis, which may result from vertical transmission of L3 via lactogenic transmission, have been reported from Asia.

Patients harboring light and moderate hookworm infections may also develop more subtle sequelae of iron deficiency. Of increasing interest is the effect of chronic moderate parasitism and iron deficiency on intellectual, cognitive, and physical growth of hookworm-infected children.[40]

PATHOGENESIS AND IMMUNITY

Infective larval migrations through tissues usually do not cause severe visceral lesions, although heavy infections can result in hookworm pneumonitis.[8] However, the inflammation associated with skin entry is pronounced and is probably exacerbated by the release of eicosanoids and hydrolytic enzymes from migrating L3 larvae.[41–44] Hookworm larvae also release a family of proteins known as the *Ancylostoma*-secreted proteins (ASPs) of unknown function, which contain amino acid sequences homologous to plant proteins, insect venom allergens, and other members of the pathogenesis-related protein superfamily.[6,45,46] The ASPs include ASP-1, a 45-kDa protein, and ASP-2, a 22-kDa protein.[45,46] The ASPs are released in vitro in response to a low-molecular-weight factor found in serum as well as glutathione and glutathione derivatives.[15] Continuous release requires the presence of the hostlike stimulus. It is believed that the parasites release the ASPs during the early stages of host entry. CLM occurs when *A. braziliense* L3 larvae fail to penetrate the basement membrane of the epidermal–dermal junction and migrate laterally in the skin.

Hookworm-induced blood loss occurs at the site of adult parasite intestinal attachment. Hookworms use their teeth (*A. duodenale*) or cutting plates (*N. americanus*) to fasten onto the mucosa and submucosa, where they secrete a battery of pharmacologically active polypeptides that prevent blood from clotting and downregulate the host inflammatory response.[4,47–53] Among the peptides identified, cloned and expressed from the adult dog hookworm *A. caninum* (but presumably also released by *A. duodenale*), are a family of serine protease inhibitors that inhibit clotting factor Xa and tissue factor VIIa.[47,48] Work is in progress to develop the hookworm anticoagulants as therapeutic agents for cardiovascular disease as well as the disseminated intravascular coagulation that occurs during Ebola virus infection.[54] Another macromolecule released by adult hookworms is neutrophil inhibitory factor (NIF).[55] NIF binds to the A domain of the integrin Mac-1 (CD11b/CD18) and probably downregulates several types of invading leukocytes. Adult hookworms also release hydrolytic enzymes.[56–59] The destruction of mucosal capillaries and the resultant extravasation of anticoagulated blood account for hookworm-associated blood loss leading to iron-deficiency anemia. Some of the red blood cells are lysed and the released hemoglobin is degraded by an orchestrated cascade of hemoglobinases that line the hookworm gut.[59,60] Chronic iron deficiency is particularly detrimental in childhood and may directly impair cognitive and intellectual abilities by interfering with the development of dopaminergic neurons and the biosynthesis of brain enzymes with iron prosthetic groups.[61–63]

The human immune responses to hookworms are not well characterized. Immunoepidemiologic studies and observations with self-administered *N. americanus* infections suggest that humoral antibodies and cellular responses to hookworm antigens often are not linked to resistance to reinfection.[64–66] It has been hypothesized that hookworms are immunosuppressive and may promote susceptibility to other infections, including malaria and HIV/AIDS.[2,67–69] In the laboratory, however, immunity to canine hookworm infections has been produced by administering repeated doses of living larvae or larvae attenuated by ionizing radiation.[70,71] Hookworm immunity generated by living larval vaccines is not sterile but manifests by reduced worm burdens and decreased egg fecundity of the adult hookworms.[71] Evidence suggests that the protective effect offered by living larval hookworm vaccines may be reproduced by immunization with genetically engineered recombinant ASP polypeptides.[6,72,73]

DIAGNOSIS

Severe hookworm anemia clinically resembles iron-deficiency anemia. The physical signs and symptoms have been outlined previously. A peripheral blood smear from a heavily infected patient will demonstrate the presence of microcytic hypochromic red blood cells. Measurement of hemoglobin concentration will also help to confirm the diagnosis. Eosinophilia is often a prominent feature of the complete blood count. In many endemic areas, other causes of anemia should be excluded, including malaria, HIV/AIDS, and hemoglobinopathies. Hookworm will also exacerbate anemia in patients with underlying nutritional deficiencies. Occasionally, a patient will be diagnosed early in the clinical course of hookworm infection because of a characteristic rash, pruritus, and pulmonary symptoms.

A definitive diagnosis of hookworm infection is established by identifying hookworm eggs from feces under light microscopy. Fecal concentration techniques are not required to diagnose moderate or heavy infections, or even most light infections. Quantitative egg counts are sometimes useful for determining the intensity of infection; this is essential to epidemiologic investigations since prevalence determination provides superficial information. Common quantitative techniques include the Kato–Katz, Beaver direct egg count, Stoll dilutional egg count, and McMaster techniques.[74] Hookworm eggs are easily differentiated from other common human intestinal nematodes, such as *Ascaris* and *Trichuris*. However, the eggs of *A. duodenale* and *N. americanus* are not usually distinguishable by light microscopy. Species assignment of eggs using the polymerase chain reaction is under investigation.[75] Currently, however, species assignment usually requires either recovery of the adult worms from patients treated with an anthelminthic agent or rearing L3 larvae from eggs by fecal cultures.[74] It is cautioned, however, that the benzimidazole anthelminthic drugs frequently cause adult worm degeneration, making species assignment difficult. Characteristic features that distinguish *N. americanus* L3 larvae from *A. duodenale* include a prominent buccal spear and conspicuous transverse striations present on the sheath in the tail regions in the former. L3 larvae of *Strongyloides* have a characteristic notched tail not found in hookworm L3 larvae.

Human *A. caninum* infections that result in eosinophilic enteritis usually result in negative fecal examinations. Often, a single male or nongravid female adult hookworm living in an ectopic gastrointestinal site can cause eosinophilic enteritis. Therefore, definitive diagnosis may require identification of the parasite by either upper endoscopy or sigmoidoscopy. CLM is most often diagnosed clinically and must be differentiated from scabies.[37] Unlike patients with CLM, the mite *Sarcoptes scabiei* or its eggs can be demonstrated from skin scrapings. Patients with CLM may not have eosinophilia or a rise in IgE titer as they frequently do in systemic helminthic infections (see Chapter 103).[37]

TREATMENT AND PROGNOSIS

The benzimidazole anthelminthic drugs, mebendazole and albendazole, are the current treatment of choice for removing adult hookworms from the gastrointestinal tract.[76] Both agents act on the microtubules of the parasite. Mebendazole is given either in a single 500-mg dose or 100 mg twice daily for 3 days; albendazole is given 400 mg once.[76] The benzimidazoles are teratogenic and embryotoxic in experimental animals and have not been rigorously tested in young children or in pregnancy. However, increasing experience with these agents given during mass chemotherapy programs in developing countries indicates that they are probably safe in children older than 1 year of age and therefore should be given to hookworm-infected preschool children, as well as pregnant women in their second and third trimesters.[77,78] In at least one anecdotal report from Papua New Guinea, thousands of children were treated with mebendazole and albendazole with no side effects.[79] Occasional adverse effects of the benzimidazoles include diarrhea, abdominal pain, and the induction of adult *Ascaris* worm migrations to ectopic sites.[76] Rarely, the benzimidazoles will cause leukopenia, alopecia, and an increase in serum transaminases.[76] As second-line agents, pyrantel pamoate, levamisole, bephenium hydroxynaphthoate, metrifonate, and even tetrachloroethylene must be used in developing countries. However, because albendazole and mebendazole are now available as low-cost generic medicines, these other agents are no longer commonly used.

The World Health Organization has advocated the use of single-dose albendazole or mebendazole for mass treatment programs of school-age children with STH infections.[77] Both agents will reduce hookworm burdens below the threshold that would otherwise result in disease. Mass treatment of school-age children offers a number of health- and non-health-related benefits to children, including improvement in iron and hemoglobin status, physical growth, cognition, educational achievement, and school absenteeism.[2,80] However, in areas of intense transmission, hookworm-infected children can be expected to reacquire their infections to pretreatment levels approximately 4 to 12 months after receiving albendazole or mebendazole.[5] In addition, one study noted diminishing efficacy of mebendazole with repeated use, possibly because of emerging anthelmintic drug resistance.[81,82] There is also no direct evidence that benzimidazole will eradicate populations of arrested, hypobiotic larvae in human tissues. Therefore, patients with latent *A. duodenale* infections could theoretically have positive fecal examinations months after curative treatment, even in non-endemic areas. The prognosis of hookworm infection is dependent on its chronicity, its intensity, and the iron reserves and diet of the host. Many of the sequelae of hookworm anemia are potentially reversible with anthelminthic drugs and iron supplementation.[83,84] However, severe hookworm iron-deficiency anemia in infancy may cause irreversible effects.[61] The majority of patients with CLM are cured by oral administration of albendazole (400 mg daily for 3 days) or ivermectin (200 μg per kg daily for 1 or 2 days).

PREVENTION AND CONTROL

Since there are no animal reservoir hosts for *A. duodenale* or *N. americanus*, effective sanitation should interrupt hookworm transmission and prevent reinfection. However, by itself, the effect of sanitation in terms of reducing community hookworm prevalence and intensity is often not realized for decades.[2,85] Economic development with improvement in living standards and the introduction of piped water supplies, water-borne sewage systems, mechanized agriculture, and replacement of human feces with chemical fertilizers will control endemic hookworm and are largely responsible for the control of hookworm infection in North America, Europe, Japan, and Korea. Presumably, these measures would be effective in many developing countries. Health education to advise on the proper use of sanitation facilities and to avoid using uncomposted human manure is also an essential component of control.[86]

Because of the health and educational benefits of albendazole and mebendazole outlined previously, and because they have become available as low-cost generic drugs, there has been interest in using them to control STH infections worldwide. At the World Health Assembly in 2001, a resolution was put forward (resolution 54.19) urging endemic countries to control STH infections and regularly treat at least 75% of all at-risk school-age children with albendazole or mebendazole (as well as praziquantel in schistosomiasis endemic regions) by 2010 (www.who.int/wormcontrol).[77,80] It has been further proposed that, wherever possible, the schools provide the infrastructure for anthelminthic health care delivery, with trained teachers responsible for administering the drugs.[77] Because *Ascaris*, *Trichuris*, and *Schistosoma* worm burdens are highest among school-age children, there is optimism that implementation of resolution 54.19 will have a significant impact on these infections and possibly help to reduce transmission. However, because hookworm disease burdens are frequently concentrated among adult populations (including pregnant women), and preschool children are vulnerable to permanent intellectual and cognitive deficits from iron deficiency,[61] there is concern that such school-based programs could fail to effectively target vulnerable hookworm-infected populations.[6,80] School-based deworming will also not reduce hookworm transmission. Moreover, where high-intensity endemic hookworm occurs, reinfection will occur within months necessitating, in some cases, thrice yearly treatments.[80–82] There is further concern that such frequent administration of benzimidazoles may promote the emergence of drug resistance.[80–82] For these reasons, there is great interest in developing new tools and strategies to control hookworm infection in developing countries. A first-generation recombinant vaccine for human necator infection has been developed and is scheduled for phase 1 clinical trials.[2,6,80]

REFERENCES

1. De Silva N, Brooker S, Hotez P, et al: Soil-transmitted helminth infections: Updating the global picture. Trends Parasitol 19:547–551, 2003.
2. Brooker S, Bethony J, Hotez PJ: Human hookworm infection in the 21st century. Adv Parasitol 58:197–288, 2004.
3. Bundy DAP, Chan MS, Savioli L: Hookworm infection in pregnancy. Trans R Soc Trop Med Hyg 89:521–522, 1995.
4. Hotez PJ, Pritchard DI: Hookworm infection. Sci Am 272:68–75, 1995.
5. Albonico M, Smith PG, Ercole E, et al: Rate of reinfection with intestinal nematodes after treatment of children with mebendazole or albendazole in a highly endemic area. Trans R Soc Trop Med Hyg 89:538–541, 1995.
6. Hotez PJ, Zhan B, Bethony JM, et al: Progress in the development of a recombinant vaccine for human hookworm disease: The human hookworm vaccine initiative. Int J Parasitol 33:1245–1258, 2003.
7. Hoagland KE, Schad GA: *Necator americanus* and *Ancylostoma duodenale*: Life history parameters and epidemiological implications of two sympatric hookworms on humans. Exp Parasitol 44:36–49, 1978.
8. Hotez P: Human hookworm infection. In Farthing MJG, Keusch GT, Wakelin D (eds): Enteric Infection 2: Intestinal Helminths. London, Chapman & Hall, 1995, pp 129–150.
9. Stiles CW: A new species of hookworm (*Uncinaria americana*) parasitic in man. Am Med 3:777–778, 1902.
10. Crosby WH: The deadly hookworm. Why did the Puerto Ricans die? Arch Intern Med 147:577–578, 1987.
11. Roche M, Layrisse M: Nature and causes of hookworm anemia. Am J Trop Med Hyg 15:1031–1102, 1966.
12. Komiya Y, Yasuroaka Y: The biology of hookworms. Prog Med Parasitol Jpn 3:4–114, 1966.
13. Smith G, Schad GA: *Ancylostoma duodenale* and *Necator americanus*: Effect of temperature on egg development and mortality. Parasitology 99:127–132, 1989.
14. Hotez PJ, Hawdon J, Schad GA: Hookworm larval infectivity, arrest and amphiparatenesis: The *Caenorhabditis elegans* Daf-c paradigm. Parasitol Today 9:23–26, 1993.
15. Hawdon JM, Hotez PJ: Hookworm: Developmental biology of the infectious process. Curr Opin Genet Dev 6:618–623, 1996.
16. Looss A: On the penetration of *Ancylostoma* larvae into the human skin. Zentralbl Hyg Umweltmed 29:733–739, 1901.
17. Schad GA, Chowdhury AF, Dean CG, et al: Arrested development in human hookworm infections: An adaptation to a seasonally unfavorable external environment. Science 180:502–504, 1973.
18. Nawalinski TA, Schad GA: Arrested development in *Ancylostoma duodenale*: Course of self-induced infection in man. Am J Trop Med Hyg 23:895–898, 1974.
19. Nawalinski T, Schad GA, Chowdhury AB: Population biology of hookworms in children in rural West Bengal. I. General parasitological observations. Am J Trop Med Hyg 27:1152–1161, 1978.
20. Schad GA: *Ancylostoma duodenale*: Maintenance through six generations in helminth-naive pups. Exp Parasitol 47:246–253, 1979.
21. Schad GA, Murrell KD, Fayer R: Paratenesis in *Ancylostoma duodenale* suggests possible meat-borne infection. Trans R Soc Trop Med Hyg 78:203–204, 1984.

22. Schad GA, Anderson RM: Predisposition to hookworm infection. Science 228:1537–1540, 1985.
23. Schad GA: Hypobiosis and related phenomena in hookworm infection. In Schad GA, Warren KS (eds): Hookworm Disease, Current Status and Future Directions. London, Taylor & Francis, 1990, pp 71-88.
24. Hawdon JM, Johnston SA: Hookworm in the Americas: An alternative to trans-Pacific contact. Parasitol Today 12:72–74, 1996.
25. Yu Sen-Hai, Jiang Ze-Xiao, Xu Long-Qi: Infantile hookworm disease in China. A review. Acta Trop 59:265–270, 1995.
26. Prociv P, Croese J: Human eosinophilic enteritis caused by dog hookworm, *Ancylostoma caninum*. Lancet 335:1299–1302, 1990.
27. Croese J, Prociv P, Maguire EJ, et al: Eosinophilic enteritis presenting as surgical emergencies: A report of six cases. Med J Aust 153:415–417, 1990.
28. Croese J, Loukas A, Opdebeeck J, et al: Human enteric infection with canine hookworms. Ann Intern Med 120:369–374, 1994.
29. Croese J, Loukas A, Opdebeeck J, et al: Occult enteric infection by *Ancylostoma caninum*: A previously unrecognized zoonosis. Gastroenterology 106:3–12, 1994.
30. Loukas A, Opdebeeck J, Croese J, et al: Immunologic incrimination of *Ancylostoma caninum* as a human enteric pathogen. Am J Trop Med Hyg 50:69–77, 1994.
31. Schad GA: Hookworms: Pets to humans. Ann Intern Med 120:434–435, 1994.
32. Mabaso MLH, Appleton CC, Hughes JC, et al: The effect of soil type and climate on hookworm (*Necator americanus*) distribution in KwaZulu Natal, South Africa. Trop Med Int Health 8:722–727, 2003.
33. Hotez PJ: China's hookworms. China Q 172:1029–1041, 2002.
34. Albonico M, Stoltzfus RJ, Savioli L, et al: Epidemiological evidence for a differential effect of hookworm species *Ancylostoma duodenale* or *Necator americanus* on iron status of children. Int J Epidemiol 27:530–537, 1998.
35. Martin LK: Hookworm in Georgia. II. Survey of intestinal helminth infections in members of rural households of southeastern Georgia. Am J Trop Med Hyg 21:930–943, 1972.
36. Labiano-Abello N, Canese J, Velazquez ME, et al: Epidemiology of hookworm infection in Itagua, Paraguay: A cross-sectional study. Mem Inst Oswaldo Cruz 94:583–586, 1999.
37. Jelinek T, Maiwald H, Nothdurft HD, et al: Cutaneous larva migrans in travelers: Synopsis of histories, symptoms, and treatment of 98 patients. Clin Infect Dis 19:1062–1066, 1994.
38. Bethony J, Chen JZ, Lin SX, et al: Emerging patterns of hookworm infection: Influence of aging on the intensity of *Necator* infection in Hainan Province, People's Republic of China. Clin Infect Dis 35:1336–1344, 2002.
39. Crosby WH: What became of chlorosis? JAMA 257:2799–2800, 1987.
40. Sakti H, Nokes C, Hertanto WS, et al: Evidence for an association between hookworm infection and cognitive function in Indonesian school children. Trop Med Int Health 4:322–334, 1999.
41. Salafsky B, Fusco AC, Siddiqui A: *Necator americanus*: Factors influencing skin penetration of larvae. In Schad GA, Warren KS (eds): Hookworm Disease, Current Status and Future Directions. London, Taylor & Francis, 1990, pp 329–339.
42. Hotez PJ, Narasimhan S, Haggerty J, et al: Hyaluronidase from *Ancylostoma* hookworm larvae and its function as a virulence factor in cutaneous larva migrans. Infect Immun 60:1018–1023, 1992.
43. Kumar S, Pritchard DI: The partial characterization of proteases present in the excretory/secretory products and exsheathing fluid of the infective (L3) larva of *Necator americanus*. Int J Parasitol 22:563–572, 1992.
44. Zhan B, Hotez PJ, Wang Y, et al: A developmentally regulated metalloprotease secreted by host-stimulated *Ancylostoma caninum* third-stage infective larvae is a member of the astacin family of proteases. Mol Biochem Parasitol 120:291–296, 2002.
45. Hawdon JM, Jones BF, Hoffman D, et al: Cloning and expression of *Ancylostoma* secreted protein: A polypeptide associated with the transition to parasitism by infective hookworm larvae. J Biol Chem 271:6672–6678, 1996.
46. Hawdon JM, Narasimhan S, Hotez PJ: Ancylostoma secreted protein 2: Cloning and characterization of a second member of a family of nematode secreted proteins from *Ancylostoma caninum*. Mol Biochem Parasitol 30:149–165, 1999.
47. Stannssens P, Bergum PW, Gansemans Y, et al: Anticoagulant repertoire of the hookworm *Ancylostoma caninum*. Proc Natl Acad Sci USA 93:2149–2154, 1996.
48. Del Valle A, Jones BF, Harrison LM, et al: Isolation and molecular cloning of a secreted hookworm platelet inhibitor from adult *Ancylostoma caninum*. Mol Biochem Parasitol 129:167–177, 2003.
49. Zhan B, Badamchian M, Bo MH, et al: Molecular cloning and purification of Ac-TMP a developmentally regulated putative tissue inhibitor of metalloprotease released in relative abundance by adult *Ancylostoma* hookworms. Am J Trop Med Hyg 66:238–244, 2002.
50. Zhan B, Liu Y, Badamchian M, et al: Molecular characterization of the *Ancylostoma*-secreted protein (ASP) family from the adult stage of *Ancylostoma caninum*. Int J Parasitol 33:897–907, 2003.
51. Basavaraju S, Zhan B, Kennedy MW, et al: Ac-FAR-1, a 20 kDa fatty acid- and retinol-binding protein secreted by adult *Ancylostoma caninum* hookworms: Gene transcription pattern, ligand binding properties and structural characterization. Mol Biochem Parasitol 126:63–71, 2003.
52. Taiwo FA, Brophy PM, Pritchard DI, et al: Cu/Zn superoxide dismutase in excretory–secretory products of the human hookworm *Necator americanus*. An electron paramagnetic spectrometry study. Eur J Biochem 264:434–438, 1999.
53. Kasper G, Brown A, Eberl M, et al: A calreticulin-like molecule for the human hookworm *Necator americanus* interacts with C1q and the cytoplasmic signaling domains of some integrins. Parasite Immunol 23:141–152, 2001.
54. Geisbert TW, Hensley LE, Jahrling PB, et al: Treatment of Ebola virus infection with a recombinant inhibitor of factor VIIa/tissue factor: A study in rhesus monkeys. Lancet 362:1953–1958, 2003.
55. Moyle M, Foster DL, McGrath DE, et al: A hookworm glycoprotein that inhibits neutrophil function is a ligand of the integrin CD11b/CD18. J Biol Chem 269:1008–1015, 1994.
56. Pritchard DI, Brown A, Toutant JP: The molecular forms of acetylcholinesterase from *Necator americanus* (Nematoda), a hookworm parasite of the human intestine. Eur J Biochem 219:317–323, 1994.
57. Hotez PJ, Cappello M, Hawdon J, et al: Hyaluronidases from the gastrointestinal invasive nematodes *Ancylostoma caninum* and *Anisakis simplex*: Their function in the pathogenesis of human zoonoses. J Infect Dis 170:918–926, 1994.
58. Brown A, Burleigh JM, Billett EE, et al: An initial characterization of the proteolytic enzymes secreted by the adult stage of the human hookworm *Necator americanus*. Parasitology 110:555–563, 1995.
59. Don TA, Jones MK, Smyth D, et al: A pore-forming haemolysin from the hookworm *Ancylostoma caninum*. Int J Parasitol 34:1029–1035, 2004.
60. Williamson AL, Brindley PJ, Knox DP, et al: Digestive proteases of blood-feeding nematodes and other parasites. Trends Parasitol 19:417–423, 2003.
61. Lozoff B, Jimenez E, Wolf AW: Long-term developmental outcome of infants with iron deficiency. N Engl J Med 325:687–694, 1991.
62. Oski FA: Iron deficiency in infancy and childhood. N Engl J Med 329:190–193, 1993.
63. Stoltzfus RJ, Dreyfuss M, Hababuu MPH, et al: Hookworm control as a strategy to prevent iron deficiency. Nutrition Rev 65:153–159, 1997.
64. Maxwell C, Hussain R, Nutman TB, et al: The clinical and immunologic responses of normal human volunteers to low dose hookworm (*Necator americanus*) infection. Am J Trop Med Hyg 37:126–134, 1987.
65. Ottesen EA: Immune responses in human hookworm infection. In Schad GA, Warren KS (eds): Hookworm Disease, Current Status and Future Directions. London, Taylor & Francis, 1990, pp 404–416.
66. Pritchard DI, Quinnell RJ, Slater AFG, et al: Epidemiology and immunology of *Necator americanus* infection in a community in Papua New Guinea: Humoral responses to excretory–secretory and cuticular collagen antigens. Parasitology 100:317–326, 1990.
67. Olatunde BO, Onyemelukwe GC: Immunosuppression in Nigerians with hookworm infection. Afr J Med Sci 23:221–225, 1994.
68. Chow SC, Brown A, Pritchard D: The human hookworm pathogen *Necator americanus* induces apoptosis in T lymphocytes. Parasite Immunol 22:21–29, 2000.
69. Loukas A, Prociv P: Immune responses to hookworm infections. Clin Microbiol Rev 14:689–703, 2001.
70. Miller TA: Vaccination against the canine hookworm diseases. Adv Parasitol 9:153–183, 1971.
71. Miller TA: Industrial development and field use of the canine hookworm vaccine. Adv Parasitol 17:315–384, 1978.

72. Goud GN, Zhan B, Ghosh K, et al: Cloning, yeast expression, isolation and vaccine testing of recombinant *Ancylostoma* secreted protein 1 (ASP-1) and ASP-2 from *Ancylostoma caninum*. J Infect Dis 189:919–929, 2004.
73. Bethony JM, Loukas A, Smout MJ, et al: Antibodies against a secreted protein from hookworm larvae reduce the intensity of infection in humans and vaccinated laboratory animals. Lancet, unpublished observations, 2004.
74. Pawlowski ZS, Schad GA, Stott GJ: Hookworm Infection and Anaemia. Approaches to Prevention and Control. Geneva, World Health Organization, 1991.
75. Hawdon JM: Differentiation between the human hookworms *Ancylostoma duodenale* and *Necator americanus* using PCR-RFLP. J Parasitol 82:642–647, 1996.
76. Drugs for parasitic infections. Medical Letter, April 2004.
77. World Health Organization: Prevention and control of schistosomiasis and soil-transmitted helminthiasis. Report of a WHO Expert Committee, WHO Technical Report Series 912. Geneva, World Health Organization, 2002.
78. Montresor A, Awasthi S, Crompton DWT: Use of benzimidazoles in children younger than 24 months for the treatment of soil-transmitted helminthiasis. Acta Tropica 86:223–232, 2003.
79. Biddulph J: Mebendazole and albendazole for infants. Pediatr Infect Dis J 9:373, 1990.
80. Hotez PJ, Brooker S, Bethony JM, et al: Current concepts: Hookworm infection. N Engl J Med 351:799–807, 2004.
81. Albonico M, Bickle Q, Ramsan M, et al: Efficacy of mebendazole and levamisole alone or in combination against intestinal nematode infections after repeated targeted mebendazole treatment in Zanzibar. Bull WHO 81:343–352, 2003.
82. Albonico M: Methods to sustain drug efficacy in helminth control programs. Acta Tropica 86:233–242, 2003.
83. Stephenson LS, Latham MC, Kurz KM, et al: Treatment with a single dose of albendazole improves growth of Kenyan schoolchildren with hookworm, *Trichuris trichiura*, and *Ascaris lumbricoides* infections. Am J Trop Med Hyg 41:78–87, 1989.
84. Stephenson LS, Latham MC, Kinoti SN, et al: Improvements in physical fitness of Kenyan schoolboys infected with hookworm, *Trichuris trichiura*, *Ascaris lumbricoides* following a single dose of albendazole. Trans R Soc Trop Med Hyg 84:277–282, 1990.
85. Esrey SA, Potash JB, Roberts L, et al: Effects of improved water supplies and sanitation on ascariasis, diarrhea, drancunculiasis, hookworm infection, schistosomiasis and trachoma. Bull WHO 69:609–621, 1991.
86. Asaolu SO, Ofoezie IE: The role of health education and sanitation in the control of helminth infections. Acta Tropica 86:283–294, 2003.

111

Strongyloidiasis

AFZAL A. SIDDIQUI
ROBERT M. GENTA
STEVEN L. BERK

INTRODUCTION

Strongyloidiasis is caused by *Strongyloides stercoralis*. It is the fourth most important intestinal nematode infection in the world. Although isolated pockets of low endemicity and indigenous sporadic infections have often been found in many temperate areas of the world, *S. stercoralis* infection predominantly occurs in humid tropical areas. The specific impact of chronic infection with *S. stercoralis* on human health is difficult to evaluate in populations with widespread enteric diseases, parasitoses, and malnutrition. However, strongyloidiasis is not generally believed to be one of the major causes of morbidity worldwide. Infection of humans with *S. stercoralis* usually produces an asymptomatic chronic disease of the gastrointestinal tract that can remain undetected for several decades. However, in immunocompromised patients and especially those receiving corticosteroids, hyperinfection can develop with the dissemination of larvae to extraintestinal organs and can result in mortality rates as high as 85%.

AGENT

History

In the second half of the 19th century, French troops deployed in the then French colony of Cochin China (modern Vietnam) often developed a persistent severe diarrhea that became known among military personnel as "diarrhée de la Cochinchine." In 1876 Louis Normand, a physician stationed at the Toulon Naval Hospital, discovered small worms in the stools of some of the repatriated soldiers and reported his findings to the Academy of Sciences of Paris.[1] Bavay, a colleague of Normand, named the worm *Anguillula stercoralis* (from the Latin words for "small eel" and "dung") and later provided a detailed description of the worm under the new name, *Anguillula intestinalis*. Several parasitologists became interested in the new nematode, and in 1879 Grassi established a new genus which he called *Strongyloides* (Greek *strongylos*, "round") and gave *Strongyloides stercoralis* its current name.[2] In subsequent years, the cycle was partially described, but the important issues of the free-living cycle, parthenogenesis, and the autoinfectious cycle were not fully elucidated until the experimental work of Fülleborn (1911), Kreis (1932), and Faust (1933). Although several detailed descriptions of individuals infected with *S. stercoralis* were published in the early part of this century,[3] it was not until Napier[4] conducted extensive clinical surveys of repatriated British soldiers and Galliard[5,6] performed systematic experiments in normal and immunosuppressed dogs that the clinical importance of strongyloidiasis began to be fully appreciated.

Taxonomy

The family Strongylidae (class Secernentasida, order Rhabditorida) comprises only the genus *Strongyloides*. The members of this genus, also called threadworms, are heterogenetic, with free-living and parasitic generations, and include at least 40 named species.[7] Most of these are parasites of mammals, but some can be found in birds, reptiles, and amphibians. The only species discussed here is *S. stercoralis*. *Strongyloides fuelleborni* is a parasite of primates that may also infect humans. Several other species are also important, either because they can cause disease in livestock (*Strongyloides ransomi, Strongyloides westeri, Strongyloides papillosus*) or because they can be used as models of human strongyloidiasis (*Strongyloides ratti*).[8]

Life Cycle and Morphology

The infection is acquired when filariform larvae (slender, fast-moving worms measuring approximately 50 μm in diameter and between 350 and 600 μm in length) penetrate the skin of a susceptible host, enter a venous or lymphatic channel, and are transported to the lungs. Here they break out of the capillaries into the alveoli (Fig. 111-1), migrate to the trachea as they mature, and are eventually swallowed. Parasitic females lodge in the lamina propria of the duodenum and the proximal jejunum, where they lay eggs (Fig. 111-2). From the hatching eggs emerge rhabditiform larvae. These shorter and slower worms (approximately 60 μm in diameter and 250 to 300 μm in length) migrate into the intestinal lumen and eventually pass with the feces into the external environment. There, depending on poorly understood environmental conditions, the rhabditiform larvae may either directly molt into infective (parasitic) filariform larvae able to repenetrate the skin of a suitable host or switch to a free-living cycle. In this latter, indirect (or heterogonic) cycle, four ecdyses

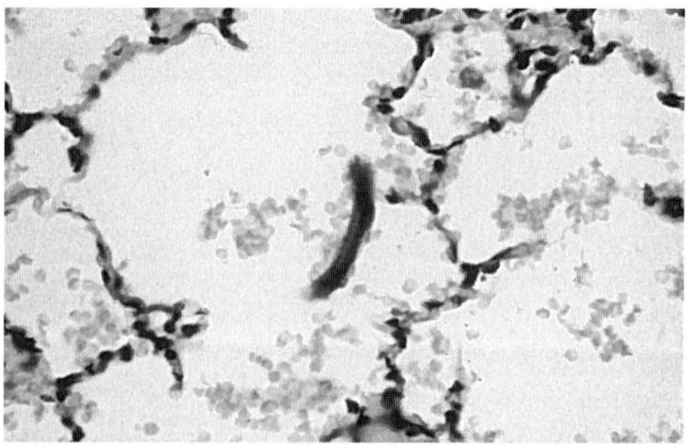

FIGURE 111-1 Fragment of a *Strongyloides stercoralis* filariform larva in the alveolar spaces of an immunocompetent host. There are scattered blood cells but no significant hemorrhage.

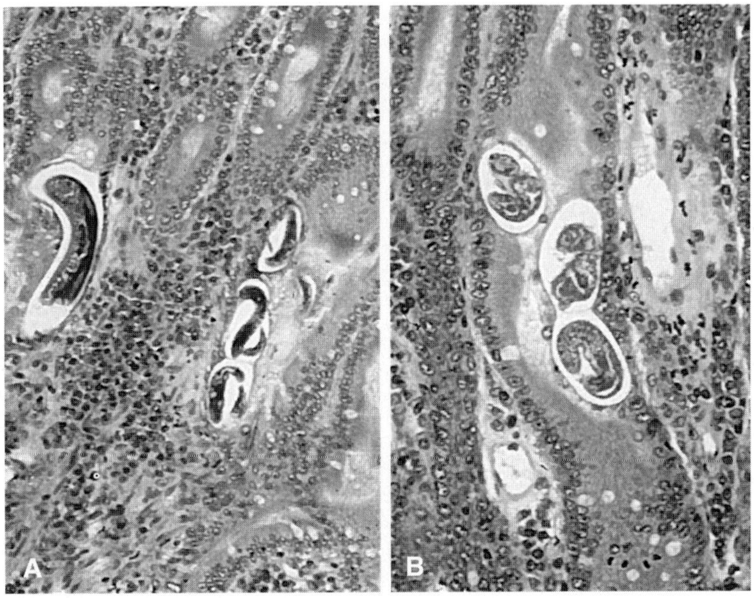

FIGURE 111-2 *A* and *B*, Section of an adult *Strongyloides stercoralis* female worm and embryonate eggs in the lamina propria of an immunocompetent subject. There is moderate mononuclear inflammation in the vicinity of the parasites.

(molts) lead to the development of adult male and female worms (Fig. 111-3). These mate and produce a generation of offspring whose filariform stage will have the ability to reenter parasitic life.[8] The characteristic of *S. stercoralis* that sets it apart from all other major human parasitic worms is that a small portion of the rhabditiform larvae molt within the host's intestine into the filariform stage. These tissue-penetrating infective larvae may penetrate the colonic wall (Fig. 111-4) or the perianal skin, complete an internal cycle, and become established as mature adult females in the small intestine. This process, known as autoinfection, is believed to represent the mechanism by which *S. stercoralis* can persist virtually indefinitely in infected hosts.[9,10]

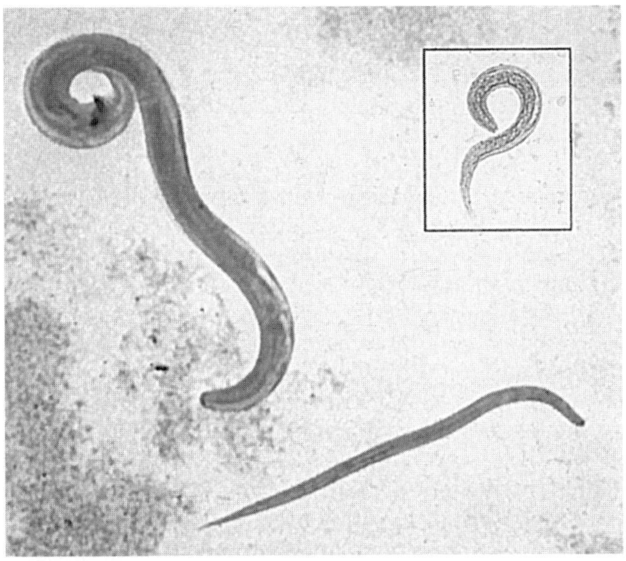

FIGURE 111-3 Filariform larva (approximately 550 μm in length) and an immature adult worm (1.3 mm) recovered from the feces of an immunocompromised dog experimentally infected with *Strongyloides stercoralis*. It is extremely rare to recover from the stools of immunocompetent patients any *S. stercoralis* stages other than the shorter (approximately 300 μm) and plumper rhabditiform larvae (*right upper corner inset*).

EPIDEMIOLOGY

The information regarding the worldwide prevalence of strongyloidiasis is inconsistent, with estimates varying between 3 million and 100 million people infected worldwide.[11] The unreliability of these estimates is further reflected in the wide range of reported prevalence rates, which vary between less than 1% and 85% in populations living in adjacent regions of the same country.[12,13] Given these limitations, *S. stercoralis* probably is present in virtually all tropical and subtropical regions of the world.[14] Areas of low endemicity (less than 1% to 3%) still exist in several countries of Europe (e.g., northern Italy, France, Spain, Switzerland, Poland), the United States (e.g., Appalachian region[15] and West Virginia[16]), Japan (Okinawa), and Australia (aboriginal populations).[14] In some areas, for example, the Valencian

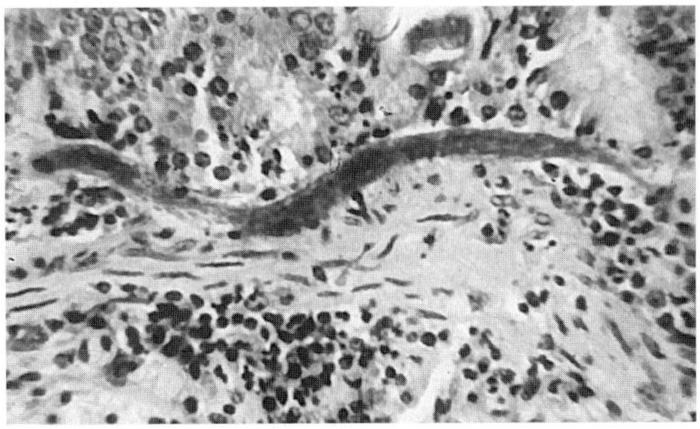

FIGURE 111-4 Intestinal muscularis mucosae and submucosa with a full-length section of a penetrating filariform larva.

Strongyloides stercoralis

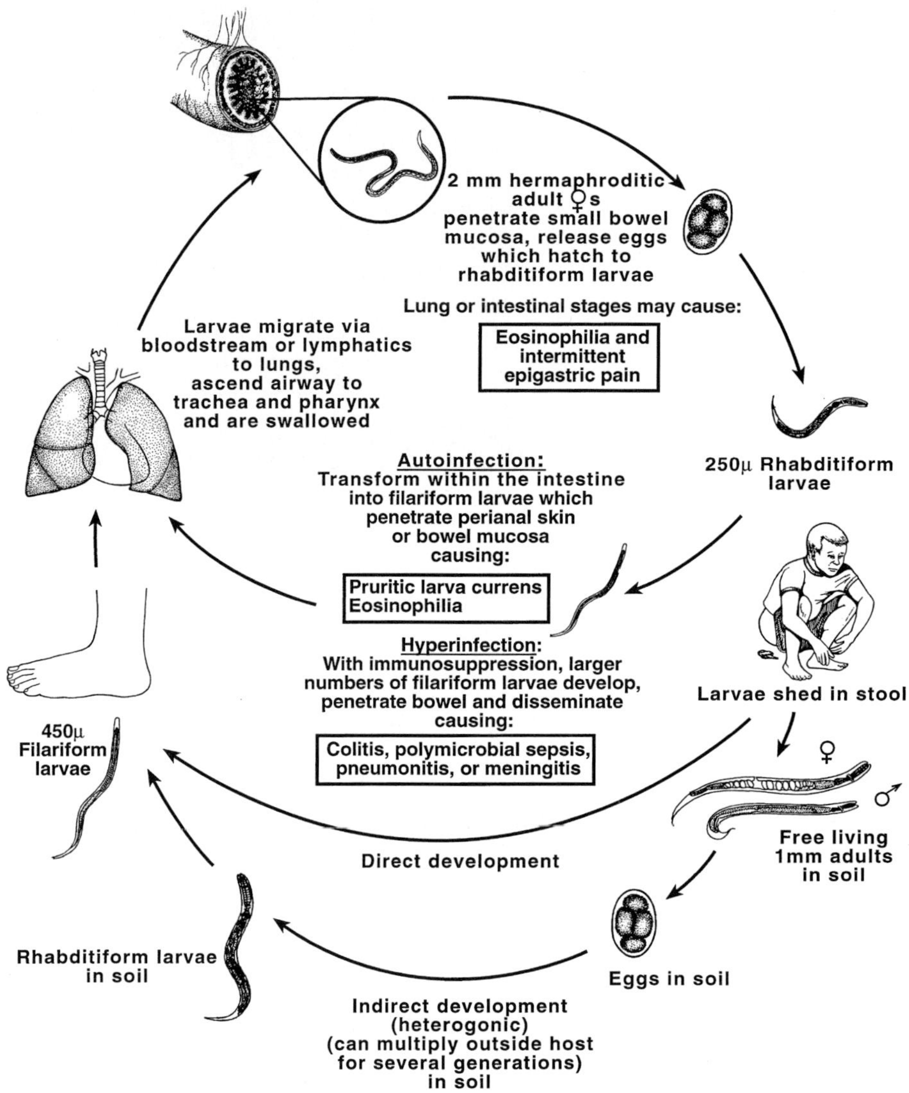

community in Spain, the high prevalence of strongyloidiasis has been attributed to the agricultural activities.[17] Strongyloidiasis has also been found intermittently in institutionalized individuals[18] as well as in patients of cancer centers[19] in several North American locations where the parasite is not endemic in the general population. The accompanying map depicts the estimated prevalence of strongyloidiasis in the world. Considering the long persistence of *S. stercoralis* in its host and its relatively high prevalence in some tropical and subtropical populations, physicians practicing in industrialized countries should consider strongyloidiasis in immigrant or refugee patients born in developing regions[20] as well as in persons from known local areas of endemicity.

PATHOGENESIS AND IMMUNITY

Chronic strongyloidiasis is probably sustained by a relatively low and stable number of adult worms that reside in harmony within their host's intestine and survive by means of well-regulated autoinfection.[21] Autoinfection is believed to be regulated by host cell–mediated immunity.[9,22,23] When immunosuppression impairs this regulatory function, increasing numbers of autoinfective larvae complete the cycle, and the population of parasitic adult worms increases (hyperinfection). Eventually, the extraordinary numbers of migrating larvae deviate from the canonical route (intestine → venous bed → lungs → trachea → intestine) and disseminate to other organs, including meningeal spaces and brain, liver, kidneys, lymph nodes, and cutaneous and subcutaneous tissues, where they cause hemorrhage and inflammation and implant gram-negative bacteria carried from fecal material. The resulting syndrome, known as disseminated strongyloidiasis, is nearly always fatal.[9,23]

The validity of the preceding model has been questioned by Schad and colleagues[24] and other investigators,[25,26] who used an experimental canine model of disseminated strongyloidiasis to show that only a few larvae could be recovered from the lungs of dogs with massive hyperinfection.

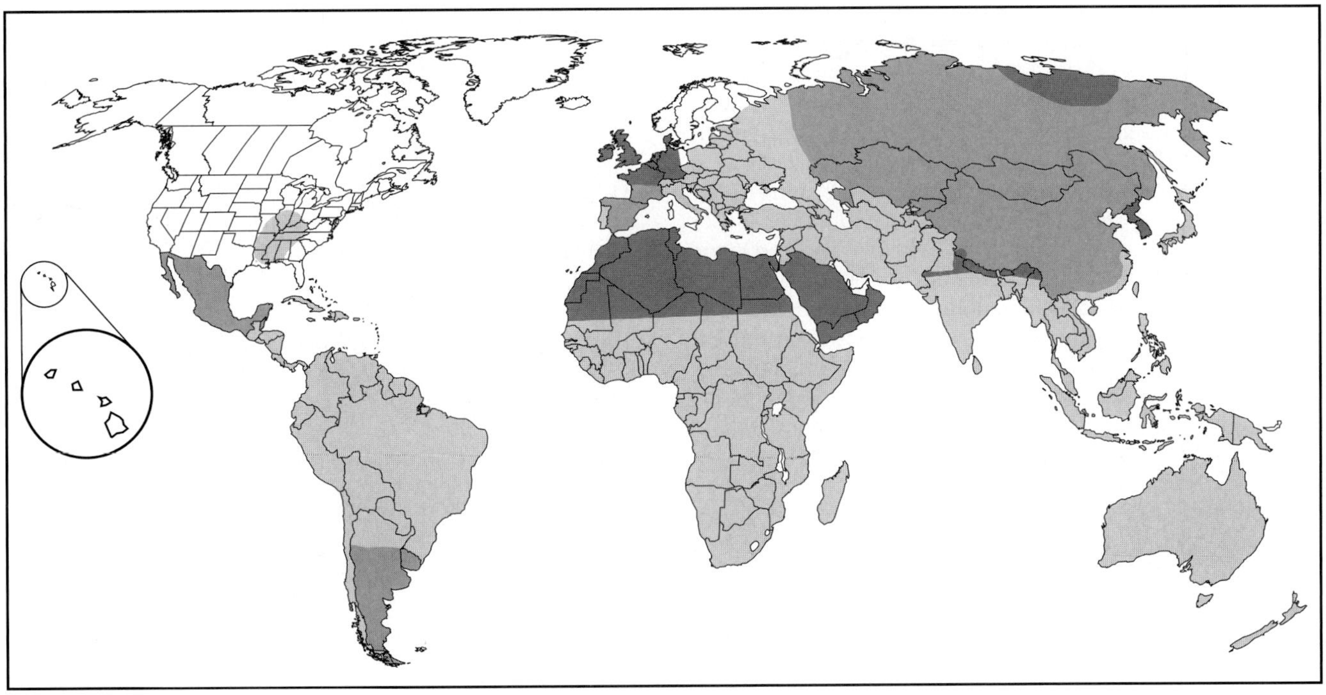

Strongyloides stercoralis

- Known endemicity
- Unknown endemicity but probably present
- Unknown endemicity but probably absent

Later, in a series of experiments based on the compartmental analysis of radiolabeled larvae and mathematical modeling, they presented convincing evidence that the tracheobronchial route in the dog was not used by the majority of the migrating larvae.[27,28] According to their model, larvae that began their migration in the skin (primary infection) or in the distal ileum (autoinfection) were not more likely to pass through the lungs than through any other organ, suggesting that the migratory pathway involved random dissemination throughout the body. However, this conclusion may not be applicable to the cycle in humans, since large numbers of larvae are frequently identified in bronchoalveolar lavage fluid from hyperinfected patients.[29,30]

Recently, the authors have challenged the accepted paradigm that host mechanisms regulate hyperinfection and dissemination.[14,21] The theory that host immunity alone controls infection fails to consider the role that parasites may play in their own regulation. The adverse impact of increased parasite density on egg production and growth has been demonstrated for several intestinal helminths. Although distinguishing between host resistance and direct parasite-to-parasite effects may be difficult, it seems clear that most parasites reach a particular population size or a critical biomass, after which yet unknown regulatory mechanisms intervene to limit the population.[28]

The authors propose that *S. stercoralis* may have the ability to reach an optimal population size in the human small intestine. If the initial infective dose of larvae is low, a higher rate of intraluminal molting (i.e., autoinfection) occurs until the "optimal" size of the adult population is reached. If *S. stercoralis*, like other nematodes, transmits its molting signal by molting hormones (ecdysteroids),[31] adult females adjust their production of ecdysteroids to levels sufficient to replace the dying adults. During the initial phase of infection, the host mounts an immune response directed at all tissue stages of the parasite.[22,32–35] These responses may not eradicate all parasites but may limit the size of the parasite population. Impaired immune responses may allow the growth of larger numbers of parasites, as reported in agammaglobulinemic patients,[36] human T-cell lymphotropic virus type I (HTLV-I)-infected subjects,[37] and severely malnourished children,[38] but total dysregulation of the parasite population does not seem to occur, since worms, in part, regulate their own growth.

The level of ecdysteroid-like substances is generally negligible in healthy subjects.[31] The administration of exogenous or endogenous corticosteroids may result in increased amounts of ecdysteroid-like substances in the host's tissues, including the intestinal wall, where adult females reside. These substances may act as molting signals for the eggs or rhabditiform larvae, which transform intraluminally into excessive numbers of filariform larvae. Available data are not sufficient to prove a dose-dependent effect, but it is indeed remarkable that patients who develop fulminating hyperinfection after only a few days of steroid administration are usually those who have received intravenous methylprednisone.[39] Once an intestinal population has become very large (e.g., 100,000 adult worms) it continues to expand rapidly, even at low molting rates, and the discontinuation of steroids is not sufficient to arrest the population growth, which leads to the host's death.

On the basis of recent observations, the authors further postulate that in *S. stercoralis* these developmental processes are regulated via a class of transcription factors that typically regulates genes in response to fat soluble hormones, such as steroids or fatty acids; as is the case for the free-living nematode *Caenorhabditis elegans*. We have recently described a gene in *S. stercoralis*[40] that showed significant homology with a number of nuclear hormone receptors including the dauer formation loci (daf) gene, daf-12 of *C. elegans*, and ecdysone receptors of insects.[40] The identification of daf-12 orthologs from *S. stercoralis* and from *Dirofilaria immitis* suggests that this component of the genetic pathway is conserved among nematodes. Daf-12 regulates the dauer diapause and developmental age in *C. elegans*, and it is possible that mechanisms similar to those acting in *C. elegans* may also regulate the development in *S. stercoralis*. Furthermore, in an animal model of *S. stercoralis*, when normal male gerbils were infected subcutaneously with 1000 infective filariform larvae, the infected animals harbored moderate numbers (83.6 ± 27.6) of adult worms at 35 days after infection.[41] More interestingly, a low-grade infection persisted for 131 days, mimicking the chronic nature of human infections. Gerbils treated weekly with 2 mg of methylprednisolone acetate developed hyperinfective strongyloidiasis, with up to 8000 autoinfective larvae occurring in these animals at postinfection day 21. Autoinfection never occurred in normal (untreated) gerbils.[41] This animal study, coupled with examples from human case reports, reinforces our argument that immune suppression per se is not the major cause of hyperinfection but rather it is the direct effect of steroid on the parasite that causes the hyperinfection.

Pathologic Changes

The pathologic lesions associated with chronic, uncomplicated *S. stercoralis* have received little attention, because only rarely have patients with such lesions come to autopsy. However, pathologic descriptions of the lesions in a few patients in whom strongyloidiasis was an incidental finding, our own experience, and animal studies[25,42,43] indicate that the worms can exist in the intestinal mucosa without causing significant inflammatory responses or tissue damage (see Fig. 111-1). The classic description of the pathologic changes in strongyloidiasis was made by De Paola and associates[44] in 1962 and later updated by Genta and Caymmi-Gomes.[45] When present, intestinal lesions range from mild mucosal congestion and abundant mucoid secretions ("catarrhal enteritis"), with a mildly increased mononuclear infiltrate in the lamina propria, to a more severe "edematous enteritis," with a grossly thickened intestinal wall. Submucosal edema, flattening of the villi, and parasites scattered throughout the lamina propria may be observed microscopically. The most severe form ("ulcerative enteritis") is almost exclusively seen in association with hyperinfection. The intestinal walls may be rigid owing to the edema and fibrosis resulting from long-standing inflammation, and the mucosa may show atrophy, erosions, and ulcerations. An abundant inflammatory infiltrate, most often consisting of neutrophils, as well as all stages of *S. stercoralis*, are present throughout the intestinal mucosa. Jejunal perforation has been reported in patients with the ulcerative enteritis form of strongyloidiasis.[46]

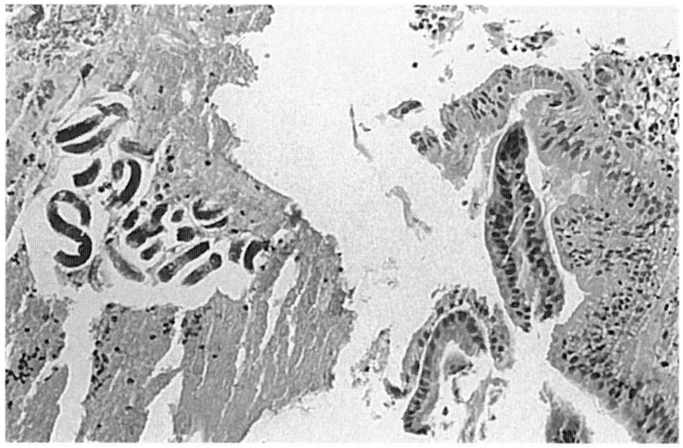

FIGURE 111-5 Gastric mucosal biopsy with numerous fragments of *Strongyloides stercoralis* larvae in a patient with AIDS and multiple opportunistic infections. The larvae were present in the mucus but were not seen penetrating the gastric mucosa itself.

Uncommonly, the mucosal damage occurs predominantly in the large intestine, simulating ulcerative colitis and pseudopolyposis.[47,48] Recently, a form of eosinophilic colitis associated with strongyloidiasis has been described in older patients.[49] *S. stercoralis* larvae have been found in the appendix, and eosinophilic appendicitis apparently caused by this parasite has been reported.[50,51] In patients with disseminated strongyloidiasis, the intestinal lesions reflect the large number of worms dwelling within the small intestinal mucosa and penetrating the intestinal walls. In addition, the stomach[52,53] (Fig. 111-5) and peritoneal cavity[50,54,55] may be invaded by migrating parasites. However, because most of these patients are receiving immunosuppressive doses of corticosteroids, the inflammatory responses are often minimal in spite of extensive tissue damage.

Migrating parasites may cause mechanical damage as well as inflammation in other organs. As larvae penetrate the large intestine, they create small breaks in the mucosa that facilitate the invasion of the bloodstream by enteric bacteria. The larvae themselves carry bacteria on their cuticle to distant sites. In human patients, the extraintestinal organ most commonly affected by this migratory damage is the lung. In severe disseminated infection, when hundreds of thousands of adult parasites dwell in the intestine and millions of larvae migrate throughout the body, alveolar microhemorrhages may result in massive pulmonary bleeding[56] (Fig. 111-6). The widespread dissemination of larvae is almost invariably associated with polymicrobial sepsis, diffuse or patchy bronchopneumonia, pulmonary and cerebral abscesses, and meningitis.[23] Filariform larvae, and occasionally rhabditiform larvae and adult worms, also may disseminate to mesenteric lymph nodes and the biliary tract, as well as the liver, pancreas, spleen, heart, endocrine glands, and ovaries.[45] In these locations the parasite may induce a granulomatous response.[57,58]

DISEASE

No other nematode has been associated with as broad a spectrum of manifestations or been implicated as the cause of so many different clinical syndromes as *S. stercoralis*.

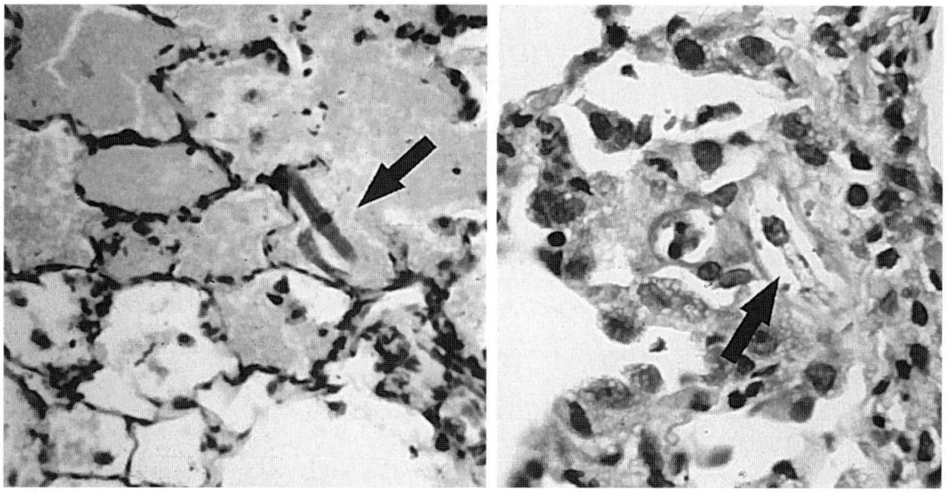

FIGURE 111-6 *Left,* severe intra-alveolar hemorrhage and fragment of a larva (*arrow*) in a patient with disseminated strongyloidiasis. In some patients, larvae may be found within the alveolar walls, where they may form granulomas. *Right,* A possible early granuloma around a fragment of larva (*arrow*).

The majority of persons with chronic infection are either asymptomatic or have mild, nonspecific symptoms. In contrast, disseminated strongyloidiasis is a catastrophic event that, if untreated, invariably results in death.

Gastrointestinal Manifestations

Epigastric abdominal pain, postprandial fullness or bloating, and heartburn are among the symptoms most commonly reported, and brief episodes of diarrhea alternating with constipation may also occur.[59,60] Occult blood is occasionally detected in the stools of subjects with chronic infections,[61] and even massive colonic[62] and gastric hemorrhage[63] have been reported. Physical examination of chronically infected patients is normal or reveals only mild abdominal tenderness on palpation. Rarely, chronic strongyloidiasis may resemble inflammatory bowel disease, particularly ulcerative colitis, and the endoscopic appearance may be that of pseudopolyposis.[47] Although malabsorption has been reported frequently in patients with strongyloidiasis,[64] a clear causal relationship between *S. stercoralis* infection and malabsorption in otherwise healthy subjects has not been established.[65]

In contrast to the usually inconsequential nature of chronic strongyloidiasis, the gastrointestinal manifestations of disseminated strongyloidiasis are almost invariably serious. Hyperinfection is often heralded by profuse diarrhea, which is a consequence of the erosions, ulcerations, and edema caused by millions of adult worms and filariform larvae in the mucosa of the small and large intestine.[23] Malabsorption, exudation, and altered motility may also result. These mucosal changes predispose the patient to bacterial enterocolitis and, after variable periods of diarrhea, paralytic ileus.[66] Possibly because of the large numbers of larvae migrating from the large intestine into the circulation,[67] polymicrobial (predominantly gram-negative) sepsis may occur and local infections and abscesses may develop in virtually any organ.[23,67] Larvae have been detected in the liver, stomach, and pancreas of patients with overwhelming infections, but their presence in these locations is not known to be associated with characteristic symptoms.[68]

Pulmonary Manifestations

Although patients with chronic obstructive pulmonary disease may have an increased risk of strongyloidiasis,[14] no respiratory signs or symptoms are associated with chronic strongyloidiasis. In these infections, the numbers of larvae passing through the lungs are probably so small that they do not cause significant tissue damage.[69] However, patients who presented with asthma (most likely unrelated to the infection) and were treated with corticosteroids later developed disseminated strongyloidiasis.[70,71] In these situations, how hyperinfection can develop is illustrated in a conceptual model shown in Figure 111-7. In summary, in patients with disseminated strongyloidiasis, pulmonary manifestations are the rule, particularly diffuse bronchopneumonia. Intra-alveolar hemorrhage, often so severe as to cause the patient's death, is frequent. Filariform larvae and at times rhabditiform larvae and even eggs may be present in respiratory secretions in those with disseminated strongyloidiasis.

Neurologic Manifestations

Uncomplicated strongyloidiasis is not associated with neurologic manifestations. Gram-negative polymicrobial meningitis is the most frequent central nervous system manifestation of disseminated strongyloidiasis, and in some cases, larvae have been identified in the cerebrospinal fluid[72] (Fig. 111-8). Less common is the formation of cerebral and cerebellar abscesses containing *S. stercoralis* larvae.[73]

Cutaneous Manifestations

Two types of cutaneous manifestations have been described in patients with chronic strongyloidiasis: urticarial rashes, possibly caused by a sensitization to parasite antigens, and a characteristic, migratory serpiginous dermatitis caused by the subcutaneous migration of filariform larvae (larva currens). The latter has been reported more often in Caucasian patients infected in the Far East.[74–76] Some patients with disseminated infection, leukopenia, and various degrees of thrombocytopenia may develop generalized or periumbilical

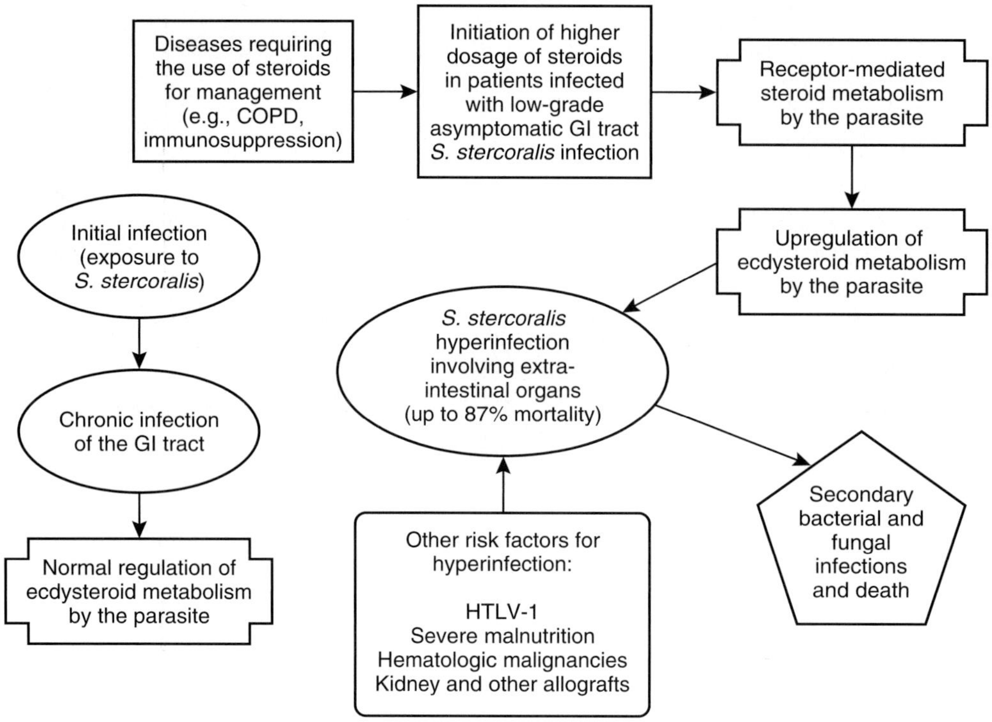

FIGURE 111-7 Conceptual model of the development of *Strongyloides stercoralis* in patients receiving corticosteroids for treatment of diseases such as chronic obstructive pulmonary disease.

cutaneous purpura,[77–80] probably related to the rupture of small vessels caused by filariform larvae migrating in the dermis.[76,79]

Other Systemic Manifestations

Arthritis is an unusual manifestation of strongyloidiasis and is associated with the local deposition of immunocomplexes containing *S. stercoralis* antigens.[81] Cardiac arrhythmias and arrest are exceedingly rare and have been attributed to direct myocardial damage caused by the migrating larvae[82] or to electrolyte imbalance precipitated by severe diarrhea.[83] The passage of larvae in semen and the presence of genital lesions[84] as well as multivisceral damage has also been attributed to strongyloidiasis.[85]

Strongyloidiasis and Diseases of the Immune System

Since disseminated strongyloidiasis is a disease of the immunocompromised, persons with either inherited or acquired immunodeficiencies would be expected to be particularly prone to this severe complication of infection.

Acquired Immunodeficiency Syndrome

Traditionally, impaired immunity was thought to be one of the main factors regulating the development of *S. stercoralis* autoinfection. Therefore, frequent and severe infections with *S. stercoralis* were expected to emerge in patients with acquired immunodeficiency syndrome (AIDS). However, this has not happened, even in areas of the world where both *S. stercoralis* and AIDS are endemic, and in general, there does not appear to be a higher incidence of chronic strongyloidiasis with AIDS (see Chapter 133).[86] Even though sporadic cases of strongyloidiasis have been reported in patients with human immunodeficiency virus (HIV),[87,88] strongyloidiasis was removed from the list of AIDS-defining illnesses by the Centers for Disease Control and Prevention. However, some conditions that cosegregate with HIV infection are known to predispose to hyperinfection syndrome, including inanition and the use

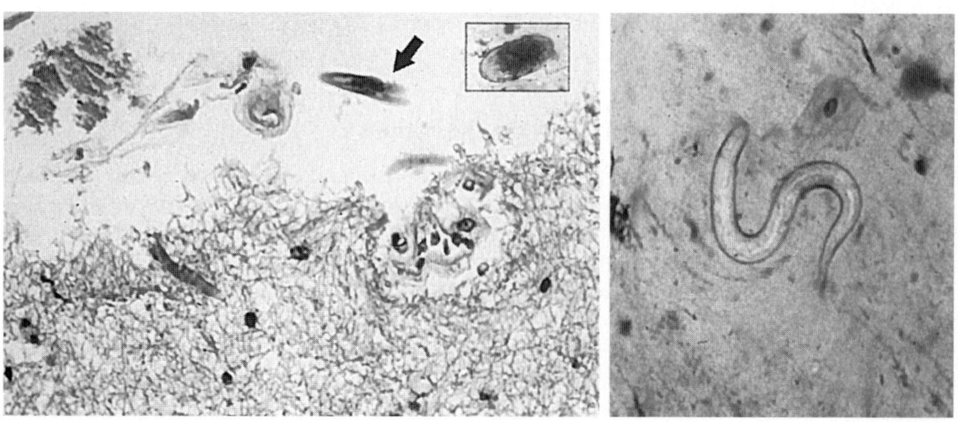

FIGURE 111-8 *Left,* fragment of larva (*arrow*) in the meninges of a man who died of disseminated strongyloidiasis. The egg in the inset was recovered from the cerebrospinal fluid when the patient was alive; this is a most unusual finding. *Right,* A larva detected during cytologic examination of a bronchoalveolar lavage specimen from the same patient.

of steroids.[89] In fact, the list of immunosuppressive diseases associated with hyperinfection are unified by the common denominator of corticosteroid therapy.[89] Nonetheless, *S. stercoralis* should be searched for and promptly treated in HIV-infected patients with a suggestive geographic history.

HTLV-1 and Leukemia

Severe strongyloidiasis has often been reported to occur in some patients infected with both *S. stercoralis* and HTLV-1 (see Chapter 76).[90] An epidemiologic association between infection with HTLV-1 and strongyloidiasis was observed on the island of Okinawa[91] and in the West Indies.[92,93] It has been suggested that HTLV-1 infection may predispose to more severe strongyloidiasis and that infection with *S. stercoralis* may promote the progression of HTLV-1 infection to leukemia.[37] Several well-documented reports have shown that patients with HTLV-1 infection and no other known predisposition to precipitating factors have developed disseminated strongyloidiasis.[94] The nature of this association remains unexplained, but physicians should be aware of it, particularly when treating patients from areas of the world where there is an epidemiologic overlap between the two infections.

Acquired Immunoglobulinopathies and Immunodeficiencies

No cases of disseminated strongyloidiasis have been reported in children with congenital immunodeficiencies. However, a few adults with acquired agammaglobulinopathy have been reported to have persistent extraintestinal *S. stercoralis* infection refractory to pharmacologic treatment. Although these individuals were producing large numbers of larvae in the stools and the sputum, they neither had symptoms that could be ascribed to strongyloidiasis nor developed the disseminated hyperinfection syndrome.[35,95,96]

DIAGNOSIS

The diagnosis of strongyloidiasis is usually accomplished by detection of larvae in the stool. However, in a majority of uncomplicated cases of strongyloidiasis, the intestinal worm load is often very low and larval output is minimal.[59,67] Eosinophilia is usually the only indication of the presence of *S. stercoralis* infection but is mild (5% to 15%) and nonspecific (see Chapter 125).[11,17,59,67,68] In more than two thirds of cases, there are no more than 25 larvae per gram of stool.[59,67] Single examination of a stool sample has been shown to be negative in up to 70% of cases. Repeated examinations of stool specimens improve the chances of finding parasites; in some studies, diagnostic sensitivity increases to 50% with three stool examinations and can approach 100% if seven serial stool samples are examined.[97] Techniques utilized to discern larvae in stool samples include direct smear of feces in saline/Lugol's iodine stain, Baermann concentration, formalin-ethyl acetate concentration, Harada-Mori filter paper culture, and nutrient agar plate cultures.[98–101]

The examination of duodenal aspirate is reportedly very sensitive; this invasive method is recommended only in children when it is necessary to achieve a rapid demonstration of parasites.[14,59] Microscopic examination of a single specimen of duodenal fluid is more sensitive than wet mount analysis of stool samples for the detection of larvae, identifying 76% of patients; the parasite was found exclusively in duodenal fluid (and not in feces) in 67% of patients.[102] The "string test," a gelatin capsule containing a string swallowed by the patient and retrieved after a few hours, enjoyed a brief period of popularity 2 decades ago but currently is used infrequently.[103] In some cases, histologic examination of duodenal or jejunal biopsy specimens may reveal *S. stercoralis* embedded in the mucosa.[14]

Detection of *S. stercoralis* larvae usually is easier in cases of hyperinfection because large numbers of worms are involved in disseminated infections.[14,59,67] The larvae can be identified in wet preparations of sputum, bronchoalveolar lavage fluid, bronchial washings and brushings, lung biopsies, and pleural fluid examined with either Gram's, Papanicolaou's, or acid-fast (Auramine O and Kinyoun) staining procedures.[14,29,67] Findings on chest films are usually variable; pulmonary infiltrates, when present, may be alveolar or interstitial, diffuse or focal, uni- or bilateral.[104] Lung consolidation, occasional cavitation, and even abscess formation have also been reported.[56] Varying chest x-ray pictures are explained by different types of bacterial superinfection, particularly gram-negative bacilli.[56,104]

A wide variety of immunodiagnostic assays have been tested over the last 2 decades with varying degrees of success. The long list includes skin testing with larval extracts, indirect immunofluorescence using fixed larvae, and radioallergosorbent testing for specific immunoglobulin E (IgE) and gelatin particle agglutination.[14,59,67,68,105–108] An enzyme-linked immunosorbent assay (ELISA) ("*Strongyloides* antibody") for detecting the serum IgG against a crude extract of the filariform larvae of *S. stercoralis* is also available at specialized centers.[105,109,110] The sensitivity and specificity of this ELISA can be improved if the sera samples are preincubated with *Onchocerca* antigens before testing.[111] The "Strongyloides antibody" test shows cross-reactivity with other helminths including filariae, *Ascaris lumbricoides*, and schistosomes, but for the general population in developed countries these are rarely in the differential diagnosis of symptomatic strongyloidiasis.[14,59,67] However, this does not hold true with respect to armed forces personnel, international travelers, immigrants, or residents of geohelminth endemic regions because they may have been exposed to "cross-reactive" antigens of other helminths in endemic areas. Furthermore, those helminths that contain "cross-reactive" antigens have the capability of long-term persistence within the host and the tendency to produce circulating antibodies that can be detected for many years after exposure. This test is unlikely to be available for wider use, because a constant supply of the *S. stercoralis* filariform larvae is needed to obtain the crude antigen preparation and because an abundant supply of *Onchocerca* antigens is required for presoaking of sera samples before an ELISA is performed. The major value of serology is the provision of a screening test that, if positive, can stimulate further searches for the parasite.[14,67] Positive ELISA serology does not distinguish prior from current infection.

In summary, stool examinations are currently the primary technique for detection of *S. stercoralis*. If special techniques are not available, several specimens collected on different days should be examined when the diagnosis is strongly suspected.

TREATMENT

Nematodes do not replicate within their definitive hosts (with the very limited exceptions of *S. stercoralis* and *Capillaria philippinensis* [see Chapter 106]). Therefore, anthelmintic treatment that reduces the worm burden for most nematodes below the level at which clinical disease can develop usually is sufficient.[14,59,68] However, in *S. stercoralis* infection, only the complete eradication of parthenogenetic adult females and autoinfective larvae removes the danger of potentially life-threatening hyperinfection.[14,59] Thus, all patients with strongyloidiasis (even asymptomatic patients) require treatment.[86] The poor sensitivity of diagnostic stool examination makes it even more difficult to determine the effectiveness of the treatment, because a true cure cannot be pronounced based on a negative follow-up stool examination.[59,67] In some instances, serologic tests and changes in eosinophil counts may serve as useful markers of treatment success.[59,67] Generally, three anthelmintics have been used to treat strongyloidiasis with varying degrees of efficacy.[86]

Ivermectin

Ivermectin is derived from β-avermectins (monocyclic lactones) that are produced by *Streptomyces avermitilis*. The mode of action of this orally administered broad-spectrum anthelmintic is through selective binding with glutamate-gated chloride ion channels in nerve and muscle cells that causes hyperpolarization of the nerve and muscle cell membranes, resulting in paralysis and death of the worm.[86] The plasma half-life of this drug is 16 hours, and it is metabolized in the liver.[86] A consensus is developing about ivermectin being the ideal drug for the treatment of intestinal and disseminated strongyloidiasis.[112–117] Ivermectin has a cure rate of 64% to 100% after a single dose.[118] Ivermectin has been registered recently as the drug of choice in the World Health Organization's Essential Drug List for the treatment of *S. stercoralis*. The standard dosage is 200 μg/kg per day, given orally (1 to 2 days), for intestinal infections.[117] The same regimen is recommended for adults and children (>15 kg). Adequate and well-controlled clinical studies have not been conducted to determine the optimal dosing regimen in immunocompromised patients or patients with the disseminated disease; it may be necessary to prolong (e.g., 7 to 10 days) or repeat the therapy.[117] Ivermectin administered as an enema may be of some benefit in patients with severe strongyloidiasis who are unable to absorb or tolerate oral therapy.[119]

Thiabendazole

Historically, thiabendazole has been the drug of choice for the treatment of strongyloidiasis, despite frequent gastrointestinal and neuropsychologic side effects and a high relapse rate. Thiabendazole has a cure rate of 50% to 94% and may not be effective in disease that is disseminated beyond the gastrointestinal tract.[19,117,118] Thiabendazole is a broad-spectrum drug for intestinal nematodes and acts by inhibiting helminth-specific mitochondrial fumarate reductase. Thiabendazole is absorbed rapidly, and peak plasma concentration is reached within 1 to 2 hours after the oral administration of a suspension.[86] The standard dosage is 50 mg/kg per day orally in two doses (maximum 3 g/day every 2 days; this dosage is likely to be toxic and may have to be decreased).[117] Pediatric dosages are same as adult dosages.[117]

Albendazole

Albendazole is an orally administered broad-spectrum anthelmintic with variable therapeutic efficacy. It is poorly absorbed from the gastrointestinal tract because of its low aqueous solubility, and it has a cure rate of 36% to 75%.[118,120] Maximal plasma concentrations of albendazole sulfoxide are achieved typically 2 to 5 hours after dosing.[86] The principal mode of action for albendazole is its inhibitory effect on tubulin polymerization, which results in the loss of cytoplasmic microtubules.[86] The standard dosage for adults (>60 kg) is 400 mg orally after meals twice a day for 3 days, 7 to 10 days for hyperinfection; for children (<60 kg), 15 mg/kg per day orally after meals in two doses for 3 days, 7 to 10 days for hyperinfection (maximum total daily dose 800 mg).[117]

For hyperinfection strongyloidiasis, the concurrent discontinuation or tapering of corticosteroids is necessary, as is appropriate antibiotic/antifungal treatment of the infections that usually accompany extraintestinal strongyloidiasis. Even with this regimen, more than two thirds of the patients with dissemination succumb to the disease.

PREVENTION AND CONTROL

Strategies for the control of strongyloidiasis in endemic areas are similar to those developed for the control of other geohelminthiases. Appropriate methods of human fecal sanitation and sewage disposal and the use of shoes are of paramount importance. For at-risk individuals, virtually all cases of fatal hyperinfection and dissemination could be prevented by suspecting, detecting, and treating chronic, well-regulated infections in patients who are candidates for immunosuppression, particularly from any form of corticosteroid therapy. Unexplained eosinophilia (see Chapter 125), prior—even remote—histories of potential exposures to contaminated soil in *Strongyloides* endemic regions, or compatible cutaneous or gastrointestinal symptoms, albeit often nonspecific, of chronic strongyloidiasis should prompt consideration of underlying strongyloidiasis prior to corticosteroid treatment.

The principal transmission mode of *S. stercoralis* is that of a geohelminthiasis, through the contamination of soil with infected feces. In ordinary hygienic conditions, human-to-human transmission does not appear to occur. Thus, the infection can be prevented by implementing public health measures aimed at ensuring proper disposal and treatment of excrement and by avoiding skin contact with contaminated soil. In institutional facilities caring for those with fecal incontinence or contamination (e.g., the mentally retarded), filariform *Strongyloides* larvae in feces can cause nosocomial or intrainstitutional spread of infection. The authors also recommend that strongyloidiasis be a reportable disease in areas of Europe and North America where autochthonous infections have been reported to ensure adequate treatment of infected patients and to maintain surveillance of the number of cases.

REFERENCES

1. Normand L: Sur la maladie dite diarrhée de la Cochinchine. (Extrait d'une lettre adressée à M. le President par le vice-admiral Jurien de la Gravière.) C R Hebdomadaires Seances Acad Sci 83:316–318, 1876.
2. Grassi GB: Sovra l'Anguillula intestinale. Rendiconti del Reale Istituto Lombardo di Scienze e Lettere 12:228–233, 1879.
3. Gage JG: A case of *Strongyloides intestinalis* with larvae in the sputum. Arch Intern Med 7:55–59, 1911.
4. Napier LE: *Strongyloides stercoralis* infection. J Trop Med Hyg 52:25–30, 1949.
5. Galliard H: Recherches sur l'infestation expérimentale à *Strongyloides stercoralis* au Tonkin. Ann Parasitol Hum Comp 25:441–473, 1951.
6. Galliard H: Les types de développement exogène de *Strongyloides stercoralis*: leur transformation par passages expérimentaux. C R Soc Biol 141:102–105, 1947.
7. Anderson RC: Nematode Parasites of Vertebrates: Their Development and Transmission, 2nd ed. Oxford and New York, CABI Publishing, 2000, pp 27–39.
8. Schad GA: Morphology and life history of *Strongyloides stercoralis*. In Grove DI (ed): Strongyloidiasis: A Major Roundworm Infection of Man. London, Taylor & Francis, 1989, pp 85–104.
9. Scowden EB, Schaffner W, Stone WJ: Overwhelming strongyloidiasis: An unappreciated opportunistic infection. Medicine (Baltimore) 57:527–544, 1978.
10. Genta RM: Immunobiology of strongyloidiasis. Trop Geogr Med 36:223–229, 1984.
11. Genta RM: Global prevalence of strongyloidiasis: Critical review with epidemiologic insights into the prevention of disseminated disease. Rev Infect Dis 11:755–767, 1989.
12. Taranto NJ, Bonomi de Filippi H, et al: Prevalence of *Strongyloides stercoralis* infection in childhood: Oran, Salta, Argentina. Bol Chil Parasitol 48:49–51, 1993.
13. Borda CE, Rea MJ, Rosa JR, et al: Intestinal parasitism in San Cayetano, Corrientes, Argentina. Bull Pan Am Health Organ 30:227–233, 1996.
14. Siddiqui AA, Genta RM, Berk SL: *Strongyloides stercoralis*. In Blaser MJ, Smith PD, Ravdin JI, et al (eds): Infections of the Gastrointestinal Tract, 2nd ed. Philadelphia, Lippincott Williams & Wilkins, 2002, pp 1113–1126.
15. Berk SL, Verghese A, Alvarez S, et al: Clinical and epidemiologic features of strongyloidiasis: a prospective study in rural Tennessee. Arch Intern Med 147:1257–1261, 1987.
16. Alcaraz CO, Adell RI, Sanchez PS, et al: Characteristics and geographical profile of strongyloidiasis in healthcare area 11 of the Valencian community (Spain). J Infect 49:152–158, 2004.
17. Kitchen LW, Tu KK, Kerns FT: *Strongyloides*-infected patients at Charleston area medical center, West Virginia, 1997–1998. Clin Infect Dis 31:E5–E6, 2000.
18. Nair D: Screening for *Strongyloides* infection among the institutionalized mentally disabled. Am Board Fam Pract 14:51–53, 2001.
19. Safdar A, Malathum K, Rodriguez SJ, et al: Strongyloidiasis in patients at a comprehensive cancer center in the United States. Cancer 100:1531–1536, 2004.
20. de Silva S, Saykao P, Kelly H, et al: Chronic *Strongyloides stercoralis* infection in Laotian immigrants and refugees 7–20 years after resettlement in Australia. Epidemiol Infect 128:439–444, 2002.
21. Genta RM: Dysregulation of strongyloidiasis: A new hypothesis. Clin Microbiol Rev 5:345–355, 1992.
22. Neva FA: Biology and immunology of human strongyloidiasis. J Infect Dis 153:397–406, 1986.
23. Igra-Siegman Y, Kapila R, Sen P, et al: Syndrome of hyperinfection with *Strongyloides stercoralis*. Rev Infect Dis 3:397–407, 1981.
24. Schad GA, Hellman ME, Muncey DW: *Strongyloides stercoralis*: hyperinfection in immunosuppressed dogs. Exp Parasitol 57:287–296, 1984.
25. Genta RM, Schad GA, Hellman ME: *Strongyloides stercoralis*: parasitological, immunological and pathological observations in immunosuppressed dogs. Trans R Soc Trop Med Hyg 80:34–41, 1986.
26. Mansfield LS, Niamatali S, Bhopale V, et al: *Strongyloides stercoralis*: Maintenance of exceedingly chronic infections. Am J Trop Med Hyg 55:617–624, 1996.
27. Schad GA, Aikens LM, Smith G: *Strongyloides stercoralis*: Is there a canonical migratory route through the host? J Parasitol 75:740–749, 1989.
28. Schad GA, Smith G, Megyeri Z, et al: *Strongyloides stercoralis*: An initial autoinfective burst amplifies primary infection. Am J Trop Med Hyg 48:716–725, 1993.
29. Berk SL, Verghese A: Parasitic pneumonia. Semin Respir Infect 3:172–178, 1988.
30. Gill GV, Beeching NJ, Khoo S, et al: A British Second World War veteran with disseminated strongyloidiasis. Trans R Soc Trop Med Hyg 98:382–386, 2004.
31. Chitwood DJ: Biochemistry and function of nematode steroids. Crit Rev Biochem Mol Biol 34:273–284, 1999.
32. Herbert DR, Nolan TJ, Schad GA, et al: The role of B cells in immunity against larval *Strongyloides stercoralis* in mice. Parasite Immunol 24:95–101, 2002.
33. Atkins NS, Conway DJ, Lindo JF, et al: L3 antigen-specific antibody isotype responses in human strongyloidiasis: Correlations with larval output. Parasite Immunol 21:517–526, 1999.
34. Kerepesi LA, Nolan TJ, Schad GA, et al: Human immunoglobulin G mediates protective immunity and identifies protective antigens against larval *Strongyloides stercoralis* in mice. J Infect Dis 189:1282–1290, 2004.
35. Siddiqui AA, Koenig NM, Sinensky M, et al: *Strongyloides stercoralis*: Identification of antigens in natural human infections from endemic areas of the United States. Parasitol Res 83:655–658, 1997.
36. Ashraf M, Gue CL, Baddour LM: Case report: Strongyloidiasis refractory to treatment with ivermectin. Am J Med Sci 311:178–179, 1996.
37. Plumelle Y, Gonin C, Edouard A, et al: Effect of *Strongyloides stercoralis* infection and eosinophilia on age at onset and prognosis of adult T-cell leukemia. Am J Clin Pathol 107:81–87, 1997.
38. Stephenson LS, Latham MC, Ottesen EA: Malnutrition and parasitic helminth infections. Parasitology 121:S23–S38, 2000.
39. Link K, Orenstein R: Bacterial complications of strongyloidiasis: *Streptococcus bovis* meningitis. South Med J 92:728–731, 1999.
40. Siddiqui AA, Stanley CS, Skelly PJ, et al: A cDNA encoding a nuclear hormone receptor of the steroid/thyroid hormone-receptor superfamily from the human parasitic nematode *Strongyloides stercoralis*. Parasitol Res 86:24–29, 2000.
41. Nolan TJ, Megyeri Z, Bhopale VM, et al: *Strongyloides stercoralis*: The first rodent model for uncomplicated and hyperinfective strongyloidiasis, the Mongolian gerbil (*Meriones unguiculatus*). J Infect Dis 168:1479–1484, 1993.
42. Grove DI, Warton A, Yu LL, et al: Light and electron microscopical studies of the location of *Strongyloides stercoralis* in the jejunum of the immunosuppressed dog. Int J Parasitol 17:1257–1265, 1987.
43. Kerlin RL, Nolan TJ, Schad GA: *Strongyloides stercoralis*: Histopathology of uncomplicated and hyperinfective strongyloidiasis in the Mongolian gerbil, a rodent model for human strongyloidiasis. Int J Parasitol 25:411–420, 1995.
44. De Paola D, Braga-Dias L, da Silva JR: Enteritis due to *Strongyloides stercoralis*. Am J Dig Dis 7:1086–1098, 1962.
45. Genta RM, Caymmi-Gomes M: Pathology. In Grove DI (ed): Strongyloidiasis: A Major Roundworm Infection of Man. London, Taylor & Francis, 1989, pp 105–132.
46. Kennedy S, Campbell RM, Lawrence JE, et al: A case of severe *Strongyloides stercoralis* infection with jejunal perforation in an Australian ex–prisoner-of-war. Med J Aust 150:92–93, 1989.
47. Carp NZ, Nejman JH, Kelly JJ: Strongyloidiasis: An unusual cause of colonic pseudopolyposis and gastrointestinal bleeding. Surg Endosc 1:175–177, 1987.
48. Al Samman M, Haque S, Long JD: Strongyloidiasis colitis: A case report and review of the literature. J Clin Gastroenterol 28:77–80, 1999.
49. Gutierrez Y, Bhatia P, Garbadawala ST, et al: *Strongyloides stercoralis* eosinophilic granulomatous enterocolitis. Am J Surg Pathol 20:603–612, 1996.
50. Nadler S, Cappell MS, Bhatt B, et al: Appendiceal infection by *Entamoeba histolytica* and *Strongyloides stercoralis* presenting like acute appendicitis. Dig Dis Sci 35:603–608, 1990.
51. Felekouras E, Kontos M, Kyriakou V, et al: *Strongyloides stercoralis* infection as a cause of acute granulomatous appendicitis in an HIV-positive patient in Athens, Greece. Scand J Infect Dis 34:856–857, 2002.
52. Kim J, Joo HS, Kim DH, et al: A case of gastric strongyloidiasis in a Korean patient. Korean J Parasitol 41:63–67, 2003.
53. Wurtz R, Mirot M, Fronda G, et al: Short report: Gastric infection by *Strongyloides stercoralis*. Am J Trop Med Hyg 51:339–340, 1994.

54. Lambroza A, Dannenberg AJ: Eosinophilic ascites due to hyperinfection with *Strongyloides stercoralis*. Am J Gastroenterol 86:89–91, 1991.
55. Lintermans JP: Fatal peritonitis, an unusual complication of *Strongyloides stercoralis* infestation. Clin Pediatr (Phila) 14:974–975, 1975.
56. Woodring JH, Halfhill H II, Reed JC: Pulmonary strongyloidiasis: Clinical and imaging features. Am J Roentgenol 162:537–542, 1994.
57. Moreira-Silva SF, Pereira FE: Intestinal nematodes, Toxocara infection, and pyogenic liver abscess in children: A possible association. J Trop Pediatr 46:167–172, 2000.
58. Lin AL, Kessimian N, Benditt JO: Restrictive pulmonary disease due to interlobular septal fibrosis associated with disseminated infection by *Strongyloides stercoralis*. Am J Respir Crit Care Med 151:205–209, 1995.
59. Liu LX, Weller PF: Strongyloidiasis and other intestinal nematode infections. Infect Dis Clin North Am 7:655–682, 1993.
60. Milder JE, Walzer PD, Kilgore G, et al: Clinical features of *Strongyloides stercoralis* infection in an endemic area of the United States. Gastroenterology 80:1481–1488, 1981.
61. Onile B, Komolafe F, Oladiran B: Severe strongyloidiasis presenting as occult gastrointestinal tract malignancy. Ann Trop Med Parasitol 79:301–304, 1985.
62. Dellacona S, Spier N, Wessely Z, et al: Massive colonic hemorrhage secondary to infection with *Strongyloides stercoralis*. NY State J Med 84:397–399, 1984.
63. Bhatt BD, Cappell MS, Smilow PC, et al: Recurrent massive upper gastrointestinal hemorrhage due to *Strongyloides stercoralis* infection. Am J Gastroenterol 85:1034–1036, 1990.
64. Alam SZ, Purohit D: A case report: Malabsorption secondary to *S. stercoralis* infestation. Med J Zambia 16:85, 1982.
65. Keiser PB, Nutman TB: *Strongyloides stercoralis* in the immunocompromised population. Clin Microbiol Rev 17:208–217, 2004.
66. Nonaka D, Takaki K, Tanaka M, et al: Paralytic ileus due to strongyloidiasis: Case report and review of the literature. Am J Trop Med Hyg 59:535–538, 1998.
67. Siddiqui AA, Berk SL: Diagnosis of *Strongyloides stercoralis* infection. Clin Infect Dis 33:1040–1047, 2001.
68. Grove DI: Human strongyloidiasis. Adv Parasitol 38:251–309, 1996.
69. Wehner JH, Kirsch CM: Pulmonary manifestations of strongyloidiasis. Semin Respir Infect 12:122–129, 1997.
70. Sen P, Gil C, Estrellas B, et al: Corticosteroid-induced asthma: A manifestation of limited hyperinfection syndrome due to *Strongyloides stercoralis*. South Med J 88:923–927, 1995.
71. Wehner JH, Kirsch CM, Kagawa FT, et al: The prevalence and response to therapy of *Strongyloides stercoralis* in patients with asthma from endemic areas. Chest 106:762–766, 1994.
72. Takayanagui OM, Lofrano MM, Araugo MB, et al: Detection of *Strongyloides stercoralis* in the cerebrospinal fluid of a patient with acquired immunodeficiency syndrome. Neurology 45:193–194, 1995.
73. Lowichik A, Ruff AJ: Parasitic infections of the central nervous system in children. 2. Disseminated infections. J Child Neurol 10:77–87, 1995.
74. Karolyi Z, Eros N, Kriston R: Cutaneous manifestations of strongyloidosis. Orv Hetil 140:191–194, 1999.
75. Amer M, Attia M, Ramadan AS, et al: Larva currens and systemic disease. Int J Dermatol 23:402–403, 1984.
76. von Kuster LC, Genta RM: Cutaneous manifestations of strongyloidiasis. Arch Dermatol 124:1826–1830, 1988.
77. Ly MN, Bethel SL, Usmani AS, et al: Cutaneous *Strongyloides stercoralis* infection: an unusual presentation. J Am Acad Dermatol 49:S157–S160, 2003.
78. Purvis RS, Beightler EL, Diven DG, et al: *Strongyloides* hyperinfection presenting with petechiae and purpura. Int J Dermatol 31:169–171, 1992.
79. Reddy TS, Myers JW: Syndrome of inappropriate secretion of antidiuretic hormone and nonpalpable purpura in a woman with *Strongyloides stercoralis* hyperinfection. Am J Med Sci 325:288–291, 2003.
80. Chaudhary K, Smith RJ, Himelright IM, et al: Case report: Purpura in disseminated strongyloidiasis. Am J Med Sci 308:186–191, 1994.
81. Brocq O, Breuil V, Agopian V, et al: Reactive arthritis induced by *Strongyloides stercoralis*. Rev Rhum Engl Ed 63:217–219, 1996.
82. Becquet R, Dutoit E, Poirriez J, et al: Cardiac form of anguillulosis. Presse Med 12:1366–1367, 1983.
83. Kane MG, Luby JP, Krejs GJ: Intestinal secretion as a cause of hypokalemia and cardiac arrest in a patient with strongyloidiasis. Dig Dis Sci 29:768–772, 1984.
84. Agbo K, Deniau M: Anguillospermia resistant to treatment: apropos of a case diagnosed in Togo. Bull Soc Pathol Exot 80:271–273, 1987.
85. Daoudal P, Ribier G, Numeric P, et al: Disseminated strongyloidiasis, a rare cause of multiple organ failure. Presse Med 31:1216–1217, 2002.
86. Siddiqui AA, Berk SL: Strongyloidiasis. Curr Treat Options Infect Dis 5:283–289, 2003.
87. Ferreira MS, Nishioka SA, Borges AS, et al: Strongyloidiasis and infection due to human immunodeficiency virus: 25 cases at a Brazilian teaching hospital, including seven cases of hyperinfection syndrome. Clin Infect Dis 28:144–155, 1999.
88. Fincham JE, Markus MB, Adams VJ: Could control of soil-transmitted helminthic infection influence the HIV/AIDS pandemic? Acta Trop 86:315–333, 2003.
89. Karp CL, Neva FA: Tropical infectious diseases in human immunodeficiency virus–infected patients. Clin Infect Dis 28:947–963, 1999.
90. Satoh M, Kiyuna S, Shiroma Y, et al: Predictive markers for development of strongyloidiasis in patients infected with both *Strongyloides stercoralis* and HTLV-1. Clin Exp Immunol 133:391–396, 2003.
91. Arakaki T, Kohakura M, Asato R, et al: Epidemiological aspects of *Strongyloides stercoralis* infection in Okinawa, Japan. J Trop Med Hyg 95:210–213, 1992.
92. Neva FA, Murphy EL, Gam A, et al: Antibodies to *Strongyloides stercoralis* in healthy Jamaican carriers of HTLV-1. N Engl J Med 320:252–253, 1989.
93. Courouble G, Rouet F, Herrmann-Storck C, et al: Epidemiologic study of the association between human T-cell lymphotropic virus type 1 and *Strongyloides stercoralis* infection in female blood donors (Guadeloupe, French West Indies). West Indian Med J 53:3–6, 2004.
94. Gabet AS, Mortreux F, Talarmin A, et al: High circulating proviral load with oligoclonal expansion of HTLV-1 bearing T cells in HTLV-1 carriers with strongyloidiasis. Oncogene 19:4954–4960, 2000.
95. Leung VK, Liew CT, Sung JJ: Strongyloidiasis in a patient with IgA deficiency. Trop Gastroenterol 16:27–30, 1995.
96. Ashraf M, Guc CL, Baddour LM: Case report: Strongyloidiasis refractory to treatment with ivermectin. Am J Med Sci 311:178–179, 1996.
97. Nielsen PB, Mojon M: Improved diagnosis of *Strongyloides stercoralis* by seven consecutive stool specimens. Zentralbl Mikrobiol 263:616–618, 1987.
98. de Kaminsky RG: Evaluation of three methods for laboratory diagnosis of *Strongyloides stercoralis* infection. J Parasitol 79:277–280, 1993.
99. Zaha O, Hirata T, Kinjo F, et al: Strongyloidiasis—progress in diagnosis and treatment. Intern Med 39:695–700, 2000.
100. Uparanukraw P, Phongsri S, Morakote N: Fluctuations of larval excretion in *Strongyloides stercoralis* infection. Am J Trop Med Hyg 60:967–973, 1999.
101. Magnaval JF, Mansuy JM, Villeneuve L, et al: A retrospective study of autochthonous strongyloidiasis in Region Midi-Pyrenees (Southwestern France). Eur J Epidemiol 16:179–182, 2000.
102. Goka AK, Rolston DD, Mathan VI, et al: Diagnosis of *Strongyloides* and hookworm infections: comparison of faecal and duodenal fluid microscopy. Trans R Soc Trop Med Hyg 84:829–831, 1990.
103. Penalba C, Deluol AM, Cenac J, et al: Value of the string test in the diagnosis of duodenal parasitosis. Bull Soc Pathol Exot Filiales 77:352–359, 1984.
104. Ansari TM, Couch L, Idell S: *Strongyloides*-induced lung disease. Emerg Med April: 127–136, 1997.
105. Gam AA, Neva FA, Krotoski WA: Comparative sensitivity and specificity of ELISA and IHA for serodiagnosis of strongyloidiasis with larval antigens. Am J Trop Med Hyg 37:157–161, 1987.
106. Sato Y, Toma H, Kiyuna S, et al: Gelatin particle indirect agglutination test for mass examination for strongyloidiasis. Trans R Soc Trop Med Hyg 85:515–518, 1991.
107. Neva FA: Biology and immunology of human strongyloidiasis. J Infect Dis 153:397–406, 1986.

108. Neva FA, Gam AA, Maxwell C: Skin test antigens for immediate hypersensitivity prepared from infective larvae of *Strongyloides stercoralis*. Am J Trop Med Hyg 65:567–572, 2001.
109. Lindo JF, Conway DJ, Atkins NS, et al: Prospective evaluation of enzyme-linked immunosorbent assay and immunoblot methods for the diagnosis of endemic *Strongyloides stercoralis* infection Am J Trop Med Hyg 51:175–179, 1994.
110. Sato Y, Kobayashi J, Shiroma Y: Serodiagnosis of strongyloidiasis: the application and significance. Rev Inst Med Trop Sao Paulo 37:35–41, 1995.
111. Conway DJ, Atkins NS, Lillywhite JE, et al: Immunodiagnosis of *Strongyloides stercoralis* infection: A method for increasing the specificity of the indirect ELISA. Trans R Soc Trop Med Hyg 87:173–176, 1993.
112. Datry A, Thellier M, Alfa-Cisse O, et al: Ivermectin, a broad spectrum antiparasitic drug. Presse Med 31:607–611, 2002.
113. Daubenton JD, Buys HA, Hartley PS: Disseminated strongyloidiasis in a child with lymphoblastic lymphoma. J Pediatr Hematol Oncol 20:260–263, 1998.
114. Adenusi AA: Cure by ivermectin of a chronic, persistent, intestinal strongyloidosis. Acta Trop 66:163–167, 1997.
115. Marti H, Haji HJ, Savioli L, et al: A comparative trial of a single-dose ivermectin versus three days of albendazole for treatment of *Strongyloides stercoralis* and other soil-transmitted helminth infections in children. Am J Trop Med Hyg 55:477–481, 1996.
116. Albonico M, Crompton DW, Savioli L: Control strategies for human intestinal nematode infections. Adv Parasitol 42:277–341, 1999.
117. Drugs for parasitic infections. Med Lett Drugs Ther 1–12, August 2004, www.medicalletter.org.
118. Salazar SA, Berk SH, Howe D, et al: Ivermectin vs thiabendazole in the treatment of strongyloidiasis. Infect Med January:50–59, 1994.
119. Tarr PE, Miele PS, Peregoy KS, et al: Case report: rectal administration of ivermectin to a patient with *Strongyloides* hyperinfection syndrome. Am J Trop Med Hyg 68:453–455, 2003.
120. Toma H, Sato Y, Shiroma Y, et al: Comparative studies on the efficacy of three anthelminthics on treatment of human strongyloidiasis in Okinawa, Japan. Southeast Asian J Trop Med Public Health 31:147–151, 2000.

112

Introduction to Tapeworm Infections

MURRAY WITTNER
A. CLINTON WHITE, Jr.
HERBERT B. TANOWITZ

Tapeworm infections are among the oldest recognized afflictions of humanity.[1,2] For example, recent phylogenetic studies[2] suggest that the ancestors of modern humans may have acquired taeniid tapeworm infections about 2 million years ago, from the animals they consumed, and eventually passed the infection on to bovine and porcine hosts about 10,000 years ago.

The Cestoda, or tapeworms, are a class in the phylum Platyhelminthes (flatworms) and except for the ciliated embryo of the order Pseudophyllidea are exclusively parasitic for their entire life.[3] In the adult stage, they live exclusively in the alimentary canal, including occasionally the bile ducts, gallbladder, and pancreatic duct. They infect members of all vertebrate classes although members of the subclass Cestodaria and several neotenic species attain adulthood in invertebrates (oligochaetes). However, cestode larvae often infect both vertebrates and invertebrates.

With few exceptions, the characteristic feature of adult tapeworms is their elongated (i.e., tapelike) dorsoventrally flattened structure. Their outer covering, or tegument, allows the passage of both nutritive and waste material. The absorptive surface of the tegument is amplified by the formation of many cytoplasmic extensions similar to microvilli of enterocytes. Numerous studies have shown that tapeworms actively take up and utilize carbohydrates from the intestinal lumen as their major, if not sole, energy source, with the production largely of lactate, proprionate, and succinate as end products. There is active uptake of α,DL amino acids across the tegumental membrane.[4] Diffusion appears to play a minor role.

Of the various orders of cestodes, there are two that include important parasites of humans and domestic and marine mammals. Their adult stage resides in the lumen of the small intestine and the larval stage in various tissues of the intermediate host. The order Pseudophyllidea is characterized by the presence of a scolex, or attachment organ, containing two sucking grooves. Examples of this group are members of the genus *Diphyllobothrium* and include *D. latum* (the broad or fish tapeworm), *D. pacificum,* and worms that infect humans only at the larval stage such as *Spirometra* (i.e., sparganosis). The order Cyclophyllidea, to which all other tapeworms that parasitize humans belong, is characterized by a scolex that possesses four suckers. This group includes those belonging to the genus *Taenia*, examples of which are the beef and pork tapeworms, *Hymenolepis, Bertiella, Dipylidium, Mesocestoides, Raillietina, Inermicapsifer,* and *Echinococcus*.

The life cycles of the Pseudophyllidea involve a minimum of three hosts. Those of the Cyclophyllidea generally require two, although in some species the definitive host can also serve as the intermediate host. Medically important tapeworms range in size from the minute dog tapeworm, *Echinococcus granulosus*, which generally consists of a scolex and three or four segments, to *Taenia saginata,* reported to reach 25 to 30 meters in length.

Adult tapeworms typically possess an anterior scolex or head that may be modified or adorned with structures or organelles that serve as organs for attachment to the small intestinal mucosa. In the Pseudophyllidea, the structures that function for attachment are termed bothria, which are two shallow sucking grooves whose gripping power is feeble.[5] Some species of Cyclophyllidea, in addition to having four sucking disks or acetabula, possess hooklets that encircle the top of the scolex or are mounted on a protrusion known as the rostellum (Fig. 112-1). In some species, such as *Hymenolepis,* the rostellum is protrusible. The distal portion of the scolex, termed the "neck," is an area of intense metabolic activity, which in most groups of tapeworms is the zone from which new segments or proglottids proliferate and form a chain of proglottids or strobila. Clinically, the scolex is highly significant since therapy is aimed at its destruction or elimination, inasmuch as failure to do so will result in regrowth of the entire tapeworm. Usually the most proximal proglottids are immature. They contain only the earliest rudiments of the organs that are present in the mature proglottids. Those further distal become mature proglottids and contain one set, and in some species two complete sets, of male and female sex organs, that is, they are hermaphroditic. The distal most segments are filled with eggs and are termed "gravid proglottids," which in cyclophyllidean cestodes the sex organs have atrophied, leaving the segment occupied largely by a uterus filled with eggs.[6]

Except for the coracidium, the tapeworm egg is the only stage that interacts with the external environment. For diagnostic purposes, eggs are characteristic. In members of the genus *Diphyllobothrium*, eggs are discharged through a muscular uterine pore and, therefore, they are regularly found in the feces. However, in many cyclophyllidean species, the gravid proglottids split and the eggs are released through rents in the proglottids. The eggs of other tapeworms, such as *Hymenolepis nana* and *H. dimunata* are found in the stool after disintegration of the gravid prognostics, whereas those of the beef tapeworm, *Taenia saginata*, are often not found in the stool because they are passed out within intact segments. In fact, a "Scotch tape" preparation, similar to that used for

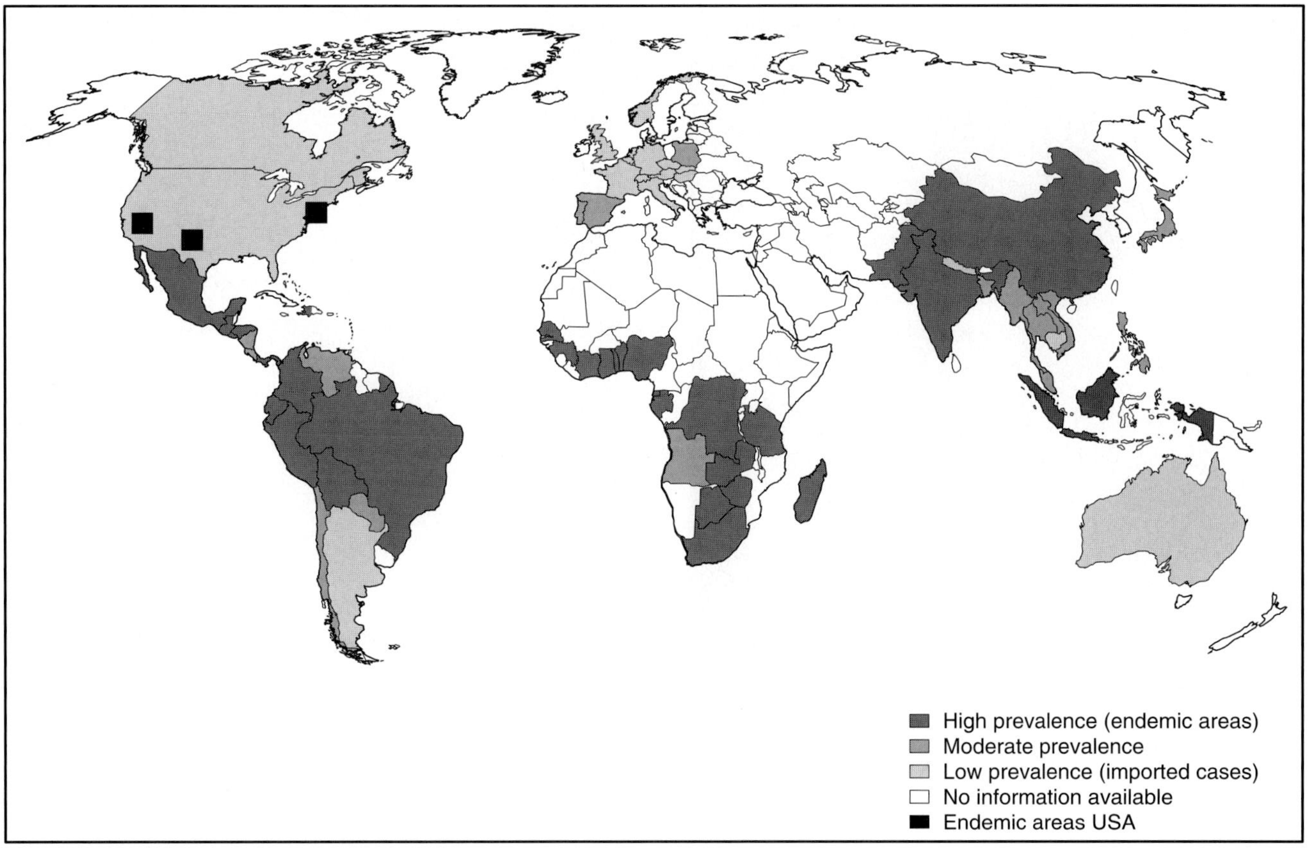

biopsies demonstrated that nearly all showed histopathologic evidence of cysticercosis.[24] For example, over half of 401 patients presenting with a single-enhancing lesion were diagnosed with NCC.[25] Neurocysticercosis is increasingly recognized in other parts of Asia including Indonesia, Southeast Asia, China, and Korea.[26]

DISEASES

The clinical presentation, pathogenesis, management, and prognosis of *T. solium* infections vary markedly depending on the location and number of cysticerci and the associated host response. Thus, neurocysticercosis should be regarded as a spectrum of illnesses rather than a single disease entity. NCC is typically separated into parenchymal and extraparenchymal disease based on whether or not there is involvement outside of the brain tissues. Extraparenchymal cases primarily include involvement of the subarachnoid space and ventricles. Pathologic studies show that many of the cysticerci found over the brain convexity are actually located in gyri, but clinically and radiologically the manifestations are indistinguishable from parenchymal cases. Extraparenchymal cases may also involve the spinal subarachnoid space, the spinal cord, or the eye. Many patients, particularly those with large numbers of parasites, will present with mixed forms. For example, most patients with subarachnoid NCC also have one or more parenchymal cysticerci.

Clinically, parenchymal neurocysticercosis usually presents with seizures and carries a favorable prognosis. Headache can also be a prominent feature. Most severe or fatal cases of NCC are due to extraparenchymal disease.[27,28] Subarachnoid and ventricular disease are often complicated by increased intracranial pressure and hydrocephalus. Thus, patients may present with symptoms of increased intracranial pressure (e.g., headache, dizziness, altered mental status, and visual changes due to papilledema). Extraparenchymal disease often requires surgical therapy and can be fatal if not managed properly. Most schemes also separate neurocysticercosis into inactive and active infection. Inactive disease does not have evidence of viable infection; disease is thought to result from the residua of prior infection. Active infection includes cases with both viable cysticerci and those with degenerating parasites. Some authors, however, propose separating degenerating (transitional) forms from viable cysticerci and using the term *active* for the latter.[29] Clinical cases are usually classified by neuroimaging studies.[29–31]

Parenchymal Neurocysticercosis

Inactive (Parenchymal Calcifications)

The characteristic of inactive neurocysticercosis on neuroimaging studies is parenchymal calcifications. The calcifications are typically 2 to 10 mm in diameter, well defined, and solid (Fig. 113-1). The calcified lesions are thought to represent

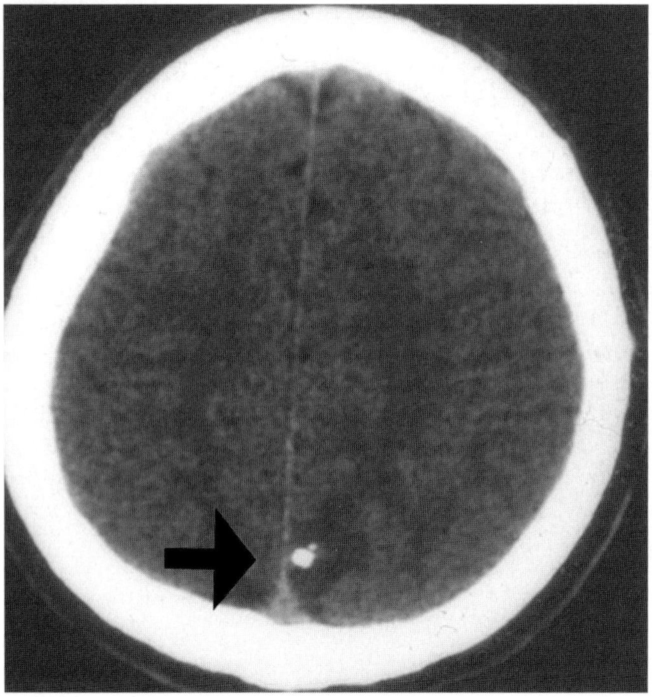

FIGURE 113-1 Calcified cysticercal lesion with surrounding edema revealed by CT scan (*arrow*).

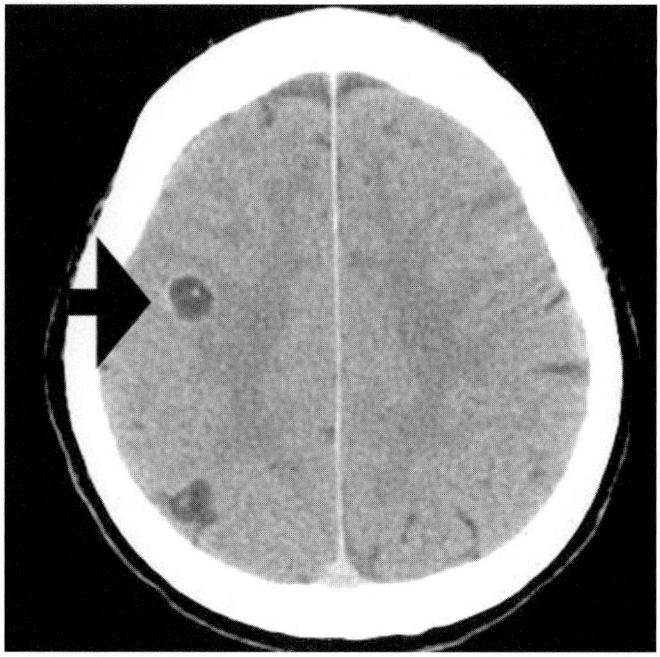

FIGURE 113-2 Parenchymal cysticercus revealed as a ring enhancing lesion (*arrow*).

fibrotic reactions to prior active infection that have calcified (calcific stage). Patients frequently present with seizures.[32] Few will have focal abnormalities on electroencephalogram (EEG) studies.[33,34] In hospital settings, patients with residual calcifications are more likely to have recurrence of seizures if antiepileptic drugs are withdrawn.[35,36] They usually should be treated with antiepileptic therapy indefinitely. Recent magnetic resonance imaging (MRI) studies have documented that some patients with NCC and seizures have calcified lesions with associated enhancement and edema.[37–40] There is no evidence that these lesions are associated with viable parasites. Instead, the enhancement may result from breakdown of the calcified granulomas with antigen release resulting in restimulation of host inflammation.[38]

Active

Active parenchymal infection is the most common form of NCC in nearly all case series. The vast majority of patients with symptomatic parenchymal NCC and seizures have neuroradiologic evidence of parasite degeneration and/or host inflammation such as edema or contrast enhancement (Fig. 113-2).[41,42] Symptoms are thought to result from the host inflammatory response, which will eventually subside. By contrast, noninflamed cysts cause few symptoms, even when they are numerous.[43] Thus, symptomatic infection likely occurs when one or more cysticerci can no longer control the host inflammatory and immune responses.

Seizures are the main clinical manifestation of parenchymal infection.[44,45] The seizures are often generalized or focal with secondary generalization, but may also be focal.[33,44–46] EEG studies for patients with active disease may reveal focal abnormalities, particularly in those with single inflamed cysticerci.[33,34] Seizures associated with active parenchymal cysts are likely caused by active parenchymal inflammation. Seizures can usually be controlled during treatment with antiepileptic drugs and often resolve after normalization of imaging studies as the inflammation subsides.[45,46] Relapse is, however, frequent.

Some patients present with large numbers of inflamed cysticerci, with diffuse cerebral edema, raised intracranial pressure, seizures, and altered mental status. This is termed *cysticercal encephalitis*.[47,48] This form is more common in children than adults and more common in women than men. Treatment is mainly directed at controlling the cerebral edema.

Extraparenchymal Neurocysticercosis

Ventricular NCC

In recent series, 10% to 20% of patients with NCC had cysticerci in the ventricles.[31,42] These cysticerci can obstruct cerebrospinal fluid (CSF) flow causing hydrocephalus. The cysticerci are found in any of the ventricles. Older series noted most of the ventricular cysticerci in the 4th ventricle, but this may have reflected more severe disease when the cysticerci are in that location. In most cases, the cysticerci cause symptoms while still viable.[49] Since viable cysticerci have thin walls with cyst fluid isodense with CSF, they may be difficult to detect. CT scanning usually only shows evidence of obstructive hydrocephalus or distortion of the shapes of the involved ventricle. Intraventricular cysticerci are frequently visible on MRI (Fig. 113-3).[50,51] However, the findings are subtle and can be missed by inexperienced observers. These patients may also have parenchymal cysticerci.

Patients with ventricular neurocysticercosis present with symptoms or signs of raised intracranial pressure. Symptoms may include nausea or vomiting, altered mental status, visual

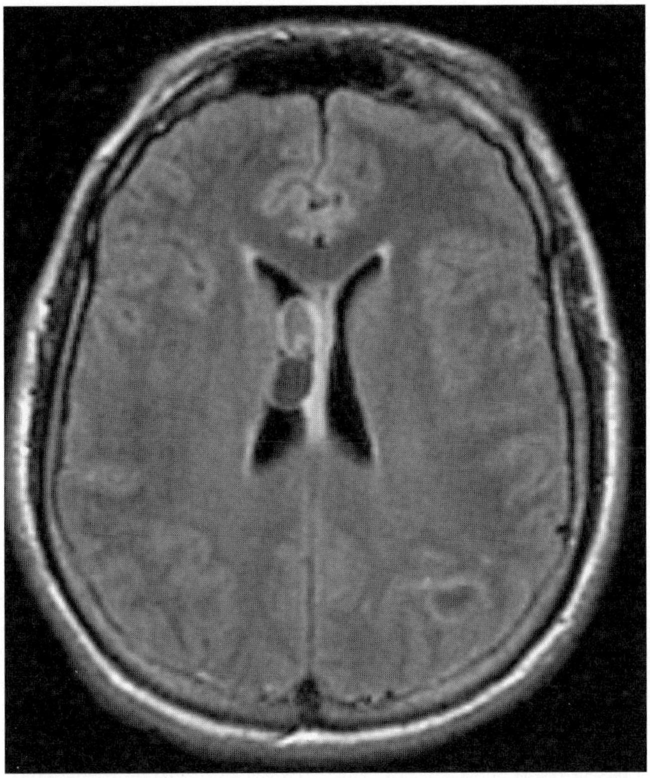

FIGURE 113-3 Two cysticerci in the lateral ventricle revealed by MRI.

changes, or dizziness. The onset varies and can be abrupt (due to acute obstruction), intermittent, or gradual. Cysticerci may form a ball valve in the foramina that may come and go with position changes. Cysticerci in the 4th ventricle have been associated with acute obstructive hydrocephalus that can lead to drop attacks.

Active Subarachnoid NCC

When patients have cysticerci in the gyri of the cerebral convexities, the radiological appearance, clinical presentation, and pathogenesis overlap with active parenchymal NCC. However, the cysts may be slightly larger and resolution is less frequent after antiparasitic chemotherapy.

Cysticerci in the fissures (especially the Sylvian fissure) can enlarge to several centimeters in diameter, termed *giant cysticerci*.[52] Isolated cysticerci in the fissures carry a similar prognosis to parenchymal cysts with symptoms resulting from parenchymal inflammation. In some cases, however, the cysts may enlarge causing mass effects such as midline shift. Frequently, giant cysticerci are accompanied by cysticerci in the parenchyma or basilar cisterns. The giant cysticerci are readily visualized by CT or MRI, but the accompanying basilar cysticerci may not be seen as easily. Cysticercosis of the basilar cisterns carries a grave prognosis. Numerous cysticerci may fill the basilar cisterns (Fig. 113-4). Patients with numerous cysticerci in the basilar cisterns can present with communicating hydrocephalus due to CSF outflow obstruction or arachnoiditis. Basilar arachnoiditis appears on imaging studies as focal or diffuse meningeal enhancement or vasculitis and can be complicated by strokes due to vasculitis.[53,54]

Inactive Extraparenchymal Neurocysticercosis

Inactive infection may also present with hydrocephalus in patients with prior arachnoiditis or granular ependimytis. The resulting obstruction of CSF flow (e.g., aqueductal stenosis) or CSF outflow obstruction can cause symptoms of hydrocephalus.

Spinal NCC

Only about 1% of patients with NCC have recognized spinal involvement.[31,42] Most cases of spinal NCC result from cysticerci in the subarachnoid space.[27] Initially, spinal subarachnoid cysticerci are free-floating, and they may move between levels. When the cysticerci degenerate, they eventually become fixed at one level. The accompanying inflammation may cause mass effect with obstruction of flow on myelogram. The clinical manifestations include radicular paresthesias or pain, which may progress to myelopathy with bowel or bladder incontinence and paraparesis. Cysticerci are rarely intramedullary, with cord compression from mass effect or accompanying inflammations.

Other Forms of Cysticercosis

Cysticercosis can involve the orbit and/or eye. The most common presentation is ptosis related to involvement of the extra-ocular muscles.[55,56] Ocular involvement is usually subretinal, but can be intravitreal or subconjunctival (Fig. 113-5).[56–59] Patients may present with altered vision. Subconjunctival cysts may spontaneously extrude. Intra-ocular disease usually requires surgical removal.

Cysticerci may involve the muscles. Only rarely do they cause more than minor symptoms. Soft tissue calcifications are frequently found in all forms of cysticercosis. Cysticerci can involve the subcutaneous tissues, where they present as a palpable, painless, and mobile cystic lesions that can be confused with sebaceous cysts. As the cysticerci degenerate, the lesions may become firm nodules or later resolve. Subcutaneous disease

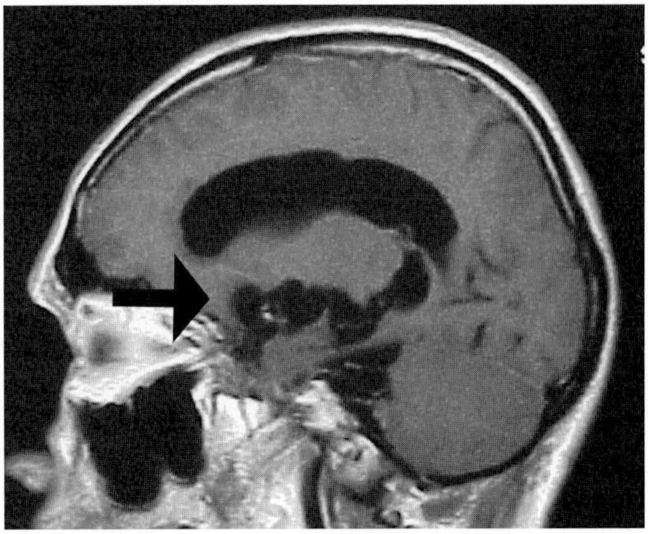

FIGURE 113-4 Cysticerci in the subarachnoid space of the basilar cisterns revealed by MRI.

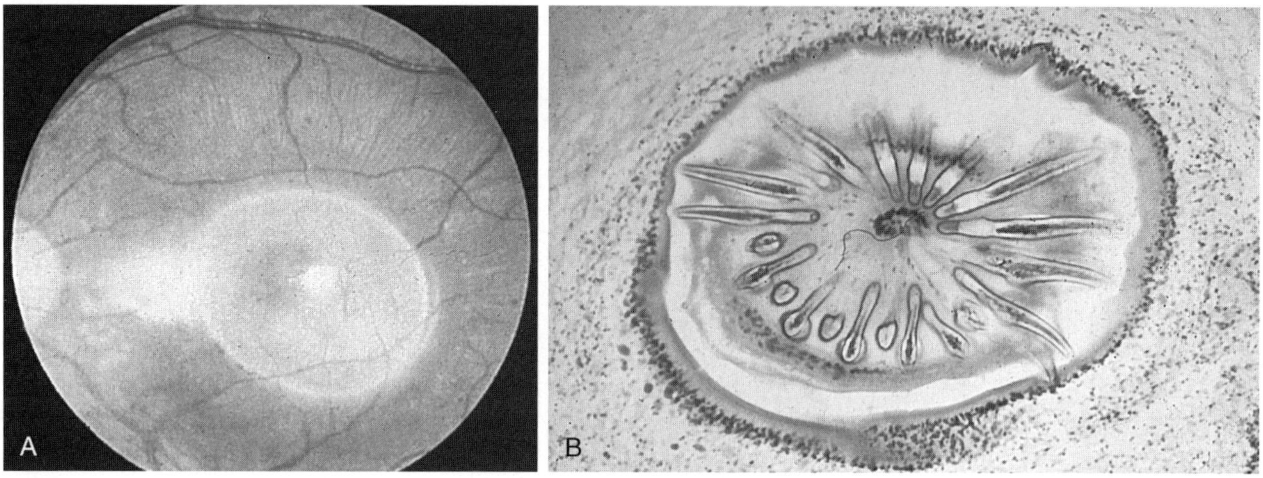

FIGURE 113-5 *A*, Subretinal cysticercosis at the macular area with overlying retinal edema. *B*, Cysticercosis of the eye. (*A*, Courtesy of Robert Ritch, MD, New York Eye and Ear Infirmary, New York, NY. From Teekhasaenee C, Ritch R, Kanchanaranya C: Ocular parasitic infection in Thailand. Rev Infect Dis 8:350–356, 1986.)

is rarely noted in the Western Hemisphere, but is commonly noted in Asia.

Mixed Forms

Clinical cases, especially those involving large numbers of cysticerci, often include more than one of the preceding forms. The pathogenesis and presentation may reflect each location. For example, patients who present with seizures will usually have parenchymal cysticerci. However, some also have cysticerci in the basilar cisterns that can progress to hydrocephalus later if not properly managed.

Other Syndromes

Headaches are common among patients with NCC and may be seen with parenchymal, ventricular, or cisternal NCC. Headaches may be hemicranial or bilateral.[60,61] The headaches can be confused with uncomplicated migraines or tension headaches. The pathogenesis is also variable. In some cases, headache is the initial symptoms of raised intracranial pressure. The association of parenchymal NCC with migraine-like headaches suggests vascular involvement.[60]

Neurocognitive defects have been described with cysticercosis.[62] Infected children are thought to suffer from learning disabilities.[63] There also appears to be an association of cysticercosis with depression and occasionally psychotic episodes.[64] By contrast, acute alterations of mental status usually reflect ongoing seizures or hydrocephalus. In our experience, altered mental status that does not resolve after a reasonable postictal period usually results from hydrocephalus.

PATHOGENESIS AND IMMUNITY

Cysticerci reach their final size within a few weeks of invasion into the central nervous system (CNS). However, there is a period of several years between infection and onset of symptoms.[20,65] In autopsy studies of individuals who died of other causes, cysticerci, when present, have an appearance similar to the viable cysticerci from pigs.[66] By contrast, cysticerci from patients who died with seizures demonstrate a prominent inflammatory infiltrate. The parasites elaborate a number of molecules that modulate or suppress the host inflammatory and immune response.[67] For example, parasite excretory proteases cleave CD4 from the surface of host lymphocytes, degrading immunoglobulin and cytokines such as interleukin (IL)-2.[68] Parasites also produce prostaglandins that modulate the host response.[69] Parasite secretory protease inhibitors block complement activation and decrease cytokine production and leukocyte chemotaxis.[70–72]

By contrast, an animal model has demonstrated that the seizures are induced by the host granulomatous response rather than the parasite per se.[73] Clinical studies suggest that after months to years, the cysticerci lose their ability to control the host response and are attacked by host inflammatory cells composed of mononuclear cells, with variable numbers of eosinophils and neutrophils.[74,75] The tissues pass through a series of stages of inflammation.[76,77] These cells elaborate type 1 cytokines such as IL-12, interferon gamma, and IL-2 as well as variable amounts of type 2 cytokines (e.g., IL-4 and IL-5).[74,75,78] Proinflammatory cytokines such as IL-1, tumour necrosis factor (TNF)-α, and IL-6 are also found in the spinal fluid from active cases.[79,80] The wall gradually degenerates, the cyst fluid increases in density and agglutinates, and the cyst cavity is invaded by inflammatory cells (colloid stage). The cysticercus subsequently is encased by fibrosis with collapse of the cyst cavity (granular-nodular stage). The fibrotic granuloma may calcify (calcified stage). Even the calcified lesions can be associated with inflammation. Interestingly, parts of the degenerating cysticercus (e.g., hooklets) may still be identified in the calcified lesion.

Imaging Findings

Similar steps in progression have been noted on neuroimaging studies.[81,82] Invasion of the central nervous system and early cysticercal development may cause focal edema or enhancement. Viable cysticerci reveal the cyst cavity as an area of decreased density, isodense with cerebrospinal fluid. The scolex may be seen as a mural nodule. The cyst wall is thin and isodense with brain parenchyma, lacks surrounding edema or contrast enhancement, and is usually not identifiable. When the cysticercus becomes inflamed, the cyst wall density increases. The cyst wall may enhance with contrast and there may be associated edema and/or enhancement in the surrounding brain parenchyma (see Fig. 113-2). Subsequently, the cyst fluid increases in density. As the cysticercus becomes fibrotic or collapses, neuroimaging studies reveal an area of focal enhancement, suggestive of a granuloma. Finally, the calcified stage is defined by focal areas of calcification. The calcifications are well demarcated, typically several millimeters in diameter. Edema and contrast enhancement often surround calcified lesions associated with symptoms (see Fig. 113-1).[37,83] Breakdown of the calcified granulomas is thought to trigger the host inflammation.

Cysticerci within the cerebral ventricles initially float in the ventricular fluid (see Fig. 113-3). They can become lodged particularly in the foramina and cause mechanical obstruction of CSF flow.[84] This type of obstruction is usually due to viable cysticerci.[49] Ependymitis and accompanying astrocytosis are associated with inflamed cysticerci or parasite remnants. The inflammation may cause the cysticerci to adhere to the ventricular walls or the inflammation may block CSF flow directly (especially in the Aqueduct of Sylvia).

Cysticerci in the basilar cisterns are associated with subarachnoid cysticercosis (see Fig. 113-4). Some of these cysticerci may enlarge to sizes up to 10 cm in diameter. These cysticerci may form clusters and without a scolex have been termed *racemose*. In fact, many of the so-called racemose cysticerci actually contain remnants of a scolex.

Subarachnoid NCC is usually accompanied by a prominent basilar arachnoiditis causing meningeal signs, communicating hydrocephalus, and/or vasculitis.[54] Hydrocephalus is thought to result from CSF outflow obstruction or blocked ventricular outflow.[84] Arachnoiditis often results in vasculitis, which may present as lacunar infarctions or, occasionally, as large vessel strokes.[53,85]

Cysticerci within the brain parenchyma typically reach a diameter of 1 to 2 cm. By contrast, cysticerci within the subarachnoid space (and particularly those in the Sylvian fissure) may expand to sizes up to 10 cm in diameter. These enlarged cysticerci may cause mass effects.[52,86,87] The mass effects are especially prominent when the cysticerci are inflamed either from spontaneous degeneration or after drug treatment.

DIAGNOSIS

Diagnosis of neurocysticercosis is problematic. The main clinical presentations (e.g., seizures or hydrocephalus) are shared with a wide spectrum of other diseases. Furthermore, the location of the parasites within the central nervous system limits the usefulness of traditional parasitologic studies. Older serologic tests were limited by poor sensitivity and specificity. Immunoblot assays, with good specificity, are not widely available. Computerized neuroimaging studies (e.g., CT and MRI) have led to a dramatic increase in case identification. However, these techniques are expensive, not readily available to populations at highest risk, and may not be diagnostic.

Despite these drawbacks, neuroimaging studies are the mainstay of diagnosis.[88] CT scanning is more sensitive than MRI at detecting calcifications and is usually used initially.[51,89] MRI is better at detecting cysticerci in the ventricles and subarachnoid space.[50,51,90,91] MRI may also reveal the scolex, which is usually not visible on CT scans.[90] Either method is adequate for imaging intraparenchymal cysticerci or hydrocephalus.

Parenchymal cystic lesions are the most common neuroradiographic manifestation of neurocysticercosis.[4,51,88,92] The number of cysticerci varies from one to several thousand. In India and the United States, the majority of cases of parenchymal NCC have only a single degenerating cyst.[4,41] By contrast, most studies from Latin America reveal multiple parasites. Whether this is due to biological differences or biases in which patients are scanned is controversial. On CT or MRI, parenchymal cysticerci appear as round cystic lesions, typically 4 to 20 mm in diameter. They are usually found in the cerebral cortex or the basal ganglia.[93] Cysts in the fissures are often larger, with a diameter of up to 10 cm. They may be either round or lobulated. For viable cysticerci, the cyst fluid is isodense with CSF. The cyst wall is thin (<1 mm thick) and is usually not visible. When identified, the scolex is a round or tubular nodule, 1 to 3 mm long on one side of the cyst wall. The presence of cystic lesions with a mural nodule is considered pathognomonic for cysticercosis, though this has never been rigorously tested.[51,89] The wall of the inflamed cyst wall is denser and may enhance with contrast (ring enhancement). The cyst fluid or surrounding tissues may also enhance. There is often edema surrounding the cysticercus, especially on T2-weighted MRI scans. Later stage cysticerci appear as focal areas of enhancement or granulomas.

Parenchymal brain calcifications are also a common CT finding in neurocysticercosis. The calcifications tend to be solid, dense, supratentorial, and 2 to 10 mm in diameter. In the absence of evidence of other illnesses, calcifications should be considered as highly suggestive of NCC. MRI scans often reveal surrounding edema and/or contrast enhancement in symptomatic cases. The latter may be associated with a residual scolex on gradient refocused echo images.[38,94]

Cysticerci in the ventricles are often poorly visualized by CT.[50,90] Most are viable cysts, with cyst fluid isodense with the cerebrospinal fluid and thin walls. The presence of ventricular cysticerci can often be inferred from distortion of the ventricular shape or the presence of obstructive hydrocephalus.[50,90] In contrast to CT, the increased resolution of MRI frequently allows visualization of the cyst walls and scolex.

Even though imaging studies detect most cases of neurocysticercosis, the appearance is not usually pathognomonic. Del Brutto and colleagues proposed diagnostic criteria based on neuroimaging studies, serologic tests, clinical history, and exposure.[95] Patients with either an absolute criterion or two major criteria alone with two minor or epidemiologic criteria were considered to have a definite diagnosis. One major criterion plus and two other criteria or three minor criteria plus exposure were considered to establish a probable diagnosis (Box 113-1).

Absolute diagnostic criteria for NCC include identification of the parasite by visualization or histology or pathognomonic neuroimaging results.[95] Traditionally, parasitologic diagnoses have depended on demonstration of the infecting parasite, but biopsy or autopsy material demonstrating *T. solium*

Box 113-1 Diagnostic Criteria for Neurocysticercosis

Absolute Criteria

Histologic demonstration of the parasite from biopsy of a brain or spinal cord lesion

Cystic lesions showing the scolex on CT of MRI

Direct visualization of subretinal parasites by fundoscopic examination

Major Criteria

Lesions highly suggestive of neurocysticercosis on neuroimaging studies

Positive serum immunoblot for the detection of anticysticercal antibodies

Resolution of intracranial cystic lesions after therapy with albendazole or praziquantal

Spontaneous resolution of small single enhancing lesions

Minor Criteria

Lesions compatible with neurocysticercosis on neuroimaging studies

Clinical manifestations suggestive of neurocysticercosis

Positive CSF ELISA for detection of anticercal antibodies or cysticercal antigens

Cysticercosis outsdie the central nervous system

Epidemiologic criteria

Evidence of a household contact with *T. solium* infection

History of frequent travel to disease-endemic areas

Individuals coming from or living in an area where cysticercosis is endemic

One major criterion and two other criteria or three minor criteria plus exposure were considered to establish a probable diagnosis.

From Del Brutto OH, Rajshekhar V, White AC Jr, et al: Proposed diagnostic criteria for neurocysticercosis. Neurology 57:177–183, 2001.

parasites are only available in a minority of cases. Parasites can occasionally be visualized directly in the eye. Neuroimaging studies revealing a cystic lesion with an associated scolex (demonstrated as a 1–3 mm mural nodule) are thought to be pathognomonic for cysticercosis.[51,89]

Neuroimaging studies highly suggestive of NCC were considered a major diagnostic criteria. These included cystic lesions, single or multiple ringlike or nodular enhancing lesions, and typical parenchymal brain calcifications. Ring or nodular enhancing lesions are also highly suggestive of neurocysticercosis, but tuberculomas, brain abscesses, and tumors can cause similar lesions. Cysticercal lesions are usually smaller than 20 mm in diameter and rarely cause midline shift.[25]

Rajshekhar and colleagues developed clinical and radiologic critieria for cysticercosis among patients who presented with seizures and single enhancing lesions.[25] The combination of a single, round, enhancing lesion, less than 20 mm in diameter, with no midline shift, in patients without increased intracranial pressure, focal neurologic deficits, or evidence of systemic disease was highly suggestive of NCC. These criteria were prospectively studied in 400 patients in India with a high sensitivity and specificity.[25] Resolution of the lesion spontaneously or after anticysticercal therapy or precipitation of symptoms by antiparasitic drugs are also supportive of the diagnosis.[96] All of these are major diagnostic criteria.[95]

Serodiagnosis is helpful in many parasitic diseases, but has proven problematic in the diagnosis of cysticercosis due to cross-reactions to other parasites and nonspecific binding. In general, assays employing unfractionated antigen have poor sensitivity and specificity.[97,98] The enzyme-linked immunotransfer blot (EITB) is an immunoblot assay employing semipurified membrane antigens.[99] Binding to any one of seven bands is considered positive. Studies have confirmed nearly 100% specificity, but the sensitivity is limited in subjects with either a single lesion or with only calcified lesions.[11,98,100,101] Interestingly, performance data suggests that the predictive value of the EITB assay for neurocysticercosis is better with serum than with CSF.[100] Other serologic tests are less accurate and are not considered major diagnostic criteria. Assays to detect parasite antigens may prove to be an important diagnostic tool.[102–107] Currently, a number of different antigen detection tests are being developed.

Minor criteria include: (1) lesions on neuroimaging studies that might be NCC, but are less suggestive (e.g., isolated basilar meningitis, hydrocephalus, or filling defects in the spinal subarachnoid space without discrete cysticerci); (2) symptoms suggestive of NCC (e.g., seizures or hydrocephalus); and (3) serologic tests for cysticercosis other than the EITB, and cysticercosis outside the nervous system (e.g., cigar-shaped muscle calcifications or subcutaneous nodules). Epidemiologic criteria include residence or prolonged visits to endemic areas or contact with a tapeworm carrier.

TREATMENT AND PROGNOSIS

Antiepileptic therapy, antiparasitic drugs, anti-inflammatory drugs, and surgical therapy are all important in the management of some neurocysticercosis patients. A key to management is that therapy should be individualized based on the pathogenesis of different forms of disease.

Symptomatic Therapy

Symptomatic therapy plays a key role in the management of NCC. Most fatalities are associated with failure to provide effective therapy for complications such as raised intracranial pressure or seizures. The key component in treatment of seizures should be effective antiepileptic drugs. Most seizures can be controlled with any of a number of antiepileptic drugs. A single first-line antiepileptic drug such as phenytoin or carbamazepime can successfully control seizures in most patients.[33,45,108] Breakthrough seizures often reflect poor adherence, subtherapeutic drugs levels, or coexisting conditions (e.g., alcohol abuse).[46] Among patients in whom neuroimaging studies normalize and seizures are controlled, antiepileptic treatment may eventually be tapered,[33,44–46] although seizures may recur in 20% to 40% of patients. In some studies, the presence of residual calcifications is a marker for high risk of recurrent seizures and is thought to be an indication for continuous antiepileptic.[35]

Hydrocephalus is primarily treated surgically. Obstructive hydrocephalus should be treated acutely by CSF diversion procedures such as ventriculoperitoneal shunting.[49] In the past, there was a high rate of shunt failure, in part due to aspiration of the cysticerci into the shunt. Recent studies have demonstrated that antiparasitic drugs and/or treatment with corticosteroids decreases the rate of shunt failure.[42,49,109–112]

Corticosteroids

Corticosteroids are used in neurocysticercosis to control inflammation and are a key component of therapy for severe forms of NCC, including cysticercal encephalitis, subarachnoid neurocysticercosis, and spinal intramedullary cysticercosis. For patients with NCC in the subarachnoid space, meningitis, vasculitis with stroke, and communicating hydrocephalus can result from the host inflammatory response and accompanying arachnoiditis. Corticosteroid therapy is an essential component in these cases. There are few data available on the optimal dose or duration of therapy. For severe disease, high doses (e.g., 1 mg/kg/d of prednisone or 0.5 mg/kg/d of dexamethasone) are often used initially. Lower doses have been used along with antiparasitic drugs to ameliorate the inflammatory reaction to the dying parasite. One randomized trial suggested that treatment with a short course of prednisolone (1 mg/kg/d for 10 days) led to a marked reduction in seizures and more rapid resolution in patients with single enhancing lesions.[113]

Antiparasitic Drugs

The role of antiparasitic drugs in the treatment of NCC has been controversial. Before CT and MRI scanning were available, the spectrum of cases diagnosed was weighted toward more severe disease. The development and dissemination of CT and MRI led to diagnosis of milder cases. Praziquantel and later albendazole were recognized as antiparasitic agents that could kill the parasites. In Latin America, initial uncontrolled trials of antiparasitic drugs were associated with resolution of neuroimaging abnormalities and improved prognosis, which was attributed to antiparasitic drug therapy.[114] In the United States, neuroimaging studies were available before antiparasitic drugs became available, and clinicians recognized that many cases (especially patients with single enhancing lesions) resolved spontaneously without antiparasitic therapy.[81,108] When antiparasitic drugs became available, reports noted worsening symptoms with treatment.[115] The first randomized, controlled trials were published in the 1990s and consensus on optimal management is only now emerging.[116]

Praziquantel was the first antiparasitic drug reported effective in neurocysticercosis. Praziquantel is absorbed well after oral administration, but has extensive first-pass metabolism, which is augmented by antiepileptic drugs (carbemazepine, phenytoin, and probably phenobarbital) as well as by corticosteroids.[117,118] This induction can be inhibited by cimetidine (e.g., 400 mg PO tid). Coadministration increases levels of praziquantel, but the effect of the increased drug levels on efficacy are unproven.[119–122] Initial dose ranging studies demonstrated greater effect at doses greater than or equal to 50 mg/kg/d in 3 daily doses for 14 days. Subsequent studies demonstrated that doses as high as 100 mg/kg/d could be given safely.[123] Studies with praziquantel in parenchymal NCC given in 3 doses of 25 mg/kg separated by only 2 hours along with cimetidine suggest similar efficacy with longer courses of therapy.[122,124,125] Adverse effects including worsening neurologic function (e.g., headaches, dizziness, seizures, increased intracranial pressure) are due to the host inflammatory response to the dying parasite. Some observers recommended use of corticosteroids along with antiparasitic drugs to decrease side effects,[115] but routine use of corticosteroids could potentially decrease efficacy of praziquantel by affecting serum levels.

Albendazole is a benzimidazole anthelminthic agent with broad-spectrum activity. Albendazole is usually used at doses of 15 mg/kg/d in 2 daily doses. Side effects include mild gastrointestinal problems and inflammatory responses to the parasites. Imaging studies demonstrated resolution of parenchymal cysticerci as good or better than those noted with praziquantel.[126,127] Controlled trials in parenchymal NCC showed no difference in neuroradiologic resolution with treatment for 7 days versus longer courses.[127–129] Albendazole was subsequently studied in cases of extraparenchymal disease and was associated with improvement.[52,109,112,130–132] However, none of these trials were controlled, due to concerns about disease progression.

Seven well-controlled studies of antiparasitic drugs have been performed in different forms of parenchymal neurocysticercosis.[46,133–138] Overall, the studies demonstrate that patients with parenchymal NCC have a more rapid radiologic response when treated with antiparasitic drugs both in cystic lesions as well as in degenerative (enhancing) lesions.

Active Parenchymal NCC with Cystic Lesions

In parenchymal cystic NCC, the clinical response is generally favorable. A recent randomized trial compared albendazole plus corticosteroids to symptomatic therapy alone and found fewer seizures in the treatment group, although the proportions of patients with at least one seizure relapse were similar.[38] While imaging studies will eventually normalize with or without antiparasitic drugs, Garcia and colleagues clearly demonstrated that spontaneous resolution of the cystic lesions was prolonged (>6 months) unless patients were treated with antiparasitic drugs.[108,133–137]

Patients present with seizures at the time of inflammation around the cyst. Thus, seizures tend to cluster in the initial weeks or months.[45,46] On the other hand, seizures are more common while there is residual parasite material present[45,46] and most studies demonstrate more rapid normalization with antiparasitic therapy.[46,134] The prognosis is thought to be worse when there are multiple lesions.[116,133] The resolution of viable and inflamed parasites may not be synchronized. Thus, most experts now argue that antiparasitic drugs improve the outcome in those with viable cysticerci and in those with multiple lesions.[43,46,116,133]

Active Parenchymal NCC with Only Enhancing Lesions

In parenchymal NCC with only enhancing lesions, the clinical response is generally favorable with or without antiparasitic therapy. Recent trials comparing albendazole plus corticosteroids[138] or just prednisolone[113] to symptomatic therapy alone in patients with single enhancing lesions demonstrated more rapid radiographic resolution and fewer seizures in follow-up in the treatment group. While there is no consensus, most experts agree that the prognosis for patients with single inflamed lesions is quite favorable with only symptomatic therapy.[108,116,133,139] However, there may be some clinical benefit of a short course of corticosteroids with or without albendazole.[113,138]

In cases with numerous inflamed lesions with associated diffuse cerebral edema (cysticercal encephalitis), antiparasitic drugs are contraindicated.[116] Instead, treatment should focus on management of cerebral edema with high-dose corticosteroids (e.g., dexamethasone).

Inactive Parenchymal NCC

Antiparasitic drugs are not recommended in inactive infection, since there are no signs of viable parasites. Patients with inactive parenchymal NCC typically present with seizures. Seizures are clustered near the time of diagnosis, but they reoccur years later.[35,44,45] Thus, these patients require chronic antiepileptic therapy. If patients maintain therapeutic levels of the drugs, the risk of recurrent seizures is very low.[33] On imaging studies, some patients will show contrast enhancement or edema around established calcified lesions.[37–39] Whether or not these patients would benefit from anti-inflammatory treatment is unclear.

Ventricular NCC

Some patients have hydrocephalus related to scarring from prior infection (e.g., aqueductal stenosis).[86] In this case, hydrocephalus can be corrected by ventriculoperitoneal shunting without the need for antiparasitic drugs. Patients with active ventricular neurocysticercosis usually present with obstructive hydrocephalus. Initial management should focus on relieving intracranial hypertension, reversing hydrocephalus, reducing the risk for recurrence, and minimizing treatment-associated morbidity.[140] In the past, removal of the cysticercus from the ventricle via an open craniotomy was the main approach. Since open brain surgery is associated with significant morbidity, alternative approaches have been tried. Recent studies have demonstrated that cysticerci can usually be removed by endoscopic surgery. When feasible, endoscopic surgery is the preferred approach, but patients should be selected carefully.[140–146] Lateral and 3rd ventricular cysts can be removed with rigid endoscopes and the 4th ventricle can be approached with flexible endoscopes. Patients with significant ependymal enhancement have not been effectively managed surgically due to adherence of the cysticerci to the ependyma. These patients may not be good candidates for endoscopic removal.[140]

An alternative approach, especially in the setting of acute decompensation, is placement of a ventriculoperitoneal shunt. Shunting is associated with a lower perioperative mortality rate than seen with an open craniotomy.[87] Up to 75% of shunts malfunction requiring shunt revision or replacement if no other treatment is given. Recent studies have demonstrated that requirement for shunt revision are infrequent among patients who are also treated with antiparasitic drugs.[41,49,109,110,112] Similarly, corticosteroids may decrease the risk of shunt obstruction.[111]

Subarachnoid NCC and Giant Cysticerci

Subarachnoid cysticercosis is a rare form associated with a poor prognosis. In one series, patients treated with only CSF diversion were noted to have a 50% mortality rate.[147] Complications include mass effect, communicating hydrocephalus, vasculitis with strokes, and basilar meningitis.[52,54,86] The basilar arachnoiditis appears to play an important role in the pathogenesis.

There are no controlled trials of management of subarachnoid NCC. Case series in which patients were treated with antiparasitic drugs, corticosteroids, and shunting for hydrocephalus have demonstrated a markedly improved prognosis compared to older studies.[27,52,131,132] Thus, most experts consider subarachnoid NCC an indication for antiparasitic therapy.[116] The optimal doses and duration of therapy have not been defined, but patients appear to require prolonged or repeated courses of antiparasitic drugs. Patients should be treated with albendazole 15 mg/kg/d for at least 28 days. They should also receive high doses of corticosteroids (e.g., prednisone 60 mg per day).

Other Forms of Neurocysticercosis

Spinal NCC can be subarachnoid or intramedullarly. There is only anecdotal evidence on the effectiveness of any therapies. Intramedullary should usually approached surgically due to the risk of paralysis from cord swelling.[116] Spinal subarachnoid cysticerci, however, may respond to antiparasitic drugs.[27] Ocular disease may also respond to antiparasitic treatment, but the standard therapy is still surgical removal.[116]

PREVENTION

Cysticercosis was hyperendemic in Europe in the 19th century. However, transmission was eliminated by improved sanitation, better animal husbandry, and meat inspection.[148,149] Porcine cysticercosis can be prevented by confining pigs and not allowing them access to human fecal material.[150] However, in most areas pigs function as scavengers cleaning up waste. By contrast, confined pigs must be fed, adding expenses to the cost of raising them. This economic pressure is a major barrier to corralling the pigs as a method of control. Human infection with adult tapeworms can also be prevented by destruction, freezing, or adequate cooking of measly pork. Meat inspection has been unsuccessful in areas where pigs are raised by peasant farmers.[151] Treatment of human tapeworm carriers could potentially eliminate the disease, but current detection methods are suboptimal. Mass chemotherapy of endemic populations results in significant decreases in human taeniasis and porcine cysticercosis, but the effects are of short duration.[148,152,153] Development of an effective vaccine against cysticercosis may provide the best potential tool toward the eradication of the disease. A recombinant vaccine has been developed for *Taenia ovis* that can provide nearly complete protection. This vaccine is currently commercially available in several countries. *T. solium* homologues have been cloned and initial studies suggest efficacy.[154]

Coenurosis

Human infection with the larval form of the canine tapeworm *Taenia multiceps (Multiceps multiceps)* is termed *coenurosis* and is reported from tropical and subtropical areas of the world.

Rarely, human disease may be caused by zoonotic infection with *Taenia serialis*.

AGENT

The definitive hosts are dogs, wolves, foxes, and coyotes, where adult *T. multiceps* or *T. serialis* are found in the small intestines.[155] The gravid proglottids passed in the feces of the canid hosts disintegrate and release eggs that are ingested by intermediate hosts including rabbits and rodents. The larval stage of *T. multiceps* usually develops in herbivores such as sheep, goats, or horses, whereas the larval stage of *T. serialis* is usually found in rabbits and squirrels. Humans may also serve as an accidental intermediate host as a consequence of ingestion of eggs released by proglottids in dog feces. As in hydatid disease, the oncospheres eventually lodge in various tissues of the body, typically the brain and spinal cord of herbivores. The cyst or bladder, about the size of a hen's egg, eventually develops. The inner membrane of the bladder develops multiple protoscolices and floating in the bladder fluid are numerous small bladders containing protoscolices or metacestodes. External bladders are also formed that remain attached by long stalks to the main bladder.

EPIDEMIOLOGY

The majority of human cases have been reported from Africa, specifically Kenya, Uganda, Nigeria, and South Africa.[156–158] Human cases have also been reported from the United Kingdom, France, and North America.[159] Subcutaneous, ocular, muscle, and CNS cysts have been commonly described, although it is unclear if all cases were due to *T. multiceps*.

DISEASE

Human coenurosis usually involves the CNS, where it presents as a cyst and acts as a space-occupying mass causing pressure necrosis as it enlarges. Intracerebral cysts may cause seizures or other localizing signs and symptoms and can be confused with neurocysticercosis and echinococosis. Intraparenchymal lesions of the spinal cord have been reported. This infection may be associated with meningitis, arteritis, arachnoiditis, ependymitis, and involvement of the eye. Subcutaneous and intramuscular cysts are reported most commonly in Africa and involve the intercostal area and anterior abdominal wall. Allergic symptoms, such as recurrent urticaria, fever, and night sweats, have also been reported.

DIAGNOSIS

Presumptive diagnosis by MRI or CT scan, as well as ultrasound, has been helpful but not definitive.[159,160] The definitive diagnosis is dependent on surgical excision and pathologic identification (Fig. 113-6). Fine-needle aspiration of a cyst has been reported to yield a diagnosis.[159] There is no reliable serologic test for this disease.

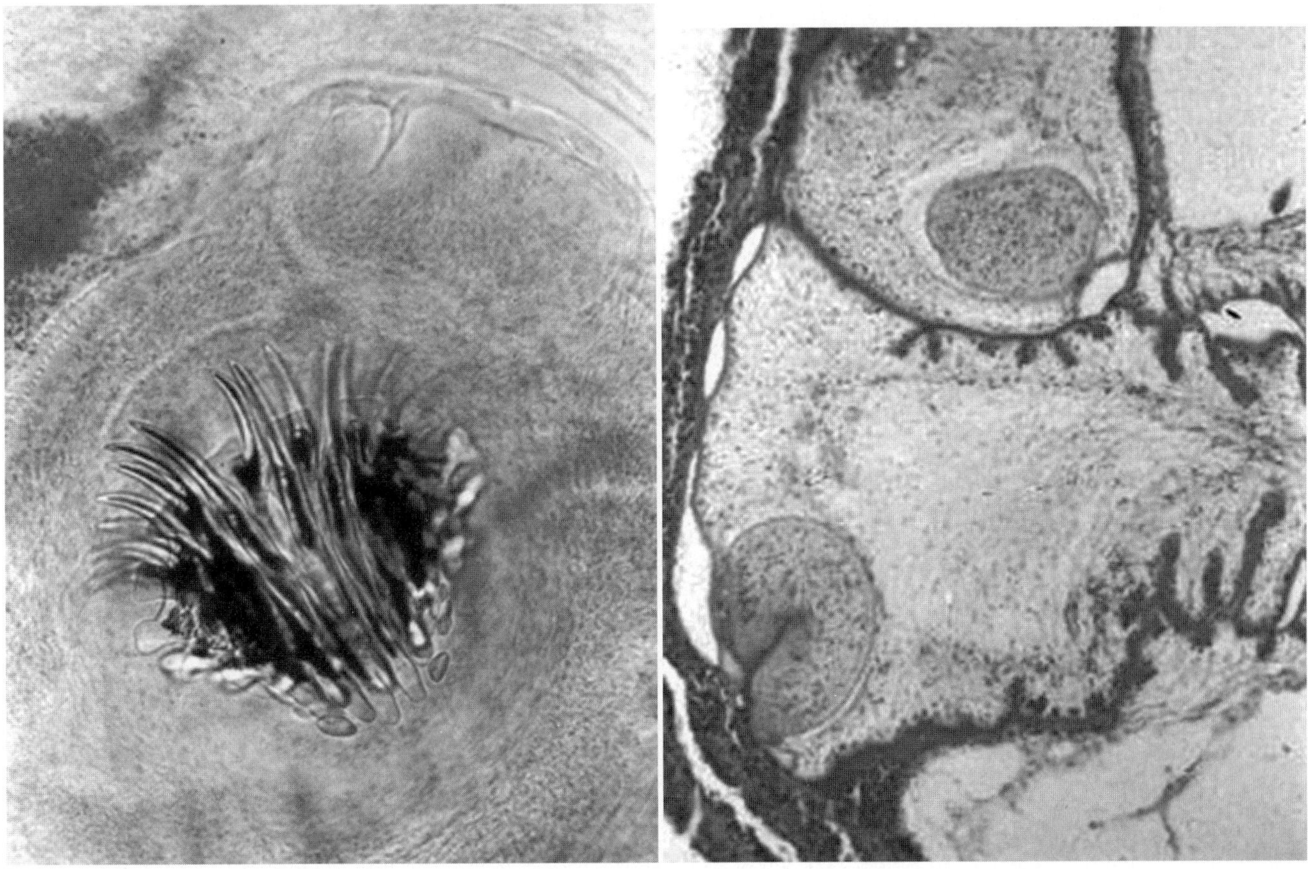

A B

FIGURE 113-6 *A* and *B*, Pathologic images of coenurosis caused by *Taenia multiceps*.

TREATMENT AND PREVENTION

Surgical intervention has been the mainstay of therapy.[161] There are no reliable data on the use of praziquantel or albendazole in this disease. Elimination of adult worms with praziquantel may reduce transmission from dogs to humans.

REFERENCES

1. Singh G, Prabhakar S: *Taenia solium* Cysticercosis: From Basic to Clinical Science. Oxford, CABI Publishing, 2002.
2. Schantz PM, Moore AC, Muñoz JL, et al: Neurocysticercosis in an Orthodox Jewish community in New York City. N Engl J Med 327:692–695, 1992.
3. Moore AC, Lutwick LI, Schantz PM, et al: Seroprevalence of cysticercosis in an Orthodox Jewish community. Am J Trop Med Hyg 53:439–442, 1995.
4. Varma A, Gaur KJ: The clinical spectrum of neurocysticercosis in the Uttaranchal region. J Assoc Physicians India 50:1398–1400, 2002.
5. Schantz PM: *Taenia solium* cysticercosis: An overview of global distribution and transmission. In Singh G, Prabhakar S (eds): *Taenia solium* Cysticercosis: From Basic to Clinical Science. Oxford, CABI Publishing, 2002, pp 63–73.
6. White AC Jr: Neurocysticercosis: Updates on epidemiology, pathogenesis, diagnosis, and management. Annu Rev Med 51:187–206, 2000.
7. Richards FO, Schantz PM, Ruiz-Tiben E, et al: Cysticercosis in Los Angeles county. JAMA 254:3444–3448, 1985.
8. Medina MT, Rosas E, Rubio-Donnadieu F, et al: Neurocysticercosis as the main cause of late-onset epilepsy in Mexico. Arch Intern Med 150:325–327, 1990.
9. Del Brutto OH, Noboa CA: Late-onset epilepsy in Ecuador: Aetiology and clinical features in 225 patients. J Trop Geogr Neurol 1:31–34, 1991.
10. Garcia HH, Gilman R, Martinez M, et al: Cysticercosis as a major cause of epilepsy in Peru. The Cysticercosis Working Group in Peru (CWG). Lancet 341:197–200, 1993.
11. Schantz PM, Sarti E, Plancarte A, et al: Community-based epidemiological investigation of cysticercosis due to *Taenia solium*: Comparison of serological screening tests and clinical findings in two populations in Mexico. Clin Infect Dis 18:879–885, 1994.
12. Bern C, Garcia HH, Evans C, et al: Magnitude of the disease burden from neurocysticercosis in a developing country. Clin Infect Dis 29:1203–1209, 1999.
13. Cruz ME, Schantz PM, Cruz I, et al: Epilepsy and neurocysticercosis in an Andean community. Int J Epidemiol 28:799–803, 1999.
14. Garcia-Noval J, Moreno E, de Mata F, et al: An epidemiological study of epilepsy and epileptic seizures in two rural Guatemalan communities. Ann Trop Med Parasitol 95:167–175, 2001.
15. Garcia HH, Gilman RH, Gonzalez AE, et al: Hyperendemic human and porcine *Taenia solium* infection in Peru. Am J Trop Med Hyg 68:268–275, 2003.
16. Druet-Cabanac M, Ramanankandrasana B, Bisser S, et al: *Taenia solium* cysticercosis in Africa. In Singh G, Prabhakar S (eds): *Taenia solium* Cysticercosis: From Basic to Clinical Science. Oxford, CABI Publishing, 2002, pp 129–137.
17. Andriantsimahavandy A, Lesbordes JL, Rasoaharimalala B, et al: Neurocysticercosis: A major aetiological factor of late-onset epilepsy in Madagascar. Trop Med Int Health 2:741-746, 1997.
18. Mafojane NA, Appleton CC, Krecek RC, et al: The current status of neurocysticercosis in Eastern and Southern Africa. Acta Trop 87:25–33, 2003.
19. Nguekam JP, Zoli AP, Zogo PO, et al: A seroepidemiological study of human cysticercosis in West Cameroon. Trop Med Int Health 8:144–149, 2003.
20. Dixon HBF, Lipscomb FM: Cysticercosis: An Analysis and Follow-up of 450 Cases, Vol. 299. (Medical Research Council special report series.) London, Her Majesty's Stationary Service, 1961.
21. Murthy JMK, Yangala R: Etiological spectrum of symptomatic localization related epilepsies: A study from South India. J Neurol Sci 158:65–70, 1998.
22. Murthy JM, Yangala R: Etiological spectrum of localization-related epilepsies in childhood and the need for CT scan in children with partial seizures with no obvious causation—A study from south India. J Trop Pediatr 46:202–206, 2000.
23. Sawhney IM, Lekhra OP, Shashi JS, et al: Evaluation of epilepsy management in a developing country: A prospective study of 407 patients. Acta Neurol Scand 94:19–23, 1996.
24. Rajshekhar V: Etiology and management of single CT lesions in patients with seizures: Understanding a controversy. Acta Neurol Scand 84:465–470, 1991.
25. Rajshekhar V, Chandy MJ: Validation of diagnostic criteria for solitary cerebral cysticercus granuloma in patients presenting with seizures. Acta Neurol Scand 96:76–81, 1997.
26. Singh G, Prabhakar S, Ito A, et al: *Taenia solium* taeniasis and cysticercosis in Asia. In Singh G, Prabhakar S (eds): *Taenia solium* Cysticercosis: From Basic to Clinical Science. Oxford, CABI Publishing, 2002, pp 111–127.
27. Bandres J, White AC Jr, Samo T, et al: Extraparenchymal neurocysticercosis: Report of five cases and review of the literature on management. Clin Infect Dis 15:799–822, 1992.
28. Estañol B, Corona T, Abad P: A prognostic classification of cerebral cysticercosis: Therapeutic implications. J Neurol Neurosurg Psychiatr 49:1131–1134, 1986.
29. Carpio A, Placencia M, Santillán F, et al: A proposal for classification of neurocysticercosis. Can J Neurol Sci 21:43–47, 1994.
30. Sotelo J, Guerrero V, Rubio F: Neurocysticercosis: A new classification based on active and inactive forms. Arch Intern Med 145:442–445, 1985.
31. Salgado P, Rojas R, Sotelo J: Cysticercosis. Clinical classification based on imaging studies. Arch Intern Med 157:1991–1997, 1997.
32. Singh G, Sachdev MS, Tirath A, et al: Focal cortical-subcortical calcifications (FCSCs) and epilepsy in the Indian subcontinent. Epilepsia 41:718–726, 2000.
33. Del Brutto OH, Santibañez R, Noboa CA, et al: Epilepsy due to neurocysticercosis: Analysis of 203 patients. Neurology 42:389–392, 1992.
34. Chayasirisobhon S, Menoni R, Chayasirisobhon W, et al: Correlation of electroencephalography and the active and inactive forms of neurocysticercosis. Clin Electroencephalogr 30:9–11, 1999.
35. Del Brutto OH: Prognostic factors for seizure recurrence after withdrawal of antiepileptic drugs in patients with neurocysticercosis. Neurology 44:1706–1709, 1994.
36. Garg RK, Karak B, Mohan Kar A: Neuroimaging abnormalities in Indian patients with uncontrolled partial seizures. Seizure 7:497–500, 1998.
37. Nash TE, Pretell J, Garcia HH: Calcified cysticerci provoke perilesional edema and seizures. Clin Infect Dis 33:1649–1653, 2001.
38. Gupta RK, Kumar R, Chawla S, et al: Demonstration of scolex within calcified cysticercus cyst: Its possible role in the pathogenesis of perilesional edema. Epilepsia 43:1502–1508, 2002.
39. Nash TE, Del Brutto OH, Butman JA, et al: Calcific neurocysticercosis and epileptogenesis. Neurology 62:1934–1938, 2004.
40. Antoniuk SA, Bruck I, Dos Santos LH, et al: Seizures associated with calcifications and edema in neurocysticercosis. Pediatr Neurol 25:309–311, 2001.
41. Shandera WX, White AC Jr, Chen J, et al: Cysticercosis in Houston, Texas: A report of 112 cases. Medicine 73:37–52, 1994.
42. White AC Jr: Neurocysticercosis: A common cause of neurologic disease worldwide. Clin Infect Dis 24:101–113, 1997.
43. Garcia HH, Del Brutto OH: Heavy nonencephalitic cerebral cysticercosis in tapeworm carriers. The Cysticercosis Working Group in Peru. Neurology 53:1582–1584, 1999.
44. Carpio A, Escobar A, Hauser WA: Cysticercosis and epilepsy: A critical review. Epilepsia 39:1025–1040, 1998.
45. Carpio A, Hauser WA: Prognosis for seizure recurrence in patients with newly diagnosed neurocysticercosis. Neurology 59:1730–1734, 2002.
46. Garcia HH, Pretell EJ, Gilman RH, et al: A trial of antiparasitic treatment to reduce the rate of seizures due to cerebral cysticercosis. N Engl J Med 350:249–258, 2004.
47. Rangel R, Torres B, Del Brutto O, et al: Cysticercotic encephalitis: A severe form in young females. Am J Trop Med Hyg 36:387–392, 1987.
48. Thomson AJG: Neurocysticercosis—Experience at the teaching hospitals of the University of Cape Town. S Afr Med J 83:332–334, 1993.
49. Kelley R, Duong DH, Locke GE: Characteristics of ventricular shunt malfunctions among patients with neurocysticercosis. Neurosurgery 50:757–761; discussion 761–762, 2002.

50. Zee C-S, Segall HD, Destain S, et al: MRI of intraventricular cysticercosis: Surgical implication. J Computer Assist Tomogr 17:932–939, 1993.
51. Zee CS, Go JL, Kim PE, et al: Imaging of neurocysticercosis. Neuroimaging Clin North Am 10:391–407, 2000.
52. Proaño JV, Madrazo I, Avelar F, et al: Medical treatment for neurocysticercosis characterized by giant subarachnoid cysts. N Engl J Med 345:879–885, 2001.
53. Barinagarrementeria F, Cantu C: Frequency of cerebral arteritis in subarachnoid cysticercosis: An angiographic study. Stroke 29:123–125, 1998.
54. Garcia HH, Del Brutto OH, Nash TE, et al: New concepts in the diagnosis and management of neurocysticercosis (Taenia solium). Am J Trop Med Hyg 72:3–9, 2005.
55. Sekhar GC, Lemke BN: Orbital cysticercosis. Ophthalmology 104:1599–1604, 1997.
56. Pushker N, Bajaj MS, Chandra M, et al: Ocular and orbital cysticercosis. Acta Ophthalmol Scand 79:408–413, 2001.
57. Cardenas F, Quiroz H, Plancarte A, et al: *Taenia solium* ocular cysticercosis: Findings in 30 cases. Ann Ophthalmol 24:25–28, 1992.
58. Chowdhary A, Bansal R, Singh K, et al: Ocular cysticercosis—A profile. Trop Doct 33:185–188, 2003.
59. Sharma T, Sinha S, Shah N, et al: Intraocular cysticercosis: Clinical characteristics and visual outcome after vitreoretinal surgery. Ophthalmology 110:996–1004, 2003.
60. Cruz ME, Cruz I, Preux P-M, et al: Headaches and cysticercosis in Ecuador, South America. Headache 35:93–97, 1995.
61. Rajshekhar V: Severe episodic headache as the sole presenting ictal event in patients with a solitary cysticercus granuloma. Acta Neurol Scand 102:44–46, 2000.
62. Levav M, Mirsky AF, Cruz ME, et al: Neurocysticercosis and performance on neuropsychologic tests: A family study in Ecuador. Am J Trop Med Hyg 53:552–557, 1995.
63. Ruiz-Garcia M, Gonzalez-Astiazaran A, Rueda-Franco R: Neurocysticercosis in children: Clinical experience in 122 patients. Childs Nerv Syst 13:608–612, 1997.
64. Forlenza OV, Filho AHGV, Nobrega JPS, et al: Psychiatric manifestations of neurocysticercosis: A study of 38 patients from a neurology clinic in Brazil. J Neurol Neurosurg Psychiatr 62:612–616, 1997.
65. de la Garza Y, Graviss E, Daver N: Epidemiology of neurocysticercosis in Houston, Texas. Am J Trop Med Hyg 2005 (in press).
66. Ridaura Sanz C: Host response in childhood neurocysticercosis. Childs Nerv Syst 3:206–207, 1987.
67. White AC Jr, Robinson P, Kuhn R: *Taenia solium* cysticercosis: Host-parasite interactions and the immune response. Chemical Immunol 66:209–230, 1997.
68. Molinari JL, Mejia H, White AC Jr, et al: *Taenia solium*: A cysteine protease secreted by metacestodes depletes human CD4 lymphocytes in vitro. Exp Parasitol 94:133–142, 2000.
69. Leid RW, McConnell LA: PGE_2 generation and release by the larval stage of the cestode, *Taenia taeniaeformis*. Prostagland Leukotr Med 11:317–323, 1983.
70. Leid RW, Suquet CM, Bouwer HGA, et al: Interleukin inhibition by a parasite proteinase inhibitor, taeniaestatin. J Immunol 137:2700–2702, 1986.
71. Leid RW, Grant RF, Suquet CM: Inhibition of equine neutrophil chemotaxis and chemokinesis by a *Taenia taeniaeformis* proteinase inhibitor, taeniaestatin. Parasit Immunol 9:195–204, 1987.
72. Leid RW, Grant RF, Suquet CM: Inhibition of neutrophil aggregation by taeniaestatin, a cestode proteinase inhibitor. Int J Parasitol 17:1349–1353, 1987.
73. Stringer JL, Marks LM, White AC Jr, et al: Epileptogenic activity of granulomas associated with murine cysticercosis. Exp Neurol 183:532–536, 2003.
74. Restrepo BI, Llaguno P, Sandoval MA, et al: Analysis of immune lesions in neurocysticercosis patients: Central nervous system response to helminth appears Th1-like instead of Th2. J Neuroimmunol 89:64–72, 1998.
75. Restrepo BI, Alvarez JI, Castano JA, et al: Brain granulomas in neurocysticercosis patients are associated with a Th1 and Th2 profile. Infect Immun 69:4554–4560, 2001.
76. Escobar A: The pathology of neurocysticercosis. In Palacios E, Rodriguez-Carbajal J, Taveras J (eds): Cysticercosis of the Central Nervous System. Springfield, IL, Charles C Thomas, 1983, pp 27–54.
77. Gutierrez Y: Cysticercosis, coenurosis, and sparganosis. In Gutierrez Y (ed): Diagnostic Pathology of Parasitic Infection with Clinical Correlation. Oxford, Oxford University Press, 2000, pp 635–674.
78. Evans CA, Garcia HH, Hartnell A, et al: Elevated concentrations of eotaxin and interleukin-5 in human neurocysticercosis. Infect Immun 66:4522–4525, 1998.
79. Rolfs A, Muhlschlegel F, Jansen-Rosseck R, et al: Clinical and immunologic follow-up study of patients with neurocysticercosis after treatment with praziquantel. Neurology 45:532–538, 1995.
80. Aguilar-Rebolledo F, Cedillo-Rivera R, Llaguno-Violante P, et al: Interleukin levels in cerebrospinal fluid from children with neurocysticercosis. Am J Trop Med Hyg 64:35–40, 2001.
81. Kramer LD, Locke GE, Byrd SE: Cerebral cysticercosis: Documentation of natural history by CT. Radiology 171:459-462, 1989.
82. Dumas JL, Visy JM, Belin C, et al: Parenchymal neurocysticercosis: Followup and staging by MRI. Neuroradiology 39:12–18, 1997.
83. Sheth TN, Lee C, Kucharczyk W, et al: Reactivation of neurocysticercosis: Case report. Am J Trop Med Hyg 60:664–667, 1999.
84. Estañol B, Kleriga E, Loyo M, et al: Mechanisms of hydrocephalus in cerebral cysticercosis: Implications for therapy. Neurosurgery 13:119–123, 1983.
85. Cantú C, Barinagarrementeria MD: Cerebrovascular complications of neurocysticercosis: Clinical and neuroimagining spectrum. Arch Neurol 53:233–239, 1996.
86. McCormick GF: Cystcercosis: Review of 230 patients. Bull Clin Neurosci 50:76–101, 1985.
87. Colli BO, Martelli M, Assitari JA, et al: Results of surgical treatment of neurocysticercosis in 69 cases. J Neurosurg 65:309–315, 1986.
88. Garcia HH, Del Brutto OH: Imaging findings in neurocysticercosis. Acta Trop 87:71–78, 2003.
89. Zee C-S, Segall HD, Ahmadi J, et al: MR imaging of neurocysticercosis. J Comput Assist Tomogr 12:927–934, 1988.
90. Jena A, Sanchetee PC, Gupta RK, et al: Cysticercosis of the brain shown by magnetic resonance imaging. Clin Radiol 39:542–546, 1988.
91. Noujaim SE, Rossi MD, Rao SK, et al: CT and MR imaging of neurocysticercosis. Am J Roentgenol 173:1485–1490, 1999.
92. Martinez HR, Rangel-Guerra R, Arrendondo-Estrada JH, et al: Medical and surgical treatment of neurocysticercosis: A magnetic resonance study of 161 cases. J Neurol Sci 130:25–34, 1995.
93. Cosentino C, Velez M, Torres L, et al: Cysticercosis lesions in basal ganglia are common but clinically silent. Clin Neurol Neurosurg 104:57–60, 2002.
94. Chawla S, Gupta RK, Kumar R, et al: Demonstration of scolex in calcified cysticercus lesion using gradient echo with or without corrected phase imaging and its clinical implications. Clin Radiol 57:826–834, 2002.
95. Del Brutto OH, Rajshekhar V, White AC Jr, et al: Proposed diagnostic criteria for neurocysticercosis. Neurology 57:177–183, 2001.
96. Rajshekhar V: The story behind solitary cysticercal granuloma. In Singh G, Prabhakar S (eds): *Taenia solium* Cysticercosis: From Basic to Clinical Science. Oxford, CABI Publishing, 2002, pp 241–250.
97. Ramos-Kuri M, Montoya RS, Padilla A, et al: Immunodiagnosis of neurocysticercosis: Disappointing performance of serology (ELISA) in an unbiased sample of neurologic patients. Arch Neurol 49:633–636, 1992.
98. Proaño-Narvaez JV, Meza-Lucas A, Mata-Ruiz O, et al: Laboratory diagnosis of human neurocysticercosis: Double-blind comparison of enzyme-linked immunosorbent assay and electroimmunotransfer blot assay. J Clin Microbiol 40:2115–2118, 2002.
99. Tsang VCW, Brand JA, Boyer AE: An enzyme-linked immunoelectrotransfer blot assay and glycoprotein antigens for diagnosing human cysticercosis (*Taenia solium*). J Infect Dis 159:50–59, 1989.
100. Wilson M, Bryan RT, Fried JA, et al: Clinical evaluation of the cysticercosis enzyme-linked immunoelectrotransfer blot in patients with neurocysticercosis. J Infect Dis 164:1007–1009, 1991.
101. Gekeler F, Eichenlaub S, Mendoza EG, et al: Sensitivity and specificity of ELISA and immunoblot for diagnosing neurocysticercosis. Eur J Clin Microbiol Infect Dis 21:227–229, 2002.
102. Garcia HH, Harrison LJ, Parkhouse RM, et al: A specific antigen-detection ELISA for the diagnosis of human neurocysticercosis. The Cysticercosis Working Group in Peru. Trans R Soc Trop Med Hyg 92:411–414, 1998.

103. Garcia HH, Parkhouse RM, Gilman RH, et al: Serum antigen detection in the diagnosis, treatment, and follow-up of neurocysticercosis patients. Trans R Soc Trop Med Hyg 94:673–676, 2000.
104. Garcia HH, Gonzalez AE, Gilman RH, et al: Circulating parasite antigen in patients with hydrocephalus secondary to neurocysticercosis. Am J Trop Med Hyg 66:427–430, 2002.
105. Espindola NM, Vaz AJ, Pardini AX, et al: Excretory/secretory antigens (ES) from in-vitro cultures of *Taenia crassiceps* cysticerci, and use of an anti-ES monoclonal antibody for antigen detection in samples of cerebrospinal fluid from patients with neurocysticercosis. Ann Trop Med Parasitol 96:361–368, 2002.
106. Pardini AX, Vaz AJ, Dos Ramos Machado L, et al: *Cysticercus* antigens in cerebrospinal fluid samples from patients with neurocysticercosis. J Clin Microbiol 39:3368–3372, 2001.
107. Das S, Mahajan RC, Ganguly NK, et al: Detection of antigen B of *Cysticercus* cellulosae in cerebrospinal fluid for the diagnosis of human neurocysticercosis. Trop Med Int Health 7:53–58, 2002.
108. Mitchell WG, Crawford TO: Intraparenchymal cerebral cysticercosis in children: Diagnosis and treatment. Pediatrics 82:76–82, 1988.
109. Proaño JV, Madrazo I, Garcia L, et al: Albendazole and praziquantel treatment in neurocysticercosis of the fourth ventricle. J Neurosurg 87:29–33, 1997.
110. Cuetter A, Garcia-Bobadilla J, Guerra L, et al: Neurocysticercosis: Focus on intraventricular disease. Clin Infect Dis 24:157–164, 1997.
111. Suastegui Roman R, Soto-Hernandez J, Sotelo J: Effects of prednisone on ventriculoperitoneal shunt function in hydrocephalus secondary to cysticercosis: A preliminary study. J Neurosurg 84:629–633, 1996.
112. Zhu L, Weng X, Shi Y, et al: CSF-VP shunt placement and albendazole therapy for cerebral cysticercosis. Chin Med J (Engl) 115:936–938, 2002.
113. Mall RK, Agarwal A, Garg RK, et al: Short course of prednisolone in Indian patients with solitary cysticercus granuloma and new-onset seizures. Epilepsia 44:1397–1401, 2003.
114. Del Brutto OH, Sotelo J, Roman GC: Therapy for neurocysticercosis: A reappraisal. Clin Infect Dis 17:730–735, 1993.
115. De Ghetaldi LD, Norman RM, Couville AW: Cerebral cysticercosis treated biphasically with dexamethasone and praziquantel. Ann Intern Med 99:179–181, 1983.
116. Garcia HH, Evans CA, Nash TE, et al: Current consensus guidelines for treatment of neurocysticercosis. Clin Microbiol Rev 15:747–756, 2002.
117. Vazquez ML, Jung H, Sotelo J: Plasma levels of praziquantel decrease when dexamethasone is given simultaneously. Neurology 37:1561–1562, 1987.
118. Bittencourt PR, Gracia CM, Martins R, et al: Phenytoin and carbamazepine decreased oral bioavailability of praziquantel. Neurology 42:492–496, 1992.
119. Dachman WD, Adubofour KO, Bikin DS, et al: Cimetidine-induced rise in praziquantel levels in a patient with neurocysticercosis being treated with anticonvulsants. J Infect Dis 169:689–691, 1994.
120. Yee T, Barakos JA, Knight RT: High-dose praziquantel with cimetidine for refractory neurocysticercosis: A case report with clinical and MRI follow-up. West J Med 170:112–115, 1999.
121. Jung H, Medina R, Castro N, et al: Pharmacokinetic study of praziquantel administered alone and in combination with cimetidine in a single-day therapeutic regimen. Antimicrob Agents Chemother 41:1256–1259, 1997.
122. Lopez-Gomez M, Castro N, Jung H, et al: Optimization of the single-day praziquantel therapy for neurocysticercosis. Neurology 57:1929–1930, 2001.
123. Bittencourt PR, Gracia CM, Gorz AM, et al: High-dose praziquantel for neurocysticercosis: Efficacy and tolerability. Eur Neurol 30:229–234, 1990.
124. Pretell EJ, Garcia HH, Custodio N, et al: Short regimen of praziquantel in the treatment of single brain enhancing lesions. Clin Neurol Neurosurg 102:215–218, 2000.
125. Del Brutto OH, Campos X, Sanchez J, et al: Single-day praziquantel versus 1-week albendazole for neurocysticercosis. Neurology 52:1079–1081, 1999.
126. Sotelo J, Escobedo F, Penagos P: Albendazole vs praziquantel for therapy for neurocysticercosis: A controlled trial. Arch Neurol 45:532–534, 1988.
127. Sotelo J, Del Brutto OH, Penagos P, et al: Comparison of therapeutic regimens of anticysticercal drugs from parenchymal brain cysticercosis. J Neurol 237:69–72, 1990.
128. Garcia HH, Gilman RH, Horton J, et al: Albendazole therapy for neurocysticercosis: A prospective double-blind trial comparing 7 versus 14 days of treatment. Cysticercosis Working Group in Peru. Neurology 48:1421–1427, 1997.
129. Singhi P, Dayal D, Khandelwal N: One week versus four weeks of albendazole therapy for neurocysticercosis in children: A randomized, placebo-controlled double blind trial. Pediatr Infect Dis J 22:268–272, 2003.
130. Del Brutto OH, Sotelo J: Albendazole therapy for subarachnoid and ventricular neurocysticercosis. J Neurosurg 72:816–817, 1990.
131. Del Brutto OH, Sotelo J, Aguirre R, et al: Albendazole therapy for giant subarachnoid cysticerci. Arch Neurol 49:535–538, 1992.
132. Del Brutto OH: Albendazole therapy for subarachnoid cysticerci: Clinical and neuroimaging analysis of 17 patients. J Neurol Neurosurg Psychiatr 62:659–661, 1997.
133. Singhi P, Ray M, Singhi S, et al: Clinical spectrum of 500 children with neurocysticercosis and response to albendazole therapy. J Child Neurol 15:207–213, 2000.
134. Baranwal AK, Singhi PD, Khandelwal N, et al: Albendazole therapy in children with focal seizures and single small enhancing computerized tomographic lesions: A randomized, placebo-controlled, double blind trial. Pediatr Infect Dis J 7:696–700, 1998.
135. Padma MV, Behari M, Misra NK, et al: Albendazole in neurocysticercosis. Natl Med J India 8:255–258, 1995.
136. Padma MV, Behari M, Misra NK, et al: Albendazole in single CT ring lesions in epilepsy. Neurology 44:1344–1346, 1994.
137. Carpio A, Santillán F, León P, et al: Is the course of neurocysticercosis modified by treatment with antihelminthic agents? Arch Intern Med 155:1982–1988, 1995.
138. Kalra V, Dua T, Kumar V: Efficacy of albendazole and short-course dexamethasone treatment in children with 1 or 2 ring-enhancing lesions of neurocysticercosis: A randomized controlled trial. J Pediatr 143:111–114, 2003.
139. Del Brutto OH: Single parenchymal brain cysticercus in the acute encephalitic phase: Definition of a distinct form of neurocysticercosis with a benign prognosis. J Neurol Neurosurg Psychiatry 58:247–249, 1995.
140. Bergsneider M, Nieto JH: Endoscopic management of intraventricular cysticercosis. In Singh G, Prabhakar S (eds): *Taenia solium* Cysticercosis: From Basic to Clinical Science. Oxford, CABI Publishing, 2002, pp 399–410.
141. Anandh B, Mohanty A, Sampath S, et al: Endoscopic approach to intraventricular cysticercal lesions. Minim Invasive Neurosurg 44:194–196, 2001.
142. Bergsneider M: Endoscopic removal of cysticercal cysts within the fourth ventricle. Technical note. J Neurosurg 91:340–345, 1999.
143. Cudlip SA, Wilkins PR, Marsh HT: Endoscopic removal of a third ventricular cysticercal cyst. Br J Neurosurg 12:452–454, 1998.
144. Neal JH: An endoscopic approach to cysticercosis cysts of the posterior third ventricle. Neurosurgery 36:1040–1043, 1995.
145. Bergsneider M, Holly LT, Lee JH, et al: Endoscopic management of cysticercal cysts within the lateral and third ventricles. J Neurosurg 92:14–23, 2000.
146. Psarros TG, Krumerman J, Coimbra C: Endoscopic management of supratentorial ventricular neurocysticercosis: Case series and review of the literature. Minim Invasive Neurosurg 46:331–334, 2003.
147. Sotelo J, Marin C: Hydrocephalus secondary to cysticercotic arachnoiditis: A long-term follow-up review of 92 cases. J Neurosurg 66:686–689, 1987.
148. Gonzalez AE, Garcia HH, Gilman RH, et al: Control of *Taenia solium*. Acta Trop 87:103–109, 2003.
149. Schantz PM, Cruz M, Sarti E, et al: Potential eradicability of taeniasis and cysticercosis. Bull Pan Am Health Org 27:397–401, 1993.
150. Vazquez-Flores S, Ballesteros-Rodea G, Flisser A, et al: Hygiene and restraint of pigs is associated with absence of *Taenia solium* cysticercosis in a rural community of Mexico. Salud Publica Mex 43:574–576, 2001.
151. Cysticercosis Working Group in Peru: The marketing of cysticercotic pigs in the Sierra of Peru. Bull World Health Org 71:223–228, 1993.
152. Sarti E, Schantz PM, Avila G, et al: Mass treatment against human taeniasis for the control of cysticercosis: A population-based intervention study. Trans R Soc Trop Med Hyg 94:85–89, 2000.
153. Cruz M, Davis A, Dixon H, et al: Operational studies on the control of *Taenia solium* taeniasis/cysticercosis in Ecuador. Bull World Health Org 67:401–407, 1989.

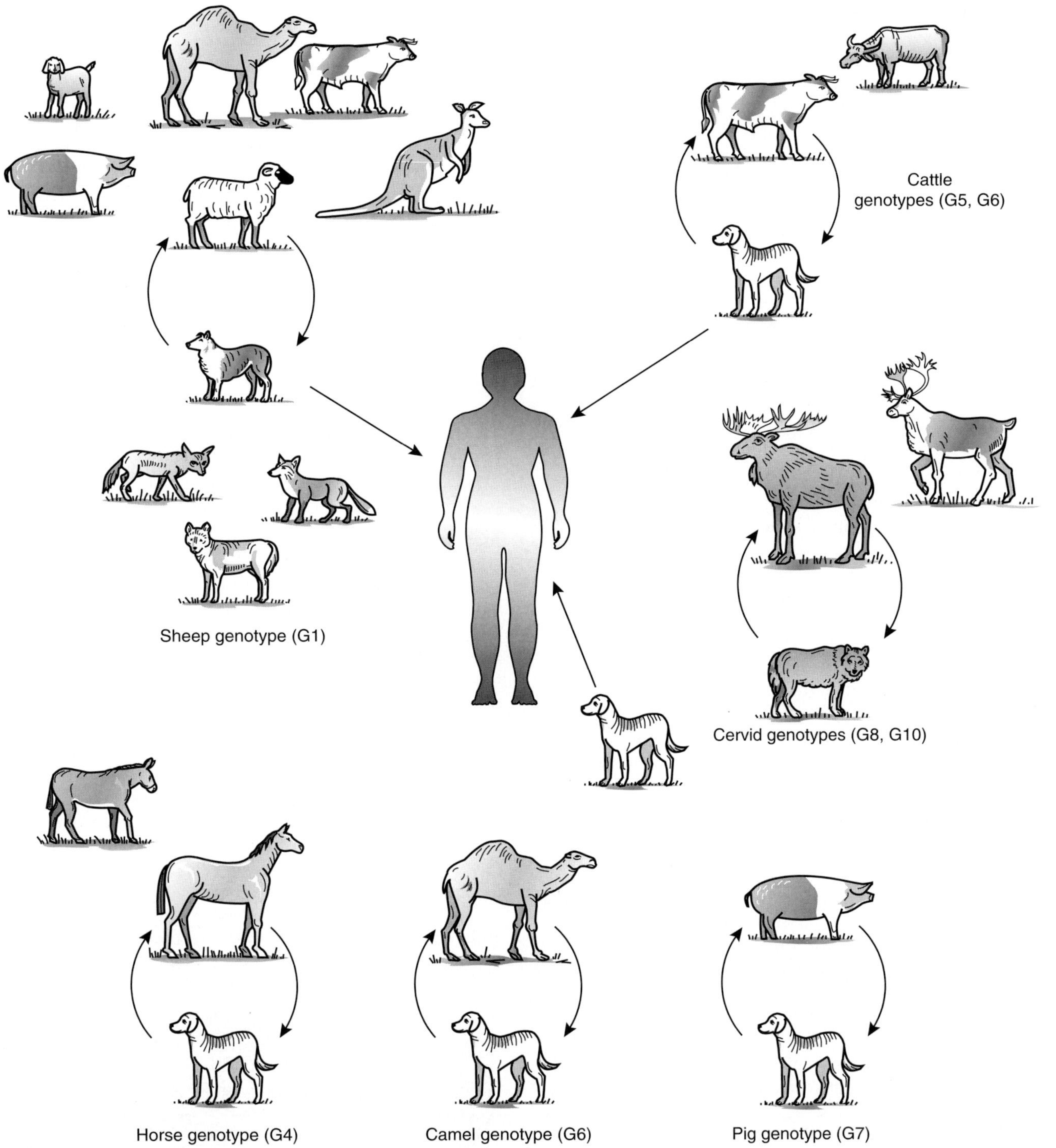

FIGURE 114-1 Life cycle patterns of principal genotypic variants of the *Echinococcus granulosus* complex and infectivity to humans. Curved arrows designate principal and alternative definitive and intermediate hosts. Straight arrows designate those variants known to infect humans. (See Table 114-1 for complete listing.) (Modified from Schantz PM, Chai J, Craig PS, et al: Epidemiology and control. In Thompson RCA, Lymbery AJ, [eds]: Echinococcosis and Hydatid Disease. London, CAB, 1995.)

isolates from human patients thus far characterized by genotype have been of the sheep genotype (G1), and this and the worldwide epidemiologic association of high endemicity with sheep raising confirm the paramount public health importance of the sheep genotype.

Comparative details of maturation and growth rates of most of the *E. granulosus* genotypic variants are not available, and the following description applies primarily to genotype G1 in sheep and canid hosts. The adult intestinal forms of *E. granulosus* genotypic variants are small tapeworms approximately 3 to 7 mm in length when fully mature; they attach firmly to the small intestine of the canine host (Fig. 114-2). Following infection by ingestion of protoscolices originating from fertile hydatid cysts, sexual maturity of adult-stage

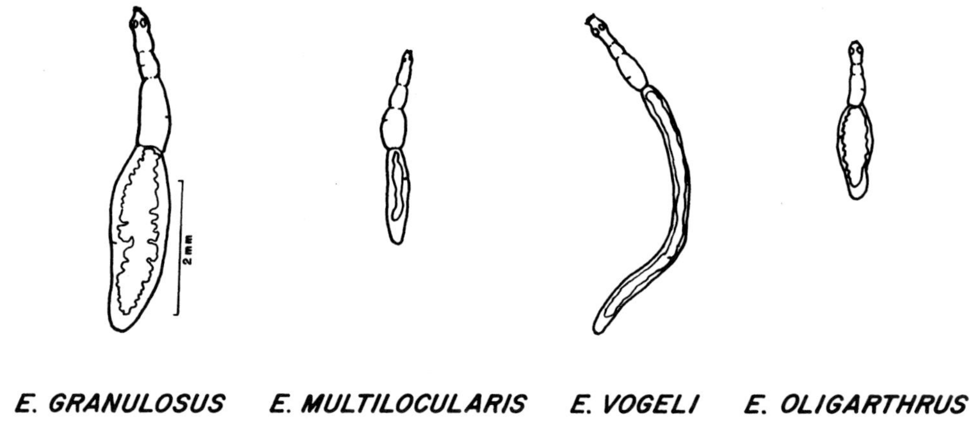

FIGURE 114-2 Comparative morphology of adult-stage *Echinococcus* species. (From Rausch RL, Bernstein JJ: *Echinococcus vogeli* sp.n [Cestodea: Taeniidae] from the bush dog *Speothos venaticus* [Lund]. Tropenmed Parasitol 23:25, 1972.)

tapeworms is reached within 4 to 7 weeks. Development from ovum to the oncosphere or hexacanth embryo takes place in utero in the adult *Echinococcus*. The oncosphere measures approximately 0.018 mm and is bilaterally symmetrical, possessing three pairs of hooks (hexacanth), muscle fibers, and glands, which aid it in penetration and locomotion within the intermediate host. The oncosphere and its surrounding membranes (0.030 to 0.036 mm in diameter) are often referred to as the cestode egg. Eggs are shed with the feces into the external environment, and when ingested by a suitable intermediate host, the oncospheres hatch and become activated. Lytic secretions may facilitate the passage of the motile oncosphere through the intestinal mucosa and into the host's circulatory system (via venous and lymphatic pathways). They are distributed to other sites via the host's circulatory system, where postoncospheral development continues. Within a few days after the oncospheres reach their preferred site, cystic development begins. This process involves degeneration of the oncospheral stage and emergence of the vesicular metacestode stage, which grows expansively by concentric enlargement. In general, hydatid cysts increase in diameter from 1 to 5 cm each year, depending on unknown factors. Protoscolex formation occurs as early as 4 months in white mice, but it may require more than 1 year in sheep and other intermediate hosts.

The fully developed metacestode (hydatid or hydatid cyst) of *E. granulosus* is typically fluid-filled and unilocular, but multiple chambers may also occur. Structurally, the cyst consists of an inner germinative layer of cells supported externally by a characteristic acidophilic-staining, acellular, laminated membrane of variable thickness (Fig. 114-3). Cytoplasmic extensions of the germinative layer unite to form a syncytium, which is differentiated into numerous microtriches. The microtriches project peripherally into the laminar layer toward the host tissues surrounding the cyst. Surrounding the parasitic cyst is a host-produced, granulomatous, adventitial reaction of extremely variable intensity. Small secondary cysts, called brood capsules, bud internally from the germinative layer and, by polyembryony, produce multiple protoscolices. A protoscolex is a scolex with the rostellum and suckers deeply withdrawn into the postsucker region. In humans, the slowly growing hydatid cysts may attain a volume of many liters and contain many thousands of protoscolices.

TRANSMISSION, EPIDEMIOLOGY, AND GEOGRAPHIC DISTRIBUTION

Dogs and other definitive hosts become infected upon ingesting organs of other animals that contain hydatid cysts or protoscolices released from recently ruptured cysts. *Echinococcus granulosus* has remarkable biologic potential; there may be as many as 40,000 tapeworms in a heavily infected dog, and each tapeworm sheds approximately 1000 eggs every 2 weeks. Dogs infected with *Echinococcus* tapeworms pass eggs in their feces, and humans become infected through fecal–oral contact, particularly in the course of playful and intimate contact between children and dogs. Eggs adhere to hairs around the infected dog's anus and are also found on the muzzle and paws. Indirect means of contact via soil, water, and contaminated vegetables, or through the intermediary of flies and other arthropods, may also result in human infections. Eggs of *E. granulosus* are capable of surviving snow and freezing conditions, remaining viable for at least 1 year on pasture, but they are susceptible to desiccation and will become incapable of hatching after only a few hours when exposed to direct sunlight. People of both sexes and all ages appear susceptible and opportunities for exposure are mainly related to direct

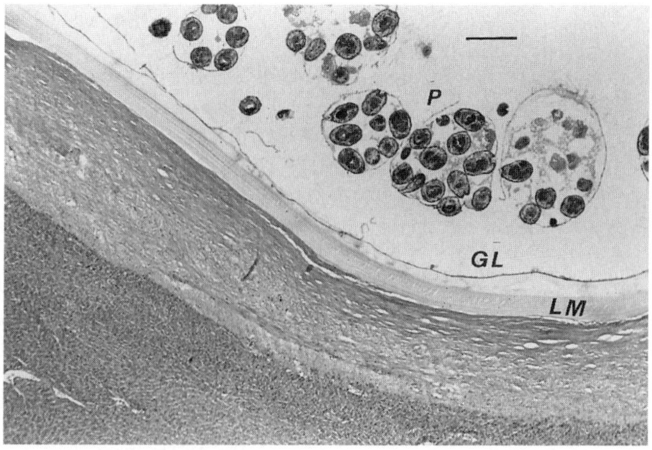

FIGURE 114-3 Hydatid cyst of *Echinococcus granulosus* in liver of sheep showing protoscolices (P) in brood capsules, germinative layer (GL), and laminated membrane (LM). (H&E; bar = 100 μm)

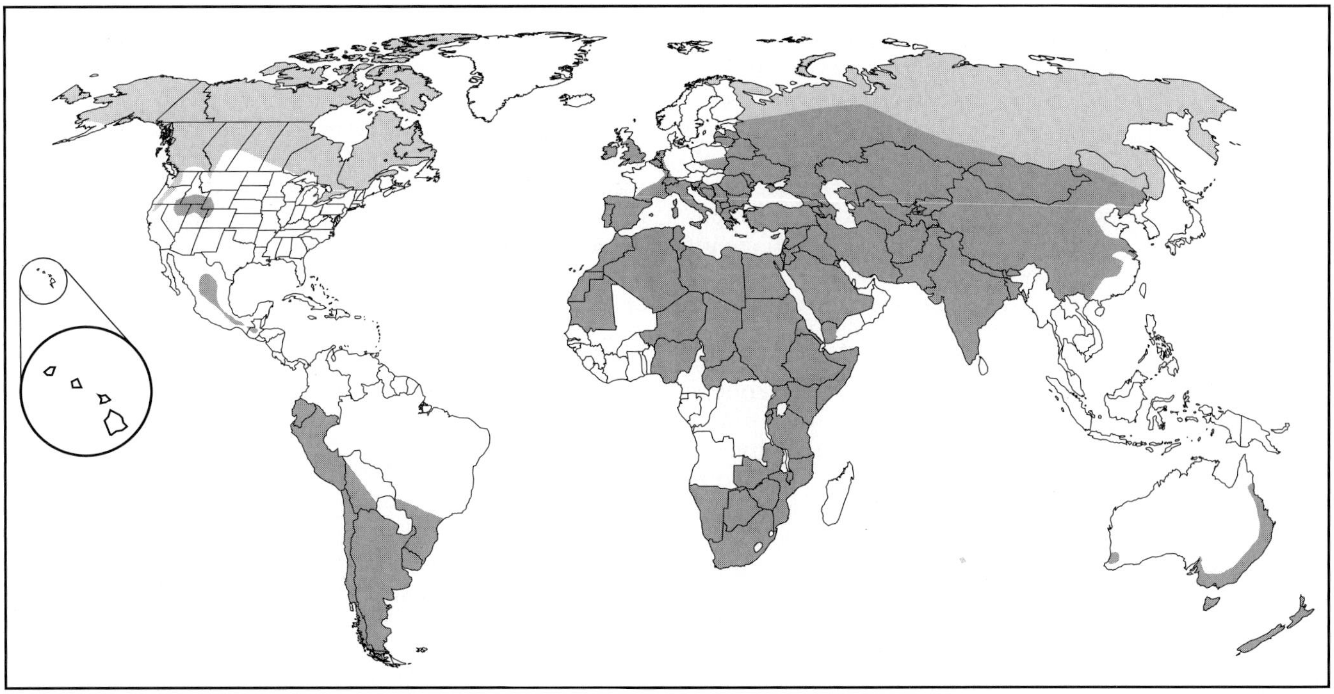

Echinococcus granulosus

- Cervid strain
- Sheep and other pastoral strains

and indirect contact with infected dogs. Socioeconomic and cultural characteristics are among the best defined risk factors for human infection: uncontrolled dogs living closely with people, uncontrolled slaughter of livestock, and insanitary living conditions.[9] Whether it be among Arabs in Tunisia, Quechua Indians in Peru, Turkana tribesmen in Kenya, or Tibetans in China, these common factors are readily discernible. When dogs at risk of infection are maintained close to the family home, all members of the family may be exposed, or, as in certain cultural situations, one sex or the other may take responsibility for feeding and handling the dogs, thus favoring exposure of people of that sex.[10,11] Cystic echinococcosis imposes serious medical and economic disabilities on affected communities through the economic burden associated with infection in livestock as well as the disability and treatment costs associated with infection in humans.[12,13]

The greatest prevalence of CE in humans and nonhuman animals is found in countries of the temperate zones, including southern South America, the entire Mediterranean littoral, the southern and central areas of the former Soviet Union, Central Asia, China, Australia, and areas of Africa (reviewed in Schantz and others[9]). Consistently, highest prevalence is found among populations involved with sheep raising, thus emphasizing the overwhelming public health importance of the sheep genotype *E. granulosus* (G1). In certain regions of the former Soviet Union (e.g., Kazakhstan and Kyrghyzstan), changing agricultural practices and disruptions in regulatory policies have led to increased transmission in both lower animal and human hosts.[13,14] The cervid genotypes (G7 and G8) also commonly infect humans in northern North America and Eurasia; as with the sheep genotype cestode, it is the synanthropic link through the dog that results in most human exposure.

In many countries of these regions, national diagnostic incidence rates have been reported to range from 5 to 20 per 100,000 population.[9] "National" rates are misleading, however, because most urban populations are at low risk; in rural endemic areas diagnostic incidence is manyfold higher. Furthermore, surveys of local populations using ultrasound imaging diagnostic techniques often measure CE prevalences of 2% to 6%.[12,13] In the United States, most infections are diagnosed in immigrants from countries in which hydatid disease is highly endemic; historically, this was mainly Italians and Greeks, but in recent years increasing numbers of cases have been diagnosed in people of Middle Eastern and Asian origin.[9] Sporadic autochthonous transmission is currently recognized in Alaska, Arizona, and New Mexico.

DISEASE

There are numerous descriptions of the diverse clinical manifestations of CE (hydatid disease) in the medical and surgical literature.[15–17] Many human infections remain asymptomatic; hydatid cysts are frequently observed as incidental findings at autopsy or detected by abdominal ultrasound screening at rates much higher than the reported local morbidity rates. The severity and nature of the signs and symptoms produced by larval cestodes are extremely variable and never pathognomonic. The particular manifestations are determined by the site of localization of the cysts, their size, and their condition.

The incubation period of human hydatid infections is highly variable and often prolonged for several years. Cysts localized in the liver or lung may grow for many years before obtaining enough mass to cause symptoms; in contrast, those located in the brain or eye need reach only very small size before clinical symptoms appear. Age-specific prevalence of liver and pulmonary hydatid cysts increases gradually with age, suggesting that new infections continue to be acquired throughout the human life span. Most primary infections in humans consist of a single cyst; however, 20% to 40% of patients have multiple cysts or multiple organ involvement. The liver is the most common site of cyst localization (65%), followed by the lungs (25%); hydatid cysts are less frequently seen in the spleen, kidneys, heart, bone, and central nervous system. Cysts of the cervid (G7), or northern sylvatic, form localize predominantly in the lungs; however, the disease caused by this variant has been described as usually more benign and uncomplicated than that caused by the sheep strain.[7] In secondary echinococcosis, new cysts develop from released protoscolices after spontaneous or trauma-induced cyst rupture or during invasive treatment procedures.

The slowly growing hydatid cyst is well tolerated by the human host until it becomes large enough to cause dysfunction. Cyst rupture, often resulting from trauma, may cause a variety of immediate or delayed sequelae. Mild to severe anaphylactoid reactions (and, occasionally, death) may follow the sudden massive release of cyst fluid. In the lungs, ruptured cyst membranes may be evacuated entirely through the bronchi or retained to serve as a nidus for bacterial infection. Dissemination of protoscolices incidental to surgical treatment may result in multiple secondary disease. In one study of 106 patients, the rate of postoperative recurrence within 3 years was 11%[15]; however, postsurgical chemotherapy reduces this risk (discussed later).

Hydatid cysts of the liver may become relatively large before producing symptoms because of the large size and the distensible nature of the organ. Signs and symptoms may include hepatic enlargement with or without a palpable mass in the right upper quadrant, right epigastric pain, nausea, and vomiting. Rupture or leakage usually results in acute or intermittent allergic manifestations. Urgent complications existing at the time of initial presentation in 7% of Australian patients with hepatic cysts include traumatic or spontaneous rupture, thoracobilia, and biliary fistula.[16]

Intact hydatid cysts in the lungs may cause no symptoms, but leakage or rupture causes chest pain, coughing, dyspnea, and hemoptysis. Hydatid membranes may be coughed up, sometimes resulting in spontaneous cure. Emergency complications existing at the time of initial presentation include cyst rupture and secondary bacterial infection. Twenty percent to 40% of patients with pulmonary hydatidosis can be shown to have liver involvement as well.[15–17]

In most surgical series, 5% to 10% of the cases involve organs other than the lungs or liver.[17,18] The clinical manifestations of cysts in unusual localizations often present special difficulties and delays in diagnosis. The first symptom of cerebral cysts may be raised intracranial pressure or focal epilepsy, whereas kidney cysts may be manifested by loin pain or hematuria. Bone cysts are often asymptomatic until pathologic fractures occur, and because of the resemblance, they are often misdiagnosed as tuberculous lesions. Cysts in the heart are especially dangerous because they may rupture and cause systemic dissemination of the protoscolices, anaphylaxis, or cardiac tamponade.

Although mortality rates associated with hydatid disease may appear low in comparison to those for some other infectious diseases, the morbidity associated with each case is considerable. Patients with hydatid disease often require multiple surgical interventions. Extensive secondary hydatid disease often becomes inoperable. Economic losses to affected families include surgical and hospital expenses as well as loss of income.[12] In Uruguay, it was shown that 60% of surgical patients were unable to return to normal activities for 4 months after leaving the hospital, and 40% were incapacitated for 6 months or longer.[19]

PATHOGENESIS AND IMMUNITY

Intermediate hosts mount an early immune response to infection with *Echinococcus* larvae as evidenced by the specific antibody and cellular responses and protective immunity generated by a primary infection.[20] The immune response may be separated into two phases: The first is that directed against the hatched oncospheres attempting to penetrate the gut mucosa and establish themselves in the host tissues. The second phase is aimed at the established metacestode at the site of election. Immune effector mechanisms of the first phase are more successful in destroying the parasites than those of the second because established metacestodes have evolved highly effective mechanisms for evading the host's defenses. Evidence suggests that early oncospheres are highly vulnerable to attack by host defenses, but only briefly, and a race between parasite development and the host response occurs in the critical first few days of infection.[21] The explanation for the ability of larvae to persist indefinitely in the tissues of immunologically competent hosts has been of great interest to parasitologists; but understanding is incomplete.[20,21]

Antibody-mediated, complement-dependent destruction of oncospheres in the gut or at the tissue site of development is the most effective mechanism of host defense. Specifically activated B lymphocytes, eosinophils, neutrophils, and macrophages migrate to and concentrate in the vicinity of the developing larvae; however, the exact roles of cellular mechanisms in the immune response are not known. Once established in the tissues, the metacestode appears well protected from the host immune response. Although direct exposure to complement and immune serum readily causes lysis of protoscolices and other metacestode tissues, in vivo they somehow evade or counteract these effects. For *E. granulosus* cysts, this protective state appears related to sequestration of the parasite by the laminated and germinative membranes and host capsule, which greatly limit the exchange of high-molecular-weight substances between host and parasite. The host's capacity for developing a parasite-specific cellular response able to eliminate the parasite may be modulated by parasite-derived effector substances. Anticomplementary factors released by the metacestode may contribute to the evasion by causing complement depletion at the host–parasite interface. Larval cestodes may also induce a disturbance of normal immune function. Mice chronically infected with *E. granulosus* exhibit an alteration of the T cell populations resulting in suppression of normal immune responsiveness; these include a polyclonal B cell activation, a marked decrease in mean T cell percentage but increase in suppressor cell activity, direct splenic T lymphocyte cytotoxicity to the metacestode, and impairment of the host defense potential by the formation of antihuman leukocyte antigen-reactive host antibodies. Other hypotheses proposed to account for prolonged survival of metacestodes include membrane fixation of blocking antibodies, which could interfere sterically with the attachment of protective antibodies or specifically sensitized cells. Several mechanisms may contribute to the parasite's defense simultaneously or at a different stage of the infection.[21]

Progress in developing effective vaccination against infection with oncospheres and immunotherapy of the metacestode have been reviewed by Lightowlers and colleagues.[22] The protoscolex appears to contain antigens that may be useful in immunotherapy, whereas the oncosphere contains antigens useful for vaccination against tissue-invading oncospheres. Antigens cloned from messenger RNA isolated from *E. granulousus*-hatched and -activated oncospheres successfully immunized lambs against challenge with infective eggs; vaccines based on these antigens may ultimately provide an additional tool for control and prevention of this infection. Possible immunotherapeutic molecules may be those involved with anticomplementary activity, those inducing changes in the host effector cell attack on metacestodes, and possible hidden antigens of the metacestode, such as serine proteases, cysteine proteases, or aspartyl proteases; however, immunotherapy is still experimental.

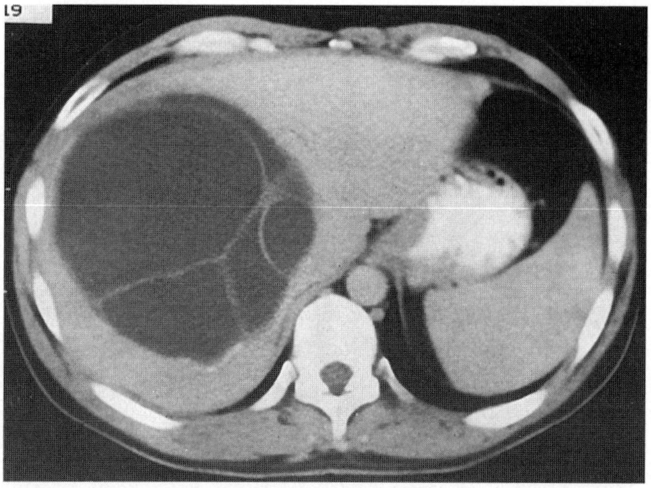

FIGURE 114-4 Abdominal computed tomography scan showing large primary hydatid cyst (*Echinococcus granulosus*) in the right lobe of the liver. Note multiple internal septations indicating secondary (daughter) cyst formation. (Courtesy of Dr. D. Rubin, New York.)

DIAGNOSIS

The presence of a cyst-like mass in a person with a history of exposure to sheepdogs in areas in which *E. granulosus* is endemic supports the diagnosis of CE; noninvasive confirmation of diagnosis can usually be obtained by ultrasound or radiologic imaging and immunologic techniques.[17] Cystic echinococcosis must be differentiated from nonparasitic cysts, cavitary tuberculosis, mycoses, abscesses, and benign or malignant neoplasms.

Radiography permits the detection of hydatid cysts in the lungs; however, in other organ sites, calcification is necessary for visualization. Computed tomography (CT), magnetic resonance imaging (MRI), and ultrasound imaging are all useful for detecting and defining the extent and condition of avascular fluid-filled cyst(s) in most organs[23,24] (Fig. 114-4). These noninvasive imaging techniques have proved valuable for diagnosis and preoperative evaluation by staging the condition of the lesion (intact, unilocular, ruptured, complicated with daughter cysts, or calcified), the extent of the lesion in reference to other organs and vital structures, and identifying the presence of additional, occult lesions. Because of its relatively low cost and portability, ultrasonography has been used widely for screening, clinical diagnosis, and monitoring of treatment of liver and intra-abdominal cysts.[24] WHO/IWGE proposed a standard ultrasound classification of echinococcal cysts based on their ultrasound appearance consistent with the natural history of the disease and response to treatment that is useful for defining the extent and condition of the cyst(s)[25] (Fig. 114-5). The standardized classification scheme is intended to promote uniform standards of diagnosis and treatment and may be applied to clinical management of patients as well as to field diagnostic surveys.

Serologic tests are useful for confirming presumptive imaging diagnoses; however, the limitations of serodiagnosis in CE must be understood to correctly interpret the findings. False-positive reactions, which, with tests using whole hydatid cyst fluid antigens, occur relatively frequently in people with other helminthic infections, cancer, and chronic immune disorders, may be misleading. Detectable specific immune responses have been associated with the location, integrity, and vitality of the larval cyst. Hepatic cysts are more likely to elicit an immune response than pulmonary cysts; nearly 50% of patients with single intact hyaline cysts of the lungs may be seronegative. Cysts in the brain and spleen are associated with lowered serodiagnostic reactivity, whereas those in bone appear to more regularly stimulate detectable antibody. Because fissuring or rupture of cysts is followed by an abrupt rise in titer of antibodies, it appears that the sensitivity of serologic tests is inversely related to the degree of sequestration of the hydatid antigens inside cysts, regardless of the location. Enzyme-linked immunosorbent assay (ELISA) and the indirect hemagglutination test are highly sensitive procedures for the initial screening of serum; diagnostic sensitivity varies from 60% to 90%, depending on the characteristics of the cases. Specific confirmation of reactivity can be obtained by demonstrating echinococcal antigens by immunodiffusion (arc 5) procedures or immunoblot assays (8-, 16-, and 21-kDa bands).[26,27] These latter serodiagnostic markers are the most *E. granulosus*-specific criteria described, but even they may be detected in serum of patients with other forms of echinococcosis and 5% to 10% of patients with *Taenia solium* cysticercosis. Circulating antigens are detectable in serum of many patients with CE. The sensitivity of antigen assays is relatively low in comparison with rates of antibody detection. However, since circulating antigens may be detectable in serum of some patients with negative or borderline antibody titers, antigen assays may be useful as a secondary test for

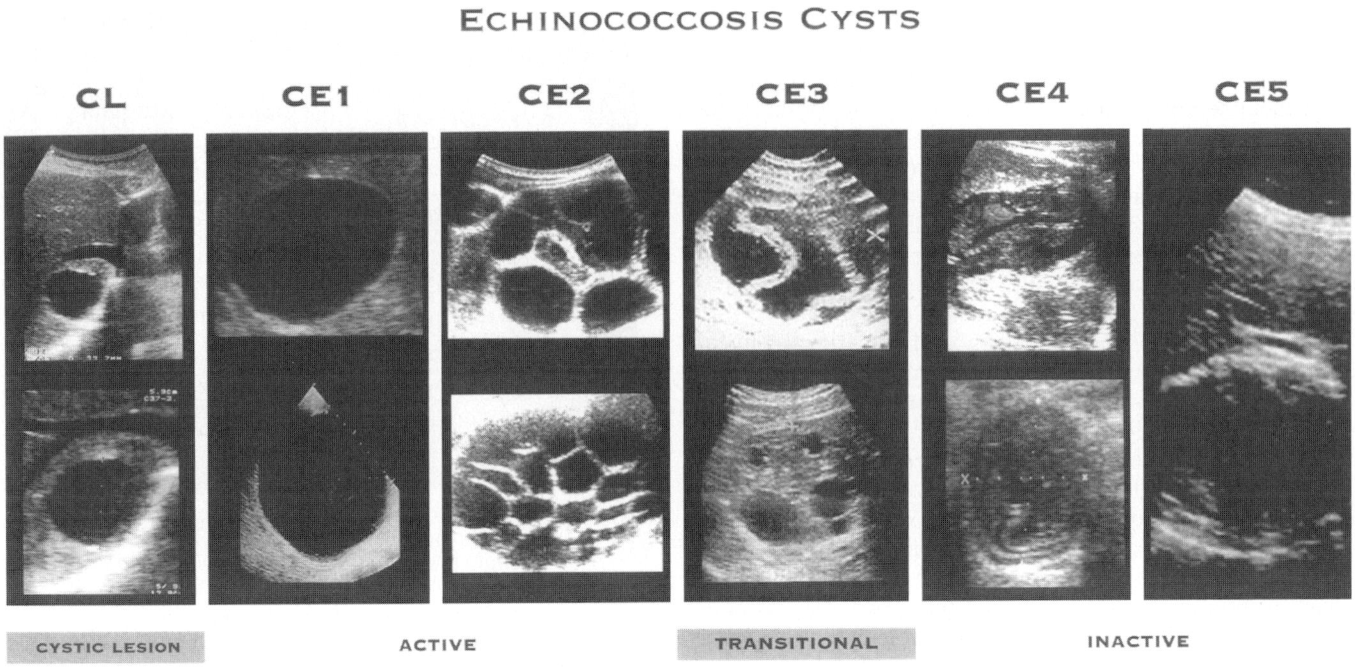

FIGURE 114-5 World Health Organization/Informal Working Group on Echinococcosis (WHO/IWGE) classification of ultrasound images of cystic echinococcosis. There are six types of cysts: CL are cysts whose parasitic nature cannot be discerned, thus requiring further diagnostic tests to reveal their identity; CE1 and CE2 are active, usually fertile echinococcal cysts; CE3 are transitional in that their membrane integrity has been compromised either by the host reaction or by therapy and may reactivate to CE2 (active) or continue to regress to inactivity, types CE4 and CE5, which are solid cysts, with calcified rim in the latter. (From WHO/IWGE: International Classification of Ultrasound Images of Cystic Echinococcosis. Reproduced with the permission of WHO.)

clinical diagnosis.[28] Antigen assays are also useful for testing fluid from cysts of unknown origin.

In seronegative patients, a presumptive diagnosis may be confirmed by demonstrating specific antigens,[28] protoscolices, or hydatid membranes in the liquid obtained by percutaneous aspiration of the cyst. Closed aspiration may result in leakage of cyst contents with attendant risks of anaphylaxis or secondary hydatidosis; however, these risks can be minimized if the procedure is guided by ultrasound or CT and followed by benzimidazole treatment. Protoscolices released from cysts can sometimes be demonstrated in aspirates, sputum, or bronchial washings; identification of hooklets is facilitated by acid-fast stains. Eosinophilia is present in fewer than 25% of infected people. Although not widely available in clinical centers, polymerase chain reaction (PCR) techniques exist that are capable of differentiating genomic *E. granulosus* DNA from that of other species of *Echinococcus* and other infectious agents.[29]

TREATMENT AND PROGNOSIS

Until recently, surgery was the only option for treatment of echinococcal cysts. However, chemotherapy with benzimidazole compounds and, more recently, cyst *p*uncture, percutaneous *a*spiration, *i*njection of chemicals, and *r*easpiration (PAIR) are increasingly used to supplement or even replace surgery as the preferred treatment.[30]

Surgery

Surgical removal of intact hydatid cysts, when possible, has the potential to remove cysts and lead immediately to complete cure. The aim of surgery is total removal of the cyst while avoiding the adverse consequences of spilling its contents. Pericystectomy is the usual preferred procedure, but simple drainage, capitonnage, marsupialization, and resection of the involved organ may be used depending on the location and condition of the cyst(s).[15–17,31,32] The more radical the intervention, the higher the operative risk but the lower the likelihood of relapse, and vice versa. Surgery is the preferred treatment when liver cysts are complicated or located in certain organs—that is, the brain, lung, or kidney.[31,32] Surgery is contraindicated in patients who refuse, are pregnant, have pre-existing medical conditions that put them at risk, or in those with multiple cysts that are difficult to access. Surgical risks include those associated with any surgical intervention (e.g., anesthesia and infections) and those unique to echinococcosis (e.g., anaphylaxis and secondary recurrence). Operative mortality varies from 0.5% to 4.0% but increases with repeated interventions and in conditions of inadequate facilities.

Traditional surgical management of CE involves injection of protoscolicidal chemical solutions into the cyst(s), followed by evacuation, prior to further manipulations and extirpation of cysts. The use of formalin is no longer acceptable for intracystic injection because of the danger of resultant sclerosing cholangitis.[33] Currently used compounds, including 70% to 90% ethyl alcohol and 15% to 20% hypertonic saline, have relatively low risk, but all have been reported to cause some complications. Few of these compounds are registered for parenteral or intraoperative use, and it is often difficult to accurately estimate the volume of cysts or determine if an intrabiliary communication exists. Given these considerations, and the current alternatives of peri- or postoperative chemotherapy[34] or both, perioperative injection of protoscolicidal chemicals should not be practiced as a routine procedure.

Chemotherapy

Documentation of experience with chemotherapy with benzimidazole compounds is extensive, and the medical approach can be recommended for many patients. Approximately one-third of patients treated with benzimidazole drugs have been cured of their disease (e.g., collapse or solidification of cysts), and higher proportions (30% to 50%) have responded with significant regression of cyst size and alleviation of symptoms.[35–39] However, between 20% and 40% of cases do not respond favorably. In general, small (<7 mm diameter) isolated cysts, surrounded by minimal adventitial reaction, respond best, whereas complicated cysts with multiple compartments or daughter cysts, or with thick or calcified surrounding adventitial reactions, are relatively refractory to treatment. Both albendazole 10 to 15 mg/kg body weight per day and mebendazole, 40 to 50 mg/kg body weight per day for 3 to 6 months have demonstrated efficacy. Some investigators who have compared both drugs concluded that albendazole has slightly greater efficacy in terms of rates of complete cure and improvement; the more consistent response obtained with albendazole may be related to its superior pharmacokinetic profile that favors intestinal absorption and penetration into the cyst(s).[36,39] Adverse reactions (neutropenia, liver toxicity, alopecia, and others), reversible on cessation of treatment, have been noted in a minority of patients treated with both drugs. The reported variability in response to medical treatment suggests that the details of treatment, such as dosage, duration, and length of follow-up, must be determined individually for each case; it seems that a minimum duration of treatment is 3 months. The long-term prognosis in individual patients is difficult to predict; therefore, prolonged follow-up with ultrasound or other imaging procedures is needed to determine the eventual outcome.[37,38]

Another important use of chemotherapy is as adjunct to surgery. Albendazole has been administered to patients prior to surgery for the intended purpose of facilitating the safe surgical manipulation of the cyst(s) by inactivating protoscolices, altering the integrity of cyst membranes, and reducing the turgidity of the cysts. Experimental studies support this rationale.[17] Benzimidazole therapy is recommended for prevention of recurrent disease secondary to the spillage of contents of cysts after spontaneous or accidental rupture. Following such accidents, preventive treatment recommendations are 1 to 3 months continuously of mebendazole or albendazole.[37] Praziquantel 40 mg/kg body weight also has high protoscolicidal activity and may be useful for postspillage preventive therapy[34] or as a protoscolicidal agent in the PAIR procedure[38] (discussed later). Although praziquantel has shown significant destructive activity on cyst germinal membranes in vitro and in vivo, sometimes greater than that of benzimidazoles, the drug has not been consistently efficacious against established hydatid cysts.[37] Combining praziquantel with albendazole was superior to albendazole alone as preoperative therapy.[40]

Contraindications to chemotherapy include patients with chronic hepatic disease and bone marrow depression. Since benzimidazole drugs are teratogenic, they should never be administered to pregnant women. Treatment of pregnant women, unless their disease is life-threatening, probably should be aimed at reducing discomfort until term, after which they can be treated with one of the previously discussed approaches.

PAIR

Another option for the treatment of hydatid cysts in the liver and some other locations is percutaneous puncture using sonographic guidance, aspiration of substantial amounts of the liquid contents, and injection of a protoscolicidal agent (e.g., 95% ethanol or 15% to 20% hypertonic saline) for at least 15 minutes, followed by reaspiration (PAIR).[41,42] Reported experiences with this approach suggest good results in terms of efficacy and safety.[43–51] Clinical consultants of the WHO/IWGE have prepared a practical guide to the PAIR procedure.[48]

PAIR is indicated for patients with single or multiple cysts in the liver, abdominal cavity, spleen, and kidney. Echinococcal cysts with ultrasound appearances of "liquid cysts" (ultrasound image types CE1 and CE3 with detached endocyst)[25] (see Fig. 114-5) respond favorably to the procedure.[48] PAIR is contraindicated for inaccessible or superficially located liver cysts, in those with multiple daughter cysts ("honeycomb" appearance on imaging), for inactive or calcified cystic lesions, and for cysts with biliary communication. To avoid sclerosing cholangitis, this procedure must not be performed in patients whose cysts have biliary communication; the presence of the latter can be determined by testing the cyst fluid for the presence of bilirubin by endoscopic retrograde cholangiopancreatography (ERCP) or, preferably, by injection of contrast medium following aspiration and prior to injection of the protoscolicidal agent. Complications have included secondary infection of the cavity, acute allergic reactions, and recurrence[47]; however, these have been managed successfully. Applications of PAIR to pulmonary cysts, employed as an alternative in patients who have failed medical therapy, have been associated with frequent complications.[49]

The physician must be prepared to treat an allergic reaction should it occur. The possibility of secondary hydatidosis resulting from accidental spillage during this procedure can be minimized by concurrent treatment with benzimidazoles; indeed, a report suggests that combined treatment (PAIR with albendazole) may improve the results in comparison with either chemotherapy or PAIR alone.[50] The recommended treatment course is 4 days prior to and 1 month (albendazole) or 3 months (mebendazole) after the PAIR procedure. For treatment of uncomplicated cysts in the liver, Khuroo and coworkers[51] reported that, in comparison with patients who underwent surgical intervention (cystectomy), patients treated by PAIR followed by 8 weeks of albendazole chemotherapy had comparable rates of cyst disappearance (88% vs. 72%) but had reduced hospital stay (4 vs. 13 days) and reduced risk of complications (32% vs. 84%).

Conventional PAIR, using fine needles, is less effective in treating multivesicular cysts (WHO CE2 and "solid" CE3; see Fig. 114-5) than univesicular cysts (CE1 and CE3 with detached endocyst); recurrent cyst growth is common following treatment of these former types of cysts with PAIR.[47] Alternative percutaneous approaches to treatment have been proposed for these types of cysts, including trocar aspiration/drainage of the cyst matrix using large bore catheters or trocar devices[52,53] or inactivation of the germinal layer using a thermal treatment similar to that used for treatment of neoplasms.[54] Data on the long-term outcome of percutaneous treatment of these complex-type hydatid cysts are limited, and long-term follow-up is needed to evaluate effectiveness.

The PAIR procedure should only be performed by experienced physicians with adequate surgical backup support to deal with complications. The procedure is minimally invasive and less expensive than surgery.[55] Reported experiences with this approach suggest good results in terms of the absence of acute complications and recurrence. A meta-analysis concluded that in comparison to conventional surgical treatment, PAIR plus chemotherapy was associated with greater clinical and parasitologic efficacy, fewer recurrences, lower morbidity and mortality, as well as shorter hospital stays.[56] The development and use of ultrasound imaging technology for clinical diagnosis and population screening has provided significant improvements for abdominal forms of echinococcosis and has provided new information on the natural history of the disease. It is now clear that many, if not the majority of cases of CE have a benign prognosis. This knowledge has led to new, unanswered questions about the necessity for, criteria for, and selection of appropriate treatments. Further long-term observations and multicenter comparative trials of various interventions and placebo are required to answer these questions.

Monitoring Results of Treatment

It has been observed that in echinococcosis, it is easier to prove treatment failure than treatment success[17]; however, noninvasive methods for monitoring cyst size, consistency, and integrity have substantially improved our ability to assess viability of hydatid cysts. The occult nature of the hydatid cyst confounds post-treatment evaluation. Objective response to treatment, whether surgery or chemotherapy or both, is best assessed by repeated evaluation of cyst(s) size and consistency at 3-month intervals with ultrasound imaging or at longer intervals with CT or MRI. Since the time of appearance of recurrence is extremely variable, monitoring should be continued for 3 or more years. Changes in titers of serologic tests have not by themselves been able to define the outcome of chemotherapy[36] or PAIR, presumably because of continued antigenic stimulation from parasitic tissue. In contrast, following successful radical surgery, antibody titers decline and sometimes disappear; titers rise again if secondary hydatid cysts develop.[18,57]

PREVENTION AND CONTROL

Echinococcus granulosus has been viewed as highly vulnerable to the implementation of preventive measures, at least in theory. When only synanthropic hosts under human control are involved, the cestode cycle can be interrupted if dogs are prevented from consuming infected viscera from sheep and other domestic ungulates. Indeed, there are a number of successful examples of echinococcosis control, achieved on a national or regional scale, that confirm that *E. granulosus* is relatively unstable in synanthropic hosts and responds readily to comprehensive and consistently applied measures of intervention.[9]

The earliest successful program was that in Iceland initiated nearly 130 years ago when cystic hydatid disease was recognized as affecting approximately one of every six Icelanders.[9] A uniquely effective health education campaign sensitized the entire population to the disease, and subsequent measures virtually eliminated home slaughter of sheep; the result was gradual elimination of transmission. By the 1950s, echinococcosis was considered eradicated from Iceland. Programs initiated in New Zealand (1959) and Tasmania (1965) were primarily based on education of rural populations and motivating them to change their practices. Strict control and prohibition of farm slaughter were key features in these programs. The initially voluntary nature of the programs was reinforced by legislative acts and strengthened efforts at enforcement as the programs progressed. This policy proved highly successful: The number of infected dogs declined steadily throughout the campaigns. The decline in canine infection preceded decreases in the prevalence of infection in sheep and young cattle and a reduced number of cases in humans diagnosed annually. In New Zealand, the first year when no dogs were found infected was 1985–1986, and hydatid cysts in sheep are now rare. No new human cases of hydatid disease have been reported in children or adults younger than 19 years old since 1977. CE has been declared provisionally eradicated in both Tasmania and New Zealand. A program in Cyprus benefited from very aggressive stray dog elimination and strict control of working dogs and those kept as pets. All used diagnostic purging of dogs with arecholine as a surveillance technique for monitoring the effectiveness of the program and identifying problem farms. Tasmania quarantined infected dogs and infected sheep flocks. Regional programs in Argentina (1970) and Chile (1978) benefited from the advent of the highly effective echinococcicidal drug praziquantel. Monitoring of surveillance data in all these programs documented the reduction of prevalence in dogs, animal intermediate hosts, and humans.[9]

The epidemiologic characteristics associated with the transmission of echinococcosis in the endemic regions where control interventions have been successful were varied, as were the events leading to official commitments to undertake control efforts and the specific technical measures employed. Nevertheless, sustained implementation of control measures resulted in a successful interruption of transmission, and it seems that the fundamental requirements for effective control are now tried and proven in a variety of epidemiologic situations.[58] Control measures with proven usefulness include health education, stray dog control, registration of owned dogs, routine diagnostic testing and treatment of dogs, restrictions or controls on commercial and home slaughter of sheep and other livestock, and enactment and enforcement of legislation supporting the other measures. Since the available technology has improved throughout the years, the degree and the rapidity of demonstrable progress have, in part, reflected the degree of sophistication of the technology. Future progress in technology (e.g., the development of a vaccine for sheep[22]) will further improve the technical possibilities for effective control. The immediate prospects for further progress in control of hydatid disease depend on the development of adequate surveillance systems and careful documentation of the disease in all important hosts in order to characterize the quantitative dynamics of transmission and the costs and benefits of different control strategies.[58,59]

It must be noted that the positive achievements of successful control programs, however significant at the local level, have not markedly changed the global distribution and public health importance of hydatid disease. In most endemic areas, effective control has not been achieved or even attempted. Much remains to be done.

Alveolar Echinococcosis (*Echinococcus multilocularis*)

AGENT

The causative agent of AE was first recognized by Virchow in 1855 as being the larval stage of an *Echinococcus* cestode, but the relationship of this organism to the adult form in canids and its taxonomic designation remained unresolved for more than 100 years. Rausch and Schiller[59] described the life cycle and morphologic characteristics of an Alaskan cestode that was distinct from *E. granulosus*, and they named this organism *Echinococcus sibiricensis*. In Germany, Vogel[60] demonstrated that this cestode was identical to the causative agent of alveolar hydatid disease in Eurasia and confirmed Leuckart's earlier designation of *E. multilocularis* as having priority.

Although there is suggestive evidence of variation in morphology, pathogenicity, developmental characteristics, and host specificity between populations of *E. multilocularis* from Europe, Alaska, and central North America, few comparative data are available and the existence of distinct strains remains unconfirmed.[1] Rausch and Richards[61] did extensive morphologic studies and experimental infection trials and concluded that, except for indications of differences in the ability of the larvae to develop in rodents of various species, the cestode in central North America appears to be indistinguishable from that of the northern tundra zone. In comparison to the genetic variability in *E. granulosus*, direct genomic variation in different geographic populations of *E. multilocularis* is minor.[2,62]

Postoncospheral development of larval *E. multilocularis* in susceptible rodent hosts is fundamentally the same as that of *E. granulosus*, except that the primary vesicle gives rise to others by continuous exogenous budding, to produce a larval mass composed of hundreds of contiguous vesicles that may occupy more than one-half of the invaded hepatic lobe (Fig. 114-6).

There is no limiting membrane of host or parasite origin. Growth of the larva from the single primary vesicle to the compound multivesicular stage with infective protoscolices may be completed in as short a period as 2 months or as long a time as 7 months, depending on conditions for growth in the host. The rapid rate of development of *E. multilocularis* compared with that of *E. granulosus* is an adaptation to the short-lived rodent intermediate hosts. The number of protoscolices within a larval mass derived from a single embryo is

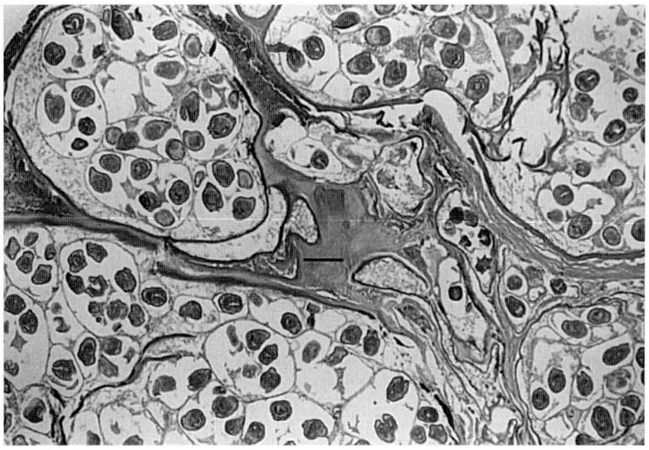

FIGURE 114-6 *Echinococcus multilocularis* in liver of infected rodent showing characteristic alveolar-like microvesicles with protoscolices. (H&E; bar = 100 μm)

highly variable within and between species of hosts but may number several thousand.

TRANSMISSION, EPIDEMIOLOGY, AND GEOGRAPHIC DISTRIBUTION

The life cycle of *E. multilocularis* involves foxes, coyotes, and arvicolid rodents; *Ochotona* sp., a small lagomorph, is an important intermediate host in Central Asia (Fig. 114-7). Domestic dogs and cats also become infected; cats are less efficient definitive hosts, however, and develop fewer, less fecund adult worms in comparison with dogs.[63]

Infection rates in the natural hosts, both intermediate and definitive, are influenced by the numerical densities of these mammals as well as the kind of predator–prey relationship that exists between them. In the northern tundra zone, a strongly defined predator–prey relationship exists between arctic foxes and microtine rodents. The arctic fox feeds almost exclusively on microtine rodents. In studies carried out during different years, infection rates in foxes and voles ranged from 40% to 100% and from 2% to 16%, respectively.[59,64] The variations correlated closely with fluctuations in the host populations; the parasites were least numerous when the populations of hosts were reduced, but infection rates were additionally influenced by habitat and climatic season. The number of worms in infected arctic foxes usually exceeds 100,000 to 200,000 per animal, but they apparently cause no adverse effects. Most worms are eliminated spontaneously 3 or 4 months after infection, although some may remain for 7 months or longer; however, these are senescent and can no longer produce eggs.[61]

Being largely confined to life cycles involving foxes and arvicolid rodents, in ecosystems generally separate from humans, exposure of humans to *E. multilocularis* is relatively less common than exposure of humans to *E. granulosus,* the cause of cystic echinococcosis.[9] Fox trappers and other people who work with foxes or their fur would appear to be relatively frequently exposed to eggs of *E. multilocularis,* but these occupations have not been associated with higher rates of infection.[65–67] In most endemic areas, there are few well-defined

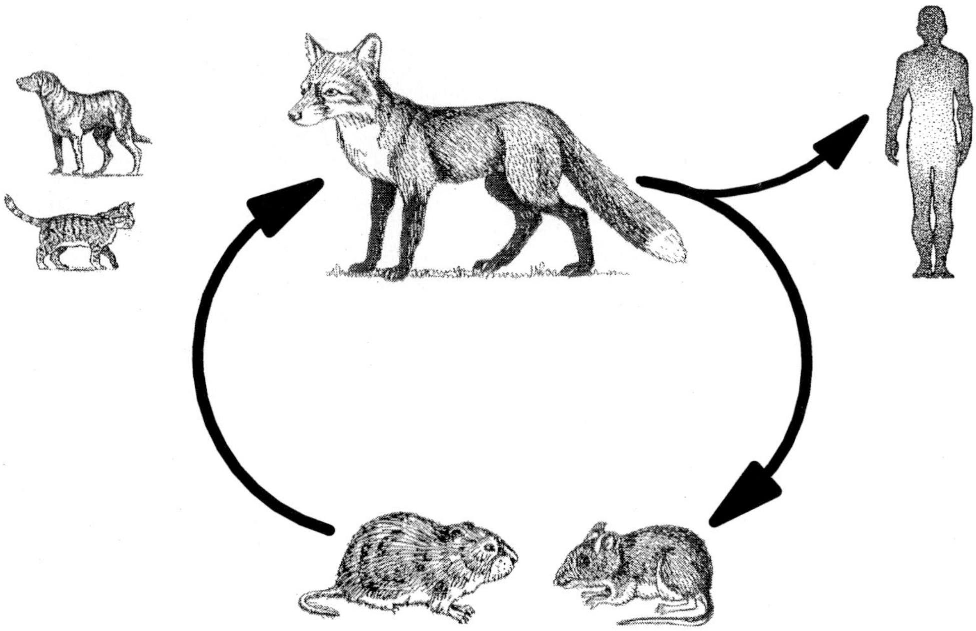

FIGURE 114-7 Life cycle and principal and alternative hosts for *Echinococcus multilocularis*.

individual risk factors for infections; however, infection rates are highest in people resident in rural areas where the cestode is endemic. There is ecological overlap to humans because domestic dogs or cats may become infected when they eat infected wild rodents, and infected pets are an important source of infection for humans.[66–68] It remains unclear whether genetic factors in humans play a role. Associations between MHC polymorphism and clinical presentation have been demonstrated.[69,70]

Hyperendemic foci have been described in some Native American villages of the North American tundra[61,68] (now largely disappeared) and in China,[10,11,71] where local dogs regularly feed on infected commensal rodent and lagomorph intermediate hosts. In these circumstances, indirect or direct contamination from feces of infected dogs appears to be the most important source of infection, and human infection prevalence may reach 2% to 6%.[10,11]

Echinococcus multilocularis has an extensive geographic range in the Northern Hemisphere, widespread and increasing in Europe, most of northern Eurasia, from Bulgaria and Turkey through most of Russia, and the newly independent nations of the former Soviet Union, extending eastward to several of

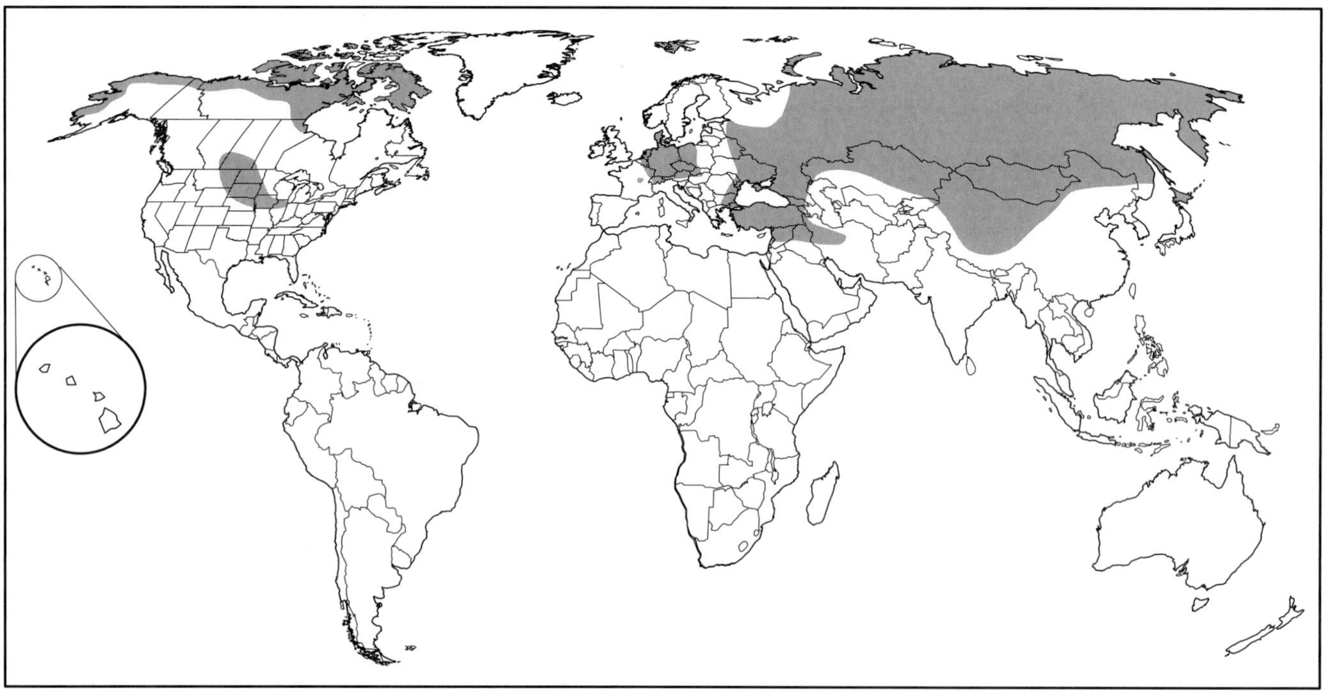

Echinococcus multilocularis

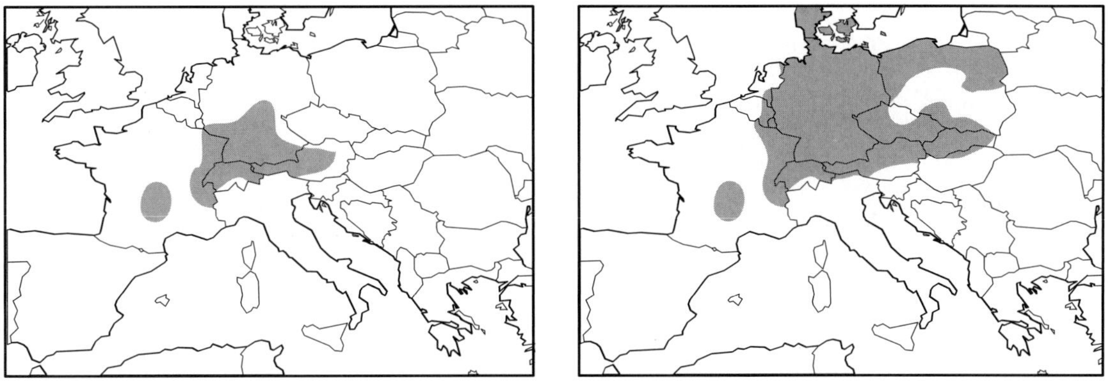

the Japanese islands.[9] In North America, the cestode is found throughout the northern tundra zone and in a discontinuous zone to the south. In the Middle East, *E. multilocularis* is reported in eastern Turkey and Iran. One human case has been reported in northern India.[72] The report of human cases from a mountainous region of northern Tunisia was the first indication of the occurrence of *E. multilocularis* in North Africa.[73]

Recent surveys in Central Europe have extended the known distribution of *E. multilocularis* from four countries at the end of the 1980s to at least 11 countries in 1999. The incidence of diagnosed disease in humans remains low, between 0.02 and 1.4 per 100,000 for entire countries or larger regions of endemicity.[74] Between 1982 and 2000, 559 cases of alveolar echinococcosis in humans were reported voluntarily from nine European countries to the European Echinococcosis Registry.[75] The cestode appears to have spread eastward in Europe in association with increased populations of foxes, and this may herald the emergence of AE in humans in central Eastern Europe. Surveys of foxes in Germany and France carried out in the mid-1990s compared recent data with that collected in the 1970s and 1980s and documented higher fox densities as well as increased prevalences of *E. multilocularis* infection.[76,77] New human cases have been reported during the past 10 years in several European countries previously considered nonendemic: Belgium, The Netherlands, Luxembourg, Czech Republic, Slovak Republic, Poland, Italy, Slovenia, Hungary, Bulgaria, and Romania.[74] Increasing fox populations, increasing encroachment of foxes into urban areas, and spillover of *E. multilocularis* infection from wild carnivores to domestic dogs and cats might presage increased public health risks of AE.[78,79]

The known distribution and prevalence of infection in foxes and coyotes have increased in central North America. Before 1964, there were no reports of *E. multilocularis* in North America south of the Arctic tundra zone, but in that year it was reported in foxes and rodents in North Dakota.[80] By 1969, parasitologic surveys revealed that the cestode was established in cycles involving red foxes, coyotes, and deer mice in North and South Dakota, Minnesota, Montana, and Iowa and the Canadian provinces of Manitoba, Saskatchewan, and Alberta.[61,81] The known range was further extended in the 1970s and 1980s by reports from Wyoming, Nebraska, Wisconsin, Illinois, Indiana, Michigan, and Ohio.[82–85] Exposure of humans appears to be rare. To date, only two people are known to have acquired their infections in the endemic region in central North America: a 54-year-old man from Manitoba, Canada, and a 60-year-old woman from Minnesota[67]; however, the potential exists for a more serious public health problem.[9,65]

DISEASE

After ingestion, cestode eggs hatch and release embryos (oncospheres) in the small intestine. Penetration through the mucosa leads to blood-borne distribution to the liver and other sites, where larval development begins. The primary infection in humans is in the liver, but direct extension to contiguous organs, as well as hematogenous metastases to the lungs and brain, is not uncommon. Alveolar echinococcosis in humans is comparable to that in the natural intermediate hosts (viz., the primary larval lesion develops in the liver) but differs in that the larval mass is inhibited by the host from completing its development and remains in the proliferative stage indefinitely. The larval mass resembles a malignancy in appearance and behavior; thus, it continues to invade and destroy the hepatic parenchyma and surrounding tissues, and retrogressive stages within the mass result in necrosis of the central portion (Fig. 114-8). In chronic AE infections, the

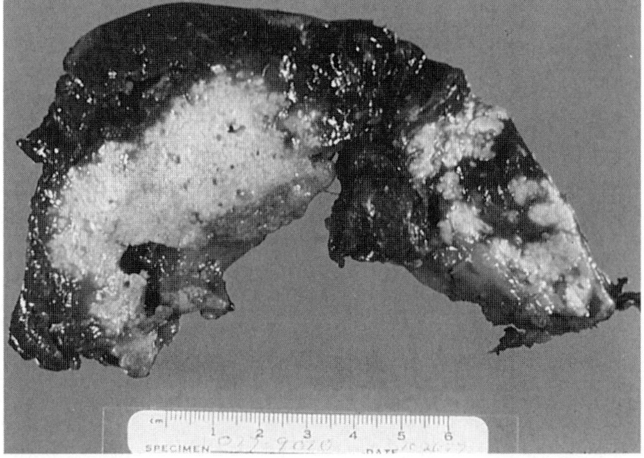

FIGURE 114-8 Alveolar echinococcosis lesion involving the left lobe of the liver following surgical resection. Note extensive destruction of the hepatic parenchyma and the necrosis producing a central abscess. (Courtesy of Dr. W. A. Gamble, Minneapolis.)

lesion consists of a central necrotic cavity filled with a white amorphous material that is covered with a thin peripheral layer of dense fibrous tissue.[86] There are focal areas of calcification and extensive infiltration by proliferating vesicles. Protoscolices are rarely observed in infections of humans. Host tissue is directly invaded by extension of the budding and proliferating cyst wall, causing a pressure necrosis of surrounding host tissue (Fig. 114-9). A fibrous tissue reaction usually surrounds the larval mass, and a moderate inflammatory reaction is restricted to active lesions. Symptoms are often vague, with presenting complaints of right upper quadrant discomfort or pain, weight loss, and malaise. Occasionally, symptoms related to pulmonary or cerebral metastases may constitute the presenting symptoms.[87]

Cases of AE are typically characterized by an initial asymptomatic incubation period of 5 to 15 years and a subsequent chronic course. Because of the natural history of the disease, the nonspecificity of early symptoms, and perhaps because health-care providers may not be familiar with the disease, diagnosis is often delayed until an advanced and inoperable stage. Alveolar echinococcosis is a serious disease; although some *E. multilocularis* infections in humans resolve spontaneously in the early stages of the disease,[88] the death rate in progressive, clinically manifest cases is high. With or without surgery, reported mortality rates have ranged between 50% and 75%.[17] Screening of populations at risk by abdominal imaging (ultrasound or CT scans) followed by specific immunodiagnostic techniques detects cases in the early stages of alveolar echinococcosis and, consequently, improves the prognosis by reducing complications, morbidity, and mortality.[74] A clinical classification system for human AE has been proposed and designated as the PNM system (P, primary lesion; N, involvement of neighboring organs, including lymph nodes; and M, metastases). The PNM classification follows closely the TNM classification of hepatocellular carcinoma and allows an anatomical description of the lesion at initial presentation as well as a prospective staging of the disease (stage I to stage IV).[89] The PNM system aids a precise description of the disease at diagnosis, providing a baseline for evaluation of treatment strategies.

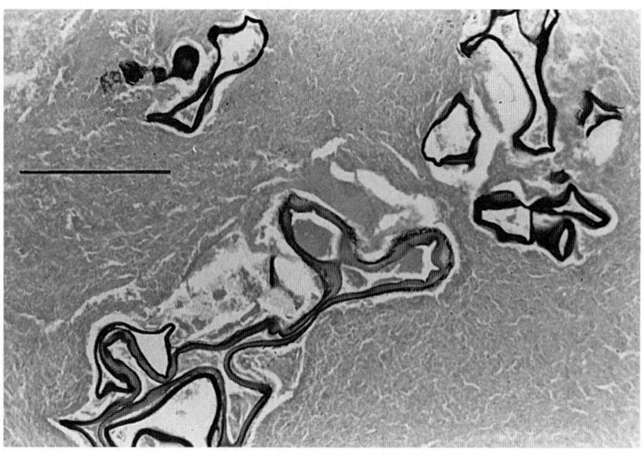

FIGURE 114-9 *Echinococcus multilocularis* larvae in liver tissue of infected patient. Irregular cuticular vesicles are prominently stained by the positive acid-Schiff reaction. (Bar = 100 μm)

PATHOGENESIS AND IMMUNITY

Immunologic or constitutional resistance to infection or immunologic resistance to disease following infection may be common features.[90] Although high levels of parasite-specific antibodies are characteristic of infections, antibodies do not appear to restrict the growth of the metacestode. In contrast, T lymphocyte interactions are of great immunopathologic significance. Periparasitic granulomas—mainly composed of macrophages, myofibroblasts, and T cells—contain a large number of CD4+ lymphocytes in patients with so-called abortive or died-out lesions, whereas in patients with active metacestodes, the number of CD8+ cells is increased.[91] An association between lymphoproliferative responsiveness and mechanisms of resistance or susceptibility to *E. multilocularis* infections has also been suggested by comparative in vitro lymphocyte stimulation assays in patients with different courses of disease. Interleukin-5 and interleukin-10 were shown to be the predominant cytokines produced by peripheral blood mononuclear cells in patients with AE, indicating the activation of Th2 immune responses in disease.[92–94] Whereas the innate immune system seems to be highly activated, there is no specific memory T cell response detectable in the chronic state of the disease.[95,96] It seems that viable larvae efficiently suppress specific cellular immune responses.

Clinical observations have allowed discrimination between two groups of people infected with *E. multilocularis*: those who develop disease, thus reflecting susceptibility to unlimited metacestode proliferation, and those in whom metacestode proliferation has ceased, who harbor intrahepatic died-out lesions, and thus reflect resistance to disease. A third group of people demonstrating putative immunologic resistance to infection has become evident in seroepidemiologic surveys. Many apparently exposed people (as evidenced by seroconversion to specific *E. multilocularis* antigen, i.e., Em2) do not permit postoncospheral parasite development and are assumed to be resistant.[90]

Murine models of AE have shown that a pre-existing larval infection can prevent or suppress the development of a secondary infection, but once a primary infection is established in susceptible laboratory rodents, the initial *E. multilocularis* metacestode appears well protected from the host immune response.[97] Depletion of T cells enhances metastasis formation in mice. Activated macrophages appear to be key participants in the immune response because they adhere to the metacestode; the cestode grows and metastasizes despite a marked lymphoproliferative activity in the B and T cell areas of lymphoid tissue. The parasite may survive by actively impairing cellular mechanisms of recognition and neutrophil chemotaxis in experimentally infected mice. Susceptibility and resistance to infection with *E. multilocularis* metacestodes may depend on genetically based immunologic factors, as evidenced by marked differences in susceptibility to infection in different mouse strains.

DIAGNOSIS

Clinical onset of AE typically occurs in people of advanced age. In the large European Registry, mean age at first diagnosis was 52.5 years, with a range of 5 to 86 years and a gender ratio of 1:1.2.[75] The disease closely mimics hepatic carcinoma and is a challenge to diagnose, even in endemic regions. The most frequent morphological profile of AE is an intrahepatic heterogeneous, infiltrative, and destructive mass, with irregular outlines, and an avascular and necrotic center that appears on abdominal ultrasound as a hypoechoic lesion with a hyperechoic rim. The usual CT image of the same lesion is a hypodense structure with a density of 0 to 25 Hounsfield units, often showing characteristic hyperdense, plaque-like calcifications.[98] The multivesicular pattern of the lesion is most clearly demarcated on T1-weighted MRI images, whereas the nonhomogeneous character of the lesion is appreciated on T2-weighted images (Fig. 114-10). Fluoro-desoxyglucose positron emission tomography (FDG-PET) was reported to be a reliable method for the determination of metabolic activity in and around *E. multilocularis* liver lesions, thereby allowing the "functional imaging" of infectious lesions.[99,100]

Most patients with AE respond to infection with synthesis of parasite-specific antibodies, including all isotypes of immunoglobulins.[90] Serologic tests are usually positive at high titers; highly specific antigens[101–103] have been identified and synthesized that, when used in serologic assays, are highly sensitive and specific for diagnosis of AE and can distinguish this infection from CE (*E. granulosus*) and other forms of echinococcosis.

As in CE, serologic tests are more useful for evaluating prognosis following surgery than for determining outcome of chemotherapy.[104] Antibodies persist indefinitely in the serum of patients treated by chemotherapy; however, negative seroconversion occurs within 1 year in patients whose lesion is completely extirpated by surgery. Antibodies of the IgG1 and IgG4 isotypes are the most sensitive IgG responses in AE, and monitoring of these isotypes tended to correlate with active vs. inactive disease and successful treatment.[105]

In seronegative patients, PCR reactions for detection of echinococcal-specific RNA or DNA in closed or open biopsy specimens have been developed and may confirm the diagnosis.[106–108] Exploratory laparotomy, sometimes performed to confirm the diagnosis and delineate the size and extent of the invasive lesion, should be avoided because of potential spread of larval tissue into the peritoneal cavity.

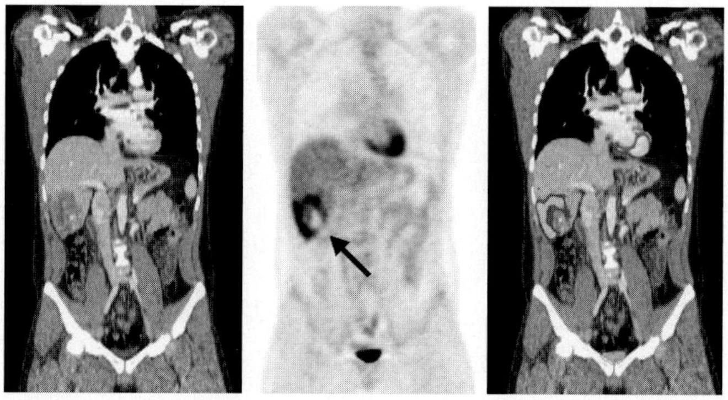

FIGURE 114-10 Images of alveolar echinococcosis, coronal views. *Left,* Computed tomographic (CT) image of liver of a patient with alveolar echinococcosis. *Middle,* The same lesion visualized by 18-fluor-desoxyglucose positron emission tomography (FDG-PET). Note enhancement of the periphery of the image indicating enhanced metabolic activity of host cells in response to the viable *E. multilocularis* larvae (*arrow*). *Right,* PET-CT; the coloration indicates different intensities of metabolic activity.

TREATMENT

Clinicians familiar with this disease emphasize that management of AE, characterized by a malignant-like proliferating cestode, is extremely difficult and usually requires radical surgery, ideally at an early stage, and long-term or lifelong chemotherapy with benzimidazoles.[17,37,109] Choosing from the variety of treatment options requires specific clinical experience; therefore, patients should be referred to recognized national or regional AE treatment centers.[37] Experience in AE screening programs in Japan and elsewhere has shown that early diagnosis reduces morbidity and mortality. Surgical treatment usually requires extensive resection of host tissue (i.e., partial or total resection of the affected hepatic lobe) and should only be performed if a safety margin of 2 cm can be achieved.[110] In cases that are inoperable, in which resection is incomplete or partial, or in cases in which there are metastases to the brain or lungs, surgery must be followed by benzimidazole chemotherapy. In clinical trials with patient follow-up of many years, mebendazole administered continuously for up to 10 years at doses of 40 to 50 mg/kg body weight per day inhibited progression of AE and reduced lesion size in approximately half of treated cases.[111,112] In patients administered albendazole for repeated periods of 28 days at doses of 10 mg/kg body weight per day with treatment-free intervals of 14 days or given continuously, the results were similar to those described with mebendazole.[112–114] Benzimidazole treatment enhanced length and quality of life. In most cases, chemotherapy with either drug was not parasiticidal; however, there are some indications that parasite death may occur after treatment for many years.[37,111,114] In Europe, postoperative chemotherapy for 2 years is routinely carried out after radical resection, with careful monitoring of the patient for a minimum of 10 years for possible recurrence.[115]

Liver transplantation is not recommended as a treatment option since larval infiltration of the transplant from the surrounding tissue is frequent. However, in patients with terminal liver disease, transplantation may prolong survival.[116]

PREVENTION AND CONTROL

In regions where the infection is enzootic in sylvatic cycles, emphasis should be placed on personal preventive measures, including avoiding contact with foxes and other potentially infected definitive hosts and carefully washing and cooking vegetables and other fresh produce. Control of working and pet dogs and cats must be practiced to prevent them from preying on rodents and, thereby, becoming infected.[9,66] Infections in dogs and cats that are liable to eat infected rodents can be prevented by prophylactic treatments with praziquantel (5 mg/kg body weight); under conditions of intense transmission, prophylactic treatments would have to be given at intervals no longer than 30 days (the prepatent period of the cestode) to most effectively prevent excretion of eggs. People living in areas where *E. multilocularis* is enzootic should be educated about the potential dangers, to promote better personal hygiene and sanitation and to motivate them to take effective measures to prevent their pets from eating rodents.

Active intervention for control of *E. multilocularis* presents special difficulties because the primary cycle is almost always sylvatic. In most regions where *E. multilocularis* is enzootic, controlling the cestode by eliminating its sylvatic hosts would be impractical for economic and logistic reasons or unacceptable for ecological reasons.[9] Two approaches to control of infection in sylvatic hosts, one mainly of historical interest and the other experimental, are described next. Where exposure of humans is mainly related to cycles involving synanthropic hosts (i.e., dogs), protection might be achieved by regular taeniacidal treatments of dogs; one such demonstration project is described here.

Control in Sylvatic Life Cycles

Approximately 25 years after its introduction in foxes translocated from the Kuril islands, *E. multilocularis* was eliminated from Rebun Island in Japan by eliminating the cestode's hosts. Between 1950 and 1955, 2026 foxes and 3224 dogs were captured and killed; without adequate numbers of definitive hosts *E. multilocularis* was soon eliminated. This is the only known instance in which *E. multilocularis* has been eradicated from an area where it was previously enzootic. However, *E. multilocularis* continues to spread on Hokkaido Island and threatens to become established on the mainland of Japan.[117]

Increases in the fox populations in areas of Europe have led to introduction of *E. multilocularis* into urban environments. Although this has not been associated with apparent increases in infections in humans, it has raised public health concerns. In Zurich, Switzerland, monthly distribution of praziquantel-containing baits during a 16-month period resulted in significantly decreased prevalence in foxes (from 39% to 67% to 1.8% to 5.5%), whereas infection in foxes remained the same in nonbaited control areas.[118]

Control in Synanthropic Cycles

Where it is determined that dogs frequently become infected by preying on commensal rodents, thus contributing significantly to local environmental contamination with eggs and potential human exposure, periodic mass echinococcidal treatments of dogs is one approach to reducing the risk of human infection. This was evaluated in a 10-year field trial in a village on St. Lawrence Island, Alaska, where *E. multilocularis* was hyperendemic.[119] All dogs in this village were given praziquantel 5 mg/kg body weight at monthly intervals. This was effective in reducing egg contamination as evidenced by an average 83% reduction in infection prevalence in voles during the course of the trial; prevalence in locally captured voles declined from an average of 29% at the beginning of the trial to less than 5% at the end. Fluctuations in the annual incidence of infection in voles appeared to be related to the degree that dog owners cooperated in making their pets available for treatment. This control method, which is relatively costly, may be applicable to other regions where synanthropic cycles create a high risk for local human populations; such areas may include recently described endemic foci in Gansu, Qinghai, and Sichuan provinces, China, where surveys showed high rates of infection in domestic dogs.[10,11] The costs and benefits of this approach require further evaluation.

Polycystic Echinococcosis (*Echinococcus vogeli* and *Echinococcus oligarthrus*)

AGENTS

Echinococcus vogeli was first described by Rausch and Bernstein[120] in 1972 from adult specimens recovered from a bush dog, *Speothos venaticus*, captured in the province of Esmeraldas, Ecuador. *Echinococcus oligarthrus* was first described by Diesing in 1863 from strobilate specimens recovered from a Brazilian puma. The larval cyst from the Brazilian agouti was named *Echinococcus cruzi* by Brumpt and Joyeux in 1924 but was subsequently shown to be that of *E. oligarthrus*.[121] *Echinococcus vogeli* is the principal cause of the polycystic form of echinocccosis in humans.[122,123] Both species utilize the same intermediate hosts (hystricognath rodents), in which the macroscopic appearance of the larval cysts is similar; however, differentiation of *E. vogeli* and *E. oligarthrus* (as well as other species of *Echinococcus*) can be made on the basis of the length and proportions of the rostellar hooks.[124] Because *E. oligarthrus* is known to infect humans, both are considered to be causes of PE. The metacestode of *E. vogeli* is fluid-filled, with a tendency to form multichambered conglomerates (polycystic); the predilection site in the intermediate host is the liver.[122,123] Endogenous proliferation and convolution of both germinal and laminated layers leads to the formation of secondary subdivisions of brood capsules and protoscolices.[124,125] The *E. oligarthrus* metacestode is similar; however, there is less subdivision into secondary chambers and the laminated layer is significantly thinner than that of *E. vogeli*. In lower animal hosts and in humans, *E. oligarthrus* metacestodes tend to be localized in the muscles or other extrahepatic sites (Fig. 114-11).

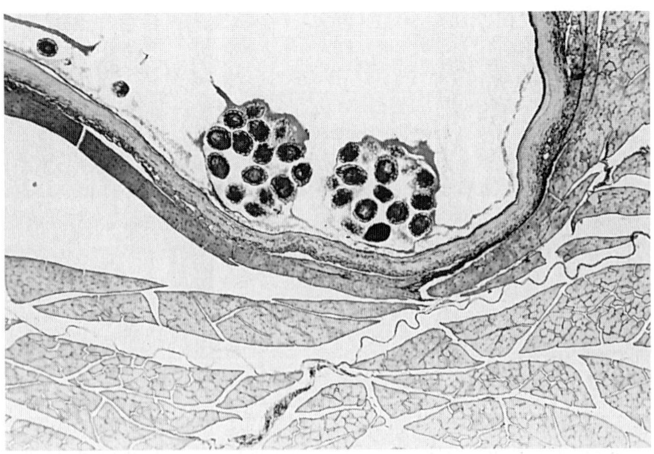

FIGURE 114-11 Hydatid cyst of *Echinococcus oligarthrus* from intramuscular connective tissue of an infected rodent. (H&E; magnification about ×1000) (Courtesy of Dr. O. E. Sousa, Panama City, Panama.)

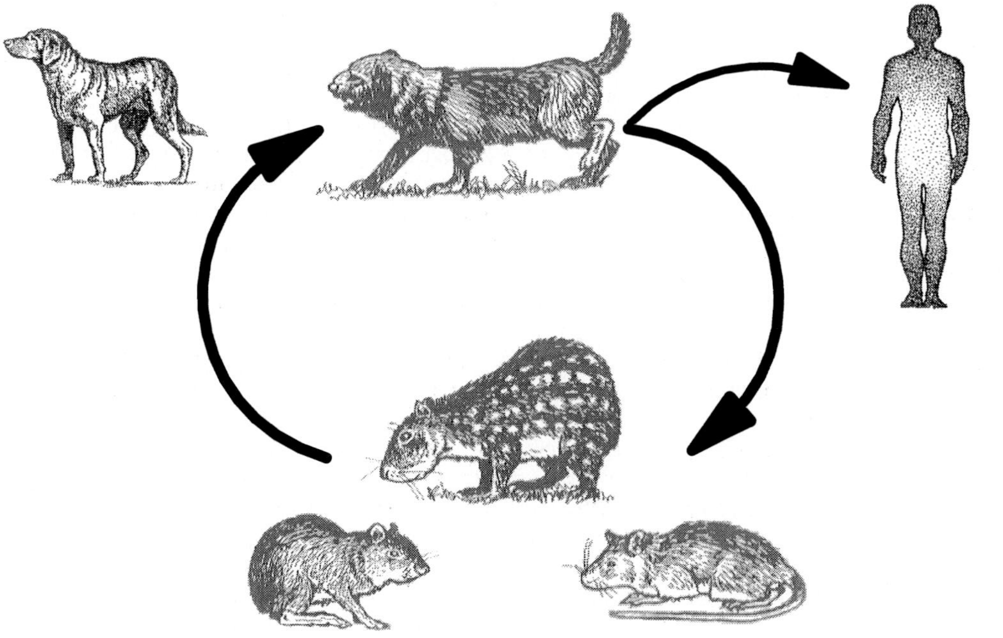

FIGURE 114-12 Life cycle and principal and alternative hosts for *Echinococcus vogeli.*

TRANSMISSION, EPIDEMIOLOGY, AND GEOGRAPHIC DISTRIBUTION

The life cycle of *E. vogeli* involves the bush dog and the paca, *Cuniculus paca*, as definitive and intermediate hosts, respectively (Fig. 114-12). Domestic dogs are also suitable definitive hosts. *Echinococcus vogeli* larvae have also been found in agoutis (*Dasyprocta* spp.) and spiny rats (*Proechimys* spp.).[122,123] Very little is known about the circumstances associated with infection with this species. Bush dogs are rare and avoid human beings, and therefore probably play little role in direct exposure of humans. In endemic areas, human infections are probably acquired from the feces of domestic dogs that become infected when they ingest viscera of infected pacas; this practice has been reported commonly by patients.[122,123]

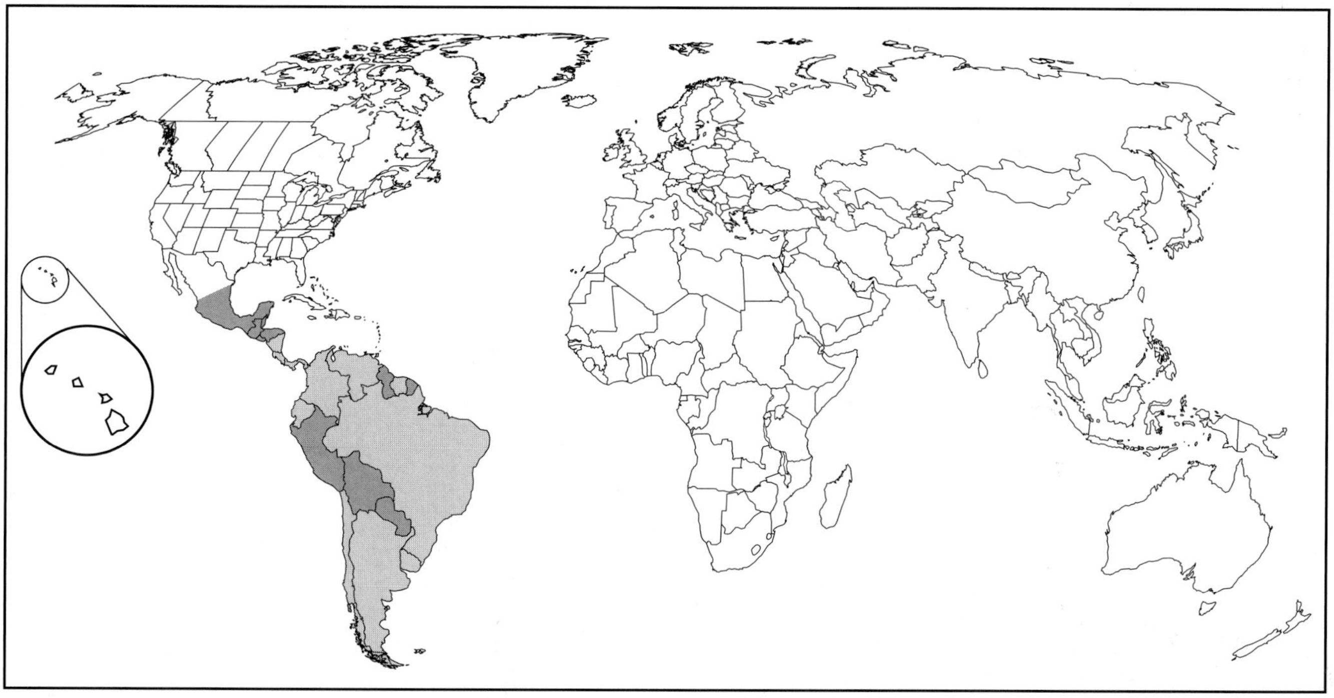

Echinococcus vogeli and *Echinococcus oligarthrus*

▪ Countries in which cases of polycystic echinococcosis in humans have been documented.

▪ Countries in which *E. vogeli* and *E. oligarthrus* are known to occur in animal hosts.

Polycystic echinococcosis due to *E. vogeli* infection has been reported in most countries within the cestode's known range in neotropical America, including Costa Rica, Panama, Colombia, Argentina, Ecuador, Brazil, Bolivia, and Venezuela.[122,123] Some cases of PE are mistakenly assumed to be *E. granulosus* infection. The natural hosts of *E. vogeli* range throughout neotropical areas of Central and South America, and as local awareness and availability of diagnostic capability increase, it is probable that increasing numbers of cases will be recorded.

The infected bush dog, from which the specimens originally identified as *E. vogeli* were recovered,[126] was housed temporarily in the "children's area" of the Los Angeles Zoo adjacent to an enclosure that housed a variety of infant higher primates, including gorillas, gibbons, orangutans, and chimpanzees. The primates were exposed to eggs in feces of the infected canid and many of them became infected, with at least 15 of them dying of polycystic hydatid disease during the ensuing 10 years.[127] No infections in zoo employees or visitors were ever identified, but this incident illustrates the potential public health hazards associated with housing wild-caught animals that are potential hosts of *Echinococcus* spp.

Echinococcus oligarthrus is the only species of *Echinococcus* that characteristically uses wild felids as definitive hosts (Fig. 114-13). Naturally acquired infections have been demonstrated in the puma, the jaguarundi, the jaguar, the ocelot, the pampas cat, and Geoffroy's cat.[1] The larval forms of *E. oligarthrus* have been described in agoutis, pacas, spiny rats, and rabbits (*Sylvilagus floridianus*). Human infection with *E. oligarthrus* is extremely rare; only three human cases are documented.[127–129] Presumably, the remote behavior of the definitive hosts limits human exposure. The documented range of *E. oligarthrus* extends from northern Mexico to southern Argentina[128]; however, one of the definitive hosts of this species, the puma, ranges from Canada to Tierra del Fuego so that this cestode may be found through the Americas. The three confirmed cases of human disease caused by *E. oligarthrus* were reported from Venezuela and Brazil.[127–129]

DISEASE

Approximately 80 human cases of PE have been recorded, mainly (more than 85%) from Brazil, Colombia, Ecuador, and Argentina.[122,123,130,131] Patients' ages at diagnosis have ranged from 6 to 78 years (median, 44), and the most common signs at presentation were hepatomegaly, palpable peritoneal masses, and jaundice. Polycystic echinococcosis has characteristics intermediate between the cystic and alveolar forms. Of cases in which the causative agent was speciated, the ratio of *E. vogeli* to *E. oligarthrus* was approximately 10:1. The primary localization of *E. vogeli* infections is the liver, but cysts often invade contiguous sites. In humans and other higher primates, the *E. vogeli* metacestode proliferates by means of a unique process after which extensive spread into the peritoneal cavity and other organs usually occurs.[125] Hepatomegaly or tumor-like masses in the liver have been typical findings. The lungs are involved in approximately 15% of cases. The clinical findings may be suggestive of malignancy, and the disease may lead to progressive deterioration of hepatic function, portal hypertension, and biliary cirrhosis. The prognosis for PE caused by *E. vogeli* is poor; approximately 14% of patients die from complications of biliary obstruction and portal hypertension. The three known cases of *E. oligarthrus* infection have involved the eyes (two cases) and the heart.[127,128]

Macroscopically, the larva of *E. vogeli* appears as a whitish-gray polycystic structure that contains a yellow fluid or gel.[132] The entire cyst may measure only 10 mm in diameter or may form vesicular aggregates that replace most of the liver. The protoscolex with its four circular suckers and rostellum with hooks can be seen in wet mount preparations and tissue sections. The large hooks are 38 to 46 μm in length, and the small hooks measure 30 to 37 μm. Microscopically, there are multiple vesicles, varying in size from a few millimeters to centimeters. The vesicles are partitioned by septa formed from the hyaline laminated membrane that is 8 to 65 μm thick and stains intensely by the periodic acid-Schiff technique. The internal surface of the septa is lined with a germinal membrane that is 3 to 13 μm thick and contains calcareous corpuscles.

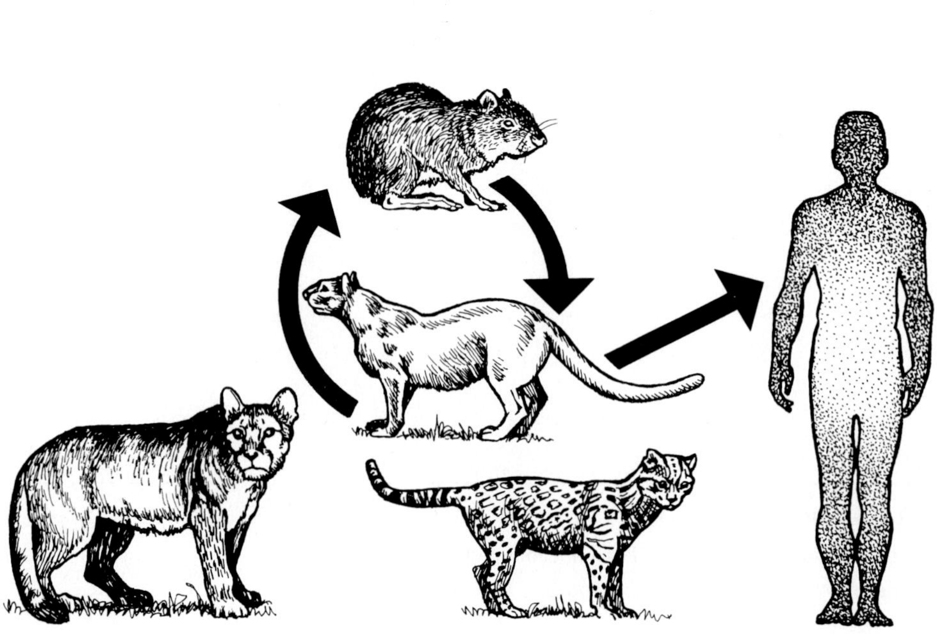

FIGURE 114-13 Life cycle and principal and alternative hosts for *Echinococcus oligarthrus*.

The brood capsules bud internally from the germinal epithelium. Externally, the cyst is surrounded by fibrous tissue, with only slight cellular infiltration. Portions of these cysts are frequently necrotic and mineralized, and the only remains of *Echinococcus* may be the hooks and calcareous corpuscles.

DIAGNOSIS

The diagnosis of PE should be considered in patients who present with abdominal masses and who live or previously lived in rural Central or South American regions where the cestode agents are known to occur.[122] Radiologic imaging (radiograph, ultrasound, or CT) is very useful for demonstrating polycystic structures and diffuse mineralization in the liver or other sites (Fig. 114-14). Serologic tests are often, but not invariably, useful for confirming the diagnosis. Specific *E. vogeli* antigens may differentiate hydatid disease due to *E. vogeli* from that caused by *E. granulosus* but not from *E. multilocularis*; however, tests using *E. vogeli*-specific antigens are not widely available.[133]

TREATMENT

Experience in the treatment of PE is limited. The principles of management of CE and AE also apply to PE. Because the lesions are so extensive, surgical resection may be difficult and usually incomplete. A combination of surgery with albendazole treatment is most likely to be successful.[122] Approximately 40% of patients with *E. vogeli* PE improved (reduction or disappearance of cysts for 10 to 30 months) after receiving albendazole 10 mg/kg/day for different lengths of time from weeks to months.[122,130]

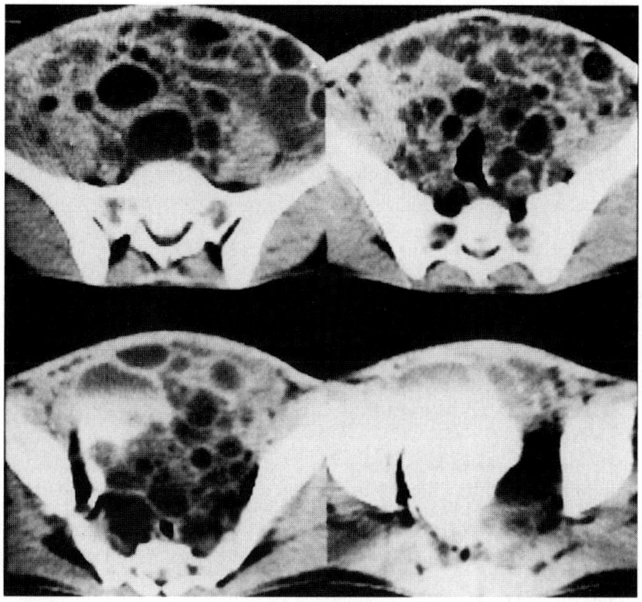

FIGURE 114-14 Abdominal computed tomography scans showing multiple *Echinococcus vogeli* larvae (polycystic echinococcosis). The lesions are hypodense, round or oval, and scattered in the liver, spleen, and abdominal cavity. (Courtesy of Dr. V. G. Meneghelli, São Paulo, Brazil.)

PREVENTION AND CONTROL

In regions where *E. vogeli* and *E. oligarthrus* are enzootic in sylvatic cycles, emphasis should be placed on personal preventive measures, including avoiding contact with wild canids and felids. Raw viscera of animals killed in hunting should not be given to dogs and cats. Control of pet dogs and cats must be practiced to prevent them from preying on rodents and thereby becoming infected. For dogs or cats that cannot be controlled and that habitually prey on local rodents, prophylactic treatment with praziquantel 5 mg/kg body weight can be given. People living in areas where *E. vogeli* and *E. oligarthrus* are enzootic should be educated about the potential dangers, to promote better personal hygiene and sanitation and to motivate them to take effective measures to prevent their pets from becoming infected.

No experiences have been reported on active intervention to limit transmission in any area.

REFERENCES

1. Thompson RCA, McManus DP: Toward a revised nomenclature of *Echinococcus*. Trends Parasitol 18:452, 2002.
2. McManus DP, Thompson RCA: Molecular epidemiology of cystic echinococcosis. Parasitology 127:S37, 2003.
3. Xiao N, Qiu J, Nakao M, et al: *Echinococcus shiquicus*: A new species of hydatid parasite from the Tibetan Plateau. Int J Parasitol 35:693, 2005.
4. Eckert J, Gemmel MA, Meslin F-X, et al (eds): WHO/OIE Manual on Echinococcosis in Humans and Animals: A Public Health Problem of Global Concern. Paris, World Health Organization/ World Organization for Animal Health, 2001.
5. Haag KL, Araujo AM, Gottstein B, et al: Breeding systems in *Echinococcus granulosus* (Cestoda, Taeniidae): Selfing or outcrossing? Parasitology 118:63, 1998.
6. Pawlowski Z, Stefaniak J: The pig strain of *Echinococcus granulosus* in humans: A neglected issue? Trends Parasitol 19:439, 2003.
7. Wilson JF, Diddams AC, Rausch RL: Cystic hydatid disease in Alaska. A review of 101 autochthonous cases of *E. granulosus* infection. Am Rev Respir Dis 98:1, 1968.
8. Lavikkainen A, Kehtinen J, Meri T, et al: Molecular genetic characterization of the Fennoscandian cervid strain, a new genotypic group (G10) of *Echinococcus granulosus*. Parasitology 127:S207, 2003.
9. Schantz PM, Chai J, Craig PS, et al: Epidemiology and control. In Thompson RCA, Lymbery AJ (eds): Echinococcosis and Hydatid Disease. London, CAB, 1995, p 233.
10. Schantz PM, Wang H, Qiu J, et al: Echinococcosis on the Tibetan Plateau: Prevalence and risk factors for cystic and alveolar echinococcosis in Tibetan populations in Qinghai Province, China. Parasitology 127:S109, 2003.
11. Wang Q, Qiu J, Schantz P, et al: Investigation of risk factors for development of human hydatidosis among households raising livestock in Tibetan areas of Western Sichuan Province. Chin J Parasit Dis 19:93, 2001.
12. Torgerson PR: Economic effects of echinococcosis. Acta Trop 85:113, 2003.
13. Torgerson PR, Budke CM: Echinococcosi—An international public health challenge. Res Vet Sci 74:191, 2003.
14. Shaikenov BS, Torgerson, PR, Usenbayev KK, et al: The changing epidemiology of echinococcosis in Kazakhstan due to transformation of farming practices. Acta Trop 85:287, 2003.
15. Amir-Jahed AK, Fardin R, Farzad A, et al: Clinical echinococcosis. Ann Surg 82:541, 1975.
16. Little JM: Hydatid disease at Royal Prince Alfred Hospital 1964–1974. Med J Aust 1:903, 1976.
17. Morris DL, Richards KS: Hydatid Disease: Current Medical and Surgical Management. Oxford, Butterworth-Heineman, 1992.
18. Kammerer WS, Schantz PM: Echinococcal disease. Infect Dis Clin North Am 7:605, 1993.
19. Purriel P, Schantz PM, Beovide H, et al: Human echinococcosis (hydatidosis) in Uruguay: A comparison of indices of morbidity and mortality, 1962–1971. Bull World Health Organ 49:395, 1974.

20. Holman B, Heath D: The early stages of *Echinococcus granulosus* development. Acta Trop 64:5, 1997.
21. Heath DD: Immunobiology of *Echinococcus* infections. In Thompson RCA, Lymberry AJ (eds): The Biology of *Echinococcus* and Hydatid Disease. London, Allen & Unwin, 1996, p 169.
22. Lightowlers MW, Lawrence SB, Gauci CG, et al: Vaccination against hydatidosis using a defined recombinant antigen. Parasite Immunol 18:457, 1996.
23. Suwan Z: Sonographic findings in hydatid disease of the liver: Comparison with other imaging methods. Ann Trop Med Parasitol 89:261, 1996.
24. Macpherson CNL, Bartholomot B, Frider B: Application of ultrasound in diagnosis, treatment, epidemiology, public health and control of *Echinococcus granulosus* and *E. multilocularis*. Parasitology 127:S21, 2003.
25. Anonymous: International classification of ultrasound images in cystic echincoccosis for application in clinical and field epidemiological settings. Acta Trop 85:253, 2003.
26. Maddison SE, Slemenda SB, Schantz PM, et al: A specific diagnostic antigen of *Echinococcus granulosus* with an apparent molecular weight of 8 Kda. Am J Trop Med Hyg 40:377, 1989.
27. Moro PL, Gilman RH, Wilson M, et al: Immunoblot and double diffusion (DD5) tests for hydatid disease cross-react with sera from patients with cysticercosis. Trans R Soc Trop Med Hyg 86:422, 1992.
28. Devi CS, Parija SC: A new serum hydatid detection test for diagnosis of cystic echinococcosis. Am J Trop Med Hyg 69:525, 2003.
29. Gottstein B, Mowatt MR: Sequencing and characterization of an *Echinococcus multilocularis* DNA probe and its use in the polymerase chain reaction. Mol Biochem Parasitol 44:183, 1991.
30. Pawlowski ZS, Eckert J, Vuitton DA, et al: Echinococcosis in humans: Clinical aspects, diagnosis and treatment. In Eckert J, Gemmel MA, Meslin F-X, et al (eds): WHO/OIE Manual on Echinococcosis in Humans and Animals: A Public Health Problem of Global Concern. Paris, World Health Organization/World Organization for Animal Health, 2001, p 20.
31. Menezes da Silva A: Hydatid cyst of the liver—Criteria for the selection of appropriate treatment. Acta Trop 85:237, 2003.
32. Buttenschoen K, Buttenschoen DC: *Echinococcus granulosus* infection: The challenge of surgical treatment. Langenbecks Arch Surg 388:218, 2003.
33. Prasad J, Bellamy PR: Instillation of scolicidal agents into hepatic hydatid cysts: Can it any longer be justified? N Z Med J 104:336, 1991.
34. Dautovic-Krkic S, Huskic J, Cengic D, et al: Praziquantel in the prevention of recurrence of human echincoccosis. Medicinski Arhiv 56:263, 2002.
35. Gil-Grande LA, Rodriguez-Cabeiro F, Prieto JG, et al: Randomised controlled trial of efficacy of albendazole in intra-abdominal hydatid disease. Lancet 342:1269, 1993.
36. Franchi C, DiVico B, Teggi A: Long-term evaluation for patients with hydatidosis treated with benzimidazole carbamates. Clin Infect Dis 29:304, 1999.
37. Horton J: Albendazole for the treatment of echinococcosis. Fundam Clin Pharmacol 17:205, 2003.
38. Kern P: *Echinococcus granulosus* infection: Clinical presentation, medical treatment and outcome. Langenbecks Arch Surg 388:413, 2003.
39. Chai J, Menghebat, Jiao W, et al: Clinical efficacy of albendazole emulsion in treatment of 212 cases of liver cystic hydatidosis. Chin Med J 115:1809, 2002.
40. Cobo F, Yarnoz C, Sesma B, et al: Albendazole plus praziquantel versus albendazole alone as a pre-operative treatment in intra-abdominal hydatidosis caused by *Echinococcus granulosus*. Trop Med Int Health 3:462, 1998.
41. Filice C, Strosselli M, Brunetti E, et al: Percutaneous drainage of hydatid liver cysts. Radiology 184:579, 1992.
42. Giorgio A, Tarantino L, Francia G, et al: Unilocular hydatid liver cysts: Treatment with US-guided, double percutaneous aspiration and alcohol injection. Radiology 184:705, 1992.
43. Akhan P, Ozmen MN, Dincer A, et al: Liver hydatid disease: Long-term results of percutaneous treatment. Radiology 198:259, 1996.
44. Salama H, Farid Abdel-Wahab M, Strickland GT: Diagnosis and treatment of hepatic hydatid cysts with the aid of echo-guided percutaneous cyst puncture. Clin Infect Dis 21:1372, 1995.
45. Filice C, Brunetti E: Use of PAIR in echinococcosis. Acta Trop 64:95, 1997.
46. Akhan P, Ozmen MN, Dincer A, et al: Percutaneous treatment of pulmonary hydatid cysts. Cardiovasc Intervent Radiol 17:271, 1994.
47. Giorgio A, Tarantino L, de Stefano G, et al: Hydatid liver cyst: An 11-year experience of treatment with percutaneous aspiration and ethanol injection. J Ultrasound Med 20:729, 2001.
48. World Health Organization: Puncture, aspiration, injection, reaspiration—An option for the treatment of cystic echincoccosis. WHO Informal Working Group on Echinococcosis (WHO-IWGE), WHO/CDC/CSR/APH 6, 2001, p 40.
49. Mawhorter S, Temeck B, Chang R, et al: Nonsurgical therapy of pulmonary hydatid cyst disease. Chest 112:1432, 1997.
50. Khuroo MS, Dar MY, Yattoo GN: Percutaneous drainage versus albendazole therapy in hepatic hydatidosis: A prospective, randomized study. Gastroenterology 104:1452, 1993.
51. Khuroo MS, Wani NA, Javid G, et al: Percutaneous drainage compared with surgery for hepatic hydatid cysts. N Engl J Med 337:881, 1997.
52. Haddad MC, Sammak BM, Al-Karawi M: Percutaneous treatment of heterogeneous predominantly solid echopattern echinococcal cysts of the liver. Cardiovasc Intervent Radiol 23:21, 2000.
53. Schipper HG, Lameris JS, van Delden OM, et al: Percutaneous evacuation (PEVAC) of multivesicular echinococcal cysts with or without cystobiliary fistulas which contain non-drainable material: First results of a modified PAIR method. Gut 50:718, 2002.
54. Brunetti E, Filice C: Radiofrequency thermal ablation of echinococcal liver cysts. Lancet 358:1464, 2001.
55. Pelaez, V, Kugler C, Del Carpio M, et al: Estudio de costos de los diferentes tratamientos de quistes hidatidicos hepaticos. Arch Inter Hidat 33:387, 1999.
56. Smego RA Jr, Bhatti S, Khaliq AA, et al: Percutaneous aspiration–injection–reaspiration drainage plus albendazole or mebendazole for hepatic cystic echinococcosis: A meta-analysis. Clin Infect Dis 37:1073, 2003.
57. Rigano R, Ioppolo S, Ortona E, et al: Long-term serological evaluation of patients with cystic echinococcosis treated with benzimidazole carbamates. Clin Exp Immunol 129:485, 2002.
58. Gemmell MA, Roberts MG, Beard TC, et al: Formulating effective and cost-effective policies in the planning phase for permanent control of *Echinococcus granulosus*. In Eckert J, Gemmel MA, Meslin F-X, et al (eds): WHO/OIE Manual on Echinococcosis in Humans and Animals: A Public Health Problem of Global Concern. Paris, World Health Organization/World Organization for Animal Health, 2001, p 209.
59. Rausch RL, Schiller EL: Studies on the helminth fauna of Alaska. XXV. The ecology and public health significance of *Echinococcus sibiricensis* Rausch and Schiller, 1954, on St. Lawrence Island. Parasitology 46:395, 1956.
60. Vogel H: Über den *Echinococcus multilocularis* Süddeutschlands. Tropenmed Parasitol 8:404, 1957.
61. Rausch RL, Richards SH: Observations on parasite–host relationships of *Echinococcus multilocularis* Leuckart, 1863, in North Dakota. Can J Zool 49:1317, 1971.
62. Rinder R, Rausch RL, Takahashi K, et al: Limited range of genetic variation in *Echinococcus multilocularis*. J Parasitol 83:1045, 1997.
63. Thompson RCA, Deplazes P, Eckert J: Observations on the development of *Echinococcus mutilocularis* in cats. J Parasitol 89:1086, 2003.
64. Rausch RL, Fay FH, Williamson FSL: The ecology of *Echinococcus multilocularis* (Cestoda: Taeniidae) on St. Lawrence Island, Alaska. II. Helminth populations in the definitive host. Ann Parasitol Hum Comp 65:131, 1990.
65. Hildreth MB, Sriram S, Gottstein B, et al: Failure to identify alveolar echinococcosis in trappers from South Dakota in spite of high prevalence of *Echinococcus multilocularis* in wild canids. J Parasitol 86:75, 2000.
66. Kern P, Ammon A, Dron M, et al: A case–control study to identify risk factors for alveolar echincoccosis in humans. Emer Infect Dis 10:2088, 2004.
67. Gamble WG, Segal M, Schantz PM, et al: Alveolar hydatid disease in Minnesota. First human case acquired in the contiguous United States. J Am Med Assoc 241:904, 1979.
68. Stehr-Green JA, Stehr-Green PA, Schantz PM: Risk factors for infection with *Echinococcus multilocularis* in Alaska. Am J Trop Med Hyg 38:380, 1988.
69. Eirmann TH, Bettens F, Tiberghien P, et al: HLA and alveolar echinococcosis. Tissue Antigens 52:124,1998.
70. Zhang S, Penfornis A, Harraga S, et al: Polymorphisms of the TAP1 and TAP2 genes in human alveolar echinococcosis. Eur J Immunogenet 30:133, 2003.

71. Craig PS, Liu D, Macpherson CNL, et al: A large focus of alveolar echinococcosis in central China. Lancet 340:826, 1992.
72. Aikat BK, Bhusnurmath SR, Cadersa M: *Echinococcus multilocularis* infection in India. Trans R Soc Trop Med Hyg 72:619, 1978.
73. Zitouna MM, Boubaker S, Dellagi K, et al: Alveolar echinococcosis in Tunisia. Apropo of 2 cases. Bull Soc Pathol Exot 78:723, 1985.
74. Eckert J, Deplazes P: Biological, epidemiological, and clinical aspects of echinococcosis, a zoonosis of increasing concern. Clin Microbiol Rev 17:107, 2004.
75. Kern P, Bardonnet K, Renner E, et al: European Echinococcosis Registry: Human alveolar echinococcosis, Europe, 1982–2000. Emer Infect Dis 9:133, 2003.
76. Romig T, Kratzer W, Kimming P, et al: An epidemiologic survey of human alveolar echinococcosis in southwestern Germany. Romerstein Study Group. Am J Trop Med Hyg 61:566, 1999.
77. Giraudoux P, Craig PS, Delattre P, et al: Interactions between landscape changes and host communities can regulate *Echinococcus multilocularis* transmission. Parasitology 127:S121, 2003.
78. Deplazes P, Hegglin D, Gloor S, et al: Wilderness in the city: The urbanization of *Echinococcus multilocularis*. Trends Parasitol 20:77, 2004.
79. Gottstein B, Saucy F, Deplazes P, et al: Is high prevalence of *Echinococcus multilocularis* in wild and domestic animals associated with disease incidence in humans? Emer Infect Dis 7:408, 2001.
80. Leiby PD, Olsen OW: The cestode *Echinococcus multilocularis* in North Dakota. Science 145:1066, 1964.
81. Leiby PD, Carney WP, Woods CE: Studies on sylvatic echinococcosis. III. Host occurrence and geographic distribution of *Echinococcus multilocularis* in the north central United States. J Parasitol 56:1141, 1970.
82. Ballard NB, Vande Vusse FJ: *Echinococcus multilocularis* in Illinois and Nebraska. J Parasitol 69:790, 1983.
83. Storandt ST, Kazacos KR: *Echinococcus multilocularis* identified in Indiana, Ohio, and east-central Illinois. J Parasitol 79:301, 1993.
84. Storandt ST, Kazacos KR: *Echinococcus multilocularis* in Wisconsin. J Parasitol 70:844, 1984.
85. Storandt ST, Virchow DR, Dryden MW, et al: Distribution and prevalence of *Echinococcus multilocularis* in wild predators in Nebraska, Kansas, and Wyoming. J Parasitol 89:420, 2002.
86. Wilson JF, Rausch RL: Alveolar hydatid disease: A review of clinical features of 33 indigenous cases of *Echinococcus multilocularis* infection in Alaskan Eskimos. Am J Trop Med Hyg 29:1340, 1980.
87. Aydin Y, Barlas O, Yolas C, et al: Alveolar hydatid disease of the brain. J Neurosurg 65:115, 1986.
88. Rausch RL, Wilson JF, Schantz PM, et al: Spontaneous death of *Echinococcus multilocularis*: Cases diagnosed serologically and clinical significance. Am J Trop Med Hyg 36:576, 1987.
89. Pawlowski ZS, Eckert J, Vuitton DA, et al: Echinococcosis in humans: Clinical aspects, diagnosis, and treatment. In Eckert J, Gemmel MA, Meslin F-X, et al (eds): WHO/OIE Manual on Echinococcosis in Humans and Animals: A Public Health Problem of Global Concern. Paris, World Health Organization/World Organization for Animal Health, 2001, p 48.
90. Gottstein B, Hemphill A: Immunopathology of echincoccosis. Chem Immunol 66:177, 1997.
91. Vuitton DA, Bresson-Hadni S, Laroche K, et al: Cellular immune response in *Echinococcus multilocularis* infection in humans. II. Natural killer cell activity and cell subpopulations in the blood and in the periparasitic granuloma of patients with alveolar echinococcosis. Clin Exp Immunol 78:67, 1989.
92. Sturm D, Menzel J, Gottstein B, et al: Interleukin-5 is the predominant cytokine produced by peripheral blood mononuclear cells in alveolar echinococcosis. Infect Immun 63:1688, 1995.
93. Godot V, Harraga S, Deschaseaux M, et al: Increased basal production of interleukin-10 by peripheral blood mononuclear cells in human alveolar echinococcosis. Eur Cytokine Net 8:401, 1997.
94. Kilwinski J, Jenne L, Jellen-Ritter A, et al: T lymphocyte cytokine profile at a single cell level in alveolar echinococcosis. Cytokine 11:373, 1999.
95. Manfras BJ, Reuter S, Wendland T, et al: Increased activation and oligoclonality of peripheral CD8(+) T cells in the chronic human helminth infection alveolar echinococcosis. Infect Immun 70:1168, 2003.
96. Manfras BJ, Reuter S, Wendland T, et al: Impeded Th1 CD4 memory T cell generation in chronic-persisting liver infection with *Echinococcus multilocularis*. Int Immunol 16:43, 2004.
97. Gottstein B, Wunderlin E, Tanner I: *Echinococcus multilocularis*: Parasite-specific humoral and cellular immune response subsets in mouse strains susceptible (AKR, C57B1/6J) or "resistant" (C57B1/10) to secondary alveolar echinococcosis. Clin Exp Immunol 96:245, 1994.
98. Reuter S, Nussle K, Kolokythas O, et al: Alveolar liver echinococcosis: A comparative study of three imaging techniques. Infection 29:119, 2001.
99. Reuter S, Schirrmeister H, Kratzer W, et al: Pericystic metabolic activity in alveolar echinococcosis: Assessment and follow-up by positron emission tomography. Clin Infect Dis 29:1157, 1999.
100. Reuter S, Buck A, Manfras B, et al: Structured treatment interruption in patients with alveolar echinococcosis. Hepatology 39:509, 2004.
101. Gottstein B, Jacquier P, Bresson-Hadni S, et al: Improved primary immunodiagnosis of alveolar echinococcosis in humans by an enzyme-linked immunosorbent assay using Em2plus antigen. J Clin Microbiol 31:373, 1993.
102. Helbig M, Frosch P, Kern P, et al: Serological differentiation between cystic and alveolar echinococcosis by use of recombinant larval antigens. J Clin Microbiol 31:3211, 1993.
103. Ito A, Sako Y, Yamasaki H, et al: Development of Em18-immunoblot and Em18-ELISA for specific diagnosis of alveolar echinococcosis. Acta Trop 85:173, 2003.
104. Gottstein B, Tschudi K, Eckert J, et al: EM2-ELISA for the follow-up of the alveolar echinococcosis after complete surgical resection. Trans R Soc Trop Med Hyg 83:389, 1989.
105. Wen H, Craig PS, Ito A, et al: Immunoblot evaluation of IgG and IgG-subclass antibody responses for immunodiagnosis of human alveolar echinococcosis. Ann Trop Med Parasitol 89:485, 1995.
106. Kern P, Frosch P, Helbig M, et al: Diagnosis of *Echinococcus multilocularis* infection by reverse-transcription polymerase chain reaction. Gastroenterology 109:596, 1995.
107. Dinkel A, von Nickisch-Rosenegk M, Bilger B, et al: Detection of *Echinococcus multilocularis* in the definitive host: Coprodiagnosis by PCR as an alternative to necropsy. J Clin Microbiol 36:1871, 1998.
108. Myjak P, Nahorski W, Pietkiewicz H, et al: Molecular confirmation of human alveolar echincoccosis in Poland. Clin Infect Dis 37:e121, 2003.
109. Reuter S, Jensen B, Buttenschoen K, et al: Benzimidazoles in the treatment of alveolar echinococcosis: A comparative study and review of the literature. J Antimicrob Chemother 46:451, 2000.
110. Buttenschoen K, Schorcht P, Reuter S, et al: Surgical therapy of alveolar echinococcosis and long-term outcome (In German). Chirurg 72:566, 2001.
111. Ammann RW, Hirsbrunner R, Cotting J, et al: Recurrence rate after discontinuation of long-term mebendazole therapy in alveolar echinococcosis. Am J Trop Med Hyg 43:506, 1990.
112. Wilson JF, Rausch RL, McMahon BJ, et al: Parasiticidal effect of chemotherapy in alveolar hydatid disease: Review of experience with mebendazole and albendazole in Alaskan Eskimos. Clin Infect Dis 15:234, 1992.
113. Cokmez A, Aydede H, Gur S, et al: Long-term albendazole treatment in one case of alveolar echinococcosis. Case report. Acta Gastro-Enterol Belg 66:255, 2003.
114. Wen H, Pei-Fan Z, Wen-Guang Y, et al: Albendazole chemotherapy for human cystic and alveolar echinococcosis in north-western China. Trans R Soc Trop Med Hyg 88:340, 1994.
115. Ammann RW, Ilitsch N, Marincek B, et al: Effect of chemotherapy on the larval mass and the long-term course of alveolar echinococcosis. Hepatology 3:735, 1994.
116. Bresson-Hadni S, Miguet JP, Mantion G, et al: Orthotopic liver transplantation for incurable alveolar echinococcosis of the liver report: Report of 17 cases. Hepatology 13:1061, 1991.
117. Kamiya Y, Sato H, Ihama Y, et al: Epidemiology of echinococcosis in Aomori Prefecture, Japan. Parasitol Inter 49(suppl):83, 2000.
118. Hegglin D, Ward PI, Deplazes P: Anthelmintic baiting of foxes against urban contamination with *Echinococcus multilocularis*. Emerg Infect Dis 9:1266, 2003.
119. Rausch RL, Wilson JF, Schantz PM: A program to reduce the risk of infection by *Echinococcus multilocularis*: The use of praziquantel to control the cestode in a village in the hyperendemic region of Alaska. Ann Trop Med Parasitol 84:239, 1990.
120. Rausch RL, Bernstein JJ: *Echinococcus vogeli* spp. n. (Cestoda: Taeniidae) from the bush dog, *Speothos venaticus* (Lund). Tropenmed Parasitol 23:25, 1972.

121. Rausch RL, D'Alessandro A, Ohbayashi M: The taxonomic status of *Echinococcus cruzi*. Brumpt and Joyeux, 1924 (Cestode: Taeniidae) from an agouti (Rodentia: Dasyproctidae) in Brazil. J Parasitol 70:295, 1984.
122. D'Alessandro A, Rausch RL, Cuello C, et al: *Echinococcus vogeli* in man with a review of human cases of polycystic hydatid disease in Colombia and neighboring countries. Am J Trop Med Hyg 28:303, 1979.
123. D'Alessandro A: Polycystic echinococcosis in Tropical America: *Echinococcus vogeli* and *E. oligarthrus*. Acta Trop 67:43, 1997.
124. Rausch RL, Rausch VR, D'Alessandro A: Discrimination of the larval stages of *Echinococcus oligarthrus* (Diesing, 1863) and *E. vogeli* Rausch and Berstein, 1972 (Cestoda: Taeniidae). Am J Trop Med Hyg 27:1195, 1978.
125. Rausch RL, D'Alessandro A: Histogenesis in the metacestode of *Echinococcus vogeli* and mechanism of pathogenesis in polycystic hydatid diseases. J Parasitol 85:410, 1999.
126. Howard EB, Gendron AP: *Echinococcus vogeli* infection in higher primates at the Los Angeles zoo. In Montali RJ, Migaki G (eds): Comparative Pathology of Zoo Animals. Washington, DC, Smithsonian Institution Press, 1980, p 379.
127. Lopera RD, Melendez RD, Fernandez I, et al: Orbital hydatid cyst of *Echinococcus oligarthrus* in a human in Venezuela. J Parasitol 75:467, 1989.
128. D'Alessandro A, Ramirez LE, Chapadeiro E, et al: Second recorded case of human infections by *Echinococcus oligarthrus*. Am J Trop Med Hyg 52:29, 1995.
129. Schantz P, Colli C: *Echinococcus oligarthrus* (Diesing, 1863) from Geoffroy's cat (*Felis geoffroyi* D'Orbigny & Gervais) in temperate South America. J Parasitol 59:1138, 1973.
130. Meneghelli UG, Martinelli ALC, Llorach Velludo MAS, et al: Polycystic hydatid disease (*Echinococcus vogeli*). Clinical, laboratory and morphologic findings in nine Brazilian patients. J Hepatol 14:203, 1992.
131. Ferreira MS, Nishioka SA, Rocha A, et al: *Echinococcus vogeli* polycystic hydatid disease: Report of two Brazilian cases outside the Amazon region. Trans R Soc Med Hyg 89:286, 1995.
132. Rausch RL, D'Alessandro A, Rausch VR: Characteristics of the larval *Echinococcus vogeli*, Rausch and Bernstein, 1972 in the natural intermediate host, the paca, *Cuniculus paca* L. (Rodentia: Dasyproctidae). Am J Trop Med Hyg 30:1043, 1981.
133. Gottstein B, D'Alessandro A, Rausch RL: Immunodiagnosis of polycystic hydatid disease/polycystic echinococcosis due to *Echinococcus vogeli*. Am J Trop Med Hyg 53:558, 1995.

115

Taenia and Other *Tapeworms*

MURRAY WITTNER
HERBERT B. TANOWITZ

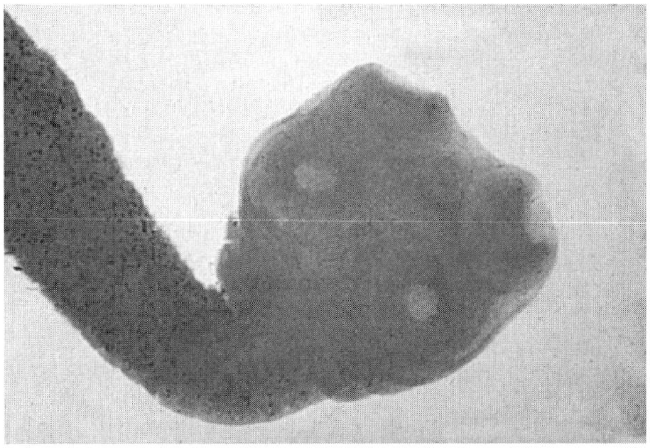

FIGURE 115-2 *Taenia saginata* scolex. Note the four suckers and no hooks. (From Zaiman H [ed]: Pictorial Presentation of Parasites. Audiovisual. Valley City, ND, Mercy Hospital, 1900–1982.)

Taeniasis

INTRODUCTION

The pork tapeworm, *Taenia solium*, and the beef tapeworm, *Taenia saginata*, are parasites of man that have been known since ancient Greece.[1] Taeniasis occurs whenever infected insufficiently cooked beef or pork is consumed.[2,3] However, it was not until 1782 that Goeze differentiated the two species. The larval stage was clearly described by Aristotle and Aristophenes from the tongue of hogs, but it remained for Leukart (1856) and Kuchenmeister (1855) to prove that human infection with the adult worm resulted from eating pork containing viable larvae.[1,2]

AGENT

Taenia saginata adult worms vary in size from 4 to 12 m and may be composed of 1000 to 2000 proglottids. When mature proglottids become gravid, the testes, ovaries, and other reproductive organs degenerate and are replaced by the enlarging egg-filled uterus (Fig. 115-1). The scolex of *T. saginata* is distinctive, being approximately 1.5 to 2.0 mm wide and possessing four simple sucking disks, and is "unarmed" (i.e., without hooklets; Fig. 115-2). In contrast, *T. solium* is somewhat smaller, varying from 2 to 8 m, with a total of approximately 1000 proglottids. The scolex possesses a well-developed crown or rostellum upon which is a double row of hooklets—that is, it is "armed"[3] (Fig. 115-3).

These tapeworms generally are attached by their scolex to the jejunal mucosa. The strobila, which is not fixed in position, moves frequently, even against the peristaltic stream. Gravid proglottids contain thousands of spherical thick-walled eggs, which are radially striated and contain a mature six-hooked (hexacanth) embryo called an oncosphere. The eggs are 30 to 40 μm in diameter and are similar and essentially indistinguishable in all members of the genus (Fig. 115-4). Cattle or hogs become infected by ingesting mature eggs contaminating low-lying pastures or barnyards. In endemic areas, pigs acquire the infection rapidly since they actively seek and eat human stools at defecation sites or latrines.[4] Hatching is initiated by the action of gastric juice,

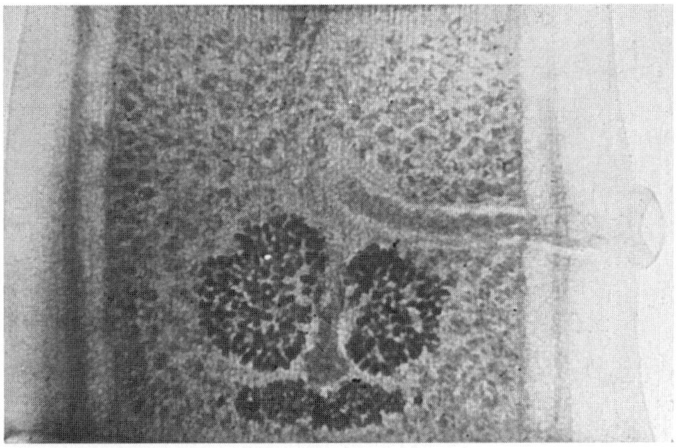

FIGURE 115-1 *Taenia solium* proglottid. (From Zaiman H [ed]: Pictorial Presentation of Parasites. Audiovisual. Valley City, ND, Mercy Hospital, 1900–1982.)

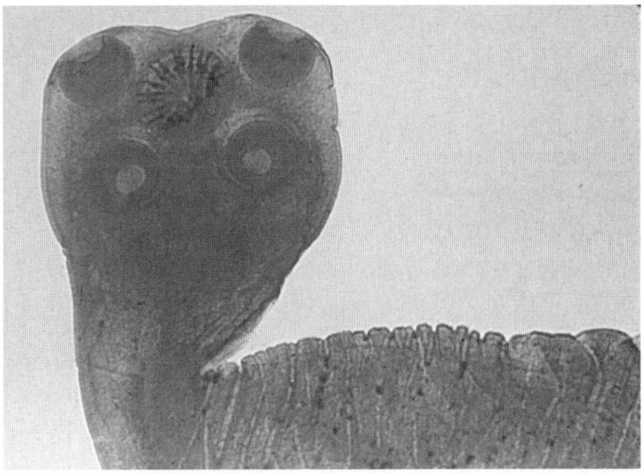

FIGURE 115-3 *Taenia solium* scolex. Four suckers and hooks are seen. (From Zaiman H [ed]: Pictorial Presentation of Parasites. Audiovisual. Valley City, ND, Mercy Hospital, 1900–1982.)

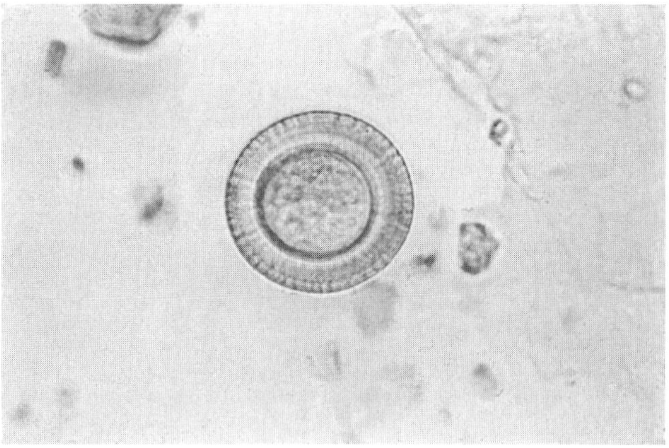

FIGURE 115-4 *Taenia* ovum. (From Zaiman H [ed]: Pictorial Presentation of Parasites. Audiovisual. Valley City, ND, Mercy Hospital, 1900–1982.)

intestinal enzymes, and bile on the eggs. Liberated embryos penetrate the intestinal mucosa of cattle or hogs, enter the circulation, and are transported throughout the body. *Taenia saginata* oncospheres produce excretory-secretory peptidases, including serine and cysteine endopeptidases, and aminopeptidase, which may play a role in invasion of the intestinal mucosa.[5] Larval encystment usually occurs in striated muscle and the central nervous system, and within 8 to 11 weeks the larvae, termed *Cysticercus solium (cellulosae)* in hogs and *Cysticercus bovis* in cattle, become infectious. Cysticerci are ellipsoid, translucent bladder-like cysts in which an inverted scolex has developed. In humans who ingest infective eggs of *T. solium*, cysticerci develop similarly.

On consumption of infected raw or inadequately cooked beef or pork, the cysticercus is activated by gastric juices and bile salts, which stimulate evagination of the scolex. It then attaches to the jejunal wall, and *T. solium* becomes a mature tapeworm in 5 to 12 weeks, whereas it takes approximately 10 to 12 weeks for *T. saginata*. The adult tapeworm may live for 25 years or more.[3] Molecular approaches in the study of *Taenia* have led to a number of potentially important findings that may aid in the diagnosis and therapy of *Taenia* infections.[6–8]

EPIDEMIOLOGY

Both infections have worldwide distribution, but there are no reliable statistics with regard to their prevalence. *Taenia saginata* is commonly found in the United States, Europe, South America, and Africa. *Taenia solium* is common in Mexico, Central and South America, Africa, Eastern Europe, China, Pakistan, and India.[9–12] Additional discussion of the epidemiology of *T. solium* and cysticercosis can be found in Chapter 113.

Humans are the obligatory definitive host for both of these tapeworms. Whereas infection with the pork tapeworm is uncommon in the United States, cysticercosis of hogs is not uncommon. Currently, *T. solium* infections are reported from a relatively small number of nations, especially Mexico, Central and South America, the Balkan countries, East Africa, India, China, and Indonesia. However, the extent of the endemicity of the infection is largely unknown. For example, it was reported that more than 13% of the pigs examined in abattoirs in Tanzania had cysticercosis,[13] and wherever adult pork tapeworm infection is encountered, human cysticercosis is not unusual.

A third form of human *Taenia* infection is due to *Taenia asiatica*, which has been reported in Taiwan, Korea, Indonesia, Vietnam, and China. Molecular approaches indicate that *T. asiatica* is more closely related to *T. saginata* than to *T. solium*.[14,15]

Taenia saginata infection occurs among those who prefer to eat raw or insufficiently cooked beef. *Taenia saginata* infection is a "true zoonosis" in which man is the mandatory definitive host who disseminates the infection to bovine intermediate hosts. More commonly, transmission occurs through fecal contamination of low-lying grazing lands, cattle feed, and also by birds and flies.[16] A solid acquired immunity to the oncosphere and postoncosphere stage develops in intermediate hosts (pigs and cattle) following ingestion of relatively few eggs and is maintained for months to years without further exposure. This limits the number of cysts in the host with regard to subsequent exposures. Low and high temperature extremes (−70° to +40°C) as well as desiccation are important environmental factors that affect survival of the ova. Dipteran flies may also increase the dispersion of eggs in the environment.[16]

DISEASE

Following the ingestion of viable metacestodes (cysticerci) in improperly cooked or raw beef or pork, the scolex evaginates and attaches to the upper jejunum by its well-developed holdfast organs, and strobilation occurs. Infection with adult tapeworms causes few pathologic changes. However, intestinal mucosal biopsies in patients harboring *T. saginata* have shown a minimal inflammatory reaction, suggesting that the worms can have an "irritative" effect, perhaps causing clinical symptoms.

Most people who harbor *T. solium* or *T. saginata* are either asymptomatic or have mild to moderate complaints. Occasionally, these infections can result in serious, life-threatening illness from intestinal,[17] biliary, or pancreatic obstruction (Fig. 115-5). Rarely, an individual may regurgitate

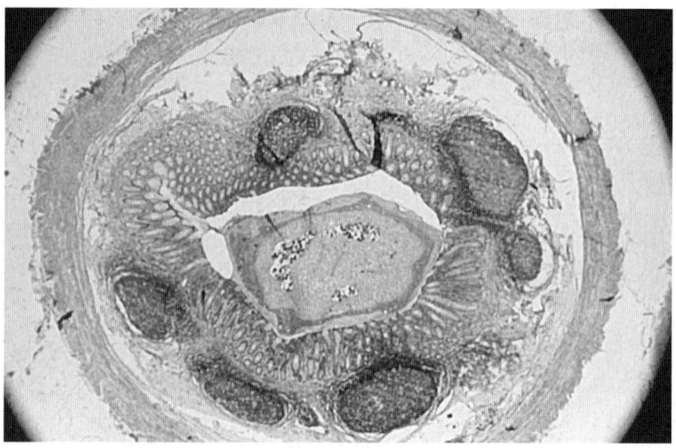

FIGURE 115-5 *Taenia* proglottid in intestine.

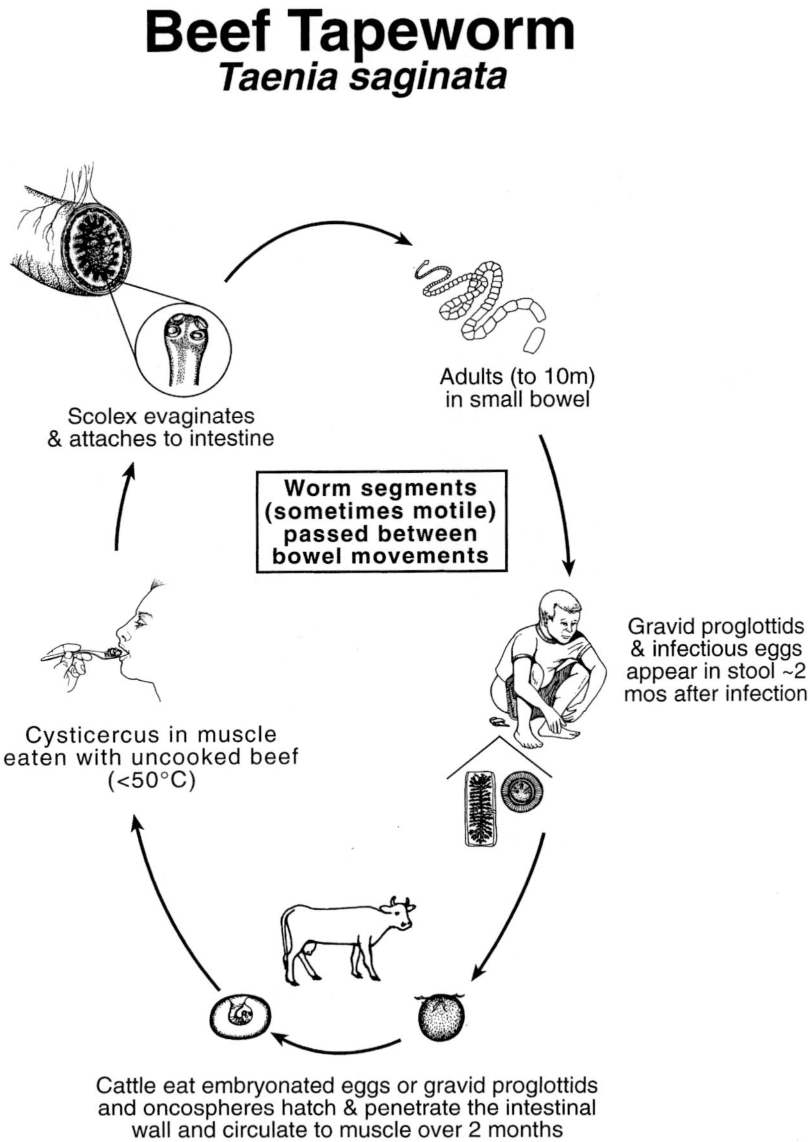

and aspirate a proglottid. The most frequently reported sign of adult *T. saginata* infection is spontaneous egress of proglottids per rectum. Infection with either species may be associated with abdominal pain, nausea, weakness, loss of appetite, increased appetite, headache, constipation, dizziness, diarrhea, pruritis ani, and hyperexcitability. Abdominal pain and nausea are reported to be more common in the morning and characteristically relieved by small amounts of food. Children are more frequently symptomatic than adults. Eosinophilia is often present and rarely levels can rise to more than 50% but are usually 5 to 15%. Serum immunoglobulin E (IgE) levels may be increased.

DIAGNOSIS

The presence of *Taenia* eggs in the stool is not sufficient to differentiate species; a gravid proglottid must be obtained for this purpose.[18] Identification of proglottids is done by pressing the segment between two glass microscope slides and counting the main lateral branches on one side of the uterus. *Taenia solium* has fewer primary branches, usually 7 to 13 on each side; *T. saginata* usually has more than 15 lateral primary branches per side[18] (Fig. 115-6). Stool examination may be unrewarding in the case of *T. saginata* infection since gravid proglottids often emerge spontaneously per anus, depositing eggs on the perianal and perineal region. Thus, anal swabs, such as the "Scotch tape" method, as usually done for the diagnosis of pinworm (see Chapter 107), are recommended to recover the ova. It has been demonstrated that using an electrolyte-polyethyleneglycol solution as a purge enhances the recovery of the scolex and proglottids, which could aid in species identification.[19]

In recent years, a number of immunodiagnostic and molecular approaches have been developed for the diagnosis of taeniasis.[8,10,20–22] These tests have included the detection of coproantigens, copro-DNA, and serum antibodies to

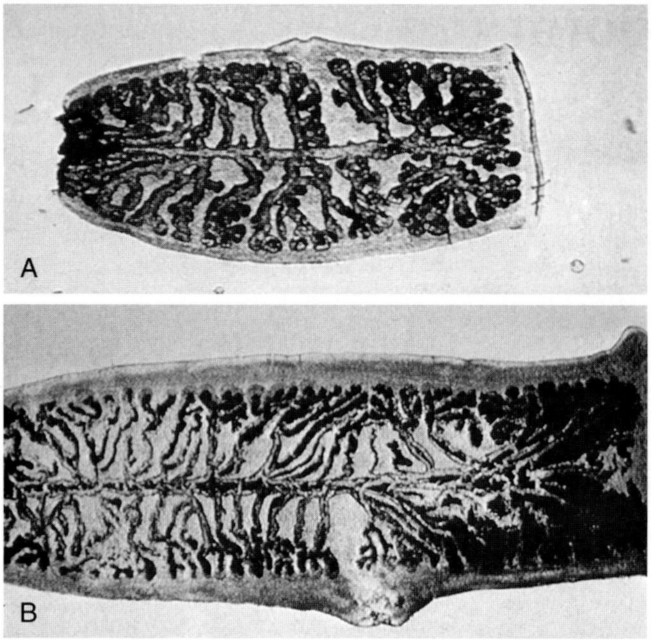

FIGURE 115-6 *A, Taenia solium* proglottid (India ink-stained). *B, Taenia saginata* proglottid (India ink-stained).

adult-stage antigens. Some of these methods were shown to be highly sensitive and specific. A multiplex polymerase chain reaction[20] has been developed for use on both feces and parasites that can differentiate among the *Taenia* species and is based on cestode mitochondrial DNA. This method may also prove to be useful for molecular epidemiology studies.

TREATMENT AND PROGNOSIS

The treatment of both tapeworm infections is similar. Praziquantel can be administered as a single dose of 10 to 20 mg/kg.[23] For the treatment of *T. solium*, precautions should be taken to prevent autoinfection or dissemination to others. Thus, drugs that induce vomiting should be avoided since retrograde peristalsis may raise gravid proglottids into the gastroduodenal area, resulting in their digestion followed by egg hatching and penetration of the intestine, leading to disseminated cysticercosis. In addition, since praziquantel kills the worm (Fig. 115-7) but does not inactivate the eggs released from the disintegrating gravid segments, cysticercosis is theoretically possible following treatment. It is also unknown whether larvae released from eggs in the colon are capable of penetrating the intestinal wall. However, no cases of cysticercosis have been reported by this mechanism. Post-treatment follow-up stool examination should be performed after approximately 5 weeks in the case of *T. solium* and 3 months for *T. saginata* infections. The prognosis of treated taeniasis is excellent.

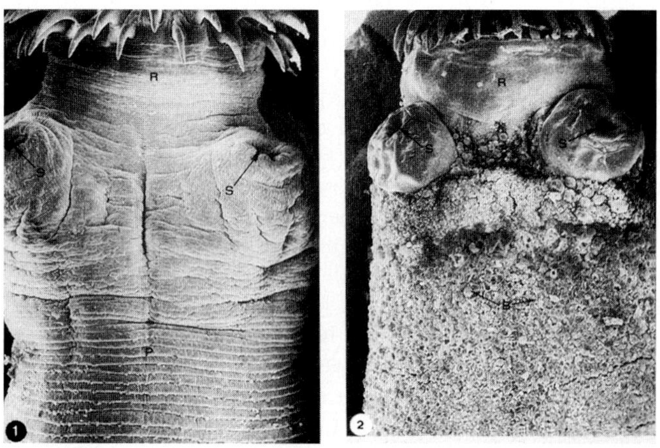

FIGURE 115-7 Scanning electron microscopy of *Taenia solium* scolex, showing effect of praziquantel. (From Thomas H, Andrews P, Mehlhorn H: New results on the effect of praziquantel in experimental cysticercosis. Am J Trop Med Hyg 31:803–810, 1982.)

PREVENTION AND CONTROL

Education is an important aspect of the prevention of taeniasis.[11] Beef and pork tapeworm infection can be prevented by adequate cooking or freezing of beef and pork. *Cysticercus solium (cellulosae)* is killed by moderate temperatures of 65°C (150°F) or if the pork is frozen at −20°C (−38°F) for at least 12 hours. Pickling in brine or salting pork is not always an adequate method. *Cysticercus bovis* is killed by thorough cooking at 56°C (131°F) or freezing at −10°C for 5 days. Pickling of beef in 25% brine for 5 or 6 days is said to render the beef safe. Treatment of all infected people would eliminate the source of soil and sewage pollution with *Taenia* eggs and therefore reduce porcine and bovine infection. Meat inspection would help reduce transmission to humans who fail to properly prepare meat. Investigations are under way to develop an effective vaccine against cysticercosis in pigs. Encouraging results have been obtained.[24]

TAENIA CRASSICEPS

Taenia crassiceps is a tapeworm of canids that is rarely transmitted to humans by the oral-fecal route. Since humans are not the usual hosts, it presents as a cysticercus in the brain, eye, or subcutaneous tissue.[25–28] Medical therapy has been disappointing. Interestingly, Chuck and colleagues[29] reported a case of subretinal *T. crassiceps* managed by surgery (Plate 115-1).

Diphyllobothriasis

INTRODUCTION

Diphyllobothrium latum is a frequent human intestinal parasite in many areas where uncooked freshwater fish is consumed.[30–34]

AGENT

The distinction between *D. latum*, the broad or fish tapeworm, and *Taenia* appears to have been well-known to medieval physicians, and it was the earliest pseudophyllidean tapeworm to be scientifically recognized (Linnaeus, 1758).[1]

The life cycle of *D. latum* requires three hosts: (1) The definitive hosts are humans and fish-eating carnivores, (2) the first intermediate hosts are a large number of copepod species (crustaceans), and (3) the second intermediate hosts are freshwater fish. It is a large tapeworm, often consisting

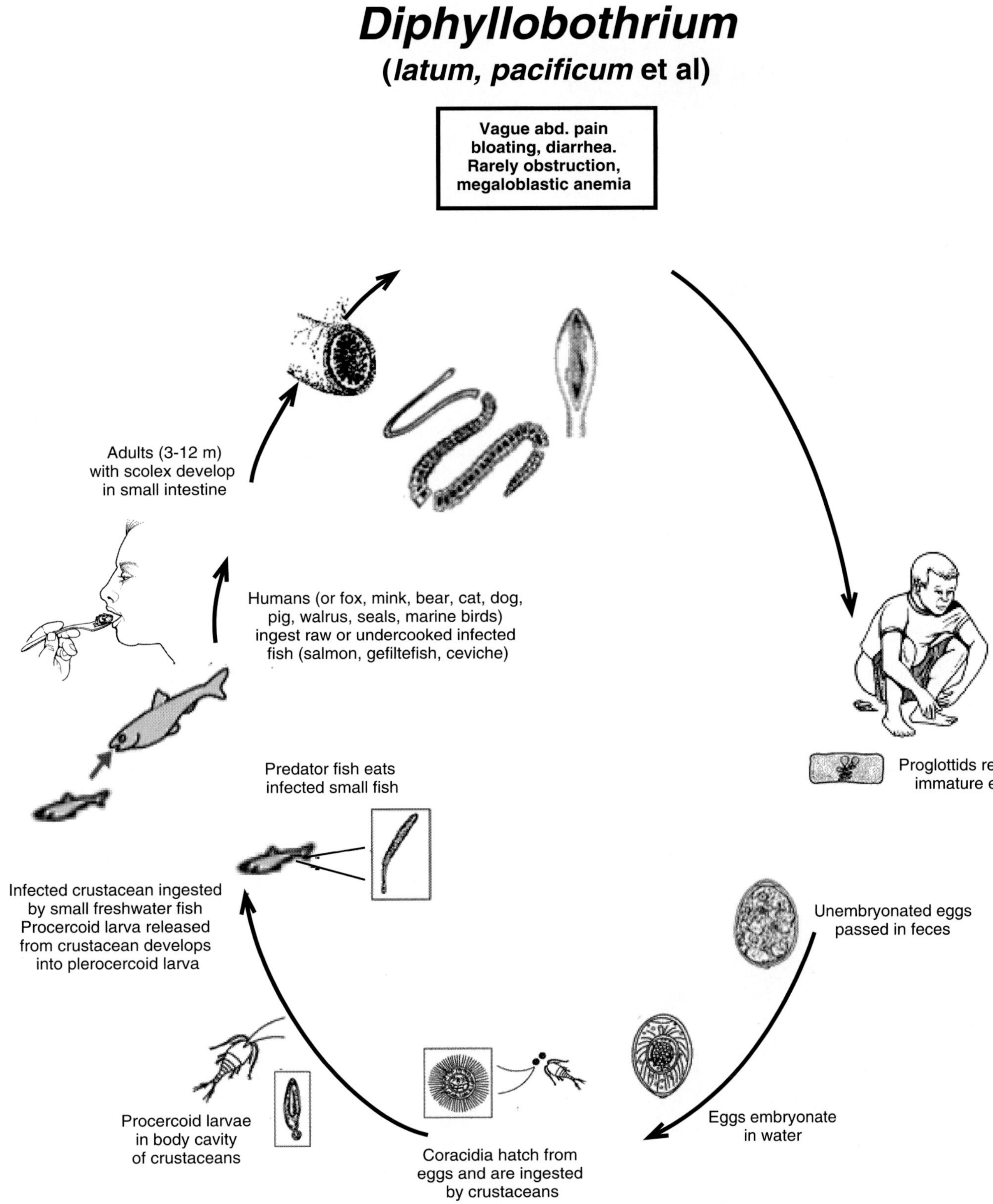

of 3000 to 4000 segments or proglottids measuring from 3 to 12 m, that inhabits the ileum and jejunum. It possesses a scolex that is characteristically elongate or spoon-shaped with a ventral and dorsal sucking groove or bothrium (Fig. 115-8). Most of this tapeworm consists of mature or maturing proglottids. Egg production usually takes place in many proglottids simultaneously over a relatively extended period. The mature proglottid is broader than it is long and contains both male and female reproductive organs. In the center of the mature proglottid is a characteristic dark rosette—that is, the egg-filled uterus that aids in its recognition (Fig. 115-9). The uterus leads to a muscular

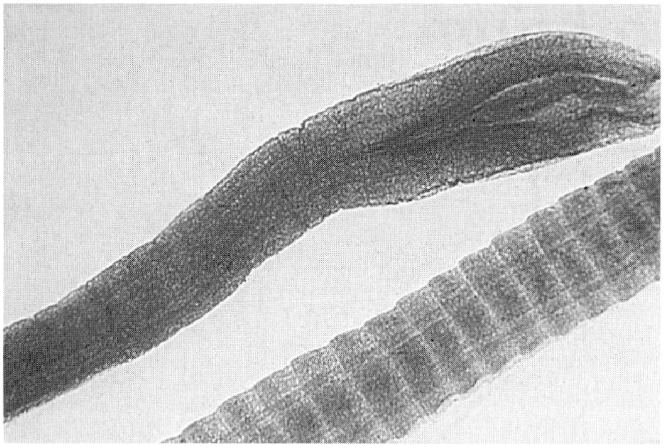

FIGURE 115-8 *Diphyllobothrium latum*. Immature proglottids and scolex. The scolex bears grooves. (From Zaiman H [ed]: A Pictorial Presentation of Parasites. Valley City, ND, Mercy Hospital, 1900–1982.)

uterine pore on the ventral surface of the segment through which the eggs pass into the feces. Typically, proglottids do not break off and migrate out of the body, as occurs in taeniasis, but upward of a million eggs per day are extruded into the small intestinal lumen by contractions of the uterine pore. Spent proglottids eventually disintegrate and pass out of the body. Occasionally, a long chain of proglottids is passed with the stool.[18]

The characteristic light-yellow eggs are 42 to 50 μm × 59 to 75 μm, with an operculum or lid at one end and a characteristic tiny knob at the abopercular end (Fig. 115-10).[7] In fresh water, the unembryonated egg requires approximately 10 days to 2 weeks to mature at 15°C to 25°C. After the operculum opens, a ciliated hexacanth, or six-hooked, embryo (coracidium) emerges; the swimming embryo must be ingested within 6 to 12 hours by one of several crustacean species of copepods or perish (*Cyclops* sp. and *Diaptomus* sp.). The larva penetrates the midgut and enters the hemocoel of the copepod and in 10 to 21 days transforms into an elongated procercoid larva, reaching approximately 0.5 mm in length. It remains in the copepod until ingested by one of many species of small freshwater plankton-eating fish (second intermediate host). The procercoid larva next makes its way through the tissues of the fish and settles between the muscle fibers, where it transforms into a plerocercoid (sparganum) larva. The latter has the characteristic rudiments of a scolex but is unsegmented. Next, these fish are eaten by larger carnivorous fish, such as rainbow trout, walleyed pike, or the burbot (paratenic or transport hosts). The plerocercoid larvae reinvade the muscles of these fish and if consumed raw or inadequately cooked by a suitable host (i.e., humans), the larva attaches to the wall of the small intestine and becomes a mature tapeworm in approximately 5 or 6 weeks.

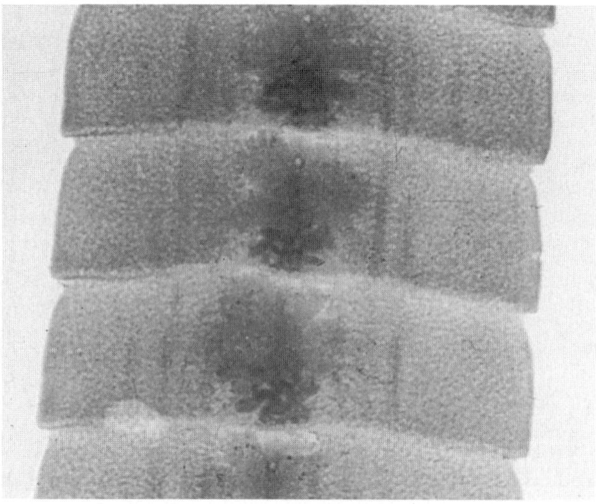

FIGURE 115-9 *Diphyllobothrium latum*. Proglottid. Note the rosette shape of the uterus. (From Zaiman H [ed]: A Pictorial Presentation of Parasites. Valley City, ND, Mercy Hospital, 1900–1982. Courtesy of Dr. J. F. Mueller.)

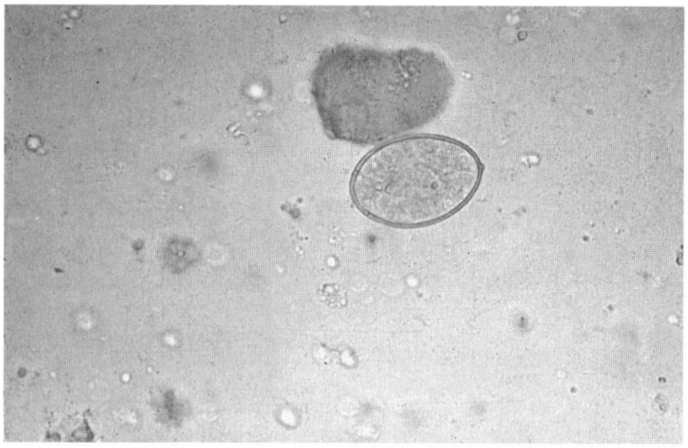

FIGURE 115-10 *Diphyllobothrium latum*. Ovum.

Other adult diphyllobothriid species, normally parasites of fish-eating mammals, have occasionally been found in humans, dogs, and cats in China: *Diplogonoporus grandis*, a whale parasite, found on rare occasions in humans in Japan; *Diphyllobothrium dendriticum*, found commonly in piscivorous birds and mammals in the Northern Hemisphere; and *Diphyllobothrium pacificum*, found in seals (its natural host) and marine fish (its intermediate host) in Peru and Chile.[35]

EPIDEMIOLOGY

Diphyllobothrium latum biotypes are mostly shallow freshwater littorals with vegetation favoring the development of copepods and fish. Infection with this parasite is most prevalent in areas of the North Temperate and sub-Arctic zones, where freshwater fish are commonly consumed.[36]

The prevalence of diphyllobothriasis has decreased in many areas of the world. The estimated worldwide prevalence is approximately 9 to 10 million people. In North America, highly endemic foci have been found among Native Americans in Alaska and Canada and particularly in the smaller lakes of the Great Lakes region. In the United States, fish from the lakes of the north-central region, especially Minnesota and Michigan, and from Florida and California are found infected. In the highly endemic regions of Finnish and Russian Karelia, prevalence has ranged from 25% to 100%.[33] In North America, there has been a decline in human cases, whereas in South America there have been increased reports from fish, especially salmonids. Transmission has been brought under control in Western Europe, and only a few cases occur in Finland, where nearly 20% of the country was infected in the 1950s. In addition, areas of Sweden, France, Switzerland, northwestern Russia, the Danube and lower Volga basins, and the lake regions of northern Italy and Switzerland contain infected fish. Freshwater lakes in many areas of Africa, including Madagascar, and in the People's Republic of China, Taiwan, Japan, Turkey, Ireland, Israel, Papua New Guinea, Australia, the Philippines, Argentina, and southern Chile may contain infected fish. Humans are the primary definitive host and most important reservoir of infection. Other definitive and reservoir hosts are fish-eating mammals, such as the fox, mink, bear, domestic and wild cat, dog, pig, walrus, and seal. Secondary intermediate hosts are many species of brackish and freshwater fish, including anadromous fish that spawn in fresh water (e.g., salmon). Salmon has been the cause of the transmission of this parasite in Japan and the West Coast of the United States where sushi has been prepared with infected salmon.[34] Important factors that have contributed to the spread of infection are the emigration of infected populations, the construction of dams and other water projects, and the practice of allowing untreated sewage to enter freshwater lakes. Cases of diphyllobothriasis sometimes occur outside endemic areas as a result of infected fish being shipped under refrigeration to be sold in markets in large urban centers.

Eating raw, insufficiently cooked, or lightly pickled fish or fresh roe is common among many ethnic groups, which consider it a delicacy. For example, for many years in New York City, infected freshwater fish, transported on ice, was the main source of this tapeworm infection among Jewish housewives who made gefilte fish. Typically, small amounts of raw fish were sampled in order to season this ethnic delicacy to taste. In northern Minnesota and Michigan, where large numbers of people of Scandinavian background live, raw and pickled fish are still eaten and infection with *D. latum* is not uncommon. Women who taste raw fish while preparing it for cooking also have higher prevalence rates. There are other diphyllobothriids that cause disease. *Diphyllobothrium pacificum* has been reported from Japan and is endemic in coastal areas of Peru. Unlike *D. latum*, infection with this parasite is acquired from eating marine fish that have been prepared in lime juice (e.g., ceviche). *Diplogonoporus grandis*, another member of this group, is found in Japan and thought to be acquired by consumption of raw anchovies and sardines. Other species of *Diphyllobothrium*, such as *Diphyllobothrium dendriticum*, *Diphyllobothrium klebaanovskii*, *Diphyllobothrium cordatum*, *Diphyllobothrium dalliae*, *Diphyllobothrium ursi*, and *Diphyllobothrium nihonkaiense*, are found as occasional human parasites.[35] Restriction fragment length polymorphism studies between *D. nihonkaiense* and *D. latum* recombinant DNA failed to show any variations, suggesting their very close identity.[37] Their usual definitive hosts are various marine mammals, carnivores, or marine birds.

DISEASE

Harboring this large tapeworm is usually associated with surprisingly few symptoms or pathologic changes in the intestinal mucosa. Often, the infection is first recognized in an asymptomatic patient as a result of a stool examination carried out for other reasons. However, some patients complain of vague abdominal pain and others describe the sensation that "something is moving inside." Others describe bloating, sore tongue, sore gums, allergic symptoms, headache, hunger pains, loss of appetite, or increased appetite. Rarely, mechanical intestinal obstruction may occur as a result of several worms becoming entangled. Diarrhea may also occur. Almost all patients become aware of the infection when spontaneously passing a large section of the spent proglottids; most often this startling event brings the patient to the office or clinic. Unlike the proglottids of *T. saginata*, those of *D. latum* do not spontaneously crawl through the anus.[38]

In a very small number of patients, a megaloblastic pernicious anemia has been shown to be caused by infection with *D. latum* ("bothriocephalus anemia" or "tapeworm anemia"). When fully manifest, this anemia is a hyperchromic, macrocytic, megaloblastic anemia with thrombocytopenia and mild leukopenia. The development of pernicious anemia is usually associated with high attachment of the tapeworm within 145 cm of the mouth. In this situation, more than 80% of vitamin B_{12} is absorbed by the worm, with a differential absorption pattern of 1000:1 in favor of the worm. For unknown reasons, the anemia associated with diphyllobothriasis is most frequently encountered in Scandinavia. In the United States, people of Scandinavian background are most frequently affected.

Approximately 40% of people harboring the worm have reduced serum vitamin B_{12} levels, but fewer than 2% develop anemia. Neurologic lesions due to vitamin B_{12} deficiency include subacute combined degeneration of the dorsal and lateral columns and peripheral nerve degeneration. In the spinal cord, the posterior and lateral columns are involved. The anemia and neurologic manifestations respond to vitamin B_{12} and do not recur after the worm has been expelled.

DIAGNOSIS

The infection can be diagnosed readily by finding characteristic ova in the feces (see Fig. 115-10).[18] Concentration methods are usually unnecessary since the numbers of eggs present are often so great that direct examination of a small amount of the patient's feces in a drop of saline is usually sufficient. Molecular methods have been explored for the diagnosis of *Diphyllobothrium* sp.[37] Tapeworm-induced anemia may be associated with free hydrochloric acid in the gastric juice; in contrast, pernicious anemia is associated with achlorhydria. There is no reliable serologic test to aid in diagnosis. It is not uncommon to find an eosinophilia of 5% to 10% in patients with *D. latum* infection accompanied by a minimal leukocytosis.

TREATMENT AND PROGNOSIS

The treatment of choice is praziquantel, which is administered as a single dose of 5 to 10 mg/kg for both adults and children.[23,39] Niclosamide is given as a 2-g dose once for adults and 50 mg/kg for children. The prognosis for treated individuals is excellent.

PREVENTION AND CONTROL

Careful cooking of freshwater fish would eliminate all possibility of human infection. The sale of fish originating in heavily infected lakes should be regulated because freezing at −10°C for 24 hours suffices to kill the plerocercoid larva. In the United States, smoked salmon is usually brined before smoking and is not considered a source of infection. Other control measures include the education of cooks regarding the sampling of raw fish during preparation. In addition, sanitary sewage disposal rather than the dumping of raw sewage into freshwater lakes also would prevent viable eggs from contaminating various intermediate hosts. In highly endemic areas, human infection should be detected by survey and treated.

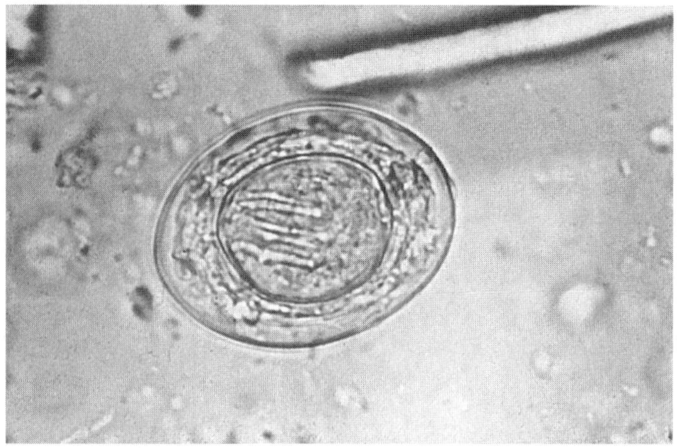

FIGURE 115-12 *Hymenolepis nana* ovum. (From Zaiman H [ed]: Pictorial Presentation of Parasites. Audiovisual. Valley City, ND, Mercy Hospital, 1900–1982.)

Hymenolepiasis

INTRODUCTION

There are two species of *Hymenolepis* that infect humans: *Hymenolepis nana* and *Hymenolepis diminuta.* Both are cosmopolitan in their distribution, but the former is more common in warmer climates and the latter is a common parasite of rats and mice and only occasionally infects humans.[40,41]

AGENT

The adult *H. nana* is approximately 0.5 cm long and is found attached to the mucosa of the ileum by a scolex that has four suckers and a retractable, armed rostellum (Fig. 115-11). The entire worm usually consists of a scolex and approximately 200 proglottids. The uterus in a gravid proglottid contains approximately 100 to 200 mature eggs that are 30 to 60 μm in diameter (Fig. 115-12).[17,40,41] An intermediate host is not required to complete the life cycle. The eggs are passed in the feces and ingested by a new human or the same host (autoinfection). The embryo hatches in the small intestine and penetrates a villus, where it becomes a cysticercoid larva (Fig. 115-13). Upon maturation, in 3 or 4 days, it emerges from the tissue and attaches to the intestinal mucosa by its scolex. In 2 or 3 weeks, the new worm is producing eggs. Hyperinfection can occur when eggs liberated in the small intestine hatch and immediately penetrate a villus to undergo a new cycle. As a result of hyperinfection, children may harbor many hundreds or even thousands of adult worms. The entire life history from ingestion of the egg to adulthood requires approximately 10 days to 2 weeks. Eggs are first seen in the stools in approximately 25 to 30 days. *Hymenolepis nana* is regarded as a hand-to-mouth infection and, as a result, is most frequently encountered in children, institutions, and families. Certain strains of *H. nana* may undergo larval development in various fleas and mealworms, and these larvae have developed to adults in mice; human infection with murine strains is unusual.

The closely related species, *H. diminuta*, which commonly parasitizes the rat and mouse, infrequently infects humans.[41] Most of the more than 200 reported human infections have been in children younger than 3 years of age. The adult worm is 10 to 60 cm × 3 to 5 mm and possesses a club-shaped scolex that has a rudimentary apical unarmed rostellum with four small suckers. The ova are spherical and 60 to 86 μm in diameter.[18]

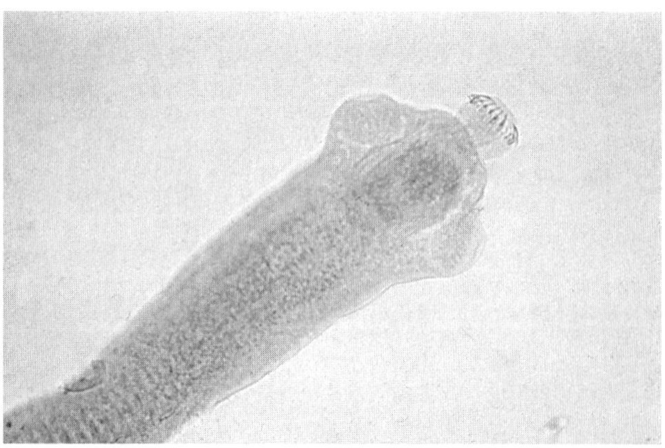

FIGURE 115-11 *Hymenolepis nana* scolex and proglottids. (From Zaiman H [ed]: Pictorial Presentation of Parasites. Audiovisual. Valley City, ND, Mercy Hospital, 1900–1982.)

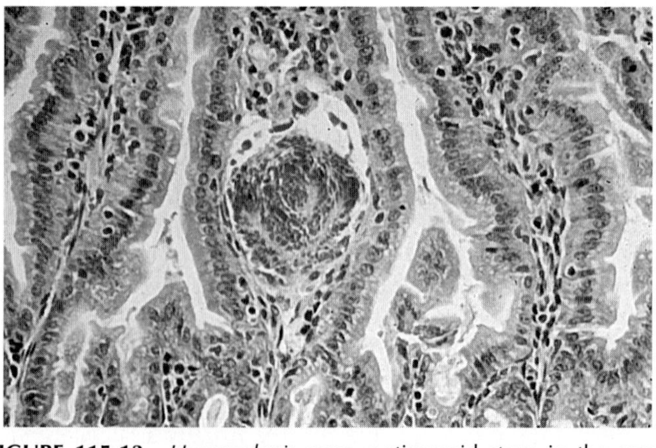

FIGURE 115-13 *Hymenolepis nana* cysticercoid stage in the small intestine. (Original photo by B. Gueft, MD, from a specimen by M. Yoelli, MD. From Zaiman H [ed]: Pictorial Presentation of Parasites. Audiovisual. Valley City, ND, Mercy Hospital, 1900–1982.)

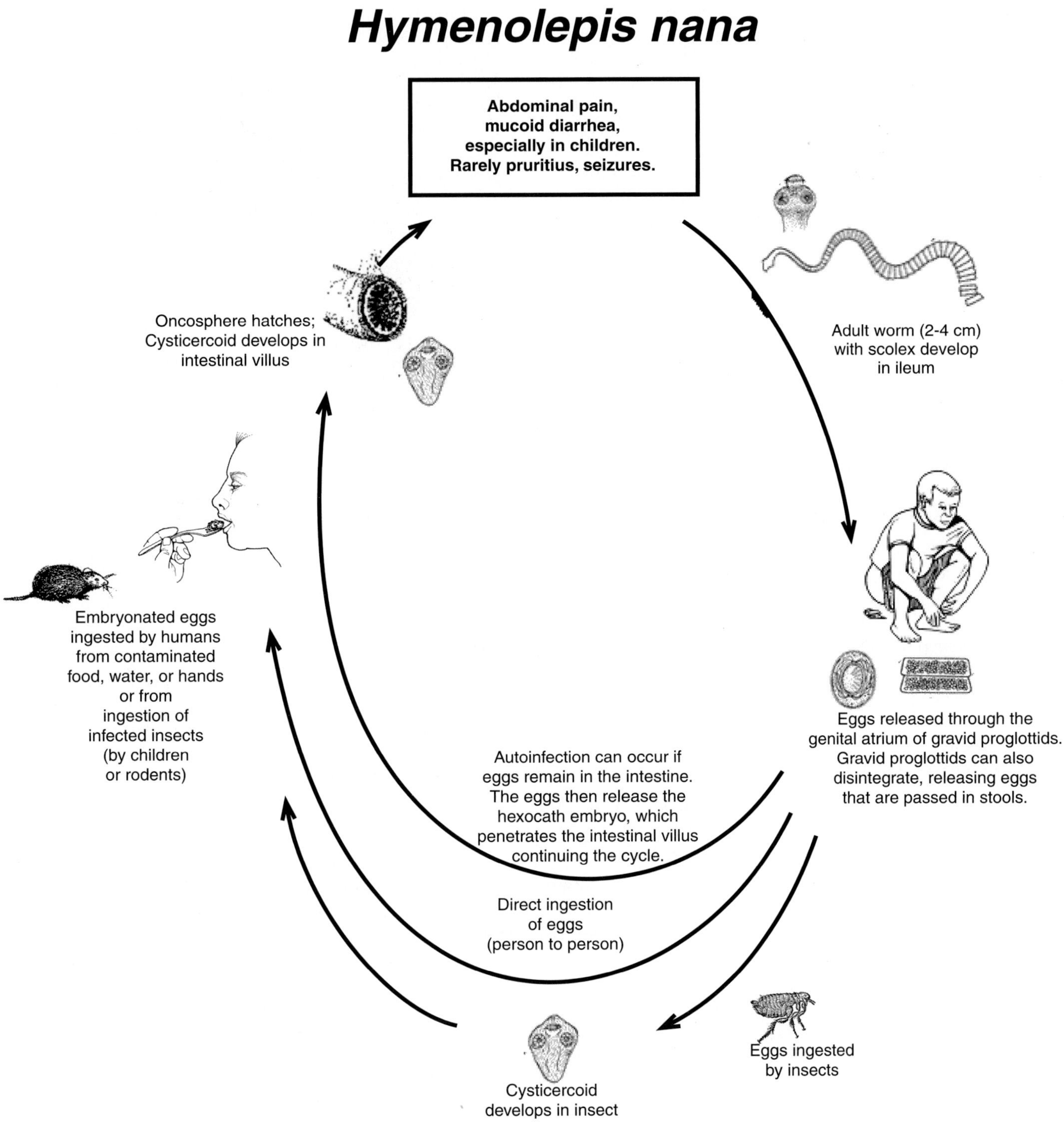

In contrast to the eggs of *H. nana*, there are no polar filaments. Development of this tapeworm requires an intermediate host. Presumably, infected rat fleas (*Nosopsyllus* and *Xenopsylla*) and mealworms (*Tenebrio*) are accidentally ingested, and the mature adult develops in approximately 3 weeks. Cockroaches may also serve as intermediate hosts and become infected by ingesting eggs passed in rodent feces. A related helminth in rodents, *Rhodentolepis* (=*Hymenolepis*) *microstoma*, has been reported in humans.[42] Molecular approaches have been applied to the epidemiology and diagnosis of *Hymenolepis* infections.[43,44] Studies indicate a role for the immune system in the expulsion of this parasite from rodent hosts.[45–47]

EPIDEMIOLOGY

The dwarf tapeworm, *H. nana*, is found in most warm regions of the world. It is the most common cestode infection in the southeastern United States and Latin America, and it is common throughout southern Europe, Russia and the former Soviet republics, and the Indian subcontinent.[41,48–50]

DISEASE

Young children are particularly troubled with *H. nana* infections, especially when many worms are present.[50]

These patients commonly have loose bowel movements or occasionally frank diarrhea with mucus but no blood. Diffuse, persistent abdominal pain is the most common complaint. Pruritus ani and nasi are occasionally encountered. Many children have sleep and behavioral disturbances that clear after successful therapy. Serious neurologic disturbances such as seizures have been reported. Many patients with hymenolepiasis have a moderate eosinophilia of 5% to 10% and skin eruptions.[51] A patient with acquired immunodeficiency syndrome (AIDS) was diagnosed with invasive lethal infection with *H. nana*.[52]

DIAGNOSIS

The diagnosis of hymenolepiasis rests on finding the characteristic ova by stool examination. Stools of the entire family must be checked before therapy is initiated because other members of a household are commonly infected, and they must also be treated for therapy to be successful. As in all tapeworm infections, post-treatment stool examinations should be done after 5 weeks and again after 3 months.[1–3]

TREATMENT AND PROGNOSIS

Praziquantel is the drug of choice for the treatment of hymenolepiasis and is highly effective in a single dose of 15 mg/kg. It not only eliminates adult worms but also, unlike other anthelmintics, is efficiently absorbed and kills the larval stages (cysticercoids) in the submucosa.[2] Praziquantel has not been approved for this indication by the U.S. Food and Drug Administration. Treated individuals have an excellent prognosis.

PREVENTION AND CONTROL

This infection is a hand-to-mouth disease and therefore extremely difficult to control. Education in hygiene is probably the only practical way to reduce the incidence.

Dipylidiasis

INTRODUCTION

The dog tapeworm, *Dipylidium caninum*, is also a frequent parasite of cats and wild carnivores worldwide. It is an occasional parasite of the small intestine of humans.

AGENT

The adult worm is approximately 15 to 20 cm long and usually has approximately 60 to 175 proglottids. The scolex is characteristic, being rhomboid with four oval suckers and an armed retractable conical rostellum containing 30 to 150 thorn-shaped hooks arranged in transverse rows (Fig. 115-14). The proglottids have a double set of reproductive organs with genital pores midway on each lateral margin (Fig. 115-15). The gravid proglottids are packed with 15 to 25 eggs. Each egg is 35 to 60 μm in diameter and contains an oncosphere with six hooklets. The strobila can migrate several inches per hour and pass out of the anus spontaneously or with the feces. Eggs are expelled by contraction or disintegration of the proglottid.[53]

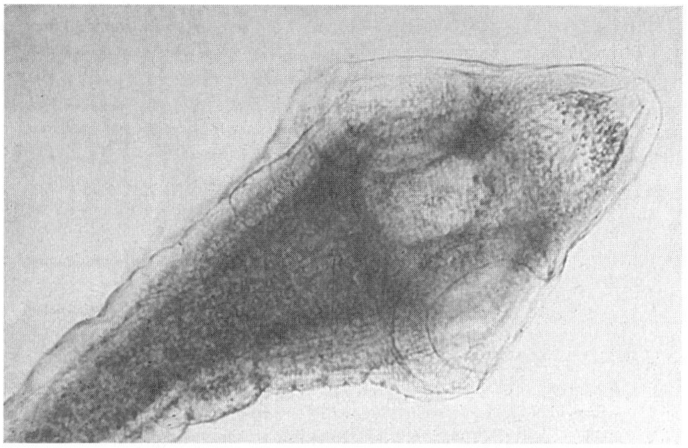

FIGURE 115-14 *Dipylidium caninum* scolex. Three of the four suckers and the retracted armed rostellum can be seen. (From Zaiman H [ed]: Pictorial Presentation of Parasites. Audiovisual. Valley City, ND, Mercy Hospital, 1900–1982.)

EPIDEMIOLOGY

Most infections occur in children younger than 8 years old as well as infants younger than 6 months of age.[54–57] The ova of *Dipylidium* are ingested by the larval dog or cat flea, in which they become cysticercoid larvae. Infection occurs following accidental ingestion of the infected flea.

DISEASE

Infection is often asymptomatic, although some children have intestinal disturbances, including abdominal pain and diarrhea (Fig. 115-16).[54–57] Allergic manifestations such as urticaria and pruritus ani have been reported; intestinal obstruction has been a rare complication.[1,2]

TREATMENT AND PREVENTION

Treatment is with 5 to 10 mg/kg of praziquantel once for both adults and children. An alternative therapy is 2 g of niclosamide once for adults and 25 mg/kg once for children. Children should not be allowed to fondle and

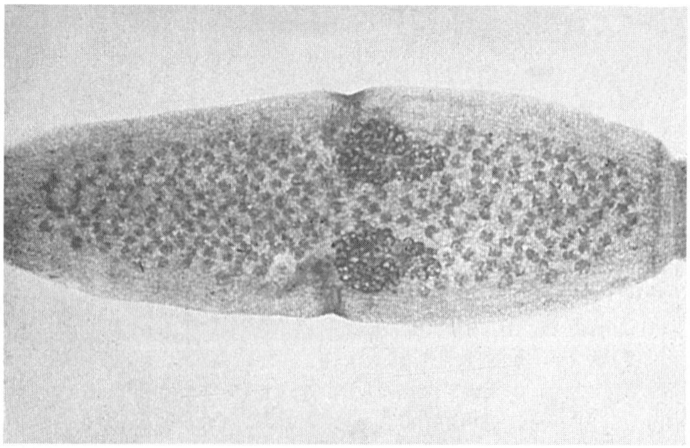

FIGURE 115-15 *Dipylidium caninum* proglottid. Note the two genital pores and the massing of the ova. (From Zaiman H [ed]: Pictorial Presentation of Parasites. Audiovisual. Valley City, ND, Mercy Hospital, 1900–1982.)

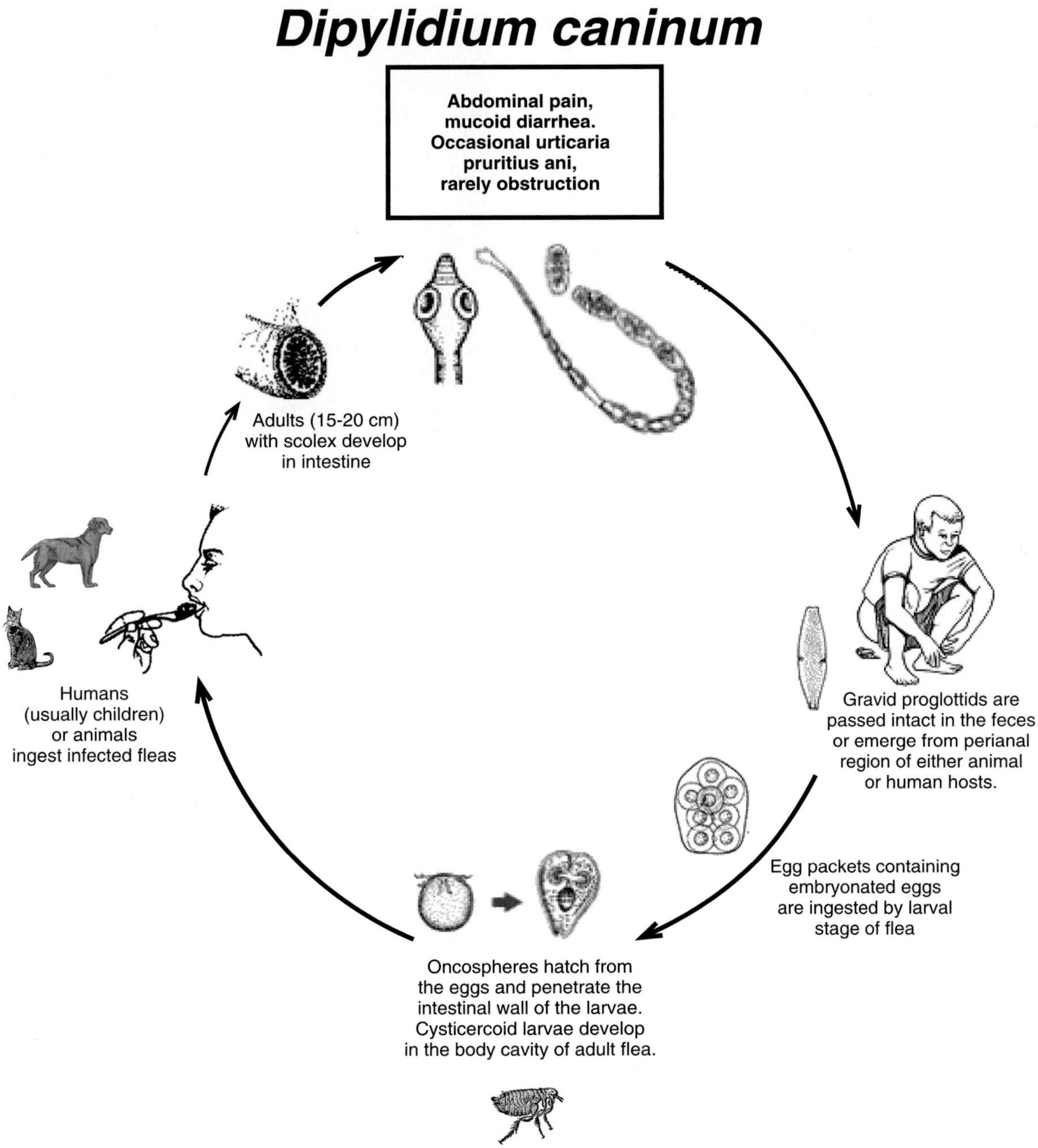

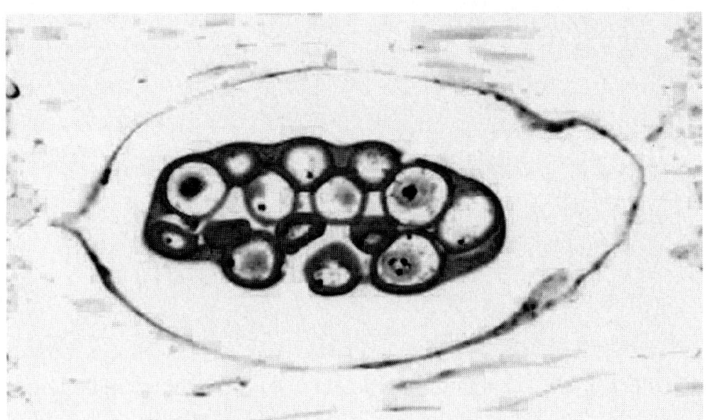

FIGURE 115-16 Egg pockets of *Dipylidium caninum* in an infant. (Courtesy of Dr. Patrick Adegboyega, Department of Pathology, University of Texas Medical Branch, Galveston, TX.)

kiss dogs and cats. Periodic treatment of pets for tapeworm infection and periodic use of insecticides to kill ectoparasites will control the spread of this infection.

Sparganosis

INTRODUCTION

Sparganosis is an uncommon parasitic infection usually caused by the migration of larval tapeworms of the genus *Spirometra*.

AGENT

Human sparganosis may occur following ingestion of species of *Cyclops* that are infected with the procercoid larva of various pseudophyllidean tapeworms of the species *Spirometra*.[1,58] The procercoid penetrates the intestinal wall and migrates to various sites, including subcutaneous tissues, the central nervous system, and muscle, where they develop to second-stage larvae or plerocercoids. This condition is called sparganosis. Ingestion, either deliberately or accidentally, of infected uncooked flesh of an amphibian, reptile,[59] bird, or mammal harboring plerocercoid larvae may also be a source of infection. Spargana also develop in hogs and it has been shown that human sparganosis can be acquired from this source. All the spargana are morphologically indistinguishable. Since these worms cannot mature in humans, they migrate into the tissues and remain as plerocercoid larvae. However, in the few instances in which the larvae were allowed to complete their life cycle in dogs or cats, they were identified as members of the genus *Spirometra*. In some cases in the United States, they were identified as *Spirometra mansoni*. Molecular approaches have been applied to this parasite that may aid in the diagnosis of this infection.[60]

EPIDEMIOLOGY

Sparganosis is reported in many areas of the world, including China, Japan, Southeast Asia, and South and Central America, and has occasionally been reported in various areas of the United States and Europe.[61,62]

DISEASE

The presence of plerocercoids in subcutaneous tissues is typically associated with a nodular mass consisting of tissue necrosis and a granulomatous inflammation with lymphocytes, plasma cells, and eosinophils (Fig. 115-17).[63–65] Swelling and edema are often painful (Fig. 115-18). Any part of the body may be involved, including the neck, breast, scrotum, and pleura.[64,66–70] Raw amphibian poultices harboring plerocercoid larvae applied to the eye have also been a cause of ocular sparganosis and may impair vision.[71,72]

Cerebral sparganosis is a rare complication of this infection. In the brain, the presence of the parasite evokes an intense inflammatory response (Fig. 115-19). Pathological and

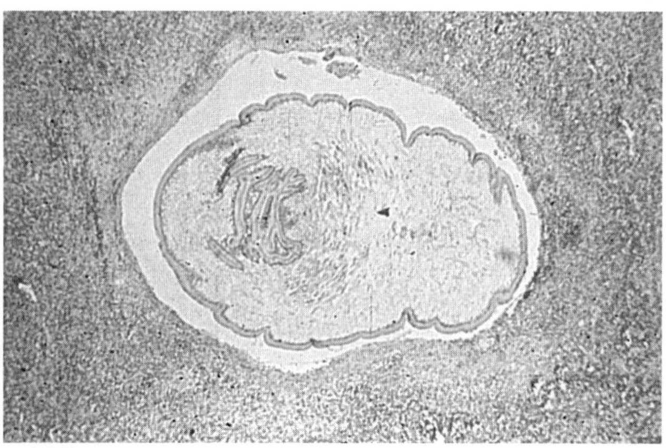

FIGURE 115-17 Sparganum: Abscess in muscle. (From Zaiman H [ed]: Pictorial Presentation of Parasites. Audiovisual. Valley City, ND, Mercy Hospital, 1900–1982.)

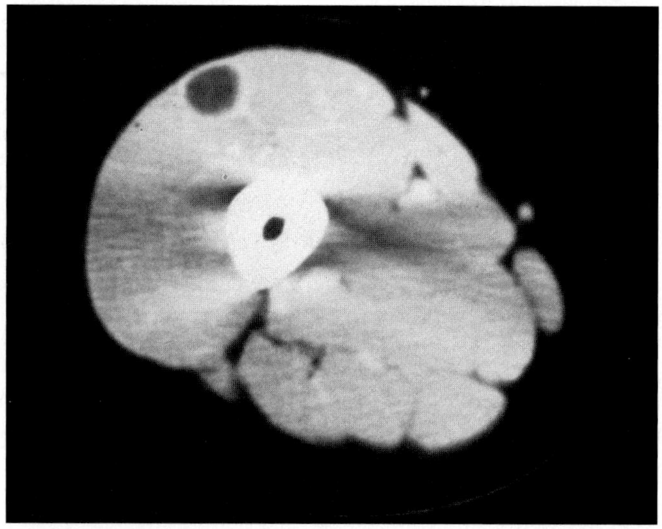

FIGURE 115-18 Sparganosis: Computed tomography scan of the thigh showing a circular hyperlucent lesion with inflammatory response of adjacent tissues. (From Zaiman H [ed]: Pictorial Presentation of Parasites. Audiovisual. Valley City, ND, Mercy Hospital, 1900–1982.)

radiographic (computed tomography and magnetic resonance imaging) studies demonstrate white matter degeneration, cortical atrophy, ventricular dilatation, punctuate calcifications, irregular or nodular enhancement, vasculitis, and hemmorhage.[73–81]

An unusual manifestation of sparganosis is a condition known as sparganum proliferum, in which larvae of a pseudophyllidean tapeworm of unknown genus and species proliferate in the tissues as independent organisms. In several instances, thousands of spargana have been found in the subcutaneous tissues.[58]

DIAGNOSIS

In general, the diagnosis is based on pathological examination of biopsy or autopsy specimens and/or direct visualization of the parasite (see Fig. 115-19). In the case of

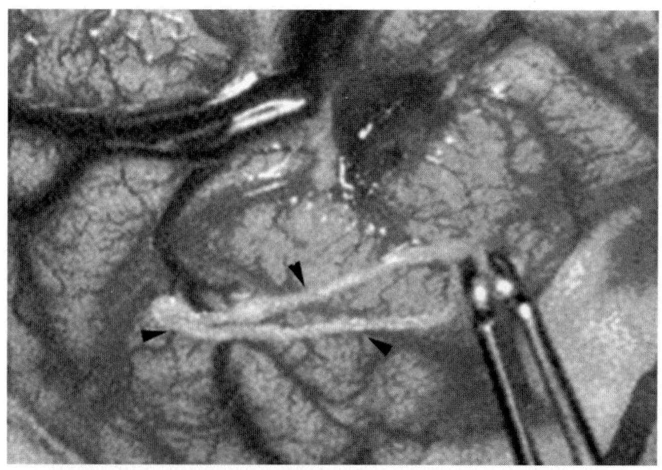

FIGURE 115-19 Sparganum removed from the right occipital cortex. (From Kim DG, Paek SH, Chang KH, et al: Cerebral sparganosis: Clinical manifestations, treatment, and outcome. J Neurosurg 85:1066–1071, 1996, with permission of the Journal of Neurosurgery and the authors.)

cerebral sparganosis, magnetic resonance imaging is most helpful in the diagnosis and is usually followed by stereotactic biopsies.[77,80] Serodiagnosis using monoclonal antibodies in a competition enzyme-linked immunosorbent assay (ELISA) has been reported.[82,83] False-positive results may occur when *Clonorchis* and *Paragonimus* infections are present.

TREATMENT AND PREVENTION

Treatment of sparganosis has been surgical removal of the larvae. Ocular sparganosis is sometimes treated by killing the larvae and allowing the organisms to resorb, although surgical removal has come into favor. Mebendazole, albendazole, and praziquantel have not been demonstrated to be useful. Spargana are destroyed by flash freezing at −10°C for 24 hours.[59]

REFERENCES

1. Grove DI: A History of Human Helminthology. Wallingford, UK, CAB, 1990.
2. Tanowitz HB, Weiss LM, Wittner M: Tapeworms. Curr Inf Dis Rep 3:77–84, 2001.
3. Wardle RA, McLeod JA: The Zoology of Tapeworms. New York, Hafner, 1968.
4. Flisser A: Neurocysticercosis in Mexico. Parasitol Today 4:131–134, 1998.
5. White AC, Baig S, Robinson P: *Taenia saginata* onchosphere excretory/secretory peptidases. J Parasitol 82:7–10, 1996.
6. Maravilla P, Souza V, Valera A: Detection of genetic variation in *Taenia solium*. J Parasitol 89:1250–1254, 2003.
7. Nakao M, Saka Y, Ito A: The mitochondrial genome of the tapeworm *Taenia solium*: A finding of the abbreviated stop condon U. J Parasitol 89:633–635, 2003.
8. Ito A, Craig PS: Immunodiagnostic and molecular approaches for the detection of taeniid cestode infections. Trends Parasitol 19:377–381, 2003.
9. Garcia HH, del Brutto OH: *Taenia solium* cysticercosis. Inf Dis Clin North Am 14:97–119, 2000.
10. Verastegui M, Gilman RH, Garcia HH: Prevalence of antibodies to unique *Taenia solium* onchosphere antigens in Taeniasis and human and porcine cysticercosis. Am J Trop Med Hyg 69:438–444, 2003.
11. Gonzalez AE, Garcia HH, Gilman RH: Control of *Taenia solium*. Acta Trop 87:103–109, 2003.
12. Zoli A, Shey-Njila O, Assana E, et al: Regional status, epidemiology and impact of *Taenia solium* cysticercosis in western and Central Africa. Acta Trop 87:35–42, 2003.
13. Boa ME, Bogh HO, Kassuku AA, et al: The prevalence of *Taenia solium* metacestodes in Tanzania. J Helminthol 69:113–117, 1996.
14. Ito A, Nakao M, Wandra T: Human taeniasis and cysticercosis in Asia. Lancet 362:1918–1920, 2003.
15. Bowles J, McManus DP: Genetic characterization of the Asian *Taenia*, a newly described taeniid cestode of humans. Am J Trop Med Hyg 50:33–44, 1994.
16. Torgerson PR, Pilkigton J, Gulland FMD, et al: Further evidence for the long distance dispersal of taeniid eggs. Int J Parasitol 25:265–267, 1995.
17. Demiriz M, Gunhan O, Celasun B, et al: Colonic perforation caused by taeniasis. Trop Geogr Med 47:180–182, 1995.
18. Ash LR, Orihel TC: Parasites, a Guide to Laboratory Procedures and Identification. Chicago, ASCP Press, 1987.
19. Jeri C, Gilman RH, Lescano AG: Species identification after treatment for human Taeniasis. Lancet 363:949–950, 2004.
20. Yamasaki H, Allan JC, Sato MO: DNA differential diagnosis of taeniasis and cysticercosis by multiplex PCR. J Clin Microbiol 42:548–553, 2003.
21. Nunes CM, Lima LG, Pereira RN, et al: *Taenia saginata*: Polymerase chain reaction for teaniasis in human fecal samples. Exp Parasitol 104:67–69, 2003.
22. Mayta H, Talley A, Gilman RH, et al: Differentiating *Taenia solium* and *Taenia saginata* infections by simple hematoxylin-eosin staining and PCR-restriction enzyme analysis. J Clin Microbiol 38:133–137, 2000.
23. Drugs for Parasitic Infections, August, 2004, www.medicalletter.org
24. Sciutto E, Fragoso G, Manoutcharian K, et al: New approaches to improve a peptide vaccine against porcine *Taenia solium* cysticercosis. Arch Med Res 33:371–378, 2002.
25. Shea M, Maberly AL, Walters J, et al: Intraocular *Taenia crassiceps (Cestoda)*. Trans Am Acad Opthalmol Otol 77:778–783, 1973.
26. Arocker-Mettinger E, Huber-Spitzy V, et al: *Taenia crassiceps* in the anterior chamber of the human eye. A case report. Klin Monatsbl Augenheilkd 201:34–37, 1992.
27. Klinker H, Tintelot K, Joeres R, et al: *Taenia crassiceps* infection in AIDS. Dtsch Med Wochenschr 117:133–138, 1992.
28. Francois A, Favenne L, Cambon-Michot C, et al: *Taenia crassiceps* invasive cysticercosis: A new human pathogen in acquired immunodeficiency syndrome? Am J Surg Pathol 22:488–492, 1998.
29. Chuck RS, Olk R, Weil GJ, et al: Surgical removal of a subretinal proliferating cysticercus of *Taenia crassiceps*. Arch Ophthalmol 115:562–563, 1997.
30. Diphyllobothriasis associated with salmon—United States. MMWR 30:331–338, 1981.
31. Von Bonsdorff B, Bylund G: The ecology of *Diphyllobothrium latum*. Ecol Dis 1:21–26, 1982.
32. Von Bonsdorff B: The broad tapeworm story. Acta Med Scand 204:241–247, 1978.
33. Dick TA, Nelson PA, Choudhury A: Diphyllobothriasis: Update on human cases, foci patterns and sources of human infections and future considerations. Southeast Asian J Trop Med Pub Health 32(Suppl 2):59–76, 2001.
34. Hutchinson JW, Bass JW, Demers DM, et al: Diphyllobothriasis after eating raw salmon. Hawaii Med J 56:176–177, 1997.
35. Revenga JE: *Diphyllobothrium dendriticum* and *Diphyllobothrium latum* in fishes from southern Argentina: Association, abundance, distribution, pathological effects, and risk of human infection. J Parasitol 79:379–383, 1993.
36. Curtis MA, Bylund G: Diphyllobothriasis: Fish tapeworm disease in the circumpolar north. Arctic Med Res 50:18–25, 1991.
37. Matsuura T, Bylund G, Sugane K: Comparison of restriction fragment length polymorphism of ribosomal DNA between *Diphyllobothrium nihonkaiense* and *D. latum*. J Helminthol 66:261–266, 1992.
38. Von Bonsdorff B: Diphyllobothriasis in Man. London, Academic Press, 1977.
39. Ohnishi K, Murata M: Praziquantel for the treatment of *Diphyllobothrium nihonkaiense* infections in humans. Trans R Soc Trop Med Hyg 88:580, 1994.
40. Beaver PC, Jung RC, Cupp EW: Clinical Parasitology, 9th ed. Philadelphia, Lea & Febiger, 1984.
41. Arai HP: Biology of the Tapeworm *Hymenolepis diminuta*. New York, Academic Press, 1980.
42. Macnish MG, Ryan UM, Behnke JM, et al: Detection of the rodent tapeworm *Rhodentolepis (=Hymenolepis) microstoma* in humans. A new zoonosis? Int J Parasitol 33:1079–1085, 2003.
43. Macnish MG, Morgan-Ryan UM, Monis PT, et al: A molecular phylogeny of nuclear and mitochondrial sequences in *Hymenolepis nana* (Cestoda) supports the existence of a cryptic species. Parasitology 125:567–575, 2002.
44. Le TH, Blair D, McManus DP: Mitochondrial genomes of parasitic flatworms. Trend Parasitol 18:206–213, 2002.
45. Ito A: Basic and applied immunology in cestode infections: From Hymenolepis to Taenia and Echinococcus. Int J Parasitol 27:1203–1211, 1997.
46. Andreassen J, Bennet-Jenkins EM, Bryant C: Immunology and biochemistry of *Hymenolepis diminuta*. Adv Parasitol 42:223–227, 1999.
47. McKay DM, Khan WI: STAT-6 is an absolute requirement for murine rejection of *Hymenolepis dimuta*. J Parasitol 89:188–189, 2003.
48. Biswash H, Arora RR, Sehgal S: Epidemiology of *Hymenolepis nana* infections in a selected rural community. J Commun Dis 10:170–174, 1978.
49. Mason PR, Patterson BA: Epidemiology of *Hymenolepis nana* infections in primary schoolchildren in urban and rural communities in Zimbabwe. J Parasitol 80:245–250, 1994.
50. Khalil HM, el Shimi S, Sarwat MA, et al: A recent study of *Hymenolepis nana* infection in Egyptian children. J Egypt Soc Parasitol 21:293–300, 1991.
51. Di Lernia V, Ricci C, Albertini G: Skin eruption associated with *Hymenolepis nana* infection. Int J Dermatol 43:357–359, 2004.

52. Olson PD, Voder K, Fajardo LF, et al: Lethal invasive cestodiasis in immunosuppressed patients. J Infect Dis 187:1962–1966, 2003.
53. Neafie RC, Marty AM: Unusual infections in humans. Clin Microbiol Rev 6:34–56, 1993.
54. Maksimova TLU, Oshevskaia ZA, Chemburova NA: Dipylidiasis in a child in Tula Province. Med Parazitol (Mosk) 2:59–60, 1995.
55. Wijesundera MD: The use of praziquantel in human infection with *Dipylidium*. Trans Soc Trop Med Hyg 83:383, 1989.
56. Chappel CL, Penn HM: *Dipylidium caninum*, an underrecognized infection in infants and children. Pediatr Infect Dis J 9:745–747, 1990.
57. Molina CP, Ogburn J, Adegboyega P: Infection by *Dipylidium caninum* in an infant. Arch Pathol Lab Med 127:e157–e159, 2003.
58. Beaver PC, Malek EA, Little MD: Proliferating larval cestode in a man in Paraguay. A case report and review. Am J Trop Med Hyg 30:625–637, 1981.
59. Milllan JM, Purdie JL, Melville LF: Public health risks of farmed crocodiles. Rev Sci Tech 16:605–608, 1996.
60. Miyadera H, Kokaze A, Kuramochi T, et al: Phylogenetic identification of *Sparganum proliferum* as a pseudophyllidean cestode by the sequence analyses on mitochondrial COI and nuclear sdhB genes. Parasitol Int 50:93–104, 2001.
61. Taylor RL: Sparganosis in the United States. Report of a case. Am J Clin Pathol 66:560–564, 1976.
62. Pampiglione S, Fioravanti ML, Rivasi F: Human sparganosis in Italy. Case report and review of the European cases. APMIS 111:349–354, 2003.
63. Campbell EW, Beals C: Striking eosinophilia in sparganosis. Case report. Postgrad Med 62:138–140, 1977.
64. Chung SY, Park KS, Lee Y, et al: Breast sparganosis: Mammographic and ultrasound features. J Clin Ultrasound 237:447–451, 1995.
65. Tsou MH, Huang TW: Pathology of subcutaneous sparganosis: Report of two cases. J Formos Med Assoc 92:649–653, 1993.
66. Chae SW, Choi JH, Lee DJ, et al: Sparganosis presenting as a lateral neck mass. Head Neck 25:74–76, 2003.
67. Sim S, You J-K, Lee I-Y, et al: A case of breast sparganosis. Korean J Parasitol 40:187–189, 2002.
68. Jeong HJ: Fournier's gangrene associated with sparganosis in the scrotum. Urology 63:176–177, 2004.
69. Ishii H, Mukae H, Inoue Y, et al: A rare case of eosinophilic pleuritis due to sparganosis. Intern Med 40:783–785, 2001.
70. Sakamoto T, Gutierrez C, Rodriquez A, et al: Testicular sparganosis in a child from Uruguay. Acta Trop 88:83–86, 2003.
71. Ausayakhun S, Siriprasert V, Morakote N, et al: Ocular sparganosis in Thailand. Southeast Asian J Trop Med Public Health 24:603–606, 1993.
72. Botterel F, Bourée P: Ocular sparganosis: A case report. J Travel Med 10:245–246, 2003.
73. Holodniy M, Almenoff J, Loutit J, et al: Cerebral sparganosis: Case report and review. Rev Infect Dis 13:155–159, 1991.
74. Kradel J, Drolshagen LF, MacDade A: MR and CT findings in cerebral sparganosis. J Comput Assist Tomogr 17:989–990, 1993.
75. Mineura K, Mori T: Sparganosis of the brain. J Neurosurg 52:588–590, 1980.
76. Munckhof WJ, Grayson ML, Susil BJ, et al: Cerebral spargaganosis in an East Timorese refugee. Med J Aust 161:263–264, 1994.
77. Tsai MD, Chang CN, Ho YS, et al: Cerebral sparganosis diagnosed and treated with stereotactic techniques. Report of two cases. J Neurosurg 78:129–132, 1993.
78. Wong CW, Ho YS: Intraventricular haemorrhage and hydrocephalus caused by intraventricular parasitic granuloma suggesting cerebral sparganosis. Acta Neurochir (Wien) 129:205–208, 1994.
79. Jeong SC, Bae JC, Hwang SH, et al: Cerebral sparganosis with intracerebral hemorrhage: A case report. Neurology 50:503–506, 1998.
80. Kim DG, Paek SH, Chang KH, et al: Cerebral sparganosis: Clinical manifestations, treatment, and outcome. J Neurosurg 85:1066–1071, 1996.
81. Han S-R, Park J-K, Kim Y-I, et al: Posterior cerebral artery infarction caused by cerebral sparganosis-induced vasculitis. Eur Neurol 46:105–107, 2001.
82. Nishiyama T, Ide T, Himes SR, et al: Immunodiagnosis of human sparganosis mansoni by micro-chemiluminescence enzyme-linked immunosorbent assay. Trans Soc Trop Med Hyg 88:663–665, 1994.
83. Yeo IS, Yong TS, Im K: Serodiagnosis of human sparganosis by a monoclonal antibody-based competition ELISA. Yonsei Med J 35:43–48, 1994.

116

Schistosomiasis

CHARLES H. KING

INTRODUCTION

Schistosomiasis remains one of the most prevalent helminthic infections in the world. It is found in tropical and subtropical areas of South America, Africa, the Middle East, East Asia, and the Philippines.[1,2] Recent World Health Organization (WHO) estimates indicate that more than 200 million people are infected worldwide, with over 600 million people at risk of infection.[1,2] Schistosomiasis is associated with renal and bladder dysfunction (*Schistosoma haematobium*) or liver and intestinal disease (*Schistosoma mansoni, Schistosoma japonicum, Schistosoma mekongi,* and *Schistosoma intercalatum*) in endemic areas, and it also is a contributing cause of anemia and growth retardation.

Schistosomiasis is acquired through the skin while wading or bathing in freshwater when the human host comes into contact with the infectious, free-living, cercarial larvae that are released by the parasite's intermediate hosts—aquatic or amphibious snails.[2] Patterns of water supply, sanitation, and human water use are, therefore, critical factors in determining the risk of infection.[3] In addition, the geographic distribution of the different *Schistosoma* species is entirely dependent on the distribution of the distinct snail species that serve as intermediate hosts. Climate, water quality, and other ecologic factors that regulate these snail populations also determine the distribution of schistosomiasis on a district as well as national level.[3]

Readily available animal models of schistosome infection have allowed intensive study of the immunology and molecular biology of schistosomiasis. Detailed analysis of host responses to these complex multicellular parasites has provided significant insight into the regulation of cell-mediated and humoral immunity,[4] as well as the resistance pathways available for elimination of macroparasites.[5] Molecular studies of the parasite[6] have provided information on novel modes of genetic expression, as well as leads for the development of vaccines[7] and new pharmaceuticals for control of this widespread chronic infection.

AGENT

Schistosomiasis is an ancient human disease. Parasites and their eggs have been identified in early Egyptian mummies and the symptoms described in early papyrus records. In modern times, the parasite cause of schistosomiasis was identified by Theodor Bilharz in 1852 and later by Patrick Manson.

Five species of schistosomes infect humans. The three major species are *S. haematobium,* found in Africa and the Middle East; *S. mansoni,* found in Africa, the Middle East, the Caribbean, and South America; and *S. japonicum,* found in China, Southeast Asia, and the Philippines. Human infection also occurs with *S. intercalatum,* which is found in central and West Africa, and *S. mekongi,* which is found only in the Mekong river basin of Southeast Asia.

Species differences are distinguished by differences in morphology, both in the parasite stages and in their eggs. The characteristic feature of the *S. mansoni* egg is its lateral spine; of the *S. haematobium* egg, its terminal spine; and of the *S. japonicum* egg, its limited, inconspicuous spine.[2] Further species distinction is made by the species of intermediate host snails found to be supporting transmission of the parasite. These are *Biomphalaria* species snails for *S. mansoni, Bulinus* species snails for *S. haematobium,* and *Oncomelania* species snails for *S. japonicum.*[3]

Given the geographic differences reported in local susceptibility to antiparasitic drugs, there undoubtedly are *Schistosoma* subspecies, as well as intraspecies strain differences that exist between continents and within individual countries.[8,9] Recent epidemiologic studies in Kenya have focused on significant differences in the pathogenicity of *S. mansoni* infection in different areas of the country.[8] Clinical evidence had suggested that there might be distinct strains of *S. mansoni,* centered in discrete geographic areas, that result in significantly different levels of morbidity when local human populations are infected. Molecular biologic studies are underway confirming the genetic similarities and differences between geographic strains of *S. mansoni* in Brazil and other endemic areas.[10] Significant differences have also been reported between the clinical aspects of *S. japonicum* infection in China and *S. japonicum* infection in the Philippines. Recent completion of the *S. mansoni* and *S. japonicum* genome projects will shed further light.[11,12]

EPIDEMIOLOGY

In endemic areas, schistosome infection is acquired in childhood. Infection increases in prevalence and intensity with age, peaking in the age group of 15 to 20 years. In older people, a drastic decline in intensity, but not in prevalence, has been demonstrated.[13–15] The debate is still active over whether the decline represents acquired immunity, a change in water contact, a change in egg production by adult worms, or a combination of these factors.[16] Schistosome infections in the human populations of endemic areas follow an overdispersed pattern, in which most infected persons show low egg counts, and a small percentage (1% to 5%) harbor extremely heavy infection. Susceptibility to high-intensity infection may reflect water exposure patterns or may be related to certain human genetic characteristics.[17] The epidemiology of schistosomiasis is further regulated by the duration of the parasite life span (3 to 7 years) and the multiple immunologic and nonimmunologic responses of the host that participate in regulating infection and disease.

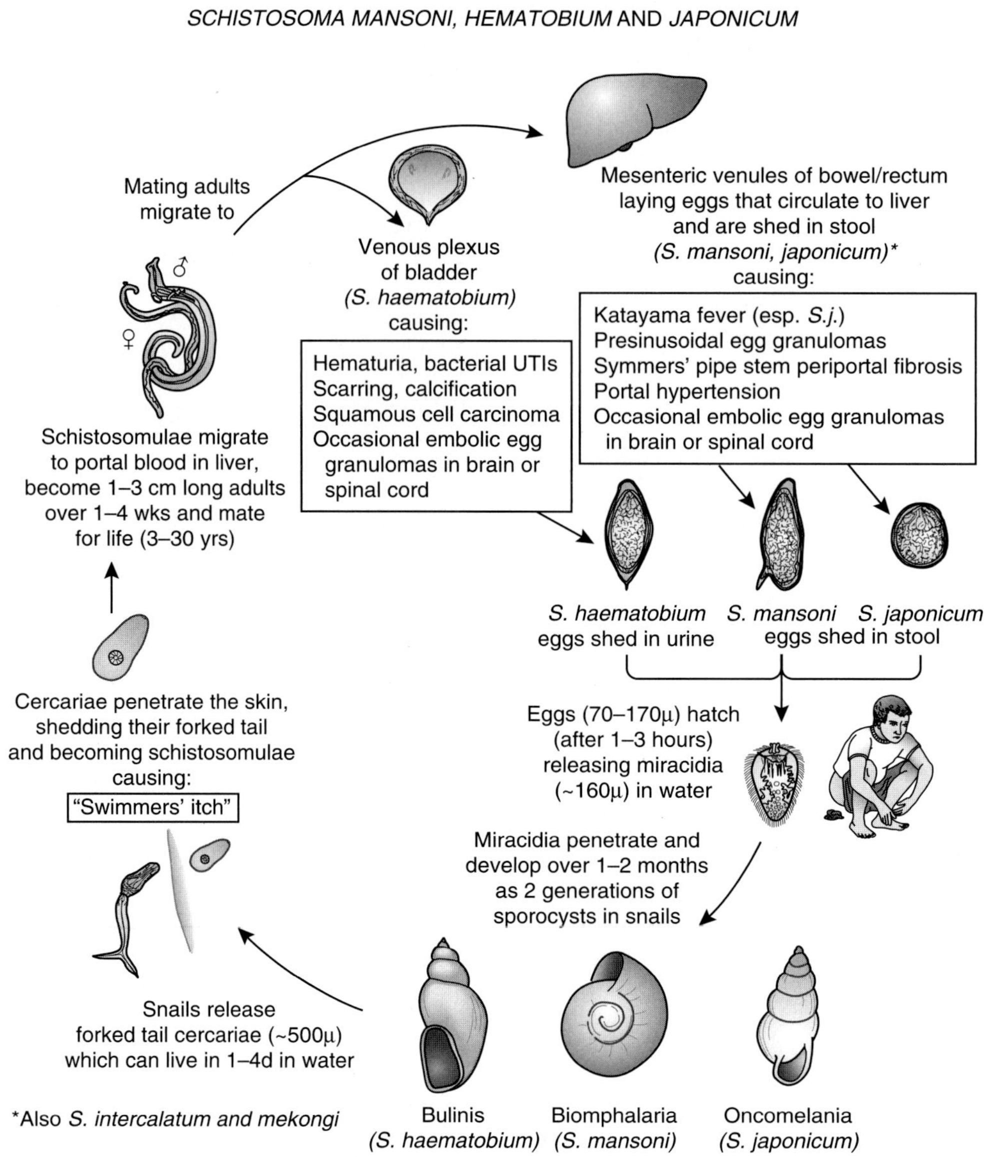

Expression of disease due to schistosome infection is similarly complex. Although adult schistosomes do not replicate in the mammalian host, they produce eggs throughout their life span. These parasite eggs elicit host immunopathologic reactions, which are responsible for most disease manifestations.[18] Pathogenesis may be related, therefore, to intensity of infection and certainly to factors that regulate host response, including genetic influences.[19]

Mathematical modeling that describes schistosome prevalence, intensity, and transmission patterns has been developed.[20,21] Central to these studies is the concept of quantification of infection, which is possible in helminthic infections because adult worms do not replicate in mammalian hosts. Access to quantitative data on schistosomiasis is mainly based on egg counts in feces or urine. Despite these limitations, however, useful mathematical models have been constructed for infection, its transmission, and its disease sequelae.[21]

DISEASE

Illness due to *Schistosoma* infection differs between the early, or acute, stages of infection and the later disease caused by chronic infection.[22] Early manifestations include dermatitis and acute schistosomiasis (Katayama or "snail" fever). These are caused by initial entry of the parasite's cercarial forms into the skin, which causes a localized dermatitis, then subsequent migration of the developing schistosomulum through the lung and hepatic circulation during its development into a mature schistosome worm. The chronic disease of schistosomiasis, which is much more prevalent in endemic areas, is due to a granulomatous response to parasite eggs, resulting in

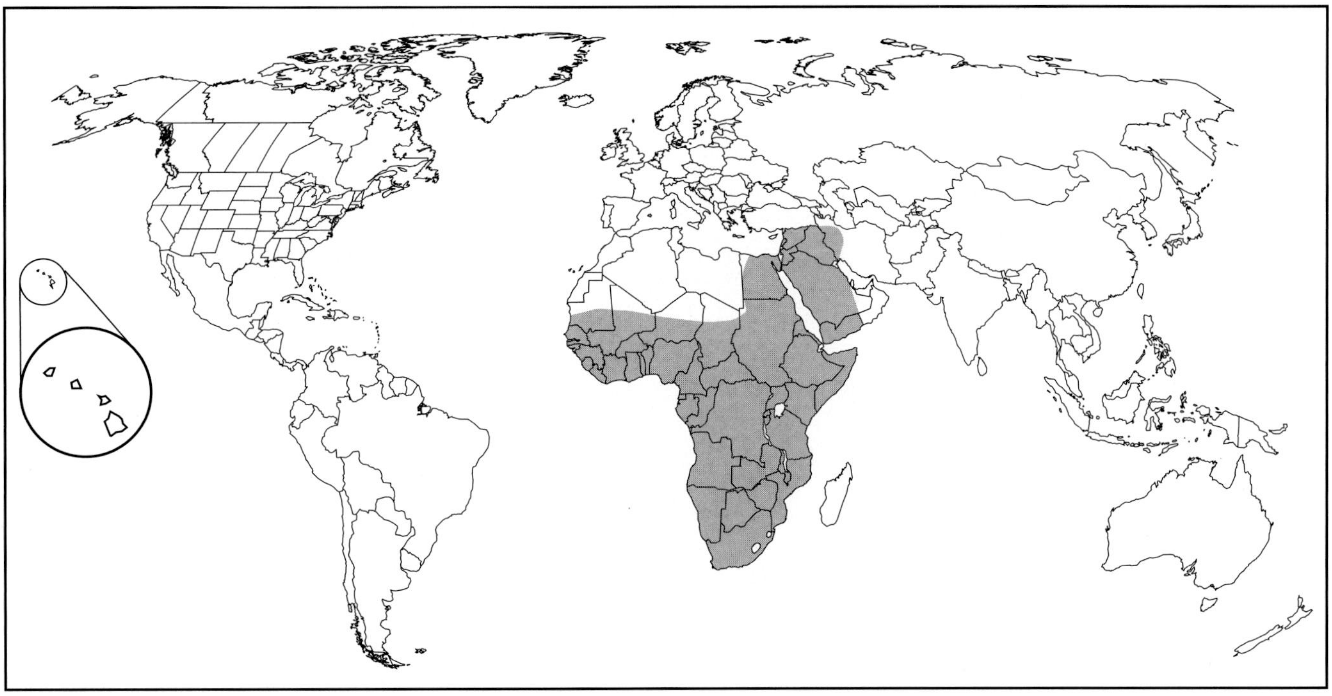

Schistosoma haematobium

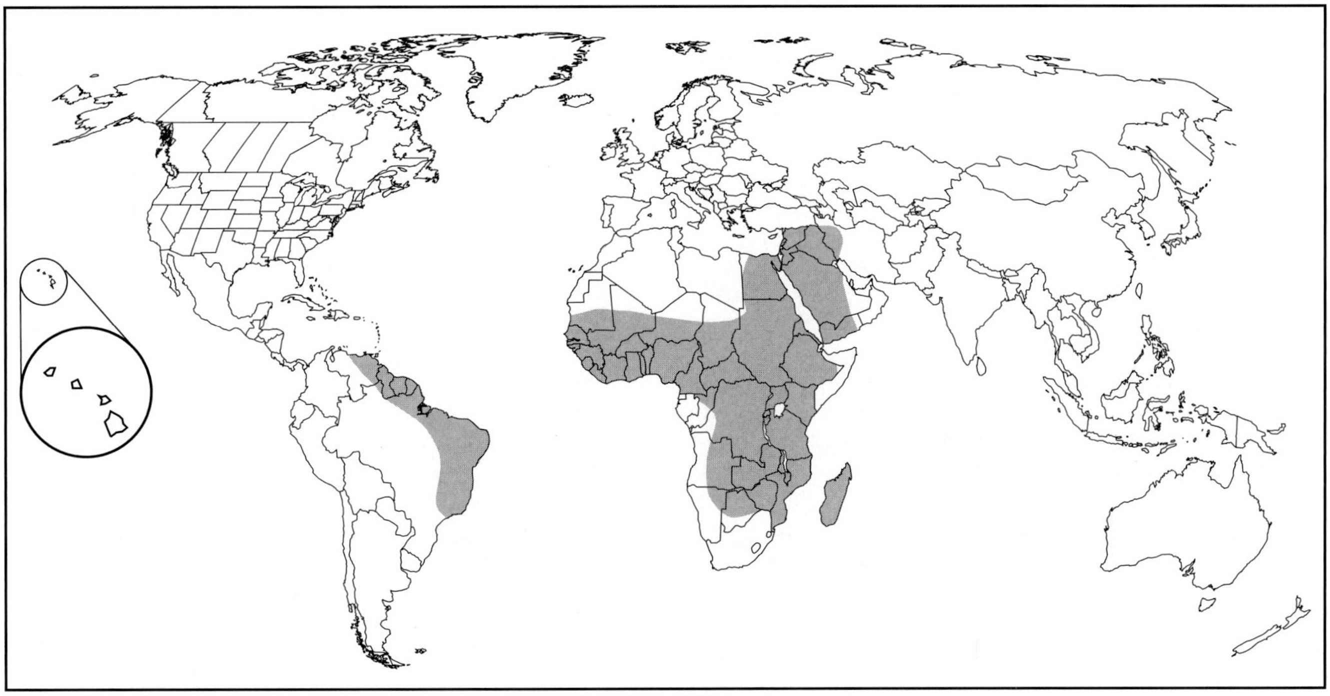

Schistosoma mansoni

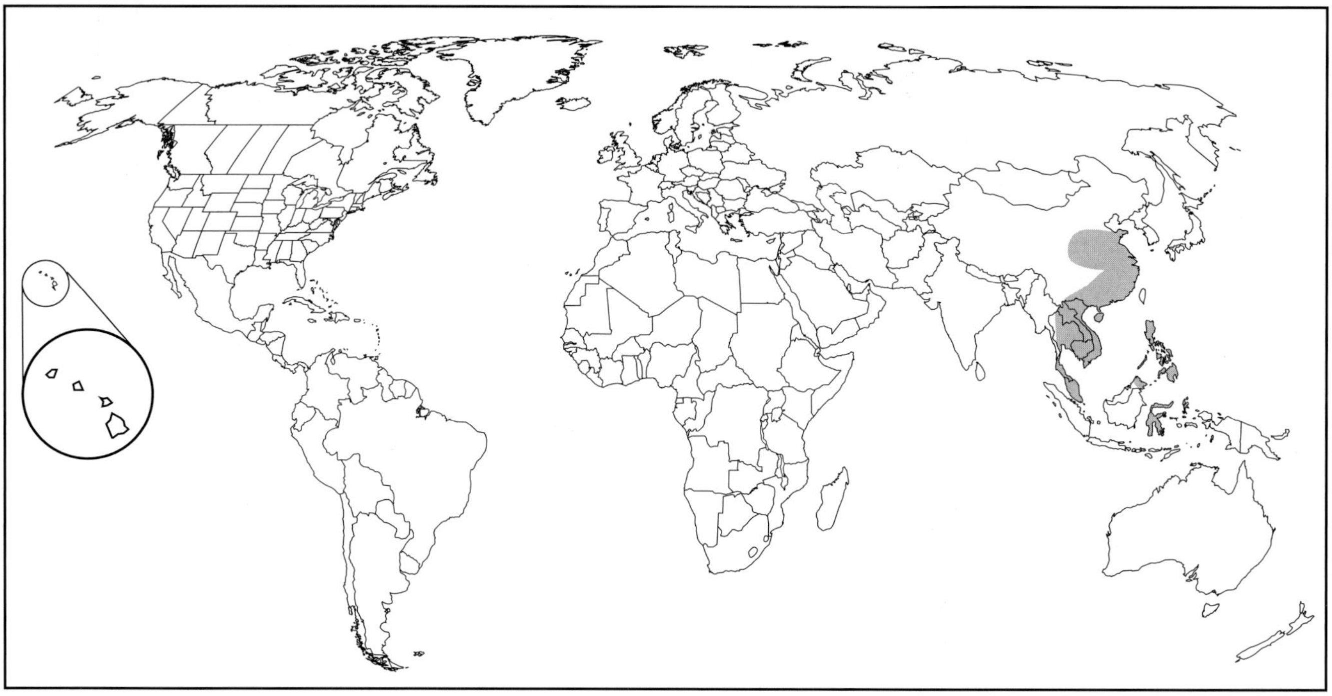

Schistosoma japonicum

chronic fibro-obstructive sequelae in the intestine or portal veins (*S. mansoni, S. japonicum, S. mekongi,* and *S. intercalatum*) or the urinary tract (*S. haematobium*).[22]

Cercarial dermatitis is a pruritic, papular rash found on skin exposed to cercaria-containing waters. In northern climates, cercarial dermatitis is the cause of "swimmer's itch," an eruption that occurs after abortive skin penetration by cercariae of bird schistosomes (*Trichobilharzia* and *Bilharziella*). In areas endemic for human schistosomiasis, cercarial dermatitis is most common in *S. mansoni* and *S. haematobium* transmission areas. It occurs within 24 hours after exposure, appearing as pruritic red papules on the surface of the skin. Because exposure typically occurs by walking or wading in infected ponds or rivers, the rash is usually located on the lower legs. The duration of symptoms depends on the intensity of the local cutaneous inflammatory response.

Acute schistosomiasis develops in some persons with heavy exposure to *S. japonicum* or *S. mansoni* infection. It is rarely seen in *S. haematobium* infection. Originally described in the Katayama Valley of southern Japan, acute schistosomiasis is most likely to occur in the traveler or new immigrant to an endemic area.[23] While symptoms usually resolve over several weeks, intense infection may result in death. Symptoms develop between 4 and 8 weeks after exposure, coinciding with the maturation of the infecting schistosome and the beginning of oviposition. Symptoms include fever, sweats, chills, cough, and headaches. Physical findings include lymphadenopathy and hepatosplenomegaly, and there is associated eosinophilia on laboratory examination. Early in the course of acute schistosomiasis, when egg production is just beginning, routine parasitologic diagnosis may be falsely negative due to the limited number of eggs in the stool. Biopsy or serologic testing may be required to establish the diagnosis. In fatal cases, large numbers of eggs are found in the liver and intestines, and massive infection is the rule.

Chronic schistosomiasis, as seen in endemic areas, is a less dramatic, progressive illness resulting from repeated prolonged tissue injury and fibrosis from deposition of parasite eggs in affected organs: the intestine and liver for *S. mansoni, S. japonicum, S. mekongi,* and *S. intercalatum,* and the bladder, ureters, and kidneys for *S. haematobium.*[2]

The patient with intestinal schistosomiasis may complain of fatigue, abdominal pain, diarrhea, or dysenteric bloody diarrhea caused by granuloma and ulcer formation in the bowel wall.[24] Granulomatous inflammation may result in polyp formation, which can be detected on barium contrast studies or endoscopy. Ulceration and chronic bleeding may lead to the development of moderate or severe iron deficiency anemia.[25]

In *S. mansoni, S. mekongi,* and *S. japonicum* infections, a significant number of parasite eggs are retained in the body and travel to the liver via the portal circulation. These eggs lodge in presinusoidal radicles of the portal vein, where they elicit a granulomatous reaction.[16] Venous flow is affected, first by the presence of the living egg and the surrounding granuloma formation, and later by local scar formation resulting from fibrosis. The net result is portal vein hypertension and the development of portosystemic collateral blood flow. The earliest sign of chronic schistosomiasis is hepatomegaly. As infection progresses, and liver damage becomes more severe, splenomegaly is also seen.[13,26] Portal pressures are markedly elevated, whereas the wedge hepatic pressure remains normal. Liver perfusion is maintained by an increase in arterial flow from the hepatic arteries. Consequently, hepatocellular function remains intact until late in the course of infection, unless alcoholism or coinfection with hepatitis B or C virus also is present.[2]

The major manifestations of *S. haematobium* infection are seen in children and young adults living in endemic areas.[14] Deposition of schistosome eggs around the lower end of ureters and in the wall of the urinary bladder results in hematuria, dysuria, and urinary frequency. In contrast to the species causing intestinal schistosomiasis, the symptoms and signs of *S. haematobium* infection are seen in a considerable percentage of those infected. The functional consequence of *S. haematobium* infection is bladder neck obstruction with back pressure causing hydroureter and hydronephrosis. Urinary schistosomiasis usually creates a setting for repeated bacterial infection, compromised kidney function, and finally renal failure.[27] In several endemic areas, *S. haematobium* infection is epidemiologically associated with squamous cell bladder carcinoma.[28,29] The relationship is such that the International Agency for Research on Cancer has classified *S. haematobium* as a human carcinogen.[30] While the sequence of events in *S. haematobium*–related disease seems clear, the natural history and outcome are poorly understood because of the lack of longitudinal long-term population-based studies.

Other clinical manifestations of intestinal and urinary schistosomiasis constitute important aspects of infection and disease. Among the most significant are pulmonary, central nervous system (CNS), renal, and cutaneous manifestations.[31–33] Pulmonary schistosomiasis results from parasite egg deposition in the pulmonary vasculature followed by granuloma formation and obstruction of blood flow.[31] The pathophysiologic consequence is pulmonary hypertension and the features of cor pulmonale. This course of events may occur during *S. haematobium* infection (because of the anatomic location of the adult worm) or during chronic intestinal schistosomiasis when eggs may pass to the pulmonary circulation via portosystemic collaterals.

CNS schistosomiasis causes grand mal epilepsy in 1% to 2% of persons with *S. japonicum* infection. Transverse myelitis is the usual disease entity detected in those with *S. mansoni* or *S. haematobium* infection. Disease usually occurs in chronically infected persons but may happen during the acute phase.[32]

PATHOGENESIS AND IMMUNITY

Schistosome infection presents the host with a complex challenge. Adult worms do not replicate in the host but produce hundreds of eggs over a life span of 4 to 7 years. Eggs retained in the host tissue survive for up to 6 weeks. Host reactions are therefore complicated by these overlapping parasite factors, which result in a myriad of immunologic and nonimmunologic responses.[16,24] Central to the cause of disease is the cell-mediated granuloma formation and multiple humoral and cellular regulatory circuitry.[16] Resistance to infection with any schistosome species is both innate and acquired.[7,34] The role of each in regulating parasite populations is still being examined. Population-based studies suggest strongly that acquired immunity exists in humans.[20] The challenge is to examine such a phenomenon to understand its mechanisms and ultimately succeed in inducing resistance.

DIAGNOSIS

The "gold standard" for identifying an established schistosome infection is to demonstrate parasite eggs in the patient's stool (*S. mansoni, S. japonicum, S. mekongi,* and *S. intercalatum*) or urine (*S. haematobium*).[35] Sensitivity of detection is improved by concentration and clarification techniques. Intensity of infection can be determined by quantitative sampling of defined quantities of stool (Kato template technique) or urine (syringe filtration). It should be noted that parasite eggs are deposited in the wall of the bowel or bladder and may pass into the lumen only some time later. The presence of a patent, active infection is associated with viable eggs (as determined by miracidial hatching when the eggs are placed in freshwater), whereas remote or treated infection is associated with passage of only nonviable eggs. In very heavy infections, the anatomical distribution of eggs may not be typical—that is, *S. haematobium* eggs may be found in the stool, and *S. mansoni* eggs may be found in the urine.

Infection is also defined when parasite eggs are identified in tissues obtained on rectal, intestinal, liver, prostatic, or bladder biopsy. Unfortunately, standard fixation and staining may not be able to distinguish the viability of these eggs, and it may not be certain whether the infection is current or remote. In ectopic infections (e.g., skin or CNS), or very light infections, the biopsy may be the first clue to the presence of schistosome infection.

Serologic tests have been developed to detect the presence of specific antischistosome antibodies in patients suspected of infection. Species-specific antigens have been identified on Western blotting, allowing some confidence in the determination of the infecting parasite.[36] However, a positive serology does not distinguish between current and past infection. In endemic populations, serology is sensitive but not specific for active infection and is therefore most useful for its negative predictive value—that is, negative serology is useful in excluding infection.[2] However, among travelers from nonendemic areas who have only a recent, brief, defined exposure to the parasite, and most often a low intensity of infection, positive serology strongly suggests an active infection, even in the presence of negative stool and urine parasitologic examinations.

A valuable approach to disease quantification in endemic areas has been ultrasound imaging by means of portable, generator-powered machines.[37] For *S. mansoni* and *S. japonicum* infection, imaging of the liver allows identification of characteristic periportal fibrosis and defines the level of disease associated with parasite infection. In *S. haematobium* infection, ultrasound examination of the kidneys and bladder allows identification of granulomas, hydronephrosis, and other inflammatory changes strongly associated with this parasite.

Recent studies have focused on alternative means of identifying active parasite infection. Workers in the Netherlands have identified two parasite antigens (CCA and CAA) that circulate in the blood during the course of active, patent infection in experimental animal models.[36] In subsequent studies in human populations, the level of circulating antigen was roughly correlated with the intensity of infection, suggesting that antigen detection may be a useful means of identifying and quantifying active infection. To improve participation in antigen testing, research is progressing on the use of dot-ELISA (enzyme-linked immunosorbent assay) techniques, which can be performed using a single drop of blood obtained by the fingerstick method. Studies are also progressing on antigen detection in urine, particularly for patients infected with *S. haematobium*.[38]

Important operational research is in progress on the use of observed macro- or microhematuria or even symptom questionnaires as surrogates for the diagnosis of *S. haematobium* infection.[39] Prior experience has identified the labor and material costs of parasitologic screening as significant factors in raising the cost of control programs for this parasite. Further, incomplete compliance with screening limits the participation of a significant proportion of infected persons with the later treatment phase of a control program. Studies in *S. haematobium*–endemic areas have identified that close to 100% of subjects under age 12 years with gross or microscopic hematuria are infected with the parasite. Treatment strategies based on urine dipstick diagnosis of hematuria are being validated in follow-up studies, with expected implementation in other heavily infected endemic areas.

TREATMENT AND PROGNOSIS

Praziquantel is currently the treatment of choice for all forms of schistosomiasis.[40] Praziquantel is a well-tolerated, broad-spectrum oral anthelmintic agent that is given as a single dose of 40 mg/kg for treatment of *S. haematobium, S. mansoni,* and *S. intercalatum* infections, and as two separate 30 mg/kg doses (spaced at least 3 hours apart) for *S. japonicum* and *S. mekongi* infections. Cure rates in field studies have typically been equal to or greater than 85%. Those with infection still remaining typically have their infection intensity reduced by more than 99%, as measured by reduction in parasite egg counts in stool or urine samples. Some side effects are directly drug-induced (vomiting, dysphoria, abdominal pain), while others are proportionate to the intensity of the parasite load and appear to be related to the host immune response to the dying parasites (abdominal pain, urticaria, diarrhea).[41] Among younger patients, completion of therapy is associated with reductions in egg output, as well as reduced blood loss (gastrointestinal with *S. mansoni* and urinary with *S. haematobium* infection),[42] and regression of granulomatous inflammation in the liver (*S. mansoni* and *S. japonicum* infection) or bladder (*S. haematobium* infection). These latter effects can result in reduction of portal pressure and reversal of hydronephrosis. In older people with more advanced fibrotic tissue injury, *Schistosoma*-associated lesions may not be able to be reversed. Likewise, in patients with the late findings of esophageal varices or cor pulmonale, therapy may or may not improve their hemodynamic values. Symptomatic "ectopic" infection, as in the CNS, may initially worsen with therapy because it provokes a strong local inflammatory response. Coinfection with human immunodeficiency virus (HIV)-1 does not alter the efficacy of praziquantel therapy for schistosomiasis.

A World Health Organization (WHO) expert panel has recently reexamined the issue of praziquantel safety during pregnancy and lactation and has determined that minimal risk is associated with treatment.[43] WHO's recommendations are that women of child-bearing years should *not* be routinely excluded from mass treatment campaigns, and further, given the potential risks of infection-associated anemia during pregnancy, that schistosome-infected pregnant women and lactating women should be offered immediate treatment whenever the infection is diagnosed.

Several, sometimes less expensive, second-line drugs are in use for treatment of specific schistosome species. Metrifonate is an older agent for treatment of *S. haematobium* infection. It is given as a single oral dose of 10 mg/kg. Metrifonate efficacy for parasitologic cure varies from 60% to 80%. Repeated use in the same area may be associated with decreased efficacy over time.[44] Oxamniquine is a second-line drug used for treatment of *S. mansoni* infection. Given in doses of 40 to 60 mg/kg as a single oral dose, it has a reported efficacy of approximately 80% in achieving parasitologic cure in most areas. *S. mansoni* resistance to oxamniquine has been documented in both Brazil and Kenya. There are currently no second-line drugs for *S. japonicum* infection.[2]

PREVENTION AND CONTROL

Given the complex nature of the *Schistosoma* life cycle, there are, in theory, a number of different ways to prevent transmission of infection or reduce the likelihood of heavy infection.[1,3] These include (1) reduction or elimination of intermediate host snails; (2) elimination of snail habitats; (3) sanitation measures to prevent human excreta from contaminating local water sources; (4) provision of safe freshwater supplies to reduce contact with snail-infested water sources (this may include provision of communal baths, laundries, and swimming facilities)[45]; (5) use of protective footwear or clothing, or use of protective medicated salves to prevent cercariae from reaching the skin; and (6) use of periodic drugs to limit infection intensity in exposed populations.[21,27] If applied on a population-wide or targeted subpopulation basis to achieve coverage of the most heavy excreters of eggs, this last approach also results in a significant reduction in parasite transmission as a result of a substantial reduction in parasite eggs reaching transmission sites.

Each of these approaches has been tested under field conditions. Long-term eradication of schistosome transmission has been achieved in Japan and Venezuela, where water improvements and sanitation measures associated with development have eliminated transmission of *S. japonicum* and *S. mansoni,* respectively. Similarly, water supply projects, including provision of communal swimming pools, were associated with a significant reduction in *S. haematobium* prevalence in southern Iraq before the onset of the first Persian Gulf War. A head-to-head comparison of snail vector control, drug therapy, and water and sanitation measures for control of *S. mansoni* was performed over a 10-year period on the island of Saint Lucia in the Caribbean.[45] Although all modalities were effective in reducing infection, drug therapy was the most effective and least expensive, while provision of piped water was nearly as effective but much more expensive, requiring provision of individual household taps, as well as communal baths and laundries, to achieve comparable levels of control.

At present, the most practical approaches to control appear to be, in the short term, provision of periodic drugs to limit intensity of infection and morbidity,[46] and in the long term, provision of safe water supplies,[47] with continuing integrated health-care education[48] to limit high-risk exposure. Repeated drug therapy reduced the prevalence of severe morbidity in longitudinal studies. However, in some cases, particularly with *S. japonicum,* suspension of control measures runs the risk of rapid reemergence of infection prevalence and increased risk of hepatic morbidity.[49] Sustainability is an essential feature of any planned schistosomiasis control program. This may be difficult to achieve without assistance from developed nations owing to the relatively high per capita cost of medication and sometimes the low priority assigned to control of a disease perceived as minimally lethal. Nevertheless, schistosomiasis has a significant impact on chronic morbidity, including malnutrition, anemia, retardation of growth and development, loss of exercise or work capacity, and either urinary tract or intestinal and hepatic disease.[50] Recent social science and health-care delivery research is focusing on developing more effective ways to raise awareness of schistosomiasis as a significant health problem and on developing means to incorporate schistosomiasis control into primary health-care delivery.

REFERENCES

1. Chitsulo L, Engels D, Montresor A, et al: The global status of schistosomiasis and its control. Acta Trop 77:41, 2000.
2. Ross AGP, Bartley PB, Sleigh AC, et al: Current Concepts: Schistosomiasis. N Engl J Med 346:1212, 2002.
3. King CH: Epidemiology of schistosomiasis: Determinants of transmission of infection. In Mahmoud AAF (ed): Schistosomiasis. London, Imperial College Press, 2001.
4. Mitchell GF, Garcia EG, Rivera PT, et al: Evidence for and implications of anti-embryonation immunity in schistosomiasis. Exp Parasitol 79:546, 1994.
5. Butterworth AE, Curry AJ, Dunne DW, et al: Immunity and morbidity in human schistosomiasis mansoni. Trop Geogr Med 46:197, 1994.
6. Simpson AJG, Dias Neto E, Johnston DA, et al: Recent molecular approaches to the study of schistosome genetics. Exp Parasitol 77:376, 1993.
7. McManus DP: The search for a vaccine against schistosomiasis—a difficult path but an achievable goal. Immunol Rev 171:149, 1999.
8. Thiongo FW, Madsen H, Ouma JH, et al: Host-parasite relationships in infections with two Kenyan isolates of *Schistosoma mansoni* in NMRI mice. J Parasitol 83:330, 1997.
9. Brouwer KC, Ndhlovu PD, Wagatsuma Y, et al: Urinary tract pathology attributed to *Schistosoma haematobium:* Does parasite genetics play a role? Am J Trop Med Hyg 68:456, 2003.
10. Rodrigues NB, Coura Filho P, de Souza CP, et al: Populational structure of *Schistosoma mansoni* assessed by DNA microsatellites. Int J Parasitol 32:843, 2002.
11. Hu W, Yan Q, Shen DK, et al: Evolutionary and biomedical implications of a *Schistosoma japonicum* complementary DNA resource. Nat Genet 35:139, 2003.
12. Verjovski-Almeida S, DeMarco R, Martins EA, et al: Transcriptome analysis of the acoelomate human parasite *Schistosoma mansoni*. Nat Genet 35:148, 2003.
13. Siongok TKA, Mahmoud AAF, Ouma JH, et al: Morbidity in schistosomiasis mansoni in relation to intensity of infection: Study of a community in Machakos, Kenya. Am J Trop Med Hyg 55:273, 1976.
14. King CH, Keating CE, Muruka JF, et al: Urinary tract morbidity in schistosomiasis haematobia: Associations with age and intensity of infection in an endemic area of Coast Province, Kenya. Am J Trop Med Hyg 39:361, 1988.
15. Hagan P, Chandiwana S, Ndhlovu P, et al: The epidemiology, immunology and morbidity of *Schistosoma haematobium* infections in diverse communities in Zimbabwe. Trop Geogr Med 46:227, 1994.
16. Warren KS: Regulation of prevalence and intensity of schistosomiasis in man: Immunology or ecology? J Infect Dis 127:595, 1973.
17. Abel L, Demenais F, Prata A, et al: Evidence for the segregation of a major gene in human susceptibility resistance to infection by *Schistosoma mansoni*. Am J Hum Genet 48:959, 1991.
18. King CL: Initiation and regulation of disease in schistosomiasis. In Mahmoud AAF (ed): Schistosomiasis. London, Imperial College Press, 2001.
19. Dessein AJ, Hillaire D, El Wali NE, et al: Severe hepatic fibrosis in *Schistosoma mansoni* infection is controlled by a major locus that is closely linked to the interferon-gamma receptor gene. Am J Hum Genet 65:709, 1999.
20. Anderson RM: Mathematical studies of parasitic infection and immunity. Science 264:1884, 1994.
21. Chan MS, Guyatt HL, Bundy DAP, et al: Dynamic models of schistosomiasis morbidity. Am J Trop Med Hyg 55:52, 1996.
22. King CH: Acute and chronic schistosomiasis. Hosp Prac 26:117, 1991.
23. Cheever AW: Schistosomiasis: infection versus disease and hypersensitivity versus immunity. Am J Pathol 142:699, 1993.
24. Strickland GT: Gastrointestinal manifestations of schistosomiasis. Gut 35:1334, 1994.
25. Stephenson L: The impact of schistosomiasis on human nutrition. Parasitology 107:S107, 1993.
26. Gryseels B, Stelma FF, Talla I, et al: Epidemiology, immunology and chemotherapy of *Schistosoma mansoni* infections in a recently exposed community in Senegal. Trop Geogr Med 46:209, 1994.
27. King CH, Muchiri EM, Ouma JH: Age-targeted chemotherapy for control of urinary schistosomiasis in endemic populations. Mem Inst Oswaldo Cruz 87(Suppl 4):203, 1992.
28. Lemmer LB, Fripp PJ: Schistosomiasis and malignancy. S Afr Med J 84:211, 1994.
29. Badawi AF, Mostafa MH: Possible mechanisms of alteration in the capacities of carcinogen-metabolizing enzymes during schistosomiasis and their role in bladder cancer induction. J Int Med Res 21:281, 1993.
30. World Health Organization, International Agency for Research on Cancer (IARC) Monographs: Schistosomiasis, Liver Flukes and *C. pylori* 60:1–270. IARC, Geneva, 1994.
31. King C: Schistosomiasis. In Mahmoud AAF (ed): Parasitic Lung Disease. New York, Marcel Dekker, 1997, p 135.
32. Scrimgeour EM, Gajdusek DC: Involvement of the central nervous system in *Schistosoma mansoni* and *Schistosoma haematobium* infection: A review. Brain 68:1023, 1985.
33. Barsoum RS: Schistosomal glomerulopathies. Kidney Int 44:1, 1993.
34. Capron M, Capron A: Immunoglobulin E and effector cells in schistosomiasis. Science 264:1876, 1994.
35. Peters PAS, Kazura JW: Update on diagnostic methods for schistosomiasis. In Mahmoud AAF (ed): Balliere's Clinical Tropical Medicine and Communicable Disease, Vol 2. Philadelphia, Saunders, 1987, p 419.
36. Al-Sherbiny MM, Osman A, Hancock K, et al: Application of immunodiagnostic assays: Detection of antibodies and circulating antigens in human schistosomiasis and correlation with clinical findings. Am J Trop Med Hyg 60:960, 1999.
37. Hatz C: The use of ultrasound in schistosomiasis. Adv Parasitol 48:225, 2001.
38. Kahama AI, Odek AE, Kihara RW, et al: Urine circulating soluble egg antigen in relation to egg counts, hematuria, and urinary tract pathology before and after treatment in children infected with *Schistosoma haematobium* in Kenya. Am J Trop Med Hyg 61:215, 1999.
39. Guyatt H, Brooker S, Lwambo NJ, et al: The performance of school-based questionnaires of reported blood in urine in diagnosing *Schistosoma haematobium* infection: Patterns by age and sex. Trop Med Int Health 4:751, 1999.
40. King CH, Mahmoud AAF: Drugs five years later: praziquantel. Ann Intern Med 110:290, 1989.
41. Olds GR, King CH, Hewlett J, et al: Double-blind placebo controlled study of concurrent administration of albendazole and praziquantel in school children with schistosomiasis and geohelminths. J Infect Dis 179:996, 1999.
42. King CH, Muchiri E, Ouma JH, et al: Chemotherapy-based control of schistosomiasis haematobia. 4. Impact of annual chemotherapy on prevalence and intensity of *Schistosoma haematobium* infection in an endemic area of Kenya. Am J Trop Med Hyg 45:498, 1991.
43. World Health Organization: Report of the WHO Informal Consultation on the use of praziquantel during pregnancy/lactation and albendazole/mebendazole in children under 24 months. Geneva, WHO/CDS/CPE/PVC 2002.4, 2003.
44. King CH, Muchiri EM, Ouma JH: Evidence against rapid emergence of praziquantel resistance in *Schistosoma haematobium,* Kenya. Emerg Infect Dis 6:585, 2000.
45. Jordan P: The St. Lucia Project. Cambridge, UK, Cambridge University Press, 1982.

46. Mahmoud AAF, Siongok TKA, Ouma JH, et al: Effect of targeted mass treatment on intensity of infection and morbidity in schistosomiasis mansoni: Three year follow up of a community in Machakos Kenya. Lancet 1:849, 1983.
47. El Kholy H, Arap Siongok TK, Koech D, et al: Effects of borehole wells on water utilization in *Schistosoma haematobium*–endemic communities in Coast Province, Kenya. Am J Trop Med Hyg 41:212, 1989.
48. Kloos H: Human behavior, health education and schistosomiasis control: A review. Soc Sci Med 40:1497, 1995.
49. Cioli D, Pica-Mattoccia L, Archer S: Antischistosomal drugs: Past, present and future. Pharmacol Ther 68:35, 1995.
50. Parraga IM, Assis AM, Prado MS, et al: Gender differences in growth of school-aged children with schistosomiasis and geohelminth infection. Am J Trop Med Hyg 55:150, 1996.

117

Liver, Lung, and Intestinal Fluke Infections

J. DICK MACLEAN
JOHN CROSS
SIDDHARTHA MAHANTY

INTRODUCTION

The trematodes that infect liver, lung, and intestine are all food-borne. Freshwater fish, crustaceans, and aquatic vegetation are the sources of human infection. Fluke diseases also are all zoonoses with reservoirs in a wide range of domestic and wild animals. It is estimated that more than 40 million people are infected with flukes, approximately 21 million with lung flukes, 20 million with liver flukes, and unknown millions with intestinal flukes.[1] The geographic distribution is worldwide, but the highest prevalences are in East and Southeast Asia. Distribution is determined as much by local eating habits as by the presence of the obligatory freshwater snail, crustacean, fish, or edible aquatic plant intermediate hosts. Any of these flukes can produce serious clinical disease, especially when infections are heavy. The site of preference of adult flukes for liver, lung, and intestine; the migration of the fluke larvae to these sites; the intensity of infection; and the longevity of the parasite are the major determinants of clinical disease. A most remarkable clinical feature of food-borne trematodes is the causal association between liver fluke infection and cholangiocarcinoma of the liver.

These flukes are hermaphroditic, bilaterally symmetrical, and flattened dorsoventrally with an anterior oral and a ventral sucker. Different species measure from 1 mm to 12 cm in length and have been described as spatulate, piriform, lanceolate, or leaflike in shape (Fig. 117-1).

Life cycles of the different fluke species have common features. Adult flukes in the mammalian host produce eggs that, when passed in feces or sputum, are ingested by, or hatch as, ciliated miracidia and penetrate appropriate first-intermediate-host snails, within which asexual multiplication through sporocyst, redia, and cercaria stages occurs. Free-swimming cercaria leave the snail and penetrate fish or shellfish or attach to aquatic vegetation to encyst as metacercaria. When eaten by the mammalian final host, the metacercaria excyst, migrate to liver or lungs, or stay in the small intestine and develop into adults.

LIVER FLUKES

Human liver flukes are members of two families, the Opisthorchiidae and the Fasciolidae, distinguished by differences in life cycle and pathogenesis. In human Opisthorchiidae there are three major species (*Clonorchis sinensis* in East Asia, *Opisthorchis viverrini* in Southeast Asia, and *Opisthorchis felineus* in countries of the former Soviet Union) and two minor species (*Opisthorchis guayaquilensis* in North and South America and *Metorchis conjunctus* in North America). In the Fasciolidae the species are *Fasciola hepatica,* which has a worldwide distribution, and *Fasciola gigantica* in South Asia, Southeast Asia, and Africa.

OPISTHORCHIASIS AND CLONORCHIASIS

AGENTS

The three major Opisthorchiidae species—*C. sinensis, O. viverrini,* and *O. felineus*—have similar life cycles and pathogenic processes. Differentiation among species is usually based on adult fluke morphology or geographic distribution, as differences in egg morphologies are small.[2,3] Adults, which live in the intrahepatic bile ducts of their host, are flat, spatulate to lanceolate, aspinous, and reddish to brown in color. *C. sinensis* is the largest (10 to 25 mm × 3 to 5 mm), in contrast to the smaller *O. viverrini* (5 to 10 mm × 1 to 2 mm) and *O. felineus* (7 to 12 mm × 2 to 3 mm; Fig. 117-2A). The adults produce ovoid eggs that are yellowish-brown, have opercula, and are of such overlapping and variable size (*O. viverrini,* 30 μm × 12 μm; *O. felineus,* 30 μm × 12 μm; *C. sinensis* 28 to 35 μm × 12 to 19 μm) that speciation is very difficult (Fig. 117-2B).

The eggs, if deposited in fresh water and ingested by the appropriate snail, hatch as miracidia and metamorphose into sporocysts and then redia. These then transform into free-swimming cercaria on leaving the snail and penetrate and then encyst as metacercaria in susceptible freshwater fish species. These metacercaria, in uncooked fish, are ingested by the final human host, excyst in the duodenum, mature rapidly into adults, and migrate through the sphincter of Oddi and up the common bile duct to become wedged in the intrahepatic biliary radicles. The prepatent period is 3 to 4 weeks, and the life span in the human host can be as long as 30 years.

EPIDEMIOLOGY

C. sinensis is endemic in China, Japan, Korea, Taiwan, Vietnam, and Asian Russia. In China, infection is endemic in 24 provinces, with prevalence rates between 1% and 57%; the greatest number of cases is in the southeastern province of Guangdong and the southern region of Guangxi Zhuangzu.[4] Hong Kong is not an endemic area for the parasite; infections are acquired by eating fish imported from the mainland of China. In Korea rates of 8% to 22% were reported in the past, while prevalence rates in the 1990s dropped to 2%. People living along river basins are more commonly infected. This parasitosis is reported from all areas of Taiwan, with the highest infection rates of 52% to 57% from three widely separated

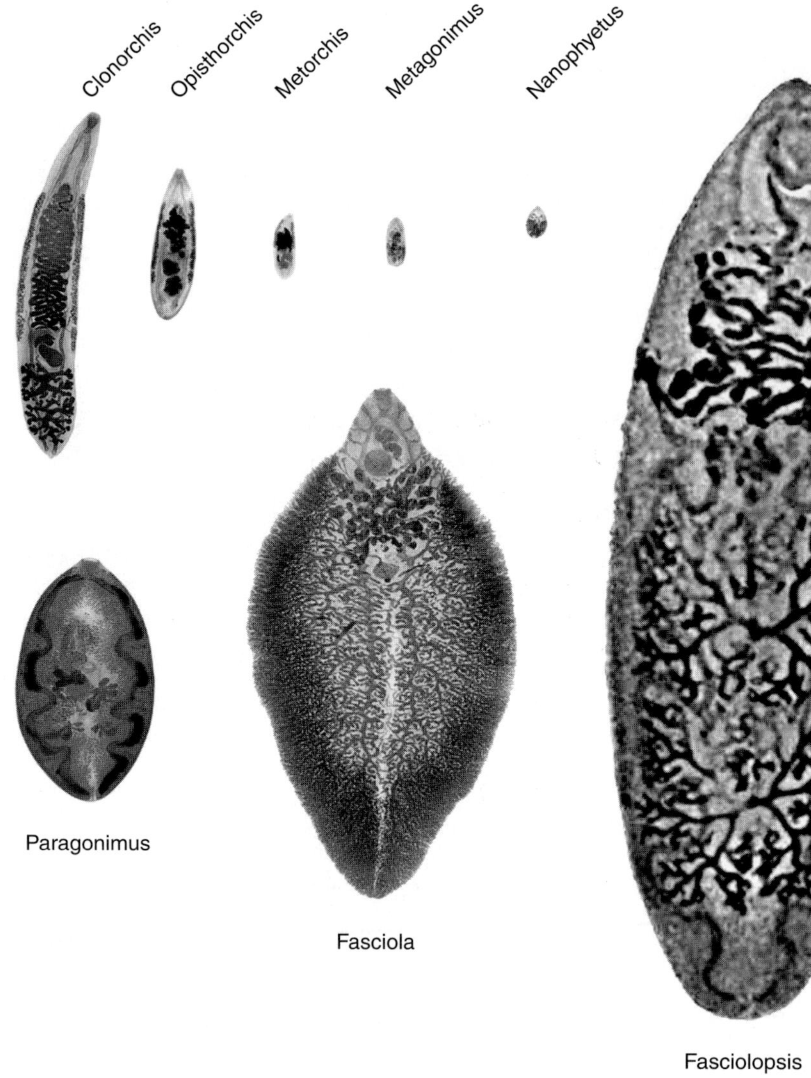

FIGURE 117-1 Threefold magnification of selected flukes illustrating relative sizes. Actual lengths: *Metagonimus yokogawai* 1.0 to 2.5 mm, *Nanophyetus salmincola* 0.8 to 2.5 mm, *Metorchis conjunctus* 1.5 to 7.0 mm, *Opisthorchis viverrini* 5 to 10 mm, *Paragonimus westermani* 7 to 16 mm, *Clonorchis sinensis* 10 to 25 mm, *Fasciola hepatica* 20 to 30 mm, *Fasciolopsis buski* 20 to 75 mm. (*Metagonimus yokogawai* image from Centers for Disease Control and Prevention, Division of Parasitic Diseases, Atlanta, GA; *Nanophyetus salmincola* and *Fasciolopsis buski* images courtesy of Steve J. Upton, Kansas State University; *Opisthorchis viverrini* image from Ash LR, Orihel TC: Atlas of Human Parasitology. Chicago, ASCP Press, 1990, plate 73, #2, p. 213; *Paragonimus westermani, Clonorchis sinensis,* and *Fasciola hepatica* images from Orihel TC, Ash LR: Parasites in Human Tissues. Chicago, ASCP Press, 1995, figures 72, 60, and 58, pp. 272, 268, and 264.)

areas in northern, central, and southern counties of the island.[5] Although clonorchiasis was found in up to 3% of the Japanese population prior to 1960, by 1991 the disease had almost disappeared. Endemic areas in Russia are in the Amur River area.

O. viverrini is highly endemic in the northeastern region of Thailand and Laos, where prevalence rates of more than 24% and 40% to 80%, respectively, are reported.[1,6] There are reports of occurrence from Vietnam with rates of 0.3% to 37%.[7]

O. felineus has been reported from an estimated 16 million people in the former USSR, with endemic foci in western Siberia, the Russian Federation, Kazakhstan, and Ukraine; prevalences range from 40% to 95%.[1]

Other opisthorchiids reported from humans are *Opisthorchis guayaquilensis* (*Amphimerus pseudofelineus*) and *Metorchis conjunctus*. These have been reported from animals and humans in Latin America and North America. An epidemic of metorchiasis occurred in 19 persons in Canada who had eaten freshly caught white suckers (*Catostomus commersoni*) near Montreal.[8]

A variety of hydrobid snails serve as first intermediate hosts for *C. sinensis, O. viverrini,* and *O. felineus. Bithynia fuchsiana, Parafossarulus manchouricus,* and *Simisulcospica libertina* are important vectors of *C. sinensis* in most endemic areas, while *Bithynia siamensis* is a vector of *O. viverrini* in Thailand; *Melanoides tuberculatus* is an important vector in Vietnam[7]; and *Codiella inflata, Codiella troscheli,* and *Codiella leachi* are vectors of *O. felineus* in the former USSR. These snails are found in freshwater bodies and are abundant in fish-raising ponds in China, Taiwan, and Thailand.

Over 100 species of fish, many of them synonyms, are reported as second-intermediate hosts of *C. sinensis*. Most are carps of the family Cyprinidae; *Ctenopharyngodon idellus* in China, *Cyprinus carpio* in Japan, and *Pseudoraspora parva* in Korea are often eaten raw. Many of the fish are cultivated in ponds inhabited by snail hosts, and the ponds are contaminated or intentionally fertilized with human and animal feces. Fifteen species of cyprinoid fish such as *Cyclocheiclichthys* spp. and *Puntius* spp. are sources of infections in Thailand, and *Carassius carassius* and seven other species are sources in Vietnam.

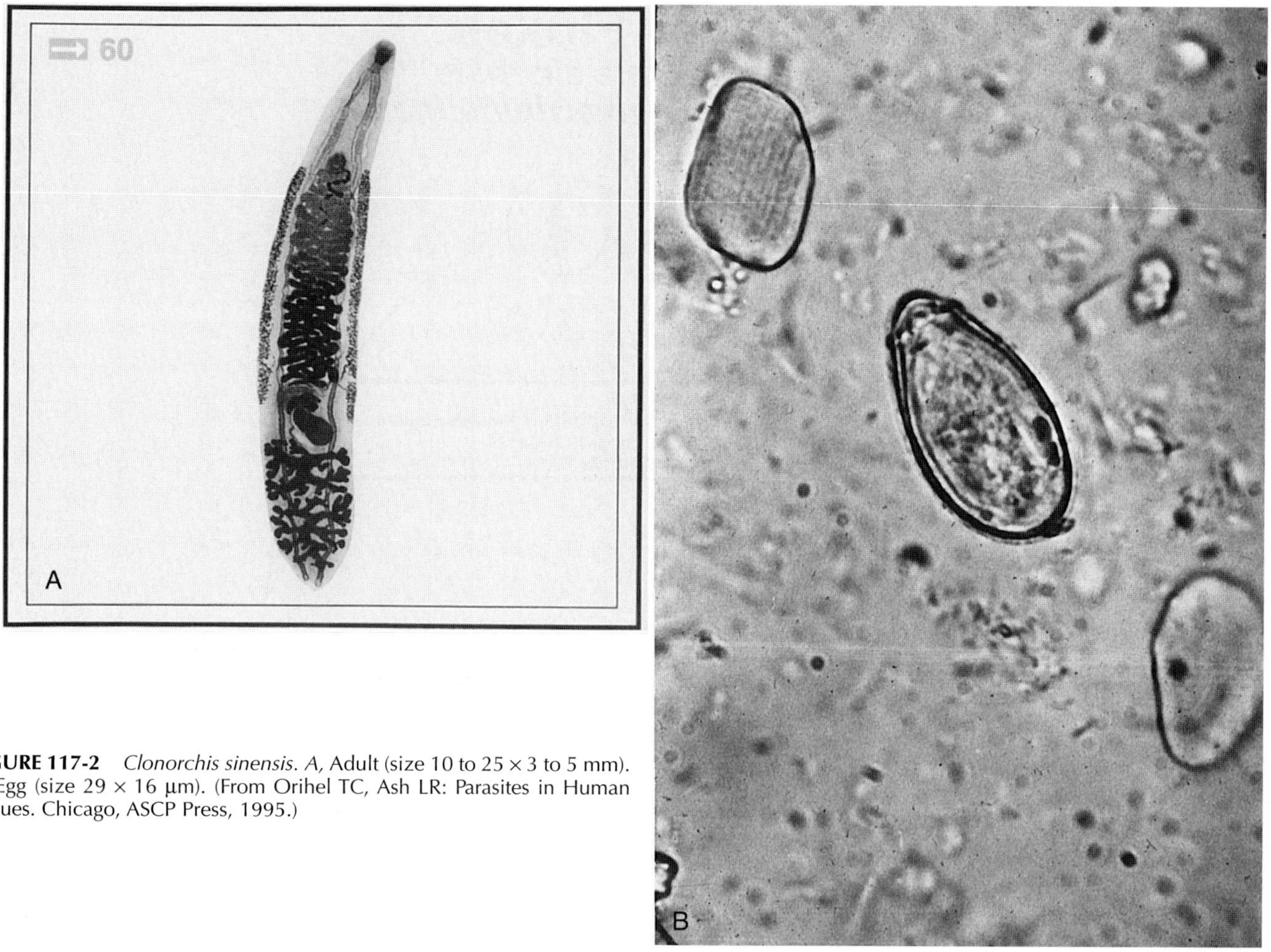

FIGURE 117-2 *Clonorchis sinensis. A,* Adult (size 10 to 25 × 3 to 5 mm). *B,* Egg (size 29 × 16 µm). (From Orihel TC, Ash LR: Parasites in Human Tissues. Chicago, ASCP Press, 1995.)

Cultured fish, as well as fish from natural sources, are infected, and as the streams dry up, fish clustering in shallow waters are easily caught and eaten raw. Twenty-two species of cyprinids are intermediate hosts for *O. felineus* in the former USSR. The fish, such as *Barbus barbus* and *Tinca tinca,* may be eaten raw, dried, salted, and sometimes frozen.

In endemic areas of opisthorchiid liver fluke infections, a myriad of mammalian hosts such as dogs, cats, pigs, rats, rabbits, and other wild fish–eating animals serve as reservoir hosts.

DISEASES

There is consensus that the biologic and pathologic characteristics of *Opisthorchis* and *Clonorchis* are the same. Variations in clinical presentations seen in different geographic areas are thought to reflect the duration and intensity of infection as well as the genetics and nutrition of the host rather than parasite-specific characteristics.[9] Acute disease has been recognized most frequently in *O. felineus* infections in Russia. The risk of cholangiocarcinoma appears greatest in *O. viverrini* infections in northern Thailand. Intrahepatic pigment stones are reported more frequently in association with *C. sinensis.*[9] Chronic infections are usually asymptomatic, although symptoms may occur in heavier infections. The complications of chronic infection include acute cholangitis, frequently bacterial, and cholangiocarcinoma.

Acute Opisthorchiasis and Clonorchiasis

Acute illness due to new infections with *C. sinensis* has rarely been reported except for a large outbreak of acute clonorchiasis in Shanghai in the 1940s.[10,11] The illness lasted several weeks and was characterized by persistent fever, abdominal pains, fatigue, an enlarged and tender liver, high eosinophil counts, and opisthorchiid eggs in the stool after 3 to 4 weeks.[10] In Russia acute opisthorchiasis has been seen frequently in migrant populations settling in regions endemic to *O. felineus.*[12,13] The presentation is fever, abdominal pain, and urticaria. In Canada an outbreak of acute illness due to *M. conjunctus* reported upper abdominal pain, moderate fever, anorexia, high eosinophil counts, and opisthorchiid eggs in the stool late in the second week of illness.[8]

Chronic Opisthorchiasis and Clonorchiasis

Light to moderate infections, lasting for years or decades, are almost always asymptomatic.[14] Case-control and

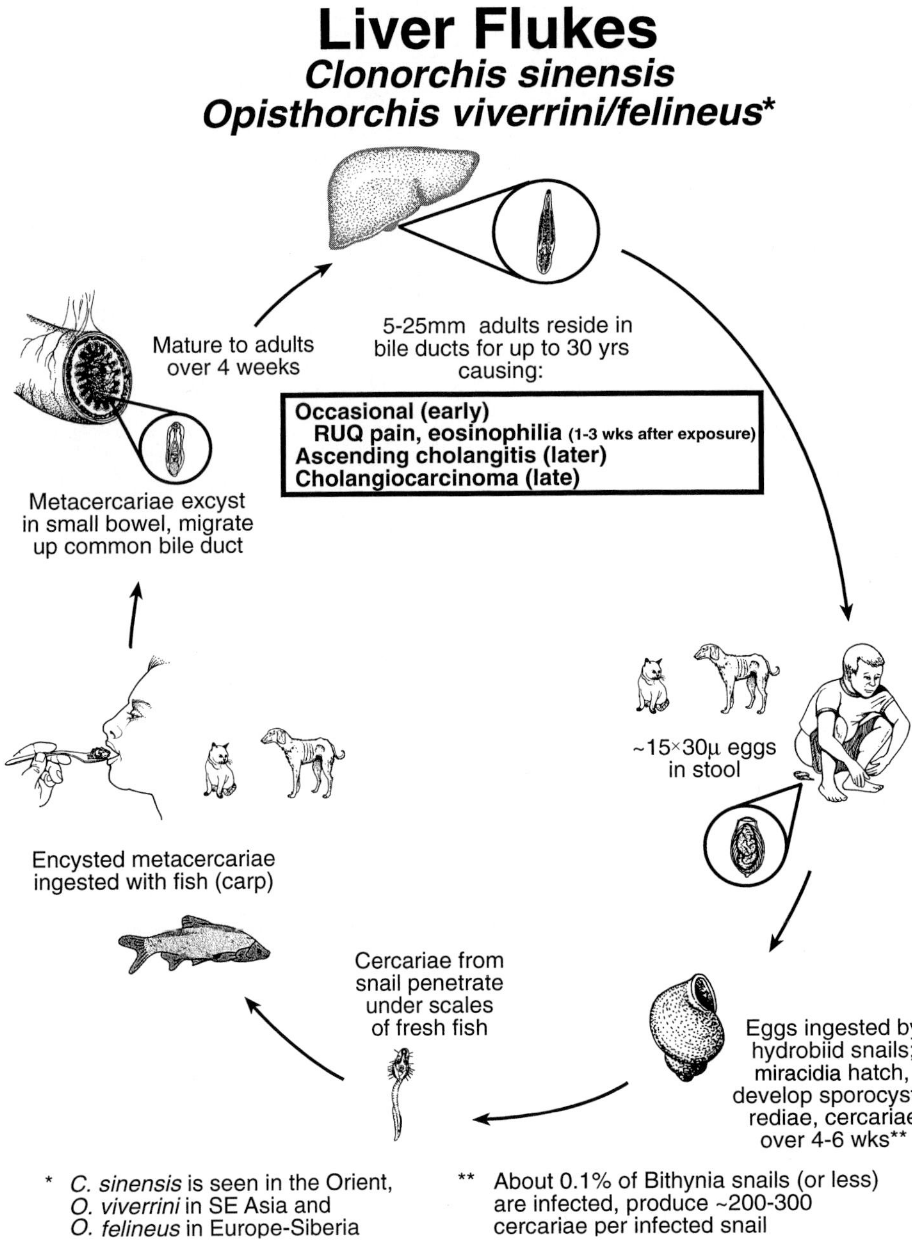

community-based studies have revealed no differences in the signs, symptoms, or laboratory findings between light infections and uninfected controls, but cases with heavy infections (more than 10,000 eggs per gram) show significantly more abdominal pain, fatigue, dyspepsia, and hepatomegaly.[15–18] There is a correlation between stool egg counts, adult fluke counts, and host disease in *Opisthorchis* infection. But even in heavily infected persons, abdominal symptoms occur in only 10%.[9,19–23] Such studies are difficult to interpret because raw fish consumption in many communities is frequent and reinfection likely.[15,18,24,25]

Many uncontrolled hospital-based studies in endemic regions demonstrate a variety of intermittent symptoms that increase in frequency in those with heavy infections.[26,27] These symptoms include intermittent fatigue, abdominal pain and fullness, anorexia, weight loss, and diarrhea. In these studies, physical signs, such as liver enlargement and tenderness, are more frequent in the heavily infected, and eosinophil counts are higher. Uncontrolled treatment trials with praziquantel have demonstrated a decrease in symptoms of upper abdominal pain, diarrhea, distention, dizziness, fatigue, and insomnia from 72% to 45%.[28]

Ultrasonographic studies have revealed a high frequency of gallbladder enlargement, sludge, dysfunction, and stones in asymptomatic moderately to heavily infected patients. Treatment appears to reverse these parasite-associated gallbladder abnormalities.[19,29,30]

Pathologic changes observed on necropsy and biopsy relate to intensity and duration of infection. Early infections reveal bile duct proliferation and pseudostratification of the

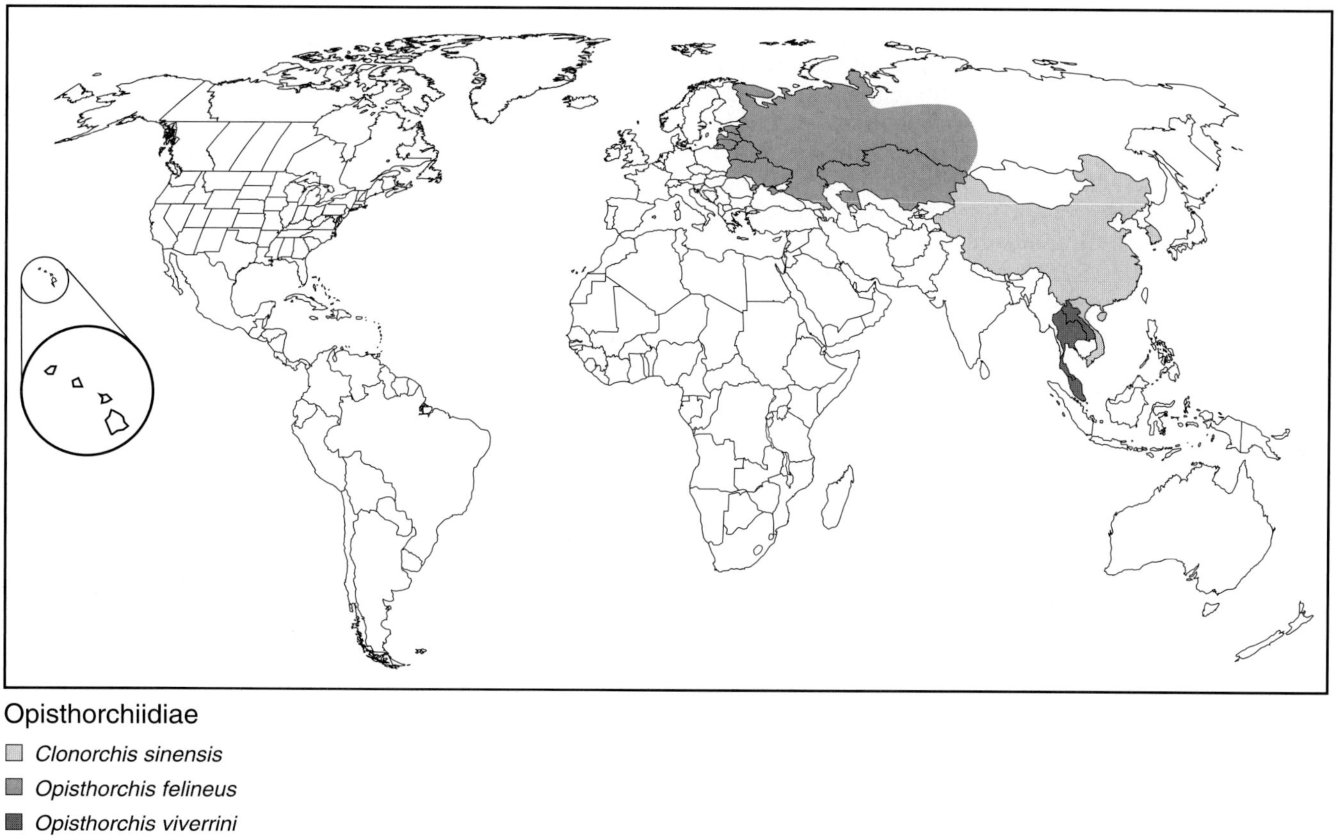

biliary epithelium. Later, metaplastic squamous cells and glandular proliferation appear, suggesting adenomatous hyperplasia.[31] A small percentage of patients with chronic infection will develop complications, which include recurrent ascending cholangitis, pancreatitis, and cholangiocarcinoma.

Recurrent Ascending Cholangitis and Pancreatitis

Recurrent ascending cholangitis is characterized by repeated episodes of fever, chills, jaundice, right upper quadrant pain, gram-negative sepsis, and leukocytosis. Soft, muddy pigment stones are found in the biliary radicles and common bile duct and are associated with dilated intrahepatic bile ducts, ectasia, strictures, and multiple pyogenic abscesses, most notably of the left lobe of the liver.[32] Recurrent exacerbations and remissions can occur over years.[33,34] Pancreatitis at times is found on endoscopic retrograde cholangiopancreatography (ERCP), or at the time of surgery or autopsy, but it is rarely symptomatic or found in isolation without liver involvement.[35,36]

Cholangiocarcinoma

An increased frequency of cholangiocarcinoma of the liver is seen in northern Thailand, where case-control studies reveal a fivefold increased risk in those infected.[37] The risk increases to 15-fold in persons with heavier infections. In one endemic province of Thailand, the rate of cholangiocarcinoma in males and females was ten- and sixfold higher, respectively, than in a nonendemic area.[37,38] In animal studies, nitrosamines increase the incidence of cholangiocarcinoma in *Opisthorchis*-infected animals.[39–41] High levels of such substances have been noted in the northern Thai diet.[42]

PATHOGENESIS AND IMMUNITY

The pathologic changes seen in the liver and biliary system in clonorchiasis and opisthorchiasis are believed to be the result of mechanical injury by the suckers of the flukes and host interactions with their secreted metabolic products.[43–45] Dilated hyperplastic bile ducts have been associated with excess proline production by adult flukes.[46] The eggs probably serve as nidi for biliary stones in the bile ducts and gallbladder.[31,47] Immunohistochemical studies indicate that the excretory-secretory proteins from the digestive and excretory organs (i.e., the intestines and bladder) are the most potent antigens and likely induce the dominant immunologic response.[4] Periductal infiltration with eosinophils and round cells with fibrosis of portal areas—a common finding—suggests that immune-mediated tissue damage is involved in the pathogenesis of disease.[4] The local reactions to eggs and migrating parasites are driven by T-lymphocyte effector mechanisms and are regulated by the CD4+ subset of T lymphocytes.[48] The presence of apparently uninfected persons in endemic regions with significantly higher levels of parasite-specific IgM, IgG, and IgA than egg-excreting persons has been used as evidence of protective immunity.[44,49,50]

DIAGNOSIS

Asymptomatic infections with Opisthorchiidae are diagnosed by the presence of characteristic findings on ultrasound, computed tomography (CT), or magnetic resonance imaging (MRI) or by the detection of eggs in stool. On ultrasound of the liver, the combination of cystic or mulberry-like dilations of intrahepatic bile ducts is pathognomonic of opisthorchiasis. With M-mode ultrasound, numerous spotty echoes and thin linear and moving intraductal echoes may be seen.[35,51,52] Examination of multiple stool specimens may be necessary in lighter infections, but in infections of less than 20 adult flukes, no eggs may be found.[22] While egg counts in stools are relatively stable over time and such egg counts have prognostic significance, low egg counts may be seen in the heaviest infections because of blockage of biliary radicles or because pyogenic ascending cholangitis has killed the adults.[21,22,53] The eggs of *Clonorchis, Opisthorchis,* and *Metorchis* are essentially indistinguishable from one another by routine microscopy and can be confused with other fluke eggs as well. A definitive diagnosis may be made by examining the adult flukes in the stool immediately after a praziquantel treatment and purge or at the time of surgery.[20,53,54]

The diagnosis of acute infection is based on a history of raw freshwater fish consumption (salted, fermented, or smoked fish, fish sauces, fish condiments), followed within several weeks by upper abdominal pain, high-grade eosinophilia, liver enzyme elevation, and the appearance of compatible eggs in the stool.

Immunodiagnosis

Immunologic tests generally complement parasitologic testing and until recently have not had a primary role in the diagnosis of opisthorchiasis and clonorchiasis. These tests are not widely available in endemic regions and do not distinguish active infections from past exposure or cured infections.[55] Intradermal tests using crude extracts of adult flukes have been used for detection of infection in epidemiologic surveys and have proved very sensitive (92%), showing no cross-reactions with other nematode infections.[4] However, these tests remain positive for many years after exposure to the parasite. The preferred assay for immunodiagnosis is the determination of antibody levels by enzyme-linked immunosorbent assay (ELISA). When compared with egg-positive stools, sensitivity can be high (79% to 96%).[4] However, ELISA using crude worm extracts is handicapped by significant lack of specificity; antibody positivity is seen in cases of paragonimiasis (33%), schistosomiasis japonica (5% to 25%), cysticercosis, hepatitis, liver cancer, and tuberculosis.[56,57] Specificity can be enhanced somewhat by using immune affinity–purified antigens.[58] More recently, the use of monoclonal antibodies in an ELISA inhibition test has proved to be sensitive (77%) and more specific (virtually no cross-reactivity with other trematode infections) than the ELISA using crude worm extracts.[4] Approaches used to refine and improve specificity of ELISA assays have included the use of excretory-secretory (ES) antigens as plate antigens.[59] A number of proteins have been identified as major components of ES preparations of *C. sinensis*, including cysteine proteases and glutathione-S-transferase.[60] The modifications to ELISAs have been reported to achieve sensitivities and specificities of greater than 95% in smaller serologic surveys, but their utility in large-scale surveillance is yet to be proved.[61] After treatment, antibody levels return to normal by 6 months in more than half of cases.[4,62] Circulating antigen detection with a monoclonal antibody–based capture ELISA has been found to detect as little as 30 ng/mL of *C. sinensis* antigen in serum. Antigen positivity is seen in 95% of antibody-positive infected patients. This test was reported to be positive in 95% of seropositive infected patients, declining to undetectable levels after 3 months in 81% of those parasitologically cured.[63,64] Stool antigen detection techniques show similar promise.[65]

TREATMENT

Praziquantel has been the drug of choice for opisthorchiasis and clonorchiasis since the 1970s because of ease of administration, lack of side effects, and demonstrated effectiveness. The recommended dosage of 25 mg/kg three times daily for 2 days has produced cure rates up to 100%, but patients with heavy infections (more than 5000 eggs per gram of stool) and some geographic regions where praziquantel cure rates are low (North Vietnam) may require retreatment.[4,31,66,67]

Albendazole has produced cure rates of 93% to 100% at a dosage of 10 mg/kg daily for 7 days.[4,68] Although some studies have suggested that it may not be as effective as praziquantel, it has fewer side effects.

Treatment success is defined by the disappearance of fluke-induced symptoms and fecal egg output, reduction in liver size, and a reversal of biliary tract abnormalities.[19] Recurrent pyogenic cholangitis is primarily a surgical problem, requiring relief of intrahepatic obstructions due to strictures, stones, and sludge, and drainage of the associated abscesses. Antibiotics may be necessary to treat the associated sepsis, and praziquantel is used to eradicate the remaining flukes.[69]

FASCIOLIASIS

Among the Fasciolidae there are two human flukes: *Fasciola hepatica,* the most common and widely distributed, and *Fasciola gigantica,* a fluke of much more focal distribution. Both have similar life cycles and produce similar human disease, but *F. gigantica* can be recognized by its larger adult and egg sizes.

AGENTS

The adult *F. hepatica* is a large fluke (30 mm long × 15 mm wide), flat and leaflike along the margins, with a cephalic cone (Fig. 117-3A). As for other flukes, size, shape, and integumental and internal morphology are species-defining features. The adult fluke lives in the common and hepatic bile ducts of the human or animal host, and eggs reach the exterior via the sphincter of Oddi and the intestine. The eggs are large (130 to 150 μm × 60 to 90 μm), ovoid, and inconspicuously operculate (Fig. 117-3B). In water, miracidia hatch from the eggs and penetrate suitable snail hosts where, after multiplying as sporocysts and redia, they leave the snail as free-living cercaria.

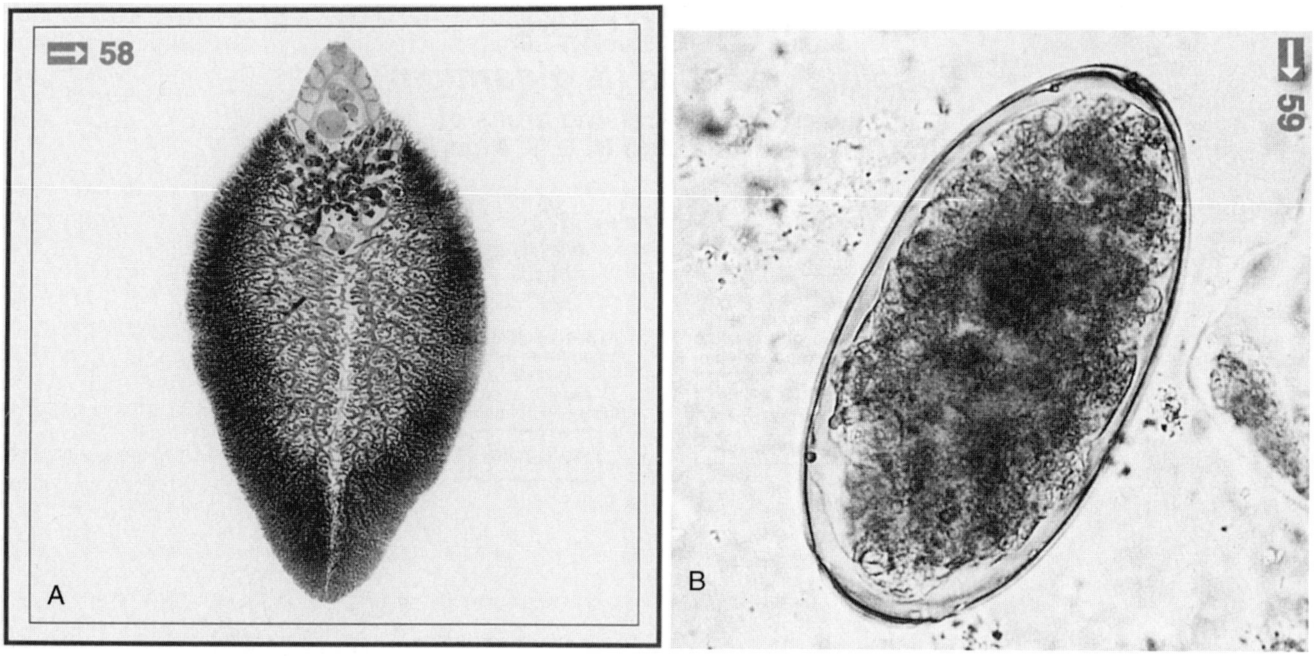

FIGURE 117-3 *Fasciola hepatica. A,* Adult (size 30 × 15 mm). *B,* Egg (size 130 to 150 × 60 to 90 μm). (From Orihel TC, Ash LR: Parasites in Human Tissues. Chicago, ASCP Press, 1995.)

These attach to suitable plants, evolve into metacercarial cysts, and when ingested by the human final host, excyst in the duodenum. The larvae migrate through the small intestinal wall and through the peritoneal cavity where they penetrate the liver capsule and slowly migrate to the large hepatic ducts. This prepatent period lasts 3 to 4 months. Anecdotal reports suggest that the life span in the human host can be up to 10 years.

EPIDEMIOLOGY

F. hepatica has been reported from 61 countries worldwide, especially in sheep-raising areas.[70] More than 2 million people are infected, mostly in Bolivia, Peru, Iran, Egypt, Portugal, and France. A variety of freshwater plants upon which metacercariae encyst, such as watercress, water lettuce, mint, and parsley, are important sources of human infection because they are often eaten raw in salads.[71] Over 25 species of amphibious lymnaeid snails serve as the first intermediate host for *F. hepatica.* The most important is *Lymnaea truncatula,* which lives in wet mud along the shoreline, rarely in fast-moving or deep waters. The major natural reservoirs for *F. hepatica* are cattle, sheep, goats, buffalo, camels, llamas, deer, pigs, horses, rabbits, and other wild animals. It is not uncommon to find high levels of infection with *F. hepatica* or *F. gigantica* in domestic and wild ruminants of endemic areas; prevalence rates of 25% to 92% are seen in Bolivia, 20% to 40% in Ecuador, 10% to 100% in Peru, and 20% to 40% in Iran. In humans, stool- or antibody-positive prevalence rates in these countries can be similarly high (65% to 92% in Bolivia, 24% to 53% in Ecuador, 2% to 17% in Egypt, and 10% in Peru).[1]

DISEASE

The clinical presentation of infection with *F. hepatica* reflects its peregrinations in the human host. Hepatic transit, variably called the hepatic, larval, invasive, or acute stage, lasts several months. This is followed by the biliary, adult, or chronic stage, which can persist for years. Where repeated ingestion of metacercaria occurs over an extended period, these two stages can overlap.[72]

Acute Hepatic (Invasive) Stage

Within 6 to 12 weeks of ingestion of metacercariae, symptoms occur that reflect larval migration through the small intestinal wall, the peritoneal cavity, and liver capsule.[73] This acute stage can last for 2 to 4 months. One large study revealed typical findings of fairly marked eosinophilia (95%), abdominal pain (65%), intermittent fever (60%), malaise and weight loss (35%), urticaria (20%), and cough, dyspnea, and chest pain (15%). A change in bowel habits, anorexia, and nausea may occur.[74,75] The abdominal pain may be generalized but frequently becomes localized to the right hypochondrium.[76,77] Hepatomegaly is a variable finding, and the liver may be tender on palpation. In some cases, mild elevations of hepatic enzymes are noted. The pulmonary symptoms may be associated with right-sided pleural effusions, which, on aspiration, reveal increased eosinophils.[78] Anemia has been reported.[79,80]

Ultrasound examination of the liver in the acute stage is usually normal although small amounts of ascites have been found.[78] CT scans frequently reveal single or, more frequently, multiple small hypodense lesions 2 to 10 mm in diameter.[74] In addition, tunnel-like, branching, hypodense lesions (best delineated with contrast), most frequently situated peripherally

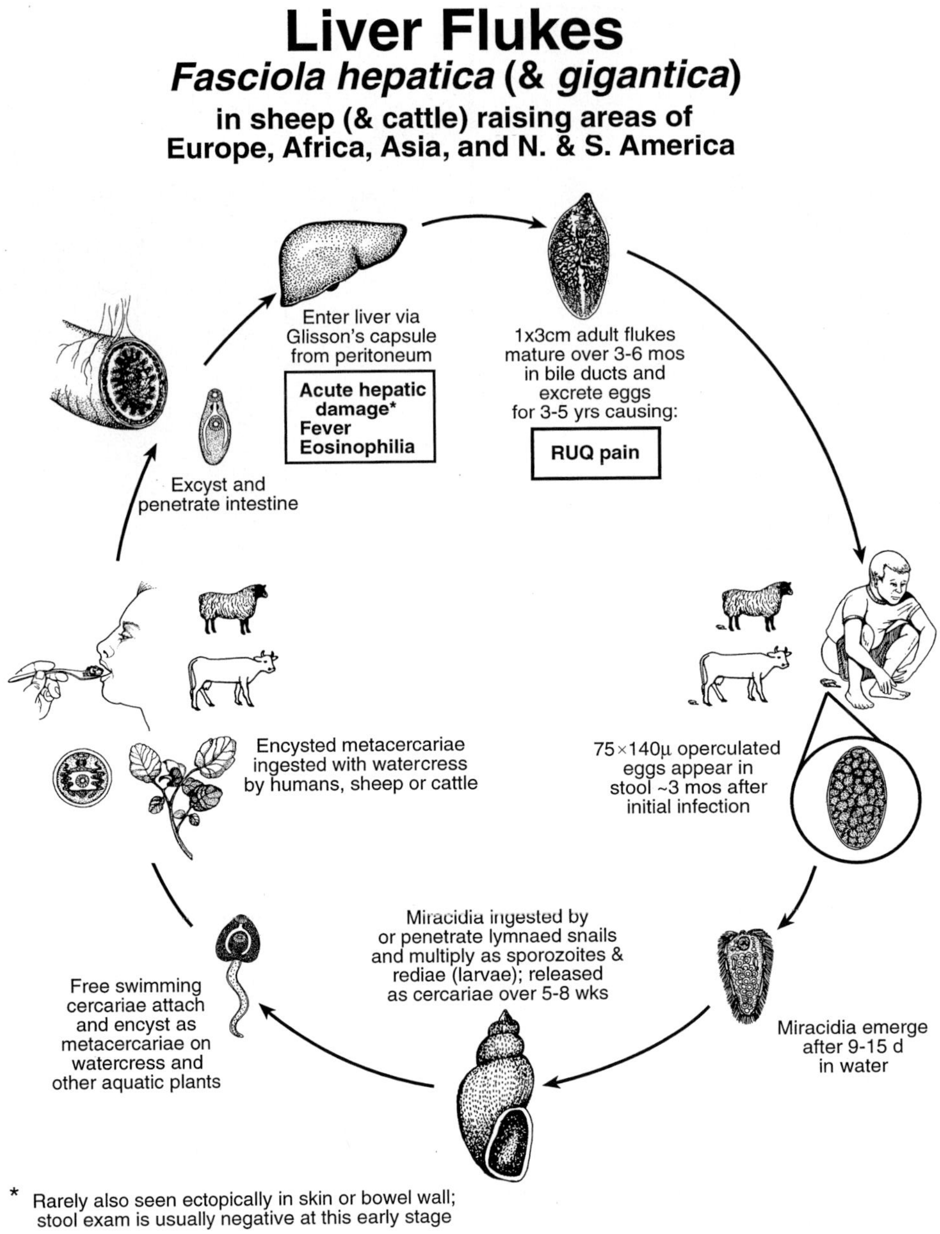

within the liver, are relatively specific for fascioliasis, representing the pathologic changes created by the migration of the immature fluke through the liver.[81] The hepatic lesions are remarkable in that, on sequential CT scans, the position, attenuation, and shape of the lesions change over time.[82] On laparoscopy, multiple gray-white and yellow nodules 2 to 20 mm in diameter and short vermiform cords are noted on the liver surface and at times on the adjacent peritoneal surface.[83] Liver biopsies reveal microabscesses and tunnel-like areas of parenchymal necrosis surrounded by inflammatory infiltrates containing abundant eosinophils.[81,84] Necropsies reveal multiple subscapular cavities 5 to 10 mm in diameter filled with necrotic material from which necrotic tracts radiate. Increasing fibrosis is seen in older lesions.[84,85]

Rarely, immature flukes may migrate to nonhepatobiliary locations such as the skin, lung, intestinal wall, brain, and genitourinary tract, where granulomatous nodules or small abscesses lead to local clinical findings. Migrating erythematous 1.5- to 6.0-cm cutaneous nodules are another form of cutaneous larva migrans.[72,74,85,86]

Chronic Biliary (Obstructive) Stage

F. hepatica has a propensity to migrate to the lumen of the common bile duct, where it reaches maturity. Eggs appear in the stool after a prepatent period of 3 to 4 months. Clinical findings reflect this new luminal location in that the liver-destructive phase of the infection ends. Fever, anorexia, and abdominal pain resolve, and the patient may become asymptomatic. Eosinophilia is infrequent. An unknown percentage of these cases develop the complication of intermittent biliary obstruction with symptoms that can include intermittent pain

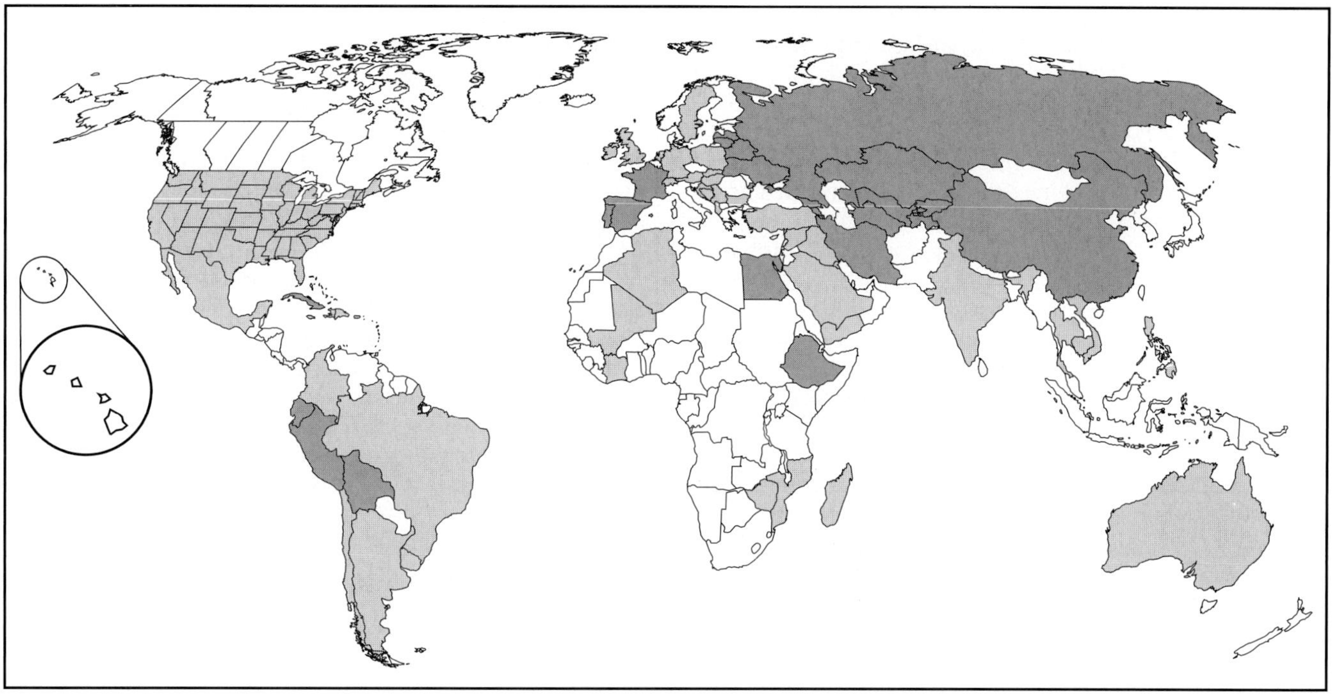

Fasciolidae

Fasciola endemic

Fasciola sporadic

in the epigastrium or right hypochondrium, mimicking biliary colic or acute cholecystitis. At times the presentation is that of ascending cholangitis with fever, jaundice, and upper abdominal pain.

Ultrasound examination (more effective than CT examination at this stage) often reveals a soft intraluminal mass obstructing the extrahepatic biliary tree. Lithiasis of the common bile duct and gallbladder is a common sequela.

PATHOGENESIS AND IMMUNITY

Morbidity from *F. hepatica* is dependent on the number of worms and stage of infection.[87] The characteristic hepatic (and extrahepatic) changes of fascioliasis result largely from the anatomic location and large size of the parasite, a foreign body that induces eosinophilic and mononuclear infiltration around the eggs and adult worms.[43] As in other tissue-invasive helminthic infections, fascioliasis is associated with prominent eosinophilia, particularly in the early stages of infection.[74,87] As with most helminths, immune responses to *F. hepatica* appear to be regulated by a subpopulation of T-helper cells designated as subtype 2 (Th2) cells, characterized by secretion of interleukin (IL)-4, IL-5, and IL-10.[88,89] This pattern of T-helper cell response also appears to regulate granuloma formation and liver disease in schistosomiasis.[48,90,91] However, the roles of T-cell- and other non-antibody-mediated effector systems in killing of the parasite and in the development of pathologic changes are not well understood.[92,93] The role of eosinophils in parasite killing is also unclear, although it has been noted that the invasive phase in the liver is associated with peripheral eosinophilia and eosinophilic infiltrates around the sites of parasites and eggs in the liver.[72,84] Recombinant parasite-derived molecules have been used to vaccinate the host before challenge with infective stages of the parasite.

Immune evasion mechanisms are likely to play an important role in the survival of this long-lived parasite, and several evasion strategies have been proposed.[94] The surface glycocalyx may mediate immune evasion in several ways. First, the glycocalyx changes in composition during development of the parasite. Second, the glycocalyx is continuously sloughed off by the maturing juvenile worm, by one estimate every 3 hours, thus presenting a moving target.[95] Third, glycocalyx released from the surface can mop up circulating antibodies, interfering with immune effector functions that involve them, such as antibody-dependent cellular toxicity (ADCC).[96] Other relevant strategies include migration away from inflammatory cells, inhibition of oxygen radical generation by macrophages and inhibition of T-cell function.[97] Natural resistance to fatal infection with *F. hepatica* has been observed in sheep and several strains of mice. Relative resistance to infection in mice correlates with type 1 (IFN-γ) responses, whereas type 2 responses are associated with susceptibility.[94] Protection from challenge infection in mice and rats can be transferred by passive transfer of serum, but this protective effect is limited to sera collected 7 to 8 weeks post–donor infection; after 25 weeks, serum from infected rats gave no protection, presumably owing to a decline in titers that accompanies the entry of the parasite into bile ducts.[95] Several potential vaccine antigens have been identified from animal models of *F. hepatica* infection. Defined antigens that are targets of antibody responses include fatty acid-binding proteins, glutathione-S-tranferase (GST), cathepsin-L, and fluke hemoglobin.[97–99] Two molecules have been shown to confer partial resistance to infection in experimental infections. One is a GST, and the second is a 14.7-kD polypeptide (Fh15) that has significant homology to, and cross-reacts with, *Schistosoma mansoni* fatty acid–binding protein.[100–102] The *F. hepatica* GST has been shown to protect sheep against experimental infection.[93] Overall, vaccine studies, using cocktails of recombinant antigens in animal models of fascioliasis, have shown that significant reductions in worm burdens (31% to 72%) and egg production (69% to 98%) can be achieved.[93,103]

DIAGNOSIS

F. hepatica eggs are not found in stool specimens during the acute phase. The diagnosis must be based on the clinical findings of persistent pain and tenderness in the right hypochondrium or epigastrium, altered intestinal function, mild to moderate fever, and blood eosinophil counts in the thousands per microliter.[82] CT scans (ultrasound is less sensitive) contribute to the diagnosis, since the majority of symptomatic patients have visible hypodense lesions and tracts in the liver and over time these lesions change in position and contour. The differential diagnosis of this clinical and radiologic syndrome includes visceral larva migrans caused by *Toxocara canis,* which usually also shows pulmonary symptoms. Needle biopsies of the liver have not been used for diagnosis. Laparoscopy may reveal elongated nodules in the liver capsule.

In the acute invasive period, lasting 3 to 4 months, immunologic techniques are valuable diagnostic tools. Skin tests using adult worm antigens or purified fractions of *F. hepatica* were used in the 1960s and 1970s; these tests were sensitive but not very specific.[104,105] Other tests have been employed with varying success, including complement fixation (CF), immunofluorescent (IF) assays, indirect hemagglutination (IHA), countercurrent electrophoresis (CEP), and ELISA.[72,106–111] ELISAs have largely replaced other techniques because they are sensitive, rapid, and quantitative.[109,111,112] The preferred ELISAs employ excretory-secretory products of the adult worm as an antigen.[112–114] Antibodies to excretory-secretory antigens are elevated early in infection (based on studies in animal models) and remain elevated for years after infection although successful treatment correlates with a decline in ELISA titers.[71,115]

More recently, the Falcon assay screening test–ELISA (FAST-ELISA), a simple and rapid assay based on the ELISA and enzyme-linked immunoblot transfer assay, has been used for serodiagnosis, achieving sensitivities of 95% to 100% compared with parasitologic diagnosis.[111,116] However, the specificity of this test is not known and may limit its utility.[74]

An ELISA antigen capture technique to detect circulating antigens has demonstrated a sensitivity of 100% and specificity of 98%.[117] Antigen detection techniques can detect parasite antigens in stool specimens 3 to 4 weeks before the appearance of eggs.[80] Immunodiagnostic tests continue to evolve, and the use of genus-specific antigens is likely to improve diagnostic accuracy.[74,118,119] Other attempts to improve the specificity of immunodiagnosis have used IgG subtype antibody levels instead of total IgG. Subtype analysis of antibody responses to excretory-secretory antigens such as the cathepsin protease (cathepsin L1) demonstrated that the predominant subtypes induced in human infections are IgG_1 and IgG_4, consistent with a predominant type 2 T-cell response.[120–124] The detection of subtype-specific antibodies in ELISAs may improve the specificity of the diagnostic immunoassays and make it possible to distinguish recent from remote infections.[125]

In chronic biliary fascioliasis, the diagnosis is made on finding *F. hepatica* eggs in stool specimens or at the time of surgery for bile duct obstruction when eggs or adult flukes are removed from the biliary tree. Because egg production tends to be low, it is advisable to examine multiple stool specimens. The formalin–ethyl acetate concentration technique appears to be less sensitive than the AMS iii (Tween 80) method or the Weller-Dammin modification method.[72,126] Eggs of *F. hepatica* can be confused with those of the intestinal flukes *Fasciolopsis buski* and echinostomes. Recovery of adults after anthelmintic treatment will allow species identification. False-positive "spurious" stool results can occur after consumption of liver of infected animals and can be ruled out by repeated stool examinations.

TREATMENT AND VACCINATION

Triclabendazole, a benzimidazole, is now the drug of choice as a single 10 mg/kg oral dose or two doses 12 hours apart. Bioavailability is increased when triclabendazole is taken with food.[127,128] Efficacy has been as high as 92% in humans, but significant resistance has been seen both in animal and in vitro studies and repeat treatment may be necessary.[129–131] The most frequent side effect was colicky abdominal pain between days 3 and 7 posttreatment, compatible with fluke expulsion through the bile ducts.

Unlike other trematodes, *F. hepatica* is frequently resistant to praziquantel, although some studies have shown effectiveness.[74,87,94,132–136] Animal studies show a lack of effectiveness of praziquantel against both immature and adult flukes in cattle and sheep. In the past bithionol has been considered the drug of choice at a dosage of 30 to 50 mg/kg/day in three divided doses on alternate days for 10 to 15 days.[137–139] More than one course may be necessary. Side effects are mild and include anorexia, nausea, vomiting, abdominal pain, and pruritus.

Acute ascending cholangitis must be treated with antibiotics and surgery. A patient with a severe acute hepatic stage may benefit from the short-term use of systemic steroids.[140] Other drugs used in the past include emitine, dehydroemetine, chloroquine, albendazole, and mebendazole, but all have been dropped because of toxicity or lack of effectiveness.[72,77]

Fasciola is one of few trematodes for which vaccines have been developed and used to protect against veterinary disease. The *F. hepatica* cathepsin-L protein, an important virulence determinant that was identified as a dominant antigen in excreted-secreted proteins, is a first-generation vaccine.[141] There have been a number of trials using this molecule in cattle and sheep, with protection against challenge infection ranging from 38% to 79%.[94,141–143] In natural and experimental infections, *F. hepatica* induces a polarized Th2 response as evidenced by the generation of IgG_1 but little or no IgG_2 antibody subtypes, whereas vaccination induces antibody responses to cathepsin-L, the immunogen, that include high titers of both IgG_1 and IgG_2, indicating a mixed Th1/Th2 response.[94,124,144] These observations have been interpreted to indicate that protection is associated with a Th1 or a mixed Th1/Th2 response.[94,124] However, some vaccine trials with the same antigen have demonstrated little or no protection, suggesting that other factors, such as adjuvant and antigen formulation, may be important in generating protective immune responses.[145] No vaccines have yet been developed for human infections.

LUNG FLUKES

INTRODUCTION

Lung flukes are members of the genus *Paragonimus* and while more than 40 species have been described, only eight are presently considered of human importance. Most of the 40 species are parasites of animals, and some may be synonymous. Twenty-eight are considered distinct species, with 21 from Asia, 2 from Africa, and 5 from the Americas; most are in tropical areas.[146]

P. westermani is the best-known species and is found in humans and animals throughout the East, from India to Japan and the Philippines. *P. heterotremus* is reported from China and Southeast Asia, *P. skrjabini* and *P. hueitungensis* from China, *P. miyazakii* from Japan, *P. uterobilateralis* and *P. africanis* from central and western Africa, *P. mexicanus* from Central and South America, and *P. kellicotti* from North America.[1,147,148]

AGENT

P. westermani was first found in a Bengal tiger that died in an Amsterdam zoo and was named after the zoo director, G. F. Westerman. The first human infection was found in a Portuguese sailor who died in Taiwan in 1879. He had earlier been a patient of Patrick Manson's in Amoy, China, and Manson later concluded that the hemoptysis seen in this man and his Chinese patients was due to this parasite.[149]

Adult *P. westermani* is reddish-brown in color, coffee bean–shaped, 7 to 16 mm in length, 4 to 8 mm in width, and 5 mm thick. The integument is spiny, and the anterior and ventral suckers are of equal size (Fig. 117-4A).

The eggs are yellow-brown in color, thick-shelled with a large operculum, and measure 80 to 120 μm × 50 to 65 μm (Fig. 117-4B). The eggs embryonate in water, and the miracidia hatch in 3 weeks and search for specific snail hosts. Development in snails yields free-swimming cercariae, which penetrate a crab or crayfish second intermediate host and encyst as metacercariae. When these are eaten raw, partially cooked, pickled, or salted, the metacercariae excyst and penetrate the intestinal wall of the definitive hosts and enter the peritoneal cavity. The larval worms remain here for several days, then cross the diaphragm, and enter the pleural cavity and eventually the lung parenchyma to mature to adults in 2 months. A fibrotic cyst wall develops around paired (or tripled) adults, but eggs that are produced escape through cyst-bronchial fistulas and are coughed up in sputum or swallowed and passed in the feces.

Other species of *Paragonimus* have life cycles similar to *P. westermani* but develop in different snail and crustacean intermediate hosts. Species differentiation is based on adult fluke rather than egg morphology.

EPIDEMIOLOGY

Paragonimus transmission occurs most notably in China (*P. westermani, P. skrjabini, P. heterotremus,* and *P. hueitungensis*), Korea (*P. westermani*), Japan (*P. westermani, P. miyazakii*), Vietnam (*P. heterotremus*), Cameroon (*P. africanus* and *P. uterobilateralis*), Ecuador (*P. mexicanus*), and Peru (*P. mexicanus*).[1] Yet the range of each of the species includes

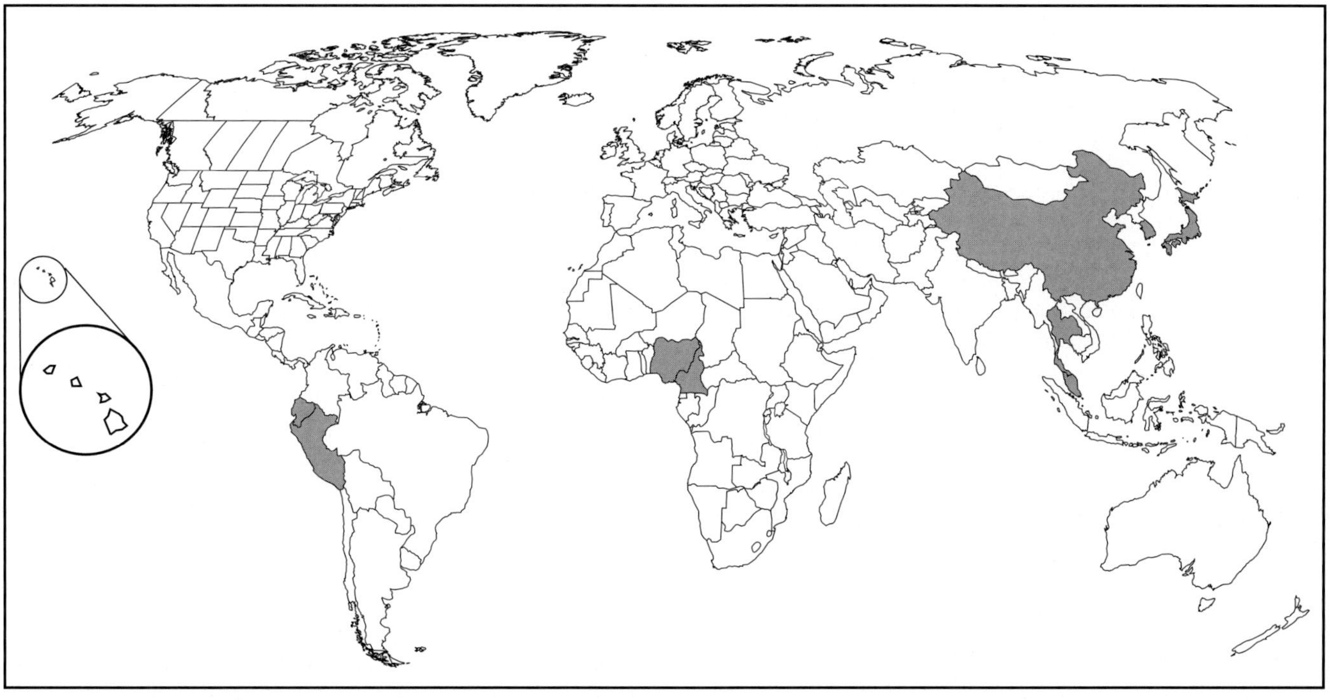

Paragonimus spp.

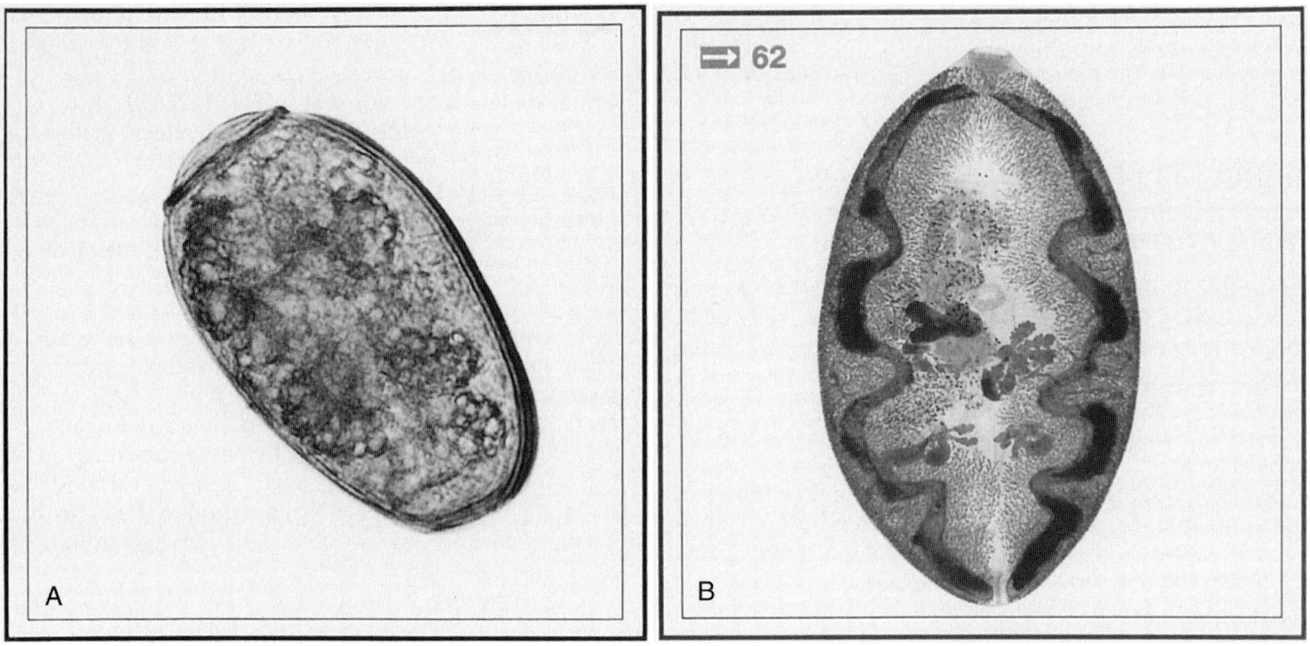

FIGURE 117-4 *Paragonimus westermani. A,* Adult (size 7 to 16 × 4 to 8 mm). *B,* Egg (size 80 to 120 × 50 to 60 μm). (From Orihel TC, Ash LR: Parasites in Human Tissues. Chicago, ASCP Press, 1995.)

many other countries. As an example, *P. westermani* is endemic to China, Japan, Korea, Taiwan, and the Philippines, and the parasite has also been found in Nepal, Bangladesh, Myanmar, Laos, Kampuchea, Vietnam, Thailand, Papua New Guinea, and the former USSR.[146,147] *P. uterobilateralis,* while most prevalent in Cameroon, is found from Zambia west to Guinea. *P. mexicanus* is found from Mexico south to Peru and Ecuador.[1]

In China, human disease caused by *P. westermani, P. skrjabini,* and *P. heterotremus* has been reported from 21 provinces with prevalences of up to 10.4% in some areas. Stool examination surveys of 146,698 people from seven prefectures between 1954 and 1968 yielded an egg-positive rate of 10.4%. Control programs in China had reduced the parasitosis to an estimated 1000 persons infected in 1991. In Korea, a national skin test survey revealed an overall prevalence of 13% in 1959. Control measures, disruption of the ecosystem, and pollution have reduced crab and crayfish populations, and only 16 of 16 million stools were egg-positive in 1990.[1] Taiwan had several endemic foci in the past, but today human infections are rare owing to changes in eating habits and the effect of water pollution and industrialization on the intermediate hosts.[150] Fewer than 300 human cases of paragonimiasis have been reported from a few areas of the Philippines, although infected crustaceans are easily found in endemic areas.[147] Little epidemiologic information is available from other countries reporting this parasitosis. Despite the reductions in Southeast and East Asia, it has been estimated that there are 20.5 million cases worldwide.[1,70]

More than 15 species of snails in the families Hydrobiidae, Thiaridae, and Pleurocercidae serve as the first intermediate hosts of *P. westermani.* The important second intermediate hosts are crabs in the genera *Eriocheir, Potamon,* and *Sundathelphusa,* and crayfish of the genus *Cambaroides.* Individuals become infected by eating these crustaceans raw or insufficiently cooked. The range of culinary artistry is wonderful. In China there is wine-soaked freshwater crab, crayfish curd, raw crab juice, and crab jam; in Thailand, raw freshwater shrimp salad or crab sauce; in Korea, raw crab in soy sauce; in the Philippines, roasted or raw crabs and crab juice seasoning. Crabs and crab juice have been used for medicinal purposes.[148]

Paragonimus species can infect many mammalian species, but some will not mature in these hosts beyond the larval stage. When humans consume these paratenic hosts, the larvae survive stomach acid and penetrate the small intestine wall, completing their life cycle in the human host. Paratenic wild boars have served as a source of infection when eaten raw.[151]

DISEASE

The different *Paragonimus* species each appear to have a different disease spectrum. *P. westermani* represents one clinical pole, with, most commonly, pleuropulmonary disease and relatively infrequent extrapulmonary disease. *P. heterotremus, P. africanus,* and *P. uterobilateralis* appear to be similar in presentation to *P. westermani.*[151–154] The other clinical pole, represented by *P. skrjabini,* is mainly extrapulmonary, with cutaneous lesions the most frequent clinical presentation. Pulmonary disease tends to be caused by adult flukes and cutaneous disease by immature flukes. It is thought that host-fluke species compatibility helps determine which clinical pole a particular species will produce.[1,155,156]

Acute Paragonimiasis

After an incubation period of between 2 and 15 days, the initial symptoms are diarrhea and abdominal pain, followed several days later by fever, chest pain, fatigue, urticaria, eosinophilia, or cough, or any combination of these, lasting several weeks.[155,157]

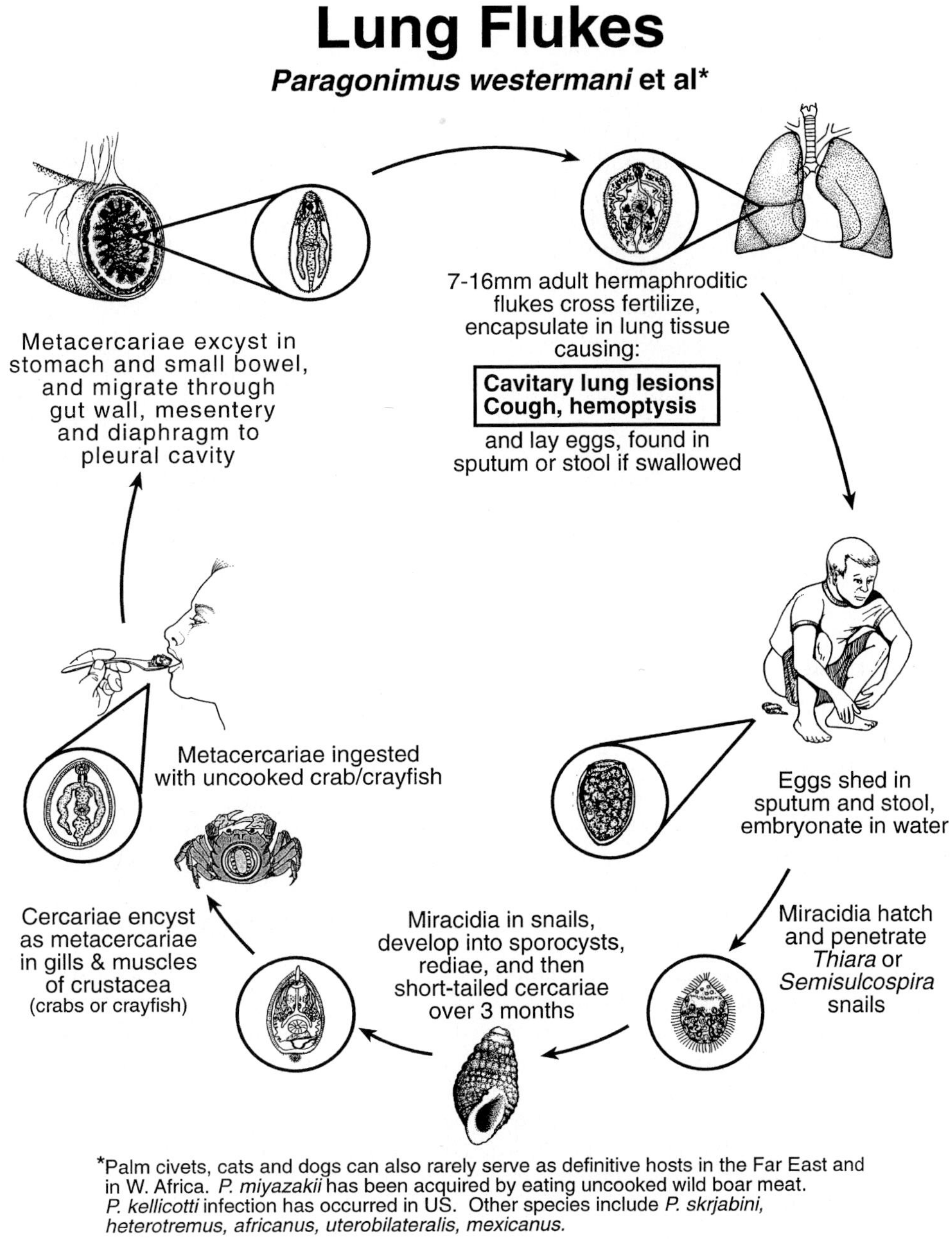

Pleuropulmonary Paragonimiasis

Although acute paragonimiasis may occur, most infections are either silent or insidious in onset. The initial clinical presentation occurs early in the 5- to 10-year life span of the adult fluke, but in some cases it may occur many years after acquisition of the infection.[158,159]

In *P. westermani* infections, the initial presentation is often an abnormal chest film in an asymptomatic patient. Early clinical symptoms include cough or chest pain. The cough, initially dry, often becomes productive of viscous and rusty-colored or blood-tinged sputum and appears to be worsened by exertion.[160] The sputum may be peppered with rusty-brown flecks consisting of clumps of eggs.[2] Charcot-Leyden crystals are frequent. Occasionally there is profuse hemoptysis following paroxysmal coughing. The chest pain is often pleuritic. Fevers are infrequent and in spite of a prolonged clinical history the patient's health usually remains relatively unimpaired. Eosinophilia may be present initially but is usually absent in chronic infections.

Radiographic findings include pulmonary lesions such as focal, segmental, or lobar air space consolidation, small cysts (5 to 30 mm), calcified spots, linear opacities, or nodules. The earliest infiltrates and nodules may show some limited migration.[158,161] About 10% to 40% of egg-positive patients will have normal chest films.[158] As the fluke matures, cavitary lesions of 1- to 4-cm diameter are seen; as the fibrotic reaction increases with time they appear as nodules, but their cavitary nature and associated burrow tracts of 0.5- to 1.0-cm diameter can be visualized by CT scan. Eventually these lesions are replaced by oval to round calcifications.[158] Bronchoscopy, other than as a means of retrieving eggs, does not reveal any diagnostic findings.[158]

Pleural lesions have been found in 5% to 71% of patients in different clinical series of *P. westermani* infections and include effusions, hydropneumothorax, and pleural thickening, which can be bilateral.[158,159,162] The frequency of pleural disease appears to be greatest in *P. skrjabini* infections.[155] Pleural fluid is sterile, contains a leukocyte count over 1000/μL, many eosinophils, and elevated protein and lactate dehydrogenase (LDH) and decreased glucose values. Eggs are rarely found in sputum or pleural fluid.

Excised pulmonary lesions reveal a wide variety of histopathologic changes characterized by the presence of adult worms within fibrous cysts up to 1.5 cm in size, juxtaposed and often communicating with bronchioles or bronchi. Egg-induced granulomas are easily confused with tuberculosis. Adjacent to the cysts are bronchiectases, various pneumonic processes, and vasculitis. Both acute and chronic cellular reactions can coexist within the same lesions.[159,160,163]

Extrapulmonary Paragonimiasis

A percentage of patients with paragonimiasis will develop lesions in locations other than the lung. The frequency is dependent on the species of *Paragonimus,* the intensity of the infection, and possibly the duration. The diagnosis of these ectopic infections depends on the organ involved; cerebral infection produces the most frequent morbidity.

Cerebral Paragonimiasis

Cerebral paragonimiasis is the most frequent form of extrapulmonary disease diagnosed, possibly reflecting the sensitivity of the central nervous system (CNS) to such an insult rather than a predilection of the parasite for that site. Cerebral involvement occurs in less than 1% of cases in community-based studies and up to 24% in hospital-based studies.[164] Cerebral paragonimiasis most often occurs in younger age groups; 90% of patients are less than 30 years of age.[165] Clinical findings in cerebral paragonimiasis are extremely varied, since they are dependent on the location of the parasite. They reflect parasite-induced meningitis, arachnoiditis, and cerebral and spinal space-occupying lesions. Meningitis tends to be acute in onset and to be the initial presentation of cerebral paragonimiasis in up to a third of cases. Intracerebral lesions occur usually in occipital or temporal lobes, or both. The clinical presentation, which tends to be insidious in onset, includes a history of seizures (80%), visual disturbances (60%), headache (55%), motor weakness (48%), sensory disturbances (40%), and vomiting (33%). Seizures are often focal motor initially, progressing to grand mal as the disease evolves.[165,166] Physical findings include ophthalmologic abnormalities (75%), a decline in mental function (70%), hemiparesis (60%), and hemihypoesthesia (45%). Pulmonary paragonimiasis is seen in the majority of cases of CNS disease and, in fact, precedes CNS involvement in two thirds of patients.

Plain films show calcifications and characteristically aggregated, round or cyst-like soap bubbles in more than 40% of patients. Common CT and MRI findings are conglomerated, multiple ring-shaped enhancing lesions with surrounding edema, described as grape clusters.[142] These rings are usually smooth and round, but may, at times, be irregular in outline. They are usually 1 to 3 cm in diameter and have contents with a density equal to or slightly greater than that of cerebrospinal fluid (CSF). At times hemorrhages up to 4 cm in diameter are associated with the ringlike structures, or the lesions may be nodular. Calcifications can be punctate, round, cystic, or amorphous and will increase in frequency with the duration of disease.[164,165,167]

Cutaneous Paragonimiasis

Although a cutaneous presentation is uncommon in *P. westermani* infections, it has been reported to occur in 80% of infections due to other species of *Paragonimus* (e.g., *P. skrjabini, P. miyazakii*). The cutaneous presentation, which has been called trematode larva migrans, consists of painless and migratory subcutaneous swellings or subcutaneous nodules on the trunk and proximal extremities.[168,169] There is often a peripheral blood eosinophilia, which can be extreme.

Miscellaneous Sites

Flukes, usually immature, may come to rest in ectopic intra-abdominal sites such as the liver, spleen, peritoneum, intestinal wall, or mesenteric lymph nodes. The clinical picture reflects the site and can include abdominal pain, diarrhea, and even dysentery.

PATHOGENESIS AND IMMUNITY

As with other tissue-dwelling trematodes, infection with *P. westermani* is also associated with eosinophilia and leukocytosis in the early stages of infection, reflecting activation of the immune system. Eosinophil infiltration around the sites of egg deposition is a consistent pathologic feature, as is eosinophilia and an elevated IgE level, indicative of a Th2 cell-regulated response.[170] IgG_4 antibodies predominate among anti-*Paragonimus* antibodies. However, it remains to be determined whether Th2 lymphocytes play an important role in resistance to the parasite.[170] In rodent models, excreted-secreted products of *Paragonimus* appear to regulate the innate and adaptive immune response in the host, by mechanisms such as attenuating the survival and function of eosinophils, and secreting pro-inflammatory cytokines and chemokines.[171–174] However, these immune mechanisms have been studied only in rodent and bovine models of paragonimiasis, and their roles in human infections have not been elucidated.

DIAGNOSIS

Pulmonary paragonimiasis must be suspected in persons from known endemic areas when a chronic cough is present; the most important differential diagnoses are tuberculosis, bronchiectasis, and chronic bronchitis. The diagnosis is almost always made by finding the characteristic eggs in sputum, stool, gastric aspirates, or tissue. Examination of blood-streaked sputum is the most productive. Egg detection in sputum may require repeated examinations, and a 24-hour sputum collection can increase the sensitivity.[175] This collection is centrifuged, the sediment dissolved in 3% sodium hydroxide, and then examined for eggs.[147] In children and the elderly, in whom sputum swallowing is more frequent, the examination of stool and gastric aspirate specimens can be more productive. Ziehl-Neelsen stains of specimens for mycobacteria may destroy the fluke eggs, making separate examinations necessary.[161] In patients who have pleural or CNS involvement, it is very uncommon to find eggs in pleural fluid or CSF aspirates.

Immunodiagnosis

Most immunologic tests used in the diagnosis of paragonimiasis employ crude extracts of flukes.[114] The CF test has been a standard test for years. This test is sensitive and becomes negative 6 to 12 months after cure, making it useful for following therapy.[176,177] Some cross-reactivity with other trematode parasites has been noted, particularly in the chronic phase of paragonimiasis.[178] A skin test using extracts of adult *Paragonimus* is useful for screening in epidemiologic surveys because of its high sensitivity (80% to 90%), but it remains positive 10 to 20 years after cure.[179] ELISAs for detection of antibodies to *P. westermani* are both sensitive (92%) and highly specific (greater than 90%), but require longer (4 to 24 months) to become positive after infection and longer to normalize after cure.[180–183] Crude worm extracts do not provide an acceptably specific ELISA.[184,185] Consequently, the most sensitive ELISA to date has been developed by Centers for Disease Control and Prevention (CDC; sensitivity, 96%; specificity, 100%), using an 8-kD component of *P. westermani* as the antigen.[186] Recently, antigen detection assays have been developed that utilize mixtures of monoclonal antibodies to capture *P. westermani* antigens from serum, with a sensitivity approaching 100% and specificity greater than 95%.[187,188] The utility of these assays in the field remains to be evaluated, but they would likely provide as sensitive a measure of active infections in field surveys as is found in individuals.

TREATMENT

Praziquantel is the drug of choice because of minimal side effects and the short course of administration. A treatment of 75 mg/kg/day in three divided doses for 2 days is 90% to 100% effective.[158,160,189,190] Symptoms improve within 2 to 3 days, although radiologic findings may worsen for the first 10 days.[161] Adverse effects are mild and include headache, intestinal symptoms, and transient urticaria. Large pleural effusions may require drainage. Surgical intervention may be required for long-standing effusions (years) or empyemas (months).[158]

Triclabendazole, a drug recently introduced as therapy for fascioliasis, successfully treats pulmonary paragonimiasis at a dosage of 5 mg/kg daily for 3 days or 10 mg/kg bid for one day.[191] Bithionol, available in the recent past, could cure 92% of pulmonary cases at a dosage of 40 mg/kg/day on alternate days for 10 to 15 doses.[192] Gastrointestinal side effects in 70%, dermatologic side effects in 21%, and the duration of treatment are recognized limitations.

Untreated pulmonary paragonimiasis can resolve in 5 to 10 years, leaving dysfunction commensurate with the degree of scar tissue produced in the pleura or lungs.[158]

INTESTINAL FLUKES

About 70 trematode species are reported to inhabit the human intestinal tract. Knowledge of their clinical presentation is limited even for those that affect relatively large populations.[1,193] The best known are *Fasciolopsis buski*; the Heterophyidae, including *Heterophyes heterophyes* and *Metagonimus yokogawai*; and several *Echinostoma* species. The intestinal flukes are thought to produce no symptoms except when present in very large numbers, which is a rare occurrence. Few cause serious disease, but community-based and case-control studies have yet to be done. Most of these flukes occur in Asia, but foci of these infections occur in other populations throughout the world. They are usually localized in areas where there are freshwater snail vectors and animal reservoir hosts and occur in people with particular dietary habits.[194]

FASCIOLOPSIS BUSKI

AGENT

F. buski, the giant intestinal fluke, was first found, by Busk, in an Indian sailor in London in 1843. The parasite is found in China, Taiwan, Thailand, Laos, Bangladesh, India, Indonesia, Vietnam, Myanmar, and Kampuchea. The worm is elongated, oval, and fleshy, measuring 20 to 75 mm × 8 to 20 mm × 0.5 to 3.0 mm. Eggs are large, operculate, and unembryonated when passed, and measure 130 to 140 μm × 80 to 85 μm. The miracidia develop in several weeks, hatch from the eggs, and infect planorbid snail intermediate hosts. After development in the snail, cercariae emerge and encyst as metacercariae on aquatic plants. When the plant is eaten, the attached metacercariae excyst and attach to the small intestinal mucosa. The prepatent period is 3 months, and the worms are known to live for 6 or more months in the human. Pigs and dogs act as reservoirs (see following discussion).

EPIDEMIOLOGY

Several planorbid snails serve as the first intermediate host of *F. buski*; these usually live in muddy ponds and streams, including those found adjacent to slaughterhouses where feces from pigs contaminate the waters. Snails and edible water plants also flourish in these waters. The metacercaria of *F. buski* can attach to most aquatic plants, including water caltrop (*Trapa bicornis, Trapa natans*), water chestnut (*Eliocharis tuberosa*), water bamboo (*Zizania aquatic*), water hyacinth (*Eukhornia crassipes*), water morning glory (*Ipomoea aquatic*), watercress (*Nasturtium officinale*), lotus (*Nymphaea lotus*), and others.[1,195] These plants may be cultivated near homes in water contaminated accidentally or fertilized intentionally with human or pig feces. Pigs are a major reservoir host, but there are some areas where humans are infected while pigs are not. Both ingested plants and water contaminated with detached metacercariae are sources of infection. Children eating plants during play, especially in rural areas, have the highest prevalence rates.

DISEASE

This large fluke attaches to the duodenal and jejunal mucosa and produces focal inflammation, ulceration, and small abscesses at the sites of attachment. However, community-based studies reveal no clinical or biochemical differences between lightly to moderately infected cases and controls.[196] Early symptoms, which begin 30 to 60 days after exposure, are epigastric pain, mimicking peptic ulcer disease, and diarrhea.[197] Hunger or anorexia, nausea, and vomiting may occur. Rarely, in heavy infections, edema of the face, abdominal wall, and legs; ascites; and severe prostration have been described.[198] The cause of these is not understood. Large numbers of flukes may cause focal ileus or intermittent obstruction. Eosinophilia is variable but may be marked.[199]

HETEROPHYIDS (HETEROPHYES SPP., METAGONIMUS SPP., ETC.)

There are a large number of small intestinal flukes less than 2.5 mm long in humans, other mammals, and birds in the families Heterophyidae, Plagiorchiidae, Lecithodendridae, Microphallidae, and others. The flukes in the Heterophyidae are the most prevalent and best studied.

AGENTS

Of at least 10 human species of intestinal fluke in the family Heterophyidae the three most prevalent are *Heterophyes heterophyes, H. nocens,* and *Metagonimus yokogawai.* Bilharz described the first, *H. heterophyes,* at the autopsy of a native of Cairo. These are the smallest of the human flukes. They measure 1 to 2 mm in length, are oval to pear-shaped, and have spiny integuments. The eggs are operculate, ovoid, and yellowish in color, measure 27 to 30 μm × 15 to 17 μm, and are very difficult to speciate. The eggs are embryonated when passed and are ingested by a snail intermediate host. Cercariae from the snail enter freshwater fish, encyst as metacercariae, and, when eaten raw, excyst and complete their development to adult flukes within 1 to 2 weeks in the small intestine of humans, other mammals, and fish-eating birds. The prepatent period is only 9 days and the parasite may live for a few months to a year in the final host.

EPIDEMIOLOGY

The highest infection rates for *H. heterophyes* have been reported in Egypt, Iran, and Sudan; for *M. yokogawai,* in Korea, China, Taiwan, Indonesia, Russia, and Japan; and for *H. nocens,* in Korea and Japan. However, there have been reports of these and other heterophyid species in scattered locations around the world, the greatest number occurring in Asia and Southeast Asia. Distributions of the different Heterophyidae greatly overlap. In Korea, of 19 different intestinal flukes reported in humans, 12 are different heterophyid species.[200] The heterophyids are parasites of fish-eating mammals and birds, which, like humans, acquire the infection by eating raw or incompletely cooked freshwater or brackish water fish.

The overall prevalence of *M. yokogawai* in Japan is low (0.2% to 0.3%), but in some areas the prevalence is high (51% to 75%).[201] In Korea, *M. yokogawai* infection rates of 1% to 2% have been reported for the population as a whole, reaching 29% along some coastal streams.[200] Infection rates of *M. yokogawai* in Taiwan and the Philippines are around 1%.[202]

H. heterophyes infects the gray mullet *Mugil cephalus* in the brackish lagoons of Egypt's Nile delta. Infection rates can reach 65% in children in villages where these fish are traditionally eaten raw.

DISEASE

Nine days on average following ingestion of the metacercaria, dyspepsia, colicky abdominal pain, diarrhea, and eosinophilia may occur.[203,204] A mild focal inflammatory reaction and superficial erosions are produced at the site of attachment.[2] The flukes appear to live for less than a year. The fluke may penetrate the mucosa, and eggs may embolize from these intramucosal sites via lymphatics to the systemic vascular system. Eggs of three different heterophyid species have been recovered from capillaries of brain, heart, lungs, spleen, and liver, where space-occupying granulomatous lesions induce clinical pathology.[204–207] Myocarditis can follow the occlusion of myocardial vessels by eggs and the resultant granulomatous and fibrotic host reaction. Thickened mitral valves containing ova have been reported.[208]

ECHINOSTOMA SPECIES

AGENT

These trematodes are primarily parasites of birds and mammals but are common among certain populations of Asia. Fifteen species have been reported in humans. The parasites are elongate, tapered at both ends, and 5 to 15 mm × 1 to 2 mm in size. The name derives from a collar of spines in two rows surrounding the oral sucker. The anterior integument is also provided with tiny spines. Eggs are operculate, thin-shelled, and vary in size (83 to 130 μm × 58 to 90 μm).[47] The eggs embryonate in freshwater in 14 days, and the miracidia enter the snail host. Cercariae emerge from the snail and encyst in the same snail from which they emerged or in other snails, clams, fish, or tadpoles, which serve as second intermediate hosts. Any of these, if eaten uncooked, infect the human final host.[209]

EPIDEMIOLOGY

The most common of the 15 reported *Echinostoma* species in humans are *E. ilocanum* in the Philippines and Thailand, and both *E. malayanum* and *E. revolutum* in Thailand.[1,210] In northern Luzon in the Philippines, *E. malayanum* infection rates have averaged 10% of surveyed populations, with highs of over 40%.[150] In northern Thailand, a variety of echinostomes infect humans with prevalence rates as high as 50%.[211] These and the other species are found at lower prevalences in Southeast Asia, eastern and South Asia, and also in Egypt and Central and South America.[193] The major source of infection with *E. ilocanum* is the snail *Pila conica,* which is eaten uncooked in parts of the Philippines. Other sources of infections are clams, tadpoles, frogs, and fish, all serving as second intermediate hosts for echinostomes. Rats, dogs, cats, birds, and other fish-eating animals are reservoirs of infection.

DISEASE

These flukes attach to small intestinal mucosa, producing inflammatory lesions and shallow ulcers at the sites of attachment. A self-infection by ingestion of 113 metacercaria of *Echinochasmus japonicus* resulted, after 10 days, in abdominal pain and diarrhea.[1,212] There are no clinical epidemiology studies, but it is generally accepted that symptoms are rare in any but the heaviest infections (approximately 500 flukes), which are uncommon.[47,213] The presentation may include colicky abdominal pain and loose bowel movements and at times diarrhea and eosinophilia.

MISCELLANEOUS INTESTINAL FLUKES

There are many other intestinal flukes within the preceding families—Fasciolidae, Heterophyidae, and Echinostomatidae. They have more limited distributions and are less well studied. Two flukes in two other families, Troglotrematidae and Paramphistomatidae, are worth mentioning.

Nanophyetus salmincola is a small fluke found in eastern Siberia and the northwestern coast of North America. It belongs to the same family, Troglotrematidae, as does *Paragonimus.* Adults are 0.8 to 2.5 mm × 0.3 to 0.5 mm, and eggs are 64 to 97 μm × 34 to 55 μm in size. Fish, such as salmon, are the second intermediate hosts. Intestinal symptoms can occur with heavy infections in a manner similar to that of other intestinal flukes. More unusually, this fluke is a vector for the rickettsial organism *Neorickettsia helminthoeca,* which produces a fatal illness in dogs ("salmon poisoning").[214,215]

Gastrodiscoides hominis is a piriform intestinal fluke that is 8 to 14 mm × 5 to 8 mm in size and produces eggs that measure 150 μm × 60 to 70 μm. It is widely distributed from India to the Philippines and north to Kazakhstan. The human colon can be colonized, with resultant mucoid diarrhea. Pigs and rodents appear to be the reservoir.

DIAGNOSIS

Since clinical presentations are nonspecific, indications that infections are present are, at times, eosinophilia, a particular dietary history, and the time interval since possible infection; *H. heterophyes* and *M. yokogawai* do not survive in the intestine for more than a year. The diagnosis is made on stool examination or by tissue biopsy or necropsy. Egg identification can be very difficult because many of the intestinal fluke eggs have similar morphology and overlapping sizes. Overlapping "small" fluke eggs include *H. heterophyes* (28 to 30 μm × 15 to 17 μm), *M. yokogawai* (26 to 28 μm × 15 to 17 μm), *C. sinensis* (28 to 35 μm × 12 to 19 μm), and *O. viverrini* (30 μm × 12 μm). Overlapping "large" fluke eggs are *Fasciolopsis buski* (130 to 140 μm × 80 to 85 μm), *Echinostoma* spp. (83 to 130 μm × 58 to 90 μm), and *Fasciola hepatica* (130 to 150 μm × 60 to 90 μm). As well, there are many other less common intestinal flukes with focal distribution that produce similarly sized eggs.

Examination of stools for expelled adult flukes after treatment with praziquantel is necessary to make a definitive diagnosis. Although praziquantel may damage the integument of the adult fluke, it is still often possible to make a species identification.

TREATMENT

Evidence from limited trials suggests that praziquantel is highly effective against intestinal flukes at 15 to 25 mg/kg given in a single dose.[1,216] The new benzimidazole, triclabendazole, at 5 mg/kg twice daily after a meal at a 6- to 8-hour interval for 1 day, shows promise in the treatment of intestinal flukes.[1] Alternative drugs include for *F. buski,* niclosamide 40 mg/kg/day for 1 to 2 days (maximum daily dose of 4 g); for *H. heterophyes,* niclosamide 1000 mg in a single dose; and for *Echinostoma* spp., albendazole 400 mg twice daily for 3 days.[47,204,217]

PREVENTION AND CONTROL

Prevention and control of food-borne trematode infections require changes in habits that have been in practice for generations.[218] These habits are variably dependent on attitudes, education, poverty, environmental degradation, food security, and other factors, and control strategies will have to take all these into account. Education can change habits. Such education should include understanding of the impact of the use of human and animal feces as fertilizer for aquatic plants and fishponds. Methods of food preservation must be addressed, since many foods deteriorate quickly in the tropics, and smoking, pickling, and fermentation methods often do not destroy metacercariae. Irradiation may offer an alternative.[219] Preservation by cooking can be difficult in many heavily populated regions where fuel is scarce. On the other hand, some populations prefer to eat raw food, aware of the nutritional value of raw foods.[1]

National strategies are necessary to control these parasites. Health education and appropriate regulations, both for water bodies used for pisciculture and aquatic plant crops, can have an impact. Mass treatment programs using praziquantel or triclabendazole may be beneficial but require more experience.[220] Molluscicide or elimination of the animal host reservoirs does not appear to be realistic over the long term.[1]

REFERENCES

1. Control of Foodborne Trematode Infections: Report of a WHO Study Group. WHO Technical Report Series No. 849. Geneva, World Health Organization, 1995.
2. Beaver PC, Jung RC, Cupp EW: Clinical Parasitology, 9th ed. Philadelphia, Lea & Febiger, 1984.
3. Wykoff DE, Harinasutra C, Juttijudata P, et al: *Opisthorchis viverrini* in Thailand—The life cycle and comparison with *O. felineus.* J Parasitol 51:207, 1965.
4. Chen M, Lu Y, Hua X, et al: Progress in assessment of morbidity due to *Clonorchis sinensis.* Trop Dis Bull 91:R9, 1994.
5. Chen ER: Clonorchiasis in Taiwan. Southeast Asian J Trop Med Public Health 22(suppl):184, 1991.
6. Ramasoota T: Current status of food-borne parasitic zoonoses in Thailand. Southeast Asian J Trop Med Public Health 22(suppl):23, 1991.

7. De NV, Murrell KD, Cong LD, et al: The foodborne trematode zoonoses of Vietnam. Southeast Asian J Trop Med Public Health 34(suppl 1):12, 2003.
8. MacLean JD, Arthur JR, Ward BJ, et al: Common-source outbreak of acute metorchiasis due to the North American liver fluke *Metorchis conjunctus*. Lancet 347:154, 1996.
9. Sithithaworn P, Haswell-Elkins MR, Mairiang P, et al: Parasite-associated morbidity: Liver fluke infection and biliary duct cancer in north-east Thailand. Int J Parasitol 24:833, 1994.
10. Koenigstein RP: Observations of the epidemiology of infections with *Clonorchis sinensis*. Trans R Soc Trop Med Hyg 42:503, 1949.
11. Zhipiao X, Huilan Z, Weiji C: Acute clonorchiasis: Report of 2 cases. Chin Med J (Engl) 92:423, 1979.
12. Bronshtein AM, Ozeretskovskaya NN: First trials of praziquantel for the treatment of patients with acute or chronic *Opisthorchis felineus*. Med Parazitol (Mosk) 5:31, 1985.
13. Mel'nikov VI, Skarednov NI: The clinical picture of acute opisthorchiasis in the immigrant population of the northern Ob' region. Med Parazitol (Mosk) 48:12, 1979.
14. Attwood HD, Chou ST: The longevity of *Clonorchis sinensis*. Pathology 10:153, 1978.
15. Upatham ES, Viyanant V, Kurathong S, et al: Relationship between prevalence and intensity of *Opisthorchis viverrini* infection, and clinical symptoms and signs in a rural community in north-east Thailand. Bull World Health Organ 62:451, 1984.
16. Upatham ES, Vivanant V, Kurathong S, et al: Morbidity in relation to intensity of infection in opisthorchiasis viverrini: study of community in Khon Kaen, Thailand. Am J Trop Med Hyg 31:1156, 1982.
17. Strauss WG: Clinical manifestations of clonorchiasis: a controlled study of 105 cases. Am J Trop Med Hyg 11:625, 1962.
18. Wykoff DE, Chittayasothorn K, Winn MW: Clinical manifestations of *Opisthorchis viverrini* infections in Thailand. Am J Trop Med Hyg 15:914, 1966.
19. Mairiang E, Haswell-Elkins MR, Mairiang P, et al: Reversal of biliary tract abnormalities associated with *Opisthorchis viverrini* infection following praziquantel treatment. Trans R Soc Trop Med Hyg 87:194, 1993.
20. Elkins DB, Sithithaworn P, Haswell-Elkins M, et al: *Opisthorchis viverrini*: Relationships between egg counts, worms recovered and antibody levels within an endemic community in Northeast Thailand. Parasitology 102:283, 1991.
21. Sithithaworn P, Tesana S, Pipitgool V, et al: Quantitative post-mortem study of *Opisthorchis viverrini* in man in north-east Thailand. Trans R Soc Trop Med Hyg 85:765, 1991.
22. Sithithaworn P, Tesana S, Pipitgool V, et al: Relationship between faecal egg count and worm burden of *Opisthorchis viverrini* in human autopsy cases. Parasitology 102:277, 1991.
23. Pungpak S, Harinasuta T, Bunnag D, et al: Fecal egg output in relation to worm burden and clinical features in human opisthorchiasis. Southeast Asian J Trop Med Public Health 21:275, 1990.
24. Upatham ES, Viyanant WY, Brockelman S, et al: Rate of re-infection by *Opisthorchis viverrini* in an endemic northeast Thai community after chemotherapy. Int J Parasitol 18:643, 1988.
25. Changbumrung S, Tungtrongchitr R, Hongtong K, et al: Food patterns and habits of people in an endemic area for liver fluke infection. J Nutr Assoc Thail 23:133, 1989.
26. Rim H-J: The current pathobiology and chemotherapy of clonorchiasis. Korean J Parasitol 24:1, 1986.
27. Pungpak S, Chalermrut K, Harinasuta T, et al: *Opisthorchis viverrini* infection in Thailand: Symptoms and signs of infection—A population-based study. Trans R Soc Trop Med Hyg 88:561, 1994.
28. Chen M-G, Hua X-J, Wan Z-R, et al: Praziquantel in 237 cases of clonorchiasis sinensis. Chin Med J (Engl) 96:935, 1983.
29. Dhiensiri Y, Eua-Ananta Y, Bunnag D, et al: Roentgenographically controlled healing of gallbladder lesions in opisthorchiasis after praziquantel treatment. Drug Res 34:1175, 1984.
30. Pungpak S, Sornmani S, Suntharasamai P, et al: Ultrasonographic study of the biliary system in opisthorchiasis patients after treatment with praziquantel. Southeast Asian J Trop Med Public Health 20:157, 1989.
31. Rim H-J: Clonorchisis in Korea. Korean J Parasitol 28(suppl):63, 1990.
32. Hou PC: The pathology of *Clonorchis sinensis* infestation of the liver. J Pathol Bacteriol 70:53, 1995.
33. Carmona RH, Crass R, Lim RC, et al: Oriental cholangitis. Am J Surg 148:117, 1984.
34. Seel DJ, Park YK: Oriental infestational cholangitis. Am J Surg 146:366, 1983.
35. Lim JH: Radiologic findings of clonorchiasis. Am J Roentgenol 155:1001, 1990.
36. Mcfadzean AJS, Yeung RTT: Acute pancreatitis due to *Clonorchis sinensis*. Trans R Soc Trop Med Hyg 60:466, 1966.
37. Haswell-Elkins MR, Mairiang E, Mairiang P, et al: Cross-sectional study of *Opisthorchis viverrini* infection and cholangiocarcinoma in communities within a high-risk area in Northeast Thailand. Int J Cancer 59:505, 1994.
38. Vatanasapt V, Tangvoraphonchai V, Titapant V, et al: A high incidence of liver cancer in Khon Kaen Province, Thailand. Southeast Asian J Trop Med Public Health 21:382, 1990.
39. Thamavit W, Bharmarapravati N, Sahaphong S, et al: Effects of dimethylnitrosamine on induction of cholangiocarcinoma in *Opisthorchis viverrini*–infected Syrian Golden Hamsters. Cancer Res 38:1634, 1978.
40. IARC Working Group: Schistosomes, Liver Flukes and *Helicobacter pylori*. Vol 61. Lyon, France, IARC Monographs on the Evaluation of Carcinogenic Risks to Humans, 1994.
41. Okuda K, Nakanuma Y, Miyazaki M. Cholangiocarcinoma: Recent progress. 1. Epidemiology and etiology. J Gastroenterol Hepatol 17:1049, 2002.
42. Mitacek EJ, Brunnemann KD, Suttajit M et al: Exposure to *N*-Nitroso compounds in a population of high cancer regions in Thailand: Volatile Nitrosamine (VNA) levels in Thai food. Food Chem Toxicol 37:297, 1999.
43. Haswell-Elkins MR, Elkins DB: Food-borne trematodes. In Cook CC (ed): Manson's Tropical Medicine, 20th ed. London, WB Saunders, 1992, p. 1457.
44. Haswell-Elkins MR, Sithithaworn P, Elkins D: *Opisthorchis viverrini* and cholangiocarcinoma in Northeast Thailand. Parasitol Today 8:86, 1992.
45. Haswell-Elkins MR, Satarug S, Elkins DB: *Opisthorchis viverrini* infection in Northeast Thailand and its relationship to cholangiocarcinoma. J Gastroenterol Hepatol 7:538, 1992.
46. Isseroff H, Sawma JT, Reino D: Fascioliasis: Role of proline in bile duct hyperplasia. Science 198:1157, 1977.
47. Harinasuta T, Bunnag D: Liver, Lung and intestinal trematodiasis. In Warren KS, Mahmoud AF (eds): Tropical and Geographic Medicine Vol 2. New York, McGraw-Hill, 1990, p. 473.
48. Finkelman FD, Pearce EJ, Urban JF Jr, et al: Regulation and biological function of helminth-induced cytokine responses. Immunol Today 12:A62, 1991.
49. Akai PS, Pungpak S, Kitikoon V, et al: Possible protective immunity in human opisthorchiasis. Parasite Immunol 16:279, 1994.
50. Haswell-Elkins MR, Sithithaworn P, Mairiang E, et al: Immune responsiveness and parasite-specific antibody levels in human hepatobiliary disease associated with *Opisthorchis viverrini* infection. Clin Exp Immunol 84:213, 1991.
51. Morikawa P, Ishida H, Niizawa M, et al: Sonographic features of biliary clonorchiasis. J Clin Ultrasound 16:655, 1988.
52. Palmer PES, Reeder MM: Clonorchiasis and other liver fluke disease. In: The Imaging of Tropical Diseases. Baltimore, Williams & Wilkins, 2001, pp. 11, 194.
53. Elkins DB, Haswell-Elkins M, Anderson RM: The epidemiology and control of intestinal helminths in the Pulicat Lake region of Southern India. Trans R Soc Trop Med Hyg 80:774, 1986.
54. Radomyos P, Bunnag D, Harinasuta T: Worms recovered in stools following praziquantel treatment. Drug Res 34:1215, 1984.
55. Sirisinha S, Chawengkirttikul R, Haswell-Elkins MR, et al: Evaluation of a monoclonal antibody–based enzyme linked immunosorbent assay for the diagnosis of *Opisthorchis viverrini* infection in an endemic area. Am J Trop Med Hyg 52:521, 1995.
56. Qiu LS, Xue HC, Zhu ZX, et al: Diagnosis of clonorchiasis by dot-ELISA. Chin J Infect Dis 7:32, 1989.
57. Hahm JH, Lee JS, Rim HJ: Comparative study on the indirect immunofluorescence antibody test, complement fixation test and ELISA in the diagnosis of human clonorchiasis. Korea Univ Med J 21:177, 1984.
58. Lee S, Chai JY, Seo M, et al: Control of foodborne trematode infections. Report of a WHO Study Group. Two cases of *Gymnophalloides seoi* infection accompanied by diabetes mellitus. World Health Organ Tech Rep Ser 849:1, 1995.
59. Choi MH, Ryu JS, Lee M, et al: Specific and common antigens of *Clonorchis sinensis* and *Opisthorchis viverrini* (Opisthorchidae, Trematoda). Korean J Parasitol 41:155, 2003.

60. Hong ST, Kho WG, Lee M, et al: Immunoblot patterns of clonorchiasis. Korean J Parasitol 35: 87, 1997.
61. Yong TS, Yang HJ, Park SJ, et al: Immunodiagnosis of clonorchiasis using a recombinant antigen. Korean J Parasitol 36:183, 1998.
62. Wang J, Lu ZY, Wang W, et al: Changes in antibody levels in clonorchiasis patients before and after treatment. Chung Kuo Chi Sheng Chung Hsueh Yu Chi Sheng Chung Ping Tsa Chih 3:60, 1985.
63. Chen YT, Liu YH, Wang QN, et al: Detection of circulating antigen in sera from clonorchiasis sinensis patients by ELISA double sandwich method. Chin Med J (Engl) 101:92, 1987.
64. Lin YL, Chen ER, Yen CM: Antibodies in serum of patients with clonorchiasis before and after treatment. Southeast Asian J Trop Med Public Health 26:114, 1995.
65. Wen PE, Li GP, Wang ZR, et al: Counter immuno-electrophoresis in detection of *Clonorchis sinensis* antigens in the stool for diagnosis of clonorchiasis. Chin J Parasitol Dis Control 3:238, 1990.
66. Bunnag D, Harinasuta: Studies on the chemotherapy of human opisthorchiasis in Thailand. 1. Clinical trial of praziquantel. Southeast Asian J Trop Med Public Health 11:528, 1980.
67. Tinga N, De N, Vien HV et al. Little effect of praziquantel or artemisin on clonorchiasis in Northern Vietnam: A pilot study. Trop Med Int Health 4: 814, 1999.
68. Liu YH, Wang XG, Gao P, et al: Experimental and clinical trial of albendazole in the treatment of clonorchiasis sinensis. Chin Med J (Engl) 104:27, 1991.
69. Fan ST, Choi TK, Wong J: Recurrent pyogenic cholangitis: Current management. World J Surg 15:248, 1991.
70. Mott KE, Nuttal I, Desjeur P, et al: New geographical approaches to the control of some parasitic zoonoses. Bull World Health Organ 73:247, 1995.
71. Bjorland J, Bryan RT, Strauss W, et al: An outbreak of acute fascioliasis among Aymara Indians in the Bolivian Altiplano. Clin Infect Dis 21:1228, 1995.
72. Chen MG, Mott KE: Progress in assessment of morbidity due to *Fasciola hepatica* infection: A review of recent literature. Trop Dis Bull 87:R1, 1990.
73. Knobloch J, Delgado E, Alvarez A, et al: Human fascioliasis in Cajamarca/Peru. 1. Diagnostic methods and treatment with praziquantel. Trop Med Parasitol 36:88, 1985.
74. Arjona R, Riancho JA, Aguado JM, et al: Fascioliasis in developed countries: A review of classic and aberrant forms of the disease. Medicine (Baltimore) 74:13, 1995.
75. Giraudet J: Réflections sur une épidémie de distomatose hépatique humaine: étude de 50 observations en milieu hospitalier. Presse Med 76:189, 1968.
76. Facey RV, Marsden PD: Fascioliasis in man: An outbreak in Hampshire. BMJ 2:619, 1960.
77. Hardman EW, Jones RLH, Davies AH: Fascioliasis—A large outbreak. BMJ 3:502, 1970.
78. Pulpeiro JR, Armesto V, Varela J, et al: Fascioliasis: Findings in 15 patients. Br J Radiol 64:798, 1991.
79. Acuna-Soto R, Braun-Roth G: Bleeding ulcer in the common bile duct due to *Fasciola hepatica*. Am J Gastroenterol 82:560, 1987.
80. Jones EA, Kay JM, Milligan HP, et al: Massive infection with *Fasciola hepatica* in man. Am J Med 63:836, 1977.
81. Serrano MAP, Vega A, Ortega E, et al: Computed tomography of hepatic fascioliasis. J Comput Assist Tomogr 11:269, 1987.
82. MacLean JD, Grawme-Cook FM: Case 12-2002-CPC, Massachusetts General Hospital: A 50-year-old man with eosinophilia and fluctuating hepatic lesions. NEJM 346:1232, 2002.
83. Uribarrena R, Borda F, Munoz M, et al: Laparoscopic findings in eight cases of liver fascioliasis. Endoscopy 17:137, 1985.
84. Acosta-Ferreira W, Vercelli-Retta J, Falconi LM: *Fasciola hepatica* human infection: Histopathological study of sixteen cases. Virchows Arch 383:319, 1979.
85. Naquira-Vildosa F, Marcial-Rojas RA: In Marcial-Rojas (ed): Pathology of Protozoal and Helminthic Diseases. Baltimore, Williams & Wilkins, 1971, p. 477.
86. Ruggieri F, Correa AJE, Martinez E: Cerebral distomiasis: Case report. J Neurosurg 27:268, 1967.
87. Price TA, Tuazon CU, Simon GL: Fascioliasis: Case reports and review. Clin Infect Dis 17:426, 1993.
88. Brown WC, Davis WC, Dobbelaere DA, et al: CD4+ T-cell clones obtained from cattle chronically infected with *Fasciola hepatica* and specific for adult worm antigen express both unrestricted and Th2 cytokine profiles. Infect Immun 62:818, 1994.
89. Brown WC, Woods VM, Chitko-McKown CG, et al: Interleukin-10 is expressed by bovine type 1 helper, type 2 helper, and unrestricted parasite-specific T-cell clones and inhibits proliferation of all three subsets in an accessory-cell–dependent manner. Infect Immun 62:4697, 1994.
90. Capron A, Dessaint JP: Immunologic aspects of schistosomiasis. Annu Rev Med 43:209, 1992.
91. Wynn TA, Jankovic D, Hieny S, et al: IL-12 enhances vaccine-induced immunity to *Schistosoma mansoni* in mice and decreases T helper 2 cytokine expression, IgE production, and tissue eosinophilia. J Immunol 154:4701, 1995.
92. Keegan PS, Trudgett A: *Fasciola hepatica* in the rat: Immune responses associated with the development of resistance to infection. Parasitol Immunol 14:657, 1992.
93. Sexton JL, Wilce MC, Colin T, et al: Vaccination of sheep against *Fasciola hepatica* with glutathione-*S*-transferase: Identification and mapping of antibody epitopes on a three-dimensional model of the antigen. J Immunol 152:1861, 1994.
94. Mulcahy G, O'Connor F, McGonigle S, et al: Correlation of specific antibody titre and avidity with protection in cattle immunized against *Fasciola hepatica*. Vaccine 16:932,1998.
95. Hanna RE: *Fasciola hepatica*: glycocalyx replacement in the juvenile as a possible mechanism for protection against host immunity. Exp Parasitol 50:103, 1980.
96. Duffus WP, Franks D: In vitro effect of immune serum and bovine granulocytes on juvenile *Fasciola hepatica*. Clin Exp Immunol 41:430, 1980.
97. Muro A, Ramajo V, Lopez J, et al: *Fasciola hepatica*: Vaccination of rabbits with native and recombinant antigens related to fatty acid binding proteins. Vet Parasitol 69:219, 1997.
98. Paykari H, Dalimi A, Madani R: Immunization of sheep against *Fasciola gigantica* with glutathione S-transferase. Vet Parasitol 105:153, 2002.
99. Morrison CA, Colin T, Sexton JL, et al: Protection of cattle against *Fasciola hepatica* infection by vaccination with glutathione S-transferase. Vaccine 14:1603, 1996.
100. Howell MJ, Board PG, Boray JC: Glutathione-*S*-transferases in *Fasciola hepatica*. J Parasitol 74:715, 1988.
101. Sexton JL, Milner AR, Panaccio M, et al: Glutathione-*S*-transferase: novel vaccine against *Fasciola hepatica* infection in sheep. J Immunol 145:3905, 1990.
102. Rodriguez-Perez J, Rodriguez-Medina JR, Garcia-Blanco MA, et al: *Fasciola hepatica*: Mmolecular cloning, nucleotide sequence, and expression of a gene encoding a polypeptide homologous to a *Schistosoma mansoni* fatty acid–binding protein. Exp Parasitol 74:400, 1992.
103. Spithill TW, Piedrafita D, Smooker PM: Immunological approaches for the control of fascioliasis. Int J Parasitol 27:1221, 1997.
104. Smithers SR: Fascioliasis and other trematode infections. In Cohen S, Warren KS (eds): Immunology of Parasitic Infections, 2nd ed. Oxford, Blackwell Scientific, 1982, p. 608.
105. Stork MG, Venables GS, Jennings SMF, et al: An investigation of endemic fascioliasis in Peruvian village children. J Trop Med Hyg 76:231, 1973.
106. Abdul-Fattah MM, Yousef SM, Nasr ME, et al: Indirect fluorescent antibody test in diagnosis of acute fasciolytic syndrome. J Egypt Soc Parasitol 22:261, 1992.
107. Cornelissen JB, de Leeuw WA, van der Heijden PJ: Comparison of an indirect haemagglutination assay and an ELISA for diagnosing *Fasciola hepatica* in experimentally and naturally infected sheep. Vet Q 14:152, 1992.
108. Adam R, Sithithaworn P, Pipitgool V, et al: Studies on metacercariae from Naiads in northeast Thailand. Southeast Asian J Trop Med Public Health 24:701, 1993.
109. Guobadia EE, Fagbemi BO: Time-course analysis of antibody response by EITB and ELISA before and after chemotherapy in sheep infected with *Fasciola gigantica*. Vet Parasitol 58:247, 1995.
110. Qureshi T, Wagner GG, Drawe DL, et al: Enzyme-linked immunoelectrotransfer blot analysis of excretory-secretory proteins of *Fascioloides magna* and *Fasciola hepatica*. Vet Parasitol 58:357, 1995.

111. Hillyer GV, Soler de Galanes M, Rodriguez-Perez J, et al: Use of the Falcon assay screening test–enzyme-linked immunosorbent assay (FAST-ELISA) and the enzyme-linked immunoelectrotransfer blot (EITB) to determine the prevalence of human fascioliasis in the Bolivian Altiplano. Am J Trop Med Hyg 46:603, 1992.
112. Espino AM, Finlay CM: Sandwich enzyme-linked immunosorbent assay for detection of excretory secretory antigens in humans with fascioliasis. J Clin Microbiol 32:190, 1994 [erratum in J Clin Microbiol 32:860, 1994].
113. Rivera Marrero CA, Santiago N, Hillyer GV: Evaluation of immunodiagnostic antigens in the excretory-secretory products of *Fasciola hepatica*. J Parasitol 74:646, 1988.
114. Ikeda T: Cystatin capture enzyme-linked immunosorbent assay for immunodiagnosis of human paragonimiasis and fascioliasis. Am J Trop Med Hyg 59:286, 1998.
115. Santiago de Weil N, Hillyer GV: Antibody profiles by EITB and ELISA of cattle and sheep infected with *Fasciola hepatica*. J Parasitol 74:810, 1988.
116. Apt W, Aguilera X, Vega F, et al: Treatment of human chronic fascioliasis with triclabendazole: drug efficacy and serological response. Am J Trop Med Hyg 52:532, 1995.
117. Shaheen HI, Kamal KA, Farid Z, et al: Dot–enzyme-linked immunosorbent assay (DOT-ELISA) for the rapid diagnosis of human fascioliasis. J Parasitol 75:549, 1989.
118. Santiago de Weil N, Hillyer GV, Pacheco E: Isolation of *Fasciola hepatica* genus–specific antigens. Int J Parasitol 14:197, 1984.
119. O'Neill SM, Parkinson M, Strauss W, et al: Immunodiagnosis of *Fasciola hepatica* infection (fascioliasis) in a human population in the Bolivian Altiplano using purified cathepsin L cysteine proteinase. Am J Trop Med Hyg 58:417, 1998.
120. Brady CP, Dowd AJ, Tort J, et al: The cathepsin L-like proteinases of liver fluke and blood fluke parasites of the trematode genera *Fasciola* and *Schistosoma*. Biochem Soc Trans 2:740, 1999.
121. O'Neill SM, Parkinson M, Dowd AJ, et al: Short report: immunodiagnosis of human fascioliasis using recombinant *Fasciola hepatica* cathepsin L1 cysteine proteinase. Am J Trop Med Hyg 60:749, 1999.
122. Carnevale S, Rodriguez MI, Guarnera, EA, et al: Immunodiagnosis of fasciolosis using recombinant procathepsin L cystein proteinase. Diag Microbiol Infect Dis 41:43, 2001.
123. Carnevale S, Rodriguez MI, Santillan G, et al: Immunodiagnosis of human fascioliasis by an enzyme-linked immunosorbent assay (ELISA) and a micro-ELISA. Clin Diag Lab Immunol 8:174, 2001.
124. Mulcahy G, Joyce P, Dalton JP: Immunology of Fasciola hepatica infection. In Dalton, JP (ed): Fasciolosis. New York, CABI Publishing, 1999, pp. 341–366.
125. Dalton J: Fascioliasis. Wallington, UK, CAB International, 1999.
126. Akahane H, Oshima T, Shimazu T, et al: Diagnosis of fascioliasis. 1. Comparison of the efficacy of various concentration techniques of ova in stool. Jpn J Parasitol 24:55, 1975.
127. Graham CS, Brodie SB, Weller P: Imported *Fasciola hepatica* infection in the United States and treatment with triclabendazole. Clin Infect Dis 33:1, 2001.
128. Lecaillon JB, Godbillon J, Campestrini, et al: Effect of food on the bioavailability of triclabendazole in patients with fascioliasis. Br J Clin Pharmacol 45:601, 1998.
129. Millan JC, Mull R, Freise S, et al: The efficacy and tolerability of triclabendazole in Cuban patients with latent and chronic *Fasciola hepatica* infection. Am J Trop Med Hyg 63:264, 2000.
130. Moll L, Gaasenbeek CP, Vellema P, et al: Resistance of *Fasciola hepatica* against triclabendazole in cattle and sheep in the Netherlands. Vet Parasitol 91:153, 2000.
131. Robinson MW, Trudgett A, Hoey EM, et al: Triclabendazole-resistant *Fasciola hepatica* beta-tubulin and response to in-vitro treatment with triclabendazole. Parasitology 124:325, 2002.
132. Schiappacasse RH, Mohammadi D, Christie AJ: Successful treatment of severe infection with *Fasciola hepatica* with praziquantel. J Infect Dis 52:1339, 1985.
133. Patrick KM, Isaac-Renton J: Praziquantel failure in treatment of *Fasciola hepatica*. Can J Infect Dis 3:33, 1992.
134. Farid Z, Trabolsi B, Boctor F, et al: Unsuccessful use of praziquantel to treat acute fascioliasis in children. J Infect Dis 154:920, 1986.
135. Le Bras M, Beylot J, Bressy H, et al: Traitement de la fasciolose humaine par le triclabendazole. Med Chir Dig 18:477, 1989.
136. Loutan L, Bouvier M, Rajanawisut B, et al: Single treatment of invasive fascioliasis with triclabendazole. Lancet 2:383, 1989.
137. Bassiouny HK, Soliman NK, El-Daly SM, et al: Human fascioliasis in Egypt: effect of infection and efficacy of bithionol treatment. J Trop Med Hyg 94:333, 1991.
138. Bacq Y, Besnier J-M, Duong T-H, et al: Successful treatment of acute fascioliasis with bithionol. Hepatology 14:1066, 1991.
139. Drugs for parasitic diseases. Medical Letter, www.medicalletter.org, August 2004.
140. Farid Z, Kamal M, Woody J: Treatment of acute toxaemic fascioliasis. Trans R Soc Trop Med Hyg 82:299, 1988.
141. Dalton JP, Neill SO, Stack C, et al: Fasciola hepatica cathepsin L-like proteases: biology, function, and potential in the development of first generation liver fluke vaccines. Int J Parasitol 33:1173, 2003.
142. Piacenza L, Acosta D, Basmadjian I, et al: Vaccination with cathepsin L proteinases and with leucine aminopeptidase induces high levels of protection against fascioliasis in sheep. Infect Immun 67:1954, 1999.
143. Wijffels GL, Salvatore L, Dosen,M, et al: Vaccination of sheep with purified cysteine proteinases of *Fasciola hepatica* decreases worm fecundity. Exp Parasitol 78:132, 1994.
144. Hoyle DC, Rattray M, Jupp R, et al: Making sense of microarray data distributions. Bioinformatics 18:576, 2002.
145. Spithill TW, Smooker PM, Sexton J, et al: Development of vaccines against *Fasciola hepatica*. In Dalton JP (ed): Fasciolosis. New York, CABI, 1999, p. 377.
146. Miyasaki I: Helminthic Zoonoses. Tokyo, International Medical Foundation of Japan, 1991.
147. Cabrera BD: Paragonimiasis in the Philippines: Current status. Arzneimittelforschung 34:1188, 1984.
148. Miyasaki I, Hirose H: Immature lung fluke found in the muscle of a wild boar in Japan. J Parasitol 62:835, 1976.
149. Grove DI: A History of Human Helminthology. Oxford, CAB International, 1990.
150. Cross JH: Changing patterns of some trematode infections in Asia. Arzneimittelforschung 34:1224, 1984.
151. Kum PN, Nchinda PN: Pulmonary paragonimiasis in Cameroon. Trans R Soc Trop Med Hyg 76:768, 1982.
152. Nwokolo C: Outbreak of paragonimiasis in eastern Nigeria. Lancet 1:32, 1972.
153. Ogakwu M, Nwokolo C: Radiological findings in pulmonary paragonimiasis as seen in Nigeria: a review based on one hundred cases. Br J Radiol 46:699, 1973.
154. Vanijanonta S, Bunnag D, Harinsuta T: Radiological findings in pulmonary paragonimiasis heterotremus. Southeast Asian J Trop Med Public Health 15:122, 1984.
155. Chung HL, Ho LY, Hsu CP, et al: Recent progress in studies of *Paragonimus* and paragonimiasis control in China. Chin Med J (Engl) 94:483, 1981.
156. Hu X, Feng R, Zheng Z, et al: Hepatic damage in experimental and clinical paragonimiasis. Am J Trop Med Hyg 31:1148, 1982.
157. Huei-lan, Wei-chi: *Paragonimus westermani* (Szechuan variety) and a new species of lung fluke—*Paragonimus szechuanensis*. 2. Studies on clinical aspects of paragonimiasis szechuanensis—A new clinical entity. Chin Med J (Engl) 81:419, 1962.
158. Shim Y-S, Cho S-Y, Han Y-C: Pulmonary paragonimiasis: A Korean perspective. Semin Respir Med 12:35, 1991.
159. Yokogawa M: *Paragonimus* and paragonimiasis. Adv Parasitol 3:99, 1965.
160. Choi DW: *Paragonimus* and paragonimiasis in Korea. Korean J Parasitol 28(suppl):79, 1990.
161. Barrett-Conner E: Parasitic pulmonary disease. Am Rev Respir Dis 126:558, 1982.
162. Im J-G, Whang HY, Kim WS, et al: Pleuropulmonary paragonimiasis: radiological findings in 71 patients. Am J Roentgenol 159:39, 1992.
163. Chung CH: Human paragonimiasis (pulmonary distomiasis, endemic hemoptysis). In Marcial-Rojas RA (ed): Pathology of Protozoal and Helminthic Diseases. Baltimore, Williams & Wilkins, 1971, p. 504.
164. Oh SJ: The rate of cerebral involvement in paragonimiasis: an epidemiological study. Jpn J Parasitol 18:211, 1969.
165. Kusner DJ, King CH: Cerebral paragonimiasis. Semin Neurol 13: 201, 1993.
166. Higashi K, Aoki H, Tatebayashi K, et al: Cerebral paragonimiasis. J Neurosurg 34:515, 1971.
167. Udaka F, Okuda B, Okada M, et al: CT findings of cerebral paragonimiasis in the chronic state. Neuroradiology 30:31, 1988.

168. Zhi-Biao X: Studies on clinical manifestations, diagnosis and control of paragonimiasis in China. In Cross JH (ed): Emerging Problems in Food-borne Parasitic Zoonosis: Impact on Agriculture and Public Health. Bangkok, Thai Watana Panich Press, 1991, p. 345.
169. Ch'i-Nan W, Lui J, Ting-Feng C, et al: The clinical manifestations and bithionol therapy of paragonimiasis in Szechuan Province. Chin Med J 83:163, 1964.
170. Wilson RA: Immunity and immunoregulation in helminth infections. Curr Opin Immunol 5:538, 1993.
171. Shin MH: Excretory-secretory product of newly excysted metacercariae of *Paragonimus westermani* directly induces eosinophil apoptosis. Korean J Parasitol 38:17, 2000.
172. Shin MH: Excretory-secretory product of *Paragonimus westermani* newly excysted metacercariae inhibits superoxide production of granulocytes stimulated with IgG. Korean J Parasitol 38:103, 2000.
173. Shin MH, Kita H, Park HY, Seoh JY: Cysteine protease secreted by *Paragonimus westermani* attenuates effector functions of human eosinophils stimulated with immunoglobulin G. Infect Immun 69:1599–1604, 2001.
174. Shin MH, Seoh JY, Park HY, et al: Excretory-secretory products secreted by *Paragonimus westermani* delay the spontaneous cell death of human eosinophils through autocrine production of GM-CSF. Int Arch Allergy Immunol 132:48, 2003.
175. Singh TS, Mutum SS, Razaque MA: Pulmonary paragonimiasis: clinical features, diagnosis and treatment of 39 cases in Manipur. Trans R Soc Trop Med Hyg 80:967, 1986.
176. Miyazadki I, Yokogawa M: Paragonimiasis. In Steele JH (ed): CRC Handbook Series in Zoonoses. Section C: Parasitic Zoonoses, Vol 3. Boca Raton, FL, CRC Press, 1982, p. 123.
177. Yokogawa M: *Paragonimus* and paragonimiasis. In Morishita K, Komiya Y, Matsubayashi H, et al (eds): Progress of Medical Parasitology in Japan. Vol 1. Tokyo, Meguro Parasitological Museum, 1964, p. 63.
178. Harinasuta T, Pungpak S, Keystone JS: Trematode infections: Opisthorchiasis, clonorchiasis, fascioliasis, and paragonimiasis. Infect Dis Clin North Am 7:699, 1993.
179. Sadum EH, Buck AA: Paragonimiasis in South Korea: Immunodiagnosis, epidemiologic, clinical, roentgenographic and therapeutic studies. Am J Trop Med Hyg 9:562, 1960.
180. Waikagul J: Serodiagnosis of paragonimiasis by enzyme-linked immunosorbent assay and immunoelectrophoresis. Southeast Asian J Trop Med Public Health 20:243, 1989.
181. Imai J: Evaluation of ELISA for the diagnosis of paragonimiasis westermani. Trans R Soc Trop Med Hyg 81:3, 1987.
182. Kirobloch J: Application of different paragonimus antigens to immunodiagnosis of human lung fluke infection. Arzneimittelforschung 34:208, 1984.
183. Voller A, Bidwell DE, Bartlett A, et al: A comparison of isotopic and enzyme-immunoassays for tropical parasitic diseases. Trans R Soc Trop Med Hyg 71:431, 1977.
184. Ikeda T, Oikawa Y, Nishiyama T: Enzyme-linked immunosorbent assay using cysteine proteinase antigens for immunodiagnosis of human paragonimiasis. Am J Trop Med Hyg 55:435, 1996.
185. Kong Y, Ito A, Yang HJ, et al: Immunoglobulin G (IgG) subclass and IgE responses in human paragonimiases caused by three different species. Clin Diag Lab Immunol 5:474, 1998.
186. Slemenda SB, Maddison SE, Jong EC, et al: Diagnosis of paragonimiasis by immunoblot. Am J Trop Med Hyg 39:469, 1988.
187. Zhang ZH, Zhang YJ, Shi ZS, et al: Diagnosis of active *Paragonimus westermani* infections with a monoclonal antibody–based antigen detection assay. Am J Trop Med Hyg 49:329, 1993.
188. Zhang Z, Zhang Y, Liu L, et al: Antigen detection assay to monitor the efficacy of praziquantel for the treatment of *Paragonimus westermani* infections. Trans R Soc Trop Med Hyg 90:43, 1996.
189. Udonsi JK: Clinical field trials of praziquantel in pulmonary paragonimiasis due to *Paragonimus uterobilateralis* in endemic populations of Igwun Basin, Nigeria. Trop Med Parasitol 40:65, 1989.
190. Johnson RJ, Jong EC, Dunning SB, et al: Paragonimiasis: Diagnosis and the use of praziquantel in treatment. Rev Infect Dis 7:200, 1985.
191. Calvopiña M, Guderian RH, Paredes W, et al: Treatment of human pulmonary paragonimiasis with triclabendazole: Clinical tolerance and drug efficacy. Trans R Soc Trop Med Hyg 92:566, 1998.
192. Kim JS: Treatment of *Paragonimus westermani* infections with bithionol. Am J Trop Med Hyg 19:940, 1970.
193. Sen-Hai Y, Mott KE: Epidemiology and morbidity of food-borne intestinal trematode infections. Trop Dis Bull 91:R125, 1994.
194. Harinasuta T, Bunnag D, Radomyos P: Intestinal fluke infections. In Pawlowski Z (ed): Bailliere's Clinical Tropical Medicine and Communicable Diseases, Vol 2. London, Bailliere Tindall, 1987, p. 695.
195. Manning GS, Brockelman WY, Viyanant V: An analysis of the prevalence of *Fasciolopsis buski* in central Thailand using catalytic models. Am J Epidemiol 93:353, 1971.
196. Plaut AG, Kampanart-Sanyakorn C, Manning GS: A clinical study of *Fasciolopsis buski* in Thailand. Trans R Soc Trop Med Hyg 63:470, 1969.
197. Rim H-J: Fasciolopsis. In Steele JH (ed): CRC Handbook Series in Zoonoses. Section C: Parasitic Zoonoses, Vol 3. Boca Raton, FL, CRC Press, 1982, p. 89.
198. Sadun EH, Maiphoom C: Studies on the epidemiology of the human intestinal fluke *Fasciolopsis buski* (Lankester) in central Thailand. Am J Trop Med Hyg 2:1070, 1953.
199. Jaroonvisama N, Charoenlarp K, Areekul S: Intestinal absorption studies in *Fasciolopsis buski* infection. Southeast Asian J Trop Med Hyg 17:582, 1986.
200. Chai J-Y, Lee S-H: Food-borne intestinal trematode infections in the Republic of Korea. Parasitol Int 51:129, 2002.
201. Kobayashi A: Changing patterns of parasitic infections in Japan. In Croll NA, Cross JH (eds): Human Ecology and Infectious Disease. New York, Academic Press, 1983, p. 137.
202. Cross JH, Basaca-Sevilla V: Intestinal parasitic infections in Southeast Asia. Southeast Asian J Trop Med Public Health 12:262, 1974.
203. Cho S-Y, Kang S-Y, Lee J-B: Metagonimiasis in Korea. Drug Res 34:1121, 1984.
204. Sheir ZM, Aboul-Enein ME: Demographic, clinical and therapeutic appraisal of heterophyiasis. J Trop Med Hyg 73:148, 1970.
205. Africa CM, Garcia EY, de Leon W: Intestinal heterophyiasis with cardiac involvement. Philipp J Public Health 2:1, 1935.
206. Africa CM, de Leon W, Garcia EY: Heterophyiasis. 5. Ova in the spinal cord of man. Philipp J Sci 62:393, 1937.
207. Tantachamrun T, Kliks M: Heterophyid infection in human ileum: Report of three cases. Southeast Asian J Trop Med Public Health 9:228, 1978.
208. Velasquez CC: Paragonimiasis. In Steele JH (ed): CRC Handbook Series in Zoonoses. Section C: Parasitic Zoonoses, Vol 3. Boca Raton, FL CRC Press, 1982, p. 99.
209. Yamashita J: Echinostome. In Morishita K, Komiya Y, Matsubayashi H, et al (eds): Progress of Medical Parasitology in Japan, Vol 1. Tokyo, Meguro Parasitological Museum, 1964, p. 289.
210. Radomyos P, Bunnag D, Harinasuta T: *Echinostoma ilocanum* (Garrison, 1908) Odhner, 1911, infection in man in Thailand. Southeast Asian J Trop Med Public Health 13:265–269, 1982.
211. Sornmani S: Echinostomiasis in Thailand: A review. In Schistosomiasis and Other Snail Transmitted Helminthiasis: Proceedings of the Fourth Southeast Asian Seminar on Parasitology and Tropical Medicine, Seameo Tropmed Project, 1969. Southeast Asian J Trop Med Public Health 1:171, 1969.
212. Lin JX, Chen YZ, Liang CZ, et al: Epidemiological investigation and experimental infection of *Echinochasmus japonicus*. Chi Sheng Chung Hsueh Yu Chi Sheng Chung Ping Tsa Chi 3:89, 1985.
213. Huffman JE, Fried B: *Echinostoma* and echinostomiasis. Adv Parasitol 29:215, 1990.
214. Millemann RE, Knapp SE: Biology of *Nanophyetus salmincola* and "salmon poisoning" disease. Adv Parasitol 8:1, 1970.
215. Eastburn RL, Fritsche TR, Terhune CA: Human intestinal infection with *Nanophyetus salmincola* from salmonid fishes. Am J Trop Med Hyg 36:586, 1987.
216. Bunnag D, Radomyos P, Harinasuta T: Field trial on the treatment of fasciolopsiasis with praziquantel. Southeast Asian J Trop Med Public Health 14:216, 1983.
217. Pungpak S, Bunnag D, Harinasuta T: Albendazole in the treatment of opisthorchiasis and concomitant intestinal helminthic infections. Southeast Asian J Trop Med Hyg 15:44, 1984.
218. Rim H-J, Farag HF, Sornmani S, et al: Foodborne trematodes: Ignored or emerging? Parasitol Today 10:207, 1994.
219. Loaharanu P, Murrell D: A role for irradiation in the control of foodborne parasites. Trends Food Sci Technol 5:190, 1994.
220. Jongsuksuntigul P, Imsomboon T: The impact of a decade-long opisthorchiasis control program in northeastern Thailand. Southeast Asian J Trop Med Public Health 28:551, 1997.

118

Arthropods, Tongue Worms, Leeches, and Arthropod-borne Diseases

JEROME GODDARD

INTRODUCTION

Arthropods (phylum Arthropoda), characterized by a chitinous exoskeleton, segmented bodies, and jointed appendages, may negatively affect human health in a number of ways. There may be direct effects, such as bites and stings; indirect effects, such as disease transmission; and perceived effects, such as entomophobia or delusions of parasitosis (see Chapter 135). Only a small percentage of all arthropod species are medically important, most being benign in their association with humans. An even smaller percentage are true human parasites—a few mite and lice species. However, especially in tropical regions, many human illnesses are either caused by or transmitted by arthropods.

Nothing better exemplifies the dynamic nature of the natural world than do the diseases transmitted by insects and other arthropods—the vector-borne diseases. For example, malaria, once on the decline, now affects hundreds of millions of people annually. In fact, the malaria situation is worsening due to development of insecticide resistance in mosquitoes and drug resistance in parasites. Dengue fever is expanding geographically and inflicts pain and suffering on millions of people annually (see Chapter 72). There are even new or emerging vector-borne diseases. Lyme disease was virtually unknown 30 years ago but now occurs at the rate of about 20,000 reported cases per year in the United States alone. Human tick-borne ehrlichiosis in the United States was first reported in 1986. There have been at least 1000 cases since then. Recent evidence indicates that there may be several *Ehrlichia* and tick species involved in this disease.

To understand and control outbreaks of these diseases requires knowledge of ecology and medical entomology not commonly encountered in today's world of molecular biology and medical specialization. This chapter provides classic medical entomology information in a brief, but readily accessible form.

PARASITIC ARTHROPODS

Although most bloodsucking arthropods (e.g., mosquitoes, ticks) could be considered "parasites" since they derive nourishment at the expense of other organisms, in this discussion the term *parasitic arthropods* is limited to human parasites that live most of their lives on or in the host. Lines of demarcation are not clear, but the parasites chosen to be included here are the human lice, a couple of skin-inhabiting mites, and a few flesh-dwelling fly larvae.

Lice

Two species of sucking lice (insect order Phthiraptera, previously known as Anoplura) are parasites of humans—head and body lice both being varieties of one species, *Pediculus humanus,* and pubic lice, *Phthirus pubis* (Figs. 118-1 and 118-2). Neither head nor pubic lice are involved in disease transmission, but body lice may carry the agents of epidemic typhus, trench fever, and louse-borne relapsing fever.[1] Body and head lice look almost identical, but head lice remain more or less on the scalp and body lice on the body or in clothing. Head and body lice are tiny (1 to 4 mm long), elongated, soft-bodied, light-colored, wingless insects with gradual metamorphosis—that is, the young look like the adults, only smaller. They are dorsoventrally flattened (top to bottom, as opposed to fleas, which are flattened side to side), with an angular ovoid head, and a nine-segment abdomen. The head bears a pair of simple lateral eyes and a pair of short five-segment antennae. Head lice live on the skin among the hairs of the patient's head. Eggs (nits) are laid at the base of shafts of hair. Body lice live primarily in the clothing of infested persons, but move to the body occasionally for a blood meal.

Head lice are transmitted among humans by close contact such as hugging or sharing of personal items such as hats, scarfs, or combs. Body lice are transmitted also by close contact, but more so by sharing infested clothing. Since neither head nor body lice usually survive more than 24 to 48 hours off their hosts, pesticidal fogging or spraying of entire homes and schools is not indicated. Pediculicidal lotions or shampoos, combined with washing of garments and bedding, will usually eliminate the infestation.

Pubic lice (crab lice) occur almost exclusively in the pubic or perianal areas, rarely on eyelashes, eyebrows, or other coarse-haired areas. They are not as active as head or body lice, being attached more often to the skin. Thus, pubic lice may often be confused with nymphal (immature) ticks. Pubic lice generally cannot survive more than 24 to 48 hours off their human hosts and therefore do not inhabit rugs, carpets, pets, or bathrooms. Although it is theoretically possible to obtain the infestation from inanimate objects such as toilet seats, most transmission occurs from sexual contact. In fact, pediculosis pubis is rightly categorized as a sexually transmitted disease (see Chapter 132). One study reported that

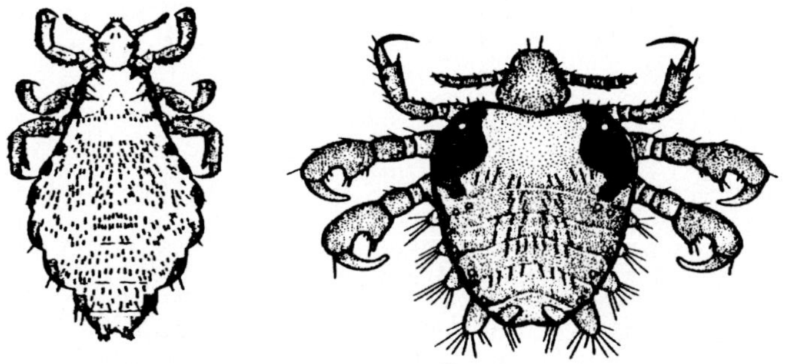

FIGURE 118-1 Head louse (*left*) and pubic louse (*right*). (From U.S. Department of Health, Education, and Welfare, Public Health Service, Centers for Disease Control and Prevention, pictorial keys.)

one-third of patients with pubic lice may have other sexually transmitted diseases.[2] Treatment involves pediculicidal lotions and shampoos for the patient, as well as all family members and sexual contacts of the patient.[3]

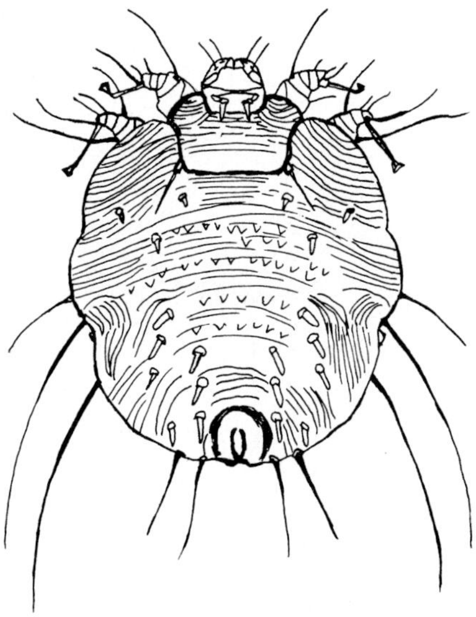

FIGURE 118-3 Scabies mite.

Mites

Scabies mites (acarine order Astigmata), *Sarcoptes scabiei*, infest human skin causing intense itching and sometimes a generalized rash. Scabies occurs worldwide, affecting all races and socioeconomic classes. The mites are very tiny (0.2 to 0.4 mm long), oval, saclike, eyeless specimens with rudimentary legs (Fig. 118-3). Scabies mites are transmitted by close human-to-human contact with infested persons. The mites burrow under the skin, leaving tiny open sores and linear serpiginous burrows (tracts) that contain the mites and their eggs. Sensitization is the cause of the itching, erythema, and rash.

Scabies should be confirmed by finding the mites in a skin scraping, since other forms of dermatitis may resemble scabies. Finding the mites is often not as easy as it seems and an experienced dermatologist may be needed. Treatment involves scabicidal creams or lotions applied per package instructions. Some commonly used products today are lindane (Kwell), permethrin (Elimite), and crotamiton (Eurax).[1] For crusted or Norwegian scabies developing in immunocompromised patients (see Chapter 133), therapy is with a single dose of ivermectin given at 200 μg/kg orally and repeated after 2 weeks, if needed.[4] Ivermectin may have specific utility in treating scabies in institutional or community outbreaks.[3,5] Since the mites cannot live off a human host for more than 24 hours or so, pesticidal treatment of rooms, schools, and so on is unnecessary.

Dog or horse scabies is also caused by races of *S. scabiei*, but these mites cannot complete their life cycle in human skin. Humans can acquire dog scabies, causing itching and papular or vesicular lesions, primarily on the waist, chest, or forearms. However, removal or treatment of the source of infestation (i.e., infested dog or horse) will lead to gradual resolution of the human case.

Follicle mites (acarine order Prostigmata) are minute, wormlike mites that infest humans. Two species may be found. *Demodex folliculorum* lives in the hair follicles and *Demodex brevis* in the sebaceous glands. Although some researchers have attributed various pathologic conditions to *Demodex* infestation, the mite is basically a harmless saprophyte. The mites are approximately 0.1 to 0.4 mm long, have vestigial legs, and transverse striations over much of the body. They most commonly occur on the forehead, the malar areas of the cheeks, the nose, and the nasolabial fold, but may occur anywhere on the face or around the ears. Most people acquire *Demodex* from maternal contacts in early childhood.

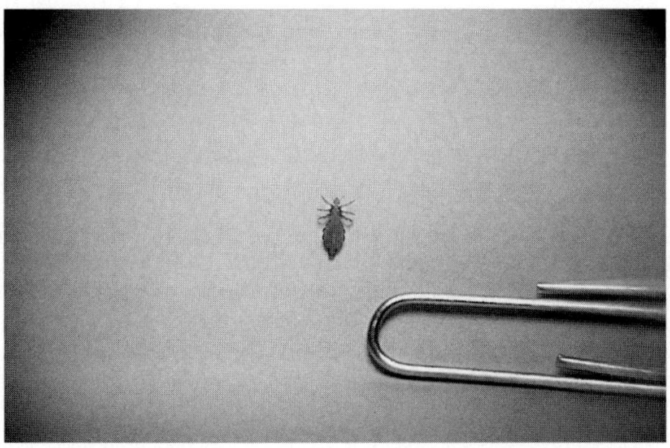

FIGURE 118-2 Body louse next to paper clip.

Parasitic Fly Larvae

Myiasis is the infestation of human or animal tissues by fly larvae (insect order Diptera). It may be accidental (e.g., eating eggs or larvae), facultative (e.g., eggs laid on malodorous or festering wounds), or obligate (e.g., necessary for fly development—true parasitism).[6] Accidental myiasis is mostly a benign event, but the larvae could possibly survive temporarily, causing stomach pains, nausea, or vomiting. Facultative myiasis may result in considerable pain and tissue damage as fly larvae leave necrotic tissues and invade healthy tissues. Obligate myiasis can be serious or even fatal, as fly larvae feed in healthy tissues.

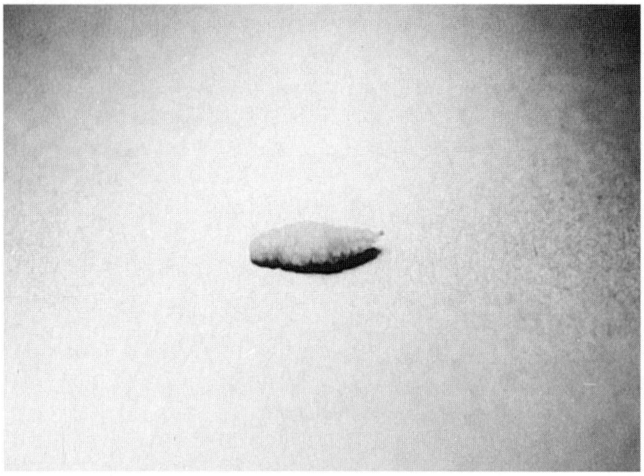

FIGURE 118-4 Syrphid fly larva involved in a case of urinary myiasis. (From Goddard J: Direct injury from arthropods. Lab Med 25:365–371, 1994. Copyright © American Society of Clinical Pathologists.)

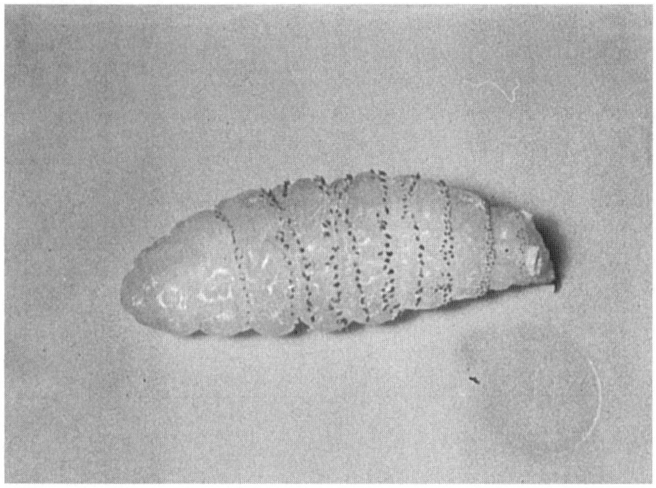

FIGURE 118-6 Third-stage *Dermatobia hominis* larva. (Courtesy of Dr. Tom Brooks.)

Species Involved in Facultative Myiasis

Numerous species of house flies (Muscidae), blow flies (Calliphoridae), and flesh flies (Sarcophagidae)—all in the insect order Diptera—have been implicated in facultative myiasis (Fig. 118-4). Some notorious offenders are the blow fly, *Phaenicia sericata,* the rat-tailed maggot, *Eristalis tenax,* the black blow fly, *Phormia regina,* and the house fly, *Musca domestica.*[7] In addition, the latrine fly, *Fannia scalaris,* has often been associated with urinary or rectal myiasis.

Species Involved in Obligate Myiasis

The human bot fly, *Dermatobia hominis,* is a parasite of humans, cattle, swine, cats, dogs, horses, sheep, and other mammals and a few birds in Mexico and Central and South America. The larvae feed under the skin, causing often episodically painful, swollen, draining cutaneous lesions with a typical air-pore. Although this parasite does not occur in the United States, numerous cases are seen by U.S. physicians as a result of people returning from cruises or vacations to endemic areas (see Chapter 126).

The adult fly (about 15 mm long) resembles a large bluish blow fly (Fig. 118-5). It has a yellowish or brown head and legs. Adult bot flies catch various bloodsucking flies (often a mosquito) and attach eggs to their sides. The carrier flies subsequently feed on a human, cow, or other host at which time the newly hatched bot fly larvae penetrate the host skin. The larvae vary in appearance depending upon stage of development (Figs. 118-5 and 118-6), usually do not move laterally within the skin, and may feed for 4 to 10 weeks. When mature, larvae exit the lesion, drop to the soil, and pupate. Treatment involves direct removal of the maggots (by excision or otherwise) and antibiotics to prevent or control secondary infection.

Screwworm flies are also obligate parasites of living flesh, feeding for the entire larval period inside a host. Natural hosts include domestic and wild mammals, as well as humans. Human infestations have resulted from the flies ovipositing on or near a wound, or sometimes inside the nostril while a person sleeps in the daytime. Upon hatching, the larvae begin feeding, causing extensive tissue destruction. There is an Old World species, *Chrysomyia bezziana,* a species of tropical Africa and Asia, and a New World species, *Cochliomyia hominivorax,* which at one time was distributed from the southern United States to southern Brazil (Fig. 118-7). Fortunately, due to a sterile male release program, the New World species no longer occurs in the United States. Treatment of screwworm myiasis involves removal of the larvae. Surgery may be

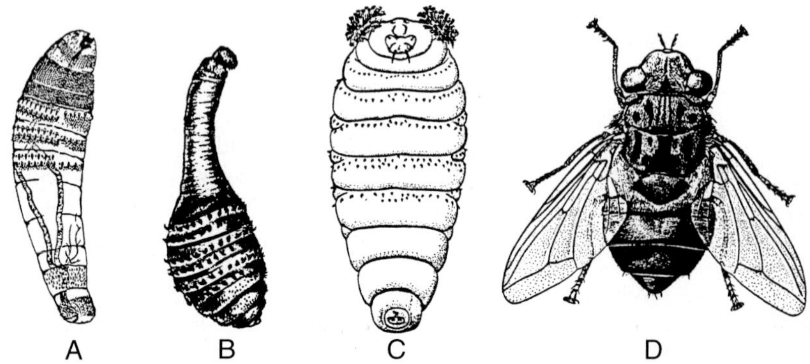

FIGURE 118-5 Human bot fly. *A,* First-stage larva. *B,* Second-stage larva. *C,* Third-stage larva. *D,* Adult fly. (From U.S. Department of Agriculture, Miscellaneous Publication No. 631.)

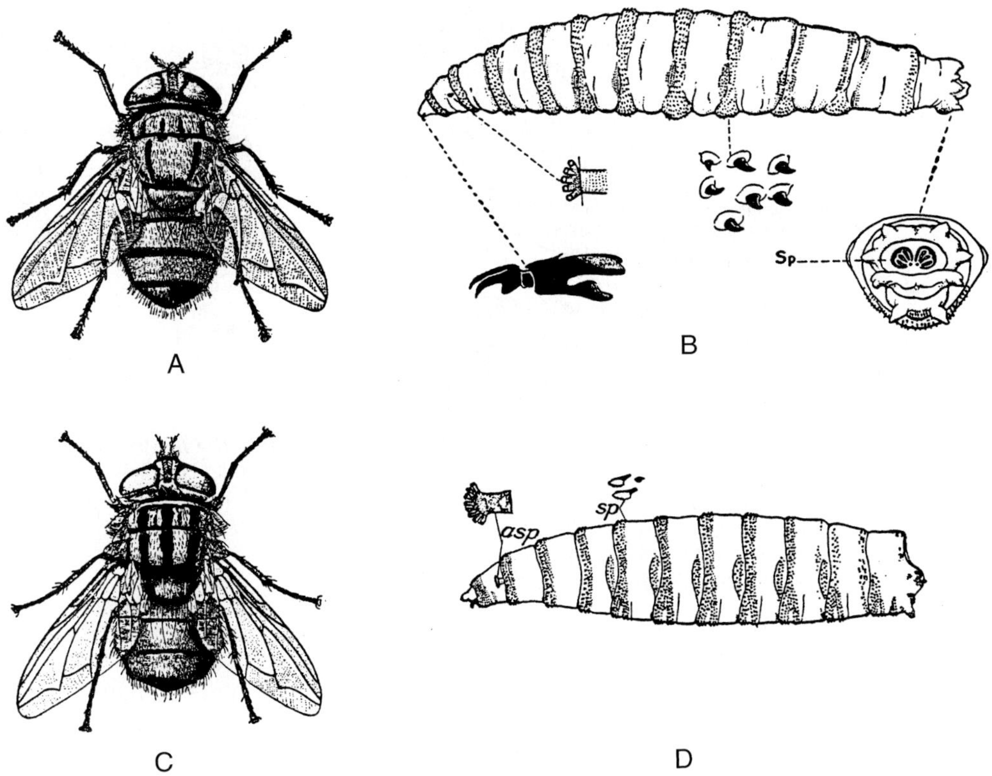

FIGURE 118-7 Screwworm flies. *A,* Adult female *Chrysomya bezziana. B,* Larva of *C. bezziana. C,* Adult female *Cochliomyia hominivorax. D,* Larva of *C. hominivorax.* (From U.S. Department of Agriculture, Miscellaneous Publication No. 631.)

required if larvae cannot be removed via natural orifices. Since eggs are laid in batches, there could be tens or even hundreds of maggots in a wound.

The Tumbu fly, *Cordylobia anthropophaga,* is a major cause of cutaneous myiasis in tropical Africa. The larvae burrow into subcutaneous tissues creating a boil-like lesion with a serous exudate. Children are most commonly affected, with lesions occurring on areas of the body covered with clothing since the flies oviposit on soiled clothing. The adult fly has a yellow-brown body and is about 6 to 12 mm long. Full-grown larvae are 13 to 15 mm long. The larvae exit their furuncular lesions after about 8 to 10 days. Treatment involves direct removal of the maggots, surgically if necessary, and treatment to prevent or control secondary infection. *Wohlfahrtia magnifica,* one of the sarcophagid flies, is an obligate parasite in the wounds and natural orifices of mammals, including humans. It occurs over the warmer parts of Europe, Asia, northern Africa, the Middle East, and the Mediterranean region. *Wohlfahrtia* behavior is similar to that of a screwworm fly, in that it oviposits—actually depositing larvae instead of eggs—on tiny skin lesions such as scratches, tick bites, and such or mucous membranes. The developing larvae feed for 5 to 7 days, exit the host, fall to the ground, and pupate. *Wohlfahrtia* flies look similar to flesh flies (Sarcophagidae), but instead of a checkerboard patten on the abdomen they have round spots. *W. magnifica* occurs over the warmer parts of Europe, Asia, northern Africa, the Middle East, and the Mediterranean region.

W. magnifica infestations are difficult to treat because of the (usually) numerous aggressively feeding larvae within the nose or existing wounds. Irrigation or possible surgical exploration to remove the larvae is needed.

INJURIOUS ARTHROPODS

Stinging Arthropods

The insect order Hymenoptera contains ants, wasps, and bees.[8] Most stinging wasps and some bees are solitary or subsocial insects; they primarily use their stings to subdue prey. Rarely does this offensive use of stinging and venom lead to human envenomization. These venoms do not cause much pain or swelling. Social wasps, bees, and ants, however, sting for defensive purposes, and their venom causes intense pain. Workers of these groups instinctively defend their nests and readily sting intruders coming too close to their nests. Social hymenopterans include yellow jackets, honeybees, paper wasps, and fire ants (Figs. 118-8 and 118-9). All stings generally cause pain, itching, wheal, flare, and other symptoms, which resolve in a couple of hours unless there are enough stings (several hundred) to produce a direct toxic reaction. Allergic systemic reactions include cutaneous manifestations (e.g., urticaria, angioedema), bronchospasm, edema of the upper airway, and hypotensive shock, and range from mild to life-threatening.[9] Even if a person is not allergic to the venom, toxic effects from hundreds of stings can occur, including histamine release (nonallergic), contraction of smooth muscle, increase in capillary permeability, vasodilation with accompanying drop in blood pressure, and hemolysis.[10]

Some caterpillars can sting. Both mechanical irritation and injection of venom by the caterpillar spines or hairs contribute to the urticarial response in humans. Upon exposure, these structures may be broken, allowing venom to either be injected into the skin or to ooze out onto abraded skin. I reported observations from a caterpillar sting case that included erythema, small papules, throbbing pain, and axillary

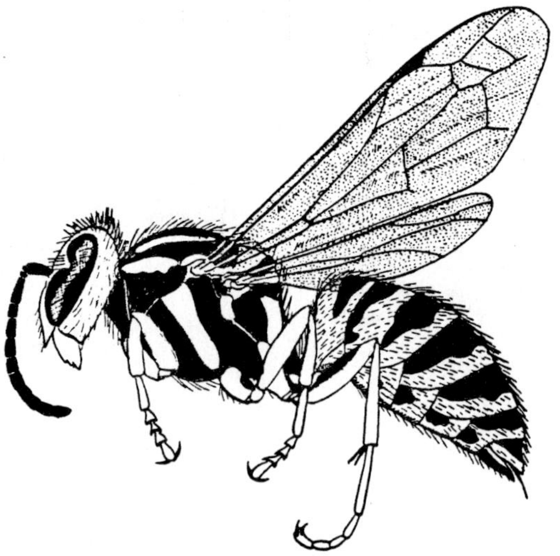

FIGURE 118-8 Typical stinging insect (yellow jacket). (From U.S. Department of Health, Education, and Welfare, Public Health Service, Centers for Disease Control and Prevention, pictorial keys.)

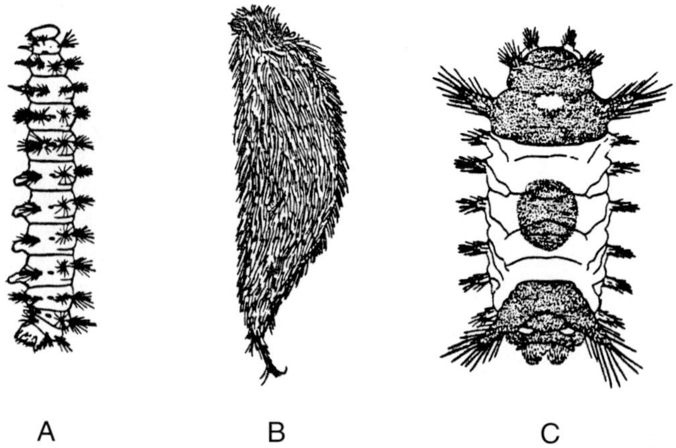

FIGURE 118-10 Some stinging caterpillars. *A*, Lo moth. *B*, Puss caterpillar. *C*, Saddleback caterpillar. (Adapted from U.S. Department of Health, Education, and Welfare, Public Health Service, Centers for Disease Control and Prevention, pictorial keys.)

pain resulting from venom travel to local lymph nodes.[11] Allergic reactions from caterpillars may occur just like those from other stinging arthropods.[12]

Urticating caterpillars include the Io moth, *Automeris io;* the brown-tail moth, *Euproctis chrysorrhoea;* the buck moth, *Hemileuca maia;* the puss caterpillar, *Megalopyge opercularis;* the saddleback caterpillar, *Sibine stimulea,* and many others (Fig. 118-10). Treatment may include ice packs and oral administration of antihistamines to relieve the itching and burning sensation. Acute urticarial lesions may be relieved by application of topical corticosteroids. For severe pain associated with stings, meperidine HCl, morphine, or codeine is sometimes used. Systemic allergic reactions such as hypotension and bronchospasm are usually treated with epinephrine, antihistamines, and other supportive measures.

Scorpions (arachnid order Scorpiones) are eight-legged, generally flattened arthropods with two apparent body regions—a broad seven-segment mesosoma and a narrow five-segment metasoma terminating in a sting (Fig. 118-11). Many scorpions pose no serious health hazard, but several species have venom sufficiently toxic to kill a human (outright, not an allergic reaction). Systemic effects from such stings include drowsiness, spreading partial paralysis, muscle twitching, profuse salivation, perspiration, hypertension, tachycardia, and convulsions. In the United States, the only dangerous species, with the exception of allergic reactions to the venom, is *Centruroides exilicauda* (formerly *C. sculpturatus*) of the southwestern United States, especially Arizona. The fat-tailed

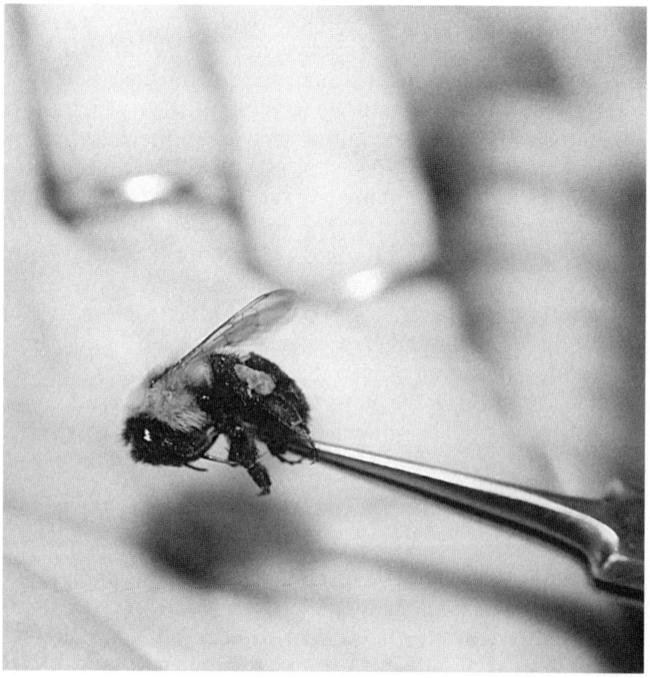

FIGURE 118-9 Bumblebee.

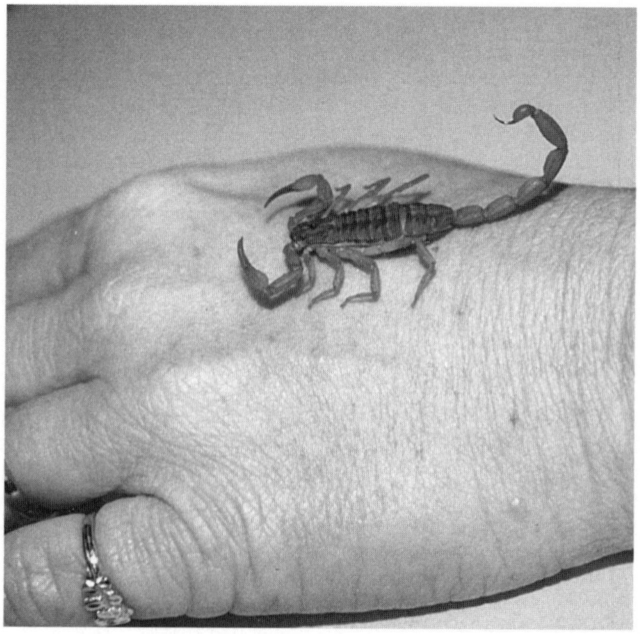

FIGURE 118-11 Typical scorpion.

scorpion, *Androctonus australis,* is a notoriously dangerous scorpion of northern Africa and the Middle East. *Buthus occitanus* is a widely distributed, dangerous scorpion composed of several subspecies that is found in southern France, Spain, Italy, Greece, several Mediterranean islands, Israel, Jordan, and northern Africa. Treatment of scorpion stings is somewhat controversial.[13] For the dangerous species, some advocate prompt use of antivenin. Others take a wait-and-see approach since many scorpion sting cases resolve on their own in a few hours. Severe cases usually occur in children and are characterized by agitation and other systemic symptoms. Hospitalization for close monitoring and supportive care is required in such cases.

Allergic Reactions to Insect Stings

Some people develop hypersensitivity to arthropod venoms; allergic reactions to stings can be roughly grouped into two categories—large local and systemic reactions.[9] Large local reactions are characterized by painful, pruritic swelling of at least 5 cm in diameter and may involve an entire extremity. However, there are no systemic symptoms far removed from the sting site. Usually only about 5% of those people who experience large local reactions will develop anaphylaxis upon future stinging events. Systemic reactions produce symptoms in areas other than the sting site. These are serious clinical manifestations characterized by urticaria, angioedema, respiratory difficulty, gastrointestinal distress, and hypotension. Sometimes a severe allergic reaction results in anaphylactic shock within 15 to 30 minutes. Persons who experience a generalized allergic reaction (even mild) may be at risk of a severe reaction and possible death upon the next sting, days, weeks, or months later. For this reason, persons who have any type of large local or systemic reaction to a sting (or bite, for that matter) should see an allergist for possible immunotherapy and prescription of autoinjectable epinephrine.[9]

Biting Arthropods

The bed bug (insect order Hemiptera), *Cimex lectularius,* is a bloodsucking human pest that causes itching and inflammation from its bites (Fig. 118-12). Bed bugs have occasionally been found that are naturally infected with disease organisms such as those causing anthrax, plague, and typhus. However, they are not considered vectors of these disease agents.[14] Adult bugs are oval-shaped (approximately 5 mm long), flattened insects that somewhat resemble immature cockroaches. They are reddish-brown in color; the immature bed bugs are yellowish-white. Bed bugs are found in temperate regions worldwide. A related species, *Cimex hemipterous,* occurs in the tropics. The bugs hide in cracks and crevices during the day, usually on or near the host's bed, and feed at night, taking blood from their host for 5 to 10 minutes. Bites from bed bugs are generally self-limited and require little specific treatment other than antiseptic or antibiotic creams or lotions to prevent infection.

Horse flies and deer flies (insect order Diptera) are notorious pests of horses, cattle, deer, dogs, and humans. They have scissors-like mouthparts and can inflict painful bites. Although no human illnesses have been associated with horse flies, deer flies can transmit the agents of tularemia and loiasis in Africa (see Chapter 99).[6]

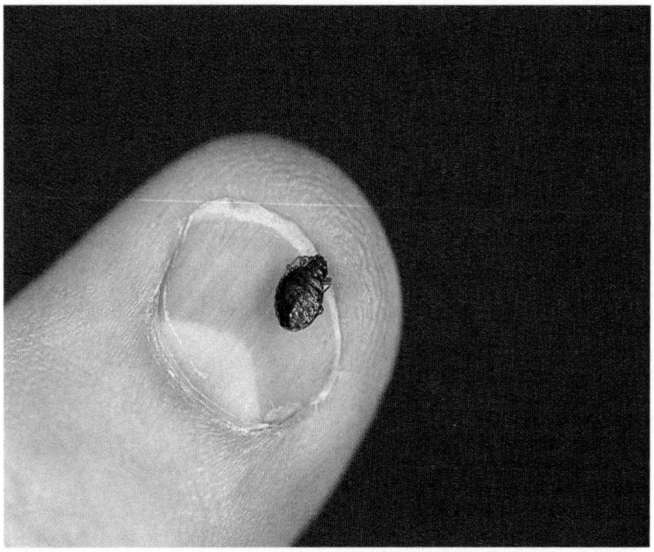

FIGURE 118-12 Bed bug. (Copyright © 2002 by Jerome Goddard, PhD, Mississippi Department of Health, Jackson, MS.)

Horse flies look like giant, robust house flies (15 to 25 mm long) with large prominent eyes (Figs. 118-13 and 118-14). Deer flies, also in the family Tabanidae, are much smaller (8 to 15 mm long) and have dark patterned wings. Many deer fly species have a gray or yellow-gray body with various arrangements of spots on the abdomen. Numerous species of both groups occur almost worldwide, where they breed in moist or semiaquatic sites such as margins of ponds, damp earth, or other sites containing mud and water. The wormlike larvae spend their entire developmental time in these muddy habitats. Adult females seek a blood meal, whereas males may feed on flower nectar. Except for secondary infections, requiring appropriate antibiotics, horse fly and deer fly bites are generally few and self-limited. Biting midges (insect order Diptera) are extremely small, delicate flies that bite people, especially near coastal areas. They are also sometimes referred to as "no-see-ums," "punkies," or "biting gnats." The midges are so small that people often remark, "something is biting me, but I can't see what it is." Other than the severe biting nuisance,

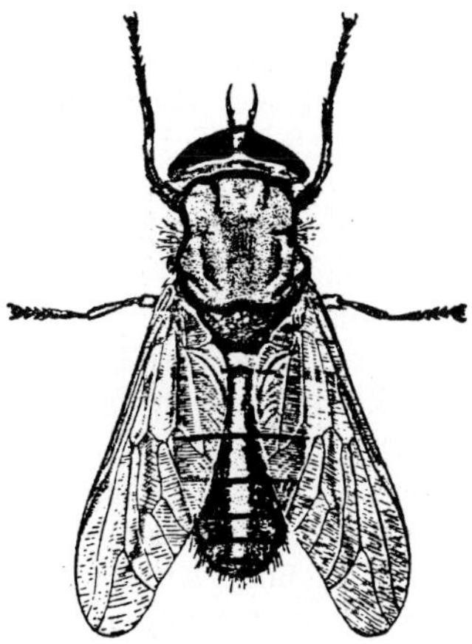

FIGURE 118-13 Adult horse fly. (From Yearbook of Agriculture, Washington, DC, U.S. Dept of Agriculture, 1952.)

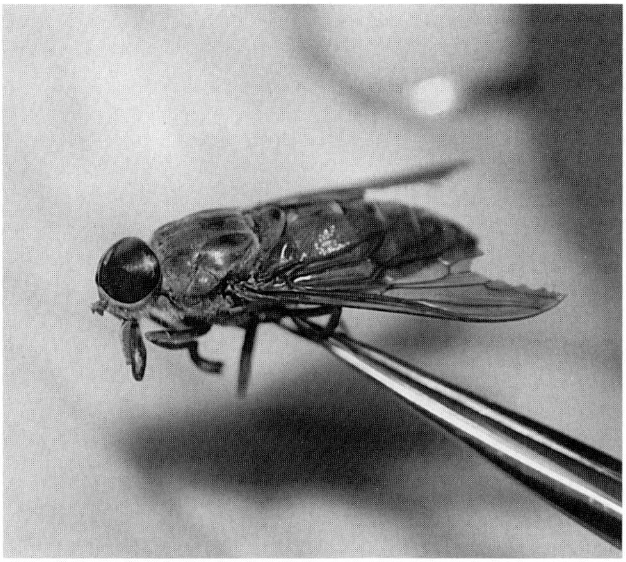

FIGURE 118-14 Horse fly.

biting midges are generally of no medical significance to humans. Numerous species of biting midges occur in temperate and tropical areas over much of the world. A notorious pest, *Culicoides furens,* is a vicious biter, occurring near salt marshes along the Atlantic, Pacific, and Gulf Coasts. In California, *Leptoconops torrens* and *Leptoconops carteri* are very bothersome. Biting midges are usually gray in color and extremely small (0.6 to 1.5 mm). They may have clear or hairy wings which fold scissors-like over the abdomen at rest. Larval stages of biting midges develop in organic detritus along the bottom of shallow areas of water or in water-saturated soil. Adults are generally active only in the warmer months of the year. Simple antipruritics are generally the only treatment needed for biting midge bites. Avoidance of midge-infested areas at or near dark (e.g., salt marshes), and repellents containing DEET are the best course of action for those affected by biting midges.[15,16]

Numerous species of spiders (arachnid order Araneae) bite people, but the hobo spiders, violin spiders, and widow spiders may be a significant medical threat.[1,17] Violin spiders have a necrotic venom affecting cutaneous tissues. The brown recluse spider, *Loxosceles reclusa,* is perhaps the most important member of the group, although other violin spiders producing necrotic lesions also occur in the United States and elsewhere. Brown recluse spider bites are usually localized, sometimes producing considerable necrosis that may result in an unsightly scar (Figs. 118-15 and 118-16). The bite may be painless at first, but becomes very painful within 8 hours. Healing may require several months. Systemic reactions to brown recluse spider bites may occur, including hematuria, anemia, rash, fever, coma, and cyanosis. Death may occur but is rare. The adult spider is tan to dark brown with a 2- to 4-cm leg span (Fig. 118-17). Six eyes, arranged in a semicircle of three pairs, are on top of the head and a characteristic violin-shaped marking (base forward) extends from the eyes to the beginning of the abdomen. The brown recluse spider may be found from Minnesota to Maine, south to Florida, and west to Arizona and Wyoming. It is most common in the south-central United States. The spider is frequently found indoors in bathrooms, bedrooms, cellars, attics, cardboard boxes, and storage areas. Outdoors, it may occur in sheds or barns and in piles of rocks or firewood. Treatment of brown recluse spider bites is symptomatic and quite controversial. Current therapies include ice, antibiotics, and the leukocyte inhibitor dapsone.[1,18–20] Controlled studies are lacking and dapsone may produce hemolysis, so it should be used under careful supervision.

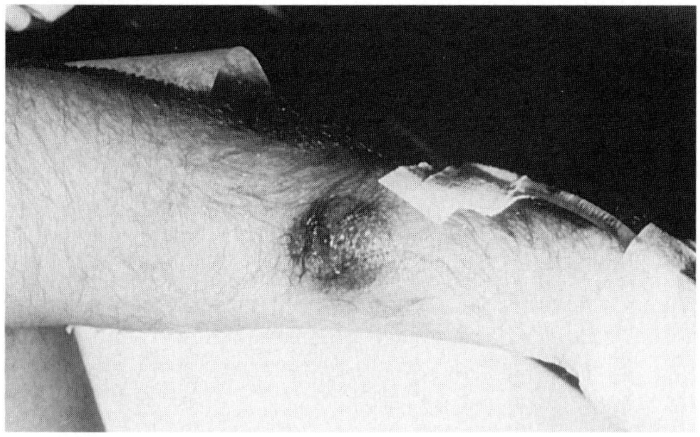

FIGURE 118-15 Brown recluse spider bite in early stages of necrosis. (From Goddard J: Physician's Guide to Arthropods of Medical Importance, 4th ed. Boca Raton, FL, CRC Press, 2002.)

Widow spiders, in contrast to violin spiders, have a neurotoxic venom that produces systemic pain, weakness, tremor, muscle spasm, and tightness in the chest. Often patients exhibit a rigid, boardlike abdomen. There is rarely a significant lesion at the bite site. Paralysis, stupor, and convulsions may occur in severe cases, with an occasional fatality. Several widow spiders occur in North America—all with similar appearance. *Latrodectus mactans* is the species most generally associated with the name "black widow spider" and the female has a red

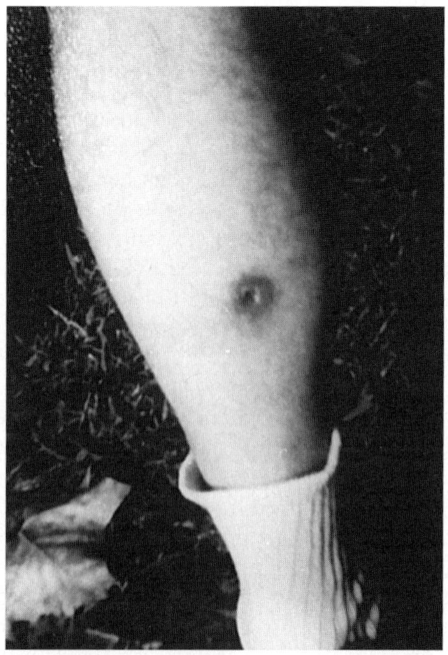

FIGURE 118-16 Brown recluse spider bite approximately 3 months post bite. (From Jarratt JH, Gaydon DG, and Goddard J, Mississippi Cooperative Extension Service, Publication No. 2154, Mississippi State, MS.)

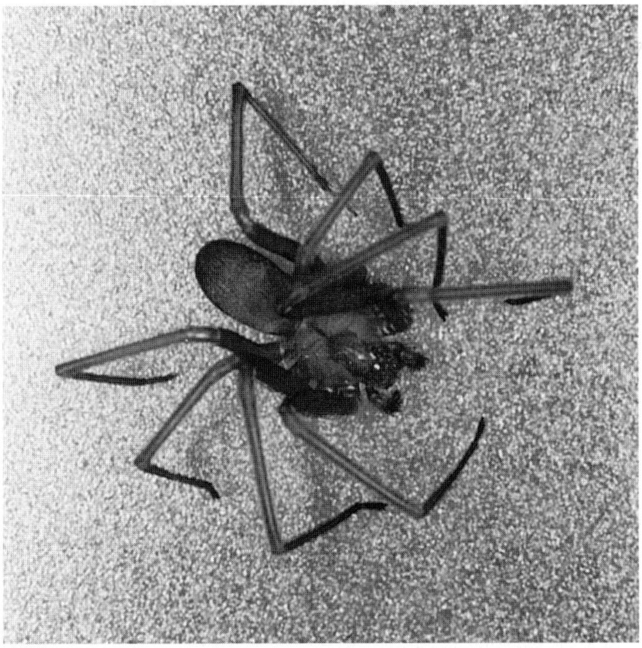

FIGURE 118-17 Adult brown recluse spider. (Courtesy of Dr. James Jarratt, Mississippi Cooperative Extension Service, Mississippi State, MS.)

or orange hourglass-shaped marking on the underside of the abdomen (Fig. 118-18). There is considerable variation in these red markings, with some species having red dots or hash marks on the top and bottom of the abdomen. Widow spiders are found in protected places such as water or gas meter housings and piles of rocks, boards, bricks, or firewood. Inside, they are often found in garage corners; dark, undisturbed cabinets; or underneath appliances. Treatment of *Latrodectus* envenomization includes application of ice, symptomatic treatment of muscle spasms and pain, and (possibly) antivenin in severe cases. Children, the elderly, and persons with other medical conditions of risk may need hospitalization and close monitoring.

Centipedes (arthropod class Chilopoda), sometimes called "hundred-leggers," are long multisegmented arthropods with one pair of legs per body segment (Fig. 118-19). They are flattened, fast-moving creatures that can inflict a painful bite. Bites are generally harmless, but often produce two red and swollen puncture wounds. Rarely, systemic symptoms such as anxiety, vomiting, irregular pulse, dizziness, and headache may occur. Most of the smaller centipede species are harmless, but larger species (especially in the genus *Scolopendra*) in the southern United States and tropics can inflict a painful bite. Treatment includes washing the bite site with soap and water, application of ice, and analgesics for pain.

Numerous mite species (arachnid subclass Acarina), while not parasitic on humans, will bite, causing itch or dermatitis (Fig. 118-20). Examples are the bird and rat mites, which will bite if in close proximity to people. People may also be bitten as a result of occupational exposure to products containing chicken mites, straw mites, or grain mites. The tropical rat mite, *Ornithonyssus bacoti,* is an ectoparasite of rats that is widely distributed on most continents. The tropical fowl mite, *Ornithonyssus bursa,* is similar in habits to the tropical rat mite, except it is found on domestic and wild birds. One of the most common mites causing human dermatitis in poultry houses, farms, ranches, and markets where chickens are sold is the chicken mite, *Dermanyssus gallinae.* The chicken mite occurs worldwide and may also infest English sparrows, starlings, and other birds. Straw itch mites, *Pyemotes tritici,* will bite people as they come into contact with infested straw, hay, grasses, oats, or peas. The grain and flour mites (several species) may cause grocer's itch, copra itch (coconuts), and other itches. Grain and flour mites occur worldwide. Treatment of mite bites primarily involves alleviation of symptoms, and avoidance or eradication of the mites. Since none of these mite species take up permanent residence on human

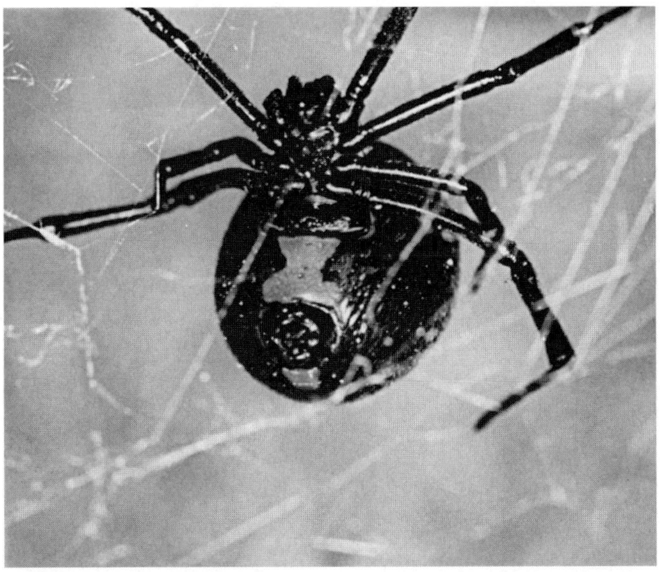

FIGURE 118-18 Female black widow spider underside showing hourglass-shaped marking. (Courtesy of Dr. James Jarratt, Mississippi Cooperative Extension Service, Mississippi State, MS.)

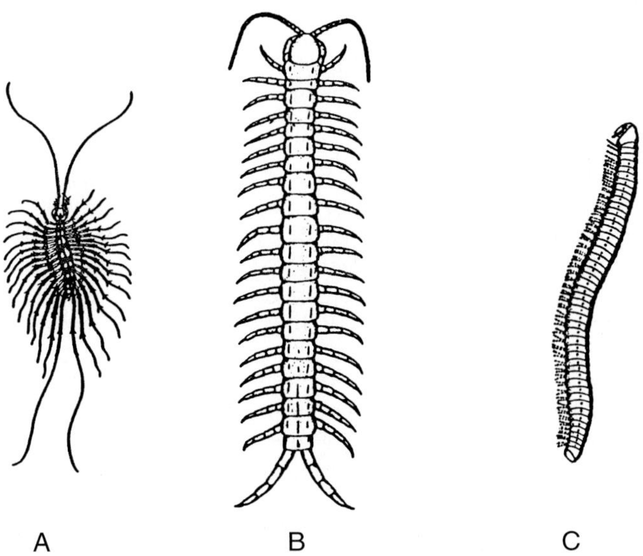

FIGURE 118-19 Centipedes and millipede. *A,* House centipede. *B,* Large southwestern United States centipede. *C,* Millipede. (From U.S. Department of Health, Education, and Welfare, Public Health Service, Centers for Disease Control and Prevention, pictorial keys.)

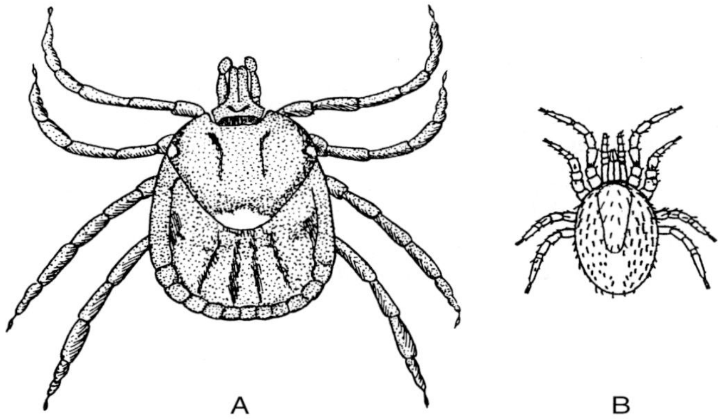

FIGURE 118-20 *A*, Tick. *B*, Mite. (From U.S. Department of Health, Education, and Welfare, Public Health Service, Centers for Disease Control and Prevention, pictorial keys.)

skin, elimination of the source of mite exposure should be the main objective. Competent pest control operators (exterminators) are often helpful in finding and eliminating bird's nests or rat's burrows in and around the home.

Chigger mites (acarine order Prostigmata), also sometimes called "harvest mites" or "red bugs," although not truly parasitic on humans, are actually the six-legged larval stage of trombiculid mites. The adults do not bite. Chiggers cause intense itching and irritation, and some species are involved in the transmission of the scrub typhus rickettsia (see Chapter 52) in the Far East.[1] Chigger larvae are very tiny (0.2 mm long), round mites with numerous setae. Although barely visible to the human eye, they look orangish or reddish when placed on a white background. Numerous chigger species occur in various parts of the world, where they utilize a wide range of vertebrate hosts. They reach their hosts by crawling up on blades of grass or leaves. On humans, they generally crawl into and attach to where clothing fits snugly or where flesh is tender. They do not actually bite, but insert their mouthparts at a pore or base of a hair follicle where they feed for a couple of days. The feeding process is irritating and produces erythematous itchy patches on affected areas of skin. Treatment often includes an antiseptic, hydrocortisone, anesthetic (benzocaine) solutions, or ointments to minimize itching and reduce the possibility of secondary infection.

Other Forms of Injury

Blister beetles (insect order Coleoptera) may cause blistering on human skin when touched or handled. The beetles contain the blistering agent cantharidin in their body fluids, which is released when they sense danger. Cantharidin penetrates human skin readily, producing blisters in a matter of hours. Many species of blister beetles exist in the United States, most in the family Meloidae, although a few beetles in the Staphylinidae family cause blisters. Three of the most common are the ash gray and striped blister beetles in the central and southeastern United States, and the oil beetles (consisting of several species) in the southwestern states. In Europe, three important blister beetles are *Paederus limnophilus, Paederus gemellus,* and *Lytta vesicatoria,* the Spanish fly of southern Europe. Blisters resulting from blister beetle exposure are usually not serious, with reabsorption occurring in a few days if the blisters are unruptured.[21] The skin may flake if the blisters have ruptured, leaving an area of mild erythema for a week or so.[19] Affected areas should be washed with soap and water and bandaged until the blisters reabsorb. Antibiotic ointments or creams may help prevent secondary infection.

Millipedes (arthropod class Diplopoda), also sometimes called "thousand-leggers," are slow-moving elongate, wormlike arthropods (see Fig. 118–19*C*). They are somewhat similar to centipedes except they have two pairs of legs on most body segments and are generally rounded instead of flattened. Millipedes are commonly found in soft, decomposing plant materials. Although millipedes neither bite nor sting, some species secrete defensive body fluids that may discolor and burn human skin. Treatment involves washing the exposed area with copious amounts of water as soon as possible. Some medical personnel have recommended using solvents such as ether or alcohol to remove the noxious fluids. Eye exposure requires a thorough irrigation with warm water and consultation with an ophthalmologist.

House dust mites (acarine order Astigmata) indirectly affect human health by producing allergic reactions in some people. The mites do not bite or sting, but a considerable amount of allergic rhinitis, asthma, and childhood eczema is attributable to their presence in the human environment.[22] Adult house dust mites are whitish, plump, very tiny (0.5 mm) mites with fine striations on their cuticle. They are most often associated with furniture on which people spend a lot of time—mattresses, sofas, and recliners. House dust mite allergy is often managed by immunotherapy using mite extracts and by minimizing the level of mites in the patient's home.[22] Carpets may need to be replaced with tile or wood floors. Feather pillows should be replaced with synthetic ones. Plastic covers are available for mattresses.

ARTHROPOD VECTORS OF DISEASE

Arthropods that are capable of transmitting disease organisms to vertebrate hosts are called vectors. For example, mosquitoes in the genus *Anopheles* are vectors of malaria (see Chapter 90). Interestingly, no other mosquitoes are able to acquire and transmit the malaria parasites. In disease outbreaks there are primary vectors (the main species involved in disease transmission) and secondary vectors (the species that may occasionally become involved under certain conditions). An understanding of how disease agents are acquired and transmitted by arthropods is crucial to preventing and managing vector-borne diseases. Mechanical transmission of disease agents occurs when arthropods just physically carry pathogens from one place or host to another host—often via body parts. For example, flies and cockroaches have numerous hairs, spines, and setae on their bodies which collect contaminants as the insects feed on dead animals or excrement (Fig. 118-21). When they subsequently walk on food or food preparation surfaces, mechanical transmission occurs. Mechanical transmission may also occur if a blood-feeding arthropod has its feeding interrupted. For example, if a mosquito feeds briefly on a viremic bird and is interrupted, a subsequent feeding (if immediate) on a second bird may result in virus transmission.

In biologic transmission, there is either multiplication or development of the pathogen in the arthropod, or both (Fig. 118-22). Biologic transmission is often classified into three types. In *cyclodevelopmental transmission* the pathogen

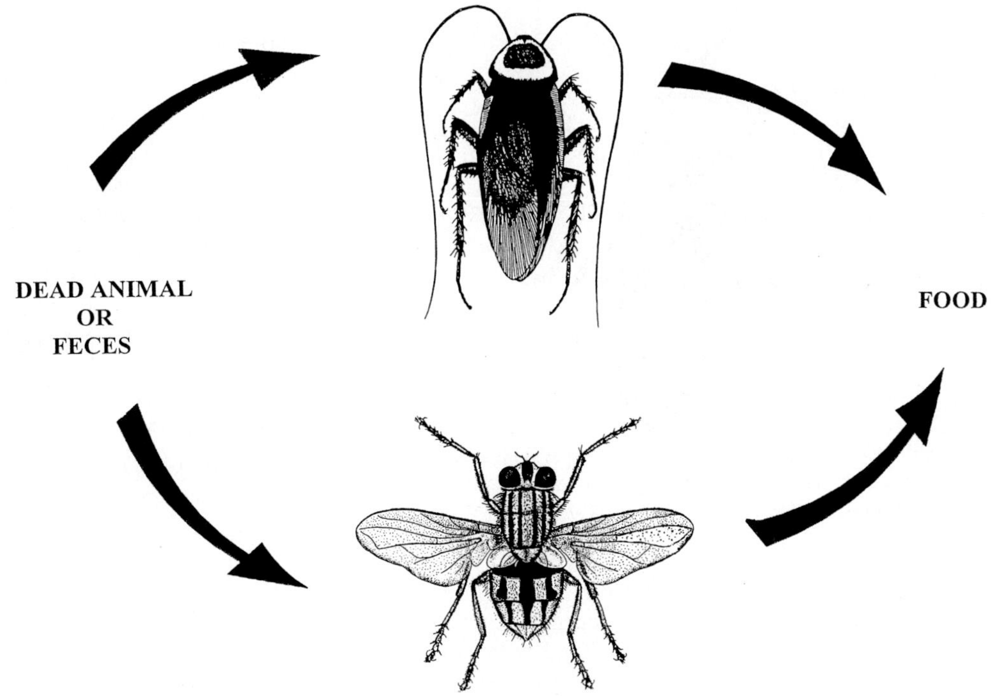

FIGURE 118-21 One example of mechanical transmission of disease organisms.

must undergo a cycle of development within the arthropod vector, but no multiplication. For example, the filarial worm that causes bancroftian filariasis (see Chapter 98), when first ingested by mosquitoes, is not infective to a vertebrate host; it must undergo a period of development. *Propagative transmission* means the pathogen must undergo multiplication before transmission can occur. There is no cyclic change or development of the organisms—plague bacteria in fleas, for example (see Chapter 42). Finally, in *cyclopropagative transmission* the pathogen must undergo both cyclic changes and multiplication. The classic example is malaria plasmodia in *Anopheles* mosquitoes (see Chapter 90). The following discussion relates to some of the arthropod species involved in biologic transmission of disease agents.

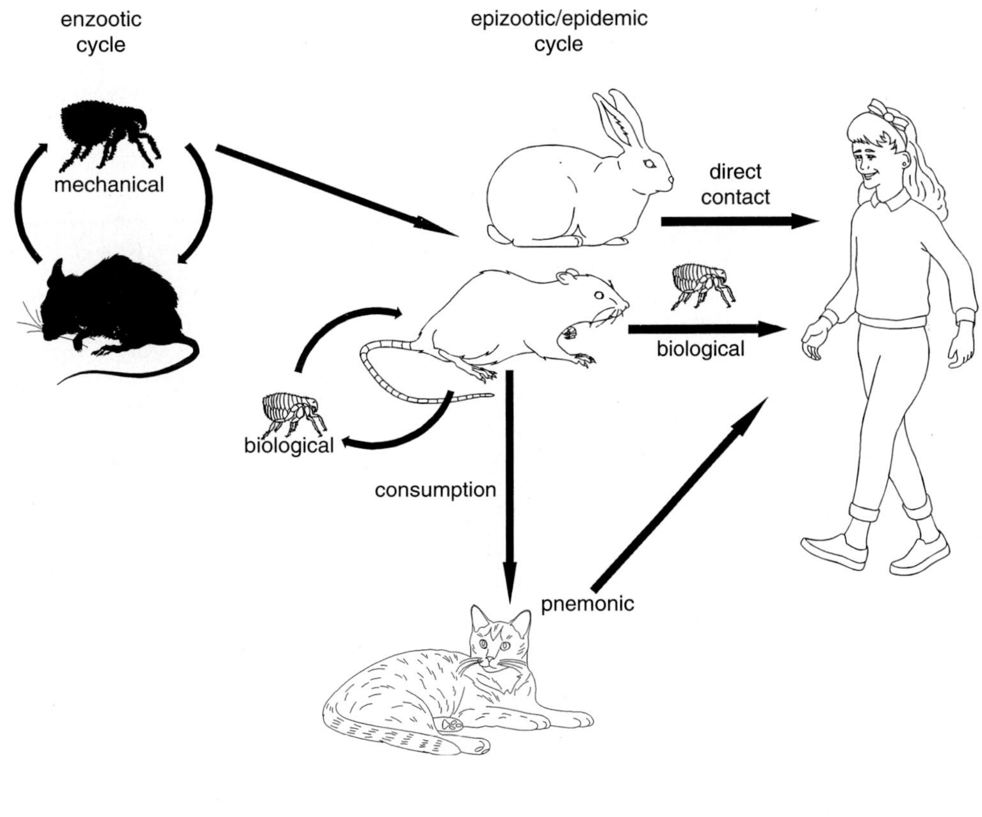

FIGURE 118-22 Biologic transmission: enzootic and epizootic transmission cycles of plague bacillus. (U.S. Air Force drawing courtesy of Dr. Chad P. McHugh.)

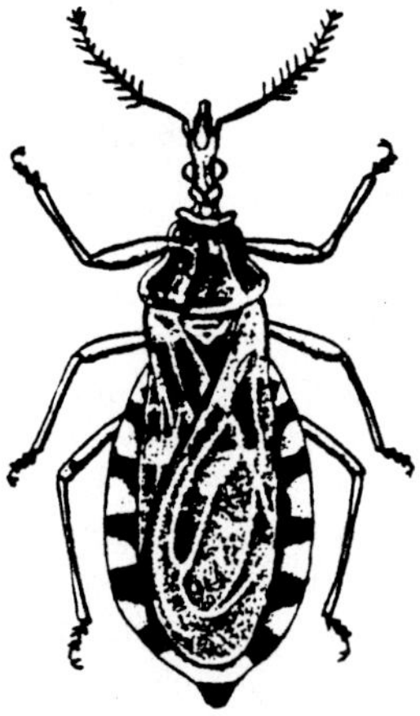

FIGURE 118-23 Kissing bug. (From U.S. Department of Health, Education, and Welfare, Public Health Service, Centers for Disease Control and Prevention, pictorial keys.)

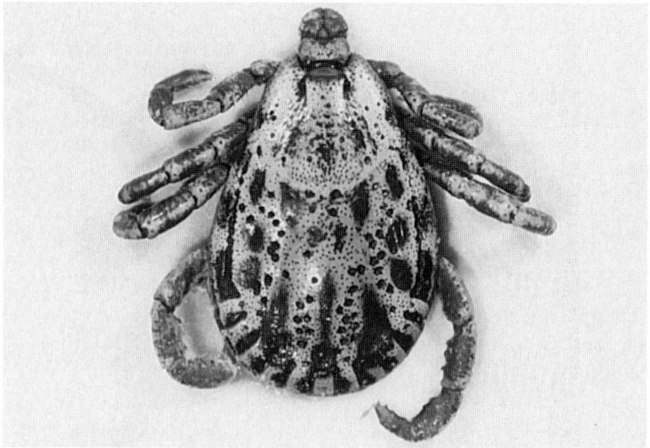

FIGURE 118-24 Male hard tick showing ornamentation. (U.S. Air Force photograph courtesy of Bob Burnes.)

Kissing bugs (insect order Hemiptera) have an elongate, cone-shaped head and are often called "cone-nose bugs" (Fig. 118-23). They are called kissing bugs because their blood meals are occasionally taken near the lips at night. Other sites of frequent attack are the hands, arms, and feet. Kissing bugs may transmit the causative agent of Chagas' disease, or American trypanosomiasis (*Trypanosoma cruzi*) in Mexico and Central and South America (see Chapter 93). Several species of kissing bugs are capable of transmitting the agent. However, four are considered principal vectors: *Panstrongylus megistus, Rhodnius prolixus, Triatoma infestans,* and *Triatoma dimidiata.* These bugs occur most commonly in poor, underdeveloped areas with dilapidated or poorly constructed huts or shacks. Infection is not by salivary secretions associated with the bite but by fecal contamination of the bite site. Treatment of kissing bug bites involves washing the bite site with soap and water, and application of topical palliatives. Oral antihistamines may help relieve itching.[23] Occasionally, systemic allergic reactions result from kissing bug bites. Those cases may be treated like any other sting or bite allergic reaction.

Ticks (acarine order Ixodida) are efficient vectors of bacteria, viruses, rickettsiae, and protozoans. At least 14 human diseases are caused or transmitted by ticks (Table 118-1). The most recent addition to this list—American boutonneuse fever—was only recently discovered as a "disease within a disease" because the new clinical entity was apparently hidden within cases diagnosed as Rocky Mountain spotted fever (RMSF).[24,25] Major tick-borne diseases in the United States are Lyme disease (approximately 20,000 cases per year; see Chapter 45), Rocky Mountain spotted fever (approximately 600 cases per year; see Chapter 50), and ehrlichiosis (approximately 100 cases per year). Two types of tick-borne ehrlichiosis (see Chapter 53) are now recognized—human monocytic ehrlichiosis (HME), caused by *Ehrlichia chaffeensis*, and human granulocytic anaplasmosis (HGA), caused by *Anaplasma phagocytophilum*.

Two families of ticks occur over much of the world: the hard ticks, Ixodidae, and the soft ticks, Argasidae. Hard ticks resemble huge mites and have anteriorly attached mouthparts visible dorsally (see Fig. 118-20A). They often have white or shiny markings (Fig. 118-24); they attach firmly to their hosts

Table 118-1 Major Tick-borne Diseases

Disease	Causative Agent	Tick Vectors
Lyme disease	Spirochete	*Ixodes ricinus* complex
Human monocytic ehrlichiosis	Rickettsia	*Amblyomma americanum*
Human granulocytic anaplasmosis	Rickettsia	*Ixodes scapularis*, others
Rocky Mountain spotted fever	Rickettsia	*Dermacentor variabilis, Dermacentor andersoni*, others
American boutonneuse fever	Rickettsia	*Amblyomma maculatum*, others
American babesiosis	Protozoan	*I. scapularis*
Colorado tick fever	Virus	Primarily *D. andersoni*
Tularemia	Bacterium	*A. americanum, D. variabilis, Dermacentor nuttalli, I. ricinus*
Boutonneuse fever	Rickettsia	*Rhipicephalus sanguineus, Rhipicephalus appendiculatus*, others
Tick paralysis	Salivary toxin	*D. andersoni, D. variabilis, Ixodes holocyclus*
Tick-borne encephalitis	Virus	*I. ricinus, Ixodes persulcatus, Dermacentor marginatus*, others
Relapsing fever	Spirochete	Several soft tick *Ornithodoros* spp.
Crimean-Congo hemorrhagic fever	Virus	*Hyalomma marginatum, Hyalomma anatolicum*, others
Siberian tick typhus	Rickettsia	Primarily *D. marginatus, Dermacentor silvarum, D. nuttalli*

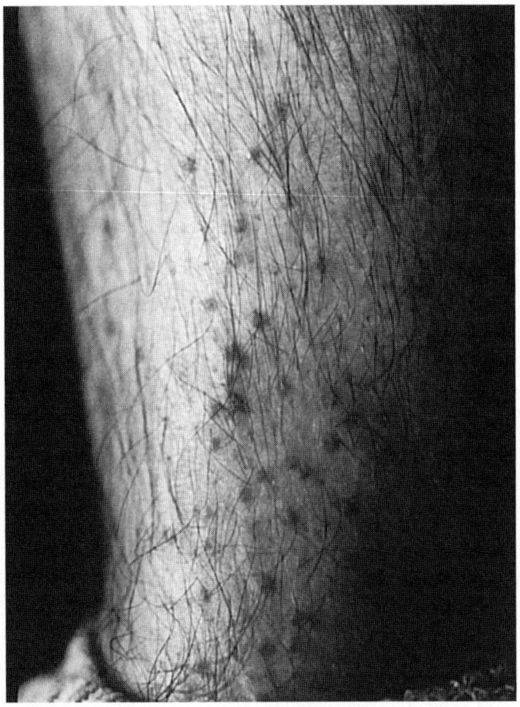

FIGURE 118-25 Seed tick bites, 4 days post attachment. (From Goddard J: Physician's Guide to Arthropods of Medical Importance, 4th ed. Boca Raton, FL, CRC Press, 2002.)

for several days. The females are capable of enormous expansion. Soft ticks are leathery without hardened plates, and their mouthparts are not visible dorsally. They do not remain firmly attached to their hosts (as larvae sometimes do), but instead feed only for approximately 15 to 30 minutes. Soft ticks are reclusive and not commonly seen or recognized by people. There are three motile life stages of hard ticks: larva, nymph, and adult. Larvae are extremely small (1 mm) and are often called seed ticks. Seed ticks of some species, especially *Amblyomma americanum* and *Amblyomma cajennense,* will feed on a wide variety of animal hosts and often get on people by the thousands, causing itching and irritation (Fig. 118-25). Nymphs (approximately 2 mm in size) also require a blood meal and some species will feed on humans. Adult ticks feed on various vertebrates, depending upon the tick species; some are specific to a certain host, whereas others are indiscriminate.

The Lone Star tick, *A. americanum,* is an important species distributed from central Texas, east to the Atlantic Coast, and north to approximately Iowa and New York. It also occurs in the northern states of Mexico. Other than nuisance effects from biting, the Lone Star tick is a known vector of the agents of tularemia and ehrlichiosis (HME).

The deer tick, *Ixodes scapularis,* is the principal vector of *Borrelia burgdorferi,* the causative agent of Lyme disease in the eastern United States. It also transmits anaplasmosis (HGA) and babesiosis. Most tick researchers now consider *Ixodes dammini* (occurring in the Northeast and upper Midwest) the same as *I. scapularis.* Thus all references to the northern form now use *I. scapularis.*[26]

The American dog tick, *Dermacentor variabilis,* is another species of medical importance in the United States. It is the primary vector of the agent of RMSF in the East, a vector of tularemia, and may cause tick paralysis. The American dog tick occurs throughout the United States except in parts of the Rocky Mountains region.

Generally, no treatment is needed for tick bites other than palliatives after tick removal. Tick removal methods vary greatly. A study by J.H. Theis[27] advocated tick removal by the use of tweezers or protected fingers using a steady retracting pressure. Needham[28] evaluated five methods commonly used for tick removal: (1) petroleum jelly, (2) fingernail polish, (3) 70% isopropyl alcohol, (4) a hot kitchen match, and (5) forcible removal with tweezers. He found that the commonly advocated methods are either ineffective, or, worse, actually created greater problems. If petroleum jelly or some other substance causes the tick to back out on its own (and most often it does not), the cement used for attachment surrounding the mouthparts remains in the skin where it continues to cause irritation. Touching the tick with a hot match may cause it to burst, increasing the risk of disease germ exposure. Furthermore, hot objects may induce ticks to salivate or regurgitate infected fluids into the wound. "Unscrewing" a tick is likely to leave broken mouthparts in the host's skin. Needham recommended the following procedure for tick removal: (1) use blunt forceps or tweezers; (2) grasp the tick as close to the skin surface as possible (Fig. 118-26) and pull upward with steady, even pressure; (3) take care not to squeeze, crush, or puncture the tick; (4) do not handle the tick with bare hands because infectious agents may enter via mucous membranes or a break in the skin; (5) after removing the tick, thoroughly disinfect the bite site and wash hands thoroughly with soap and water.[28]

Mosquitoes (insect order Diptera) are the most significant, medically important arthropods worldwide, causing annoyance and transmitting disease to humans and a host of other animals (Fig. 118-27). Besides the disease threat, the nuisance effect of mosquito bites can be unbearable, leaving many geographic areas undeveloped. Only a relatively few of the 3000 or so mosquito species are significant vectors of human disease, but mosquito-borne diseases are major health problems (Table 118-2). Mosquitoes are small flies with long, 15-segment antennae, a long proboscis for bloodsucking, and scales on their wings. Due to the pattern of wing scales, some mosquitoes may appear to have spots on their wings (Fig. 118-28). Female mosquitoes take a blood meal and subsequently lay eggs on or at a water source. The water source varies, depending on the mosquito species, but includes swamps, flooded areas, tree holes, and artificial containers such as cans, discarded tires, and the like. The larvae develop in their aquatic habitat for one or more weeks after which they pupate and eventually emerge as adult mosquitoes.

Numerous species in the genus *Anopheles* are vectors of the malaria organism. Notorious members of the genus are the *A. gambiae* complex in Africa, *A. albimanus* in Central and South America, and the *A. minimus* complex in Southeast Asia.[1] There are at least three efficient malaria vectors in the United States—*A. quadrimaculatus, A. hermsi,* and *A. freeborni.* Other major mosquito-borne diseases are yellow fever, dengue fever, filariasis, and numerous encephalitis viruses. *Aedes albopictus* and *Aedes aegypti* are the primary vectors of yellow fever and dengue. Various species in the genera *Culex,*

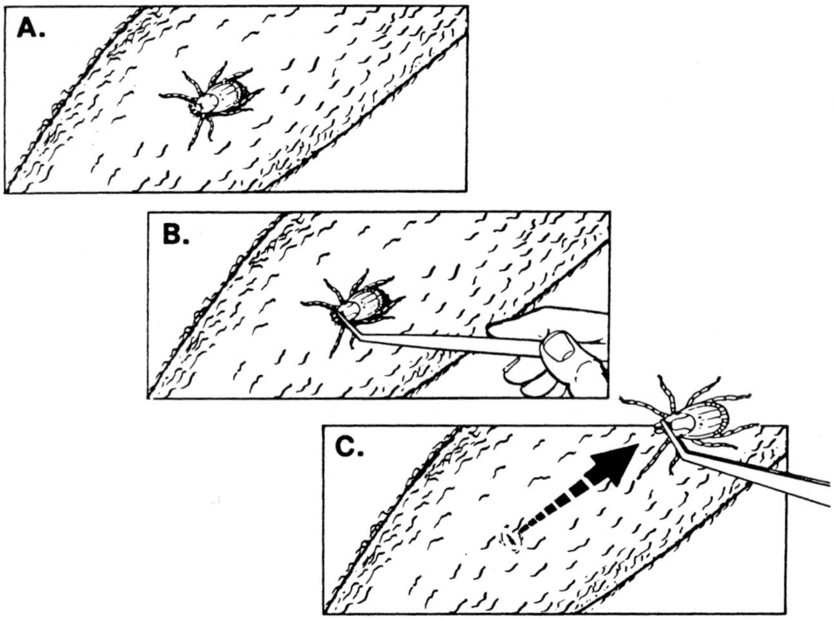

FIGURE 118-26 Recommended method of tick removal. (From U.S. Air Force Publication No. USAF-SAM-SR-89-2.)

Mansonia, Psorophora, and others transmit the agents of filariasis and mosquito-borne encephalitis, such as West Nile virus.

Other than the disease transmission threat, treatment of mosquito bites is generally unnecessary. Exceptions may include topical corticosteroids or antibiotic creams to prevent secondary infection (especially in children), and hypersensitivity reactions to the bites themselves. People highly sensitive to mosquito bites may safely reduce the cutaneous reactions to bites by prophylactic treatment with nonsedating antihistamines such as cetirizine[29] and DEET-containing insect repellants are effective.[15,16]

Fleas (insect order Siphonaptera) constitute a major human health threat because of their ability to transmit the causative agents of plague (see Chapter 42) and murine typhus (see Chapter 51). They may also serve as intermediate hosts of the dog tapeworm, *Dipylidium caninum.* Fleas are small, laterally flattened, wingless insects that take a blood meal from a wide variety of animal hosts. Some species are extremely host-specific, only biting a particular rodent or bat, or other animal. Others are indiscriminate, feeding on most any mammal (some attack birds also). The cat flea, *Ctenocephalides felis,* is one of the most important fleas in North America, feeding on several domestic and wild animal species, causing severe annoyance. Most fleas found on dogs in the United States are cat fleas. The oriental rat flea, *Xenopsylla cheopis,* is an ectoparasite of Norway rats and roof rats and is the primary vector of plague and murine (endemic) typhus. The cosmopolitan human flea, *Pulex irritans,* occurs on a wide range of host animals, especially pigs. The chigoe flea, *Tunga penetrans,* burrows into the skin (especially toes) of people in tropical and subtropical regions. Flea bites may be treated with topical corticosteroids and antibiotics if secondary infection is a problem. Tungiasis (tropics) may require excision of the embedded fleas.

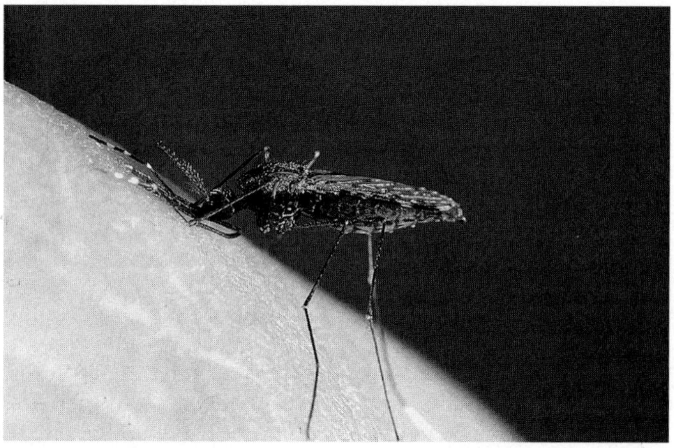

FIGURE 118-27 Female mosquito taking bloodmeal. (Centers for Disease Control and Prevention photo, Atlanta, GA)

Sand flies (insect order Diptera) are small, delicate bloodsucking flies that somewhat resemble tiny mosquitoes. Though not commonly recognized by most people, sand flies are significant vectors of the disease agents of leishmaniasis (see Chapter 94), bartonellosis (see Chapter 40), and sand fly fever (see Chapter 69). Sand flies are tiny (3 mm), golden, brown, or gray long-legged flies. They hold their wings in a V when at rest. Instead of scales (like mosquitoes) on the wing margins, these flies have hairs. Numerous species occur almost worldwide. *Phlebotomus caucasicus, Phlebotomus papatasii, Phlebotomus longipes,* and *Phlebotomus pedifer* are efficient sand fly vectors of dermal leishmaniasis in the Old World. *Phlebotomus argentipes* is the chief vector of visceral leishmaniasis in many parts of the Old World. *Lutzomyia longipalpis* is a major vector in the New World. Sand fly fever vectors are primarily *P. papatasii* and *Phlebotomus sergenti.* Bartonellosis is transmitted by *Lutzomyia verrucarum.* Other than disease transmission concerns, treatment of sand fly bites generally only involves palliative antipruritic lotions or creams.

Tsetse flies (insect order Diptera), including several species in the genus *Glossina,* are vectors of trypanosomes of

Table 118-2 Some Major Mosquito-borne Diseases

Disease	Causative Agent	Mosquito Vectors
Malaria	Protozoan (4 species)	Numerous *Anopheles* spp.
Dengue fever	Virus	*Aedes aegypti, Aedes albopictus*
Filariasis	Nematode	Various *Culex* spp., *Anopheles, Mansonia*
Yellow fever	Virus	Mainly *A. aegypti*
West Nile encephalitis	Virus	Numerous *Culex* spp.
St. Louis encephalitis	Virus	*Culex quinquefasciatus, Culex tarsalis, Culex nigripalpus,* others
Western equine encephalitis	Virus	Mainly *C. tarsalis*
Eastern equine encephalitis	Virus	*Ochlerotatus sollicitans, Coquillettidia perturbans,* others
La Crosse encephalitis	Virus	Mainly *Ochlerotatus triseriatus*
Venezuelan equine encephalitis	Virus	*Psorophora columbiae,* others
Japanese encephalitis	Virus	*Culex tritaeniorhychnus,* others

humans and animals in Africa. The Gambian form (*Trypanosoma brucei gambiense*) of African trypanosomiasis, or sleeping sickness (see Chapter 92), is transmitted by *Glossina palpalis, Glossina fuscipes,* and *Glossina tachinoides.* The East African form (*Trypanosoma brucei rhodesiense*) is primarily transmitted by *Glossina morsitans, Glossina swynnertoni,* and *Glossina pallidipes* Tsetse flies (7 to 13 mm long) are yellow, brown, or black, and fold their wings scissors-like over their back at rest (Fig. 118-29). They superficially resemble honeybees. Contrary to popular belief, people are not the preferred hosts of tsetse flies; these flies feed on a wide variety of mammals and a few reptiles. The effects of their bites are generally self-limited (aside from the disease transmission threat), but hypersensitive persons may react to the saliva, and subsequent bites produce welts and extensive swelling.

Black flies (insect order Diptera), also known as buffalo gnats or turkey gnats, are small, humpbacked flies that are important as disease vectors and nuisance pests. The causative agent of onchocerciasis, *Onchocerca volvulus,* is transmitted by black flies in tropical areas of Africa and Central America (see Chapter 100). Black flies may attack in swarms, biting viciously. Black flies (2 to 5 mm) are smaller than mosquitoes and are black with a humpbacked appearance. They breed in shallow, fast-flowing streams, mainly in upland regions. *Prosimulium mixtum* is a serious pest of people and animals in much of the United States, as are *Simulium vittatum* and *Simulium venustum.* In Africa, members of the *Simulium damnosum* complex are important vectors of onchocerciasis. Black fly bites may be itchy and slow in healing.

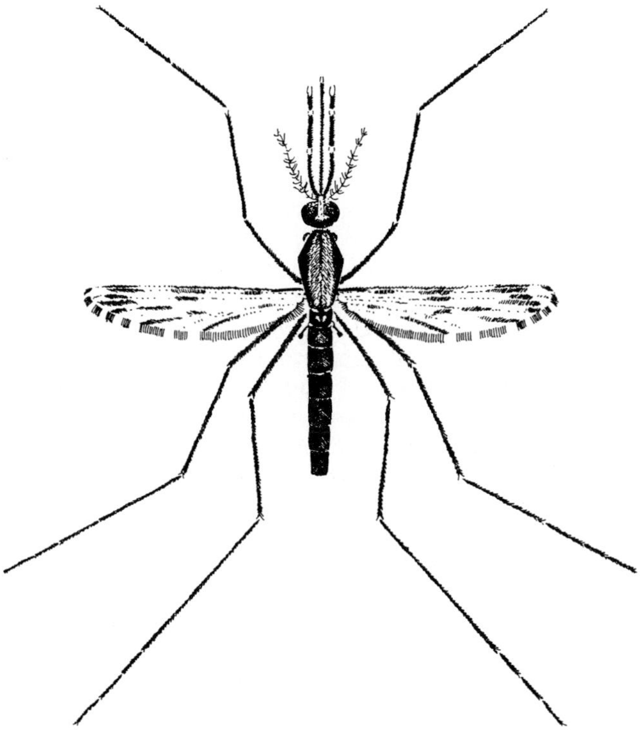

FIGURE 118-28 Some *Anopheles* mosquitoes appear to have spotted wing patterns. (From Goddard J: Physician's Guide to Arthropods of Medical Importance, 4th ed. Boca Raton, FL, CRC Press, 2002.)

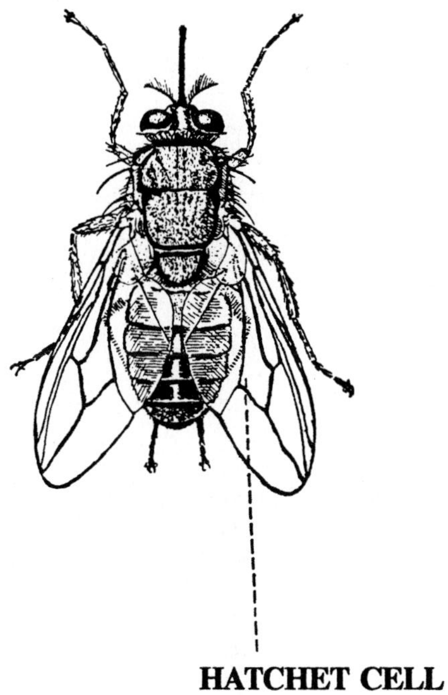

FIGURE 118-29 Adult tsetse fly. (From Yearbook of Agriculture. Washington, DC, U.S. Dept of Agriculture, 1952.)

Occasionally, people experience systemic reactions to black fly bites such as hives, wheezing, and leukocytosis.

TONGUE WORMS AND LEECHES

Tongue Worms

Pentastomes (phylum Pentastomida), sometimes also classified as members of the Arthropoda because of their chitinous exoskeleton, are wormlike parasites that are found mainly in the respiratory tracts of carnivorous mammals, reptiles, and birds.[30] Almost half of the genera parasitize snakes. Human parasitism by pentastomes is called pentastomiasis and may occur in the viscera, where nymphs develop in the liver, spleen, lungs, eyes, and other organs, or in the nasopharyngeal area. Nasopharyngeal pentastomiasis involves infestation of the nasal passages, larynx, or eustachian tubes. Most infestations are asymptomatic and only found by radiography, surgery, or autopsy.

The worms vary in color and shape, depending upon the species, but are generally colorless to yellow, ringed organisms with no apparent legs or body regions. The body may be cylindrical or flattened. Females may be up to 130 mm long and 10 mm wide; males are smaller, being up to 30 mm long. On either side of the mouth are two pairs of hollow, fanglike hooks, which can be retracted into grooves like the claws of a cat. Two species account for 99% of the infections in humans.[30,31] The tongue worm, *Linguatula serrata,* which occurs worldwide, is often found in the nasal passages and frontal sinuses of several host animals, but especially dogs (Fig. 118-30). Human infestations may result in discomfort in the throat, paroxysmal coughing, and sneezing. *Armillifer armillatus* (see Fig. 118-30) ordinarily inhabits the respiratory tract of certain snakes in central Africa. In humans, the free-moving larvae may migrate through many tissues and organs. Encysted larvae are often found in the mesenteries.

The life cycle of *Linguatula serrata* is provided as an example of pentastomid biology.[32] Adults are often found in the nasal passages and frontal sinuses of canines and felines. Eggs are produced and pass out of their host in nasal discharges that are deposited in water or on vegetation. An intermediate host (e.g., rabbit or sheep) swallows contaminated water or vegetation and the eggs hatch into primary larvae, which penetrate the intestinal wall and become lodged in the liver, lungs, or mesenteric nodes. The larvae then pass through two molts resulting in a pupa-like stage. Up to seven more molts may occur before the nymphal stage develops (sometimes called an infective larva). The nymphs then migrate to the abdominal or pleural cavity of the intermediate host where they become encysted. When a definitive host (dog or cat) eats the intermediate host, the nymphs escape rapidly and migrate anteriorly, subsequently clinging to the lining within the host's mouth. From this point they migrate to the nasal cavities where they develop into adults. The adult stage may survive for up to 2 years.

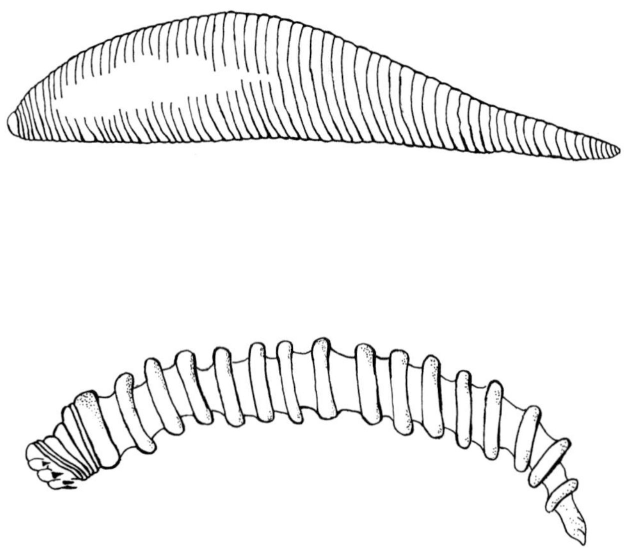

FIGURE 118-30 Pentastomids: tongue worm, *Linguatula serrata* (*top*), and *Armillifer armillatus,* a common species (*bottom*).

Treatment of pentastomiasis is usually not necessary, but in symptomatic cases surgical removal of the parasites may be needed.[30,31]

Leeches

Most leeches (annelid class Hirudinea) are bloodsucking parasites that attach themselves to vertebrate hosts, bite through the skin, and suck out a quantity of blood. Other than the nuisance effect of their biting, their medical significance is generally minimal. On feeding, leeches secrete an anticoagulant (hirudin) that aids in securing a full blood meal. Leeches vary in shape from elongated cylindrical to broadly ovoid, and may be black, brightly colored, or mottled; they have muscular suckers at both their anterior and posterior ends. Their dorsal side is convex and the ventral side is flattened. Leeches have external annulation (segments) like other annelids, but differ in having neither setae nor appendages. They are hermaphroditic. Length varies from minute (5 mm long) to giant (45 cm long).

Several different groups or types of leeches occur worldwide. The familiar freshwater leeches parasitize people or animals visiting muddy-bottomed rivers or ponds. This external attachment of leeches is often called external hirudiniasis. The famous medicinal leech, *Hirudo medicinalis,* a freshwater worm about 10 cm long, was often used in the 18th century as a means of bloodletting. Bloodthirsty land leeches inhabit warm moist areas of South America and Southeast Asia. Land or terrestrial leeches commonly live in tropical rain forests where they may be found on stones, shrubs, and leaves. Some leeches attach internally when people drink contaminated water, infesting the upper digestive or respiratory tract. "Horse leeches" may attach inside the pharynx or nasal passages of horses or people drinking water from infested pools or streams in the Middle East or North Africa. The internal leech, *Limnatis nilotica,* is found in southern Europe, northern Africa, and western Asia, where it may become attached to the mucous membranes of the pharynx, nasopharynx, and esophagus. Persons with *L. nilotica* infestation often present with epistaxis, hemoptysis, or hematemesis.

Treatment of leech infestation generally involves only mechanical removal of the worms. This is often done by the victim without medical consultation. However, leech infestation of the nasopharynx, respiratory tract, or esophagus is usually remedied by endoscopic removal.

REFERENCES

1. Goddard J: Physician's Guide to Arthropods of Medical Importance, 4th ed. Boca Raton, FL, CRC Press, 2002.
2. Chapel TA, Katta T, Kuszmar T: *Pediculosis pubis* in clinic for treatment of sexually transmitted disease. Sex Transm Dis 6:257, 1979.
3. Heukelbach J, Feldmeier H: Ectoparasites—The underestimated realm. Lancet 363:889, 2004.
4. Drugs for parasitic infections. Med Lett, 2004.
5. Wendel K, Rompalo A: Scabies and pediculosis pubis: An update of treatment regimens and general review. Clin Infect Dis 35(suppl 2): S146, 2002.
6. Harwood RF, James MT: Entomology in Human and Animal Health, 7th ed. New York, Macmillan, 1979.
7. James MT: The flies that cause myiasis in man. U.S. Dept, of Agriculture miscellaneous publication No. 631. Washington, DC, U.S. Dept. of Agriculture, 1947.
8. Borror DJ, Triplehorn CA, Johnson NF: An Introduction to the Study of Insects, 6th ed. Philadelphia, WB Saunders, 1989.
9. Moffit JE, Goldon DB, Reisman RE, et al: Stinging insect hypersensitivity: A practice paramenter. J Allergy Clin Immunol 103:963, 1999.
10. Murray JA: A case of multiple bee stings. Cent Afr J Med 10:249, 1964.
11. Goddard J: Stings by the puss caterpillar. Am Fam Physician 52:86, 1995.
12. Everson GW, Chapin JB, Normann SA: Caterpillar envenomations: A prospective study of 112 cases. Vet Hum Toxicol 32:114, 1990.
13. Polis GA: The Biology of Scorpions. Stanford, CA, Stanford University Press, 1990.
14. Goddard J: Bed bugs bounce back—But do they transmit disease? Infect Med 20:473, 2003.
15. Insect repellants. Med Lett 45:41, 2003.
16. Schultze HA: Department of Defense doctrine and material for protecting personnel from biting arthropods. J Trav Med 8:133, 2001.
17. Necrotic arachnism—Pacific Northwest. MMWR 45:433, 1996.
18. King LE Jr: Spider bites. Arch Dermatol 123:41, 1987.
19. DeLozier JB, Reaves L, King LE Jr, et al: Brown recluse spider bites of the upper extremity. South Med J 81:181, 1988.
20. Rees R, Campbell D, Rieger E, et al: The diagnosis and treatment of brown recluse spider bites. Ann Emerg Med 16:945, 1987.
21. Frazier CA, Brown FK: Insects and Allergy and What to Do About Them. Norman, OK, University of Oklahoma Press, 1980.
22. Arlian LG, Platts-Mills TAE: The biology of dust mites and the remediation of mite allergens in allergic disease. J Allergy Clin Immunol 107:406, 2001.
23. Moffitt JE, Venarske D, Goddard J, et al: Allergic reactions to Triatoma bites. Ann Allergy Asthma Immunol 91:122, 2003.
24. Paddock CD, Sumner JW, Comer JA, et al: *Rickettsia parkeri*: A newly recognized agent of spotted fever rickettsiosis in the United States. Clin Infect Dis 38:805, 2004.
25. Goddard J: American boutonneuse fever: A new spotted fever richettsiosis. Infect Med 21:207, 2004.
26. Oliver JH Jr, Owsley MR, Hutcheson HJ, et al: Conspecificity of the ticks *Ixodes scapularis* and *I. dammini*. J Med Entomol 30:54, 1993.
27. Theis JH: Mechanical removal of *Rhipicephalus sanguineus* from the dog. J Am Vet Assoc 153:433, 1968.
28. Needham GR: Evaluation of five popular methods for tick removal. Pediatrics 75:997, 1985.
29. Fradin MS: Mosquitoes and mosquito repellents: A clinician's guide. Ann Intern Med 128:931, 1998.
30. Drabick JJ: Pentastomiasis. Rev Infect Dis 9:1087, 1987.
31. Binford CH, Conner DH: Pathology of Tropical and Extraordinary Diseases, Vol. 2. Washington, DC, Armed Forces Institute of Pathology, 1976.
32. Hobmaier A, Hobmaier M: On the life cycle of *Linguatula rhinaria*. Am J Trop Med 20:199, 1940.

SECTION III

Practice: Approach to the Patient in the Tropics

119

Distinguishing Tropical Infectious Diseases from Bioterrorism

JUAN P. OLANO
C. J. PETERS
DAVID H. WALKER

MICROORGANISMS AND TOXINS CAUSING TROPICAL DISEASES WITH POTENTIAL USE AS BIOTERROR AGENTS

Bioterrorism can be defined as the intentional use of infectious agents or microbial toxins with the purpose of causing illness and death leading to fear in human populations. The dissemination of infectious agents with the purpose of attacking livestock and agricultural resources has similar motives. Many of the agents that could potentially be used in bioterror (BT) attacks are also responsible for naturally occurring infectious diseases in the tropics. As such, naturally occurring outbreaks must be differentiated from BT attacks for public health, forensic, and security reasons. If a BT attack occurs in tropical underdeveloped countries, owing to their weak public health infrastructure, the public health implications would be even more dramatic than in developed countries. An outbreak of smallpox due to a BT attack would probably require vaccination and mandatory quarantine of millions of people in order to control the outbreak and quell global public unrest. This chapter will concentrate on selected infectious agents that have the potential to be used as bioterror agents in human populations.

The first step in managing the damage from a covert biological dissemination is recognition of the attack and the organism(s). As in most emerging infections, we predict that in bioterrorist attacks the etiological diagnosis will be made by a clinician or pathologist and the recognition of a bioterrorist event will be through geographical and epidemiological anomalies. We have very limited environmental detection capability at this time, and there are no comprehensive point-of-care diagnostics for most of the high-impact BT agents. Some diseases such as inhalational anthrax or smallpox may be relatively readily recognized by an alert clinician because of their very distinctive presentation in many cases. However, the leading edge of a BT epidemic may arrive on a pathologist's doorstep without prior suspicion. For example, individual cases of pneumonic plague as the earliest harbingers of an attack will presumably present as community-acquired pneumonia and probably die without clinical diagnosis. Given the short window available for successful treatment, the recognition of these earliest cases is paramount. Sartwell[1] has demonstrated empirically that incubation periods follow a log-normal distribution, which results in "front-loading" of cases (Fig. 119-1). Delay in recognizing the epidemic through reliance on syndromic surveillance or other surrogates will likely result in most of the cases of diseases such as plague and tularemia being well into their disease course and perhaps unsalvageable.[2]

Bioterrorist events will enlarge our knowledge of tropical diseases. For example, inhalational anthrax and several viral hemorrhagic fevers (VHF) thought to be transmitted mainly by aerosol[3] are under-represented in naturally occurring case series, and a BT attack would provide an opportunity to answer questions about the underlying host factors

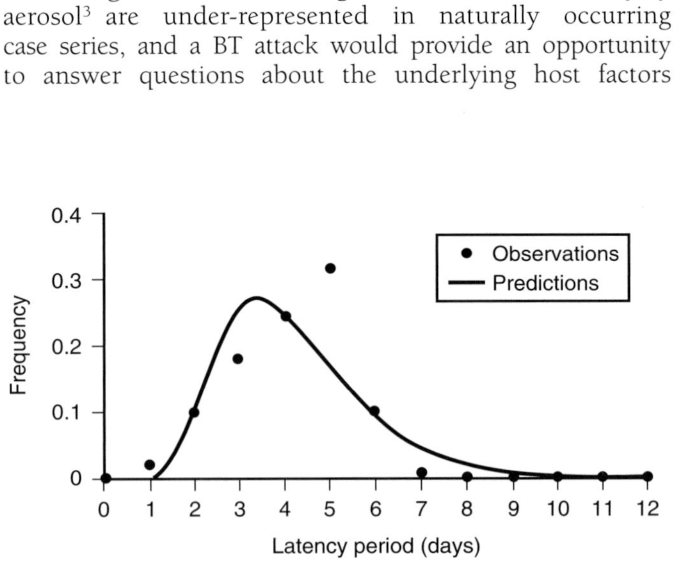

FIGURE 119-1 Log-normal distribution of incubation periods. (From Sartwell P: The distribution and incubation periods of infectious diseases. Am J Hyg 51:310–318, 1950.)

and pathogenesis. Indeed, the extension of the risk population to include children, the elderly, and the immunosuppressed is likely to provide considerable insight into these often-understudied groups. It is also likely that our lack of information about them will challenge our current diagnostic algorithms.

In October 2001, anthrax spores were distributed covertly in the U.S. postal service, leading to 22 cases of human anthrax and billions of dollars spent on controlling the potentially devastating effects of a small inhalational anthrax epidemic.[4,5] This attack was by no means the first intentional attempt to use infectious agents as weapons of terror. Ever since the times of the ancient Greeks and Romans, humans have tried to inflict damage by the use of contagion on other populations.[6,7] Less than 4% of the people or groups responsible for terrorist attacks on human populations take responsibility for their actions.[8] Therefore, the use of biological weapons is ideal to conduct covert attacks. In addition, it has been estimated that to kill the same number of human beings with biological weapons as compared to chemical or nuclear weapons, the cost is far less with biological weapons ($2/human casualty) compared with chemical ($2000/human casualty) and nuclear ($2,000,000/human casualty) weapons.[6] Hypothetical BT attacks would range from an overt attack of a large city with a bomb containing several kilograms of an agent (weaponized bacteria, viruses, or toxins) to discrete or covert intentional release of the infectious agent through a delivery system, such as spray devices, postal service, ventilation ducts, water supplies, and food supply.

Based on transmissibility, severity of morbidity and mortality, and likelihood of use (availability, stability, weaponization), potential BT agents are divided into three categories (Table 119-1). This chapter will concentrate on selected agents from categories A and B and on the diagnostic challenges posed by illnesses caused by such agents.

Table 119-1 Potential Bioterror Agents

Categories/Agent	Disease
Category A	
Viruses	
Smallpox	Variola major
Ebola, Marburg, CCHF, RVF, Lassa, Machupo, and Junin viruses	Viral hemorrhagic fevers
Bacteria	
Francisella tularensis	Tularemia
Yersinia pestis	Plague
Toxins	
C. botulinum toxins	Botulism
Category B	
Viruses	
Alphaviruses (VEE, EEE, WEE)	Various encephalitides
Bacteria	
Rickettsia prowazekii	Epidemic typhus
R. rickettsii	Rocky Mountain spotted fever
Brucella spp.	Brucellosis
Coxiella burnetii	Q fever
Burkholderia mallei	Glanders
Burkholderia pseudomallei	Melioidosis
Toxins	
Ricin	
SEB	

EPIDEMIOLOGY

All infectious agents described in Table 119-1 are capable of producing illness under natural circumstances. Therefore, the first challenge is to identify the infectious agent responsible for a certain disease correctly, followed by a thorough epidemiologic and microbiologic analysis of the epidemic or outbreak. In some circumstances, the identification of a BT attack would be obvious. A case of smallpox in any human population is an international emergency that would trigger a massive response of the public health systems around the world. Sophisticated epidemiological investigations would follow in order to characterize the outbreak, identify the source, and possibly label it "intentional." In other cases, the identification of the outbreak as secondary to intentional dissemination of an infectious agent will require the use of sophisticated epidemiological and molecular tools, especially for diseases endemic to the area where the outbreak occurs. The need to use genetic sequences as markers has spawned a new discipline referred to as microbial forensics, sister to phylogenetics and "molecular epidemiology."

Differentiation between natural infections and a biological warfare attack rests firstly on disease patterns given by several epidemiological clues. They include presence of disease outbreaks of the same illness in noncontiguous areas, disease outbreaks with zoonotic impact, different attack rates in different environments (indoor versus outdoor), presence of large epidemics in small populations, increased number of unexplained deaths, unusually high severity of a disease for a particular pathogen, unusual clinical manifestations owing to route of transmission for a given pathogen, presence of a disease (vector-borne or not) in an area not endemic for that particular disease, multiple epidemics with different diseases in the same population, a case of a disease by an uncommon agent (smallpox, viral hemorrhagic fevers, inhalational anthrax), unusual strains of microorganisms when compared to conventional strains circulating in the same affected areas, and genetically homogenous organisms isolated from different locations.[9,10] These are a few guidelines that could prove helpful when investigating an outbreak, but it has to be kept in mind that the deduction will not be based on any single finding but rather the pattern seen in its totality. First and foremost, the possibility of an attack must be ever in mind, or differentiation of a covert BT attack and a natural outbreak of an infectious disease may not be made. In fact, the outbreak of salmonellosis in Oregon in 1984 was due to a covert attack planned by the Rajneeshee leadership and accompanied by distinctive epidemiological clues. It was not labeled as intentional until somebody came forward with the information leading to the responsible group; as in most of medicine, the unsuspected diagnosis is the easiest to miss.[11]

An increasing number of public health departments are now acquiring the technology necessary to perform syndromic surveillance. This new method of surveillance is based on syndromic disease rates such as respiratory, gastrointestinal, and neurological syndromes or analysis of other health-related activities such as laboratory test requests and results, purchasing rates for certain pharmaceutical agents, unexplained death rates, and veterinary surveillance.[2,10,11] The purpose of syndromic surveillance is to detect a BT attack as early as possible by analyzing the previously mentioned variables by extracting and analyzing data through computer networks. The rationale behind syndromic surveillance is the nonspecific nature of early signs and symptoms of many of the illnesses caused by BT agents. Examples of proposed syndromes are as follows: gastroenteritis of any apparent infectious etiology, pneumonia with the sudden death of a previously healthy adult, widened mediastinum in a febrile patient, acute neurologic illness with fever, and advancing cranial nerve impairment with weakness.[12] A key component of this system is the continuous analysis of health-care variables to establish thresholds for all variables being analyzed. It is worth mentioning that one of the first flags raised by the human immunodeficiency virus (HIV) pandemic in its early stages in the United States was the increased number of orders for pentamidine from the Centers for Disease Control and Prevention (CDC) to treat several patients in California for *Pneumocystis carinii* pneumonia. As of May 2003, syndromic surveillance systems had been established in approximately 100 sites. One of the best known systems is the so-called Electronic Surveillance System for the Early Notification of Community-based Epidemics (ESSENCE II) being developed by the Johns Hopkins University Applied Biophysics Laboratory.[12] This project is sponsored by the Defense Advanced Research Projects Agency (DARPA) for use in the Department of Defense Global Emerging Infections System. The first system developed (ESSENCE I) is already in use at all U.S. military treatment facilities.[12] ESSENCE II uses the following syndromes for analysis: respiratory, gastrointestinal, fever, dermatological hemorrhagic, dermatological infectious, neurological, and coma.

Factors affecting syndromic surveillance include selection of data sources, definition of syndrome categories, selection of statistical detection thresholds, availability of resources for follow-up, recent experiences with false alarms, and criteria for initiating investigations. It must be emphasized that these systems are experimental and not yet of proven value in managing BT attacks. They are expensive, require follow-up confirmation, have unproven sensitivity and specificity, and ultimately depend on the clinician.[2] They may prove to be more useful in managing an event than in expeditiously detecting one.

Conventional epidemiological investigations are by no means obsolete with the availability of more sophisticated methods to study possible BT attacks. They include the confirmation of an outbreak once it is suspected. Confirmation is based in many cases on laboratory analysis of patients' samples or autopsy material. A case definition is constructed to increase objectivity of the data analyzed and to enable determination of the attack rate. Other variables are included in the analysis, such as time and place, and an epidemiological curve can be constructed.[10] Epidemiological curves are an important tool to analyze epidemics and suggest the mode of transmission and propagation. A point source epidemic curve is classically log-normal in distribution[1] and would suggest a common exposure of a population to an infectious agent. Of course, there can be variations depending on the presence of susceptible subpopulations (e.g., children, immunosuppressed, aged) and on varying doses of the agent. Propagative curves are more characteristic of highly communicable agents such as smallpox.

A short description of selected category A and B agents follows. All these pathogens are addressed as naturally occurring disease agents in other chapters of this book.

CATEGORY A

Bacterial Agents

Bacillus anthracis (Anthrax)

B. anthracis (see Chapter 39) is without a doubt the microorganism that has received the most attention as a BT agent due to its high lethality (inhalational form), ease of propagation, and high environmental stability. Fortunately, the disease is not transmitted from person to person. However, the first three characteristics make it one of the ideal bioweapons.

Anthrax presents in humans as four different clinical syndromes, depending on the portal of entry: cutaneous (the most common form of the disease resulting from contact with infectious animal products), gastrointestinal and oral/oropharyngeal (both secondary to ingestion of contaminated meat), and inhalational (woolsorter's disease), secondary to inhalation of spores from the environment. In the event of a bioterror attack, either overt or covert, the clinical presentation of the patients affected by the attack would be that of inhalational anthrax. This form of anthrax is so rare that a single case of inhalational anthrax should raise immediate suspicion, as dramatically demonstrated during the BT attacks in the fall of 2001.[13–15] During those attacks, 50% of cases were cutaneous anthrax thought to be secondary to handling of anthrax-laced mail envelopes or environmental surface contamination in the presence of minor cutaneous lesions, providing a portal of entry for the spores.[5] An outbreak of inhalational anthrax also took place in Sverdlovsk (former Soviet Union) as a result of an accidental release into the air of *B. anthracis* spores from a facility producing anthrax for the bioweapons program in the USSR.[5,16–18]

Inhalational anthrax should be suspected clinically in any individual presenting with fever and a widened mediastinum on chest radiograph (due to hemorrhagic mediastinitis).[19,20] The incubation period is normally 3 to 5 days, but in some cases it can be as short as 2 days and as long as 60 days depending on inoculum and the time of germination of the spore.[17] Based on research performed on rhesus monkeys, the LD_{50} is estimated to be 8000 to 10,000 spores.[21–23] However, as few as 1 to 3 spores may be capable of producing a fatal outcome in approximately 1% of those exposed to these quantities.[24] The initial symptoms are nonspecific and consist of fever, malaise, anorexia, fatigue, and dry cough. These symptoms are followed in 3 to 4 days by an abrupt onset of respiratory insufficiency, stridor, diaphoresis, and cyanosis. The subsequent clinical course is rapid, and patients usually die within 24 to 36 hours after clinical deterioration. Mortality is 100% without antibiotic therapy.[20,25–27] Early diagnosis, aggressive treatment with antimicrobial agents to which the bacteria are susceptible, and aggressive supportive therapy decreased the mortality to 40% in the 2001 attacks.[5] Pathologic studies performed on the Sverdlovsk victims confirmed some of the findings in animal models of inhalational anthrax, such as hemorrhagic lymphadenitis and mediastinitis. However, many patients also developed hematogenous hemorrhagic pneumonia. Pleural effusions were usually large and frequently led to severe lung atelectasis. In about half of cases, hemorrhagic meningitis developed, leading rapidly to central nervous system (CNS) manifestations terminating in coma and death.[16,28,29]

Yersinia pestis (Plague)

Y. pestis (see Chapter 42) is a gram-negative, aerobic, nonsporulating coccobacillus, member of the Enterobacteriaceae with a wide host range, including rodents, felines, and humans.[30] The most important reservoirs are urban rats, and its main vector is the rat flea. In rural epizootics, reservoirs include prairie dogs and squirrels in the United States.[31] *Y. pestis* has been responsible for some of the most devastating pandemics in human history in the preantibiotic era (6th, 14th, and 19th centuries).[32] Public health measures have made this disease a rarity in the United States (around 20 cases/year) and around the world, although approximately 1000 cases are reported to the World Health Organization (WHO) every year (countries reporting plague include Madagascar, Tanzania, and Peru, among others).

Clinical presentation in naturally acquired infections takes five forms, namely bubonic, septicemic, pneumonic, cutaneous, and meningeal. The pneumonic form is the most likely presentation in a case of plague due to a BT attack. It is worth mentioning that plague has already been used as a BT agent when Japan dropped thousands of *Y. pestis*–infected fleas over China leading to small outbreaks of bubonic plague in continental China during World War II.[33,34]

The incubation period for pneumonic plague is short, ranging from 2 to 3 days. It is the rarest form in natural infections (1% or less) but has the highest mortality, reaching 100% in untreated patients. The initial presentation is nonspecific and consists of cough, fever, and dyspnea. Cough may be productive (bloody, purulent, or watery in the initial phases). This is followed by a rapid clinical course leading to respiratory failure and the patient's demise if not treated with antibiotics early in the course of the disease.[30,31,35]

The factors that led to the severe Manchurian pneumonic plague outbreaks in the early 20th century are unknown, but weather, hygiene, and crowding were important factors. More recent outbreaks worldwide and particularly in the United States have been much smaller and readily controlled. Pneumonic cases are common in the United States, but secondary transmission has been rare in the last 50 years. Modeling of pneumonic transmission using eight small outbreaks to derive the parameters find average of secondary cases per primary case (Ro) to be approximately 1.3 prior to any control measures.[36]

Francisella tularensis (Tularemia)

This is one of the most scientifically neglected microorganisms with BT potential. Tularemia is a zoonotic infection caused by a strictly aerobic, gram-negative, nonsporulating small coccobacillus. Two subspecies are recognized, namely *F. tularensis* subspecies *holarctica* (Jellison type B) and *F. tularensis* subspecies *tularensis* (Jellison type A).[37] Type A is by far the more virulent and is present only in North America. Of the bacteria with potential as BT agents, *F. tularensis* has by far the widest host range, including wild and domestic animals, humans, fish, reptiles, and birds. Vectors are also numerous and include ticks, fleas, mosquitoes, and biting flies.[37,38] This is an impressive range for any human pathogen.

In contrast to other diseases described in this chapter, tularemia does not have the remarkable history that some of the other pathogens have. In Europe, tularemia was first described in 1532; in the United States, it was first described in 1911 in California in the aftermath of the San Francisco earthquake.[38]

In natural infections, the most common source of infection is a tick bite and manipulation of infected animals such as wild rabbits. Six different clinical syndromes have been described as follows: ulceroglandular, glandular, oculoglandular, pharyngeal, pneumonic, and typhoidal. Marked overlap exists among all these forms, and for practical purposes two syndromes (ulceroglandular and typhoidal) have been proposed.[39–41] As a BT agent, *F. tularensis* will most likely cause a disease with a primary pulmonary component with secondary dissemination (typhoidal/systemic). In natural infections, both ulceroglandular and typhoidal forms can have a hematogenous pulmonary component, although it is more common in typhoidal forms. Pulmonary features include cough, pleural effusions, and multifocal bronchopneumonic infiltrates. If not treated promptly, patients usually develop adult respiratory distress syndrome leading to respiratory insufficiency and the patient's demise. Case-fatality rate approaches 30% if not treated with appropriate antibiotics.[41]

Viral Agents

Smallpox Virus (Variola Major)

Smallpox eradication remains the single most important victory in the war against infectious diseases. Smallpox (see Chapter 58) is the only disease so far eradicated from the face of the earth due to human intervention. The WHO declared smallpox eradicated in 1980 after the last case of natural disease was diagnosed in Somalia in 1977,[42] and vaccination ceased around the world, rendering humankind vulnerable to reintroduction of the virus.[43–45] A laboratory accident was responsible for two more cases in 1978 in England. This accident prompted the WHO to restrict the frozen virus to two places in the world: the CDC in Atlanta, Georgia, and the Institute for Polyomyelitis and Viral Encephalitides in Moscow, later moved to NPO VECTOR, Novosibirisk, Russia. However, it is suspected that secret military repositories exist after the fragmentation of the Soviet Union and the subsequent exodus of scientists involved in its bioweapons program (Biopreparat).[46,47] The agent responsible for this disease is an orthopox virus with no known animal reservoir, but high aerosol infectivity, stability, and mortality. Although not a category A agent, monkeypox is responsible for outbreaks in Africa and is the only other member of the orthopox genus capable of producing systemic disease in humans. The clinical disease is potentially indistinguishable from smallpox, where mortality rates in tropical Africa are around 10% to 15%. In May and June 2003, an outbreak of monkeypox occurred in the United States.[48] Thirty-seven infections were laboratory-documented and involved humans exposed to infected prairie dogs that had become infected because of contact with infected Gambian rats and dormice, two animal species shipped from Africa earlier that year. Infected humans included veterinarians, exotic pet dealers, and pet owners. The clinical spectrum in this outbreak ranged from asymptomatic seroconversions to febrile illness with papulovesicular rash. No deaths were associated with this outbreak. However, phylogenetic analysis of the virus placed it in the West Africa clade as opposed to the Central Africa clade which carries the previously mentioned case-fatality rate of 10% to 15%.

A single case of smallpox would trigger a massive public health response in order to contain the outbreak. An outbreak in Germany in 1970 resulted in 19 cases with 100,000 people vaccinated to contain the infection. In 1972, Yugoslavia underwent an epidemic with a total of 175 cases (35 deaths) and a vaccination program that included 20 million people in order to contain the outbreak and obtain international confidence. Vaccination with the vaccinia virus (a related orthopox virus) is the most effective way to prevent the disease and can be administered up to 4 days after contact with ill patients. Strict quarantine with respiratory isolation for 17 days is also mandatory. The newer generation of antivirals that have been developed after the disease was eradicated has never been tested in human populations, but in vitro data and experiments in animal models of poxvirus disease suggest some antiviral activity for the acyclic nucleoside phosphonates such as cidofovir.[49] The only vaccine available in the United States is Dryvax, and sufficient doses have been manufactured to cover the entire U.S. population. However, newer vaccines that may have fewer side effects are being developed.

The clinical presentation is characteristic. The incubation period ranges from 10 to 12 days. The initial phase is nonspecific, common to other viral syndromes, and is characterized by abrupt onset of fever, fatigue, malaise, and headaches. During this prodromal phase in 10% of patients with fair complexion, a discrete erythematous rash appears on the face, forearms, and hands. The typical smallpox rash has a centrifugal distribution (that is, more abundant on the face and extremities than on the trunk and abdomen). An enanthem also develops with presence of oral ulcerations by the time the exanthem appears. Systemic manisfestations begin to subside once the rash appears and can reappear with superinfection of skin lesions or superimposed bacterial bronchopneumonia. Progression of the lesions is synchronous (maculopapules, vesicles, pustules). After pustules rupture, scabs form and detach in 2 to 3 weeks, leaving depigmented, scarred areas. This form of the disease, called variola major, is fatal in up to 30% of unvaccinated patients and 3% of vaccinated individuals. Various hemorrhagic forms exist. In some cases, the rash progresses very slowly and hemorrhage develops into the base of the lesions, which remain flat and soft instead of tense, carrying a bad prognosis. In some other cases, the disease is hemorrhagic from the beginning, leading to death 5 to 7 days after the initial symptoms appear (case-fatality rate: 100%). Finally, in some cases, a severe and overwhelming illness is followed by dusky skin lesions; these patients have a large quantity of virus and are extremely dangerous epidemiologically. Previously vaccinated individuals usually develop a milder disease that consists of a mild pre-eruptive phase followed by few skin lesions that appear more superficial, evolve more rapidly, and are not as synchronous as the classical type.[50]

Viral Hemorrhagic Fevers

Viral hemorrhagic fever (VHF; see Chapter 65) is caused by a heterogenous group of RNA viruses that belong to several different families. The CDC identified filoviruses (Ebola and Marburg viruses), arenaviruses (Lassa, Junin, Machupo, Guanarito, and Sabia), and bunyaviruses (Crimean-Congo hemorrhagic fever [CCHF] and Rift Valley fever [RVF]).[51–53]

The common denominator in these infections is the increased vascular permeability in the microcirculation leading to hemorrhagic diathesis and systemic manifestations such as pulmonary edema and cerebral edema related to leaky capillaries.[54] These viruses usually have a very narrow geographic range determined by their natural reservoirs and vectors. Humans are accidental hosts. These diseases have caught great public attention due to their high mortality. This, combined with their aerosol infectivity, has led to the use of biosafety level 4 laboratories in their study.

Clinical presentation is usually nonspecific and consists of fever and malaise, followed by signs of increased vascular permeability and circulatory compromise. VHF usually terminates in shock, generalized mucocutaneous hemorrhages, and multiorgan failure. Differences exist among the clinical details and pathogenesis of the different viruses (see Chapter 65 for an overview and the individual chapters for details). For example, VHF due to filoviruses usually have prominent hemorrhagic manifestations and disseminated intravascular coagulation (DIC) as a terminal event. RVF virus leads to liver damage, DIC, and hemorrhagic manifestations in approximately 1% of patients with severe disease. CCHF also behaves like the filoviral infections with prominent hemorrhagic manifestations. Lassa fever has few neurologic or hemorrhagic manifestations. The South American arenaviral hemorrhagic fevers usually have hemorrhagic and neurologic components.

Diseases Caused by Toxins

Toxins in the context of BT agents are substances of biologic origin that are capable of producing human illness. Toxins are usually proteins synthesized by living bacteria, fungi, or plants. Toxins are generally less dangerous than infectious agents. The most potent biological toxin is that from *Clostridium botulinum* and it is 10-fold or more less lethal than anthrax on a weight basis. Other toxins such as ricin are more than a 1000-fold less toxic than botulinum toxin and sarin is 30-fold less toxic than ricin.

Clostridium botulinum Toxins (Botulism)

There are seven similar toxins produced by seven different serotypes of *C. botulinum* (A to G), all leading to the same clinical manifestations and with the same lethality. The toxins have a molecular weight of approximately 150 kDa and block neurotransmission at the presynaptic level in cholinergic neurons including the neuromuscular junction, leading to progressive palsies of cranial nerves and skeletal muscle. Botulinal toxins are among the most lethal substances known to mankind with LD_{50} of 0.001 μg/g of body weight when administered parenterally.[25,55,56] The aerosol route decreases its lethality 80 to 100 times. Both aerosol attacks and contamination of food supplies are potential BT scenarios.

Clinical manifestations consist of progressive bulbar and skeletal paralysis in the absence of fever, including diplopia, dysphagia, blurred vision, ptosis, dysarthria, dysphonia, mydriasis, dry mucosae, and descending paralysis.[25,56] The cause of death in lethal cases is respiratory insufficiency due to paralysis of respiratory muscles. Onset of symptoms is variable and depends on the inoculum, ranging from 24 hours to several days after exposure. Most cases of naturally occurring intoxication are related to consumption of improperly sterilized canned food or ingestion of preserved fish. Rare cases of inhalational botulism were documented in Germany in the early 1960s due to accidental laboratory exposure. The rapid absorption through the respiratory tract may offer a different pathogenesis and it is not known if antitoxin is useful in therapy, although animal models show efficacy in prophylaxis.

CATEGORY B AGENTS

All the agents in category A are generally recognized as serious threats for causing extensive casualties. Categories B and C are much more heterogeneous. They were considered to provide significant threat potential but there are continuing reassessments.

Viral Agents

Viral Encephalitides

These conditions are caused by the genus *Alphavirus*, family Togaviridae (eastern, western, and Venezuelan equine encephalitis [VEE] viruses; see Chapter 74). Natural infections are usually transmitted by mosquitoes, but aerosol transmission is the notorious cause of numerous laboratory infections and is the basis of its historic weaponization.[52,57] Most of these viruses cause systemic illness characterized by fever, myalgias, and prostration.

Clinically apparent involvement of the central nervous system is present in some cases and varies among the different viruses. Eastern equine encephalitis (EEE) is by far the most virulent, leading to case-fatality rates of 50% to 75%, and survivors usually have severe neurologic sequelae.[58,59] VEE, in contrast, leads to CNS manifestations in no more than 4% of cases and almost all VEE infections are symptomatic even in the absence of CNS involvement.[60–62]

Bacterial Agents

Rickettsia prowazekii (Epidemic Typhus) and *R. rickettsii* (Rocky Mountain Spotted Fever)

Typhus (see Chapter 51) is another disease that has played a historic role in human populations.[63–66] Millions of people perished in World War I and World War II due to epidemic, louse-borne typhus. Large outbreaks of the disease still occur in tropical regions around the world in areas stricken by war, famine, and poverty. Rocky Mountain spotted fever (RMSF), on the other hand, is transmitted by tick bites and occurs endemically in South and Central America as well as North America. Rickettsiae target the microvascular endothelium leading to leaky capillaries systemically.[67] The main causes of morbidity and mortality are noncardiogenic pulmonary edema and cerebral edema leading to diffuse alveolar damage and meningoencephalitis. Clinical manifestations are nonspecific and include fever, malaise, headache, myalgias/arthralgias, cough, nausea, vomiting, confusion, stupor, and coma in severe cases. Skin rash ranges from maculopapular to petechial, depending on the severity, and is observed in around 90% of patients with RMSF and 2% to 100% of cases of epidemic typhus, depending on the darkness of cutaneous pigmentation. Rickettsiae are remarkably underestimated biothreats as they are highly infectious by low-dose aerosol exposure, possess a stable extracellular form, and are resistant to most empirically administered antibiotics, including β-lactams, aminoglycosides, and macrolides, and are exacerbated by sulfonamides. Case-fatality rates can be as high as 40% to 50% without antibiotic therapy and 3% to 5% with adequate antibiotic coverage. Lethal cases are usually due to delayed diagnosis.[64,65,68]

These rickettsiae are highly infectious by aerosol and are potent BT agents. They are often discounted because of their susceptibility to tetracycline and chloramphenicol. However, the severity of the illness, the exhaustion of antibiotics in the face of a mass attack, and the existence of antibiotic-resistant organisms suggest they are still formidable players.

Coxiella burnetii (Q Fever)

This gram-negative, obligately intracellular bacterium has a high degree of infectivity (one organism is capable of causing infection by inhalation) and low lethality.[69–72] The distribution of Q fever is worldwide and results from exposure to animals such as sheep, cattle, goats, cats, rabbits, and others. *C. burnetii* has spore-like characteristics that can withstand harsh environmental conditions and be transported by wind to other places. In natural infections, 60% of cases are asymptomatic and are diagnosed by seroconversion. In symptomatic cases, the presentation is nonspecific and includes malaise, fever, myalgias, cough, chills, headaches, anorexia, weight loss, and in some cases pleuritic chest pain. Hepatomegaly and splenomegaly are sometimes observed, although not frequently.

Brucella spp. (Brucellosis; Other Names: Undulant Fever, Mediterranean Fever, Malta Fever)

Four species of these gram-negative, aerobic, non-spore-forming coccobacilli are pathogenic to humans: *B. abortus, B. melitensis, B. suis,* and *B. canis* (see Chapter 41). Host ranges include goats and sheep (*B. melitensis*), swine and horses (*B. suis*), cattle, bison, elk, horses (*B. abortus*), and dogs (*B. canis*).

Transmission occurs by exposure to infected animal products (meat, milk). Less common routes of infection are inhalational and cutaneous. The clinical presentation of brucellosis is highly variable, even after inhalational exposure. The clinical spectrum ranges from asymptomatic seroconversion to severe acute systemic disease. Intermediate forms include undulant fever or chronic disease, characterized by presence of *Brucella* in virtually any organ. Acute systemic disease is highly incapacitating with high fever, headache, nausea, vomiting, chills, severe sweating, and, in very severe cases, delirium, coma, and death. Undulant fever is characterized by relapses of fever, weakness, generalized aching, and headache. Chronic infections may have manifestations related to several organ systems such as the gastrointestinal and genitourinary tracts, CNS, joints, and bones.[73–75]

Food and Waterborne Pathogens

Developing countries with insufficient water treatment and food security are more vulnerable to enteric BT attack. These agents include *Shigella dysenteriae, Salmonella* spp., enterohemorrhagic *E. coli, Vibrio cholerae,* and *Cryptosporidium parvum.*

Shigella and *Salmonella* have in fact already been used as agents of biorevenge or biopolitics in small-scale attacks: one (*Shigella*) in an office setting by a disgruntled employee and one in Oregon by a religious sect that led to nearly 1000 cases of *Salmonella*-related gastroenteritis.[11,76] These agents are indeed ideal for small-scale attacks since large-scale attacks would require contamination of large water supplies which, because of enormous dilution factors and susceptibility of all these agents (except for *C. parvum*) to standard chlorinating procedures, would decrease the number of bacteria to below that required to infect large numbers of people.[69]

Occasional outbreaks of nontyphoidal *Salmonella* and *Shigella* infections occur in the United States. *Shigella* is a highly infectious organism that requires very low numbers (10^2–10^3 organisms) to provoke clinical disease. The illness caused by *Shigella* and enterohemorrhagic *E. coli* is explosive and starts with fever, vomiting, severe abdominal cramping, bloody diarrhea, and systemic manifestations such as hypotension, and circulatory collapse if not treated rapidly. Both microorganisms produce an exotoxin responsible for most of the systemic manifestations associated. A distinct complication, hemolytic uremic syndrome, occurs in a small percentage of cases, being more common in children younger than 10 years of age, leading to renal failure and hemolysis. *Salmonella* is less infectious and less explosive than *Shigella*, and leads to fever, vomiting, diarrhea, abdominal cramping, and in some cases to typhoidal manifestations. Imported cases of *V. cholerae* have been diagnosed in the United States in the past. However, the disease occurs in southern Asia and Latin America as large outbreaks. The clinical illness is characterized by explosive watery diarrhea that leads to rapid dehydration and circulatory collapse.

C. parvum infections are characterized by watery diarrhea and abdominal cramping for 2 to 3 weeks. The disease is self-limited except in patients with acquired immunodeficiency syndrome (AIDS) or other conditions of compromise, in whom illness can last for months or years if immune function is not restored. *C. parvum* is resistant to standard chlorine concentrations in water supplies.[77] The largest outbreak in this country occurred in Milwaukee in the early 1990s and was responsible for thousands of cases and increased mortality among those with AIDS.[69,78,79]

Category B Toxins

This section addresses other toxins considered of potential BT use, such as staphylococcal enterotoxin B (SEB) and ricin toxin (derived from castor beans, which in turn are the fruit of the *Ricinus communis* plant).

Ricin Toxin (Castor Beans from *Ricinis communis* Plants)

The ricin toxin is composed of two glycoproteins of approximately 66,000 kDa.[80] The toxin inhibits protein synthesis by blocking elongation factor 2 (EF2) at the ribosomal level. Ricin toxin is not a weapon of mass destruction since its lethal dose in humans is much higher than previously believed. However, the use of the toxin in small BT attacks is possible in the tropics because of its ready availability and relatively easy extraction from the beans. Clinical presentation depends on the route of administration as does the LD_{50}. In cases where large amounts of the toxin are ingested, the manifestations include nausea, vomiting, severe abdominal cramping, rectal hemorrhage, and diarrhea. As the clinical course progresses, anuria, mydriasis, severe headaches, and shock supervene leading to the patient's demise in 2 to 3 days. Clinical manifestations usually appear within 10 hours after ingestion of the toxin. Inhalational exposure leads to prominent pulmonary manifestations 8 to 28 hours after exposure and fever, dyspnea, progressive cough, cyanosis, and death. Histologically, there is widespread necrosis of pulmonary parenchyma and pulmonary edema. A single case of parenteral intoxication was documented. A defector from Bulgaria was injected with a pellet containing ricin from a weapon disguised in an umbrella, resulting in local necrosis, regional lymphadenopathy, gastrointestinal hemorrhage, liver necrosis, nephritis, and DIC.[81]

Staphylococcus aureus Enterotoxin B

Staphylococcus aureus enterotoxin B (SEB) is a 28-kDa, heat-stable exotoxin produced by certain strains of *S. aureus* and is responsible for food poisoning after ingestion of the preformed exotoxin in improperly handled food. In BT scenarios, exposure can occur either by inhalation or ingestion leading to SEB food poisoning or SEB respiratory syndrome. The toxin is highly incapacitating and not very lethal. The dose that causes symptoms in half of exposed persons and LD_{50} differ by a magnitude of 5 log scales for inhalational exposure.[82] Thus, it is thought of as an incapacitating agent.

Incubation time after ingestion is short (4–12 hours) followed by explosive vomiting that persists for several hours. Weaponization of the toxin as an aerosol is possible due to its high stability. Manifestations after inhalation of the SEB are related to the respiratory system and consist of fever, cough, chills, myalgias, chest pain, and pulmonary insufficiency due to alveolar edema. General symptoms and signs are universal and consist of multiorgan failure secondary to a cytokine storm.[25] These toxins are superantigens due to their ability to bind to major histocompatibility complex (MHC) class II molecules on large numbers of lymphocytes and macrophages, leading to a hyperactivation of the immune system and massive cytokine release including interferon-gamma (IFN-γ), tumor necrosis factor-alpha (TNF-α), interleukin (IL-6), and other mediators such as leukotrienes and histamine.[82]

DIAGNOSIS

The role of the clinical laboratory in the diagnosis of possible cases related to a BT attack is of utmost importance.[83,84] On the one hand, standard clinical microbiology laboratories will be receiving specimens for diagnostic purposes, and communication with clinicians regarding their suspicions is critical. Certain isolates in the laboratory are not pursued further (*Bacillus* spp. is a classic example) unless specifically requested due to the frequent isolation of contaminants with similar characteristics. In addition, handling of certain specimens will require added biosafety level requirements due to their infectivity (Table 119-2). Certain samples will have to be shipped to highly specialized laboratories for initial or further work-up. Environmental testing is challenging due to the complexity of the samples to be analyzed.[85,86] This type of testing takes place in highly specialized laboratories and is not undertaken by the standard clinical microbiology laboratory.

Conventional and Molecular Diagnosis of Potential BT Agents

General Principles

The bacterial diseases caused by the BT agents outlined in this chapter, with the exception of *C. burnetii* and *Rickettsia* spp., can be diagnosed by standard isolation techniques in clinical microbiology laboratories. Isolation of rickettsiae and the BT viruses requires specialized laboratories with BSL-3 or BSL-4 biocontainment.[87] Serological assays are available for detection of antibodies against all BT agents. However, for many organisms serological assays require the presence of rising antibody titers, and therefore the serologic diagnosis is usually retrospective in nature. For some viral diseases, a reliable diagnosis can be established based on elevation of immunoglobulin M (IgM) titers in the acute phase of the disease.

With the advent of molecular techniques, rapid and sensitive diagnostic tests are becoming available for BT agents during the acute phase of the disease.[88–90] This is of utmost importance in a BT event since identification of the first cases would be critical for a rapid and effective public health response. In addition, treatment and prophylactic measures can also be initiated as quickly as possible. Molecular diagnostic techniques can be applied to potential BT agents in an additional setting: as part of the epidemiological and forensic investigations that a BT attack would immediately trigger. Postmortem diagnosis is also possible by analysis of frozen or paraffin-embedded tissues by immunohistology or nucleic acid–based amplification techniques.

Rapid diagnosis of the initial case (cases) in a BT event requires a high degree of clinical suspicion from the physicians having contact with such patients in the emergency room or outpatient setting. The clinical laboratories would then play a critical role in detecting the suspected agent and/or referring the appropriate specimens to higher level laboratories for specialized testing (Table 119-3).[83,85,91]

Several of the agents discussed in this chapter are zoonotic diseases. Therefore, diagnosis of certain zoonotic diseases in animals may be important in identifying some BT attacks. In such situations, animals could be seen as either direct victims of the attack or as sentinel events in a human outbreak. There are currently efforts to establish a network of laboratories dedicated to diagnosis of veterinary agents.[85]

Table 119-2 Biosafety in Microbiologic and Biomedical Laboratories

Level	Definition	Examples
BSL-1	Suitable for work involving well-characterized agents not known to cause disease in healthy adult humans and of minimal potential hazard to laboratory personnel and the environment.	*Bacillus subtilis* *Naegleria gruberi* Canine hepatitis virus
BSL-2	Suitable for work involving agents of moderate potential hazard to personnel and the environment. Laboratory personnel have specific training in handling pathogenic agents and are directed by competent scientists; access to the laboratory is limited when work is being conducted; extreme precautions are taken with contaminated sharp items; and certain procedures in which infectious aerosols or splashes may be created are conducted in biological safety cabinets or other physical containment equipment.	Measles virus *Salmonella* spp. Toxoplasma spp. Hepatitis B virus
BSL-3	Suitable for work with infectious agents which may cause serious or potentially lethal disease as a result of exposure by the inhalation route. In addition to the requirements described for work in BSL-2 environment, all procedures are conducted within biological safety cabinets, or other physical containment devices, and by personnel wearing appropriate personal protective clothing and equipment. Laboratory should be located in a separate building or an isolated zone within a building. Laboratories are equipped with double door entry, directional inward flow, and single-pass air.	*Coxiella burnetii* *Rickettsia* spp. *M. tuberculosis* Alphaviruses
BSL-4	Required for work with dangerous and exotic agents that pose a high individual risk of aerosol-transmitted laboratory infections and life-threatening disease. Members of the laboratory staff have specific and thorough training in handling extremely hazardous infectious agents. They are supervised by competent scientists who are trained and experienced in working with these agents. Access to the laboratory is strictly controlled by the laboratory director. The facility is either in a separate building or in a controlled area within a building, which is completely isolated from all other areas of the building. All activities are confined to Class III biological safety cabinets, or Class II biological safety cabinets used with one-piece positive pressure personnel suits ventilated by a life support system. The Biosafety Level 4 laboratory has special engineering and design features to prevent microorganisms from being disseminated into the environment.	Filoviruses Arenaviruses

Table 119-3 Laboratory Response Network for Bioterrorist Attacks

Level	Functions
A	Community level laboratories that should recognize the clues of a possible bioterrorist agent and be able to package samples and ship them for confirmation at the upper-level laboratories.
B	State and county public health laboratories with capacity to work with BSL-2 and some with BSL-3 agents. Capable of isolation of some of the agents, presumptive level testing, and antibiotic susceptibility profiles.
C	Greater BSL-3 capabilities than level B and molecular testing capabilities for rapid identification.
D	Highest level of containment (BSL-4) for isolation and identification of highly pathogenic viruses.

Diagnosis of Specific BT Agents

Bacillus anthracis

The diagnosis of inhalational anthrax is based on isolation and identification of *B. anthracis* from a clinical specimen collected from an ill patient. In cases of inhalational anthrax, samples of sputum, blood, or cerebrospinal fluid (CSF) may yield growth of the agent. Demonstration of *B. anthracis* from nasal swabs has more epidemiological and prophylactic implications than clinical importance. Standard diagnostic techniques are based on visualization and isolation in the clinical microbiology laboratory and serological demonstration of antibodies against *B. anthracis*.[92–96]

Visualization of *B. anthracis* from clinical specimens (blood cultures, CSF, and cutaneous lesions) by Gram stains is not difficult. *B. anthracis* appears as large gram-positive, spore-forming rods with a bamboo appearance. Isolation is achieved by inoculating standard sheep blood agar plates, and colonies appear as small, gray-white, nonhemolytic colonies. A selective medium (polymyxin-lysozyme-EDTA-thallous acetate agar) is available mostly for environmental samples and inhibits the growth of other *Bacillus* spp., such as *B. cereus*. Growth is rapid (24–48 hours).[93] Confirmatory tests include γ-phage lysis, detection of specific cell wall and capsular antigens, and polymerase chain reaction (PCR) amplification of DNA followed by sequencing.[90]

Serological tests available for clinical diagnosis are based on detection of antibodies directed against protective antigen (PA). Cross-reactive antibodies decrease the specificity of this test. Assays based on toxin detection are available in specialized centers and are based on capture of anthrax toxins by using antibodies. Antibody-coated immunomagnetic beads are then analyzed by electrochemiluminescence technology. The analytical sensitivity of this technique for detection of anthrax toxin is at the picogram to femtogram level (10^{-12} to 10^{-15}).[97,98] Immunoliposomal technology combined with real-time PCR (for a DNA reporter sequence) is also in the early stages of development for several toxins (ricin, cholera, and botulinum) and appears promising with analytical sensitivity in the attomolar to zeptomolar (10^{-18} to 10^{-21}) range for cholera toxin.[99] The specificity of this assay is given by the toxin-capturing antibody.

Nucleic acid amplification techniques (PCR) are also available both in standard format and real-time format. Extraction of DNA from spores is challenging and requires modification of DNA extraction protocols in order to facilitate release of DNA from spores or induction of germination prior to DNA extraction.[90] Real-time PCR tests have been developed by Applied Biosystems (TaqMan 5' nuclease assay) and Roche Applied Science (LightCycler).[100–102] The analytical sensitivity of both techniques is extremely high, and testing times have been decreased to 1 to 2 hours. Portable PCR instruments are being developed for rapid deployment to the field.[103] Examples include the rugged advanced pathogen identification device (RAPID),[100] the Smartcycler (Cepheid, CA),[101] and the miniature analytical thermal cycler instrument (MATCI) developed by the Department of Energy's Lawrence Livermore National Laboratory.[104] This instrument later evolved into the advanced nucleic acid analyzer (ANAA) and handheld advanced nucleic acid analyzer (HANAA).[105]

Molecular subtyping of *B. anthracis* is also possible by using the 16S ribosomal RNA (rRNA) subunit gene, multiple-locus vari-able number tandem repeat analysis of eight genetic loci, and amplified fragment length polymorphism (AFLP) techniques.[106,107]

Environmental testing also plays a role in the investigation of a BT event. In this setting, detection of *B. anthracis* relies heavily on molecular techniques for confirmation of potentially contaminated samples (e.g., surfaces, air).[108,109]

Postmortem diagnosis is also possible by using Gram stains on paraffin-based tissues or immunohistochemical procedures using polyclonal or monoclonal antibodies against various anthrax antigens.

Yersinia pestis

Diagnosis of *Y. pestis* is based on demonstration of the bacillus in blood or sputa from patients. Standard diagnostic techniques in the laboratory include visualization of gram-negative coccobacilli, which by Giemsa, Wright, or Wayson stains reveal a "safety pin" appearance. Isolation is performed in blood and McConkey agar plates on which colonies appear as nonlactose fermentors. The organisms are identified preliminarily by direct immunofluorescent assay with *Y. pestis*–specific antibodies, with final identification based on biochemical profiles in clinical microbiology laboratories.[110]

Molecular diagnostic techniques based on real-time PCR have become available in recent years and involve detection of *Y. pestis* genes such as plasminogen activator (*pla*), genes coding for the Yop proteins and the capsular F1 antigen, and the 23S rRNA gene, which allows distinction from other *Yersinia* spp.[111–113] Assays have been developed to detect resistance to particular antibiotics. The importance of these diagnostic techniques in a disease such as plague is evident. The log-normal epidemic curve with a narrow dispersion of the incubation periods (see Fig. 119-1) and the short interval for successful antibiotic therapy mandate recognition of the earliest cases if the bulk of the exposed are to be saved. Molecular subtyping of *Y. pestis* is also possible by analyzing polymorphic sites in order to identify the origin of strains in the event of a BT attack.

Francisella tularensis

Diagnosis is made in the clinical laboratory by demonstration of the microorganisms in secretions (sputa, exudates) by direct immunofluorescence or immunohistochemically in biopsy specimens. Isolation in the clinical laboratory may be achieved by using regular blood agar plates, posing a risk to laboratory personnel not employing BSL-3 facilities and procedures.

The procedure for isolation of *F. tularensis* in the laboratory is very similar to that described for *Y. pestis*. Final identification in the clinical laboratory is based on the biochemical profile.[114] Molecular diagnostic techniques are based on PCR detection of *F. tularensis* by using primers for different genes such as outer membrane protein (*Fop*) or *tul4* and real-time detection systems.[90,115,116]

Smallpox Virus

Diagnosis of variola major is suggested by its clinical presentation and the visualization of Guarnieri bodies in skin biopsy samples. Preliminary confirmation requires visualization of the typical brick-shaped orthopox virus by electron microscopy, followed by isolation from clinical specimens and accurate molecular identification to differentiate it from the morphologically (and sometimes clinically) similar monkeypox virus. Confirmation of this diagnosis is performed only under BSL-4 containment facilities at the CDC.[47]

Molecular techniques are based on PCR amplification using real-time or standard technology followed by sequencing or use of restriction fragment length polymorphism (RFLP) for accurate identification.[117] Technologies so far developed for smallpox molecular testing include Taqman- and LightCycler-based assays with primers designed for the hemagglutinin gene and A-type inclusion body proteins.[118–121]

Sequencing of the smallpox genome has been completed for some Asian strains of variola major and one of variola minor. Other strains are being sequenced and will provide more information for probe design and treatment targets.[90]

Viral Hemorrhagic Fevers

Diagnosis of these diseases is performed in highly specialized centers in the United States because special isolation procedures and highly contained laboratories are required.

Initial diagnosis of these diseases is suspected on clinical and epidemiologic grounds. Laboratory diagnosis involves isolation, electron microscopy, and serological assays. Immunohistochemical detection of hemorrhagic fever viral antigens in paraffin-embedded tissues is also performed in highly specialized centers such as the CDC.[122–126]

Molecular diagnostic techniques have also improved dramatically during the last few years. Serum or blood is the most common specimen used for reverse transcriptase–PCR amplification of viral nucleic acids. Both standard and real-time techniques are available.

Design of primers for this heterogenous group of RNA viruses that are highly variable is one of the limitations.[90] Therefore, multiplex PCR techniques are required to detect as many targets as possible in a single assay.[127,128] Real-time PCR based on detection of the target sequence using fluorescent probes therefore limits the number of targets that can be identified because of the limited wavelength range for fluorescent applications (usually only four different wavelengths can be detected at the same time).[128–130] The use of microchips containing several thousands of oligonucleotides from all viruses known to be pathogenic to humans is an encouraging development. In fact, the rapid identification and characterization of the novel human coronavirus responsible for the SARS outbreak in 2003 is an excellent example of the power of hybridization-based microchips.

The creation of an automated and easily deployable instrument capable of detecting all possible potential BT agents based on highly sensitive techniques such as electrochemoluminescence (ECL) or PCR would be ideal. The nonspecific nature of presenting symptoms is a major problem with several of the agents. The rapid recruitment of cases into the infected cohort requires that an early diagnosis of the epidemic be established, particularly for organisms such as *Y. pestis* in which there is only a short window for successful treatment. In fact, such projects are already in the making. An example of this system is the Automated Biological Agent Testing System (ABATS) that combines the techniques mentioned previously.[86] The system is the result of integrating several commercially available technologies into a single automated and robotized instrument for detection of viruses, bacteria, and parasites considered potential BT agents. The technologies incorporated into this "super system" include automated specimen preparation (both nucleic acid–based and protein-based such as immunodiagnostics), thermocyclers for PCR detection, chemiluminescent detectors for immunobased assays, sequencers, and software programs for sequence analysis.

Category B Agents

Rickettsia prowazekii (Epidemic Typhus) and *R. rickettsii* (Rocky Mountain Spotted Fever)

Diagnosis of these infections in the clinical microbiology laboratory currently rests on the identification of antibodies in serum during the acute and convalescent period in order to demonstrate seroconversion or rising titers. The diagnosis is therefore retrospective.[131,132] Detection of rickettsial DNA from blood or skin samples during the acute phase of the disease is possible via PCR assays. However, these assays are not standardized and are not commercially available. Primers have been designed for amplification of several rickettsial genes including citrate synthase, 17-kDa protein gene, OmpA, and OmpB.[132–136] The clinical sensitivity and specificity of standard or real-time PCR techniques have not been determined. Most likely real-time PCR is superior due to the higher analytical sensitivity of this technique and low risk of sample contamination with DNA amplicons when compared to standard PCR amplification methods.

Isolation of rickettsiae from clinical specimens is performed in very few specialized laboratories in the nation and requires the use of cell monolayers, embryonated eggs, or animals. Detection of rickettsial antigens or whole bacteria in blood specimens is theoretically possible by using ultrasensitive methods, but such assays are currently only in the early phases of development. Immunohistochemical detection of rickettsiae in paraffin-embedded tissue has also been applied to tissue samples obtained pre- or postmortem.[137–139]

Salmonella spp., *Shigella dysenteriae*, *Vibrio cholerae*, and *Cryptosporidium parvum* (Acute Enteric Syndromes)

Diagnosis of *Salmonella*, *Shigella*, and *Vibrio* infections is based on isolation of the offending agent on standard microbiological media in the clinical laboratory, followed by specialized confirmatory tests to identify the specific serotype involved.[140] Diagnosis of *C. parvum* is based on visual identification of the protozoan in fecal specimens by using modified trichrome stain.[140]

Coxiella burnetii (Q Fever)

The diagnosis rests on serological demonstration of antibodies by immunofluorescent assay (IFA) or enzyme-linked immunosorbent assay (ELISA). Antibodies remain elevated for years after the acute infection, and therefore a fourfold rise in titers is the gold standard for diagnosis. PCR detection of *C. burnetii* DNA from blood or tissues also yields a diagnosis of Q fever.[88]

Brucella spp.

Diagnosis of brucellosis requires a high degree of clinical suspicion due to the protean manifestations related to this disease. Laboratory diagnosis is based on isolation of the microorganism from blood, bone marrow, or other tissue samples. Isolation is not easy due to the slow-growth of *Brucella* spp. Colonies usually appear after 4 to 6 weeks, and therefore communication with the clinical laboratory is important so that appropriate media will be used and the cultures will be held long enough for colonies to be detected.[90] Serologic assays for demonstration of rising antibody titers are available, although the diagnosis is retrospective. PCR detection is promising, but it is not standardized.[141–143]

Alphaviruses (Encephalitic Syndromes: Venezuelan, Eastern, and Western Equine Encephalomyelitis)

Diagnosis is based on isolation of the virus from serum or brain (postmortem specimens) in a BSL-3 environment. PCR detection of viral sequences is also possible. Serologic diagnosis is based on demonstration of antibodies in acute and convalescent sera.[144–146]

Botulinum Toxins

The diagnosis of botulism relies heavily on clinical parameters. An afebrile patient with signs and symptoms of progressive bulbar palsies and descending neuromuscular paralysis is highly suspected of having botulism. Demonstration of the toxin in cases of botulism due to ingestion of contaminated food is made from gastric samples, feces, blood, and urine. However, detection of minute amounts of toxin (and contacts with samples from cases may prove fatal due to the toxin's potency) would be difficult by current immunoassay systems such as ELISA platforms.[146] Detection techniques based on electrochemiluminescence and immunoliposomes are currently under development.[99,147] PCR assays can be performed in cases of ingestion of contaminated food in order to detect the genetic material present in *C. botulinum*. If weaponized toxin is used in the absence of *C. botulinum* organisms, detection of the genetic material would be difficult and would rely on the presence of residual DNA after toxin purification procedures. If inhalational botulism is suspected, respiratory secretions and nasal swabs should be obtained as early as possible. Postmortem samples of liver and spleen can be used for detection of botulinum toxins.

Ricin Toxin

Diagnosis is also based on clinical presentation and requires a high index of suspicion due to the nonspecific nature of the signs and symptoms. Laboratory diagnosis rests on detection of the toxin in body fluids by immunoassays (capture ELISA and IgG ELISA).[146] A new generation of tests using more sensitive detection methods is under development (see preceding discussion).

Staphylococcal Enterotoxin B

Diagnosis is also suspected on clinical grounds and confirmed by demonstration of the toxin in nasal swabs early in the disease process, feces, and, in fatal cases, from kidney and lung tissue. Serum can be analyzed by ELISA, and PCR can be performed for detection of toxin genes of *S. aureus* if present.[146]

REFERENCES

1. Sartwell P: The distribution and incubation periods of infectious diseases. Am J Hyg 51:310–318, 1950.
2. Buehler JW, Berkelman RL, Hartley DM, et al: Syndromic surveillance and bioterrorism-related epidemics. Emerg Infect Dis 9:1197–1204, 2003.
3. Khan AS, Ksiazek T, Peters CJ: Viral hemorrhagic fevers. Semin Pediatr Infect Dis 8:64–73, 1997.
4. Hughes JM, Gerberding JL: Anthrax bioterrorism: Lessons learned and future directions. Emerg Infect Dis 8:1013–1014, 2002.
5. Jernigan DB, Raghunathan PL, Bell BP, et al: Investigation of bioterrorism-related anthrax, United States, 2001: Epidemiologic findings. Emerg Infect Dis 8:1019–1028, 2002.
6. Marty AM: History of the development and use of biological weapons. In Marty AM (ed): Laboratory Aspects of Biowarfare. Philadelphia, WB Saunders, 2001, pp 421–434.
7. Christopher GW, Cieslak TJ, Pavlin JA, et al: Biological warfare. A historical perspective [see comment]. JAMA 278:412–417, 1997.
8. Marty AM: Preface. In Marty AM (ed): Laboratory Aspects of Biowarfare. Philadelphia, WB Saunders, 2001, pp xv–xvii.
9. Pavlin JA: Epidemiology of bioterrorism. Emerg Infect Dis 5:528–530, 1999.
10. Burkle FM Jr: Mass casualty management of a large-scale bioterrorist event: An epidemiological approach that shapes triage decisions. Emerg Med Clin North Am 20:409–436, 2002.
11. Torok TJ, Tauxe RV, Wise RP, et al: A large community outbreak of salmonellosis caused by intentional contamination of restaurant salad bars. JAMA 278:389–395, 1997.

12. Lombardo J, Burkom H, Elbert E, et al: A systems overview of the Electronic Surveillance System for the Early Notification of Community-Based Epidemics (ESSENCE II). J Urban Health 80:i32–i42, 2003.
13. Bales ME, Dannenberg AL, Brachman PS, et al: Epidemiologic response to anthrax outbreaks: Field investigations, 1950–2001. Emerg Infect Dis 8:1163–1174, 2002.
14. Jernigan JA, Stephens DS, Ashford DA, et al: Bioterrorism-related inhalational anthrax: The first 10 cases reported in the United States. Emerg Infect Dis 7:933–944, 2001.
15. Traeger MS, Wiersma ST, Rosenstein NE, et al: First case of bioterrorism-related inhalational anthrax in the United States, Palm Beach County, Florida, 2001. Emerg Infect Dis 8:1029–1034, 2002.
16. Grinberg LM, Abramova FA, Yampolskaya OV, et al: Quantitative pathology of inhalational anthrax I: Quantitative microscopic findings. Mod Pathol 14:482–495, 2001.
17. Meselson M, Guillemin J, Hugh-Jones M, et al: The Sverdlovsk anthrax outbreak of 1979. Science 266:1202–1208, 1994.
18. Walker DH, Yampolska O, Grinberg LM: Death at Sverdlovsk: What have we learned? Am J Pathol 144:1135–1141, 1994.
19. Inglesby TV, Henderson DA, Bartlett JG, et al: Anthrax as a biological weapon: Medical and public health management. Working Group on Civilian Biodefense [see comment; erratum appears in JAMA 283(15):1963, 2000]. JAMA 281:1735–1745, 1999.
20. Inglesby TV, O'Toole T, Henderson DA, et al: Anthrax as a biological weapon, 2002: Updated recommendations for management [see comment; erratum appears in JAMA 288:1849, 2002]. JAMA 287:2236–2252, 2002.
21. Fritz DL, Jaax NK, Lawrence WB, et al: Pathology of experimental inhalation anthrax in the rhesus monkey. Lab Invest 73:691–702, 1995.
22. Zaucha GM, Pitt LM, Estep J, et al: The pathology of experimental anthrax in rabbits exposed by inhalation and subcutaneous inoculation. Arch Pathol Lab Med 122:982–992, 1998.
23. Vasconcelos D, Barnewall R, Babin M, et al: Pathology of inhalation anthrax in cynomolgus monkeys (*Macaca fascicularis*). Lab Invest 83:1201–1209, 2003.
24. Barakat LA, Quentzel HL, Jernigan JA, et al: Fatal inhalational anthrax in a 94-year-old Connecticut woman [see comment]. JAMA 287:863–868, 2002.
25. Franz DR, Jahrling PB, Friedlander AM, et al: Clinical recognition and management of patients exposed to biological warfare agents. JAMA 278:399–411, 1997.
26. Mayer TA, Bersoff-Matcha S, Murphy C, et al: Clinical presentation of inhalational anthrax following bioterrorism exposure: Report of 2 surviving patients [see comment]. JAMA 286:2549–2553, 2001.
27. Nalin DR: Recognition and treatment of anthrax [comment]. JAMA 282:1624–1625, 1999.
28. Abramova FA, Grinberg LM, Yampolskaya OV, et al: Pathology of inhalational anthrax in 42 cases from the Sverdlovsk outbreak of 1979. Proc Natl Acad Sci USA 90:2291–2294, 1993.
29. Guarner J, Jernigan JA, Shieh WJ, et al: Pathology and pathogenesis of bioterrorism-related inhalational anthrax [see comment]. Am J Pathol 163:701–709, 2003.
30. Butler T: *Yersinia* species, including plague. In Mandell G, Bennett JE, Dolin R (eds): Principles and Practice of Infectious Diseases. Philadelphia, Churchill Livingstone, 2000, pp 2406–2414.
31. Butler T: *Yersinia* infections: Centennial of the discovery of the plague bacillus [see comment]. Clin Infect Dis 19:655–661; quiz 662–663, 1994.
32. McEvedy C: The bubonic plague. Sci Am 258:118–123, 1988.
33. Harris S: Factories of Death. London, Routledge, 1994.
34. Franz DR, Jahrling PB, McClain DJ, et al: Clinical recognition and management of patients exposed to biological warfare agents. Clin Lab Med 21:435–473, 2001.
35. Inglesby TV, Dennis DT, Henderson DA, et al: Plague as a biological weapon: Medical and public health management. Working Group on Civilian Biodefense [see comment]. JAMA 283:2281–2290, 2001.
36. Gani R, Leach S: Epidemiologic determinants for modeling pneumonic plague outbreaks. Emerg Infect Dis 10:608–614, 2004.
37. Chu MC, Weyant R, Robbin S: *Francisella* and *Brucella*. In Murray PR, Jorgensen JH, Pfaller MA, et al (eds): Manual of Clinical Microbiology, 8th ed. Washington, DC, ASM Press, 2003, pp 789–808.
38. Martin G, Aileen M: Clinicopathologic aspects of bacterial agents. In Marty AM (ed): Laboratory Aspects of Biowarfare. Philadelphia, WB Saunders, 2001, pp 513–548.
39. Dennis DT, Inglesby TV, Henderson DA, et al: Tularemia as a biological weapon: Medical and public health management [see comment]. JAMA 285:2763–2773, 2001.
40. Evans ME: *Francisella tularensis*. Infect Control 6:381–383, 1995.
41. Evans ME, Gregory DW, Schaffner W, et al: Tularemia: A 30-year experience with 88 cases. Medicine 64:251–269, 1985.
42. Deria A, Jezek Z, Markvart K, et al: The world's last endemic case of smallpox: Surveillance and containment measures. Bull World Health Org 58:279–283, 1980.
43. Arita I: Virological evidence for the success of the smallpox eradication programme. Nature 279:293–298, 1979.
44. Arita I, Wickett J, Nakane M: Eradication of infectious diseases: Its concept, then and now. Japan J Infect Dis 57:1–6, 2004.
45. Fenner F, Arita I, Jezek Z, et al: Smallpox and Its Eradication. Geneva, World Health Organization, 1988.
46. O'Toole T: Smallpox: An attack scenario [see comment]. Emerg Infect Dis 5:540–546, 1999.
47. Henderson DA, Inglesby TV, Bartlett JG, et al: Smallpox as a biological weapon: Medical and public health management. Working Group on Civilian Biodefense. JAMA 281:2127–2137, 1999.
48. Guarner J, Johnson BJ, Paddock CD, et al: Monkeypox transmission and pathogenesis in prairie dogs. Emerg Infect Dis 10:426–431, 2004.
49. Baker RO, Huggins JW: Potential antiviral therapeutics for smallpox, monkeypox, and other orthopox virus infections. Antiviral Res 57:13–23, 2003.
50. Dixon C: Smallpox. Boston, J & A Churchill, 1962.
51. Bausch DG, Ksiazek TG: Viral hemorrhagic fevers including hantavirus pulmonary syndrome in the Americas. Clin Lab Med 22:981–1020, 2002.
52. Bronze MS, Huycke MM, Machado LJ, et al: Viral agents as biological weapons and agents of bioterrorism. Am J Med Sci 323:316–325, 2002.
53. Borio L, Inglesby T, Peters CJ, et al: Hemorrhagic fever viruses as biological weapons: Medical and public health management [see comment]. JAMA 287:2391–2405, 2002.
54. Peters CJ, Zaki SR: Role of the endothelium in viral hemorrhagic fevers. Crit Care Med 30:S268–S273, 2002.
55. Sellin LC: The action of botulinum toxin at the neuromuscular junction. Med Biol 59:11–20, 1981.
56. Middlebrook JF: Botulinum toxins. In Sidell FR, Takafuji ET, Franz DR (eds): Medical Aspects of Chemical and Biological Warfare. Washington, DC, Borden Institute, 1997, pp 643–654.
57. Weaver SC, Ferro C, Barrera R, et al: Venezuelan equine encephalitis. Ann Rev Entomol 49:141–174, 2004.
58. Hart KL, Keen D, Belle EA: An outbreak of eastern equine encephalomyelitis in Jamaica, West Indies. I: Description of human cases. Am J Trop Med Hyg 13:331–334, 1964.
59. Hayes R: Eastern and western equine encephalitis. In Beran G (ed): Handbook Series in Zoonoses: Viral Zoonoses. Boca Raton, FL, CRC Press, 1981, p 29.
60. Franck PT, Johnson KM: An outbreak of Venezuelan equine encephalomeylitis in Central America. Evidence for exogenous source of a virulent virus subtype. Am J Epidemiol 94:487–495, 1971.
61. Martin DH, Eddy GA, Sudia WD, et al: An epidemiologic study of Venezuelan equine encephalomyelitis in Costa Rica, 1970. Am J Epidemiol 95:565–578, 1972.
62. Johnson KM, Martin DH: Venezuelan equine encephalitis. Adv Vet Sci Comparative Med 18:79–116, 1974.
63. Zinsser H: Rats, Lice and History. Boston, Little, Brown 1935.
64. Walker DH, Dumler JS: Rickettsial infections. In Lack EE (ed): Pathology of Infectious Diseases. Stamford, CT, Appleton & Lange, 1997, pp 789–799.
65. Walker DH: Rocky Mountain spotted fever and other rickettsioses. In Medoff G (ed): Mechanisms of Microbial Disease. Baltimore, Williams & Wilkins, 1998, pp 268–274.
66. Patterson KD: Typhus and its control in Russia, 1870–1940. Med Hist 37:361–381, 1993.
67. Walker DH, Popov VL, Wen J, et al: *Rickettsia conorii* infection of C3H/HeN mice. A model of endothelial-target rickettsiosis. Lab Invest 70:358–368, 1994.
68. Raoult D, Roux V: Rickettsioses as paradigms of new or emerging infectious diseases. Clin Microbiol Rev 10:694–719, 1997.
69. Moran G: Threats in bioterrorism II: CDC category B and C agents. Emerg Med Clin North Am 20:311–330, 2002.

70. Raoult D, Tissot-Dupont H, Foucault C, et al: Q fever 1985–1998. Clinical and epidemiologic features of 1,383 infections [see comment]. Medicine 79:109–123, 2000.
71. Maurin M, Raoult D: Q fever. Clin Microbiol Rev 12:518–553, 1999.
72. Tissot-Dupont H, Raoult D, Brouqui P, et al: Epidemiologic features and clinical presentation of acute Q fever in hospitalized patients: 323 French cases [see comment]. Am J Med 93:427–434, 1992.
73. Young EJ: Human brucellosis. Rev Infect Dis 5:821–842, 1983.
74. Young EJ: An overview of human brucellosis. Clin Infect Dis 21:283–289; quiz 290, 1995.
75. Hoover DFA: Brucellosis. In Sidell FR, Takafuji ET, Franz DR (eds): Medical Aspects of Chemical and Biological Warfare. Washington, DC, Borden Institute, 1997, pp 513–521.
76. Kolavic SA, Kimura A, Simons SL, et al: An outbreak of *Shigella dysenteriae* type 2 among laboratory workers due to intentional food contamination. JAMA 278:396–398, 1997.
77. Brasseur P, Uguen C, Moreno-Sabater A, et al: Viability of *Cryptosporidium parvum* oocysts in natural waters. Folia Parasitol 45:113–116, 1998.
78. Kramer MH, Herwaldt BL, Craun GF, et al: Surveillance for waterborne-disease outbreaks—United States, 1993–1994. MMWR Surveill Summ 45:1–33, 1996.
79. Cicirello HG, Kehl KS, Addiss DG, et al: Cryptosporidiosis in children during a massive waterborne outbreak in Milwaukee, Wisconsin: Clinical, laboratory and epidemiologic findings. Epidemiol Infect 119:53–60, 1997.
80. Franz DJ: Ricin toxin: In Sidell FR, Takafuji ET, Franz DR (eds): Medical Aspects of Chemical and Biological Warfare. Washington, DC, Borden Institute, 1997, pp 631–642.
81. Crompton R, Gall D: Georgi Markor—Death in a pellet. Med Leg J 48:51–62, 1980.
82. Ulrich RS, Taylor TJ: Staphylococcal enterotoxin B and related pyrogenic toxins. In Sidell FR, Takafuji ET, Franz DR (eds): Medical Aspects of Chemical and Biological Warfare. Washington, DC, Borden Institute, 1997, pp 621–630.
83. Klietmann WF, Ruoff KL: Bioterrorism: Implications for the clinical microbiologist. Clin Microbiol Rev 14:364–381, 2001.
84. Jortani SA, Snyder JW, Valdes R Jr: The role of the clinical laboratory in managing chemical or biological terrorism. Clin Chem 46:1883–1893, 2000.
85. Pavlin JA, Gilchrist MJ, Osweiler GD, et al: Diagnostic analyses of biological agent-caused syndromes: Laboratory and technical assistance. Emerg Med Clin North Am 20:331–350, 2002.
86. Byrne KM, Fruchey IR, Bailey AM, et al: Automated biological agent testing systems. Expert Rev Mol Diagn 3:759–768, 2003.
87. Richmond JY, McKinney RW: Health Biosafety in Microbiological and Biomedical Laboratories, 4th ed. Washington, DC, U.S. Department of Health and Human Services, Public Health Service, 1999.
88. Krafft AE, Kulesh DA: Applying molecular biological techniques to detecting biological agents. Clin Lab Med 21:631–660, 2001.
89. Henchal EA, Teska JD, Ludwig GV, et al: Current laboratory methods for biological threat agent identification. Clin Lab Med 21:661–678, 2001.
90. Firmani MA, Broussard LA: Molecular diagnostic techniques for use in response to bioterrorism. Expert Rev Mol Diagn 3:605–616, 2003.
91. Gilchrist MJ: A national laboratory network for bioterrorism: Evolution from a prototype network of laboratories performing routine surveillance. Mil Med 65(7 Suppl 2):28–31, 2000.
92. Turnbull PC: Definitive identification of *Bacillus anthracis*—A review. J Appl Microbiol 87:237–240, 1999.
93. Logan NT: PC *Bacillus* and other aerobic endospore-forming bacteria. In Murray PR, Baron EJ, Jorgensen JH, et al (eds): Manual of Clinical Microbiology. Washington, DC, ASM Press, 2003, pp 445–460.
94. Kozel TR, Murphy WJ, Brandt S, et al: mAbs to *Bacillus anthracis* capsular antigen for immunoprotection in anthrax and detection of antigenemia. Proc Natl Acad Sci USA 101:5042–5047, 2004.
95. Quinn CP, Semenova VA, Elie CM, et al: Specific, sensitive, and quantitative enzyme-linked immunosorbent assay for human immunoglobulin G antibodies to anthrax toxin protective antigen. Emerg Infect Dis 8:1103–1110, 2002.
96. Biagini RE, Sammons DL, Smith JP, et al: Comparison of a multiplexed fluorescent covalent microsphere immunoassay and an enzyme-linked immunosorbent assay for measurement of human immunoglobulin G antibodies to anthrax toxins. Clin Diagn Lab Immunol 11:50–55, 2004.
97. Rivera VR, Merrill GA, White JA, et al: An enzymatic electrochemiluminescence assay for the lethal factor of anthrax. Anal Biochem 321:125–130, 2003.
98. Yu H: Comparative studies of magnetic particle-based solid phase fluorogenic and electrochemiluminescent immunoassay. J Immunol Methods 218:1–8, 1998.
99. Mason JT, Xu L,Sheng ZM, et al: High-sensitivity detection of biological toxins. In Department of Defense Military Health Research Forum, 2004. San Juan, Puerto Rico, U.S. Army Medical Research and Materiel Command, 2004, p 30.
100. Higgins JA, Cooper M, Schroeder-Tucker L, et al: A field investigation of *Bacillus anthracis* contamination of U.S. Department of Agriculture and other Washington, DC, buildings during the anthrax attack of October 2001. Appl Environ Microbiol 69:593–599, 2003.
101. Higgins JA, Ibrahim MS, Knauert FK: Sensitive and rapid identification of biological threat agents. Ann NY Acad Sci 894:130–148, 1999.
102. Bell CA, Uhl JR, Hadfield TL, et al: Detection of *Bacillus anthracis* DNA by LightCycler PCR [see comment]. J Clin Microbiol 40:2897–2902, 2002.
103. Higgins JA, Nasarabadi S, Karns JS, et al: A handheld real time thermal cycler for bacterial pathogen detection. Biosens Bioelectron 18:1115–1123, 2003.
104. Ibrahim MS, Lofts RS, Jahrling PB, et al: Real-time microchip PCR for detecting single-base differences in viral and human DNA. Anal Chem 70:2013–2017, 1998.
105. Belgrader P, Benett W, Hadley D, et al: Rapid pathogen detection using a microchip PCR array instrument. Clin Chem 44:2191–2194, 1998.
106. Dalton R: Genetic sleuths rush to identify anthrax strains in mail attacks. Nature 413:657–658, 2001.
107. Sacchi CT, Whitney AM, Mayer LW, et al: Sequencing of 16S rRNA gene: A rapid tool for identification of *Bacillus anthracis*. Emerg Infect Dis 8:1117–1123, 2002.
108. Teshale EH, Painter J, Burr GA, et al: Environmental sampling for spores of *Bacillus anthracis*. Emerg Infect Dis 8:1083–1087, 2002.
109. Sanderson WT, Stoddard RR, Echt AS, et al: *Bacillus anthracis* contamination and inhalational anthrax in a mail processing and distribution center. J Appl Microbiol 96:1048–1056, 2004.
110. Bockemuhl J, Wong JD: *Yersinia*. In Murray PR, Baron EJ, Jorgensen JH, et al (eds): Manual of Clinical Microbiology. Washington, DC, ASM Press, 2003, pp 673–683.
111. Trebesius K, Harmsen D, Rakin A, et al: Development of rRNA-targeted PCR and in situ hybridization with fluorescently labelled oligonucleotides for detection of *Yersinia* species. J Clin Microbiol 36:2557–2564, 1998.
112. Higgins JA, Ezzell J, Hinnebusch BJ, et al: 5' nuclease PCR assay to detect *Yersinia pestis*. J Clin Microbiol 36:2284–2288, 1998.
113. Perry RD, Fetherston JD: *Yersinia pestis*—Etiologic agent of plague. Clin Microbiol Rev 10:35–66, 1997.
114. Chu MC, Weyant RS: *Francisella* and *Brucella*. In Murray PR, Baron EJ, Jorgensen JH, et al (eds): Manual of Clinical Microbiology. Washington, DC, ASM Press, 2003, pp 789–808.
115. Higgins JA, Hubalek Z, Halouzka J, et al: Detection of *Francisella tularensis* in infected mammals and vectors using a probe-based polymerase chain reaction. Am J Trop Med Hyg 62:310–318, 2000.
116. Emanuel PA, Bell R, Dang JL, et al: Detection of *Francisella tularensis* within infected mouse tissues by using a hand-held PCR thermocycler. J Clin Microbiol 41:689–693, 2003.
117. Ropp SL, Jin Q, Knight JC, et al: PCR strategy for identification and differentiation of small pox and other orthopoxviruses. J Clin Microbiol 33:2069–2076, 1995.
118. Olson VA, Laue T, Laker MT, et al: Real-time PCR system for detection of orthopoxviruses and simultaneous identification of smallpox virus. J Clin Microbiol 42:1940–1946, 2004.
119. Meyer H, Ropp SL, Esposito JJ: Gene for A-type inclusion body protein is useful for a polymerase chain reaction assay to differentiate orthopoxviruses. J Virol Methods 64:217–221, 1997.
120. Ibrahim MS, Esposito JJ, Jahrling PB, et al: The potential of 5′ nuclease PCR for detecting a single-base polymorphism in orthopoxvirus. Mol Cell Probes 11:143–147, 1997.
121. Espy MJ, Cockerill IF, Meyer RF, et al: Detection of smallpox virus DNA by LightCycler PCR. [Erratum appears in J Clin Microbiol 40(11):4405, 2002.] J Clin Microbiol 40:1985–1988, 2002.
122. Hooper P, Zaki S, Daniels P, et al: Comparative pathology of the diseases caused by Hendra and Nipah viruses. Microbes Infect 3:315–322, 2001.

TRAVELERS' DIARRHEA

S. L. Gorbach wrote that "travel expands the mind and loosens the bowels."[73] Several studies have shown that diarrhea is the most frequent health impairment among travelers to developing countries, affecting one- to two-thirds of all travelers.[74–77] Among those who become ill, 30% will remain in bed and another 40% will have to curtail their activities.[73] In general, countries with higher standards of living present lower risks of travelers' diarrhea.[76–79] Although all age groups are at risk, the incidence is highest among the very young, presumably due to increased fecal-oral contamination[80]; those with decreased gastric acidity[81]; and those in the 15- to 29-year-old age group, probably because of their adventurous lifestyle and ingestion of larger amounts of potentially contaminated foods.[76,82,83] Bacterial pathogens are the most frequent cause of travelers' diarrhea, particularly enterotoxigenic *Escherichia coli* (ETEC), enteroadherent *E. coli* (EAEC), and *Shigella, Salmonella,* and *Campylobacter* species[84] (see Table 120-1). However, the prevalence of each organism varies according to season and destination. For example, *Campylobacter* (increasingly fluroquinolone resistant) is the most frequent cause of travelers' diarrhea in areas of Southeast Asia, notably Thailand, whereas ETEC is the most frequent cause of diarrhea in most other developing destinations.[79] When counseling travelers about diarrhea, several issues must be considered: food and water precautions, chemoprophylaxis, self-treatment of illness, and immunization.[61]

Food and Water Precautions

Unpeeled fruits, uncooked vegetables, and food that has been cooked or stored at insufficiently hot or cold temperatures, respectively, are believed to be the main sources of enteric pathogens for the traveler. An additional important source is unpurified water and ice cubes made from it. Tap water and ice cubes should be avoided unless there are strong assurances of proper treatment. Organisms in contaminated ice will survive concentrations of alcohol found in drinks mixed with tequila and whisky.[85] Since swallowed water can lead to infection, swimming in water that is contaminated by sewage should also be avoided.[86]

Tea or coffee is safe if consumed hot. Commercially bottled, carbonated beverages are highly recommended since carbonation results in an acid pH that will effectively kill bacteria over a period of several days.[86] Unpasteurized milk and milk products should be avoided.[87] If safe beverages are not available, travelers may need to disinfect water from potentially contaminated sources. Since almost all enteropathogens are readily killed at 100°C, bringing water to a boil is sufficient for disinfection.[88] Tap water "too hot to touch" has not been shown to be reliably disinfected; even in situations in which a low inoculum of organisms may be transmitted, such as in toothbrushing, bottled water is to be preferred.

Although not effective for resistant cysts such as *Cryptosporidium,* chemical disinfection with the halogens iodine or chlorine is an otherwise effective method of water purification. Two drops (0.1 mL) of 5% chlorine bleach or four drops of 2% tincture of iodine should be added to a liter of water and allowed to stand for 30 minutes at room temperature (20°C) before using.[86] Commercial tablets and iodine crystals serve the same purpose; however, it is important to note that colder water temperature and turbidity will inhibit the purification process, necessitating a longer contact time.[88,89] Various new products containing, for example, chlorine dioxide (Pristine), appear to be more effective and better tolerated than standard halides and, with sufficient contact time, will eradicate *Cryptosporidium* cysts.[90]

Unlike the straightforward approaches to water and beverage precautions, avoidance of contaminated food entails considerably more restrictions. Raw foods are best avoided. Not only should food be well cooked but also it should be served hot. Reheated foods may not be safe because of the presence of preformed heat-stable toxins. Since vegetables are not infrequently grown in "night soil" (human excrement used for fertilizer) or washed with fecally contaminated water before display, they should be well cooked or treated adequately. Only fruit that can be peeled by the traveler should be eaten. Pastries are an excellent source of substrates for bacterial proliferation.

It should be noted that the location where meals are taken is important. Studies from Mexico have shown that the incidence of travelers' diarrhea is higher when food is purchased from street vendors or restaurants or eaten at the homes of locals than when travelers prepare their own meals.[91]

Unfortunately, many studies have shown that education regarding food and water precautions has a decidedly low efficacy in the prevention of travelers' diarrhea. In one study, stricter observance of precautions was associated with a greater likelihood of acquiring diarrhea, explained by a recall bias.[92] In a subsequent prospective study, 98% of international travelers committed dietary indiscretions within 3 days; the incidence of diarrhea was proportional to the number of "mistakes" made.[93] If one considers the standard precautions outlined previously, it is clear that flawless observance may be virtually impossible, particularly among vacationers, who, wanting to relax and indulge in local cuisine, are more likely to be noncompliant with food precautions. For this reason, the concepts of chemoprophylaxis and self-treatment have gained popularity in recent years. One particularly insightful colleague noted, "Boil it, peel it, cook it, or forget it—easy to remember, impossible to do" (Lawrence Green, personal communication, 1995).

Chemoprophylaxis

Given the high risk of travelers' diarrhea and the difficulty in maintaining food and water precautions, a variety of pharmacologic interventions have been evaluated to prevent this illness. Since bacterial pathogens account for the majority of episodes of travelers' diarrhea,[94–96] antibiotics and bismuth subsalicylate (BSS) have been the focus of testing for its prevention (Table 120-3).

BSS, an insoluble salt of bismuth and salicylic acid, is hydrolyzed in the stomach to bismuth oxychloride and salicylate. The exact mechanism of its action is not completely understood, but it appears to involve both antimicrobial activity linked to the bismuth moiety and antisecretory activity associated with the salicylate portion.[97,98] Studies of BSS have shown a protective effect of up to 65% with the liquid form, 60 mL four times per day (4.2 g/day), or tablet form, two tablets four times per day (2.1 g/day).[99] BSS is generally safe but should be avoided in those with salicylate hypersensitivity or in those

Table 120-3 Antimicrobial and Nonantimicrobial Prophylaxis of Travelers' Diarrhea

Drug	No.	Dose	Location	Protection (%)
Antibiotics				
TMP-SMX	87	1 DS mg qd	Mexico	71–95
Trimethoprim	145	200 mg qd	Mexico	59
Doxycycline	44	100 mg qd	Mexico	68
Mecillinam	22	200 mg qd	Honduras	76
Bicozamycin	30	500 mg qd	Egypt	100
Norfloxacin	120	400 mg qd	Mexico	88
Norfloxacin	127	200 mg qd	Mexico	
			Africa, Asia, Latin America	68
Norfloxacin	222	400 mg qd	Eqypt	93
Ciprofloxacin	54	500 mg qd	Tunisia	94
Ciprofloxacin	21	250 mg qd	Asia	100
Nonantibiotics				
Bismuth subsalicylate	120	60 mL or 2 tablets qid	Mexico	65
Lactobacillus GG	160	2 × 10^9 CFU	Morocco	39
Saccharomyces boulardii	350	6.7 × 10^9 CFU	Africa, Asia, Middle East	26

CFU, colony-forming units; DS, double-strength tablet (trimethoprim 160 mg/sulfamethoxozole 800 mg); TMP-SMX, trimethoprim-sulfamethoxazole.

already taking salicylates, anticoagulants, or antihyperuricemic drugs. Also, BSS interferes with absorption of doxycycline, which may be used for malaria, rickettsial, and leptospiral chemoprophylaxis and for treatment. Studies of the use of lactobacilli to prevent travelers' diarrhea have shown minimal or no efficacy.[100–103] The protective efficacy of antibiotics for travelers' diarrhea varies with the season and geographic area visited, which in turn determine the likely pathogens and degree of antibiotic resistance.[104] The widespread use and abuse of antimicrobial agents globally has resulted in the emergence of resistant organisms, particularly enteric pathogens.[79] Previously used antibiotics for the prophylaxis of travelers' diarrhea, such as doxycycline and trimethoprim sulfa, are no longer recommended due to significant bacterial resistance in most areas of the world.

In view of their activity against most bacterial enteropathogens, quinolone antibiotics—notably ciprofloxacin, gatifloxacin, levofloxacin, and ofloxacin—have become the agents of choice for the prevention and treatment of travelers' diarrhea. Protective efficacy has ranged from 88% to 94% in various areas of the world.[105–107] However, reports of quinolone resistance are increasing. In Thailand and Egypt, approximately 90% and 50%, respectively, of *Campylobacter* isolates were resistant to ciprofloxacin but sensitive to azithromycin.[108,109] Quinolone resistance rates among travelers with diarrhea, however, were markedly lower.[84] Although toxicity from quinolones remains low, these agents can cause central nervous system symptoms, which potentially could be aggravated by antimalarials such as chloroquine or mefloquine and may augment xanthine or theophylline toxicity. Also, they are not recommended for children or pregnant women. However, a number of travel medicine and pediatric infectious disease experts use very short-term quinolone regimens for self-treatment in children who develop travelers' diarrhea. Rifaximin, a nonabsorbable antibiotic, was approved by the U.S. Food and Drug Administration (FDA) for use as treatment for bacterial diarrhea.[110,111] Comparative trials have shown that rifaximin is equally effective as quinolone antibiotics for this use.[112] There is no approved indication for use of this drug for the prophylaxis of travelers' diarrhea, although some consider it useful, especially since a significant number of travelers may suffer from prolonged postinfectious irritable bowel syndrome.[113–115]

The indications for antibiotic prophylaxis of travelers' diarrhea are controversial since it is well established that self-treatment regimens are highly effective in shortening the course of illness.[116,117] Routine use of antibiotic prophylaxis in travelers' diarrhea has not been endorsed by the National Institute of Health Consensus Development Conference,[74] and this view was reiterated at a meeting of travelers' diarrhea experts. Even strong advocates of chemoprophylaxis do not recommend its routine use.[118–121] Prophylaxis with BSS, a quinolone antibiotic, or rifaximin may be considered for less than 3 weeks' duration for the following groups of travelers: those who repeatedly develop diarrhea during their travels, those with diminished protective gastric acidity, those who cannot afford incapacity for even 1 day (e.g., athletes, military personnel, and businesspeople), and those with an underlying medical disorder for whom travelers' diarrhea may be poorly tolerated (e.g., those suffering from inflammatory bowel disease, brittle insulin-dependent diabetes mellitus, chronic renal failure, or AIDS, although the last group should take extra care to avoid such potentially devastating infections as cryptosporidiosis, not prevented by antimicrobial agents). Vaccine development against travelers' diarrhea has focused on preventing ETEC since it is responsible for the majority of cases. Because of the similarity between the cholera toxin and heat-labile toxin of ETEC, efficacy studies of the oral cholera B subunit whole-cell vaccine to prevent travelers' diarrhea have been performed. Field trials showed an overall protective efficacy of 23%, which increased to 52% when ETEC was isolated and to 60% when ETEC was associated with another pathogen. This cross-protection was extremely short-lived, lasting less than 3 months.[122] However, those receiving this cholera vaccine must still use food and water precautions and carry an antibiotic for self-treatment of diarrhea due to other pathogens.

Self-Treatment

The overriding principle in the management of travelers' diarrhea is the maintenance of an adequate fluid and electrolyte balance. Rehydration can be achieved with tea with sugar,bottled soft drinks, juices, or electrolyte-containing oral rehydration solutions such as those formulated by WHO.[123,124] Because of damage to the intestinal lactase-producing cells by enteric pathogens, dairy products should be avoided during illness.

When dysenteric symptoms are absent, nonantibiotic preparations alone may be useful in the management of travelers' diarrhea. BSS 30 mL every 30 minutes for eight doses reduces diarrhea by 25%.[125] Loperamide up to 16 mg/24 hours reduces the duration of diarrhea by 42%[126] and is more effective than BSS[127] for diarrhea reduction and abdominal pain but less effective for nausea. However, loperamide should be avoided during bouts of dysentery, pragmatically defined as diarrhea with fever and/or blood admixed to the stools, unless used with an antibiotic. Kaolin- and pectin-containing agents are not very effective.[128] Therapy with lactobacilli or other probiotics has not been shown to be effective in modifying the course of travelers' diarrhea.[129]

Few would disagree that most travelers should carry an antimotility agent and an antibiotic for self-treatment of diarrhea that occurs during travel.[130,131] Many studies have shown that antimicrobial therapy leads to symptomatic improvement and a reduction in the duration of illness, particularly in those infected with ETEC and *Shigella*[116,117,132] (Table 120-4). Antimicrobial therapy of nontyphoidal salmonellosis remains controversial because of the potential for antibiotics to prolong convalescent excretion of the organism[133]; however, the duration of illness is decreased with the use of quinolones.[116] A theoretical concern remains that travelers may inadvertently self-treat with antibiotics when they have illness due to *E. coli* O157, but this organism rarely is a cause of travelers' diarrhea.

Quinolones, and in some cases azithromycin, have become the antibiotics of choice for self-treatment. Studies have shown single-dose therapy and 3- to 5-day courses to be equally effective, except when *Shigella dysenteriae* is the offending pathogen.[117,132,134–137] Loperamide does not appear to enhance the effect of ciprofloxacin.[117,138] A study of U.S. soldiers in Thailand has led to concern about the continued usefulness of quinolone antibiotics for the management of travelers' diarrhea because of *Campylobacter* resistance.[109] Although azithromycin was an efficacious alternative, the drug was less effective than ciprofloxacin against other pathogens. Two different studies in Mexico showed that rifaximin and azithromycin were as effective as ciprofloxacin for treatment of travelers' diarrhea.[112,139] More data are needed to confirm these results in different geographic areas.

Table 120-4 Treatment of Travelers' Diarrhea

Drug	Dose	Duration (Days)
Standard dose		
TMP-SMX	1 DS bid	3–5
Norfloxacin	400 mg bid	3–5
Ciprofloxacin	500 mg qd/bid	1–5
Ofloxacin	300 mg bid	3
Levofloxacin	500 mg qd	3
Azithromycin	500 mg qd	3
Bismuth subsalicylate	30 mL q 30 min for 8 doses	
Single dose		
Standard therapy		
TMP-SMX	4 DS	
Norfloxacin	800 mg	
Ciprofloxacin	500 mg–1 g	
Fleroxacin	400 mg	

TMP-SMX (DS, double strength), trimethoprim 160 mg/sulfamethoxazole 800 mg.

MALARIA

More than 30,000 North American and European travelers develop malaria each year.[140] Studies have shown that the majority of travelers who acquire malaria are VFRs.[141–143] They visit travel clinics infrequently for pretravel health advice and usually do not follow recommendations concerning antimalarial chemoprophylaxis. However, they often visit high-risk malarious areas, particularly sub-Saharan Africa. The risk of malaria per month of stay without prophylaxis is highest in sub-Saharan Africa and Oceania (1:50 to 1:1000) and during the past decade has increased more than fivefold in travelers to Kenya. The risk is intermediate (1:1000 to 1:12,000) in travelers to Haiti and the Indian subcontinent, and it is low (<1:50,000) in travelers to Southeast Asia and to Central and South America.[144] Of the 1200 to 1500 cases of malaria reported annually in the United States, most of those due to *Plasmodium falciparum* occur in travelers returning or immigrating from Africa and Oceania.[145] With the worldwide increase in chloroquine- and multidrug-resistant falciparum malaria, decisions on chemoprophylaxis have become more difficult. In addition, the spread of malaria due to primaquine- and chloroquine-resistant strains of *Plasmodium vivax* has added further complexity to the issue of malaria prevention and treatment.[146,147] Compliance with antimalarial chemoprophylaxis regimens and the use of personal protection measures to prevent mosquito bites are keys to prevention.[141] Several studies indicate that only approximately 50% of travelers adhere to basic recommendations for malaria prevention.[148–150] Travelers must be educated about the risk of malaria, personal protection measures against mosquito bites, appropriate chemoprophylaxis, symptoms of the disease, and measures to be taken in case of suspected malaria during travel. This approach is outlined in the checklist for travelers to malarious areas (Box 120-1). In order to make the previously discussed determinations, travel medicine advisors must conduct a careful review of the itinerary, including whether urban or rural areas will be visited, the length of stay, styleof travel, and a medical history, including allergies, previous experience with antimalarials, and the likelihood of pregnancy.

Personal Protection Measures

Anopheles mosquitoes, the vectors of malaria, are exclusively nocturnal in their feeding habits; protection from mosquito bites from dusk to dawn is highly effective in reducing the risk of

Box 120-1 Checklist for Advising Travelers to Malarious Areas: Key Issues to Be Considered

Risk of Malaria and the Presence of Drug-Resistant* Plasmodium falciparum *in the Area of Destination

- Antimosquito measures
  - Insect repellants
  - Knockdown insecticides
  - Bed nets
  - Long-sleeved shirts, trousers
- Chemoprophylaxis
  - Contraindications to use of antimalarials
  - Appropriate drug regimen
  - Need to start drug before travel, during exposure, and for 4 weeks after leaving the malaria-endemic area
  - If necessary, need for self-treatment
  - Adverse effects of antimalarials
  - Warning that malaria may develop despite chemoprophlaxis
  - Warning that fellow travelers or locals may recommend alternative drug regimens that may be less effective
- In case of illness, travelers should be informed about
  - Symptoms of malaria (unexplained fever, with or without headache, muscle aches, chills, weakness, vomiting, or diarrhea)
  - Need for prompt medical help if malaria is suspected since it may be fatal if treatment is delayed; for diagnosis, a blood sample should be examined on one or more occasions
  - Self-treatment in special circumstances, the need to take it only if prompt medical care is not available, and the need to seek medical advice as soon as possible after self-treatment

Adapted from World Health Organization: International Travel and Health. www.who.int.

infection (although *Aedes* mosquitoes carrying dengue fever virus bite during the day). When practical, travelers should wear protective clothing, such as long-sleeved shirts and long pants, when outside during evening hours. The most effective method of preventing mosquito bites is to combine a pesticide such as permethrin on clothing with an insect repellent containing DEET (diethymetaltoluamide) to exposed skin.[151] Although all concentrations of DEET (from 10% to 99.9%) are equally efficacious in preventing mosquito bites, the duration of action is proportional to the concentration (e.g., 30% DEET lasts 4 to 6 hours, whereas 99% DEET provides 8 to 10 hours of protection). Newer controlled-release formulations with lower concentrations of DEET provide prolonged protection.[152] DEET is well tolerated, but serious adverse reactions such as toxic encephalopathy have rarely occurred in very young children who were exposed to excessive amounts for extended periods.[153–156] The Environmental Protection Agency and the American Academy of Pediatrics have recommended that 30% DEET may be used in children 2 months of age or older.[157] This recommendation is not uniformly accepted by experts in all countries.[158] Also, DEET has been shown to be safe during the second and third trimesters of pregnancy.[159] Insect repellents should be applied sparingly to intact skin and washed off when there is no longer a risk of mosquito bites. Although the cosmetic product Skin-So-Soft has some repellent activity, it requires frequent (hourly) reapplication.[154,160] Picaridin has been shown to be equally effective as DEET.[161–163]

Efficacy rates of up to 80% in the prevention of malaria have been shown by using bed nets impregnated with permethrin.[164,165] A pyrethroid-based flying insect spray should be used to clear the bed net and room of mosquitoes. Where bed nets are not available, mosquito coils and other preparations of vaporized pyrethrum flowers have been shown to reduce mosquito bites.[166] A number of herbal products that have far less efficacy than DEET are sold in stores or on the Internet.

Chemoprophylaxis

Personal protective measures greatly reduce but do not eliminate the risk of malaria. Antimalarials are only suppressives, and they act on the hepatic or erythrocytic stage of the parasite, thereby preventing the clinical symptoms of disease but not infection. No drug guarantees protection against malaria. For this reason, travelers must be informed that any febrile illness that occurs during or soon after travel to a malaria-endemic area should be evaluated immediately by a health-care professional for malaria. Since in only one-third of patients in the United States and Canada who died from malaria was the diagnosis considered before death, it is incumbent upon travelers to inform their health-care provider of the risk of malaria and the need to have it ruled out regardless of the malaria prophylactic used.[167,168]

The choice of a drug regimen for chemoprophylaxis will be dependent on the individual's itinerary, length of stay, age, pregnancy status, use of other medications, general medical history (including previous experience with antimalarials), cost, and the estimation of the risk of drug side effects compared with the risk of developing malaria.[169–171] Antimalarials should be started 1 day to 2 weeks prior to entry to a malarious area, during exposure, and for some period of time after departure. Beginning some antimalarials early ensures an adequate blood concentration of the drug and enables travelers to change to alternative drugs should adverse effects occur. The postexposure period of prophylaxis for antimalarials such as chloroquine, mefloquine, and doxycycline is particularly important to enable the antimalarial to eradicate any organisms that are released from the liver into the bloodstream after departure from a malarious area. This may not apply to *P. vivax* and *Plasmodium ovale* infections, which often have dormant hypnozoites in the liver that may be released many months after the onset of infection. With other medications, such as atovaquone/proguanil and primaquine, this postexposure period may be shortened considerably because these drugs act on the hepatic phase.

The development of resistance to antimalarial drugs has seriously hampered the ability to prevent and treat infections.[172] Chloroquine-resistant *P. falciparum* infections have spread throughout the world except in areas of Central America, Haiti, and the Middle East[173] (see maps). Along the Thailand-Cambodia and Thailand-Myanmar borders, *P. falciparum* malaria is resistant to chloroquine and mefloquine.[174,175] Reports from the Indonesian archipelago and Oceania indicate considerable chloroquine-resistant *P. vivax* and *Plasmodium malariae*.[176,177] However, because of chloroquine-resistant *P. falciparum* in these areas, the problem of *P. vivax* resistance does not affect current recommendations for chemoprophylaxis.

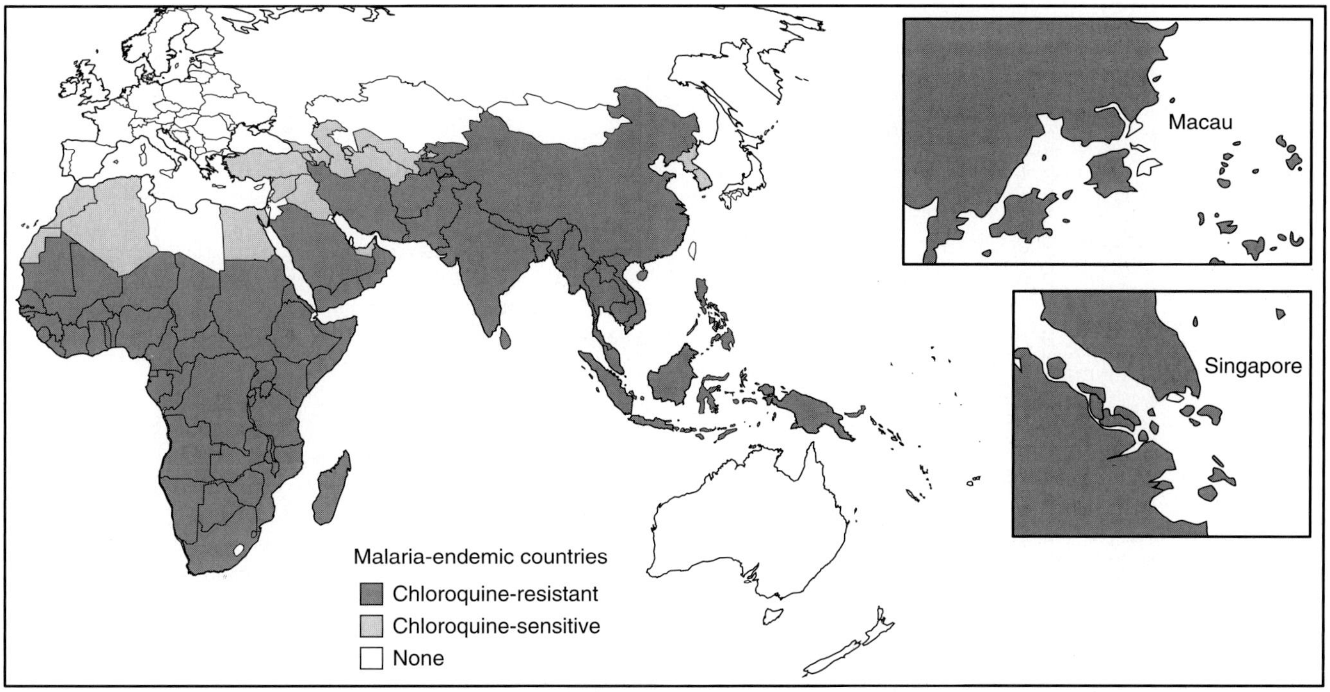

ANTIMALARIAL DRUGS

Table 120-5 lists the drugs, doses, and adverse effects of available drugs for malaria chemoprophylaxis and self-treatment.[178–180]

Chloroquine

Chloroquine is a 4-aminoquinolone that acts by inhibiting heme polymerase.[181] Although formulated as chloroquine phosphate in North America, it is used as a sulfate and hydrochloride salt elsewhere. Chloroquine is well tolerated and in appropriate doses may be safely used by young children and pregnant women.[182] Transient nausea or vomiting are seen in a small proportion of individuals and may usually be reduced by taking the drug with food. Occasionally, headaches or blurred vision are reported. Intense pruritus is well documented, almost exclusively in black Africans.[183,184] Although long-term chloroquine use can produce keratic precipitates, irreversible keratopathy does not occur in the

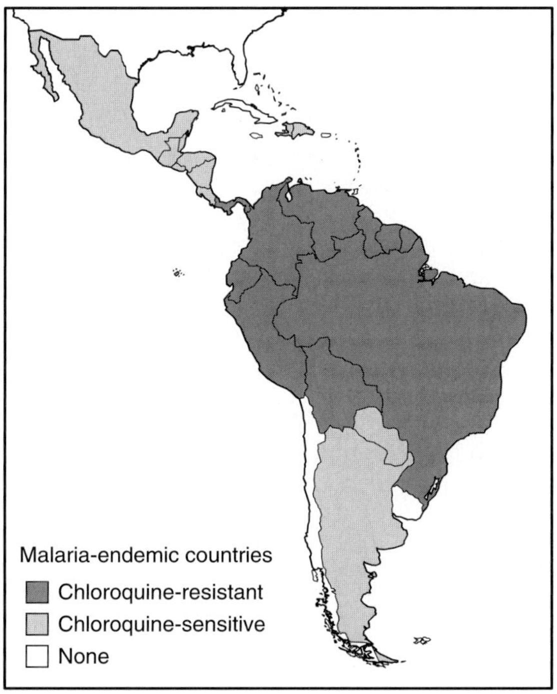

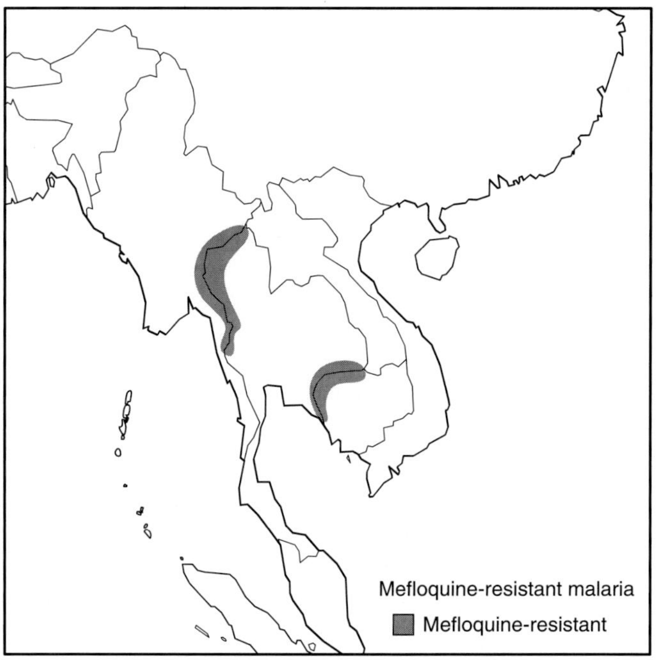

Table 120-5 Antimalarial Drugs for Chemoprophylaxis and Self-Treatment

Drug	Tablet Size	Adult Dose	Pediatric Dose	Side Effects
Prevention				
Atovaquone plus proguanil (Malarone) pediatric tablets	250 mg atovaquone plus 100 mg proguanil 62.5 mg atovaquone plus 25 mg proguanil	1 tablet daily —	11–20 kg: 1 pediatric tablet 21–30 kg: 2 pediatric tablets 31–40 kg: 3 pediatric tablets >40 kg: 4 pediatric tablets	Frequent: GI upset, headache Occasional: fever, rash, cough, insomnia
Chloroquine phosphate (Aralen)	150 mg base (250 mg salt) or 300 mg base (500 mg salt)	300 mg base (500 mg salt) once weekly	<1 yr: 37.5 mg base 1–3 yr: 75 mg base 4–6 yr: 100 mg base 7–10 yr: 150 mg base 11–16 yr: 225 mg base once weekly	Frequent: pruritis, nausea, headache Occasional: skin eruptions, reversible, corneal opacity, partial alopecia
Hydroxycholoroquine sulfate (Plaquenil sulfate)	310 mg base (400 mg salt)	310 mg base once weekly	5 mg/kg base	See above
Doxycycline	100 mg	100 mg once daily	<8 yr: contraindicated ≥8 yr: 2 mg/kg once daily (maximum 100 mg/day)	Frequent: gastrointestinal upset, vaginal candidiasis, photosensitivity Occasional: azotemia in renal disease Rare: allergic reactions, blood dyscrasias
Mefloquine (Lariam)	250 mg base	250 mg base once weekly	<15 kg: ~1/8 tablet 15–19 kg: ~1/4 tablet 20–30 kg: 1/2 tablet 31–45 kg: 3/4 tablet	Frequent: dizziness, nausea, diarrhea, headache, insomnia, strange dreams Occasional: depression, anxiety, irritability Rare: seizures, psychosis
Primaquine				
Prevention of *Plasmodium vivax* relapse	15 mg base	30 mg base/day for 14 days	0.5 mg base/kg/day for 14 days	Occasional: gastrointestinal upset, hemolysis secondary to glucose-6-phosphate dehydrogenase deficiency, methemoglobinemia
Prophylaxis	15 mg base	30 mg base/day	0.5 mg/kg/day	
Self-treatment				
Mefloquine	250 mg base	15 mg/kg in 2 divided doses 12 hr apart (or 1250 mg in 1 dose)	Same as adults	
Atovaquone plus	250 mg	500 mg bid × 3 days		Frequent: gastrointestinal upset, headache Occasional: fever, skin rash, cough
Proguanil (Atovaquone + proguanil = Malarone)	100 mg	200 mg/day × 3 days		Occasional: anorexia, nausea, diarrhea, mouth ulcers Rare: hematuria

doses used for malaria chemoprophylaxis. Chloroquine should be avoided in people with a history of epilepsy.[185] Chloroquine should be stored in childproof containers because as little as a single tablet can be fatal to an infant; overdosages should be reported to a physician immediately.

Mefloquine

Mefloquine is a 4-quinoline methanol compound that has a prolonged half-life of approximately 30 days[186]; steady-state levels are not reached for approximately 7 weeks, unless a loading dose is used. Comparative studies among travelers have shown that mefloquine is less well tolerated than other antimalarials, although only 5% of users have to stop the drug due to adverse events.[187,188] A study of malaria chemoprophylaxis in nonimmune travelers to sub-Saharan Africa showed that 40% of mefloquine and chloroquine/proguanil users suffered side effects that were significant enough to interfere with daily activities compared with approximately 30% for doxycycline or atovaquone/proguanil.[187] With mefloquine use, seizures and acute psychosis occur in 1:10,000 to 1:13,000 users.[189–192] Mefloquine is safe during the second half of pregnancy, and there is increasing evidence that it is safe during the first trimester as well.[193–196] However, due to increasing concerns about the neuropsychiatric adverse events, the FDA has required that all health providers distribute drug information with all mefloquine prescriptions.

Mefloquine is currently recommended for all age groups, including infants, at a dose of 5 mg/kg weekly (maximum, 250 mg).[197–199] Mefloquine is contraindicated in those with a history of seizures or psychiatric disorder, including depression or anxiety reaction. The drug should be used cautiously in anyone with a history of such problems. These adverse events tend to occur more frequently among women,[199–201] and they appear to be less common in children.[202] Although mefloquine has traditionally been advised with caution to those who require fine coordination and spatial discrimination, such as airline pilots, mountain climbers, and perhaps divers, there are no data in the literature to substantiate the need for this precaution. The drug should be used with caution in those who have a known cardiac conduction disturbance. It should not be used in those taking chloroquine or quinine-like drugs, including halofantrine.

Doxycycline

Doxycycline is a tetracycline derivative with a half-life of approximately 16 hours. Its major benefit is that it is effective against multidrug-resistant *P. falciparum* as well as *P. vivax*.

The most common adverse reactions to doxycycline are gastrointestinal disturbances and phototoxicity (exaggerated sunburn).[203,204] The former can be reduced by taking the drug with extra fluids and meals, and the latter can be reduced by using a sunscreen that absorbs ultraviolet (UV) A as well as UVB radiation. It is estimated that 2% to 15% of those using doxycycline will develop phototoxicity. Doxycycline should not be ingested while in the supine position because of the risk of esophageal ulceration caused by lodgment of the tablet in the distal esophagus. BSS (Pepto-Bismol) and antacids decrease doxycycline bioavailability. In addition, vaginal candidiasis is a very common and troublesome problem in female travelers; some advisors suggest carrying fluconazole for self-treatment as necessary. The drug is contraindicated in pregnant women and children younger than the age of 8 years.

Proguanil

Proguanil is a dihydrofolate reductase inhibitor that is not commercially available in the United States. In conjunction with chloroquine, it provides suboptimal protection in East Africa and even less in West Africa.[205] The drug has been used as an alternative to chloroquine in chloroquine-sensitive areas of the world. When combined with sulfisoxazole, it was very effective in preventing multidrug-resistant malaria in Thailand.[206,207] Side effects from proguanil include gastrointestinal upset and mouth ulcers, which occur in approximately 35% of users.[208]

Primaquine

Primaquine is an 8-aminoquinolone that has been shown to be a good second-line alternative for the prevention of all forms of malaria.[209] It has slightly lower protective efficacy against *P. falciparum* compared with the first-line agents (e.g., it has been shown to have 85% to 95% protective efficacy in studies in East Africa, Colombia, and Irian Jaya, Indonesia[205,210–214]). Unlike chloroquine, doxycycline, and mefloquine, primaquine acts on the primary exo-erythrocytic stage in the liver and eradicates dormant hypnozoites. For this reason, the drug may be discontinued soon after leaving the malarious area.

Primaquine may also be used as terminal prophylaxis to prevent relapses of *P. vivax* malaria when taken after departure from a malarious area. It is effective for this indication because it eradicates dormant hypnozoites in the liver. Terminal prophylaxis should be reserved for those who have had prolonged intense exposure outside of sub-Saharan Africa where there is little *P. vivax,* such as missionaries, overseas volunteers, and relief workers.

Primaquine is a potent oxidizing agent that causes hemolysis in people with glucose-6-phosphate dehydrogenase (G6PD) deficiency. The drug has been shown to produce mild (below toxic levels) methemoglobinemia when used for prolonged periods as prophylaxis in those with normal enzyme levels.[213] G6PD levels should be measured before primaquine is used, especially in those who are likely to be at risk for this enzyme deficiency (blacks, southern Europeans, and Asians). Gastrointestinal side effects may be reduced by taking the drug with food. Primaquine is contraindicated during pregnancy.

Atovaquone/Proguanil (Malarone)

The most recent addition to the armamentarium for the prophylaxis and treatment of malaria is the fixed combination or atovaquone and proguanil (250 mg of atovaquone/100 mg proguanil).[215–217] Atovaquone acts by interfering with the parasite mitochondrial membrane potential at the cytochrome *b–c1* complex.[218] Proguanil is metabolized to cycloguanil, which acts as a folate antagonist, and appears to act by enhancing the collapse of the malarial mitochondrial membrane. [219] Like primaquine, atovaquone/proguanil targets the liver and blood stages, but it does not eradicate the dormant hypnozoites. For this reason, the drug may be discontinued soon after leaving the malarious area. This combination is highly efficacious and is equivalent to mefloquine or doxycyline.[220–223] Adverse events include headache, gastrointestinal upset, insomnia, dizziness, and rash. Side effects are lowest among current recommended antimalarials; 0.2% to 1.2% of users discontinued the drug compared with 5% for mefloquine and 2% for chloroquine/proguanil.[187,188,224] The high cost of this excellent antimalarial is prohibitive for some users, especially for those visiting friends and relatives and for long-term travelers.

Recommended Regimens

Table 120-5 lists the recommended antimalarial drug regimens for travelers to malaria-endemic areas. For travel to chloroquine-sensitive areas, chloroquine is the drug of choice. Any of the other first-line drugs may be used as alternatives. However, many travelers prefer atovaquone/proguanil because it may be discontinued soon after departure. For travel to chloroquine-resistant *P. falciparum* areas, atovaquone/proguanil, doxycycline, and mefloquine are the first-line drugs of choice. Primaquine is a second-line drug for these travelers because of the need for a G6PD level prior to its use. For travel to chloroquine- and mefloquine-resistant areas (the Thailand-Cambodia and Thailand-Myanmar borders), atovaquone/proguanil and doxycycline are the drugs of choice. Regardless of the chemoprophylactic regimen recommended, it is important for travel health advisors to indicate to travelers that globally there is no uniformity concerning recommendations for malaria chemoprophylaxis and therefore they are likely to meet fellow travelers and health-care providers overseas who give conflicting advice as to the optimal regimen. Also, in many developing countries, particularly those in Africa, malaria is often overdiagnosed among travelers due to a high rate of false positivity of blood films.[225,226] Travelers should be advised to continue their antimalarial regimen even if they are told they have developed malaria while taking a recommended regimen. Travelers are advised not to purchase antimalarials in developing countries due to high rates of the manufacture and sales of counterfeit drugs.

Self-Treatment

People who are unable to tolerate effective antimalarials, who are in an area where drug resistance is frequent, or who are unable to obtain medical care in less than 48 hours may consider a self-treatment regimen. In many European countries, malaria chemoprophylaxis is not generally prescribed for travelers to most areas of Asia and Latin America wherever low endemicity prevails; instead, self-treatment regimens are routinely recommended. Unfortunately, however, there is evidence that those who carry self-treatment regimens often use them inappropriately.[227] Also, there is evidence that travelers who use the rapid diagnostic drug kits for malaria do not use them effectively.[228–230]

Few recommend a self-treatment drug in addition to chemoprophylactic medication. Drugs used for self-treatment should be different from the agent used for prophylaxis. Most travel medicine advisors recommend atovaquone/proguanil as the drug of choice for self-treatment. If atovaquone/proguanil is being used for prophylaxis and there is a high degree of suspicion for malaria, mefloquine or the combination of quinine and doxycycline may be used for self-treatment. Although the artemisinin derivatives are not available in North America, they are the most widely used and effective drugs for the treatment of malaria.

The global spread of drug-resistant malaria has stimulated the search for new approaches to the prevention and treatment of malaria. Several drugs are in the clinical trial stage and are promising alternatives to the current armamentarium. For example, on the horizon is a primaquine analogue, tafenoquine.[231] This drug has a long half-life and is 12 times more potent than primaquine as an antimalarial. A study in semiimmunes showed that three daily doses provided more than 90% protection for more than 3 months.[232,233] However, like primaquine, it is a potent oxidizing agent for which a G6PD level will be required prior to use. Unfortunately, a malaria vaccine for travelers, an ideal preventive strategy, is many years away.[234]

SEXUALLY TRANSMITTED DISEASES AND BLOOD-BORNE PATHOGENS

During international travel, people often feel a sense of anonymity, may be less sexually inhibited, and may therefore put themselves at greater risk for the acquisition of sexually transmitted diseases (STDs).[235–237] In a survey of 354 British travelers, 4.8% admitted to having casual sex while abroad compared with 6.4% of 484 Swiss travelers.[238] In another study, 5.6% of short-term travelers to Peru had casual sexual contact; only 70% were protected by condoms.[239] A Canadian study revealed that between 5% and 15% engaged in sex with a new partner during travel lasting approximately 1 month.[44] Long-term overseas workers appear to put themselves at even greater risk of acquiring STDs. Among Belgian men working in central Africa, 51% and 31% reported casual sex with local women or prostitutes, respectively.[240] In a study of 2000 Dutch expatriates working in sub-Saharan Africa, 31% of males and 13% of females had casual sexual contacts with African partners; consistent condom use was reported by fewer than 25% of those surveyed.[241]

The most effective ways to avoid STDs during travel are to abstain from sexual activity, have sexual relations with a well-known partner, or use safer sexual practices. These practices will only succeed in preventing infection if applied in each and every sexual encounter, especially when different partners are involved. The highest risk activity is with prostitutes; 90% of prostitutes in Nairobi and more than 50% of those in Bangkok are HIV infected.[242] Since precautions may fail because of condom breakage, having "safe sex" with a high-risk partner may still be dangerous. Some of the STDs that are very common in the developing world include gonorrhea, syphilis, chancroid, chlamydia infection, trichomoniasis, and viral infections such as hepatitis B, C, and HIV-1, HIV-2, and human T-cell lymphotropic virus type I.[236,237,243]

Since several of the pathogens mentioned previously may also be transmitted by exposure to blood and secretions, safer sexual practices are not the only way to avoid infection. People requiring injections overseas (e.g., travelers requiring updating of their immunizations or those with diabetes mellitus) should carry their own needles and syringes, particularly long-stay travelers who plan to visit remote areas. Those who plan to carry medical equipment should be aware that such items may be misconstrued by foreign officials as tools for illegal drug use. A note from a physician indicating why the items are being carried may prevent an uncomfortable or embarrassing situation at a border post. In case of serious accident or injury, all travelers should know their blood type, particularly if they are traveling with a group, which is considered to be a "safe" source of blood for transfusion. Although no guarantee of safety, blood received from expatriates or staff at embassies, consulates, or international agencies may be less risky with regard to HIV infection. In a study of U.S. travelers to developing countries, it was noted that medical care was sought by 8% of all travelers, of whom 17% received an injection.[46] The significance of this as a risk factor was highlighted by data that showed that in Southeast Asia and in the eastern Mediterranean approximately 80% of injections were given using nonsterile equipment.[45] Furthermore, there appear to be an increasing number of individuals who travel to developing countries for the purpose of having surgical procedures performed. Although the cost is often far less and the availability of donor tissue for transplants is far greater, these procedures are fraught with health hazards. For management of illnesses, surgery, or trauma that is not life threatening, but where blood products may be necessary, transportation to the home country or nearest developed country should be considered in situations in which blood cannot be accurately screened prior to transfusion. Travelers may wish to purchase insurance before departure to cover the enormous cost of being transported home or to specialized medical centers.

The HIV-Infected Traveler

The HIV-infected traveler is at increased risk of serious infections from a number of pathogens that may be more prevalent at travel destinations than at home. However, the degree of risk depends almost entirely on the state of the immune system at the time of travel. People with AIDS and others with immunodeficiency require special counseling before travel.[244–246]

Several countries continue to deny entry to HIV-positive people, even though there are no data that show that these restrictions decrease rates of transmission of the virus. In general, HIV testing has been required of those people who intend to stay longer than 3 months or who intend to work or study abroad. Some countries accept an HIV serologic test done within 6 months of departure, whereas others require that the test be done at the time of arrival.

Health insurance is highly recommended for HIV-positive travelers. Such policies should include trip cancellation and evacuation insurance in the event of illness.

Immunizations

In general, live attenuated vaccines are contraindicated for people with immune dysfunction. Exceptions to this rule include measles and yellow fever vaccines for those who must travel to high-risk areas. The HIV-infected person whose CD4 count is less than 200/μL should be discouraged from traveling to areas endemic for yellow fever.

Gastrointestinal Illness

Travelers' diarrhea is especially problematic in HIV-infected people because of decreased levels of gastric acid and abnormal gastrointestinal mucosal immunity. Salmonellosis, shigellosis, and campylobacterosis are likely to be more frequent, more severe, and more difficult to treat.[247–249] Both isosporiasis and cryptosporidiosis are greater risks in developing countries. Because of these potential problems, the HIV-infected traveler must take stringent food and water precautions.

Other Travel-Related Infections

Reports strongly suggest that HIV infection predisposes to more severe malaria infection, which may stimulate HIV replication. [250,251] There are few data on the interactions between antimalarial drugs and antiretroviral drugs, even though protease inhibitors share common hepatic pathways (e.g., cytochrome P-450). One unpublished study of healthy volunteers suggested that plasma levels of ritonavir decreased with concomitant use of mefloquine. Other vector-borne diseases, such as visceral leishmaniasis and Chagas' disease, may cause serious illness in HIV-infected travelers.[252–254] Precautions to avoid sandfly bites in the case of leishmaniasis and reduviid bug bites in the case of Chagas' disease should be undertaken. Tuberculosis is not usually of concern to the short-term HIV-infected traveler. However, histoplasmosis from caves and coccidioidomycosis in endemic areas are of concern because of their greater morbidity and mortality among HIV-infected people.[255,256]

Special Health Considerations for Travelers

Issues of chronic illness, disability, pregnancy, and travel with young children are beyond the scope of this article. However, excellent reviews of these subjects have been published.[257,258]

Mortality

Despite the emphasis on pretravel advice on prevention of infection, deaths from infection are relatively uncommon.[5–9] In a study of 421 deaths among Australian travelers, only 10 (2.4%) were attributed to infection, and in a Scottish study involving 952 people who died abroad, infection occurred in only 34 (3.6%).[8,9] Cardiovascular disease is the most common cause of death in travelers, accounting for 35% to 69% of deaths.

Motor Vehicle Accidents and Injuries

Trauma is by far the most important preventable cause of death in travelers.[5–9] Injury deaths, particularly from motor vehicle accidents, account for 21% to 26% of deaths that occur during travel. As expected, when those with cardiovascular disease are compared with those who had injuries or accidents, there is a marked preponderance of older people in the former group and younger people in the latter. Motor vehicle accidents can be reduced by advising travelers to avoid travel by road in rural areas at night, overcrowded public vehicles, and riding on motorcycles.

Bites and Stings

Arthropods and Insects

Although malaria is the most important vector-borne infection in travelers, there are others that require attention. Of these, dengue is an increasing problem. The past decade has seen a dramatic rise globally in dengue, particularly in the Caribbean, Central and South America, and Southeast Asia.[259–261] This has been reflected by a marked increase in travelers.[262] In fact, a study from Sweden reported that 1:3500 travelers to the Malay peninsula become infected.[263] The infection is transmitted by the *Aedes* mosquito, which prefers an urban and often indoor habitat. This mosquito bites during the day, particularly in the hours of the early morning and late afternoon. In addition to insect precautions, some vector-borne diseases can be prevented by prophylactic medication. For example, loaiasis can be prevented by taking 300 mg (adult dose) of diethylcarbamazine once each week while in a very heavily infested area, such as Central or West Africa.[264] Unfortunately, diethylcarbamazine is no longer available in the United States, except from the CDC drug service, which will provide it to clinicians who are treating documented cases. Tick- and mite-borne typhus, relapsing fever, bartonellosis, and plague can be prevented by using doxycycline prophylaxis 100 mg/day during exposure.[265] For the most part, prophylaxis of these infections is not recommended except for a very select group of individuals at high risk. Chagas' disease, transmitted by the night-biting reduviid bug, can be prevented by the use of a bed net and by avoiding sleeping in thatched huts and/or those with mud and stick walls.

Travelers who walk through undergrowth or have close contact with animals are at risk of tick infestation. Tick-transmitted diseases include Lyme disease, ehrlichiosis, relapsing fever, tularemia, typhus, and Congo-Crimean hemorrhagic fever. The risk of a tick bite can be reduced by wearing long sleeves and pants, tucking the latter into socks, and by using effective insect repellents such as DEET. Permethrin clothing spray will protect against tick bites for 2 weeks or more. Finally, a "tick check" of the entire skin should be performed each night by the traveler.

Venomous scorpions are found in many areas of the developing world. Children are at particular risk of dying from a scorpion bite.[266,267] The risk of a scorpion sting can be reduced by shaking out boots, shoes, blankets, sleeping bags, and clothing before use; consistently and properly using a mosquito net; wearing shoes when walking at night; not putting one's hands blindly into ground holes, wood piles, and so on; wearing gloves when cleaning rocks or debris; and removing debris from around housing and camping areas.

Animal and Snakebites

Although many travelers worry most about bites from snakes and spiders, it is the dog bite that is a much more common and potentially fatal problem. Mouth flora from domestic animals may cause overwhelming infections (e.g., *Pasturella multocida*) in those who are splenectomized. Consideration should be given to providing such travelers with an antibiotic that may be used in the event of a bite. In many countries, a significant proportion of stray dogs carry rabies, a uniformly fatal disease.[64] In addition to receiving preexposure rabies immunization, the more practical approach is to avoid petting or touching animals, particularly dogs, in rabies-endemic areas. Animal bites, licks, or scratches require prompt and careful management.

Snakebites are a major problem among populations forced to live and work, relatively unprotected, within the snake's chosen environment.[268] By avoiding high-risk situations, most travelers can avoid being bitten. Snake charmers should be observed at a considerable distance. Travelers should be advised not to disturb, corner, or attempt to handle a snake; even a severed head can strike. Walking in undergrowth or deep sand without boots, socks, and long trousers should be avoided. Flashlights should be used at night; unlit paths are particularly dangerous after rainstorms. Other prohibitions include the collection of firewood or movement of logs or boulders with bare hands and putting one's hand or a stick into burrows, holes, or crevices.

Diseases Transmitted by Soil and Water

Schistosomiasis is a helminthic disease that infects more than 200 million people worldwide in areas of South America, the Caribbean, Africa, the Middle East, and Southeast Asia. To avoid schistosomiasis, travelers should be advised to stay out of freshwater in most developing countries. Swimming in the ocean or freshwater pools without snails is safe. Travelers who cannot control their urge to swim in freshwater should confine themselves to the middle of a lake. After emerging from potentially contaminated water, travelers should dry off quickly in an attempt to prevent skin penetration by the parasite. By allowing infested water to stand for 48 hours, the infectivity of the schistosome larvae in the water will be eliminated. Studies strongly suggest that DEET in a lipid formulation prevents cercarial penetration and therefore may be a practical approach in the prevention of infection when schistosome-infested water cannot be avoided.[269–271]

Leptospirosis is another risk associated with freshwater flooding and ecotourism. Infection can be prevented in unavoidable high-risk situations by taking doxycycline 200 mg per week.[272]

Walking barefoot exposes the traveler to a variety of hazards, including tungiasis (the sand flea), snakebites, cutaneous larva migrans from larvae of the dog and cat hookworm, human hookworm infection, and strongyloidiasis. Sandals provide only partial protection.

Adaptation to the Environment

Excessive sun exposure can cause erythema and sunburn, chemical hypersensitivity, eye damage, bleaching of skin, and predisposition to skin cancers, including malignant melanoma.[273,274] The effects of UV irradiation can be minimized by the use of sunscreens that either absorb or block harmful UV light. UVB radiation (290- to 320-nm wavelength) is the major cause of sunburn and chronic skin damage, whereas UVA radiation (320 to 400 nm) is the cause of most sensitivity reactions. The efficacy of a sunscreen in the prevention of UVB damage may be determined by the sun protection factor (SPF) assigned to it. The SPF indicates how long one can stay in the sun without burning. Although sunscreens with an SPF 15 offer 93% protection, travelers are advised to use higher SPF values because of the tendency to apply too little, too late.[275–279] Data are conflicting concerning the effect of concomitant use of sunscreens and insect repellents. One study showed a 33% decrease in sun protection,[280] whereas another showed no effect of sunscreen on insect repellent efficacy.[281]

Travelers who are taking drugs such as a tetracycline or sulfonamides, which can cause photosensitivity reactions, should use a sunscreen that contains benzophenones or protects

226. Holtz TH, Onikpo F, Lama M, et al: Malaria microscopy in eight secondary health care facilities in Oueme, Abstract 546 P 332. Meeting of the American Society of Tropical Medicine and Hygiene, November 11–15, 2001, Atlanta, GA.
227. Schlagenhauf P, Steffen R, Tschopp A, et al: Behavioural aspects of travellers in their use of malaria presumptive treatment. Bull World Health Organ 73:215–221, 1995.
228. Moody A: Rapid diagnostic tests for malaria parasites. Clin Microbiol Rev 15:66–78, 2002.
229. Whitty CJM, Armstrong M, Behrens RH: Self-testing for falciparum malaria with antigen-capture cards by travelers with symptoms of malaria. Am J Trop Med Hyg 63:295–297, 2000.
230. Jelinek T, Grobusch MP, Nothdurft HD: Use of dipstick tests for the rapid diagnosis of malaria in nonimmune travelers. J Travel Med 7:175–179, 2000.
231. Shanks GD, Oloo AJ, Aleman GM, et al: A new primaquine analogue, tafenoquine (WR 238605), for prophylaxis against *Plasmodium falciparum* malaria. Clin Infect Dis 33:1968–1974, 2001.
232. Lell B, Faucher JF, Missinou MA, et al: Malaria chemoprophylaxis with tafenoquine: A randomised study. Lancet 355:2041–2045, 2000.
233. Hale BR, Owusu-Agyei S, Fryauff DJ, et al: A randomized, double-blind, placebo-controlled, dose-ranging trial of tafenoquine for weekly prophylaxis against *Plasmodium falciparum*. Clin Infect Dis 36:541–549, 2003.
234. Webster D, Hill AV: Progress with new malaria vaccines. Bull World Health Organ 81:902–909, 2003.
235. Picot N, Gorijon C, Sylvestre P, et al: What risks are travellers in fear of? Presented at the Fourth International Conference on Travel Medicine, Acapulco, Mexico, April 23–27, 1995, Abstract 197.
236. Etkind P, Ratelle S, George H: International travel and sexually transmitted disease. Emerg Infect Dis 9:1654–1656, 2003.
237. Memish ZA, Osoba AO: Sexually transmitted diseases and travel. Int J Antimicrob Agents 21:131–134, 2003.
238. Gillies P, Slack R, Stoddart N, et al: HIV-related risk behaviour in U.K. holiday makers. AIDS 6:339–342, 1992.
239. Cabada MM, Montoya M, Echevarria JI, et al: Sexual behavior in travelers visiting Cuzco. J Travel Med 10:214–218, 2003.
240. Bonneux L, Van der Stuyft P, Taelman H, et al: Risk factors for infection with human immunodeficiency virus among European expatriates in Africa. BMJ 297:581–584, 1988.
241. Houweling H, Coutinho RA: Risk of HIV infection among Dutch expatriates in sub-Saharan Africa. Int J STD AIDS 2:252–257, 1991.
242. Estébanez P, Fitch K, Najera R: HIV and female sex workers. Bull World Health Organ 71:397–412, 1993.
243. Piot P, Tezzo R: The epidemiology of HIV and other sexually transmitted infections in the developing world. Scand J Infect Dis Suppl 69:89–97, 1990.
244. Castelli F, Pizzocolo C: The traveler with HIV. In Keystone JS, et al (eds): Travel Medicine. St. Louis, CV Mosby, 2004.
245. Ostrowski M, Tessier D, Keystone JS: Information for the patient: Travelling with HIV. Can J Infect Dis 6:291–295, 1995.
246.. Castelli F, Patroni A: The human immunodeficiency virus-infected traveler. Clin Infect Dis 31:1403–1408, 2000.
247. Baskin DH, Lax JD, Barenberg D: *Shigella* bacteremia in patients with acquired immunodeficiency syndrome. Am J Gastroenterol 82:338–341, 1987.
248. Sperber SJ, Schleupner CH: Salmonellosis during infection with human immunodeficiency virus. Rev Infect Dis 9:925–934, 1987.
249. Perlman DM, Ampel NM, Schifman RB, et al: Persistent *Campylobacter jejuni* infection in patients infected with HIV. Ann Intern Med 108:540–546, 1988.
250. Bates I, Fenton C, Gruber J, et al: Vulnerability to malaria, tuberculosis, and HIV/AIDS infection and disease. Part 1: Determinants operating at individual and household level. Lancet Infect Dis 4:267–277, 2004.
251. Harms G, Feldmeier H: HIV infection and tropical parasitic diseases—Deleterious interactions in both directions? Trop Med Int Health 7:479–488, 2002.
252. Fernandez-Guerrero ML, Robles P, Rivas P, et al: Visceral leishmaniasis in immunocompromised patients with and without AIDS: A comparison of clinical features and prognosis. Acta Trop 90: 11–16, 2004.
253. Russo R, Laguna F, Lopez-Velez R, et al: Visceral leishmaniasis in those infected with HIV: Clinical aspects and other opportunistic infections. Ann Trop Med Parasitol 97(suppl 1):99–105, 2003.
254. Rocha A, de Meneses AC, da Silva AM, et al: Pathology of patients with Chagas' disease and acquired immunodeficiency syndrome. Am J Trop Med Hyg 50:261–268, 1994.
255. Karimi K, Wheat LJ, Connolly P, et al: Differences in histoplasmosis in patients with acquired immunodeficiency syndrome in the United States and Brazil. J Infect Dis 186:1655–1660, 2002.
256. Ampel NM, Wieden MA, Galgiani J: Coccidioidomycosis: Clinical update. Rev Infect Dis 11:897–911, 1989.
257. Keystone JS, Kozasky E, Freedman DO, et al: Travel Medicine. St. Louis, CV Mosby, 2004.
258. Ericsson CD: Travellers with pre-existing medical conditions. Int J Antimicrob Agents 21:181–188, 2003.
259. Sung V, Brown GV, Torresi J: Dengue fever in travelers returning from Southeast Asia. J Travel Med 10:208–213, 2003.
260. Sutherst RW: Global change and human vulnerability to vector-borne diseases. Clin Microbiol Rev 17:136–173, 2004.
261. Gubler DJ: The changing epidemiology of yellow fever and dengue, 1900 to 2003: Full circle? Comp Immunol Microbiol Infect Dis 27:319–330, 2004.
262. Jelinek T, Muhlberger N, Harms G, et al; European Network on Imported Infectious Disease Surveillance: Epidemiology and clinical features of imported dengue fever in Europe: Sentinel surveillance data from TropNetEurop. Clin Infect Dis 35:1047–1052, 2002.
263. Lindback H, Lindback J, Tegnell A, et al: Dengue fever in travelers to the tropics, 1998 and 1999. Emerg Infect Dis 9:438–442, 2003.
264. Nutman TB, Miler KD, Mulligan M, et al: Diethylcarbamazine prophylaxis for human loaiasis: Results of a double-blind study. N Engl J Med 319:752–756, 1988.
265. Twartz JC, Shirai A, Selvaraju G: Doxycycline prophylaxis for scrub typhus. J Infect Dis 146:811–818, 1982.
266. Steen CJ, Carbonaro PA, Schwartz RA: Arthropods in dermatology. J Am Acad Dermatol 50:819–842, 2004.
267. LoVecchio F, McBride C: Scorpion envenomations in young children in central Arizona. J Toxicol Clin Toxicol 41:937–940, 2003.
268. Gold BS, Dart RC, Barish RA: Bites of venomous snakes. N Engl J Med 347:347–356, 2002.
269. Salafsky B, Ramaswamy K, He YX, et al: Development and evaluation of LIPODEET, a new long-acting formulation of *N,N*-diethyl-*m*-toluamide (DEET) for the prevention of schistosomiasis. Am J Trop Med Hyg 61:743–750, 1999.
270. Ramaswamy K, He YX, Salafsky B, et al: Topical application of DEET for schistosomiasis. Trends Parasitol 19:551–555, 2003.
271. Jackson F, Doherty JF, Behrens RH: Schistosomiasis prophylaxis in vivo using *N,N*-diethyl-*m*-toluamide (DEET). Trans R Soc Trop Med Hyg 97:449–450, 2003.
272. Takafuji ET, Kirkpatrick JW, Miller RN, et al: An efficacy trial of doxycycline chemoprophylaxis against leptospirosis. N Engl J Med 310:497–500, 1984.
273. Bickers DR: Sun-induced disorders. Emerg Med Clin North Am 3:659–676, 1985.
274. Taylor CR, Gober AJ: Sun exposure and skin diseases. Annu Rev Med 47:181–191, 1996.
275. Council on Scientific Affairs: Harmful effects of ultraviolet radiation. JAMA 262:380–384, 1989.
276. Almahroos M, Kurban AK: Sun protection for children and adolescents. Clin Dermatol 21:311–314, 2003.
277. Morison WL: Photoprotection by clothing. Dermatol Ther 16:16–22, 2003.
278. Rosen CF: Topical and systemic photoprotection. Dermatol Ther 16:8–15, 2003.
279. Ramirez R, Schneider J: Practical guide to sun protection. Surg Clin North Am 83:97–107, 2003.
280. Montemarano AD, Gupta RK, Burge JR, et al: Insect repellents and the efficacy of sunscreens. Lancet 349:1670–1671, 1997.
281. Murphy ME, Montemarano AD, Debboun M, et al: The effect of sunscreen on the efficacy of insect repellent: A clinical trial. J Am Acad Dermatol 43:219–222, 2000.
282. Rigel DS, Friedman RJ, Kopf AW: The incidence of malignant melanoma in the United States: Issues as we approach the 21st century. J Am Acad Dermatol 34:839–847, 1996.

283. MacLennan R, Green AC, McLeod GR, et al: Increasing incidence of cutaneous melanoma in Queensland, Australia. J Natl Cancer Inst 84:1427–1432, 1192.
284. Moseley PL: Mechanisms of heat adaptation: Thermotolerance and acclimatization. J Lab Clin Med 123:48–52, 1994.
285. Khosla R, Guntupalli KK: Heat-related illnesses. Crit Care Clin 15:251–263, 1999.
286. Comperatore CA, Krueger GP: Circadian rhythm, desynchronosis, jet lag, shift lag and coping strategies. Occup Med 5:323–341, 1990.
287. Reynolds NC Jr, Montgomery R: Using the Argonne diet in jet lag prevention: Deployment of troops across nine time zones. Military Med 167:451–453, 2002.
288. Daan S, Lewy AJ: Scheduled exposure to daylight: A potential strategy to reduce "jet lag" following transmeridian flight. Psychopharmacol Bull 20:566–568, 1984.
289. Wever RA: Phase shifts of human circadian rhythms due to shifts of artificial zeitgebers. Chronobiologica 7:303–327, 1980.
290. Czeisler CA, Kronauer RE, Allen JS, et al: Bright light induction of strong (type O) resetting of the human circadian pacemaker. Science 244:1328–1332, 1989.
291. Seidel WF, Roth T, Roehrs T, et al: Treatment of a 12 hour shift of sleep schedule with benzodiazepines. Science 224:1262–1264, 1984.
292. Bixler EO, Kales A, Manfredi RL: Next day memory impairment with triazolam use. Lancet 337:827–831, 1991.
293. Suhner A, Schlagenhauf P, Hofer I, et al: Effectiveness and tolerability of melatonin and zolpidem for the alleviation of jet lag. Aviat Space Environ Med 72:638–646, 2001.
294. Herxheimer A, Petrie KJ: Melatonin for preventing and treating jet lag. Cochrane Database Syst Rev. 1:CD001520, 2001. [Update in Cochrane Database Syst Rev 2:CD001520, 2002]
295. Caspi O: Melatonin for the prevention and treatment of jet lag. Altern Ther Health Med 10:74–78, 2004.
296. Jamieson AO, Zammit GK, Rosenberg RS, et al: Zolpidem reduces the sleep disturbance of jet lag. Sleep Med 2:423–430, 2001.
297. Awada A, Kojan S: Neurological disorders and travel. Int J Antimicrob Agents 21:189–192, 2003.
298. Parry BL: Jet lag: Minimizing it's effects with critically timed bright light and melatonin administration. J Mol Microbiol Biotechnol 4:463–466, 2002.
299. Lathrop NJ, Lentz M: Melatonin, light therapy, and jet lag. Air Med J 20:30–34, 2001.
300. Zisapel N: Circadian rhythm sleep disorders: Pathophysiology and potential approaches to management. CNS Drugs 15:311–328, 2001.
301. Hackett PH, Roach RC: High-altitude illness. N Engl J Med 345:107–114, 2001.
302. Gallagher SA, Hackett PH: High-altitude illness. Emerg Med Clin North Am 22:329–355, viii, 2004.
303. Basnyat B, Murdoch DR: High-altitude illness. Lancet 361: 1967–1974, 2003.
304. Barry PW, Pollard AJ: Altitude illness. BMJ 326:915–919, 2003.
305. Brundrett G: Sickness at high altitude: A literature review. J R Soc Health 122:14–20, 2002.
306. Rodway GW, Hoffman LA, Sanders MH: High-altitude-related disorders—Part II: Prevention, special populations, and chronic medical conditions. Heart Lung 33:3–12, 2004.
307. Rodway GW, Hoffman LA, Sanders MH: High-altitude-related disorders—Part I: Pathophysiology, differential diagnosis, and treatment. Heart Lung 32:353–359, 2003.
308. Ellsworth AJ, Larson EB, Strickland DA: Randomized trial of dexamethasone and acetazolamide for acute mountain sickness prophylaxis. Am J Med 83:1024–1030, 1987.
309. Reid LD, Carter KA, Ellsworth A: Acetazolamide or dexamethasone for prevention of acute mountain sickness: A meta-analysis. J Wilderness Med 5:34–38, 1994.
310. Basnyat B, Gertsch JH, Johnson EW, et al: Efficacy of low-dose acetazolamide (125 mg BID) for the prophylaxis of acute mountain sickness: A prospective, double-blind, randomized, placebo-controlled trial. High Alt Med Biol 4:45–52, 2003.
311. Rabold MB: Dexamethasone for prophylaxis and treatment of acute mountain sickness. J Wilderness Med 3:54–60, 1992.
312. Bernhard WN, Schalick LM, Gittelsohn A: Dexamethasone for prophylaxis against mountain sickness during rapid ascent to 5334 m. J Wilderness Med 5:331–338, 1994.
313. Zell SC, Goodman PH: Acetazolamide and dexamethasone in the prevention of acute mountain sickness. West J Med 148:541–545, 1988.
314. Bärtsch P, Maggiorini M, Ritter M, et al: Prevention of high altitude pulmonary edema by nifedipine. N Engl J Med 325:1284–1289, 1991.
315. Bartsch P, Swenson ER, Maggiorini M: Update: High altitude pulmonary edema. Adv Exp Med Biol 502:89–106, 2001.
316. Gertsch JH, Basnyat B, Johnson EW, et al: Randomised, double blind, placebo controlled comparison of ginkgo biloba and acetazolamide for prevention of acute mountain sickness among Himalayan trekkers: The Prevention of High Altitude Illness Trial (PHAIT). BMJ 328:797, 2004.
317. Gertsch JH, Seto TB, Mor J, et al: Ginkgo biloba for the prevention of severe acute mountain sickness (AMS) starting one day before rapid ascent. High Alt Med Biol 3:29–37, 2002.
318. Dumont L, Mardirosoff C, Tramer MR: Efficacy and harm of pharmacological prevention of acute mountain sickness: Quantitative systematic review. BMJ 321:267–272, 2000.
319. Brown TP, Shuker LK, Rushton L, et al: The possible effects on health, comfort and safety of aircraft cabin environments. J R Soc Health 121:177–184, 2001.
320. Jacobson BF, Munster M, Smith A, et al: The BEST study—A prospective study to compare business class versus economy class air travel as a cause of thrombosis. S Afr Med J 93:522–528, 2003.
321. Ferrari E, Chevallier T, Chapelier A, et al: Travel as a risk factor for venous thromboembolic disease: A case–control study. Chest 115:440–444, 1999.
322. Kraaijenhagen RA, Haverkamp D, Koopman MM, et al: Travel and risk of venous thrombosis. Lancet 356:1492–1493, 2000.
323. Samama MM: An epidemiologic study of risk factors for deep vein thrombosis in medical outpatients: The Sirius study. Arch Intern Med 160:3415–3420, 2000.
324. Schwarz T, Siegert G, Oettler W, et al: Venous thrombosis after long-haul flights. Arch Intern Med 163:2759–2764, 2003.
325. Scurr JH, Machin SJ, Bailey-King S, et al: Frequency and prevention of symptomless deep-vein thrombosis in long-haul flights: A randomised trial. Lancet 357:1485–1489, 2001.
326. ten Wolde M, Kraaijenhagen RA, Schiereck J, et al: Travel and the risk of symptomatic venous thromboembolism. Thromb Haemost 89:499–505, 2003.
327. Paganin F, Bourde A, Yvin JL, et al: Venous thromboembolism in passengers following a 12-h flight: A case–control study. Aviat Space Environ Med 74:1277–1280, 2003.
328. Arya R, Barnes JA, Hossain U, et al: Long-haul flights and deep vein thrombosis: A significant risk only when additional factors are also present. Br J Haematol 116:653–654, 2002.
329. Adi Y, Bayliss S, Rouse A, et al: The association between air travel and deep vein thrombosis: Systematic review & meta-analysis. BMC Cardiovasc Disord 4:7, 2004.
330. Bagshaw M: Traveller's thrombosis: A review of deep vein thrombosis associated with travel. The Air Transport Medicine Committee, Aerospace Medical Association. Aviat Space Environ Med 72:848–851, 2001.
331. Cesarone MR, Belcaro G, Brandolini R, et al: The LONFLIT4-Venoruton Study: A randomized trial—Prophylaxis of flight-edema in venous patients. Angiology 54:137–142, 2003.
332. Suh KN, Keystone JS: Antibiotics for travelers: What's good and what's not. Curr Infect Dis Rep 6:13–21, 2004.
333. Stauffer WM, Konop RJ, Kamat D: Traveling with infants and young children. Part I: Anticipatory guidance: Travel preparation and preventive health advice. J Travel Med 8:254–259, 2001.
334. Ryan ET, Kain KC: Health advice and immunizations for travelers. N Engl J Med 342:1716–1725, 2000.
335. Spira AM: Preparing the traveller. Lancet 361:1368–1381, 2003.
336. Spira AM: Assessment of travellers who return home ill. Lancet 361:1459–1469, 2003.
337. Ryan ET, Wilson ME, Kain KC: Illness after international travel. N Engl J Med 347:505–516, 2002.
338. Keystone JS, Kozarsky PE, Freedman DO: Internet and computer-based resources for travel medicine practitioners. Clin Infect Dis 32:757–765, 2001.
339. Horvath LL, Murray CK, DuPont HL: Travel health information at commercial travel websites. J Travel Med 10:272–278, 2003.

121

Migrant, Immigrant, and Refugee Health

SUSAN A. MALONEY
LUIS S. ORTEGA
MARTIN S. CETRON

INTRODUCTION

The global migration landscape has undergone substantial changes in the past quarter century, and the number of population groups contributing to global mobility is steadily rising. The volume of global migrants more than doubled between 1975 and 2000, from 84 million in 1975 to 175 million in 2000. The International Organization for Migration (IOM) estimates that the number of global migrants in 2050 will reach 230 million.[1] Migration is truly a major social phenomenon, with many complex links to economic, trade, social, security, and health policies. In the dynamic relationship between migration and health, immigration has long been recognized to have a large impact on disease epidemiology and the use of health services in migrant receiving nations[2,3] For example, the impact of immigration on disease epidemiology is demonstrated by the global epidemiology of tuberculosis. Tuberculosis (TB) is a major global cause of infectious disease morbidity and mortality; however, rates of TB in most regions of the developing world are many times higher than those in the developed world (the TB prevalence gap) and are decreasing at a much slower rate.[4] Many migration-receiving countries in the developed world have had stable or increased migration of persons from regions with high TB prevalence, while at the same time having successfully decreased TB incidence in their native-borne population, further exacerbating the prevalence gap. Consequently, the majority of TB cases in migration-receiving countries such as the United States and Canada are now being diagnosed in foreign-born populations from high-prevalence source countries.[5,6] (Fig. 121-1).

Many immigration-receiving countries have prearrival medical examination requirements and protocols for entering migrants, which vary both by the types of populations screened and by the diseases for which examination is required. The health conditions tested through the medical examination procedures required by countries such as Canada, Australia, New Zealand, and the United States are determined on the basis of the risk or danger that these conditions can represent to public health and safety and the additional costs that may be incurred by national public services expenditures.[7–11] In general, these medical examination procedures include a review of the past medical history, a physical examination, and tests that include a chest radiograph and laboratory analyses. The diseases most frequently tested to determine visa eligibility or admissibility of a migrant are infectious diseases such as tuberculosis, sexually transmitted diseases, and mental or behavioral conditions. Immigration regulations

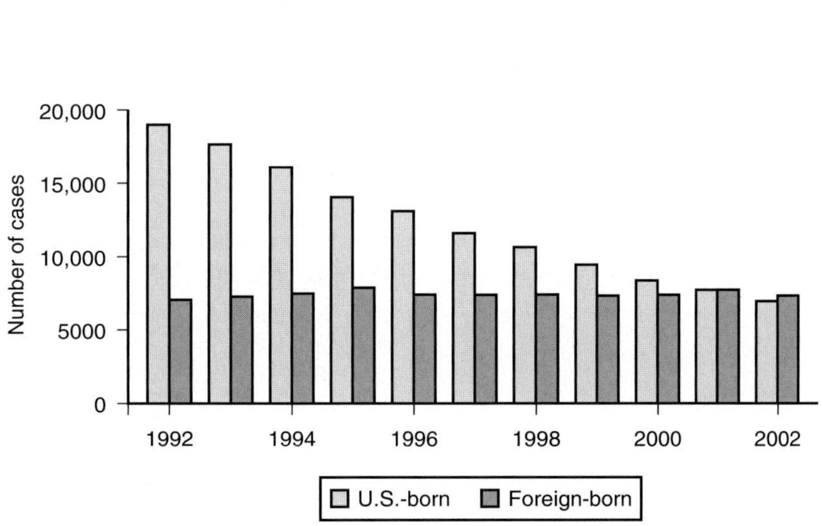

FIGURE 121-1 Number of tuberculosis cases in U.S.-born vs. foreign-born persons, United States, 1992–2002. (Data from the Division of Tuberculosis Elimination, Centers for Disease Control and Prevention.)

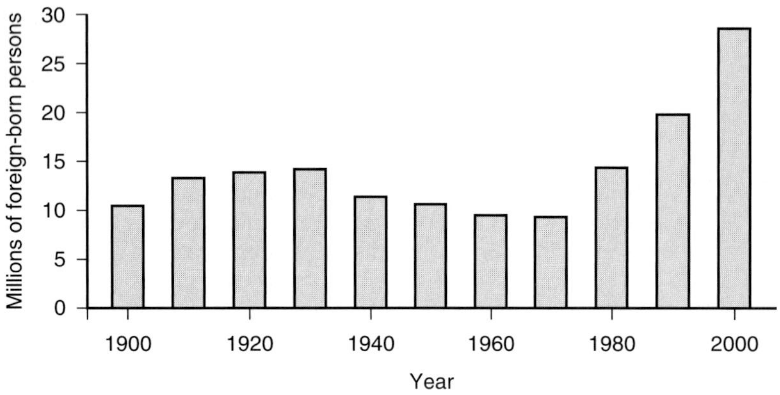

FIGURE 121-2 Number of foreign-born persons living in the United States, 1900–2000. (Data from the Center for Immigration Studies, Washington, D.C.)

in these countries do allow for the consideration of medical waivers to inadmissible health conditions. Although many immigration-receiving countries in Europe either do not require prearrival health evaluations or have fewer requirements and only limited grounds for refusal of admission based on health grounds, most have provisions for notification and inspection if a communicable or serious health condition is recognized or suspected.[12,13]

U.S. MIGRATION AND HEALTH SCREENING POLICIES

The number of foreign-born persons living in the United States, approximately 28 million, is greater than ever before in the nation's history[14] (Fig. 121-2). In 2004, the foreign-born proportion of the total U.S. population reached approximately 12%, a proportion comparable to the peak reached during the great immigration wave at the turn of the 20th century. In contrast to the previous 20th century U.S. immigration wave, which was dominated by Eastern Europeans who were driven from their countries of origin by such factors as persecution and poverty (so-called "push factors"), the 21st century immigration wave, which began in the 1970s, is characterized predominantly by Hispanic followed by Asian migrants who are attracted to the United States for economic opportunities (or "pull factors"). In both waves of migration, migrants have brought with them not only skills and cultural traditions that enriched the U.S. economic and social fabric, but also diseases and disease exposures that were different from those existing in U.S.-receiving communities. In addition, 21st century migrants are more mobile and remain connected to their countries of birth, typically making several back and forth journeys to visit friends and relatives (VFR). New immigrants and refugees, who cross disease prevalence gaps and frequently travel to visit friends and relatives, constitute potentially high-risk populations for translocating communicable diseases of public health significance.

The U.S. Department of Homeland Security has reported that approximately 60,500,000 migrants enter the United States annually (Table 121-1).[15] These migrants include immigrants, refugees, migrants adjusting their visa status, persons with nonimmigrant visas, persons in short-term transit status, and other groups that entered the United States without inspection, including undocumented migrants. The majority of these migrants are not required to undergo health screening prior to U.S. entry (see Table 121-1). Given the immense numbers of persons crossing U.S. borders and finite resources for evaluation and surveillance, U.S. migrant health screening policy focuses on migrants planning to establish permanent U.S. residence, since this group has the largest potential long-term impact both on disease epidemiology and health care resource utilization. Currently, the U.S. Immigration and Nationality Act (INA) requires that medical screening examinations be performed overseas for all U.S.-bound immigrants and refugees, and in the United States for migrants applying to adjust their visa status to permanent residence ("green cards").[10,11,16,17]

Table 121-1 Categories and Number of Migrants Entering the United States by Medical Screening Requirements, 2002

Category	Annual No.	Medical Screening	Screening Site	Screening Location
Immigrants	384,427	Yes	Panel physicians	Overseas
Refugees	26,839*	Yes	Panel physicians	Overseas
Status adjusters	679,305	Yes	Civil surgeons	United States
Nonimmigrants	27,907,139	No	—	—
Short-term transit	~30,000,000	No	—	—
Others†	~1,500,000	No	—	—
Total	**~60,500,000**			

*Numbers are below traditional annual arrivals because of new security requirements following 9/11/2001.
†Others include migrants who entered the United States without inspection, including those who entered with and without proper documentation.
Data from U.S. Department of Homeland Security, Washington, D.C.

In 2002, more than 1,000,000 immigrants, refugees, and migrants seeking visa status adjustment underwent medical screening examinations. The remainder of this chapter covers U.S. medical screening issues for immigrants and refugees.

REQUIRED OVERSEAS MEDICAL SCREENING EXAMINATIONS FOR U.S.-BOUND IMMIGRANTS AND REFUGEES

Over 400,000 immigrants and refugees arrive in the United States annually; immigrants make up approximately 90% of arrivals, and refugees close to 10%.[15] Trends in the number and regions of origin for U.S.-arriving immigrants and refugees are presented in Figures 121-3 and 121-4. From 1997 to 2002, more than 2.4 million immigrants arrived in the United States; the number of arrivals and regions of origin remained relatively stable over the 6 years examined. Between 357,000 and 410,000 immigrants arrived annually: 43% from Asia/Oceania, 26% from the Americas (with the majority [roughly 60%] from Mexico), 13% from the Caribbean, 12% from Europe, and 7% from Africa. From 1997 to 2004 (projected), close to 480,000 refugees arrived in the United States; in contrast to immigrants, the number of arrivals and regions of origins have changed markedly over the 8 years examined. From 1997 through 2001, the number of refugees entering the United States remained stable at approximately 70,000 per year. However, after the September 11th terrorist attacks on the United States, increased security requirements delayed some refugee processing, and therefore the number of refugees arriving in 2002 and 2003 decreased to 30,000 or less. It is projected that between 50,000 and 70,000 refugees will arrive in the United States by the end of 2004. The number and proportions of arriving refugees from different regions of the world also changed over the 8 years examined. In 1997, the majority (70%) of arriving refugees were from Europe and Central Asia, with only 9% from Africa. In contrast, in 2004, it is projected that more than 35% (approximately 25,000 refugees) will be from Africa. These trends have important implications for medical evaluation and treatment of refugees, both overseas and stateside, since refugees from Africa have relatively high rates of certain diseases, including immunodeficiency virus (HIV) infection, TB, malaria, intestinal helminth infections, and other tropical diseases (e.g., schistosomiasis) and likely lack routine vaccination coverage.

All immigrants and refugees migrating to the United States are required to have a medical screening examination overseas, which are performed by local physicians (panel physicians) appointed by the local U.S. embassy.[10,11] The mandated medical examination focuses primarily on detecting diseases determined to be inadmissible conditions for the purposes of visa eligibility. These diseases include certain serious infectious diseases such as infectious tuberculosis, HIV infection, syphilis and other sexually transmitted infections, and infectious Hansen's disease. Other diseases designated as inadmissible conditions include mental disorders associated with harmful behavior and substance abuse. For the purposes of determining the inadmissibility of an applicant, medical conditions are categorized as class A or B. Class A conditions are defined as those conditions that preclude an immigrant or refugee from entering the United States. Class A conditions require approved waivers for U.S. entry and immediate medical follow-up upon arrival. These conditions include communicable diseases of public health significance, a physical or mental disorder associated with violent or harmful behavior, and drug abuse

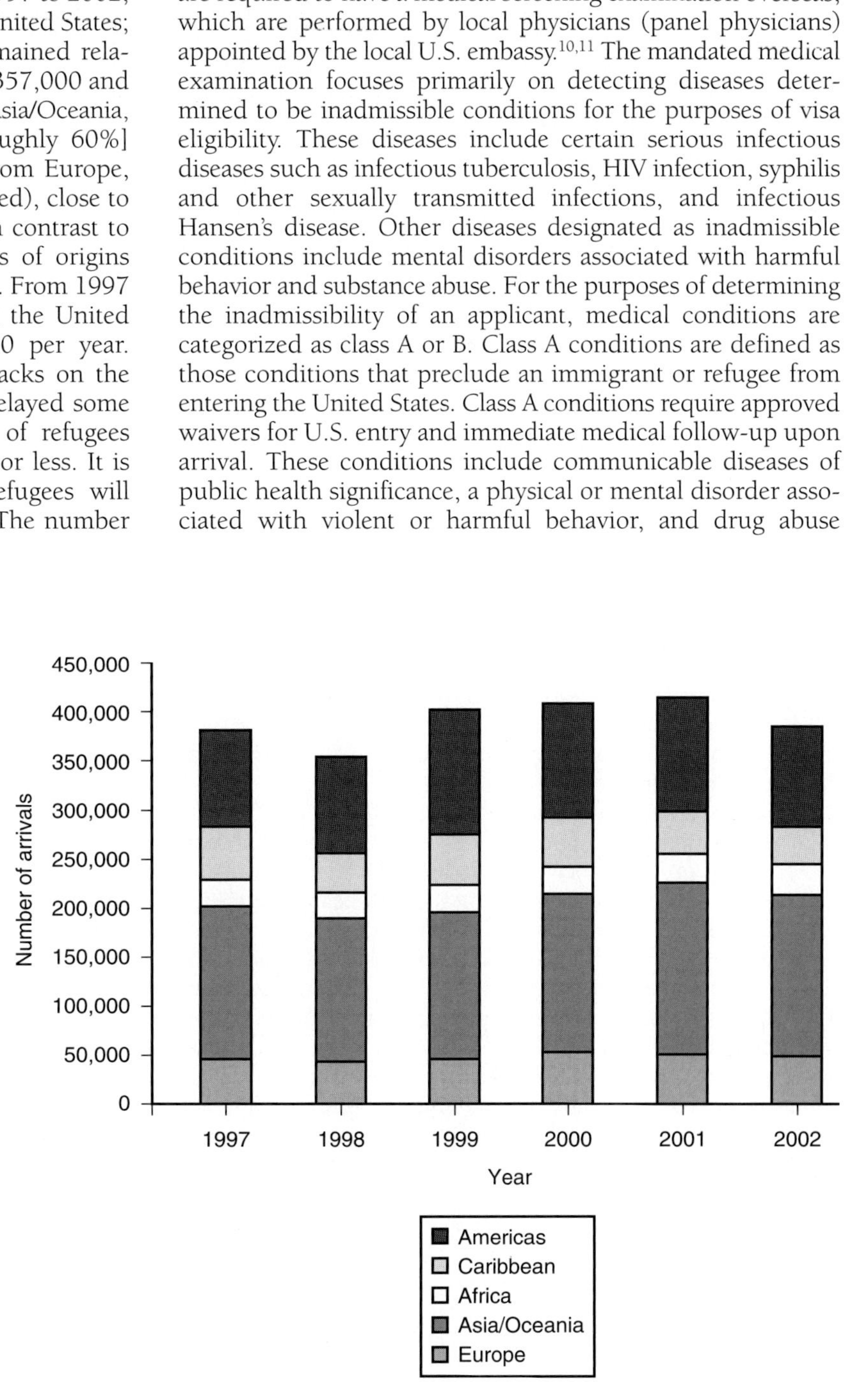

FIGURE 121-3 U.S. immigrant arrivals, 1997–2002. (Data from the U.S. Department of Homeland Security, Washington, D.C.)

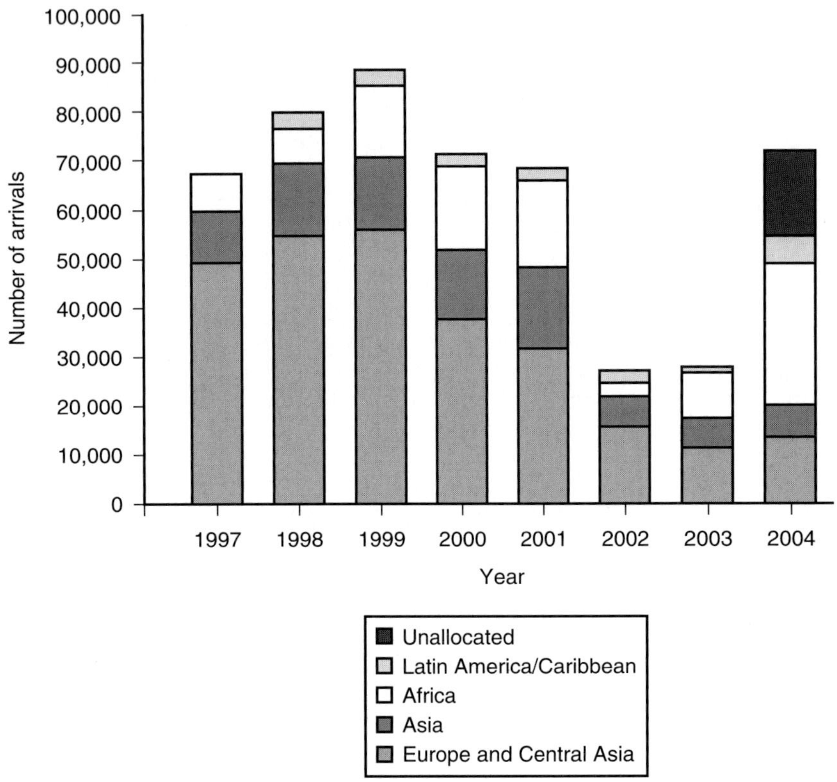

FIGURE 121-4 U.S. refugee arrivals, 1997–2004. (Data from the U.S. Department of Homeland Security, Washington, D.C.)

or addiction. Class B conditions are defined as significant health problems: physical or mental abnormalities, diseases, or disabilities serious in degree or permanent in nature amounting to a substantial departure from normal well-being. Follow-up evaluation soon after U.S. arrival is recommended for migrants with class B conditions. If an immigrant or refugee is found to have an inadmissible condition that may make them ineligible for a visa, a visa may still be issued after the illness has been adequately treated or after a waiver of the visa eligibility has been approved by the U.S. Department of Homeland Security.

In 1996, a new subsection was added to the INA requiring that persons seeking immigrant visas for permanent residency show proof of receipt of at least the first dose of all vaccination series recommended by the American Committee for Immunization Practices (ACIP). Although these regulations apply to all adult immigrants and most immigrant children, internationally adopted children who are younger than 10 years of age have been exempted from the immunization requirements as a consequence of strong objections posed by advocacy groups, who cited safety concerns over immunization practices in several origin countries. Refugees are not required to meet the INA immunization requirements at the time of initial entry into the United States but must show proof of vaccination at the time they apply for permanent U.S. residence, typically within 3 years of U.S. arrival.

The U.S. Centers for Disease Control and Prevention (CDC), Division of Global Migration and Quarantine (DGMQ), is responsible for providing technical guidance to the panel physicians performing the overseas medical screening examination.[16] The testing modalities recommended for the medical examination are outlined in Table 121-2, and the algorithm for the required overseas medical screening examination is presented in Figure 121-5. The CDC DGMQ is also responsible for monitoring the quality of the overseas medical examination process at more than 650 panel physician sites (health care staff, radiology facilities, and laboratories) worldwide, through its Quality Assurance Program (QAP). Owing to limited resources, not all panel physician sites can be visited and assessed annually. Sites are prioritized for monitoring based on the number of immigrant and refugee visas processed and

Table 121-2 Testing for Required Overseas Medical Screening Examination

Health Condition	Testing
Tuberculosis	Chest radiograph; AFB smear if chest radiograph is positive
HIV	Serology
Syphilis	Serology
Other sexually transmitted diseases	Physical examination
Hansen's disease	Physical examination
Mental disorders with associated harmful behavior	History
Drug abuse or addiction	History, physical examination
Vaccinations	History/vaccination records Serology

Data from Division of Global Migration and Quarantine, Centers for Disease Control and Prevention.

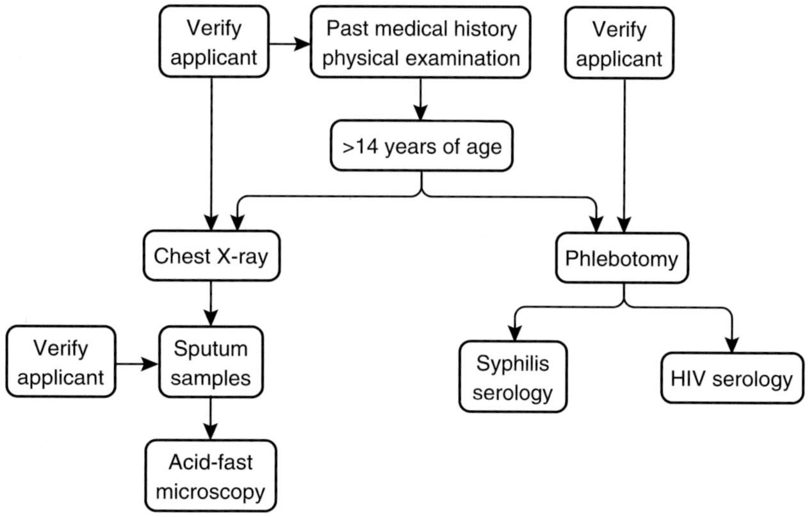

FIGURE 121-5 Required overseas medical screening examination from the Division of Global Migration and Quarantine, Centers for Disease Control and Prevention.

country-specific prevalence of such diseases as TB and HIV. In addition, DGMQ performs remediation visits when medical screening examination deficiencies have been identified.

The CDC DGMQ is also responsible for notifying state and local health departments of all arriving refugees and those immigrants with health conditions who are resettling in their jurisdiction and need follow-up evaluation and possible treatment in the United States.[10,11] Under the current system, forms summarizing the results of the overseas medical examination, including classification of health conditions, are manually collected at U.S. ports of entry. This information is transmitted to state and local health departments through the U.S. mail. State and local health departments are asked to report to DGMQ the results of these U.S. follow-up evaluations and also any significant public health conditions occurring among recently arrived immigrants and refugees.

HEALTH CONDITIONS IDENTIFIED THROUGH REQUIRED OVERSEAS MEDICAL SCREENING EXAMINATIONS

The number and types of health conditions identified through required overseas medical screening examinations among the approximately 2 million immigrants and 280,000 refugees who arrived in the United States from 1999 through 2003 are summarized in Table 121-3. For both refugees and immigrants, the most frequent conditions identified were suspected active and inactive tuberculosis.

The underlying objective of the overseas TB screening process is to limit the entry of persons seeking long-term U.S. residence who have infectious (defined as acid-fast bacilli [AFB] smear–positive) active TB and who therefore pose an immediate public health risk, and to refer others with suspected active and inactive TB for further evaluation and treatment in the United States, where diagnostic facilities and mycobacterial culture capability are generally more readily available and treatment can more easily be monitored and supervised. Suspected active TB (classes A and B1) was identified in 0.96% of immigrants and 0.77% of refugees examined overseas from 1999 through 2003. Previous studies have reported that during U.S. follow-up, pulmonary TB disease was diagnosed in 3.3% to 14.0% of immigrants and refugees classified overseas as having suspected active TB.[18–24] If these estimates are used to calculate expected rates of active TB among newly arrived U.S. immigrants and refugees with suspected active TB, the expected rates of pulmonary TB disease for immigrants would be between 29 and 134 per 100,000 persons and for refugees between 23 and 208 per 100,000 persons. These rates are as high and likely higher than the reported TB rate among all foreign-born persons in the United States in 2002 (23.6 per 100,000).[5] Furthermore, compared with the U.S. native-born TB rates (2.8 per 100,000), these expected rates are higher by several orders of magnitude.[5]

These data underscore the importance of assuring timely and appropriate U.S. follow-up evaluation of immigrants and refugees with suspected active TB, since the yield for TB case

Table 121-3 *Number of Health Conditions Identified Through Overseas Medical Screening Examination Among Immigrants and Refugees, 1999–2003*

Health Conditions	Immigrants	Refugees	Total
Infectious (AFB^+) active TB: class A	29	7	36
Not infectious (AFB^-) active TB: class B1	19,206	2140	21,346
Not active TB: class B2	17,026	8025	25,051
HIV	102	735	837
Syphilis	209	62	271
Hansen's disease	13	4	17
Mental disorder associated with harmful behavior	39	18	57
Drug abuse or addiction	5	1	6
Total	36,629	10,992	47,621

Data from Division of Global Migration and Quarantine, Centers for Disease Control and Prevention.

finding is high. Although rates of follow-up for immigrants and refugees identified overseas as class B1 or B2 are relatively high (63% to 99%),[18] problems exist with late or lost arrival notifications in up to 30% of notifications (CDC, unpublished data, 2002). These deficiencies in the current manual notification process can delay the evaluation and treatment of TB cases among immigrants and refugees after arrival in the United States and can potentially contribute to increased TB morbidity and mortality and disease transmission. A CDC initiative to develop an electronic disease notification system for arriving refugees and immigrants is under way to address these deficiencies and is discussed in the following sections.

The number of HIV infections identified during the overseas medical screening examination is relatively small. Early identification of HIV infections among immigrants and refugees is important to assure appropriate notification and linkages to medical services in resettlement communities. Current regulations require that syphilis infections be treated before departure to the United States. During 1999–2003, less than 300 immigrants and refugees infected with syphilis were identified overseas. In reference to other inadmissible conditions listed in Table 121-3, fewer than 20 cases of Hansen's disease, fewer than 60 cases of mental disorder associated with harmful behavior, and only six cases of drug abuse or addiction were identified among U.S.-bound immigrants and refugees.

NEW HEALTH SCREENING PROGRAM INITIATIVES TO IMPROVE IMMIGRANT AND REFUGEE HEALTH

Electronic Disease Notification System

DGMQ has recently embarked on a long-term, multiyear initiative to develop a comprehensive electronic disease notification system to communicate with both national and international partners about diseases and disease outbreaks occurring among mobile populations entering the United States. Such mobile populations include immigrants, refugees, migrants, and international travelers (including temporary visitors). The system, called the Electronic Disease Notification (EDN) system, will integrate data from multiple sources and surveillance systems and will include modules dedicated to specific populations and disease entities of public health importance such as tuberculosis. The EDN-Tuberculosis (EDN-TB) module was prioritized for implementation because of the crucial role it can play in enhancing tuberculosis control and prevention efforts among arriving immigrants and refugees, and it is currently being tested in several U.S. states. The objectives of the EDN-TB module are to (1) use the CDC secure data network to electronically notify health departments of newly arriving immigrants and refugees with class A and class B tuberculosis, (2) provide an electronic system for health departments to inform other health departments of secondary migration of immigrants and refugees with TB conditions within the United States, (3) provide health departments with an electronic system to record and evaluate the outcome of domestic follow-up examinations (4) provide federal and state public health officials with data to evaluate the effectiveness of follow-up of immigrants and refugees with suspect tuberculosis, and (5) allow comparison of overseas health assessments with domestic follow-up outcomes as part of a comprehensive quality assessment program for overseas TB screening examinations.

Enhanced Refugee Health Program Initiative

It has long been recognized that immigrants and refugees may carry significant disease burdens, which are determined by geographic origin, ethnicity, and living and health conditions in countries of origin or departure.[25] These migrants can suffer from a multitude of health conditions, including infectious diseases (such as tuberculosis and many tropical and parasitic diseases), malnutrition, reproductive health needs, and mental health disorders, often caused by tenuous circumstances in their countries of origin or departure.[25–31] Such disease burdens can seriously hamper migrants' ability to successfully integrate and optimally contribute to their resettlement communities and may cause strain on health and social services systems in the United States.[28] Most of these health conditions are not addressed during the required overseas medical examination process. Refugees do receive stateside evaluation and treatment, usually conducted at state or local health departments, within 3 months of U.S. arrival, but currently there is no standardized nationwide protocol for postarrival health assessment, and therefore the content of postarrival refugee health evaluations varies from state to state, and funding sources are often noted to be inadequate to provide comprehensive services. Further, both refugees and immigrants often have other daily demands to achieve integration into their new living environment that may compete with their need for health evaluations and treatment. Optimizing migrant health prior to resettlement and addressing migrant health needs early in the migration process can be cost-effective and prevent larger expenditures later.[23,32–35] Realization of this fact has led to the development of the U.S. Enhanced Refugee Health Program (ERHP), an initiative aimed at achieving integration of the health needs of migrant populations with facilities of the host and receiving countries. The CDC developed the initiative, in collaboration with the U.S. Bureau of Population and Migration (PRM), the International Organization for Migration (IOM), and U.S. state and local health departments, to begin to comprehensively address health care needs of U.S.-destined refugees while they are still overseas, and to facilitate and promote appropriate stateside evaluation and treatment. The ERHP currently focuses on refugees for a number of reasons: (1) refugees are vulnerable populations, exposed to a variety of harsh environmental conditions and diverse diseases, with limited access to health care; (2) a unique opportunity exists to address refugee health concerns during required overseas health assessments; (3) the language and charge of the U.S. Refugee Act provide more latitude to address conditions of public health concern among refugees (in addition to inadmissible conditions); and (4) lessons learned from a focus on the smaller number of refugees may be potentially applicable to the larger numbers of immigrants or other migrant groups.

The ERHP strategy is to utilize the required overseas medical examination process as a unique opportunity to assess and improve the health status of refugees overseas, and to incorporate both required screening components for inadmissible conditions and additional expanded components, which are tailored to specific refugee population needs and targeted to diseases of public health importance. The program first ensures quality staffing and infrastructure in the field, evaluating, training, and lending resources to support the capacity currently in place when necessary. Extending health services in the country of origin or transit allows patients to be served by health-care providers who are closer geographically and often culturally to the patients' circumstances and health needs. Furthermore, through the development of enhanced and electronic data exchange systems, ERHP promotes more timely transmission of population-based health and medical examination data acquired overseas to U.S. health departments in resettlement communities, facilitating appropriate follow-up and treatment of refugees after arrival in the United States. In the future, ERHP will strive to support and standardize follow-up evaluation and treatment of refugees after U.S. arrival by state and local health departments and other community health-care providers.

Since 1997, the CDC has undertaken enhanced refugee health programs for at least eight large-scale, emergent movements of refugee populations and one U.S.-based intervention for the Lost Boys and Girls of Sudan (Fig. 121-6). These programs have included components to provide presumptive predeparture treatment for malaria, intestinal parasites, and other tropical diseases, expanded TB diagnosis and treatment, HIV services, appropriate immunizations, dental and mental health assessments, chronic disease evaluations, and postarrival treatment for schistosomiasis and strongyloides infection (Table 121-4). These programs have successfully prevented thousands of cases of intestinal parasitosis, malaria, and vaccine-preventable diseases and hundreds of cases of TB and other communicable diseases among U.S.-bound refugees.[36–40] Other integral components of the ERHP initiative have been efforts to provide linkages to U.S. programs in host countries, such as the Global AIDS Program (GAP), which can provide diagnostic, treatment, and prevention services to refugees awaiting U.S. resettlement. Such efforts are aimed at assuring refugees access to needed health-care services in a prompt manner even while still in asylum countries prior to U.S. resettlement, and to reduce the burden placed on host country resources, since overseas interventions can decrease refugee health utilization once in the United States, reduce treatment costs, and avoid overburdening the domestic health system. Finally, some more recent ERHP programs have included enhanced surveillance and response for emerging infectious diseases, including vector-borne and vaccine-preventable diseases, and most recently, H5N1 avian influenza in Asia. As part of the EHRP for Liberian refugees in Côte d'Ivoire, field staff were able to identify Onong n'yong fever, an emerging infectious disease in West Africa, and prevent its importation.[40]

Vaccine-preventable diseases are a source of significant morbidity and mortality in developing countries, and refugees are known to be undervaccinated owing to collapsing public health infrastructure in countries of origin or departure and lack of access to health care.[41] In addition, outbreaks of measles, rubella, and varicella among U.S.-bound Liberian refugees in Côte d'Ivoire and varicella among the Somali Barawans in Kenya in 1997, Somali Bantu refugees in Kenya in 2003 and 2004, and Hmong refugees in Thailand in 2004 were identified and controlled during ERHP programs (unpublished data, CDC).[42] As a result of these and other disease outbreaks, the movement of refugees has frequently been significantly delayed and necessitated substantial additional per capita investments in the resettlement process (e.g., last-minute cancellation of nonrefundable commercial airline tickets and the need for dedicated refugee charter flights), not to mention

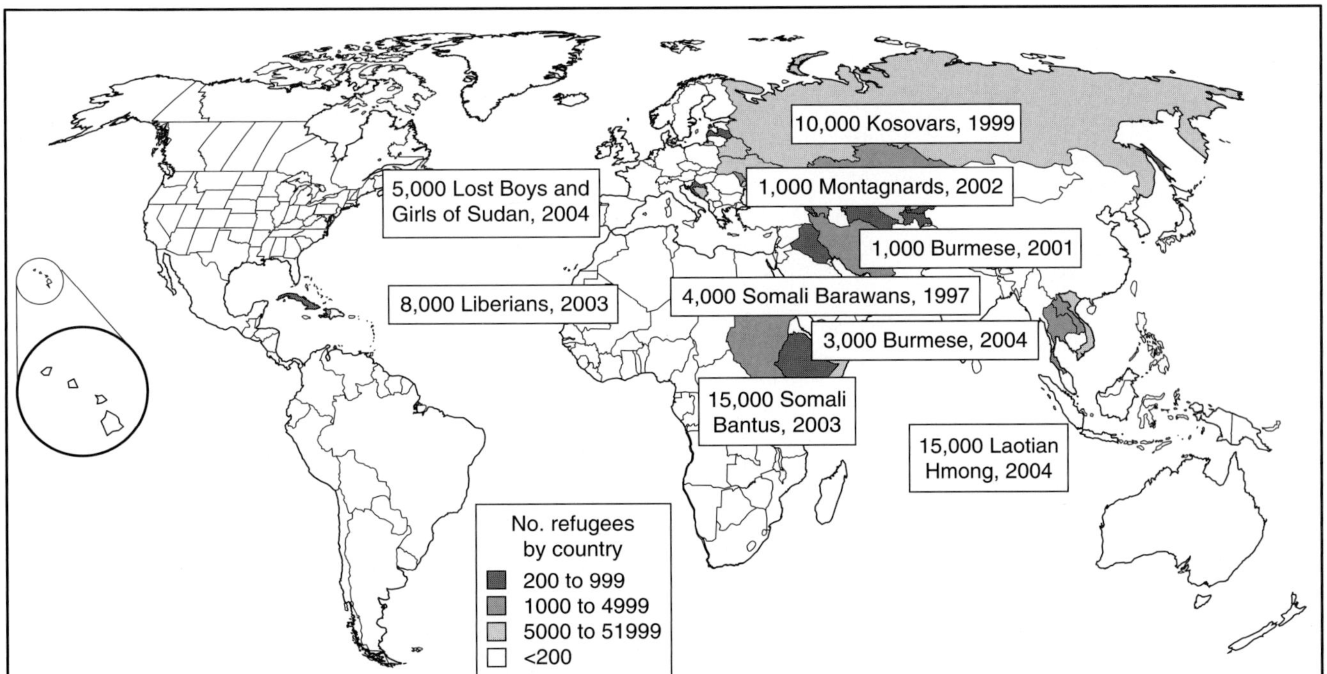

FIGURE 121-6 Enhanced refugee health programs from the Centers for Disease Control and Prevention.

Table 121-4 *Enhanced Refugee Health Programs, by Population Group and Program Components, 1997–2004*

	Population Group, Year, (n)								
Program Components	**Somali Barawans, 1997 (4000)**	**Kosovars, 1999 (10,000)**	**Burmese, 2001 (1000)**	**Vietnamese Montagnards, 2002 (1000)**	**Somali Bantu, 2003 (15,000)**	**Liberians, 2003 (8000)**	**Burmese, 2004 (3000)**	**Laotian Hmong, 2004 (15,000)**	**Lost Boys of Sudan, 2004 (5000)**
Overseas									
Predeparture treatment									
Malaria	X				X	X			
Intestinal parasites	X			X	X	X	X	X	
Screening/targeted treatment									
Malaria	X			X			X	X	
Schistosomiasis	X								
Immunizations (emergent)	X				X	X		X	
Immunizations (routine)			X	X			X	X	
Expanded tuberculosis diagnosis and treatment		X		X		X	X	X	
Expanded HIV services			X			X	X	X	
Emergent disease surveillance					X	X	X	X	
Outbreak response					X	X		X	
Enhanced notification and data transmission	X	X	X	X	X	X	X	X	
Electronic notification and data transmission						X			
United States/Stateside									
Postarrival treatment for									
Malaria				X					
Schistosomiasis									X
Strongyloides									X
Scabies		X							
Acute and primary care		X							
Chronic disease evaluation		X							
Mental health		X							
Dental health		X							
Immunizations (routine)		X		X					
Expanded TB evaluation		X		X			X	X	
Hepatitis screening				X					
Outbreak response		X				X		X	X

Data from Centers for Disease Control and Prevention.

in the isolation of *Ehrlichia chaffeensis*, the causative agent of human monocytic ehrlichiosis in 1990.[50] A prospective serological study of 1194 U.S. military personnel following a training exercise in Arkansas indicated a 2.5% seroconversion rate to spotted fever group ricksettsia (SFGR) and a 1.3% seroconversion rate to *Ehrlichia* species, although most infections were not associated with symptoms (73% of SFGR seroconvertors and 67% of the *Ehrlichia* species seroconvertors did not report symptoms).[51] The use of permethrin-treated uniforms is thought to decrease the risk of tick-borne infections; however, only 35% of the soldiers reported using this preventive measure.

These rates of infection have importance beyond the health of the individual soldier. In 1997, 10 U.S. National Guard members in Iowa presented with symptoms consistent with tickborne diseases shortly after a two-week training exercise in Arkansas.[52] Several of these soldiers, along with others in their unit, had donated blood shortly before becoming ill. Among the 377 blood donors, 12 individuals were found to have confirmed or probable infection with Rocky Mountain spotted fever or ehrlichiosis. Sixty (16%) donors had evidence of asymptomatic seroconversion. A total of 320 units of platelets or packed red blood cells were transfused into 129 recipients in nine states. Seven hundred units were recalled. Ten recipients received units from ill soldiers, although none became ill.

Sporadic cases of SFGR and *Ehrlichia* species infections have been reported in troops deployed abroad. In 2000, a U.S. soldier who had been living in Korea for 3 months presented with fever, rash, leucopenia, and thrombocytopenia. Acute serum obtained on admission demonstrated the presence of IgM antibody to *Ehrlichia chaffeensis*.[53] A U.S. soldier returning from duty in Somalia in 1993 was diagnosed with Mediterranean spotted fever caused by *R. conorii*.[54]

Tickborne disease can affect the operational readiness of an entire unit. In 1992, a large outbreak of African tick bite fever occurred in an U.S. airborne unit that had deployed to Botswana for 2 weeks.[55] Eighteen percent (31/169 soldiers) were clinically ill and had lab confirmation consistent with *Rickettsia africae* infection. Personal protection measures were not fully utilized.

Scrub typhus is an important disease entity to rural and military populations throughout Southeast Asia, Korea, and Japan. Since 1934, outbreaks have been described among U.S. and Japanese troops training in a camp near Mt. Fuji, Japan. Recent outbreaks among U.S. forces were reported in 1995, 2000, and 2001.[56] Attack rates of 1% were observed in each incident. Scrub typhus was once common in north Queensland, Australia, but cases had not been reported for 30 years until 1996.[57] At that time, a soldier was diagnosed with scrub typhus and an investigation followed. Seventeen additional cases were identified. One year later, another outbreak involving 11 cases occurred at the same training site. Based on seroconversion rates, Thai soldiers working near the Thai-Cambodian border during 1992 had an estimated 2.66% annual infection rate.[58]

Infections caused by the protozoan parasite *Leishmania* (see Chapter 94) can cause significant morbidity to military forces worldwide. Numerous outbreaks of cutaneous leishmaniasis (CL) have been associated with military units deployed to jungle training centers. The incubation period of CL varies widely from a few days to many years, but the majority of lesions appear within the first few months after exposure. For short-term training missions, most cases occur after re-deployment to their home base. Training related outbreaks have occurred in Belize,[59] French Guiana, the Brazilian Amazon,[60–62] and at the U.S. Army–operated Jungle Operations Training Center (JOTC) in Panama.[63] Attack rates (AR) can be surprisingly high in nonimmune soldiers with 80% to 90% reported from French Guiana.[64] A striking example is a report from 1990 of 17 cases of CL seen in 27 Canadian paratroopers (63% AR) on the ground for 6 hours in British Guyana.[65] CL is a serious morale problem for Latin American military organizations. Overall infection rates of 1% to 2%, with much higher epidemic outbreaks in small units are not uncommon in units stationed in remote areas to counter antigovernment insurgencies or narco-trafficking.

CL caused by *L. major* was described in soldiers with Middle East peacekeeping duty associated while serving in the Multinational Force and Observers (MFO) in the Sinai desert.[66,67] Both Israeli and Jordanian soldiers have suffered epidemic outbreaks of CL caused by *L. major* while assigned to duties near the Jordan River valley and the Negev desert.[68,69]

Prior to the deployment of troops to Iraq and Afghanistan for Operation Iraqi Freedom (OIF) and Operation Enduring Freedom (OEF), the U.S. military experience with CL was predominately related to training missions in Central America, especially Panama.[70–72] The recent deployment to Iraq has resulted in the largest outbreak of CL in U.S. forces since WWII.[73–75] Over 700 cases of CL caused by *L. major* have been described to date. The majority of cases were acquired in Iraq with a few cases of CL caused by *L. tropica* acquired in Afghanistan.

Recent military experience with visceral leishmaniasis (VL) is more limited, most likely due to the fact that military operations have not occurred in areas of the world at highest risk for VL, such as the Ganges River drainage in India, Nepal, and Bangladesh, and the southern Sudan. In addition, clinically apparent disease is much less common than inapparent infection in otherwise healthy, nonimmune adults. Sporadic cases of VL in have been described in Chad,[76] and in four U.S. soldiers, two cases acquired in Iraq and two in Afghanistan.[73,77,78] VL may present differently in healthy nonimmune adults with lower parasite burdens, making parasitological diagnosis more difficult, and more atypical symptoms.[79] For example, 12 cases of systemic illness caused by *L. tropica*, a parasite usually associated with CL, were described in U.S. soldiers following the first Gulf War in 1991.[80,81] None of these patients presented with typical signs and symptoms of VL and instead presented with fatigue, malaise, gastrointestinal symptoms, adenopathy, transient hepatosplenomegaly, and mild laboratory abnormalities. The syndrome was called "viscerotropic" because parasites were isolated from bone marrow, liver tissue, or lymph nodes.

There are large groups of American military personnel and their families who live in *Leishmania* endemic areas of the world. The U.S. Navy has a naval air station in Sigonella, Sicily. This is an area long known to be endemic for a zoonotic cycle of *L. infantum*, canine reservoirs, and local sand fly vectors. Occasional cases of infantile kala-azar are seen in children of assigned military personnel. Infection rates in humans are not known, but a study in companion pet dogs showed a 75% subclinical infection rate.[82] This much higher than expected infection rate in companion dogs would indicate subclinical human infection occurs, perhaps at much higher rates than expected.

Prevention of *Leishmania* infection in military populations relies on vector personal protection measures (PPMs). The use of permethrin-impregnated uniforms is recommended, but clinical trial data to support such use is limited. Four of 143 (3%) Colombian soldiers wearing impregnated uniforms acquired CL, while 18 of 143 (18%) wearing control uniforms acquired CL.[83] The success in Colombia was not seen in a clinical trial in Iran.[84] Practical insect avoidance measures, combined with treated bed nets and DEET based repellants, can achieve high protection against biting arthropods.[84]

DISEASES TRANSMITTED BY THE FECAL-ORAL ROUTE

Diarrheal diseases continue be an important cause of illness in modern military forces. Rates and etiologies reflect regional and seasonal distributions of enteric pathogens. During a training exercise in southern China in 1997, medical officials reported a diarrheal attack rate of 7.3% among 2636 members of the People's Liberation Army during a 20-day observation period.[85] Enterotoxigenic *Esherichia coli* was the predominant pathogen isolated (35%). *Shigella* species were the major bacterial pathogen (40%) among Peruvian soldiers training in the Amazon River basin in 2002.[86] *Campylobacter* infections were a leading cause of diarrhea in U.S. troops training in Thailand during the 1990s as quinolone-resistant strains became more prevalent in that area.[87]

Port visits have been linked to shipboard outbreaks. Twenty-one percent of surveyed U.S. naval personnel ($n = 500$) reported having acute diarrhea during or shortly after departing Alexandria, Egypt, in 1988.[88] An outbreak of cryptosporidiosis occurred on a U.S. Coast Guard cutter that had filled its tank with city water while docked at Milwaukee, Wisconsin, in March, 1993.[89] A massive outbreak was later reported among city inhabitants.[90]

During conflict or a time of rapid buildup of forces, toilet facilities can be primitive consisting of open trenches or wooden latrines. Fly control may not be established and adequate levels of personal hygiene and sanitation are difficult to maintain. These factors, together with crowded living conditions, increase the transmission potential of pathogens transmitted by the fecal-oral route.

In 1990 during the initial months of Operation Desert Shield, outbreaks of watery diarrhea occurred in U.S. troops.[91] This was followed by outbreaks of more severe, bloody diarrhea in the second month. More than 50% of 2022 U.S. combatants surveyed reported at least one episode of diarrhea and 20% of affected combatants reported that it interfered with their work and resulted in a medical visit.[91] In a separate survey, microbiologic studies showed that half of the diarrhea in combatants seeking medical care was of bacterial origins, mostly enterotoxigenic *E. coli* and *Shigella* species.[91] Susceptibility testing showed many multidrug resistant strains reflecting the patterns observed among the endemic population. Empiric antibiotic treatment regimens were altered in response to these resistance patterns. Many of the outbreaks were attributed to ingestion of raw vegetables, especially lettuce, that were procured from countries outside the United States.

Diarrhea control measures among U.S. forces were strongly enforced during Operation Restore Hope in Somalia, 1992–1993. A comprehensive medical surveillance system that included over 85% of all deployed forces was instituted and found that less than 1% of the force each week sought care for diarrhea during the first 2 months.[44] No large diarrhea outbreaks were observed. *Shigella* species (33%) and enterotoxigenic *E. coli* (16%) were the predominant bacterial pathogens isolated.

An early report about self-reported disease prevalence during Operation Iraqi Freedom and Operation Enduring Freedom (Aghanistan) indicated that diarrhea rates may have been high during the initial phase of deployment.[92] Seventy percent of 2389 volunteers reported at least one episode of diarrhea and 56% reported multiple episodes. Seventeen percent of those with diarrhea reported being on bed rest for a median of 2 days.

Diarrhea rates during deployments on humanitarian missions can be high. British ($n = 36$) and Australian ($n = 75$) medical teams working among the Kurdish refugees in 1991 had different rates of diarrhea during the first 5 weeks in northern Iraq.[93] Diarrhea rates were higher among the British force (69%), which did not use doxycycline for malaria prophylaxis and did not enforce hand- and plate-washing procedures, than the Australian group (36%) who did. In 1994 among a 131-person Dutch military unit serving in the refugee camps in Goma, Zaire, 20% reported diarrhea during the first 3 weeks.[94] On the day of departure, 102 servicemen ate at a local hotel and 59% developed diarrhea shortly after returning home.

Diarrhea continues to be an important disease affecting operational readiness in the military despite having preventive measures which can minimize attack rates. Vaccine development for major bacterial causes of diarrhea in troops is a major area of research for the military.

Norovirus outbreaks are being increasingly recognized among military forces. While outbreaks among civilian ships have received publicity, at least 60% to 80% of cases occur on land.[95] Outbreaks of vomiting were reported in Operation Desert Shield/Storm among American forces and an attack rate of 4% to 9% occurred over a 5-month period in one Marine unit.[96] Ninety-nine soldiers in an Army trainee unit (12%) were hospitalized during an outbreak at El Paso, Texas, in 1998.[97] In May 2002, eleven British soldiers were air-evacuated from Afghanistan when the initial patients presented with a severe acute illness characterized by headache, neck stiffness, photophobia, obtundation, and gastrointestinal symptoms.[98] Two patients required ventilatory support and one patient's illness progressed to disseminated intravascular coagulation. Norovirus infection was later confirmed by laboratory analyses in England.

Explosive outbreaks have occurred on U.S. Navy vessels with several hundred sailors becoming ill in a short time period.[99] For the deployed forces, this infection causes a major diagnostic dilemma. Currently, there are no rapid diagnostic field tests to identify norovirus infection from an unknown chemical or biological attack that produces similar clinical symptoms and attack rates.

ZOONOTIC DISEASES

Thousands of cases of Q fever (see Chapter 54) have been reported in military units throughout history. An outbreak of Q fever occurred among British and Czech soldiers deployed as part of the United Nations Stabilization Force in Bosnia-Herzegovina during May and June, 1997.[100] Approximately 4% (26/610 personnel) became infected and over half exhibited clinical symptoms. A flu-like illness was the predominant presentation and three soldiers had atypical pneumonias. A sheep farm was located 100 meters from one of the bases. It was thought that exposure occurred when infectious aerosols were generated during lambing season by the approach and landing of helicopters.

A few cases of Q fever have also been identified in U.S. forces during the recent past. In Operation Desert Storm/Shield, one case of Q fever–related meningoencephalitis, one case of pneumonia, and three individuals who were epidemiologically linked to the pneumonia case and seroconverted were identified.[101] During 2003 in Operation Iraqi Freedom, eight soldiers with pneumonia were diagnosed by serology retrospectively.[102]

It is likely that the incidence of Q fever among soldiers is severely underestimated. Most infections present as a flu-like illness and are self-limited. The most common clinical presentation is pneumonia and is commonly misdiagnosed as a community-acquired pneumonia. Even if primary health-care providers suspected Q fever, confirmation is difficult and requires specimens be sent to a reference laboratory.

Hemorrhagic fever with renal syndrome (HFRS), a rodent-borne disease (see Chapter 68), has caused significant casualties during military conflicts. The war in the Balkans during the 1990s was no exception. In Bosnia, more than 300 military and civilian cases were treated in a single hospital during a 1-year period.[103] In 1995, large outbreaks of HFRS occurred at several sites in Croatia. Of the 129 reported cases, 120 were Croatian Army soldiers. Two of the soldiers died.[104] Severe clinical manifestations were reported in many patients. These infections were caused by a newly described hantavirus, Dobrava, rather than the Puumala virus, which also circulates in this area but causes a milder illness.

The association of rodent-borne diseases and war comes as no surprise. Improperly stored food and garbage in military camps can contribute to an increase in the size of rodent populations. However, military outbreaks have also occurred during field training when the rodent's natural habitat is disturbed. In January 1990, U.S. troops camping in southern Germany during training maneuvers had 16 cases of HFRS for an attack rate in one unit of 8.5%.[105]

In Korea, HFRS affects both civilian and military populations. From 1980 to 1985, over 3000 cases were diagnosed.[106] Approximately 24% of these cases were Korean soldiers, but only 22 cases occurred among American soldiers. An outbreak occurred in 1986 among 3754 U.S. Marines who had participated in a 5-week joint training exercise with Korean troops.[107] Fourteen cases occurred; two died. Of note, eight of the cases became symptomatic after leaving Korea. Infection can occur without exposure to a field setting. Recently, a case occurred in a soldier in which it appeared that the infection was acquired on base in an urban environment.[108]

Leptospirosis (see Chapter 46) is an occupational hazard for soldiers operating in swampy environments. In the early 1980s, some U.S. military units training in Panama had attack rates of 2% to 8%. In response, military researchers tested and demonstrated the efficacy of weekly doxycycline for chemoprophylaxis.[109] In 1987, two clusters of cases occurred in U.S. military personnel serving in Okinawa, Japan, with attack rates of 47% and 18%.[110] In 1999, 193 Peruvian military recruits trained for 2 weeks in the high jungles near Pichanaqui, Peru.[111] During the subsequent 4 weeks, 78 recruits became ill with an acute undifferentiated febrile illness. Laboratory testing was negative for dengue, Oropuche, Venezuela equine encephalitis, Mayaro, yellow fever, group C bunyaviruses, rickettsia, ehrlichia, and malaria; however, 92% of the cases were positive for leptospirosis by microscopic agglutination test. Like Q fever, this disease is probably under-reported because physicians are unfamiliar with its clinical presentation and difficulty in obtaining laboratory confirmation.

DISEASES TRANSMITTED THROUGH EXPOSURE TO SOIL AND DUST

Military forces working or training in areas endemic to mycoses that can be transmitted through inhalation are at particular risk of acquiring these infections. Certain field activities that produce dust, such as the driving of vehicles, digging ditches, or cleaning of abandoned buildings, increase the risk for exposure. For American forces, there are at least 10 major military bases located in the southwest desert of the United States where coccidioidomycosis (see Chapter 80) is endemic.[112] Sporadic cases, as well as outbreaks of this disease, occur in military populations.[112–116] From 1981 to 1994, 113 U.S. sailors and Marines were hospitalized in Navy medical facilities for coccidioidomycosis, with primary pulmonary disease representing the most common form (72%).[115] Failure to obtain an adequate travel history and unfamiliarity with this disease has led to delayed or missed diagnoses.[113,116] In 1992, a 27-man Marine reserve unit from Tennessee trained for 3 weeks at Vandenberg Air Force Base, California.[116] A week after returning, one of the reservist developed symptoms of pneumonia and, despite treatment with tetracycline and amoxicillin, his illness persisted. Later during his hospitalization, coccidioidomycosis was diagnosed. Other members of the group (26%) had symptoms consistent with coccidioidomycosis infection. All had sought medical intervention, but only two were diagnosed correctly. Misdiagnoses are not infrequent. During the fall of 2001, elite Navy Special Forces personnel ($n = 23$) trained for 6 weeks in Coalinga, California.[113] Six presented to a local medical clinic during the exercise with cough, fever, chills, night sweats, and malaise, but were diagnosed with a "viral illness".[113] Because of persistent symptoms, one Navy Seal was evaluated at a military hospital 6 weeks later and a diagnosis of coccidioidomycosis was made. An investigation of the group found that 45% of the team had serologic evidence of acute coccidioidomycosis and all were symptomatic. In summary, physicians attending to any ill military personnel must be vigilant for this disease. Large numbers of personnel train in desert warfare at Fort Irwin, California, and may present with their illness thousands of miles away from this endemic area. Early detection and treatment can prevent progression to disseminated disease and complications.

Melioidosis (see Chapter 34) is an important infectious disease for military personnel because of its multiple modes of transmission, the severity of illness, latent infections that become clinically apparent years after initial exposure, its intrinsic resistance to many antibiotics, and its high relapse rate.[117]

It is a bacterial disease which is highly endemic throughout Southeast Asia and caused several hundred hospitalizations in U.S forces during the Vietnam conflict.[118] U.S. military personnel have presented with disease years after exposure in Vietnam.[119] Between 1987 and 1994, 23 acute cases were diagnosed in the Singapore Armed Forces.[120] Unlike patients from endemic areas who frequently have underlying illnesses or are elderly, soldiers are usually fit. The disease is probably underdiagnosed in soldiers as well as endemic populations because of failure of medical personnel to recognize its many clinical presentations and the lack of access to microbiologic assays.[117]

Parasitic infections that are transmitted by contact with contaminated soil, such as hookworm and strongyloides (see Chapters 110 and 111), have long been associated with deployed soldiers. During World War II, there were 23,300 hospitalizations of U.S. troops attributed to hookworm.[121] In a study of 500 American soldiers returning from Vietnam in 1965, 15% were infected with intestinal parasites (55% had hookworm, 19% had strongyloides, and 14% had both).[122] During 1983 after military intervention in Grenada, over 200 soldiers in different U.S. Army units reported signs and symptoms consistent with soil-transmitted helminthic infections.[123] Hookworm was confirmed in 8.3% of soldiers in one survey. Outbreaks of hookworm and strongyloides infections occurred repeatedly in U.S. troops training at the JOTC in Panama during the 1980s and 1990s.[124] In 1993, 566 soldiers from an infantry battalion trained for 3 weeks in Panama. Approximately 3 weeks after returning home, soldiers began to seek medical care for abdominal pain, nausea, vomiting, and diarrhea. An investigation identified hookworm infection in 12% of 75 soldiers who submitted a single stool sample and strongyloides in 3%. Eosinophilia (>7%) was detected in 129 of 473 blood samples, suggesting helminthic infection in 27% of the soldiers. These outbreaks demonstrated the importance of considering helminthic infections in troops exposed to muddy, contaminated soil. Many will present with gastrointestinal symptoms several weeks after exposure, but before eggs are observed in the stool. Soldiers should have a complete blood count with differential to document eosinophilia and uncover asymptomatic infections. Of particular concern to the long-term health of infected soldiers is the ability to detect strongyloides infections, which, if untreated, can lead to life-long infection and the possibility of life-threatening hyperinfection if the soldier/veteran becomes immunosuppressed.

CONCLUSION

Not all infectious diseases that have been reported in modern military forces were discussed in this chapter. There was not enough space to present all the published evidence for the diseases that were included in the chapter. Individual cases of unique parasitic diseases that have been described in military personnel and sexually transmitted diseases and HIV infections were also not reviewed.

Although modern war has evolved substantially, and today's battlefield is quite different from previous conflicts, infectious diseases remain a major threat to deployed troops. Presently, large numbers of military personnel from many countries are sent to areas with high incidences of infectious diseases. When their working and living conditions are crowded or unhygienic, particularly in times of war and conflict, their risk of infection increases. When appropriate public health and preventive measures are implemented, the incidence of infectious diseases can be greatly reduced. When military and civilian physicians who care for ill soldiers recognize their illnesses and institute appropriate therapies promptly, morbidity from infectious diseases can be lessened. However, even in these optimal circumstances, infectious diseases still occur.

When appropriate preventive measures are not instituted and treatment providers are not adequately prepared, attack rates from malaria, diarrheal diseases, acute respiratory infections, and other contagious infectious diseases can be quite high and deaths do result. Many nations do not have the resources to implement sound public health measures in their troops or to deploy sophisticated medical care. Although developed nations, such as the United States, may have the means to prevent and treat infectious diseases even in the most austere conditions, sometimes they do not implement the most effective preventive and curative services. Furthermore, with the speed of today's travel, deployed troops incubating an infectious illness may return home and present to garrison-based or civilian physicians. All physicians, whether they are with deployed troops or caring for those who returned home, need to be mindful of the exposures to infectious diseases and the illnesses that can occur in military settings. The ill soldier or veteran represents a high risk traveler that may have been exposed to various pathogens in many different countries.

REFERENCES

1. Gray GC, Callahan JD, Hawksworth AW, et al: Respiratory diseases among U.S. military personnel: Countering emerging threats. Emerg Infect Dis 5:379, 1999.
2. Centers for Disease Control and Prevention: Two fatal cases of adenovirus-related illness in previously healthy young adults—Illinois, 2000. MMWR 50:553, 2001.
3. United States Army Center for Health Promotion and Preventive Medicine: Influenza among soldiers in Advanced Individual Training, Aberdeen Proving Ground, Maryland, December 1996. Medical Surveillance Monthly Report 3:12, 1997. Accessed on November 28, 2004, at amsa.army.mil/1MSMR/1997/v03_n02.pdf#page=12.
4. United States Army Center for Health Promotion and Preventive Medicine: Influenza among immunized members of an aviation squadron, US Navy, Hawaii. Medical Surveillance Monthly Report 4:10, 1998. Accessed on November 28, 2004, at amsa.army.mil/1MSMR/1998/v04_n02.pdf#page=10.
5. United States Army Center for Health Promotion and Preventive Medicine: An outbreak of parainfluenza type 1 acute respiratory illnesses among basic trainees, Fort Sill, Oklahoma, June 1998. Medical Surveillance Monthly Report 4:12, 1998. Accessed on November 28, 2004, at amsa.army.mil/1MSMR/1998/v04_n08.pdf#page=14.
6. Crum NF, Wallace MR, Lamb CR, et al: Halting a pneumococcal pneumonia outbreak among United States Marine Corps trainees. Am J Prev Med 25:107, 2003.
7. Centers for Disease Prevention and Control: Outbreak of group A streptococcal pneumonia among Marine Corps recruits—California, November 1–December 20, 2002. MMWR 52:106, 2003.
8. Sanchez JL, Craig SC, Kolavic S, et al: An outbreak of pneumococcal pneumonia among military personnel at high risk: Control by low-dose azithromycin postexposure chemoprophylaxis. Mil Med 168:1, 2003.
9. DiStasio AJ, 2nd, Trump DH: The investigation of a tuberculosis outbreak in the closed environment of a U.S. Navy ship, 1987. Mil Med 155:347, 1990.

10. Houk VN, Baker JH, Sorensen K, et al: The epidemiology of tuberculosis infection in a closed environment. Arch Environ Health 16:26, 1968.
11. Lamar JE, 2nd, Malakooti MA: Tuberculosis outbreak investigation of a U.S. Navy amphibious ship crew and the Marine expeditionary unit aboard, 1998. Mil Med 168:523, 2003.
12. Brundage JF, Ryan MA, Feighner BH, et al: Meningococcal disease among United States military service members in relation to routine uses of vaccines with different serogroup-specific components, 1964–1998. Clin Infect Dis 35:1376, 2002.
13. Bergman BP, Hayton JC, Green AD: Effectiveness of the meningococcal vaccination programme for British Armed Forces recruits. Commun Dis Public Health 3:298, 2000.
14. Gdalevich M, Mimouni D, Eldad A, et al: Secular trends in the epidemiology of major infectious diseases among Israeli soldiers. Public Health Rev 27:297, 1999.
15. Spiegel A, Quenel P, Sperber G, et al: [Evaluation of systematic anti-meningococcal vaccination strategy in French military recruits]. Sante 6:383, 1996.
16. United States Army Center for Health Promotion and Preventive Medicine: Meningococcal meningitis, Fort Bliss, TX. Medical Surveillance Monthly Report 1:7, 1995. Accessed November 28, 2004, at amsa.army.mil/1MSMR/1995/v01_n08.pdf.
17. Farr W, Gonzalez MJ, Garbauskas H, et al: Suspected meningococcal meningitis on an aircraft carrier. Mil Med 169:684, 2004.
18. United States Army Center for Health Promotion and Preventive Medicine: Rubella outbreak in German troops at Fort Bragg. Medical Surveillance Monthly Report 1:2, 1995. Accessed on November 28, 2004, at amsa.army.mil/1MSMR/1995/v01_n02.pdf#page=2.
19. Ziebold C, Hassenpflug B, Wegner-Brose H, et al: An outbreak of rubella aboard a ship of the German Navy. Infection 31:136, 2003.
20. D'Amelio R, Biselli R, Fascia G, et al: Measles-mumps-rubella vaccine in the Italian armed forces. JAMA 284:2059, 2000.
21. Sanchez JL, Bendet I, Grogl M, et al: Malaria in Brazilian military personnel deployed to Angola. J Travel Med 7:275, 2000.
22. Migliani R, Josse R, Hovette P, et al: [Malaria in military personnel: The case of the Ivory Coast in 2002–2003]. Med Trop (Mars) 63:282, 2003.
23. Hopperus Buma AP, van Thiel PP, Lobel HO, et al: Long-term malaria chemoprophylaxis with mefloquine in Dutch marines in Cambodia. J Infect Dis 173:1506, 1996.
24. Sergiev VP, Baranova AM, Orlov VS, et al: Importation of malaria into the USSR from Afghanistan, 1981–1989. Bull World Health Org 71:385, 1993.
25. Park JW, Klein TA, Lee HC, et al: Vivax malaria: A continuing health threat to the Republic of Korea. Am J Trop Med Hyg 69:159, 2003.
26. United States Army Center for Health Promotion and Preventive Medicine: *P. vivax* malaria acquired by US soldiers in Korea: Acquisition trends and incubation period characteristics, 1994–2000. Medical Surveillance Monthly Report 7:7, 2001. Accessed on November 28, 2004, at amsa.army.mil/1MSMR/2001/v07_n01.pdf.
27. United States Army Center for Health Promotion and Preventive Medicine: Malaria among active duty US soldiers, January-December 2000. Medical Surveillance Monthly Report 7:2, 2001. Accessed on November 28, 2004, at amsa.army.mil/1MSMR/2001/v07_n01.pdf.
28. Wallace MR, Sharp TW, Smoak B, et al: Malaria among United States troops in Somalia. Am J Med 100:49, 1996.
29. Newton JA, Jr., Schnepf GA, Wallace MR, et al: Malaria in US Marines returning from Somalia. JAMA 272:397, 1994.
30. Smoak BL, DeFraites RF, Magill AJ, et al: *Plasmodium vivax* infections in U.S. Army troops: Failure of primaquine to prevent relapse in studies from Somalia. Am J Trop Med Hyg 56:231, 1997.
31. Peragallo MS, Sabatinelli G, Majori G, et al: Prevention and morbidity of malaria in non-immune subjects: A case-control study among Italian troops in Somalia and Mozambique, 1992–1994. Trans R Soc Trop Med Hyg 91:343, 1997.
32. Kitchener SJ, Auliff AM, Rieckmann KH: Malaria in the Australian Defence Force during and after participation in the International Force in East Timor (INTERFET). Med J Aust 173:583, 2000.
33. Edgcomb JH, Arnold J, Yount EH, Jr., et al: Primaquine, SN 13272, a new curative agent in vivax malaria; a preliminary report. J Natl Malar Soc 9:285, 1950.
34. Jelinek T, Nothdurft HD, Von Sonnenburg F, et al: Long-term efficacy of primaquine in the treatment of vivax malaria in nonimmune travelers. Am J Trop Med Hyg 52:322, 1995.
35. Archambeault C: Mass antimalarial therapy in veterans returning from Korea. JAMA 154:1411, 1954.
36. Garrison PL, Hankey DD, Coker WG, et al: Cure of Korean vivax malaria with pamaquine and primaquine. JAMA 149:1562, 1952.
37. Clyde DF, McCarthy VC: Radical cure of Chesson strain vivax malaria in man by 7, not 14, days of treatment with primaquine. Am J Trop Med Hyg 26:562, 1977.
38. Baird JK, Rieckmann KH: Can primaquine therapy for vivax malaria be improved? Trends Parasitol 19:115, 2003.
39. Clayman CB, Arnold J, Hockwald RS, et al: Toxicity of primaquine in Caucasians. JAMA 149:1563, 1952.
40. Hockwald RS, Arnold J, Clayman CB, et al: Toxicity of primaquine in Negroes. JAMA 149:1568, 1952.
41. Baird JK, Hoffman SL: Primaquine therapy for malaria. Clin Infect Dis 39:1336, 2004.
42. Trofa AF, DeFraites RF, Smoak BL, et al: Dengue fever in US military personnel in Haiti. JAMA 277:1546, 1997.
43. Gambel JM, Drabick JJ, Swalko MA, et al: Dengue among United Nations mission in Haiti personnel, 1995: Implications for preventive medicine. Mil Med 164:300, 1999.
44. Sharp TW, Wallace MR, Hayes CG, et al: Dengue fever in U.S. troops during Operation Restore Hope, Somalia, 1992–1993. Am J Trop Med Hyg 53:89, 1995.
45. Peragallo MS, Nicoletti L, Lista F, et al: Probable dengue virus infection among Italian troops, East Timor, 1999–2000. Emerg Infect Dis 9:876, 2003.
46. Chungue E, Burucoa C, Boutin JP, et al: Dengue 1 epidemic in French Polynesia, 1988–1989: Surveillance and clinical, epidemiological, virological and serological findings in 1752 documented clinical cases. Trans R Soc Trop Med Hyg 86:193, 1992.
47. Kitchener S, Leggat PA, Brennan L, et al: Importation of dengue by soldiers returning from East Timor to north Queensland, Australia. J Travel Med 9:180, 2002.
48. Durand JP, Bouloy M, Richecoeur L, et al: Rift Valley fever virus infection among French troops in Chad. Emerg Infect Dis 9:751, 2003.
49. United States Army Center for Health Promotion and Preventive Medicine: Ross River virus disease ("epidemic polyarthritis"), Exercise Tandem Thrust 97, Queensland, Australia, March 1997. Medical Surveillance Monthly Report 3:7, 1997. Accessed on November 28, 2004, at amsa.army.mil/1MSMR/1997/v03_n07.pdf#page=13.
50. Dawson JE, Anderson BE, Fishbein DB, et al: Isolation and characterization of an *Ehrlichia* sp. from a patient diagnosed with human ehrlichiosis. J Clin Microbiol 29:2741, 1991.
51. Yevich SJ, Sanchez JL, DeFraites RF, et al: Seroepidemiology of infections due to spotted fever group rickettsiae and *Ehrlichia* species in military personnel exposed in areas of the United States where such infections are endemic. J Infect Dis 171:1266, 1995.
52. Arguin PM, Singleton J, Rotz LD, et al: An investigation into the possibility of transmission of tick-borne pathogens via blood transfusion. Transfusion-Associated Tick-Borne Illness Task Force. Transfusion 39:828, 1999.
53. United States Army Center for Health Promotion and Preventive Medicine: *Ehrlichia chaffeensis* infection in an active duty soldier stationed in Korea. Medical Surveillance Monthly Report 6:9, 2000. Accessed on November 28, 2004, at amsa.army.mil/1MSMR/2000/v06_n10.pdf.
54. Williams WJ, Radulovic S, Dasch GA, et al: Identification of *Rickettsia conorii* infection by polymerase chain reaction in a soldier returning from Somalia. Clin Infect Dis 19:93, 1994.
55. Smoak BL, McClain JB, Brundage JF, et al: An outbreak of spotted fever rickettsiosis in U.S. Army troops deployed to Botswana. Emerg Infect Dis 2:217, 1996.
56. Jiang J, Marienau KJ, May LA, et al: Laboratory diagnosis of two scrub typhus outbreaks at Camp Fuji, Japan in 2000 and 2001 by enzyme-linked immunosorbent assay, rapid flow assay, and Western blot assay using outer membrane 56-kD recombinant proteins. Am J Trop Med Hyg 69:60, 2003.
57. McBride WJ, Taylor CT, Pryor JA, et al: Scrub typhus in north Queensland. Med J Aust 170:318, 1999.
58. Frances SP, Eamsila C, Strickman D: Antibodies to *Orientia tsutsugamushi* in soldiers in northeastern Thailand. Southeast Asian J Trop Med Public Health 28:666, 1997.
59. Hepburn NC, Tidman MJ, Hunter JA: Cutaneous leishmaniasis in British troops from Belize. Br J Dermatol 128:63, 1993.

60. Silveira FT, Ishikawa EA, De Souza AA, et al: An outbreak of cutaneous leishmaniasis among soldiers in Belem, Para State, Brazil, caused by *Leishmania (Viannia) lindenbergi* n. sp. A new leishmanial parasite of man in the Amazon region. Parasite 9:43, 2002.
61. Brandao-Filho SP, de Brito ME, Martins CA, et al: [American cutaneous leishmaniasis in a military training center located in Zona da Mata, Pernambuco, Brazil]. Rev Soc Bras Med Trop 31:575, 1998.
62. de Oliveira Guerra JA, Talhari S, Paes MG, et al: [Clinical and diagnostic aspects of American tegumentary leishmaniosis in soldiers simultaneously exposed to the infection in the Amazon Region]. Rev Soc Bras Med Trop 36:587, 2003.
63. Sanchez JL, Diniega BM, Small JW, et al: Epidemiologic investigation of an outbreak of cutaneous leishmaniasis in a defined geographic focus of transmission. Am J Trop Med Hyg 47:47, 1992.
64. Banzet S: [Epidemics of cutaneous leishmaniasis in military personnel working in French Guiana]. Med Trop (Mars) 60:297, 2000.
65. Martin S, Gambel J, Jackson J, et al: Leishmaniasis in the United States military. Mil Med 163:801, 1998.
66. Norton SA, Frankenburg S, Klaus SN: Cutaneous leishmaniasis acquired during military service in the Middle East. Arch Dermatol 128:83, 1992.
67. Fryauff DJ, Modi GB, Mansour NS, et al: Epidemiology of cutaneous leishmaniasis at a focus monitored by the multinational force and observers in the northeastern Sinai Desert of Egypt. Am J Trop Med Hyg 49:598, 1993.
68. Giladi M, Danon YL, Greenblatt C, et al: Keziot—A new endemic site of cutaneous leishmaniasis in Israel. An epidemiological and clinical study of a non-immune population entering an endemic area. Trop Geogr Med 37:298, 1985.
69. Jumaian N, Kamhawi SA, Halalsheh M, et al: Short report: Outbreak of cutaneous leishmaniasis in a nonimmune population of soldiers in Wadi Araba, Jordan. Am J Trop Med Hyg 58:160, 1998.
70. Chulay JD, Oster CN, McGreevy PB, et al: American cutaneous leishmaniasis: Presentation and problems of patient management. Rev Soc Bras Med Trop 21:165, 1988.
71. Walton BC, Person DA, Bernstein R: Leishmaniasis in the U.S. military in the Canal Zone. Am J Trop Med Hyg 17:19, 1968.
72. Aronson NE, Wortmann GW, Johnson SC, et al: Safety and efficacy of intravenous sodium stibogluconate in the treatment of leishmaniasis: Recent U.S. military experience. Clin Infect Dis 27:1457, 1998.
73. Wiena PJ, Neafie RC, Wortmann G, et al: Old World leishmaniasis: An emerging infection among deployed US military and civilian workers. Clin Infect Dis 39:1674, 2004.
74. Centers for Disease Prevention and Control: Cutaneous leishmaniasis in U.S. military personnel—Southwest/Central Asia, 2002–2003. MMWR 52:1009, 2003.
75. Centers for Disease Prevention and Control: Update: Cutaneous leishmaniasis in U.S. military personnel—Southwest/Central Asia, 2002–2004. MMWR 53:264, 2004.
76. Djidingar D, Chippaux JP, Gragnic G, et al:. [Visceral leishmaniasis in Niger: six new parasitologically confirmed cases]. Bull Soc Pathol Exot 90:27, 1997.
77. Halsey ES, Bryce LM, Wortmann GW, et al: Visceral leishmaniasis in a soldier returning from Operation Enduring Freedom. Mil Med 169:699, 2004.
78. Centers for Disease Prevention and Control: Two cases of visceral leishmaniasis in U.S. military personnel—Afghanistan, 2002–2004. MMWR 53:265, 2004.
79. Most H, Lavietes P: Kala-azar in American military personnel. Medicine 26:221, 1947.
80. Magill AJ, Grogl M, Gasser RA, Jr., et al: Visceral infection caused by *Leishmania tropica* in veterans of Operation Desert Storm. N Engl J Med 328:1383, 1993.
81. Magill AJ, Grogl M, Johnson SC, et al: Visceral infection due to *Leishmania tropica* in a veteran of Operation Desert Storm who presented 2 years after leaving Saudi Arabia. Clin Infect Dis 19:805, 1994.
82. Orndorff GR, Cooper BA, Smith W, et al: Canine visceral leishmaniasis in Sicily. Mil Med 165:29, 2000.
83. Soto J, Medina F, Dember N, et al: Efficacy of permethrin-impregnated uniforms in the prevention of malaria and leishmaniasis in Colombian soldiers. Clin Infect Dis 21:599, 1995.
84. Asilian A, Sadeghinia A, Shariati F, et al: Efficacy of permethrin-impregnated uniforms in the prevention of cutaneous leishmaniasis in Iranian soldiers. J Clin Pharm Ther 28:175, 2003.
85. Bai Y, Dai YC, Li JD, et al: Acute diarrhea during army field exercise in southern China. World J Gastroenterol 10:127, 2004.
86. Jones FR, Sanchez JL, Meza R, et al: Short Report: High incidence of shigellosis among Peruvian soldiers deployed in the Amazon River basin. Am J Trop Med Hyg 70:663, 2004.
87. Sanders JW, Isenbarger DW, Walz SE, et al: An observational clinic-based study of diarrheal illness in deployed United States military personnel in Thailand: Presentation and outcome of *Campylobacter* infection. Am J Trop Med Hyg 67:533, 2002.
88. Haberberger RL, Scott DA, Thornton SA, et al: Diarrheal disease aboard a U.S. Navy ship after a brief port visit to a high risk area. Mil Med 159:445, 1994.
89. Moss DM, Bennett SN, Arrowood MJ, et al: Enzyme-linked immunoelectrotransfer blot analysis of a cryptosporidiosis outbreak on a United States Coast Guard cutter. Am J Trop Med Hyg 58:110, 1998.
90. Mac Kenzie WR, Hoxie NJ, Proctor ME, et al: A massive outbreak in Milwaukee of *Cryptosporidium* infection transmitted through the public water supply. N Engl J Med 331:161, 1994.
91. Hyams KC, Bourgeois AL, Merrell BR, et al: Diarrheal disease during Operation Desert Shield. N Engl J Med 325:1423, 1991.
92. Sanders JW, Putnam SD, Riddle MS, et al: The epidemiology of self-reported diarrhea in operations Iraqi Freedom and Enduring Freedom. Diagn Microbiol Infect Dis 50:89, 2004.
93. Rudland S, Little M, Kemp P, et al: The enemy within: Diarrheal rates among British and Australian troops in Iraq. Mil Med 161:728, 1996.
94. Bruins J, Bwire R, Slootman EJ, et al: Diarrhea morbidity among Dutch military service men in Goma, Zaire. Mil Med 160:446, 1995.
95. Centers for Disease Prevention and Control: Norovirus activity—United States, 2002. MMWR 52:41, 2003.
96. Hyams KC, Malone JD, Kapikian AZ, et al: Norwalk virus infection among Desert Storm troops. J Infect Dis 167:986, 1993.
97. Arness MK, Feighner BH, Canham ML, et al: Norwalk-like viral gastroenteritis outbreak in U.S. Army trainees. Emerg Infect Dis 6:204, 2000.
98. Centers for Disease Prevention and Control: Outbreak of acute gastroenteritis associated with Norwalk-like viruses among British military personnel—Afghanistan, May 2002. MMWR 51:477, 2002.
99. McCarthy M, Estes MK, Hyams KC: Norwalk-like virus infection in military forces: Epidemic potential, sporadic disease, and the future direction of prevention and control efforts. J Infect Dis 181(suppl 2): S387, 2000.
100. Splino M, Beran J, Chlibek R: Q fever outbreak during the Czech Army deployment in Bosnia. Mil Med 168:840, 2003.
101. Byrne WR: Q fever. In Sidell FR, Takfuji ET, Franz DR (eds): Medical Aspects of Chemical and Biological Warfare. Textbook of Military Medicine. Washington, DC, Office of the Surgeon General and Borden Institute, 1997, p 524.
102. Smoak B, Personal communication.
103. Hukic M, Kurt A, Torstensson S, et al: Haemorrhagic fever with renal syndrome in north-east Bosnia. Lancet 347:56, 1996.
104. Mulic R, Ropac D: Epidemiologic characteristics and military implications of hemorrhagic fever with renal syndrome in croatia. Croat Med J 43:581, 2002.
105. Clement J, Underwood P, Ward D, et al: Hantavirus outbreak during military manoeuvres in Germany. Lancet 347:336, 1996.
106. Lee HW: Hemorrhagic fever with renal syndrome in Korea. Rev Infect Dis 11(suppl 4):S864, 1989.
107. Pon E, McKee KT, Jr., Diniega BM, et al: Outbreak of hemorrhagic fever with renal syndrome among U.S. Marines in Korea. Am J Trop Med Hyg 42:612, 1990.
108. Sachar DS, Narayan R, Song JW, et al: Hantavirus infection in an active duty U.S. Army soldier stationed in Seoul, Korea. Mil Med 168:231, 2003.
109. Takafuji ET, Kirkpatrick JW, Miller RN, et al: An efficacy trial of doxycycline chemoprophylaxis against leptospirosis. N Engl J Med 310:497, 1984.
110. Corwin A, Ryan A, Bloys W, et al: A waterborne outbreak of leptospirosis among United States military personnel in Okinawa, Japan. Int J Epidemiol 19:743, 1990.
111. Russell KL, Montiel Gonzalez MA, et al: An outbreak of leptospirosis among Peruvian military recruits. Am J Trop Med Hyg 69:53, 2003.
112. Crum NF, Lederman ER, Hale BR, et al: A cluster of disseminated coccidioidomycosis cases at a US military hospital. Mil Med 168:460, 2003.

113. Crum N, Lamb C, Utz G, et al: Coccidioidomycosis outbreak among United States Navy SEALs training in a *Coccidioides immitis*–endemic area—Coalinga, California. J Infect Dis 186:865, 2002.
114. Gibbs BT, Neff RT: A 22-year-old Army private with chest pain and weight loss. Mil Med 169:157, 2004.
115. Gray GC, Fogle EF, Albright KL: Risk factors for primary pulmonary coccidioidomycosis hospitalizations among United States Navy and Marine Corps personnel, 1981–1994. Am J Trop Med Hyg 58:309, 1998.
116. Standaert SM, Schaffner W, Galgiani JN, et al: Coccidioidomycosis among visitors to a *Coccidioides immitis*–endemic area: An outbreak in a military reserve unit. J Infect Dis 171:1672, 1995.
117. White NJ: Melioidosis. Lancet 361:1715, 2003.
118. Moore WL, Jr.: Section II. Melioidosis. In Ognibene AJ, Barrett ON Jr. (eds): Internal Medicine in Vietnam, vol II: General Medicine and Infectious Diseases. Washington, DC, Office of the Surgeon General, US Government Printing Office, 1982, p 197.
119. Koponen MA, Zlock D, Palmer DL, et al: Melioidosis. Forgotten, but not gone! Arch Intern Med 151:605, 1991.
120. Lim MK, Tan EH, Soh CS, et al: *Burkholderia pseudomallei* infection in the Singapore Armed Forces from 1987 to 1994—An epidemiological review. Ann Acad Med Singapore 26:13, 1997.
121. Reister FA (ed): Medical Statistics in World War II. Washington, DC, Office of the Surgeon General, US Government Printing Office, 1975, p 410.
122. Sheehy TW: Digestive disease as a national problem. VI. Enteric disease among United States troops in Vietnam. Gastroenterology 55:105, 1968.
123. Kelley PW, Takafuji ET, Wiener H, et al: An outbreak of hookworm infection associated with military operations in Grenada. Mil Med 154:55, 1989.
124. Stoute JA, Brundage JF, Petruccelli BP, et al: Outbreak of eosinophilia and gastrointestinal illness in soldiers returning from jungle training in Panama. Washington, DC, Epidemiology Consultant Service (EPICON) Report on file, Office of the Surgeon General, 1995.

123

Gastrointestinal Symptoms

LUIS M. VALDEZ
EDUARDO GOTUZZO
NATHAN M. THIELMAN
HERBERT L. DUPONT

Box 123-1 Important Aspects of the History in Patients from Tropical Areas

Environment

Travel history (knowledge of epidemic or endemic diseases in the area)
Insect bites
Occupational or recreational exposures
Contact with animals (domestic and wild)
Dietary history (type and source of food and water)

Host

Recent contact with infected persons
Previous infections
Vaccination status
History of sexually transmitted diseases and risk factors for HIV infection

INTRODUCTION

We live in a changing world where the effects of rural-to-urban migration and international travel to and from tropical areas of the world underscore the importance of recognizing and understanding tropical infections. Because most developing countries are in the tropics, the poor sanitary conditions that exist in these areas favor the acquisition of infections in which the gastrointestinal tract is an important portal of entry for microbes. These infections may manifest in different ways, with signs and symptoms that may or may not be related to the gastrointestinal tract. Although gastrointestinal symptoms are many times nonspecific, it is important to recognize them in the context of the patient's environment, exposures, and immune status. The last in particular has become increasingly important in tropical areas, as the burden of human immunodeficiency virus (HIV) infection is linked to the social disorganization and increasing poverty seen in the tropical developing countries. It is estimated that greater than 90% of the world's acquired immunodeficiency syndrome (AIDS) cases occur in resource-poor regions, many of which are in the tropics.[1]

When assessing patients with gastrointestinal symptoms, it is important to remember that although these symptoms are usually related to enteric infections, they may be secondary to systemic infections or to complications from a previously acquired infection. For example, malaria may often present with diarrhea and mislead critical diagnostic evaluation. It is thus essential to obtain a careful history, with emphasis on environmental exposures, dietary habits, contacts, and immunizations (Box 123-1). Gastrointestinal symptoms in the tropics are diverse, and although some may be related to "nontropical" conditions, it is also important to remember that some tropical enteric infections may present with predominantly systemic symptoms.

SYMPTOMS AND SYNDROMES

In tropical enteric infections, the presence of symptoms relates to organism virulence, the degree of infestation or inflammation caused by the infecting organism, and the host immune response. In the case of some enteric infections, especially in children living in endemic areas, the presence of pathogenic organisms may not correlate with the existence of symptoms.[2] In studies in Egypt, looking at children with *Giardia* infection, the protozoan was found in symptomatic and asymptomatic children, and there was a failure to show an association between infection and symptomatic illness.[3] The same has been described in longitudinal studies in Peruvian children, where no association was found between a variety of enteropathogens and persistent diarrhea.[4] This argues against diagnosing and treating microbe-specific infections in areas where the risk of reinfection is high, although increasing evidence suggests that asymptomatic infections with organisms such as enteroaggregative *Escherichia coli*[5] and *Cryptosporidium*[6] may be associated with impaired growth, probably because of inflammatory responses and/or malnutrition caused by these pathogens. Studies looking at adult subjects with documented enteric parasitic infections corroborate the fact that symptoms may be absent, particularly in subjects from tropical areas who have migrated to areas where these infections are uncommon.[7,8]

We have classified gastrointestinal symptoms in the tropics into seven syndromes (Table 123-1), and it is important to consider that certain microorganisms may cause more than one syndrome. In many infections, specific therapies are available (Table 123-2), but in some diseases, when the symptoms are a result of the host response to the infection, antimicrobial agents are ineffective.

Although systemic symptoms may be even nonspecific, it is important to recognize that some enteric tropical infections may present without a predominance of enteric symptoms. Such is the case, for example, of *Cyclospora cayetanensis* infections, where symptoms of profound fatigue, anorexia, and weight loss often predominate over the diarrheal symptoms.[9]

Enteric Fever

Enteric infections can cause clinical syndromes in which fever is predominant, sometimes associated with abdominal pain, in a protean clinical picture distinctive from other acute

Table 123-1 *Syndromes (and Their Most Common Causes) in Patients with Gastrointestinal Symptoms in the Tropics*

Syndrome	Agent/Condition	Organisms	Differential Diagnosis
Enteric fever	Bacteria	Typhoid fever (*Salmonella typhi*) Salmonellosis (non-S. *typhi*) Brucellosis Yersiniosis (rare) *Campylobacter* (rare)	Tuberculosis Acute schistosomiasis Malaria Septicemic plague Abdominal anthrax
Oral lesions	Bacteria	Noma (children), syphilis (primary or secondary), actinomycosis, oral anthrax	
	Mycobacteria	Tuberculosis, leprosy	
	Fungi	Paracoccidioidomycosis Histoplasmosis, candidiasis	
	Protozoa	Mucocutaneous leishmaniasis	
	Viruses	Herpes simplex	
Dysphagia	Protozoa	Trypanosomiasis	Esophageal cancer
	Fungi	Candidiasis (AIDS)	
	Viruses	Herpes simplex (AIDS) Cytomegalovirus (AIDS)	
Bleeding	Upper gastrointestinal bleeding	Esophageal varices: chronic schistosomiasis, cirrhosis (hepatitis B and C)	Stomach cancer
	Peptic ulcer disease	*Helicobacter pylori* infection	
	Lower gastrointestinal bleeding	Typhoid fever, nonspecific colitis Tuberculosis (rare), amebiasis (rare)	Polyps, colon cancer Diverticulosis
Abdominal pain	Peptic ulcer disease	*H. pylori*	Appendicitis
	Intestinal parasitosis	*Ascaris lumbricoides, Strongyloides stercoralis, Angiostrongylus costaricensis, Anisakis marina, hookworm*	Complicated hernia Intussusception
	Bacteria	Tuberculosis Typhoid (perforation)	
Abdominal mass	Bacteria	Tuberculosis, actinomycosis	Colon cancer, lymphoma
	Parasites	Ameboma, *Angiostrongylus*	
	Fungi	Histoplasmosis	
Diarrhea	Watery diarrhea and gastroenteritis	ETEC, EAEC, *Vibrio cholerae* O1 and non-O1, *Salmonella, Shigella, Campylobacter, Staphylococcus aureus and Bacillus cereus* (toxin-mediated), *Cryptosporidium parvum, Cyclospora cayetanensis, Isospora belli,* viruses (rotavirus and others)	
	Inflammatory diarrhea	*Shigella, Salmonella, Campylobacter, Entamoeba histolytica, Balantidium coli*	
	Persistent diarrhea	EAEC, tuberculosis, *Giardia lamblia, C. parvum, Cyclospora, I. belli, S. stercoralis, Capillaria philippinensis*	Tropical sprue, Brainerd diarrhea Lymphoma
	Traveler's diarrhea	ETEC, EAEC, *Shigella, Campylobacter jejuni, Aeromonas, Plesiomonas shigelloides, Salmonella, Giardia, Cryptospordium, Cyclospora*	

AIDS, acquired immunodeficiency syndrome; EAEC, enteroadherent *Escherichia coli*; ETEC, enterotoxigenic *E. coli*.

enteric processes. Usually the portal of entry in these infections is the gastrointestinal tract, but the differential diagnosis includes other infections and some noninfectious conditions. The classic infections causing enteric fever include typhoid fever, caused by *Salmonella typhi*, and the nontyphoid salmonellosis, brucellosis, yersiniosis, and *Campylobacter* infections. What characterizes these infections is the gastrointestinal portal of entry and the intracellular nature of the infection, where the organisms multiply in the lymphoid tissue before disseminating.

Typhoid fever caused by *S. typhi* is the classic prototype of enteric fever and still represents an important cause of morbidity and mortality in areas where it is endemic.[10] It is estimated that there are 16.6 million cases of typhoid fever each year with 600,000 deaths.[11] Although the syndrome classically is characterized as an acute illness with fever, headache, and abdominal pain, the symptoms are relatively nonspecific and the differential diagnosis, especially when there is associated splenomegaly, should include malaria, brucellosis, amebic liver abscess, visceral leishmaniasis, and viral syndromes such as dengue, depending on the geographic area from which the patient comes. Delays in the diagnosis of typhoid fever should be avoided, since complications can ensue. The complications in typhoid fever may be related directly to dissemination of *S. typhi* (meningitis, endocarditis, bone lesions), to the systemic inflammatory

*Table 123-2 Recommended Antimicrobial Therapy for Adults Infected by Selected Organisms Causing Gastrointestinal Disease in the Tropics**

Organisms	Therapy
Typhoidal syndrome	Ciprofloxacin 500 mg po bid × 10–14 days *or* Ceftriaxone 2.0 g IV × 10–14 days *or* Chloramphenicol 50 mg/kg/day po qid (max daily dose 3 g) × 14 days *or* Ofloxacin 15 mg/kg po qd × 7 days *or* Cefixime 200 mg po q12h × 14 days
Brucellosis	Doxycycline 100 mg po bid × 6 wk + streptomycin 1 g qd IM × 2 wk
Helicobacter pylori	Clarithromycin 500 mg po bid + omeprazole 40 mg po qd × 14 days *or* Metronidazole (250 mg po tid) + amoxicillin (500 mg po qid) + bismuth subsalycilate (2 × 262-mg tablets qid) × 14 days
Vibrio cholerae O1	Tetracycline 500 mg po qid *or* doxycycline 100 mg po × 3 days *or* Doxycycline 300 mg po × 1 *or* Ciprofloxacin 250 mg po q12h × 3 days
V. cholerae, non-O1	Tetracyclines *or* ciprofloxacin Resistant to furazolidone and trimethoprim-sulfamethoxazole
Shigella	Ciprofloxacin 500 mg q12h × 3 days *or* Norfloxacin 400 mg q12h × 3 days
Campylobacter	Erythromycin 500 mg po qid × 5 days *or* other macrolides as above
Salmonella	Therapy not indicated unless severe or in a host susceptible to bacteremic complications; fluroquinolones × 7–10 days
Giardia lamblia	Metronidazole 250 mg po tid × 5 days *or* Tinidazole 2.0 g × 1 dose *or* Quinacrine 100 mg po tid × 5 days
Entamoeba histolytica	Metronidazole 750 mg po tid (500 mg IV q6h) × 10 days *or* Tinidazole 1.0 g po q12h × 3 days *or* Tetracycline 500 mg po qid × 14 days All followed by iodoquinol 650 mg po tid × 20 days
Cyclospora cayetanensis	Trimethoprim-sulfamethoxazole 1 double-strength bid po × 3–7 days
Cryptosporidium parvum	No effective therapy demonstrated in adults Paromomycin 500 mg po qid (partial response, used in patients with AIDS) Nitazoxanide 500–1000 mg bid × 14 days (response in some patients with AIDS)
Isospora belli	Trimethoprim-sulfamethoxazole 1 double-strength po qid × 10 days then bid × 3 wk
Balantidium coli	Tetracycline 500 po qid × 10 days *or* Metronidazole 750 mg po tid × 5 days *or* Paromomycin 500 mg po tid × 7 to 10 days
Ascaris lumbricoides	Mebendazole 100 mg po bid × 3 days *or* Pyrantel pamoate 11 mg/kg po qd × 3 days *or* Albendazole 400 mg po single dose
Strongyloides stercoralis	Thiabendazole 22 mg/kg po bid × 2 days *or* Albendazole 400 mg po qd × 3 days *or* Ivermectin 200 μg/kg/day × 2 days

*Duration of therapy for nonimmunocompromised patients. Duration of therapy will be prolonged in patients with AIDS.

response secondary to the infection (typhoid state), or to direct involvement of the gut resulting in hemorrhage, perforation, and ileus.[12] Other salmonella (especially *S. paratyphi* A and B, *S. choleraesuis*, and other *Salmonella* serotypes) may also cause a typhoidal clinical syndrome.[13]

Acute brucellosis is another cause of enteric fever in which systemic symptoms predominate over those symptoms related to the gastrointestinal tract. In a recent fever surveillance study in Egypt, 87% of patients with brucellosis were actually diagnosed with and treated for typhoid.[14] Anorexia, abdominal pain, vomiting, and diarrhea or constipation are some of the complaints elicited in patients with brucellosis if the patient is carefully questioned.[15] In areas where brucellosis is endemic, it is important to obtain a detailed history assessing ingestion of unpasteurized milk or cheese, as well as occupational exposures.

Yersinia enterocolitica infections, although found in tropical areas, are rarely a cause of tropical diarrhea,[16] and the septicemic disease is seen mostly in patients with underlying predisposing factors and chronic diseases.

Some zoonoses, such as plague and anthrax, can occasionally present with a clinical picture suggestive of enteric fever, so epidemiologic information is essential to the diagnosis of these conditions. Septicemic plague, for example, can sometimes present with prominent gastrointestinal symptoms (nausea, vomiting, diarrhea, and abdominal pain), symptoms that may precede the development of a bubo, or even be part of septicemic plague, in which no bubo is recognized. In a review of 71 human plague cases, gastrointestinal symptoms occurred in 57% of the patients, with nausea and vomiting being the most common symptoms and diarrhea and abdominal pain occurring less often (28% and 17% of patients, respectively).[17] In disease caused by *Bacillus anthracis* following the ingestion of contaminated food, abdominal anthrax will present after an incubation period of 2 to 11 days.[18] Symptoms initially may be nonspecific, with fever, anorexia, nausea, and vomiting. As the disease progresses, abdominal pain, hematemesis, and bloody diarrhea will often develop.

Two other conditions that have to be considered in the differential diagnosis of fever and enteric symptoms are tuberculosis and schistosomiasis. In patients with intestinal tuberculosis, although they may have associated pulmonary disease, some series have found evidence of active or remote pulmonary tuberculosis in as few as 25% of cases, the diagnosis being an unexpected finding at exploratory laparotomy.[19] Patients with acute schistosomiasis (Katayama fever) may also present with an enteric fever syndrome. Typically, this occurs in subjects who are not residents of endemic areas, and it is believed to be in relationship to the host response to the parasite.[20] The history of swimming in freshwater during the previous month in areas in which schistosomiasis is endemic also favors this diagnosis.

It is important to recognize the endemicity of certain tropical diseases in order to recognize infections like typhoid fever and those that are unusual in other geographic settings. When approaching patients with enteric fever, it is thus essential to obtain a complete history and to do a complete physical examination looking for clinical clues that may suggest one process or another. Microbiologic diagnosis should be attempted whenever possible, but in some tropical areas this may not be feasible and in the case of typhoid the diagnosis may rely on serologic methods (Widal's test) and a suggestive clinical picture.[21] In an Indian study, Widal's test was acceptable as a diagnostic tool, with a high specificity and positive predictive value when an O-antigen 1:160 dilution defined a positive result in the presence of a suggestive clinical picture.[22] In the same study, the same titer was observed in 10.2% of patients with other febrile illnesses of known cause and in 1.8% of normal children. Studies in nonendemic areas also show that the test can give a significant number of false positives.[23] The diagnosis of typhoid fever by Widal's test alone is prone to error and there are no universally applicable criteria for the serologic diagnosis. In areas where microbiologic diagnosis is not possible, Widal's test should only be considered a sensitive and specific "fever screen" for typhoid, but it has to be recognized that it will not identify all cases and may give some false positives. In areas where malaria is endemic, false positives have been described; in one study, Widal's test was found to be positive in 15% and 10% of malaria patients for salmonella O- and H-antigen titers, respectively.[24] In areas where malaria is also endemic, typhoid fever and malaria always have to be considered in the differential diagnosis of an acute febrile illness, so a thick smear in addition to cultures for *Salmonella* should be obtained. For the microbiologic diagnosis of typhoid fever, blood and stool cultures have been recommended traditionally for the isolation of *S. typhi*, but bone marrow cultures and duodenal string cultures (duodenal string-capsule culture) provide a higher yield. In a Peruvian study in adult patients with documented *S. typhi* infection, duodenal content cultures were as sensitive as bone marrow in providing a diagnosis (86% and 75% sensitivity, respectively) compared with blood (42%) and stool (26%) cultures.[25] Bone marrow and duodenal string cultures also remain positive for a longer period despite antibiotic therapy, and thus may be useful in patients who have received empirical antibiotic therapy and in whom a microbiologic diagnosis is needed.[25,26] In older pediatric patients, the duodenal string method has also been shown to be better than blood cultures,[27] but in smaller children it may not be practical.[27,28]

The treatment of patients with acute enteric fever syndromes should be based on an etiologic diagnosis, but at times empirical therapy may be necessary while awaiting culture results. In the case of typhoid fever, delays in diagnosis and treatment should be avoided because of the impact of therapy on disease mortality and on the incidence of intestinal hemorrhage.[12] When treating patients with typhoid fever one has to consider that strains of *S. typhi* that are resistant to the three first-line antibiotics (chloramphenicol, amoxicillin, and trimethoprim-sulfamethoxazole) have been described in many tropical countries,[29] so it is essential to know the local resistance patterns in each endemic area. These multiresistant organisms are typically susceptible to third-generation cephalosporins and to the fluoroquinolones,[30,31] but responses have been slower with the cephalosporins. In an open study comparing ceftriaxone (2 g per day for 5 days) with fleroxacin (400 mg once a day for 7 days), the mean fever clearance times were 160 hours and 81 hours, respectively, and there were two failures in the ceftriaxone group and none in the fleroxacin group.[32] In another study comparing ceftriaxone (3 g per day for 7 days) with ciprofloxacin (500 mg twice a day for 7 days), there were six failures (out of 22 patients) in the ceftriaxone group and none in the ciprofloxacin group.[33] Oral cefixime has been studied in children with multidrug-resistant typhoid in Pakistan, but failures were reported in 3 of 50 patients (6%).[34] Fluoroquinolones are currently considered the drugs of choice for patients with multidrug-resistant typhoid, although there have been reports of ciprofloxacin resistance from India and in travelers returning to the United Kingdom after travel to the Indian subcontinent.[35,36] Fluoroquinolone-resistant strains, which are often multidrug-resistant are best treated with either azithromycin (which also covers quinolone-resistant *Campylobacter*) or cephalosporins.[37] Short courses of fluoroquinolones have been used in Vietnam for the treatment of typhoid. In one of the studies, involving 438 patients (286 were younger than 14 years old), two short-course regimens of ofloxacin (15 mg/kg per day for 3 days vs. 10 mg/kg per day for 5 days) were assessed and there was only one failure in one patient who took only one dose.[38] Table 123-2 summarizes the most accepted regimens for treating typhoid, and the antibiotics should be used based on the knowledge of the local patterns of resistance, cost, compliance, and safety. Although short-course treatments using fluoroquinolones may improve compliance and reduce costs, these short-course treatments should also be evaluated in other geographic areas before they can be recommended elsewhere.

Oropharyngeal Lesions

Bacterial, fungal, parasitic, and viral infections can all give rise to oropharyngeal lesions. The first three types present with increased frequency in the tropics.

Among the bacterial infections causing oral lesions seen in tropical areas, one seen with an increased incidence in West Africa is noma (cancrum oris), a severe gangrene of the soft and hard tissues of the mouth, face, and neighboring areas.

Fusobacterium necrophorum, along with other organisms, has been implicated in its pathogenesis. These opportunistic pathogens invade oral tissues in children whose immune system is weakened by malnutrition, acute necrotizing gingivitis, debilitating conditions, trauma, and other oral mucosal ulcers.[39]

Considering the increasing prevalence rates for sexually transmitted diseases in developing countries, orogenital contact can result in oral and oropharyngeal lesions of syphilis. Secondary syphilis can also present with painful oral ulcerations or oral condyloma lata lesions.[40,41] In contrast with the oral lesions of primary syphilis, which tend to be solitary, painless, indurated, and punched-out ulcers, oral lesions of secondary syphilis are typically painful and multiple and are accompanied by a generalized rash.

Actinomycosis, anthrax, tuberculosis, and leprosy can also present with oral lesions. Actinomycotic infections of the cervicofacial area are rare, and the most common presentation is an acute painful swelling associated with a soft tissue abscess secondary to dental lesions.[42] Rare cases of oral actinomycosis may mimic neoplasms of the tongue.[43] Oral anthrax is characterized by a mucosal lesion in the oral cavity or oropharynx which can progress to pseudomembranous necrosis, and to cervical adenopathy and edema.[44] Primary tuberculosis of the mouth may present with painless ulcerations of long duration and enlargement of the regional lymph nodes.[45] Lepromatous leprosy can cause oral lesions in 20% to 60% of patients. Oral lesions are often an extension of disease in the nasal mucous membranes. Oral lesions are characterized as hemorrhagic sessile nodules involving the maxillary incisive papilla, lips, tongue, soft palate, uvula, and glossopharyngeal arches.[46]

Among the fungal infections in the tropics, paracoccidioidomycosis (South American blastomycosis), histoplasmosis, and candidiasis can present with oral lesions. Oral lesions may be the first sign of paracoccidioidomycosis. Patients may present with chronic, proliferative, mulberry-like ulcerated oral lesions. Typically the gingiva or alveolar process is affected, but lesions can be seen on the palate and lip. Most patients with oral lesions have detectable pulmonary involvement.[47] In disseminated histoplasmosis, lesions of the oral mucosa may be found in 30% to 50% of cases. Oral lesions may involve the lips, tongue, gingiva, and palate.[48] Oral candidiasis can be associated with malnutrition and debilitating diseases, but within the current AIDS epidemic its presence should raise the possibility of HIV infection.

Among the protozoan infections, mucocutaneous leishmaniasis can present with oral lesions. Patients with infection by *Leishmania viannia braziliensis* in Latin America may develop mucosal lesions of the nose, mouth, pharynx, or larynx months to years after the primary infection.[49] Other protozoal and helminthic infections may be associated on very rare occasions.[50]

Dysphagia

Many of the conditions causing oral lesions in tropical areas can present with dysphagia. In this section, we concentrate on infectious processes that may affect primarily the esophagus.

In areas where *Trypanosoma cruzi* infection (Chagas' disease) is endemic, esophageal symptoms like dysphagia and regurgitation may be secondary to motor disorders related to this parasitic disease.[51] The involvement of the esophagus encompasses a spectrum with megaesophagus at the most severe end to milder variants without evidence of esophageal dilation in subjects who have documented serologic evidence of infection with *T. cruzi*.

Dysphagia and odynophagia may present secondary to infectious esophagitis, a condition known to occur with increased frequency in patients with HIV infection.[52] *Candida* esophagitis is by far the most common cause of esophageal symptoms in patients with HIV infection, accounting for 50% to 100% of symptomatic patients, and may occur in asymptomatic patients. After *Candida*, the most common causes of esophageal disease in symptomatic patients are cytomegalovirus (CMV), herpes simplex, and idiopathic esophageal ulcers.

Among the noninfectious pathologic conditions, esophageal cancer is unevenly distributed within the tropical regions; its prevalence rate is higher in East and South Africa and in the Far East. In these areas, this must be a consideration when assessing patients with esophageal symptoms.[53]

Gastrointestinal Bleeding

Apart from the usual noninfectious causes of gastrointestinal bleeding, some infectious conditions in the tropics may present in this way. For example, enterohemorrhagic *E. coli* (EHEC) can cause bloody diarrhea in the tropics as in increasing outbreaks in industrialized temperate areas.

In schistosomiasis, the existence of periportal fibrosis leads to portal hypertension and varices with the resultant risk of gastrointestinal bleeding, representing an important cause of morbidity and mortality in endemic areas due to the large number of infected subjects.[54] In a field study in an area of the Sudan endemic for *Schistosoma mansoni*, the prevalence of esophageal varices in subjects undergoing esophagoscopy ranged between 54% and 67%. The varices were usually asymptomatic, with symptomatic varices (with a positive history of hematemesis) occurring in 3% to 4% of subjects with sonographic evidence of liver periportal fibrosis.[55] Abdominal ultrasound can accurately measure liver and spleen size and configuration and detect and grade periportal fibrosis and portal hypertension, and these findings can predict the risk of variceal bleeding in patients with complicated schistosomiasis.[56]

Another infectious condition that may present with gastrointestinal bleeding is typhoid fever, typically resulting from necrotic erosion of a Peyer's patch into an enteric vessel.[37] If untreated, it may result in passage of gross blood in the feces or melena in 10% to 20% of patients, with severe gastrointestinal bleeding occurring in 2% of patients late in the course of the disease.[12] Early treatment of typhoid fever will reduce the frequency of this complication, so in endemic areas for typhoid rapid diagnosis and therapy should be established.

Gastrointestinal tuberculosis on rare occasions can present with gastrointestinal bleeding. There have been case reports describing upper gastrointestinal bleeding from a tuberculous gastric ulcer and from esophageal tuberculosis.[57,58]

Reports of massive rectal bleeding from colonic tuberculosis have also been published.[59,60] Amebiasis, which commonly presents with bloody stools, on rare occasions may present with massive gastrointestinal bleeding requiring surgical therapy.[61]

In patients with lower gastrointestinal bleeding, colonoscopic examination may provide the diagnosis in a majority of patients. In a study of lower gastrointestinal bleeding carried out in a tropical area of India, predominant lesions in 138 adults were nonspecific colitis and ulcers (58%), polyps (19%), cancer (10%), rectal varices (4%), and tuberculosis (3%), with most lesions involving the left colon. Diffuse lesions were seen when nonspecific colitis and ulcers were the source of bleeding.[62] In another study from India, of 166 patients who underwent colonoscopy, a diagnosis could be made in 85%. Major causes of lower gastrointestinal bleeding included idiopathic ulcerative colitis (19.3%), acute colitis (12.0%), colonic polyps (10.2%), radiation colitis (9.0%), solitary rectal ulcer (7.8%), and colonic carcinoma (7.2%). Among the infectious conditions, colonic tuberculosis was found in 4.2% and enteric fever in 3.0%.[63]

Abdominal Pain

The causes of abdominal pain are diverse, and enteric tropical infections certainly represent a definite group in the differential diagnosis in patients from tropical areas. Abdominal pain can be acute or chronic, and sometimes be part of an acute abdominal syndrome that may require a surgical approach. It is thus essential to recognize the common tropical diseases that may present with abdominal pain within the different tropical areas of the world.

Epigastric abdominal pain of gastric or duodenal origin can be linked to *Helicobacter pylori* infection, and there is definite evidence of a link between this organism and peptic ulcer disease and chronic gastritis, and epidemiologic evidence supporting its role in gastric cancer and lymphoma.[64] Gastric *H. pylori* infection is very common throughout the tropics, as evidenced by serologic surveys, yet active gastric infection does not always correlate with the incidence of serious upper gastrointestinal changes.[65] In a study in patients examined by gastroscopy for dyspepsia in northern Nigeria, 176 (92%) of 193 with acceptable biopsies had gastritis. *H. pylori* was present in 161 of 192 patients (84%): in 31 of 41 (75%) with chronic gastritis and in 130 of 135 (96%) with active gastritis.[66] Considering the role of *H. pylori* in gastritis, dyspepsia, peptic ulcer disease, and possibly gastric cancer, eradication of this infection should be attempted, although the cost of therapy may be difficult to justify in developing tropical areas.

Abdominal pain can also be a nonspecific symptom of intestinal parasitosis,[67] and in travelers to exotic areas the absence of symptoms should not preclude examination of the stools looking for parasites.[8] Although ascariasis is rarely a cause of abdominal pain, in a study in Nigeria assessing 865 patients with suspected peptic ulcer disease, 175 patients (20%) were found to have *Ascaris* infection, and their symptoms resolved after the use of anthelmintics.[68] Interestingly, the diagnosis of ascariasis was done radiologically as part of the workup for the diagnosis of peptic ulcer disease. The authors proposed that in areas with a high prevalence of ascariasis, a stool examination should be part of the assessment in patients with uncomplicated suspected peptic ulcer disease. Hookworm may also be associated with abdominal pain and eosinophilia in the tropics, presenting several weeks before ova are shed to aid in the diagnosis.[69]

Among the causes of chronic abdominal pain in the tropics, when there is an association with ascites, the possibility of tuberculous peritonitis should be considered. The presentation of peritoneal tuberculosis is quite insidious, with most patients having symptoms for weeks or months before seeking medical attention. Marshall,[70] in a review of tuberculosis of the gastrointestinal tract and peritoneum, summarized data from six large series in the literature (two from tropical countries). In his review, abdominal pain was present 58% of the time, and the most common symptom was abdominal distention (about 82% of the cases). Other common symptoms included fever and weight loss. The ascitic fluid is an exudate with a lymphocytic predominance in the white blood cell differential count. The diagnostic yield from smears and cultures from the ascitic fluid is very low, although Singh and colleagues[71] reported 83% positive cultures when culturing 1 L of fluid concentrated by centrifugation. Currently, the best diagnostic test is laparoscopic biopsy of the peritoneum. Simply the gross appearance of the peritoneal cavity during laparoscopy allows a presumptive diagnosis in 85% to 95% of patients, and caseating granulomas are found from the biopsy specimens in 85% to 90% of cases.[70,72] The measurement of adenosine deaminase activity (ADA) has been reported as a sensitive way of making a presumptive diagnosis.[73]

Abdominal pain can also be the presenting symptom of an acute abdomen, and in the tropics, apart from the usual pathologic changes seen in other areas, certain infectious conditions should be considered in the differential diagnosis.

In the case of appendicitis, the most common abdominal surgical emergency in nontropical areas, pathologic studies in tropical areas have shown that in a few cases infection can be detected. In a pathologic study of 2921 appendectomies in a tropical area over a 25-year period, 70 (2.3%) specimens showed typical evidence of tuberculosis. Parasitic infestation was detected in 75 (2.5%), including enterobiasis (1.4%), amebiasis (0.5%), ascariasis (0.5%), ascariasis with trichuriasis (0.05%), and taeniasis (0.05%).[74]

Intestinal obstruction in patients living in tropical areas can be caused by external hernia, sigmoid volvulus, intussusception (particularly in children), and ascariasis.[75,76] In a prospective evaluation of acute intestinal obstruction in 3550 consecutive patients in Africa, the majority of patients (75%) had an external hernia.[75] However, *Ascaris* infection in children, volvulus of the sigmoid colon in adults, and intussusception in both children and adults were significant causes of abdominal obstruction in 18% of the patients. In highly parasitized children, a mass of *Ascaris* adult worms can cause acute small bowel obstruction, although in most cases the obstruction is not complete and conservative measures and anthelmintic therapy can obviate the need for surgery.[77] *Strongyloides stercoralis* has also been reported, presenting as a subacute intestinal obstruction in two patients from Iraq.[78] Gastrointestinal tuberculosis can sometimes present with a subocclusive or obstructive picture. In a series of 300 cases of abdominal tuberculosis that required surgical therapy,

Bhansali[79] found that of the 139 patients that presented with abdominal pain, 92 had abdominal obstruction, 23 had perforation, and 19 presented with peritonitis. In 56 of the patients, the acute episode was the first manifestation of abdominal tuberculosis, while the other 83 had a previous history of chronic abdominal pain for a period of time that ranged from 1 month to more than 10 years. Only 10% of the patients had active pulmonary or pleural tuberculosis, and another 12% gave a history of previous tuberculosis, or their chest films showed a past, healed focus. Obstruction can be secondary to narrowing of the lumen by hyperplastic cecal tuberculosis, strictures of the small intestine, adhesions, or be related to extrinsic compression of the bowel by mesenteric lymph nodes. In approaching patients with abdominal pain in tropical areas where tuberculosis is prevalent, this diagnostic possibility should always be considered.

One of the most lethal complications of typhoid fever is ileal perforation, which should be considered if an acute abdomen develops in a patient with prolonged fever. The most important sign is pneumoperitoneum on plain abdominal film. This complication requires surgical therapy, usually consisting of simple closure and irrigation of the peritoneal cavity.[80] In a review of the literature published after 1960 on typhoid perforation in different developing countries, information was obtained on a total of 1990 cases of typhoid perforation in 66,157 patients with typhoid fever, published in 52 reports from all over the world.[81] The overall frequency of intestinal perforation in typhoid fever was 3% with an overall mortality rate of 39.6%. In a recent report from Turkey,[82] mortality decreased significantly, from 28% to 10%, with the institution of aggressive fluid resuscitation and appropriate antibiotic therapy in the preoperative period, and total parenteral nutrition to provide adequate metabolic support during the postoperative period. Apart from specific antibiotic therapy against *S. typhi*, broad-spectrum antibiotics should be added to cover enteric flora (mainly anaerobes and gram-negative organisms).

The tropical spectrum of generalized peritonitis is different from the Western spectrum. In a study in India, of a total 155 cases of generalized peritonitis that were surgically treated, the most common cause of peritonitis was peptic ulcer perforation followed by typhoid perforation. Other causes of peritonitis in the same study were appendicular perforations, tubercular perforations (sometimes with a previous history of subacute intestinal obstruction and evidence of pulmonary tuberculosis), and ruptured amebic liver abscess.[83] Amebic perforation of the colon has also been described in patients presenting with an acute abdomen and a past history of fever, pain, and diarrhea.[84]

It is important in tropical areas to identify nonsurgical infectious causes of abdominal pain that may mimic an acute abdomen. *Angiostrongylus costaricensis* is found in areas of Central and South America and infections in children caused by this organism may present with fever, anorexia, vomiting, and right lower quadrant or flank pain or mass, suggesting a classic case of appendicitis. In a study in Costa Rica, more than three fourths of children found to have *A. costaricensis* underwent surgery.[85] Ileocecal tuberculosis, amebiasis, and salmonellosis may also mimic appendicitis, although a more prolonged story of pain or fever may differentiate them from acute appendicitis. Patients with mesenteric adenitis may also have an illness clinically indistinguishable from acute appendicitis, although this condition has been reported mostly in nontropical areas. Anisakiasis, although not typical of tropical areas, is a disease caused by the larval nematode *Anisakis marina* ("herring worm") and is associated with eating raw fish. It is a recognized public health problem in Japan, and cases have been reported in Europe. The intestinal burrowing of the larval form causes acute abdominal symptoms clinically resembling acute appendicitis.[86]

Abdominal Mass

Among the infectious conditions that can present with an abdominal mass, tuberculosis should be in the differential diagnosis. Primary intestinal tuberculosis may present with abdominal pain, fever, and a tender, fixed palpable mass in the ileocecal area.[87] Bhansali,[79] in his series of patients with tuberculosis requiring surgery, found 96 patients who had a palpable mass on physical examination, and all of these patients had a chronic presentation. In 75 of these patients, the mass was caused by hyperplastic cecal tuberculosis, in 19 it was due to a mass of enlarged lymph nodes, and in the remaining 2 it was related to rolled-up omentum. Common symptoms in these patients were fever, weight loss, altered bowel habits, and chronic abdominal pain. Although uncommon in nonimmunocompromised persons, tuberculosis can involve the mesenteric lymph nodes and present with abdominal pain, fever, a palpable mass, or symptoms of partial small bowel obstruction.[88] In contrast, in patients with AIDS tuberculosis, mesenteric lymphadenitis is more common and generally more extensive.[89]

Another infectious condition that may present with a mass is abdominal actinomycosis. The cecal area is most frequently the site of abdominal actinomycosis, and it can present as an abscess or as a firm-to-hard mass lesion that is often fixed to the underlying tissue. Sinus tracts may develop, draining through the abdominal wall or perianal region.[90] Amebiasis can present as a chronic localized infection termed *ameboma*. An ameboma presents as a painful abdominal mass that occurs more commonly in the cecum or the ascending colon.[91]

Other tropical infectious disease conditions that may present with an abdominal mass are histoplasmosis[92] and *A. costaricensis* infection (described previously). Histoplasmosis involving the gastrointestinal tract usually occurs with disseminated disease. Gastrointestinal histoplasmosis differs from other forms of disseminated histoplasmosis in that pulmonary symptoms are uncommon and gastrointestinal symptoms predominate. Common symptoms, although they may be absent in as many as 50% of cases, include diarrhea, weight loss, abdominal pain, and fever. Clinically, patients may also present with generalized lymphadenopathy and hepatosplenomegaly. Histoplasmosis involving the gastrointestinal tract most frequently is characterized by ulcerations or an intestinal mass, especially when there is involvement of the terminal ileum, cecum, or colon.[92]

Diarrhea

Diarrheal diseases, despite major scientific advances, are a major cause of morbidity, and their frequency in the tropical areas of the world underscores the global impact of tropical diseases.[93] In these areas, diarrhea is a common cause of infant mortality, and diarrheal morbidity and mortality are linked with the poverty and sanitary deficiencies commonly seen in developing areas. For people from nontropical developed areas visiting the tropics, it also represents an important cause of morbidity, since it can affect 20% to 50% of travelers.[94]

When approaching patients with diarrhea, it is important to obtain a good history and to define the clinical syndrome: acute watery diarrhea (small bowel disease), profuse vomiting (gastroenteritis), dysenteric disease, or persistent diarrhea.

Acute Watery Diarrhea

Acute watery diarrhea is characterized by the presence of large-volume stools and is usually associated with a small bowel secretory process. The causes of acute watery diarrhea are different in temperate climates compared with tropical areas. In temperate climates, the usual causative organisms are largely undefined, although viruses are suspected in many cases. In the tropics, where most adults live in areas with poor sanitation, several other agents can cause acute noninflammatory diarrhea. Of particular importance are enterotoxigenic *Escherichia coli* (ETEC) diarrhea and cholera. Enteroaggregative *E. coli* (EAEC) is an enteric pathogen showing increasingly recognized importance as a cause of worldwide diarrhea mediated by intestinal inflammatory mechanisms causing watery, nonbloody diarrhea. EAEC is an important cause of persistent diarrhea in infants in the developing world, travelers' diarrhea, and AIDS-associated diarrhea in many regions.

The seventh pandemic, caused by *Vibrio cholerae* biotype El Tor, has affected most of the continents of the Eastern Hemisphere, including Asia, Africa, and the Mediterranean region of Europe. In 1991, the organism appeared in Peru and spread throughout Latin America.[95] Peru alone reported 322,562 cases, half of which occurred during the first 12 weeks of the epidemic. A new strain of the non-O1 serogroup, *V. cholerae* O139 synonym Bengal, was seen in late 1992, beginning in Madras, India, and rapidly spreading to Calcutta and Bangladesh in 1993, causing epidemic cholera gravis.[96,97] This may represent the beginning of an eighth pandemic.[98] The hallmark of this disease is a secretory diarrhea induced by an enterotoxin, commonly referred to as cholera toxin, which produces water and electrolyte losses in the intestinal lumen resulting in dehydration ranging from mild to severe. In endemic areas, the differential diagnosis in cases of mild to moderate disease should include infections produced by ETEC, food poisoning, and viruses such as rotavirus (especially in children).

Other bacterial pathogens, such as *Shigella, Salmonella*, and *Campylobacter jejuni*, which typically cause inflammatory diarrhea, may occasionally present with a clinical picture of acute watery diarrhea. Because it is not possible to differentiate between these infections solely on clinical grounds, the assistance of a microbiology laboratory is advised, although in remote areas in the tropics it is not always possible to obtain a properly equipped and staffed laboratory facility. To make the diagnosis of cholera bacteriologically, one should culture stool specimens onto thiosulfate-citrate-bile salts-sucrose (TCBS) agar.

Initial management of these patients should include adequate fluid replacement, preferably orally with glucose electrolyte solutions, or if unable to tolerate oral fluids or if severely dehydrated, intravenously with isotonic fluids. Oral rehydration therapy, in conjunction with educational programs on its effective use, allowed Peruvian physicians to achieve a survival rate of more than 99% in the more than 300,000 cholera patients seen during the first year of the outbreak in Peru.[99] Antibiotic therapy with tetracyclines and quinolones is effective in decreasing the duration and severity of the disease and in eradicating the infecting organism.[100,101]

Among the parasitic diseases capable of causing acute noninflammatory diarrhea, two coccidians are becoming increasingly important, especially because of the fact that water-borne outbreaks in the case of *Cryptosporidium parvum*[102] and food and water-borne outbreaks caused by *Cyclospora cayetanensis*[9] have been recognized with increasing frequency, and because both are capable of causing significant disease in immunocompromised hosts, particularly those suffering from AIDS.[103,104] The fact that chlorination is ineffective in eliminating these organisms adds to their impact.

Cryptosporidiosis can cause acute, noninflammatory, self-limited diarrhea. Although not limited to tropical areas, this parasite can be easily transmitted in areas with poor sanitation, with transmission rates similar to other highly infectious enteric pathogens such as *Shigella* species.[105] This coccidian parasite is particularly important in malnourished children and immunocompromised hosts, causing a more severe and prolonged clinical picture than in immunocompetent hosts. In a study in Guinea-Bissau, cryptosporidiosis was associated with excess mortality in children independent of malnutrition, socioeconomic factors, hygienic considerations, or breastfeeding.[106] *Cryptosporidium* has been found in as many as 50% of patients with AIDS and diarrhea in developing countries.[107] The diagnosis is made by the microscopic detection of oocysts in stools using acid-fast stains. Newer methods based on enzyme-linked immunosorbent assay (ELISA) or immunofluorescence are also available, and a recent study showed that all methods (including acid-fast staining) were equally sensitive and specific in detecting oocysts,[108] but the threshold of detection may not be optimal.[109] Therapy is problematic. Paromomycin has been shown to decrease oocyst excretion and the number of stools in patients with AIDS and cryptosporidiosis,[110] but is rarely curative. Recently approved for pediatric use in the United States, nitazoxanide was found to improve cryptosporidial diarrhea in one study of patients with AIDS in Mexico[111] and in HIV-negative children in Zambia.[112] The most effective intervention in this circumstance, however, remains immunologic recovery mediated by highly active antiretroviral therapy.[113]

Cyclospora cayetanensis has been described in Central and South America, the Caribbean, India, South Africa, Southeast Asia, eastern Europe, and recently from several outbreaks in the United States.[9] The disease seems to be endemic in areas of Nepal, Haiti, and Peru, and coincides with the rainy season in those areas. Although diarrhea is a common manifestation of *Cyclospora* infection, it may not be the presenting or predominant symptom in immunocompetent patients with this condition. A flulike syndrome may precede the onset of diarrhea. *Cyclospora* has been described as a cause of prolonged diarrhea in patients with HIV infection.[104]

The diagnosis of *Cyclospora* infection is based on the microscopic detection of oocysts from fecal specimens. Like *Cryptosporidium, Cyclospora* oocysts should be stained using acid-fast techniques such as the modified Ziehl-Neelsen stain or the Kinyoun acid-fast stain. *Cyclospora* oocysts are autofluorescent, appearing neon-blue when seen under an ultraviolet fluorescence microscope. Trimethoprim-sulfamethoxazole is the drug of choice for treating *Cyclospora* infection.[114]

In general, the management of acute, noninflammatory diarrhea in adults consists primarily of rehydration. If glucose or sucrose accompanies the isotonic fluid taken orally, the coupled absorption of sodium and water is often sufficient to replace fluid loss. In the absence of a significant febrile or inflammatory process, low doses of antimotility agents may offer some relief with minimum risk if cramping is severe. Symptomatic treatment is more often used in industrialized regions to improve symptoms, allowing persons to return to work or school. In tropical regions drugs play a minor role in the treatment of acute diarrhea. In selected cases, the use of antibiotics may provide a faster resolution of the symptoms.

Gastroenteritis

The syndrome of acute nausea and vomiting, or "viral gastroenteritis" due to rotaviruses or noroviruses, commonly occurs in winter months in temperate climates, whereas this syndrome occurs year-round in tropical areas. The syndrome may also be caused by ingestion of preformed toxins of *Staphylococcus aureus* and *Bacillus cereus*. In a recent study from Taiwan, 20% and 15% of food-poisoning outbreaks were caused by *S. aureus* and *B. cereus*, respectively.[115]

Acute staphylococcal food poisoning typically occurs in food-borne epidemics. Patients will present initially with nausea, vomiting, and acute salivation, followed by abdominal cramps and diarrhea. The short incubation period (2 to 7 hours) and the existence of similar cases from a common source (meal) will suggest the diagnosis. The diarrhea usually is watery, but rarely can contain mucus and blood. Management consists of rehydration and monitoring and replacement of fluid and electrolyte losses. The symptoms usually resolve after a few hours. The potentially contaminated food should be examined for the presence of *S. aureus* (culture and Gram's stain) and enterotoxin. Meat, poultry, or their products (with ham and chicken most frequently implicated) are among the most common vehicles, but other foods, including fish and shellfish and milk and milk products, have also been implicated.[116]

Outbreaks of food-borne disease caused by *B. cereus* have been reported from tropical and nontropical areas. The organism produces an emetic or diarrheal syndrome induced by an emetic toxin and enterotoxin, respectively.[117] The emetic syndrome has a shorter incubation time (1 to 7 hours) and mimics staphylococcal food poisoning. Typically, the illness is associated with the ingestion of contaminated rice. The diarrheal syndrome has a longer incubation time (10 to 14 hours) and is usually related to the consumption of meat or vegetables. The diarrhea is profuse, lasting 12 to 24 hours, and is associated with abdominal pain, tenesmus, and nausea. *B. cereus* food-borne disease is self-limited, and again treatment is symptomatic, with rehydration provided as needed.

Many forms of diarrheal disease present with both watery diarrhea and vomiting. This form of gastroenteritis may be caused by enteropathogens that infect the upper gastrointestinal tract, including enteric viruses, bacterial pathogens such as diarrheogenic *E. coli, Shigella* spp., *Salmonella* spp., noncholera vibrios, *Campylobacter jejuni, Aeromonas* spp., and the protozoal parasites.

Acute Inflammatory Diarrhea

Acute inflammatory diarrhea is characterized by the passage of many small-volume stools often containing blood and mucus. The causes of acute inflammatory diarrhea include several specific distal small bowel and colonic infections such as shigellosis, salmonellosis, campylobacteriosis, and amebiasis as the most representative organisms. Enteroinvasive *E. coli* has also been described as a cause of inflammatory diarrhea in tropical areas, but data on its prevalence are scarce.[118,119]

Shigella infection is characterized by the occurrence of an invasive bacterial colitis. It is estimated that *Shigella* spp. are responsible for over 163 million infections annually in developing countries, resulting in 1.1 million deaths.[120] The disease can present with acute bloody diarrhea with high fever and systemic manifestations of malaise, headache, and abdominal pain. The incubation period ranges from 8 hours to 9 days but is usually between 14 and 72 hours, and a very low inoculum is required for its transmission, facilitating its spread. This syndrome may be particularly severe in malnourished children, in whom the mortality can be as high as 11%.[121] *Campylobacter* enteritis has been associated with ingestion of contaminated water, raw milk, or poultry, and typically occurs in young children or in travelers visiting tropical areas, and it is recognized as a common pathogen during the rainy seasons.[122]

Entamoeba histolytica is an important cause of inflammatory diarrhea (although fecal leukocytes may be pyknotic or absent). It is estimated that infection by *E. histolytica* results in 50 million cases of invasive enteric disease and liver abscess and up to 100,000 deaths per year. High rates of infection occur in the Indian subcontinent, southern and western Africa, in the Far East, and in the tropical areas of Central and South America. Patients with amebic colitis typically present with a 1- to 2-week history of abdominal pain, tenesmus, and frequent loose watery stools containing blood and mucus. Fever can be present, and on occasion the disease can be severe enough to cause extensive colitis with colonic perforation.[123] The diagnosis of intestinal amebiasis is based on examination of the stools or biopsy of mucosal tissue. A direct saline wet mount will reveal motile trophozoites, some containing red blood cells, suggesting invasive disease. In 90% of the cases, three separate stool examinations are required for the diagnosis. Rapid stool antigen detection kits have been developed based on antilectin antibodies, differentiating between *E. histolytica* and the nonpathogenic *Entamoeba dispar* (which morphologically are indistinguishable) in stool specimens.[124] Metronidazole is the drug of choice for the treatment of invasive colitis. A luminal agent is recommended (usually iodoquinol) after nitroimidazole therapy of invasive amebiasis.

Balantidium coli is another protozoan capable of causing inflammatory diarrhea in tropical areas of the world.[125] The most common reservoir is swine, and in tropical areas, monkeys. Like *E. histolytica*, this parasite invades the terminal ileum and colon, and may cause appendicitis or a dysenteric syndrome with rectosigmoid ulceration. The diagnosis is made by examination of wet preparations. Tetracycline is the drug of choice, but metronidazole is also active against this ciliated protozoan.[126]

In the management of patients with acute inflammatory diarrhea, it is necessary to perform a stool culture and a parasitologic examination, based on the organisms prevalent in each tropical area. Antimicrobials are essential to those with severe shigellosis and amebiasis, and empirical antimicrobial therapy is indicated in patients with diarrhea who have high fever and systemic toxicity or dysenteric disease.

Persistent and Chronic Diarrhea

Most diarrheal episodes acquired in the tropics subside spontaneously within a few days, but in some patients diarrhea may persist for more than 2 weeks.[127] Classic causes of persistent diarrhea include *Giardia lamblia*, EAEC, and *Cryptosporidium* (which can also cause acute disease as described previously). *Cyclospora* can also cause persistent diarrhea.[128] Tuberculosis can also present with chronic diarrhea.[70]

Infection with *G. lamblia* ranges from asymptomatic cyst passage to a chronic syndrome of diarrhea with malabsorption and weight loss. Symptomatic giardiasis is characterized by the acute onset of diarrhea, abdominal cramps, bloating, and flatulence. Initially, stools may be profuse and watery, but later are commonly greasy and foul-smelling. Patients may present with periods of diarrhea alternating with periods of constipation or normal bowel habits, and the disease may wax and wane over months until therapy is given or spontaneous resolution occurs. For the diagnosis of giardiasis, repeated stool examinations may be necessary. Immunofluorescent- and ELISA-based methods have also been developed for the diagnosis of giardiasis. The drugs of choice for the treatment of giardiasis are metronidazole and tinidazole. Nitazoxanide, which is available as a liquid and given for 3 days, is another treatment option for children.

Isospora belli infection appears to occur more commonly in tropical and subtropical climates, and although diarrhea due to *I. belli* infection is typically acute and self-limited in the immunologically normal host, prolonged diarrhea can occur in certain patients.[129] In immunocompromised hosts, including patients with AIDS, isosporiasis can be protracted, with profuse diarrheal disease. Laboratory diagnosis is done by examination of stained stool specimens by the modified Ziehl-Neelsen method. *I. belli* infection responds promptly to trimethoprim-sulfamethoxazole therapy and recurrent disease can be prevented with either trimethoprim or sulfamethoxazole.

Among the nematodes, *Strongyloides stercoralis, Capillaria philippinensis, Trichuris trichiura*, and *Schistosoma* have been reported as causing diarrhea.[130] *Strongyloides* can be associated with persistent diarrhea, cramping abdominal pain, and weight loss, particularly when there is hyperinfection or disseminated strongyloidiasis. Eosinophilia is a prominent feature of this infection. Occasionally some patients may complain of nausea, vomiting, and weight loss with evidence of malabsorption or of protein-losing enteropathy. *C. philippinensis* is a nematode that can also cause chronic diarrhea and malabsorption. The infection is seen in the Philippines and Thailand, and has also been reported in India and Egypt. *T. trichiura* can also be a cause of diarrhea (chronic dysentery) in highly parasitized patients. In schistosomiasis, diarrhea may occur due to the resulting granulomatous inflammation of the colon seen during the chronic phase in patients with heavy infections, or during acute schistosomiasis in unexposed patients (Katayama fever). In the latter case, the pathologic findings are completely different from those seen in the chronic form and are likely to be related to a hypersensitivity reaction.

Postinfective malabsorption (tropical sprue or "tropical enteropathy") was a common cause of chronic small bowel diarrhea, malabsorption, and weight loss in adults, especially in India, East Asia, and Central America. Small bowel bacterial overgrowth seems to play a role in the pathogenesis of tropical sprue. The treatment of tropical sprue with tetracycline and folate for up to 6 months seems to be most effective in symptom resolution and cure of diarrhea, with promotion of weight gain. *Tropical enteropathy* is a term used to describe an increasingly recognized syndrome of reduced absorption (with villous flattening) that is seen in many who live in tropical, developing areas (including Peace Corps volunteers)[131] and in many infections (ranging from *Cryptosporidium, Cyclospora,* or microsporidia to viral enteropathies).[132]

A form of persistent diarrhea showing worldwide distribution is Brainerd diarrhea. This is an idiopathic secretory process wherein the gut mucosa may show focal chronic inflammatory cells. The source is characteristically unpasteurized milk or untreated (well or surface) water. The prognosis is good, with diarrhea generally subsiding after 6 months to 1 year.

Traveler's Diarrhea

Traveler's diarrhea is a syndrome characterized by a twofold or greater increase in the frequency of unformed bowel movements, associated with one or more signs or symptoms of enteric infection occurring during or shortly after a trip away from home. The tropical areas of Latin America, Africa, and southern Asia are considered the high-risk areas for traveler's diarrhea.[133] Attack rates are variable, but average approximately 40% for travel from an industrialized region to one of the high-risk areas.

Bacterial enteropathogens cause most cases of traveler's diarrhea regardless of the specific area of risk. Enterotoxigenic *E. coli* is the single most common bacterial pathogen isolated, followed by *Shigella* spp., *Campylobacter jejuni, Aeromonas* spp., *Plesiomonas shigelloides, Salmonella* spp., and noncholera vibrios. Parasites such as *G. lamblia* and *Cryptosporidium parvum* occur in approximately 2% to 3% of cases of traveler's diarrhea. In 20% to 50% of episodes of traveler's diarrhea, no agents can be identified despite complete microbiologic assessment. Most of this undefinable illness appears to be bacterial in origin in view of the favorable response to antimicrobial therapy.

The management of patients with traveler's diarrhea involves adequate rehydration, followed by dietary management and symptomatic treatment.[94] For rehydration, the consumption of potable fruit juices, caffeine-free soft drinks, or flavored mineral water, coupled with a source of sodium chloride (e.g., saltines) is usually enough for hydrating most ill travelers. For adequate dietary management, staple foods such as cereals (wheat, rice, or oats), potatoes, noodles, crackers, and bananas are recommended during the acute phase of the illness. Patients should resume their usual diet once stools retain their shape. Drinks or food containing caffeine or lactose should be avoided while stools are unformed, since they may prolong diarrhea. Commonly used symptomatic drugs include bismuth subsalicylate and the antimotility synthetic opiate drugs such as loperamide. These agents are useful for the symptomatic treatment of mild to moderate cases of traveler's diarrhea.

Antimicrobial therapy shortens the duration of traveler's diarrhea from an average of 59 to 93 hours to 16 to 30 hours. This therapy is indicated in moderate to severe cases or when enteric symptoms persist for 48 hours or longer. Fluoroquinolones, or in South Asia, newer macrolides like azithromycin, are the preferred agents because of their activity against enteric pathogens in most high-risk parts of the world. Rifaximin, a poorly absorbed oral rifamycin derivative, was recently approved by the FDA for the treatment of traveler's diarrhea caused by noninvasive *E. coli*. Its use in patients with fever or blood in the stool and for those infected with *Campylobacter jejuni* is discouraged.

With regard to prevention, travelers to high-risk areas should be educated as to the safe foods and beverages to consume. Antimicrobial prophylaxis will prevent 70% to 80% of the disease that would occur without prophylaxis. If the traveler has an important underlying health impairment, or the trip will be ruined if the traveler has a brief illness that might force a change in itinerary, antimicrobial prophylaxis may be considered. An effective antibacterial drug for prevention of traveler's diarrhea is poorly absorbed rifaximin.[135] However, it is ineffective for treatment of invasive enteritis like Shigellosis. Bismuth subsalicylate has also been used as a prophylactic agent, preventing up to 65% of the cases of diarrhea that would occur during travel to high-risk areas if prophylaxis were not employed.[136] Travelers should begin taking the drug to be used for prophylaxis on their first day in the country they are visiting and should continue to take it for 1 or 2 days after leaving the country. However, pathogens such as *Cryptosporidium,* which may be devastating in immunocompromised patients, are prevented only by strict food and water precautions.

REFERENCES

1. UNAIDS. AIDS Epidemic Update: December 2003. Geneva, UNAIDS, 2003.
2. Cook GC: The clinical significance of gastrointestinal helminths—A review. Transact R Soc Trop Med Hyg 80:675–685, 1986.
3. Sullivan PS, DuPont HL, Arafat RR, et al: Illness and reservoirs associated with *Giardia lamblia* infection in rural Egypt: The case against treatment in developing world environments of high endemicity. Am J Epidemiol 127:1272–1281, 1988.
4. Lanata CF, Black RE, Maurtua D, et al: Etiologic agents in acute vs. persistent diarrhea in children under three years of age in peri-urban Lima, Peru. Acta Paediatr 381(Suppl):32–38, 1992.
5. Steiner TS, Lima AA, Nataro JP, et al: Enteroaggregative *Escherichia coli* produce intestinal inflammation and growth impairment and cause interleukin-8 release from intestinal epithelial cells. J Infect Dis 177:88–96, 1998.
6. Checkley W, Gilman RH, Epstein LD, et al: Asymptomatic and symptomatic cryptosporidiosis: Their acute effect on weight gain in Peruvian children. Am J Epidemiol 145:156–163, 1997.
7. Speelman P, Ljungstrom I: Protozoal enteric infections among expatriates in Bangladesh. Am J Trop Med Hyg 35:1140–1145, 1986.
8. Fryatt RJ, Teng J, Harries AD, et al: Intestinal helminthiasis in expatriates returning to Britain from the tropics. A controlled study. Trop Geogr Med 42:119–122, 1990.
9. Soave R: *Cyclospora*: An overview. Clin Infect Dis 23:429–437, 1996.
10. Gupta FP, Gupta MS, Bhardwaj S, et al: Current clinical patterns of typhoid fever: A prospective study. J Trop Med Hyg 88:377–381, 1985.
11. Pang T, Bhutta ZA, Finlay BB, et al: Typhoid fever and other salmonellosis: A continuing challenge. Trends Microbiol 3:253–255, 1995.
12. Rowland HAK: The complications of typhoid fever. Trop Med Hyg 64:143–152, 1961.
13. Saphra I, Winter JW: Clinical manifestations of salmonellosis in man. An evaluation of 7779 human infections identified at the New York Salmonella Center. N Engl J Med 256:1128–1134, 1957.
14. Crump JA, Youssef FG, Luby SP, et al: Estimating the incidence of typhoid fever and other febrile illnesses in developing countries. Emerg Infect Dis 9:539–544, 2003.
15. al-Aska AK: Gastrointestinal manifestations of brucellosis in Saudi Arabian patients. Trop Gastroenterol 10:217–219, 1989.
16. Carniel E, Butler T, Hossain S, et al: Infrequent detection of *Yersinia enterocolitica* in childhood diarrhea in Bangladesh. Am J Trop Med Hyg 35:370–371, 1986.
17. Hull HF, Montes JM, Mann JM: Plague masquerading gastrointestinal illness. West J Med 145:485–487, 1986.
18. Kunanusont C, Limpakarnjanarat K, Foy HM: Outbreak of anthrax in Thailand. Ann Trop Med Parasitol 84:507–512, 1990.
19. Jakubowski A, Elwood RK, Enarson DA: Clinical features of abdominal tuberculosis. J Infect Dis 158:687–692, 1988.
20. Rocha MO, Pedroso ER, Lambertucci JR, et al: Gastrointestinal manifestations of the initial phase of schistosomiasis mansoni. Ann Trop Med Parasitol 89:271–278, 1995.
21. Petit PL, Wamola IA: Typhoid fever: A review of its impact and diagnostic problems. East Afr Med J 71:183–188, 1994.
22. Rasaily R, Dutta P, Saha MR, et al: Value of a single Widal test in the diagnosis of typhoid fever. Indian J Med Res 97:104–107, 1993.
23. Koeleman JG, Regensburg DF, van Katwijk F, et al: Retrospective study to determine the diagnostic value of the Widal test in a non-endemic country. Eur J Clin Microbiol Infect Dis 11:167–170, 1992.
24. Jhaveri KN, Nandwani SK, Mehta PK, et al: False positive modified Widal test in acute malaria. J Assoc Physicians India 43:754–755, 1995.
25. Benavente L, Gotuzzo E, Guerra J, et al: Diagnosis of typhoid fever using a string capsule device. Trans R Soc Trop Med Hyg 78:404–406, 1984.
26. Gasem MH, Dolmans WMV, Isbandrio BB, et al: Culture of *Salmonella typhi* and *Salmonella paratyphi* from blood and bone marrow in suspected typhoid fever. Trop Geogr Med 47:164–167, 1995.
27. Antony TJ, Patwari AK, Anand VK, et al: Duodenal string test in typhoid fever. Indian Pediatr 30:643–647, 1993.
28. Vallenas C, Hernandez H, Kay B, et al: Efficacy of bone marrow, blood, stool and duodenal contents cultures for bacteriologic confirmation of typhoid fever in children. Pediatr Infect Dis 4:496–498, 1985.
29. Mirza SH, Beeching NJ, Hart CA: Multidrug resistant typhoid: A global problem. J Med Microbiol 44:317–319, 1996.
30. Soe GB, Overdurf GD: Treatment of typhoid fever and other systemic salmonellosis with cefotaxime, ceftriaxone, cefoperazone and other newer cephalosporins. Rev Infect Dis 9:719–736, 1987.
31. DuPont HL: Quinolones in *Salmonella typhi* infection. Drugs 45(Suppl 3): 119–124, 1993.
32. Hien TT, Duong NM, Ha HD, et al: A randomised comparative study of fleroxacin and ceftriaxone in enteric fever. Trans R Soc Trop Med Hyg 88:464–465, 1994.
33. Wallace MR, Yousif AA, Mahroos GA, et al: Ciprofloxacin versus ceftriaxone in the treatment of multiresistant typhoid fever. Eur J Clin Microbiol Infect Dis 12:907–910, 1993.
34. Bhutta ZA, Khan IA, Molla AM: Therapy of multi-drug resistant typhoid fever with oral cefixime vs intravenous ceftriaxone. Pediatr Infect Dis 13:990–994, 1994.
35. Daga MK, Sarin K, Sarkar R: A study of culture positive multi-drug resistant enteric fever—Changing patterns and emerging resistance to ciprofloxacin. J Assoc Physicians India 42:599–600, 1994.
36. Rowe B, Ward LR, Threlfall EJ: Ciprofloxacin-resistant *Salmonella typhi* in the UK. Lancet 346:1302, 1995.

37. Parry CM, Hien TT, Dougan G, et al: Typhoid fever. N Engl J Med 347:1770–1782, 2002.
38. Hien TT, Bethell DB, Hoa NTT, et al: Short course of ofloxacin for treatment of multi-drug resistant typhoid. Clin Infect Dis 20:917–923, 1995.
39. Enwonwu CO: Noma: A neglected scourge of children in sub-Saharan Africa. Bull World Health Organ 73:541–545, 1995.
40. Junkins-Hopkins JM: Multiple painful oral ulcerations. Secondary syphilis. Arch Dermatol 131:833–836, 1995.
41. de Swaan B, Tjiam KH, Vuzevski VD, et al: Solitary oral condylomata lata in a patient with secondary syphilis. Sexual Transm Dis 12:238–240, 1985.
42. Samuels RH, Martin MV: A clinical and microbiological study of *Actinomycetes* in oral and cervicofacial lesions. Br J Oral Maxillofac Surg 26:458–463, 1988.
43. Ficarra G, Di Lollo S, Pierleoni F, et al: Actinomycosis of the tongue: A diagnostic challenge. Head Neck 15:53–55, 1993.
44. Sirisanthana T, Navachareon N, Tharavichitkul P, et al: Outbreak of oral-oropharyngeal anthrax: An unusual manifestation of human infection with *Bacillus anthracis*. Am J Trop Med Hyg 33:144–150, 1984.
45. Dimitrakopoulos I, Zouloumis L, Lazaridis N, et al: Primary tuberculosis of the oral cavity. Oral Surg Oral Med Oral Pathol 72:712–715, 1991.
46. Fitch HB, Alling CC: Leprosy, oral manifestations. J Periodontol 33:40–44, 1962.
47. Sposto MR, Scully C, de Almeida OP, et al: Oral paracoccidioidomycosis. A study of 36 South American patients. Oral Surg Oral Med Oral Pathol 75:461–465, 1993.
48. Zislis T, Adrian JC, Cutright DE: Oral manifestations of tropical infectious diseases of Central and South America. Part II: Bacterial and mycotic infections. Mil Med 145:529–534, 1980.
49. Pearson RD, de Queiroz Souza A: Clinical spectrum of leishmaniasis. Clin Infect Dis 22:1–13, 1996.
50. Zislis T, Adrian JC, Cutright DE: Oral manifestations of tropical infectious diseases of Central and South America. Part I: Protozoan and helminthic infections. Mil Med 145:525–528, 1980.
51. de Oliveira RB, Filho JR, Dantas RO, et al: The spectrum of esophageal motor disorders in Chagas' disease. Am J Gastroenterol 90:1119–1124, 1995.
52. Laine L, Bonacini M: Esophageal disease in human immunodeficiency virus infection. Arch Intern Med 154:1577–1582, 1994.
53. Gendron Y, Courbil LJ, Aubry P: Esophageal cancer in the tropical environment. Med Trop 43:253–262, 1983.
54. Strickland GT: Gastrointestinal manifestations of schistosomiasis. Gut 35:1334–1337, 1994.
55. Saad AM, Homeida M, Eltom I, et al: Oesophageal varices in a region of the Sudan endemic for *Schistosoma mansoni*. Br J Surg 78: 1252–1253, 1991.
56. Abdel-Wahab MF, Esmat G, Farrag A, et al: Ultrasonographic prediction of esophageal varices in *Schistosomiasis mansoni*. Am J Gastroenterol 88:560–563, 1993.
57. Weissman D, Gumaste VV, Dave PB, et al: Bleeding from a tuberculous gastric ulcer. Am J Gastroenterol 85:742–744, 1990.
58. Newman RM, Fleshner PR, Lajam FE, et al: Esophageal tuberculosis: A rare presentation with hematemesis. Am J Gastroenterol 86:751–755, 1991.
59. Monkemuller KE, Lewis JB Jr: Massive rectal bleeding from colonic tuberculosis. Am J Gastroenterol 91:1439–1441, 1996.
60. Pozniak AL, Dalton-Clark HJ, Ralphs DN: Colonic tuberculosis presenting with massive rectal bleeding. Tubercle 66:295–299, 1985.
61. Eggleston FC, Verghese M, Handa AK: Amebiasis causing massive gastrointestinal bleeding. Arch Surg 113:1472, 1978.
62. Bhargava DK, Rai RR, Dasarathy S, et al: Colonoscopy for unexplained lower gastrointestinal bleeding in a tropical country. Trop Gastroenterol 16:59–63, 1995.
63. Goenka MK, Kochhar R, Mehta SK: Spectrum of lower gastrointestinal hemorrhage: An endoscopic study of 166 patients. Indian J Gastroenterol 12:129–131, 1993.
64. Fennerty MB: *Helicobacter pylori*. Arch Intern Med 154:721–727, 1994.
65. Holcombe C, Omotara BA, Eldridge J, et al: The commonest bacterial infection in Africa. *Helicobacter pylori*: A random serological survey. Am J Gastroenterol 87:28–30, 1992.
66. Holcombe C, Umar H, Lucas SB, et al: Low incidence of clinically significant gastroduodenal pathology despite a high incidence of *Helicobacter pylori* infection. Trans R Soc Trop Med Hyg 88:569–571, 1994.
67. Singh S, Raju GV, Samantaray JC: Parasitic gut flora in a north Indian population with gastrointestinal symptoms. Trop Gastroenterol 14:104–108, 1993.
68. Hamed AD, Akinola O: Intestinal ascariasis in the differential diagnosis of peptic ulcer disease. Trop Geogr Med 42:37–40, 1990.
69. Anyaeze CM: Reducing burden of hookworm disease in the management of upper abdominal pain in the tropics. Trop Doct 33:174–175, 2003.
70. Marshall JB: Tuberculosis of the gastrointestinal tract and peritoneum. Am J Gastroenterol 88:989–999, 1993.
71. Singh MM, Bhargava AN, Jain KP: Tuberculous peritonitis: An evaluation of pathogenetic mechanisms, diagnostic procedures and therapeutic measures. N Engl J Med 281:1091–1094, 1969.
72. Rai S, Thomas WM: Diagnosis of abdominal tuberculosis: The importance of laparoscopy. J R Soc Med 96:586–588, 2003.
73. Dwivedi M, Misra SP, Misra V, et al: Value of adenosine deaminase estimation in the diagnosis of tuberculous ascites. Am J Gastroenterol 85:13–15, 1990.
74. Gupta SC, Gupta AK, Keswani NK, et al: Pathology of tropical appendicitis. J Clin Pathol 42:1169–1172, 1989.
75. Otu AA: Tropical surgical abdominal emergencies: Acute intestinal obstruction. Afr J Med Med Sci 20:83–88, 1991.
76. Holcombe C: Surgical emergencies in tropical gastroenterology. Gut 36:9–11, 1995.
77. Pinus J: Surgical complications of ascariasis. Prog Pediatr Surg 15:79–86, 1982.
78. al-Bahrani ZR, al-Saleem T, al-Gailani MA: Sub-acute intestinal obstruction by *Strongyloides stercoralis*. J Infect 30:47–50, 1995.
79. Bhansali SK: Abdominal tuberculosis. Am J Gastroenterol 67:324–336, 1977.
80. Bitar R, Tarpley J: Intestinal perforation in typhoid fever: A historical and state-of-the-art review. Rev Infect Dis 7:257–271, 1985.
81. van Basten JP, Stockenbrugger R: Typhoid perforation. A review of the literature since 1960. Trop Geogr Med 46:336–339, 1994.
82. Akgun Y, Bac B, Boylu S, et al: Typhoid enteric perforation. Br J Surg 82:1512–1515, 1995.
83. Sharma L, Gupta S, Soin AS, et al: Generalized peritonitis in India—The tropical spectrum. Jpn J Surg 21:272–277, 1991.
84. Eggleston FC, Verghese M, Handa AK: Amoebic perforation of the bowel: Experiences with 26 cases. Br J Surg 65:748–751, 1978.
85. Loria-Cortes R, Lobo-Sanahuja JF: Clinical abdominal strongyloidiasis: A study of 116 children with intestinal eosinophilic granuloma caused by *Angiostrongylus costaricensis*. Am J Trop Med Hyg 29:538–544, 1980.
86. Kark AE, McAlpine JC: Anisakiasis ("herring worm disease") as a cause of acute abdominal crisis. Br J Clin Pract 48:216–217, 1994.
87. Davis AA: Hypertrophic intestinal tuberculosis. Surg Gynecol Obstet 56:907, 1933.
88. Gilinsky NH, Marks IN, Kotler RE, et al: Abdominal tuberculosis. A 10 year review. S Afr Med J 64:849–857, 1983.
89. Radin DR: Intraabdominal mycobacterial tuberculosis vs *Mycobacterium avium-intracellulare* infection in patients with AIDS: Distinction based on CT findings. AJR 156:487–491, 1991.
90. Berardi R: Abdominal actinomycosis. Surg Gynecol Obstet 149:257–266, 1979.
91. Ravdin JI: Amebiasis. Clin Infect Dis 20:1453–1466, 1995.
92. Capell MS, Mandell W, Grimes MM, et al: Gastrointestinal histoplasmosis. Dig Dis Sci 33:353–360, 1988.
93. Guerrant RL: Twelve messages from enteric infections for science and society. Am J Trop Med Hyg 51:26–35, 1994.
94. DuPont HL, Ericsson CD: Prevention and treatment of travelers diarrhea. N Engl J Med 328:1821–1827, 1993.
95. Gotuzzo E, Cieza J, Estremadoyro L, et al: Cholera. Lessons from the epidemic in Peru. Infect Dis Clin North Am 8:183–205, 1994.
96. Ramamurthy T, Garg S, Sharma S, et al: Emergence of a novel strain of *Vibrio cholerae* with epidemic potential in southern and eastern India. Lancet 341:703–704, 1993.
97. Cholera Working Group: Large epidemic of cholera-like disease in Bangladesh caused by *Vibrio cholerae* O139 synonym Bengal. Lancet 342:387–390, 1993.
98. Swerdlow DL, Ries AA: *Vibrio cholerae* non-O1—The eighth pandemic? Lancet 342:382–383, 1993.
99. Carpenter CCJ: The treatment of cholera: Clinical science at the bedside. J Infect Dis 166:2–14, 1992.

100. Swerdlow DL, Ries AA: Cholera in the Americas: Guidelines for the clinician. JAMA 267:1495–1499, 1992.
101. Gotuzzo E, Seas C, Echevarria J, et al: Ciprofloxacin for the treatment of cholera: A randomized, double blind, controlled clinical trial of a single daily dose in Peruvian adults. Clin Infect Dis 20:1485–1490, 1995.
102. MacKenzie WR, Hoxie NJ, Proctor ME, et al: A massive outbreak in Milwaukee of *Cryptosporidium* infection transmitted through the public water supply. N Engl J Med 331:161–167, 1994.
103. Blanshard C, Jackson AM, Shanson DC, et al: Cryptosporidiosis in HIV-seropositive patients. Q J Med 85:813–823, 1992.
104. Pape JW, Verdier RI, Boncy J, et al: *Cyclospora* infection in adults infected with HIV. Clinical manifestations, treatment and prophylaxis. Ann Intern Med 121:654–657, 1994.
105. Newman RD, Zu S, Wuhib T, et al: Household epidemiology of *Cryptosporidium parvum* infection in an urban community in Northeast Brazil. Ann Intern Med 120:500–505, 1994.
106. Molbak K, Hojlyng N, Gottschau A, et al: Cryptosporidiosis in infancy and childhood mortality in Guinea-Bissau, West Africa. BMJ 307:417–420, 1993.
107. Colebunders R, Francis H, Mann JM, et al: Persistent diarrhea strongly associated with HIV infection in Kinshasha, Zaire. Am J Gastroenterol 82:859–864, 1987.
108. Kehl KS, Cicirello H, Havens PL: Comparison of four different methods for detection of *Cryptosporidium* species. J Clin Microbiol 33:416–418, 1995.
109. Weber R, Bryan RT, Bishop HS, et al: Threshold detection of *Cryptosporidium* oocysts in human stool specimens: Evidence for low sensitivity of current diagnostic methods. J Clin Microbiol 29:1323–1327, 1991.
110. White AC, Chappell CL, Hayat CS, et al: Paromomycin for cryptosporidiosis in AIDS: A prospective, double-blind trial. J Infect Dis 170:419–424, 1994.
111. Rossignol JF, Hidalgo H, Feregrino M, et al: A double-'blind' placebo-controlled study of nitazoxanide in the treatment of cryptosporidial diarrhoea in AIDS patients in Mexico. Trans R Soc Trop Med Hyg 92:663–666, 1998.
112. Amadi B, Mwiya M, Jusuku J, et al: Effect of nitazoxanide on morbidity and mortality in Zambian children with cryptosporidiosis: A randomized controlled trial. Lancet 360:1375–1380, 2002.
113. Carr A, Marriott D, Field A, et al: Treatment of HIV-1-associated microsporidiosis and cryptosporidiosis with combination antiretroviral therapy. Lancet 351:256–261, 1998.
114. Hoge CW, Shlim DR, Ghimire M, et al: Placebo-controlled trial of co-trimoxazole for *Cyclospora* infections among travelers and foreign residents in Nepal. Lancet 345:691–693, 1995.
115. Pan TM, Chiou CS, Hsu SY, et al: Food-borne disease outbreaks in Taiwan, 1994. J Formos Med Assoc 95:417–420, 1996.
116. Wieneke AA, Roberts D, Gilbert RJ: Staphylococcal food poisoning in the United Kingdom, 1969–90. Epidemiol Infect 110:519–531, 1993.
117. Drobniewski FA: *Bacillus cereus* and related species. Clin Microbiol Rev 6:324–338, 1993.
118. Taylor DN, Bodhidatta L, Echeverria P: Epidemiologic aspects of shigellosis and other causes of dysentery in Thailand. Rev Infect Dis 13(Suppl 4):S226–S230, 1991.
119. Mandal BK, Schofield PF: Tropical colonic diseases. Gut 305:638–641, 1992.
120. Kotloff KL, Winickoff JP, Ivanoff B, et al: Global burden of Shigella infections: Implications for vaccine development and implementation of control strategies. Bull World Health Organ 77:651–666, 1999.
121. Bennish ML, Wojtyniak BJ: Mortality due to shigellosis: Community and hospital data. Rev Infect Dis 13(Suppl 4):S245–S251, 1991.
122. Pazzaglia G, Bourgeois AL, Araby I, et al: *Campylobacter*-associated diarrhoea in Egyptian infants: Epidemiology and clinical manifestations of disease and high frequency of concomitant infections. J Diarrhoeal Dis Res 11:6–13, 1993.
123. Wanke C, Butler T, Islam M: Epidemiologic and clinical features of invasive amebiasis in Bangladesh: A case-control comparison with other diarrheal diseases and postmortem findings. Am J Trop Med Hyg 38:335–341, 1988.
124. Haque R, Neville LM, Hahn P, et al: Rapid diagnosis of *Entamoeba* infection by using *Entamoeba* and *Entamoeba histolytica* stool antigen detection kits. J Clin Microbiol 33:2558–2561, 1995.
125. Ogunba EO: The prevalence of human intestinal protozoa in Ibadan, Nigeria. J Trop Med Hyg 80:187–191, 1977.
126. Garcia-Laverde A, de Bonilla L: Clinical trials with metronidazole in human balantidiasis. Am J Trop Med Hyg 24:781–783, 1975.
127. Cook GC: Persisting diarrhoea and malabsorption. Gut 35:582–586, 1994.
128. Berlin OGW, Noval SM, Porschen RK, et al: Recovery of *Cyclospora* organisms from patients with prolonged diarrhea. Clin Infect Dis 18:606–609, 1994.
129. Pape JW, Johnson WD Jr: *Isospora belli* infections. Prog Clin Parasitol 2:119–127, 1991.
130. Genta RM: Diarrhea in helminthic infections. Clin Infect Dis 16(Suppl 2): S122–S129, 1993.
131. Lindenbaum J, Kent TH, Sprinz H: Malabsorption and jejunitis in American Peace Corps volunteers in Pakistan. Ann Intern Med 65:1201–1209, 1966.
132. Guerrant RL, Thielman NM: Emerging enteric protozoa: *Cryptosporidium, Cyclospora,* and Microsporidia. In Scheld WM, Armstrong D, Hughes JM (eds): Emerging Infections. Washington, DC, ASM Press, 1998, pp 233–245.
133. Black RE: Epidemiology of travelers' diarrhea and relative importance of various pathogens. Rev Infect Dis 12(Suppl 1):S73–S79, 1990.
134. Medical Letter 46:74–76, September 2004.
135. DuPont HL, Jiang ZD, Okhuysen PC, et al: A randomized, double-blind, placebo-controlled trial of rifaximin to prevent travelers' diarrhea. Ann Intern Med 142:805–812, 2005.
136. DuPont HL, Ericsson CD, Johnson PC, et al: Prevention of travelers' diarrhea by the tablet formulation of bismuth subsalicylate. JAMA 257:1347–1350, 1987.

124

Fever and Systemic Symptoms

MARY E. WILSON
RICHARD D. PEARSON

Box 124-1 Key Concepts in the Evaluation of the Febrile Patient

- Fever after travel may be unrelated to exposures during travel.
- A history of fever in a person exposed to malaria should prompt evaluation for malaria, even if the patient is afebrile at the moment seen.
- Always look for malaria. Look again if exposures and clinical findings are consistent with that diagnosis.
- Exposure to many widely distributed infections is more common during travel than during life at home.
- Unfamiliar infections can follow exposures in temperate areas.
- Re-examine the febrile patient if the initial evaluation does not suggest a specific diagnosis.
- Keep in mind the public health implications. Should the infection be reported? Do contacts need treatment or special attention? Are special isolation techniques required?
- Use electronic networks to supplement and update information from other sources.

INTRODUCTION

Fever in the tropics and after travel is a common response to microbial invasion. Fever can presage rapidly progressive disease or indicate a trivial self-limited infection. Early symptoms of self-limited and lethal infections can be indistinguishable. Several features make evaluation of fever a major and continuing challenge: the causes include diverse infectious and noninfectious diseases; similar signs and symptoms characterize infections caused by unrelated pathogens requiring different interventions; and timing of onset of fever after exposure to a pathogen can range from hours to decades. Interventions may be lifesaving if applied in good time.

This chapter describes the causes of fever in persons with tropical and other diverse geographic exposures. The discussion focuses on recognizing possible causes of fever and on reaching a specific diagnosis and omits details of treatment, which can be found elsewhere in this book. Although the differential diagnosis for the febrile international traveler who has visited an area briefly and the febrile resident of the tropics may be similar, the relative likelihood of specific diseases and their consequences may differ greatly, thus mandating flexibility in the approach to the initial evaluation. Foreign-born residents of industrialized countries and their children who visit relatives and friends in developing countries may receive no pretravel prophylaxis and often have intense local exposures, placing them at greater risk for a wider range of infections than the usual vacationer or business traveler.[1] Several key concepts that underlie the evaluation of the febrile patient are listed in Box 124-1.

PATHOGENESIS

The complex interactions of endogenous pyrogens and neural pathways in the pathogenesis of fever are reviewed in recent publications.[2–4] Pyrogenic cytokines, such as interleukin (IL)-1β, IL-6, and tumor necrosis factor–α, which result from stimulated mononuclear phagocytes, interact directly with the anterior hypothalamus, which coordinates thermoregulation through a hierarchy of neural structures. Prostaglandin E_2 is a proximal mediator in the preoptic-anterior hypothalamic area. Direct neural pathways from the periphery to the brain also may be involved.[2]

EPIDEMIOLOGY

Fever is a common reason for seeking medical care during and after travel. Although risks and types of infection vary greatly depending on the circumstances of travel and the specific time and place, available studies provide general estimates of the likelihood of fever during and after travel. In the classic studies by Steffen and colleagues,[5] 152 of 7886 (almost 2%) of Swiss short-term travelers to developing countries reported "high fevers over several days" on questionnaires completed between 4 and almost 7 months after return from travel. Among those reporting fever, 39% said they had fevers only while abroad, 37% had fevers abroad and at home, and 24% had fevers at home only. In a study of 784 American travelers who spent 3 months or less in developing countries, 3% reported fever unassociated with other symptoms.[6] Among more than 20,000 ill returned travelers who were seen at 27 different clinical sites as part of the global GeoSentinel surveillance network, 22.2% had fever as a chief complaint.[7]

The risk of infection is strongly related to the geographic location of exposure. In recent years, risk of dengue was highest in parts of Asia, falciparum malaria in sub-Saharan Africa, and enteric fever in the Indian sub-continent. Among German travelers who acquired dengue fever in tropical areas in 2002, incidence rate per 100,000 travelers ranged from 27.9 for Thailand to 2.1 for the Greater Antilles islands in the Caribbean.[8] The snapshot of returning travelers is only part of the picture of the disease burden experienced by travelers. Many infections begin and are treated abroad. In one study that analyzed malaria in travelers to Africa, about half of the cases were treated abroad.[9] Activities of travelers and types of accommodations also influence risk. Studies by Steffen and co-workers[10,11] estimated the incidence rate of hepatitis A to be 3 to 6 per 1000 per month of stay in a developing country in unprotected travelers. The risk may rise to 20 per 1000 per month in persons living under poor hygienic conditions.

Useful information can be gathered from studies that have defined the causes of fever after travel. MacLean and colleagues[12] found malaria was the most common diagnosis (present in 32%)

in evaluation of 587 persons seen between 1981 and 1988 in Montreal with fever after tropical travel. In Switzerland, among 336 travelers and migrants who were seen at an outpatient clinic with a history of fever or malaise, 29% of those who had blood tested for malaria had confirmed malaria.[13] Of 195 consecutive patients hospitalized with fever between November 1992 and April 1993 at the London Hospital for Tropical Diseases, malaria was the most common diagnosis, accounting for 42% of admissions.[14] An additional two recent studies of hospitalized febrile returned travelers, one from Australia[15] and the other from Italy,[16] also found malaria as the most common diagnosis. Among 153 hospitalized febrile returned pediatric travelers in the UK, diarrheal disease and malaria were the most common diagnoses.[17] Recent papers also highlight the growing importance of dengue fever in tropical areas,[18–20] and as a cause of hospitalization after travel, second only to malaria in one series of patients seen in Israel.[21] It was the most common arboviral infection diagnosed in Swedish travelers in 1989 and 1990.[22]

It is worth noting that in the series of MacLean and associates[12] and Doherty and coworkers,[14] of the top 10 most common causes of fever after tropical travel, more than half are diseases with broad or worldwide distribution (respiratory infections, hepatitis, diarrheal illness, urinary tract infections, pharyngitis). Box 124-2 lists the most common causes of fever after tropical travel as described in published series. Many categories define a body site of infection and not a specific pathogen. In the series of MacLean and colleagues and Doherty and associates, the cause of about one fourth of the fevers was undefined. Among the patients with a specific etiologic agent defined, the most common were malaria, dengue, hepatitis A, rickettsial infection, streptococcal pharyngitis, typhoid fever, *Campylobacter, Salmonella, Shigella,* and amebic liver abscess.

Patterns of infectious disease are dynamic and will continue to change, influenced substantially by international travel and trade.[23,24] Several factors can lead to changes in the types and relative frequencies of diseases diagnosed in persons visiting tropical regions: shifts in the epidemiology of disease; the rising resistance of infections to drugs; changes in popular destinations for travelers; the availability and wide use of effective preventive strategies (e.g., vaccines against hepatitis A and B); and new knowledge and techniques that facilitate diagnosis.

Studies that describe causes of fever in specific geographic areas help define the infectious disease profile for a region or country. They are most relevant to clinicians when the populations studied have included both local residents and visitors to that region. In the end, information about which infections occur and where is collected from anecdotal cases, published data on residents, and reports of outbreaks among travelers.[25] Often the available information is incomplete, unrepresentative, and out-of-date. The capacity to share information through electronic networks has improved the flow of information.[26] Regularly updated references,[27–28] Web sites, and tropical disease textbooks are good sources of information.

Exposures differ among travelers, long-term visitors (such as missionaries and Peace Corps workers), local residents, and military troops, but studies from these groups can be useful. Several studies looked at U.S. troops in Vietnam. The most frequently made diagnoses in 524 U.S. Marines in South Vietnam with acute fevers lasting at least 4 days included leptospirosis (20.1%), scrub typhus (11.6%), Japanese encephalitis (6.8%), and infectious mononucleosis (5.4%).[29] Another study in Vietnam of febrile American troops (with a negative malaria smear) found dengue the cause of fever in 29%, chikungunya in 9%, scrub typhus in 8%, and malaria in 7%.[30] While these studies provide a general idea of the pathogens in that region, most troops have a level of exposure to water, soil, and arthropods unmatched by the usual traveler (see Chapter 122).

Series of evaluations of febrile residents in other countries give some suggestion as to the heterogeneity of causes and geographic variation. For example, of 1629 febrile patients hospitalized in rural Malaysia, scrub typhus was the most common diagnosis (19.3% of all illnesses), followed by typhoid and paratyphoid fevers (7.4%), flavivirus infection (7.0%), leptospirosis (6.8%), and malaria (6.2%).[31] In Jakarta, Indonesia, in 1971–1972, bacteremic salmonella infections (predominantly *Salmonella enterica* serotype typhi) were the most common infections documented in patients hospitalized with fever.[32] In 876 consecutive febrile adults seen at a general hospital in Nepal in 2001, enteric fever and pneumonia were the most common clinical diagnoses.[33] A putative pathogen was identified in 37%, with the most common specific diagnoses being typhoid and paratyphoid fevers, murine typhus, pneumococcal infection, scrub typhus, and leptospirosis. The most common diagnoses in 505 adults in Spain with unexplained fever (with negative chest films and without localizing signs or symptoms) lasting 1 to 3 weeks were Q fever (21%), brucellosis (19%), spotted fever (murine typhus and boutonneuse fever; 15%), and mononucleosis syndrome (9%).[34]

In northern Thailand, melioidosis, caused by the gram-negative organism *Burkholderia pseudomallei*, is a major cause of community-acquired sepsis.[35] During a 1-year period from October 1986 through September 1987, 63 cases of septicemic melioidosis and 206 patients with other community-acquired septicemias were documented. Melioidosis accounted for about 20% of all documented cases of sepsis and about 40% of all deaths from community-acquired sepsis. As a cause of positive

Box 124-2 Common Causes of Fever After Tropical Travel*

- Malaria
- Respiratory tract infections (including pneumonia)
- Diarrheal illness
- Hepatitis
- Urinary tract infection
- Dengue fever
- Enteric fever
- Rickettsial infection
- Infectious mononucleosis
- Pharyngitis

*Among the patients with a specific etiologic agent defined, the most common causes were malaria, dengue, hepatitis A, rickettsial infection, streptococcal pharyngitis, typhoid fever, *Campylobacter, Salmonella,* and *Shigella* infections, and amebic liver abscess.

Data from MacLean JD, Lalonde RG, Ward B: Fever From the Tropics, section 5. Travel Medicine Advisor. Atlanta, American Health Consultants, 1994, p 27.1; and Doherty JF, Grant AD, Bryceson AD: Fever as the presenting complaint of travelers returning from the tropics. Q J Med 88:277, 1995.

with ehrlichiosis caused by *Ehrlichia chaffeensis* and include altered mental status, lymphocytic pleocytosis, and elevated CSF protein.[172] Many clinicians are familiar with Lyme disease and ehrlichiosis but may be unaware that they occur in many countries outside the United States.[173,174]

Few helminthic infections cause fever and neurologic findings. The presence of eosinophilia should suggest one of these infections (see Chapter 125). Angiostrongyliasis due to *Parastrongylus (Angiostrongylus) cantonensis* can cause fever, headache, and eosinophilia in CSF and peripheral blood. In 2000, an outbreak of eosinophilic meningitis occurred in travelers who had visited Jamaica and had shared a meal.[175] Disseminated strongyloidiasis in compromised hosts can be associated with bacteremias and meningitis, sometimes years or decades after the host has left the endemic region. Other helminths that reach the CNS (e.g., cysticercosis) are not associated with an acute febrile illness. When trichinellosis[176] and schistosomiasis cause fever and CNS findings, it is typically in the setting of other systemic findings, including eosinophilia.

The differential diagnosis of a patient with fever and unexplained meningitis should include the possibility of drug-induced meningitis. Among the drugs that have been implicated are trimethoprim-sulfamethoxazole (TMP-SMX) and several nonsteroidal anti-inflammatory agents, drugs that are used widely and may be obtained without a prescription in many parts of the world.

Fever and Respiratory Symptoms

The respiratory tract is a common site of infection during and after travel, though the specific cause often remains undefined.[6] Among approximately 22,000 ill returned travelers who presented to a GeoSentinel site for medical evaluation (from September 1997 through August 2001), almost 8% had respiratory tract infections.[177] In a study of American travelers,[6] 26% reported respiratory tract symptoms during travel and 10% following travel. Patients with pneumonia after travel should be evaluated for common pathogens, such as *Streptococcus pneumoniae, Staphylococcus aureus, Haemophilus influenzae*, and *Mycoplasma pneumoniae*. Outbreaks and sporadic cases of influenza occur in travelers, including on cruise ships[178] and in pilgrims to the Hajj.[179] One well-studied outbreak documented the spread of influenza on an aircraft.[180] Recent outbreaks of avian influenza in Asia have heightened worries that a highly pathogenic strain could become more transmissible in humans.[181] Probable person-to-person transmission was noted in Thailand in 2004.[182] The clinical spectrum may include diarrhea and CNS changes.[183] Outbreaks of SARS in 2002–2003 caused more than 8000 cases and almost 800 deaths and disrupted global travel.[184] Fever is prominent in SARS, often preceding the development of respiratory findings. Transmission also occurred on aircraft.[185] Several clusters have highlighted the acquisition of Legionnaires' disease during travel in many regions of the world.[186,187] Between 45% and 65% of cases of Legionnaires' disease in England and Wales have been travel-related.

Melioidosis is a common cause of pneumonia, especially in parts of Asia, as described previously. The fungal infections coccidioidomycosis and histoplasmosis have caused recent outbreaks in travelers in the Americas.[188–190] Q fever is a common cause of pneumonia in some areas, including Spain.[34]

Risk of infection with *Mycobacterium tuberculosis* is increased by travel to areas highly endemic for tuberculosis, especially with prolonged stays.[191,192] Transmission can also occur on long flights. Infection may manifest months or years after travel.

Other infections that can produce prominent pulmonary findings include hantaviruses, plague, tularemia, and anthrax. In patients with amebic liver abscess, extension of the process to the diaphragmatic surface of the liver may cause pulmonary findings.[102] Severe malaria may be complicated by acute respiratory distress syndrome. Pulmonary infiltrates may be present during the pulmonary migration phase of several helminths, including hookworm, ascaris, and strongyloides (see Chapter 125). Acute schistosomiasis (Katayama syndrome) may cause fever and pulmonary infiltrates.[193] Pulmonary emboli and infarction can cause fever and pulmonary findings that can mimic respiratory infections including pneumonia.

Fever and Diarrhea

Many infections are acquired via ingestion of contaminated food or drink. The gastrointestinal tract may be the portal of entry and the initial or primary site of infection. Enteric infections, such as campylobacteriosis and salmonellosis, may produce an illness with just fever and no, few, or delayed gastrointestinal symptoms. Workup of the febrile patient with diarrhea should include studies for *Clostridium difficile*. This infection has been reported after many antimicrobials, including doxycycline taken for malaria chemoprophylaxis.[194] Diarrhea and other gastrointestinal symptoms can also be found as part of systemic infections (e.g., malaria, dengue fever, rickettsial infections), hence the workup of the febrile patient with diarrhea should not focus exclusively on enteric pathogens. Persons with an amebic liver abscess may give a history of diarrhea, but many deny diarrhea at the time they seek medical care for fevers. In a series of 52 patients with amebic liver abscess in Cairo, 25% gave a history of diarrhea and 6% reported dysentery.[195] Fever and right upper quadrant pain were the most common manifestations. In this series, 42% had an acute illness, characterized by high fever, vomiting, and leukocytosis, and 58% had a more chronic illness, often with low-grade fever, weight loss, and anemia.[195]

Systemic infections can involve the gut and be associated with gastrointestinal symptoms and fever. Some of these include visceral leishmaniasis, histoplasmosis, tuberculosis, nontuberculous mycobacteria, and Whipple's disease.[196]

Fever and Hepatitis

Hepatitis A traditionally has been the most common form of hepatitis after travel to developing countries. In Swedish travelers who did not receive immunoglobulin in a study that was done before hepatitis A vaccine was available, the risk of hepatitis A was 1 in 100 to 150 after travel to tropical Asia or Africa.[197] Hepatitis A is extremely uncommon in persons who have recently received immunoglobulin. Available studies with the hepatitis A vaccines suggest a protective efficacy of greater than 95%. A relapsing form of hepatitis A has been described, though fever has not been a prominent finding.[198,199] Hepatitis B assumes a more important role in persons with prolonged stays in developing areas and those who have close contact, including sexual contact, with local residents, receive injections, or have other parenteral exposures.[200]

Among American troops in Korea (1983 to 1985) hospitalized with acute hepatitis, 75% had hepatitis B and 25% had hepatitis A. Immunoglobulin was used, but hepatitis B vaccine was not available at the time the study was done. Serologic studies suggested that 6% of American troops stationed in Korea for 4 to 12 months became infected with hepatitis B. Among those with acute hepatitis B, 83% gave a history of Korean sexual partners.[130]

Hepatitis D virus (HDV) infection, which requires a helper function from hepatitis B virus (HBV), is a risk for persons already infected with HBV or who become coinfected with HBV and HDV. Hepatitis D can be expressed in the absence of detectable hepatitis B surface antigen (HBsAg).[201] Acute infection can be confused with yellow fever in tropical regions where both can occur. HDV has been a cause of severe and frequently fulminant hepatitis in outbreaks in South America (Amazon Basin).[202] Other geographic areas reported to have a high incidence of infection include parts of Africa, the Middle East, and islands of the South Pacific.[203] Rates of hepatitis D infection in HBsAg carriers range from 30% to 90% in these areas. In Europe, high rates of infection have been reported primarily in the Mediterranean basin, the Balkan peninsula, and in the European part of the former Soviet Union. In North America, Australia, and other parts of Europe, hepatitis D is largely a problem in intravenous drug users.

Travelers occasionally acquire hepatitis E.[204–206] Outbreaks have occurred in many areas, including Mexico, Asia,[204–207] and Africa. The manifestations of HEV are similar to those of HAV except in pregnant women, who are at substantial risk of developing severe or fulminant hepatitis with HEV.

Of 328 North American missionaries, 78% of whom served in sub-Saharan Africa, 5.8% seroconverted showing evidence of infection with hepatitis A, 8.5% with hepatitis B, 0.6% with hepatitis C, and 0% with hepatitis E viruses. The study period was between 1967 and 1984. Their average period of service was 7.3 years.[208]

In the evaluation of patients with fever and marked abnormalities of liver function, treatable infections such as leptospirosis, Q fever, brucellosis, and rickettsial diseases should be considered. Many viral infections, including yellow fever, cause prominent hepatic dysfunction.

Fever and Rash

Skin findings are visible clues that may help suggest or exclude specific diagnoses[209–211] (see also Chapter 126). The distribution of a rash, the nature of the lesions, the time of onset relative to other symptoms, and its evolution over time may be helpful pieces of information. The astute clinician will repeat careful examinations of the skin when a patient has persistent fever of uncertain cause. Rashes are not a clinical feature of malaria; thus, the presence of a rash excludes malaria as the cause of fever unless the patient has a rash for another reason. A careful history of drugs, including over-the-counter agents, is essential in any patient with a rash. Skin lesions secondary to insect bites, hypersensitivity reactions to topical agents, and dermatitis related to water-associated infestations may occur in patients with an acute systemic infection causing fever. The presence of skin lesions from an unrelated process can sometimes misdirect the initial evaluation to focus only on infections that cause skin lesions.

Petechial lesions and hemorrhagic findings herald life-threatening diseases and should prompt a search for one of the hemorrhagic fevers (see previous discussion). Initial skin lesions in these infections may not be hemorrhagic. In the series of patients with African tick-bite fever described by Raoult and coworkers, 4% of patients with rash had purpuric lesions.[114] A local skin lesion may reflect the portal of entry of the pathogen, for example, tache noire in rickettsial infection, erythema migrans, cutaneous diphtheria, the eschar of anthrax, chagoma in American trypanosomiasis (Chagas' disease), and the chancre in African trypanosomiasis.[212] Diffuse rashes are seen in many bacterial (including rickettsial) and viral infections. Few are sufficiently distinctive to allow a definitive diagnosis on the basis of the skin findings alone. Characteristic skin lesions, such as those described in many rickettsial infections and the rose spots of typhoid fever, may appear late or not at all.[213] Their absence should not lead the clinician to reject the diagnosis if findings are otherwise typical. Rashes that mimic the diffuse erythema of staphylococcal and streptococcal toxic shock syndrome have been reported in other infections, such as dengue fever and ehrlichiosis. Rubella and measles viruses remain endemic in many countries, and these infections can be acquired during travel.[214]

Among the more common infections causing high fevers after tropical exposures, dengue produces a rash in 30% to 50% of cases,[215,216] typhoid fever is associated with rose spots (though they may be evanescent) in 30% to 50%, and the rashes of rickettsial infections vary with the infecting rickettsial species. Ross River fever, also known as epidemic polyarthritis and found in South Pacific islands and Australia, is associated with a maculopapular rash in 40% to 78% of cases.[217,219] Although dengue has become increasingly recognized as a common infection in travelers, all that resembles dengue is not dengue. During a 1984 dengue outbreak in Mexico, Bustos and colleagues[220] found that 10% of patients with the clinical diagnosis of dengue had serologic evidence of acute rubella infection. Rickettsial infections can also mimic dengue fever. During a 1993 study of dengue fever in Mexico, 50 patients with clinical findings suggestive of dengue fever but negative serologic tests for dengue infection underwent further study. Twenty (40%) had IgM antibodies reactive with spotted fever group rickettsiosis.[221] Other treatable infections that can cause skin lesions include leptospirosis, relapsing fever, rat-bite fever, syphilis, Q fever, psittacosis, bartonellosis,[222] brucellosis,[223] and tularemia.

Vesicular and vesiculopustular rashes that can resemble varicella are seen in rickettsial infections[224,225] including rickettsialpox.[226] Among 55 patients with African tick-bite fever with rash (46% of the total cases), lesions were maculopapular in 51%, vesicular in 45%, and purpuric in 4%.[114] A number of viral infections, some widespread (e.g., parvovirus, enteroviruses) and others focal (e.g., monkeypox, Ockelbo, Sinbis viruses), can cause vesicular rashes. In one study, of 29 travelers who had swum in freshwater pools in the Dogon area of Mali, West Africa, 28 became infected with schistosomiasis. Of those, 10 (36%) had cercarial dermatitis and 15 (54%) later developed Katayama fever.[51]

Erythema nodosum and other skin lesions may be present in acute coccidioidomycosis and histoplasmosis.[185] Urticarial skin lesions in the person with fever in addition to hypersensitivity reactions related to drugs should bring to mind early hepatitis B and several helminthic infections (e.g., acute schistosomal infection or Katayama syndrome, fascioliasis, trichinosis, loiasis, and others). Fever is not a prominent finding in many helminthic infections, but of 20 patients with acute fascioliasis diagnosed at a university hospital in Spain, 12 (60%) had fever and 4 (20%) had urticaria. Although patients with fascioliasis can have undifferentiated fever, the presence of abdominal or right upper quadrant pain and eosinophilia are findings that can suggest this infection.[227] Vasculitic skin manifestations are associated with a variety of infections, collagen vascular diseases, and antimicrobial drugs.[228]

Fever and Lymphadenopathy

The presence and location of any enlarged lymph nodes should be noted on initial and follow-up examinations. Localized lymphadenopathy frequently appears adjacent to the entry of a pathogen. Generalized lymphadenopathy more often suggests systemic infection though it does not necessarily indicate infection of lymphoid tissue. Prominent local enlargement of nodes in tularemia, leishmaniasis, plague, cat-scratch disease (*Bartonella*), syphilis, primary herpes simplex, lymphogranuloma venereum (LGV), and some rickettsial infections may suggest a nearby portal of entry through the skin or genital tract. Generalized lymphadenopathy is found in many viral infections (including infectious mononucleosis and acute HIV infection), rickettsial infections,[229] leptospirosis, brucellosis, and relapsing fever, among others. Of 22 patients with rickettsiosis imported to Germany, lymphadenopathy was found in 14 (64%); an eschar was noted in 55% of patients with *Rickettsia conorii* infection and in one patient with scrub typhus.[230]

Lymphadenopathy can be found in several protozoan infections—trypanosomiasis (both African and American), leishmaniasis, and toxoplasmosis—but not malaria. Acute lymphangitis, lymphadenitis, orchitis, and epididymitis are characteristic features of filariasis.[47] These episodes frequently are recurrent. Local lymphadenopathy can precede the development of skin lesions in *Leishmania braziliensis* infections.

Persistent and Relapsing Fevers

Persisting and recurring fevers present a clinical challenge. Reviews since 1961 of persons in the United States with fevers of unknown origin (typically defined as fevers lasting 3 weeks or longer), excluding persons with HIV infection or other immunocompromising conditions, have found infections in 30% to 36%, neoplasms in 10% to 31%, collagen-vascular diseases in 9% to 16%, and miscellaneous causes in 18% to 25%.[231–234] In these series, 7% to 12% remained undiagnosed. An analysis of causes of fever of undetermined origin in 129 patients hospitalized in Cairo, Egypt, in 1971 to 1973 found that infections accounted for the majority (60%) of the fevers and neoplasms for only 14%. In that setting, the most commonly diagnosed infections were enteric fevers (salmonellosis), tuberculosis, pyelonephritis, sepsis, endocarditis, brucellosis, visceral leishmaniasis, and amebic hepatitis.[235] A 1990 Egyptian study of 133 patients with undiagnosed fever lasting at least 3 weeks again found infectious diseases in the majority (56%).[236]

Among 43 pediatric patients (age 1 to 14 years) in Egypt with fever lasting at least 3 weeks, 30 (69.7%) had parasitic infections. Schistosomiasis (23.3%), visceral leishmaniasis (16.3%), toxoplasmosis (11.6%), and malaria (4.7) were the most commonly diagnosed parasitic infections. In addition, more than 10% of patients had a parasitic infection in association with another infection or disease. The most commonly identified bacterial infections were typhoid fever (11.6%), tuberculosis (7.0%), and urinary tract infection (4.7%).[237]

Viral infections occupy a less important role in chronic than in acute fevers. Perhaps the most common viral cause of prolonged fever is CMV infection.[238] EBV and HIV can also cause prolonged fever, often associated with atypical lymphocytosis. Among 41 patients with acute illness associated with HIV seroconversion, the most common symptoms were fever, sore throat, fatigue, weight loss, and myalgia. The median duration of symptoms was 14 days though symptoms persisted 4 weeks or longer in 32%.[129] Physical findings in patients with acute HIV infection often include rash (70%) and lymphadenopathy (77%).[239] In the evaluation of a person with prolonged fever, it is important to determine the HIV status, since the range of infections and the probabilities of each will be altered if the person is HIV infected.

Causes of chronic or persistent fevers include protozoa, e.g., malaria, amebic liver abscess, trypanosomiasis (American and African), and visceral leishmaniasis; chronic bacterial infections such as brucellosis,[240] tuberculosis, bartonellosis, and melioidosis; fungal infections, such as histoplasmosis, coccidioidomycosis, and paracoccidioidomycosis;[241] and a few helminthic infections, such as visceral larva migrans, fascioliasis, and schistosomiasis.

Visceral leishmaniasis is an important cause of chronic fevers that can be acquired in some temperate as well as tropical areas of the world.[242–244] For example, of 89 patients with visceral leishmaniasis in France in 1986–1987, 70 (79%) had acquired the infection in France. Imported cases came primarily from other Mediterranean countries.[242] In recent years visceral leishmaniasis has emerged as an important opportunistic infection in persons with acquired immunodeficiency syndrome (AIDS) living in southern France, Spain, and Italy.

Melioidosis is an infection that can have an acute and fulminant, subacute, or chronic course and can reactivate years after the initial exposure. Manifestations are protean. Infection can involve lung, skin, and soft tissues and any part of the body via bacteremic spread. Pulmonary changes, including cavitation, can mimic tuberculosis.[245,246] In a series of 602 patients seen in one hospital in Thailand over a 5-year period, in-hospital mortality was 42%. Among 118 adult patients with long-term follow-up, 23% had culture-proven relapses, occurring 1 to 290 weeks after discharge (median, 21 weeks).[247] The adequacy of initial antimicrobial treatment influenced the probability of relapse. Recrudescent infection has been reported as long as 26 years after initial infection.[248]

Ehrlichiosis is another potentially treatable cause of prolonged fever. In a series of 41 cases of human ehrlichiosis identified between 1989 and 1993, six patients manifested protracted fever as the principal finding.[249] The reported duration of fevers ranged from 17 to 51 days.

Chronic or recurrent fevers can be the result of uncommon complications of an infection, sometimes related to hematogenous seeding of tissues, for example, Q fever endocarditis, brucella osteomyelitis or endocarditis, and splenic or liver abscesses secondary to melioidosis.[250] In a prospective study of 530 patients with brucellosis in Spain followed for at least a year after treatment, 86 patients relapsed (97 relapse episodes). The mean interval between completion of therapy to relapse was 69.1 days (range, 7 to 350 days). Among recognized relapses, 95% occurred within 6 months of the end of therapy.[251] Less effective initial therapy appeared to be an important risk factor for relapse.

Relapsing fevers are commonly seen with relapsing fever due to *Borrelia*[252–256] and with malaria. They can also occur with cholangitis (which can be associated with parasites as well as with stones and other biliary disease), chronic meningococcemia,[257] rat-bite fever (*Streptobacillus moniliformis*), brucellosis, filariasis, infective endocarditis, visceral leishmaniasis, trypanosomiasis, Hodgkin's disease, Whipple's disease,[196] and many other diseases.[258,259] Pyomyositis can cause undifferentiated fever in its early stages. It is usually seen in persons who have lived in tropical areas.

The fever that accompanies acute schistosomiasis (Katayama fever) and fascioliasis[227] can persist for weeks. In an outbreak of schistosomiasis among travelers, 15 of 29 who were infected developed Katayama syndrome with typical symptoms being fever, drenching sweats, myalgia, and prostration. The median duration of symptoms was 12 days with a range of 4 to 46 days.[51] Visceral larva migrans[260] can cause prolonged or intermittent fevers. The associated findings of leukocytosis, eosinophilia, and enlarged liver suggest the diagnosis.

Box 124-6 lists some of the more common causes of persisting and intermittent or relapsing fevers. The timing of onset of symptoms relative to exposures can be important in choosing the infection for greatest attention.

Box 124-6 Persistent and Relapsing Fevers*

Bacterial
Bartonellosis
Brucellosis
Ehrlichiosis
Endocarditis (multiple causes)
Leptospirosis
Lyme disease
Melioidosis
Q fever
Relapsing fever
Rickettsial infections (several)
Syphilis
Tuberculosis and nontuberculous mycobacteriosis
Tularemia
Typhoid fever

Fungal
Blastomycosis
Coccidioidomycosis
Cryptococcosis
Histoplasmosis
Paracoccidioidomycosis
Penicilliosis (*Penicillium marneffei*)

Protozoan
Amebic liver abscess
Babesiosis
Leishmaniasis (visceral)
Malaria
Toxoplasmosis
Trypanosomiasis

Viral
Cytomegalovirus infection
Human immunodeficiency virus infection

Helminthic
Angiostrongyliasis due to *Angiostrongylus costaricensis*
Fascioliasis
Filariasis
Clonorchiasis
Gnathostomiasis
Loiasis
Opisthorchiasis
Paragonimiasis
Schistosomiasis
Toxocariasis
Trichinellosis

*List includes infections that may cause fevers with duration exceeding 3 weeks. Infections unrelated to tropical exposures (e.g., endocarditis, cholangitis, Hodgkin's disease, others) also can be associated with chronic and relapsing fevers.

Fevers and Remote Residence in Tropical Areas

Some infections can become clinically manifest years or decades after a person has left the place of acquisition. Late manifestations also may result from chronic sequelae of an earlier infection, even if active infection no longer is present. Persons with long residence in tropical areas are more likely to have acquired infections with late sequelae (Box 124-7). Some infections may require repeated exposure to produce symptomatic infection. The mechanisms by which remotely acquired infections can cause disease are several. Latent infection may reactivate, causing fevers and focal or systemic symptoms. Examples include tuberculosis, histoplasmosis, melioidosis, and leishmaniasis. Low-grade, persistent infections may expand (recrudesce), causing symptoms leading to diagnosis (e.g., malaria, Brill-Zinsser disease). The balance between host and microbe may tip in favor of the microbe in persons whose immunity has been altered by disease, drugs, or age. *Strongyloides* larvae may disseminate widely outside their usual gastrointestinal habitat, for example, in persons with cell-mediated immunosuppression, particularly those taking corticosteroids or coinfected with HTLV-1.

Salmonella enterica serotype typhi may be carried in the biliary tree and remain inapparent unless mechanical (e.g., biliary obstruction) or other factors alter the local milieu. Worms with long life spans may breach a tissue barrier or cause chronic inflammatory changes leading to acute symptoms. Migration of ascaris can provoke acute pancreatitis or cause biliary obstruction.

Remote infection may cause scarring, obstruction, or alteration in structure that may predispose to superimposed infections or affect function. Scarring associated with renal tuberculosis can increase the risk of urinary tract infection with *E. coli* and other uropathogens, even if tuberculosis is inactive or has been treated and cured. Scarring of the urinary tract secondary to *Schistosoma haematobium* can be associated with bacterial infections and an increased risk of bladder cancer. Late sequelae of schistosomiasis may include portal and

Box 124-7 Sequelae of Infections Acquired More Than 10 Years Earlier: Mechanisms and Examples

Reactivation of Latent Infection or Recrudescence of Inapparent Infection

Brill-Zinsser disease (*Rickettsia prowazekii*)
CNS Chagas' disease
Coccidioidomycosis
Histoplasmosis
Leishmaniasis
Malaria (*Plasmodium malariae)*
Melioidosis
Paracoccidioidomycosis
Strongyloidiasis
Toxoplasmosis
Tuberculosis

Persistent Infection and Recurrent Symptoms or Progressive Disease

Chagas' disease
Filariasis
Leprosy
Loiasis
Onchocerciasis
Syphilis

Mechanical Effects; Loss of Normal Function; Scarring, Fibrosis, Tissue Destruction

Cysticercosis
Echinococcal cysts
Liver flukes
Onchocerciasis (blindness)
Schistosomiasis
Tuberculosis (e.g., cavities and bronchiectasis in lungs; scarring and obstruction in urinary tract; adrenal insufficiency)

Malignancy*

Bladder cancer (*Schistosoma haematobium*)
Epstein-Barr virus
Hepatitis B and hepatitis C viruses (hepatocellular carcinoma)
Human immunodeficiency virus
Human T-cell lymphotropic virus type-I
Liver flukes

Allergic, Hypersensitivity Reactions

Rupture of echinococcal cyst

*Papillomaviruses are also associated with cancers, but fever is not a feature of these infections.

pulmonary hypertension and polyps and fistulas of the bowel. Echinococcal cysts can impinge on the biliary tree, causing acute obstructive symptoms, or erode into the biliary tree and cause symptoms of acute cholangitis. Rupture of an echinococcal cyst can cause acute allergic symptoms, even anaphylaxis. Seizures can occur in patients with cysticercosis, even if parasites are no longer viable. Late complications of Chagas' disease typically do not include fever unless progression of infection occurs (e.g., in persons with AIDS or immunocompromised transplant patients).[261–263]

Clinical findings of hepatocellular malignancy related to remotely acquired, persistent infection with hepatitis B or hepatitis C virus may include fever secondary to tissue necrosis and the effects of the tumor.

Processes Other Than Infection Causing Fever After Travel

Travel itself may predispose to problems that cause fever. Already noted is the possibility of fever related to drugs taken for prophylaxis, empirical therapy, or for documented infection. Dependent edema of the lower extremity following prolonged travel may predispose to acute streptococcal cellulitis. Pulmonary emboli after prolonged air flights (dubbed the economy class syndrome because of the immobility imposed by cramped quarters[264]) may be associated with fever.[265]

Noninfectious diseases also cause fevers and should be considered if studies do not document infection.[259,266,267] Biopsy may be necessary to confirm a diagnosis in processes such as inflammatory bowel disease, malignancies, and lymphadenopathy of Kikuchi.[268,269] Hyperthyroidism may present with fever and diarrhea.

Special Patients (HIV-infected, Immunocompromised, Pregnant)

Many infections are more common, are more severe, or have altered clinical expression in persons who are immunocompromised. Opportunistic infections, such as tuberculosis, visceral leishmaniasis,[270] American trypanosomiasis, and histoplasmosis and other fungal infections may reactivate and become clinically apparent long after the infection was acquired. The person may be unaware of the initial event. An evaluation of 50 HIV-infected patients in Spain with unexplained fever lasting at least 4 weeks found the most frequent diagnoses were tuberculosis (42%), visceral leishmaniasis (14%), and disseminated *Mycobacterium avium* complex (14%).[271] Both host factors and exposure influence the relative proportions of various infections in different areas. Disseminated infection with the fungus *Penicillium marneffei* is occasionally seen in travelers, typically persons immunocompromised by HIV infection or other disease.[272] In its endemic area in Thailand and Southeast Asia it is an important opportunistic pathogen.[273] Clinical findings can be nonspecific and include fever, cough, malaise, and hepatosplenomegaly. Skin lesions may be present.[273]

It is important to know during the evaluation whether a woman patient is pregnant. The cause of fever may threaten the pregnancy, diagnostic tests and therapies may be harmful to the fetus, some infections can be transmitted transplacentally, and others infection, such as malaria and hepatitis E, are more severe in pregnant than in nonpregnant women.

EVALUATION OF THE PATIENT WITH FEVER

Patients with fever and recent tropical exposures always deserve careful evaluation even though similar symptoms might be treated casually in a person without a history of travel. It is helpful to construct a differential diagnosis encompassing potential bacterial, viral, parasitic and fungal pathogens based on initial history, geographic exposures, and clinical findings. Patients with confusion, hypotension, hypoxemia, or hemorrhagic skin rash need immediate attention and care. A more leisurely pace may be appropriate in patients with subacute or chronic fevers. Any patient with a potential exposure to malaria who is febrile or gives a history of fevers or chills must

Box 124-8 Approach to Patient with Fever and History of Tropical Exposure

Initial Evaluation of Acute Fever

- Complete blood count with differential
- Liver enzymes and function tests
- Blood culture—bacterial, viral, fungal (rarely)
- Urinalysis (culture if abnormal)
- Blood smears for malaria
- Other tests
  - Serologic tests (save acute serum)
  - Urinary antigens (e.g., *Legionella* species)
  - Blood smears for *Babesia, Borrelia* causing relapsing fever
  - Bone marrow aspiration/biopsy: pathology and culture

Tests to Consider for Focal Symptoms and Findings

- Cough: chest film; sputum Gram's stain, acid-fast stain, stains for fungi; cultures for bacteria, mycobacterial species, fungi; wet preparation for ova (Paragonimus species) or larvae (hyperinfection with Strongyloides stercoralis); bronchoscopy
- Diarrhea: examination for fecal leukocytes (lactoferrin where available); blood (stool guaiac); toxin and culture for *Clostridium difficile;* ova and parasites, stool cultures; fecal antigens; endoscopy
- Sore throat: rapid streptococcal antigen test, culture, infectious mononucleosis absorption test (Monospot) (in appropriate clinical setting)
- Skin lesions: aspirate, scrapings, biopsy, Gram's stain, acid-fast stain, fungal stain, Wright-Giemsa stain (leishmania); culture for bacteria, fungi, mycobacteria, leishmania
- Lymphadenopathy: aspirate or biopsy, acid-fast stain, fungal stain, Wright-Giemsa stain (trypanosomes); culture
- Genital lesions or symptoms: pelvic examination, dark-field examination of ulcers, cultures for *Neisseria gonorrhoeae* and *Chlamydia trachomatis,* wet preparation for white blood cells, *Trichomonas vaginalis, Candida albicans,* and clue cells (bacterial vaginosis)
- CNS: CT scan, MRI, lumbar puncture with opening pressure and examination of CSF for cells, protein, glucose, bacterial antigens; cultures for bacteria, *Mycobacterium tuberculosis,* fungi, viruses; India ink for *Cryptococcus neoformans* and cryptococcal antigen; VDRL, PCR for specific antigens; rarely, brain biopsy
- Abdominal pain: liver enzymes, amylase, stool examination (see above), abdominal radiographic series, CT scan, MRI
- Arthritis: aspirate—examine fluid for cells, protein, crystals; stains and cultures for bacteria, fungi, *Mycobacterium* species.
- Cardiac findings: echocardiogram (transesophageal or transthoracic), blood cultures (at least three sets), serology for Q-fever and brucellosis

be evaluated for malaria.[274–277] In general, most infections with the potential for rapid progression and fulminant course (e.g., falciparum malaria, hemorrhagic fevers, meningococcemia, plague, rickettsial infections) become manifest within a month of exposure. In thinking about the causes of fever in a person with diverse geographic exposures, one should always think first about possible diagnoses had the person not traveled, and then expand the differential diagnosis to include infections that may be related to exposures during travel. Omitting the first step can lead to pursuit of obscure or exotic diseases when the patient has a common readily treatable infection, such as acute pyelonephritis or streptococcal pharyngitis.

Initial studies will generally include a complete blood count (CBC) with a differential leukocyte and platelet estimate, thick and thin malaria smears, blood cultures, urinalysis, and liver function tests. Serum should be saved early in the course in the event serologic studies are indicated. Chest radiographs should be obtained in patients with pulmonary symptoms or signs and in persons with persistent, unexplained fever. Legionnaires' disease, for example, can cause undifferentiated fever in the absence of cough. Serologic studies for HIV infection should be requested in persons with persistent fevers and those with possible exposures during travel. Studies that may yield useful information if initial studies are unrevealing include repeated malaria smears, blood cultures, serial CBCs, differentials, and liver function testing. Repeated physical examinations may yield new information with the development of new skin findings, lymphadenopathy, or a tender liver or spleen. Although many of these findings may not give the diagnosis, they may help refine the list of considerations, allowing a more focused and efficient path to the diagnosis. Occasionally a patient will have two unrelated infections, both requiring specific interventions.[278,279] Box 124-8 outlines an approach to patients with fever and a history of tropical exposures.

SOURCES OF ASSISTANCE

Electronic communication networks bring resources to clinicians throughout the world and provide linkages to colleagues who can provide information unavailable in textbooks. Physicians who regularly care for persons who have lived or traveled in other parts of the world need access to several kinds of information: current data about the epidemiology of diseases in specific geographic regions, assistance with the diagnosis of rare diseases, assistance with public health support, sources of and information about rarely used drugs, and names of drugs and translations of drug names that patients may have received in other parts of the world. Some of this information can be obtained through regular communications from the CDC and World Health Organization (WHO) and through electronic networks such as ProMED[26] and those available to members of the American Society of Tropical Medicine and Hygiene and the International Society of Travel Medicine.

226. Kass EM, Szaniawski WK, Levy H, et al: Rickettsialpox in a New York City hospital, 1980 to 1989. N Engl J Med 331:1612, 1994.
227. Arjona R, Riancho JA, Aguado JM, et al: Fascioliasis in developed countries: a review of classic and aberrant forms of the disease. Medicine (Baltimore) 74:13, 1995.
228. Somer T, Finegold SM: Vasculitides associated with infections, immunizations, and antimicrobial drugs. Clin Infect Dis 20:1010, 1995.
229. Marschang A, Nothdurft HD, Kumlien S, et al: Imported rickettsioses in German travelers. Infection 23:94, 1995.
230. Berman KS, Kundin WD: Scrub typhus in South Vietnam: a study of 87 cases. Ann Intern Med 79:26, 1973.
231. Petersdorf RB, Beeson PB: Fever of unexplained origin: a report on 100 cases. Medicine (Baltimore) 40:1, 1961.
232. Jacoby GA, Swartz NM: Fever of unknown origin. N Engl J Med 289:1407, 1973.
233. Larson EB, Featherstone HJ, Petersdorf RG: Fever of undetermined origin: Diagnosis and follow-up of 105 cases, 1970–1980. Medicine (Baltimore) 61:269, 1982.
234. Kazanjian PH: Fever of unknown origin: review of 86 patients treated in community hospitals. Clin Infect Dis 15:968, 1992.
235. Hassan A, Farid Z: Fever of unknown origin in Cairo. N Engl J Med 290:807, 1974.
236. Farid Z, Kilpatrick ME, Kamal M: Cryptogenic tuberculosis—1990, Cairo, Egypt. J Trop Med 2:31, 1993.
237. Aboul-Hassan S, El-Shazly AM, Farag MK, et al: Epidemiological, clinical and laboratory studies on parasitic infections as a cause of fever of undetermined origin in Dakahlia Governorate, Egypt. J Egypt Soc Parasitol 27:47, 1997.
238. Schmitz H, Kern P, Dietrich M: High risk of cytomegalovirus mononucleosis in adult Europeans visiting tropical areas. Lancet 2:503, 1985.
239. Clark SJ, Saag MS, Decker WD, et al: High titers of cytopathic virus in plasma of patients with symptomatic primary HIV-1 infection. N Engl J Med 324:954, 1991.
240. Arnow PM, Smaron M, Ormista V: Brucellosis in a group of travelers to Spain. JAMA 251:505, 1984.
241. Manns BJ, Baylis BW, Urbanski SJ, et al: Paracoccidioidomycosis: case report and review. Clin Infect Dis 23:1026, 1996.
242. Geraci JE, Wilson WR, Thompson JH: Visceral leishmaniasis (kala-azar) as a cause of fever of unknown origin. Mayo Clin Proc 55:455, 1980.
243. Maru M: Clinical and laboratory features and treatment of visceral leishmaniasis in hospitalized patients in northwestern Ethiopia. Am J Trop Med Hyg 28:15, 1979.
244. Jeannel D, Tuppin P, Brucker G, et al: Imported and autochthonous kala-azar in France. BMJ 303:336, 1991.
245. Dhiensiri T, Puapairoj S, Susaengrat W: Pulmonary melioidosis: clinical-radiologic correlation in 183 cases in northeastern Thailand. Radiology 166:711, 1988.
245. Ip M, Osterberg LG, Chau PY, et al: Pulmonary melioidosis. Chest 108:1240, 1995.
247. Chaowagul W, Suputtamongkol Y, Dance DAB, et al: Relapse in melioidosis: incidence and risk factors. J Infect Dis 168:1181, 1993.
248. Mays EE, Ricketts EA: Melioidosis: recrudescence associated with bronchogenic carcinoma twenty-six years following initial geographic exposure. Chest 68:261, 1975.
249. Roland WE, McDonald G, Caldwell CW, et al: Ehrlichiosis—a cause of prolonged fever. Clin Infect Dis 20:821, 1995.
250. Vatcharapreechasakul T, Suputtamongkol Y, Dance DAB, et al: *Pseudomonas pseudomallei* liver abscesses: a clinical, laboratory, and ultrasonographic study. Clin Infect Dis 14:412, 1992.
251. Ariza J, Curredoira J, Pallares R, et al: Characteristics of and risk factors for relapse of brucellosis in humans. Clin Infect Dis 20:1241, 1995.
252. Barbour AG: Antigenic variation in relapsing fever *Borrelia* species. Annu Rev Microbiol 44:155, 1990.
253. Barclay AJ, Coulter JB: Tick-borne relapsing fever in central Tanzania. Trans R Soc Trop Med Hyg 84:852, 1990.
254. Colebunders R, De Serrano P, Van Comple A, et al: Imported relapsing fever in European tourists. Scand J Infect Dis 25:533, 1993.
255. Flanigan TP, Schwan TG, Armstrong C, et al: Relapsing fever in the US Virgin Islands: a previously unrecognized focus of infection. J Infect Dis 163:1391, 1991.
256. Southern PM Jr, Sanford JP: Relapsing fever: a clinical and microbiological review. Medicine (Baltimore) 48:129, 1969.
257. Benoit FL: Chronic meningococcemia: case report and review of the literature. Am J Med 35:103, 1963.
258. Knockaert DC, Vaneste LJ, Bobbaers JH: Recurrent or episodic fever of unknown origin: review of 45 cases and review of the literature. Medicine (Baltimore) 72:184, 1993.
259. Drenth J, Haagsma C, Van der Meer J: Hyperimmunoglobulinemia D and periodic fever syndrome: the clinical spectrum of a series of 50 patients. Medicine (Baltimore) 73:133, 1994.
260. Schantz PM, Glickman LT: *Toxocara* visceral larva migrans. 298:436, 1978.
261. Kirchhoff LV, Neva FA: Chagas' disease in Latin American immigrants. JAMA 254:3058, 1985.
262. Rocha A, De Meneses ACO, Da Silva AM, et al: Pathology of patients with Chagas' disease and acquired immunodeficiency syndrome. Am J Trop Med Hyg 50:261, 1994.
263. Tanowitz HB, Kirchhoff LV, Simon D, et al: Chagas' disease. Clin Microbiol Rev 5:400, 1992.
264. Cruickshank JM, Gorlin R, Jennett B: Air travel and thrombotic episodes: the economy class syndrome. Lancet 2:497, 1988.
265. Murray HG, Ellis GC, Blumenthal DS, et al: Fever and pulmonary thromboembolism. Am J Med 67:232, 1979.
266. Carsons SE: Fever in rheumatic and autoimmune disease. Infect Dis Clin North Am 10:67, 1996.
267. Simon HB, Daniels GH: Hormonal hyperthermia: endocrinologic causes of fever. Am J Med 66:257, 1979.
268. Sweet RD: An acute febrile neutrophilic dermatosis. Br J Dermatol 76:349, 1964.
269. Pearl D, Strauchen JA: Kikuchi's disease as a cause of fever of unknown origin. N Engl J Med 320:1147, 1989.
270. Cummins D, Amin S, Halil O, et al: Visceral leishmaniasis after cardiac surgery. Arch Dis Child 73:235, 1995.
271. Miralles P, Moreno S, Perez-Tascon M, et al: Fever of uncertain origin in patients infected with the human immunodeficiency virus. Clin Infect Dis 20:872, 1995.
272. Duong TA: Infection due to *Penicillium marneffei*, an emerging pathogen: review of 155 reported cases. Clin Infect Dis 23:125, 1996.
273. Kok I, Veenstra J, Rietra PF, et al: Disseminated *Penicillium marneffei* infection as an imported disease in HIV-1 infected patients: description of two cases and a review of the literature. Neth J Med 44:18, 1994.
274. Greenwood B: Fever and malaria. Lancet 348:280, 1996.
275. Humar A, Keystone J: Evaluating fever in travelers returning from tropical countries. BMJ 312:953, 1996.
276. Jelinek T, Nothdurft H-D, Loscher T: Malaria in nonimmune travelers: a synopsis of history, symptoms, and treatment in 160 patients. J Travel Med 1:199, 1994.
277. Svenson JE, Gyorkos TW, MacLean JD: Diagnosis of malaria in the febrile traveler. Am J Trop Med Hyg 53:518, 1995.
278. Gopinath R, Keystone JS, Kain KC: Concurrent falciparum malaria and salmonella bacteremia in travelers: report of two cases. Clin Infect Dis 20:706, 1995.
279. Shaket Y, Maier MK, Samra P: Relapsing fever and salmonella bacteremia simultaneously affecting a healthy young man. J Infect 13:308, 1986.

125

Eosinophilia

MARY E. WILSON
PETER F. WELLER

INTRODUCTION

Eosinophilia develops as an immunologically mediated response in association with diverse processes, including allergic, neoplastic, and infectious diseases (Box 125-1). Eosinophilia is a hematologic marker that warrants attention and serves as a clue to help direct a diagnostic workup. Although many diseases are associated with eosinophilia, the presence of eosinophilia in a person with tropical exposures suggests the possibility of specific parasitic infections. Eosinophilia is notably common in association with multicellular, helminthic parasites, especially those in tissues.[1] Before embarking on an exhaustive search for parasitic infections in a patient with eosinophilia, however, it is prudent to consider common noninfectious causes of eosinophilia, such as allergic diseases and drug-induced hypersensitivity reactions.[2]

Eosinophilia in parasitic infections is the result of dynamic interactions that are influenced by host factors, the stage of parasite development, the location of the parasite within the human host, and the parasite burden, among other factors. Eosinophilia may wax and wane. Parasites often associated with eosinophilia may not provoke an identified eosinophilic response in all patients or at all times. Parasites may elicit a localized eosinophilic tissue response that is not reflected by an increase in peripheral blood eosinophil numbers. This chapter describes the immunobiology of the eosinophil, the causes of eosinophilia with special attention to parasitic infections, and the evaluation of the patient with eosinophilia.

OVERVIEW

Most unicellular pathogens do not provoke an eosinophilic response.[1,2] In contrast, presentation of antigenic material from multicellular parasites, notably helminths, is a common and potent stimulus to eosinophilia (Box 125-2). Relative to most bacterial and viral pathogens, helminths are large and have a long life span, often measured in years or even decades.[1] Unlike viral and bacterial pathogens that multiply in human hosts, most helminths cannot undergo their complete reproductive cycles in humans; hence the numbers of adults are limited by the number of eggs or larval forms acquired by the human. Prolonged or repeated exposures may be required for a human to acquire sufficient parasites to cause symptomatic infection. Many helminthic infections cause few or no symptoms or only intermittent findings. For instance, of 303 persons who had serologic evidence of current or past schistosome infection after visiting or living in Malawi, 62% had no symptoms.[3] In addition, because of the lengthy developmental period and longevity of helminthic parasites, symptoms may begin months or years after exposures in endemic regions. For example, in 6 of 20 Peace Corps workers who developed loiasis during a 2-year stay in Gabon, only one had demonstrable disease within the first year.[4] Thus, the time period between possibly relevant exposures and the onset of clinical or other evidence of infection is much longer than usually considered in obtaining a medical history for most clinical evaluations.

Most protozoan infections are not associated with eosinophilia. Exceptions are *Isospora belli*[5] and possibly *Dientamoeba fragilis*,[6] which have been reported to be associated

Box 125-1 Eosinophil-associated Diseases and Disorders

"Allergic" Diseases

Atopic and related diseases
Medication-related eosinophilias

Infectious Diseases

Parasitic infections, mostly with helminths
Specific fungal infections
Other infections—infrequent

Hematologic and Neoplastic Disorders

Hypereosinophilic syndrome
Leukemia, variants of the M-4 phenotype of acute myelomonocytic leukemia
Lymphomas, especially nodular sclerosing Hodgkin's; some T- and B-cell lymphomas
Tumor-associated: on occasion with large cell non-keratinizing cervical tumors, large cell undifferentiated lung carcinomas, squamous carcinomas (vagina, penis, skin, nasopharynx), adenocarcinomas (stomach, large bowel, uterine body), and transitional bladder cell carcinoma
Mastocytosis

Diseases with Specific Organ Involvement

Skin and subcutaneous diseases (e.g., blistering diseases, bullous pemphigoid, pemphigus vulgaris, dermatitis herpetiformis, herpes gestationis, and drug-induced lesions)
Pulmonary diseases (e.g., acute or chronic eosinophilic pneumonia, allergic bronchopulmonary aspergillosis)
Gastrointestinal diseases (e.g., eosinophilic gastroenteritis)
Neurologic diseases (e.g., eosinophilic meningitis)
Rheumatologic diseases (e.g., Churg-Strauss vasculitis)
Cardiac diseases (e.g., endomyocardial fibrosis)
Renal diseases (e.g., drug-induced interstitial nephritis, eosinophilic cystitis, dialysis)

Immunologic Reactions

Specific immunodeficiency diseases (hyper-IgE syndrome, Omenn's syndrome)
Transplant rejection

Endocrine

Hypoadrenalism

Other

Atheroembolic disease
Irritation of serosal surfaces
Inherited

Modified from Weller PF: Eosinophilia and eosinophil-related disorders. In Adkinson NF Jr, Yunginger JW, Busse WW, et al (eds): Allergy: Principles and Practice, 6th ed. St. Louis, Mosby–Year Book, 2003, p 1105.

Box 125-2 Key Concepts: Eosinophils in Parasitic Infections

- Elevation is caused primarily by helminthic parasites that reside in tissues. Most protozoan parasitic infections are not associated with eosinophilia.
- Eosinophils may be prominent during only one stage of parasite development. Migration of parasites within tissues is often associated with high-grade eosinophilia. Chronic parasitic infections in antigenically sequestered sites (e.g., echinococcal cysts) or solely within the gut lumen (e.g., adult *Ascaris* or tapeworms) may not provoke an eosinophilic response. Release of antigenic material when parasites die or when walls protecting parasites are breached may lead to increased eosinophilia.
- Eosinophil levels may wax and wane; many factors unrelated to the helminthic infection influence the level of blood eosinophilia. Acute bacterial, viral, and protozoal (e.g., malaria) infections suppress eosinophilia.
- High-grade eosinophilia and symptoms may be prominent during the prepatent period and before the diagnosis can be confirmed by finding eggs or diagnostic forms of the parasite in tissues. Serologic tests may help in early diagnosis.
- The degree of eosinophilia and other clinical manifestations caused by helminthic infections may differ between long-term residents of endemic regions and short-term visitors, being more prominent in the latter.
- Many infections associated with eosinophilia cause no or intermittent symptoms; first symptoms may develop months or years after exposure. Many helminths are long-lived with life spans that can exceed a decade.
- Multiple infections may be present, especially in long-term residents of tropical areas. Finding intestinal eggs or certain parasites does not confirm that they are the cause of the eosinophilia. In a patient with *Ascaris* eggs and moderate or high-grade eosinophilia, the search for the cause of eosinophilia should continue.
- Absence of eosinophilia does not exclude a parasitic infection typically associated with eosinophilia.

with increases in eosinophils. In some reports of these infections, other causes of eosinophilia had not been excluded. Eosinophilia and acute symptomatic eosinophilic myositis has been found in association with the coccidian parasite *Sarcocystis*.[7,8] In Malaysia, the parasite was found in 21% of routine autopsies when tongues were carefully examined.[9] More studies are needed to define whether or how often *Sarcocystis* causes eosinophilia. In general, however, the finding of eosinophilia in a patient with a protozoan infection should prompt a search for another, principally helminthic, infection or an alternative noninfectious process to explain the eosinophilia.

Only a few bacterial, viral, and fungal infections are associated with eosinophilia (Box 125-3). As noted in the following sections, acute bacterial or viral infections characteristically produce eosinopenia.[10] Likewise, acute protozoan infections, including malaria,[11,12] will suppress eosinophilia, including that caused by helminthic infections, during the intercurrent infection. It is likely that bacterial superinfections that complicate hyperinfection strongyloidiasis contribute to suppression of eosinophilia that might otherwise be an obvious clue to the presence of strongyloidiasis. When eosinophilia is observed in bacterial infections, it is in the resolving phase, as occurs with

Box 125-3 Infections Associated with Eosinophilia

Bacterial

Streptococcal—resolving scarlet fever

Viral

Human immunodeficiency virus (may be associated with skin eruption)

Fungal

Aspergillus—only with allergic bronchopulmonary aspergillosis

Coccidioides immitis—acute and sometimes later disseminated infections

Protozoan

Isospora belli

Dientamoeba fragilis

Helminthic

Many (see Table 125-1)

Infestations

Scabies

Myiasis

scarlet fever, or is attributable to a hypersensitivity reaction to a drug used for treatment. Two fungal diseases are associated with eosinophilia: aspergillosis, in the form of allergic bronchopulmonary aspergillosis,[13] and coccidioidomycosis.[14] Blood eosinophilia, peaking during the second or third week of illness, occurs with primary coccidioidomycosis.[15] Eosinophilia, at times prominent, also may develop with disseminated coccidioidomycosis.[16,17] A few reports note eosinophilia in patients with infestations caused by myiasis[18] and scabies.[19]

PATHOGENESIS

Eosinophils are bone marrow–derived leukocytes. Eosinophilia develops when specific cytokines, granulocyte-macrophage colony–stimulating factor (GM-CSF), interleukin (IL)-3, and IL-5 stimulate enhanced eosinophilopoiesis. Of these three eosinophil growth factor cytokines, IL-5 is principally responsible for increases in eosinophilopoiesis and eosinophilia in helminthic, allergic, and other diseases.[20] In humans, enhanced eosinophilopoiesis within the marrow requires over a week to increase blood eosinophilia. IL-5 also acts more rapidly to increase blood eosinophilia by mobilizing a marginated pool of preformed eosinophils resident within the marrow. IL-5 is a cytokine produced by Th2-like CD4+ T lymphocytes (as well as other cells, including eosinophils); and eosinophilia is frequent with immune responses characterized by Th2-like T-cell activation, including those elicited by helminthic parasite infections and associated with allergic diseases.[21] In both of these, enhanced IgE production is usually present.[21] In other diverse diseases associated with eosinophilia (see Box 125-1), the mechanisms leading to eosinophilia are not yet delineated. GM-CSF, IL-3, and IL-5 also act on mature eosinophils to prolong their survival by antagonizing apoptosis and to enhance their effector functions.

Although Th2-like T-cell responses lead to eosinophilia, it remains uncertain how specific parasitic or allergic diseases characteristically stimulate Th2-type responses. Some findings, such as the capacity of Sephadex beads embolized into the lungs to elicit eosinophilia, suggest that eosinophilia may develop not in response to specific antigens, such as those of helminths, but rather from the immune response to large particulate objects. Nevertheless, it remains possible, but not yet defined, that specific features of helminthic antigens, as well as their particulate presentation, influence the initial antigen presentation process that leads to Th2-like lymphocyte responses and consequent eosinophilia. As noted in the following discussion, eosinophilia is most prominent with helminthic infections when parasites are migrating through or beginning to localize within tissues.

IMMUNOBIOLOGY

Eosinophils are primarily tissue-dwelling leukocytes normally distributed within specific tissues. Eosinophils are several hundred–fold more abundant in tissues than in blood, and eosinophil numbers are greatest in those tissues with a mucosal epithelial interface with the environment, including the respiratory, gastrointestinal, and lower genitourinary tracts. The life span of eosinophils is longer than that of neutrophils. Eosinophils probably survive for weeks within tissues.

In patients with eosinophilia of parasitic and other causes, blood eosinophils often exhibit morphologic and functional alterations consequent to being "activated" in vivo. These changes include increased metabolic activity, diminished density ("hypodense"), enhanced antibody-mediated cytotoxicity, and enhanced leukotriene C_4 formation. Morphologic changes include cytoplasmic vacuolization, alterations in granule numbers and size, and increased lipid body formation, all visible by light microscopy, and losses within specific granules of the matrix or eosinophil major basic protein (MBP)–containing cores, visible only by electron microscopy.[22] This phenotypic alteration can be reproduced in vitro by exposure of eosinophils to the eosinophil growth factor cytokines, GM-CSF, IL-3, and IL-5. While these eosinophil growth factor cytokines contribute to eosinophil "activation," these cytokines alone do not elicit all measures of eosinophil activation. Other cytokines or tissue- or extracellular matrix–derived activating stimuli are likely to be involved in augmenting the functional capabilities of eosinophils.

The immunologic functions of eosinophils remain the subject of intense investigation. In addition to functioning as endstage effector leukocytes, eosinophils likely have additional roles in interacting with lymphocytes and other cells. As effector cells, eosinophils are capable of releasing specific lipid mediators, such as leukotriene C_4, and are a source of a range of granule-stored cytokines. In addition, eosinophils uniquely contain specific, highly positively charged ("cationic") proteins within their cytoplasmic granules. These eosinophil granule cationic proteins include MBP and eosinophil cationic protein (ECP). The release of these granule proteins can damage host tissues. A beneficial effect of these granule proteins is that they can contribute to the killing of helminthic parasites. The extent to which eosinophils are involved in the immune responses to helminthic parasites, and especially their early larval forms, to help kill these parasites in vivo is still not certain.[21,23]

In patients with marked eosinophilia, eosinophils may cause organ damage, most notably to the heart. The damage to the heart, ranging from early necrosis to subsequent endomyocardial thrombosis and fibrosis, is the same with varied eosinophilic conditions. Thus, endomyocardial thrombosis and fibrosis develop with eosinophilia associated with the hypereosinophilic syndromes,[24] carcinomas and lymphomas, and parasitic infections, including trichinellosis, visceral larva migrans, loiasis, or other filarial infections.[25–29] Pathologically, eosinophilic endomyocardial fibrosis, originally described by Löffler,[30] is identical to tropical endomyocardial fibrosis.[31,32] While diverse eosinophilic diseases can cause identical forms of cardiac disease, many patients with sustained eosinophilia never develop cardiac disease. Thus, the pathogenesis of eosinophil-mediated cardiac damage involves both the presence of increased eosinophils and other, as yet ill-defined, stimuli for recruitment or activation of these leukocytes.

HOST FACTORS THAT INFLUENCE EOSINOPHIL RESPONSES

Several evaluations of the upper limits of normal blood eosinophil numbers have been published, and based on these, blood eosinophilia is clearly present when eosinophils are in excess of 450 cells per microliter of blood. Published studies use cutoffs that range from 350 to 500 cells per microliter of blood. Increased percentages, but not absolute numbers, of blood eosinophils (pseudoeosinophilia) due to leukopenia in another white blood cell line can be misleading.

Many host factors and other stimuli influence peripheral blood eosinophil levels (Box 125-4). Blood eosinophil numbers vary diurnally, with levels being highest in the early morning and lowest at about noon. Levels are higher in the neonatal period and decline with age. Eosinophil levels fall during pregnancy; during the stress of delivery they almost disappear from the peripheral circulation.[33] Epinephrine causes a sharp fall in circulating eosinophils, after a transient increase. The β-adrenergic blocker propranolol increases counts by about 30% and can block the effect of epinephrine.[34] Injection of 100 mg hydrocortisone is followed by a decrease in peripheral eosinophils to 35% of control levels within 1 hour, and blood eosinophils are nearly absent 4 hours after the steroid administration.[34,35] Corticosteroids inhibit tissue accumulation of eosinophils, probably by several mechanisms, including promoting eosinophil apoptosis ("programmed cell death").[36] Acute pyogenic infections, including bacterial and viral infections, as noted previously, and other processes causing acute inflammation are associated with a decline in blood eosinophils.[34,35,37] This can transiently erase a peripheral blood eosinophilia. Eosinophils drop during acute malaria, even if previously elevated.[11,12] Depression of eosinophils in malaria persisted beyond the clearance of fever and parasitemia, and was followed by an increase in eosinophils in convalescence.[12] When it is important to know whether a patient has eosinophilia, a blood differential count should be repeated after a patient has recovered from an acute intercurrent infection.

Box 125-4 Factors That Lower Eosinophil Counts

- Acute bacterial and viral infections; acute malaria
- Corticosteroids—endogenous and exogenous
- Acute stress
- Pregnancy (counts especially low during stress of delivery)
- Immunosuppressive states (also less elevation of IgE; sensitivity of serologic tests may be lower)
- Epinephrine (sharp fall after initial transient rise; can be inhibited by β-blockers)

PATTERNS

Characteristics of the eosinophil response that may be useful in assessing more likely causes of eosinophilia include level, duration, pattern (constant vs. intermittent), and associated symptoms. If a person has had tropical exposures, the timing of onset of eosinophilia in relation to those exposures may help in the evaluation. Eosinophilia should be characterized by level, not simply as present or absent. Absolute eosinophil counts of greater than 3000 per microliter are categorized as marked or high grade eosinophilia. Several different patterns of eosinophilia may be seen in relation to parasitic infections. Factors that influence these patterns include the type of parasite, the stage of parasite development, the location within the human host, the integrity of barriers between parasite and host, and the viability of the parasite, as well as many attributes of the host (Table 125-1).[1] In some parasitic infections, eosinophilia is

Table 125-1 Helminthic Infections and Eosinophilia

Parasitic Infection	Main Body Site	Diagnosis
Angiostrongyliasis cantonensis	CNS	Larvae in CSF
Angiostrongyliasis costaricensis	GI	Tissue biopsy (ileum, colon)
Anisakiasis	GI	Parasite via endoscopy or biopsy
Ascariasis	GI, lung (larvae)	Stool examination; sputum examination or BAL for early infection (larvae)
Capillariasis hepatica	Hepatobiliary	Biopsy of liver
Capillariasis philippinensis	GI	Eggs, larvae, adults: stool, duodenal or jejunal aspirate, biopsy
Clonorchiasis	Hepatobiliary	Stool examination, duodenal aspirate; serology
Coenurosis	Many, including CNS	Parasite in tissue
Cysticercosis	Many, including CNS, soft tissues	Tissue examination, serology
Dicrocoeliasis	GI	Eggs in stool, duodenal aspirate, bile
Dirofilariasis	Lung, subcutaneous	Morphology in biopsied tissue
Dracunculiasis	Soft tissues, skin	Morphology of worm
Echinococcosis	Liver, lung, CNS, other	Morphology in tissue or aspirate; serology
Echinostomiasis	GI	Eggs in stool
Enterobiasis	GI, perianal	Eggs or worms in perianal area
Fascioliasis	Hepatobiliary	Eggs in stool, duodenal aspirate
Fasciolopsiasis	GI	Eggs in stool
Filariasis		
Lymphatic: *Wuchereria, Brugia*	Blood, lymphatics	Microfilariae in blood; worm in tissue
Loiasis	Subcutaneous, eye	Removed worm; microfilariae in blood
Mansonellae		
M. ozzardi	Blood, skin, body cavities	Microfilariae: blood, skin biopsy
M. perstans	Blood, body cavities	Microfilariae: blood, fluids; adult in tissue
M. streptocerca	Skin, subcutaneous tissues	Microfilariae: skin biopsy, snips; adult in tissue
Onchocerciasis	Skin, subcutaneous tissues, eye	Microfilariae: skin snips, blood, eyes; adults: tissue
Tropical pulmonary eosinophilia	Lung	Serology
Gnathostomiasis	Subcutaneous, other tissues	Morphology in surgical specimen
Heterophyiasis	GI	Eggs in stool
Hookworm	Skin (transient), GI, lung (larvae)	Eggs in stool
Hymenolepiasis	GI	Eggs in stool
Metagonimiasis	GI	Eggs in stool
Opisthorchiasis	Hepatobiliary	Eggs in stool, duodenal aspirate, bile
Paragonimiasis	Lung, CNS, subcutaneous	Eggs: sputum, BAL, feces, pleural fluid
Schistosomiasis		
Schistosomal dermatitis	Skin	Morphology on biopsy
S. haematobium	Urinary tract, rarely CNS	Eggs in urine, tissue biopsy; serology
S. intercalatum	Liver, GI (venules of bowel), rarely CNS	Eggs in stool, biopsy
S. japonicum	Liver, GI (venules of bowel), rarely CNS	Eggs in stool, biopsy; serology
S. mansoni	Liver, GI (venules of bowel), rarely CNS	Eggs in stool, biopsy; serology
Sparganosis	Subcutaneous, multiple sites	Parasite in surgical specimen
Strongyloidiasis	GI, lung (larvae), skin (episodic)	Larvae in stool, duodenal aspirate; serology
Trichinellosis	GI (early), muscle, CNS	Muscle biopsy; serology
Trichostrongyliasis	GI	Eggs in stool or duodenal aspirate
Trichuriasis	GI	Eggs in stool, worms on protoscopy
Visceral larva migrans		
Toxocara canis, Toxocara cati	Liver, eye, lung (larvae)	Larvae in tissue; serology
Bayliscaris procyonis	CNS, eye, other	Identification of larva

BAL, bronchoalveolar lavage; CNS, central nervous system; CSF, cerebrospinal fluid; GI, gastrointestinal.

Table 125-2 Common Parasitic Causes of Marked Eosinophilia

Parasite/Disease	Magnitude	Comment
Angiostrongyliasis	High early	
Ascariasis	Moderate to high (larval migration)	Often absent with adult worms
Clonorchiasis	High early	May wax and wane in chronic infection
Fascioliasis	High early	May wax and wane in chronic infection
Fasciolopsiasis	High early	
Filarial infections		
Loiasis	High	Especially in expatriates
Mansonellosis	Can be high	
Onchocerciasis	Can be high	Normal eosinophil counts in up to 30%
Tropical pulmonary eosinophilia	High	
Gnathostomiasis	May be high	Wax and wane in chronic infection
Hookworm	High during larval migration	Persistent low to moderate
Opisthorchiasis	High early	
Paragonimiasis	High in early infection	Low or absent late
Schistosomiasis	High during early infection	Low or absent in chronic infection
Strongyloidiasis	High during larval migration	Low to moderate in chronic infection
Trichinellosis	High during acute infection	Absent late
Visceral larva migrans	High to moderate	May persist months or longer

prominent only during one stage of parasite development. An example is the common intestinal parasite *Ascaris lumbricoides*, which provokes eosinophilia principally during the stage of larval migration through the lungs (see Chapter 109). Adult worms residing in the lumen of the gut typically do not cause an eosinophilic response. Some parasites, such as the tapeworms *Diphyllobothrium latum* and *Taenia saginata*, whose entire life in the human host takes place in the lumen of the gut, cause little or no eosinophilic response even though they can grow to impressive lengths and survive for decades. Table 125-1 lists the many helminthic infections associated with eosinophilia and the main body site affected by each.

Several parasites may induce high-grade eosinophilia during one stage of development (Table 125-2) followed by chronic low-to-moderate levels of eosinophilia. Acute schistosomiasis (Katayama syndrome)[38,39] (see Chapter 116) and the larval migration stage of *Ascaris*[40] and hookworms[41] may provoke high-grade eosinophilia, which declines during the chronic stages of infection. In experimental hookworm infections, blood eosinophilia increases progressively after 2 to 3 weeks of infection and peaks between 5 and 9 weeks before gradually diminishing. In recipients of 45 to 50 infective larvae, peak eosinophil counts ranged from 1350 to 3828 cells per microliter in one study.[41] In untreated hookworm infections, eosinophilia slowly diminishes but can persist for several years after experimental infection.[42] Persistence of eosinophilia has been attributed to the attachment of adult worms to the intestinal mucosa, causing mild tissue damage and a continuing stimulus to eosinophilia, especially in heavy infections.[43] The blood and pulmonary eosinophilia, so often characterized as "transient," associated with the pulmonary migration phase of intestinal parasites (*Ascaris*, hookworms) typically persists for weeks or months.[40,44,45] The eosinophilia with strongyloidiasis (see Chapter 111) often fluctuates over time, being high during pulmonary migration and low to moderate during chronic infection. During hyperinfection syndromes, eosinophilia can be prominent or absent, influenced by host characteristics and suppression due to corticosteroids or concomitant bacterial infection.[46] The dramatic eosinophilia seen with acute trichinellosis usually disappears when a fibrous capsule forms around the larvae in muscles (except with the nonencapsulating species *Trichinella pseudospiralis*, which may cause a prolonged eosinophilic myositis[47]) (see Chapter 104). Parasites encysted in tissues, such as echinococcal cysts and cysticercosis, and physically isolated from the host by cyst walls, typically cause no eosinophilia unless disruption of the barrier allows leakage of antigen-rich material. Intermittent leakage of fluids from echinococcal cysts can transiently stimulate increases in blood eosinophilia and elicit allergic (urticaria, bronchospasm) or anaphylactic reactions.[48,49] Breaching of these barriers or disintegration with death of the parasite can lead to intense tissue reactions, increased eosinophilia, and acute symptoms in the host.

Adult parasites that live and migrate in tissues, such as *Loa loa* and *Gnathostoma spinigerum*, provide an ongoing stimulus to eosinophils.[28,50] Many filarial infections cause persistent eosinophilia (see Chapters 98 through 100).

The magnitude of eosinophilic responses and the presence and intensity of other symptoms may vary greatly depending on age at first exposures, the immunologic state of the host, and the number and timing of subsequent exposures. Temporary residents and long-term residents of endemic regions have different patterns of response to a number of helminths.[51] Loiasis in temporary residents of endemic regions is characterized by immunologic hyperresponsiveness, high-grade eosinophilia, and severe symptoms not seen in long-term residents of the same area.[28] Short-term residents are more likely to have Calabar swellings (95% vs. 16% for residents) and less likely to have detectable microfilaremia (10% vs. 90%) than the native population.[28,52] With schistosome infections, previously unexposed and nonimmune persons, and not long-term residents of endemic areas, may experience the Katayama fever syndrome in acute schistosomal infection.[38,39,53]

EPIDEMIOLOGY

Published studies give some clues as to the more common infections associated with eosinophilia in persons who have visited or resided in tropical regions.[54] In a study from London (Hospital for Tropical Disease), 261 patients with eosinophilia (defined as $>0.5 \times 10^9$ mL) from October 1997 to March 2002 were evaluated according to a standard protocol and with all diagnostic studies done at one laboratory.[55] A diagnosis related to tropical exposures was made in 64%, with the most common diagnoses being schistosomiasis (33%), strongyloidiasis (25%), hookworm (5.3%), onchocerciasis (4.2%), loiasis (2.3%), ascariasis (2.3%), and trichuriasis (2.3%). More than one parasitic infection was found in 17%. The predominant diagnoses varied by geographic areas of exposure. Schulte and colleagues in Germany found blood eosinophilia (defined as ≥8% of total WBC count) in 4.8% of 14,298 patients who were evaluated after return from developing countries.[56] The majority (73.6%) were born in Europe, and the median duration of travel was 35 days. One-third of those studied were asymptomatic. A definite diagnosis was made in 36%. In 18.9%, a specific helminth infection was found, with the most common helminth infections being schistosomiasis, hookworm, cutaneous larva migrans, strongyloidiasis, filariasis, and ascariasis. Travelers to Africa were more likely to have eosinophilia than those who visited the Indian subcontinent and Latin America. In returned travelers with higher levels of eosinophils (>16%), a helminth infection was found in 46.6%. In Belgium, of more than 8000 consultations for tropical diseases in 1991, 378 patients were found to have eosinophil levels greater than 450/μL. Specific diagnoses were made in 170 patients, and parasites were detected 107 times, most commonly intestinal helminths and filarial and schistosomal species. When serologic tests and the Mazzotti test (see Chapter 100) were added as diagnostic criteria, intestinal helminthic infections were diagnosed in 19%, filarial infections in 13%, and schistosomal infections in 10% of patients.[57] In Indochinese refugees with persistent eosinophilia whose initial comprehensive screening failed to reveal a cause for the eosinophilia, the most commonly implicated infections after further investigation were hookworm (55%) and *Strongyloides* (38%) infections.[58] In this study, all patients with greater than 1000 eosinophils per microliter and 88% of those with greater than 500 eosinophils per microliter had documented infection with at least one helminth species. Of 40 patients assessed serologically by enzyme-linked immunosorbent assay (ELISA) for *Strongyloides* infection, 34 had a positive titer. Of the 34, *Strongyloides* larvae were found on a single stool examination in only 24 (71%).[58]

The prevalence of various helminthic causes of eosinophilia will vary from one population to another depending on their geographic origins, their long-term residence or shorter-term exposures in previously unexposed visitors, and their exposure-related activities. Although eosinophilia is a useful marker that suggests the possible presence of certain parasitic infections, many patients with these infections do not have eosinophilia when evaluated.[59] The absence of eosinophilia does not exclude the possibility of schistosomiasis, strongyloidiasis, and other infections commonly associated with eosinophilia. In a study of 1107 travelers with schistosomiasis seen in the UK, eosinophilia was present in only 44%.[60] In the study by Schulte and colleagues, 45% of 92 returned travelers with schistosomiasis had eosinophilia.[56] When persons are known to have had intense exposure to parasites, such as schistosomes, screening tests for these infections are warranted in the absence of eosinophilia or specific symptoms.[59] Many helminthic infections persist for years or even decades in the human host (Box 125-5).

In contrast to persons who have not left temperate areas, persons with tropical exposures are more likely to have an infection as the cause of eosinophilia. Although infections associated with eosinophilia, such as visceral larva migrans, trichinellosis, or even strongyloidiasis, can be acquired in temperate regions, these infections account for a small percentage of cases of eosinophilia in nontravelers. Eosinophilia in most temperate regions is more likely to be caused by a process other than infection. As a rule of thumb, one should think first of parasitic infections in persons with eosinophilia and extensive tropical exposures and look first for nonparasitic infections in persons who have always lived in temperate climates.

Many infections associated with eosinophilia are seen primarily in persons with repeated or prolonged exposures. In general, cysticercosis, onchocerciasis, loiasis, lymphatic filariasis, paragonimiasis, and clonorchiasis are rare in persons with brief exposures (e.g., a few weeks or less). Although most persons with loiasis have had exposures in endemic regions lasting months or years, occasional infections have been documented in persons with less than one month of exposure.[61] In evaluating patients, it is useful to consider the prerequisites of symptomatic infection. Repeated exposures to a parasite may be required for the establishment of sufficient burden to cause symptomatic infections, for example, hookworm infections. Where a single exposure can lead to infection, the probability of infection in a visitor depends on how widespread and

Box 125-5 Eosinophilia and Remote Tropical or Other Exposures*

- Clonorchiasis
- Coenurosis
- Cysticercosis
- Echinococcosis
- Fascioliasis (rarely >10 years)
- Gnathostomiasis
- Hookworm (rarely 10 years or longer)
- Hymenolepiasis
- Loiasis
- Mansonelliasis
- Onchocerciasis
- Opisthorchiasis (up to 10 years)
- Paragonimiasis
- Schistosomiasis
- Sparganosis (at least 9 years)
- Strongyloidiasis (autoinfection enables persistence for decades)
- Tropical pulmonary eosinophilia (filarial)
- Visceral larva migrans

*Parasitic infections that can be associated with eosinophilia 10 years or more after exposures in tropical areas. Eosinophilia may wax and wane.

accessible the areas of risk are. Development of acute schistosomiasis after a single brief exposure to infested water has been described repeatedly.[38,53] Because of differences in the immunologic response to parasites, as noted previously, a nonimmune visitor to an endemic region may develop severe symptoms and more marked eosinophilia with a small parasite burden relative to that in residents of the region.

COMMON CAUSES

Strongyloides

Among the helminths, the principal parasite that needs to be considered is *Strongyloides* since it frequently elicits eosinophilia of varying magnitudes; is often difficult to detect on stool examination; can persist for decades, even without causing major symptoms; and, importantly, can cause a disseminated, often fatal, disease (hyperinfection syndrome) in patients unsuspectingly given immunosuppressive corticosteroids (see Chapter 111).[46] In a study from Toronto General Hospital, of 51 consecutive individuals with *Strongyloides stercoralis* larvae documented in fecal specimens (and no other parasites found), 83% had eosinophilia (absolute eosinophil count >400 cells/μL) with a mean eosinophil count of 890 cells/μL.[62] Infection was longstanding in many; 22% had immigrated to Canada more than 10 years before diagnosis. Among 76 patients with strongyloidiasis 25% were asymptomatic, 42% had gastrointestinal symptoms, and 22% had skin complaints (primarily urticaria or pruritus).[62] In a study from the United Kingdom, eosinophilia was found in 88% (36/41) of travelers and 76% (44/58) of immigrants with larvae on fecal examination.[63] While low-level or varying eosinophilia may be the only clue to strongyloidiasis, at times the magnitude of hypereosinophilia suggests a hypereosinophilic syndrome.[64]

The capacity of *Strongyloides* larvae to mature within the host into filariform larvae which invade the mucosa of the colon or penetrate the skin (usually in the perianal region) means that ongoing reinfection enables the parasite to persist for the lifetime of the host. Illustrative of this potential chronicity of clinically unrecognized strongyloidiasis was the experience with US, UK, and Australian former World War II prisoners in Asia. For instance, in American ex-prisoners of war, who acquired strongyloidiasis while working on the Burma-Thailand railroad in the 1940s, 37% had evidence of previously unrecognized, but persisting, *Strongyloides* infections.[65] In this group, more than 90% were symptomatic with intermittent creeping eruption (larva currens), gastrointestinal symptoms, or urticaria,[65] but in other patients with persisting strongyloidiasis, eosinophilia may be the sole sentinel finding.[66]

The importance of deliberately considering *Strongyloides* infections, especially in those with eosinophilia, is based on the additional capacity of this infection to develop into disseminated, potentially fatal, disease (hyperinfection syndrome) if patients subsequently receive corticosteroids or become immunocompromised.[46] Thus, clinicians should carefully assess the probability of past exposure to *Strongyloides* in persons who will be given steroids or other immunosuppressive agents or who develop diseases associated with immunosuppression.[46] Rarely, disseminated strongyloidiasis has been reported in apparently immunocompetent persons.[67] Persons infected with human T-cell lymphotropic virus type I (HTLV-I) are significantly more likely to be infected with *Strongyloides* than those who are uninfected with HTLV-I. Although certain groups of immunocompromised patients (especially those with hematologic malignancies, or on steroids, or with severe malnutrition) appear to be at increased risk for the *Strongyloides* hyperinfection syndrome, this has not been a frequently reported complication in human immunodeficiency virus serotype 1 (HIV-1)–infected persons in areas such as Brazil and sub-Saharan Africa, where both HIV-1 and *Strongyloides* infections are common. As discussed in the following sections, fecal examinations are insensitive, and ELISA serology is useful in detecting strongyloidiasis even when fecal examinations are unrevealing.[58]

Schistosomes

Eosinophilia frequently accompanies schistosomiasis (see Chapter 116). Travelers from endemic areas may present with acute schistosomiasis, with less acute symptoms, or even without symptoms.[68] Many reports document sporadic cases and clusters of nonimmune persons with acute schistosomiasis after brief exposures in endemic regions.[39,53] Typical findings are spiking fevers, sweating, diarrhea, and dry cough that can persist for a month or longer. Pulmonary symptoms were noted in 8 of 60 nonimmune travelers seen in Israel with acute schistosomiasis, occurring 3 to 6 weeks after exposure.[69] Chest radiographs showed multiple small nodules and diffuse interstitial infiltrate.[69] Among 31 patients with acute schistosomiasis mansoni in Brazil, 90% had fever, 94% had diffuse abdominal pain, and liver enzymes were elevated in 38%.[70] Cough was reported by 81% and dyspnea by 52%.[70] All had eosinophilia.[70] In one study of 15 patients with Katayama syndrome, the median duration of illness was 12 days (range, 4 to 46 days).[39] Ten of 12 patients in this series had eosinophilia during the first 10 weeks of infection.[39] Other symptomatic presentations of schistosomiasis in travelers can include hematuria, hematospermia, or, uncommonly, transverse myelitis.[71–73] Infections can occur after a brief stay,[74] but for many schistosomiasis develops only after longer-term exposures in endemic regions. A British study of 173 expatriates with schistosomiasis acquired primarily in Africa found that the mean duration of stay in an endemic area was 7 years (range, 3 to 41 years) for those who were infected vs. 3 years for an uninfected control population returning from similar endemic regions.[75] A study of expatriates and visitors to Malawi found that serologic evidence of current or past schistosome infection increased directly with the length of stay in Malawi.[3] Seroprevalence was 48% in people resident 4 years or longer in contrast to 11% for those resident 1 year or less. Recreational freshwater exposure in Lake Malawi was an important source of infection.[3]

Filariae

Eosinophilia is common in infections caused by the various filarial parasites (see Chapters 98 through 100), which differ by geographic region and are transmitted by biting insects (e.g., mosquito, black fly, or midge). In general, these infections are transmitted inefficiently and only rarely acquired after brief stays in tropical regions. For lymphatic filariasis, early manifestations may include filarial fevers with lymphangitis.[76,77] With loiasis, reactions to adult worms are more common, especially in nonimmune short-term residents.[28,52]

Human Immunodeficiency Virus Type 1

Occasional reports have noted increased levels of eosinophils in HIV-1–infected persons.[78] In a study of 855 HIV-infected persons in New York examined over 4 years, however, no single, consistent cause of eosinophilia could be identified.[78] Increased eosinophil levels appeared to result from a relative preservation of the eosinophil cell line (while other cell lines declined as the CD4 count decreased) in some patients and in others from the presence of truly increased eosinophils.[78] Increased eosinophil levels in HIV-infected subjects were more commonly associated with rashes, including eosinophilic folliculitis,[79] atopic dermatitis, and prurigo nodularis, in another study that suggested no extensive evaluation for eosinophilia was warranted.[80] Although some HIV-infected patients with eosinophilia have a definable cause, such as adverse drug reactions or adrenal insufficiency due to cytomegalovirus and other infections, in most instances no obvious cause can be identified, indicating that HIV infection may be associated at times with increased levels of eosinophils. While case reports have documented the occurrence of various eosinophilic syndromes in those infected with HIV,[81–83] these hypereosinophilic disorders are uncommon and likely not related to underlying HIV infection. A recent report has correlated the presence of eosinophilia, likely due to schistosomiasis, with the progression to active tuberculosis in HIV-1–infected Ugandans,[84] but the implications of this finding remain to be ascertained.

COMMON SYNDROMES

Pulmonary

Eosinophilic lung diseases are a heterogeneous group of disorders characterized by a common presence of increased eosinophils in inflammatory infiltrates in the airways or parenchyma of the lungs. The clinical presentation of pulmonary eosinophilia usually consists of symptoms referable to the respiratory system accompanied by an abnormal chest radiograph and blood or sputum (or bronchoalveolar lavage) eosinophilia. While the pathogenic mechanisms underlying many of the disorders are undefined, we have classified the pulmonary eosinophilias based on recognized etiologic agents and distinct clinical and pathologic patterns[2] (Box 125-6). Several helminthic infections can cause eosinophilic lung diseases, and these can be categorized based on the behavior of the parasites.

Box 125-6 Pulmonary Eosinophilia

1. Drug- and toxin-induced eosinophilic lung diseases
2. Helminthic infection–related eosinophilic lung diseases
   Transpulmonary passage of larvae (Löffler's syndrome): *Ascaris,* hookworm, *Strongyloides*
   Pulmonary parenchymal invasion: mostly helminths, paragonimiasis, echinococcosis
   Heavy hematogenous seeding with helminths: trichinellosis, disseminated strongyloidiasis, cutaneous and visceral larva migrans, schistosomiasis
   Tropical pulmonary eosinophilia: filaria
3. Fungal-related eosinophilic lung diseases
   Allergic bronchopulmonary aspergillosis
4. Chronic eosinophilic pneumonia
5. Acute eosinophilic pneumonia
6. Churg-Strauss syndrome—vasculitis
7. Other: neoplasia, idiopathic hypereosinophilic syndrome, bronchocentric granulomatosis

Modified from Weller PF: Eosinophilia and eosinophil-related disorders. In Adkinson NF Jr, Yunginger JW, Busse WW, et al (eds): Allergy: Principles and Practice, 6th ed. St. Louis, Mosby–Year Book, 2003, p 1105.

Transpulmonary Passage of Helminth Larvae

This category, the true Löffler's syndrome, arises from reactions elicited by developing larvae that pass through the lungs as part of the parasite's initial developmental cycle in the human. For three helminthic intestinal parasites (*Ascaris,* hookworms, and *Strongyloides*), infecting larvae pass through the lungs, entering via the bloodstream, penetrating into alveoli, and then ascending the airway to transit down the esophagus into the small bowel. Löffler, who first described this syndrome of migratory pulmonary infiltrates and blood eosinophilia in Swiss patients, subsequently implicated *Ascaris* infection, acquired from the use of contaminated "nightsoil" (human excrement) as fertilizer, as the cause of this syndrome.[85] *Ascaris* is especially capable of eliciting eosinophilic inflammatory responses and is prevalent in regions where human feces contaminate soil or are used as fertilizer. Although infecting hookworm and *Strongyloides* larvae likewise traverse the lungs, these larvae rarely elicit symptoms of pulmonary eosinophilia in natural or experimental infections.[86]

Since Löffler's syndrome occurs only when developing larvae are transiting the lungs, about 9 to 12 days after ingestion of *Ascaris* eggs, this cause of pulmonary eosinophilia should be considered only in those with a recent exposure to *Ascaris* eggs (see Chapter 109). In symptomatic patients, common complaints are an irritating, nonproductive cough and burning substernal discomfort, and over half of patients have rales and wheezing. Acute symptoms generally subside within 5 to 10 days. Chest radiographs show unilateral or bilateral nonsegmental densities with indefinite borders ranging in size from several millimeters to several centimeters. Infiltrates are generally transient and migratory and clear over one or more weeks. Blood eosinophilia increases after several days of symptoms and resolves over many weeks. *Ascaris* pneumonia is diagnosed at the time of pneumonic involvement only by detecting *Ascaris* larvae in respiratory secretions or gastric aspirates.[86] At least 40 days must elapse before the larvae responsible for pulmonary infiltrates have matured sufficiently to produce eggs detectable in the stool. Negative stool examinations during or soon after an episode of pneumonitis do not exclude *Ascaris* as the cause nor do positive stool examinations for *Ascaris* eggs during the stage of pulmonary involvement establish the cause, as these eggs reflect infection acquired 2 to 24 months earlier.

Pulmonary Parenchymal Invasion with Helminths

In contrast to the parasites mentioned previously that transit through the lungs, a few helminths, such as *Paragonimus* lung flukes (see Chapter 117) and echinococcal species (see Chapter 114), have a predilection to localize within the pulmonary parenchyma, and these may elicit eosinophil-enriched inflammatory reactions.[86] *Paragonimus* larvae undergo maturation in the lungs. Larval flukes can leave hemorrhagic, necrotic tracts; their eggs provoke a granulomatous response. Infection is endemic throughout much of Southeast Asia and is seen in the United States in immigrants from those areas. Because the chronic cavitary lesions of paragonimiasis can mimic tuberculosis, and many adults from Southeast Asia have positive tuberculin tests, patients may be misdiagnosed as having tuberculosis.[87] Echinococcal infection can also involve the lungs, though encysted parasites typically do not elicit a peripheral eosinophilia.

Heavy Hematogenous Seeding with Helminths

This disease category includes the eosinophilic pulmonary responses elicited by helminthic larvae or eggs that are carried into the lungs hematogenously in an aberrant fashion. Thus, in contrast to the "normal" transpulmonary migration noted previously, etiologic helminths include abnormal numbers of nonhuman hookworms or ascarids causing cutaneous or visceral larva migrans,[88,89] abnormal numbers of hematogenous larvae in heavy trichinellosis infections,[86] and abnormal spread following chemotherapy of schistosomal parasites via collateral vessels into the lungs.[86,90] Also included in this category is disseminated strongyloidiasis, which develops when the *Strongyloides* autoinfection cycle becomes unbridled, often in association with corticosteroid or cytotoxic drug administration (see Chapter 111). Large numbers of larvae traverse the lungs eliciting pulmonary findings. Adult parasites can develop in the bronchial tree causing bronchospasm mimicking asthma.[91] In disseminated strongyloidiasis, filariform larvae can be found in many sites, including the stool, sputum, and bronchoalveolar washings. The usual eosinophilia of strongyloidiasis can be suppressed in disseminated disease because of concomitant pyogenic infection or steroid administration.

Tropical Pulmonary Eosinophilia

This form of eosinophilic pneumonia results from a distinct immune response to the normally blood-borne microfilarial stages of lymphatic filariae, *Wuchereria bancrofti,* and, less commonly, *Brugia malayi* (see Chapter 98).[92,93] The disease is prevalent in regions where these filariae are endemic, and residents or immigrants from these regions are those who may experience tropical pulmonary eosinophilia. Males are affected more often than females in a ratio of about 4:1. Dyspnea, wheezing (especially at night), and chest discomfort may be accompanied by weight loss and malaise. Asthma may be the presenting complaint.[94] In addition to blood eosinophilia, features specific to tropical pulmonary eosinophilia include high levels of serum IgE and antifilarial antibodies. Bloodstream microfilariae are almost never found. Abnormalities on chest radiographs may be subtle and include diffuse miliary lesions 1 to 3 mm in size, patchy consolidations, cavitation, reticulonodular infiltrates of the lower lung zones, and an interstitial nodular pattern.[95] Tropical pulmonary eosinophilia is an immunologically mediated disorder with microfilariae trapped in the lungs. Microfilariae are detected in inflammatory foci in biopsies from the lung, liver, and lymph nodes. A related, nonfilarial syndrome of tropical pulmonary eosinophilia of uncertain cause has been recognized.[96]

Other Pulmonary Eosinophilias

At least 10 cases of severe acute pneumonitis with elevated eosinophils (peripheral and pulmonary) occurred in US military personnel deployed to Southwest Asia in 2003.[97] The etiology was not determined; an association with recent initiation of smoking was noted.

Among the drugs reported to cause pulmonary eosinophilia are ones sometimes taken for malaria prophylaxis and hence pertinent in patients who will have had tropical exposures. These include pyrimethamine and dapsone.[98,99]

Eosinophilic pleural effusions (Box 125-7) can have multiple causes.[100] In the setting of someone with potential infectious exposures, several helminthic infections, including toxocariasis,[101] tropical pulmonary eosinophilia,[102] paragonimiasis,[103] loiasis,[104] and anisakiasis,[105] can cause eosinophilic pleural effusions.

Abdominal Pain or Diarrhea

The gut is the primary or sole residence in the human host for many helminthic parasites. Symptoms from these parasitic infections may result from several mechanisms, including attachment of the parasite to, or penetration of, the gut mucosa, causing irritation and inflammation; migration through the wall or to other adjacent sites (such as biliary and pancreatic ducts); intraluminal obstruction by a bolus of worms; and

Box 125-7 Eosinophilic Pleural Effusions

Helminthic Infections

Anisakiasis (rare)
Echinococcosis
Gnathostomiasis
Loiasis
Paragonimiasis
Strongyloidiasis (disseminated infection; may also find larvae in fluid)
Toxocariasis
Trichinellosis (early weeks of infection)
Tropical pulmonary eosinophilia

Other Infections

Coccidioidomycosis
Tuberculosis

Other Causes

Hemothorax
Hypersensitivity reactions, including drug reactions
Malignancy
Pneumothorax, including from thoracentesis
Pulmonary infarct
Rheumatologic diseases

Box 125-8 Parasites Causing Eosinophilia and Abdominal Pain or Diarrhea

Helminths

Ancylostoma caninum (eosinophilic enteritis)
Anisakis spp. and other genera (anisakiasis)
Angiostrongylus costaricensis
Ascaris lumbricoides
Capillaria philippinensis
Clonorchis sinensis
Echinococcus
Enterobius vermicularis (eosinophilic colitis)
Fasciola hepatica
Fasciolopsis buski
Gnathostoma
Hookworm (Heavy Infection)
Schistosomes
Strongyloides
Trichinella spiralis
Toxocara canis, Toxocara cati, other (visceral larva migrans)

Protozoa

Dientamoeba fragilis
Isospora belli

Other Causes

Eosinophilic gastroenteritis
Dermatitis herpetiformis
Periarteritis nodosa, especially Churg-Strauss syndrome
Regional enteritis
Ulcerative colitis
Lymphoma
Solid tumors
Drug reaction (e.g., eosinophilic colitis from naproxen)
Hypereosinophilic syndrome
Allergy (e.g., cow's milk, soy protein in infants)

entry into the appendix, among others. Helminths and other processes associated with eosinophilia and abdominal pain and diarrhea are listed in Box 125-8. The canine hookworm *(Ancyclostoma caninum)* has been associated with a syndrome of abdominal pain, sometimes acute and severe, and peripheral eosinophilia.[106] The main pathologic finding is a focal or diffuse eosinophilic inflammation, which seems to be caused by a hypersensitivity response to secreted antigens from the canine hookworm. Larvae of the pinworm *Enterobius vermicularis* have also been reported to cause eosinophilic colitis and enteritis.[107] Helminth-elicited disease must be distinguished from often idiopathic eosinophilic gastroenteritis.[108,109]

Skin

Intermittent and migratory lesions of the skin and subcutaneous tissues can reflect migration of parasites in human tissues (see Chapter 126). Parasites associated with lesions of the skin and soft tissues are listed in Table 125-3. Skin lesions associated with gnathostomiasis (see Chapter 106) may begin as early as 3 to 4 weeks after ingestion of the parasite or may be delayed until months or even years later. The third-stage larvae cause localized swellings that typically last 1 to 2 weeks and are associated with edema, pain, itching, and variable erythema. Swellings may recur off and on for 10 to 12 years. Because a single gnathostome can cause symptoms, cases have occurred after a brief stay in an endemic area or after eating foods, usually raw fish, from those areas. Disease has been most often reported from Southeast Asia. An increase in cases in Mexico, Peru, and Ecuador has been noted in recent years.[110,111] In addition to causing cutaneous disease, the worm can also migrate to tissues throughout the body, causing pulmonary, gastrointestinal, genitourinary, central nervous system (CNS), ocular, and other localized disease.[50] Loiasis, another disease causing migratory lesions and eosinophilia, follows exposures to *L. loa* in west-central Africa (see Chapter 99).[61] Symptoms typically do not appear until at least 4 months after exposure and can first appear more than 5 years after exposure. Classic findings are localized areas of angioedema (Calabar or fugitive swellings), which may be warm, red, itchy, or painful.[28,52] They usually disappear within a few days and may recur multiple times per year. Fever may accompany migration of worms. Worms migrating at a rate up to 1 cm per minute may be visible crossing the conjunctivae or bridge of the nose. Adult worms can survive more than 10 years.

A pruritic skin rash is a common feature of onchocerciasis (see Chapter 100). Swelling of an extremity should suggest obstruction of lymphatics caused by one of the filarial parasites. Patients may experience recurrent lymphangitis (often with retrograde progression) lasting 3 to 7 days, which may be associated with fever.[77] Orchitis and epididymitis are also characteristic features. Although eosinophilia can occur in patients with cutaneous larva migrans caused by the hookworm *Ancylostoma braziliense* and related nematodes, in one series only 20% had at least 7% blood eosinophilia.[112]

Penetration of schistosomal cercariae is typically followed by the development of an itchy, erythematous, papular rash.[113] Exposures to avian schistosomes elicit a similar skin reaction (swimmer's itch).[113,114] Skin biopsy is characterized by infiltration of eosinophils, though peripheral eosinophilia may be absent.

Hepatobiliary

Several parasites reside in the biliary tree and cause localized inflammatory changes and can obstruct the bile or pancreatic ducts leading to a clinical picture that can mimic acute cholangitis or cholecystitis (see Chapter 117). Other parasites, such as *Ascaris*, can wander from their usual habitat within the gut lumen to enter pancreatic or biliary ducts causing acute symptoms (see Chapter 109). In fascioliasis, the young fluke penetrates the capsule of the liver and migrates through liver parenchyma causing local necrosis and inflammation before it enters the bile ducts where it matures and produces eggs that are released into bile and passed in feces.[115,116] Eosinophilia may wax and wane when infection becomes chronic. Clonorchiasis, endemic in eastern and southeastern Asia, and opisthorchiasis, acquired mainly in Southeast Asia, are other parasites that reside in bile ducts (see Chapter 117). Among 17 immigrants who were found have ova of *Opisthorchis* spp. or *Clonorchis sinensis* in fecal specimens when evaluated in the US Midwest, 88% had eosinophilia (defined as absolute eosinophil counts >500/μL). Clinical symptoms included vague right upper abdominal discomfort; 24% of those infected had been in the United States at least 5 years.[117] Other helminths as

Table 125-3 Helminths Associated with Eosinophilia and Skin and Soft Tissue Changes

Parasite/Disease	Manifestation
Ascariasis	Urticaria
Coenurosis	Subcutaneous nodules, usually solitary
Cutaneous larva migrans*	Characteristic serpiginous lesions
Cysticercosis	Rubbery, painless cysts; often multiple
Dracunculiasis	Papules, vesicles; rupture and discharge larvae
Echinococcosis	Soft, subcutaneous cysts, varying sizes; urticaria
Fascioliasis	Urticaria; rare painful or itchy subcutaneous nodules
Filariasis	
Brugia zoonotic filariae	Local lymphadenopathy
Zoonotic dirofilariasis	Subcutaneous nodule
Loiasis	Pruritic 5–10-cm Calabar swellings; urticaria; papulovesicular lesions
Onchocerciasis	Subcutaneous nodules; papules and severe itching; urticaria; lizard skin
Wuchereria bancrofti	Recurrent retrograde lymphangitis and lymphadenitis; scrotal mass; hydrocele, elephantiasis
Brugia malayi, Brugia timori	Recurrent retrograde lymphangitis and lymphadenitis; scrotal mass; hydrocele, elephantiasis
Gnathostomiasis	Urticarial, edematous, recurrent, migratory subcutaneous swellings; creeping eruption; panniculitis
Hookworm	Urticaria; itchy maculopapular rash; may be vesicular
Paragonimiasis	Urticaria (early); subcutaneous nodules
Schistosomiasis	Urticaria, itchy maculopapules (early); papules (ectopic egg deposition)
Sparganosis	Edematous, painful migratory swellings secondary to worm migration
Strongyloidiasis	Itchy papular and migratory serpiginous lesions at points of penetration and dermal migration (larva currens); urticaria; papulovesicular lesions; petechiae and purpuric lesions in hyperinfection syndrome
Trichinellosis	Urticaria; periorbital edema; splinter hemorrhages
Visceral larva migrans	Urticaria; nodules

*Eosinophilia usually low grade or absent.

well are associated with eosinophilia and hepatic dysfunction (Box 125-9).

Fever

The clinical picture of undifferentiated fever and eosinophilia can be seen in acute schistosomiasis,[39,118] toxocaral visceral larva migrans,[119] trichinellosis,[120] fascioliasis,[115] gnathostomiasis,[50] and some other parasitic infections.[121] In many instances, focal findings will develop (e.g., localized subcutaneous swellings, lymphangitis, cough and pulmonary infiltrates, abdominal pain, and others) that will give clues as to the organ systems involved. The combination of exposure history (when, where, and what activities) along with clinical findings can help the clinician to focus on more likely diagnoses. Box 125-10 lists helminthic infections causing eosinophilia and prominent fever.

Box 125-9 Infections Causing Eosinophilia and Hepatic Dysfunction

- Angiostrongyliasis cantonensis (infrequent hepatic involvement)
- Ascariasis (mechanical obstruction of bile ducts by migrating worm)
- Capillariasis due to *Capillaria hepatica*
- Clonorchiasis
- Dicrocoeliasis
- Echinococcosis (eosinophilia may be absent with intact cysts; liver function may remain normal despite multiple cysts)
- Fascioliasis
- *Metorchis conjunctus*
- Opisthorchiasis
- Schistosomiasis
- Strongyloidiasis (with hyperinfection)
- Taeniasis (*Taenia saginata*; rare obstruction of bile ducts)
- Visceral larva migrans (toxocariasis)

Central Nervous System Findings

Larvae of *Angiostrongylus cantonensis* migrate to the brain, spinal cord, and eye, where the larvae and young adults provoke an intense inflammatory response and cause the clinical picture of eosinophilic meningoencephalitis (see Chapter 105).

Box 125-10 Helminthic Infections Causing Eosinophilia and Prominent Fever*

- Clonorchiasis
- Fascioliasis
- Gnathostomiasis (early, episodic)
- Onchocerciasis
- Schistosomiasis (Katayama fever)
- Trichinellosis
- Visceral larva migrans (toxocariasis)

*Acute, early ascaris, hookworm, or strongyloides may be associated with fever.

Box 125-11 Causes of Eosinophilia in Cerebrospinal Fluid

Helminths

Nematode (Roundworm) Infections with Migrating Larvae Inherently Neurotropic

Angiostrongylus cantonensis
Gnathostoma spinigerum
Baylisascaris procyonis

Cestode (Tapeworm) Infection with Cysts Developing in the CNS

Cysticercosis
Echinococcosis
Coenurosis

Trematode (Fluke) Infection with Ectopic CNS Localization

Paragonimus westermani
Schistosomiasis
Fascioliasis

Miscellaneous Infectious Causes

Coccidioidomycosis
Cryptococcus neoformans
Toxocariasis (*Toxocara canis*)
Trichinellosis
Myiasis (larvae of cattle botflies)

Noninfectious Causes

Ventriculoperitoneal shunts
Leukemia or lymphoma with CNS involvement (Hodgkin's)
Drug hypersensitivity reactions: nonsteroidal anti-inflammatory agents, antibiotics (e.g., sulfonamides, ciprofloxacin, vancomycin), phenytoin; myelography contrast agents
Idiopathic hypereosinophilic syndrome
Sarcoidosis

Although most cases and outbreaks have been reported from Southeast Asia and the Pacific basin, in 2000, 12 US travelers developed eosinophilic meningitis after travel to the Caribbean (Jamaica) where they had shared a meal.[122] Peripheral eosinophilia was present in 44% of patients on initial evaluation, though it eventually developed in all 9 who were hospitalized. A number of other parasites or their eggs can be associated with an eosinophilic tissue response and with variable eosinophils in the spinal fluid. Cysticercosis, which commonly involves the CNS, typically causes focal neurologic findings, including seizures (see Chapter 113). The cerebrospinal fluid (CSF) may be acellular and peripheral eosinophilia absent. In addition to helminthic parasites, other infections, drug reactions, and other processes can induce an eosinophilic meningitis[123,124] (Box 125-11).

NONINFECTIOUS DISEASES

Many processes, as outlined in Box 125-1, are associated with eosinophilia and may need to be considered if helminthic infections do not explain a patient's eosinophilia. Because drug hypersensitivity reactions are relatively common, drugs should always be considered as a potential cause of eosinophilia even in persons who have visited or lived in tropical regions (Box 125-12). The presence of a characteristic rash may suggest a hypersensitivity reaction, but drug-associated eosinophilia can occur in the absence of skin changes. In addition to peripheral eosinophilia, drug reactions may be associated with pathologic changes and dysfunction of other tissues and organs (Table 125-4). Any of these findings may predominate, or a combination of several may be seen at the same time or in staggered development. Rechallenge of patients with the drug may cause an accelerated reaction. Because of the striking blood or tissue eosinophilia, some drug reactions can mimic parasitic infections.

EVALUATION OF PATIENTS WITH EOSINOPHILIA

Several key concepts are relevant to the evaluation of a patient with eosinophilia after tropical exposures:

- Multiple parasitic infections may be present.
- Excretion of eggs may be in small numbers or intermittent.
- Examination of stool for eggs is useless during the prepatent period. Symptoms such as fever and eosinophilia may be present for two weeks or more before the products of the adult parasite (e.g., eggs or larvae) are passed in the stool.
- Eosinophilia is most prominent with tissue-dwelling helminths, and many of these never enter the intestinal tract. Stool examinations will not detect tissue-dwelling helminths or exclude their presence as a cause of eosinophilia.
- Serologic tests may be negative early in the symptomatic period.

It is necessary to have some idea of the possible infections that might be present in order to focus the evaluation and determine which tests to do and which tissues to examine. Even if the patient is entirely asymptomatic and the physical examination is unremarkable, the presence of eosinophilia should lead to a workup to identify treatable diseases that could cause future problems. Eosinophilia, however, need not be present.[59] Knowledge of the geographic distribution of various parasites and the characteristic time interval between exposure and onset of symptoms and the presence of diagnostic forms of parasites or eggs in tissue or fluids is an essential part of the evaluation[1] (Box 125-13). For example, microfilariae of *W. bancrofti* will not be present on blood smears until about one year after exposure. A period of 4 to 6 weeks must pass after exposure to hookworm larvae before eggs can be found in the stool.

Whetham and colleagues outline a general strategy for evaluating returned tropical travelers with eosinophilia based on geographic areas.[55] They would do microscopic examinations of concentrated stool and *Strongyloides* culture and serology on all. For travelers to Africa, they would add schistosomal serology, terminal urine microscopy, and filarial serology. When travel or prior residence included West Africa, filtration and examination of blood for microfilaria was added. Whether skin snips were done depended on symptoms and filarial serology.[55]

Diagnosis of strongyloidiasis is often missed if the clinician relies on routine stool examinations. Although larvae can be found in stool samples, the sensitivity of the stool examination is low (see Chapter 111). In published series, estimates of positivity with a single stool examination range from 0% to 66%. Therefore, serologic tests that detect IgG antibodies to antigens of *Strongyloides* larvae are helpful in detecting strongyloidiasis.[46,58]

Box 125-12 Drugs Often Associated with Eosinophilia

Antimicrobial Agents
Amoxicillin
Ampicillin*
Cephalosporins
Ciprofloxacin
Clarithromycin
Erythromycin
Fluconazole
Imipenem-cilastin
Isoniazid
Macrodantin*
Minocycline*
Moxalactam
Nitrofurantoin*
Penicillins (also methicillin, nafcillin)
Sulfonamides
Rifampin
Tetracycline
Tobramycin
Trimethoprim-sulfamethoxazole*
Vancomycin

Cardiovascular Agents
Captopril*
Enalapril
Heparin
Lovastatin
Methyldopa
Ticlopidine
Quinidine

Gastrointestinal Agents
Cimetidine
Ranitidine
Sulfasalazine

Illicit Drugs
Cocaine (inhaled)*
L-Tryptophan

Neurologic Agents, Including Antidepressants, Antiepileptics
Carbamazepine*
Clozapine
Divalproex
Fluoxetine*
Levodopa
Phenytoin*
Valproic acid

Nonsteroidal Anti-Inflammatory Agents
Aspirin
Ibuprofen*
Naproxen*
Piroxicam
Sulindac*

Other
Granulocyte-macrophage colony–stimulating factor
Interleukin-3 and interleukin-2 (used in trials)
Isotretinoin
Iodides and iodinated contrast dyes
Rheumatologic agents
Allopurinol
Gold*

*Reported to be associated with pulmonary changes.
Based on published reports and reports of adverse reactions to the Food and Drug Administration.

Table 125-4 Examples of Drug-associated Reactions with Eosinophilia

Drug Reactions	Examples
Cytokine-mediated	GM-CSF, IL-2
Pulmonary infiltrates	NSAIDs
Pleuropulmonary	Dantrolene
Interstitial nephritis	Semisynthetic penicillins, cephalosporins
Necrotizing myocarditis	Ranitidine
Hepatitis	Semisynthetic penicillins, tetracyclines
Hypersensitivity vasculitis	Allopurinol, phenytoin
Gastroenterocolitis	NSAIDs
Asthma, nasal polyps	Aspirin
Pharmacologic	β-Blockers
Eosinophilia-myalgia syndrome	L-Tryptophan contaminant
Asymptomatic	Ampicillin, penicillins, cephalosporins

GM-CSF, granulocyte-macrophage colony–stimulating factor; IL-2, interleukin-2, NSAIDs, nonsteroidal anti-inflammatory agents.
Modified from Weller PF: Eosinophilia and eosinophil-related disorders. In Adkinson NF Jr, Yunginger JW, Busse WW, et al (eds): Allergy: Principles and Practice, 6th ed. St. Louis, Mosby-Year Book, 2003, p. 1105.

Studies have reported sensitivities ranging from 80% to 90%. A study from London found serology was positive in 73% (22/30) of travelers and 98% (45/46) of immigrants with larvae found on stool examination.[63] In a study in Toronto of 76 patients with *Strongyloides* larvae found in fecal specimens, the *Strongyloides* enzyme immunoassay (EIA) done at the Centers for Disease Control and Prevention had a sensitivity of 94.5%.[62] Antibody titers declined slowly over many months after therapy.

Timing of Tests

Even when sensitive and specific serologic tests are available, they may be negative early in the course of infection. In a study of patients with acute schistosomiasis, serologic results were negative in 3 of 8 persons tested during the first week of illness.[39] If suspicion is high, serologic tests should be repeated if initially negative. During the prepatent period, serologic studies may be the only way to confirm the diagnosis.[125]

Timing of obtaining blood to search for microfilariae needs to be done cognizant of the potential periodicity exhibited by

Box 125-13 Eggs or Parasites in Tissues or Fluids

In Urine

Dioctophymosis (eggs; rare infection)
Filariasis (microfilariae, e.g., *Wuchereria bancrofti, Loa loa*)
Gnathostomiasis (parasite passed in urine; rare)
Schistosome eggs *(Schistosoma haematobium)*
Strongyloidiasis (larvae, rare)

In Sputum

Ascariasis (larvae during early migration)
Echinococcosis (fragments of larvae and free scolices after rupture of cyst into bronchus; rare)
Gnathostomiasis (rarely coughed-up worm)
Hookworm (larvae, early)
Paragonimiasis (eggs in sputum)
Schistosomiasis (eggs)
Strongyloidiasis (filariform larvae, and rarely eggs and adults, in sputum in hyperinfection syndrome)

In Pleural Fluid

Paragonimiasis (eggs)
Strongyloidiasis (filariform larvae)

On Blood Smears

Microfilariae of filariasis (e.g., *W. bancrofti, Brugia malayi, L. loa, Mansonella perstans, Mansonella ozzardi*)
Trichinellosis (rarely observed on blood smears)

In CSF

Angiostrongyliasis due to *Angiostrongylus cantonensis* (larvae in CSF)

On Perirectal Skin (Tape Test)

Pinworm eggs
Tapeworm proglottids

In Feces*

Strongyloidiasis (20%–30% positive with a single examination; 60%–70% with three or more; 40%–90% positive on duodenal sample or endoscopic aspirate)
Several intestinal nematodes, trematodes, and cestodes

*Eggs and parasites are not found in feces in patients with many helminthic infections, such as echinococcosis, toxocaral visceral larva migrans, and trichinellosis; stool examinations are often negative at the time of earliest symptoms in patients with many infections, including schistosomiasis, ascariasis, and hookworm infections.

the species and strains of filariae (see Chapters 98 and 99). In a study in Brazil, Dreyer and associates[126] found that microfilariae of *W. bancrofti* in both venous and capillary blood showed a nocturnal periodicity pattern, with the fewest microfilariae in the capillary bed of the skin when the biting activity of the local *Culex* vector was at its lowest level. Carriers with higher levels of microfilariae (at least one microfilaria per 20- or 60-μL blood smear at night) could be identified during daytime hours by a filtration technique using 1 mL of venous blood. Routine blood films did not identify persons with low levels of parasitemia, even if done at night. Box 125-14 lists examples of useful diagnostic tissues to sample.

In general, it is preferable to diagnose infection by identification of eggs, larvae, adults, or other parasitic stages or products in tissues, fluids, or stool. Sometimes diagnostic material is unavailable or its retrieval would entail serious risk to the patient (e.g., brain biopsy, liver biopsy, major surgical intervention). When parasites, eggs, or other products are unavailable, serologic tests are useful in some infections (Table 125-5). Problems with serologic tests may include lack of sensitivity, availability, standardization and quality control, and low specificity. Cross-reactivity to related parasites is common for many of the tests.

Acid-fast techniques stain schistosome eggs and hooklets of *Echinococcus granulosus*. Most helminths can be seen on hematoxylin and eosin–stained sections, but special stains, such as Weigert's iron hematoxylin or Russel-Moval pentachrome, can demonstrate the exoskeleton of helminths and improve visualization of characteristic morphology.[127]

Box 125-14 Identification of Parasite or Its Products by Morphology, Staining Characteristics, and Appearance

- Skin biopsy: schistosome eggs
- Skin snips: microfilariae of *Onchocerca volvulus* and *Mansonella streptocerca*
- Rectal biopsy: for eggs of *Schistosoma japonicum, Schistosoma mansoni*
- Bladder biopsy: for eggs of *Schistosoma haematobium*
- Muscle biopsy: for *Trichinella* larvae
- Liver biopsy: larvae of *Toxocara*
- Excision of masses or biopsy of other tissues with pathologic changes (e.g., cysts or soft tissue masses caused by infections such as cysticercosis, gnathostomiasis, sparganosis, echinococcosis, others; filarial epididymal mass). In loiasis, the adult worm is found in subcutaneous tissue.

Table 125-5 *Serologic Tests and What They Detect*

Infection	Serologic Tests Detect
Clonorchiasis	Antibody
Cysticercosis	Antibody, antigen
Echinococcosis	Antibody (can be negative even with established cysts), antigen
Fascioliasis	Antigen
Filariasis	Antibody, antigen
Gnathostomiasis (possibly useful)	Antibody
Onchocerciasis	Antigen
Paragonimiasis (possibly useful)	Antibody
Schistosomiasis	Antibody (IFA, IHA, ELISA), antigen
Strongyloidiasis	Antibody (ELISA IgG to *Strongyloides stercoralis* antigen, 80%–90%; IFA, up to 90%)
Toxocariasis	Antibody, antigen
Trichinellosis	Antibody (may not be positive to 3rd week of infection)

ELISA, enzyme-linked immunosorbent assay; IFA, indirect fluorescent antibody (test); IHA, indirect hemagglutination antibody (test).

RESPONSE TO TREATMENT

Several key points should be kept in mind when treating patients with helminthic infections:

- Treatment may not be curative; efficacy may vary depending on the stage of the parasite.
- Symptoms may worsen, usually only transiently, with therapy.
- The level of eosinophilia may be a poor predictor of whether treatment has cured infection.
- Relapses can occur late.

Even when parasitic infections are recognized and treated, anthelmintic drugs may fail to cure infection. In a study of loiasis, 38% of patients were considered cured after a single course of diethylcarbamazine (DEC), increasing to 59% after one to three courses.[128] Although most relapses occurred within the first year after treatment, relapses occurring up to eight years after therapy have been reported, reflecting the long life span of the worms. Of 22 travelers treated for acute schistosomiasis after exposures in West Africa, eight still had evidence of active infection during 52 weeks of follow-up, though in two cases the possibility of reinfection could not be excluded.[39] Of 18 patients in Brazil with acute *Schistosoma mansoni* infection followed for two years, 14 (77.8%) were considered parasitologically cured. In that series, children had more intense clinical manifestations, were cured less often, and had slower resolution of symptoms than did adults.[129]

A temporary rise in eosinophilia after treatment has been observed in a number of helminthic infections.[130,131] The magnitude of the post-treatment eosinophilia correlates with the parasite burden prior to therapy.[132] This may be associated with other symptoms, such as pruritus, dermatitis, arthralgia, and myalgia in patients with loiasis.[128] Patients with schistosomiasis may develop respiratory symptoms and new pulmonary infiltrates in association with therapy.[90,131,132] Severe symptoms have been reported when treatment is given early (during Katayama fever).[130] These worsening symptoms and the rise in eosinophils may reflect the host immune response to antigens released or exposed from dead or dying larvae or worms. In patients with loiasis treated with DEC, levels of eosinophils usually returned to normal within six months.[128] This occurred even in patients who had late relapses of infection.[128] Thus, normalization of levels of eosinophils after treatment does not necessarily indicate that infection has been eradicated. Conversely, however, the persistence of eosinophilia likely indicates that infections persist.

When ivermectin was used to treat 43 microfilaremic patients with bancroftian filariasis in Brazil, adverse clinical reactions, usually fever, headache, weakness, and myalgia, occurred in almost all patients but generally disappeared within 24 to 48 hours. Post-treatment eosinophilia was common and proportional to pretreatment microfilarial levels. After treatment, 38% of patients developed transient pulmonary dysfunction, 23% developed liver enzyme abnormalities, and 22% had hematuria.[133]

Timing of treatment may be important. Praziquantel, for example, is thought to be less active against the larval forms of schistosomes; schistosomes that have not reached the adult stage when treatment is given may survive.[39] Oral mebendazole, which is not well absorbed systemically, may have limited efficacy against developing hookworm larvae still in the lungs.

Box 125-15 outlines an approach to the evaluation of the patient with eosinophilia.

Box 125-15 Evaluation of the Patient with Eosinophilia

Eosinophil Determinations

Confirm that the eosinophil count is elevated.

Estimate the absolute blood eosinophil count: normal, ≤350 eosinophils per μL; elevated, >450 eosinophils per μL.

Categorize eosinophilia as low (<1000/μL), moderate (1000–3000/μL), or high (>3000/μL) (see Table 125-2)

Medical History

Eosinophil history: Inquire from history or medical records if eosinophil counts were previously normal or elevated, and if so for how long.

Medication history: Review drug exposure history for recent or current drugs that may be associated with eosinophilia. Discontinue any drugs that are commonly associated with eosinophilia and make a complete list of other medications, vitamins, supplements, or herbal preparations that the patient is taking. If patient is taking drugs that have been associated with eosinophilia, assess for associated serious organ involvement. Note any history of allergies to drugs or otheragents.

Disease history: Review the medical history for diseases typically associated with eosinophilia (see Box 125-1). Given their prevalence, allergic and atopic disorders should be noted, although new onset of some allergic manifestations (e.g., urticaria [see Table 125-1], bronchospasm, wheezing) may be secondary to helminthic infections.

Geographic history: Review history of past residence and travel in other countries or regions. Relevant are time periods extending even decades before. Especially relevant are exposures in tropical regions and those with poor sanitation. Note places, dates, and duration of exposures. Some helminths have discrete geographic distributions (e.g., *Clonorchis* in the Far East; *Angiostrongylus cantonensis,* a cause of eosinophilic meningitis, principally, but not exclusively, in the Pacific Basin; *Loa loa* in central-west Africa; *Onchocerca volvulus* in equatorial Africa and elevated regions in Central America). Even nontropical geographic histories are relevant to some helminths and other agents, e.g., the southwestern United States for coccidiodomycosis. Exposures in sheep-rearing areas are pertinent to *Echinococcus granulosus.*

Continued

Box 125-15 Evaluation of the Patient with Eosinophilia—Cont'd

Activity history: Review occupational and recreational exposures. Histories of swimming in or contact with freshwater in areas where schistosomiasis occurs are pertinent. Contact with fresh- or saltwater followed by a rash on water-exposed skin suggests schistosome dermatitis (avian schistosome species). Skin contact with soil potentially contaminated with human or dog feces, walking barefoot, or occupational (military or job-related) exposures, are pertinent to the acquisition of cutaneous larva migrans, hookworm, and *Strongyloides* infections.

Dietary history: Dietary histories are pertinent to several helminthic infections, including anisakiasis (raw fish), fish tapeworm (fish), *Nanophyetus salmincola* (salmon), *Taenia solium* (pork), *Taenia saginata* (beef), fascioliasis (watercress), fasciolopsiasis (water chestnut), gnathostomiasis (freshwater fish, eels, frogs, snakes, and poultry and pigs fed on fish), *Angiostrongylus cantonensis* (land snails or slugs, freshwater shrimp, crabs, some marine fish), and trichinosis (pork, boar, bear, horse, walrus, warthog).

Other epidemiologic history: Helpful in the evaluation is knowledge of whether the patient traveled with others and whether others developed similar illnesses—relevant to common-source water exposures (e.g., schistosomiasis) or food-borne illness (e.g., trichinellosis). In concert with geographic exposures, histories of exposures to insect vectors are pertinent (e.g., filarial infections).

General history: Do a careful review of systems for any current or recent symptoms, including a history of fevers (see Box 125-10), skin lesions (see Table 125-3) that may have cleared, and gastrointestinal illnesses (see Box 125-8).

Physical Examination

Do a careful physical examination paying close attention to skin and soft tissue for nodules or masses.

Initial Laboratory Evaluation

The presence of specific clinical symptoms and physical findings, as well as other information from the history, may begin to direct laboratory testing.

As needed, check routine studies to assess organ involvement (e.g., liver function tests, renal function tests, urinalysis, chest radiograph [CXR]).

Further Diagnostic Evaluations

Symptomatic patient with localizing findings: The evaluation will be guided by the nature of the historical information and results from the physical examination and initial laboratory tests based on the focal findings:

Skin: skin snips, skin biopsy, excision of mass

CNS: Computed tomography (CT) and magnetic resonance imaging (MRI); cerebrospinal fluid (CSF) examination (cell counts, differential, protein, glucose; larvae)

Pulmonary findings or abnormal CXR: sputum examination (routine, acid-fast bacteria, ova and parasites [O&P]), CT or MRI to better define lesions, including those not seen on CXR

Stool O&P; urine O&P; rectal biopsy, other tests (see Table 125-5; Boxes 125-13 and 125-14)

Eosinophilia in a patient without other findings:

Stools for O&P (×3 as needed)

Strongyloides serology (if stools negative); *Toxocara* serology

If exposures are relevant, check studies (Table 125-5; Boxes 125-13 and 125-14) for schistosomiasis, filariasis, onchocerciasis.

REFERENCES

1. Wilson ME: Eosinophilia. In A World Guide to Infections. Diseases, Distribution, Diagnosis. New York, Oxford University Press, 1991, p 164.
2. Weller PF: Eosinophilia and eosinophil-related disorders. In Adkinson NF Jr, Yunginger JW, Busse WW, et al (eds): Allergy: Principles and Practice, 6th ed. St Louis, Mosby–Year Book, 2003, p 1105
3. Cetron MS, Chitsulo L, Sullivan JJ, et al: Schistosomiasis in Lake Malawi. Lancet 348:1274, 1996.
4. Nutman TB, Reese W, Poindexter RW, et al: Immunologic correlates of the hyperresponsive syndrome of loiasis. J Infect Dis 157:544, 1988.
5. Junod C: *Isospora belli* coccidiosis in immunocompetent subjects (a study of 40 cases seen in Paris). Bull Soc Pathol Exot 81:317, 1988.
6. Cuffari C, Oligny L, Seidman EG: *Dientamoeba fragilis* masquerading as allergic colitis. J Pediatr Gastroenterol Nutr 26:16, 1998.
7. Van den Enden E, Praet M, Joos R, et al: Eosinophilic myositis resulting from sarcocystosis. J Trop Med Hyg 98:273, 1995.
8. Arness MK, Brown JD, Dubey JP, et al: An outbreak of acute eosinophilic myositis attributed to human *Sarcocystis* parasitism. Am J Trop Med Hyg 61:548, 1999.
9. Wong KT, Pathmanathan R: High prevalence of human skeletal muscle sarcocystosis in South-east Asia. Trans R Soc Trop Med Hyg 86:631, 1992.
10. Bass DA: Behavior of eosinophil leukocytes in acute inflammation. II. Eosinophil dynamics during acute inflammation. J Clin Invest 56:870, 1975.
11. Shanks GD, Wilairatanaporn C: Eosinophilic response to falciparum malaria infections. Southeast Asian J Trop Med Public Health 23:795, 1992.
12. Davis TM, Ho M, Supanaranond W, et al: Changes in the peripheral blood eosinophil count in falciparum malaria. Acta Trop 48:243, 1991.
13. Bergner RK, Bergner A: Marked peripheral eosinophilia: A clue to allergic bronchopulmonary aspergillosis in office practice. N Engl Regul Allergy Proc 6:367, 1985.
14. Echols RM, Palmer DL, Long GW: Tissue eosinophilia in human coccidioidomycosis. Rev Infect Dis 4:656, 1982.
15. Koepke A, Albus C, Barth A, et al: Coccidioidomycosis—Differential diagnosis of lung infiltrates with peripheral eosinophilia. Dtsch Med Wochenschr 114:218, 1989.
16. Schermoly MJ, Hinthorn DR: Eosinophilia in coccidioidomycosis. Arch Intern Med 148:895, 1988.
17. Harley WB, Blaser MJ: Disseminated coccidioidomycosis associated with extreme eosinophilia. Clin Infect Dis 18:627, 1994.
18. Starr J, Pruett JH, Yunginger JW, et al: Myiasis due to *Hypoderma lineatum* infection mimicking the hypereoosinophilic syndrome. Mayo Clin Proc 75:755, 2000.
19. Deshpande AD: Eosinophilia associated with scabies. Practitioner 231:455, 1987.
20. Rothenberg ME: Eosinophilia. N Engl J Med 338:1592, 1998.
21. Klion AD, Nutman TB: The role of eosinophils in host defense against helminth parasites. J Allergy Clin Immunol 113:30, 2004.

22. Weller PF, Dvorak AM: Human eosinophils: Development, maturation and functional morphology. In Busse WW, Holgate ST (eds): Asthma and Rhinitis, 2nd ed. Boston, Blackwell Scientific, 2000, p 351.
23. Maizels RM, Balic A: Resistance to helminth infection: The case for Interleukin-5-dependent mechanisms. J Inf Dis 190:427, 2004.
24. Weller PF, Bubley GJ: The idiopathic hypereosinophilic syndrome. Blood 83:2759, 1994.
25. Andy JJ, O'Connell JP, Daddario RC, et al: Trichinosis causing extensive ventricular mural endocarditis with superimposed thrombosis. Evidence that severe eosinophilia damages endocardium. Am J Med 63:824, 1977.
26. Andy JJ, Bishara FF, Soyinka OO, et al: Loiasis as a possible trigger of African endomyocardial fibrosis: A case report from Nigeria. Acta Trop 33:179, 1981.
27. Andy JJ: Helminthiasis, the hypereosinophilic syndrome and endomyocardial fibrosis: Some observations and an hypothesis. Afr J Med Med Sci 12:155, 1983.
28. Nutman TB, Miller KD, Mulligan M, et al: *Loa loa* infection in temporary residents of endemic regions: Recognition of a hyperresponsive syndrome with characteristic clinical manifestations. J Infect Dis 154:10, 1986.
29. Ive FA, Willis AJP, Ikeme AC, et al: Endomyocardial fibrosis and filariasis. Q J Med 36:495, 1967.
30. Löffler W: Endocarditis parietalis fibroplastica mit Bluteosinophilie. Ein eigenartiges Krankheitsbild. Schweiz Med Wochenschr 17:817, 1936.
31. Chew CY, Ziady GM, Raphael MJ, et al: Primary restrictive cardiomyopathy. Non-tropical endomyocardial fibrosis and hypereosinophilic heart disease. Br Heart J 39:399, 1977.
32. Roberts WC, Buja LM, Ferrans VJ: Löffler's fibroplastic parietal endocarditis, eosinophilic leukemia, and Davies' endomyocardial fibrosis. The same disease at different stages? Pathol Microbiol (Basel) 35:90, 1970.
33. Fleming AF: Haematological changes in pregnancy. Clin Obstet Gynecol 2:269, 1975.
34. Beeson PB, Bass DA: The Eosinophil. Philadelphia, WB Saunders, 1977.
35. Bass DA: Behavior of eosinophil leukocytes in acute inflammation. I. Lack of dependence on adrenal function. J Clin Invest 55:1229, 1975.
36. Meagher LC, Cousin JM, Seckl JR, et al: Opposing effects of glucocorticoids on the rate of apoptosis in neutrophilic and eosinophilic granulocytes. J Immunol 156:4422, 1996.
37. Gil H Magy N Mauny F Dupond JL: Inflammatoires: Un " vieux" marqueur revisite [Value of eosinopenia in inflammatory disorders: An "old" marker revisited]. Rev Med Interne 24:431, 2003.
38. Chapman PJ, Wilkinson PR, Davidson RN: Acute schistosomiasis (Katayama fever) among British air crew. BMJ 297:1101, 1988.
39. Visser LG, Polderman AM, Stuiver PC: Outbreak of schistosomiasis among travelers returning from Mali, West Africa. Clin Infect Dis 20:280, 1995.
40. Gelpi AP, Mustafa A: Seasonal pneumonitis with eosinophilia: A study of larval ascariasis in Saudi Arabia. Am J Trop Med Hyg 16:646, 1967.
41. Maxwell C, Hussain R, Nutman TB, et al: The clinical and immunologic responses of normal human volunteers to low dose hookworm (*Necator americanus*) infection. Am J Trop Med Hyg 37:126, 1987.
42. Ball PAJ, Bartlett A: Serological reactions to infection with *Necator americanus*. Trans R Soc Trop Med Hyg 63:362, 1969.
43. Beaver PC: Observations on *Necator* infection resulting from exposure to three larvae. Rev Iberica Parasitol 1:1, 1955.
44. Bean WJ: Recognition of ascariasis by routine chest or abdomen roentgenograms. AJR 94:379, 1965.
45. Phills JA, Harrold AJ, Whiteman GV, et al: Pulmonary infiltrates, asthma and eosinophilia due to *Ascaris suum* infestation in man. N Engl J Med 286:965, 1972.
46. Keiser PB, Nutman TB: *Strongyloides stercoralis* in the immunocompromised population. Clin Microbiol Rev 17:208, 2004.
47. Jongwutiwes S, Chantachum N, Kraivichian P, et al: First outbreak of human trichinellosis caused by *Trichinella pseudospiralis*. Clin Infect Dis 26:111, 1998.
48. Mooraki A, Rahbar MH, Bastani B: Spontaneous systemic anaphylaxis as an unusual presentation of hydatid cyst: Report of two cases. Am J Trop Med Hyg 55:302, 1996.
49. Arora VK, Gowrinath K, Johri A: Recurrent bronchospasm due to an unusual cause. Indian J Chest Dis Allied Sci 36:27, 1994.
50. Rusnak JM, Lucey DR: Clinical gnathostomiasis: Case report and review of the English-language literature. Clin Infect Dis 16:33, 1993.
51. McCarthy JS, Ottesen EA, Nutman TB: Onchocerciasis in endemic and nonendemic populations: differences in clinical presentation and immunologic findings. J Infect Dis 170:736, 1994.
52. Klion AD, Massougbodji A, Sadeler BC, et al: Loiasis in endemic and nonendemic populations: Immunologically mediated differences in clinical presentation. J Infect Dis 163:1318, 1991.
53. Doherty JF, Moody AH, Wright SG: Katayama fever: An acute manifestation of schistosomiasis. BMJ 313:1071, 1996.
54. Moore TA, Nutman TB: Eosinophilia in the returning traveler. Infect Dis Clin North Am 12:503, 1998.
55. Whetham J, Day JN, Armstrong M, et al: Investigation of tropical eosinophilia: Assessing a strategy based on geographical area. J Infect 46:180, 2003.
56. Schulte C, Krebs B, Jelinek T, et al: Diagnostic significance of blood eosinophilia in returning travelers. Clin Infect Dis 34:407, 2002.
57. Van den Ende J, van Gompel A, van den Enden E, et al: Hypereosinophilia after a stay in tropical countries. Trop Geogr Med 46:191, 1994.
58. Nutman TB, Ottesen EA, Ieng S, et al: Eosinophilia in Southeast Asian refugees: Evaluation at a referral center. J Infect Dis 155:309, 1987.
59. Fryatt RJ, Teng J, Harries AD, et al: Intestinal helminthiasis in expatriates returning to Britain from the tropics: A controlled study. Trop Geogr Med 42:119, 1990.
60. Whitty CJM, Mabey D, Armstrong M, et al: Presentation and outcome of 1107 cases of schistosomiasis from Africa diagnosed in a non-endemic country. Trans R Soc Trop Med Hyg 94:531, 2000.
61. Rakia RM, White AC Jr, Kielhofner MA: *Loa loa* infection as a cause of migratory angioedema: Report of three cases from the Texas Medical Center. Clin Infect Dis 17:691, 1993.
62. Loutfy MR, Wilson M, Keystone JS, et al: Serology and eosinophil count in the diagnosis and management of strongyloidiasis in a non-endemic area. Am J Trop Med Hyg 66:749, 2002.
63. Sudarshi S, Stumphle R, Armstrong M, et al: Clincial presentation and diagnostic sensitivity of laboratory tests for *Strongyloides stercoralis* in travelers compared with immigrants in a non-endemic country. Trop Med Int Health 8:728, 2003.
64. Savage D, Foadi M, Haworth C, et al: Marked eosinophilia in an immunosuppressed patient with strongyloidiasis. J Intern Med 236:473, 1994.
65. Pelletier LL: Chronic strongyloidiasis in World War II Far East ex-prisoners of war. Am J Trop Med Hyg 33:55, 1984.
66. Gill GV, Baily JW: Eosinophilia as a marker for chronic strongyloidiasis—Use of a serum ELISA test to detect asymptomatic cases. Ann Trop Med Parasitol 83:249, 1989.
67. Husni RN, Gordon SM, Longworth DL, et al: Disseminated *Strongyloides stercoralis* infection in an immunocompetent patient. Clin Infect Dis 23:663, 1996.
68. Day JH, Grant AD, Doherty JF, et al: Schistosomiasis in travellers returning from sub-Saharan Africa. BMJ 313:268, 1996.
69. Schwartz E, Rozenmann J, Perelman N: Pulmonary manifestations of early Schistosoma infection among nonimmune travelers. Am J Med 109:718, 2000.
70. Ribeiro de Jesus A, Silva A, Santana LB, et al: Clinical and immunologic evaluation of 31 patents with acute schistosomiasis mansoni. J Infect Dis 185:98, 2001.
71. Ueki K, Parisi JE, Onofrio BM: *Schistosoma mansoni* infection involving the spinal cord. Case report. J Neurosurg 82:1065, 1995.
72. Corachan M, Valls ME, Gascon J, et al: Hematospermia: A new etiology of clinical interest. Am J Trop Med Hyg 50:580, 1994.
73. Nixon A, Nacey J, Russell G, et al: Schistosomiasis: A review of cases in Wellington 1993–4. N Z Med J 109:7, 1996.
74. Istre GR, Fontaine RE, Tarr J, et al: Acute schistosomiasis among Americans rafting the Omo river, Ethiopia. JAMA 251:508, 1984.
75. Harries AD, Fryatt R, Walker J, et al: Schistosomiasis in expatriates returning to Britain from the tropics: A controlled study. Lancet 1:86, 1986.
76. Bean B, Ellman MH, Kagan IG: Acute lymphatic filariasis in an American traveler. Diagn Microbiol Infect Dis 15:345, 1992.
77. Weller PF, Arnow PM: Paroxysmal inflammatory filariasis. Filarial fevers. Arch Intern Med 143:1523, 1983.
78. Cohen AJ, Steigbigel RT: Eosinophilia in patients infected with human immunodeficiency virus. J Infect Dis 174:615, 1996.
79. Basarab T, Russell Jones R: HIV-associated eosinophilic folliculitis: Case report and review of the literature. Br J Dermatol 134:499, 1996.
80. Skiest DJ, Keiser P: Clinical significance of eosinophilia in HIV-infected individuals. Am J Med 102:449, 1997.

81. Drabick JJ, Magill AJ, Smith KJ, et al: Hypereosinophilic syndrome associated with HIV infection. Military Medical Consortium for Applied Retroviral Research. South Med J 87:525, 1994.
82. Paganelli R, Scala E, Mezzaroma I, et al: Immunologic aspects of hyperimmunoglobulinemia E-like syndrome in patients with AIDS. J Allergy Clin Immunol 95:995, 1995.
83. Kaplan MH, Hall WW, Susin M, et al: Syndrome of severe skin disease, eosinophilia, and dermatopathic lymphadenopathy in patients with HTLV-II complicating human immunodeficiency virus infection. Am J Med 91:300, 1991.
84. Elliott AM, Kyosiimire J, Quigley MA, et al: Eosinophilia and progression to active tuberculosis in HIV-1-infected Ugandans. Trans R Soc Trop Med Hyg 97:477, 2003.
85. Löffler W: Transient lung infiltrations with blood eosinophilia. Int Arch Allergy Appl Immunol 8:54, 1956.
86. Weller PF: Parasitic pneumonias. In Pennington JE (ed): Respiratory Infections: Diagnosis and Management, 3rd ed. New York, Raven Press, 1994, p 695.
87. Johnson RJ, Johnson JR: Paragonimiasis in Indochinese refugees. Roentgenographic findings with clinical correlations. Am Rev Respir Dis 128:534, 1983.
88. Schaub NA, Perruchoud AP, Buechner SA: Cutaneous larva migrans associated with Löffler's syndrome. Dermatology 205:207, 2002.
89. Inoue K, Inoue Y, Arai T, et al: Chronic eosinophilic pneumonia due to visceral larva migrans. Intern Med 41:478, 2002.
90. Davidson BL, el-Kassimi F, Uz-Zaman A, et al: The "lung shift" in treated schistosomiasis. Bronchoalveolar lavage evidence of eosinophilic pneumonia. Chest 89:455, 1986.
91. Nwokolo C, Imohiosen EAE: Strongyloidiasis of the respiratory tract presenting as "asthma." BMJ 2:153, 1973.
92. Ottesen EA, Nutman TB: Tropical pulmonary eosinophilia. Annu Rev Med 43:417, 1992.
93. Udwadia FE: Tropical eosinophilia: A review. Respir Med 87:17, 1993.
94. Jiva TM, Israel RH, Poe RH: Tropical pulmonary eosinophilia masquerading as acute bronchial asthma. Respiration 63:55, 1996.
95. Sandhu M, Mukhopadhyay S, Sharma SK: Tropical pulmonary eosinophilia: A comparative evaluation of plain chest radiography and computed tomography. Australas Radiol 40:32, 1996.
96. Rocha A, Dreyer G, Poindexter RW, et al: Syndrome resembling tropical pulmonary eosinophilia but of non-filarial aetiology: Serological findings with filarial antigens. Trans R Soc Trop Med Hyg 89:573, 1995.
97. Centers for Disease Control and Prevention: Severe acute pneumonitis among deployed U.S. military personnel—Southwest Asia, March-August 2003. MMWR 36:587, 2003.
98. Begbie S, Burgess KR: Maloprim-induced pulmonary eosinophilia. Chest 103:305, 1993.
99. Davidson AC, Bateman C, Shovlin C, et al: Pulmonary toxicity of malaria prophylaxis. BMJ 297:1240, 1988.
100. Kalomenidis I, Light RW: Eosinophilic pleural effusions. Curr Opin Pulm Med 9:254, 2003.
101. Jeanfaivre T, Cimon B, Tolstuchow N, et al: Pleural effusion and toxocariasis. Thorax 51:106, 1996.
102. Boornazian JS, Fagan JM: Tropical pulmonary eosinophilia associated with pleural effusions. Am J Trop Med Hyg 34:473, 1985.
103. Romeo DP, Pollock JJ: Pulmonary paragonimiasis: Diagnostic value of pleural fluid analysis. South Med J 79:241, 1986.
104. Klion AD, Eisenstein EM, Smirniotopoulos TT, et al: Pulmonary involvement in loiasis. Am Rev Respir Dis 145:961, 1992.
105. Matsuoka H, Nakama T, Kisanuki H, et al: A case report of serologically diagnosed pulmonary anisakiasis with pleural effusion and multiple lesions. Am J Trop Med Hyg 51:819, 1994.
106. Croese J, Loukas A, Opdebeeck J, et al: Human enteric infection with canine hookworms. Ann Intern Med 120:369, 1994.
107. Liu LX, Chi J, Upton MP, et al: Eosinophilic colitis associated with larvae of the pinworm *Enterobius vermicularis*. Lancet 346:410, 1995.
108. Ettinghausen SE: Collagenous colitis, eosinophilic colitis, and neutropenic colitis. Surg Clin North Am 73:993, 1993.
109. Talley NJ, Shorter RG, Phillips SF, et al: Eosinophilic gastroenteritis: A clinicopathological study of patients with disease of the mucosa, muscle layer, and subserosal tissues. Gut 31:54, 1990.
110. Chappuis F, Farinelli T, Loutan L: Ivermectin treatment of a traveler who returned from Peru with cutaneous gnathostomiasis. Clin Infect Dis 33:e17, 2001.
111. Rojas-Molina N, Pedraza-Sanchez S, Torres-Bibiano B, et al: Gnathostomiasis, an emerging foodborne zoonotic disease in Acapulco, Mexico. Emerging Infect Dis 5:264, 1999.
112. Jelinek T, Maiwald H, Nothdurft HD, et al: Cutaneous larva migrans in travelers: Synopsis of histories, symptoms, and treatment of 98 patients. Clin Infect Dis 19:1062, 1994.
113. Gonzalez E: Schistosomiasis, cercarial dermatitis, and marine dermatitis. Dermatol Clin 7:291, 1989.
114. de Gentile L, Picot H, Bourdeau P, et al: La dermatite cércarienne en Europe: Un problème de santé publique nouveau? Bull World Health Organ 74:159, 1996.
115. Arjona R, Riancho JA, Aguado JM, et al: Fascioliasis in developed countries: A review of classic and aberrant forms of the disease. Medicine (Baltimore) 74:13, 1995.
116. Graham CS, Brodie SB, Weller PF: Imported *Fasciola hepatica* infection in the United States and treatment with triclabendazole. Clin Infect Dis 33:1, 2001.
117. Stauffer WM, Sellman JS, Walker JF: Biliary liver flukes (opisthorchiasis and clonorchiasis) in immigrants in the United States: Often subtle and diagnosed years after arrival. J Travel Med 11:157, 2004.
118. Rocha MO, Pedroso ER, Greco DB, et al: Pathogenetic factors of acute schistosomiasis mansoni: Correlation of worm burden, IgE, blood eosinophilia and intensity of clinical manifestations. Trop Med Int Health 1:213, 1996.
119. Bhatia V, Sarin SK: Hepatic visceral larva migrans: Evolution of the lesion, diagnosis, and role of high-dose albendazole therapy. Am J Gastroenterol 89:624, 1994.
120. McAuley JB, Michelson MK, Schantz PM: *Trichinella* infection in travelers. J Infect Dis 164:1013, 1991.
121. Mahanty S: Febrile illness caused by parasites. Pediatr Ann 23:398, 1994.
122. Slom TJ, Cortese MM, Gerger SI, et al: An outbreak of eosinophilic meningitis caused by *Angiostrongylus cantonensis* in travelers returning from the Caribbean. N Engl J Med 346:668, 2002.
123. Weller PF: Eosinophilic meningitis. Am J Med 95:250, 1993.
124. Lo Re V, Gluckman SJ: Eosinophilic meningitis. Am J Med 114:217, 2003.
125. Pitkanen YT, Peltonen M, Lahdevirta J, et al: Acute schistosomiasis mansoni in Finnish hunters visiting Africa: Need for appropriate diagnostic serology. Scand J Infect Dis 22:597, 1990.
126. Dreyer G, Pimentael A, Medeiros Z, et al: Studies on the periodicity and intravascular distribution of *Wuchereria bancrofti* microfilariae in paired samples of capillary and venous blood from Recife, Brazil. Trop Med Int Health 1:264, 1996.
127. Woods GL, Walker DH: Detection of infection or infectious agents by use of cytologic and histologic stains. Clin Microbiol Rev 9:382, 1996.
128. Klion AD, Ottesen EA, Nutman TB: Effectiveness of diethylcarbamazine in treating loiasis acquired by expatriate visitors to endemic regions: Long-term follow-up. J Infect Dis 169:604, 1994.
129. Rabello ALT, Garcia MMA, Pinto da Silva RA, et al: Humoral immune responses in patients with acute *Schistosoma mansoni* infection who were followed up for two years after treatment. Clin Infect Dis 24:405, 1997.
130. Harries AD, Cook GC: Acute schistosomiasis (Katayama fever): Clinical deterioration after chemotherapy. J Infect 14:159, 1987.
131. Pedroso ERP, Lambertucci JR, Greco DB, et al: Pulmonary schistosomiasis mansoni: Post-treatment pulmonary clinical-radiological alterations in patients in the chronic phase: A double-blind study. Trans R Soc Trop Med Hyg 81:778, 1987.
132. Ottesen EA, Weller PF: Eosinophilia following treatment of patients with *Schistosomiasis mansoni* and Bancroft's filariasis. J Infect Dis 139:343, 1979.
133. Coutinho AD, Dreyer G, Medeiros Z, et al: Ivermectin treatment of bancroftian filariasis in Recife, Brazil. Am J Trop Med Hyg 50:339, 1994.

126

Cutaneous Lesions

STEVEN D. MAWHORTER
DAVID L. LONGWORTH

INTRODUCTION

International travel exposes the traveler to a number of potential health risks. Although most visits to developing countries are uneventful, 15% to 37% of travelers experience some health concern, usually diarrheal.[1,2] Dermatoses occur in up to 12.4% of overseas travelers.[1–3] In nearly all surveys of returning travelers, skin lesions are one of the top five medical concerns.[1–6] The majority of lesions develop prior to return home and only rarely require hospitalization, although they often lead to medical evaluation.[4–6] The skin also represents the largest organ of the body and the most accessible to direct examination and observation. As a result, it is often a sentinel for many infectious diseases by being the primary site of involvement; the entry site of parasitic or bacterial pathogens; or by demonstrating lesions that result from toxin-, inflammatory-, or vascular-mediated changes associated with infection.[7]

Specific pathogens and the clinical manifestations of diseases commonly found in people residing in, or traveling to, tropical areas are discussed in detail elsewhere in this book. This chapter begins with a discussion of the pathophysiology of tropical and parasite-associated skin reactions, and then focuses on the approach to the patient who presents with cutaneous manifestations, to assist in the generation of a thoughtful differential diagnosis.

THE SKIN AS TARGET ORGAN—PATHOGENETIC MECHANISMS

Although many pathogens can produce cutaneous manifestations, the skin has a limited number of responses to inflammatory or infectious processes. In general, the pathogenesis of skin manifestations of infectious diseases can be considered under six broad categories. The first category involves blood-borne dissemination of the actual infectious agent.[8,9] This category can be further subdivided into two areas based on whether the etiologic agent engages in direct interaction with the skin and dermal appendages to produce the cutaneous manifestations or mediates the interaction through cellular, humoral, or other immune mechanisms. Examples of organisms that directly involve the skin include *Neisseria meningitidis*, *Rickettsia* spp., endocarditis-related bacterial embolization (e.g., Janeway lesions and Osler's nodes), *Pseudomonas* spp. and other gram-negative ecthyma lesions, *Bacillus anthracis*, and *Candida* spp. In this setting, Gram's stain of the skin lesion may reveal the offending organism.[10,11] Viral pathogens, such as varicella-zoster virus and many enteroviruses, may cause direct cutaneous findings following viremic seeding of the skin.[9]

Examples of immune reactions involving the skin to blood-borne organisms include *Salmonella* spp. (rose spots), *N. meningitidis* and *Neisseria gonorrhoeae*, measles, and rubella.[9] In these cases, cutaneous manifestations are typically due to local cutaneous immune vasculitis or dermal immune responses, including, but not limited to, immune complex deposition. Since the skin changes are largely immune complex mediated, direct smears of the lesions are much less likely to reveal a pathogen. Consistent with the bacteremic or viremic pathogenesis of this first category, many of the diseases associated with this mechanism of cutaneous involvement are often severe and occasionally life-threatening.[9]

The second category involves the local reaction to parasites that gain access to the body elsewhere and migrate to the skin but are not blood-borne. They can also elicit a direct or indirect immunologic response to produce the observed cutaneous changes. This category includes lymphatically borne agents such as the filarial parasites *Onchocerca volvulus* (onchocerciasis) and *Loa loa* (loiasis).[12,13] The nodules of both onchocerciasis and loiasis often contain adult worms (direct mechanism). However, generalized pruritus and maculopapular eruptions appear to be mediated by immune reactions to dermal-based microfilariae (indirect mechanism).[14] Other helminthic examples include the cutaneous nodules of *Dracunculus medinensis* (guinea worm) and *Spirometra* spp. (sparganosis).[12,15]

A third category involves the cutaneous immune reaction to direct penetration of the organism, which may or may not proceed to the further development of active deep-seated infection. Here, the examples are primarily parasitic, including human hookworm "ground itch," which occurs at the site of primary penetration.[16] When nonhuman helminths, such as feline or canine hookworms, penetrate the skin, they are unable to complete their life cycle. As a result, they persistently migrate through the epidermis with characteristic serpiginous tracks, called cutaneous larva migrans, created by the worm and the local host immune reaction. "Swimmer's itch," caused by avian schistosome cercariae penetrating the skin of sensitized people, is another example of an abortive helminthic infection.[17,18] The immunologic nature of the response (IgE-mediated histamine response in this case) is shown by the absent or minimal reaction in previously unexposed people.[19,20] Similar pruritic reactions occur in human schistosomiasis at the time of cercarial penetration, prior to the subsequent development of a productive infection.[18] Myiasis (see Plate 126-2C) and arthropod infestations, such as scabies and lice, are further examples in this category.[21–24] Arthropod bite and sting reactions are similar in that they usually represent a local immune reaction to deposited salivary contents that many vectors use to facilitate their blood meal. Mosquito saliva-specific IgE antibodies have been detected in humans after experimental bite exposure.[25,26] Although repetitive mosquito bites increase the chance of disease transmission, the actual immune reaction to mosquito bites is significantly diminished after repetitive heavy exposure, consistent with desensitization of IgE-mediated immune reactions.[27]

The fourth pathogenetic category involves dissemination to the skin of toxins produced by infectious agents.[8] The causative microorganisms are typically localized and distant from the skin. Representative examples are toxic shock syndrome, streptococcal scarlet fever, and staphylococcal scalded skin syndrome.[8,28] Depending on the specific agent involved and the host response, diffuse erythema or vesiculobullous lesions can be seen. Significant hemodynamic instability is often produced by the toxins as well.

The fifth category relates to the mechanical disruption of normal cutaneous homeostatic mechanisms resulting in pathologic changes in the skin and its supporting structures. Lymphatic filariasis, with its inflammatory and physical distortion of the normal lymphatic structures, is a good example of this category.[29,30] The resulting lymphedema and increased susceptibility to infection both contribute to the skin changes that can occur over time. Similarly, lesions that form ulcers significantly increase the likelihood of secondary bacterial infection, usually prevented by an intact dermal–epidermal layer. This is often compounded by the limited hygiene available in many developing countries to both natives and travelers.

A sixth category is less well understood but involves an apparently systemic immunologic pathogenesis. Examples include erythema nodosum (Fig. 126-1), classic erythema multiforme, and Stevens-Johnson syndrome (referred to by some as erythema multiforme major or exudativum; Plate 126-1). In some cases of erythema multiforme, herpes simplex virus or *Mycoplasma pneumoniae* organisms have been found in the skin of such lesions, but most cases in this category do not show cutaneous antigen localization or toxin production.[31–38] Infectious, noninfectious, and idiopathic causes are seen in this category. Infectious agents associated with erythema nodosum (Box 126-1) and erythema multiforme (Box 126-2) include bacteria, mycobacteria, fungi, viruses, and helminths. In addition, most serious cutaneous manifestations due to medications are mediated through this mechanism.[39–41] This is especially important in the context of traveling patients since most have been given new medications for prophylactic or empiric use, and many take medications chronically.

Owing to the varied nature of medication-related cutaneous reactions, it is useful to consider drug reactions as a separate category, although some overlap exists with the aforementioned categories. A section has been included at the end of this chapter to document the spectrum of cutaneous reactions reported with medications commonly prescribed for people traveling to developing or tropical countries.

Box 126-1 Differential Diagnosis of Erythema Nodosum in the Traveler

Bacteria

Bartonella spp. (cat-scratch disease)
Brucella spp.
Chlamydia trachomatis (lymphogranuloma venereum)
Chlamydia psittaci (psitticosis)
Streptococcal infections
Francisella tularensis
Yersinia spp., *Campylobacter* spp., *Salmonella* spp. (diarrheal diseases)

Mycobacteria

Mycobacterium tuberculosis
Mycobacterium leprae
Mycobacterium marinum

Viruses

Cytomegalovirus
Epstein-Barr virus
Hepatitis C virus
Vaccinia (smallpox inoculation agent)

Fungi

Blastomycosis
Cryptococcosis
Coccidioidomycosis
Histoplasmosis
Trichophyton: deep-seated infection

Protozoa

Giardia lamblia

Helminths

Ascaris lumbricoides
Filariases (especially *Wuchereria bancrofti*)
Trypanosomiasis, African

Drugs

Noninfectious: systemic lupus erythematosus, sarcoid, pregnancy, Crohn's disease, ulcerative colitis, and Behçet's syndrome
Idiopathic (Up to 40%)

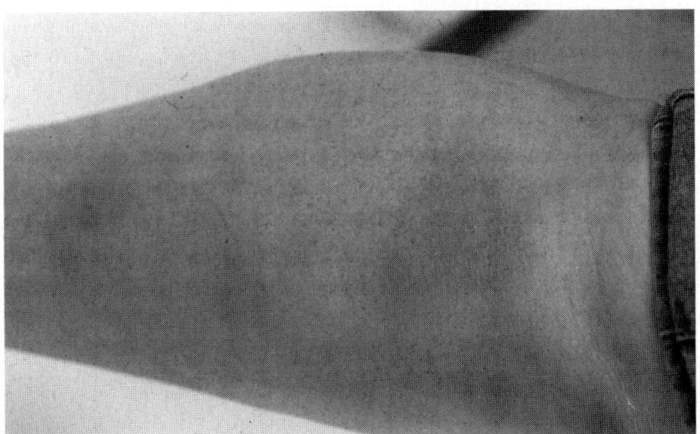

FIGURE 126-1 Erythema nodosum. (Courtesy of Kenneth J. Tomecki, MD, Cleveland, OH.)

GENERAL APPROACH TO THE PATIENT

In approaching patients with rash and tropical exposure, there are three important steps to help define the diagnostic possibilities. First, the patient's general medical and exposure history needs to be obtained.[42] Second, the rash should be accurately defined based on morphology (e.g., macule, papule, vesicle, and nodule), location, and distribution.[43,44] Third, associated clinical information gathered from a complete medical history and physical examination needs to be integrated. Such information includes a medication list, any sensations associated with the rash, pigmentation, migratory nature, duration, and changes in the rash over time. Ancillary clinical information not directly related to the rash must also be considered,

Box 126-2 Causes of Erythema Multiforme in the Traveler*

Bacteria
Chlamydia spp.
Proteus spp.
Francisella tularensis
Salmonella spp.
Staphylococcus spp.
Streptococci, hemolytic
Vibrio spp.
Yersinia spp.
Mycoplasma pneumoniae

Mycobacteria
Mycobacterium tuberculosis

Viruses
Herpes simplex virus types 1 and 2 (commonly associated)
Epstein-Barr virus
Adenovirus
Coxsackievirus (especially B5)
Orf virus

Fungi
Histoplasmosis
Coccidioidomycosis

Parasites
Cutaneous larva migrans
Trichomonas

Drugs
Nonsteroidal anti-inflammatory agents
Antituberculosis drugs
Sulfonamides

Case Reports
Mebendazole
Mefloquine
Albendazole
Streptococcal toxic shock syndrome

Idiopathic (Up to 50%)

*Important to differentiate from giant urticaria and Stevens-Johnson syndrome (erythema multiforme major).

including other organ system involvement and the results of laboratory tests.

Patients often present to health care providers with a specific rash, which provides a starting point for the evaluation and subsequent construction of the differential diagnosis.[45,46] The importance of careful characterization of the rash cannot be overemphasized. This chapter is organized to provide important general information regarding the evaluation of patients with rash who have international exposure and includes tables organized by the character of the specific lesion or primary associated symptom to facilitate the practical usefulness of the information. The primary focus is on parasite-associated skin conditions and those nonparasitic conditions that are more prevalent in tropical and subtropical climates. The reader is encouraged to refer to standard dermatology texts for additional information on rash-associated disorders when tropical exposure is deemed to represent an incidental component of the medical history.[47] In addition, important ancillary information has been included in the expanded tables to allow for more rapid review of the differential diagnosis. Efforts have been made to include the most common and most differentiating information to facilitate diagnosis in individual cases. It is hoped that the information will help focus the subsequent evaluation. When the disease listed refers to another table, this indicates that the condition is less commonly associated with the specific dermatologic presentation covered in that table compared with the listings with full text.

Most of the tables based on presenting manifestation in this chapter (see Tables 126-6 and 126-8 to 126-11) include information about the geographic distribution of the disease entities. They also provide acquisition and incubation information together with parasite survival times to help assess which diagnoses fit the medical history of exposure. Common associated findings are included since cutaneous findings are often not the sole problem but, rather, one aspect of a multisystem disorder. The presence or absence of specific associated findings may also help the provider to focus further evaluation by knowing what other things to look for to rule in or rule out a specific diagnostic consideration. The additional information column is intended to comment on helpful details associated with a specific condition or unique findings that may lead to a diagnosis apart from other possibilities.

This chapter focuses on evaluation and the approach to patients with cutaneous manifestations of travel or tropically acquired conditions and does not include expanded information on the details of specific diseases. Common diseases found primarily in the developed world are often not included for the sake of focus and brevity. We have also left discussions of prognosis and treatment to the chapters in this book dealing with the various diseases.

History

A detailed history is the essential starting point in the evaluation of a patient with a skin rash or cutaneous lesion who has traveled abroad. Box 126-3 outlines important points to consider when performing a history in this setting. In broad terms, the history has three main components. First is information about the patient, second is information about the patient's exposure to possible pathogens, and third is a detailed history regarding the rash.[47] As a general rule, travel within the past 3 months is more likely to be relevant to the diagnosis of an acute illness than more remote travel.[47,48]

The age of the patient is important because it has implications regarding disease prevalence, vaccine status, and types of exposures. Moreover, the character of the rash produced by a pathogen may differ depending on the age of the patient. For example, congenital toxoplasmosis and adult-acquired toxoplasmosis have different skin manifestations when rash is present. The skin lesions of congenital disease are usually papular or hemorrhagic with occasional petechial, nodular, bullous, or erythrodermic changes.[49] In adult-acquired disease, rash is much less common, but when present it is frequently maculopapular with centripetal spread. Rare lichenoid, purpuric, vesiculobullous, and urticarial presentations have been described.[50,51]

Box 126-3 Important Historical Aspects in the Traveler with Rash

Patient Demographics

Age
Sex
Occupation
Reason for travel (vacation vs. business vs. other)
Medications, allergies, immunizations
Pretravel evaluation (compliance with pretravel recommendations?)
Medical conditions that may alter immune status
Time interval from travel dates to onset of symptoms

Exposure

Geographic location
Description of location
Duration of exposure
Vector exposure (precautions taken?)
Animal exposure (wild vs. domestic)
List of items purchased (e.g., animal hide rugs, nickel-containing jewelry)
Sexual contact with new partners
Parenteral exposure (e.g., vaccine or injection abroad, acupuncture, tattoos, poultices on open sores)
Immigrant?
- Country of origin
- Age on arrival in developed country
- Frequency and duration of return visits

Rash-related information
- Prodromal symptoms
- Character
- Distribution
- Progression
  - Speed
  - Physical pattern
- Relation to fever
- Previous treatment and efficacy

The underlying immune status of the patient also has important implications regarding the differential diagnosis. Immunosuppressed travelers may be at increased risk of acquiring intestinal protozoa, including *Giardia lamblia*, *Isospora belli*, *Entamoeba histolytica*, and *Cryptosporidium parvum*.[52,53] Once infected, several reports document a more prolonged and more symptomatic infection in patients with altered cellular or humoral immunity.[54–57] Common organisms in the environment, such as *Candida* spp., *Cryptococcus neoformans*, *Pneumocystis carinii*, and *Mycobacterium tuberculosis*, are also a greater threat to travelers with weakened immune systems. Interestingly, there is little evidence that human immunodeficiency virus (HIV) infection increases the rate of helminthic infection or decreases the efficacy of treatment, with the limited exception of strongyloidiasis.[58] Immunosuppressed patients who have a history of international travel may have acquired long-lived and latent organisms such as toxoplasmosis that may lead to possible dissemination and symptomatic reactivation long after the time of travel.[59,60] Examples of other developing-world diseases with the potential for reactivation or dissemination include coccidioidomycosis, histoplasmosis, hepatitis B, leishmaniasis, strongyloidiasis, and *Trypanosoma cruzi* infection.[61] In addition, the high prevalence and intrinsically persistent nature of members of the herpesvirus family (herpes simplex virus, cytomegalovirus, Epstein-Barr virus, and varicella-zoster virus) result in frequent reactivation during immunosuppression.[62] Herpesvirus reactivation may also be triggered by sun exposure and stress, both of which can increase with travel to developing countries.[63]

Current, chronic, and travel-related medication use and vaccine status are crucial demographic data that may help to reveal a cause (e.g., drug reaction) or tailor the differential diagnostic considerations for the traveler with a new rash. For example, in a patient with petechiae after travel to central Africa, the level of compliance with antimalarials or whether meningococcal vaccination was performed prior to travel can significantly influence the weighting of the considerations in the differential diagnosis.

Details related to the specific exposures of an individual patient are a crucial aspect of the history. Issues to elucidate include potential exposure to the etiologic agent directly, the vectors that may harbor the pathogen, and personal behavior(s) that alters the likelihood of exposure to a given agent. In most cases, these issues involve overlapping considerations, as discussed later.

The possibility of direct exposure is usually higher if travel includes significant rural exposure. A travel itinerary that includes only short stays in first-class hotels in major urban centers is less likely to result in the acquisition of a tropical disease than extended treks in underdeveloped areas of the country. However, the food preparer at a first-class resort may come from an impoverished area where hepatitis A is highly prevalent and may inadvertently contaminate the food prepared in such settings.[64]

Casual sexual contact is an example of potential direct exposure in which choice of protection use controls the relative risk of disease acquisition. Because sexually transmitted diseases (STDs) rank high on lists of disease prevalence in travelers, a sexual history is an essential part of the exposure evaluation.[1,65] Moreover, many STDs, such as primary HIV, secondary syphilis, and the group of genital ulcerative conditions, have prominent cutaneous findings (Table 126-1 and Plate 126-2D). A survey of malaria and sexual preventive measures found equivalent knowledge of the risks of malaria, HIV, and other STDs. However, whereas 87% of travelers adhered to malaria chemoprophylaxis recommendations, 50% of travelers engaged in casual sexual encounters abroad, with 38% of those unprotected.[66] Of note, those who engaged in high-risk sexual practices were not the same group that were noncompliant with malaria protective measures.

Vector exposure related to geography, types of vectors present, and intensity of exposure all need to be considered. Many tropical diseases have a very defined distribution, making geographic exposure very important. The risk of malaria and its pattern of drug resistance can vary greatly, even within a country such as Thailand or Kenya.[67] Malaria is uncommon in most urban centers, whereas yellow fever can be found there, reflective of the breeding patterns of the specific mosquito vectors transmitting malaria and yellow fever, respectively.[68] In addition to location, the duration and intensity of vector and pathogen exposure are also important. Some diseases, such as schistosomiasis, may be readily acquired after a single

Table 126-1 Dermatologic Manifestations of Sexually Transmitted Diseases

Disease	Ulcer	Nodule	Maculopapular	Pigment Change	Lymphadenopathy	Other
Chancroid	X (p)				X (p, L)	
Donovanosis	X (nt)					
Gonorrhea			Dissem disease			
Granuloma inguinale	X (nt)	X			Pseudobubo	Occasional painful necrotic ulcer
HIV			1°		X (nt, G)	
Herpes simplex virus	X (p)					Vesicle ulcerates
Lymphogranuloma venereum	X (nt)	X			X (p, L)	
Syphilis, endemic (bejel)	X (nt)	X		↓ (late)	X (G)	
Syphilis, venereal	X (nt)		2°		2° (L, G)	Occasional oropharyngeal mucous patches
Yaws	X (nt)		X	↓ (late)	X (L)	
Scabies		X	X			

G, generalized lymphadenopathy; HIV, human immunodeficiency virus; L, localized lymphadenopathy; nt, nontender; p, painful; 1°, primary disease; 2°, secondary disease; ↓, hypopigmented.

exposure to an infected water source. Other diseases, such as malaria or lymphatic filariasis, usually require repetitive mosquito exposure since even in endemic areas the vast majority of mosquitoes are not infectious.[69,70] If closed shoes are consistently worn, the likelihood of acquiring cutaneous penetrating helminths, such as hookworm or *Strongyloides stercoralis*, is greatly reduced.[16,71]

Recent exposure is typically most important, especially exposure within the past 3 months. However, as noted in the tables, malaria, many helminths, and other tropically acquired pathogens can persist for months to years in the human host, requiring their consideration in selected clinical settings well beyond the actual time of travel.[42] In such cases, the presentation is typically subacute or chronic, although it may be punctuated by acute episodic illness. For example, vivax malaria has a typical incubation period of 2 weeks but may first present 8 months after leaving a malarious area. In addition, recrudescence may occur up to 5 years later in untreated patients.[72] Another example is lymphatic filariasis, which may have a relatively asymptomatic early phase but later can present with either subacute or chronic lymphedema or secondary cellulitis related to the disrupted lymphatics. The importance of understanding the life cycles of common parasitic pathogens and their impact on the patient's history is illustrated by *L. loa* infection. *Loa loa*-associated symptoms often require at least 6 months to appear and can first present as late as 18 months after the last possible exposure.[73] This is because microfilarial production typically takes 6 or more months to commence and the host immune response is primarily directed against the microfilariae rather than the adult worms. Adult worms in lymphatic filariasis and *L. loa* can persist for up to 10 years without reexposure.[74] Because of an autoinfective cycle, *S. stercoralis* infections acquired decades earlier can result in risk to people who require immunosuppression many years after their disease exposure and acquisition.[75,76]

Another exposure-related issue is whether the patient is a lifelong resident of a developed world country or has emigrated to a developed country recently or remotely. Expatriates are much more likely to have an allergic or hypersensitivity form of *L. loa* infection compared to the local population.[77] The frequency and duration of return visits to tropical areas may be very important information in creating the proper differential diagnosis. Malaria may be significantly more severe in people who have returned to an endemic area after several years away. In addition, people traveling to visit family in developing countries may be less rigorous about seeking pretravel advice and using prophylactic medication, incorrectly believing that their prior exposures are protective. Rarely, the "traveler" may not be the index patient one is evaluating but, rather, a friend or worker who has significant contact with the patient. For example, reports of cysticercosis in Orthodox Jewish community members in New York who had not traveled outside the United States were associated with employing a housemaid or cook from endemic areas in Central America.[78]

The occupation of the traveler is an important aspect of the history as well. For example, development workers are much more likely to be exposed to soil-, water-, and arthropod-borne diseases than a businessperson with an urban itinerary. Compliance with preventive precaution instructions is important since proper use of protective footwear and avoiding swimming in areas endemic for schistosomiasis, for example, essentially rule out the disease as a diagnostic possibility. Animal exposure will help establish the relative risk of zoonoses for a particular patient.[79]

Questioning the patient about unusual situations or risky behaviors may uncover certain events, such as ingestion of raw seafood or questionable medical interventions, that are relevant. Acupuncture with unsterilized needles carries a risk of hepatitis and HIV transmission. A peculiar route of acquisition of sparganosis is seen when raw frog flesh is used as a poultice. Frogs can function as an intermediate host of this normally feline or canine tapeworm. The pathogen has worldwide distribution.[15] Physicians unaware of alternative medical practices of some immigrant populations usually do not consider such a route of exposure when obtaining a history. Asking about souvenirs purchased may reveal exposure to animal products (e.g., animal skin rugs) that carry the risk of disease transmission, such as brucellosis or anthrax, or to new materials (e.g., nickel-containing jewelry) that can result in allergic contact skin reactions.[80]

Occasionally, the careful history may also help to point to an obsessional concern about the presence of parasites without other evidence to support such a diagnosis. Patients with this preoccupation often present to physicians with a variety of cutaneous lesions described as parasite "tracks" and may bring containers filled with "parasites."[81] Many of these patients have attempted to extract the parasite themselves to present it to the physician. In reality, the dermatoses are self-inflicted injuries. Although cutaneous arthropod infestations can be protean in presentation and very challenging to diagnose, when faced with the presenting constellation noted previously, the possibility of delusional parasitosis should be considered.[82,83]

Specific questions about the rash and any associated clinical symptoms, such as fever pattern, weight loss, diarrhea, and response to treatment, if attempted, are also important for complete evaluation. The symptoms related to the rash may, at times, provide important diagnostic clues. For example, patients with myiasis, produced by cutaneous invasion by larvae of the botfly in Latin America or tumbu fly in Africa, often present with papules, nodules, and subcutaneous swellings and will frequently describe a sensation of movement and intermittent pain at the site of the lesion.

Box 126-4 Important Aspects of the Physical Examination in the Traveler with Rash

Vital signs
General appearance
- Level of toxicity to establish tempo of evaluation and therapy

Primary character of the rash
- Petechial or hemorrhagic
- Macular
- Papular
- Migratory
- Urticarial
- Nodular
- Ulcerative

Secondary character of the rash
- Shape (linear vs. circular vs. irregular)
- Size
- Scale on surface
- Other

Location of primary lesion, if any
Distribution of rash
Direction of spread (centripetal or centrifugal)
Mucosal or conjunctival involvement
Genital involvement
Associated physical findings
- Visible parasite at the site of the rash
- Lymphadenopathy
- Splenomegaly or hepatosplenomegaly

Physical Examination

The physical examination is central to the evaluation of the patient with rash and tropical exposure. A complete examination is important since cutaneous manifestations may be only one component of a systemic disorder. Since the pattern of the rash may be important, the entire skin should be examined with attention to the elements listed in Box 126-4. Repeat examination over time may be necessary. The rapidity of spread can have implications regarding the aggressiveness of the evaluation. The general level of toxicity and the nature and tempo of the pattern of the rash dictate the initial evaluation and therapeutic approach. Although only 7% of cases with petechiae and fever will turn out to be meningococcemia,[84] the life-threatening nature of meningococcal disease requires an aggressive evaluation and often empirical therapy when this diagnosis is a consideration.[7,8]

The classification of the rash is often the focal entry point into the creation of a differential diagnosis.[4–6] As a result, the primary and secondary character of the rash should be carefully determined (see Box 126-4). Diagnostic considerations based on the information obtained are discussed under Characterizing the Rash. Some rashes are fleetingly present, such as *Salmonella* spp. rose spots. Other rashes may evolve in relatively unique patterns over time, such as anthrax, Rocky Mountain spotted fever (RMSF), and dengue.[21,85–89] Cutaneously acquired anthrax characteristically evolves from a papule to a vesicle with surrounding brawny, gelatinous edema, and occasional satellite vesicles[85,86] (Fig. 126-2). The lesion then progresses to hemorrhage and necrosis, eventually turning into an eschar. RMSF skin changes are often absent in the first few days of clinical illness. Then a macular rash typically starts on the wrists and ankles with centripetal spread.[21] During progression, the rash usually becomes petechial or purpuric or both (Fig. 126-3). Dengue fever rash often begins as a transient macular exanthem approximately 24 hours after the abrupt onset of fever. Three or 4 days later, a generalized maculopapular truncal rash appears, with centripetal spread, sparing the palms and soles (Fig. 126-4). This rash may become petechial and may even desquamate.[87–89]

The original and subsequent distribution of the rash, consideration of mucosal (enanthem) or genital involvement, and

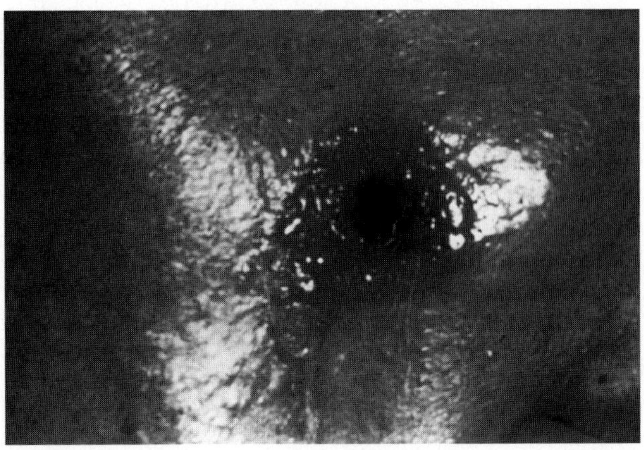

FIGURE 126-2 Cutaneous anthrax showing characteristic central eschar with surrounding edema and vesicles. (Courtesy of Kenneth J. Tomecki, MD, Cleveland, OH.)

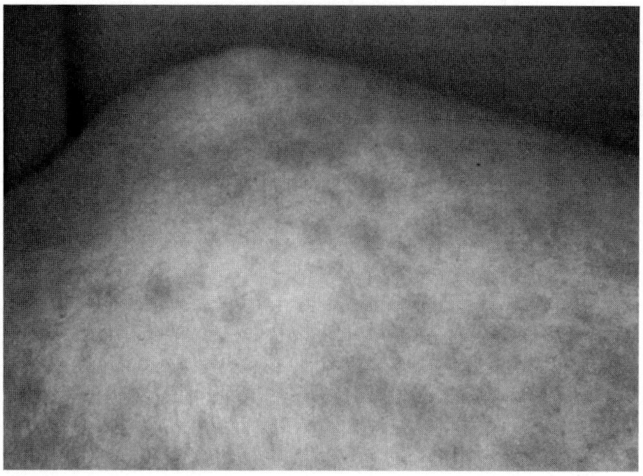

FIGURE 126-3 Early macular rash of Rocky Mountain spotted fever. Papular and petechial changes are often seen. The rash typically begins around the wrists and ankles.

other associated physical findings may be helpful in establishing a diagnosis. The presence of lymphadenopathy (Box 126-5) and splenomegaly or hepatosplenomegaly (Box 126-6) are examples of findings that may help focus the evaluation. If a primary lesion or an inoculation site can be determined, it should be given careful attention. For example, an eschar would indicate rickettsial disease or anthrax (Table 126-2), whereas periorbital swelling in a child soon after a visit to rural Brazil would focus the evaluation on Chagas' disease. The presence of a visible parasite at the site of the rash is also quite helpful in narrowing the differential diagnosis. For example, in some patients with myiasis who present with papular or nodular lesions that may resemble boils, a central opening termed a breathing pore is sometimes present from which larvae of the botfly or the tumbu fly may emerge. In some patients with dracunculiasis, the visible presence of the worm protruding from the skin establishes the diagnosis. Patients with tungiasis, produced by the female jigger or sand flea, *Tunga penetrans*, often present with nodules on the feet with a central dark punctum, which represents the flea's posterior abdominal segments. Despite these examples in which the appearance of the rash can point to the diagnosis, the appearance of the rash is often not pathognomonic of a single disease entity.

Characterizing the Rash

The careful identification of the primary and secondary character of the rash will facilitate the creation of a differential diagnosis, especially when integrated with the clinical history and other associated physical findings. After defining the rash, the reader should refer to the table related to that characteristic to help with diagnosing the individual patient. The role of tropical exposure is highlighted here.

Significant medical conditions with prominent cutaneous manifestations may be due to common pathogens with worldwide distribution despite exposure to specific tropical pathogens. For example, although petechiae in the recently returned febrile traveler may represent malaria, dengue, or even Lassa fever, it is still crucial to consider meningococcemia, rickettsial disease, and other diagnoses. Table 126-3 identifies life-threatening diagnoses with cutaneous manifestations that are seen throughout the temperate and tropical world.[7,8]

Hemorrhage and Petechiae

Hemorrhagic or petechial rashes (Table 126-4) must be considered of life-threatening importance and evaluated rapidly.[7,8,21] Although many nonlethal rashes have this presentation, it is difficult, if not impossible, to rule out serious pathogens at the initial evaluation. Worldwide, meningococcemia is the most important cause of life-threatening disease presenting with fever and hemorrhage or petechiae. It is endemic in central Africa and sporadically epidemic in Brazil, India, Nepal, and Saudi Arabia (especially at the Hajj). Vaccination is available and efficacious.[90] Infection-mediated petechial or purpuric

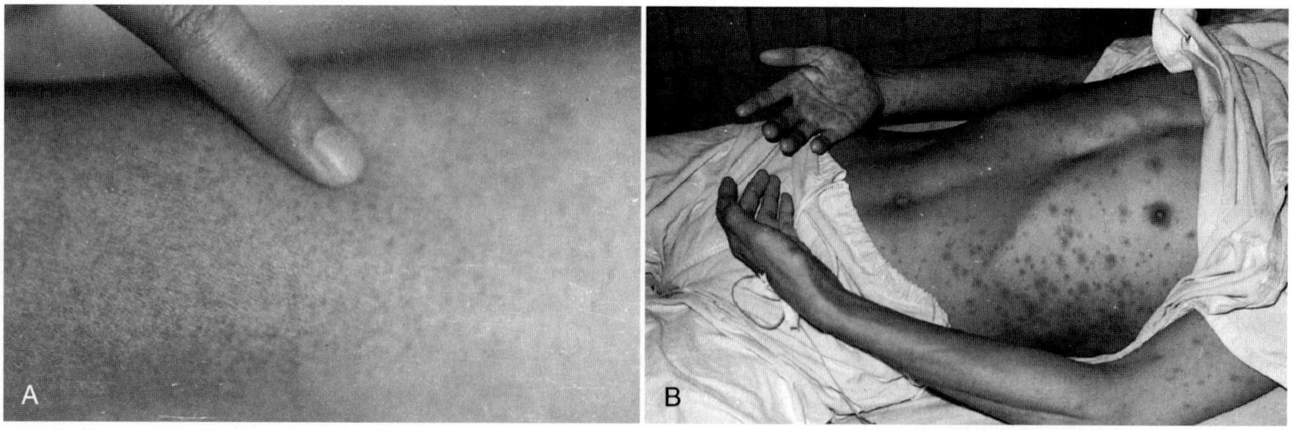

FIGURE 126-4 Cutaneous manifestations of dengue. *A*, Early maculopapular nonpruritic rash usually seen at the time of defervescence. *B*, Late hemorrhagic and purpuric skin changes of a patient with dengue hemorrhagic fever. (Courtesy of James H. Maguire, MD, Centers for Disease Control and Prevention, Atlanta, GA.)

Box 126-5 Differential Diagnosis of Rash with Lymphadenopathy in the Traveler

Helminths

Lymphatic filariasis
- *Brugia malayi*
- *Brugia timori*
- *Wuchereria bancrofti*

Loiasis
Mansonelliasis
Onchocerciasis
Opisthorchiasis
Schistosomiasis (Katayama fever)

Protozoa

Leishmaniasis
- Cutaneous and mucocutaneous
- Visceral

Toxoplasmosis
Trypanosomiasis
- African
- American

Fungi

Coccidioidomycosis
Chromomycosis
Cryptococcosis
Histoplasmosis
Lobomycosis
Paracoccidioidomycosis
Penicilliosis marneffei
Sporotrichosis

Bacteria

Numerous

Viruses

Numerous, including primary human immunodeficiency virus

lesions may arise directly from infected emboli or via an indirect immunologic mechanism. Thrombocytopenia from a variety of causes may also lead to purpuric or petechial lesions. Excellent data on the severity and mortality of severe adverse drug reactions, including hemorrhagic or petechial presentations, are found in a review.[39]

Macules and Papules

Macules are flat lesions with altered pigmentation less than 1 cm in size. A *patch* is a macule greater than 1 cm in diameter. A *papule* is a solid elevated lesion less than 1 cm, whereas a *plaque* is used to describe a similar lesion larger than 1 cm or a group of confluent papules.

In general, macules, papules, and maculopapular eruptions are the most common cutaneous manifestations of infectious diseases and imply an inflammatory response to the inciting pathogen. Viral and bacterial diseases are the most common causes (Table 126-5).[91] Some specific tropical bacterial and viral disorders associated with macular, papular, or maculopapular rashes include anthrax, bartonellosis (Fig. 126-5), brucellosis, glanders, leptospirosis, Lyme disease, melioidosis, plague, relapsing fever, *Rickettsia* infections (especially typhus and trench fever), tularemia, yaws, meningococcemia, dengue, rat-bite fever, secondary syphilis, tuberculosis, and *Vibrio vulnificus* infection. Many other viral pathogens acquired in the tropics are commonly associated with maculopapular eruptions. Most of the viral hemorrhagic fevers progress from macular exanthems to a maculopapular form prior to developing a hemorrhagic appearance.[87,89,92] Although often unappreciated, the acute illness associated with HIV seroconversion may be accompanied by a transient maculopapular dermatitis in approximately 50% of patients.[93,94] Protozoan parasites rarely cause macular or papular rashes.

Box 126-6 Differential Diagnosis of Rash with Splenomegaly or Hepatosplenomegaly in the Traveler

Organomegaly commonly associated
- Brucellosis
- Ehrlichiosis
- Epstein-Barr virus infection
- Glanders (*Burkholderia mallei*)
- Leishmaniasis, visceral
- Penicilliosis (*Penicillium marneffei*)
- Q fever
- Relapsing fever (*Borrelia recurrentis*)
- Schistosomiasis (*Schistosoma mansoni, Schistosoma japonicum*)
- Trypanosomiasis (*Trypanosoma cruzi*)

Organomegaly occasionally associated
- Cytomegalovirus infection
- Histoplasmosis
- Leptospirosis
- Malaria
- Psittacosis
- Rocky Mountain spotted fever (*Rickettsia rickettsii*)
- Typhoid fever
- Scrub typhus (*Rickettsia tsutsugamushi*)

Organomegaly rarely associated
- Babesiosis
- Drug reaction
- Serum sickness

***Table 126-2** Diagnostic Considerations in the Traveler with an Eschar*

Pathogen	Condition (Vector)
Rickettsia africae	African tick bite fever
Rickettsia akari	Rickettsialpox (mite)
Rickettsia australis	Queensland coastal fever (tick)
Rickettsia conorii	Mediterranean spotted fever (tick)
Rickettsia sibirica	North Asian tick typhus
Rickettsia tsutsugamushi	Scrub typhus (mite)
Bacillus anthracis	Anthrax*
Loxosceles reclusa	Brown recluse spider bite

*Usually transmitted by contact with infected animals or their products, rarely mechanically via biting flies or insects.

Table 126-3 Life-Threatening Conditions with Cutaneous Manifestations

Cutaneous Manifestation	Pathogen	Time to Appearance (after Onset of Illness)	Pathophysiology
Peripheral gangrene	Gram-negative bacteria	12–36 hr	Vascular thrombosis due to shock
Scattered, multiple petechiae and purpura	*Neisseria meningitidis* *Rickettsia rickettsii* Gram-negative bacteria	12–36 hr (later for *Rickettsia*)	Vascular invasion (?) Schwartzman reaction
Ecthyma gangrenosum	*Pseudomonas* spp. Gram-negative bacteria	Days	Vascular invasion, mostly venous
Asymmetrical scattered maculopapular rash	*N. meningitidis* *Neisseria gonorrhoeae*	3–10 days	Immune vasculitis due to immune complex deposition
Polymorphous lesions	*N. meningitidis* *N. gonorrhoeae* *Salmonella* spp.	3–10 days	Immune vasculitis
Rose spots	*Salmonella* spp.	5–10 days	Immune vasculitis
Osler's nodes; small (<1 cm) painful nodular erythema	*Staphylococcus aureus*	Days to weeks	Emboli from endocarditis with microabscesses
Janeway lesions: small or large (>1 cm) painless, purpuric or pustular, infarcted lesions	*Streptococcus* spp.	Days to weeks	Emboli from endocarditis
Diffuse toxic erythema	*S. aureus* *Streptococcus pyogenes*	Minutes	Vascular toxin with peripheral vasodilation
Macronodules	*Candida* spp.	Several days	Vascular invasion of dermis
Progressive petechiae and purpura (distinctive periumbilical purpura)	*Strongyloides stercoralis* (hyperinfection syndrome)	Hours to days from immunosuppression	? Larval skin penetration ? Immune vasculitis
Petechiae, purpura, hemorrhage	Viral hemorrhagic fevers	Within 3 wk of exposure	Immune vasculitis (disseminated intravascular coagulation) Thrombocytopenia Decreased clotting factor synthesis

The exceptions are toxoplasmosis, African trypanosomiasis, and some forms of both cutaneous and visceral leishmaniasis[51,95–98] (Fig. 126-6). Fungal infections usually manifest a nodular or ulcerative appearance (Plate 126-2E)[99]; however, coccidioidomycosis may have a maculopapular presentation.[100] Helminthic infections rarely have a papular or macular appearance, although some forms of chronic onchocerciasis occasionally present this way.[12,101,102] Arthropod bites (e.g., mosquito bites) and infestations (e.g., scabies), together with water-related exposures to some diatoms, venomous fish, jellyfish, or sea urchins, commonly result in a toxin-mediated papular eruption.[17,21,22] This type of rash is also common in

Table 126-4 Differential Diagnosis of a Petechial or Purpuric Rash after Travel or Tropical Exposure

Organism	Disease	Comment
Bacteria		
Borrelia spp.	Relapsing fever	
Enterococcus and viridans steptococci	Endocarditis	HACEK organisms as well
Haemophilus influenzae, Haemophilus aegyptius	Brazilian purpuric fever	Purulent conjunctivitis; mostly children ages 1–4 yr
Leptospira interrogans		
Neisseria meningitidis	Meningococcemia	
Neisseria gonorrhoeae	Gonococcemia	
Burkholderia pseudomallei	Melioidosis	
Pseudomonas aeruginosa	Ecthyma gangrenosum	
Streptobacillus moniliformis	Rat-bite fever	Different from *Spirillum minus*
Treponema pallidum	Syphilis (especially congenital)	
Yersinia pestis	Plague (septicemic)	"Black death" referred to purpura
Rickettsia prowazekii	Epidemic typhus	
Rickettsia typhi	Murine typhus	
Rickettsia rickettsii	Rocky Mountain spotted fever	Often on wrists and ankles
Vibrio vulnificus		

Continued

Table 126-4 Differential Diagnosis of a Petechial or Purpuric Rash after Travel or Tropical Exposure—Cont'd

Organism	Disease	Comment
Viruses		
Alphaviruses		
Enteroviruses		
Cytomegalovirus		Especially congenital
Colorado tick fever		
Measles	Atypical measles	
Lassa fever		
Dengue		
Junin	Argentine hemorrhagic fever	
Machupo	Bolivian hemorrhagic fever	
Chikungunya		
Crimean–Congo hemorrhagic fever		Tick bite; contact with infected blood
Ebola		
Hantavirus	Hemorrhagic fever with renal syndrome	Aerosol from rodent excreta
Kyasanur Forest		
Marburg		
Omsk hemorrhagic fever		
Rift Valley fever		Mosquito bite; aerosol or contact with fresh carcasses of infected animals
Yellow fever		
Protozoa		
Plasmodium falciparum	Malaria	
Toxoplasma gondii	Toxoplasmosis	Especially congenital
Helminths		
Trichinella spiralis	Trichinellosis	

the setting of drug hypersensitivity reactions.[39] Note that some arthropod bites/exposures may persist for weeks as immunologic reactions (e.g., papular urticaria) beyond the actual exposure, without indicating persistence of the organism. Fever is seen with many, although not all, skin reactions manifesting as macules or papules, possibly reflective of the systemic immune mechanism responsible for many maculopapular rashes.

Migratory Rash

Migratory lesions are somewhat unique to parasites (Table 126-6). They represent a common cause of cutaneous lesions in travelers to tropical countries.[5] In some cases, such as cutaneous and visceral larva migrans,[103] humans are accidental hosts. The parasite is hence unable to complete its normal life cycle, resulting in continued wandering of the infecting larva through the skin.[85] Cutaneous larva migrans (CLM) (Fig. 126-7A and B) due to canine and feline hookworm species is the classic presentation; a differential diagnosis of this subset of migratory dermatoses is presented in Table 126-7.[16,104–107] Human hookworm (Fig. 126-7C) and strongyloidosis will occasionally manifest skin changes during initial or reinfective cutaneous penetration.[16,104] *Dracunculus medinensis* may produce superficial migratory skin lesions at the completion of its life cycle, prior to expulsion of the adult through the skin.[12] Parasite-associated eosinophilia is primarily related to the tissue migratory phase of the life cycle. As a result, parasitic conditions characterized by migratory lesions often have an especially intense eosinophilia.[108–110] Lyme disease is a nonparasitic disease that may present with an expanding macular rash—erythema chronicum migrans.[111]

Pruritus and Urticaria

A common manifestation of inflammatory skin conditions is pruritus (Table 126-8). Often, the inciting pathogen, drug, or irritant causes an immune response characterized by IgE production and subsequent histamine release by mast cells in sensitized people. As a result, pruritus is often accompanied by urticarial lesions. Classic syndromes include the intense itching seen following exposure to avian schistosome cercariae in IgE-sensitized people (swimmer's itch)[17,18] and the pruritic migratory angioedema seen with *L. loa* infections[77] (Fig. 126-8). Most helminthic parasites are capable of inducing an urticarial response, although it is uncommon. Helminthic infections in which humans are accidental hosts, such as CLM, gnathostomiasis, and sparganosis, are very likely to present this way due to the continued presence of the parasite in the skin. Human helminthic infections with cutaneous penetrating or cutaneous resident parasites, such as hookworm, strongyloidiasis, onchocerciasis, and loiasis, also frequently cause pruritus and urticaria. Hence, there is overlap with many of the migratory parasites. Some myiasis infestations are pruritic, especially when the larvae move.[112,113] Pruritus and/or urticaria are rare presentations of *Giardia lamblia*, but its worldwide distribution

Table 126-5 Differential Diagnosis of Macular and Maculopapular Rashes after Travel or Tropical Exposure

Organism/Agent	Disease
Epstein-Barr virus	Mononucleosis
Dengue virus	Dengue fever*
Lassa fever virus	Lassa fever
Marburg virus	
West Nile virus	West Nile fever†
Rickettsia typhi	Endemic (murine) typhus
Rickettsia prowazekii	Epidemic (louse) typhus
Rickettsia quintana	Trench fever
Coxiella burnetii	Q fever
Bacillus anthracis	Anthrax*
Spirillum minus	Rat-bite fever
Streptobacillus moniliformis	Rat-bite fever
Leptospira spp.	Leptospirosis
Yersinia pestis	Plague
Salmonella typhi	Typhoid fever (rose spots)
Borrelia burgdorferi	Lyme disease Erythema chronica migrans
Borrelia recurrentis	Relapsing fever
Bartonella bacilliformis	Bartonellosis
Brucella spp.	Brucellosis
Treponema pallidum	Syphilis (secondary syphilis)
Coccidioides immitis	Coccidioidomycosis
Toxoplasma gondii	Toxoplasmosis
Strongyloides stercoralis	Strongyloidiasis
Onchocerca volvulus	Onchocerciasis
Leishmania spp.	Leishmaniasis (some visceral forms, rare cutaneous forms)
Ancylostoma duodenale and *Necator americanus*	Hookworm disease
Human immunodeficiency virus (HIV)	Primary HIV infection
Drug	

*Only at onset; later, hemorrhage.
†50% rash late in course of 3 to 6 day fever.

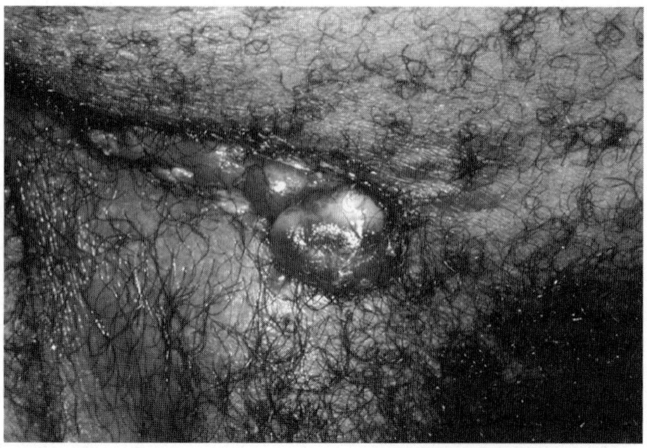

FIGURE 126-5 Bacillary angiomatosis in a patient with HIV infection. Typical friable, exophytic papulonodular changes and violaceous hue are noted. (Courtesy of Karim A. Adal, MD, Minneapolis, MN.)

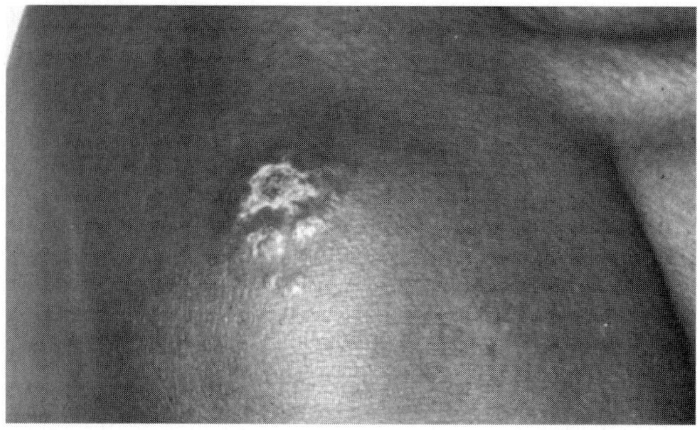

FIGURE 126-6 Cutaneous leishmaniasis lesion demonstrating characteristic painless papular, nodular, and ulcerative lesions with serum crusting.

and relative prevalence reinforce the need for consideration of this parasite in the differential diagnosis. Humans have been shown to develop specific IgE antibodies to mosquito saliva and some people may benefit from prophylactic administration of antihistamines, resulting in less intense bite reactions.[25] Nonspecific skin inflammation can also result in pruritus in association with other lesions. Travelers to tropical climates may experience a noninfectious condition known as miliaria rubra (prickly heat) with characteristic itchy papules or vesicles on an erythematous base that are concentrated on the trunk and in flexure areas.[99]

Nodules and Ulcers

A *nodule* is a palpable solid lesion greater than 0.5 to 1.0 cm in diameter. Nodules larger than 2.0 cm are classified as tumors. Most nodules are dermal in location, although occasionally they can arise from the epidermis (Table 126-9). Adult worms of *O. volvulus* typically reside in dermal lymphatics and develop into nodules due to chronic inflammation (Fig. 126-9).[14] Nodules are typically nearer the head in South and Central American disease, but they tend to involve the hips in African onchocerciasis. This difference in nodule location is attributable to preferred biting sites of the vectors. Some helminthic infections, such as dracunculiasis, need to leave the human host via the skin to complete their life cycle; hence, they form a nodule prior to extrusion.[12] In other examples, such as echinococcosis, CLM, sparganosis, and dirofilariasis, humans represent accidental intermediate hosts, which results in developmental arrest of the parasite at the larval stage, typically in skin or muscle tissue. An inflammatory nodule forms around the larva.[114,115] Humans can be the definitive (intestinal) and intermediate host (cysticercosis) for *Taenia solium.* In cysticercosis, subcutaneous nodules are occasionally part of the clinical manifestations.[116]

Although nodules and ulcers are separate dermatologic entities and can arise individually, there is often an association between the two lesions. In many cases, nodular lesions undergo eventual ulceration if the inflammatory process is intense enough to result in destruction of the overlying epidermis. *Ulcers* are defined as skin defects with loss of the epidermis and the

Text continued on page 1514

Table 126-6 Differential Diagnosis of Migratory Skin Lesions

Cause of Migratory Lesions	Distribution	Acquisition	Incubation	Parasite Survival	Common Associated Findings	Additional Information
Cutaneous larva migrans ("creeping eruption") Larval movement of zoonotic nematodes	Worldwide (especially tropics, subtropics)	Skin contact with contaminated soil (especially beaches)	Usually 2–3 days (range, 1–6 days)	Weeks to months	Transient eosinophilia; serpiginous skin lesions can migrate up to several centimeters per day	Dog and cat hookworm; zoonotic *Strongyloides*; humans incidental host; larvae cannot mature, wander in skin
Dracunculiasis Movement of adult worm just below dermis before eruption	Sub-Saharan Africa and India, Pakistan	Ingestion of copepod in drinking water	~1 yr	12–18 mo	Eosinophilia during tissue migration; can see dead calcified worms on radiograph	Adults exit via skin; blisters with eosinophils; rarely ulcerates; reinfection can occur
Fascioliasis Migratory inflammatory lesions	Worldwide except Oceania; sheep and cattle raising areas mostly	Ingestion of metacercariae on watercress or other in-water plants	3–4 mo	≥10 yr	Eosinophilia, abnormal LFT, anemia Early: fever, RUQ pain, jaundice, diarrhea, hepatomegaly Chronic: usually asymptomatic	Rare extrabiliary migration; nodules up to 6 cm; duodenal aspirate may help diagnosis; serology available
Gnathostomiasis Migratory inflammatory lesions	Asia (especially Thailand and Japan); sporadic worldwide	Ingestion of larva in undercooked or raw meat; ingestion of infected copepod in water; rare skin penetration	GI symptoms: 1–2 days; soft tissue swelling in 3–4 wk Other symptoms: months to years	≥10 yr	Eosinophilia common; can migrate anywhere, including CNS	Humans incidental host; larva cannot mature yet migrates in tissues, move 1 cm/hr, or faster when subcutaneous
Hookworm Larval movement during inoculation	Worldwide (especially tropics, subtropics)	Skin contact with contaminated soil	Local skin symptoms: 1–2 days Pulmonary symptoms: 1–3 wk GI symptoms: ~4 wk	*Ancylostoma duodenale:* 1 yr *Necator americanus:* 2–6 yr	Eosinophilia during tissue migration; anemia	Gross or occult blood in stools; eggs appear in 4–6 wk; rare reports of parasite survival for 15–20 yr (? hypobiosis of *A. duodenale*)
Loiasis Migratory inflammatory swellings	Central and West Africa	Bite of infected *Chrysops* fly	~1 yr (range, 4 mo–8 yr)	10 yr	Eosinophilia, increased IgE; expatriates have more hypersensitivity symptoms; microfilariae peak numbers in blood near noon	5–6 mo until microfilariae seen in blood; serology available

Continued

Table 126-6 Differential Diagnosis of Migratory Skin Lesions—Cont'd

Cause of Migratory Lesions	Distribution	Acquisition	Incubation	Parasite Survival	Common Associated Findings	Additional Information
Paragonamiasis Subcutaneous migratory swelling or subcutaneous nodules	Sub-Saharan and southern Africa Americas: all except temperate climates; East and Southeast Asia	Ingestion of metacercariae in raw or undercooked crustaceans	Pulmonary symptoms: 6 mo CNS symptoms: 12–16 mo	≤ 10 yr	Eosinophilia 80%; sputum may have Charcot-Leyden crystals; CXR can have almost any appearance (including 20% normal)	Eggs in sputum, feces, pleural or spinal fluid, first appear in 10 wk
Sparganosis Larval movement	Worldwide (especially tropics; most cases Southeast Asia)	Ingestion of infected copepod in water; ingestion of raw or undercooked meat; use of infected flesh as poultice on open wound	Depends on route of acquisition	≥9 yr	Eosinophilia and leukocytosis during migration	Humans are incidental hosts, hence larva cannot mature; larva can migrate anywhere, including CNS
Strongyloidiasis (*Strongyloides stercoralis*) Migratory, serpiginous lesions of larva (larva currens)	Worldwide (especially tropics, subtropics)	Skin or mucous membrane contact with contaminated soil	Skin and pulmonary symptoms: days Other symptoms: days to decades	Indefinite (autoreinfection possible)	Eosinophilia; skin changes (larva currans) common even in chronic infection; can migrate up to 5–10 cm/hr	Some institutions for mentally impaired may have high rates of infection; ex-POWs can carry asymptomatically for decades
Myiasis Visible movement of maggot(s) or larva(e)	Worldwide (especially tropics)	Many mechanisms depending on fly species; contact with infected arthropods, vegetation, food, clothes; direct inoculation	Depends on fly: *Cordylobia anthropophaga* 7–10 days; *Dermatobia bominis* 5–12 wk	≥2 mo	Occasional eosinophilia; visible movement of maggot(s) within the lesion may be noted; larvae of some Diptera (e.g., *Hypoderma*) migrate in soft tissues	Adult leaves host when mature

CNS, central nervous system; CXR, chest x-ray film; GI, gastrointestinal; LFT, liver function test(s); RUQ, right upper quadrant.

Table 126-7 Causes of Cutaneous Larva Migrans–like Rash

Pathogen	Condition	Usual Host
Common		
Ancylostoma braziliense	Cutaneous larva migrans	Dog and cat hookworm
Ancylostoma caninum		Dog hookworm
Ancylostoma duodenale	Ground itch	Human hookworm
Necator americanus		Human hookworm
Strongyloides stercoralis	Larva currens	Human nematode
Uncommon		
Strongyloides myopotami		Zoonotic *Strongyloides*
Gnathostoma spinigerum		Nematode of dog, cats
		Deep, broad tunnels
Unicinaria stenocephala		Hookworm of European dogs
Bunostomum phlebotomum		Hookworm of cattle
Spirometra sp.	Sparganosis	Tapeworm of dogs, cats
		More commonly visceral than cutaneous
Spirurina sp.	Creeping eruption	?Marine birds or mammals
		Raw fish, squid, shrimp, or turtles may transmit
		Thin, narrow tunnels
		Eosinophilia uncommon

Data from references 16, 104–107.

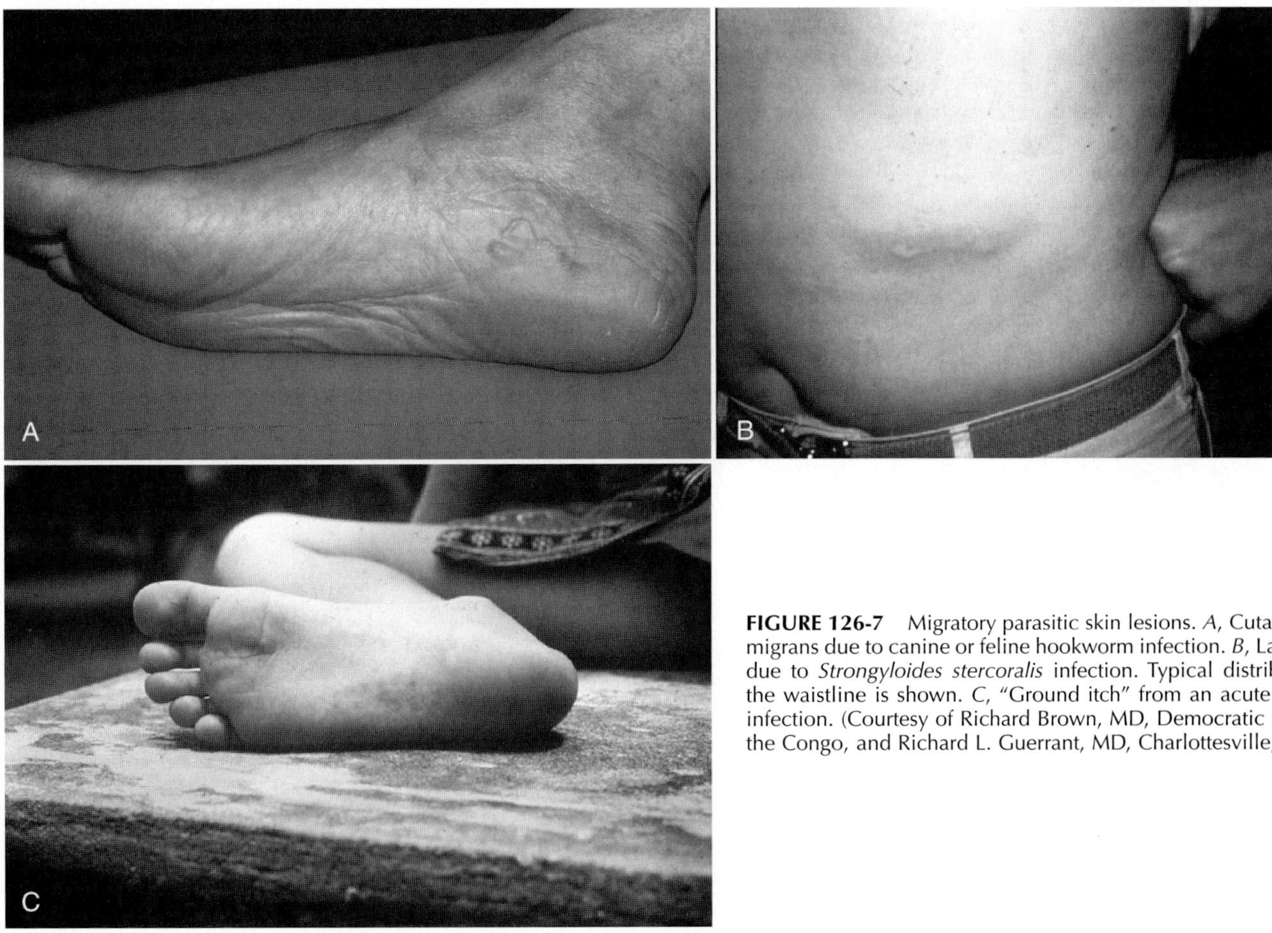

FIGURE 126-7 Migratory parasitic skin lesions. *A*, Cutaneous larva migrans due to canine or feline hookworm infection. *B*, Larva currens due to *Strongyloides stercoralis* infection. Typical distribution near the waistline is shown. *C*, "Ground itch" from an acute hookworm infection. (Courtesy of Richard Brown, MD, Democratic Republic of the Congo, and Richard L. Guerrant, MD, Charlottesville, VA.)

Table 126-8 Differential Diagnosis of Pruritic and Urticarial Skin Lesions

Cause of Pruritic Lesions	Distribution	Acquisition	Incubation	Organism Survival	Common Associated Findings	Additional Information
Helminthic						
Cercarial dermatitis; avian schistosome dermatitis	Worldwide (for all species salt- and freshwater)	Skin contact with cercariae in water	Hours	Unable to survive in human host		Avian and small mammal schistosomes; symptoms increase in severity with repeated exposure
Cutaneous larva migrans	See Table 126-6					
Dracunculiasis	See Table 126-6					
Gnathostomiasis Migratory inflammatory lesions	Asia (especially Thailand and Japan); sporadic worldwide	Ingestion of larva, undercooked or raw meat; ingestion of copepod in water; rare skin penetration	GI symptoms: 1–2 days; soft tissue swelling in 3–4 wk; other symptoms: months to years	≥10 yr	Eosinophilia common; can migrate anywhere, including CNS	Humans incidental host; larvae cannot mature yet migrate in tissues; move 1 cm/hr, or faster when subcutaneous
Hookworm Larval movement during inoculation	Worldwide (especially tropics, subtropics)	Skin contact with contaminated soil	Local skin symptoms: 1–2 days GI symptoms: ~4 wk Pulmonary symptoms: 1–3 wk	*Ancylostoma duodenale:* 1 yr *Necator americanus:* 2–6 yr	Eosinophilia during tissue migration; anemia	Gross or occult blood in stools; eggs appear in 4–6 wk; rare reports of parasite survival for 15–20 yr (? hypobiosis of *A. duodenale*)
Loiasis Migratory inflammatory swellings	Central and western Africa	Bite of infected *Chrysops* fly	~1 yr (range, 4 mo–8 yr)	10 yr	Eosinophilia, increased IgE; expatriates have more hypersensitivity symptoms; microfilariae peak numbers in blood near noon	5–6 mo until microfilariae seen in blood; serology available
Onchocerciasis Severe, persistent pruritus	Sub-Saharan Africa, Mexico, Central and tropical South America, Yemen, Saudi Arabia	Bite of infected black fly	1–2 yr	Microfilariae: 2–3 yr Adult: 10–15 yr	Eosinophilia Skin nodules common Africa: mostly near hips South America: mostly near head	Microfilariae reside in skin; need skin snip to help diagnose; slitlamp may show microfilariae in anterior chamber of eye
Pinworms ("pruritus ani") Adult worm movement near anus	Worldwide	Ingestion of infective eggs	4–6 wk	≥Months; autoreinfection common	Nocturnal perianal itching; eosinophilia only with rare tissue invasion; eggs in stool ≤5%; often no associated rash	Diagnosis by tape test; women may develop vulvovaginitis
Schistosomiasis (early)	Asia, Africa, Caribbean, tropical South America	Skin contact with cercariae in water	Skin symptoms: hours Katayama fever* 2–10 wk	3–10 yr	Eosinophilia early; hepatosplenomegaly with chronic infection	Consider rectal snip to diagnose if stool and urine for eggs negative; rare ectopic egg deposition to unusual locations, including CNS

Strongyloidiasis (*Strongyloides stercoralis*) Migratory, serpiginous lesions of larva (larva currens)	Worldwide (especially tropics, subtropics)	Skin or mucous membrane contact with contaminated soil	Skin and pulmonary symptoms: days Other symptoms: days to decades	Indefinite (autoreinfection possible)	Eosinophilia; skin changes (larva currens) common even in chronic infection; can migrate up to 5–10 cm/hr	Some institutions for mentally impaired may have high rates of infection; ex-POWs can carry asymptomatically for decades
Trypanosomiasis, African	Sub-Saharan and southern Africa; scattered foci in east, central, and West Africa	Bite of infected tsetse fly	2–3 wk to fever	Years	Chancre at bite site starts in 2–3 days, lasts 2–4 wk; rash common, mostly on trunk; episodic/recurrent fevers last 1–6 days separated by weeks; generalized lymphadenopathy; anemia common; splenomegaly; chronic infection	Diagnosis difficult; elevated IgM seen in both serum and CSF when CNS involved; treatment toxic
Trichinellosis	Worldwide	Ingestion of raw or undercooked meat with larvae	10–20 days (range, 1–76 days)	Cysts viable in muscle 5–10 yr	1st week: diarrhea, abdominal pain, vomiting 2nd week: fever, myalgia, periorbital edema, marked eosinophilia CNS involvement 10%–20%	Antibody level low before 3rd week, then helpful; encysted larvae do *not* cause symptoms; humans are incidental host; most cases asymptomatic; smoking, salting, drying meat does not kill larvae
Protozoan						
Amebiasis	Worldwide	Cyst ingestion of fecally contaminated food or water	1–3 wk (range, 3 days–months)	Months		Rare presentation
Giardiasis	Worldwide	Cyst ingestion of fecally contaminated food or water; as few as 10 cysts can produce infection	1–3 wk (range, 1 day–6 wk)	Weeks–months	Malabsorption symptoms predominate; self-limited diarrhea; occasional chronic GI symptoms; increased in patients with immunodeficiency, especially hypogammaglobulinemia	Rare presentation; stool examination difficult; stool antigen test good sensitivity; most common cause of chronic diarrhea after travel; survives up to 2–3 mo in cool weather
Bacterial						
Relapsing fevers (*Borrelia* spp. infections)	Louse: Africa, South America, Asia Tick: worldwide except Caribbean and Oceania	Contact with infected louse (hemolymph of crushed louse); tick bite	7–8 days (range, 2–18 days)	Months	Relapsing fevers last 4–10 days separated by approximately 1 wk; relapses milder Louse: 1–5 relapses (mean, 1) Tick: 1–13 relapses (mean, 3)	Louse: case fatality in epidemics 40% Louse and tick: mortality with treatment 2%–5%

Continued

Table 126-8 Differential Diagnosis of Pruritic and Urticarial Skin Lesions—Cont'd

Cause of Pruritic Lesions	Distribution	Acquisition	Incubation	Organism Survival	Common Associated Findings	Additional Information
Pinta	Central and South America	Close contact with an infected person	7–21 days (range, 8–60 days)	≥10 yr	Slowly enlarging papules over weeks to months; often see regional lymphadenopathy; papulosquamous rash 3–12 mo later with generalized lymphadenopathy; depigmented macules seen months to years later with atrophic scars	50% of infections subclinical; VDRL and FTA-ABS used as with syphilis
Typhus fever (*Rickettsia prowazekii*)	Worldwide	Infected louse feces enter mucosal surface or break in skin	10–14 days (range, 5–23 days)	Lifetime of host	Characteristic symptoms: fever, severe headache, myalgias; fever lasts 8–20 days untreated; rash (maculopapular) starts on trunk on day 4–7, spreads to extremities	Infection occurs in endothelial cells→ widespread vasculitis; Brill-Zinsser disease (recrudescent infection): Milder symptoms Fever 7–12 days Much less rash Serology available
Secondary syphilis	Worldwide	Direct contact with infectious lesions; usually sexually transmitted	2–4 wk from onset of primary lesion (range, 10 days–years)	Lifetime of host	Chancre early; skin and mucous membrane lesions appear weeks to months later	Protean manifestations; HIV infection may affect serology; can be transmitted by blood transfusion
Rat-bite fever (*Spirillum minus*)	Worldwide	Bite or close contact with infected rat	1–3 wk (range, 5–40 days)	Months	Bite site heals, then suppurates/ulcerates; rash in 75%, most prominent near bite, reddish brown to purple	Can cause false-positive VDRL: organism best seen by darkfield examination; animal inoculation most sensitive test
Plague	Worldwide except Australia	Bite of infected flea or infected animal; inhalation of fomites from an infected patient	2–3 days pneumonic, 2–7 days bubonic (range, 1–14 days)	No long-term carriage	Abrupt onset of fever, chills, headache, and GI symptoms; hours later buboes form (no buboes if septicemic form); WBC may reach 50,000; CXR shows diffuse interstitial infiltrate; infarcts, hemorrhagic and necrotic nodules common	Fleas infectious for months; can contact disease without travel; hunting and skinning animals a risk
Viral						
Hepatitis B	Worldwide	Sexual and intimate contact; blood and blood-contaminated objects (e.g., needles); mucous membrane contact with infected material; transplacental	2–3 mo	Usually weeks; uncommon chronic carriage	Usually asymptomatic; jaundice, anorexia, diarrhea; 5%–10% of cases show urticarial rash with arthralgia or arthritis	Chronic infection increases risk of hepatocellular cancer; vaccine safe and effective

Arthropod Bite and Infestations						
Myiasis (Diptera fly larva)	Worldwide	Deposition of eggs directly, or via arthropod or inanimate vector	Days–weeks	2 mo; larvae leave host when adult	Local swelling and redness; occasional secondary bacterial infection	Some forms cause local tissue necrosis
Tungiasis (*Tunga penetrans*)	Tropical Central and South America, Caribbean, Africa, Asia (including India)	Skin penetration by larva of female sand flea	8–12 days	Up to 1 mo (flea dies after laying eggs)	Local pain and swelling usually on feet; tiny black spot at site of penetration	Inflammatory reaction to dead flea can persist; can result in tetanus and (rarely) gas gangrene
Fleas	Worldwide	Flea bite (usually unnoticed)	Hours–days	NA	Urticarial papules; papulovesicles/bullae (can persist days to weeks)	Skin lesions often found in clusters
Lice (*Pediculus humanus*, *Phthirus pubis*)	Worldwide	Close physical contact with infected person	Days–weeks	Months† (life cycle: 3–4 wk)	Papular urticaria; nits (eggs) found on hair shaft; excoriations common; blue-gray macules at bite site	Shaving affected area may facilitate treatment
Mosquitoes	Worldwide	Bite of female mosquito	Immediate and 24 hr	NA	Immediate wheal (IgE + histamine–mediated); delayed (24 hr) papule	Repeated exposure alters cutaneous response
Bedbugs	Worldwide	Bite of *Cimex lectularius*	Hours	NA	Papular urticaria	
Kissing bugs	South America	Bite of *Triatoma sanguisuga*	Hours	NA	Papular urticaria; occasional nodular lesion	Walls of mud homes
Scabies	Worldwide	Skin-to-skin contact with infected person; scabies mite acquisition from infected source (live 2 days on clothing/bedding)	Primary infection: 1 mo Repeat infection: hours–days	Months† (life cycle: 3–4 wk)	Severe generalized pruritus; burrows; occasional vesicles or nodules	Hypersenitivity to mite and mite products; nodules often need steroid injections to heal
Tick granuloma	Worldwide	Bite of uninfected tick	Few hours	NA	After removal of tick a pruritic, red, papule/plaque seen; lasts 1–2 wk; occasionally firm nodule "tick granuloma" seen	At times need intralesional steroid or surgery for relief of pruritus

CNS, central nervous system; CSF, cerebrospinal fluid; CXR, chest x-ray film; FTA-ABS, fluorescent treponemal antibody absorption (test); GI, gastrointestinal; HIV, human immunodeficiency virus; NA, not available; VDRL, Venereal Disease Research Laboratories; WBC, white blood cells.

*Katayama fever is characterized by fever, chills, cough, malaise, hepatosplenomegaly, diarrhea, eosinophilia, occasional urticaria, and lymphadenopathy. Symptoms last days to 3–4 months.

†Symptoms persist from reinfection until treatment given.

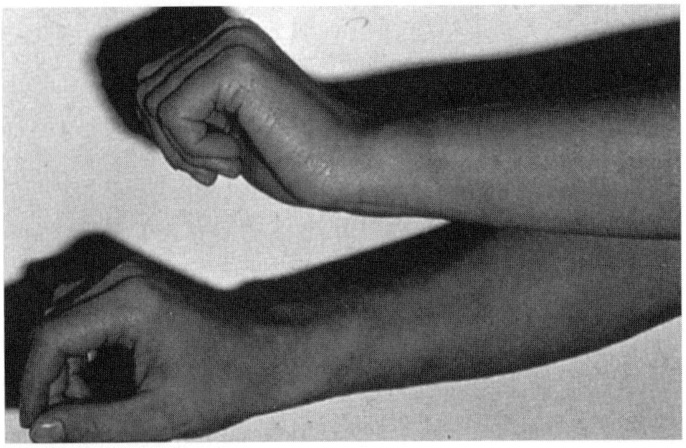

FIGURE 126-8 Calibar swelling in the left (upper) forearm of an expatriate patient with loiasis. Eosinophilia of 60% was coincident with this rash.

papillary layer of the dermis (Table 126-10; Plates 126-2A and 126-2B). Although ulcers often develop from nodules, the reverse is rarely ever seen. Fungal skin lesions are typical of infections that show a spectrum of nodular and ulcerative presentations and hence are listed in a separate table[98,117] (Table 126-11). The time sequence of fungal skin lesions is indicated in Table 126-11 by the designation *I* for initial lesions and *S* for secondary ulceration. Anthrax, cutaneous leishmaniasis, and cutaneous mycobacterial diseases (*M. marinum* and *M. ulcerans*) are typical examples of lesions that progress through a nodular phase to develop ulcers in most patients[85,118–120] (Fig. 126-10). Chancroid and syphilitic chancres are examples of lesions that directly develop painless ulcers, without a primary nodular phase. Tularemia also presents with an ulcer at the inoculation site, which typically is intensely painful. Because *Francisella tularensis* can survive prolonged freezing, it is possible that imported meat may result in an infection distant in time and place from the source.[121]

When pyoderma gangrenosum is the leading diagnostic consideration for an ulcerative lesion, it is important to consider infectious etiologies. Travel-related possibilities include deep fungal infections, herpes simplex type 2, cutaneous tuberculosis, amebiasis cutis, and brown recluse spider bites.

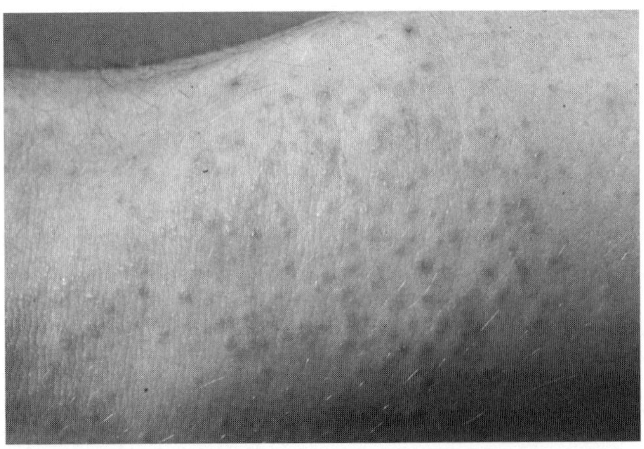

FIGURE 126-9 Onchocercal dermatitis demonstrating characteristic pruritic papules due to cutaneous microfilaria.

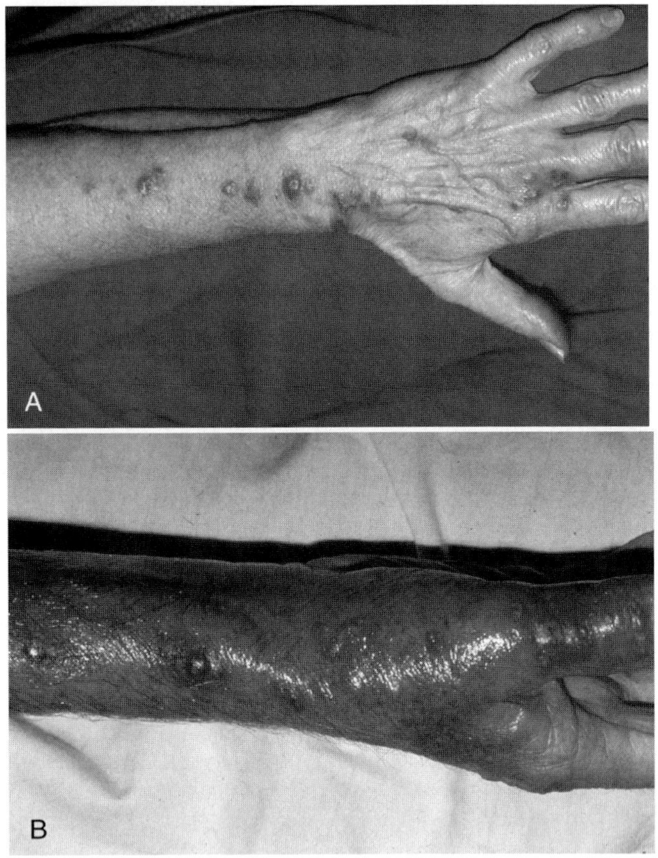

FIGURE 126-10 *A*, Sporotrichoid rash of *Mycobacterium marinum* infection showing typical location on the superficial cooler body tissues of the extremities. *B*, A similar rash in a patient with classical sporotrichosis due to the fungal pathogen *Sporothrix schenckii*.

Cysts

Cysts are similar to nodules but contain fluid. Overall, nodules are much more common than true cysts among tropical-associated infections. In echinococcosis and coenurosis, a true cyst is formed as part of the developmental process of the parasite. However, cutaneous and subcutaneous disease is rare with both of these infections. Some patients with *Gnathostoma spinigerum* form cysts around the parasite as part of the host immune response.[105] Among the filarial parasites, loiasis and onchocerciasis have skin nodules that harbor the adult parasites and occasionally appear cystic due to fluid accumulation around the nodule. Lymphatic filariasis occasionally results in lymphatic obstruction of the scrotal lymphatics in men, resulting in the development of a cystic hydrocele as the presenting manifestation.[122]

Vesicles

There are three broad categories of vesicular lesions (Table 126-12). The first and most common is single or localized lesions.[9] An example is anthrax, with its evolving cutaneous lesion from painless papule to ulcer with surrounding vesicles. Other examples include herpes simplex and varicella-zoster, contagious ecthyma (orf and parapoxvirus), milker's

Text continued on page 1528

Table 126-9 *Differential Diagnosis of Nodular Skin Lesions*

Cause of Nodular Lesions	Distribution	Acquisition	Incubation	Organism Survival	Common Associated Findings	Additional Information
Helminthic						
Coenurosis	North America, South America, Europe, Africa, Asia	Ingestion of eggs in food, water, or on feces; contaminated hands	Months	≥15 yr	Usually no eosinophilia; neurologic symptoms if CNS involved; painless mass lesion ~2–6 cm cyst	Very rare infection, <100 cases reported; hematogenous spread before encystment
Cysticercosis Cysts, may be multiple	Worldwide	Ingestion of eggs in food, water, or on feces; contaminated hands	2 yr to onset of symptoms (range, months–30 yr)	10–15 yr	Usually no eosinophilia; abnormal head CT with cysts + multiple punctate calcifications; 25%–53% have intestinal *Taenia solium*	Symptoms can start after parasite dead; human is incidental host in this form of *T. solium* infection
Dirofilariasis	Worldwide (rare in Africa)	Bite of infected mosquito	2–3 mo	Months–years	No symptoms; rare hemoptysis; occasional subcutaneous nodules; coil lesion on CXR	Human is incidental host
Dracunculiasis Movement of adult worm just below dermis before eruption	Sub-Saharan Africa and India and Pakistan	Ingestion of copepod in drinking water	~ 1 yr	12–18 mo	Eosinophilia during tissue migration; can see dead calcified worms on radiograph	Adults exit via skin; blister with eosinophils, rarely ulcerates; reinfection can occur
Echinococcosis	Worldwide (*Echinococcus multilocularis*) Northern Hemisphere only)	Ingestion of eggs with food, fluid, or on fingers	Few years	Up to lifetime of host	Eosinophilia <35%; cyst wall may be calcified; liver > lung disease; symptoms due to mass effect or immune reaction	Humans are incidental intermediate host; hematogenous and lymphatic dissemination; serology available often negative with lung inf.
Filariasis (*Wuchereria bancrofti; Brugia malayi*) Mass in scrotum	*W. bancrofti*: tropics and subtropics of Africa, Asia, Pacific islands, Central and South America, Carribbean *B. malayi*: South and East Asia	Bite of infected mosquito	5–18 mo	8–10 yr	Hydrocele (scrotal mass); lymphedema, lymphadenitis, elephantiasis, eosinophilia and increased IgE; microfilariae in blood peak near midnight	Rare tropical pulmonary eosinophilia syndrome (1%), serology available
Gnathostomiasis Migratory inflammatory lesions	Asia (especially Thailand and Japan); sporadic worldwide	Ingestion of larva or undercooked or raw meat; ingestion of copepod in water; rare skin penetration	GI symptoms: 1–2 days Soft tissue swelling in 3–4 wk; other symptoms months to years	≥10 yr	Eosinophilia common; can migrate anywhere, including CNS	Humans incidental host; larvae cannot mature yet migrate in tissues, move 1 cm/hr, or faster when subcutaneous
Loiasis Migratory inflammatory swellings	Central and western Africa	Bite of infected *Chrysops* fly	~1 yr (range, 4 mo–8yr)	10 yr	Eosinophilia, increased IgE, expatriates have more hypersensitiviy symptoms; microfilariae peak in blood near noon	5–6 mo until microfilariae seen in blood; serology available

Continued

Table 126-9 Differential Diagnosis of Nodular Skin Lesions—Cont'd

Cause of Nodular Lesions	Distribution	Acquisition	Incubation	Organism Survival	Common Associated Findings	Additional Information
Onchocerciasis Severe, persistent pruritus	Sub-Saharan Africa, Mexico, Central and tropical South America, Yemen, Saudi Arabia	Bite of infected black fly	1–2 yr	Microfilariae: 2–3 yr Adult: 10–15 yr	Eosinophilia Skin nodules common: Africa: mostly near hips South America: mostly near head	Microfilariae reside in skin, need skin snip to help diagnosis; slit lamp may show microfilariae in anterior chamber of eye
Paragonimiasis Subcutaneous migratory swelling or subcutaneous nodules	Africa: Sub-Saharan and southern Americas: All except temperate climates East and Southeast Asia	Ingestion of metacercariae in raw or undercooked crustaceans	Pulmonary symptoms: 6 mo CNS symptoms: 12–16 mo	≤10 yr	Eosinophilia 80%; sputum may have Charcot–Leyden crystals; CXR can have almost any appearance (including 20% normal)	Eggs in sputum, feces, pleural or spinal fluid first appear in 10 wk
Schistosomiasis (early)	Asia, Africa, Caribbean + tropical South America	Skin contact with cercariae in water	Skin symptoms: hours Katayama fever* 2–10 wk	3–10 yr	Eosinophilia early; HSM with chronic infection	Consider rectal snip to diagnose if stool and urine for eggs negative; rare ectopic egg deposition to unusual locations, including CNS
Sparganosis Larval movement	Worldwide (especially tropics; most cases Southeast Asia)	Ingestion of infected copepod in water; ingestion in raw or undercooked meat; use of infected flesh as poultice on an open wound	Depends on route of acquisition	≥9 yr	Eosinophilia and leukocytosis during migration	Humans are incidental hosts, hence larva cannot mature; larva can migrate anywhere, including CNS
Visceral larva migrans Due to *Toxocara canis* and other nematodes	Worldwide (need contact between human and dogs)	Ingestion of embryonated eggs from contaminated soil	≥1 mo (range, weeks–years)	10 yr	Eosinophilia: marked persistent Leukocytosis; fever, cough, wheeze, myalgia, abdominal pain, tender hepatomegaly CXR infiltrate 4%–33%	Serology available Eye disease uncommon: No eosinophilia Causes focal eye symptoms
Protozoan						
Amebiasis, cutaneous	Worldwide	Cyst ingestion in fecally contaminated food or water; uncommon sexual transmission	1–3 wk (range 2 days–months)	Months–years	Mucous membrane lesions of vagina, anus, or penis similar to carcinomas; cutaneous amebiasis is rare; painful granulation tissue or ulcers on presentation	Cysts can remain viable in environment up to 2 mo
Leishmaniasis, cutaneous and mucocutaneous	Scattered: Africa, South and Central America, Caribbean, Asia (middle and western, central and southern), U.S.–Mexico border	Infected sandfly bite	Weeks–2 mo; strain-dependent; may take months to years for correct diagnosis	Months–years	Papule → nodule with central crust; crust falls off to reveal painless ulcer with raised border; heals slowly with scar; single lesion to cluster to widespread	Presentation varies from self-limited to disfiguring; infection can be subacute, chronic, or relapsing; biopsy best diagnostic

					papules, nodules, plaques: mucocutaneous more ulcerative and erosive; cutaneous more nodular	test—need to suspect or easy to miss
Leishmaniasis, visceral	Africa, Mexico, South and Central America, Mediterranean area, Asia	Infected sandfly bite; rare blood transfusion	2–6 mo (range, 10 days–1 yr)	Years	Bite papule/nodule may persist for months; insidious onset of fever, malaise, weight loss, and sweats; diarrhea and cough may be prominent; nontender HSM and LN seen; post kala-azar dermal disease (≤20 %) starts 1–20 yr after apparent cure, as nodular infiltration of skin	Can see profound decrease in CD4 T cells without HIV; serology can be helpful, but often negative if also HIV-infected
Trypanosomiasis, African	Africa, East, Central, West	Bite of infected tsetse fly	2–3 wk (range, 2 days–months)	Years	Bite "chancre"; starts 2–3 days after bite; lasts 2–4 wk; red/purple, indurated several centimeters in diameter; painless to tender; lymphadenopathy common (posterior cervical LN = Winterbottom's sign); occasional red, circinate patches on trunk that wax and wane; splenomegaly in chronic infection	Elevated IgM typical; systemic symptoms common; neurologic changes start months to years after primary infection
Trypanosomiasis, American	Central and South America	Bite of infected triatomine bug; blood transfusion; ingestion of food contaminated by triatomine feces; ingestion of uncooked meat of infected animal	Few days → chagoma; 2–3 wk → systemic symptoms (days–years)	Lifetime of human host	*Acute:* fever, LN, HSM, and HA Chagoma at bite site: 1–3 cm red indurated lesion (25%); Romaña's sign (periorbital chemosis) in 50% of children. *Chronic infection:* arrhythmia, CHF, megacolon, megaesophagus	Disease range asymptomatic to fatal; disease acute, subacute, or chronic; abnormal ECG (43%); antibody test may be helpful
Bacterial						
Bartonellosis	South America: along the western slope of the Andes below 3200 m, and Guatemala	Bite of infected sandfly	3 wk to fever; 1–2 mo to eruptive stage	Weeks–years	Multiple nodules, may be verrucous; fever, rigor, myalgia, arthralgias; skin lesions last 3–4 mo (range, 1 mo–2 yr); jaundice; variable HSM; generalized tender lymphadenopathy and pancytopenia; Salmonella bacteremia up to 40% coinfection	Fever irregular or remittent; lasts 3–4 wk; low-grade *Bartonella* bacteremia can last years; mortality 10%–50% in untreated acute disease; mortality <5% in eruptive stage; skin lesion may worsen with steroid treatment; can see organism in tissue section of skin lesions

Continued

Table 126-9 Differential Diagnosis of Nodular Skin Lesions—Cont'd

Cause of Nodular Lesions	Distribution	Acquisition	Incubation	Organism Survival	Common Associated Findings	Additional Information
Cat-scratch disease	Worldwide	Scratch, lick, or bite of infected cat (90%), or dog	5–7 days to primary skin lesion (range, 3–10 days); 3 wk to adenopathy (range, 3–50 days)	Months	Local lymphadenopathy; papule or pustule at inoculation site; malaise, headache, weight loss, sore throat; ESR often elevated	Risk kitten > cat; cats can have chronic asymptomatic bacteremia; rare encephalitis; angiomatous nodules in AIDS patients
Glanders	Sporadic in Asia, Africa, South America	Inhalation of aerosolized organism; direct inoculation of mucous membrane; ingestion of contaminated meat or drink	5–14 days (range, 1 day–3 wk): aerosol shorter; skin, mucous membrane longer	Weeks–years	CXR can show nodular, lobar, or peribronchial infiltration, *Inhalation:* fever, chills, myalgia, pleurisy, lymphadenopathy common; splenomegaly common. *Percutaneous:* nodular lesion; local lymphangitis may progress to ulcer, gangrene *Mucous membrane:* local inflammation *Disseminated:* papular/pustular eruption	Usually equine disease; pathogen is *Burkholderia mallei*; can have latent infection; chronic infection → multiple subcutaneous and intramuscular abscesses with sinus tract formation; highly variable clinical presentation, from mild to rapidly fatal
Granuloma inguinale (genital) (*Calymmatobacterium granulomatis*)	Worldwide	Sexual contact	7–30 days (range, 3 days–6 mo)	Years in human host	Insidious onset, papule → nodule → ulcer; lesion painless; tissue response characterized by acanthosis and pseudoepitheliomatous changes	Borders of lesions well-defined and irregular; organisms visible in macrophages with Wright's or Giemsa stain (Donovan bodies)
Mycetoma Mixed bacterial and fungal infection; begins as subcutaneous nodule	Worldwide (especially in tropics)	Percutaneous inoculation	Weeks–months	Years (up to 25 yr untreated)	Granules may be discharged from wound; sinus tracts common; nodules slowly enlarge and become phlegmonous	Systemic symptoms usually absent; male: female ratio 4:1; local bone invasion in 33%; radiograph may show cortical erosion, lytic lesions; tendons spared; pathology: granuloma around purulent center
Lymphogranuloma venereum (genital) (*Chlamydia trachomatis*)	Worldwide (especially tropics and subtropics)	Direct contact (usually sexual) with infected person	7–10 days to primary lesion (range, 3–30 days); 10–30 days to inguinal bubo (range months)	Weeks–years	Painless papule → vesicle → ulcer; heals without scar; prominent, painful, fluctuant inguinal adenopathy (bubo); rectal infection → proctitis with blood, tenesmus, and mucoid discharge; fever, chills, HA, malaise, lymphadenopathy	Male:female ratio 6:1; rare presentation with FUO; rare distant problems (e.g., arthritis, hepatitis, pericarditis, and erythema nodosum)

Rhinoscleroma (*Klebsiella rhinoscleromatis*)	Worldwide sporadic	Uncertain	Uncertain	Months–decades	Nodular nose lesions; usually painless; slow local progression; enlarged cervical lymphadenopathy; can see destruction of bone and cartilage	Pathology: chronic histiocytic granulomatous changes Characteristic: Mikulicz's cell (large, vacuolated macrophage)
Syphilis, endemic; bejel (*Treponema pallidum* subsp. *endemicum*)	Focal: Africa (Sahal), Asia (western), Australia	Exposure to contaminated utensils	Weeks (range, 2 wk–3 mo)	Months–years	Primary lesion rarely seen (<1%); secondary lesion: papillomas at corner of mouth; mucous patch on oropharynx, tongue, buccal region, later disseminated papillomas; generalized lymphadenopathy; late painful osteoperiostitis of tibia and fibula (15 %)	Not transmitted by direct or sexual contact; infection usually acquired in childhood; untreated lesions often resolve in 1 yr, but may relapse
Mycobacteriosis Due to *Mycobacterium ulcerans* (begins as nodule)	Focal distribution: Africa, Southeast Asia, Papua New Guinea, Australia, South and Central America	Percutaneous inoculation	6 wk (range, 3 wk–3 mo)	Years	Lesions single (98%) and extremity (90%) or trunk; nodule at onset can be pruritic; nodule → ulcer that enlarges over 1–4 mo; extensive undermined edges and necrotic base; usually no redness, LN, or systemic symptoms	Toxin-mediated process → extensive subQ necrosis BCG: limited protection Mostly found in vegetation in swampy lowlands; bony involvement < 1%
Leprosy	Worldwide (especially tropics and subtropics)	Person–person fomite	3–5 yr	Lifetime of host	Mostly subclinical; 75% with single skin lesion heal spontaneously; spectrum of disease from tuberculoid (TT) to lepromatous (LL): TT—few anesthetic asymmetrical macules/ papules with red rim + hypopigmented center LL—many bilateral symmetrical lesions (macules, papules, plaques, or nodules) Iritis and keratitis common	50%–70% with no known contact of patient with leprosy; erythema nodosum seen occasionally; may worsen with pregnancy; anesthesia → trauma → deformity; ANA, RF, VDRL; may be false positive
Mycobacterium marinum	Worldwide	After trauma in infected water or from infected fish/ crustaceans	2–3 wk	NA	Papule → larger nodule with blue/purple hue → suppuration → ulceration; sporotrichoid pattern; usually confined to superficial, cooler body tissue of extremities	Grows best at 25–32°C; pathologic findings range from pus to granulomas
Leptospirosis	Worldwide (especially tropics)	Ingestion of water or food contaminated by animal urine	7–12 days (range, 2–26 days)	Blood: 3 mo Urine: 11 mo	Pretibial, red, tender nodules 1–5 cm seen with serotype *Leptospira autumnalis*	Organism can survive weeks to months in soil and water; symptomatic infection lasts >2 wk (40%), 1 mo (7%)

Continued

Table 126-9 Differential Diagnosis of Nodular Skin Lesions—Cont'd

Cause of Nodular Lesions	Distribution	Acquisition	Incubation	Organism Survival	Common Associated Findings	Additional Information
Yaws (*Treponema pallidum* subsp. *partenue*)	Focal warm, humid, rural areas; Africa, Asia, Central and South America, Caribbean, Oceania	Direct contact with person with infected lesion	3–5 wk (range, 10 days–3 mo)	Years–decades	Painess papule at start enlarges to 1–3 cm papillomatous raspberry-like lesion; can ulcerate → fluid teeming with spirochetes; some regional lymphadenopathy; primary lesion heals without scar in 6 mo; secondary lesions months later are disseminated papillomas in moist areas; late lesions years later cause tissue destruction and scarring	Latent infection:active disease ratio 5:1; variable presentation: self-limited to destructive chronic
Fungal All invasive fungal infections can cause nodular skin lesions (see Table 126-11)						
Viral						
Orf (*Parapoxvirus*)	All goat and sheep raising countries	Close contact with infected animals with skin break	3–6 days (range. 2–7 days)	Weeks	Papule at entry site → nodule → 1–2 cm plaque/vesicle; weeping ulcer with crust develops; lesions single or multiple; usually painful; local lymphadenopathy, fever seen	Associated with exposure to sheep and goats; heals spontaneously over weeks
Pseudocowpox (*Parapoxvirus*) Milker's nodule	Dairy herds worldwide	Close contact with cow lesion and skin break	5–7 days (range, 5–14 days)	Weeks	Papules → 0.5–2.0 cm nodule; firm, cherry red to red/blue, painless; regional lymphadenopathy seen; no systemic symptoms	Associated with milking cows; heals spontaneously over 4–6 wk without scar
Arthropod						
Myiasis	Worldwide (especially tropics)	Many mechanisms depending on fly species; contact with infected arthropods, vegetation, food, clothes, or direct inoculation	Depends on fly: *Cordylobia anthropophaga* 7–10 days; *Dermatobia bominis* 5–12 wk	≥2 mo	Occasional eosinophilia; visible movement of maggot(s) within the lesion may be noted; larvae of some Diptera (e.g., *Hypoderma*) migrate in soft tissues	Adult leaves host when mature

Scabies	Worldwide	Skin-to-skin contact with infected person; scabies mite acquisition from infected source (live 2 days on clothing/bedding)	Primary infection: 1 mo Repeat infection: hours/days	Months (life cycle 3–4 wk)	Severe generalized pruritus; burrows; occasional vesicles or nodules	Hypersensitivity to mite and mite products; nodules often need steroid injections to heal
Tick granuloma	Worldwide	Bite of uninfected tick	Few hours	NA	After removal of tick, a pruritic, red, papule/plaque; lasts 1–2 wk; occasionally firm nodule "tick granuloma"	At times need intralesional steroid or surgery for relief of pruritus
Tungiasis (*Tunga penetrans*)	Tropical Central and South America, Carribbean, Africa, Asia (including India)	Skin penetration by larva of female sand flea	8–12 days	Up to 1 mo (flea dies after laying eggs)	Local pain and swelling usually on feet; tiny black spot at site of penetration	Inflammatory reaction to dead flea can persist; can result in tetanus and rarely gas gangrene

AIDS, acquired immunodeficiency syndrome; ANA, antinuclear antibody; BCG, bacille Calmette-Guérin; CHF, congestive heart failure; CNS, central nervous system; CT, computed tomography; CXR, chest x-ray film; ECG, electrocardiogram; ESR, erthyrocyte sedimentation rate; FUO, fever of unknown origin; GI, gastrointestinal; HA, headache; HIV, human immunodeficiency virus; HSM, hepatosplenomegaly; LN, lymph node; NA, not available; RF, rheumatoid factor; VDRL, Venereal Disease Research Laboratories.

*See Table 126-4.

Table 126-10 *Differential Diagnosis of Ulcerative Skin Lesions*

Entity	Distribution	Acquisition	Incubation	Organism Survival	Common Associated Findings	Additional Information
Bacterial						
Anthrax (*Bacillus anthracis*)	Worldwide, sporadic; Asia, Africa, especially with animal care	Contact with infected animals or their products via skin break, inhalation, or ingestion of contaminated meat; rare biting fly transmission	2–5 days (range, 12 hr–7 days)	Duration of acute illness in human host; spores persist years in soil	Cutaneous entry (90%) → papule→ vesicular with surrounding brawny, gelatinous edema; satellite lesions seen; lesion becomes hemorrhagic → necrotic → eschar; low-grade fever, malaise common	Variable disease: subclinical to rapidly fatal; toxin mediates many symptoms; 10% develop septicemic form: hemorrhagic meningitis then common, severe GI symptoms also common
Chancroid (*Haemophilus ducreyi*)	Worldwide (especially tropics)	Sexual contact with infected person	3–10 days (range, 2–21 days)	Weeks to months	Papule/pustule ulcerates in 1–2 days (1–2 cm); edges irregular, undermined; painful ulcer; multiple ulcers (67%); unilateral/bilateral LN (40%) painful, prone to rupture	Autoinoculation can occur; 2% urethritis
Diphtheria, cutaneous (*Corynebacterium diphtheriae*)	Worldwide	Close contact with infected person (fomite + direct contact); rarely in contaminated unpasteurized milk	2–5 days (range, 1–10 days)	Usually <2 wk; rare carriers 6 mo	Deep, punched-out ulcers covered by easily removed membrane; can look like impetigo or infected insect bite; nasopharynx infected in 20% of patients with skin infection; cardiac arrhythmias common; cranial + peripheral neuropathies seen and can persist 2–3 mo	Toxin mediates most of disease process; adults immunized as children often lack immunity (25%–75%); can superinfect other skin sores
Glanders (*Burkholderia mallei*)	Sporadic in Asia, Africa, South America	Inhalation of aerosolized organism; direct inoculation of mucous membrane; ingestion of contaminated meat or drink	5–14 days (range, 1 day–3 wk); aerosol shorter; skin, mucous membrane longer	Weeks–years	CXR can show nodular, lobar, or peribronchial infiltration *Inhalation:* fever, chills, myalgia, pleurisy, lymphadenopathy common; splenomegaly common *Percutaneous:* nodular lesion; local local lymphangitis may progress to ulcer, gangrene *Mucous membrane:* local inflammation *Disseminated:* papular/ pustular eruption	Usually equine disease: can have latent infection; chronic infection → multiple subcutaneous and intramuscular abscesss with sinus tract formation; highly variable clinical presentation form mild to rapidly fatal
Granuloma inguinale (genital) (*Calymmato-bacterium granulomatis*)	Worldwide	Sexual contact	7–30 days (range, 3 days–6 mo)	Years in human host	Insidious onset, papule → nodule → ulcer; lesion painless; tissue response characterized by acanthosis and pseudoepitheliomatous changes	Borders of lesions well-defined and irregular; organisms visible in macrophages with Wright's or Giemsa stain (Donovan bodies)
Leprosy	See Table 126-9				Neuropathic ulcers, especially in later tuberculoid leprosy	

Melioidosis (*Barkholderia pseudomallei*)	Tropics and subtropics; endemic Southeast Asia	Direct contact with contaminated water or soil via skin break; aspiration of contaminated water	2 days–3 wk (range, 1 day–years)	Decades	Percutaneous entry → cellulitis, lymphangitis, bacteremia; pustular rash then due to bacteremic spread; can see chronic suppurative changes in skin, bones, CNS, liver, spleen, others; acute disease → many systemic symptoms	Pulmonary infiltrates on CXR Upper lobes 90% Cavitation 60% Disease can be acute or chronic
Mycetoma	See Table 126–9					
Mycobacteriosis Due to *Mycobacterium ulcerans* (begins as nodule)	Focal distribution: Africa, Southeast Asia, Papua New Guinea, Australia, South and Central America	Percutaneous inoculation	6 wk (range, 3 wk–3 mo)	Years	Lesions single (98%) and extremity (90%) or trunk; nodule at onset can be pruritic; nodule → ulcer that enlarges over 1–4 mo; extensive undermined edges and necrotic base; usually no redness, LN, or systemic symptoms	Toxin-mediated process → extensive subcutaneous necrosis BCG: limited protection Mostly found in vegetation in swampy lowlands; bony involvement < 1%
Plague (*Yersinia pestis*)	Worldwide except Australia	Bite of infected flea; inhalation of airborne bacilli from a patient; bite or scratch of infected animal (e.g., cat)	2–7 days bubonic; 2–3 days pneumonic (range, 1–14 days)	No carrier state known	Abrupt onset with severe systemic symptoms; painful swollen mass/LN (bubo) seen in hours, groin > axilla; red/purple skin lesions; GI symptoms (>70%)	High mortality if untreated; septicemic form may have no bubo formation
Rickettsia*						
Syphilis, veneral (*Treponema pallidum*)	Worldwide	Direct contact with infected lesion, usually sexually; transplacental; blood transfusion	2–4 wk to primary lesion	Lifetime of human host	Primary lesion: painless ulcer with indurated edge Secondary lesions: protean skin and mucous membrane lesions seen after asymptomatic interval	Serologic tests do not distinguish among treponemes; disease can be acute, subacute, latent, or chronic
Tropical ulcer (mixed bacteria including *Fusobacterium nucleatum*)	Worldwide (especially tropics)	? Minor trauma may play a role	?	Months	Papule/pustule/vesicle → painful ulcer 1–6 cm diameter; circular raised edge and surrounding edema; deeply penetrating and destructive	Male > female; can see tetanus and gas gangrene; multiple and recurrent ulcers seen
Tuberculosis, primary cutaneous	Worldwide	Unusual direct cutaneous inoculation	Months	Lifetime of human host	Inoculation papule can ulcerate	Rare form of tuberculosis
Tularemia	North America, Europe, Asia (scattered)	Bite of infected arthropod or animal; contact with infected animal tissue; inhalation; ingestion of contaminated meat or water	3–5 days (range, 1–25 days)	2–4 wk in human host; organism can survive prolonged freezing	Clinical symptoms reflect portal of entry; skin inoculation → local, painful ulcer followed by painful regional lymphadenopathy, fever; rare erythema nodosum	Disease range is asymptomatic to fatal; ulceroglandular form of disease most common (75%–85%); chronic/recurrent fevers and lymphadenopathy seen (15% untreated); vaccine for high-risk persons

Continued

Table 126-10 *Differential Diagnosis of Ulcerative Skin Lesions—Cont'd*

Entity	Distribution	Acquisition	Incubation	Organism Survival	Common Associated Findings	Additional Information Yaws
Yaws	See Table 126-9					
Fungal	See Table 126-11				All invasive fungal infections can cause ulcerative skin lesions	Deep abscesses and sinus tracts may form
Helminthic						
Dracunculiasis	See Table 126-6				Ulcer at site of eruption of worm	
Protozoan						
Amebiasis, cutaneous Painful, rapidly growing ulcers; necrotic	Worldwide	Infectious cyst ingestion in fecally contaminated food or water	1–3 wk (range, 2 days–months)	Months–years	When cutaneous, painful, rapid-growing ulcers with necrosis; genital and anal mucous membrane lesions similar to carcinoma; diarrhea/colitis most common presentation; 1%–10% liver abscess	Infection more prevalent in crowded unsanitary conditions; infection more severe in infants, pregnant women, people on steroids; uncommon sexual transmission: anal > vaginal intercourse
Leishmaniasis, cutaneous and mucocutaneous	See Table 126-9					
Viral						
Orf (*Parapoxvirus*)	All goat and sheep-raising countries	Close contact with infected animals with skin break	3–6 days (range, 2–7 days)	Weeks	Papule at entry site → nodule → 1–2 cm plaque/vesicle; weeping ulcer with crust develops; lesions single or multiple; usually painful; local lymphadenopathy, fever	Associated with exposure to sheep and goats; heals spontaneously over weeks
Herpes simplex	Worldwide	Type 1: direct contact with infected oral secretions Type 2: contact with genital secretions	2–12 days	Lifetime in human host	Grouped vesicles on erythematous base ulcerate; lesions painful; moderate to severe generalized systemic symptoms with primary infection; local adenopathy common	Recurrence due to latent virus in neural cells; autoinoculation possible
Arthropod						
Brown recluse spider bite (*Loxosceles reclusa*)	?	Spider bite	Immediate–hours	NA	Bite → mild sting followed by intense pain in 2–8 hr, bullae + erythema, local ischemic necrosis, deep ulceration Occasional fever, myalgias, and generalized morbilliform rash 24–48 hr after bite	Parenteral steroid use in first 24 hr controversial; heals spontaneously though scars common Can be confused with pyoderma gangrenosum
Myiasis	See Table 126-8					Untended ulcers, e.g., neurotropic ulcer in homeless is potential egg deposition site
Tungiasis	See Table 126-8					

BCG, bacille Calmette-Guérin; CNS, central nervous system; CXR, chest x-ray film; GI, gastrointestinal; NA, not available; LN, lymph node.
*Several rickettsial infections are associated with an ulcerative eschar; see Table 126-2.

Table 126-11 *Differential Diagnosis of Nodular and Ulcerative Fungal Infections*

Entity	Distribution	Acquisition	Incubation	Organism Survival	Common Associated Findings: Nodule	Common Associated Findings: Ulcer	Additional Information
Primary skin infections							
Chromomycosis (several agents)	Worldwide, especially tropics and subtropics	Skin inoculation of nonintact skin	Weeks–months	Years	I + + + +	S + + +	Lymphatic involvement seen, including elephantiasis and lymphedema; starts as local papule → painless, irregular, papule → nodule
Entomophthoromycosis (*Basidiobolus baptosporus*)	Tropical Africa, rarely elsewhere	Percutaneous inoculation of nonintact skin	?	Years	Painless subcutaneous nodule → expanding woody swelling Nodule: I + + + +	Ulcer: None	Rare systemic symptoms or dissemination
Lobomycosis (*Loboa loboi*)	Tropical Central and South America	Percutaneous inoculation of nonintact skin	1–2 yr	Years	Starts as painless, small, mobile nodules Nodule: I + + + +	Ulcer: S +	Autoinoculation seen; spontaneous regression is rare; disease only seen in humans and dolphins; histopathology characteristic
Mycetoma Mixed bacterial and fungal infection; begins as subcutaneous nodule	Worldwide (especially tropics)	Percutaneous inoculation	Weeks–months	Years (up to 25 yr untreated)	Granules may be discharged from wound; sinus tracts common; nodules slowly enlarge and become phlegmonous Nodule: I + + +	Ulcer: S + +	Systemic symptoms usually absent; male–female ratio 4:1; local bone invasion 33%; radiograph may show cortical erosion, lytic lesions; tendons spared; pathology: granuloma around purulent center
Pityriasis (tinea) versicolor (*Malassezia furfur*)	Worldwide	Direct inoculation of fungal elements	?	?	Circumscribed hypo- or hyper- (brown) pigmented scaly lesions; usually upper chest and back Nodule: None	Ulcer: None	Superficial stratum corneum infection; enzyme of fungus produces pigment changes
Sporotrichosis (*Sporothrix schenckii*)	Worldwide	Direct percutaneous inoculation	3–8 wk	Months–years	Papule → painless; nodule → may ulcerate; secondary nodules along lymphatic channels Nodule: I + + + +	Ulcer: S + +	25% extracutaneous lung, bone, joints
Tinea imbricata (*Trichophyton concentricum*)	Asia: East, South, Middle; South Pacific islands; Mexico, Central and South America	Direct contact with infected person	10 days	Lifetime of host	Concentric rings 0.3–1.25 cm apart; no systemic symptoms except pruritus Nodule: None	Ulcer: None	Hypopigmentation more than hyperpigmentation; covers up to 70% of body

Continued

Table 126-11 Differential Diagnosis of Nodular and Ulcerative Fungal Infections—Cont'd

Entity	Distribution	Acquisition	Incubation	Organism Survival	*Common Associated Findings* Nodule	Ulcer	Additional Information
Primary nasal and oropharyngeal infections							
Entomophthoromycosis (*Conidiobolus coronatus*)	Tropical Africa; rarely elsewhere	Inhalation of spore usually onto nasal turbinate	?	Years	Painless indurated mass → local insidious spread Nodule I + + + +	Ulcer None	Male–female ratio 8:1
Rhinosporidiosis (*Rhinosporidium seeberi*)	Worldwide (sporadic); highly endemic foci in India and Sri Lanka	Direct inoculation of fungus	Weeks–months	Years–decades	Characteristic, friable, vascular, sessile growth or polyps on mucosal surfaces; lesions painless Nodule I + + + +	Ulcer None	Treatment surgical, but recurrence common
Primary respiratory infections							
Blastomycosis (*Blastomyces dermatitidis*)	North America (most); sporadic in Central and South America, Africa, Poland, India, Middle East	Inhalation of infectious conidia; rare percutaneous inoculation; rare STD from men with genitourinary infection	1–2 mo inhaled; 2 wk cutaneous	~15 yr in human host	Nodule I + + +	Ulcer S + +	Mostly hematogenous to skin; 20%–80% of patients disseminated to skin, bone, genitourinary tract (male > female), CNS; soil contact increases risk; male: female ratio 3–9:1
Coccidioidomycosis (*Coccidioides immitis*)	Southwest U.S., Mexico, Central and South America	Inhalation of infectious arthroconidia; rare cutaneous inoculation	2 wk	Years	Primary disease; fever, cough, chest pain, malaise Hypersensitivity reactions (15%–20%): erythema nodosum, generalized erythema, maculopapular rash, arthralgias, urticaria, rare erythema multiforme Nodule +	Ulcer +	Extrapulmonary disease rare (<1 %): bone, skin, lymphadenopathy, CNS, joints, genitourinary, gastrointestinal, eye; eosinophilia common in primary infection; frequent dressing changes if open wound to prevent formation of infectious arthroconidia
Cryptococcosis (*Cryptococcus neoformans*)	Worldwide	Inhalation of infectious conidia	?	?	Mostly pulmonary; mostly asymptomatic; skin lesions 10% (hematogenous papule → nodule → ulcer) Nodule I + +	Ulcer S + +	Can cause CNS, bone, prostate, liver, eye, heart, kidney infections rarely

Histoplasmosis (*Histoplasma capsulatum*)	Worldwide (but focal and sporadic)	Inhalation of infectious spores	2 wk	Years	Mostly pulmonary; mostly asymptomatic; can see skin changes (especially erythema nodosum) with hypersensitivity reaction to primary infection Nodule: I; Often oropharynx; + Ulcer: I; Oropharynx; +	Rare dissemination: 15%–20% metastatic skin lesions Disseminated disease can affect any organ
Histoplasmosis, African (*Histoplasma capsulatum*, var. *duboisii*)	Tropical Africa	Uncertain; suspect inhalation of infected spores	?	Years	Common skin lesions from skin *and* from underlying bony disease; skin lesions painless Nodule: I; + + + Ulcer: I; + + +	Lytic bony lesions common
Paracoccidioido-mycosis (*Paracoccidioides brasiliensis*)	Central and South America	Inhalation of infectious spores	Months–years	Years–decades	Initial respiratory infection usually asymptomatic; common mucocutaneous lesions of oropharynx due to hematogenous dissemination (60%) Nodule: I; + + + Ulcer: I; + +	Ratio of disease in males and females 9:1, though skin test–positive ratio is 1:1; overall skin test only 50% sensitive; isolated CNS or adrenal involvement seen
Penicilliosis (*Penicillium marneffei*)	East and Southeast Asia	Inhalation/ ingestion of infectious spores; rare percutaneous inoculation	9 days–1 mo	Years	Nodules actually multiple subcutaneous abscesses; ulcers from necrosis of nodules/papules Nodule: I; + + + Ulcer: S; + +	Most patients (86%) disseminate; immunodeficiency favors ulcer formation

CNS, central nervous system; I, initial lesion; S, secondary lesion; STD, sexually transmitted disease; +, scale (1–4) based on frequency when skin lesions present: +, rare; + +, uncommon; + + +, occasional; + + + +, frequent.

Table 126-12 Differential Diagnosis of a Vesicular Rash after Travel or Tropical Exposure

Organism/Agent	Disease	Comment
Bacteria		
Bacillus anthracis	Anthrax	Often associated with enlarging ulcer
Brucella spp.	Brucellosis	
Mycobacterium tuberculosis	Papulonecrotic tuberculids	Rare
Mycoplasma spp.	—	
Rickettsia akari	Rickettsialpox	
Rickettsia tsutsugamushi (?)	—	
Streptococcus pyogenes (?)	Impetigo	
Vibrio vulnificus		
Viruses		
Alphaviruses (chikungunya, O'nyong-nyong, Ross River, Sindbis)		
Enteroviruses (coxsackievirus, echovirus, enterovirus 71)		
Measles	Atypical measles	
Mumps (??)		
Monkeypox		
Herpes simplex (type 1 and type 2)		Latent virus with recurrence
Varicella-zoster	Chickenpox	Latent virus with recurrence
Vaccinia	Progressive vaccinia Eczema vaccinatum Accidental remote inoculation	Occasionally close contact of vaccine recipient
Variola	Smallpox	
Orf	Ecthyma contagiosum	
Tanapox		
Parasitic		
Leishmania braziliensis	American cutaneous leishmaniasis	
Necator americanus	Hookworm	At site of skin penetration
Noninfectious		
Toxic epidermal necrolysis	Drug-related	
	Vaccine-related	Rare case reports with: Bacille Calmette-Guérin Diphtheria toxoid Measles Poliomyelitis Tetanus toxoid
Plant dermatitis	Poison ivy	
Drug hypersensitivity		

nodule (pseudocowpox), tanapox, and papulonecrotic tuberculids. In addition, secondarily infected skin lesions with phage group 2 toxin-producing staphylococci can produce bullous impetigo. Noninfectious plant toxin contact, such as with poison ivy, typically results in a vesicular reaction.[123]

The second category consists of generalized lesions with greatest concentration on the head and scalp. Varicella (chickenpox) is the prototype of this vesicular presentation. The third group includes generalized lesions with greatest concentration on the extremities. Although predominantly peripheral, rickettsialpox lesions are noted to spare the palms and soles.[21] In contrast, coxsackievirus has a very characteristic predilection for those areas, resulting in the name hand-foot-and-mouth disease to describe this combination of exanthem and enanthem. Disseminated gonococcal infection is associated with painful peripheral lesions that mature into vesicles, often on a hemorrhagic base (Fig. 126-11). Toxic epidermal necrolysis and some drug hypersensitivity reactions can produce

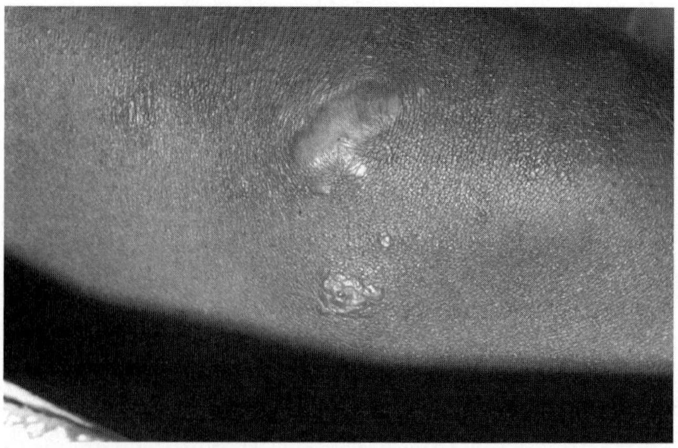

FIGURE 126-11 Disseminated gonococcal infection. Cutaneous lesions showing characteristic discrete pustules and papules with subcutaneous hemorrhage. (Courtesy of Kenneth J. Tomecki, MD, Cleveland, OH.)

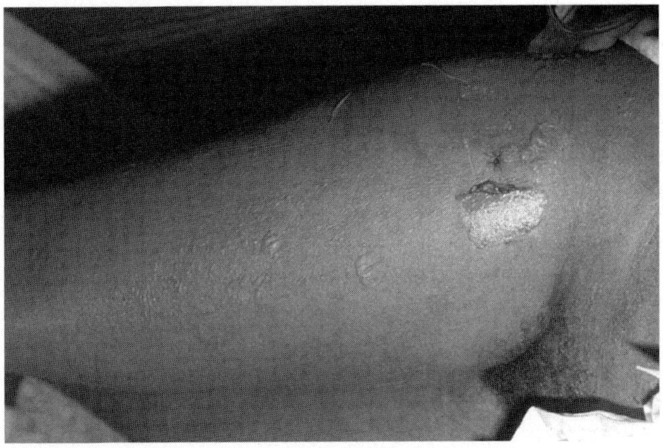

FIGURE 126-12 Toxic epidermal necrolysis showing large, flaccid bullae and characteristic ruptured bullae with separation of sheets of skin (Nikolsky's sign); can occur with toxin producing *S. aureus*, drug reaction, and viral illnesses. (Courtesy of Kenneth J. Tomecki, MD, Cleveland, OH.)

vesicles (Fig. 126-12). Bullae (large vesicles) are occasionally seen with gram-negative bacteria (especially *Pseudomonas aeruginosa*)-associated ecthyma lesions.[7,32]

Changes in Pigmentation

Changes in skin pigmentation are usually immunologically mediated. The lesions are commonly either hypo- or hyperpigmented. In addition, they can be focal, scattered, generalized, or a combination thereof. Finally, the lesion may be noted early or late in the disease process. Table 126-13 summarizes these findings for tropically acquired conditions associated with altered pigmentation of the skin. In general, pigmentation changes early in a disease process are more likely to result in hyperpigmentation, whereas later changes more commonly result in decreased pigmentation. This information is occasionally helpful in differentiating the underlying cause. Pinta is an example in which papulosquamous skin lesions are usually red at onset and then shift to a spectrum of blue, gray, violaceous, yellow, black, and brown, referred to as dyschromic lesions. Over many months to years, the skin lesions become depigmented macules associated with atrophic scars.[124]

Cutaneous jaundice is occasionally seen in patients related to hepatic involvement with various pathogens (Box 126-7). The major pathogen causing jaundice in travelers is hepatitis A. The annual incidence of hepatitis in travelers is 11 to 87 per 1000 people exposed in developing countries.[1,125] The agents associated with jaundice have a wide geographic distribution. The incubation period can be an important clue to the cause. Yellow fever symptoms usually begin within 2 weeks of exposure, whereas the incubation period for the hepatitis viruses is 2 to 6 weeks. Due to extensive exposure to water among triathletes and eco-challenge participants, they represent a high-risk group for water-borne illness, especially leptospirosis.

Owing to vaccine availability and excellent efficacy, the vaccination status of the traveler provides important information in formulating the differential diagnosis of the jaundiced traveler.[126] Rarely, both pigment alteration (e.g., erythroderma) and jaundice (e.g., immune-mediated hepatic involvement of drug hypersensitivity) can be medication related.[39]

Table 126-13 Alterations in Pigmentation

	Location			***Time***	
	Focal	**Scattered**	**Generalized**	**Early**	**Late**
Decreased pigmentation					
Leishmaniasis, visceral	+ + (face)	+			+ (untreated)
Leprosy	+	+		+	+
Onchocerciasis	+ (pretibial)				+
Pinta	+	+	+		+
Pityriasis (tinea) versicolor				+	
(*Malassezia furfur*)		+			
Syphilis, venereal, secondary	+ + (neck)				+
Yaws	+ (inoculation site)	+ (hand, wrist, feet)		+	
Yaws					
Increased pigmentation					
Erythrasma (*Corynebacterium minutissimum*)	+			+	
Pinta	+	+	+	+	+
Loiasis	+			+	
Pityriasis (tinea) versicolor (*Malassezia furfur*)		+		+	
Leishmaniasis, visceral (especially India)			+		+

+, present; ++, common.

Box 126-7 Diagnostic Concerns in the Traveler with Jaundice

Diseases in Which Jaundice Is Common	
Yellow fever	Symptom onset less than 2 weeks
Hepatitis A–E	Incubation to symptoms varies from 2 to 6 weeks
Rift Valley fever	Zoonotic hepatitis pathogen (arbovirus) Seen throughout Africa Transmission: mosquito, airborne, unpasteurized milk
Diseases in Which Jaundice Is Uncommon	
Leptospirosis	Animal urine (especially rats) contaminates environment worldwide Organism can survive weeks to months in soil and water (? triathlete/eco-challenge) Incubation period 7–12 days Symptoms last 2–4 weeks
Dengue fever	Usually in setting of severe disease
Malaria	
Epstein-Barr virus	
Q fever	
Syphilis	
Drug reactions	

TRAVEL-RELATED MEDICATIONS

The care of patients who travel to or live in the tropics often involves the use of medications not usually prescribed by physicians in the developed world. Although medication reactions are rare, these agents represent a significant new exposure for many travelers to tropical and subtropical climates. Drug reactions can take many forms, with mechanisms both direct and immunologic. Hypersensitivity reaction types 1 to 4 have been documented with various pharmacologic agents.[71] The actual dermatologic presentation can take any form, from maculopapular to urticarial, vesiculobullous, or vasculitic. Other less frequent manifestations of drug eruptions include toxic epidermal necrolysis, erythema nodosum, and lichenoid reactions.[127,128] With few exceptions, the information related to the cutaneous reactions associated with medications in this setting comes from case reports. Table 126-14 is organized by application of the medications (e.g., antimalarials and antidiarrheals). The reactions listed for each medication appear in the approximate order of their reported incidence.

Chloroquine can occasionally induce a pruritic reaction without cutaneous changes, which can be moderately severe in up to 90% of cases. There appears to be an increased risk of a reaction to chloroquine in blacks and in people with a family history of pruritus.[129] If another option exists for malaria prophylaxis, it should be considered in such patients. Symptomatic patients

Table 126-14 Cutaneous Reactions to Travel Medications

Medication	Reactions	Factors That May Increase Reactions
Antimalarials		
Chloroquine	Hair blanching	Dosing ≥1 yr Hair exposed to light
	Pruritus without rash	Black race Family history of reaction
	Photosensitivity	Long-term usage Increased age Female > male
	Worsens psoriasis	
	Rare: hypo- or hyperpigmentation of skin, blue-brown nail bed changes, erythema annulare centrifugum, bullous erythema, toxic epidermal necrolysis (TEN), erythema nodosum	Pyrimethamine use Renal failure
Mefloquine	Rare: itching, varied nonspecific rashes, Stevens-Johnson syndrome	
Proguanil	Rare: mild urticaria, phototoxic reactions, exanthems, periorbital papules	
	Hair loss	Female > male
	Scaling of palms/soles	2 of 6 patients receiving concurrent chloroquine
Primaquine	None reported	
Doxycycline	Photosensitivity	
	Rare: photo-onycholysis, exanthematous pustulosis, urticaria, angioedema, purpura, anaphylaxis, serum sickness	
Quinine	Urticaria, papular rash, scarlatilniform rash, erythema multiforme	
	Rare: fixed drug eruption; urticaria; flushing, sweating, facial edema; photosensitivity	
Halofantrine	Pruritus post-treatment	Incidence 0.3%–2.3% Black race Family member with history of pruritus post-treatment

Continued

Table 126-14 Cutaneous Reactions to Travel Medications—Cont'd

Medication	Reactions	Factors That May Increase Reactions
Antidiarrheals		
Pepto-Bismol	Salicylate hypersensitivity, erythematous rash, bismuth reaction, transient darkening of tongue	
Trimethoprim–sulfamethoxazole	Diffuse maculopapular rash, allergic/toxic dermatitis	Overall incidence 2.2%;
	Rare: erythema multiforme	HIV/AIDS higher incidence
	Exfoliative eczema exanthems	~1/200.000 doses
	Stevens-Johnson syndrome	~1/200.000 doses
	TEN	
Ciprofloxacin	Generalized skin rash	Incidence of 1.1%
	Rare: pruritus, urticaria, photosensitivity, flushing, angioedema, hyperpigmentation, erythema nodosum, fixed drug eruption, pustulosis, TEN	
Ofloxacin*	Generalized skin rash, pruritus, eczema	Incidence up to 14% of patients
	Rare: hypersensitivity vasculitis, phototoxic dermatitis, photo-onycholysis	
Metronidazole	Hypersensitivity reaction, flushing, ± erythematous rash	Alcohol ingestion
	Rare: pityriasis rosea, fixed drug eruption	
Furazolidone	Maculopapular eruptions, vesicular-morbilliform, hypersensitivity reaction, pruritic rash, contact dermatitis, erythema multiforme	0.5 % incidence rate overall (based on evaluation of 10,433 patients)
Anthelminthics		
Albendazole	Hair loss (reversible)	High-dose chronic therapy
	Rash and pruritus	
	Stevens-Johnson syndrome	
Diethylcarbamazine (DEC)	Hypersensitivity reaction (Mazzotti reaction)	Onchocerciasis >> *Loa* > other filariae
Ivermectin	Rash and pruritus	
Biting arthropod repellent		
Diethyltoluamide (DEET)	Rare: local irritant reaction, scarring bullous dermatitis	

*The newer quinolones sparfloxacin and levofloxacin have photosensitivity reaction rates of 6% to 8%.
Data from references 120–131, 133–148.

often desire treatment to relieve this bothersome reaction. Chloroquine pruritus is usually not responsive to antihistamines, although a study on chlorpheniramine showed efficacy when given 3 hours after ingestion of chloroquine in 70% of patients compared with 40% when given concomitantly.[130] Prednisolone 5 mg or niacin 50 mg also significantly reduced the pruritus intensity time curve in another study. Chloroquine may also exaggerate existing psoriasis; hence, psoriasis should be considered a relative contraindication to the use of chloroquine. The mechanism is possibly mediated through stimulation of a lower lymphocyte transformation. Bleaching of the hair can be seen, although usually after use longer than 1 year.[131]

In patients traveling to tropical and subtropical climates, there is almost always increased exposure to sunlight in both time of exposure and intensity of exposure. Sunscreens are an important part of the cutaneous hygiene in such travelers. In addition, certain medications given to travelers carry potential photosensitization as a side effect, especially doxycycline, quinine, proguanil, ciprofloxacin, and ofloxacin.[71,132–135] Nonsteroidal anti-inflammatory agents can also photosensitize, and sedentary travelers who are physically active during foreign travel may use them frequently.[136] Travelers who require these medications should be reminded to be especially vigilant about using sunscreens with high sun protection factor ratings.

For many years, diethylcarbamazine (DEC) has been the drug of choice for the treatment and occasional prophylaxis of most filarial infections, but it can induce a significant hypersensitivity reaction in certain patients. People with onchocerciasis or loiasis are particularly at risk of developing the Mazzotti reaction.[137] The Mazzotti reaction is thought to be an IgE-mediated hypersensitivity reaction to dying microfilariae and is characterized by rapid onset of itching followed within hours by edema and swelling, which may progress to a generalized anaphylactoid reaction with fever, tachycardia, and hypotension. Eosinophilia, lymphadenopathy, and myalgias and arthralgias are also common. Because of the potential severity of this reaction, the first dose of DEC is often given under medical observation, especially when onchocerciasis or a high microfilarial count with *L. loa* infection are diagnosed. Administration of corticosteroids with DEC is usually effective in minimizing the inflammatory response due to the Mazzotti reaction.[74] Concurrent corticosteroid therapy may theoretically reduce the efficacy of DEC, although the factors influencing the ultimate clinical response to DEC are complex. In general, antihistamines have not been of great value, although broad antihistamines, such as diphenhydramine (Benadryl) and hydroxyzine (Atarax), may be more efficacious than selective H_1 histamine blockers.

Very rarely, travelers will develop serum sickness or serum sickness-like reactions to vaccines or antibiotics administered for travel-related disease prevention.[39] As a type of immune complex disease, a spectrum of reactions can be seen, from mild morbilliform maculopapular eruptions to multisystem organ involvement arising from systemic (including cutaneous) vasculitis.[128] A more common presentation of serum sickness is fever, urticaria, arthralgias, and lymphadenopathy approximately 1 to 3 weeks after primary antigen exposure or 3 days after reexposure.[138] Rare case reports have described this reaction to bacille Calmette-Guérin, measles, and poliomyelitis vaccines, as well as to tetanus and diphtheria antitoxins.[90] Antibiotics such as penicillin and sulfa-containing drugs can also act as the foreign antigen initiating a cascade immune response very similar to serum sickness.[139] Another rare, but potentially severe, cutaneous reaction is seen with sulfadoxine pyrimethamine (Fansidar) use in malaria prophylaxis or treatment. Both Stevens-Johnson syndrome and toxic epidermal necrolysis have been reported. Development of rash during use is considered an indication to discontinue this medication.

ACKNOWLEDGMENTS

We are indebted to Dr. Mary Wilson[42] for gathering an enormous amount of data related to the practical information that bears on the clinical care of patients with health concerns related to international and tropical medicine. We also acknowledge Kenneth Tomecki, MD, for his helpful review and comments. In addition, we thank Vicki Grosh for significant assistance in the preparation of the tables.

REFERENCES

1. Steffen R, Rickenbach M, Wilhelm U, et al: Health problems after travel to developing countries. J Infect Dis 156:84–91, 1987.
2. Reid D, Cossar JH: Epidemiology of travel. Br Med Bull 49:257–268, 1993.
3. Salata RA, Blauton RE, King CH, et al: Illnesses in returning travelers and immigrants from developing countries. In Lobel HO, Steffan R, Kozarsky PE (eds): Travel Medicine, 2. Proceedings of the Second Conference on International Travel Medicine. Atlanta, International Society of Travel Medicine, 1991, pp 74–76.
4. Caumes E, Carriere J, Guermonprez G, et al: Dermatoses associated with travel to tropical countries: A prospective study of the diagnosis and management of 269 patients presenting to a tropical disease unit. Clin Infect Dis 20:542–548, 1995.
5. Caumes E, Brucker G, Brousse G, et al: Travel-associated illness in 838 French tourists in Nepal in 1984. Travel Med Int 9:72–76, 1991.
6. Shlim DR: Learning from experience: Travel medicine in Katmandu. In Lobel HO, Steffen R, Kozarsky PE (eds): Travel Medicine, 2. Proceedings of the Second Conference on International Travel Medicine. Atlanta, International Society of Travel Medicine, 1991, pp 40–42.
7. Weber DJ, Cohen MS: The acutely ill patient with fever and rash. In Mandell GL, Bennett JE, Dolin R (eds): Principles and Practice of Infectious Diseases. New York, Churchill-Livingstone, 1995, pp 549–561.
8. Kingston ME, Mackey D: Skin clues in the diagnosis of life-threatening infections. Rev Infect Dis 8:1–11, 1986.
9. Cherry JD: Cutaneous manifestations of systemic infections. In Feigin RD, Cherry JD (eds): Textbook of Pediatric Infectious Diseases. Philadelphia, WB Saunders, 1987, pp 786–817.
10. Fanning WL, Aronson M: Osler node, Janeway lesions, and splinter hemorrhages: Occurrence with an infected arterial catheter. Arch Dermatol 113:648–649, 1977.
11. Hill WR, Kinney TD: The cutaneous lesions in meningococcemia: A clinical and pathologic study. JAMA 134:513–518, 1947.
12. Elgart ML: Onchocerciasis and dracunculosis. Dermatol Clin 7:323–330, 1989.
13. Davis BR: Filariases. Dermatol Clin 7:313–322, 1989.
14. Ottesen EA: Immunological aspects of lymphatic filariasis and onchocerciasis in man. Trans R Soc Trop Med Hyg 78:9–18, 1984.
15. Beaver PC, Rolon FA: Proliferating larval cestode in a man in Paraguay. A case report and review. Am J Trop Med Hyg 30:625–637, 1981.
16. Chaudhry AZ, Longworth DL: Cutaneous manifestations of intestinal helminthic infections. Dermatol Clin 7:275–290, 1989.
17. Gonzales E: Schistosomiasis, cercarial dermatitis and marine dermatitis. Dermatol Clin 7:291–300, 1989.
18. Arner M: Cutaneous schistosomiasis. Dermatol Clin 12:713–717, 1994.
19. Millikan LE: Papular urticaria. Semin Dermatol 12:53–56, 1993.
20. Snyman JR, Sommers DK, Gregorowski MD: Influence of histamine receptor antagonists on the dynamics of the cutaneous hypersensitivity reaction in patients infected with *Schistosoma haematobium*. Eur J Pharmacol 44:467–471, 1993.
21. Myers SA, Sexton DJ: Dermatologic manifestations of arthropod-borne diseases. Infect Dis Clin North Am 8:689–712, 1994.
22. Millikan LE: Mite infestations other than scabies. Semin Dermatol 12:46–52, 1993.
23. Arosemena R, Booth SA, Su WP: Cutaneous myiasis. J Am Acad Dermatol 28:254–256, 1993.
24. Noutsis C, Millikan LE: Myiasis. Dermatol Clin 12:729–736, 1994.
25. Reunala T, Lappalainen P, Brummer-Korvenkontio H, et al: Cutaneous reactivity to mosquito bites: Effect of cetirizine and development of anti-mosquito antibodies. Clin Exp Allergy 2:617–622, 1991.
26. Brummer-Korvenkontio H, Lappalainen P, Reunala T, et al: Detection of mosquito saliva-specific IgE and IgG antibodies by immunoblotting. J Allergy Clin Immunol 93:551–555, 1994.
27. McKeil JA, West AS: Nature and causation of insect bite reactions. Pediatr Clin North Am 8:795–815, 1961.
28. Toffe RW, Williams DN: Clinical and laboratory manifestations of toxic shock syndrome. Ann Intern Med 96:843–847, 1982.
29. Witte MH, Jamal S, Williams WH, et al: Lymphatic abnormalities in human filariasis as depicted by lymphangioscintigraphy. Arch Intern Med 153:737–744, 1993.
30. Freedman DO, Almeida F, Braga C, et al: Lymphoscintigraphic analysis of lymphatic abnormalities in symptomatic and asymptomatic human filariasis. J Infect Dis 170:927–933, 1994.
31. Weston WL: What is erythema multiforme? Pediatr Ann 25:106–109, 1996.
32. Meseguer MA, de Rafael L, Vidal ML: Stevens-Johnson syndrome with isolation of *Mycoplasma pneumoniae* from skin lesions. Eur J Clin Microbiol 5:167–168, 1986.
33. Ajonuma LC, Chika LC: Outbreak of Stevens-Johnson syndrome among Filipino overseas contract workers using mebendazole for helminthiasis prophylaxis. Trop Doctor 30:57, 2000.
34. Vaughan TK, English JC 3rd: Cutaneous larvae migrans complicated by erythema multiforme. Cutis 62:33–35, 1998.
35. Dewerdt S, Machet L, Jan-Lamy V, et al: Stevens-Johnson syndrome after albendazole. Acta Derm Venereol 77:411, 1997.
36. Peterson CM, Schuppert K, Kelly PC, et al: Coccidioidomycosis and pregnancy [Review]. Obstet Gynecol Surg 483:149–156, 1993.
37. Van den Enden E, Van Gompel A, Colebunders R, et al: Mefloquine-induced Stevens-Johnson syndrome. Lancet 337:683, 1991.
38. March CH: Erythema multiforme bullosum associated with *Trichomonas* infection. Arch Dermatol 92:674–675, 1965.
39. Roujeau JC, Stern RS: Severe adverse cutaneous reactions to drugs. N Engl J Med 331:1272–1285, 1994.
40. Steiger U, Weber M: Usual etiology of erythema nodosum, pleural effusion and reactive arthritis: *Giardia lamblia*. Schweiz Rund Med Praxis 91:1091–1092, 2002.
41. Lammintausta K, Kotilainen P, Hohenthal U, et al: A patient with a mucocutaneous eruption and intestinal giardiasis. Acta Dermato-Venereol 81:310–311, 2001.
42. Wilson ME: Gathering the history. In: A World Guide to Infections: Diseases, Distribution, Diagnosis. New York, Oxford University Press, 1991, pp 23–41.
43. Fitzpatrick TB, Bernard JD: The structure of skin lesions and fundamentals of diagnosis. In Jeffers JD, Scott E, White J (eds): Dermatology in General Medicine. Textbook and Atlas, ed 3. New York, McGraw-Hill, 1987, pp 20–49.
44. Valman HB: Common rashes. BMJ 283:970–971, 1981.
45. Mackey SL, Wagner KF: Dermatologic manifestations of parasitic disease. Infect Dis Clin North Am 8:713–743, 1994.
46. Colven RM, Prose NS: Parasitic infestations of the skin. Pediatr Ann 23:436–442, 1994.

47. Gawkrodger DJ: Dermatology, 2nd ed. New York, Churchill-Livingstone, 1997.
48. Lockwood DN, Keystone JS: Skin problems in returning travelers. Med Clin North Am 76:1393–1411, 1992.
49. Jester JD, Saenz RE, Nesbitt LT, et al: Protozoan and helminth infections. In Sanders CV, Nesbitt LT (eds): The Skin and Infection. Baltimore, Williams & Wilkins, 1995, pp 217–219.
50. Pinkerton H, Henderson RG: Adult toxoplasmosis: A previously unrecognized disease entity simulating the typhus-spotted fever group. JAMA 116:807–814, 1941.
51. Mawhorter SD, Effron D, Blinkhorn R, et al: Cutaneous manifestations of toxoplasmosis. Clin Infect Dis 14:1084–1088, 1992.
52. Ament ME, Rubin CE: Relation of giardiasis to abnormal intestinal structure and function in gastrointestinal immunodeficiency syndromes. Gastroenterology 62:216–226, 1972.
53. Heyworth MF: Immunology of *Giardia* and *Cryptosporidium* infections. Infect Dis 166:465–472, 1992.
54. LoGalbo PR, Sampson HA, Buckley RH: Symptomatic giardiasis in three patients with agammaglobulinemia. J Pediatr 101:78–80, 1982.
55. Ganguly NK, Mahajan RC, Gill NJ, et al: Kinetics of lymphocyte subpopulations and their functions in cases of amoebic liver abscess. Trans R Soc Trop Med Hyg 75:807–810, 1981.
56. Kanani SR, Knight R: Relapsing amoebic colitis of 12 years' standing exacerbated by corticosteroids. BMJ 2:613–614, 1969.
57. DeHovitz JA, Pape JW, Boncy M, et al: Clinical manifestations and therapy of *Isopora belli* infection in patients with the acquired immunodeficiency syndrome. N Engl J Med 315:87–90, 1986.
58. Bentwich Z, Weisman Z, Moroz C, et al: Immune dysregulation in Ethiopian immigrants in Israel: Relevance to helminth infections? Clin Exp Immunol 103:239–243, 1996.
59. Israelski D, Remington J: Toxoplasmosis in the non-AIDS immunocompromised host. Curr Clin Top Infect Dis 13:322–356, 1993.
60. Luft BJ, Remington JS: AIDS commentary. Toxoplasmic encephalitis. J Infect Dis 157:1–6, 1988.
61. Morrow RH, Colebunders RL, Chin J: Interactions of HIV infection with endemic tropical diseases. AIDS 3(suppl):S79–S87, 1989.
62. Straus SE: Introduction to Herpesviridae. In Mandell GL, Bennett JE, Dolin R (eds): Principles and Practice of Infectious Diseases. New York, Churchill-Livingstone, 1995, pp 1330–1336.
63. Hay RJ: Skin disease. Br Med Bull 49:440–453, 1993.
64. Koff RS: Preventing hepatitis A infections in travelers to endemic areas. Am J Trop Med Hyg 53:586–590, 1995.
65. Bras L, Mazaudier E, Bigaignon-Receveur MC, et al: Epidemiology and clinical aspects of imported tropical diseases. J Rev Med Interne 13:205–210, 1992.
66. Gagneux OP, Blochliger CU, Tanner M, et al: Malaria and casual sex: What travelers know and how they behave. J Travel Med 3:14–21, 1996.
67. Phillips-Howard PA, Radalowicz A, Mitchell J, et al: Risk of malaria in British residents returning from malarious areas. BMJ 300:499–503, 1990.
68. Monath TP: Yellow fever: A medically neglected disease. Report on a seminar. Rev Infect Dis 9:165–175, 1987.
69. Manual on Practical Entomology in Malaria. Geneva, World Health Organization, 1975.
70. Encarnacion CF, Giordano MF, Murray HW: Onchocerciasis in New York City. Arch Intern Med 154:1749–1751, 1994.
71. Kelsall BL, Pearson RD: Evaluation of skin problems. Infect Dis Clin North Am 6:441–472, 1992.
72. Jotte RS, Scott J: Malaria: Review of features pertinent to the emergency physician. J Emerg Med 11:729–736, 1993.
73. Nutman TB, Miller KD, Mulligan M, et al: Diethylcarbamazine prophylaxis for human loiasis. Results of a double-blind study. N Engl J Med 319:752–756, 1988.
74. Ottesen EA: Filarial infections. Infect Dis Clin North Am 7:619–633, 1993.
75. Pelletier LL Jr: Chronic strongyloidiasis in World War II Far East ex-prisoners of war. Am J Trop Med Hyg 33:55–61, 1984.
76. Neva FA: Biology and immunology of human strongyloidiasis. J Infect Dis 153:397–406, 1986.
77. Nutman TB, Miller KD, Mulligan M, et al: *Loa loa* infection in temporary residents of endemic regions: Recognition of a hyperresponsive syndrome with characteristic clinical manifestations. J Infect Dis 154:10–18, 1986.
78. Moore AC, Lutwick LI, Schantz PM, et al: Seroprevalence of cysticercosis in an Orthodox Jewish community. Am J Trop Med Hyg 53:439–442, 1995.
79. Parish LC, Schwartzman RM: Zoonoses of dermatological interest. Semin Dermatol 12:57–64, 1993.
80. Anthrax contamination of Haitian goatskin products. MMWR 30:338, 1981.
81. Driscoll MS, Rothe MJ, Grant-Kels JM, et al: Delusional parasitosis: A dermatologic, psychiatric, and pharmacologic approach. J Am Acad Dermatol 29:1023–1033, 1993.
82. Lynch PJ: Delusions of parasitosis. Semin Dermatol 12:39–45, 1993.
83. Wykoff RF: Delusional parasitosis: A review. Rev Infect Dis 9:433–437, 1987.
84. Baler RC, Sequin JH, Leslie N, et al: Fever and petechiae in children. Pediatrics 84:1051–1055, 1989.
85. Singh RS, Sridhar MS, Sekhar PC, et al: Cutaneous anthrax—A report of ten cases. J Assoc Physicians India 40:46–49, 1992.
86. Natori N: A case of cutaneous anthrax. Tohoku J Exp Med 176:187–190, 1995.
87. Cobra C, Rigau-Perez JG, Kuno G, et al: Symptoms of dengue fever in relation to host immunologic response and virus serotype, Puerto Rico, 1990–1991. Am J Epidemiol 142:1204–1211, 1995.
88. Henchal EA, Putnak JR: The dengue viruses. Clin Microbiol Rev 3:376–396, 1990.
89. Lange WR, Beall B, Denny SC: Dengue fever: A resurgent risk for the international traveler. Am Fam Physician 45:1161–1168, 1992.
90. ACP Taskforce on Adult Immunization: Guide for Adult Immunization. Philadelphia, American College of Physicians, 1994, pp 71–142.
91. Monath TP, Tsai TF: Flaviviruses. In Richman DD, Whitley RJ, Hayden FG (eds): Clinical Virology. New York, Churchill Livingstone, 1997, p 1133.
92. Edmond RTD, Smith H, Welsby PD: Assessment of patients with suspected viral haemorrhagic fever. BMJ 1:966–967, 1978.
93. Hulesbosch HJ, Clasessen FAP, Van Ginkel CJW, et al: Human immunodeficiency virus exanthem. J Am Acad Dermatol 23:483–486, 1990.
94. Cooper DA, Maclean P, Finlayson R, et al: Acute AIDS retrovirus infection: Definition of a clinical illness with seroconversion. Lancet 1:537–540, 1985.
95. McGovern TW, Williams W, Fitzpatrick JE, et al: Cutaneous manifestations of African trypanosomiasis. Arch Dermatol 131:1178–1182, 1995.
96. Richman TB, Kerdel FA: Amebiasis and trypanosomiasis. Dermatol Clin 7:301–312, 1989.
97. Melby PC, Kreutzer RD, McMahon-Pratt D, et al: Cutaneous leishmaniasis: Review of 59 cases seen at the National Institutes of Health. Clin Infect Dis 15:924–937, 1992.
98. Amichai B, Finkelstein E, Grunwald MH, et al: Think cutaneous leishmaniasis. Aust Fam Physician 22:1213–1214, 1217, 1993.
99. Wilson ME: Other clinical clues. In: A World Guide to Infections. New York, Oxford University Press, 1991, pp 146–163.
100. Hobbs ER: Coccidioidomycosis. Dermatol Clin 7:227–239, 1989.
101. Murdoch ME, Hay RJ, Mackenzie CD, et al: A clinical classification and grading system of the cutaneous changes in onchocerciasis. Br J Dermatol 129:260–269, 1993.
102. Okello DO, Ovuga EB, Ogwal-Okeng JW: Dermatological problems of onchocerciasis in Nebbi District, Uganda. East Afr Med J 72:295–298, 1995.
103. Hotez PJ: Visceral and ocular larva migrans [Review]. Semin Neurol 13:175–179, 1993.
104. Gordon SM, Gal AA, Solomon AR, et al: Disseminated strongyloidiasis with cutaneous manifestations in an immunocompromised host. J Am Acad Dermatol 31:255–259, 1994.
105. Rusnak JM, Lucey DR: Clinical gnathostomiasis: Case report and review of the English-language literature [Review]. Clin Infect Dis 16:33–50,1993.
106. Deshpande VV: Subcutaneous sparganosis—A rare infection in man. J Assoc Physicians India 41:685, 1993.
107. Taniguchi Y, Ando K, Shimizu M, et al: Creeping eruption due to larvae of the suborder Spirurina—A newly recognized causative parasite. Int J Dermatol 33:279–281, 1994.
108. Neva RA, Ottesen EA: Tropical (filarial) eosinophilia. N Engl J Med 298:1129–1131, 1978.
109. Weller PF: The immunobiology of eosinophils. N Engl J Med 324:1110–1118, 1991.

110. Philpott J, Keystone JS: Eosinophilia: An approach to the problem in the returning traveler. Travel Med Int 1:51–56, 1987.
111. Trevisan G, Cinco M: Lyme disease. Int J Dermatol 29:1–8, 1990.
112. Jelinek T, Nothdurft HD, Rieder N, et al: Cutaneous myiasis: Review of 13 cases in travelers returning from tropical countries. Int J Dermatol 34:624–626, 1995.
113. Vennos E, Burke E, Johns C, et al: Tungiasis. Cutis 56:206–207, 1995.
114. Herzberg AJ, Boyd PR, Gutierrez Y: Subcutaneous dirofilariasis in Collier County, Florida, USA. Am J Surg Pathol 19:934–939, 1995.
115. Bresson-Hadni S, Humbert P, Paintaud G, et al: Skin localization of alveolar echinococcosis of the liver. J Am Acad Dermatol 34:873–877, 1996.
116. Kamal MM, Grover SV: Cytomorphology of subcutaneous cysticercosis. A report of 10 cases. Acta Cytol 39:809–812, 1995.
117. Tomecki KJ, Stech WD, Hall GS, et al: Subcutaneous mycoses. J Am Acad Dermatol 21:785–790, 1989.
118. Marsden PD, Nonata RR: Mucocutaneous leishmaniasis—A review of clinical aspects. Rev Soc Bras Med Trop 9:309–326, 1975.
119. Gart GS, Forstall GJ, Tomecki KJ: Mycobacterial skin disease: Approaches to therapy. Semin Dermatol 12:352–356, 1993.
120. Sehgal VN, Bhattacharya SN, Jain S, et al: Cutaneous tuberculosis: The evolving scenario. Int J Dermatol 33:97–104, 1994.
121. Penn RL: *Francisella tularensis* (tularemia). In Mandell GL, Bennett JE, Dolin R (eds): Principles and Practice of Infectious Diseases. New York, Churchill Livingstone, 1995, pp 2060–2068.
122. Noroes J: Ultrasonographic evidence of abnormal lymphatic vessels in young men with adult *Wuchereria bancrofti* infection in the scrotal area. Urology 155:409–412, 1996.
123. Juckett G: Plant dermatitis. Possible culprits go far beyond poison ivy. Postgrad Med 100:159–163, 167–171, 1996.
124. Dominguez-Soto L, Hojyo-Tomoka T, Vega-Memije E, et al: Pigmentary problems in the tropics. Dermatol Clin 12:777–784, 1994.
125. Hadler SC: Global impact of hepatitis A virus infection changing patterns. In Hollinger FB, Lemon SM, Margolis H (eds): Viral Hepatitis and Liver Disease. Baltimore, Williams & Wilkins, 1991, pp 14–20.
126. Innis BL, Snitbhan R, Kunasol P, et al: Protection against hepatitis A by an inactivated vaccine. JAMA 271:1328–1364, 1994.
127. Bigby M, Jick S, Jick H, et al: Drug-induced cutaneous reactions: A report from the Boston collaborative drug surveillance program on 15,438 consecutive inpatients, 1975–1982. JAMA 256:3358–3363, 1986.
128. Wintroub BU, Stern RS, Arndt K: Cutaneous reactions to drugs. In Fitzpatrick TB, Even AZ, Wolff K, et al (eds): Dermatology in General Medicine. New York, McGraw-Hill, 1987, pp 1353–1366.
129. Okor RS: Responsiveness of chloroquine-induced pruritus to antihistamine therapy—A clinical survey. J Clin Pharmacol Ther 15:147–150, 1990.
130. Okor RS: Onset of pruritogenicity of chloroquine and the implication for the timing of suppressive therapy. J Clin Pharmacol Ther 16:463–465, 1991.
131. Marriott P, Borrie PF: Pigmentary changes following chloroquine. Proc R Soc Med 68:535–536, 1975.
132. Chetelat AA, Albertini S, Gocke E: The photomutagenicity of fluoroquinolones in tests for gene mutation, chromosomal aberration, gene conversion and DNA breakage (Comet assay). Mutagenesis 11: 497–504, 1996.
133. Bjellerup M, Ljunggren B: Differences in phototoxic potency should be considered when tetracyclines are prescribed during summertime: A study of doxycycline and lymecycline in human volunteers, using an objective method for recording erythema. Br J Dermatol 130: 356–360, 1994.
134. Scully JE, Neu HC, Parry MF, et al: Oral ciprofloxacin therapy of infections due to *Pseudomonas aeruginosa*. Lancet 1:819–822, 1986.
135. Shah PM, Mulert R: Safety profile of quinolones. Eur Urol 17(suppl 1):-46–51, 1990.
136. Kaidby KH, Mitchell FN: Photosensitizing potential of certain non-steroidal anti-inflammatory agents. Arch Dermatol 125:783–786, 1989.
137. Bryceson AD, Warrell DA, Pope HM: Dangerous reactions to treatment of onchocerciasis with DEC. BMJ 1:742–744, 1977.
138. Kniker WT, Cochrane CG: The location of circulating immune complexes in experimental serum sickness: The role of vasoactive amines and hydrodynamic forces. J Exp Med 127:119–136, 1968.
139. Chambers HF, Nev HC: Penicillins. In Mandell GL, Bennett JE, Dolin R (eds): Principles and Practice of Infectious Diseases. New York, Churchill Livingstone, 1995, p 23.
140. Van den Enden E, Van Gompel A, Golebunders R, et al: Mefloquine-induced Stevens-Johnson syndrome. Lancet 537:683, 1991.
141. Eriksson B, Bjorknau A, Keisu M: How safe is proquanil? A post-marketing investigation of side effects. Scand J Infect Dis 23:489–493, 1991.
142. Bateman DN, Dyson EH: Quinine toxicity adverse drug reaction. Acute Poisoning Rev 5:215–233, 1986.
143. DuPont HL, Ericson CD, Johnson PC, et al: Prevention of travelers' diarrhea by the tablet formulation of bismuth subsalicylate. JAMA 257:1347–1350, 1987.
144. Maize JC, Tomecki KJ: Pityriasis rosea-like drug eruption secondary to metronidazole. Arch Dermatol 113:1457–1458, 1977.
145. Knowles S, Choudhury T, Shean NH: Metronidazole hypersensitivity. Ann Pharmacother 28:325–326, 1994.
146. Altamirano A, Bondani A: Adverse reactions to furazolidone and other drugs: A comparative review. Scand J Gastroenterol 169(suppl): 70–80, 1989.
147. Horton RJ: Chemotherapy of echinococcal infections in man with albendazole. Trans R Soc Trop Med Hyg 83:97–102, 1989.
148. Awadzi K, Aziz MA, Schulz-Key H, et al: The chemotherapy of onchocerciasis XI: A double-blind comparative study of ivermectin. Ann Trop Med Parasitol 80:433–442, 1986.

127

Hepatobiliary Disease

JOHANNA P. DAILY
JAMES H. MAGUIRE

INTRODUCTION

The hepatobiliary tract is the target of a wide variety of tropical infections. Some diseases, such as chronic hepatitis and biliary ascariasis, are important causes of morbidity and mortality among residents of the tropics in many parts of the world. Others, such as hepatitis A, pose a greater threat to the expatriate traveler. Among the millions of persons in the tropics with the acquired immunodeficiency syndrome (AIDS), opportunistic infections with even once obscure pathogens have become important causes of hepatobiliary disease.

DIAGNOSTIC CONSIDERATIONS

For patients with known or suspected hepatobiliary disease, categorizing the problem into one of several clinical syndromes narrows the list of diagnostic possibilities. Hence, the first step is to determine whether there is parenchymal disease of the liver (hepatitis, cirrhosis, granulomatous and other infiltrative processes, space-occupying lesions), biliary disease (biliary obstruction, other causes of jaundice), vascular disease, or splenomegaly. Priority should be given to life-threatening but treatable conditions such as hepatic abscess, cholangitis, and falciparum malaria, and to diseases that threaten the public health, such as hepatitis A and several of the viral hemorrhagic fevers. It is important to rule out diseases that are also common in temperate climates, such as cholecystitis and pancreatic carcinoma, and noninfectious processes that occur more frequently in the tropics, such as veno-occlusive disease.

The spectrum of hepatobiliary infections differs among residents of the developing world, immigrants from these areas, and the expatriate traveler.[1–9] Acute hepatitis A is common among travelers returning to temperate zones, who typically lack prior exposure and immunity, while it is rare among immigrants and adult residents of the tropics, who experienced infection during childhood.[10] Biliary ascariasis is familiar to clinicians in the developing world, where a large proportion of the population harbors adult worms (see Chapter 109).[11–14] Although ascariasis is not uncommon among immigrants from the tropics, the risk of hepatobiliary complications decreases rapidly during the first year after arrival, because the worms die and are not replaced.

Routine evaluation of the patient begins with a clinical history that may help distinguish between disease processes and point to a diagnosis. There should be questions about the pace of illness, right upper quadrant pain or discomfort, indigestion, jaundice, dark urine, pruritus, fever, anorexia, and other constitutional symptoms. A history of underlying conditions, medications, vaccinations, and an epidemiological history of exposures should be taken. Examination should evaluate the size, consistency, and tenderness of the liver, spleen, and gallbladder. The presence of jaundice, ascites, dilated periumbilical veins, spider angiomata, or other stigmata of liver disease should be ascertained. Measurements of serum bilirubin, liver enzymes, and alkaline phosphatase are part of routine screening for hepatobiliary disease. Depending on their availability, further studies such as measurements of serum albumin and prothrombin time, serologic tests, imaging studies, cholangiography, and liver biopsy may be indicated.

Ultrasonography (US) is more widely available in tropical areas than computed tomography (CT) or magnetic resonance imaging (MRI). US is useful for detecting gallstones, dilated biliary ducts, thickened gallbladder walls, masses within and around the liver, periportal fibrosis, hepatosplenomegaly, and evidence of portal hypertension. US can distinguish solid lesions from abscesses and cysts and can demonstrate certain helminths within the hepatobiliary tree.[15–17]

In the sections to follow, diseases of the hepatobiliary tree are discussed according to clinical syndromes and manifestations. Emphasis is on differential diagnosis and the approach to diagnosis.

ACUTE HEPATITIS

The clinical spectrum of acute hepatitis ranges from asymptomatic illness to fulminant, massive hepatic necrosis. In typical symptomatic cases, there is vague discomfort and tenderness in the right upper quadrant, nausea, anorexia, jaundice, and fever. The broad differential diagnosis is outlined in Figure 127-1. In all cases, a history of exposure to toxins and drugs that cause damage to the liver should be sought.

Elevation of hepatic enzymes and bilirubin also occurs in response to a number of systemic infections, including bacterial sepsis, pneumonia, typhoid fever, and malaria, even when the pathogen does not directly infect liver tissue.[1,18] Cholestasis and frank jaundice are prominent in such cases and may take days to several weeks to resolve after the responsible infection is cleared. In malaria, hepatomegaly without evidence of hepatocellular injury can occur as a consequence of vascular congestion and Kupffer cell hyperplasia.

The most common causes of hepatitis throughout the world are hepatitis viruses A through E (see Chapter 64). In many developing regions, hepatitis A virus (HAV) infection occurs in the first years of life through fecal-oral transmission and is usually asymptomatic.[19] In areas where the quality of drinking water has improved, however, the prevalence of hepatitis A in children has decreased in recent years.[20] Hepatitis A infection is one of the most common causes of illness among travelers to the tropics, occurring at a rate of 3 to 6 per 1000 persons per month in one study and accounting for 60% of cases of hepatitis in returning travelers.[21] Appropriate use of hepatitis A vaccine or pooled serum immunoglobulin reduces the risk of infection among travelers to less than 5% and 15%, respectively.[22]

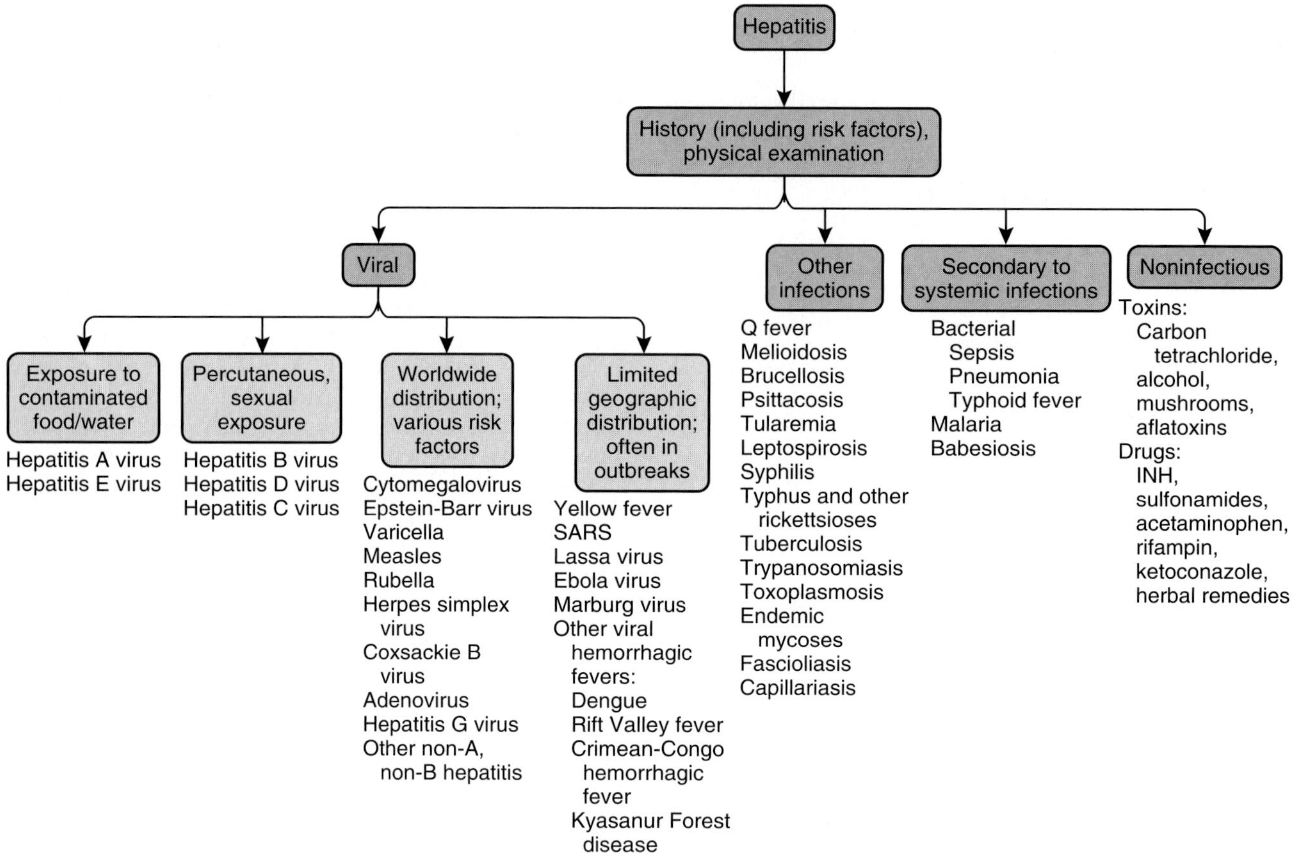

FIGURE 127-1 Differential diagnosis of acute hepatitis.

The prevalence of hepatitis B surface antigenemia varies from less than 1% in Mexico and temperate South America to as high as 15% in parts of Africa, Southeast Asia, China, the Philippines, Pacific islands, Middle East, and the Amazon basin.[23,24] Residents of such areas generally acquire asymptomatic infections in the perinatal and early childhood periods. Acute hepatitis B is four to five times less common than hepatitis A among travelers to the tropics.[25] Expatriates at high risk for hepatitis B include health-care professionals, persons receiving inoculations or dental treatment, and those who engage in unprotected sexual contact or share needles.[26] Only persons infected with hepatitis B virus (HBV) are at risk for superinfection with delta virus (hepatitis D virus, HDV). Direct person-to-person contact of HDV has been responsible for the high number of cases of fulminant hepatitis in the Amazon region (Lábrea hepatitis), northern Colombia (hepatitis of the Sierra Nevada of Santa Marta), and remote Amerindian settlements in Venezuela, rather than percutaneous needle exposure, which is the usual route in other parts of the world.[27–29]

Acute hepatitis C virus (HCV) infection occurs usually via the parenteral route, or less commonly via sexual transmission. It is endemic worldwide with high prevalence in Japan and the Mediterranean countries of Europe, Africa, and the Middle East, where it causes significant morbidity, but is rare among returning travelers.[30–32] High rates of hepatitis C infection in Egypt are attributed to use of inadequately sterilized needles for administration of tartar emetic during mass treatment campaigns to control schistosomiasis in the 1960s through the 1980s.[33] Another virus transmitted via the fecal-oral route, hepatitis E, has caused outbreaks in India, Nepal, Pakistan, the former Soviet Union; parts of Africa, Mexico, and China; and the Middle East. Sporadic cases have been reported among travelers.[34–36]

Distinguishing the different types of hepatitis on clinical grounds alone is difficult. The incubation periods of hepatitis A and B are 2 to 6 weeks and 6 weeks to 6 months, respectively. The hepatic manifestations of HBV infection may be preceded by rash, arthralgia, and arthritis. Mortality due to fulminant hepatitis occurs in 0.15% of persons with HAV infection (and in 2% to 3% of those over the age of 40 years), in fewer than 1% of those with HBV infection, in up to 50% of those with HDV co-infection, and in up to 20% of pregnant women during the third trimester who become infected with hepatitis E virus (HEV).

There are specific immunoglobulin M (IgM) antibody tests for hepatitis A, D, and E. Acute hepatitis B is diagnosed using assays for hepatitis B surface antigen or anti-HBV core antigen.[37,38] Diagnosis of acute hepatitis C requires detection of HCV RNA, since anti-HCV antibodies are usually slow to develop. Household contacts of patients with hepatitis A should receive serum immunoglobulin, and precautions to prevent enteric spread should be taken. Hepatitis B immune globulin and immunization are effective in preventing infection of sexual partners and neonates born to infected mothers.

Other viruses that cause acute hepatitis are listed in Figure 127-1.[39] Diagnosis is made by serologic tests, microscopic examination of biopsy specimens, and viral cultures of liver tissue, blood, urine, and other fluids. In the forested areas of sub-Saharan Africa and South America, yellow fever occurs in epidemics or as sporadic cases among unvaccinated persons, including the occasional traveler (see Chapter 71). Only 10% to 20% of cases of infection with the yellow fever virus lead to the classic syndrome of biphasic fever, jaundice, hemorrhage, and hepatic necrosis. Other agents of viral hemorrhagic fever that involve the liver include the tick-borne Kyasanur Forest disease in India and Crimean-Congo hemorrhagic fever in Africa and Asia; Lassa fever in West Africa; Marburg virus disease in Uganda, Kenya, and Zimbabwe; and Ebola virus disease in Zaire and Sudan (see Chapters 65–67, and 70).[40] Because transmission of the highly lethal Lassa fever, Marburg, and Ebola viruses is by direct contact with blood and excreta, strict isolation and infection control precautions are indicated. Hepatic necrosis has been reported also with dengue hemorrhagic fever and Rift Valley fever. Hepatic impairment and elevated levels of transaminases in the serum that occur in up to 60% of persons with the severe acute respiratory syndrome (SARS) are due to infection of the liver with the SARS-associated coronavirus.[41]

Hepatomegaly and, at times, clinically apparent hepatitis are seen in nonviral infections such as leptospirosis, relapsing fever, and early syphilis (see Chapters 44–46). Hepatitis is rare in Lyme borreliosis. In leptospirosis, the elevation of serum bilirubin is usually out of proportion to that of the hepatic enzymes. Leptospirosis is enzoonotic throughout the tropics, and outbreaks among residents and travelers in the tropics have followed contact with contaminated water or moist soil.[42,43]

Pulmonary involvement and a history of contact with livestock or parturient cats clinically distinguishes the hepatitis of acute Q fever from that of viral hepatitis. Hepatomegaly or hepatitis occurs frequently in typhoid fever, acute brucellosis, tularemia, meloidosis, and psittacosis, as well as in rickettsioses.[44,45] Massive hepatic necrosis may complicate miliary tuberculosis.[46]

A mild increase in serum transaminases can be seen in cases of acute acquired toxoplasmosis. Mild hepatomegaly during acute Chagas' disease results from infection of hepatocytes and Kupffer cells and the host's immune response (see Chapter 93). Approximately 2 months after ingestion of watercress containing metacercariae of *Fasciola hepatica,* immature flukes migrate through the liver, causing right upper quadrant pain, nausea, and fever (see Chapter 117). Tender hepatomegaly and elevated serum hepatic enzymes are suggestive of viral hepatitis, but a marked peripheral blood eosinophilia and urticarial eruptions point to the proper diagnosis. Hypoechoic and hypodense lesions of the liver detected by US and CT correspond to the track of the parasite as it burrows through the liver.[16,47] Diagnosis of acute fascioliasis is made by serologic tests because symptoms precede egg-laying by weeks.[48] Rare human cases of *Capillaria hepatica* have been reported from Africa, Asia, and Latin America (see Chapter 106).[49] Acutely, there may be tender hepatomegaly and anorexia. The diagnosis is suggested by peripheral blood eosinophilia and confirmed by demonstration of worms and eggs in the liver by biopsy or at autopsy. Hepatomegaly in acute schistosomiasis results from egg deposition in the liver and the immune response to worm and egg antigens (see Chapter 116).[50] Specific serologic tests become positive several weeks before eggs can be found in the stool.

CHRONIC HEPATITIS AND OTHER CAUSES OF DIFFUSE HEPATOMEGALY

Chronic active hepatitis in the tropics is caused most commonly by HBV and HCV (see Chapter 64). Co-infection with HDV may accelerate the course of chronic HBV infection. While failure to resolve infection with these agents may lead to cirrhosis or hepatoma, persons with chronic hepatitis may remain asymptomatic for years, despite persistently elevated hepatic enzymes. Serologic testing and liver biopsy confirm the diagnosis.

Macronodular or "postnecrotic" cirrhosis develops in up to 25% of chronic hepatitis B surface antigen carriers and in over 20% of persons infected with HCV for over 20 years. The process may be clinically silent for several years before the appearance of symptoms and signs of hepatocellular dysfunction and portal hypertension such as jaundice, encephalopathy, ascites, and bleeding from esophageal varices. The liver is firm, nodular, and shrunken.

The periportal or "pipe stem" fibrosis of chronic schistosomiasis gives the liver a nodular appearance which resembles that of cirrhosis. True cirrhosis in schistosomiasis, however, is usually due to coinfection with HBV or HCV, or other chronic liver disease, and only occasionally is it seen in the absence of other hepatic lesions.[51] Cirrhosis has been reported as a consequence of visceral leishmaniasis.

Chronic alcoholism is a common cause of micronodular cirrhosis in the tropics. African or Bantu cirrhosis is thought to be related in part to chronic iron overload and hemochromatosis, whereas Indian childhood cirrhosis may be related to high copper intake as well as genetic factors.[52] Many cases of cirrhosis in the tropics remain undiagnosed. The differential diagnosis of hepatomegaly is shown in Box 127-1.

Granulomatous Disease

Systemic infections may infiltrate the liver and induce granuloma formation. Usually, both the liver and spleen are enlarged, and the alkaline phosphatase is elevated. In visceral leishmaniasis, disseminated tuberculosis, atypical mycobacterial infections, histoplasmosis, disseminated *Penicillium marneffei* infection, and other fungal infections, organisms invade Kupffer cells and other cells of the reticuloendothelial system. Disseminated infections of this sort are common in advanced human immunodeficiency virus (HIV) disease, but because of impaired immunity there may be little or no granulomatous reaction on histologic examination. Diagnosis is made by microscopic examination of biopsied liver tissue and culture of tissue and blood.

In chronic schistosomiasis mansoni and schistosomiasis japonica, granulomas form around eggs trapped in portal venules. Typically, the left lobe of the liver is enlarged more than the right lobe. As infection progresses, the size of the liver decreases as the diameter of the granulomas is reduced by immunomodulation. Periportal fibrosis, a specific finding in hepatosplenic schistosomiasis, is detected by US, CT, and MRI. In *Schistosoma japonicum* infection, calcified eggs in the liver

Box 127-1 Differential Diagnosis of Hepatomegaly

Infiltrating or Granulomatous Infections

Q fever
Melioidosis
Psittacosis
Brucellosis
Granuloma inguinale
Tularemia
Listeriosis
Syphilis
Bartonellosis
Tuberculosis
BCG vaccination or immunotherapy
Leprosy
Cryptococcosis
Histoplasmosis and other endemic fungi
Visceral leishmaniasis
Schistosomiasis
Microsporidiosis
Strongyloidiasis
Ascariasis
Toxocariasis
Capillariasis
Baylisascaris infection
Fascioliasis
Viral infections (CMV, EBV)

Abscesses and Cysts

See Figure 127-3

Response to Systemic Infection

See Figure 127-1

Acute Hepatitis

See Figure 127-1

Portal Hypertension

Schistosomiasis
Cirrhosis
Chronic liver disease
Portal vein thrombosis
Veno-occlusive disease
Noncirrhotic portal fibrosis
Clonorchiasis

Noninfectious Causes

Lymphoma
Leukemia
Metastatic carcinoma
Hepatocellular carcinoma
Fatty changes
Polycystic disease
Heart failure
Amyloidosis
Alcoholic cirrhosis
Siderosis and septal fibrosis
Bantu cirrhosis

BCG, bacille Calmette-Guérin; CMV, cytomegalovirus; EBV, Epstein-Barr virus

produce a characteristic "turtle-back" pattern on MRI. In severe cases, portal hypertension may lead to gastroesophageal varices, but jaundice, ascites, and hepatic encephalopathy are only seen in "decompensated" cases in which there is hepatocellular damage as well as portal hypertension. The diagnosis of chronic schistosomiasis is made by finding eggs in specimens of stool. Serologic tests are useful for screening travelers, who often have light and asymptomatic infections. Hepatosplenomegaly and early periportal fibrosis may regress after treatment with praziquantel.

Granulomas may form around migrating filariform larvae of *Strongyloides* during hyperinfection and dissemination. Granulomas form around *Ascaris* eggs trapped in liver tissue when adult worms enter the biliary tree. Hepatic granulomas around adult worms, larvae, and eggs are characteristic of chronic *Capillaria hepatica* infection. In visceral larva migrans due to *Toxocara canis* or *Baylisascaris procyonis,* migrating larvae provoke an eosinophilic granulomatous response.[53] Hepatomegaly, fever, and peripheral blood eosinophilia prompt a clinical diagnosis, which can be confirmed by serologic tests.

Space-Occupying Lesions of the Liver

Symptoms of mass lesions in the liver produce abdominal discomfort from distention of Glisson's capsule, an increase in abdominal girth, obstruction of the biliary system, or rupture into the peritoneum, pericardium, or pleural space or through the abdominal wall. Asymptomatic lesions occasionally are detected by imaging procedures during evaluation of unexplained fever or weight loss. The characteristics of lesions imaged by US, CT, or MRI may yield a precise diagnosis of certain helminthic infections such as schistosomiasis, acute fascioliasis, or echinococcosis, but the cause of most lesions is determined by serologic tests, blood cultures, or culture and microscopic examination of specimens obtained by aspiration or biopsy.

Liver abscesses, whether amebic or bacterial, may present subacutely with low-grade fever, weight loss, and localized pain, or acutely with temperatures above 102°F and signs of toxicity. Jaundice is unusual in the absence of biliary obstruction, and the alkaline phosphatase may be the only hepatic enzyme that is elevated.

Certain features may help differentiate amebic and bacterial abscesses[54] (Fig. 127-2). Amebic abscesses occur frequently in Mexico, Central America, northern South America, West and South Africa, and India. Most persons with amebic abscesses do not have dysentery, and stool examination does not show trophozoites or cysts in 50% of those tested. Serologic tests for antiamebic antibodies become positive in 99% of persons after 7 days of symptoms. Antibodies may persist for years, however, and the specificity of serologic tests may be low in endemic areas. Aspiration of the abscess usually is not necessary for diagnosis; abscess fluid typically contains few or no amebae, rare white blood cells, and no bacteria. A trial of metronidazole or tinidazole confirms a clinical diagnosis if patients defervesce or show symptomatic improvement within a few days.[55] Aspiration is indicated in cases of pending rupture or in cases with uncertain diagnoses that do not respond to medical treatment.[56] Treatment with metronidazole or tinidazole should be followed by a course of a luminal amebicide such as paromomycin, iodoquinol, or diloxanide furoate.

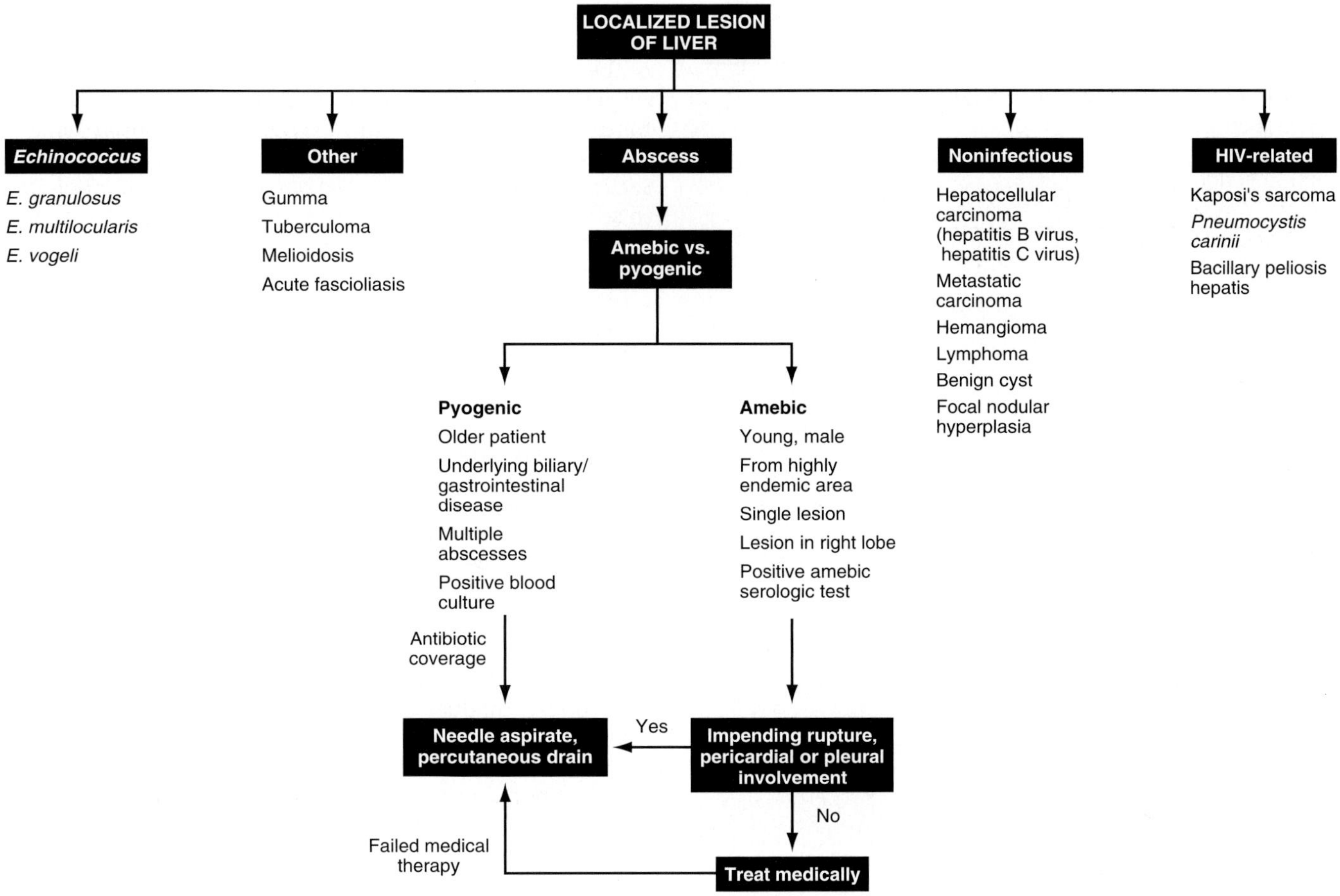

FIGURE 127-2 Differential diagnosis of space-occupying lesions of the liver.

Pyogenic liver abscesses most commonly are caused by enteric organisms, streptococci, and *Staphylococcus aureus*.[57] Blood cultures and cultures of abscess fluid are positive in about 50% and 73% of persons, respectively.[58] In the tropics, *Salmonella typhi, Brucella* species, and *Burkholderia (Pseudomonas) pseudomallei* occasionally cause hepatic abscesses. Occasional causes of large space-occupying lesions in the liver include tuberculosis, gummatous syphilis, and, in persons with AIDS, bartonellosis (peliosis hepatis), and *Pneumocystis jiroveciii.* During acute fascioliasis, CT or MR often show hypodense lesions in the liver measuring 1 cm or more in diameter that move to different parts of the liver over the course of several weeks. These lesions correspond to the tortuous and branching linear tracks of necrotic tissue and eosinophilic inflammatory infiltrates along the path of larval migration.[59]

Hydatid cysts of the liver (see Chapter 114) may be distinguished from simple hepatic cysts when US, CT, or MRI shows intracystic septations indicative of daughter cysts. Otherwise, a history of residence in a sheep raising or other endemic area or a history of urticarial or anaphylactic reactions may suggest the diagnosis of hydatid disease. A highly sensitive enzyme-linked immunosorbent assay (ELISA) and confirmatory immunoblot for antibodies to *Echinococcus granulosus* are available.[60] Microscopic examination of cyst fluid taken by needle aspiration or at surgery usually shows diagnostic protoscolices, hooklets, and calcareous bodies.[61] Treatment includes high-dose albendazole and either careful surgery or percutaneous drainage with inactivation of cysts.[62,63] Less common cestodes that cause mass lesions in the liver include *Echinococcus multilocularis* in northern regions of the world and *Echinococcus vogeli* and *Echinococcus oligarthrus* in Central and South America.[64] Hepatic cysticercosis is unusual.

Vascular Disease

Chronic passive congestion of the liver due to heart failure may produce chronic hepatomegaly and eventually cardiac cirrhosis. In tropical areas, important causes include chronic Chagas' cardiomyopathy, rheumatic heart disease, restrictive pericarditis from tuberculosis, and endomyocardial fibrosis. Veno-occlusive disease involving hepatic venules causes rapidly progressive tender hepatomegaly, ascites, and death from variceal bleeding or liver failure. It is associated with ingestion of pyrrolizidine alkaloids in herbal teas in Jamaica and parts of Africa and Asia.[65]

Splenomegaly

The spleen is enlarged in many of the same infections in which the liver is enlarged (Box 127-2). Massive splenomegaly may be seen in visceral leishmaniasis, chronic

Box 127-2 Differential Diagnosis of Splenomegaly*

Infiltrating or Granulomatous Infections
Visceral leishmaniasis
Tuberculosis
Viral infection
Fungal infection

Abscesses and Cysts
Brucellosis
Salmonellosis
Other bacterial abscesses
Echinococcosis
Melioidosis

Response to Systemic Infection
Malaria
Acute Chagas' disease
African trypanosomiasis
Endocarditis
Typhus
Bartonellosis
Rickettsial disease
Viral disease
Salmonellosis

Portal Hypertension
Schistosomiasis
Cirrhosis
Chronic liver disease
Portal vein thrombosis
Veno-occlusive disease
Noncirrhotic portal fibrosis
Clonorchiasis

Noninfectious Causes
Lymphoma
Leukemia
Metastatic carcinoma
Sickle cell disease
Thalassemia
Thrombocytopenic purpura
Felty's syndrome
Heart failure
Amyloidosis

*Many of the infectious diseases listed in Box 127-1 can also cause splenomegaly.

malaria (tropical splenomegaly syndrome), and myeloproliferative disorders.[66] Splenomegaly secondary to portal hypertension occurs with schistosomiasis, cirrhosis, and many other severe chronic liver diseases. Unusual causes of splenomegaly in the tropics include abscesses due to *Salmonella typhi, Brucella* species (especially *B. suis*), and *Burkholderia (Pseudomonas) pseudomallei*. Hypoechogenic lesions in the spleen have been detected by ultrasonography in persons with loiasis.[67]

JAUNDICE

Tropical infectious diseases produce jaundice by several mechanisms (Fig. 127-3). Hemolysis leading to predominantly unconjugated hyperbilirubinemia and depressed serum haptoglobin levels is the result of direct infection of red blood cells by *Plasmodia, Babesia,* and *Bartonella bacilliformis*. It also may occur via indirect mechanisms such as disseminated intravascular coagulation accompanying a variety of systemic infections or the hemolytic-uremic syndrome associated with *Escherichia coli* O157-H7. Mixed conjugated and unconjugated hyperbilirubinemia is seen with infections that produce hepatitis by directly or indirectly damaging hepatocytes, as discussed earlier. Typically, there is an element of intrahepatic cholestasis in addition to impaired uptake and conjugation of bilirubin.

Obstruction of biliary ducts by stones, tumors, strictures, and certain infections produces marked elevation of the serum conjugated bilirubin and serum alkaline phosphatase, 5-nucleotidase, and γ-glutamyltranspeptidase. US, CT, and endoscopic cholangiography assist in the identification of the cause of obstruction.

BILIARY OBSTRUCTION

Obstruction of the biliary or cystic duct leads to biliary colic with right upper quadrant pain or pressure of sudden onset that radiates to the shoulder (Table 127-1). Persistence and progression of the pain, frequently with nausea, vomiting, localized peritoneal signs, and low-grade fever suggest cholecystitis. High fevers, shaking chills, leukocytosis, and jaundice suggest cholangitis, which may lead to septicemia and shock. Gradual obstruction of the common bile duct leads to painless jaundice, often with pruritus.

Obstruction of the biliary tract in the tropics is frequently caused by parasitic infections. Biliary ascariasis (see Chapter 109)

***Table 127-1** Causes of Obstructive Biliary Disease in the Tropics*

Infectious	Noninfectious
Leptospirosis	Neoplasma
Salmonellosis	Metastatic disease
Tuberculosis	Hepatoma
Syphilis	Cholangiocarcinoma associated with *Clonorchis* or *Opisthorchis* infection
Actinomycosis	Pancreatitis
Helminthic infections	Lymphadenopathy
Nematodes	Gallstones
Ascaris lumbricoides	
Strongyloides stercoralis	
Capillaria hepatica	
Cestodes	
Echinococcus spp.	
Trematodes	
Clonorchis sinensis	
Opisthorchis viverrini	
Opisthorchis felineus	
Fasciola hepatica	
Fasciola gigantica	
Paragonimus spp.	
Protozoa	
Cryptosporidium parvum	
Isospora belli	
Cyclospora cayetanensis	
Giardia lamblia	
Microsporidia	

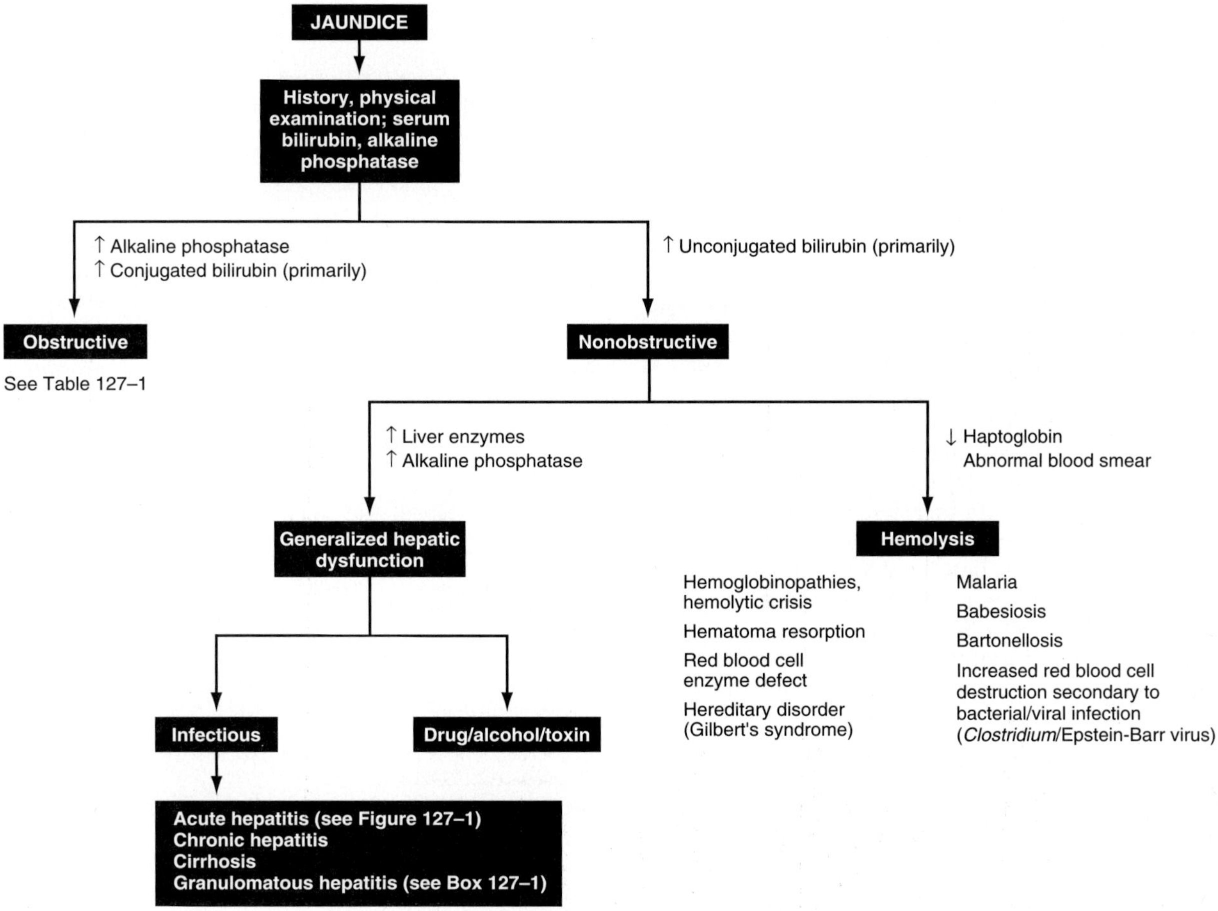

FIGURE 127-3 Differential diagnosis and evaluation of jaundice.

complicates chronic ascariasis in fewer than 0.1% of cases, but the huge number of infected persons makes the condition an important cause of hepatobiliary disease.[11] When individual adult worms enter and exit the bile ducts, symptoms of biliary colic are intermittent, but when worms fail to exit the duct, pyogenic cholangitis, hemorrhagic pancreatitis, or liver abscesses may result. Worms that die in the biliary tree may form the nidus of gallstones.[68] In a series of 500 patients with biliary and pancreatic ascariasis in India, 56% had biliary colic, 24% had acute cholangitis, 13% had acute cholecystitis, 6% had pancreatitis, and 1% had liver abscesses.[14] The diagnosis is made by US, CT, cholangiography, or endoscopic retrograde cholangiopancreatography (ERCP) and may demonstrate worms in the biliary or pancreatic ducts or gallbladder.[69,70] Treatment consists of extraction of worms during ERCP or anthelmintic treatment, preferably with pyrantel pamoate, which acts rapidly and paralyzes the worms. Nasogastric suction, antispasmodics, analgesics, and intravenous fluids usually obviate the need for surgery.

Clonorchiasis and opisthorchiasis (see Chapter 117) are common infections in Southeast Asia, China, and other parts of Asia where carp is consumed without proper cooking.[71,72] Most persons are asymptomatic, but small numbers of persons with long-standing infection develop recurrent episodes of cholangitis or cholangiocarcinoma.[73] Adult flukes that inhabit the bile ducts and gallbladder are responsible for hyperplasia of the ductal epithelium and occasionally biliary stones or pancreatitis. Chronic infections with adult *Fasciola hepatica* and *Fasciola gigantica* may remain asymptomatic for years before adult worms cause cholecystitis and cholangitis.[74] Hemobilia from ulceration of biliary epithelium, sclerosing cholangitis, and biliary stones are unusual complications of chronic fascioliasis.[75] The diagnosis of chronic clonorchiasis, opisthorchiasis, and fascioliasis is made by identifying eggs in the stool or bile or identifying adult worms by cholangiography or visually at the time of surgery. US and CT may demonstrate adult *Fasciola*. *Paragonimus* has been reported to cause obstructive granulomas involving the biliary tree resulting in biliary cirrhosis (see Chapter 117).[76]

Hydatid cysts of the liver (see Chapter 114) cause biliary obstruction by compressing biliary radicals as they grow or by rupturing into the biliary tree and causing blockage with daughter cysts and cyst membranes.[77] Cyst rupture can be provoked by trauma and may lead to bacterial cholangitis, liver abscess, and anaphylactic reactions to the highly antigenic cyst contents.

Other parasitic causes of biliary diseases include *Cryptosporidium parvum* (see Chapter 88) and microsporidia (see Chapter 96) in persons with AIDS. Findings are similar to those of primary sclerosing cholangitis, with diffuse involvement of intrahepatic or extrahepatic bile ducts, or both, strictures, ampullary stenosis, and pancreatic duct involvement.

ERCP defines the lesions anatomically, and examination of feces or bile for oocysts of cryptosporidia or *Isospora* or spores of microsporidia are diagnostic. AIDS-associated cholangiopathy may also be caused by cytomegalovirus, *Mycobacterium avium* complex, *Mycobacterium tuberculosis,* and *Histoplasma capsulatum.*[78–81]

Acalculous cholecystitis may be provoked by organisms that infect the gallbladder in the absence of stones. Leptospirosis, salmonellosis, and giardiasis have been implicated in immunocompetent persons, and the same agents that cause AIDS-associated cholangiopathy occasionally cause acalculous cholecystitis in HIV-infected persons. Acalculous cholecystitis has been seen in association with systemic infections such as actinomycosis, tuberculosis, and syphilis.

Cholelithiasis has become more common in some developing areas as residents have adopted a westernized diet.[1] In addition, gallstones result from chronic hemolytic states such as sickle cell anemia and other hemoglobinopathies and malaria. Recurrent pyogenic cholangitis is a condition of unknown cause in the Far East in which there is formation of pigment stones and sludge. It has been suggested that parasites such as *Clonorchis, Opisthorchis,* and *Ascaris* act as the nidus for stone formation in this condition, but dietary deficiencies that alter bile salt metabolism may be more important.

HIV INFECTION AND HEPATOBILIARY DISEASE

HIV infection, which is highly prevalent in many parts of the tropics (see Chapters 76 and 133), may alter the natural history, clinical presentation, diagnosis, and management of infections involving the liver and biliary tract. For example, HIV infection may lead to unusual clinical syndromes, such as cholangitis caused by cytomegalovirus, intestinal coccidia, microsporidia, and mycobacteria, or bacterial peliosis due to *Bartonella.* HIV co-infection has been associated with decreased egg excretion in persons with *S. mansoni* due to impaired granuloma formation and increased trapping of eggs in tissue. Serologic tests for the diagnosis of visceral leishmaniasis may yield false negative results in HIV-infected patients, but recovery of parasites from the peripheral blood is enhanced. Treatment of certain infections of the hepatobiliary tract in persons infected with HIV may present difficult challenges, such as the high rate of relapse of visceral leishmaniasis following standard therapy. Importantly, highly active antiretroviral therapy (HAART) may play a key role in preventing progression of latent diseases, reducing the rate of relapse, and enhancing efficacy of treatment.[82,83]

REFERENCES

1. Cook GC: Gastroenterological emergencies in the tropics. Baillieres Clin Gastroenterol 5:861–886, 1991.
2. Gyr KE, Barz A: Imported gastrointestinal diseases in industrialized nations. Baillieres Clin Gastroenterol 1:425–445, 1987.
3. Steffen R, Rickenbach M, Wilhelm U, et al: Health problems after travel to developing countries. J Infect Dis 156:84–91, 1987.
4. Wilson M: World Guide to Infections: Diseases, Distribution, Diagnosis. Oxford, Oxford University Press, 1991.
5. Keystone J, Kozarsky P, Freedman D, et al: Travel Medicine. Philadelphia, CV Mosby, 2003.
6. Liu LX, Weller PF: Approach to the febrile traveler returning from Southeast Asia and Oceania. Curr Clin Top Infect Dis 12:138–164, 1992.
7. Wyler DJ: Evaluation of cryptic fever in a traveler to Africa. Curr Clin Top Infect Dis 12:329–347, 1992.
8. Oster CN, Tramont EC: Fever in a recent visitor to the Middle East. Curr Clin Top Infect Dis 13:57–73, 1993.
9. Maguire JH: Epidemiologic considerations in the evaluation of undifferentiated fever in a traveler returning from Latin America or the Caribbean. Curr Clin Top Infect Dis 13:26–56, 1993.
10. Gust ID, Ruff TA: Hepatitis in the tropics. Med J Aust 159:691–695, 1993.
11. Crompton DWT, Nesheim MC, Pawlowski ZS (eds): Ascariasis and Its Prevention and Control. London, Taylor & Francis, 1989.
12. Pawlowski Z: Ascariasis. Clin Trop Med Common Dis 2:595, 1987.
13. Schuster DI, Belin RP, Parker JC Jr, et al: Ascariasis—Its complications, unusual presentations and surgical approaches. South Med J 70:176–178, 1977.
14. Khuroo MS, Zargar SA, Mahajan R: Hepatobiliary and pancreatic ascariasis in India. Lancet 335:1503–1506, 1990.
15. el-Tahir MI, Omojola MF, Malatani T, et al: Hydatid disease of the liver: Evaluation of ultrasound and computed tomography. Br J Radiol 65:390–392, 1992.
16. Takeyama N, Okumura N, Sakai Y, et al: Computed tomography findings of hepatic lesions in human fascioliasis: Report of two cases. Am J Gastroenterol 81:1078–1081, 1986.
17. Richter J, Hatz C, Haussinger D: Ultrasound in tropical and parasitic diseases. Lancet 362:900–902, 2003.
18. Gilles HM, Warrell DA, Bruce-Chwatt, LJ: Bruce-Chwatt's Essential Malariology, 3rd ed. London, Edward Arnold, 1993.
19. Abdool Karim SS, Coutsoudis A: Sero-epidemiology of hepatitis A in black South African children. S Afr Med J 83:748–750, 1993.
20. Innis BL, Snitbhan R, Hoke CH, et al: The declining transmission of hepatitis A in Thailand. J Infect Dis 163:989–995, 1991.
21. Steffen R: Risk of hepatitis A in travellers. Vaccine 10(suppl 1): S69–S72, 1992.
22. Koff RS: Preventing hepatitis A infections in travelers to endemic areas. Am J Trop Med Hyg 53:586–590, 1995.
23. Perrillo RP: Hepatitis B: Transmission and natural history. Gut 34:S48–S49, 1993.
24. Moyer LA, Mast EE: Hepatitis B: Virology, epidemiology, disease, and prevention, and an overview of viral hepatitis. Am J Prev Med 10(suppl):45–55, 1994.
25. Steffen R: Risks of hepatitis B for travellers. Vaccine 8(suppl):S31–S32; discussion S41–S43, 1990.
26. Struve J, Norrbohm O, Stenbeck J, et al: Risk factors for hepatitis A, B and C virus infection among Swedish expatriates. J Infect 31:205–209, 1995.
27. Buitrago B, Hadler SC, Popper H, et al: Epidemiologic aspects of Santa Marta hepatitis over a 40-year period. Hepatology 6:1292–1296, 1986.
28. Hadler SC, De Monzon M, Ponzetto A, et al: Delta virus infection and severe hepatitis. An epidemic in the Yucpa Indians of Venezuela. Ann Intern Med 100:339–344, 1984.
29. Bensabath G, Hadler SC, Soares MC, et al: Hepatitis delta virus infection and Lábrea hepatitis. Prevalence and role in fulminant hepatitis in the Amazon Basin. JAMA 258:479–483, 1987.
30. Sharara AI: Chronic hepatitis C. South Med J 90:872–877, 1997.
31. Tibbs CJ: Tropical aspects of viral hepatitis. Hepatitis C. Trans R Soc Trop Med Hyg 91:121–124, 1997.
32. Ray Kim W: Global epidemiology and burden of hepatitis C. Microbes Infect 4:1219–1225, 2002.
33. Rao MR, Naficy AB, Darwish MA, et al: Further evidence for association of hepatitis C infection with parenteral schistosomiasis treatment in Egypt. BMC Infect Dis 2:29, 2002.
34. Bader TF, Krawczynski K, Polish LB, et al: Hepatitis E in a U.S. traveler to Mexico. N Engl J Med 325:1659, 1991.
35. Centers for Disease Control and Prevention: Hepatitis E among US travelers, 1989–1992. JAMA 269:845–846, 1993.
36. Emerson SU, Purcell RH: Hepatitis E virus. Rev Med Virol 13:145–154, 2003.
37. DeGuzman LJ, Pitrak DL, Dawson GJ, et al: Diagnosis of acute hepatitis E infection utilizing enzyme immunoassay. Dig Dis Sci 39:1691–1693, 1994.
38. Kumar S, Pound DC: Serologic diagnosis of viral hepatitis. Postgrad Med 92:55–62, 65, 68, 1992.
39. Teichmann D, Gobels K, Niedrig M, et al: Dengue virus infection in travellers returning to Berlin, Germany: Clinical, laboratory, and diagnostic aspects. Acta Trop 90:87–95, 2004.

40. Speed BR, Gerrard MP, Kennett ML, et al: Viral haemorrhagic fevers: Current status, future threats. Med J Aust 164:79–83, 1996.
41. Chau TN, Lee KC, Yao H, et al: SARS-associated viral hepatitis caused by a novel coronavirus: Report of three cases. Hepatology 39:302–310, 2004.
42. van Crevel R, Speelman P, Gravekamp C, et al: Leptospirosis in travelers. Clin Infect Dis 19:132–134, 1994.
43. Sejvar J, Bancroft E, Winthrop K, et al: Leptospirosis in "Eco-Challenge" athletes, Malaysian Borneo, 2000. Emerg Infect Dis 9:702–707, 2003.
44. Zaidi SA, Singer C: Gastrointestinal and hepatic manifestations of tickborne diseases in the United States. Clin Infect Dis 34:1206–1212, 2002.
45. Memish ZA, Balkhy HH: Brucellosis and international travel. J Travel Med 11:49–55, 2004.
46. Asada Y, Hayashi T, Sumiyoshi A, et al: Miliary tuberculosis presenting as fever and jaundice with hepatic failure. Hum Pathol 22:92–94, 1991.
47. Han JK, Choi BI, Cho JM, et al: Radiological findings of human fascioliasis. Abdom Imaging 18:261–264, 1993.
48. Hillyer GV, Soler de Galanes M: Initial feasibility studies of the fast-ELISA for the immunodiagnosis of fascioliasis. J Parasitol 77:362–365, 1991.
49. Guttierrez Y: Diagnostic Pathology of Parasitic Infections with Clinical Correlations. New York, Oxford University Press, 2000.
50. Lambertucci JR: A new approach to the treatment of acute schistosomiasis. Mem Inst Oswaldo Cruz 84(suppl 1):23–30, 1989.
51. Lichtenberg V: Consequences of infections with schistosomes. In Rollinson D, Simpson AJG (eds): Biology of Schistosomes from Genes to Latrines. London, Academic Press, 1987, p 185.
52. Scheinberg IH, Sternlieb I: Is non-Indian childhood cirrhosis caused by excess dietary copper? Lancet 344:1002–1004, 1994.
53. Glickman LT, Magnaval JF: Zoonotic roundworm infections. Infect Dis Clin North Am 7:717–732, 1993.
54. Barnes PF, De Cock KM, Reynolds TN, et al: A comparison of amebic and pyogenic abscess of the liver. Medicine (Baltimore) 66:472–483, 1987.
55. Sharma MP, Rai RR, Acharya SK, et al: Needle aspiration of amoebic liver abscess. BMJ 299:1308–1309, 1989.
56. Singh JP, Kashyap A: A comparative evaluation of percutaneous catheter drainage for resistant amebic liver abscesses. Am J Surg 158:58–62, 1989.
57. Rubin RH, Swartz MN, Malt R: Hepatic abscess: Changes in clinical, bacteriologic and therapeutic aspects. Am J Med 57:601–610, 1974.
58. McDonald MI, Corey GR, Gallis HA, et al: Single and multiple pyogenic liver abscesses. Natural history, diagnosis and treatment, with emphasis on percutaneous drainage. Medicine (Baltimore) 63:291–302, 1984.
59. MacLean JD, Graeme-Cook FM: Case records of the Massachusetts General Hospital. Weekly clinicopathological exercises. Case 12–2002. A 50-year-old man with eosinophilia and fluctuating hepatic lesions. N Engl J Med 346:1232–1239, 2002.
60. Donovan SM, Mickiewicz N, Meyer RD, et al: Imported echinococcosis in southern California. Am J Trop Med Hyg 53:668–671, 1995.
61. Filice C, Di Perri G, Strosselli M, et al: Parasitologic findings in percutaneous drainage of human hydatid liver cysts. J Infect Dis 161:1290–1295, 1990.
62. Bret PM, Fond A, Bretagnolle M, et al: Percutaneous aspiration and drainage of hydatid cysts in the liver. Radiology 168:617–620, 1988.
63. Filice C, Brunetti E, Bruno R, et al: Percutaneous drainage of echinococcal cysts (PAIR—puncture, aspiration, injection, reaspiration): Results of a worldwide survey for assessment of its safety and efficacy. WHO-Informal Working Group on Echinococcosis-Pair Network. Gut 47:156–157, 2000.
64. Kammerer WS, Schantz PM: Echinococcal disease. Infect Dis Clin North Am 7:605–618, 1993.
65. MacGregor FB, Abernethy VE, Dahabra S, et al: Hepatotoxicity of herbal remedies. BMJ 299:1156–1157, 1989.
66. Hutt MS, Lowenthal MN: Chronic splenomegaly in the tropics. Trop Doct 4:51–55, 1974.
67. Schuurkamp GJ, Kereu RK, Bulungol PK, et al: Diethylcarbamazine in the control of splenomegaly associated with *Bancroftian filariasis* in the Ok Tedi area of Papua New Guinea. Trans R Soc Trop Med Hyg 86:531–536, 1992.
68. Pilankar KS, Amarapurkar AD, Joshi RM, et al: Hepatolithiasis with biliary ascariasis—A case report. BMC Gastroenterol 3:35, 2003.
69. Filice C, Marchi L, Meloni C, et al: Ultrasound in the diagnosis of gallbladder ascariasis. Abdom Imaging 20:320–322, 1995.
70. Rocha Mde S, Costa NS, Costa JC, et al: CT identification of ascaris in the biliary tract. Abdom Imaging 20:317–319, 1995.
71. Mairiang E, Mairiang P: Clinical manifestation of opisthorchiasis and treatment. Acta Trop 88:221–227, 2003.
72. Chan HH, Lai KH, Lo GH, et al: The clinical and cholangiographic picture of hepatic clonorchiasis. J Clin Gastroenterol 34:183–186, 2002.
73. Sithithaworn P, Haswell-Elkins MR, Mairiang P, et al: Parasite-associated morbidity: Liver fluke infection and bile duct cancer in northeast Thailand. Int J Parasitol 24:833–843, 1994.
74. Harinasuta T, Pungpak S, Keystone JS: Trematode infections. Opisthorchiasis, clonorchiasis, fascioliasis, and paragonimiasis. Infect Dis Clin North Am 7:699–716, 1993.
75. Acuna-Soto R, Braun-Roth G: Bleeding ulcer in the common bile duct due to *Fasciola hepatica*. Am J Gastroenterol 82:560–562, 1987.
76. Okuda K, Kuratomi S, Moriyama M, et al: Biliary cirrhosis secondary to extrapulmonary paragonimiasis. Digestion 2:347–353, 1969.
77. Atlas DH, Kamenear H: Rupture of echinococcus cysts into the bile ducts simulating stones in the common duct. Am J Med 13:384–386, 1952.
78. Morrow RH, Colebunders RL, Chin J: Interactions of HIV infection with endemic tropical diseases. AIDS 3(suppl 1):S79–S87, 1989.
79. Tarimo DS, Killewo JZ, Minjas JN, et al: Prevalence of intestinal parasites in adult patients with enteropathic AIDS in north-eastern Tanzania. East Afr Med J 73:397–399, 1996.
80. Amarapurkar DN, Chopra KB, Phadke AY, et al: Tuberculous abscess of the liver associated with HIV infection. Indian J Gastroenterol 14:21–22, 1995.
81. Houston S: Tropical respiratory medicine. 3. Histoplasmosis and pulmonary involvement in the tropics. Thorax 49:598–601, 1994.
82. de la Rosa R, Pineda JA, Delgado J, et al: Influence of highly active antiretroviral therapy on the outcome of subclinical visceral leishmaniasis in human immunodeficiency virus–infected patients. Clin Infect Dis 32:633–635, 2001.
83. Pintado V, Martin-Rabadan P, Rivera ML, et al: Visceral leishmaniasis in human immunodeficiency virus (HIV)–infected and non-HIV-infected patients. A comparative study. Medicine (Baltimore) 80:54–73, 2001.

128

Approach to the Patient in the Tropics with Pulmonary Disease

GREGORY J. MARTIN

Pulmonary disease is one of the leading causes of morbidity and mortality throughout the world and respiratory tract infections are the most frequent infections of humans.[1] As represented in Box 128-1, four of the ten leading causes of global death reported to the World Health Organization (WHO) are attributable to some form of acute or chronic pulmonary disease.[2] The viral, bacterial, fungal, and protozoal etiologies of worldwide lung disease are protean. Tropical pulmonary disease includes most temperate climate etiologies as well as a greater incidence and prevalence of tuberculosis (TB), human immunodeficiency virus (HIV)-related disease, and helminthic infections. Diverse factors such as poverty, crowding, malnutrition, and proximity to animals are responsible for a range of diseases that are infrequently encountered outside the tropics.

As developing nations make economic transitions, smoking and unregulated occupational and environmental exposures become significant risk factors for previously uncommon pneumoconioses and respiratory malignancies.[3,4] Conversely, as travel between industrialized and tropical nations increases, agents responsible for localized outbreaks of disease in remote, undeveloped areas have been more frequently imported to the industrialized world. Most notably, in China and Southeast Asia in 2003, the ability of a zoonotic coronavirus (later designated SARS CoV) to infect humans led to the severe acute respiratory syndrome (SARS). SARS quickly became a major public health emergency not only in much of Asia but also in Canada and, to a lesser extent, in the United States and Europe. Novel influenza viruses have commonly been first discovered in tropical Asian populations where animals, especially chickens, ducks, and pigs, are often kept in close proximity to humans. As outbreaks of avian (and swine) influenza occur in these areas, sporadic cases of these same strains occur in humans, creating the potential for human-zoonotic recombinations and the possibility of returning travelers presenting with these "exotic" strains.

Box 128-1 Ten Leading Causes of Death Worldwide, 2002

1. Ischemic heart disease 12.6%
2. Cerebrovascular disease 9.6%
3. Lower respiratory infections 6.6%
4. HIV/AIDS 4.9%
5. Chronic obstructive pulmonary disease 4.8%
6. Perinatal conditions 4.3%
7. Diarrheal diseases 3.1%
8. Tuberculosis 2.8%
9. Trachea, bronchus, lung cancers 2.2%
10. Malaria 2.1%

Mathers CD, Bernard C, Moesgaard Iburg K, et al: Global burden of diseases in 2002: Data sources, methods and results. WHO Global Programme on Evidence for Health Policy Discussion Paper No. 54, 2003.

The following overview is designed as a starting point in developing a differential diagnosis for patients presenting with pulmonary complaints who have had exposure in the tropics. Emphasis will be given to those entities found exclusively or more commonly in the tropics. In Table 128-1, parasitic etiologies associated with respiratory disease from the tropics and their geographic distributions are shown and demonstrates the diversity of pathogens that must be considered.[5] The specific disease entities and treatment are fully described in the individual pathogen chapters of the text.

Clinicians evaluate patients' illnesses in geographic areas differently depending on the resources available and the local prevalence of diseases. In developing a differential diagnosis for respiratory complaints, it is helpful to consider patients in three relatively distinct groups that have considerable differences in their exposure to various risk factors:

1. Lifelong denizens of the tropics (as well as those from the tropics who have recently immigrated to a temperate area)
2. Travelers who have returned from the tropics after short (less than 1 month) visits
3. Expatriates from temperate areas who are currently living in or have just returned from the tropics.

Even when coming from (or living in) the same region, the etiologies and diagnostic approaches to each of these groups may be quite different as the intensity of their exposures, potential contact with infected individuals, and access to medical care (and advanced diagnostics) may be significantly diverse. For example, a patient who presents with hemoptysis in most industrialized nations has a high likelihood of having a lung neoplasm, whereas natives of the tropics with hemoptysis are much more likely to have tuberculosis, and the differential diagnosis for an expatriate living in the tropics falls somewhere between these two groups.[6]

ACUTE RESPIRATORY TRACT INFECTIONS, INCLUDING PNEUMONIA

Acute respiratory tract infections (ARIs) include a spectrum of illnesses from colds and influenza to streptococcal pharyngitis and pneumococcal pneumonia. As such, they may be little more than an annoyance or they may be associated with a fulminant course and significant morbidity and mortality.

Upper respiratory illnesses (URIs) are the most common infections in humans in both temperate and tropical climates and are primarily viral in etiology. The frequency of respiratory

Table 128-1 Parasites Associated with Respiratory Illness

Parasite	Distribution
Nematodes	
Roundworms	
Ascaris spp.	Worldwide
Toxocara canis & *T. cati*	
Hookworms	
Necator americanus	SE Asia, West and Central Africa
Ancyclostoma duodenale	S. Europe, N. Africa, India, China, Japan
Ancyclostoma caninum	S. USA, Mexico, Africa, Asia, S. America
Necator brasiliense	S. America, Caribbean
Filariae	
Loa loa	West and Central Africa
Wuchereria bancrofti	Pacific, Asia, Africa, China, Americas
Brugia malayi	Southeast Asia
Dirofilaria immitis	SE Asia, America, S. Africa, Australia
Other	
Gnathostoma spinigerum	India, Philippines, Thailand
Strongyloides stercoralis	Worldwide
Trichinella spiralis	Worldwide
Trematodes	
Schistosomes	
Schistosoma mansoni	Africa, S. Arabia, S. America, Caribbean
S. haematobium	Africa, Middle East
S. japonicum	Far East
S. intercalatum	West and Central Africa
Liver flukes	
Paragonimus westermanii	Far East, China, Japan, Philippines
P. africanus	Africa
P. caliensis	South and Central America
Cestodes	
Hydatid disease	
Echinococcus granulosus	Australia, Africa (endemic)
E. multilocularis	Worldwide
Protozoa	
Entamoeba histolytica	Worldwide
Plasmodium falciparum	Africa, South and Central America, Asia
Pneumocystis jaroveci	Worldwide
Toxoplasma gondii	Worldwide
Leishmania donovani	Africa, Middle East, S. America, Asia

Modified from Savani DM, Sharma OP: Eosinophilic lung disease in the tropics. Clin Chest Med 23:377, 2002.

infections among children is much greater than in adults.[7] Although the frequency of URIs in the tropics appears to be no higher than in temperate climates, children in the tropics often suffer from chronic malnutrition. Undernourished children experience respiratory infections, coupled with bouts of diarrhea, intestinal helminth infection, epidemic measles, and more. These co-morbidities make what might be a mild respiratory illness in an otherwise healthy child significantly more serious in children living in the tropics (Table 128-2).[8]

Table 128-2 Annual Childhood Deaths Associated with ARI

Region	Total Deaths	ARI Deaths	Due to ARI
Africa	3,608,000	800,000	22%
Americas	436,000	60,000	14%
Eastern Med	1,345,000	261,000	19%
Europe	217,000	24,000	11%
South East Asia	3,274,000	606,000	19%
Western Pacific	979,000	132,000	13%
Total	9,901,000	1,880,000	19%

ARI, acute respiratory infection.
Modified from Williams BG, Gouws E, Boschi-Pinto C, et al: Estimates of world-wide distributions of child deaths from acute respiratory infections. Lancet Infect Dis 2:25, 2002.

The role of viral URIs, particularly influenza and respiratory syncytial virus, in predisposing individuals to subsequent bacterial infection, predominantly with *Streptococcus pneumoniae* and *Hemophilus influenzae* has emphasized the importance of controlling epidemic influenza in developing nations where vaccines have been historically underutilized.[9]

Acute lower respiratory infections cause most of the respiratory disease–associated deaths and, in terms of years of life lost (YLL) in sub-Saharan Africa, ranks second only to diarrheal diseases.[10] The most common etiologies of childhood pneumonia in developing countries are summarized in Box 128-2.[11]

Box 128-2 Etiologies of Childhood Pneumonia in the Tropics

Main Bacterial Etiologies

Streptococcus pneumoniae
Haemophilus influenzae

Other Bacterial Etiologies

Salmonella and other enteric bacteria
Staphylococcus aureus
Streptococcus spp.
Moraxella spp.

Viral Etiologies

Respiratory syncytial virus (RSV)
Influenza A and B
Parainfluenza
Adenovirus
Herpes simplex
Rubeola (measles)

Others

Chlamydia spp.
Mycoplasma spp.
Ureaplasma spp.
Pneumocystis jaroveci (formerly *P. carinii*)

Outbreak Associated

Hantaviruses
Lass, Ebola, other hemorrhagic fever viruses
SARS Coronavirus

Modified from Adegbola RA, Obaro SK: Diagnosis of childhood pneumonia in the tropics. Ann Trop Med Parasitol 94:197, 2000.

ESTIMATES OF THE PERCENTAGE OF CHILDREN WHO DIE FROM ACUTE LOWER RESPIRATORY INFECTION BY COUNTRY, 2000

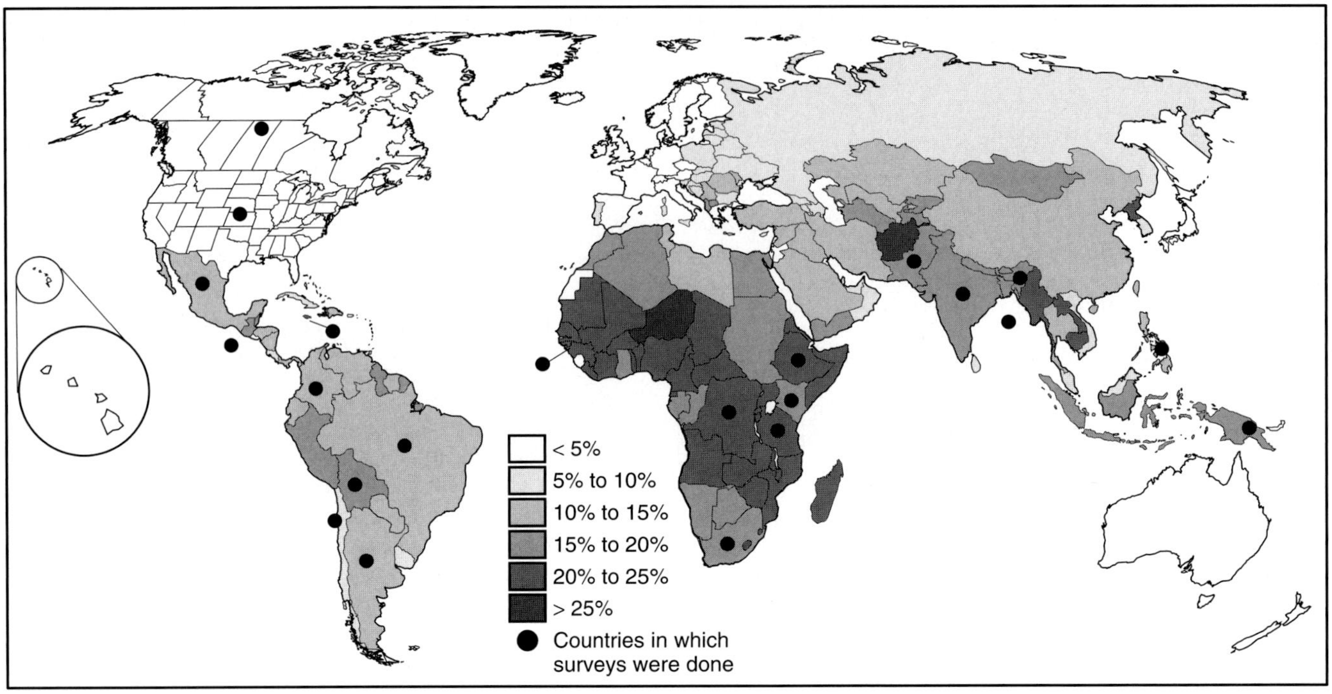

Although all age groups have some deaths associated with lower respiratory infections, the greatest burden is borne by children, especially those younger than 5 years old, with an estimated 3 to 4 million deaths annually.[12,13] Data from WHO reveal a marked difference in the proportion of deaths in children less than 5 years old caused by ARIs in Europe (11%) and the Americas (14%) versus Africa (22%) and Southeast Asia (19%).[1] Most developed nations of Europe and North America report less than 5% of childhood deaths due to ARIs. Africa not only bears the burden of very high childhood mortality, but also has nations with more than 25% of childhood deaths due to ARIs.[1] The role of co-infection with HIV and/or malnutrition in ARI-associated deaths cannot be overemphasized. Recent WHO data from Botswana, currently the nation with the highest prevalence of HIV infection, revealed that aproximately 60% of childhood deaths due to HIV/acquired immunodeficiency virus (AIDS), often associated with respiratory coinfections.[14]

S. pneumoniae and *H. influenzae* remain the most important bacterial causes of pneumonia in young children, accounting for 70% of the deaths from pneumonia and neonatal sepsis.[11] The use of *H. influenzae B* and, more recently, pneumococcal conjugate vaccines has dramatically decreased the frequency of these infections in developed countries but, due to their cost, they remain underutilized in the developing nations.[9]

Bacterial antimicrobial resistance has become an increasing problem worldwide, including in the tropics. Lack of antibiotic availability in some areas has led to low prevalence of resistant organisms. Conversely, poorly controlled access to antibiotics and inappropriate use has led to very high levels of resistance in other areas. One study in Uganda identified 95% of *S. pneumoniae* as penicillin-resistant and 75% of *H. influenzae* as β-lactamase producing. Despite this resistance, there was a good clinical response to ampicillin even among HIV-infected individuals.[15]

Availability of antibiotics in developing nations is quite variable: Many nations have access to less expensive penicillin, ampicillin, chloramphenicol, erythromycin, tetracycline and aminoglycosides, but the more expensive third-generation cephalosporins, fluoroquinolones, and newer macrolides that are commonly used in developed nations are often unavailable.

Common causes of atypical pneumonia, such as *Mycoplasma pneumoniae, Chlamydia pneumoniae,* and *Legionella* spp., are probably as common in the tropics as they are in temperate areas but have been poorly studied due to difficulty in culturing and the expense of serology. Outbreaks of Legionnaires' disease associated with travel, especially among the elderly, have been reported on numerous occasions. Nearly half the cases of *Legionella* pneumonia in the United Kingdom are travel-associated.[16]

Measles (rubeola) is the most important viral respiratory disease. Measles is associated with significant morbidity and mortality in much of the developing world, with an estimated 40 million annual cases and 800,000 deaths per year, half of which occur in Africa. Most unvaccinated children in endemic areas are infected by age 5.[17] Since the introduction of measles vaccination in 1963, there has been a marked decrease in measles cases and, as of March 2005, no indigenous transmission of measles has occurred in the Americas for over 2 years; WHO has a goal of worldwide eradication by 2015.[17] Death from measles is usually associated with either a primary viral pneumonia or secondary bacterial infection with *S. pneumoniae, H. influenzae, Staphylococcus aureus,* or secondary viral infection with herpes simplex or adenovirus.

Numerous studies from the 1930s to the present have demonstrated a marked reduction in morbidity and mortality associated with measles infections after initiation of childhood vitamin A supplementation. This is especially evident in refugee settings where malnutrition and a measles outbreak may be the leading cause of death.[18]

Particular settings in the tropics may suggest the role of certain bacterial organisms: Examples are staphylococcal pneumonia complicating measles and varicella, pertussis in areas with inadequate childhood immunization, and *Klebsiella* pneumonia in lower socioeconomic rural settings where alcoholism and malnutrition may play a role. Chronic cavitary upper lobe infiltrates in a patient from Southeast Asia may be misidentified as tuberculosis but actually represent melioidosis, a chronic infection of *Burkholderia pseudomallei*, a soil saprophyte endemic to Southeast Asia and part of Australia (see Chapter 34). Melioidosis is the most common cause of fatal, community-acquired pneumonia at a regional referral hospital in the Northern Territory of Australia. In a series of 252 cases of melioidosis in Australia, half presented with pneumonia and one-quarter were bacteremic, 15% presented with pneumonia and septic shock, and 84% of the septic individuals died.[19] Melioidosis is well documented to occur months to years after exposure and it should remain in the differential diagnosis for those with appropriate exposure who present with chronic, subacute or acute pulmonary disease that may appear to be tuberculosis.[20]

Occupational exposures may suggest an etiology for unusual bacterial pneumonias such as anthrax, Q fever, tularemia, and leptospirosis. Outbreaks associated with Hantaviruses, pneumonic plague, influenza, and SARS corona-virus are all potential etiologies that should be considered. Since all of these rarer causes of pneumonia can be found nearly worldwide to varying degrees, it may be most helpful to query WHO (www.who.int/csr/outbreaknetwork/en/) or CDC (www.cdc.gov/travel/outbreaks.htm) websites to get updates about outbreaks of diseases in different countries.

CHRONIC COUGH

Cough, a common symptom of URIs, is also frequently associated with pneumonia, chronic obstructive pulmonary disease, bronchiectasis, sinusitis, and asthma. URIs are the most common illnesses of travelers to the tropics. Patients will often assume the worst, that they have developed SARS, tuberculosis, or pneumonia, and seek medical evaluation earlier than they may have if they became ill without traveling. Patients usually do not seek medical attention for cough until it has persisted for more than 5 to 7 days and most cough lasting less than two months is associated with relatively benign viral or bacterial etiologies, but may be associated with recent infection with *Ascaris*, hookworm, *Strongyloides*, or schistosomes. Cough persisting for more than 2 months is considered chronic, and a far wider differential diagnosis should be considered, especially in individuals in the tropics or returning from the tropics.[21,22] Table 128-3 lists some considerations for the differential diagnosis of chronic cough. Many of the infectious etiologies for cough are fully described in other chapters.

In developing a differential diagnosis for chronic cough, in-depth inquiry into the patient's travel background and exposure history must be obtained. A knowledge of which diseases and infectious agents are endemic to the area is also crucial. A short-term traveler to an urban area of the tropics may have only a remote opportunity to have encountered helminths or tuberculosis, whereas those with a long-term travel history to remote areas, and extensive exposure to the local population, have probably had ample opportunity to be exposed to the wide range of infectious agents endemic in the tropics. Some of these same exposure considerations should be applied to those who live in the tropics; an urban office worker is much less likely to have had the constant animal, insect, and freshwater contact of a rice farmer in rural areas.

Tuberculosis should nearly always be considered in the differential of chronic cough if there is associated fever, weight loss, and pulmonary infiltrates, particularly in infants and young children. Schistosomiasis and intestinal helminths should be considered in "eco-tourists," campers, and those who report freshwater exposure as well as rural denizens. Endemic mycoses, melioidosis, and environmental toxins are potential etiologies that should be entertained in the context of the appropriate geographic region and exposure history. Chest radiographs and serology, as well as sputa and stool microscopy, will usually confirm these diagnoses if they have been considered in the evaluation.

A complete blood count with differential should always be obtained, as cough associated with a parasitic infection may have a normal total leukocyte count but a significantly elevated eosinophil count that would guide the diagnostic evaluation (see Chapter 125). Radiographs of the chest are also indicated in evaluation of chronic cough as characteristic radiologic findings are seen with many of the diagnoses. Abnormal chest radiographs in resource-rich nations are often further evaluated

Table 128-3 Common Etiologies of Cough of More than 2 Months Duration That Occur Worldwide and Those More Commonly Associated with Exposure in the Tropics

Worldwide	Tropics
• Allergic and nonallergic rhinitis	• Tuberculosis
• Reactive airways disease (asthma)	• Loeffler's syndrome (helminthic pulmonary transmigration)
• Chronic obstructive pulmonary disease	• Schistosomiasis (acute or late stage disease)
• Bronchiectasis	• Tropical pulmonary eosinophilia (filarial infection with hypersensitivity reaction)
• Congestive heart failure	• Paragonimiasis
• Gastroesophageal reflux	• Penicilliosis marneffei
• Angiotensin-converting enzyme inhibitors	• Paracoccidioidomycosis
• Eosinophilic bronchitis	• Melioidosis
• Recurrent aspiration	
• Interstitial lung disease	
• Sarcoidosis	
• Neoplasm	
• Tuberculosis	
• Pneumoconioses	
• Endemic mycoses	
• HIV-associated opportunistic infections	

by computed tomography (CT) scan. Although readily available in most developed nations, CT scanners are not available in 40% of the sub-Saharan countries and are not readily available in many other areas as well.[23] Similarly, availability of bronchoscopic evaluation is variable outside developed nations but should be considered if the etiology of cough cannot be determined with less invasive testing. Sputum examination is generally available in most areas. Sputum examination is most important to rule out tuberculosis (TB) and, in contrast to some other diagnostic modalities, microscopists in the developing world are often quite experienced and skilled in reading stains for acid-fast bacteria, protozoa, and helminths. In temperate areas, routine sputa and even bronchoscopic samples are often not examined for fungi, mycobacteria, and parasites. These etiologies, more common in the tropics, should nearly always be considered in the diagnostic evaluation.

HEMOPTYSIS

Regardless of tropical or temperate exposure, the development of significant hemoptysis nearly always warrants diagnostic evaluation. While trivial hemoptysis with scant streaks of blood is not uncommon with bronchitis, the differential diagnosis should remain broad, especially in those with tropical exposure. While studies of the etiology of hemoptysis vary significantly depending on geographic location and decade of publication, hemoptysis often indicates an underlying serious disease.

Although bronchiectasis and neoplasia are the most common causes of hemoptysis in developed nations, tuberculosis may exceed these noninfectious etiologies in developing nations. Understanding the prevalence of TB in the area where the patient was traveling (or living) is crucial in developing the differential diagnosis. In a 1997 study from Israel of 208 patients presenting with hemoptysis, only 3 (1.4%) were associated with TB.[24] Similarly, in an older U.S. study from Boston in 1952, only 2 (1.9%) of 105 cases of hemoptysis were attributed to tuberculosis.[25] Conversely, in a 2002 study from Turkey of 108 cases of hemoptysis, 18 (17.4%) were associated with tuberculosis[26] and in a 2001 study of 52 patients with hemoptysis from Kuwait, 17 (32.7%) of the cases were attributed to either "old" or active pulmonary TB.[27] A similar study performed in an area with much higher TB rates, such as Afghanistan or sub-Saharan Africa, might find TB in an even greater percentage of patients presenting with hemoptysis than the relatively less affected Turkey and Kuwait.

Table 128-4 Etiologies of Hemoptysis Worldwide and Those More Commonly Associated with Exposure in Developing Nations

Worldwide	Developing Nations
• Bronchiectasis	• Tuberculosis
• Bronchogenic neoplasm	• Endemic mycoses
• Bronchitis	• *Echinococcus*
• Congestive heart failure	• *Paragonimus*
• Blood dyscrasias	• *Entamoeba histolytica*
• Tuberculosis	• Leptospirosis
• Endemic mycoses	• Melioidosis

The role of other infectious etiologies such as *S. pneumoniae, Haemophilus* spp., melioidosis, endemic fungi, amoeba, and helminthic agents (ascaris, hookworm, *Strongyloides, Echinococcus,* and *Paragonimus*) should all be considered in the differential diagnosis based on the location of the exposure and are summarized in Table 128-4.

Work-up of hemoptysis should start with chest radiographs but may require CT scan or bronchoscopy with biopsies to make a definitive diagnosis. Again, informing the microbiology and pathology laboratories of the potential for fungal, mycobacterial, and parasitic disease will ensure that appropriate stains and cultures are performed.

EOSINOPHILIA ASSOCIATED WITH PULMONARY COMPLAINTS

Patients presenting for medical attention in the tropics, or after returning from a trip to the tropics, not uncommonly (up to 5%) are found incidentally to have eosinophilia.[28] Although generally not considered to be clinically significant until reaching an absolute eosinophil count of greater than 1000, a relative increase in eosinophils on a complete blood count will often lead to pulmonary or infectious diseases consultation. The differential diagnosis and evaluation of eosinophilia is thoroughly reviewed in Chapter 125.

Evaluation of patients with eosinophilia can be very difficult, especially in the absence of significant symptoms to help guide the assessment. A thorough account of both domestic and tropical travel must be included in the history as well as a detailed inquiry into use of prescription drugs, over-the-counter drugs, and supplements as the etiology may be a hypersensitivity reaction as opposed to an infection. There are a host of nonparasitic and even noninfectious etiologies that should be considered in the evaluation and these are considered in Chapter 125. Furthermore, multiple infections with a number of helminths from a shared exposure occur quite commonly. Stool, sputa, and serologic assays are frequently negative during the larval stages in the pulmonary vasculature.

The intestinal helminths most commonly associated with transmigration of their larvae through the lung leading to the eosinophilia, frequently referred to as Loeffler's syndrome, are *Ascaris, Strongyloides,* and the hookworms *Necator* and *Ancyclostoma*.[29] Larvae penetrate into the alveolar spaces, are coughed into the mouth and then swallowed, thereby completing their journey to the intestinal tract where the adult stages live. *Ascaris* are most likely to be associated with development of significant pulmonary symptoms; hookworm and *Strongyloides* usually cause minimal inflammation during pulmonary transmigration. Loeffler's syndrome occurs 10 to 12 days after ingestion of *Ascaris* eggs (or 5–10 days after penetration of hookworm or *Strongyloides* larva) and, if there are any symptoms, is characterized by development of 5 to 10 days of nonproductive cough, burning substernal chest pain, and, frequently, wheezing and rales. Chest radiograph reveals ill-defined, patchy, homogenous consolidation or, occasionally, a fine miliary pattern. Infiltrates may be unilateral or bilateral, have indefinite borders, and range from a few millimeters to 2 to 3 cm.[23]

The migration of the larvae of *Toxocara canis* or *T. cati* in pulmonary tissues as a manifestation of visceral larva migrans (see Chapter 103) is associated with high levels of eosinophilia, and may be associated with fever, hepatosplenomegaly, and transient reticulonodular infiltrates.[30]

Schistosomes may be associated with eosinophilia and chest symptoms (see Chapter 116). Especially in nonimmune travelers, acute schistosomiasis (3–8 weeks after schistosome penetration) may be associated with headache, malaise, dyspnea, wheezing, and nonproductive cough, especially while recumbent in bed. These pulmonary symptoms may coincide with the fever (Katayama fever) associated with acute infection, but more commonly present a few weeks after resolution of fever and are associated with marked eosinophilia (approximately 30%–50%), mild to moderate leukocytosis, and liver enzyme abnormalities.[31] Since schistosomes pass through the lung shortly after penetration (5–7 days), the pulmonary symptoms are likely an immune effect triggered in the lung while the organism has become established elsewhere in the host, similar to established intestinal helminths that may also cause pulmonary infiltrates.[32] Chronic pulmonary disease is a complication of established schistosomal infections as ectopic migration of schistosome eggs occurs. This becomes more common in late disease as portal hypertension leads to portacaval shunts and deposition of eggs in the pulmonary vasculature. The granulomatous response to eggs in the pulmonary vessels leads to pulmonary hypertension and eventually cor pulmonale. Finally, some helminths (most importantly *Paragonimus* spp. and *Echinococcus* spp.) establish their adult stage in the lung and may be associated with years of waxing and waning eosinophilia[30] (see Chapters 114 and 117).

PLEURAL EFFUSION

The etiologies for pleural effusion are protean and include a wide variety of infectious agents from bacterial and viral to protozoal and helminthic. Common noninfectious etiologies such as malignancies, heart or liver failure, collagen vascular diseases, and others predominate in temperate areas. The differential diagnosis of pleural effusion after exposure in the tropics is skewed due to the high prevalence of tuberculosis and HIV-associated disease and the increased incidence of helminthic, protozoal, and fungal infections. In one study from Zimbabwe of 100 consecutive patients with pleural effusion of unknown etiology, TB was ultimately determined as the final diagnosis in 58 of the patients after pleural biopsy was performed.[33] Temperate areas with a high incidence of tuberculosis may also have TB as a common cause of pleural effusion. For example, a large study of 642 pleural effusions in Spain (in an area with high incidence of TB—95 per 100,000) found TB responsible for 25%, neoplasia for 23%, and congestive heart failure for 18%.[34,35] In areas with a low prevalence of TB, pleural effusions are rarely associated with tuberculosis and are much more commonly a sign of malignancy. Table 128-5 summarizes etiologic considerations for pleural effusion worldwide and in a patient with potential exposure in the tropics.

Evaluation of pleural effusion should involve consideration of multiple aspects of the clinical setting. Bilateral pleural effusion in a patient with underlying heart disease returning from the tropics is still likely a pleural transudate related to heart failure. Presence of fever, pleuritic chest pain, and leukocytosis are obvious indicators of potential infectious etiologies and are indications that thoracentesis is indicated.

Table 128-5 Etiology of Pleural Effusion with Additional Considerations from the Tropics

Worldwide	Frequency Diagnosed	Additional Etiologies Tropical Regions
Heart failure		
Malignancy		
Pulmonary embolus	Common	
Parapneumonic	↑	Tuberculosis
Cirrhosis	│	Paragonimiasis
Tuberculosis	│	Cryptococcosis
Endemic fungi	│	Histoplasmosis
Nephrotic syndrome	│	Sparganosis
Idiopathic	│	Toxocariasis
Hypothyroidism	↓	Echinococcosis
Drug hypersensitivity	Infrequent	Amebiasis
Asbestosis		
Collagen vascular diseases		
Pancreatitis		

In addition to cell count, differential, pH, chemistries, Gram stain, and bacterial culture that are routinely obtained, additional consideration of mycobacterial or fungal disease should prompt appropriate stains and cultures.[36] If chest radiographs or the clinical scenario are consistent with possible TB, then a large volume of pleural fluid (at least 10 mL) should be centrifuged and the pellet examined with acid-fast (and fungal) stains and culture to increase the diagnostic yield. Adenosine deaminase levels in the pleural fluid, pleural biopsy, and tuberculin skin testing may also be considered.

An effusion with an eosinophilic pleocytosis at pleurocentesis appropriately prompts consideration of helminthic or other exotic etiologies. Although estimates are that 5% to 16% of pleural effusions are eosinophilic (more than 10% of nucleated cells are eosinophils), only a minority of eosinophilic effusions are due to infectious etiologies, and even fewer are due to helminths or protozoa. In most studies, blood or air in the pleural space is most commonly associated with eosinophilic pleural effusions, but malignancy, infection, pulmonary embolus, drug-induced, and asbestos-associated are all frequent.[37,38] The etiology of eosinophilic pleural effusions is summarized in Table 128-6.[38,39] Patients in or from the tropics presenting with eosinophilic pleural effusion (who do not have an identified etiology for the effusion) should also have a sputum examination and culture for fungi and mycobacteria. Sputa and stool should be examined for ova and parasites as well. Bronchoscopy and/or lung biopsy are considerations if the less invasive diagnostic evaluation is unrevealing. If biopsies are performed, it is important to consider evaluating tissue for fungi, mycobacteria, and parasitic etiologies in the microbiology and pathology labs.

Of all the parasitic etiologies, *Paragonimus* spp. infections are the most likely to be associated with a significant eosinophilic pleural effusion. Asian studies have found approximately 50% of cases of paragonimiasis are associated with pleural effusions.[40,41] Findings of pleural pH less than 7.1 and pleural fluid glucose less than 60 are characteristic.[38] Sputum exam with *Paragonimus* spp. ova will then confirm the diagnosis. Further information on *Paragonimus* spp. is included in Chapter 117.

Table 128-6 Etiology and Clinical Features of Eosinophilic Pleural Effusions

Etiology	Clinical Features
Chest trauma or thoracic medical procedure	Presence of air or blood in the pleural cavity Pleural fluid is bloody or straw-colored
Malignancy, either primary pulmonary or pleural or metastatic	Increased eosinophils, even in nonbloody effusions
Parapneumonic effusions	Eosinophils appear a month or more after resolution of infiltrate Gram's stain and culture are negative for bacteria
Tuberculosis, either pleural TB or associated with pulmonary infiltrates or nodule(s)	Although eosinophils are rarely associated with TB the frequency of pleural effusion due to TB is common in the tropics
Endemic fungi such as coccidioidiomycosis, histoplasmosis, cryptococcisis, penicilliosis	If living in or traveling from an endemic area
Parasitic infections Paragonimiasis, ascariasis, strongyloidiasis, echinococcosis, filariasis, loiasis, toxocariasis, dracunculiasis, amebiasis, cutaneous myiasis	Travel to or living in endemic areas Pleural fluid exam reveals ova, larva or fragments Paragonimiasis is the most common parasitic etiology (associated with pleural pH < 7.1 and glucose < 60 mg/dL)
Medication associated Nitrofurantoin, isotretinoin, fluoxetine, warfarin, dantrolene, glipizide, mesalamine, bromocriptine	Usually weeks to months after drug administration but may be as short as hours or as long as years.
Pulmonary embolism	18% of pleural effusions are eosinophilic Pleuritic chest pain and dyspnea greater than would be expected with size of effusion
Asbestosis or other pneumoconiosis	History of occupational exposure, Pleural effusion is usually the sole radiographic abnormality Up to 50% of asbestos-associated effusions are eosinophilic
Idiopathic	Most commonly in middle-aged males with small to moderate, unilateral effusion. May be longstanding but associated with a good prognosis. Should prompt consideration of undiagnosed parasitic infections.

Modified from Kalomenidis I, Light RW: How to approach a patient with an eosinophilic pleural effusion. J Respir Dis 24:247, 2003.

Despite aggressive evaluation, as many as one-third of eosinophilic pleural effusions remain undiagnosed, but the prognosis for these individuals even if the effusion has been prolonged has been shown to be excellent. There is some suggestion that asbestos-associated pleural effusion is the etiology in many of these undiagnosed cases. This may be even more common in the tropics where occupational exposures may be substantial and personal protective measures may be minimal; patients may not even be aware of their occupational exposure to asbestos.

TUBERCULOSIS

A discussion of pulmonary disease in the tropics cannot escape the overwhelming impact of tuberculosis on the lives of those in the developing world. Although TB is addressed in-depth in Chapter 36, the importance of including TB in the differential diagnosis of nearly all pulmonary complaints from the tropics cannot be overemphasized.

Approximately 80% of the 8 million new TB cases in the world are from 20 countries, mostly in the developing world. In pediatrics the numbers are even more staggering, with 90% of the cases and 95% of the deaths from TB occurring in developing nations.[2,14] Many of these same nations are also burdened with the highest HIV infection rates. As the two infections act synergistically to cause progression of each, the effects have been devastating, especially in sub-Saharan Africa (see Chapters 76 and 133).

The incidence of multidrug resistance has been a further, relatively recent complication of TB in the tropics. Inadequate treatment and follow-up has led to gradually increasing levels of drug resistance, thus requiring not only expensive sensitivity testing but also more expensive, and potentially more toxic, therapy.

Numerous studies have documented the frequency of TB in those who have immigrated to developed nations from the tropics. Concerns about travelers visiting areas of high TB endemicity and potential exposures during air travel are frequently raised. The risk of acquiring TB infection among short-term travelers and on flights is actually quite low.[42] Despite commonly held misconceptions about aircraft air systems, the fairly rapid filtering of air released overhead and leaving the cabin near the floor close to the same row removes and dilutes most infectious particles. Despite hundreds of thousands of flights annually, transmission of TB on aircraft has rarely been reported.[42]

In contrast to short-term travelers, those who remain in areas with a high prevalence of TB have rates of infection that approach that of the local population. This was seen most dramatically in long-term Dutch travelers to Africa, Asia, and Latin America, where their risk of infection increased from approximately 10 infections per 100,000 person-years to approximately 2000 infections per 100,000 person-years. Health-care workers with direct patient contact had more than threefold greater risk of TB than other travelers.[43] Obviously, in considering the possibility of tuberculosis in a returning traveler, a new immigrant or a patient in the tropics, it is critical to know the prevalence of TB in the nation of concern as well as contacts with TB, the living situation, and the activity of the individual evaluated.

There is little evidence to support the use of either routine bacillus Calmette-Guérin (BCG) immunization prior to travel or tuberculin skin testing (TST) before and after. Again, consideration of the length of travel, the prevalence of TB in the area, and the activities planned by the individual may make either BCG immunization or TST reasonable recommendations for some individuals.[44,45]

Individuals who immigrate to developed nations have been documented in numerous studies to have a much higher incidence of TB disease than natives of developed nations. Over 50% of cases of TB in the United States and the United Kingdom occur in people born overseas, and the incidence of disease is more than 3 times greater in foreign-born than U.S.-born individuals.[46,47] Approximately 25% of foreign TB cases diagnosed in the United States present within the first year of presentation. The incidence of active TB among political asylum seekers in London was 241 per 100,000, a level 20 times greater than the overall incidence in England.[48] Clearly individuals from developing nations who present with pulmonary complaints, especially chronic cough associated with hemoptysis, weight loss, and night sweats, should have TB considered as one of the more likely etiologies on a differential diagnosis and have chest radiography, possibly a TST, and sputa examination as part of the evaluation. In some cases, the index of suspicion may be so high that empiric therapy with four antituberculous drugs, preferably with directly observed therapy, should be instituted. Since the prevalence of multidrug-resistant TB is significantly higher in many developing nations, use of four drugs and mycobacterial sensitivity profiles should always be used.[49]

PLASMODIUM-ASSOCIATED PULMONARY FINDINGS

Plasmodium falciparum and, to a lesser extent, *P. vivax* have been associated with significant pulmonary involvement in only a minority of infected patients (see Chapter 90). In contrast to older literature that described "bronchitic" and "pneumonitic" malaria, there is no evidence that malarial infections are associated with a true pneumonitis. More recent studies have demonstrated the development of pulmonary edema during the treatment of falciparum malaria, especially more severe cases. Malaria-associated pulmonary edema is noncardiogenic (high cardiac index and low systemic vascular resistance) and is considered by most authorities to be consistent with the acute respiratory distress syndrome (ARDS) and related to the malaria-associated increase in pulmonary permeability.[50]

While pulmonary edema occurs in less than 1% of all cases of falciparum malaria, it was found in 42% of a series of U.S. soldiers in the Second World War who died of severe malaria.[51] More recently, three of five Marines who returned from Liberia in 2003 with more than 10% falciparum parasitemia developed ventilatory failure and an ARDS-like presentation 48 to 72 hours after initiation of antimalarial treatment and clearance of parasitemia (unpublished personal data). Malaria-associated pulmonary disease should be considered in the differential diagnosis of those returning from a malarious region with unexplained pulmonary edema.

HIV-ASSOCIATED PULMONARY DISEASE

Like tuberculosis, the prevalence of HIV in many areas of the tropics, especially sub-Saharan Africa, make it an important consideration in the differential diagnosis of pulmonary disease. HIV infection is fully addressed in Chapter 76 and HIV-associated opportunistic infections in Chapter 133.

As stated previously, TB coinfection is clearly the greatest threat to HIV-infected individuals in the tropics. The WHO reports rates of TB/HIV co-infection greater than 250 per 100,000 in a number of sub-Saharan nations.[52]

Table 128-7 *Selected Pathological Findings by Age and HIV Status of Children Dying of Respiratory Illness in Zambia*

	Age Group								
	HIV-1-Positive				HIV-1-Negative				
Pathologic Finding	0–5 Months	6–11 Months	12–17 Months	18 Months–<16 Years	0–5 Months	6–11 Months	12–17 Months	18 Months–<16 Years	Total
Acute pyogenic pneumonia	18	20	10	26	8	15	11	8	116
Pneumocystis carinii pneumonia	39	6	2	5	6	0	0	0	58
Tuberculosis	11	4	7	10	3	3	7	9	54
CMV	32	5	2	1	2	0	0	1	43
Interstitial pneumonia	5	3	3	4	7	2	1	5	30
Shock lung	11	3	3	7	1	0	0	2	27
Pulmonary edema	4	2	3	1	2	3	2	2	19
Lymphocytic interstitial pneumonitis	2	0	2	5	0	0	0	1	10
Measles	1	1	1	2	0	2	0	0	7

From Chintu C: Lung disease at necropsy in African children dying from respiratory illnesses: A descriptive necropsy study. Lancet 360:985, 2002.

Although *Pneumocystis jaroveci* (formerly *P. carinii*) pneumonia (PCP) remains an important pathogen in HIV-associated pulmonary disease, it is not as common in the HIV-infected patients in the tropics as in temperate zones. However, in a study of African children dying from respiratory illness in Zambia, PCP was exceeded only by acute pyogenic pneumonia as the cause of death in children infected with HIV who were under a year old. CMV, TB, and interstitial lung disease were all common findings (Table 128-7).[53]

As described in Chapter 133, the etiology of HIV-associated pulmonary disease in the tropics includes all those seen in temperate areas but the variety of pathogens is more extensive. A few notable geographic considerations are the prevalence of *Penicillium marneffei* and melioidosis in Southeast Asia and Australia, paracoccidioidomycosis in South America, and blastomycosis in areas of Africa, South America, and Asia. These diseases are often erroneously attributed to TB, even in the areas where they are most common. With the frequency of multiple simultaneous pulmonary infections in HIV infection, even in those diagnosed with TB the possibility of additional diagnoses should be considered.

NONINFECTIOUS ETIOLOGIES OF TROPICAL RESPIRATORY DISEASE

Tobacco Use in Developing Nations

Estimates are that a half billion of the world's current population will be killed by tobacco, with increasing numbers of deaths in the developing world.[54,55] It is estimated that the prevalence of male smoking exceeds 50% in many parts of Asia and Latin America.[54] Thus, a change in approach to the patient in the tropics with pulmonary complaints will need to occur as more tobacco-related diseases emerge.

Rheumatic Heart Disease Presenting with Pulmonary Symptoms

Rheumatic heart disease (RHD) continues to be a very common heart problem in the developing world. Incidence rates of RHD as high as 206 per 100,000 and prevalence rates as high as 18.6 per 1000 are described.[56] Pulmonary complaints and fever in the tropics may represent acute rheumatic carditis or bacterial endocarditis complicating prior rheumatic heart damage. Fever, cough, hemoptysis, and shortness of breath may often lead to an incorrect diagnosis of a primary pulmonary infection. Pulmonary hypertension or congestive heart failure with pulmonary edema due to rheumatic heart damage is not uncommonly seen in impoverished countries, where secondary prophylaxis to prevent recurrent RHD episodes is difficult to administer and valve replacements are prohibitively expensive.

Pulmonary Diseases Caused by Occupational and Environmental Exposures

Discussion of pulmonary disease in the tropics cannot ignore the significant role of environmental exposures in acute and chronic lung disease. Poorly regulated working conditions in agriculture and mining have resulted in substantial burdens of occupationally related and environmental lung disease in many regions.[57] Although good prevalence data are lacking, it is likely that there are millions of cases of silicosis worldwide[58] and possibly comparable numbers of other lung disorders due to cotton dust (byssinosis),[59] extrinsic allergic alveolitis caused by microbial contamination of agricultural products such as sugar cane, and airway injury from indiscriminant use and poor control of indoor and outdoor air pollutants.[3,60]

There is a dramatic increase in both TB risk and virulence in populations with silicosis, and probably also people with exposure to silica without overt silicosis. In areas where large portions of the (male) population have been historically recruited into mining, as in southern Africa, this risk factor is very broadly disseminated and may account in part for the astronomical rates of TB in that region of the world. In a study of 304 men from Botswana who had been employed in South African mines for a mean of 15 years, 30% had pneumoconiosis and 6.8% had progressive massive fibrosis, and additionally 26% had a history of, or current, tuberculosis.[61]

While adult males are the primary victims of occupational exposures, children and women face increased risk from indoor, nonoccupational exposures due to the use of dung and other biomass fuels for cooking and heating huts and homes. When combusted, these materials emit everything from silica and other minerals to hazardous air pollutants such as oxides of sulfur and nitrogen, resulting in various clinical problems, including silicosis (so-called hut lung in this setting), chronic bronchitis, asthma, and increased risk of respiratory tract infection.[4,60] The most severely affected regions are those with colder climates, such as the sierra region of South America, the mountainous regions of central Asia, and the high plains of Africa.

Ambient air pollution due to rapid urbanization has resulted in levels of ozone, oxides of nitrogen, and other irritants (photo-oxidant pollution) that are much higher than even in the worst cities in Europe and North America. Data from Latin America, India, and China suggest that very high rates of respiratory infection and asthma may be resulting.[3]

SUMMARY

To summarize, developing a differential diagnosis for a patient presenting with pulmonary complaints after exposure in the tropics requires clinicians to consider a range of infectious and noninfectious etiologies that is extraordinarily broad. Narrowing the differential is possible only with careful review of the exposure history and geographical areas coupled with knowledge of the available diagnostic resources and treatments.

ACKNOWLEDGMENTS

I appreciate the input of Dr. Michelle Barry who, as author of this chapter in the first edition, provided significant material for this edition and the editing provided by Lori Martin.

REFERENCES

1. Williams BG, Gouws E, Boschi-Pinto C, et al: Estimates of world-wide distributions of child deaths from acute respiratory infections. Lancet Infect Dis 2:25, 2002.

2. Mathers CD, Bernard C, Moesgaard Iburg K, et al: Global burden of diseases in 2002: Data sources, methods and results. WHO Global Programme on Evidence for Health Policy Discussion Paper No. 54, 2003.
3. Romieu I, Samet JM, Smith KR, et al: Outdoor air pollution and acute respiratory infections among children in developing countries. J Occup Environ Med 44:640, 2002.
4. Ezzati M, Kammen DM: Indoor air pollution from biomass combustion and acute respiratory infections in Kenya: An exposure-response study. Lancet 358:619, 2001.
5. Zumla AI, James DG: Immunologic aspects of tropical lung disease. Clin Chest Med 23:283, 2002.
6. Spira AM: Assessment of travelers who return home ill. Lancet 361:1459, 2003.
7. Monto AS: Epidemiology of viral respiratory infections. Am J Med 112(Suppl 6A):4S, 2002.
8. WHO: Integrated management of the sick child. Bull World Health Organ 73:735, 1995.
9. Peltola VT, McCullers JA: Respiratory viruses predisposing to bacterial infections: Role of neuraminidase. Pediatr Infect Dis J 23:S87, 2004.
10. Wurthwein R, Gbangou A, Sauerborn R, et al: Measuring the local burden of disease. A study of years of life lost in sub-Saharan Africa. Int J Epidem 30:501, 2001.
11. Adegbola RA, Obaro SK: Diagnosis of childhood pneumonia in the tropics. Ann Trop Med Parasitol 94:197, 2000.
12. Mulholland K: Magnitude of the problem of childhood pneumonia. Lancet 354:590, 1999.
13. Duke T, Michael A, Mgone J, et al: Etiology of child mortality in Goroka, Papua, New Guinea: A prospective two-year study. Bull World Health Organ 80:16, 2002.
14. Mathers C, Shibuya K, Stein C: Global Health: Today's challenges. In: The World Health Report 2003: Shaping the Future. Geneva, Switzerland, World Health Organization, 2003, p 13.
15. Yoshimine H, Oishi K, Mubiru F, et al: Community-acquired pneumonia in Ugandan adults: Short-term parenteral ampicillin therapy for bacterial pneumonia. Am J Trop Med Hyg 64:172, 2001.
16. Habib NA, Behrens RH: Respiratory infections in the traveler. Curr Opin Pulm Med 6:246, 2000.
17. deQuadros CA: Can measles be eradicated globally? Bull World Health Org 82:134, 2004.
18. Ross DA: Recommendations for vitamin A supplementation. J Nutr 132:2902S, 2002.
19. Currie BJ, Fisher SA, Howard DM, et al: Endemic melioidosis in tropical Northern Australia: A 10-year prospective study and review of the literature. Clin Infect Dis 31:981, 2000.
20. Weller PF: Case records of the Massachusetts General Hospital, Case 40. N Engl J Med 327:1081, 1992.
21. Irwin RS, Madison JM: The diagnosis and treatment of cough. N Engl J Med 343:1715, 2000.
22. Curie GP, Gray RD, McKay J, et al: Chronic cough. BMJ 326:261, 2003.
23. Tshibwabwa ET, Richenberg JL, Aziz ZA: Lung radiology in the tropics. Clin Chest Med 23:309, 2002.
24. Hirshberg B, Biran I, Glazer M, et al: Hemoptysis: Etiology, evaluation, and outcome in a tertiary referral hospital. Chest 112:440, 1997.
25. Souders CR, Smith AT: The clinical significance of hemoptysis. N Engl J Med 247:790, 1952.
26. Fidan A, Ozdogan S, Oruc O, et al: Hemoptysis: A retrospective analysis of 108 cases. Respir Med 96:677, 2002.
27. Abal AT, Nair PC, Cherian J: Haemoptysis: Aetiology, evaluation and outcome—a prospective study in a third-world country. Respir Med 95:548, 2001.
28. Whetham J, Day JN, Armstrong M, et al: Investigation of tropical eosinophilia; Assessing a strategy based on geographical area. J Infect 46:180, 2003.
29. Culley FJ, Brown A, Girod N, et al: Innate and cognate mechanisms of pulmonary eosinophilia in helminth infections. Eur J Immunol 32:1376, 2002.
30. Savani DM, Sharma OP: Eosinophilic lung disease in the tropics. Clin Chest Med 23:377, 2002.
31. Schwartz E: Pulmonary schistosomiasis. Clin Chest Med 23:433, 2002.
32. Schwartz E, Rozenman J, Perelman M: Pulmonary manifestations of early schistosome infection among nonimmune travelers. Am J Med 109:718, 2000.
33. Sinzobahamvya N, Bhakta HP: Pleural exudate in a tropical hospital. Eur Respir J 2:145, 1989.
34. Valdes L, Alvarez D, Valle JM, et al: The etiology of pleural effusions in an area with a high incidence of tuberculosis. Chest 109:159, 1996.
35. Porcel JM, Vives M: Etiology and pleural fluid characteristics of large and massive pleural effusions. Chest 124:978, 2003.
36. Maskell NA, Butland RJ, et al, for the British Thoracic Society: BTS guidelines for the investigation of a unilateral pleural effusion in adults. Thorax 58(Suppl 2):8, 2003.
37. Kalomenidis I, Light RW: How to approach a patient with an eosinophilic pleural effusion. J Respir Dis 24:247, 2003.
38. Rubins JB, Bloomfield Rubins H: Etiology and prognostic significance of eosinophilic pleural effusions: A prospective study. Chest 110:1271, 1996.
39. Jeanfaivre T, Cimon B, Tolstuchow N, et al: Pleural effusion and toxocariasis. Thorax 51:106, 1996.
40. Nakamura-Uchiyama F, Mukae H, Nawa Y: Paragonimiasis: A Japanese perspective. Clin Chest Med 23:409, 2002.
41. Mukae H, Taniguchi H, Matsumoto M, et al: Clinicoradiologic features of pleuropulmonary *Paragonimus westermani* on Kyusyu Island, Japan. Chest 120:514, 2001.
42. Rieder HL: Risk of travel-associated tuberculosis. CID 33:1393, 2001.
43. Cobelens FGJ, van Deutekom H, Draayer-Jansen IWE, et al: Risk of infection with *Mycobacterium tuberculosis* in travelers to areas of high tuberculosis endemicity. Lancet 356:461, 2000.
44. Lifson AR: Prevention of travel-associated tuberculosis in the high-risk traveler. CID 34:1163, 2002.
45. Lifson AR: *Mycobacterium tuberculosis* infection in travelers: Tuberculosis comes home. Lancet 356:442, 2000.
46. CDC: Reported Tuberculosis in the United States, 2002. Atlanta, GA, U.S. Department of Health and Human Services, CDC, 2003.
47. CDC: Tuberculosis morbidity among U.S.-born and foreign-born populations, United States, 2000. MMWR 51:101, 2002.
48. Callister MEJ, Barringer J, Thanabalasingam ST, et al: Pulmonary tuberculosis among political asylum seekers screened at Heathrow Airport, London, 1995-9. Thorax 57:152, 2002.
49. CDC: Treatment of tuberculosis. CDC, ATS and IDSA guidelines. MMWR 52:1, 2003.
50. Taylor WRJ, White NJ: Malaria and the lung. Clin Chest Med 23(2):457, 2002.
51. Sheehy TW, Reba RC: Complications of falciparum malaria and their treatment. Ann Intern Med 66:807, 1967.
52. UNAIDS/WHO: AIDS Epidemic Update, December 2003. Geneva, UNAIDS/WHO, 2003.
53. Chintu C, Mudenda V, Lucas S, et al: Lung diseases at necropsy in African children dying from respiratory illnesses: A descriptive study. Lancet 360:985, 2002.
54. Peto R, Lopez AD, Boreham J, et al: Mortality from smoking worldwide. Brit Med Bull 52:12, 1996.
55. Barry M: The influence of the U.S. tobacco industry on the health, economy, and environment of developing countries. N Engl J Med 324:917, 1991.
56. Eisenberg MJ: Rheumatic heart disease in the developing world: Prevalence, prevention and control. Eur Heart J 14:122, 1993.
57. Cullen MR: Occupational hazards in the international setting. In Fleming LE, Herystein J, Bunn WB (eds): Issues in International Occupational and Environmental Medicine. OEM Press, Beverly, MA, 1997.
58. Li YR: Prevention and treatment of pneumoconiosis in China. Biomed Environ Sci 8:211, 1995.
59. Wang XR, Eisen EA, Zhang HX, et al: Respiratory symptoms and cotton dust exposure; Results of a 15-year follow up observation. Occup Environ Med 60:935, 2003.
60. Mohamed N, Ng'ang'a L, Odhiambo J, et al: Home environment and asthma in Kenyan school children: A case-control study. Thorax 50:74, 1995.
61. Steen TW, Gyi KM, White NW, et al: Prevalence of occupational lung disease among Botswana men formerly employed in the South African mining industry. Occup Environ Med 54:19, 1997

129

Ocular Disease

EDWARD T. RYAN
MARLENE DURAND

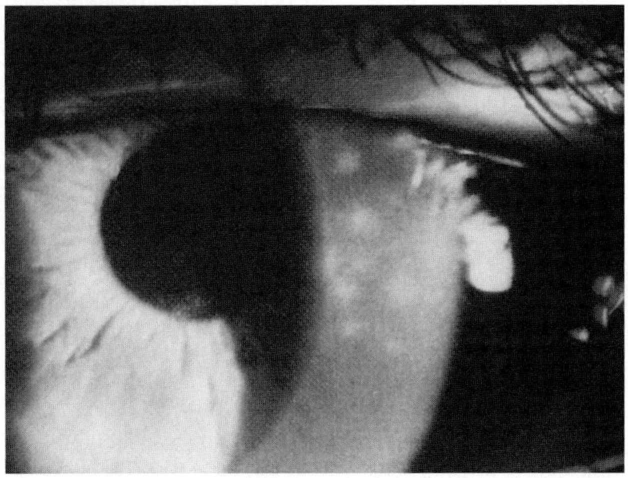

FIGURE 129-1 Adenoviral keratoconjunctivitis. Note punctate opacities in the cornea. (From Sandford-Smith J: Eye Diseases in Hot Climates, 2nd ed. Oxford, Wright Publishers, Butterworth Heinemann, 1990, plate 4e.)

INTRODUCTION

Many tropical infectious diseases have ocular manifestations. A number of such infections (i.e., trachoma, onchocerciasis, measles/xerophthalmia, leprosy) are the cause of significant visual loss and blindness worldwide.[1–3] Ocular involvement by tropical infectious diseases may manifest as conjunctivitis, keratitis, uveitis, retinitis, optic neuritis, lesions of the adnexa including ulcerative lesions of the eyelid, or Parinaud's oculoglandular syndrome (an ulceronodular conjunctival/corneal lesion with associated preauricular adenopathy). Tropical infections may also present as proptosis (a forward bulging of the eye itself) or as a conjunctival, intraocular, or orbital "worm."

VIRAL INFECTIONS

Adenovirus

Worldwide, adenovirus is probably the most common cause of viral ocular infection.[4–6] Over 40 serotypes of adenovirus have been identified (see Chapter 59). Ocular involvement by adenovirus usually manifests as one of three clinical syndromes: nonspecific follicular conjunctivitis, pharyngoconjunctival fever, or epidemic keratoconjunctivitis. Nonspecific follicular conjunctivitis is the most common manifestation of ocular adenoviral infection. It has been reported with many adenoviral serotypes and is most often mild, self-limited, and nonspecific. Adenoviral conjunctivitis may include petechiae or may more rarely present as hemorrhagic conjunctivitis.[7] Pharyngoconjunctival fever is also a self-limited disease.[8] It is most commonly associated with serotypes 3, 4, and 7. It manifests as acute follicular conjunctivitis that is associated with an upper respiratory tract infection, regional lymphadenopathy, and fever. Mild punctuate keratitis may appear. The illness spontaneously resolves over 1 to 2 weeks and is most frequently reported in children.

Epidemic keratoconjunctivitis has the most severe ocular manifestations. It manifests as acute follicular conjunctivitis with a diffuse, superficial, fine "pinpoint" epithelial keratitis. Because of the involvement of the cornea, ocular pain is a prominent feature. Preauricular lymphadenopathy may be present. By the second week of infection, focal or punctate epithelial keratitis can occur (Fig. 129-1).[6] By the second to third week of infection, subepithelial corneal infiltration may be present in 30% to 80% of affected persons.[6] The infiltrates are thought to represent an immunologic reaction, can persist for months to years, and can result in significant visual disturbances if located within the visual axis. Epidemic keratoconjunctivitis is most frequently associated with adenovirus serotypes 3, 8, 10, 19, 21, and 37.[6] Rarely, a large corneal erosion or conjunctival pseudomembrane can occur.[6,9] Diagnosis is usually one of clinical recognition. Viral cultures, immunofluorescence studies, serologic examinations, and molecular techniques can be employed.[6,7] Treatment is usually symptomatic.[10] Topical steroids should be used only to treat severe and symptomatic subepithelial corneal involvement in epidemic keratoconjunctivitis or if extensive pseudomembrane formation has occurred (and only after concomitant herpetic ocular involvement has been excluded).[6] Adenoviral ocular involvement can be explosively epidemic. Adenoviruses may persist on fomites for as long as 2 months. Contact precautions and disinfection of contaminated equipment and surfaces are required.

Enterovirus

The enterovirus group includes enterovirus, poliovirus, coxsackievirus, and echovirus (see Chapter 60). Over 70 enteroviruses, 30 echoviruses, and 20 coxsackieviruses have been identified. Ocular manifestations of enteroviral infections include acute hemorrhagic conjunctivitis, cranial nerve dysfunction in acute enteroviral neuropathy, and possibly retinitis.[11]

Acute Hemorrhagic Conjunctivitis

Acute hemorrhagic conjunctivitis was first recognized as a clinical entity in Africa in 1969. The entity is highly contagious, and a pandemic ensued.[12] Enterovirus 70 and coxsackievirus 24 have been established as major etiologic agents.[12,13] The viruses are spread by hand-to-hand and fomite-to-hand transfer. Respiratory spread may occur. The illness has an incubation period of only 1 to 2 days. Presentation is one of acute conjunctivitis with eyelid edema and lacrimation. Ten percent to 70% of affected persons have some conjunctival hemorrhages, usually bulbar.[12] Hemorrhagic involvement may be either petechial or involve the entire conjunctiva (Plate 129-1).[12] Mild follicular inflammatory changes can be present. Mild, self-resolving, punctate, epithelial keratitis can occur in a small minority of patients.[12] Preauricular lymphadenopathy is frequent, and mild iritis has been reported. The syndrome is usually short in duration, with resolution beginning within 2 to 4 days of onset and continuing for 1 to 2 weeks. Mild systemic manifestations may include headache, pharyngitis, and coryza in a minority of patients. There are usually no long-term ocular sequelae. Enterovirus-70 acute hemorrhagic conjunctivitis, however, is associated with the subsequent development of polio-like radiculomyelitis.[13]

The neurologic syndrome often presents with lancinating pain, fever, and malaise. The radiculomyelitis occurs 2 to 60 days after the onset of the conjunctivitis and most often presents acutely.[12] Involvement results in flaccid weakness and paralysis that is asymmetrical and areflexic.[12,13] Pleocytosis of the cerebral spinal fluid is present. Cranial nerves can be affected. Extraocular palsies can result. The polio-like syndrome can resolve over months but often results in permanent deficits.[12] By analogy to what is observed in clinical poliomyelitis, the neurologic syndrome has a predilection to occur in limbs that have received an intramuscular injection.[14]

Box 129-1 Causes of Selected Types of Conjunctivitis

Hyperacute Conjunctivitis*

Neisseria gonorrhoeae†
Neisseria meningitidis†
Corynebacterium diphtheriae
Streptococcus species

Membranous/Pseudomembranous Conjunctivitis

Corynebacterium diphtheriae†
Pneumococci
Streptococcus species
Neisseria species
Chlamydia species
Mycoplasma species (Stevens-Johnson syndrome–associated)
Adenovirus†
Enterovirus
Candida species

Hemorrhagic Conjunctivitis

Enterovirus type 70†
Coxsackievirus A24†
Pneumococci
Neisseria species
Haemophilus species
Chlamydia species
Borrelia species
Rickettsia species
Adenovirus
Herpesvirus
Newcastle virus
Hemorrhagic fever virus (e.g., Ebola virus)
Trichinella spiralis

*Hyperacute conjunctivitis is defined as a rapidly progressive conjunctivitis with copious purulence.
†Common or classic ocular manifestation of infection.

Intramuscular injections should therefore be avoided in the treatment of patients with acute hemorrhagic conjunctivitis.

Diagnosis of acute hemorrhagic conjunctivitis is one of clinical recognition (usually during an epidemic). Viral cultures or serologic assays can be performed. Systemic antibody responses are rarely prominent. It should be recalled that "hemorrhagic conjunctivitis" has been associated with a number of nonenteroviral infectious agents (Box 129-1), including pneumococci, *Neisseria* species, *Haemophilus* species, chlamydia, herpesvirus, and the poultry-associated Newcastle disease virus. Treatment of acute hemorrhagic conjunctivitis associated with enterovirus-7 and coxsackievirus-24 is symptomatic. Strict handwashing procedures and sterilization of equipment should be performed.

Poliovirus

Ocular manifestations of poliomyelitis are rare, but they do occur (see Chapter 60). Bulbar poliomyelitis is associated with paralysis of muscle groups innervated by cranial nerves. Five percent to 35% of persons with paralytic poliomyelitis experience bulbar involvement. Although involvement of the IXth and Xth cranial nerves (with pharyngeal paralysis) is most frequent, over 10% of patients with bulbar poliomyelitis have cranial nerve involvement that affects the eyes, orbital musculature, or both. Ocular palsies, ptosis, pupillary disturbances, and ophthalmoplegia can occur. Therapy is supportive.

Influenza

The most common ocular manifestation due to infection with influenza virus (see Chapter 59) is anterior uveitis that may occur during acute illness or during convalescence. Conjunctivitis, dacryoadenitis, mild keratitis, chorioretinitis, retinal hemorrhages, retinal edema, cranial nerve dysfunction, and optic neuritis may also occur during influenza, although many of the reports describing such associations predate the availability of confirmatory viral studies. Treatment of influenza is usually symptomatic. Oral amantadine, rimantadine, or selective neurominadase inhibitors may be employed in the treatment of certain debilitated patients. Ocular manifestations are usually mild and self-limited. Topical steroids may be used in the treatment of anterior uveitis. Effective yearly vaccines are available. Aggregation of split virion particles in certain influenza vaccine preparations may cause a self-limited oculorespiratory syndrome that manifests as mild conjunctivitis following parenteral immunization.[15]

Measles

Keratitis occurs in all persons with measles (see Chapter 55).[16] Such keratitis occurs within a few days of the outbreak of the skin rash and may persist for months. Slit-lamp examination discloses punctuate epithelial erosions even in patients with measles without eye symptoms. Conjunctivitis with tearing and eyelid edema is also common and usually resolves without any lasting sequelae.[16]

Vitamin A deficiency results in xerophthalmia (conjunctival/corneal epithelial irregularities and xerosis; Fig. 129-2). Acute vitamin A deficiency can be induced by measles in persons with marginal vitamin A stores.[17] Results can be catastrophic.

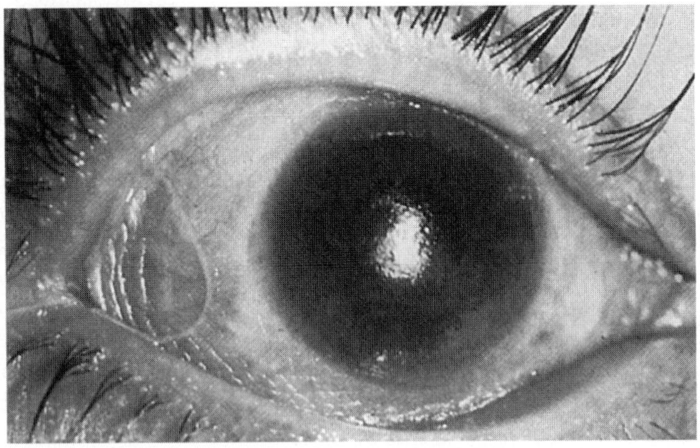

FIGURE 129-2 Early xerophthalmia. Corneal and conjunctival xerosis secondary to vitamin A deficiency. (From Sandford-Smith J: Eye Diseases in Hot Climates, 2nd ed. Oxford, Wright Publishers, Butterworth Heinemann, 1990, plate 12a.)

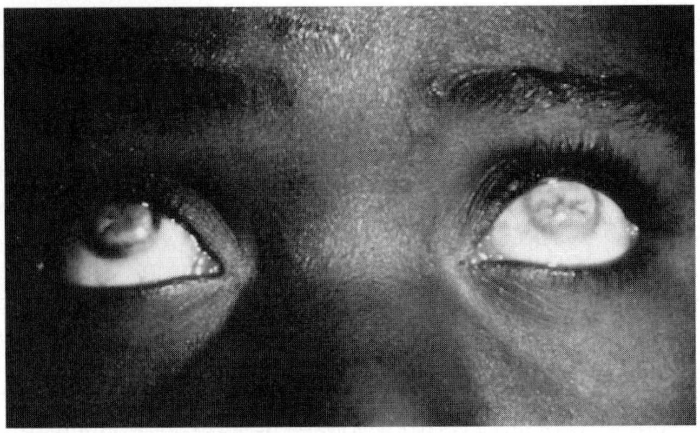

FIGURE 129-4 Child blinded from corneal scarring secondary to measles and xerophthalmia. (From Sandford-Smith J: Eye Diseases in Hot Climates, 2nd ed. Oxford, Wright Publishers, Butterworth Heinemann, 1990, cover.)

Without adequate vitamin A, the punctuate epithelial keratitis of measles can coalesce into larger epithelial ulcers (Plate 129-2). Such erosions can become secondarily infected with bacteria or fungi. Corneal scarring may result. Reactivation of herpes simplex keratitis and corneal ulceration may occur.[18] The application of traditional eye medicines or poultices can result in additional ocular damage. Keratomalacia, a marked weakening of the corneal stroma that can result in total melting of the cornea, can occur in persons who are markedly deficient in vitamin A (Fig. 129-3). Worldwide, measles-associated corneal ulceration and scarring result in significant visual loss and blindness (Fig. 129-4).[19,20]

Posterior ocular disease associated with measles includes retinopathy, retinal vessel attenuation, retinal edema, and retinal hemorrhages.[21] Retinal pigmentary changes may persist.[21] Visual acuity may be markedly decreased and, even after resolution of the acute illness, loss of vision may be severe.[21] Involvement of the central nervous system with measles-associated acute encephalitis or subacute sclerosing panencephalitis can be associated with papilledema, chorioretinitis,

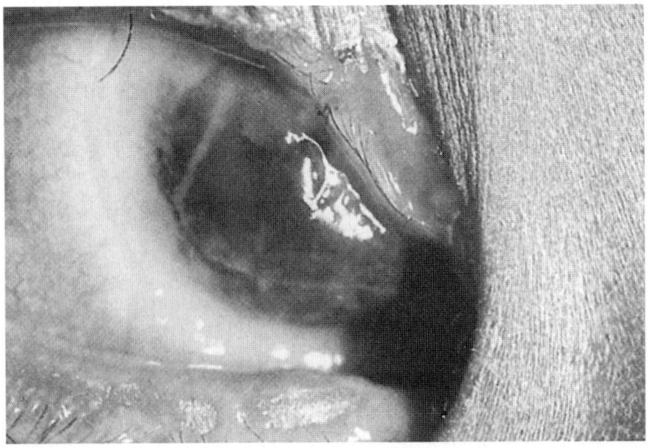

FIGURE 129-3 Measles-associated keratomalacia in a child with vitamin A deficiency. The cornea has completely melted away and only a thin sheet of fibrin covers the iris. (From Sandford-Smith J: Eye Diseases in Hot Climates, 2nd ed. Oxford, Wright Publishers, Butterworth Heinemann, 1990, plate 12d.)

optic neuritis, optic atrophy, and extraocular palsies.[21] Congenital measles is associated with pigmentary retinopathy and with cataract formation.

Diagnosis of measles is usually one of clinical recognition. Viral culture and antigenic studies can be performed on tissue scrapings or samples in atypical cases. Treatment of uncomplicated measles is usually supportive. A number of studies in the developing world have demonstrated that the routine administration of vitamin A to patients with measles (both among hospitalized individuals and in the community) can lead to a 30% to 80% reduction in measles-associated mortality as well as to a marked reduction in measles-associated morbidity (see Chapter 55).[22,23] A number of dosing regimens have been shown to be equally efficacious.[22,23] Specific ocular therapy should be directed toward preventing the progression and superinfection of corneal ulcers. Antibiotic eye drops/ointments and eye patching may be employed. Uncomplicated cases of measles rarely require specific ocular therapy beyond the use of artificial tears or cold compresses.

Rubella

Infection with rubella virus can be either acquired or congenital. Acquired rubella often manifests as a systemic viral illness with mild exanthem and lymphadenopathy. The most common ocular manifestation during acquired rubella infection is conjunctivitis, which occurs in 70% of symptomatic patients.[24] Epithelial keratitis occurs in 5% to 10% of infected patients.[24] Corneal stromal involvement, iritis, retinitis, and vasculitis have been reported.[25] Rubella infection that occurs in a susceptible woman in her first trimester of pregnancy has an 80% chance of affecting the fetus.[26] Ocular manifestations may occur in over half of all such neonates with congenital rubella.[27] Retinopathy is the most common manifestation and is characterized by patchy black retinal pigmentary changes.[21,28] Visual acuity is often preserved. Cataracts affect 15% of persons with the congenital rubella syndrome and may be either unilateral or bilateral.[29] Microphthalmia, glaucoma, buphthalmos, retinal neovascularization, and nystagmus can occur.[21] Diagnosis is usually one of clinical recognition. Serological conversion or isolation of virus can confirm the diagnosis.[21] Therapy is supportive. Acute rubella retinitis appears to respond to systemic steroids.[30] The treatment of ocular manifestations of congenital rubella syndrome may include cataract extraction and antiglaucoma therapy.

Mumps

Mumps classically presents as parotitis and fever. Orchitis, oophoritis, and pancreatitis can also occur. The most common ocular manifestation is dacryoadenitis, which may occur in up to 20% of persons with acute mumps.[31] Dacryoadenitis may present as edema and erythema of the superotemporal lid and conjunctiva. The gland may be visibly enlarged. Involvement is usually bilateral. Optic neuritis, disciform keratitis, iritis, uveitis, scleritis, and acute glaucoma have been reported.[31] Diagnosis is one of clinical recognition and serology. Therapy is usually supportive. Steroid therapy may be of benefit in optic neuritis, iritis, and acute glaucoma.

Herpes Simplex Virus

Worldwide, herpes simplex virus (HSV) infection of the eye is a leading cause of visual impairment.[32,33] Ocular involvement can result from infection with either HSV-1 or HSV-2 (see Chapter 57). Primary ocular involvement in children and adults is usually due to HSV-1. Such involvement usually presents as follicular conjunctivitis that may be associated with epithelial keratitis. Vesicular formation on the eyelid and ulcerative blepharitis can occur.[34] Primary ocular involvement in neonates is usually due to HSV-2, usually the result of infection during passage through the birth canal. Ocular manifestations can occur in 15% to 20% of infected neonates and usually develop 2 to 14 days after birth.[21] Almost all HSV-infected neonates with ocular findings have some evidence of skin involvement/vesiculation. Neonatal ocular HSV disease usually presents as nonfollicular conjunctivitis.[35] Keratitis, chorioretinitis, acute necrotizing retinitis, optic neuritis, and iritis can occur. Cataracts, chorioretinal scarring, optic atrophy, and micro-ophthalmia may result.[21]

Non-neonatal ocular involvement by HSV can be due to primary infection as described earlier or can be the result of viral reactivation. The most common manifestation of recurrent HSV ocular disease is epithelial keratitis that coalesces to form a thin-branching, dendritic, ulcerative pattern (Plate 129-3).[34] Lacrimation, photophobia, pain, and blurring of vision are common. The corneal ulceration usually heals within 1 to 3 weeks (more quickly if antiviral therapy is used). Some epithelial ulcers do not completely heal and may undergo recurrent breakdown, despite the inability to document persistence of the virus. These "metaherpetic" ulcers are thought to be multifactoral in origin and can lead to frank corneal perforation. Involvement of the corneal stroma during HSV ocular disease can lead to interstitial keratitis, which may lead to scarring. Neovascularization, limbic vasculitis, corneal "ring" immunologic reactions, disciform keratitis, iridocyclitis, corneal anesthesia, and secondary glaucoma can occur.[34]

Posterior ocular HSV disease is more rare than anterior disease. HSV retinitis can include perivascular sheathing, retinal hemorrhages and edema, vascular occlusion, papilledema, optic neuritis, and the most common manifestation, acute retinal necrosis.[36] HSV-associated encephalitis or meningoencephalitis can result in papilledema, cranial nerve dysfunction, extraocular palsies, and visual disturbances. HSV retinitis can occur concurrently with HSV encephalitis.[21]

Compared with what is the case in the developed world, ocular HSV disease in the developing world is more likely to present with larger geographic or amoeboid corneal epithelial ulcerations than with classic, thin-branching, dendritic, ulcerative patterns; is more likely to present with bilateral ocular involvement; and is more likely to involve non-neonatal children.[37] These differences may be related to differences in nutritional status and to delay in seeking medical attention. The occurrence of HSV ocular disease has also been well associated with concurrent measles and malaria, possibly because of fever-induced reactivation of HSV disease, concurrent immunologic alterations, or both.

Diagnosis of ocular herpetic involvement is usually one of clinical recognition. The classic corneal dendritic epithelial ulceration pattern may be visualized with fluorescein or rose bengal staining and is most frequently associated with HSV (although it may also occur with varicella zoster virus infection). Viral antigenic assays, molecular techniques, and cultures can be performed.[38] Tzanck preparation of an epithelial scraping can disclose multinucleated giant cells. Seroconversion during primary infection can aid in diagnosis, as can the presence of anti-HSV immunoglobulin M (IgM) antibodies in neonates; however, interpretation of antibody levels in recurrent disease is problematic.[21] A number of antiviral agents are available for the treatment of ocular HSV disease, including trifluridine, idoxuridine, vidarabine, bromovinyldeoxyuridine, and acyclovir. The application of topical antiviral agents combined with gentle débridement or interferon therapy can be employed in the therapy of simple epithelial HSV involvement.[10,39] Treatment with oral acyclovir alone is as effective in most cases. Patients with HSV necrotizing keratitis, interstitial keratitis, disciform keratitis, metaherpetic ulceration, iridocyclitis, and retinitis all require more intensive therapy that may include the use of systemic antiviral agents or steroids.[34] It should be stressed, however, that for most HSV ocular disease, steroid use is contraindicated. Steroids are limited to a number of specific HSV-ocular entities and should be employed only by an eye specialist.[34]

Varicella Zoster Virus

Infection with varicella zoster virus (VZV) can present in one of two classic patterns: *varicella* (chickenpox) or *zoster* (shingles; see Chapter 57).

Varicella (Chickenpox)

Ocular involvement during acute varicella is usually one of vesicular lid eruption, conjunctivitis, and keratitis. Approximately 4% of children with varicella experience some ocular involvement. Varicella vesicles can form on the conjunctiva itself and may be associated with marked edema and injection (Fig. 129-5).[8,40] Keratitis may be dendritic. Deep ocular involvement can occur. Disciform keratitis, stromal keratitis, and uveitis have been reported. Rarely, optic neuritis, retinopathy, and cranial nerve palsies can occur. Varicella encephalitis can be complicated by papilledema and extraocular palsies. Congenital varicella infection is rare; however, chorioretinitis, cataracts, and microphthalmia can occur.

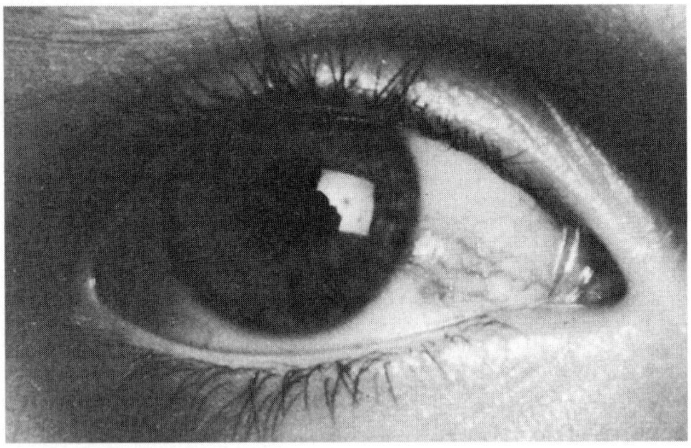

FIGURE 129-5 Chickenpox-associated limbic varicella pock. Note surrounding localized injection. (From Jordan DR, Noel LP, Clarke WN, et al: Ocular involvement in varicella. Clin Pediatr 23:435, 1984.)

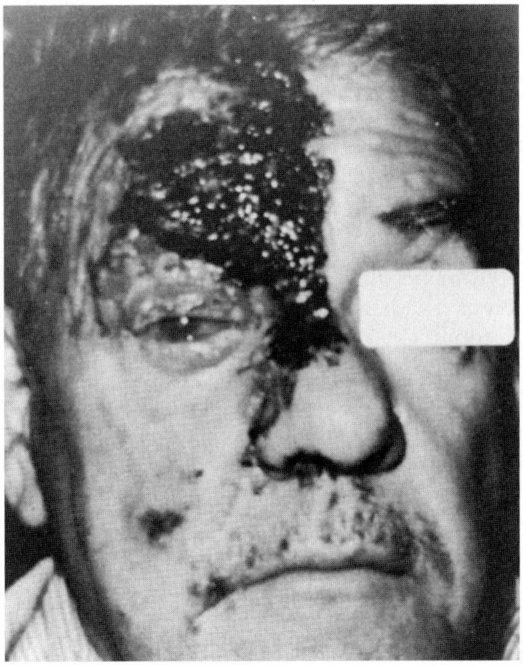

FIGURE 129-6 Severe, hemorrhagic zoster eruption involving the frontal branch of the trigeminal nerve. (From Pavan-Langston D: Varicella-zoster ophthalmicus. Int Ophthalmol Clin 15:177, 1975.)

Diagnosis of acute varicella is usually one of clinical recognition. Tzanck preparation of epithelial scrapings of the base of vesicles can disclose multinucleated giant cells. Viral antigenic assays or culture can be employed in unclear cases. Therapy is usually supportive. Systemic antiviral agents should be employed in immunocompromised persons and adults because the incidence of severe complications is increased in these populations. Antiviral agents include acyclovir, valacyclovir, and famciclovir. Anterior ocular involvement in varicella is usually treated symptomatically. Monitoring for bacterial superinfection should be performed, and epithelial ulcers should be treated with topical antibiotic drops or ointments. Anterior uveitis and deep stromal involvement may be treated with topical steroids, and iridocyclitis should be treated with cycloplegia to lessen the incidence of synechial formation. Retinitis and deep ocular disease should be treated with systemic antivirals, usually intravenously.

Zoster

The varicella virus can remain dormant in sensory ganglionic neurons. When the virus reactivates along a nerve distribution, it is called shingles or zoster. Reactivation is most frequent in thoracic or trigeminal nerve distributions and is most common in older or immunocompromised persons.[40] Involvement of the ophthalmic branch of the trigeminal nerve (V_1) is called zoster ophthalmicus. Such involvement is associated with ocular manifestations in 50% to 70% of affected persons (Figs. 129-6 and 129-7). Involvement of the nasociliary branch of V_1 can produce vesicles on the lateral aspect of the tip of the nose (Hutchinson's sign). Such involvement is associated with ocular manifestations in 85% of affected patients. As in varicella, most ocular disease in zoster involves the anterior segment of the eye. Eyelid involvement can lead to lid scarring with retraction and complicating ectropion, exposure keratitis, or both. Papillary conjunctivitis, epithelial keratitis, stromal infiltrative keratitis, and disciform keratitis can occur.[40] Corneal anesthesia may be pronounced and persistent. Such involvement can predispose affected persons to complicating corneal infections and ulcerations.[40] Corneal scarring can occur (Fig. 129-8). Iridocyclitis (with secondary iris atrophy and secondary glaucoma), optic neuritis, vitritis, and retinitis have been reported.[21,40,41] Acute and postherpetic neuralgia can be debilitating.[34]

The retinitis associated with zoster may be more frequent in immunocompromised persons, especially among those with acquired immunodeficiency syndrome (AIDS).[42] The retinitis can be necrotic and can lead to the syndrome of acute retinal necrosis (ARN).[43] VZV is associated with vasculitis, and much of the necrosis, retinitis, and optic neuritis associated with VZV infection is thought to be vascular. Branch artery inclusion can occur.[44] Rare persons can experience ocular VZV involvement in zoster without cutaneous involvement. In such persons, pain in the V_1 nerve distribution may be present. Zoster may be the presenting feature of infection with human immunodeficiency virus (HIV), especially in young persons.

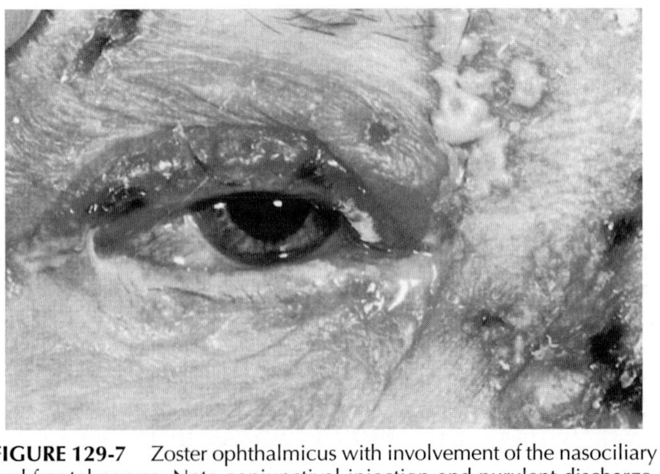

FIGURE 129-7 Zoster ophthalmicus with involvement of the nasociliary and frontal nerves. Note conjunctival injection and purulent discharge. (From Liesegang TJ: The varicella-zoster virus: Systemic and ocular features. J Am Acad Dermatol 11:170, 1984.)

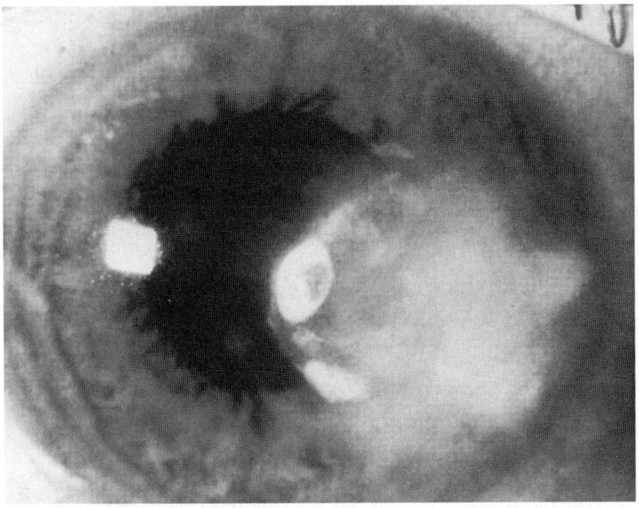

FIGURE 129-8 Residual corneal scarring, lipid deposition, and corneal thinning after zoster ophthalmicus. (From Liesegang TJ: The varicella-zoster virus: Systemic and ocular features. J Am Acad Dermatol 11:172, 1984.)

Diagnosis is usually one of clinical recognition. Tzanck preparation of an epithelial scraping, culture, or viral antigenic studies can be performed in unclear cases. Topical antiviral agents may be applied. Systemic acyclovir, valacyclovir, and famciclovir can decrease the time to healing and may lessen the pain associated with zoster. Foscarnet may also be of benefit.[42] Intravenous therapy should be considered in immunocompromised patients and should be employed in patients with retinitis, ARN, or disseminated zoster.[21,34] Topical steroids can be employed for the treatment of deep anterior inflammatory ocular disease. Cycloplegia can aid in preventing synechial formation. Patients with corneal epithelial defects should receive topical antimicrobial agents to prevent bacterial or fungal superinfection. Systemic analgesia is often required for pain control.

Acute Retinal Necrosis

ARN is a syndrome characterized by retinal vasculitis, retinal necrosis, and vitritis. The syndrome may present with decreased vision, uveitis, or ocular pain.[21,43,45] It has been most frequently associated with herpes family viruses, most commonly with VZV and HSV. Visual loss can be severe, and involvement can be bilateral. Prolonged systemic acyclovir should be employed, with initial therapy being administered intravenously.[45] Systemic steroids are sometimes employed.[45] Surgery is often required to treat retinal detachments secondary to vitreal retractions. Patients immunocompromised with HIV may have a similar syndrome of progressive outer retinal necrosis associated with herpetic involvement. Uveitis and vitritis are usually much less pronounced in such persons.[45]

Cytomegalovirus

Cytomegalovirus (CMV; see Chapter 57) infection is usually subclinical and can be acquired either congenitally or during later life. Approximately 40% of newborn infants born to mothers who sustain primary CMV infection during pregnancy acquire congenital infection. Ten percent to 15% of such newborns have clinical manifestations, and approximately 20% to 30% of infants with severe cytomegalic inclusion disease have chorioretinitis.[46] Optic atrophy and, rarely, anophthalmia may occur.[21,46]

Acute infection acquired after gestation in immunocompetent persons is most often asymptomatic. A mononucleosis-like syndrome can occur and can be associated with mild, nonspecific conjunctivitis.[47] Rare cases of retinitis have been reported.[48] Most symptomatic disease, however, occurs in immunocompromised persons, especially in those with AIDS. AIDS-associated CMV ocular disease occurs almost exclusively in persons whose CD4 cell count is less than or equal to 50 cells/mL.[49] In such persons, CMV classically involves the eye with hemorrhagic necrotizing chorioretinitis (Fig. 129-9). The retinitis often follows a perivascular distribution. The retinitis is progressive and can be bilateral. Retinal detachments are frequent. Optic neuritis can occur and can result in optic atrophy.[21] Punctate keratitis and iridocyclitis can occur. Up to 40% of individuals with untreated AIDS will develop ocular CMV disease.

Diagnosis of ocular CMV disease is usually one of clinical recognition. Systemic CMV disease can be diagnosed by viral antigenic assays, serologic or molecular assays, and culture. CMV retinitis needs to be distinguished from acute retinal necrosis, VZV retinitis, progressive outer retinal necrosis, and toxoplasmosis-associated retinitis, among other entities. CMV retinitis in immunocompromised patients is progressive without therapy. The antiviral agents ganciclovir, valganciclovir, foscarnet, and cidofovir are the mainstays of therapy. These agents are virostatic and, after an initial course of induction therapy, maintenance therapy must be continued. Even after an initially favorable clinical response is achieved, reactivation of CMV chorioretinitis almost always occurs if the severe immunocompromised state continues.[50] In the case of CMV retinitis associated with advanced HIV disease, immune reconstitution following initiation of antiretroviral therapy has been associated with an immune recovery uveitis.[51] Maintenance anti-CMV treatment has been successfully discontinued in individuals with HIV whose CD4 count

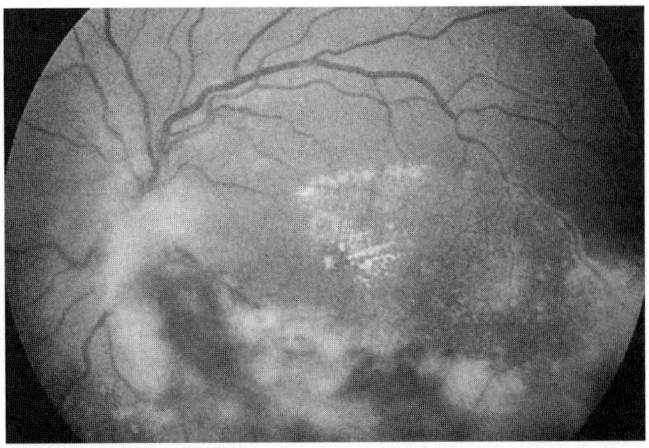

FIGURE 129-9 Cytomegalovirus-associated retinitis. Note hemorrhagic necrosis of the retina with exudates and periphlebitis. (From Rao NA: Acquired immunodeficiency syndrome and its ocular complications. Indian J Ophthalmol 42:57, 1994.)

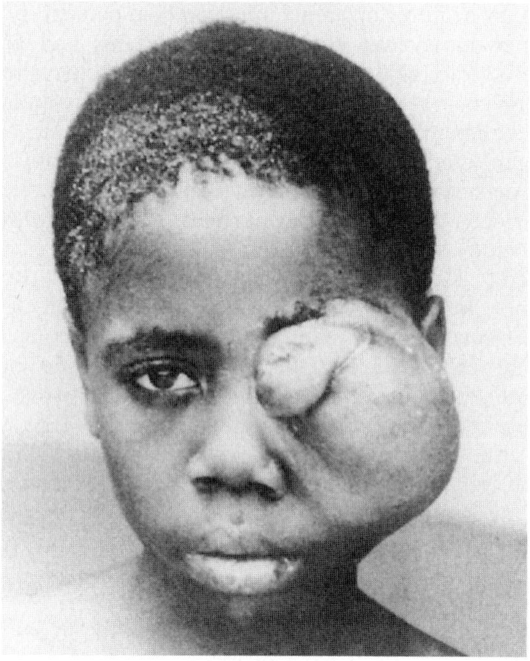

FIGURE 129-10 A child with Epstein–Barr virus–associated Burkitt's lymphoma involving the left orbit and maxilla. (From Sandford-Smith J: Eye Diseases in Hot Climates, 2nd ed. Oxford, Wright Publishers, Butterworth Heinemann, 1990, p 210.)

increases to at least 75 × 10^6 cells/mL who have been taking highly active antiretroviral treatment for at least 18 months.[52]

Oral valganciclovir may be used for maintenance therapy, as can a sustained-release ganciclovir intraocular implant.[53,54] Repetitive intravitreal injections of ganciclovir can also be employed in both induction and maintenance therapies of CMV retinitis.[55] Such local modalities of therapy, however, result in minimal if any systemic drug levels. In addition, such therapies neither prevent nor treat ocular disease in the contralateral eye (or systemic CMV disease). Management of retinal detachment in CMV retinitis may entail primary vitrectomy and installation of silicon oil to act as a tamponade (with or without scleral buckling).[56]

Epstein–Barr Virus

Epstein–Barr virus (EBV) is worldwide in distribution (see Chapter 57). Persons in developing nations are most often infected as children.[21] While most infections are relatively asymptomatic, EBV is the leading cause of infectious mononucleosis. The most common ocular manifestation of EBV infection is transient mild conjunctivitis that is often follicular, can be unilateral, and occurs in 2% to 40% of persons with infectious mononucleosis. Superficial and stromal keratitis have also been reported.[57] EBV may also play a role in the dry eye of Sjögren's syndrome and in the lymphocytic infiltration of corneal endothelium in the iridocorneal endothelial syndrome.[57] EBV infection may be associated with uveitis, iritis, retinitis, choroiditis, optic neuritis, papilledema, dacryoadenitis, cranial nerve palsies, and Parinaud's oculoglandular syndrome.[57–60] EBV associated with Burkitt's lymphoma, a disorder most frequently reported in children in sub-Saharan Africa (but worldwide in distribution), most often manifests as a maxillary/orbital mass and can present with proptosis (Fig. 129-10).

Heterophile or monospot antibody assays can be employed in the diagnosis of acute EBV, and serologic assays to various EBV antigens can be employed in unclear or in chronic cases.[21] Treatment of infectious mononucleosis is usually supportive. Optimal therapy for ocular manifestations is unclear. Antiviral agents do not appear to alter the clinical course substantially. Extensive inflammation has been treated with steroid preparations.

Human Immunodeficiency Viruses

HIV-1 and HIV-2 are the causative agents of AIDS (see Chapter 76). The majority of patients with untreated AIDS have ocular manifestations. HIV has been isolated from tears, conjunctiva, cornea, retina, retinal vessel endothelium, and vitreous.[21] Ocular manifestations of HIV infection can be due to HIV itself or to secondary opportunistic ocular infections. The most common ocular involvement resulting from HIV itself is HIV retinopathy (Fig. 129-11). HIV retinopathy occurs in over two-thirds of patients with untreated AIDS; is characterized by the formation of retinal cotton wool spots, microaneurysms, and hemorrhages; and appears to be due to a microvasculopathy.[61,62] Cotton wool spots represent areas of ischemia in the nerve fiber layer and are usually oriented along vascular arcades. The pathogenesis of the vasculopathy is not well understood. The frequency of HIV retinopathy increases as the level of immunologic suppression increases, but HIV retinopathy usually remains asymptomatic as long as the macula is not affected. Some persons infected with HIV develop large-vessel vasculopathy for unclear reasons. The consequent, retinal vaso-occlusion can involve central or branch retinal veins and visual loss can be severe. HIV infection can also be associated with a primary optic neuropathy and an infiltrative lymphocytosis syndrome.[63]

Compared with what occurs with primary HIV eye involvement, HIV-induced ocular opportunistic infections (see Chapter 133) are often symptomatic, may be the presenting feature of infection by HIV, and can result in severe

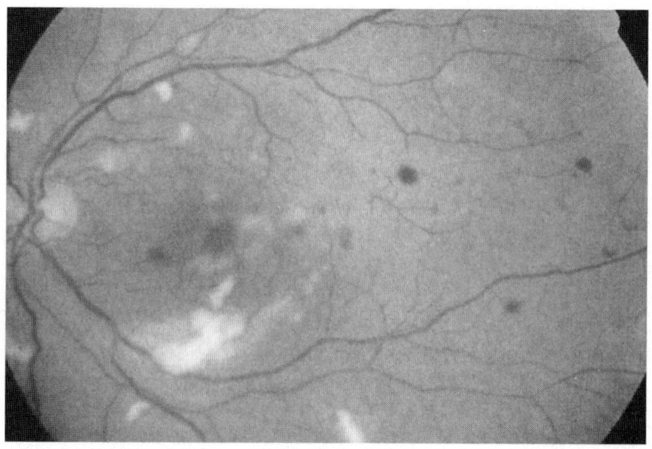

FIGURE 129-11 Human immunodeficiency virus–associated retinopathy. Note retinal cotton wool spots and hemorrhages. (From Rao NA: Acquired immunodeficiency syndrome and its ocular complications. Indian J Ophthalmol 42:57, 1994.)

visual loss or blindness. The frequency of specific ocular opportunistic infections varies by geographic location and patient population but may include such entities as CMV, toxoplasmosis, tuberculosis, syphilis, cryptococcosis, histoplasmosis, and HSV infection, among others.[64–66] Such infections can result in chorioretinitis, uveitis, optic neuritis, and keratitis. AIDS-associated meningitis or encephalitis may also be associated with cranial nerve dysfunction and ocular palsies. Involvement of the central nervous system or orbit by HIV-associated lymphoma may result in papilledema or proptosis, respectively.

A number of distinct ocular entities also appear to occur in persons infected with HIV. Infectious multifocal choroiditis is a term used to describe a choroidal infection, usually caused by a systemic opportunistic infection with *Pneumocystis jiroveci* (previously *Pneumocystis carinii*), *Cryptococcus neoformans*, *Mycobacterium tuberculosis*, *Histoplasma capsulatum*, or *Mycobacterium-avium-intracellulare* complex, among others (see Chapter 133). Progressive outer retinal necrosis is a posterior ocular syndrome that occurs in patients with AIDS and is thought to be related to herpes viral infection.[67] There is no effective treatment and visual outcome is usually dismal. An ocular vasculopathy that occurs in patients with AIDS may also be associated with conjunctival microvascular changes that may manifest as dilated, short segments of conjunctival vessels. Coinfection with *Molluscum contagiosum* virus can also lead to follicular conjunctivitis. Ocular involvement in patients with AIDS can be extensive and bilateral. Kaposi's sarcoma of the eyelid, conjunctiva, and orbit has also been reported in patients with AIDS. Ocular surface squamous neoplasia may also be associated with HIV infection.[68] Treatment of HIV retinopathy is directed toward systemic anti-HIV therapy, and treatment of opportunistic ocular infections is targeted to the specific pathogenic entity.

Human T-Cell Lymphotropic Virus Type I

Human T-cell lymphotropic virus type I (HTLV-I) infection is usually asymptomatic; however, a minority of persons infected with HTLV-I develop adult T-cell leukemia/lymphoma (ATCLL) or tropical spastic paraparesis/HTLV-I–associated myelopathy (TSP/HAM; see Chapter 76). A number of ocular manifestations have been reported in patients symptomatically or asymptomatically infected with HTLV-I.[69] Similar to what is observed in persons infected with HIV, asymptomatic retinal cotton wool spots and transient retinal exudates and hemorrhages have been observed.[70] Uveitis and interstitial keratitis are the most frequent symptomatic ocular manifestation of HTLV-I infection.[69–72] The uveitis appears to be due to the presence of virally infected T cells in the eye, is often unilateral, and can be anterior, posterior, or panuveal.[69] Keratoconjunctivitis sicca, vitritis, retinal vasculitis, retinal exudates, and retinal hemorrhages have been reported.[69,71,73] Ocular involvement in persons with TSP/HAM can include uveitis and vasculitis as well as neurophthalmologic manifestations. Ocular involvement in persons with ATCLL can include direct lymphomatous or leukemic involvement of the eye. Lymphoma/leukemia of the eyelid, orbit, retina, and vitreous, as well as a lymphoma/leukemia that diffusely infiltrates all ocular structures have been reported.[70] Patients with ATCLL often die of opportunistic infections, and CMV retinitis has been reported in patients with HTLV-I and ATCLL.[70] Diagnosis of HTLV-I infection is usually based on a serologic antibody assay (although viral studies may also be performed).[69] No treatment is indicated in persons with asymptomatic HTLV-I infection. Topical or systemic steroids can be employed in persons with HTLV-I uveitis.[69] Opportunistic infection should be treated. Antiretroviral agents are not effective.

Viral Encephalitis

Encephalitis can be caused by a number of viruses, including herpesviruses and arboviruses, the latter including West Nile virus, Venezuelan equine encephalitis virus, western equine encephalitis virus, Japanese encephalitis virus, Murray Valley encephalitis virus, Rocio virus, and Oropouche virus, among others (see Chapters 57, 72, and 74). Ocular manifestations during encephalitis are rarely reported; however, elevated intracranial pressure can result in papilledema. Encephalitis involving brainstem structures can result in disorders of ocular motility, and diffuse encephalitis can result in cortical visual disturbances.

Specific ocular involvement is associated with Rift Valley fever virus (see Chapter 67).[74] The majority of patients with Rift Valley fever present with an acute influenza-like illness that may be biphasic. In 1% to 5% of affected persons, however, hemorrhagic manifestations, encephalitis, or chorioretinitis can occur. Ocular involvement may be immunologically mediated. Clinical features of hemorrhagic fever, encephalitis, and retinitis usually do not overlap in the same individual. Ocular disease includes retinal vasculitis, retinal hemorrhages, and retinitis. Retinal detachment, optic atrophy, vitreal hemorrhages, and blindness can occur.[74] Involvement may be unilateral or bilateral.[74] Conjunctivitis, keratitic precipitates, and uveitis have been reported.[74] Diagnosis is usually one of clinical recognition of community-level symptoms of fever, hemorrhage, encephalitis, and blindness, often with a simultaneous occurrence of an epizoonosis in livestock such as sheep, cattle, or camels. Serologic assays are available, and viral cultures can be performed. Treatment is usually supportive.

West Nile virus infection has been associated with multifocal chorioretinitis, occlusive retinal vasculitis, optic neuritis, uveitis, and vitritis.[75–79] Acute flaccid paralysis of facial and ocular muscles can result in diplopia.[80]

Viral Hemorrhagic Fevers

Infections with a number of viruses can lead to hemorrhagic manifestations. In some persons, Rift Valley fever can itself present with hemorrhagic manifestations as opposed to being associated with encephalitis or retinopathy. Other hemorrhagic fever viruses include dengue fever, yellow fever, Lassa fever, Kuyasanur Forest disease, Congo–Crimean hemorrhagic fever, Junin, Machupo, hantaviruses, and Marburg and Ebola viruses, among others (see Chapters 65–73). Ocular involvement in hemorrhagic fevers is usually a manifestation of a systemic bleeding diathesis. Endothelial vascular and rheologic abnormalities can lead to hemorrhagic involvement of the conjunctivae and retina. Nonspecific eye pain may be a prominent presenting feature of dengue fever, and hemorrhagic conjunctivitis has been reported in patients infected with Ebola virus.[81] A specific ocular association has been recognized with Puumala virus in the Scandinavian hantavirus-associated hemorrhagic fever and renal syndrome, nephropathia epidemica.[82] Transient myopia is the most frequent ocular manifestation and relates to forward movement of the ocular anterior diaphragm and thickening of the lens.[83] Eyelid edema, chemosis, conjunctival injection, conjunctival hemorrhage, iritis, acute glaucoma, and retinal edema and hemorrhages have also been reported.[84] Diagnosis can be made by serologic antibody assay. Ocular involvement in nephropathia epidemica usually resolves spontaneously.[82]

Hepatitis Viruses

Hepatitis can be caused by a number of viral entities and can lead to jaundice (see Chapter 64). The conjunctiva is one of the most sensitive areas of the body for detecting jaundice. Acute viral hepatitis B can itself be associated with immune-complex deposition during the icteric phase of illness, and posthepatitis polyneuritis has been reported (including Guillain–Barré syndrome). Cranial nerves involved by neuritis can result in extraocular palsies. Retrobulbar optic neuritis has been reported in a patient recovering from hepatitis B. Immune-complex deposition resulting from chronic active hepatitis B or C infections can result in a variety of clinical vasculitic entities. Uveitis associated with chronic active hepatitis B may occur. Chronic hepatitis C infection is associated with a dry eye syndrome similar to a Sjögren's syndrome and/or ischemia retinopathy caused by hepatitis C–induced vasculitis or treatment with interferon.[85,86] Diagnosis of acute and chronic hepatitis is usually based on serologic antibody assays or detection of virus. Acute viral hepatitis is treated supportively; chronic active hepatitis may respond to antiviral agents and systemic interferon therapy, the latter itself associated with formation of cotton wool spots, retinal flame hemorrhages, and intraocular hemorrhages.[87,88] Patients with diabetes may be most susceptible to interferon-associated retinopathy and permanent visual loss during treatment for hepatitis C infection.[86]

Rabies

Ocular structures may be involved during rabies (see Chapter 75). Rabies secondary to animal bites of the face may be associated with facial paralysis and mydriasis. Retinitis and retinal vasculitis can occur with direct viral destruction of retinal ganglion cells and inflammation of the ciliary bodies and choroid have been reported. Human-to-human transmission of rabies has only occurred through corneal transplantation.[89] There is no specific treatment for rabies. Effective active and passive immunization is available for postexposure prophylaxis.

Lymphocytic Choriomeningitis Virus

Lymphocytic choriomeningitis virus (LCM) is excreted into the urine and feces of infected rodents. Infection in humans may be influenza-like with concomitant meningitis. Evaluation of cerebrospinal fluid usually discloses a lymphocytic pleocytoses; hypoglycorrhacia may be present. Chorioretinitis may be present. Congenital infection with LCM may result in a chorioretinopathy (that mimics that seen in toxoplasmosis) and neurological sequelae.[68,90] Diagnosis is usually based on serologic or molecular techniques. Treatment is supportive.

BACTERIAL INFECTIONS

Chlamydiae

There are three chlamydial species that are currently recognized to infect humans: *Chlamydia trachomatis, C. pneumoniae*, and *C. psittaci* (see Chapters 47–49). On the basis of antigenic differences, *C. trachomatis* is divided into various immunotypes. Immunotypes A to C are most commonly associated with trachoma. Immunotypes D to K are most commonly associated with genital tract disease (and less frequently with neonatal ocular infections and adult inclusion conjunctivitis). Immunotypes L_1, L_2, and L_3 are responsible for lymphogranuloma venereum (LGV).

Trachoma

Trachoma, caused by *C. trachomatis* A to C, is the leading infectious cause of blindness worldwide (see Chapter 47).[47] *C. trachomatis* A to C is transmitted by direct contact. Spread of disease is often intrafamilial. Unhygienic practices, aridity, crowding, low socioeconomic status, and the presence of flies have all been identified as important epidemiologic risk factors for developing trachoma. Trachoma occurs predominantly in rural communities of developing nations.

Active trachoma is predominantly a disease of children. Following direct deposition, the organism infects columnar epithelial cells of the conjunctiva. After an incubation period of 5 to 7 days, chronic follicular conjunctivitis of varying severity can result (Figs. 129-12B and 129-12C). Inflammation may be intense, with marked conjunctival edema, conjunctival papillae, and lymphoid folliculitis. Preauricular lymphadenopathy rarely is present. Superficial keratitis can occur. Rupture and scarring of limbic follicles can lead to a semilunar pattern known as Herbert's pits. Untreated infection may resolve over weeks to months. Long-term ocular sequelae from a single episode of *C. trachomatis* A to C conjunctivitis are often minimal. Ocular pathology and morbidity are due to recurrent episodes of conjunctival infection.[91–93] The upper tarsal conjunctiva is most severely affected. Recurrent infectious episodes can lead to eyelid scar formation and cicatrization (Fig. 129-12D). The inflammation and scarring can impede lacrimal tear production and can lead to a decrease in the number of mucus-producing goblet cells. The resultant corneal dryness can lead to additional epithelial breakdown. The cicatrization may lead to retraction of the eyelids inward (entropion; Fig. 129-13). Eyelashes can then sweep directly over the cornea and conjunctival surfaces (trichiasis; see Figs. 129-12E and 129-13). Trichiasis can lead to epithelial breakdown, erosion, ulcerations, inflammatory responses, pannus formation, neovascularization, and scarring (Figs. 129-12F and 129-14). This corneal scarring is the primary cause of trachoma-associated blindness.[92] The World Health Organization's categorization system delineates the various stages/manifestations of

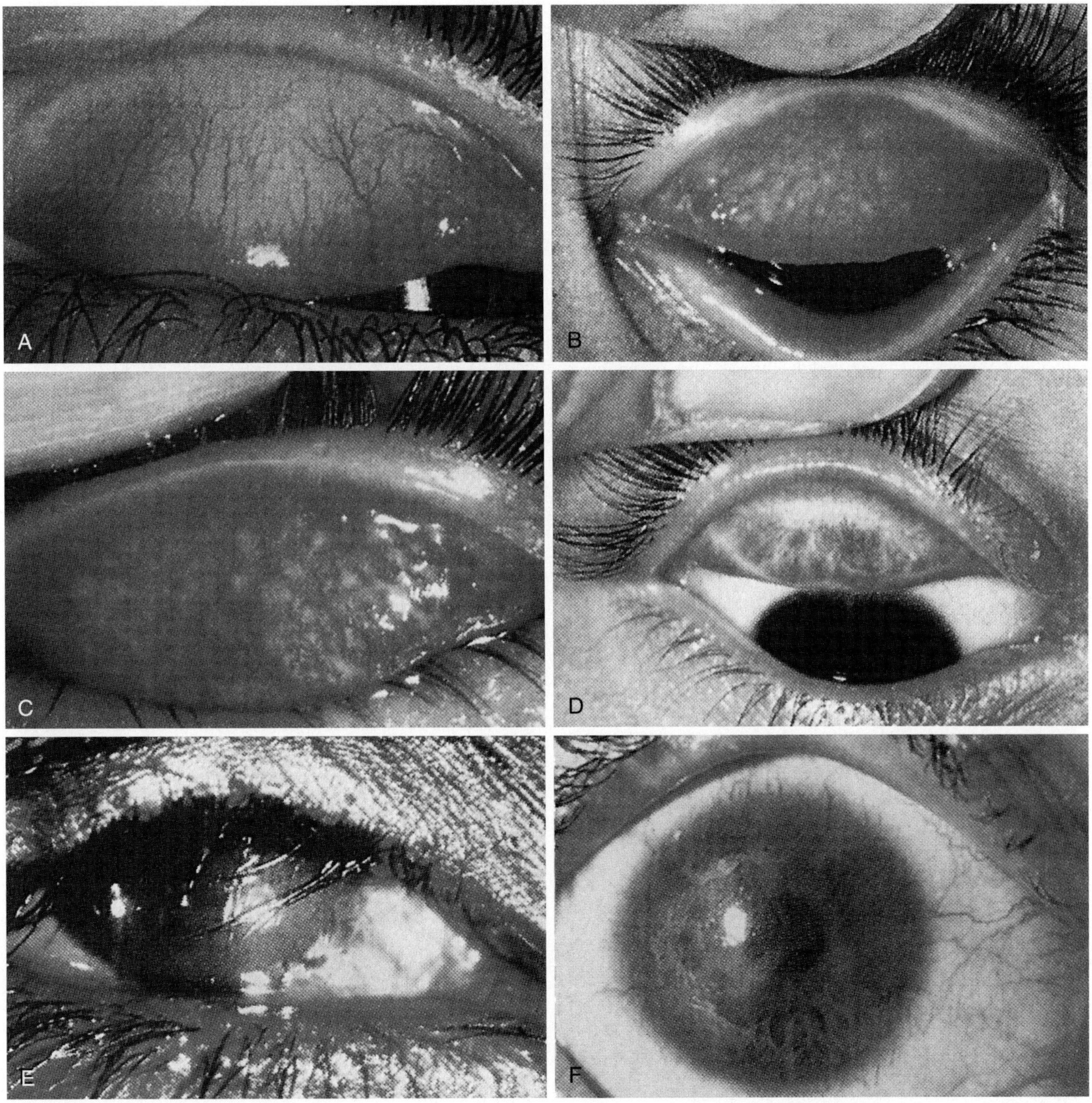

FIGURE 129-12 Trachoma—World Health Organization classification system. *A,* Normal tarsal conjunctiva. *B,* Trachomatous inflammation—follicular (TF). *C,* Trachomatous inflammation—intense (TI). *D,* Trachomatous scarring (TS). *E,* Trachomatous trichiasis (TT). F, Corneal opacity (CO). (From Thylefors B, Dawson CR, Jones BR, et al: A simple system for the assessment of trachoma and its complications. Bull World Health Org 65:481, 1987.)

ocular involvement during trachoma (Box 129-2 and Fig. 129-12).

Although most active ocular infections occur during childhood or adolescence, most visual loss and blindness occurs in adults (because of the chronic nature of the ocular damage and the requirement for repetitive acute infections; Fig. 129-15). Bacterial superinfection is not uncommon. Diagnosis is usually one of clinical recognition. Laboratory confirmation can be obtained. Culture is the gold standard of diagnosis of chlamydial infections but requires mammalian cell lines, is often impractical, and is often negative when performed on patients with end-stage trachomatous damage. Giemsa staining can be performed on conjunctival scrapings and can disclose *Chlamydia*-associated inclusion bodies in epithelial cells, but this method is insensitive in trachoma. Monoclonal antibodies have been developed that react with chlamydial antigens. Immunofluorescent assays and enzyme-linked immunosorbent assays (ELISAs) are available.

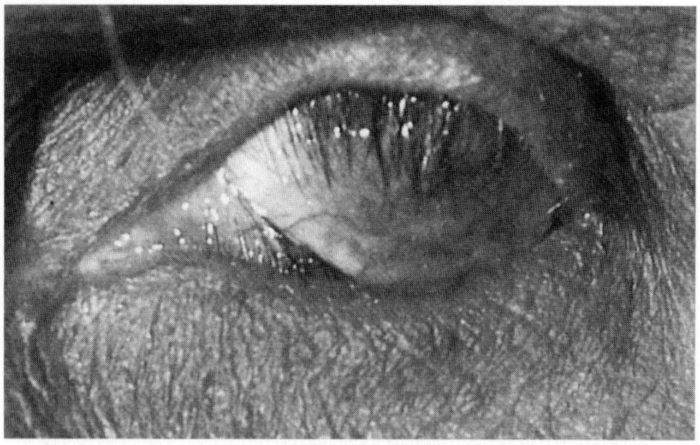

FIGURE 129-13 Trachoma-associated entropion and trichiasis. Note inturning of the upper and lower eyelids. The eyelashes of the lower eyelid are present, but completely inturned. (From Sandford-Smith J: Eye Diseases in Hot Climates, 2nd ed. Oxford, Wright Publishers, Butterworth Heinemann, 1990, plate 7b.)

Molecular techniques are also available.[94] Compared with culture techniques, these assays have over 90% sensitivity and specificity. Serologic evaluation for the presence of antichlamydial antibodies can also be employed on blood or tissue samples but is more frequently employed in nontrachomatous chlamydial infection. Tear antibody evaluations may have their greatest utility in late-stage trachomatous disease. It is important to note, however, that many persons with clinical evidence of trachoma do not have laboratory evidence confirming the presence of chlamydial organisms. This is the case even in patients with early trachomatous disease, underscoring the role that the inflammatory response plays in the clinical manifestations of trachoma.

Treatment of trachoma can be directed toward an individual patient or at a community–mass treatment level. Community education in hygienic and behavioral modifications can prevent the chronic and repetitive infections. Individuals and the community can be treated with a number of treatment regimens. Although prolonged topical therapy is efficacious, compliance is often poor.[10,95] Studies have demonstrated that single-dose oral azithromycin, 20 mg/kg, is equivalent to topical therapeutic regimens.[95–97] The complications of established trachoma can be treated by surgical correction of inturned eyelids.[98] This simple surgical technique can be performed by persons without formal medical training.[99] Epilation of eyelashes may exacerbate the problem because the regrowing eyelash stubs can be abrasive to the corneal surface. Cauterization of the follicular stub may prevent regrowth. For established corneal scars or blindness, corneal transplantation is theoretically possible but often impractical. The degree of conjunctival/corneal scarring and destruction

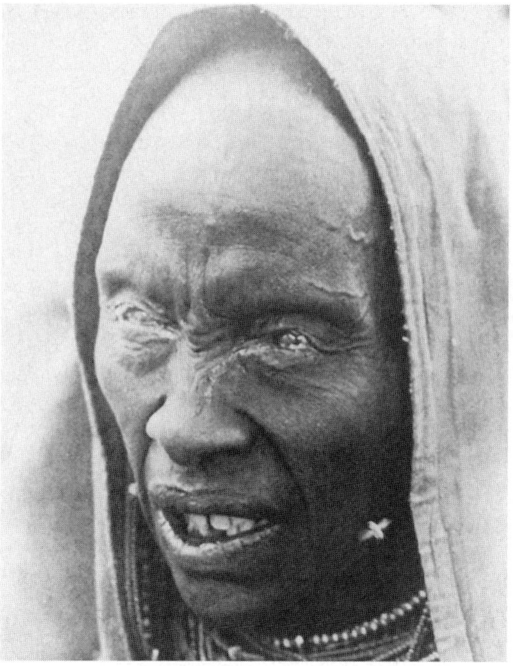

FIGURE 129-15 An adult with entropion, trichiasis, corneal ulceration, pyogenic infection, and blindness due to lifelong trachoma. (From Schwab L, Whitfield R Jr, Ross-Degnan D, et al: The epidemiology of trachoma in rural Kenya. Ophthalmology 102:476, 1995.)

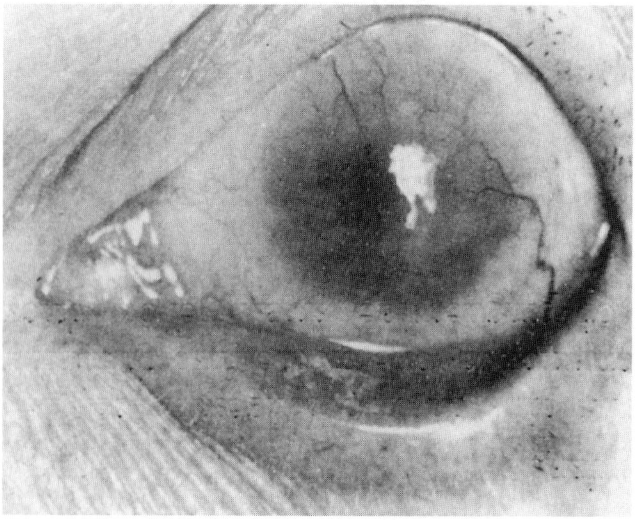

FIGURE 129-14 Trachoma-associated corneal pannus formation and neovascularization. (From Choyce DP: Tropical eye disease. Int Ophthalmol Clin 7:473, 1967.)

Box 129-2 Trachoma: World Health Organization Categorization

Trachomatous inflammation—follicular (TF): Presence of at least five follicles in the upper tarsal conjunctiva (see Fig. 129-12B)
Trachomatous inflammation—intense (TI): Obscuring of at least half of the normal deep tarsal vessels by a pronounced inflammatory thickening of the upper tarsal conjunctiva (see Fig. 129-12C)
Trachomatous scarring (TS): Scarring of the tarsal conjunctiva (see Fig. 129-12D)
Trachomatous trichiasis (TT): At least one eyelid rubbing on an eyeball (or evidence of self-epilation due to trichiasis) (see Fig. 129-12E)
Corneal opacity (CO): Visible corneal opacity over the pupil (see Fig. 129-12F)

also limits its utility. If part of the cornea remains clear and unscarred, a partial iridectomy may restore vision.

C. trachomatis Nontrachoma Ocular Disease

Ophthalmia Neonatorum

C. trachomatis immunotypes D to K, common causes of genital disease, including urethritis, cervicitis, and epididymitis (see Chapter 48), can also cause ocular disease. Neonates can be infected during passage through the birth canal, and *C. trachomatis* is one of the most common causes of ophthalmia neonatorum (along with *Neisseria gonorrhoeae*). Other causes of ophthalmia neonatorum include *Streptococcus*, *E. coli*, and other gram-negative organisms.[100] Ophthalmia neonatorum occurs in 1% to 2% of newborns in developed nations, and in 10% to 20% of infants born in developing nations that do not employ prophylactic measures.[101,102] Prophylaxis can be achieved with application at the time of birth of topical silver nitrate or tetracycline and can reduce the incidence of ophthalmia neonatorum by 60% to 70%.[101,102] Approximately 20% to 30% of neonates exposed to *C. trachomatis* during birth develop conjunctivitis, and 10% to 20% develop pneumonitis.[103] The conjunctival presentation is one of a diffuse papillary reaction with lacrimation that occurs between 5 and 14 days after birth. Eyelids are swollen, and hyperemia is present. Discharge may be purulent, and pseudomembranes can form.[104] The conjunctivitis is nonfollicular because the immature immune system of neonates is unable to generate follicles. After 6 to 8 weeks, follicles can form, and chronic infection may present at this time as follicular conjunctivitis.[104] Keratitis has been reported. Conjunctival scars and corneal neovascularization can occur.

C. trachomatis is not only present in ocular structures of affected neonates but may also be found in the nasopharynx, vagina, and rectum. The systemic nature of the infection (and the risk of developing pneumonitis or autoreinocculation) negates topical therapy as a sole therapeutic intervention. Untreated, the ocular disease slowly resolves over weeks to months. Diagnosis may be confirmed by conjunctival scrapings with culture and Giemsa staining. Giemsa staining for the detection of chlamydial inclusion bodies may have a sensitivity of over 90% in ophthalmia neonatorum. Immunofluorescent or ELISA antigenic assays are usually performed.[102] Molecular techniques may also be employed. Serology is often not helpful.[105] Tear antibody assays may be of benefit.[106] Tetracyclines are contraindicated in infants. Erythromycin is usually employed. Topical therapy may be added. Repeated courses of therapy may be required. The mother and her sexual partners require systemic therapy, even if asymptomatic.

Adult Inclusion Conjunctivitis

C. trachomatis D to K can also cause inclusion conjunctivitis in children, adolescents, and adults. Ocular involvement results from direct inoculation of infectious genital secretions. Genital infection is most frequently asymptomatic. Ocular involvement is often unilateral. Conjunctival involvement is usually follicular, and onset is usually acute. Preauricular adenopathy may be present. Discharge is minimal, and pseudomembranes that may be present in neonates do not form in adults.[104] Epithelial keratitis, subepithelial opacities, anterior uveitis and corneal vascularization can occur. Untreated, the conjunctivitis may be chronic and usually resolves over months. Diagnosis can be made by culture or Giemsa staining of conjunctival scrapings; however, a direct immunofluorescent assay is usually employed. Molecular techniques are also available.[107] Examination of the genital tract for chlamydial infection and other concomitant sexually transmitted diseases must be performed. Sexual partners need to be appropriately evaluated and treated. Treatment is systemic, with doxycycline or tetracycline employed in nonpregnant adults.[10] Children and pregnant women should be treated with systemic erythromycin. Concomitant sexually transmitted diseases need to be treated, and follow-up evaluation should be performed.

Lymphogranuloma Venereum

LGV is a sexually transmitted disease caused by *C. trachomatis* immunotypes L_1, L_2, or L_3 (see Chapter 48). Ocular involvement during LGV is rare but described. Keratoconjunctivitis may include fleshy vascularization of the conjunctiva or marginal cornea. Parinaud's oculoglandular syndrome with preauricular adenopathy, and small corneal ulcerations, episcleritis, iridocyclitis, uveitis, and optic neuritis may occur.[104,108,109] Granulomas may involve the orbit or eyelid, and scarring and blockage of lymphatic drainage may result in eyelid elephantiasis.[104] Diagnosis may occasionally be confirmed by culture; however, LGV is usually diagnosed by serologic assay employing complement fixation or microimmunofluorescence.[110] Therapy involves systemic doxycycline, tetracycline, or erythromycin, and prolonged courses may be required.[110]

Chlamydia psittaci

C. psittaci is the cause of psittacosis or ornithosis (see Chapter 49). Uncommon ocular manifestations have included follicular conjunctivitis, uveitis, and keratitis that may be epithelial or interstitial. Serologic assay of antibody levels, including complement fixation titers, is usually employed for diagnosis. *C. psittaci* should be treated with systemic tetracycline or doxycycline.

Reiter's Syndrome

The classic triad of Reiter's syndrome includes conjunctivitis, urethritis, and arthritis. Characteristic skin, mucous membrane, and bone lesions can occur. The syndrome may be accompanied by keratoderma blennorrhagica (red-brown papular/vesicular/pustular skin lesions that usually occur on the feet) or balanitis circinata (moist, well-demarcated erosions with raised borders involving the penis). The syndrome is thought to be immunologically mediated and appears to be initiated by a number of infectious processes. Chlamydial urethritis appears to be a frequent precipitating factor. Ocular manifestations during Reiter's syndrome include the classic conjunctivitis, which is usually nonfollicular. Keratitis, iridocyclitis, corneal ulcerations, hypopyon, intraocular hemorrhages, posterior uveitis, and optic neuritis may also occur. Diagnosis is usually one of clinical recognition. Many clinicians would evaluate for chlamydial involvement of the genitourinary system. If there is evidence of a sexually transmitted disease, sexual partners should also be evaluated and treated. Treatment of individuals with Reiter's syndrome involves the use of nonsteroidal anti-inflammatory agents for the arthritis. Systemic steroids are neither required nor helpful. Topical steroids may be employed in the treatment of anterior uveitis.

Mycobacteria

Leprosy

Ocular involvement in leprosy, caused by *Mycobacterium leprae* (see Chapter 38), is common; and, worldwide, leprosy is a leading infectious cause of visual loss.[111,112] Between 30% and 80% of patients with leprosy have ocular involvement.[113] Between 1% and 30% of patients with leprosy have an optimal visual acuity of less than 20/200, and 250,000 patients with leprosy have an optimal visual acuity of less than 20/400.[114]

Ocular involvement in leprosy can be due to direct mycobacterial involvement of the eye or to secondary immunologic or inflammatory manifestations. The eye may be involved during all forms of leprosy, but ocular involvement occurs most frequently during lepromatous leprosy (Fig. 129-16).[115] *M. leprae* prefers the cool temperatures of the anterior chamber of the eye, and ocular disease is usually anterior in nature. The eye can act as a chronic nidus of inflammation and infection. Involvement of the Vth and VIIth cranial nerves during type I lepra reactions can lead to corneal anesthesia and lagophthalmos (the inability to fully close the eyelids). Such involvement can predispose affected persons to corneal ulcerations, suppurative keratitis, corneal perforation, corneal scarring, and blindness. Staphyloma, a marked bulging of the anterior eye through a weakened corneal wall, may result (Fig. 129-17).

Persons with lepromatous leprosy may also experience erythema nodosum leprosum (type II reactions).[116] This form of the disease appears to be immune complex–mediated and

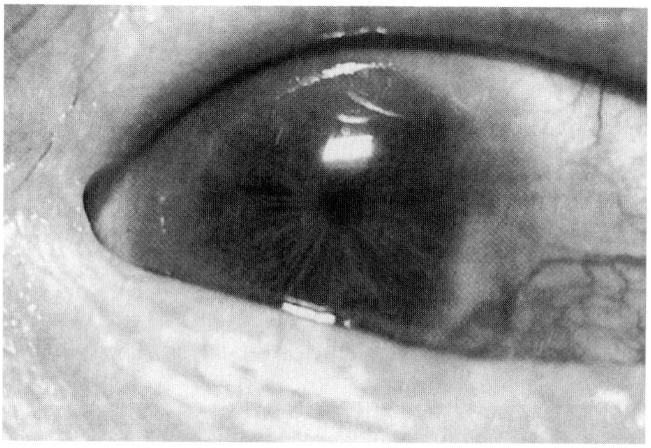

FIGURE 129-16 Ocular involvement in lepromatous leprosy. Interstitial keratitis is shown by the white appearance of the margin of the cornea. Episcleritis is shown by the dilated episcleral vessels. There is chronic iritis with constriction of the pupil. Note also the loss of eyelashes. (From Sandford-Smith J: Eye Diseases in Hot Climates, 2nd ed. Oxford, Wright Publishers, Butterworth Heinemann, 1990, plate 22f.)

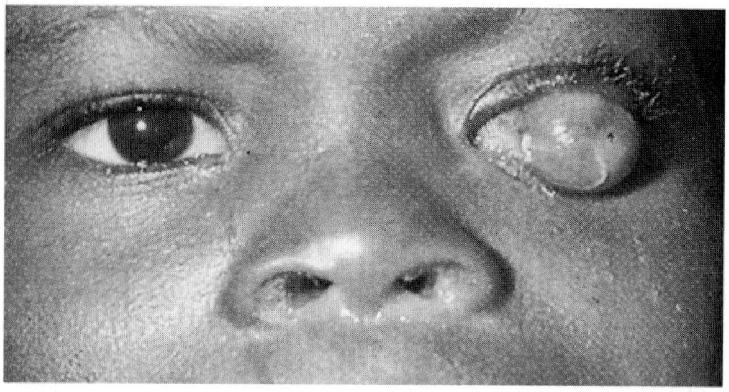

FIGURE 129-17 Staphyloma secondary to marked weakening of the cornea and sclera. The damage is irreversible. (From Sandford-Smith J: Eye Diseases in Hot Climates, 2nd ed. Oxford, Wright Publishers, Butterworth Heinemann, 1990, plate 9.)

may manifest as a serum sickness–type reaction with fever, myalgias, diffuse subcutaneous nodule formation, and arthritis. Iridocyclitis and episcleritis can occur. The iridocyclitis can become chronic and can lead to iris atrophy, persistent myosis, and posterior synechiae.[117]

Adnexal ocular involvement during leprosy is common. *Madarosis* is the term used to describe leprosy-associated loss of eyelids and eyelashes (the lateral third of the eyelids is most commonly lost). Madarosis is most common in multibacillary leprosy. Lagophthalmos may be due to either type I reactions in paucibacillary disease or to chronic nerve infiltration and inflammation in multibacillary disease. Lagophthalmos may be associated with paralytic ectropion of the lower eyelid.[115] Multibacillary disease may be associated with a marked thickening of the eyelids and can lead to excessive folds of skin (blepharochalasis) and apparent ptosis.

Lepromatous forms of leprosy may be associated with limbic lepromas (focal, nodular mycobacterial lesions). Corneal sensation can be decreased or absent in both tuberculoid and lepromatous forms of leprosy: the former from acute reversal reactions involving the Vth cranial nerve, the latter from direct mycobacterial invasion and chronic low-grade inflammation of corneal nerve fibers. Loss of corneal sensation may precede any other ocular manifestation of leprosy.[118] Beading of corneal nerves, punctate keratitis, interstitial keratitis, and pannus formation may occur. Giant lepromas have been reported. Involvement of the lacrimal gland can lead to dacryoadenitis and keratoconjunctivitis sicca. Nasal collapse in multibacillary disease can lead to obstruction of the nasal lacrimal duct with resulting epiphora (excessive tearing).[115]

Acute or chronic iridocyclitis can occur in multibacillary disease. Iris pearls represent iris edge leproma that may be miliary or nodular. Atrophy of the dilatory muscle eventually leads to nonreactive pinpoint pupils and posterior synechiae. Intraocular pressure is often lowered during leprosy. Cataract formation may occur in patients with leprosy.[114] It is controversial whether chronic iridocyclitis predisposes to their formation.[114] Posterior ocular involvement during leprosy is infrequent but has been reported. Lepromatous choroiditis, retinal pearls, and optic neuritis have all been reported.

Diagnosis of leprosy rests on clinical recognition and involves demonstration of acid-fast bacilli in skin smears or skin/nerve biopsies. An ocular manifestation can be the presenting feature of leprosy. Treatment of leprosy requires multidrug treatment involving dapsone, rifampin, and clofazimine. Specific ocular therapy is tailored to the given clinical manifestation. Type I reactions of less than 6 months' duration (including involvement of cranial nerves such as V and VII) indicate the need for immediate institution of systemic steroids. High-dose clofazimine may also be employed. Erythema nodosum leprosum reactions (with associated iridocyclitis) can be treated with systemic steroids, clofazimine, and thalidomide (contraindicated in women of childbearing age). Iridocyclitis, episcleritis, and scleritis can be treated with topical steroids.[115] Cycloplegics should be employed in acute iritis. Mydriatics should be employed in chronic iritis.[115] Chronic ocular manifestations such as lagophthalmos and ectropion may require surgical management, including tarsorrhaphy (suturing of the lateral eyelids together to protect the exposed cornea) and lid suspension.[119] Recognition of ocular involvement, corneal anesthesia, and lagophthalmos should prompt measures to prevent exposure keratitis and progressive ocular disease. Education, eye patches, protective glasses, repeated conscious blinking, antibiotic eye drops, and surgery should all be considered.[115]

Tuberculosis

Ocular involvement occurs in less than 1% of persons with tuberculosis, caused by *Mycobacterium tuberculosis* (see Chapter 36).[120] Ocular structures can be involved during pulmonary tuberculosis, during systemic extrapulmonary tuberculosis, or as isolated ocular involvement.[120] The choroid is most frequently involved during ocular tuberculosis, perhaps because of its tremendous vascularity and numerous reticuloendothelial cells. The most common manifestation of ocular tuberculosis is multifocal choroiditis (Fig. 129-18). Involvement may also manifest as choroidal tuberculomas (Fig. 129-19), iritis, or iridocyclitis.[121] Involvement of the ciliary body can result in secondary glaucoma.[121] Choroidal tuberculomas can present as small miliary nodules or, more rarely, as large solitary masses (see Fig. 129-18). Choroidal tuberculomas represent hematogenous dissemination, and

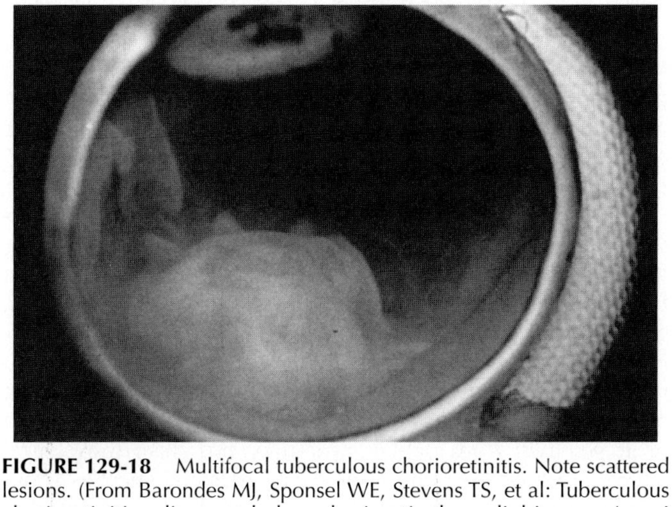

FIGURE 129-18 Multifocal tuberculous chorioretinitis. Note scattered lesions. (From Barondes MJ, Sponsel WE, Stevens TS, et al: Tuberculous chorioretinitis diagnosed by chorioretinal endiobiopsy. Am J Ophthalmol 112:460, 1991.)

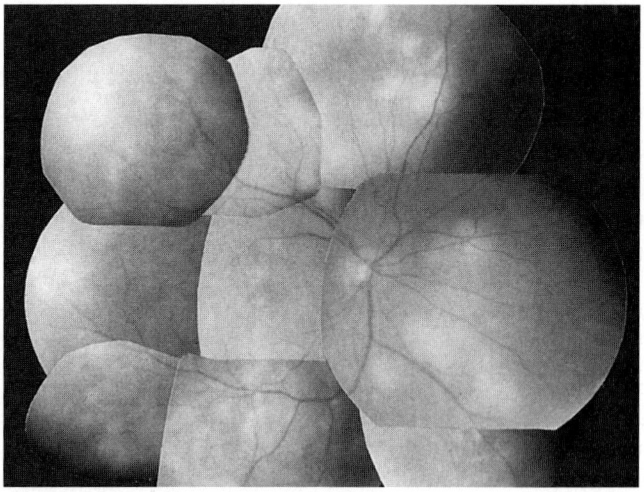

FIGURE 129-19 Choroidal tuberculoma. Gross section of the left globe. (From Lyon CE, Grimsen BS, Peiffer RL Jr, et al: Clinicopathological correlation of a solitary choroidal tuberculoma. Ophthalmology 92:847, 1985.)

miliary choroidal tuberculomas are often found with miliary tuberculosis. Serpiginous choroiditis and choroidal hemorrhages may occur.[122] When the eye itself is the site of direct infection of *M. tuberculosis*, disease is most often limited to conjunctival or corneal structures. Conjunctival involvement may be ulcerative, granulomatous, or miliary.[121] Preauricular adenopathy is common, and involvement is usually unilateral. Tuberculoid eyelid abscesses can occur from direct deposition or from contiguous spread from sinus structures.[121] Phlyctenular keratoconjunctivitis can occur (Plate 129-4). A phlyctenula first appears as a raised nodule with surrounding hyperemia that becomes necrotic and then sloughs. It is thought to be an immune response to microbial proteins and is associated with a number of infectious processes, including tuberculosis.[121] Involvement is usually at or near the limbus. Infection with *M. tuberculosis* can also result in interstitial keratitis and corneal ulceration. Involvement of the retina is rare and most frequently associated with choroidal involvement.[121] Retinal vasculitis may occur. Mild vitritis has also been reported. Tuberculosis may be associated with the development of Eales' disease, an inflammatory vasculitis that predominantly affects the peripheral retina of adults. Its classic description is of a syndrome of retinal perivasculitis, peripheral retinal nonperfusion, and neovascularization. Retinal and vitreal hemorrhages can occur. The disorder has frequently been reported in South Asia.[123] Many causes have been postulated, including a hypersensitive reaction to the microbial products of *M. tuberculosis*.[121,123] Orbital tuberculosis can result from hematogenous dissemination or contiguous spread, is often unilateral, may present as proptosis, and may be associated with the formation of fistulae. Panophthalmitis may also occur.

Diagnosis of isolated ocular tubercular disease can be problematic.[121] Skin testing, history of exposure to tuberculosis, and chest radiography can all assist in diagnosis; however, the diagnosis is usually one of clinical recognition. The presence of choroidal tuberculomas is often helpful. Persons with AIDS and tuberculosis may have positive blood cultures.[124] Ocular tuberculosis responds well to standard systemic multidrug chemotherapeutic regimens. Ethambutol therapy itself, however, may cause optic neuritis.[121]

Atypical Mycobacteria

Atypical mycobacteria are rare causes of ocular infection, although atypical mycobacterial keratitis following LASIK (laser assisted in situ keratomileusis) surgery is being increasingly recognized (see Chapter 36). *M. fortuitum* and *M. chelonae* are the atypical mycobacteria that most frequently affect the eye.[125] Keratitis, corneal ulceration, orbital granulomas, scleral abscesses, iritis, and endophthalmitis have been reported. Such involvement is usually associated with trauma or surgery or occurs in persons who wear contact lenses. Such involvement is thought to be secondary to the direct deposition of organisms. *M. gordonae, M. marinum*, and *M. flavescens* have more rarely been associated with keratitis. *M. avium-intracellulare/M. avium* complex (MAI/MAC) has been associated with corneal ulcerations, preseptal cellulitis, endophthalmitis, and choroiditis (the latter being associated with coinfection with HIV).[125]

Diagnosis of atypical mycobacterial infection of the eye is based on demonstration of organisms by acid-fast staining and culture. Persons with HIV disease and disseminated MAI/MAC infection may have positive blood cultures. Atypical mycobacteria are often resistant to the chemotherapeutic agents that are used in the treatment of tuberculosis. Clarithromycin may be effective. Topical therapy with amikacin and a second or third topical agent such as a fourth-generation fluoroquinolone antibiotic (such as moxifloxacin or gatifloxacin) or clarithromycin (depending on sensitivity assays of the specific organism) is usually effective for keratitis.[126] Surgical extirpation is usually required.[126] Disseminated MAI/MAC disease should be treated with systemic therapy.

Spirochetes

Treponematoses

Syphilis. Syphilis is caused by *Treponema pallidum* (see Chapter 44). The eye can be involved during all stages of congenital or acquired syphilis. During primary acquired syphilis, chancres of the eyelid, conjunctiva, and lacrimal gland have been reported. During the rash of secondary syphilis, conjunctivitis and blepharitis can occur. Approximately 10% of persons with secondary syphilis have ocular involvement. Madarosis (loss of eyelashes and eyebrows) has been reported. Keratitis, iritis, iris hyperemia (roseolae), iris nodules, episcleritis, and scleritis can also occur. Anterior uveitis is the most common ocular finding during secondary syphilis. Keratitis may be unilateral. Chorioretinitis (that may be placoid), peripapillary neuroretinitis, pigmentary retinitis, retinal vasculitis, and vitritis may also occur. Retinal detachment and a "salt-and-pepper" retinopathy can result. During tertiary syphilis, the eyelid, lacrimal glands, and deep ocular structures can be involved with destructive gummatous lesions. Orbital bones may be involved with periostitis that can be bilateral. Chronic interstitial keratitis is not infrequent (Fig. 129-20). The most common ocular manifestations of syphilis are uveitis and optic neuritis, although iritis, episcleritis, scleritis, chorioretinitis, papillary neuroretinitis, vitritis, and retinal vasculitis can occur. Occlusive retinal vascular disease, neovascularization, aneurysm formation, retinal detachments, and pigmentary retinopathy can also occur.

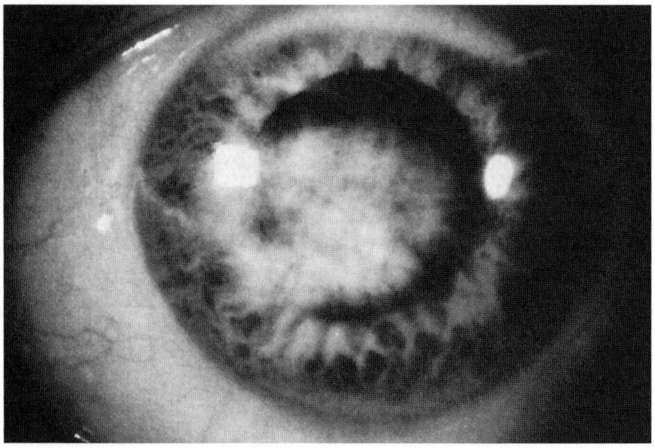

FIGURE 129-20 Central stromal scarring and ghost vessel formation secondary to late latent syphilitic interstitial keratitis. (From Brooks AMV, Weiner JM, Robertson IF: Interstitial keratitis in untreated latent [late] syphilis. Aust NZ J Ophthalmol 14:128, 1986.)

Neurosyphilis can occur during any stage of clinical disease. Meningovascular syphilis can be associated with neurophthalmic complications. Nerve palsies can result in ocular dysmotilities. The classic Argyll Robertson pupil may be visible in meningovascular syphilis. It manifests as a small, irregular pupil that reacts normally to accommodation but not to light. Papilledema can also occur. Neurophthalmic findings are possible with parenchymous neurosyphilis, but they are rare. Argyll Robertson pupil and optic atrophy can be seen in tabes dorsalis.

Ocular involvement during congenital syphilis may be mild or even asymptomatic. Clinically evident involvement during the first few months of life can include conjunctivitis, iridocyclitis, uveitis, optic neuritis, salt-and-pepper chorioretinitis, extraocular paresis, and neurophthalmic manifestations. Disease often becomes quiescent, with only pigmentary retinopathy being subsequently evident. The disease can reactivate, however, and an affected patient can present with chronic interstitial keratitis as an adolescent or as an adult. Such involvement is usually bilateral and is most often misdiagnosed. Chronic inflammation can lead to scarring, neovascularization, and residual "ghost vessel" formation. Hutchinson's triad includes malformed Hutchinson's teeth, deafness (from VIIIth nerve involvement during neurosyphilis), and interstitial keratitis. Iritis or keratouveitis may occur and can result in secondary glaucoma. Chronic retinitis and pigmentary retinopathy may be evident.

Ocular syphilitic involvement in neurosyphilis appears to be common during concurrent infection with HIV.[127] Involvement is possible even in patients previously treated for syphilis.[127] Conjunctivitis, iridocyclitis, uveitis, retinitis, neuroretinitis (Fig. 129-21), vitritis, papillitis, optic perineuritis (Fig. 129-22), and retrobulbar neuritis have all been reported.[127] Standard therapeutic regimens for the treatment of syphilis assume an intact immunologic system. Eradication of *T. pallidum* from ocular structures and from the central nervous system in immunodeficient persons, such as those coinfected with HIV, requires higher doses and longer duration of penicillin therapy.[127]

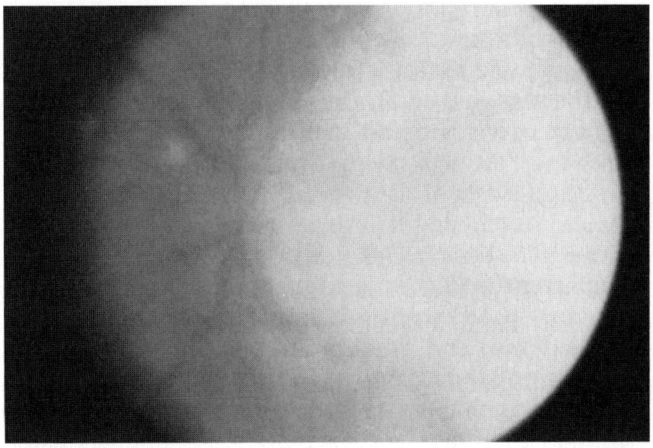

FIGURE 129-21 A large wedge-shaped area of syphilitic neuroretinitis with small cotton wool spots. (From McLeish WM, Pulido JS, Holland S, et al: The ocular manifestations of syphilis in the human immunodeficiency virus type 1–infected host. Ophthalmology 97:198, 1990.)

Diagnosis is usually based on clinical recognition and serologic examination. A lumbar puncture should be performed to evaluate for concomitant neurosyphilis. Independent of the evaluation of the central nervous system, all persons with ophthalmic manifestations of syphilis should be treated with a 10- to 14- day course of intravenous high-dose penicillin therapy. Certain immunocompetent persons with an isolated primary chancre of the eyelid or periorbital area could be treated with short, low-level therapy. Follow-up serologic analysis should be performed to monitor post-therapy resolution of disease. Follow-up analysis of cerebrospinal fluid should be performed in patients with neurosyphilitic involvement. Topical steroids, mydriatics, and cycloplegics may also be employed for anterior syphilitic inflammatory ocular disease, including keratitis and uveitis. Sexual partners of affected persons need to be appropriately evaluated and treated.

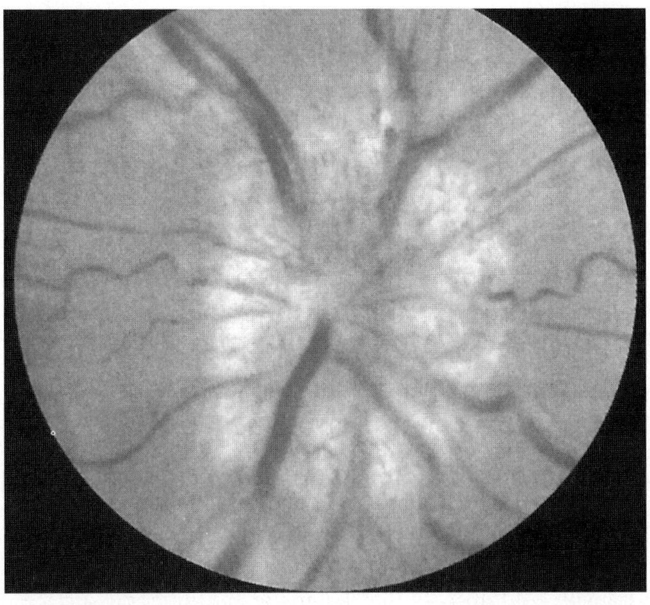

FIGURE 129-22 Syphilitic optic perineuritis with disk swelling. (From McLeish WM, Pulido JS, Holland S, et al: The ocular manifestations of syphilis in the human immunodeficiency virus type 1–infected host. Ophthalmology 97:198, 1990.)

Endemic Treponematoses

Nonvenereal Endemic Syphilis: Bejel. Syphilis (bejel) is a nonvenereal treponematosis caused by a variant of *T. pallidum* that is morphologically and serologically indistinguishable from that which causes venereal syphilis (see Chapter 44). Endemic syphilis is rarely, if ever, sexually transmitted, has not been associated with congenital infection, and is rarely, if ever, associated with late cardiac or neurologic manifestations. A number of ocular manifestations, including anterior uveitis, choroiditis, and chorioretinitis have been postulated to be a late manifestation of bejel.[128] Diagnosis is one of clinical recognition in an appropriate demographic setting. Serologic assays cannot distinguish between venereal and nonvenereal syphilis, so it is clinically impossible to firmly ascribe isolated ocular disease to venereal and nonvenereal syphilis. The treatment of nonvenereal syphilis is penicillin. Active uveitis resolves on penicillin therapy alone.[128]

Yaws. Yaws (pian, framboesia) is caused by *Treponema pertenue*. The infection is found in warm tropical areas throughout the world, is spread by bodily contact, and has distinct early, latent, and late-stage manifestations (see Chapter 44). Yaws has been associated with neurophthalmic abnormalities (including Argyll Robertson–type pupillary responses), sheathing of retinal vessels, perivascular pigmentation, and optic atrophy. Spirochetes have been identified in the anterior chamber, and iritis has been reported. Acute skin lesions can involve the eyelid and may result in catarrhal conjunctivitis. Scarred/healed skin lesions of the face may result in ectropion. Massive destruction of the nasal mucosa can result in saddle-nose, and central facial necrosis (yaws gangosa) can result in destruction of the eye and orbit. Serologic assays cannot distinguish yaws from syphilis.

Pinta. Pinta (mal de pinto) is caused by *Treponema carateum* (see Chapter 44). No ocular abnormality has definitely been associated with pinta except for scarring skin lesions that have involved the eyelids.[129]

Leptospirosis

Leptospirosis can be caused by a number of *Leptospira* species (see Chapter 46). During the acute leptospiremic phase, a retro-orbital headache can occur. Conjunctival suffusion and photosensitivity are common. During the immune phase, meningitis can occur that may be associated with cranial nerve paresis and optic neuritis. If the severe form of leptospirosis, Weil's disease, develops, scleral jaundice and conjunctival and retinal hemorrhages can occur. Uveitis is the most frequent ocular manifestation after conjunctival suffusion. The uveitis may present from 10 days to many months after the initial infection.[130] The initial infection may even have been clinically asymptomatic. Uveitis, often acute and bilateral, usually presents as anterior uveitis and iridocyclitis. Anterior chamber involvement, hypopyon, elevated intraocular pressure, and synechiae can occur. Posterior uveitis, vitreal clouding, retinal exudates, and retinal hemorrhages may also occur. Diagnosis involves serologic assay for antibodies. Treatment of leptospirosis involves systemic penicillin, tetracycline, or doxycycline. Leptospiral anterior uveitis may be treated with topical steroids and mydriatics. Systemic steroids may rarely be required.

Relapsing Fever

Epidemic relapsing fever is caused by louse-borne *Borrelia recurrentis*; endemic relapsing fever is caused by tick-borne *B. duttoni* (see Chapter 45). Ocular manifestations during acute relapsing fever include photophobia, eye pain, and conjunctivitis. During severe episodes of relapsing fever, bleeding diathesis can occur, and conjunctivitis and conjunctival and intraocular hemorrhages can result. Meningoencephalitis and cranial neuritis can occur. Involvement of the VIth and VIIth cranial nerves can result in disorders of ocular motility and ptosis. Optic neuritis can occur. Uveitis may be the most frequent ocular manifestation associated with relapsing fever and can occur after several relapses of the disorder. Iridocyclitis is most common, and posterior synechial formation can result. Posterior uveitis, vitritis, vitreal exudates, and retinal venous occlusion have all been reported. The febrile episodes can precipitate reactivation of latent herpes simplex keratitis. Diagnosis usually involves demonstrating spirochetes in peripheral blood during acute illness. Relapsing fever-associated uveitis may occur late in the disease course, and demonstration of *Borrelia* organisms may then be problematic. Acridine-orange fluorescent stain and analysis of bone marrow samples may be helpful. Serologic antibody and antigenic assays and molecular diagnostic techniques are available.

Rickettsia

Louse-borne epidemic typhus is caused by *Rickettsia prowazeki*. Flea-borne endemic typhus is caused by *R. mooseri*. The clinical manifestations of endemic typhus are similar to those of epidemic typhus but are usually less severe (see Chapter 51). Ocular manifestations are predominantly visible during epidemic typhus. During acute epidemic typhus, conjunctival suffusion may occur and can predate the appearance of the body rash. The rash itself may be associated with small, oval, pink-purple, conjunctival lesions. Persons with typhus may appear to have a glassy-eyed “drugged look.” Keratoconjunctivitis has been reported, and hemorrhagic manifestations can lead to conjunctival and intraocular hemorrhages. The vascular damage induced by rickettsial infection can lead to vascular thrombosis, retinal vasculitis, retinal hemorrhages, and possibly uveitis.

Tick-borne rickettsial spotted fevers can be caused by many *Rickettsia* species, including *R. rickettsii* (the cause of Rocky Mountain spotted fever), *R. conorii* (the cause of boutonneuse fever), and *R. africae* (the cause of African tick fever; see Chapter 50). Mite-borne scrub typhus is caused by *R. tsutsugamushi* (see Chapter 52). An eschar may be evident at the site of the tick or mite bite in boutonneuse fever/African tick fever or scrub typhus, respectively. Eschars can involve the lid and periocular structures. Conjunctival suffusion and photophobia may occur in acute cases of rickettsial spotted fevers or in scrub typhus. Direct ocular inoculation of infectious blood from crushed ticks can result in conjunctivitis, corneal ulceration, and preauricular adenopathy (Parinaud's ocular glandular syndrome).[131,132] Bilateral anterior uveitis, papilledema, retinal vein engorgement, retinal hemorrhage, retinal vein occlusion, papillitis, and optic neuritis can occur.[133] Meningoencephalitis can result in cranial nerve dysfunction and in ocular palsies. Diagnosis involves specific serologic assays and molecular techniques.

Mycoplasma

Mycoplasma pneumoniae

Mycoplasma pneumoniae is associated with the development of Stevens–Johnson syndrome/erythema multiforme major (SJS/EMM). With SJS, vesicles and bullae can involve mucocutaneous surfaces, including conjunctivae. Conjunctival involvement is present in 50% to 80% of patients with SJS/EMM. Catarrhal conjunctivitis, pseudomembranous conjunctivitis, and membranous conjunctivitis can occur. Anterior uveitis has been reported. The residual scarring can lead to keratitis sicca, lid retraction, corneal pannus formation, corneal opacifications, corneal ulcerations, and corneal perforations. Trichiasis and lagophthalmos can occur. Epiphora can result from scarring of lacrimal puncta and canaliculi. Late ocular complications are directly related to the severity of the primary SJS.[134] *M. pneumoniae*–associated SJS has a male predominance and tends to occur in younger patients.

Diagnosis of *M. pneumoniae* infection is usually based on clinical recognition. Cold agglutinins may be present. *M. pneumoniae*–specific antibody serologic assays, antigenic assays, and molecular techniques are available. Treatment involves tetracycline, macrodides, and certain fluoroquinolone antibiotics. The role of steroids in the treatment of SJS/EMM is controversial. Secondary complications may require surgical intervention.[135] Ocular lubrication and protection of the cornea and the visual axis should be primary goals.

Mycoplasma hominis/Ureaplasma urealyticum

M. hominis may be present in genital secretions and may be associated with mild neonatal conjunctivitis. *Ureaplasma urealyticum* may be associated with the development of conjunctivitis as part of the presentation of Reiter's syndrome.

Actinomyces

Actinomycosis

Actinomycosis can be caused by a number of species of *Actinomyces*. The organisms are worldwide in distribution and are part of the mouth flora. Ocular manifestations are usually due to *Actinomyces israelii* and is due to direct deposition of organisms or contiguous spread.[136] Actinomycosis can cause canaliculitis and can involve the lacrimal sac. The chronic inflammation can lead to obstruction of tear drainage, epiphora, and chronic conjunctivitis. Lacrimal sac involvement can lead to laminated concretions that obstruct normal tear drainage.

Orocervicofacial actinomycosis is characterized by an expansile cold abscess that begins at the mucosal surface of the oropharynx and does not respect anatomic borders. Sinus tract formation and fistula formation/drainage are common. Infection can involve sinuses, and direct extension into orbital tissues can occur. *Actinomyces* species may also be introduced into ocular structures during ocular surgery or through trauma.[137] Diagnosis of actinomycotic infection is confirmed by culture. Examination of tissue samples or secreted granules can disclose the characteristic stellate radiations of the organism. Isolated canaliculitis may be treated with local antibiotics. Expression of lacrimal duct concretions should be attempted in order to reestablish normal tear flow. Curettage and irrigation may be required. Prolonged high-dose penicillin therapy is required for deep involvement. Tetracycline and erythromycin may also be effective. Percutaneous drainage of an abscess or surgical intervention may be required.

Nocardia

Nocardia species are soil organisms that are worldwide in distribution. Nocardial ocular infections are rare, but they do occur. Ocular involvement in immunocompetent persons is usually related to trauma, introduction of foreign bodies, or surgical manipulation. Involvement in immunocompromised persons is usually secondary to hematogenous dissemination (usually from a pulmonary focus). Dacrocystis or canaliculitis with concretions (similar to that associated with actinomycosis) can occur. Preseptal cellulitis, catarrhal conjunctivitis, keratitis, or corneal ulcerations may all occur after contaminating inoculation.[138] Regional lymphadenopathy may be present.[138] Nocardial uveitis, iritis, necrotizing chorioretinitis, and endophthalmitis can occur in immunocompromised persons.[139] Retinal detachment and endophthalmitis can occur. Diagnosis is usually based on culture results. Treatment should be systemic for intraocular disease and usually includes a sulfonamide, often administered as trimethoprim–sulfamethoxazole. Amikacin may be added.[139] Prolonged therapy may be required. Nocardial canaliculitis may be treated with topical sulfacetamide drops. Nocardial keratitis in immunocompetent persons may be treated with local application of trimethoprim–sulfamethoxazole or amikacin.

Whipple's Disease

Whipple's disease is caused by *Tropheryma whippelii*, a gram-positive, non–acid fast, periodic acid-Schiff (PAS)–positive bacillus with a characteristic trilamellar plasma membrane surrounded by a cell wall. It is related to *Actinomycetes* and is probably fairly ubiquitous in soil. The organism can be identified in the saliva of 10% to 30% of healthy individuals. In certain individuals (usually Caucasian males), the organism is able to cause deep systemic infection. In these individuals, there is a marked absence of any immune or cytotoxic response and organisms replicate freely within foamy macrophages. The classic manifestations of Whipple's disease include a large joint arthritis, diarrhea, weight loss, and abdominal pain. Rash and neurological and ocular manifestation are common. Ocular manifestation includes uveitis and ocular movement disorder; ocular movement manifestations pathogenomic for Whipple's disease include oculomasticatory myoryhthmia (continuous rhythmic movements of eye convergence with concurrent contractors of masticatory muscles) and oculofacial-skeletal myorhythmia.[140–142] These abnormalities are usually accompanied by supranuclear vertical gaze palsy. Posterior uveitis may be present.[143] Diagnosis is usually based on identification of organisms on pathology specimens or using molecular techniques. Treatment should be systemic and prolonged and usually involves trimethoprim–sulfamethoxazole or penicillin. Retinal Jarisch–Herxheimer reactions have been reported.[144] Relapses are common.

Brucellosis

Brucellosis in humans may be caused by *Brucella melitensis, B. suis, B. abortus,* or *B. canis* (see Chapter 41). Ocular manifestations during the acute/early stage of infection include endophthalmitis and optic neuritis. There may be marked pain on eye movement. Involvement of the meninges during *Brucella* meningoencephalitis can result in ocular palsies and in papilledema. Ocular manifestations during the more chronic phase of infection may include uveitis, which may be granulomatous, episcleritis, and nummular keratitis.[145] Isolated iridocyclitis or choroiditis may occur.[145] Uveitis may be the only apparent manifestation of brucellosis and may occur after appropriate antibrucellosis therapy has been employed.[145] Less common manifestations may include dacroadenitis, conjunctivitis, corneal ulceration, retinal detachment, papillitis, and retrobulbar optic neuritis.[146] Optic atrophy may result.

Diagnosis is usually based on a serologic assay. Direct culture of infected material may be helpful during the early stage of infection. Therapy of brucellosis involves prolonged administration of a combination of antimicrobial agents. Doxycycline and rifampin or trimethoprim–sulfamethoxazole are often employed. Streptomycin or other aminoglycosides are often coadministered for severe infections. Ocular manifestations during early disease usually respond best to systemic antibrucellosis therapy. Optic neuritis has been treated with systemic steroids and systemic antibrucellosis therapy. Late manifestations of disease may in part be immunologically mediated. Anterior uveitis may be treated with topical steroids, mydriatics, and systemic antimicrobial agents.[145]

Tularemia

Tularemia is caused by *Francisella tularensis*. Ocular manifestations usually result from deposition of the organism either through direct inoculation of infectious material on or around ocular structures or through aerolization. The disease may be bilateral. Deposition on the conjunctivae may result in an ulceronodular conjunctivitis that is usually painful.[147,148] Chemosis, injection, and excessive lacrimation may be present. Painful, local lymphadenopathy may be prominent. Tularemia is a leading cause of Parinaud's oculoglandular syndrome.[147] Nodal suppuration, corneal ulceration, and dacryocystitis can occur.[148] Although the organism may be cultured, the diagnosis is usually confirmed with antibody-based serologic assays. Streptomycin is the treatment of choice. Gentamicin may also be effective.

Bartonella Infections

Trench Fever

A number of *Bartonella* species can cause disease in humans (see Chapter 40). *Bartonella quintana* is the cause of trench fever. Ocular manifestations occur only as part of the systemic illness. The headache of trench fever is often localized at the front of the head and behind the eyes. Conjunctival injection and congestion can occur. Diagnosis is usually based on antibody-based serologic assay. Culture and molecular analyses are also available.

Bacillary Angiomatosis

B. quintana and *B. henselae* can cause bacillary angiomatosis (see Chapter 40). The vascular proliferative lesions of bacillary angiomatosis may involve the conjunctiva, eyelid, and anterior orbit.[149] Lesions may appear superficially similar to those of Kaposi's sarcoma. Diagnosis is usually based on histologic examination of biopsy samples. Treatment usually involves erythromycin or doxycycline, often with an aminoglycoside.

Cat-Scratch Disease

B. henselae is also a cause of cat-scratch disease (see Chapter 40). Ocular manifestations due to *Bartonella* species infections are most frequently associated with cat-scratch disease. Parinaud's oculoglandular syndrome with unilateral conjunctivitis and adjacent preauricular lymphadenopathy is the most common ocular manifestation of bartonellosis (Fig. 129-23). Conjunctival involvement may be granulomatous. Cat-scratch disease may also be associated with encephalopathy that may result in cranial nerve dysfunction and in ocular palsies or dysmotilities. Optic neuritis and stellate macular retinitis may also occur (Fig. 129-24).[150] The latter entity is called Leber's stellate neuroretinitis and may present as a painless, unilateral (rarely bilateral) loss of vision, with a central scotoma, optic disk swelling, and macular star formation. Inflammation and occlusion of retinal vessels may occur.[151] Disciform keratitis, orbital masses, and retinal detachments have also been reported. The retinal star is related to exudative leakage of optic nerve capillaries. Diagnosis of *B. henselae* infection during cat-scratch disease is usually based on serologic assay. Culture and molecular assays may also be employed. Treatment is of uncertain benefit, but, if administered, usually involves clarithromycin, azithromycin, erythromycin, tetracycline, rifampin, sulfonamides, or quinolones. Systemic steroids are also sometimes administered to individuals with cat-scratch disease–associated optic neuritis or neuroretinitis.[152]

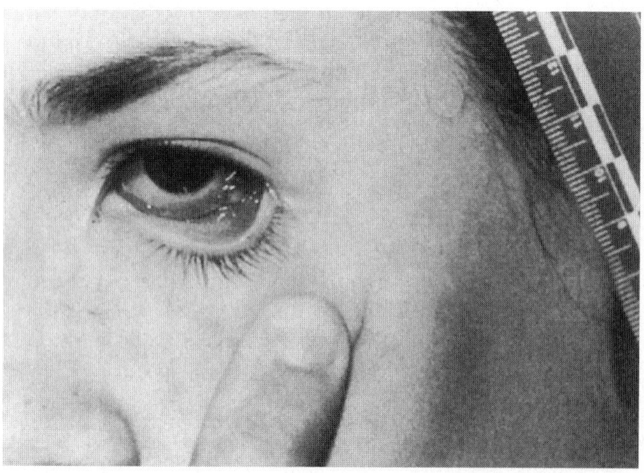

FIGURE 129-23 Parinaud's oculoglandular syndrome secondary to *Bartonella (Rochalimaea) henselae* infection. Note the oval, granulomatous lesion of the eyelid conjunctiva and the ipsilateral preauricular adenopathy delineated by the ruler. (From Bass JW, Vincent JM, Person DA: The expanding spectrum of *Bartonella* infection: II. Cat scratch disease. Pediatr Infect Dis J 16:170, 1997.)

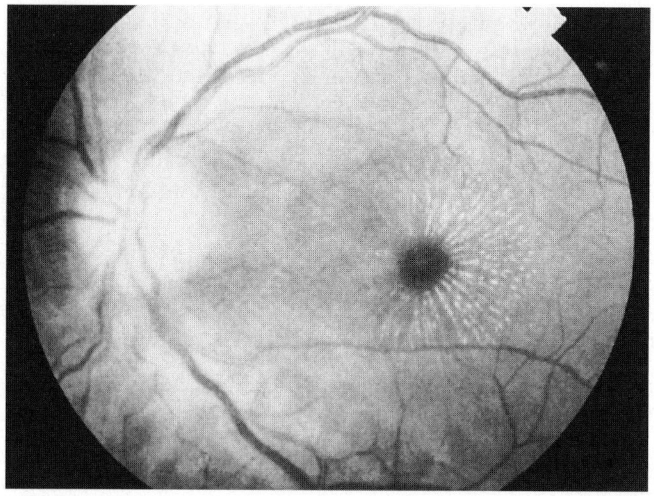

FIGURE 129-24 *Bartonella* infection–associated Leber's stellate macula retinitis. (From Bass JW, Vincent JM, Persen DA: The expanding spectrum of *Bartonella* infection: II. Cat scratch disease. Pediatr Infect Dis J 16:171, 1997.)

Carrion's Disease

B. bacilliformis is the cause of Carrion's disease, which during its early stage may manifest as Oroya fever and during its late stage may manifest as verruca peruana (see Chapter 40). Verruca peruana is associated with the formation of vascular proliferative nodular lesions, which are similar to those observed in bacillary angiomatosis. The skin is the most frequently involved site, but mucous membranes (including the conjunctiva) may also be affected. Diagnosis during Oroya fever is usually based on culture or microscopic examination of peripheral blood for erythrocyte-adherent bacteria. Diagnosis of verruca peruana is usually based on histologic examination. Treatment may include chloramphenicol, penicillin, tetracycline, fluoroquinolones, or macrolides.

Q Fever

Q fever is caused by *Coxiella burnetii* (see Chapter 54). Ocular manifestations are rare; however, cranial nerve palsies and optic neuritis have been reported.[153] Diagnosis usually involves serologic assay, although culture analysis may be employed. Optic neuritis may be treated with antibiotics and systemic steroids. Even with appropriate therapy, optic atrophy and residual visual loss are frequent.[153]

Anthrax

Anthrax is caused by *Bacillus anthracis* (see Chapter 39). The eye and periocular structures may be involved by the eschar and edema of cutaneous anthrax.[154] Preseptal cellulitis can occur.[155] Extensive eyelid scarring can lead to severe ectropion. Diagnosis is usually based on clinical appearance, microscopic examination, or culture. Molecular and antigen assays are available.

Diphtheria

Diphtheria is caused by *Corynebacterium diphtheriae* (see Chapter 35). Ocular diphtheria may occur after or concurrently with nasopharyngeal diphtheria, oropharyngeal diphtheria, or cutaneous diphtheria.[156] Ocular diphtheria can also occur independently of other diphtheric manifestations.[157] Ocular diphtheria usually presents as membranous or pseudomembranous conjunctivitis, nonspecific purulent conjunctivitis, or a corneal process. Affected eyelids and conjunctivae are "hardened," tender, and erythematous. Pain and preauricular adenopathy may be pronounced, and discharge is initially minimal. Conjunctival membranes or pseudomembranes may then appear. Such membranes represent necrotic material/cellular debris and are leather-like and pale gray in appearance. Subepithelial petechiae may be present.[156] Vascular necrosis is common. If the adherent membrane is removed, punctate hemorrhages appear. The membrane eventually sloughs with extensive exudation. Granulation tissue then appears. Healing can lead to extensive scar formation, with such secondary ocular sequelae as entropion, trichiasis, and xerosis.[157] The cornea may also be involved in acute disease. Corneal erosions and a punctate keratitis may occur.[156] Corneal ulceration can lead to total destruction of the cornea within hours of presentation.[157] Diphtheria toxin that is systemically absorbed from any site (e.g., nasopharyngeal, oropharyngeal) can lead to demyelinating neuritis. Cranial nerve paralysis can then occur and can result in disorders of ocular motility and ciliary function.

Diagnosis is usually one of clinical recognition and culture analysis. If the diagnosis of diphtheria is considered, treatment with systemically administered antitoxin should begin immediately, prior to culture confirmation. Prevention or minimization of such catastrophic complications as carditis and neuritis are associated with early administration of systemic antitoxin. It should be recalled, however, that the presence of membranous or pseudomembranous conjunctivitis is not pathognomonic for ocular diphtheria (see Box 129-1). Such membranes may be seen with conjunctival infections due to pneumococci, *Streptococcus* species, *Neisseria* species, certain enteroviruses, and adenovirus 8.[156] A Gram stain may be helpful; however, large gram-positive rods may be commensal conjunctival organisms (e.g., *Corynebacterium xerosis*).[156] Treatment of diphtheria is twofold. Primary therapy involves the administration of equine diphtheria antitoxin. Allergic testing should precede systemic administration because 5% to 10% of persons are allergic to equine antiserum. Antibiotics should also be administered and usually involve the use of penicillin or erythromycin. Topical antibiotics may be used to supplement the systemic regimen. Affected persons should be placed in isolation. Long-term sequelae of ocular diphtheria (such as entropion) may require surgical intervention.

Botulism

Botulism is caused by neurotoxins produced by *Clostridium botulinum*. Blurred vision secondary to mydriasis is often the presenting clinical feature of botulism.[158] Autonomic dysfunction may also manifest as paresis of accommodation and as dry eye.[158] Involvement of cranial nerves may result in ptosis, diplopia, ophthalmoplegia, and nystagmus.[159–162] Pupillary abnormalities may be present and may persist for months.[159] Ocular manifestations may vary, depending on the type of botulism toxin being produced.[161] Diagnosis is usually based on antigenic assays for toxin, culture, and electrophysiologic studies. Therapy involves administration of equine antitoxin with preliminary skin testing. Intestinal purgatives or lavage may be employed if contaminated food is thought to be still present within the intestinal lumen. Persons with wound botulism should undergo débridement. Botulism toxin could be used as an agent of bioterrorism and the simultaneous presentation of many individuals with blurred vision should prompt consideration of intentional or inadverdent intoxication.[163] Systemic penicillin or metronidazole is often coadministered. Administration of antitoxin only limits or prevents additional neuronal damage. Established and developing neuronal dysfunction should be managed supportively, including the possible use of respiratory support.

Tetanus

Tetanus is caused by the neurotoxins of *Clostridium tetani* (see Chapter 43). Ocular manifestations can occur during any manifestation of tetanus (generalized, localized, cephalic, and neonatal) but are most frequently observed during cephalic tetanus. Cephalic tetanus usually results from production of toxin from a local head or neck infection. Cephalic tetanus is associated with cranial nerve dysfunction.[164,165] Ocular involvement during tetanus may include ptosis, ocular palsies, ophthalmoplegia, saccadic eye movements, and supranuclear palsies.[165–168] Facial palsies may also occur.[169] Ocular structures may themselves also be directly infected by *C. tetani* organisms, usually in the setting of traumatically introduced foreign bodies.[170] Orbital cellulitis, corneal infection, and panophthalmitis have all been reported. Diagnosis is one of clinical recognition. Strychnine poisoning needs to be excluded. Treatment involves the use of passive immunization with human tetanus immunoglobulin. Débridement of wounds is required. Systemic metronidazole or penicillin is usually employed. The respiratory status and autonomic instability of affected persons need to be appropriately managed. Benzodiazepines and intensive supportive care are required. An effective vaccine is available. Active immunization with the vaccine should be employed even in persons who have survived clinical tetanus.

Neisseria Species

Neisseria meningitidis

N. meningitidis can involve the eye in a number of ways (see Chapter 25). Primary purulent conjunctivitis can occur.[171] The conjunctivitis is hyperacute, with production of extensive purulent discharge (Fig. 129-25).[171] Involvement is usually unilateral and may include subconjunctival hemorrhages.[171] Keratitis can occur, and corneal ulceration and endophthalmitis may result.[171] Ocular structures may also be involved during meningococcemia or meningococcal meningitis.[37,172] Conjunctival petechiae and hemorrhages, iritis, hypopyon, vitritis, endophthalmitis, panophthalmitis, and orbital cellulitis may then occur. Diagnosis rests on clinical recognition

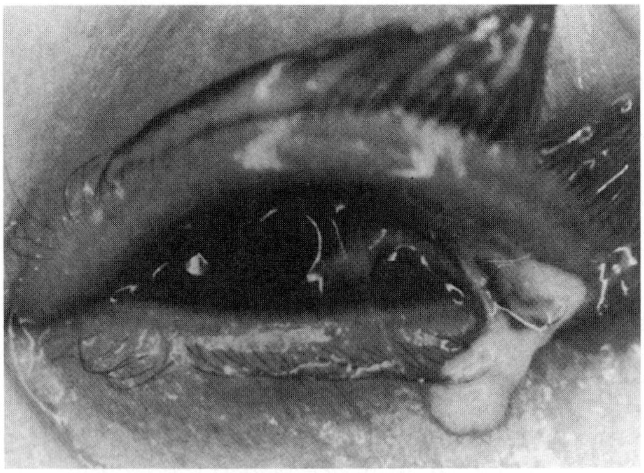

FIGURE 129-25 *Neisseria meningitidis* hyperacute conjunctivitis. (From Al-Mutlaq F, Byrne-Rhodes KA, Tabbara KF: *Neisseria meningitidis* conjunctivitis in children. Am J Ophthalmol 104:281, 1987.)

and culture. Gram stain of conjunctival scrapings may disclose the presence of gram-negative diplococci.[171] Treatment should be systemic, even in isolated conjunctival disease. Such an approach has been shown to lessen the incidence of subsequent systemic dissemination.[171]

Neisseria gonorrhoeae

N. gonorrhoeae is a more common cause of hyperacute purulent conjunctivitis (see Fig. 129-25) than is *N. meningitidis* (see Chapter 26). Keratitis, corneal ulceration/perforation, iritis, panophthalmitis, and lid abscesses can occur. Involvement is usually unilateral. Lymphadenopathy may be present. The disease not only involves sexually active persons, but also affects neonates. Gonococcal ophthalmia neonatorum usually begins between 1 and 13 (usually 2 to 5) days after birth, is often bilateral, and is often markedly purulent.[102,104] Corneal ulceration and perforation can occur. Corneal scarring, neovasculization, and blindness may result.[173] Diagnosis is based on microscopic examination of conjunctival smears and culture. Treatment should be systemic. Ceftriaxone may be employed. The mother of an affected infant, the mother's sexual partner(s), and adults with *N. gonorrhoeae*–associated conjunctivitis should be examined for the presence of additional sexually transmitted diseases and appropriately treated. Local irrigation and removal of conjunctival purulent material should be performed. Topical therapy may supplement systemic therapy. Prophylactic regimens of topical silver nitrate, tetracycline, and erythromycin should be used at the time of birth to prevent or diminish the chance of ophthalmia neonatorum.[173]

Brazilian Purpuric Fever

Brazilian purpuric fever is caused by *Haemophilus influenzae* biogroup *aegyptius* (previously known as *H. aegyptius*; see Chapter 28).[174] The disorder may manifest as a purpura fulminans, with high fever, abdominal pain, vomiting, vascular collapse, purpura, and necrosis.[174] The disorder occurs 3 to 15 days after an episode of purulent conjunctivitis caused by a specific strain/clone of *H. influenzae* biogroup *aegyptius*. Blood cultures are often positive during the severe illness.[175] The disorder mimics meningococcemia. Treatment of Brazilian purpuric fever involves systemic antibiotics and supportive care. Mortality can approach 70%. The disease occurs even in persons in whom topical antibacterial agents have been employed in the therapy of purulent conjunctivitis.

Chancroid

Chancroid is a sexually transmitted disease caused by *Haemophilus ducreyi* (see Chapter 27). Ocular involvement is rare but has been reported, presumably secondary to ocular inoculation of contaminating secretions.[104] Involvement of the eyelid, conjunctiva, or both has been reported. The chancroid papule forms a shallow, painful, purulent ulcer. Conjunctivitis can occur. Marked enlargement of preauricular lymph nodes can occur. Diagnosis is usually based on clinical recognition, the presence of characteristic "schools of fish" gram-negative bacilli on Gram stain of ulcer secretions, and, rarely, culture. Treatment is systemic.

Cholera

Cholera is caused by *Vibrio cholerae* O1 and *V. cholerae* O139 (see Chapter 21). Ocular manifestations during cholera are directly related to the severe volume loss and osmotic/electrolyte disturbances that occur in affected persons. Severe dehydration leads to the characteristic "sunken" eyes of patients with cholera (Fig. 129-26). There is a decrease in tear production and in spontaneous blinking. Conjunctivitis and exposure keratitis with subsequent corneal ulceration may result. Fluid and osmotic shifts may result in corneal edema and can precipitate the sudden development of bilateral cataracts.

Typhoid

Typhoid due to *Salmonella enterica* serovar Typhi can involve ocular structures (see Chapter 17). Rose spots can involve the conjunctiva, and conjunctivitis has been reported. Involvement of the central nervous system during typhoid

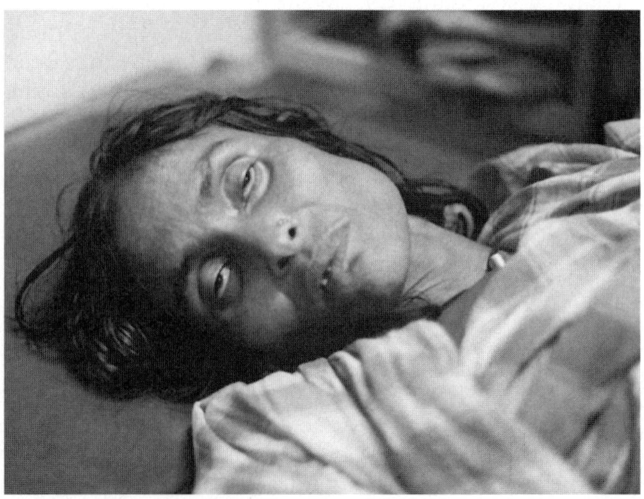

FIGURE 129-26 Woman with severe dehydration from cholera. Note the sunken and unclosed eyes.

can result in cranial nerve dysfunction, pupillary disturbances, and extraocular palsies. Severe dehydration and osmotic shifts can lead to cataract formation.

Bacillary Dysentery

Bacillary dysentery is classically associated with shigellosis, although it may also be caused by a number of other infectious agents (see Chapters 16, 18, 19, and 20). Direct ocular deposition of *Shigella* species can result in conjunctivitis, keratitis, and corneal ulceration. Diffuse orbital inflammation of unclear etiology may occur.

The conjunctivitis associated with Reiter's syndrome may be precipitated by an episode of dysentery-type diarrhea caused by *Shigella* species, *Salmonella* species, *Campylobacter* species, and *Yersinia* species, among others. Such involvement can occur 1 to 4 weeks after resolution of the dysenteric symptoms.[176] Uveitis and iridocyclitis may be observed. Synechial formation may occur. Nonshigellosis dysenteric pathogens may also more rarely be associated with direct infection of ocular tissues and can result in a conjunctivitis, keratitis, Parinaud's oculoglandular syndrome, and endophthalmitis. Diagnosis is one of clinical recognition and historical questioning. Cultures are often unrevealing in cases of postdysenteric ocular disease, although they are helpful in infective ocular cases. Treatment involves systemic antibiotics for infective cases. Postdysentery immunologically mediated ocular reactions may be managed with topical steroids.[176]

Melioidosis and Glanders/Farcy

Melioidosis is caused by *Burkholderia pseudomallei* (see Chapter 34). Ocular involvement may occur after direct traumatic deposition of the organism or from hematogenous dissemination. Necrotic scleral nodules and orbital abscesses may present with chemosis and exophthalmos. Chronic untreated infections may be associated with the development of a mild iritis. Intracerebral abscesses may form and can lead to papilledema. Diagnosis is usually made by culture.

Glanders is a systemic disease with a primary pulmonary component caused by *Burkholderia mallei*. *Farcy* is the term used to describe infection by *B. mallei* that presents predominantly with ulcerative lesions of the skin with lymphadenopathy. The disease is predominantly a disorder of equines. Infection in humans can occur from direct deposition of organisms on mucous membranes. Conjunctival deposition can result in a mucopurulent conjunctival discharge with preauricular lymphadenopathy. An ulcerative granulomatous lesion can occur, which may present as Parinaud's oculoglandular syndrome. Photophobia and lacrimation may be pronounced. Diagnosis is usually confirmed by culture.

Bacterial Keratitis and Conjunctivitis

Bacterial keratitis may be caused by a number of organisms, including *Streptococcus* species, pneumococci, *Staphylococcus aureus, Haemophilus influenzae, Moraxella* species, *Neisseria* species, *Pseudomonas* species, and Enterobacteriaceae (including *Escherichia coli* and *Klebsiella* species), among others (Fig. 129-27 and Boxes 129-3 through 129-8).[177–179] Keratitis of bacterial origin is a leading cause of visual loss in the developing world.[180,181] Such conditions as trauma, introduction of foreign bodies, epithelial defects from xerophthalmia/measles, herpetic keratitis, exposure keratitis, and entropion with trichiasis all predispose affected persons to the development of suppurative keratitis. Corneal scarring, neovascularization, and corneal ulceration/perforation may result (Figs. 129-27 and 129-28).[177] Diagnosis should include a Gram stain and culture of conjunctival or corneal scrapings.[181]

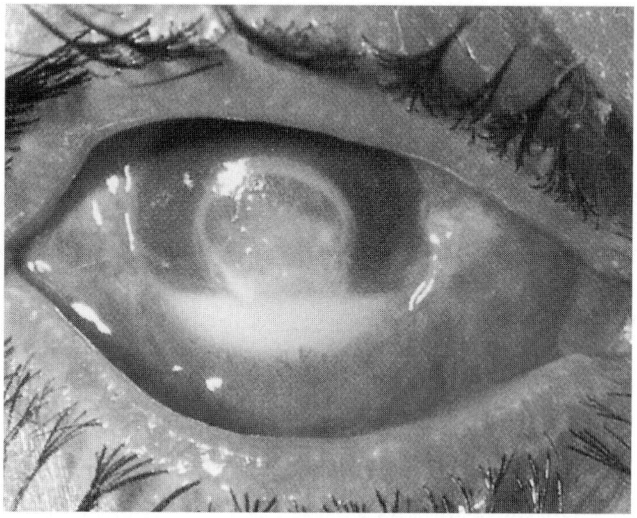

FIGURE 129-27 Suppurative keratitis with a large hypopyon and corneal ulceration. (From Sandford-Smith J: Eye Diseases in Hot Climates, 2nd ed. Oxford, Wright Publishers, Butterworth Heinemann, 1990, plate 8.)

Treatment of bacterial keratitis needs to be urgent and intense. Topical fluoroquinolones or topical cefazolin and gentamicin or tobramycin are usually employed.[10,182] Careful clinical monitoring is required. If the Gram stain or culture result discloses fungal forms or if the keratitis is progressive despite the use of topical antibacterial agents, a topical antifungal agent (such as amphotericin, miconazole, or natamycin) should be employed.[179,183] A mydriatic/cycloplegic is often employed in persons with suppurative keratitis.[10]

The most common causes of acute bacterial conjunctivitis are *Staphylococcus aureus*, streptococci, and *Haemophilus influenzae*. Bacterial conjunctivitis usually resolves spontaneously over 7 to 10 days. Topical application of an antibiotic speeds resolution.

Bacterial Endophthalmitis

Exogenous bacterial endophthalmitis may result from introduction of organisms through trauma, surgery, or a perforated corneal ulcer. Endogenous bacterial endophthalmitis is secondary to hematogenous dissemination of a systemic infection (Plate 129-5).[184,185] Therapy of endophthalmitis must include intravitreal installation of antibiotics (usually vancomycin and a third generation cephalosporin or amikacin).[10,186] Vitrectomy is beneficial in severe cases. The role of systemic antibiotics in isolated endophthalmitis without systemic infection is controversial.

Bacterial Orbital Cellulitis

Bacterial orbital cellulitis results from infection/inflammation that occurs within the bony orbit. Orbital cellulitis may result

Box 129-3 Infectious Causes of Conjunctivitis

Viral
Adenovirus*
Coxsackievirus*
Measles virus*
Herpes simplex virus
Herpes zoster virus
Molluscum contagiosum
Rubella virus
Mumps virus
Cytomegalovirus
Epstein–Barr virus
Rift Valley fever virus

Bacterial
*Streptococcus pyogenes**
Pneumococci*
*Staphylococcus aureus**
*Haemophilus influenzae**
*H. influenzae aegypticus**
Moraxella species*
Neisseria species*
Corynebacterium diphtheriae
*Francisella tularensis**
Brucella species
Bartonella species
Shigella species
Burkholderia mallei
Burkholderia pseudomallei
Actinomyces species
Nocardia species
Treponema pallidum
Treponema pertenue
Leptospira species
Borrelia species
Mycoplasma species
*Chlamydia trachomatis**
Chlamydia psittaci
Rickettsia species
Coxiella burnetii
Mycobacterium tuberculosis

Fungal
Candida species
Coccidioides immitis
Aspergillus species
*Sporothrix schenckii**
*Rhinosporidium seeberi**

Parasitic
Microsporidia species*
Loa loa
Dirofilaria species
Mansonella species
Thelazia species*
Trichinella spiralis
*Gnathostoma spinigerum**
Ascaris lumbricoides
Wuchereria bancrofti/B. malayi/B. timori
Dracunculus medinensis
Cysticercus cellulosae
Spirometra species (sparganosis)*
Echinococcus species
Schistosoma species
Myiasis*

*Common or classic ocular manifestation of infection.

Box 129-4 Infectious Causes of Keratitis

Viral
Adenovirus*
Herpes simplex virus*
Herpes zoster virus*
Mumps virus
Measles virus*
Rubella virus
Enterovirus
Rift Valley fever virus

Bacterial
Streptococcus species
Staphylococcus species*
*Haemophilus influenzae**
Moraxella species*
Klebsiella species*
Corynebacterium diphtheriae
Neisseria species*
Pseudomonas species*
Brucella species
Shigella species
Rickettsia species
Treponema pallidum
Actinomyces species
Nocardia species
Vibrio cholerae (exposure keratitis)
*Mycobacterium leprae**
Mycobacterium tuberculosis
Atypical mycobacteria*
*Chlamydia trachomatis** (secondary keratitis)
Chlamydia psittaci

Fungal
Aspergillus species*
Candida species*
Curvularia species*
Mucorales species*
Sporothrix schenckii
Coccidioides immitis
Fusarium species*
Penicillium species*
Cephalosporium species*
Phaeohyphomycosis
*Cryptococcus neoformans**

Parasitic
Microsporidia species*
Acanthamoeba species*
Trypanosoma species
Ancylostoma species
*Onchocerca volvulus**
Thelazia species
Echinococcus species
Coenuriasis* (exposure keratitis)
Myiasis

*Common or classic ocular manifestation of infection.

Box 129-5 Infectious Causes of Posterior Uveitis, Anterior Uveitis, or Both

Viral

Cytomegalovirus*
Herpes simplex virus*
Herpes zoster virus*
Rubella virus
Mumps virus
Epstein–Barr virus
Enterovirus
Influenza virus
Rift Valley fever virus
Hantavirus
Hepatitis viruses
Human T-cell lymphotropic virus I

Bacterial

*Francisella tularensis**
Brucella species*
Coxiella burnetii
Burkholderia pseudomallei
Neisseria species
Bartonella henselae
*Mycobacterium leprae**
*Mycobacterium tuberculosis**
*Treponema pallidum**
Treponema pertenue
Tropheryma whippelii
Leptospira species
Borrelia species
Rickettsia species
Chlamydia trachomatis
Chlamydia psittaci

Fungal

Aspergillus species
Candida species
*Cryptococcus neoformans**
*Histoplasma capsulatum**
Blastomyces dermatitidis
Paracoccidioides brasiliensis
Sporothrix schenckii
*Pneumocystis jiroveci**

Parasitic

*Toxoplasma gondii**
Trypanosoma brucei species
*Onchocerca volvulus**
Toxocara species
Loa loa
Dirofilaria species
Gnathostoma spinigerum
Coenuriasis
Schistosoma species*
Myiasis
Pentastomiasis (Lingulata serrata)

*Common or classic ocular manifestation.

Box 129-6 Infectious Causes of Ulcerative Lesions of the Eyelid

Viral

Herpes simplex virus
Herpes zoster virus
Measles virus

Bacterial

Treponema pallidum
Treponema pertenue
Mycobacterium tuberculosis
Haemophilus ducreyi
Rickettsia species (eschar)
Bacillus anthracis (eschar and edema)

Fungal

Blastomyces dermatitidis
Paracococcidioides brasiliensis
Sporothrix schenckii

Parasitic

Leishmania species
Entamoeba histolytica

Box 129-7 Infectious Causes of Parinaud's Oculoglandular Syndrome

Viral

Adenovirus
Enterovirus
Epstein–Barr virus
Mumps virus

Fungal

*Sporothrix schenckii**
*Blastomyces dermatitidis**
*Coccidioides immitis**
Paracoccidiodes brasiliensis

Parasitic

*Trypanosoma cruzi**

Bacterial

Bartonella species*
*Francisella tularensis**
Corynebacterium diphtheriae
Pasteurella species
Yersinia species
Burkholderia mallei
Haemophilus ducreyi
Chlamydia trachomatis
Rickettsia conorii
Treponema pallidum
*Mycobacterium tuberculosis**
Actinomyces species

*Common or classic ocular manifestation of infection.

Box 129-8 Infectious Causes of Proptosis

Viral
Epstein–Barr virus–associated Burkitt's lymphoma
Bacterial
Orbital cellulitis
Orbital abscess
Fungal
Mucorales species
Aspergillus species
Histoplasma capsulatum var. *duboisii*
Orbital abscess
Parasitic
Angiostrongylus cantonensis
Gnathostoma spinigerum
Echinococcus species
Cysticercus cellulosae
Spirometra species (sparganosis)
Coenuriasis

from contiguous spread from adjacent sinuses, from direct inoculation/trauma, or rarely from hematogenous dissemination. Involvement can result in extensive orbital edema, chemosis, proptosis, endophthalmitis, cavernous sinus thrombosis, meningitis, and brain abscess formation. Subperiosteal and orbital abscesses may be present. Ocular palsies and ophthalmoplegia may result. Treatment involves systemic antimicrobial agents.[10] Abscesses often require surgical drainage. Concomitant sinusitis needs to be excluded and, if present, treated appropriately.

FUNGAL INFECTIONS

Fungal Keratitis

The cornea is the most common site of fungal infection of the eye. Fungal keratitis (keratomycosis) can lead to corneal ulceration, corneal scarring, visual loss, and blindness.[178] In the tropics, 25% to 50% of all cases of suppurative keratitis are fungal in origin.[178,187–189] The most common causes of fungal keratitis are *Aspergillus* species and *Fusarium* species. Others include *Curvularia* species, *Candida* species, *Penicillium* species, and *Cephalosporium* species, among others (see Box 129-3).[177,179,181,183,190,191] Keratomycosis may occur after minor corneal trauma, especially trauma involving vegetable matter. The fungal corneal infiltrate typically has a feathery border and satellite lesions.[183] Corneal scrapings by an ophthalmologist should be performed in all cases of suppurative keratitis. Gram stain and potassium hydroxide wet-mount preparations are economic and effective means of preliminarily establishing whether keratitis is bacterial or fungal in origin and in directing initial treatment. Suppurative keratitis of either mycotic or bacterial origin is an ophthalmic emergency, and therapy should be instituted immediately (see Fig. 129-27). Definitive therapy may be guided by culture results of corneal scrapings. If a preliminary Gram stain does not disclose fungal forms but the corneal lesion is progressive despite the administration of appropriate topical antibacterial agents, strong consideration should be given to the empirical addition of an antifungal agent. Treatment of keratomycosis should be intense and include hourly eye drops with topical amphotericin B (0.15%) and/or topical natamycin. Therapy of keratitis due to *Candida* species may include topical amphotericin or fluconazole. Topical and oral flucytosine or oral fluconazole may be used as supplemental therapy in the management of candidal keratitis.[183] For keratitis caused by *Aspergillus* species, topical amphotericin or natamycin may be supplemented with oral itraconazole or voriconazole. Topical natamycin should be used in keratitis caused by such organisms as *Fusarium* species, *Penicillium* species, and *Cephalosporium* species. Topical silver sulfadiazine has also been used in the treatment of keratomycosis, especially that caused by *Fusarium* species.[183] The use of steroids should be avoided. Débridement may improve ocular penetration of drugs. Surgical intervention, including cryotherapy, cauterization, penetrating keratoplasty, or conjunctival flaps may be required.[183]

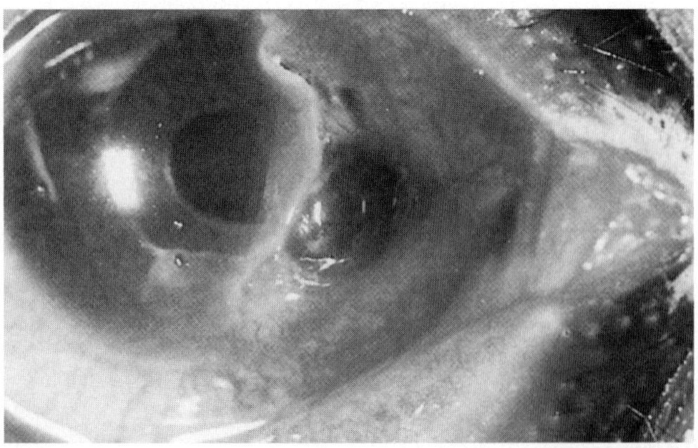

FIGURE 129-28 Corneal perforation secondary to ulceration. Note prolapse of the iris. (From Sandford-Smith J: Eye Diseases in Hot Climates, 2nd ed. Oxford, Wright Publishers, Butterworth Heinemann, 1990, plate 4e.)

Aspergillosis

Aspergillosis can be caused by a number of *Aspergillus* species. Ocular involvement by *Aspergillus* species may result in conjunctivitis that may involve the canalicular lacrimal duct and can result in tear-flow obstruction.[192] Scleritis with ulceration may occur.[193] Keratitis with extensive corneal ulceration may occur.[183] Endophthalmitis may result from posterior progression of keratitis, from traumatic or surgical inoculation, or from hematogenous dissemination (the latter usually occurring in immunocompromised persons or in intravenous drug abusers).[194] Such involvement may present with loss of vision. Iritis, chorioretinitis, retinal hemorrhages, retinal detachment, vitritis, endophthalmitis, perivasculitis, and optical neuritis may occur.[195] Ocular aspergillosis can rarely present as an isolated anterior chamber expansile mass. *Aspergillus* species can involve sinus structures, and such an infection can extend into the orbit. Acute invasive fungal sinusitis can be caused by *A. fumigatus* (although more commonly by fungi of the order Mucorales), usually in immunocompromised persons. Orbital involvement with proptosis and chemosis can occur. A more chronic form of invasive fungal sinusitis, often due to *A. fumigatus*, may occur in immunocompetent or immunocompromised persons and is associated with the development of orbital apex syndrome: ptosis, proptosis, ophthalmoplegia, neuralgia of the ophthalmic division of the trigeminal nerve, and visual loss.[196] A more chronic, indolent fungal sinusitis, often caused by *A. flavus* and called granulomatous invasive fungal sinusitis, is most commonly reported in Africa and South Asia.[196,197] Involvement is usually in immunocompetent persons, who often present with unilateral proptosis. Surgical intervention, supplemented by amphotericin B, caspofungin, or voriconazole is required.[196] Diagnosis of ocular involvement by *Aspergillus* species is usually based on microscopic examination of tissue preparations and cultures. Topical (0.15%), intravitreal, and systemic antifungal agents (or combinations) are employed, depending on the location of the *Aspergillus* infection.[193] Penetrating keratoplasty may be required for keratomycosis caused by *Aspergillus*; vitrectomy with installation of intravitreal amphotericin is required for endophthalmitis caused by *Aspergillus*.[193,198] Systemic administration of antifungal agents is usually required.

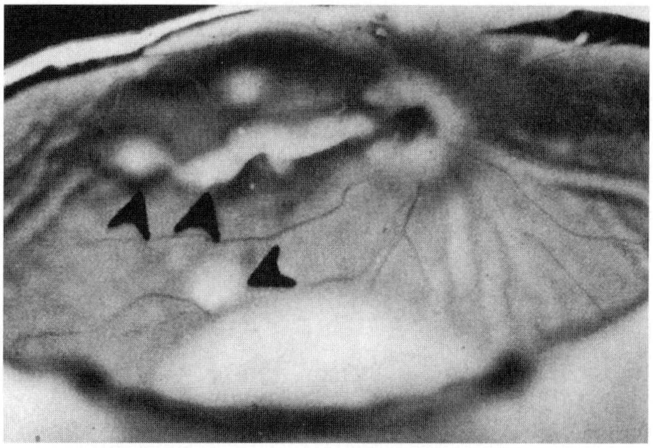

FIGURE 129-30 Chorioretinal candidal lesions of the posterior fundus *(arrowheads)*. The optic disk is edematous. Gross specimen, right eye. (From Edwards JE Jr, Foos RY, Montgomerie JZ, et al: Ocular manifestations of *Candida* septicemia: Review of seventy-six cases of hematogenous *Candida* endophthalmitis. Medicine [Baltimore] 53:48, 1974.)

Candidiasis

Candidiasis can be caused by a number of *Candida* species, of which the most commonly reported is *C. albicans* (see Chapter 83). Ocular involvement by *Candida* species most commonly manifests as chorioretinitis complicating hematogeneous dissemination (usually in an immunocompromised host); other manifestations include choroiditis, chorioretinitis, vitritis, endophthalmitis, uveitis, iridocyclitis, keratitis, and infection of the lacrimal system or eyelids[183] (Figs. 129-29 and 129-30). Involvement of superficial ocular structures usually occurs after epithelial disruption, trauma, or surgical manipulation. Patients who successfully recover from candidal chorioretinitis may be at risk for subsequent choroidal neovascularization. Diagnosis is based on microscopic analysis and fungal culture of scraping or tissue samples. Blood cultures may be positive in persons with candidemia. Candidal keratitis should be treated with topical amphotericin or, if *Candida albicans*, topical fluconazole and oral fluconazole. Candidal chorioretinitis will respond to systemic amphotericin. Candidal endophthalmitis should be treated with vitrectomy and intravitreal amphotericin B (irregardless of *Candida* species) and systemic fluconazole (if *Candida albicans*). Systemic flucytosine may be employed during the initial stage of therapy.

Cryptococcosis

Cryptococcosis is caused by *Cryptococcus neoformans* (see Chapter 80). Ocular involvement during cryptococcal infection usually occurs in the setting of disseminated cryptococcosis, usually with cryptococcal meningitis. Thirty percent to 40% of persons with cryptococcal meningitis have ocular signs or symptoms. The organism can spread directly along the optic nerve sheet and can result in direct cryptococcal invasion of the optic nerve. Papilledema and visual loss are common (Fig. 129-31). Optic atrophy usually results if the

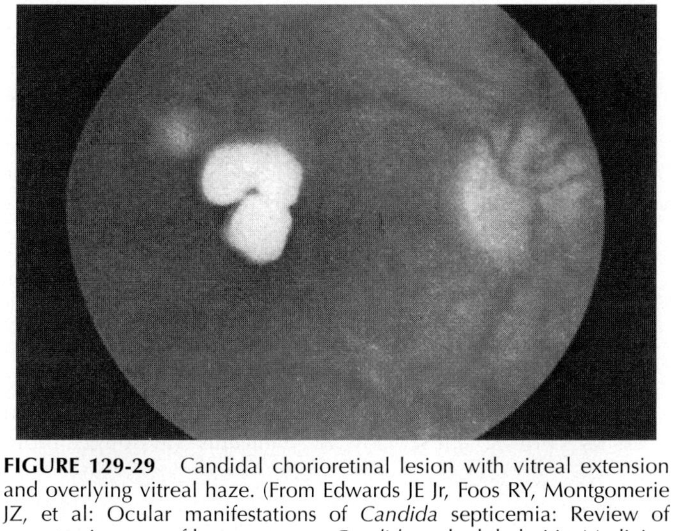

FIGURE 129-29 Candidal chorioretinal lesion with vitreal extension and overlying vitreal haze. (From Edwards JE Jr, Foos RY, Montgomerie JZ, et al: Ocular manifestations of *Candida* septicemia: Review of seventy-six cases of hematogenous *Candida* endophthalmitis. Medicine [Baltimore] 53:48, 1974.)

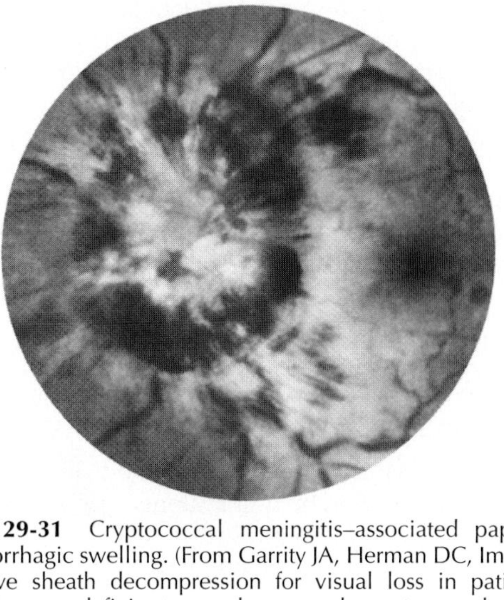

FIGURE 129-31 Cryptococcal meningitis–associated papilledema. Note hemorrhagic swelling. (From Garrity JA, Herman DC, Imes R, et al: Optic nerve sheath decompression for visual loss in patients with acquired immunodeficiency syndrome and cryptococcal meningitis with papilledema. Am J Ophthalmol 116:47, 1993.)

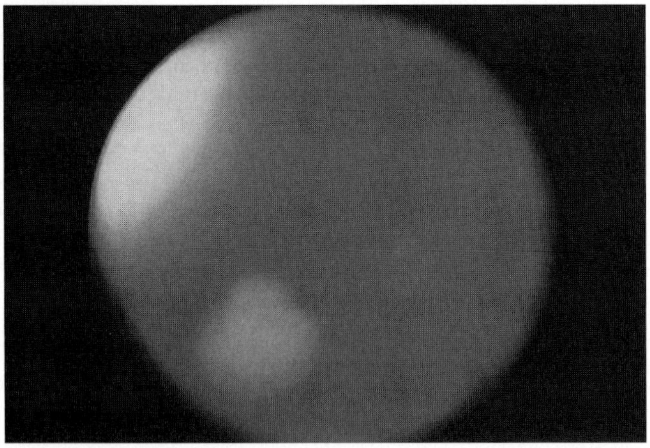

FIGURE 129-32 Cryptococcal retinovitreal abscess along the inferotemporal arcade, right eye. (From Hiss PW, Shields JA, Augsberger JJ: Solitary retinovitreal abscess as the initial manifestation of cryptococcosis. Ophthalmology 95:162, 1988.)

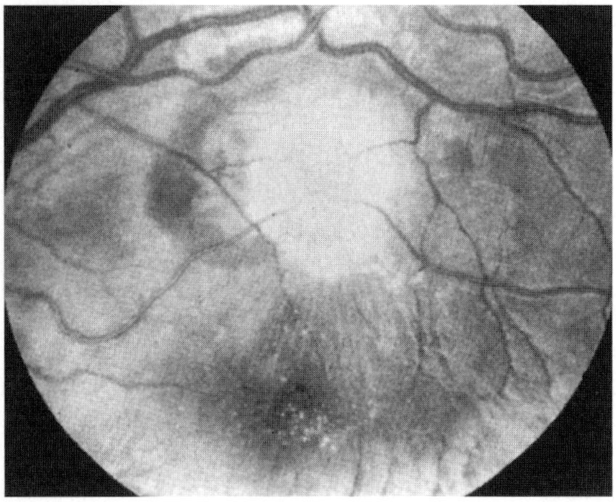

FIGURE 129-33 Acute *Histoplasma capsulatum* choroidal granuloma. (From McMillan TA, Lashkari K: Ocular histoplasmosis. Int Ophthalmol Clin 36:180, 1996.)

patient survives an acute infection complicated by cryptococcal papilledema. Involvement of the central nervous system during cryptococcosis may result in cranial nerve dysfunction and extraocular muscle paresis.

Hematogenous spread usually involves the posterior pole of the eye and usually occurs in immunocompromised persons, such as those with AIDS or those on steroid immunosuppression. Immunocompetent persons, however, may also be affected. Involvement may be focal or multifocal and may be bilateral. Isolated ocular involvement can occur and may precede systemic manifestations.[199–201] Posterior involvement includes choroiditis, chorioretinitis, neuroretinitis, and endophthalmitis (Fig. 129-32).[200,201] More rarely, anterior uveitis, iridocyclitis, and an iris mass occur.[202] Direct intraocular inoculation of organisms following trauma or surgery may result in rare cases of keratitis and cryptococcal endophthalmitis.

Diagnosis rests on microscopic and culture analysis of aqueous or vitreal samples. Persons with disseminated cryptococcosis may have positive blood cultures, and cryptococcal antigen assays of blood, cerebrospinal fluid, or urine may be positive.[201] Treatment involves fluconazole and/or intravitreal and systemic amphotericin B. Flucytosine may be added during acute management. Repetitive (daily) lumbar punctures with removal of cerebrospinal fluid to control intracranial hypertension are often required. Surgical intervention may be required. Once the infection is controlled, oral fluconazole may be employed. Recrudescence is common, especially in immunocompromised persons. Maintenance fluconazole may be required.

Histoplasmosis

Histoplasma capsulatum

Ocular involvement due to *H. capsulatum* can take one of three forms, depending on the immunologic status of the affected person: chorioretinal granuloma formation, disseminated histoplasmosis, and presumed ocular histoplasmosis syndrome (POHS).[203] Involvement of the eye by *H. capsulatum* occurs predominantly during hematogenous dissemination (see Chapter 80). Immunocompetent persons may present with a focal chorioretinal granuloma (Fig. 129-33). Such a lesion can present as a tumor-like intraocular mass or as a diffusely infiltrating granulomatous lesion. Conjunctival granulomata have also been reported.[204] Ocular involvement during widely disseminated histoplasmosis is most common among immunocompromised persons, such as those with AIDS.[205] Choroiditis, chorioretinitis, retinitis, optic neuritis, endophthalmitis, iritis, scleritis, and conjunctivitis can occur. Fungal invasion of the central retinal vein has been reported. Inflammatory responses may be minimal in such severely immunocompromised persons.

POHS is thought to occur in persons with strong immunity to *H. capsulatum*.[203,206] It is thought that a previous, perhaps even asymptomatic, episode of histoplasmosis leads to multiple foci of choroidally deposited *H. capsulatum* organisms. A prompt and potent immune response leads to destruction of the organisms and to resultant disciform scar formation (Fig. 129-34). The presumed ocular histoplasmosis syndrome includes the findings of peripapillary or peripheral chorioretinal scars and disciform macular lesions.[203] There is no evidence of active vitreal or aqueous inflammation. A histoplasmin

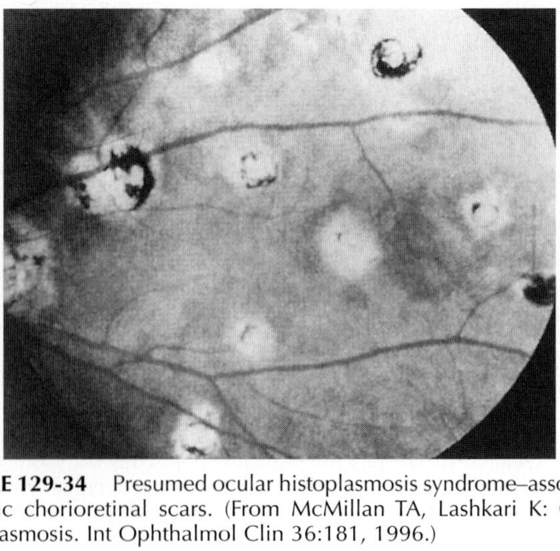

FIGURE 129-34 Presumed ocular histoplasmosis syndrome–associated atrophic chorioretinal scars. (From McMillan TA, Lashkari K: Ocular histoplasmosis. Int Ophthalmol Clin 36:181, 1996.)

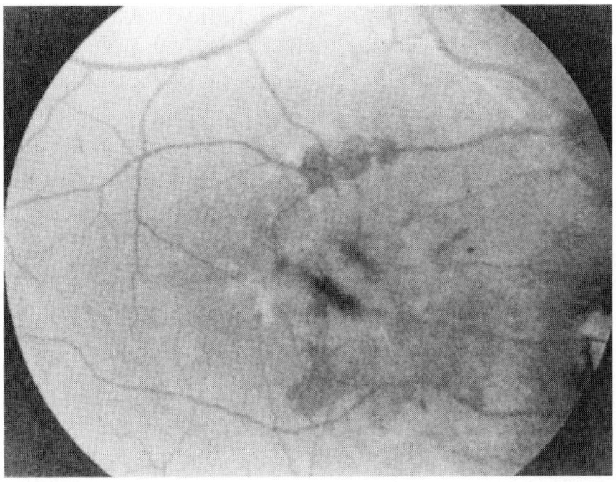

FIGURE 129-35 Presumed ocular histoplasmosis syndrome–associated choroidal neovascular membrane, macular. (From McMillan TA, Lashkari K: Ocular histoplasmosis. Int Ophthalmol Clin 36:182, 1996.)

skin test result is often positive, although evidence of active histoplasmosis is absent. Patients with POHS are at risk for neovascularization that may be complicated by retinal hemorrhages (Fig. 129-35).[203] Loss of vision may be pronounced.

Diagnosis of granulomatous or disseminated ocular histoplasmosis usually rests on demonstration of the organism. *H. capsulatum* may be cultured from the blood in severely immunocompromised persons. Diagnosis of POHS usually rests on funduscopic findings and serologic or skin test evaluations. Treatment of active ocular histoplasmosis includes the use of systemic amphotericin B. Intravitreal therapy may also be employed. Itraconazole has poor intraocular penetration and should be used only after control of the active infection has been achieved. Immunocompromised persons may require maintenance suppressive therapy. In POHS, antifungal therapy is not administered. Laser photocoagulation has been demonstrated to lessen loss of vision secondary to choroidal neovascular membrane formation (when such lesions are nonfoveal).[203,206] Careful ophthalmic monitoring of patients with POHS is required. It is controversial whether steroids are of benefit, but they are sometimes employed in the treatment of foveal POHS lesions.[203,207]

H. capsulatum variety *duboisii*

Infection with *H. capsulatum* var. *duboisii* has been reported from Africa and causes a clinically distinct form of histoplasmosis called African histoplasmosis (see Chapter 80).[208] Involvement is usually of the skin, soft tissue, and bone. Lesions are chronic and may present as nodules or expansile cold abscesses. Involvement may present as an isolated lesion or, more rarely, as a systemic infection. Involvement of bones is common. Ocular involvement has been reported due to orbital spread from the bones of the face (Fig. 129-36).[209] Diagnosis is based on microscopic and culture analysis of tissue specimens or abscess contents.[209] Treatment of ocular *H. capsulatum* var. *duboisii* has involved surgical intervention supplemented by systemic antifungal agents.[209]

Coccidioidomycosis

Coccidioidomycosis is caused by *Coccidioides immitis* (see Chapter 80). Eye involvement may occur during acute coccidioidomycosis but may remain asymptomatic. Funduscopic examination in such persons may disclose healed inactive chorioretinal scars that are similar to, but distinct from, those associated with previous histoplasmosis. Symptomatic involvement usually occurs during disseminated disease or during chronic coccidioidomycosis. Primary pulmonary coccidioidomycosis may be associated with phlyctenular conjunctivitis, scleritis, episcleritis, or keratoconjunctivitis.[210] Such manifestations may well represent hypersensitivity reactions and may occur in the presence of erythema nodosum.[210] Immunocompromised persons with disseminated disease may present with conjunctivitis and preauricular adenopathy. Granulomas of the eyelid may occur in disseminated disease.[210] Intraocular involvement during progressive systemic coccidioidomycosis may include iridocyclitis, iris nodule formation, choroiditis, chorioretinitis, and endophthalmitis (Figs. 129-37 and 129-38).[210] Involvement is often granulomatous.[211] Choroidal involvement may present as whitish yellow, slightly raised nodular lesions (see Fig. 129-38). Such involvement of deeper ocular structures may rarely occur in the absence of apparent systemic coccidioidomycosis.[210,211] Involvement of the central nervous system can result in papilledema and

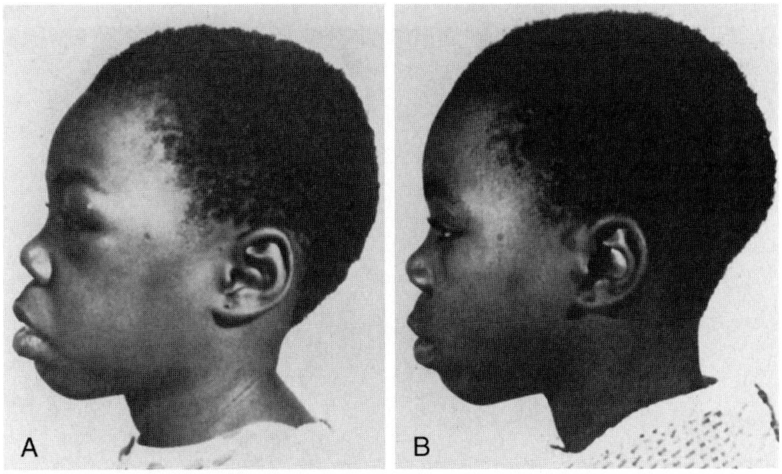

FIGURE 129-36 Left orbital extension of *Histoplasma capsulatum* var. *duboisii* from facial and orbital bones. *A,* Pretreatment, showing periorbital swelling. *B,* Six months after surgery and amphotericin B treatment. (From Olurin O, Adetokunbo O, Lucas MD, et al: Orbital histoplasmosis due to *Histoplasma duboisii*. Am J Ophthalmol 68:15, 1969.)

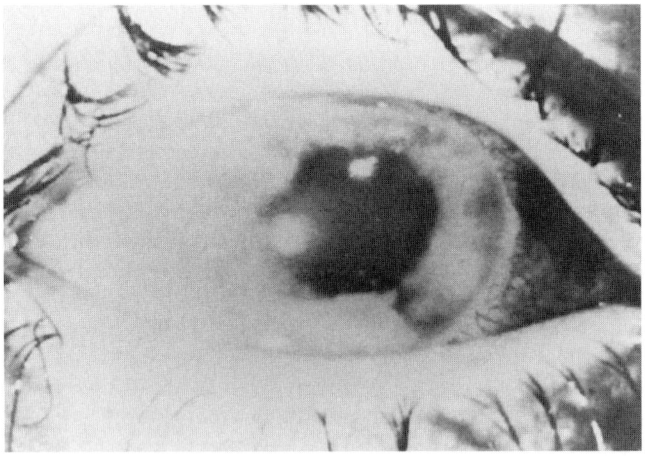

FIGURE 129-37 Iris nodules due to *Coccidiodes immitis*. (From Rodenbiker HT, Gansley JP: Ocular coccidioidomycosis. Surv Ophthalmol 24:275, 1980.)

cranial nerve dysfunction.[210] Involvement of the optic nerve may also result in optic atrophy.[210] Choroidal coccidioidomycosis does not appear to be associated with the development of choroidal neovascularization.[210]

Diagnosis is usually confirmed through clinical recognition with histologic examination and culture of tissue specimens, or both.[211] Skin tests and serologic assays are also available. Ocular involvement usually occurs in disseminated disease, and therapy is usually systemically administered. Intraocular involvement should be treated with systemic antifungal agents, usually amphotericin B.[211] After control of the acute infection, systemic fluconazole or itraconazole may be employed. Surgical intervention may be required. Chronic suppressive therapy may be required in immunocompromised persons, such as those with AIDS.

Blastomycosis

Blastomycosis is caused by *Blastomyces dermatitidis* (see Chapter 80). Ocular involvement during blastomycosis is rare. Most often, involvement of the eye by *B. dermatitidi* manifests as a blastomycotic skin lesion involving the eyelid. The sclera, conjunctiva, and cornea may be involved. Scarring can lead to ectropion. Hematogenous dissemination may result in direct ocular deposition of organisms, usually in the choroid. Choroidal granulomas may present as small subretinal masses or as diffuse granulomatous lesions with vitritis. Iritis, iris nodules, choroiditis, endophthalmitis, or panophthalmitis may occur.[212] Orbital involvement has been reported. Ocular involvement usually occurs in patients with disseminated blastomycosis, although rare persons may present with apparently isolated ocular involvement. The incidence of the disease does not appear to be increased among immunocompromised persons with AIDS. Diagnosis is confirmed by histologic examination or culture of tissue samples, often of skin lesions.[212] Due to the systemic nature of the infection, ocular blastomycosis should normally be treated with systemic antifungal agents, usually amphotericin B. Once control of the acute infection is achieved, systemic itraconazole or fluconazole may be employed.

Paracoccidioidomycosis (South American Blastomycosis)

Paracoccidioidomycosis, also known as South American blastomycosis, is caused by *Paracoccidioides brasiliensis* (see Chapter 81). Ocular involvement by *P. brasiliensis* usually involves contiguous spread of an ulceronodular skin lesion that rarely involves the eyelid. Parinaud's oculoglandular syndrome has been reported. Disease is often systemic, and choroidal granulomatous lesions have been reported.[213] Chorioretinitis may occur. Involvement of the central nervous system can lead to granulomatous meningoencephalitis or mass lesions, with resultant cranial nerve dysfunction and ocular palsies. The optic nerves and chiasm may also be involved.[213] Diagnosis is usually one of clinical recognition, histologic examination, and culture analysis. Serologic assays are available. The incidence of *P. brasiliensis* infection is apparently not increased in immunocompromised persons, including those with AIDS.

Sporotrichosis

Sporotrichosis is caused by *Sporothrix schenckii* (see Chapter 84). Involvement of the eye usually entails conjunctival, adnexal, or eyelid disease. Orbital infection of deeper ocular structures may occur. Ocular involvement may occur

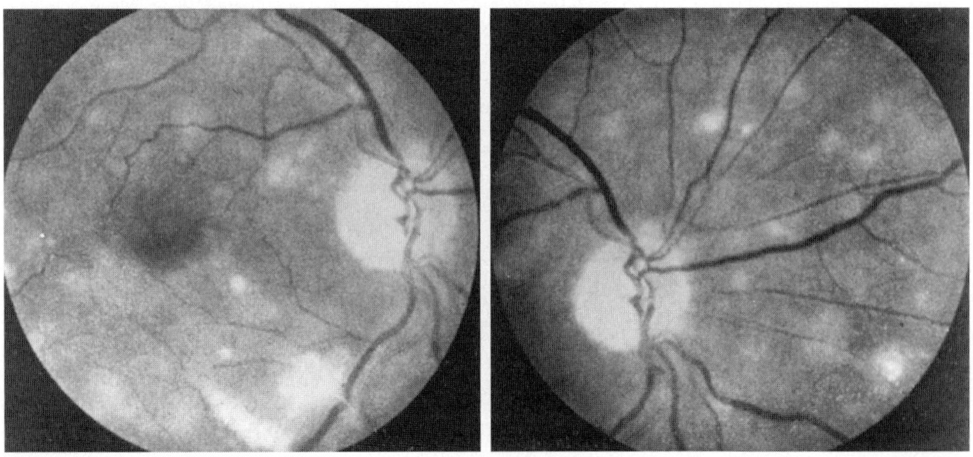

FIGURE 129-38 Ocular choroidal coccidioidomycosis. Fundus photograph of right eye. *Left,* Small, round, perimacular lesions and large diffuse lesion inferotemporal to the optic disk. *Right,* Typical scattered, discrete, round choroidal lesions nasal to the optic disk. (From Rainin EA, Little HL: Ocular coccidioidomycosis: A clinicopathologic case report. Trans Am Acad Ophthalmol Otolaryngol 76:646, 1972.)

with hematogenous dissemination, after trauma (especially that involving vegetable matter/thorns), or after surgical manipulation.[214] Involvement of sinuses and facial bones can lead to contiguous orbital spread. Scleritis, keratoconjunctivitis, corneal perforation, iridocyclitis, iris nodule formation, necrotizing granulomatous chorioretinitis, granulomatous uveitis, optic neuritis, vitritis, endophthalmitis, and panophthalmitis may occur.[214,215] Regional lymphadenopathy may be present. Parinaud's ulceroglandular syndrome may occur. The necrotizing chorioretinitis may mimic that occurring in toxoplasmosis; however, the degree of overlying vitreal inflammation may be less pronounced in sporotrichosis. Hematogenously disseminated sporotrichosis may present with isolated ocular disease. Diagnosis is usually confirmed by microscopic analysis and culture of superficial lesions, intraocular aspirates, or tissue samples. The organism is difficult to grow in culture. Therapy of cutaneous sporotrichosis with external ocular disease may sometimes be treated with systemic itraconazole, potassium iodide, or amphotericin B. Systemic sporotrichosis with deep ocular disease requires intravitreal and systemic amphotericin B.[214] Surgical débridement, enucleation, or both are often required.[214]

Mucormycosis

Rhino-orbital-cerebral mucormycosis is a clinical entity that may be caused by a number of *Mucorales* fungi, including *Mucor* species, *Rhizopus* species, and *Absidia* species, among others. The same organisms can also rarely be a cause of isolated post-traumatic keratitis in immunocompetent persons. Rhino-orbital-cerebral mucormycosis is characterized by necrotizing sinusitis, usually in a person with insulin-depenent diabetes or who is immunocompromised. Ocular involvement results from contiguous spread of the necrotizing and rapidly progressing fungal process. Orbital cellulitis is the most frequent ocular presentation. Chemosis, proptosis, ptosis, ophthalmoplegia, uveitis, optic neuritis, hypoesthesia of the forehead (cranial nerve V_1), central retinal artery inclusion, cavernous sinus thrombosis, and orbital apex syndrome may occur.

Diagnosis is usually one of clinical recognition followed by biopsy of intranasal or orbital tissues. An eschar of the hard pallet may be evident. Intranasal examination usually reveals a black eschar due to necrosis of the mucosa/turbinates. Definitive diagnosis rests on microscopic and cultural analysis of tissue samples or discharge. Treatment is urgent and requires aggressive systemic amphotercin B and surgical intervention.[216] If the eye is involved, exenteration of orbital contents may be required (but may sometimes be avoided).[217] Even in preserved eyes, visual loss is usually pronounced and permanent.

Isolated post-traumatic keratitis due to *Mucorales* species may be treated as mycotic keratitis. Systemic therapy and corneal transplantation may be required.

Entomophthoramycosis

Entomophthoramycosis can be caused by *Conidiobolus* species or *Basidiobolus* species (see Chapter 84). When entomophthoramycosis involves the face, it is characterized by a slowly progressive subacute infiltrative process that usually involves the nose and perinasal sinus areas (Fig. 129-39).[218,219] The infiltrative process can become periocular and can result in inability to open the eyelids. Diagnosis is usually one of clinical recognition and pathologic/culture analysis of subcutaneous tissue samples. Optimal therapy is not known. Oral ketoconazole, amphotericin B, and trimethoprim–sulfamethoxazole may be employed. Surgical resection of infected tissue is often required.

Facial Mycotic Infections and Fungal Sinusitis

Rare reports of infiltrative or ulceronodular fungal facial lesions have also been reported with chromoblastomycosis, mycetoma, and lobomycosis (see Chapters 78, 79, and 84). Facial involvement may result in eyelid, conjunctival, or lacrimal canal involvement. Phaeohyphomycosis (see Chapter 79) has rarely been associated with keratitis, corneal ulceration, and endophthalmitis after trauma or epitheal disruption. Fungal sinusitis may be caused by phaeohyphomycosis and *Aspergillus* species, *Scedosporium* species, *Fusarium* species, and *Penicillium* species. Fungal sinusitis may also occur with mucormycosis, blastomycosis, coccidioidomycosis, histoplasmosis, and paracoccidioidomycosis, among others. Fungal sinusitis may lead to orbital involvement, which can lead to proptosis, diplopia,

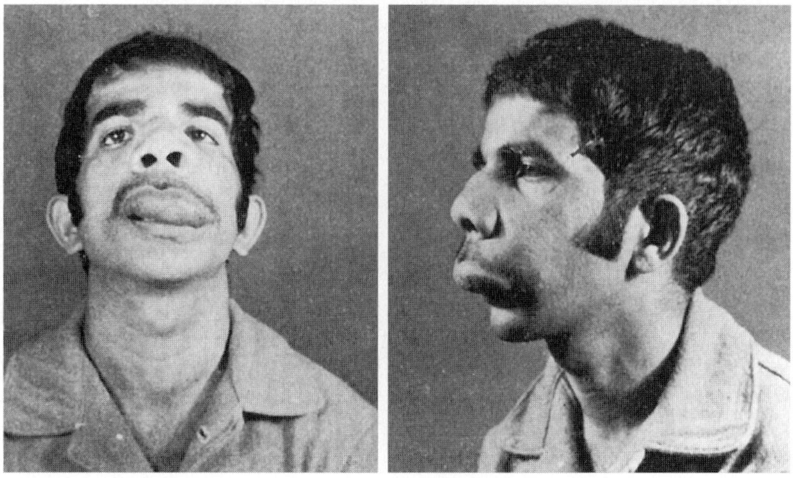

FIGURE 129-39 Facial rhinoentomophthoromycosis. Facial involvement can extend to the periorbital area and lead to inability to open the eyelids. (From Singh D, Kochlar RR, Seth HN: Rhinoentomophthoromycosis. J Laryngol Otolaryngol 90:872, 1976.)

ptosis, epiphora, or an orbital mass. Diagnosis usually rests on culture analysis of tissue samples. Surgical management supplemented by amphotericin B and azole agents such as voriconazole is often required.

Rhinosporidiosis

Rhinosporidiosis, caused by *Rhinosporidium seeberi* (see Chapter 84), is usually associated with a polypoid (often pedunculated) lesion of the nasal mucosa. The conjunctival mucosa may also be affected (Plate 129-6). Conjunctival involvement is usually unilateral. Scleral melting may result. Lacrimal glands may be involved. Keratitis has been reported.[220] Diagnosis is usually based on histologic examination of resected polyps. Treatment has involved surgical excision and basal cauterization. Adjunctive topical or systemic amphotericin B or dapsone has also been employed.[220]

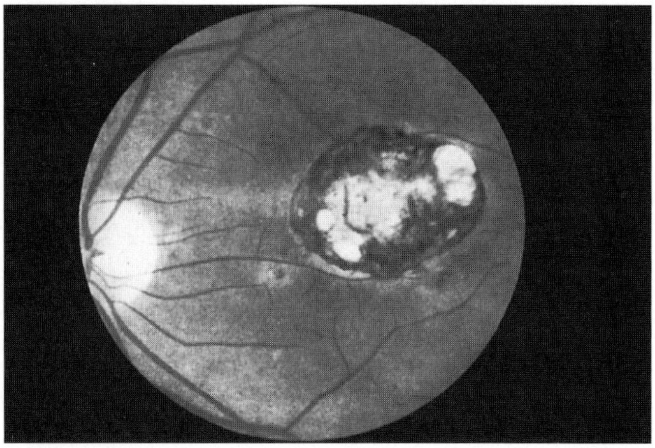

FIGURE 129-41 A lesion of toxoplasmic chorioretinitis showing a cotton-like patch with hemorrhage. (From Kean BH, Sun TS, Ellsworth DM (eds): Color Atlas of Ophthalmic Parasitology. New York, Igaku-Shoin, 1991, p 17.)

PARASITIC INFECTIONS

Microsporidial Infections: Microsporidiosis

Microsporidiosis may be caused by *Encephalitozoon* species, *Enterocytozoon* species, *Nosema* species, *Vittaforma* species, and *Pleistophora* species (see Chapter 96). *Nosema* and *Vittaforma* species can result in stromal keratitis and keratoconjunctivitis after trauma and direct inoculation of organisms in immunocompetent persons.[221] Such involvement usually results in a prominent inflammatory response.[222] Ocular involvement during disseminated microsporidiosis can occur in immunocompromised patients, especially those with AIDS, and is usually due to *Encephalitozoon hellem*.[223,224] Ocular involvement in disseminated microsporidiosis usually presents as a superficial keratitis with fine to coarse epithelial opacities, mild conjunctivitis, or both (Fig. 129-40).[222] Endophthalmitis has been reported.[225] Diagnosis rests on microscopic identification of organisms in corneal/conjunctival scrapings. In disseminated microsporidiosis, the organism may also be present in urine, stool, and nasal mucosal tissue samples. Treatment of ocular microsporidiosis secondary to *E. hellem* in HIV-infected persons has included fumagillin eye drops and systemic albendazole. Ocular involvement by *Vittaforma cornea* and other microsporidia is less responsive to therapy, and surgical intervention/debridement may be required.

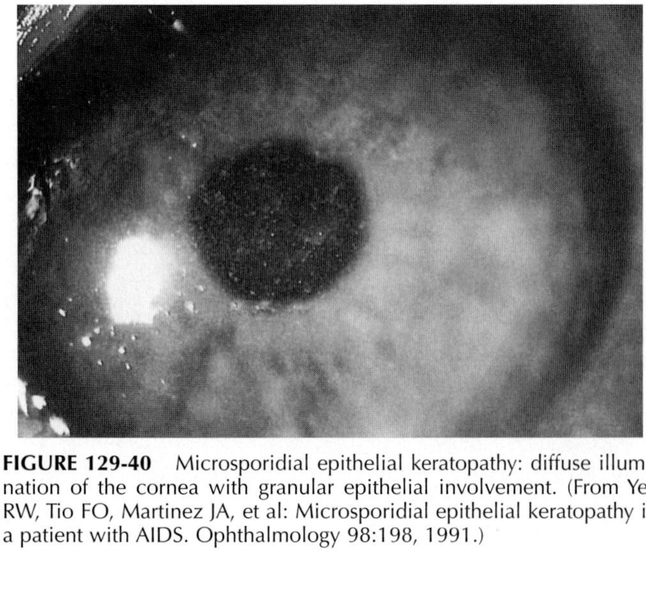

FIGURE 129-40 Microsporidial epithelial keratopathy: diffuse illumination of the cornea with granular epithelial involvement. (From Yee RW, Tio FO, Martinez JA, et al: Microsporidial epithelial keratopathy in a patient with AIDS. Ophthalmology 98:198, 1991.)

Protozoal Infections

Toxoplasmosis

Toxoplasmosis is caused by *Toxoplasma gondii* (see Chapter 97). Ocular toxoplasmosis usually presents as unilateral and painless posterior uveitis with a white-yellow necrotic retinal lesion with uneven pigmentation (Fig. 129-41). Vitreal inflammation may be pronounced in active disease, and retinal tears, hemorrhages, and detachment may occur.[226,227] Satellite lesions may surround a central larger lesion. Vitritis, panuveitis, scleritis, secondary glaucoma, and optic neuritis have been reported.[228] Once the active inflammation subsides, a hypopigmented "punched out" scar with a surrounding area of retinal hyperpigmentation may be present.

Congenital toxoplasmosis is evident in the minority of infected neonates. Ocular involvement in such infections may be bilateral and severe. Chorioretinitis, vitritis, glaucoma, nystagmus, strabismus, ocular muscle palsies, and microphthalmia may occur.[226,229] Infants with congenital toxoplasmosis that is clinically silent at birth often develop clinically evident reactivation chorioretinitis by their second or third decade of life.[230] Reactivation usually occurs along the borders of old lesions or at previously uninvolved sites.

Chorioretinal involvement may be severe, bilateral, and multifocal in immunocompromised persons.[231] In such persons, toxoplasmosis can cause vitritis, uveitis, scleritis, and optic neuritis; involvement of the central nervous system can produce space-occupying lesions that may result in ocular palsies, nystagmus, and visual field defects.

The diagnosis of ocular toxoplasmosis is usually clinical, based on the appearance of the eye. No treatment is required if isolated ocular disease is quiescent and asymptomatic. There is controversy as to whether to treat all immunocompetent persons with isolated active ocular disease if lesions are small and peripherally based because disease activity is self-limited.[230] Anti–*T. gondii* therapy and concomitant steroids, however, have been shown to decrease the size of active lesions and to result in smaller retinal scar formation. Affected immunocompromised patients, patients with centrally located lesions, and patients with large retinal lesions, pronounced vitritis, or both should all receive systemic anti–*T. gondii* therapy.[230] Therapy should be continued beyond the resolution of active disease. Therapy may need to be long-term or lifelong in immunocompromised persons. The use of concomitant systemic steroids in ocular toxoplasmosis is controversial. Immunocompetent persons often have extensive inflammation and may benefit from the anti-inflammatory effects of steroids. Necrosis is predominantly organism-mediated in immunocompromised patients and steroid use does not appear to benefit such persons.

Malaria

Ocular involvement during malaria occurs predominantly during infection with *Plasmodium falciparum* (see Chapter 90). The ability of this parasite to cause erythrocyte sludging, vascular congestion, local cytokine release, and local tissue hypoxemia is thought to account for its ability to affect the eye.[232] Such involvement of retinal vessels can lead to retinal sludging, hemorrhage, edema, and exudates. Involvement may be most prominent in the macular area (Figs. 129-42 and 129-43).[233–237] Involvement of ophthalmic and cerebral vessels can result in intraocular ischemia, infarction, hemorrhages, optic neuritis, papilledema, ocular palsies, and cortical blindness. Papilledema during malaria is associated with a marked increase in mortality.[235] An episode of malaria may be complicated by reactivation of herpes simplex keratitis. Diagnosis usually rests on microscopic identification of the parasite in blood. Treatment is systemic (see Chapter 70). Chronic, inappropriate use of the antimalarial agent cholorquine (which is available "over the counter" in much of the world) can produce a characteristic "bull's-eye" retinal pigmentary maculopathy. Visual acuity is often decreased.[238]

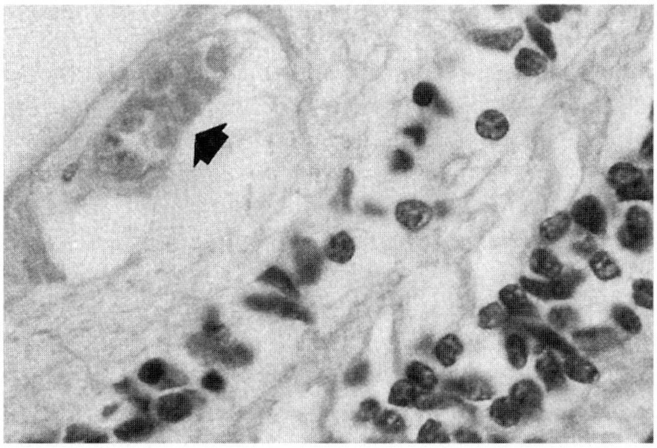

FIGURE 129-42 *Plasmodium falciparum* malarial involvement of a retinal capillary *(arrowhead)*. Note almost complete occlusion of the vessel lumen by parasitized erythrocytes. (H&E stain; original magnification ×750.) (From Hidayat AA, Nalbanian RM, Sammens DW, et al: The diagnostic histopathologic features of ocular malaria. Ophthalmology 100:1184, 1993.)

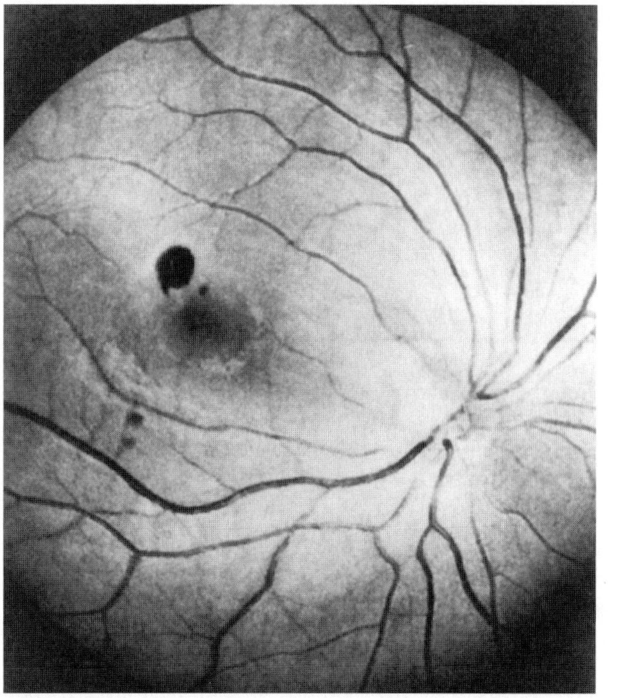

FIGURE 129-43 Four deep retinal hemorrhages (two close to the macula, two below and temporal to the optic disk) in a patient with *Plasmodium falciparum* malaria. (From Davis TME, Supputtamongkol Y, Spencer JL, et al: Measures of capillary permeability in acute falciparum malaria: Relation to severity of infection and treatment. Clin Infect Dis 15:261, 1992.)

African Trypanosomiasis (Sleeping Sickness)

African trypanosomiasis is caused by *Trypanosoma brucei gambiense* and *T. b. rhodesiense* (see Chapter 92). Ocular involvement during African trypanosomiasis is secondary to trypanosomal infiltration of ocular tissues and can result in mild eyelid edema, conjunctival injection, interstitial keratitis, and uveitis.[239] Stromal opacification and deep neovascularization may occur. Papilledema, ptosis, ophthalmoplegia, and optic neuritis may complicate neuroencephalitis. Diagnosis rests on identification of trypanosomes in blood, in tissue sections, in aspirated lymph node fluid, or in cerebrospinal fluid. Serologic evaluation may be of benefit, especially in persons infected with *T. b. gambiense*. Treatment is systemic (see Chapter 92).

American Trypanosomiasis (Chagas' Disease)

The most common and well-recognized ocular feature of American trypanosomiasis, caused by *Trypanosoma cruzi* (see Chapter 93), is Romaña's sign: a painless, unilateral, pronounced periorbital edema and conjunctivitis that persists for days (Fig. 129-44). Romaña's sign results from conjunctival inoculation and penetration of infective trypomastigotes from reduviid bug feces. Lacrimal gland involvement and preauricular and regional lymphadenopathy may occur. Romaña's sign occurs with acute Chagas' disease, and its appearance

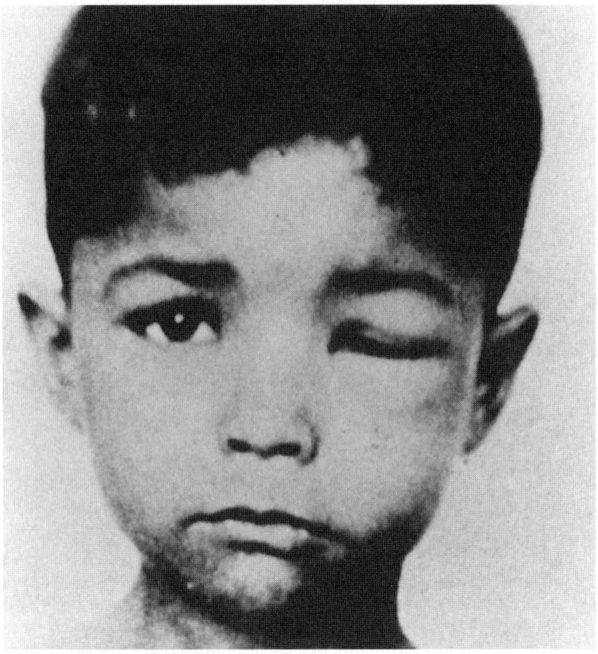

FIGURE 129-44 Romaña's sign (painless, nonpitting periorbital edema) secondary to *Trypanosoma cruzi* in acute Chagas' disease. (Courtesy of Dr. Braulio Luna, Institute de Coração, São Paulo, Brazil.)

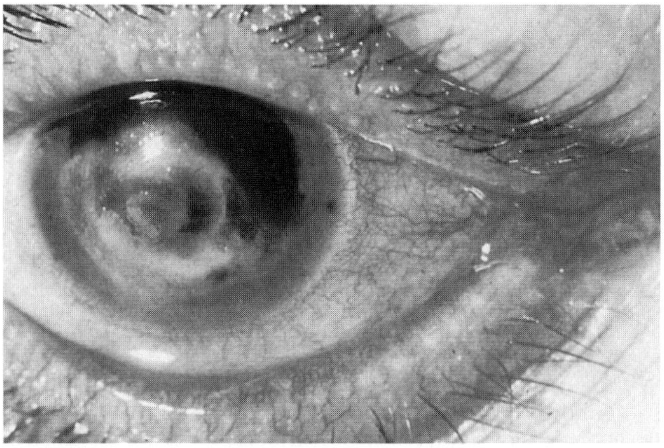

FIGURE 129-45 *Acanthamoeba* keratitis. Note chemosis, double concentric ring of the corneal infiltrate, and a central corneal epithelial defect. (From Hirst LW, Green WR, Merry W, et al: Management of *Acanthamoeba* keratitis. Ophthalmology 91:1106, 1984.)

necessitates the institution of systemic benznidazole or nifurtimox therapy.

Leishmaniasis

Leishmaniasis is caused by a number of *Leishmania* species (see Chapter 94). Ocular involvement can occur during visceral, cutaneous, or mucocutaneous leishmaniasis. Ocular involvement during visceral leishmaniasis is rare. Keratitis, iritis, papillitis, chorioretinitis, and retinal hemorrhages have all been reported during visceral leishmaniasis and have been noted to improve after the initiation of antileishmanial therapy; however, direct leishmanial involvement of ocular tissues has not been documented.[240,241] Bilateral anterior uveitis and secondary glaucoma have rarely been reported after completion of antileishmanial therapy.[240] Ocular involvement during cutaneous and mucocutaneous leishmaniasis usually results from direct extension of a leishmanial lesion and usually involves a nodular or ulcerative lesion of the eyelid that can extend into the lacrimal gland or onto the conjunctiva.[242–244] Dacryocystitis may also occur.[245] Total ocular destruction may complicate severe cases of mucocutaneous leishmaniasis. Diagnosis is usually based on clinical recognition and microscopic identification of organisms in tissue scrapings or samples. Treatment varies, depending on the type, location, and severity of leishmanial involvement and may be systemic or topical (see Chapter 94).

Acanthamoebiasis

Acanthamoebiasis may be caused by a number of *Acanthamoeba* species (see Chapter 95). Ocular involvement is usually one of keratitis that follows trauma or contact lens wear. Acanthamoebic keratitis is characterized by pain out of proportion to eye findings.[246] The keratitis is progressive and is often originally misdiagnosed as being herpetic in origin.[247] The corneal stroma often discloses a ring corneal infiltrate (Fig. 129-45). There may be a sterile inflammatory reaction in the anterior chamber. Diagnosis is made by microscropic analysis and culture of corneal scrapings.[182] Treatment is with topical polyhexamethylene biguanide (Baquacil) or topical propamidine isethionate (Brolene, 0.1%).[247] A dibromopropamide isethionate 0.15% ointment may be applied at night.[182,248] Corneal transplantation is often required, but should be deferred until the keratitis is inactive.[182,247]

Amebiasis

Documented ocular involvement during amebiasis (see Chapter 86) is rare but usually involves an expansile ulcerative lesion of the face. The most frequent site of ocular involvement is the eyelid, but total ocular destruction can occur. Space-occupying amebic lesions of the central nervous system may result in papilledema, ocular palsies, and visual loss. Invasive amebiasis has been associated with keratitis, small retinal hemorrhages, and pigmentary and cystlike changes in the choroid. Such ocular involvement has been reported to improve after the initiation of specific antiamebic therapy; however, direct involvement of the eye by *E. histolytica* in such cases has not been documented. Diagnosis involves molecular or microscopic identification of organisms in stool, intestinal samples, or aspirates of tissue collections. Treatment is systemic (see Chapter 86). Invasive disease requires metronidazole.

Giardiasis

Direct parasitic involvement of ocular structures during giardiasis (see Chapter 87) has never been documented. Iridocyclitis, choroiditis, retinal and subretinal hemorrhages, and macular changes have been reported in persons with giardiasis and have been noted to improve or resolve after anti–*Giardia lamblia* therapy is initiated, but causality has never been established. Such involvement may represent immunologically mediated reactions or may be secondary to nutritional deficiencies due to *Giardia*-induced malabsorption.

Box 129-9 "Worms" That Involve the Conjunctiva*

Nematodes
Loa loa†
Dirofilaria species†
Thelazaria species†
Ascaris lumbricoides
Mansonella perstans
Dracunculus medinensis
Wuchereria bancrofti/Brugia malayi/Brugia timori

Cestodes
Spirometra species (sparganosis)†
Cysticercus cellulosae (cystic involvement)
Taenia multiceps, T. serialis (coenuriasis; cystic involvement)
Gnathostoma spinigerum

Trematodes
Paragonimus species

Ectoparasites
Myiasis†

*This list includes ectoparasites and nonmicrofilarial helminths.
†Common or classic ocular manifestation of infection.

Box 129-11 "Worms" That Involve the Orbital Space/Cavity*

Nematodes
Angiostrongylus cantonensis†
Gnathostoma spinigerum†
Loa loa
Dirofilaria species
Mansonella perstans

Cestodes
Cysticercus cellulosae (cystic involvement)†
Spirometra species (sparganosis)†
Echinococcus species (cystic involvement)
Taenia multiceps, T. serialis (coenuriasis; cystic involvement)

Trematodes
Paragonimus species†

Ectoparasites/Pentastomids
Lingulata serrata†
Myiasis†

*This list includes ectoparasites and nonmicrofilarial helminths.
†Common or classic ocular manifestation of infection.

Helminthic Infections: Nematodes

See Boxes 129-9 through 129-11.

Onchocerciasis

Ocular involvement is a major clinical manifestation of onchocerciasis (see Chapter 100), which is one of the five leading causes of blindness worldwide. Microfilariae can migrate freely within the cornea, anterior chamber, vitreous, retina, choroid, and optic nerve. Dead or dying microfilariae provoke a prominent inflammatory response either relating to microfilarial antigens themselves or to antigens of the endosymbiont *Wolbachia*. Live microfilariae provoke a limited inflammatory response. Ocular onchocerciasis may be anterior (keratitis and iritis) or posterior (chorioretinitis, papillitis, and optic atrophy). The type of ocular disease may depend in part on parasitic strain and variability. Involvement of the anterior eye can result in punctate keratitis with "fluffy snowflake" corneal opacities that represent local responses to dead or dying microfilariae (Fig. 129-46). Such lesions clear without any residua and occur most commonly in young persons. Punctate keratitis can occur spontaneously or after the initiation of anti-onchocercal therapy. Chronic, recurrent, ongoing inflammation may result in a more serious sclerosing

Box 129-10 "Worms" That Involve Intraocular Structures*

Nematodes
Toxocara species†
Baylisascaris procyonis†
Angiostrongylus cantonensis†
Gnathostoma spinigerum†
Loa loa
Dirofilaria species
Wuchereria bancrofti/Brugia malayi/B. timori

Cestodes
Cysticercus cellulosae (cystic involvement)†
Spirometra species (sparganosis)†
Echinococcus species (cystic involvement)
Taenia multiceps, T. serialis (coenuriasis; cystic involvement)

Trematodes
Paragonimus species†
Schistosoma species

Ectoparasites/Pentastomids
Lingulata serrata†
Myiasis†

*This list includes ectoparasites and nonmicrofilarial helminths.
†Common or classic ocular manifestation of infection.

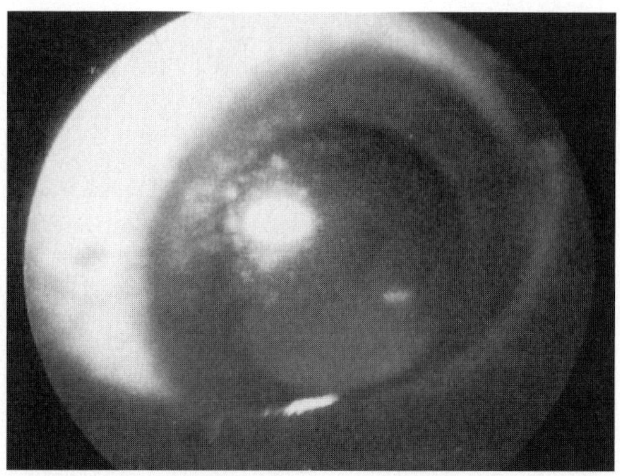

FIGURE 129-46 Punctate keratitis secondary to onchocerciasis. (Courtesy of Armed Forces Institute of Pathology, Washington, DC, negative No. 75–1622.)

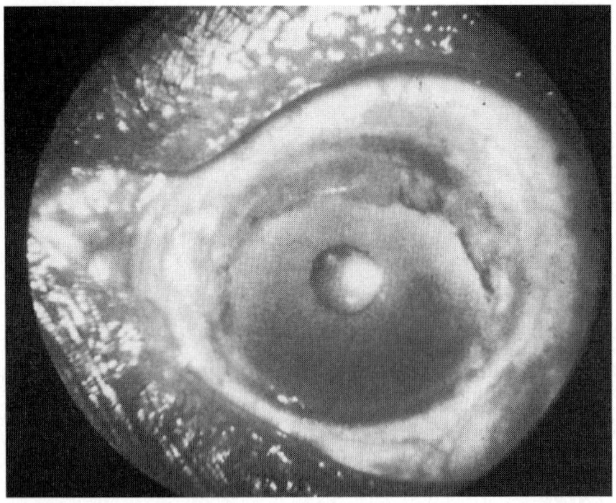

FIGURE 129-47 Moderately advanced sclerosing keratitis secondary to onchocerciasis. (Courtesy of Armed Forces Institute of Pathology, Washington, DC, negative No. 75–1624.)

keratitis, which usually affects older persons and can result in total loss of vision. Sclerosing keratitis is characterized by a pannus of inflammatory cells and neovascularization that encroaches from the lower, medial, and temporal borders of the cornea (Figs. 129-47 and 129-48). Residents of the hyperendemic Sudano-Guinean savannah are particularly susceptible to this process. Fifty percent of populations who have sustained heavy onchocercal infections for decades may be rendered blind before death.[249] Anterior inflammation may also include iritis. Secondary glaucoma, cataracts, and synechiae may result. The risk of sclerosis, keratitis, or iritis has been associated with the presence and load of microfilariae in the anterior chamber, cornea, and outer canthus of the eyelid.

The pathophysiology of posterior ocular involvement is less well understood. Chorioretinitis and atrophic changes may occur. Atrophic changes have been associated with filarial load and may be the result of low-level, ongoing host-parasite interactions. Chorioretinitis may be severe, may be unilateral, and may often involve the temporal retina and spare the macula in early disease. Pigmentary hyperplasia and

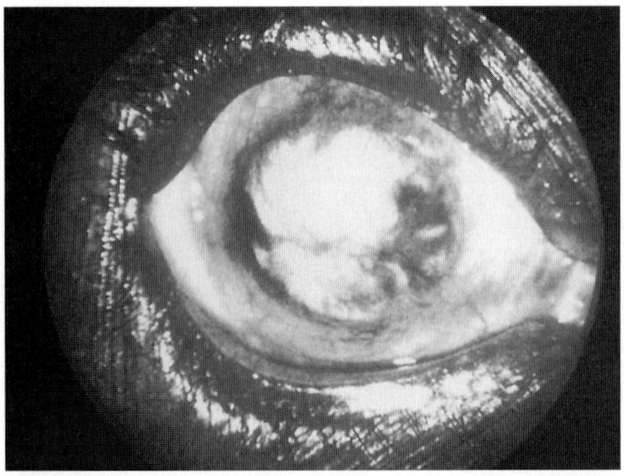

FIGURE 129-48 Advanced sclerosing keratitis secondary to onchocerciasis. (Courtesy of Armed Forces Institute of Pathology, Washington, DC, negative No. 75–1626.)

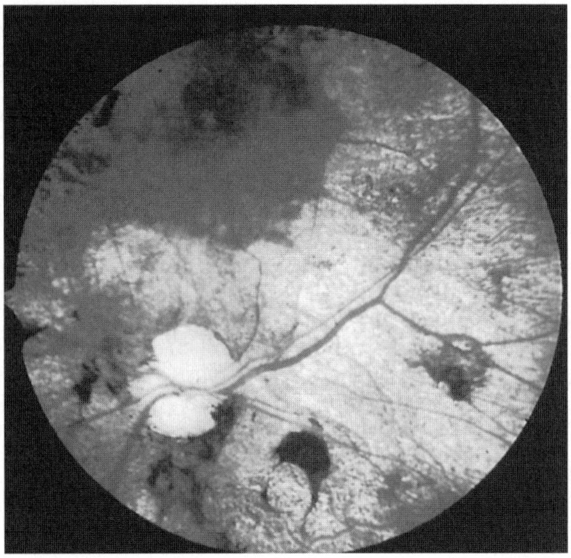

FIGURE 129-49 Extensive chorioretinal degeneration secondary to onchocerciasis with sparing of the macula and optic atrophy. (Courtesy of Armed Forces Institute of Pathology, Washington, DC, negative No. 75–1632.)

atrophy, fibrosis, and neovascularization may be present (Fig. 129-49). Chorioretinitis has not been associated with filarial load. Optic atrophy may be the result of optic neuritis or secondary glaucoma from iridocyclitis.

Diagnosis often involves clinical recognition, skin snip analysis, or serological assays[250] (see Chapter 100). Surgical nodulectomy and identification of the adult worm may also be employed. Ophthalmic diagnosis rests on slit-lamp and funduscopic examination. Visualized living microfilariae are curved, motile, and transparent and are visible in the anterior chamber and cornea. Dead microfilariae are straight and opacified. Optimal treatment for onchocerciasis involves ivermectin (see Chapter 100).

Loiasis

Ocular manifestations of loiasis, caused by *Loa loa* (see Chapter 99), relate to migration of adult worms into and around the eyes. Subconjunctival migration is most common (Fig. 129-50). Conjunctival migration results in a foreign-body sensation and conjunctival injection. The worm moves approximately 1 cm/minute. Periorbital swelling and pruritus may occur. Migration of the worm can result in Calabar swelling of the eyelid (Fig. 129-51). Adult worms may rarely migrate across or through the anterior chamber, vitreous, or retina.

Diagnosis rests on visualization of subconjunctival worms, a history of Calabar swellings, or demonstration of microfilariae in blood (see Chapter 99). Eosinophilia may be striking, especially in persons nonendemic to the area of infection. Surgical removal of the adult worm is not necessary, but if performed, may involve the application of a topical conjunctival anesthetic, such as lidocaine to numb the conjunctiva and slow or halt the movement of the worm. After a single small conjunctival incision is made, the adult worm may then be grasped gently with forceps and a small suture may be

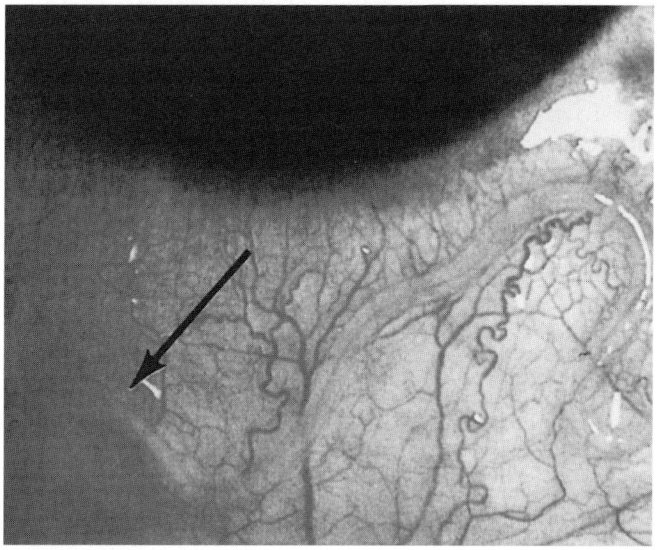

FIGURE 129-50 Adult worm of *Loa loa* visible under the conjunctiva *(arrow)*. (From Kean BH, Sun TS, Ellsworth DM [eds]: Color Atlas of Ophthalmic Parasitology. New York, Igaku-Shoin, p 127. Courtesy of Armed Forces Institute of Pathology, Washington, DC, negative No. 73–6654.)

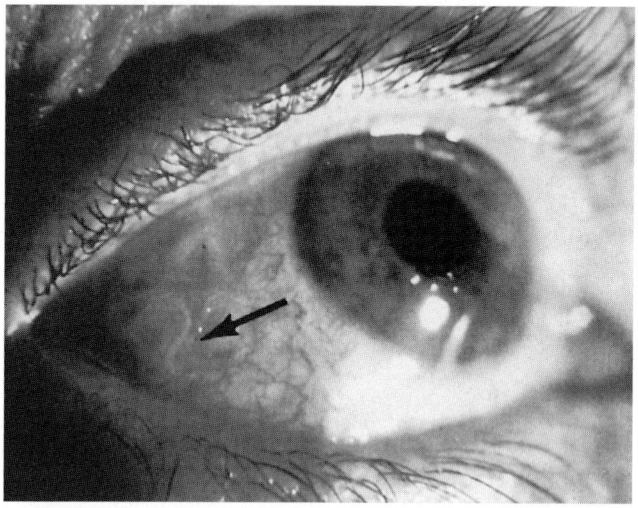

FIGURE 129-52 A subconjunctival female worm of *Dirofilaria tenuis (arrow)*. (From Kean BH, Sun TS, Ellsworth DM (eds): Color Atlas of Ophthalmic Parasitology. New York, Igaku-Shoin, 1991, p 133. Courtesy of Armed Forces Institute of Pathology, Washington, DC, negative No. 74–6351–2.)

passed beneath the worm and carefully tied. The worm may then be removed by dissection. Systemic therapy usually involves diethylcarbamazine (see Chapter 99). It should be recalled that areas endemic for *L. loa* and *O. volvulus* overlap. The possibility of coinfection should be considered.

Dirofilariasis

Dirofilariasis may be caused by a number of *Dirofilariae* species (see Chapter 101). Ocular involvement is most frequently associated with dirofilarial species associated with subcutaneous migration and nodule formation: *Dirofilaria repens, D. ursi*, and *D. tenuis* (previously, *D. conjunctiva*).[251] Ocular dirofilariasis usually involves a migrating worm that most frequently invades the eyelid or subconjunctiva or, more rarely, intraocular structures (Fig. 129-52). Inflammatory reactions and nodule formation, foreign-body sensation, eyelid swelling, ptosis and pruritus, uveitis, and glaucoma have all been reported. Diagnosis is usually based on pathologic examination of a cystlike or inflammatory ocular lesion. Treatment involves surgical removal of the worm.

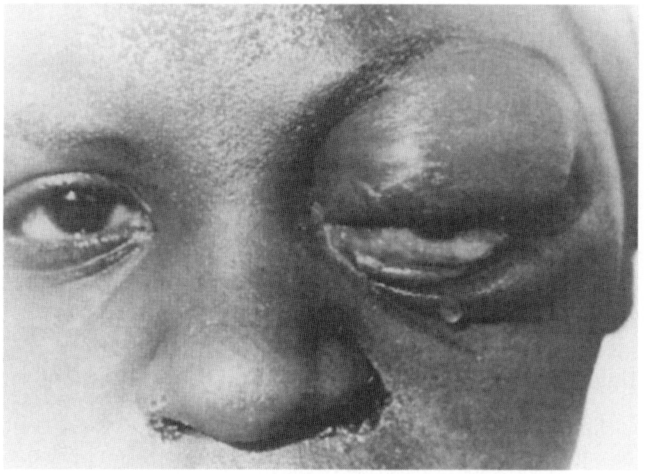

FIGURE 129-51 *Loa loa*–associated Calabar swelling of periocular structures. (From Sandford-Smith J: Eye Diseases in Hot Climates, 2nd ed. Oxford, Wright Publishers, Butterworth Heinemann, 1990, p 185.)

Mansonellaiasis

Migrating adult *M. perstans* organisms have been found in subcutaneous tissues and can present with *L. loa*–like Calabar swellings (see Chapter 98). Involvement of ocular structures by immature adult *M. perstans* worms can result in conjunctival nodule formation, eyelid swelling, and proptosis.[252] Retinal masses have been reported.[253] Diagnosis involves pathologic identification of adult or immature worms after surgical resection or morphologic identification of microfilariae in blood. Ocular disease has been surgically treated.[252] *Mansonella ozzardi* infections have been associated with keratitis presumably, from migratory microfilariae.[254]

Bancroftian and Brugian Filariasis (Lymphatic Filariasis)

Lymphatic filariasis may be caused by *Wuchereria bancrofti, Brugia malayi*, or *Brugia timori* (see Chapter 98). Ocular involvement during lymphatic filariasis usually results from aberrant adult worm migration to the conjunctiva, resulting in chemosis, pain, and foreign-body sensation. Adult and maturing worms have also been reported in the lacrimal gland, eyelid, anterior chamber, iris, and subretina. Blocked lymphatic drainage may result in chronic elephantiasis of the eyelids. Microfilariae, although usually confined to blood, have also been isolated from the lacrimal gland, anterior chamber, iris, lens, choroid, and retina. Diagnosis involves identification of microfilariae in blood.

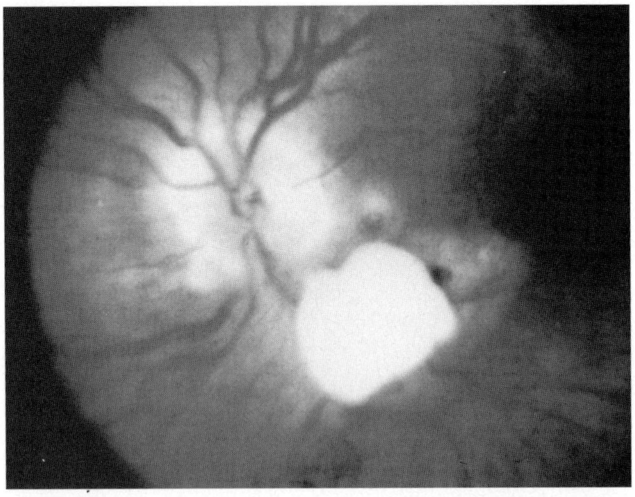

FIGURE 129-53 A toxocaral granuloma *(center)* visible on the eye ground. (From Kean BH, Sun TS, Ellsworth DM [eds]: Color Atlas of Ophthalmic Parasitology. New York, Igaku-Shoin, 1991, p 112.)

Toxocariasis

Toxocariasis is usually caused by the canine ascarid *Toxocara canis* but may also be caused by the feline ascarid *T. cati* (see Chapter 103). Toxocariasis may present as visceral larva migrans or as ocular larva migrans, perhaps depending on the load of infecting organisms. Ocular larva migrans results from infection with only one or a few larvae. It is most common in older children and, more rarely, in adults. Ocular involvement relates to the migration of a wandering larva and the granulomatous-inflammatory host response that it provokes (Figs. 129-53 and 129-54).[255] Peripherally based ocular inflammatory masses may result in visual field defects. Centrally located ocular inflammatory masses can lead to a marked decrease in visual acuity. Retinal inflammation and edema may be severe. Migrating larvae can produce retinal scarring and retinal "track" formation. Retinal traction, retinal hemorrhages, and retinal detachment may occur. Rupture of retinally based inflammatory masses or active migration of larva out of the retina and into the vitreous may result in severe, painless endophthalmitis. Migratory larvae can also result in granulomatous uveitis and secondary glaucoma, keratitis, and optic neuritis. Ocular larva migrans due to toxocariasis often presents as a unilateral, painless, white, retinally based mass in a child and thus must be distinguished from retinoblastoma. The manifestations and approaches to the diagnosis and treatment of ocular larva migrans are more fully considered in Chapter 103.

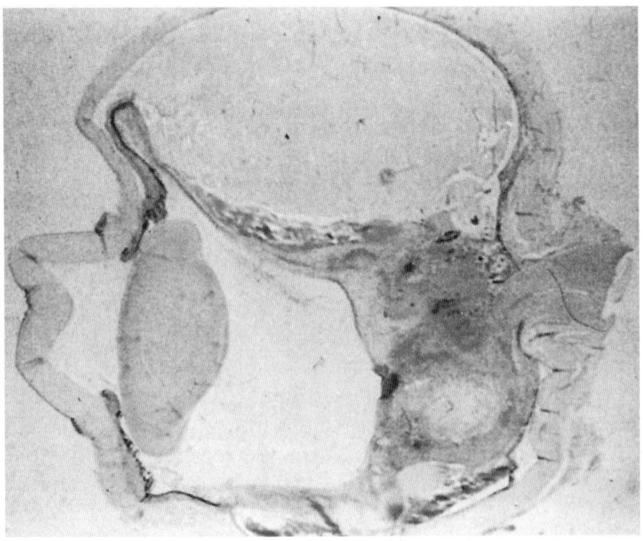

FIGURE 129-54 A sagittal section of an eye showing a large toxocaral granuloma. (H&E stain; original magnification ×25.) (From Kean BH, Sun TS, Ellsworth DM [eds]: Color Atlas of Ophthalmic Parasitology. New York, Igaku-Shoin, 1991, p 112.)

Baylisascariasis

Baylisascariasis is caused by the racoon ascarid *Baylisascaris procyonis* (see Chapter 106). Baylisascariasis may present with involvement of the central nervous system with severe neurological sequelae. Isolated ocular involvement may also occur and is one of ocular larval migrans.[256] Larval migration in the eye can cause diffuse unilateral neuroretinitis and multiple choroidal infiltrates, a granulomatous retinal mass, retinal and subretinal track formation, retinal scars, retinal hemorrhages, chorioretinitis, vitritis, and uveitis.[257–259] Diagnosis of ocular disease is one of clinical recognition upon viewing the moving larva. Neurological involvement usually involves serologic evaluation employing *Baylisascaris*-specific antigens.[260] Optimal therapy for *Baylisascaris*-associated ocular larval migrans is not known.[260] Photocoagulation and surgical extraction have been successfully employed.[257]

Ascariasis

Ascariasis is caused by *Ascaris lumbricoides* (see Chapter 109). Ocular involvement by *A. lumbricoides* is extremely rare, but young adult *A. lumbricoides* worms have been recovered from the nasolacrimal duct, presumably after migration up the esophagus into the nasopharynx.[261,262] Treatment of facial/ocular ascariasis involves mechanical removal of the worm; however, systemic therapy should be employed to treat concomitant intestinal involvement.

Hookworm

Humans may act as a definite host in hookworm infection caused by *Necator americanum* or *Ancylostoma duodenale* or as a dead-end host for canine hookworms such as *A. braziliense* or *A. caninum* (see Chapter 110). Infectious filariform larvae of the latter species can migrate throughout the host and can result in a syndrome of cutaneous larva migrans (see Chapter 103). Migratory hookworm larvae have been reported to involve ocular structures, including the cornea.[263,264]

Thelaziasis

Thelaziasis is caused by *Thelazia callipaeda* (the oriental eyeworm) or *T. californiensis* (see Chapter 106). The worms inhabit the conjunctival sac and lacrimal system of various mammals.[265] Humans occasionally become infected.[266,267] Adult worms residing in the conjunctival sac of mammalian hosts release eggs that are ingested by flies. After maturing in the insect vector, worms are regurgitated during a subsequent ocular secretion meal. Adult worms are approximately 2 cm in length. Ocular involvement in humans results in excessive lacrimation, foreign-body sensation, and local discomfort.[268] Corneal and conjunctival scarification can result.[266] Diagnosis rests on identification of recovered worms. Treatment of the disease in humans involves mechanical removal of the worms.[266]

Dracunculiasis

Dracunculiasis is caused by *Dracunculis medinensis*, the Guinea worm (see Chapter 102). The older literature reported orbital involvement during dracunculiasis; however, the only confirmed case of *D. medinensis* involving ocular structures entailed the isolation of an adult female worm from the conjunctiva of a patient with extensive lacrimation and conjunctival irritation.[269] Therapy of ocular disease involves mechanical removal of the worm.[269]

Angiostrongyliasis

Angiostrongyliasis is caused by *Angiostrongylus cantonensis (Parastrongylus cantonensis)*, the rat lungworm (see Chapter 105). Ocular angiostrongyliasis results from ocular migration of worms in various stages of development.[270] Worms can migrate through the anterior chamber and the vitreous and subretinal space, and then can cause eyelid edema, blepharospasm, inflammation of the anterior chamber, iridocyclitis, retinal detachment, and vitritis (Fig. 129-55). Vitreal migration can lead to vitreal fibrosis and resultant retinal distortion and detachment (Fig. 129-56).[271] Angiostrongyliasis-associated eosinophilic meningoencephalitis may be associated with papilledema (often unilateral) and optic neuritis. Cranial nerve dysfunction can result in ocular palsies and ptosis.[272–274] Orbital involvement may result in extraocular palsies and exophthalmos.[272] Intraocular angiostrongyliasis may occur without associated meningitis.[271,275,276] Diagnosis is usually based on the diagnosis of eosinophilic meningoencephalitis or pathologic examination of migratory worms. Cerebral angiostrongyliasis is usually self-limited. Steroids, analgesics, and repeated removal of cerebral spinal fluid may relieve symptoms. Ocular angiostrongyliasis has been treated with surgical removal of the worm.[272]

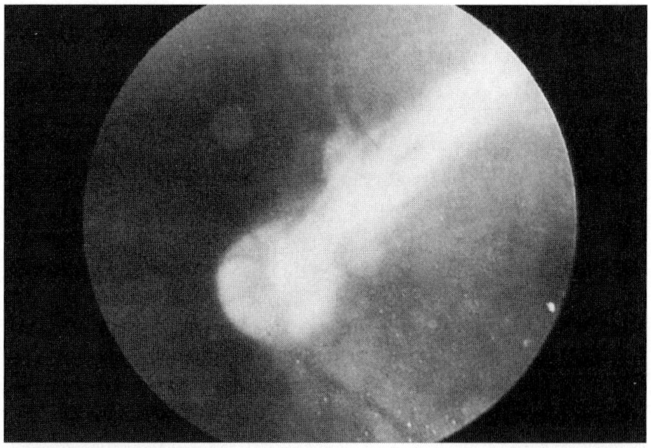

FIGURE 129-56 *Angiostrongylus cantonensis*: fibrous tract formation from the optic head into the vitreous cavity. (From Teekhasaenee C, Ritch R, Kanchanaranya C: Ocular parasitic infection in Thailand. Rev Infect Dis 8:352, 1986.)

Gnathostomiasis

Gnathostomiasis in humans is usually caused by *Gnathostoma spinigerum* (see Chapter 106). Ocular gnathostomiasis usually results from direct invasion of the eye or surrounding tissues by a migratory larva (Fig. 129-57). Direct invasion of ocular tissue may result in corneal ulceration, iris perforation, subretinal hole formation, optic neuritis, and retinal artery occlusion. The inflammatory response may be pronounced, and uveitis, vitreal hemorrhage, vitritis, and secondary glaucoma can occur.[277,278] Edema and hemorrhage of the eyelid and orbital inflammation may also be prominent (Fig. 129-58). Fibrous reactions and scarring along worm

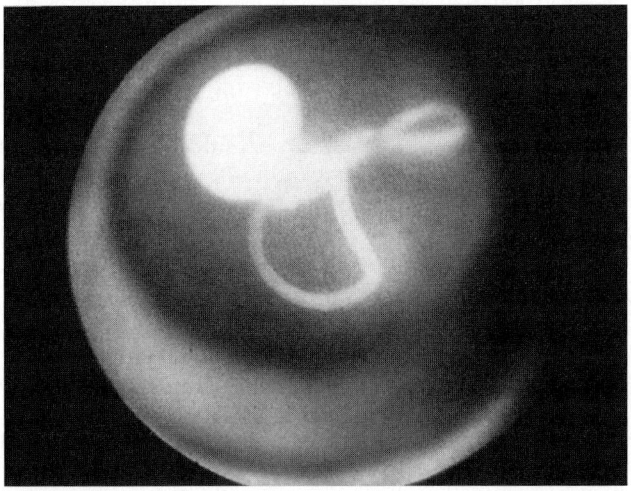

FIGURE 129-55 *Angiostrongylus cantonensis* in the vitreous cavity. (From Teekhasaenee C, Ritch R, Kanchanaranya C: Ocular parasitic infection in Thailand. Rev Infect Dis 8:352, 1986.)

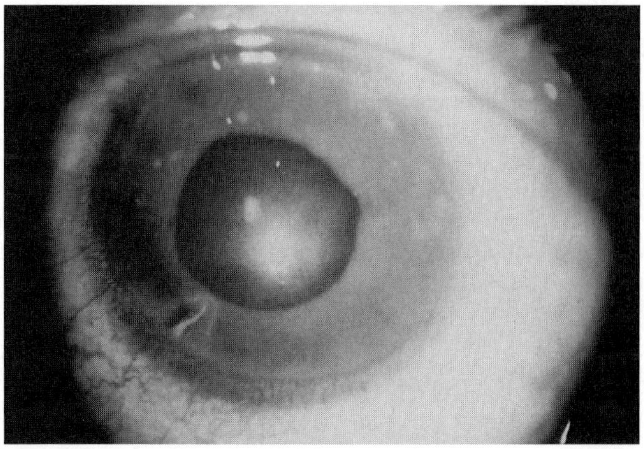

FIGURE 129-57 Intraocular gnathostomiasis. *Gnathostoma spinigerum* worm in the anterior chamber with the head end attached to the cornea. (From Biswas J, Gopal L, Sharma T, et al: Intraocular *Gnathostoma spinigerum*. Clinicopathologic study of two cases with review of literature. Retina 14:440, 1954.)

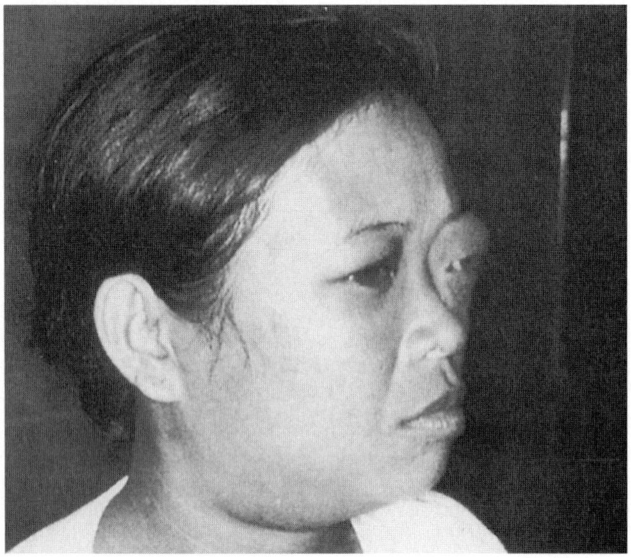

FIGURE 129-58 Ocular gnathostomiasis in a patient with marked periorbital edema. (From Kean BH, Sun TS, Ellsworth DM [eds]: Color Atlas of Ophthalmic Parasitology. New York, Igaku-Shoin, 1991, p 155.)

tracks can result in vitreal fibrosis. Retinal distortion and detachment may result.[272,279] Worms may invade the central nervous system and may provoke eosinophilic meningoencephalitis. Papilledema and cranial nerve palsies may result.[280] Specific diagnosis may be difficult. Inflammation is usually severe. Serologic assays may cross-react with tests for other helminths.[279] Although optimal therapy is not known, systemic disease has been treated with albendazole, mebendazole, and ivermectin. Ocular disease is usually treated with mechanical removal of the worm. Such a procedure not only treats the ophthalmic disease itself but also prevents subsequent penetration of the worm into brain parenchyma.[272,279] In an attempt to decrease inflammation, corticosteroids may be of benefit when used concurrently with surgical intervention.[279]

Trichinellosis

Trichinellosis is caused by *Trichinella spiralis* and related species (see Chapter 104). Ocular involvement in trichinellosis usually occurs during the invasive larval stage and usually manifests as bilateral palpebral edema. Invasion of ocular musculature and structures by larvae may result in conjunctival chemosis and hemorrhage, photophobia, retinal hemorrhages, optic neuritis, and optic edema. Pain on eye movement may be prominent. Trichinellosis should be considered in any person presenting with bilateral palpebral edema, myalgias, and eosinophilia. Diagnosis is usually one of clinical recognition, serologic assay, or muscle biopsy.

Helminthic Infections: Cestodes

Cysticercosis

Cysticercosis is a disseminated infection caused by the larval stage (metacestode: *Cysticercus cellulosae*) of the pork tapeworm, *Taenia solium* (see Chapter 113). Ocular involvement in cysticercosis relates to the intraocular or periocular presence of cysticerci (Fig. 129-59).[281,282] The posterior segment of the eye is most frequently involved symptomatically in ocular cysticercosis. Subretinal cysticerci may be quiescent or may provoke prominent inflammatory responses.[272] Retinal edema, hemorrhage, and detachments may occur. Rupture into the vitreal cavity can occur, as can chorioretinitis, vitritis, and vasculitis. Freely floating cysticerci have been noted in the anterior and posterior chambers, and cysticerci may embed on the ciliary body, iris, or optic nerve. Cysticerci may also develop in the conjunctiva, lacrimal glands, and periorbital musculature. Cysticerci within the central nervous system may result in papilledema, cranial nerve dysfunction, and ocular palsies. Diagnosis and treatment of ocular cysticercosis and neurocysticercosis are considered in Chapter 113.

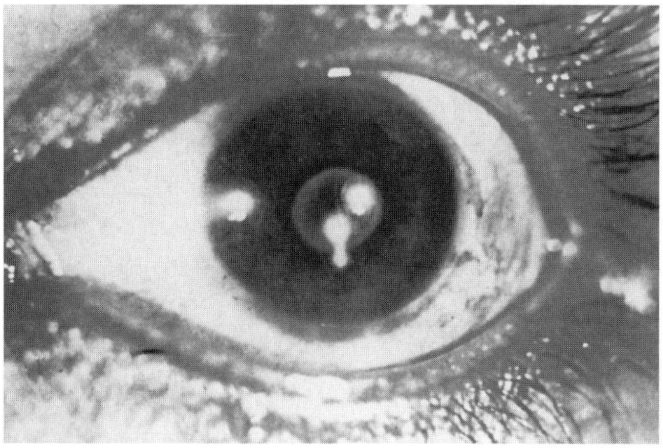

FIGURE 129-59 Ocular cysticercosis. Three cysticerci, one of them evaginated, are visible in the eye. (From Kean BH, Sun TS, Ellsworth DM [eds]: Color Atlas of Ophthalmic Parasitology. New York, Igaku-Shoin, 1991, p 180.)

Sparganosis

Sparganosis is caused by migratory plerocercoid larvae of *Spirometra* species (see Chapter 115). Migratory worms can involve ocular structures. The application of fresh flesh (usually frog or snake flesh) as traditional eye poultices can lead to direct ocular deposition of larvae. Invasion of periocular structures in the anterior chamber may occur; however, ocular worms are usually found in the subconjunctiva. Inflammation may be pronounced and proptosis, lacrimation, periocular edema, pain, and pruritus may be intense (Fig. 129-60). Diagnosis involves pathologic identification of removed worms. Ocular therapy involves surgical removal of the worm. No systemic antiparasitic agent has been shown to be of benefit.

Echinococcosis

Echinococcosis may be caused by *Echinococcus granulosus* (cystic hydatid disease), *E. multilocularis* (alveolar hydatid disease), or related, less common, species (see Chapter 114). Ocular involvement in cystic hydatid disease usually relates to enlargement of a hydatid cyst in the orbital cavity, usually arising from bony structures (Fig. 129-61). Proptosis, exposure keratitis, corneal ulcerations, extensive lacrimation, conjunctival chemosis and injection, impairment of extraocular mobility,

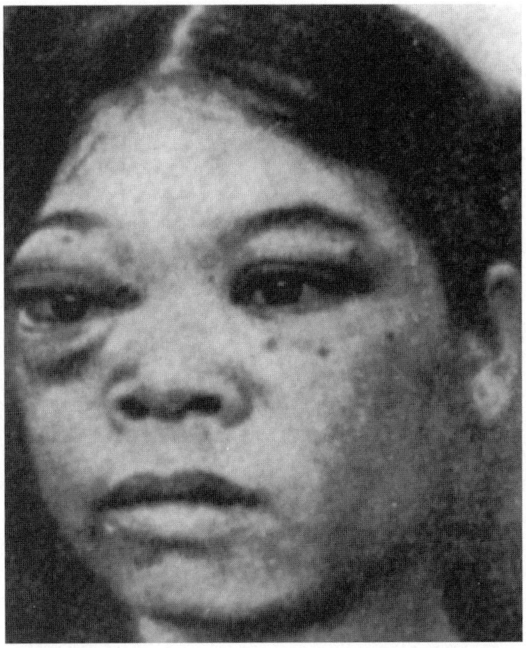

FIGURE 129-60 Ocular sparganosis with unilateral periorbital edema and chemosis. (From Zhong HL, Shao L, Lian DR: Ocular sparganosis-caused blindness. Chin Med J [Engl] 96:74, 1983.)

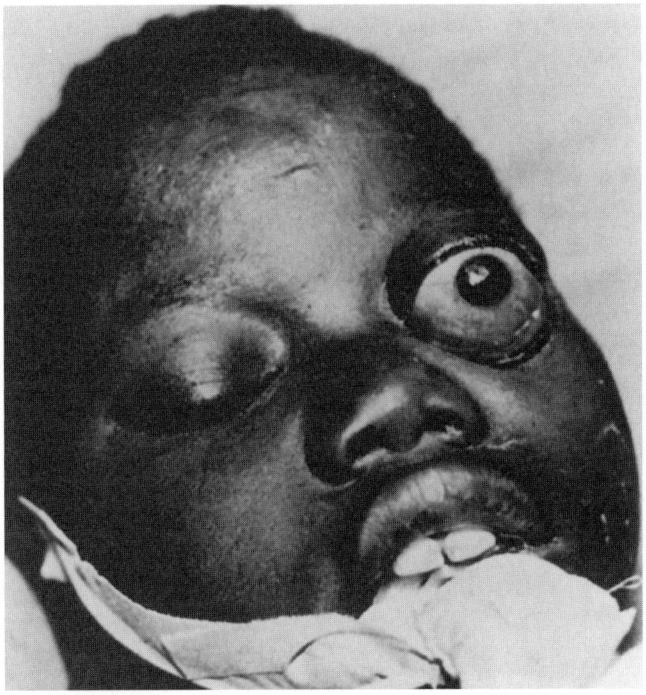

FIGURE 129-61 Orbital hydatid *(Echinococcus granulosus)* disease with proptosis and conjunctival hyperemia. (From Chana HS, Klauss V, Shah A: Orbital hydatid disease in Kenya. Am J Trop Med Hyg 35:992, 1986.)

optic atrophy, and orbital bone erosion may result.[283] Replacement of the vitreous by intraocular cysts has also been reported. Hydatid disease of the central nervous system can result in papilledema.[283] Intraocular disease due to invasive alveolar hydatid disease has also been reported. Diagnosis involves clinical recognition, imaging studies, and serologic assays.[284] Systemic therapy is considered in Chapter 114. Ocular cystic and alveolar hydatid disease should be treated surgically.

Coenuriasis

Coenuriasis is caused by the cystic larval stage of dog *Taenia* species tapeworms (see Chapter 115). *Taenia multiceps* and *T. serialis* appear to have a tropism for ocular structures and for the central nervous system. Ocular involvement is usually one of a space-occupying cystic lesion. Ocular cysts may occur in the eyelids, conjunctiva, and extraocular muscles. Intraocular cysts may be located subretinally or intravitreally. Proptosis, exposure keratitis, and corneal ulceration may occur. Older and ruptured cysts can provoke a prominent inflammatory response. Panophthalmitis and blindness may result. Diagnosis involves clinical recognition, imaging studies, and histologic examination. Ocular disease is treated with surgery.[285]

Helminthic Infections: Trematodes

Schistosomiasis

Schistosomiasis is caused by various *Schistosoma* species (see Chapter 116). During acute schistosomiasis (Katayama fever), eyelid edema may be present. Direct ocular involvement in later disease can be due to egg deposition from portosystemic shunting, passive egg transfer via the vesicovertebral-central nervous system venous plexus, or by an aberrantly migrating worm pair. Ocular eggs elicit a granulomatous response that may be pronounced. Most confirmed cases of ocular involvement in schistosomiasis have involved conjunctival or lacrimal gland egg-related granuloma formation.[286,287] Choroidal egg-related granulomatous lesions have been reported, and involvement of the optic nerve can lead to optic atrophy.[288–290] Ocular involvement is most frequently reported with *S. haematobium* infection. Aberrantly migrating worms have been found in the superior ophthalmic vein and in the anterior chamber.[291] Diagnosis and treatment of schistosomiasis are considered in Chapter 116. Ocular involvement should be treated systemically.

Paragonimiasis

Paragonimiasis can be caused by a number of *Paragonimus* species (see Chapter 117). Ocular involvement usually involves aberrantly migrating worms. Mechanical damage can be extensive. Ocular pain due to an actively migrating worm is usually severe and recurrent, but the pain often spontaneously resolves within an hour of onset.[292] Worms can migrate through the eyelid, anterior chamber, and orbit. Retinal hemorrhages and subluxation of the lens can occur. Prominent inflammatory responses can result in hypopyon, uveitis, and secondary glaucoma. Cerebral involvement can result in cranial nerve palsies and papilledema.[293] Diagnosis and treatment is considered in Chapter 117. Ocular disease should be surgically treated.

Ectoparasites

Pentastomiasis

Pentastomal infection in humans ("tongue worm") can be caused by *Lingulata serrata* (see Chapter 118). Ocular involvement in pentastomiasis involves migratory nymphs that have been recovered from the anterior chamber. Iritis and secondary glaucoma have been reported.[294] Diagnosis involves histologic examination of recovered specimens. Therapy for ocular disease involves surgical removal of the pentastomid.

Myiasis

Ocular involvement by the larvae of flies is called ophthalmomyiasis (see Chapter 118). Ocular involvement in humans has been reported with a number of fly species, including *Oestrus ovis* ("sheep bot fly"), *Gasterophilidae* ("horse bot fly" or "horse warble fly"), *Wohlfahrtia magnifica* ("sheep maggot fly"), *Chrysomyia bezziana* ("screw worm fly"), *Cordylobia anthropophaga* ("tumbu fly"), and *Dermatobia hominis*, among others.[295,296] Ocular disease occurs from deposition of eggs by flies or by secondary vectors, such as mosquitoes. Larvae emerge and penetrate the periocular and ocular tissues. Ocular involvement of the orbit, eyelid, or conjunctiva is called "ophthalmomyiasis externa."[297,298] "Ophthalmomyiasis interna" implies that larvae have invaded deep ocular structures (Fig. 129-62). Such involvement may be either anterior or posterior.[299] Larval migration can result in conjunctivitis, keratitis, scleritis, iritis, vitritis, subluxation of the lens, uveitis, and vitreal hemorrhage.[295,300] Subretinal involvement may result in retinal detachment and hemorrhages. Retinal scarring and "track" formation may result. Involvement may be bilateral.

Specific diagnosis is confirmed by pathologic examination of recovered larvae or of subsequently matured flies.

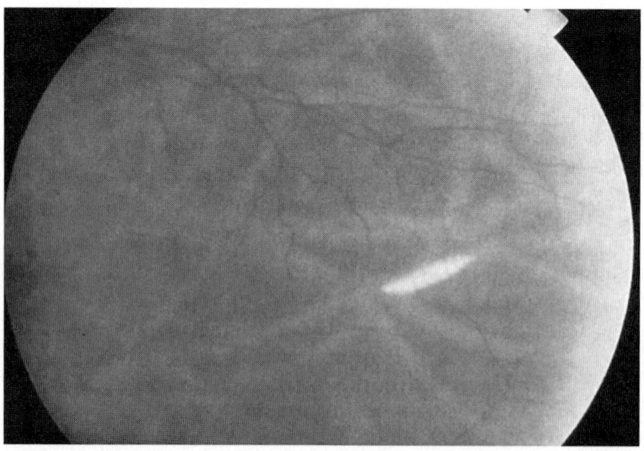

FIGURE 129-62 Internal ophthalmomyiasis. Funduscopic examination showing a segmented fly larva. Note depigmented, subretinal epithelial tracks. (From Currier RW, Johnson WA, Rowley WA, et al: Internal ophthalmomyiasis and treatment by laser photocoagulation: A case report. Am J Trop Med Hyg 52:312, 1995.)

Treatment of ophthalmomyiasis externa involves mechanical removal of the larva(e) with careful searching for the presence of additional intranasal or intraocular larvae. Ophthalmomyiasis interna may be treated with laser photocoagulation or with surgery.[295,301–303] Topical and systemic steroids may be used to minimize local inflammatory reactions.[302,303]

BLINDNESS AND NONINFECTIOUS TROPICAL OCULAR PATHOLOGY

The World Health Organization estimates that approximately 40 million persons are currently blind worldwide and that over 100 million persons have markedly decreased vision and are at substantial risk of becoming blind. Leading causes of blindness worldwide include cataract formation, trachoma, glaucoma, onchocerciasis, xerophthalmia, diabetic retinopathy, and age-related macular degeneration.[180] Trauma is a leading cause of unilateral blindness worldwide. Blindness due to thermal or chemical burns to the eye may be accidental or intentional. The application of traditional eye medicines and poultices in much of the developing world often exacerbates initial ocular pathology. End-stage ocular damage may result in formation of a markedly shrunken, useless eye (phthisis bulbi; Fig. 129-63). End-stage ocular damage may also result in a marked anterior bulging of the cornea due to a severely weakened cornea and sclera (staphyloma; see Fig. 129-17).

Sunlight can cause a number of ophthalmologic conditions. Intensive prolonged ultraviolet exposure may be associated with cortical cataract formation. Exposure to ultraviolet sunlight is linked to the development of climatic droplet keratopathy, a degenerative condition in which corneal opacifications form in the superficial corneal stroma. This condition may also be associated with extensive puffiness of the eyelids. Formation of a pterygium (a "fleshy wing" of conjunctival/subconjunctival tissue that encroaches on the cornea laterally and medially) may be related to ultraviolet irradiation. Intense, acute exposure to ultraviolet light may also lead to corneal/conjunctival epithelium damage that can present as photophobia, lacrimation, and ocular pain. Direct observation of the sun or exposure to excessive reflective glare can also result in macular damage that may be permanent.

A number of other conditions that may occur in the tropics may also result in ocular manifestations. Deficiency of

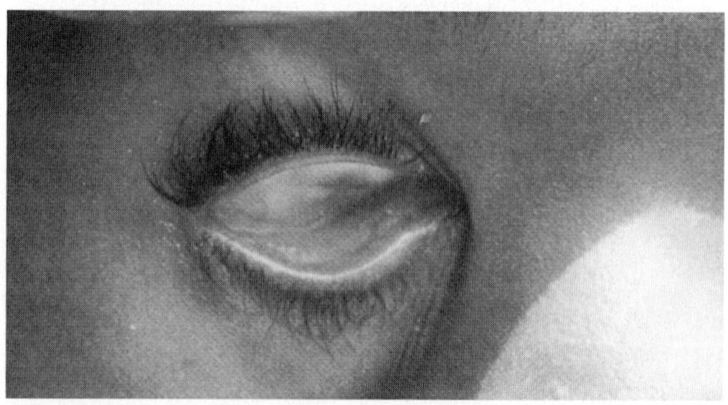

FIGURE 129-63 Phthisis bulbi. Note shrunken, scarred, blind, end-stage eye. Damage is irreversible. (From Sandford-Smith J: Eye Diseases in Hot Climates, 2nd ed. Oxford, Wright Publishers, Butterworth Heinemann, 1990.)

vitamin A may result in xerophthalmia. Deficiency of vitamin B complex may result in optic neuropathy. Snake venom from spitting cobras may result in conjunctivitis, keratitis, or both that may be blinding. Argemone–poppy oil intoxication may result in glaucoma and optic nerve atrophy in India and Bangladesh. Local reactions to secretions of blister beetles, millipedes, and centipedes may result in painful conjunctivitis. Improperly prepared cassava can cause cyanide-related peripheral neuritis and optic neuropathy. The vasculopathy of sickle cell disease may result in ocular vascular changes, hemorrhages, scarring, and neovascularization. Reaction to an unknown allergen may result in vernal keratoconjunctivitis, a disorder that is most common in children and results in papillary conjunctivitis involving the tarsal conjunctiva and limbal region.[304,305]

REFERENCES

1. Muhit M, Gilbert C: A review of the epidemiology and control of childhood blindness. Trop Doct 33:197, 2003.
2. Roodhooft JM: Leading causes of blindness worldwide. Bull Soc Belge Ophtalmol 283:19, 2002.
3. Whitcher JP, Srinivasan M, Upadhyay MP: Corneal blindness: A global perspective. Bull World Health Org 79:214, 2001.
4. Chang CH, Lin KH, Sheu MM, et al: The change of etiological agents and clinical signs of epidemic viral conjunctivitis over an 18-year period in southern Taiwan. Graefes Arch Clin Exp Ophthalmol 241:554, 2003.
5. Altemeier WA III: The importance of adenoviral infections in pediatrics. Pediatr Ann 30:439, 452, 2001.
6. Viswalingam NS: Adenovirus keratoconjunctivitis: An enigma. Eye 7(pt. 3 suppl):5 1993.
7. Chang CH, Sheu MM, Lin KH, et al: Hemorrhagic viral keratoconjunctivitis in Taiwan caused by adenovirus types 19 and 37: Applicability of polymerase chain reaction–restriction fragment length polymorphism in detecting adenovirus genotypes. Cornea 20:295, 2001.
8. Harley D, Harrower B, Lyon M, et al: A primary school outbreak of pharyngoconjunctival fever caused by adenovirus type 3. Commun Dis Intell 25:9, 2001.
9. Chodosh J, Miller D, Stroop WG, et al: Adenovirus epithelial keratitis. Cornea 14:167, 1995.
10. Donahue SP, Khoury JM, Kowalski RP: Common ocular infections: A prescriber's guide. Drugs 52:526, 1996.
11. Haamann P, Kessel L, Larsen M: Monofocal outer retinitis associated with hand, foot, and mouth disease caused by coxsackievirus. Am J Ophthalmol 129:552, 2000.
12. Wolken SH: Acute hemorrhagic conjunctivitis. Surv Ophthalmol 19:71, 1974.
13. Kono R, Miyamura K, Tajiri E, et al: Virological and serological studies of neurological complications of acute hemorrhagic conjunctivitis in Thailand. J Infect Dis 135:706, 1977.
14. Phuapradit P, Roongwithu N, Limsukon P, et al: Radiculomyelitis complicating acute haemorrhagic conjunctivitis. A clinical study. J Neurol Sci 27:117, 1976.
15. Scheifele DW, Duval B, Russell ML, et al: Ocular and respiratory symptoms attributable to inactivated split influenza vaccine: Evidence from a controlled trial involving adults. Clin Infect Dis 36:850, 2003.
16. Deckard PS, Bergstrom TJ: Rubeola keratitis. Ophthalmology 88:810, 1981.
17. Hussey GD, Klein M: A randomized controlled trial of vitamin A in children with severe measles. N Engl J Med 323:160, 1990.
18. Sachs U, Marcus M: Bilateral herpetic keratitis during measles. Am J Ophthalmol 91:796, 1981.
19. Titiyal JS, Pal N, Murthy GV, et al: Causes and temporal trends of blindness and severe visual impairment in children in schools for the blind in North India. Br J Ophthalmol 87:941, 2003.
20. Kello AB, Gilbert C: Causes of severe visual impairment and blindness in children in schools for the blind in Ethiopia. Br J Ophthalmol 87:526, 2003.
21. Yoser SL, Forster DJ, Rao NA: Systemic viral infections and their retinal and choroidal manifestations. Surv Ophthalmol 37:313, 1993.
22. Sommer A: Vitamin A, infectious disease, and childhood mortality: A 2 cent solution? J Infect Dis 167:1003, 1993.
23. Semba RD: Vitamin A, immunity and infection. Clin Infect Dis 19:489, 1994.
24. Hara J, Fujimoto F, Hishibashi T: Ocular manifestations of the 1976 rubella epidemic in Japan. Am J Ophthalmol 57:642, 1979.
25. Riikonen RS: Retinal vasculitis caused by rubella. Neuropediatrics 26:174, 1995.
26. Freij BJ, South MA, Sever JL: Maternal rubella and the congenital rubella syndrome. Clin Perinatol 15:247, 1988.
27. Vijayalakshmi P, Kakkar G, Samprathi A, et al: Ocular manifestations of congenital rubella syndrome in a developing country. Indian J Ophthalmol 50:307, 2002.
28. Slusher MM, Tyler ME: Rubella retinopathy and subretinal neovascularization. Ann Ophthalmol 14:292, 1982.
29. Eckstein M, Vijayalakshmi P, Killedar M, et al: Aetiology of childhood cataract in south India. Br J Ophthalmol 80:628, 1996.
30. Gerstle C, Zinn KM: Rubella-associated retinitis in an adult: Report of a case. Rev Infect Dis 3:1151, 1981.
31. Riffenburn RS: Ocular manifestations of mumps. Arch Ophthalmol 66:739, 1961.
32. Cook SD: Herpes simplex virus in the eye. Br J Ophthalmol 76:365, 1992.
33. Ronday MJH, Stilma JS, Barbe RF, et al: Aetiology of uveitis in Sierra Leone, West Africa. Br J Ophthalmol 80:956, 1996.
34. Chang EJ, Dreyer EB: Herpesvirus infections of the anterior segment. Int Ophthalmol Clin 36:17, 1996.
35. Mets MB: Eye manifestations of intrauterine infections. Ophthalmol Clin North Am 14:521, 2001.
36. Tan JCH, Byles D, Stanford MR, et al: Acute retinal necrosis in children caused by herpes simplex virus. Retina 21:344, 2001.
37. Yorston D, Foster A: Herpetic keratitis in Tanzania: Association with malaria. Br J Ophthalmol 76:582, 1992.
38. Pramod NP, Thyagarajan SP, Mohan KV, et al: Polymerase chain reaction in the diagnosis of herpetic keratitis: Experience in a developing country. Can J Ophthalmol 35:134, 2000.
39. Wilhelmus KR: Interventions for herpes simplex virus epithelial keratitis. Cochrane Database Syst Rev CD002898, 2003.
40. Ostler HB, Thygeson P: The ocular manifestations of herpes zoster, varicella, infectious mononucleosis and cytomegalovirus disease. Surv Ophthalmol 21:148, 1976.
41. Marsh RJ, Easty DL, Jones BR: Iritis and iris atrophy in herpes zoster ophthalmicus. Am J Ophthalmol 78:255, 1974.
42. Johnston WH, Holland GN, Engstrom RE Jr, et al: Recurrence of presumed varicella-zoster virus retinopathy in patients with acquired immunodeficiency syndrome. Am J Ophthalmol 116:42, 1993.
43. Walters G, James TE: Viral causes of the acute retinal necrosis syndrome. Curr Opin Ophthalmol 12:191, 2001.
44. Zamora RL, Del-Priore LV, Storch GA, et al: Multiple recurrent branch retinal artery occlusions associated with varicella zoster virus. Retina 16:399, 1996.
45. Freilich JM, Ryan EA, Lou PL, et al: Acute retinal necrosis syndrome: findings, management, and differential diagnosis. Int Ophthalmol Clin 36:141, 1996.
46. Weller TH, Hanshaw JB: Virologic and clinical observations on cytomegalic inclusion disease. N Engl J Med 266:1233, 1962.
47. Garau J, Kabins S, DeNosago S: Spontaneous cytomegalovirus mononucleosis with conjunctivitis. Arch Intern Med 137:1631, 1977.
48. England IAC, Miller SA, Maki DG: Ocular findings of acute cytomegalovirus infection in an immunologically competent adult. N Engl J Med 307:94, 1982.
49. Kuppermann BD, Petty BD, Richmann DD, et al: Correlation between CD4+ counts and prevalence of cytomegalovirus retinitis and human immunodeficiency virus-related noninfectious retinal vasculopathy in patients with acquired immunodeficiency syndrome. Am J Ophthalmol 115:575, 1993.
50. Holbrook JT, Jabs DA, Weinberg DV, et al: Visual loss in patients with cytomegalovirus retinitis and acquired immunodeficiency syndrome before widespread availability of highly active antiretroviral therapy. Arch Ophthalmol 121:99, 2003.
51. Song MK, Azen SP, Buley A, et al: Effect of anti-cytomegalovirus therapy on the incidence of immune recovery uveitis in AIDS patients with healed cytomegalovirus retinitis. Am J Ophthalmol 136:696, 2003.

52. Jouan M, Saves M, Tubiana R, et al: Discontinuation of maintenance therapy for cytomegalovirus retinitis in HIV-infected patients receiving highly active antiretroviral therapy. AIDS 15:23, 2001.
53. Drew WL, Ives D, Lalezari JP, et al: Oral ganciclovir as maintenance treatment for cytomegalovirus. N Engl J Med 333:615, 1995.
54. Martin DF, Parks DJ, Mellow SD, et al: Treatment of cytomegalovirus retinitis with an intraocular sustained-release ganciclovir implant. Arch Ophthalmol 112:1531, 1994.
55. Engstrom RE, Holland GN: Local therapy of cytomegalovirus retinopathy. Am J Ophthalmol 333:615, 1995.
56. Garcia RF, Flores-Aguilar A, Quiceno JI, et al: Results of rhegmatogenous retinal detachment repair in cytomegalovirus retinitis with and without scleral buckling. Ophthalmology 102:236, 1995.
57. Pflugfelder SC, Crouse CA, Atherton SS: Ophthalmic manifestations of Epstein-Barr virus infection. Int Ophthalmol Clin 33:95, 1993.
58. Gardner BP, Margolis TP, Mondino BJ: Conjunctival lymphocytic nodule associated with the Epstein-Barr virus. Am J Ophthalmol 112:567, 1991.
59. Yamamoto M, Ohga S, Ohnishi Y, et al: Optic disk vasculitis associated with chronic active Epstein-Barr virus infection. Ophthalmologica 216:221, 2002.
60. Rhem MN, Wilhelmus KR, Jones DB: Epstein-Barr virus dacryoadenitis. Am J Ophthalmol 129:372, 2000.
61. Furrer H, Barloggio A, Egger M, et al: Retinal microangiopathy in human immunodeficiency virus infection is related to higher human immunodeficiency virus-1 load in plasma. Ophthalmology 110:432, 2003.
62. Padhani DH, Manji KP, Mtanda AT: Ocular manifestations in children with HIV infection in Dar es Salaam, Tanzania. J Trop Pediatr 46:145, 2000.
63. Kestelyn P, Lepage P, Karita E, et al: Ocular manifestations of infection with the human immunodeficiency virus in an African pediatric population. Ocul Immunol Inflamm 8:263, 2000.
64. Moraes HV Jr: Ocular manifestations of HIV/AIDS. Curr Opin Ophthalmol 13:397, 2002.
65. Biswas J, Fogla R, Gopal L, et al: Current approaches to diagnosis and management of ocular lesions in human immunodeficiency virus positive patients. Indian J Ophthalmol 50:83, 2002.
66. Biswas J, Kumar AA, George AE, et al: Ocular and systemic lesions in children with HIV. Indian J Pediatr 67:721, 2000.
67. Brezin AP, Thulliez P, Cisneros B, et al: Lymphocytic choriomeningitis virus chorioretinitis mimicking ocular toxoplasmosis in two otherwise normal children. Am J Ophthalmol 130:245, 2000.
68. Pola EC, Masanganise R, Rusakaniko S: The trend of ocular surface squamous neoplasia among ocular surface tumour biopsies submitted for histology from Sekuru Kaguvi Eye Unit, Harare between 1996 and 2000. Cent Afr J Med 49:1, 2003.
69. Machizuki M, Ono A, Ikeda E, et al: HTLV-I uveitis. J AIDS Human Retrovirol 13:S50, 1996.
70. Ohba N, Matsumoto M, Sameshima M, et al: Ocular manifestations in patients infected with human T-lymphotropic virus type I. Jpn J Ophthalmol 33:1, 1989.
71. Merle H, Cabre P, Olindo S, et al: Ocular lesions in 200 patients infected by the human T-cell lymphotropic virus type 1 in Martinique (French West Indies). Am J Ophthalmol 134:190, 2002.
72. Merle H, Cabre P, Merle S, et al: A description of human T-lymphotropic virus type I–related chronic interstitial keratitis in 20 patients. Am J Ophthalmol 131:305, 2001.
73. Nakao K, Ohba N: Human T-cell lymphotropic virus type 1–associated retinal vasculitis in children. Retina 23:197, 2003.
74. Siam AL, Meegan JM, Gharbaw KF: Rift Valley fever ocular manifestations: Observations during the 1977 epidemic in Egypt. Br J Ophthalmol 64:366, 1980.
75. Anninger WV, Lomeo MD, Dingle J, et al: West Nile virus–associated optic neuritis and chorioretinitis. Am J Ophthalmol 136:1183, 2003.
76. Kaiser PK, Lee MS, Martin DA: Occlusive vasculitis in a patient with concomitant West Nile virus infection. Am J Ophthalmol 136:928, 2003.
77. Kuchtey RW, Kosmorsky GS, Martin D, et al: Uveitis associated with West Nile virus infection. Arch Ophthalmol 121:1648, 2003.
78. Vandenbelt S, Shaikh S, Capone A Jr, et al: Multifocal choroiditis associated with West Nile virus encephalitis. Retina 23:97, 2003.
79. Bains HS, Jampol LM, Caughron MC, et al: Vitritis and chorioretinitis in a patient with West Nile virus infection. Arch Ophthalmol 121:205, 2003.
80. Miller AH, Liang IE: Diplopia: A focal neurologic presentation of West Nile meningoencephalitis. Ann Emerg Med 42:413, 2003.
81. Sureau PH: Firsthand clinical observation of hemorrhagic manifestations in Ebola hemorrhagic fever in Zaire. Rev Infect Dis 11(suppl 4):790, 1989.
82. Kontkanen MI, Puustjarvi TJ, Lahdevirta JK: Intraocular pressure changes in nephropathia epidemica. Ophthalmology 102:1813, 1995.
83. Kontkanen M, Puustjarvi T, Lahdevirta J: Myopic shifts and its mechanism in nephropathia epidemica or Puumala virus infection. Br J Ophthalmol 78:903, 1994.
84. Parssinen O, Klemetti A, Rossi-Rautiainen E, et al: Ophthalmic manifestations of epidemic nephropathy. Acta Ophthalmol 338:1353, 1993.
85. Perez-Alvarez AF, Jimenez-Alonso J, Reche-Molina I, et al: Retinal vasculitis and vitreitis in a patient with chronic hepatitis C virus. Arch Intern Med 161:2262, 2001.
86. Zegans ME, Anninger W, Chapman C, et al: Ocular manifestations of hepatitis C virus infection. Curr Opin Ophthalmol 13:423, 2002.
87. Kuga K, Hasumura S, Nagamori S, et al: Intraocular hemorrhage developing during interferon therapy. Intern Med 35:15, 1996.
88. Schulman JA, Liang C, Kooragayala LM, et al: Posterior segment complications in patients with hepatitis C treated with interferon and ribavirin. Ophthalmology 110:437, 2003.
89. Hogan RN, Cavanagh HD: Transplantation of corneal tissue from donors with diseases of the central nervous system. Cornea 14:547, 1995.
90. Mets MB, Barton LL, Khan AS, et al: Lymphocytic choriomeningitis virus: An underdiagnosed cause of congenital chorioretinitis. Am J Ophthalmol 130:209, 2000.
91. Mecaskey JW, Knirsch CA, Kumaresan JA, et al: The possibility of eliminating blinding trachoma. Lancet Infect Dis 3:728, 2003.
92. Thylefors B, Dawson CR, Jones BR, et al: A simple system for the assessment of trachoma and it complications. Bull World Health Org 65:477, 1987.
93. Grayston JT, Wang S-P, Yeh L-J, et al: Importance of reinfection in the pathogenesis of trachoma. Rev Infect Dis 7:717, 1985.
94. Bird M, Dawson CR, Schachter JS, et al: Does the diagnosis of trachoma adequately identify ocular chlamydial infection in trachoma-endemic areas? J Infect Dis 187:1669, 2003.
95. Tabbara KF, Abu El-Asrar AM, Al-Omar O, et al: Single-dose azithromycin in the treatment of trachoma. A randomized, controlled study. Ophthalmology 103:842, 1996.
96. Bailey RL, Arullendran P, Whittle HC, et al: Randomised controlled trial of single-dose azithromycin in treatment of trachoma. Lancet 342:453, 1993.
97. Dawson CR, Schachter J, Sallam S, et al: A comparison of oral azithromycin with topical oxytetracycline/polymyxin for the treatment of trachoma in children. Clin Infect Dis 24:363, 1997.
98. Bowman RJ, Faal H, Myatt M, et al: Longitudinal study of trachomatous trichiasis in the Gambia. Br J Ophthalmol 86:339, 2002.
99. Reacher MH, Huber MJE, Camarearatnam R, et al: A trial surgery for trichiasis of the upper lid from trachoma. Br J Ophthalmol 4:109, 1990.
100. Mohile M, Deorari AK, Satpathy G, et al: Microbiological study of neonatal conjunctivitis with special reference to Chlamydia trachomatis. Indian J Ophthalmol 50:295, 2002.
101. Laga M, Plummer FA, Piot P: Prophylaxis of gonococcal and chlamydial ophthalmia neonatorum. A comparison of silver nitrate and tetracycline. N Engl J Med 318:653, 1988.
102. Chandler JW, Rapoza PA: Ophthalmia neonatorum. Int Ophthalmol Clin 30:36, 1990.
103. Alexander ER, Harrison HR: Role of *Chlamydia trachomatis* in perinatal infection. Rev Infect Dis 5:713, 1983.
104. Ostler HB: Oculogenital disease. Surv Ophthalmol 20:233, 1976.
105. Schachter J, Grossman M, Azimi PH: Serology of *Chlamydia trachomatis* in infants. J Infect Dis 146:530, 1982.
106. Hammerschlag MR, Roblin PM, Gelling M, et al: Use of polymerase chain reaction for the detection of *Chlamydia trachomatis* in ocular and nasopharyngeal specimens from infants with conjunctivitis. Pediatr Infect Dis J 16:293, 1997.
107. Kowalski RP, Uhrin M, Karenchak LM, et al: Evaluation of the polymerase chain reaction test for detecting chlamydial DNA in adult chlamydial conjunctivitis. Ophthalmology 102:1016, 1995.
108. Macnie JP: Ocular lymphogranuloma venereum. Arch Ophthalmol 25:255, 1941.

109. Meyer GP, Reber J: A case of corneal ulcer associated with lymphogranuloma venereum. Am J Ophthalmol 24:161, 1941.
110. Buus DR, Pflugfelder SC, Schacter J, et al: Lymphogranuloma venereum conjunctivitis with a marginal corneal perforation. Ophthalmology 95:799, 1988.
111. Courtright P, Daniel E, Sundarrao, et al: Eye disease in multibacillary leprosy patients at the time of their leprosy diagnosis: Findings from the Longitudinal Study of Ocular Leprosy (LOSOL) in India, the Philippines and Ethiopia. Lepr Rev 73:225, 2002.
112. Singhi MK, Kacchawa D, Ghiya BC: Ocular involvement in leprosy. Indian J Ophthalmol 50:355, 2002.
113. Schipper A, Lubbers WJ, Hogeweg M, et al: Disabilities of hands, feet and eyes in newly diagnosed leprosy patients in eastern Nepal. Lepr Rev 65:239, 1994.
114. Waddell KM, Saunderson PR: Is leprosy blindness avoidable? The effect of disease type, duration, and treatment on eye damage in Uganda. Br J Ophthalmol 79:250, 1995.
115. Ostler HB: Hansen's disease. Int Ophthalmol Clin 30:42, 1990.
116. Dhaliwal U, Mohanty S, Bhattacharya SN: Erythema nodosum leprosum and orbital involvement. Int J Lepr Other Mycobact Dis 71:10, 2003.
117. Espiritu CG, Gelber R, Ostler HB: Chronic anterior uveitis in leprosy: An insidious cause of blindness. Br J Ophthalmol 75:273, 1991.
118. Hieselaar LCJM, Hogeweg M, de Vries CL: Corneal sensitivity in patients with leporosy and in controls. Br J Ophthalmol 79:993, 1995.
119. Thompson KJ, Brand M: Temporary tarsorrhaphy: A valuable procedure in Hansen disease. Arch Ophthalmol 121:149, 2003.
120. Biswas J, Badrinath SS: Ocular morbidity in patients with active systemic tuberculosis. Int Ophthalmol 19:293, 1996.
121. Helm CJ, Holland GN: Ocular tuberculosis. Surv Ophthalmol 38:229, 1993.
122. Gupta V, Gupta A, Arora S, et al: Presumed tubercular serpiginouslike choroiditis: Clinical presentations and management. Ophthalmology 110:1744, 2003.
123. Das T, Diswas J, Kumar A, et al: Eale's disease. Indian J Ophthalmol 42:3, 1994.
124. Beare NA, Kublin JG, Lewis DK, et al: Ocular disease in patients with tuberculosis and HIV presenting with fever in Africa. Br J Ophthalmol 86:1076, 2002.
125. Turner L: Atypical mycobacterial infections in ophthalmology. Trans Am Ophthalmol Soc 68:667, 1970.
126. Huang SCM, Soong HK, Liang YS: Non-tuberculous mycobacterial keratitis: A study of 22 cases. Br J Ophthalmol 80:962, 1966.
127. Katz DA, Berger JR: Neurosyphilis in acquired immunodeficiency syndrome. Arch Neurol 46:895, 1989.
128. Tabbara KF, Al Kaff AS: Ocular manifestations of endemic syphilis (bejel). Ophthalmology 96:1087, 1989.
129. Smith JL, David NJ, Indgin S, et al: Neuro-ophthalmological study of late yaws and pinta: II. The Caracas project. Br J Vener Dis 47:226, 1971.
130. Watt G: Leptospirosis as a cause of uveitis. Arch Intern Med 150:1130, 1990.
131. Espejo E, Bella F, Espaulella J, et al: Mediterranean spotted fever presenting as oculoglandular syndrome. Trans R Soc Trop Med Hyg 82:642, 1988.
132. Pinna A, Sotgiu M, Carta F, et al: Oculoglandular syndrome in Mediterranean spotted fever acquired through the eye. Br J Ophthalmol 81:172, 1997.
133. Nagaki Y, Hayasaka S, Kadoi C, et al: Branch retinal vein occlusion in the right eye and retinal hemorrhage in the left in a patient with classical Tsutsugamushi disease. Jpn J Ophthalmol 45:108, 2001.
134. Kompella VB, Sangwan VS, Bansal AK, et al: Ophthalmic complications and management of Stevens-Johnson syndrome at a tertiary eye care centre in south India. Indian J Ophthalmol 50:283, 2002.
135. Gomes JA, Santos MS, Ventura AS, et al: Amniotic membrane with living related corneal limbal/conjunctival allograft for ocular surface reconstruction in Stevens-Johnson syndrome. Arch Ophthalmol 121:1369, 2003.
136. Nithyanandam S, D'Souza O, Rao SS, et al: Rhinoorbitocerebral actinomycosis. Ophthalmol Plast Reconstr Surg 17:134, 2001.
137. Garelick JM, Khodabakhsh AJ, Josephberg RG: Acute postoperative endophthalmitis caused by *Actinomyces neuii*. Am J Ophthalmol 133:145, 2002.
138. Hunter LR, Krinsky AH, Fleener CH: Preseptal cellulitis caused by *Nocardia brasiliensis*. Am J Ophthalmol 114:372, 1992.
139. Phillips WB, Shields CL, Shields JA, et al: *Nocardia* choroidal abscess. Br J Ophthalmol 76:694, 1992.
140. Durand DV, Lecomte C, Cathebras P, et al: Whipple disease. Clinical review of 52 cases. The SNFMI Research Group on Whipple Disease. Societe Nationale Francaise de Medecine Interne. Medicine (Baltimore) 76:170, 1997.
141. Lee AG: Ocular Whipple's disease. Ophthalmology 109:1952, 2002.
142. Rickman LS, Freeman WR, Green WR, et al: Brief report: Uveitis caused by *Tropheryma whippelii* (Whipple's bacillus). N Engl J Med 332:363, 1995.
143. Nishimura JK, Cook BE Jr, Pach JM: Whipple disease presenting as posterior uveitis without prominent gastrointestinal symptoms. Am J Ophthalmol 126:130, 1998.
144. Playford RJ, Schulenburg E, Herrington CS, et al: Whipple's disease complicated by a retinal Jarisch-Herxheimer reaction: A case report. Gut 33:132, 1992.
145. Walker J, Sharma OP, Rao NA: Brucellosis and uveitis. Am J Ophthalmol 114:374, 1992.
146. Gungur K, Bekir NA, Namiduru M: Ocular complications associated with brucellosis in an endemic area. Eur J Ophthalmol 12:232, 2002.
147. Halperin SA, Gast T, Ferrieri P: Oculoglandular syndrome caused by *Francisella tularensis*. Clin Pediatr 24:520, 1985.
148. Hanna C, Lyford JH: Tularemia infection of the eye. Ann Ophthalmol 3:1321, 1971.
149. Tsai PS, DeAngelis DD, Spencer WH, et al: Bacillary angiomatosis of the anterior orbit, eyelid, and conjunctiva. Am J Ophthalmol 134:433, 2002.
150. Gass JDM: Diseases of the optic nerve that may simulate macular disease. Trans Am Acad Ophthalmol 83:763, 1977.
151. Gray AV, Michels KS, Lauer AK, et al: *Bartonella henselae* infection associated with neuroretinitis, central retinal artery and vein occlusion, neovascular glaucoma, and severe vision loss. Am J Ophthalmol 137:187, 2004.
152. Golnik KC, Marotto ME, Fanous MM, et al: Ophthalmic manifestations of *Rochalimaea* species. Am J Ophthalmol 118:145, 1994.
153. Schuil J, Richardus JH, Baarsma GS, et al: Q fever as a possible cause of bilateral optic neuritis. Br J Ophthalmol 69:580, 1985.
154. Chovet M, Ducam M, Negrel AD, et al: Late aspects of palpebral anthrax. Med Trop 39:91, 1979.
155. Soysal HG, Kiratli H, Recep OF: Anthrax as the cause of preseptal cellulitis and cicatricial ectropion. Acta Ophthalmol Scand 79:208, 2001.
156. Rysselaere M, Vanneste L: Diphtheria of the eye—A forgotten diagnosis. Bull Soc Belge Ophthalmol 201:89, 1982.
157. Chandler JW, Milam DF: Diphtheria corneal ulcers. Arch Ophthalmol 96:53, 1978.
158. Konig H, Gassman HB, Jenzer G: Ocular involvement in benign botulism B. Am J Ophthamol 80:430, 1975.
159. Cherington M: Botulism: Ten-year experience. Arch Neurol 30:432, 1974.
160. Hedges TR III, Jones A, Stark L, et al: Botulin ophthalmoplegia. Clinical and oculographic observations. Arch Ophthalmol 101:211, 1983.
161. Terranova W, Palumbo JN, Breman JG: Ocular findings in botulism type B. JAMA 241:475, 1979.
162. Ying S, Shuyan C: Botulism in China. Rev Infect Dis 8:984, 1997.
163. Caya JG: *Clostridium botulinum* and the ophthalmologist: A review of botulism, including biological warfare ramifications of botulinum toxin. Surv Ophthalmol 46:25, 2001.
164. Abde VW, Dekate MP: Cephalic tetanus. J Indian Med Assoc 74:111, 1980.
165. Vakil BJ, Singhal BS, Pandya SS: Cephalic tetanus. Neurology 10:1091, 1973.
166. Biglan AW, Ellis FD, Wade TA: Supranuclear oculomotor palsy and extropia after tetanus. Am J Ophthalmol 86:666, 1978.
167. Meienberg O, Burgunder JM: Saccadic eye movement disorder in cephalic tetanus. Eur Neurol 24:182, 1985.
168. Saltissi S, Hankin RN, Pearce J: Ophthalmoplegia in tetanus. BMJ 1:437, 1976.
169. Mayo J, Berciano J: Cephalic tetanus presenting with Bell's palsy. J Neurol Neursurg Psychiatry 48:290, 1985.
170. Iyer MN, Kranias G, Daun ME: Post-traumatic endophthalmitis involving *Clostridium tetani* and *Bacillus* spp. Am J Ophthalmol 132:116, 2001.

171. Barquet N, Gasser I, Domingo P, et al: Primary meningococcal conjunctivitis: Report of 21 patients and review. Rev Infect Dis 12:838, 1990.
172. Gartaganis SP, Eliopoulou MJ, Georgakopoulos CD, et al: Bilateral panophthalmitis as the initial presentation of meningococcal meningitis in an infant. J AAPOS 5:260, 2001.
173. Laga M, Meheus A, Piot P: Epidemiology and control of gonococcal ophthalmia neonatorum. Bull World Health Org 87:471, 1989.
174. Harrison LH, Broome CV: Report of a symposium: Brazilian purpuric fever. Pediatr Infect Dis J 237, 1989.
175. Brazilian Purpuric Fever Study Group: Brazilian purpuric fever: Epidemic purpura fulminans associated with antecedent purulent conjunctivitis. Lancet 2:757, 1987.
176. Ford DK: The clinical spectrum of Reiter's syndrome and similiar postenteric arthropathies. Clinical Orthop Relat Res 143:59, 1979.
177. Dunlop AA, Wright ED, Howlader SA, et al: Suppurative corneal ulceration in Bangladesh—A study of 142 cases examining the microbiological diagnosis, clinical and epidemiological features of bacterial and fungal keratitis. Aust NZ J Ophthalmol 22:105, 1994.
178. Williams G, Billson F, Husain R, et al: Microbiological diagnosis of suppurative keratitis in Bangladesh. Br J Ophthalmol 71:315, 1987.
179. Gopinathan U, Garg P, Fernandes M, et al: The epidemiological features and laboratory results of fungal keratitis: A 10-year review at a referral eye care center in South India. Cornea 21:555, 2002.
180. Tabbara K, Ross-Degnan D: Blindness in Saudi Arabia. JAMA 255:3378, 1986.
181. Hagan M, Wright E, Newman M, et al: Causes of suppurative keratitis in Ghana. Br J Ophthalmol 79:1024, 1995.
182. Durand M, Adamis A, Baker AS: Infections of the eyelid, lacrimal system, conjunctiva, and cornea. Curr Clin Top Infect Dis 16:125, 1996.
183. Abad J-C, Foster CS: Fungal keratitis. Int Ophthalmol Clin 36:1, 1996.
184. Jackson TL, Eykyn SJ, Graham EM, et al: Endogenous bacterial endophthalmitis: A 17-year prospective series and review of 267 reported cases. Surv Ophthalmol 48:403, 2003.
185. Wong JS, Chan TK, Lee HM, et al: Endogenous bacterial endophthalmitis: An east Asian experience and a reappraisal of a severe ocular affliction. Ophthalmology 107:1483, 2000.
186. Durand ML, Heier JS: Endophthalmitis. Curr Clin Top Infect Dis 20:271, 2000.
187. Kotigadde S, Ballal M, Jyothirlatha, et al: Mycotic keratitis: A study in coastal Karnataka. Indian J Ophthalmol 40:31, 1992.
188. Agrawal V, Biswas J, Madhavan HN: Current perspectives in infectious keratitis. Indian J Ophthalmol 42:171, 1994.
189. Leck AK, Thomas PA, Hagan M, et al: Aetiology of suppurative corneal ulcers in Ghana and south India, and epidemiology of fungal keratitis. Br J Ophthalmol 86:1211, 2002.
190. Kumari N, Xess A, Shahi SK: A study of keratomycosis: Our experience. Indian J Pathol Microbiol 45:299, 2002.
191. Garg P, Gopinathan U, Choudhary K, et al: Keratomycosis: Clinical and microbiologic experience with dematiaceous fungi. Ophthalmology 107:574, 2000.
192. Brightbell FS, Fraser LK: Unilateral keratoconjunctivitis with canalicular obstruction by *Aspergillus fumigatus*. Arch Ophthamol 91:421, 1974.
193. Rodriguez-Ares MT, de Rojas Silva MV, Pereiro M, et al: *Aspergillus fumigatus* scleritis. Acta Ophthalmol Scand 73:467, 1995.
194. Feman SS, Nichols JC, Chung SM, et al: Endophthalmitis in patients with disseminated fungal disease. Trans Am Ophthalmol Soc 100:67, 2002.
195. Choi MY, Bae IH, Lee JH, et al: Aspergillosis presenting as an optic neuritis. Korean J Ophthalmol 16:119, 2002.
196. deShazo RD, Chapin K, Swain RE: Fungal sinusitis. N Engl J Med 337:254, 1997.
197. Milosev B, el-Mahgoub S, el-Hassan AM, et al: Primary aspergilloma of paranasal sinuses in the Sudan: A review of seventeen cases. Br J Surg 56:132, 1969.
198. Dhiwakar M, Thakar A, Bahadur S: Invasive sino-orbital aspergillosis: Surgical decisions and dilemmas. J Laryngol Otolaryngol 117:280, 2003.
199. Schulman JA, Leveque C, Coats M, et al: Fatal disseminated cryptococcosis following intraocular involvement. Br J Ophthalmol 72:171, 1988.
200. Hiss PW, Shields JA, Augsburger JJ: Solitary retinovitreal abscess as the initial manifestation of cryptococcosis. Ophthalmology 95:163, 1988.
201. Crump JRC, Elner SG, Elner VM, et al: Cryptococcal endophthalmitis: Case report and review. Clin Infect Dis 14:1069, 1992.
202. Bisseru B, Bajaj A, Carruthers RH, et al: Pulmonary and bilateral retinochoroidal cryptococcosis: Current status. Br J Ophthalmol 67:157, 1983.
203. McMillan TA, Lashkari K: Ocular histoplasmosis. Ophthalmology 36:179, 1996.
204. Knox DL, O'Brien TP, Green WR: Histoplasma granuloma of the conjunctiva. Ophthalmology 110:2051, 2003.
205. Gonzales CA, Scott IU, Chaudhry NA, et al: Endogenous endophthalmitis caused by *Histoplasma capsulatum* var. *capsulatum*: A case report and literature review. Ophthalmology 107:725, 2000.
206. Ciulla TA, Piper HC, Xiao M, et al: Presumed ocular histoplasmosis syndrome: Update on epidemiology, pathogenesis, and photodynamic, antiangiogenic, and surgical therapies. Curr Opin Ophthalmol 12:442, 2001.
207. Rechtman E, Allen VD, Danis RP, et al: Intravitreal triamcinolone for choroidal neovascularization in ocular histoplasmosis syndrome. Am J Ophthalmol 136:739, 2003.
208. Cockshott WP, Lucas AO: *Histoplasma duboisii*. Q J Med 33:223, 1964.
209. Bansal RK, Suseelan AV, Gugnani HC: Orbital cyst due to *Histoplasma duboisii*. Br J Ophthalmol 61:70, 1977.
210. Rodenbiker HT, Ganley JP: Ocular coccidioidomycosis. Surv Ophthalmol 24:263, 1980.
211. Moorthy RS, Rao NA, Sidikaro Y, et al: Coccidioidomycosis iridocyclitis. Ophthalmology 101:1923, 1994.
212. Gottlieb JL, McAllister IL, Guttman FA, et al: Choroidal blastomycosis: A report of two cases. Retina 15:248, 1995.
213. Dantas AM, Yamane R, Camara AG: South American blastomycosis: Ophthalmic and oculomotor nerve lesions. Am J Trop Med Hyg 43:386, 1990.
214. Witherspoon CD, Kuhn F, Owens SD, et al: Endophthalmitis due to *Sporothrix schenckii* after penetrating ocular injury. Ann Ophthalmol 22:385, 1990.
215. Curi AL, Felix S, Azevedo KM, et al: Retinal granuloma caused by *Sporothrix schenckii*. Am J Ophthalmol 136:205, 2003.
216. Talmi YP, Goldschmied-Reouven A, Bakon M, et al: Rhino-orbital and rhino-orbito-cerebral mucormycosis. Otolaryngol Head Neck Surg 127:22, 2002.
217. Luna JD, Ponssa XS, Rodriquez SD, et al: Intraconal amphotericin B for the treatment of rhino-orbital mucormycosis. Ophthalmic Surg Lasers Imaging 27:706, 1996.
218. Ochoa LF, Duque CS, Velez A: Rhinoentomophthoromycosis. Report of two cases. J Laryngol Otolaryngol 110:1154, 1996.
219. Lithander J, Louon A, Worthing E, et al: Orbital entomophthoramycosis in an infant: Recovery following surgical debridement, combination antifungal therapy and use of hyperbaric oxygen. Br J Ophthalmol 85:374, 2001.
220. Bhomaj S, Das JC, Chaudhuri Z, et al: Rhinosporidiosis and peripheral keratitis. Ophthalmic Surg Lasers Imaging 32:338, 2001.
221. Chan CM, Theng JT, Li L, et al: Microsporidial keratoconjunctivitis in healthy individuals: A case series. Ophthalmology 110:1420, 2003.
222. Rastrelli PD, Didier E, Yee RW: Microsporidial keratitis. Ophthalmol Clin North Am 7:617, 1994.
223. Metcalfe TW, Doran RM, Rowlands PL, et al: Microsporidial keratoconjunctivitis in a patient with AIDS. Br J Ophthalmol 76:177, 1992.
224. Schwartz DA, Visvesvara GS, Diesenhouse MC: Pathologic features and immunofluorescent antibody demonstration of ocular microsporidiosis in seven patients with acquired immunodeficiency syndrome. Am J Ophthalmol 115:285, 1993.
225. Yoken J, Forbes B, Maguire AM, et al: Microsporidial endophthalmitis in a patient with acute myelogenous leukemia. Retina 22:123, 2002.
226. de Jong PTVM: Ocular toxoplasmosis: Common and rare symptoms and signs. Int Ophthalmol 13:391, 1989.
227. Silveira C, Belfort R Jr, Muccioli C, et al: A follow-up study of *Toxoplasma gondii* infection in southern Brazil. Am J Ophthalmol 131:351, 2001.
228. Suhardjo, Utomo PT, Agni AN: Clinical manifestations of ocular toxoplasmosis in Yogyakarta, Indonesia: A clinical review of 173 cases. Southeast Asian J Trop Med Public Health 34:291, 2003.
229. Perry DD, Merritt JC, Greenwood RS, et al: Congenital toxoplasmosis associated with acquired oculomotor nerve (CN III) palsy. J Pediatr Ophthalmol Strabismus 19:265, 1982.

230. Hay J, Dutton GN: *Toxoplasma* and the eye. BMJ 310:1021, 1995.
231. Peacock JE, Greven CM, Cruz JM, et al: Reactivation toxoplasmic retinochoroiditis in patients undergoing bone marrow transplantation: Is there a role for chemoprophylaxis? Bone Marrow Transplant 15:983, 1995.
232. Lewallen S, White VA, Whitten RO, et al: Clinical-histopathological correlation of the abnormal retinal vessels in cerebral malaria. Arch Ophthalmol 118:924, 2000.
233. Looareesuwan S, Warrel DA, White NJ, et al: Retinal hemorrhage, a common sign of prognostic significance in cerebral malaria. Am J Trop Med Hyg 35:911, 1983.
234. Hidayat AA, Nalbandian RM, Sammons DW, et al: The diagnostic histopathologic features of ocular malaria. Ophthalmology 100:1183, 1993.
235. Lewallen S, Bakker H, Taylor TE, et al: Retinal findings predictive of outcome in cerebral malaria. Trans R Soc Trop Med Hyg 90:144, 1996.
236. Kochar DK, Shubhakaran, Kumawat BL, et al: Prognostic significance of eye changes in cerebral malaria. J Assoc Physicians India 48:473, 2000.
237. Beare NA, Lewis DK, Kublin JG, et al: Retinal changes in adults with cerebral malaria. Ann Trop Med Parasitol 97:313, 2003.
238. Sassani JW, Brucker AJ, Cobbs W, et al: Progressive chloroquine retinopathy. Ann Ophthalmol 15:19, 1983.
239. Lam S: Keratitis caused by leishmaniasis or trypanomiasis. Ophthalmol Clin North Am 7:635, 1995.
240. DeChant W, Rees PH, Kager PA: Post kala-azar uveitis. Br J Ophthalmol 64:680, 1980.
241. Montero JA, Ruiz-Moreno JM, Sanchis E: Intraretinal hemorrhage associated with leishmaniasis. Ophthalmic Surg Lasers Imaging 34:212, 2003.
242. Nandy A, Addy M, Chowdhury AB: Leishmanial blepharo-conjunctivitis. Trop Geogr Med 43:303, 1991.
243. Oliveira-Neto MP, Martins VJ, Mattos MS, et al: South American cutaneous leishmaniasis of the eyelids: Report of five cases in Rio de Janeiro State, Brazil. Ophthalmology 107:169, 2000.
244. Abrishami M, Soheilian M, Farahi A, et al: Successful treatment of ocular leishmaniasis. Eur J Dermatol 12:88, 2002.
245. Baddini-Caramelli C, Matayoshi S, Moura EM, et al: Chronic dacryocystitis in American mucocutaneous leishmaniasis. Ophthalmol Plast Reconstr Surg 17:48, 2001.
246. Srinivasan M, Burman S, George C, et al: Non-contact lens related *Acanthamoeba* keratitis at a tertiary eye care center in south India: Implications for eye care programs in the region. Med Sci Monit 9:CR125, 2003.
247. Illingworth CD, Karabatasas CH, Easty DL: *Acanthamoeba* keratitis: Risk factors and outcome. Br J Ophthalmol 79:1078, 1995.
248. Kumar R, Lloyd D: Recent advances in the treatment of *Acanthamoeba* keratitis. Clin Infect Dis 35:434, 2002.
249. Taylor HR: Onchocerciasis. Int Ophthalmol 14:189, 1990.
250. Enk CD, Anteby I, Abramson N, et al: Onchocerciasis among Ethiopian immigrants in Israel. Isr Med Assoc J 5:485, 2003.
251. Sekhar HS, Srinivasa H, Batru RR, et al: Human ocular dirofilariasis in Kerala, Southern India. Indian J Pathol Microbiol 43:77, 2000.
252. Baird JK, Neafie RC, Connor DH: Nodules in the conjunctiva, bung-eye, and bulge-eye in Africa caused by *Mansonella perstans*. Am J Trop Med Hyg 38:553, 1988.
253. Bregani ER, Ceraldi T, Rovellini A, et al: Case report: Intraocular localization of *Mansonella perstans* in a patient from south Chad. Trans R Soc Trop Med Hyg 96:654, 2002.
254. Garrido C, Campos M: First report of presumed parasitic keratitis in Indians from the Brazilian Amazon. Cornea 19:817, 2000.
255. Gillespie SH, Dinning WJ, Voller A, et al: The spectrum of ocular toxocariasis. Eye 7:415, 1993.
256. Kazacos KR, Vestre WA, Kazacos EA: Racoon ascarid larvae (*Baylisascaris procyonis*) as a cause of ocular larva migrans. Invest Ophthalmol Vis Sci 25:1177, 1984.
257. Goldberg MA, Kazacos KR, Boyce WM, et al: Diffuse unilateral subacute neuroretinitis. Morphometric, serologic, and epidemiologic support for *Baylisascaris* as a causative agent. Ophthalmology 100:1695, 1993.
258. Kuchle M, Knorr HL, Medenblik-Frysch S, et al: Diffuse unilateral subacute neuroretinitis syndrome in a German most likely caused by the raccoon roundworm, *Baylisascaris procyonis*. Graefes Arch Clin Exp Ophthalmol 231:48, 1993.
259. Mets MB, Noble AG, Basti S, et al: Eye findings of diffuse unilateral subacute neuroretinitis and multiple choroidal infiltrates associated with neural larva migrans due to *Baylisascaris procyonis*. Am J Ophthalmol 135:888, 2003.
260. Cunningham CK, Kazacos KR, McMillan JA, et al: Diagnosis and management of *Baylisascaris procyonis* infection in an infant with nonfatal meningoencephalitis. Clin Infect Dis 18:868, 1994.
261. Hui JY, Woo PC, Kan PS, et al: Ultrasonographic features of pseudotumorous form of ascariasis. Eur J Radiol 39:188, 2001.
262. Balasubramaniam M, Sudhakar P, Subhashini M, et al: *Ascaris lumbricoides* in the lacrimal passage. Indian J Ophthalmol 48:53, 2000.
263. Baldone JA, Clark WB, Jung RC: Nematode ophthalmitis: Report of two cases. Am J Ophthalmol 57:763, 1964.
264. Nadbath RP, Lawlor PP: Nematode (ancylostoma) in the cornea. A case report. Am J Ophthalmol 59:486, 1965.
265. Bhaibulaya M, Prasertsilpa S, Vajrasthira S: *Thelazia callipaeda* Railliet and Henry, 1910, in man and dog in Thailand. Am J Trop Med Hyg 19:476, 1970.
266. Mahanta J, Alger J, Bordoloi P: Eye infestation with *Thelazia* species. Indian J Ophthalmol 44:99, 1996.
267. Koyama Y, Ohira A, Kono T, et al: Five cases of thelaziasis. Br J Ophthalmol 84:441, 2000.
268. Kirschner BI, Dunn JP, Ostler HB: Conjunctivitis caused by *Thelazia californiensis*. Am J Ophthalmol 110:573, 1990.
269. Verma AK: Ocular dracontiasis. Int Surg 50:508, 1968.
270. Dissanaike AS, Ihalamulla RL, Naotunne TS, et al: Third report of ocular parastrongyliasis (angiostrongyliasis) from Sri Lanka. Parasitologia 43:95, 2001.
271. Toma H, Matsumura S, Oshiro C, et al: Ocular angiostrongyliasis without meningitis Symptoms in Okinawa, Japan. J Parasitol 88:211, 2002.
272. Teekhasaenee C, Ritch R, Kanchanaranya C: Ocular parasitic infection in Thailand. Rev Infect Dis 8:350, 1986.
273. Scrimgeour EM, Chambers BR, Kaven J: A probable case of ocular angiostrongyliasis in New Britain, Papua New Guinea. Trans R Soc Trop Med Hyg 76:538, 1982.
274. Nelson RG, Warren RC, Scotti FA: Ocular angiostrongyliasis in Japan: A case report. Am J Trop Med Hyg 38:130, 1988.
275. Prommindaroj K, Leelawongs N, Pradatsundarasar A: Human angiostrongyliasis of the eye in Bangkok. Am J Trop Med Hyg 1:759, 1962.
276. Ketsuwan P, Pradatsundarasar A: Second case of ocular angiostrongyliasis in Thailand. Am J Trop Med Hyg 15:50, 1966.
277. Xuan lT, Rojekittikhun W, Punpoowong B, et al: Case report: Intraocular gnathostomiasis in Vietnam. Southeast Asian J Trop Med Public Health 33:485, 2002.
278. Baquera-Heredia J, Cruz-Reyes A, Flores-Gaxiola A, et al: Case report: Ocular gnathostomiasis in northwestern Mexico. Am J Trop Med Hyg 66:572, 2002.
279. Biswas J, Gopal L, Sharma T, et al: Intraocular *Gnathostoma spinigerum*. Clinicopathologic study of two cases with review of literature. Retina 14:438, 1994.
280. Schmutzhard E, Boongird P, Vejjajiva A: Eosinophilic meningitis and radiculomyelitis in Thailand, caused by CNS invasion of *Gnathostoma spinigerum* and *Angiostrongylus cantonensis*. J Neurol Neurosurg Psychiatr 51:80, 1988.
281. Malik SRK, Gupta AK, Choudhry S: Ocular cysticercosis. Am J Ophthalmol 11:68, 1968.
282. Pushker N, Bajaj MS, Betharia SM: Orbital and adnexal cysticercosis. Clin Exp Ophthalmol 30:322, 2002.
283. Sami A, Achouri M, Harouch M, et al: Intra-orbital hydatid cysts 10 cases. Neurochirurgie 41:398, 1995.
284. Ba'assiri A, Jabi A: Computerized tomography in orbital echinococcosis. Br J Radiology 57:270, 1984.
285. Pau A, Perria C, Turtas S: Long-term follow-up of the surgical treatment of intracranial coenurosis. Br J Neurosurg 4:39, 1990.
286. Welsh NH: Bilharzial conjunctivitis. Am J Ophthalmol 65:774, 1968.
287. Sparrow CH: Bilharziasis in the human eye: Report of a case. Cent Afr J Med 12:55, 1966.
288. Orefice F, Jimal CJR, Pittella JEH: Schistosomatic choroiditis, I. Funduscopic changes and differential diagnosis. Br J Ophthalmol 69:294, 1985.
289. Pittella JEH, Orefice F: Schistosomatic choroiditis. Report of first case. Br J Ophthalmol 69:300, 1985.

290. Creed TD: Unilateral optic atrophy presumed secondary to schistosomiasis of the optic nerve. J Am Optometric Assoc 64:440, 1993.
291. Newton JC, Kanchananaranya C, Previte LR Jr: Intraocular *Schistosoma mansoni*. Am J Ophthalmol 65:774, 1968.
292. Wang WJ, Xin YJ, Robinson NL, et al: Intraocular paragonimiasis. Br J Ophthalmol 68:85, 1984.
293. Oh JS: Ophthalmological signs in cerebral paragonimiasis. Trop Geogr Med 20:13, 1968.
294. Rendtorff RC, Deweese MW, Murrah W: The occurrence of *Linguatula serrata*, a pentastomid, with the human eye. Am J Trop Med 11:764, 1962.
295. Chodosh J, Clarridge J: Ophthalmomyiasis: A review with special reference to *Cochliomyia hominivorax*. Clin Infect Dis 14:444, 1992.
296. Cameron JA, Shoukrey NA, Al-Garni AA: Conjunctival ophthalmomyiasis caused by the sheep nasal botfly (*Oestrus ovis*). Am J Ophthalmol 112:331, 1991.
297. Grammer J, Erb C, Kamin G, et al: Ophthalmomylasis externa due to the sheep botfly *Oestrus ovis* (Diptera: Oestridae) in southwest Germany. German J Ophthalmol 4:188, 1995.
298. Risco JM, Al-Dosari F, Millar L: Sheep nasal botfly (*Oestrus ovis*) larvae infestation of the conjunctiva. Arch Ophthalmol 113:529, 1995.
299. Edwards KM, Meredith TA, Hagler WS, et al: Ophthalmomyiasis interna causing visual loss. Am J Ophthalmol 97:605, 1984.
300. Gozum N, Kir N, Ovali T: Internal ophthalmomyiasis presenting as endophthalmitis associated with an intraocular foreign body. Ophthalmic Surg Lasers Imaging 34:472, 2003.
301. Forman AR, Cruess AF, Benson WE: Ophthalmomyiasis treated by argon-laser photocoagulation. Retina 4:163, 1984.
302. Currier RW, Johnson WA, Rowley WA, et al: Internal ophthalmomyiasis and treatment by laser photocoagulation: A case report. Am J Trop Med Hyg 52:311, 1995.
303. Gjotterberg M, Ingemansson SO: Intraocular infestation by the reindeer warble fly larva: An unusual indication for acute vitrectomy. Br J Ophthalmol 72:420, 1988.
304. Ukponmwan CU: Vernal keratoconjunctivitis in Nigerians: 109 consecutive cases. Trop Doct 33:242, 2003.
305. Kosrirukvongs P, Vichyanond P, Wongsawad W: Vernal keratoconjunctivitis in Thailand. Asian Pac J Allergy Immunol 21:25, 2003.

130

Neurologic Disease

TOM SOLOMON
MUSTAPHA DANESI
FRANK J. BIA
THOMAS P. BLECK

INTRODUCTION

Neurologic presentations are more common in the tropics than in other regions and offer particular diagnostic and management challenges. A variety of factors contribute to this increased incidence, including a climate that favors transmission of insect-borne pathogens (e.g., malaria, arthropod-borne viruses, trypanosomiasis); the increased incidence of vaccine-preventable diseases (e.g., tetanus, diphtheria, polio); the impact of human immunodeficiency virus (HIV) on central nervous system (CNS) infections, particularly tuberculous meningitis; and the poverty, overcrowding, and poor sanitation that are risk factors for so many tropical diseases (e.g., cysticercosis, typhoid). Although this chapter focuses on infectious neurologic diseases, noncommunicable neurologic diseases are also more common in the tropics (e.g., motor vehicle collisions and other forms of trauma). The patterns of cerebrovascular disease in many parts of the tropics are catching up with those in the developed world.

DIAGNOSTIC APPROACHES

Taking a careful history and performing a detailed neurologic and general medical examination are even more important in the tropics than elsewhere because in many tropical settings the availability of diagnostic tools—particularly imaging—is limited. This section concentrates on the approach to the comatose patient, which is often the greatest challenge.

History

Compared with seeing a patient in more developed nations, getting a history from a patient with a neurologic problem in the tropics can be especially difficult. The patient may have traveled a great distance over many days to arrive at the health facility, and the person accompanying the patient may not know the original history. In addition, it may not be clear what drugs were administered along the way; for example, anticonvulsants given at a clinic on the way to hospital. Obtaining an accurate history about possible seizures is particularly difficult because of the range of terms used in different settings and the ways in which abnormal movements are interpreted. Remember that in many settings seizures may be regarded as a sign of mental illness or even of possession by evil spirits.[1] Communication problems are often further compounded by language and translation difficulties. It is worth making a special effort to inquire about possible remedies given by a traditional healer. In many parts of the world, the traditional healer is the first port of call, and referral to conventional health-care systems is very much a last resort.

Examination

It is common to be faced with a comatose patient for whom little reliable history is available. There may be important clues to the cause on examination: check the pockets for any drugs or other information about past medical history; examine the skin for rash, bites (e.g., snakebite), marks of intravenous drug abuse, a healed dog bite (rabies), chancre (for trypanosomiasis); examine the ears and nose carefully for blood or cerebrospinal fluid (CSF) leak consistent with head trauma; feel for lymphadenopathy, particularly in the posterior cervical triangle (Winterbottom's sign in African trypanosomiasis); and smell the breath for alcohol or ketones.

In the neurologic examination, determine the level of consciousness, check for neck stiffness and other signs of meningism (including Kernig's sign—with the patient supine, and the hip and knee flexed, extension of the knee causes pain and neck flexion), and Brudzinski's sign (with the patient supine, flexion of the neck causes spontaneous flexion of the hip and knee); focus on whether there is hemiparesis, brainstem abnormalities (particularly of the pupils, eye movements (spontaneous or elicited), the breathing pattern, or other focal signs.

It should be possible to classify comatose patients into one of four groups (which may overlap):

1. Diffuse encephalopathy (i.e., a reduction in consciousness) with no focal neurologic signs. If the patient is febrile or has a history of fever, think of CNS infection (e.g., cerebral malaria) or a metabolic cause of coma (e.g., diabetic coma, drugs, toxins) with secondary infection such as aspiration pneumonia
2. Encephalopathy with meningism (neck stiffness, or positive Kernig's sign). If the patient is febrile, a CNS infection (especially bacterial meningitis) is likely, but subarachnoid hemorrhages or posterior fossa vascular disorders should also be considered, especially if the onset was sudden
3. Encephalopathy with lateralizing neurologic signs (e.g., hemiparesis). This often indicates supratentorial focal damage; think of abscess, tuberculoma, meningitis with a subdural collection, stroke, or if the history is more insidious, tumor
4. Encephalopathy with brainstem signs. This may indicate pathology within the brainstem itself (caused, for example, by a local infection) or herniation of the brainstem secondary to raised intracranial pressure due to any of the preceding causes.

Laboratory Investigations

Examination of the cerebrospinal fluid is the single most important investigation for diagnosis of a CNS infection. In industrialized nations, if a patient has deep coma or focal neurologic signs, a computed tomographic (CT) scan is usually performed before a lumbar puncture to ensure there is no intracranial abscess or other significant type of raised intracranial pressure, since if there is incipient herniation of the brain stem, a lumbar puncture can worsen this situation. However, if CT scanning is not readily available, particularly in patients with deep coma or focal neurologic signs, the benefits of a lumbar puncture in terms of obtaining an accurate diagnosis are often felt to outweigh the risks.[2]

A definitive diagnosis may require radiographic confirmation of a neurologic lesion with skull or sinus films, CT scans, magnetic resonance imaging (MRI) or angiographic studies, myelography, electroencephalography (EEG), electromyography (EMG), nerve conduction studies, or histologic study of muscle biopsy specimens. Infections such as bacterial meningitis can be confirmed by Gram's stain and culture of the infecting organisms obtained from CSF, though pretreatment with antibiotics before patients come to hospital is common. In suspected bacterial meningitis, treatment should not be delayed because a lumbar puncture cannot be performed quickly. Blood cultures should be obtained regardless of whether a lumbar puncture is performed, since they may reveal the cause of the meningitis. Parasitic infection may be confirmed by examination of blood films, sputum, stool, or in some cases, CSF obtained for the identification of adult parasites, larvae, or ova. Serologic studies of peripheral blood or CSF can be useful in confirming certain bacterial or viral infections. Simple rapid diagnostic kits are becoming available for a variety of infections. Many viral CNS infections are now diagnosed by using the polymerase chain reaction, particularly encephalitis caused by herpes simplex virus.

SYNDROME-BASED DIAGNOSIS

Syndrome-based differential diagnosis is a convenient way to organize the large number of neurologic infections encountered in tropical medicine. Box 130-1 and Table 130-1 present detailed information on the diagnosis of parasitic infections of the CNS.[3–6]

Meningitides

The various forms of meningitis usually present with fever, headache, photophobia, mental confusion, or seizures. Physical examination shows a febrile patient with neck stiffness on flexion and other indications of meningeal irritation. Signs of raised intracranial pressure, such as papilledema, may be found in some. For infants and very young children, signs of meningeal irritation may not be obvious, and it may present with either seizures in the setting of fever, mildly impaired consciousness or drowsiness, and occasionally a bulging anterior fontanel. Acute bacterial meningitis generally has a rapid onset and progression. In the tropics, meningococcal meningitis usually occurs in epidemics, affecting mainly children and young adults living within arid geographic regions such as sub-Saharan Africa.[7]

Pneumococcal meningitis can present with markedly raised intracranial pressure and coma. It usually occurs in adults and is particularly common in patients with sickle cell hemoglobinopathy, HIV infection, and functional or anatomic asplenia. *Haemophilus influenzae* meningitis occurs in unvaccinated children or older adults and is associated commonly with seizures linked with fever in children. Complications of bacterial meningitis include cranial nerve palsies, deafness, and subdural effusion in children. The presentations of viral meningitis are typically less fulminant or severe; the infection is commonly due to enteroviruses, such as poliovirus or echovirus. In recent years, there have been large outbreaks of human enterovirus 71 causing aseptic meningitis, and other CNS complications, in the Asia Pacific area.[8]

Subacute and chronic meningitis due to CNS tuberculosis, fungi, or late chronic neurosyphilis have a less fulminant onset and a slow disease progression.[9] However, aseptic meningitis in secondary syphilis mimics acute viral disease and additionally may cause cranial nerve palsies, particularly in HIV-infected patients. In the early phase of tuberculous meningitis, symptoms may be vague with complaints of headache, insomnia, and body pains. Unless there is a high level of suspicion, the diagnosis could be missed at an early stage of the disease, particularly in adults. Later stages are associated with cranial nerve palsies due to basilar meningitis, though presentations with dementia are not unknown. Characteristically, chronic inflammation occurring at the base of the brain also entraps cerebral blood vessels and may lead to vascular compromise and stroke. Hemiplegia is a potential outcome. Focal tuberculous infections (tuberculomas) present as mass lesions and may be mistaken for brain tumors.[10]

Parasitic disease such as acute amebic meningoencephalitis usually presents with features similar to acute bacterial meningitis but with an associated characteristic olfactory involvement based on presumed entry of the organism through the cribriform plate.[11] Seizures and coma rapidly progress in this disease, even in previously healthy persons. *Naegleria fowleri,* the causative organism, is found in warm, freshwater streams and pools, and obtaining a history of such exposure is highly relevant. Motile flagellated amebic trophozoites may be identified during microscopic examination of a wet CSF preparation. *Acanthamoeba* species are more commonly identified as causative organisms in debilitated, immunosuppressed persons, usually producing a subacute or chronic encephalitis. Angiostrongyliasis and gnathostomiasis may cause eosinophilic meningitis, as well as multiple brain abscesses with focal neurologic signs. Strongyloidiasis occurs in specific populations of immunosuppressed persons such as patients given corticosteroids, transplant recipients, or those infected with human T-cell lymphotropic virus type I (HTLV-I). Paragonimiasis may involve the CNS in young children with severe consequences of chronic meningoencephalitis. Trichinosis occasionally involves the CNS, causing seizures, meningoencephalitis, or hemorrhagic infarction from larval invasion of the microvasculature. Cerebral edema and death from brainstem herniation may occur.[3]

Encephalopathies

Encephalopathy means a reduction in consciousness level, and when this is due to inflammation of the brain substance, the term encephalitis is used. The signs and symptoms of encephalitis include headache, lethargy, stupor, delirium, seizures, hyperreflexia, and spasticity with a positive Babinski sign. Coma and

Box 130-1 Tropical Infections and Infectious Disease with Major Neurologic Presentations

Meningitides and Meningoencephalitides

- Acute bacterial meningitis
  - *Haemophilius influenzae* type b meningitis
  - Meningococcal meningitis
  - Pneumococcal meningitis
  - *Listeria monocytogenes* meningitis
- Subacute bacterial meningitis
  - Secondary syphilis with asceptic meningitis
  - Borreliosis
- Tuberculous meningitis
- Fungal meningitis
  - *Candida* spp. meningitis
  - Coccidioidal meningitis
  - Cryptococcal meningitis
- Viral meningitides and meningoencephalitides
  - Cytomegalovirus
  - Epstein-Barr virus
  - Enteroviruses
  - Mumps virus
  - Herpes simplex and varicella-zoster viruses
  - Human immunodeficiency virus
  - Arboviruses (e.g., Japanese B encephalitis virus)
  - Rabies
  - Rubeola

Postviral and Postimmunization Meningoencephalitides

- Measles, rubella, varicella-zoster
- Measles vaccine, rabies vaccine, yellow fever vaccine

Parasitic Meningitides and Meningoencephalitides

- Amebic meningoencephalitis (*Naegleria* and *Acanthamoeba* spp.)
- Strongyloidiasis
- Paragonimiasis
- *Angiostrongylus cantonensis*
- *Gnathostoma spinigerum*
- Trichinosis
- *Toxocara canis* (visceral and ocular larva migrans)
- Trypanosomiasis
  - *Trypanosoma gambiense*
  - *Trypanosoma rhodesiense*
- *Loa loa* (filarial)

Brain Abscesses

- Bacterial (also causing subdural empyema and epidural abscess)
  - Anaerobic bacteria (e.g., mouth flora)
  - Gram-negative enteric and nosocomial organisms
  - *Streptococcus intermedius*
  - Staphylococci
- Fungal
  - Immunologically normal host
    - Coccidioidomycosis
  - Immunologically impaired host
    - Aspergillosis
    - Candidiasis
    - Zygomycosis (e.g., mucormycosis in diabetic ketoacidosis)
- Parasitic mass lesion of the central nervous system (CNS)
  - Cysticercosis
  - Echinococcus (hydatid cysts)
  - Schistosomiasis (*Schistosoma japonicum*)
  - Amebiasis (*Entamoeba histolytica*)
  - Toxoplasmosis

Infections with Minimal CNS Inflammation

- Borreliosis
- Brucellosis
- Ehrlichiosis
- Leptospirosis
- Malaria
- Rickettsial infections

Infections Producing Brain Stem and Spinal Cord Syndromes

- Bacterial
  - Spinal epidural abscess
- Viral
  - Human T-cell lymphotropic virus type I–associated tropical spastic paraplegia
  - Poliomyelitis
  - Rabies
- Parasitic
  - *Diphyllobothrium latum* (megaloblastic anemia, vitamin B_{12} deficiency)
  - *Dracunculus medinensis*
  - Schistosomiasis (*Schistosoma mansoni* and *Schistosoma haematobium*)
  - Paragonimiasis

Infections Involving the Peripheral Nerves and Muscles

- Leprosy
  - Acute inflammatory polyneuropathy
  - Viruses (e.g., Epstein-Barr virus, varicella, etc)
  - Bacteria (e.g., *Campylobacter*)
- Toxin-mediated
  - Tetanus
  - Botulism
- Muscle infection
  - Trichinosis
  - Tropical pyomyositis
  - Diabetes-associated and human immunodeficiency virus–associated pyomyositis
  - Necrotizing fasciitis

signs of raised intracranial pressure may be present. There may be clinical clues to the particular virus; for example, tremors, rigidity spasms, and other movement disorders suggest involvement of the basal ganglia, which is often seen in encephalitis caused by flaviviruses such as Japanese encephalitis virus and West Nile virus.[12] Alphaviruses such as Eastern equine encephalitis can cause a similar syndrome.

In herpes simplex type 1 encephalitis, a focal neurologic disorder of the temporal lobe is almost always documented on brain imaging, and characteristic periodic complexes are often observed in the EEG. In African trypanosomiasis, somnolence alternating with insomnia is characteristic, and these patients have a course that evolves to manifestations of abnormal movement and gait, total indifference, and eventually stupor.[13]

Table 130-1 Parasitic Infections of the Central Nervous System

	Distribution	Exposure	Major Manifestations
Protozoan			
Toxoplasma gondii	Worldwide	Rare meat, cat feces	Focal findings, occasionally diffuse encephalopathy, meningoencephalitis in immunocompromised hosts
Plasmodium falciparum malaria	Tropics	Female *Anopheles* mosquitoes	Coma, obtundation, personality changes, movement disorders, focal findings (cerebrospinal fluid usually unremarkable)
Entamoeba histolytica	Worldwide	Fecal-oral	Brain abscess
PAM and GAE			
Naegleria fowleri	Worldwide	Freshwater lakes (nasal, via cribriform plate)	Fulminant and rapidly fatal
Acanthamoeba spp.	Worldwide	Brackish warm water (respiratory, eyes, skin)	Chronic granulomatous necrotizing encephalitis in immunocompromised hosts
Balamuthia mandrillaris	Peru, Venezuela, Mexico	?River	Meningoencephalitis
Helminthic			
Neurocysticercosis (*Taenia solium*)	Worldwide	Fecal-oral (ova) (pork meat tapeworm only)	Seizures, hydrocephalic meningitis, cord lesions
Echinococcosis (hydatid disease)			
Echinococcus granulosus	South-central Europe, Middle East, South America, Africa, Australia, New Zealand	Fecal-oral from dogs, foxes, etc.	Fewer, larger cysts
Echinococcus multilocularis	North America		
Echinococcus vogeli	South and Central America		Invasive polycystic disease (extramedullary >brain)
Trichinella spiralis	Worldwide	Rare pork, bear, horse meat	Focal infections, inflammation, infarction, or hemorrhage
Strongyloides stercoralis	Worldwide	Skin, autoinfection	Immunosuppression causes hematogenous spread of larvae causing brain abscesses, microinfarcts, granuloma formation, or meningitis
Schistosoma japonicum	Orient, Southeast Asia	Swimming in freshwater containing infected snails	Encephalitis, seizures, focal findings
Schistosoma haematobium	Africa, South America		Myelopathy, seizures
Schistosoma mansoni	Asia, Africa, Latin America		Rare cord compression, spinal artery occlusion, myelitis
Paragonimus westermani	Asia	Eating raw freshwater crustaceans	"Soap-bubble" central nervous system (CNS) calcifications with cavitary lung lesions, occasional seizures, meningitis, focal findings
Paragonimus mexicanus	Costa Rica	Crustaceans	Focal CNS hemorrhage
Helminthic causes of eosinophilic meningitis:			
Angiostrongylus cantonensis	Southeast Asia	Freshwater crustaceans (infected from domestic rat)	Usually self-limited meningitis
Gnathostoma spinigerum	Southeast Asia	Freshwater fish, frogs, snakes, and paratenic poultry, ducks	Meningitis with residual neurologic deficits (45%)
Toxocara canis	Worldwide	Pica, puppy feces	Rare meningoencephalitis
Baylisascaris procyonis	Worldwide	Tree bark contaminated by raccoon feces	Rare meningoencephalitis

GAE, granulomatous amebic encephalitis; PAM, primary amebic meningoencephalitis.

Cerebral malaria is a complication of severe *Plasmodium falciparum* infection and is particularly common in children and pregnant women living in endemic areas.[14] Cerebral malaria often rapidly progresses to seizures and coma in febrile patients who go undiagnosed.[15] Prevention is of particular importance for nonimmune adult visitors, who are at even greater risk for this complication of severe malaria. They must receive prophylaxis or presumptive therapy that covers potentially resistant strains of *P. falciparum.* Severe malaria may also cause hypoglycemia and mimic the early symptoms of cerebral malaria. Quinine administration can accentuate this problem by enhancing insulin release from the pancreas and contributing to hypoglycemia.

Postimmunization and Postinfectious Encephalitides

Postimmunization encephalitis has occurred following immunization against yellow fever or rabies, especially in the past when earlier vaccines were utilized.[16] Newer vaccines produced from cell culture are less likely to cause such complications. Postviral encephalitis is well described following measles vaccination in older children. It is characterized by a reduced level of consciousness and multifocal neurologic signs, including hemiparesis and paraparesis.

Brain Abscess and Other Intracranial Mass Lesions

Brain abscess presents with features of raised intracranial pressure, seizure disorders, and focal neurologic deficits but not necessarily with fevers. Brain abscesses are often caused by mixed anaerobic bacteria, but gram-negative organisms are commonly isolated after middle ear or sinus infections and trauma. Hematogenous dissemination of bacteria such as *Staphylococcus aureus* to the CNS may also result in staphylococcal brain abscess formation. Subdural empyema may present with headache, fever, altered mental status, seizures, nuchal rigidity, and focal neurologic deficits. Most subdural empyemas occur as a consequence of contiguous spread from sinusitis, otitis media, or mastoiditis. Rupture of a CNS tuberculoma to produce meningitis is particularly common in the tropics, and there may be coexistent reactivation of pulmonary tuberculosis.

Neurocysticercosis may produce cystic parenchymal lesions and also causes chronic inflammation of the subarachnoid space with resultant hydrocephalus. Amebic brain abscess from *Entamoeba histolytica* occurs generally in a setting of disseminated disease with concomitant liver abscess. Paragonimiasis can produce mass lesions, chronic meningitis, cerebral infarction, and hemorrhage. Hydatid cyst disease causes local inflammation as well as mechanical obstruction of CSF flow with resulting hydrocephalus.

It is useful to characterize some of the more common clinical scenarios associated with parasitic infections of the CNS, since these syndromes often generate requests for tropical medicine consultation from other practitioners. It is relatively easy to produce a rather long list of diagnostic possibilities when a patient comes in with what appears to be a possible mass lesion of the CNS, but discerning one entity from another on a clinical basis in order to direct the remainder of the diagnostic workup is a challenging task for any consultant. The following clinical paradigms can be considered in sorting out just such cases when they present for evaluation.

Neurocysticercosis

Neurocysticercosis often presents with a new seizure disorder.[17] In the developing world, cysticercosis is one of the most common causes of seizures. In the tropics, patients are often children, who suffer concomitant injuries, such as burns, when seizures occur near open fires.

Pork ingestion is not necessary for the development of cysticercosis. Human ingestion of the ova produced by pork tapeworms poses the threat of neurocysticercosis. Most commonly, the disease is acquired by ingestion of ova that contaminate foodstuffs grown in soil. Rarely, the source of these ova can be the patients themselves, who may have previously acquired pork tapeworm infection by eating undercooked pork containing the larvae of *Taenia solium*. The ova passed in their stools are produced by adult tapeworms and are potentially infectious to both themselves (autoinfection) and others in the immediate household environment. Within communities of the developed world, where food may be prepared by *T. solium*–infected persons who have recently migrated from endemic areas, employers and families are at risk of acquiring this disease.

Larvae-containing cysticerci infecting the CNS do not result in any single disease pattern. The clinical presentation depends on the intensity of infection; the number, size, and localization of cysts; and the intensity of the immunologic responses to their presence. The cysts expand slowly, and larvae within these cysts eventually die. Inflammation follows, sometimes associated with seizures. The lesions ultimately calcify. If an intraventricular cyst suddenly blocks the flow of CSF, causing obstructive hydrocephalus, rapid deterioration or death may occur. Ocular infections (which may occur in about 20% of cases) should be ruled out before the institution of any antiparasitic therapy to prevent further irreparable ocular damage from additional inflammatory responses. If evidence of ocular infection is present, corticosteroids should be administered prior to the antiparasitic agent.

In the diagnostic workup of patients with suspected neurocysticercosis, CT and MRI have enhanced our ability to diagnose these disorders and have delineated different patterns of disease in adults and children. Adults from an endemic area are more likely to have older calcified lesions, which show very little contrast enhancement on CT scanning. These patients generally will *not* have demonstrable *Taenia* ova in their stools. In contrast, children are more likely to have acute lesions with contrast enhancement secondary to host inflammatory responses. These reactions represent immune responses to degeneration of the parasites themselves and account for the acute presentations with seizures. The therapeutic decisions surrounding the use of antiparasitic agents, and the potential use of corticosteroids during treatment of acute lesions, are based on these differences.

Echinococcosis (Hydatid Disease)

Although echinococcosis is also characterized by cystic lesions of the CNS, which can be difficult to distinguish from those of cysticercosis, the epidemiology of human infections and clinical presentations differ considerably from those of neurocysticercosis. Echinococcal cysts tend to be larger and fewer in number, and unlike cysticercosis, echinococcal cysts are not usually found in cerebral parenchyma. They are more likely to infect and destroy vertebral bone, resulting in spinal cord compression from their continuous expansion. Hydatid disease of the CNS only occurs in 1% to 2% of human echinococcosis cases, and CNS infections are more common in children. Compression of the spinal cord is the most common CNS manifestation of this disease.

When children or adults with CNS echinococcosis also have a history of contact with dogs or sheep in areas endemic for this disease, the diagnosis of hydatid disease should be considered. The sequence of infection first involves one of several species of cestodes of the genus *Echinococcus* infecting carnivores, such as dogs. Within the canine gastrointestinal tract, the parasites grow into adult tapeworms, and humans become infected by accidental ingestion of ova excreted by the infected dog, as in the case of the most common species of parasite infecting humans, *Echinococcus granulosus*.

CT scanning or MRI is useful for demonstrating typical extramedullary cord compression and vertebral involvement. As serologic diagnosis becomes more sensitive and specific, a positive antibody titer in conjunction with a typical appearance of cysts on CT scanning or MRI, or vertebral radiographs demonstrating osseous lesions and the appearance of motheaten vertebrae, with a supportive epidemiologic history, should suggest the diagnosis once spinal cord and vertebral involvement by large cystic lesions is confirmed.

Cerebral Paragonimiasis

The pulmonary presentation of infections with the lung fluke *Paragonimus westermani* is easily mistaken for tuberculosis. The appearance of multiple cavitary lesions in a young patient with chronic hemoptysis and CNS symptoms mimics the spread of pulmonary tuberculosis to the CNS associated with tuberculous meningitis. This picture can be even more confusing when the disease occurs in a population that has a high incidence of positive tuberculin skin test reactivity.

However, when a patient is from an endemic area for paragonimiasis, such as Southeast Asia, where crustaceans or their juices are commonly eaten raw, there is the potential for the complex life cycle of this parasite to involve the human host. Children are particularly susceptible to ectopic cerebral infections with these migrating flukes, particularly if infected early in life, since most cerebral infections occur before 10 years of age. The most common neurologic symptoms include seizure disorders, headache, and visual disturbances; the majority of patients in various clinical series of cerebral paragonimiasis have abnormal eye findings. They include impaired visual acuity, homonymous hemianopsia, optic atrophy, papilledema, nystagmus, and pupillary abnormalities.

A clue to the presence of cerebral paragonimiasis may often be found in plain skull films obtained on patients who have cerebral infection with the adult lung flukes. As the ectopic adult flukes degenerate, skull films may show punctate or nodular calcifications, or even advanced lesions with a "soap-bubble" appearance. *Paragonimus* ova can be found in sputum, feces, pleural and peritoneal fluid, or biopsy tissue.

Hence, any clinical presentation that suggests chronic cavitary pulmonary tuberculosis in a young patient with apparent CNS infection, and particularly ocular involvement, might lead to further questioning to obtain the appropriate epidemiologic data indicating that the patient had been at risk for paragonimiasis. Radiologic evaluation with skull films or CT scanning, observation of typical ova, and confirmatory serologic testing aid in diagnosis.

Several patterns of parasitic infections of the CNS lead to rapid consideration of other potential parasitic causes of CNS infections. Patients with intestinal *amebiasis* caused by *E. histolytica* generally do *not* develop a brain abscess unless there is a generalized and disseminated amebic infection. It is extremely unusual to have an amebic brain abscess develop without an antecedent liver abscess in patients with amebiasis. Even in the presence of an amebic liver abscess, the incidence of brain abscess is usually less than 10%.

Prior to the current acquired immunodeficiency syndrome (AIDS) pandemic, abscess formation due to *Toxoplasma gondii* infection was rare. It was most likely to occur as reactivation of a latent *Toxoplasma* infection in a compromised host receiving chemotherapy for a disease such as lymphoma, which compromised cell-mediated immunity. However, with the emergence of AIDS, toxoplasmosis became the most common opportunistic CNS infection early in the epidemic, and it has been documented in at least 25% of patients. Because the organisms are sensitive to folic acid antagonists, which are now the drugs of choice for prophylaxis against *Pneumocystis carinii* pulmonary infections, the incidence of *Toxoplasma* reactivation has diminished considerably. Previously infected but asymptomatic patients not receiving prophylaxis, whose HIV infections are not under intensive therapy and who present with multiple ring-enhancing lesions on CT scanning or MRI, are likely to have reactivated this infection.

Many anticipated that the AIDS pandemic would result in large numbers of patients chronically infected with *Strongyloides stercoralis* succumbing to disseminated infections. Filariform larvae reach the CNS via hematogenous spread and would occlude small vessels, resulting in microinfarcts, abscesses, or bacterial meningitis (from carriage of bacteria within the larvae). In some cases, the larvae traverse the perivascular spaces to cause granuloma formation in the meninges or parenchyma, as they have in immunocompromised patients such as transplant recipients. To date, this has not been a major problem, with only about 20 such instances described. However, clinicians should be aware of the increasing recognition of disseminated *Strongyloides* infections that occur together with HTLV-I infections and their associated lymphomas. The presence of disseminated strongyloidiasis in a patient with HIV infections should lead to a consideration of potential coinfection with HTLV-I.

Infections Involving the Brainstem and Spinal Cord

These infections cause paraparesis, paraplegia, or tetraparesis and occasionally cranial nerve dysfunction. In acute transverse myelitis associated with viral infections, fever, backache, leg weakness, sensory disturbances, and sphincter dysfunction may occur. During the acute phase of illness, flaccid paralysis, with absent or reduced tendon reflexes, is observed. Spasticity and hyperactive tendon reflexes occur later in the course of the disease. A sensory level is usually identified at the involved level of the cord. Transverse myelitis may be a nonspecific complication following a number of viral infections. However, some viruses specifically attack the anterior horn cells of the spinal cord to confer an acute flaccid paralysis in which there may be few sensory symptoms and signs. Poliovirus is the classic cause of this syndrome, but other enteroviruses (e.g., human enterovirus 71) and flaviviruses (e.g., Japanese encephalitis and West Nile virus) can also cause a polio-like syndrome.[18]

Cord compression from an epidural abscess produces similar symptoms and signs to transverse myelitis, but MRI or myelography demonstrates evidence of the cord compression. Most patients with a spinal epidural abscess present with focal spinal back pain aching or tenderness at the level of infection, followed by nerve root pain radiating from the spinal level of involvement. Subsequently, paraparesis with bladder involvement may progress to complete paraplegia.

In spinal tuberculosis, granulomatous arachnoiditis may arise at any level and subsequently cause radiculomyelopathy. Patients present with a combination of nerve root and cord compression. Tuberculous granulomatous masses or abscess formation may be confined to the epidural space and produce cord compression. However, involvement of vertebral bodies, that is, tuberculous spondylitis, may lead to vertebral collapse with spinal cord compression. *Schistosoma mansoni* and *Schistosoma haematobium* may also cause true granulomatous inflammation of the spinal cord associated with spastic paraplegia and anesthetic sensory levels.[19]

Tropical spastic paraplegia is common in some parts of the tropics, such as Jamaica or southern Japan, where HTLV-I infections are more common, and can evolve into a chronic inflammatory disease of the spinal cord. This is a slowly progressive paraparesis with both increased tendon reflexes and Babinski signs, sphincter dysfunction, and sensory impairment. Paraparesis has been reported in paralytic (dumb) rabies, varicella-zoster infections, and herpes simplex myelitis.

Infections Affecting Peripheral Nerves and Muscles

Acute Paralysis

Acute inflammatory polyneuropathy (Guillain-Barré syndrome) occurs in children and adults following a wide variety of microbial infections; examples include Epstein-Barr virus, other herpesviruses, and bacteria-causing enteritis, such as *Campylobacter jejuni.* Symmetric weakness of the lower limbs progresses rapidly to involve the upper limbs and later the trunk and the intercostal, cervical, and cranial nerves. Weakness progresses to paralysis and absent tendon reflexes. Disturbances of autonomic functions may occur. In botulism, the clostridial toxins interfere with release of acetylcholine at the neuromuscular junction and cause acute paralysis.[20] Botulism frequently, but not always, produces diplopia and failure of pupillary constriction, which are rarely seen in the Guillain-Barré syndrome. Diphtheria presents as an acute flaccid paralysis weeks to months after a patient has recovered from the acute illness.[21] It is more common in those whose acute illness was severe, with myocarditis, but can occur in patients whose initial illness was so mild they did not seek medical attention; such cases will be diagnosed only by taking a careful history about a preceding sore throat.

Chronic Neuropathy

Gradually evolving neuropathy in tropical countries is often due to leprosy, a result of direct invasion of nerves by *Mycobacterium leprae.* In tuberculoid leprosy, where few organisms are present in nerves, patches of superficial sensory loss and granulomatous enlargement of subcutaneous nerves, such as the ulnar, median, peroneal, posterior auricular, and facial nerves, occur in association with sensory or motor deficits. In lepromatous leprosy, lack of resistance to intracellular bacterial growth causes widespread mycobacterial invasion of cutaneous sensory nerves and a symmetrical pattern of pain and temperature loss with anesthesia involving most of the cutaneous surfaces. Since small sensory fibers are predominantly involved, tendon reflexes are usually preserved, but anesthesia leads to widespread tissue injuries and trophic changes that result from loss of innervation.

Myositis and Other Muscle Diseases

In tetanus, persistent spasms of the skeletal muscles occur owing to the effects of tetanus toxin on the normally inhibitory spinal neurons (e.g., Renshaw cells) which usually function to inhibit the activity of motor neurons.[22] Reflex muscle spasm occurs in response to various visual, tactile, or auditory stimuli. Spontaneous muscle spasms occur in severe cases, and death from respiratory arrest or laryngeal spasm may occur. In trichinosis parasitic muscle invasion causes deposition of larvae in muscle with considerable muscle pain, periorbital edema, and eosinophilia. Staphylococci and streptococci can directly invade muscle to cause bacterial myositis, often a disease of patients with diabetes mellitus but which is now being seen more frequently in association with HIV infection.

THERAPEUTIC APPROACHES

Initial Approach

The initial approaches to emergent problems are outlined in Table 130-2.

Table 130-2 Initial Approaches to Emergent Problems in Patients with Neurologic Dysfunction

Problem	Approach
Suspected bacterial meningitides	Location- and age-specific appropriate empirical antibiotic therapy
Increased intracranial pressure	Mannitol 0.25 g/kg; hyperventilation to $PaCO_2$ near 30 torr; corticosteroids (e.g., dexamethasone 10 mg)
Shock	Intravenous fluid support (e.g., saline) and vasopressor support (e.g., norepinephrine, phenylephrine, epinephrine)
Seizures or status epilepticus	If acute treatment required, begin with an intravenous benzodiazepine (e.g., lorazepam or clonazepam), followed by intravenous phenytoin 20 mg/kg
Acute paraplegia or quadriplegia	Consider high-dose methylprednisolone 30 mg/kg
Acute respiratory failure	Endotracheal intubation and mechanical ventilation; if elevated ICP is suspected, premedicate with either intravenous lidocaine 1.0 to 1.5 mg/kg or thiopental 3 to 5 mg/kg

ICP, intracranial pressure; $PaCO_2$, arterial carbon dioxide tension.

Specific Conditions

In *meningitis,* appropriate treatment with antibiotics should be started immediately to minimize neurologic complications and should not be delayed to await imaging studies. The choice of empirical antibiotics depends on the age of the patient, the clinical features, the CSF Gram's stain, and current local epidemiologic factors. The most commonly utilized antibiotic agents include penicillins and second- or third-generation cephalosporins. In children, dexamethasone is often given intravenously (0.6 mg/kg/day) to reduce inflammation, though they were shown to have no benefit in one study in Africa.[23] In *tuberculous meningitis,* corticosteroids are used to minimize complications arising from chronic inflammation and arachnoiditis, particularly at the base of the brain, and have recently been shown to reduce the risk of death.[24] In an accessible *brain abscess,* CT- or MRI-guided aspiration and antibiotics are the treatment of choice. Anaerobic coverage is usually indicated, since mixed anaerobic infections are often the cause of such abscesses and may not be recovered from the abscess for technical reasons. Surgical drainage and excision of the abscess cavity may be necessary when aspiration is not feasible or is contraindicated. Long-term therapy with antibiotics is usual and in rare cases may be the only treatment required.

In *cerebral malaria,* intravenous antimalarials, such as quinine or quinidine, are often used, though drugs such as artemether, based on the Chinese herb qinghaosu, are being used increasingly.[25] Concomitant glucose infusions are important in preventing drug-induced hypoglycemia, which could easily be confused with cerebral malaria. In *cerebral neurocysticercosis,* both oral praziquantel and albendazole treatment are effective in reducing the number and size of brain cysts. Adjunctive treatment is largely symptomatic; *epilepsy* is treated with anticonvulsants, *hydrocephalus* by ventricular shunting, and *cerebral edema* with dexamethasone. *Postinfection* or *postimmunization encephalomyelitis* usually responds incompletely to corticosteroids. *Acute paraplegia* resulting from transverse myelitis due to viral infections or specifically, HTLV-I, may respond to treatment with corticosteroids. *Tuberculous radiculomyelitis* responds to antituberculous chemotherapy, but *psoas abscess* or *vertebral collapse* may also require drainage, laminectomy, and decompression of the spinal cord. *Tetanus* is treated with tetanus immunoglobulin to neutralize the toxin, metronidazole, wound treatment to kill the causative bacteria, and large doses of intravenous benzodiazepines to relax the involved muscles. In severe cases, tracheostomy, neuromuscular junction blockade, and mechanical ventilation may be necessary.

Whatever the cause of CNS infection, in addition to treating the specific condition attention should be paid to the nonspecific complications and sequelae. In particular, secondary pneumonias are common in patients with reduced consciousness; bedsores, spasticity, and contractures are problems in patients bed-bound for any length of time. Good nursing care and physiotherapy can make an enormous difference to the eventual outcome.

REFERENCES

1. Fadiman A: The spirit catches you and you fall down: A Hmong child, her American doctors, and the collision of two cultures. New York, Farrar, Straus & Giroux, 1998.
2. Shakir RA, Newman PK, Poser CM (eds): Tropical Neurology. London, WB Saunders, 1996.
3. Patterson TF, Patterson JE, Barry M, et al: Parasitic infections of the central nervous system. In Schlossberg D (ed): Infections of the Nervous System. New York, Springer-Verlag, 1990, pp 234–261.
4. Bia FJ: Parasitic diseases of the nervous system. Semin Neurol 13:131–237, 1993.
5. Scaravilli F: Tropical diseases: a historical perspective. Brain Pathol 7:561–711, 1997.
6. Reed RP, Cooke-Yarborough CM, Jaquiery AL, et al: Fatal granulomatous amoebic encephalitis caused by *Balamuthia mandrillaris.* Med J Aust 167:82–84, 1997.
7. Gray F: Bacterial infections. Brain Pathol 7:629–648, 1997.
8. McMinn PC: An overview of the evolution of enterovirus 71 and its clinical and public health significance. FEMS Microbiol Rev 26:91–107, 2002.
9. Chimelli L, Maher-Araújo MB: Fungal infections. Brain Pathol 7:613–628, 1997.
10. Danesi MA, Arigbabu SO, Mordi PN, et al: Intracranial tuberculoma in Lagos, Nigeria. Trop Geogr Med 37:279–280, 1985.
11. Martinez AJ, Visvesvara GS: Free-living, amphizoic, and opportunistic amebas. Brain Pathol 7:583–598, 1997.
12. Solomon T: Current Concepts—Flavivirus encephalitis. N Engl J Med 351:370–378, 2004.
13. Chimelli L, Scaravilli F: Trypanosomiasis. Brain Pathol 7:599–612, 1997.
14. Hamer DH, Wyler DJ: Cerebral malaria. Semin Neurol 13:180–188, 1993.
15. Turner G: Cerebral malaria. Brain Pathol 7:569–582, 1997.
16. Bleck TP, Rupprecht CE: Rhabdoviruses. In Richman DD, Whitley RJ, Hayden FG (eds): Clinical Virology, 2nd ed. Washington, DC, ASM Press, 2002, pp 857–873.
17. de Bittencourt PR, Adamolekum B, Bharucha N, et al: Epilepsy in the tropics: 1. Epidemiology, socioeconomic risk factors, and etiology. Epilepsia 37:1121–1127, 1996.
18. Solomon T, Willison H: Infectious causes of acute flaccid paralysis. Curr Opin Infect Dis 16:375–381, 2003.
19. Pittella JEH: Neuroschistosomiasis. Brain Pathol 7:649–662, 1997.
20. Bleck TP: Clostridium botulinum. In Mandell GM, Bennett JE, Dolin R (eds): Principles and Practice of Infectious Diseases, 6th ed. New York, Churchill Livingstone, 2004, pp 2822–2828.
21. White NJ, Hien TT: Diphtheria. In Cook G (ed): Manson's Tropical Diseases, 20th ed. London, WB Saunders, 1996, pp 931–935.
22. Bleck TP, Brauner JS: Tetanus. In Scheld WM, Whitley RJ, Marra CM (eds): Infections of the Central Nervous System, 3rd ed. New York, Lippincott Williams & Wilkins, 2004, pp 625–648.
23. Molyneux EM, Walsh AL, Forsyth H, et al: Dexamethasone treatment in childhood bacterial meningitis in Malawi: A randomised controlled trial. Lancet 360:211–218, 2002.
24. Thwaites GE, Nguyen DB, Nguyen HD, et al: Dexamethasone for the treatment of tuberculous meningitis in adolescents and adults. N Engl J Med 351:1741–1751, 2004.
25. van Hensbroek MB, Onyiorah E, Jaffar S, et al: A trial of artemether or quinine in children with cerebral malaria. N Engl J Med 335:69–75, 1996.

131

Approach to the Patient in the Tropics with Anemia

GEOFFREY PASVOL
SAAD H. ABDALLA

INTRODUCTION

Anemia is a major problem in tropical areas largely because of interactions among three factors peculiar to these geographic regions[1–3]: (1) a high prevalence of infections and infestations capable of causing anemia, especially those caused by malaria, helminths, tuberculosis, and human immunodeficiency virus (HIV); (2) the common presence of dietary deficiencies; and (3) a high frequency of inherited red blood cell (RBC) disorders that result in anemia. Added to these adverse prevailing conditions is the scarcity or absence of resources for the investigation and treatment of anemia, which leads the practicing physician to place more reliance on observational and clinical skills rather than complex laboratory tests. This chapter outlines a rational approach to the diagnosis and management of anemia in these most challenging and diverse settings.

DEFINITION

Anemia can be defined simply as a hemoglobin (Hb) value below the reference range for age, sex, and ethnic origin. A reference range is normally determined for a given population using specific standardized and rigorous methods of measurement. In the case of tropical countries, reference ranges are difficult to define because of the common occurrence of concomitant disease and inherited RBC disorders. Ideally, a reference range should be established by measuring Hb in healthy volunteers not seeking medical help. The definition of a healthy volunteer is difficult in this setting because the perception of health is relative and because a definition that excludes asymptomatic subjects who may have a parasite infection or an inherited RBC disorder is difficult, especially under conditions in which these groups constitute a large proportion of the population.

The World Health Organization (WHO) has devised a definition of anemia[1]:

In children

- 6 months to 2 years, and Hb less than 11 g/dL
- 2 to 12 years, and Hb less than 12 g/dL

In adults

- 13 g/dL for males
- 12 g/dL for nonpregnant females
- 11 g/dL for pregnant females

A definition of anemia incorporated with a more practical approach for use in a tropical setting is shown in Table 131-1. In addition, consideration needs to be given as to whether these anemias develop acutely or over a more prolonged period (chronic). Acute anemias may demand more immediate intervention, such as blood transfusion, whereas compensatory mechanisms may render these interventions unnecessary in the chronic anemias.

PATHOPHYSIOLOGY

Anemia leads to a reduction in oxygen-carrying capacity and to a reduction in work performance of potentially important economic consequence to the individual and to society. Examples of the socioeconomic importance of anemia in the tropics have been well demonstrated using different methodologies in various settings involving, for example, sugar cutters in Guatemala,[4] latex tappers in Indonesia,[5] and tea pickers in Sri Lanka.[6] In all three examples, the reduction in work capacity was reversed by correction of the anemia. When more severe, anemia can lead to morbidity and sometimes death from heart failure.

The interactions between anemia, its treatment, and susceptibility to infection are complex and subject to controversy. A full description cannot be provided here, but three major arguments emerge[2]:

1. Anemia increases the risk of infection. This has been demonstrated in iron-deficient subjects by several epidemiologic and clinical studies. Other studies have also shown an increased incidence of infections (gastrointestinal, respiratory, and malaria) in subjects with megaloblastic anemia, but it can be argued that infected subjects utilize or lose folate more rapidly and the association is that of increased need in these subjects rather than increased susceptibility. Several studies have demonstrated a reduction in cell-mediated immunity in iron and in folate deficiency.[2]

Table 131-1 Practical Definition of Anemia Severity

Degree	Possible Consequences	Hb Level (g/dL)
Mild anemia	Minimal or no work or exercise intolerance	>10
Moderate anemia	Some impairment but still able to function	7–10
Severe anemia	Marked impairment of function but not at rest	4–7
Life-endangering anemia	Impending cardiac decompensation, dyspnea at rest	<4

2. Correction of anemia may have a deleterious effect on infection (i.e., the converse of No. 1). This concept has been put forward as a possible cause of exacerbation of malaria in malnourished patients when refed. This may be due to the resultant reticulocytosis, leading to an increase in the invasion of RBCs by parasites rather than a direct effect of replenishment of serum iron. Other factors may also play a role, such as the higher incidence of malaria and bacterial infections in refugees, which may be due to displacement and exposure to pathogens to which they have no immunity. The subject is complex, but for a review see Abdalla.[7]
3. Anemia may act as a nonspecific protective response to infection or perhaps be a by-product of that response. This view has been put forward in particular in the context of the anemia of chronic disease (ACD, anemia of inflammation, and secondary anemia). The inflammatory response to infection is important as a nonspecific protective mechanism but also results in ACD.[3]

In clinical practice, it is important to place the pathophysiology of anemia in perspective and to tailor investigations and treatment to the degree of anemia.

Box 131-1 Major Causes of Anemia in the Tropics

Infection/Infestation
Bacteria
  Severe acute or chronic bacterial sepsis
  Tuberculosis
Viruses
  Human immunodeficiency virus infection
  Parvovirus (in the presence of hemolytic anemia)
Protozoa
  Malaria
  Amebiasis
  Leishmaniasis
  Trypanosomiasis
Helminths
  Hookworm
  Schistosomiasis
  Trichuriasis

Dietary Deficiency
Iron deficiency
Folate deficiency
Vitamin B_{12} deficiency
Protein/calorie malnutrition

Inherited Disorders
Hemoglobinopathies
  Hemoglobin variants: Hb S, C, D, E, etc.
  α- and β-thalassemia
Red blood cell enzyme deficiency
  Glucose-6-phosphate dehydrogenase deficiency
Red blood cell membrane defects (minor decrease in Hb only)
  Elliptocytosis, spherocytosis
  Southeast Asian (band III) ovalocytosis

MECHANISM AND CLASSIFICATION OF ANEMIA

There are several ways that anemias can be classified. The three major etiologic factors in anemia in the tropics are (1) infections or infestations, (2) dietary deficiency, and (3) inherited disorders (Box 131-1). With some agents, pathogenesis may be multifactorial, as in HIV infection, ACD, and malaria. A more practical laboratory-oriented method is to classify anemias as to whether they are hypochromic and microcytic, normocytic, or macrocytic.

CLINICAL APPROACH

The recognition of severe anemia is often easy on clinical grounds. Iron deficiency and malaria are the two most common causes of anemia in the tropics. However, there are a number of important points in the history and clinical examination that often enable the clinician to further narrow the diagnostic possibilities.

History

The geographic locality is obviously important with regard to the prevalence of specific infections and infestations. Such information is particularly pertinent to malaria, hookworm infestation, tuberculosis, HIV infection, and other important but less frequently occurring causes of anemia, such as visceral leishmaniasis and trypanosomiasis. The physician also needs to know local dietary practices and information such as

- The hematinic, protein, and vitamin contents of common staple local foods and their seasonal variation and availability
- Local restrictive diets, such as vegetarianism and veganism
- The feeding practices for infants and young children (e.g., the age at weaning and the weaning foods)

The clinician needs to be aware of the local prevalence of Hb and other genetic RBC disorders, particularly the more common variants, such as sickle cell anemia (SCA), thalassemia, glucose-6-phosphate dehydrogenase (G6PD) deficiency, and RBC membrane defects (e.g., Southeast Asian ovalocytosis). Knowledge of the local epidemiology of malaria as well as drug-resistance patterns of this parasite is important.

A specific question that needs to be asked is whether the anemia has been present from birth, suggesting an inherited disorder, or is of recent onset. A detailed gastrointestinal history, particularly with regard to diet and abdominal pain, as well as the color and frequency of the stool, is important. A history of high fevers in the previous few weeks may suggest malaria. The anemia of malaria is particularly common in primigravidas and in children younger than the age of 5 years. Mild jaundice may be present in hemolytic conditions. It is important to determine whether the jaundice is intermittent and whether precipitating factors are present, as occurs in G6PD-deficient patients given oxidant drugs. A family history of anemia may be relevant. Bone and joint pains suggest sickling disorders. In women of childbearing age, it is particularly important to determine parity and previous menstrual history. HIV infection should be considered in those in relevant risk groups. People with HIV infection are susceptible to anemia, which may be exacerbated by drugs such as antifolates.[8]

Physical Examination

The clinical examination often yields little apart from pallor of the nail beds, palms, and mucous membranes of the mouth and conjunctivae. There may be other features that reveal an etiologic diagnosis. The presence of a high-grade fever in children is especially suggestive of malaria. Koilonychia (spoon-shaped nails) may suggest severe iron deficiency anemia, as may less commonly occurring esophageal and pharyngeal webs. Angular or atrophic stomatitis is most frequently seen in vitamin B_{12} or folate deficiency, but it is not specific and may occur in a variety of other vitamin deficiencies. Atrophic glossitis with mild jaundice may be observed in megaloblastic anemias. Hemolytic anemias are also associated with mild to moderate degrees of jaundice often exacerbated by infection but may be confused with viral hepatitis. Signs of peripheral neuropathy are suggestive of vitamin B_{12} deficiency.

Splenomegaly, especially in the presence of fever, is suggestive of acute malaria or typhoid fever. Varying splenomegaly occurs in a number of other conditions, including visceral leishmaniasis, hyperreactive malarial splenomegaly, hemoglobinopathies, thalassemia, and lymphomas. Associated features of HIV disease, including cachexia, oral candidiasis, generalized lymphadenopathy, and thrombocytopenia, may provide clues to this diagnosis.

The basic laboratory requirements for the diagnosis of anemia in the primary health care setting should include facilities to measure or carry out the following relatively simple tests:

1. Hb estimation using a spectrophotometric method will confirm the presence of anemia, quantitate the degree of severity according to the criteria described previously (see Table 131-1), and facilitate the monitoring of treatment.
2. Blood film examination is one of the most useful, relatively simple tests to carry out in the investigation of anemia, but it requires investment of two types: the acquisition of a microscope of reasonable quality with an adequate light source and a person with sufficient basic training capable of recognizing the more important common changes. Examination of blood smears (including a thick film) remains the gold standard in the diagnosis of malaria, identification of the infecting species, and assessment of the degree of parasitemia. Occasionally, trypanosomes, microfilariae, or spirochetes may be seen on the film. The thin blood film provides a starting point in the diagnostic algorithm because it can be used to divide anemia into a number of useful diagnostic categories:
   a. *Microcytic hypochromic anemia:* The RBCs are small or there is an increase in the normal area of central pallor in the cells (normal, up to one-third of the cell diameter). Microcytic hypochromic anemia is most commonly seen in iron deficiency (Fig. 131-1), thalassemia (Fig. 131-2), and, occasionally, ACD.
   b. *Normocytic, normochromic anemia* is often found in ACD, which in a tropical setting is most often due to infection rather than inflammatory or neoplastic conditions. It is also seen in acute blood loss, hypersplenism, certain hemolytic anemias, and anemias due to the underproduction of RBCs (e.g., aplastic anemia and bone marrow infiltration).
   c. *Macrocytic anemias* may be of two major types. Oval macrocytes and hypersegmented neutrophils (neutrophils with more than five lobes or 5% with five lobes) are suggestive of a megaloblastic anemia, such as vitamin B_{12} or folate deficiency, whereas round macrocytes without hypersegmented neutrophils occur in the nonmegaloblastic macrocytic anemias seen in alcoholism, liver disease, hypothyroidism, and other disorders (Fig. 131-3).

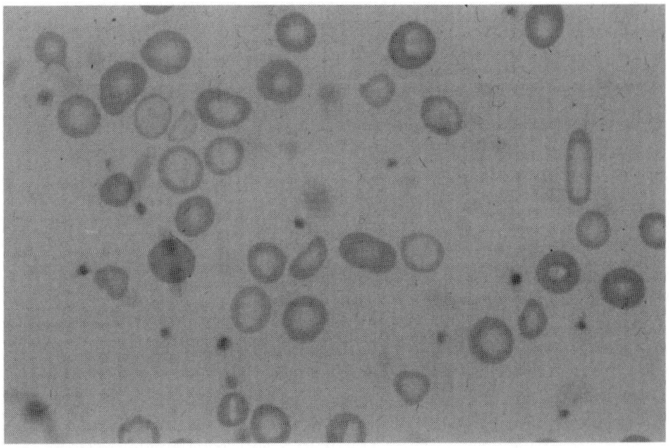

FIGURE 131-1 Severe iron deficiency anemia. Peripheral blood film obtained after partial treatment with oral iron. Note the population of normally hemoglobinized red blood cells and another with extreme hypochromia. Note also the single elongated red blood cell sometimes referred to as a "pencil cell."

Considerable additional practical information may be obtained from the blood film, such as the following:

   a. *Polychromasia:* The presence of polychromasia (diffuse bluish discoloration of the RBCs) correlates with the presence of reticulocytes. Polychromasia suggests that the marrow is responding appropriately to anemia in conditions such as hemorrhage, hemolysis, and hematinic replacement. The absence of polychromasia in the face of anemia suggests a dietary deficiency state or marrow suppression as a result of some other cause (e.g., infection or drugs).
   b. *Abnormal RBC shape:* Abnormally shaped RBCs may be found, such as sickle cells in SCA, spherocytes in spherocytosis, or irregularly contracted RBCs suggestive of oxidant damage as in acute hemolysis

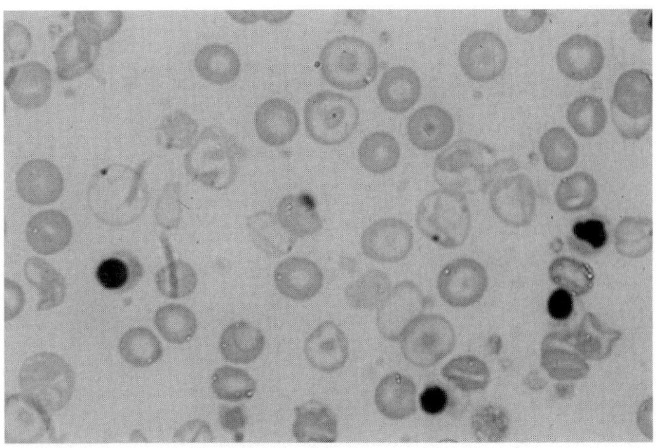

FIGURE 131-2 Thalassemia major. Blood film from an inadequately transfused patient with numerous nucleated red blood cells. There are a small number of poorly hemoglobinized red blood cells and some target cells, but the majority of red blood cells are normal ones from the transfusion.

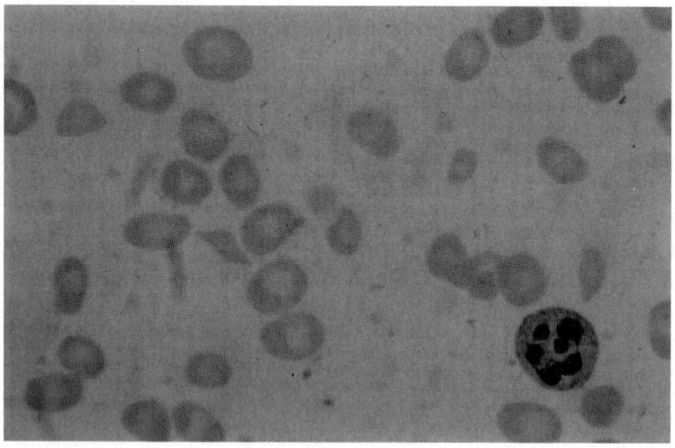

FIGURE 131-3 Severe megaloblastic anemia. Peripheral blood film showing poikilocytosis and an oval macrocyte. The single neutrophil has a nucleus with six lobes and is hypersegmented.

following infection or oxidant drug treatment in patients with G6PD deficiency. RBC fragments may be seen in microangiopathic hemolyic anemias (Fig. 131-4). Other abnormal cells include elliptocytes (in hereditary elliptocytosis), pencil cells (in iron deficiency), and teardrop cells (in thalassemias and bone marrow infiltration such as myelofibrosis or bone marrow secondaries).

3. *Microscopic examination of the stool* for cysts and ova of parasites is important to exclude worm infestation, especially hookworm and *Trichuris* spp. infestations.
4. *Tests for fecal occult blood* can be carried out to exclude gastrointestinal hemorrhage as a cause of the anemia.
5. *A therapeutic trial:* Where resources are limited, it may often be cost-effective or necessary to embark on a therapeutic trial in the management of anemia that may help establish an etiologic diagnosis. Such a trial may involve, for example, an antimalarial, iron, or both.

Further Investigations

In the primary health care setting with limited facilities, undiagnosed or unresponsive cases, or those requiring special treatment such as blood transfusion, may be referred to a center with access to facilities for further investigation. Investigations may include the following:

1. *Electronic cell count:* An electronic cell counter will provide RBC indices: mean corpuscular volume (MCV), RBC count, mean corpuscular hemoglobin (MCH), mean corpuscular hemoglobin concentration (MCHC), a white blood cell count (with or without a differential), and platelet count. The RBC indices will confirm whether the anemia is microcytic, hypochromic; normocytic or normochromic; or macrocytic.
2. *Examination of the bone marrow:* The bone marrow examination needs to be interpreted by someone who has special training in the field. The information obtained may not always be diagnostic but will assist in defining the cellularity of the marrow and provide a semiquantitative estimate of body iron stores. The marrow will indicate whether erythropoiesis is microcytic, micronormoblastic, megaloblastic, or dysplastic. Marrow infiltrations, for example, by malignancy or infection such as leishmaniasis, can be detected. Marrow examination will also help define the maturation of the myeloid and megakaryocytic series. The bone marrow findings in some of the more common conditions are as follows:

a. *Microcytic hypochromic anemias*
   - Iron deficiency demonstrates micronormoblasts with absent iron stores on Perls' staining (an iron-specific reagent) and no hemosiderin granules in erythroblasts (Fig. 131-5).
   - In the thalassemias, the erythroblasts show poor hemglobinization with hemosiderin granules present in erythroblasts, sometimes both large and excessive in number.
   - ACD may be hypochromic with an increase in storage iron but an absence of hemosiderin granules in erythroblasts—the so-called iron utilization block.
   - Sideroblastic anemias show increased iron stores with characteristic "ring sideroblasts."

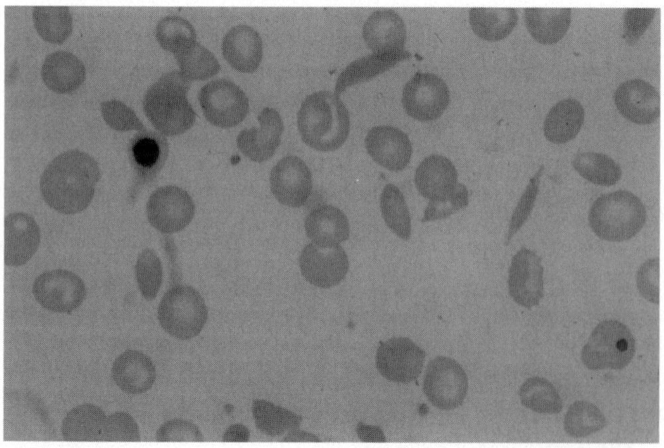

FIGURE 131-4 Sickle cell anemia. Peripheral blood film showing elongated red blood cells that have pointed ends and no central pallor. Not all cells have the classic curved sickle shape. Note the nucleated red blood cells and the Howell–Jolly body, indicative of hyposplenism.

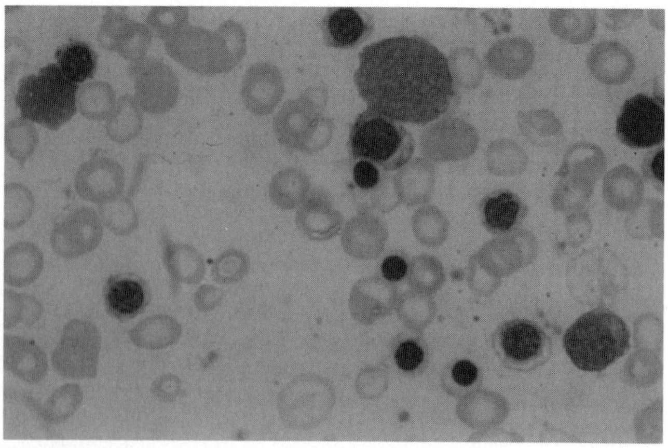

FIGURE 131-5 Severe iron deficiency anemia. Bone marrow film. Red blood cell precursors show micronormoblastic erythropoiesis. The changes are seen in intermediate and late erythroblasts and consist of cells that are smaller than normal with poor irregular hemoglobinization and, in one case, basophilic stippling.

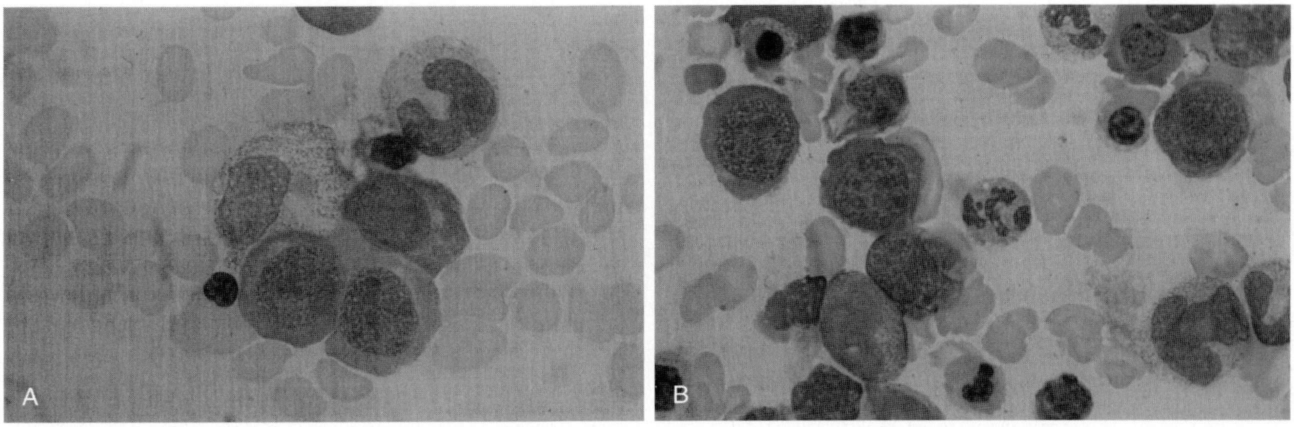

FIGURE 131-6 Severe megaloblastic anemia. Bone marrow films showing megaloblastic changes of the erythroid series consisting of erythroblasts that are larger than normal, asynchrony of maturation in which the cytoplasm is more mature than the nucleus, and a rather grainy erythroblast nucleus (*A*). In addition, there is a giant metamyelocyte that is twice the size of a normal metamyelocyte and has a contorted nucleus (*B*).

b. *Macrocytic anemias:* Macrocytic anemias (as judged from the blood film) can be classified on the basis of the bone marrow appearance:
   - Megaloblastic anemia, with megaloblastic changes in the erythroblasts and giant metamyelocytes due to vitamin B_{12} or folate deficiency (Fig. 131-6).
   - Normoblastic hemopoiesis, as occurs in liver and thyroid disease and alcoholism.

c. *Normocytic anemias:* In normocytic anemias, it is important to establish whether the cellularity of the bone marrow is low, normal, or increased with regard to erythroblasts and incidental other cell types:
   - A hypocellular bone marrow is characteristic of aplastic anemia consequent to drugs such as chloramphenicol or following hepatitis B infection.
   - A selective reduction in erythropoiesis but with normal myelopoiesis is found in parvovirus infection and other more rare causes, such as selective RBC aplasia.
   - A normocellular bone marrow is found in a variety of anemias, including ACD.
   - A hypercellular bone marrow is found in hemolytic anemias, leukemias, megaloblastic anemias, and dyserythropoietic anemias, congenital or acquired (Fig. 131-7).

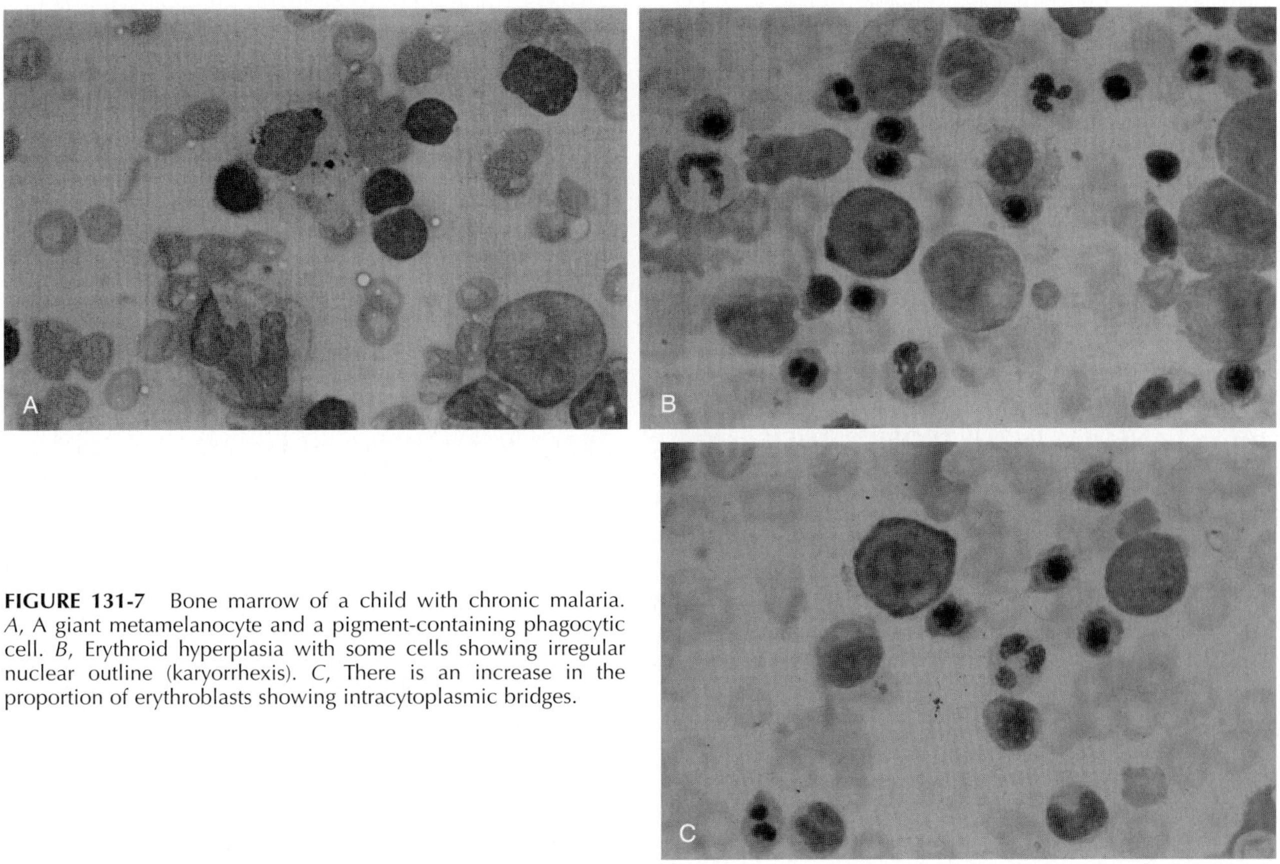

FIGURE 131-7 Bone marrow of a child with chronic malaria. *A,* A giant metamelanocyte and a pigment-containing phagocytic cell. *B,* Erythroid hyperplasia with some cells showing irregular nuclear outline (karyorrhexis). *C,* There is an increase in the proportion of erythroblasts showing intracytoplasmic bridges.

3. *Investigation of hemoglobinopathies:* Investigation of hemoglobinopathies is important in geographic areas where Hb disorders are common. Tests include the following:
   a. The sickle solubility test (using sodium metabisulfite) is a simple test based on the insolubility of Hb S in the reagents used. It is advisable to carry out Hb electrophoresis in cases with a positive solubility test to distinguish between patients with sickle cell trait (AS), SCA, or other compound heterozygotes such as S-β-thalassemia and SC. The limitation of the sickle solubility test is that it may not detect sickle Hb at low levels (<20%) and is therefore of no use in screening neonates and infants up to 6 months of age when the concentration of HbS is low.
   b. Hb electrophoresis will confirm the presence of Hb S and other major structural Hb variants, such as Hb C, D, and E, and also distinguish between hetero- and homozygotes. Hb electrophoresis will also detect fetal hemoglobin (Hb F) levels higher than approximately 2%.
   c. Quantitation of Hb F using an alkali denaturation method is important in the diagnosis of β-thalassemia major and intermedia.
   d. Quantitation of Hb A2 using a column elution method is important to diagnose β-thalassemia trait because it is higher than 3.5% in carriers. Accurate diagnosis is relevant in areas where genetic counseling is an important strategy in preventing β-thalassemia major.
4. *Serum ferritin or serum iron and transferrin:* A low serum ferritin or a low serum iron with a raised transferrin suggests an iron deficiency anemia, whereas a low serum iron and low transferrin suggest a secondary anemia (e.g., to infections or inflammation).
5. *Vitamin B_{12} and RBC folate assays:* Serum vitamin B_{12} levels are usually low in megaloblastic anemias due to vitamin B_{12} deficiency, but they can be low without anemia in vegans. RBC folate is a more stable measure of storage folate than labile serum folate and shows a moderate to severe reduction in folate deficiency. Care must be taken in interpreting the results because folate can be reduced in vitamin B_{12} deficiency.
6. HIV testing is crucial because a positive test will have considerable management implications.

IMPORTANT ANEMIAS IN THE TROPICS, THEIR DIAGNOSES, AND THEIR MANAGEMENT

Anemia of Malaria

In areas of high endemicity, severe anemia associated with malaria most commonly occurs in children up to 5 years of age, in whom it can be severe and sometimes fatal.[9,10] Severe anemia most commonly occurs in a younger age group (often <2 years) than in those suffering from cerebral malaria. In contrast, in areas where the occurrence of malaria is epidemic rather than endemic, the age distribution of malarial anemia is less well defined and it may also occur in adult semi-immune people, especially in primigravidas. The importance of anemia as a cause of death in malaria may well be underestimated because of the difficulty in diagnosis.[11] Attributing malaria as the cause of anemia in a tropical setting is often difficult. Some sources have included a minimal arbitrary Hb and parasitemia (<5g/dL in the presence of parasitemia >10,000/μL) to define severe malarial anemia. However, this definition should be regarded as being for research rather than clinical purposes.

The pathogenesis of the anemia of malaria is both complex and multifactorial but is largely due to hemolysis of infected and uninfected RBCs because the decline in Hb is often far in excess of what can be accounted for by the loss of infected RBCs alone.[12] It is usually normochromic, normocytic.

Two clinical patterns predominate in the development of anemia in malaria: severe acute malaria in which anemia supervenes[13] and anemia that has developed insidiously.[9] In the first, patients suffering a severe acute attack of malaria, and who are seen early after the onset of clinical symptoms, are initially not anemic, nor do they have splenomegaly. However, anemia may develop dramatically during the course of infection, which has been associated with a shortened survival of uninfected RBCs, sometimes well after parasites have disappeared from the blood film.[14] The cause of anemia in malaria in these acute episodes is probably multifactorial and may include inhibition of erythropoietin secretion, which is low and associated with an initial poor reticulocyte response.[15]

The second pattern of malarial anemia in the context of malaria occurs particularly in endemic areas.[9] These patients, usually children, become gradually anemic, often without a clear history of repeated attacks of malaria.[16] The history may be one of intermittent fevers and general symptoms of ill health occurring insidiously over weeks rather than days. Splenomegaly of varying degree may be present and the peripheral blood film may show minimal parasitemia with only the presence of gametocytes and malarial pigment within phagocytic cells as evidence of a past infection. The bone marrow often shows the picture of dyserythropoiesis,[9] with multinuclearity of erythroid precursors, mitotic figures, and intercytoplasmic bridging between dividing cells (see Fig. 131-7). In functional terms, these appearances are associated with ineffective erythropoiesis (i.e., the marrow is active but not producing functional red cells). Unlike the acute situation, erythropoietin levels are increased.[17]

Great difficulty remains in attributing the relative roles of each mechanism that contributes to the development of the anemia of malaria, such as intravascular hemolysis, extravascular clearance of RBCs, and marrow dysfunction. The major mechanisms are those of RBC destruction and decreased RBC production. The former includes loss of infected cells by rupture or phagocytosis, removal of uninfected cells due to antibody sensitization or other physicochemical membrane changes, and increased reticuloendothelial activity, particularly in organs such as the spleen and bone marrow.[9,10] Shortened RBC survival may persist well after parasite clearance[14] and may be related to reduced RBC deformability.[18] Decreased production tends to predominate in acute infections and dyserythropoiesis in more prolonged infections.[19] Successful eradication of the malarial parasite is paramount in the management of this anemia. Malaria on its own does not result in iron or folate deficiency, although there is evidence that children given iron but not folate at the time of an acute attack have higher mean

Hb levels at follow-up.[20] Blood transfusion may occasionally be required in selected severe cases, although most patients have a brisk increase in Hb levels once the malaria has been successfully treated.[21] There is insufficient evidence concerning whether giving blood routinely to children with severe anemia reduces death.[22] A suggested guideline for transfusion in severe malarial anemia, based on Hb level, a safe blood supply, and the presence of severe complications (notably respiratory distress), has been proposed.[23] Insecticide-treated bed nets may have a role to play in the reduction of malaria, especially in infants and young children.[24,25]

Anemia of Human Immunodeficiency Virus Infection

Anemia is common in patients with HIV infection and present in almost all patients with acquired immunodeficiency syndrome (AIDS), but it is often only mild (>10 g/dL).[8,26] The anemia is often normochromic and normocytic, with low reticulocyte counts and erythropoietin levels but normal or increased iron stores and serum ferritin levels. The cause is multifactorial and complex. The anemia may be even more severe in the presence of mycobacterial infections (*Mycobacterium tuberculosis* and *Mycobacterium avium* complex), fungal infections (e.g., cryptococcal), persistent parvoviral B19 infection, lymphoma, and as a result of many of the drugs used in treatment. Particularly important drugs in the cause of anemia in HIV infection are the antiviral drugs such as zidovudine but also numerous other antiinfective agents, such as dapsone, sulfonamides, primaquine, isoniazid, rifampicin, pyrimethamine, and trimethoprim. Blood loss and microcytosis occur when the gastrointestinal tract is involved with Kaposi's sarcoma, cytomegalovirus, or lymphoma.

Nutritional Anemias

Nutritional anemias result from the discrepancy between the supply of and the demand for specific nutritional elements. The causes may be dietary or may be due to excessive loss or increased demand for these substances.

Iron Deficiency Anemia

Iron deficiency is probably the most common cause of anemia worldwide[27]; the major causes of iron deficiency in the tropics are shown in Box 131-2. This deficiency predominates because of the extremely tight regulation of iron absorption by the intestinal mucosa and because of the generally poor bioavailability of iron from most diets in tropical areas. In addition, local factors may contribute to negative iron balance, such as hookworm, schistosomiasis, and other gut infestations. Iron status and iron deficiency may be evaluated using a number of indicators (see Box 131-2).

The differential diagnosis of a hypochromic anemia may require additional investigations, such as Hb A_2 estimation (to exclude β-thalassemia trait) or Hb F estimation (supportive of a diagnosis of β-thalassemia major or intermedia), or by bone marrow examination (Table 132-2). The true incidence of iron deficiency in the population may be overestimated or underestimated according to the measures used to define iron deficiency.

Box 131-2 Causes of Iron Deficiency in the Tropics

Reduced Intake

- Late weaning
- Poor diet

Increased Demand

- Growth
  - Childhood
  - Adolescence
  - Pregnancy
- Blood loss
  - Menstruation
  - Gastrointestinal
    - Hookworm
    - Schistosomiasis
    - *Helicobacter pylori* infection
    - Trichuriasis
- Other causes found worldwide
  - Hiatal hernia
  - Peptic ulcer
  - Aspirin
  - Hemorrhoids
  - Malignancy

Reduced Absorption

- Malabsorption
  - Tuberculosis
  - Lymphoma
  - Giardiasis
  - Bacterial overgrowth
  - Celiac disease (uncommon)

In general, using a single indicator is often unreliable and extensive studies in different areas of the world are difficult to carry out. Often, a therapeutic trial relying on the knowledge that iron deficiency may be the most common anemia in the population is the only practical management strategy.

Folate Deficiency

Folate is found in most foodstuffs, especially in liver, other meats, green vegetables, and some fruits, and it is destroyed by prolonged boiling. Absorption occurs throughout the small intestine.[2] Folate deficiency is therefore rarely due to dietary deficiency and may be due to increased utilization, as occurs in pregnancy, lactation, and malabsorption states. Folate is essential for metabolic functions involved in methyl group transfer and is utilized in nucleic acid synthesis. Deficiency manifests as megaloblastic anemia and also leads to mucosal atrophy.

Serum folate is labile and reflects a transit pool of folate that may be depressed to very low levels within a few weeks on a deficient diet. RBC folate, on the other hand, represents a storage pool formed during erythropoiesis and therefore changes more slowly after deprivation than serum folate. Folate stores usually last 4 or 5 months, after which deficiency occurs. The diagnosis of anemia due to folate deficiency is based on the presence of a macrocytic anemia with oval macrocytes and hypersegmented neutrophils on the blood film and a megaloblastic bone marrow together with a low RBC folate.

Table 131-2 Differential Diagnosis of Hypochromic Anemia in the Tropics

Indices	IDA	ACD	Thalassemia Trait (α or β)
Degree of anemia	Any	Rarely <9 g/dL	Mild
MCV	Reduced (<76 fL or μ³)	Normal or reduced	Very reduced
MCH, MCHC	Reduced	Reduced	Reduced
RBC count	Normal or reduced	Normal or reduced	Increased
RDW	Increased	Normal or increased	Normal or increased
Blood film	Microcytic, hypochromic	Microcytic, hypochromic; may be normochromic, normocytic	Microcytic, hypochromic; teardrop cells, basophilic stippling, target cells
Serum iron	Reduced	Normal or reduced	Normal
Serum transferrin	Increased	Reduced	Normal
Iron-binding saturation (%)	Very low	Low	Normal
Serum ferritin	Reduced	Normal or increased	Normal
Bone marrow	Mildly hypocellular	Normocellular or hypocellular	Mildly hypercellular
	Micronormoblastic erythropoiesis	Hypercellular when neutrophil leukocytosis is present	Some dyserythropoiesis
	Absent marrow iron	Marrow iron present	Present
Serum transferring receptor	Specific for iron deficiency	Normal	Normal
Response to therapeutic trail of iron replacement	Good	None except when IDA and ACD coexist	Potential iron overload
Other		Raised ESR	

ACD, anemia of chronic disease; ESR, erythrocyte sedimentation rate; IDA, iron deficiency anemia; MCH, mean corpuscular hemoglobin; MCHC, mean corpuscular hemoglobin concentration; MCV, mean corpuscular volume; RBC, red blood cell; RDW, red blood cell distribution width (index).

Folate deficiency may arise acutely during pregnancy, during acute alcohol intake with a poor diet, and in patients in intensive care in whom severe deficiency may occur with pancytopenia but with normal levels of RBC folate. This picture may also be seen when patients with borderline folate stores are given antifolate drugs, which include sulfonamides and antimalarials such as pyrimethamine and proguanil. Folate deficiency is easily treated with 5 mg/day of folic acid. This pharmacologic dose is easily absorbed and should correct any deficiency. Prophylactic folate should be given to pregnant women and patients with chronic hemolytic anemias such as SCA in which there is increased RBC turnover.

Vitamin B_{12} Deficiency

Vitamin B_{12} deficiency is not generally considered to be a major problem in the tropics. However, there are some situations in which the recognition of vitamin B_{12} deficiency is important. These include areas where veganism is common for religious or other reasons, because vitamin B_{12} is found only in food from animal sources. Vitamin B_{12} deficiency may also occur in abdominal tuberculosis when the terminal ileum is involved and leads to malabsorption. Pernicious anemia is said to be rare in tropical countries, especially in the Indian subcontinent. There are no major systematic studies of pernicious anemia in Africa, but there are numerous case reports that suggest that the condition may occur at a much earlier age than in northern Europe, where the youngest patient recorded was 16 years of age.[28]

Deficiency of vitamin B_{12} can lead to a megaloblastic anemia, symmetrical polyneuropathy, and, less frequently, gonadal dysfunction and glossitis. Subacute degeneration of the cord may ensue if the deficiency is not treated. The combination of anemia and neurological symptoms should alert the physician to the possibility of pernicious anemia.

Anemia of Chronic Disease

ACD describes a normocytic anemia or sometimes a mildly to moderately microcytic, hypochromic anemia that occurs in patients with infectious, inflammatory, or neoplastic disease.[3,29–31] The important causes of ACD in the tropics include acute infections such as pneumonia or septicemia, chronic infections such as tuberculosis and HIV infection, and only rarely autoimmune disorders such as rheumatoid arthritis and systemic lupus erythematosus.

Pathogenesis

ACD is characterized by underproduction of RBCs; the reticulocyte count is usually low. The bone marrow is either normocellular or initially hypocellular, but occasionally it can be hypercellular due to increased granulocytic activity (see Table 131-2). The pathogenesis of ACD is complex; the main mechanism appears to be a block in the incorporation of iron into erythroblasts with an increase in macrophage iron possibly due to the release of proinflammatory cytokines.[3] These include interleukin (IL)-1, IL-6; interferons-α, -β, and -γ; and tumor necrosis factor-α. ACD can lead to diagnostic difficulties, especially when there is coexistent iron deficiency.

Management

ACD resolves after successful treatment of the underlying condition. In untreatable conditions or where there is limited response to treatment or in the initial phases of treatment, other approaches can be used to alleviate the anemia, such as blood transfusion. Despite low serum iron, administration of iron is of limited or no benefit. ACD has been shown to respond to administration of recombinant erythropoietin,[30] but this treatment is less likely to be available where resources are limited.

Inherited Red Blood Cell Disorders

There is a high prevalence of genetic disorders affecting RBCs in tropical areas where malaria is or has been endemic. It is thought that carriers of these disorders are protected against malaria even though people fully affected may suffer severe consequences if they contract malaria. The malaria hypothesis proposes that the protective benefit from the carrier state leads to a better survival advantage than either the normal or affected homozygote.

The majority of these disorders lead to hemolytic anemia in affected people, either in the steady state or under conditions of stress. The most important of these disorders are the sickling disorders, the thalassemia syndromes, and G6PD deficiency.

Sickling Disorders

SCA is a major cause of morbidity and mortality in children in rural Africa, where the condition is common.[32–34] A single DNA base substitution leads to an amino acid substitution from valine to glutamic acid in position 6 of the β globin chain. This substitution causes a major change in the solubility of Hb S under conditions of low oxygenation, leading to the formation of "tactoids"—elongated crystalline structures that lead to the formation of classic sickle cells, which can lead to irreversible RBC sickling. SCA occurs when the condition is inherited in the homozygous state. The precipitating factors for sickling episodes include infections, hypoxia, and dehydration, but in many patients there may not be an obvious precipitating cause. At birth, the amount of Hb S is too low to cause problems because the predominant Hb is Hb F.

Other sickling disorders include the coinheritance of Hb S with β^+- or β^0-thalassemia (i.e., Hb S β-thalassemia) or Hb C trait (Hb SC) or Hb D (Hb SD). These cases may be milder than SCA. There is thus major variability in the clinical picture in sickling disorders from individual to individual due to the interaction of a variety of genotypes, the level of Hb F, interaction with α-thalassemia, unknown genetic factors, and

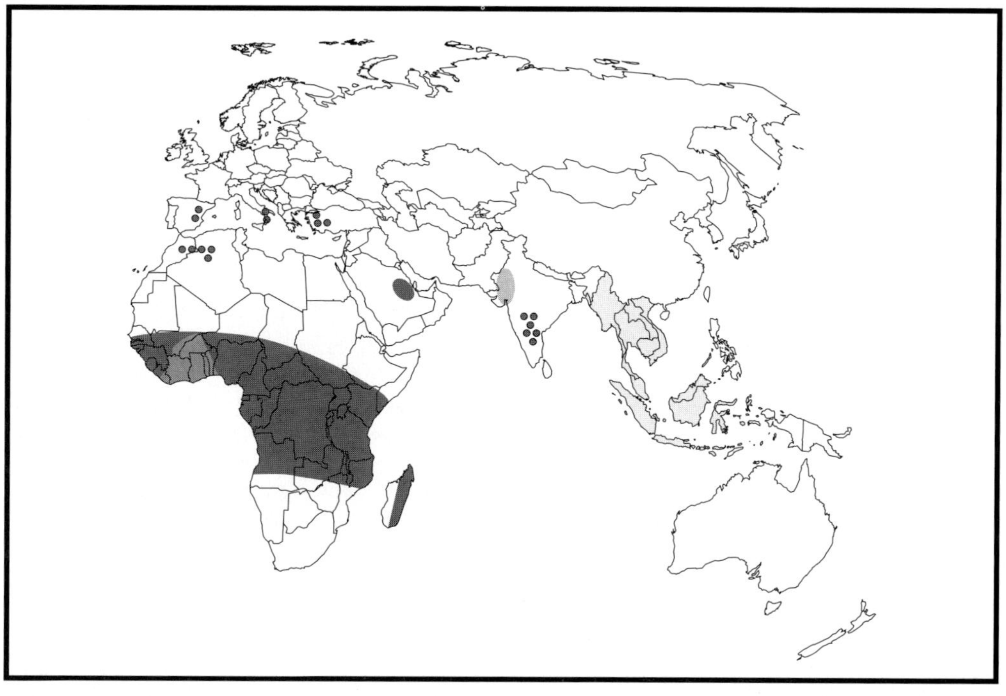

environmental factors (e.g., altitude). It is thought that the gene arose on four independent genetic backgrounds, as shown by the variety of β-globulin haplotypes. The effects of the sickle Hb from these haplotypes are similar, although inheritance of certain haplotypes may be associated with mild clinical disease.

The first manifestation of the disease usually occurs after 6 months of life, when the most common presentation is that of a dactylitis (Box 131-3). As the child grows older, other manifestations include painful crises due to vascular occlusion in bone and sometimes other organs, such as the brain, gastrointestinal tract, and lung. The typical crisis that occurs is due to multiple microinfarcts in bone leading to severe disabling pain. More serious complications include sequestration crises in the lungs, spleen, or, less commonly, the brain, ranging from minor strokes to repeated infarcts and major cerebral infarcts. In rural areas, children frequently die at an early age from SCA, often from malaria or sepsis, but with careful medical attention they may survive to adulthood. Patients with SCA are especially susceptible to infection with *Streptococcus pneumoniae* and *Salmonella* spp. Patients with sickle cell trait (Hb S) are not anemic and rarely symptomatic, except when they have painful crises in unphysiologic conditions such as in unpressurized aircraft and during anesthesia.

Box 131-3 Clinical Manifestations of Sickle Cell Anemia

Bone Marrow and Bone

Expansion of hematopoiesis leading to
- Dactylitis (hand and foot syndrome), especially at 4 to 6 months of age
- Prognathism
- Bossing of the skull

Chronic hemolytic anemia
Painful crises due to microinfarction of bone
Osteomyelitis, often due to *Salmonella* spp.

Lungs

Acute chest syndrome with breathlessness, reduced oxygen saturation (<70%), and radiographic changes
Lung infections often complicated; if hypoxia results, this may precipitate a crisis
Ultimately may lead to pulmonary fibrosis and cor pulmonale

Heart

Cardiomegaly due to chronic anemia
Congestive cardiac failure in later life

Spleen

Hypoactivity leading to susceptibility to infection, including encapsulated organisms and malaria
Acute sequestration crisis with rapid enlargement and anemia, especially in infancy, and which tends to recur
Chronic splenic enlargement with hypersplenism (anemia, leukopenia, and thrombocytopenia)

Liver and Gallbladder

Acute liver sequestration
Gallstones

Kidneys

Renal tubular defect leads to inability to concentrate urine, leading to enuresis
Dehydration, which may precipitate crises
Tubular necrosis
Intermittent hematuria
Chronic renal failure

Brain

Recurrent cerebral infarction (may be silent)
Stroke

Skin

Chronic leg ulcers (seen especially in Jamaica)

Management. In general, treatment of acute crises involves ensuring adequate hydration, oxygenation, and analgesia; vigorous treatment of the underlying infection; keeping patients warm in cold weather; and reversal of acidosis. More severe complications, such as acute anemia due to splenic sequestration, increased hemolysis, parvovirus infection, or lung sequestration, are treated with top-up transfusion when the Hb falls below 6 g/dL. Where the Hb is higher and in the presence of certain complications, such as chest syndrome, priapism, and severe abdominal sickling, exchange transfusions are advocated to reduce the Hb S percentage to less than 20% and to continue by monthly transfusion thereafter. Pain management is particularly important. The pain is often very severe and may necessitate the use of opiate analgesia at frequent intervals. The particular opiate used (e.g., pethidine, diamorphine, or morphine) is dependent on local preference. Opiates have the disadvantage of a depressive effect on respiratory drive, which may worsen existing hypoxia, and potential addiction in those requiring opiates for repeated attacks. A study in Jamaica showed that, using pulse oximetry, a considerable degree of hypoxia may be found in patients with sickling disorders in the steady state.[35] Nonsteroidal anti-inflammatory drugs may be useful for bone pain provided there are no contraindications to their use.

Prevention of Complications. Prevention of the complications of SCA rests on the recognition and avoidance of precipitating factors of acute attacks, such as exposure to cold (e.g., swimming), dehydration, infections, altitude, travel in nonpressurized aircraft, anesthesia, and extremes of physical activity. Parents and patients should be taught to recognize early the manifestations of disease, such as dactylitis or splenic sequestration, which may begin with symptoms of listlessness and signs of pallor. Because these patients have effectively been autosplenectomized, they should receive pneumococcal, *Haemophilus influenzae* type b (Hib), and meningococcal vaccinations as well as prophylactic antimalarials, impregnated bed nets, and early treatment of malaria. Hepatitis B vaccination should be considered, especially when patients require transfusion and donors are not screened. Folate 5 mg/day should also be given because of the high RBC turnover.

Hydroxycarbamide (previously known as hydroxyurea) reduces the frequency of painful crisis, chest syndrome, and transfusion requirements in both adults and children with severe sickle cell disease. It also appears to improve growth and possibly prevent hyposplenism in children. It has not been proven to prevent stroke or avascular necrosis in joints, and it is the subject of ongoing trials in Europe and North America.[36] Caution is advised, however, because its long-term profile in terms of toxicity, mutagenicity, teratogenicity, and leukemogenic potential is unknown. Careful discussion of these issues with patients prior to commencing hydroxyurea is essential. For guidelines on the use of hydroxyurea in sickle cell disease, see Box 131-4.

Box 131-4 Hydroxycarbamide (Hydroxyurea) in Sickle Cell Disease

Patient Exclusion Criteria

Regular transfusion regime
Abnormal liver function tests (AST or ALT >2× upper limit of normal)
Inability to attend clinic regularly for follow-up

Patient Eligibility

Patients (Hb SS or Sβ^0-thalassemia, not Hb SC) with a severe clinical course may be offered hydroxyurea, i.e., with
- Three admissions with painful crisis within 1 year, or
- Frequent days of pain at home, leading to a lot of time off work, or
- Recurrent acute chest syndrome

The following predict a more severe clinical course and are additional reasons to consider offering hydroxyurea:
- Steady-state values
  - Hb < 7g/dL
  - WBC > 15 × 10^9/L
  - HbF < 6%
- Renal insufficiency due to sickle cell disease

Dose and Monitoring

Start at 15 mg/kg/day (to the nearest 500 mg/day). If no or poor response, increase dose by increments of 5 mg/kg/day every 4 weeks (max: 30 mg/kg/day)
Monitor FBC, Hb F %, and reticulocytes every 1 or 2 weeks initially, then every 4 weeks when on a stable dose
Monitor biochemistry profile (hydroxyurea has renal excretion and hepatic toxicity)

Thalassemia Syndromes

The thalassemias are a group of disorders in which there is reduced production of one of the two main types of globin chains, α or β, leading to α- or β-thalassemia, respectively. These conditions are widely distributed throughout areas of Africa, the Mediterranean, the Middle East, the Indian subcontinent, and Southeast Asia. β-Thalassemia is especially common in the tropics in areas such as northern Thailand, Laos, and Vietnam. In these areas, there are complex interactions between these disorders and Hb E, a β-chain variant that is also underexpressed leading to a thalassemia-like phenotype. In Africa, β-thalassemia occurs in the northern areas of West African countries such as Ghana.

The underlying molecular genetic abnormalities of these disorders are complex. Each normal individual has four functioning α genes and two β genes. In α-thalassemia, one, two, or three of the α globin genes may be nonfunctional. Deletion of a single gene in one chromosome is labeled α^+ thalassemia and of two on the same chromosome as α^0. Homozygotes for α^0 (deletion of all four genes) lead to intrauterine or neonatal death from hydrops fetalis. In Hb H disease, α^0/α^+ double heterozygotes, three of the α globin genes are nonfunctional. In β-thalassemia, output from each β globin allele may be reduced (β^+) or absent (β^0). The underproduction of Hb leads to microcytic, hypochromic RBCs. Globin chain imbalance results in the formation of tetramers of β chain (Hb H) in α-thalassemia or γ chain (Bart's Hb) in the fetus and neonate. In addition to microcytosis, anemia is made worse by ineffective erythropoiesis because of globin chain imbalance in β-thalassemia and by hemolysis in Hb H disease since Hb H is unstable.

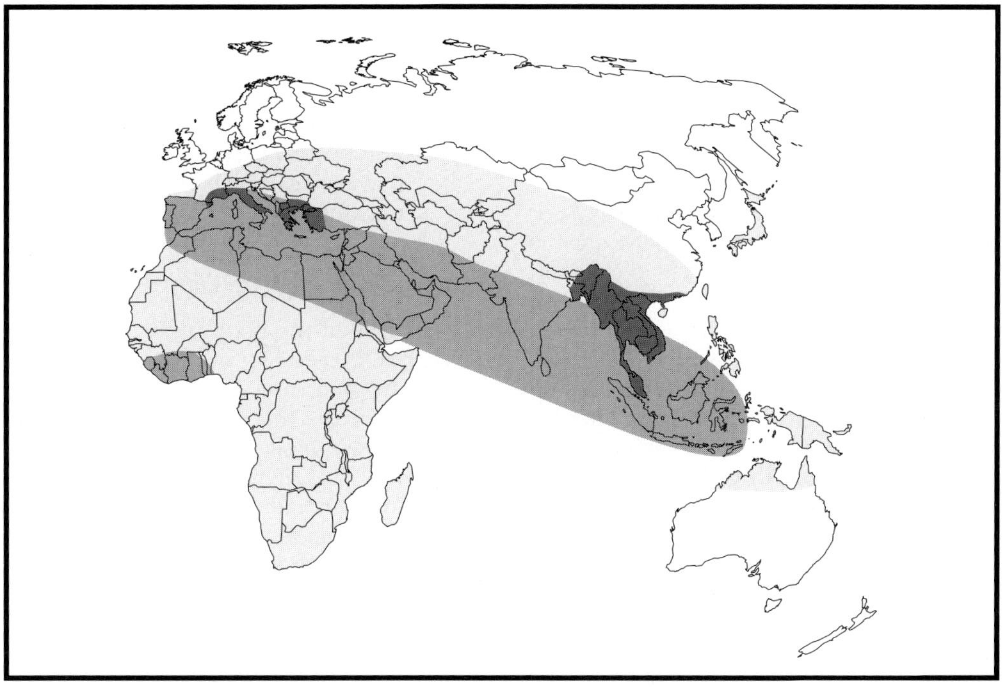

Thalassemias

- ■ α-Thalassemia, two α gene deletions (α–/α–)
- ■ β-Thalassemia
- □ α-Thalassemia, single α gene deletion (α–)

Underexpression of α chains in α-thalassemia is commonly caused by deletions involving one or more of the α genes (two on each chromosome 16) but sometimes also involving gene expression control regions. In contrast, the majority of β chain defects are caused by single base pair mutations usually resulting in reduced or absent gene expression (β^+- or β^0-thalassemia) from the single β gene on each chromosome 11. Whatever the cause, underproduction of adult Hb leads to the formation of hypochromic, microcytic RBCs with reduced MCH. The other main thalassemic indices include an elevated RBC count, a low MCV and MCH, and a relatively less reduced MCHC.

Clinically, the thalassemias may be grouped into three entities—minor, intermedia, and major:

1. In thalassemia minor, there is only a minor degree of hypochromic anemia (Hb 9 to 11 g/dL) in the absence of physiologic stress. Some patients, however, may develop a more clinically significant anemia in certain circumstances, such as pregnancy or other physiologic stress. Subjects generally appear clinically normal. Examples are α^+ hetero- and homozygotes, α^- heterozygotes, β-thalassemia trait, and the Hb $A^{\text{Constant spring}}$ heterozygote. Diagnosis is made on routine RBC count, most commonly because of the low MCV, which may be confused with iron deficiency (see Table 131-2).
2. In thalassemia intermedia, there is a moderate hypochromic, microcytic anemia but the patient is not normally transfusion dependent. Patients may become transfusion dependent intermittently when exposed to stress, such as pregnancy or intercurrent infection. Examples of thalassemia intermedia include Hb H disease and interaction between β^0-thalassemia and Hb E trait and between β^0- and β^+-thalassemia. Splenomegaly is a common feature in the thalassemia intermedia syndrome and hypersplenism may complicate the clinical picture. Patients may have cardiomegaly and in later life suffer from cardiac failure. Even in the absence of transfusion, iron overload may result from increased dietary iron absorption because of the increased erythropoiesis.
3. In thalassemia major (β^0 homozygotes) there is little or no production of Hb A, and there is progressive anemia from a few months of age leading to an Hb of less than 4 g/dL in the absence of transfusion. In untreated or inadequately treated patients, there is an expansion of erythropoiesis causing expansion of medullary bone, leading to features such as prognathism and bossing of the skull as well as hepatosplenomegaly. There is severe growth retardation and pathologic fractures. In untreated cases, death may occur in the first few years of life. Patients who are transfused may survive longer but develop iron overload with hypogonadism and secondary deposition of iron in the myocardium, pancreas, and liver, leading to death due to cardiac failure, diabetes mellitus, or liver failure, unless intensive iron chelation is used.

Management. The cornerstones of management are as follows:

1. *Counseling and advice:* In thalassemia trait the main clinical problems are the differential diagnosis from iron deficiency to avoid unnecessary and potentially harmful iron therapy and provision of proper counseling regarding prevention of pregnancy with a thalassemia major child.
2. *Transfusion:* In Hb H disease, a chronic hemolytic state, episodes of acute hemolysis may occur, necessitating transfusion. In the case of thalassemia intermedia, monitoring is required perhaps at 6-month intervals in childhood and yearly intervals in adult life,[37] and transfusion may be needed during periods of stress. In thalassemia major, regular transfusions to maintain an Hb higher than 10 g/dL are needed from an early age to maintain normal growth and prevent bony deformities. However, repeated transfusion carries the risk of iron overload, sensitization to white blood cells causing febrile reactions, and the possibility of transmission of infections such as hepatitis B and C and HIV.
3. *Iron chelation with subcutaneous desferrioxamine infusion together with vitamin C:* Continuous iron chelation is also needed to prevent cardiac, hepatic, and endocrine organ deposition of iron leading to dysfunction of these organs and ultimately death. This treatment regimen, in addition to being expensive, requires special motivation for effective compliance.
4. *Splenectomy:* Some patients with either thalassemia intermedia or thalassemia major may develop hypersplenism consisting of splenic enlargement accompanied by increasing anemia, leukopenia, and thrombocytopenia. These patients may require splenectomy. Indications for splenectomy include a requirement for transfusion in a patient who previously did not require transfusion, increasing transfusion requirements in those who are transfusion dependent, clinically significant thrombocytopenia, and the mechanical effects of the large spleen. However, splenectomy should be considered carefully in a tropical environment.
5. Some patients may develop cardiomegaly with compromised myocardial function leading to cardiac failure in the fifth or sixth decade of life. Monitoring with chest radiography in the first instance and echocardiography, if available, may be helpful. Such patients may require transfusion.

Glucose-6-Phosphate Dehydrogenase Deficiency

All cells of the body contain G6PD, an enzyme that catalyzes the breakdown of glucose-6-phosphate to 6-phosphogluconate producing reduced NADPH from oxidized NADP and leading to the five-carbon sugar ribose necessary for nucleotide synthesis. Reduced NADPH is essential to maintaining several intracellular protein and membrane sulfhydryl groups in their reduced state (e.g., glutathione). The RBC is particularly susceptible to the deleterious effect of oxidant stress because of its function in oxygen carriage, and for this reason the effects of enzyme deficiency leading to hemolysis are most commonly observed in red cells.[38]

G6PD deficiency is sex linked and affects mainly males. The enzyme is a protein consisting of 515 amino acids and has a molecular weight of 59 kDa. There are many variants of G6PD, and the majority of these are the result of a single base mutation in the genes causing a single amino acid substitution. The substitution may have no or a minor effect on the function

Table 131-3 Examples of the Most Common Glucose-6-Phosphate Dehydrogenase (G6PD) Variants

Type	Characteristics	G6PD Activity (%)	Distribution
B	Slower electrophoretic mobility than A	100	Common wild type worldwide
A	Faster electrophoretic mobility than B	70–90	Africa
Deficient variants			
A⁻	Drug and infection induced; hemolysis self-limited	15–20	Africa
Mediterranean	Severe, sometimes fatal hemolysis	<10	Mediterranean
Mahidol	Severe hemolysis	<10	Thailand, Southeast Asia
Canton	Severe hemolysis	<10	Orientals

of the enzyme, producing functionally normal variants, or may have a moderate or severe effect. Using previously agreed WHO methodology, including electrophoretic mobility, kinetics, and other properties, 299 variants of G6PD have been described but only a few are encountered frequently in clinical practice (Table 131-3). Using more specific DNA characterization, 60 enzyme variants have been identified. Deficiency of G6PD is mostly seen in hemizygous males and less frequently in homozygous females. The gene frequency of G6PD mutations is particularly high in certain populations, such as Kurdish Jews (0.70) and black Americans (0.1 to 0.11), black Africans, and some Asians.

Clinical Picture

G6PD deficiency may present with a wide spectrum of clinical manifestations. The generally accepted broad classification is as follows: class 1, the most severe, characterized by a chronic nonspherocytic hemolytic anemia; class 2 deficiency, such as G6PD Mediterranean (Gd Med), in which there is significant hemolysis with exposure to oxidants; and class 3, in which there is only mild to moderate deficiency, such as Gd A⁻ found in Africa. Class 1 variants are rare and usually not found as a polymorphism in areas where malaria is endemic. In contrast, class 2 and 3 variants are common in malaria-endemic areas. The following are the most common manifestations of G6PD deficiency:

- *Infection-induced hemolysis:* This is one of the most common manifestations of G6PD deficiency observed in tropical areas and is seen in conditions such as viral hepatitis, typhoid, malaria, lobar pneumonia, and severe sepsis in which the release of oxygen radicals and nitric oxide may lead to hemolysis. Patients with G6PD deficiency are more likely to develop intravascular hemolysis mimicking blackwater fever with falciparum malaria. The hemolysis seen in G6PD deficiency with viral hepatitis is unexplained.
- *Drug-induced hemolysis:* The range of drugs causing hemolysis in the tropics in G6PD-deficient people may be more limited because of the milder forms of deficiency present in these areas.[38] The issue of antimalarial drugs is important. The schizonticidal drugs chloroquine and quinine are considered safe in normal therapeutic doses. The combination drugs containing sulfonamide, dapsone, or pyrimethamine should be avoided; dapsone may cause hemolysis even in non-G6PD-deficient subjects. Primaquine is one of the major drugs that should be avoided. The manufacturers of the aminoquinoline drugs, such as ciprofloxacin and ofloxacin, advise caution in their use in G6PD deficiency.
- *Neonatal jaundice:* This is a common and potentially serious complication of G6PD deficiency in Asia, Greece, and Africa that can lead to kernicterus. Anemia is not always present and may be due to hepatocyte rather than RBC deficiency of the enzyme. A history of neonatal jaundice may assist in the diagnosis of G6PD deficiency in later life.
- *Food-induced jaundice:* Some foods and additives are known to contain oxidants that may cause hemolysis in G6PD deficiency. The best known of these are fava beans and a food coloring in Nigeria called suya. Favism is a hemolytic anemia associated with the ingestion of fava beans seen mainly in G6PD deficiency but which will vary according to the type of bean, the way the beans are cooked, whether the beans are dried or fresh, and the metabolism of the individual.

Diagnosis

The blood film is normal in patients with G6PD deficiency in the steady state. However, during a hemolytic crisis changes may be seen in the peripheral blood, including irregularly contracted RBCs called "hemighosts" (Plate 131-1A). In cases in which there is overwhelming hemolysis or in patients who are hyposplenic, a supravital stain will reveal the presence of Heinz bodies, which are denatured Hb or globin precipitates associated with red cell membrane (Plate 131-1B).

There are several methods available commercially for the detection of G6PD deficiency; all utilize the reduction of NADP to NADPH in the presence of excess G6PD and red cell lysate. Reduced NADPH is then detected either by fluorescence under ultraviolet light or by an electron transfer reaction involving tetrazolium compounds that are reduced by NADPH to insoluble forms.

G6PD deficiency of all types can be detected easily in this manner in male hemizygotes in the steady state and in homozygotes with the more severe class of enzyme deficiencies (e.g., Gd Med). Difficulties may arise in the less severe types of deficiencies (class 3, especially Gd A minus [A⁻]), in which reticulocytes and young RBCs, relatively rich in enzymes, tend to restore levels to the normal range. This relatively normal G6PD level in otherwise deficient people explains why these milder deficiencies cause self-limited hemolysis even in the presence of continued use of the drug or infection. Diagnosis of heterozygotes is more problematic. An intermediate range in the enzyme assay may be diagnostic of heterozygosity in females, but a considerable number of females will fall within the normal range. Genetic studies using DNA analysis are being increasingly used to diagnose G6PD deficiency and the carrier state, but they are not routinely available in the tropics.

Management

Acute management of G6PD deficiency during a hemolytic crisis includes adequate hydration, maintenance of urinary output, withdrawal of the offending drug or agent responsible for the hemolysis, and transfusion of RBCs if necessary. In neonatal jaundice, phototherapy or exchange transfusions may be required according to bilirubin levels. Deficient patients should be counseled to (1) avoid agents that are potentially hemolytic; (2) report early for treatment in case of infections, especially infections in children; and (3) report the onset of jaundice or pallor early, especially in children.

REFERENCES

1. WHO: Nutritional Anaemias. Geneva, WHO, 1968.
2. Hercberg S, Galan P: Nutritional anaemias. Bailliere's Clin Haematol 5:143–168, 1992.
3. Kent S, Weinberg E, Stuart-Macadam P: The aetiology of the anaemia of chronic disease and infection. J Clin Epidemiol 47:23–33, 1994.
4. Viteri F, Torun B: Anaemia and physical work capacity. Clin Haematol 3:609–625, 1974.
5. Basta SS, Soekirman, Karyadi D, et al: Iron deficiency anemia and the productivity of adult males in Indonesia. Am J Clin Nutr 32:916–925, 1979.
6. Edgerton VR, Gardner GW, Ohira Y, et al: Iron-deficiency anaemia and its effect on worker productivity and activity patterns. BMJ 2:1546–1549, 1979.
7. Abdalla SH: Iron and folate in malaria. In Abdalla SH, Pasvol G (eds): Malaria: A Hematological Perspective. London, Imperial College Press, 2004, pp 97–128.
8. Holland H, Spivak J: Haematological manifestations of acquired immune deficiency syndrome. Bailliere's Clin Haematol 3:103–114, 1990.
9. Abdalla S, Weatherall D, Wickramasinghe S, et al: The anaemia of *P. falciparum* malaria. Br J Haematol 46:171–183, 1980.
10. Phillips RE, Pasvol G. Anaemia of *Plasmodium falciparum* malaria. Bailliere's Clin Haematol 5:315–330, 1992.
11. Brabin B, Premji Z, Verhoef F: An analysis of anemia and child mortality. Am Soc Nutr Sci 131:636S–648S, 2001.
12. McDevitt MA, Xie J, Gordeuk V, et al: The anemia of malaria infection: Role of inflammatory cytokines. Curr Hematol Rep 3:97–106, 2004.
13. Phillips RE, Looareesuwan S, Warrell DA, et al: The importance of anaemia in cerebral and uncomplicated falciparum malaria: Role of complications, dyserythropoiesis and iron sequestration. Q J Med 58:305–323, 1986.
14. Looareesuwan S, Merry AH, Phillips RE, et al: Reduced erythrocyte survival following clearance of malarial parasitaemia in Thai patients. Br J Haematol 67:473–478, 1987.
15. Burgmann H, Looareesuwan S, Kapiotis S, et al: Serum levels of erythropoietin in acute *Plasmodium falciparum* malaria. Am J Trop Med Hyg 54:280–283, 1996.
16. Newton C, Warn P, Winstanley P, et al: Severe anaemia in children living in a malaria endemic area of Kenya. Trop Med Int Health 2:165–178, 1997.
17. Burchard G, Radloff P, Philipps J, et al: Increased erythropoietin production in children with severe malarial anemia. Am J Trop Med Hyg 53:547–551, 1995.
18. Dondorp AM, Angus BJ, Chotivanich K, et al: Red blood cell deformability as a predictor of anemia in severe falciparum malaria. Am J Trop Med Hyg 60:733–737, 1999.
19. Abdalla SH, Pasvol G: Malaria: A Hematological Perspective. London, Imperial College Press, 2004.
20. van Hensbroek M, Morris-Jones S, Meisner S, et al: Iron, but not folic acid, combined with effective antimalarial therapy promotes haematological recovery in African children after acute falciparum malaria. Trans R Soc Trop Med Hyg 89:672–676, 1995.
21. English M, Ahmed A, Ngando C, et al: Blood transfusion for severe anaemia in a Kenyan Hospital. Lancet 359:494–495, 2002.
22. Meremikwu M, Smith HJ: Blood transfusion for treating malarial anaemia. Cochrane Database Syst Rev 2;2000:CD001475.
23. Pasvol G, Abdalla SH: Definition, epidemiology, diagnosis and management of the anemia of malaria. In Abdalla SH, Pasvol G (eds): Malaria: A Hematological Perspective. London, Imperial College Press, 2004, pp 29–60.
24. ter Kuile FO, Terlouw DJ, Kariuki SK, et al: Impact of permethrin-treated bed nets on malaria, anemia, and growth in infants in an area of intense perennial malaria transmission in western Kenya. Am J Trop Med Hyg 68(suppl 4):68–77, 2003.
25. Leenstra T, Phillips-Howard PA, Kariuki SK, et al: Permethrin-treated bed nets in the prevention of malaria and anemia in adolescent schoolgirls in western Kenya. Am J Trop Med Hyg 68(suppl 4):86–93, 2003.
26. Doweiko J: Hematologic aspects of HIV infection. AIDS 7:753–757, 1993.
27. Cook JD, Skikne BS, Baynes RD: Iron deficiency: The global perspective. Adv Exp Med Biol 356:219–228, 1994.
28. Abdalla S, Corrah P, Mabey D: Severe megaloblastic anaemia due to vitamin B_{12} deficiency in the Gambia. Trans R Soc Trop Med Hyg 80:557–562, 1986.
29. Kranz S: Pathogenesis and treatment of anemia of chronic disease. Am J Med Sci 307:307–359, 1994.
30. Means R, Krantz S: Progress in understanding the pathogenesis of anemia of chronic disorders. Blood 80:1639–1647, 1992.
31. Fuchs D, Hausen A, Reibnegger G: Immune activation and the anaemia associated with chronic inflammatory disorders. Eur J Haematol 46:65–70, 1991.
32. Sergeant G: Sickle Cell Disease. Oxford, Oxford University Press, 1989.
33. Sergeant G: The clinical features of sickle cell disease. Bailliere's Clin Haematol 6:93–115, 1993.
34. Fleming A (ed): Sickle Cell Disease. A Handbook for the General Clinician. London, Churchill Livingstone, 1982.
35. Homi J, Levee L, Higgs D, et al: Pulse oximetry in a cohort study of sickle cell disease. Clin Lab Haematol 19:17–22, 1997.
36. Amrolia PJ, Almeida A, Halsey C, et al: Therapeutic challenges in childhood sickle cell disease. Part 1: Current and future treatment options. Br J Haematol 120:725–736, 2003.
37. Piomelli S: Management of Cooley's anaemia. Bailliere's Clin Haematol 6:287–298, 1993.
38. Beutler E: G-6-PD deficiency. Blood 84:3613–3636, 1994.

132

Sexually Transmitted and Urinary Tract Infections

ARLENE C. SEÑA
ALLAN RONALD
KIMBERLEY K. FOX
MYRON S. COHEN

INTRODUCTION

Sexually transmitted infections (STIs) are a major global public health problem; they are responsible for serious and sometimes fatal complications, and facilitate the transmission of the human immunodeficiency virus (HIV). Approximately 340 million new cases of the five curable STIs—gonorrhea, chlamydia, syphilis, chancroid, and trichomoniasis—were estimated to have occurred worldwide in 1999.[1] In the developing world, it is estimated that STIs, excluding acquired immunodeficiency syndrome (AIDS), are the second leading cause of healthy life lost among women between 15 and 44 years of age.[2] With the continued epidemic of HIV/AIDS, the control of other STIs has gained greater significance due to the established links between STIs and HIV transmission.

Though South and Southeast Asia had the largest number of new cases of STIs estimated in 1999, sub-Saharan Africa had the highest STI prevalence among the developing regions (119 cases per 1000 population).[1] The reliability and completeness of STI data from developing countries are inconsistent due to lack of surveillance systems and the extent of asymptomatic infections in the population, which are usually not detected or reported. Trichomoniasis continues to be the most common STI worldwide, with an estimated 76 million new cases in South and Southeast Asia in 1999.[1] However, the prevalence of herpes simplex virus type 2 (HSV-2) is increasing and is now the major cause of genital ulcer disease (GUD) throughout the world. High rates of HSV-2 are seen in sub-Saharan Africa and the Caribbean, with serological prevalences over 50% reported among adults from Kenya, Zambia, and Cameroon.[3]

Many ecological and behavioral factors contribute to the epidemic of STIs. Factors which vary widely among societies include male circumcision traditions, condom use, spermicide and other contraception practices, and patterns of alcohol or illicit drug use that influence sexual behaviors.[4] Factors contributing to the high rate of STIs in the tropics include changes in population density (e.g., urbanization); stages of demographic transition (e.g., a high proportion of young people at risk); migration and travel (e.g., increased mobility); and the accessibility, quality, and use of STI health services (e.g., inadequate health facilities).

Contact with sex workers is an important risk factor for STI acquisition and is reported as the probable source of infection by 40% to 80% of male patients in Africa.[5,6] Other STI risk factors include young age, unmarried status, residence in an urban area, multiple sexual partners, and a history of prior STIs.[7] Several STI-related syndromes are caused by a multitude of viruses and bacteria (Table 132-1). Complications of STIs such as pelvic inflammatory disease (PID), ectopic pregnancy, infertility, epididymitis, urethral strictures, neonatal conjunctivitis, and congenital syphilis occur frequently in tropical settings, presumably in part due to the lack of effective diagnostic and therapeutic interventions. In the absence of screening programs, the extent of asymptomatic disease associated with most STIs contributes to delays in diagnosis and treatment. Complications may be especially common in patients coinfected with HIV/AIDS.

Utilization of standardized protocols adapted to local epidemiological and antimicrobial susceptibilities of organisms is generally recommended in STI management. Treatment of STIs based on laboratory diagnosis is theoretically desirable, but is neither necessary nor possible in most settings. Therefore, algorithms (also called flowcharts or decision trees) have been developed as guides for STI management based on clinical signs and symptoms.[8–10] Promoted by the World Health Organization (WHO), the syndromic approach allows health-care providers to manage STIs without determining etiology with laboratory tests or specialized techniques. The advantages of syndromic management are the immediate treatment of patients and avoidance of laboratory costs. These must be balanced against the disadvantages, which include failure to detect atypical or subclinical infections, and the costs and risks associated with treatment of uninfected persons.[11] Flowcharts for the management of STI syndromes in men and PID and genital ulcers in women have proven diagnostic validity in various clinical settings; however, flowcharts for the management of vaginal discharge tend to have low sensitivity and specificity in clinically differentiating between cervical and vaginal infections.[9,10,12,13] These algorithms can be improved with a risk profile approach whereby selected symptoms and signs, as well as demographic and behavioral characteristics, are chosen for their likelihood of association with the STI under consideration.[10]

Urinary tract infections (UTIs) can have similar clinical presentations to STIs. The global incidence of UTIs exceeds 150 million annually and these infections are common everywhere. The epidemiology of UTI in developing countries has not been well studied, and extrapolation from studies in industrialized societies is required to estimate the extent and burden of illness. UTIs are categorized as either "uncomplicated," when they occur in a normal urinary tract with no structural, functional, or underlying host illness to account for the infection, or "complicated," when an underlying abnormality is believed to have enabled the infection to occur.

Table 132-1 Common Sexually Transmitted Infection-Related Syndromes and Etiologic Agents

Syndrome	Major Etiologic Agents
Genital ulcer disease	
Chancroid	*Haemophilus ducreyi*
Syphilis	*Treponema pallidum*
Genital herpes	Herpes simplex virus
Granuloma inguinale	*Calymmatobacterium granulomatosis*
Lymphogranuloma venereum	*Chlamydia trachomatis* (L serovars)
Nonulcerative genital lesions	
Genital warts	Human papillomavirus
Molluscum contagiosum	Molluscum virus
Scabies	*Sarcoptes scabiei*
Pediculosis*	*Phthirus pubis*
Vaginal discharge	
Vaginitis	*Trichomonas vaginalis, Candida albicans*
Bacteria vaginosis	*Gardnerella vaginalis, Mycoplasma hominis,* peptostreptococci, *Bacteroides* species, *Mobiluncus* species
Endocervicitis	*Neisseria gonorrhoeae, Chlamydia trachomatis,* herpes simplex virus
Endocervicitis	*Trichomonas vaginalis,* herpes simplex virus
Urethritis (women)	*Neisseria gonorrhoeae, Chlamydia trachomatis*
Urethritis (men)	*Neisseria gonorrhoeae, Chlamydia trachomatis, Ureaplasma urealyticum, Mycoplasma genitalium, Trichomonas vaginalis,* herpes simplex virus
Pelvic inflammatory disease	*Neisseria gonorrhoeae, Chlamydia trachomatis, Mycoplasma hominis, Mycoplasma genitalium,* anaerobic bacteria
Epididymitis	*Neisseria gonorrhoeae, Chlamydia trachomatis*
Proctitis	*Neisseria gonorrhoeae, Chlamydia trachomatis,* herpes simplex virus
Pharyngitis	*Neisseria gonorrhoeae, Chlamydia trachomatis*
Conjunctivitis	*Neisseria gonorrhoeae, Chlamydia trachomatis* (including L serovars)
Hepatitis	Hepatitis A virus, hepatitis B virus, hepatitis C virus, cytomegalovirus

*Pediculosis (pubic lice infestation) may be mistaken for genital lesions.

GENITAL ULCERS

GUD occurs more frequently in tropical countries than in other areas of the world, accounting for 10% to 30% of STI clinic visits in Asia and Africa compared with 2% to 5% in western Europe and North America.[14] The STIs resulting in GUD include chancroid, syphilis, genital herpes, granuloma inguinale or donovanosis, and lymphogranuloma venereum (LGV). The male-to-female ratio for GUD in tropical areas is at least 4:1.[15] This may be due to the greater visibility of the male genitalia, resulting in a higher rate of diagnosis in men, or prostitution, resulting in a higher number of cases in men. *Haemophilus ducreyi* has traditionally been the most common cause of GUD in the tropics, previously reported among 60% to 70% of genital ulcers in men,[16] and 50% of genital ulcers in women.[17] The increasing prevalence of HSV-2 in developing countries, including South Africa, Peru, and the Dominican Republic, has now made genital herpes the most common cause of GUD worldwide.[3,18,19] Granuloma inguinale occurs most frequently in western Papua New Guinea, India, the Caribbean, and among Australian aborigines.[20,21] LGV is endemic in parts of Africa, India, Asia, South America, and the Caribbean. Though only 10% of cases of LGV are noted to have a primary lesion at the time of the initial presentation, this disease should be included in the differential diagnosis of GUD.

GUD usually begins as a papule or pustule on the skin or mucous membranes, followed by ulceration and development of inguinal and/or femoral lymphadenopathy. *Treponema pallidum* penetrates through either abraded skin or intact mucous membranes within hours to days after exposure, subsequently enters the bloodstream, and disseminates.[22] HSV enters the epidermis and dermis, followed by replication in nerve ganglia and migration via peripheral sensory nerves, potentially (but rarely) leading to development of lesions distant from the primary site of exposure.[23] The other bacterial STIs that cause GUD typically result in localized disease; disseminated disease is rare but has been reported with donovanosis.

Clinical Manifestations

The manifestations of STIs associated with GUD are outlined in Table 132-2. The clinical features may help differentiate GUD etiology. Chancroid is the most likely disease in a patient presenting with one or more painful genital ulcers accompanied by an inguinal bubo (a group of tender, matted lymph nodes). The pain associated with the ulcer is perhaps the most distinguishing feature of this disease. The ulcers have ragged, undermined borders, a purulent base, and no induration; they may coalesce to form giant lesions. They are most frequently located on the coronal sulcus and prepuce in circumcised and uncircumcised men, respectively. In men, painful inguinal lymphadenopathy occurs in over half of patients; it occurs less commonly in women. The lymphadenitis of chancroid is usually unilateral; the bubo can become fluctuant and rupture, resulting in a draining abscess.

Table 132-2 Typical Clinical Features in the Differential Diagnosis of Genital Ulcer Disease Caused by Sexually Transmitted Infections

Feature	Chancroid	Primary Syphilis	Genital Herpes	Granuloma Inguinale	Lymphogranuloma Venereum
Incubation period	3–7 days	2–4 weeks	2–7 days	1–4 weeks	10–14 days
Number of lesions	Usually 1–3	Usually 1	Multiple	Single or multiple	Usually 1
Genital lesion					
Appearance	Deep, defined or irregular ulcer	Defined ulcer	Superficial, grouped vesicles or ulcerations	Defined or irregular ulcer; hypertrophic or verrucous	Papule, pustule, vesicle, or ulcer (transient)
Base	Yellow-gray, rough	Red, smooth, shiny	Red, smooth	Red, beefy, rough, usually friable	Variable
Induration	Soft	Firm	None	Firm	None
Pain	Common	None	Common*	Rare	Variable
Inguinal lymphadenopathy	Unilateral or bilateral; tender; may suppurate	Unilateral or bilateral; nontender; no suppuration	Bilateral; tender*	None; inguinal swelling	Unilateral or bilateral; tender, may suppurate
Constitutional symptoms	Rare	Rare	Common	Rare	Frequent

*Occurs more commonly in primary episodes of genital herpes than in recurrences.

In comparison, a patient presenting with a painless solitary ulcer accompanied by nontender unilateral or bilateral inguinal lymphadenopathy most likely has primary syphilis. The ulcer is typically indurated with a defined, raised border, a clear, granular base, and a serous exudate. Though a solitary painless chancre is the hallmark of primary syphilis, almost half of patients have more than one lesion.[24] Syphilitic chancres are most frequently located on the inner or outer side of the foreskin or coronal sulcus in men, and the labia in women. As many as 10% of primary chancres may be extragenital.[24] Approximately one-third of homosexual men with primary syphilis will present with an anorectal lesion. Patients with secondary syphilis may also present with anogenital ulcers; however, these are usually accompanied by exanthema of the skin and mucous membranes.

A patient with grouped vesicles or ulcers on an erythematous base, especially with a history of similar episodes, has a high likelihood of having herpes. Genital herpes in the tropics is usually caused by HSV-2. A prodrome of paresthesias around the outbreak site usually precedes the appearance of lesions by 12 to 48 hours. The grouped vesicles are considered the hallmark of genital herpes; they subsequently rupture resulting in shallow, painful ulcerations with crusting. These lesions are usually located on the prepuce, the glans, and the shaft of the penis in men, and on the labia minora, labia majora, and cervix in women. The cervix may appear diffusely or locally erythematous, with superficial erosions and sometimes necrosis. Homosexual men may have lesions in the anorectal area, which may be accompanied with symptoms of proctitis. A patient with associated symptoms of low-grade fever, chills, malaise, tender bilateral lymphadenopathy, and severe pain or paresthesias is probably experiencing a primary first episode of genital herpes (e.g., there is no pre-existing antibody to HSV-1 or HSV-2). The duration of disease is longer during primary infection. Vesicles can last 10 to 12 days before forming ulcers, which can persist for another 1 to 2 weeks. Symptoms tend to be milder during the nonprimary first episode of HSV infection, when there are pre-existing antibodies to the heterologous HSV type (in the tropics, over 90% of adults have had previous HSV-1 infection). Patients with recurrent disease, when detectable antibodies are present to the infecting HSV type, usually have fewer symptoms lasting no more than 10 days. Persistent, painful genital ulceration due to HSV-2 is extremely common in immunosuppressed HIV-infected patients in regions of high prevalence.

A patient with one or more nonpainful genital ulcers with inguinal swelling (pseudobubo) may have granuloma inguinale, also called donovanosis. This infection is caused by *Calymmatobacterium granulomatis,* a gram-negative bacillus. The patient may report the appearance of one or more firm, painless papules or nodules, which subsequently ulcerate. The predominant sites of involvement are the distal penis for men and the introitus for women; the inguinal area is affected in 10% of cases. Granuloma inguinale may take many forms, including an ulcerative or ulcero-granulomatous lesion (a nontender, beefy-red ulcer with a granulated base); a hypertrophic or verrucous lesion with profuse granulation and friability; a necrotic, painful lesion with a foul-smelling exudate; or a sclerotic bandlike lesion with fibrous tissue formation.

A patient with tender inguinal lymphadenopathy or a suppurating bubo without a visible genital ulcer may have LGV. This syndrome is caused by infection with the serovars L1, L2, and L3 of *Chlamydia trachomatis*. The lesion is transient and frequently goes unnoticed; it precedes the development of unilateral or bilateral lymphadenitis by 7 to 30 days. The lesion appears as a small, painless papule, pustule, or herpetiform ulcer. It is located most commonly on the coronal sulcus, prepuce, glans of the penis, or the urethral meatus in men, and on the vulva, vaginal wall, or cervix in women. The most easily recognized clinical feature of LGV in men is the "groove sign," or the enlargement of nodes above and below the inguinal ligament. However, a groove sign can also be found in patients with chancroid. The inguinal buboes of LGV may become fluctuant and rupture, or form a hard inguinal mass with suppuration. Women may present with enlarged pelvic nodes and associated pelvic pain, or with symptoms of proctitis due to lymphatic spread to the rectal mucosa.

Diagnosis

The medical history should determine the suspected time of exposure, the nature and duration of the lesions, the presence of pain, and the presence of constitutional symptoms such as fever or malaise. The physical examination should include the skin, oral cavity, external genitalia, the inguinal or femoral lymph nodes, and the anorectal area. In women, a pelvic examination should be performed whenever possible.

The diagnosis of GUD can be problematic without laboratory testing, since several studies have demonstrated the unreliability of clinical etiologic diagnosis.[25,26] One study found that the clinical diagnosis of GUD was accurate in only 68% of cases where single infections were detected. The accuracy was highest (80%) for the most common etiology, chancroid, and least for other causes: 55% for primary syphilis, 27% for LGV, and 22% for genital herpes.[26] Diagnostic techniques for the specific agents associated with GUD are outlined in Table 132-3. Ideally, the diagnostic workup should include darkfield examination for *T. pallidum,* culture for *H. ducreyi,* culture for HSV, and serologic tests for syphilis. Cultures should be obtained from the base of the ulcer after washing the lesion with saline. If buboes are present, a diagnostic and therapeutic aspiration should be performed. Unfortunately, false negative tests are frequently encountered in the evaluation of GUD, due to the low sensitivity of available tests. Though darkfield microscopy can provide a definitive diagnosis of syphilis, a negative result does not exclude syphilis since the accuracy of the test depends on the quality of the specimen and the experience of the individual performing the procedure. Sufficient organisms may not be present following self-medication. Nontreponemal blood tests for syphilis, such as the rapid plasma reagin (RPR) test or the Venereal Disease Research Laboratory (VDRL) tests, are positive in approximately 80% of primary syphilis cases.[27] Furthermore, positive syphilis serologies may reflect past infection, and false positive results may occur for a variety of reasons. Confirmation with a specific treponemal test (fluorescent treponemal antibody absorption test or FTA-ABS; the microhemagglutinin assay–*T. pallidum* or MHA-TP; or the *T. pallidum* passive agglutination assay or TP-PA) is therefore important. The FTA-ABS has the highest sensitivity among the treponemal tests (86% to 100% for primary syphilis).[27]

Table 132-3 Diagnostic Tests and Treatment for the Most Common Causes of Genital Ulcer Disease

	Definitive Diagnosis	Probable Diagnosis	Recommended Treatment Regimes
Chancroid	Culture	Clinical presentation	Azithromycin 1.0 g PO × 1; or ciprofloxacin 500 mg PO bid × 3 days; or erythromycin 500 mg PO tid or qid × 7 days (Alternative: ceftriaxone 250 mg IM × 1) (Pregnancy: erythromycin or ceftriaxone as above)
Primary syphilis	Darkfield examination; direct immunofluorescence	Clinical presentation; serology	Benzathine penicillin G 2.4 million units IM × 1 (Alternatives: procaine penicillin 1.2 million units IM × 10 days; or doxycycline 100 mg PO bid or tetracycline 500 mg PO qid × 14 days) (Pregnancy: penicillin as above)
Genital herpes	Viral culture	Clinical presentation; antigen detection by immunofluorescence or enzyme immunoassay; serology	Acyclovir 200 mg PO 5 ×/day, or acyclovir 400 mg PO tid, or famciclovir 250 mg PO tid, or valaciclovir 1.0 g PO bid × 7 days* (Pregnancy: oral acyclovir as above)
Granuloma inguinale	"Donovan bodies" in tissue smears or biopsy specimens	Clinical presentation	Azithromycin 1.0 g × 1, then 500 mg PO every day; or doxycycline 100 mg PO bid for a minimum of 14 days (Alternatives: erythromycin 500 mg PO qid, or tetracycline 500 mg PO qid, or trimethoprim (80 mg)–sulfamethoxazole (400 mg) 2 tablets PO bid for a minimum of 14 days) (Pregnancy: erythromycin as above)
Lymphogranuloma venereum	Isolation in cell culture	Clinical presentation; serology	Doxycycline 100 mg PO bid × 14 days; or erythromycin 500 mg PO qid × 14 days (Alternative: tetracycline 500 mg PO qid × 14 days) (Pregnancy: erythromycin as above)

*Recommended for the primary episode of genital herpes. For recurrent genital herpes, the recommended regimens are acyclovir 800 mg PO bid × 5 days, famciclovir 125 mg PO bid × 5 days, valacyclovir 500 mg PO bid or 1.0 g PO daily × 5 days.

Other tests in the laboratory diagnosis of GUD have important limitations. The identification of gram-negative coccobacilli in parallel rows or in a clustered "school of fish" appearance is reported to be characteristic of *H. ducreyi*, but is no longer recommended due to its poor sensitivity and specificity. Culture for chancroid is considered to be the definitive test, but is difficult to perform and has an estimated sensitivity of 75% compared to nucleic acid amplification detection from genital ulcer swabs.[14] If a diagnosis of genital herpes is not certain from the clinical presentation, a culture can provide the most sensitive and specific test when available. The sensitivity of herpes culture approaches 100% for vesicular lesions, but decreases to 33% during the ulcer stage.[28] If the culture for HSV is not available, the Tzanck smear can provide a probable diagnosis of HSV; this is performed by scraping the base of the lesion, staining a slide of the material with Wright stain, and looking for multinucleated giant cells. The sensitivity of the Tzanck smear for genital herpes is approximately 67% in the vesicular stage and 50% in the ulcer stage.[29] Type-specific HSV serologies that detect antibodies to HSV glycoproteins have become available and can support a diagnosis of genital herpes in patients with atypical presentations.[30] When granuloma inguinale is suspected, a Giemsa stain or Wright stain of crushed tissue smears or biopsy specimens looking for Donovan bodies (bacillary organisms within histiocytes) should be performed. Donovan bodies can be demonstrated in only 60% to 80% of cases from either direct smears or biopsy specimens. The isolation of *C. trachomatis* in cell culture provides definitive diagnosis of LGV, but the recovery rate is only 50%.[31] Serologic testing with complement fixation (CF) or microimmunofluorescence (MIF) can assist the diagnosis when performed in the appropriate clinical setting, but does not distinguish among infections with other *Chlamydia* species. Positive titers greater than 1:256 with CF or greater than 1:128 with MIF are strongly indicative of LGV, although invasive genital infections with the *C. trachomatis* serovars D–K can also give rise to high serum titers.[32]

Coinfection with more than one pathogen has been reported in 5% to 10% of all GUD cases[33]; most commonly encountered are coexistent syphilis and chancroid. In one-fourth to one-half of GUD cases, no cause can be found by simple laboratory testing.[13,33] Nucleic acid amplification involving polymerase chain reaction (PCR) for *T. pallidum*, *H. ducreyi*, and HSV have been applied in research studies as a more sensitive detection method than traditional tests for the diagnosis of genital lesions.[20,21,34,35] Rapid diagnostic tests for *T. pallidum* are being investigated and may assist in future GUD diagnostic efforts by enabling immediate diagnosis at the first visit.[36]

Other causes of genital ulceration to consider in the differential include abrasions and trauma, contact dermatitis, fixed drug eruptions, Reiter's syndrome, Behçet's syndrome, and carcinoma. Infectious diseases such as systemic fungal diseases and cutaneous leishmaniasis, if endemic in the area, may also confuse the diagnosis. Atypical presentations of GUD associated with STIs must always be considered and are often seen in the tropics as a result of coinfections, coexistent HIV/AIDS, ineffective self-treatment, use of traditional remedies, superinfections, and other complications due to long-standing disease.

Management

Algorithms for the management of genital ulcers depend on the local prevalence of causal agents. One example of an algorithm for the syndromic management of genital ulcers is the WHO flowchart provided in Figure 132-1. A similar algorithm whereby all patients with GUD were treated for syphilis and chancroid has reported cure rates of 69% for females and 83% for males.[37] Empirical therapy for both *T. pallidum* and *H. ducreyi* infections should be considered for all patients with GUD in areas like sub-Saharan Africa, where syphilis and chancroid are common. Otherwise, treatment regimens should be directed, usually during the initial visit, towards the most likely diagnosis determined from the clinical presentation and available laboratory studies (see Table 132-3).

In selecting therapy for chancroid, it should be noted that there is widespread resistance of *H. ducreyi* to penicillins (PCNs) and tetracyclines in all geographic areas[38,39]; therefore, these drugs should not used as part of any treatment regimens. Azithromycin, ciprofloxacin, erythromycin, and ceftriaxone should be used for chancroid treatment, as noted in Table 132-3. Drainage of fluctuant buboes may be necessary. HIV-positive patients may fail single-dose therapy for

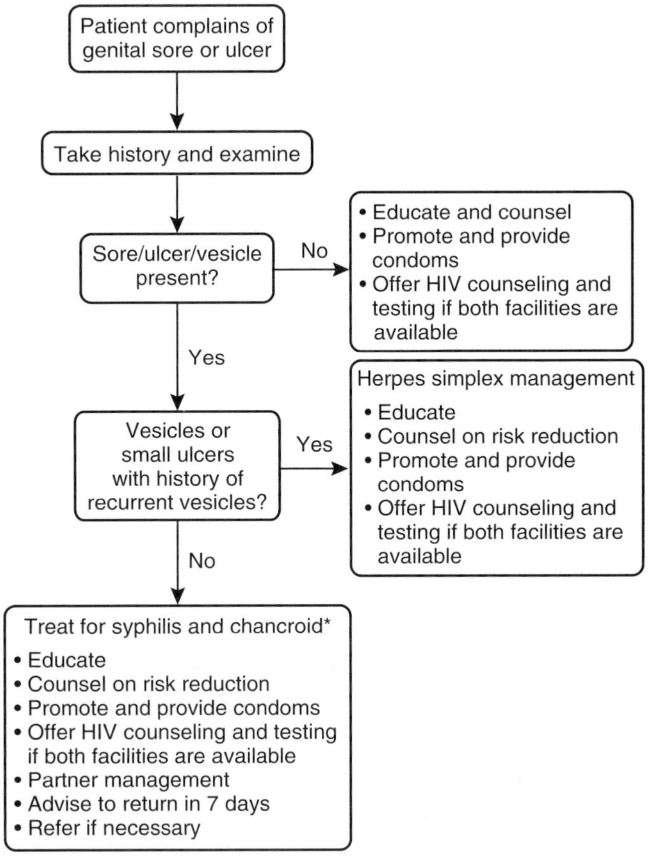

*Needs adaptation to local epidemiological situation.

FIGURE 132-1 World Health Organization flowchart for the syndromic management of patients with a genital sore or ulcer. (Redrawn from Guidelines for the Management of Sexually Transmitted Infections [WHO/HIV-AIDS/2001.01]. Geneva, World Health Organization, 2001.)

chancroid,[40] and may have increased likelihood of coinfections with syphilis or genital herpes.

Whereas actual resistance of *T. pallidum* to PCN is not known to occur, a significant proportion of patients in the early stages of syphilis fail to demonstrate serologic cure after standard therapy.[41] Serologic cure for syphilis is defined by a fourfold decrease (two or more dilutions) in nontreponemal titers within 6 months after treatment.[42] Serologic treatment failure for primary syphilis has been reported in 5% of HIV-negative patients and 22% of HIV-infected patients at 6 months after standard therapy.[41] Primary syphilis unresponsive to a single dose of PCN should be re-treated with benzathine PCN 2.4 million units intramuscularly (IM), administered weekly for 3 weeks. Alternative regimens for PCN-allergic patients with early syphilis are doxycycline 100 mg orally twice a day or tetracycline 500 mg orally four times a day for 14 days.[7] Oral therapy with azithromycin at 2.0 g orally in a single dose is a potential alternative for treatment of early syphilis.[43] However, there have been a few reported treatment failures with this regimen,[44] especially among HIV-infected persons, underscoring the importance of close follow-up until its treatment efficacy has been fully investigated. Pregnant women with syphilis who are allergic to PCN should be desensitized in a hospital setting, as alternative therapies are inadequate in preventing congenital syphilis. Treatment regimens for HIV-infected persons with early syphilis are the same as for non-HIV-infected persons. However, examination of cerebrospinal fluid should be considered in HIV-positive patients regardless of their stage of syphilis due to their increased risk for early neurosyphilis. Persons with early syphilis should be re-evaluated clinically and serologically using a nontreponemal test after 6 months to assess response to therapy. Repeat evaluations after 6 months and after 12 months may be indicated based on response to therapy and local resources. Re-treatment should be considered for persons with persistent or recurrent clinical signs or symptoms of active syphilis, or persons with a confirmed fourfold (two dilution) increase in the nontreponemal test titers.

There is no known cure for genital herpes, but treatment with acyclovir or its analogues initiated as soon as possible after the onset of symptoms reduces the development of new lesions, the duration of pain, and viral shedding (see Table 132-3). Patients with recurrent herpes should be advised to seek treatment or to start medications during their prodrome phase or within 1 day after onset of lesions in order to benefit from therapy. Patients with recurrent genital herpes (e.g., six or more recurrences per year) are candidates for daily suppressive therapy with acyclovir 400 mg orally twice a day, famciclovir 250 mg orally twice a day, or valaciclovir 500 mg or 1.0 g orally once daily for 6–12 months,[45] followed by reassessment of the need for continued therapy after that period. The safety and efficacy of suppressive therapy with acyclovir has been assessed up to 5 years; more than 20% of patients on suppressive therapy were reported to be recurrence free during this 5-year period.[46] Patients infected concomitantly with HIV can benefit from chronic suppression. However, they may develop thymidine-kinase deficient virus from suppressive therapy, resulting in difficulties with long-term management.

Patients with granuloma inguinale should be given azithromycin or doxycycline, with the addition of gentamicin at 1.0 mg/kg intravenously every 8 hours considered in difficult cases involving HIV-infected persons. Relapses of granuloma inguinale are frequent and may require a second course of antibiotics. Other drugs which have been reported to be efficacious for this disease include erythromycin, tetracycline, ciprofloxacin, and streptomycin.[33] LGV should be treated with doxycycline or erythromycin for 14 days. However, some patients with advanced disease may require a longer duration of treatment and surgery may be required for sequelae such as strictures and/or fistula.

Medical management of sexual contacts of patients with GUD should include an examination for lesions and empirical treatment in all cases because of the high likelihood of infection. Sexual contacts of patients with genital herpes are an exception, since the infection is not curable and therapy is provided primarily for palliation of symptoms. In addition, education and counseling are critical.

NONULCERATIVE GENITAL LESIONS

Several STDs may appear as nonulcerative lesions in the genital area (see Table 132-1). Human papillomavirus (HPV) infection resulting in genital warts is frequently encountered in the tropics.[47,48] A cross-sectional study of women attending an STD clinic in Jamaica found that 29% were HPV-positive using Southern blot hybridization techniques on cervicovaginal lavage specimens.[49] HPV in the tropics has been increasingly recognized due to the association of certain "high-risk" HPV types (especially types 16, 18, 31, 33, and 35) with cervical and penile carcinoma. The preceding HPV types are usually associated with subclinical infection in the premalignant phase, while HPV types 6 and 11 cause benign exophytic warts. Concomitant HIV and high-risk HPV may lead to invasive cervical cancer in young women.[50] The pathogenesis of HPV infection involves the squamous epithelium, in which there is viral entry and replication associated with increased proliferation of all the epidermal layers except the basal layer. Effective host defenses are important in the resolution of HPV infections, but these defenses are poorly understood.

Molluscum contagiosum is caused by a large DNA virus of the Poxviridae family resulting in a superficial cutaneous infection of children and young adults. Molluscum is usually a benign condition which may be transmitted through sexual or other close contact, but can occur as an opportunistic infection in patients with AIDS. Scabies should be included in the differential diagnosis of papular lesions in the genital area, as a condition that can also be transmitted through sexual or other close contact. Scabies is caused by *Sarcoptes scabiei* var. *hominis* and is discussed in greater detail in Chapter 118.

Clinical Manifestations

A patient complaining of vulvar or penile nonulcerative lesions in the absence of other symptoms may have genital warts. Warts are typically multiple, but may be solitary. Genital warts can appear as rough, slightly pigmented papules, flat keratotic plaques, or as soft, fleshy, exophytic lesions called condylomata acuminata. Papular warts usually have the same color as that of the surrounding epithelium; if gray or brown discoloration is present, dysplasia should be suspected. Genital warts may be located on the penile shaft, perineum, labia, or cervix, or in the urethra. Cervical HPV lesions may occasionally present as classic condylomata acuminata, but are more likely to be subclinical. Intra-anal warts are common among men and women who practice receptive anal intercourse.[51] Most patients with genital warts are asymptomatic. Men with genital warts may complain of penile pruritus or bloody ejaculate due to the presence of intraurethral condylomas.

A patient found to have small (2–5 mm), dome-shaped papules with characteristic central umbilication likely has molluscum contagiosum. These lesions are usually pearly white, but can be flesh-colored or yellow. They are typically multiple and may be noted in the inguinal area or inner thighs or in extragenital sites such as the palms, soles, eyelids, and conjunctivae. There may be extensive involvement of the face and torso in AIDS patients.

A patient presenting with highly pruritic polymorphic papules should arouse suspicion of scabies. In early lesions, a tiny dot representing the buried mite may be seen at one end of the papule. The lesions can become excoriated, eczematous, and secondarily infected. When sexually transmitted, the lesions are typically found over the lower abdomen, buttocks, inner thighs, and genitalia. Lesions due to scabies can also appear on the finger webs, ventral wrist fold, and underneath the breasts in women.

Diagnosis

The diagnosis of genital warts is made primarily on clinical grounds. Physical examination assisted by bright light and magnification is the recommended approach to primary diagnosis.[52] Histopathology of suspicious lesions should be performed in some cases to rule out malignancies. Pelvic examination with cervical and Papanicolau (Pap) smears is recommended for women suspected of HPV infection. Abnormal cervical lesions should be biopsied for pathologic examination. Condyloma acuminata should be distinguished from the condyloma lata of secondary syphilis, which can form large fleshy masses that frequently erode and have thick secretions loaded with spirochetes. The differential diagnosis of atypical lesions includes genital herpes, molluscum contagiosum, lichen planus, benign neoplasms, genital squamous cell cancer, and Bowen's disease.

Molluscum contagiosum is also diagnosed based on the clinical appearance of the papules. If confirmation is needed, smears of the caseous material expressed from the lesions or a histologic specimen can be examined for characteristic intracytoplasmic inclusions. The differential diagnosis of these lesions is similar to that for genital warts.

The diagnosis of scabies can be made by identifying the typical elongated burrows within the papules, which may be more visible after application of ink. Scrapings of the lesions can be visualized microscopically for the presence of adult mites, larvae, eggs, or fecal pellets. Scabies may be confused with secondary syphilis, atopic or contact dermatitis, drug eruption, and impetigo.

Management

No therapy has been demonstrated to eradicate HPV once acquired. However, external genital warts can be removed if the patient desires with excisional curettage, electrosurgery, or weekly cryotherapy with liquid nitrogen. Other treatment regimens can be provider or patient administered. Provider-administered therapies which require careful application to external warts include podophyllin in a 10% to 25% solution or trichloroacetic acid in an 80% to 90% solution applied weekly for up to 6 weeks. Podofilox (a compound purified from podophyllin) in a 0.5% solution may be applied by the patient twice daily for 3 days, followed by 4 days of no treatment, for up to 4 weeks. Imiquimod is a patient-administered immunotherapy for external genital and perianal warts that can be used as a 5% cream applied three times a week for as long as 16 weeks; it may have the advantage of reducing recurrence rates and causing less discomfort to the patient than traditional therapies.[53] Cryotherapy or podophyllin can be used for genital warts located in the vagina or penile urethra. Exophytic cervical warts should be evaluated for dysplasia before initiation of therapy. During pregnancy, the removal of visible warts is advocated because they tend to proliferate and become friable; podophyllin, podofilox, and imiquimod are not recommended as treatment options in pregnancy.

Molluscum contagiosum rarely requires treatment, but for cosmetic reasons or minor symptoms, excisional curettage or cryotherapy is usually effective. Scabies may be treated with 5% permethrin cream or 1% lindane lotion applied to the body for 8 hours and repeated in 1 week. Pregnant women should not be treated with lindane. Bedding and clothing of affected persons should be decontaminated in hot water or a clothes dryer.

Treatment of sexual contacts is not necessary for genital warts or molluscum contagiosum. However, sexual partners to persons with genital warts should be counseled regarding their exposure and risk for disease. Female partners should have a cervical Pap smear. Sexual and other close contacts of patients with scabies should be examined and treated appropriately.

VAGINAL DISCHARGE

Three general syndromes result in a vaginal discharge: vaginitis or vaginosis, endocervicitis, and ectocervicitis. The type of epithelium present and other factors such as the pH in the microenvironment determine the susceptibility of each site to specific pathogens. The etiologic agents associated with each syndrome are provided in Table 132-1. Trichomoniasis is reported to be the most common nonviral STI worldwide, with reported infection rates as high as 31% among female students and 25% to 38% among pregnant women screened in Nigeria.[54–56] Bacterial vaginosis (BV) is also widely prevalent; in parts of Africa, up to 60% of women presenting with a vaginal discharge have been reported to have BV.[57,58] BV is a clinical syndrome resulting from a disequilibrium of the normal vaginal flora, which consists predominantly of lactobacilli. In BV, there is a massive overgrowth of *Gardnerella vaginalis, Mobiluncus* species, and other anaerobes. The role of sexual transmission in BV is controversial[54]; sexual activity may increase the risk for BV through mechanisms such as alteration of vaginal pH. Factors associated with vulvovaginal candidiasis (VVC) include pregnancy, uncontrolled diabetes mellitus, young age, and recent antimicrobial therapy.[58,59] Sexual transmission of candidiasisis is infrequent.

While vaginitis and vaginosis are the most common causes of vaginal discharge, cervical infections are more important from a public health standpoint because of their potential complications, including PID, infertility, and neonatal disease.

Trichomoniasis and BV have recently been implicated as causes of obstetric complications (e.g., premature rupture of membranes, low birth weight) and PID. [60–62] However, the association of gonorrhea and chlamydial infection with upper genital tract disease and adverse obstetric and neonatal outcomes is more strongly supported by epidemiologic and biologic data (see the later discussion of PID). Subclinical PID, defined by the presence of histologic endometritis, has been reported among 26% of women infected with *Neisseria gonorrhoeae* and 27% of women infected with *C. trachomatis* in the lower genital tract.[63] Unfortunately, the majority of women infected with *N. gonorrhoeae* and *C. trachomatis* are asymptomatic, making efforts directed at disease detection and prevention challenging.

Gonorrhea has been the most prevalent STI in the tropics. Among low-risk populations attending antenatal or family planning clinics, the prevalence of gonorrhea in tropical countries ranges from 2.0% in India[64] to 3.6% in Tanzania.[65] Among symptomatic women, the prevalence of gonorrhea in Africa has been reported as high as 17.1% in Malawi.[66] Chlamydial infection has a reported prevalence ranging from 1.8% in Brazil[67] to 39.3% in Jamaica[68] among women tested in antenatal or family planning clinics. *N. gonorrhoeae* primarily affects the mucous epithelium of the lower genital tract, resulting in a vigorous neutrophilic response, development of submucosal microabscesses, and exudation of pus. Gonorrhea can also affect the rectum, oropharynx, and conjunctivae, and is discussed in further detail in Chapter 26. The trachoma biovar of *C. trachomatis* primarily affects the squamocolumnar epithelial cells of the endocervix, urethra, rectum, and conjunctiva.[69] Marked inflammation in the upper genital tract of infected women leading to ectopic pregnancy and infertility may be associated with the presence of serum antibodies reactive with the *C. trachomatis* heat-shock protein.[70]

Coinfection with both gonorrhea and chlamydia occurs frequently and should be a consideration in the management of patients with cervicitis. Mucopurulent cervicitis (MPC) is an STI syndrome that is a diagnosis of exclusion. It has been defined as cervical inflammation that is not secondary to *N. gonorrhoeae*[71]; it may be associated with *C. trachomatis* or less frequently with HSV, but in most cases no pathogen is found by routine testing.

Clinical Manifestations

Symptoms of vaginitis may include discharge, odor, external dysuria, and itching of the vulva and perivaginal mucosa. Patients may also complain of vaginal soreness, irritation, discomfort, and dyspareunia. Unfortunately, the symptoms of vaginitis are nonspecific and differentiation of syndromes cannot be based on these findings alone (Table 132-4). A patient with BV may present with a "fishy" white, homogenous vaginal discharge in the absence of irritative symptoms. A patient with trichomoniasis may also have a malodorous discharge, but usually have accompanying signs of vulvovaginal irritation such as pruritus and dysuria.[72] A patient presenting with a curdlike vaginal discharge and pruritus of the vulva and perivaginal mucosa is more likely to have VVC.

Both gonococcal and chlamydial cervicitis produce few if any symptoms. When symptoms do occur, they include vaginal discharge, dysuria, and occasionally minor bleeding. Pelvic examination may reveal a purulent, mucopurulent, or bloody cervical discharge, with edema, erythema, or friability of the cervical os. An obvious endocervical discharge or a purulent vaginal discharge originating from the cervix is present in only 10% to 20% of women with gonorrhea.[73] MPC is characterized by the presence of a yellow-green endocervical exudate when viewed on a white cotton swab, or easily induced cervical bleeding when the swab is placed in the endocervix. The presence of mucopurulent discharge along with ulcerations and erythema of the ectocervix should arouse suspicion for HSV.

Diagnosis

The medical history should include the nature and duration of symptoms, the sexual history (including recent new sex partners), history of prior STDs, past therapy, and response to therapy. The physical examination should include inspection and palpation of the inguinal lymph nodes, vulva, vaginal vestibule, and anorectal area. The color, consistency, volume, and odor of the vaginal secretions should be noted. A speculum examination should be performed when possible to evaluate the vaginal mucosa and cervix for erythema, petechiae, ulceration, edema, atrophy, and adherent discharge.

Table 132-4 Differential Diagnosis or Vaginitis or Vaginosis

Feature	Trichomoniasis	Bacterial Vaginosis	Vulvovaginal Candidiasis
Discharge	Thin; gray to yellow-green frothy; mild to fishy odor	Thin; gray to white homogenous; fishy odor	Thick; white; often curdlike; minimal odor
Vaginal examination	Vulvovaginal erythema	Minimal or no vulvovaginal erythema	Vulvovaginal erythema; mucosal swelling
Cervical examination	Ectocervical erythema; rare punctate hemorrhages ("strawberry cervix")	Normal	Occasional ectocervical erythema
Wet mount	Trichomonads; increased PMNs	Clue cells; few PMNs	Budding yeast; pseudohyphae; few PMNs
KOH slide	Positive "whiff" test* in some cases	Positive "whiff" test*	Allows clearer view of yeast
pH of discharge	pH > 4.5	pH > 4.5	pH normal (4.0–4.5)

PMN, polymorphonuclear leukocytes.
*Intensification of foul fishy odor upon addition of KOH to a sample of vaginal discharge.

The differential diagnosis of vaginitis is presented in Table 132-4. Whenever possible, a clinical examination should be accompanied by a wet mount, potassium hydroxide preparation (KOH), and pH determination of the vaginal discharge. The wet mount, performed by mixing vaginal fluid with normal saline on a slide, is examined for polymorphonuclear neutrophils (PMNs), motile trichomonads, and clue cells. Trichomonads are ovoid and slightly larger than PMNs. Clue cells are exfoliated vaginal squamous epithelial cells covered with bacteria, giving the cells a granular or stippled appearance and masking the cell borders. Increased numbers of PMNs (ratio greater than 1:1 relative to epithelial cells) are seen in trichomoniasis, as well as in gonorrhea, chlamydia, and HSV infection. The absence of trichomonads on a wet mount does not exclude the diagnosis since the sensitivity is only 60% to 70% compared with culture, which detects 95% of *T. vaginalis* infections.[74] A wet mount has a sensitivity of 40% to 60% for VVC.[57] The sensitivity can be improved by adding a few drops of 10% KOH to vaginal fluid on a slide to dissolve cellular matter, making yeast forms more visible. The finding of pseudohyphae or budding yeast supports the diagnosis of yeast vaginitis in the setting of appropriate symptoms; however, budding yeast may be part of the normal flora if present in small numbers.

Diagnosis of BV requires three of the following four criteria: (1) a homogeneous, white noninflammatory discharge that adheres to the vaginal walls; (2) the presence of clue cells on microscopic examination; (3) vaginal fluid pH greater than 4.5; and (4) a positive whiff test (a fishy odor before or after addition of 10% KOH to a sample of vaginal discharge).[42] A scoring system based on Gram stain of the vaginal discharge (Nugent criteria) can provide a standardized method for the diagnosis of BV, with a sensitivity of 89%.[75,76] In this scoring system, the absence of lactobacilli, along with the presence of small and curved gram-variable rods (representing *G. vaginalis, Bacteroides* species, and *Mobiluncus* species), is most predictive of BV.

Patients suspected of or likely to have cervical infection should be tested for *N. gonorrhoeae* and *C. trachomatis*. The most widely available test for gonorrhea is culture on selective media, which has a reported sensitivity of 86% to 96%.[77] Tissue culture for *C. trachomatis* has a sensitivity of 70% to 80% in experienced laboratories, with a specificity close to 100%,[78,79] but is of limited utility because of its exacting requirements. The sensitivities of both the enzyme immunoassay (EIA) and direct fluorescent antibody (DFA) test for *C. trachomatis* vary, depending on the population being evaluated and skill of the laboratorian. The reported sensitivities range from 73% to 95% for EIA of cervical specimens,[80,81] and 50% to 81% for DFA.[82,83] The specificity of EIA is usually greater than 95%.[84] The specificity of DFA depends on the experience and reliability of the laboratory performing the test. A DNA probe test is also available for the detection of *N. gonorrhoeae* and *C. trachomatis*. The detection of *N. gonorrhoeae* with this test is comparable to culture, and the test has the advantage of requiring only one specimen for identifying both organisms.[85–87] PCR for *N. gonorrhoeae* and *C. trachomatis* using endocervical and urethral specimens provides greater sensitivity and specificity than traditional tests.[88,89] Self-inserted vaginal swabs for PCR detection are also acceptable methods for specimen collection.[90] Urine-based PCR for gonorrhea and chlamydia has the advantage of being noninvasive and has sensitivities almost equivalent to PCR from endocervical and urethral specimens, but requires first-voided urine specimens for maximum recovery of organisms. However, the cost and the infrastructure required to perform these detection methods may limit their utility in tropical settings.

A Gram stain of the cervical discharge may be helpful in choosing empirical therapy, but should be interpreted with caution owing to the limitations of the technique. Increased PMNs, especially greater than 30 per high-power field (HPF), may be correlated with gonococcal or chlamydial infection. When read by an experienced microscopist, the presence of intracellular gram-negative diplococci is 50% to 60% sensitive and highly specific for gonorrhea, while extracellular diplococci may represent normal genital flora. However, the absence of diplococci on an endocervical smear does not exclude gonococcal infection.

In patients with a vaginal discharge but no obvious infectious cause, the differential diagnosis should include chemical or allergic vulvovaginitis, which can result from contact with deodorants, douches, or spermicides, or the presence of a foreign body in the vagina. Cervical, vaginal, and vulvar neoplasias often cause a minor discharge.

Management

For settings in which a speculum and bimanual examination cannot be performed, the WHO recommends an algorithm for vaginal discharge or vulval itching/burning based on the presence of an abnormal discharge, lower abdominal tenderness, and a risk assessment adapted to the local social, behavioral, and epidemiological situation. When the patient has an abnormal discharge and a positive risk assessment, this algorithm recommends empiric treatment for gonococcal, chlamydial and trichomonal infections, and BV.[8] An algorithm for the syndromic management of patients presenting with a vaginal discharge is provided as an example in Figure 132-2. This algorithm requires a risk assessment and a speculum examination and was found to be 84% sensitive and 40% specific for the presence of a cervical infection in a Jamaican STD clinic.[12] Recommended therapies for vaginitis and cervicitis are provided in Table 132-5. The single oral dose of 2 g metronidazole for trichomoniasis has a cure rate of 82% to 88%.[91] Due to the occurrence of *T. vaginalis* with resistance to metronidazole, infections that do not respond to the single-dose regimen should be re-treated with metronidazole 500 mg twice a day for 7 days. If treatment failure recurs, the patient should be treated with metronidazole 2 g orally once daily for 3 to 5 days. The single-dose regimen of 2 g metronidazole for BV has clinical response rates comparable to the standard regimen, but higher recurrence rates have been reported.[92,93] Pregnant women who have symptomatic BV can be treated with metronidazole at 250 mg orally three times a day for 7 days, or with a single 2-g dose. Alternative therapies in pregnancy include topical metronidazole gel and oral clindamycin. There are several topical antimycotic agents for VVC with similar clinical efficacies. Oral therapy for VVC with fluconazole 150 mg as a one-time dose is superior to these topical therapies; however, fluconazole is expensive and should be avoided in pregnancy. Recurrent VVC, usually defined as three or more episodes per year, occurs in a minority of patients with risk factors such as immunosuppression or corticosteroid use.

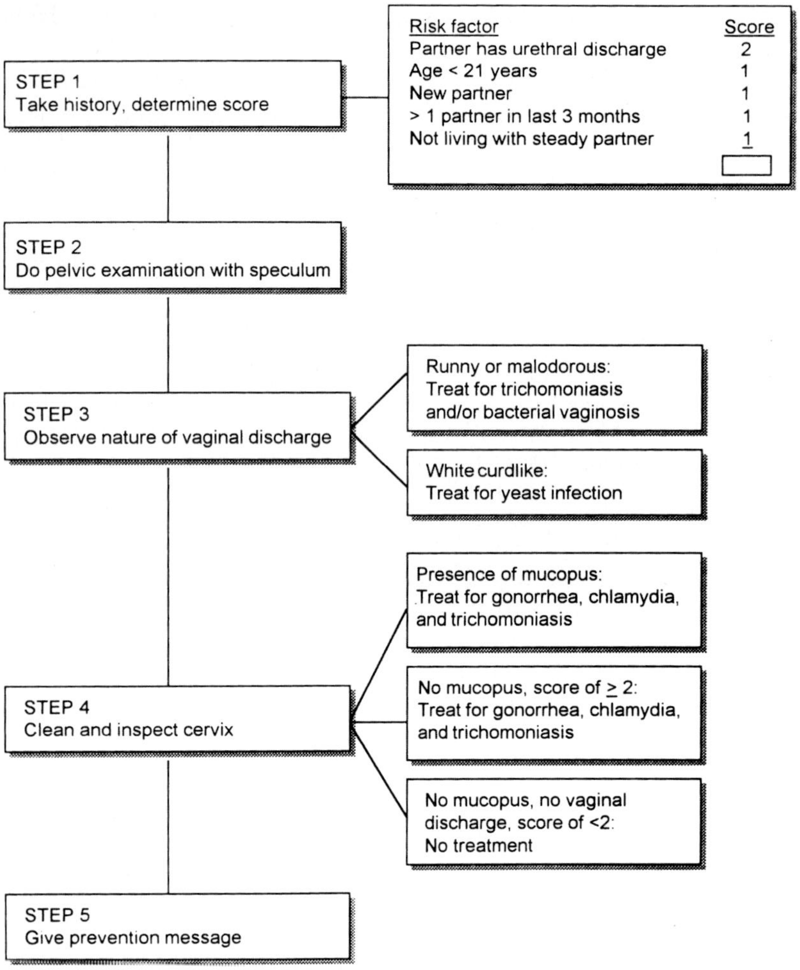

FIGURE 132-2 Example of a flowchart for the management of patients with a vaginal discharge. (From Behets PMT, Williams Y, Brathwaite A, et al: Management of vaginal discharge in women treated at a Jamaican sexually transmitted disease clinic: Use of diagnostic algorithm versus laboratory testing. Clin Infect Dis 21:1450, 1995.)

Table 132-5 Recommended Treatment Regimens for Vaginitis, Cervicitis, and Urethritis

Trichomonas vaginitis/ urethritis	Metronidazole 2 g PO × 1 dose; or tinidazole 2 g PO × 1 dose (Alternatives: metronidazole 500 mg PO bid × 7 days; or tinidazole 500 mg PO bid × 5 days) (Pregnancy: metronidazole 2 g dose as above)	
Bacterial vaginosis	Metronidazole 500 mg PO bid × 7 days (Alternatives: metronidazole 2 g PO × 1 dose; or metronidazole gel 0.75% 5 g intravaginally bid × 5 days; or clindamycin 300 mg PO bid × 7 days; clindamycin cream 2% 5 g intravaginally at bedtime × 7 days) (Pregnancy: metronidazole 250 mg PO tid × 7 days or the 2 g dose, metronidazole gel or clindamycin as above)	
Candida vaginitis	Miconazole or clotrimazole 200 mg intravaginally every day × 3 days; or clotrimazole 500 mg PO intravaginally × 1 dose; or fluconazole 150 mg PO × 1 dose; (Alternative: nystatin 100,000 IU intravaginally every day × 14 days) (Pregnancy: any 7-day topical treatment)	
Gonococcal cervicitis/ urethritis*	Ciprofloxacin 500 mg PO × 1 dose†‡§#; or ofloxacin 400 mg PO × 1 dose†‡; levofloxacin 250 mg PO × 1 dose†‡; cefixime 400 mg PO × 1 dose‡; or ceftriaxone 125 mg IM × 1 dose‡§#; or spectinomycin 2 g IM × 1 dose‡# (Pregnancy: cefixime, ceftriaxone, or spectinomycin as above)	plus treatment for *C. trachomatis*
Chlamydial cervicitis/ urethritis*	Doxycycline 100 mg PO bid × 7 days; or azithromycin 1 g PO × 1 dose; (Alternatives: amoxicillin 500 mg PO tid × 7 days; erythromycin base 500 mg PO qid × 7 days; ofloxacin 300 mg PO bid × 7 days; tetracycline 500 mg PO qid × 7 days) (Pregnancy: amoxicillin or erythromycin as above)	
Nongonococcal urethritis	Doxycycline 100 mg PO bid × 7 days; or azithromycin 1 g PO × 1 dose; or erythromycin base 500 mg PO qid × 7 days	

*Regimen is for uncomplicated cervicitis or urethritis only.
†Knowledge of local resistance patterns is recommended due to increasing fluoroquine resistance.
‡Regimens recommended for anorectal infections.
§Regimens recommended for treatment of gonococcal pharyngitis.
#Regimens recommended for treatment of adult gonococcal conjunctivitis.

The frequency of episodes can be reduced with a regimen of ketoconazole 100 mg orally once daily or fluconazole 100 mg orally once weekly for 6 months.[94] Chronic suppressive therapy may be required for patients with HIV/AIDS who may have severe episodes of VVC and frequent relapses.

Treatment regimens for gonorrhea and chlamydial infection require several considerations, including antimicrobial resistance of *N. gonorrhoeae,* concurrent infection, and involvement of the upper genital tract. Resistance of *N. gonorrhoeae* to PCN and tetracycline has been well recognized in developing countries, with more than 50% of strains in Africa reported to be penicillinase-producing.[95,96] Resistance to *N. gonorrhoeae* has also been reported for spectinomycin.[97] Fluoroquinolone resistance is common in much of southeast Asia and is increasingly recognized in other parts of the world.[98,99] Alternative regimens with kanamycin or trimethoprim–sulfamethoxazole is recommended only for countries with low in vitro resistance in which patients treated with these regimens can be closely monitored.[7] Because of the high likelihood of coinfection, persons treated for gonorrhea should also receive treatment that is effective against *C. trachomatis.* Doxycycline and azithromycin have similar efficacy against *C. trachomatis;* the choice of regimen depends on cost and expected patient compliance. Azithromycin is administered as a single-dose regimen and may be more cost-effective since successful therapy with doxycycline requires compliance with a 7-day course. Empirical treatment of both gonorrhea and chlamydial infection should be considered for patients with mucopurulent cervicitis, especially in populations with a high prevalence of these infections and when laboratory testing is not available.

Treatment and counseling should be provided for sex partners of patients with trichomoniasis, gonococcal, or chlamydial infection. There is an increased cure rate of trichomoniasis in women following treatment of their male sexual partners.[100] In the absence of definitive laboratory diagnosis, patients should be told that an infection with an STI is possible but not proven, requiring treatment of the patient and all sex partners. Treatment of sex partners is not required for BV or VVC.

URETHRAL SYNDROMES AND URINARY TRACT INFECTIONS IN WOMEN

Urethral syndromes in women may present as urethritis caused by STIs or cystitis caused by urinary tract pathogens. The causative organisms associated with urethritis in women include *N. gonorrhoeae, C. trachomatis,* and HSV infection. The microbiology of UTIs is the same worldwide. Most uncomplicated infections, usually over 80%, are due to *Escherichia coli.* Between 5% and 10% of infections, particularly in females, are due to *Staphylococcus saprophyticus* and the remainder are due to a variety of aerobic organisms. Complicated UTIs are also most commonly due to *E. coli.*, but the strains are often more resistant to antimicrobial agents and occur following selection within an institutional environment or secondary to the effects of repeated courses of antibacterial therapy. *Klebsiella* spp., *Proteus* spp., *Pseudomonas aeruginosa, Enterococcus* spp., and *Candida* spp. occur much more frequently in patients with underlying structural or functional abnormalities and in patients who have acquired infection nosocomially. Anaerobes and more fastidious organisms are rarely responsible for UTIs and are found in fewer than 3% of patients.

In tropical countries, *Salmonella* spp., particularly *S. typhimurium,* are common causes of UTI. In Egypt, *Salmonella* may account for 10% to 20% of the complicated urinary infections.[101] *Salmonella* spp. are also very common in patients who have concomitant infection with *Schistosoma haematobium.*[101] These patients may have bladder calculi so that management can be complex and require careful treatment of infection, as well as dissolution of calculi.

Mycobacterium tuberculosis urinary infection is common in tropical countries and must be considered in all patients who present with symptoms of UTI with pyuria and otherwise "sterile" urine cultures. Genitourinary tuberculosis is discussed elsewhere. *Brucella* spp. can cause chronic urinary infection with granulomatous pyelonephritis or cystitis.

Clinical Manifestations

Women with urethritis secondary to STIs may present with dysuria, urinary frequency, and lower abdominal pain, and concomitant symptoms associated with cervicitis or vaginitis. Urethritis should be differentiated from acute cystitis, which may also present with dysuria, frequency, and lower abdominal pain, and be accompanied by urinary urgency and/or gross hematuria. Additional symptoms of fever, chills, flank pain, and systemic complaints should raise suspicion for pyelonephritis. In about one-fourth of women with pyelonephritis, subsequent bacteremia can lead to the "sepsis syndrome." Asymptomatic bacteriuria occurs commonly with a prevalence of 3% to 10% in otherwise healthy adult women. Pregnant women with asymptomatic bacteriuria are predisposed to developing invasive pyelonephritis and other complications; therefore, these women should be routinely screened for urinary tract disease.

Diagnosis

Women with urethral symptoms should have a urinalysis, a urine culture, a sexual risk assessment, and a pelvic examination whenever possible to differentiate urinary infection from the various STI syndromes.

The laboratory diagnosis of gonococcal, chlamydial, and HSV infections are discussed in previous sections. Laboratory diagnosis of UTI requires demonstration of pyuria and bacteriuria. A clean-catch midstream urine specimen with 10 or more leukocytes per high-power field (HPF) supports the diagnosis of infection if no other cause of pyuria is present. Leukocyte esterase and nitrite strips can be used to screen urine for evidence of infection, but the sensitivity is usually less than 90% and specificity about 80%.[102] A presumptive diagnosis of UTI may be achieved with a microscopic examination revealing 5 to 10 organisms per oil immersion field on Gram stain. Quantitative urine cultures should be requested on clean-voided midstream urine and quickly transported to the laboratory. However, if an immediate culture is not feasible, storage for 24 hours at 4°C in a refrigerator maintains bacterial stability. Urine cultures are of no value if specimens have been improperly collected and stored, as bacteria grow readily in urine and urine cultures will be falsely positive. Urine is cultured on blood agar and selective media (such as MacConkey's agar) with a quantitative loop that enables an estimation of the bacterial count (colony-forming units, CFU).

Determination of the antimicrobial susceptibilities of the bacterial isolates may be important in patients with complicated infections. Pyuria is almost invariably present in patients with symptomatic urinary infections. Of note, between 10% and 50% of patients with acute symptoms will have bacterial counts of less than 10^8 CFU/L or less than 10^5 CFU/mL.[103] "Low count" bacteriuria is a real entity; in both males and females with symptoms, it usually portends infection. On the other hand, asymptomatic bacteriuria in females should usually be diagnosed only if at least two urine cultures have counts of greater than 10^8 CFU/L (10^5 CFU/mL).

For women who are prone to UTIs and have had multiple recurrences, symptomatic episodes should be managed with as little investigation as possible. A urinalysis may be all that is required for diagnosis.

Management

Management of women with suspected STIs has been discussed previously. Treatment of acute cystitis has been standardized to a 3-day oral regimen with trimethoprim 160 mg and sulfamethoxazole 800 mg twice daily or cephalexin 500 mg four times daily. If resistance among *E. coli* strains to these agents is widespread in the community, the fluoroquinolones are effective treatment choices. Most *E. coli* strains that cause acute uncomplicated cystitis are now resistant to amoxicillin.

Women who present with presumed acute pyelonephritis require urgent attention. Alternative diagnoses, particularly surgical conditions, acute PID, ectopic pregnancy, and other illnesses, need to be excluded. About one-third of patients initially diagnosed as having acute pyelonephritis are found to have other illnesses. Women should have urine and blood cultures and be treated immediately with an effective regimen. Ampicillin and gentamicin are appropriate for initial parenteral therapy; oral regimens may then be prescribed for 2 weeks. The fluoroquinolones are satisfactory oral choices for patients with acute pyelonephritis if the infecting pathogen is susceptible.

Recurrence of infection should be anticipated in women with UTIs. Recurrent symptomatic cystitis is best managed by continuous low-dose prophylaxis or with intermittent prophylaxis taken with intercourse.[104] Trimethoprim–sulfamethoxazole or a fluoroquinolone is the most effective prophylactic agent. Women with recurrent UTIs may be given medication to initiate self-treatment when their symptoms recur. Postmenopausal women may respond to local vaginal estrogens with dramatic reductions in the number of recurring episodes of cystitis.[105] Recurring renal infection mandates studies to exclude abnormalities in the upper tract. Some women will require continuous suppression to prevent recurring symptoms.

All pregnant women should be screened for infection with a urinalysis and a urine culture. Asymptomatic bacteriuria should be treated; this will prevent over 80% of acute episodes of pyelonephritis in pregnancy and will also prevent 10% to 20% of premature deliveries. All pregnant women who have a urinary infection should be followed with frequent urinalysis throughout their pregnancy. Asymptomatic infections are usually treated in children but not in adults or in individuals with indwelling catheters unless there is evidence of invasive disease.

URETHRAL SYNDROMES AND URINARY TRACT INFECTIONS IN MEN

Urethral syndromes in men are classified as urethritis, epididymitis, prostatitis, cystitis, and pyelonephritis. In sexually active men, *N. gonorrhoeae* and *C. trachomatis* are the most common causes of urethritis and epididymitis. The prevalence of gonorrhea among males presenting with a urethral discharge varies from 50% to 60% in Africa.[106,107] In comparison, the prevalence of chlamydial infection among males presenting with a urethral discharge varies from 12.3% in parts of Africa to 53.4% in Jamaica.[66,108] Approximately one-half to three-fourths of cases of nongonococcal urethritis (NGU) are caused by other pathogens, including *Ureaplasma urealyticum, Mycoplasma genitalium, T. vaginalis,* or HSV. *M. genitalium* has gained increased recognition as a causative agent of acute and chronic NGU and appears to act independently of *C. trachomatis* with approximately the same frequency.[109] *T. vaginalis* may be a particularly important cause of urethritis in some tropical areas such as Africa, where 19% of males presenting with urethral discharge were diagnosed with *T. vaginalis.*[110,111]

E. coli and other urinary tract pathogens can also present as urethritis, epididymitis, and prostatitis; an initial empirical treatment regimen should include all of these organisms in its spectrum. UTIs occur with an incidence of about 1 per 100 during the first year of life in boys. These infections are often associated with underlying congenital anomalies. The presence of a foreskin increases the incidence of UTIs in boys and in adult men by two- to threefold.[112] During adult life, the annual incidence is approximately 3 per 1000, which increases dramatically during the seventh decade with the onset of prostatic disease.

Clinical Manifestations

A patient with urethritis may present with a urethral discharge, dysuria, or itching at the meatus. Gonorrhea typically develops 2 to 6 days after exposure, whereas NGU may take 1 to 5 weeks from exposure to the onset of symptoms. Gonococcal and NGU can be differentiated by the clinical manifestations in up to three-fourths of cases. A profuse, yellow-green discharge with an acute onset is suggestive of gonococcal origin, while a mucopurulent or mucoid discharge noted only after urethral stripping or in the morning before voiding is likely to be nongonococcal in etiology. However, atypical presentations may occur as a result of self-medication, a common practice in the tropics.[113] Crusting at the urethral meatus may be the only manifestation of NGU in some men. Dysuria is present in both conditions, but the presence of dysuria without a urethral discharge is a very good predictor of NGU. A profuse mucoid discharge with severe dysuria suggests HSV, especially if accompanied by regional lymphadenopathy and external genital lesions.

Urinary frequency, urgency, and hematuria are not generally part of the urethritis syndrome in men, and suggest the presence of prostatitis, cystitis, or other disorders. Asymptomatic bacteriuria is less common in men, usually occurring with the onset of prostatic hypertrophy or cancer and urinary tract obstruction. Prostatitis usually presents with perineal and lower abdominal pain, fever, burning, frequency, and occasionally with a sepsis-like syndrome.

Diagnosis

A Gram stain should be performed on the urethral discharge and examined for the presence of greater than 4 PMNs per HPF as objective evidence of urethritis. When the discharge is minimal or absent, a thin endourethral swab should be inserted 2 to 4 cm into the urethra and rolled onto a glass slide. The finding of gram-negative intracellular diplococci is highly specific for gonococcal urethritis (95% sensitivity, 98% specificity), but a negative smear does not exclude gonorrhea, particularly in cases where self-medication is suspected. If PMNs are present but no intracellular organisms are seen, a tentative diagnosis of NGU should be made. Additional tests should be obtained for *N. gonorrhoeae* and *C. trachomatis* when possible. In areas with limited laboratory resources, the leukocyte esterase test can be performed on the first-voided portion of urine from symptomatic men with urethritis; this dipstick measurement has a reported sensitivity of 76% and specificity of 80% for the presence of gonorrhea or chlamydia in one study involving STD clinic patients.[114] Trichomonads may occasionally be found on Gram stain or on a wet mount of urethral discharge. Testing for *U. urealyticum* is seldom clinically useful since the organism frequently colonizes the urethra. In the patient with symptoms suggestive of urethritis but with less than 4 PMNs per HPF on the Gram stain, a second examination may be helpful. After several hours without micturition, urethral stripping may produce a small amount of discharge which can be examined microscopically.

Males with UTI are often investigated to exclude congenital or acquired abnormalities.[115] An intravenous pyelogram or an ultrasound examination should be combined with a cystoscopic study. Since the majority of adult men will not have an underlying anatomic abnormality as a predisposing factor for their UTIs, the recurrence of infection is an excellent indicator for men who require further investigation. Men with chronic prostatitis should have a culture performed on expressed prostatic secretions to identify the bacterial etiology.

Management

The WHO flowchart (Fig. 132-3) is provided as an example of the syndromic management of patients presenting with a urethral discharge; it is a simple flowchart recommending treatment of gonorrhea and NGU for every man with evidence of a urethral discharge. Use of a similar algorithm whereby all men with a urethral discharge were treated with either ceftriaxone or ciprofloxacin combined with doxycycline resulted in 92% clinical success in primary health clinics in Côte d'Ivoire.[22] In areas with a high prevalence of gonococcal and chlamydial infection, or where tests are not available, empirical treatment aimed at both *N. gonorrhoeae* and *C. trachomatis* for all patients with urethritis can be a cost-effective option. The recommended therapies for urethritis are given in Table 132-5. Because of the high cost of some medications, alternative therapies such as gentamicin and kanamycin for gonorrhea may be reasonable options in some settings depending on local antimicrobial susceptibilities.[116] Men with persistent or recurrent urethritis despite appropriate therapy may be given erythromycin 500 mg orally four times a day for 14 days as treatment for presumptive tetracycline-resistant *U. urealyticum* or metronidazole 2 g orally once for trichomoniasis. Recurrence of NGU days to weeks after therapy may be due to a prostatic focus of infection and may be treated with a 3- to 6-week course of doxycycline, erythromycin, or azithromycin. Sex partners of patients with trichomoniasis, gonorrhea, chlamydial infection, or NGU require presumptive treatment and counseling.

Males of all ages with lower tract infection should be treated with a 14-day course of an effective antibacterial regimen.

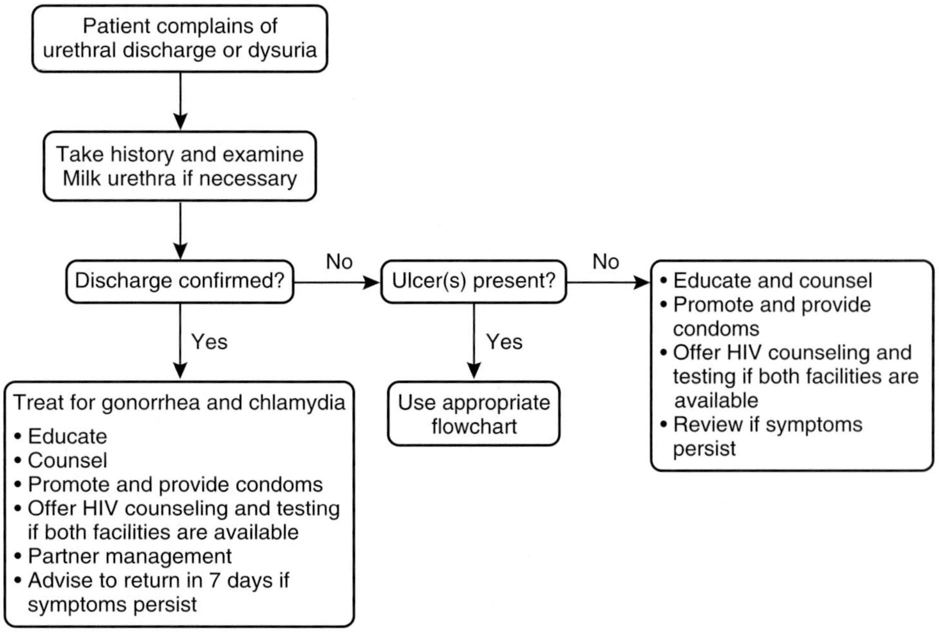

FIGURE 132-3 World Health Organization flowchart for the syndromic management of patients with a urethral discharge or dysuria. (Redrawn from Guidelines for the Management of Sexually Transmitted Infections [WHO/HIV-AIDS/2001.01]. Geneva, World Health Organization, 2001.)

Trimethoprim–sulfamethoxazole is an acceptable initial regimen. Patients with symptoms of prostatitis and patients who have recurrence after an initial 14-day course of treatment should be given trimethoprim–sulfamethoxazole for at least 6 weeks. Long courses are necessary to eradicate infection in some men. Men with acute pyelonephritis should be treated initially with parenteral regimens; continuing treatment for 14 days should be prescribed with an oral regimen such as trimethoprim–sulfamethoxazole or a fluoroquinolone. These drugs achieve satisfactory levels within prostatic tissue and are more likely to eradicate the organism from this site.

Chronic prostatitis is a problematic diagnosis since proof of bacterial infection is necessary. For men with relapsing chronic prostatitis, continuous therapy may be necessary to prevent recurrences.

LOWER ABDOMINAL PAIN

Sexually active women presenting with lower abdominal pain should be evaluated for PID or an ascending infection of the uterus, fallopian tubes, and adjacent pelvic structures resulting in endometritis, salpingitis, pelvic peritonitis, or tuboovarian abscess. The long-term sequelae of undetected disease include infertility, ectopic pregnancy, and chronic pelvic pain. In sub-Saharan Africa, the majority of cases (85%) of infertility are due to bilateral tubal occlusion resulting from PID.[117] PID is frequently encountered in tropical countries, where the annual incidence in urban women aged 15 to 35 years has been estimated to be 1% to 3%.[118] Most cases of PID are caused by *N. gonorrhoeae*, *C. trachomatis*, and anaerobic flora of the gastrointestinal and genital tracts (e.g., *Bacteroides* spp.). Approximately 30% to 40% of cases are associated with mixed infections of both aerobic and anaerobic organisms.[119–121] Organisms associated with bacterial vaginosis contribute to some cases of PID,[122] while in 20% of cases no cause has been found.[119] *Mycoplasma genitalium* has been recently associated with PID.[123,124] Predisposing factors for PID include young age, multiple sex partners, use of intrauterine devices, douching, and prior history of PID.[125,126]

Clinical Manifestations

A patient presenting with lower abdominal pain accompanied by an abnormal vaginal discharge should be suspected of having PID. Other symptoms suggestive of PID include abnormal uterine bleeding, dysuria, dyspareunia, menometrorrhagia, pain associated with menses, nausea, vomiting, and fever. Gonococcal PID is more likely when there is an abrupt onset of symptoms such as fever and abdominal pain. Physical examination may reveal a purulent cervical discharge, cervical motion, and adnexal tenderness. A patient presenting with symptoms of PID and pleuritic upper abdominal pain should raise suspicion for perihepatitis and peritonitis due to extension of the infection to the subphrenic and subdiaphragmatic space, a condition known as the Fitz-Hugh–Curtis syndrome.

Diagnosis

The diagnosis of PID is usually based on the minimum clinical criteria of lower abdominal pain together with cervical motion and adnexal tenderness. Laparoscopic visualization has been considered the gold standard but is usually not warranted. The mimimum criteria for PID has a reported sensitivity of 83% compared to endometrial sampling, in comparison with a 95% sensitivity for adnexal tenderness.[127] Additional criteria which may increase the specificity of diagnosis include fever, abnormal discharge, and laboratory documentation of cervical infection. A pelvic examination should be performed to determine the presence of any cervical discharge, uterine, adnexal, or cervical motion tenderness, or masses. Endocervical specimens should be obtained and tested for *N. gonorrhoeae* and *C. trachomatis*. Laboratory examination for other organisms associated with PID is not useful since they are often part of the normal flora in healthy women. The differential diagnosis of acute lower abdominal pain in women includes pregnancy, appendicitis, ovarian cyst, diverticular disease, urinary tract infections, and enteric illnesses.

Management

Empirical therapy for PID should be instituted in the presence of the minimum clinical criteria and in the absence of another established cause of the patient's symptoms. Because of the difficulty in determining the exact infectious cause of PID, treatment should be directed at all potential pathogens and should be broad-spectrum in nature. Effective inpatient and outpatient regimens for PID are presented in Table 132-6. Antibiotic therapy should be continued for

Table 132-6 Recommended Treatment Regimens for Pelvic Inflammatory Disease

Inpatient regimens	Cefoxitin 2 g IV every 6 hours (hrs); or cefotetan 2 g IV every 12 hrs; or ceftriaxone 250 mg IM × 1 q day* *Plus* doxycycline 100 mg IV or PO every 12 hrs × 14 days *Plus* metronidazole 500 mg IV or PO bid × 14 days
	Clindamycin 900 mg IV every 8 hrs *plus* gentamicin 1.5 mg/kg IV every 8 hrs*†
Outpatient regimens	Ceftriaxone 250 mg IM × 1 dose, or cefoxitin 2 gm IM with probenecid 1 gm PO × 1 dose *Plus* doxycycline 100 mg PO bid or tetracycline 500 mg PO qid × 14 days *Plus* metronidazole 500 mg PO bid × 14 days
	Ofloxacin 400 mg PO bid × 14 days; or levofloxacin 500 mg PO once daily × 14 days *Plus* metronidazole 500 mg PO bid × 14 days

*These regimens should be continued for at least 48 hours after clinical improvement and then followed by an oral regimen to complete 14 days of therapy.
†After discontinuation, this regimen should be followed by either doxycycline 100 mg PO bid or tetracycline 500 mg PO qid to complete 14 total days of therapy.

a 10- to 14-day course; the clinical efficacy of these regimens ranges from 81% to 94%.[128,129] Azithromycin as a single dose is effective for chlamydial endocervicitis but has not been studied in the treatment of PID. Hospitalization is required in a substantial but ill-defined proportion of women with PID in developing countries.[118] Hospitalization is generally recommended when the diagnosis is uncertain, the possibility of a surgical emergency cannot be excluded, a pelvic abscess is suspected, the patient is pregnant or immunocompromised, severe illness precludes outpatient management, the patient cannot tolerate an outpatient regimen, or the patient has failed to respond to outpatient therapy. Reassessment of the patient after 72 hours is recommended to evaluate the response to outpatient treatment. Removal of an intrauterine device, which is a risk factor for the development of PID, is recommended after initiation of antimicrobial therapy. Because of the risk of reinfection, sex partners of women with PID should be evaluated and empirically treated with regimens that are effective against both *N. gonorrhoeae* and *C. trachomatis*. Bed rest, avoidance of sexual intercourse during therapy, and evaluation of the male sexual partner are integral components of PID management. The woman and her partner(s) should be counseled appropriately; when a definite laboratory diagnosis is not possible, patients should be told that an STI is suspected, requiring treatment of the woman and all partners.

SCROTAL SWELLING

Men presenting with scrotal swelling should be evaluated for epididymitis, an acute inflammation of the epididymis which is usually a complication of gonococcal or chlamydial urethritis in men less than 35 years of age. Unlike PID, ascending infection from *N. gonorrhoeae* or *C. trachomatis* to the epididymis is uncommon except in areas where treatment facilities are inadequate or nonexistent. Extension of the infection to involve the adjacent testicle results in epididymo-orchitis. In older men, epididymitis is more commonly associated with enteric organisms (e.g., *E. coli*, *Klebsiella* spp.). Other organisms that should be considered as a cause of epididymitis include *Mycobacterium tuberculosis, Brucella* spp., and blastomycosis, which is usually accompanied by orchitis or disease elsewhere such as in the lungs or bones.

Clinical Manifestations

The presence of acute scrotal swelling with scrotal and inguinal pain suggests the possibility of epididymitis. Testicular torsion can manifest with similar symptoms and must be differentiated because it is a surgical emergency. Symptoms of epididymitis usually begin unilaterally, but may soon progress to a bilateral epididymo-orchitis. Physical examination may reveal a swollen, tender epididymis and vas deferens, and a red, edematous scrotum. Symptoms of urethritis may also be present. Approximately half of patients presenting with epididymitis of gonococcal origin have a urethral discharge.

Diagnosis

Simple laboratory tests can help with the diagnosis of epididymitis. A urethral smear revealing greater than 4 PMNs per HPF provides objective evidence of urethritis, and supports the diagnosis of epididymitis in a man with scrotal pain. A urethral swab or urine specimen should be obtained and tested for *N. gonorrhoeae* and *C. trachomatis*. Urinalysis and urine culture can determine the presence of an associated urinary tract infection. The differential diagnosis of scrotal swelling includes testicular torsion, orchitis secondary to non–sexually transmitted pathogens, hydrocele, spermatocele, and testicular carcinoma.

Management

Empirical therapy of epididymitis is recommended while awaiting test results. Patients suspected of having an STI should be treated for both *N. gonorrhoeae* and *C. trachomatis,* using ceftriaxone 125 mg IM in a single dose plus doxycycline for 10 days. Ofloxacin 300 mg orally twice a day for 10 days is an alternative regimen that is effective against both organisms, as well as against gram-negative bacilli which may be associated with a UTI. Bed rest with scrotal elevation and application of ice packs may assist in decreasing local inflammation and swelling. Sex partners of men with epididymitis thought to be of gonococcal or chlamydial etiology should be evaluated and treated.

OTHER CLINICAL PRESENTATIONS OF SEXUALLY TRANSMITTED INFECTIONS

STIs can present less commonly as other clinical syndromes including proctitis, pharyngitis, conjunctivitis, and hepatitis, depending on the site of exposure or the propensity of the organism to affect certain organ systems (see Table 132-1). Patients with proctitis may present with a rectal discharge, anorectal pain, or tenesmus. In sexually active individuals, especially men who have sex with men who engage in receptive anal intercourse, empiric treatment with ceftriaxone 125 mg IM and doxycycline for 7 days should be considered when an anorectal exudate or PMNs on a Gram stain of the anorectal secretions is found on examination. Patients with a history of oral sexual activity, especially fellatio, may present with a sore throat, acute pharyngitis, or tonsillitis secondary to gonorrhea. Chlamydial infection of the pharynx is unusual; however, empiric therapy should be directed towards both pathogens when gonococcal pharyngitis is suspected since co-infections can occur. Conjunctivitis in adults secondary to STIs may result from oculogenital contact, as well as direct or indirect contact from digits or fomites from infected persons. Patients with conjunctivitis secondary to gonorrhea may present with an acute mucopurulent discharge of the conjunctiva, redness, or swelling. The presentation and management of viral hepatitis are presented in greater detail in Chapter 64. Sexual activity is a significant risk factor for acquisition of hepatitis A, hepatitis B, hepatitis C, and cytomegalovirus infections.

SEXUALLY TRANSMITTED INFECTIONS–HUMAN IMMUNODEFICIENCY VIRUS INTERACTIONS

The epidemiologic and biologic associations between STIs and HIV infection underscore the importance of integrating STI/HIV management in clinical settings. Many STIs appear to serve as cofactors facilitating HIV transmission, while HIV infection itself appears to alter the natural history and therapeutic response of some STIs. Biological studies have shown that persons with STIs have increased susceptibility to HIV by the presence of increased inflammatory cells and disruptions in their genital mucosa, and that the presence of other STIs in HIV-infected persons facilitates shedding of the virus in their genital tracts, thereby promoting HIV infectiousness.[130–132]

Among the STIs, GUD has been found to have the strongest association with HIV.[133] Studies have also shown associations between HIV infection and gonorrhea,[134,135] chlamydial infection,[136] trichomoniasis,[134] bacterial vaginosis,[137] and genital warts,[138] independent of other risk factors for HIV infection, including sexual behavior. The higher prevalence of nonulcerative STIs makes them equally important as GUD as cofactors for HIV transmission. Therefore, prompt and appropriate treatment of STIs is important in limiting the spread of HIV infection. HIV voluntary testing and counseling should be offered to patients presenting with STIs. HIV-positive persons may have rapid progression or severe manifestations of STIs such as syphilis, HSV, or HPV. Patients with HIV infection may be less responsive to standard antibiotic therapy for chancroid, [139] syphilis,[41,140] genital HSV,[141] and HPV.[142]

CONTROL OF SEXUALLY TRANSMITTED INFECTIONS

Effective STI control cannot be achieved solely on the basis of correct diagnosis and prompt treatment of symptomatic patients. Primary prevention programs including culturally appropriate sex education through schools and religious institutions, encouragement of delay in sexual debut among adolescents, programs to encourage gender respect and equity including educational opportunities for girls, supportive sex-worker interventions, marriage support initiatives, prenatal screening programs, and condom access programs are all important to provide a foundation on which to build secondary control programs. Behavioral change plays a crucial part in the control of STIs and should be addressed through individual counseling or comprehensive health education programs emphasizing safe sex practices and condom use. In developing countries, public health interventions targeting groups with the highest rates of sex partner change (e.g., commercial sex workers) may improve the cost-effectiveness of HIV and other STI prevention efforts. In addition to strategies on the individual level, community-oriented approaches to STI control may be helpful in settings where STIs are highly prevalent.[143–145]

Partner notification and screening among at-risk individuals are integral components of secondary STI control programs due to the fact that a significant proportion of persons infected with STIs, especially women, have no symptoms. Partners of patients with STIs should be contacted for evaluation and treatment to decrease the reservoir of potentially infectious persons. STI screening should be considered in areas of high prevalence or among high-risk groups, depending on available laboratory techniques and resources. Screening of pregnant women for STIs, especially syphilis, is important and should be performed at the first prenatal visit and again in the third trimester for individuals at high risk for exposure. The promotion of condom use and other barrier methods is imperative and can decrease the rate of transmission of STIs and HIV. Though nonoxynol-9 was not found to reduce male-to-female transmission of STIs,[146,147] efforts are continuing to develop safe and acceptable topical microbicides that could inactivate STIs including HIV.

REFERENCES

1. World Health Organization, Global Programme on AIDS: Global Prevalence and Incidence of Selected Curable Sexually Transmitted Diseases: Overview and Estimates. Geneva, World Health Organization, 1999.
2. World Bank: World Development Report, 1993: Investing in Health. New York, Oxford University Press, 1993.
3. Weiss HA, Buvé A, Robinson NJ, et al: Study Group on Heterogeneity of HIV Epidemics in African Cities. The epidemiology of HSV-2 infection and its association with HIV infection in four urban African populations. AIDS 15:S97, 2001.
4. Holmes KK: Human ecology and behavior and sexually transmitted bacterial infections. Proc Natl Acad Sci USA 91:2448, 1994.
5. Adler MW: Sexually transmitted diseases control in developing countries. Genitourin Med 72:83, 1996.
6. D'Costa IJ, Plummer FA, Bowmer L, et al: Prostitutes are a major reservoir of sexually transmitted diseases in Nairobi, Kenya. Sex Transm Dis 12:64, 1985.
7. Piot P, Meheus AZ: Épidémiologic des maladies sexuellement transmissibles dans les pays en développement. Ann Soc Belg Med Trop 63:87, 1983.
8. World Health Organization: Guidelines for the Management of Sexually Transmitted Infections (WHO/HIV-AIDS/2001.01). Geneva, World Health Organization, 2001.
9. Vuylsteke B, Laga M, Alary M, et al: Clinical algorithms for the screening of women for gonococcal and chlamydial infection: Evaluation of pregnant women and prostitutes in Zaire. Clin Infect Dis 17:82, 1993.
10. Behets FMT, Williams Y, Brathwaite A, et al: Management of vaginal discharge in women treated at a Jamaican sexually transmitted disease clinic: Use of diagnostic algorithms versus laboratory testing. Clin Infect Dis 21:1450, 1995.
11. Ryan CA, Holmes KK: How should clinical algorithms be used for syndromic management of cervical and vaginal infections? (Editorial) Clin Infect Dis 21:1456, 1995.
12. Behets FM-T, Desormeaux J, Joseph D: Control of sexually transmitted diseases in Haiti: Results and implications of a baseline study among pregnant women living in Cité Soleil shantytowns. J Infect Dis 172:764, 1995.
13. Vishwanath S, Talwar V, Prasad R, et al: Syndromic management of vaginal discharge among women in a reproductive health clinic in India. Sex Transm Infect 76:303, 2000.
14. Lewis DA: Chancroid: Clinical manifestations, diagnosis, and management. Sex Transm Infect 79:68, 2003.
15. Mroczkowski TF, Martin DH: Genital ulcer disease. Dermatol Clin 12:753, 1994.
16. Dangor Y, Fehler G, Exposto FD, et al: Causes and treatment of sexually acquired genital ulceration in southern Africa. S Afr Med J 76:339, 1989.
17. Plummer FA, D'Costa LJ, Nsanze H, et al: Clinical and microbiologic studies of genital ulcers in Kenyan women. Sex Transm Dis 12:193, 1985.
18. O'Farrell N: Increasing prevalence of genital herpes in developing countries: Implications for heterosexual HIV transmission and STI control programmes. Sex Transm Infect 75:377, 1999.
19. Sanchez J, Volquez C, Totten PA, et al: The etiology and management of genital ulcers in the Dominican Republic and Peru. Sex Transm Dis 29:559, 2002.
20. Joseph AK, Rosen T: Laboratory techniques used in the diagnosis of chancroid, granuloma inguinale, and lymphogranuloma venereum. Dermatol Clin 12:1, 1994.
21. La Ruche G, Lorougnon F, Digbeu N: Therapeutic algorithms for the management of sexually transmitted diseases at the peripheral level in Côte d'Ivoire: Assessment of efficacy and cost. Bull World Health Org 73:305, 1995.
22. Tramont EC: *Treponema pallidum*. In Mandell GL, Bennett JE, Dolin R (eds): Principles and Practice of Infectious Diseases. Philadelphia, Churchill Livingstone, 2000, p 2474.
23. Corey L: Herpes simplex virus. In Mandell GL, Bennett JE, Dolin R (eds): Principles and Practice of Infectious Diseases. Philadelphia, Churchill Livingstone, 2000, p 1564.

24. Chapel TA: The variability of syphilitic chancres. Sex Transm Dis 5:68, 1978.
25. Fast MW, D'Costa LJ, Nsanze H, et al: The clinical diagnosis of genital ulcer disease in the tropics. Sex Transm Dis 11:72, 1984.
26. Dangor Y, Ballard RC, da L Exposto F, et al: Accuracy of clinical diagnosis of genital ulcer disease. Sex Transm Dis 17:184, 1990.
27. Larsen SA, Steiner BM, Rudolph AH: Laboratory diagnosis and interpretation of tests for syphilis. Clin Microbiol Rev 8:1, 1995.
28. Mosley RC, Corey L, Benjamin D, et al: Comparison of viral isolation, direct immunofluorescence, and indirect immunoperoxidase techniques for detection of genital herpes simplex virus infection. J Clin Microbiol 13:913, 1981.
29. Solomon AR, Rasmussen JE, Varani J, et al: The Tzanck smear in the diagnosis of cutaneous herpes simplex. JAMA 251:633, 1984.
30. Wald A, Ashley-Morrow R: Serological testing for herpes simplex virus (HSV)-1 and HSV-2 infection. Clin Infect Dis 35(Suppl 2):S173, 2002.
31. Joseph AK, Rosen T: Laboratory techniques used in the diagnosis of chancroid, granuloma inguinale, and lymphogranuloma venereum. Dermatol Clin 12:1, 1994.
32. Mabey D, Peeling RW: Lymphogranuloma venereum. Sex Transm Infect 78:90, 2002.
33. Schmid GP: Approach to the patient with genital ulcer disease. Med Clin North Am 74:559, 1990.
34. Orle KA, Gates CA, Martin DH, et al: Simultaneous PCR detection of *Haemophilus ducreyi, Treponema pallidum,* and herpes simplex virus types 1 and 2 from genital ulcers. J Clin Microbiol 34:49, 1996.
35. Liu H, Rodes B, Chen CY, et al: New tests for syphilis: Rational design of a PCR method for detction of *Treponema pallidum* in clinical specimens using unique regions of the DNA polymerase I gene. J Clin Microbiol 39:1941, 2001.
36. World Health Organization: The Sexually Transmitted Diagnostics Initiative (SDI). Special Programme for Research and Training in Tropical Diseases (TDR). Geneva, World Health Organization, 2003.
37. Hanson S, Sunkutu RM, Kamanga J, et al: STD care in Zambia: An evaluation of the guidelines for case management through a syndromic approach. Int J STD AIDS 7:324, 1996.
38. Rutanarugsa A, Vorachit M, Polnikorn N, et al: Drug resistance of *Haemophilus ducreyi.* Southeast Asian J Trop Med Public Health 21:185, 1990.
39. van Dyck E, Bogaerts J, Smet H, et al: Emergence of *Haemophilus ducreyi* resistance to trimethoprim-sulfamethoxazole in Rwanda. Antimicrob Agents Chemother 38:1647, 1994.
40. Tyndall M, Malisa M, Plummer FA, et al: Ceftriaxone no longer predictably cures chancroid in Kenya. J Infect Dis 167:469, 1993.
41. Rolfs RT, Joesoef MR, Hendershot EF, et al: A randomized trial of enhanced therapy for early syphilis in patients with and without human immunodeficiency virus infection. N Engl J Med 337:307, 1997.
42. Centers for Disease Control and Prevention: 2001 Guidelines for treatment of sexually transmitted diseases. MMWR 42, 2001.
43. Hook EW, Martin DH, Stephens J, et al: A randomized, comparative pilot study of azithromycin versus benzathine penicillin G for treatment of early syphilis. Sex Transm Dis 29:486, 2002.
44. Centers for Disease Control and Prevention. Brief report: Azithromycin treatment failures in syphilis infections—San Francisco, California, 2002–2003. MMWR 53:197, 2004.
45. Kaplowitz LG, Baker D, Gelb L, et al: Prolonged continuous acyclovir treatment of normal adults with frequently recurring genital herpes simplex virus infection. The Acyclovir Study Group. JAMA 265:747, 1991.
46. Goldberg LH, Kaufman R, Kurtz TO, et al: Long-term suppression of recurrent genital herpes with acyclovir. Arch Dermatol 129:582, 1993.
47. Latif A: Sexually transmitted diseases in Africa. Genitourin Med 69:352, 1993.
48. Law CL, Merianos A, Grace J, et al: Clinical and virological associations between external anogenital warts and cervical HPV infection in an STD clinic population. Int J STD AIDS 2:30, 1991.
49. Figueroa JP, Ward E, Luthi TE, et al: Prevalence of human papillomavirus among STD clinic attenders in Jamaica: Association of younger age and increased sexual activity. Sex Transm Dis 22:114, 1995.
50. Maiman M, Fruchter RG, Guy L, et al: Human immunodeficiency virus infection and invasive cervical carcinoma. Cancer 71:402, 1993.
51. Sonnex C, Schofield JH, Kocjan G, et al: Anal human papillomavirus infection in heterosexuals with genital warts: Prevalence and relation with sexual behavior. BMJ 303:1243, 1991.
52. Wiley DJ, Douglas J, Beutner K, et al: External genital warts: Diagnosis, treatment, and prevention. Clin Infect Dis 35:S210, 2002.
53. Edwards L, Ferenczy A, Eron L, et al: Self-administered topical 5% imiquimod cream for external anogenital warts. HPV Study Group. Arch Dermatol 134:25, 1998.
54. Hillier SL, Holmes KK: Bacterial vaginosis. In Holmes KK, Mardh P-A, Sparling PF, et al (eds): Sexually Transmitted Disease. New York, McGraw-Hill, 1989, p 313.
55. Holst E, Wathne B, Hovelius B, et al: Bacterial vaginosis: Microbiological and clinical findings. Eur J Clin Microbiol 6:536, 1987.
56. Joesoef MR, Wiknjosasatro GG, Norojono W: Coinfection with chlamydia and gonorrhea among pregnant women and bacterial vaginosis. Int J STD AIDS 7:61, 1996.
57. Fehler HG, Duncan MO, Bilgeri YR, et al: Sexually transmitted diseases amongst urban black women. S Afr J Sex Transm Dis 4:48, 1984.
58. Pochoe E, Crewe-Brown HH, Adam A, et al: Microbiology of vaginal discharge. S Afr J Epidemiol Infect 1:91, 1986.
59. Eckert LO, Hawes SE, Stevens CE, et al: Vulvovaginal candidiasis: Clinical manifestations, risk factors, management algorithm. Obstet Gynecol 92:757, 1998.
60. Hillier SL, Nugent RP, Eschenbach DA, et al: Association between bacterial vaginosis and preterm delivery of a low-birth-weight infant. The Vaginal Infections and Prematurity Study Group. N Engl J Med 333:1737, 1995.
61. Purwar M, Ughade S, Bhagat B, et al: Bacterial vaginosis in early pregnancy and adverse pregnancy outcome. J Obstet Gynaecol Res 27:175, 2001.
62. Moodley P, Wilkinson D, Connolly C, et al: *Trichomonas vaginalis* is associated with pelvic inflammatory disease in women infected with human immunodeficiency virus. Clin Infect Dis 34:519, 2002.
63. Wiesenfeld HC, Hillier SL, Krohn MA, et al: Lower genital tract infection and endometritis: Insight into sublinical pelvic inflammatory disease. Obstet Gynecol 100:456, 2002.
64. Luthra UK, Murthy NS, Sehgal A, et al: Reproductive tract infections in India: The need for comprehensive reproductive health policy and programs. In Germain A, Holmes KK, Piot P, et al (eds): Reproductive Tract Infections. New York, Plenum Press, 1992, p 317.
65. Mwakagile D, Swai AB, Sandstrom E, et al: High frequency of sexually transmitted diseases among pregnant women in Dar es Salaam, Tanzania: Need for intervention. East Afr Med J 73:675, 1996.
66. Costello DC, Wangel AM, Hoffman IF, et al: Validation of the WHO diagnostic algorithm and development of an alternate scoring system for the management of women presenting with vaginal discharge in Malawi. Sex Transm Inf 74(Suppl 1):S50, 1998.
67. Faundes A, Tanaka AC: Reproductive tract infections in Brazil: Solutions in a difficult economic climate. In Germain A, Holmes KK, Piot P, et al (eds): Reproductive Tract Infections. New York, Plenum Press, 1992, p 253.
68. King SD, Dowe G, Wynter HH, et al: Chlamydial infections in selected populations in Jamaica. West Indian Med J 42:136, 1992.
69. Jones RB, Batteiger BE: *Chlamydia trachomatis.* In Mandell GL, Bennett JE, Dolin R (eds): Principles and Practice of Infectious Diseases. Philadelphia, Churchill Livingstone, 2000, p 1989.
70. Brunham RC, Peeling R, Maclean I, et al: *Chlamydia trachomatis*–associated ectopic pregnancy: Serologic and histologic correlates. J Infect Dis 165:1076, 1992.
71. Centers for Disease Control and Prevention. Case definitions for infections conditions under public health surveillance. MMWR 46:50, 1997.
72. Swygard H, Sena AC, Hobbs MM, et al: Trichomoniasis: Clinical manifestations, diagnosis, and management. Sex Transm Infect 80:91, 2004.
73. Judson FN: Gonorrhea. Med Clin North Am 74:1353, 1990.
74. Krieger JN, Tam MR, Stevens CE, et al: Diagnosis of trichomoniasis: Comparison of conventional wet-mount preparation with cytological studies, cultures, and monoclonal antibody staining of direct specimens. JAMA 259:1223, 1988.
75. Nugent RP, Krohn MA, Hillier SL: Reliability of diagnosing bacterial vaginosis is improved by a standardized method of Gram stain interpretation. J Clin Microbiol 29:297, 1991.
76. Schwebke JR, Hillier SL, Sobel JD, et al: Validity of the vaginal Gram stain for the diagnosis of bacterial vaginosis. Obstet Gynecol 88:573, 1996.
77. Ehrer JM, Judson FN: Gonorrhea. In Wentworth BB, Judson FN, Gilchrist MJR (eds): Laboratory Methods for the Diagnosis of Sexually Transmitted Diseases. Washington, DC, American Public Health Association, 1991, pp 53–94.

78. Schachter J: Biology of *Chlamydia trachomatis*. In Holmes KK, Mardh PA, Sparling PF, et al (eds): Sexually Transmitted Diseases. New York, McGraw-Hill, 1984, p 243.
79. Scanam WE: Laboratory diagnosis of chlamydia infection. In Bowie WR, Caldwell HD, Jones RP, et al (eds): Chlamydial Infections. Cambridge, UK, Cambridge University Press, 1990, p 460.
80. Blanding J, Hirsch L, Stranton N, et al: Comparison of the Clearview Chlamydia, the PACE 2 assay, and culture for detection of *Chlamydia trachomatis* from cervical specimens in a low-prevalence population. J Clin Microbiol 31:1622, 1993.
81. Stratton NJ, Hirsch L, Harris E, et al: Evaluation of the rapid Clearview Chlamydia test for direct detection of chlamydia from cervical specimens. J Clin Microbiol 29:1551, 1991.
82. Gann PH, Hermann JE, Candib L, et al: Accuracy of *Chlamydia trachomatis* antigen detection methods in a low-prevalence population in a primary care setting. J Clin Microbiol 28:1580, 1990.
83. Iwen PC, Blair TMH, Woods GL: Comparison of the Gen-probe PACE 2 system, direct fluorescent-antibody, and cell culture for detecting *Chlamydia trachomatis* in cervical specimens. J Clin Pathol 95:578, 1991.
84. Woods GL: Update on laboratory diagnosis of sexually transmitted diseases. Clin Lab Med 15:665, 1995.
85. Panke ES, Yang LI, Leist PA, et al: Comparison of Gen-probe DNA probe test and culture for the detection of *Neisseria gonorrhoeae* in endocervical specimens. J Clin Microbiol 29:883, 1991.
86. Vlaspolder F, Mutsaets JAEM, Biog E, et al: Value of a DNA probe assay (Gen-Probe) compared with that of a culture for diagnosis of gonococcal infection. J Clin Microbiol 31:107, 1993.
87. Limberger RJ, Biega R, Evancoe A, et al: Evaluation of culture and the Gen-probe Pace 2 assay for detection of *Neisseria gonorrhoeae* and *Chlamydia trachomatis* in endocervical specimens transported to a state health laboratory. J Clin Microbiol 30:1162, 1992.
88. Crotchfelt KA, Welsh LE, DeBonville D, et al: Detection of *Neisseria gonorrhoeae* and *Chlamydia trachomatis* in genitourinary specimens from men and women by a coamplification PCR assay. J Clin Microbiol 35:1536, 1997.
89. Centers for Disease Control and Prevention. Screening tests to detect *Chlamydia trachomatis* and *Neisseria gonorrhoeae* infections—2002. MMWR 51:1, 2002.
90. Schachter J, McCormack WM, Chernesky MA, et al: Vaginal swabs are appropriate specimens for diagnosis of genital tract infection with *Chlamydia trachomatis*. J Clin Microbiol 41:3784, 2003.
91. Hager WD, Brown ST, Kraus SJ, et al: Metronidazole for vaginal trichomoniasis: Seven day vs. single dose regimens. JAMA 244:1219, 1980
92. Eschenbach DA, Critchlow CW, Watkins H, et al: A dose duration study of metronidazole for the treatment of nonspecific vaginosis. Scand J Infect Dis Suppl 40:73, 1983.
93. Swedberg J, Steiner JF, Deiss F, et al: Comparison of a single-dose vs. one-week course of metronidazole for symptomatic bacterial vaginosis. JAMA 254:1046, 1985.
94. Sobel JD: Pathogenesis and treatment of recurrent vulvovaginal candidiasis. Clin Infect Dis 14:S148, 1992.
95. Van Dyck E, Crabbe F, Nkila N, et al: Increasing resistance of *Neisseria gonorrhoeae* in West and Central Africa. Sex Transm Dis 24:32, 1997.
96. West B, Changalucha J, Grosskurth H, et al: Antimicrobial susceptibility, auxotype and plasmid content of *Neisseria gonorrhoeae* in northern Tanzania: Emergence of high level plasmid mediated tetracycline resistance. Genitourin Med 71:9, 1995.
97. Joesoef MR, Knapp JS, Idajadi A, et al: Antimicrobial susceptibilities of *Neisseria gonorrhoeae* strains isolated in Surabaya, Indonesia. Antimicrob Agents Chemother 38:2530, 1994.
98. Fox KK, Knapp JS: Antimicrobial rsistance in *Neisseria gonorrhoea*. Curr Opin Urol 9:65, 1999.
99. Kam KM, Wong PW, Cheung MM, et al: Quinolone-resistant *Neisseria gonorrhoeae* in Hong Kong. Sex Transm Dis 23:103, 1996.
100. Lyng J, Christensen J: A double-blind study of the value of treatment with a single dose tinidazole of partners to females with trichomoniasis. Acta Obstet Gynecol Scand 60:199, 1981.
101. Neves J, Raso P, Marinko PP: Prolonged septicemic salmonellosis intermittent with schistosomiasis mansoni infection. J Trop Med Hyg 74:9, 1971.
102. Semeniul H, Church D: Evaluation of the leukocyte esterase and nitrite urine dispstick screening tests for detection of bacteriuria in women with suspected uncomplicated urinary tract infections. J Clin Micro 37:3051, 1999.
103. Kunin CM: Urinary tract infections in females. Clin Infect Dis 18:1, 1994.
104. Stapleton A, Latham R, Johnson C, et al: Randomized, double-blind, placebo-controlled trial post-coital antimicrobial prophylaxis for recurrent UTI. JAMA 264:703, 1990.
105. Raz R, Stamm WE: A controlled trial of intravaginal estriol in postmenopausal women with recurrent urinary tract infections. N Engl J Med 329:753, 1993.
106. Ismail SO, Ahmed HJ, Grillner L: Sexually transmitted diseases in men in Mogadishu, Somalia. Int J STD AIDS 1:102, 1990.
107. Sehgal SC: Epidemiology of male urethritis in Nigeria. J Trop Med Hyg 93:151, 1990.
108. Ballard RC, Fehler HG, Bilgeri YR, et al: A clinical and microbiological evaluation of the treatment of urethritis with minocycline. S Afr J Epidemiol Infect 1:19, 1986.
109. Taylor-Robinson D: *Mycoplasma genitalium*—An update. Int J STD AIDS 13:145, 2002.
110. Hoosen AA, Coetzee KD, van den Ende J: A microbiological study of failed penicillin therapy for gonococcal urethritis in Durban. S Afr Med J 78:189, 1990.
111. Pillay DG, Hoosen AA, Vezi B, et al: Diagnosis of *Trichomonas vaginalis* in male urethritis. Trop Geogr Med 46:44, 1994.
112. Spach DH, Stapleton AE, Stamm WE: Lack of circumcision increases the risk of urinary infection in young men. JAMA 267:679, 1992.
113. Nichter M: Self-medication and STD prevention. Sex Transm Dis 23:353, 1996.
114. Tyndall MW, Nasio J, Maitha G, et al: Leukocyte esterase urine strips for the screening of men with urethritis—Use in developing countries. Genitourin Med 70:3, 1994.
115. Lipsky BA: Urinary tract infections in men: Epidemiology, pathophysiology, diagnosis, and treatment. Ann Intern Med 110:138, 1989.
116. Lule G, Behets FM, Hoffman IF, et al: STD/HIV control in Malawi and the search for affordable and effective urethritis therapy: A first field evaluation. Genitourin Med 70:384, 1994.
117. Cates W, Farley TMM, Rowe PJ: Worldwide patterns of infertility: Is Africa different? Lancet 2:596, 1985.
118. Over M, Piot P: HIV infection and sexually transmitted diseases. In Jarnison DT, Mosley WH, Measham AR, et al (eds): Disease Control Priorities in Developing Countries. New York, Oxford University Press, 1993, p 455.
119. Brunham RC, Binns B, Guijon F, et al: Etiology and outcome of acute pelvic inflammatory disease. J Infect Dis 158:510, 1988.
120. Soper DE, Brockwell NJ, Dalton HP: Microbial etiology of urban emergency department acute salpingitis: Treatment with ofloxacin. Am J Obstet Gynecol 167:653, 1992.
121. Wasserheit JN, Bell TA, Kiviat NB, et al: Microbial causes of proven pelvic inflammatory disease and efficacy of clindamycin and tobramycin. Ann Intern Med 104:187, 1986.
122. Weisenfeld HC, Hillier SL, Krohn MA, et al: Lower genital tract infection and endometritis: Insight into subclinical pelvic inflammatory disease. Obstet Gynecol 100:456, 2002.
123. Cohen CR, Manhart LE, Bukusi EA, et al: Association between *Mycoplasma genitalium* and acute endometritis. Lancet 359:765, 2002.
124. Simms I, Eastick K, Mallinson H, et al: Associations between *Mycoplasma genitalium, Chlamydia trachomatis* and pelvic inflammatory disease. Sex Transm Infect 79:154, 2003.
125. Washington AE, Aral SO, Wolner-Hanssen P, et al: Asssessing risk for pelvic inflammatory disease and its sequelae. JAMA 266:2581, 1991.
126. McCormack WM: Pelvic inflammatory disease. N Engl J Med 330:115, 1994.
127. Peipert JF, Ness R, Blume J, et al: Clinical predictors of endometritis in women with symptoms and signs of pelvic inflammatory disease. Am J Obstet Gynecol 184:856, 2001.
128. Peterson HB, Walker CK, Kahn JG, et al: Pelvic inflammatory disease. Key treatment issues and options. JAMA 266:2605, 1991.
129. Waiker CK, Kahn JG, Washington AE, et al: Pelvic inflammatory disease: metaanalysis of antimicrobial regimen efficacy. J Infect Dis 168:969, 1993.
130. Royce RA, Sena A, Cates W, et al: Sexual transmission of HIV. N Eng J Med 336:1072, 1997.

131. Fleming DT, Wasserheit JN: From epidemiological synergy to public health policy and practice: The contribution of other sexually transmitted diseases to sexual transmission of HIV infection. Sex Transm Inf 75:3, 1999.
132. Cohen MS, Hoffman IF, Royce RA, et al: Reduction of concentration of HIV-1 in semen after treatment of urethritis: Implications for prevention of sexual transmission of HIV-1. Lancet 349:1868, 1997.
133. Cameron DW, Simonsen JN, D'Costa LJ, et al: Female to male transmission of human immunodeficiency virus type 1: Risk factors for seroconversion in men. Lancet 2:403, 1989.
134. Weir SS, Feldblum PJ, Roddy RE, et al: Gonorrhea as a risk factor for HIV acquisition. AIDS 8:1605, 1994.
135. Laga M, Manoka A, Kivuvu M, et al: Non-ulcerative sexually transmitted diseases as risk factors for HIV-1 transmission in women: Results from a cohort study. AIDS 7:95, 1993.
136. Plummer F, Simonsen JN, Cameron W, et al: Co-factors in male-female transmission of human immunodeficiency virus type 1. J Infect Dis 163:233, 1991.
137. Cohen CR, Duerr A, Pruithithada N, et al: Bacterial vaginosis and HIV seroprevalence among female commercial sex workers in Chiang Mai, Thailand. AIDS 9:1093, 1995.
138. Quinn TC, Gasser D, Cannon RO, et al: Human immunodeficiency virus infection among patients attending clinics for sexually transmitted diseases. N Engl J Med 318:197, 1988.
139. Cameron DW, Simonsen JN, D'Costa LJ, et al: Prediction of HIV infection by treatment failure for chancroid, a genital ulcer disease. Presented at the Fourth International Conference on AIDS, Stockholm, Sweden, June 12–16, 1988, abstract 7637.
140. Berry CD, Hooton TM, Collier AC, et al: Neurologic relapse after benzathine penicillin therapy for secondary syphilis in a patient with HIV infection. N Engl J Med 316:1587, 1987.
141. Erlich KS, Mills J, Chatis P, et al: Acyclovir-resistant herpes simplex virus infections in patients with acquired immunodeficiency syndrome. N Engl J Med 320:293, 1989.
142. McMillan A, Bishop PE: Clinical course of anogenital warts in men infected with human immunodeficiency virus. Genitourin Med 65:225, 1989.
143. Holmes KK, Johnson DW, Kvale PA, et al: Impact of a gonorrhea control program, including selective mass treatment, in female sex workers. J Infect Dis 174:230, 1996.
144. Grosskurth H, Mosha F, Todd I, et al: Impact of improved sexually transmitted diseases on HIV infection in rural Tanzania: Randomised controlled trial. Lancet 346:530, 1995.
145. Wawer MJ, Sewankambo NK, Serwadda D, et al: Control of sexually transmitted diseases for AIDS prevention in Uganda: A randomized community trial. Rakai Project Study Group. Lancet 353:525, 1999.
146. Roddy RE, Zekeng L, Ryan KA, et al: A controlled trail of nonoxynol 9 film to reduce male-to-female transmission of sexually transmitted diseases. N Engl J Med 339:504, 1998.
147. Wilkinson D, Ramjee G, Tholandi M, et al: Nonoxynol-9 for preventing vaginal acquisition of sexually transmitted infections by women from men. Cochrane Database Syst Rev 4:CD003939, 2002.

133

Approach to the Patient with HIV and Coinfecting Tropical Infectious Diseases

CHRISTOPHER L. KARP
ROBERT COLEBUNDERS

All ... fall into one of two categories: Infected with HIV or at risk for HIV infection.

Mary E. Wilson[1]

INTRODUCTION

The morbidity, mortality, and social disruption due to the global acquired immunodeficiency syndrome (AIDS) pandemic weigh disproportionately upon resource-poor areas of the tropics.[2] Because these are the very areas where "tropical" infectious diseases continue to hold greatest sway, the potential for interactions between human immunodeficiency virus (HIV) infection and other tropical infectious diseases is great.

Such interactions are marked by epidemiologic complexity. The AIDS pandemic is best described as the sum of discontinuous and overlapping epidemics of disease among populations of variable and varying risk (see Chapter 76). The predominant modes of transmission of HIV (perinatal, sexual, and parenteral) result in a bimodal distribution of disease, with peaks among young children and young adults. The risk of infection or disease due to tropical pathogens varies widely with differences in ecological, political, and socioeconomic conditions (including access to medical care); related specific host factors such as age of exposure, pregnancy, behavior, and nutrition; and host genetics. Disease due to a coinfecting pathogen may be due to primary infection, recurrent infection, or the reactivation of latent infection. For some pathogens, the risk factor responsible for the acquisition of HIV may also be the risk factor responsible for the acquisition of the coinfecting pathogen. As a consequence of this epidemiologic complexity, both the prevalence and the expression of coinfection are likely to be variable across ecological, economic, political, behavioral, and cultural divides.

There is also, of course, considerable biologic and clinical complexity in the interaction of agents of tropical diseases with HIV. Either pathogen has the potential for altering the natural history, immune response, or response to therapy of the other.[3,4]

EFFECTS OF HIV ON TROPICAL COINFECTIONS

Infection with HIV has the ability to influence the natural history of infection with other pathogens through (1) facilitating infection, (2) altering the incidence of disease by increasing the ratio of disease to infection, (3) changing the presentation of disease, or (4) exacerbating the course of disease.[4] Such effects are presumed to be primarily the result of the immunosuppression associated with HIV infection.

Abnormalities of immune function are found in essentially every cellular and functional compartment of the immune system in AIDS, although profound defects in cell-mediated immunity (CMI) appear to be of greatest clinical importance.[5] In vitro correlates include functional abnormalities of

- CD4+ T cells, with progressive failure of proliferation, interleukin (IL)-2 and interferon-γ (IFN-γ) production,[6,7] dysregulated expression of molecules essential for T-cell/antigen presenting cell interactions,[8] abnormal activation-induced apoptosis,[9,10] and expansion of a subset of CD4+ T cells (CD4+CD25+ regulatory T cells) that are potent inhibitors of immune responses both to self and to pathogens[11,12]
- Monocyte/macrophages, with decreased chemotaxis and intracellular microbicidal activity and abnormal cytokine production[5,6]
- Dendritic cells, with reduced ability to present antigen and activate T cells (along with efficient transfer of HIV infection to CD4+ T cells)[13]
- CD8+ T cells, with decreased cytotoxic T-lymphocyte (CTL) function[5] and abnormal activation-induced apoptosis[10]
- Natural killer (NK) cells, with decreased proliferation and IFN-γ production[14]

Dysregulation of humoral immunity, marked by polyclonal B-cell activation, is also seen.[5] Functionally, abnormalities of CD4+ T cell, monocyte/macrophage, and dendritic cell function have been thought to be paramount to the suppression of CMI and the opportunistic infections seen in patients with AIDS. In addition to the direct effects of HIV infection, the immune system of HIV-seropositive people may also be compromised in clinically significant ways by profound nutritional and metabolic derangements (e.g., wasting or "slim disease"), therapeutic interventions (e.g., corticosteroids used for the treatment of *Pneumocystis* pneumonia), and the immune abnormalities associated with secondary infections (e.g., the suppression of CMI seen in visceral leishmaniasis).

The list of infectious diseases that are exacerbated by HIV coinfection[5] includes many that are predictable from data demonstrating the important role of CMI in protection from the etiologic agent. Several pathogens for which immunity has been presumed to depend on CMI do not appear to be exacerbated by HIV coinfection, however. The HIV "experiment of nature" has caused a reexamination of the immunology of such "missing infections" in AIDS.[15]

HIV infection can also influence the therapeutic response of patients with presumed tropical infection. The ability to diagnose and monitor coinfection may be compromised by aberrant serologic responses, including false positives due to polyclonal B-cell activation, false negatives due to blunted antigen-specific antibody responses to newly acquired pathogens in late HIV disease, and false serologic reversion after treatment in late HIV disease.[5] Diagnosis may also be hindered by unusual presentations of disease with coinfecting pathogens. Finally, a plethora of intercurrent pathologic conditions may lead to a dulling of Ockham's razor during the evaluation of disease in AIDS patients. A single pathogen, multiple pathogens, HIV infection, side effects of therapeutic drugs, or a combination of these may be responsible for the presenting complaints. Given the suboptimal response to the chemotherapy of many infections in the presence of profound immunosuppression, drugs may need to be given in greater numbers or for a longer duration. With many pathogens, in the absence of immune reconstitution resulting from highly active antiretroviral therapy (HAART), lifelong suppressive therapy is necessary. Drug therapy in the HIV-infected patient may be complicated further by increased rates of drug allergy as well as by untoward drug interactions in the setting of polypharmacy.[16] Prophylaxis against coinfections may be compromised by substandard vaccination responses.[17–19] Finally, the presence of HIV coinfection can complicate the public health consequences of tropical diseases. AIDS may increase the transmissibility of secondary infections and provide fertile soil for the development of drug resistance. Public health resources devoted to the AIDS pandemic may divert resources away from the control and prevention of other infectious diseases.

The presence of HIV coinfection can lead to disease of markedly greater incidence or severity [the standard definition of an opportunistic infection (OI)][20] with some tropical infectious diseases, such as leishmaniasis and American trypanosomiasis (Chagas' disease). Coinfection has also been demonstrated to have subtle effects on the course of disease with other tropical agents, such as *Schistosoma mansoni*. No identified alteration has been found in the natural history of many tropical infections, including most nematodes.

With organisms in the latter groups, the current absence of evidence of significant effects of HIV on the expression of disease or the response to treatment should not be construed as strong evidence for the absence of such effects. Most research resources have been spent on understanding the clinical and epidemiologic manifestations of the HIV pandemic in industrialized countries, where tropical infectious diseases are obviously underrepresented.[4,21] Where coinfections with HIV and endemic tropical diseases are marked by low prevalence, subtlety of interaction, diagnostic difficulty, or low research priority, the presence and significance of any interaction are likely to be missed. For example, despite the research priority among tropical infections accorded to malaria, a significant interaction with HIV infection—the lack of a benefit of increasing parity in the control of malaria in pregnant women—was only discovered 15 years after the AIDS epidemic was recognized.[22] With less heavily studied pathogens, comparatively subtle interactions will likely emerge over time as research resources are appropriately directed.

Focusing on OIs may help to highlight some of the clearest data on the clinical expression of AIDS in the tropics. Of the more than 100 agents known to cause OIs in AIDS patients, several are classic tropical pathogens.[20] These are mostly found among the intracellular protozoans, bacteria, and endemic fungi; there is a marked absence of metazoans. Overall, the clinical expression of AIDS in many resource-poor areas of the tropics appears to involve a different spectrum of OIs than those common in North America and Europe. In place of the high incidences of *Pneumocystis carinii* pneumonia (PCP), disseminated *Mycobacterium avium*, and cytomegalovirus (CMV) found in the resource-rich north, the clinical expression of AIDS in much of the tropics has been marked by frequent tuberculosis (the most common serious AIDS OI in the world), chronic diarrhea, wasting, chronic fever without an obvious localizing source, and pulmonary disease.[23]

The contribution of predominantly tropical pathogens to these latter common syndromes is unclear, which illuminates the problems with much of the available data on HIV disease in the tropics. Understanding the spectrum of AIDS-associated OIs in any given area depends on the presence of adequate surveillance systems, which are often lacking in resource-poor regions of the tropics. In the presence of inadequate infrastructures, limited financial resources, and difficult access to medical care on the part of the socially disadvantaged, surveillance is likely to be sporadic and to involve mainly the sampling of subgroups of AIDS patients at late stages of disease.[21] Where resources are limited, diagnostic reporting is likely to be biased in favor of OIs that are inexpensive to diagnose (or misdiagnose).[21] Even the common impression that the progression of AIDS is more rapid in sub-Saharan Africa than in industrialized countries[24–27] rests on data that are less than robust.[28] A more rapid observed course (presumed due to a higher frequency and virulence of coinfection and problems of nutrition and access to medical care) may represent in large part a systematic bias in favor of later initial diagnosis of HIV infection and AIDS.[21,23] Conversely, it has been suggested that the burden of illness and mortality in early HIV disease (often unrecognized as such) due to high-grade pathogens, such as *Streptococcus pneumoniae, Mycobacterium tuberculosis*, and the salmonellae, may rival that due to the OIs of late-stage AIDS in the tropics.[29,30]

HIV has shed light on many previously obscure human pathogens. Some, such as the enteric microsporidians, were unknown as agents of human disease prior to the AIDS epidemic. Others, such as *Cryptosporidium parvum*, were underappreciated as causes of disease in normal hosts until their prevalence in AIDS patients led to systematic study in normal hosts. The list of agents causing OIs in AIDS patients is bound to expand. It is reasonable to expect that tropical regions will be prime locations for the identification of further such agents.

EFFECTS OF TROPICAL INFECTIONS ON HIV COINFECTION

There are theoretical and experimental reasons to believe that coinfection can significantly alter the course of HIV pathogenesis. The central role of ongoing viral replication in HIV pathogenesis is firmly established, and the set point concentration of plasma viremia correlates well with long-term clinical outcome.[31] It is presumed that any increases in viral replication have the potential for accelerating the course of disease. Efficient replication of HIV in CD4+ T cells is dependent on cellular activation. Similarly, activation of monocyte/macrophages and dendritic cells can stimulate HIV replication by increasing transcription factor binding to the HIV long terminal repeat region (LTR), enhancing LTR-directed transcription. Coinfecting pathogens can stimulate such immune cell activation either directly (e.g., stimulating signaling through pathogen recognition receptors such as Toll-like receptors[32] or upregulating transcription factor transactivation in coinfected immune cells) or indirectly (e.g., promoting the generation of proinflammatory cytokines such as tumor necrosis factor-α [TNF-α] or activating CD4+ T cells as part of the adaptive immune response). Immune activation can also lead to upregulation of the expression of HIV coreceptors,[33] thereby facilitating the infection of fresh cells.

Immunologic responses to pathogens, as well as to purified vaccine antigens, clearly have the potential for enhancing the dynamic burden of HIV replication. In vitro studies with diverse pathogens have provided mechanistic support for this idea.[34–36] Experimental evidence has also suggested that immune activation-driven augmentation of the HIV viral burden can occur in vivo.[37–44] There is also circumstantial evidence that such immune activation may enhance HIV pathogenesis.[45,46] Both points remain somewhat controversial, however.[47] Whether immune activation-related increases in viral load actually accelerate the pathogenesis of HIV may depend on whether the changes are transient (as with immunization or with treated acute infection) or chronic (as with untreated or untreatable infection, or through a resetting of the set point of plasma viremia by a particular coinfection).[48]

Direct equation of immune activation with upregulation of HIV replication is simplistic, however. With CD4+ T cells, the mechanism of activation appears to be critical to whether viral replication is induced or suppressed.[49,50] Furthermore, activation of proinflammatory cytokine production with positive effects on HIV replication goes hand in hand with activation of anti-inflammatory cytokine production that can inhibit HIV replication.[51] More generally, proinflammatory responses reliably induce counterregulatory responses that suppress subsequent immune activation.[52] It thus should not be surprising that in vitro studies have provided mechanistic support for the ability of coinfecting pathogens to suppress HIV replication.[53–56] Indeed, the overall effect of acute coinfection with some pathogens, including measles virus, dengue virus, and *Orientia tsutsugamushi,* may be a decrease in HIV viral load.[57–59]

In addition to the viral sequelae of generalized immunologic activation, induction of specific alterations in the immunoregulatory environment of the host by ubiquitous tropical pathogens has been postulated to accelerate the course of HIV. Cross-regulating subsets of CD4+ T cells have been distinguished by their cytokine profiles and functional activities: Th1 cells (producing IFN-γ and IL-2, among other cytokines) are important in classical macrophage activation, the development of CMI, and the generation of humoral responses involving complement-fixing antibody isotypes; Th2 cells (producing IL-4, IL-5, and IL-13, among other cytokines) are important in alternative macrophage activation, the generation of immunoglobulin E (IgE) responses, eosinophilia, mast cell responses, and atopy. The immunologic response to most helminthic parasites is dominated by the production of Th2 cytokines. Evidence from murine systems shows that helminth-driven Th2 polarization can shift the immunologic response to heterologous antigens and pathogens from a Th1- to a Th2-dominant pattern, as well as significantly suppress CD8-mediated viral clearance.[60,61] Such responses have also been found to impair antigen-specific Th1 immune responses in both mice and humans.[60,62] Helminthic infection is chronic and widespread in the tropics. The resultant Th2 "priming" of the immune system may favor progression of HIV disease.[63] Several mechanisms have been postulated. First, a Th2-polarized immune system may directly suppress CD8 T cell–mediated anti-HIV responses.[61] Second, HIV may preferentially replicate in Th2 cells.[64] Third, T cells from HIV-seropositive people undergo abnormal activation-induced apoptosis,[9,10] which is thought to play a role in the depletion of both CD4+ and CD8+ T cells over time. Th2 cytokines can amplify such activation-induced apoptosis.[65] Fourth, Th2 cytokines can upregulate HIV coreceptor expression by CD4+ T cells and monocyte/macrophages.[66,67] Of note, it has been demonstrated that peripheral blood cells from patients with intestinal helminth infection are more susceptible to in vitro infection with HIV than are cells from helminth-uninfected patients.[68,69]

Although intriguing, the hypothesis that endemic helminth coinfection leads to acceleration of the disease course of HIV remains unproven. A study in Ethiopia indicated that HIV viral load was significantly higher in individuals with various helminthic infections than in individuals without helminths, correlating positively with the parasite load as well as decreasing after elimination of the worms by antiparasitic treatment.[70] However, similar studies performed in Uganda and examining larger numbers of patients convincingly failed to replicate these findings.[71,72] These latter studies strongly suggest that helminth coinfection is not associated with faster progression of HIV disease.

Other effects of coinfection are perhaps more concrete. Tropical diseases may lead directly to an increased risk of infection with HIV. Treatment of the severe anemia induced by malaria has led to the HIV infection of countless children by transfusion.[73] Genital schistosomiasis, like other genital inflammatory conditions, may increase the efficiency of HIV transmission.[74]

CLINICAL SUSPICION OF COINFECTION

Lewis Thomas wrote that infectious disease "usually results from inconclusive negotiations for symbiosis."[75] In this light, most tropical pathogens lead to high infection:disease ratios. Whether disease is present or not, sterile immunity is not thought to be achieved after infection with most intracellular protozoans. This is as much the case with the tropical and subtropical agents of leishmaniasis and Chagas' disease as it is with the ubiquitous agent of toxoplasmosis. These are thus lifelong infections, with serious disease often resulting when an HIV-infected host defaults on his or her side of these immunologic "negotiations." From the point of view of the clinician in a nonendemic area, this necessitates obtaining a lifetime travel history for all HIV-infected patients. From the perspective of the clinician from either endemic or nonendemic areas, it is equally necessary to have an appropriate index of suspicion for HIV coinfection when contemplating the possibility of a tropical infectious disease. In the process of giving this important virus its diagnostic due, however, it is critical to avoid letting the presence or suspicion of HIV infection distract from the careful consideration of etiologic agents that present and respond similarly in HIV-seronegative and HIV-seropositive people.

The basic biology of HIV; the progression, diagnosis, and treatment of HIV disease; and the epidemiology of HIV/AIDS in the tropics are discussed in Chapter 76. This chapter focuses on the natural history, diagnosis, treatment, and prevention of tropical diseases and OIs in the HIV patient. Distinguishing tropical from other pathogens has its artificial side. Measles, not usually thought of as a tropical disease, causes significant mortality only in the tropics today. Tuberculosis, a pandemic infection, is the principal AIDS-related OI in the tropics. Given the historical preoccupation of the field of tropical medicine with parasitic infections, such infections receive close attention here. For practical reasons, OIs that are common in the industrialized world are not discussed in depth unless there are compelling clinical or epidemiologic reasons for doing so. Multiple references are available via the Internet that discuss these cosmopolitan OIs in detail.[76–79] Further information on all of the specific organisms discussed here can also be found in the relevant chapters of this book.

The diagnostic, prophylactic, and therapeutic recommendations discussed here describe an approach to the HIV patient that is not limited by scarce medical resources. As such, like many strategies for dealing with HIV disease that have evolved in affluent industrialized countries (including HAART, high-technology diagnostics, and multidrug chemoprophylaxis), many of these recommendations may not easily be translated to resource-poor areas of the tropics.

PATHOGENS

Protozoan Infections

Malaria

Malaria (see chapter 90) remains one of the most important infectious diseases in the world today, causing 100 to 200 million new cases and 1 to 2 million deaths each year. Evidence from both murine and human studies suggests an important role for CD4+ T cells in protective immunity to blood-stage malaria. With large areas of shared endemnicity and prevalence, a medically significant interaction between HIV and malaria was thus expected and feared.[80] Initial studies were negative; falciparum malaria did not appear be an OI or to accelerate the progression of HIV disease.[80–85] However, follow-up studies have revealed significant bidirectional interactions between *Plasmodium falciparum* and HIV.

HIV replication in peripheral blood cells is enhanced by exposure to *P. falciparum* antigens in vitro, in part through induction of TNF-α.[86] Increased HIV replication in dendritic cells has also been seen after the in vivo infection with *Plasmodium chabaudi* of mice transgenic for the HIV genome in a process that appears to be dependent on CD4+ T-cell activation.[87] The production of TNF-α during malarial paroxysms,[88] along with the antigenic exposure of parasitemia, might thus reasonably be expected to increase HIV viral load. Indeed, clinical studies from Malawi have shown that *P. falciparum* infection is associated with increased HIV viral burden in peripheral as well as placental blood.[89,90] Treatment was associated with a reduction in viral load, although it remained elevated compared to controls for the 4-week duration of the study.[89] Whether or not malaria-mediated increases in HIV replication accelerate the course of HIV disease remains to be determined.

The first significant clinical effect of HIV on malaria was found in the setting of pregnancy. In areas of high malarial endemnicity, the high degree of immunity that women of childbearing age have developed to severe malaria is compromised by pregnancy. The placental vasculature shields parasitized erythrocytes from the systemic immune response, allowing localized erythrocytic replication of the parasite. Placental parasitemia has been associated with low birth weight and, hence, increased infant mortality. Local uteroplacental immune responses do restrict parasite replication, however, and the effectiveness of these local responses increases in subsequent pregnancies under pressure of recurrent malarial exposure. In 1996, a study performed in rural Malawi demonstrated that the beneficial effects (maternal, placental, and neonatal) of parity in the control of parasitemia during pregnancy were markedly attenuated in the face of HIV coinfection.[22] Since then, multiple studies performed in sub-Saharan Africa have probed the effects of coinfection on the outcome of pregnancy.[90–100] Such studies have shown that (1) HIV infection is associated with increased rates and levels of peripheral and placental parasitemia, clinical malaria, and maternal anemia in pregnant women, and (2) coinfection is associated with a higher risk of low birth weight, preterm birth, intrauterine growth retardation, and postnatal infant mortality.[101] Although placental parasitemia is associated with increased placental HIV viral loads in coinfected patients,[90] it remains unclear as to whether malaria infection increases the risk of mother-to-child transmission of HIV. Conflicting results (enhancement, protection, and no effect) have been published.[96,97,100] A World Health Organization (WHO) technical consultation has recommended that HIV-infected pregnant women who are at risk for malaria should always have protection with insecticide-treated bed nets, along with (according to HIV stage) either intermittent preventive treatment with sulfadoxine/pyrimethamine or daily trimethoprim–sulfamethoxazole (cotrimoxazole; TMP–SMX) prophylaxis.[102]

HIV infection is associated with an increased incidence of parasitemia, the risk of clinical malaria is significantly higher in HIV-infected adults, and this risk increases with decreasing CD4 cell count.[103–105] Notably, HIV infection has also been found to be a risk factor for severe malaria in nonimmune populations (in an area of unstable transmission).[106] Finally, although early studies found no evidence that the treatment or prophylaxis of malaria was altered by HIV coinfection,[81,83] the risk of malaria treatment failure has recently been found to be higher in CD4-depleted HIV positive individuals.[107,108]

HIV protease inhibitors currently used for HAART have understudied interactions with a variety of drugs used for malaria prophylaxis and treatment. A variety of protease inhibitors, as well as the nonnucleoside reverse transcriptase inhibitors delaviradine and efavirenz, inhibit hepatic cytochrome P-450 enzymes. Principal effects are on the CYP3A4 isoform (with ritonavir being the most potent inhibitor), although the CYP2D6 isoform may also be affected.[109,110] Nevirapine and efavirenz cause secondary induction of CYP3A4, an effect of ritonavir and nelfinavir as well.[109,110] Most antimalarial agents are largely metabolized via P-450 enzymes. Mefloquine appears to be no exception, although the details remain poorly understood.[111] Proguanil and chloroquine metabolism appears to be largely by the CYP2C19 and CYP2D6 isoforms, respectively.[112–115] Chloroquine also undergoes appreciable renal excretion, whereas doxycycline largely avoids these pathways in vivo. A detailed understanding of atovaquone metabolism appears to be lacking.

Actual published pharmacokinetic data suggest that (1) there are no significant drug–drug interactions between nelfinavir or indinavir and mefloquine[116]; (2) ritonavir has minimal effects on mefloquine pharmacokinetics, whereas mefloquine suppresses ritonavir plasma levels[117]; and (3) atovaquone increases serum zidovudine (AZT) levels by approximately 30%, although AZT has no effect on the pharmacokinetics of atovaquone.[118] In summary, the actual pharmacokinetics are not easily predictable from theoretical considerations, and there is a paucity of data. Based on the current data, mefloquine, doxycycline, chloroquine, and malarone (atovaquone + proguanil) are likely to be safe and to retain efficacy for prophylaxis of sensitive strains of malaria.

Among other malaria treatment options, quinidine, quinine, and β-artemether are all predominantly metabolized through CYP3A4 isoforms.[110] Large (more than threefold) increases in the area under the curve (AUC) for quinidine are expected for ritonavir.[119] As a result, quinidine has been considered to be contraindicated for those on ritonavir,[119] and this likely applies to quinine as well. There are no actual data, however. Whether there are clinically relevant effects of these protease inhibitors on the metabolism of artemisinin compounds (dependent at least in part on CYP3A4) remains unknown. Uncomplicated malaria can probably be safely treated with chloroquine (if sensitive), pyrimethamine/sulfadoxine, or mefloquine. Use of quinine, quinidine, or artemisinin compounds remains essential for the parenteral therapy of severe chloroquine-resistant malaria. For those on ritonavir (and/or other protease inhibitors, delaviridine, or efavirenz), the normal loading dose of quinine or quinidine should probably be given, along with some reduction of the maintenance infusion dose. Obviously, careful monitoring needs to be done for the potentially fatal arrhythmic consequences of quinine/quinidine overdosage in this setting. Given the lack of data, however, underdosing may also be a potential problem. The "washout" period for the metabolic effects of ritonavir is thought to be 24 to 48 hours.

A higher incidence of allergic responses to sulfonamides makes pyrimethamine–sulfadoxine (Fansidar) less attractive as a malaria therapy in HIV-seropositive patients, at least in North American populations.[120] Furthermore, Stevens–Johnson syndrome and related adverse mucocutaneous reactions to the long-acting sulfa compound, sulfadoxine, have contraindicated its benefits for use in malaria prophylaxis in developed countries.[121]

The presence of HIV infection alters the predictive value of fever in the empirical diagnosis of malaria. In areas with a high prevalence of both HIV and malaria, the common practice of empirically treating febrile adults for malaria leads to gross overestimation and overtreatment of malaria.[103] Finally, treatment of severe anemia due to malaria is one of the most common reasons for blood transfusion in sub-Saharan Africa. Malaria thus provides an indirect but very important risk factor for the acquisition of HIV infection by children where the blood supply is not well screened.[73]

Babesiosis

The genus *Babesia* contains more than 70 known species of tick-borne intraerythrocytic protozoans that parasitize wild and domestic vertebrates, predominantly in tropical and subtropical areas. Human babesial disease has been reported mostly from temperate climates (see Chapter 91). A significant clinical interaction with HIV infection has been suggested for *Babesia microti,* raising the possibility that disease with tropical babesial species may be a risk for AIDS patients and providing the rationale for the current discussion. There are five reported cases of babesiosis due to *B. microti* in HIV-infected people.[122–126] Two cases occurred in splenectomized patients; in one, chronic low-level hemolysis due to *Babesia* prior to splenectomy was likely. Patients with intact spleens presented with fevers of unknown origin (FUOs) in the face of CD4 counts less than 200/μL. In one, the FUO lasted for months and was associated with night sweats, dry cough, weight loss, and dyspnea on exertion. Persistent parasitemia after clinically successful chemotherapy led to the need for chronic suppressive therapy. In another patient, recurrent disease led to retreatment 8 months after initial therapy. Quinine plus clindamycin and atovaquone plus azithromycin both have therapeutic efficacy in acute disease.[127] In HIV-infected patients, chronic suppressive therapy appears to be indicated. As with all vector-borne diseases, vector avoidance is the most efficient way to prevent disease. Significant interactions with HIV infection remain to be described for European bovine *Babesia* species (*Babesia bovis* and *Babesia divergens*) and the emerging agents of human babesiosis (WA_1, CA_1, MO_1) in North America.

Leishmaniasis

With the exception of *Toxoplasma gondii, Leishmania* is the most common tissue protozoan causing OI in patients with AIDS (see Chapter 94). This is not surprising because cellular immune responses (in particular, Th1-mediated immune responses) are critical for protection from *Leishmania.* The competence of the Th1 axis of cellular response becomes increasingly compromised during the progression of HIV-related immunosuppression, providing a favorable environment for disease due to *Leishmania* species. Furthermore, in vitro evidence suggests that coinfection of macrophages with HIV and *Leishmania* can directly upregulate parasite replication.[128] In vivo, the overall loss of immunological control of parasite infection is reflected by often aberrant manifestations of visceral leishmaniasis (VL) in AIDS, including peripheral parasitemia (found in more than 50% of coinfected people) and parasite dissemination to unusual body compartments.[129] An AIDS-related OI occurring at low CD4+ T-cell counts, leishmaniasis may be due either to primary *Leishmania* infection or to the reactivation of clinically latent infection.[130,131] Although the published data on the interaction of HIV and *Leishmania* focus largely on the effects of HIV on leishmanial infection and disease, it should be noted that there is also both in vitro and in vivo evidence that *Leishmania* can augment HIV replication.[132–135]

Although leishmaniasis has a worldwide distribution in the tropics and subtropics, it normally requires an arthropod vector, the sandfly, to move the organism from its sylvatic (zoonotic) cycle to the human host. With certain species of *Leishmania (Leishmania tropica* and *Leishmania donovani)* and in some locations (e.g., Syria and India, respectively), an anthroponotic human-to-human cycle via the sandfly can exist. In situations in which intravenous drug use is practiced, transmission is simplified even further by direct person-to-person transfer via contaminated needles and syringes. Generally, however, leishmaniasis is a rural or periurban zoonosis.

The experience with VL complicating HIV/AIDS in Mediterranean countries indicates that many, perhaps most, of the leishmanial infections are acquired with HIV or after HIV infection has already occurred. The transmission of both agents that occurs by sharing of needles and syringes by intravenous drug users could theoretically be reduced by an aggressive program of education and provision of clean needles and syringes. An effective program of sandfly vector control will interrupt transmission from heavily infected human reservoirs to other humans as well as the more usual cycle of infected dogs to humans. Vector control is also the only way to prevent coinfection with *Leishmania* in those who acquire HIV sexually.

From the relatively high prevalence of latent leishmanial infections, it would appear that reactivation of latent infections could account for the increasing numbers of HIV–*Leishmania* coinfections; however, this concept is not always supported by epidemiologic evidence. A greater variability in zymodemes (enzyme markers) has been found in parasite isolates from HIV-infected than -uninfected patients. In one series, five isolates were recovered from HIV-infected patients that had previously not been encountered in immunocompetent people with either VL or cutaneous leishmaniasis (CL).[136] The finding that certain strains of *Leishmania* typically causing cutaneous disease are being recovered from the bone marrow of coinfected patients could support either the primary or the reactivation hypothesis.[137]

Normally, the age distribution of VL caused by *L. donovani* includes adults as well as children. In contrast, VL due to *Leishmania infantum* affects children predominantly, often age 5 years or younger. In Spain, where intravenous drug use accounts for the majority of HIV–*Leishmania* coinfections, the age distribution of VL has been reversed, with most cases occurring in young adult males.[138] The fact that 50% of coinfected patients have demonstrable organisms in peripheral blood smears[139] and the fact that sandflies can readily be infected by feeding on coinfected patients[140] provide evidence for an additional anthroponotic cycle of transmission in this setting.[137] In summary, although reactivation of latent leishmanial infection is difficult to exclude, increasing evidence—in southern Europe, at least—favors primary infection by certain strains of *Leishmania* as the main mechanism for coinfection with HIV/AIDS.

With the spread of the HIV pandemic, there is increasing epidemiological overlap of areas in which HIV and leishmania occur, particularly in eastern Africa, India, Brazil, and Europe. Cases have been reported from approximately 40 countries, although the bulk of cases have been reported from southern Europe.[129–131,137,141,142] Of note, relatively few cases of American mucocutaneous leishmaniasis have been recognized in HIV-infected subjects.[143,144] The propensity for disseminated disease in the presence of HIV appears to be limited to certain species of *Leishmania*. The bulk of the information on VL complicating HIV infection involves *L. infantum* in the Mediterranean region. Presumably, the ability to visceralize under the influence of HIV also applies to *L. donovani* in southern Asia and Africa and to *L. chagasi* in Latin America; however, documentation for this is still somewhat meager, one of the possible reasons being the poor overlap between geographic distribution of leishmaniasis caused by these species and the distribution, as well as prevalence, of HIV infection. The species of *Leishmania* that cause CL have been implicated only rarely as OIs in HIV/AIDS. In one instance, *L. braziliensis* was recovered from the bone marrow of a patient with a CD4+ T-cell count of less than 10/μL,[145] but the main clinical picture in this case, as well as in others,[146–148] including a patient infected with *Leishmania major*,[149] has been one of multiple cutaneous lesions resembling diffuse CL.

A febrile illness of longer than 2 weeks' duration in an HIV-infected person with a lifetime history of travel to *Leishmania*-endemic regions of the world should certainly raise suspicion of leishmaniasis complicating HIV infection. If the patient is an intravenous drug user, travel to southern Europe, especially Spain, France, and Italy, would be particularly pertinent. Clinical diagnosis of VL in leishmania–HIV coinfected people may be difficult. Only 75% of HIV-infected patients, as opposed to 95% of non-HIV-infected patients, exhibit the characteristic clinical pattern, namely fever, splenomegaly, and hepatomegaly.[130,131,137,142,150] With increasing immunosuppression, clinically evident ectopic localization of parasites becomes common.[151] Gastrointestinal, laryngeal, pulmonary, and peritoneal involvement has been reported.[151–158] Single and multiple cutaneous forms and/or mucosal and mucocutaneous lesions have also been described in AIDS patients worldwide.[148,153,159]

In immunocompetent people, tests for antileishmanial antibodies have been very useful in the diagnosis of VL because B cell activation is prominent, with large amounts of both specific and nonspecific antibody being produced. In contrast, approximately 50% of coinfected patients lack detectable antibody levels.[130,131,150,160] The situation may be different in instances in which leishmanial infection has preceded HIV infection and the impaired immune response that ensues. Gradoni and associates[161] suggested that this type of serologic data could be used as an indicator of the sequence of acquisition of the two infections. Support for this concept is provided by a report from Ethiopia of seven cases of VL with HIV coinfection, all with highly elevated antileishmanial antibody titers.[162] All patients had lived for many years in a leishmaniasis-endemic area of Ethiopia.[162] The recombinant antigen rK-39 appears to be highly sensitive and specific for immunodiagnosis of VL due to *L. donovani* and *L. chagasi* in patients without complicating HIV infection; however, the sensitivity of rK-39 for immunodiagnosis of cutaneous cases from Turkey was greatly reduced compared with most cases of VL.[163] The utility of rK-39-based diagnostics is not clear in HIV-seropositive people. The peripheral parasitemia displayed by many HIV coinfected individuals allows the detection of parasites from the blood in approximately 50% of cases. Cultures and polymerase chain reaction (PCR) of buffy-coat preparations are positive in 70% and up to 100%, respectively.[130,131,164]

There is abundant evidence that successful treatment of leishmanial disease, regardless of the drugs used, ultimately requires intact CMI. The coinfected patient is the victim of a double insult to the immune system. VL is associated with antigen-specific T-cell unresponsiveness[165] and dysfunctional cytokine responses.[166] This situation is further compounded by the immunologic abnormalities associated with HIV infection.

Therapy for VL in the face of HIV coinfection remains controversial, largely due to a lack of firm data. The same drugs used for treatment of VL in normal hosts (including pentavalent antimonials and amphotericin B preparations) have utility in the treatment of HIV coinfected patients, albeit with significantly less efficacy.[150] Amphotericin B is a conventional drug for all forms of leishmaniasis, including visceral disease. Liposomally encapsulated amphotericin has the theoretical advantage of being targeted to monocyte/macrophages, host cells for leishmanial parasites. Between 40% and 65% of coinfected patients have initial parasitological cure after treatment with pentavalent antimonials, amphotericin B deoxycholate, or amphotericin B lipid complex.[150,167,168] Among these options, treatment with lipid formulations of amphotericin B appears to have similar efficacy, but less severe toxicity, than the other drugs. However, the experience with lipid formulations of amphotericin B in coinfected patients remains meager.[168] These lipid formulations are also quite expensive. Trials aimed at optimizing the therapy of VL in AIDS are clearly needed.[168] Even with initial cure, relapse is predictable over time, occurring in up to 80% of coinfected individuals within 1 year.[150,167,169] The optimal drug for secondary prophylaxis remains unclear. Pentamidine given once every 3 or 4 weeks[170] and liposome-encapsulated amphotericin every 2 weeks[171] or 3 weeks[169] have been used for secondary prophylaxis.

Miltefosine, an oral agent that is safe and effective for the treatment of Indian patients with VL,[172] has shown some promise in early compassionate-use treatments for VL in HIV-infected subjects.[173] Further optimization of treatment and suppressive regimens of miltefosine in HIV patients may establish roles for this new antileishmanial agent for therapy and suppressive prophylaxis of VL in HIV-infected patients.

The fact that significant reductions in the incidence of AIDS-related VL have been seen in southern Europe after the advent of HAART,[174,175] along with the fact that HAART-related immune reconstitution has allowed the discontinuance of secondary prophylaxis for other OIs, has raised hope that HAART will allow for safe discontinuance of secondary prophylaxis for VL. Details of the levels of immunological and virological responses needed for termination of such secondary prophylaxis remain to be determined.[176–178]

American Trypanosomiasis (Chagas' Disease)

American trypanosomiasis, or Chagas' disease (see Chapter 93), is a well-recognized OI in AIDS.[179] The causative organism, *Trypanosoma cruzi,* and the blood-sucking vector (triatomine) bugs that transmit this protozoan are restricted to the Western Hemisphere but are widely distributed from the United States to Chile and Argentina. Because the HIV-related Chagas' disease reported to date largely represents reactivation of chronic infection during the course of HIV-induced immunosuppression and not primary infection in the face of AIDS (which is not surprising given the differing patterns of epidemiological risk for these infections: largely rural for *T. cruzi* and largely urban for HIV), this OI can be expected to appear outside these geographic bounds. It should be noted that activation of latent *T. cruzi* infection, as well as exacerbated primary infection (transmitted by blood transfusion), is also well described in the face of the iatrogenic immunosuppression used for solid organ transplantation and therapy for hematological malignancies.

Available data suggest that clinical *T. cruzi* reactivation in the face of HIV coinfection occurs largely in those with CD4+ T-cell counts less than 200/μL. Clinically, such reactivation most commonly involves the central nervous system.[179,180] *Trypanosoma cruzi* was probably late in being recognized as an opportunistic pathogen in those with HIV infection because the most prominent features of central nervous system disease are similar to those of toxoplasmic meningoencephalitis. Enlargement of hemorrhagic foci can produce mass effects simulating brain tumors. Lesions are often multiple, with computed tomographic (CT) scans and magnetic resonance imaging (MRI) showing ring enhancement and preferential involvement of the white matter. Toxoplasmic encephalitis may also be present in the same patient.[181] The cerebrospinal fluid (CSF) findings include a slight pleocytosis, increased protein, slightly decreased glucose in some patients, and the presence of trypanosomes. Histologically, the brain lesions show necrotic foci with hemorrhage and infiltration of inflammatory cells. Amastigote forms of the parasite are abundant in glial cells and macrophages and only occasionally in neuronal cells. Myocarditis is a common autopsy finding in those dying of AIDS-related *T. cruzi* meningoencephalitis.[178] Such myocarditis is often clinically silent. Clinical manifestations, when present, involve arrhythmias and congestive heart failure.[179,182,183] Correct diagnosis of reactivated *T. cruzi* infection depends, first, on considering the possibility based on the geographic origin of the patient and on an appreciation of the clinical picture. If neurologic signs are present, performing a CT scan or MRI is key.[184] The imaging pattern of central nervous system (CNS) *T. cruzi* infection is indistinguishable from that of toxoplasmic encephalitis. Direct microscopic examination of centrifuged sediment of CSF will often show motile trypanosomes. If fever and other systemic signs are present, direct examination of the buffy coat from the microhematocrit tube may also show motile trypanosomes. Since serum antibodies to *T. cruzi* indicate previous infection with the parasite, this test is only useful for ruling out reactivated infection if it is negative. If other tests are inconclusive, biopsy of a brain lesion to demonstrate characteristic organisms can be done. PCR on blood or CSF requires research laboratory facilities.

Clinically, differentiating HIV-related reactivation of Chagas' disease reactivation from chronic chagasic disease may be difficult. HIV-related reactivation is associated with high parasitemia, however, whereas the parasitemia of chronic disease is very low.[185] Indeed, even in the absence of overt, clinical reactivation, chronic Chagas' disease is associated with a higher percentage and level of parasitemia in those coinfected with HIV (independent of CD4 count) than in HIV seronegatives.[186] The effects of coinfection appear to be bidirectional. HIV viral load was carefully documented to increase simultaneously with an asymptomatic increase in *T. cruzi* parasitemia, subsequently returning to baseline in the face of successful antiparasitic treatment.[187] Nifurtimox and benznidazole, both of which have moderate antitrypanosomal activity, are the standard drugs recommended for treatment of Chagas' disease. There simply is not enough experience to evaluate the effectiveness of these drugs in the treatment of *T. cruzi* infections complicating HIV or AIDS, especially in cases with meningoencephalitis. No information is available on the penetration of these drugs into the CNS, and the survival time of reported cases of coinfection has been short. A patient reported by Nishioka and coworkers[188] survived for 92 days, with disappearance of trypanosomes from the blood and CSF as well as clearance of a brain lesion while being treated with benznidazole at a dose of 8 mg/kg/day for 80 days. Clinical improvement and reduction in size of a brain lesion were attributed to treatment with benznidazole plus, later, itraconazole and fluconazole in another patient with coinfection who survived for at least

6 months.[189] Although there is no other reported experience with the use of itraconazole or fluconazole in the treatment of American trypanosomiasis in humans, itraconazole was reported to be very effective in experimental infections.[190] Infected mice given as little as 15 mg/kg/day were protected against death, and concentrations of itraconazole as low as 0.001 μg/mL inhibited replication of the parasites in macrophages. It has been recommended that treatment of *T. cruzi* infection in HIV-positive individuals be started early in the reactivation process, when parasitemia is detectable, but before irreversible end-organ damage has occurred.[187] Such a strategy would hinge on serological identification of those at risk, something indicated in all HIV-infected individuals with appreciable risk of *T. cruzi* infection. Although data are lacking, it should be noted that immunological reconstitution through HAART therapy is likely to provide considerable prophylactic and therapeutic benefit in this disease.

African Trypanosomiasis

No significant interactions between the agents of African trypanosomiasis (see Chapter 92) and HIV have been delineated. Although T cell and macrophage responses are not thought to be important in the protective host response to trypanosomiasis, trypanosomiasis can suppress cellular immune responses, so a biologic interaction between the two is plausible. No significant epidemiologic association between *Trypansoma brucei gambiense* and HIV has been found.[191–194] Whether HIV alters the clinical course of either West or East African trypanosomiasis is unclear.[193] There is anecdotal evidence that HIV may complicate the therapy of West African trypanosomiasis, however. Of 18 patients treated with melarsoprol in a rural hospital in the Congo, all 14 HIV-negative patients recovered, whereas 3 of 4 HIV-positive patients died during treatment (likely due to treatment-related encephalopathy) and the fourth failed to respond to therapy.[195]

Other Trypanosomatids

In addition to the two genera, *Leishmania* and *Trypanosoma,* known to cause disease in humans, the Trypanosomatidae family includes other genera of protozoa that parasitize other vertebrates, insects, and plants. There have been three reports of HIV-infected individuals presenting with symptoms typical of visceral leishmaniasis in which ultrastructural, isoenzyme, and/or kinetoplast DNA analyses of the isolated lesional parasites have indicated that the responsible organism actually belongs to one of these latter genera.[196] The strong implication is that HIV-related immunosuppression can render humans vulnerable to normally nonpathogenic lower trypanosomatids.

Toxoplasmosis

Toxoplasma gondii is a ubiquitous parasite of mammals throughout the world (see Chapter 97). Latent infection lasts for the lifetime of the host. Maintenance of latency is dependent on CMI responses. Reactivation of latent infection is common with increasing immunosuppression in AIDS. The principal manifestation of such reactivation, toxoplasmic encephalitis (TE), is thus a common OI in AIDS patients throughout the world. The incidence of TE is proportional to the prevalence of latent infection in the population at risk of or with AIDS.[197] In the United States, the rate of latent infection varies between 10% and 40%; in Paris, the rate is 90%.[197] Acquisition of *Toxoplasma* infection is age dependent, but there is wide variation in infection rates even over narrow geographic areas.[198,199] Prevalence rates in the tropics vary from 0% to 90%, with most measured communities falling in a broad middle range.[200–206]

In the United States, prior to the advent of HAART, one-third of *Toxoplasma*-seropositive AIDS patients developed TE in the absence of prophylaxis,[207] 90% of such cases were in patients with less than 200 CD4+ T cells/μL and 70% in those with less than 100 CD4 T cells/μL.[208] The prevalence of TE in AIDS patients in the tropics is unclear, but the burden is thought to be immense and underdiagnosed. Autopsy series that have included examination of the brain have suggested disease prevalence rates in late-stage AIDS patients of 15% in Abidjan, Côte d'Ivoire,[209] 25% in Mexico City,[210] and 36% in Kampala, Uganda.[211]

The presumptive diagnosis of TE is based on clinical presentation, positive *Toxoplasma* serologies, and characteristic neuroradiologic features.[212] A final clinical diagnosis is made based on the clinical and radiographic response to specific chemotherapy. Less common manifestations of toxoplasmosis in AIDS include pneumonia, retinochoroiditis, myocarditis, orchitis, and gastrointestinal involvement. The reader is referred to one of many excellent reviews on *Toxoplasma* in AIDS for information on the clinical management of this cosmopolitan OI.[76–79]

Five percent of TE occurs not as reactivation but as an acute infection.[207] Preventing the transmission of *T. gondii* to *Toxoplasma*-seronegative, HIV-infected people has two facets: (1) avoiding the ingestion of tissue cysts of other intermediate mammalian hosts (i.e., cooking meat well) and (2) avoiding the oocysts of the definitive host, the cat. Avoiding cat feces in and around dwellings is probably not sufficient because the oocysts are viable for up to 18 months in moist soil. Contamination of fresh vegetables may be a common method of human infection, and such foodstuffs should probably be washed well or cooked or both.

Primary prophylaxis (TMP–SMX is preferred)[213] should be taken by all *Toxoplasma*-seropositive HIV patients with a CD4+ T-cell count less than 100/μL. It is safe to discontinue both primary and secondary prophylaxis after HAART-related immune reconstitution (sustained CD4+ T-cell counts >200/μL).[76–79]

Free-Living Amebae

Free-living amebae of the *Acanthamoeba* and *Balamuthia* genera (see Chapter 95) are rare causes of opportunistic encephalitis and cutaneous disease in late-stage AIDS. Most case reports have been from the United States, but the worldwide environmental distribution of these ubiquitous protozoans and the fact that diagnosis is often postmortem suggest that underdiagnosis is widespread in the tropics and elsewhere.

Granulomatous amebic encephalitis (GAE), a subacute to chronic disease of compromised hosts caused by multiple species of *Acanthamoeba* as well as *Balamuthi mandrillaris,* generally causes death in weeks to months. Clinical and pathologic data, as well as animal models, suggest that the pathogenesis of GAE involves hematogenous dissemination to the brain from initial upper or lower respiratory (or perhaps cutaneous) sites of infection.[214] Pathologic changes, in the form of necrotizing granulomatous inflammation, are found predominantly in the posterior neuraxis.

Acanthamoeba and *Balamuthia* have been isolated from soil, water (including tap water, bottled water, chlorinated pools, and natural sources of fresh- and seawater), and air throughout the world.[215] The isolation of *Acanthamoeba* from the nasopharynx of healthy adults indicates that these organisms may be a common constituent of normal flora.[216] Cellular immunity, along with antibody and complement, appears to be critical to protective immunity to *Acanthamoebae*.[217] Invasive disease occurs in the immunocompromised and debilitated.[214] Occasionally, encephalitis with *Balamuthia mandrillaris* has occurred in apparently normal hosts.[218,219]

More than 20 cases of GAE have been reported in AIDS patients.[214,220–229] Implicated *Acanthamoeba* organisms include *Acanthamoeba castellani, Acanthamoeba culbertsoni, Acanthamoeba polyphaga, Acanthamoeba rhysodes,* and *Acanthamoeba divionensis*. Disseminated cutaneous disease [subacute granulomatous dermatitis (SGD)] has been a feature of many of these cases and has preceded clinical cerebral involvement by weeks or months in some. SGD has been the sole manifestation of invasive disease in some patients.[230–234] Reported CD4+ T-cell counts have been less than 250/μL (median, 24/μL) at the time of presentation. Where CD4 counts have not been reported, the histories reveal clinical evidence of late-stage AIDS.[214,234]

GAE in AIDS patients is marked by a more rapid course (with death in 3 to 40 days)[214] and a paucity of well-formed granulomas in comparison to other hosts with the disease.[214,233] Symptomatic involvement of the nasopharynx, paranasal sinuses, or the skin prior to development of GAE is common in AIDS patients.[214] Cutaneous lesions are usually nodular, with subsequent enlargement, ulceration, and metastatic spread. Such lesions can be quite pleomorphic (pustules, plaques, eschars, and cellulitis), however, and have been confused with cat-scratch disease, cryptococcosis, sporotrichosis, bacillary angiomatosis, mycobacterial infections, and vasculitis.[214] The most common presentation of cerebral disease is that of fever and headache.[214,232] Focal neurologic deficits and profound changes in mental status are also frequent. Neuroradiologic findings mimic those of toxoplasmic encephalitis, with multiple enhancing mass lesions and surrounding edema. CSF findings are quite variable.[214,232]

A high index of suspicion and tissue or microbiologic diagnosis is key to the antemortem identification of disseminated *Acanthamoeba* infection. Wet mounts of CSF are occasionally useful. Both trophozoites and cysts can be found in tissue biopsies. Cysts have been mistaken for the sporangia of *Rhinosporium* or *Prototheca* or for cryptococci; trophozoites have been mistaken for tissue macrophages.[214] *Acanthamoebae* can be isolated by culture on *Escherichia coli*–seeded non-nutrient agar or in tissue culture medium.[214,232] Identification of species (and even differentiation of *Acanthamoeba* from *Balamuthia*) is not possible morphologically. Immunofluorescence techniques can differentiate *Acanthamoeba* to the group level in tissue section or with cultured organisms. Treatment of disseminated disease due to these organisms is difficult. No chemotherapeutic regimen is clearly efficacious. Agents with possible clinical utility in combination therapy include pentamidine, 5-fluorocytosine, sulfamethazine, sulfadiazine, fluconazole, itraconazole, ketoconazole, macrolides, phenothiazines, and rifampin.[214,228,229,231] There may be value in testing clinical isolates for drug sensitivities. With isolated cerebral lesions, there may be a role for surgical excision.[229]

In a possible foreshadowing of a newly emerging OI, a case of primary amebic meningoencephalitis due to an apparently newly recognized ameba and not associated with thermally polluted water was reported in a patient with late-stage AIDS in Spain.[235,236]

Enteric Coccidiosis (*Isospora, Cryptosporidium,* and *Cyclospora*)

A trio of coccidian protozoa—*Isospora belli, Cryptosporidium* spp., and *Cyclospora (Eimeria) cayetanensis*—are all prominent causes of self-limited, small bowel diarrhea in immunologically normal hosts as well as causes of chronic, severe disease in the face of HIV coinfection. All are cosmopolitan infections. Infection with a fourth organism, *Sarcocystis hominis,* responsible for both enteric and disseminated coccidioisis in humans, does not appear to have been reported in HIV-infected individuals.

***Cryptosporidium* spp.** (see Chapter 88). In addition to the most common human pathogen *Cryptosporidium hominis* (previously *Cryptosporidium parvum* human genotype, or genotype 1), a variety of zoonotic species also infect humans, including *Cryptosporidium parvum* (previously bovine genotype, or genotype 2), *Cryptosporidium canis, Cryptosporidium felis, Cryptosporidium meleagridis,* and *Cryptosporidium muris*.[237–239] Zoonotic species may cause more severe human disease and may occur more commonly in immunocompromised people. Because of the high prevalence of disease and the lack of effective specific treatment, cryptosporidiosis is a particularly common and severe problem as an OI throughout the world. Chronic infection and disease are most frequent with CD4+ T cell counts less than 180/mL[240] and are associated with increased mortality. [241–243] The use of HAART therapy has led to a decreasing prevalence of cryptosporidial disease in HIV-infected individuals.[244,245]

Four clinical syndromes of cryptosporidial diarrheal disease in patients with AIDS have been limned: chronic diarrhea (36%), cholera-like disease (33%), transient diarrhea (15%), and relapsing illness (15%). The severe end of the spectrum is seen largely in those with CD4+ T-cell counts less than 180/μL.[246,247] Less commonly, extraintestinal sites are secondarily involved, including biliary tract, stomach, pancreas, lung, paranasal sinuses, and middle ear.[246–249] Of these, biliary tract involvement (presenting with right upper quadrant pain, nausea, vomiting, and fever) represents the most common, clinically important site, being found in up to one-fourth of patients with AIDS-related intestinal disease prior to the use of HAART.[250] Individuals with CD4+ T-cell counts less than 50/μL are at a particular risk for development of symptomatic biliary disease.[250]

No antimicrobial agent has demonstrable, consistent efficacy in HIV-related cryptosporidiosis. Immune reconstitution with HAART should be pursued.[251,252] If HAART fails or is not available, a variety of antimicrobial agents (including nitazoxanide, azithromycin, paromomycin, and atovaquone) may be tried. Supportive treatment with fluids, nutrition, and antimotility agents plays an obvious therapeutic role.[76–79]

Isospora belli (see Chapter 88). Disease due to *Isospora* is less cosmopolitan than that due to *Cryptosporidia,* being most common in tropical and subtropical areas.[253] Isosporiasis usually presents with chronic watery diarrhea and weight loss, with or without vomiting, abdominal pain, and fever.[254] Invasion of gallbladder tissue, similar to that described with *Cryptosporidium,* has been described, along with disseminated involvement of mesenteric and tracheobronchial lymph nodes, in the setting of HIV coinfection.[254,255] Prominent tissue eosinophilia of the involved lamina propria is often present.[253] Diagnostic and therapeutic issues are covered in Chapter 88. TMP–SMX provides effective therapy.[256] Pyrimethamine (with leucovorin) provides a second option.[257] Clinical response is usually rapid, but relapses are common. In the absence of immune reconstitution, suppressive therapy is indicated.[76–79]

Cyclospora* (Eimeria) *cayetanensis (see Chapter 89). The clinical picture of enteric infection with *C. cayetanensis* in AIDS appears to be similar to that due to other coccidia.[258] It is of interest that biliary tract involvement—as evidenced by right upper quadrant pain, elevated alkaline phosphatase, and thickened gallbladder by ultrasound—has also been described in *Cyclospora* infection.[259] Thus, all three of the enteric coccidia of humans are capable of invading the gallbladder. Diagnostic and therapeutic issues are covered in Chapter 89. As with isosporiasis, cyclosporiasis in AIDS is treatable with TMP/SMX.[258] Subsequent suppressive therapy is indicated.[76–79]

Microsporidiosis

Microsporidia are intracellular protozoans that, due to HIV and AIDS, have emerged from their relative obscurity as pathogens of insects, fish, and laboratory animals to occupy a new role as important OIs of humans. These cosmopolitan emerging pathogens of the immunosuppressed (including *Enterocytozoon bienusi, Enterocytozoon [Septata] intestinalis, Enterocytozoon cuniculi, Enterocytozoon hellem,* as well as pathogens from several other genera) are considered in Chapter 96.

Other Protozoan Infections

Entamoeba histolytica. This intestinal parasite (see Chapter 86) was initially associated with HIV because of its high prevalence in men who have sex with men (MSM). Despite considerable evidence that immunity in amebiasis requires the participation of CMI, there is no evidence that patients with HIV infection or AIDS are more likely to develop invasive disease.

Giardia lamblia. As with *E. histolytica,* a high prevalence of infection with *G. lamblia* (see Chapter 87) was found in the 1980s among MSM.[260] A study of MSM performed at that time revealed no increased prevalence or severity of giardiasis in patients with AIDS.[261] Since then, no evidence has been found of a significant effect of HIV coinfection. Although some studies have indicated a higher prevalence of giardiasis in HIV seropositives, this has not been a consistent finding. Therapy of giardiasis in people with AIDS is usually successful. Some patients, immunocompromised as well as immunocompetent, are refractory to standard therapeutic regimens for giardiasis. It may well be that such refractoriness to standard therapy is found more commonly in the face of HIV coinfection.[262]

Blastocystis hominis. Controversy continues to exist as to the role of this organism as a cause of diarrheal disease in either immunocompetent patients or HIV-infected people.[263] *Blastocystis hominis* has a cosmopolitan distribution; there is no association with the tropics.

Balantidium coli. No information is available as to whether this organism can serve as an OI in HIV-infected people.

Helminthic Infections

Trematodes

There is no evidence that any trematode infection is more severe or difficult to treat in HIV-infected people. More subtle interactions have been explored in schistosomiasis (see Chapter 116). Study of car washers working on the shores of Lake Victoria in Kenya, a population with a high intensity of exposure to *S. mansoni* and an HIV seroprevalence of approximately 30%, has provided insights into the bidirectional effects of coinfection.[264] The CD4+ T cell–dependent granulomatous response to schistosome eggs has been shown to be important in egg migration from venules to the lumen of the intestine in mouse models of disease.[264] As might thereby be expected, a significant suppression of egg excretion efficiency, controlled for the degree of infection, was found in *S. mansoni*–infected patients in the presence of HIV coinfection and low CD4+ T-cell counts.[265] Although successful therapy of *S. mansoni* infection with praziquantel may depend on the host antibody response, praziquantel was efficacious in treating schistosomiasis in this HIV-infected cohort.[266] Given that schistosome infection likely preceded HIV infection in these individuals, whether praziquantel will have equal efficacy in individuals infected with HIV first remains an open question. Notably, despite similar responses to therapy, individuals with HIV coinfection and low CD4+ T cell counts showed increased susceptibility to reinfection after therapy,[267] a response that appears to correlate with blunted immunological responses to successful drug therapy (and the resultant release of parasite antigen) in such individuals.[268] A study of HIV/*S. haematobium* coinfection in Zambia led to findings that mirror these findings with *S. mansoni*: (1) Coinfected individuals had lower egg excretion, and (2) praziquantel retained efficacy in the face of HIV coinfection.[269] No alteration in resistance to reinfection with *S. haemotobium* was seen in the face of HIV infection, but CD4+ T-cell counts were not performed in this cohort lacking evident HIV-related disease. It thus remains possible that, as with *S. mansoni* infection, resistance to reinfection with *S. haematobium* is decreased with progression of HIV/AIDS.

As for effects of schistosomiasis on HIV, there is evidence suggesting that genital schistosomiasis due to *S. haematobium* infection is a risk factor for HIV transmission.[269–271] As with a variety of sexually transmitted diseases, the mucosal (vulval, vaginal, and cervical) inflammatory lesions associated with female genital schistosomiasis are likely to compromise the antiviral barrier of the mucosa, provide a cellular milieu that allows for efficient viral transmission and replication, and enhance viral shedding.[270,271] Correspondingly, male genital schistosomiasis is also likely to be associated with an increased risk of HIV transmission. In Madagascar, *S. haematobium* caused inflammation of the prostate and of the seminal vesicles in most adolescent and adult male patients.[272] By analogy to bacterial urethritis, such chronic inflammation is likely to be associated with increased viral shedding in the semen in HIV-coinfected individuals.

Schistosomiasis is a prime example of a chronic tropical infection that has been postulated to enhance the pathogenesis of HIV. *Schistosoma mansoni* infections act as powerful inducers of Th2 polarization in both murine models and humans.[60–62] The type 2 cytokine environment induced by *S. mansoni* eggs can significantly suppress CD8 T cell–mediated viral clearance in experimental models[61] and has been found to impair antigen-specific Th1 immune responses in both mice and humans.[61,66] Type 2–dominant immunologic responses have also been postulated to favor HIV progression due to preferential replication of HIV in Th2 cells,[64] amplification of activation-induced apoptosis in lymphocytes by type 2 cytokines,[9,10] and upregulation of expression of the HIV coreceptors CCR5 and CXCR4 by CD4+ T cells and monocyte/macrophages.[66,67] Finally, the antigenic exposure of schistosomiasis may lead to sustained upregulation of HIV replication via the effects of chronic immune activation.[60] These considerations remain theoretical. Indeed, treatment of *S. mansoni* infection does not appear to reduce plasma HIV load in coinfected individuals.[273,274]

Cestodes

A few unusual manifestations of cestode infection have been reported in AIDS patients. A rapidly expanding, invasive, and ultimately lethal abdominal mass in a patient with a CD4+ T-cell count less than 100/μL was found by ribosomal DNA amplification and sequencing to be due to an as yet uncharacterized cestode.[275] Whether this represents merely the fortuitous concurrence of an unusual pathologic finding with dramatic improvements in diagnostic technology (previous rare cases in normal hosts having occurred in the absence of diagnosis) or the recognition of a new disease because its expression is facilitated or dependent on immunosuppression (AIDS patients serving as "sentinel chickens" for the population at large) is unclear. The latter interpretation is favored by a previous similar case report of presumably disseminated cestode infection in the face of immunosuppression due to Hodgkin's disease and its therapy.[276]

Four cases of exuberant subcutaneous disease due to the larval form of *Taenia crassiceps* have been reported in AIDS patients.[277–280] As this bests by one the previous number of case reports of human infection with *T. crassiseps,* the suggestion is that HIV infection is a risk for disease with this cestode. A case of hepatic alveolar echinococcal disease in a 6-year-old child with AIDS has been described.[281] Uncommon features of this case include the remarkably young age and hence short incubation period for disease and the complete lack of demonstrable parasite-specific humoral or cellular immune responses.

Finally, 10 cases of neurocysticercosis have been reported in HIV-infected patients,[282–286] a number that is sure to increase given the increasing rates of HIV infection in endemic areas. The frequency of giant cysts and racemose forms of disease is remarkably elevated in these reported cases, again perhaps a reflection of the role of CD4+ T cells in tissue immunity to *T. solium*. Further clinical data on the interaction between HIV and cestode infections are awaited.

Nematodes

Strongyloides stercoralis. The only nematode implicated as a cause of an OI in the presence of HIV coinfection is the intestinal parasite, *Strongyloides stercoralis* (see Chapter 111). *S. Stercoralis* appeared to qualify as an OI because it is one of the few nematodes capable of actually multiplying in, especially immunocompromised, human hosts. *Capillaria philippinensis,* for which humans are not the natural host, can also multiply internally, but *C. philippinensis* is rare, quite limited in its geographic distribution, and has not been reported as a coinfection in HIV-seropositive people (see Chapter 106).

One way in which immunosuppression enhances *Strongyloides* infection is by permitting or stimulating an increased degree of the normal process of autoinfection.[287] In this process, first-stage rhabditiform larvae (L1) produced by the adult female worm in the upper small bowel are transformed into infective filariform larvae (L3) that can reinvade the intestinal wall of the colon or the perianal or perineal areas. Massive upregulation of the autoinfective process results in the hyperinfection syndrome, with the development of many more adult worms, and the production of large numbers of larvae that disseminate to all organs. The clinical picture is dominated by gram-negative bacterial sepsis, meningitis, or pneumonia.

Hyperinfection is usually associated with immunosuppression, particularly the administration of corticosteroids. In fact, the list of immunosuppressive diseases, both malignant and benign, associated with hyperinfection is unified by having corticosteroids as a common denominator of treatment,[287] but steroids do much more than alter T-cell function, both in the host and in the organism. The defense mechanisms necessary for control of *S. stercoralis* in humans have not been identified. Even direct effects of steroids on the female worms' reproductive efficiency have been postulated.[287,288] The data are meager.

Strongyloides was initially designated as an AIDS OI on its past record of causing hyperinfection in the immunosuppressed.[289] Five years later, when it became apparent that hyperinfection syndrome was not being encountered frequently in patients with AIDS, it was removed from the list of OIs indicative of AIDS.[290] Given the low but appreciable rate (3.9%) of strongyloidiasis among men attending a venereal disease clinic in New York City in 1981,[291] the AIDS epidemic in the United States that developed in the 1980s should have provided some clinical evidence of any predisposition of AIDS patients to hyperinfection. This did not occur. The available evidence makes it extremely unlikely that misdiagnosis or underreporting are the relevant factors here; severe strongyloidiasis or hyperinfection syndrome has prominent clinical features and is often fatal if untreated, and it is not likely that the association would escape notice. Few cases of hyperinfection syndrome have been reported in the English-language literature.[292–301] Even among these cases, the presence of hyperinfection is poorly documented in many.

Diagnosis of (as opposed to suspicion of) hyperinfection syndrome depends on the demonstration of markedly increased numbers of filariform larvae in the stool or multiple such larvae in the sputum. The mere presence of filariform larvae in the sputum only indicates the existence of autoinfection. (It should also be noted that the presence of rhabditiform larvae in the sputum points to neither autoinfection nor hyperinfection but to the presence of adult female worms in the lung.) Unfortunately, confusion of gastrointestinal disease with hyperinfection syndrome is embedded in the literature.

It is possible that the frequency of severe strongyloidiasis complicating HIV infection is much higher in certain areas of the tropics where both infections are prevalent and medical facilities are lacking; however, an absence of such an association has been noted from just such areas.[15] Petithory and Derouin[302] pointed out that clinical studies of AIDS patients in central Africa, where the prevalence of strongyloidiasis varies from 26% to 48%, did not mention extraintestinal strongyloidiasis. Similarly, a report from Brazil estimated a 1% or 2% prevalence of *Strongyloides* infection in the population of São Paulo, finding the parasite in 10% of 100 AIDS patients, who showed no evidence of systemic strongyloidiasis.[303] Similar results have been found in Zambia.[304,305] A survey of urban adults in Kinshasa (Congo, formerly Zaire) detected *S. stercoralis* in 20% by intensive fecal examinations of single specimens, and it estimated a 50% infection rate in the same population on the basis of positive serologies. There were no significant differences in infection rates in those seropositive or seronegative for HIV (F. Neva, unpublished observations).

Taken together, these data suggest that the presence and severity of clinical disease due to *S. stercoralis* are not significantly increased in patients with HIV infection or AIDS alone. A recent study has shed light on the subject.[306] Careful quantitation of the numbers and proportions of free-living adult worms and directly developing L3 larvae in stool cultures revealed a surprising negative correlation between CD4+ T-cell count and the proportions of adult worms in individuals infected with HIV. Thus, advancing immunosuppression due to HIV is associated, paradoxically, with suppression of the direct development of L3 larvae.[306]

More subtle interactions, such as an increased mean gastrointestinal parasite burden or slower response to therapy, may have been missed. Also, some conditions that cosegregate with HIV/AIDS are known to predispose to the hyperinfection syndrome, including the use of steroids (given for pneumocystis pneumonia and lymphoma in AIDS), inanition (seen in patients with chronic diarrhea, untreated oropharyngeal or esophageal candidiasis, and slim disease), and coinfection with human T-cell lymphotropic virus type I (HTLV-I; see Chapter 76). Strongyloidiasis is an important OI in individuals infected with HTLV-1, and *Strongyloides* infection has been suspected to be a cofactor in the development of acute T-cell leukemia and tropical spastic paraparesis in asymptomatic carriers of HTLV-I.[307,308] Notably, intravenous drug use is a risk factor for infection with both HTLV-I and HIV.

Intestinal helminthiasis. Intestinal helminth infection is ubiquitous in low-income tropical countries. Although such helminths do not appear to act as OIs in AIDS, it has been hypothesized that the immune dysregulation associated with geohelminthic infections may alter the natural history of HIV infection in an unfavorable manner. Such hypotheses are founded on the presence of chronic immune activation and Th2 polarization during chronic helminthic infection. Indeed, it has been demonstrated that peripheral blood cells from patients with intestinal helminth infection[68] (and filarial infection[69]) are more susceptible to in vitro infection with HIV than are cells from helminth-uninfected patients. The overall hypothesis remains unproven, however. An initial study from Ethiopia indicated that HIV viral load was significantly higher in individuals with various helminthic infections than in individuals without helminths, correlating positively with the parasite load as well as decreasing after elimination of the worms by antiparasitic treatment.[70] However, similar studies performed in Uganda and examining far larger numbers of patients have convincingly failed to replicate these findings.[71,72] These latter studies strongly suggest that helminth coinfection is not associated with faster progression of HIV disease.

Onchocerca volvulus. Among the filaria, the effect of HIV coinfection has been studied in a large cohort of patients with *Onchocerca volvulus* infection. No significant epidemiological association was found between the two infections, nor was there any difference in the efficacy of ivermectin treatment in HIV-infected compared with -uninfected patients.[309]

Arthropods

Sarcoptes scabiei var. *hominis* stands alone among the arthropod and crustacean infestations of humans as a cause of exacerbated disease in the presence of HIV infection. In normal hosts, scabies is usually manifest as a markedly pruritic, papular, and vesicular dermatitis, with pathognomonic burrows harboring gravid females. Excoriations, nodules, and eczematous or impetiginized plaques may also be found. Relatively few adult mites are normally present.

Norwegian or crusted scabies is seen in neurologically impaired or immunosuppressed patients. Pruritus is often absent or mild. Lesions consist of widespread hyperkeratotic, crusted, scaling, fissured plaques. The nails are frequently involved. Patients tend to be heavily infested, with thousands of adult mites (see Chapter 118). Crusted scabies has been reported as a complication of HIV infection. CD4+ T-cell counts in reported cases have been less than 500/μL.[310–312] Both typical and atypical presentations are seen, the latter including the "pruritus of AIDS," crusting with pruritus, pruritic papular dermatitis, and mimics of Darier's disease and psoriasis.[311] Secondary sepsis and death have been reported.[313] In the face of this clinical variability, the diagnosis of crusted scabies in HIV-seropositive people rests on appropriate clinical suspicion and the demonstration of heavy infestation by microscopic examination of skin scrapings. With such extraordinary mite loads, these patients are remarkably contagious.[314,315] Combination therapy with ivermectin 200 μg/kg and topical benzyl benzoate (or perhaps permethrin) appears be the treatment of choice.[312] Single-dose ivermectin is also effective at preventing transmission in close contacts. Despite speculation early in the AIDS pandemic, there is no evidence of transmission of HIV by arthropod vectors.

Pruritic papular eruptions associated with HIV infection are common in sub-Saharan Africa. The etiology of these intensely pruritic lesions has been attributed to exaggerated immune responses to arthropod bites in HIV-infected individuals.[316]

Fungal Infections

Penicillium marneffei

Disseminated infection with *P. marneffei*, a dimorphic fungus endemic to Southeast Asia and southern China (see Chapter 82), has emerged as an important OI in AIDS patients. It is the third most common OI in HIV disease in northern Thailand, after extrapulmonary tuberculosis and cryptococcal meningitis.[316] First isolated in 1956, infection with *P. marneffei* was a rare event before the arrival of the AIDS pandemic in Southeast Asia.[316] Since then, thousands of cases have been diagnosed, primarily in southern China, northern Thailand, Hong Kong, Taiwan, Malaysia, Vietnam, Singapore, Indonesia, and Myanmar.[316–320] The overwhelming majority of cases have been in AIDS patients, although normal hosts are also known to develop systemic disease with this fungus.[316,318,321] There is a pronounced intracountry variation in infection rates. In northern Thailand, up to one-fourth of AIDS patients suffer disease with it, whereas in southern Thailand the prevalence is 10-fold less.[320] The environmental reservoir for *P. marneffei* is unknown, but the organism has been isolated from the organs, feces, and burrows of three species of bamboo rats. The geographic range of these rodents overlaps the previously mentioned known areas of endemicity for disease with *P. marneffei*[317–319] and suggests the likelihood that this fungus is also endemic in Laos, Cambodia, and Malaysia.[316] Whether bamboo rats are important reservoirs for human infection or just another natural host is unclear. There is no evidence of transmission between rats and humans. The seasonal distribution of the diagnosis of disseminated disease in AIDS patients suggests that the reservoir for *P. marneffei* expands during the rainy season.[317] Exposure to soil appears to be a key factor.[322]

The pathogenesis of disease due to *P. marneffei* is presumed by analogy with other endemic systemic mycoses to involve transmission by inhalation, with secondary systemic dissemination. Like *Histoplasma capsulatum, P. marneffei* is an intracellular parasite of monocyte/macrophages.[318] A murine model of pulmonary and disseminated infection shows that T cells play a central role in controlling infection.[323] In AIDS patients, disseminated disease is associated with CD4+ T-cell counts less than 100/μL.[316,324]

The largest clinical series reported to date of AIDS patients with disseminated *P. marneffei* infection provided detailed information on 80 patients.[316] The onset of symptoms was generally sudden and intense. The most common presenting symptoms and signs were fever (92%), anemia (77%), weight loss (76%), and skin lesions (71%). Other frequent signs and symptoms included cough (49%), generalized lymphadenopathy (58%), hepatomegaly (51%), and diarrhea (31%). The most common cutaneous manifestation (87%) was a generalized papular rash with central umbilication that resembled the lesions of molluscum contagiosum. These were predominantly found on the face, scalp, and upper extremities but occurred throughout the body, including the palate. Other cutaneous lesions included papules without umbilication, a maculopapular rash, subcutaneous nodules, acne-like lesions, and folliculitis. Chest films were frequently abnormal, with diffuse reticulonodular or localized alveolar infiltrates the most common.

The mean duration of illness prior to presentation in this study was 4 weeks. The incubation period for disseminated disease is unclear, as is the percentage of patients whose disease is a result of reactivation of latent infection, as opposed to new infection or reinfection. The fact that reactivation with increasing immunosuppression occurs is supported by the several cases of disseminated disease reported from nonendemic areas in AIDS patients who had a distant history of travel to endemic areas.[324,325] Many such patients had spent little time in endemic areas, indicating that infection with *P. marneffei* can occur rapidly. The development of clinically active disease within weeks of exposure in endemic areas[326] and the reports of children with vertically transmitted HIV infection developing disease in the first months and years of life[327] demonstrate that primary infection can quickly lead to disseminated disease. Finally, the pronounced seasonal variation in disease incidence implies an important role for exogenous reinfection in the expression of disease with *P. marneffei* in AIDS patients in endemic areas.[317]

The mortality rate of patients with disseminated *P. marneffei* infection is very high in the absence of prompt treatment. Diagnosis depends on a high index of suspicion, including a careful history to assess possible residence or travel in an endemic area. The differential diagnosis includes tuberculosis, other endemic fungi, and cryptococcosis. Cutaneous lesions may mimic those of AIDS-related molluscum contagiosum, *Histoplasma capsulatum* and *Cryptococcus neoformans*. An absence of cutaneous lesions may retard diagnosis. In this regard, a characteristic syndrome of hepatic disease in the absence of skin lesions (fever, hepatomegaly, and markedly elevated serum alkaline phosphatase levels) should be noted.[328] A presumptive diagnosis can be made by the examination of a Wright's-stained bone marrow aspirate, lymph node aspirate, or touch preparations of skin biopsy specimens.[316,318,329] Intracellular and extracellular basophilic elliptic yeast-like organisms with central septation (as opposed to the budding of *H. capsulatum*) are characteristic. Indirect fluorescent antibody reagents have been developed that may prove useful for differentiating *P. marneffei* from *H. capsulatum* and *C. neoformans* in tissue.[330] Characteristic intracellular organisms have been detected on routine blood smears.[331] In the previously discussed series, definitive diagnosis was performed by culture of *P. marneffei* from blood (76%, even in the absence of routine lysis-centrifugation culture), skin biopsy (90%), bone marrow (100%), and sputum (34%). Diagnostic antigenemia tests that may prove valuable for rapid diagnosis have been developed.[332,333] Quantitation of urinary antigen by enzyme immunoassay (employing rabbit hyperimmune IgG) is especially promising: High sensitivity and specificity were demonstrated in an area of high endemnicity.[334] Of note, *P. marneffei* infection is a known cause of false-positive reactions in the *H. capsulatum* polysaccharide antigen immunoassay.[335] Current serologic assays are unlikely to be helpful in the diagnosis of AIDS patients but, with improved sensitivity, may provide a useful index of infection.[330,336]

Amphotericin B, 0.6 mg/kg/day for 2 weeks, followed by itraconazole, 200 mg twice a day for 10 weeks, is safe and effective.[337] In mild to moderately ill patients, primary therapy with itraconazole may be reasonable. Secondary prophylaxis is mandatory, given relapse rates of 50% within 6 months in its absence.[338] A placebo-controlled, double-blind randomized trial showed that secondary prophylaxis with itraconazole (200 mg once daily) is safe and effective.[78,339] With immune reconstitution as a result of a successful response to HAART, discontinuation of secondary prophylaxis is probably safe.[340] A controlled, double-blind trial of primary prophylaxis with itraconazole (200 mg once daily) in Thai patients with AIDS and CD4+ T-cell counts less than 200/μL showed that the regimen was well tolerated and effective at preventing both cryptococcosis and penicilliosis.[341] No survival benefit was found, but the study was not powered to detect a survival advantage.[341]

United States and Europe have a higher frequency of MAC isolation, however, and economic conditions may lead to greater exposure to MAC-containing droplets via showerheads in economically developed countries[445,446,464]; such differences, however, are unlikely to lead to an essentially total absence of disease in countries such as Uganda. Exposure to different *M. avium* serovars or strains may well be important. Data on serotyping of African clinical strains are scarce. Preliminary data suggest that African clinical isolates are distinguishable from European and American isolates by restriction fragment length polymorphism analysis.[465] The possibility of underlying genetic differences in host susceptibility is belied by the similar rates of disseminated *M. avium* infection as a presenting diagnosis in African and non-African AIDS patients in a London clinic.[380] Greater acquired immunity to mycobacterial disease through BCG vaccination[441] or prior infection with *M. tuberculosis* may exist, but the reported BCG coverage (50%) and PPD reactivity (82%) in Uganda seem unlikely to explain the lack of any disseminated MAC disease.[456] Earlier death due to a greater environmental presence of, or greater latent infection with, more virulent pathogens may occur. This is unlikely to be the entire explanation because patients in many of the previously mentioned studies had clinical late-stage AIDS. Finally, the design of several of the previous studies makes the assertion that the central problem is one of a lack of diagnostic sophistication untenable. Further data are awaited.

Mycobacterium leprae

Mycobacterium leprae, the causative agent of leprosy (see Chapter 38), is an incredibly slow-growing parasite of monocyte/macrophages. For comparative purposes, it may be useful to recall that *Leishmania,* which infects similar cells, is a prominent opportunistic pathogen for patients with HIV infection. The importance of CMI in leprosy and leishmaniasis was emphasized by Turk and Bryceson[466] in their detailed comparison of skin lesions and histopathology of both diseases. Moreover, the immunopathology of both infections is very similar. In view of the widespread prevalence of leprosy in the tropics and subtropics, the immunosuppressive effects of HIV or AIDS on leprosy would be expected to become readily apparent, but there is little or no evidence of this interaction. In fact, in a comprehensive analysis of the possible interaction between HIV/AIDS and leprosy, Lucas concluded that leprosy appears to be another "missing infection in AIDS."[15]

There is no quantitative measure of immune unresponsiveness in leprosy, such as the CD4 count in AIDS, as an indicator of clinical progression; however, there is general agreement that the tuberculoid form of disease is characterized by a well-organized granuloma on biopsy of a skin lesion or the lepromin reaction, with very few or no organisms (paucibacillary). Patients with lepromatous leprosy have a negative lepromin skin test, and biopsies of their skin lesions lack a granulomatous response and show large numbers of organisms (multibacillary). Some of the ways in which the adverse effects of HIV infection on leprosy could be manifested include an increase in the disease:infection ratio, a shift toward multibacillary disease, or an altered response to antileprosy chemotherapy. Of course, the presence of leprosy may also enhance HIV infection.

Several studies have examined positive serology for HIV in newly diagnosed leprosy cases. One report from a rural hospital in Zambia found a higher prevalence of reactors compared with blood donors and surgical patients (6 of 18 vs. 9 of 105), but the numbers were small and the controls were not adequately matched.[467] A larger study of HIV seroprevalence in northwest Tanzania of 93 new leprosy cases compared with more than 4000 controls found that the presence of HIV antibody was significantly associated with multibacillary disease.[468] The fact that this association was based on only five HIV-positive cases with multibacillary disease illustrates the complexity of epidemiologic analysis in a disease such as leprosy. Another comparison of seropositivity for HIV was carried out among 189 new cases of leprosy matched for age, sex, and district of residence with 481 controls in Uganda. No significant difference in overall positive rates was found (12% in cases vs. 18% in controls), but again, positive HIV reactions were more frequent among multibacillary cases.[469] A different clinical association was noted in Zambia in leprosy patients with active neuritis, which suggested that HIV-positive cases had poorer recovery of nerve function than controls after treatment with steroids.[470]

A factor that should be considered in evaluating reports of HIV/AIDS in leprosy patients is the greater likelihood of false-positive serologic reactions. One or more positive bands to HIV antigens in Western blots were commonly found in several hundred sera from northern India in the absence of positive enzyme-linked immunosorbent assays (ELISAs).[471] Another report claimed that 3 of 75 (4%) sera from Indonesia and 6 of 100 (6%) sera from Somalia gave positive HIV ELISAs but negative Western blots.[472] These were attributed to leprosy.

There appears to be no striking evidence that HIV infection has an adverse effect on the course of leprosy. There is a suggestion from several of the reports cited previously that multibacillary disease may develop under the influence of HIV infection; however, there are several features of leprosy that may tend to obscure an interaction with HIV infection. Both infections are chronic and slow in their progression, so it may simply take more time to recognize an influence of one on the other. Leprosy is predominantly a rural infection involving people not yet caught up with the ravages of HIV and AIDS. Patients with AIDS in the tropics may not survive long enough to display interactions with leprosy. Finally, patients in the early stages of leprosy have relatively subtle clinical manifestations with which physicians in the urban environment may not be familiar. Therefore, there may be more going on out there than we realize. It has been noted that HAART-associated immune reconstitution may trigger injurious inflammatory reactions in treated patients coinfected with leprosy.[473–475]

Other Nontuberculous Mycobacteria

Disease due to *Mycobacterium genavense* (see Chapter 36) mimics that due to *M. avium,* causing disseminated disease in AIDS patients with very low CD4+ T-cell counts (mean, <50/μL). The pathogenesis appears to involve initial gastrointestinal colonization followed by dissemination.[476,477] The important environmental reservoirs are unclear, but pet birds can have extensive gastrointestinal tract involvement.

The organism may also be present in tap water.[478] The geographic range of disease is only beginning to be defined. Cases have been reported from North America, Europe, and Australia.[476] The most common presenting symptoms and signs are fever, weight loss, abdominal pain, chronic diarrhea, lymphadenopathy, hepatosplenomegaly, "pseudo-Whipple's disease," and anemia.[476,479,480] Imaging of the spleen may suggest splenic abscesses[481]; diffuse nodular infiltrates may be seen in the lung.[482] Pathologically, involved organs are filled with histiocytes that are packed with acid-fast bacilli. The diagnosis can be established by the isolation of *M. genavense* from normally sterile sites (blood, bone marrow, lymph node, and spleen). Specific diagnosis is confounded by the fastidious growth requirements of the organism. Primary isolation on solid media is difficult, and growth in liquid broth may have only 50% sensitivity. Definitive identification demands PCR techniques.[476] The clear implication is that a significant percentage of cases ascribed to disseminated *M. avium* are likely due to *M. genavense*.[479] Data on treatment are all retrospective, but therapy appears to be associated both with improvement in symptoms and with survival. Multidrug regimens that include clarithromycin appear to be associated with the best clinical responses.[483,484]

Before the AIDS pandemic, *Mycobacterium kansasii* was known primarily as a cause of chronic pulmonary disease, resembling tuberculosis in lungs with underlying damage. *Mycobacterium kansasii* is second to MAC among nontuberculous mycobacteria as a cause of disease in HIV-infected patients in the United States.[485] Although *M. kansasii* has been reported as a cause of pulmonary disease in most areas of the world, most case reports of HIV coinfection are from North America and Europe. However, coinfection may be especially prevalent in the gold mines of the Transvaal in South Africa.[486] In HIV-infected individuals, disease due to *M. kansasii* and *M. tuberculosis* has very similar clinical and radiological characteristics.[487] A major difference (with epidemiological and prognostic implications) is that *M. kansasii* disease tends to occur later in the course of HIV infection. The mean CD4+ T-cell count at the time of presentation is approximately 50 to 60/μL[487–489]; 60% to 90% present with pulmonary disease alone and 20% to 35% with disseminated disease.[489,490] The incidence in industrialized countries has plummeted in the HAART era.[491] With all nontuberculous mycobacteria, differentiation between colonization, contamination, and disease can be problematic. Mere colonization of the respiratory tract with *M. kansasii* appears to be infrequent in AIDS patients, however. All pulmonary isolates should be taken seriously.[488,490] Despite relative in vitro resistance to isoniazid,[491] the recommended therapy is isoniazid, rifampin, and ethambutol. Therapy clearly alters survival in patients with pulmonary disease.[489,490,492] Disseminated disease has a particularly poor prognosis.

First described in 1977, *Mycobacterium malmoense* is an uncommon cause of pulmonary disease resembling tuberculosis. The environmental reservoir is unknown. Person-to-person transmission has never been documented. Multisystem disease with bacteremia has rarely occurred in the presence of profound immunosuppression, including several patients with AIDS and low CD4+ T-cell counts. Pulmonary and gastrointestinal disease, along with bacteremia, is usual.[493,494] In vitro susceptibility testing does not correlate well with clinical response.[495] The best regimen for pulmonary disease in the nonimmunosuppressed patient appears to be isoniazid, rifampin, and ethambutol.[495] Optimal therapy in AIDS patients is unclear.

Mycobacterium haemophilum causes localized lymphadenitis in immunologically healthy children and cutaneous, osteoarticular, and, more rarely, pulmonary or disseminated disease in immunocompromised patients. Several cases have been reported in AIDS patients.[496–500] Cutaneous lesions include furuncles, abscesses, papules, vesicles, and deep ulcers. Such lesions are usually diffuse, most often on the extremities. Culture (at 30° to 32°C) demands supplementation of media with an iron source. In vitro susceptibility data and scattered clinical reports suggest that rifampin plus ciprofloxacin is reasonable empirical therapy. Other agents with good activity include amikacin, ciprofloxacin, and clarithromycin.[498] The environmental source and mode of infection are unclear.

Several other mycobacteria have been demonstrated or suspected to cause opportunistic disease in AIDS patients, including *Mycobacterium fortuitum* (primary pulmonary disease,[501] disseminated disease,[502] cervical lymphadenitis,[502] and meningitis[503]), *Mycobacterium marinum* (disseminated cutaneous and systemically disseminated disease[504,505]), *Mycobacterium celatum* (pulmonary and disseminated disease[506,507]), *Mycobacterium xenopi* (disseminated disease, pulmonary disease, and pulmonary colonization[508–510]), *Mycobacterium gordonae* (pulmonary, cutaneous, and disseminated disease[511–513]), *Mycobacterium scrofulaceum* (disseminated disease[514]), *Mycobacterium bovis* (disseminated disease), and *Mycobacterium simiae* (disseminated disease[515,516]). Although a smattering of case reports have suggested that HIV does not exacerbate disease due to *M. ulcerans*, the causative agent of Buruli ulcer,[517] a case report has called this into question.[518]

Spirochetal Infections

Along with other genital inflammatory or ulcerative diseases, syphilis (see Chapter 44) has been implicated as a cofactor in HIV transmission. Many case reports have suggested that HIV infection can alter the course of disease with *Treponema pallidum*. In the presence of concurrent HIV infection, syphilis has been thought to (1) progress more frequently and rapidly to neurosyphilis,[519,520] (2) lead to an increased incidence of meningitic manifestations of neurosyphilis,[521] (3) lead to an increased frequency of "malignant secondary syphilis" with ulcerating lesions and prominent systemic symptoms,[522] and (4) be less amenable to successful therapy with standard regimens as assessed by clinical or serologic measures (including a lack of appropriate nontreponemal titer reduction or a serologic relapse).[523–527] Such concerns, based largely on case reports and retrospective studies, were amplified by the disconcerting finding of *T. pallidum* invasion of the CNS in early syphilis in HIV-infected patients. Such early invasion of the CNS occurs equally frequently in HIV-seropositive and -seronegative people, however,[528] and the "atypical" courses of syphilis described previously were well-known in the pre-AIDS era. Knowledge of the actual frequency and relative significance of such events has awaited well-designed prospective studies. Three studies now provide evidence that the clinical presentation and clinical and serologic responses to treatment of syphilis may not be appreciably altered by HIV coinfection.[529–531] A major caveat of these studies is that the mean level of immunosuppression in the patients in these studies, as assessed by CD4+ T-cell counts, was not severe. Furthermore, the number of patients involved was relatively small. Thus, the clinical course of syphilis in the face of severe HIV-induced immunosuppression may in fact be exacerbated, and the response to conventional therapy may lead to the infrequent occurrence of serious adverse treatment outcomes.[531] The clinical approach to the HIV patient infected with this cosmopolitan sexually transmitted disease (STD) has been thoroughly discussed elsewhere[76–79,532,533] and will likely continue to evolve.

Whether HIV infection has a deleterious effect on the course of the nonvenereal, endemic treponematoses (see Chapter 44) is unknown, but such an effect has been postulated by analogy with syphilis.[534] No effects of HIV on concurrent infection with the *Borrelia* species that cause relapsing fever have been reported (see Chapter 45). Whether Lyme disease follows an unusual course in HIV-infected people is unclear.[535,536] Finally, initial observations suggest that leptospirosis (see Chapter 46) runs a similar course in patients coinfected with HIV.[537,538]

Rickettsial and Ehrlichial Infections

Among the rickettsiae and related organisms, only *Coxiella burnetii* and *Ehrlichia* organisms have been suspected of being exacerbated by concurrent HIV infection. Notably, these pathogens are obligate intracellular parasites of monocyte/macrophages.

Q fever (see Chapter 54) has a worldwide distribution. The responsible pathogen, *C. burnetii,* lives and multiplies in the phagolysosomes of monocyte/macrophages. As with other such parasites, host defense against infection appears to depend on specific T-cell activation of the microbicidal effector functions of infected cells.[539] Radiation, cyclophosphamide, corticosteroids, and pregnancy have led to reactivation of disease in animal models.[539] Case series have suggested that patients with immunocompromise due to a variety of causes (including leukemia, Hodgkin's disease, bone marrow and renal transplantation, and alcoholism) are more susceptible to both symptomatic acute and relapsing or chronic disease with *C. burnetii.*[540–542] The rationale for expecting more frequent or serious disease in the HIV-infected patient is clear. The data are less so. A study from southern France demonstrated a threefold higher prevalence of antibodies to *C. burnetii* in HIV-seropositive people.[543] This suggestion of an increased rate of transmission in HIV-infected people has not been found in other seroprevalence studies from Paris, Spain, or the Central African Republic.[544–546] Given the differential prevalence of risk factors for the acquisition of HIV infection between the studies, the contradictory data strongly suggest that *C. burnetii* can be blood-borne and that intravenous drug use is a risk for its transmission. Two studies from southern Europe have further suggested that HIV infection leads to a higher disease-infection ratio with *C. burnetii.*[543,547] A retrospective serologic study of 520 patients with acute Q fever from an area of Spain with a high incidence of both HIV and *C. burnetii* infection revealed no overrepresentation of HIV-infected people, however.[546] The clinical features of Q fever do not appear to vary between HIV-infected and -uninfected hosts.[543,545–547] However, definitive statements await prospective studies in severely immunosuppressed AIDS patients.

Human monocytic ehrlichiosis (HME), caused by the tick-borne *Rickettsia*-like agent *E. chaffeensis,* is an acute febrile illness associated with leukopenia, thrombocytopenia, and hepatic enzyme abnormalities. Most case reports of infection with *E. chaffeensis* (see Chapter 53) have been from the United States. A report of infection in Mali supports a much wider distribution of disease, however.[548] HME appears to be an AIDS-related OI.[549] Reported hospitalized cases have had a high rate of complications and a mortality of approximately 30%[549] (compared with an estimated case fatality rate for HME in the absence of HIV of <3%[550]). Patients with fatal disease had CD4+ T-cell counts less than 200/μL; in patients with less than 100/μL, the mortality rate was more than 50%. Of eight reported cases of disease caused by *E. ewingii,* a related tick-borne agent, seven occurred in patients with immune deficiencies, including four with HIV infection.[549,550] The suspicion is thus strong that *E. ewingii* is an opportunistic pathogen in the setting of HIV infection.[551] No cases of infection with the tick-borne agent of human granulocytic ehrlichiosis[552] in the face of HIV infection appear to have been reported.

There is no evidence implicating any of the spotted fever or typhus group of rickettsiae as having a clinically significant interaction with HIV. Although neither the mortality nor the morbidity of Rocky Mountain spotted fever are changed by HIV coinfection, this infection should not be overlooked in favor of defined OIs in the differential diagnosis of febrile illness in HIV-seropositive patients. A prospective study on scrub typhus [due to *Orientia* (formerly *Rickettsia*) *tsutsugamushi*] revealed no increase in clinical severity at time of presentation in HIV-infected patients with a median CD4+ T-cell count of 70/μL.[553] Interestingly, rickettsemia occurred significantly less often in the HIV-seropositive patients. Neither the relative prevalence of infection nor the response to treatment was addressed in this study.

Bacterial Infections

Brucella

A cause of systemic disease worldwide, *Brucella* species are facultative intracellular parasites that infect and multiply in macrophages (see Chapter 41). CMI responses, particularly the activation of monocyte/macrophages by antigen-specific T cells, are important in host resistance. Despite this, the meager published data on coinfection do not support a significant effect of HIV on infection with *Brucella* and, in fact, prior to the AIDS pandemic, only two cases of brucellosis in immunocompromised hosts (hairy cell leukemia and IgM deficiency) had been reported.[554,555] A retrospective seroprevalence study found no significant association between *Brucella* serology and HIV serology in a cohort of female sex workers in Kenya.[556] The prevalence of antibodies to each pathogen was high (HIV, 65%; *Brucella,* 35%). The clinical course of brucellosis in the 18 reported cases with concurrent HIV infection was not outside the spectrum of disease seen in normal hosts.[556–560] Definitive data on the interaction between these two pathogens await careful prospective studies.

Burkholderia pseudomallei

Melioidosis (see Chapter 34) does not appear to behave as an AIDS-related OI. The disease is endemic in Southeast Asia, particularly in northern Thailand, where the prevalence of AIDS is high. Only one case of fatal, recrudescent, bacteremic disease in an HIV-seropositive person has been reported, however.[561] Clinical series from Thailand are silent with regard to the presence of melioidosis in AIDS patients,[374,375,561–563] and a 10-year study of bloodstream infections in a hospital in northern Thailand reported a similar proportion of *B. pseudomallei* isolates in HIV-infected and -uninfected patients.[564]

Enteric Bacteria

Several enteric bacterial infections have been reported to cause disease of greater severity, invasiveness, chronicity, or recurrence in the presence of HIV coinfection. Enterotoxigenic *E. coli* has not been described as causing more severe disease in HIV-seropositive patients, but *Shigella* species, *Salmonellae, Campylobacter,* and *Listeria monocytogenes* have all been implicated as causes of more severe or relapsing disease in the presence of HIV. Data from the tropics on enteric bacterial pathogens are scant. Studies of slim disease (enteropathic AIDS) have not revealed an enteric bacterial cause in most cases.[304,458,459] The prevalence of certain enteric pathogens such as *Campylobacter,* vibrios, and enteropathogenic *E. coli* in the tropics has not been accurately assessed because their detection requires the use of special media and experienced laboratory personnel. In the case of less fastidious organisms that are easier to detect, such as *Salmonella* spp., the phenomenon of bacteremia with nontyphoid organisms has been noted in tropical Africa.[29] Since bacteremia with *Shigella* spp. probably occurs more commonly in patients with HIV disease,[565] this association may be expected to occur in the tropics as well. There is no reported evidence to suggest that cholera is altered in the presence of HIV, although the gastric secretory failure that occurs commonly in AIDS may lead to a greater susceptibility to infection to *Vibrio cholerae.*[566,567] It should be noted that although the live oral cholera vaccine is considered to be contraindicated in people with HIV infection by the USPHS–IDSA working group,[213] it has been shown to be safe and immunogenic in HIV-infected adults in Mali.[568] Further details on the association of HIV and enteric bacterial infections, including therapy, are presented in Chapters 16 through 21 and in reviews elsewhere.[76,77]

Other Bacteria

Although the data on HIV infection and epidemic meningococcal meningitis have not provided evidence for a significant interaction,[569] studies suggest that HIV infection may be a risk factor for sporadic meningococcal disease.[570,571] Interactions between HIV and *Bacillus anthracis* or *Yersinia pestis* have not been reported. The globally endemic *Bartonella* species, *Bartonella henselae* and *Bartonella quintana* (see Chapter 40), cause acute and persistent bacteremia as well as localized tissue infection (including bacillary angiomatosis, bacillary peliosis, microscopic abscess formation, and lymphadenitis), primarily in AIDS patients and other immunocompromised people.[572] The closely related species *Bartonella bacilliformis,* which is geographically restricted to Andean river valleys, causes a similar spectrum of disease (including acute and persistent bacteremia and hemangiomatous nodules resembling those seen in bacillary angiomatosis) in immunologically normal hosts (see Chapter 40). Cases of coinfection with HIV and *B. bacilliformis* do not appear to have been reported.

Viral Infections

Hemorrhagic Fever Viruses, Arboviruses, and Others

None of the viruses that, along with parasites, have formed the traditional focus of the Anglo-American specialty of tropical medicine have been reported to cause uniquely prevalent, severe, or unusual disease in people infected with HIV. No significant interactions have been well documented between HIV and bunyaviruses, hantaviruses, phleboviruses, arenaviruses, alphaviruses, or filoviruses. In part, of course, this may be a function of a lack of sufficient experience with coinfection with these agents. Among the flaviviruses, (1) two uncontrolled series of patients with St. Louis encephalitis in Texas have suggested the possibility that the ratio of disease to infection, but not the course of symptomatic disease, is worsened in the presence of HIV infection,[573,574] and (2) there are insufficient data to determine whether HIV alters the course of yellow fever (no case reports; 20% to 50% mortality in the absence of coinfection[575]), West Nile virus infection (single case report[576]), or dengue infection (single case report[577]). Interestingly, the case report of dengue coinfection suggests that dengue fever, like acute measles and scrub typhus, may lead to a reversible suppression of HIV replication.[577]

Should the live-attenuated yellow fever vaccine be given to those infected with HIV? There are theoretical risks of vaccine-induced encephalitis and/or hepatic damage due to prolonged viremia in the immunodeficient.[575] A handful of cases of post-vaccinial encephalitis or multiple organ failure (yellow fever vaccine-associated viscerotropic disease [YEL-AVD]) have been reported in presumably immunocompetent patients (against a denominator of approximately 400 million people vaccinated).[575] Of note, 4 of 23 vaccinees who developed YEL-AVD had undergone thymectomy for thymomas, raising the concern that deficient thymic function may permit fatal vaccine-induced viral infections.[578] A single case has also been reported of fatal myeloencephalitis after vaccination in a Thai man with asymptomatic HIV infection, albeit a low CD4+ T-cell count and a high viral load.[579] Approximately 100 asymptomatic HIV-seropositive U.S. military personnel received yellow fever vaccination prior to the introduction of routine HIV screening; no adverse effects were detected (R. Redfield, personal communication, 1997). Small published series of travelers have suggested safety and variable efficacy of the 17D yellow fever vaccine in HIV seropositives without severe immunosuppression.[580–582] The immunogenicity of yellow fever vaccination has been noted to be severely reduced, again in the absence of significant adverse events, in HIV-infected children in Côte d'Ivoire[583] (T. Tsai, personal communication, 1997). WHO recommendations are to use yellow fever vaccine in HIV-seropositive patients who are asymptomatic. It remains a part of the WHO EPI.[443] Pending further studies, yellow fever vaccine is not recommended for symptomatic HIV-infected patients by WHO.[443] The ACIP recommends that HIV-infected people without AIDS or other symptomatic manifestations of HIV infection, who have laboratory-established verification of adequate immune function, and who cannot avoid potential exposure to yellow fever be offered the choice of vaccination.[584] Given apparent reduced vaccination efficiency, neutralizing antibody titers should probably be measured prior to travel. If travel requirements (as opposed to actual risk of infection) are the only reason for vaccination of an asymptomatic HIV-infected person, a vaccination waiver letter (which may not be accepted at some borders) should be obtained.[584] For all travelers, avoidance of areas of transmission and, if travel to such areas is essential, conscientiously avoiding mosquito exposure is prudent.

Measles Virus

Measles virus (see Chapter 55) causes an annual mortality in the tropics far in excess of that due to the "traditional" tropical disease viruses. In fact, the worldwide yearly mortality due to measles is rivaled among single pathogens only by falciparum malaria, tuberculosis, and AIDS. This mortality is predominantly in sub-Saharan Africa. Similar to AIDS, infection with measles virus is accompanied by marked abnormalities of CMI that contribute to the increased susceptibility to secondary infections that account for much of the morbidity and mortality of the disease.[585–589]

Measles is exacerbated in the presence of HIV coinfection.[590–602] The mortality rate in North American case series and reports of measles in HIV-positive children and adults has been 40%, far higher than the usual 0.1% case fatality rate seen in the United States.[509–599] Although the presentation of disease has been normal in many, up to 40% have had no rash. In these reports, giant cell pneumonitis has been the principal complication and the prime cause of death, although fatal subacute measles encephalitis has also been described. CD4+ T-cell counts have not been reported in many of these cases, but where they have been reported they have generally been less than 500/µL. Such case reports and series are obviously likely to be biased toward the severe end of the spectrum of disease, however. Three substantial studies have investigated HIV–measles coinfection in sub-Saharan Africa.[600–602] A study of children hospitalized with measles in Kinshasa showed similar mortality rates among HIV-seropositive (31.3%) and -seronegative (28%) children.[600] The fact that only severely ill patients, with complications, were hospitalized likely obviated the ability to detect differential mortality in this study. An initial study of children with measles in Lusaka revealed a significantly higher mortality rate in HIV seropositives (28%) than seronegatives (8.3%).[601] A second prospective study in hospitalized children in Lusaka that distinguished between HIV infection and HIV seropositivity found few differences in the clinical presentation, complications, or mortality of HIV-infected compared to -uninfected children with measles.[602] However, enrollment was based on a clinical diagnosis of measles, which would be expected to minimize the ability to detect differences in clinical presentation; there was a bias against enrollment of critically ill children and those dying soon after admission; and there was significantly greater mortality among HIV-infected compared with -uninfected children among those with clinically diagnosed as opposed to confirmed measles.[602] Early death prior to mounting diagnostic measles IgM titers in the face of severe immunosuppression was suspected to be confounding. Other positive findings in this study included a higher proportion of HIV infection among children hospitalized with measles than expected from (maternal) population prevalence rates, a greater proportion of coinfected patients hospitalized with measles younger than the age of 9 months, and a longer duration of illness before hospitalization and longer hospitalization in coinfected children.[602] Follow-up studies have shown that coinfected patients have a higher risk (90.9% vs. 52.8%) for prolonged (30 to 61 days after rash onset) shedding of measles virus[603]; and that in vivo HIV replication appears to be suppressed during acute measles.[604]

No therapies have been rigorously studied. Vitamin A, which has been shown to be protective in severe measles in malnourished children,[605] may be of benefit, especially given the marginal nutritional status of many with HIV infection. Ribavirin has been shown to reduce the severity of measles in normal hosts.[606] Reports of its use in HIV-positive patients with measles pneumonitis have suggested some efficacy, although rigorous data are lacking.[591,592,594,595,598] Intravenous use is probably most effective. Intravenous immune globulin (IVIG) may also be of benefit.[592]

Given the severity of measles in HIV patients, prevention is key. Postexposure prophylaxis with intramuscular immune globulin attenuates disease in normal hosts. It is recommended by the ACIP[607] in symptomatic HIV patients (and in those with CD4+ T-cell counts <200/µL) regardless of measles serostatus, but it may have limited efficacy in these and other immunosuppressed patients.[595,608] The recommended dose is 0.5 mL/kg (15 mL maximum), given intramuscularly within 6 (or, better, 3) days. Such postexposure prophylaxis is also recommended by the American Academy of Pediatrics (AAP) for all HIV-infected children and adolescents, and for all children of unclear infection status born to HIV-infected women, regardless of measles immunization status or degree of immunosuppression.[609] Preexposure prophylaxis with monthly IVIG has been advocated for HIV-positive children with documented measles vaccine nonresponsiveness during community outbreaks of measles,[595] but this is not likely to be an economically viable option in the resource-poor areas of the tropics where measles is heavily endemic.

Vaccination remains the principal strategy for preventing measles in HIV-infected people. In normal hosts, the protective efficacy of measles vaccination is greater than 95%.[610] Vaccination efficacy data in HIV-seropositive people is lacking, but seroconversion data are available. This is a less than ideal surrogate. In general, there is a strong correlation between levels of neutralizing antibody and protection, but the failure of postexposure prophylaxis with immune serum globulin in preventing fatal giant cell pneumonia in patients with the cellular immunodeficiencies noted previously provides compelling evidence that CMI mechanisms, whether specific or nonspecific, are important even in protection from initial infection. In adults with HIV infection, there appears to be no waning of measles antibody titers with increasing immunosuppression.[611–613] Unfortunately, there are no clear data on the response to vaccination in those adults who lack antibodies to measles.[614] In children, the situation is different. HIV-infected infants have a markedly lower rate of seroconversion after measles vaccination, generate lower titers of antibody on seroconversion, and have a high rate of secondary vaccine failure, with antibody titers that decrease with time and with increasing immunosuppression.[615] Variable, but generally poor, responses to second doses of vaccine have been reported.[615]

There may be a benefit to vaccinating early (at 6 to 9 months of age) to take advantage of the fact that there is less HIV-related immunosuppression at this early age. Early vaccination may also be valuable because both HIV-positive and HIV-negative infants born to HIV-infected mothers have lower titers of maternal antimeasles antibody.[616] In a study in Kenya, the risk of acquiring measles before vaccination at 9 months of age (the standard age of vaccination in Africa at the time) was 3.8 times higher (95% confidence interval, 1.2 to 13.2) in infants born to HIV-seropositive mothers.[616] High-titer measles vaccines may be more immunogenic in HIV-infected children[617,618] but have been discontinued for safety reasons in all children.

Safety concerns have obviously been of great importance in the use of this live-attenuated vaccine in HIV patients. Although the use of measles vaccine had appeared to be quite safe in HIV-infected children and adults,[619] two reports have emphasized the need for some caution. A 20-year-old man with no HIV-related symptoms but a CD4+ T-cell count "too few to enumerate" received a second dose of measles vaccine prior to entry into college. One year after vaccination, he developed progressive, vaccine-associated measles pneumonitis.[620] A study of the effect of HIV on measles mortality in 356 children hospitalized with measles in Lusaka, Zambia, is also troubling.[601] Previous studies have suggested that when prior measles vaccination does not prevent disease, it can reduce the severity of infection.[600] In HIV-seronegative boys hospitalized for measles, prior measles vaccination did lead to a significantly lower case fatality rate.[601] Although case fatality rates were not significantly lower in vaccinated HIV-seropositive boys or HIV-seronegative girls than in their unvaccinated controls, there was a trend toward a lower case fatality rate in the vaccinees. Surprisingly, however, the case fatality rate was higher in measles-vaccinated than in unvaccinated HIV-seropositive girls. Although this did not reach statistical significance, it is reminiscent of the experience with the high-titered Edmonston–Zagreb (EZ) vaccine. Use of high-titered EZ vaccine at less than 9 months of age was associated with a delayed excess mortality in several study sites.[621–623] This occurred exclusively in female infants for reasons that remain unclear. It is notable that in the Zambian study noted previously, the highest mortality was seen in the youngest, vaccinated HIV-seropositive girls. However, in regions where there is measles transmission, risk–benefit analysis clearly favors measles immunization of all children regardless of HIV status.[615] In regions where measles transmission does not occur and where immune status can be monitored, withholding of measles vaccine from HIV-infected children with severe immune compromise is wise.[615] WHO recommends measles vaccination for all children in developing countries regardless of HIV infection or symptom status because of the high risk and severity of measles in general in such countries.[443,624]

In the United States, the USPHS–IDSA working group and the ACIP recommend measles vaccination for HIV-infected people according to the schedule and conditions for normal hosts if they are not severely immunocompromised.[213,610] In addition, the risks and benefits of vaccination or immune globulin prophylaxis should be weighed in severely immunocompromised patients who are at increased risk due to travel or outbreaks.[213,607] AAP recommendations for HIV-infected infants to young adults in the United States include

- No immunization in the face of severe immunosuppression
- Use of the measles–mumps–rubella (MMR) vaccine at 12 months of age, with a second dose given as soon as 28 days after the first dose
- With measles transmission in the community, vaccination of infants as young as 6 months old with MMR or monovalent measles vaccine, and revaccination with MMR at 12 months
- Vaccination of all measles-susceptible household members of an HIV-infected person
- Use of immune globulin prophylaxis as noted previously[609]

Few data are available on other paramyxoviruses in AIDS. With respiratory syncytial virus infection, pneumonia may be more common than bronchiolitis with wheezing, and viral carriage may also be prolonged.[625–628] Copathogens may occur more frequently than in normal hosts.[626] Ribavirin appears to be efficacious in both children and adults.

Rabies

Most human rabies (see Chapter 75) occurs in tropical countries where canine rabies is still endemic. The presentation of rabies does not appear to be altered by HIV infection.[629] HIV-infected children and adults clearly have substandard responses to rabies vaccination, however.[630–632] WHO recommendations for postexposure prophylaxis in the face of HIV infection include mandatory use of rabies immune globulin, use of intramuscular vaccine, and monitoring of neutralizing antibody titers.[633] Revaccination may be necessary. Even multiple-site, double-dose postexposure vaccination has led to poor responses in the face of HIV coinfection.[632]

Poliomyelitis

Great strides have been made in worldwide polio eradication (see Chapter 60). Most of the remaining burden of poliomyelitis is in the tropics outside the Western Hemisphere. There is no evidence that HIV infection alters the outcome of infection with poliovirus. It has been estimated that more 500,000 HIV-infected children have received live oral polio vaccine (OPV).[615] Only two cases of vaccine-associated paralytic poliomyelitis in HIV-infected children have been reported.[615] If there is greater risk of vaccine-associated disease in the face of HIV infection, the attributable risk is thought to be very low.[615] OPV remains part of the WHO EPI for all children.[443] In the United States, the OPV is supported by the ACIP as the only vaccine recommended for polio eradication where there still is transmission of wild-type polio.[634] ACIP recommendations have replaced OPV with inactivated polio vaccine for all vaccinees in the United States.[634]

Other Enteric Viruses

Chronic diarrhea is a common problem in AIDS patients throughout the world. Although no definite pathogenic role has been ascribed to enteric viruses (small round structured viruses, enteric adenoviruses, and coronaviruses) in AIDS-related diarrhea in either North America or Africa,[635,636] there are some preliminary data suggesting greater disease severity in children coinfected with HIV and astroviruses[637] and an association of picobirnaviruses with diarrhea in HIV-coinfected patients.[638] In non-cholera-endemic areas of the tropics, rotavirus is probably the principal cause of diarrheal deaths in HIV-uninfected infants.[639] Rotavirus diarrhea does not appear to be an opportunistic pathogen in children with HIV coinfection. In a large study in Malawi, no differences in the severity of rotavirus gastroenteritis were found between HIV-infected and -uninfected children.[640] Interestingly, rotavirus was less frequently detected in HIV-infected children with gastroenteritis. Despite equal resolution of clinical disease, however, the frequency of death after hospital discharge was significantly greater in coinfected children.[640]

Hepatitis Viruses

Infection with hepatitis A virus (HAV) (see Chapter 64) occurs worldwide. In resource-poor countries, especially in the tropics, HAV is hyperendemic, and exposure to the virus (usually subclinical) is essentially universal by the age of 10 years. Virtually all adults are immune. HIV/HAV coinfection appears to be associated with a higher HAV serum viral load, a longer duration of viremia, and lower elevations in serum alanine aminotransferase levels[641] but a similar disease course.[641–643] Vaccination against HAV is safe in HIV-infected patients.[644–646] Efficacy wanes with increasing immunosuppression.[645,646] Some recommend vaccination for all those at risk (defined by a negative serology).[76]

Infection with hepatitis E virus (HEV) (see Chapter 64) is more localized, with sporadic and epidemic disease being reported in Mexico; North and West Africa; the Middle East; and South, Southeast, and East Asia. Clinical disease occurs in both adults and children. HEV has not been implicated as having any significant interaction with HIV.

With the cosmopolitan hepatitis viruses that are capable of causing chronic disease, however, several potentially important interactions with HIV have been described. The prevalence of coinfection is furthered by the fact that these viruses share routes of transmission with HIV. For hepatitis B virus (HBV) (see Chapter 64), CMI responses are thought to be important both for the resolution of acute disease and for the production of hepatic inflammation in chronic disease. HIV infection has been reported to lead to

- At least a threefold increase in risk of the development of a chronic HBV carrier state (with an inverse correlation with the CD4 count), without a significant change in the severity of acute disease[647,648]
- Potential reactivation of quiescent HBV infection[649,650]
- Increased HBV replication and decreased inflammation in those with[647,649] or without[651] chronic hepatitis
- A decreased response to HBV vaccination[652]
- Loss of HBV antibody over time[652,653]
- A 15-fold increase in liver-related mortality in HBV-infected individuals[654]

Vaccination against HBV has reasonable efficacy in HIV-seropositive populations. Interestingly, however, the highest reported rate of development of the chronic carrier state in adults (56% to 80%) occurred in HIV-infected people who were vaccinated at the same time that they developed HBV infection.[648] HBV does not appear to have a significant effect on the clinical course of HIV infection.[655]

With hepatitis C virus (HCV) infection (see Chapter 64), HIV coinfection is associated with an increased risk of progression to chronic infection.[656] Documented interactions between the two viruses[657] include (1) an increase in HCV viral load[658,659]; (2) an increase in vertical[660] and male-to-female sexual transmission[659] of HCV, probably due to higher viral load; (3) a more severe clinical and histopathologic course[661,662]; and (4) a high percentage of indeterminate HCV immunoblot assays, with frequent HCV seroreversion.[656] Whether HCV infection has a significant effect on the natural history of HIV infection or the response to HAART therapy remains controversial.[663–667] Maternal HCV infection appears to be associated with an increased risk of HIV vertical transmission.[668] Treatment of both HIV/HCV and HIV/HBV infection has been reviewed recently.[657]

The data on hepatitis D virus (HDV) are more meager. HDV replication may be prolonged or reactivated in the presence of HIV coinfection.[669,670]

Herpesviruses

As in the industrial world, herpes zoster is quite common in adult AIDS patients in the tropics. A history of shingles is reported by more than 10% of AIDS patients in Africa.[671] In areas of Africa with a high seroprevalence for HIV, the positive predictive value of a history of shingles for HIV infection is greater than 90%.[671] As elsewhere, zoster tends to develop early in HIV disease, and recurrence is common.[671,672]

Chronic genital herpes simplex lesions are common throughout the world in patients with sexually transmitted HIV infection. CMV infection is ubiquitous in most of the tropics.[673] The reported incidence of severe disease due to CMV in AIDS in Africa and Asia (although not Latin America and the Caribbean) has lagged behind that of the industrial north, however, likely because of greater mortality at earlier stages of disease.[674,675] The natural history, diagnosis, and therapy of disease due to coinfection with these cosmopolitan herpesviruses have been discussed elsewhere.[76–79]

Endemic (central Africa), AIDS-related, "classic," and post-transplant Kaposi's sarcoma are all closely associated with human herpesvirus 8 (HHV8) (see Chapter 57).[676] In the AIDS era, Kaposi's sarcoma has become one of the leading malignancies in areas of sub-Saharan Africa.[677] The epidemiology, clinical manifestations, and therapy of HHV8 infection and Kaposi's sarcoma (a disease that the industrialized world had considerable experience with early in HIV pandemic) have been reviewed elsewhere.[76,77,678,679]

Other Viruses

Although data remain somewhat limited, the cosmopolitan influenza virus appears to cause more severe disease in HIV coinfected patients, with prolongation of symptoms and a higher risk for complications, hospitalization, and death.[680] Influenza vaccination is safe and recommended by the ACIP for HIV-infected patients.[680] Such vaccination has been shown to have good efficacy in a study in individuals with a mean CD4+ T-cell count of 200/μL.[681] With advanced HIV, vaccination may not generate protective antibody titers.[682]

The single case report of severe acute respiratory syndrome (SARS) coronavirus infection in the face of HIV coinfection was within the described clinical spectrum of this newly emerging virus.[683]

SPECIAL ISSUES

HIV and Eosinophilia

The association of blood (or tissue) eosinophilia with tissue exposure to helminthic parasites can be of considerable diagnostic utility in non-HIV-infected populations (see Chapter 125). Data suggest that this utility may be lessened by the presence of HIV infection. Both relative and absolute eosinophilia occur for nonparasitic reasons with considerable frequency in HIV-infected populations. A relative eosinophilia commonly occurs with progressive HIV disease, at least in North American adult AIDS patients,[684,685] due to a sparing of absolute blood eosinophil concentrations in the face of decreasing concentrations of all other granulocytic and mononuclear leukocyte populations.[685] This effect becomes marked with CD4+ T-cell counts less than 200/μL.[685] Nonhelminth-related absolute eosinophilia also occurs with regularity with advancing HIV disease. Absolute eosinophilia in North American HIV-seropositive adults has most frequently been associated with pruritic cutaneous disease, particularly the diagnoses of eosinophilic pustular folliculitis, atopic dermatitis, and prurigo nodularis.[686] Most such patients have CD4 counts less than 100/μL.[686] It remains unclear in these patients whether the eosinophilia is primary with secondary cutaneous manifestations or an allergic response to a predominantly cutaneous antigen. A few AIDS patients have presented with what appears to be a variant of the hypereosinophilic syndrome with prominent cutaneous manifestations[687,688] or a hyper-IgE-like syndrome.[689] Rare causes of tissue or blood eosinophilia in AIDS patients have included acute eosinophilic pneumonia[690] and high-grade B-cell lymphomas.[691] Adverse reactions to various prophylactic and therapeutic agents may also elicit eosinophilia in AIDS patients. Other causes of secondary blood eosinophilia appear to be quite uncommon in North American AIDS patients.[691] This includes adrenal insufficiency, despite the high prevalence of adrenalitis at autopsy in AIDS patients.[692] The upshot of these reports is that the diagnostic specificity of blood eosinophilia for tissue helminthic infection is probably poorer in HIV-infected than in HIV-free adult patients in the industrial north (a conclusion somewhat undermined by the low population prevalence of helminthic disease in the studies cited previously). It is probably reasonable, however, to avoid an extensive workup for parasitic and other causes of eosinophilia in adult eosinophilic AIDS patients with cutaneous disease from the industrial world; however, in populations at higher risk of helminthiasis, such a conclusion is unwarranted in the absence of prospective studies of eosinophil levels in AIDS patients with tissue helminthiasis.[693] Such eosinophilia with advancing HIV disease has not been noted in children in the industrial world.[694,695]

The data from the tropics are dramatically at variance with the reports from the industrial world. A study of patients with tuberculosis in Burkina Faso reported lower eosinophil levels in HIV-seropositive people compared with seronegative people, with a strong correlation between CD4+ T-cell and eosinophil counts.[696] A follow-up study in Faso reported that in helminth noninfected HIV patients, eosinophil counts were higher in CDC stage B patients than in controls but were severely decreased in CDC stage C patients.[697] Mean eosinophil counts in a cohort of 611 HIV-infected patients in Cote d'Ivoire, with a mean CD4+ T-cell count of 115 cells/μL, were in the normal range for HIV-uninfected populations in areas of the world with a low prevalence of helminth infection.[698] Finally, a case report from England of HAART-related immune reconstitution in a schistosome-infected woman from southeast Africa is intriguing.[699] The patient presented with a CD4+ T-cell count less than 200/μL and an eosinophil count of 300/μL. Immune reconstitution was accompanied by the development of robust eosinophila (1500/μL) that decreased with praziquantel treatment. Taken together, these findings suggest that late HIV disease in the tropics, as opposed to the industrial world, is associated with a suppression of blood eosinophil levels. The mechanism(s) responsible for these divergent findings remains unclear.

Prevention of Opportunistic Infections

The USPHS–IDSA working group has updated guidelines for preventing OIs in HIV-infected people in industrialized countries.[213] The data on 19 OIs frequent in North American HIV-infected populations were reviewed. Factors considered in these evaluations were

- Disease incidence
- Disease severity in terms of morbidity and mortality
- The level of immunosuppression at which disease is most likely to occur
- The feasibility, efficacy, and cost of preventive measures
- The impact of intervention on quality of life
- Toxicities, drug interactions, and the potential for drug resistance
- The quality of the evidence supporting each recommendation[213]

The prevention of each OI was evaluated from the standpoint of prevention of exposure, prevention of the first episode of disease by immuno- or chemoprophylaxis (primary prophylaxis), prevention of disease recurrence (secondary prophylaxis), and discontinuance of prophylaxis in those whose CD4+ T-cell counts had risen in response to HAART.[213]

Specific recommendations for prevention of exposure were made for several agents, including *T. gondii, C. parvum, M. tuberculosis,* bacterial enteric agents, *Bartonella,* herpes simplex virus (HSV), varicella zoster virus (VZV), CMV, HHV8, human papillomavirus, and HCV.[213] For adults and adolescents, prophylaxis to prevent the first episode of opportunistic disease was strongly recommended as a standard of care for *P. carinii, M. tuberculosis* (in the face of tuberculin skin test reactivity or contact with a case of active tuberculosis), *T. gondii, M. avium* complex, and VZV (with exposure to chickenpox or shingles in patients without a history of such, or with negative serologies for VZV [varicella Zoster immunoglobulin (VZIG)]. Primary prophylaxis against HBV, HAV, influenza virus, and *S. pneumoniae* was generally recommended. Although evidence exists for efficacy, primary prophylaxis against *C. neoformans, H. capsulatum,* CMV, and bacterial infection (in the face of neutropenia) was not routinely recommended. For two of these agents (*P. carinii* and *M. avium*), primary prophylaxis has been shown to confer a survival benefit.[700,701] Secondary prophylaxis to prevent recurrent disease was strongly recommended as the standard of care for *P. carinii, T. gondii, M. avium* complex, CMV, *C. neoformans, H. capsulatum, C. immitis,* and nontyphi *Salmonella* species. Such prophylaxis was recommended for HSV and *Candida* only if subsequent episodes are frequent or severe.[213]

For children, primary prophylaxis was strongly recommended as a standard of care for *P. carinii, M. tuberculosis,*

M. avium complex, and VZV (VZIG); generally recommended for *T. gondii*, VZV (immunization in the absence of immunosuppression), and influenza virus; and recommended only in unusual circumstances for invasive bacterial infection (hypogammaglobulinemia, IVIG), *C. neoformans* (severe immunosuppression), *H. capsulatum* (severe immunosuppression, endemic geographic area), and CMV (CMV antibody positivity and severe immunosuppression). Primary prophylaxis was also addressed through review of the recommendations for routine immunization schedules in HIV-infected children. In addition to standard schedules for immunization against HBV, HAV, polio, *H. influenzae* type b, diphtheria, tetanus, and pertusis, altered schedules for vaccination against *S . pneumoniae* (use of the heptavalent pneumococcal conjugate vaccine beginning at 2 months, followed by 23-valent pneumococcal polysaccharide vaccine at 2 years), influenza (yearly dose recommended), MMR (no administration to severely immunosuppressed children), and VZV (administration only to asymptomatic, nonimmunosuppressed children) were reviewed. Recommendations for secondary prophylaxis were similar to recommendations for adults, with the addition of a recommendation for use of TMP–SMX or IVIG to prevent invasive bacterial infection in the presence of more than two such infections in a 1-year period.[213]

These recommendations are likely to find broad applicability in the industrial world, where the OI spectrum, health-care priorities, and available prevention options are similar. The applicability to much of the tropics is less clear, however, given differing spectra of OIs, differences in antibiotic resistance patterns, and differences in sociocultural acceptability or feasibility of preventive measures. Limits in the availability of health-care resources (including not just an inability to support the cost of many prevention regimens but also an inability to diagnose HIV disease early enough for preventive measures to be effective, to reliably stage the degree of HIV-associated immunosuppression, and to definitively diagnose OIs) also directly influence the range of prevention options and priorities. It should also be noted that compared with HAART therapy (or prevention of HIV infection), the benefit of OI prevention in reducing HIV-related morbidity and mortality may be somewhat modest.[702] Adequate global provision of HAART represents an ongoing, immense challenge, however, and wide implementation of simple, cheap, effective OI prevention strategies provides an opportunity to rapidly and widely reduce morbidity and mortality.[675] The wide availability of affordable and effective regimens may also encourage people to seek HIV testing.[675]

In 1996, Kaplan and colleagues argued that effective research on OI prevention strategies in the tropics will require an integrated approach, including the area-specific determination of OI spectra, determination of environmental reservoirs of opportunistic pathogens and feasible ways to reduce exposure, assessment of immuno- and chemoprophylaxis against such pathogens, and improvement in the ability to identify and inexpensively stage HIV infection.[20] Since then, data on the efficacy of some OI prevention strategies in resource-poor countries of the tropics have accrued.

First, as noted previously, primary preventive therapy against tuberculosis (TB) with isoniazid has been shown be effective in HIV-infected individuals, regardless of tuberculin status.[423,424,675] WHO and UNAIDS recommendations are for primary preventive therapy to be given to PPD-positive, HIV-infected individuals who do not have active TB.[425] In settings where it may not be feasible to do PPD testing, the recommendations are for primary preventive therapy to be considered for those living in populations with a prevalence of tuberculous infection estimated to be more than 30%, health-care workers, household contacts of TB patients, prisoners, miners, and other groups at high risk of acquisition or transmission of TB.[425]

Second, TMP–SMX—a cheap, widely available antibiotic with activity against a plethora of OIs (including PCP, nontyphoid salmonellosis, pneumococcal disease, and toxoplasmosis) and malaria—has been shown to reduce morbidity and mortality in HIV-infected adults[675,702–705] and children.[401,706] WHO/UNAIDS recommendations are that TMP–SMX should be used for prophylaxis in adults and children living with HIV/AIDS in Africa as a minimum package of care.[707] For adults in Africa (defined as those older than the age of 13 years), such prophylaxis should be offered to all people with symptomatic HIV disease, those who are asymptomatic with a CD4 count of 500/μL or less (or total lymphocyte equivalent), and pregnant women after the first trimester.[707] WHO/UNAIDS/UNICEF recommendations are that all HIV-exposed children (born to HIV-infected mothers) should get TMP–SMX from the age of 4 to 6 weeks, as should any child identified as HIV infected with any clinical signs or symptoms suggestive of HIV, regardless of age or CD4+ T-cell count.[708] It is further recommended that TMP–SMX should be discontinued (1) in HIV-exposed children only once HIV infection has confidently been excluded (and the mother is no longer breastfeeding); (2) in HIV-infected children on antiretroviral therapy only when evidence of immune restoration has occurred; and (3) in those with severe cutaneous, renal, hepatic, or hematological toxicity.[708] It has been noted that such mass prophylaxis strategies entail some as yet to be quantified risks, principally of increasing rates of drug-resistant bacteria and malaria.[709] Studies to examine such risks should be performed.

Third, a large, randomized, double-blind, placebo-controlled trial of the 23-valent pneumococcal polysaccharide vaccine in HIV-infected Ugandan adults showed no protective effect (with invasive pneumococcal disease as the primary endpoint).[710] Surprisingly, increased rates of pneumococcal disease were seen in vaccine recipients. The potential mechanism(s) remains unclear; not surprisingly, the study remains controversial.

Fourth, among the specifically tropical OIs, a controlled, double-blind trial of primary prophylaxis with itraconazole in Thailand showed efficacy in preventing penicilliosis (and cryptococcosis).[340] There are little or no data available on the prophylaxis of other tropical OIs, such as leishmaniasis and American trypanosomiasis, although the utility of avoiding exposures to the vectors of the agents of these diseases should be clear.

More generally, certain options for preventing or reducing exposure to opportunistic pathogens are likely to be broadly useful, including avoiding unboiled water, raw or undercooked foods, and unpasteurized milk to prevent enteric bacterial and protozoan infections as well as *T. gondii* exposure and also avoiding contact with patients with TB, for example, in patient-care settings. Avoidance of exposure to the opportunistic agents of disseminated fungal disease is likely to be impractical in most settings.

The HIV-Infected Traveler in the Tropics

It is clear that for many people, HIV infection is more an inducement than a hindrance to travel.[711] For HIV-infected patients from the industrial world, travel to the tropics leads to an increased risk of exposure to a variety of ubiquitous as well as geographically focal infectious diseases (see Chapter 120). The principal concerns are enteric, respiratory, and vector-borne infections. STDs deserve special mention, however. Despite the AIDS pandemic, studies continue to document a high frequency of unprotected sexual encounters among travelers to the tropics.[712,713] For the HIV-infected traveler, it bears remembering that spread of the AIDS pandemic has been along the routes of human travel and migration.[712] HIV-infected travelers should notify sexual partners of their HIV status, observe safe sex practices, refrain from donating fluids or tissue, inform health-care providers of the need for blood precautions, and avoid the sharing or recreational use of needles. For travelers who are not infected with HIV, pretravel counseling should be given on strategies to minimize the risk of HIV acquisition during travel, including

- Avoiding sex with new partners
- Using latex condoms if having sex (remembering that condom quality varies throughout the world)
- Taking a supply of sterile needles and syringes if routine or frequent injections are required (e.g., for insulin-dependent diabetes) or if a prolonged stay in remote areas is planned
- Avoiding all skin-piercing procedures (e.g., tattooing, acupuncture, and shaving by barbers) and avoiding invasive medical and dental procedures if possible
- Being cognizant of the risks of motor vehicle travel because motor vehicle injuries are not just among the greatest health threats to travelers in the tropics but also provide a major risk factor for needing emergency blood transfusion in countries where HIV screening of the blood supply is not routine

These are also important educational points for HIV-infected travelers.

There are recent reviews of medical issues in the HIV-infected tropical traveler from the industrial world[714,715] and information is available from www.cdc.gov/travel/hiv. trav.htm. Careful, timely pretravel advice and planning can help HIV-infected patients minimize the unavoidable risks of travel to the tropics. Issues to cover include

- Providing an adequate supply of currently used medications
- Identifying optimal sources of medical care in planned destinations (and obtaining adequate medical insurance to cover such care)
- Discussing potential legal restrictions on travel
- Providing education on avoiding food-, water-, and vector-borne disease
- Providing vaccination, chemoprophylaxis, and antimicrobial agents as appropriate reviewing the medical geography of the route and planned activities to identify any special risks
- Providing for adequate medical follow-up on return from travel

Prior to travel, those at risk of HIV infection should be screened for infection as part of the routine pretravel evaluation. Those known or found to be HIV infected should have their disease staged by CD4 count and viral load because the level of immunosuppression will influence the travel medical recommendations given. Therapy with HAART can complicate tropical travel.[715] For those already on HAART, concerns include

- The problem of appropriate clinical and laboratory monitoring—for those planning extended residence in places lacking appropriate clinical or laboratory services, it would be prudent to schedule two or three trips per year for medical follow-up to a country where such services are available
- Difficulties with compliance with complicated HAART regimens during the dislocations and changing daily schedules of travel
- The fact that approximately 50 countries currently restrict the entry of those infected with HIV, especially long-term visitors such as students and workers, despite compelling arguments against the utility and for the counterproductive nature of such policies

An unofficial listing of country requirements is available at http://travel.state.gov/trvel/HIVtestingregs.html. Because possession of HAART medications may reveal the traveler's HIV infection, a potential solution is to remove or cover drug labels. Clearly, this is not without its own risks, which demand that careful records (medication names, dosages, frequencies, and physical appearance) be kept in more than one safe place by the traveler. Finally, there is the problem of untoward drug interactions with protease inhibitors. When initial HIV infection diagnosis and/or staging occurs during pretravel evaluation, the traveler may be newly recognized to fall into a group for whom HAART therapy is recommended. For those planning short-term travel, initiation of HAART just prior to departure is probably unwise due to the risk of developing significant side effects—many of which tend to be worse with initiation of therapy and some of which are intensified by stress—in the absence of close contact with a knowledgeable provider. For those in this situation who are planning long-term residence in the tropics, departure should probably be postponed until the traveler is stably on HAART therapy, unless close, timely follow-up can be achieved in the destination country. A critical variable, as ever in the rapidly changing field of HIV clinical care, is adequate, ongoing experience. Travel physicians without extensive, current experience in the care of those with HIV/AIDS should be in close consultative contact with physicians who possess this expertise: Today's verities rapidly become out of date. Textbooks of HIV care with frequent Web-based updates are also valuable resources.[76,77]

Sufficient quantities of currently used medications, along with replacement prescriptions, are essential. Patients should be counseled to seek medical attention promptly when ill. Although the current communication revolution allows a growing number of traveling patients to stay in close contact with their HIV and travel medicine physicians at home via e-mail, the prior identification of physicians with significant HIV experience in countries of planned travel is prudent. Obtaining medical insurance to cover such care is wise.

Another basic consideration, especially for those with advancing HIV-related disease, is the buying of trip cancellation and/or repatriation insurance.

Enteric pathogens are a major threat to the HIV-infected traveler to the tropics. In addition to the fact that many tropical travel-associated enteric bacterial infections are more severe in the presence of HIV coinfection, the achlorhydria that occurs in AIDS may markedly lower the amount of inoculum needed for the establishment of infection.[566,567] Precautions recommended for all travelers should be followed assiduously. Foods and beverages may be contaminated, particularly raw, unpeeled fruits and vegetables; raw or undercooked eggs; meats; seafood; tap water; ice; unpasteurized dairy products (beware of soft cheeses); and food purchased from street vendors.[213] Steaming hot foods, meat cooked until brown throughout, water brought to a boil for 1 minute, bottled (especially carbonated) beverages, very hot beverages, beer and wine, and fruits and vegetables peeled by the traveler are generally safe.[213] In addition to preventing enteric disease, following these precautions will also lower the risk of infection with *T. gondii*. Treating water with iodine or chlorine may be done, preferably in conjunction with filtration, when boiling is not practical. Filtration of water, using reverse osmosis or sub 1 micron filters, is efficacious in removing *Cryptosporidia* from water.[716] All tap water should be avoided, even small amounts used for brushing teeth. Recreational water exposure also carries a risk. Obviously, fecally contaminated water should be avoided altogether. Swallowing water while swimming should be avoided.[213] Direct contact with soil and sand should be avoided in places where fecal contamination is likely; hands should be washed frequently. Antimicrobial prophylaxis for enteric pathogens is not routinely recommended for HIV-uninfected

Table 133-1 *Immunizations for HIV-Infected Adults Who Are Traveling to the Tropics*

Vaccine	Recommendation	Comments
Routine immunizations*		
Tetanus–diphtheria	Boost every 10 yr	
Pneumococcus	Use 23-valent polysaccharide vaccine; boost at 5 yr	Recommended by USPHS–IDSA
Influenza		Recommended by ACIP, USPHS–IDSA Year-round infection in the tropics Southern Hemisphere: April through September; repeat annually
Hepatitis B	3 doses of Recombivax HB or Engerix B	
Measles†	Single dose of measles vaccine or MMR for susceptible persons who are not severely immunosuppressed; in the face of severe immunosuppression, consider immunoglobulin	
Standard travel immunizations		
Hepatitis A	Single dose 2 wk prior to travel; boost at 6–12 mo	
Poliomyelitis	Single dose of enhanced inactivated vaccine	Oral (live) vaccine is contraindicated and discouraged in close contacts
Typhoid	Single dose of polysaccharide vaccine at least 2 wk prior to travel; boost at 2 yr Alternately, two doses (separated by at least 1 mo) of inactivated vaccine; boost at 3 yr	Side effects lessened with polysaccharide vaccine; live oral vaccine is contraindicated
Yellow fever†		Contraindicated by the ACIP; recommended for those with asymptomatic HIV infection by WHO; considered for those with asymptomatic HIV infection who cannot avoid potential exposure, by USPHS, IDSA
Special travel immunizations		
Cholera	Two doses, at least 1 wk apart; boost at 6-mo intervals	Rarely indicated, given low risk of disease and limited effectiveness of vaccine; live vaccine contraindicated
Meningococcus	Single dose (A/C/Y/W-135)	
Plague	Three doses (one each at 0, 1, and 3–6 mo), with boost at 1 or 2 yr	
Rabies	See text	Avoid giving HDCV given intradermally, given potentially weaker response
Japanese encephalitis	Three doses, one each on days 0, 7, and 30; boost, based on antibody levels, at 1–3 yr	

*Routine primary series of immunization for diphtheria–tetanus, MMR, and polio is assumed.
†Absolutely or relatively contraindicated in some circumstances.

travelers. For HIV-infected travelers, such prophylaxis may be considered, however, depending on the level of immunosuppression, the risk of infection, and the duration of travel.[213] Fluoroquinolones are probably the drugs of choice. All HIV-infected travelers should carry antimicrobials (with or without antimotility agents) for an empirical treatment course in case diarrhea develops. Ciprofloxacin 500 mg twice a day for 3 to 7 days is a reasonable choice. Alternatives such as TMP–SMX or azithromycin should be used for children and pregnant women. Medical attention should quickly be sought if empirical therapy fails, if shaking chills or hematochezia occur, or if dehydration develops.[213]

Contact with arthropod vectors should be reduced through the careful use of insect repellents, wearing clothes that cover the arms and legs when outdoors, sleeping in well-screened areas or under a bed net, and avoiding outdoor exposure between dusk and dawn (see Chapter 120). The threat of sandfly transmission of visceral leishmaniasis (see Chapter 94) deserves special mention and education.

Malarial chemoprophylaxis is essential, where indicated, for all travelers. The HIV protease inhibitors currently used for HAART have understudied interactions with a variety of drugs used for malaria prophylaxis and treatment. Based on current data, mefloquine, doxycycline, chloroquine, and malarone (atovaquone + proguanil) are likely to be safe and to retain efficacy for malaria prophylaxis. The provision of empiric, standby treatment doses (e.g., of malarone) seems prudent.

Recommendations for the immunization of HIV-seropositive travelers to the tropics are summarized in Table 133-1. Preparation for travel should include a careful review of routine vaccinations in addition to both routine and special travel vaccinations. Vaccine response rates, as measured by antibody titers, tend to decline with increasing HIV-related immunosuppression. This gives impetus, especially for "routine" vaccinations, to early identification of the need for vaccination. Essentially all live bacterial and viral vaccines are considered to be contraindicated in the presence of HIV infection,[213] including oral polio vaccine, oral typhoid vaccine (Ty21a), and BCG. The special cases of measles and yellow fever vaccines are considered in the "pathogen-centered" discussions earlier in the chapter and in Table 133-1.

The risk of acquisition of tuberculosis is much higher in most tropical countries than in the United States, although the risk of becoming infected during short-term travel is low. As noted previously, the ACIP and the USPHS–IDSA working group consider the administration of BCG to be contraindicated because of the risk of dissemination, although it is recommended by WHO for those with asymptomatic HIV infection in areas with a high prevalence of TB infection. All HIV-infected people should receive PPD testing. Follow-up testing after return from the tropics (or during travel or residence in the tropics, if extended) should be performed. With a positive PPD (>5 mm induration) or a known high-risk exposure, HIV-infected people with no evidence of active TB, or history of treatment for latent or active TB, should be treated for latent TB.[213] Whether primary chemoprophylaxis should be recommended for travel in areas with a high population prevalence of TB is unclear.

The endemic systemic fungi carry considerable risk for HIV-infected travelers. Where the environmental sources are known, the risk of infection may be reduced somewhat by attempting to minimize exposure. Such measures include avoiding soil exposure, especially during the rainy season, in southern China and Southeast Asia (*P. marneffei*); avoiding exposure to disturbed soil and dust in lower Sonoran life zones of the Americas (*C. immitis*); and avoiding caves and soil and dust exposure in areas with heavy avian and bat excrement (*H. capsulatum*). Most often, the reservoirs are either unknown or too widespread to allow for avoidance. Primary prophylaxis with itraconazole (200 mg daily) may have merit for short-term prophylaxis during travel in areas with a high incidence of systemic fungal infection.[340,717]

Finally, it may be wise to avoid some areas of high potential risk by changing the planned travel itinerary or activities, especially for those people with advanced HIV disease. In this regard, it should be noted that many of the tropical infectious diseases of special concern here, such as yellow fever, have a fairly focal pattern of risk within endemic countries.

REFERENCES

1. Wilson ME: Travel and HIV infection. In Jong EC, McMullen R (eds): The Travel and Tropical Medicine Manual. Philadelphia, WB Saunders, 1995, p 166.
2. UNAIDS: AIDS epidemic update: 2004. www.unaids.org/wad2004/report_pdf.html.
3. Smith PG, Morrow RH, Chin J: Investigating interactions between HIV infection and tropical diseases. Int J Epidemiol 17:705, 1988.
4. Morrow RH, Colebunders RL, Chin J: Interactions of HIV infection with endemic tropical diseases. AIDS 3:S79, 1989.
5. Dybul M, Connors SM, Fauci AS: Immunology of HIV infection. In Paul WE (ed): Fundamental Immunology, 5th ed. Philadelphia, Lippincott, Williams & Wilkins, 2003, p 1285.
6. Chehimi J, Starr SE, Frank I, et al: Impaired interleukin-12 production in human immunodeficiency virus-infected patients. J Exp Med 179:1361, 1994.
7. Roos MTL, Miedema F, Koot M, et al: T cell function in vitro is an independent progression marker for AIDS in HIV-infected asymptomatic subjects. J Infect Dis 171:531, 1995.
8. Zhang R, Fichtenbaum CJ, Hildemann DA, et al: CD40 ligand dysregulation in HIV-associated dysfunction of antigen-presenting cells. J Immunol 172:2678, 2004.
9. Groux H, Torpier G, Monte D, A et al: Activation-induced death by apoptosis in $CD4^+$ T cells from human immunodeficiency virus-infected asymptomatic individuals. J Exp Med 175:331, 1992.
10. Sarin A, Clerici M, Blatt SP, et al: Inhibition of activation-induced programmed cell death and restoration of defective immune responses of HIV^+ donors by cysteine protease inhibitors. J Immunol 153:862, 1994.
11. Aandahl EM, Michaelsson J, Moretto WJ, et al: Human CD4+CD25+ regulatory T cells control T-cell responses to human immunodeficiency virus and cytomegalovirus. J Virol 78:2454, 2004.
12. Weiss L, Donkova-Petrini C, Caccavelli L, et al: Human immunodeficiency virus-driven expansion of CD4+CD25+ regulatory T cells, which suppress HIV-specific CD4 T-cell responses in HIV patients. Blood 104:3249, 2004.
13. Cameroun PU, Freudenthal PS, Barker JM, et al: Dendritic cells exposed to human immunodeficiency virus type-1 transmit a vigorous cytopathic infection to CD4+ T cells. Science 257:383, 1992.
14. Chehimi J, Starr S, Frank I, et al: Natural killer (NK) cell stimulatory factor increases the cytotoxic activity of NK cells from both healthy donors and human immunodeficiency virus-infected patients. J Exp Med 175:789, 1992.
15. Lucas SB: Missing infections in AIDS. Trans R Soc Trop Med Hyg 84:S34, 1990.
16. Gazzard BG: Problems of chemotherapy in multiply-infected AIDS patients. Trans R Soc Trop Med Hyg 84:S25, 1990.
17. Kroon FP, vanDissel JT, Labadie J, et al: Antibody response to diphtheria, tetanus, and poliomyelitis vaccines in relation to the number of $CD4^+$ lymphocytes in adults infected with human immunodeficiency virus. Clin Infect Dis 21:1197, 1995.

18. King JC, Vink PE, Farley JJ, et al: Comparison of the safety and immunogenicity of a pneumococcal conjugate with a licensed polysaccharide vaccine in human immunodeficiency virus and non-human immunodeficiency virus-infected children. Pediatr Infect Dis J 15:192, 1996.
19. Kroon FP, vanDissel JT, Rijker GT, et al: Antibody response to *Haemophilus influenzae* type b vaccine in relation to the number of CD4+ T lymphocytes in adults infected with human immunodeficiency virus. Clin Infect Dis 25:600, 1997.
20. Kaplan JE, Masur H, Holmes KK, et al: USPHS/IDSA guidelines for the prevention of opportunistic infections in persons infected with human immunodeficiency virus: Introduction. Clin Infect Dis 21:S1, 1995.
21. Kaplan JE, Hu DJ, Holmes KK, et al: Preventing opportunistic infections in human immunodeficiency virus-infected persons: Implications for the developing world. Am J Trop Med Hyg 55:1, 1996.
22. Steketee RW, Wirima JJ, Bloland PB, et al: Impairment of a pregnant woman's acquired ability to limit *Plasmodium falciparum* by infection with human immunodeficiency virus type-1. Am J Trop Med Hyg 55:42, 1996.
23. Morgan D, Maude GH, Malamba SS, et al: HIV-1 disease progression and AIDS-defining disorders in rural Uganda. Lancet 350:245, 1997.
24. N'Galy B, Ryder RW, Bila K, et al: Human immunodeficiency virus infection among employees in an African hospital. N Engl J Med 319:1123, 1988.
25. Nagelkerke NJD, Plummer FA, Holton D, et al: Transition dynamics of HIV disease in a cohort of African prostitutes: A Markov model approach. AIDS 4:743, 1990.
26. Colebunders RL, Latif AS: Natural history and clinical presentation of HIV-1 infection in adults. AIDS 5(suppl 1):S103, 1991.
27. Mulder DW, Nunn AJ, Wagner HU, et al: HIV-1 incidence and HIV-1-associated mortality in a rural Ugandan population cohort. AIDS 8:87, 1994.
28. Morgan D, Mahe C, Mayanja B, et al: HIV-1 infection in rural Africa: Is there a difference in median time to AIDS and survival compared with that in industrialized countries? AIDS 16:597, 2002.
29. Gilks CF, Brindle RJ, Otieno LS, et al: Life-threatening bacteremia in HIV-1 seropositive adults admitted to hospital in Nairobi, Kenya. Lancet 336:545, 1990.
30. Gilks CF, Otieno LS, Brindle RJ, et al: The presentation and outcome of HIV-related disease in Nairobi. Q J Med 297:25, 1992.
31. Mellors JW, Rinaldo CR, Gupta P, et al: Prognosis of HIV-1 infection predicted by the quantity of virus in plasma. Science 272:1167, 1996.
32. Bafica A, Scanga CA, Schito M, et al: Influence of coinfecting pathogens on HIV expression: Evidence for a role of Toll-like receptors. J Immunol 17:1123, 2004.
33. Secor WE, Shah A, Mwinzi PMN, et al: Increased density of human immunodeficiency virus type 1 coreceptors CCR5 and CXCR4 on the surfaces of CD4+ T cells and monocytes of patients with *Schistosoma mansoni* infection. Infect Immun 71:6668, 2003.
34. Zhao C, Papadopoulo B, Tremblay MJ: *Leishmania infantum* promotes replication of HIV type 1 in human lymphoid tissue cultured ex vivo by inducing secretion of the proinflammatory cytokines TNF-α and IL-1α. J Immunol 172:3086, 2004.
35. Xiao L, Owen SM, Rudoph DL, et al: *Plasmodium falciparum* antigen-induced human immunodeficiency virus type 1 replication is mediated through induction of tumor necrosis factor-α. J Infect Dis 177:437, 1998.
36. Puri A, Riley JL, Ritchey DW, et al: Influenza virus upregulates CXCR4 expression in CD4+ cells. AIDS Res Hum Retroviruses 16:19, 2000.
37. Mole L, Ripich S, Margolis D, Holodniy M: The impact of active herpes simplex infection on human immunodeficiency virus load. J Infect Dis 176:766, 1997.
38. Donovan RM, Bush CE, Markowitz NP, et al: Changes in virus load markers during AIDS-associated opportunistic diseases in human immunodeficiency virus-infected persons. J Infect Dis 174:401, 1996.
39. Sulkowski MS, Chaisson RE, Karp CL, et al: The effect of acute infectious illnesses on plasma human immunodeficiency virus (HIV) type 1 load and the expression of serologic markers of immune activation among HIV-infected adults. J Infect Dis 178:1642, 1998.
40. Berhe N, Wolday D, Hailu A, et al: HIV viral load and response to antileishmanial chemotherapy in co-infected patients. AIDS 13:1921, 1999.
41. Hoffman IF, Jere CS, Taylor TE, et al: The effect of *Plasmodium falciparum* malaria on HIV-1 RNA blood plasma concentration. AIDS 13:487, 1999.
42. Goletti D, Weissman D, Jackson RW, et al: Effect of *Mycobacterium tuberculosis* on HIV replication: Role of immune activation. J Immunol 157:1271, 1996.
43. Staprans SI, Hamilton BL, Follansfee SE, et al: Activation of virus replication after vaccination of HIV-1-infected individuals. J Exp Med 182:1727, 1995.
44. Couch RB: Editorial response: Influenza, influenza virus vaccine, and human immunodeficiency virus infection. Clin Infect Dis 28:548, 1999.
45. Youle MS, Gassard BG, Johnson MA, et al: Effects of high-dose oral acyclovir on herpesvirus disease and survival in patients with advanced HIV disease: A double-blind, placebo-controlled study. AIDS 8:641, 1994.
46. Whalen C, Horsburgh CR, Hom D, et al: Accelerated course of human immunodeficiency virus infection after tuberculosis. Am J Respir Crit Care Med 151:129, 1995.
47. Day JH, Grant AD, Fielding KL, et al: Does tuberculosis increase HIV load? J Infect Dis 190:1677, 2004.
48. Golden MP, Sajjad Z, Elgart L: Influenza and human immunodeficiency virus infection: Absence of HIV progression after acute influenza infection. Clin Infect Dis 32:1366, 2001.
49. Carroll RG, Riley JL, Levine BL, et al: Differential regulation of HIV-1 fusion cofactor expression by CD28 costimulation of CD4+ T cells. Science 276:273, 1997.
50. Roederer M, Raju PA, Mitra DK, et al: HIV does not replicate in naive CD4 T cells stimulated with CD3/CD28. J Clin Invest 99:1555, 1997.
51. Ancuta P, Bakri Y, Chomont N, et al: Opposite effects of IL-10 on the ability of dendritic cells and macrophages to replicate primary CXCR4-dependent HIV-1 strains. J Immunol 166:4244, 2001.
52. Wills-Karp M, Santeliz J, Karp CL: The germless theory of allergic disease: Revisiting the hygiene hypothesis. Nat Rev Immunol 1:69, 2001.
53. Asada H, Klaus-Kovtun V, Golding H, et al: Human herpesvirus 6 infects dendritic cells and suppresses human immunodeficiency virus type 1 replication in co-infected cultures. J Virol 73:4019, 1999.
54. Pinto LA, Blazevic V, Patterson BK, et al: Inhibition of human immunodeficiency virus type 1 replication prior to reverse transcription by influenza virus stimulation. J Virol 74:4505, 2000.
55. Goletti D, Carrara S, Vincenti D, et al: Inhibition of HIV-1 replication in monocyte-derived macrophages by *Mycobacterium tuberculosis*. J Infect Dis 189:624, 2004.
56. Verani A, Sironi F, Siccardi AG, et al: Inhibition of CXCR4-tropic HIV-1 infection by lipopolysaccharide: Evidence of different mechanisms in macrophages and T lymphocytes. J Immunol 168:6388, 2002.
57. Moss WJ, Ryon JR, Monze M, et al: Suppression of human immunodeficiency virus replication during acute measles. J Infect Dis 185:1035, 2002.
58. Watt G, Kantipong P, Jongsakul K: Decrease in human immunodeficiency virus type 1 load during acute dengue fever. Clin Infect Dis 36:1067, 2003.
59. Watt G, Kantipong P, de Souza M, et al: HIV-1 suppression during acute scrub-typhus infection. Lancet 356:475, 2000.
60. Kullberg MC, Pearce EJ, Hieny SE, et al: Infection with *Schistosoma mansoni* alters Th1/Th2 cytokine responses to a nonparasite antigen. J Immunol 148:3264, 1992.
61. Actor JK, Shirai M, Kullberg MC, et al: Helminth infection results in decreased virus-specific CD8+ cytotoxic T cell and Th1 cytokine responses as well as delayed virus clearance. Proc Natl Acad Sci USA 90:948, 1993.
62. Sabin EA, Araujo MI, Carvalho EM, et al: Impairment of tetanus toxoid-specific Th1-like immune responses in humans infected with *Schistosoma mansoni*. J Infect Dis 173:26, 1996.
63. Bentwich Z, Kalinkovich A, Weisman Z: Immune activation is a dominant factor in the pathogenesis of African AIDS. Immunol Today 16:187, 1995.
64. Maggi E, Mazzetti M, Ravina A, et al: Ability of HIV to promote a Th1 to Th0 shift and to replicate preferentially in Th2 and Th0 cells. Science 265:244, 1994.
65. Clerici M, Sarin A, Coffman RL, et al: Type 1/type 2 cytokine modulation of T-cell programmed cell death as a model for human immunodeficiency virus pathogenesis. Proc Natl Acad Sci USA 91:11811, 1994.
66. Wang J, Harada A, Matsushita S, et al: IL-4 and a glucocorticoid up-regulate CXCR4 expression on human CD4+ T lymphocytes and enhance HIV-1 replication. J Leukoc Biol 64:642, 1998.

67. Secor WE, Shah A, Mwinzi PMN, et al: Increased density of human immunodeficiency virus type 1 coreceptors CCR5 and CXCR4 on the surfaces of CD4+ T cells and monocytes of patients with *Schistosoma mansoni* infection. Infect Immun 71:6668, 2003.
68. Shapira-Nahor O, Kalinkovich A, Weisman Z, et al: Increased susceptibility to HIV-1 infection of peripheral blood mononuclear cells from chronically immune-activated individuals. AIDS 12:1731, 1998.
69. Gopinath R, Ostrowski M, Justement SJ, et al: Filarial infection increases susceptibility to human immunodeficiency virus infection in peripheral blood mononuclear cells in vitro. J Infect Dis 182:1804, 2000.
70. Wolday D, Mayaan S, Mariam ZG, et al: Treatment of intestinal worms is associated with decreased HIV plasma viral load. J AIDS 31:56, 2002.
71. Elliott AM, Mawa PA, Joseph S, et al: Associations between helminth infection and CD4+ T cell count, viral load and cytokine responses in HIV-1-infected Ugandan adults. Trans R Soc Trop Med Hyg 97:103, 2003.
72. Brown M, Kizza M, Watera C, et al: Helminth infection is not associated with faster progression HIV disease in co-infected adults in Uganda. J Infect Dis 190:1869, 2004.
73. Greenberg AE, Nguyen-Dinh P, Mann JM, et al: The association between malaria, blood transfusions, and HIV seropositivity in a pediatric population in Kinshasa, Zaire. JAMA 259:545, 1988.
74. Feldmeier H, Krantz I, Poggensee G: Female genital schistosomiasis as a risk factor for the transmission of HIV. Int J STD AIDS 5:368, 1994.
75. Thomas L: The Lives of a Cell: Notes of a Biology Watcher. New York, Viking Press, 1974.
76. Bartlett JG: Medical Management of HIV Infection: 2004 Edition. Baltimore, Johns Hopkins Medicine Health Publishing Business Group, 2004. Available at www.hopkins-aids.edu.
77. Cohen PT, Sande MA, Voberding PA: The HIV inSite Knowledge Base. http://hivinsite.ucsf.edu/InSite.
78. Centers for Disease Control and Prevention: Treating opportunistic infections among HIV-infected adults and adolescents: Recommendations from CDC, the National Institutes of Health, and the HIV Medicine Association/Infectious Diseases Society of America. MMWR 53:1, 2004.
79. Centers for Disease Control and Prevention: Treating opportunistic infections among HIV-infected children: Recommendations from CDC, the National Institutes of Health, and the HIV Medicine Association/ Infectious Diseases Society of America. MMWR 53:1, 2004.
80. Butcher GA: HIV and malaria: A lesson in immunology? Parasitol Today 8:307, 1992.
81. Colebunders R, Bahwe, Nekwei W, et al: Incidence of malaria and efficacy of oral quinine in patients recently infected with human immunodeficiency virus in Kinshasa, Zaire. J Infect 21:167, 1990.
82. Müller O, Moser R: The clinical and parasitological presentation of *Plasmodium falciparum:* Malaria in Uganda is unaffected by HIV-1 infection. Trans R Soc Trop Med Hyg 84:336, 1990.
83. Greenberg AE, Nsa W, Ryder RW, et al: *Plasmodium falciparum* malaria and perinatally acquired human immunodeficiency virus type 1 infection in Kinshasa, Zaire. N Engl J Med 325:105, 1991.
84. Taha TET, Canner JK, Dallabetta GA, et al: Childhood malaria parasitaemia and human immunodeficiency virus infection in Malawi. Trans R Soc Trop Med Hyg 88:164, 1994.
85. Kalyesubula I, Musoke-Mudido P, Marum L, et al: Effects of malaria infection in human immunodeficiency virus type 1-infected Ugandan children. Pediatr Infect Dis J 16:876, 1997.
86. Xiao L, Owen SM, Rudolph DL, et al: *Plasmodium falciparum* antigen-induced human immunodeficiency virus type 1 replication is mediated through induction of tumor necrosis factor-a. J Infect Dis 177:437, 1998.
87. Freitag C, Chougnet C, Schito M, et al: Malaria infection induces virus expression in human immunodeficiency transgenic mice by CD4 T cell-dependent immune activation. J Infect Dis 183:1260, 2001.
88. Kwiatkowski D, Cannon JG, Manogue KR, et al: Tumour necrosis factor production in falciparum malaria and its association with schizont rupture. Clin Exp Immunol 77:361, 1989.
89. Hoffman IF, Jere CS, Taylor TE, et al: The effect of *Plasmodium falciparum* malaria on HIV-1 RNA blood plasma concentration. AIDS 13:487, 1999.
90. Mwapasa V, Rogerson SJ, Molyneux ME, et al: The effect of *Plasmodium falciparum* malaria on peripheral and placental HIV-1 RNA concentrations in pregnant Malawian women. AIDS 18:1051, 2004.
91. Bloland PB, Wirima JJ, Steketee RW, et al: Maternal HIV infection and infant mortality in Malawi: Evidence for increased mortality due to placental malaria infection. AIDS 9:721, 1995.
92. Parise ME, Ayisi JG, Nahlen BL, et al: Efficacy of sulfadoxine-pyrimethamine for prevention of placental malaria in an area of Kenya with a high prevalence of malaria and human immunodeficiency virus infection. Am J Trop Med Hyg 59:813, 1998.
93. Verhoeff FH, Brabin BJ, Hart CA, et al: Increased prevalence of malaria in HIV-infected pregnant women and its implications for malaria control. Trop Med Int Health 4:5, 1999.
94. van Eijk AM, Ayisi JG, Feiko O, et al: Human immunodeficiency virus seropositivity and malaria as risk factors for third-trimester anemia in asymptomatic pregnant women in western Kenya. Am J Trop Med Hyg 65:623, 2001.
95. Ladner J, Leroy V, Simonon A, et al: HIV infection, malaria, and pregnancy: A prospective cohort study in Kigali, Rwanda. Am J Trop Med Hyg 66:56, 2002.
96. Brahmbhatt H, Kigozi G, Wabwire-Mangen F, et al: The effects of placental malaria on mother-to-child HIV transmission in Rakai, Uganda. AIDS 17:2539, 2003.
97. Inion I, Mwanyumba F, Gaillard P, et al: Placental malaria and perinatal transmission of human immunodeficiency virus type 1. J Infect Dis 188:1675, 2003.
98. Ticconi C, Mapfumo M, Dorrucci M, et al: Effect of maternal HIV and malaria infection on pregnancy and perinatal outcome in Zimbabwe. J Acquir Immune Defic Syndr 34:289, 2003.
99. Ayisi JG, van Eijk AM, ter Kuile FO, et al: The effect of dual infection with HIV and malaria on pregnancy outcome in western Kenya. AIDS 17:585, 2003.
100. Ayisi JG, van Eijk AM, Newman RD, et al: Maternal malaria and perinatal HIV transmission, western Kenya. Emerg Infect Dis 10:643, 2004.
101. ter Keuile FO, Parise ME, Verhoeff FH, et al: The burden of co-infection with human immunodeficiency virus type 1 and malaria in pregnant women in sub-Saharan Africa. Am J Trop Med Hyg 7(suppl 2):41, 2004.
102. WHO: Malaria and HIV/AIDS. Interactions and implications: Conclusions of a technical consultation convened by WHO, 23–25 June, 2004. Available at http://mosquito.who.int/malariacontrol.
103. Whitworth J, Morgan D, Quigley M, et al: Effect of HIV-1 and increasing immunosuppression on malaria parasitemia and clinical episodes in adults in rural Uganda: A cohort study. Lancet 356:1051, 2000.
104. Francesconi P, Fabiani M, Dente MG, et al: HIV, malaria parasites, and acute febrile episodes in Ugandan adults: A case–control study. AIDS 15:2445, 2001.
105. French N, Nakiyingi J, Laguda E, et al: Increasing rates of malarial fever with deteriorating immune status in HIV-1-infected Ugandan adults. AIDS 15:899, 2001.
106. Grimwade K, French N, Mbatha DD, et al: HIV infection as a cofactor for sever falciparum malaria in adults living in a region of unstable malaria transmission in South Africa. AIDS 18:547, 2004.
107. van Geertruyden JP, Mwananyanda L, Chalwe V, et al: Higher risk of antimalarial treatment in HIV positive than HIV negative individuals with clinical malaria. HIV and Emerging Diseases Congress, Toulon, June 2004.
108. Kamya MR, Kigonya CN, McFarland: HIV infection may adversely affect clinical response to chloroquine therapy for uncomplicated malaria in children. AIDS 15:1187, 2001.
109. Malaty LI, Kuper, JJ: Drug interactions of HIV protease inhibitors. Drug Safety 20:147, 1999.
110. Flockhart D: Cytochrome p450 Drug Interaction Database. http://medicine.iupui.edu/flockhart/table.htm.
111. Bangchang KN, Karbwang J, Back DJ: Mefloquine metabolism by human liver microsomes. Effect of other antimalarial drugs. Biochem Pharmacol 43:1957, 1992.
112. Adedoyin A, Frye RF, Mauro K, et al: Chloroquine modulation of specific metabolizing enzymes activities: Investigation with selective five drug cocktail. Br J Clin Pharmacol 46:215, 1998.
113. Masimirembwa CM, Hasler JA, Johansson, I: Inhibitory effects of antiparasitic drugs on cytochrome P450 2D6. Eur J Clin Pharmacol 48:35, 1995.
114. Coller JK, Somogyi AA, Bochner F: Comparison of (S)-mephenytoin and proguanil oxidation in vitro: Contribution of several CYP isoforms. Br J Clin Pharmacol 48:158, 1999.
115. Birkett DJ, Rees D, Andersson T, et al: In vitro proguanil activation to cycloguanil by human liver microsomes is mediated by CYP3A isoforms as well as by S-mephenytoin hydroxylase. Br J Clin Pharmacol 37:413, 1994.

116. Schippers EF, Hugen PWH, den Hartigh J, et al: No drug–drug interaction between nelfinavir or indinavir and mefloquine in HIV-1-infected patients. AIDS 14:2794, 2000.
117. Kahliq Y, Gallicano K, Tisdale C, et al: Pharmacokinetic interaction between mefloquine and ritonavir in healthy volunteers. Br J Clin Pharmacol 51:591, 2001.
118. Lee BL, Tauber MG, Goldstein D, et al: Atovaquone inhibits the glucuronidation and increases the plasma concentrations of zidovudine. Clin Pharmacol Ther 59:14, 1996.
119. Norvir package insert. Abbott Laboratories, 2004.
120. Fansidar-associated fatal reaction in an HIV-infected man. MMWR 37:571, 1988.
121. Current trends: Adverse reaction to Fansidar and updated recommendations for its use in the prevention of malaria. MMWR 33:713, 1985.
122. Benezra D, Brown AE, Polsky B, et al: Babesiosis and infection with human immunodeficiency virus (HIV). Ann Intern Med 107:944, 1987.
123. Ong KR, Stavropoulos C, Inada Y: Babesiosis, asplenia, and AIDS (letter). Lancet 336:112, 1990.
124. Machtinger L, Telford SR, Inducil C, et al: Treatment of babesiosis by red blood cell exchange in an HIV-positive splenectomized patient. J Clin Apheresis 8:78, 1993.
125. Falagas ME, Klempner MS: Babesiosis in patients with AIDS: A chronic infection presenting as fever of unknown origin. Clin Infect Dis 22:809, 1996.
126. Froberg KM, Dannen D, Bakken JS: Babesiosis and HIV. Lancet 363:704, 2004.
127. Krause PJ, Lepore T, Sikand VK, et al: Atovaquone and azithromycin for the treatment of babesiosis. N Engl J Med 343:1454, 2000.
128. Wolday D, Berhe Nm Akuffo H, Britton S: Leishmania–HIV interaction: Immunopathogenic mechanisms. Parasitol Today 15:182, 1999.
129. Rosenthal E, Marty P, le Fichoux Y, et al: Clinical manifestations of visceral leishmaniasis associated with HIV infection: A retrospective study of 91 French cases. Ann Trop Med Parasitol 94:37, 2000.
130. WHO: Leishmania/HIV co-infection: Epidemiological analysis of 692 retrospective cases. Wkly Epidemiol Rec 8:49, 1997.
131. Leishmania/HIV co-infection, southwestern Europe, 1990–1998. Wkly Epidemiol Rec 44:365, 1999.
132. Bernier R, Barbeau B, Tremblay MJ, et al: The lipophosphoglycan of *Lesihmani donovani* up-regulates HIV-1 transcription in T cells through the nuclear factor-kB elements. J Immunol 160:2881, 1998.
133. Wolday D, Akuffo H, Demisse A, et al: Role of *Leishmania donovani* and its lipophosphoglycan in CD4+ T-cell activation-induced human immunodeficiency virus replication. Infect Immun 67:5258, 1999.
134. Berhe N, Wolday D, Hailu A, et al: HIV viral load and response to antileishmanial chemotherapy in co-infected patients. AIDS 13:1921, 1999.
135. Zhao C, Papadopoulou B, Tremblay MJ: *Leishmania infantum* promotes replication of HIV type 1 in human lymphoid tissue cultured ex vivo by inducing secretion of the proinflammatory cytokines TNF-α and IL-1α. J Immunol 172:3086, 2004.
136. Gramiccia M, Fradoni L, Troiani M: Heterogeneity among zymodemes of *Leishmania infantum* from HIV-positive patients with visceral leishmaniasis in South Italy. FEMS Microbiol Lett 128:33, 1995.
137. Alvar J, Cañavate C, Gutierrez-Solar B, et al: *Leishmania* and human immunodeficiency virus co-infection: The first 10 years. Clin Microbiol Rev 10:98, 1997.
138. Alvar J: Leishmaniasis and AIDS co-infection. The Spanish example. Parasitol Today 10:160, 1994.
139. Medrano FJ, Jimenez-Mejias E, Calderon C, et al: An easy and quick method for the diagnosis of visceral leishmaniasis in HIV-1-infected individuals. AIDS 13:1399, 1993.
140. Molina R, Cañavate C, Cercenado E, et al: Indirect xenodiagnosis of visceral leishmaniasis in ten patients with HIV infection using colonized *Phlebotomus perniciosus*. AIDS 8:277, 1994.
141. Berhe N, Hailu A, Wolday D, et al: Ethiopian visceral leishmaniasis patients co-infected with human immunodeficiency virus. Trans R Soc Trop Med Hyg 89:205, 1995.
142. Desjeux P: Global control and leishmania HIV co-infection. Clin Dermatol 17:317, 1999.
143. Rabello A, Orsini M, Disch J: Leismania/HIV co-infection in Brazil: An appraisal. Ann Trop Med Parasitol 97(suppl 1):17, 2003.
144. Mattos M, Caiza A, Fernandes O, et al: American cutaneous leishmaniasis associated with HIV infection: Report of four cases. J Eur Acad Dermatol Venereol 10:218, 1998.
145. Hernandez DE, Oliver M, Martinez C, et al: Visceral leishmaniasis with cutaneous and rectal dissemination due to *L. braziliensis* in acquired immunodeficiency syndrome (AIDS). Int J Dermatol 34:114, 1995.
146. Machado ES, Braga M, daCruz AM, et al: Disseminated American muco-cutaneous leishmaniasis caused by *Leishmania braziliensis braziliensis* in a patient with AIDS: A case report. Mem Inst Oswaldo Cruz 87:487, 1992.
147. Nogueira-Castañon MCM, Pereira CAC, Fustado T: Unusual association of American cutaneous leishmaniasis and acquired immunodeficiency syndrome. Int J Dermatol 35:295, 1996.
148. Mattos M, Caiza A, Fernandes O, et al: American cutaneous leishmaniasis associated with HIV infection: Report of four cases. J Eur Acad Dermatol Venereol 10:218, 1998.
149. Gillis D, Klaus S, Schnur LF, et al: Diffusely disseminated cutaneous *Leishmania major*. Pediatr Infect Dis 14:247, 1995.
150. Pintado V, Martin-Rabadan P, Rivera ML, et al: Visceral leishmaniasis in human immunodeficiency virus (HIV)-infected and non-HIV-infected patients. A comparative study. Medicine (Baltimore) 80:54, 2001.
151. Rosenthal E, Marty P, del Giudice, et al: HIV and *Leishmania* co-infection: A review of 91 cases with focus on atypical locations of *Leishmania*. Clin Infect Dis 31:1093, 2000.
152. Laguna F, Garcia-Samaniego J, Soriano V, et al: Gastrointestinal leishmaniasis in human immunodeficiency virus-infected patients: Report of five cases and review. Clin Infect Dis 19:48, 1994.
153. Chehter EZ, Longo MA, Laudanna AA, et al: Pancreatic involvement in co-infection of visceral leishmaniasis and HIV: Histological and ultrastructural aspects. Rev Inst Med Trop Sao Paulo 43:75, 2001.
154. Gonzalez-Anglada MI, Pena JM, Barbado FJ: Two cases of laryngeal leishmaniasis in patients infected with HIV. Eur J Clin Microbiol Infect Dis 13:509, 1994.
155. Heudier P, Taillan B, Garnier G, et al: Pulmonary site of visceral leishmaniasis in HIV infection. Presse Med 22:1060, 1993.
156. Munoz-Rodriguez FJ, Padro S, Pastor P, et al: Pleural and peritoneal leishmaniasis in an AIDS patient. Eur J Clin Microbiol Infect Dis 16:246, 1997.
157. Dauden E, Penas PF, Rios L, et al: Leishmaniasis presenting as a dermatomyositis-like eruption in AIDS. J Am Acad Dermatol 35:316, 1996.
158. Colebunders R, Depraetere K, Verstaeten T, et al: Unusual cutaneous lesions in two patients with visceral leishmaniasis and HIV infection. J Am Acad Dermatol 41:847, 1999.
159. Grasa JM, Lorente J, Crego F, et al: Nasal leishmaniasis in an HIV-positive patient. Acta Otorrinolaringol Esp 51:169, 2000.
160. Medrano FJ, Canavate C, Leal M, et al: The role of serology in the diagnosis and prognosis of visceral leishmaniasis in patients co-infected with human immunodeficiency virus type-1. Am J Trop Med Hyg 59:155, 1998.
161. Gradoni L, Scalone A, Gramiccia M: HIV–*Leishmania* co-infections in Italy: Serological data as an indication of the sequence of the two infections. Trans R Soc Trop Med Hyg 87:94, 1993.
162. Berke N, Hailu A, Wolday D, et al: Ethiopian visceral leishmaniasis patients co-infected with human immunodeficiency virus. Trans R Soc Trop Med Hyg 89:205, 1995.
163. Qu JQ, Zhong L, Masoon-Yasinzai M, et al: Serodiagnosis of Asian leishmaniasis with a recombinant antigen from the repetitive domain of a *Leishmania* kinesin. Trans R Soc Trop Med Hyg 88:543, 1994.
164. Dereure J, Pratlong F, Reynes J, et al: Haemoculture as a tool for diagnosing visceral leishmaniasis in HIV-negative and HIV-positive patients: Interest for parasite identification. Bull World Health Organ 76:203, 1998.
165. Sacks DL, Lal SL, Shrivastava SN, et al: An analysis of T cell responsiveness in Indian kala azar. J Immunol 138:908, 1987.
166. Karp CL, el-Safi SH, Wynn TA, et al: In vivo cytokine profiles in patients with kala azar. Marked elevation of both IL-10 and IFN-γ. J Clin Invest 91:1644, 1993.
167. Laguna F, Lopez-Velez R, Pulido F, et al: Treatment of visceral leishmaniasis in HIV-infected patients: A randomized trial comparing meglumine antimoniate with amphotericin B. AIDS 13:1063, 1999.
168. Laguna F, Videla S, Jimenez-Mejias ME, et al: Amphotericin B lipid complex versus meglumine antimoniate in the treatment of visceral

leishmaniasis in patients infected with HIV: A randomized pilot study. J Antimicrob Chemother 52:464, 2003.
169. Lopez-Velez R, Videla S, Marquez M, et al: Amphotericin B lipid complex versus no treatment in the secondary prophylaxis of visceral leishmaniasis in HIV-infected patients. J Antimicrob Chemother 53:540, 2004.
170. Pérez-Molina JA, López-Vélez R, Montilla P, et al: Pentamidine isethionate as secondary prophylaxis against visceral leishmaniasis in HIV-positive patients. AIDS 10:237, 1996.
171. López M, Gil A, Lavilla P, et al: Efficacy of liposomal amphotericin B in the treatment and secondary prophylaxis of visceral leishmaniasis in HIV-infected patients: Report of two cases. J Antimicrob Chemother 32:657, 1993.
172. Sundar S, Jha TK, Thakurr CP, et al: Oral miltefosine for Indian visceral leishmaniasis. N Engl J Med 347:1739, 2002.
173. Sindermann H, Engel KR, Fischer C, et al: Oral miltefosine for leishmaniasis in immunocompromised patients: Compassionate use in 39 patients with HIV infection. Clin Infect Dis 39:1520, 2004.
174. Lopez-Velez R: The impact of highly active antiretroviral therapy (HAART) on visceral leishmaniasis in Spanish patients who are co-infected with HIV. Ann Trop Med Parasitol 97(suppl 1):143, 2003.
175. Casado JL, Lopez-Velez R, Pintado V, et al: Relapsing visceral leishmaniasis in HIV-infected patients undergoing successful protease inhibitor therapy. Eur J Clin Microbiol Infect Dis 20:202, 2001.
176. del Giudice R, Mary-Krause M, Pradier C, et al: Impact of highly active antiretroviral therapy on the incidence of visceral leishmaniasis in a French cohort of patients infected with human immunodeficiency virus. J Infect Dis 186:1366, 2002.
177. Berenguer J, Cosín J, Miralles P, et al: Discontinuation of secondary anti-*Leishmania* prophylaxis in HIV-infected patients who have responded to highly active antiretroviral therapy. Aquir Immune Defic Syn 14:2946, 2000.
178. Mira JA, Corzo JE, Rivero A, et al: Frequency of visceral leishmaniasis relapses in human immunodeficiency virus-infected patients receiving highly active antiretroviral therapy. Am J Trop Med Hyg 7:298, 2004.
179. Ferreira MS, Nishioka SA, Silvestre MTA, et al: Reactivation of Chagas' disease in patients with AIDS: Report of 3 new cases and review of the literature. Clin Infect Dis 25:1397, 1997.
180. Silva N, O'Bryan L, Medeiros E, et al: *Trypanosoma cruzi* menignoencephalitis in HIV-infected patients. J Acquir Immune Defic Syndrome Hum Retrovir 20:342, 1999.
181. Yoo TW, Mlikotic A, Cornford ME, et al: Concurrent cerebral American trypanosomiasis and toxoplasmosis in a patient with AIDS. Clin Infect Dis 39:e30, 2004.
182. Sartori AMC, Shikanai-Yasuda MA, Neto VA, et al: Follow-up of 18 patients with human immunodeficiency virus infection and chronic Chagas' disease, with reactivation of Chagas' disease causing cardiac disease in three patients. Clin Infect Dis 26:177, 1998.
183. Sartori AMC, Lopes MH, Benvenuti LA, et al: Reactivation of Chagas' disease in a human immunodeficiency virus-infected patient leading to severe heart disease with a late positive direct microscopic examination of the blood. Am J Trop Med Hyg 59:784, 1998.
184. diLorenzo GA, Pagano MA, Taratuto AL, et al: Chagas' granulomatous encephalitis in immunosuppressed patients. Computed tomography and magnetic resonance imaging findings. J Neuroimaging 6:94, 1996.
185. Perez-Ramirez L, Barnabe C, Sartori AMC, et al: Clinical analysis and parasite genetic diversity in human immunodeficiency virus/Chagas' disease co-infections in Brazil. Am J Trop Med Hyg 61:198, 1999.
186. Sartori AMC, Neto JE, Nunes EV, et al: *Trypanosoma cruzi* parasitemia in chronic Chagas' disease: Comparison between human immunodeficiency virus (HIV)-positive and HIV-negative patients. J Infect Dis 286:872, 2002.
187. Sartori AMC, Caiaffa-Filho HH, Bezerra RC, et al: Exacerbation of HIV viral load simultaneous with asymptomatic reactivation of chronic Chagas' disease. Am J Trop Med Hyg 67:521, 2002.
188. Nishioka S deA, Ferreira MS, Rocha A, et al: Reactivation of Chagas' disease successfully treated with benznidazole in a patient with AIDS. Mem Inst Oswaldo Cruz 88:493, 1993.
189. Solari A, Saavedra H, Sepulveda C, et al: Successful treatment of *Trypanosoma cruzi* encephalitis in a patient with hemophilia and AIDS. Clin Infect Dis 16:255, 1993.
190. McCabe RE, Remington JS, Araujo FG: In vitro and in vivo effects of itraconazole against *Trypanosoma cruzi.* Am J Trop Med Hyg 35:280, 1986.
191. Noireau F, Brun-Vezinet F, Larouze B, et al: Absence of relationship between human immunodeficiency virus 1 and sleeping sickness. Trans R Soc Trop Med Hyg 81:1000, 1987.
192. Louis KP, Moulia-Pelat JP, Jannin J, et al: Absence of epidemiological inter-relations between HIV infection and African human trypanosomiasis in Central Africa. Trop Med Parasitol 42:155, 1991.
193. Pepin J, Ethier L, Kazadi C, et al: The impact of human immunodeficiency virus infection on the epidemiology and treatment of *Trypanosoma brucei gambiense* sleeping sickness in Nioki, Zaire. Am J Trop Med Hyg 47:133, 1992.
194. Meda HA, Doua F, Laveissière C, et al: Human immunodeficiency virus infection and human African trypanosomiasis: A case–control study in Côte d'Ivoire. Trans R Soc Trop Med Hyg 89:639, 1995.
195. Blum J, Nkunku S, Burri C: Clinical description of encephalopathic syndromes and risk factors for their occurrence and outcome during melarsoprol treatment of human African trypanosomiasis. Trop Med Int Health 6:390, 2001.
196. Chicharro C, Alvar J: Lower trypanosomatids in HIV/AIDS patients. Ann Trop Med Parasitol 97(suppl 1):S75, 2002.
197. Luft BJ, Remington JS: Toxoplasmic encephalitis in AIDS. Clin Infect Dis 15:211, 1992.
198. Sousa OE, Saenz RE, Frenkel JK: Toxoplasmosis in Panama: A 10-year study. Am J Trop Med Hyg 38:315, 1988.
199. Etheredge GD, Frenkel JK: Human *Toxoplasma* infection in Kuna and Embera children in the Bayano and San Blas, eastern Panama. Am J Trop Med Hyg 53:448, 1995.
200. Morakote N, Thamasonthi W, Charachinda K, et al: Prevalence of *Toxoplasma* antibodies in Chiang Mai population. Southeast Asian J Trop Med Public Health 15:80, 1984.
201. Zumla A, Savva D, Wheeler RB, et al: *Toxoplasma* serology in Zambian and Ugandan patients infected with the human immunodeficiency virus. Trans R Soc Trop Med Hyg 85:227, 1991.
202. Ndumbe PM, Andela A, Nkemnkeng-Asong J, et al: Prevalence of infections affecting the child among pregnant women in Yaounde, Cameroon. Med Microbiol Immunol 181:127, 1992.
203. Guimaraes AC, Kawarabayashi M, Borges MM, et al: Regional variation in toxoplasmosis seronegativity in the São Paulo metropolitan region. Rev Inst Med Trop Sao Paulo 35:479, 1993.
204. al-Amari OM: Prevalence of antibodies to *Toxoplasma gondii* among blood donors in Abha, Asir Region, southwestern Saudi Arabia. J Egypt Public Health Assoc 69:77, 1994.
205. Doehring E, Reiter-Owona I, Bauer O, et al: *Toxoplasma gondii* antibodies in pregnant women and their newborns in Dar es Salaam, Tanzania. Am J Trop Med Hyg 52:546, 1995.
206. Ledru E, Diagbouga S, Ledru S, et al: A study of *Toxoplasma* and cytomegalovirus serology in tuberculosis and in HIV-infected patients in Burkina Faso. Acta Trop 59:149, 1995.
207. Luft BJ, Remington JS: Toxoplasmic encephalitis. J Infect Dis 157:1, 1988.
208. Porter SB, Sande MA: Toxoplasmosis of the central nervous system in the acquired immunodeficiency syndrome. N Engl J Med 327:1643, 1992.
209. Lucas SB, Hounnou A, Peacock C, et al: The mortality and pathology HIV infection in a West African city. AIDS 7:1569, 1993.
210. Mohar A, Romo J, Salido F, et al: The spectrum of clinical and pathological manifestations of AIDS in a consecutive series of autopsied patients in Mexico. AIDS 6:467, 1992.
211. Lucas SB, Odida M, Wabinga H: The pathology of severe morbidity and mortality caused by HIV infection in Africa. AIDS 5:S143, 1991.
212. Luft BJ, Hafner R, Korzun AH, et al: Toxoplasmic encephalitis in patients with the acquired immunodeficiency syndrome. N Engl J Med 329:995, 1993.
213. CDC: Guidelines for preventing opportunistic infections among HIV-infected persons—2002. MMWR 51:1, 2002.
214. Sison JP, Kemper CA, Loveless M, et al: Disseminated *Acanthamoeba* infection in patients with AIDS: Case reports and review. Clin Infect Dis 20:1207, 1995.
215. Bottone EJ: Free-living amebas of the genera *Acanthamoeba* and *Naegleria:* An overview and basic microbiologic correlates. Mt Sinai J Med 60:260, 1993.
216. Wang SS, Feldman HA: Isolation of *Hartmannella* species from human throats. N Engl J Med 277:1174, 1967.
217. Cursons RTM, Brown TJ, Keys EA, et al: Immunity to pathogenic free-living amoebae: Role of cell-mediated immunity. Infect Immun 29:408, 1980.

218. Riestra-Castaneda JM, Riestra-Castaneda R, Gonzalez-Garrido AA, et al: Granulomatous amebic encephalitis due to *Balamuthia mandrillaris* (leptomyxiidae): Report of four cases from Mexico. Am J Trop Med Hyg 56:603, 1997.
219. Fettz TR, Sawyer MH, Billman G, et al: Successful treatment of *Balamuthia* amebic encephalitis: Presentation of 2 cases. Clin Infect Dis 37:1304, 2003.
220. Miyamato EK, Duane GB: *Acanthamoeba* meningoencephalitis: Diagnosis by squash preparation of brain biopsy specimen. Cytopathology 131:1, 1985.
221. Gonzalez MM, Gould E, Dickinson G, et al: Acquired immunodeficiency syndrome associated with *Acanthamoeba* infection and other opportunistic organisms. Arch Pathol Lab Med 110:749, 1986.
222. Wiley CA, Safrin RE, Davis CE, et al: *Acanthamoeba* meningoencephalitis in a patient with AIDS. J Infect Dis 155:130, 1987.
223. Anzil AP, Rao C, Wrzolek MA, et al: Amebic meningoencephalitis in a patient with AIDS caused by a newly recognized opportunistic pathogen. Leptomyxid ameba. Arch Pathol Lab Med 115:21, 1991.
224. Gardner HAR, Martinez AJ, Visvesvara GS, et al: Granulomatous amebic encephalitis in an AIDS patient. Neurology 41:1993, 1991.
225. diGregorio C, Rivasi F, Mongiardo N, et al: *Acanthamoeba* meningoencephalitis in a patient with acquired immunodeficiency syndrome. Arch Pathol Lab Med 116:1363, 1992.
226. Friedland LR, Raphael SA, Deutsch ES, et al: Disseminated *Acanthamoeba* infection in a child with symptomatic human immunodeficiency virus infection. Pediatr Infect Dis J 11:404, 1992.
227. Gordon SM, Steinbert JP, duPuis MH, et al: Culture isolation of *Acanthamoeba* species and leptomyxid amebas from patients with amebic meningoencephalitis, including two patients with AIDS. Clin Infect Dis 15:1024, 1992.
228. Tan B, Weldon-Linne M, Rhone DP, et al: *Acanthamoeba* infection presenting as skin lesions in patients with the acquired immunodeficiency syndrome. Arch Pathol Lab Med 117:1043, 1993.
229. Martinez MS, Gonzlez-Mediero G, Santiago P, et al: Granulomatous amebic encephalitis in a patient with AIDS: Isolation of *Acanthamoeba* sp. group II from brain tissues and successful treatment with sulfadiazine and fluconazole. J Clin Microbiol 38:3892, 2000.
230. May LP, Sidhu GS, Buchness MR: Diagnosis of *Acanthamoeba* infection by cutaneous manifestations in a man seropositive to HIV. J Am Acad Dermatol 26:352, 1992.
231. Helton J, Loveless M, White CR Jr: Cutaneous *Acanthamoeba* infection associated with leukocytoclastic vasculitis in an AIDS patient. Am J Dermatopathol 15:146, 1993.
232. Park CH, Iyengar V, Hefter L, et al: Cutaneous *Acanthamoeba* infection associated with acquired immunodeficiency syndrome. Lab Med 25:386, 1994.
233. Hunt SJ, Reed SL, Mathews WC, et al: Cutaneous *Acanthamoeba* infection in the acquired immunodeficiency syndrome: Response to multidrug therapy. Cutis 56:285, 1995.
234. Murakawa GJ, McCalmont T, Altman J, et al: Disseminated acanthamebiasis in patients with AIDS. Arch Dermatol 131:1291, 1995.
235. Clavel A, Franco L, Letona S, et al: Primary amebic meningoencephalitis in a patient with AIDS: Unusual protozoological findings. Clin Infect Dis 23:1314, 1996.
236. Jonckheere JF, Brown S: Primary amebic meningoencephalitis in a patient with AIDS: Unusual protozoological findings. Clin Infect Dis 25:943, 1997.
237. Xiao L, Morgan UM, Fayer R, et al: *Cryptosporidium* systematics and implications for public health. Parasitol Today 16:287, 2000.
238. Gatei W, Greensill J, Ashford RW, et al: Molecular analysis of the 18S rRNA gene of *Cryptosporidium* parasites from patients with or without human immunodeficiency virus infections living in Kenya, Malawi, Brazil, the United Kingdom, and Vietnam. J Clin Microbiol 41:1458, 2003.
239. Cama VA, Bern C, Sulaiman LM, et al: *Cryptosporidium* species and genotype in HIV-positive patients in Lima, Peru. J Eukaryot Microbiol 50(suppl):531, 2003.
240. Flanigan T, Whalen C, Turner J, et al: *Cryptosporidium* infection and CD4 counts. Ann Intern Med 116:840, 1992.
241. Manabe YC, Clark DP, Moore RD, et al: Cryptosporidiosis in patients with AIDS: Correlates of disease and survival. Clin Infect Dis 27:536, 1998.
242. Chaisson RE, Gallant JE, Keruly JC, et al: Impact of opportunistic disease on survival in patients with HIV infection. AIDS 12:29, 1998.
243. Colfod JM, Tager IB, Hirozawa AM, et al: Cryptosporidiosis among patients infected with human immunodeficiency virus. Factors related to symptomatic infection and survival. Am J Epidemiol 144:807, 1996.
244. Le Moing V, Bissuel F, Costagliola D, et al: Decreased prevalence of intestinal cryptosporidiosis in HIV-infected patients concomitant to the widespread use of protease inhibitors. AIDS 12:1395, 1998.
245. Kim LS, Hadley WK, Stansell J, et al: Declining prevalence of cryptosporidiosis in San Francisco. Clin Infect Dis 27:655, 1998.
246. Chen XM, Keithly JS, Paya CV, et al: Cryptosporidiosis. N Engl J Med 346:1723, 2002.
247. Clark DP: New insights into human cryptosporidiosis. Clin Microbiol Rev 12:554, 1999.
248. Dunand VA, Hammer SM, Rossi R, et al: Parasitic sinusitis and otitis in patients infected with human immunodeficiency virus: Report of five cases and review. Clin Infect Dis 25:267, 1997.
249. French AL, Beaudet LM, Benator DA, et al: Cholecystectomny in patients with AIDS: Clinicopathologic correlations in 107 cases. Clin Infect Dis 21:852, 1995.
250. Vakil NB, Schwartz SM, Buggy BP, et al: Biliary cryptosporidiosis in HIV-infected people after the waterborne outbreak of cryptosporidiosis in Milwaukee. N Engl J Med 334:19, 1996.
251. Miao YM, Awad-El-Kariem FM, Franzen C, et al: Eradication of cryptosporidia and microsporidia following successful antiretroviral therapy. J Acquir Immune Defic Syndr 25:124, 2000.
252. Treatment of HIV-associated microsporidiosis and cryptosporidiosis with combination antiretroviral therapy. Lancet 351:256, 1998.
253. Lindsay DS, Dubey JP, Blagburn BL: Biology of *Isospora* spp. from humans, nonhuman primates, and domestic animals. Clin Microbiol Rev 10:19, 1997.
254. DeHovitz JA, Pape JW, Boncy M, et al: Clinical manifestations and therapy of *Isospora belli* infection in patients with the acquired immunodeficiency syndrome. N Engl J Med 314:87, 1986.
255. Benator DA, French AL, Beaudet LM, et al: *Isospora belli* infection associated with acalculous cholecystitis in a patient with AIDS. Ann Intern Med 121:663, 1994.
256. Pape JW, Verdier RI, Johnson WD: Treatment and prophylaxis of *Isospora belli* infection in patients with the acquired immunodeficiency syndrome. N Engl J Med 320:1044, 1989.
257. Weiss LM, Perlman DC, Sherman J, et al: *Isospora belli* infection: Treatment with pyrimethamine. Ann Intern Med 109:474, 1988.
258. Pape JW, Verdier RI, Boney M, et al: *Cyclospora* infection in adults infected with HIV. Clinical manifestations, treatment, and prophylaxis. Ann Intern Med 121:654, 1994.
259. Sifuentes-Osornio J, Porras-Cortés G, Bendall RP: *Cyclospora cayetanensis* infection in patients with and without AIDS: Biliary disease as another clinical manifestation. Clin Infect Dis 21:1092, 1995.
260. Quinn TC, Stamm WE, Goodell SE, et al: The polymicrobial origin of intestinal infections in homosexual men. N Engl J Med 309:576, 1983.
261. Laughon BE, Druckman DA, Vernon A, et al: Prevalence of enteric pathogens in homosexual men with and without acquired immunodeficiency syndrome. Gastroenterology 94:984, 1988.
262. Nash TE, Ohl CA, Subramanian G, et al: Treatment of patients with refractory giardiasis. Clin Infect Dis 33:22, 2001.
263. Hailemariam G, Kassu A, Abebe G, et al: Intestinal parasitic infections in HIV/AIDS and HIV seronegative individuals in a teaching hospital, Ethiopia. Jpn J Infect Dis 57:41, 2004.
264. Secor WE, Karanja DMS, Colley DG: Interactions between schistosomiasis and human immunodeficiency virus in western Kenya. Mem Inst Oswaldo Cruz 99(suppl 1):93, 2004.
265. Karanja DMS, Colley DG, Nahlen BL, et al: Studies on schistosomiasis in western Kenya. I. Evidence for immune-facilitated excretion of schistosome eggs from patients with *Schistosoma mansoni* and HIV co-infections. Am J Trop Med Hyg 56:515, 1997.
266. Karanja DMS, Boyer AE, Strand M, et al: Studies on schistosomiasis in western Kenya: II. Efficacy of praziquantel for treatment of schistosomiasis in persons co-infected with human immunodeficiency virus-1. Am J Trop Med Hyg 59:307, 1998.
267. Karanja DM, Hightower AW, Colley DG, et al: Resistance to reinfection with *Schistosoma mansoni* in occupationally exposed adults and effect of HIV-1 co-infection on susceptibility to schistosomiasis: A longitudinal study. Lancet 360:592, 2002.

268. Joseph S, Jones FM, Laidlaw ME, et al: Impairment of the *Schistosoma mansoni*-specific immune responses elicited by treatment with praziquantel in Ugandans with HIV-1 co-infection. J Infect Dis 190:613, 2004.
269. Mwanakasale V, Vounatsou P, Sukwa TY, et al: Interactions between *Schistosoma haematobium* and human immunodeficiency virus type 1: The effects of co-infection on treatment outcomes in rural Zambia. Am J Trop Med Hyg 69:420, 2003.
270. Poggensee G, Feldmeier H, Krantz I: Schistosomiasis of the female genital tract: Public health aspects. Parasitol Today 15:378, 1999.
271. Poggensee G, Kiwelu I, Weger V, et al: Female genital schistosomiasis of the lower genital tract: Prevalence and disease-associated morbidity in northern Tanzania. J Infect Dis 181:1210, 2000.
272. Leutscher PDC, Behets F, Rousset D, et al: Sexual behavior and sexually transmitted infections in men living in rural Madagascar. Sex Transm Dis 30:262, 2003.
273. Lawn SD, Karanja DM, Mwinzi P, et al: The effect of treatment of schistosomiasis on blood plasma HIV-1 RNA concentration in co-infected individuals. AIDS 14:2437, 2000.
274. Elliott AM, Mawa PA, Joseph S, et al: Associations between helminth infection and CD4+ T cell count, viral load and cytokine responses HIV-1-infected Ugandan adults. Trans R Soc Trop Med Hyg 97:103, 2003.
275. Santamariá-Fríes M, Fajardo LF, Sogin MI, et al: Lethal infection by a previously unrecognized metazoan parasite. Lancet 347:1797, 1996.
276. Connor DH, Sparks AK, Strano AJ, et al: Disseminated parasitosis in an immunosuppressed patient. Arch Pathol Lab Med 100:65, 1976.
277. Klinker H, Tintelnot K, Joeres R, et al: *Taenia-crassiceps*-Infektion bei AIDS. Dtsch Med Wochensehr 117:133, 1992.
278. Chermette R, Bussiéras J, Marionneau J, et al: Cysticercose envahissante à *Taenia crassiceps* chez un patient atteint de sida. Bull Acad Natl Med 4:777, 1995.
279. Francois A, Favennec L, Cambon-Michot C, et al: *Taenia crassiceps* invasive cysticercosis: A new human pathogen in acquired immunodeficiency syndrome? Am J Surg Pathol 22:488, 1998.
280. Maillard H, Marionneau J, Prophette B, et al: *Taenia crassiceps* cysticercosis and AIDS. AIDS 12:1551, 1998.
281. Sailer M, Boelder B, Allerberger F, et al: Alveolar echinococcosis of the liver in a six-year-old girl with AIDS. J Pediatr 130:320, 1997.
282. Delobel P, Signate A, El Guedj M, et al: Unusual form of neuro-cysticercosis associated with HIV infection. Eur J Neurol 11:55, 2004.
283. Soto-Hernandez JL, Ostorsky-Zeichner L, Tavera G, et al: Neurocysticercosis and HIV infection: Report of two cases and review. Surg Neurol 45:57, 1996.
284. White AC Jr, Dakik H, Diaz P: Asymptomatic neurocysticercosis in a patient with AIDS and cryptococcal meningitis. Am J Med 99:101, 1995.
285. Thornton CA, Houston S, Latif AS: Neurocysticercosis and human immunodeficiency virus infection. Arch Neurol 49:963, 1992.
286. Moskowitz LB, Hensley GT, Chan JC, et al: The neuropathology of acquired immune deficiency syndrome. Arch Pathol Lab Med 108:867, 1984.
287. Keiser PB, Nutman TB: *Strongyloides stercoralis* in the immunocompromised population. Clin Microbiol Rev 17:208, 2004.
288. Genta RM: Dysregulation of strongyloidiasis: A new hypothesis. Clin Microbiol Rev 5:345, 1992.
289. Anonymous: Update: Acquired immunodeficiency syndrome (AIDS) in the United States. MMWR 31:508, 1982.
290. Anonymous: Revision of the CDC surveillance case definition for acquired immunodeficiency syndrome. MMWR 36:35, 1987.
291. Phillips SC, Mildvan D, William CD, et al: Sexual transmission of enteric protozoa and helminths in a venereal disease clinic population. N Engl J Med 305:603, 1981.
292. Maayan S, Wormser GP, Widerhorn J, et al: *Strongyloides stercoralis* hyperinfection in a patient with the acquired immunodeficiency syndrome. Am J Med 83:945, 1987.
293. Armignacco O, Capecchi A, deMori P: *Strongyloides stercoralis* hyperinfection and the acquired immunodeficiency syndrome. Am J Med 86:258, 1989.
294. Dutcher JP, Marcus SL, Tanowitz HB: Disseminated strongyloidiasis with central nervous system involvement diagnosed antemortem in a patient with acquired immunodeficiency syndrome and Burkitt's lymphoma. Cancer 66:2417, 1990.
295. Kramer MR, Gregg PA, Goldstein M, et al: Disseminated strongyloidiasis in AIDS and non-AIDS immunocompromised hosts: Diagnosis by sputum and bronchoalveolar lavage. South Med J 83:1226, 1990.
296. Gompels MM, Todd J, Peters BS, et al: Disseminated strongyloidiasis in AIDS: Uncommon but important. AIDS 5:329, 1991.
297. Harcourt-Webster JN, Scarvilli F, Darwish AH: *Strongyloides stercoralis* hyperinfection in an HIV-positive patient. J Clin Pathol 44:346, 1991.
298. Lessnau KD, Can S, Talavera W: Disseminated *Strongyloides stercoralis* in human immunodeficiency virus-infected patients: Treatment failure and a review of the literature. Chest 104:119, 1993.
299. Torres JR, Isturiz R, Murillo J, et al: Efficacy of ivermectin in the treatment of strongyloidiasis complicating AIDS. Clin Infect Dis 17:900, 1993.
300. Celedon JC, Mathur-Wagh U, Fox J, et al: Systemic strongyloidiasis in patients infected with the human immunodeficiency virus: A report of 3 cases and review of the literature. Medicine (Baltimore) 73:256, 1994.
301. Cahill KM, Shevehuk M: Fulminant, systemic strongyloidiasis in AIDS. Ann Trop Med Parasitol 90:313, 1996.
302. Petithory JC, Derouin F: AIDS and strongyloidiasis in Africa. Lancet 1:921, 1987.
303. Neto VA, Pasternak J, Moreira AAB, et al: *Strongyloides stercoralis* hyperinfection in the acquired immunodeficiency syndrome. Am J Med 87:602, 1989.
304. Conlon CP, Pinching AJ, Perera CY, et al: HIV-related enteropathy in Zambia: A clinical, microbiological, and histological study. Am J Trop Med Hyg 42:83, 1990.
305. Hunter G, Bagshawe AF, Baboo KS, et al: Intestinal parasites in Zambian patients with AIDS. Trans R Soc Trop Med Hyg 86:543, 1992.
306. Viney ME, Brown M, Omoding NE, et al: Why does HIV infection not lead to disseminated strongyloidiasis? J Infect Dis 190:2175, 2004.
307. Sato Y, Shiroma Y: Concurrent infections with *Strongyloides* and T cell leukemia virus and their possible effect on the immune response of the host. Clin Immunol Immunopathol 52:214, 1989.
308. Marsh BJ: Infectious complications of human T cell leukemia/ lymphoma virus type I infection. Clin Infect Dis 23:138, 1996.
309. Fischer P, Kipp W, Kabwa P, et al: Onchocerciasis and human immunodeficiency virus in western Uganda: Prevalences and treatment with ivermectin. Am J Trop Med Hyg 53:171, 1995.
310. Orkin M: Scabies in AIDS. Semin Dermatol 12:9, 1993.
311. Schlesinger I, Oelrich DM, Tyring SK: Crusted (Norwegian) scabies in patients with AIDS: The range of clinical presentations. South Med J 87:352, 1994.
312. Meinking TL, Taplin D, Hermida JL, et al: The treatment of scabies with ivermectin. N Engl J Med 333:26, 1995.
313. Hulbert TV, Larsen RA: Hyperkeratotic (Norwegian) scabies with gram-negative bacteremia as the initial presentation of AIDS. Clin Infect Dis 14:1164, 1992.
314. Corbett EL, Crossley I, Holton J, et al: Crusted ("Norwegian") scabies in a specialist HIV unit: Successful use of ivermectim and failure to prevent nosocomial transmission. Genitourin Med 72:115, 1996.
315. Portu JJ, Santamaria JM, Zubero Z, et al: Atypical scabies in HIV-positive patients. J Am Acad Dermatol 34:915, 1996.
316. Supparatpinyo K, Khamwan C, Vaosoung V, et al: Disseminated *Penicillium marneffei* infection in southeast Asia. Lancet 344:110, 1994.
317. Chariyalertsak S, Sirisanthana T, Supparatpinyo K, et al: Seasonal variation of disseminated *Penicillium marneffei* infections in northern Thailand: A clue to the reservoir? J Infect Dis 173:1490, 1996.
318. Duong TA: Infection due to *Penicillium marneffei,* an emerging pathogen: Review of 155 reported cases. Clin Infect Dis 23:125, 1996.
319. Phillips P: *Penicillium marneffei*: Part of southeast Asian AIDS. JAMA 276:86, 1996.
320. Hung C-C, Hsueh P-R, Chen M-Y, et al: Invasive infection caused by *Penicillium marneffei*: An emerging pathogen in Taiwan. Clin Infect Dis 26:202, 1998.
321. Supparatpinyo K, Chiewchanvit S, Hirunsri P, et al: *Penicillium marneffei* infection in patients infected with human immunodeficiency virus. Clin Infect Dis 14:871, 1992.
322. Chariyalertsak S, Sirisanthana T, Supparatpinyo K, et al: Case–control study of risk factors for *Penicillium marneffei* infection in HIV-infected patients in northern Thailand. Clin Infect Dis 24:1080, 1997.
323. Kudeken N, Kawakami K, Kusano N, et al: Cell-mediated immunity in host resistance against infection caused by *Penicillium marneffei.* J Med Vet Mycol 34:371, 1996.

324. Kok I, Veenstra J, Rietra PJGM, et al: Disseminated *Penicillium marneffei* infection as an imported disease in HIV-1 infected patients. Neth J Med 44:18, 1994.
325. Kronauer CM, Schär G, Barben M, et al: Die HIV-assoziierte *Penicillium-marneffei*-infektion. Schweiz Med Wschenschr 123:385, 1993.
326. Peto TEA, Bull R, Millard PR, et al: Systemic mycosis due to *Penicillium marneffei* in a patient with antibody to human immunodeficiency virus. J Immunol 16:285, 1988.
327. Sirisanthana V, Sirisanthana T: *Penicillium marneffei* infection in children infected with human immunodeficiency virus. Pediatr Infect Dis J 12:12021, 1993.
328. Kantipong P, Panich V, Pongsurachet V, et al: Hepatic penicilliosis in patients without skin lesions. Clin Infect Dis 26:1215, 1998.
329. Chaiwan B, Khunamornpong S, Sirivanichai C, et al: Lymphadenopathy due to *Penicillium marneffei* infection: Diagnosis by fine needle aspiration cytology. Mod Pathol 15:939, 2002.
330. Kaufman L, Standard PG, Anderson SA, et al: Development of specific fluorescent antibody test for tissue form of *Penicillium marneffei*. J Clin Microbiol 33:2136, 1995.
331. Supparatpinyo K, Sirisanthana T: Disseminated *Penicillium marneffei* infection diagnosed on examination of a peripheral blood smear of a patient with human immunodeficiency virus infection. Clin Infect Dis 18:246, 1994.
332. Kaufman L, Standard PG, Jalbert M, et al: Diagnostic antigenemia tests for penicilliosis marneffei. J Clin Microbiol 34:2503, 1996.
333. Wong SSY, Wong KH, Hui WT, et al: Differences in clinical and laboratory diagnostic characteristics of *Penicilliosis marneffei* in human immunodeficiency virus (HIV)- and no-HIV-infected patients. J Clin Microbiol 39:4535, 2001.
334. Desakaron V, Smith BD, Walsh AL: Diagnosis of *Penicilliosis marneffei* infection by quantitation of urinary antigen by using an enzyme immunoassay. J Clin Microbiol 37:117, 1999.
335. Wheat J, Wheat H, Connolly P, et al: Cross-reactivity in *Histoplasma capsulatum* variety *capsulatum* antigen assays of urine samples from patients with endemic mycoses. Clin Infect Dis 24:1169, 1998.
336. Yuen K, Wong SS, Tsang DN, et al: Serodiagnosis of *Penicillium marneffei* infection. Lancet 344:444, 1994.
337. Sirisanthana T, Supparatpinyo K, Perriens J, et al: Amphotericin B and itraconazole for treatment of disseminated *Penicillium marneffei* infection in human immunodeficiency virus-infected patients. Clin Infect Dis 26:1107, 1998.
338. Supparatpinyo K, Nelson KE, Merz WG, et al: Response to antifungal therapy by human immunodeficiency virus-infected patients with disseminated *Penicillium marneffei* infections and in vitro susceptibilities of isolates from clinical specimens. Antimicrob Agents Chemother 37:2407, 1993.
339. Supparatpinyo K, Perriens J, Nelson KE, et al: A controlled trial of itraconazole to prevent relapse of *Penicillium marneffei* infection in patients infected with human immunodeficiency virus. N Engl J Med 339:1739, 1998.
340. Chariyaleertsak S, Supparatpinyo K, Sirisanthana T, et al: A controlled trial of itraconozaole as primary prophylaxis for systemic fungal infections in patients with advanced human immunodeficiency virus infection in Thailand. Clin Infect Dis 34:277, 2002.
341. Hung C-C, Chen M-Y, Hsieh S-M, et al: Discontinuation of secondary prophylaxis for *Penicilliosis marneffei* in AIDS patients responding to highly active anti-retroviral therapy. AIDS 16:672, 2002.
342. Brummer E, Castaneda E, Restrepo A: Paracoccidioidomycosis: An update. Clin Microbiol Rev 6:89, 1993.
343. Mota NGS, Rezkallah-Iwasso MT, Peracoli MTS, et al: Correlation between cell-mediated immunity and clinical forms of paracoccidioidomycosis. Trans R Soc Trop Med Hyg 79:765, 1985.
344. Bava AJ, Mistchenko AS, Palacios MF, et al: Lymphocyte subpopulations and cytokine production in paracoccidioidomycosis patients. Microbiol Immunol 35:167, 1991.
345. Goldani LZ, Sugar AM: Paracoccidioidomycosis and AIDS: An overview. Clin Infect Dis 21:1275, 1995.
346. Bernard G, Duarte AJS: Paracoccidioidomycosis: A model for evaluation of the effects of human immunodeficiency virus infection on the natural history of endemic tropical diseases. Clin Infect Dis 31:1032, 2000.
347. Silva-Vergara ML, Teixeira AC, Curi VGM, et al: Paracoccidioido-mycosis associated with human immunodeficiency virus infection. Med Mycol 41:259, 2003.
348. Nishioka Sde A: Paracoccidioidomycosis and AIDS. Clin Infect Dis 22:1132, 1996.
349. Carme B, Ngolet A, Ebikili B, et al: Is African histoplasmosis an opportunistic fungal infection in AIDS? Trans R Soc Trop Med Hyg 84:293, 1990.
350. Peeters P, Depre G, Richaert F, et al: Disseminated African histoplasmosis in a white heterosexual male patient with the acquired immune deficiency syndrome. Mycoses 10:449, 1987.
351. Arendt V, Coremans-Pelseneer J, Gottlob R, et al: African histoplasmosis in a Belgian AIDS patient. Mycoses 34:59, 1991.
352. Carme B, Ngaporo AI, Ngolet A, et al: Disseminated African histoplasmosis in a Congolese patient with AIDS. J Med Vet Mycol 30:245, 1992.
353. Geffray L, Veyssier P, Cevallos R, et al: Histoplasmose africaine: Aspects cliniques et thérapeutiques-relations avec le SIDA. Ann Med Interne (Paris) 145:424, 1994.
354. Manfredi R, Mazzoni A, Nanetti A, et al: Histoplasmosis capsulati and duboisii in Europe: The impact of the HIV pandemic, travel and immigration. Eur J Epidemiol 10:675, 1994.
355. Chandenier J, Goma D, Moyen G, et al: African histoplasmosis due to *Histoplasma capsulatum* var. *duboisii:* Relationship with AIDS in recent Congolese cases (in French). Sante 5:227, 1995.
356. Al-Tawfiq JA, Wools KK: Disseminated sporotrichosis and *Sporothrix schenkii* fungemia as the initial presentation of human immunodeficiency virus infection. Clin Infect Dis 26:1403, 1998.
357. Rocha MM, Dassin T, Lira R: Sporotrichosis in patient with AIDS: Report of a case and review. Rev Iberoam Micol 18:133, 2001.
358. Kauffman CA: Sporotrichosis. Clin Infect Dis 29:231, 1999.
359. Kauffman CA, Hajjeh R, Chapman SW: Practice guidelines for the management of patients with sporotrichosis. For the Mycoses Study Group. Infectious Diseases Society of America. Clin Infect Dis 30:684, 2000.
360. Wheat LJ, Kauffman CA: Histoplasmosis. Infect Dis Clin North Am 17:1, 2003.
361. Pappas PG: Blastomycosis in the immunocompromised patient. Semin Respir Infect 12:243, 1997.
362. Chiller TM, Galgiani JN, Stevens DA: Coccidioidomycosis. Infect Dis Clin North Am 17:41, 2003.
363. Wheat J: Endemic mycoses in AIDS: A clinical review. Clin Microbiol Rev 8:146, 1995.
364. Wheat LJ, Connolly-Stringfield PA, Baker RL, et al: Disseminated histoplasmosis in the acquired immune deficiency syndrome: Clinical findings, diagnosis and treatment, and review of the literature. Medicine (Baltimore) 69:361, 1990.
365. Baily GG, Robertson VJ, Neill P, et al: Blastomycosis in Africa: Clinical features, diagnosis, and treatment. Rev Infect Dis 13:1005, 1991.
366. diSalvo AF: The ecology of *Blastomyces dermatitidis*. In al-Doory Y, diSalvo AF (eds): Blastomycosis. New York, Plenum Press, 1992, p 43.
367. Pappas PG, Pottage JC, Powderly WG, et al: Blastomycosis in patients with the acquired immunodeficiency syndrome. Ann Intern Med 116:847, 1992.
368. Tan G, Kaufman L, Peterson EM, et al: Disseminated atypical blastomycosis in two patients with AIDS. Clin Infect Dis 16:107, 1993.
369. Bonnimann DA, Adam RD, Galgiani JN, et al: Coccidioidomycosis in the acquired immunodeficiency syndrome. Ann Intern Med 106:372, 1987.
370. Singh VR, Smith DK, Lawerence J, et al: Coccidioidomycosis in patients infected with human immunodeficiency virus: Review of 91 cases at a single institution. Clin Infect Dis 23:563, 1996.
371. Chuck SL, Sande MA: Infections with *Cryptococcus neoformans* in the acquired immunodeficiency syndrome. N Engl J Med 321:794, 1989.
372. Powderly WG: Current approach to the acute management of cryptococcal infections. J Infect 41:18, 2000.
373. Diamond RD: The growing problem of mycoses in patients infected with the human immunodeficiency virus. Rev Infect Dis 13:480, 1991.
374. Thongcharoen P, Vithayasai P, Vithayasai V, et al: Opportunistic infections in AIDS/HIV infected patients in Thailand. Thai AIDS J 4:117, 1992.
375. Swasdisevi A: Clinical study of HIV disease in the lower area of northern Thailand in 1994. J Med Assoc Thai 77:440, 1994.
376. Karstaedt AS: AIDS—The Baragwanath experience. III. HIV infection in adults at Baragwanath Hospital. S Afr Med J 82:95, 1992.

377. Piot P, Quinn TC, Taelman H, et al: Acquired immunodeficiency syndrome in a heterosexual population in Zaire. Lancet 22:65, 1984.
378. Odio W, Kapita B, Mbendi N, et al: Le syndrome d'immunodéficience acquise (SIDA) à Kinshasa, Zaire: Observations cliniques et épidémiologiques. Ann Soc Belg Med Trop 65:357, 1985.
379. Desmet P, Kayembe KD, deVroey C: The value of cryptococcal serum antigen screening among HIV-positive/AIDS patients in Kinshasa, Zaire. AIDS 3:77, 1989.
380. delAmo J, Petruckevitch A, Phillips AN, et al: Spectrum of disease in Africans with AIDS in London. AIDS 10:1563, 1996.
381. Volkow P, Ponce deLeón S, Calva J, et al: Transfusion associated AIDS in Mexico. Clinical spectrum, conditional latency distribution, and survival. Rev Invest Clin 45:133, 1993.
382. Daley CL: Pulmonary infections in the tropics: Impact of HIV infection. Thorax 49:370, 1994.
383. Ministerio da Saude do Brasil: Dados e pesquisa em DST e AIDS. Coordenacao do programa nacional de DTS/AIDS. Brasilia, 2002. www.aidsgov.br.
384. Ellis DH, Pfeiffer TJ: Natural habitat of *Cryptococcus neoformans* var. *gatti*. J Clin Microbiol 28:1642, 1990.
385. Levitz SM: The ecology of *Cryptococcus neoformans* and the epidemiology of cryptococcosis. Rev Infect Dis 13:1163, 1991.
386. Lopez-Martinez R, Soto-Hernandex JL, Ostrosky-Zeichner L, et al: *Cryptococcus neoformans* var. *gatti* among patients with cryptococcal meningitis in Mexico. First observations. Mycopathology 134:61, 1996.
387. Peglow SL, Smulian AG, Linke MJ, et al: Serologic responses to *Pneumocystis carinii* antigens in health and disease. J Infect Dis 161:296, 1990.
388. Smulian AG, Sullivan DW, Linke MJ, et al: Geographic variation in the humoral response to *Pneumocystis carinii*. J Infect Dis 167:1243, 1993.
389. Lee C-H, Lu J-J, Bartlett MS, et al: Nucleotide sequence variation in *Pneumocystis carinii* strains that infect humans. J Clin Microbiol 31:754, 1993.
390. Kaplan JE, Hanson D, Dworkin MS, et al: Epidemiology of human immunodeficiency virus-associated opportunistic infections in the United States in the era of highly active antiretroviral therapy. Clin Infect Dis 30(suppl 1):S5, 2000.
391. Morris A, Lundgren JD, Masur H, et al: Current epidemiology of *Pneumocystis* pneumonia. Emerg Infect Dis 10:1713, 2004.
392. McLeod DT, Neill P, Gwanzura L, et al: *Pneumocystis carinii* pneumonia in patients with AIDS in Central Africa. Respir Med 84:225, 1990.
393. M'boussa J, Kaoudi E, Kokolo J, et al: Pneumocystoses observées au Congo chez les malades atteints de SIDA. Rev Pneumol Clin 47:39, 1991.
394. Abouya YL, Beaumel A, Lucas S, et al: An uncommon cause of death in African patients with acquired immunodeficiency syndrome. Am Rev Respir Dis 145:617, 1992.
395. Aderaye G, Bruchfeld J, Olsson M, et al: Occurrence of *Pneumocystis carinii* in HIV-positive patients with suspected pulmonary tuberculosis in Ethiopia. AIDS 17:435, 2003.
396. Carme B, M'boussa J, Andzin M, et al: *Pneumocystis carinii* is rare in AIDS in Central Africa. Trans R Soc Trop Med Hyg 85:80, 1991.
397. Batungwanayo J, Taelman H, Lucas S, et al: Pulmonary disease associated with the human immunodeficiency virus in Kigali, Rwanda. Am J Respir Crit Care Med 149:1591, 1994.
398. Malin AS, Gwanzura LKZ, Klein S, et al: *Pneumocystis carinii* pneumonia in Zimbabwe. Lancet 346:1258, 1995.
399. Ansari NA, Kombe AH, Kenyon TA, et al: Pathology and causes of death in a group of 128 predominantly HIV-positive patients in Botswana, 1997–1998. Int J Tuberc Lung Dis 6:55, 2002.
400. Stansell JD, Osmond DH, Charlebois E, et al: Predictors of *Pneumocystis carinii* pneumonia in HIV-infected persons. Pulmonary complications of HIV infection study group. Am J Respir Crit Care Med 155:60, 1997.
401. Mahdi SA, Cutland C, Ismail K, et al: Ineffectiveness of trimethoprim-sulfamethoxazole prophylaxis and the importance of bacterial and viral co-infections in African children with *Pneumocystis carinii* pneumonia. Clin Infect Dis 35:1120, 2002.
402. Newell ML, Coovadia H, Cortina-Borja M, et al: Mortality of infected and uninfected infants born to HIV-infected mothers in Africa: A pooled analysis. Lancet 364:1263, 2004.
403. Graham SM: HIV and respiratory infections in children. Curr Opin Pulm Med 9:215, 2003.
404. Simonds RJ, Lindegren ML, Thomas P, et al: Prophylaxis against *Pneumocystis carinii* pneumonia among children with perinatally acquired human immunodeficiency virus infection in the United States. N Engl J Med 332:786, 1995.
405. Thomas CF, Limper AH: *Pneumocystis* pneumonia. N Engl J Med 350:2487, 2004.
406. Vartivarian SE, Anaissie EJ, Bodey GE: Emerging fungal pathogens in immunocompromised patients: Classification, diagnosis, and management. Clin Infect Dis 17:S487, 1993.
407. Perfect JR, Schell WA: The new fungal opportunists are coming. Clin Infect Dis 22:S112, 1996.
408. Narain FP, Raviglione MC, Kochi A: HIV-associated tuberculosis in developing countries: Epidemiology and strategies for prevention. Tuber Lung Dis 73:311, 1992.
409. Harries AD, Hargreaves NJ, Kemp J, et al: Deaths from tuberculosis in sub-Saharan African countries with a high prevalence of HIV-1. Lancet 357:1519, 2001.
410. Mocroft A, Vella S, Benfield TL, et al: Changing patterns of mortality across Europe in patients infected with HIV-1. EuroSIDA Study Group. Lancet 352:1725, 1998.
411. Ellner JJ: Tuberculosis in the time of AIDS—The facts and the message. Chest 98:1051, 1990.
412. Martin DJ, Sim JGM, Sole GJ, et al: CD4+ lymphocyte count in African patients co-infected with HIV and tuberculosis. J Acquir Immune Defic Syndr Hum Retrovirol 8:386, 1995.
413. Goletti D, Weissman D, Jackson RW, et al: Effect of *Mycobacterium tuberculosis* on HIV replication. J Immunol 157:1271, 1996.
414. Tossi Z, Mayanja-Kizza H, Hirsch CS, et al: Impact of tuberculosis (TB) on HIV-1 activity in dually infected patients. Clin Exp Immunol 123:233, 2001.
415. Morris L, Martin DJ, Helba Bredell, et al: Human immunodeficiency virus-1 RNA levels and CD4 lymphocyte counts, during treatment for active tuberculosis, in South African patients. J Infect Dis 187:1967, 2003.
416. Lawn SD, Shatock RJ, Acheampong JW, et al: Sustained plasma TNF-α and HIV-1 load despite resolution of other parameters of immune activation during treatment of tuberculosis in Africans. AIDS 13:2231, 1999.
417. Wolday D, Hailu B, Girma M, et al: Low CD4+ T-cell count and high HIV viral load precede the development of tuberculosis disease in a cohort of HIV-positive Ethiopians. Int J Tuberc Lung Dis 7:110, 2003.
418. Alpert PL, Munsiff SS, Fourevitch MN, et al: A prospective study of tuberculosis and human immunodeficiency virus infection: Clinical manifestations and factors associated with survival. Clin Infect Dis 24:661, 1997.
419. Badri M, Ehrlich R, Wood R, et al: Association between tuberculosis and HIV disease progression in a high tuberculosis prevalence area. Int J Tuberc Lung Dis 5:225, 2001.
420. Perneger TV, Sudre P, Lundgren JD, et al: Does the onset of tuberculosis in AIDS predict shorter survival? Results of a cohort study in 17 European countries over 13 years. BMJ 311:1468, 1995.
421. del Amo J, Perez-Hoyos S, Hernandez AI, et al: Impact of tuberculosis on HIV disease progression in persons with well-documented time of HIV seroconversion. J Acquir Immune Defic Syndr 33:184, 2003.
422. Crampin AC, Floyd S, Glynn JR, et al: Long-term follow-up of HIV-positive and HIV-negative individuals in rural Malawi. AIDS 16:1545, 2002.
423. Wilkinson D, Squire SB, Garner P: Effect of preventive treatment for tuberculosis in adults infected with HIV: Systematic review of randomised placebo controlled trials. BMJ 317:625, 1998.
424. Bucher HC, Griffith LE, Guyatt GH, et al: Isoniazid prophylaxis for tuberculosis in HIV infection: A meta-analysis of randomized controlled trials. AIDS 13:501, 1999.
425. Anonymous: Preventive therapy against tuberculosis in people living with HIV. Policy statement. Weekly Epidem Rec 46:385, 1999.
426. Gordin F, Chaisson RE, Matts JP, et al: Rifampin and pyrazinamide vs. isoniazid for prevention of tuberculosis in HIV-infected persons. JAMA 283:1445, 2000.
427. Halsey NA, Coberly JS, Desormeaux J, et al: Randomised trial of isoniazid versus rifampin and pyrazinamide for prevention of tuberculosis in HIV-1 infection. Lancet 351:786, 1998.

428. Mwinga A, Hosp M, Godfrey-Faussett P, et al: Twice weekly tuberculosis preventive therapy in HIV infection in Zambia. AIDS 12:2447, 1998.
429. Anonymous: Update: Fatal and severe liver injuries associated with rifampicin and pyrazinamide for latent tuberculosis infection, and revisions in American Thoracic Society/CDC recommendations—United States, 2001. MMWR 50:733, 2001.
430. Gordin FM, Cohn DL, Matts JP, et al: Hepatotoxicity of rifampin and pyrazinamide in the treatment of latent tuberculosis infection in HIV-infected persons: Is it different than in HIV-uninfected persons? Clin Infect Dis 39:561, 2004.
431. Burman WJ, Jones BE: Treatment of HIV-related tuberculosis in the era of effective antiretroviral therapy. Am J Respir Crit Care Med 164:7, 2001.
432. American Thoracic Society/Centers for Disease Control and Prevention/Infectious Diseases Society of America: Treatment of tuberculosis. Am J Respir Crit Care Med 167:603, 2003.
433. Anonymous: Disseminated *Mycobacterium bovis* infection from BCG vaccination of a patient with acquired immunodeficiency syndrome. MMWR 34:227, 1985.
434. Ninane J, Grymonprez A, Burtonboy G, et al: Disseminated BCG in HIV infection. Arch Dis Child 63:1268, 1988.
435. Weltman AC, Rose DN: The safety of bacille Calmette–Guérin vaccination in HIV infection and AIDS. AIDS 7:149, 1993.
436. Talbot EA, Perkins MD, Fagundes S, et al: Disseminated bacille Calmette–Guérin disease after vaccination: Case report and review. Clin Infect Dis 24:1139, 1997.
437. Colebunders RL, Lebughe I, Musampu M, et al: BCG vaccine abscesses are unrelated to HIV infection (letter). JAMA 259:352, 1988.
438. Lallemant-leCoeur S, Lallemant M, Cheynier D, et al: Bacillus Calmette–Guérin immunization in infants born to HIV-1-seropositive mothers. AIDS 5:195, 1991.
439. O'Brien KL, Ruff AJ, Louis MA, et al: Bacillus Calmette–Guérin complications in children both to HIV-1-infected women with a review of the literature. Pediatrics 95:414, 1995.
440. Bhat GJ, Diwan VK, Chintu C, et al: HIV, BCG and TB in children: A case control study in Lusaka, Zambia. J Trop Pediatr 39:219, 1993.
441. Marsh BJ, von Reyn CF, Edwards J, et al: The risks and benefits of childhood bacille Calmette–Guérin immunization among adults with AIDS. AIDS 11:669, 1997.
442. Garly ML, Martins CL, Bale C, et al: BCG scar and positive tuberculin reaction associated with reduced child mortality in West Africa. A non-specific bacterial effect of BCG? Vaccine 21:2782, 2003.
443. WHO: The safety of EPI-recommended vaccines in HIV-infected individuals. www.who-int/vaccines-disease/diseases/HIV.shtml, 2004.
444. Advisory Council for the Elimination of Tuberculosis and the Advisory Committee on Immunization Practices: The role of BCG vaccine in the prevention and control of tuberculosis in the United States. A joint statement by the Advisory Council for the Elimination of Tuberculosis and the Advisory Committee on Immunization Practices. MMWR 45:1, 1996.
445. Inderlied CB, Kemper CA, Bermudez LEM: The *Mycobacterium avium* complex. Clin Microbiol Rev 6:266, 1993.
446. von Reyn CF, Waddell RD, Eaton T, et al: Isolation of *Mycobacterium avium* complex from water in the United States, Finland, Zaire, and Kenya. J Clin Microbiol 31:3227, 1993.
447. Horsburgh CR Jr, Cohn DL, Roberts RB, et al: *Mycobacterium avium–M. intracellulare* isolates from patients with or without AIDS. Antimicrob Agents Chemother 30:955, 1986.
448. Tsang AY, Denner JC, Brennan PJ, et al: Clinical and epidemiological importance of typing of *Mycobacterium avium* complex isolates. J Clin Microbiol 30:479, 1992.
449. Ellner JJ, Goldberger MJ, Parenti DM: *Mycobacterium avium* infection and AIDS: A therapeutic dilemma in rapid evolution. J Infect Dis 163:1326, 1991.
450. Nightingale SD, Byrd LT, Southern PM, et al: Incidence of *Mycobacterium avium–intracellulare* complex bacteremia in HIV-positive patients. J Infect Dis 165:1082, 1992.
451. Jacobson MA, Hopewell PC, Yajko DM, et al: Natural history of disseminated *Mycobacterium avium* complex infection in AIDS. J Infect Dis 164:994, 1991.
452. Havlik JA Jr, Metchock B, Thompson SE III, et al: A prospective evaluation of *Mycobacterium avium* complex colonization of the respiratory and gastrointestinal tracts of persons with HIV infection. J Infect Dis 168:1045, 1993.
453. Chin DP, Hopewell PC, Yajko DM, et al: *Mycobacterium avium* complex in the respiratory or gastrointestinal tract and the risk of *M. avium* complex bacteremia in patients with HIV infection. J Infect Dis 169:289, 1994.
454. Wong B, Edwards FF, Kiehn TE, et al: Continuous high-grade *Mycobacterium avium–intracellulare* bacteremia in patients with AIDS. Am J Med 78:35, 1985.
455. Okello DO, Dewankambo N, Goodgame R, et al: Absence of bacteremia with *Mycobacterium avium–intracellulare* in Ugandan patients with AIDS. J Infect Dis 162:208, 1990.
456. Morrissey AB, Aisu TO, Falkinham JO, et al: Absence of *Mycobacterium avium* complex disease in patients with AIDS in Uganda. J Acquir Immune Defic Syndr Hum Retrovirol 5:477, 1992.
457. Vugia DJ, Kiehlbauch JA, Yeboue K, et al: Pathogens and predictors of fatal septicemia associated with human immunodeficiency virus infection in Ivory Coast, West Africa. J Infect Dis 168:564, 1993.
458. Sewankambo N, Mugerwa RD, Goodgame R, et al: Enteropathic AIDS in Uganda. An endoscopic, histological and microbiological study. AIDS 1:9, 1987.
459. Colebunders R, Lusakumuni K, Nelson AM, et al: Persistent diarrhoea in Zairian AIDS patients: An endoscopic and histological study. Gut 29:1687, 1988.
460. Gilks CF, Brindle RJ, Mwachari C, et al: Disseminated *Mycobacterium avium* infection among HIV-infected patients in Kenya. J Acquir Immune Defic Syndr Hum Retrovirol 8:195, 1995.
461. Jessurum J, Angeles-Angeles A, Gasman N: Comparative demographic and autopsy findings in acquired immune deficiency syndrome in two Mexican populations. J Acquir Immune Defic Syndr Hum Retrovirol 3:579, 1990.
462. Barreto JA, Palaci M, Ferrazoli L, et al: Isolation of *Mycobacterium avium* complex from bone marrow aspirates of AIDS patients in Brazil. J Infect Dis 168:777, 1993.
463. von Reyn CF, Barber TW, Arbeit RD, et al: Evidence of previous infection with *Mycobacterium avium–Mycobacterium intracellulare* complex among healthy subjects: An international study of dominant mycobacterial skin test reactions. J Infect Dis 168:1553, 1993.
464. duMoulin GC, Stottmeier KD, Pelletier PA, et al: Concentration of *Mycobacterium avium* by hospital hot water systems. JAMA 260:1599, 1988.
465. McFadden JJ, Kunze ZM, Portaels F, et al: Epidemiological and genetic markers, virulence factors and intracellular growth of *Mycobacterium avium* in AIDS. Res Microbiol 143:423, 1992.
466. Turk JL, Bryceson ADM: Immunological phenomena in leprosy and related diseases. Adv Immunol 13:209, 1971.
467. Meeran K: Prevalence of HIV infection among patients with leprosy and tuberculosis in rural Zambia. BMJ 298:364, 1989.
468. Borgdorff MW, vandenBroek J, Chum HJ, et al: HIV-1 infection as a risk factor for leprosy: A case–control study in Tanzania. Int J Lepr 61:556, 1993.
469. Kawuma HJS, Bwire R, Adatu-Engwau F: Leprosy and infection with the human immunodeficiency virus in Uganda: A case control study. Int J Lepr 62:521, 1994.
470. Vreeburg AEM: Clinical observations on leprosy patients with HIV-1 infection in Zambia. Lepr Rev 63:134, 1992.
471. Shiv Raj L, Patil SA, Girdhar A, et al: Antibodies to HIV-1 in sera from patients with mycobacterial infections. Int J Lepr 56:546, 1988.
472. Nuti M, deFelici A, vonAxel-Castrelli I, et al: False HIV positivity in leprosy (abstract). Int J Lepr 57:S366, 1989.
473. Pereira GA, Stefani MM, Araujo Filho JA, et al: Human immunodeficiency virus type 1 (HIV-1) *and Mycobacterium lepra* co-infection: HIV-1 subtypes and clinical, immunologic, and histopathologic profiles in a Brazilian cohort. Am J Trop Med Hyg 71:679, 2004.
474. Couppie P, Abel S, Voinchet H, et al: Immune reconstitution inflammatory syndrome associated with HIV and leprosy. Arch Dermatol 140:997, 2004.
475. Pignatoaro P, Rocha a Ada S, Nery JA: Leprosy and AIDS: Two cases of increasing inflammatory reactions at the start of highly active antiretroviral therapy. Eur J Clin Microbiol Infect Dis 23:408, 2004.
476. Böttger EC: *Mycobacterium genavense:* An emerging pathogen. Eur J Clin Microbiol Infect Dis 13:932, 1994.
477. Dumonceau J-M, Fonteyne P-A, Realini L, et al: Species-specific *Mycobacterium genavense* DNA in intestinal tissues of individuals not infected with HIV. J Clin Microbiol 33:2514, 1995.

478. Hillebrand-Haverkort ME, Kolk AH, Kox LF, et al: Generalized *Mycobacterium genavense* infection in HIV-infected patients: Detection of the mycobacterium in hospital tap water. Scand J Infect Dis 31:63, 1999.
479. Perchère M, Opravil M, Wald A, et al: Clinical and epidemiologic features of infection with *Mycobacterium genavense.* Arch Intern Med 155:400, 1995.
480. Albrecht H, Rüsch-Gerdes S, Stellbrink H, et al: Disseminated *Mycobacterium genavense* infection as a cause of pseudo-Whipple's disease and sclerosing cholangitis. Clin Infect Dis 25:742, 1997.
481. Gaynor CD, Clark RA, Koontz FP, et al: Disseminated *Mycobacterium genavense* infection in two patients with AIDS. Clin Infect Dis 18:455, 1994.
482. Monill JM, Franquet T, Sambeat MA, et al: *Mycobacterium genavense* infection in AIDS: Imaging findings in eight patients. Eur Radiol 11:193, 2001.
483. Bessesen MT, Shlay J, Stone-Venohr B, et al: Disseminated *Mycobacterium genavense* infection: Clinical and microbiological features and response to therapy. AIDS 7:1357, 1993.
484. Matsioka-Bernard P, Ghierry D, deTruchis P, et al: *Mycobacterium genavense* infection in a patient with AIDS who was successfully treated with clarithromycin. Clin Infect Dis 20:1565, 1995.
485. Horsburgh CR Jr, Selik RM: The epidemiology of disseminated nontuberculous *Mycobacterium* infection in AIDS. Am Rev Respir Dis 139:4, 1989.
486. Corbett EL, Blumberg L, Churchyard GJ, et al: Nontuberculous mycobacteria: Defining disease in a prospective cohort of South African miners. Am J Respir Crit Care Med 160:15, 1999.
487. Canueto-Quintero J, Callero-Granado J, Herrero-Romero M, et al: Epidemiological, clinical, and prognostic differences between the diseases caused by *Mycobacterium kansasii* and *Mycobacterium tuberculosis* in patients infected with human immunodeficiency virus: A multicenter study. Clin Infect Dis 37:584, 2003.
488. Levine B, Chaisson RE: *Mycobacterium kansasii:* A cause of treatable pulmonary disease associated with advanced HIV infection. Ann Intern Med 114:861, 1991.
489. Campo RE, Campo CE: *Mycobacterium kansasii* disease in patients infected with HIV. Clin Infect Dis 24:1233, 1997.
490. Witzig RS, Fazal BA, Mera RM, et al: Clinical manifestations and implications of co-infection with *Mycobacterium kansasii* and HIV type 1. Clin Infect Dis 21:77, 1995.
491. Manfredi R, Nanetti A, Valenti R, et al: Epidemiological, clinical and therapeutic features of AIDS-related *Mycobacterium kansasii* infection during the HIV pandemic: An 11-year follow-up study. HIV Med 5:431, 2004.
492. Carpenter JL, Parks JM: *Mycobacterium kansasii* infections in patients positive for HIV. Rev Infect Dis 13:789, 1991.
493. Zaugg M, Salfinger M, Opravil M, et al: Extrapulmonary and disseminated infections due to *Mycobacterium malmoense:* Case report and review. Clin Infect Dis 16:540, 1993.
494. Fakih M, Chapalamadugu S, Ricart A, et al: *Mycobacterium malmoense* bacteremia in two AIDS patients. J Clin Microbiol 34:731, 1996.
495. Banks J, Jenkins PA, Smith AP: Pulmonary infection with *Mycobacterium malmoense*—A review of treatment and response. Tubercle 66:197, 1985.
496. Saubolle MA, Kiehn TE, White MH, et al: *Mycobacterium haemophilum:* Microbiology and expanding clinical and geographic spectra of disease in humans. Clin Microbiol Rev 9:435, 1996.
497. Kristjansson M, Bieluch VM, Byeff PD: *Mycobacterium haemophilum* infection in immunocompromised patients: Case report and review of the literature. Rev Infect Dis 13:906, 1991.
498. Kiehn TE, White M: *Mycobacterium haemophilum:* An emerging pathogen. Eur J Clin Microbiol Infect Dis 13:925, 1994.
499. Soubani AO, al-Marri M, Forlenza S: Successful treatment of disseminated *Mycobacterium haemophilum* infection in a patient with AIDS (letter). Clin Infect Dis 18:475, 1994.
500. Paech V, Lorenzen T, von Krosigk A, et al: Remission of cutaneous *Mycobacterium haemophilum* infection as a result of antiretroviral therapy in a human immunodeficiency virus-infected patient. Clin Infect Dis 34:1017, 2002.
501. Lambert GW, Baddour LM: Right middle lobe syndrome caused by *Mycobacterium fortuitum* in a patient with HIV infection. South Med J 85:767, 1992.
502. Smith MB, Schnadiz VJ, Boyars, et al: Clinical and pathologic features of *Mycobacterium fortuitum* infections: An emerging pathogen in patients with AIDS. Am J Clin Pathol 116:225, 2001.
503. Smith MB, Boyars MC, Woods GL: Fatal *Mycobacterium fortuitum* meningitis in a patient with AIDS. Clin Infect Dis 23:1327, 1996.
504. Lambertus MW, Mathisen GE: *Mycobacterium marinum* infection in a patient with cryptosporidiosis and AIDS. Cutis 42:38, 1988.
505. Tchornobay A-M, Claudy AL, Perrot J-I, et al: Fatal disseminated *Mycobacterium marinum* infection. Int J Dermatol 31:286, 1992.
506. Tortoli E, Piersimoni C, Bacosi D, et al: Isolation of the newly described species *Mycobacterium celatum* from AIDS patients. J Clin Microbiol 33:137, 1995.
507. Piersimoni C, Tortoli E, deLalla F, et al: Isolation of *Mycobacterium celatum* from patients infected with HIV. Clin Infect Dis 24:144, 1997.
508. Jiva TM, Jacoby HM, Weymouth LA, et al: *Mycobacterium xenopi:* Innocent bystander or emerging pathogen? Clin Infect Dis 24:226, 1997.
509. Kerkiriou L, Ustianowski A, Johnson MA, et al: Human immunodeficiency virus type 1-related pulmonary *Mycobacterium xenopi* infection: A need to treat? Clin Infect Dis 37:1250, 2003.
510. Gazzola L, Cesari M, Slaerno F, et al: Clinical and therapeutic management of pulmonary *Mycobacterium xenopi* infection in HIV-positive patients. Clin Infect Dis 38:1642, 2004.
511. Barber TW, Craven DE, Farber HW: *Mycobacterium gordonae:* A possible opportunistic respiratory tract pathogen in patients with advanced HIV, type 1 infection. Chest 100:716, 1991.
512. Weinberger M, Berg SL, Feuerstein IM, et al: Disseminated infection with *Mycobacterium gordonae:* Report of a case and critical review of the literature. Clin Infect Dis 14:1229, 1992.
513. Rusconi S, Gori A, Vago L, et al: Cutaneous infection caused by *Mycobacterium gordonae* in a human immunodeficiency virus-infected patient receiving antimycobacterial treatment. Clin Infect Dis 25:1490, 1997.
514. Sanders JW, Walsh AD, Snider RL, et al: Disseminated *Mycobacterium scrofulaceum* infection: A potentially treatable complication of AIDS. Clin Infect Dis 20:549, 1995.
515. Huminer D, Dux S, Smara Z, et al: *Mycobacterium simiae* infection in Israeli patients with AIDS. Clin Infect Dis 17:508, 1993.
516. Anonymous: Disseminated infection with *simiae–avium* group mycobacteria in persons with AIDS—Thailand and Malawi, 1997. MMWR 51:501, 2002.
517. Allen S: Buruli ulcer and HIV infection. Int J Dermatol 31:7445, 2002.
518. Johnson RC, Ifebe D, Hans-Moevi A, et al: Disseminated *Mycobacterium ulcerans* disease in an HIV-positive patient: A case study. AIDS 16:1704, 2002.
519. Musher DM: Syphilis, neurosyphilis, penicillin, and AIDS. J Infect Dis 163:1201, 1991.
520. Gordon SM, Eaton ME, George R, et al: The response of symptomatic neurosyphilis to high-dose intravenous penicillin G in patients with HIV infection. N Engl J Med 331:1469, 1994.
521. Katz DA, Berger JR, Duncan RC: Neurosyphilis. A comparative study of the effects of infection with HIV. Arch Neurol 50:243, 1993.
522. Schöfer H, Imhof M, Thoma-Greber E, et al: Active syphilis in HIV infection: A multicentre retrospective survey. Genitourin Med 72:176, 1996.
523. Johns DR, Mierney M, Felsenstein D: Alteration in the natural history of neurosyphilis by concurrent infection with HIV. N Engl J Med 316:1569, 1987.
524. Musher DM, Hamill RJ, Baughn RE: Effect of HIV infection on the course of syphilis and on the response to treatment. Ann Intern Med 113:872, 1990.
525. Telzak EE, Greenberg MSZ, Harrison J, et al: Syphilis treatment response in HIV-infected individuals. AIDS 5:591, 1991.
526. Malone JL, Wallace MR, Hendrick BB, et al: Syphilis and neurosyphilis in a HIV type-1 seropositive population: Evidence for frequent serologic relapse after therapy. Am J Med 99:55, 1995.
527. Yinnon AM, Coury-Coniger P, Polito R, et al: Serologic response to treatment of syphilis in patients with HIV infection. Arch Intern Med 156:321, 1996.
528. Lukehart SA, Hood EW III, Baker-Zander SA, et al: Invasion of the central nervous system by *Treponema pallidum:* Implications for diagnosis and treatment. Ann Intern Med 109:855, 1988.
529. Gourevitch MN, Selwyn PA, Davenny K, et al: Effects of HIV infection on the serologic manifestations and response to treatment of syphilis in intravenous drug users. Ann Intern Med 118:350, 1993.

530. Goeman J, Kivuvu M, Nzila N, et al: Similar serologic response to conventional therapy for syphilis among HIV-positive and HIV-negative women. Genitourin Med 71:275, 1995.
531. Rolfs RT, Joesoef MR, Hendershot EF, et al: A randomized trial of enhanced therapy for early syphilis in patients with and without HIV infection. N Engl J Med 337:307, 1997.
532. Lynn WA, Lightman S: Syphilis and HIV: A dangerous combination. Lancet Infect Dis 4:456, 2004.
533. Sexually transmitted diseases treatment guidelines—2002. MMWR 51:1, 2002. www.cdc.gov/mmwr/preview/mmwrhtml/rr5106a1.htm.
534. Noordhoek GT, vanEmbden JDA: Yaws, an endemic treponematosis reconsidered in the HIV era. Eur J Clin Microbiol Infect Dis 10:4, 1991.
535. Garcia-Monco JC, Frey HM, Villar BF, et al: Lyme disease concurrent with HIV infection. Am J Med 87:325, 1989.
536. Cordolani F, Vignon-Pennamen MD, Assous MV: Atypical Lyme borreliosis in an HIV-infected man. Br J Dermatol 137:437, 1997.
537. daSilva MV, Batista L, Camargo ED, et al: Leptospirosis in patients with anti-HIV antibodies: Report of 2 cases. Rev Soc Bras Med Trop 23:229, 1990.
538. Neves Ede S, Pereira MM, Galhardo MC, et al: Leptospirosis patient with AIDS: The first case reported. Rev Soc Bras Med Trop 27:39, 1994.
539. Kazar J: Immunity in Q fever. Acta Virol 32:358, 1988.
540. Heard SR, Ronalds CJ, Heath RB: *Coxiella burnetii* infection in immunocompromised patients. J Infect 11:15, 1985.
541. Raoult D, Brouqui P, Marchou B, et al: Acute and chronic Q fever in patients with cancer. Clin Infect Dis 14:127, 1992.
542. Brouqui P, Dupont HT, Drancourt M, et al: Chronic Q fever. Ninety-two cases from France, including 27 cases without endocarditis. Arch Intern Med 153:642, 1993.
543. Raoult D, Levy P-Y, duPont JT, et al: Q fever and HIV infection. AIDS 7:81, 1993.
544. Bélec L, Ekala MT, Gilquin J: *Coxiella burnetii* infection among HIV-1-infected people living in Paris, France (letter). AIDS 7:1136, 1993.
545. Bélec L, Grésenguet G, Ekala MT, et al: *Coxiella burnetii* infection among subjects infected with HIV type 1 in the Central African Republic. Eur J Microbiol Infect Dis 12:775, 1993.
546. Montes M, Cilla G, Marimon J, et al: *Coxiella burnetii* infection in subjects with HIV infection and HIV infection in patients with Q fever. Scand J Infect Dis 27:344, 1995.
547. Boschini A, Di Perri G, Legnani D, et al: Consecutive epidemics of Q fever in a residential facility for drug abusers: Impact on persons with human immunodeficiency virus infection. Clin Infect Dis 28:866, 1999.
548. Uhaa IJ, Maclean JD, Breene CR, et al: A case of human ehrlichiosis acquired in Mali: Clinical and laboratory findings. Am J Trop Med Hyg 46:161, 1992.
549. Paddock CD, Folk SM, Shore GM, et al: Infections with *Ehrlichia chaffeensis* and *Ehrlichia ewingii* in persons co-infected with human immunodeficiency virus. Clin Infect Dis 33:1586, 2001.
550. Paddock CD, Suchard DP, Grumbach KL: Fatal seronegative ehrlichiosis in a patient with HIV infection. N Engl J Med 329:1164, 1993.
551. Buller RS, Arens M, Hmiel SP, et al: *Ehrlichia ewingii*, a newly recognized agent of human ehrlichiosis. N Engl J Med 341:148, 1999.
552. Bakken JS, Dumler JS, Chen SM, et al: Human granulocytic ehrlichiosis in the upper Midwest United States: A new species emerging? JAMA 272:212, 1994.
553. Kantipong P, Watt G, Jongsakul K, et al: Infection with human immunodeficiency virus does not influence the clinical severity of scrub typhus. Clin Infect Dis 23:1168, 1996.
554. Oksenhendler E, Morinière B, Rouveix E: Brucellosis in hairy cell leukaemia. Trans R Soc Trop Med Hyg 82:336, 1988.
555. Raziuddin S, Bilal N, Benjamin B: Transient T cell abnormality in a selective IgM-immunodeficient patient with *Brucella* infection. Clin Immunol Immunopathol 46:360, 1988.
556. Paul J, Gilks C, Batchelor B, et al: Serological responses to brucellosis in HIV-seropositive patients. Trans R Soc Trop Med Hyg 89:228, 1995.
557. Pedro-Botet J, Coll J, Auguet T, et al: Brucellosis and HIV infection: A casual association? (letter) AIDS 6:1039, 1992.
558. Galle C, Struelens M, Leisnard C, et al: *Brucella melitensis* osteitis following craniotomy in a patient with AIDS. Clin Infect Dis 24:1012, 1997.
559. Moreno S, Ariza J, Espinosa FJ, et al: Brucellosis in patients infected with the human immunodeficiency virus. Eur Clin Microbiol Infect Dis 17:319, 1998.
560. Ibarra V, Blanco JR, Metola L, et al: Relapsing brucellosis in a patient infected with the human immunodeficiency virus (HIV). Clin Microbiol Infect 9:1259, 2003.
561. Tanphaichitra D: Tropical disease in the immunocompromised host: Melioidosis and pythiosis. Rev Infect Dis 11(suppl 7):S1629, 1989.
562. Kanai K, Kurata T, Akksilp S, et al: A preliminary survey for human immunodeficiency virus (HIV) infections and melioidosis patients in Ubon Tatchathani, Thailand. J Med Sci Biol 45:247, 1992.
563. Kityaporn D, Tansuphaswadikul S, Kohsomboon P, et al: Survival of AIDS patients in the emerging epidemic in Bangkok, Thailand. J Acquir Immune Defic Syndr Hum Retrovirol 11:77, 1996.
564. Chierakul W, Rajanumong A, Wuthiekanum V, et al: The changing pattern of bloodstream infection associated with the rise in HIV prevalence in northern Thailand. Trans R Soc Trop Med Hyg 98:678, 2004.
565. Angulo FJ, Swerdlow DL: Bacterial enteric infections in persons infected with human immunodeficiency virus. Clin Infect Dis 21(suppl 1):584, 1995.
566. Giannella RA, Broitman SA, Zamcheck N: Influence of gastric acidity on bacterial and parasitic enteric infections. A perspective. Ann Intern Med 78:271, 1973.
567. Lake-Bakaar G, Quadros E, Beidas S, et al: Gastric secretory failure in patients with the acquired immunodeficiency syndrome (AIDS). Ann Intern Med 109:502, 1988.
568. Perry RT, Plowe CV, Koumare B, et al: A single dose of live oral cholera vaccine CVD 103-HgR is safe and immunogenic in HIV-infected and HIV-noninfected adults in Mali. Bull World Health Organ 76:63, 1998.
569. Kipp W, Kamugisha J, Rehle T: Meningococcal meningitis and HIV infection: Results from a case-control study in western Uganda. AIDS 6:1557, 1992.
570. Stephens DS, Hajjeh RA, Baughman WS, et al: Sporadic meningococcal disease in adults: Results of a 5-year population-based study. Ann Int Med 123:937, 1995.
571. Couldwell DL: Invasive meningococcal disease and HIV co-infection. Commun Dis Intell 25:278, 2001.
572. Regnery RL, Childs JE, Koehler JE: Infections associated with *Bartonella* species in persons infected with human immunodeficiency virus. Clin Infect Dis 21(suppl 1):S94, 1995.
573. Okhuysen PC, Crane JK, Pappas J: St. Louis encephalitis in patients with human immunodeficiency virus infection. Clin Infect Dis 17:140, 1993.
574. Wasay M, Diaz-Arrastia R, Suss RA, et al: St. Louis encephalitis: A review of 11 cases in a 1995 Dallas, Texas epidemic. Arch Neurol 57:114, 2000.
575. Monath TP, Cetron MS: Prevention of yellow fever in persons traveling to the tropics. Clin Infect Dis 34:1369, 2002.
576. Szilak I, Minamoto GY: West Nile viral encephalitis in an HIV-positive woman in New York. N Engl J Med 342:59, 2000.
577. Watt G, Kantipong P, Jongsakul K: Decrease in human immunodeficiency virus type 1 load during acute dengue fever. Clin Infect Dis 36:1067, 2003.
578. Eidex RS for the Yellow Fever Vaccine Safety Working Group: History of thymoma and yellow fever vaccination. Lancet 364:936, 2004.
579. Kengsakul K, Sathirapongsasuti K, Punyagupta S: Fatal myeloencephalitis following yellow fever vaccination in a case with HIV infection. J Med Assoc Thai 85:131, 2002.
580. Tattevin P, Departureaux G, Chapplain JM, et al: Yellow fever vaccine is safe and effective in HIV-infected patients. AIDS 18:825, 2004.
581. Receveur MC, Thiebaut R, Vedy S, et al: Yellow fever vaccination of human immunodeficiency virus-infected patients: Report of 2 cases. Clin Infect Dis 31:e7, 2000.
582. Goujon C, Touin M, Feuillie V, et al: Good tolerance and efficacy of yellow fever vaccination among carriers of human immunodeficiency virus. J Travel Med 2:145:1995.
583. Sibailly TS, Wiktor SZ, Tsai TF, et al: Poor antibody response to yellow fever vaccination in children. Pediatr Infect Dis J 16:1177, 1997.
584. Advisory Committee on Immunization Practices: Yellow fever vaccine: Recommendations of the Advisory Committee on Immunization Practices (ACIP), 2002. MMWR 51(RR-17):1, 2002.

585. Karp CL, Wysocka M, Wahl LM, et al: Mechanism of suppression of cell-mediated immunity by measles virus. Science 273:228, 1996.
586. Atabani SF, Byrnes AA, Jaye A, et al: Natural measles causes prolonged suppression of interleukin-12 production. J Infect Dis 184:1, 2001.
587. Schlender J, Schnorr JJ, Spielhofer P, et al: Interaction of measles virus glycoproteins with the surface of uninfected peripheral blood lymphocytes induces immunosuppression in vitro. Proc Natl Acad Sci USA 93:13194, 1996.
588. Marie JC, Kehren J, Trescol-Biemont MC, et al: Mechanism of measles virus-induced suppression of inflammatory immune responses. Immunity 14:69, 2001.
589. Slifka MK, Homann D, Tishon A, et al: Measles virus infection results in suppression of both innate and adaptive immune responses to secondary bacterial infection. J Clin Invest 111:805, 2003.
590. Markowitz LE, Chandler FW, Roldan EO, et al: Fatal measles pneumonia without rash in a child with AIDS. J Infect Dis 158:480, 1988.
591. Krasinski K, Borkowsky W: Measles and measles immunity in children infected with HIV. JAMA 251:2512, 1989.
592. Ross LA, Kim KS, Mason WH, et al: Successful treatment of disseminated measles in a patient with AIDS: Consideration of antiviral and passive immunotherapy (letter). Am J Med 88:313, 1990.
593. Nadel S, McGann K, Jokinka RL, et al: Measles giant cell pneumonia in a child with HIV infection. Pediatr Infect Dis J 10:542, 1991.
594. Kaplan LJ, Daum RS, Smaron M, et al: Severe measles in immunocompromised patients. JAMA 267:1237, 1992.
595. Palumbo P, Hoyt L, Demasio K, et al: Population-based study of measles and measles immunization in HIV-infected children. Pediatr Infect Dis J 11:1008, 1992.
596. Mustafa MM, Weitman SD, Winick NJ, et al: Subacute measles encephalitis in the young immunocompromised host: Report of two cases diagnosed by polymerase chain reaction and treated with ribavirin and review of the literature. Clin Infect Dis 16:654, 1993.
597. Stogner SW, King JW, Black-Payne C, et al: Ribavirin and intravenous immune globulin therapy for measles pneumonia in HIV infection. South Med J 86:1415, 1993.
598. Forni AL, Schluger NW, Roberts RB: Severe measles pneumonitis in adults: Evaluation of clinical characteristics and therapy with intravenous ribavirin. Clin Infect Dis 19:454, 1994.
599. laCroix C, Blanche S, Dussiax E, et al: Acute necrotizing measles encephalitis in a child with AIDS. J Neurol 242:249, 1995.
600. Sension MG, Quinn TC, Markowitz LE, et al: Measles in hospitalized African children with HIV (letter). Am J Dis Child 142:1271, 1988.
601. Oshitani H, Suzuki H, Mpabalwani ME, et al: Measles case fatality by sex, vaccination status, and HIV-1 antibody in Zambian children (letter). Lancet 348:415, 1996.
602. Moss WJ, Monze M, Ryon JJ, et al: Prospective study of measles in hospitalized human immunodeficiency virus (HIV)-infected and HIV-uninfected children in Zambia. Clin Infect Dis 35:189, 2002.
603. Permar SR, Moss WJ, Ryon JR: Prolonged measles virus shedding in human immunodeficiency virus-infected children, detected by reverse transcriptase-polymerase chain reaction. J Infect Dis 183:532, 2001.
604. Moss WJ, Ryon JR, Monze M: Suppression of human immunodeficiency virus replication during acute measles. J Infect Dis 185:1035, 2002.
605. Hussey GD, Klein M: A randomized, controlled trial of vitamin A in children with severe measles. N Engl J Med 323:160, 1990.
606. Banks G, Fernandez H: Clinical use of ribavirin in measles: A summarized review. In Smith RA, Knight V, Smith JAD (eds): Clinical Applications of Ribavirin. Orlando, Fla, Academic Press, 1984, p 203.
607. Advisory Committee on Immunization Practices: Update: Vaccine side effects, adverse reactions, contraindications, and precautions. Recommendations of the Advisory Committee on Immunization Practices (ACIP). MMWR 45:1, 1996.
608. Kay HEM, Rankin A: Immunoglobulin prophylaxis of measles in acute lymphoblastic leukaemia. Lancet 2:901, 1984.
609. Committee on Infectious Diseases and Committee of Pediatric AIDS, American Academy of Pediatrics: Measles immunization in HIV-infected children. Pediatrics 103:1057, 1999.
610. Centers for Disease Control and Prevention: Measles, mumps, and rubella—Vaccine use and strategies for elimination of measles, rubella, and congenital rubella syndrome and control of mumps: Recommendations of the Advisory Committee on Immunization Practices (ACIP). MMWR 47:1, 1998.
611. Sha BE, Harris AA, Benson CA, et al: Prevalence of measles antibodies in asymptomatic HIV-infected adults. J Infect Dis 164:973, 1991.
612. Kemper CA, Zolopa AR, Hamilton JR, et al: Prevalence of measles antibodies in adults with HIV infection: Possible risk factors of measles seronegativity. AIDS 6:1321, 1992.
613. Zolopa AR, Kemper CA, Shiboski S, et al: Progressive immunodeficiency due to infection with HIV does not lead to waning immunity to measles in a cohort of homosexual men. Clin Infect Dis 18:636, 1994.
614. Sprauer MA, Markowitz LE, Nicholson JKA, et al: Response of HIV-infected adults to measles-rubella vaccination. J Acquir Immune Defic Syndr Hum Retrovirol 6:1013, 1993.
615. Moss WJ, Clements CJ, Halsey NA: Immunization of children at risk of infection with human immunodeficiency virus. Bull World Health Org 81:61, 2003.
616. Embree JE, Datta P, Stackiw W, et al: Increased risk of early measles in infants of HIV type 1-seropositive mothers. J Infect Dis 165:262, 1992.
617. lePage P, Dabis F, Msellati P, et al: Safety and immunogenicity of high-dose Edmonston–Zagreb measles vaccine in children with HIV-1 infection. A cohort study in Kigali, Rwanda. Am J Dis Child 146:550, 1992.
618. Cutts FT, Mandala K, St. Louis M, et al: Immunogenicity of high-titer Edmonston–Zagreb measles vaccine in HIV-infected children in Kinshasa, Zaire. J Infect Dis 167:1418, 1993.
619. Moss WJ, Cutts F, Griffin DE: Implications of the human immunodeficiency virus epidemic for control and eradication of measles. Clin Infect Dis 29:106, 1999.
620. Anonymous: Measles pneumonitis following measles–mumps–rubella vaccination of a patient with HIV infection, 1993. MMWR 45:603, 1996.
621. Garenne M, Leroy O, Beau JP, et al: Child mortality after high-titre measles vaccines: Prospective study in Senegal. Lancet 338:903, 1991.
622. Aaby P, Knudsen K, Whittle H, et al: Long-term survival after Edmonston Zagreb measles vaccination in Guinea-Bissau: Increased female mortality rate. J Pediatr 122:904, 1993.
623. Holt EA, Moulton LH, Biberry GK, et al: Differential mortality by measles vaccine titer and sex. J Infect Dis 168:1087, 1993.
624. World Health Organization: HIV-infected children should be immunized against measles. World Health Forum 10:288, 1989.
625. Murphy D, Rose RC III: Respiratory syncytial virus pneumonia in a HIV-infected man (letter). JAMA 261:1147, 1989.
626. Chandwani S, Borkowsky W, Krasinski K, et al: Respiratory syncytial virus infection in HIV-infected children. J Pediatr 117:251, 1990.
627. Sriskandan S, Shaunak S: Respiratory syncytial virus infection in an adult with AIDS (letter). Clin Infect Dis 17:1065, 1993.
628. King JC, Burke AR, Clemens JD, et al: Respiratory syncytial virus illnesses in human immunodeficiency virus-infected and -noninfected children. Pediatr Infect Dis 12:733, 1993.
629. Adle Biassette H, Bourhy H, Gisselbrecht M, et al: Rabies encephalitis in a patient with AIDS: A clinicopathological study. Acta Neuropathol 92:415, 1996.
630. Jaijaroensup W, Tantawichen T, Khawplod P, et al: Postexposure rabies vaccination in patients infected with human immunodeficiency virus. Clin Infect Dis 28:913, 1999.
631. Thisyakorn U, Pancharoenn C, Ruxrungtham K, et al: Safety and immunogenicity of postexposure rabies vaccination in children infected with human immunodeficiency virus type 1. Clin Infect Dis 30:218, 2000.
632. Tantawichen T, Jaijaroensup W, Khawplod P, et al: Failure of multiple-site intradermal postexposure rabies vaccination in patients infected with human immunodeficiency virus with low CD4+ lymphocyte counts. Clin Infect Dis 33:e122, 2001.
633. Rabies vaccine: www.who.int/wer/pdf/2002/wer7714.pdf, 2004.
634. Prevots DR, Burr RK, Sutter RW, et al: Poliomyelitis prevention in the United States. Updated recommendations of the Advisory Committee on Immunization Practice (ACIP). MMWR 49:1, 2000.
635. Grohmann GS, Glass RI, Pereira HG, et al: Enteric viruses and diarrhea in HIV-infected patients. N Engl J Med 329:14, 1993.
636. Thea DM, Glass R, Grohmann, GS, et al: Prevalence of enteric viruses among hospital patients with AIDS in Kinshasa, Zaire. Trans R Soc Trop Med Hyg 87:263, 1993.
637. Cunliffe NA, Dove W, Gondwe JS, et al: Detection and characterization of human astroviruses in children with acute gastroenteritis in Blatyre, Malawi. J Med Virol 67:563, 2002.

638. Giordano MO, Martinez LC, Rinaldi D, et al: Detection of picobirnavirus in HIV-infected patients with diarrhea in Argentina. J Acquir Immune Defic Syndr Hum Retrovirol 18:380, 1998.
639. Shukry S, Zaki AM, duPont HL, et al: Detection of enteropathogens in fatal and potentially fatal diarrhea in Cairo, Egypt. J Clin Microbiol 24:959, 1986.
640. Cunliffe NA, Gondwe JS, Kirkwood CD, et al: Effect of concomitant HIV infection on presentation and outcome of rotavirus gastroenteritis in Malawian children. Lancet 358:550, 2001.
641. Ida S, Tachikawa N, Nakajima A, et al: Influence of human immunodeficiency virus type 1 infection on acute hepatitis A virus infection. Clin Infect Dis 34:379, 2002.
642. Fonquernie L, Meynard JL, Charrois A, et al: Occurrence of acute hepatitis A in patients infected with human immunodeficiency virus. Clin Infect Dis 32:297, 2001.
643. Setsuko I, Tachikawa N, Kikuchi Y, et al: Rate of subclinical hepatitis A virus infection in adult HIV-1-infected patients. Jpn J Infect Dis 54:31, 2001.
644. Bodsworth NJ, Neilsen GA, Donovan B: The effect of immunization with inactivated hepatitis A vaccine on the clinical course of HIV-1 infection: 1-year follow-up. AIDS 11:747, 1997.
645. Wallace MR, Brandt CJ, Earhart KC, et al: Safety and immunogenicity of an inactivated hepatitis A vaccine among HIV-infected subjects. Clin Infect Dis 39:1207, 2004.
646. Kemper CA, Haubrich R, Fran I, et al: Safety and immunogenicity of hepatitis A vaccine in human immunodeficiency virus-infected patients: A double-blind, randomized, placebo-controlled trial. J Infect Dis 187:1327, 2003.
647. Bodsworth NJ, Cooper DA, Donovan B: The influence of HIV type 1 infection on the development of the hepatitis B virus carrier state. J Infect Dis 163:1138, 1991.
648. Hadler SC, Judson FN, O'Malley PM, et al: Outcome of hepatitis B virus infection in homosexual men and its relationship to prior HIV infection. J Infect Dis 163:454, 1991.
649. Krogsgaard K, Lindhardt Bö, Nielsen JO, et al: The influence of HTLV-III infection on the natural history of hepatitis B virus infection in male homosexual HBsAg carriers. Hepatology 7:37, 1987.
650. Lazizi Y, Grangeot-Kedos L, delFraissy J-F, et al: Reappearance of hepatitis B virus in immune patients infected with HIV type 1. J Infect Dis 158:666, 1988.
651. Housset C, Pol S, Carnot F, et al: Interactions between human immunodeficiency virus and hepatitis B virus infections in 260 chronic carriers of hepatitis B virus. Hepatology 15:578, 1992.
652. Collier AC, Corey L, Murphy VL, et al: Antibody to HIV and suboptimal response to hepatitis B vaccination. Ann Intern Med 109:101, 1988.
653. Biggar RJ, Goedert JJ, Hoofnagle J: Accelerated loss of antibody to hepatitis B surface antigen among immunodeficient homosexual men infected with HIV (letter). N Engl J Med 316:630, 1987.
654. Thio CL, Seaberg EC, Skolasky R, et al: HIV-1, hepatitis B virus, and risk of liver-related mortality in the Multicenter Cohort Study (MACS). Lancet 360:1921, 2002.
655. Scharschmidt B, Held M, Hollander H, et al: Hepatitis B in patients with HIV infection: Relationship to AIDS and patient survival. Ann Intern Med 117:837, 1992.
656. Thomas DL, Astemborski J, Rai RM, et al: The natural history of hepatitis C virus infection: Host, viral, and environmental factors. JAMA 284:450, 2000.
657. Sulkowski MS, Thomas DL: Hepatitis C in the HIV-infected person. Ann Intern Med 138:197, 2003.
658. Eyster ME, Fried MW, diBisceglie AM, et al: Increasing hepatitis C virus RNA levels in hemophiliacs: Relationship to HIV infection and liver disease. Blood 84:1020, 1994.
659. Thomas DL, Shih JW, Alter HJ, et al: Effect of HIV on hepatitis C virus infection among injecting drug users. J Infect Dis 174:690, 1996.
660. Zanetti AR, Tanzi E, Paccagnini S, et al: Mother-to-infant transmission of hepatitis C virus. Lancet 345:289, 1995.
661. Eyster ME, Diamondstone LS, Lien J-M, et al: Natural history of hepatitis C virus infection in multitransfused hemophiliacs: Effect of co-infection with HIV. J Acquir Immune Defic Syndr Hum Retrovirol 6:602, 1993.
662. Soto B, Sánchez-Quijano A, Rodrigo L, et al: HIV infection modifies the natural history of chronic parenterally-acquired hepatitis C with an unusually rapid progression to cirrhosis. J Hepatol 26:1, 1997.
663. Piroth L, Duong M, Quantin C, et al: Does hepatitis C co-infection accelerate clinical and immunological evolution of HIV-infected patients? AIDS 12:381, 1998.
664. Greub G, Ledergerber B, Battegay M, et al: Clinical progression, survival, and immune recovery during antiretroviral therapy in patients with HIV-1 and hepatitis C virus co-infection: The Swiss HIV Cohort Study. Lancet 356:1800, 2000.
665. Sulkowski MS, Moore RD, Mehta SH, et al: Hepatitis C and progression of HIV disease. JAMA 288:199, 2002.
666. Staples CT Jr, Rimland D, Dudas D: Hepatitis C in the HIV Atlanta VA Cohort Study: The effect of co-infection on survival. Clin Infect Dis 29:150, 1999.
667. Chung RT, Evans SR, Yang Y, et al: Immune recovery is associated with persistent rise in hepatitis C virus RNA, infrequent liver test flares, and is not impaired by hepatitis C virus in co-infected subjects. AIDS 16:1915, 2002.
668. Hershow RC, Riester KA, Lew J, et al: Increased vertical transmission of HIV from hepatitis C virus-co-infected mothers. J Infect Dis 176:414, 1997.
669. Shattock AG, Finlay H, Hillary IB: Possible reactivation of hepatitis D with chronic antigenaemia by HIV. BMJ 294:1656, 1987.
670. Castillo I, Bartolomé J, Medejón A, et al: Hepatitis delta virus RNA detection in chronic HBsAg carriers with and without HIV infection. Digestion 48:149, 1991.
671. Colebunders R, Mann JM, Francis H, et al: Herpes zoster in African patients: A clinical predictor of human immunodeficiency virus infection. J Infect Dis 157:314, 1988.
672. van de Perre P, Bakkers E, Batungwanayo J, et al: Herpes zoster in African patients: An early manifestation of HIV infection. Scand J Infect Dis 20:277, 1988.
673. Krech U: Complement-fixing antibodies against cytomegalovirus in different parts of the world. Bull World Health Organ 49:103, 1973.
674. Kestelyn P: The epidemiology of CMV retinitis in Africa. Ocul Immunol Inflamm 7:173, 1999.
675. Grant AD, Kaplan JE, de Cock KM: Preventing opportunistic infections among human immunodeficiency virus-infected adults in African countries. Am J Trop Med Hyg 65:810, 2001.
676. Cathomas G: Kaposi's sarcoma-associated herpesvirus (KHHV)/human herpesvirus 8 (HHV-8) as a tumour virus. Herpes 10:72, 2003.
677. Dedicoat M, Newton R: Review of the distribution of Kaposi's sarcoma-associated herpesvirus (KHSV) in Africa in relation to the incidence of Kaposi's sarcoma. Br J Cancer 88:1, 2003.
678. Hengge UR, Ruzicka T, Tyring SK, et al: Update of Kaposi's sarcoma and other HHV8 associated diseases. Part 1: Epidemiology, environmental predispositions, clinical manifestations, and therapy. Lancet Infect Dis 2:281, 2002.
679. Henke-Gendo C, Schulz TF: Transmission and disease association of Kaposi's sarcoma-associated herpesvirus: Recent developments. Curr Opin Infect Dis 17:53, 2004.
680. Harper SA, Fukuda K, Uyeki TM, et al: Prevention and control of influenza. Recommendations of the Advisory Committee on Immunization Practices (ACIP). www.cdc.gov/mmwr/preview/mmwrhtml/rr53061.htm, 2004.
681. Tasker SA, O'Brien WA, Treanor JJ, et al: Effects of influenza vaccination in HIV-infected adults: A double-blind, placebo-controlled trial. Vaccine 16:1039, 1998.
682. Kroon FP, van Dissel JT, de Jong JC, et al: Antibody response after influenza vaccination in HIV-infected individuals: A consecutive 3-year study. Vaccine 18:3040, 2000.
683. Wong AT, Tsang OT, Wong MY, et al: Coronavirus infection in an AIDS patient. AIDS 18:829, 2004.
684. Smith KJ, Skelton HG, Drabick JJ, et al: Hypereosinophilia secondary to immunodysregulation in patients with HIV-1 disease. Arch Dermatol 130:119, 1994.
685. Cohen AJ, Steigbigel RT: Eosinophilia in patients infected with human immunodeficiency virus. J Infect Dis 174:615, 1996.
686. Skiest DJ, Keiser P: Clinical significance of eosinophilia in HIV-infected individuals. Am J Med 102:449, 1997.
687. May LP, Kelly J, Sanchez M: Hypereosinophilic syndrome with unusual cutaneous manifestations in two men with HIV infection. J Am Acad Dermatol 23:202, 1990.
688. Drabick JJ, Magill AJ, Smith KJ, et al: Hypereosinophilic syndrome associated with HIV infection. South Med J 87:525, 1994.

689. Paganelli R, Scala E, Mezzaroma I, et al: Immunologic aspects of hyperimmunoglobulinemia E-like syndrome in patients with AIDS. J Allergy Clin Immunol 95:995, 1995.
690. Mayo J, Collazos J, Martinez E, et al: Acute eosinophilic pneumonia in a patient infected with the human immunodeficiency virus. Tuber Lung Dis 76:77, 1995.
691. Samoszuk M, Ravel J, Ramzi E: Epstein–Barr virus and interleukin-5 mRNA in acquired immunodeficiency syndrome-related lymphomas with eosinophilia. Hum Pathol 23:1355, 1992.
692. Scharnbelan M, Grumfeld C: Endocrine abnormalities associated with HIV infection and AIDS. In Broder S, Merigan TC, Bolognesi D (eds): Textbook of AIDS Medicine. Baltimore, Williams & Wilkins, 1994, p 629.
693. Colebunders R, Van Den Eynde C, Tolo A, et al: Eosinophilia in patients infected with human immunodeficiency virus. J Infect Dis 174:615, 1997.
694. Bacot BK, Paul ME, Navarro M, et al: Objective measures of allergic disease in children with human immunodeficiency virus infection. J Allergy Clin Immunol 100:707, 1997.
695. Onorato J, Esposito S, Scovena E, et al: Eosinophil involvement and serum IgE level in HIV-1-infected children. J Allergy Clin Immunol 104:245, 1999.
696. Ledru E, Diagbouga S, Tranchot-Diallo J, et al: Eosinophils: A putative marker of immunodepression in HIV-infected African patients with tuberculosis? Trans R Soc Trop Med Hyg 88:117, 1994.
697. Diagbouga S, Aldebert D, Fumoux F, et al: Relationship between interleukin-5 production and variations in eosinophil counts during HIV infection in West Africa: Influence of *Mycobacterium tuberculosis* infection. Scand J Immunol 49:203, 1999.
698. Chorba TL, Nkengasong J, TH Roels, et al: Assessing eosinophil count as a marker of immune activation among human immunodeficiency virus-infected persons in sub-Saharan Africa. Clin Infect Dis 34:1264, 2002.
699. Fernando R, Miller R: Immune reconstitution eosinophilia due to schistosomiasis. Sex Transm Infect 78:76, 2002.
700. Fischl MA, Dickinson GM, laVoie L: Safety and efficacy of sulfamethoxazole and trimethoprim chemoprophylaxis for *Pneumocystis carinii* pneumonia in AIDS. JAMA 259:1185, 1988.
701. Pierce M, Crampton S, Henry D, et al: A randomized trial of clarithryomycin as prophylaxis against disseminated *Mycobacterium avium* complex infection in patients with advanced acquired immunodeficiency syndrome. N Engl J Med 335:384, 1996.
702. Mocroft A, Vella S, Benfield TL, et al: Changing patterns of mortality across Europe in patients infected with HIV-1. EuroSIDA Study Group. Lancet 352:1725, 1998.
703. Grimwade K, Swingler G: Cotrimoxazole prophylaxis for opportunistic infections in adults with HIV. Cochrane Database Syst Rev 3:CD003108, 2003.
704. Feikin DR, Feldman C, Schuchat A, et al: Global strategies to prevent bacterial pneumonia in adults with HIV disease. Lancet Infect Dis 4:445:2004.
705. Mwaungulu FBD, Floyd S, Crampin AC, et al: Cotrimoxazole prophylaxis reduces mortality in human immunodeficiency virus-positive tuberculosis patients in Karonga District, Malawi. Bull World Health Org 82:354, 2004.
706. Chintu C, Bhat GJ, Walker AS, et al: Co-trimoxazole as prophylaxis against opportunistic infections in HIV-infected Zambian children (CHAP): A double-blind randomised placebo-controlled trial. Lancet 364:1865, 2004.
707. WHO/UNAIDS: Provisional WHO/UNAIDS Secretariat recommendations on the use of cotrimoxazole prophylaxis in adults and children living with HIV/AIDS in Africa. www.unaids.org/EN/other/functionalities/Search.asp, 2004.
708. WHO/UNAIDS/UNICEF: Joint WHO/UNAIDS/UNICEF statement on use of cotrimoxazole as prophylaxis in HIV exposed and HIV infected children. www.who.int/entity/3by5/mediacentre/en/Cotrimstatement.pdf, 2004.
709. Gill CJ, Sabin LL, Tham J, et al: Reconsidering empirical cotrimoxazole prophylaxis for infants exposed to HIV infection. Bull World Health Org 82:290, 2004.
710. French N, Nakiyingi J, Carpenter LM, et al: 23-Valent pneumococcal polysaccharide vaccine in HIV-1-infected Ugandan adults: Double-blind, randomised and placebo controlled trial. Lancet 355:2106, 2000.
711. Kemper CA, Linett A, Kane C, et al: Travels with HIV: The compliance and health of HIV-infected adults who travel. Int J STD AIDS 8:44, 1997.
712. Mulhall BP: Sex and travel: Studies of sexual behaviour, disease and health promotion in international travellers—A global review. Int J STD AIDS 7:455, 1996.
713. Matteelli A, Carosi G: Sexually transmitted diseases in travelers. Clin Infect Dis 32:1063, 2001.
714. Karp CL: Preparation of the HIV-infected traveler to the tropics. Curr Infect Dis Rep 3:50, 2000.
715. Colebunders R, Nachega J, Van Gompel A: Antiretroviral treatment and travel to developing countries. J Travel Med 6:27, 1999.
716. Centers for Disease Control and Prevention: Preventing cryptosporidiosis: A guide to water filters and bottled water. www.cdc.gov/ncidod/parasites.cryptosporidiosis/factsht_crypto_preventwter.htm, 2004.
717. McKinsey DS, Wheat LJ, Cloud GA, et al: Itraconazole prophylaxis for fungal infections in patients with advanced human immunodeficiency virus infection: Randomized, placebo-controlled, double-blind study. Clin Infect Dis 28:1049, 1999.

134

Travel-Related Health Concerns Associated with Extremes of Environment

DAVID A. BOBAK
PAUL S. AUERBACH

INTRODUCTION

In addition to a variety of infectious diseases confronting travelers to tropical areas, there are other health concerns that can arise from exposure to the environment. Without adequate preventive measures, a traveler may develop a serious illness or exacerbation of an underlying medical problem. In this chapter, we address certain travel-related health disorders caused by extremes or changes in the environment.

HEAT-RELATED ILLNESS

Background

In most circumstances, humans are extremely tolerant of heat, an attribute most likely reflecting the common evolutionary origin of our species from tropical Africa. However, on exposure to excessively hot and humid conditions, unacclimatized people or people with certain underlying medical problems can be especially prone to develop serious heat-related illnesses, such as heatstroke. Furthermore, despite dramatic improvements in cooling methods used for the treatment of heatstroke, there has been little real decrease in mortality or morbidity due to this illness in the past few decades.[1] For these reasons, understanding the basic principles of prevention, diagnosis, and management of heat-related illness is important for health-care providers who offer pretravel counsel or onsite care to travelers to tropical countries.

Health disturbances related to heat are conveniently, although somewhat arbitrarily, divided into minor disorders, such as prickly heat, heat cramps, heat edema, heat syncope, and heat exhaustion, and the much more severe disorder known as heatstroke. Heatstroke is further categorized into "classic" and so-called exertional forms based primarily on epidemiologic criteria.[1–7] The clinical descriptions of the common heat disorders are discussed in this chapter as relatively discrete clinical entities, but in reality these distinctions are frequently blurred and heat-exposed patients may present with multiple or mixed syndromes.

Thermoregulation

Core body temperature is the net result of a variety of internal and external factors, each working to increase or lower body temperature. This observation is clinically relevant; for example, the most important pathophysiologic defect underlying the development of the life-threatening disorder of heatstroke is the loss of the body's ability to maintain normal thermoregulation.[1–3,7] Humans have internal homeostatic mechanisms that normally act to preserve a preset equilibrium between heat production and heat loss. By this means, body temperature is maintained within a relatively narrow temperature range. Net heat production results from the heat absorbed from external sources and that generated from internal metabolic processes.

The major mechanisms of heat transfer in humans include radiation, conduction, convection, and evaporation.[2,4,6] Radiation is the process of heat transfer via electromagnetic waves. A person placed in an environment in which the air temperature is lower than the body temperature will lose heat predominantly by radiation. In contrast, a person placed in an environment in which the air temperature is much greater than the body's temperature will actually gain heat by the same process of radiation. In the process of conduction, heat is transferred directly from warmer to cooler objects by physical contact. In normal circumstances, only a small amount of heat loss from the body occurs by conduction. However, if a person is immersed in cool water, heat loss by conduction is markedly increased, a phenomenon that has therapeutic implications for the treatment of heatstroke. Convection is the loss of heat into the molecules of air and water vapor circulating around an object. In this way, heat is dissipated into moving, cooler air passing over a warmer object such as a person's body. As might be expected, the efficiency of heat loss by convection is dramatically influenced by both wind speed and air temperature.

Finally, heat is lost when a liquid is converted into a gas, a process known as evaporation. Evaporation is an extremely important mechanism for heat loss in humans, especially for people exposed to a high ambient temperature. When the ambient temperature exceeds 35°C (95°F), almost all of a person's heat loss occurs by evaporation. The efficiency of evaporation is influenced considerably by the level of ambient humidity. As humidity increases (particularly above 75%), the efficacy of evaporation decreases markedly. This is the reason why even a profusely sweating person will lose little heat under conditions of high ambient humidity.

Predisposing Factors

Loss of normal thermoregulation is caused by a combination of several factors: excessive exogenous heat gain, increased endogenous heat production, decreased heat loss, or a combination of these.[1–4,6] Excessive exogenous heat gain typically occurs when a person enters an environment of high ambient temperature and high humidity. Endogenous heat production can be increased by exertion, pharmacologic agents, or clinical syndromes such as febrile illnesses, seizures, and hyperthyroidism. In a cyclic fashion, endogenous heat production can increase basal metabolism and generate increased endogenous heat. Tricyclic antidepressants, amphetamines, cocaine, and phencyclidine are examples of drugs that can induce hyperthermia through an increase or dysregulation of muscular activity.[7] Sympathomimetic drugs can also cause hyperthermia, probably by altering hepatic metabolism.[7]

A variety of other factors can serve to impair the body's ability to dissipate heat.[1–4,6] Dehydration and volume depletion are important risk factors for hyperthermia. These factors cause decreased sweating and alter the compensatory cardiovascular responses normally triggered by hyperthermia. For these same reasons, people with significant cardiovascular disease are also at increased risk of heat-related illness. Because the major cooling mechanisms of the body use the cutaneous vascular system, abnormal regulation of blood flow can dramatically inhibit the efficacy of heat loss. Examples of conditions that result in circulatory inefficiency include congestive heart failure, atherosclerotic coronary vascular disease, and peripheral vascular disease, as well as ingestion of medications that may alter cardiovascular function (e.g., diuretics, β-blockers, and calcium channel blockers). In addition to being at greater risk of acquiring heat illness, patients with circulatory insufficiency are also at higher risk of developing heat stress–induced medical illnesses, such as myocardial infarction, congestive heart failure, cardiac dysrhythmias, and stroke.

Patients with significant abnormalities of the skin, such as scleroderma, or metabolic diseases, such as cystic fibrosis, have a defect in heat dispersion efficiency and are also at higher risk of developing heat-related illness.[2,6,8] Obese people have several factors that increase their risk of heat-related illness: ineffective heat dispersion because of increased insulation, a large surface area-to-mass ratio, and impaired cardiovascular conditioning. In addition, acute and chronic alcohol use are associated with an increased susceptibility to heat illness. The ingestion of alcohol impairs recognition of heat stress, inhibits normal compensatory behavioral responses, causes peripheral vascular dilation, and inhibits antidiuretic hormone.

Finally, it is important to recognize that infants and the elderly are particularly susceptible to heat-related illness. Normal thermal regulatory and sweating mechanisms are underdeveloped in neonates and infants. In addition, children have a larger surface area-to-mass ratio, sweat less, and have a higher metabolism than adults—all factors that can inhibit effective heat loss.[5,9] Many factors have been identified to explain the predisposition of the elderly to heat illness: relative cardiovascular inefficiency, reduced sweat production, lessened physical conditioning, a higher likelihood of underlying cardiovascular disease, and increased use of drugs that may interfere with cardiovascular or sweating responses to heat.

Minor Heat-Related Disorders

Prickly Heat. Prickly heat, or heat rash, is a maculopapular, pruritic, and erythematous rash that most commonly appears over clothed areas of the body.[6,10] Prickly heat occurs when sweat pores are blocked, leading to inflammation of the sweat ducts. The predominant clinical feature of this condition is intense itching. Effective treatment involves exposing the rash to cool, dry air and the administration of antihistamines. Prickly heat can frequently be prevented by wearing loose-fitting clothing. Complications of prolonged heat rash can include secondary cutaneous infections (most commonly with *Staphylococcus aureus*) or the development of chronic dermatitis.

Heat Cramps. Heat cramps are caused by involuntary and painful contraction of skeletal muscles.[4,6,11–13] The muscles most frequently affected are those that are most commonly used, such as the musculature of the shoulders, thighs, and calves. Heat cramps usually occur when physically unfit or heat-unacclimatized people exercise in a hot environment. Clinically, patients with this disorder generally present with acute and severe muscle pain. Importantly, the patient's temperature and other vital signs are usually normal. How heat cramps occur is not exactly known, but the pathophysiology likely involves disordered fluid and electrolyte balance at the level of the individual muscles. The risk of developing heat cramps appears to be increased in people who combine prolonged exercise in a hot environment with hypotonic fluid (e.g., water) replacement. In rare instances, a patient may exhibit evidence of heat- and exertion-induced rhabdomyolysis. With rhabdomyolysis, muscle pain is generally out of proportion to the other physical findings observed on physical examination. Laboratory investigation (e.g., urinalysis and muscle enzyme levels) is needed to clearly differentiate the serious disorder of heat-induced rhabdomyolysis from the benign disorder of heat cramps.

Heat cramps are generally benign and generally respond to massage, rest, and rehydration. For mild cases, treatment consists of massage and oral rehydration with a 0.1% or 0.2% saline solution or one of many commercially available electrolyte drinks. For severe cases, intravenous rehydration with normal saline solution can provide dramatic resolution of symptoms. When physical exertion in a hot environment is anticipated, maintaining adequate hydration will frequently prevent heat cramps. Fluid replacement with water alone appears to be satisfactory for mild to moderate exercise of short duration (30 minutes or less). With vigorous exercise for longer time periods, or in an extremely hot and humid setting, an appropriate electrolyte-containing solution should be used as fluid replacement.

Heat Edema. Heat edema is characterized by swelling and tightening of the hands and feet, usually within the first few days of exposure to a hot environment.[6,13] Unacclimatized or elderly patients are especially prone to this disorder. Not uncommonly, otherwise healthy travelers originating from a colder climate develop heat edema within a few days after arrival in a tropical area. The edema is usually mild; signs and symptoms of other systemic causes of edema are absent. Excessive orthostatic pooling of interstitial fluid in the extremities secondary to cutaneous vasodilation appears to be the major mechanism of heat edema formation. No treatment is usually necessary and the edema gradually responds within hours to days. Occasionally, however, edema may last for up to 4 to 6 weeks, and in these cases, leg elevation and support stockings may hasten resolution. Diuretics should not be used for the treatment of heat edema because they are ineffective and can actually predispose the patient to developing more serious heat-related disorders by causing dehydration.

Heat Syncope. Normally, hyperthermia induces shunting of blood to peripheral tissues to hasten cooling. In some

Table 134-1 World's 20 Largest Metropolitan Populations, 2004 (Estimates)

City	Population
Tokyo	28,000,000
Mexico City	18,100,000
Mumbai (Bombay)	18,000,000
Sao Paulo	17,700,000
New York City	16,600,000
Shanghai	14,173,000
Lagos	13,500,000
Los Angeles	13,100,000
Calcutta	12,900,000
Buenos Aires	12,400,000
Seoul	12,200,000
Beijing	12,000,000
Karachi	11,800,000
Delhi	11,700,000
Dhaka	11,000,000
Manila	10,800,000
Cairo	10,700,000
Osaka	10,600,000
Rio de Janeiro	10,500,000
Tianjin (China)	10,300,000

Data from Top 100 cities of the world. *www.worldatlas.com/citypops.htm*, 2004; and Th. Brinkoff. Principal agglomerations of the world. *http://citypopulation.de/cities.html*, 2004.

sunscreens have been reported to directly or indirectly cause one or more of the sun-related cutaneous reactions discussed in this chapter. Therefore, pretravel testing with a minute amount of sunscreen on a small area of skin can be helpful in avoiding disturbing chemical hypersensitivity.

ILLNESS CAUSED BY ATMOSPHERIC POLLUTION

Essentially all travelers entering tropical countries will spend at least some time in a medium or large city. Most of the largest metropolitan areas in the world are located in underdeveloped or developing countries (Table 134-1).[59,60] Because air pollution laws and regulations in most developing countries are generally lax, travel-associated morbidity secondary to exposure to atmospheric pollution is a real concern for most travelers to such cities. Health hazards due to atmospheric pollution thus represent one category of medical problems shared by industrialized and developing nations.

Fossil fuel combustion and industries produce photochemical smog, carbon dioxide, carbon monoxide, suspended particulates, acid aerosols, and a variety of toxic pollutants, including lead, other heavy metals, and trace organics.[61–66] These agents have been associated with a variety of health problems in healthy adults as well as in patients with underlying cardiopulmonary problems, and they are associated with increased risk of morbidity and mortality among exposed populations (Table 134-2).[61–83] Cities with particularly notorious

Table 134-2 Medically Important Atmospheric Pollutants

Pollutant	Populations at Risk	Range of Health Effects
Particulates	Healthy adults and children Patients with asthma, COPD, CLD, CHD	Increased respiratory symptoms Impaired lung function Increased airway reactivity/inflammation Increased respiratory illnesses Increased mortality in CHD, CLD patients
Tropospheric ozone	Healthy adults and children Outdoor workers Athletes Patients with asthma, COPD	Increased respiratory symptoms Impaired lung function Decreased exercise capacity Increased airway reactivity/inflammation Increased hospitalizations Effects worsened in combination with acid aerosols and particulates
Sulfur dioxide	Healthy adults and children Patients with asthma, COPD	Increased respiratory symptoms Impaired lung function Increased hospitalizations Increased respiratory infections
Nitrogen dioxide	Healthy adults and children Patients with asthma, COPD	Increased respiratory symptoms Impaired lung function Increased airway reactivity Increased respiratory infections
Carbon monoxide	Healthy adults and children Patients with IHD	Decreased exercise capacity Increased ischemic episodes and mortality in IHD patients
Lead, heavy metals	Healthy adults and children	Altered neurologic function Altered behavioral function Hematologic toxicity Increased incidence of hypertension Highest risk in countries allowing leaded gasoline
Acid aerosols	Healthy adults and children Patients with asthma, CLD	Increased respiratory symptoms Impaired lung function Impaired mucociliary clearance

CHD, chronic heart disease (all types); CLD, chronic lung disease (all types); COPD, chronic obstructive pulmonary disease; IHD, ischemic heart disease.
Data from references 61–63, 71–75.

levels of air pollutants include Mexico City, cities along the Pacific basin of the Americas (e.g., Los Angeles), many cities within eastern Europe, Beijing, and most large cities in Asia. In many low-lying cities, temperature inversions can exacerbate the effects of air pollution. In addition, natural sources of particulates, such as sandstorms, can combine with extreme heat and artificial contaminants to cause increased respiratory health risks in many areas of North Africa and the Middle East.

Components of photochemical smog include sulfur dioxide, ozone, and nitrogen oxide. Exposure of people to elevated levels of sulfur dioxide in the atmosphere is associated with a measurable decrease in pulmonary function. As sulfur dioxide levels increase, exacerbation of disease in patients with underlying pulmonary disease is frequently seen. Patients with asthma and chronic obstructive pulmonary disease (COPD) appear to be particularly at risk of symptomatic flare secondary to high levels of sulfur dioxide and particulates. Ozone is another important component of photochemical smog. Elevated levels of ozone cause chest discomfort and eye irritation in normal adults and children. With high levels of tropospheric ozone, pulmonary dysfunction, bronchospasm, and inflammatory pulmonary exudates can be noted, even in otherwise healthy people. The third major component of photochemical smog is nitrogen oxide. This pollutant likely causes fewer acute or serious illnesses than the other agents, but at higher levels it has been associated with the induction of bronchospasm, decreased pulmonary function, and increased respiratory infection, primarily in patients with asthma or COPD. In cities with congested freeways and aging, poorly repaired automobiles, exposure to significant levels of carbon monoxide is a continual concern. In people with chronic exposure to low or medium levels of carbon monoxide, elevated carboxyhemoglobin levels, impaired cognition, and other symptoms of carbon monoxide toxicity may be observed. The diagnosis and treatment of carbon monoxide toxicity are summarized elsewhere.[76,77]

People who must go outdoors during peak episodes of atmospheric pollution should minimize the time of exposure, avoid exercise, and consider wearing particle-filtering masks. For patients with asthma or COPD, prophylactic treatment with oral antihistamines and aerosolized ipratropium bromide may be helpful. Finally, the risk of exposure to environmental allergens should always be considered when traveling, especially if the traveler has a history of atopic disease, asthma, or COPD.

HIGH-ALTITUDE ILLNESS

Background

The term *high-altitude illness* usually invokes images of technical mountaineering performed under arctic-like conditions. However, exposure to high altitude occurs in large numbers of travelers visiting tropical or subtropical countries every year. For example, trekking to the Mt. Everest base camp (5366 m/17,600 ft) or to the summit of Mt. Kilimanjaro in Africa (5891 m/19,321 ft) is a common tourist activity. This section provides an overview of some of the more common medical illnesses associated with travel to high altitude. For detailed discussions of the epidemiology, physiology, and pathophysiology of medical complications of high-altitude exposure, the reader is directed to recent journal reviews and book chapters.[55,84–95]

Pathophysiology

Much of the understanding of the pathophysiology of altitude-related illnesses has come from the experiences of mountain climbers and high-altitude balloonists.[96,97] In addition, more recent use of high-altitude field testing and research stations has dramatically improved our understanding of the pathogenesis, presentation, and treatment of many altitude-related diseases. The unifying finding from almost all of these venues is that hypoxia represents the primary environmental stress responsible for the pathophysiology of most altitude-related illness.

At sea level, the partial pressure of oxygen is approximately 149 Torr (1 Torr = a unit of pressure sufficient to support a 1-mm column of mercury at 0°C) and results in a partial pressure of alveolar oxygen (PaO_2) of approximately 100 Torr. Because the percentage of oxygen in the atmosphere is constant at 21%, the decreased barometric pressure at high altitude results in a decreased atmospheric partial pressure of oxygen. At an altitude of 4572 m (15,000 ft), the partial pressure of inspired oxygen decreases to approximately 80 Torr, which results in PaO_2 of approximately 43 Torr. *High altitude* is generally defined as an altitude higher than 2500 m (approximately 8200 ft), *very high altitude* as 3500 to 5500 m (approximately 11,500 to 18,000 ft), and *extreme altitude* as higher than 5500 m (approximately 18,000 ft; Table 134-3).[55,89–95] Mild forms of altitude sickness are relatively common at high altitude. Acclimatization is required to avoid medical complications when ascending to very high altitude. Serious medical problems are commonly associated with ascent to extreme altitude, even with appropriate periods of prior acclimatization.

Table 134-3 Association of Symptoms with High-Altitude Exposure

M	FT	Comments
2500	8,200	
3000	9,840	High altitude is 2500–3500 m; mild acute mountain sickness is common
3500	11,480	
4000	13,120	Very high altitude is 3500–5500 m; moderate altitude-related illness is frequent; serious problems commonly occur in unacclimatized people
4500	14,760	
5000	16,400	Mt. Everest base camp is 5366 m (17,600 ft)
5500	18,040	Extreme altitude is greater than 5500 m; altitude-related illness is universal, even in acclimatized people; a significant risk of serious medical problems is associated with extended stays at extreme altitude
6000	19,680	Mt. Kilimanjaro is 5891 m (19,321 ft)
6500	21,320	
7000	22,960	
7500	24,600	
8000	26,240	
8500	27,880	
8850	29,028	Altitude of Mount Everest

Data from references 55, 84, 85, 89.

Acute Mountain Sickness

Acute mountain sickness (AMS) is the most benign form of altitude-related illness.[55,84–89,91–93,98] This syndrome affects thousands of travelers and trekkers each year as they ascend to altitudes higher than 2500 m. Symptoms include headache, anorexia, nausea, vomiting, sleep disturbance, lethargy, and dyspnea on exertion. Symptoms most commonly occur when people undergo rapid ascent to altitudes higher than 2500 m. The severity of symptoms in AMS is increased by physical exertion, higher attained altitude, and more rapid ascent. The susceptibility to AMS varies dramatically among people and is often difficult to predict.[99–101] No consistent correlation has been found between the likelihood or severity of AMS and such factors as age, level of physical fitness, or sex. One report suggests that younger, less physically fit people living at low altitude had a higher risk of developing AMS.[102] Another study indicated that obese men exhibited higher AMS scores than nonobese men when subjected to a simulated ascent to 3658 m.[103] One factor that appears to be strongly associated with an increased risk of AMS is a previous history of altitude-related illness, especially when such people perform a rapid ascent.[91–93] For most people, the development of AMS is not associated with serious complications or sequelae. A minority of patients, however, can progress from the relatively benign syndrome of AMS to more serious illnesses, such as high-altitude pulmonary edema or high-altitude cerebral edema.

In most people, acclimatization to a certain altitude occurs over 2 or 3 days, after which symptoms of AMS usually decrease markedly.[55,84–89,91–93,98] For a mild case of AMS, rest and acclimatization to the presently held altitude are frequently all that is needed. More troublesome symptoms can be relieved by treatment with a variety of drugs. In particular, administration of acetazolamide reduces the symptoms of AMS and improves pulmonary gas exchange and function (Table 134-4).[55,84–89,91–93,98] Acetazolamide therapy does not appear to interfere with the process of acclimatization. In patients with a previous history of AMS, acetazolamide therapy can reduce the severity of AMS if it is initiated immediately prior to ascent. Recommended dosing for acetazolamide varies by authors and ranges from 250 mg at evening to 250 mg every 8 hours.[55,84,91–93] We generally recommend 125 to 250 mg twice a day, depending on severity of symptoms and efficacy of response. Most authors recommend that acetazolamide be used for only a few days to facilitate acclimatization. Dexamethasone therapy also lessens the symptoms of AMS, especially in people who rapidly ascend to high altitudes.[55,84–89,91–93,98,104] Although dexamethasone is as good as or better than acetazolamide at relieving many of the symptoms of AMS, it has no measurable beneficial effect on pulmonary function. Therefore, most authors do not routinely recommend dexamethasone for either prophylaxis or as first-line therapy for the treatment of AMS.[91–93] In more severe cases of AMS, the combination of acetazolamide with dexamethasone should be considered, especially when descent is not an option.[55,85,91–93,105] Because acetazolamide is a sulfonamide, there has been general reluctance to prescribe this medication for a patient who gives a history of allergy to sulfonamide antibiotics. Strom and colleagues retrospectively analyzed a large general practice patient database in the United Kingdom and found that history of an allergy to penicillin

Table 134-4 Treatment Guidelines for Serious Forms of High-Altitude Illness

Syndrome	Treatment	Comments
Acute mountain sickness (AMS)	Discontinue ascent Increase fluids Acetaminophen prn Acetazolamide 250 mg q8–12h *or* Dexamethasone 4 mg q6h If *severe:* supplemental O_2 and acetazolamide 500 mg q8h and dexamethasone 4–8 mg q6h	If prophylaxis is indicated More gradual ascent Acetazolamide 250 mg qhs or q12h (start day before ascent and continue for 3–5 days) *or* Dexamethasone 2–4 mg q6h (start day before ascent and continue for 3–5 days) Nifedipine not effective as prophylaxis for AMS; theophylline may be beneficial Nifedipine is also effective as a prophylactic agent
High-altitude pulmonary edema	Discontinue ascent Bed rest Supplemental O_2 If *moderate to severe:* above and furosemide (titrated prn) and morphine (titrated prn) and nifedipine (10 mg sl, then 20 mg PO q6h or 30 mg SR PO q12h) and immediate descent or hyperbaric therapy if unable to descend	Inhaled NO or beta-agonists (e.g., salmeterol) or sildenafil may be beneficial for prophylaxis or treatment based on small studies Dexamethasone does not benefit pulmonary function
High-altitude cerebral edema	Immediate descent and evacuation if possible or hyperbaric therapy if descent is not possible Supplemental O_2 Dexamethasone 4–8 mg q4h	

sl, sublingual; SR, sustained release.
Data from references 55, 84–89, 91–95, 104, 109, 124, 125, 130, 131, 136, 137.

was actually associated with a greater risk of allergy with administration of acetazolamide than was a history of an allergy to a sulfonamide antibiotic.[106] The authors concluded that an allergic history to "sulfa" drugs incurred only a small risk for developing an allergic reaction in response to acetazolamide. If there is no history of anaphylaxis and there is a strong medical need for use of acetazolamide, a small test dose of acetazolamide should still be carefully tried prior to travel before prescribing a full prophylactic or treatment regimen. Even then, acetazolamide use should be considered only when no other viable options (i.e., descent) are available.

Effective alternative agents for AMS are as yet unproven, although some preliminary studies are encouraging. Although spironolactone has been advised as a prophylactic agent, experience with this agent is limited and its routine use cannot be recommended at this time. Agents such as furosemide and nifedipine have been used successfully to treat patients with high-altitude pulmonary edema. However, there is no evidence that therapy with either of these agents is beneficial in the treatment or prophylaxis of AMS. Ginkgo biloba has been promoted as an effective and healthy alternative to acetazolamide for the prophylaxis of AMS. However, randomized, double-blind, placebo-controlled study of nonnative trekkers in Nepal found ginkgo ineffective in reducing either the severity or the incidence of AMS. In contrast, acetazolamide at 250 mg twice a day was very effective and displayed few adverse effects.[107] In a few small studies, prophylactic use of theophylline has been shown to have some efficacy in decreasing the severity or duration of AMS.[108,109]

A nonpharmacologic treatment for AMS involves use of a portable pressurization chamber.[110] Initial uncontrolled studies demonstrated that use of this apparatus in patients with AMS was associated with rapid and marked relief of symptoms.[111,112] Recent controlled studies indicate that there is indeed a greater short-term relief of symptoms (within 1 or 2 hours) using this apparatus.[113–116] However, there was no decrease in symptoms noted at later time points for patients treated with the pressurization apparatus compared with control patients placed in the apparatus but maintained at ambient atmospheric pressure. Evidence suggests that portable pressurization chamber treatment may slightly delay the onset of AMS but does not prevent AMS or decrease the severity of symptoms.[113–117] Use of portable pressurization devices should never substitute for descent when feasible. An empiric trial of use can be justified in the patient with a serious form of altitude illness who is unable to descend because of medical or logistical issues. Further studies are needed to elucidate the specific indications and potential benefits of the current, newer models of portable pressurization chambers.

It must be emphasized that the best and most effective therapy for AMS, as for all forms of altitude-induced illness, is descent to a sufficiently lower altitude.[55,84,85,89,91–93,98] In patients with moderate to severe symptoms of AMS, descent in combination with drug therapy as outlined previously should always be seriously considered. In addition, any symptoms that suggest the development of more serious complications, such as high-altitude pulmonary edema or high-altitude cerebral edema, mandate an attempt at descent. Prevention is often the best form of therapy. A slow and gradual ascent is probably the best way to prevent or at least reduce the severity of symptoms associated with AMS. Relevant to this point, travelers are often at the mercy of schedules that may lack sufficient time allocation for gradual ascent. In these instances, travelers are encouraged to seek the guidance of a travel medicine advisor to obtain appropriate counsel as to the symptoms and treatment of AMS.

High-Altitude Pulmonary Edema

High-altitude pulmonary edema (HAPE) is a potentially life-threatening condition that typically occurs in young, otherwise healthy people after rapid ascent to an altitude of 2500 m or higher.[55,84–88,91–95] Some individuals, however, can develop HAPE at moderate altitude (<2400 m). This appears to be more common than generally appreciated.[118] Symptoms of HAPE usually develop within 1 to 3 days following ascent and consist of orthopnea, dyspnea, and a cough productive of frothy, pink sputum. Patients with HAPE usually present with cyanosis, tachypnea, tachycardia, and rales. Development of HAPE appears to be more common in young males and has been associated with pre-existing lower respiratory tract infection, cold weather, history of previous episodes, and vigorous physical activity. The pathophysiology of HAPE most likely represents a variant of noncardiac pulmonary edema.[90–95,119–125] Pulmonary artery hypertension in the setting of normal pulmonary capillary wedge pressure is the characteristic finding. Most of these findings appear to be due to an excessive pulmonary vascular vasoconstrictive response to hypoxia. Earlier evidence indicated a prominent inflammatory component to HAPE, but this reaction may be coincidental rather than causal. Most current information regarding the pathophysiology of HAPE supports alteration of cardiopulmonary circulatory regulatory pathways, acid–base function, endothelial cell function, and vasoregulatory factors such as nitric oxide, atrial natriuretic peptide, and the renin–angiotensin system.[90–95,119–125] Further evidence indicates that genetic polymorphisms in some of these pathways may predispose certain individuals to HAPE.[126–129]

The mainstays of treatment of HAPE include immediate descent and oxygen therapy.[55,84–86,88,90] Certain drugs useful in other forms of pulmonary edema (e.g., furosemide and morphine) are also helpful in the treatment of HAPE. Acetazolamide, nifedipine, inhaled nitric oxide, salmeterol, and sildenafil have all been shown in clinical studies to improve both clinical symptoms and oxygenation defects associated with HAPE (see Table 134-4).[55,84–86,88,91–95,124,125,130,131] The reader is referred to detailed reviews and studies regarding specific treatment options for this disorder.[91–95,124,125]

High-Altitude Headache

The hypoxia associated with ascent to high altitude can also cause a variety of neurologic problems. High-altitude headache is extremely common and usually seen in combination with other symptoms associated with AMS.[91–93,132–134] High-altitude headache tends to be more severe in patients who are younger, female, and have a high frequency of headaches at their baseline altitude of residence. In addition to the treatment for AMS, as outlined previously, placebo-control studies have indicated that treatment with aspirin or ibuprofen is highly effective for high-altitude headache.[133,134] Mild cognitive defects have been noted in conjunction with

AMS. Most of the changes appear to be mild and resolve after descent and symptomatic recovery from AMS.

High-Altitude Cerebral Edema

The most serious neurologic problem associated with altitude is high-altitude cerebral edema (HACE).[55,91–93,135–137] This condition was formerly believed to occur only during ascent to extreme altitudes. However, HACE has been occasionally reported at modest altitudes, so travelers at risk should be familiar with the symptoms and clinical course of this syndrome. Initially, symptoms of HACE closely resemble those of AMS. With HACE, there is a relatively rapid progression of neurologic and cognitive defects, including severe malaise, weakness, dizziness, impaired memory, altered judgment, excessive drowsiness, visual disturbances, and hallucinations. Clinical signs suggestive of HACE include disorientation, somnolence, obtundation, paralysis, ataxia, and seizures. Retinal hemorrhages are not uncommon. A variety of pathophysiologic disturbances have been described for HACE: high brain capillary pressure with edema and vascular leakage, osmotic cell swelling, focal ischemia, and angiogenesis.[55,91–93,135–139] Cerebral pathologic changes noted on autopsy from patients with HACE include petechial hemorrhage, thrombosis, and gross edema.

Occasionally, clinical differentiation between moderately severe AMS and full-blown HACE is difficult. If there is any question of the presence of HACE, an attempt at immediate descent is mandatory. The presence of neurologic abnormalities, such as ataxia, obtundation, excessive somnolence, or confusion, should raise strong concern that the patient is suffering from HACE. In addition to rapid and immediate evacuation to a lower altitude, adjunctive therapies with oxygen and dexamethasone are known to be helpful and potentially lifesaving in this syndrome (see Table 134-4).[55,91–93]

High-Altitude Retinopathy

Heavy physical exertion and a rapid ascent to very high altitude predispose the patient to develop high-altitude retinal hemorrhage.[140–142] The reported incidence of this syndrome is approximately 5% at 14,000 ft, 50% at 17,000 ft, and 100% at 21,000 ft. High-altitude retinal hemorrhage is generally asymptomatic, although macular visual field defects occasionally occur. Clinical findings include flame-shaped retinal hemorrhages, cotton wool exudates, and vitreous hemorrhages. Resolution is usually spontaneous with minimal sequelae following descent to a lower altitude, and most physical findings resolve within a few weeks. Although high-altitude retinal hemorrhage is not considered a serious problem, it is frequently associated with the presence of HACE or HAPE. The development of this form of retinopathy, therefore, must be an indication to carefully monitor the patient for further development of more serious altitude-related illnesses. Certain preexisting ocular problems may also be exacerbated by ascent to high altitude. For more serious conditions, consultation with an ophthalmalogist may be warranted.[143]

Other Problems

Ascent to high altitude may exacerbate problems in patients with underlying medical conditions.[91–93,144,145] In general, any disease that can be worsened by hypoxia can also be worsened by ascent to high altitude. Patients with respiratory illness such as asthma or COPD appear to be at increased risk of exacerbation of their disease and development of altitude-related medical illness. However, there are few studies that assess the specific risk for such patients who ascend to the types of moderate or high altitudes generally associated with tourist travel. Patients with any form of pulmonary hypertension are likely to be especially prone to the effects of altitude. It would therefore seem advisable to recommend avoidance of travel to high or very high altitude for patients with significant respiratory illnesses unless absolutely necessary. In addition, patients who elect to undertake treks or travel to high altitude should travel with a person who understands the symptoms and signs of, and therapeutic options for, altitude-associated illnesses. Furthermore, these patients should be especially careful to program gradual ascent into any trip that requires even a short stay at moderately high, or higher, altitudes.

Similarly, patients with significant cardiac disease (congestive heart failure, coronary artery disease, dysrhythmias, etc.) and patients with severe hypertension are also theoretically at risk of increased problems at high altitude. A few small studies and anecdotal reports indicate that patients with well-controlled angina or otherwise stable cardiovascular disease can ascend to moderately high altitude without adverse effects.[87,88,91–93,100,102,145] However, no controlled studies of travelers have been performed. Therefore, patients with significant but stable cardiovascular disease must be carefully counseled as to risks and potential therapeutic interventions when considering a trip involving exposure to moderate or high altitude.

JET LAG

Most living organisms have evolved mechanisms enabling them to sense the day–night cycle.[146–149] Humans are no exception, and many of our physiologic values appear to have circadian patterns. The relationship between exogenous environmental clues and endogenous physiologic rhythms results in a carefully regulated cycle of most of these physiologic functions.[146–149] When there is a conflict between perceived external cues and ongoing internal rhythms, a variety of unpleasant symptoms are produced. A common form of conflict exists when a traveler crosses several time zones, resulting in a syndrome known as jet lag or "time zone fatigue."[146–151] Body rhythms that are tightly regulated by environmental cues such as cycles of light and dark can adjust relatively rapidly after arrival in a new time zone. On the other hand, strong endogenous and light-insensitive internal rhythms may take much longer to readjust. It is known that the syndrome of jet lag is associated with actual change of time zone and not merely air travel because jet lag is only observable with east–west travel across time zones. Jet lag per se does not occur even with lengthy north–south travel.

The most common symptoms of jet lag include difficulty falling asleep, altered states of wakefulness, fatigue, lightheadedness, mild disorientation, anorexia, and mild to moderate forms of gastrointestinal upset.[146–149] In general, travel from west to east is associated with more severe symptoms than travel in the opposite direction. Acclimatization to the new time zone depends on the number of time zones crossed in travel. In general, a decrease in symptoms and improvement of normal sleep–wake phases usually occur within 1 to 4 days. Time acclimatization can be accelerated by certain behavioral changes, such as outdoor activity in sunlight.

Evidence suggests that it may be possible to alleviate many of the symptoms of jet lag by resetting certain aspects of normal circadian rhythm pharmacologically.[146,147,149,151] The use of a short-acting and relatively nonsedating hypnotic agent (such as zolpidem 10 mg or temazepam 15 mg at bedtime) for a few days after arrival can be helpful in alleviating transient insomnia associated with jet lag.[152,153] Some researchers have suggested the use of the hormone melatonin in alleviating jet lag symptoms and rapidly enhancing time zone acclimatization. Melatonin is an important regulator of the sleep–wake cycle, and most studies have indicated that nightly administration of 3 to 5 mg of melatonin begun just before or on the day of arrival can significantly reduce the severity and duration of jet lag.[153–158] Nearly all of these studies were performed using pharmaceutical formulations of melatonin available in Europe. Melatonin is marketed in the United States only as a nutritional supplement. Therefore, although the use of melatonin at bedtime for 3 to 5 days beginning on the night of arrival has possible benefit for jet lag, the complete safety and efficacy of the formulations available in the United States have not been determined.

NATURAL DISASTERS

Extreme variations in the climate can have sudden, severe, and long-lasting effects on the health of the resident and transient populations of the affected areas.[159–164] The most commonly recognized forms of natural disasters occur yearly in many diverse areas of the world (Box 134-2). Although the impact of such disasters occurs globally, the worst damage and loss of life are often greatest in the poorest and most underdeveloped countries. The public health impact of such events is usually far-reaching and ranges from disruption of infrastructure to outbreaks of communicable diseases.[159–164]

On December 26, 2004, a magnitude 9.0 earthquake occurred under the Indian Ocean near the Indonesian island of Simelulue. It was the largest magnitude earthquake recorded in the world since 1964.[165] The force generated from the earthquake spawned a series of tsunamis that devastated coastal areas and islands of many countries, including Indonesia, Thailand, India, and Sri Lanka. Damaging effects of tsunami wave action were observed as far away as Kenya and South Africa. As of January 2005, more than 225,000 people were reported dead; millions of others were injured, became ill, or were displaced from their homes. This event is recognized as the deadliest tsunami in recorded history. Although the data are not yet available, it is very likely that more world travelers from industrialized countries will have died or become injured or ill from the results of this single event in 2005 than from all other forms of travel-related illnesses combined.

Health hazards due to tsunamis are numerous and known to occur in many other types of natural disasters as well.[159–166] The initial impact is due to loss of life from drowning, flooding, and destruction of homes, buildings, and vehicles. To compound matters, disruption of communication, transportation, and health-care delivery systems means that many injured or ill will die of otherwise treatable conditions. In the days following the event, damage to water and sanitation systems leads to the risk of waterborne diseases, such as viral gastroenteritis, cholera, dysentery, typhoid, and hepatitis A. In tropical and even temperate areas, flooding and disruption of water reservoirs can provide new breeding areas for insects, potentially promoting outbreaks of serious mosquito-borne diseases, such as malaria, yellow fever, and viral encephalitides. Although commonly labeled as high-risk sources of communicable disease outbreaks, the actual risk of disease associated with decomposing animal or human corpses appears to be minimal.[167,168] The sickest victims are often transported to cities outside the damage zone, increasing the risk of epidemic spread of certain forms of diseases. Because tsunamis, as well as most other types of natural disasters, can occur in otherwise low-risk and well-developed resort areas within tropical countries, all travelers need to be aware of the potentially lethal effects of natural disasters, even though the risk of occurrence is low.[169]

Box 134-2 Natural Disasters Associated with Risks to Public Health

- Avalanches
- Cyclones and hurricanes
- Extreme cold
- Extreme heat and drought
- Floods
- Landslides
- Tornadoes
- Tsunamis
- Volcanic eruptions
- Wildfires

REFERENCES

1. Bouchama A: Heatstroke: A new look at an ancient disease. Intensive Care Med 21:623, 1995.
2. Bouchama A, Knochel JP: Heat stroke. N Engl J Med 346:1978, 2002.
3. Epstein Y, Sohar E, Shapiro Y: Exertional heatstroke: A preventable condition. Isr J Med Sci 31:454, 1995.
4. Hubbard RW, Gaffin SL, Squire DL: Heat-related illness. In Auerbach PS (ed): Wilderness Medicine, 3rd ed. St. Louis, Mosby-Year Book, 1995, p 167.
5. Gutierrez G: Solar injury and heat illness: Prevention and treatment in children. Phys Sports Med 23:43, 1995.
6. Lugo-Amador NM, Rothenhaus T, Moyer P: Heat-related illness. Emerg Med Clin North Am 22:315, 2004.
7. Martinez M, Devenport L, Saussy J, et al: Drug-associated heat stroke. South Med J 95:799, 2002.
8. Cheshire WP, Freeman R: Disorders of sweating. Semin Neurol 23:399, 2003.
9. Bar-Or O: Climate and the exercising child. In Bar-Or O (ed): Pediatric Sports Medicine for the Practitioner. New York, Springer-Verlag, 1983, p 259.
10. Scott J: Heat-related illnesses. Postgrad Med 85:154, 1989.
11. Ladell WSS: Heat cramps. Lancet 2:836, 1949.
12. Talbott JH: Heat cramps. N Engl J Med 302:777, 1935.
13. Yarbrough B: Heat illness. In Rosen P, Barkein RM, Braen GR, et al (eds): Emergency Medicine: Concepts and Clinical Practice, 3rd ed. St. Louis, Mosby Yearbook, 1992, p 944.
14. Stolwijk JA: Responses to the thermal environment. Fed Proc 36:1655, 1977.

15. Collings GH, Shoudy LA, Shaffer FE: The clinical aspects of heat diseases. Ind Med 12:728, 1943.
16. Dematte JE, O'Mara K, Buescher J, et al: Near-fatal heat stroke during the 1995 heat wave in Chicago. Ann Intern Med 129:173, 1998.
17. Anonymous: Impact of heat waves on mortality—Rome, Italy, June–August 2003. MMWR 53:369, 2004.
18. Anonymous: Heat-related deaths—Chicago, Illinois, 1996–2001, and United States, 1979–1999. MMWR 52:610, 2003.
19. Ghaznawi HI, Ibrahim MA: Heatstroke and heat exhaustion in pilgrims performing the Haj in Saudi Arabia. Ann Saudi Med 7:323, 1987.
20. Anonymous: Heatstroke—United States. MMWR 30:277, 1981.
21. Anonymous: Heat-related deaths—United States, 1993. MMWR 42:558, 1993.
22. Anonymous: Heatstroke—Philadelphia and the United States, 1994. MMWR 43:453, 1994.
23. Sonna LA, Wenger CB, Flinn S, et al: Exertional heat injury and gene expression changes: A DNA microarray analysis study. J Appl Physiol 96:1943, 2004.
24. Sminia P, van der Zee J, Wondergem J, et al: Effect of hyperthermia on the central nervous system: A review. Int J Hyperthermia 10:1, 1994.
25. Shapiro Y, Seidman DS: Field and clinical observations of exertional heatstroke patients. Med Sci Sports Exerc 22:6, 1990.
26. Costrini AM, Pitt HA, Gustafson AB, et al: Cardiovascular and metabolic manifestations of heatstroke and severe heat exhaustion. Am J Med 66:296, 1979.
27. Beard MEJ, Hickton CM: Haemostasis in heat stroke. Br J Haematol 52:269, 1982.
28. Shibolet S, Fisher S, Gilat T, et al: Fibrinolysis and hemorrhages in fatal heatstroke. N Engl J Med 266:169, 1962.
29. Lin YF, Wang JY, Chou TC, et al: Vasoactive mediators and renal haemodynamics in exertional heat stroke complicated by acute renal failure. QJM 96:193, 2003.
30. Bouchama A, al-Sedairy S, Siddiqui S, et al: Elevated pyrogenic cytokines in heatstroke. Chest 104:1498, 1993.
31. Hammami MM, Bouchama A, Alsedairy S, et al: Concentrations of soluble tumor necrosis factor and interleukin-6 receptors in heatstroke and heatstress. Crit Care Med 25:1314, 1997.
32. Akhtar MJ, al-Nozha M, al-Harthi S, et al: Electrocardiographic abnormalities in patients with heatstroke. Chest 104:411, 1993.
33. Costrini A: Emergency treatment of exertional heatstroke and comparison of whole body cooling techniques. Med Sci Sports Exerc 22:15, 1990.
34. Cooper JK: Preventing heat injury: Military versus civilian perspective. Military Med 162:55, 1997.
35. Weiner JS, Khogali M: A physiological body-cooling unit for treatment of heatstroke. Lancet 1:507, 1980.
36. Taylor CR, Sober AJ: Sun exposure and skin disease. Annu Rev Med 47:181, 1996.
37. Gould JW, Mercurio MG, Elmets CA: Cutaneous photosensitivity diseases induced by exogenous agents. J Am Acad Dermatol 33:551, 1995.
38. Gonzalez E, Gonzalez S: Drug photosensitivity, idiopathic photodermatoses, and sunscreens. J Am Acad Dermatol 35:871, 1996.
39. Yashar SS, Lim HW: Classification and evaluation of photodermatoses. Dermatol Ther 16:1, 2003.
40. Ferguson J: Diagnosis and treatment of the common idiopathic photodermatoses. Austr J Dermatol 44:90, 2003.
41. Harth Y, Rapoport M: Photosensitivity associated with antipsychotics, antidepressants, and anxiolytics. Drug Saf 14:252, 1996.
42. Cardullo AC, Ruszkowski AM, DeLeo VA: Allergic contact dermatitis resulting from sensitivity to citrus peel, geraniol, and citral. J Am Acad Dermatol 21:395, 1989.
43. Wagner AM, Wu JJ, Hansen RC, et al: Bullous phytophotodermatitis associated with high natural concentrations of furanocoumarins in limes. Am J Contact Dermatol 13:10, 2002.
44. Weber IC, Davis CR, Greeson DM: Phytophotodermatitis: The other "lime" disease. J Emerg Med 17:235, 1999.
45. Nigg HN, Nordby HE, Beier RC, et al: Phototoxic coumarins in limes. Food Chem Toxicol 31:331, 1993.
46. Soter NA: Acute effects of ultraviolet radiation in the skin. Semin Dermatol 9:11, 1990.
47. Tsien A: Solar urticaria. Cutis 57:87, 1996.
48. Bech-Thomsen N, Thomsen K: Solar pruritus. Acta Dermatol Venereol 75:488, 1995.
49. Goodless DR, Eaglstein WH: Brachioradial pruritus: Treatment with topical capsaicin. J Am Acad Dermatol 29:783, 1993.
50. Walcyk PJ, Elpern DJ: Brachioradial pruritus: A tropical dermopathy. Br J Dermatol 115:177, 1986.
51. Knight TE: Solar (brachioradial) pruritus—Response to capsaicin cream. Int J Dermatol 33:206, 1994.
52. Ros A, Wennersten G: Current aspects of polymorphous light eruption in Sweden. Photodermatology 3:215, 1986.
53. Fesq H, Ring J, Abeck D: Management of polymorphous light eruption: Clinical course, pathogenesis, diagnosis and intervention. Am J Clin Dermatol 4:399, 2003.
54. Wittenberg S: Solar radiation and the eye: A review of knowledge relevant to eye care. Am J Optom Physiol Optics 63:676, 1986.
55. Hackett PH, Roach RC: High-altitude medicine. In Auerbach PS (ed): Wilderness Medicine, 3rd ed. St. Louis, Mosby-Year Book, 1995.
56. Young AR: Cumulative effects of ultraviolet radiation in the skin: Cancer and photoaging. Semin Dermatol 9:25, 1990.
57. Armstrong BK, Kricker A: How much melanoma is caused by sun exposure. Melanoma Res 3:395, 1993.
58. Fitzpatrick TB: The validity and practicality of sun-reactive skin types I through VI. Arch Dermatol 124:869, 1988.
59. UN Center for Human Settlements: Global Report on Human Settlements. Nairobi, Kenya, UN Center for Human Settlements, 1995.
60. Anonymous: Cities as disease vectors. Science 270:1125, 1995.
61. Bates DV: Particulate air pollution. Thorax 51(suppl 2):S3, 1996.
62. Bascom R, Bromberg PA, Costa DA, et al: Health effects of outdoor air pollution (pt 1). Am J Respir Crit Care Med 153:3, 1996.
63. Bascom R, Bromberg PA, Costa DA, et al: Health effects of outdoor air pollution (pt 2). Am J Respir Crit Care Med 153:477, 1996.
64. Fox DL: Air pollution. Anal Chem 69:1, 1997.
65. Finlayson BJ, Pitts JN: Tropospheric air pollution-ozone, airborne toxins, polycyclic aromatic hydrocarbons, and particles. Science 276:1045, 1997.
66. Haines A, Patz JA: Health effects of climate change. JAMA 291:99, 2004.
67. Barnes PJ: Air pollution and asthma—Molecular mechanisms. Mol Med Today 1:149, 1995.
68. Little R: Public health in central and eastern Europe and the role of environmental pollution. Annu Rev Public Health 19:153, 1998.
69. Katsouyanni K, Pershagen G: Ambient air pollution exposure and cancer. Cancer Causes Control 8:284, 1997.
70. Brunekreef B: Air pollution and life expectancy—Is there a relation? Occup Environ Med 54:781, 1997.
71. Krishna MT, Chauhan AJ: Air pollution and health. J R Coll Physicians London 30:448, 1996.
72. Krishna MT, Mudway I, Kelly FJ, et al: Ozone, airways, and allergic airways disease. Clin Exp Allergy 25:1150, 1995.
73. Rusznak C, Devalia JL, Wang JH, et al: Pollution-induced airway disease and the putative underlying mechanisms. Clin Rev Allergy Immunol 15:205, 1997.
74. Moolgavkar SH, Luebeck EG: A critical review of the evidence on particulate air pollution and mortality. Epidemiology 7:420, 1996.
75. Lebowitz MD: Epidemiological studies of the respiratory effects of air pollution. Eur Respir J 9:1029, 1996.
76. Braun R, Krishel S: Environmental emergencies. Emerg Med Clin North Am 15:451, 1997.
77. Balzan MV, Agius G, Galea A: Carbon monoxide poisoning: Easy to treat but difficult to recognize. Postgrad Med J 72:470, 1996.
78. Sunyer J, Basagana X, Belmonte J, et al: Effect of nitrogen dioxide and ozone on the risk of dying in patients with severe asthma. Thorax 57:687, 2002.
79. McConnell R, Berhane K, Gilliland F, et al: Prospective study of air pollution and bronchitic symptoms in children with asthma. Am J Respir Crit Care Med 168:790, 2003.
80. Samet JM, Dominici F, Curriero FC, et al: Fine particulate air pollution and mortality in 20 U.S. cities, 1987–1994. N Engl J Med 343:1742, 2000.
81. Wong GW, Lai CK: Outdoor air pollution and asthma. Curr Opin Pulm Med 10:62, 2004.
82. Brook RD, Brook JR, Urch B, et al: Inhalation of fine particulate air pollution and ozone causes acute arterial vasoconstriction in healthy adults. Circulation 105:1534, 2002.
83. Routledge HC, Ayres JG, Townend JN: Why cardiologists should be interested in air pollution. Heart 89:1383, 2003.
84. Coote JH: Medicine and mechanisms in altitude sickness. Sports Med 20:149, 1995.
85. Hsia CCW: Southwestern internal medicine conference: Pulmonary complications of high-altitude exposure. Am J Med Sci 307:448, 1994.

86. Jerome EH, Severinghaus JW: High altitude pulmonary edema (editorial). N Engl J Med 334:662, 1996.
87. Peacock AJ: High altitude pulmonary oedema: Who gets it and why? Eur Respir J 8:1819, 1995.
88. Richalet JP: High altitude pulmonary oedema: Still a place for controversy? Thorax 50:923, 1995.
89. Ward M, Milledge J, West J: High Altitude Medicine and Physiology, 2nd ed. London, Chapman & Hall, 1994.
90. Hultgren HN: High-altitude pulmonary edema—Current concepts. Annu Rev Med 47:267, 1996.
91. Barry PW, Pollard AJ: Altitude illness. BMJ 326:915, 2003.
92. Basnyat B, Murdoch DR: High-altitude illness. Lancet 361:1967, 2003.
93. Hackett PH, Roach RC: High-altitude illness. N Engl J Med 345:107, 2001.
94. Hackett P, Rennie D: High-altitude pulmonary edema. JAMA 287:2275, 2002.
95. Voelkel NF: High-altitude pulmonary edema. N Engl J Med 346:1606, 2002.
96. Doherty MJ: James Glaisher's 1862 account of balloon sickness: Altitude, decompression injury, and hypoxemia. Neurology 60:1016, 2003.
97. Huey RB, Eguskitza X, Dillon M: Mountaineering in thin air. Patterns of death and of weather at high altitude. Adv Exp Med Biol 502:225, 2001.
98. Hackett PH, Rennie D, Levine HD: The incidence, importance, and prophylaxis of acute mountain sickness. Lancet 2:1149, 1976.
99. Hohenhaus E, Paul A, McCullough RE, et al: Ventilatory and pulmonary vascular response to hypoxia and susceptibility to high altitude pulmonary oedema. Eur Respir J 8:1825, 1995.
100. Roach RC, Houston CS, Honigman B, et al: How well do older persons tolerate moderate altitude? West J Med 162:32, 1995.
101. Austin D, Sleigh J: Prediction of acute mountain sickness. BMJ 311:989, 1995.
102. Honigman B, Theis MK, Koziol-Mclain J, et al: Acute mountain sickness in a general tourist population at moderate altitudes. Ann Intern Med 118:587, 1993.
103. Ri-Li G, Chase PJ, Witkowski S, et al: Obesity: Associations with acute mountain sickness. Ann Intern Med 139:253, 2003.
104. Levine B, Yoshimura K, Kobayashi T, et al: Dexamethasone in the treatment of acute mountain sickness. N Engl J Med 321:193, 1989.
105. Bernhard WN, Schalick LM, Delaney PA, et al: Acetazolamide plus low-dose dexamethasone is better than acetazolamide alone to ameliorate symptoms of acute mountain sickness. Aviat Space Environ Med 69:883, 1998.
106. Strom BL, Schinnar R, Apter AJ, et al: Absence of cross-reactivity between sulfonamide antibiotics and sulfonamide nonantibiotics. N Engl J Med 349:1628, 2003.
107. Gertsch JH, Basnyat B, Johnson EW, et al: Randomised, double blind, placebo controlled comparison of ginkgo biloba and acetazolamide for prevention of acute mountain sickness among Himalayan trekkers: The prevention of high altitude illness trial (PHAIT). BMJ 328:797, 2004.
108. Fisher R, Lang SM, Steiner U, et al: Theophylline improves acute mountain sickness. Eur Respir J 15:123, 2000.
109. Fisher R, Lang SM, Leiti et al: Theophylline and acetazolamide reduce sleep-disordered breathing at high altitude. Dur Respir J 23:47, 2004.
110. Gamow RI, Geer GD, Kasic KF, et al: Methods of gas-balance control to be used with a portable hyperbaric chamber in the treatment of high altitude illness. J Wilderness Med 1:165, 1990.
111. Robertson JA, Shlim DR: Treatment of moderate acute mountain sickness with pressurization in a portable hyperbaric (Gamow) bag. J Wilderness Med 2:268, 1991.
112. King SJ, Greenlee RR: Successful use of the Gamow hyperbaric bag in the treatment of altitude illness at Mount Everest. J Wilderness Med 1:193, 1990.
113. Bartsch P, Merki B, Hofstetter D, et al: Treatment of acute mountain sickness by simulated descent: A randomised controlled trial. BMJ 306:1098, 1993.
114. Keller HR, Maggiorini M, Bartsch P, et al: Simulated descent v. dexamethasone in treatment of acute mountain sickness: A randomized trial. BMJ 310:1232, 1995.
115. Harry JP, Jean D, Kayser B, et al: Effect of a 3-h recompression at 220 mbar on AMS during climbing Mount Blanc. Int J Sports Med 13:83, 1992.
116. Kayser B, Jean D, Herry JP, et al: Pressurization and acute mountain sickness. Aviat Space Environ Med 64:928, 1993.
117. Pollard AJ: Treatment of acute mountain sickness (letter). BMJ 311:629, 1995.
118. Gabry AL, Ledoux X, Mozziconacci M, et al: High-altitude pulmonary edema at moderate altitude (<2,400 m; 7,870 feet): A series of 52 patients. Chest 123:49, 2003.
119. Naeije R: Pulmonary circulation at high altitude. Respiration 64:429, 1997.
120. Arnett FC: High-altitude pulmonary edema—An immunogenetically mediated disease. Circulation 97:1111, 1998.
121. Maggiorini M: Cardio-pulmonary interactions at high altitude. Pulmonary hypertension as a common denominator. Adv Exp Med Biol 543:177, 2003.
122. Swenson ER, Maggiorini M, Mongovin S, et al: Pathogenesis of high-altitude pulmonary edema: Inflammation is not an etiologic factor. JAMA 287:2228, 2002.
123. Busch T, Bartsch P, Pappert D, et al: Hypoxia decreases exhaled nitric oxide in mountaineers susceptible to high-altitude pulmonary edema. Am J Respir Crit Care Med 163:368, 2001.
124. Ghofrani HA, Reichenberger F, Kohstall MG, et al: Sildenafil increased exercise capacity during hypoxia at low altitudes and at Mount Everest base camp: A randomized, double-blind, placebo-controlled crossover trial. Ann Intern Med 141:169, 2003.
125. Sartori C, Allemann Y, Duplain H, et al: Salmeterol for the prevention of high-altitude pulmonary edema. N Engl J Med 346:1631, 2002.
126. Mortimer H, Patel S, Peacock AJ: The genetic basis of high-altitude pulmonary oedema. Pharmacol Ther 101:183, 2004.
127. Aldashev AA, Sarybaev AS, Sydykov AS, et al: Characterization of high-altitude pulmonary hypertension in the Kyrgyz: Association with angiotensin-converting enzyme genotype. Am J Respir Crit Care Med 166:1396, 2002.
128. Droma Y, Hanaoka M, Ota M, et al: Positive association of the endothelial nitric oxide synthase gene polymorphisms with high-altitude pulmonary edema. Circulation 106:826, 2002.
129. Hotta J, Hanaoka M, Droma Y, et al: Polymorphisms of renin-angiotensin system genes with high-altitude pulmonary edema in Japanese subjects. Chest 126:825, 2004.
130. Oelz O, Maggiorini M, Ritter M: Nifedipine for high altitude pulmonary oedema. Lancet 2:1241, 1989.
131. Scherrer U, Vollenweider L, Delabays A, et al: Inhaled nitric oxide for high-altitude pulmonary edema. N Engl J Med 334:624, 1996.
132. Silber E, Sonnenberg P, Collier DJ, et al: Clinical features of headache at altitude: A prospective study. Neurology 60:1167, 2003.
133. Broome JR, Stoneham MD, Beeley JM, et al: High altitude headache: Treatment with ibuprofen. Aviat Space Environ Med 65:19, 1994.
134. Burtscher M, Likar R, Nachbauer W, et al: Ibuprofen versus sumatriptan for high-altitude headache. Lancet 346:254, 1995.
135. Hornbein TF, Townes BD, Schoen RB, et al: The cost to the central nervous system of climbing to extremely high altitude. N Engl J Med 321:1714, 1989.
136. Hamilton AJ, Cymerman A, Bloch M: High altitude cerebral edema. Neurosurgery 19:841, 1986.
137. Severinghous JW: Hypothetical roles of angiogenesis, osmotic swelling, and ischemia in high-altitude cerebral edema. J Appl Physiol 79:375, 1995.
138. Schoch HJ, Fischer S, Marti HH: Hypoxia-induced vascular endothelial growth factor expression causes vascular leakage in the brain. Brain 125:2549, 2002.
139. Kinsey CM, Roach R: Role of cerebral blood volume in acute mountain sickness. Adv Exp Med Biol 543:151, 20003.
140. Lubin JR, Rennie D, Hacket P, et al: High altitude retinal hemorrhage: A clinical and pathological case report. Ann Ophthalmol 14:1071, 1982.
141. Sutton JR: High altitude retinal hemorrhage. Semin Respir Med 5:159, 1983.
142. McFadden DM, Houston CS, Sutton JR, et al: High altitude retinopathy. JAMA 245:581, 1981.
143. Mader TH, Tabin G: Going to high altitude with pre-existing ocular conditions. High Alt Med Biol 4:419, 2003.
144. Johnson AO: Chronic obstructive pulmonary disease: Fitness to fly with COPD. Thorax 58:729, 2003.
145. Wyss CA, Koepfli P, Fretz G, et al: Influence of altitude exposure on coronary flow reserve. Circulation 108:1202, 2003.
146. Wetterberg L: Light and biological rhythms. J Intern Med 235:5, 1994.

147. Brown GM: Day–night rhythm disturbance, pineal function, and human disease. Horm Res 37(suppl 3):105, 1992.
148. Honma K, Hashimoto S, Nakao M, et al: Period and phase adjustments of human circadian rhythms in the real world. J Biol Rhythms 18:261, 2003.
149. Reid KJ, Chang AM, Zee PC: Circadian rhythm sleep disorders. Med Clin North Am 88:631, 2004.
150. Waterhouse J, Reilly T, Atkinson G: Jet-lag. Lancet 350:1611, 1997.
151. Caldwell JL: The use of melatonin: An information paper. Aviat Space Environ Med 71:238, 2000.
152. Roth T, Roehrs T, Vogel G: Zolpidem in the treatment of transient insomnia: A double-blind, randomized comparison with placebo. Sleep 18:246, 1995.
153. Jamieson AO, Zammit GK, Rosenberg RS, et al: Zolpidem reduces the sleep disturbance of jet lag. Sleep Med 2:423, 2001.
154. Spitzer RL, Terman M, Williams JB, et al: Jet lag: Clinical features, validation of a new syndrome-specific scale, and lack of response to melatonin in a randomized, double-blind trial. Am J Psychiatr 156:1392, 1999.
155. Suhner A, Schlagenhauf P, Hofer I, et al: Effectiveness and tolerability of melatonin and zolpidem for the alleviation of jet lag. Aviat Space Environ Med 72:638, 2001.
156. Chase JE, Gidal BE: Melatonin—Therapeutic use in sleep disorders. Ann Pharmacol 31:1218, 1997.
157. Herxheimer A, Petrie KJ: Melatonin for the prevention and treatment of jet lag. Cochrane Database Syst Rev 2:CD001520, 2002.
158. Petrie K, Dawson AG, Thompson L, et al: A double-blind trial of melatonin as a treatment for jet lag in international cabin crew. Biol Psychiatr 33:526, 1993.
159. Hunter PR: Climate and waterborne and vector-borne diseases. J Appl Microbiol 94(suppl):37S, 2003.
160. Haines A, Patz JA: Health effects of climate change. JAMA 291:99, 2004.
161. Euripidou E, Murray V: Public health impacts of floods and chemical contamination. J Public Health (Oxford) 26:376, 2004.
162. Young S, Balluz L, Malilay J: Natural and technologic hazardous material releases during and after natural disasters: A review. Sci Total Environ 322:3, 2004.
163. Mozsynski P: Extreme weather worsens global hunger. News. BMJ 329:473, 2004.
164. Noji EK: Public health issues in disasters. Crit Care Med 33:S29, 2005.
165. "Indian Ocean Earthquake." Wikipedia online encyclopedia 2005. http:en.wikipedia.org/wiki/2004_Indian_Ocean_earthquake.
166. Chou YJ, Huang N, Lee CH, et al: Who is at risk of death in an earthquake? Am J Epidemiol 160:688, 2004.
167. Morgan O: Infectious disease risks from dead bodies following natural disasters. Pan American J Public Health 15:307, 2004.
168. Gottlieb S: Dead bodies do not pose health risk in natural disasters. BMJ 328:1336, 2004.
169. Seynaeve G, Archer F, Fisher J, et al: International standards and guidelines on education and training for the multi-disciplinary health response to major events that threaten the health status of a community. Prehospital Disaster Med 19:S17, 2004.

135

Delusional Parasitosis

KATHRYN N. SUH
JAY S. KEYSTONE

INTRODUCTION

Delusional parasitosis (DP) is a rare disorder in which affected individuals have the mistaken but unshakable belief (delusion) that they are infected by "bugs": parasites, worms, bacteria, mites, or other living organisms. As with all delusions, this belief is unfounded and irrational but cannot be corrected by reasoning, persuasion, or logical argument. The spectrum of symptoms leading to consideration of the diagnosis of DP can be broad and may encompass a range of symptoms and beliefs. Some individuals are quite functional and merely have the feeling that they are infested, others may experience the sensation of crawling or moving insects in their skin (formication), and yet others may have true delusions of parasitic infection that interfere with their usual activities to varying degrees.[1]

Delusional parasitosis is known by many names. Other English terms that have been used include Ekbom syndrome (not to be confused with Wittmaack-Ekbom syndrome, or restless legs), delusory parasitosis, psychogenic parasitosis, delusional infestation, delusional ectoparasitosis, formication, chronic tactile hallucinosis, dermatophobia, parasitophobia, and cocaine bugs.

HISTORICAL PERSPECTIVE

The first reported case of what is now referred to as DP is credited to George Thibierge, who coined the term acarophobia in his 1894 description of patients who were convinced they were infected with mites.[2] In 1938, Karl Ekbom described a similar clinical picture that he called "praeseniler Dermatozoenwahn" (presenile dermatozoic delusion),[3] subsequently referred to as Ekbom syndrome. He postulated that abnormal sensations experienced by his and several other patients subsequently led to delusions that parasites were present. This theory was supported over 30 years later by Berrios, who also suggested that the initial sensation *as if* something is crawling on the patient's skin leads to the conviction that something really *is* crawling on the skin.[4]

In 1946, Wilson and Miller described a total of 45 cases reported up to that time in addition to six cases of their own and introduced the term "delusional parasitosis."[5] Bers and Conrad proposed the term "chronic tactile hallucinosis" in 1954, because the similarities they observed with alcohol included hallucinosis.[6] Munro suggested that DP was in fact a form of monosymptomatic hypochondriasis or monosymptomatic hypochondriacal psychosis (MHP), a fixed, single hypochondriacal belief that exists when no other disorder of thought is present.[7] By 1995, in an extensive review of the topic, Trabert[8] had identified 1223 cases in the literature. Many additional case reports and case series have since been reported.

PSYCHIATRIC PERSPECTIVE

The interaction between psychiatric symptoms and dermatologic conditions has been well described.[9–11] It is estimated that 30% to 40% of patients seen in dermatology clinics have some psychiatric symptoms.[12] This is not to suggest, however, that psychiatric illness is the *cause* of dermatologic symptoms in all such patients. Koo has described three forms of psychodermatologic conditions in which disorders of skin and mind may be intermingled[9]: psychophysiologic disorders, in which the patient's mental state can directly affect the condition of an underlying skin disease (e.g., eczema worsened by stress); primary psychiatric disorders such as DP, in which cutaneous symptoms or findings can be directly attributed to an underlying psychiatric disease; and secondary psychiatric disorders, such as anxiety or depression, that may result from an intractable disfiguring skin condition (e.g., alopecia, ichthyosis).

In its truest form, DP is a delusional disorder of the somatic type: "delusions that the person has some physical defect of general medical condition."[13] Nonexistent disease or alteration of the body forms the basis of a somatic (or somatoform) delusional disorder. Delusions of parasitosis are classified as an MHP and are the most common form of this disorder; others include delusions of dysmorphism and delusions of body odor or halitosis.

The etiology of somatic disorders such as DP and the mechanisms of its persistence in affected individuals are unknown. One hypothesis is that for some individuals, distressing symptoms become amplified and are then perpetuated following the result of newly acquired knowledge or awareness of a disease, new or renewed public health interest, or intense media coverage, for example.[14] Fleeting pruritus following an encounter with an individual with scabies may not be uncommon, but for some the pruritus might worsen as they learn more about scabies. The reasons for this degree of symptom amplification are unclear. Some individuals may truly believe that they are sick, others may behave this way because they think that is how they are expected to behave, and others may be seeking secondary gains.[14,15] Regardless, symptoms are continuously intensified with the resulting perception that the individual is now suffering from a serious disease. Patients may also develop a heightened awareness of and misinterpret new sensations or symptoms that they were previously oblivious to, reaffirming their beliefs that they must be sick, and perpetuating the cycle. As with dermatologic disease, stress can also exacerbate other somatic complaints, and the stress induced by the severity of the perceived illness may also act to augment it further.

CLASSIFICATION OF DELUSIONAL PARASITOSIS

No definitive classification of DP exists.[16] However, in broad terms, three different forms can be described based on published accounts.[17] Primary psychotic DP exists when the delusion of parasitic infection is the only manifestation of disease; that is, no other psychiatric or psychological disorder is present. Secondary DP may occur in the presence of underlying psychiatric disease, such as schizophrenia or depression. Delusions of parasitosis may also be features of underlying medical illnesses and intoxication or substance abuse (e.g., cocaine), and rarely have been described as adverse effects of some prescription medications.

Primary Delusional Parasitosis

As noted previously, primary DP refers to a somatic delusional disorder. By definition, patients with delusional disorders do not meet all criteria required for the diagnosis of schizophrenia.[13] Specifically, hallucinations, disorganized speech, schizophrenic behavior, and other "negative" symptoms should be absent, although hallucinations that are clearly related to the delusional theme (i.e., tactile hallucinations) may be present. Sufferers of DP and other forms of MHP generally have intact mental function, lack other manifestations of psychiatric disease, and have otherwise normal behavior. Their delusions are limited in scope and generally do not encroach on personal and professional aspects of their lives. Criteria for the diagnosis of delusional disorders are shown in Table 135-1.

Strictly speaking, DP differs from hypochondriasis in that individuals with the latter condition recognize that fear of illness or disease is unfounded, and it differs from phobias in that patients with DP do not have a fear of becoming ill—they believe they *are* ill. Underlying psychiatric disorders, including schizophrenia and mood disorders, and pre-existing medical conditions (including true parasitic infections!), substance abuse, and drug side effects must be ruled out prior to establishing a diagnosis of primary DP. Other mood disorders (e.g., anxiety, depression) may be present with primary delusions of parasitosis, but they must clearly be secondary to the delusional disorder in order to classify the delusional disorder as primary DP.

Table 135-1 Diagnostic Criteria for Delusional Disorder

- Patient has nonbizarre delusions involving situations that occur in real life, lasting longer than 1 month
- Patient does not meet all criteria for diagnosis of schizophrenia
- Patient's function is otherwise not markedly impaired
- Patient's mood episodes, if concurrent, are brief compared with duration of delusions
- Substance abuse, medication side effects, and medication use in general must be ruled out

Adapted from American Psychiatric Association: DSM-IV-TR: Diagnostic and Statistical Manual of Mental Disorderss, 4th ed., Text Revision. Washington, D.C., American Psychiatric Association, 2000, pp 323–329.

Secondary Delusional Parasitosis

Delusions of parasitosis may occur in conjunction with other psychiatric symptoms. Some patients with DP are clearly schizophrenic. Others have varying degrees of psychiatric illness including anxiety, depression, obsessive-compulsive disorder, schizophreniform disorder, bipolar disorder, or a family history of psychiatric illness.[15,18,19] One case has been described in the setting of post-traumatic stress disorder.[20] Delusions of parasitosis in the setting of underlying psychiatric disease must be distinguished from primary DP because the management differs; however, differentiating these conditions may be challenging, particularly for the family physician or dermatologist, who is most likely to encounter such patients. Phobias and hypochondriasis may present with apparent delusions of parasitosis and may be considered secondary delusional parasitosis by some.[18]

Delusions of Parasitosis Associated with Underlying Medical Conditions

Up to 25% of cases of DP have been attributed to underlying medical diseases.[8,21] Establishing whether delusions are related to an associated medical disorder, drug, or toxin may be critical, since treatment of the condition (or withdrawal of the offending agent) may lead to resolution of delusional symptoms.

Central nervous system (CNS) disorders appear to be the most common underlying medical conditions associated with DP. Delusions have been described in the setting of dementia of various etiologies,[21,22] head injury,[23] cerebrovascular accidents,[23,24] multiple sclerosis,[23] multiple system atrophy,[25] and CNS infections including encephalitis, meningitis, and neurosyphilis.[21]

In addition, DP has been associated with diseases of most other organ systems including the hematopoietic,[23] pulmonary,[23] cardiac,[5,26] renal,[23] gastrointestinal,[23] and endocrine.[22,23,27] Nutritional deficiencies including vitamin B_{12},[23,28] folate,[21,23] and pellagra[23,29] have also been reported as causes of DP. Delusions of parasitosis may also be a manifestation of a variety of malignancies[21,27,30] or systemic infections such as human immunodeficiency virus infection,[31] tuberculosis,[5] and leprosy.[22]

Substance abuse is another precipitant of parasitic delusions and should be considered, particularly when DP presents in younger age groups.[19,23] In such instances, the delusions are usually transient and of inadequate duration to meet the criteria for delusional disorder. Cocaine, alcohol, and amphetamines (e.g., Ritalin) are common precipitants.[32] Rarely, prescription drugs may induce delusions of parasitosis; DP has been reported with the use of phenelzine,[33,34] pargyline,[34] ketoconazole,[35] and corticosteroids.[21] Drug-induced DP generally resolves once the offending drug is discontinued. A more thorough list of medical conditions and drugs/toxins associated with DP is shown in Table 135-2.

EPIDEMIOLOGY

Delusional disorders in general are rare.[36] The incidence and prevalence of delusional disorders have been estimated to be 0.7 to 3.0 and 24 to 30 cases per 100,000 population (upper limits of 0.003% and 0.03%), respectively,[37] although

Table 135-2 Medical Conditions Associated with Delusional Parasitosis

Neurologic disorders	Dementia Alzheimer's disease Multi-infarct Huntington's disease Head trauma Infarction Meningitis, encephalitis Human immunodeficiency virus Neurosyphilis Multiple sclerosis Pernicious anemia Tumors of the central nervous system
Endocrine disorders	Diabetes mellitus Hyperthyroidism
Hematologic disorders	Severe anemia Leukemia Polycythemia vera
Cardiopulmonary disease	Congestive heart failure Hypertension Asthma
Infectious diseases	Human immunodeficiency virus Leprosy Tuberculosis Prior infestation
Malignancy	Lymphoma Solid organ: breast, colon, lung
Nutritional deficiency	B_{12}, folate, thiamine deficiency Pellagra
Other disorders	Arthritis Hepatitis Stasis dermatitis Vitiligo
Drugs or toxins	Alcohol Amphetamines including methylphenidate Cocaine
Prescription medications	Corticosteroids Ketoconazole Pargyline Phenelzine

Adapted from Slaughter JR, Zanol K, Rezvani H, et al: Psychogenic parasitosis: A case series and literature review. Psychosomatics 1998; 39:491–500; and Johnson GC, Anton RF: Delusions of parasitosis: Differential diagnosis and treatment. South Med J 1985;78:914–918.

the rates in this study were not determined using currently accepted diagnostic criteria. Males and females are almost equally affected, with delusional disorders being slightly more common in women.

The exact rates of DP are even more difficult to determine. A retrospective study of almost 10,500 psychiatric outpatients in China identified 86 (0.83%) with delusional disorders, two of whom had unspecified somatic delusions.[38] In a Norwegian study of over 3000 psychiatric admissions to hospital, 0.4% of patients with paranoid psychoses had hypochondriacal delusions.[39] However, because patients with DP insist that their symptoms do not have a psychiatric basis and hence refuse to seek psychiatric help, the true incidence and prevalence of this disorder may be greatly underestimated in the psychiatric literature. Trabert estimated the incidence and prevalence of DP to be 16.6 and 83.2 cases per million population per year, respectively, in southwest Germany.[40] Although the number of reported cases of DP in the literature continues to increase, it remains extremely uncommon. Based on Lyell's retrospective survey,[23] Lynch estimated that a practicing dermatologist could expect to see one patient with DP for every 7 years in practice.[1] Most cases have been reported from centers in North America and Europe and more recently from Asia.

CLINICAL FEATURES AND PRESENTATION

General characteristics of patients with DP are fairly consistent based on data reported in two physician surveys[23,26] and several case series.[8,19,21,22] Delusional parasitosis can affect patients of all ages but is more common in older age groups (>50 years).[8,26] The mean age of onset in 802 patients for whom this was recorded in Trabert's review of 1228 cases was 57 years[8]; 84% of patients were over age 50. The age of onset does not differ significantly between men and women, although men tend to be slightly younger.[8] In all age groups, the disorder appears to be more common in women; overall, women outnumber men by roughly a 2–3:1 ratio.[8,22,23] Although the sex distribution is almost equal in early adulthood, the preponderance of women in older age groups is striking, with the female-to-male ratio exceeding 3:1 in individuals over 50 years of age.[8,23] Patients in younger age groups are more likely to have an underlying cause for their delusions, notably, head injuries, substance abuse, and schizophrenia, and are more likely to be involved in shared delusions.[19,23]

Patients with primary DP are usually otherwise functional individuals who do not have an antecedent history of psychiatric illness. For some patients, the delusions may be triggered by an event in which possible exposure to parasites may have occurred, (e.g., sleeping in unclean bedsheets or borrowing someone else's clothes).[1] Travel to and receipt of gifts from exotic destinations have precipitated DP.[41,42] Documented parasitic infections predate the development of DP in only 2% of cases.[23] Patients may be from any socioeconomic background. Many affected individuals are highly functional and highly educated; in Lyell's survey,[23] several of the 282 patients described were professionals, including physicians and psychologists. Despite this, they are, by definition, unable to appreciate their delusional state, although in some cases of primary DP, the unfounded basis of the patient's delusions has become apparent to the individual during the course of pharmacologic treatment.[32]

Many patients are single and have been categorized as "loners."[7,43] In Trabert's series, only 21% of the 67 patients for whom social interactions were described were considered to have "good and stable social contacts"; 54% were considered "socially isolated."[8] Social isolation appears to be a premorbid state rather than a consequence of illness.[8] A higher-than-expected prevalence of personality disorders has also been observed in some case series.[21,23]

Patients with DP often have a long history of dermatologic complaints including rashes, pruritus, and sensations of stinging, biting, and formication. The onset is usually insidious, and most patients have symptoms for at least 6 months and often many years before the diagnosis is made.[8,22] In Trabert's review, the average duration of symptoms was 3 years and the median duration 1 year.[8] Typically, patients have sought the help of multiple physicians (most commonly primary care physicians and dermatologists, sometimes infectious diseases physicians, rarely psychiatrists) or entomologists, usually with little satisfaction. Those who attribute their illness to household pets may have visited veterinarians repeatedly, seeking treatment for their pets. Many patients have received repeated courses of dermatologic and antiparasitic therapies, despite the lack of an objective diagnosis. They often bring in specimens for examination that they have picked from their skin—the "matchbox sign,"[44] which more recently has been aptly referred to as the "Ziploc bag sign."[18] Occasionally, these containers will contain parts of nonpathogenic insects, but most often they will harbor normal skin flakes or dust, hair, or other "flotsam of normal life."[15]

Patients may provide bizarre and unlikely stories concerning their infestation, including exhaustive descriptions and diagrams of the parasites' appearance, habitat, entry and egress to and from various body cavities, and reproductive cycles. Patients can often enumerate the parasites and provide details of their activities. Many have repeatedly called exterminators into their homes, consulted pest-control services, and sprayed themselves and their homes with potentially toxic pesticides and other chemicals to eradicate the bugs. Those driven to extremes may move or rid themselves of some or all of their belongings in the hopes of ending the problem. The fear of contagion and transmission of disease to others may or may not be present.

Other persons occasionally are drawn into the patient's delusional system; 8% to 25% of delusions of parasitosis may be shared.[21,23,45,46] Delusions are most often shared with one other person (folie à deux), usually a partner or spouse, or less commonly with offspring,[23] and usually are induced by a woman.[46] On occasion, trios (folie à trois) or even larger groups, such as entire families or groups of occupational colleagues, have developed shared delusions.

Apart from the firm belief that they suffer from a parasitic infection, the behavior of affected patients is usually unremarkable. Physical examination is often unrevealing apart from ulcers, excoriations, and scars that result from attempts to remove the organisms from the skin by using fingernails, knives, pins, or other objects. On exposed skin, lesions may be asymmetric, reflecting the increased range of the patient's dominant hand; this may be particularly evident over the shoulders and scapulae.[23] Contact or irritant dermatitis resulting from excessive cleaning or the use of abrasive soaps or chemicals may be present.

MANAGEMENT

Approach to the Patient with Delusional Parasitosis

The diagnosis of DP should be suspected when an individual has an irrational, fixed belief that he or she is infected with internal or external parasites despite reassurance and ample evidence to the contrary. Clearly, it is important to determine the following: (1) is the belief founded in reality? (i.e., is the patient really infected?); (2) if infection can be reliably excluded, is the patient truly delusional, or is the belief "shakable"? (is the patient merely hypochondriacal and can the patient possibly be convinced that he or she may not be infected?); and (3) if the patient is delusional, which form of DP is present? (i.e., primary DP, secondary DP, or DP associated with underlying medical illness or medications/toxins). Therapy differs markedly depending on the answers to these three questions. Clearly, treatment of a previously undiagnosed parasitic infection or of an underlying medical condition (if possible) is indicated if either is present. If the patient is truly delusional and an organic cause can be ruled out, the major challenge is to determine whether the patient has a primary delusional disorder (i.e., MHP) or an underlying psychiatric illness (i.e., secondary delusions of parasitosis). A psychiatric opinion is invaluable in such instances, but it is often never obtained, since patients with DP usually refuse a psychiatric assessment.

One key to the management of patients with DP is the development of a strong, therapeutic relationship. A significant proportion of these patients, if not the majority, express dissatisfaction with previous physicians, whom they believe are incompetent and uncaring. As a result, patients often fail to attend follow-up appointments and receive inadequate or no therapy, whereas many could benefit from readily available and effective therapy if only they would take it. A sympathetic ear, a nonjudgmental approach, acknowledgment that the patient's symptoms are real, and empathetic exploration into the effects of their symptoms on their daily lives can instill a sense of trust into the relationship.[47] It has been debated whether the physician should overtly agree or disagree with the patient's beliefs,[15] but many authors suggest a conservative and nonconfrontational approach.[1,15,48,49] Use of phrases such as, "I cannot see any parasites today" rather than "there are no parasites,"[23] and acknowledgment that the problem *may* have resulted from a previous infection[18] (perhaps even stating that the persistent symptoms are due to a "chemical imbalance") may accomplish this while at the same time gaining the patient's trust. It is important not to dismiss patients' complaints as trivial, even when it is obvious that they are delusional, but probably equally important not to overtly support their beliefs and feed into their delusional system. Reassurance that they can be helped also is valuable.

Initial assessments should focus on the patient's primary complaints, attempting to rule out true infection and organic causes of symptoms. A thorough history, including use of prescription and illicit drugs, and review of systems should be obtained. Listening carefully to the patient's answers sometimes provides clues to underlying psychiatric or medical illness. A complete physical examination is warranted, with particular attention paid to the skin, since most patients have cutaneous symptoms. Careful assessment of any skin lesions is essential; in a small number of cases, patients believed to have DP in fact have a true parasitic infection. Evaluation by a dermatologist, if not already performed, can be beneficial to the primary care physician and may also provide reassurance to patients that their symptoms are being taken seriously. If the patient has brought in specimens, reassure the patient that they will be sent to a proper laboratory or entomologist for examination. To avoid the argument that the "parasites" have been or will be missed because of improper preservation, provide the patient with specimen bottles containing preservative for subsequent samples. Skin biopsies may rarely be indicated in some instances; skin scrapings or other cutaneous specimens may be more appropriate and can be readily obtained during an office visit. Negative results, especially from repeated examinations of submitted specimens, can eliminate the possibility of a real parasitic infection.

Possible organic causes of DP may be evident from the history or physical examination (e.g., hyperthyroidism, neurologic disease). Blood work should be obtained to complete the assessment. Appropriate initial investigations include a complete blood count and differential, electrolytes, urea, creatinine, liver function tests, fasting blood sugar, thyroid-stimulating hormone level, and B_{12} and folate levels, as well as a chest radiograph. Based on the individual's risk factors, additional tests such as serology for human immunodeficiency virus infection, tuberculosis skin testing, VDRL or rapid plasma reagin test, or other radiologic imaging (e.g., computed tomography or magnetic resonance imaging of the brain), may be indicated. Those with organic diseases may be better managed by referral to an appropriate specialist (e.g., internist, neurologist). By means of a thorough history and physical examination and some basic investigations, true infestation and the more commonly reported medical conditions associated with DP can be eliminated.

Over the course of several visits, serial examination of skin lesions can be performed and additional specimens (or other investigations) obtained as required. In addition, follow-up visits provide the opportunity for the patient to develop more trust in the physician. Trust in the physician is crucial if a psychiatric referral is likely to be required. Repeated assessments of the patient are helpful in determining whether the patient has a shakable belief (hypochondriasis) rather than true delusions; he or she may eventually question whether the problem might be imaginary or "in his or her head," or ask the physician's opinion of the problem.[18] Such shakable beliefs are often associated with anxiety or depression;[18] supportive therapy and anxiolytic or antidepressant therapy are required for these patients. In contrast, antipsychotic therapy is usually indicated for patients with primary delusional parasitosis.

Treatment of Organic Causes of DP

Any real infestation should be treated appropriately. If an underlying organic cause is diagnosed, treatment may lead to resolution of the delusions[29]; input from other specialists may be indicated. Any medications or toxins that may be implicated should be discontinued as soon as possible if this is feasible.

Psychiatric Assessment

Once true infestation has been excluded, a psychiatric referral is warranted. Effective therapies are available for both primary and secondary DP, but they differ. Delusions of parasitosis associated with underlying psychiatric disorders such as schizophrenia or depression require treatment of the underlying disorder; this is probably best managed by a psychiatrist and is not discussed further. Although delusions in some patients who have organic causes of DP may improve or resolve with treatment of the underlying condition, these individuals may also benefit from psychiatric care. Gould and Gragg[50] suggest that psychiatric evaluation is appropriate only for selected patients with DP (such as those with schizophrenia) and that many others can be adequately managed by primary care physicians or dermatologists lest they be lost to medical care altogether by the suggestion that they see a psychiatrist. However, many authors suggest that a psychiatrist at least be consulted at some point in the patient's care.[18,19,32] Regardless of the approach, the treating physician's credibility often dissipates at the mention of the need for psychiatric consultation or therapy.

A thorough psychiatric assessment can provide confirmation of (or establish) the diagnosis; this is perhaps the most important reason for referral, and it allows determination of the most appropriate form of therapy. Another reason for psychiatric referral is that family physicians and dermatologists generally are neither trained nor prepared to provide the psychotherapy and pharmacotherapy that can benefit both the hypochondriacal patient (without true delusions) and the patient with primary or secondary DP. Many hypochondriacal patients will agree to a psychiatric assessment, but most patients with DP will not; therefore, tact and careful strategy are required.

Convincing patients with DP of the need for and importance of a psychiatric referral is extremely difficult. Gradual introduction of the topic over the course of several office visits, with emphasis on the need for expert guidance to manage the effects that DP has had on the patient's life, may result in greater success. Acceptance of psychiatric referral is likely to be higher if an on-site psychiatrist is present to perform an immediate assessment, such as in a dermatology-psychiatry liaison clinic, rather than asking the patient to attend a separate appointment in a different place,[18,32,50] but a significant proportion of patients will refuse even in this setting.[32] Furthermore, this arrangement often is not practical for physicians practicing outside of academic centers. At a minimum, if a psychiatric evaluation cannot be obtained for any reason, the case should be discussed with a psychiatrist prior to commencement of any therapy.

Treatment of Primary Delusional Parasitosis

Psychotherapy, psychosurgery, and electroconvulsive therapy have had relatively little success in the treatment of DP.[30] Psychotherapy has been successful in only 10% of cases, similar to the rate of resolution in untreated patients.[15] Antidepressant and anxiolytic medications may be beneficial if delusions are attributable to a pre-existing depressed or anxious state but have little or no role in the treatment of primary DP. Secondary mood disorders (i.e., those that are a consequence of the delusional state) may be improved, but delusions will persist. Prior to the introduction of effective neuroleptic therapy, DP was considered to be a progressive disorder with a low rate of spontaneous remission.

Treatment of primary DP was revolutionized by the advent of atypical antipsychotic medications. However, no clinical trials have examined the efficacy of neuroleptic medications for the treatment of DP. Nonetheless, if the diagnosis has been established with certainty, antipsychotics are now the mainstay of therapy. Convincing patients to take these medications provides yet another obstacle in the management of this disorder. Even if patients agree to start medication, adherence may be a problem. Occasionally, bargaining with a patient might work, whereby the physician agrees to a patient's request (e.g., treatment with an antiparasitic agent) on condition that the patient also takes antipsychotic medication.[18] Patients often refuse to try such drugs as risperidone or pimozide if they discover that they are antipsychotic agents. The physician can warn the patient that the agent is commonly used for schizophrenia and indicate that "of course, you are not schizophrenic!"

Patients are more likely to agree to take medication for treatment of a "chemical imbalance" than for a psychiatric problem. The physician can provide examples of other medications that have multiple indications for their use, such as aspirin for pyrexia and coronary artery disease, or amitriptyline for depression and neuritis. Some, particularly those insistent on knowing whether medication will cure their problem, may be persuaded to try medication if they are told that other patients with similar conditions have experienced great relief from symptoms and improvement in their well-being.

Before the introduction of atypical antipsychotics (such as ziprasidone, clozapine, risperidone, olanzapine, and quetiapine), pimozide was frequently used as first-line therapy for DP. However, today, many psychiatrists would choose the newer antipsychotics over pimozide because of their better safety profile and more specific actions.

Pimozide

Pimozide has been the most extensively used antipsychotic agent and has had the greatest reported success rate for treatment of DP. The first reports of successful treatment of MHP were published in 1975.[51,52] Shortly thereafter, small case series of patients with DP who were successfully treated with pimozide were published.[7,53] Subsequent case series have documented the effectiveness of pimozide, with up to 87% of patients demonstrating some response (33% to 52% complete, 28% to 35% partial), although such data should be interpreted with caution as they are observational only.[21,54] In the two retrospective physician surveys, pimozide was reported to induce a clinical response in 73% and 81% of treated patients,[8,23,26] with a full remission in 50%[8,23] although, like other retrospective studies, these results are prone to inherent bias. One placebo-controlled, double-blind trial with 10 patients[55] and another double-blind, crossover trial with 11 patients[56] both demonstrated efficacy of greater than 90%.

Pimozide is an oral diphenylbutylpiperidine antipsychotic agent. It is related in structure to butyrophenones, of which haloperidol is the most well known. The mechanism of action is selective blockade of dopamine type 2 receptors; it has minimal effect on other CNS neurotransmitters, although its antagonistic effects on opiate receptors may contribute to reducing the sensations of pruritus and formication.[55] Other pharmacologic effects of pimozide include a mild anticholinergic effect, blockage of calcium channels and of some adrenergic receptors, and induction of prolactin secretion. The most common adverse effects of pimozide when used at therapeutic doses are extrapyramidal reactions (tremor, bradykinesia, shuffling gait), which occur in up to 15% of patients.[19] Prolongation of the QT interval with the possibility of fatal arrhythmias may occur, particularly with higher doses of the drug; therefore, a baseline electrocardiogram is recommended prior to starting pimozide and periodically during therapy to monitor the QT interval duration. Increase of the QT interval by 25% or more from baseline, or a QT interval of greater than 520 msec, warrants temporary cessation of the drug and a subsequent dose reduction. Acute dystonic reactions, akathisia, anticholinergic effects, orthostatic hypotension, and galactorrhea are other side effects of pimozide.

Doses between 1 and 12 mg daily are usually effective for treatment of DP. Pimozide should be instituted at a low dose (0.5 to 1 mg daily) and increased gradually (e.g., by 1 mg weekly) either until the desired clinical effect is achieved[19] or to the maximum recommended dose of 20 mg/day. The lowest effective dose of pimozide should be used to minimize the risk of adverse events, ideally no more than 10 mg/day. Once a satisfactory response has been obtained, which may require several weeks of therapy, the patient should be maintained on the same dose for at least one and preferably several months.[19,57] The dose should then be tapered gradually (by 1 mg every 1 to 2 weeks) until it is discontinued, with careful observation for relapse.[19,57] If relapse occurs, it often responds to reinstitution of the drug; some patients will require prolonged therapy in order to control symptoms.

Other Antipsychotic Agents

Neuroleptic agents other than pimozide have been used with success in the treatment of DP but have not been reported to the same extent. In view of the cardiotoxic effects of pimozide, however, other agents may be preferable, particularly in the elderly and those with known cardiac disease. Furthermore, a more recent small case series has questioned the effectiveness of pimozide for treatment of delusional disorders such as DP.[58]

Haloperidol, similar in structure to pimozide, has been used successfully.[18,32,59] Risperidone has been effective in small numbers of patients, including some for whom haloperidol and pimozide have not been effective.[60–63] Serotonin is believed to play a significant role in psychosis[64]; risperidone is one of several atypical antipsychotic agents that preferentially blocks serotonin receptors while still maintaining some activity against dopamine receptors. Because of its lower toxicity compared with pimozide, some authors consider risperidone to be the first-line therapy for treatment of DP.[65] Between 0.25 and 5 mg daily, administered in one or two doses, have been required for clinical response.[60,61,63] Adverse effects including extrapyramidal reactions can occur, but overall risperidone appears to be safer and better tolerated than pimozide.[65]

Other antipsychotic agents that have been used with success include chlorpromazine,[66] olanzipine,[67,68] perphenazine,[27] quetiapine,[63] sertindole,[69] sulpiride,[70] thioridazine,[71] and trifluoperazine.[66]

OUTCOME AND PROGNOSIS

Delusional parasitosis was previously considered a progressive disorder with little chance of spontaneous improvement; only 10% to 30% of cases would remit spontaneously prior to the use of neuroleptics.[8,15]

The duration of symptoms is directly associated with the outcome of therapy; the longer the duration of symptoms, the less likely the patient will achieve a full remission.[8] Regardless, the use of effective pharmacotherapy has improved the prognosis for patients with DP. In Trabert's retrospective case series, 52% of patients who were followed after 1960 (i.e., after the introduction of neuroleptics for treatment) had a sustained remission during follow-up, compared with 33% who were diagnosed before 1960.[8] Outcomes related specifically to neuroleptic use were not addressed in this study, however. Other case series have demonstrated high rates of full recovery using pimozide, with 50% to 90% of patients achieving a sustained remission.[54,72] An additional one-third of patients may respond well but without achieving full remission.[23,54] The relapse rate is difficult to determine, but relapses appear to be common[23]; however, they do tend to respond well to reinstitution of therapy, regardless of the neuroleptic agent used.[18,23,27]

REFERENCES

1. Lynch PJ: Delusions of parasitosis. Semin Dermatol 1993;12:39–45.
2. Thibierge G : Les acaraphobes. Rev Gén Clin Thér 1894;8:373–376.
3. Ekbom KA: Der praeseniler dermato-zoenwahn. Acta Psychiatrica et Neurologica Scandinavica 1938;12:227–259.
4. Berrios GE: Tactile hallucinosis: Conceptual and historical aspects. J Neurol Neurosurg Psychiatry 1982;45:285–293.
5. Wilson JW, Miller HE: Delusions of parasitosis. Arch Dermatol Syphilol 1946;54:39–56.
6. Bers N, Conrad K: Die chronische tactile Halluzinose. Fortschr Neurol Psychiatr 1954;22:254–270.
7. Munro A: Monosymptomatic hypochondriacal psychosis manifesting as delusions of parasitosis: A description of four cases successfully treated with pimozide. Arch Dermatol 1978;114:940–943.
8. Trabert W: 100 years of delusional parasitosis: Meta-analysis of 1,223 case reports. Psychopathology 1995;28:238–246.
9. Koo J: Psychodermatology: The mind and skin connection. Am Fam Phys 2001;64:1873–1878.
10. Koo J, Gambla C, Fried R: Pseudopsychodermatologic disease. Dermatol Clin 1996;14:525–530.
11. Woodruff PWR, Higgins EM, du Vivier AWP, et al: Psychiatric illness in patients referred to a dermatology-psychiatry clinic. Gen Hosp Psychiatry 1997;19:29–35.
12. Hughes KE, Barraclough BM, Jamblin LG, et al: Psychiatric symptoms in dermatology patients. Br J Psychiatry 1983;143:51–54.
13. American Psychiatric Association: DSM-IV-TR: Diagnostic and Statistical Manual of Mental Disorders, 4th ed., Text Revision. Washington, D.C., American Psychiatric Association, 2000, pp 323–329.
14. Barsky AJ, Borus JF: Functional somatic syndromes. Ann Intern Med 1999;130:910–921.
15. Wykoff RF: Delusions of parasitosis: A review. Rev Infect Dis 1987;9:433–437.
16. Musalek M, Bach M, Passweg V, et al: The position of delusional parasitosis in psychiatric nosology and classification. Psychopathology. 1990;23:115–124.
17. Freinhar JP: Delusions of parasitosis. Psychosomatics 1984;25:47–53.
18. Zanol K, Slaughter J, Hall R: An approach to the treatment of psychogenic parasitosis. Int J Dermatol 1998;37:56–63.
19. Driscoll MS, Rothe MJ, Grant-Kels JM, et al: Delusional parasitosis: A dermatologic, psychiatric, and pharmacologic approach. J Am Acad Dermatol 1993;29:1023–1033.
20. Oruc L, Bell P: Multiple rape trauma followed by delusional parasitosis: A case report from the Bosnian war. Schizophr Res 1995;16:173–174.
21. Skott A: Delusions of infestation. Reports from the Psychiatric Research Center. No. 13. Göteborg, Sweden, St. Jörgen's Hospital, University of Göteborg, 1978.
22. Bhatia MS, Jagawat T, Choudhary S: Delusional parasitosis: A clinical profile. Int J Psychiatry Med 2000;30:83–91.
23. Lyell A: Delusions of parasitosis. Br J Dermatol 1983;108:485–499.
24. Nagaratnam N, O'Neile L: Delusional parasitosis following occipito-temporal cerebral infarction. Gen Hosp Psychiatry 2000;22:129–132.
25. Kumbier E, Kornhuber M: Dermatozoenwahn bei Multisystematrophie. Nervenarzt 2002;73:380–383.
26. Reilly TM, Batchelor DH: The presentation and treatment of delusional parasitosis: A dermatological perspective. Int Clin Psychopharmacol 1986;1:340–353.
27. May WW, Terpenning MS: Delusional parasitosis in geriatric patients. Psychosomatics 1991;32:88–94.
28. Pope FM: Parasitophobia as the presenting symptom of vitamin B_{12} deficiency. Practitioner 1970;204:421–422.
29. Aleshire I: Delusions of parasitosis: Report of successful care with antipellagrous treatment. JAMA 1954;155:15–17.
30. Berrios G: Delusional parasitosis and physical disease. Compr Psychiatry 1985;26:395–402.
31. Alciati A, Fusi A, D'Arminio Monforte A, et al: New-onset delusions and hallucinations in patients infected with HIV. J Psychiatry Neurosci 2001;26:229–234.
32. Slaughter JR, Zanol K, Rezvani H, et al: Psychogenic parasitosis: A case series and literature review. Psychosomatics 1998;39:491–500.
33. Aizenberg D, Schwartz B, Zemishlany Z: Delusional parasitosis associated with phenelzine. Br J Psychiatry 1991;159:716–717.
34. Liebowitz MR, Nuetzel EJ, Bowser AE, et al: Phenelzine and delusions of parasitosis: A case report. Am J Psychiatry 1978;135:1565–1566.
35. Finkelstein E, Amichai B, Halevy S: Paranoid delusions caused by ketoconazole. Int J Dermatol 1996;35:75.
36. Manschreck TC: Delusional disorder and shared psychotic disorder. In Sadock BJ, Sadock VA (eds): Comprehensive Textbook of Psychiatry, 7th ed. Philadelphia, Lippincott Williams & Wilkins, 1999, pp 1243–1264.
37. Kendler KS: Demography of paranoid psychosis (delusional disorder): A review and comparison with schizophrenia and affective illness. Arch Gen Psychiatry 1982;39:890–902.
38. Hsiao MC, Liu CY, Yang YY, et al: Delusional disorders: Retrospective analysis of 86 Chinese outpatients. Psychiatry Clin Neurosci 1999;53:673–676.
39. Retterstol N: Paranoid psychoses with hypochondriacal delusions as the main delusion. Acta Psychiatr Scand 1968;44:334–353.
40. Trabert W: Zur Epidemiologie des Dermatozoenwahns. Nervenarzt 1991;62:165–169.
41. Gill CJ, Hamer DH: "Doc, there's a worm in my stool": Munchausen parasitosis in a returning traveler. J Travel Med 2002;9:330–332.
42. Schwartz E, Witztum E, Mumcuoglu KY: Travel as a trigger for shared delusional parasitosis. J Travel Med 2001;8:26–28.
43. Reilly TM: Monosymptomatic hypochondriacal psychosis: Presentation and treatment. Proc R Soc Med 1977;70(suppl 10):39–42.
44. The matchbox sign. [Letter.] Lancet 1983;2:261.
45. Trabert W: Shared psychotic disorder in delusional parasitosis. Psychopathology 1999;32:30–34.
46. Musalek M, Kutzer E: The frequency of shared delusions in delusions of infestation. Eur Arch Psychiatr Neurol Sci 1990;239:263–266.
47. Gould WM, Gragg TM: Delusions of parasitosis: An approach to the problem. Arch Dermatol 1976;112:1745–1748.
48. Aw DCW, Thong JY, Chan HL: Delusional parasitosis: Case series of 8 patients and review of the literature. Ann Acad Med Singapore 2004;33:89–94.
49. Winsten M: Delusional parasitosis: A practical guide for the family practitioner in evaluation and treatment strategies. J Am Osteopath Assoc 1997;97:95–99.
50. Gould WM, Gragg TM: A dermatology-psychiatry liaison clinic. J Am Acad Dermatol 1983;9:73–77.
51. Riding BE, Munro A: Pimozide in monosymptomatic psychosis. [Letter.] Lancet 1975;1:400–401.
52. Reilly TM: Pimozide in monosymptomatic psychosis. [Letter.] Lancet 1975;1:1385–1386.
53. Reilly TM, Jopling WH, Beard AW: Successful treatment with pimozide of delusional parasitosis. Br J Dermatol 1978;98:457–459.
54. Zomer SF, de Wit FRE, van Bronswijk JEH, et al: Delusions of parasitosis: A psychiatric disorder to be treated by dermatologists? An analysis of 33 patients. Br J Dermatol 1998;138:1030–1032.
55. Ungvari G, Vladar K: Pimozide treatment for delusions of infestation. Act Nerv Super (Praha) 1986;28:103–107.
56. Hamann K, Avnstorp C: Delusions of infestation treated by pimozide: A double-blind crossover clinical study. Acta Dermatol Venereol 1982;62:55–58.
57. Koo J, Gambla C: Delusions of parasitosis and other forms of monosymptomatic hypochondriacal psychosis: General discussion and case illustrations. Dermatol Clin 1996;14:429–438.
58. Silva H, Jerez S, Ramirez A, et al: Effects of pimozide on the psychopathology of delusional disorder. Prog Neuropsychopharmacol Biol Psychiatry 1998;22:331–340.
59. Andrews E, Bellard J, Walter-Ryan WG: Monosymptomatic hypochondriacal psychosis manifesting as delusions of infestation: Case studies of treatment with haloperidol. J Clin Psychiatry 1986;47:188–190.
60. De Leon OA, Furmaga KM, Canterbury AL, et al: Risperidone in the treatment of delusions of infestation. Int J Psychiatry Med 1997; 27:403–409.

61. Safer D, Wenegrat B, Roth WT: Risperidone in the treatment of delusional parasitosis: A case report. J Clin Psychopharmacol 1997;17:131–132.
62. Gallucci G, Beard G: Risperidone and the treatment of delusions of parasitosis in an elderly patient. Psychosomatics 1995;36:578–580.
63. Wenning MT, Davy LE, Catalano G, et al: Atypical antipsychotics in the treatment of delusional parasitosis. Ann Clin Psychiatry 2003;15:233–239.
64. King BH: Hypothesis: Involvement of the serotonergic system in the clinical expression of monosymptomatic hypochondriasis. Pharmacopsychiatry 1990;23:85–89.
65. Elmer KB, George RM, Peterson K: Therapeutic update: Use of risperidone for the treatment of monosymptomatic hypochondriacal psychosis. J Am Acad Dermatol 2000;43:683–686.
66. Srinivasan TN, Suresh TR, Jayaram V, et al: Nature and treatment of delusional parasitosis: A different experience in India. Int J Dermatol 1994;33:851–855.
67. Nakaya M: Olanzipine treatment of monosymptomatic hypochondriacal psychosis. Gen Hosp Psychiatry 2004;26:164–169.
68. Freudenmann RW: Ein Fall von Dermatozoenwahn bei schwerer Herzinsuffizienz. Nervenarzt 2003;74:591–595.
69. Yorston G: Treatment of delusional parasitosis with sertindole. Int J Geriatric Psychiatry 1997;12:1127–1128.
70. Takahashi T, Ozawa H, Inuzuka S, et al: Sulpiride for treatment of delusion of parasitosis. Psychiatry Clin Neurosci 2003;57: 552–553.
71. Freyne A, Wrigley M: Delusional infestation in an elderly population. Ir Med J 1994;87:86–88.
72. Hamann K, Avnstorp C: Delusions of infestation treated by pimozide: A double-blind crossover clinical study. Acta Der Venereol 1982;62:55–58.

136

Tropical Infectious Disease Concerns in Pregnancy

RAUL E. ISTURIZ
EDUARDO GOTUZZO

Tropical infectious diseases that occur during pregnancy, an otherwise healthy, life-affirming state, pose special risks to the mother and fetus. Furthermore, many diagnostic, therapeutic, and preventive measures often must be modified during pregnancy because of their potential for serious side effects. This chapter discusses tropical infectious diseases that, during pregnancy, are especially important to mother or fetus, or that are more common or severe when associated with gestation. The reader must bear in mind that every diagnostic, therapeutic, or preventive strategy applied to a pregnant woman must be individually weighted against the possible side effects both to her and to her developing infant once instituted.

Worldwide, approximately eight million women suffer complications related to their pregnancies every year, and over half a million maternal deaths result. Maternal and neonatal morbidity and mortality show a stark divide between developing and developed countries. In some tropical areas, such as sub-Saharan Africa and central South Asia, one woman in 16 may die of pregnancy-related complications. This compares unfavorably with an average of one in 2800 in developed countries. These figures may be an underestimation since the World Health Organization (WHO) estimates that maternal deaths are under-reported by as much as 50%. Tragically, motherless children are 10 times more likely to die in childhood than children whose mothers survive. Although maternal infectious diseases in the tropics have an important contributing effect on maternal and childhood morbidity and mortality, their actual impact is unknown.

Based on anecdotal clinical observations and perhaps rooted in a need to explain maternal tolerance of intrauterine fetal tissues, physicians have perceived that the maternal immune response must to some extent be suppressed during gestation. Other than diminished T- and NK-cell function, no measurable suppression has been found in maternal immunity. Neutrophil numbers and function, B-cell counts and subsets, immunoglobulin G (IgG), IgM, and IgA concentrations, antibody-dependent cellular cytotoxicity (ADCC), and complemet have been found within the normal limits. Nevertheless, the mild immunosuppression that may accompany pregnancy but that does not last postpartum may play an as yet undefined role in maternal infectious morbidity and mortality by the diseases described in this chapter. The importance of direct or indirect exposure of pregnant women to microorganisms derived from poor tropical areas cannot be overemphasized.

Table 136-1 Risk Categories of Selected Antimicrobial Agents in Pregnant Women

Agent	Pregnancy Category*
Atovaquone-proguanil	C
Artemisinin	N/A
Azithromycin	B
Aztreonam	B
Chloroquine	N/A (C?)
Chloramphenicol	N/A (C?)
Clarithromycin	C
Cefoperazone	B
Cefotaxime	B
Ceftriaxone	B
Cycloserine	N/A (C)
Clindamycin	B
Dapsone	C
Doxycycline	D
Erythromycin	B
Ethambutol	C
Ethionamide	C
Halofantrine	N/A
Isoniazid	C
Mefloquine	C
Pyrazinamide	C
Quinine	N/A
Rifabutin	B
Rifampicin	C
Rifapentine	C
Spiramycin	N/A
Streptomycin	D
Sulfadoxine	N/A

N/A, not available.
*See Table 136-2.

Furthermore, the potential risks of anti-infective drugs in pregnancy also complicate the management of important tropical infectious diseases in pregnant and newborn individuals. The U.S. Food and Drug Administration (FDA) risk category definitions and assignments for selected antimicrobial agents are shown in Tables 136-1 and 136-2. As considered below, for malaria infections that are life-threatening to mother and fetus, the benefits of antimalarial agents and the lack of significant documented human toxicities for chloroquine, mefloquine, atovaquone-proguanil, and quinine, mandate their use.

BRUCELLOSIS

Although teratogenicity has not been described, *Brucella* has been isolated from placental, fetal, and newborn tissues, demonstrating vertical transmission.[1–3] Epidemiologic evidence suggests that *Brucella* species, and *B. melitensis* in particular, can produce preterm and intrauterine fetal death followed by spontaneous abortions in humans, probably more frequently than do other bacterial infections.[4] An increased incidence of fetal loss among infected pregnant women with brucellosis has been repeatedly described.[4–6] In their review of 92 pregnant women with brucellosis in endemic Saudi Arabia, Khan and colleagues note that "although comparative

Table 136-2 *U.S. FDA Use-in-Pregnancy Ratings*

Category	Interpretation	Comments
A	Controlled studies show no risk	No demonstration of risk to the fetus in any trimester
B	No evidence of risk in humans	The chance of fetal harm is remote, but remains a possibility
C	Risk cannot be ruled out	There is a chance of fetal harm, but the potential benefits may outweigh the potential risk
D	Positive evidence of risk	Fetal risk demonstrated, potential benefits may outweigh the risk
X	Contraindicated in pregnancy	Positive evidence of fetal abnormalities or risk that clearly outweighs any possible benefit

data are limited, the incidence of abortion from 10% to 42% in patients with active brucellosis exceeds that observed in patients infected with other organisms, such as *Campylobacter* species and *Salmonella* species, and suggests that *Brucella* species may indeed produce human abortions more frequently than do other bacterial pathogens." They also recommend prompt antimicrobial therapy in pregnant women with brucellosis.[4]

The absence of erythritol in the human placenta, and anti-*Brucella* activity in human amniotic fluid, may explain why brucellosis causes fewer spontaneous abortions in humans than in farm animals, especially bovine species.[7] *Brucella* has also been isolated from human breast milk and from vaginal swabs from nonpregnant females, but the relevance of these findings remains uncertain.[8–12]

The clinical presentation of brucellosis during pregnancy has prognostic implications for fetal survival. In the Saudi study, during the first and second trimesters, vaginal bleeding with or without febrile illness was associated with spontaneous abortion in all cases of brucellosis, but patients who were treated because they presented with a predominantly febrile illness had no spontaneous abortions.[4] Of 11 patients who were treated because of febrile brucellosis presenting preterm during the third trimester, one spontaneous abortion was observed. Also one spontaneous abortion was documented out of 14 patients that presented with febrile brucellosis at term. The presence of bacteremia or high brucella agglutinin antibody titers did not correlate with the incidence of abortion. In this series, antibiotics used for treatment were trimethoprim–sulfamethoxazole (TMP-SMX) and rifampin.

In a series of studies in Peru, 97 pregnant women with brucellosis have been treated in Lima over a 25-year period.[13,14] Several presented with jaundice, one patient died of hepatic failure in her third trimester, and 7 had spontaneous abortions. Of 22 patients that were admitted to the hospital with threatened abortion, 6 had premature deliveries and 16 eventually delivered a term infant. In this series, rifampin was given for 6 weeks plus an aminoglycoside for the first 2 weeks. Treated patients had no abortions.

Combination treatment of brucellosis is effective,[15–17] but tetracycline is contraindicated in pregnancy. Antepartum treatment with active antibiotics prevents spontaneous abortion and current information seems enough to recommend treatment of all cases. During pregnancy, combination therapy with rifampin plus TMP-SMX provides the best therapeutic balance to cure the disease, prevent relapses, and protect the developing infant.

CHOLERA

In endemic areas, but especially during epidemics and pandemics, adult individuals including pregnant women can and do acquire cholera.[18–20]

Among pregnant women, cholera is associated with diarrhea and dehydration of such severity that intrauterine suffering and death may occur. In 1892, 57% of pregnant women with cholera died and the abortion rate was estimated around 54%. Conversely, during a 1979–1980 cholera outbreak in Ile-Ife (Nigeria), where 61 pregnant patients were identified, cholera appeared to be less severe and to have a lower mortality in pregnant than in nonpregnant women.[19]

Cholera, a toxin-mediated disease without hematogenous spread or placental invasion, is not transmitted vertically, but intrafamilial transmission from adults with diarrhea is possible in the neonatal period. In Peru, among 626 children with cholera, isolation of *Vibrio cholerae* O1 was possible in 310 (49%), more commonly in children older than 24 months of age.

In a retrospective review of the records of 32 pregnant women treated for cholera of less than 24-hour duration, dehydration was moderate in 62.5% and severe in 37.5%.[21] Two fetal deaths occurred among the patients with severe dehydration, one on arrival and one within 8 hours of emergency room care. This series underscored the immediate favorable outcome for mother and fetus of prompt and vigorous hydration. This was accomplished initially intravenously and after 4 hours orally using the WHO oral rehydration solution (ORS). In another Peruvian series from a university hospital, of 8690 patients with cholera treated, 84 (0.96%) were pregnant women.[22] Eighty-one were treated using a standard rehydration protocol, 20 required hospitalization because of the clinical severity of dehydration, and 64 were treated and discharged from the emergency ward to complete treatment as outpatients. In this series, fetal deaths occurred in 7.7% of first trimester pregnancies, 6.9% in second trimester pregnancies, and 3.6% during the third trimester. Younger pregnant women (<20 years) were more frequently hospitalized (50%) than older mothers and had a higher rate of fetal death associated with the disease. Remarkably, there were no maternal deaths; three patients suffered transitory renal failure that recovered without dialysis.[22]

Treatment for pregnant patients with cholera consists of the rapid and adequate replacement of fluids, electrolytes, and base. There is conclusive evidence that solutions may be given orally and that the WHO ORS is safe and effective for pregnant women.

The rationale for the use of antibiotics for the treatment of cholera is that the duration and volume of fluid loss can be diminished and that clearance of *V. cholerae* from the stools can be hastened. Tetracycline, doxycycline, and quinolones have many more weaknesses than strengths in pregnancy and are not recommended. Ampicillin, TMP-SMX, and erythromycin are safer and can be substituted, provided susceptibility is assured.

Oral cholera vaccines have been available outside of the United States (see Chapter 21), but there are no data on the use of any cholera vaccine during pregnancy. Intrafamilial spread occurs but does not appear to play a major role in transmission to pregnant women.

DENGUE FEVER AND DENGUE HEMORRHAGIC FEVER

Intrauterine transmission of dengue viruses appears to be confirmed by several case reports and small series, but the exact mechanisms of transmission and the fetal pathogenesis have not been elucidated.[23–27] No significant increase in prevalence or in severity of the disease has been noted associated with pregnancy. The review of many small studies of women with clinical diagnosis of dengue fever during pregnancy strongly suggests that the risk of premature birth and fetal death are increased as a consequence of the disease, as are the risks of thrombocytopenia and hemorrhage for both mother and newborn.[23,25,28–30]

Fever is the most common presenting symptom in the mother, and when it occurs near term, the likelihood of hemorrhage is higher.[23] Neonates appear healthy at birth but develop symptoms after 3 to 7 days.[31,32] They should be thoroughly observed even if the mothers are clinically doing well. Maternal monitoring and treatment are as described for nonpregnant individuals. When cesarean section is indicated, platelet transfusions may be necessary.

VIRAL HEPATITIS

Infection by the hepatotropic viruses designated A, B, C, D, E, and G constitutes the most common cause of jaundice during pregnancy.[33] Hepatitis A and B viruses are responsible for most of the cases in developing and developed countries, and documentation of infection is most common during the third trimester. The severity and prognosis of maternal acute hepatitis A, B, C, and D does not seem to be affected by pregnancy. Prematurity and perinatal death may be slightly increased, but no increase in congenital malformations, abortion, low birth weight (LBW), or intellectual disabilities has been noted. Maternal management is not altered in any major way by the coexistence of pregnancy.

Hepatitis A

In utero transmission of hepatitis A is not recognized, and transmission by fecal contamination during delivery is rare. Infection during pregnancy or delivery does not appear to result in increased complications in the mother or increased clinical disease in the newborn.[34] Acute hepatitis A in the pregnant woman requires supportive care and recovery is expected; fulminant hepatitis has been observed in less than 1% of the cases. For newborn infants of infected mothers, immunoglobulin (Ig) is given as prophylaxis in postexposure situations.[34] Pregnant women may wish to avoid travel to endemic areas, and when nonimmune to hepatitis A, can receive immunization or Ig prophylaxis when needed.

Hepatitis B

Hepatitis B infection is highly prevalent in the tropics, where large segments of the population are not exposed to universal vaccination programs. Areas such as sub-Saharan Africa, the Amazon basin, most Pacific islands and some Caribbean islands, parts of the Middle East, and China have the highest prevalence of hepatitis B virus (HBV) infection. High prevalence can be expected in these areas during reproductive years.

Acute hepatitis B occurs in approximately 1 to 2 per 1000 pregnancies,[33] and it does not seem to pose special risks to the mother when compared to background rates for the general population. However, perinatal exposure poses great risk for acquisition of HBV by the infants born to hepatitis B surface antigen (HB_sAg)–seropositive mothers. The frequency of chronic hepatitis B in pregnancy is higher (approximately 5–15 per 1000) and also constitutes a risk for vertical transmission. Data from the Centers for Disease Control and Prevention (CDC) analyzed in 1996 estimated that 22,000 children are born to HBV-positive mothers every year in the United States alone. In highly endemic areas, the risk to the neonate to become perinatally infected and to develop chronic infection is very high.[35,36] Therefore, all pregnant women should be screened for HB_sAg during prenatal visits. Transmission rates are higher if the mother is also hepatitis B e antigen (HB_eAg)–positive.[34] Intrauterine infection occurs as evidenced by the fact that 2.5% of infants born to infected mothers have hepatitis B antigenemia during the neonatal period, but in most cases antigenemia appears later, suggesting transmission at delivery. Maternal blood, amniotic fluid, or feces may contain HBV, but cesarean section delivery and avoidance of breastfeeding do not prevent transmission. Most vertically infected infants carry HB_sAg by 2 to 5 months of age, but in some detection may take longer. Up to 20% of infants born to HB_sAg-positive mothers may become infected, and up to 90% of infants infected by their HB_eAg-positive mothers may become chronically infected if untreated. Gestational age, birth weight, and viral subtype do not appear to predict the likelihood of the baby becoming a chronic carrier. Although HB_sAg has been found in breast milk, breastfeeding does not appear to be a major risk factor for transmission. Most cases of HBV infection during pregnancy are asymptomatic, and when symptomatic the illness is similar to that of the general nonpregnant population. Fulminant hepatitis B[37] has been described at a rate of approximately 1%.

The diagnosis and management of hepatitis B during pregnancy is similar to that of nonpregnant patients. Hepatitis B vaccination is not contraindicated during pregnancy or lactation. Women of unknown HB_sAg status who present in labor or after delivery should be considered potentially infected. Infants born to HB_sAg-positive mothers or mothers with unknown HB_sAg status must receive monovalent hepatitis B vaccine along with 0.5 mL of hepatitis B immunoglobulin (HBIg) at a different anatomical site within 12 hours of birth, and complete a total of four or five doses regardless of gestational age.[38] The series can be completed using combination vaccines. Adoptees should be tested for HB_sAg. All children must be vaccinated. Postvaccination testing and revaccination are beyond the scope of this chapter but have been recently investigated.[39]

The management of hepatitis D coinfection during pregnancy does not differ from the management of hepatitis B. Perinatal transmission has been reported. Neonatal prophylaxis as described for HBV may prevent transmission of HDV.

Hepatitis C

A major problem worldwide, infection with the hepatitis C virus (HCV) has not been shown to affect fertility or increase rates of abortion, prematurity, LBW, or obstetric interventions compared to control subjects. There is, however, a risk of transmission from mother to infant of approximately 5%. Although the risk of perinatal transmission and the severity of the maternal disease must be considered, there is no contraindication for pregnancy in HCV-infected females. Vertical transmission in utero and during birth canal passage occurs, especially when high maternal viral loads are present[40] and when the expectant mother is an IV drug user and or is coinfected with HIV.[41] Nonviremic mothers (gravidas) rarely transmit HCV, but viremia at delivery reaches 55% to 75% rates. Current treatment options for hepatitis C such as pegylated interferon plus ribavirin are not used during pregnancy because of the unknown efficacy for treatment and prevention and the risk for potential side effects for mother and fetus. Delivery by cesarean section and avoidance of breastfeeding may decrease transmission, but data are inconclusive[42] and no formal evidence-based recommendation can be given at this time. Routine screening of all pregnant women is not recommended. Testing can be recommended for high-risk women and their offspring and for potential adoptees. Anti-HCV antibodies are usually present by age 1 year and PCR can detect HCV earlier.

Hepatitis E

There are data that suggest that infection with the hepatitis E virus (HEV), found most commonly in endemic areas of the Indian subcontinent, the Middle East, Southeast Asia, and Latin America, can be associated with higher mortality from fulminant disease during pregnancy,[43] especially when acute disease develops in the third trimester. Intrauterine death has been associated with severe disease and hypoglycemia. Perinatal transmission may occur more commonly than initially estimated[44] and may cause infant mortality as well. Immunoglobulin pooled from patients in endemic areas may prove beneficial.

Hepatitis G

In HIV-1-infected women, hepatitis G virus (HGV) coinfection is common,[45] and HGV can be transmitted sexually. Children born to HGV RNA–positive women coinfected with HIV are also likely to be HGV infected. Transmission appears to occur antenatally. Children remain infected and asymptomatic for long periods.

HUMAN IMMUNODEFICIENCY VIRUS AND ACQUIRED IMMUNODEFICIENCY SYNDROME

Globally, women represent approximately 60% of the total population of human immunodeficiency virus (HIV)–infected individuals, and the more efficient heterosexual, male-to-female transmission constitutes their greatest exposure risk. Younger women have the highest risk of infection. In areas of sub-Saharan Africa, HIV infection rates in pregnant women may exceed a staggering 25%. The disparity in the delivery of interventions to halt the deleterious effects of HIV and acquired immunodeficiency syndrome (AIDS) between developed and developing countries is very large and growing.

HIV infection is transmitted from an infected mother to her fetus during pregnancy, during delivery, and by breastfeeding. The timing of infection has been estimated and is schematically represented and simplified in Table 136-3. Determinants of transmission efficiency include social factors, concurrent sexually transmitted diseases (STDs), CD4 count and viral load, antiretroviral therapy (ART), as well as obstetric factors and feeding choices. Currently, with the vanishing exception of a few surviving children infected by blood products decades ago, virtually all HIV infections in children less than 13 years of age have been transmitted vertically from their infected mothers. In the United States alone, approximately 7000 HIV-positive women give birth each year. Worldwide, the number of HIV-infected mothers delivering infants is increasing dramatically, mainly in developing areas, while a major decrease has been noted in industrial countries.

Given no comorbidities, and accepting imperfections in the published studies, HIV infection appears to have little if any effect on pregnancy and pregnancy has little if any effect on HIV disease progression. Anemia, LBW, and prolonged labor are more frequently reported from areas where women have more advanced or untreated disease, malnutrition, and coinfections, but pregnancy does not adversely influence survival except in women with very advanced disease.[46,47]

Recurrent vaginal candidiasis is a common presenting complaint during pregnancy in HIV-infected women. With the exception of Kaposi's sarcoma, more common in men, the rates and patterns of symptoms, opportunistic infections, and malignancies are similar in nonpregnant and pregnant women. A somewhat greater predisposition to suffer esophageal candidiasis and bacterial pneumonia has been suggested in the literature. The diagnosis of HIV infection during pregnancy

Table 136-3 *Timing of HIV Transmission from Mother to Infant (n = 100)*

Gestational Age (in weeks)	Number Infected
≤14	1
14–36	4
36–labor	12
Intrapartum	8
Breastfeeding	Variable
Total developed countries	14–32%
Total developing countries	25–48%

Modified from Kourtis AP, Bulterys M, Nesheim SR, et al: Understanding the timing of HIV infection from mother to infant. JAMA 285:709–712, 2001 and several other authors.

is made in the same manner as in nonpregnant females. Shortcomings of the use of ELISA and Western blot tests in pregnant women must be kept in mind. Once diagnosed, a number of interventions to prevent or minimize mother-to-child transmission of HIV become vitally important. In the United States, aiming at the maintenance of the health of the patient and at interventions that sharply reduce vertical transmission, published guidelines recommend voluntary counseling and HIV testing to all pregnant women as early in pregnancy as possible.[48] Counseling must be based on testing that provides definitive information. In the developing world, in many areas of Africa, Asia, India, Latin America, and the Caribbean, very large numbers of pregnant women do not recognize the need for prenatal care, have difficulties accessing health facilities and personnel, and receive no or suboptimal diagnostic, prophylactic, and therapeutic interventions. This situation must change. Expert monitoring for health maintenance during pregnancy and for HIV-related issues must be assured. HIV-related monitoring must include timely testing, the prevention and treatment of opportunistic infections including tuberculosis, the use of pregnancy-specific individualized combination ART,[49] the timely election (or not) of the cesarean section, and discouraging (or not) of breastfeeding. These are all desirable, but not always or seldom possible in poor regions.

Current criteria for recommendation of combination ART in females in general apply to pregnant women. During pregnancy, individualization becomes more important and decisions about the initiation, continuation, and choice of treatment include fetal factors. Combination ART offers greater protection against perinatal transmission and should be considered even if the mother does not fulfill criteria for initiation of ART. Zidovudine (ZDV) should be included when possible. A single dose of nevirapine to mothers with HIV, when added to oral ZDV, has recently been proven highly efficacious in reducing vertical transmission of HIV,[50] but resistance mutations may appear in mother and baby.[51] In pregnant HIV-positive women, reverse transcriptase inhibitors (RTIs) may be responsible for more frequent and pronounced lactic acidosis and even hepatic steatosis. Protease inhibitors (PIs) may worsen insulin resistance and hyperglycemia. Hemolysis, elevated liver function tests, and low platelets, the so-called HELLP syndrome described in late pregnancy in otherwise healthy HIV-infected women, may also be more common with use of RTIs and PIs. Efavirenz is contraindicated in pregnancy because of simian embryopathy. Stavudine and dideoxyinosine (ddI) in combination with either PIs or nevirapine must be avoided or discontinued in pregnancy. An Antiretroviral Pregnancy Registry (www.apregistry.com) has been designed to better understand the strengths and weaknesses of the use of ART during pregnancy and may become an important international tool.

Elective cesarean section reduces the risk of perinatal transmission of HIV even in women who are taking antiretroviral drugs and even at low maternal viral loads,[52] but maternal morbidity is a consideration. With undetectable maternal viral loads, no evidence exists to guide a recommendation at this time.[53] Breastfeeding is discouraged in areas where infant formula is available, but extremely controversial in poor parts of the world where over 95% of HIV-infected women reside[54] who for social, economic, and other reasons will continue to lactate.

To control HIV infection and AIDS in women, pregnant women, and children, major global efforts will be required that close the growing standard of care gap between rich and poor and to ensure that the huge medical advances of the last decades reach as many people as possible.

HUMAN T-LYMPHOTROPIC VIRUS TYPE I

Human T-lymphotropic virus type 1 (HTLV-I) infection, a frequently ignored but important disease, is hyperendemic in the south of Japan and endemic in Africa, the Caribbean, and Latin America. Based on small studies, the clinical course of pregnancy does not seem to be altered by the presence of infection by HTLV-I and babies appear normal at birth. Vertical transmission does occur in 6% to 35% of newborns, usually postpartum via breast milk.[55] There is a threefold increased risk of transmission with breastfeeding for more than 6 months; from less than 10% to almost 35%. When breastfeeding was continued for more than one year, the proportion of infected children rose to almost 40% (E. Gotuzzo, unpublished data, 2005). Mothers with strongyloidiasis seem to transmit HTLV-I with enhanced efficiency, in contrast with asymptomatic mothers or those suffering tropical spastic paraparesis. Intrauterine and intrapartum transmissions also occur, but together they account for approximately 5% of vertical transmission. Perinatally transmitted HTLV-I infection poses a risk for the development of adult T-cell leukemia/lymphoma.[56]

Routine combination HTLV-I/II antibody testing of blood products is a strategy implemented in the United States since 1997, and in countries where the prevalence of infection in pregnant women exceeds 2% to 4%, screening of all pregnant mothers and formula feeding of infants of infected mothers is a logical strategy that is in use in Japan.[57] It may reduce childhood infection rates by nearly 90% and is a strategy that requires further study in less developed tropical countries. There is no therapy or vaccine available.

LEPTOSPIROSIS

Leptospira survives well in tropical nonsaline waters and leptospirosis is common in several tropical settings.[58,59] In certain endemic areas, up to 5% to 10% of patients who present to academic or research institutions may have leptospirosis. Data about leptospirosis occurring during gestation are scarce and come from small case series and reviews, case reports, and anecdotal information.[60–65] Little is known about the mutual effects of pregnancy and leptospirosis when they coincide in the same woman. Transplacental transmission is thought to occur and leptospira have been found in infected organs of mother and fetus. In a series of 11 cases diagnosed by culture or serology in French Guyana, fetal death occurred in over 50% of the cases.[64] In another report of one case from Israel and a review of 15 previous cases, eight pregnancies terminated in abortions, four newborns had neonatal leptospirosis and four were uninfected and appeared normal at birth.[61] During the early months of pregnancy, leptospirosis is more likely to result in spontaneous abortion, and during the last trimesters, more premature deliveries and neonatal disease result. Leptospirosis may present with jaundice and pulmonary abnormalities in a higher percentage of pregnant than nonpregnant women but these observations have not been confirmed.[60] Maternal mortality seems not affected compared to the background of nonpregnant women. Early diagnosis and antibiotic treatment of leptospirosis during pregnancy is essential. High-dose penicillin or ceftriaxone is associated with faster maternal recovery and improved fetal prognosis. Doxycycline is contraindicated during pregnancy. The Jarisch– Herxheimer reaction occurs rarely.[66]

LISTERIOSIS

Pregnancy is a risk factor for infection with *Listeria monocytogenes*.[67] Listeriosis among pregnant patients mainly affects women who have no comorbidities; cell-mediated immunity depression attributed to pregnancy itself has been cited as a predisposing factor. The incidence of listeriosis is estimated to increase from approximately 0.7 per 100,000 in the general population to approximately 12 per 100,000 in pregnant women, and intrauterine infection has been clearly associated with placental colonization, chorioamnionitis, spontaneous abortion, stillbirth, preterm labor, prematurity, and neonatal infection (including granulomatosis infantisepticum) and significant mortality.[67,68] In humans, there are no convincing data to link the past history of listeriosis with repeated spontaneous abortions.

Maternal infection, which can occur at any gestational age, presents clinically as a mild to moderate febrile illness, but a flulike syndrome is also a common presentation.[67] Maternal infection can occasionally be severe and meningitis has been reported. A high index of suspicion is essential to obtain specimens for microbiological confirmation of diagnosis. Specimens that are useful for culture of the organisms include maternal blood, placenta, amniotic fluid, cervical secretions, stool, and urine. Blood cultures should be performed to evaluate fever and/or flulike symptoms in pregnant women because they can detect the organism in some 35% of the cases. Gram stains of the placenta, as well as frozen sections when available, can produce a rapid presumptive diagnosis.

Early gestational listeriosis may result in bacteremia and seeding of the uterine contents. Fetal prognosis, worse in early pregnancy, is guarded throughout. Treatment of the disease at early stages is associated with better pregnancy outcomes. Approximately 20% of pregnancies complicated with listeriosis result in fetal death, and approximately two-thirds of the surviving infants develop neonatal disease. Early-onset neonatal listeriosis (<5 days) is predominantly septic and with correct treatment carries a high (approximately 30%) mortality rate; late onset (>5 days) is predominantly meningitic and mortality is lower (approximately 10%) with therapy.[69] A common differential diagnosis is with group B streptococcal sepsis. Disseminated neonatal disease is extremely serious and, if associated with prematurity, has a mortality rate that may approach 90%. Neurologic sequelae have been reported in survivors of neonatal disease. Furthermore, even neonates who do not develop clinically apparent listeriosis but who are born to mothers who suffered listeriosis during their pregnancy may have prolonged hospital stays.

During pregnancy, high-dose ampicillin, considered superior to penicillin for this indication, is felt to be the treatment of choice; adding gentamicin is synergistic and its use must be evaluated in special situations in light of the potential side effects to the fetus. Cephalosporins and clindamycin are not effective. No risk-free alternative exists during pregnancy and when penicillin hypersensitivity is suspected or reported, allergy testing and/or desensitization should be considered. TMP-SMX, active against listerosis but avoided during pregnancy, may—as is the case with brucellosis—offer benefits that exceed risks in certain cases. Prevention of listeriosis during pregnancy relies on the same principles that prevent listeriosis in general. They should be stressed as most important for women of reproductive capacity and risk factors during pregnancy.[70]

MALARIA

Malaria, the most significant parasitic disease worldwide, remains a major cause of maternal morbidity and mortality.[71] Globally, the pathological effects of infection during gestation and the negative implications for fetal development and survival are underscored by the fact that about 40% of the world's pregnant women (approximately 1 billion) are exposed to the risks of malaria while pregnant. LBW, a common consequence of gestational malaria, is an important risk factor for infant and childhood mortality.[72] In Africa alone, malaria-induced LBW may kill nearly 400,000 infants each year. Recent studies have demonstrated that the frequency and severity of placental malaria and consequential newborn disease and LBW are greater in pregnant women with concomitant HIV infection.

The negative impact of plasmodial infection during pregnancy varies predictably according to maternal immunity, a consequence of the intensity of transmission, and the parasite species. In areas of unstable transmission, where malaria is uncommon except during epidemics and immunity is rare, pregnant women suffer high-level parasitemia with more severe, acute complications including anemia, hypoglycemia, pulmonary edema, the acute respiratory distress syndrome, cerebral malaria, and death. Fetal distress, premature labor, stillbirth, or LBW result.[73] Fetal and perinatal losses have been estimated to be as high as 60% to 70% in nonimmune pregnant woman. This situation is similar in pregnant women from nonendemic areas or travelers to malarious zones. In contrast, adults who are long-term residents of areas of moderate or high malaria transmission exhibit high-level immunity and infection is usually asymptomatic or mild. But during gestation, this immunity is altered. Infection is still frequently oligo- or asymptomatic and severe disease is uncommon,[73] but it is associated with accumulation of parasitized erythrocytes in the placental microcirculation. In these areas, up to three doses of presumptive intermittent treatment during the duration of gestation has been shown to decrease the risk of severe maternal anemia. Sequestration of *Plasmodium falciparum*–infected red blood cells in the placenta is due to parasite adhesion molecules expressed on the surface of erythrocytes binding to host receptors such as chondroitin sulfate A (CSA). Parasite ligands also mediate placental adhesion. Thus, by invading the placenta,[74] malaria parasites cause more severe maternal anemia and LBW babies. These complications tend to be more common in primi-and secundigravida women with *P. falciparum* infection (weight reduction, approximately 170 g) and in multigravida women with *P. vivax* infection (weight reduction, approximately 100 g).

Congenital malaria is acquired from the infected, usually nonimmune mother pre- or perinatally in less than 5% of newborns. The transmission efficacy and the clinical severity are functions of the parasite species (more commonly observed with *P. vivax* and *P. malariae* but possible with all human plasmodia) and their density in maternal blood and placenta. In fact, placental malaria is significantly associated with stillbirth regardless of parity. A serious problem in tropical areas, it is rarely reported in the United States. Congenital infection is an important cause of intrauterine growth retardation, premature birth, abortion, miscarriage, stillbirth, and neonatal and infant death. The clinical manifestations can be apparent from the first day after birth to about 1 month later (commonly 10–30 days). They include fever, restlessness, pallor, obtundation, poor feeding, diarrhea, and vomiting. Signs include jaundice, cyanosis, and hepatosplenomegaly. Hypoglycemia is associated with increased mortality and neurologic sequelae.

The clinical features of malaria in obstetric patients, including laboratory and image findings, can be quantitatively more severe and qualitatively unique, but are essentially the same as described in detail for nonpregnant individuals.[75] Features indicating a poor prognosis must always be investigated. Special attention to physical exam, including level of consciousness, blood pressure, urine output, hemoglobinuria, hemoglobin and hematocrit, leukocytes, coagulation tests, arterial blood gases and blood glucose and lactate levels, creatinine, aminotransferases, bilirubin, muscle enzymes, and urate levels as well as chest radiography, is warranted. In serious cases, this is best done in intensive care unit (ICU) settings until clinical stability/improvement. An HIV test is commonly indicated.

Early diagnosis of malaria in pregnancy is extremely important because successful specific treatment can impact mother and child. The diagnosis rests, as in nonpregnant individuals, on the demonstration of asexual plasmodial forms in thick and thin stained smears of peripheral blood. Fluorescent microscopy, rapid detection tests, and polymerase chain reaction (PCR) are described in Chapter 90. Parasitemias can be very high. Serology has mainly epidemiological uses.

Malaria during pregnancy must be treated with antiparasitic agents, but optimal therapy is difficult to select because there are no reliable clinical data for most oral or parenteral antimalarial drugs to be declared safe for use in pregnant women. The agent or agents of choice and the route of administration also depend on the suspected or demonstrated infecting species and the likelihood of drug resistance. The geographic distribution of drug-resistant malaria parasites can be found elsewhere in this book. Antimalarials with special importance during pregnancy are briefly described here and their administration schedules are found in Chapter 90; drug doses may need to be altered depending on the stage of pregnancy. In pregnancy, the persistence of *P. falciparum* in the placenta after apparently effective treatment has been described.[76]

Chloroquine is generally well tolerated and considered safe in pregnancy[77] and continues to be the drug of choice for all *P. ovale* and *P. malariae* infections and for susceptible *P. falciparum* and *P. vivax* infections.

With the exception of the possibility of stillbirth and LBW, mefloquine, used for treatment and prophylaxis, appears safer for the fetus during any trimester of pregnancy than many other drugs and has been used extensively.[78] In the expectant mother, the drug may produce neuropsychiatric side effects and possibly cardiotoxicity. Combination with halofantrine, not available in the United States, produces prolongation of QTc interval. Tetracyclines and doxycycline are contraindicated during pregnancy; clindamycin (see later discussion) is an alternative. Dapsone in combination with other drugs might provide an alternative to treatment of resistant *P. falciparum* malaria, as suggested by a recent review of 924 pregnancies,[79] but there is no information on hemolytic effects to mother or fetus with or without glucose-6-phosphate dehydrogenase (G6PD) deficiency.

The combination of atovaquone (250 mg) and proguanil (100 mg) is highly effective against chloroquine- and mefloquine-resistant *P. falciparum* malaria, but data in pregnancy are scarce. Combined with artesunate, the combination has been useful and well tolerated in Thailand[80] as rescue treatment of multidrug-resistant *P. falciparum* malaria in pregnant women without recorded maternal or fetal toxicity.

Quinine and quinidine have been given in therapeutic doses to pregnant women throughout gestation[77]; continuous monitoring of vital signs, blood glucose, and EKG are recommended. Quinine is preferred but availability accounts for greater use of quinidine in North America. Quinine at the intravenous doses used to treat malaria does not induce oxytocic effects. There are concerns about maternal cardiac side effects and tolerance, especially gastrointestinal.

Pyrimethamine-sulfadoxine and clindamycin have also been used in pregnancy with consistent good results; fears of development of kernicterus with the former and colitis with the latter have not materialized. Clindamycin has been used routinely in combination with quinine to treat pregnant patients with multidrug-resistant *P. falciparum* in Brazil for two decades; other than vomiting, no significant side effects have been observed in mothers or fetuses. It should not be used alone because of its slow antimalarial activity.

Artemisinin-derived antimalarials and combinations have considerably faster parasitic clearance rates and shorter half-lives and may be as effective as quinine in treating severe malaria. They can be used orally, intravenously, and rectally. Small studies suggest good tolerance during pregnancy and no evidence of adverse fetal effects.[80] Birth outcomes are similar to community rates for abortion, stillbirth, and congenital anomalies or mean gestation age at delivery. There is a risk of potential teratogenicity if used in the first trimester.

The use of intravenous antimalarials in combination with exchange transfusions with careful monitoring should be considered in selected cases of severe complicated malaria in pregnant women.

We recommend hospitalization for pregnant women with suspected malaria at lower levels of severity than for nonpregnant counterparts. This is true for ward and ICU admission. When *P. falciparum* is suspected or demonstrated, or when disease is moderate to severe, hospitalization is always strongly recommended. *P. falciparum* treatment is administered when the organism is demonstrated or suspected (even if not demonstrated) for all infections where one suspects infection with more than one organism, and for severely ill patients.

Chloroquine alone, or with proguanil, remains the preferred drug for chemoprophylaxis for pregnant women in malarial areas where it is still effective. In chloroquine-resistant areas, mefloquine may be used instead.

Doxycycline, atovaquone-proguanil, and primaquine are not used for prophylaxis. Intermittent preventive treatment (IPT) with pyrimethamine-sulfadoxine in areas of parasite susceptibility is a common option. Recently, the use of a double dose was associated with a decrease of maternal parasitemia and newborns with malaria, among nulliparous and primiparous pregnant women in Mozambique. The safety of other prophylactic agents has not been established. Pregnant women from nonmalarial areas should not visit malarial zones, but when unavoidable, antivector strategies cannot be overemphasized.

Women become resistant to pregnancy-associated malaria over successive pregnancies as they acquire antibodies that recognize placental parasites, suggesting that protection by a vaccine during pregnancy is feasible.

TETANUS

Maternal tetanus is an extremely serious disease with high morbidity and mortality. It is not communicable, but may be acquired by ways unrelated to pregnancy, such as dirty wounds, or pregnancy-related, such as contaminated delivery or abortion. Tetanus neonatorum, the most common form of tetanus in developing tropical countries, is caused by contamination of the umbilical stump with spores, typically from application of animal dung to the umbilical stump. Virtually all affected are not properly immunized. Symptoms develop after 3 to 14 days. Even with specific treatment, maternal and neonatal tetanus have high mortality rates.

The clinical picture in mother and infant is secondary to the potent tetanospasmin exotoxin produced during anaerobic growth of *Clostridium tetani* at the site of injury and has been described elsewhere. The diagnosis is clinical, and aggressive treatment, performed in intensive care settings, includes life-sustaining methods, sedation, passive and active immunization, and antibiotics. Tetanus is preventable with the use of one of the safest available immunization products. Immunization of the susceptible pregnant woman should be routine[81,82] and include at least two doses of tetanus toxoid, 4 to 8 weeks apart, at least two 2 before delivery. A booster is indicated for pregnant women immunized more than 10 years previously. Partially immunized women should complete a three-dose series. Clean practices for caring for the umbilical stump are clearly to be enforced.

TOXOPLASMOSIS

The incidence of toxoplasmosis during pregnancy is estimated to be similar to that of nonpregnant women of the same age group, and most infections are asymptomatic. A minority of infected patients, calculated around 20%, develops clinical signs and symptoms of a usually self-limited and rarely prolonged disease.[83] The diagnosis may be made at consultation with symptoms or when specific serological tests are performed after conception.

When infection by *Toxoplasma gondii* is acquired by a woman near the time of conception or during gestation,[84] the organism may be transmitted to the fetus through the placenta. This happens in about one-third of the cases. The incidence of congenital toxoplasmosis in the United States is estimated in 1/1000 to 1/8000 live births or 400 to 4000 infants per year.

The parasite reaches the placenta after hematogenous spread of tachyzoites released from ingested cysts or oocysts after release of bradyzoites or sporozoites that have invaded the maternal intestinal epithelium. In placental tissue, tachyzoites (demonstrated by Wright, Giemsa, and immunoperoxidase) replicate and cause tissue damage evidenced by chronic inflammation and cysts. From the placenta, hematogenous spread and establishment of a persistent infection with potential for lifelong reactivation and further disease occurs in the fetus.

Before conception, the likelihood of vertical transmission increases from about 6 months to the establishment of pregnancy. Once established, the age of gestation at the time of infection is a critical factor in transmission and fetal outcome. Infections occurring during the first trimester have the lowest vertical transmission (approximately 15%), but the resulting neonatal disease is more severe. The presence of HLA-DQ3 can worsen the prognosis of the fetus when infected in this period. During the third trimester, transmission is greatest (approximately 65%), but clinically apparent neonatal disease is less common or severe. The differences may be explained by placental or immunologic factors.

In severe prenatal infections, intrauterine fetal death may be the consequence of fetal multiorgan failure secondary to parasitic invasion. Acute congenital toxoplasmosis is characterized by intrauterine growth retardation and prematurity, anemia thrombocytopenia and jaundice, hepatosplenomegaly, hydrocephalus, microcephaly, and intracranial calcifications. Surviving congenitally infected babies, including untreated asymptomatic neonates, most often exhibit neurological sequelae such as chorioretinitis (and visual impairment), seizures, and learning disabilities later in childhood and by adolescence.[83,85–87] Clinical manifestations are often similar in monozygotic and different in dizygotic twins. In the latter instance, diagnosis of severe toxoplasmosis in one twin can suggest subclinical disease in the other. Early and appropriate treatment may allow for clinical cure and normal development and is of critical importance.

When clinical manifestations of toxoplasmosis in the pregnant woman become apparent, they do not differ from those described for immune competent nonpregnant individuals. Single or multiple, usually nontender cervical lymphadenopathy[88]; nonspecific flulike symptoms such as headache, malaise, fatigue, fever, sore throat, abdominal discomfort, and pain; a maculopapular rash; and meningoencephalitis have been well described. More rarely, lung, pericardium and myocardium, brain, and striated muscles can be affected.

The efficient diagnosis of toxoplasmosis during pregnancy can be extremely challenging. In practice, serologic tests are the most commonly used, but they require experience to be interpreted correctly.[83] Acute *Toxoplasma* infection can be diagnosed by the isolation of the parasite in blood or body fluid cultures from the mother and any fluid or tissue from the fetus or neonate. Immediate intraperitoneal inoculation of processed blood, body fluids, or tissues into mice, and periodic examination of mouse peritoneal fluid looking for tachyzoites, takes several days; examination of surviving inoculated mice with detectable antibody for brain cysts takes about 6 weeks. Reinoculation of mouse tissues into other mice is even more cumbersome and time consuming. Thus, cultures are difficult and expensive and, in pregnancy, may not provide a useful window of diagnostic opportunity.

In a pregnant woman with lymphadenopathy, characteristic histological features can support a clinical diagnosis of acute toxoplasmosis.[88] Histologic and histochemical examination of biopsy specimens, bone marrow aspirates, cerebrospinal fluid (CSF), amniotic fluid, and other specimens is rarely performed during pregnancy but can demonstrate tachyzoites. More than one staining method (including immunoperoxidase) is necessary. In the mother, tissue cysts are diagnostic, but the duration of infection cannot be ascertained. Cysts in the placenta or fetal/newborn tissues represent congenital infection.

In broad terms, recent *Toxoplasma* infection can be diagnosed by the presence of *Toxoplasma*-specific IgM antibody, by the simultaneous presence of specific IgM and IgG antibodies, or by demonstration of seroconversion of repeated IgG antibody titers. The presence of IgA antibodies suggests recent infection. A wide range of serologic tests is available commercially, and experience with their utilization varies among laboratories and societies. Systematic serologic screening of all women preconception, during pregnancy, and intra-partum is strongly advised, but in tropical countries this is seldom performed.

IgM-based diagnosis is based on the rapid—few days—rise and fall—weeks to months—of antibodies. It includes the utilization of the IgM indirect fluorescent antibody (IgM-IFA) test, the double-sandwich enzyme-linked immunosorbent assay (ELISA), and the immunosorbent agglutination assay (ISAGA). All tests are sensitive and specific. The ELISA is more sensitive and specific than the IgM-IFA test, circumvents the false positive results from rheumatoid factor in the mother and the false negative results from transferred maternal IgG in the newborn, and has been used to detect infection in pregnant women. The ISAGA avoids false-positive results from the presence of rheumatoid factor and antinuclear antibodies. ISAGA IgM is detected earlier, with higher sensitivity, and for a longer time than with the ELISA test. An IgA ELISA is even more sensitive for detection of acute infection in some pregnant women and congenital infection in newborns, but may remain elevated for months to years. A simple, accurate, and inexpensive French agglutination test is available in Europe.

IgG titers can be detected in low levels as early as 1 to 2 weeks after infection, peak with high titers (≥1:1000) after 6 to 8 weeks, and decline to a new individual low level (1:4–1:64) to persist for life. The Sabin-Feldman dye test, the IgG-IFA, and the ELISA are sensitive and specific and have been in sustained clinical use.

Other serology-based diagnostics include the differential agglutination (HS/SC) test, which may be especially useful to exclude remote infection in pregnant women, the avidity test, and the indirect hemagglutination test (IHA). The IHA should not be relied upon for diagnosis of acute infection during pregnancy because it may remain negative for a prolonged period after infection.

During the acute phase of toxoplasmosis during pregnancy, antigen present in serum samples can be detected by PCR. PCR performed in amniotic fluid is the diagnostic test of choice for congenital fetal infection.[89,90] Timing at 18 weeks of pregnancy is preferred because of optimal sensitivity. A reference laboratory should confirm the diagnosis of acute toxoplasmosis during pregnancy.

Ultrasonography is also useful for fetal diagnosis. Combined with amniocentesis for PCR, a sensitivity of 97% and specificity of 100% for fetal infection is reached.

Appropriate treatment of a woman who acquires *Toxoplasma* infection during pregnancy[84] has been shown to reduce placental invasion and prevent congenital infection of the fetus carried in that pregnancy. Spiramycin (1 g taken every 8 hours by mouth on an empty stomach) is started as soon as possible[87] to prevent fetal infection, because it decreases vertical transmission (from approximately 60% to approximately 20%). When fetal infection seems highly probable or severe and when diagnosis of fetal infection is certain, combination therapy with pyrimethamine (50 mg PO once daily) and sulfadoxine (2 g PO twice daily) are given with folinic acid (10 mg PO once daily). During the first trimester, when pyrimethamine can be teratogenic, spiramycin is substituted and no folinic acid is needed.

No treatment is needed in subsequent pregnancies or for infections acquired over 6 months before any conception provided maternal immunocompetence, but previously infected immunosuppressed women should be given spiramycin for the duration of each pregnancy. In pregnant HIV-infected women, as a reasonable, albeit theoretical approach, spiramycin can be used for the first 17 weeks of gestation followed by pyrimethamine (at a higher dose of 75 mg PO once daily), sulfadoxine, and folinic acid until delivery. Clindamycin (1.2 g IV every 6 hours) can be used instead of sulfadoxine.

There is no *Toxoplasma* vaccine. Women who do not exhibit specific antibodies against *T. gondii* must be counseled. Avoiding raw meats and contact with cat excreta have proven preventive efficacy. All women not previously tested must have serologic screening at the first prenatal visit and during delivery.

TUBERCULOSIS AND MULTIDRUG-RESISTANT TUBERCULOSIS

The increasing burden of tuberculosis (TB) during pregnancy affects the health of large numbers of mothers and infants.[91] Diagnostic, therapeutic, and prophylactic constraints during gestation include the dangers of x-rays and the intrinsic difficulties in testing anti-TB drugs.

Untreated pulmonary and particularly extrapulmonary TB (other than lymphadenitis) in pregnant women increase the risk for prematurity, fetal growth retardation, LBW, and perinatal mortality.[92,93] The most common mechanism of infection in the newborn is airborne transmission from an adult with pulmonary TB. Congenital TB is rare. It is more likely to be transmitted vertically after primary infection than after reactivation of previous infection. It may occur from a placental lesion through the umbilical vein, from which bacilli reach the fetal liver where a primary focus may be established for hematogenous spread to several organs. In the lungs, oxygenation and pulmonary circulation after birth increase and activate dormant bacilli. A less frequent mechanism is aspiration of infected amniotic fluid. Newborns show signs of TB after the second postnatal week; these are nonspecific and resemble other forms of neonatal sepsis. Fever, respiratory distress, irritability, ear discharge, abdominal symptoms, pulmonary infiltrates, and hilar or generalized lymphadenopathy are common. Up to 50% of infants develop meningitis. Frequently, the mother's disease is discovered as a consequence of the diagnosis in the newborn. The infant's purified protein derivative (PPD) becomes positive after 1 to 3 months. *M. tuberculosis* can be isolated from middle ear drainage, bone marrow, tracheal aspirate, and liver biopsy, rarely from CSF. Mortality is higher with delayed diagnosis.

Because untreated TB is harmful to both the mother and the fetus, because it represents a great danger to the infant after delivery, and because the disease can be transmitted to others, TB in pregnant women always should be treated without delay. Consensus treatment guidelines have been produced by the American Thoracic Society (ATS), the Infectious Diseases Society of America (IDSA), the CDC,[94] WHO,[95] and the International Union against Tuberculosis and Lung Diseases (IUATLD).[96] The following discussion on anti-TB drug use by pregnant women will closely follow the guidelines. Dosages are individualized during pregnancy and a general discussion can be found in Chapter 36.

The initial regimen, provided no multidrug resistance (MDR) is suspected, consists of isoniazid (INH), rifampin (RIF), and ethambutol (EMB) for a minimum duration of 9 months and with pyridoxine. INH, RIF, and EMB cross the placental barrier but have elicited no teratogenicity.[97] Streptomycin should not be substituted for EMB because it interferes with the development of the ear and hearing loss or vestibular defects may affect the developing fetus (approximately 1–3 per 6 live births) at any period throughout gestation.[98] Presumably, other aminoglycosides such as kanamycin, amikacin, and capreomycin share the ototoxicity potential. The safety of pyrazinamide in pregnancy has not been established and the drug is not recommended for routine use in the United States. Pyrazinamide is listed among the recommendations of the WHO[95] and the IUATLD[96] and has been used without reported adverse events by some public health jurisdictions in the United States. Para-aminosalicylic acid (PAS) was frequently used in combination with isoniazid (INH); no indication of teratogenicity was encountered in children of women who used them during pregnancy. The safety of cycloserine and ethionamide is untested; one report suggested human teratogenicity from ethionamide,[99] a drug that causes birth defects and spontaneous abortion when used in high doses in animals. The fluoroquinolones are avoided in pregnancy because of animal teratogenicity, but may need to be used during pregnancy for treatment of MDR TB infections unresponsive to other drugs.[97] Levofloxacin has been used more often than moxifloxacin for treatment of adults and children, and switching from levofloxacin to moxifloxacin, which may be more active against *M. tuberculosis*, after delivery seems an appropriate option. When anti-TB drugs are to be used during pregnancy, the expectant mother should be counseled concerning the known and unknown risks to the developing fetus of all treatment offered.

High-risk or symptomatic pregnant mothers should be tested with a tuberculin skin test. The PPD or "Mantoux" (5TU) tuberculin test is the most specific and sensitive standardized screening skin test for TB and is preferred. Pregnancy does not measurably affect the response of PPD and there has been no observed evidence of adverse events on women or their children from skin testing. All pregnant women not known previously to be skin reactors and many women of reproductive capacity and high risk (symptomatic, exposed, HIV, diabetes, high prevalence, caretaker, etc.) should ideally be tested.[100] Subsequent investigation of skin reactors facilitates the identification of infected individuals and the treatment of tuberculosis.

Although INH is not teratogenic, the treatment of latent TB infection (LTBI) is often deferred until after delivery, when there may be an increased risk of disease, because of concerns of isoniazid-associated hepatitis, which could be more frequent and/or severe during pregnancy. There might be an exception for pregnant women who have been infected recently; INH in that situation could be started after the first trimester. Mothers with LTBI do not need to be separated from their infants after delivery and the child needs no special evaluation or treatment provided he or she remains asymptomatic. No treatment is recommended for women with inactive TB if they received adequate treatment in the past.

The diagnosis of maternal TB at delivery requires rapid and thorough evaluation of mother and child. If chest radiography and positive sputum smear confirm the diagnosis, additional steps, such as INH, skin testing follow-up, and rarely separation from the mother are necessary to protect the infant. An HIV test is also indicated.[101]

Because the concentrations of first-line antituberculosis drugs in human breast milk are low, breastfeeding should not be discouraged in nursing mothers treated with them.[102] The risk of toxicity can be minimized if the mother takes her medication after breastfeeding and substitutes saved milk or a bottle for the next feeding. The small concentrations that a baby receives during feeding are not effective as treatment for LTBI or active infection.

TYPHOID FEVER

Studies from the early 1900s, when typhoid fever (TF) was extremely prevalent around the world, suggested an increased severity of TF when it affected pregnant women. In the pre-antibiotic era, two-thirds of pregnancies complicated by TF resulted in abortion.[103] In one series from the Philippines,[104] mortality rates were 32% and 25% as infection occurred while pregnancy progressed from the first to the third trimester, compared to an accepted general mortality rate of less than 15% to 20% for the general untreated population. Additionally, fetal prognosis was found to be quite poor, with rates around 60% for fetal demise and 35% for premature labor. Since then, small series, literature reviews, and case reports have produced contradictory reports of more severe vs. equally severe clinical manifestations of TF in pregnant women when compared to nonpregnant females. Some of the largest case series of 100 cases from Chile,[105] 81 cases from Mexico,[106] and 129 cases from Peru,[107] though incomplete, are consistent with the notion of increased severity of TF during pregnancy and unequivocal in showing improvement of maternal and fetal prognosis with early antibiotic treatment. They also underscore the continuous presence in tropical and subtropical areas of a disease that has been all but eradicated in societies that have achieved adequate sanitation.

Salmonella typhi causes sepsis of intestinal origin and colonization of reticuloendothelial tissues such as liver, spleen, lymph nodes, and bone marrow and crosses the placental barrier causing chorioamnionitis and villitis. In autopsy specimens, microscopy has revealed numerous colonies of gram-negative bacilli within the fibrin between the placental villi. Vertical transmission can also occur in late pregnancy and the the perinatal period. Interestingly, cases of chorioamnionitis and transplacental and perinatal infection of a fetus by nontyphoidal *Salmonella* strains have also been described. The neonatal disease begins after an asymptomatic period of 1 to 3 days after birth. Vomiting, diarrhea, abdominal distention, and fever are common. Seizures may occur. Anorexia and weight loss, hepatomegaly, and jaundice may be severe. Prompt treatment is effective. Maternal long-term asymptomatic carriers may pose a risk for disease in the newborn, and elimination of such state with treatment (15 of 99 in a Japanese study) may prevent infection in the newborn, but no controlled studies exist. The treatment of the carrier state in pregnancy is not known.

In the mother, prolonged fever and gastrointestinal or abdominal symptoms, at times following a nonspecific flulike prodrome, is characteristic but nonspecific for pregnancy. Rose spots, hepatosplenomegaly, and relative bradycardia are very useful when present. Gastrointestinal perforation and hemorrhage are late complications that acutely risk the lives of mother and fetus. Sustained bacteremia without endocarditis is a characteristic of typhoid fever that has three major deleterious consequences: (1) a severe activation and hyperplasia of reticuloendothelial organs, typically the intestinal and mesenteric lymph nodes, the liver, and the spleen; (2) metastatic seeding; and (3) immune complex disease. All have been described in pregnant women. Relapses and long-term carriers have also been seen in pregnancy.

S. typhi can be found in breast milk (5 of 26 in Chile and 3 of 23 in Peru), but treatment with amoxicillin has been effective in eradicating the organism in 1 to 3 days. Other drugs have no proof of efficacy and resistance makes this information difficult to interpret.

Whether or not TF is more severe during pregnancy, the disease must be treated to avoid morbidity and mortality in mother and fetus and to decrease transmission.[105–107] Currently, due to the appearance of resistance,[108–110] two drugs, ciprofloxacin and ceftriaxone,[111] are considered first-line and one, azithromycin, is considered alternative. Ciprofloxacin use in pregnancy is controversial and at present not advisable, particularly if there are alternatives, but ceftriaxone has demonstrated safety and efficacy in a series of 25 pregnant patients from French Guiana.[112] Provided susceptibility is assured and in spite of cost considerations, it is the drug of choice during all trimesters. Cefotaxime and cefoperazone are reasonable alternatives, but first- and second-generation cephalosporins, aminoglycosides, and aztreonam are not. Azithromycin use in pregnancy is permitted, but efficacy for treatment of TF is unknown.

Chloramphenicol is not recommended in pregnancy because of *Salmonella* resistance, the fetal risk of gray syndrome, and potential bone marrow toxicity for mother and fetus. Nevertheless, the emergence of quinolone and ceftriaxone resistance,[110] the possible re-emergence of susceptibility to chloramphenicol, and the absence of hematologic side effects or gray syndrome in some series, suggest a need to re-evaluate the issue.

No trials of corticosteroids in pregnancy have been performed, but their use may be justified in severe cases.

There are no data reported on the use of typhoid vaccines among pregnant women. The CDC advises to avoid vaccinating during pregnancy, but vaccination should be considered in some women (for example, those allergic to cephalosporins traveling to an endemic area) if actual risk of disease and probable benefits of effective nonlive vaccine (such as the Vi vaccine) outweigh theoretical risks (especially the effect of live bacteria) to the fetus.

Screening with stool cultures of pregnant women seems unjustified in areas of low prevalence. In a large UK study of 30,471 mothers over 9 years, only 60 (0.2%) yielded *Salmonella*[113] and 43 (72%) were asymptomatic. Seven of the 60 neonates (12%) excreted *Salmonella* with similar characteristics as their mothers, but no individual suffered invasive disease. However, in other areas like Tuscany (where 7431 pregnant women were studied), stool cultures may be cost effective in late summer and fall.[114] In developing tropical countries, the question is unanswered. The reader is referred to Chapter 17 on TF for detailed discussions of antibiotic dosage and prevention measures.

YELLOW FEVER

The course and severity of yellow fever do not seem affected by pregnancy, but no studies exist to confirm this assessment. Yellow fever is a very severe disease with high mortality and no specific treatment; therefore, in the general population emphasis has been placed on prevention with an easy-to-use, economical, available, safe, and very effective vaccine.

The safety of yellow fever vaccination, a live virus vaccine, has not been established during pregnancy. Studies of infants who were born to mothers that had been vaccinated with the YF17D immunogen during their pregnancies have been analyzed.[115–118] Infection of the fetus with the vaccine strain was documented in one newborn and no congenital abnormalities were observed.[117] In women vaccinated with YF17D early in pregnancy, the relative risk for spontaneous abortion was 2.3, but the difference with unvaccinated cases was not statistically significant. Seventy-four prospectively enrolled cases were analyzed; pregnancies ended in 46 births, five voluntary and seven spontaneous abortions; three newborns had minor and two major defects.[115] Although the samples are small, and the follow-up incomplete, these data, plus limited clinical trials in Africa and Europe, suggest that the risk of vaccination of pregnant women who are likely to be exposed to infection with the yellow fever flavivirus in endemic areas is less than the risk of contracting yellow fever. There is a theoretical but unproved risk of transmission of the YF17D strain in human milk during breastfeeding. Small studies from Brazil[116] and Trinidad[117] stress the need for caution. Therefore, pregnant and lactating women who must travel to endemic areas can be offered the vaccine with clear explanations of the risk/benefit ratio as understood at the time of consultation, if the risk of contracting yellow fever is high. Pregnant women who have been inadvertently vaccinated should be reassured. Seroconversion rates during pregnancy can be lower,[118] and immunity should probably be verified.

OTHER INTRAUTERINE INFECTIONS

Cytomegalovirus

Primary cytomegalovirus (CMV) infection during pregnancy may be transmitted to the fetus in 25% to 75% of cases. Reinfection with a different strain may have lower potential for transmission. CMV can persist in a latent stage after primary infection, and reactivate during pregnancy to be transmitted to the fetus. Deleterious developmental outcomes have been observed in infants.[119] Treatment with ganciclovir has not been evaluated in pregnancy and is being studied for symptomatic congenital infection.[120]

Herpes Simplex Virus 1 and 2

Genital infection by either herpes simplex virus 1 or 2 is rarely transmitted in utero to the fetus, but it is more commonly transmitted intrapartum to the newborn. It can also be transmitted later unrelated to pregnancy. Transmission occurs even in asymptomatic women, more efficiently in primary than in reactivated infections. Data on the safety of acyclovir, valacyclovir, and famciclovir are not complete but many specialists recommend its use during pregnancy in several situations.[121] Neonatal disease is very serious, potentially lethal, and has a high risk of severe sequelae and early treatment with intravenous acyclovir reduces but does not eliminate morbidity and mortality.[114] Delivery by cesarean section is advocated to prevent neonatal herpes, but this does not totally eliminate the risk.

Rubella

Rubella remains prevalent in some areas of the developing world where vaccination programs have not reached the population. The rubella virus interferes with critical steps in fetal organ development during early pregnancy and causes the congenital rubella syndrome (CRS), a disease of poor prognosis and severe sequelae. Global immunization programs and individual vaccination of women before their first pregnancy can prevent CRS.[122]

Syphilis

The risk of syphilis during pregnancy parallels the rates of syphilis in women of childbearing age in a given population. All pregnant women should have a syphilis detection test at the first prenatal visit, and in many instances the test should be repeated one or more times to the time of delivery.[123] All seropositivity should be considered infection unless appropriate treatment can be documented and antibody concentrations decline. Since treatment in pregnancy both prevents and treats fetal infection, it is recommended without delay and consists of the penicillin regimen appropriate for the stage of syphilis diagnosed. Safe and effective alternatives to penicillin are not documented.[124]

REFERENCES

1. Carbajo-Ferreira AJ, Ochoa-Sangrador C, Canut-Blasco A, et al: Neonatal brucellosis. Pediatr Infect Dis J 14:406, 1995.
2. Giannacopoulos I, Eliopoulou MI, Ziambaras T, et al: Transplacentally transmitted congenital brucellosis due to *Brucella abortus*. J Infect 45:209, 2002.
3. Singer R, Amitai Y, Geist M, et al: Neonatal brucellosis possibly transmitted during delivery. Lancet 338:127, 1991.
4. Khan MY, Mah MW, Memish ZA: Brucellosis in pregnant women. Clin Infect Dis 32:1172, 2001.
5. Zavala-Trujillo I, Nava-Zavala A, Guerra-Cáceres J, et al: Brucellosis. Infect Dis Clin North Am 8:225, 1994.
6. Malone FD, Athanassiou A, Nores LA, et al: Poor perinatal outcome associated with maternal *Brucella abortus* infection. Obstet Gynecol 90:674, 1997.
7. Keppie J, Williams AE, Witt K, et al: The role of erythritol in the tissue localization of the *Brucellae*. Br J Exp Pathol 46:104, 1965.
8. al-Eissa YA: Probable breast-milk borne brucellosis in a young infant. Ann Trop Paediatr 10:305, 1990.
9. Palanduz A, Palanduz S, Guler K, et al: Brucellosis in a mother and her young infant: Probable transmission by breast milk. Int J Infect Dis 4:55, 2000.
10. Ibrahim AIA, Award R, Shetty SD, et al: Genito-urinary complications of brucellosis. Br J Urol 61:294, 1988.
11. Odeh M, Olivera A: Acute brucellosis associated with massive proteinuria. Nephron 72:688, 1996.
12. Young EJ: *Brucella* species. In Mandell GL, Bennet JE, Dolin R (eds): Mandell, Douglas, and Bennett's Principles and Practices of Infectious Diseases, 4th ed. New York, Churchill Livingstone, 1995, p 2053.
13. Espinoza M: Brucelosis y Gestación. Tesis de Bachiller, Facultad de Medicina Alberto Hurtado. Lima, Universidad Peruana Cayetano Heredia, 1985.
14. D'Onadío G: Brucelosis y Gestación: Cuadro Clínico y Pronóstico Materno-fetal. Tesis de Bachiller, Facultad de Medicina Alberto Hurtado. Lima, Universidad Peruana Cayetano Heredia, 2003.
15. Acocella G, Bertrand A, Beytout J, et al: Comparison of three different regimens in the treatment of acute brucellosis: A multicenter multinational study. J Antimicrob Chemother 23:433, 1989.
16. Solera J, Martinez-Alfaro E, Saez L: Meta-analysis of the efficacy of the combination of rifampicin and doxycycline in the treatment of human brucellosis. Med Clin Barc 102:731, 1994.
17. Hall WH: Modern chemotherapy for brucellosis in humans. Rev Infect Dis 12:1060, 1990.
18. Cholera in the Americas. Bull Pan Am Health Org 25:267, 1991.
19. Ayangade O: The significance of cholera outbreak in the prognosis of pregnancy. Int J Gynaecol Obstet 19:403, 1981.
20. Seas C, Miranda J, Gil AI, et al: New insights on the emergence of cholera in Latin America during 1991: The Peruvian experience. Am J Trop Med Hyg 62:513, 2000.
21. Grados P, Battilana CA:Tratamiento de la diarrea coleriforme durante la gestación. Bol Oficina Sanit Panam 116:198, 1994.
22. Saona P, Astudillo J, Figueroa M, et al: Cólera en gestantes en el Hospital Nacional Cayetano Heredia, Lima-Perú. Rev Med Hered 2:112, 1991.
23. Janjindamai W, Pruekprasert P: Perinatal dengue infection: A case report and review of literature. Southeast Asian J Trop Med Public Health 34:793, 2003.
24. Kerpanich A, Watanaveeradej V, Samakoses R, et al: Perinatal dengue infection. Southeast Asian J Trop Med Public Health 32:488, 2001.
25. Chye JK, Lim CT, Ng KB, et al: Vertical transmission of dengue. Clin Infect Dis 25:1374, 1997.
26. Chotigeat U, Kalayanorooj S, Nisalak A: Vertical trensmission of dengue infection in Thai infants: Two case reports. J Med Assoc Thai 86:S628, 2003.
27. Boussemart T, Babe P, Sibile G, et al: Prenatal transmission of dengue: Two new cases. J Perinatol 21:255, 2001.
28. Carles G, Talarmin A, Peneau C, et al: Dengue fever and pregnancy. A study of 38 cases in french Guiana. J Gynecol Obstet Biol Reprod (Paris) 28:758, 2000.
29. Carles G, Peiffer H, Talarmin A: Effects of dengue fever during pregnancy in French Guiana. Clin Infect Dis 28:637, 1999.
30. Restrepo BN, Isaza DM, Salazar CL, et al: Prenatal and postnatal effects of dengue infection during pregnancy. Biomedica 23:416, 2003.
31. Thaithumyanon P, Thisyakorn U, Deerojnawong J, et al: Dengue infection complicated by severe hemorrhage and vertical transmission in a parturient woman. Clin Infect Dis 18:248, 1994.
32. Witayathawornwong P: Parturient and perinatal dengue hemorrhagic fever. Southeast Asian J Trop Med Public Health 34:479, 2003.
33. Dinsmoor MJ: Hepatitis in the obstetric patient. Infect Dis Clin North Am 11:77, 1977.
34. Snyder JD, Pickering LK: Viral hepatitis. In Behrman RE, Kliegman RM, Jenson HB (eds): Nelson Textbook of Pediatrics, 17th ed. Philadelphia, WB Saunders, 2004, p 1124.
35. Ranger-Rogez S, Denis F: Hepatitis B mother-to-child transmission. Expert Rev Anti Infect Ther 2:133, 2004.
36. Boxall EH, Sira J, Standish RA, et al: Natural history of hepatitis B in perinatally infected carriers. Arch Dis Child Fetal Neonatal Ed 89:F456, 2004.
37. Yang YB, Li XM, Shi ZJ, et al: Pregnant woman with fulminant hepatic failure caused by hepatitis B virus infection: A case report. World J Gastroenterol 10:2305, 2004.

38. Thomson R: Hepatitis B. In Thomson R (ed): Travel and Routine Immunizations. Milwaukee, Shoreland, 2003, p 36.
39. Bracebridge S, Irwin D, Millership S: Prevention of perinatal hepatitis B transmission in a health authority area: An audit. Commun Dis Public Health 7:138, 2004.
40. Resti M, Manelli F, Moriondo M, et al: Mother to child transmission of hepatitis C virus: Prospective study of risk factors and timing of infection in children born to women seronegative for HIV-1. Tuscany Study Group on Hepatitis C Virus Infection. BMJ 317:437, 1998.
41. Lima MP, Pedro RJ, Rocha MD: Mother to infant transmission of hepatitis C virus (HCV) in Brazil. J Trop Pediatr 50:236, 2004.
42. Gibb G, Goodal RL, Dunn DT, et al: Mother to child transmission of hepatitis C virus: Evidence for preventable peripartum transmission. Lancet 356:904, 2004.
43. Rab MA, Bile MK, Mubarik MM, et al: Water-borne hepatitis E virus epidemic in Islamabad, Pakistan: A common source outbreak traced to the malfunction of a modern water treatment plant. Am J Trop Med Hyg 57:151, 1997.
44. Khuroo MS, Kamili S, Jameel S: Vertical transmission of hepatitis E virus. Lancet 345:1025, 1995.
45. De Martino M, Azzari C, Resti M, et al: Hepatitis G virus infection in human immunodeficiency virus type-1 infected mothers and their children. J Infect Dis 178:862, 1998.
46. French R, Brocklehurst P: The effect of pregnancy on survival in women infected with HIV: A systematic review of the literature and meta-analysis. Br J Obstet Gynaecol 105:827, 1998.
47. Weisser M, Rudin C, Mattegay M, et al: Does pregnancy influence the course of HIV infection? Evidence from two large Swiss cohort studies. J Acquir Immune Defic Syndr Human Retrovirol 17:404, 1998.
48. Centers for Disease Control and Prevention: Sexually transmitted diseases treatment guidelines. MMWR 51:10, 2002.
49. Minkoff H, Ahdieh L, Watts H, et al: The relationship of pregnancy to the use of highly active antiretroviral therapy. Am J Obstet Gynecol 184:1221, 2001.
50. Lallemant M, JourdainG, Le Coeur S, et al: Single dose perinatal nevirapine plus standard zidovudine to prevent mother-to-child transmission of HIV-1 in Thailand. New Engl J Med 351:217, 2004.
51. Herzmann C: Nevirapine plus zidovudine to prevent mother-to-child transmission of HIV. New Engl J Med 351:2013, 2004.
52. Ioannidis JP, Abrams EJ, Amman A, et al: Perinatal transmission of human immunodeficiency virus type-1 by pregnant women with RNA viral loads of 1000 copies/ml. J Infect Dis 183:539, 2001.
53. Read JS, Tuomala R, Kpamegan E, et al: Mode of delivery and post-partum morbidity among HIV-infected women: The women and infants transmission study. J Acquir Immune Defic Syndr 26:236, 2001.
54. Cotton D: Human immunodeficiency virus infection in women. In Gorbach SL, Bartlett JG, Blacklow NR (eds): Infectious Diseases, 3rd ed. Philadelphia, Lippincott Williams & Wilkins, 2004, p 1090.
55. Fujino T, Nagata Y: HTLV-I transmission from mother to child. J Reprod Immunol 47:197, 2000.
56. Takima K, Cartier L: Epidemiological features of HTLV-I and adult T cell leukemia. Intervirology 38:238, 1995.
57. Hino S, Katamine S, Miyata H, et al: Primary prevention of HTLV-I in Japan. J Acquir Immune Defic Syndr Hum Retrovirol 13(Suppl 1):S199, 1996.
58. Bharti AR, Nally JE, Ricaldi JN, et al: Peru–United States Leptospirosis Consortium: Leptospirosis: A zoonotic disease of global importance. Lancet Infect Dis 3:757, 2003.
59. Vinetz JM: Leptospirosis. Curr Opin Infect Dis 14:527–538, 2001.
60. Trevejo RT, Rigau-Perez JG, Ashford DA, et al: Epidemic leptospirosis associated with pulmonary haemorrhage—Nicaragua, 1995. J Infect Dis 178:1457, 1998.
61. Shaked Y, Shpilberg O, Samra D, et al: Leptospirosis in pregnancy and its effect on the fetus: Case report and review. Clin Infect Dis 17:241, 1993.
62. Chedraui PA, San Miguel G: A case of leptospirosis and pregnancy. Arch Gynecol Obstet 269:53, 2003.
63. Tramoni G, Clement HJ, Lopez F, et al: [An unusual case of postpartum haemorrhage: Leptospirosis infection.] Ann Fr Anesth Reanim 22:363, 2003.
64. Carles G, Montoya E, Joly F, et al: [Leptospirosis and pregnancy. Eleven cases in French Guyana.] J Gynecol Obstet Biol Reprod (Paris) 24:418, 1995.
65. Coghlan JD, Bain AD: Leptospirosis in human pregnancy followed by death of the foetus. BMJ 25:228, 1969.
66. Emmanouilides CE, Kohn OF, Garibaldi R: Leptospirosis complicated by the Jarisch-Herxheimer reaction and adult respiratory distress syndrome. Clin Infect Dis 18:1004, 1994.
67. Mylonakis E, Paliou M, Hohmann E, et al: Listeriosis during pregnancy: A case series and review of 222 cases. Medicine (Baltimore) 81:260, 2002.
68. Benshushan A, Tsafrir A, Arbel R, et al: *Listeria* infection during pregnancy: A 10-year experience. Israel Med Assoc J 4:776, 2002.
69. Baltimore R: *Listeria monocytogenes*. In Behrman RE, Kliegman RM, Jensen HB (eds): Nelson Textbook of Pediatrics, 17th ed, Philadelphia, WB Saunders, 2004, p 890.
70. Guevara RE, Gallagher AM, Mascola L: An 11-year retrospective study on listeriosis in Los Angeles County, 1992–2002. Proc IDSA, San Diego, California, 2003, Abstract # 866.
71. Nosten F, Rogerson SJ, Beeson JG, et al: Malaria in pregnancy and the endemicity spectrum: What can we do? Trends Parasitol 20:425, 2004.
72. Guyat HL, Snow RW: Impact of malaria during pregnancy on low birth weight in sub-Saharan Africa. Clin Microbiol Rev 17:760, 2004.
73. Shulman CE, Dorman EK: Importance and prevention of malaria in pregnancy. Trans R Soc Trop Med Hyg 97:30, 2003.
74. Mayengue PI, Rieth H, Khattab A, et al: Submicroscopic *Plasmodium falciparum* infections and multiplicity of infection in matched peripheral, placental and umbilical cord blood samples from Gabonese women. Trop Med Int Health 9:949, 2004
75. Maitra N, Joshi M, Hazra M: Maternal manifestations of malaria in pregnancy: A review. Indian J Matern Child Health 4:98, 1993.
76. Procop GW, Jessen R, Hyde SR, et al: Persistence of *Plasmodium falciparum* in the placenta after apparently effective quinidine/clindamycin therapy. J Perinatol 21:128, 2001.
77. McGready R, Thwai KL, Chot T, et al: The effects of quinine and chloroquine antimalarial treatment in the first trimestrer of pregnancy. Trans R Soc Trop Med Hyg 96:180, 2002.
78. Adam I, Ali DA, Alwaseila A, et al: Mefloquine in the treatment of *falciparum* malaria during pregnancy in Eastern Sudan. Saudi Med J 25:1400, 2004.
79. Brabin BJ, Eggelte TA, Parise M, et al: Dapsone therapy for malaria during pregnancy: Maternal and fetal outcomes. Drug Safety 27:633, 2004.
80. McGready R, Keo NK, Villegas L, et al: Artesunate-atovaquone-proguanil rescue treatment of multidrug-resistant *Plasmodium falciparum* malaria in pregnancy: A preliminary report. Trans R Soc Trop Med Hyg 97:592, 2003.
81. Centers for Disease Control and Prevention: Recommended Adult Immunization Schedule by Age Group and Medical Conditions, United States, 2003–2004. www.cdc.gov/nip/recs/adult-schedule.pdf.
82. Gall SA: Maternal immunization. Obstet Gynecol Clin N Am 30:623, 2003.
83. McLeod R, Remington JS: Toxoplasmosis. In Gorbach SL, Bartlett JG, Blacklow NR: Infectious Diseases, 3rd ed. Philadelphia, Lippincott Williams & Wilkins, 2004, p 1508.
84. Vogel N, Kirisits J, Michael E, et al: Congenital toxoplasmosis transmitted from an immunologically competent woman infected before conception. Clin Infect Dis 63:1055, 1996.
85. Wilson CB, Remington JS, Stagno S, et al: Development of adverse sequelae in children born with subclinical congenital *Toxoplasma* infection. Pediatrics 66:767, 1980.
86. Koppe JG, Loewer-Sieger DH, de Toever-Bonnet H: Results of 20-year follow up of congenital toxoplasmosis. Lancet 1:254, 1986.
87. Hohlfeld P, Daffos F, Thulliez P, et al: Fetal toxoplasmosis: Outcome of pregnancy and infant follow up after in utero treatment. J Pediatr 115:765, 1989.
88. McCabe RE, Brooks RG, Dorfman RF, et al: Clinical spectrum in 107 cases of toxoplasmic lymphadenopathy. Rev Infect Dis 9:754, 1987.
89. Grover CM, Thulliez P, Remington JS, et al: Rapid prenatal diagnosis of congenital *Toxoplasma* infection by using polymerase chain reaction and amniotic fluid. J Clin Microbiol 28:2297, 1990.
90. Romand S, Wallon M, Franck J, et al: Prenatal diagnosis using polymerase chain reaction on amniotic fluid for congenital toxoplasmosis. Obstet Gynecol 97:296, 2001.
91. Pillay T, Khan M, Moodley J, et al: The incresing burden of tuberculosis in pregnant women, newborns and infants under 6 months of age in Durban, KwaZulu-Natal. S Afr Med J 91:983, 2001.
92. Figueroa-Damian R, Arredondo-Garcia JL: Neonatal outcome of children born to women with tuberculosis. Arch Med Res 32:66, 2001.

93. Jana N, Vasishta K, Jindal SK, et al: Perinatal outcome in pregnancies complicated by pulmonary tuberculosis. Int J Gynaecol Obstet 44:119, 1994.
94. Centers for Disease Control and Prevention: Treatment of tuberculosis. MMWR 52:1, 2003.
95. World Health Organization: Treatment of Tuberculosis: Guidelines for National Programmes, 2nd ed. Geneva, Switzerland, WHO,1997.
96. Enarson DA, Rieder HL, Arnodittir T, et al: Tuberculosis Guide for Low-Income Countries, 4th ed. Paris, International Union Against Tuberculosis and Lung Diseases, 1996.
97. Briggs GG, Feldman RK, Yaffe SJ (eds): Drugs in Pregnancy and Lactation, 5th ed. Baltimore, Williams & Wilkins, 1998.
98. Varpela E, Hietalalahti J, Aro M: Streptomycin and dihidrostreptomycin during pregnancy and their effects on the child's inner ear. Scand J Respir Dis 50:101, 1969.
99. Potworowska M, Sianozecko E, Szuflodowica R: Ethionamide treatment and pregnancy. Polish Med J 5:1153, 1966.
100. Bergeron KG, Bonebrake NG, Gray CJ: Tuberculosis in pregnancy: Current recommendations for screening and treatment in the USA. Expert Rev Anti Infect Ther 2:589, 2004.
101. Pillay T, Khan M, Moodley J, et al: Perinatal tuberculosis and HIV-1: Considerations for resource limited settings. Lancet Infect Dis 4:155, 2004.
102. Snider DE, Powell KE: Should women taking antituberculous drugs breast-feed? Arch Intern Med 144:589, 1984.
103. Cohen JL, Bartlett JA, Corey GR: Extra-intestinal manifestations of *Salmonella* infections. Medicine (Baltimore) 66:349, 1987.
104. Villarama A, Galang JS: Typhoid fever in pregnancy. Phillippine Islands Med Assoc 10:311, 1930.
105. Zunino E, Olea P: Fiebre tifoidea y embarazo. Rev Chil Infect 3:112–228, 1986.
106. Olivares-Lopes F et al: Tifoidea yembarazo. Rev Med IMSS (Mex) 27:23–26, 1989.
107. Gotuzzo E: Unpublished.
108. Rowe B, Ward LR, Threlfall EJ: Multidrug-resistant *Salmonella typhi*: A worldwide epidemic. Clin Infect Dis 24(Suppl 1):S106, 1997
109. Jesudason MV, John R, John TJ: The concurrent prevalence of chloramphenicol-sensitive and multi-drug resistant *Salmonella typhi* in Vellore, S. India. Epidemiol Infect 116:225, 1996.
110. Gupta A, Swarnkar NK, Choudhary SP: Changing antibiotic sensitivity in enteric fever. J Trop Pediatr 47:369, 2001.
111. Ti TY, Monteiro EH, Lam S, et al: Ceftriaxone therapy in bacteremic typhoid fever. Antimicrob Agents Chemother 28:540, 1985.
112. Carles G, Montoya Y, Seve B, et al: Typhoid fever and pregnancy. J Gynecol Obstet Biol Reprod 31:495, 2002.
113. Roberts C, Wilkins EG: *Salmonella* screening in pregnant women. J Hosp Infect 10:67, 1987.
114. Citernesi A, Spinelli G, Piazzesi G, et al: Screening for *Salmonella* in pregnancy. Minerva Ginecol 46:681, 1994.
115. Robert E, Vial T, Schaefer C, et al: Exposure to yellow fever vaccine in early pregnancy. Vaccine 17:283, 1999.
116. Nishioka Sde A, Nunes-Araujo FR, Pires WP, et al: Yellow fever vaccination during pregnancy and spontaneous abortion: A case control study. Trop Med Int Health 3:29, 1998.
117. Tsai TF, Paul R, Lynberg MC, et al: Congenital yellow fever virus infection after immunization in pregnancy. J Infect Dis 168:1520, 1993.
118. Nasidi A, Monath TP, Vandenberg J, et al: Yellow fever vaccination and pregnancy: A four-year prospective study. Trans R Soc Trop Med Hyg 87:337, 1993.
119. Noyola DE, Demmier GJ, Nelson CT, et al: Early predictors of neurodevelopmental outcome in symptomatic congenital cytomegalovirus infection. J Pediatr 138:325, 2001.
120. Whitley RJ, Cloud G, Gruber A, et al: Ganciclovir treatment of symptomatic congenital cytomegalovirus infection: Results of a phase II study. J Infect Dis 175:1080, 1997.
121. Kimberlin DW, Lin CY, Jacobs RF, et al: Natural history of neonatal herpes simplex virus infections in the acyclovir era. Pediatrics 108:223, 2001.
122. Plotkin SA: Rubella eradication. Vaccine 19:3331, 2001.
123. Sanchez PJ, Wendel GD: Syphilis in pregnancy. Clin Perinatol 24:71, 1997.
124. Centers for Disease Control and Prevention: Sexually transmitted diseases treatment guidelines. MMWR 51:25, 2002.

INDEX

Page numbers followed by b, f, or t indicate boxes, figures, or tables, respectively.

F

P

U

V